Principles of Internal Medicine

Principles of
INTERNAL MEDICINE

Editors

T. R. HARRISON, A.B., M.D.
Professor of Medicine, The Medical College of the University of Alabama, Birmingham

RAYMOND D. ADAMS, B.A., M.A., M.D., M.A. (HON.)
Bullard Professor of Neuropathology, Harvard Medical School

IVAN L. BENNETT, JR., A.B., M.D.
Baxley Professor of Pathology and Director of the Department of Pathology,
Johns Hopkins University School of Medicine

WILLIAM H. RESNIK, PH.B., M.D.
Clinical Professor of Medicine, Yale University School of Medicine

GEORGE W. THORN, M.D., M.A. (HON.), LL.D. (HON.), SC.D. (HON.)
Hersey Professor of the Theory and Practice of Physic, Harvard Medical School

M. M. WINTROBE, B.A., M.D., B.SC. (MED.) PH.D., D.SC. (HON.)
Professor and Head, Department of Medicine, and Director, Laboratory for Study of
Hereditary and Metabolic Disorders, University of Utah College of Medicine, Salt Lake City

Fourth Edition

The Blakiston Division

McGRAW-HILL BOOK COMPANY, INC.

New York   Toronto   London

PRINCIPLES OF INTERNAL MEDICINE

III

To all those who have taught us,
and especially to our younger colleagues
who continue to teach and inspire us

Contributors

RAYMOND D. ADAMS, B.A., M.A., M.D., M.A. (HON.)
Bullard Professor of Neuropathology, Harvard Medical School; Chief of Neurology Service and Neuropathologist, Massachusetts General Hospital, Boston.

JEAN N. ANGELO, B.S., M.D.
Resident, New England Center Hospital; Research Fellow in Psychiatry, Tufts University School of Medicine, Boston.

KARL-ERIK ÅSTRÖM, M.D.
Assistant Professor in Neuropathology, Karolinska Institutet, Stockholm, Sweden.

HENRY T. BAHNSON, M.D.
Professor of Surgery, Johns Hopkins University School of Medicine, Baltimore.

PAUL B. BEESON, M.D.
Ensign Professor of Medicine, Yale University School of Medicine, New Haven, Connecticut.

ALBERT R. BEHNKE, B.A., M.D., M.S. (HON.)
Formerly Radiological Medical Director, U.S. Naval Radiological Defense Laboratory, San Francisco.

IVAN L. BENNETT, JR., A.B., M.D.
Baxley Professor of Pathology and Director of the Department of Pathology, Johns Hopkins University School of Medicine and Pathologist-in-Chief, Johns Hopkins Hospital, Baltimore.

DANIEL S. BERNSTEIN, M.D.
Research Associate, Robert Breck Brigham Hospital, Boston.

STUART BONDURANT, M.D.
Associate Professor of Medicine, Director, Heart Research Center, Indiana University Medical Center, Indianapolis.

PHILIP K. BONDY, B.A., M.D.
Professor of Medicine, Yale University School of Medicine, New Haven, Connecticut.

BEN V. BRANSCOMB, M.D.
Associate Professor of Medicine, The Medical College of the University of Alabama, Birmingham.

ABRAHAM I. BRAUDE, M.D.
Professor of Medicine, University of Pittsburgh; Director of Microbiology, Presbyterian-University Hospital, Pittsburgh.

RALPH W. BRAUER, A.B., M.SC., PH.D.
Head, Pharmacology Branch, Biological and Medical Sciences Division, U.S. Naval Radiological Defense Laboratory, San Francisco.

JOSEPH J. BUNIM, M.D.
Clinical Director, National Institute of Arthritis and Metabolic Diseases, National Institutes of Health, Bethesda, Md.; Associate Professor of Medicine, Johns Hopkins University School of Medicine, Baltimore.

CHARLES H. BURNETT, M.D.
Professor of Medicine and Chairman, Department of Medicine, University of North Carolina School of Medicine; Chief of Medical Service, North Carolina Memorial Hospital, Chapel Hill.

GEORGE F. CAHILL, JR., B.S., M.D.
Associate in Medicine and Tutor in Medical Sciences, Harvard Medical School; Senior Associate in Medicine, Peter Bent Brigham Hospital, Boston.

GEORGE E. CARTWRIGHT, B.A., M.D.
Professor of Medicine, University of Utah College of Medicine, Salt Lake City.

E. CHERASKIN, M.D., D.M.D.
Professor of Dentistry and Head of Section on Oral Medicine and Surgery, The University of Alabama School of Dentistry, Birmingham.

LEIGHTON E. CLUFF, M.D.
Associate Professor of Medicine and Head, Division of Allergy and Infectious Disease, Department of Medicine, Johns Hopkins University School of Medicine, Baltimore.

LEWIS L. CORIELL, M.A., PH.D., M.D., F.A.A.P.
Associate Professor of Pediatrics, University of Pennsylvania School of Medicine, Philadelphia; Medical Director, Camden Municipal Hospital for Contagious Diseases, Camden, N.J.; Senior Physician, The Children's Hospital, Philadelphia.

EUGENE P. CRONKITE, M.D.
Head, Division Experimental Pathology, Medical Research Center, Brookhaven National Laboratory, Upton, New York.

PRAFUL M. DALAL, M.D.
Teaching Fellow in Neurology, Harvard Medical School, Boston; Tutor in Medicine, T. M. Medical College, B.Y.L. Nair Charitable Hospitals, Bombay, India.

GUSTAVE J. DAMMIN, B.A., M.A., M.D.
Elsie T. Friedman Professor of Pathology, Harvard Medical School; Pathologist-in-Chief, Peter Bent Brigham Hospital, Boston.

WILLIAM J. DARBY, M.D., PH.D.
Professor of Biochemistry, Assistant Professor of Medicine, and Director of the Division of Nutrition, Vanderbilt University School of Medicine, Nashville, Tennessee.

LEWIS DEXTER, M.D.
Clinical Professor of Medicine and Tutor in Medicine, Harvard Medical School; Physician, Peter Bent Brigham Hospital, Boston.

JOSEPH F. DINGMAN, M.D.
Director of Medical Research, Lahey Foundation, Boston.

WILLIAM DOCK, B.S., M.D.
Professor of Medicine, State University of New York Downstate Medical Center; Attending Physician, Kings County Hospital, University Division, Brooklyn.

PHILIP R. DODGE, M.D.
Associate Neurologist and Associate Physician, Children's Service, Massachusetts General Hospital; Associate in Neurology, Harvard Medical School, Boston.

HENRI VANDER EECKEN, H.M., M.D.
Professor of Medical Psychology and Agrégé in Neurology, Faculty of Medicine, University of Ghent, Ghent, Belgium.

KENDALL EMERSON, JR., B.S., M.D.
Assistant Professor of Medicine, Harvard Medical School; Physician, Peter Bent Brigham Hospital; Visiting Physician, Boston Lying-in Hospital, Boston.

FRANKLIN H. EPSTEIN, M.D.
Associate Professor of Medicine, Yale University School of Medicine, New Haven, Connecticut.

HARRY A. FELDMAN, A.B., M.D.
Professor and Chairman, Department of Preventive Medicine, State University of New York Upstate Medical Center at Syracuse, New York.

ALTO E. FELLER, B.S., M.D.
Professor and Chairman, Department of Microbiology; Professor of Medicine, University of Virginia School of Medicine, Charlottesville.

C. MILLER FISHER, M.D.
Assistant Clinical Professor of Neurology, Harvard Medical School, Boston.

PETER H. FORSHAM, M.A., M.D.
Professor of Medicine and Pediatrics, Chief of Endocrinology and Metabolism, Department of Medicine, and Director, Metabolic Research Unit, University of California School of Medicine, San Francisco.

DONALD S. FREDRICKSON, M.D.
Clinical Director, National Heart Institute, National Institutes of Health, Bethesda.

LAWRENCE R. FREEDMAN, M.D.
Assistant Professor of Medicine, Yale University School of Medicine, New Haven, Connecticut.

FRANK H. GARDNER, M.D.
Assistant Professor of Medicine, Harvard Medical School; Senior Associate in Medicine, Peter Bent Brigham Hospital, Boston.

ALAN GOLDFIEN, A.B., M.D.
Associate Professor of Medicine (Obstetrics and Gynecology); Staff Member of the Cardiovascular Research Institute, University of California Medical School, San Francisco.

SEYMOUR J. GRAY, B.A., M.D., PH.D.
Associate Clinical Professor of Medicine, Harvard Medical School; Physician, Peter Bent Brigham Hospital, Boston.

T. R. HARRISON, A.B., M.D.
Professor of Medicine, The Medical College of the University of Alabama, Birmingham.

LLOYD L. HEFNER, B.S., M.D.
Associate Professor of Medicine, The Medical College of the University of Alabama, Birmingham.

ALBERT HEYMAN, B.S., M.D.
Professor of Neurology, Duke University School of Medicine, Durham, North Carolina.

S. RICHARDSON HILL, JR., B.A., M.D.
Associate Professor of Medicine, The Medical College of the University of Alabama, Birmingham.

FREDERIC L. HOCH, M.D.
Associate in Medicine, Harvard Medical School; Senior Associate in Medicine, Peter Bent Brigham Hospital, Boston.

PAUL D. HOEPRICH, M.D.
Assistant Professor of Internal Medicine and Assistant Research Professor of Pathology, University of Utah College of Medicine, Salt Lake City.

EDWARD W. HOOK, M.D.
Associate Professor of Medicine, Cornell University Medical College, New York.

JUSTIN M. HOPE, B.S., M.D.
Professor of Clinical Psychiatry, Tufts University School of Medicine; Chief of Psychiatric Service, New England Center Hospital, Boston.

RICHARD B. HORNICK, M.D.
Assistant Professor of Medicine, Division of Infectious Diseases, University of Maryland School of Medicine, Baltimore.

FRANZ J. INGELFINGER, B.A., M.D.
Professor of Medicine, Boston University School of Medicine, Boston.

LEONARD W. JARCHO, A.B., M.A., M.D.
Associate Professor and Chairman of the Division of Neurology; Associate Professor of Medicine, Uni-

versity of Utah College of Medicine; Chief of Neurology Service, Veterans Administration Hospital, Salt Lake City.

DALTON JENKINS, M.A., M.D.
Associate Professor of Medicine, Head of the Division of Endocrinology, University of Colorado, School of Medicine, Denver.

MICHEL JÉQUIER, M.D.
Professeur de Neurologie, Faculté de Médecine Université de Lausanne, Lausanne, Switzerland.

RICHARD J. JOHNS, M.D.
Associate Professor of Medicine, Johns Hopkins University School of Medicine, Baltimore.

WILLIAM M. M. KIRBY, B.S., M.D.
Professor of Medicine, University of Washington School of Medicine, Seattle.

JULIAN I. KITAY, A.B., M.D.
Assistant Professor of Medicine and Physiology, School of Medicine, University of Virginia, Charlottesville, Virginia.

GERALD KLATSKIN, M.D.
Professor of Medicine, Yale University School of Medicine, New Haven, Connecticut.

JOHN H. KNOWLES, A.B., M.D.
Chief, Pulmonary Disease Unit, and Assistant Physician, Massachusetts General Hospital; Associate in Medicine, Harvard Medical School, Boston.

W. EUGENE KNOX, M.D.
Assistant Professor of Biological Chemistry, Harvard Medical School; The New England Deaconess Hospital, Boston.

JOHN C. LAIDLAW, M.A., PH.D., M.D., F.R.C.P. (C).
Associate Professor of Medicine, University of Toronto; Senior Physician, Toronto General Hospital, Toronto, Canada.

DEAN M. LAIRD, B.S., M.D.
Clinical Instructor in Psychiatry, Tufts University School of Medicine; Assistant Psychiatrist, New England Center Hospital, Boston.

GUSTAF E. LINDSKOG, B.S., M.D., M.A. (HON.)
William H. Carmalt Professor of Surgery, Yale University School of Medicine, New Haven, Connecticut.

CHAMP LYONS, A.B., M.D.
Professor and Chairman, Department of Surgery, The Medical College of the University of Alabama, Birmingham.

FRED R. McCRUMB, JR., M.D.
Director, Section of Infectious Diseases, University of Maryland School of Medicine, Baltimore.

VICTOR A. McKUSICK, M.D.
Professor of Medicine and Chief, Division of Medical

Genetics, Department of Medicine, Johns Hopkins University School of Medicine, Baltimore.

ALBERT I. MENDELOFF, M.D.
Associate Professor of Medicine, Johns Hopkins University School of Medicine; Physician-in-Chief, Sinai Hospital of Baltimore, Baltimore.

JOHN P. MERRILL, A.B., M.D.
Assistant Professor of Medicine, Harvard Medical School; Senior Associate in Medicine, Peter Bent Brigham Hospital; Investigator of the Howard Hughes Medical Institute, Boston.

JOST MICHELSEN, M.D.
Instructor in Neurology, Harvard Medical School; Clinical Associate in Neurosurgery, Massachusetts General Hospital, Boston.

EDWARD S. MILLER, M.D.
Assistant Clinical Professor in Medicine, University of Colorado School of Medicine, Denver.

WILLIAM R. MILNOR, A.B., M.D.
Associate Professor of Medicine, Johns Hopkins University School of Medicine; Physician, Johns Hopkins Hospital, Baltimore.

CARL A. MOYER, B.A., M.S., M.D.
Bixby Professor of Surgery, Washington University School of Medicine; Barnes Hospital, St. Louis.

DON H. NELSON, M.D.
Associate Professor of Medicine, University of Southern California School of Medicine, Los Angeles.

ELLIOT V. NEWMAN, M.D.
Joe and Morris Werthan Professor of Experimental Medicine, Vanderbilt University School of Medicine, Nashville, Tennessee.

VINCENT PERLO, A.B., M.D.
Instructor in Neurology, Harvard Medical School; Associate Neurologist, Massachusetts General Hospital, Boston.

ROBERT G. PETERSDORF, M.D.
Associate Professor of Medicine, University of Washington School of Medicine; Physician-in-Chief, King County Hospital, Seattle.

SIR GEORGE PICKERING, M.A., M.D., F.R.C.P., F.R.S.
Regius Professor of Medicine, University of Oxford, Oxford, England.

DONALD M. PILLSBURY, M.D., D.SC.
Professor and Chairman, Department of Dermatology, University of Pennsylvania School of Medicine, Philadelphia.

CHARLES H. RAMMELKAMP, JR., B.A., M.D., D.SC. (HON.)
Professor of Medicine and Associate Professor of Preventive Medicine, Western Reserve University School

of Medicine; Director, Department of Medicine and Research Laboratories, Cleveland Metropolitan General Hospital, Cleveland.

T. J. REEVES, M.D.
Associate Professor of Medicine, The Medical College of the University of Alabama, Birmingham.

EDWARD C. REIFENSTEIN, JR., B.A., M.D.
Senior Associate Medical Director, Clinical Research Division, The Squibb Institute for Medical Research, E. R. Squibb & Sons Division, Olin Mathieson Chemical Corporation; Assistant Clinical Professor of Medicine, New York Medical College, Flower and Fifth Avenue Hospitals, New York.

ALBERT E. RENOLD, M.D.
Assistant Professor of Medicine, Harvard Medical School; Senior Associate in Medicine, Peter Bent Brigham Hospital; Director, Baker Clinic Research Laboratory, New England Deaconess Hospital, Boston.

WILLIAM H. RESNIK, PH.B., M.D.
Clinical Professor of Medicine, Yale University School of Medicine; Consultant Physician, Grace-New Haven Community Hospital, New Haven; Consultant Physician, Stamford Hospital, Stamford, Connecticut.

EDWARD P. RICHARDSON, JR., A.B., M.D.
Assistant Professor of Neuropathology, Harvard Medical School; Associate Neurologist and Neuropathologist, Massachusetts General Hospital, Boston.

EUGENE ROBIN, M.D.
Associate Professor of Medicine, University of Pittsburgh Medical School, Pittsburgh.

RAFAEL RODRIGUEZ-MOLINA, B.S., M.D., D.SC. (INT. MED.)
Associate Chief of Staff for Research, Veterans Administration Hospital; Clinical Professor of Medicine, University of Puerto Rico School of Medicine–School of Tropical Medicine, San Juan, Puerto Rico.

DAVID E. ROGERS, M.D.
Professor of Medicine, Department of Medicine, Vanderbilt University School of Medicine; Physician-in-Chief, Vanderbilt University Hospital, Nashville, Tennessee.

ROBERT S. SCHWAB, A.B., B.A., M.A., M.D.
Associate Clinical Professor of Neurology, Harvard Medical School; Neurologist and Director of the Brain Wave Laboratory, Massachusetts General Hospital, Boston.

HERBERT A. SELENKOW, M.D.
Clinical Associate in Medicine and Tutor in Medical Science, Harvard Medical School; Senior Associate in Medicine, Peter Bent Brigham Hospital, Boston.

ARNOLD M. SELIGMAN, M.D.
Associate Professor of Surgery, Johns Hopkins University School of Medicine; Surgeon-in-Chief, Sinai Hospital, Baltimore.

WALTER B. SHELLEY, PH.D., M.D.
Professor of Dermatology, University of Pennsylvania School of Medicine, Philadelphia.

LAWRENCE E. SHULMAN, M.D., PH.D.
Assistant Professor of Medicine, Johns Hopkins University School of Medicine, Baltimore.

MARVIN H. SLEISENGER, M.D.
Associate Professor of Clinical Medicine, Cornell University Medical College; Chief, Gastrointestinal Clinic, New York Hospital–Cornell Medical Center; Associate Attending Physician, New York Hospital–Cornell Medical Center, New York.

J. E. SMADEL, A.B., M.D., M.S. (HON.), D.SC. (HON.)
Chief, Laboratory of Virology and Rickettsiology, Division of Biologics Standards, National Institutes of Health, Bethesda.

J. LAWTON SMITH, M.D.
Assistant Professor of Ophthalmology, Duke University School of Medicine, Durham, North Carolina.

WESLEY W. SPINK, B.A., M.D., D.SC. (HON.)
Professor of Medicine, University of Minnesota Hospitals and Medical School, Minneapolis.

EUGENE A. STEAD, JR., B.S., M.D.
Professor and Chairman, Department of Medicine, Duke University School of Medicine; Physician-in-Chief, Duke Hospital, Durham, North Carolina.

JOHN H. TALBOTT, M.D.
Editor, Journal of the American Medical Association, Chicago.

MELVIN L. TAYMOR, M.D.
Clinical Associate in Gynecology, Harvard Medical School, Boston.

GEORGE W. THORN, M.D., M.A. (HON.), LL.D. (HON.), SC.D. (HON.)
Hersey Professor of the Theory and Practice of Physic, Harvard Medical School; Physician-in-Chief, Peter Bent Brigham Hospital, Boston.

ANSGAR TORVIK, M.D.
Research Fellow in Neuropathology, Harvard Medical School, Boston; on leave from Department of Pathology, Ullevaal Hospital, Oslo, Norway.

PHILIP A. TUMULTY, M.D.
Associate Professor of Medicine, Johns Hopkins University School of Medicine, Baltimore.

FRANK H. TYLER, B.A., M.D.
Professor of Medicine, University of Utah College of Medicine, Salt Lake City.

BERT L. VALLEE, B.S., M.D., M.A. (HON.)
Associate Professor of Medicine, Harvard Medical

School; Physician, Peter Bent Brigham Hospital, Boston; Research Associate, Department of Biology, Massachusetts Institute of Technology, Cambridge, Massachusetts.

MAURICE VICTOR, M.D.
Assistant Clinical Professor of Neurology, Harvard Medical School; Neurologist, Massachusetts General Hospital, Boston.

RICHARD W. VILTER, M.D.
Professor of Medicine and Director, Department of Internal Medicine, University of Cincinnati College of Medicine, Cincinnati.

WARREN E. WACKER, M.D.
Associate in Medicine, Harvard Medical School, Boston.

ROBERT R. WAGNER, M.D.
Associate Professor of Microbiology and Assistant Dean, Johns Hopkins University School of Medicine, Baltimore.

FRANK B. WALSH, M.D.
Professor of Ophthalmology, Johns Hopkins University School of Medicine, Baltimore.

JOHN N. WALTON, M.D., M.R.C.P.
Neurologist, Newcastle-upon-Tyne General Hospital and Newcastle Regional Hospital Board; Assistant Physician in Neurology, Royal Victoria Informary, Newcastle-upon-Tyne, England.

HENRY deF. WEBSTER, M.D.
Instructor in Neurology, Harvard Medical School; Assistant Neurologist and Assistant Neuropathologist, Massachusetts General Hospital, Boston.

LOUIS WEINSTEIN, M.S., PH.D., M.D.
Professor of Medicine, Tufts University School of Medicine; Lecturer on Infectious Disease, Harvard Medical School, Lecturer in Medicine, Boston University School of Medicine, Boston.

LOUIS G. WELT, A.B., M.D.
Professor of Medicine, University of North Carolina School of Medicine, Chapel Hill.

M. M. WINTROBE, B.A., M.D., B.SC. (MED.) PH.D., D.SC. (HON.)
Professor and Head, Department of Medicine, and Director, Laboratory for Study of Hereditary and Metabolic Disorders, University of Utah College of Medicine, Salt Lake City.

SUMNER WOOD, JR., M.D.
Associate Professor of Pathology, Johns Hopkins University School of Medicine, Baltimore.

T. E. WOODWARD, M.D.
Professor of Medicine and Head, Department of Medicine, University of Maryland School of Medicine, Baltimore.

GEORGE W. WRIGHT, B.S., M.D.
Head of Medical Research, Department of Medicine, St. Luke's Hospital; Associate Clinical Professor of Medicine, Western Reserve University School of Medicine, Cleveland.

Preface

From the inception of this work, its basic idea has been that a medical text must remain abreast of medical teaching; this in turn depends on scientific progress in medicine. Our concern has been not only with content but particularly with concept; not with mere "what" but more especially with the "why" of disease—in short, with education rather than didacticism. Our experience as teachers of medicine at undergraduate, graduate, and postgraduate levels, in addition to our exciting but not always painless adventures as editors during almost two decades, have confirmed the conviction that *Principles of Internal Medicine* should recapitulate the life-long educational process of a physician.

A primary requisite in the educational process is the development of a high sense of responsibility toward patients and a sensitivity to the significance of illness. Part One, The Physician and the Patient, summarizes our views concerning the attitudes and obligations involved in this relationship.

Progress in internal medicine during the present century has been influenced largely by unraveling of the basic mechanisms of disease. Modern methods of teaching have incorporated this progress by introducing the student to manifestations and mechanisms before taking up specific diseases. In the present day, it is not sufficient for the physician to have *memorized knowledge* of the common causes of symptoms; he also needs an *understanding* of the mechanisms which produce them. Such an understanding, which involves a familiarity with the abnormalities of both structure and function, serves to narrow the gap between clinical medicine and the preclinical sciences. The etiologic and morphologic approaches to disease, appropriate as they were in the nineteenth century, are not sufficient in the twentieth. These considerations are responsible for our decision to devote a major portion of the book (Part Two) to Cardinal Manifestations of Disease.

The symptoms of which patients complain not only afford the initial clues to the nature of the disease process, but they offer the optimal means for the establishment of a proper relationship with the patient.

Furthermore, patients do not come to physicians bearing labels of their diseases. Rather, like Joseph, they wear coats of many colors, each hue indicating a specific manifestation and the whole representing a *symptom complex or syndrome* which may have multiple causes. The search for the underlying disease is greatly facilitated by the initial recognition of a clinical pattern. Thus the approach to disease through an understanding or appreciation of manifestations and syndromes becomes in large measure the consideration of those common manifestations of disease which the physician encounters daily. Furthermore, to cite an example, the recognition that a patient is suffering from a syndrome such as pericardial effusion with tamponade furnishes not only a guide to treatment but also leads to further diagnostic procedures which will aid the search for the specific causative disorder.

The discussion of syndromes offers the additional advantage that it becomes unnecessary in the description of a single disease to elaborate in detail on features which are common to others. Thereby it becomes possible to limit such discussions to those features which have a relatively high degree of specificity and to achieve a concise consideration of the most characteristic aspects of that particular disease. Diagnostic and therapeutic problems which are common to a number of disorders, such as the recognition of the underlying cause of the nephrotic symptom complex or the management of respiratory, renal, or cardiac failure, can often be considered best when these conditions are approached as syndromes rather than as diseases.

Part Three, Biologic Considerations, is concerned with certain broad principles of genetics, of electrophysiology, and of the regulation of the internal chemical environment. Comprehension of these concepts is essential for the physician who desires to bring to his patients the practical benefits of advances in the biologic sciences.

The Parts which follow have been prepared along more or less conventional lines and therefore need no explanation.

Since the study of medicine is a life-long process, this book has been planned for all students of internal medicine, whether they be undergraduates, young physicians receiving advanced training, busy practitioners, or preclinical or clinical teachers. However, each of these groups may prefer to use the volume in a somewhat different manner.

The *first or second year medical student* will find Part Two especially useful as a means of comprehending the relation of the basic sciences to clinical medicine. The *preclinical teacher* may find that this portion of the book aids in creating interest in these sciences, because the basic principles are presented in a clinical framework.

The *third year medical student* should read those areas in which are discussed the specific syndromes and diseases which apply to the patients he encounters. The emotional impact associated with the problems of an individual patient will thus tend to fix in his mind the significance of what he reads. At the same time he should study again those manifestations and mechanisms of disease which his patients present. The *fourth year student* should continue this process and also should begin to narrow the gaps in his knowledge by learning about those less common diseases which he has not yet personally encountered. Thus he will supplement his understanding of principles and his clinical experience by additional factual knowledge.

The *clinical teacher,* who emphasizes that his students must know what phenomena are likely to be present in a given disease but that they must also gain an understanding of the functional distortions which produce clinical phenomena, is far more likely to be successful than his colleague who teaches by rote rather than by reason. It is well to recall the statement of Plato, "Knowledge which is acquired under compulsion obtains no hold on the mind." In the educational process, the digestion of knowledge is even more important than its ingestion.

The *young physician* who, already having considerable experience, wishes to use the book as an aid toward qualifying examinations, will find especially helpful a review of those early Parts (Two and Three), which deal with the common manifestations and the more important mechanisms of disease. In most instances, five or more years will have elapsed since his basic science courses were completed, and he will need to refresh his knowledge by reviewing the more recent advances in pathophysiology.

It is our hope that the volume will prove a helpful source of quick reference for all of these groups, and especially for the *practicing physician* when an unfamiliar manifestation or disorder is encountered or when specific information about a disease or a new therapeutic procedure is desired. We trust that the index, which we have personally prepared, will be an effective guide for rapid reference.

Extensive changes have been made in the fourth edition. Most of it has been completely rewritten. The areas devoted to renal, pulmonary, gastrointestinal, and muscular and cutaneous disorders have been expanded. A chapter on Ocular Manifestations of Disease has been introduced. The previously long chapters on cardiac disease have been subdivided into shorter ones to make their contents more readily accessible. A short chapter on Principles of Physical Signs Referable to the Heart has been added. Introductory discussions, explaining the arrangement and indicating the common problems, have been inserted at the beginning of the several sections dealing with diseases of the various organ systems.

A deliberate attempt has been made to avoid long bibliographies. Rather, the references are limited to reviews and monographs which contain comprehensive bibliographies, together with an occasional reference to older works of unusual historical significance and, at times, a recent publication presenting important new information.

It is hoped that, as the result of the increasing availability of this textbook in different countries and in multiple languages, faculties of medicine outside of North America will have an opportunity to become familiar with the method of teaching internal medicine used on this continent, thereby permitting them to appropriate those techniques which seem good while retaining those methods of their own which have proved especially effective in their own environments.

Once again, we wish to express appreciation to our authors for their willingness to modify their chapters in response to editorial suggestions. We continue to be indebted to numerous colleagues and friends for invaluable criticisms. Among them are: Drs. Samuel P. Asper, F. Robert Fekety, John Eager Howard and Richard Ross of Baltimore; Drs. John Balint and Walter Frommeyer of Birmingham; Drs. Stanley Cobb, Mandel E. Cohen, A. Price Heusner, Erich Lindemann and Roe E. Wells of Boston; Dr. H. M. Spiro of New Haven; Dr. Clark Millikan of Rochester, Minnesota; and Drs. Jerome E. Cohn, Edwin Englert, Hans H. Hecht, John A. Linfoot, Charles A. Nugent, Gerald T. Perkoff, Attilio D. Renzetti and John R. Ward of Salt Lake City.

The preparation of a new edition would have presented insuperable problems without the loyal and effective aid of our several secretarial coworkers. We are especially indebted to: Mrs. Norma Nicewonger and Mrs. Ann Zurek of Baltimore; Miss Minnie Mae Tims of Birmingham; Mrs. Margaret Elinor Adams, Miss Eulalia Grzebieniowska, Mrs. Ruth Rae Simmonds and Mrs. Barbara Wood Zimmers of Boston; Miss Ruth Compton of New York; Miss Alida Woolley of Salt Lake City, and Mrs. Dolores Ready of Stamford.

Our relations with the McGraw-Hill Company, particularly with its Blakiston Division, have been cordial and friendly rather than merely agreeable and satisfactory.

R.D.A.,   I.L.B.,   T.R.H.,   W.H.R.,   G.W.T.,   M.M.W.

Contents

PART THREE

Biologic Considerations

PART FOUR

Metabolic and Endocrine Disorders

Appendix

Color Plates

PART ONE
The Physician and the Patient

Section 1: Approach to the Patient

1 APPROACH TO THE PATIENT

The Editors

No greater opportunity, responsibility, or obligation can fall to the lot of a human being than to become a physician. In the care of the suffering he needs technical skill, scientific knowledge, and human understanding. He who uses these with courage, with humility, and with wisdom will provide a unique service for his fellow man, and will build an enduring edifice of character within himself. The physician should ask of his destiny no more than this; he should be content with no less.

In the practice of medicine the physician employs a discipline which seeks to utilize scientific methods and principles in the solution of its problems, but it is one which, in the end, remains an art. It is an art in the sense that rarely, if ever, can the individual patient be considered the equivalent of an experiment so completely controlled that it is possible to exclude judgment and experience from the interpretation of the patient's reactions. It is an art, too, in the sense that the practicing physician can never be content with the sole aim of endeavoring to clarify the laws of nature; he cannot proceed in his labors with the cool detachment of the scientist whose aim is the winning of the truth, and who, theoretically, is uninterested in the practical outcome of his work. The practicing physician must never forget that his primary and traditional objectives are utilitarian—the prevention and cure of disease and the relief of suffering, whether of body or mind.

Today, with periodic health, preemployment, and insurance examinations, the scope of the physician has been enlarged. He must be accomplished in the study of presumably well people in addition to those who are ill. With the latter group the history is of great value; with those who are well, objective methods of study are all important, for patients tend to emphasize different facts, depending on whether they seek employment, pensions, disability, or insurance. It is obvious that the same symptoms will rarely be described in the same way by the soldier desiring release from military duty, by the prospective employee seeking certification of his fitness for work, or by the patient who is alarmed because of fear of a serious ailment. The approach to the patient, therefore, must be varied to correspond with the conditions which bring physician and patient together. Yet there are fundamental considerations which underlie all sound practice.

In every case the physician must have in mind three responsibilities. First comes the search for the underlying causes of all symptoms noted by the patient or his family, and the cure or alleviation of the disorder producing these symptoms. Next comes the detection of latent disease or of potential sources of disability, and the acquainting of the patient with steps to be taken in order to maintain his health and to protect others if his illness is communicable. Finally, the physician must understand and evaluate the environmental stresses and the patient's probable reaction to them. All these responsibilities are of immediate importance in those who are not acutely ill or in people sent for examinations by insurers or employers. In those confined to bed the latter two responsibilities become urgent only on convalescence, save when contagion, or the occupational or psychogenic origin of the disease, is demonstrable. The approach to the patient, therefore, begins by determining what the urgent, immediate issues are, and what can properly be studied more effectively at a later date.

Since intelligent treatment depends primarily on a knowledge of the cause, diagnosis becomes the foundation on which the art of medical practice rests. Diagnosis implies the discovery of all the various factors that are responsible for the illness. It involves an estimation of the extent and severity of the functional and anatomic changes produced by the disorder, and it necessitates an insight into the rate of progress and the probable outcome. To this end are correlated and integrated the facts obtained from the history, the physical examination, and the laboratory investigations.

HISTORY

The history aims to embody all the facts that may have influenced the patient in a medical way up to the time he consults the physician. Most important of all, in the case of the patient who is ill, the history contains an account of the symptoms that have impelled him to seek advice. The history can never be the mere mechanical recording of data. Each statement must be scrutinized for its possible bearing on the present status of the patient, and, more particularly, for any light it may throw on the symptoms of which he now complains. The mind of the physician must be constantly alert to the possibility that any event related by the pa-

3

tient, any symptom, however trivial or remote, may yet hold the key to the solution of a medical problem. In the main, we are dealing with subjective manifestations filtered through the consciousness of individuals who vary in their capacity to observe and describe; who differ widely in their responses to the same stimuli; whose accounts are colored, consciously or unconsciously, by fears and misconceptions as to the nature and significance of their disorders. Added to these difficulties, one occasionally encounters the barrier of language, so that it is not surprising if even the careful physician becomes somewhat impatient with the arduous task of collecting data that cannot be accurately weighed or measured but that have value only in so far as they can be considered to represent more or less close approximations of the truth.

Despite these shortcomings, the taking of the history, by and large, constitutes the most important part of the examination. A skillfully taken history, carefully interpreted, will provide important information regarding the emotional and psychologic background of the patient which may be of utmost value in the solution of his problem. At the same time an interested sympathetic interview constitutes the foundation for a successful patient-physician relationship.

It is the subjective symptom that usually calls the attention of the patient to his departure from good health; for him, that is sufficient reason that the meaning of the symptom be thoroughly explored. It is the symptom that determines the physician's line of inquiry to the end that from the various possible causes for the symptom there will emerge a pattern or clinical picture that will permit the physician to draw at least a tentative conclusion as to the nature of the malady. In some instances so clear a picture will be drawn, as when a classic story of angina pectoris is obtained, that the diagnosis may be largely established from the symptoms alone, regardless of the outcome of the physical and laboratory examinations. In most cases the history will not be so decisive, but it will have so limited the diagnostic possibilities that a logical program of investigation will be suggested. It is usually from the history that one can estimate most accurately the speed and evolution of the disease. It is in the taking of the history and in the analysis and interpretation of the data contained therein that the skill, knowledge, and experience of the physician are most frequently and rigorously tested.

Because the symptom is a subjective manifestation, one that is not readily corroborated or measured, there is too often a disposition to value it lightly, or even to disregard it when it cannot be explained on the basis of our present-day knowledge. Credulity is to be avoided; but only less zealously must one steer away from an attitude of such rigid skepticism that one refuses to entertain the possibility that a core of truth may be contained in an odd or unfamiliar phenomenon described by the patient. "Disease often tells its secrets in a casual parenthesis." The demonstration that the virtue of cod-liver oil was something more than an old wives' fancy, and the discovery of the leaf of the foxglove as a therapeutic agent in heart failure may be cited as examples of the beneficent effect of listening with an open mind.

PHYSICAL EXAMINATION

Little need be said regarding the importance of the physical examination, for early in his training the physician becomes impressed with the diagnostic value of physical signs, objective and verifiable evidence of pathologic change. Regardless of the confusion of data obtained from the history, regardless of the inconsistencies of statement voiced by the patient, the physical sign has an indisputable value as solid evidence in the case. Symptoms and signs have varying clinical value in proportion to the extent to which they narrow the field of possible diagnosis. From this point of view, the value of physical signs is beyond question. Skill in physical diagnosis is acquired with experience. But it is not experience merely in the technique of physical examination that determines how successful one may be in eliciting the signs that provide the clues to the correct diagnosis. Detection of a few scattered petechiae or of a faint diastolic murmur or of a small mass in the abdomen is not accomplished because the trained clinician has eyes, ears, or fingers that are more acute than those of his colleagues. Usually these diagnostic signs have been revealed because the observer has been prepared by other features of the history or examination to search for them.

All investigations of the body should be regarded as part of the physical examination. The use of various instruments such as the ophthalmoscope, sphygmomanometer, galvanometer, or roentgen tube may be necessary to study certain structures and functions of the patient, but all these methods of study are part of the physical examination, and all of them may be used by physicians practicing internal medicine. Tests made on fluids or tissues removed from the patient are laboratory examinations, and, since it is so obvious that it is too often forgotten, it should be stated that the proper collection of material is as important as its correct study.

INSTRUMENTAL AND LABORATORY EXAMINATIONS

The last century has witnessed the introduction of newer methods of instrumental and laboratory investigation of ever-increasing precision and refinement, and inevitably there has been a drift toward reliance on knowledge gained from these special means of study in the solution of clinical problems. No one can view the enormous advances that have been made in these past several decades without recognizing that they have come from the use of techniques of exactitude that were unavailable in earlier times. These newer methods of examination should be accepted with gratitude; yet one hears, from time to time, lamentations regarding the neglect that is accorded the older traditional sources of information gained from the history and the use of the unaided senses. But what force can these lamentations have when it has been so abundantly demonstrated that roentgenologic inspection of the chest will reveal changes that are completely beyond the perceptions of even the most skilled exponent of the art of physical diagnosis; when similar methods of examination of the digestive tract uncover with certainty what may only dimly be surmised from the history and the routine physical examination; when differentiation of many infectious diseases can be placed on a sure footing only by exact bacteriologic and immunologic technique; and when only by more or less intricate methods of chemical analysis can diseases of metabolism be studied? The need is neither to stress the value nor to deplore the use of these special methods of examination; rather is it to recognize their limitations and their proper use in the practice of medicine. By virtue of their impersonal quality and the complexity of the techniques involved in obtaining them, data secured by instrumental and laboratory methods are frequently surrounded by an aura of authority, without heed to the fact that the data are collected by fallible human beings who are capable of committing errors of technique, or who may misinterpret the most precise evidence. Too great emphasis may be placed on minor deviations that may yet lie well within the range of normality. These and other possible errors serve to indicate that even these data cannot release the physician from the necessity of careful observation and study of the patient. The wise physician is he who understands the merits and limitations of each source of information, whether it be derived from the history, or the physical examination, or the laboratory investigations. Barring those exigencies that make careful study impracticable or impossible, the history and physical examination should be thorough and painstaking, and the special examinations and laboratory tests should be adequate to furnish what additional information may be necessary. In some cases, it will suffice to use merely the simple tests that should be at the disposal of every practicing physician; in the more obscure cases the full resources of the most advanced teaching hospital may be essential for the successful unraveling of the clinical problem. The physician should weigh carefully not only the hazards but also the expense involved in every test that he demands. Every procedure that does not have a specific purpose toward contributing to the management of the patient's illness is a pretentious economic waste resulting from ignorance or callousness or plain charlatanism. Scientific study of a clinical problem does not consist merely of filling a patient's record with endless data. Discrimination in the ordering of laboratory procedures, judgment in appraising the risk and expense of a procedure as against the value of the information to be derived from it are among the criteria by which one estimates the manner in which the art and science of medicine have been fused by the physician.

THE ART OF MEDICINE

Despite the constantly increasing application of scientific methods to the problems of medicine, there remain large areas that are as yet insusceptible of solution by the use of precise methods. To extract the telltale clue from a maze of confusing symptoms, to determine from a mass of conflicting physical signs and laboratory data the ones that are of crucial significance, to know in a borderline case when to initiate and when to refrain from a line of treatment —these decisions are not usually the outcome of laboratory study alone. In the end, these decisions are expressions of judgment acquired through "assimilated experience."

Concerning the more personal relations with the patient and the understanding and capacity to peer beyond surface motivations and behavior, no instruction or training can entirely replace an intuitive talent and maturing wisdom. The astute physician will recognize when the casual mention of an apparently trivial complaint is the device for seeking reassurance regarding a feared disorder such as cancer or heart disease. He will know or suspect how profitable it will be to continue probing the more intimate aspects of the patient's life, when to overcome a reluctance to discuss them, and when to permit them to remain undiscussed. Knowing when to express a bright and reassuring prognosis and when and how to utter doubt and caution requires more than a knowledge of disease.

No problem can be more distressing than that presented by the patient with incurable disease, particularly when death is imminent and inevitable. There should be no iron-clad, inflexible rule that the patient must be told "everything." All patients do not have the courage or faith or stoicism that the advocates of this conviction think they may or should have. "One thing is certain: it is not for you to don the black cap and, assuming the judicial function, take hope away from any patient . . . hope that comes to us all." (William Osler) The proponents of this principle do not really adhere to their philosophy when they tell the "truth" in such a manner that the kernel of the truth is not conveyed to the patient. How much, for example, is communicated to the patient when the physician says to the patient who has leukemia: "You have more white corpuscles in your blood than is normal, but we have found no evidence that any damage has been done." Nor can one conscientiously follow the opposite rule of never telling the patient the truth. How much the patient is to be told will depend on his religious convictions, the wishes of his family, the state of his affairs, and his own desires and character. But even this platitude solves nothing, since it is not merely the recognition of these factors but the physician's wisdom in assessing the relative importance of each that determines how complete a discussion of the facts will best serve the interests of the patient. The younger physician may extract some small measure of consolation from the knowledge that his older and more experienced colleague has no simple and easy formula for meeting the question.

I do not know that I have anything to reproach in my conduct, and certainly nothing in my feelings and intentions towards the dead. But it is a moment when we are apt to think that, if this or that had been done, such event might have been prevented. (Letter to Shelley from Lord Byron on the death of his daughter.)

These words express the feelings of guilt that almost invariably afflict the members of a family when parent or child or spouse has died. The doctor must be prepared to tender what assurance is possible that no fault need be attached to the living.

Somewhat related to this problem is the expiatory attitude of the family when a member becomes gravely or hopelessly ill. The meager resources that may represent the savings of a lifetime of toil may be dissipated in weeks or months in the payment for needlessly expensive rooms, private nursing services, and consultations. It is difficult for the physician to oppose these futile gestures too strenuously for they serve more to bring consolation to the family than to assuage the distress of the patient.

THE MIDDLE ZONE

In clinical medicine it is common practice to think of disease in terms of "organic" and "functional," and to imply by the latter expression a disturbance due solely to emotional instability or nervous strain. It is recognized, of course, that there are a vast number of bodily derangements which are due to functional dislocations that often are based neither on structural disease nor on primary

psychogenic disorder: shock due to extracellular fluid deficit, diabetic ketosis, and paroxysmal auricular tachycardia are examples. These may be considered disorders of the middle zone. There are other less dramatic forms of nonpsychogenic functional disturbances that so frequently resemble malfunctions due to psychic influence, and that often are so intricately woven with emotional components that it may be forgotten that other factors may be playing an important or even predominant role. A palpitation that is clearly not due to organic disease and that may readily be attributed to "nerves" may actually be due to hypoglycemia brought on by faulty diet. Chronic indigestion or diarrhea or recurrent headache may be ascribed to emotional disturbance when exhaustive investigation has revealed no structural disorder or other tangible basis for the ailment; yet a specific intolerance to foods may turn out to be the chief cause of the trouble. Statements so trite in theory would hardly deserve mention, were they not so often forgotten in practice.

THE PATIENT AND HIS ENVIRONMENT

Over and beyond the obligation of the physician to consider the psychic as well as the physical problems of the patient lies his responsibility to relate the individual to a wider sphere. He must deal with all the circumstances, whether environmental, genetic, occupational, or social, that may ultimately have a bearing on the health of his patient and, through this patient, on the health of his family and immediate associates. The practice implied by this concept may be termed *clinical epidemiology*, but it does not represent the realm of still another specialist in medicine. Rather, it has traditionally been identified as an area of medicine peculiarly adapted to conscientious and intelligent family practice.

MANAGEMENT OF THE PATIENT

The art of medicine lies in establishing *all* the diagnoses in each case, and in instituting the most effective management, even though absolute accuracy of diagnosis of many conditions is often impossible. The restoration of the patient's comfort and confidence should begin with his initial contact with the physician and his assistants. Gentle, thorough, and interested interrogation and examination prepare the way for more painful procedures that may be essential. Even the patients who experience relief from the propitiatory nature of suffering expect and need consideration and humane, affectionate care from their families, their physicians, and their nurses or other attendants. There must, however, be firmness in obtaining cooperation in study and management, both of which should be carried out with minimal discomfort or risk to the patient. Disease often profoundly alters personality and makes skill in handling the patient as important as familiarity with diagnostic procedures, and the nature, seats, and causes of disease.

Tact, sympathy, and understanding are expected of the physician, for the patient is no mere collection of symptoms, signs, disordered functions, damaged organs, and disturbed emotions. He is human, fearful, and hopeful, seeking relief, help, and reassurance. To the physician, as to the anthropologist, nothing human is strange or repulsive. The misanthrope may become a smart diagnostician of organic disease, but he can scarcely hope to succeed as a physician. The true physician has a Shakespearean breadth of interest in the wise and the foolish, the proud and the humble, the stoic hero and the whining rogue. He cares for people.

2 THE PHYSICIAN'S RESPONSIBILITY
The Editors

THE PATIENT AS A PERSON

The student receives much expert coaching in the methods of physical and laboratory diagnosis, and it is in these areas that he will most easily develop the skills which permit him to be comfortable with the patient. Mastery of the more intangible psychologic aspects of medicine is not so easily learned, however. The skills essential here depend not simply on instruction but on emotional maturity, manifested by sensitive self-cultivation of the capacity to see deeply and accurately the problems of another human being. The challenge is further magnified by the fact that the examining physician is himself a human instrument, subject to error due to the events in his own biography. The irritability and exasperation of even the kindest and most conscientious physician may sometimes represent not the legitimate protest at the patient's lack of cooperativeness but a basic and not wholly conscious sense of his own insecurity. The successful management of the patient properly begins with the development of emotional maturity on the part of the physician.

Just as the physical growth of each person depends on an adequate and balanced supply of appropriate foodstuffs, so does emotional growth depend on the receipt of proper psychologic nutrients. Although each individual is born with manifold potentialities determined by his genes, the emotional climate in which he grows and develops will shape his eventual character and abilities just as surely as foodstuffs will modify his physique. Just as invading bacteria influence multitudinous bodily reactions, so do emotions possess the capacity to exert force and thereby alter behavior, including certain of the biochemical processes of the body.

Any departure from good health carries a potential threat of physical disintegration or crippling disability, and even the most intelligent and best-informed patient should not be considered immune to forebodings just because he refrains from mentioning them. It is especially important that these fears be borne in mind when dealing with the elderly patient, who is rarely unmindful that "the trap is laid" and death is always near.

The attitude of the patient approaching the doctor must always be tinged—for the most part unconsciously—with distaste and dread; its deepest desire will tend to be comfort and relief rather than cure, and its faith and expectation will be directed towards some magical exhibition of these boons. Do not let yourselves believe that however smoothly concealed by education, by reason, and by confidential frankness these strong elements may be, they are ever in any circumstances altogether absent. (Wilfred Trotter)

In the long development of growth from infancy to adult life, there is a progressive change in social relationships, from one of complete dependence on parent, family, and teacher to one of relative independence. At the same time, the process of maturation requires the partial suppression of egocentric drives to the point that the affairs of other members of one's family and social group assume increasing importance. These trends and their modification during the life experience are part of the elaborate theory of personality development to be found in the writings of psychologists, particularly those of the psychoanalytically related schools. Deviations in these natural developments have been shown to prevent satisfactory social adjustment and to result in neuroticism.

Illness constitutes a threat not only to the physical integrity of the individual but also to his status in his social group, a fact that is soon learned by every thoughtful physician. Prolonged invalidism during childhood tends invariably to leave behind an excessive egocentricity, which may become the basis of a life-long neurosis. In the adult, illness often enforces a return to a posture of dependency, a change usually accompanied by feelings of apprehension and discouragement, sometimes leading to frank anxiety and depression. It is for these reasons that many adults in positions of responsibility express greater concern about the economic and social implications of their illness than about the illness itself. This explains a number of common psychologic defenses which the patient exercises against illness. He may refuse medical aid or if he summons the courage to consult a physician, he may minimize or even fail to mention the very symptom about which he is most deeply concerned. On the other hand, there are individuals whose attainment of maturity has been tenuous and uncertain, so that the position of dependency imposed by illness comes as a welcome relief from adult responsibility. They appear to enjoy illness and to resent anything that menaces their state of invalidism. Lesser degrees of this tendency are to be noted among those who consult the physician at the appearance of every new symptom and who are continuously preoccupied with their past illnesses and operations.

It is not easy to keep these basic facts in mind when examining a draped patient in the relatively neutral domain of the hospital ward or even in the private examining room. There are potent obstacles that stand in the way of the physician's making an adequate study of the patient's emotional life. Organic lesions have a way of compelling attention to themselves, and it is less exhausting to limit one's focus to the sphere of physical disease. More time, energy, and experience are necessary to view the patient as an active participant in an enormous moving pageant which includes the personal eccentricities of his forebears, his own fears and patterns of reaction, as well as the hopes for his children's future. It is not enough to know that poverty, insecurity, and perhaps poor vocational and domestic relations are now keeping the patient unhappily depressed, for all too often it is apparent that present socioeconomic (external) factors are not crucial determinants in the contemporary scene. To explain many of the manifestations of illness, it is necessary to view the patient more deeply as an organism with a vast repository of past experiences dating from the earliest days of life, many of which are vaguely remembered, yet have become the foundation of its current system of meeting daily problems. Under the threat of disease, defensive attitudes, which were useful in infancy and childhood but inappropriate in adult life, have a way of reasserting themselves; one of the oldest, the state of readiness for fight or flight (Cannon), may be a precipitating cause of illnesses such as peptic ulcer or hypertension when called upon too frequently.

The young physician usually finds himself inadequate in his dealings with the patient, for not only does he experience an inevitable sense of insecurity with respect to the patient's problems, but he feels equally uneasy about his newly acquired role of authority and responsibility. Moreover, both he and his older colleague often find it difficult to control their own reactions: disinterest because the patient presents no fascinating problem of organic disease, irritation at his verbosity and lack of clarity and consistency in the recital of the history, annoyance because the patient's illness fails to respond to treatment in the expected manner. The physician can hardly expect to achieve a deep appreciation of the patient's psychologic problems unless he learns to recognize and control his own.

More broadly stated, the physician has a special function in society because he should be a trained biologist in human behavior as well as in human diseases. He brings highly technical knowledge and skills to bear upon the problems of his patient as a person as well as upon the patient's physiologic functioning. He should bring to the suffering patient a quiet humanity, a confidence and security based upon the conviction that all will be done that can be done. The patient must feel that his unique individuality is recognized and appreciated and that his life's problems are meaningful. This is important in patients with well-defined organic disease as well as in the "stress" syndromes largely due to emotional pressures expressed through the body. If we can accept the principle of causality in human behavior, we can, with patience and diligence, learn to fathom the large outlines of a person's motivations even though many of the details very often remain obscure.

"Let me see in the sufferer the man alone. . . . Let me be intent upon one thing, O Father of Mercy, to be always merciful to Thy suffering children." (Maimonides)

IATROGENIC DISORDERS

Every physician, however rational and objective, must feel a measure of frustration and defeat when the patient's illness defies his most earnest efforts. Far more distressing to the physician, however, is the knowledge that on a person entrusted to his care he has inflicted an iatrogenic disorder. This term refers to adverse effects induced by the physician in caring for his patients: not only the direct injuries that may result from therapeutic and diagnostic measures, but also the hurt that can be inflicted by words or actions. The term generally carries with it the connotation of an untoward effect that could have been avoided by exercise of reasonable care and knowledge on the part of the physician.

Every medical procedure, whether diagnostic or therapeutic, contains within it the potentiality of harm, and it would be impossible to afford the patient all the benefits of modern scientific medicine if every legitimate step in diagnosis and therapy were withheld because of the possible risks involved. "Legitimate" here implies that the physician has weighed the pros and cons for a procedure and has concluded on rational grounds that it is advisable or essential for the relief of discomfort or the cure or amelioration of disease. An iatrogenic disorder in the sense that it is here considered is one that is deemed to have ensued when the deleterious effects of the physician's action exceed any advantages that could have reasonably been anticipated.

Not only are there unavoidable risks in the use of many of the newer and more potent therapeutic agents, even when employed with the utmost caution and intelligence, but the task of the physician is multiplied because the rate at which these new agents are introduced is usually more rapid than the pace at which contraindications become clear and understood. Even when the need for a drug is indisputable, its harmful effects can hardly be viewed with complacence, but they are all the more deplorable when a better understanding of the patient's illness and an appreciation of the dubious or negligible indications for the use of a drug or other procedure would have prevented the accident. None of the antibiotics is free from disturbing and sometimes dangerous side effects. A persistent diarrhea due to a proctitis caused by a broad-spectrum antibiotic may be far more distressing than the trivial respiratory infection for which it is prescribed. The use of cortisone in a patient with relatively mild arthritis may cause a serious gastric hemorrhage or perforation, the activation of a latent tuberculosis, or a fatal adrenal crisis if a relatively mild stress is imposed shortly after the withdrawal of the drug. Death may occur following an operative procedure when cortisone has been given and then withdrawn just prior to operation. It is known that in spite of tropic hormone administration (thyroid-stimulating, adrenal-cortical-stimulating, or follicle-stimulating hormone) several weeks are required before a hypofunctioning gland is restored to normal. Fatal homologous serum jaundice may follow the needless transfusions of plasma or blood, and serious depression of the bone marrow may result from a large variety of drugs. It is difficult to condone these and other catastrophes when the advantages expected of the offending agents could hardly have been commensurate with the risks inherent in their use. Too often a serious accident has followed the use of a therapeutic agent when the physician, at a loss for a diagnosis or a logical program of management, has simply decided upon an ill-advised "therapeutic trial." These hazards are likely to increase as patients become more and more informed of the miracles of modern research, widely heralded in newspapers, radio, and television, and more likely to demand that new discoveries be made available to them.

Ill effects have been known to ensue from the injudicious administration of excessive doses of vitamins. Fortunately, the widespread use of vitamin mixtures, fortified with minerals and other substances in ludicrously microscopic quantities, usually involves nothing more serious than a waste of money. But estrogens, cleverly advertised in even the most reputable medical journals to relieve almost every complaint occurring in a middle-aged woman, may cause uterine bleeding, which, aside from being serious in itself, inevitably raises the question of possible malignancy and the necessity for a diagnostic curettage. Thyroid extract, often given without justification and in doses far exceeding the endogenous level of secretory activity of a normal person, may precipitate ectopic rhythms or even congestive failure. Increasing evidence to incriminate the role of radiation in causing cancer and leukemia should make us wary of blithely ordering x-ray therapy for enlarged thymus, bursitis, annoying but harmless skin disorders, and even for diagnostic procedures, especially when repeated without sound reason.

There is one long-standing "iatrogenic" disorder that deserves particular mention: habituation to opiates. Too often the administration of an opiate to a susceptible patient may initiate a lifelong problem, all the more tragic when the need for sedation and relief of pain might have been met successfully by other measures. Added caution must be employed in the care of professional associates who have ready access to these drugs. The same warning applies to the use of synthetic derivatives of morphine or related substances which are sometimes glibly quoted as being relatively free from the danger of habituation.

It is equally important to consider the harm which physicians may do to patients through ill-considered or unjustified remarks. No matter what the constitutional make-up of the patient may be, he approaches the physician with at least some degree of fear and concern. His anxiety can be enhanced by a too serious demeanor, a flippant remark, or an impressive conference. Particularly is it true that untoward remarks or actions have had ill effects in relation to heart disease. Many persons have been crippled by cardiac neurosis because a physician has misinterpreted the significance of a heart murmur or an electrocardiographic finding. Even when organic heart disease is present, the patient may be more severely disabled by an unjustified statement regarding prognosis, or the imposition of too strict limitation of activity. The physician's manner and behavior are important in their implications to the patient. A spirited bedside discussion regarding the interpretation of auscultatory findings may give the false impression that serious heart disease exists. Conversely, a solemn-appearing conclave just out of earshot may cause the patient to conclude erroneously that his prognosis is grave or hopeless. Sometimes the patient's pride is unwittingly offended because of his misinterpretation of terms overheard, such as "degenerative process" or "neurosis." Similar-sounding medical words have been confused; e.g., a patient heard the word "leukopenia" and concluded that he had leukemia.

The good physician appreciates the fact that he is always in a position where he may cause injury by his treatment, by his words, and by his behavior. Skill in handling of patients cannot be taught; all that one can do is to emphasize the importance of tact, caution, judgment, and wisdom—ideals to be striven for but never fully attained. Better than words are the examples of thoughtfulness and understanding that are exhibited by the medical teacher or senior staff physician in his ward or clinic conferences with students and younger colleagues. But even if it were possible finally to achieve the goal—a generation of flawless physicians with infallible judgment and infinite wisdom—there would still be the patients who have uncanny capacity for misinterpreting the most innocent remarks and the most cautiously expressed opinions. In the end, "iatrogenic" illness is largely a matter of incomplete knowledge and fallacious judgment on the part of the physician, conjoined with the fears and anxieties of the patient. So long as medicine remains an art, "iatrogenic" illness will remain. The best hope for diminishing its incidence will come from a ceaseless consideration by the physician of the wisdom of each of his decisions and acts and from a greater appreciation of the mood and attitude of the person who consults the physician.

PART TWO
Cardinal Manifestations of Disease

Section 1: Pain

3 GENERAL CONSIDERATIONS OF PAIN

Raymond D. Adams and
William H. Resnik

Pain, it has been said, is one of "Nature's earliest signs of morbidity." Few will deny that it stands preeminent among all the sensory experiences by which man judges the existence of disease within himself. There are relatively few maladies that do not have their painful phases, and in many of them pain is a characteristic without which diagnosis must always be in doubt. It seems appropriate, therefore, to begin a section on the cardinal manifestations of disease with a discussion of the more general aspects of pain.

The painful experiences of the sick pose manifold problems for the practitioner of medicine, and the student should know something of these problems in order to prepare himself properly for the task ahead. He must be ready to diagnose disease in patients who have felt only the first rumblings of discomfort, before other symptoms and signs of disease have appeared. To cope effectively with problems of this type requires a sound knowledge of the sensory supply of the viscera and a familiarity with the typical symptoms of many diseases. He will be consulted by some patients who seek treatment for pains that appear to have no obvious structural basis, and further inquiry will disclose that worry, fear, and other troubled emotional states may have aggrandized relatively minor aches and pains. To understand problems of this type requires insight into the psychologic factors which influence behavior and a knowledge of psychiatric disease. Next, he must manage the "difficult pain cases," in which no amount of investigation will bring to light either medical disease or psychiatric illness, and it is here that he will sense the need of a sound and assured clinical approach to the pain problem. Finally, he must care for the patients with intractable pain, often from an established and incurable disease, who demand relief either by drug or the "less moderate means of surgery." The possibilities of the latter require a comprehension of the anatomic pathways of pain.

END ORGANS, AFFERENT TRACTS, AND NUCLEI OF TERMINATION OF PAIN PATHWAYS

Pain is now regarded by most physiologists and psychologists as a sensation which depends on its own specific sensory apparatus. The receptors in the skin and deep structures are fine, freely branching nerve endings, which form an intricate network. A single primary pain neurone, with its cell body in the posterior root ganglion, subdivides into many small peripheral branches to supply an area of skin of at least several square millimeters. The cutaneous area of each neurone overlaps with those of other neurones, so that every spot of skin is within the domain of from two to four sensory neurones. These free nerve endings are also found in many of the other specialized sensory receptors in the skin, such as the Krause end-bulbs, the Ruffinian plumes, and Pacinian corpuscles, which may account for the extremes of hot, cold, and pressure sensation becoming painful. However, the whole subject of specific nerve endings for each modality of sensation is being reinvestigated, and a final statement cannot be made at this time. It appears now that free nerve endings themselves may serve as receptors for other types of sensation. They are the only end organ in the cornea where touch, temperature, and pain are felt.

The sensory nerve fibers for pain course through somatic and visceral nerves, where they are mixed with motor fibers, and they enter the spinal cord and brain stem through the posterior roots and the cranial nerves, respectively. The fibers are of two sizes, one very small, 2 to 4 μ in diameter, with a slow conducting velocity, the other somewhat larger, 6 to 8 μ, with more rapid transmission rates. As the posterior root fibers enter the spinal cord they terminate in the posterior horn of gray matter, where they synapse with the secondary sensory neurone, the axone of which ascends and crosses the anterior commissure of the spinal cord within three or four segments to find its place in the anterolateral spinothalamic tract. Some of the nerve cells in the posterior horns send their axones to the central gray matter and anterior horn cells of the same segment and adjacent segments and subserve such reflex functions as the flexor reflex, of which the Babinski sign is but a part. The anterolateral spinothalamic tract continues upward to the posterolateral nucleus of the thalamus. This tract lies in the anterior part of the lateral and the anterior funiculi of the spinal cord and passes through the retroolivary part of the medulla and the dorsolateral parts of the pons and midbrain (Fig. 3-1, see also Fig. 28-3). The most superficial fibers are those from the opposite foot and leg and the successively deeper ones from the trunk, arm, neck, and face. Before reaching the thalamus, collateral branches are given off to other segmental structures, such as

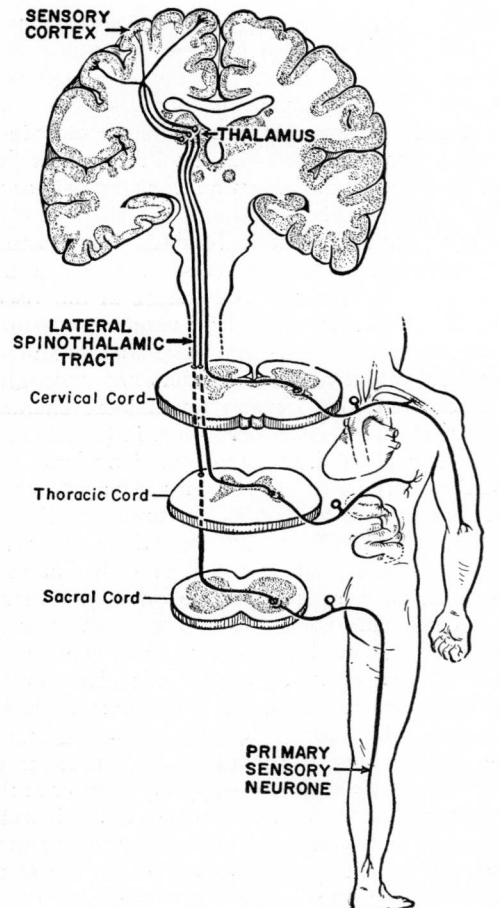

SENSORY
CORTEX

THALAMUS

LATERAL
SPINOTHALAMIC
TRACT

Cervical Cord

Thoracic Cord

Sacral Cord

PRIMARY
SENSORY
NEURONE

FIG. 3-1. Diagram of pain pathways. Stimuli acting on free nerve endings in the skin, muscles, blood vessels, and viscera give rise to sensory impulses which are transmitted along the primary sensory neurones into the posterior horn of the spinal cord. The secondary sensory neurones cross to the opposite side of the spinal cord almost immediately, within one or two segments, and combine to form the lateral spinothalamic tract, which terminates in the posterolateral nucleus of the thalamus. The third sensory neurone conveys the impulse from the thalamus to the cortex of the postcentral convolution. Visceral pain fibers, although they pass through the sympathetic ganglions en route to the spinal cord, do not differ from other somatic pain fibers.

the reticular formation of the brain stem and the hypothalamus. In addition there appears to be a great diminution in the number of fibers as one pursues the tract upward, which means that many of the ascending fibers are terminating in structures located in the brain stem. The thalamic termination of the spinothalamic tracts along with the secondary trigeminothalamic tracts synapse with the third sensory neurones, which project to the cortex in the

parietal lobes. Physiologists are not agreed, however, as to the cortical terminus, for electrical stimulation of the cortex in the conscious human being does not produce a painful sensation but only a tingling as a rule, nor do parietal lobe lesions cause central pain. Nearly all pain fibers from the periphery cross to the contralateral half of spinal cord, brain stem, and thalamus, but a few are believed to ascend ipsilaterally, at least for a considerable distance. This point is still being studied.

The pain-sensitive structures in the viscera and integuments of the body, the mechanisms of their excitation, and the peripheral nervous pathways are now fairly well established. The skin and mucous membranes are sensitive to pain, as are also many of the mesodermal tissues. As a means of quick orientation it should be remembered that the facial structures and anterior cranium are the field of the trigeminal nerves; the back of head, second cervical; the neck, third cervical; epaulet area, fourth cervical; deltoid area, fifth cervical; the thumb, sixth cervical; the index finger, seventh cervical; middle finger, eighth cervical; the little finger, first thoracic; the nipple segment, fifth thoracic; the umbilicus, tenth thoracic; the groin, first lumbar; the medial side of knee, third lumbar; the great toe, fifth lumbar; the little toe, first sacral; the back of thigh, second sacral; and genitosacral areas, third, fourth, and fifth sacrals (Figs. 28-1 and 28-2). The first to fourth thoracic nerves are the important dermatomes for the intrathoracic viscera, and the sixth, seventh, and eighth thoracic segments for the upper abdominal organs (see Figs. 28-1 and 28-2). The student should memorize these facts just as he has the multiplication table.

The stimuli that are effective in arousing the sensation of pain vary to some degree for each tissue. The very existence of pain impulses arising from viscera was debated until it was demonstrated that the adequate stimuli for pain originating in the heart or digestive tract, for example, are different from those which cause pain in the skin. The latter is sensitive to pricking, cutting, and burning, whereas these same forms of stimulation give rise to no distress when applied to the stomach or intestine. Pain in the gastrointestinal tract is produced by local trauma of an engorged or inflamed mucosa, distention or spasm of smooth muscle, and traction upon the mesenteric attachment. Severe pain may be induced in voluntary muscles by ischemia, the basis for the condition known as *intermittent claudication*, and also by the injection of water or irritating solutions. Also, prolonged contraction of muscles is a source of pain. Joints are insensitive to pricking, cutting, or cautery, but the synovial membrane responds to hypertonic saline solution and inflammation. Ischemia, the only proved cause of pain in the heart muscle, is responsible for the pain of angina pectoris and myocardial infarction. Arteries give rise to pain when punctured with a needle, when induced to pulsate excessively, as in migraine, and in certain diseases affecting their walls, such as temporal arteritis. Distortion of cranial vessels by traction, displacement, or distention is a common cause of headache.

PHYSIOLOGY AND PSYCHOLOGY OF PAIN

Superficial Pain. There are distinct differences in the characteristics of pain arising in the skin and that originating in the viscera. The effective stimulus for pain in the skin and superficial structures may be mechanical, thermal, chemical, or electrical. At their lowest levels these stimuli may evoke sensations of touch, pressure, warmth, or cold. Only when they reach a certain intensity, usually approaching tissue destruction, does pain develop, and the resulting experience is thereafter a mixed one, combining pain with the original sensation. Wolff points out that the threshold for burning pain with a thermal stimulus is approximately two thousand times the threshold for warmth. Tissue damage is believed to be a common effect of all pain stimuli, a fact from which our concept of the fundamental biologic or self-preservation value of pain derives much of its plausibility.

The threshold for the perception of pain is defined as the lowest intensity of stimulus which is recognized as pain. It is approximately the same in all persons. The pain threshold is lowered by inflammation of the peripheral nerve endings and is raised by local anesthetics (such as procaine), lesions of the peripheral and cerebral nervous system, centrally acting analgesic drugs, and distraction or suggestion. Neurotic patients in general have the same pain threshold as normal subjects, but their reaction may be excessive or abnormal. The threshold in the frontal-lobotomized patient is undiminished, but he no longer reacts to his pain. The intensity of the pain stimulus bears a roughly quantitative relationship to the reported degree of sensory experience. The ratio between the two is expressed by the Weber-Fechner law, which states that when a series of progressively increasing stimuli is applied, in order for minimal sensory differences to be perceived, the new stimulus must be increased by a constant fraction of the previously effective one.

Pain arising in the skin has a pricking or burning quality and is localized with a high degree of precision. Pricking pain has a more rapid rate of conductivity than burning pain, being transmitted by the larger pain fibers. Together they constitute the "double response" of Lewis. A painful stimulus to the toe produces first a pricking pain and about 2 sec later a burning pain. Ischemia of the nerve subserving

an area of skin produced by application of a tourniquet abolishes pricking pain before burning pain.

In the skin, localization of the pain stimulus is achieved by the simultaneous stimulation of multiple overlapping sensory neurones. Analgesia results from the interruption of all sensory neurones, and hypalgesia from the interruption of a few leaving others intact.

Deep (Including Visceral) Pain. The existence of visceral pain was long disputed, but it is now generally accepted that pain arising in the viscera does occur, provided that the stimuli are adequate. There is sound evidence that pain from viscera and deep skeletal structures is mediated through a common sensory apparatus and that the character and behavior of both are essentially the same. Hence, when we discuss visceral pain, the same principles will apply to deep skeletal pain. The pain is recognized by the patient as being "deep," i.e., deep to the skin; it is dull and aching in quality (although occasionally burning, as in the heartburn of esophageal disorders and rarely in anginal pain); the double response is absent; the pain is poorly localized and its borders are only vaguely delineated. It is probable that the high threshold and poor localization of deep pain are related, in part at least, to the relatively sparsely occurring sensory endings in the deep structures, in contrast to the closely distributed and overlapping terminals in the skin where pain threshold is low and accurately localized. Probably the most important characteristics are its relatively crude segmental localization beneath the surface of the body and its frequent reference to certain areas of the body. The simplest explanation for these latter phenomena is that suggested by Lewis:

If we suppose that certain tissues are represented in great detail in the sensorium, we can also understand that pain arising in these tissues may be localized with accuracy. But in other tissues having only a massive cerebral representation, localization may be expected to be less accurate. Segmental reference of deep pain may mean no more than that, centrally, the deep tissues supplied by a given cord segment have a general but little detailed representation. Thus, the impulses received whether these are derived from a viscus or from a deep somatic tissue, would tend to awaken very similar sensory impressions, and to be localized over a general sphere having no precise margins. And it may be regarded as natural enough that the general reference should be to regions that are relatively superficial, regions from which we are habitually receiving sensory impressions, and which are endowed with some positional sense.

The above concept implies that when pain originates in a viscus or deep skeletal tissue, the sensorium recognizes and localizes the pain as arising not in the exact region wherein it occurs but roughly in any or all structures innervated by cord segments subserving the affected viscus or deep somatic tissue. The pain appears to be projected toward the body surfaces supplied by these segments. For example, the sensory fibers from the heart terminate in the first through the fourth thoracic cord segments (possibly in some cases the fifth thoracic); and pain arising in the heart as the result of ischemia is not localized specifically in the region of the heart or in the precise region of the injured myocardium but in those superficial and deep structures whose sensory nerves also end in the first through the fourth thoracic spinal segments (see Fig. 3-2, showing theoretic distribution of heart pain in the first through fourth thoracic segments). Unfortunately, from the standpoint of diagnosis, the same cord segments receive fibers from the aorta, pulmonary artery, esophagus, and skeletal structures, which explains why pain arising in them may resemble that of myocardial infarction.

Referred Pain. All that has been said about segmental localization of deep pain applies also to referred pain, a term used in clinical medicine to indicate the appearance of pain in a location of the body some distance from the viscus in which the pain originates. According to the hypothesis of Lewis and Kellgren, presented above, the referred pain is an integral part of the phenomenon of visceral pain. Thus, with cardiac pain in which sensory impulses enter mainly the left half of the first through fourth thoracic cord segments, the reference of pain to the arms is explained by the anatomic fact that the first thoracic segment supplies the inner surface of the arm as well as the thorax and heart. Thus it is just as natural for heart pain to appear in the characteristic location in the left arm as it is in the anterior midchest.

This view of visceral and referred pain is obviously incomplete. It does not explain why, in the total area bounded by the first through fourth thoracic myotomes, heart pain should so commonly appear only in the anterior midline. Possibly this is related to the fact that the anterior surfaces of the body are more profusely supplied with sensory fibers. It does not explain, also, why in exceptional cases the pain may be experienced only in some unusual part of the "normal" area, for example, an anginal pain occurring only in the interscapular region of the chest. Nor do we know why visceral pain may sometimes overflow into territories completely unrelated to the known innervation of the involved viscus, for example, the appearance of anginal pain in the jaws. Clinical experience teaches us that spread of pain beyond the limits that are "normal" is due in some cases to an unusual intensity of pain; thus an anginal pain that is ordinarily confined to the midsternal region (second through

fourth thoracic nerves) may spread to the neck and shoulders (third through seventh cervical nerves). In other cases, extension of pain outside the normal boundaries may be due to coexistent lesions in structures with innervation not too distant from the cord segments primarily involved in the cardiac pain. Thus an anginal pain may be localized high in the epigastrium (seventh and eighth thoracic nerves) when peptic ulcer or gallbladder disease is also present. This may be because of summation of stimuli reaching the affected cord segments. We do not know why visceral pains overflowing into neighboring cord segments beyond the limits that are normal for the viscus tend preferentially to wander into higher rather than lower segments, except that cephalad structures have a more abundant representation in consciousness than do caudad ones.

Deep Skeletal Pain. Since there is sound experimental evidence for the view that visceral pain and deep skeletal pain are mediated through a common deep sensory system, it is not surprising that their characteristics should be similar and that on occasion differentiation between the two may be extremely difficult. Thus a small tear or injury in a lumbar muscle or ligament innervated by the twelfth thoracic or first lumbar nerve may give rise to a pain whose quality and localization, including radiation into the groin and scrotum, are indistinguishable from those of pain caused by renal colic. A similar injury in the right upper rectus muscle may cause a pain that mimics closely the pain of gallbladder colic; and a lesion in a muscle or ligament deep in the chest wall may cause pain with radiation to the left arm, identical in localization with that of angina. Under these circumstances, differentiation of somatic from visceral pain must be made on grounds other than the location and reference of pain.

Hyperalgesia, Hyperpathia, and Involuntary Muscle Spasm. Superficial pain is often accompanied by hyperalgesia (increased sensitivity) of the skin, and deep pain by hyperalgesia of the subcutaneous tissue and muscle in the corresponding dermatomes and myotomes. This phenomenon of excessive sensitivity or soreness may be due to either hyperalgesia or hyperpathia. The former refers to a lowering of the pain threshold and is often induced by inflammations not only in the skin but also in the mucous membrane of the nose, stomach, colon, bladder, or esophagus. Hyperpathia refers to an alteration in the sensory experience without reduction in the sensory threshold, in which instance stimuli evoke a more intense and persistent sensation than usual. Unlike other sensory experiences, pain from deep structures may also cause involuntary spasm in skeletal muscles supplied by the same or adjacent segments of the spinal cord, e.g., spasm of the right upper rectus muscle with a gallstone impacted in the cystic duct or of the pectoral muscles in myocardial infarction.

Pain sensation may be induced by stimulation of the receptors or by irritation of peripheral nerves or roots, and in certain areas of the body it may be abolished by diseases which affect the peripheral or cerebral nervous system or by a surgical procedure which may accomplish the same result. Pain in a circumscribed region may be terminated by section of the nerve which supplies that region (neurotomy) or the spinal roots (posterior rhizotomy); pain in a limb or one side of the trunk may be interrupted by section of the anterolateral spinothalamic tract (lateral spinal tractotomy in the spinal cord or lateral medullary tractotomy in the medulla).

Perception of Pain. The arrival of pain impulses at the thalamocortical level of the nervous system is attended by conscious awareness of the pain stimulus. Clinical study has not informed us of the exact localization of the nervous apparatus for this mental process. It is not entirely abolished by a total hemispherectomy including the thalamus on one side. It is often said that impulses reaching the thalamus create awareness of the attributes of sensation and that the parietal cortex is necessary for the appreciation of the intensity and localization of the sensation. This seems an oversimplification. Probably a close and harmonious relationship between thalamus and cortex must exist in order for a sensory experience to be complete. The traditional separation of sensation (in this instance awareness of pain) and perception (awareness of the painful stimulus) has been abandoned in favor of the view that sensation, perception, and the various conscious and unconscious responses to a pain stimulus comprise an indivisible process.

Although similar to other sensory or perceptive phenomena in certain respects, such as predictable response to given intensity of stimulus, pain differs in other ways. One of its most remarkable characteristics is the strong feeling tone, or affect, with which it is endowed, nearly always one of unpleasantness. Furthermore, pain does not appear to be subject to negative adaptation. Most stimuli, if applied continuously, soon cease to be effective, whereas pain may persist as long as the stimulus is operative and, by establishing a central excitatory state, may even outlast the stimulus.

Psychologic Aspects of Pain. A discussion of this problem could hardly be complete without some reference to the influence of emotional states or to the importance of racial, cultural, and religious factors on the pain response, especially the overt expressions. It is common knowledge that some individuals, by virtue of training, habit, or phlegmatic character, are relatively stoical and that others are excessively responsive to pain. Rarely one encounters individuals who are totally incapable of experiencing pain throughout their lifetime, not from any lack of sensory endings or peripheral sensory apparatus but from some peculiarity of central reception.

Lastly, it is important to keep in mind the devastating effects of chronic pain. As Ambroise Paré is alleged to have said, "There is nothing that abateth so much the strength as paine." Continuous pain can be observed to have an adverse effect on the entire nervous system. There is increased irritability, fatigue, troubled sleep, poor appetite, and loss of emotional stability. Courageous men are reduced to a whimpering, pitiable state that may arouse only the scorn of a healthy person. They are irrational about illness and may make unreasonable demands of family and physician. Of course the effect of narcotic drugs often complicates the picture. This state, which may be termed *pain shock,* once established, requires delicate but firm management.

CLINICAL APPROACH TO THE PATIENT WITH PAIN AS THE PREDOMINANT SYMPTOM

One of the most frequent errors is to think of pains always in terms of the severe, intractable pains of disease, overlooking the fact that there are thousands of other pains which are part of the daily sensory experience of otherwise healthy individuals. To mention but a few, there is the momentary, hard pain over an eye, in the temporal region, or in the ear or jaw, which strikes with alarming suddenness; the more persistent ache which arises in some fleshy part such as the shoulder, neck, thigh, or calf; the darting pain in an arm or leg; the fleeting precordial discomfort that arouses momentarily the thought of heart disease; the breath-taking catch in the side; the cluster of abdominal pains with their associated intestinal rumblings; and the brief discomfort upon movement of a joint. These *"normal pains,"* as they should be called, occur at all ages, tending to be brief and to depart as obscurely as they came. They acquire medical significance only when elicited by the inquiring physician or when presented as a complaint by the worried patient; and of course they must always be distinguished from the *abnormal pains* of disease.

When pain by its intensity, duration, and the circumstance of its occurrence appears to be abnormal or constitutes one of the principal symptoms of disease, an attempt should be made by careful analysis of it to reach a tentative decision as to its cause and the mechanism of its production. This can usually be accomplished by a very thorough interrogation of the patient in which he is encouraged to relate as accurately as possible the main characteristics of the pain. This is followed by a physical

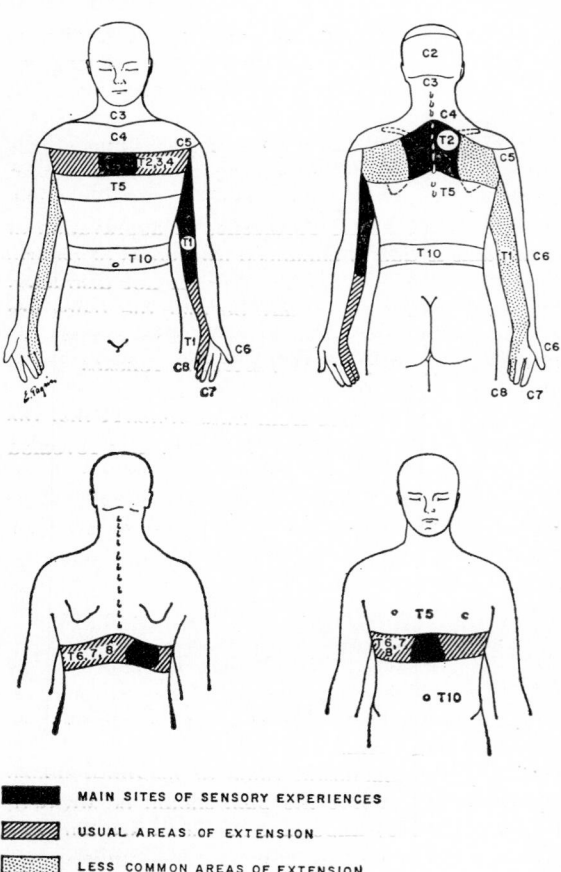

MAIN SITES OF SENSORY EXPERIENCES

USUAL AREAS OF EXTENSION

LESS COMMON AREAS OF EXTENSION

FIG. 3-2. Radiation and sites of reference of cardiac pain (*upper*); gallbladder pain (*lower*).

examination and not infrequently by special laboratory tests, of which there has been much refinement in recent years.

Location of Pain. When the pain is caused by a superficial lesion, the cause and effect are usually so obvious that no problem is posed. It is the deep lesion, whether involving somatic or visceral structures, that causes trouble, and here exact localization becomes especially important. We have already seen that pain originating from such tissues no longer is sensed as coming from them but is instead roughly segmental, i.e., within the territory of the cord segments innervating the structure. The identification of the segments involved is of value, for it sets the limit on the diagnostic possibilities that must be considered, i.e., to those structures having a corresponding innervation. Thus an epigastric or subxiphoid pain or one in the opposite region in the back obliges one to search for its cause in all those structures innervated by the sixth through eighth thoracic cord segments, i.e., the esophagus, stomach, duodenum, pancreas, biliary tract, the upper retroperitoneal structures, as well as the deep

somatic tissues in this region. Also one must consider the possibility that a lesion in a viscus innervated by spinal segments above or below the sixth through eighth thoracic cord segments may at times be the source of pain that has spread outside its normal boundaries and involved the epigastrium (Fig. 3-2).

Provoking and Relieving Factors. These factors are of greater value than quality of pain in providing important data concerning its mechanism. Pain related to breathing, swallowing, and defecation focuses attention on the respiratory apparatus, the esophagus, and the lower bowel, respectively. A pain coming on a few minutes after the beginning of general bodily movement and relieved within a few minutes by rest indicates ischemia as the probable cause. Pain occurring several hours after meals and relieved by food or alkali suggests the irritative effect of acid on the raw lining of the stomach or duodenum. Pain that is brought on or relieved by certain movements or postures of parts of the body is usually due to the activity of diseased skeletal structures (bones, muscles, ligaments). Pain that is enhanced by cough, sneeze, and strain is usually radicular in origin or arises in ligamentous structures. Pain that is increased or altered by cutaneous stimuli is due to disease in sensory tracts in the peripheral or central nervous system. These are a few examples illustrating the paramount importance of determining with the greatest possible accuracy the factors that influence the appearance or relief of pain.

Quality and Time-Intensity Characteristics of the Pain. These features are of importance. However, too much stress should not be laid on the adjectives that the patient uses to describe his pain. His choice of words will depend, in part at least, on his vocabulary and on what he imagines is taking place. "Crushing" or "squeezing" are commonly employed to describe an anginal pain, and this implication of pressure does have some significance, since the pain may depend on an associated involuntary contraction of the pectoral muscles. Another patient with the same disease, however, may describe the pain as "exploding" or "burning." Far more important than the adjective used is the information that the pain is steady and does not fluctuate. Similarly, the ulcer pain is frequently designated as "gnawing"; but again, the deep, steady quality is more important than the word used to denote it. Gallbladder colic and renal colic are misnomers, if by colic is meant a "paroxysmal abdominal pain due to spasm, obstruction or distention of any of the hollow viscera." *In both these disorders, the pain is steady.* The aching quality of all deep pains is usually characteristic, but there are in addition several other informative attributes. A true colicky pain, one that is rhythmic and cramping, suggests an obstructive lesion in a hollow viscus. If the patient is a woman and has had children, it is a good idea to ask whether her "cramp" resembles the pains she had during childbirth. A pain that is steady and varies little or not at all from moment to moment means that the stimulus to pain is steady and unwavering, as in angina pectoris and peptic ulcer. Thus a pain in the anterior midsternal region whose intensity fluctuates appreciably within the space of a minute or two is not due to angina, even though the history may appear to suggest a relation to exertion. Similarly, a high epigastric pain appearing several hours after a meal and even apparently relieved by food is not caused by an ulcer if the pain fluctuates perceptibly within seconds or a few minutes. The stimulus to ulcer pain does not quickly vary in intensity. A throbbing pain indicates that an arterial pulsation is giving rise to painful stimuli. Sharp, transitory pain is caused by disease of nerve roots or ganglions, as exemplified by tic douloureux or tabes, or by some disorder in a somatic tissue such as a tear of a muscle or ligament; and often there is a background of dull, aching pain. Particularly noteworthy here is the abrupt intensification of the dull ache of root pain by cough, sneeze, or strain which momentarily increases the intraspinal pressure and stretches or alters the position of the root.

Mode of Onset of the Pain. This factor is also important. A pain reaching its full intensity almost immediately after its appearance suggests a rupture of tissue. The pain of a dissecting aortic aneurysm often develops in this manner. In fact, the suddenness and the severity of the pain, reaching a peak of intensity within seconds or minutes, sometimes provides the first clue differentiating this type of chest pain from that caused by myocardial infarction. A similarly rapid accession of pain may occur with the rupture of a peptic ulcer.

Duration of the Pain. This is another important attribute. Anginal pain rarely lasts less than 2 or 3 min or more than 10 or 15 min. Ulcer pain may continue for an hour or more, unless terminated by the ingestion of food or alkali or a tumbler of water.

Severity of Pain. In any given disease, the severity of pain is subject to wide variation, and also patients differ in their tolerance to it. Therefore one cannot judge the gravity of an illness by the intensity of the pain. As a rule, pains that completely interrupt work and pleasurable activity, require opiates for relief, enforce bed rest, and awaken the patient from sound sleep are to be taken more seriously than those which have the opposite characteristics.

Time of Occurrence. An accurate determination must be made of the time of occurrence. The relationship of ulcer pain to the preceding meal has already been described. Postural aches come after prolonged activity and disappear with rest, whereas arthritic pains are usually most severe during the first movements after prolonged inactivity. The mechanism for this latter phenomenon is not known; nor do we understand why painful lesions of the bone, such as those caused by metastatic cancer, are likely to be most disturbing during the night. It is possible that the occurrence or aggravation of such pains is due to enhanced awareness of painful stimuli at a time when the mind is not distracted by other stimuli; or it may be that the pains are now more easily evoked by unconscious movements made during sleep when protective reflexes are in abeyance.

It should be obvious from these remarks that the full significance of a pain is usually not revealed by any one single characteristic. It is only by combining all these data that one can determine its anatomic site and its mechanism. In general, *the most important and revealing clues are obtained from the answers to the questions: What brings on the pain? What relieves it?* Pain is a subjective manifestation, not a state to be observed or measured. The accuracy of our data depends on the skill with which we frame our questions and on the powers of observation and memory of the person answering them.

Finally the diagnostic value of measures which *reproduce* and *relieve the pain* should be stressed. Not only are they important for diagnosis, but they convince the patient that the physician understands and can control the mechanism of his pain and the illness behind it. Climbing several flights of stairs under the physician's supervision may settle the question of the presence or absence of angina pectoris. An injection of procaine into a tender area in the chest wall or some other skeletal structure with complete disappearance of the pain may establish a skeletal origin and exclude the possibility of visceral disease. Reproducing the distress sometimes caused by aerophagia merely by distending the esophagus or stomach with air, or reproducing the vague but sometimes alarming sensation of pressure in the chest caused by unconscious hyperventilation by having the patient hyperventilate are other examples of how the principle of the reproduction of pain may be usefully employed.

A systematic interrogation of the patient will not lead to accurate diagnosis in every instance, but the habit of searching for the identifying characteristics of pain will enable the physician to increase his skill in this difficult field. Furthermore, after becoming familiar with the customary responses to these questions, he becomes more alert to the anxious, the hysterical, or the depressed patient who while complaining of pain seems incapable of describing any of its details, or unwilling to do so. Instead, there is preoccupation with theories of what is wrong or with the treatments or mistreatments already given. Finally, there will always be cases that defy solution, when the physician can proceed only by repeatedly reexamining the patient, explaining the need for continued observation, and enlisting his aid and forbearance during this trying period. Asking the patient to tolerate a certain amount of pain without the use of powerful analgesics is usually effective, particularly when the possibility of drug addiction is explained to him.

INTRACTABLE PAINS

In the relatively rare circumstances when all manner of investigation has failed to throw light on the cause and mechanism of the pain, demands for pain-relieving surgery may become increasingly insistent. The physician may in desperation turn to measures which are more dangerous than the disease. Here the commonest source of error is to operate unnecessarily on the hysterical patient (see Chap. 43), only to discover too late that each operative procedure leaves a new pain, often at a higher level than the first. Or, a depressive psychosis may masquerade as a painful state, and electric shock therapy may dramatically terminate the illness. Sometimes a half dozen or more operations are unsuccessfully performed on a single patient. The safest rule to follow in these cases is not to use opiates continuously or to recommend operation for the relief of pain unless a reasonable diagnosis has been made. For the pains of metastatic cancer, the thalamic pain of vascular disease of the brain, and other incurable diseases, the relative advantages of the controlled use of opiates versus lateral spinothalamic tractotomy or frontal lobotomy must be carefully weighed in each patient. The age of the patient, life expectancy, and mental state are all of importance in selecting the treatment procedure. Too often today an operation on the spinal cord or brain is chosen in preference to narcotics and the controlled use of drugs. Forgotten is the fact that many patients with cancer were formerly kept relatively comfortable and active by the judicious use of morphine and its analogues and were never subjected to costly operations or deprived of any of those qualities of mind and character which are so treasured by their families.

Superficial pain arising in integumentary structures rarely presents a problem in therapy. Acetylsalicylic acid, 0.30 to 0.60 Gm orally every 4 hr, usually suffices. Acetophenetidin may be added. These two drugs are a particularly effective combination when one element of pain is integumentary. Commercial proprietary preparations of these drugs containing caffeine or amphetamine such as A.S.A., Empirin compound, or Edrisal are available in most pharmacies. The caffeine or amphetamine is particularly useful if there is central nervous system depression. When this type of pain is not effectively controlled by nonnarcotic analgesics, codeine should be given. Usually the addition of small amounts (8 to 30 mg) of codeine phosphate to the standard dose of acetylsalicylic acid and acetophenetidin is effective. A preparation containing codeine phosphate 8 to 30 mg, acetylsalicylic acid 0.23 Gm, acetophenetidin 0.16 Gm, and caffeine 0.032 Gm is commercially available (Empirin compound with codeine phosphate). Codeine, 30 to 45 mg every 3 hr, gives maximal analgesia with minimal side effects. Adequate rest and relief of muscle tension should also be encouraged. The application of heat, especially moist heat, is usually beneficial. Occasionally, cold applications are preferred; but with the exception of cooling packs applied to an inflamed, burning skin or to a causalgia, cold is more likely to aggravate than to soothe the painful condition.

Occasionally integumental and deep pains of skeletal structures are of such severity as to require more powerful narcotic analgesics, such as meperidine hydrochloride (Demerol) in doses of 50 to 100 mg orally or intramuscularly, methadone hydrochloride 5 to 10 mg orally or subcutaneously, or dihydromorphine hydrochloride (Dilaudid) 1.0 to 2.0 mg orally or subcutaneously. These drugs are most useful in conditions when sedation is not required. When pain is unusually severe and some degree of euphoria is desired, morphine is the ideal drug. It should be given in doses of 8.0 to 15.0 mg orally or subcutaneously. Frequently a dose as small as 4.0 to 6.0 mg will relieve pain without causing undesirable nausea and vomiting. If the original dose is too small, a second dose of the same or slightly larger size can be given in 2 hr. This divided dose is less likely to induce nausea and vomiting than the larger single dose, because the stimulating effect of the first dose is insufficient to produce these symptoms and the depressant effect which follows reduces the sensitivity of the vomiting mechanism or renders it refractory to the second dose. Since all these narcotic analgesics are, for the most part, detoxified by the liver, they either should not be used or should be given in only half the usual dose in cases of liver disease, myxedema, adrenal insufficiency, and other states in which the metabolic rate is reduced. Morphine and related narcotic analgesics tend to cause pruritus and therefore should be used with care in patients with skin irritability. The possibility of initiating addiction in susceptible individuals must be carefully evaluated in every instance.

If the patient exhibits mental tension, insomnia, and restlessness, a sedative drug such as phenobarbital or sodium barbital may be given with the analgesic agents. Sedative medication, especially the quick-acting barbiturates, should not be used alone for the control of pain, because they sometimes cause excitement and confusion under these circumstances.

Visceral pain originating in the stomach, gallbladder, intestines, or heart is usually very poorly controlled by the nonnarcotic analgesics. Various combinations of acetylsalicylic acid and acetophenetidin usually prove to be ineffective unless given with sedatives. The narcotic analgesics are the agents of choice, but of course should never be given until the physician is certain that the relief of the pain will not mask the state of his patient. If sedation is not desirable, and if constipation is a troublesome problem, the newer synthetic analgesics, meperidine in doses of 50 to 100 mg orally or intramuscularly or methadone 5 to 10 mg by mouth or subcutaneously every 4 to 6 hr, are recommended. Like morphine, these drugs are habit-forming, but they do not share with morphine the properties of strong analgesia, sedation, and euphoria. Patients with severe visceral pain who are also anxious or fearful and unable to relax or sleep should be given morphine sulfate in doses of 8 to 15 mg subcutaneously. The well-known spasmogenic effects of morphine are partially counteracted by atropine sulfate, 0.3 to 0.4 mg. Aminophylline, 0.5 Gm intravenously, overcomes much of this undesirable spastic action; a rectal suppository of 0.5 Gm, although less effective, may be substituted.

Intractable pain due to incurable diseases such as metastatic carcinoma is one of the most difficult of therapeutic problems. As a rule, one resorts to narcotic drugs because of their strong analgesic action, and habituation is accepted as the lesser of two evils. An alternative is "pain-relieving surgery." Section of peripheral nerves, the lateral spinothalamic tracts in the spinal cord (cordotomy), or the lateral part of the medulla and lobotomy are relatively safe procedures which have advantages in certain cases over the continuous use of opiates.

REFERENCES

Cohen, H.: The Mechanism of Visceral Pain, Trans. Med. Soc. London, 64:35, 1944.

Feindel, W. H., G. Weddell, and D. C. Sinclair: Pain Sensibility in Deep Somatic Structures, J. Neurol., Neurosurg. Psychiat., 11:113, 1948.

Hardy, J. D., H. G. Wolff, and H. Goodell: "Pain Sensations and Reactions," Baltimore, The Williams & Wilkins Company, 1952.

Lewis, T.: "Pain," New York, The Macmillan Company, 1942.

Ryle, J. A.: "The Natural History of Disease," London, Oxford University Press, 1936.

White, J. C., and W. H. Sweet: "Pain, Its Mechanisms and Neurosurgical Control," Springfield, Ill., Charles C Thomas, Publisher, 1955.

4 HEADACHE
George Pickering

Interpreted literally, headache signifies ache or pain located anywhere in the head; but its meaning has been narrowed by long usage to signify ache or pain experienced in the region of the cranial vault.

Headache is thus an experience or sensation which can be described. As in other forms of pain, its description can be analyzed into certain components—namely, quality, location, intensity, time relations, and the manner in which it is influenced by other events in the immediate environment of the patient. These characteristics, the associated sensations, and the presence of certain physical signs are the means whereby it is possible to decide which disorder is responsible for headache in a given instance. The characteristics of headache may now be discussed briefly in general terms.

Quality. The quality of pain is often described in terms of past experience, actual or imagined. Such descriptions are of limited value in deciding the origin of pain. There is strong evidence for the belief that if associated sensations are excluded, the subject can recognize only two types of pain by its quality: superficial pain arising from the skin, which is sharp and burning in character; and deep pain arising from all structures deep to the skin, which is dull or aching. With very few exceptions, headache is a dull, aching pain, and thus of the type that arises from structures deep to the skin.

Location. Pain arising from the skin is localized fairly precisely to its point of origin. Pain arising from structures deep to the skin is less accurately localized the farther the point of origin is beneath the surface, and both pain arising from really deep somatic structures and pain from visceral tissues are referred in a segmental pattern. These same principles apply to headache. Thus pain arising from a localized lesion not far beneath the surface, such as temporal arteritis, may be fairly well localized over the lesion itself. But with deep extracranial lesions, such as those affecting the accessory sinuses of the nose and the upper cervical vertebras and their joints and ligaments, pain may be more widely referred in an area that is not directly over the lesion; still more is this true of intracranial lesions. Although headache is not necessarily located directly over the lesion, the reference of pain arising from the various structures from which it may arise is fairly constant from one subject to another, and is thus of some diagnostic value.

Intensity. The intensity of pain is notoriously hard to assess. Patients' statements on intensity are not of themselves of much value, for it is not unusual to find that the most extravagant epithets are applied to pains for which there is little organic basis, and where the physician is forced to conclude that the major disturbance is not of the body but of the mind. The sensitivity to pain varies with different individuals, and with the same individual under different circumstances. Intensity may be judged by other criteria. Thus headache which wakens the patient at night and, to a lesser extent, headache which prevents sleep are nearly always of organic origin. Severe headaches again are often accompanied by vomiting, but this is more common in those of intracranial than of extracranial origin. The severest headaches are probably those associated with meningitis, and here the patient may frequently sweat with the pain and be obliged to cry out.

Time-Intensity Curve. Very rarely is headache a momentary flash of severe pain, and then usually it is due to trigeminal neuralgia affecting the supraorbital division of the nerve. More usually the pain lasts minutes or hours, and the duration of pain may be of assistance, diagnostically. Thus in cerebral tumor the pain occurs at first in paroxysms lasting several minutes. In many forms of headache of extracranial origin and of little pathologic import, the pain may at the outset last for some days. Some pains, though continuous, wax and wane with the pulse beat, and it is clear that in such instances of throbbing pain the pain arises from a structure which is moved by the arterial pulse.

Relationship of Headache to Other Events in the Environment. In many instances of organic headache, the tissue disturbance which leads to the excitation of the pain nerves is influenced by events in the environment. Thus exposure to cold may act as a trigger to that ill-defined process that will be considered under nodular or fibrositic headache. In cerebral tumor, circumstances influencing the inflow or outflow of blood from the cranial cavity may precipitate headache. The headache of hypertensive disease is most frequent on waking in the morning, as is that of cerebral tumor, and that of infection of the nasal accessory sinuses may recur at certain hours of the day with almost astronomic regularity. Other examples will be found later, but these instances serve to show that an analysis of this feature of headache is of considerable value from the diagnostic aspect, and the facts so elicited must, of course, be accounted for in any hypothesis that seeks to explain the mechanism of pain.

Pain-sensitive Structures. The structures which may give rise to headache are, in general, those of the cranial cavity, the cranium itself, the covering of the skull, and other adjacent structures such as the orbital contents, the accessory nasal sinuses, and the deep structures of the neck close to the occipital region of the skull. Of intracranial structures, the brain itself is insensitive. Its pial covering is likewise insensitive except over the great vessels of the circle of Willis, and their chief branches such as the anterior, posterior, and middle cerebral, for a variable distance from their origin. Pain from these structures is referred to the same side of the head, if far from the midline, or bilaterally, if near the midline. From the anterior and middle cerebral arteries the pain is referred to the forehead and temple, from basilar to the occiput. The parietal dura mater is sensitive only along the course of the main arteries such as the middle meningeal, from which pain is referred to the temple on the same side, and along the course of the large venous sinuses such as the superior longitudinal sinus, where the cerebral veins enter. Deflection of the falx, or of the tentorium, also produces pain. Pain from the superior longitudinal sinus and straight sinus is referred to behind or above the eye, from the lateral part of the lateral sinus to the ear. Deflection of the tentorium produces supraorbital pain. The periosteum of the skull is sensitive but the bone not so. Of superficial structures, the galea, muscles, ligaments, arteries, and skin are all sensitive to pain. Pain arising from the more superficial of these deep structures—that is, the coverings of the cranial vault over most of its extent—is referred fairly well to the point stimulated. But with the deeper ligaments, muscles, and tendons of the occipital region, reference over the upper cervical segments is found. The nerves conveying sensory impulses are the trigeminal, particularly the ophthalmic division from structures above the tentorium; from structures below the tentorium the glossopharyngeal and the upper cervical spinal nerves.

Fatigue and Psychologic Disturbance. It is not infrequent for headache to develop in otherwise healthy individuals during times of great mental or emotional stress or when their tolerance is lowered by infection or other debilitating agents. Such a tendency may be enhanced by such common disturbances of the mind as anxiety, fear, conflict, and fatigue. In such cases headache tends to occur toward the end of the day and to be experienced as a dull ache in the forehead which may spread to the temples or occiput; it is not usually throbbing and usually is relieved by sound sleep. There has been a tendency to assume that this headache is feigned or imagined or determined by psychologic factors, but this seems an unlikely explanation. It is accepted that fear and worry may accentuate pain by focusing attention on it, but it is held that the pain itself nearly always has as its basis the stimulation of pain nerves. It is suggested that many such cases result from excessive and maintained contraction of the muscles of facial expression, particularly the frontalis and the muscles of the scalp and neck. It may often be observed in such persons that the forehead is unusually deeply furrowed, and this type of headache can sometimes be abolished by conscious relaxation of the muscles of the forehead and scalp.

A sensation of pressure on the head, particularly on the vertex—as of a tightly fitting hat—is also met with in psychologic disorders, but while this is often described as headache, it is not true pain. It seems that in those with a disorder limited to the mind, the symptoms referred to the head are not so much simple sensations as expressions of the disordered personality.

Aside from the importance of fatigue and psychologic disorders as primary causes of headache, these factors are of great secondary importance in precipitating and aggravating headache due to almost any other primary cause. It is important that the physician should bear this consideration in mind, for if he does not he will be unable to assess the relative parts played in the production of the symptom by local disturbances of the body, and by the mind. On such assessment must depend his whole therapeutic approach.

VARIETIES OF HEADACHE

In perusing the following account of headache as we know it today, the reader should realize that the experimental method was used for the first time in the study of headache less than 30 years ago. He will realize that our knowledge is by no means complete and that both the classification presented and the explanations offered may require modification as knowledge advances. The classification to follow is presented from the standpoint of logical arrangement rather than clinical importance, and hence such frequent causes of headache as migraine and fever are not discussed first. The main classification used here is (1) headache arising from cranial and extracranial structures, (2) headache arising from intracranial structures, and (3) headache which cannot as yet be classified in this way.

From Cranial and Extracranial Structures

By their peculiar structure and function the viscera naturally interest the student and practitioner much more than the body wall, and in the case of headache the idea of an intracranial cause occurs most readily. But it is very probable that the cause of headache lies outside the skull at least as frequently as inside.

From Arteries or Their Neighborhood. As will be discussed later, there is evidence that dilatation of the temporal arteries, with stretching of surrounding sensitive structures, is responsible for most of the pain in migraine and some of the pain in febrile headache. In addition, the temporal or occipital arteries may rarely be the seat of a subacute inflammation involving the periarterial tissues

and the arterial wall, often leading to occlusion of the vessel ("temporal arteritis"). Pain begins in the region of the affected vessel and, as it becomes more severe, spreads more widely over that side of the head; sometimes pain is more or less bilateral throughout, though it is not yet certain whether in such cases arteries are affected bilaterally. The pain is dull, with or without a throbbing or shooting element. It is often severe, sometimes interfering with sleep, and commonly lasts for weeks or months. The disease affects individuals over the age of fifty-five, and other arteries—retinal, cerebral, and the major branches of the aorta—may be affected. Disturbances of vision, particularly blindness, which is usually permanent, and transient diplopia are common, and periods of disorientation are not infrequent. Blindness is due to obstruction of the ophthalmic artery or of the central retinal artery or one of its branches, and lesions of these may be seen on ophthalmoscopic examination. Other evidences of a constitutional upset may be found, such as fever, malaise, anorexia, night sweats, a raised sedimentation rate, and anemia. The affected arteries of the scalp are always tender, and the overlying skin may be reddened; the arterial pulse distal to the lesion is usually lost for a while.

Associated with Myofibrositis. In certain cases of headache, tender nodules may be felt near the cranial insertion of the sternomastoids; in muscles near their insertions to the superior and inferior nuchal lines; in the occipitalis, frontalis, and trapezius muscles; or in the temporalis and the galea aponeurotica. The pathologic basis of these nodules, as of those in myofibrositis of the trunk, is obscure, and it is also uncertain whether the tenderness of these nodules signifies that pain arises from them or is a secondary consequence of pain. It is thus possible that the tenderness of these nodules and the pain itself are referred from a distant and deep-seated focus, for nodules may be felt in the absence of pain or tenderness, and pain of deep origin is widespread and accompanied by deep tenderness in the area of the pain. The pain, which is of the deep aching type, often begins in a localized area in the forehead, temple, or nape of neck, and spreads to involve one or both sides of the head. It is often precipitated by exposure to cold or draft, and intense paroxysms may be added to an ache which may continue for weeks or months at a lower level of intensity. The pain may be severe but rarely keeps the patient awake at night. It can be abolished in many cases by massage applied to the nodules, but massage may make the pain worse at first. The frequency of this type of headache is disputed; by some it is said to be the commonest of all, but the general opinion seems to be that it is rather uncommon.

From Ligaments and Deep Structures Attached to the Occiput and Upper Cervical Vertebras. If hypertonic saline solution is injected into ligament, muscle, tendon, fascia, periosteum, or periarticular tissue situated deep in the neck near the occiput, pain is referred to the back of the head and the nape of the neck on the same side. One of the commonest causes of pain in these areas is cervical osteoarthritis. A similar pain may be seen in spondylitis ankylopoietica and in rheumatoid arthritis affecting the cervical spine. This pain is often produced or increased by movement of the head, and may be found to disappear when ankylosis becomes virtually complete. These structures are also subject to trauma, and occasionally headache initially occipital in distribution is found to follow a sudden flexion, extension, or torsion of the head on the neck. The pain may last days or weeks. Headache arising from these deep cervical structures is not uncommon, but it is often difficult to elucidate the causal lesion.

The Nasal Accessory Sinuses. Acute or subacute suppuration in the maxillary antrum gives pain over the antrum or in the forehead. In suppuration of the frontal ethmoid and sphenoid sinuses, the pain is around the eyes on one or both sides, but it may be in the vertex or other part of the cranium, especially in disease of the sphenoid sinuses. In all cases, pain may be associated with tenderness of the skin in the same distribution. Other signs are usually present, such as nasal or postnasal discharge of pus, fever, and opacity of the sinuses to transillumination or x-ray. Unless such clinical evidence of infection is present, headache is unlikely to be due to sinusitis. The pain may have two remarkable properties: (1) when throbbing, it may be abolished by compressing the carotid artery on the same side; (2) it tends to recur and get better at the same hours on successive days, most frequently occurring when the patient wakes, and disappearing after the patient gets out of bed. These time relations are generally ascribed to the sinuses filling up during the night and discharging after the erect posture has been assumed. The pain can usually be abolished by inhaling vasoconstrictors such as amphetamine (Benzedrine) or by anesthetizing the orifices of the sinuses. Although some believe that sinus pain arises chiefly at the nasal orifices of the sinuses, it is generally assumed that the headache arises from the mucous membrane lining the sinus, and that the pain nerves are stimulated by tension. If so, it seems probable that sinus headache, like earache, is usually due to suction on the mucous membrane when aeration is impeded by block; it is then relieved when aeration is effected. During airplane flight both earache and sinus headache tend to occur on descent when the relative pressure in

the blocked viscus falls, rather than on ascent when such pressure tends to rise.

Eyestrain. Errors of refraction of the eyes are a well-recognized cause of headache. In such cases pain tends to be referred to the orbit, forehead, and temple, does not throb with the pulse, and tends to occur during intensive use of the eyes as in reading or close work, and to persist for some time afterward. It is particularly obtrusive toward evening and if the subject is fatigued. There is evidence to show that, in the presence of refractive error, use of the eyes produces sustained contraction of the extraocular muscles of the orbit and of the frontal, temporal, and even occipital muscles, and it is suggested that the pain results from this contraction. A similar mechanism is postulated for the headache of glaucoma. The relief of such refractive errors by use of the correct spectacles abolishes the headache. Headache from eyestrain is probably not so frequent as would be indicated by the number of spectacles prescribed for its relief. Hyperopic astigmatism is a more frequent cause than myopia.

Osteitis. Syphilitic osteitis of the skull, now rare, Paget's disease, and metastases from primary tumors elsewhere may all produce headache, which is sometimes severe.

From Intracranial Structures

Histamine Headache. Although opinions vary concerning the existence and frequency of spontaneous headache due to histamine, the relation of the drug to the symptom is, nevertheless, of some interest, since it was the first kind of headache in which the mechanism of the pain was demonstrated. The headache can be produced easily in a normal subject by quick intravenous injection of 0.1 mg

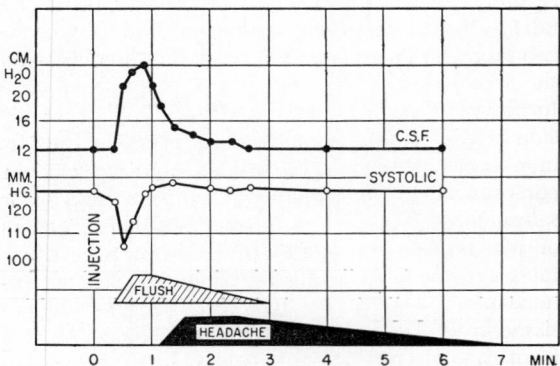

FIG. 4-1. Chart showing the course of the cerebrospinal fluid (CSF) pressure, the systolic blood pressure, the facial flush, and the headache following intravenous injection of 0.1 mg histamine. (*Pickering: Clin. Sci.,* 1:82, 1933.)

histamine acid phosphate. Headache begins about a minute after the injection, as the facial flush is beginning to fade, is maximal at about the second minute when the flush is nearly gone, and disappears about the eighth minute (Fig. 4-1). At first, it throbs conspicuously with each beat of the pulse but is felt in both sides of the forehead, and at its height it extends to the vertex and occiput. It can be established that:

1. Headache does not arise from an extracranial structure, because arrest of the circulation to the scalp before injection of histamine does not prevent the pain.

2. Headache arises from a structure innervated by the trigeminal nerve, since it does not occur on that side of the head when the sensory root has been severed or the ganglion injected with alcohol.

3. It probably arises from structures in the meninges, as it is greatly increased by shaking the head gently, and the meninges are the structures which will be chiefly strained in this movement.

4. It arises from the territory supplied by the internal carotid artery, since injection of histamine into the internal carotid produces headache, but injection into the external carotid does not.

The most striking events following the intravenous injection of histamine are consequences of vasodilatation; thus the face flushes, the blood pressure falls, and the cerebrospinal fluid pressure rises. Curiously enough, headache begins only when these signs of vasodilatation are subsiding, and, in fact, is prevented from appearing by the phenomena occurring during the phase of obvious vasodilatation. Thus, when histamine is slowly infused into a vein, headache does not usually appear until after the infusion is stopped; and an established headache is temporarily relieved at the moment the face flushes after a second injection of histamine. It can further be shown that any event which leads to a fall in arterial pressure tends to relieve the histamine headache, as does any event which tends to increase the cerebrospinal fluid pressure. Thus the headache throbs with the pulse and is abolished on the same side of the head by digital obliteration of the common carotid artery. The headache is relieved by compression of the jugular veins, or by injecting saline solution into the subarachnoid space, both of which raise cerebrospinal fluid pressure. These facts are most easily explained by supposing that headache results from stretching of pain-sensitive tissue around the large intracranial arteries derived from the internal carotid, such as the anterior and middle cerebral. It is supposed that these arteries are relaxed by histamine but that the headache does not occur when they are prevented from expanding by low blood pressure and high intracranial pressure.

It is probable that a similar mechanism is concerned in producing the headache of fever.

The injection of histamine is being increasingly used as a diagnostic method, but caution should be used in interpreting the results. The reproduction of a patient's headache by histamine probably points to an abnormality in the structures concerned but does not necessarily mean that histamine is the cause. Thus the localized headache of cerebral tumor can be reproduced, and the localized headaches of trauma and the generalized headache of fever increased, by histamine.

A rather peculiar syndrome reproduced in this way has been termed *histamine cephalagia* or *paroxysmal nocturnal orbital cephalagia*. The patients are usually adult males and are awakened from sleep by an intense pain in and around the orbit, which reaches a peak of severity within a few minutes and after 15 to 45 min subsides. The pain is accompanied by lacrimation, blockage of the nostril, sweating, and sometimes by swelling over the temporal vessels on the same side of the head. The attacks may occur every day or night for weeks or months and then subside completely, only to recur in exactly the same locality at some later time. The attacks may also occur by day, but this is less frequent. The attacks themselves may be cut short by inhalation of oxygen or by intravenous injection of ergot alkaloids as described for migraine (p. 29).

Lumbar Puncture Headache. A very characteristic headache occasionally occurs a few hours to a few days following lumbar puncture, particularly if the patient has been allowed up or if several attempts have been made to enter the spinal theca. The headache is usually, but not always, throbbing and is felt chiefly in the occiput but also widely over the cranial vault; the pain may spread into the neck and back. It may be accompanied by vomiting and neck rigidity and other signs of meningeal irritation. The most characteristic feature of the headache is its very conspicuous increase when the patient sits up and its relief on lying down. The headache is caused by a leakage of cerebrospinal fluid along the tract left at lumbar puncture. For if, when the headache is present, a second lumbar puncture is performed with the patient horizontal, the pressure of cerebrospinal fluid is found to be zero, and if the pressure is restored by the injection of normal saline solution into the theca, the headache is abolished, though it usually returns after some hours, presumably because the leakage continues. The headache is increased by compression of the jugular veins and is usually unaffected by digital obliteration of one carotid artery. From these facts it seems probable that the headache results from the tension exerted on some pain-sensitive structure by the caudad displacement of the brain, consequent on the emptying of cerebrospinal fluid from the subarachnoid space. Tension on the venous attachments of the brain to the great dural venous sinuses seems the most likely mechanism.

The occasional occurrence of headaches following lumbar puncture has led some to adopt the point of view that all patients should be kept in the recumbent position, preferably prone, following the procedure. Headache following cisternal puncture is rare.

A similar headache syndrome sometimes occurs after straining or a fall on the buttocks. Presumably, there is a tear in the arachnoid membrane, with a leakage of cerebrospinal fluid. The pressure of the cerebrospinal fluid is low and there may be a slight pleocytosis. The condition subsides spontaneously within a few days to weeks.

Raised Intracranial Pressure. Headache is an outstanding symptom in a number of diseases in which intracranial pressure becomes elevated, and the suggestion has been widely accepted that such headache results from stretching the pain-sensitive parietal dura mater. This hypothesis must now be rejected for the following reasons:

1. It is difficult to see how the parietal dura mater, supported as it is by the bony skull, can be stretched by a rise in intracranial pressure, except at the various foramens of the skull.

2. The cerebrospinal fluid pressure may be raised to very high levels (500 or 600 mm H_2O) by injecting saline solution into the subarachnoid space at lumbar puncture or by jugular compression, without headache resulting.

3. A critical examination of the behavior of headache in several diseases reveals facts which cannot be reconciled with the hypothesis. These facts will be described separately, under the several diseases.

Meningitis. One of the most severe headaches is that associated with meningitis—particularly the acute inflammations produced by the pyogenic microbes, the meningococcus, streptococcus, pneumococcus, and staphylococcus; in the less acute tuberculous meningitis, headache is often less intense. The headache is more or less generalized over the calvarium and may be throbbing or not; it is associated with rigidity of the neck muscles, so that when the head is flexed the neck muscles contract strongly and pain is felt in the occiput and neck; Kernig's and Brudzinski's signs may also be present but are less reliable. The patient commonly lies on his side with the head extended and the hips and knees flexed, and he shuns the light. This headache is very greatly increased by shaking the head, and the patient may resent any movement of his bed.

In all forms of meningitis the cerebrospinal fluid pressure is commonly raised, sometimes to very high levels of over 600 mm H_2O, and it is not infrequent to find that removal of cerebrospinal fluid

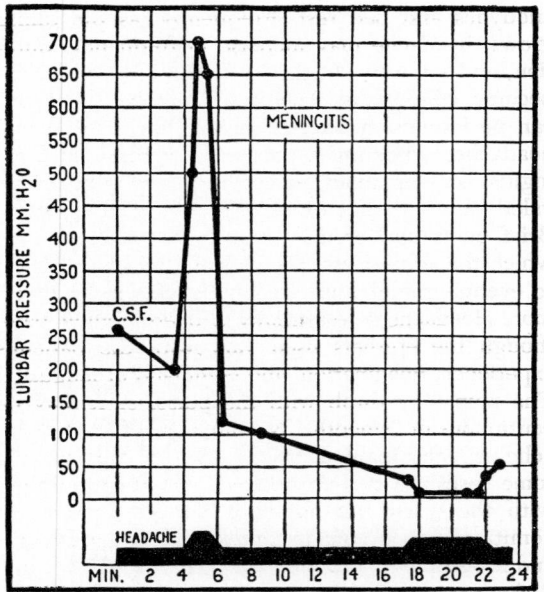

FIG. 4-2. Chart showing the relationship of headache to cerebrospinal fluid pressure in a case of meningococcal meningitis in which the pressure was altered by withdrawal of cerebrospinal fluid and injection of saline solution through the lumbar puncture needle. (*Pickering: Brit. Med. J.*, 1:907, 1939.)

by lumbar puncture relieves the pain (Fig. 4-2). Nevertheless, it is found that if the pressure is reduced still further—below the normal level—pain is increased, to be relieved by reinjection of fluid and restoration of pressure to normal. It seems probable that in this instance pain is due to a chemical irritation of the pain nerve endings of the meninges, consequent on the tissue damage of bacterial action, and that mechanical distortion of these inflamed tissues, as by distention or depletion of the subarachnoid space, may further increase pain. The mechanism of pain thus is probably identical with that occurring in acute inflammatory conditions elsewhere, such as those affecting the pulp of the finger and the peritoneum.

Cerebral Tumor. Headache is the outstanding symptom of cerebral tumor. Its features are very variable, and while there are certain features of headache which strongly suggest tumor, these features will not be found in all cases. Headache in cerebral tumor at first occurs in attacks lasting only a few seconds to 3 hr, and typically about 1 hr. The paroxysms may be precipitated by any activity, especially such as involves abrupt changes in position of the head, and they diminish in frequency when the patient is kept in bed. With the patient at rest the attacks often occur when the patient wakes in the morning. Usually no simple event is found to abolish the pain, and relief is sought from anodynes and bed rest. Frequently, as the tumor grows, headache may increase in frequency, duration, and intensity. In the later stages the pain may become continuous. The pain may be slight but can be intolerably severe. In fact, the most severe headaches occurring in disease are those of meningitis, subarachnoid hemorrhage, and tumor, rivaled only by that of intrathecal air insufflation. Brief paroxysms of most intense headache, during which the subject writhes in agony and is oblivious to events around him, are highly suggestive of tumor. Headache is essentially a deep, aching pain, though the epithets used vary with the patient's experience, imagination, and command of language. The pain may throb with the pulse, or it may be continuous or "smooth." Not infrequently the headache is accompanied by nausea or vomiting. In some cases the two are related, vomiting occurring with the worst but not with the least pain; but vomiting also occurs in tumor without headache, and it occurs without preceding nausea. (See Chap. 286.)

Most frequently in tumor, headache is bilateral and frontal, but there is some relation between sites of pain and tumor, in the absence, but not in the presence, of papilledema. Thus occipital headache is more frequent with tumors below than with those above the tentorium, and when headache is unilateral the tumor is on the same side in about 90 per cent of cases. Sometimes headache is localized to an area roughly 5 cm in diameter, which may correspond fairly closely to the site of the tumor. Headache is more frequent in quickly growing tumors, such as gliomas, than in the slower-growing varieties, such as meningiomas. It is also more frequent and begins earlier when the mass is smaller in tumors involving the ventricles, or below the tentorium, than when the frontal or parietal lobes are involved; tumors of the temporal and occipital lobes occupy an intermediate position with respect to time of onset and severity of headache.

It may be accepted that the afferent impulses responsible for tumor headache arise within the cranial cavity for, as will be mentioned, pain can be induced and relieved by procedures which affect only the cranial content; also that the stimulus is mechanical, for the common effect of such procedure is to alter the stresses and strains inside the skull. The stimulus is probably not stretching of the parietal dura mater by raised intracranial pressure, because:

1. The parietal dura mater is firmly suffixed by the skull.

2. In a given case, cerebrospinal fluid pressure measured in the presence of headache is not significantly higher than in its absence.

3. Lumbar puncture may relieve, but it may also increase or induce, headache.

4. Raising intracranial pressure by jugular compression, or by intrathecal injection of saline solution, may relieve as well as increase headache in cerebral tumor.

5. It has been shown at operation under local anesthesia that headache may sometimes be reproduced by emptying or distending the ventricles on the same or opposite side.

From these experimental findings, as well as from the clinical features of headache, it seems that sudden changes of intracranial pressure, either up or down, may precipitate pain. Two ideas of the origin are widely entertained: that it arises from the arteries at the base of the brain and that it arises from tension on the dural attachments of, and supports for, the brain. The first explanation finds support in the observation that histamine may, in a given patient, reproduce precisely the headache of tumor, even when this has a highly individual localization. The second explanation is not easily compatible with certain details of observations made on individual cases, though it agrees with much of the evidence; for it is well known that tumor gives rise to distortions of the intracranial septums and that such distortions can give rise to pain, presumably, by tension on the pain-sensitive tissues around the dural sinuses. That headache is due to such distortion would be in harmony with many of the facts about tumor headache, namely, that it may be either relieved or increased by lowering cerebrospinal fluid pressure, that the headache may frequently be relieved by intravenous or rectal injections of hypertonic solutions, and that the headache may disappear following operations for decompression. Moreover, this hypothesis would be compatible with its high incidence in posterior fossa and rapidly growing tumors.

Subarachnoid Hemorrhage. Headache is a constant feature of spontaneous subarachnoid hemorrhage resulting from rupture of a miliary aneurysm of the circle of Willis or its main branches, and the stories given by such patients indicate that headache must begin at about the time when the aneurysm ruptures. Thus, a patient who up to that time has been perfectly well is seized abruptly with the most severe generalized headache, and a few moments later sinks to the ground unconscious. The headache is invariably severe when the patient recovers consciousness and lasts for some days or weeks afterward. It has been supposed that the headache arises, as does that of meningitis, from inflammation of the meninges evoked by the presence of blood, and it is true that neck rigidity is a constant feature of subarachnoid hemorrhage, as it is in meningitis. Pain may also arise from the pain-sensitive tissue in the region of the aneurysmal sacs; and it is possible that sudden stretching of the perivascular tissue, with consequent headache, may precede the actual rupture into the subarachnoid space. However, it is to be noted that accounts of pain produced at operation by stimulating the great vessels at the base of the brain describe pain as unilateral, while in subarachnoid hemorrhage it is nearly always bilateral. Moreover, there is evidence from intracranial aneurysm that headache from the region of the artery is more localized, for in unruptured aneurysms headache occurring in paroxysms restricted to the same side of the head is common. (See Chap. 284.)

Vascular Lesions. Headache occurs seldom if ever in cerebral embolism and very uncommonly in cerebral thrombosis. Intracerebral rupture of an artery, as in atheroma or hypertension, usually produces loss of consciousness at once and often results in death. If the patient recovers consciousness, he often complains of severe headache and may show neck rigidity, as in subarachnoid hemorrhage. Blood may be present in the cerebrospinal fluid. The idea that the imminence of cerebral hemorrhage can be foretold by headache is, in general, entirely without foundation but has obvious commercial value and appeals to the intellectually feeble or the morally unscrupulous.

Migraine

Manifestations. Classic migraine presents a dramatic sequence of events. On waking in the morning the patient may feel slightly confused and unable to see quite clearly. Within a few minutes bright spots appear in one-half of his field of vision, arrange themselves as a zigzag pattern which subsequently fragments and fades, to be followed by blackness of that visual field. As sight gradually returns, headache begins as a dull, boring, throbbing pain usually in the opposite but sometimes in the ipsilateral temple, gradually increasing in intensity until the whole of the same side of the head is affected. The patient is now pale and prostrate and can get relief only by lying down in a quiet and darkened room where, after some time, he falls into a deep sleep from which he awakens well. In most attacks nausea and vomiting occur either throughout or at the height of the headache, which may, in fact, be relieved by vomiting. Much variation occurs. Thus any of the three components —aura, headache, or vomiting—may be absent. The aura may be different from that described. Visual forms are commonest, but they differ much in detail; numbness and tingling of the tongue or fingers, often restricted to one side, are not uncommon; transient aphasia may occur, and transient hemiplagia has been described (though the author would doubt that this accompanies true migraine). Disturbance of the mind is not uncommon; excitement is sometimes present, but mental confusion, depression, and extreme irritability are more common. Headache, though classically unilateral ("migraine" is derived from *hemicrania*), may be bilateral. Its situation is not always the same in different attacks. During the attack, as is nearly always true when vomiting occurs, the patient may be pale, cold, and sweating and may seem ill.

Pathogenesis. Over a century and a half ago Parry observed that the headache of migraine could be relieved temporarily by compressing the common carotid artery in the neck on the same side. In 1867 Mollendorf wrote:

If the common carotid artery be compressed on the painful side at the level of the thyroid cartilage during the hemicranial paroxysm so that the pulse in the temporal artery begins to fail, the headache vanishes as if by magic. . . . With the intermission of the compression, with the first full pulse wave the pain begins afresh and, indeed, the first pulsation will be felt to be much more painful. . . . Conversely, compression of the other side enhances the pain.

In certain cases complete relief of pain is obtained by digital obliteration of the temporal or occipital arteries or both; in others it is not, and complete relief can be attained only by compression of the common carotid. It seems, therefore, that in many cases of migraine, headache arises entirely from stretching of the walls of the large arteries of the scalp—temporal, occipital, or frontal —and it can be shown (1) that a similar pain can be evoked by stretching the walls of these arteries exposed surgically and (2) that ligature of the arteries may abolish the attacks of headache. In other cases, however, it must be presumed that at least some of the pain must originate similarly from dilatation of the middle meningeal artery. The headache of migraine often may be relieved quickly by intravenous injection of ergotamine tartrate, or aborted if the injection is made before headache starts, and it has been shown that the drug constricts the scalp arteries. Although some writers believe that cerebral vasoconstriction is responsible for the aura, the available evidence favors the view that the headache of migraine is due to expansion of walls of arteries, chiefly extracranial. However, so far, no other superficial arteries have been shown to give rise to pain when they expand. How this expansion is brought about in migraine, why it should not be produced by physiologic measures such as heat, and what its relationship is to the presumably intracranial events responsible for the aura, are unknown. That emotional disturbances are of great importance as precipitating factors cannot be doubted; that they are the underlying cause remains to be demonstrated. Many believe allergy to be the dominant factor; for this there is little evidence.

Migraine usually begins in childhood or in adolescence; as age advances it tends to become less severe and finally to disappear. Sometimes the aura persists without the headache, and vice versa. It tends to disappear during pregnancy. It is probably due to an inherited abnormality, since a strong family history of migraine is common.

Wolff has shown that water, sodium, and potassium are retained during the prodromal phase and excreted during the headache phase.

Diagnosis. The classical migraine already described should give rise to no difficulty in diagnosis, provided a good history is obtained; and patients with migraine are usually intelligent.

The real difficulty comes from two sources: (1) it is known that even in the classical case, aura, headache, or vomiting may cease to occur as time passes, leaving only one or two of the original three; (2) there is much variation in the character of the headache.

Briefly the situation is as follows:

1. There are certain conditions which resemble migraine but have a defined organic basis. The best known is ophthalmoplegic migraine, in which oculomotor palsies accompany, and may outlast, the headache; these attacks are usually due to leakage from a congenital aneurysm of the internal carotid or anterior cerebral artery.

2. Attacks indistinguishable from migraine may occur in patients with high blood pressure or cerebral tumor.

3. Paroxysms of headache not hemicranial in distribution, not preceded by an aura, and not accounted for by other known cause may or may not be migraine. Unfortunately the controversy as to where migraine begins and ends is of the armchair type which settles nothing. Favoring the diagnosis of migraine are a family history of it and response of the headache to the ergot derivatives.

4. A variety of episodic attacks have been described as migraine equivalents: attacks of abdominal pain, associated with nausea, vomiting, and diarrhea (abdominal migraine); pain localized in the thorax, pelvis, or extremities; bouts of fever; transient disturbances in mood (psychic equivalent of migraine). The only advantage of such a practice is that it protects some patients from unnecessary surgical intervention. But it may prevent necessary surgery, and the writer prefers not to prejudge the issue by applying a term for which there is at present no scientific justification and which serves as a rather threadbare cloak for ignorance.

Treatment. Migraine may require no treatment other than an explanation to the patient and a reassurance that it will do him no harm. Some patients know, or allege to know, that certain acts induce attacks; these acts should be avoided. In certain persons correction of an error of refraction,

or of a personality defect by psychotherapy, has banished the attacks. However, it is difficult, because of the natural history of the disease and its variability, to assess the general value of such methods.

Treatment is rarely required during the phase of the aura, but it is said that the inhalation of amyl nitrite will abolish, temporarily at least, the visual disturbance. It is, however, the headache and its associated vomiting that distress the patient most. The milder attacks usually respond to the usual analgesics, acetylsalicylic acid 0.6 to 0.9 Gm (10 to 15 gr) with or without the addition of caffeine citrate (25 mg) and codeine (60 mg). More severe attacks respond only to the ergot preparations ergotamine and dihydroergotamine. In most patients with migraine the attacks can be cut short by intravenous injection of 1 mg dihydroergotamine methane sulfonate or 0.5 mg ergotamine tartrate, the former being less likely to induce vomiting than the latter; the injection may be repeated in an hour if necessary. The drugs raise arterial pressure, and care should be taken with their use in the presence of left ventricular failure or angina pectoris. So used they abort the attack if given within an hour of its onset in some 90 per cent of patients. They are less effective by intramuscular injection and least effective by mouth. The most effective oral treatment of an attack is by tablets containing 1 mg ergotamine tartrate and 100 mg caffeine; two tablets are taken at once and a third after half an hour if the headache has not stopped; if the patient has nausea or vomiting, suppositories containing 2 mg ergotamine and 100 mg caffeine are used in the same way instead. They are said to be effective in some 80 per cent of patients.

Other Forms of Headache

From Hypertension. Hypertension is now a diagnosis so commonly made, and carrying with it in the public mind such fear of its consequences, that many of its symptoms are to be attributed not so much to the disease as to the state of mind that its diagnosis engenders. Headache is not a common complaint of patients with mild hypertension prior to diagnosis; occurring in such patients after diagnosis, the headache has no peculiar features. But in severe hypertension a characteristic headache is common and is frequently the symptom bringing the patient to the doctor. It may be troublesome and may be severe. Characteristically, the pain is occipital, and is noticed on waking in the morning, to improve as the day advances; it may last an hour or longer. The headache may be associated with nausea and vomiting. Over a large series of cases there is some relationship between intensity of headache and intensity of hypertension, and the severest headaches are thus commonly found in hypertension of the malignant type. As papilledema also occurs in malignant hypertension, and cerebral thrombosis is by no means rare in that condition, a mistaken diagnosis of cerebral tumor may be made unless the level of the blood pressure and the total clinical picture are taken into consideration.

The precise mechanism of headache in hypertension remains obscure. The cerebrospinal fluid pressure is raised in rough proportion to the diastolic arterial pressure, but is the same in the presence and absence of headache. That the headache may have an intracranial source is indicated by its often being increased by withdrawal of cerebrospinal fluid at lumbar puncture. Evidence has been produced to show that headache of hypertension is often due to stretching of the walls of extracranial arteries. Thus the headache is said to be relieved by compression of the superficial arteries supplying the scalp, and abolished by tying these arteries. Pain is often uninfluenced by carotid artery compression, nor is its morning incidence dependent on whether the patient sleeps with one or several pillows.

From Fever. Headache occurs in many diseases in which the temperature rises—for example, acute tonsilitis, typhoid fever, malaria, and sandfly fever. The pain may be throbbing with the pulse or steady and may be frontal, occipital, or generalized. The headache is very much like the histamine headache in being relieved on the same side by carotid artery compression, on both sides by compression of the jugular veins, or by the injection of saline solution into the subarachnoid space; it is increased by shaking the head. Like histamine headache, pain is temporarily relieved by injection of histamine or amyl nitrite during the time the arterial pressure is lowered and the cerebrospinal pressure raised by these drugs. It seems probable, therefore, that the headache arises in the same way as that following histamine—namely, from stretching of pain-sensitive tissue around the large arteries at the base of the brain. In certain cases, however, pain may be lessened by compression of temporal or angular arteries, and in these a component of the headache seems to be derived from the walls of extracranial arteries, as in migraine.

From Anemia. Some patients suffering from severe anemia experience headache which is abolished when the hemoglobin content of the blood is restored by treatment. The headache is usually frontal or generalized, and may or may not be throbbing. It tends to occur toward evening. This headache has been insufficiently investigated to reveal its mechanism. Headache is, however, a common experience after exposure to high altitudes and thus to oxygen lack, and it is tempting to suppose that the two may be related. Curiously enough, if exposure to a high altitude (over 14,000 ft) is brief —say 4 hr—headache is experienced not during the exposure, but afterward. The explanation of this curious fact is unknown. Likewise, the explanation for the headache which may occur in patients with polycythemia is uncertain.

Posttraumatic. After head injury, especially one that has caused loss of consciousness, over 50 per cent of patients suffer from headache. Other associated symptoms are dizziness, amounting to a sense of instability rather than to true vertigo, and mental change, of which loss of memory and inability to concentrate are the chief signs. (See Chap. 285.)

Considerable divergence of opinion exists as to the mechanism of headache in such cases. In a small series with dull pain more or less localized to the area of injury and persisting up to 8 years afterward, Penfield recorded localized changes in the subarachnoid and subdural spaces revealed by air insufflation into the spinal theca. He also described the relief of headache after such insufflation. In cases not so relieved, he reported success from dividing adhesions formed near the site of injury between the dura and piarachnoid. Consequently, he ascribed the headache in these cases to tension set up in these adhesions between the brain and its coverings, the adhesions being formed when the brain was out of place due to the local tissue reaction to injury. The fuller experience of the Second World War suggests that headache of this type and origin is uncommon. More usually, the headache is bilateral, frontal, or generalized, often throbbing, and usually occurring in paroxysms or liable to paroxysmal exacerbations. The paroxysms may be induced by stooping, physical exertion, noise, and excitement. The pain may be increased by lying down and relieved by raising the head on pillows, or relieved by recumbency, and is worst in the erect posture. These observations suggest an organic cause for the headache, but the nature of this has not been worked out. The headaches usually pass off with the improvement of the patient, consequent on modern rehabilitation management, and are relieved by the ordinary anodynes.

The evolution of posttraumatic headache is often complicated by the presence of economic problems in relation to compensation.

APPROACH TO THE PATIENT WITH HEADACHE

From the foregoing account it will be appreciated that certain forms of headache may be diagnosed and others suspected, when a lucid description of the pain has been obtained from the patient. Headache occurring toward the end of the day and relieved by sound sleep may be due to fatigue or eyestrain; that due to a disturbed mind is less often relieved by sleep. Paroxysmal headache, often unilateral, preceded by an aura and accompanied by vomiting is recognizable as migraine. Occipital headache occurring on waking, and declining as the day wears on, usually is due to hypertension, but may be due to cerebral tumor. Headache persisting without remission for weeks or months, and unaccompanied by other manifestations of disease, is commonly due to an affection of the deep structures of the neck and head, such as myofibrositis; occasionally, its abrupt onset following sudden movement indicates a traumatic lesion. Following head injury, headache is common and often associated with dizziness, inability to concentrate, and impaired memory. Headache recurring over short periods, at a definite hour of the day, suggests a sinus infection. Headache that is accompanied by symptoms of fever and acute infection probably is due to a febrile illness; when meningitis is present, the headache is very severe and neck rigidity is almost invariable. Headache occurring in brief and severe paroxysms, becoming recently longer and more frequent, is suggestive of cerebral tumor; the headache has localizing value. Sudden severe headache, followed by loss of consciousness, suggests a subarachnoid hemorrhage. After lumbar puncture, headache may develop when the patient sits up and may be relieved when the patient lies down.

These points in the history which have been noted are very important; but they are often no more than pointers as to which investigations should be carried out in a specific case. Many of the conditions named have physical signs that should be sought.

The central nervous system, the eyes, the ears, nose, and throat, the skull, the scalp, the neck, the blood pressure, and the urine should be examined in all cases, particular attention being paid to the fundus oculi. Anemia and syphilis may have to be excluded, and an x-ray examination of the head and neck may be needed. Other special examinations particularly relevant to the cranial content should be done if there are clear indications for them. It is equally important that the physician should try to assess the contribution made by disturbances of the mind. While mental disturbance per se produces a feeling of pressure or confinement of the head rather than ache or pain, pain may arise from secondary effects on the muscles of the head and neck, and any pains, however trivial, may appear severe to a mind that is tormented with fear or doubt.

REFERENCES

GENERAL

Kellgren, J. H.: On the Distribution of Pain Arising from Deep Somatic Structures with Charts of Segmental Pain Areas, Clin. Sci., 4:35, 1939.

Lewis, T.: "Pain," New York, The Macmillan Company, 1942.
—— and W. Hess: Pain Derived from the Skin and the Mechanism of Its Production, Clin. Sci., 1:39, 1933.

HEADACHE

Graham, J. R., and H. G. Wolff: The Mechanism of Migraine Headache and Action of Ergotamine Tartrate, Arch. Neurol. Psychiat., 39:737, 1938.
Horton, B. T.: Use of Histamine in Treatment of Specific Types of Headache, J.A.M.A., 116:377, 1941.
Northfield, D. W. C.: Some Observations on Headache (Especially That of Cerebral Tumor), Brain, 61:133, 1938.
Penfield, W.: Chronic Meningeal (Post-traumatic) Headache and Its Specific Treatment by Lumbar Air Insufflation, Surg. Gynecol. Obstet., 45:747, 1927.
Pickering, G. W.: Experimental Observations on Headache, Brit. Med. J., 1939, I:907.
——: Observations on the Mechanism of Headache Produced by Histamine, Clin. Sci., 1:77, 1933.
Wolff, H. G., et al.: "Pain," Baltimore, The Williams & Wilkins Company, 1943.

5 PAIN IN THE CHEST
T. R. Harrison, William H. Resnik, and T. J. Reeves

The common problem in patients who complain of chest pain involves the distinction of trivial disorders from coronary disease, which is attended by the threat of sudden death. There is little parallelism between the severity of the pain and the gravity of its cause. An incorrect positive diagnosis of a hazardous condition such as angina pectoris is likely to have harmful psychologic and economic consequences. In no field of medicine is accurate diagnosis more important or, at times, more difficult.

The apparently bizarre radiation of pain arising in the thoracic viscera can usually be explained in terms of the known facts concerning nerve supply. These have been considered in the third chapter. One occasionally sees a patient with extension of pain to a location which cannot be logically explained. In most instances, such an individual will be found to have more than one disorder capable of causing pain in the chest. The presence of the second and often silent condition may affect the radiation of the pain produced by the primary disorder. Thus when the pain of angina pectoris extends to the back, the patient will usually be found to have also a significant degree of spinal arthritis. Similarly, the radiation of anginal pain to the abdomen commonly occurs only in individuals who have some upper abdominal disorder, such as hiatal hernia, disease of the gallbladder, pancreatitis, or peptic ulcer. When such instances are excluded, there is only an occasional patient who presents a distribution of pain which cannot be logically explained in terms of the known facts about nerve supply.

The common tendency to assume that the presence of an objective abnormality, such as a hiatal hernia or right bundle branch block, necessarily means that an atypical chest pain is arising in the stomach or the heart is to be strongly condemned. Such an assumption is justified only provided that the careful history indicates that the behavior of the pain is entirely compatible with the site of origin which is suggested by the objective finding.

The Left-arm Myth. There is a long tradition, widely accepted by physicians and laymen, that pain in the left arm, especially when appearing in conjunction with chest pain, has a unique and ominous significance as being almost certain evidence of the presence of ischemic heart disease. This is a myth that has neither a theoretic nor clinical foundation. From a theoretic standpoint, *any* disorder involving the deep afferent fibers of the upper thoracic region should be capable of causing pain in either area, both areas, or neither area (p. 18). Hence a pain of trivial significance arising in skeletal tissues innervated by upper (first to fourth) thoracic nerves would be expected to produce left-arm-area pain. These expectations are exactly in accord with clinical observation. Almost any condition which is capable of causing pain in the chest may induce radiation to the left arm. Such localization is common not only in patients with coronary disease but also in those with numerous other types of chest pain. Neither the location, radiation, nor quality of pain is of crucial diagnostic significance. Rather, it is the careful history of the behavior of the pain, in terms of the conditions which induce it and relieve it.

Only the more important or more common conditions listed in Table 5-1 will be considered in the text. No attempt has been made to enumerate all the causes of chest pain.

PAIN DUE TO OXYGEN DEFICIENCY OF THE MYOCARDIUM

Physiologic Considerations of the Coronary Circulation. Pain due to myocardial ischemia occurs when the oxygen supply to the heart is deficient in relation to the oxygen need. The oxygen consumption of this organ is closely related to the physiologic effort made during contraction or the "tension-time index" (the area under the ventricular pressure curve.) Thus the oxygen consumption depends not

Table 5-1. CLASSIFICATION OF CHEST PAIN

I. Heart
  A. Myocardium: oxygen deficiency
    1. Infarction (permanent anoxia)
    2. Angina pectoris (temporary hypoxia)
    3. Preinfarctional angina (usually combining some features of both 1 and 2, above)
  B. Pericardium: inflammation
  C. Periapical pain and precordial ache (these are really varieties of chest wall pain and are not of cardiac origin)
II. Aorta: dissecting aneurysm (the pain of saccular aneurysm is usually due to pressure on surrounding structures)
III. Other thoracic organs
  A. Pleura (including pleuritis, pneumothorax, and pleurodynia)
  B. Mediastinum (emphysema, inflammation, masses)
  C. Esophagus (esophagitis, spasm, carcinoma, diverticulum)
IV. Chest wall (musculoskeletal pain—the commonest cause of pain in the chest)
  A. Primary, with no associated cardiovascular disease
    1. "Rheumatic"
    2. Psychogenic
  B. Secondary (indirectly induced by underlying visceral disease usually cardiac; the shoulder-hand syndrome is the classic example)
    1. Shoulder-hand syndrome
    2. Pectoral syndrome
  C. Associated (not initially caused by cardiovascular disease but conditioned and aggravated by it)
V. Abdominal disorders causing chest pain:
  A. Stomach: aerophagia and pouches (especially hiatal hernia, rarely diverticulum)
  B. Splenic flexure
  C. Gallbladder, duodenum, and pancreas (rare causes of anterior chest pain, except when radiation is conditioned by coexisting coronary disease)
VI. Rare and miscellaneous

only on the energy involved in expelling blood but also on the "wasted" isometric energy required to raise the ventricular pressure sufficiently to open the semilunar valves. When other factors remain constant, an elevation of stroke volume produces an efficient type of response because it leads to increase in ejection work only, the isometric factor per minute remaining relatively constant. Thus a rise in flow load causes less increment in myocardial oxygen consumption than does a comparable increase in cardiac work per minute, brought about either by elevation of pressure or of heart rate. The two latter conditions are both associated with increase in the total isometric work per minute. However, the net effects of these hemodynamic variables depend not on oxygen need alone but rather

EFFECT OF HEART RATE AND OF
MECHANICAL LOAD ON CORONARY BLOOD FLOW

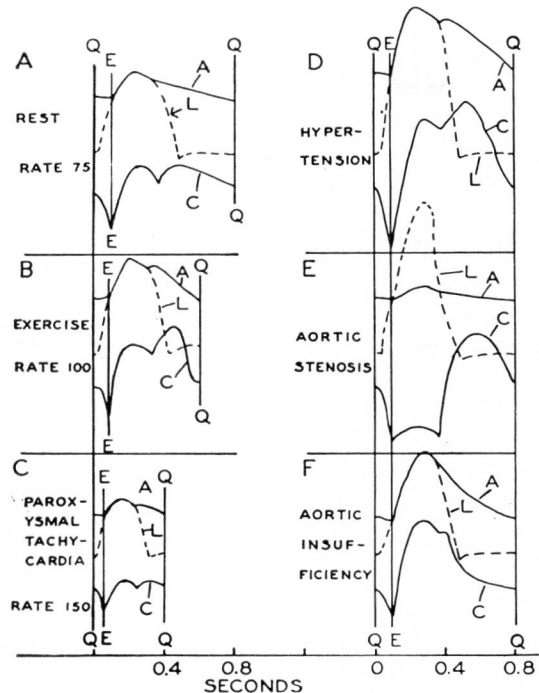

FIG. 5-1. (A) and (L) indicate aortic and left ventricular pressure curves, respectively. (C) designates coronary blood flow.

The diagram illustrates the total coronary flow. The wide differences between the two ventricles and between the deep and superficial parts of the left ventricle (see text) are not indicated.

A. Rest. After excitation (Q) but before ejection (E), there is a sharp decline in flow because the intramural resistance is increasing but the aortic perfusion (diastolic) pressure is still falling. During ejection the rapid rise in aortic pressure increases flow, even though the intramural resistance is still high. Early in diastole the sudden decline in resistance as relaxation occurs leads to a second peak in perfusion, which then gradually declines as aortic pressure diminishes. Total diastole per minute is 33 sec.

B. Exercise with increased upstroke volume and heart rate. Despite the shortening of diastole the flow per cycle is maintained at a normal level because of slightly higher systolic pressure and reflex coronary dilatation. Total diastole per minute is 28 sec.

C. Extreme tachycardia with decreased stroke volume. The systolic flow is decreased because the aortic pressure is low. The shortening of diastole causes marked curtailment of diastolic flow. Total diastole per minute is 24 sec.

D. Hypertension. The exaggerated decline of flow before ejection is balanced by a rise during ejection and diastole because of elevated aortic pressure. Thus

on the balance between the demand and the supply of oxygen.

Continued activity of a muscle causes increased local acidity and a shift to the right of the oxygen dissociation curve of the blood passing through it (Bohr effect). Hence the oxygen is more readily given up by the hemoglobin. Since the heart is always active, the coronary venous blood is normally much more desaturated than that from other areas of the body. Thus the removal of more oxygen from a unit of blood, which is one of the two adjustments commonly utilized by exercising skeletal muscle, is already employed in the "resting" heart. Therefore, this organ has only one effective means of obtaining the additional oxygen required for greater work, and this is by increase in the coronary blood flow.

It follows, from Poiseuille's equation (p. 94), that the flow of blood through the coronary arteries is proportional to the gradient between the aortic and intramural (during systole) or intraventricular (during diastole) pressures, but is proportional to the *fourth power of the radius* of the coronary arteries. Thus a relatively slight alteration in coronary diameter will produce a large change in coronary flow, provided that other factors remain constant.

The phasic variations of flow during the cardiac cycle are different in the different portions of the myocardium. The systolic pressure in the subendocardial portions of the left ventricle is approximately the same as that in the aorta and effectively closes the coronary branches in this area. Therefore, the chief flow to the subendocardial part of the left ventricle occurs during diastole. The pressure in the wall of the *subepicardial* part of the left ventricle undergoes less rise during systole, and this portion receives blood throughout the cycle, as does the right ventricle with its lower intramural systolic pressure. The net effect of these variables on total coronary perfusion is illustrated in Fig. 5-1A. During isometric contraction there is a sharp decrease in flow because intramural pressure is rising rapidly. This effect is balanced during ejection by the elevation in aortic pressure, and coronary flow increases. A second rise occurs as relaxation reduces intramural resistance.

---

coronary perfusion keeps pace with increased cardiac work.

E. Aortic stenosis. The systolic flow is markedly diminished because the increased intramural resistance is not balanced, as in D, by rising perfusion pressure. Angina will result unless coronary dilatation during diastole is sufficient to compensate for reduced systolic flow.

F. Aortic insufficiency. The flow is increased during systole and reduced during diastole because of the wide variation in aortic pressure.

A given increment in external cardiac work is accomplished at a cost of less rise in myocardial oxygen consumption when due to augmented stroke volume than when brought about by either elevation of pressure or increase of rate. Thus, although each condition is associated with increased coronary flow, the more efficient response is that of increased stroke volume (Fig. 5-1*B* and *C*). During exercise in healthy persons, the coronary flow tends to keep pace with the oxygen demand of the heart. Very rarely, under the condition of maximal effort, an apparently healthy young individual may have typical anginal pain and may even suddenly succumb. This is probably the result of inability of coronary flow to keep up with the extreme oxygen needs of the myocardium. It is likely, although unproved, that early atheromatous changes or congenital anomalies are present in the coronary arteries of all such persons. This rare disorder might properly be called the Pheidippides syndrome, after the Greek athlete who, having raced from the battlefield of Marathon to Athens with the news of the victory over the Persians, suddenly expired.

Tachycardia with diminished stroke volume exerts only harmful effects. It increases the myocardial need for oxygen and tends to reduce the supply. Hence electrocardiographic evidence of ischemia is frequently encountered, and anginal pain sometimes occurs during bouts of paroxysmal tachycardia in young persons who have no clinical evidence of coronary disease, although it is possible that subclinical narrowing might be present.

The coronary dilatation associated with increased stroke volume which normally compensates for the tachycardia of exercise is impaired when there is fixed coronary narrowing. Thus physical exertion, or any other condition which increases heart rate, tends to precipitate anginal attacks. Bradycardia usually has the opposite effects, and this apparently explains the rarity of angina in persons with complete heart block, even when this disorder is caused by coronary disease. However, extreme bradycardia is associated with pronounced decline in diastolic pressure, which may reduce the coronary flow.

The relation between blood pressure, coronary flow, and anginal pain is complex. Hypertension favors the development of coronary atheromatous narrowing and thus of angina. However, in the absence of such narrowing the rise in blood pressure, although causing increased intramural systolic resistance, augments perfusion and also tends to widen the coronary vessels (Fig. 5-1*D*). Thus angina does not ordinarily occur in patients with hypertension unless there is coexistent atheroma.

A fall in blood pressure not only decreases the perfusing pressure but also tends to reduce coronary caliber. However, unless there is either structural disease of the coronary arteries or marked tachycardia, anginal pain and electrocardiographic changes of ischemia are absent. The decreased rate of flow consequent to shock or hemorrhage predisposes to thrombosis in patients with atheromatous narrowing of the coronary vessels.

Many patients with angina have attacks of pain starting during sleep. In a few instances this appears to be due to reabsorption, in the recumbent position, of excess extracellular fluid from the legs. However, in many instances the reason for the nocturnal attacks is unknown.

There are two points of view concerning the mechanism of the beneficial action of nitrites in patients with ischemic heart disease. However, the evidence for the "decreased cardiac work" concept is decidedly unconvincing. In all probability the generally accepted view, which ascribes the benefit to dilatation of coronary branches, is correct.

Causes of Myocardial Hypoxia. By far the most frequent underlying cause is disease of the coronary arteries. This is usually the result of atheroma, which is often complicated by blood clots. Much less frequently, narrowing of the coronary orifices due to luetic aortitis or to distortion by a dissecting aneurysm may be responsible. A drug, such as ergot, which causes constriction of the coronary arteries, may occasionally induce anginal attacks in the absence of organic disease. There is no evidence that vasoconstriction or increased cardiac work (rise in rate or blood pressure, or liberation of catecholamines) due to emotion can precipitate angina unless there is also structural narrowing of the vessels. However, when this is present it is likely that reflex vasoconstriction from abdominal or other disorders, as well as emotional vasoconstriction, may precipitate episodes.

Aside from conditions which narrow the lumen of the coronary arteries, the only other frequent causes of myocardial hypoxia are disorders, such as aortic stenosis, which cause a marked disproportion between the perfusion pressure and the ventricular work. Under such conditions the systolic rise in left ventricular pressure is not, as in hypertensive states, balanced by corresponding elevation of aortic pressure (Fig. 5-1*E*), and most of the coronary flow occurs in diastole. Therefore, increase in heart rate is especially harmful because it shortens diastole more than systole and thereby decreases the total available perfusion time per minute.

Patients with marked right ventricular hypertension may have exertional pain which is, in most respects, identical with that of the common type of angina. It is likely that this discomfort results from relative ischemia of the right ventricle brought about by the increased oxygen need and by the elevated intramural resistance, with sharp reduction of the normally large systolic perfusion of this chamber.

In persons with syphilitic aortitis, angina is not uncommon and the relative roles of aortic insufficiency and of coronary ostial narrowing are difficult to assess. However, the latter factor is absent in patients with rheumatic aortic insufficiency, and unless there is coexistent stenosis angina is exceptional. Apparently, the reduction in diastolic perfusion pressure (Fig. 5-1F) is usually balanced by the greater systolic perfusion due to coronary dilatation. Angina may be severe when marked regurgitation is associated with a relatively slight degree of stenosis.

The importance of tachycardia, decline in blood pressure, or diminution in arterial oxygen content will be apparent from the above discussion. However, these are precipitating and aggravating rather than underlying causes of angina.

The Effects of Myocardial Hypoxia. The most important of these is *anginal pain,* which is considered in some detail in Chap. 254. The exact mechanism of the pain stimulus is still unknown. The evidence that oxygen deficiency is in some way responsible appears to be overwhelming, but the precise mechansim of its action has not been established.

As a rule, myocardial infarction is associated with a pain similar in quality and distribution to that of angina but of greater intensity and much longer duration. It is not relieved by coronary dilator drugs. Occasionally, the pain is minimal or even completely absent. In such instances, it is probable that preexisting long-standing myocardial ischemia has caused damage to the nerve fibers which would otherwise conduct the pain impulses.

A second effect of myocardial ischemia is often seen in the *electrocardiogram.* Most persons with angina have normal tracings between attacks, and the record may even remain normal during the seizures. However, in many instances, depression of the S-T segments appears in leads I, II, AVL, or in those from the left precordium. There is strong experimental evidence that such depressions, as well as the elevations which are usually seen in patients with infarction and are observed in a few patients during anginal attacks, are related to alterations in ionic balance. These changes affect the diastolic base-line (T-P) potential and thus produce relative depression (low plasma potassium or high plasma sodium) or elevation (low sodium or high potassium) of the S-T segment. It would appear that the net effect of very severe ischemia is to produce S-T elevation, while less marked ischemia has the reverse effect. However, in many patients myocardial hypoxia sufficient to produce severe pain is associated with either no electrocardiographic change or with such minor alterations as may be produced in healthy subjects by tachycardia or by emotional stress. The value and limi-

tation of electrocardiographic changes occurring after exercise in the diagnosis of angina pectoris is discussed in Chap. 254.

A third effect of myocardial hypoxia is alteration in contraction. It has been shown that the pulmonary capillary (wedge) pressure may rise during anginal attacks. This indicates *temporary left ventricular failure,* which is presumably induced by the decreased contractility of the ischemic areas. Further evidence of the frequent occurrence of temporary ventricular failure during anginal attacks is the exaggeration of atrial forces (Fig. 5-2) which often appears during the ischemic episodes in records of precordial motion (kinetocardiogram) and which is similar to the change seen in patients with congestive heart failure.

Nitroglycerin relieves the pain of angina and may or may not cause reversal of the electrocardiographic changes. Occasionally, one observes the paradoxical combination of clinical benefit with worsening of the electrocardiogram. However, the relief of pain is associated with evidence of im-

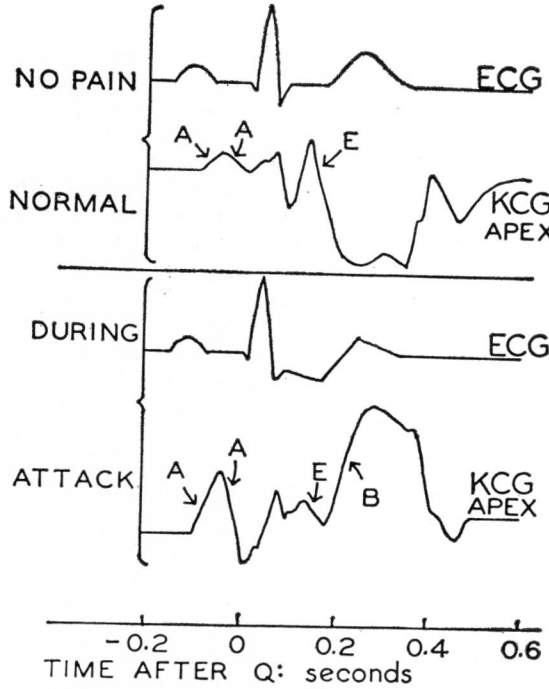

FIG. 5-2. During the anginal episode the ECG exhibits a depressed and downsloping S-T segment. The apex record displays three striking changes during the attack: (1) Exaggeration of atrial motions (*A*) due to rise in ventricular end-diastolic pressure and increased atrial stretch. (2) Decreased size of the ejection inward motion (*E*). (3) The appearance of a large midsystolic outward bulge (*B*). This is ascribed to loss of contractility and ballooning of the ischemic area as the healthy muscle contracts vigorously.

proved contractility. It has been shown in animals that occlusion of a coronary vessel results, in a few beats, in *systolic bulging* of the ischemic region. There is ample evidence that a similar bulge often occurs during anginal attacks (Fig. 5-2). These temporary ischemic bulges, which can actually be felt in a minority of the patients and recorded in many instances, are regularly abolished by glyceryl trinitrate (nitroglycerin). The transient left ventricular failure (i.e., elevated pulmonary capillary pressure) is also relieved by this drug. The different concepts of its mechanism of action have already been mentioned.

Another characteristic effect of myocardial hypoxia is *liability to sudden death*. This may never occur, despite hundreds of anginal episodes. However, it may supervene early in the disease and even in the first attack. Under exceptional circumstances, when the conducting system is involved, the patient may expire because of atrioventricular block, with standstill of the ventricle. However, the usual mechanism is ventricular fibrillation, which can often be seen to occur in animals following ligation of a coronary artery.

Pericarditis. Experimental studies made on man indicate that the visceral and the internal surface of the parietal pericardium are ordinarily insensitive to pain, although when the latter is sufficiently inflamed, painful stimuli may originate from it. The most highly sensitive region is the lower part of the external surface of the parietal layer, and the pain associated with inflammation of the remaining part usually arises in the adjacent pleura. These observations explain why noninfectious pericarditis (that associated with uremia and with myocardial infarction) with relatively mild inflammation is usually painless or accompanied rarely with very mild pain, whereas infectious pericarditis, being nearly always more intense and spreading to the neighboring pleura, is usually associated with typical pleuritic pain (i.e., aggravated by breathing, coughing, etc.). Since the central part of the diaphragm receives its sensory supply from the phrenic nerve, which arises from the third to fifth cervical segments of the spinal cord, pain arising from the lower parietal pericardium and central tendon of the diaphragm is felt characteristically at the tip of the shoulder, the adjoining trapezius ridge, and the neck. Involvement of the more lateral part of the diaphragmatic pleura, supplied by branches from the intercostal nerves (sixth to ninth thoracic), causes pain not only in the anterior chest but also in the upper abdomen and corresponding region of the back, thus sometimes simulating the pain of acute cholecystitis or pancreatitis.

Pericarditis causes three distinct types of pain. By far the most common is the pleuritic pain, related to respiratory movements and always aggra-vated by cough or deep inspiration, sometimes brought on by swallowing, because the esophagus lies just beyond the posterior portion of the heart, sometimes by change of bodily position. This type of pain is due to the pleuritic component of the pleuropericarditis so commonly present in the infectious forms. The next most common pericardial pain is the steady, crushing substernal pain identical with that of acute myocardial infarction; if the pleuritic component is absent, differentiation on the basis of the pain alone is impossible. The mechanism of this steady substernal pain is not certain, but it is probable that it arises from the highly inflamed inner parietal surface of the pericardium or from the irritated afferent cardiac nerve fibers lying in the periadventitial layers of the superficial coronaries. The third type of pain, one that a priori should appear to be the most common and characteristic, is actually quite uncommon. This pain is synchronous with the heart beat and is felt at the left border of the heart and left shoulder. Rarely, all three types may be present simultaneously.

The painful syndromes which may follow operations on the heart ("postcommissurotomy syndrome"), myocardial infarction, or trauma to the heart are discussed in later chapters (pp. 1441 and 1468). Such pains often but not always arise in the pericardium.

Pleural pain is very common and may be identical with that of pericarditis. However, its sharp superficial quality (p. 15) and its aggravation by each breath readily distinguishes it from the deep dull steady unwavering pain of myocardial ischemia. The pain of mediastinitis or of mediastinal emphysema (p. 1567) usually resembles that of pleuritis but is more likely to be maximal in the substernal region, and the associated feeling of constriction may cause confusion with myocardial infarction.

APPROACH TO THE PATIENT WITH PAIN IN THE CHEST

Most individuals with this complaint will fall into one of two general groups. The first consists of persons with prolonged and often severe pain without obvious initiating factors. Such persons will frequently be gravely ill. The problem is that of differentiating such serious conditions as myocardial infarction, dissecting aneurysm, and pulmonary embolism from each other and from less grave causes. In some such instances, the careful history will provide significant clues, while objective evidence of crucial importance will appear within the subsequent two or three days. Thus, when the initial examinations are not decisive, a watch and wait policy, with repeated electrocardiograms coupled with measurements of the transaminase, sedimentation rate, etc., will commonly provide the correct answer.

The second group of patients comprises those who have brief episodes of pain, with otherwise apparently excellent health. Here, the resting electrocardiogram will rarely supply decisive information, but records taken after exercise will often reveal characteristic changes (p. 1448). However, in many instances it is the study of the subjective phenomenon, i.e., of the pain itself, that will lead to the diagnosis. Of the several methods of investigation which are available for such patients, three are of cardinal importance.

A detailed and *meticulous history* of the behavior of the pain is the most important method. The location, radiation, quality, intensity, and, especially, the duration of the episodes are important. Even more so is the story of the aggravating and alleviating factors. Thus a history of sharp aggravation by breathing, coughing, or other respiratory movements will usually point toward the pleura, pericardium (because of the associated pleuropericarditis), or mediastinum as the site, although chest wall pain is likewise affected by respiratory motions. Similarly, a pain which regularly appears on rapid walking and vanishes within a few minutes upon standing still will usually mean angina pectoris, although here, once again, a similar story will rarely be obtained from patients with skeletal disorders.

When the history is inconclusive, the *study of the patient at the time of the spontaneous episode* will often supply crucial information. Thus the electrocardiogram, which may be normal both at rest and after exercise in the absence of pain, will occasionally demonstrate striking changes when recorded during an anginal episode. Similarly, x-ray of the esophagus or of the stomach may show no evidence of cardiospasm or of hiatal hernia except when the observation is made during the pain.

The third method of study represents the *attempt to produce and alleviate the pain at will*. This procedure is necessary only when doubt exists following the history or when needed for psychotherapeutic purposes. Thus the demonstration that a localized pain, which can be reproduced by pressure on the chest, is completely relieved by local infiltration with novocaine will often be of conclusive importance in convincing the patient that the heart is not the site. The discomfort due to distention of the stomach or of the splenic flexure with air is frequently mistaken by the patient, and occasionally by the physician, for pain of cardiac origin. The simple demonstration, by passing a tube to the appropriate area and inflation with air, that the pain can be exactly reproduced may be not only of diagnostic but also of psychotherapeutic value. However, the demonstration that such procedures will reproduce the patient's pain may be misleading in persons who have angina in addition to another disorder. It may, therefore, be necessary to study also the effect of exercise on the pain and on the electrocardiogram.

When, as is not rarely the case, the history is atypical, the correct diagnosis of angina pectoris will often depend in large measure on the response to nitroglycerin. Here, a number of pitfalls should be avoided. If the patient has previously had the drug, careful questioning may be necessary to avoid errors. Thus disappearance after its sublingual administration does not necessarily prove that there is a cause and effect relationship. It is necessary to be certain that the pain vanishes more rapidly (usually within 5 min) and more completely when the drug is used than when it is not employed. A false negative impression concerning the effect of nitroglycerin may be the result of the use of a deteriorated preparation which has been exposed to light. It is thus necessary to be sure that the dosage used is sufficient to induce a pharmacologic effect in the form of a slight flush or a mild pounding headache. In doubtful instances, repeated exercise tests, with and without preceding administration of nitroglycerin, are necessary. The demonstration that the time required for a given exercise to produce pain is consistently and considerably longer when it is undertaken within a few minutes after a sublingual nitroglycerin pill than after a placebo may, in some instances, represent the sole method for accurate recognition of angina pectoris. A completely negative response to such repeated tests constitutes almost conclusive evidence against angina.

CLINICAL ASPECTS OF SOME OF THE MORE COMMON CAUSES OF CHEST PAIN

Some of the features of pericarditis have already been described, and those of the more serious causes of chest pain such as myocardial ischemia (angina pectoris and infarction), dissecting aneurysm, and disorders of the pleura, esophagus, stomach, duodenum, and pancreas are considered in the appropriate chapters dealing with these problems. Here, we are concerned with the discussion of those causes which are not considered in more detail elsewhere.

Pain Arising in the Chest Wall or Upper Extremity. This may develop as a result of muscle or ligament strains brought on by unaccustomed exercise and felt in the costochondral or chondrosternal junctions or in the chest wall muscles. We mention the upper extremities and especially the left because of the deeply ingrained legend that pain in the left arm has a specific significance in indicting the heart. Another cause is spinal arthritis.

Finally, pains in the upper extremity (shoulder-hand syndrome) and in the pectoral muscles may, through unknown mechanisms, follow acute myocardial infarction.

Skeletal pains in the chest wall or shoulder girdles or arms are usually recognized quite easily. Localized tenderness of the affected area is usually present, and the pain is sometimes clearly related to movements involving the painful locus. Thus deep breathing, turning or twisting of the chest, movements of the shoulder girdle and arm will elicit and duplicate the pain of which the patient complains. The pain may be very brief, lasting only a few seconds, or dull and aching and enduring for hours. The duration is, therefore, likely to be either longer or shorter than untreated anginal pain, which usually lasts for only a few minutes. Occasionally, one sees a patient with a pain due to violent cramp of the intercostal muscles, lasting a few seconds to a minute. It is usually felt in the anterior axillary region, and its quality is identical with that of the "night cramp" in the muscles of the calves.

These skeletal pains often have a sharp or sticking quality. In addition, there is frequently a feeling of tightness which is probably due to associated spasm of intercostal or pectoral muscles. This may produce the "morning stiffness" seen in so many skeletal disorders. The discomfort is unaffected by nitroglycerin but often abolished by infiltration of the painful areas with procaine (Novocain).

When chest wall pain is of recent origin and follows some unusual activity involving the pectoral muscles, it presents no problem in diagnosis. However, *long-standing skeletal pain is frequent in persons who also have angina pectoris.* This association is sometimes coincidental, because both disorders are very common. In other instances, it seems that the coronary disease is responsible for the chest wall pain, the exact mechanism being uncertain but similar to that responsible for the well-known shoulder-hand syndrome. This coexistence of the two different types of chest pain in the same patient is a frequent cause of a confusing history because in the patient's mind the anginal needle may be hidden in the skeletal haystack. Thus every middle-aged or elderly patient who has long-standing anterior chest wall pain merits careful study.

Detailed questioning will sometimes reveal that what was originally thought by the patient to be a single type of discomfort actually comprises two different pains which, though similar in quality and area, differ as regards duration and initiating factors. When the history is inconclusive, the postexertional electrocardiogram may furnish decisive information. However, both false positive and false negative tracings may be obtained, according to whether they are interpreted loosely or critically (p. 1446). It may thus be necessary to study the

pain itself and to learn by direct observations whether exercise alone or postprandial exertion, or even postprandial effort undertaken holding an ice cube, is capable of producing it. Repeated tests may be required, the effects of preceding placebos, as compared to nitroglycerin, on the amount of exertion required to induce the pain being compared. *The confusion created by the presence of innocent skeletal pain impairs the reliability of the history and is probably the commonest cause of errors—both positive and negative—in the diagnosis of angina pectoris.*

Emotional disorders are also common causes of chest wall pain. Usually, the discomfort is experienced as a sense of "tightness," sometimes called "aching," and occasionally, it may be sufficiently severe as to be designated as a pain of considerable magnitude. Since the discomfort has almost always the additional quality of tightness or constriction and, furthermore, since it is often localized across the sternum, although it may be felt in other areas of the anterior chest, it is not surprising that this type of pain is frequently confused with that of myocardial ischemia. Ordinarily, it lasts for a half hour or more and may persist for a day or less with slow fluctuation of intensity. The association with fatigue or emotional strain is usually clear, although it may not be recognized by the patient until called to his attention. The pain probably develops through unconscious and prolonged increase of muscle tone (as in frowning in the face, or as can be quickly produced in the hand by tightly clinching the fist), often enhanced by an accompanying hyperventilation (by causing a contraction of the chest wall muscles similar to the painful tetany of the extremities). When the hyperventilation and/or the associated adrenergic effect due to anxiety also causes innocent changes in the T waves and S-T segments, the confusion with coronary disease is strengthened. However, the long duration of the pain, the lack of any relation to exertion but rather to fatigue or tension, and the usual periodic occurrence on successive days without any limitation of capacity for exercise usually make the differentiation from ischemic pain quite clear.

As compared to these two causes (the chest wall muscle and ligament strains and the contraction of the pectoral muscles due to reflex influences, fatigue, or tension) the various other conditions that may cause skeletal discomfort are uncommon and readily recognized after appropriate observation: spinal arthritis, herpes zoster, anterior scalene and hyperabduction syndromes, malignant disease of the ribs, etc.

The several *abdominal disorders* which may at times mimic anginal pain may usually be suspected from the history, which ordinarily will indicate some relationship to swallowing, eating, belching, the expulsion of flatus, etc. Occasionally, as in some patients with hiatal hernia, the gastrointestinal x-ray will be of crucial significance. Rarely, it may be necessary to inflate the stomach or the splenic flexure with air, in order to satisfy both the doctor and the patient that one of these organs is responsible for a tight pain in the lower chest. It should be emphasized again that the demonstration of the presence of a coexistent abdominal disorder such as hiatal hernia does not constitute proof that the chest pain of which the patient complains is due to this. Such disorders are frequently asymptomatic and are not at all uncommon in patients who also have angina pectoris.

SUMMARY

The location of a pain in the chest has little diagnostic import. The concept that radiation from the anterior chest to the left arm necessarily indicates coronary disease as a cause is an old wives' tale. The several thoracic viscera and the chest wall have nerve fibers which pass by a final common pathway to the pain receptive areas of the brain. One can no more identify the cause of the pain by its location alone than one can hear the ring of a telephone and know the city from which the call originated. Differences in the quality and duration of pain may be of diagnostic value. However, the most important aspect of the history in the diagnosis of *brief and recurrent chest pain is the relationship to various precipitating and alleviating factors*. The observation of the effect of exercise on the electrocardiogram and on the pain is often conclusive. In many instances the study of the effect of nitroglycerin on the amount of exercise required to produce pain is of crucial import.

In the spontaneously arising pains of long duration, as in myocardial infarction, dissecting aneurysm, pulmonary embolism, acute pericarditis, gallbladder colic, incarcerated hiatal hernia, acute pancreatitis, in all of which the pain may be identical in location, severity, character, and sites of reference, it is often the corollary data, clinical and laboratory, that finally determine the diagnosis.

Reproducing and alleviating the discomfort is not only sometimes of value in establishing the diagnosis but of immense psychologic benefit to the patient when he learns that an apparently mysterious and disturbing disorder can be mimicked and relieved at will.

When, as will occasionally occur, the thorough examination leaves one in doubt, observation over a period of time will often clarify the question, at least to the extent of establishing or excluding the more serious causes of the pain. Under such circumstances the patient should be advised to follow the same exertional and dietary regime which one would advise in any healthy middle-aged person, because this is essentially the same as that advised for a person with minimal myocardial ischemia (p. 1447). At the same time, fear can be alleviated by the reassurance that this regime is aimed not at treatment of an existing condition but at preventing future vascular disease.

REFERENCES

Capps, J. A.: Pain from the Pleura and Pericardium, A. Research Publs. Assoc. Research Nervous Mental Disease (1942) 23:263, 1943.

Edwards, W. L. Jack: Musculoskeletal Pain Following Myocardial Infarction, Am. Heart. J., 49:713, 1955.

Gorlin, R., N. Brachfeld, C. MacLeod, and P. Bopp: Effect of Nitroglycerine on the Coronary Circulation in Patients with Coronary Disease of Increased Left Ventricular Work, Circulation, 19:705, 1959.

Harrison, T. R., Some Clinical Aspects of Angina Pectoris, Bull. Johns Hopkins Hosp., 104:275, 1959.

Hoing, C. R., S. M. Tenney, and P. V. Gobel: The Mechanism of Cardiovascular Action of Nitroglycerine, Am. J. Med., 19:910, 1960.

Keefer, C. S., and W. H. Resnik: Angina Pectoris: A Syndrome Caused by Anoxemia of the Myocardium, Arch. Internal Med., 41:769, 1928.

Müller, O., and K. Rørvik: Haemodynamic Consequences of Coronary Heart Disease with Observations during Anginal Pain and on the Effect of Nitroglycerine, Brit. Heart J., 20:302, 1958.

Prinzmetal, M., and R. A. Massumi: Anteoir Chest Wall Syndrome: Chest Pain Resembling Pain of Cardiac Origin, J.A.M.A., 159:177, 1955.

Sarnoff, S. J., R. B. Case, P. E. Waithe, and J. P. Isaacs: Insufficient Coronary Flow and Myocardial Failure as Complicating Factor in Late Hemorrhagic Shock, Am. J. Physiol., 176:439, 1954.

6   ACUTE ABDOMINAL PAIN
Carl A. Moyer

ABDOMINAL PAIN

Abdominal pain may be defined as a consciousness of distress in the abdomen. Under certain conditions this manifests itself as indigestion, which will be considered later. It may have a parenchymatous, metabolic, or neurogenic origin. The etiologic classification in Table 6-1, while not complete, includes the important causes of this symptom.

The differentiation of abdominal pain is difficult. The location of the pain, its type (colicky, steady, boring), its mode of onset, its rate of change in intensity, its relationship to eating and to evacuation of bowel and bladder are historically important in the determination of cause. The degree and lo-

Table 6-1. ETIOLOGIC CLASSIFICATION
OF ABDOMINAL PAIN

I. Pain associated with parenchymatous disease
   A. Pain referred to the abdomen from extraabdominal disorders (i.e., from thorax, spine, or genitalia)
   B. Pain having its origin within the abdomen
      1. Incident to disturbances of function or obstruction of hollow organs
         - Bowel
         - Bile ducts
         - Ureter
         - Bladder
         - Pancreatic duct
      2. Incident to peritoneal inflammation
         a. Chemical
            - Gastric juice
            - Pancreatic juice
            - Urine
            - Bile
            - Blood extravasation from a parenchymatous organ* (liver, spleen, kidney, ovary)
         b. Bacterial
            - Gastrointestinal contents
            - Bacterial invasion of uterus and oviducts
            - Rupture of abscesses into the remaining free peritoneal cavity
            - Invasion of peritoneal cavity from the blood stream— primary peritonitis
      3. Incident to disturbances in blood supply
         a. Pressure or torsional occlusion
            - Volvulus
            - Strangulated hernias
            - Twisted pedunculated cysts
            - Uterine fibroids
         b. Embolism and thrombosis
            - Arterial
            - Venous
         c. "Inflammatory" (e.g., visceral angiitis)
      4. Incident to disruption of a viscus (e.g., rupture of a viscus or tearing apart of arterial walls)
      5. Incident to an increase in tension upon supporting elements
         a. Traction on mesenteries
         b. Rapid swelling of capsules (e.g., congested liver, carcinomatous lymph nodes)
         c. Rapid separations of leaves of mesenteries
            - New growths
            - Rupture of vessels
      6. Incident to disease of muscle
         a. Traumatic myopathy
         b. Infectious myositis
            - Viral
            - Bacterial
            - Parasitic
II. Pain associated with metabolic disease
   A. Endogenous
      1. Toxic (uremia, diabetic coma, porphyria)
      2. Allergic

* Blood introduced into the peritoneal cavity through a needle or from torn mesenteric vessels usually produces no pain.

Table 6-1. ETIOLOGIC CLASSIFICATION
OF ABDOMINAL PAIN (*Continued*)

   B. Exogenous
      1. Toxic (e.g., lead poisoning)
      2. Biologic (e.g., bite of the black widow spider)
III. Central or neurogenic pain
   A. Organic
      1. Lesions of the central nervous system (postapoplectic pain)
      2. Root pain (including the "lightning" pain of tabes dorsalis)
      3. Causalgia
   B. Ideogenous ("mind pain," "psychogenic pain")

cation of muscle spasm, changes in the pattern of breathing, the location of tenderness to percussion and to steady increase in pressure, the threshold of counter pain necessary to remove abdominal pain from consciousness, and the determination of changes in cutaneous sensitivity are signs of importance in the differentiation of abdominal pain.

Of Parenchymatous Origin

Referred Abdominal Pain. This type of pain is the enigma of the surgeon, for he recognizes that the lower thoracic cavity and the upper abdomen are neurologically and lymphatically one unit. For example, early acute lobar pneumonia, with basilar pleurisy, may be attended by severe abdominal pain and a degree of "spasm" of the abdominal muscles so intense as to lead one to think that a duodenal ulcer has perforated or that the gallbladder has ruptured and peritonitis is present. To make matters more confusing, the abdominal pain of pneumonia may be present before any physical or roentgenologic signs of pneumonia are detectable. Conversely, acute cholangitis and acute subphrenic abscesses are often associated with pleuritic pain in the lower right chest and signs of fluid in or atelectasis of the lower lobe of the lung. Coronary occlusive disease and acute cholecystitis, with cystic duct obstruction, may also be mistaken one for the other.

The differentiation of referred abdominal pain from that arising within the abdominal cavity may depend solely upon the course that the illness takes during a brief period of careful observation. However, a tentative opinion of the probable anatomic location of the primary difficulty can often be made from the elucidation of a few clinical signs.

Abdominal pain referred from within the chest is usually associated with alterations in breathing, lag and restriction of motion of the lower thoracic segment that are much more apparent than those associated with pain of intraabdominal origin. In addition, pain that accompanies intraabdominal inflammatory processes (exclusive of those limited to the lesser omental cavity) is generally associated with spasm of the abdominal muscles that *does not* perceptibly relax during the inspiratory phase of the respiratory cycle; whereas the spasm occasioned by the referred type does relax during inspiration. Evidently the reciprocal inhibition of the abdominal muscles, which are expiratory muscles, that normally takes place during inspiration still occurs with referred abdominal pain but does not occur with that of peritonitis. Another point of difference that may be of help is that steady, gentle pressure over the painful area does not materially increase, and may actually relieve, the pain if it is referred, but generally increases it if it is of intraabdominal inflammatory origin.

It is especially important that referred and intraabdominal inflammatory pain be differentiated, because the latter often indicates immediate surgical intervention. Intrathoracic diseases more commonly associated with abdominal pain are lobar pneumonia, coronary occlusive disease, infectious pericarditis, and "cardiospasm." The routine careful search for specific clinical signs of their existence will often lead to the correct inference as to the origin of pain that appears superficially to be of abdominal origin. However, it is well to remember that diseases may be coexistent, and the existence of intrathoracic or intraabdominal disease before the acute disease develops, even though it may be "asymptomatic," may result in unusual areas of reference of the acute pain. For example, a painless healed abdominal incision, especially if it is recent, often becomes the point of reference for pain arising from widely separated organs within the abdomen. Though it has not as yet been proved, it is thought that the same principle may explain the peculiar references of pain with acute gallbladder disease to the left shoulder, if coronary occlusive disease exists; and the radiation of the pain of myocardial infarction to the epigastrium or right upper quadrant of the abdomen, if preexisting, though asymptomatic, gallbladder or duodenal disease is present.

Referred pain arising from the testis is acutely intensified by light testicular pressure, and that arising from the seminal vesicle is usually relieved by expression of its contents. That arising from vertebral disease often has the characteristics of root pain.

The commonest causes of abdominal pain having their origins within that cavity are disturbances in the function of hollow organs, intraabdominal inflammation, and increase in tension of supporting elements.

Pain Associated with Disturbances in Function of Hollow Organs. This pain is, at least initially, intermittent or colicky. It is generally associated with definite organic disease but may occasionally accompany variations in physiologic function without visible organic disease. Anyone who has observed the terrific colic of acute coccal food poisoning or who, having made a diagnosis of acute intestinal obstruction, has had the misfortune of performing a celiotomy upon an individual who is actually suffering from porphyria, and has seen the unbelievable contortions performed by the intestine, is convinced that severe colic can be associated solely with changes in physiologic function.

Pain which is incident to disturbances in the function of various hollow organs has certain relatively specific areas of reference. That associated with obstruction of the cystic duct or distention of the gallbladder is referred most commonly to the epigastrium, then to the right posterior chest about the scapula, and occasionally to the left lower quadrant of the abdomen. Sudden common bile duct or pancreatic duct obstruction by stone produces pain that is felt in the epigastrium and in the upper lumbar region of the back. The colicky pain of midgut obstructive origin, or in other words, terminal duodenal, small intestinal, appendiceal, ascending and proximal transverse colonic obstructive origin, is generally supraumbilical or circaumbilical. That associated with lesions in the flexures of the colon is felt in the region of these structures. Obstructive lesions of the lower descending and sigmoid colon produce pain that is felt most often in the left iliac region and over the sacrum.

Obstruction of the ureter from below the ureteropelvic junction to its intravesical portion is productive of pain that is initially felt directly over the point of obstruction, but after spasm of lumbar and flank muscles develops, the pain becomes diffuse and tends to cover the flanks. Acute occlusion of the intravesicular portion of the ureter, and of the proximal urethra, tends to produce pain which is referred to the shaft of the penis, the scrotum, and the inner surface of the thigh in the male, to the inner surface of the thigh in the female, and to the suprapubic regions of both sexes.

Rapid distention of the bladder is productive of suprapubic pain. Obstruction of the ureteropelvic junction is associated with pain in the costovertebral angle.

Pain Incident to an Inflammatory Process Involving a Parietal Peritoneal Surface. Pain of this sort is located over the area involved and is steady and aching in character. The rate of its development and intensity are dependent upon the amount and character of the chemical substances which impinge upon a given surface per unit of time. For example, a milliliter of highly acid sterile gastric juice or a milliliter of sterile alkaline pancreatic juice (which, in addition to their acidity and alkalinity, are enzymatically potent) in the peritoneum is immediately productive of much more intense inflammation and pain than is a milliliter of bac-

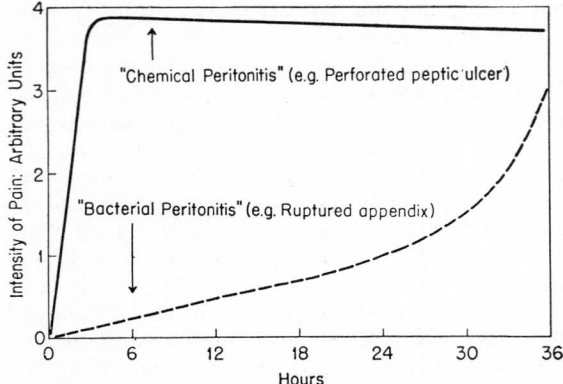

FIG. 6-1. The time-intensity curve of pain due to peritonitis depends on the underlying cause. When enzymatic digestion of the peritoneum is responsible, the pain rapidly reaches a maximal degree of intensity. When bacterial inflammation is responsible, the progression is much slower and is apparently related to the rate of bacterial growth.

teria-laden, neutral, enzymatically impotent liquid feces from the ascending colon.

Ultimately, as the bacteria multiply and elaborate irritants, the peritoneal surface over which the organisms spread becomes severely inflamed and painful. The differentiation between inflammatory processes of bacterial chemical and body chemical origin is primarily dependent upon the analysis of progression of the inflammation or pain (Fig. 6-1).

Another factor that must be considered in the analysis of the severity of the pain that accompanies an inflammatory process is the rate of change in the intensity of the stimulus. If the rate of change in the intensity of a stimulus is sufficiently slow, no sensation of pain will be felt, even if a very intense, widespread inflammatory reaction is present (e.g., tuberculous peritonitis); if the rate of change is very rapid, the pain is intense (e.g., ruptured duodenal ulcers). In general, the intensity of pain is more intimately related to the rate of change in strength of stimulus than it is to the area to which the stimulus is applied.

The location and extent of tonic muscle spasm, which usually occurs with peritonitis, is fundamentally dependent upon the surface area involved in the process. The intensity of the spasm is usually related directly to the rate of development of the inflammation and is related inversely to the functional integrity of the central nervous system. The latter relationship is especially important. A severely ill or a dying man will not show spasm of the abdominal muscles, even if his stomach or gallbladder ruptures. Degenerated psychotic (schizophrenic) patients, those suffering from advanced Parkinson's disease and from extensive multiple sclerosis, have been observed in whom the acute

rupture of a viscus (gallbladder or duodenum) with widespread generalized peritonitis has been unattended by any significant degree of muscle spasm.

The pain incident to inflammation is aggravated by pressure on the abdomen.

Abdominal pain that attends vascular occlusive disease is characteristically rapid in onset, and agonizing, if the process is at all extensive. It tends to be constant and diffuse. If it is not complicated by coexistent inflammatory pain, the tonic spasm of muscles is much less in relation to the severity of the pain than is the muscle spasm associated with an acute peritoneal inflammation.

The pain attending the rupture of a viscus (except those containing potent chemicals) is a sudden, sharp, terrifying pain that is quickly over. The pains of rupture of the gravid uterus, of the spleen, or of the distended, obstructed appendix are of this type.

Pain Frequently Associated with Increase in Tension upon Supporting Elements of Organs (Capsules, Ligaments, and Mesentery). This pain tends to be steady and aching in character, increased by muscular activity, and relieved by rest and may vary considerably with change of posture. It may be absent in the morning, following a well-slept night, but increases gradually during the activities of the day. It is not well localized; it tends to be circaumbilical and supraumbilical if the organ involved lies in the abdominal cavity and infraumbilical, suprapubic, and in the low-back region if the organ involved is located in the pelvis. Gentle percussion with the closed fist or pressure over the organ involved aggravates this type of pain. The area of tenderness to percussion shifts with position if the organ involved is mobile (e.g., lymph nodes in the mesentery). Abdominal muscle spasm is usually minimal if present at all.

Abdominal pain associated with generalized myositis of infectious origin mimics that of pain of intraabdominal inflammatory origin. It is constant, aching, aggravated by movement and pressure, and associated with tonic muscle spasm. The main differential point between the pain of myositis and the pain of peritoneal inflammation is the presence, in the former, of tenderness and spasm of muscle masses not innervated by the nerves supplying the peritoneum and, in the latter, limitation of muscle spasm and tenderness to their areas of distribution.

Abdominal pain of "metabolic" origin may mimic all other types, and its recognition depends upon the constant awareness on the part of the doctor that it may simulate early small intestinal obstruction, appendicitis, cholecystitis, ruptured ulcer, etc.

The abdominal pain with sickle-cell anemia tends to migrate, and the areas of tenderness likewise tend to shift within brief periods of time (1 to 3 hr).

That associated with diabetes and uremia has no specific characteristics.

The bite of the black widow spider is productive of severe pain and rigidity, not only in the abdominal muscles but also in the long muscles of the back (sacrospinalis), a region rarely affected by pain of intraabdominal origin.

The abdominal crisis of chronic porphyria mimics acute intestinal obstruction and is characteristically attended by unusually prominent signs of increased peristaltic activity.

The pain of lead colic has no specific characteristics.

Ileus, or obstruction of the intestine, may accompany all types of abdominal pain. (See Chap. 276.)

Of Neurogenic or Central Origin

Pain associated with abnormalities of the spinal nerves and roots such as tumors and degenerative diseases (diabetic and syphilitic) or incident to impingement of bone (arthritis and fractures of the spine) or soft tissue (ruptured nucleus pulposis) upon nerve roots or elements of the cauda equina are usually localized. Cord and root pains tend to have a sudden onset (lightning pains) and a lancinating character and are often limited to a few neural segments. They have no consistent relationship to eating. The abdominal pain arising from the impingement of bone or a ruptured nucleus upon nerve roots is aggravated by movements of the spine. Muscle spasm is often intense, but it is not particularly increased by gentle pressure on the abdomen. Changes in nerve thresholds are common (hyperesthesia, hypesthesia). Distention of the abdomen is uncommon, and persistent changes in breathing are not seen often.

Causalgia (Peripheral Type). This quality of pain is usually limited to areas of distribution of peripheral nerves that have been partially severed or have partially regenerated after complete severance or pressure block. Its quality is variable; usually the person cannot describe it with clarity and precision; it is most troublesome during periods of rest.

In persons with causalgic pain the respiration and muscle tonus are normal; the threshold of counter pain necessary to remove abdominal causalgic pain from consciousness is low; the light touch of a pinpoint to the forehead is frequently enough. The geographic distribution of cutaneous pain spots is grossly altered in the painful area. These spots are very irregularly spaced, with frequent gaps of a centimeter between them. In fact, disturbance in pain-spot distribution may be the only significant clue that a pain is causalgic. In general, peripheral causalgia seems to be fundamentally related to a change in the relationships of the various cutaneous sensory stimuli that simultaneously impinge upon the skin and deep structures.

For example, feeling a rough surface is not a painful experience, but it may be if the ulnar or median nerves are partially severed. The recognition that a surface is rough is dependent upon a pattern of stimuli arising in touch, pressure, and pain endings. Unequal interference with the receptive capacity of various sensory endings or fibers so changes the central appreciation of feeling a rough surface as to make it distressful to the individual. The painful sensations that accompany the stepping on a "sleeping" foot are similar to causalgia, and the differential disturbances of various peripheral sensory components are relatively easily demonstrable.

Psychogenic Pain. This pain is characterized by indefiniteness of onset, diffuseness of location, and casual definition of type, with little or no relationship to meals or evacuation. Generally, irregularly cyclic muscle spasms may be felt, and many bizarre types of change in the character of breathing may be seen. The commonest type of change in breathing is a restriction of the depth of inspiration without accentuation of the speed of expiration. The expiratory accessory muscles of respiration may be tonically (not rhythmically) active. If generalized abdominal muscle spasm is present, the abdomen will be protuberant in the lateral view and normal or narrow in the anterior view. Generally speaking, no persistent localized point of tenderness will be present excepting when the abdomen is scarred. The physical signs of central psychogenic pain can be obliterated by the suppression of consciousness [drowsiness or sleep or with thiopental (Pentothal) N_2O "analgesia"], or by inducing a powerful stimulation of breathing with 10 per cent carbon dioxide.

The foregoing chapter has been concerned, in the main, with the more severe types of abdominal pain. The milder types of abdominal discomfort will be considered in Chap. 16, in the section dealing with Indigestion.

REFERENCES

Association for Research in Nervous and Mental Disease: "Pain: Proceedings of the Association, December 18 and 19, 1942," Baltimore, The Williams & Wilkins Company, 1943 (Research Publications, vol. 23, 1942).

Bishop, G. H.: Response to Electrical Stimulation of Single Sensory Units of Skin, J. Neurophysiol., 6:361, 1943; The Peripheral Unit of Pain, ibid., 7:71, 1944; The Structural Identity of the Pain Spot in Human Skin, ibid., 7:185, 1944.

Fine, J., B. M. Banks, and L. Hermanson: The Treatment of Gaseous Distention of the Intestine by the Inhalation of 95 Per Cent Oxygen, Ann. Surg., 103:375, 1936.

Lewis, T.: "Pain," New York, The Macmillan Company, 1942.

Olivecrona, H.: Inhibition Ileus (Paralytic), chap. 23, pp. 425–442, in "Intestinal Obstruction," 2d ed., O. H. Wangensteen (Ed.), Springfield, Ill., Charles C Thomas, Publisher, 1942.

Wangensteen, O. H.: "Therapeutic Problem in Bowel Obstructions," Springfield, Ill., Charles C Thomas, Publisher, 1937.

7 PAIN IN THE BACK

Raymond D. Adams, Michel Jequier, and Jost Michelsen

Painful afflictions of the back are considered apart from other algesic states for the reason that they offer unusual difficulties in diagnosis and require a number of special techniques of examination.

Each part of the spine has its own anatomic peculiarities and is subject to some diseases more than others. The following remarks are directed to the lower back since it is most frequently the site of disabling pain. A few additional comments concerning pain in the neck will be added. Certain aspects of painful affections of the thoracic spine are presented in Chaps. 82 and 301.

The major problem created by painful conditions in the lower back relates essentially to frequent failure to ascertain the cause and nature of the pain and inability, therefore, to learn from past clinical experience. The lower spine and pelvis, with their many muscular and tendinous attachments, are relatively inaccessible to palpation and also to inspection, even through the medium of x-ray. Moreover, the lack of complete knowledge of the physiologic mechanisms whereby pain is produced in these structures proves to be a further hindrance in diagnosis. For want of reliable physical signs and laboratory tests, it is often necessary to depend on the patient's description of his pain, which may not be altogether accurate, and his behavior during the execution of certain maneuvers. Seasoned clinicians, for these reasons, come to appreciate the need of a systematic clinical approach, the description of which will be one of the main purposes of this chapter.

ANATOMY AND PHYSIOLOGY OF THE LOWER BACK

The student is referred to any one of the standard textbooks of orthopedics for a detailed account of the applied anatomy of the spine. It is sufficient for our purposes to indicate merely that the spine is roughly divisible into two parts: an anterior column of articulated vertebral bodies and intervertebral disks held together by the anterior and posterior longitudinal ligaments, which together constitute the supporting pillar of the body; and a posterior segment consisting of pedicles and laminas, fused to form the walls of the spinal canal, and which provides protection for the spinal cord and also points of attachment of paravertebral muscles.

The stability of the spine depends on two types of supporting structures, the ligamentous (passive) and muscular (active). Active muscular support and movement are contributed by the erectores spinae, abdominal, glutei maximus, psoas, and hamstring muscles.

The vertebral and paravertebral structures derive their innervation from the recurrent branches of the spinal nerves. Pain endings and fibers have been demonstrated in the ligaments, muscles, periosteum of bone, annulus fibrosus, and synovia of the articular facets. The sensory fibers from these structures and the sacroiliac and lumbosacral joints join to form the sinovertebral nerves which pass via the recurrent branches of the spinal nerves of the first sacral and the fifth to first lumbar vertebras into the gray matter of the corresponding segments of the spinal cord. Efferent fibers emerge from these segments and extend to the muscles through the same nerves. The sympathetic nerves contribute only to the innervation of blood vessels and appear to play no part in voluntary and reflex movement, though they do contain sensory fibers.

The parts of the back that possess the greatest freedom of movement, hence are most frequently subject to injury, are the lumbar and cervical. The majority of these movements are reflex and are the basis of posture.

GENERAL CLINICAL CONSIDERATIONS

Types of Low Back Pain. Of the several symptoms of disease of the spine (pain, stiffness or limitation of movement, and deformity), pain is of foremost importance by virtue of its frequency and disabling effects. Four types of pain may be differentiated: local, referred, radicular, and that arising from secondary (protective) muscular spasm. One must identify these several types of pain by the patient's description, and here reliance is placed mainly on the character, location, and the conditions which modify them. The mechanism of the several types of pain has already been described in Chap. 3.

Local pain is caused by any pathologic process which impinges upon or irritates sensory endings. Involvement of structures which contain no sensory endings is painless. The substance of the vertebral body may be destroyed by tumor, for example, without evocation of pain, whereas lesions of periosteum, synovial membranes, muscles, annulus fibrosus, and ligaments are often exquisitely painful. Although painful states are often accompanied by swelling of the affected tissues, this is not apparent if a deep structure of the back is the site of disease. Local pain is steady, of the aching type, and rather diffuse but is always felt in or near the affected part of the spine. Often there is involuntary splinting of the spine segments by paravertebral muscles, and certain movements or postures which alter the position of the injured tissues aggravate or relieve the pain. Firm pressure upon superficial structures in the region of the involved structure usually evokes tenderness which is of aid in identifying the site of the abnormality.

Referred pain is of two types, that projected from the spine into regions lying within the area of the lumbar and upper sacral dermatones and that projected from the pelvic and abdominal viscera to the spine. Pain due to diseases of the upper lumbar spine is usually referred to the anterior aspects of the thighs and legs; and that from the lower lumbar spine is referred to the gluteal regions, posterior thighs, and calves. Pain of this type tends also to be deep, of aching quality, and rather diffuse. In general the referred pain parallels in intensity the local pain in the back. In other words, maneuvers which alter local pain have a similar effect on referred pain, though not with such precision and immediacy as in "root pain." Pain from visceral disease usually is felt within the abdomen or flanks and may be modified by the state of activity of the viscera. Its character and temporal relationships are those of the particular visceral structure involved, and posture and movement of the back have relatively little effect, either on the local pain or that referred to the back.

Radicular or "*root*" *pain* has some of the characteristics of referred pain but differs in its greater intensity, distal radiation, circumscription to the territory of a root, and the factors which excite it. The mechanism is distortion, stretching, irritation, or compression of a spinal root, most often at the intervertebral foramen but sometimes central to this point. The pain is sharp, often quite intense, and nearly always radiates from a central position near the spine to some part of the lower extremity. It is usually superimposed on the dull ache of referred pain. Cough, sneeze, and strain characteristically evoke this sharp radiating pain, though these maneuvers may also jar or move the spine and enhance local pain. Any motion which stretches the nerve, i.e., forward bending with the knees extended or "straight-leg raising," excites radicular pain; and jugular vein compression, which raises intraspinal pressure and may cause a shift in the position of

the root, has a similar effect. The fourth and fifth lumbar and first sacral roots, which form the sciatic nerve, if involved in disease, cause pain which extends mainly down the posterior aspect of thigh, the postero- and anterolateral aspects of the leg, and into the foot, in the distribution of this nerve—so-called "sciatica." Tingling, paresthesias, and numbness or sensory impairment of the skin, soreness of the skin, and tenderness along the nerve usually accompany radicular pain. Also reflex loss, weakness, atrophy, fascicular twitching, and often stasis edema may occur if motor fibers are involved in the anterior roots.

Pain resulting from muscular spasm is usually mentioned in relation to local pain, but it deserves separate consideration. As stated above, muscle spasm is associated with most conditions which result in local pain. Muscles in a state of persistent tension pull on their periosteal attachments and give rise to a dull ache which Smith-Petersen has called "secondary pain." One can feel the tautness of the erector spinae and gluteal muscles and demonstrate by palpation that the pain is localized to them.

Other pains often of undetermined origin are sometimes described by patients with chronic disease of the lower back. In the legs drawing, pulling, cramping sensations (without involuntary muscle spasm), tearing, throbbing, or jabbing pains, feelings of burning or coldness are difficult to interpret and, like paresthesias and numbness, should always suggest the possibility of nerve or root disease.

Since it is often difficult to obtain physical or laboratory confirmation of painful disease of the lower spine, the importance of an accurate history and description of symptoms cannot be overemphasized. Frequently the most important lead comes from knowledge of the mode of onset and circumstances which initiated the pain. Inasmuch as many painful affections of the back are the result of injury incurred during work or in an accident, the possibility of exaggeration or prolongation of pain for personal reasons, or even hysteria or malingering, must always be kept in mind.

The Examination of the Lower Back. *Inspection* of the spine, buttocks, and legs when standing erect, walking, stooping, and squatting is of value. The patient's resting posture should be noted because faulty posture, whether from congenital abnormalities or other diseases, predisposes to strain of the lumbosacral and sacroiliac regions. With sciatica the lumbar spine is often scoliotic, with the convexity toward the normal side, though the converse may occur. Also, flattening or even a slight flexion of the lumbar lordosis is common with acute painful states. The presence of a definite kyphosis usually signifies deformity of one of the vertebral bodies, e.g., fracture. Spasm of paravertebral muscles on one or both sides is often obvious during inspection. One may also notice a hypotonia of the glutei on the affected side, with drooping of the gluteal fold.

The next step in the examination is observation of the spine, hips, and legs during certain motions. During the procedure it is well to remember that no advantage accrues from trying to find out how much the patient can be hurt. Instead, it is much more important to determine when and under what conditions the pain commences. The natural motions of the patient should be observed as he disrobes and while he is standing, sitting, and reclining, except when certain positions cannot be tolerated because of pain. When standing, the motion of forward bending normally produces flattening and reversal of the lumbar lordotic curve and exaggeration of the dorsal curve. With lesions of the lumbosacral region which involve the posterior ligaments, articular facets, or erector spinae, the patient attempts to avoid stretching these structures. As a consequence, the erectores spinae remain taut and prevent motion in the lumbar spine. Forward bending then occurs at the hips and at the lumbar-thoracic junction. With disease of the lumbosacral joints and spinal roots, the patient bends in such a way as to avoid tensing the hamstring muscles and putting leverage upon the pelvis. In unilateral "sciatica," with its increased curvature toward the side of the lesion, lumbar and lumbosacral motions are splinted and bending is mainly at the hips; at a certain point the knee on the affected side is flexed to relieve hamstring spasm and tilting of the pelvis, which stretch the roots and sciatic nerve.

Lateral bending is usually less instructive than forward bending. However, in unilateral ligamentous or muscular sprain, bending to the opposite side aggravates the pain by stretching the damaged tissues. Moreover, in lateral disk lesions, bending of the spine may be fuller toward the opposite side.

In diseases of the lower spine, flexion while sitting can normally be performed easily, even to the point of bringing the knees in contact with the chest. The reason for this is that knee flexion relaxes the hamstring muscles and the principal motion is then at the hips. The lumbar and lumbosacral joints and the normal curve of the spine need not be altered under these conditions. On the other hand, if the knees are extended, the same impedance of movement noted during forward bending, while standing with the legs straight, is observed.

The study of motions in the reclining position yields the same information as those in the standing and sitting positions, with the difference that they may also be performed passively by the examiner. Passive lumbar flexion is like active forward bending in the standing position. With lumbosacral lesions and sciatica, it causes little pain and is not limited as long as the hamstrings are relaxed (knee flexed). With lumbosacral and lumbar spine disease (e.g., arthritis), passive flexion of the hips is free, whereas flexion of the lumbar spine is impeded and painful. Passive straight-leg raising (possibly up to 90° except in those who are congenitally stiff), like forward bending in the standing posture with the leg straight, places the sciatic nerve and its roots, also the hamstrings, under tension, thereby producing pain. Consequently, in diseases of the lumbosacral joints and of the lumbosacral roots, this movement is limited on the affected side and, to a lesser extent, the opposite side. Lasègue's sign (pain and limitation of movement during elevation of the leg when the knee is extended) is but a variation of this test, as are Golthwaite's sign (limited extension at the knee after the thigh has been flexed on the trunk) and Lewin's sign (snapping back of the knee into flexion when released). The evoked pain is always referred to the diseased side, no matter which leg is flexed. In disease of the lumbosacral joints there may also be slight limitation of straight-leg raising, though rarely to the degree seen in disease of the lumbosacral roots.

The motion of hypertension is best performed with the patient standing or lying prone. If the condition causing back pain is acute, it may be difficult to extend the spine in the standing position. A patient with lumbosacral sprain can usually extend or hyperextend the spine without aggravation of pain, since this motion tenses the iliopsoas and thereby rotates the ilium forward, relieving the pull on the lumbosacral and to some extent the sacroiliac joints. If involved in an active inflammatory or other acute process, however, tightening of the iliopsoas muscles lateral to the sacroiliac joints will exert pressure upon these joints. Also, if there is ligamentous sprain, no enhancement of pain occurs because the posterior segments of the spine are relaxed during extension. The converse is true if there is sprain of extensor muscles, for hyperextension places the muscular attachments to the periosteum under tension. Although disease of articular facets may limit extension, little or no pain is produced. In lumbar disk disease, extension of the spine is usually tolerated well, though in some patients with a displaced disk fragment situated posterolaterally pain is evoked by extension rather than flexion. A reversed Lasègue's sign (limitation in the hyperextension of straight leg while in prone position) suggests spinal nerve involvement at the midlumbar level or a lesion of the lumbosacral joint.

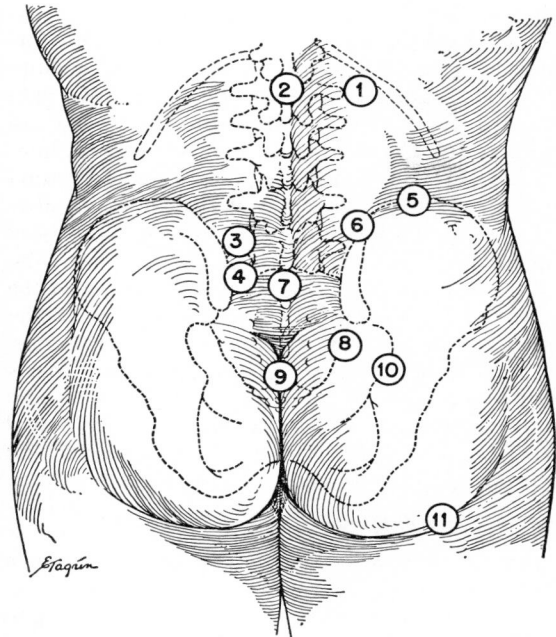

Fig. 7-1. (1) Costovertebral angle. (2) Spinous process and interspinous ligament. (3) Region of articular fifth lumbar to first sacral facet. (4) Dorsum of sacrum. (5) Region of iliac crest. (6) Iliolumbar angle. (7) Spinous processes of fifth lumbar to first sacral vertebras (tenderness = faulty posture or occasionally spina bifida occulta). (8) Region between posterior superior and posterior inferior spines. Sacroiliac ligaments (tenderness = sacroiliac sprain; often tender with fifth lumbar to first sacral disk). (9) Sacrococcygeal junction (tenderness = sacrococcygeal injury, i.e., sprain or fracture). (10) Region of sacrosciatic notch (tenderness = fourth to fifth lumbar disk rupture and sacroiliac sprain). (11) Sciatic nerve trunk (tenderness = ruptured lumbar disk or sciatic nerve lesion).

Inspection of the patient in action is not complete unless his lower back and every joint in the lower extremities are seen through a full range of motion.

Palpation and percussion of the spine are the last steps in the examination. The approach must always be gentle since rough percussion of the designated area of pain only confuses the physician and antagonizes the patient. It is preferable to palpate first those regions which are the least likely to evoke pain. At all times the examiner should know what structures are being palpated (see Fig. 7-1). Localized tenderness, if pronounced, means a lesion of that region, but it is more apt to be significant in disease of the spine because the involved structures are so deep that they less often give rise to surface tenderness. Mild superficial and poorly localized tenderness signifies only a disease process within the affected segment of the body.

Tenderness over the costovertebral angle often indicates genitourinary disease, adrenal disease (Rogoff's sign), or an injury to the transverse process of the first lumbar vertebra [Fig. 7-1(1)]. Hypersensitivity on palpation of the transverse processes of the other lumbar vertebras as well as the overlying erector spinae muscles may signify fracture of the transverse process or a sprain of muscle attachments.

Upon palpation of the spinous processes and interspinous ligaments any deviation in the anteroposterior or lateral plane must be particularly noted. Such a deviation usually indicates a fracture of the spinous processes or of the vertebral bodies or other disease of these structures. Tenderness of the interspinous ligaments is indicative of acute sprain or strain [Fig. 7-1(2)].

Tenderness in the region of the articular facets between the fifth lumbar and first sacral vertebras is consistent with a lumbosacral sprain from a hyperflexion or hyperextension injury or from strain due to faulty posture [Fig. 7-1(3)]. It is also not infrequent in disease of the lumbar disks with nerve root involvement.

Pain or tenderness referable to the dorsum of the sacrum is usually due to an exaggerated congenital lordosis with a postural and muscular strain and protective muscle spasm [Fig. 7-1(4)].

Tenderness in the region of the iliac crests may signify muscle sprain at the origin of the iliocostalis muscle [Fig. 7-1(5)]. Most commonly this point is used as a landmark in locating the spinous process of the third lumbar interspace. A useful sign of radicular involvement is radiation of pain in a nerve root distribution upon pressure lateral to the affected vertebra, over the point of exit of the spinal nerve.

Upon palpating the iliolumbar angles, the transverse process of the fifth lumbar vertebra, the iliolumbar ligaments, and the erector spinae are the structures under the probing finger [Fig. 7-1(6)]. Tenderness at this point suggests possible fracture of the transverse process, strain of the iliolumbar ligaments due to faulty posture, as well as an acute sprain of the same structure of the erector spinae. A unilateral sacralized transverse process of the fifth lumbar vertebra sometimes gives rise to tenderness and pain referable to the iliolumbar angle.

Rectal and pelvic examination constitute an essential part of the diagnostic study of all cases of low back pain and sciatica.

Upon completion of the examination of the back a search for motor, reflex, and sensory changes (see Syndrome of Ruptured Disk, p. 49), particularly in the lower extremities, should be made.

Special Laboratory Procedures. Laboratory tests often aid in diagnosis. Depending on the circumstances, these may include measurement of the serum proteins, phosphatases (alkaline and acid), calcium, phosphorus, or uric acid. X-rays should be taken in every case of low back pain and sciatica in the anterior-posterior, lateral, and oblique planes of the lumbar spine and, at times, the thoracic spine. Stereoscopic or laminographic films may provide further information, if the regular x-rays show abnormalities. In many cases of low back pain with neurologic manifestations, examination of the spinal canal with a contrast medium (myelogram) is necessary. This study can be combined with tests of dynamics of the cerebrospinal fluid, and a sample of the fluid should always be removed for cytologic and chemical examination prior to the installation of the contrast medium (Pantopaque, Myodil, or air). Injection and removal of Pantopaque require special skill and should not be attempted without previous experience with the procedure. If done properly, the procedure is harmless. Injection of contrast medium directly into the intervertebral disk (diskograms) has recently become popular. The technique of this procedure is more complicated than that of myelographic examination, and the risk of damage to nerve roots or the introduction of infection is not inconsiderable. In the authors' opinion, the results do not warrant the risk involved.

PRINCIPAL CONDITIONS WHICH GIVE RISE TO DISABLING PAIN IN THE LOWER BACK

Congenital Anomalies of the Lumbar Spine

Anatomic variations of the spine are not at all infrequent, and although not of themselves the source of pain and functional derangement, they may be of importance because they dispose to strain by permitting excessive mobility or the adoption of abnormal postures.

There may be a lack of fusion of the laminas of the neural arch—a spina bifida—of one or several of the lumbar vertebras, or of the sacrum. Hypertrichosis or hyperpigmentation in the sacral area may betray the condition, but it may remain entirely occult until disclosed by x-ray. The anomaly induces pain only when accompanied by malformation of vertebral joints or stretching and distortion of nerve roots. The anomaly may also condition the spine in such fashion as to encourage postural low back pain. A *filum terminale syndrome* (cf. Chap. 285), due to fixation of the spinal cord and interference with its ascent during the growth period, may be induced by violent flexion of the lumbar spine and injury to caudal roots.

Spondylolysis, another important anomaly, consists of a bony defect in the pars interarticularis which is replaced by cartilage, permitting a forward displacement of the vertebral body (spondylolisthesis), usually the fifth lumbar. Although of congenital origin, the first symptoms of disordered function (low back pain radiating to the thighs, tightness of back muscles, and signs of involvement of spinal roots—paresthesias and sensory loss, muscle weakness, and reflex impairment) may not appear until later in life and are often precipitated by an injury.

Articular facets of the vertebras may be set in an unusual plane, either oblique or frontal, rather than the sagittal one as in the normal lumbar spine; they are then unusually susceptible to injury. There may also be an abnormality of the number of mobile lumbar vertebras (either six or four). The lowest vertebra, if asymmetrical in its relation to the sacrum, may give rise to chronic back pain.

Traumatic Afflictions of the Lower Back

Trauma constitutes the most frequent cause of low back pain. The nature and direction of the mechanical forces imparted to the spine determine its severity. Pain may follow minor sprains or strains to the ligaments and muscles. It may also be caused by disturbances of alignment, usually associated with previous fractures of bony structures, and by extrusions of intervertebral cartilage. Trauma may be superimposed on and incite the initial symptoms of preexisting asymptomatic conditions, such as osteoporosis, a frayed annulus fibrosus, spondylolisthesis, and other bony or vascular abnormalities.

In severe acute injuries, the examining physician must be careful to avoid further damage. In tests of motility, all movements must be kept to a minimum until an approximate diagnosis has been made and adequate measures have been instituted for the proper care of the patient. If the patient complains of pain in his back and cannot move his legs, his spine may have been fractured. The prone position is then most advantageous, and his neck should not be flexed nor should he be allowed to sit up. (See Chap. 285 for further discussion of spinal cord injury.)

Sprains and Strains. The terms *strain* and *sprain* are used loosely by most physicians. The word strain should designate a minor injury which does not produce gross structural damage. The abnormal mechanical force may be acute, as in heavy lifting, or mild and persistent, due to maintenance of an abnormal posture. The latter is often occupational. Rest and relaxation promptly alleviate the discomfort, attesting to the lack of major structural change. Sprain, properly speaking, refers to an injury of joints, muscles, tendons, and ligaments (i.e., annulus fibrosus). In other words, definite structural damage has occurred. Both strains and sprains of the back are caused by lifting heavy objects, with the spine in a position of imperfect mechanical balance, as when lifting and turning at the same time. Sudden unexpected motion is particularly dangerous.

The diagnosis of strains and sprains of the various structures of the lower back depends upon the description of the injury, the localization of the pain by the patient, the finding of localized tenderness, and the augmentation of pain when tension is exerted on the involved muscles, ligaments, and joints by the appropriate maneuvers. The prompt alleviation of the pain by rest and relaxation indicates the existence of a strain. Sprain of the back responds less rapidly to such simple measures. It may, however, be relieved by local infiltration of an anesthetic agent, a finding which is also helpful in diagnosis.

Damage to interspinous or supraspinous ligaments may result from sudden flexion injuries (with or without associated fractures or intervertebral disk injuries). With this condition there is a sharp pain at the time of the injury. Localized tenderness, limitation of flexion, and abolition of discomfort on infiltration with procaine are diagnostic.

The patient suffering from an injury or sprain of the lumbosacral joint has pain in the lumbosacral region, deep tenderness in this area, and usually very little spasm of the lower lumbar back muscles. A great deal of discomfort is experienced upon extending the spine from a fully flexed position. Before reaching a diagnosis of lumbosacral strain, disk herniation must be excluded. Obviously, damage to the intervertebral disk at this level will produce disorganization of the lumbosacral joint. Simple lumbosacral strain is a much less common cause of low back pain than is "diskogenic" disease at this level.

Sacroiliac sprain, once so popular as an explanation of unilateral back pain, is now highly controversial. Because of their irregular surfaces the sacroiliac bones are interlocked, joint movement is minimal and is further restricted by strong sacroiliac ligaments. Only violent injury could derange this well-protected and stable joint. When the joint is injured, the principal symptom is a localized ache which is made worse by rotatory movements of the pelvis, local percussion, and reverse Lasègue sign. It must be remembered that involvement of a spinal nerve root (fifth lumbar or first sacral) associated with injury to the disk is the more common cause of pain and local tenderness in the area of the sacroiliac joint.

Vertebral Fractures. Fractures of the lumbar vertebral body are usually the result of flexion injuries. Spasm of the lower lumbar muscles, limitation of movements of the lumbar spine, and the x-ray appearance of the damaged portion of the lumbar spine (with or without neurologic abnormalities) are the basis of clinical diagnosis. The pain is usually immediate, though occasionally it may be delayed for days, and some patients are found to have had crushed fractures of the vertebral body without being able to recall any traumatic episode.

Fractured transverse processes, which are almost always associated with tearing of the psoas muscle, are diagnosed by the finding of deep tenderness at the site of the injury, local muscle spasm on one side, and limitation of all movements which stretch the lumbar muscles. Radiologic evidence provides the final confirmation.

Protrusion of Lumbar Intervertebral Disks. This is now recognized as the major cause of severe and chronic or recurrent low back and leg pain. This condition is most likely to occur between the fifth lumbar and first sacral vertebras and with lessening frequency between the fourth to fifth lumbar, the third to fourth lumbar, the second to third lumbar, and the first to second lumbar vertebras. Almost nonexistent in the thoracic spine, it is next most frequent at the sixth to seventh and fifth to sixth cervical vertebras. The cause is usually a flexion injury, but in a considerable proportion of cases no trauma is recalled. Degeneration and minor trauma of posterior longitudinal ligaments and the annulus fibrosus, which occurs in many adults of middle and advanced years, may have taken place silently or have been manifested by mild, recurrent lumbar ache. A sneeze, lurch, or other trivial injury may then cause the nucleus pulposus to extrude through the frayed ligament (Fig. 7-2).

The fully developed syndrome of ruptured intervertebral disk consists of a combination of orthopedic and neurologic abnormalities. The orthopedic symptoms and signs comprise backache, abnormal posture, and limitation of motion of the spine (particularly flexion). The neurologic manifestations are those of nerve root involvement and include radicular pain, sensory disturbances (paresthesias, hyper- and hyposensitivity in dermatome pattern), motor abnormalities (weakness and atrophy, coarse twitching and fasciculation, and muscle spasms), and impairment of tendon reflexes. Since herniation of the intervertebral lumbar disks most often occurs between the fourth and fifth lumbar vertebras and the fifth lumbar and first sacral vertebras with irritation and compression of the fifth lumbar and first sacral roots, respectively, it is important to recognize the clinical characteristics of lesions of these two roots. *Lesions of the fifth lumbar* root produce pain in the region of the hip, groin, posterolateral thigh, lateral calf to the external malleolus, dorsal surface of the foot, and the first or second and third toes. Paresthesias may be in the entire territory or only the distal parts of these territories. The tenderness is in the lateral gluteal region and near the head of the fibula. Weakness, if present, involves the extensor of the big toe and of the foot. Either the knee or ankle reflex may be diminished, but these reflexes are usually unchanged. Walking on the heels may be more uncomfortable than walking on the toes. In *lesions of the first sacral* root the pain is felt in the midgluteal region, posterior thigh, posterior calf to the heel, and the plantar surface of the foot and fourth and fifth toes. Tenderness is most pronounced over the midgluteal region (sacroiliac joint), posterior thigh, and calf. Paresthesias and sensory loss are mainly in the lower leg and outer toes, and weakness, if present, involves the flexor muscles of the foot and toes, abductors of the toes, and hamstring muscles. The ankle reflex is diminished to absent in the majority of cases. Walking on the toes is more uncomfortable than on the heels. Straight-leg raising during the acute, painful stages is present with lesions of either root.

The rarer *lesions of the fourth and third lumbar roots* give rise to pain in the anterior part of the thigh and knee, with corresponding sensory loss. The knee-jerk is diminished or abolished. An inverted Lasègue sign is positive when the third lumbar root is affected.

The syndrome is usually unilateral. Only with massive derangements of the disks do bilateral symptoms and signs occur, and these may then be associated with paralysis of the sphincters. The pain may be mild or severe. All or part of the above syndrome may be present. There may be back pain with little or no leg pain; rarely leg pain may be experienced without pain in the back. The rupture of multiple lumbar or lumbar and cervical disks is not infrequent, attesting to a basic disorder of the annulus fibrosus.

When all parts of the syndrome are present, both the skeletal as well as the neurologic components, the diagnosis is easy; when only one part is present, particularly backache, it may be difficult, especially if there has been no accident. Since similar symptoms may occur without demonstrable disk rupture, other diagnostic procedures are required. Plain x-rays usually show no abnormality or at most a narrowing of the intervertebral space; hence one must resort to Pantopaque myelography. This will reveal in most cases an indentation of the lumbar subarachnoid space or deformity of the root sleeve. Unfortunately, a small ruptured disk may not show. The electromyogram is helpful in showing denervation of leg muscles (see p. 530). The protein of the cerebrospinal fluid is elevated in some instances.

Tumor of the spinal canal, epidural or intradural, may produce a syndrome similar to that of ruptured disk (see Chap. 286).

Arthritis

Arthritis will be discussed more fully elsewhere. It need only be mentioned that hypertrophic arthritis is much more frequent than rheumatoid and that the latter may take two forms, one in which the spine involvement is but a part of a generalized arthritis, often with other signs of "connective tissue disease," and the other limited almost exclusively to the spine, sacroiliac joints, and hips (rheumatoid spondylitis or Marie-Strümpell arthritis) (p. 1915). An extreme form of hypertrophic arthritis in the cervical region, sometimes leading to spinal cord or nerve compression, is called spondylosis (see Chap. 301).

Rheumatoid spondylitis, which often begins with involvement of the sacroiliac joints, induces continuous aching pain and stiffness in the back or in the buttocks and thighs. Rarely, however, the disease reaches an advanced degree without pain. Acute painful exacerbations are probably due to involvement of the apophyseal joints. The pain is centered in the spine and is worse on movement, especially after the patient has been inactive. Pain during the night or in the early morning hours is another common feature. It may be partially relieved by activity and is often aggravated by seasonal and barometric changes. The effect of salicylates, which usually alleviate the pain to some degree, may be taken as another diagnostic feature. Signs of root involvement are incompatible with the diagnosis of rheumatoid arthritis.

In *hypertrophic arthritis*, by contrast, pain in the spine may or may not be accompanied by the motor, reflex, or sensory changes of root involvement. The pain in the spine is of the same type as in rheumatoid spondylitis and is also accompanied by a sense of stiffness and limitation of movement. It differs slightly in being more clearly aggravated by motion, more readily relieved by rest, and less pronounced at night. The severity of the pain is not clearly related to the degree of the process as seen in the x-ray. X-ray evidence of the disease in the spine is found in a majority of individuals beyond the age of fifty as is also clicking in the neck on head movement. The presence of such changes should not be accepted as establishing an arthritic source of a severe and progressive pain, since it may be due to a more serious unrelated condition, such as a neoplasm.

Injury may exacerbate the pain of both rheumatoid and hypertrophic arthritis. (See Chap. 301 for further discussion of spondylitis.)

Destructive Diseases

These may be neoplastic, infectious, or metabolic. Metastatic carcinoma (breast, bronchus, prostate, thyroid, hypernephroma, stomach, uterus), multiple myeloma, and lymphoma are the common tumors which involve the spine; tuberculosis and pyogenic osteomyelitis are the most frequent infections, though brucellosis, typhoid fever, actinomycosis, and blastomycosis are known to occur.

Special mention should be made of the spinal *epidural abscess* (usually staphylococcal), which necessitates urgent surgical treatment. The symptoms are a localized pain, spontaneous as well as on percussion and palpation, often with radicular irradiation, and a rapidly developing flaccid paraplegia appearing in a febrile patient.

Destructive lesions of any type may develop silently, i.e., without any pain, as long as they are limited to the osseous tissue. Upon spreading to the periosteum or to the adjacent spinous structures, however, they become the source of much pain of both local and referred type, and often one or more spinal roots are implicated as well, with the typical radicular type being added to the clinical picture. Pain caused by neoplasms of the spine is of aching character and more or less steady, though occasionally waxing and waning. It is especially severe at night, seeming to be only slightly benefited by rest; yet activity during the day also worsens the pain. As the disease progresses, the pain increases in duration and severity. It may then be of a throbbing character. The most important physical finding, which should lead one to suspect a destructive lesion, is an intensification of the pain by jarring the spine, by percussing the spinous processes gently with the fist or a reflex hammer, or by exerting a steady pressure upon these parts. Axial compression (downward pressure exerted on the head or falling on the heels) may also serve to intensify the pain. Nocturnal pain, spinal ache, and percussion sensitivity are also characteristic of Pott's disease and osteomyelitis. The establishment of the cause of the pain is often delayed because the first x-rays may not disclose the lesion. If these are negative, they should be repeated after an interval of a few weeks. Other laboratory data such as white blood count and smear, sedimentation rate, and levels of globulin, acid and alkaline phosphatase in the serum are helpful.

In so-called metabolic bone diseases (osteoporosis of either the postmenopausal or senile type or osteomalacia) a considerable degree of demineralization may occur without any symptoms whatsoever. Many such patients do, however, complain of aching in the lumbar or thoracic area. This is most likely to occur following an injury, sometimes of trivial degree, which leads to collapse or wedging of a vertebra. Certain movements greatly enhance the pain, and certain positions relieve it. One or more spinal roots may then be involved. Paget's disease of the spine is nearly always painless. The

recognition of these bone disorders is discussed in some detail elsewhere (Chaps. 77 to 82).

Referred Pain from Visceral Disease

The pain of disease of the pelvic, abdominal, or thoracic viscera is often felt in the region of the spine; i.e., it is referred to the more posterior parts of the spinal segment which innervates the diseased organ. Occasionally back pain may be the first and only sign. The general rule is that pelvic diseases are referred to the sacral region, lower abdominal disease to the lumbar region (centering around the second to fourth lumbar vertebrae), and upper abdominal diseases to the lower thoracic spine (eighth thoracic to the first and second lumbar vertebrae). Characteristically there are no local signs, no stiffness of the back, and motion is of full range without augmentation of the pain. However, some positions, e.g., flexion of the lumbar spine in the lateral recumbent position, may be more comfortable than others.

Low Thoracic and Upper Lumbar Pain in Abdominal Disease. Peptic ulceration or tumor of the wall of the stomach and of the duodenum most typically induces pain in the epigastrium (see Chaps. 16 and 272); but if the posterior wall is involved and particularly if there is retroperitoneal extension, the pain may be felt in the region of the spine. Usually the pain is central in location or is more intense on one side. If very intense it may seem to encircle the body. It tends to retain the characteristics of pain from the affected organ; e.g., if due to peptic ulceration it is relieved by food and soda and appears about 2 hr after a meal.

Diseases of the pancreas (peptic ulceration with extension to the pancreas, cholecystitis with pancreatitis, tumor) are apt to cause pain in the back, being more to the right of the spine if the head of the pancreas is involved and to the left if the body and tail are implicated.

Diseases of retroperitoneal structures, e.g., lymphomas, sarcomas, and carcinomas, may evoke pain in this part of the spine with some tendency toward radiation to the lower abdomen, groins, and anterior thighs. A secondary tumor of the ileopsoas region on one side often produces a unilateral lumbar ache with radiation toward the groin and labia or testicle; there may also be signs of involvement of the upper lumbar spinal roots. An aneurysm of the abdominal aorta may induce a pain which is localized to this region of the spine but may be felt higher or lower, depending on the location of the lesion.

Lumbar Pain with Lower Abdominal Diseases. Inflammatory diseases of segments of the colon (colitis, diverticulitis) or tumor of the colon cause pain which may be felt in the lower abdomen between the umbilicus and pubis, or in the midlumbar region, or in both places; and if very intense it may have a beltlike distribution around the body. A lesion in the transverse colon or first part of the descending colon may be central or left-sided, and its level of reference to the back is to the second to third lumbar vertebras. If the sigmoid colon is implicated the pain is lower, in the upper sacral region and anteriorly in the midline suprapubic region or left lower quadrant of the abdomen.

Sacral Pain in Pelvic (Urologic and Gynecologic) Diseases. Although gynecologic disorders may manifest themselves by back pain, the pelvis is seldom the site of a disease which causes obscure low back pain. For the most part the diagnosis of painful pelvic lesions is not difficult, for a thorough palpation of structures by abdominal, vaginal, and rectal examination may be supplemented by methods (sigmoidoscopy, barium enema, pyelography) which adequately visualize all these parts.

Menstrual pain itself may be felt in the sacral region. It is rather poorly localized, tends to radiate down the legs, and is of a crampy nature. The most important source of chronic back pain from the pelvic organs, however, is the uterosacral ligaments. Endometriosis or carcinoma of the uterus (body or cervix) may invade these structures, while malposition of the uterus may pull on them. The pain is localized centrally in the sacrum below the lumbosacral joint but may be more on one side. In endometriosis the pain begins during the premenstrual phase and often continues, merging with menstrual pain. Malposition of the uterus (retroversion, descensus, and prolapse) characteristically leads to sacral pain, especially after the patient has been standing for several hours. Posture may also evoke pain here when a fibroma of the uterus pulls on the uterosacral ligaments. Carcinomatous pain due to implication of nerve plexuses is continuous, becomes progressively more severe; it tends to be more intense at night. The primary lesion may be inconspicuous, being overlooked upon pelvic examination. Papanicolaou smears and a pyelogram are the most useful diagnostic procedures. X-ray therapy of these tumors may produce sacral pain consequent to swelling and necrosis of tissue, the so-called "radiation phlegmon of the pelvis." Low back pain with radiation into one or both thighs is a common phenomenon during the last weeks of pregnancy.

Chronic prostatitis, evidenced by prostatic discharge, frequency of urination, and slight reduction in sexual potency, may be attended by a nagging sacral ache; it may be mainly on one side, with radiation into one leg if the seminal vesicle is involved on that side. Carcinoma of the prostate with metastases to the lower spine is another cause of sacral or lumbar pain. It may be present without urinary frequency or burning. Spinal nerves may be infiltrated by tumor cells, or the spinal cord itself may be compressed if the epidural space is invaded. The diagnosis is established by rectal examination, x-rays of the spine, and measurement of acid phosphatase (particularly the prostatic phosphatase fraction). Lesions of the bladder and testes are usually not accompanied by back pain. When the kidney is the site of disease, the pain is ipsilateral, being felt in the flank or lumbar region.

Visceral derangements of whatever type may intensify the pain of arthritis, and the presence of arthritis may alter the distribution of visceral pain. With disease of the spine in the lumbosacral region, for example, distention of the ampulla of the sigmoid by feces or a bout of colitis may aggravate the arthritic pain. In patients with arthritis of the cervical or thoracic spine, the pain of myocardial ischemia may radiate to the back.

OBSCURE TYPES OF LOW BACK PAIN AND THE QUESTION OF PSYCHIATRIC DISEASE

The practicing physician is consulted by many individuals who complain of low back pain of obscure origin. A safe rule is to assume that all of them have some type of primary or secondary disease of the spine and its supporting structures or of the abdominal or pelvic viscera. If the pain is of acute onset and short duration, it may be due to only a minor trauma, a "fibrositis," or some form of articular disease. If it is recurrent, the possibility of a ruptured disk, an instability of the spine due to a congenital malformity, or the effects of bad posture must be considered. If it is severe and progressive, neoplasia, a tuberculous infection, and rheumatoid spondylitis should be kept in mind. Adolescent girls are subject to an obscure form of epiphyseal disease of the spine (Scheuermann's disease) which may cause low back pain with exercise over a period of 2 to 3 years.

Postural Back Pain

Many slender asthenic individuals, some with a disposition to anxiety or neurocirculatory asthenia, have discomfort in the back. Their back aches much of the time, and the pain interferes with effective work. The physical examination is negative except for slack musculature and poor posture. The pain is diffuse in the mid or low back and characteristically is relieved by bed rest and induced by the maintenance of a particular posture over a period of time. Pain in the neck and between the shoulder blades is a common complaint among thin, tense, active women and seems to be related to taut trapezius muscles.

Psychiatric Illness

Low back pain may be encountered in compensation hysteria and malingering, in anxiety or neurocirculatory asthenia (formerly called neurasthenia), in depression and hypochondriasis, and in many nervous individuals whose symptoms and complaints do not fall within any category of psychiatric illness.

Again it is probably correct to assume that pain in the back in such patients usually signifies disease of the spine and adjacent structures, and this should always be carefully looked for. However, the pain may be exaggerated, prolonged, or woven into a pattern of invalidism or disability because of coexistent or secondary psychologic factors. This is especially true when there is the possibility of personal gain (notably compensation). The patients seeking compensation from protracted low back pain without obvious structural disease tend, after a time, to become suspicious, hostile toward the medical profession or anyone who might question the authenticity of their illness, and they are uncooperative. One notes in them a tendency to describe their pain poorly and to prefer, instead, to discuss the degree of their disability and their mistreatment in the hands of the medical profession. These features and a negative examination of the back should lead one to suspect a psychologic factor. A few patients, usually frank malingerers, adopt the most bizarre attitudes, being unable to straighten up, walking with trunk flexed at almost a right angle (camptocormia) (see Chap. 43).

The depressed and hypochondriacal patient represents a troublesome problem, and a common error is to minimize the importance of anxiety and depression or to ascribe them to worry over the illness and its social effects. The more common and minor back ailments, e.g., those due to osteoarthritis, postural ache, etc., are enhanced and rendered intolerable by the irritable moodiness and self-concern. The disability seems excessive for the degree of spinal malfunction, and misery and despair are the prevailing features of the syndrome. One of the most reliable diagnostic measures is the response to drugs which alleviate the depression (see Chap. 44).

PAIN IN THE NECK AND SHOULDER

This topic has been discussed to some extent in the chapter on thoracic pain, and further references will be found under pain in the extremities.

It is useful to distinguish here three major categories of painful disease—those of the spine, cervical plexus, and shoulder. Although the pains in these three regions of the body may overlap, the patient himself usually can indicate the site of the origin. Pain arising from the cervical spine is nearly always felt in the spine (though it may be projected to the shoulder and arm), is evoked or enhanced by certain movements or positions of the neck, and is accompanied by tenderness and limitations of motions of the neck. Similarly, pain of brachial plexus origin is experienced in and around the shoulder, is induced by the performance of certain tasks with the arm and by certain positions, and is associated with tenderness of structures above the clavicle. There may be a palpable abnormality above the clavicle (aneurysms of subclavian artery, tumor, cervical rib). The combination of circulatory symptoms and signs referable to the lower part of the brachial plexus, manifested in the hand by obliteration of pulse when the patient takes and holds a full breath with the head tilted back or turned (Adson's test), unilateral Raynaud's phenomenon, trophic changes in the fingers, sensory loss over the ulnar side of the hand with or without interosseous atrophy, completes the clinical picture. X-rays showing a cervical rib or deformed thoracic outlet or superior sulcus tumor of the lung (Pancoast syndrome) offer confirmation of the diagnosis. Shoulder pain is localized to the shoulder region, is influenced by motion, and is associated with tenderness and limitation of motions (extension, abduction, external and internal rotation). Here, the most common diseases are bursitis and tear of the rotator cuff. Spine, plexus, and shoulder pain all may radiate into the arm or hand, but sensory, motor, and reflex changes always indicate involvement of nerve roots (in disease of the spine), plexus, or nerves.

Hypertrophic arthritis of the cervical spine may cause pains which radiate into the back of the head, shoulders and arms on one or both sides of the thorax. Coincident involvement of nerve roots is manifested by paresthesias, sensory loss, weakness, or tendon reflex change. Should bony ridges form in the spinal canal (spondylosis), the spinal cord may be compressed, with resulting weakness and atrophy and sometimes sensory disturbances in the arms and spastic weakness and ataxia with loss of vibratory and position sense in the legs. A Pantopaque cervical myelogram reveals the degree of encroachment on the spinal canal and the level at which the spinal cord is affected. The authors have experienced the greatest difficulty in distinguishing spondylosis with spinal cord compression from primary neurologic diseases (syringomyelia, amyotrophic lateral sclerosis, ruptured disk, or tumor) with an unrelated hypertrophic arthritis of the cervical spine, particularly at the fifth to sixth and sixth to seventh cervical vertebras, where the disk spaces are often narrowed in the adult. A combination of nervous tension with hypertrophic arthritis

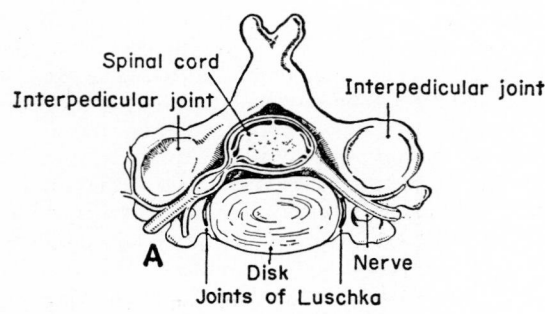

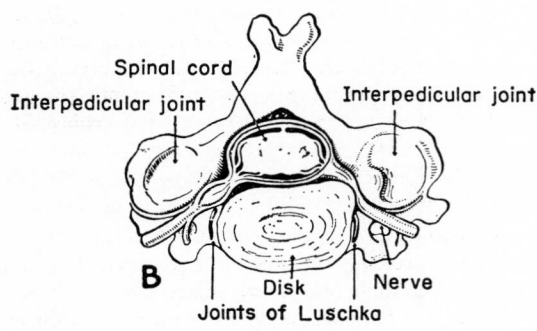

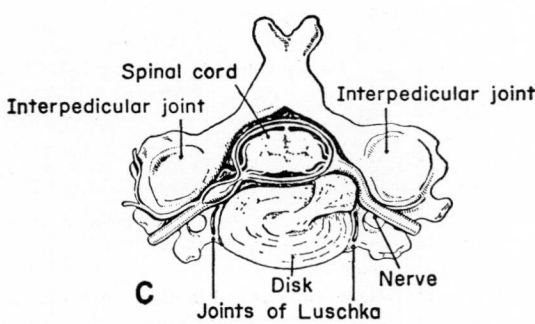

FIG. 7-2. *A.* The normal relationship between the intervertebral disk, the bony structures, and the neural elements in the lower cervical region. *B.* The mechanism of compression of one of the cervical nerve roots by osteophytic spurs. *C.* Lateral rupture of a cervical intervertebral disk with herniation of the nucleus pulposus. (*Spurling and Segerberg: J.A.M.A.,* 151:355, 1953.)

of the cervical spine or a painful injury to ligaments and muscles after an accident in which the neck is forcibly extended and flexed (e.g., whiplash injury to spine) are extremely vexatious clinical syndromes. If the pain is persistent and limited to the neck, the problem will usually prove to have been complicated by psychologic factors.

One of the most common causes of neck, shoulder, and arm pain is disk herniation in the lower cervical region. As with rupture of the lumbar disks, the syndrome includes the aforementioned disorder

of spinal function and evidence of neural involvement. It develops after a trauma which may be major or minor (sudden hyperextension of the neck, diving, forceful manipulations, chiropractic treatment, etc.). Virtually every patient exhibits an abnormality in full motion of the neck (limitation and pain). Hyperextension is the movement that most consistently aggravates the pain. With laterally situated disk lesions between the fifth to sixth cervical vertebras, the symptoms and signs are referred to the sixth cervical roots, i.e., pain felt at the trapezius ridge, tip of the shoulder, anterior upper arm, radial forearm, and often in the thumb; paresthesias and sensory impairment or hypersensitivity in the same regions; tenderness in the area above the spine of the scapula and in the supraclavicular and biceps regions; weakness in flexion of the forearm; diminished to absent biceps and supinator reflexes (triceps retained or exaggerated). With sixth to seventh cervical disk disease and involvement of the seventh cervical root, the pain is in the region of the shoulder blade, pectoral region and medial axilla, posterolateral upper arm, dorsal forearm and elbow, index and middle fingers, or all the fingers; tenderness is most pronounced over the medial aspect of the shoulder blade opposite the third to fourth thoracic spinous processes, in the supraclavicular area and triceps region; paresthesias and sensory loss are most pronounced in the second and third fingers or tips of all the fingers; weakness is in extension of the forearm (occasionally wrist drop is present) and in the hand grip; the triceps reflex is diminished to absent, and the biceps and supinator reflexes are preserved. Cough, sneeze, and downward pressure on the head in the hyperextension position exacerbate pain, and traction (even manual) tends to relieve it (Fig. 7-2).

Unlike lumbar disks, the cervical ones, if large and centrally situated, may result in compression of the spinal cord (central disk, all of the cord; paracentral disk, part of the cord, i.e., Brown-Séquard syndrome). The central disk is often nearly painless, and the cord syndrome may simulate a degenerative disease (amyotrophic lateral sclerosis, combined system disease). A common error is to fail to think of a ruptured disk in the cervical region in patients with obscure symptoms in the legs. The diagnosis of ruptured cervical disk should be confirmed by the same laboratory procedures that were mentioned under lumbar disk.

Metastases in the cervical spine may be very painful, but the problem is not different from that of secondary deposits of tumor in other parts of the spine.

Shoulder injuries (rotator cuff), subacromial or subdeltoid bursitis, the frozen shoulder (periarthritis or capsulitis), tendinitis, and arthritis may develop in patients who are otherwise well, but these conditions are more frequent in hemiplegics or in individuals suffering from coronary heart disease. The pain is often severe and extends toward the neck and down the arm into the hand. The dorsum of the latter may tingle without other signs of nerve involvement. Vasomotor changes also may occur in the hand (shoulder-hand syndrome), and after a time osteoporosis and atrophy of cutaneous and subcutaneous structures occur (Sudeck's atrophy or Sudeck-Leriche syndrome). These conditions fall more within the province of orthopedics than of medicine and will not be discussed in detail.

The carpal tunnel syndrome with paresthesias and numbness in palmar distribution of the median nerve and aching pain which extends up into the forearm may be mistaken for disease of the shoulder or neck.

MANAGEMENT OF BACK PAIN

A muscular sprain is always benign in character, and one may expect full recovery in 2 to 4 weeks. Ligamentous sprains, if severe, may last longer, from 6 to 12 weeks. The underlying principle of therapy in both is immobilization or protection in a position that relaxes and removes pressure from the injured structure. If the erector spinae are sprained the optimal position is hyperextension; the same is true of sprains of the posterior and sacroiliac ligaments. This position is best maintained by having the patient lie with a small pillow or blanket under the lumbar spine or lie face down. During the acute phase of any injury of this type, the application of cold, in the form of an ice bag or cold water bottle (ethyl chloride spray of the skin is said to give dramatic relief at times), is indicated. It reduces the circulation and consequently the swelling. After the third or fourth day, heat is desirable to improve the circulation and to relax protective muscle spasm. Analgesic medication should be given liberally during the first few days [codeine 30 mg and aspirin 0.6 Gm, meperidine (Demerol) 50 mg, or morphine 10 to 15 mg]. When ready for ambulation, after some days in bed, the patient may need protection of the injured part, preferably adhesive strapping in case of muscle sprain or a belt or brace. Plaster casts should be avoided. Ambulatory treatment is supplemented by corrective exercises designed to overcome faulty position and to increase the mobility of the spinal joints (Fig. 7-3). Only if these measures prove inadequate and the patient is partially disabled over long periods of time by an unstable, painful lower back (recurrent lumbosacral backache) should operative intervention, usually some form of fusion operation, be considered.

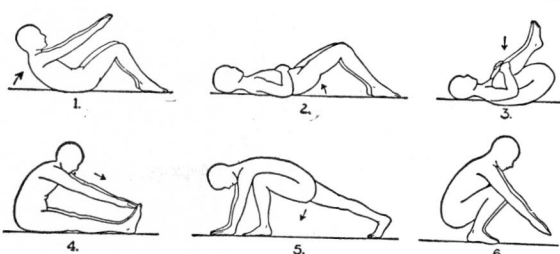

FIG. 7-3. Front of postural instruction sheet. Patient is instructed as follows:

Exercises should be taken on a padded floor. Exercise 4 should be omitted unless otherwise instructed. Start exercises by doing each one _____ times morning and evening, increasing the series one a day until you are doing each one _____ times morning and evening. Exercises are essential in obtaining a proper muscular balance but a correct posture is acquired only through conscious effort.

Remember—
1. When standing or walking, toe straight ahead and take most of your weight on heels.
2. Try to form a crease across the upper abdomen by holding the chest up and forward and elevating the front of the pelvis.
3. Avoid high heels as much as possible.
4. Sit with the buttocks "tucked under" so that the hollow in the low back is eradicated.
5. When possible, elevate the knees higher than the hips while sitting. This is especially important when driving (driver's seat forward) or riding as a passenger in an automobile.
6. Sleep on your back with knees propped up or on your side with one or both knees drawn up. Bed should be firm.
7. Do not lift loads in front of you above the waist line.
8. Never bend backward.
9. Do not bend forward with knees straight. Always "squat."
10. Avoid standing as much as possible.

Learn to Live 24 Hours a Day without a Hollow in the Lower Part of Your Back

In the treatment of an acute rupture of a lumbar or cervical disk, complete bed rest is essential and strong analgesic medication is required. Traction is of little value in lumbar disk disease, and it is best to permit the patient to find the most comfortable position. Later, traction, if of any value, keeps the patient confined to bed. In contrast, traction is of great help in rupture of cervical disks. Often the pain subsides after 2 to 3 weeks in bed, and the patient may remain free of pain upon resuming normal activities. Or he may suffer some minor recurrence but can carry on his usual activi-

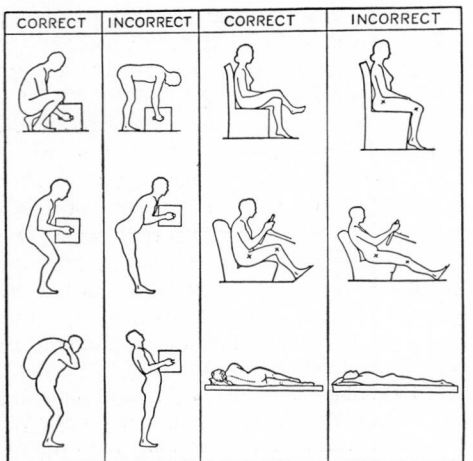

Fig. 7-4. Reverse side of postural instruction sheet showing correct and incorrect methods of lifting, sitting, and sleeping.

ties, and eventually he will recover. There is always danger of relapse. To prevent this, mild muscle strengthening exercises of the spine after the pain has subsided (see Fig. 7-3) and avoidance of activities which favor spine injury (see Fig. 7-4) are recommended. If the pain does not subside after a trial of prolonged bed rest (several weeks) and the myelogram demonstrates a large disk, an operative removal, preferably without spine fusion, should be undertaken. The final decision as to the time and necessity of surgery depends on the duration and gravity of the pain and the neurologic disorder.

For the many patients with back pain who do not fall into any one of the above categories, simple measures are beneficial. For the adolescent with a suspicion of epiphyseal disease, restricted activity (avoidance of vigorous sports) for a few months or years and a supporting garment help. Muscle strengthening exercises and a physical conditioning program are indicated for postural backache (see Fig. 7-3). Spine fusion should be reserved only for the exceptional patient with disabling and persistent pains.

Spondylosis of the cervical spine, if painful, is helped by bed rest and traction; if signs of spinal cord involvement are present, a collar to limit movement may halt the progression and even lead to improvement. Decompressive laminectomy with sectioning of denticulate ligaments is reserved for severe instances of the disease with advancing neurologic symptoms. The shoulder-hand syndrome may benefit from stellate ganglion blocks or ganglionectomy, but the basic treatment is physiotherapy, with surgical procedures being used only as measures of last resort.

8 PAIN IN THE EXTREMITIES
Eugene A. Stead, Jr.

Pain in the extremities comes from disturbances within the tissues of the extremities or from irritation at any level of the sensory nerve paths serving the extremity, or it is referred from deep somatic or visceral structures.

DISTURBANCES WITHIN THE TISSUES

Any lesion causing inflammation, swelling, ischemia, or destruction of pain-sensitive tissues of the extremity may cause pain. Burns, frostbite, and chemical injuries are painful. Arthritis, cellulitis, abscesses, osteomyelitis and hematomas, tumors, Paget's disease, and bone changes with hyperparathyroidism cause varying degrees of pain. Degeneration of nerves and trauma to nerve trunks are painful. Damage to nerves or to muscles from ischemia is painful.

IRRITATION OF SENSORY NERVES

Involvement of the nerves at any point in their course from the extremity to the spinal cord may cause pain in the extremity. The pain of cervical rib, ruptured intervertebral disk, spinal cord tumor, and tabes dorsalis falls into this group. Central pain from involvement of the spinothalamic tract and thalamus is occasionally seen.

PAIN REFERRED FROM DEEP STRUCTURES

The pain of angina pectoris and myocardial infarction frequently radiates to the inner surfaces of the arms. Pain from the hip may be referred to the knee. Pain from the deep muscles of the back or from the vertebras may be the source of pain referred to the extremity.

CAUSES OF PAIN IN THE EXTREMITIES

Pain from Trauma, Inflammation, and Swelling. The immediate response to trauma is due to mechanical stimulation of nerve endings. Pain persisting after the injury may result from chemical stimuli produced by the injured tissues. Lewis has described the reactions in skin made hyperalgesic by injury. Needle pricks too light to awaken pain in uninjured skin will arouse a response in a traumatized area. Pain is easily induced by friction or warming, and often by cooling. Distention of the skin by direct stretching or by venous congestion causes pain. If injured skin is rubbed, pain is felt immediately; this subsides and is followed in about 15 sec by a second pain which lasts a minute or more. If the circulation to the part is obstructed, the initial pain is unaltered, but the second pain rises to a greater intensity and persists until approximately 1 min after the circulation is restored. The first pain comes from direct stimulation of sensory nerves, the second from a relatively stable pain-giving substance released into, and held within, the tissue space. The chemical nature of this substance is not known. Skin made hyperalgesic by injury, regardless of the mechanism of the injury, will respond to heat and congestion with burning pain. If this reaction occurs diffusely in the skin of the extremities without obvious cause, the burning pain from warmth and congestion is called *erythromelalgia*.

The injury to the skin caused by heat is well recognized. That prolonged cold will cause tissue damage in many ways comparable to burns is less commonly realized. Prolonged immersion of the feet or prolonged exposure to cold with the feet in wet boots will cause severe tissue damage to the point of gangrene, even though actual freezing does not occur. Freezing, of course, causes tissue damage and may produce gangrene. Fibrosis and ischemic neuritis are common after any form of injury from cold and may cause persistent tenderness and pain.

In bacterial infections, the mechanical factor of rapidly forming edema increases local tissue pressure and causes pain in skin already made hyperalgesic by chemical factors associated with injury. Congestion aggravates the pain, and elevation of the part alleviates it. Less rapid edema formation usually does not cause pain, because the tissues stretch gradually. Patients with cardiac edema complain of heaviness of the legs and occasionally of diffuse tenderness. Edema associated with varicose veins may cause a sense of fullness and dull ache. In acute thrombophlebitis, pain may arise from the involved veins. It may be aggravated by ischemia secondary to sympathetic vasoconstriction resulting from the sensory stimuli from the inflamed veins. Tumor masses may cause pressure on bone or peripheral nerves.

Arthritis is a common cause of pain in the extremities. Paget's disease and pulmonary osteoarthropathy are less common causes of bone pain.

The syndrome of sore, painful shoulder with superficial and deep areas of exquisite tenderness is common. It frequently begins as wryneck and at times occurs in a number of persons closely associated with one another. Marked spasm prevents abduction of the arm at the shoulder. The entire upper extremity may feel numb and queer. There is no fever. Biopsy of the skin and muscles shows apparently normal tissues. Light freezing of the skin with ethyl chloride or procainization of the superficial and deep tender areas frequently gives dramatic relief of pain, relief which may be permanent. The mechanism of pain production in this syndrome is not known.

Pain from Ischemia, Thrombosis, Embolism, and Arteritis. Interference with blood supply may result from obliterative arterial disease or embolus or from arteriolar spasm secondary to stimulation of sensory receptors or nerves. It may be aggravated in polycythemia by the adverse effect of increased viscosity of the blood. The pain may be produced by the action on sensory nerve endings of metabolites accumulating in the muscles or by changes in the nerves themselves.

The sensations produced by ischemia to the extremity are familiar to all. When the blood supply is occluded, the part gradually becomes numb and paralyzed and we say the part has "gone to sleep." If the part is not moved, pain does not develop. The sensation at the end of the fingers becomes dulled in about 12 to 15 min. At that time, light pressure on the fingers may hurt, and stroking the finger tips causes an unpleasant sensation. Later, pain is dulled, and much later, analgesia develops. On release of the arterial occlusion, unpleasant tingling occurs, particularly in the fingers. This tingling is not the result of the inrush of blood into the fingers, because it occurs if blood is released only into the proximal part of the extremity. It results from changes in the main nerves of the arm during recovery. Stroking the fingers accentuates it. The paresthesias produced by the injury and recovery of the nerve from ischemia are similar to those produced by chronic disease processes involving the peripheral nerves or nerve roots.

If the extremity is exercised while the circulation is completely occluded, a continuous diffuse aching pain develops in the muscles because the sensory nerves are stimulated by the formation of stable metabolites. The pain is present during and between contractions. It is frequently described as a cramp, but the muscles are flaccid. If the contractions are continued, the muscles become tender. On release of the tourniquet, the pain disappears in a few seconds, probably as the result of the carrying away of readily diffusible metabolites.

If the brachial artery at the elbow or the femoral artery at the inguinal ligament is occluded by digital pressure for $1/2$ hr, instead of by application of a cuff, much less change in the circulation occurs, because collateral circulation is not stopped. Loss of sensation does not occur, and on release of the occlusion, the reactive hyperemia is much less intense than with the cuff.

In occlusive vascular disease of the vessels of the legs, a common symptom is pain with tenderness of the muscles which is relieved by rest. It is called *intermittent claudication*, and represents in the muscles of the extremities the same changes which occur in the heart with angina pectoris. The resting muscle is receiving an adequate supply of blood for normal metabolism. When muscle metabolism is increased by exercise and occlusive vascular disease prevents increase of the blood supply, metabolites accumulate in the muscles and stimulate the sensory nerve endings. The nature of the chemical substances has not been determined. The more severe the circulatory impairment, the less exercise is required to produce the pain and the more slowly the pain disappears on rest.

In occlusive vascular disease, the nerves themselves may become ischemic and cause severe and persistent pain. This pain, in certain instances, is aggravated by dependency because of stimuli resulting from congestion. In addition to Buerger's disease and arteriosclerosis, ischemic neuritis is a prominent symptom in small-vessel involvement of the type seen in periarteritis nodosa.

Embolus or thrombus in the brachial or femoral vessels frequently produces sufficient circulatory impairment to cause pain. The pain in thrombosis is indistinguishable from the pain of embolism. The pains do not occur at the site of occlusion but in the muscles and tissues distal to it. The time of onset of the pain will depend on the temperature of the part, the amount of activity, and the amount of associated vasospasm. If the part is warm and still, the limb may become numb before the muscle pain is produced. Heat applied to a limb with poor circulation may cause gangrene from (1) increased metabolism of tissue without corresponding increase in blood supply or (2) lack of cooling effect of the blood. When heat above body temperature is applied to the skin, the blood normally acts as a cooling system; in the presence of arterial occlusion, local heating causes an immediate rise in temperature of the part. If the part is exercised, the muscle pain occurs early. Twenty-four hours after an embolus has lodged, the vessel wall may be tender because of periarterial inflammation. Occlusion of small blood vessels does not cause pain unless ischemia of muscle or nerve is produced.

Normal skin hurts when warmed after severe exposure to cold. This is a response to direct injury from the cold. The white, cold fingers in Raynaud's phenomenon may be painful. In scleroderma the thickening of the connective tissue combined with spasm of the digital arteries may result in painful ulceration of the fingers and eventual loss of the terminal phalanges.

The pain from ischemia or infection is frequently altered or absent in patients with diabetes because of associated peripheral neuropathy. Whenever a painful-looking lesion of the extremity is treated casually by the patient, neuropathy should be suspected. Tabes dorsalis, leprosy, senile cortical atrophy, and syringomyelia should be considered.

The circulation to the extremities can be greatly modified by overactivity of the sympathetic nervous system. In many instances of injury, inflammation, or thrombophlebitis, sensory stimuli arising in the extremity may produce intense reflex vasoconstriction, and the resulting ischemia may cause diffuse pain. Relief of the vasoconstriction by paravertebral procaine block of the appropriate sympathetic ganglions may cause striking relief of pain. Similarly, sensory impulses arising from ischemic areas after arterial occlusion by an embolus or thrombus may stimulate sympathetic nervous system activity and reflex spasm. Paravertebral block will relieve the spasm of collateral vessels, and if circulation improves sufficiently, pain will disappear.

Pain from Neuropathy, Neuritis, Ganglionitis, and Pressure on Nerves or Nerve Roots. Involvement of the peripheral nerves frequently causes unpleasant sensations in the extremities. In diabetic neuropathy, numbness may be accompanied by diffuse pains through both lower extremities. Any combination of sensory loss and pain may occur in peripheral nerve damage from infection, poisons, or mechanical factors such as trauma or pressure. Spinal cord tumors and slipped intervetebral disks are common causes of nerve root pain. Inflammation of the dorsal root ganglions results in the syndrome of herpes zoster. The redness and blistering is attributed to antidromic vasodilatation from stimulation of the sensory nerves. Impulses arising in sensory nerves or ganglions and passing peripherally to the sensory end organs are called *antidromic*. Involvement of the dorsal root ganglions, dorsal roots, and adjacent spinal cord produces the lightning pains in the extremities typical of tabes dorsalis. Paralysis from pressure in the axilla may be caused by crutches or by sleeping with the arm thrown over the back of a chair. The latter usually occurs in alcoholic stupor and is called "Saturday night paralysis."

Pain from Immobilization, Spasm, and Cramps. Prolonged immobilization of a part results in stiffness of muscles and joints. The muscles tighten and splint the joint, and motion is prevented. An attempt to move the part produces pain. Local infiltration with procaine will frequently allow a great improvement in motility, which may be permanent. Similar spasm occurs after trauma. A painful sprain of the ankle which prevents walking may be relieved in a few minutes by procainization. Even in acute arthritis part of the pain may be secondary to spasm and may respond to curare or procaine, which relax the muscle. In acute poliomyelitis, nonparalyzed muscles may be sore and contracted. Application of hot packs gives relief.

Muscles placed in unusual positions may go into intense contraction and cause severe pain. Cramps in the foot or leg occurring at night are common. They are relieved by forcefully extending the joint so as to stretch the cramped muscles. In nocturnal cramps, pain occurs so quickly that simple ischemia would seem unlikely. They differ from the cramps of arterial disease in that the pain is not brought on by exercise. Painful muscle cramps occur in tetany and in chloride deficiency. Whether the pain of tetany is caused by ischemia from the prolonged contraction or related to damage because of the intensity of the contraction is not known.

Unaccustomed, strenuous exercise causes aching, tender muscles, tendons, and joints. The pain results from low-grade injury to the muscles from repetitive maximal contractions.

Glomus Tumor. Tumor of the glomus, the specialized arteriovenous anastomosis of the skin, produces unusual vasomotor phenomena and radiating pain. It is characteristically a small (a few millimeters in diameter), extremely painful, purplish nodule either in the skin of the extremity or under the nail. Pain is caused by contact or change of temperature and may spread to involve the entire extremity. Why these tumors are so painful is not clear. While most observers have noted an unusually rich nerve supply, others have not found it.

Pain from Causalgia. Pain in the extremity associated with signs of local circulatory dysfunction is seen in nerve injuries after amputations and in persons with coronary arterial disease with or without myocardial infarction. It occurs in the hand-shoulder syndrome. The above conditions have one thing in common: local injury sets up a reaction which at first appears to be the result of sensory stimuli from the injured part. Later changes occur in the peripheral nerves, spinal cord, or central nervous system so that the process continues after the injury has apparently healed.

Classic Causalgia. Injury to any nerve, more commonly the medial or sciatic nerve, may give rise after a few days or weeks to a burning pain. The gross injury to the nerve may have been severe or trivial. The pain will be caused by light friction; deep pressure is less painful. Heat usually provokes the pain. The skin becomes smooth and glossy and is frequently wet with sweat. It has a red or purplish tint. The temperature of the involved part is usually said to be increased. The pain is frequently relieved by sympathectomy. Causalgic pain may result from the activation of sensory fibers by sympathetic impulses. If injury links the two systems so that leakage of efferent sympathetic impulses into the sensory nerves can occur, most of the clinical phenomena of causalgia, including the relief by sympathetic block, can be explained.

The initiating mechanisms of causalgia are unknown. Several theories have been advanced: (1) The sensitivity of the skin may result from vaso-dilator substances released by repeated centrifugal impulses arising in the injured area. It is known that stimulation of the paralyzed end of a cut cutaneous nerve results in vasodilatation which may be accompanied by itching and burning pain. (2) The sensitivity of the skin may result from a summation of impulses from normal skin with those from the injured nerve.

Regardless of the local mechanism, it appears that other mechanisms central to the extremity are capable of continuing the process once the causalgia has been present for some time. At this stage, dorsal root section or sections of the spinothalamic tract may not modify the pain. Chain reactions within the short interconnecting nerves in the spinal cord have been postulated. Paravertebral block or sympathectomy should be done early before these central changes occur and before the patient becomes a drug addict. Because the patient's complaints are so bizarre and because the original injury may be mild, causalgia is frequently mistaken for a compensation neurosis.

Phantom Limb Pain. After amputation, the patient may complain of pain which he localizes in the removed part. At times this may be caused by a neuroma of the cut nerves or by the faulty construction of the stump. The stump may show vasomotor changes. In most instances, therapy directed toward the stump does not relieve the pain; at times, paravertebral block of the sympathetic ganglions does. The clinical observations suggest that, as in causalgia, pain may begin locally but that changes may take place in the central nervous system which are responsible for its continuation.

Hand-Shoulder Syndrome. Myocardial infarction is frequently complicated by persistent shoulder pain with marked limitation of motion. At times, swelling of the hand and wrist and contraction of the palmar fascia are present. The elbow is not involved. Atrophy of skin and osteoporosis may follow. Similar disturbances in shoulder and hand function have occurred in association with trauma, hemiplegia, herpes zoster, and cervical osteoarthritis. This syndrome may occur without recognized associated diseases. The exact mechanism of this fairly common syndrome is unknown.

APPROACH TO THE PATIENT

A careful history will usually yield important clues. The pain may be felt in the region of the knee when the disease is in the hip or in the foot when the knee is the seat of the disorder. Pain on first arising in the morning, particularly when associated with stiffness, suggests a disturbance of joints or muscles. When the bone is affected, there is commonly nocturnal aggravation. Pain of throbbing character usually arises in tense tissues with free blood supply and, hence, suggests bone as the source. Sharp shooting pain of brief duration, brought on by coughing or sneezing, is common with disorders of the vertebral column or of the posterior nerve roots. Relief of discomfort by elevation suggests venous obstruction; relief by dependency suggests an arterial lesion. Pain ascribed to walking may actually be due to standing and may have its source in the feet. Pain due to ischemia of muscles is characteristically induced by walking, with latency of onset and of offset. Disorders of joints are likely to be accompanied by pain on local movement, the duration of the discomfort paralleling that of the movement.

The history having suggested the responsible structure, the suspicion is confirmed or disproved by the physical findings and the appropriate special procedures. Since these are mentioned in the later chapters dealing with the disorders of the various systems of the body, they need not be cited here. However, it should be emphasized that x-ray examination, while often invaluable in the case of long-standing disease of the bones, may be entirely negative in the presence of serious skeletal disorders of recent origin. This is especially important in regard to acute osteomyelitis and to the earlier stages of metastatic neoplasms of bone.

REFERENCES

Allen, E. V., N. W. Barker, and E. A. Hines, Jr.: "Peripheral Vascular Diseases," Philadelphia, W. B. Saunders Company, 1946.

Doupe, J. C., C. H. Cullen, and G. Q. Chance: Post-traumatic Pain and the Causalgic Syndrome, J. Neurol., Neurosurg. Psychiat., 7:33, 1944.

Lewis, Thomas: "Pain," New York, The Macmillan Company, 1942.

———: "Vascular Disorders of the Limbs," New York, The Macmillan Company, 1946.

Steinbrocker, O.: Shoulder-Hand Syndrome: Associated Painful Homolateral Disability of Shoulder and Hand with Swelling and Atrophy of Hand, Am. J. Med., 3:402, 1947.

Sweet, W. H.: Pain, chap. 19, p. 459, in "Handbook of Physiology," vol. 1, sec. 1, Neurophysiology, The American Physiological Society, Washington, D.C., 1959.

Section 2: Fever

9 ALTERATIONS IN BODY TEMPERATURE

Paul B. Beeson

The mechanisms for control of body temperature are so efficient that a healthy person can engage in widely different physical activities or subject himself to the most diverse conditions of environment with only slight variation in his temperature. By contrast, a sick person lying quietly in bed may show considerable fluctuation, as if the "thermostat" had lost its sensitivity; or his temperature may be maintained at a higher than normal level, as if the adjustment of the "thermostat" had been altered. Elevation of the body temperature is, in fact, such a sensitive and reliable indication of the presence of disease that thermometry has become one of our commonest clinical procedures.

Much study has been devoted to the subject of body temperature regulation. The ways in which heat can be produced and dissipated have been elucidated, and the cerebral centers for control of body temperature have been accurately located. On the other hand, little is known about the relative importance of various kinds of stimuli to which the cerebral centers react, or about the pathogenesis of fever. In the pages to follow, after a review of some of the established facts, certain theories of the pathogenesis of fever will be considered, and various classes of febrile illness will be discussed.

The principal source of body heat is the combustion of foods. Although this occurs everywhere in the body, the greatest amount of heat is generated in two places: the liver and the voluntary muscles. Heat production in the voluntary muscles is of particular importance in temperature regulation, because the quantity can be varied according to the need. In most circumstances this variation consists of small increases and decreases in the number of nerve impulses to the muscles, causing unapparent tensing or relaxing. When, however, there is a strong stimulus for heat production, muscle activity may increase to the point of shivering, or even to a generalized rigor.

Heat is lost from the body in several ways. Small amounts are used in warming food or drink and in the evaporation of moisture from the respiratory tract. The principal heat loss takes place on the surface of the body, where radiation, convection, and evaporation all play a part. The relative importance of these processes depends upon environmental factors. When the outside temperature is equal to or above that of the body, the only possible means of heat loss is evaporation of water. The principal method of regulating heat loss is by varying the volume of blood flowing to the surface of the body. A rich circulation in the skin and subcutaneous tissues serves to carry heat from deeper portions of the body to the surface, where it can escape. In addition, sweating increases heat loss by providing water to be vaporized; this is under control of cholinergic elements of the autonomic nervous system. When the need is for conservation of warmth, adrenergic autonomic stimuli cause a sharp reduction in the blood flow to the surface. This transforms the skin and subcutaneous tissue into layers of insulation.

The control of body temperature, integrating the various physical and chemical processes for heat production or loss, is a function of cerebral centers located in the hypothalamus and brain stem. An animal whose brain stem has been sectioned loses ability to control body temperature, which consequently tends to vary with the environment. Damage to the brain above the hypothalamus leaves temperature regulation intact. The exact position of the thermoregulatory centers in monkeys and cats was worked out by Ranson and his associates. They found that stimulation of areas in the cephalic portion of the hypothalamus caused activation of mechanisms for heat loss, such as sweating and panting. Stimulation of the caudal part of the hypothalamus activated mechanisms for warming the body and conservation of heat, such as shivering and erection of hair. Clinical experience indicates that the thermoregulatory centers have similar locations in human beings. Lesions which damage the anterior portion of the hypothalamus may be associated with high levels of body temperature, whereas lesions in the posterior part may cause marked hypothermia.

It is probable that the cerebral temperature-regulating centers can be affected by more than one kind of stimulus. Experiments on animals show that variation in the temperature of the blood flowing through the brain can cause activation of the appropriate counteracting mechanisms, either for heat loss or for heat production. There is also evidence indicating that these centers may be stimulated by sensory impulses, e.g., the flushing and sweating which may occur after ingestion of highly seasoned food. That physiologic variations in endocrine function may affect the body temperature is shown by the fact that the mean body temperature of women is higher during the second half of the menstrual cycle than it is between the onset of menstruation and the time of ovulation.

A basic problem on which information is needed is the reason why the normal body temperature of warm-blooded animals is in the neighborhood of 98 to 103°F. Animals or human beings whose cervical cords have been severed maintain about the same body temperature, although fluctuations tend to be greater because of lack of neural control. There may be some intrinsic chemical regulating mechanism in the tissues.

NORMAL BODY TEMPERATURE

It is not practical to designate an exact upper level of normal body temperature, since there are small differences among normal persons. There are rare individuals whose temperatures are always elevated slightly above accepted "normal" levels. The physician must use some judgment in deciding what constitutes an abnormal temperature in a given case. In general, however, it is safest to regard an oral temperature above 98.6°F in a person who has been lying in bed as an indication of disease. A temperature above 99.0°F in a person who has been engaged in moderate activity has the same significance. The temperature may be as low as 96.5°F in healthy individuals. Rectal temperature is usually 0.5 to 1.0°F higher than oral temperature. In very hot weather the body temperature may be elevated by 0.5° or perhaps even 1.0°F.

In all persons the body temperature varies by 0.5 to 2.0°F during each 24-hr period. The highest temperature is usually attained late in the afternoon; the lowest occurs during sleep, in the early hours of the morning. The cause of this pattern of variation is not known with certainty. Many writers have attributed the higher level in the late afternoon to the combined effects of digesting food and physical activity. These, together with the temperature-lowering effect of sleep, may be the factors which cause the diurnal rhythm to be established. The rhythm persists, however, sometimes for days or weeks when the time relationships of these factors are altered, and an exaggeration of the normal diurnal pattern of variation is frequently observed in sick people confined to bed, too ill to eat.

Body temperature may be elevated temporarily to fever levels by conditions which overwhelm the mechanisms for heat loss. Examples are hot baths and strenuous muscular exercise. Children are particularly liable to slight elevations after hard play, since their temperature-regulating mechanisms are not so efficient as those of adults. Elevations such as these hardly deserve the term *fever*, which should generally be reserved for rises in body temperature due to disease.

PATHOGENESIS OF FEVER

Bedside observation of febrile patients reveals evidence that the smooth functioning of the cerebral thermoregulatory centers has been disturbed. Alternating flushing and pallor of the skin, chilling and sweating, and wide daily fluctuations are seen. The mechanism of this disturbance is obscure. Some pathogenic microorganisms produce endotoxins which are pyrogenic and appear to act centrally. However, there is reason to believe that these substances have little to do with the production of fever in most infectious diseases. Furthermore, there are many febrile disorders, e.g., myocardial infarction and hypernephroma, in which there is no invasion of the body by a pyrogen-producing parasite. Here we are forced to postulate some other mechanism of fever.

Several hypotheses have been offered regarding the mechanism of disturbed temperature regulation in noninfectious disease. Some investigators have attempted to explain fever on the basis of shifts in body water interfering with normal mechanisms for heat production and heat loss. It is true that newborn infants may exhibit fever when the fluid intake is inadequate and that their temperature elevations subside promptly when fluid is administered. In adults there are occasional instances of fever associated with extracellular-fluid deficit at times when the environmental temperature is high (above 90°F). On the other hand, "dehydration" is not ordinarily associated with fever in adults, and the clinical practice of attributing fever to this cause is to be deprecated.

Some writers have attempted to account for the phenomena of fever on the basis of alterations in endocrine function, with particular reference to the thyroid and adrenal glands. Actually there is little clinical or experimental evidence to support such a theory. Temperature regulation is normal in Addison's disease and in the Cushing syndrome. Although the level of body temperature is a little above normal in thyrotoxicosis and a little below in myxedema, these differences are in keeping with the altered metabolic rate, and there is no real evidence of impaired regulatory function in either disease.

There has been a renewal of interest in the possible role of the endocrines in the pathogenesis of fever with the finding that certain steroid compounds, e.g., etiocholanolone, can elevate the body temperature in man. Some evidence has been obtained suggesting that abnormal etiocholanolone metabolism may exist in some patients with "periodic disease."

The factor common to nearly all febrile diseases is tissue injury. The hypothesis which best fits clinical and experimental observations is that fever results from disturbance of cerebral thermoregulation brought about as an effect of a product or products of tissue injury. It has been shown experimentally that there is something in inflammatory exudates which will produce fever when these materials are injected intravenously into normal animals. Further work indicates that one source of

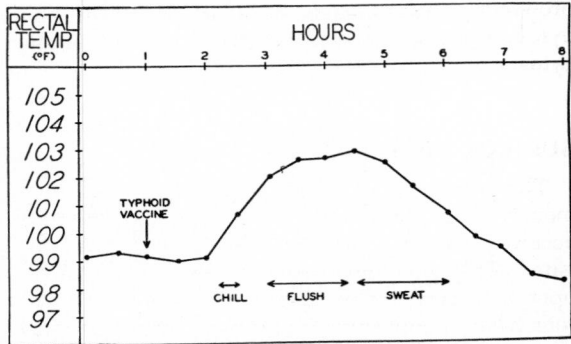

FIG. 9-1. A typical temperature response of a human being to intravenous injection of a comparatively large dose of typhoid vaccine—100,000,000 organisms.

material capable of causing such fever is the polymorphonuclear leukocyte.

While considering the pathogenesis of fever, it is worthwhile to note the sequence of events which follows intravenous injection of killed bacteria or of purified bacterial pyrogen. Figure 9-1 illustrates a typical temperature response of a human being to intravenous injection of a comparatively large dose of typhoid vaccine—100,000,000 organisms. It is to be noted that the body temperature does not begin to rise until about an hour after the intravenous injection of the pyrogen. During the interval, the patient's appearance reveals no change; furthermore, he does not complain of discomfort. Then, rather suddenly, he begins to show signs of malaise; he complains of being cold and within a few minutes is burrowing down into the bedclothes, asking for more blankets. He begins to shiver and soon is having a hard, shaking chill, which usually lasts 10 to 20 min. During this time his skin is pale, cyanotic, and cold to the touch because of intense vasoconstriction. The rectal temperature, nevertheless, is rising steeply. After subsidence of the rigor, the patient gradually begins to feel less cold, and the circulation in his skin increases. By the end of the second hour he is flushed, his skin is hot, and he now complains of feeling feverish. After an hour or so, profuse sweating occurs and the temperature begins to return to normal.

Much remains to be learned about the nature of the series of events which follows intravenous injection of a pyrogenic substance. It has been well established that bacterial pyrogen is removed from the circulation within a few minutes by cells of the reticuloendothelial system. It can be assumed too that the febrile reaction to the bacterial toxin involves some effect on the thermoregulatory centers in the hypothalamus. Experimental evidence on this point suggests that two mechanisms may be involved: a direct effect on the central nervous system by the bacterial toxin and an indirect effect by products of tissue injury such as the endogenous pyrogen contained in polymorphonuclear leukocytes.

SUBJECTIVE SYMPTOMS OF FEVER

The perception of fever by patients varies enormously. Some individuals can tell with considerable accuracy whether their body temperatures are elevated. This perception seems to depend principally upon a sensation of warmth in the skin. Other persons have no subjective symptoms of fever, even in the presence of considerable elevation. For example, patients with tuberculosis may be wholly unconscious of body temperatures as high as 103°F. As pointed out in the preceding section, during a period of rapid temperature elevation a patient may actually feel cold. Often, also, patients are not conscious of fever because of the presence of other more unpleasant symptoms such as headache and pleuritic pain.

The headache of fever is discussed on p. 25. The pain usually experienced in muscles and in the back during acute infectious diseases such as influenza and dengue seems to be due to an effect of the infectious agent and not to be a direct manifestation of fever.

DISORDERED THERMOREGULATION

As has already been mentioned, disease of the regulatory centers in the hypothalamus may affect body temperature. Cases have been observed in which there was destruction of the centers controlling heat-conserving mechanisms, with resulting hypothermia. More commonly, cerebral lesions are manifested by higher-than-normal body temperature; this may occur with tumors, infections, degenerative diseases, or vascular accidents. It is not uncommon in cerebral apoplexy for the temperature to rise to 105 to 107°F during the last few hours before death of the patient.

Heat stroke is an interesting example of fever due to interference with the controlling mechanism. Here the mechanisms for cooling the body seem suddenly to fail and the patient ceases to sweat, despite the fact that his temperature is rising. Some of the highest temperatures ever observed in human beings (112 to 113°F) have been in cases of heat stroke. A temperature higher than 114°F is not compatible with life.

Increased Heat Production. Patients with thyrotoxicosis frequently have an elevation in temperature 1 to 2°F above the normal range. This is ascribable to the increased amount of heat produced by an increase in the activity and rate of the metabolic processes. Dinitrophenol, a drug which was formerly used for weight reduction in obese persons, causes elevation of temperature; this too seems to be caused by an increased metabolic activity, produced by some mechanism outside the thyroid.

Impairment of Heat Loss. Patients with congestive heart failure nearly always have an elevation of body temperature. Usually this is only a matter of 0.5 to 1.5°F. It has been thought by many that the elevation is caused by impairment of heat dissipation as a result of diminished cardiac output, decline in cutaneous blood flow, the insulating effect of edema, and the increased heat production incident to the muscular activity of dyspnea. Others have objected to this explanation because patients with congestive heart failure are likely to have other causes of fever, such as venous thrombosis, embolism, myocardial infarction, rheumatic fever, and urinary tract infection. However, since slight fever is so regularly present even in the absence of such complications, it would appear that the circulatory disturbance may be responsible.

Patients with extensive skin diseases such as ichthyosis or with congenital absence of sweat glands may have fever in a warm environment because of inability to lose heat from the surface of the body.

Tissue Injury. Owing to the inadequacy of our knowledge about the pathogenesis of fever, most febrile diseases fall in the tissue injury group: (1) It is safe to generalize that all *infections*, whether caused by bacteria, rickettsias, viruses, or more complex parasites, may cause fever. (2) *Mechanical injury*, as in crushing injuries or extensive surgical procedures, frequently gives rise to temperature elevation. The duration of this kind of fever is rarely more than 1 or 2 days. (3) The majority of *neoplastic* diseases can cause fever. Carcinoma of the stomach or pancreas, with metastasis to the liver, is nearly always associated with temperature elevation. Hypernephroma can produce a hectic type of fever with daily chills. The lymphomatous group of diseases deserves special mention. In lymphosarcoma and Hodgkin's disease, fever may be the first manifestation or one of the prominent early manifestations. (4) Many *hematopoietic disorders* are characterized by pyrexia, examples being acute hemolytic episodes, severe pernicious anemia, and the leukemias. (5) *Vascular accidents* of any magnitude nearly always cause fever. Examples are myocardial infarction, cerebral hemorrhage or thrombosis, and peripheral vascular occlusion. The temperature elevation in these conditions is probably related to tissue injury in the area where the blood supply has been impaired. (6) *Diseases due to immune mechanisms or inflammatory diseases of uncertain etiology* constitute an important group of febrile diseases. This group includes the so-called "collagen diseases" as well as drug fevers and serum sickness. (7) Certain *acute metabolic disorders* are associated with fever, examples being gout, porphyria, and thyroid storm.

The list of febrile disorders is amplified in the chapter which follows.

CLINICAL IMPORTANCE OF FEVER

The clinical thermometer was one of the first instruments of precision to be introduced into the practice of medicine. Its objectivity and simplicity make it an immensely valuable aid to physical diagnosis. Nowadays we are so accustomed to graphic temperature charts in hospitals and the ready availability of the clinical thermometer for use in the home that we scarcely realize our great dependence upon them. Determination of the body temperature assists in estimating the severity of an illness, its course and duration, and the effect of therapy, or even in deciding whether a person has an organic illness.

A question frequently asked is whether fever is beneficial. There are a few infections of man in which pyrexia appears definitely to be beneficial to the host, examples being neurosyphilis, some gonococcal infections, and chronic brucellosis. Certain other diseases, such as uveitis and rheumatoid arthritis, sometimes improve after fever therapy. In experimental animals some pneumococcal and cryptococcal infections have been influenced in favor of the host animal by raising the body temperature. Aged and debilitated patients with infection may exhibit little or no fever, and this is generally interpreted as a bad prognostic sign. In the great majority of infectious diseases, however, there is no reason to believe that pyrexia accelerates phagocytosis, antibody formation, or other defense mechanisms.

Fever has its detrimental aspects. The greater velocity of all metabolic processes accentuates weight loss and nitrogen wastage. The work and the rate of the heart are increased. Sweating aggravates loss of fluid and salt. There may be discomfort due to headache, photophobia, general malaise, or unpleasant sensation of warmth. The rigors and profuse sweats of hectic fevers are particularly unpleasant for the patient.

Management of Fever. Since fever ordinarily does little harm and imposes no great discomfort, antipyretic drugs are rarely necessary and may obscure the effect of a specific therapeutic agent and of the natural course of the disease. There are situations, however, in which lowering of the body temperature is of vital importance: heat stroke, postoperative hyperthermia, delirium due to high pyrexia, shock associated with fever. Under these circumstances, sponging the body surface with alcohol or the application of cool compresses to the skin and forehead may be employed. When high internal temperature is combined with cutaneous vasoconstriction, as in heat stroke or postoperative hyperthermia, the cooling measures should be combined with massage of the skin in order to bring blood to the surface, where it may be cooled. Immediate immersion in a tub of ice water should be considered a lifesaving emergency procedure in patients with heat stroke if the internal body temperature is in excess of 108°F.

If antipyretic drugs, such as aspirin (0.3 to 0.6 Gm), are employed to bring about a fall in temperature, the ill effects of the unpleasant diaphoresis, sometimes associated with an alarming fall in blood pressure and the subsequent return of fever, occasionally accompanied by a chill, can be mitigated by enforcing a liberal fluid intake and by administering the drug regularly at 3- or 4-hr intervals.

Hypothermia. From the clinical standpoint, reduction of body temperature is of far less frequency and importance than is elevation. Daily variation of temperature within the "subnormal" range, i.e., 97 to 98.6°F, is observed in all healthy individuals. The temperature range may be somewhat lower than normal, i.e., 96 to 97.5°F, in patients with myxedema and during the first day or so after critical fall in temperature associated with infectious disease. Oral temperatures below 96°F are rarely encountered, as there is apparently a potent countering mechanism which opposes fall below that level. This barrier may of course be broken through by exposure to extreme cold (p. 836). Furthermore, when cerebral function has been impaired, as by alcohol or large doses of sedative drugs, less severe chilling can result in fall in body temperature. The lowered body temperature in shock may be due to impaired cerebral regulation or to inability to produce adequate heat.

One condition in which profound hypothermia may develop is myxedema with coma. Body temperature in such a patient may gradually sink to 80 to 85°F. Attending personnel may fail to recognize this because the clinical thermometer registers only as low as it has been shaken; hence a series of readings in the range of 95 to 97°F may be erroneously recorded.

REFERENCES

Atkins, E.: Pathogenesis of Fever, Physiol. Rev., 40:580, 1960.

Kappas, A., R. H. Palmer, and P. B. Glickman: Steroid Fever, Am. J. Med., 31:167, 1961.

Pickering, G. W.: Regulation of Body Temperature in Health and Disease, Lancet, 1:1 and 59, 1958.

10 DIAGNOSTIC SIGNIFICANCE OF FEVER

Paul B. Beeson

Physicians frequently have the problem of dealing with illness of unknown etiology in which fever is a prominent manifestation. As was discussed in the preceding chapter, fever is not an indication of any particular group of diseases; instead it should be looked upon merely as a reaction to injury, comparable to alterations in leukocyte count, increased erythrocyte sedimentation rate, altered protein metabolism, etc. The present chapter presents a general discussion of febrile illnesses from the standpoint of diagnostic possibilities and procedures. An attempt is made to indicate the more important probabilities to be considered in various circumstances and to suggest methods of dealing with diagnostic problems of this kind.

FEBRILE ILLNESSES OF SHORT DURATION

Acute febrile illnesses of less than 2 weeks' duration are a common occurrence in medical practice. In many instances they run their courses, progressing to complete recovery; yet the physician in attendance is never able to arrive at a precise diagnosis. In most instances, however, it is safe to assume that the illness is of infectious origin; for although short febrile illnesses can be of noninfectious origin, e.g., allergic fevers due to drugs or serums, thromboembolic disease, hemolytic crises, gout, etc., such are decidedly in the minority.

Most of these acute febrile infectious diseases in which diagnosis is obscure are probably viral infections, since diagnostic methods for bacterial infection are better, and since most bacterial infections are rapidly brought under control by the chemotherapeutic agents now in common use. It is not practicable to carry out tests needed to identify all the viruses at present known, and furthermore there must be a considerable number of as yet unidentified viruses pathogenic for man. One could speculate, for example, that measles would not yet have been differentiated from other acute viral respiratory infections except for the circumstance that it happens to be accompanied by a specific cutaneous eruption.

Although specific diagnosis of the infectious diseases of short duration is often impossible, they have certain features in common which enable the physician to recognize them as infectious diseases. The following attributes, while not restricted solely to acute infectious diseases, are nevertheless highly suggestive:

1. Abrupt onset
2. High fever, i.e., 102 to 105°F, with or without chills
3. Respiratory symptoms—sore throat, coryza, cough
4. Severe malaise, with muscle or joint pain, photophobia, pain on movement of the eyes, headache
5. Nausea, vomiting, or diarrhea
6. Acute enlargement of lymph nodes or spleen
7. Meningeal signs, with or without spinal fluid pleocytosis
8. Leukocyte count above 12,000 or below 5,000 per cu mm

To repeat, none of the symptoms or signs listed is encountered only in infection. Many of these features could be seen in acute myeloblastic leukemia or disseminated lupus erythematosus. Nevertheless in a given instance of acute febrile illness with some or all of the manifestations listed, the probabilities strongly favor infection, and the physician is able to give reasonable assurance that the patient will probably recover in a week or two, regardless of a precise diagnosis.

It is desirable of course to establish an accurate diagnosis, and the physician should take whatever steps are practicable in the circumstances to establish the etiology. Cultures of the throat, blood, urine, or feces should be obtained *before* institution of antibacterial chemotherapy. Diagnosis by means of skin tests or serologic test should be carried out. In the meantime it is a common practice to proceed with antibiotic therapy, in case the infection should happen to be caused by a susceptible microorganism.

PROLONGED FEBRILE ILLNESSES

Some of the knottiest problems in differential diagnosis in the field of internal medicine are found in cases of prolonged fever in which the diagnosis remains unsolved for weeks or even months. Eventually, however, the true nature of the illness usually reveals itself, since a disease which causes injury sufficient to evoke temperature elevations of 101°F or higher for several weeks does not often subside without leaving some clue as to its nature. As a matter of fact, prolonged fever is generally a manifestation of grave organic disease.

The elucidation of diagnostic problems of this sort calls for skillful application of all diagnostic methods —careful history, thorough physical examination, and the considered application of good laboratory examinations.

It is obviously not possible or practical in this section to mention all the known entities which may cause prolonged febrile disease, or even to give an adequate discussion of the differential diagnosis of the more frequent ones. An attempt is made, however, to indicate the breadth of the problem, to list some of the diseases which must be considered in patients with fever of obscure origin, and to mention a point or two about each which may be of assistance in directing attention toward or away from them. Additional details about the manifestations and differential diagnosis of the entities mentioned will be found elsewhere.

Infectious Diseases

The infections occupy a less prominent position among the causes of prolonged fever now than formerly, because of the common practice of administering antibiotic drugs to any patient in whom fever persists for more than a few days. Consequently, many infections are at present being eradicated by more or less "blind" therapy, without their nature or location ever accurately being determined.

Certain infections do not respond to the usual antibiotic therapy and must be thought of in differential diagnosis at the present time. In general, this does not apply to virus diseases, for although chemotherapy rarely affects them, they tend to run their courses more or less acutely and do not often cause continued illness lasting many weeks or months. The following infections must be mentioned.

Tuberculosis. This disease proves to be responsible for puzzling febrile disease with surprising frequency, despite the facts that there is a fairly effective therapy and that the simple procedure of chest x-ray is usually sufficient for diagnosis of the commonest clinical form. The drugs given as therapeutic trials may not include those with tuberculostatic activity such as streptomycin or isoniazid. Extrapulmonary forms of tuberculosis may not be easily located, e.g., disease of the bones, deep lymph nodes, genital or urinary organs. Furthermore the pulmonary lesions of miliary tuberculosis may not be detectable by x-ray until very late in the course of the disease. In considering the possibility of tuberculous infection, the skin test may be of great assistance, since negative reaction to a properly executed skin test rules out the possibility of tuberculosis except in rare instances of overwhelming disease. A positive skin reaction, on the other hand, does not prove that tuberculosis is causing the patient's illness, but in its presence the experienced physician will continue to keep tuberculosis in mind as a possibility until another cause for the fever and other symptoms are found.

Bacterial Endocarditis. In the classical subacute form of the disease, a heart murmur is nearly always present; therefore absence of murmur largely eliminates this disease from consideration. The correct diagnosis is likely to be missed in middle-aged or elderly patients, in whom the presence of a heart murmur may not be given much weight. For example, an elderly patient with subacute bacterial endocarditis may first present himself following the occurrence of a cerebral embolus and may be regarded as having had a hemorrhage or thrombosis because of arteriosclerosis. The best clinical practice is to culture the blood of *every* patient who has fever and a heart murmur. One cannot take the risk of overlooking this curable disease.

Brucellosis. The point to be emphasized is that this infection is a most unlikely possibility in an American city dweller. It has to be considered in the case of farmers, veterinarians, or slaughterhouse workers. There is a common misconception that brucellosis frequently causes arthritis. While arthralgia and myalgia are common, actual redness and swelling of joints are rare in this disease. Peripheral leukocytosis is seldom seen in brucellosis. In active febrile disease the blood culture and bone marrow culture frequently are positive, and specific agglutinins are *nearly always* present in the serum. Precise diagnosis is therefore a relatively easy matter.

Salmonella Infection. Although typhoid fever is subject to great variability and may cause fever for several weeks, it should not often be a cause of prolonged fever of obscure origin, since cultures of feces or blood will be positive, and the specific antibodies are detected in the agglutination reaction. Other salmonella organisms may, however, cause prolonged febrile illness, and these may present greater diagnostic difficulty. Routine serologic tests are not helpful, and few laboratories can or will carry out serologic tests to detect antibody responses to all possible infecting strains. Antibiotics, including chloramphenicol (Chloromycetin), may not be effective. Repeated culture of the blood or of bone marrow may yield the causative organism. There may eventually be localization of infection in a joint or the pleural cavity from which the etiologic agent can be obtained.

Pyogenic Infection. Chemotherapy does not succeed in eradicating all localized pyogenic infection, and in certain locations inflammation may be relatively asymptomatic. These infections include osteomyelitis of the vertebras or pelvic bones, abscess (subdiaphragmatic, hepatic, perinephric, renal cortical, retropharyngeal, mediastinal), cholangitis, and bronchiectasis. If these possibilities are thought of, appropriate questioning, examination, and x-ray studies will usually reveal their presence.

Amebiasis. Amebic colitis usually evokes symptoms pointing to disease of the colon. Hepatic involvement, on the other hand, may not give a distinctive clinical picture, and prolonged fever may be the principal manifestation. Some assistance may be obtained from a history of dysentery, or from the elicitation of tenderness or enlargement of the liver, and elevation of the right leaf of the diaphragm. The complement fixation test has little diagnostic value, either when positive or when negative. Therapeutic trial of an antiamebic drug, such as chloroquine or emetine, which acts on the hepatic form of amebiasis, may be justified.

Histoplasmosis. This infection is prevalent in the region of the Mississippi Valley of the United States, although in most individuals it is not clinically recognizable. The disease may, however, be manifested as a chronic febrile illness, with localizing manifestations pointing to many organ systems. Fever, leukopenia, anemia, hepatomegaly, and splenomegaly in a person who has resided in a geographic area where histoplasmosis occurs should suggest the possibility. The skin reaction to histoplasmin should be positive. The organisms may be demonstrated in biopsy or by culture of involved tissue or in bone marrow, occasionally even in the peripheral blood.

Coccidioidomycosis. This disease need be considered only in persons who have traveled through, or resided in, the Southwest part of the United States. Clinical manifestations are like those of the various forms of tuberculosis. The coccidioidin skin test and serologic reaction to this antigen are positive.

Schistosomiasis. Persons who have lived in the Caribbean islands, in Africa, or in the Far East may have prolonged febrile illness associated with this infestation. Diarrhea, bladder symptoms, cough, hepatosplenomegaly, and anemia are suggestive. Diagnosis is made by finding the ova in feces or urine or in rectal or hepatic biopsy.

Collagen Diseases

Under this term is included a broad spectrum of diseases (see p. 1883) in which there are histologic evidences of disorders of the collagen and the blood vessels. Some of these diseases are particularly important causes of prolonged febrile illness.

Disseminated Lupus Erythematosus. This disease is by no means rare, being encountered with greater frequency in American hospitals than typhoid fever. Diagnosis is relatively easy when the characteristic eruption is present over the nose and malar eminences, but this eruption may be a late manifestation and in fact is absent in about half of all cases. The possibility should receive special consideration in a young woman with fever, polyarthritis, low or low normal leukocyte count, anemia, pulmonary infiltrations or pleural involvement, and hematuria and other evidence of acute nephritis. Behavioral abnormalities, orbital edema, and salivary gland swelling are less common features. The diagnosis can be made with confidence in patients who develop the full clinical picture, or by demonstration of the LE cell or LE phenomenon. The

diseases likely to be confused with disseminated lupus erythematosus are rheumatic fever and rheumatoid arthritis.

Periarteritis Nodosa. Features which particularly point to this syndrome are febrile illness in a male of any age, with leukocytosis, eosinophilia, anemia, asthma, peripheral neuritis, arthritis or muscle pain, hypertension, and evidence of renal involvement. Lesions in medium-sized arteries can give rise to the clinical pictures of myocardial infarction, mesenteric embolism, and peripheral vascular disease. There may be a variety of cutaneous eruptions. The only conclusive method of diagnosis is biopsy of a muscle or a skin lesion or of other tissue excised at operation.

Rheumatoid Arthritis. In its earlier stages there may not be characteristic swelling and deformity of joints but only vague pains in muscles and joints, together with fever, slight anemia, and malaise. Differentiation from rheumatic fever and from disseminated lupus erythematosus may be difficult. Sometimes diagnosis cannot be made until the more characteristic picture of the disease develops.

Rheumatic Fever. Fever, with or without muscle and joint pains, may persist for weeks and months at a time. A history of preceding attacks or of an upper respiratory infection before onset of the systemic illness, the presence of a heart murmur, relative tachycardia, and prolonged P-R interval in the electrocardiogram are suggestive findings. Significant elevation of the antistreptolysin O titer is present in 80 per cent of cases.

Erythema Nodosum. The characteristic painful erythematous plaques in the skin of the shins or forearms should point to this diagnosis. However, they may be inconspicuous and may fade, although fever and arthralgia persist.

Henoch-Schönlein, or Allergic, Purpura. There may be fever, joint pains, and evidences of renal and pulmonary involvement. The results of the capillary fragility test and platelet count are normal. Differentiation from lupus erythematosus, rheumatic fever, and acute glomerulonephritis may be difficult. Diagnosis will depend on the finding of hemorrhagic occurrences, usually in the intestinal lumen or in joints.

Neoplastic Diseases

Fever is a common manifestation of malignant growth but a very rare accompaniment of benign tumors. In patients in the age range where cancer is common, unexplained fever should always suggest the possibility of neoplasm.

Carcinomas and Sarcomas. Certain malignant processes seem especially likely to cause fever. Notable are sarcomas involving bone or lymphoid tissue, hypernephroma, carcinoma of the pancreas or stomach, and metastatic cancer of the liver. Occasionally the clinical picture is strongly suggestive of pyrogenic infection, with hectic fever, chills, sweats, and marked leukocytosis; and patients have been subjected to laparotomy with preoperative diagnoses such as empyema of the gallbladder, localized peritonitis, or liver abscess.

Hodgkin's Disease. Fever may be the principal symptom and only objective finding early in the course of Hodgkin's disease, especially when the principal involvement is in the abdominal viscera. Cases with splenomegaly and vague abdominal distress have been confused with typhoid fever. The Pel-Ebstein fever seen in a minority of cases of Hodgkin's disease will be mentioned later. Diagnosis of this disorder is made by biopsy.

Hematopoietic Diseases

Disorders of blood formation or blood destruction are frequently associated with fever. This is not surprising when it is recalled that the bone marrow constitutes one of the largest and most active organs of the body.

Leukemias. It is not uncommon for acute leukemia to be mistaken for acute infection at the onset. The acute leukemias are nearly always accompanied by fever, sometimes as high as 105°F. The correct diagnosis will be suggested by rapid development of anemia and characteristic changes in peripheral blood and bone marrow. Chronic leukemia, particularly lymphatic, may be characterized by low-grade fever but, because of the typical changes in circulating leukocytes, it is not often a diagnostic problem.

Hemolytic Episodes. Most of the hemolytic diseases are characterized by bouts of fever. Acute crises of hemolysis may give rise to shaking chills and marked elevations of temperature. The difficulty sometimes encountered in differentiating sickle-cell disease from acute rheumatic fever is now well known. The presence of these hemolytic disorders is suggested by the more rapid development of anemia than occurs in other febrile illnesses and by the usual accompaniment of icterus. Diagnosis is confirmed by appropriate laboratory tests.

Fever is not characteristic of severe anemia due to external blood loss or of the anemia of uremia.

Vascular Disease

Reference has already been made to the fever of collagen diseases, all of which are accompanied by vascular lesions. In addition, certain other diseases of the blood vessels, not usually regarded as being in the same category as the collagen diseases, may cause chronic febrile illness.

Temporal, or Cranial, Arteritis. This is a disease of old people, featured by severe aching pain in the temporal area, with fever and leukocytosis. There may be accompanying visual defect or blindness due to involvement of the retinal artery. The temporal or occipital arteries may be inflamed and tender. Diagnosis is not difficult if the condition is thought of and the superficial arteries are carefully palpated.

Thromboembolic Disease. In migratory thrombophlebitis, segments of large veins become inflamed and thrombosed. There is usually local pain and swelling, but sometimes the lesions have to be searched for. Symptomless thrombosis of deep calf or pelvic veins may cause prolonged febrile illness as a result of repeated small emboli. These emboli may not be manifested by pleuritic pain or hemoptysis, but cough, dyspnea, or vague thoracic discomfort is likely to be present. Careful examination of the legs and repeated examination of the lungs should reveal the diagnosis.

Miscellaneous

A number of other conditions should be mentioned.

Liver Disease. Most patients with cirrhosis exhibit low-grade fever at times. Rarely there are chills and high fever, owing either to salmonella infection or to bacteremia due to coliform bacteria.

Sarcoidosis. Ordinarily fever is not characteristic of sarcoidosis, but in a minority of cases it does occur, especially in cases characterized by arthralgia and cutaneous lesions resembling erythema nodosum, or in those with extensive hepatic lesions. Diagnosis is suggested by lymphoid enlargement, ocular lesions, and hyperglobulinemia and is clinched by biopsy of skin, lymph nodes, or liver.

Drug Fever. Great emphasis should be placed on this category of febrile disease. One of the first things the consultant should inquire into is the matter of drug ingestion. Fever due to allergy to one of the antibiotics may become superimposed on the fever of the infection for which the drug was given, resulting in a very confusing picture. Other drugs capable of causing fever are the sulfonamides, arsenicals, iodides, thiouracils, and barbiturates. One should not forget laxative drugs in this connection, especially those containing phenolphthalein. Any question of drug fever can be resolved rapidly by discontinuing all medication. The diagnosis can be further substantiated by giving a test dose of the drug after fever has subsided, but this may result in a very unpleasant or even dangerous reaction.

Malingering. Rarely, a patient will wish to seem to be having fever. A variety of methods has been employed to cause the thermometer to register higher than the true temperature. If malingering is suspected, all that is necessary to prove it is to repeat the temperature determination immediately after a high reading has been obtained, with someone remaining at the bedside while the thermometer is in place.

PROLONGED LOW-GRADE TEMPERATURE ELEVATIONS

Not infrequently the physician is consulted because it has been observed that a patient, while not appearing acutely ill, has been subject to elevation of body temperature above the "normal" level, i.e., a level in the range of 99.0 to 100.5°F. This poses a very difficult problem, calling for searching observation and competent judgment. Prolonged low-grade fever may be a manifestation of serious illness, or it may be a matter of no real consequence. Possibly there are some individuals whose "normal" temperatures are in this range. However, there is no certain way of identifying such individuals. The possibilities which the physician has to consider in such cases vary considerably according to the age groups concerned.

In children it should not be forgotten that temperature regulation may be somewhat erratic even up to the age of twelve years. Children may therefore have slight temperature elevations when excited or after exercise. A mother may note that her child's skin feels hot when he has been playing and find his temperature slightly above the normal line. Reexamination on subsequent days may reveal the same elevation from time to time. The physician consulted about this has to decide whether the "fever" is an indication of disease or of imperfect thermoregulation. The diseases which may have to be considered include rheumatic fever, tuberculosis, recurrent urinary tract infection, etc. If the physical examination reveals no abnormality, if the appetite is good and the child is gaining weight, and if there is no anemia or urinary abnormality, it is fairly safe to advise the parent to cease taking temperatures and forget about "fever." Real harm can be done by restricting the activity of an otherwise healthy child, owing to misinterpretation of the significance of low-grade fever.

In young adults chronic low-grade temperature elevation cannot easily be imputed to imperfect thermoregulation. Here one has to consider tuberculosis, brucellosis, and rheumatic fever or other collagen disease, as well as many of the conditions mentioned in the preceding section. A special problem encountered in females of this age group is that which has been called *habitual hyperthermia*. Every experienced physician has encountered examples of the syndrome. The patient may have temperatures of 99.0 to 100.5°F regularly or intermittently for years. The patient usually has a variety of complaints characteristic of psychoneurosis, such as fatigability, insomnia, bowel distress, vague aches, and headache. Prolonged careful study and observation fail to reveal evidence of organic disease. Unfortunately, many of these people go from doctor to doctor and are subjected to a variety of unpleasant, expensive, and even harmful tests, treatments, and operations. The diagnosis of this syndrome can be made with reasonable certainty after a suitable period of observation and study, and if the patient can be convinced of it, a real service will have been rendered.

In a patient past middle age, fever, even low-grade, should always be regarded as a probable indication of organic disease. The possibilities to be considered in this age group are the same as those discussed above in the section Prolonged Febrile Illnesses.

RELAPSING AND RECURRENT FEVERS

Occasionally patients are encountered who have recurrent bouts of high fever at more or less regular intervals. The following are among the diseases which have to be considered:

Malaria. The disease has almost completely vanished from the United States and Canada, but cases are encountered occasionally in persons recently arrived from foreign countries. It is most unusual, however, for malaria to recur after a symptom-free interval of one year or more. Seizures recur at 2- or 3-day intervals, depending on the maturation cycle of the parasite. Diagnosis depends on demonstration of the parasites in the blood.

Relapsing Fever. This disease occurs in the Southwest part of the United States, extending as far east as Texas. Again the recurrences are doubtless related to some cycle in the development of the parasites. Diagnosis is by demonstration of the spirochetal organisms in stained films of the blood.

Rat-bite Fever. Two etiologic agents—*Spirillum minus* and *Streptobacillus moniliformis*—can be transmitted by the bite of a rat. Both may cause an illness characterized by periodic exacerbations of fever. The clue as to the diagnosis depends on obtaining a history of rat bite 1 to 10 weeks previous to the onset of symptoms. The etiology can be established by appropriate laboratory procedures.

Pyogenic Infection. In rare instances, localized pyogenic infections give rise to periodic bouts of fever separated by afebrile and relatively symptom-free intervals. The so-called "Charcot's intermittent biliary fever," i.e., cholangitis with biliary obstruction due to stones, is an example. The febrile attacks are usually associated with slight jaundice. There should be a history suggestive of cholelithiasis, and during the attacks tenderness can be elicited in the right upper quadrant. *Urinary tract infection*, with episodes of ureteral obstruction due to small stones or inspissated pus, can also cause recurrent fever.

Hodgkin's Disease. In perhaps 5 to 10 per cent of cases, there is seen at some time during the course of the disease the so-called "Pel-Ebstein fever"—bouts of fever lasting 3 to 10 days, separated by afebrile and asymptomatic periods of 3 to 10 days. These cycles may be repeated regularly over a period of several months. In rare instances this periodicity of the fever has been sufficiently striking to suggest the correct diagnosis before lymph node swelling or splenomegaly had become evident.

Periodic Disease. There is a rare group of disorders in which symptoms recur at intervals over periods of months or years, without apparent progression. During the afebrile phases the patients feel quite well, and no etiology is determined despite careful study. The manifestations include fever, abdominal pain, arthralgia or joint swelling, leukocytosis, or leukopenia and may occur in various combinations. Whether this condition is caused by a group of unrelated disorders which happen to have the common feature of periodicity and obscure etiology cannot be stated with certainty, but there is evidence that abnormal metabolism of the steroid compound etiocholanolone may play a role in pathogenesis, in some cases, whereas others appear to be hereditary disorders.

DIAGNOSTIC PROCEDURE

When faced with so large a number of possibilities, it is obvious that no single plan can be outlined for the systematic study of every problem in unexplained fever. One must develop the course of study according to the probabilities in a given case, depending upon leads provided by the history and the physical examination. Obviously if the features suggest the presence of infectious disease, the main dependence will be upon bacteriologic and immunologic methods of diagnosis, whereas in an obscure febrile disorder in a person in the "cancer age group" the best chance of early diagnosis may lie in x-ray studies.

Careful elicitation of the patient's past *history* and the chronologic development of his symptoms may give the important leads. In respect to infection we are interested in places of recent residence, contact with domestic or wild animals and birds, preceding acute infectious diseases such as diarrheal illness or boils, contact with persons with tuberculosis, etc. Knowledge as to drugs ingested may be important. Localizing symptoms may give a clue to an organ system affected by neoplasm or infection.

In the *physical examination,* careful search is made for skin lesions and for petechial hemorrhages in the ocular fundi, conjunctivas, nail beds, and skin. The lymph nodes are carefully palpated, with special attention to the retroclavicular and axillary areas. The finding of a heart murmur or of change in the character of a preexisting one may be important. Detection of an abdominal mass may be the first lead to diagnosis of neoplastic disease. Palpable

enlargement of the spleen suggests infection, leukemia, or lymphoma and points away from a diagnosis of cancer. Enlargement of the liver and spleen suggests lymphoma, leukemia, chronic infection, or cirrhosis. A large liver without palpable spleen would point to liver abscess or metastatic cancer. Nowadays the rectum and the female pelvic organs are sure to be examined, but the male patient's testicles may not be examined, with resulting failure to discover a teratoma or tuberculosis.

References have already been made to a variety of laboratory examinations which may be needed: cultures of blood, bone marrow, urine, or other body fluids; examination of blood smears for parasites or for evidence of hematologic disorder; tests for hemolysins, LE phenomenon; serologic studies; etc. X-ray studies are of course of the greatest assistance also. In all patients the chest should be examined early in the study, and the examination should perhaps be repeated occasionally. It may be expedient to proceed with studies of the gastrointestinal and urinary tracts even in the absence of symptoms referable to these areas, especially in the case of patients in the older age groups.

It will have been noted how often biopsy has been mentioned as the best means of definitive diagnosis. Bone marrow aspiration may be helpful, not only for the histology of the marrow but also for occasional demonstration of other disease processes such as metastatic carcinoma or granulomas and for culture. Aspiration biopsy of the liver is a very useful procedure and can be done with reasonable safety. It may be helpful not only with primary or metastatic disease of the liver, but also because of the fact that the liver may reveal existence of other diseases such as histoplasmosis, schistosomiasis, brucellosis, tuberculosis, sarcoidosis, or lymphoma. Lymph node biopsy is, of course, helpful in diagnosis of many diseases, including the lymphomas, metastatic cancer, tuberculosis, and mycotic infections. Careful examination and consideration should precede excision of a node. The inguinal nodes are notoriously unsatisfactory for biopsy, yet are too frequently chosen because of their easy accessibility. Axillary, cervical, and supraclavicular nodes are much more likely to yield helpful information, and the node excised need not necessarily be a large one. Muscle biopsy may be of assistance in the recognition of dermatomyositis, periarteritis nodosa, sarcoidosis, and trichinosis.

Exploratory laparotomy is to be recommended occasionally, since it may be the only means of finding a cryptic abscess or other remediable lesion.

THERAPEUTIC TRIALS

It is common practice to give a trial of antibiotic therapy to patients with unidentified febrile disorders. While this kind of marksmanship has had its good effects, one cannot applaud "blind" therapy. Undesirable features include drug toxicity, superinfection due to resistant pathogenic bacteria, and interference with accurate diagnosis by cultural methods. Furthermore, a coincidental fall in temperature not due to the therapy is likely to be interpreted as response to treatment, with the conclusion that one is dealing with an infectious disease. If, in spite of these disadvantages, decision is made to proceed with therapeutic trial of antibiotics, streptomycin or isoniazid should not be omitted, since they alone affect tuberculosis.

Other drugs may be given on a trial basis where there is a question of such infections as amebiasis,

schistosomiasis, malaria, and similar conditions.

One does not obtain much information from a trial of cortisone or ACTH therapy. These have an antipyretic effect, and also produce a euphoric state in many individuals, so that apparent improvement while receiving these agents tells little about the nature of the underlying disease.

REFERENCES

Geraci, J. E., L. A. Weed, and D. R. Nichols: Fever of Obscure Origin—The Value of Abdominal Exploration in Diagnosis, J.A.M.A., 169:1306, 1959.

Petersdorf, R. G., and P. B. Beeson: Fever of Unexplained Origin: Report of 100 Cases, Medicine, 40:1, 1961.

Section 3: Disorders of the Integument

11 THE SKIN AND ITS APPENDAGES

*Donald M. Pillsbury and
Walter B. Shelley*

APPROACH TO THE PATIENT WITH A DERMATOLOGIC DISORDER

Approach through the History

The *medical history* in a patient with a disease affecting the skin should be obtained with the same care that is exercised in a patient with any general medical or surgical illness. However, skin lesions are often too quickly assessed as trivial and unimportant, their precise extent is undetermined, and their general medical importance remains unsuspected.

Though it is often useful in any medical history to record the chief complaint exactly as given by the patient, this frequently is not the case with dermatologic patients. A term such as "rash" is obviously noninformative, and patients often describe their diseases in very colloquial terms. Symptoms such as pruritus or pain vary so greatly with skin lesions that often they are not helpful. It may be useful, therefore, to delay putting down the chief complaint until after the initial inspection. The initial summary of the complaint should include data on the chief type or types of lesions, whether they are localized or diffuse, whether the dermatosis is acute or chronic, and whether it is associated with symptoms or signs indicative of systemic disease.

It is also very useful to record early in the history

whether or not any *topical or systemic therapy* has been used, and, if so, what, because reactions to such medicaments are very common, and frequently greatly obscure the underlying disease. It is important to know whether *ultraviolet therapy* has been used, whether this produced an exacerbation or improvement; and whether any type of *ionizing radiation* or *corticosteroid* therapy has been employed.

Otherwise the objectives of medical history in a patient with a disease affecting the skin are precisely the same as those of any other medical history, namely, to trace the development of the disease as accurately as possible; to determine those elements of the patient's past history which may be related to the disease in question and those which are not; to establish the relation of the patient and his disease to his heredity, personal and occupational environment, psychic and emotional status, and previous medical care; and to establish a good physician-patient relationship by an attitude of kindly interest and willingness to listen. In many patients who are seen because of a localized process, such as a wart or seborrheic keratosis, there will understandably be some resistance to extensive questioning and examination. However, particularly in patients of middle age or above, requestioning may reveal that the patient has neglected himself medically, and a few simple inquiries regarding the patient's general physical state and emphasis on the value of preventive health examinations may prove highly rewarding. The authors have had numerous occasions to direct such patients to appropriate general medical care, through the small wedge of a banal skin lesion. Many patients are, curiously enough, far more inclined to seek attention for what may be a very minor visible lesion on the skin than for the vague symptoms of more serious conditions.

Family History. It is obviously of importance in patients with dermatoses which appear to be allergic to inquire concerning allergic manifestations in blood relatives. It is necessary that the more common allergic diseases such as hives, eczema, hay fever, and asthma be mentioned specifically. Other skin diseases in which a familial trend is frequent include ichthyosis, acne, baldness, rosacea, and psoriasis. Occasionally, skin tumors, such as seborrheic keratoses, may be strongly familial. Less common conditions such as neurofibromatosis, epiloia (neurocutaneous syndrome), and encephalotrigeminal angiomatosis may be genetically endowed. Disturbances of pigmentation are common in families as is hereditary hemorrhagic telangiectasia (Rendu-Osler-Weber disease). Benign or juvenile acanthosis nigricans frequently has a high family incidence. Many other examples could be cited, but most of them are uncommon or rare.

Age as a Factor in Diagnosis. As with many other diseases, certain groups of skin conditions are seen much more frequently in certain age groups. Nevertheless, great caution should be exercised, and age alone should not be allowed to become a determining factor in arriving at a diagnosis. This is particularly true of tumors. The incidence of cancer of the skin increases with age, but it is by no means rare in children (with the exception of malignant melanoma) and is moderately common in young adults. Acne reaches its height in adolescence and rosacea in middle age, but these conditions are not entirely confined to these age groups. Atrophy of the skin and keratoses are characteristic of senility, but they occur in young adults who are sensitive to sunlight and even in children (xeroderma pigmentosum). Atopic dermatitis frequently shows an age periodicity and is, fortunately, not common after late adolescence; nevertheless, it can persist indefinitely in severe or restricted forms. The common types of ringworm of the scalp are seen entirely in children, but an adult form has become endemic in the Southwest and Western United States. Older individuals are less likely to have severe contact sensitization reactions in the skin, and frequently become less troubled by sensitivities such as that to poison ivy. Aside from tumors, perhaps the single most important consideration of age in relation to diseases of the skin is the increased vulnerability of aged persons to dermatitis, ulceration, or bacterial infection of the extremities secondary to peripheral vascular disease. Destructive effects from all types of physical and chemical trauma are more severe and recovery is slower in older patients.

Race. Though many diseases affecting the skin occur more frequently in members of particular races, this consideration is rarely crucial in diagnosis. Pemphigus is more common in Jews, but it can occur in gentiles. Kaposi's sarcoma is seen more frequently in patients from southeastern Europe, but, again, this must not be a determining factor. Psoriasis is infrequent in pure-blooded Negroes, but such persons are now rare outside Africa. Pediculosis, particularly of the scalp, is uncommon in Negroes. Negroes also develop bizarre and exuberant cutaneous reactions in secondary syphilis and in sarcoid.

Geographic Origin. Some diseases affecting the skin can be acquired only under climatic and other conditions which render them contagious and endemic in certain areas. For instance, a person can almost never acquire leprosy if he has not lived for an extended period in an environment other than a Temperate Zone of Europe or of North America. Certain treponemal diseases, such as yaws, pinta, and bejel, are seen only in tropical environments; indeed, bejel is encountered only in the eastern Mediterranean area. Contact dermatitis to poison ivy does not occur in England because the plant does not grow there. However, individuals who are sensitive to poison ivy may have marked reactions to plants of the family Anacardiaceae, which have an extensive geographic distribution, e.g., the cashew nutshell, mango tree, Japanese lacquer tree, and dhobie mark tree.

While the strong geographic tendencies of some diseases are useful in making a list of diagnostic considerations more complete, they may also lead to error. If a patient states that he has spent some time in the tropics, too great emphasis may be placed on the esoteric with neglect of aggravated forms of common diseases. An individual who spends some time in a tropical climate but who is not a native is much more likely to have some very marked form of a disease commonly found in temperate climates such as miliaria or bacterial or fungous infections of the skin than he is to have a disease which is peculiarly and uniquely tropical. Moreover, it must be kept in mind that the geographic foci of many diseases are expanding and contracting, for reasons that are not immediately apparent. Coccidioidomycosis is common in the San Joaquin valley of California, but there are other areas in the United States in which it is found. Creeping eruption due to cat or dog hookworm is very common along the coastal areas of the Southeastern United States, but during suitably warm weather with beaches densely populated, may extend well into northern New Jersey. "Jungle rot" (a thoroughly nondescript term) and "monkey pox" (widespread impetigo arising on miliaria) may be seen among the "natives" of cities such as Philadelphia and Baltimore during prolonged periods of steaming humidity.

Seasonal Incidence. Certain diseases have seasonal peaks. Contact dermatitis will obviously be seen far more frequently during seasons when plants are growing. A diffuse dermatitis from airborne or ragweed pollen is invariably first seen in any particular patient during the ragweed season, but with recurrence of the disease recovery may be more and more delayed and the seasonal incidence less apparent. Photosensitization reactions are at their peak during the summer season, often occurring only in areas where there is no filtration of the sun's rays by smoke and other matter, but with recurrences the direct relation of the reaction to sunlight may become less evident. In all patients with chronic recurrent skin disorders the history of *climatic and other factors at the time of onset* is of great importance. Prolonged questioning may be required to elicit this relation in proper perspective and detail.

Many diseases, including various types of dermatitis and superficial fungous infections, become much worse during seasons of high environmental temperature. Miliaria is caused almost entirely by this factor and is rare during cold weather. Certain common diseases, such as acne, show variable responses in relation to season. Acne is ordinarily improved by exposure to sun, but it may become much worse in an environment of great heat and humidity. A patient with congenital ichthyosis or senile atrophic skin is often worse during the winter because of the low humidity of artificially heated houses and prolonged exposure of the skin to the pleasure of hot baths. Psoriasis and atopic dermatitis are ordinarily much improved during the summer months, though not invariably so. The very common disease, pityriasis rosea, shows increased incidence in the spring and fall for reasons which are a complete mystery. Erythema multiforme of the recurrent urticarial or bullous types may occur principally during the spring through factors which are likewise unknown.

Personal, Hygienic, and Occupational Factors. The skin is subjected to a wider variety of traumatic stimuli than any other organ of the body. Through a number of finely adjusted physiologic mechanisms, it performs a vital service in the life of the person which it contains. It does this with a surprising capacity to maintain its own integrity and functions. There are few diseases of the skin in which environmental factors require no consideration. In easily recognizable form they manifest themselves in the calloused hands of the workman, the whealing of the skin in a patient with dermographism, the characteristic patch of pigmented thickened skin on the neck which marks the violin player, the keratoses and skin cancers which may mark the sailor long home from the sea, the bullous reactions to trauma occurring in patients with epidermolysis bullosa, the fungous infections as a penalty for wearing shoes, and the dermatitic reactions to innumerable sensitizing and irritating occupational contactants. This list of environmental excitants of cutaneous disease can be extended to include hundreds of examples.

Approach through the Lesion

Inspection of the skin and mucous membranes is the simplest of all the procedures of physical examination. Adequate exposure, proper illumination, good vision, and thoroughness are essential. Certain sites, such as the scalp, the folds of the skin, the buccal mucous membranes (not just the pharynx), the palms and soles, the anogenital region, and the vaginal membranes are often not examined. Gross diagnostic errors may result solely from insufficient illumination. In obsolescent hospital wards and clinic quarters the natural or artificial illumination available is frequently unsatisfactory. A flashlight or, for that matter, almost any small bulb source of illumination is entirely inadequate. The physician places himself at a serious disadvantage if he makes a dermatologic examination with light sources which are glaring or produce distorted shadows. Natural daylight without glare is the best source of illumination for general inspection of the skin. An ordinary stand lamp with at least a 60-watt bulb is also very satisfactory. In offices or clinics, a wall bracket which permits positioning of the bulb is a necessity if large numbers of examinations are being done. Fluorescent lighting is generally unsatisfactory because of flickering and color distortion. Certain special surgical type lamps produce a superb shadowless, nonglaring illumination of the skin. The routine use of a hand lens or a head loupe is essential for the adequate interpretation of many small lesions of the skin, especially tumors.

The diagnosis of a disease affecting the skin often depends upon accurate classification of the individual lesions. In diseases in which only the skin is involved, where there is no systemic disturbance, and no specific information obtainable by laboratory studies, the morphologic characteristics furnish the only diagnostic clues. It is therefore important that they be described accurately. This can be done in straightforward, simple terms; there is no need to use an obsolescent or esoteric terminology. The essential facts to be noted are:

1. Distribution of the lesions
2. Physical characteristics
   a. Flat, raised, or containing fluid (serous, purulent, or sanguineous)

b. Size, shape, and color

c. If palpable, any special characteristics

Many conditions of the skin, especially chronic ones, present a variety of lesions. With few exceptions, however, a skin disease in the individual patient is characterized initially by predominance of a single type of lesion which may be pathognomonic. It is the mark of the expert in any field of medicine or surgery that he is able to sort out the presenting signs and symptoms in a complicated disorder and to determine which are representative of the underlying disease. This faculty is particularly helpful in classifying diseases of the skin. Among the debris of a chronic dermatosis the characteristic primary or initial lesion represents true diagnostic treasure. From this it is ordinarily possible to determine the chain of secondary consequential lesions.

This section outlines the various types of skin lesions with particular reference to systemic diseases in which they may occur. No reference will be made to other parts of the examination, but it is not intended to raise the classification of skin lesions to a stature more important than they deserve.

Principal Initial Lesions of Diseases Affecting the Skin. *Macule.* A macule is simply a flat, circumscribed change in the color of the skin. The term ordinarily connotes lesions of relatively small size, up to 1 or 2 cm in diameter. More extensive changes in color are ordinarily referred to as patches or areas. Macular processes are of three general types: (1) due to extrinsically derived colored materials, such as tattoo marks, or embedded material from lacerations or explosions; (2) due to intrinsically derived pigment, i.e., flat moles, petechiae, and hemorrhages, or localized increase or decrease of melanin; (3) erythematous reactions to a wide variety of pathogenic agents. In the presence of constitutional symptoms or if there are purpuric changes in the lesion, macules must be regarded as probable evidence of systemic disease. Drug reactions are commonly macular, and this possibility must always be considered.

Papule. Papules are circumscribed elevations of the skin, varying roughly from a millimeter to a centimeter in size. Larger infiltrated areas are often called plaques. *Nodules* are circumscribed, usually solid, lesions which lie deeper in the skin or subcutaneous tissue. The term is frequently applied to inflammatory processes, e.g., erythema nodosum or subcutaneous fat necrosis, but it may be applied to tumors as well. Considerable confusion exists regarding the term *tumor* which is ordinarily used to designate the larger and deeper circumscribed infiltration of the skin or subcutaneous tissue. However, it is commonly used to describe lesions which are neoplastic, regardless of size or location.

The majority of papular eruptions may be diagnosed accurately by clinical examination and appropriate laboratory studies, but in those which cannot be classified accurately, biopsy is usually mandatory. The histologic characteristics are, by and large, clear-cut. The most common dermatologic syndromes characterized by papules are tumors, psoriasis, lichen planus, viral infections, such as warts and moluscum contagiosum, some drug eruptions, xanthoma, and certain lymphomas, though there are many others. The initial lesions of smallpox may be papular and secondary syphilis is frequently so. The presence of atrophy or frank scarring immediately narrows the diagnostic considerations; uncomplicated psoriasis, for instance, never produces scarring.

Wheals (*hives*) are special types of papules. They may remain as small individual lesions but frequently enlarge to form large plaques, often with striking geographic outlines, or may produce marked swelling of the face or an extremity (angioedema). Acute urticaria is most commonly produced by foods, drugs, and insect bites. The cause of chronic recurrent urticaria is usually difficult to determine; psychosomatic influences undoubtedly play a role. Wheals are frequently a component of the eruption of erythema multiforme. Wheals ordinarily respond to antihistaminics, though large doses may be necessary. Corticosteroid therapy is usually promptly effective though the lesions recur quickly, often in more severe form, if such treatment is discontinued without removal of the primary etiologic factor.

Vesicles and Bullae. These are sharply circumscribed collections of free fluid in the skin, principally in the outer layers. The most common representatives of vesicular dermatoses are contact dermatitis, dyshidrosis of the hands and feet, and herpes simplex. In most instances the principal etiologic factor is readily determinable. Bullae, which are simply large vesicles, represent a very vigorous effort of the skin to counteract some noxious agent. Lesions may be bullous in a severe reaction to a contact allergen and, of course, chemical irritants or physical agents frequently produce a bullous reaction. Under such circumstances the cause is ordinarily readily apparent. In very extensive or chronic bullous eruptions thorough study is indicated. The more important diseases characterized by bullous lesions are pemphigus, dermatitis herpetiformis, erythema multiforme (Stevens-Johnson type). Bullae do not occur in psoriasis, in most types of dermatitis other than reactions to contactants or drug eruptions, or in acquired syphilis in the adult.

Pustules. Pustules are simply circumscribed collections of free pus, i.e., very superficial abscesses of the skin. Dermatoses showing both vesicles and pustules are very common, and vesicles frequently become pustular even in the absence of overt bacterial infection. Pustular lesions of the skin cover a very wide range of conditions. In pustular eruptions of more than a few days' duration pathogenic bacteria are frequently culturable, but it must not be assumed from this that all such organisms are necessarily acting as etiologic agents in the eruption.

Lesions Which Represent Sequential or Evolutionary Changes. *Scales.* These are simply accumulations of loose, horny fragments of stratum corneum. Certain types of scales are quite characteristic, e.g., the greasy, rather yellowish scales of chronic seborrheic dermatitis, or the silvery, piled-up scales of psoriasis. The chemical characteristics of scales vary considerably in different processes; e.g., it is possible to make a diagnosis of psoriasis in some instances by simple chemical tests of the scales. Such methods have not reached a level which is generally practical, but as knowledge of the normal and pathologic biochemistry of the skin increases, it should furnish aid in the diagnosis of obscure conditions.

Crusts (Scabs). These are the dried remains of exudate from oozing, erosive, or ulcerated skin lesions. They may consist of dried blood, serum, pus, or an admixture. Unless the diagnosis of a particular dermatosis is readily apparent, representative crusts should always be removed to see what lies underneath. One of the most characteristic of all crusts is that seen in diphtheria cutis, which produces a covering tenacious and adherent, unlike that seen in other bacterial infections.

Ulcers. Since ulcers represent a destructive process of the skin, they always require explanation. They may vary from small superficial erosions which heal without perceptible scarring to deep, sometimes widespread, lesions which involve underlying tissues or even adjacent bone. If the etiologic factor concerned is not readily apparent, such lesions deserve the most thorough study. The factors concerned may sometimes be multiple and obscure.

Scars. Scars may, of course, follow ulcers or may result from conditions in which there is no true ulceration, e.g., discoid lupus, atrophic lichen planus, stasis, or circumscribed scleroderma. As with ulcers, if the cause of the scarring is not apparent, thorough and searching study from all standpoints is indicated. The differentiation between temporarily hypertrophic scars and keloids is sometimes difficult to make; temporary hypertrophy and elevation of scars after injury is by no means uncommon and may persist for several months. Scars are frequently slightly painful or itchy. Scars from ionizing irradiation are particularly vulnerable to trauma of all types, especially sunlight. Extensive scars from whatever cause, but most particularly thermal burns, tuberculosis, and

x-ray therapy, are all prone to malignant changes.

Configuration of Lesions. Three characteristics of the *configuration* or *arrangement* of multiple lesions have considerable usefulness. They are:

Grouping. Characteristic grouped aggregations of vesicles occur in herpes simplex, zoster, and dermatitis herpetiformis. "Id" reactions in the skin to infections are sometimes grouped, i.e., in tuberculids or dermatophytids. The multicentric foci of epithelioma (*in situ* type) are frequently grouped and gradually coalesce to form a single tumor plaque.

Annularity. This is a striking feature of many dermatoses and reactions to systemic disease. Pityriasis rosea, lichen planus, superficial ringworm infections, bacterial infections, urticaria, erythema multiforme, sarcoidosis, discoid lupus, syphilis, deep fungous infections, and other processes may produce rather characteristic annular lesions.

Linearity. A linear arrangement of individual lesions may come about as part of the basic pattern of the disease, as in localized scleroderma, linear nevi, and even herpes zoster. In some diseases the skin reacts to trauma in a characteristic linear pattern as in lichen planus and psoriasis. Scars and keloids are frequently linear. Viral infections such as warts may be inoculated in the skin by a scratch.

The Primary Inoculation or Chancre Complex. The association of a lesion at the site of inoculation with regional adenopathy or with a more or less linear development of subsequent lesions is most commonly seen in acute bacterial infections (see p. 965). Syphilis produces the best known of all the chancre complexes, but this reaction is now observed rarely. Primary inoculations of tuberculosis and certain deep fungous infections such as blastomycosis, sporotrichosis, and coccidioidomycosis may follow a pattern of development of an inflammatory papule and ulcer at the site of inoculation. Regional adenopathy and the later development of inflammatory lesions along the areas of lymphatic drainage may occur. The recognition of such a mode of reaction is important in the case of tuberculosis or the deep fungous infections, as distinguished from spread of the lesions to the skin from a visceral focus, because the resistance displayed to the infection after inoculation in the skin is often very high, and such infections are usually self-limited.

Distribution of Lesion. In some diseases the *pattern of distribution of skin lesions* over the body is so characteristic as to be almost pathognomonic; in others, while one distribution pattern may be most characteristic, variations from it are frequent. The following are diseases which tend to involve certain sites.

Acne. Since acne is a disease in which the follicular orifices and sebaceous glands are affected, the lesions are concentrated in areas where these structures are most abundant, large, and active. The face is the most frequently involved site, but lesions appear on the shoulders, chest, upper back, neck, and upper arms in more extensive forms of the disease. The lack of involvement of the scalp is striking; even in the most severe cases only the scalp margins are invaded. An even more extensive distribution may be seen in so-called "tropical acne," in which the entire trunk may be affected, with lesions on the buttocks and thighs as well.

Rosacea. The lesions of rosacea occur in a highly characteristic pattern. In severe and long-standing examples, diffuse involvement of the face may be noted, but the flush areas are the sites affected initially. These are the malar prominences, the nose, the forehead, and point of the chin. Rosacea is often seen in middle-aged persons who have had acne in adolescence. There is frequently an associated seborrheic dermatitis. In the more severe forms pustules are common, but these do not characteristically derive from blackheads as does acne. The differentiation of rosacea from discoid lupus or systemic lupus erythematosus is ordinarily easily made, though, of course, the two conditions may coexist. The eyes should always be examined in rosacea, however mild, because of the infrequent but severe complication of rosacea keratitis.

Seborrheic Dermatitis. This is a third member of the common triad with acne and rosacea. In seborrheic dermatitis of moderate severity the scalp may be the only site involved, but the following areas are affected in approximate order of frequency in more extensive cases: eyebrows, skin above the bridge of the nose, sides of the nose, ears (especially the external auditory canals and retroauricular region), presternal and interscapular areas, eyelid margins (a frequent source of chronic blepharitis), intertriginous areas on any part of the body, especially the axillas, the anogenital region, and under the breasts in women. The skin of the involved areas is peculiarly susceptible to acute or chronic secondary bacterial infection; the intertriginous areas of the toes are rarely involved.

Psoriasis. A tendency to involve the scalp, knees, elbows, and back is characteristic of at least 75 per cent of all cases of psoriasis. The most common alternate distribution of psoriasis is to the seborrheic areas. Psoriasis is frequently misdiagnosed because of a failure to examine the skin carefully and to determine the presence of lesions elsewhere. This is likely if there is involvement of the nails (which is common in psoriasis), in which the condition may be wrongly diagnosed as a fungous infection; if there is involvement of the feet and hands, there may be confusion with ringworm infections and with syphilis; if there is involvement of the genitalia, it may be taken for moniliasis.

Pityriasis Rosea. The individual lesion of pityriasis rosea is annular and ovoid often with a slight border and a characteristic narrow band of moderate scaling just inside this border. In the efflorescence which follows the appearance of the primary or mother plaque the lesions tend to involve principally the trunk and upper portions of the extremities, with the long axis of the lesions strikingly arranged along the lines of cleavage. Even in examples of the disease in which the lesions themselves are unusual, namely, urticarial or more inflammatory, this distribution pattern still holds. The most common alternate distribution is a tendency for the lesions to occur distally on the extremities with relative absence of involvement of the trunk. Pityriasis rosea may involve the neck but rarely the face. It is a banal disease, though sometimes very worrisome to the patient. The course is that of a low-grade infection, though a causative organism has never been found. Second attacks occur in no more than one per cent of patients. Treatment is usually not necessary, but if the lesions are extensive, inflammatory, and pruritic, corticosteroid therapy for 3 to 4 days will usually give prompt relief.

Scabies. The female *Acarus* prefers the following sites for her burrows: the interdigital spaces of the fingers, the palms, the flexor surface of the wrists, the axillary folds, along the belt line, the buttocks, the genitalia in men, and about the areola of the breasts in women. The head is almost never involved in adults.

Atopic Dermatitis (Disseminated Neurodermatitis). The objective changes in this very chronic disease are principally the result of rubbing and excoriation; they involve the face, neck, antecubital spaces, popliteal fossae, wrists, and thighs. The condition commonly disappears after age twenty-five but sometimes persists in a more localized form such as a chronic dermatitis of the hands.

Contact Dermatitis. Reaction of the skin to external agents, which includes primary chemical irritant effects and true sensitization reactions, has a characteristic distribution involving the exposed sites in the case of industrial contactants, plants, and air-borne pollens and chemicals.

Lichen Planus. This chronic and pruritic disease is of little systemic significance. The milder forms involve the buccal surfaces of the cheek, the genitalia, the flexor surfaces of the wrists, and the trunk. In the hypertrophic form the most marked lesions may be found on the lower legs; this is the usual location of the lichen planus-like lesions of Atabrine dermatitis.

There are, of course, many other diseases with more or less characteristic patterns of distribution.

Approach through the Laboratory and Skin Testing

The laboratory aids used in general medicine are helpful in arriving at a diagnosis of a disease affecting the skin. Several special methods are useful.

Biopsy. Biopsy is an essential procedure in almost all chronic dermatoses, in all pigmented lesions which are excised, and in all lesions where there is a possibility of malignant change or serious systemic disease. The diagnosis of some lesions will require the services of a pathologist with special training in dermatopathology. Others present a clear-cut pathognomonic picture and are easily diagnosed by the general pathologist. A process involving the skin is seldom static. The skin is not bathed in a homeostatic milieu as are internal organs; it is subjected to numerous external influences which may disguise the primary process. It is the responsibility of the clinician to exercise care and judgment in the selection of the lesion to be examined, in determining which technique shall be used in obtaining the biopsy, and in providing an informative protocol. The specimen should be typical of the process and least subject to secondary trauma. Generally this is the most recently evolved lesion. Occasionally more than one biopsy may be required before the exact nature of a disease can be determined. Multiple biopsies may be needed in large lesions such as chronic ulcers evolving at the site of an old burn or in granuloma inguinale.

While consideration should be given to the cosmetic results in the procedure, it must be emphasized that an inadequate biopsy specimen benefits neither the pathologist, the physician, nor the patient. The most satisfactory procedure is removal of small lesions *in toto* (excision biopsy), and, with larger lesions, the removal of an elliptic specimen with its long axis through and at right angles to the border of the lesion. In selected instances, a 2-mm punch may provide adequate information and leave only a small inconsequential scar (see Fig. 11-1). A 5-mm biopsy punch is sometimes required. Bleeding may be stopped by pressure and the application of a small disk of gel foam or by electrodesiccation. The scar from this procedure is small and tends to contract and become more linear in the course of time.

Pathologic Patterns in the Skin. The fundamental pathologic changes in the skin are few and simple. Actually any cellular unit of the skin has but a triad of basic responses to multiple and diverse factors which cause disease. These are (1) *functional*—impairment of function in the absence of morphologic changes; (2) *inflammatory*—degenerative changes following cellular injury; and (3) *proliferative*—increase in the number of cells of given type, viz., tumors, benign or malignant.

For purposes of analysis Table 11-1 presents the units of the skin which may undergo changes and Fig. 11-2 diagrams these.

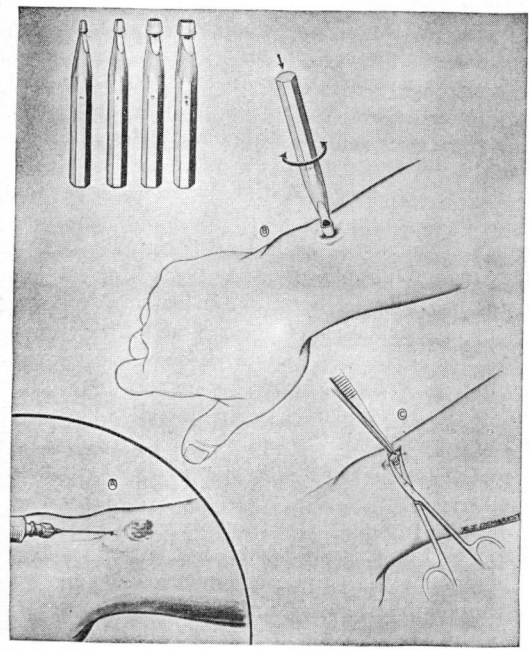

FIG. 11-1. Punch biopsy. This is a useful method for obtaining tissue from lesions in which complete excision is not feasible or when multiple biopsies may be desirable. The removal should extend to the subcutaneous fat. Punches of various diameters, 2 to 8 mm, are shown. (*D. M. Pillsbury, W. B. Shelley, and A. M. Kligman:* "Dermatology," *p. 1331, Philadelphia, W. B. Saunders Company, 1956.*)

Table 11-1. SKIN UNITS

Cells and layer		Epidermal appendages	Systems
Keratinocyte	} Epidermis	Hair	Vascular
Melanocyte		Sebaceous gland	Neural
Fibrocyte			
Histiocyte	} Dermis	Apocrine gland	Extraneous cells:
Mastocyte			
Lipocyte	Subcutaneous	Eccrine sweat gland	Myeloid
			Lymphoid

The clinician perceives three fundamental morphologic changes in the skin: in *color, mass,* or *fluid content*. The color changes (macules, plaques) usually involve the melanocyte or the vascular system. Changes in mass (papules, nodules, tumors) may result from hyperplasia of any of the units listed. Growths derived from the keratinocyte, melanocyte, and blood vessels are by far the most

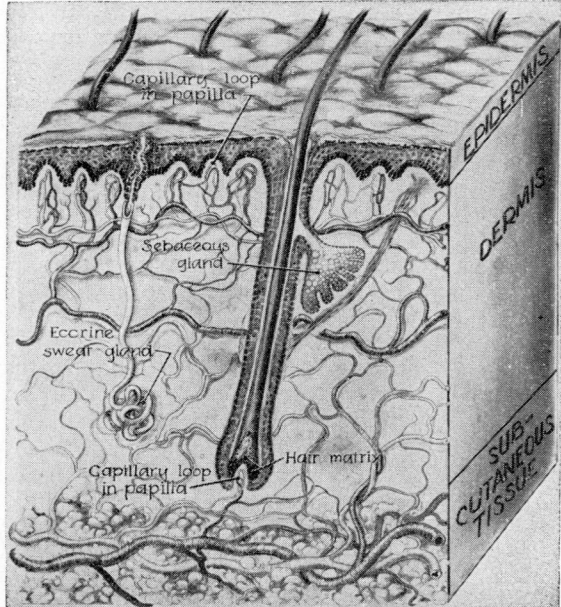

FIG. 11-2. The stratified organization of the skin. The top layer, the epidermis, is thin but solidly cellular, in contrast to the much thicker and largely fibrous corium which acts mainly as a support for the appendages, vessels, and nerves. The hair is the deepest epidermal appendage, extending down to the subcutaneous tissue, 3 to 5 mm below the surface. Just as the hair papilla is an invagination of connective tissue into the cellular hair matrix, so the papillae of the upper corium extend upward as connective tissue intrusions into the epidermis. Each papilla has a single capillary loop which nourishes the "cap" of epithelial cells overlying it (there are no blood vessels in the epidermis or hair matrix). Note that eccrine sweat is delivered directly to the surface, but sebum empties into the upper part of the follicle. (*D. M. Pillsbury, W. B. Shelley, and A. M. Kligman: "Dermatology," p. 3, Philadelphia, W. B. Saunders Company, 1956.*)

common. The change in free fluid of the epidermis (vesicle, bulla) is fundamentally a reaction of the keratinocyte to injury. In the dermis extravascular fluid masks itself clinically as a solid mass (urticaria).

Epidermis. Keratinocyte. *Keratinization is the most important function of the epidermis.* Disturbances or lack of other functions are inconvenient but rarely of crucial importance. Complete failure of keratinization is incompatible with life. In addition to the hyperkeratinization which results from chronic injury, certain genetically influenced changes may be seen, an example being congenital hyperkeratosis of the palms and soles. Psoriasis is another disease in which there is a disturbance of keratinization, with failure of the cycle to be completed. In ichthyosis the principal change appears

to be a retarded exfoliation of the stratum corneum. This may reach severe degrees and be accompanied by atrophy or absence of eccrine and sebaceous glands.

Melanocyte. This is the second important cell of the epidermis. In the albino, a genetic flaw in enzyme systems (tyrosinase) results in complete failure of pigment formation. Negro skin contains an increased amount of melanin but the same number of melanocytes as white skin. Local areas in which the melanocyte elaborates too little melanin (vitiligo, leukoderma) or too much melanin (chloasma, freckles) are frequent.

The melanin-synthesizing capacity of the skin is regulated by the melanocyte-stimulating hormone (MSH) of the anterior pituitary gland. There is a balance between this hormone and those elaborated by the adrenal cortex which furnishes an explanation for the pigmentation seen in Addison's disease and, perhaps, in pregnancy.

The melanocyte reacts to injurious stimuli by producing less or more melanin. Certain superficial inflammatory processes, e.g., seborrheic dermatitis, may produce temporary depigmentation, but the ordinary response is increased pigment. This is useful in protecting the skin from acute or chronic changes. The incidence of epithelioma is directly related to the amount of sunlight to which the skin of the patient is exposed and to a lessened ability to lay down protective melanin in the epidermis. With aging, the activity of melanocytes varies and dyspigmentation results.

Neoplastic change in the melanocyte accounts for the most common of all skin lesions, the ordinary pigmented nevus, or mole, and is the origin of the most malignant of all skin tumors (malignant melanoma). Simple hyperplasia leads to hyperpigmented, flat macules (lentigo, junction nevus), or even palpable masses. Usually brown or black, nevi may be flesh colored, indicating an absence of function in the hyperplastic cells. Not all melanocytic nevi are epidermal. Overgrowth of pigmented cells in the dermis gives a blue color (blue nevus, mongolian spot).

The interpretation of various types of pigmented lesions in the skin in terms of the possibility of malignant melanoma is a common and vexing clinical problem which is discussed in some detail later.

Corium (Dermis). The master cell of the dermis is the *fibrocyte,* the source of collagen and ground substance. Normal functioning of this cell is essential to skin repair. Unrestrained reparative activity can lead to large deposits of collagen (keloid). This condition is a steady increase in scar tissue which may continue indefinitely in some individuals, principally Negroes. Benign overgrowth of the fibrocyte produces a simple fibroma. Malignant change is rare and produces fibrosarcoma or "spindle cell" sarcoma. Cortisone prevents the normal development of collagenous tissue, and vitamin C deficiency interferes with the elaboration of normal reticulum.

Histiocytes normally phagocytize particulate matter, including melanin (melanophore), lipids (foam cell), hemosiderin, some tattoo pigments, viruses, bacteria, fungi, and protozoa. When confronted with larger masses of material (uric acid crystals, petrolatum), histiocytes commonly fuse to form multinucleated foreign-body giant cells. In xanthomas, multinucleated histiocytes filled with lipid droplets appear (Touton giant cells). In granulomas, the histiocytes change into epithelioid cells, which divide into another form of giant cell (Langhans). These are phagocytic and are distinctive of the general group of granulomas of the skin (syphilis, tuberculosis, leprosy, sarcoidosis, and deep mycoses).

The third principal type of cell in the corium is the *mast cell*. This requires special histologic methods for its demonstration and is rarely seen in routine biopsy specimens. The mast cell granules contain both heparin and histamine. The mast cells are localized about the vascular system. The signal protective role of the mast cell is shown by the fact that it releases its granules in response to any injury with production of immediate vascular changes and an outpouring of leukocytes and plasma from the blood stream. This appears to be the mechanism involved in the production of the *triple response* and in dermographism.

Overgrowth and aggregations of mast cells produce the condition known as *urticaria pigmentosa* which has been presumed to be a rare disease occurring almost entirely in childhood. However, this concept is being rapidly extended, and Table 11-2 indicates the various findings which may be encountered in this condition.

Lipocyte. In this, the chief cell of subcutaneous fat tissue, inflammatory changes are common. Nonspecific fat necrosis manifests itself in subcutaneous nodules which may or may not be tender. There is often a preceding history of trauma, including the injection of various medicinal compounds, or reactions to insect bites, or thermal injury. Occlusive peripheral vascular changes may impair circulation to the subcutaneous tissue sufficiently to result in formation of localized areas of fat necrosis.

A striking specific syndrome which involves fatty tissue is Weber-Christian disease (relapsing febrile nodular nonsuppurative panniculitis, see p. 1899).

Cytologic Smear (Tzanck Test). Cytologic examination of a fresh bulla is useful in the study of vesiculobullous eruptions. The youngest vesicular lesion present is swabbed with an alcohol sponge, the vesicle roof split with a scalpel, and the fluid sponged away with dry gauze. After the walls of the vesicle are reflected, the base of the lesion is

Table 11-2. CLINICAL AND LABORATORY FINDINGS IN THE MORE SERIOUS TYPES OF URTICARIA PIGMENTOSA (MASTOCYTOSIS)

Clinical

HISTORY: Months to years with pruritus and dermographism

AGE: Over 30 years

SEX: Either

SUBJECTIVE SYMPTOMS: Nausea, vomiting, weakness, and weight loss

SKIN MORPHOLOGY: Macular to nodular, red to brown, telangiectatic

VISCERAL: Hepatosplenomegaly

Laboratory

BIOPSY OF SKIN: Proliferation of mast cells

BONE CHANGES BY X-RAY: Generalized, osteoporotic, osteosclerotic, and thickened trabeculae of ribs, vertebras, long bones, and pelvis; when first seen it suggests miliary metastases from carcinoma, multiple myeloma, or myelofibrosis of depressed bone marrow

STERNAL MARROW: Mast cells sometimes present

BONE BIOPSY: Nests or sheets of mast cells

SPLEEN OR LIVER BIOPSY: Mast cells sometimes present

BLOOD STUDIES: Low normal or leukopenic, thrombocytopenic, and sometimes a monocytosis

SOURCE: W. R. Nickel, Urticaria Pigmentosa (Mastocytosis), A.M.A. Arch. Dermatol., 76:476–498, 1957.

scraped gently with a scalpel to remove the basal epidermal cells. The whitish material is smeared onto a clean glass slide, dried in air, fixed in methyl alcohol, and stained with a routine Giemsa stain. It can be mounted in balsam or examined directly after application of immersion oil to clear the cells. In pemphigus one sees numerous small round epithelial cells, many in isolated form. No prickle cells are seen, and there is a basic acantholysis. The nucleus is large in relation to the cytoplasm which may be condensed in a basophilic peripheral ring.

In herpes simplex, zoster, or varicella, the typical and significant cytologic findings are polymorphism and giant multinuclear epithelial cells.

Demonstration of Organisms. The most commonly employed procedure here is the study of scales, hair, and nails for the presence of fungi. Scales scraped from the periphery of a lesion are placed on a microscope slide in a drop of 10 per cent aqueous potassium hydroxide. Clearing occurs rapidly with warming, and under "high dry" magnification one may see the delicate hyphae of the organism. If the skin surface has been cleansed before making the scraping, any fungi demonstrated are significant and pathogenic. Cultures of the scales may also be made to determine the specific organism present. Such planting of scales on Sabouraud's agar is followed (in a few weeks of room temperature incubation) by the appearance of a colony, often grossly identifiable to the mycologist.

Regular bacteriologic isolation techniques and antibiotic sensitivity testing of the pathogenic staphylococci should be employed in resistant pyodermas.

The dark-field examination of material from genital and other lesions suggesting infectious syphilis is still a valuable procedure, although it is being employed with decreasing frequency.

Likewise, at times, virologic isolation procedures may be carried out by specialized laboratories. Finally smears from granulomatous lesions may be stained for the presence of Donovan bodies when granuloma inguinale is suspected.

Skin Tests. The accessibility of the skin offers an unrivaled opportunity for in vivo testing of the cutaneous effects of a wide variety of chemicals and biologic products. Nearly all these tests are done to detect the unusual or allergic response as an explanation for the appearance of disease. The universal response such as irritation of the skin from acids and alkalies can generally be recognized by the history without recourse to testing.

Patch Tests. The most commonly employed tests involve contact reactions to substances applied topically, e.g., under a Band-Aid for a period of up to 48 hr. The disease in miniature is thus produced in the sensitive person. The procedure is not so benign and simple as it might appear since all substances must be applied in a concentration such as to be without primary irritancy (for representative dilutions see the tables of Baer and Witten). It should not be used indiscriminately; in exquisitely sensitive individuals it may lead to a bullous reaction so intense as to produce depigmentation, scarring, or even a generalized reaction. It has no value in predicting which persons may later become sensitized. However, intelligently used as an adjunct to a careful history, it is valuable in tracking the specific cause of a contact dermatitis.

Intradermal Tests. An unbelievably wide array of commercially available extracts are available for scratch and intradermal skin testing. The *immediate* reaction is urticarial and erythematous, and it would seem to duplicate the disease; yet the method is of limited usefulness in clinical practice.

The prototype of the *delayed* reaction is the tuberculin skin test in which the inflammatory reaction occurs at 48 hr. This has considerable value in the assessment of lesions suspected to be allergic in nature (e.g., tuberculids). Many other biologic allergens are available, e.g., trichophytin, histoplasmin, and coccidioidin. All are used on occasion.

New agents for skin testing in cutaneous autoimmune states include erythrocytes and leukocytes. Here the reaction may be an immediate wheal type or a delayed inflammatory one.

Finally, attention is directed to the significance of the sarcoid skin test which represents a 4 to 6 week delayed skin reaction. In this instance the material is introduced intradermally (Kveim antigen, lepromin, zirconium, beryllium). A positive reaction consists of the appearance of a papule which histologically is sarcoid in nature (pure epithelioid tubercles). This appears to represent a distinctive type of delayed allergic response which reduplicates the disease *in situ*. It should receive increasing attention in the study of sarcoidosis.

Physical Allergy. Abnormal reactions to sunlight may account for a great variety of cutaneous changes. This problem of *photosensitivity* is best attacked by specific light testing procedures. Practical information can be obtained by exposing a small test site of the patient's skin to radiation from a carbon arc or hot quartz lamp. If marked photosensitivity is suspected, however, such tests should be considered very carefully. They are contraindicated in any patient suspected of having systemic lupus erythematosus.

Hypersensitivity to cold is easily demonstrated in some patients by contact of the skin with ice. Here the common reaction is an immediate urticarial one. In other individuals a general fall in skin temperature is the trigger mechanism, and testing in a cool room may be necessary.

Heat hypersensitivity likewise may be elicited either by a local or general increase in the temperature. In the local type, heating produces a local wheal, whereas in the generalized cholinergic type, exercise or a hot bath induces numerous small wheals with considerable axon reflex erythema.

Special Tests for Function of Appendages of Skin. *Sweating.* Hyperhidrosis is obvious, but detection of anhidrosis requires actual observation of the patient under a heat stimulus. A regular heat cabinet offers the best tool, but too often improvised arrangements with infrared bulbs, blankets, and hot drinks have to suffice. The most satisfactory objective recording of the response is achieved with the starch paper iodine print method of Randall.

Sebum Formation. The secretion of the sebaceous gland is generally an invisible film of oil, but at times on the face and scalp one may see droplets of sebum which simulate eccrine sweat. These two secretions can be distinguished by making a contact print with a clean glass slide or paper. Sweat rapidly evaporates, whereas sebum does not.

Hair. In addition to biopsy and mycologic studies, examination of plucked hairs under the microscope gives a valuable assessment of general health changes in the patient during the past months. The shaft diameter quickly reflects general disturbances, including radiation damage. It is also possible to prognosticate in cases of alopecia by making a count of the relative number of hairs in a quiescent nongrowing state. The resting hair

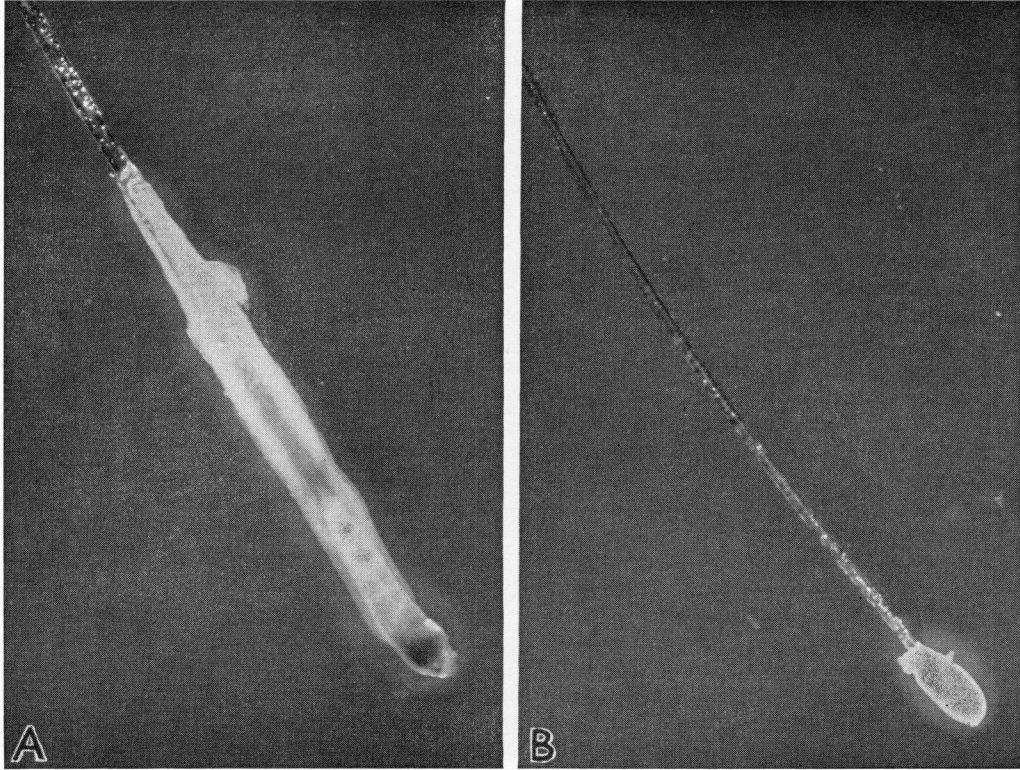

Fig. 11-3. Plucking the hair will show whether it is growing or resting (provided it does not break off). *A.* A growing hair. The hair root is surrounded by an extensive translucent sheath, and the proximal tip is deeply pigmented. The hair itself may be seen within the sheath. *B.* A resting or club hair. All that is seen is a bulbous, nonpigmented tip. There is no sheath save for an inconspicuous one limited to the very tip of the hair. Club hairs are also likely to be somewhat lighter and thinner, because pigment production and keratin synthesis diminish when the hair nears the end of the growth phase. (*D. M. Pillsbury, W. B. Shelley, and A. M. Kligman: "Dermatology," p. 42, Philadelphia, W. B. Saunders Company, 1956.*)

has an atrophic club ending quite unlike the ensheathed pigmented hair which is still growing. If the club hair percentage is above 20, this augurs further hair loss in the near future (see Fig. 11-3).

Nail. Using a small punch, biopsies may be secured of the nail plate and its underlying bed. If the matrix area is not entered, no deformity results. The most common examination, however, is of scrapings for fungi. It must not be forgotten that nail growth rates may be accurately observed by filing or cutting a transverse band at the base of the nail.

Blood Tests. Certain blood tests relate more specifically to skin disturbances. These include the serologic test for syphilis, lupus erythematosus test, demonstration of cryoglobulins, and detection of circulating cancer cells. In allergic studies, passive transfer tests may be employed occasionally.

Urine. The presence of porphyrins, melanin, or hemoglobin may herald the cutaneous signs of porphyria, malignant melanoma, or physical allergy.

COMMON DISTURBANCES OF THE SKIN

Dryness. There is probably no more universal complaint than that of dryness. Everyone from time to time experiences areas of dryness of the skin, and a host of creams and emollients are in daily use for the relief of this symptom. If we look into the causes for dryness, we come upon an interesting story which relates to the thin cellular sheath which envelops us, the epidermis. Before detailing this, it is well to note that the exquisitely sensitive tactile receptor system in the finger tips is largely responsible for our full awareness of the presence of dryness. Furthermore, dryness may be accompanied by subclinical inflammatory change so that pruritus and related sensations may arise in the area under question. Thus, major changes are usually not involved but rather a delicate change in the physicochemistry of our outermost covering. This epidermis is paper thin and composed entirely of two sets of cells. One, the keratinocyte, is concerned solely with the elaboration of a resistant fibrous coating; the other, the melanocyte, produces the light protective melanin which will be discussed in the next section.

The keratinocyte over a period of a month goes through a life cycle dedicated to the manufacture of a keratin surface made up entirely of fused dead cells. It is in this stratum corneum or outermost layer of dead keratinocytes that the changes occur which we sense as dryness. This layer is a virtual hygrometer showing physical changes which reflect the interplay of atmospheric conditions and the chemistry of the surface. When the ambient environment has a low absolute humidity, this stratum corneum loses water at a rate faster than it can be replaced from below. Once the water content drops below 10 per cent, the keratin layer becomes hard and brittle. The skin looks dry and scaly. Chapping soon ensues since this brittle membrane breaks, fissures, and cracks with every movement, much as might an old leather book binding. Dry skin is not due to absence of sebum or grease, but rather to the absence of water. A supple pliable epidermis reflects a well-hydrated stratum corneum. Without water no amount of greasing will correct the problem, and it is interesting that the most popular creams for relief of dryness contain a goodly pecentage of water.

Merely soaking the skin in water does not afford other than transient relief, and soaking actually is deleterious. Hence, *overbathing* in the winter in the northern climes is the most common cause of dryness of the skin and its later concomitants of itch and dermatitis. It removes much of the water-binding chemical system from the stratum corneum, even as do harsh organic solvents. Furthermore, the intimate relationship of the finely meshed dead cells is disrupted, leading to scaling and dryness. Many times also the underlying viable keratinocytes are damaged so that a defective or excessive stratum corneum develops as a later change. Once the defatting and dehydrating influences have been at work, it is necessary to keep the skin under optimal conditions for at least a month before normal hydration and texture will return.

In summary, dryness may reflect a low absolute humidity in the environment (winter, chemical industries) or a late effect of nonspecific damage to the epidermis. It calls for protection of the skin, mild hydrated emollients, some avoidance of bathing, and measures to increase the humidity of the air.

Pigmentary Changes. Although the melanocytes are but 5 per cent of the cell population of the epidermis, they account for the major portion of skin coloring. Pigments circulating in the blood may account for altered hues, e.g., carotenemia and jaundice, but the degree and extent of epidermal and dermal melanin dispersion are the chief determinant of skin color. Remove the melanin and one has the albino, increase it and one sees the black skin.

Melanocytes are immigrant cells of the epidermis. Stemming embryologically from the neural crest, they come into close symbiotic existence with the keratinocytes after a polar migration to the edge of the body. Those few cells which fail to reach the epidermal borders may rest in the dermis, still forming melanin. Here, in the dermis, because of optical principles, the color is blue-black rather than the brown pigment to which we are accustomed in epidermal tanning. Melanocytes retain their nerve cell anatomy with long branching dendrites which embrace the surrounding basal keratinocytes, curiously, infusing them with melanin. The degree of color is entirely controlled by the *activity* of the cell, and this hyperpigmentation does not spell an increase in the *number* of melanocytes. The cell is under precisely known hormonal and local influences (see p. 788).

Keratin coloring agents have been introduced commercially to simulate sun tan. These contain dihydroxyacetone, an intermediate in the metabolism of carbohydrates. Within hours of application of the colorless 5 per cent aqueous solution, the skin becomes a light brown and remains so for several days. The reaction occurs in the dead stratum corneum. Hair and nails are not affected since only the soft keratin reacts. Although the speed of reaction is temperature sensitive, it is in no way related to sunlight or melanin. In some patients, depigmented spots can be successfully covered by the use of this new agent.

Itching. No sensation is more uniquely cutaneous than itching. Defined as the urge to scratch, itching signals damage to the epidermis. Unlike pain, it is not a universal sensation, but is limited to the skin. It is a pathologic sensation and hence one that received little attention from the sensory physiologists. Itching cannot be elicited by atraumatic means such as pressure or temperature change. Trauma to the epidermis is necessary; yet this must be of a degree that will not destroy the filamentous intraepidermal nerve receptor network. Furthermore, individual differences are of crucial importance. Some patients are "itchish" just as others are ticklish, and there are others who are itch insensitive. These individuals may experience mosquito bites, poison ivy dermatitis, and even scabies without the itch. It is little wonder then that the clinician sees a most capricious patterning in this sensory modality.

Under ordinary testing, stimuli adequate for the elicitation of pain, heat, cold, or touch completely fail to produce pruritus. Yet these same stimuli, if applied in a punctate manner to certain specific sensitive points on the skin, will give rise to pruritus. Thus, we see that there are itch points, but that under ordinary circumstances the sensations of pain, heat, cold, or touch are prepotent inasmuch as purely spatial relationships favor these other sensations. Nevertheless, using chemical stimuli, it is possible to elicit a clear pure signal of pruritus with intensity duplicating the maddening itch seen clinically. The first such compound to be identified was histamine. Later it was learned that the histamine liberators were equally active. It would appear then that pruritus is a sensation mediated by histamine. However, this has not received full acceptance inasmuch as histamine never produces pruritus without an accompanying hive response; yet many of the most severe itches occur in skin which appears completely normal. Indeed histamine may be diluted out to a point where it elicits only wheal and flare, but no itching. Nevertheless it must be recognized that release of microquantities of histamine from the mast cell at the critical itch points might initiate pruritus without clinical whealing, even though it evades experimental demonstration as yet.

More distinctive pruritogenic stimuli are those of the proteinase group. It has been found that proteinases (endopeptidases) which act in the physiologic pH range are remarkably active in eliciting itch. In normal skin, 0.1 μg may be active, and in the sensitive skin of the atopic as little as 0.01 μg has been an effective stimulus for itching. On a molar basis, a typical pruritogenic proteinase, papain, was found to be 200 times more active than histamine. Even more significant, crystalline papain will produce pruritus in the absence of wheal and flare. Known sources are the epidermal cells (cathepsins), the blood (plasmin, erythrocyte protease, and leukoproteases), and microbiologic flora (proteinases of bacteria and fungi). Most significant is the fact that pruritus is the hallmark of the cutaneous allergic state, and allergic reactions involve the release of proteases as well as histamine. Thus it seems evident that the peripheral mechanism of clinical itch involves the participation of histamine and/or proteases.

Just what is the itch receptor? It consists of the peripheral fringe of unmyelinated fine fibers as found in increased number in certain epidermal and subepidermal loci. There are no specialized nerve endings subserving this sensation. Rather one finds a large rich nondifferentiated nerve net growing out into the epidermis. The specificity and sensitivity of the itch receptor must reside in other than peripheral neuroanatomic findings. The analysis of experimental itch would suggest, however, that itching is carried over the small fine unmyelinated or C fibers. In this and other ways, itch appears to be related to burning pain.

From the clinical standpoint any significant degree of pruritus deserves as close an examination and explanation as does pain. Probably the most common cause is dry skin. In these instances, detergents, hot water, and frequent bathing are an "unholy three" of causative factors which rarely appear except as a result of direct interrogation of the patient. It is especially common in the older individual who does not alter his life-long bathing habits to conform with the decreased resistance of his aging skin to the trauma of soap and water. Advice as to the cause and regular use of emollient creams often offer considerable relief.

Often it is difficult to ascertain if a primary dermatitis is present or not. Scratch marks, secondary bacterial infection, and contact dermatitis due to overtreatment may all be present. Sometimes a "drug holiday" must be declared for both topical and systemic preparations since these may be the very causes of the pruritus. The absence of primary skin changes suggests that some circulating agent is releasing proteinase to produce the itch signal. Allergens are a common cause. In trace amounts they can produce an almost unbearable pruritus—yet without visible skin alterations. It is both hazardous and ill-informed to dismiss such complaints as "the result of tensions." The search for causative allergens such as drugs, foods, chemicals, and inhalants must go on.

Diabetes mellitus, Hodgkin's disease, and pregnancy are three common causes of pruritus. Other instances reflect a sensitization reaction to a malignancy. Renal, hepatic, and thyroid disturbances also initiate generalized pruritus. Intestinal parasites are an unusual but definite cause. Many psychiatric disorders have an accompanying pruritus, and unquestionably there are psychogenic factors contributing to pruritus. For example, the tense individual experiences a greater problem with itching than others. Many mechanisms may be operative. In some persons, a hyperactive scratch reflex produces a hyperalgesic area of skin, and this leads to an unfortunate itch-scratch cycle. In others, autonomic nerve discharges produce sweating and miliaria. In such instances the escape of sweat into the epidermal tissue may initiate marked itching. Flushing is another mechanism since this increases the skin temperature with a consequent rise in the sensitivity of the itch network. In addition, new evidence suggests that autonomic nerves may release histamine and so induce itching. Here during an attack one can detect small urticarial wheals in good cross lighting.

Insect bites, if unnoticed by the patient, may also pass undetected by the physician since they are often completely debrided by the energetic scratch reflex. In children, sensitization reactions to the insect may occur, leading to a chronic reaction known as *papular urticaria*. Until exposure to the insect (e.g., dog or sand flea) is eliminated, the problem persists as intractable pruritus. Lice, with their regional predilections, are another cause of pruritus. Another occult parasitic cause is scabies, the illustrious "seven-year itch." It still occurs, and in the "well-washed" is hard to detect. At times these patients are subjected to lengthy allergic studies when a therapeutic trial with a modern scabicide (e.g., benzyl benzoate) would convert the process into a "seven-hour" itch.

Turning to the specific dermatologic entities or reaction patterns, allergic *contact dermatitis* is the most common acute cause of itching. Occurring on any part of the body and readily recognized with respect to nature, if not as to specific excitant, this condition is virtually always pruritic. Nevertheless, *atopic dermatitis* is the cause of the most severe chronic pruritus. Here the itch may be one of years! A constant complicating factor is that of sweat retention. Each burst of sweat may trigger a fierce burst of itching.

Actually, primary *miliaria* or prickly heat is a pruritic dermatitis purely on the basis of this sweat retention. In hot humid weather and especially in infants, it accounts for much of the pruritus. Characterized by an eruption which waxes and wanes with the temperature, miliaria responds best to a cool environment. *Urticaria* with its attendant release of histamine from the mast cell is another pruritic eruption. *Seborrheic dermatitis* is also pruritic and is an especially common cause of itching of the scalp. Among the rare dermatoses, lichen planus and dermatitis herpetiformis are the two with the most astounding and regular degree of pruritus.

Treatment of pruritus is ideally achieved by elimination of the cause. Often such an ideal is not rapidly reached, and the patient must have the benefit of symptomatic measures. Among these, topical approaches are very valuable. If left to their own devices, patients may desperately eliminate itching by actual destruction of the epidermal nerve network, e.g., steaming hot water, fingernail strippings of the skin, or application of caustic chemicals. It is safer to instruct these patients on the use of the bland cool compress. Local anesthetics are often employed, but here the danger of sensitization is ever present. Topical steroids are also effective in that they reduce the inflammatory component. At times topical antibiotics are also remarkably helpful. In some, chronic lichenified plaques may best be treated by an occlusive dressing with 3 per cent ichthammol in zinc oxide ointment. For larger areas the use of a calamine liniment or lotion with 0.1 per cent camphor and 1 per cent menthol gives considerable relief.

Systemically, the best symptomatic relief is often provided by the use of a tranquilizer, such as Temaril or Librium. There is no analgesic with a specific effect on itching, but Temaril and Librium seem to act centrally to allay pruritus or the cortical response to it. Possibly they also act by reducing autonomic activity. Papaverine and aspirin have been used by some individuals with help. Actually, systemic steroids afford the most effective treatment for the marked itching that is associated with any extensive dermatitis. The action of these agents is anti-inflammatory, and the antipruritic benefits are secondary but real. Such powerful agents must not be used for "mosquito bites" but rather reserved for the serious widespread forms of pruritus. Occasional patients benefit from systemic antibacterial agents which reduce the secondary bacterial population of infected dermatitis. Although ordinary pyodermas do not itch, in dermatitic skin, bacterial proteinases may cause considerable pruritus. In some atopics, anticholinergic compounds (Prantal) may be indicated to reduce the sweating and miliarial component responsible for itching.

Finally, the patient should be told to avoid any trauma to the skin such as might come from alcohol rubs, frequent bathing, sensitizing drugs, and woolen clothing.

Anhidrosis—Hyperhidrosis. *Anhidrosis,* as the failure to sweat, is often an elusive subtle sign of disease which must be searched out by actual testing. Many patients are unaware of the presence of this defect but come complaining of fever, heat intolerance, headaches, and fatigue. Only after observation during heat stress does the sign of anhidrosis become apparent.

The eccrine sweat glands which number over two million constitute an invisible system for thermoregulation. The obvious and rather exclusive function of the gland is to secrete water for evaporative cooling. Hence, widespread anhidrosis may make the patient completely intolerant to heat. The gland is not an excretory unit, although certain elements of the extracellular fluid are perforce excreted. Most prominent among these is sodium chloride, which may be lost in considerable amounts in profuse sweating. However, this loss is greatly reduced in the well-functioning acclimatized gland. Other elements are found in rather small amounts. In view of this, one does not see any real change in the excretory work of the kidney associated with anhidrosis. The gland itself functions in response to cholinergic impulses from the sympathetic branch autonomic nerve network. Centrally, the hypothalamic heat regulatory center controls the sweat glands through the autonomic nerves.

Clinically, the causes of anhidrosis are legion and must be reviewed in any given case. Disease or disturbance of the hypothalamus (as in surgery, heat stroke, neoplasm, or vascular accident) may well account for a generalized anhidrosis. Hysteria appears in the literature also as a cause of anhidrosis. Cord changes interfere by cutting off the efferent pathways. Such changes include multiple sclerosis, syringomyelia, and poliomyelitis. Likewise, the peripheral autonomic fibers or adenoneural junction may be affected as in leprosy, sympathectomy, or autonomic blockage. In diabetes mellitus and gout there may be destruction of the peripheral network of nerves, with postural hypotension as well as anhidrosis.

At the level of the sweat gland, anhidrosis may reflect congenital absence or dysplasia. Ichthyosis is often associated with anhidrosis. Widespread skin diseases such as psoriasis, atopic dermatitis, miliaria also show anhidrotic areas. Many of these changes are transient, but in burn scars, sweating may be permanently eliminated by the destructive effects.

Treatment ranges from the obvious attack on the primary problem to acquainting the patient with the environmental limitations which the anhidrosis imposes. By avoiding or reducing heat stresses, these patients may live normal lives. The widespread appearance of air conditioning has been an especial boon in this regard.

Hyperhidrosis is the classic sign of fever, exercise, or heating. Here the body is attempting to reduce the temperature by evaporative cooling. Less often, one may see "cold sweat" in such disturbances as motion sickness. Actually the most common form of hyperhidrosis is the localized form of excessive sweating seen as a result of emotional stimuli. This is the axillary, palmar, or plantar outpouring of sweat as a result of excitement, fear, pain, or even mental effort. Often the degree of sweating is annoying, but only rarely is it disabling. Sympathectomy has been employed with success for some examples of recalcitrant palmar hyperhidrosis. Generally, topical astringents are employed or systemic anticholinergic drugs. However, the results are not entirely satisfactory.

Odor. Although eccrine sweat is devoid of odor, it does promote the growth of bacteria which are responsible for surface odor. The distinctive axillary odor interestingly results from the growth of these surface bacteria on the apocrine sweat substrate. The apocrine sweat, coming from a unique large sweat gland appendage of the hair follicle, is both sterile and odorless. Yet on the skin surface it serves as the substrate for bacterial action forming malodorous fatty acids. This odor is restricted to the few areas of the body where the apocrine glands are found. Significantly the apocrine gland is under adrenergic innervation and responds to stress.

Seborrhea. The skin surface is continuously supplied with a thin surface film of oil or sebum which arises from the sebaceous glands. Excess oil production has received the term of seborrhea. The absence of oil production is clinically inapparent so that the condition has received scant interest and hence no real name. Many of these patients are simply described as having dry skin, since reduction in sebum production is associated with a reduction in the potential water content of the stratum corneum.

Seborrhea is common. For a closer view of its nature, we look to the sebaceous gland. This gland is under hormonal control to a degree, androgens promoting its growth and estrogens causing a reduction in size. It is thus at puberty that physiologic seborrhea becomes most evident. Unlike the eccrine sweat glands, the sebaceous glands are not randomly distributed over the skin surface, nor are they innervated. The richest supply is on the face, scalp, and chest. There is a striking diminution in size and number of the glands as one proceeds distalward, so that the gland is completely absent on the palms and soles. The sebaceous gland is holocrine in secretory activity, each cell being swept out as an oily end product of the life cycle. In the extremes of age, oil production is considerably reduced as compared with puberty. In some instances a central nervous system control appears evident, e.g., in the seborrhea of parkinsonism. The mechanism remains obscure.

Little can be done to counteract the problem of seborrhea since the growth rate of the gland (just as in the case of hair and nails) is evidence of a normal metabolic activity. However, frequent removal of the surface oil aids in preventing the complications of bacterial infection. Certainly soap and water or an alcohol pad is effective. In acne, where the sebaceous gland is a central target organ, this is especially important.

Alopecia and Hirsutism. Although strictly an atavistic organ beyond modern need, hair receives an inordinate amount of attention from the patient. As a cosmetic status symbol, hair is a primary concern of nearly everyone. Over and above this concern there are observations to be made on the hair of considerable medical significance.

Hairs arise from a specialized epidermal follicle which has a remarkable capacity for keratin synthesis. Taking the scalp hair as a prototype we find that these keratin cells continuously replace themselves, leading to a daily holocrine extrusion of cells measuring 0.35 mm in length. This intense reproductive cycle is the natural target for any toxic influence. It is especially valuable as a sensitive indicator of the toxic effects of cancer chemotherapeutic agents. One does not wait for a defluvium, but rather hairs are manually epilated and examined under magnification. Normally about 85 per cent of the hairs are growing; the remainder being in a resting phase. In illness and during cancer chemotherapy, the percentage of growing hairs drops considerably. Even more striking are the effects on the hair shaft diameter. There are marked inhibitory effects, with constriction of the hair shaft. At points of severe constriction the hairs break off. Dysplastic hair roots have also been observed in patients after prolonged application of selenium sulfide shampoo. This is in agreement with the fact that selenium sulfide shampoos may cause a reversible type of hair loss.

Certain hairs give a clue as to the hormonal status of the patient. These are the hairs of the axilla, pubes, beard, and chest, forming a secondary sex characteristic. It is the male hormone testosterone which governs these sex hairs in both women and men. In contrast, androgens are believed responsible for the loss of hair which occurs on the scalp. Male castrates never become bald, nor do they have axillary, pubic, beard, or body hair. Androgens will completely reverse this. Other hormones appear to play no primary role in hair growth.

Hair growth is cyclic in contrast to the nail where growth is continuous. In the scalp the hair may grow for 2 to 6 years or longer. The resting hair remains passively in the follicle until expelled by the infant hair of an entirely new follicle. Unlike animals who show these cycles in waves for the entire hair growth, man has a random loss of only a small amount at one time. Man has approximately 100,000 scalp hairs, so that 10,000 to 20,000 random hairs are in a resting stage. These latter hairs will all fall out day by day over the following few months. It is no wonder that man normally sheds up to 100 scalp hairs a day. In this way the hair loss is not apparent in man until large numbers of hairs go into the resting phase as in the postpartum period, in illness, or as a result of toxic drugs. By plucking hairs one can easily count the number of club (resting) hairs and prognosticate for the patient experiencing hair thinning (Fig. 11-3). Further hair loss is imminent if the club count exceeds 20 or 30 per cent.

It should be realized that the hair shaft is a dead, inert structure. No force, chemical or physical, applied solely to its surface can harm or help the regenerative hair-forming system below the skin surface. Many popular "remedies" for baldness are entirely without basis except as occupational therapy for the patient.

Alopecia may follow any deep scarring reaction in the scalp, e.g., burn, radiodermatitis, carbuncle, herpes zoster, and lupus erythematosus. It also occurs in the absence of any skin change. The most common example of this is the patterned baldness of hereditary origin which is seen in men and to a lesser degree in women. It is an aging change,

and little can be done to arrest its inexorable course. Far better in prognosis is the distinctive condition, *alopecia areata*. In this disease, patches of complete hair loss are seen, and occasionally every terminal (large coarse) hair of the body may fall out. Often associated with emotional shock, alopecia areata is usually followed by regrowth of the lost hair within months. At times systemic steroids are employed to stimulate hair regeneration. As mentioned above, debilitating diseases, especially those with high fevers, may cause diffuse or even total hair loss. In turn, heparin, thallium, vitamin A (large amounts), and cancer chemotherapy may likewise be responsible for hair loss. Some individuals pull hairs out consciously or unconsciously. Finally, in children, patchy loss of hair often spells tinea capitis.

Melanocytes in the bulb of the hair follicle are responsible for the color of the hair, and it is their failure which leads to graying. This may be the typical age change or may correspond to a congenital problem such as vitiligo. At other times gray hair may be the regrowth in a patch of alopecia areata. It has been observed that chloroquine causes loss of hair color in those patients having red, light brown, or yellow hair. Apparently these patients have a melanocyte producing pheomelanins in place of regular melanin, and the chloroquine specifically blocks this latter pathway.

Hirsutism or excessive hair is commonly a problem of females. In its idiopathic form it occurs on the chin, cheeks, upper lip, and chest of women. Much of this represents a genetic trait and appears as a racial characteristic. In a few, it may herald endocrinologic disturbances, even a masculinizing tumor of the ovary. Careful endocrinologic survey is advisable. The adrenal may be the source of the masculinizing hormones, as in Cushing's disease. The same effect may follow corticosteroid therapy or may develop during pregnancy.

In the hereditary type of hirsutism, epilation by electrolysis is the only satisfactory approach leading to permanent help. Even here, caution must be observed by an experienced operator to prevent scarring. *X-rays must not be used.* Plucking the hairs mechanically is a safe but temporary measure. Some are able to bleach the excess hairs to an unobtrusive blonde.

Nail Changes. The fingernail plate offers the clinician a quick retrospective view of the patient's general condition for the past 4 or 5 months. Actually toenail plate records history for 18 months but is less reliable because of the trauma of footgear and the common presence of fungous infection of the nail. The nail plate is a hard keratin product of the ever-active nail matrix. It is colorless and without melanin pigment; yet when the nail separates from its underlying bed it becomes whitish. The pink color of the major portion of the plate reflects the rich vascular plexus in the nail bed. The *lunula* is a semilunar white region at the proximal end of the plate, generally found in the thumb nail. It corresponds to the tip of the nail forming matrix of cells. White spots in the nail are entirely different. These *leukonychia* result from errors in keratinization, sometimes from trauma.

The nail bed forms an intimate firm union with the plate, and a unique forward and linear co-growth occurs. This can be shown by the way a hematoma under the plate gradually moves outward, eventually being swept away by the growth currents. Any foreign matter under the nail may experience the same fate. Normally the nail bed does not keratinize except at the distal end. However, in a disease such as psoriasis, subungual masses of dead soft keratin may pile up, making a bizarre dystrophic pattern.

Fine longitudinal ridges are seen in the normal plate. In the aged they appear as bold ribs, a predictable nonpathologic process marking the trail to senility. Longitudinal splitting of the nails always follows the potential cleavage planes of these natural striations. Horizontal splitting is, on the contrary, rare.

Defects in the posterior nail matrix result in surface defects of the plate. Such pitting and superficial wrinkling represent transient interference with nail synthesis. A permanent injury to a localized area of matrix understandably gives rise to a longitudinal defect in the plate seen as a ridge or groove. Likewise, a transverse depression or thinning (Beau's line) must represent a temporary pause in nail growth, usually the result of a severe systemic reaction such as a coronary thrombosis or high fever. By measuring the distance from the furrow to the cuticle, one can estimate the date of the illness, by assuming a daily growth rate of 0.1 mm. The matrix is most commonly damaged by a dermatitis of the posterior nail fold or by paronychia. Chronic eczema of the fingers accounts for much in the way of nail dystrophy. Another force to be reckoned is the effect of periarticular and osteitic processes in the terminal joint which will also affect the matrix. Synovial cysts, verrucae, and other growths may likewise produce nail plate changes.

Nail disorders of a more primary type are seen in *psoriasis* and *fungous infections*. These two cannot be clearly distinguished by clinical inspection. It is necessary to do mycologic studies to rule out onychomycosis. Thickened nails often result from trauma. Atrophy of nails may be the result of trophic vascular changes, mutilating dermatoses, or congenital influences.

Many women complain of fraying, brittle or weak nails. Some of this results from use of organic solvents to remove nail polish, detergents, soap and water, as well as heredity and aging. It is likely that a program of protection of the nails is the best treatment, although this must be persisted in for a period of over 6 months to permit the appearance of an entirely new plate. Splintered nails are often seen also in association with alopecia areata.

Actual defluvium of all the nails may occur in severe illness due to interference with nail synthesis.

REFERENCES

ALOPECIA—HIRSUTISM

Flesh, P.: Hair Growth, in "Physiology and Biochemistry of Skin," S. Rothman (Ed.), Chicago, University of Chicago Press, 1954.

ANHIDROSIS—HYPERHIDROSIS

DeTakats, G.: Surgical Treatment of Hyperhidrosis, A.M.A. Arch. Dermatol., 76:31, 1957.

Hurley, H. J., and W. B. Shelley: "The Human Apocrine Sweat Gland in Health and Disease," Springfield, Ill., Charles C Thomas, Publisher, 1960.

Shelley, W. B., P. N. Horvath, and D. M. Pillsbury: Anhidrosis: An Etiologic Interpretation, Medicine, 29:195, 1950.

DRYNESS

Blank, I. H.: Factors Which Influence the Water Content of the Stratum Corneum, J. Invest. Dermatol., 18:433, 1952.

ITCHING

Cormia, F., and J. W. Dougherty: Proteolytic Activity in Development of Pain and Itching, J. Invest. Dermatol., 35:21, 1960.

Shelley, W. B., and R. P. Arthur: The Neurohistology and Neurophysiology of the Itch Sensation in Man, A.M.A. Arch. Dermatol., 76:296, 1957.

NAIL CHANGES

Pardo-Castello, V., and O. A. Pardo: "Diseases of the Nails," 3d ed., Springfield, Ill., Charles C Thomas, Publisher, 1960.

PIGMENTARY CHANGES

Becker, S. W.: Hyperpigmentation and Depigmentation, in "Modern Dermatologic Therapy," T. H. Sternberg and V. D. Newcomer (Eds.), New York, McGraw-Hill Book Company, Inc., Blakiston Division, 1959.

Lerner, A. B., and J. D. Case: Pigment Cell Regulatory Factors, J. Invest. Dermatol., 32:211, 1959.

Maibach, H. I., and A. M. Kligman: Dihydroxyacetone: A Suntan-simulating Agent, A.M.A. Arch. Dermatol., 82: 505, 1960.

SEBORRHEA

Kligman, A. M., and W. B. Shelley: An Investigation of the Biology of the Human Sebaceous Gland, J. Invest. Dermatol., 30:99, 1958.

THE HISTORY

Pillsbury, D. M., W. B. Shelley, and A. M. Kligman: "A Manual of Cutaneous Medicine," Philadelphia, W. B. Saunders Company, 1961.

THE LABORATORY

Baer, R., and V. Witten: Allergic Eczematous Contact Dermatitis. Part II. Test Procedures, in "The Year Book of Dermatology and Syphilology," Chicago, Year Book Publishers, Inc., 1957–1958.

Blank, H., and G. Rake: "Viral and Rickettsial Diseases of the Skin, Eye and Mucous Membranes," Boston, Little, Brown & Company, 1955.

Caro, M. R.: Skin Biopsy Technique, A.M.A. Arch. Dermatol., 76:9, 1957.

Jillson, O. F., and W. L. Curwen: Phototoxicity, Photoallergy and Photoskin Tests, A.M.A. Arch. Dermatol., 80: 678, 1959.

Lever, W. F.: "Histopathology of the Skin," 3d ed., Philadelphia, J. B. Lippincott Company, 1961.

Lewis, G. M., M. E. Hopper, J. W. Wilson, and O. A. Plunkett: "An Introduction to Medical Mycology," 4th ed., Chicago, Year Book Publishers, Inc., 1958.

Van Scott, E. J., R. P. Reinertson, and R. Steinmuller: The Growing Hair Roots of the Human Scalp and Morphologic Changes Therein Following Amethopterin Therapy, J. Invest. Dermatol., 29:197, 1957.

THE LESION

Siemens, H. W.: "General Diagnosis and Therapy of Skin Diseases," Chicago, University of Chicago Press, 1958.

Stratton, E. K.: "Atlas of Regional Dermatology," Springfield, Ill., Charles C Thomas, Publisher, 1953.

Section 4: Disturbances in Circulation

12 PALPITATION
William H. Resnik

Palpitation is a subjective phenomenon and may be defined as consciousness of the beating of the heart. From the standpoint of diagnosis, it is not usually a very important symptom. Palpitation, except for certain cardiac arrhythmias, is not pathognomonic of any particular group of disorders; even when it occurs as a more or less prominent complaint, the diagnosis of the underlying malady is made largely on the basis of other associated symptoms and data, rather than by an analysis of the palpitation alone. Nevertheless palpitation frequently constitutes a symptom of considerable importance in the minds of patients. The clear association of this symptom with the function of the heart and the fear engendered by the suspicion that heart disease may be present account for the apprehension frequently inspired by consciousness of the heartbeat. This anxiety is all the more pronounced in patients who know or who have been told that they may have heart disease; to them palpitation may seem to be an omen of impending disaster.

In the following paragraphs a number of conditions will be discussed primarily from the standpoint of palpitation. It must not be inferred, however, that in all these disorders palpitation is always a symptom of great magnitude, even from the patient's standpoint. Palpitation may be absent without affecting the ultimate diagnosis; but in the various conditions discussed below, palpitation *may* be the chief source of the patient's discomfort and the outstanding complaint.

Palpitation may be expressed by the patient in various terms, such as "pounding," "fluttering," "flopping," and "skipping," and in most cases it will be obvious that the complaint is of a sensation of disturbance of the heartbeat. Not infrequently, the patient complains of throbbing in the neck or upper abdomen, when under similar circumstances most persons would refer the palpitation to the precordium.

PATHOGENESIS OF PALPITATION

Under ordinary circumstances the rhythmic heartbeat is imperceptible to the healthy individual of average or placid temperament. Palpitation may be experienced by normal persons who have engaged in strenuous physical effort or have been strongly aroused emotionally. This type of palpitation is physiologic and represents the normal awareness of an overactive heart—that is to say, a heart that is beating at a rapid rate and at the same time expelling more than the usual amount of blood with each beat. Since palpitation accompanies physiologic overactivity of the heart as well as certain pathologic forms of overactivity, such as are seen in severe anemia or thyrotoxicosis, it is commonly assumed that it is the overactivity per se or the associated increased stroke output that is responsible for the symptom. However, overactivity of the heart is associated with several alterations in cardiac function: increased stroke output, acceleration of heart rate, steeper gradient of development of intraventricular pressure during the period of isometric contraction, increased intensity of the heart sounds, especially of the first sound. Of these various factors, the last two are probably the ones chiefly concerned with the appearance of palpitation, whereas increased stroke output, both on clinical and experimental grounds, appears to play no immediate role in the causation of this symptom. For example, complete heart block is characterized by a considerably increased output per beat; in this condition palpitation is inconspicuous and occurs only when the atrial contraction precedes the ventricular by a very brief interval, thus giving rise to a loud first sound (*bruit de canon*).

On the basis of clinical experience, there seems to be a closer correlation between palpitation and intensity of the first heart sound than between this symptom and any other single phenomenon related to cardiac function. Intensity of the first heart sound depends mainly on the vigor with which the atrioventricular valve leaflets are brought into apposition by ventricular systole. In turn, the force with which the valves are snapped together depends on (1) the position of the AV valves at the onset of ventricular contraction, and (2) the rapidity with which intraventricular tension increases following the beginning of ventricular systole.

The influence of the position of the AV valves may be explained as follows. In general, when diastole is abbreviated, as after a short P-R interval or in the case of a premature beat occurring during the early filling phase of diastole, the AV valves are widely separated and pressed against the ventricular walls. When contraction starts, the valves are forced to make a maximal excursion in order to come into closure, hence the loud sound. On the other hand, after a long P-R interval or at the onset of a premature beat occurring during the phase of diastasis, the AV valves in late diastole have already floated back into a position of semiclosure. The final movement of the AV valves to closure after the onset of ventricular systole is through a reduced arc, and the first sound is correspondingly diminished in intensity.

The rate at which intraventricular pressure rises during systole also has an important effect on the abruptness and force with which the AV valves are closed, and hence on the intensity of the first sound. Thus, following the administration of epinephrine, the speed of contraction of the left ventricle increases, the duration of the isometric contraction phase is diminished (both phenomena are the result of an increased gradient of intraventricular pressure), and the intensity of the first sound is increased. It has also been suggested that this mechanism as well as the wide separation of the valve leaflets is responsible for the loud first sound after a brief P-R interval. When the AV leaflets are widely separated, more time is required to close the valves, and in the additional increment of time, more ventricular fibers are excited and contracting at the moment of closure than is normally the case. Hence, the ventricular systole is more vigorous, the ventricular pressure rises more rapidly, and vibrations of greater intensity are induced by closure of the AV valves. Experimentally, it has been demonstrated that the vibrations chiefly responsible for the intensity of the first sound occur during isometric contraction, and these vibrations increase as isometric pressure increases.

Thus, palpitation is probably a sensation accompanying an unusually rapid and forceful closure of the atrioventricular valves which gives rise to a first sound of greater than normal intensity. These circumstances prevail in any clinical condition characterized by an increased stroke volume in conjunction with a rapid rate.

These various considerations indicate that whether or not palpitation appears will often depend on the summation of numerous conflicting forces. To illustrate: In paroxysmal tachycardia the intensity of the first sound will tend to be increased by the shortening of the diastole and the quickening of the P-R interval which keep the AV valves wide open at the onset of ventricular systole. On the other hand, the diminished cardiac output tends to cause a fall in the gradient of intraventricular pressure, and this in turn diminishes the intensity of the first sound. Moreover, as myocardial fatigue supervenes and incomplete emptying of the ventricle increases the residual blood in the ventricles, the AV valves are floated back from a position of wide patency to one of semiclosure and the intensity of the first sound is thereby diminished further, an effect enhanced by the reduced velocity of ventricular contraction. In mitral stenosis the first sound is characteristically sharp and loud; yet palpitation is usually absent. The probable explanation is that the quality of the first sound in this condition is due chiefly to the altered physical characteristics (scarring) of the leaflets rather than to the force of the mitral valve closure.

Actually, there are available no carefully controlled studies undertaken to investigate the problem of palpitation, and further speculation regarding the importance of the various factors involved in the causation of the symptoms would be fruitless at present.

IMPORTANT CAUSES OF PALPITATION

It is impracticable to enumerate all the circumstances under which palpitation may occur. Hence only those disorders will be mentioned in which palpitation *may* be a prominent symptom.

Palpitation Due to Disorders of the Mechanism of the Heartbeat. *Extrasystoles.* The symptoms are fairly consistent, and in most cases the diagnosis will be suggested by the patient's story. The actual premature contraction is often described as a "flopping" or as if "the heart turns over." The pause following the premature contraction may be felt as an actual cessation of the heartbeat, in contrast to the complete unconsciousness of the pause when the heart beats normally or at a slow rate, and the patient will often magnify the duration of the interval and sometimes express apprehension as to whether the heart will actually resume its beat. The first ventricular contraction succeeding the pause may be felt as an unusually vigorous beat and will be described as "pounding" or "thudding." Any one or all three of these different symptoms initiated by the premature contraction may be experienced by the patient. It should be strongly emphasized that, *in the absence of clinical or other evidence of organic heart disease, premature beats have no significance whatever.* Usually the identification of the extrasystole as the cause of palpitation is a simple matter. When numerous extrasystoles are present, differentiation from atrial fibrillation can be made by any procedure that will bring about a definite increase in the ventricular rate; at increasingly rapid heart rates, the extrasystoles usually diminish in frequency and then disappear, whereas the irregularity of atrial fibrillation increases. Heart block, with dropped beats, is the only other common arrhythmia with which the premature contraction is likely to be confused; here, simple auscultation will reveal the absence of the premature beat prior to the pause.

The Ectopic Tachycardias. These conditions, which are considered in some detail in Chap. 250, are, with the exception of ventricular tachycardia, common and important causes of palpitation. If the patient is seen between attacks, the diagnosis of ectopic tachycardia will depend upon the history of abrupt onset and offset.

The specific type of ectopic tachycardia can often be surmised from a consideration of all the data obtained from the history, but a precise diagnosis can be made only when an electrocardiogram and observations on the effect of carotid sinus pressure are made during a seizure.

The diagnosis of paroxysmal tachycardia from the history alone, regardless of the type, depends on securing a story of abrupt onset and offset. In many cases of rapid heart action, it is difficult or impossible to determine with certainty whether there was an actual sudden onset or whether there was a preceding period of anxiety followed by the rapid, but not abrupt, development of sinus tachy-cardia. It is usually even more difficult to ascertain the exact characteristics of the offset of the tachy-cardia.

Palpitation Dependent on the Presence of Some Organic or Functional Disturbance Originating Outside the Circulatory System. Once again, only the more important and common conditions, particularly those which may not be readily recognized, will be mentioned.

Thyrotoxicosis. In its fully developed form, thyrotoxicosis will usually be evident and offers little difficulty in the way of diagnosis. It is the lesser grades, particularly those which are complicated by the presence of myocardial failure, that are likely to be overlooked. The suspicion that thyrotoxicosis is present may be aroused by the detection of any one of its characteristic features, and confirmation of the diagnosis will be obtained by the procedures mentioned in Chap. 66.

Anemia. When mild, anemia may cause palpitation during exertion; when severe, it causes palpitation at rest. In some patients the coloring of the skin may not reveal the cause of the symptom, but appropriate studies of the blood will clarify the situation.

Fever. Palpitation may be present in acute infections, particularly in the early stages; but here the symptom is merely an insignificant phenomenon in the midst of other obviously more important ones. Palpitation may be one of the more prominent symptoms in an individual suffering from one of the chronic and sometimes more obscure febrile illnesses, such as incipient tuberculosis, chronic brucellosis, subacute bacterial endocarditis, or acute rheumatic fever with carditis and relatively few or no joint manifestations. Carditis in acute rheumatic fever and subacute bacterial endocarditis cannot of course be considered causes of palpitation originating outside the heart. They are considered in this group because the presenting symptoms, including palpitation, are often only those of an infection without localizing symptoms that direct suspicion to the heart. The problem is to determine that the cause of the palpitation is an infectious illness and to carry out the usual procedures to reveal the type of infection.

Hypoglycemia. Palpitation is often a prominent feature of this condition and appears to be related to release of epinephrine. Confirmation of the diagnosis is obtained by appropriate blood sugar estimations and by prompt relief of all symptoms on the administration of glucose in one form or another (Chap. 71).

Aerophagia. Many patients who complain of "gas" and belching also complain of palpitation, possibly due in some cases to an associated anxiety state. This type of palpitation is readily recognized by the history of relief through eructation.

Tumors of Adrenal Medulla (Pheochromocytomas). Such tumors may give rise to recurrent attacks whose symptoms, including paroxysms of hypertension and palpitation, are identical with those seen following the injection of epinephrine or norepinephrine. This type of tumor is rather uncommon and is mentioned chiefly because cure may be effected by surgical removal.

Drugs. The relationship between the development of palpitation and the use of tobacco, coffee, tea, alcohol, epinephrine, ephedrine, aminophylline, atropine, or thyroid extract will usually be obvious, and further elaboration is unnecessary.

Palpitation as a Manifestation of the Anxiety State. Persons who are healthy physically and well-adjusted emotionally may have palpitation under certain circumstances. Thus during or immediately after vigorous physical exertion or during sudden emotional tension, palpitation is common and is usually associated with outspoken tachycardia. Occasionally such a person may be conscious of the heartbeat when lying on the left side, but this type of palpitation is clearly due to the better transmission of the heart sounds to the ear. Lifting the head from the pillow will bring about a striking diminution or immediate disappearance of the symptom.

In some patients, palpitation may be one of the outstanding manifestations of a transitory episode of acute anxiety which may never recur. That is, after this one episode or between infrequent bouts of increased nervous tension, he may experience no palpitation which is not normal for the otherwise healthy, well-adjusted individual. In other persons the palpitation may, with other symptoms, represent a lifelong disorder indicative of disturbed autonomic function. Whether this illness is simply an expression of a chronic, deep-seated anxiety state superimposed on a normal autonomic nervous system or depends on a constitutional or inherited autonomic instability, as some believe, is not yet entirely clear. At any rate, the clinical significance of this differentiation between the transitory and the enduring forms is that the former is often dissipated by emphatic reassurance from the physician, whereas the latter is usually resistant even to the most thorough and expert psychiatric care. In the latter case, the patient must be given constant psychologic support and should be taught to live within the limits of his physical capabilities.

This chronic form of palpitation is known by various names such as *Da Costa's syndrome, soldier's heart, effort syndrome, irritable heart, neurocirculatory asthenia,* and *functional cardiovascular disease.* Aside from palpitation, the chief symptoms are one or more of those of an anxiety state (p. 390, Anxiety).

Physical examination usually reveals the typical findings of the hyperkinetic syndrome (p. 99).

Electrocardiograms may display minor depressions of the S-T junction and inversion of T waves and so occasionally lead to a mistaken diagnosis of coronary disease; this is particularly likely to occur when these findings are associated with complaints by the patient of an aching feeling of substernal tightness, commonly present in emotional stress (Fig. 254-4). Minimal elevation of body temperature is sometimes present and may be responsible for an erroneous diagnosis of subacute rheumatic carditis (Chap. 114). A normal sedimentation rate and a tendency for the tachycardia to decrease sharply during sleep constitute strong evidence against rheumatic carditis. The two conditions may coexist. In fact, the presence of any kind of organic disease is one of the commonest causes of the underlying anxiety which frequently produces this functional syndrome.

The diagnosis of this type of anxiety state depends on the positive phenomena mentioned above. Even when a patient presents undoubted objective evidence of structural cardiac disease, a superimposed anxiety state should be considered responsible for the symptoms when the clinical picture is that which has been described. Normal values for vital capacity and for circulation time make it extremely improbable that dyspnea is due to organic cardiac disease which does not cause a sighing type of dyspnea. Pain localized to the region of the apex, lasting for hours or days, and accompanied by hyperesthesia is rarely due to structural cardiac disease but is common in the functional syndrome. Palpitation associated with organic cardiac disease is nearly always accompanied by arrhythmia or by marked tachycardia, but the symptom may exist with regular rhythm and with a heart rate of 80 or less in patients with the anxiety state. Giddiness due to this syndrome can usually be reproduced by hyperventilation (Chap. 42) or by change from the recumbent to the erect posture.

The treatment of the anxiety cardiac syndrome depends on removal of the cause. *In many instances the examination itself and the physician's attitude are the treatment.* A very thorough history followed by a detailed explanation, emphatic assurance, and instructions to take more rather than less physical exercise will produce dramatic relief in many instances. Frequently, the demonstration that the physician can reproduce not only the palpitation but many other symptoms of the anxiety state merely by the hypodermic injection of 0.5 to 1.0 ml epinephrine serves to convince the patient that his symptoms are not the result of some mysterious disorder but rather the effect of a well-understood physiologic mechanism. This is especially true when the initial anxiety has been mainly the result of fear of heart disease. When the cause is more deep-seated, or when the physician has not been able to gain the complete confidence of the patient, little or no benefit is the usual outcome. Even so, the psychiatrist may be able to do much toward emotional and economic rehabilitation.

Management of these patients is facilitated by a clear understanding on the physician's part of the mechanisms of the symptoms. The palpitation is probably related to release of epinephrine and to the lowered perception threshold. The pain probably arises in the intercostal tissues as the result of the pounding of the heart. The hyperventilation with its ensuing train of symptoms (Chap. 42) is analogous to emotional sighing. There is evidence that the entire syndrome is related to decline of the normal inhibitory effect of the cerebral cortex on those hypothalamic centers which normally control the sympathetic system ("cortical-hypothalamic imbalance"). Explanation of these physiologic mechanisms to the patient is one of the most important features of therapeutic reassurance.

The most common causes for palpitation have been enumerated and briefly discussed. Since this symptom occurs in such a wide variety of disorders which have no common or closely related under-

lying disturbance of structure or function, aside from the alterations in the intensity of the heart sounds, it is impossible to follow closely any predetermined plan of study in elucidating the significance of the symptom. The exact procedure will vary, of course, with the circumstances under which the patient is seen. Table 12-1 summarizes the main points of information that will be ascertained in the history. These questions, and others formulated according to circumstances of the individual case, will serve to suggest the additional lines of inquiry that may be necessary for analysis and appraisal of palpitation.

Two points merit special emphasis. The first is that in a person with a regular rhythm the presence of palpitation is usually good evidence against the simultaneous presence of myocardial failure. The second point is that as a rule palpitation produces anxiety and fear out of all proportion to its seriousness. When the cause has been accurately determined and its significance explained to the patient, the symptom is often ameliorated and may disappear entirely.

REFERENCES

Cohen, M. E., and P. D. White: "Life Stress and Bodily Disease," chap. 56, vol. 29, 1949, in Research Publications of the Association for Research Nervous Mental Disease, Baltimore, The Williams and Wilkins Company, 1950.

Kjellberg, S. R., V. Rudhe, and T. Sjöstrand: The Effect of Adrenaline on the Contraction of the Human Heart under Normal Circulatory Conditions, Acta Physiol. Scand., 24:333, 1952.

Lewis, J. K., and W. Dock: Origin of Heart Sounds and Their Variation in Myocardial Disease, J.A.M.A., 110:271, 1938.

Siecke, H., and H. E. Essex: Relation of the Difference in Pressure across the Mitral Valve to the Amplitude of the First Heart Sound in Dogs with Atrioventricular Block, Am. J. Physiol., 192:135, 1958.

Yu, P. N., B. J. B. Yim, and C. A. Stanfield: Hyperventilation Syndrome. Changes in the Electrocardiogram, Blood Gases, and Electrolytes during Voluntary Hyperventilation; Possible Mechanisms and Clinical Implications, A.M.A. Arch. Internal Med., 103:902, 1959.

Table 12-1

Does the palpitation occur:	If so, suspect:
As isolated "jumps" or "skips"?	Extrasystoles
In attacks, known to be of abrupt beginning, with a heart rate of 120 or over, of regular or irregular rhythm?	Paroxysmal rapid heart action
Independent of exercise or excitement adequate to account for the symptom?	Atrial fibrillation, auricular flutter, thyrotoxicosis, anemia, febrile states, hypoglycemia, anxiety state
In attacks developing rapidly though not absolutely abruptly, unrelated to exertion or excitement?	Hemorrhage, hypoglycemia, tumor of the adrenal medulla
In conjunction with the taking of drugs?	Tobacco, coffee, tea, alcohol, epinephrine, ephedrine, aminophylline, atropine, thyroid extract
On standing?	Postural hypotension
In middle-aged women, in conjunction with flushes and sweats?	Menopausal syndrome
When the rate is known to be normal and the rhythm regular?	Anxiety state

13 CIRCULATORY FAILURE

Lewis Dexter, Lloyd L. Hefner, and T. R. Harrison

The purpose of this chapter is to consider the relationship of certain clinical disorders to some general principles of physiology and of physics.

Some of these principles are germane to airflow and respiration as well as to blood flow and circulation. Actually, they can rarely be applied in a strict quantitative sense to the complex conditions existing in the body. However, they are qualitatively applicable and tend to clarify the mechanisms involved.

In general, this chapter is concerned with pathophysiology and not with diagnosis or therapy. However, the treatment of shock and of hypotension are discussed because these disorders are not considered in detail elsewhere in the book.

TYPES OF CIRCULATORY DISORDERS

Local disturbances of the vascular system are presented in those sections devoted to disease of veins or of the coronary, cerebral, renal, or peripheral arteries. This chapter deals with the *general* circulatory syndromes. These may be classified according to a number of different criteria. The *topographic* approach would separate them into peripheral and cardiac disorders, the latter group being further subdivided according to whether the myocardium, endocardium, or pericardium is primarily affected. The *clinical* classification involves viewing these disturbances according to their outstanding manifestations, and might include the states of circulatory overactivity (as in thyrotoxicosis), of shocklike states, of congestive phenomena, and of various combinations of these conditions. However, the *physiologic* approach may be preferable because all the general circulatory disorders involve changes in important functions. Thus the cardiac output is usually altered either as regards the absolute value or its level in relation to other circulatory parameters. The two functions which are of especial importance in this regard are (1) the resistance to outflow, which is closely related to the emptying load, and (2) the filling load, or the amount of blood offered to the heart. The latter may be considered to be the amount of blood which would enter a cardiac chamber during filling if its pressure were zero throughout the period.

The essential function of the circulation, which is the interchange of gases, water, and solutes with the tissues, occurs in the capillaries. Accordingly, for the purposes of the discussion to follow, *circulatory failure may be defined as a state in which this primary function is threatened or actually impaired as the result of changes in pressure and/or flow in the capillaries.* This definition includes both the peripheral and cardiac types of circulatory failure.

The classification of circulatory disorders in Table 13-1 will be utilized in the later discussion.

Before considering these specific disturbances, certain physical and physiologic principles will be discussed.

Table 13-1. CLASSIFICATION OF CIRCULATORY DISORDERS

I. Local disturbances (considered in other chapters)
II. General disturbances without circulatory failure
   A. Increased peripheral resistance. See discussions of systemic and pulmonary hypertension (Chaps. 245 and 262)
   B. Decreased peripheral resistance without impairment of venous return (physiologic hypotension)
   C. Increased venous return with adequate cardiac response ("overactive circulation," "hyperkinetic syndrome")
III. Circulatory failure
   A. Decrease in cardiac output due to defective venous return ("shock" or peripheral circulatory failure) — Disorders of filling
   B. Heart failure
      1. Due to defective filling (e.g., tamponade) — Disorders of filling — Low output failure
      2. Due to defects in emptying
         a. Diminished myocardial strength (e.g., coronary disease)
         b. Excessive resistance load (e.g., hypertension)
         c. Excessive flow load (e.g., arteriovenous fistula)

High output failure

RELATIONS BETWEEN PRESSURE, FLOW, AND RESISTANCE

Certain concepts from physics are indispensable to an understanding of the interrelationships of many of the important variables in the circulatory system. When a fluid flows in laminar fashion through a cylindrical tube, the quantity of fluid that passes per unit time is directly proportional to the difference in pressure at the two ends of the tube and inversely proportional to the various factors that hinder the flow, collectively called the resistance. This may be expressed as an equation:

$$Q = \frac{P_1 - P_2}{R}$$

where Q is the flow per unit time, P_1 and P_2 are the pressures at the two ends of the tube, and R is the resistance. This simple formula is often used to calculate the resistance to flow across certain sections of the cardiovascular system where one can determine the flow and the pressure difference, or the pressure gradient as it is often called.

The interpretation of changes in resistance often presents a formidable problem. If one is dealing with constant laminar flow through rigid cylindrical tubes, the resistance is dependent upon the viscosity of the fluid and the radius and length of the tube according to the following relationship:

$$R = \frac{8ul}{\pi r^4}$$

where R is the resistance, u is the coefficient of viscosity, l is the length of the tube, and r is the radius. It is important to note that, because the radius is raised to the fourth power, small changes in radius have a disproportionately great influence on the resistance to flow, whereas changes in viscosity or length produce only a proportionate change in resistance.

Even though the above equation for resistance is helpful conceptually, it is only crudely applicable to the complex situation existing in the circulatory system where the flows and pressures are not constant but pulsatile, the flow may not be laminar, the fluid is not homogeneous, the tubes are not rigid or necessarily cylindrical, and there is repeated branching. It is true, nevertheless, that large changes in resistance may safely be ascribed to changes in the radius of the tubes involved. Small changes in calculated resistance often cannot be interpreted. The situation is further complicated by the fact that, since the vessels involved are elastic, the radius is not an independent variable but is in part dependent on the pressure. Thus a change in caliber of a vessel may be a passive result of a change in pressure or may mean an active change in vasomotor tone.

The two equations above may be combined into a single one, called the Poiseuille equation:

$$Q = \frac{(P_1 - P_2)\pi r^4}{8ul}$$

The symbols have the same meaning as before. Note that r here refers to radius, not resistance.

The Poiseuille equation may be related in a general way, with due caution for the reasons mentioned above, to the situation as it exists in circulatory failure. By simple algebraic manipulation the equation may be written:

$$Q = \frac{P_1\pi r^4}{8ul} - \frac{P_2\pi r^4}{8ul}$$

As a conceptual aid in discussing circulatory failure, let Q be the cardiac output, P_1 the diastolic pressure just proximal to the cardiac chamber being considered, P_2 the diastolic pressure in the chamber itself, and r the effective radius of the stream of blood entering the cardiac chamber.

It is recognizable that $P_1\pi r^4/8ul$ coincides with the definition of filling load given earlier in this chapter, that is, the amount of blood which would enter a cardiac chamber if the diastolic pressure were zero. The important variables which determine filling load, then, are P_1 (the filling pressure) and r (the radius of the stream entering the chamber).

As discussed elsewhere, in all forms of heart failure the ratio cardiac output/filling load is abnormally small, but neither the numerator nor the denominator alone is adequate to define heart failure. In high output states without failure both numerator and denominator are increased, but the ratio is normal. In peripheral circulatory failure both numerator and denominator are decreased, with a normal ratio.

In left ventricular failure, e.g., in coronary artery disease, the filling load to the left ventricle is increased, but the cardiac output is normal or diminished; so the ratio is low. At the same time we conclude that left atrial failure coexists because the filling load to the left atrium is also increased, while the output of the left atrium is of course the same as that of the left ventricle. On the other hand, in heart failure due to mitral stenosis the filling load to the left ventricle $(P_1\pi r^4)/8ul$ is usually diminished because, though P_1 (left atrial pressure) is increased, r^4 is drastically diminished. In mitral stenosis, by definition, it is the left atrium which fails because the filling load is increased (P_1, pulmonary venous pressure, and r, pulmonary venous size, are both increased) while the left atrial output is normal or low.

It is instructive to compare the hemodynamics of exercise to those of heart failure. During exercise in vigorous healthy subjects the left atrial pressure may exceed 20 mm Hg, and since the pulmonary veins must also be distended by this increased pressure, the filling load actually exceeds that seen in many persons with left ventricular failure. However, the cardiac output is also greatly increased, and a normal cardiac output/filling load ratio permits the reasonable conclusion that left ventricular failure is not present.

The above discussion is intended for clarification of concepts. For reasons already mentioned, and also because the effective radius of the stream bed cannot be determined, the quantitative use of the Poiseuille equation in heart failure is not practical.

One should be careful to distinguish the volume of blood flow from the linear velocity of blood flow. For example, the linear velocity of flow in the Mississippi River is much smaller than in a mountain brook, but the volume of flow is incomparably greater, because of the enormous discrepancy between the sizes of the streams. In heart failure the discrepancy between the resting cardiac output, which is often only slightly decreased and may be normal, and the circulation time, which may be markedly prolonged, is explicable in the same way, the stream size being larger than normal in heart failure because of venous distention.

The Poiseuille equation is even less applicable to the consideration of stenotic valves than it is to other, more physiologic circumstances existing in the circulatory system. The anatomy of a stenotic valve has very little resemblance to a cylindrical tube. In addition, flow through a stenotic valve is turbulent, not laminar. For turbulent streams, the flow is proportional to the square root of the pressure gradient, rather than to the pressure gradient itself, as in the Poiseuille equation. In general, valve size may be calculated, using the following formula:

$$A = \frac{F}{K\sqrt{P_1 - P_2}}$$

where A is the area of the valve in square centimeters, F is the flow in milliliters per minute of systolic ejection (for pulmonic or aortic valve) or of diastolic filling (for mitral or tricuspid valve), K is an empirically determined constant characteristic for the particular valve being studied, and $P_1 - P_2$ is the pressure difference across the valve in millimeters Hg. A false low value for the calculated valve size will occur if the valve is insufficient, because the actual value for the flow will be underestimated.

It is important to realize that, if the flow across a valve orifice falls, the pressure gradient will also fall, so that determination of pressure gradient alone is not sufficient for determining the size of a valve orifice. One cannot compare preoperative and postoperative pressure gradients to judge the efficacy of surgery unless one also determines the simultaneous flows.

PRESSURE AND FLOW IN RELATION TO HEART FAILURE

From the point of view of bodily economy, the heart performs just two functions. It pumps a certain amount of blood (cardiac output) at a certain pressure (low for the right ventricle and high for the left). Their product is the useful work that the heart performs. Useful work = cardiac output × pressure. Other types of work—isometric, heat-producing, kinetic, etc.—are not pertinent to this discussion.

The two sides of the heart may have different outputs for a few beats at a time, as occurs during the different phases of breathing. However, the output per minute of the two ventricles is normally the same, despite the wide differences in pressure which are illustrated in Fig. 13-1.

Pressures in the right chambers of the heart and in the pulmonary artery are readily measured in the human being by cardiac catheterization. The pulmonary "capillary pressure" (wedge pressure) is measured by passing the catheter snugly into a branch of the pulmonary artery in such a way as to occlude this vessel completely.

Contractility of the normal heart is under neurohumoral control. Sympathetic stimulation, epinephrine, and norepinephrine produce more complete systolic emptying, a quicker contraction, and a more vigorous contraction. These impulses and humoral agents are largely responsible for the way in which the normal heart meets conditions of physiologic stress.

All striated muscle, including the myocardium, responds to increased stretch, at least to its physiologic limit, by an increased force of contraction. Applied to the heart, this is called *Starling's law*, which states that "the mechanical energy set free in passing from the resting to the contracted state depends on the area of chemically active surfaces, i.e., on the length of the muscle fibers." In the healthy human heart the response according to Starling's law appears to be a second line of defense, the neurohumoral mechanisms described above being the first line. As the heart fails, the importance of Starling's law in explaining the sequence of cardiac behavior becomes more and more apparent.

With the heart-lung preparation, heart rate, peripheral resistance, venous inflow, diastolic volume (as a measure of stretch of the muscle), output, and pressure can be controlled or measured. The effect of changing one of these factors on the others can readily be studied. Studies using the heart-lung preparation have demonstrated the normal response of the heart to diminished or augmented load (produced by changing either the peripheral resistance or the height of the venous reservoir) (Fig. 13-2).

If, in the heart-lung preparation, the level of the venous reservoir is lowered, the diastolic filling of the heart is reduced and the systolic output declines. If the lowering of the venous reservoir is of sufficient degree, filling and output diminish so

NORMAL CIRCULATION

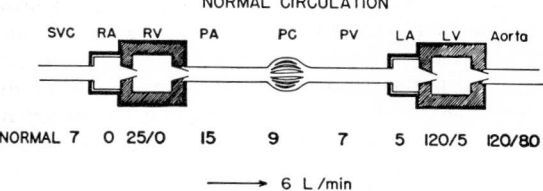

SVC	RA	RV	PA	PC	PV	LA	LV	Aorta

NORMAL 7   0 25/0   15   9   7   5 120/5 120/80

⟶ 6 L /min

FIG. 13-1. The pressure in the systemic capillaries (not shown) is about 25 mm Hg and equal to the osmotic pressure of the plasma proteins. The low pressures in the right chambers and in the pulmonary vessels are illustrated. The wide margin between the pulmonary capillary pressure, about 9 mm Hg, and the protein osmotic pressure, approximately 25 mm Hg, protects against edema of the lungs but does not interfere with gas exchange. Ventricular failure is characterized by increased ventricular diastolic pressure due to defective systolic emptying. Secondarily, there is rise in the pressures in the corresponding atrium, veins, and capillaries. Left ventricular failure leads to increase in the pulmonary arterial pressure and hence tends to cause right ventricular failure. However, because of the much greater resistance in the peripheral arterioles, the rise in capillary pressure due to right ventricular failure is not reflected in the systemic arteries.

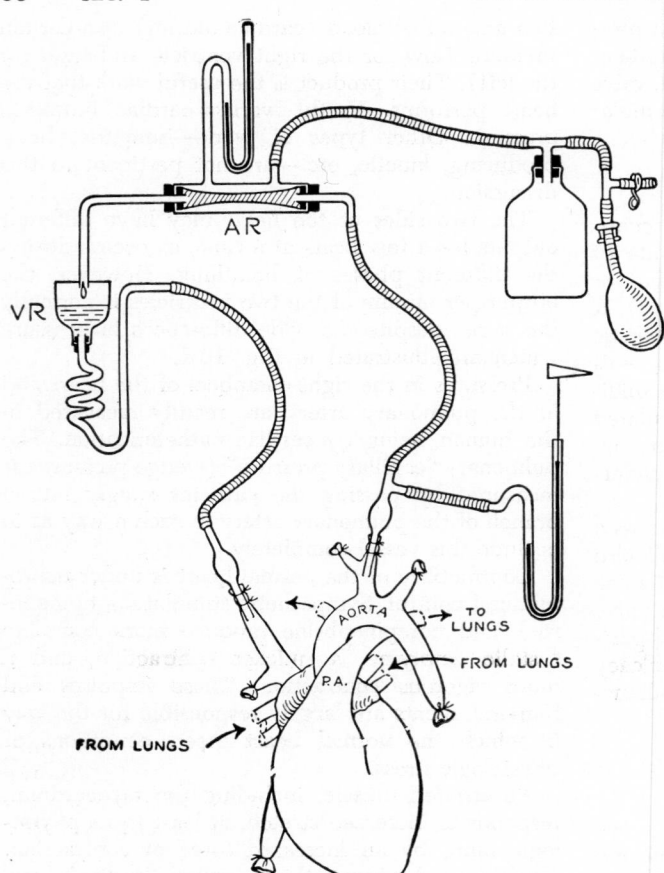

1. Excessive increase in peripheral resistance

2. Exhaustion of myocardium

3. Excessive elevation of venous reservoir

4. Excessive lowering of venous reservoir (Peripheral failure)

5. Combinations of these procedures

FIG. 13-2. Methods of producing circulatory failure in heart-lung preparation. *AR =* artificial peripheral resistance; *VR =* venous reservoir; *PA =* pulmonary artery. It should be noted that excessive lowering of the venous reservoir produces peripheral circulatory failure but not heart failure. The other procedures produce heart failure.

much that the coronary circulation becomes inadequate to supply the needs of the heart, which soon ceases to beat. Under such circumstances we are dealing with failure of the preparation not as the result of a primary disorder of the heart but as the result of a defective venous return. It will be pointed out later that this set of circumstances corresponds to peripheral circulatory failure in man.

A sudden increase of work load in the form of either output or pressure results in a *decrease of ventricular emptying,* with only part of the contents being discharged (diminished stroke output) and some of the contents remaining behind (increased residual volume). The deficient emptying, with a continuing venous return, is the basic cause of an increase of end-diastolic pressure (stretch) of the affected ventricle. If the ventricular muscle is diseased or its function is in any way impaired, it requires a greater stretch to perform a given work load, and *eventually even the normal work load may result in deficient emptying* and an increase of its diastolic pressure. Each ventricle has a different

curve, as indicated in Fig. 13-3. In the normal heart small changes of diastolic pressure are reflected by large changes in work performance. A 1-cm H_2O rise of diastolic pressure may be reflected in a 300 per cent increase of ventricular stroke work. At

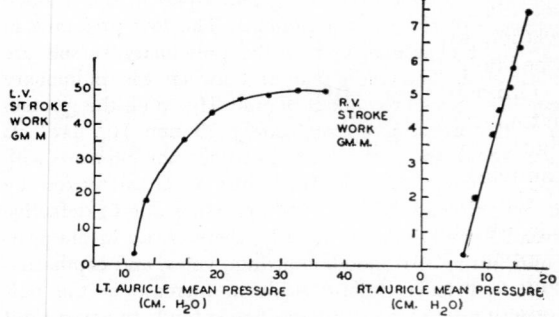

FIG. 13-3. Left and right ventricular function curves showing relation between ventricular stroke work and mean pressure in the corresponding atrium (*Sarnoff and Berglund: Circulation,* 9:706, 1954.)

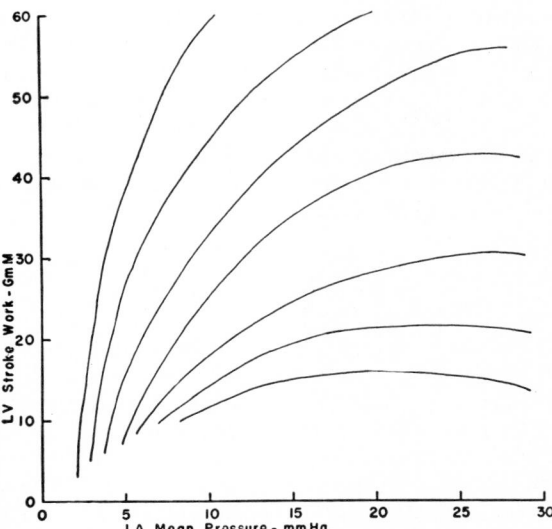

FIG. 13-4. This series of curves represents the changing relation between left ventricular diastolic pressure (represented by left atrial mean pressure) and left ventricular stroke work in dogs. The normal ventricular response follows the left-hand curve. As the ventricle fails, the curve of the myocardial response migrates to the right and downward. (*After Dexter et al.: Trans. Assoc. Am. Physicians,* 66:266, 1953.)

high filling pressures, the curve flattens off. The oft-quoted descending limb of Starling's curve does not occur in the normal dog's heart but may occur in a heart with a compromised myocardium. As the myocardial function becomes impaired by disease or experimentally by drugs, the curve relating work to diastolic pressure migrates to the right, as shown in Fig. 13-4, i.e., Starling's curve is not a single line but rather a whole family of curves, and the curve for the right ventricle is quite different from that for the left. This indicates that, as the heart fails, it requires a greater stretch to produce a given amount of work. Diastolic pressure in the *right* ventricle, atrium, and systemic veins bears no direct relation to the function of the left ventricle, and vice versa.

Ordinarily, diminished emptying and diminished output appear together. However, a person with shock may have decreased output despite increased emptying, and a patient with thyrotoxicosis or one of the other disorders causing high output failure may have increased output despite decreased emptying. In any case, it is the defective emptying, with a continued inflow from the atrium and the consequent accumulation of residual blood, which leads to the rise in end-diastolic pressure and the subsequent train of events responsible for the congestion of heart failure.

The clinical manifestations of a low cardiac out-put are loss of energy and abnormal fatigability. These symptoms are usually masked by the presence of respiratory distress which, when on a congestive basis, introduces an element of suffocation, apprehension, and inability to take in air. In fact, it is so disagreeable and alarming that most patients are not aware of their weakness and fatigue. It is only when respiratory complaints are absent that the weakness of a low cardiac output becomes an important complaint.

If the myocardium is sufficiently diseased, or if an excessive work load is placed upon it, its ventricular end-diastolic pressure rises. There is some evidence that, during relaxation, the ventricles may exert a momentary suction due to elastic recoil after systole and, therefore, that the ventricles have something to do with maintaining a low diastolic pressure. On the other hand, the ventricles have no ability to raise their own diastolic pressure. This increased pressure has its ultimate origin in the other ventricle, although dilatation or constriction of the intervening vasculature may have a profound effect in influencing the diastolic pressure rise. As myocardial function continues to deteriorate, the ventricular end-diastolic pressure rises with less and less stress, until it is finally elevated at rest.

The rise in ventricular diastolic pressure is transmitted to the corresponding atrium, which because of its thin wall is readily stretched by a relatively small increase in pressure. The atrium responds with more vigorous contraction. This relatively early sign of ventricular failure may be readily recorded from the precordial area.

In considering first the left ventricle, the extent to which its diastolic pressure can rise before serious symptoms occur is determined by the osmotic pressure of plasma. A rise of diastolic pressure in the left ventricle is associated with a similar rise in the atrium and throughout the lungs and right ventricle in systole. A moderate rise in the pulmonary capillary pressure may cause congestion without edema and hence mild dyspnea without rales. If, however, the pressure in the pulmonary capillaries exceeds the osmotic pressure of plasma (25 mm Hg is assumed for discussion), outward filtration of fluid into the alveoli will take place and the ensuing pulmonary edema will make dyspnea more severe. Any factor that lowers osmotic pressure or raises left ventricular diastolic pressure or interferes sufficiently with the drainage of lymph from the lungs predisposes to pulmonary edema.

The end-diastolic pressure of the right ventricle rises in the same manner as that of the left ventricle in response to its own stresses or to damage of its myocardium. When its end-diastolic pressure rises, there is a similar elevation of pressure in the right atrium and systemic veins. As these pressures increase, veins usually become distended (provided that they do not have an accompanying vasoconstriction, as they sometimes do), and the liver becomes congested, enlarged, and tender from stretch of its capsule. These are the two most reliable signs of right ventricular failure (see Chap. 249).

A hypertrophied ventricle can carry on much more work at a normal end-diastolic filling pressure than can a normal unhypertrophied ventricle. When, however, this hypertrophied ventricle becomes damaged or its load becomes excessive, it empties less completely and dilatation ensues. As its end-diastolic pressure rises and its work performance (usually flow) decreases, all the usual manifestations of failure of that chamber ensue.

HEART FAILURE IN RELATION TO CERTAIN CIRCULATORY FUNCTIONS

The relations of cardiac output and of intracardiac pressures to congestive failure have already been discussed.

Venous Pressure. Venous pressure is elevated in the great majority of patients with heart failure. Measurements of the pulmonary "capillary" (wedge) pressure have consistently demonstrated such increase in patients with failure of the left side of the heart. In the case of the systemic venous pressure, the initial elevation can be ascribed to the rise in the end-diastolic right ventricular pressure, but the increase in blood volume is an important although secondary factor. There is likewise evidence that venoconstriction exists in the smaller veins and possibly in the large veins, also, when heart failure sets in rapidly. The orthopneic position is an important factor in edema formation because it obviously causes marked elevation of the venous pressure in the dependent portions of the body, even though this pressure as measured at heart level may be normal.

Circulation Time and Velocity of Blood Flow. The circulation time is prolonged and the velocity of blood flow reduced in patients with heart failure due to pressure loads or to myocardial or pericardial disorders, but it may be normal when failure is induced by increased flow loads (high output failure). When the left side of the heart fails, the lung-to-tongue time is increased; with right-sided failure the arm-to-lung time is increased. Prolonged circulation time is usually associated with diminished cardiac output and widening of the stream bed resulting from cardiac dilatation and from congestion. Either factor alone may produce it.

Circulating Blood Volume. This is elevated in most patients with congestive failure. Such elevation is rarely the cause (see below) but commonly the result of the failure. Presumably, the loss of blood from the peripheral into the central vascular bed, as dilatation of the cardiac chambers and congestion in the pulmonary circuit occur, leads to a deficit of blood in those areas which regulate the production of erythrocytes and of plasma protein. Possibly, the same mechanism is concerned in the renal retention of water and electrolytes. The redistribution of blood into the central region presumably has the same effect as external hemorrhage on these regulatory areas.

THE RENAL FACTOR IN CARDIAC FAILURE

The local or tissue factors which favor the development of peripheral edema are several. The importance of the balance between capillary pressure and the protein osmotic pressure and of lymph flow have already been mentioned. The orthopneic position is of great importance because it causes a large increase in hydrostatic pressure in the dependent areas, and also tends to impair lymphatic return. These local factors can lead to distributional changes in the extracellular fluid but cannot cause an increase in its total volume unless the rate of water loss from the body is less than the rate of intake. Thus the kidney is the chief quantitative determinant of the extracellular fluid excess that occurs in edematous states. The renal mechanisms involved are considered in Chap. 21.

CAUSES AND MECHANISMS OF HEART FAILURE

Some of the particular features of heart failure due to specific disorders such as the various valvular lesions are considered in later chapters. Here, we are concerned with certain principles which are applicable to heart failure in general.

It is apparent from the preceding discussion of the heart-lung preparation that heart failure is related under all conditions to a rise in the ratio myocardial load/strength of contraction. When, as in certain forms of inflammatory or infiltrative disease, there is widespread myocardial injury, failure may occur with a normal or even diminished load on the heart. Focal ventricular injury, usually due to ischemia, is a rare cause of long-standing failure in young or middle-aged persons because of the large reserve power of the remaining healthy musculature. Lesser degrees of ischemic scarring may lead to congestive failure in older persons because of the loss of cardiac reserve normally associated with aging (p. 1378).

The effect of a *pressure load* depends on which cardiac chamber is immediately affected. Thus hypertension or aortic stenosis may be tolerated for years without symptoms because the relatively great strength of the left ventricle and, especially when it is hypertrophied, may lead to effective emptying and prevent a pressure rise in the left atrium. When the latter chamber, with its thinner wall, is primarily affected by a comparable degree of mitral stenosis, the manifestations of pulmonary congestion appear at a relatively early stage of the disease. Nevertheless, the principle is the same; i.e., a pressure load produces failure when the emptying of the affected chamber becomes inadequate.

The causes of increased *ventricular filling loads* may be *primary* (flow load) and due to increased venous return or *secondary* and due to the accumulation of blood in the atria and great veins because the corresponding ventricle does not empty normally. In either case the augmented filling load means that a greater than normal amount of blood is offered to the ventricle. In the one case, the offered blood is accepted and determines the cardiac output or *flow* load (primary filling load) and thus, taken with the pressure, is an index to the work the heart actually performs. In the other instance, that of the secondarily increased filling load, the part of the offered blood which is not accepted by the ventricle is an index to the work it should but does not do.

Among the disorders associated with increase in venous return and hence in the primary filling load are arteriovenous shunts and conditions, such as thyrotoxicosis, beriberi, or anemia, which alter the metabolism or the oxygen tension in the tissues. *Sudden increase in blood volume* increases the flow load and hence may induce or aggravate heart failure. Thus nocturnal reabsorption of edema fluid because of the recumbent position commonly precipitates acute pulmonary edema (p. 1382) in predisposed patients. Occasionally heart failure is caused in older persons by the postoperative administration of excessive quantities of intravenous fluid.

Patients with acute glomerulonephritis may have hypertension and hypervolemia with elevation of both pressure and flow loads. They may also exhibit increase in cardiac output not only actually but also relative to the oxygen consumption or metabolic needs of the body. In addition, they may have dyspnea, rales in the lungs, gallop rhythm, and cardiac enlargement. Elevation of pulmonary capillary (wedge) pressure and of the end-diastolic pressures of both ventricles may be present. Because

Table 13-2. CAUSES OF HEART FAILURE IN RELATION TO CONCEPTS OF PATHOGENESIS*

| Conditions | | Absolute decrease in CO** per minute | Decreased CO per minute relative to metabolic needs of body | | Excessive increase in ventricular load/strength ratio† | Excessive load relative to force of contraction‡ | Increased ventricular end-diastolic pressure | Increased mean atrial pressure | Decreased CO per minute relative to filling load‡ |
Main group	Subgroup		Relative to O₂ consumption	Relative to tissue O₂ tension					
Primary myocardial disease	Ischemia infiltration myocarditis, etc.	+	+	+	+	+	+	+	+
Increased pressure load	Hypertension Aortic stenosis Pulmonary hypertension Pulmonic stenosis	±	+	+	+	+	+	+	+
Stenosis of AV valves	Mitral Tricuspid	±	+	+	Ventricle − Atrium +	+	−	+	+
Pericardial tamponade	Fluid	+	+	+	−	+	+	+	+
	Thickening	+	+	+	+ If muscle is involved	+	+	+	+
Excessive venous return with failure	Thyrotoxicosis	−	+	+	+	+	+	+	+
	Anemia, AV fistula, etc.	−	−	+	+	+	+	+	+
	Primary hypervolemia (e.g., large I.V. infusions)	−	−	−	+	+	+	+	+
Coexistent cardiac and peripheral failure		+	+	+	+	+	−§	−§	+

* Not all causes included; only conditions illustrating concepts selected.
** CO = cardiac output.
† The potential contractile strength may remain normal despite impairment of the actual contractile force because of diminished filling (mitral stenosis, tamponade).
‡ Note that these are the only constantly present mechanisms.
§ In the terminal phase of peripheral failure these values may rise as heart failure occurs because of deficient coronary flow.

the cardiac output is high relative to the metabolic rate, such patients have sometimes been considered to have generalized congestion without heart failure. However, the striking improvement which some such patients exhibit when digitalis is administered would seem to constitute conclusive evidence that heart failure is present in these particular individuals. This type of failure is analogous to that which can be produced in dogs by the intravenous administration of very large quantities of fluid. Although rare, it is of conceptual importance in relation to the hemodynamic definition of heart failure (Table 13-2).

Under most circumstances, failure is associated with decline in output, either actually or in proportion to the oxygen need or oxygen tension in the tissues. However, as indicated above, the failure due to hypervolemia is exceptional in this respect.

Most heart failure is accompanied by elevated ventricular end diastolic pressure brought about by defective ventricular emptying. This in turn produces elevation of atrial pressure. However, there are exceptions. Severe hemorrhage or marked depletion of blood volume by diuretics and salt restriction may restore ventricular and atrial pressures to normal, despite the persistence of heart failure.

In heart failure, there are at least two common denominators (Table 13-2). One of these is the load on either one or both ventricles in relation to the strength of contraction. The load may be less or greater than normal. It may be excessive, as with advanced aortic stenosis. The strength of contraction may be absolutely reduced because of myocardial disease or may be relatively reduced, though absolutely strong, in such conditions as hypertension or aortic stenosis.

The other hemodynamic defect, which is present in all instances of heart failure, is the inability of the heart to handle in an adequate fashion the blood which is offered to it. The latter may be considered the filling load and may be defined as the amount of blood which would enter the cardiac chambers if their pressure remained at zero throughout filling. The inability of the ventricle to eject the venous return adequately results in heart failure.

The distinction, already mentioned, between primary and secondary causes of increased filling load should be emphasized. When atrial and venous pressure and/or volume are increased because of deficient ventricular emptying, the amount of blood offered the affected chamber and hence the filling load is secondarily increased, but the actual inflow and output are usually decreased. The discrepancy between filling load and cardiac output is appreciable, and failure exists. However, when the increase in filling load is primary, i.e., due to actual increase in venous return as in the high output states, the cardiac output remains elevated be-

cause of adequate myocardial contractility. In the presence of coexistent pressure loads or myocardial impairment, failure occurs when the filling load exceeds the ability of the ventricle to eject its contents.

There are three conditions which produce clinical manifestations identical with heart failure and yet are not due to impaired ventricular contractility— mitral stenosis, tricuspid stenosis, and pericardial tamponade. In each condition, there is obstruction to ventricular inflow—the left ventricle in mitral stenosis, the right ventricle in tricuspid stenosis, or the heart as a whole in pericardial tamponade. These are purely mechanical obstructions, and for blood to pass the obstructions in adequate amounts to maintain cardiac output and life, a rise in pressure must and does occur proximal to the obstruction. In mitral stenosis, pressure rises in the left atrium, pulmonary circuit, and right ventricle, and eventually, right ventricular failure may occur. But the manifestations of pulmonary congestion are not due to left ventricular failure but to the mechanical obstruction to blood flow at the mitral valve. When, late in the disease, right ventricular failure occurs, the manifestations are venous distention, hepatomegaly, and fluid retention.

In tricuspid stenosis, pressure rises in the right atrium and systemic veins. The pressure and flow load on the right ventricle are reduced. There is no right ventricular failure. Unlike mitral stenosis, which produces pulmonary hypertension, the rise in pressure proximal to the obstruction is never sufficient to raise the systemic arterial pressure.

In pericardial tamponade, there is inflow obstruction to both sides of the heart. The result is a rise of pressure in both venous systems (pulmonary and systemic) which tends to sustain the filling of each ventricle. The pressures in each venous system are identical and are the same or slightly higher than the intrapericardial pressure. The intracardiac pressures, as related to pericardial pressure, are quite normal but high as related to intrapleural or atmospheric pressure. This results in high pressures, i.e., those existing in the pericardium, in the pulmonary veins, capillaries and arteries, and in systemic veins. Such elevations are accompanied by the congestive features of heart failure, even though the ventricular myocardium may be normal.

Thus these three conditions lead to pulmonary and/or systemic congestion but have mechanical causes rather than being due to impaired ventricular contractility, absolute or relative, as in other types of congestive heart failure.

PERIPHERAL CIRCULATORY FAILURE OR SHOCK

The *clinical manifestations* of these several disorders vary, depending on the severity of the condition and the acuteness with which it develops. However, they are all related to the fundamental physiologic disturbance which is *defective venous return to the heart with consequent reduction in cardiac output.* Apathy and lassitude are the earliest manifestations when the condition develops slowly over a period of several hours; faintness and syncope, when it occurs acutely; sudden death may occur when there is massive hemorrhage. When peripheral failure is outspoken, the blood pressure declines, the systolic pressure being reduced before the diastolic. Reduction of pulse pressure is, therefore, one of the earlier manifestations. In the initial stages the decline in pulse pressure and the associated faintness may be manifest only in the standing or sitting position. The heart rate is usually very rapid but may be slow. The skin is either cold and clammy or dry and inelastic. Other features of the clinical picture will be discussed later.

Peripheral failure is to be sharply distinguished from heart failure, from which it differs as regards cause, mechanism, and management.

Regardless of its underlying cause and outstanding clinical picture, the immediate mechanism responsible for peripheral failure is decline in venous return, leading to decrease in cardiac output and, hence, to inadequacy of the blood flow to the tissues. When the onset is sudden, there is no time for compensatory adjustments, and the brain suffers severely—hence consciousness is lost. When the onset is more gradual, compensatory adjustment in the form of vasoconstriction in the less vital areas occurs, the cerebral blood flow is kept at a more nearly normal level, and in the absence of other complicating factors, consciousness is usually retained unless the person attempts to sit or stand.

Types

Peripheral circulatory failure may be subdivided into several types, according to which of the various functions is initially disturbed.

From the practical standpoint, it should be emphasized that emotional syncope is the most frequent of the less serious types of peripheral circulatory failure, and primary decline in blood volume is much the most common of the more serious types. The therapeutic implications are obvious.

Primary Decline in Blood Volume (Hematogenic or Oligemic Type)

This may be brought about by hemorrhage, by loss of fluid or blood into injured tissues (traumatic shock, burns, etc.), or by the development of a deficit in extracellular fluid volume as the result of reduced water intake or excessive loss of water and electrolytes from the gastrointestinal tract, kidneys, or skin. Diabetic coma is a common cause. Marked

sinus tachycardia with rates of 130 to 160 per minute is nearly always present. This is the most serious and important type of peripheral circulatory failure, and it is in this type that replacement therapy, utilizing blood, plasma, plasma substitutes, electrolytes, or water (depending on the nature of the deficit), has its greatest value.

Primary Loss of Vascular Tone (Neurogenic Type)

This may occur as the result of emotional disturbances (psychogenic syncope), of physical insults (e.g., sympathectomy or transection of the spinal cord), or of drugs (ganglionic blocking agents, spinal anesthesia). Various diseases of the spinal cord, such as diabetic myelopathy, may interfere with the postural vasoconstrictor reflex and cause syncope on standing. In such instances the decline in blood pressure is primary, and hence vasoconstrictor drugs may be of especial value. In many instances the assumption of the recumbent posture leads to immediate recovery. The heart rate may be abnormally slow as in most instances of psychogenic syncope. The marked tachycardia which occurs in the oligemic type is rarely observed when shock is of the neurogenic variety.

It is probable that the decline in blood pressure which accompanies certain grave visceral disorders such as myocardial infarction and acute pancreatitis is related, in part, to reflex vasodilation. However, other factors, such as myocardial weakness with decline in output and loss of fluid into the peritoneal cavity, are perhaps even more important in these respective disorders.

Primary Arteriolar and Capillary Dilatation (Vasogenic Type)

This is the result of chemical agents acting directly on the vessels and is probably rare. It may be produced experimentally by the administration of histamine or of nitrites and is probably involved in the mechanism of anaphylactic shock. There is some evidence that the substances having a histamine-like action may arise in injured tissues and cause local capillary damage, thereby aggravating the reduction in blood volume which is the usual initiating factor in traumatic shock.

Venous pooling likewise may lead to peripheral circulatory failure, especially when the patient is in the upright position. Such a mechanism is illustrated by the attacks of faintness and syncope in persons with varicose veins, as well as in those attacks which occur in persons with atonic muscles while they are standing still. Mechanical measures, such as bandaging the legs, are of especial value in persons with this type of peripheral failure.

*Mixed and Unknown Types
of Peripheral Circulatory Failure*

In certain patients, more than one of these several mechanisms may be active. Thus the individual with acute peritonitis resulting from perforation of a peptic ulcer may have initial reflex vascular dilatation, later complicated by further local dilatation due to the irritating effect of the gastrointestinal secretions and eventual decline of blood volume consequent to the escape of water, salts, and protein into the peritoneal cavity.

The precise mechanism responsible for the collapse which accompanies acute adrenal injury is not fully understood. The hemorrhagic necrosis of these glands, which may complicate meningococcus infections, childbirth, or (rarely) anticoagulant therapy, probably leads to arteriolar dilatation. A similar adrenal mechanism is possibly concerned in the fulminant shock sometimes associated with the invasion of the blood stream by gram-negative bacilli. The presence of a normal or elevated value for the total (not differential) count of eosinophil cells in the blood constitutes suggestive evidence that adrenal cortical deficiency may be a significant factor in the circulatory failure.

Irreversible Shock

The several conditions mentioned all lead to a decrease in blood flow to the peripheral tissues as the result of decline in cardiac output and blood pressure. When such a diminution is of sufficient duration and severity, grave consequences ensue. Impairment of oxidative mechanisms and of enzyme systems may develop. There is evidence that diminished flow of blood to the liver is of especial importance in producing the terminal irreversible state that occurs when shock is prolonged. Necrosis of the intestinal mucosa due to prolonged anoxia may allow the escape of a large volume of fluid into the gut or permit invasion of the blood stream by gram-negative bacilli and thus perpetuate a vicious cycle. The beneficial effect of hydrocortisone in many instances of severe shock would suggest that adrenal failure may be an important factor in causing the irreversible state.

The peripheral and splanchnic vasoconstriction tends to maintain the blood pressure and the coronary and cerebral flow. However, when the severity and duration of the decline in cardiac output are sufficiently great, the heart and the brain exhibit evidence of progressive impairment. Cardiac failure, with acute pulmonary edema, may appear, and in this terminal stage the administration of fluid may not only be useless but may actually aggravate the congestive failure. There is some evidence that the blood becomes more coagulable when shock is severe and that this leads to multiple venous thrombi with secondary pulmonary and hepatic embolization when fluid is infused. Heparin is said to prevent this factor in "irreversible shock." In the final moribund stage, arterial and venous constriction give way to dilatation as the vasomotor mechanisms become impaired because of prolonged anoxia. Under such conditions treatment either is entirely unavailing or, at best, offers much less likelihood of improvement. It is, therefore, of cardinal importance that peripheral failure be recognized in its incipient stages.

Complications

Recovery of the peripheral circulation does not necessarily imply that the patient will proceed to ultimate recovery. The prolonged renal ischemia resulting from local vasoconstriction may induce the syndrome of hypoxic nephrosis with oliguria or anuria. Although important advances have been made in the treatment of this disorder (p. 103), it still carries a grave prognosis. Prolonged ischemia may likewise lead to serious impairment of the liver or the colon. It is important to prevent the development of these complications by proper treatment of peripheral circulatory failure in its earliest phases.

Early Diagnosis

The classic circulatory signs do not usually develop until the venous return and the cardiac output have already undergone serious reduction. When the skin is cold and moist (clammy), it is not usually necessary to look for other signs. However, patients with diabetic coma or other dehydrated states may have dry skin despite peripheral circulatory failure. One of the earlier manifestations of shock is likely to be a decline of the blood pressure when the patient changes from the recumbent to the sitting posture. This sign is more significant in young than in elderly patients. Another relatively early sign, particularly valuable in the postoperative state, is the presence of a low urine volume— less than 25 ml per hr—despite an adequate intake of water and in the absence of significant fluid loss by extrarenal channels.

The cardiac disorders most likely to be confused with peripheral failure are painless coronary occlusion and ectopic tachycardia. These and other causes of sudden heart failure should be excluded before vigorous fluid therapy is initiated.

Another procedure that may be of aid in the detection of the earlier stages of peripheral circulatory failure is the measurement of blood volume by the dye method. Reductions of 20 to 30 per cent from the estimated normal volume may occur without the clinical manifestations of shock. Such reduction constitutes an urgent indication for replacement therapy. This procedure is of especial value in patients with internal hemorrhage.

Treatment

Peripheral circulatory failure must often be treated per se while attempts to determine and manage the underlying cause are still in progress.

General Measures. Either the flat or the Trendelenburg position may be preferred. Significant elevation of body temperature, i.e., to levels of 102°F or higher, should be combated by sponging, fans, or wet sheets. Pain should be relieved by narcotics, with the realization that absorption, destruction, and excretion of drugs are likely to be impaired. Oxygen should be administered if the patient exhibits cyanosis, dyspnea, or basilar rales.

Administration of Fluid. *The fluid employed should replace that which is lacking* and may be whole blood, plasma, plasma volume expander, or solutions of electrolytes (Chaps. 47 and 50). Intravenous administration of electrolyte-free solutions of glucose is also indicated in order to provide water for insensible loss and for urine volume. The fluids of choice are blood when shock is due to hemorrhage, plasma and saline when burns are responsible, a combination of blood and plasma when there is trauma, while the shock due to loss of extracellular fluid should be treated by the use of the appropriate protein-free electrolyte-containing fluid.

When doubt exists as to the type of solution for administration, it is well to start with blood and to change to plasma or other solutions if the hematocrit subsequently becomes abnormally high. When shock is severe, the administration of blood should be continued at the rate of about 1 liter per hr for 3 or 4 hr. The transfusion is terminated when the signs of shock have disappeared and when a free flow of urine (40 ml or more per hour) has appeared. The development of gallop rhythm, tachypnea, venous distention, increase in venous pressure, rales at the bases, or labored breathing usually contraindicate further intravenous therapy. If the shock state is still present despite these phenomena, it will usually be wise to reduce the rate of the infusion to that needed for the administration of vasopressor drugs, to add *Digitalis lanata* [1.2 to 1.6 mg lanatoside C (Cedilanid) intravenously in about 2 hr] to the infusion fluid, to elevate the patient's head, and to administer oxygen.

As soon as the state of shock has been brought under control, isotonic (6 per cent) glucose solution should be administered in order to compensate for insensible loss of water. The amount needed for this purpose is usually about 1 liter each 24 hr. Since the storage of glucose as glycogen involves the transfer of potassium to the intracellular com-

partment, it is often wise to add potassium chloride (3 Gm per liter) to the infusion fluid. However, this should not be done if oliguria is present. When shock is due to diabetic coma, potassium salts are especially important because of the migration of potassium into the cells as insulin-induced glycogenesis occurs.

Vasopressor Drugs. These are indicated in instances of acute hypotension due to primary vasodilatation (e.g., spinal anesthesia, antihypertensive drugs) and are often valuable in the shock due to such visceral disorders as myocardial infarction or pancreatitis. They are of dubious value and possibly harmful in the type due to hemorrhage or to loss of extracellular fluid, and should not be used as a substitute for fluid replacement.

Of the several vasopressor drugs, norepinephrine is the most potent vasoconstrictor. It should be given only by intravenous infusion, the utmost care being taken to avoid infiltration of the subcutaneous tissues, since necrosis and sloughing of the skin are likely to ensue [should extravasation occur, 5 mg phentolamine (Regitine) diluted in 20 ml water and infiltrated throughout the involved tissues has been found to prevent necrosis] From 5 to 15 ml of a 1:1,000 solution is added to 1 liter of infusion fluid, which is administered initially at a rate of 20 to 40 drops per minute. The rate of infusion is then varied so as to maintain the blood pressure at a level approaching the preshock level of the patient. It should be remembered that a systolic pressure of 120 mm Hg may represent serious hypotension in an elderly person with previous hypertension.

Other vasopressor drugs, enumerated in their descending order of effectiveness, may be used: metaraminol (Aramine), mephentermine (Wyamine), methoxamine (Vasoxyl), and phenylephrine (Neo-Synephrine). They may be administered subcutaneously or intramuscularly in doses of 3 to 15 mg or more, approximately every 15 min, the exact dose and frequency of administration depending on the behavior of the blood pressure; or they may be given by intravenous infusion in concentrations of 30 to 200 mg per liter.

Intravenous pressor drugs should be employed only when a physician or nurse is constantly at the bedside, watching the patient, the blood pressure, and the urine volume and altering the rate of infusion according to the response. The appearance of numerous premature beats or of ventricular tachycardia is an indication to discontinue the infusion or to reduce its rate.

Steroid Hormones. Although the importance of adrenal failure in the pathogenesis of most types of shock remains uncertain (see above), there is little doubt concerning the value of steroid therapy. This has been demonstrated by well-controlled studies on animals with severe hypotension due to hemorrhage or to the administration of bacterial endotoxin.

Regardless of the underlying cause, all patients with severe shock should receive hydrocortisone (500 to 1,000 mg) intravenously over a period of several hours. The remaining measures will depend on the initiating mechanism. When doubt exists, blood or other fluids should be administered provided there is no evidence of pulmonary edema.

HYPOTENSION

Aside from shock, acute decline in blood pressure is most commonly of the *postural type* and is a frequent cause of fainting. Its management is considered in Chap. 33. Heart failure of rapid onset, especially that due to the ectopic tachycardias, produces acute hypotension, and the respective treatment of these conditions is discussed in Chap. 250.

Chronic Hypotension

Chronic hypotension is not a disease but a manifestation. Frequently, it is a manifestation of good health rather than of a pathologic process. This is especially true when a middle-aged or elderly individual, with a favorable family history and without symptoms, is found to have a blood pressure of 100 to 110 mm Hg systolic and 60 to 75 diastolic. In this situation the hypotension calls for no treatment other than congratulations.

Even though the patient complains of nervousness and fatigability, the finding of a systolic blood pressure of about 100 mm Hg is no occasion for concern or for treatment. Perhaps one such patient in a thousand has Addison's disease, and one in ten has some organic disorder such as tuberculosis or aortic stenosis. Most of the remaining nine will present clear evidence of an emotional disorder

and this, rather than the hypotension, should be managed. Thus *persistent low blood pressure should never be treated* as such. The cause should be sought and treated.

For more detailed consideration of some of the topics mentioned in the foregoing chapter, the reader is referred to chapters dealing with Edema (p. 181), Syncope (p. 304), and Congestive Heart Failure (p. 1380).

REFERENCES

Berglund, E., J. Sarnoff, and J. P. Isaacs: Ventricular Function: Role of the Pericardium in Regulation of Cardiovascular Dynamics, Circulation Research, 3:133, 1955.

Connolly, J. E.: Use of Adrenal Cortical Compounds in Hemorrhagic Shock, J. Lancet, 79:460, 1959.

Crowell, J. W., and W. L. Read: In Vivo Coagulation—A Probable Cause of Irreversible Shock, Am. J. Physiol., 183:565, 1955.

DeFazio, V., R. C. Christensen, T. J. Regan, L. G. Baer, Y. Morita, and H. K. Hellems: Circulatory Changes in Acute Glomerulonephritis, Circulation, 20:190, 1959.

Lewis, B. M., H. E. J. Houssay, F. W. Haynes, and L. Dexter: The Dynamics of Both Right and Left Ventricles at Rest and during Exercise in Patients with Heart Failure, Circulation Research, 1:312, 1953.

McMichael, J.: Changing Views on Heart Failure, Ann. Internal Med., 51:635, 1959.

Sarnoff, S. J.: Myocardial Contractility as Described by Ventricular Function Curves: Observations on Starling's Law of the Heart, Physiol. Revs., 35:107, 1955.

Symposium on Congestive Heart Failure, Circulation, 21 (1, 2, 3):95, 1960.

Section 5: Disturbances in Respiration

14 DYSPNEA AND ALLIED MANIFESTATIONS

George W. Wright

It is the primary purpose of the respiratory apparatus, acting in conjunction with the circulatory system, to maintain an optimal partial pressure of oxygen and carbon dioxide (P_{O_2}, P_{CO_2}) throughout the tissues of the body over a wide range of metabolic activity. The respiratory apparatus can be

conveniently thought of as having three major anatomic components. The first of these, the lung, is essentially a plexus of capillaries constituting a large vascular sheet suspended in a gaseous atmosphere. The lung is contained within the second component, a musculoskeletal box capable of rhythmic changes in volume whereby a flow of air into and out of the gaseous space of the lung is induced. The muscles of the respiratory pump are under the control of the central nervous system which, with the varied connections of the respiratory center, constitutes the third anatomic portion of the respiratory apparatus.

From the point of view of function, it is also convenient to divide the act of respiration into three components. The first of these is alveolar ventilation, dependent primarily on mechanical and neuromuscular actions. The second is diffusion of oxygen and carbon dioxide between the gas and blood phase dependent upon (1) the gradient of their pressure across the alveolocapillary membrane, (2) the condition and surface area of this membrane and, (3) factors relating ventilation of the alveolus to perfusion of its capillaries. The third component is the integration of gas and blood flow at various intensities of metabolic activity. An understanding of the physiology of respiration and the way in which disease influences it is of practical assistance in the diagnosis and management of diseases involving these structures. Thus one can expect disease leading to narrowing of the tracheobronchial lumen to interfere with alveolar ventilation, diseases that destroy the pulmonary-vascular bed to limit maximal oxygen uptake, diseases causing a thickening of the alveolar membrane to lead to arterial hypoxia, and so forth.

Injury to or malfunction of the respiratory system may lead to clinical manifestations such as dyspnea, or the awareness of respiratory distress (a subjective phenomenon); breathing that appears to require more effort or to be more voluminous than customary for the circumstances; abnormal patterns of breathing; signs of unusual obstruction of the flow of air through the larynx, trachea, or bronchi, as, for example, wheezing or stridor or unusual retraction or ballooning of interspaces during respiration; cyanosis; cough; thoracic pain; limitation of thoracic motions; or other of the usual physical signs indicating abnormal anatomy within the thorax.

Experience over the past 20 years has convincingly demonstrated that these clinical manifestations of respiratory injury may at times fail to bear a precise quantitative relationship to measurable evidences of respiratory malfunction. At times the clinical manifestations do not develop until rather severe impairment of pulmonary function has occurred. This situation arises from two facts. The first is that the limiting factor for maximal sustained physical exercise in normal persons is the peripheral flow of blood and not the act of respiration. The second is the many physical aids to locomotion, so characteristic of contemporary life, which permit a subtle and progressive moderation of physical activity. For these two reasons, considerable impairment of respiratory prowess often occurs without the development of symptoms of respiratory embarrassment. The converse also occurs, with the result that we are at times faced with a complaint

of dyspnea, cough, or pain without being able to disclose any measurable evidences of respiratory malfunction. This feature occurs less often as we acquire greater knowledge of respiratory function and skill in making appropriate measurement. Nevertheless, the situation does exist.

This considerable disparity between clinical and measurable evidences of altered respiratory function forms an obstacle to the optimal management of the ill. Patients dependent upon the development of signs or symptoms for cognizance that they are ill may fail to seek the advice of a physician until after serious measurable abnormalities of respiration have occurred. Likewise, the physician who relies entirely on the history and the physical signs may overlook significant impairment of the respiratory function.

DYSPNEA

Patients with pulmonary or heart disease, anemia, or neuroses often consult a physician for the first time because they are "out of breath" or "can't get their breath." Some complain that breathing "does not satisfy them," or they "feel the air goes in only a little distance," or they use a number of similar expressions. Since this complaint often brings them to a physician, one must assume that the situation is distressing to them. These complaints characterize dyspnea. For our purposes, it is defined as "the awareness of respiratory distress" or "of unusual breathlessness." It is a subjective phenomenon and liable to all the influences of emotion, ignorance, fatigue, and other factors that make human beings such variable creatures from day to day.

The physician faces the problem of understanding and evaluating statements of the patient, who all too often finds difficulty in describing his distress. Some who make this complaint believe the feeling of breathlessness to be the same as that experienced by normal persons during intense physical exercise, but are distressed because the sensation now develops on less intense effort than previously. Others may have the same lowered threshold for the development of breathlessness, but, in addition, complain that the sensation is different. They describe it as being akin to smothering. Others speak of recurring or constant vague feelings that the act of inspiration does not satisfy. Some speak of weakness in relation to the act of breathing, especially on sustained effort. To reiterate, dyspnea is a form of breathlessness that is distressing or unusual because of the circumstances under which it develops, or because the sensation itself is unusual. It may or may not be associated with the labored breathing or other signs of respiratory embarrassment.

From where do the impulses arise that stream to the cortex and evoke the sensation of breathlessness? During rest or mild exercise, breathing does not produce any sensation, but as the respiratory apparatus is used with increasing vigor, one may become conscious of effort, of the sound and sensation of air being moved through the mouth, nose, and trachea, of the motion of the chest wall, and, finally, of a sensation best described as a feeling that there is a demand or need for increased breathing effort, or a feeling that one is not breathing "enough." It would appear that the impulses responsible for the sensation of breathlessness arise from multiple sources, including the respiratory pump itself, the various sensory endings in the periphery that are known to influence respiration, and possibly from the respiratory center also.

In normal persons, the sensation of a need for augmented breathing during heavy exercise is not a distressing one. This may be because we are accustomed to the sensations associated with the increase of respiratory drive. It may also be because of an inhibition or neutralization of respiratory drive by each act of inspiration, so that a steady state of respiratory drive exists in which each act of inspiration satisfies the demand for more air. Stretch receptors resident within the lung and chest wall may be activated by inspiration in such a manner as to inhibit the sensation of respiratory need. When, however, the act of inspiration does not sufficiently neutralize the respiratory drive, a persistent activity of the inspiratory center may accumulate and finally reach a level that in some ways sends impulses to the cortex which are recognized as "unsatisfied need for breathing." There is some experimental evidence to support this concept of the genesis of the abnormal sensations of dyspnea.

A useful approach for understanding the underlying mechanisms in some patients complaining of dyspnea is the following: One can liken the respiratory apparatus to a pump which, when used at a small percentage of its maximal capacity, performs effortlessly and without calling attention to itself. As the load is increased, evidence of strain gradually intrudes upon consciousness and becomes distressing under the circumstances discussed previously. Bearing this concept in mind, one can explore the individual who complains of dyspnea from the viewpoint of three variables: load, capacity, and the sensitivity of the cerebral cortex. The estimated load during effort would be best expressed in units of work performed by the muscles of respiration. Measurements of the relationship between volume of air flow and transthoracic or transpulmonary pressure gradient are, however, not readily available in most clinics. A usable, though not perfect, substitute for the work of breathing is the "effect" of that work, namely, the liters of air breathed per minute. The load at the time when dyspnea is experienced during exercise can, therefore, be expressed in terms of minute ventilation.

The capacity of the breathing apparatus can be measured in the same terms, namely, the maximal breathing capacity expressed in liters per minute. The ratio of the breathing load, at the time that dyspnea develops, to maximal breathing capacity expressed in liters per minute is referred to by some as the dyspnea index. The strain or sensation associated with respiratory effort will be related to this quotient, and the normal person is unaware of any strain until the "index" exceeds 0.30 to 0.35. It is apparent that the dyspnea index can exceed 0.35 at lower than normal intensities of exercise *if the maximal breathing capacity is reduced or if the minute ventilation is abnormally augmented.* If the sensations of respiration intrude upon consciousness at lesser values, one may infer that the cortex has been made more aware of or is more sensitive than normal to these sensations. Thus some persons, usually classed as neurotic, are exquisitely sensitive to the breathing sensation, while others, because of powerful or engrossing distractions, completely ignore breathing sensations.

When studying a patient who complains of dyspnea, one estimates the normality of the load by measuring the oxygen ventilation equivalent (p. 112) under circumstances provocative of dyspnea. If the O_2V is abnormally high, it can be considered to contribute to the development and sensation of dyspnea. The normality of the breathing capacity is measured in terms of the maximal breathing capacity relative to the predicted normal figure for that individual. If the maximal breathing capacity is pathologically low, one can assume that it contributes to dyspnea. Obviously, factors other than these play a role in this sensation. Fatigue of the respiratory muscles, a phenomenon probably not measured by any of our tests, undoubtedly plays a role in the sensation of dyspnea. The intensity of the sensation of dyspnea experienced by persons with cardiovascular insufficiency is sometimes out of all proportion in its severity to the abnormalities disclosed by the method just described.

Although this simple approach to dyspnea will not explain every aspect in all patients, it is of genuine help in exploring such a complaint. It also enables one to estimate rather closely the intensity of physical effort that a patient can be expected to be capable of accomplishing with comfort. It has the advantage of adding an element of objectivity to that which has heretofore been largely unmeasured and subjective.

Dyspnea can be caused by primary pulmonary or cardiovascular disease and also may exist in the absence of either of these. Regardless of its cause,

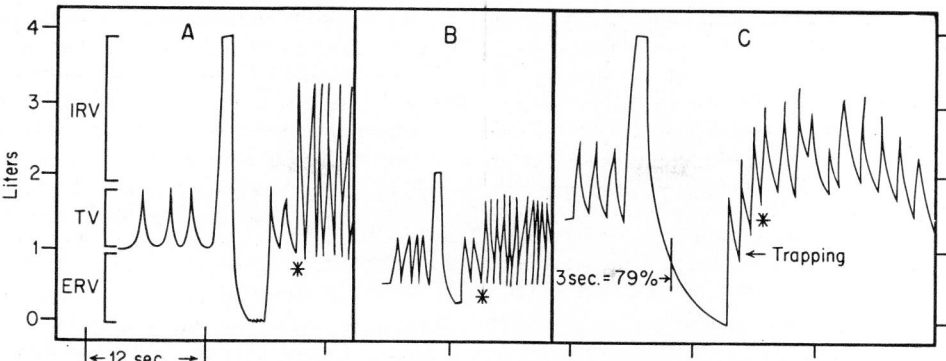

FIG. 14-1. *IRV* = Inspiratory reserve volume. *ERV* = Expiratory reserve volume. The inspiratory capacity is the sum of the inspiratory reserve and the tidal volume (*TV*). The vital capacity is the inspiratory capacity plus the expiratory reserve, or the largest expiration possible from the position of full inspiration. Each of the three spirograms begins with a few tidal breaths, followed by a vital capacity breath blown at maximal velocity. At the asterisk, each subject began to breathe as rapidly and deeply as possible (the maximal breathing capacity).

A. The spirogram of a normal person. The vital capacity is rapid and smooth and completed in less than 3 sec. The maximal breathing is not only rapid but deep.

B. The spirogram of a patient with severe diffuse interstitial fibrosis without emphysema. It is a typical record illustrating restrictive ventilatory insufficiency. Because of increased retractive force within the lungs, tidal breathing is shallow and near the position of complete expiration. Consequently, the expiratory reserve volume is small. The respiratory rate is rapid to compensate for the greater percentage of dead-space breathing. The vital capacity is small but rapidly exhaled. The maximal breathing capacity is reduced but not so severely as the vital capacity, since an increased rate partially offsets the loss of depth.

C. Spirogram characteristic of obstructive ventilatory insufficiency obtained from a patient with emphysema. Although the vital capacity is large, expiration is severely obstructed, so that only 79 per cent is exhaled in 3 sec. Trapping of air in the lungs is indicated by the shifting level of the end-expiratory position of the breath following the vital capacity effort. The maximal breathing effort is carried out near full inspiration and is irregular and severely reduced below normal.

it usually appears first during exercise and is present at rest only when impairment of function is severe. Those diseases which weaken the neuromuscular system, or reduce the mobility of the thorax or the flexibility of the lung, or increase obstruction to air flow induce dyspnea chiefly, but not entirely, by causing a loss of breathing power. Those diseases which pose an abnormal barrier to the transit of oxygen across the alveolocapillary membrane or are associated with an increase of lung rigidity induce dyspnea chiefly by causing an abnormally high load of breathing. Often, both loss of breathing power and abnormally high load of breathing coexist. In some patients, undoubted dyspnea occurs when no significant demonstrable abnormality of the respiratory or circulatory system can be demonstrated. The cerebral cortex in these patients is perhaps more sensitive then usual to the sensations associated with respiration. Perhaps some of the neuroses are in this category. The author has observed several examples of iatrogenic dyspnea. The demonstration of normal physiologic data to such patients plus encouragement and rehabilitation by exercise considerably increase their tolerance for physical exertion.

STUDY OF RESPIRATORY FUNCTION

During the past 20 years, methods of acceptable sensitivity and repeatability have been devised for the study of respiratory function. Some are available on a clinical basis, others are still too complicated or costly to be available outside the research laboratories. The application of these methods has broadened our understanding of the pathologic physiology underlying clinical manifestations of altered pulmonary function and has done much to sharpen our clinical aptitudes and to indicate the limits beyond which clinical skills cannot be presumed to go.

The simple methods of testing pulmonary function will be considered first. Although these do not pinpoint a precise locus of the abnormality of function, they do provide a useful estimate of the capacity of the respiratory apparatus to carry out its ventilatory activity. The history and physical examination are relatively insensitive methods for this purpose. Auscultation of wheezes throughout the lungs, inability to augment the normal respiratory murmur by rapid inspiration and expiration, plus the observation of limited thoracic cage motion, virtually assures a diminished ability to move air into and out of the lungs. Regional wheezing suggests localized bronchial narrowing and has a clinical significance of its own. Careful fluoroscopic examination of the chest with observation of motion of the thoracic cage and diaphragm and the changes in lung density that accompany emptying and filling of the lung during quiet breathing and during explosive forced full inspiration and expiration is a very useful maneuver for a rough estimate of the capacity for air movement into and out of the lungs. Unfortunately, this method lacks quantitation.

Measurements of Pulmonary Volumes. These are simple and valuable in assessing the integrity of the respiratory apparatus. A study of Fig. 14-1 indicates the useful information that may be gleaned from spirometry. The pulmonary volumes are static measurements and lack the element of time. The respiratory pump is capable of augmenting its action many-fold, and dynamic measurements of this function are important. A single explosive full expiratory effort started from a position of full inspiration adds the element of velocity to volume of air flow. Various segments of this expiratory act can be measured, as, for example, the peak flow rate, the maximal mid-expiratory flow rate, the maximal flow rate during the last liter of the vital capacity, and the absolute volume and proportion of total vital capacity expelled in the first second of such an effort. These single expiratory efforts fail to take into consideration the fact that respiration is a repetitive phenomenon, and for this reason plus others, a measurement of the maximal voluntary breathing capacity has some advantages. Each of these procedures measures the integrated activity of component factors governing the function of the respiratory pump discussed in some detail later. These measurements are quite sensitive to any change occurring in an individual, provided the measurement is made before and after the alteration of function occurs. Unfortunately, there is a wide range of variation in the maximal capacity for air flow among normal persons. Hence, although the test faithfully reveals the ability of the person, it will not indicate with certainty that an abnormal state exists until a reduction of capacity to approximately 75 per cent or less of the predicted normal is observed. Even so, these methods are superior to purely clinical observations.

At the end of a maximal forced expiration, a volume of gas still remains in the lung, known as the residual volume. Incomplete emptying of the lung, such as occurs in diffuse obstructive disease, will be revealed by an enlargement of the residual volume. This can be measured either by physical or by gas-rinsing procedures.

Mechanics of Respiration and Alveolar Ventilation. Movement of air into and out of the lungs arises consequent to enlargement and reduction in the size of the thorax. The force developed by contraction of the muscles of respiration is used for the following purposes:

1. Movement of the thoracic cage
2. Movement of the underlying lung structures
3. Movement of air through the tracheobronchial tree

Thus it is seen that the respiratory muscles are used to overcome resistive forces, which can be considered under three categories:

a. Elastic resistances, such as the "spring" of the ribs and stretch of the elastic tissues of the lung
b. Nonelastic resistances, such as those tissues of the chest wall and lung which have no property of recoil
c. Resistance to air flow in the tracheobronchial tree

Two of these forces, namely, those caused by resistance to air flow and motion of nonelastic tissue, can be measured only during respiratory movement, whereas elastic resistance is a static force measured in the absence of movement. The minor forces involved in overcoming inertia can be neglected.

An estimate of the total forces to be overcome by the muscles of respiration during inspiration can be made in the following way. In the anesthetized state and with the muscles of respiration paralyzed by appropriate drugs, the whole body is placed inside a respirator, the head protruding from it. The pressure gradient (transthoracic) between the mouth and the air surrounding the body in the respirator represents the force required to move the thorax and lungs against the various resistive elements. By relating this pressure change to the volume change, one can make approximate comparisons of the normal and abnormal state. For obvious reasons, these measurements have not been made in large numbers of human beings.

The resistance to movement during inspiration caused by the lung tissues plus air flow can be measured by recording the gradient between the intrapleural and oral pressures (transpulmonary pressure), and this in turn can be related to the volume changes occurring in response to this pressure gradient. Because the intraesophageal pressure reflects rather accurately the changes in intrapleural pressure, many such measurements in health and disease have been made.

One can separate the force required to overcome the elastic resistive factors from those required to overcome resistance to air flow plus nonelastic tissue in the following manner: If one measures the intrapleural pressure in a position of expiration and inspiration at moments of zero flow with the glottis open, the difference of intrapleural pressure at the two positions represents the force of the elastic resistive factors overcome in changing the degree of inflation of the lung. The ratio of volume of air inspired to the drop in intrapleural pressure is spoken of as "mechanical compliance" of the lung and is customarily expressed in liters of air per centimeter of water pressure.

If one records the moment to moment pressure change in the pleural space during the act of inspiration, it will be observed that the drop in pressure is always greater than would have been predicted on the basis of the mechanical compliance from the volume change at the precise moment. This excess in pressure drop is the force required to overcome resistance of bronchial air flow and the nonelastic resistances of the lung tissue. It will be noted that this excess of pressure difference will be augmented by increasing the speed of change in volume. This is caused by the greater pressure gradient required for an increase in rate of air flow and frictional resistance of nonelastic tissue. If one neglects the resistance caused by nonelastic tissue, an expression of the resistance to tracheobronchial air flow can be obtained by this indirect method.

It is also possible by an ingenious method using a body plethysmograph to measure directly the gradient between the oral and intraalveolar pressures at instantaneous rates of flow. Observations utilizing this technique have confirmed earlier anatomic studies demonstrating that the lumen of the tracheobronchial system becomes smaller during expiration, and, in fact, toward the end of full expiration the small radicles may become nearly closed. For this reason, airway resistance measurements must be expressed relative to the volume of the lung at the time of the measurement.

Using these various procedures, much has been learned about the effect of disease upon the ease with which the lungs can be ventilated. It is apparent, for example, that diseases which increase the rigidity of the lung parenchyma or which reduce the number of available lung units will decrease the compliance of the lung and thereby increase the work of breathing. Also, diseases which alter the elastic character of the lung in a manner such as to reduce the recoil will increase the compliance of the lung and by the same token diminish the force of the elastic recoil which is used during passive or slow expiration. While on the one hand this reduces the work of breathing during inspiration, it increases the work of breathing during expiration.

Resistance to air flow is related to three primary factors, namely, the diameter and length of the lumen of the tubes and the presence or absence of turbulent and eddy flow as contrasted with laminar flow. Disease processes leading to a reduction in the size of the lumen will increase the resistanec to flow in those areas. Moreover, anything that produces irregularities in the lumen or changes the branching angle may set up turbulent or eddy flow and, consequently, increase the resistance to transbronchial air flow. This is especially apt to occur during augmented rates of flow. During rates of flow that accompany the resting state expiration, in contrast to inspiration, is for the most part a passive phenomenon, the forces accomplishing this act arising by virtue of recoil of elastic tissue within the lung and chest wall. During greater rates of flow, however, active expiratory effort utilizing muscular contraction is required. Under these circumstances, a decrease in thoracic or lung compliance or an increase in airway resistance will require unusually augmented work of breathing.

Relatively little is known concerning the magnitude of the work of breathing because of the difficulty with which such measurements are made. Studies currently available indicate that during the resting state approximately 2 per cent of the total body oxygen uptake is utilized by the muscles of respiration. In normal persons, at the rate of ventilation developed during maximal intensity of exercise, approximately 10 to 15 per cent of the total body oxygen uptake is utilized by the respiratory muscles. This may amount to as much as 400 to 500 ml per min. In diseased states leading to a marked augmentation of the work of breathing, it seems obvious that much larger portions of the total body oxygen uptake, especially in the resting state, would be used for metabolic purposes by the respiratory muscles. This will be discussed later. It is apparent that therapeutic efforts aimed at reducing the work of breathing in pathologic situations may be very important, not only in terms of reduced stress on the respiratory muscles with consequent reduction in their oxygen need but also because of a reduction in their carbon dioxide production, which may be a large contributing factor in the maintenance of high CO_2 levels in the blood where ventilation is impaired and the work of breathing is augmented.

Disturbances of Alveolar Ventilation. The mere fact that large volumes of air can be respired does not assure optimal alveolar ventilation. If the volume respired per minute is too small to satisfy the metabolic demand, alveolar hypoventilation exists. Normally, the volume of air respired is increased in direct proportion to augmented demand for oxygen and carbon dioxide exchange during exercise, so that the partial pressure of these gases in the alveoli stays within narrow limits over a wide range of physical effort. When the respiratory apparatus cannot augment ventilation sufficiently to keep pace with the demands for gas exchange, the alveolar P_{O_2} drops and P_{CO_2} rises. A second situation leading to alveolar hypoventilation has to do with the relationship of the tidal volume to the anatomic dead space. During shallow breathing, the majority of each tidal breath moves into and out of the anatomic dead space and relatively little alveolar ventilation occurs, with the consequence that the turnover of alveolar gas is reduced and the P_{O_2} drops and P_{CO_2} rises. A third type of alveolar hypoventilation occurs when the distribution of each breath is uneven so that some clusters of alveoli are over- and others underventilated. This causes regional variations in alveolar P_{O_2} and P_{CO_2}. If the hypoventilated alveoli, either regional or generalized, are perfused with pulmonary artery blood, the natural consequence is apt to be arterial hypoxia and hypercapnia. On the other hand, the consequences of alveolar hypoventilation will vary, dependent upon whether or not the alveoli are perfused, and studies of recent years have shown that ventilation perfusion ratios can be extremely variable. This point will be discussed later.

The auscultation of wheezes or evidence of impaired respiratory mechanics of various sorts strongly suggests that alveolar hypoventilation either exists or can be made to exist under the stress of physical exercise. Methods are available for measuring the effectiveness of alveolar ventilation per se. In the presence of severe alveolar hypoventilation involving the majority of the alveoli, a sample of alveolar air will be found to have an abnormally high P_{CO_2} and low P_{O_2}. With due regard to the difficulties of obtaining true alveolar air, it can be said that terminal expired air, when sampled properly, should reveal evidences of abnormal gas constituents in the alveoli. The measurement of the CO_2 concentration in terminal expired air is now possible by means of an infrared CO_2 analyzer, and its use is recommended as a means of minimizing the clinical nonrecognition of hypoventilation states. Lesser grades of alveolar hypoventilation must be recognized by the use of a foreign or metabolically inert gas. Rising curves either of the single- or multiple-breath type utilizing helium or nitrogen are very useful in this respect.

Disturbances of Transmembrane Diffusion of O_2 and CO_2. Oxygen and carbon dioxide move between the blood and gas phases of the lung across the alveolocapillary structure because of the pressure gradient for the gases between these two media. The highly complex chemical and physical forces governing this transit will not be discussed here. In the presence of pulmonary disease, this process can become one of the chief limiting factors in physical performance. The integrity of this process can be examined, but instrumentation is needed for such studies. Two approaches can be used.

In normal persons the blood leaving the alveolar capillaries has its hemoglobin fully oxygenated, but when a sample of peripheral systemic arterial blood is examined, a measurable amount of hemoglobin will be found to be in the reduced form. This means either that some blood has perfused hypoventilated (low P_{O_2}) alveoli, and emerged with an abnormal amount of reduced hemoglobin, or that venous blood in some area of the lung has completely bypassed the alveoli and the blood from one or the other of these two sources has then contaminated the peripheral arterial sample by mixing in the left ventricle. Both situations exist to a slight degree in normal persons. It is believed that approximately 5 per cent of the blood leaving the left ventricle represents venous admixture from various sources within the lung, and this accounts for the fact that the arterial hemoglobin at sea level is only 96 to 98 per cent oxygenated.

Methods of acceptable accuracy are available for the direct measurement of P_{O_2} in the blood and, by calculation, of the P_{O_2} in the alveolar gas. As might be expected, because of the venous admixture factor, there is a higher P_{O_2} in the alveolar gas than in the arterial blood. This difference of approximately 10 ml Hg is referred to as the alveolar-arterial (A-a) gradient. The A-a gradient may be increased by disease if the alveolocapillary membrane is thickened or otherwise altered in character, or if a portion of the pulmonary artery blood flow bypasses the alveoli entirely as, for example, in arteriovenous fistula. Arterial hypoxia may occur, therefore, as a result of three entirely different conditions: alveolar hypoventilation, altered alveolocapillary membrane, and direct arteriovenous communications that bypass the alveoli. When alveolar hypoventilation is the cause, the A-a gradient will be normal or only slightly increased, but other abnormalities, discussed under the mechanics of respiration, will be disclosed. Alveolar bypass and alteration of the alveolocapillary membrane (alveolocapillary block) are associated with an increased arteriovenous gradient, and evidences of alveolar hypoventilation are usually absent.

One can distinguish between alveolocapillary block and arteriovenous fistula in most instances in the following way. If one respires a mixture containing 30 to 40 per cent oxygen, the alveolar P_{O_2} is raised sufficiently to drive the necessary molecules of oxygen across the alveolocapillary membrane and restore a normal degree of arterial hemoglobin saturation. Blood passing through an arteriovenous communication within the lung does not perfuse alveoli and, hence, will not be influenced by the elevated alveolar P_{O_2}. Raising the alveolar P_{O_2} will alter the arterial saturation only slightly, if at all, in the arterial hypoxia caused by arteriovenous fistulas. Other methods are also available for discriminating between arteriovenous shunt and alveolocapillary block as a cause of arterial hypoxia. It should be remembered that arteriovenous communications other than the so-called arteriovenous aneurysm or fistula occur, for example, in many of the diseases that cause fibrosis of the lung and in diseases leading to pulmonary artery hypertension.

A second approach to the integrity of the alveolocapillary membrane is a more direct one. The capacity of the lung to permit the transit of oxygen from the gas to the blood phase can be expressed in terms of cubic centimeters of gas per millimeter of pressure gradient per unit of time. This is commonly referred to as the D_L for O_2 and has been found to be larger during exercise than in the resting state. This property of the lung is dependent primarily upon the following factors: the effective surface area of the pulmonary capillary bed, the thickness and character (tissue components) of the membranes separating the gas from the blood phase, and the volume of blood in the capillaries to which the gas is exposed.

The D_L for other gases differs from that of O_2. Carbon dioxide, because it passes across animal membranes approximately twenty times as easily as does oxygen, has a much larger D_L. For this reason, disease involving the alveolocapillary membrane rarely interferes with carbon dioxide removal from the blood (at least to a clinically significant degree), whereas serious impediment to oxygen does occur. Because of much greater technical convenience, it is customary today to use carbon monoxide as the gas for studying these characteristics of the lung. Using this gas, it is possible to distinguish between the membrane component and the capillary blood volume component, but it is still not possible to discriminate between the effective surface area of the membrane and the nature of the membrane itself. Current experience is beginning to indicate that abnormalities of the diffusion characteristics of the lung are more common than heretofore believed and may play an important role in the symptoms and physical limitations of diseased persons.

A further discussion of arterial hypoxia and hypercapnia occurs later in this section.

Ventilation Perfusion Relationships. Alveolar hypoventilation and alveolocapillary block may occur as generalized lung phenomena in which all, or the vast majority, of the units are involved, or may oc-cur in isolated clusters of units scattered throughout the lung, or may involve chiefly one lung. The effects of scattered areas of hypoventilation are not the same as those of generalized hypoventilation because commonly the alveoli not involved by hypoventilation actually undergo hyperventilation. Since the dissociation curves of oxygen and of carbon dioxide have different shapes, clusters of hyperventilated alveoli cannot effectively augment amounts of oxygen put into the blood, but can remove significant quantities of carbon dioxide. As a consequence, the arterial blood gas findings differ in these two situations. In generalized hypoventilation, hypoxia and hypercapnia coexist, whereas in the patchy varieties of alveolar hypoventilation, hypoxia may exist without any attending hypercapnia.

The final effect of hypo- or hyperventilation of alveoli upon arterial blood gases will depend also upon the degree to which these alveoli are perfused with mixed venous blood. Diseases leading to destruction or serious impairment of alveolar function very commonly also destroy the anatomically associated vascular bed. As a result, pulmonary artery blood does not perfuse the injured alveoli and arterial hypoxia and hypercapnia are avoided. In the resting state, for reasons poorly understood, alveolar hypoventilation of the patchy type is often not associated with arterial hypoxia or hypercapnia because a reduction in capillary perfusion occurs to a degree commensurate with the hypoventilation, so that the ventilation and perfusion ratios actually are normal although the oxygen uptake and CO_2 output per lung unit are reduced. This relationship may be grossly disturbed during exercise, however. The necessity of using the stress of physical exercise to unmask abnormal conditions in the lung cannot be emphasized too greatly. Not only must one increase the metabolic demand and thus unbalance the ventilation perfusion ratio, but also it would appear that some of the arterialvenous shunt mechanisms are responsive to intravascular pressure changes and operate only during the periods of increased blood flow or the pulmonary hypertension that may accompany physical exercise.

Regional areas of hypoperfusion may also occur in the presence of normally ventilated alveoli. Two things may occur in this situation. The first is that blood is shunted away from the hypoperfused areas and there is augmented blood flow through other alveoli, with the consequence that such alveoli then become relatively hypoventilated. The second is that actual hyperventilation of these overperfused alveoli may come about by reason of increased minute ventilation, thus abolishing the relative hypoventilation. If, for example, one suddenly ligated the main pulmonary artery on one side, the tremendous increase in blood flow through the other lung would greatly augment the rate of removal of oxygen and delivery of carbon dioxide to that perfused lung. Hypoxia and hypercapnia would ensue unless these perfused alveoli were physically hyperventilated. The alveoli of the ligated lung, of course, continue to be ventilated but perform no useful function and, therefore, constitute a physiologic dead space. Although this precise circumstance rarely occurs, a similar situation involving scattered clusters of alveoli is common. This leads to a persistent hyperventilation state with abnormally large physiologically dead space.

The mechanisms whereby variations in perfusion can occur are not entirely clear. Arteriolar or capillary thrombosis or actual destruction of the tissue are obvious mechanisms. On the other hand, a reduction in perfusion paralleling that of ventilation, even to the point that perfusion virtually ceases in nonventilated portions of lung, has been observed without attending anatomic obstruction to blood flow. Studies during recent years have shown that some mechanism is available whereby alveolocapillary perfusion is diminished (presumably by narrowing or closure of these vessels) whenever the alveolar P_{O_2} is diminished by hypoventilation. The reaction is probably more complex than this. The important thing is to realize that the respiratory system exhibits a great ability to tailor its perfusion to whatever ventilation exists in various regions of the lung.

It is apparent from these comments that the pulmonary-vascular bed may undergo a considerable reduction in size as a result of intrinsic pulmonary disease, some of which is on an organic basis and some on a functional basis. This restriction of the vascular bed may lead to serious circulatory consequences that will be discussed in detail in Chap. 262.

INTEGRATION AND CONTROL OF RESPIRATION

The rate and depth of respiration are controlled directly by impulses arising within the brain stem from cells designated as the respiratory centers. The discharge of these cells is modified as to rate and intensity by a host of impulses coming to them from many parts of the body. The cerebral cortex, chemo- and pressoreceptors, thermoreceptors, muscle tension receptors, sensory bodies in the lung, pain receptors, and other less certainly established sensory bodies elsewhere in our anatomy send out such regulatory impulses. The cells of the respiratory center also vary their discharge in response to their own tissue environment. Hence, the rate of flow of blood to these cells and its chemical char-

acter in terms of pH, P_{O_2} and P_{CO_2} will modify the discharge of the respiratory center. With so many influences, one marvels that the respiratory discharge is other than chaotic. Normally, the stimuli are well integrated so that there is reciprocal stimulation and inhibition of the various parts of the center and the final discharge pattern has an orderly character. The intensity of the discharge is not the strict arithmetic sum of the various physiologic and psychologic influences.

How can one measure the output of impulses from the respiratory center and by inference the character of the stimuli that drive it? If the respiratory apparatus is mechanically capable of responding fully to the discharge from the respiratory center, a situation not always obtaining in the presence of disease, then the volume of air moved per minute must be a function of the total discharge from the respiratory center. The volume of air respired per minute can, therefore, be used as an estimate of the respiratory drive under the conditions stated. How can one know whether that drive is normal? During the "resting state" the volume of air respired per minute depends to a large measure on environmental stimuli and conscious or perhaps even subconscious activity of the cortex. Excitement, interest in surrounding events, etc., have a large influence on the pattern and rate of ventilation at rest. Because of this, our ability to recognize abnormal respiratory drive at rest is limited. If, at rest, the minute volume consistently exceeds 10 liters for men and 7 liters for women, unusual respiratory drive probably exists. In contrast, sustained physical work by a normal person under normal physiologic conditions will cause the respired minute volume to increase directly in a straight-line fashion with the measured increment of oxygen uptake. The ratio of these two measurements over a wide range of physical activity is 25 ± 5 liters of air respired for each liter of oxygen uptake in the steady state. This ratio may be termed the "oxygen ventilation equivalent" (O_2V). At the extremes of hard physical exercise, this ratio becomes increased because oxygen uptake reaches a plateau whereas the respiratory minute volume continues to rise.

On the basis of known responses of the respiratory center to various stimuli, one can predict that certain abnormalities should lead to an unusual respiratory drive. Hypoxia, hypercapnia, decrease of blood pH, increased rigidity of the thoracic cage or of the lung itself are all likely to cause an increase of respiratory drive and a consequent abnormally large O_2V. It is of more than passing interest that, in the presence of chronic abnormalities of the sort just mentioned, the respiratory center appears to adapt itself and the abnormal responses elicited by exercise are often less than one would anticipate.

The relation of the O_2V to dyspnea has already been mentioned (p. 112).

The preceding paragraphs present a brief résumé and discussion of certain aspects of the physiology of respiration in normal persons as they pertain to a better understanding of the symptoms and signs of abnormal respiratory function and the effects of disease upon the respiratory apparatus. The reader is encouraged to seek other more detailed and comprehensive literature concerning this subject, especially as to methodology.

APPROACH TO THE PATIENT WITH DYSPNEA

When muscular disorders, anemia, thyrotoxicosis, or metabolic acidosis are responsible for dyspnea, this symptom is a relatively minor phenomenon and the clinical picture is dominated by other and more specific manifestations of the underlying diseases. The problems arise in the differentiation of the psychogenic, pulmonary, and cardiac varieties of dyspnea from each other and, more especially, in evaluation of the relative significance of each of these types when two of them coexist, as they frequently do.

Emotional dyspnea is characterized by a sensation of smothering often described as "a need for more oxygen" or "my breathing does not get in enough air." Associated complaints such as numbness of the face or extremities, tightness of the chest muscles with slight pain, "drawing" of the hands, faintness, lightheadedness, "floating away," palpitation, or aerophagia with belching are usually present. In most instances the symptoms are episodic and there is little relation of dyspnea to exertion. The manifestation of panic or of the acute anxiety state (p. 390) may be pronounced. Unless there is coexistent cardiac or pulmonary disease, the various tests of respiratory function yield normal findings, although during an attack there is hypocapnia and an increased ventilation in relation to oxygen uptake.

As a general rule, dyspnea of pulmonary or cardiac origin appears initially during exertion. However, bronchial asthma and acute left ventricular failure (p. 1382) may first occur at rest. Cough of long duration is a frequent concomitant of pulmonary dyspnea, but acute episodic coughing may accompany either type. Clinical, radiologic, or electrocardiographic evidence of primary pulmonary or cardiac disease is of obvious importance.

Seizures of dyspnea which waken the patient speak for a cardiac origin, but early morning episodes associated with cough and expectoration point toward pulmonary disease.

The arm-to-tongue circulation time is usually prolonged in patients with cardiac dyspnea but normal when the distress is of pulmonary origin. A decrease in the rate of air flow (i.e., in the "timed vital capacity" or "forced expiratory volume") is more likely to signify pulmonary dyspnea. Both types of dyspnea are associated with decrease in total vital capacity, which is usually reduced less in relation to the decline in maximal breathing capacity in the pulmonary than in the cardiac disorders. This relative disproportion, which is due to airway obstruction, may, however, be present in those patients with cardiac failure who have pronounced wheezes (cardiac asthma, p. 1382).

Arterial hypoxia, which is common in patients with pulmonary disease, is absent or minimal in those with cardiac disorders, except when edema of the lungs is pronounced or some complication such as pulmonary infarction supervenes. Hypercapnia is the rule in the advanced stages of those disorders of the lungs associated with alveolar hypoventilation; it is absent in patients with cardiac failure except for those instances due to primary pulmonary disorders (cor pulmonale).

As dyspnea and limitation for physical exercise become progressively more severe, orthopnea begins to be experienced by the patient who has heart failure. In contrast, orthopnea rarely occurs in primary pulmonary disease, even though the dyspnea associated with exercise may be severe. When the pulmonary cripple begins to experience orthopnea, he is apt to be developing cor pulmonale and heart failure. Two factors may play a role. A transfer of blood from the abdomen and lower extremities to the thorax occurs when assuming the recumbent position, and the cardiac output tends to be increased. Something associated with this fluid shift, perhaps an increase in distention of the pulmonary vasculature with associated acute reduction in mechanical compliance, may induce the sensation of breathlessness. A second and probably more potent factor is that in the recumbent position the functional residual volume (position of involuntary termination of expiration) becomes suddenly markedly reduced. As a consequence, the lumen of the smaller bronchi and bronchioles is suddenly reduced, with an abrupt rise of airway resistance. If there is any tendency to the development of bronchial secretions, as by a mild attack of pulmonary edema, this effect will be augmented. A combination of these two factors of fluid shift and airway resistance increase probably accounts for the sensation of orthopnea.

For further discussion of the differentiation between pulmonary and cardiac dyspnea, the reader is referred to p. 1380.

HYPERCAPNIA AND HYPOCAPNIA

Although hypercapnia, an abnormally elevated P_{CO_2} in tissues and blood, is a relatively common clinical state as a result of pulmonary disease, it occurs only in those situations leading to alveolar hypoventilation. Alveolocapillary block does not lead to clinically significant hypercapnia because of the greater ability for carbon dioxide to traverse the membrane and the common occurrence of alveolar hyperventilation. All the conditions leading to alveolar hypoventilation discussed earlier will if severe enough lead to hypercapnia provided, of course, the hypoventilated alveoli are also perfused with pulmonary artery blood.

Hypocapnia, the development of a subnormal P_{CO_2}, in the tissues and blood, is unusual. It may occur in those pulmonary diseases which lead to hyperventilation of alveoli that are relatively well perfused with pulmonary artery blood. More often it is the result of emotional disturbances.

For further discussion of hypercapnia and hypocapnia, the reader is referred to Chap. 51.

HYPOXIA

In a broad sense, hypoxia can be defined as "oxygen deficiency in the body." It is customary to refer to hypoxia as being either localized or general and also to use modifying terms suggesting the cause of the deficiency. Most physicians are familiar with hypoxia, but it is less appreciated that a condition one might speak of as hyperoxia also does occur, although not commonly. This state of too much oxygen can have profound medical importance. Those working in high atmospheric pressures know that oxygen tensions above 1 atm may have severe central nervous system effects, a factor that contributes to the limitations for deep-sea diving. Less appreciated is the fact that elevated pressures of oxygen such as occur during therapeutic use of pure oxygen at 1 atm may have serious cytotoxic affects in the lung per se.

Oxygen utilized by the body which is supplied via the act of external respiration moves from the alveolus into the plasma solely on the basis of its partial pressure. Its movement out of the plasma into the tissues, where it is utilized chemically, is also governed solely by the gradient of pressure between plasma and the interior of the tissue cell. Under resting conditions, the quantity of oxygen extracted from 100 ml of blood as it perfuses the tissues is extremely variable, but for the body as a whole, approximately 4 to 5 ml of oxygen is removed from each 100 ml of blood during one tissue passage. The amount of oxygen that can be put into physical solution in the blood plasma in the lung when a normal man respires ambient air at sea level is only about 0.27 to 0.30 ml of oxygen per 100 ml of blood. Life could not be sustained with this meager supply were it not for the fact that a large quantity of oxygen can be stored in the hemoglobin carried in the red blood cell to be released as needed to replenish the plasma O_2 as the tissues are perfused. It is important also to note that hemoglobin becomes united with oxygen more readily (at a lower P_{O_2}) when in an alkaline medium than when in an acid medium. This, of course, favors its pickup in the lung where CO_2 is discharged and its release at the tissues where carbon dioxide is entering the red cell and combining with the hemoglobin molecule. This, the Bohr effect of hydrogen ion concentration on hemoglobin oxygen linkage, is of considerable physiologic importance.

Normally, mixed venous blood returning to the heart has a plasma P_{O_2} of approximately 40 mm Hg, and 30 per cent of its hemoglobin is in the reduced state. The shape of the hemoglobin dissociation curve (Fig. 14-2) is such that a large part of the O_2 uptake can occur without a build-up of plasma P_{O_2}. This helps to maintain a large P_{O_2} gradient across the alveolocapillary membrane during the transfer of the bulk of the O_2 uptake. The dynamics of the process of loading the hemoglobin are reasonably well understood. The delivery of oxygen to the tissues is not as well studied, largely because methods are not well developed for measuring the gradient of P_{O_2} from plasma to tissue fluid and intracellular fluid. Study of blood leaving specific organs shows a great variation in the P_{O_2} of the plasma and in the quantity of oxygen that has been removed. The importance of hemoglobin at the delivery end is obvious. At the lung, the oxygen tension of plasma is increased by reason of a reservoir of oxygen in the alveolus at high P_{O_2}. In the tissues, the plasma P_{O_2} would drop to seriously low levels very rapidly if it were not for the fact that the hemoglobin is there to supply a large amount of oxygen and thus maintain a high enough P_{O_2} in the plasma to secure a gradient into the cells.

The venous blood leaves the tissues at a P_{O_2} varying from 40 to 20 mm Hg, the actual value reached being a function of rate of blood flow and metabolism of the tissue. One can assume, therefore, that the cells are capable of functioning over a range somewhat lower than this. Without hemoglobin, the required magnitude of P_{O_2} in the tissues could not be maintained. The peculiar characteristic of hemoglobin as revealed in the dissociation curve (Fig. 14-2) serves a useful purpose here as it does in the lungs. The tissue P_{O_2} is in the precise range over which a large quantity of oxygen can be delivered from the hemoglobin to the plasma, with a small variation in oxygen tension. This circumstance permits a wide range of metabolic activity in the tissues with maintenance of optimal tissue P_{O_2}, the factor that governs movement of molecular oxygen. Also, with these facts in mind,

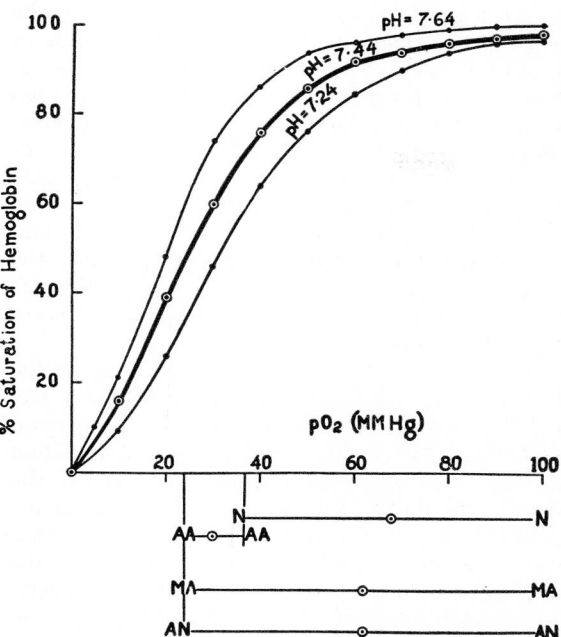

Fig. 14-2. Relationship between oxygen tension and oxygen saturation of the hemoglobin of the blood. The heavy line is for blood at pH 7.44. The curves to the right and left are for those bloods at pH 7.24 and 7.64, respectively, indicating quantitatively the magnitude of the Bohr effect for hydrogen ion concentration changes of these magnitudes.

Thus, at about the middle of the curve shown for pH 7.44, a fall in pH to 7.24 will decrease the saturation of hemoglobin by about 15 per cent, without change in oxygen tension. Hence, during severe muscular exercise the increase in tissue acidity makes oxygen more available to the muscles. At high altitudes, or under conditions which lower alveolar carbon dioxide tension, the shift in the dissociation curve upward and to the left makes it possible for the blood to take up more oxygen at a given tension. It should be realized that the Bohr effect, although of especial importance under certain conditions of adverse environment or physiologic stress, plays a significant role in oxygen exchange, even under normal resting conditions.

Beneath the abscissas are plotted the calculated arteriovenous oxygen differences, upon the presumption of the right-heart venous oxygen content normally being 5 vol per cent less than the arterial content, and with constant cardiac output in the following states: N = normal person, arterial oxygen content 20 vol per cent; AA = same person suffering from arterial hypoxia sufficient to lower the arterial oxygen content to 14.6 vol per cent (= 73 per cent saturation), but with oxygen consumption unaltered; MA = same person with 100 per cent increase in oxygen consumption; AN = anemic patient, arterial oxygen content 10 vol per cent, with arterial saturation and oxygen consumption same as in normal person. The heavy dots indicate the mean oxygen tension in each instance.

it is easy to see why blood having a subnormal amount of hemoglobin must flow at a faster rate in order to maintain the optimal tissue P_{O_2}.

The role of plasma as a potential oxygen carrier should not be dismissed. At sea level respiring pure oxygen in an open circuit, the P_{O_2} in the alveolus can approach 700 mm Hg partial pressure. At this tension, plasma can carry as much as 2 ml of oxygen per 100 ml of blood. If one-half the blood circulating through a diseased lung passes through normally acting alveoli, as much as one-fifth of the metabolically needed oxygen can be introduced by inspiring pure oxygen. This mechanism is of use in the treatment of hypoxia. When hypoxia is on the basis of alveolar hypoventilation, it is not necessary to respire pure oxygen because, under these circumstances, one only need raise the mean alveolar P_{O_2} by a few millimeters of mercury in order to restore almost normal oxygenation of the hemoglobin.

Mechanisms of Hypoxia. Hypoxic states can be divided into four main categories:

Arterial Hypoxia (Hypoxic Hypoxia). This develops consequent to insufficient oxygenation of the blood in the lungs, the chief causes of which are alveolar hypoventilation, abnormal ventilation perfusion relationships, alveolocapillary block, admixture of systemic venous blood with pulmonary vein blood via anatomic shunts, a reduction in ambient air P_{O_2}.

Anemic Hypoxia. This is tissue hypoxia resulting from a diminished concentration of total hemoglobin in the blood and a consequent inability to maintain an optimal tissue P_{O_2}. This may result

---

It should be understood that the conditions depicted in these states are exaggerated in comparison to those actually obtaining in normal persons. Thus, the consequences of the normal Bohr effect and of temperature upon the dissociation curve are ignored. In instances of arterial hypoxia, increases in circulating hemoglobin usually occur, and the venous tension is still further modified by the Bohr effect in a direction depending upon the mechanism by which the arterial unsaturation is produced. In the case of metabolic hypoxia, the effects of temperature increase and rising cardiac output lessen the degree of hypoxia which otherwise would obtain. In the case of anemia hypoxia, a rising cardiac output tends to lessen the hypoxia.

In spite of these simplifications, the diagram indicates the principles concerned in the understanding of the relative severity of hypoxia produced by different mechanisms. The quantitative lesions involved vary for each tissue, depending upon a number of factors, but chiefly upon the normal volume of blood flow per unit time per unit mass of tissue and the inherent oxygen consumption of the tissue concerned. The actual tissue tensions, in any event, are less than the corresponding capillary tensions.

from actual loss or failure to produce hemoglobin or from alterations of a portion of the hemoglobin to forms that do not carry oxygen.

Circulatory Hypoxia. This ensues from any altered relationship between peripheral blood flow and the metabolic demands of tissues. This is a highly complex form of hypoxia and is discussed in greater detail in Chap. 13. It is a normal phenomenon during severe exercise when blood flow is markedly reduced in the gut and parenchymatous organs and greatly augmented in the active muscles. In disease, a subnormal cardiac output may greatly augment this regional form of circulatory hypoxia and may cause a generalized circulatory hypoxia. Localized venous or arterial obstructions either of a physiologic or anatomic nature will cause regional circulatory hypoxia. In essence, circulatory hypoxia occurs whenever perfusion does not keep pace with metabolism and may arise whenever circulation is inadequate or metabolism excessive, or a combination of the two.

Histotoxic Hypoxia. This results from failure of utilization of oxygen because of cellular malfunction in the presence of otherwise adequate stores of molecular oxygen, usually caused by poisons such as cyanide.

Arterial Hypoxia. The most common cause of arterial hypoxia, exclusive of residence at high altitude, is alveolar hypoventilation. Alveolocapillary block and direct arteriovenous communication with alveolar bypass are less common causes. These situations refer primarily to conditions arising within the lung and commonly coexist in the same individual. Another, but less common, cause of arterial hypoxia is congenital heart disease, in which communications permitting the passage of venous blood from the right to the left side of the heart may occur. It also may occur in acquired heart disease by reason of the development of direct communications between the pulmonary artery and pulmonary vein that bypass the alveoli as, for example, in pulmonary hypertension. Pulmonary edema may also cause arterial hypoxia because the transudate leads to alveolar hypoventilation plus alveolocapillary block.

The common clinical sign suggesting arterial hypoxia is cyanosis, a condition to be discussed in greater detail later. It is imperative that one realize that "cyanosis" when caused by arterial hypoxia is a manifestation of severe hypoxia and that clinically significant grades of arterial hypoxia commonly exist without cyanosis. For this reason, one must rely on chemical determination of oxygen saturation in anaerobically collected arterial blood for the early recognition of arterial hypoxia. While, by definition, hypoxia is a subnormal P_{O_2} in the arterial blood, few laboratories are equipped to make direct measurements of oxygen tension. Because of

this, it is customary to measure the degree to which arterial hemoglobin is saturated with oxygen in order to recognize the presence of arterial hypoxia. Normally, arterial hemoglobin should be 96 to 98 per cent saturated, and anything less than this can be considered arterial hypoxia.

Methods for differentiating between the causes of arterial hypoxia have already been discussed.

A moderate grade of arterial hypoxia occurring during exercise is of clinical significance primarily as an indication that some abnormality of the lungs or heart exists. An arterial hemoglobin saturation of 85 to 94 per cent, clearly a subnormal value, has little importance in regard to causing serious tissue hypoxia. The reason for this is understood on inspection of the dissociation curve in Fig. 14-2. The major volume transfer of oxygen in the lungs and at the tissues occurs in the range of P_{O_2} between 40 and 60 mm Hg. In other words, adequate quantities of oxygen to support life and even permit rather severe exercise will go on in an entirely satisfactory manner with an arterial P_{O_2} that reaches 60 mm Hg with the hemoglobin saturation of 90 per cent by the time the blood leaves the terminal portion of alveolar capillaries. The tissues suffer little or not at all unless the arterial P_{O_2} is lower than 60 mm Hg. Arterial hypoxia occurring during the resting state is more serious because virtually without exception it becomes more severe during exercise and may reach seriously low levels.

Anemic Hypoxia. This form occurs whenever there is a reduction in the amount of available oxygen carrying hemoglobin in the circulating blood, regardless of whether this occurs by reason of a loss of total hemoglobin or a conversion of a part of the total hemoglobin to the nonoxygen combining pigment. It is identified by demonstrating a subnormal oxygen combining capacity in the arterial blood. The arterial blood will be found to have a normal P_{O_2}. However, as the anemic blood passes through the capillaries of the tissues, the usual amount (5 ml per 100 ml of blood at rest) of oxygen is removed from it, and as a consequence the tension of oxygen in the blood leaving the tissues declines to subnormal levels. The removal of the usual amount of oxygen from subnormal hemoglobin stores in the arterial blood of necessity causes a greater degree of unsaturation in the venous blood. As a consequence, the P_{O_2} of the venous blood will be subnormal and the mean P_{O_2} of the tissues of necessity will be subnormal unless some ameliorating factor, such as increase in blood flow, occurs.

The hemoglobin in simple anemia combines with oxygen according to the usual dissociation curve. In contrast, the presence of methemoglobin or carboxyhemoglobin shifts the lower part of the dissociation curve to the left so that oxygen tends to stay combined with hemoglobin with greater tenacity. As a result, in methemoglobinemia and carbon monoxide poisoning, sufficient numbers of oxygen molecules will be released to the tissue only in the presence of unusually low partial pressures of oxygen and, hence, the hypoxia of these two conditions is much more severe than in simple anemia of a commensurate degree. Because of the subnormal total quantity of oxygen available when the blood reaches the tissues in anemic hypoxia, the effects of increased metabolism in the tissues are markedly augmented. For this reason, although anemia may not lead to symptoms of hypoxia at rest, severe distress may occur during exercise.

Circulatory Hypoxia. In essence, this form of hypoxia arises within the tissues because of an imbalance between the oxygen demands of the metabolically active cells and the quantity of blood supplied per unit time to the tissues. Possible causes of this form of hypoxia have been indicated under the classification of hypoxia, and for further details the reader is referred to Chap. 13.

Histotoxic Hypoxia. Tradition requires the mention of this form of hypoxia, even though according to the strict definition subnormal oxygen tension within the tissues does not exist. This category refers to interference with the intermediary metabolism of oxygen by reason of certain poisons that act upon tissue cells and impair the function of those cells, regardless of the fact that the partial pressure of oxygen is within the limits of normal.

Effects of Hypoxia. Hypoxia has clinical significance in part because of its interference with cellular function and in part because of manifestations developed by the body's attempts to minimize its degree. While the withholding of molecular oxygen from living cells will ultimately result in their death, little is known concerning the changes in functions that may occur at specified degrees of hypoxia. The various types of cells of which the body is composed show a rather remarkable difference in their powers to maintain function in the presence of hypoxia. Nervous tissue is the least capable of withstanding oxygen deprivation. The cells of the higher centers are especially affected by hypoxia so that total deprivation from oxygen for periods of 5 to 8 min results in death of the cells of the cerebrum, and the medullary centers tend not to survive periods beyond 12 to 13 min. Even though these cells may survive lesser periods of deprivation, they may at times not function normally, following such injury. In contrast, the ciliated cells of the bronchial mucosa have been shown to survive for many hours after removal from the body, provided proper thermal and electrolyte environments are maintained.

There is abundant literature concerning the effects of various grades of hypoxia upon the component parts of the body. For the most part, these experiments and observations have been carried out in normal and sometimes exceptionally healthy individuals. Some caution must be exercised in transferring this information to individuals who become hypoxic during the course of disease because, in the latter individual, certain adaptive mechanisms are impaired.

Furthermore, in various clinical states, hypoxia is commonly associated with hypercapnia. Carbon dioxide has a marked narcotic effect upon cells of the brain, and in many situations involving hypercapnia and hypoxia at the same time, the symptoms of mental disturbance are more those of hypercapnia than those of hypoxia. A failure to realize this may be serious because therapeutic measures effective in overcoming hypoxia may at the same time abolish the hypoxic drive of the respiratory center and lead to augmentation of the hypercapnia, sometimes with fatal results (Chap. 268).

Although there is some disagreement, the consensus is that oxygen uptake remains the same in the presence of all degrees of hypoxia that are compatible with continued life. It is difficult to reconcile this with the known evidences of malfunction of the central nervous system and muscular system during severe hypoxia. Perhaps it is a matter of new balances in the various pathways of intermediary metabolism being reached requiring the same amount of oxygen, but since operation goes on at a lower P_{O_2}, optimal function is not maintained. It is known, for example, that lactic acid may accumulate and persist at a higher than normal level for the duration of the hypoxic state, thus indicating an abnormal metabolic process even though oxygen uptake is maintained. For the metabolic effects of hypoxia, the reader is referred to Chaps. 51 and 52.

The body's reaction to hypoxia can be subdivided into three categories on the basis of rapidity of onset and duration. The fulminating category is actually a form of total hypoxia or anoxia and occurs as a result of inhalation of undiluted inert gases such as may be met with accidentally. Unconsciousness, collapse, and death ensue rapidly over a period of several minutes, and there is no need to discuss this further. Acute hypoxia occurs when moderate or severe hypoxia occurs over a matter of minutes or hours and, depending on its severity, may lead to breathlessness, palpitation, headaches, mental confusion, disorientation, depression, irrationality, muscular weakness and incoordination, nausea, and sometimes disturbances in vision and hearing. It should be recalled that most of these same disturbances can be caused by hypercapnia. Chronic hypoxia is characterized by persistence of some of the symptoms just mentioned, but because the body may react in a way to ameliorate the effects, some of the symptoms are minimized and new ones are added.

When hypoxia first develops the body responds in a number of ways, attempting to minimize the effects by improving the mean P_{O_2} in the blood and the tissues. Respiration is augmented and alveolar ventilation is increased, with the result that the alveolar P_{O_2} may be elevated to a significant degree. This is especially true in alveolocapillary block but is less true in hypoxia resulting from alveolar hypoventilation. As a result of the increased alveolar P_{O_2}, the A-a gradient is increased and the alveolar capillary blood becomes more saturated in those persons having alveolocapillary block. Unfortunately, by the same token, alveolar hyperventilation leads to a further loss of carbon dioxide, causing the blood to become even more alkaline and, as a consequence, the dissociation curve is shifted to the left and delivery of oxygen at the tissues is impaired. To some extent this may be offset by the augmented lactic acid production in the tissues.

A most important effect of acute hypoxia is the increase in cardiac output brought about largely by an increase in pulse rate and venous return. In addition, as a general rule, hypoxia leads to vasodilatation in the tissues. As a result of the increased tissue flow, less hemoglobin is required to give up its oxygen and the mean tissue P_{O_2} is maintained closer to the arterial P_{O_2} level than if this circulatory adjustment did not develop.

The renal and gastrointestinal and endocrinologic effects of acute hypoxia are relatively insignificant but become important in chronic hypoxia. One other effect of acute hypoxia deserves mention because of its importance in certain disease states. In recent years it has been shown that hypoxia leads to an increase in pulmonary blood flow resistance, presumably by reason of narrowing of the arterioles or capillaries. The combination of increase in vascular resistance and elevated pulmonary blood flow consequent to hypoxia produces a significant elevation of pulmonary artery pressure and increased right ventricular work. This train of circumstances can scarcely be thought of as being beneficial in the diseased individual. Some benefit may, however, be gained in those circumstances wherein pulmonary disease leads to regional alveolar hypoventilation with a low alveolar P_{O_2}. Under these circumstances the pulmonary vessels supplying the hypoventilated alveoli apparently undergo narrowing, with a consequent elevation of resistance sufficient to shunt blood away from the hypoventilated alveoli and into more normally ventilated alveoli, with the consequence that blood perfusing the lung tends to pass through the best ventilated alveoli. In this manner, hypoxia of the arterial blood is ameliorated in the hypoventilation states.

When hypoxia persists for a matter of days or becomes chronic, other physiologic adjustments occur. There is some evidence that the cells may be able to utilize oxygen more effectively, although firm proof for this does not exist. Clinical observations indicate that with the passage of time, in the hypoxic state, mental acuity tends to improve. That this may be the result of other adaptations such as increased blood flow and polycythemia cannot be denied. Hyperventilation persists with the maintenance of this helpful adaptation that tends to promote an increase in alveolar P_{O_2}. In contrast, the respiratory center develops a considerable tolerance to hypercapnia. The respiratory alkalosis which may develop as a result of hypoxia of the nonhypoventilation varieties becomes minimized by the excretion of buffer base. This serves two useful purposes. It makes the respiratory center more sensitive to any acute increase of carbon dioxide because of the loss of buffering power of the plasma. In addition, it tends to minimize the effect of alkalosis on hemoglobin binding at the tissue level. Because of this, plus the tendency to accumulate lactic acid in the tissues and, hence, in the tissue capillaries, the delivery of oxygen at the tissue level is improved in chronic hypoxias as compared to acute hypoxia. In chronic hypoxia, the augmented cardiac output and increased blood flow persist. There is some evidence in experimental animals that the vascular bed of muscle tissue becomes increased.

One of the most striking developments in chronic hypoxia is the increase in red blood corpuscles and hemoglobin (polycythemia), thus significantly augmenting the oxygen-carrying power of the blood. The effect of this is the exact opposite of that discussed under anemic hypoxia, and as a consequence the mean tissue P_{O_2} is augmented. There is some evidence in experimental animals that there may be an increase in myoglobin as well as in hemoglobin.

At moderate levels of tissue hypoxia, most organs of the body continue to function normally. The extent to which organs such as the liver and kidney function in the presence of more severe grades of chronic hypoxia has not been clearly elucidated. One of the difficulties is that the disturbances of circulation, which may either cause or prevent the proper adaptations to chronic hypoxia, may also play an equal role in malfunction of the organ that is being studied in individuals suffering from hypoxia. At least two of the endocrine glands are known to be influenced by chronic hypoxia. The adrenal cortex is known to hypertrophy in normal animals during chronic hypoxia. Observations in this regard are not easy to evaluate in diseased persons because the disease causing the hypoxia may, by virtue of its stressing action in respect to things other than hypoxia, also influence the adrenal cortex. The gonads appear to be influenced also. There is evidence that a number of animals are virtually sterile at high altitudes. In addition, records indicate that, although the Andean natives were quite prolific, their Spanish conquerors showed a greatly lessened birth rate. Some evidence of sterility as a result of chronic carbon monoxide poisoning has been reported also.

Chronic hypoxia in the diseased person may develop and become more severe very slowly and over a long period of time. Because of this the body has ample opportunity to make the necessary adjustments, and one is often surprised at the exercise capacity of patients suffering from any of the three varieties of chronic hypoxia. Experiments creating a low alveolar P_{O_2} suddenly in a non-acclimated person (high altitude) demonstrate that, at a P_{O_2} of 25 mm Hg in the arterial blood, collapse and coma will occur in a few minutes. The author has observed patients with an arterial P_{O_2} of 25 mm Hg (alveolocapillary block and congenital heart disease) who exhibit none of the cortical abnormalities associated with hypoxia and who are comfortable at rest. Brief mild exercise, such as level walking at 2 mph, caused severe dyspnea and tachycardia without mental disturbance. Fever caused rather marked disorientation and somnolence. The ability to do hard physical work (admittedly less than at sea level) has been repeatedly demonstrated by those who climb above 20,000 ft, in which circumstances the arterial P_{O_2} is less than 40 mm Hg and hemoglobin saturation below 70 per cent. In this connection it is perhaps well to remember that great civilizations, namely, those of the Incas and Aztecs, were built in environments where everyone was chronically hypoxic from birth until death.

It will not be amiss to reiterate two points of particular clinical importance at the close of these remarks concerning hypoxia. (1) Severe disability for physical effort can exist as the result of pulmonary disease without arterial hypoxia. In this instance, mechanical defects increasing the work of and reducing the capacity for breathing are most often implicated. (2) Hypercapnia is an equally or even more serious development than hypoxia in the hypoventilation states. Since it does not lead to a specific sign such as cyanosis, it too often goes unrecognized and may even be augmented by the treatment of hypoxia with oxygen.

POLYCYTHEMIA

This term signifies an increase to abnormal levels of the total number of circulating red blood cells.

One of the most important systemic reactions to chronic hypoxia is a stimulation of the production of red cells and hemoglobin, with the development of an absolute polycythemia. The exception to this situation is that form of hypoxia caused by anemia secondary to impairment of red cell production and release. In this connection, the chemical forms of anemic hypoxia (methemoglobinemia, etc.) will produce an absolute polycythemia. The increase in circulating red cells is usually accompanied by an increase in the volume of packed red cells and in the hemoglobin. The presence of polycythemia is established by direct measurements of the volume of red blood cells in active circulation; at sea level the red cell mass is usually less than 30 ml per kg in normal persons. Because the direct determination of red cell mass is still largely a research laboratory measurement, for clinical purposes the polycythemic state is generally thought to be present when (at sea level) the hematocrit exceeds 55 per cent, when the number of erythrocytes exceeds 6,300,000 per cu mm, or when the hemoglobin concentration exceeds 18 Gm per 100 ml of blood. The various forms of polycythemia are discussed in Chap. 236.

CYANOSIS

The peculiar color of the skin, mucous membranes, and nail beds referred to as cyanosis develops by reason of an abnormal amount of reduced hemoglobin coursing through the venules and capillaries close to the skin surface. Although the color is mainly between blue and violet, the shade varies, depending upon the other pigments in the skin and the number and depth of the vessels. Metallic deposits (argyria) may simulate cyanosis, but can readily be differentiated in the skin by pressure on the skin, using a glass permitting one to see the persistence of the color in argyria and the blanching in true cyanosis. The reddish color of carboxyhemoglobin should not confuse one, but the plethoric violaceous color sometimes seen in erythremia may at times be difficult to differentiate. Substances leading to the formation of methemoglobin or sulfhemoglobin may produce a discoloration that cannot be differentiated from reduced hemoglobin and, hence, a striking cyanosis may exist as a result of these pigments.

It has been shown that, when cyanosis is visible, approximately 5 Gm or more of reduced hemoglobin will be in the blood, perfusing the capillaries and venules of the skin. Under normal circumstances, the blood entering the skin would contain less than half a gram of reduced hemoglobin, so that the blood in the capillaries and probably in the venules under conditions of normal flow would contain much less than an average of 5 Gm of reduced hemoglobin. The recognition of cyanosis apparently carries with it a rather large observer variation. It has been shown that experienced observers examining subjects exposed to various oxygen tensions in the ambient air fail to show good agreement until the arterial hemoglobin saturation is 80 per cent or less. As a useful sign of arterial hypoxia, the recognition of cyanosis leaves much to be desired.

Sufficient quantities of reduced hemoglobin can accumulate in the skin in two ways. The first of these is arterial hypoxia, where the reduced hemoglobin delivered to the skin plus that which develops by virtue of metabolism in the skin is sufficient to produce cyanosis. The second situation arises because even though the amount of reduced hemoglobin delivered to the skin may be entirely normal (absence of arterial hypoxia), the removal of oxygen from each unit of blood may be great enough to develop the necessary amount of reduced hemoglobin in the skin. Stasis or reduced blood flow thus readily causes cyanosis. Anything leading to the sluggish flow of blood in the skin is apt to produce cyanosis even in normal individuals. It is imperative, therefore, when one makes an observation that cyanosis exists, that a differentiation between arterial hypoxia and peripheral stasis be made. This can be done with certainty only by determining the amount of reduced hemoglobin in the arterial blood sample.

The influence of erythrocytosis upon the development of cyanosis is rather striking. Engorgement of the vessels produces a greater color in the skin, and the slow circulation so typical of polycythemia enhances the opportunity for the accumulation of large amounts of reduced hemoglobin in the skin. In contrast, anemia, may prevent the development of cyanosis. If the blood contains less than 5 Gm hemoglobin per 100 ml, the necessary amount of reduced hemoglobin cannot be developed in the skin. Under these circumstances, arterial or circulatory hypoxia may cause a grayish or slate-blue color because of the loss of the ordinary red background provided by larger amounts of oxygenated hemoglobin. The presence of other pigments, as for example in jaundice, plus the relative number of open capillaries and thickness of skin all modify the appearance of cyanosis.

Some of the more important points in the differentiation of the several mechanisms of cyanosis are indicated in Table 14-1.

From a practical standpoint it is useful to divide cyanosis into the *circulatory, pulmonary,* and *hematogenous* groups. The circulatory group includes cardiac and peripheral types. When cyanosis is due to acquired disease of the heart, it is usually slight in degree and is accompanied by evidence of mitral

Table 14-1. CAUSES OF CYANOSIS

I. Circulatory disorders
  A. Cardiac disease
    1. Congenital: intense cyanosis, clubbed fingers, polycythemia
    2. Acquired: slight cyanosis, no clubbed fingers, no polycythmia
  B. Peripheral circulatory failure or local obstruction: pallid or ashen cyanosis, cold extremities
II. Pulmonary disorders
  A. Acute (pneumonia, edema, infarction): no clubbing and no polycythemia
  B. Chronic (emphysema, extensive fibrosis): clubbing and polycythemia often present
III. Hematogenous disorders
  A. Polycythemia—erythrocytosis of high altitudes: cyanosis, more or less clubbing; erythremia: plum red cyanosis, usually no clubbing
  B. Abnormality in hemoglobin: no clubbing, minimal polycythemia
    1. Exogenous (acetanilid and various other aniline derivatives, e.g., sulfanilamide, carbon monoxide, etc.)
    2. "Enterogenous cyanosis" (nitrites, sulfides)

stenosis, congestive failure, or both these conditions. Cyanosis due to congenital lesions is likely to be intense and to be associated with enlargement of the heart and clubbing of the fingers. Cyanosis dependent on disorders of the peripheral circulation is either local and accompanied by evidence of arterial or venous obstruction, or general and associated with the manifestations of peripheral circulatory failure or shock (Chap. 13). Pulmonary cyanosis, whether acute or chronic, is accompanied by the clinical and radiographic evidences of the responsible process, while hematogenous cyanosis is associated with polycythemia or with abnormal pigments in the blood.

In a given patient with cyanosis the following points are likely to be especially important in arriving at a correct interpretation of the cause:

1. The history, particularly as regards the duration (cyanosis present since birth usually is due to congenital heart disease), and the possible exposure to the various drugs or poisons which may produce abnormal types of hemoglobin.

2. Objective evidence by radiographic or physical examination of disorders of the respiratory or circulatory systems.

3. The presence or absence of clubbing of the fingers. (Slight clubbing without cyanosis is frequent in patients with subacute bacterial endocarditis, and may occasionally occur in healthy persons.) Slight cyanosis of the lips and cheeks, without clubbing of the fingers, is common in well-compensated patients with mitral stenosis, and probably is due to minimal arterial hypoxia resulting from changes in the lungs secondary to long-

standing congestion. The combination of slight cyanosis and slight clubbing is frequent in many patients with chronic diseases of the lungs. Marked clubbing and marked cyanosis occur together most commonly in patients with certain types of congenital cardiac disease and are seen occasionally in persons with advanced pulmonary disorders or pulmonary arteriovenous shunts. Cyanosis due to acquired cardiac disease, to acute disorders of the lungs, or to acute intoxications is not associated with clubbed fingers.

4. Spectroscopic examination of the blood for abnormal types of hemoglobin in instances where there is a story of suitable exposure, or where examination of the circulatory and respiratory systems affords no adequate explanation for the presence of cyanosis.

REFERENCES

Arnott, W. M.: The Syndrome of Alveolar-Capillary Block and Its Functional Pathology, Progr. in Cardiovascular Diseases, 1:435, 1959.

Brisco, W. A., and A. B. Dubois: The Relationship between Airway Resistance, Airway Conductance and Lung Volume in Subjects of Different Age and Body Size, J. Clin. Invest., 37:1279, 1958.

Comroe, J. H., Jr., et al.: "The Lung," Chicago, Year Book Publishers, Inc., 1955.

Donald, K. W., P. N. Wormald, et al.: Changes in the Oxygen Content of Femoral Venous Blood and Leg Blood Flow during Leg Exercise in Relation to Cardiac Output Response, Clin. Sci., 16:567, 1957.

Forster, R. E.: Exchange of Gases between Alveolar Air and Pulmonary Capillary Blood: Pulmonary Diffusing Capacity, Physiol. Rev., 37:391, 1957.

Fishman, A. P., et al.: Polycythemia, Am. J. Med., 24:132, 1958.

Fry, D. L., R. V. Ebert, W. W. Stead, and C. C. Brown: The Mechanics of Pulmonary Ventilation in Normal Subjects and in Patients with Emphysema, Am. J. Med., 16:80, 1954.

Harvey, R. M., M. I. Ferrer, D. W. Richards, Jr., and A. Cournand: Influence of Chronic Pulmonary Disease on the Heart and Circulation, Am. J. Med., 10:719, 1951.

West, J. R., E. de F. Baldwin, A. Cournand, and D. W. Richards, Jr.: Physiopathologic Aspects of Chronic Pulmonary Emphysema, Am. J. Med., 10:481, 1951.

Wright, G. W., and G. F. Filley: Pulmonary Fibrosis and Respiratory Function, Am. J. Med., 10:642, 1951.

—— and B. V. Branscomb: The Origin of the Sensations of Dyspnea, Trans. Am. Clin. & Climatol. A., 66:116, 1954.

15 COUGH AND HEMOPTYSIS
George W. Wright and Paul B. Beeson

COUGH

There is a great variability of the concentration and character of air contaminants presented at the "breathing level" of human beings. The "self-cleansing" mechanisms of the lung (Chap. 263) can be augmented to meet intensified challenges. In general, this leads to an increase of secretions and activity of the mucociliary apparatus. When the macrophage and leukocyte responses increase, the secretions become purulent. The augmented secretions of the supralaryngeal area are removed by voluntary mechanical means. Those from the tracheobronchial system are removed by cough.

Like sneezing, cough may be a reflex mechanism, and to some degree can be inhibited voluntarily. It arises by virtue of stimulation of the mucosa or deeper structures in the major bronchi or trachea, or of the vagus nerve itself which supplies this area. Cough also can be initiated voluntarily with various degrees of violence. Accumulation of mucus on the surface or inflammation, drying, cooling, or chemical stimulation of the mucosa will initiate this reflex, or desire to cough. The mechanical details of the expulsive action of cough are complex. Cinefluorographic plus pressure studies indicate the following train of events. The intrathoracic pressure is raised against the closed glottis. When the trachea is subsequently abruptly opened, the pressure in the lumen of the tracheobronchial system falls far more rapidly than in the surrounding structures. This imbalance of pressure leads to a bronchial transmural pressure gradient that momentarily causes marked narrowing, if not complete closure, of the trachea and bronchial lumens. At the time that this narrowing occurs, air is forced from the distal parts toward the larynx at an ever-increasing velocity. These two events, namely, lumen narrowing and augmented velocity of air flow, push mucus toward the oral pharynx in the same manner that a pea is expelled far better from a close-fitting tube than from a loose-fitting one. Preliminary closure of the glottis is helpful but not absolutely essential because laryngectomized persons cough effectively through a patent tracheostomy. Studies of this sort have not confirmed the concept of a "peristaltic milking" of the tracheobronchial tree during cough.

Cough as a symptom of disease has little intrinsic value in differential diagnosis. It is, however, an important warning that disease is present and *always demands* a full exploration of possible causes, since at times cough is the earliest symptom of curable disease. No person having a cough should ever be dismissed lightly as having a "cigarette cough," even though this factor is commonly enough found to be the case.

It is not unusual for normal persons to cough several times a day, but if the pattern changes, becoming more frequent with longer paroxysms and perhaps the production of phlegm, the cause of this change should be sought for.

Anything causing inflammation or necrosis of the bronchial mucosa will lead to the symptom of coughing. In most forms of *acute bronchitis* the cough is usually nonproductive at the onset, but may become productive of purulent sputum in a day or so. Substernal burning almost always occurs, and some degree of wheezing is common. If the cough occurs as a complication of the common cold, the diagnosis is usually apparent. As a rule, the symptoms associated with acute bronchitis are not severe and the cough subsides in a few days. Cough of an acute onset may, of course, be associated with more profound evidences of infection or lung damage, and in such instances the physical examination and the chest roentgenogram will usually reveal the underlying cause. Occasionally, a *pulmonary infarction* will be associated with no other symptom than cough.

If a changed pattern of coughing persists for more than a few days, other causes must be sought. Sputum examination and x-ray are indicated. Films taken in the PA and lateral projections will usually reveal evidence of inflammatory disease such as *tuberculosis, fungous infection,* or other granulomas by the time any one of these has progressed to the stage of causing a cough. At times, however, the roentgenogram fails to reveal the cause. Bronchoscopic examination may then be necessary because localized diseases of the bronchi such as *tumors* or inflammatory disease may first be disclosed only by this procedure. Sometimes even this method of examination fails to reveal disease in the distal and nonvisualized bronchi. Cytologic studies of bronchial washings and sputum and bronchography must then be used to explore the possibility of disease of the distal bronchi. Occasionally, fluoroscopy of the lungs will demonstrate "trapping" of air in a segment whose supplying bronchus is obstructed by intrabronchial disease. Emphasis must be placed upon the fact that cough may precede any other evidence of lung disease. Hence, if cough persists and no cause is found, the entire gamut of studies must be repeated after a brief lapse of time.

There are other causes of cough which do not manifest their presence readily in the roentgenogram. *Chronic bronchitis,* a disease characterized by a productive cough of several years' duration, cough occurring *throughout* the day and especially in the morning on arising and also at night, usually associated with one or more attacks of purulent bronchitis with bronchopneumonia each winter and often ultimately associated with respiratory insufficiency is diagnosed primarily by history and exclusion of other causes of the symptoms such as bronchiectasis (see Chap. 264).

Another common but often unrecognized cause of chronic cough is *diffuse obstructive disease of the lung* (diffuse obstructive emphysema). The cough associated with this disease is not always productive, but may be paroxysmal and severe.

At times, cough of a chronic nature may be caused by *congestion of the lungs.* Mitral stenosis and left ventricular failure, especially of a slight degree, may cause a rather characteristic cough. The episodes under these circumstances are characterized by a frequently recurring single cough, at times little more than a "clearing of the throat." The cough has a particularly annoying feature in the frequency with which it is repeated, although no single episode is as a rule very prolonged or violent. In frank *pulmonary edema* the cough may, of course, be much more severe.

Cough has a protective purpose as a rule, but it can also be harmful. Distal bronchial secretions tend to be spread peripherally during cough and thus may spread disease within the lung. The exact mechanism of this is not known. Trauma to the tracheobronchial wall or larynx may occur during cough and lead to bleeding or to implantation of infection. The muscular effort involved in coughing is relatively great and may aggravate heart failure in patients who have passive congestion of the lungs.

Ribs may be fractured as a result of cough. Muscle soreness also develops from chronic prolonged cough. The pain thus induced often is a difficult problem. In a prolonged paroxysm of cough, the persistent high intrathoracic pressure may so impede venous return that cardiac output falls and cerebral ischemia occurs. Fainting or convulsions (laryngeal syncope) may occur. Such attacks developing in a person operating a mechanical device may lead to disastrous results.

HEMOPTYSIS

Bleeding from the lungs is an important and fairly common medical problem. It is, of course, important to ascertain that the blood is actually coming from the pulmonary tree, not from the gastrointestinal tract or the nasopharynx. Blood which comes from the lungs is often bright red and frothy in appearance, whereas that from the stomach may be dark red, brown, or black and may be mixed with particles of food. Vomiting of blood is usually preceded by a feeling of nausea and commonly accompanied by retching, whereas hemorrhage from the lung may begin without antecedent symptoms and usually is accompanied either by coughing or by clearing of the throat. Not infrequently patients with bleeding in the lung experience a vague sensation which enables them to tell the approximate location of the hemorrhage.

Hemoptysis Associated with Hard Coughing. Very commonly, persons who have a hard, forceful cough will produce sputum which is blood streaked. This is a result of trauma to the air passages from the force of the coughing and is of little clinical significance. This type of hemoptysis usually can be identified by the history and by inspection of the sputum, noting that the blood is streaked on the surface, not intimately mixed with it.

Allied to this is the blood spitting which occurs rarely in patients with calcified lymph nodes adjacent to large bronchi. There may be erosion of the bronchial wall by the calcified mass, with bleeding and eventual ingress of the foreign body to the bronchial lumen (broncholith). Or conceivably bleeding may be caused by tearing the mucosa during the act of coughing, owing to acute angulation of a bronchus over the unyielding node.

Pneumonia. The sputum in bacterial pneumonia nearly always contains blood; only rarely is this the case with the viral pneumonias. In pneumococcal pneumonia the sputum may be pink or red, but more commonly, because of bacterial growth, it is the color of rust or prune juice. In staphylococcal pneumonia the sputum may be "rusty" or it may be a bright cherry red. In Friedländer bacillus pneumonia the sputum is characteristically bloody and tenacious, varying in color from dark brown to bright red. In pneumonia of any etiology the sputum seldom resembles pure blood; nearly always it is a mixture of mucopurulent material with blood.

Pulmonary Infarction. Clinicians are becoming more and more aware of the frequency and seriousness of pulmonary infarction due to embolism in the pulmonary vessels. This is the commonest cause of hemoptyis which occurs in the course of a nontuberculous illness in a hospital patient. Emboli come most frequently from thromboses in the deep veins of the calves but may originate in the pelvic veins or the right side of the heart. Occlusion of a pulmonary artery by an embolus usually is followed by turgescence of the capillaries in the area of lung supplied by that artery. The influx of blood is by way of capillary anastomoses from neighboring areas and is perhaps intensified by reflex spasm of the veins draining the area. This impaired circulation leads to necrosis and to entry of blood cells and edema fluid into the alveoli of the part; it is this material which appears as sputum. The excellent studies of Hampton and Castleman have shown that the incidence of pulmonary infarction following embolism is approximately 90 per cent in patients with heart disease, contrasted with an in-

cidence of about 60 per cent in other diseases. The higher incidence in cardiac patients probably is due to the already existing congestion and slow blood flow in the pulmonary circuit.

Bronchiectasis. It is estimated that hemoptysis occurs in 50 per cent of patients with bronchiectasis, and in young persons this is one of the most frequent causes of the symptom. Erosion of the inflamed bronchial mucous membrane, by infection or the trauma of coughing, causes bleeding. Diagnosis in this type of hemoptysis is usually not difficult, in view of the history of chronic productive cough and positive findings on the bronchogram. Often, however, the bleeding point is located too far in the periphery for identification by the bronchoscopist.

Pulmonary Tuberculosis. Small hemorrhages may occur early in the exudative phase of tuberculosis, as a result of direct erosion of vessels. In chronic ulcerative tuberculosis, bleeding occurs from incompletely obliterated pulmonary vessels which run through or along the walls of cavities. In some cases the source of bleeding is an aneurysmal dilatation, and this may bleed profusely.

Although hemorrhage in pulmonary tuberculosis is seldom immediately fatal, it may have serious effects. The plugging of a large bronchus with blood may cause atelectasis. Of even greater seriousness is the widespread dissemination of the tuberculous infection which may occur. Blood from a tuberculous cavity may be heavily contaminated with tubercle bacilli, and, as discussed previously, because of its fluidity it may be widely distributed throughout the lungs by coughing.

Pulmonary Neoplasms. Adenomas of the bronchi nearly always cause hemoptysis which is likely to be profuse. In bronchogenic carcinoma, the symptom is present in 25 to 50 per cent of cases. The source of bleeding is erosion of the surface of the tumor, within the lumen of the bronchus.

Mitral Stenosis. Obstruction to the emptying of the left atrium very frequently causes blood spitting; some authors place mitral stenosis second only to tuberculosis as a cause of hemoptysis in young people. Most writers have attributed the bleeding to increased pulmonary venous pressure with diapedesis into the alveoli. Ferguson, Kobilak, and Deitrick, however, suggested that the bleeding in mitral stenosis is due in many cases to the rupture of submucous varicosities in the bronchi. By examination of lungs removed at autopsy they proved the existence of venous anastomoses between the pulmonary and bronchial veins. They found, furthermore, that in patients with mitral stenosis these anastomoses were markedly increased in size, resembling small varicose veins. It was their opinion that the increased pressure in the pulmonary veins in mitral stenosis caused the dilatation and permitted some blood to drain from the pulmonary into the bronchial venous system. This hypothesis is attractive as an explanation of the cause of the large hemorrhages which sometimes occur in mitral stenosis.

Other Causes. The diseases mentioned previously are the principal causes of pulmonary hemorrhage, although various others occasionally may be responsible. In aneurysm of the aorta there may be bleeding through an eroded bronchus. Rarely, hemoptysis occurs in patients with arterial hypertension, presumably because of rupture of a submucous artery. Abscess in the lung may cause bleeding, as may the various purpuric states. Patients with hereditary hemorrhagic telangiectasia may bleed from the lungs repeatedly.

Episodes of hemoptysis occasionally are encountered in persons without other symptoms in whom careful study fails to reveal the cause. Possibly some of these episodes are associated with small areas of bronchiectasis of such limited extent that diagnosis by present methods is impossible.

REFERENCES

Ferguson, F. C., R. E. Kobilak, and J. E. Deitrick: Varices of the Bronchial Veins as a Source of Hemoptysis in Mitral Stenosis, Am. Heart J., 28:445, 1944.

Hampton, A. O., and B. Castleman: Correlation of Postmortem Chest Teleroentgenograms with Autopsy Findings, with Special Reference to Pulmonary Embolism and Infarction, Am. J. Roentgenol., 43: 305, 1940.

Johnston, R. N., W. Lockhart, R. T. Richie, and D. H. Smith: Hemoptysis, Brit. Med. J., 1:592, 1960.

Section 6: Indigestion and Jaundice

16 INDIGESTION, DYSPHAGIA, NAUSEA, AND VOMITING

William H. Resnik

INDIGESTION

Definition. Indigestion, or dyspepsia, has no sharply defined meaning. Some authors restrict the term to a multitude of symptoms aside from outspoken pain: heartburn and acid regurgitation, nausea and vomiting, gaseous distention and belching, and the various forms of distress such as a feeling of fullness or pressure that cannot be catalogued strictly as pain. Here we shall consider indigestion as constituting any of the above symptoms which the patient attributes to a deranged digestion, including the chronic recurrent types of pain the severity and character of which fall short of placing them among the acute abdominal emergencies—a distinction not always easy to make.

Visceral Pain. The characteristics of visceral pain have been described in previous chapters (Chaps. 3 and 6). The researches of Kellgren and Lewis have demonstrated that there are two main categories of pain: *superficial,* which tends to be sharp, stinging, or burning in quality and is susceptible of accurate localization; and *deep,* which tends to be more aching, diffuse, and segmentally distributed. Abdominal pain or distress may be *somatic,* when it arises in the parietal peritoneum or dome of the diaphragm, the impulses being conveyed by the intercostal or phrenic nerves. This type of pain is of the superficial variety. Or abdominal discomfort may be of the *visceral* or *splanchnic* type, originating in certain of the viscera or closely contiguous structures such as the mesentery, the afferent impulses being carried in the sensory nerves that run in the sympathetic system. The various forms of distress associated with indigestion are almost always of the deep visceral type.

Characteristics of Visceral Pain. The importance of localization and reference of pain, of the factors that provoke and relieve it, and of its quality and severity have been discussed in Chap. 3.

There are very few types of abdominal or digestive tract pain that are so definitely characteristic as to have diagnostic significance. One exception is *heartburn* (a sensation of warmth behind the lower sternum). This has been shown to arise predominantly, if not exclusively, from irritation of the lower esophagus. *Rebound tenderness,* associated with involuntary muscular rigidity, cutaneous hyperesthesia, and localized tenderness, usually indicates irritation of the parietal peritoneum. However, occasionally no peritonitis may be present, and it is probable that the rebound tenderness is then due to intense muscle spasm, so severe that the slight distortion incidental to the sudden release of pressure is sufficient to cause a pain identical with that characteristic of peritonitis.

Obviously, the presence of other associated manifestations that have localizing value is also important: localized rigidity and tenderness of the abdominal musculature, hematemesis, melena, and

Table 16-1. DISTRIBUTION OF PAIN ON THE BASIS OF CLINICAL AND EXPERIMENTAL DATA

Origin of pain	*Location of referred pain*
Esophagus............	Behind sternum, predominantly at level of xiphoid or suprasternal notch
Stomach and first part of duodenum	High epigastrium
Gallbladder and extra-hepatic bilary ducts	High epigastrium, right side of back
Pancreas.............	High epigastrium, left side of back
Liver................	Epigastrium
Small intestine........	Region of umbilicus
Colon...............	Below umbilicus
Rectosigmoid........	Low in abdomen, just above symphysis

jaundice. An elevated sedimentation rate should serve as a warning signal in any condition presumed to be due to a functional disorder. The appraisal of abdominal pain or indigestion requires a careful consideration of all the features that have been mentioned: the location of the discomfort, its character and intensity, the circumstances provoking and relieving it, and the associated findings, as well as the data pertaining to the age, sex, and environmental factors surrounding the individual.

Common Symptoms and Syndromes Expressed as Indigestion. The digestive tract responds to abnormal stimuli by alterations in secretory and motor activity. It is abnormal motor activity which is, in large part, the cause of most of the symptoms which fall into the category of indigestion: heartburn (which is due to primary or reflex disturbances in the lower esophagus), regurgitation, and the various other symptoms mentioned below under Early Postprandial Indigestion.

Anorexia. Anorexia is a symptom which should be distinguished from satiety. There seems to be no single physiologic basis for loss of appetite. In some (probably most) cases in which correlation of gastric function with anorexia has been made, inhibition of gastric activity has been found. However, it has been shown that under certain conditions the converse may be true; loss of appetite may occur when gastric functions (secretory and motor activity) are enhanced. These contradictory findings emphasize the more complex nature of appetite as compared with hunger and indicate the large role that various psychic influences play in determining the presence or absence of appetite. In many illnesses, return of appetite after a period of anorexia is a favorable prognostic sign.

Clinically, anorexia occurs in so many conditions of ill health, both psychogenic and organic, that its diagnostic significance is small in the light of other more positive manifestations that signify the nature of the underlying disorder. In some cases loss of appetite may be the only symptom in a person in whom the history, physical examination, and routine laboratory examinations reveal no adequate cause. Under these circumstances, it is important to remember that anorexia may be the sole clue to the presence of a malignant growth in the digestive tract, particularly in the stomach or colon. Anorexia is often also the only symptom suggesting the existence of a subacute hepatitis.

Belching. This is the eructation of gas from the stomach or esophagus. It may result from ingestion of carbonated drinks or bicarbonate of soda. Usually, however, the gas is due to swallowed air or air that is sucked into the esophagus by negative intrathoracic pressure in individuals who consciously or unconsciously relax the superior esophageal sphincter. Once having gained entrance into the esophagus, part of the air is passed on into the stomach; part is eructated from the esophagus without ever entering the stomach. The gas is not due to fermentation in the stomach. Entrance of excessive quantities of air into the esophagus or stomach may occur in patients suffering from practically any form of indigestion, but the most spectacular belching occurs in neurotics who may continue the sequence of gulping and eructating for hours, in the vain effort to rid themselves of gas that they assume is being formed in the stomach in prodigious amounts. The simple device of persuading them to place a cigarette holder or pencil between the teeth often serves to convince them that the symptom is self-induced.

Another cause of aerophagia is the expiratory grunt which is so common in patients with pneumonia or other conditions associated with severe pleural pain. In such subjects the increase in intrathoracic pressure associated with the grunting expiration seems to force air into the esophagus and stomach. This is probably the cause of the abdominal distention which may constitute such a grave problem in patients with pneumonia. Relief may be obtained by the use of an indwelling tube in the stomach.

Flatulence. Flatulence, or meteorism, is due to excessive quantities of gas in the small or large intestine. To some degree it may be due to unusual bacterial action on foods or to impaired absorption of gases into the blood stream. Possibly, diffusion of gas from the blood stream into the intestinal lumen may play a role in some cases. However, it is generally agreed that most of the gas is air that has gained entrance into the stomach by the mechanisms described above and then passed on into the intestines. Gastric distention due to air swallowing is often associated with palpitation and precordial distress and not infrequently leads to fear of heart disease.

Early Postprandial Indigestion. When food is ingested by a normal individual, a prompt diminution in the tone and peristaltic activity of the gastric musculature ensues. The subsequent motor activity incidental to the process of digestion goes on below the level of consciousness. When the normal motor responses are disturbed and gastric tone is enhanced rather than relaxed by the entrance of food into the stomach, the resultant effects of the abnormal tension in the gastric wall are felt as indigestion coming on immediately or shortly after the taking of food. The symptoms appear in different forms and combinations: a feeling of pressure or fullness or actual pain, nausea and vomiting, belching of gas, heartburn (presumably due to reflex alterations in the lower esophageal wall or irritation of the esophagus by regurgitation of gastric contents), etc. These symptoms persist for a variable period of time, sometimes curtailed by vomiting, spontaneous or induced, and the subject then experiences relative or complete relief until the next meal is taken. Such early postprandial discomfort may be due to a wide variety of causes and hence has little diagnostic significance.

Late Postprandial Indigestion. In other individuals, indigestion is experienced only after a period of time has elapsed after the ingestion of food—usually 1 hr or more. As in early postprandial indigestion, the symptoms may consist of heartburn, nausea, epigastric fullness, or fluctuating symptoms in various combinations. The location of these symptoms indicates their origin to be in the esophagus, stomach, or duodenum, and they are probably due to disturbances in the muscular tension of these organs. At times the discomfort is in the distribution of colon pain, either below the umbilicus or in the region of the flexures, presumably because of an overactive gastrocolic reflex. The classic example of late postprandial indigestion is encountered in uncomplicated peptic ulcer, typically described as a deep gnawing, *steady* pain of long duration, felt high in the epigastrium.

Several hypotheses have been advanced as explanations of the mechanism of ulcer pain. The three most widely held and vigorously defended by their proponents attribute the pain to (1) increased tension in the muscular walls of the stomach or duodenal cap, (2) irritation by the acid of the gastric juice, (3) increased sensitivity of the inflammatory tissue in and around the ulcer influenced by alterations in blood flow. In all probability, all three factors play important roles in the causation of ulcer pain, and it may be a question of semantics to declare that one factor alone is the essential one. Ulcer pain has been observed in the absence of free acid; nevertheless, in the vast majority of cases, the behavior of ulcer pain *appears*

to be in accord with the concentration of acid bathing it, and from a practical standpoint this is important because (1) deep, steady pain occurring an hour or more after eating and relieved by food, alkali, or vomiting (in each instance diminishing the concentration of acid) implies the irritating effect of acid on a defective membrane of the stomach or duodenum; (2) such pain occurring during the course of ulcer treatment implies inadequate neutralization of acid.

The types of indigestion do not always divide themselves neatly into these patterns of early and late postprandial discomfort. In some instances both the early and the late forms may be seen in the same subject, as well as indeterminate types that are so irregular that they defy classification. Late postprandial indigestion of the kind described above as characteristic of ulcer pain immediately suggests benign peptic ulcer, but essentially the same pain may be witnessed in other disorders such as carcinoma of the stomach with hyperacidity, ulcerative gastritis, or duodenitis. Late postprandial indigestion that does not conform to the characteristics of ulcer pain may be due to a wide variety of other primary or reflex disturbances of the stomach.

Pyloric Obstruction. Obstruction of the pylorus due either to organic stenosis or to spasm and edema usually is associated with the early appearance of indigestion, sometimes continuous, culminating hours later in colicky epigastric pains and the retention type of vomiting.

Postgastrectomy Syndromes. Following resection of a large part of the stomach, the patient may experience early satiety and nausea following the ingestion of even small amounts of food, owing to the loss of the reservoir function of the stomach. In addition, many patients experience the "dumping" syndrome characterized by nausea, palpitation, sweating, epigastric distress, weakness—a clinical picture very much like that caused by hypoglycemia. When this group of symptoms occurs soon after eating, it has been demonstrated that alterations in blood sugar are not responsible for the syndrome, which appears to be due rather to the rapid entrance of food, containing osmotically active substances, into the gut. This brings about a transfer of fluid into the jejunum, with a consequent fall in blood volume. The appearance or absence of the dumping syndrome seems to depend on variations that different individuals display in the degree to which the blood volume declines and in the manner in which they react to these declines. However, somewhat similar symptoms occurring $1\frac{1}{2}$ to 3 hr after eating have been found to be associated with hypoglycemia, the latter being due to a reactive hyperinsulinism in response to a preceding rapid rise in blood sugar. Finally, these patients may suffer from malnutrition and inability to maintain weight, owing to the "small-stomach" symptoms and fat and nitrogen loss in stools.

Partial Intestinal Obstruction. Acute obstruction of the bowel, if complete, is an emergency of such magnitude that it cannot be considered to fall into the province of the disorders now under discussion. However, incomplete obstruction may give rise to periodic bouts of cramplike pain, nausea, and vomiting, sometimes accompanied by distention. These symptoms, when mild, may be considered "indigestion" by the patient. The characteristic picture is less likely to be evidenced in partially obstructive lesions of the large bowel, particularly in the cecum, where extensive lesions may be present without giving rise to any obstructive phenomena.

Differential Diagnosis. A detailed outline of all the causes of recurrent indigestion is obviously impossible. However, certain principles that may be used as a guide in the analysis of chronic indigestion may be discussed. In every case the following questions must be answered: (1) Are the symptoms due to organic disease outside the digestive tract, or to organic disease within the digestive tract (including the gallbladder and extrahepatic biliary passages), or to a functional disturbance? (2) If organic disease of the digestive tract is present, is the lesion malignant or benign? (3) If the disorder is functional, is its origin psychogenic or nonpsychogenic (allergy, hypoglycemia, drugs, reflex effects)? The classification of indigestion on the basis of whether the fundamental lesion is primarily in the alimentary canal or outside it must in some instances be an arbitrary one. For example, indigestion may be a prominent feature of pernicious anemia, a condition which is associated with structural alterations in the stomach that may be the actual root of the disease. Nevertheless, tradition has placed this disorder among the diseases of the hematopoietic system.

Indigestion Due to Organic Disease outside the Digestive Tract. A complete catalogue of all the conditions outside the digestive tract capable of causing indigestion would serve to do little more than call attention to the fact that diseases of practically all systems of the body may at times be accompanied by indigestion in one form or another. The presenting complaint of the patient with pernicious anemia, pulmonary tuberculosis, myocardial failure, chronic infection of the urinary tract, or disease of the pelvic organs may be dyspepsia. Migraine, epilepsy, or other disturbances of the central nervous system may manifest themselves in chronic abdominal complaints. The digestive symptoms vary in detail and severity and have no characteristics that betray the fact that they are secondary to some more remote malady.

Gastritis. In recent years the concept of gastritis has been resurrected after being long held in disfavor. A good deal of ambiguity continues to surround the subject, at least from the clinical standpoint. This is because of various reasons, the most important being the lack of a constant relationship between clinical, gastroscopic, and histologic findings and also the fact that in the same individual gastroscopic pictures of hypertrophic or atrophic gastritis may be dependent solely on the emotional status of the patient. Many poorly defined syndromes indicative of gastric dysfunction, now ascribed to functional disorders of the stomach, may have as their basis an actual gastritis. The clinician may surmise that such is the case when there is a previous history of exposure to excessive use of alcohol or tobacco or to drugs; or when "indiscreet" eating is followed by indigestion; or when there is a history somewhat suggestive of ulcer or cancer, neither of which can be demonstrated by objective methods.

Confirmation by gastroscopy lends weight to the diagnosis, but even this method is not conclusive, since mucosal alterations deviating from the normal may be transitory and caused by emotional factors. There can be no doubt that massive hematemesis may be due to gastritis, and occasionally a hypertrophic gastritis localized in the antral and prepyloric region may simulate cancer so closely that differentiation can be made only by histologic study. Conversely, patients with clear-cut gastroscopic evidence of gastritis may be free of suggestive symptoms.

Peptic Ulcer. The characteristic qualities of the pain of uncomplicated ulcer of the stomach or duodenum are its rhythmicity and periodicity. "Rhythmicity" refers to the pain-food-ease sequence, the classic prototype of the late-postprandial form of indigestion. "Periodicity" expresses the tendency for the indigestion to appear for weeks at a time and later to disappear for months, over the course of a number of years. Ulcer is far more common in the duodenum than in the stomach, and the incidence in males is higher than in females. Ulcer may develop at any decade. The usual location of the pain is in the high epigastrium or midepigastrium; vomiting occurs infrequently in the uncomplicated ulcer; pain before breakfast is practically never encountered. As complications develop, the clinical picture tends to become distorted and to lose its usually sharply drawn lines. In cases of penetration with extension into the surrounding tissue, the characteristic pain-food-ease pattern tends to be less clearly delineated; the pain becomes more continuous and radiates more widely as the nerves of the involved tissues become affected. Obstruction at the pylorus is also heralded by alteration of the classic ulcer syndrome; there is earlier onset of pain, relief of which often is no longer afforded by food and alkali, and vomiting of the retention type makes its appearance.

Carcinoma of the Stomach. The traditional history of anemia, loss of weight, strength, and appetite, and discomfort of variable intensity and form after eating usually represents an advanced carcinoma of the stomach. It is now appreciated that the early stage of carcinoma of the stomach presents a picture of considerable diversity, dependent on the location and extent of the lesion. If the growth exists at the cardia or pylorus, early obstructive phenomena may be witnessed. If the lesion is small and ulcerated and if the gastric juice contains free hydrochloric acid, the clinical picture of a benign peptic ulcer may be reproduced so perfectly in symptoms, in roentgenologic appearance, and even in temporary response to treatment, that clinical differentiation may be practically impossible. In some cases the digestive symptoms, though present, may be so mild and vague as to be hardly suggestive of the disorder. Finally, in a considerable number of instances, especially those with achylia, no gastric symptoms occur until anemia, wasting, or other changes are fully displayed. In short, not only is the indigestion of early carcinoma of the stomach lacking in any definitive features that are indicative of the causative lesion, but the entire clinical picture may be equally uninformative. *The inevitable consequence of these observations is that any indigestion in the upper abdomen not otherwise clearly accounted for, particularly when it occurs in a male over the age of forty, should be suspected of having its origin in a malignant lesion of the stomach and should be carefully studied by every available method with this possibility in mind. There are no criteria in regard to size, location of ulcer, x-ray appearance, or gastroscopic study that differentiate with certainty benign from malignant ulcers.*

Chronic Gallbladder Disease. The symptoms of chronic gallbladder disease are of two kinds, indigestion and colic. The indigestion may occur early or late after a meal and is lacking in any distinctive qualities that permit a diagnosis of the basic disorder. Intolerance of fats is sometimes described as a characteristic feature. Carefully taken histories disclose that, when the patient does have an intolerance of certain foods, nonfatty foods are frequently incriminated as well as the fatty ones, that some fats are acceptable when others are not, and that the particular fats that bring on symptoms vary with different individuals. Fat intolerance is, therefore, not a symptom that is an expression of an inability to handle fats alone but is rather one feature of a much broader food intolerance that applies to nonfatty foods as well and differs in its de-

tails from patient to patient. *It is more accurate, then, to speak of food intolerance rather than fat intolerance as a common symptom in chronic gallbladder disease.* However, this kind of food intolerance is not peculiar to gallbladder disease alone. Exactly the same intolerance of foods, fatty as well as nonfatty, is encountered in patients who suffer from functional disorders or from a variety of other organic ailments in the absence of any demonstrable disease of the biliary tract. In other words, *neither the indigestion nor the so-called fat intolerance that is sometimes ascribed to gallbladder disease is distinctive.* It may be added that, since there is no evidence that in the absence of obstructive jaundice all fats are poorly digested and tolerated, there is no justification for the common practice of severely restricting the use of all fats in the diets of patients with chronic gallbladder disease. As in patients suffering from allergic disorders, dietary restrictions should be made according to the individual problems of the patient. There is no rational basis for any diet that is applicable to all patients with chronic gallbladder disease. The relationship of an indigestion to a coexistent disorder of the gallbladder, even when proved roentgenographically, is difficult to define. In one patient, surgical removal of the diseased gallbladder may bring about complete relief of the indigestion. In other individuals, removal of the gallbladder may afford no amelioration of the indigestion, and this is especially likely to be the case when the gallbladder is merely thickened but contains no stones and when there has been no previous history of acute cholecystitis.

Apart from the indigestion, the patient with chronic gallbladder disease is often subject to more or less severe attacks of biliary colic. It is these acute attacks of pain, localized high in the epigastrium or in the right (rarely in the left) hypochondrium, radiating to the right subscapular or to the interscapular regions, or sometimes to the tip of the right shoulder, which are really suggestive of gallbladder disease; when they are associated with jaundice, the diagnosis becomes clear. The frequency of this condition renders suspect every woman over the age of twenty-five, particularly if she has borne children, and all individuals over the age of forty, complaining of indigestion. Fortunately, the diagnosis is capable of confirmation in a high percentage of cases by cholecystography and cholangiography. Biliary drainage is useful only if the gallbladder has been previously removed or if it is believed that a nonfilling gallbladder is secondary to parenchymal liver disease.

Disorders of the Pancreas. Clinically, the symptoms of pancreatitis are so similar to those of gallbladder disease as to be practically indistinguishable. Probably the most important factor in making the diagnosis of pancreatitis is to keep in mind that such a condition may be present when one would ordinarily consider gallbladder disease to be the cause of the patient's complaints. In the acute exacerbations of chronic relapsing pancreatitis, the differentiation hinges primarily on finding an increased serum amylase or serum lipase at the onset of the attack. In the chronic phases of the disorder, the recognition of its presence will depend chiefly on the discovery of steatorrhea or diabetes mellitus or x-ray demonstration of calcification or enlargement of the pancreas. Numerous studies have revealed that the classic picture of painless, progressive jaundice is not the most common form in which carcinoma of the pancreas presents itself. Jaundice occurs in about half the cases, upper abdominal pain with no definite pattern or constant form of radiation in a much higher percentage. In the absence of jaundice, diagnosis is sometimes suggested by the roentgenologic demonstration of deformity of neighboring structures by extrinsic pressure.

Diaphragmatic (Hiatal) Hernia. In recent years there has been a growing appreciation of the fact that diaphragmatic (hiatal) hernia may be responsible for a variety of clinical pictures, one of which is chronic indigestion. In the typical case, an overweight individual of middle age or over tends to have symptoms on assuming the recumbent position or on leaning forward after a full meal. The herniation may be associated with a nondescript form of indigestion or may cause a more severe attack of pain, sometimes strongly suggestive of biliary colic. At other times the pain is identical in type and distribution with that due to angina pectoris or myocardial infarction, although the characteristic relation to effort in respect to the former, or the diagnostic electrocardiographic findings in respect to the latter, are absent (Chap. 5). The diagnosis is established with certainty when an awareness of the possible existence of diaphragmatic hernia leads to confirmation by roentgenologic examination made with this condition in mind.

Disorders of the Small Intestine. When organic disease of the bowel arouses recurrent attacks of abdominal pain of the type that may be considered to fall in the category of chronic indigestion, the clue to the site of the trouble will come from the recognition of the significance of the localization of the pain in the region of the umbilicus. More exact definition of the lesion will depend primarily on x-ray examination, which should be carried out with more careful attention to the small intestine than is ordinarily given in a routine gastrointestinal series.

Chronic Disease of the Appendix (Recurrent Obstructive Disease of the Appendix). In a small number of cases, chronic disease of the appendix may be the basis for a persistent indigestion of either the early or the late postprandial type. Experimental observations have demonstrated that irritation in the colon or over the appendix may produce pain in the prepyloric region, owing to reflex peristaltic activity. The mere presence of continued pain and tenderness in the right lower quadrant does not signify chronic disease of the appendix; the most common cause of this type of pain is an irritable colon. The diagnosis of chronic disease of the appendix cannot be made with reasonable certainty until evidence of appendiceal inflammation (localization of pain in the right lower quadrant, tenderness and rigidity in McBurney's region, fever, and leukocytosis) has occurred in the midst of one or more attacks of appendiceal colic. It is worth bearing in mind that bouts masquerading as attacks of appendiceal colic may be caused by terminal ileitis (see Chap. 274).

Organic Disease of the Colon. In most cases organic disease of the colon is characterized by the appearance of one or a combination of the following symptoms: (1) diarrhea or constipation, or both; (2) bleeding from the bowel; (3) abdominal pain. The following statements regarding disease of the colon are made primarily with respect to pain and the possibility that such pain may be interpreted by the patient to be "indigestion." The character of the pain is determined by the site of the lesion, the presence or absence of obstruction, and the extent to which neighboring structures are involved. In general, pain due to disorders of the colon is referred to the lower half of the abdomen, although lesions in the hepatic or splenic flexure may give rise to pain in the upper right or left quadrants of the abdomen, respectively, while lesions in the cecum may cause periumbilical pain not infrequently mistaken for appendicitis. Obstructive phenomena, which are relatively rare in disorders of the proximal part of the colon, occur much more frequently on the left side of the colon, owing to the more solid contents of the colon in this region and also to the frequency of fibrous annular lesions due to cancer or diverticulitis, the latter two lesions often being clinically indistinguishable. Indigestion, frequently associated with nausea, is common, usually because of reflex disturbances in the stomach. The symptoms of the different organic diseases of the colon have so many features in common that exact diagnosis usually must rest on the results of the more precise methods of examination, the most important of which are x-ray and proctoscopic examination. It hardly needs to be emphasized that in every such case a careful digital examination of the rectum should be performed. Any symptom referable to the colon warrants a thorough investigation with the special aim of searching for a carcinoma. Particularly in the colon, but also in the stomach, a normal x-ray study does not rule out cancer. If symptoms fail to clear under therapy, the x-ray examination, like any other physical examination, should be repeated.

Indigestion Due to Functional Disorders of the Digestive Tract. Several circumstances afford presumptive evidence of the functional origin of chronic indigestion: clear association of symptoms with states of fatigue or emotional stress, youth of the patient, duration of the illness over a long period of time, variability of symptoms, absence of serious deterioration of health. The diagnosis may be considered established, however, only when history and physical examination, laboratory data, x-ray examination, and in appropriate cases, endoscopic examination fail to reveal organic disease, in or out of the digestive tract, that can logically explain the digestive symptoms. Even when the investigation has been carried out in the most thorough and expert manner, unavoidable error will occur in a small percentage of cases, and the passage of time will disclose organic disease not previously demonstrable.

Psychogenic factors, excessive use of tobacco, coffee, or alcohol, improper habits of eating, cathartic habituation—each alone or in combination with the others may be responsible for the faulty functioning of the digestive tract. The symptoms vary widely, sometimes mimicking organic diseases involving the stomach or colon so closely that only after the most intensive survey and prolonged observation will it be possible to conclude that no structural disease of the digestive tract is present. One needs hardly to be reminded that almost any drug taken by mouth may cause indigestion. When this indigestion is precipitated by highly alkaline drugs such as diphenylhydantoin sodium (Dilantin), the customary treatment with alkali will tend to aggravate rather than ameliorate the trouble.

Even when demonstrable structural disease exists, the symptoms may be markedly influenced by coexistent, although less apparent, emotional disturbances. When no structural disease is found, one is not justified in assuming that psychologic factors are responsible for the symptoms unless the patient presents clear evidence of emotional disturbance. Mistakes will be minimized if one bears in mind that, though psychogenic disorders are a very common cause of indigestion, it is unsafe to make such a diagnosis in an individual case unless the evidence, both positive and negative, points unequivocally toward such a conclusion (Chap. 42).

Indigestion Due to Food Intolerance. Hypersensitiveness to specific foods is a frequent cause of digestive symptoms. In some cases, the constant association of symptoms with the ingestion of certain foods, even when the recipient is unaware that the offending foods are incorporated in the diet, the personal and familial history of an allergic

background, the demonstration of positive skin tests and of antibodies that are capable of being transferred passively, the prompt cessation of symptoms on elimination of the offending foods from the diet —all these afford a chain of evidence that is incontestable. However, in a much higher percentage of cases, the proof that indigestion is caused or aggravated by a suspected food allergy rests on much more uncertain ground. This uncertainty is common to most disorders ascribed to an allergic reaction to foods. The immunologic tests may be negative, the provocation of symptoms by the offending foods may not be immediate and clear-cut, and the harmful influence of the suspected foods may have no better support than the statement of the patient himself. In the absence of objective proof, it is frequently difficult or impossible to know how much a supposed food sensitivity is attributable to a genuine food intolerance and how much to the fears and suspicions of an apprehensive patient. When the intolerance to specific foods seems real, it is again a problem to decide whether the symptoms are due to the relative indigestibility of the foods or their content of chemical irritants that may be more potent in some individuals than others, or whether an allergic reaction in the digestive tract is the basis of the disturbed function. The fact remains that, however obscure may be the mechanism by which these various food intolerances operate, there are frequent instances in which indigestion seems to be related to the specific effect of certain foods, varying for each individual case. In some persons food intolerance appears to be the sole cause of symptoms; in others it may exert its effects in conjunction with obvious psychogenic influences, while in still others the food intolerance may be expressed only when demonstrable organic disease is present.

Suspicion with regard to the allergic basis of the indigestion is aroused by a family history of allergy or a personal history, in the past or present, of some unquestionably allergic disorder such as hay fever or asthma. Frequently the patient recognizes that certain foods, such as eggs or milk, may be responsible for his symptoms but may be unmindful of the fact that these same foods are commonly used in the preparation of other articles of his diet.

For the detection of the offending foods, skin tests are so unreliable as to be usually valueless. More helpful information can be obtained from elimination diets or from a careful, time-consuming history in which the patient is questioned regarding his experience with all the common articles of a dietary. Only by testing and retesting the effects of suspected foods is it possible to arrive at a reasonably clear conclusion as to the role that specific food idiosyncrasies are playing in the particular case. It should be emphasized again that the discovery of a food intolerance and the temporary relief of symptoms by elimination of the offending substance do not prove the absence of concomitant organic disease. It is not uncommon, for example, for the indigestion of chronic gallbladder disease to be considerably relieved or completely abolished for long periods of time merely by eliminating the known food offenders.

General Diagnostic Considerations. The introduction of more exact methods of diagnosis has brought about a steady diminution in the importance of the clinical picture alone for arriving at a conclusion as to the nature of the specific disorder responsible for a malady. However varied may be the types of injury or stress, the responses of the digestive tract and the resulting symptoms are relatively limited. Accurate information regarding the localization and projection of the pain and, hence, the cord segments affected by the sensory stimuli affords an invaluable starting point from which one may consider the various structures that could be responsible for the symptoms. Additional data pertaining to the age and sex of the patient, duration of the illness, factors precipitating or relieving the symptoms, and accessory details narrow still further the diagnostic possibilities. In the main, however, a definite diagnosis will rest chiefly on the results of x-ray or direct inspection of the affected organ by endoscope or at the time of operation. The similarity of symptoms produced by a variety of lesions in the same structure or in other structures innervated from the same cord segments makes diagnosis on clinical grounds alone a hazardous undertaking, particularly in the detection of disease in its early and most remediable stages. Reliance on x-ray or endoscopic examination must be tempered with a recognition of the shortcomings of even these methods of investigation; in some cases only microscopic examination of the suspected tissues can define the character of the morbid process.

Difficulties in ascertaining the primary site of a gastrointestinal disorder are frequently aroused by the reciprocal relationships between the upper and lower digestive tract. Lesions in the upper tract, such as gallbladder disease or peptic ulcer, commonly give rise to reflex disturbance in the colon, and in some cases the symptoms referable to the irritable colon may preponderate to such an extent that they actually occupy the forefront of the patient's attention. Similarly, primary disorders in the colon may be associated with reflex alterations in the functions of the stomach, and indigestion, characterized by high epigastric distress, may be the predominant symptom, distracting the attention from the original site of the trouble.

Procedure in Investigation of Chronic Indigestion. The first step in the elucidation of chronic indigestion must cover the ground encompassed in every thorough initial examination: a painstaking and complete history and physical examination and the routine blood and urine tests. The results of this first survey and the additional special procedures that may be suggested by it will serve to indicate whether any organic disease can explain the symptoms of which the patient complains. In some cases, as in angina pectoris or myocardial failure, where the diagnosis is clearly ascertained, further investigation of the digestive tract is unnecessary.

X-ray examination of the alimentary tract and gallbladder is the cornerstone on which the diagnosis of gastrointestinal disease is built; elaboration on the importance of this procedure is unnecessary. Lesions of the stomach and colon ordinarily are readily disclosed. The standard gastrointestinal series frequently fails to reveal the small intestine in adequate detail; special studies of the small intestine should be made when involvement of this structure is suspected.

As far as indigestion is concerned, the chief value of stool examinations is in the detection of occult blood and, occasionally, microscopic detection of ova and parasites. The persistence of bleeding in a case of gastric ulcer that is being properly treated arouses the strong presumption that the lesion is malignant.

Gastric analysis no longer occupies a position of importance in the diagnosis of disorders of the stomach and duodenum. Normal individuals exhibit variations in the acidity of gastric juice that may range from complete absence of hydrochloric acid to high figures that tend to overlap those seen in disease. Moreover, aside from the measurement of the volume and acidity of the gastric juice, the information afforded by the various special test meals is ascertained more easily and accurately by x-ray examination. Nevertheless, with appreciation of its limitations, gastric analysis continues to be employed as a procedure that provides data that may be of assistance in cases where the x-ray evidence is equivocal.

Fasting gastric juice of large volume and high concentration of acid is an almost constant finding in the presence of duodenal ulcer. In benign gastric ulcer, the volume and the level of acid concentration tend to be lower, but acid is rarely completely and persistently absent. Nevertheless, even after histamine stimulation, anacidity has been present, at least for periods of time, in authenticated cases of benign peptic ulcer. On the other hand, while histamine anacidity bespeaks strongly of the malignant character of a gastric ulcer, free acid does not rule out malignant disease of the stomach. In cases of pernicious anemia, in which indigestion may be the presenting symptom, anacidity refractory to histamine is invariably present.

Proctoscopic examination and digital examination of the rectum are indicated in most conditions suggestive of organic disease of the colon and are obligatory when there is any suspicion that cancer of the rectum exists.

Gastroscopy is useful in the determination of the completeness of healing of a gastric ulcer and in disclosing lesions unseen by x-ray, notably hemorrhagic and ulcerative gastritis. Moreover, the accuracy of gastroscopic diagnosis has been enhanced by the introduction of an operating gastroscope which makes biopsy possible. However, gastroscopy is not to be considered a substitute for x-ray. A better conjecture about the status of the stomach can be made after both gastroscopic and x-ray studies than after either alone.

Cytologic examination of the gastric contents has been found, in experienced hands, to be extremely accurate in differentiating between benign and malignant disorders.

Finally, when organic disease of the digestive tract has been excluded and the possibility of an allergic disorder is entertained, elimination diets should be employed.

The question of procedure in the investigation of chronic indigestion in a patient on the wards of a large teaching hospital or at a diagnostic clinic poses no difficult problems. All the methods mentioned above may be employed; under these circumstances the patient expects and usually submits to any examination that will throw light on his illness. The problem is different in private practice, away from such institutions, and it is essentially an economic one. There would be no serious problem if the necessary examinations were as inexpensive as a blood count or a simple blood chemical analysis. A high percentage of gastrointestinal disorders seen in patients who make up the practice of the average physician are of functional origin. To subject all persons complaining of indigestion to an immediate routine survey involving all the indicated procedures would be difficult, if not impossible, from the standpoint of expediency and expense. On the other hand, the alert physician must be constantly aware of the fact that any compromise with thoroughness inevitably exposes the patient to the risk of losing the opportunity, possibly an irretrievable one, of discovering an early and curable malignant disease. For the average conscientious physician in private practice, this dilemma is well-nigh insoluble.

DYSPHAGIA

Difficulty in swallowing may be expressed either by food "sticking" some place in its passage to the stomach or by pain associated with or aggravated by the act of swallowing. Pain arising from the esophagus is described more fully in Chap. 271, p. 1583.

Dysphagia may be classified according to the three chief mechanisms causing this symptom:

1. Dysphagia due to mechanical obstruction in the esophagus
2. Dysphagia due to disturbance in the neuromuscular mechanisms of swallowing
3. Dysphagia due to lesions of the mouth, pharynx, or larynx, causing pain or mechanical hindrance to passage of food into the esophagus

Dysphagia Due to Mechanical Obstruction in the Esophagus. This group is by far the most important and comprises 90 per cent or more of all cases of dysphagia.

Carcinoma. This is the most common lesion causing mechanical obstruction in the esophagus and is responsible for 50 to 60 per cent of all cases in which the complaint is dysphagia. The condition occurs far more frequently in men than in women, usually in patients over fifty years of age. The first and most important symptom is difficulty in swallowing, usually of gradual onset, sometimes sudden, progressing steadily until softer foods, and then liquids, are unable to pass the stricture. Regurgitation and pain are usually inconspicuous or absent. X-ray examination usually reveals an irregular obstruction, with relatively little dilatation of the esophagus above. Diagnosis is made certain by esophagoscopic examination and obtaining bits of tissue for microscopic analysis.

Achalasia (Cardiospasm). This disorder is found in about 20 per cent of all cases of dysphagia. The cause is not known but is generally considered to be a disturbance of motility of the lower esophagus, with diminished tone and propulsive action of the esophageal musculature and failure of relaxation of the cardiac sphincter. The majority of cases begin in early adult life, the onset being either gradual or sudden, with either pain or dysphagia as the first symptom. Dysphagia is usually transitory, with variable intervals of practically complete freedom from this symptom intervening. Gradually, over a period of years, the difficulty in swallowing becomes more persistent and severe. Pain and regurgitation are common, the latter frequently taking place during the night and causing aspiration and infection of the respiratory tract. Aside from the history, diagnosis is made from the characteristic x-ray findings and response to parasympathomimetic drugs as determined by pressure tracings using electromagnetic transducers.

Esophageal Spasm. In some individuals, attacks of dysphagia characterized by pain and a sense of food "sticking" may occur from time to time or only for a brief time, never to recur again. Exhaustive examination may reveal no organic basis for the dysphagia, and the symptom can be attributed only to spasm, occasionally demonstrable by x-ray (*lower esophageal contractile ring*).

Esophagitis. This condition usually results from the irritating effect of regurgitated gastric juice due to persistent vomiting, or the trauma of prolonged esophageal intubation, or the combined effects of both. It occurs not infrequently after abdominal operations when both factors are present, or as the result of regurgitation of gastric juice in patients suffering from a peptic ulcer of the stomach or duodenum, or from a congenitally short esophagus. The outstanding symptom is pain on swallowing, sometimes associated with obstruction due to spasm or edema of the esophageal wall. Occasionally, serious hemorrhage may occur. Superficial erosion or deeper ulceration may be present, but the latter should be differentiated from so-called "peptic ulcer of the esophagus." In a high percentage of cases, this latter condition occurs in association with a congenitally short esophagus, and it is believed by some, though this view is not universally accepted, that the ulcer actually is present in the stomach wall which happens to lie above the diaphragm. It is also believed that an ulcer may develop in an island of ectopic gastric mucosa, but this view, too, has been questioned. Confirmation of the diagnosis of esophagitis must rest on x-ray and endoscopic examination.

Benign Stricture. In strictures following the ingestion of lye or other corrosive chemicals, the cause is clear. In others, however, the cause is uncertain and may be related to a previous episode of prolonged vomiting (as in pregnancy), with resultant reflux peptic esophagitis, while in still others the cause is unknown. It should be mentioned here that in most cases of *scleroderma* a stricture is not present, and the difficulty in swallowing is due to atony of the esophageal wall, somewhat similar to that occurring in achalasia. In most strictures the history is practically identical with that seen in carcinoma. X-ray usually reveals a smooth constriction with little or no dilatation above. When the symptoms have lasted more than 18 months or 2 years, the differentiation from carcinoma is usually not a problem, since patients with untreated carcinoma rarely survive this period of time. When the symptoms are of short duration, differentiation from carcinoma may be difficult or impossible without esophagoscopy and biopsy.

Pharyngoesophageal Diverticulum (Zenker's Diverticulum). This is a relatively uncommon cause of dysphagia. The pouch projects from the hypopharynx just above the opening of the esophagus. As the pouch enlarges and sags, because of the weight of its contents, it tends to occlude the esophagus. A common early symptom is that of "food sticking in the throat." Later, actual dysphagia and regurgitation of food that has become trapped in the pouch occur. The appearance on x-ray examination is diagnostic.

Foreign Bodies. Usually the history discloses the possibility that an accident has occurred. Pain with each swallow and dysphagia are the outstanding symptoms. X-ray examination is sometimes of value in the diagnosis. In some doubtful cases, esophagoscopy is essential.

Extraesophageal Lesions. Dysphagia may also be caused by extraesophageal disorders such as carcinoma of the thyroid, aneurysm of the aorta, mediastinal tumors, vascular anomalies of the aortic arch (aortic rings), diaphragmatic hernia, and, rarely, by the dilated left atrium of mitral stenosis.

Dysphagia Due to Disturbances in the Neuromuscular Mechanisms of Swallowing. In the act of swallowing, food is transferred from the oral cavity by contraction of the tongue against the hard palate, by the action of the pharyngeal constrictors, and by the relaxation of the pharyngoesophageal sphincter. Food is thereby prevented from being forced into the nasopharynx, and it fails to enter the larynx by virtue of the elevation of this structure beneath the protective cover of the base of the tongue. Dysphagia results when any part of this coordinated and complex series of movements is disturbed. The features witnessed in varying degree in these disorders are difficulty in maneuvering food into the esophagus in the absence of pain or mechanical hindrance, regurgitation of fluids through the nasopharynx, aspiration of food into the larynx, nasal character of the voice, and weakness of the palate. Examples of this type of dysphagia are *myasthenia gravis, bulbar palsy, diphtheritic polyneuritis, acute bulbar poliomyelitis, cerebral vascular accidents, hepatolenticular degeneration (Wilson's disease)*, and *botulism*. The *Plummer-Vinson syndrome* may also be listed here, since the difficulty of swallowing in this condition resembles that due to a neuromuscular disorder, although pain may be an additional disturbing feature. The actual mechanism of the dysphagia is not entirely clear but is due sometimes to esophageal webs, membranous structures stretching across the esophagus and partially occluding it. At other times, no web can be demonstrated and the dysphagia may then be caused by atrophic changes in the pharynx, possibly associated with disturbances of the intrinsic nervous apparatus in the pharyngeal wall. *Dermatomyositis* is another muscular disorder that causes dysphagia by involvement of the pharyngeal and hypopharyngeal musculature.

Dysphagia Due to Lesions of the Mouth, Pharynx, or Larynx, Causing Pain or Mechanical Hindrance to Passage of Food into the Esophagus. In most cases the cause of trouble in this group is obvious, and detailed consideration of the various lesions is unnecessary; examples are acute tonsillitis, peritonsillar abscess, infiltrating carcinoma of the tongue, and angioneurotic edema of the tongue or pharynx.

Differential Diagnosis. A common complaint, not to be confused with dysphagia, is *globus hystericus.* This symptom consists of a sense of constriction in the throat; the patient usually believes there is a lump in the throat that is not visible. He is likely to be fearful that the imagined tumor may interfere with swallowing, although careful questioning reveals that there is actually no dysphagia. This fear is naturally enhanced if any enlargement of the thyroid coexists. Globus hystericus is always a manifestation of emotional stress or fatigue. The symptom is usually considered to be due to increased tonus of the hypopharyngeal musculature, although this is rarely demonstrable by x-ray. It is, of course, important to reassure the patient of the benign nature of the symptom, but it is equally mandatory not to overlook an organic disturbance of which the vague sense of dysphagia may be the early manifestation.

Determination of the basic mechanism responsible for the dysphagia is usually a simple matter, but identification of the exact disorder is not infrequently quite difficult. For example, cancer of the esophagus sometimes presents a sudden rather than a gradual onset, and the roentgenogram may have the smooth, symmetric appearance more commonly seen with benign stricture or cardiospasm; even esophagoscopy may be inconclusive, and biopsy may yield deceptive results if the bit of tissue happens to contain no neoplastic cells. Similarly, mediastinal disorders causing mechanical obstruction may be difficult to classify, and the same is true of the neurologic disturbances interfering with swallowing.

Certain symptoms associated with dysphagia have diagnostic value. Hiccups, together with difficult swallowing, indicate a lesion at the terminal portion of the esophagus, such as carcinoma, achalasia, or hiatal hernia. Dysphagia, followed after an interval of some duration by hoarseness, usually means extension of a malignant growth beyond the walls of the esophagus and the involvement of a recurrent laryngeal nerve. When the hoarseness comes first and the dysphagia later, the primary lesion is almost always in the larynx. Dysphagia and unilateral wheezing practically always indicate a mediastinal mass involving the esophagus and a main or large bronchus. Coughing with each swallow of food or drink means a fistulous communication between the esophagus and the trachea. Coughing occurring some time after swallowing may be due to regurgitation of food, most common in achalasia and pharyngeal pouch.

Procedure. Examination of the mouth and pharynx should disclose those lesions the effect of which is to impede the transfer of food from the mouth to the esophagus, either because of pain or mechanical interference. When lesions of the hypopharynx (e.g., chronic abscess secondary to tuberculosis of the spine) or of the larynx (e.g., tuberculosis or carcinoma) are suspected, examination with a mirror is necessary.

The investigation of mechanical obstructions in the esophagus is accomplished mainly by x-ray examination and, in doubtful cases, by esophagoscopy and biopsy of the suspected tissue. Barium mixtures should not be used in cases of suspected foreign body, since the latter may be obscured; nor should a thick barium mixture be employed when the history indicates the presence of an almost complete obstruction, since complete occlusion may be precipitated. In cases of obstruction at the cardiac orifice, a large thick-walled stomach tube should be introduced. If the tube enters the stomach without difficulty, cardiospasm or some other neuromuscular disorder such as scleroderma may be assumed to be present; otherwise, a benign or malignant stricture is responsible for the obstruction.

Studies of esophageal motility with the aid of tiny electromagnetic transducers have been found to contribute information of great value in problems of disturbed esophageal function when the usual methods of examination are indecisive. Cytologic studies are important when malignancy is suspected.

When a neuromuscular disturbance of the pharynx is thought to be the cause of dysphagia, this can be demonstrated most readily by fluoroscopic examination When barium mixture is swallowed, some of the opaque material will be seen to cling to the pharyngeal walls and in the pyriform sinuses, and almost invariably a small amount of the barium will trickle into the trachea. If there is a question of myasthenia gravis being present, a mixture of 1.5 mg neostigmine and 0.6 mg atropine is given intramuscularly, which should bring about very striking relief of dysphagia within 30 min in cases of myasthenia gravis, and little or no improvement in other forms of neuromuscular dysphagia. Similar dissipation of the dysphagia of myasthenia gravis can be effected within 2 min by intravenous administration of 10 mg edrophonium chloride (Tensilon).

NAUSEA AND VOMITING

Nausea and vomiting may each occur independently, but they are so closely allied that they may be conveniently treated as one symptom. Commonly, nausea precedes vomiting. This symptom is usually associated with a diminution of the functional activity of the stomach, alterations of the motility of the duodenum, and other evidences of autonomic activity: pallor of the skin, increased perspiration, salivation, and the occasional association of hypotension and bradycardia (vagal stimulation). Anorexia is also present, and it is assumed that the loss of appetite and nausea are devices developed in the course of evolution to protect the organism against the ingestion and absorption of harmful materials.

Vomiting is a more complicated symptom, depending on the coordinated activity of a number of structures: closure of the glottis, contraction and then fixation of the diaphragm in the inspiratory position, closure of the pylorus and relaxation of the rest of the stomach including the cardiac orifice, and contraction of the abdominal muscles. It is the latter act that is primarily responsible for the expulsion of the gastric contents, the stomach playing a relatively passive role. When vomiting is prolonged and forceful, reverse peristalsis in the small intestine may force bile-stained duodenal contents, or even material from lower levels of the small bowel, into the stomach.

These various activities involved in the act of vomiting are controlled and coordinated in the proper sequence by the vomiting center, which lies in the dorsal portion of the lateral reticular formation of the medulla. This center receives afferent stimuli from emetic receptor sites in the periphery of the body as well as from the brain, and then, if adequately stimulated, sends out efferent impulses to the appropriate structures: larynx, diaphragm, stomach, abdominal muscles.

It was long held that vomiting stimuli fell into two main groups: those that acted primarily by enhancing the activity of the vomiting center ("central" vomiting) and those that arose in the peripheral parts of the body and were then conveyed to the vomiting center ("reflex" vomiting). Newer evidence has modified this concept of the vomiting mechanism. It has been demonstrated that in addition to the vomiting center there exists an accessory medullary center that is responsive to chemical stimuli such as apomorphine and digitalis, but which mediates also the vestibular impulses responsible for motion sickness. In other words, the "central" vomiting due to apomorphine and digitalis is not due to direct stimulation of the vomiting center, but rather to stimulation of the medullary chemoreceptor trigger zone, which then forwards impulses to the vomiting center. Indeed, it is now believed that no drug, or other circulating emetic agent such as occurs in infections and uremia, causes "central" vomiting in the old sense, through direct stimulation of the vomiting center. All emetic stimuli originate at peripheral or central receptor sites. These latter are not autonomous since, when they are stimulated, vomiting can occur only if an intact vomiting center is present.

Probably all sensory nerves, cranial and peripheral as well as autonomic, are capable of transmitting emetic impulses. Any stimulus, if sufficiently painful, may be associated with nausea and vomiting: the "sickening" pain of a blow to the testis is an example. However, pain associated with abdominal disorders is far more likely to be associated with nausea and vomiting than is pain due to extraabdominal disturbances. In the abdomen, afferent stimuli are carried by the vagus and sympathetic nerves. Experimental work on structures subserved by both sets of nerves shows that the vagi are usually the more important in this respect. Cortical stimuli as a result of psychic disturbances, disagreeable sights, odors, or tastes, stimuli from the labyrinth and pharynx, as well as impulses from the digestive and biliary tracts, peritoneum, and urinary and pelvic organs, are common causes of nausea and vomiting. In addition, vomiting may result from the action of drugs and poisons introduced into the body, as well as from toxic substances generated in the organism. In the latter category are the "toxins" of acute infectious diseases and, presumably, the retention products responsible for the vomiting of uremia.

Although the general principles concerned with the mechanism of vomiting appear to be clear, the precise application of these principles in the elucidation of vomiting as it appears in specific clinical conditions is not always possible. In many instances multiple factors may be operative, and it is difficult to estimate the part played by each. In others, the stimuli to vomiting are unknown, and we are uncertain whether their effect is peripheral or central. For example, the cause of vomiting in uremia is still a matter of conjecture. It has been variously attributed to the irritating effect on the gut of ammonium salts converted by bacterial action from urea; to the retention of guanidine, phenol, and other as yet unknown "toxic" substances; to ulceration of the intestinal mucosa; and to dehydration and electrolyte disturbances. Further enumeration of the uncertainties of our knowledge is unnecessary to stress the point that in many clinical conditions the mechanism of vomiting is complex and imperfectly understood.

There is one form of vomiting that occurs in conditions associated with increased intracranial pressure and is quite distinctive—the so-called "projectile" vomiting. This is characterized by a sudden unexpected and sometimes violent ejection of gastric contents. The reason for its chief peculiarity, absence of nausea, is unknown.

Effects of Vomiting. As is true in any condition accompanied by profuse loss of water and salts, excessive vomiting may lead to a state of deficiency of sodium, potassium, and chloride, and hence to a loss of extracellular fluid volume (Chap. 50) and plasma volume, and finally to acute peripheral circulatory failure (Chap. 13). However, vomiting is distinctive in that the loss of chloride is greater than the loss of base. Normally, hydrochloric acid is formed in the stomach by removing the chloride ion from the blood. When, as the result of vomiting, there is excessive loss of hydrochloric acid from the body, a characteristic chemical pattern develops in the blood. This is characterized by deficiency of chloride and excess of bicarbonate (formed from the base no longer balanced by chloride), and elevation of nonprotein nitrogen as the result of prerenal deviation (Chap. 19). This chemical pattern is most typically seen in persons with pyloric or intestinal obstruction but may be observed whenever there is excessive vomiting (Chap. 50).

Classification. Vomiting is so common a manifestation of bodily dysfunction, and its mode of origin so uncertain in many disorders, that a simple, logical classification, according to either mechanism or etiology, is impossible. The one given below has no special merit and serves only as a basis for brief comments on certain specific conditions.

Acute Infectious Diseases. In children nausea and vomiting may be encountered at the onset or during practically any acute infection of a severity sufficient to cause the usual constitutional symptoms. In adults, nausea and vomiting are likely to occur when the infectious process is one primarily involving the gastrointestinal tract, the liver (e.g., acute infectious hepatitis, probably due to an associated duodenitis), or the meninges (in the latter case, the vomiting may be of the projectile type).

Acute Abdominal Emergencies ("Surgical Abdomen"). All the various disorders that fall into this category, and that need not be enumerated, are associated with nausea and vomiting. When the biliary tract is involved, these symptoms are far more intense in obstructions of the common duct than when the gallbladder alone is affected. In general, the most severe and persistent vomiting is seen in acute peritonitis and in acute obstructions of the small bowel (including paralytic ileus).

In certain cases of acute appendicitis, pain may be minimal and vomiting outspoken, although the reverse relationship is more common.

Chronic Indigestion. Spontaneous and frequent nausea and vomiting are uncommon in uncomplicated peptic ulcer; more often, vomiting is induced by the patient to relieve pain. The regular appearance of nausea and the vomiting of copious quantities of material a number of hours after eating indicate the presence of pyloric obstruction due to either a benign or a malignant lesion. Unexplained nausea and loss of appetite may be the earliest symptoms of a carcinoma of the stomach or of almost any type of diffuse disease of the liver.

Diseases of the Heart. Congestive heart failure is frequently associated with nausea and vomiting, which may be the chief complaints of the patient. Under such circumstances these symptoms may result from drugs (more especially from digitalis, opiates, and xanthines), from congestion of the abdominal viscera, or from the frequently associated uremia, sometimes due to salt depletion.

Metabolic Disorders. During the crises of hyperthyroidism, in hypoparathyroidism as well as acute hyperparathyroidism, in the course of Addison's disease (especially during the acute phases), and at the onset of diabetic acidosis, nausea and vomiting may be prominent symptoms. Anorexia and, less commonly, vomiting may result from disorders of the pituitary gland (Simmonds' disease). The familiar morning sickness of the early weeks of pregnancy is listed here because there is some evidence that this phenomenon, so frequent as to be considered physiologic by some, is due to endocrine metabolic alteration initiated by the implantation of the fertilized ovum—possibly to the increased production of estrogens. Psychogenic factors undoubtedly play a role in some cases, and in the more severe form (pernicious vomiting of pregnancy) there are superimposed additional causes of vomiting due to the effects of the prolonged vomiting itself: starvation, dehydration, etc. Reference has already been made to the sometimes severe and persistent nausea and vomiting of uremia, which are to be differentiated from the somewhat similar manifestations that may occur in acute nephritis or hypertensive disease, without nitrogen retention (pseudouremia). In this latter condition the symptoms have long been considered to be due to cerebral edema or spasm of the cerebral vessels; in some cases the symptoms are actually due to thrombosis in the cerebral vessels.

Disorders of the Nervous System. Meningitis, migraine, and tabetic crises are associated with nausea and vomiting, sometimes severe and prolonged. Occasionally, nausea and vomiting may be the predominant or only symptoms in migraine. The projectile vomiting caused by lesions associated with increased intracranial pressure has already been mentioned. The coexistence of nausea, vomiting, and well-marked vertigo is suggestive of a labyrinthine disturbance such as occurs in motion sickness and in the characteristic seizures of Ménière's syndrome.

Drugs and Poisons. Since the majority of these substances are capable of inducing vomiting which subsides after withdrawal of the offending substance, detailed comment is unnecessary.

Pharyngeal Irritation. A prosaic but common and sometimes disturbing cause of morning vomiting is the irritating effect of a postnasal discharge, frequently due to excessive smoking.

Psychogenic Vomiting. This term is applied to the nausea and vomiting that may occur as transitory phenomena, the result of some emotional upset, or persistent as a consequence of a more profound psychic disturbance. The condition known as *anorexia nervosa,* in which, as the result of an emotional disturbance, the patient may suffer from a profound loss of appetite and may vomit after every meal, with consequent rapid weight loss, constitutes one example of this type of vomiting. More commonly, patients with emotional disorders and vomiting maintain a relatively normal state of nutrition, because only a relatively small fraction of the ingested food is vomited.

Differential Diagnosis. Vomiting is to be differentiated from regurgitation, which implies the expulsion from the esophagus of undigested food retained because of some obstruction such as occurs with cardiospasm or esophageal diverticulum, or the expulsion of gastric contents without preceding nausea. Regurgitation is caused by the intrinsic activity of the esophagus or stomach and is not accompanied by the forceful contraction of the abdominal muscles (retching) that characterizes vomiting.

The character of the vomitus and the circumstances under which vomiting occurs are sometimes of importance in estimating the significance of this symptom. When several hundred milliliters of material are vomited regularly a number of hours after the preceding meal, and particularly when particles of undigested food can be recognized, pyloric obstruction is a practical certainty. If this vomitus contains free hydrochloric acid, the obstruction may be due either to ulcer or to carcinoma; absence of free hydrochloric acid suggests a malignant growth. Fecal odor after protracted vomiting indicates the presence of low obstruction of the small bowel or of peritonitis. Streaks of blood have no significance. Large quantities of blood, either bright red or dark brown (when it has been chemically altered by the acid of gastric juice), usually denote an intragastric lesion or a ruptured esophageal varix. Bile is commonly present in the gastric contents whenever vomiting is prolonged. It has no significance unless constantly present in large quantities, when it may signify an obstructive lesion below the ampulla of Vater.

In general, nausea and vomiting due to lesions or functional derangement of the stomach bear some definite relationship to eating. Unfortunately, this statement is less helpful than would appear at first glance. Indigestion associated with nausea and vomiting, especially occurring shortly after eating, may be caused by a functional disturbance of the stomach dependent on an obscure lesion such as a

chronic infection in the urinary tract or pelvic organs. Vomiting, practically always self-induced, which relieves an epigastric pain of the postprandial type and often occurring during the night, is highly suggestive of a peptic ulcer.

Vomiting which is entirely unrelated to eating is often due to exogenous (drugs) or endogenous (uremia, hepatic and diabetic coma) intoxication, to disorders of the nervous system, or to the various metabolic disturbances which have been mentioned. Vomiting occurring before breakfast in a young woman is commonly due to pregnancy.

Nausea and vomiting are symptoms too widespread to be investigated by any definite program of study. In most cases the associated symptoms are of more value in defining the cause of the underlying disorder. It may be well, however, to mention some of the conditions in which the cause of the nausea and vomiting may not be readily apparent: carcinoma of the stomach in an early stage, chronic indigestion due to lesions remote from the stomach, diabetic acidosis, uremia, Addison's disease, pregnancy, tabetic crises, migraine when the headache is brief and overshadowed by the nausea and vomiting, acute hepatitis at the onset and before jaundice appears, or the acute epidemic infectious disease whose only manifestation is nausea and vomiting (epidemic nausea and vomiting).

REFERENCES

DYSPHAGIA

Benedict, E. B., and G. L. Nardi: "The Esophagus," Boston, Little, Brown & Company, 1958.

Kramer, P., and F. J. Ingelfinger: Esophageal Sensitivity to Mecholyl in Cardiospasm, Gastroenterology, 19:242, 1951.

Wynder, E. L., and J. H. Fryer: Etiologic Considerations of Plummer-Vinson (Patterson-Kelly) Syndrome, Ann. Internal Med., 49:1106, 1958.

INDIGESTION

Bloomfield, A. L.: Mechanism of Pain with Peptic Ulcer, Am. J. Med., 17:165, 1954.

Hobsley, M., and L. P. LeQuesne: The Dumping Syndrome. II. Cause of the Syndrome and the Rationale of Its Treatment, Brit. Med. J., 1:147, 1960.

Kinsella, V. J.: Pain in Chronic Gastric Ulcer: Basic Anatomy and Mechanism, Lancet, 2:353, 1953.

Palmer, W. L.: Mechanism of Pain with Peptic Ulcer: A Reply, Am. J. Med., 18:513, 1955.

Smith, A. W. M.: The Pain of Peptic Ulceration, Quart. J. Med., 24:293, 1955.

The above papers of Bloomfield, Palmer, Kinsella, and Smith present concise expositions of the leading theories regarding the mechanism of peptic ulcer pain: disturbed motility, acid irritation, and local inflammatory reaction, respectively.

Maddock, W. G.: The Importance of Air in Gastro-Intestinal Distention, Surg. Clin. North Am., 32:71, 1952.

Wolf, S., and H. G. Wolff: "Human Gastric Function," 2d ed., New York, Oxford University Press, 1947.

NAUSEA AND VOMITING

Borison, H. L., and S. C. Wang: Physiology and Pharmacology of Vomiting, Pharmacol. Rev., 5:193, 1953.

Cummins, A. J.: Nausea and Vomiting, Am. J. Digest. Diseases, 3:710, 1958.

Wolf, S., and H. G. Wolff: "Human Gastric Function," 2d ed., New York, Oxford University Press, 1947.

17 CONSTIPATION AND DIARRHEA

Albert I. Mendeloff

Diarrhea and *constipation* are terms given to alterations in the normal pattern of human defecation habits. There is no standard definition by which patients or physicians may classify strictly the deviation from normal; the range of variation in bowel habits among apparently healthy persons is extraordinarily wide, so that the deviation must, in the last analysis, be compared with each patient's own previous habit pattern rather than with that characterizing the mean, the median, or the mode of the population. Such comparisons involve so many associated functions that it will suffice for the purposes of this discussion to define diarrhea as the frequent passage of unformed stools, and constipation as an undue delay in the evacuation of feces. It is the task of the physician to understand enough of the normal and disturbed physiology of digestion, absorption, and propulsive motility that he may ask pointed questions of the patient which serve to define more precisely the locus, the nature, and the severity of the disturbance. Since the gastrointestinal tract is a primitive organ upon which all manner of stimuli, from hunger to fear, rage, fever, and fatigue, from grossly infected or chemically toxic ingesta to the most subtly allergenic refined foods, exert effects productive of disturbed function, this task is rarely simple.

When one considers that a north-woods lumberjack may consume several kilograms of foodstuffs per day, furnishing him nearly 6,000 cal, and yet produce a stool which weighs only 100 to 200 Gm, of which nearly three-quarters is water, the efficiency of the gut becomes clearly evident. Just as slight changes in renal function may result in abnormal amounts of urine being excreted, so relatively minor deviations in the absorption of water,

in intestinal tone, in propulsive motility, or in rectal sensitivity may result in dramatic changes in the caliber and consistency of the stools. On a normal mixed diet the stomach is nearly empty several hours after food is ingested; the chyme has entered the duodenum, stimulated the production from the stomach and duodenal mucosa of hormones which cause the gallbladder to contract and the pancreas to pour out its digestive juice, and become admixed with these secretions as well as with those of the small bowel itself. Gastric muscular contraction passes across the pylorus to activate strong contractions of the duodenum; intraluminal contents are fairly rapidly passed along the jejunum, then are slowed down in the ileum. Contractions of the small intestine are usually classified as either rhythmical segmenting contractions or propulsive peristaltic movements. By x-ray techniques the bolus is seen to proceed very rapidly for 10 to 25 cm, then to stop and undergo segmentation for many minutes. When coordinated waves suddenly become continuous, a "mass peristalsis" results, with sudden propulsion of the bolus for distances as great as 150 cm. By the time the head of the food column reaches the ileocecal valve, 99 per cent of the carbohydrate, 99 per cent of the protein, and 97 per cent of the fats have been broken down into absorbable form and entered the portal venules and the lacteals.

When the intestinal bolus reaches the terminal ileum, it tends to proceed very sluggishly unless the stomach empties; the so-called "gastroileal reflex" causes the ileum to empty into the cecum by a rapid series of small squirts. The ileocecal valve is a puzzling structure which offers no resistance to the oncoming ileal bolus, but is supposed to prevent regurgitation, at least of gas, from the cecum into the ileum. The ileal contents reaching the cecum daily comprise a volume of less than 500 ml, a slurry thoroughly churned in the right colon by segmental contractions of the haustra. Every now and then a coordinated wave involving a short length of colon pushes the soggy mass along into the next area; reflexes brought on by eating sweep from duodenum or stomach to the colon, and an occasional movement occurs by means of which a fairly large section of colon is emptied of its contents, and the left colon fills with a more desiccated mass. Defecatory reflexes originate from the rectal walls, which normally are approximated around a small lumen empty of feces; when sigmoid contraction distends the rectal musculature, the defecatory reflex center in the sacral cord causes the levatores ani to pull the lower rectum and both sphincters up and almost around or over the descending fecal mass; forced expiration and contraction of abdominal muscles supply the additional pressure required to force the stool past the external sphincter.

However, if the sphincter is voluntarily contracted, the sigmoid colon relaxes, and the fecal mass slips back up into the rectosigmoid.

Symptoms. Exaggerations of the motor components of normal gastrointestinal activity constitute the most important early symptoms of gastrointestinal diseases. In the small intestine rapid propulsive motility may be associated with dyssynergy, the combination giving rise to cramping contractions. Because of the rather imprecise character of man's system for the detection and recognition of the sources of visceral pain, these cramps are usually projected to the midline—if they originate in the duodenum, to the epigastrium; if from the jejunum, to the umbilicus; if from the lower ileum, to the area just below the umbilicus. In the colon, dyssynergic activity is rarely projected to the midline but usually is lateralized along the general course of the offending organ. Since the colon is large, festooning the abdomen, and full of fluid and partially compressible gas, contractions in one or another area of the bowel may force the contents back toward the cecum; a simultaneous dyssynergic contraction anywhere else in the colonic wall may trap gas in the area intervening, distending a relaxed but otherwise innocent portion of the bowel so that discomfort is referred to the distended site, often in the splenic or hepatic flexure. Excessive gas results entirely from air swallowed with food or drink or from such "tics" as sighing or forced belching. Sharp, unpleasant contractions in the left lower quadrant associated with straining at stool, and partially relieved by defecation, are called *tenesmus.* A sensation of urgent need to defecate—*rectal urgency*—is an extremely distressing symptom associated with irritability of the rectum. Sharp pain in the anal area is made worse by defecation and is usually associated with an inflammatory response in the skin of the anus—*anal pain.*

After establishing the presence or absence of these deviations, the physician must find out whether or not eating or defecation exacerbates or relieves them, whether the patient tries to mitigate the discomfort by moving about or lying still, or by holding the abdominal wall immobilized with his hands or against the mattress. Although the general topography of the area of distress may localize findings to large or small intestines, relief by defecation is a feature of disturbance of the left colon, as exacerbation by eating is a feature of malfunction of the small intestine or right colon. Restlessness occurs with colic; peritoneal irritation tends to immobilize the patient. All these disturbances originate as increases in the tone of the bowel wall, and pressure relationships between adjacent segments of intestine determine not only the tension exerted against the wall but also the speed and character of the flow of the fluid contents along the

lumen. As increased tension may compress the vessels nourishing the gut wall, so disease or contraction of the nourishing vasculature may deprive the wall of its ability to contract, to absorb, or to secrete. Unabsorbed residue or unduly large volumes of secretions attract more fluid into the lumen, further distending the gut; if large volumes of swallowed air cannot be passed quickly along the small bowel to the cecum, as is usual, the movements of the air-fluid mixture in the small intestine become loud enough to be noticed by the patient; such borborygmi are heard normally in the colon. Sudden changes in volume of the abdomen—distention—occur when the intraluminal volume of small or large bowel increases, because of paralysis of neuromuscular elements, abnormal handling of gas, or mechanical obstruction behind which muscular contractile activity is greatly increased. Bowel sounds may be absent if the wall is paralyzed, faint if the injury is submaximal, or increased if a viable area is forced to raise its intraluminal pressure in order to drive fluid past an obstructed segment. Sudden changes in pain reference occurring during the course of an illness usually indicate that the peritoneal surfaces have become involved, with more accurate cerebral localization of the underlying disturbance, and perhaps with associated development of spasm or guarding of the overlying musculature.

Diarrhea. Acute disturbances of bowel function are relatively common and usually manifest themselves as diarrhea. The sudden onset of loose stools in a previously healthy person commonly is due to an active infection, and much less often to the ingestion of preformed toxins, poisonous chemicals, or drugs or to acute radiation sickness. When the patient is first seen, the history will usually point toward the source of the trouble: the eating of a particular meal or food in company with others who have also become similarly ill within 24 hr of eating the suspected food is prima-facie evidence that a preformed toxin has been ingested; diarrhea developing in a number of patients within 28 to 72 hr after a common meal should make one suspect a salmonella infection. The presence of fever, malaise, muscle aching, and profound epigastric or periumbilical discomfort with severe anorexia suggests an inflammatory disease of the small intestine. The stools are characteristically watery, often accompanied by the explosive passage of gas; there is no rectal urgency or tenesmus and little hypogastric cramping. On physical examination one finds a generally tender abdomen without guarding, and one hears "whooshing" peristaltic sounds. A variant of the syndrome consists only of severe periumbilical pain and vomiting. The hemogram usually is within normal limits. Such an entity is commonly produced by infection with a virus, of which a number of species have been identified. The disease is called *viral gastroenteritis,* runs an acute course for 2 to 3 days, then gradually subsides.

The stool in viral gastroenteritis never contains recognizable exudate—it is singularly free of inflammatory cells, blood, or fibrin. Culture of the stool is usually nonproductive. By contrast, inflammatory diseases of the colon almost always result in leukocytic exudate and fibrin in the feces; stools may give cultures positive for organisms of the genus *Salmonella* or *Shigella* or may on microscopic examination show motile forms and/or cysts of various parasites, the most important of which in the United States is *Endamoeba histolytica.* Colonic infections usually are accompanied by hypogastric cramping, tenesmus, and rectal urgency. The patient may not have true anorexia but may be afraid to eat because eating stimulates the urge to defecate. There is usually fever and leukocytosis.

The physician must remember that an acute diarrhea may be the presenting symptom of any type of systemic infection or of a hitherto-silent chronic gastrointestinal disease, of which the most well-defined are regional enteritis and ulcerative colitis; the latter may occasionally begin with fulminant dysentery, the former more often presents as a tender mass in the right lower quadrant with mild diarrhea. Generalized cramping and diarrhea may follow use of a parasympathomimetic drug. Tenesmus, urgency, and left-sided hypogastric tenderness and cramping are classical symptoms of diverticulitis; the stool may contain pus, blood, or both, usually with much mucus. A fecal impaction may make a patient have rectal urgency, ask for a bedpan or visit the toilet often, but expel only a little watery exudate, or nothing. Short-circuiting operations on the intestine and stomach usually result in at least mild diarrhea for months after the operation.

Differential diagnosis of these varied entities is made by history, physical examination, gross and microscopic appearance of the stools, appropriate bacteriologic studies, and proctoscopy. It is important to see the excreta put out by the patient, not just to rely on his description or on that of a third party. Toilets are not distinguished for satisfactory lighting, nor upset patients for careful observation, and even trained personnel seldom display a curiosity sufficient to overcome the unpleasantness of a stool held close enough for accurate appraisal. Since fluid and electrolyte losses in diarrhea may be so great as to be life threatening, the patient is given supportive care until studies indicate specific treatment. If no definitive etiologic agent can be identified, barium enema and upper gastrointestinal x-rays should be carried out. Upper gastrointestinal films may be very misleading when the barium meal is fed within the first few days of an acute enteritis or colitis, and should be reserved for a time when the whole disease has become more quiescent.

Chronic Diarrhea. A history of bouts of loose stools extending over a period of months or years, usually intermittent in character, calls for painstaking investigation. One particularly wants to know the circumstances of the first such bout—did it follow an acute infection, an operation, an emotional upset of severe degree? The number of days or weeks lost by the patient from his daily occupation on account of the illness, changes in weight and strength, and the appearance of the patient give important leads as to the nature and severity of the underlying disease. By the time the patient sees a physician the presenting symptoms may not be diarrhea, but rather those of serious malnutrition, since any long-continued illness of this type may interfere with appetite, as well as with the absorptive and digestive functions of the gastrointestinal tract. Associated signs and symptoms may reveal that the diarrhea and malnutrition are due to a generalized disorder which may involve the intestines functionally or structurally—hyperthyroidism, tuberculosis, lymphosarcoma, to name a few. More often, no such disorder will be found, and the physician must consider another, more specifically gastrointestinal disease.

A long history of intermittent diarrhea unaccompanied by fever, weight loss, blood in the stools, or significant loss of working capacity suggests a disturbance of emotional or, less commonly, of allergic origin, and associated symptoms should be elicited (Chaps. 42, 232). A detailed dietary history is important in such cases, in order to establish the adequacy of the nutrient intake and to allow the patient a chance to ventilate his ideas on the relationship of food and eating to his symptoms. In such disordered functional states, the patient usually has a fairly formed stool on arising in the morning but then has one or two loose stools within the next hour. A similar pattern may occur after the evening meal. The stool caliber is usually small, and there may be mild discomfort, relieved by defecation, in the left lower quadrant of the abdomen. Such a triad of symptoms makes up the diarrheal component of the "irritable colon" syndrome, an extremely common disorder in anxious, nervous people, in which the symptoms result from exaggeration of normal colonic function.

When the history suggests that the diarrheal episodes have been characterized by blood in the stools, or by fever, malaise, anorexia, and weight loss in addition, one suspects a chronic inflammatory process involving either or both small bowel and colon. Regional enteritis may attack any portion of the intestine, producing an encroachment on the lumen and episodes of partial obstruction, ulcerations of the mucous membrane, or local abscesses and fistulas to the abdominal or anal skin, to the bladder, or to other loops of bowel. On proctoscopic examination the rectum is found to be uninvolved and the stools show little microscopic exudate although they are often positive for occult blood, gross bleeding being infrequently encountered. Tuberculosis and lymphosarcoma of the intestine can give similar symptoms and may be impossible to differentiate, although usually the roentgenologic appearances are dissimilar. The involvement may be primarily colonic, the most important disease entity being ulcerative colitis, whether idiopathic or due to amebic infestation, venereal lymphogranuloma, or chronic bacillary dysentery. Here the feces show pus cells and red cells when the disease is active, and proctoscopy is usually diagnostic. Stool cultures and examinations for parasites on numerous occasions are important aspects of the medical investigation.

When the patient presents with diarrhea of more than a few months' duration, without fever, blood in the stools, or cramping pain, but with weight loss, weakness, and symptoms of nutritional deficiency diseases (Chaps. 62; 279), one focuses attention on the small intestine. In children celiac disease and cystic fibrosis of the pancreas are the important disorders to be differentiated; in older patients the same distinction between an absorptive defect and a digestive disorder must still be made in order to distinguish idiopathic steatorrhea from chronic pancreatitis. Occasionally an adult with such a syndrome will give a history of having had celiac disease as a child or of having celiac siblings. In adults the finding of anemia, macrocytic early in the disease, hypochromic and microcytic later, suggests a malabsorption syndrome. A low serum carotene concentration and diminished uptake of a labeled fat or fat-soluble vitamin suggest a defect in fat absorption. Gross inspection and properly performed microscopic study of the stools for fat may make the diagnosis; stool analyses for fat and nitrogen (in borderline cases after at least a 4-day balance study) confirm a diagnosis of steatorrhea if more than 8 per cent of the ingested fat reaches the stool and establish an excessive nitrogen loss if more than 2.5 Gm of nitrogen is found in the 24-hourly stool. Thus one establishes the presence of the absorptive defect, but does not identify its cause, although it is unusual to have large nitrogen losses in idiopathic steatorrhea. Fat-soluble vitamin deficiencies are common and may be the presenting symptom; hypoprothrombinemia in particular may be a fatal complication of steatorrhea, particularly if antibacterial agents have been added to the therapeutic regimen. Glucose tolerance test results are of diabetic type often in chronic pancreatic insufficiency, whereas they are normal or "flat" in primary intestinal malabsorption. Previous surgery on the biliary tract suggests biliary fistulas or chronic pancreatitis as possible causes for the fecal nitrogen loss; sudden and dramatic weight loss always results from gastrocolic fistulas. A long history of diabetes with or without peripheral neuropathy may be accompanied by the development of autonomic visceral neuropathy, with low tonus of the small bowel and frequent diarrhea, particularly when the patient is in bed. Such patients usually do not excrete abnormal amounts of fat and nitrogen in the stools, but show marked debility because of fluid loss and complications of diabetes and neuropathy. Occasionally partial mechanical obstruction of the ileum may cause steatorrhea; neoplasms and granulomas are the usual offenders, but recurrent volvulus and adhesive bands may be responsible. Visible peristalsis in a patient with marked weight loss points to this diagnosis.

A history of progressive disease characterized by arthritis, abdominal pain, diarrhea, and weight loss in middle-aged males suggests the diagnosis of intestinal lipodystrophy (Whipple's disease), in which abnormal deposits of glycoproteins accumulate in the lacteal system of the mesentery and small focal granulomas develop in the viscera and lymph nodes. Lymphosarcomas of low degrees of malignancy may produce malabsorption syndromes by blockage of lymphatic channels from the small bowel; loops of intestine made "blind" by surgery or by the healing of lesions of regional enteritis can produce syndromes of severe macrocytic anemia and diarrhea. Rarer causes of diarrhea are the enormous hypersecretion of gastric juice due to endocrine tumors (Zollinger-Ellison syndrome) and the cramping diarrhea associated with high circulating levels of serotonin (see Chap. 90).

Special techniques are often needed to define clearly all these abnormalities, and isotopic labeling of nutrients has been very helpful in this respect. Duodenal intubation and analysis of digestive juices for pancreatic enzymes is a procedure of considerable importance in ruling out primary disease of the pancreas. Nevertheless, the aid of the skilled radiologist is probably more useful than any test in interpreting all but the earliest manifestations of these syndromes. Pancreatic calcification, fistulas, distortions of the duodenal loop, diffuse granulomatous diseases of the small bowel, diverticula, polyps, ulcerated areas, stenosis, and obstruction—all these can be identified by modern radiologic techniques, which provide in addition base-line data for evaluating the natural history of the disease and response to therapy.

Constipation. Whereas diarrhea may be a dangerous symptom per se, with its accompaniment of dehydration and loss of cations, constipation of itself is not debilitating, although mild abdominal discomfort and straining at stool are not salutary and tend to increase the severity of preexisting ano-rectal lesions. The acute onset of severe obstipation in an apparently normal person signifies that something has disturbed the neural, vascular, or muscular integrity of the gut or associated defecatory reflexes and muscles. Such disturbances may result from severe infections, particularly of the central nervous system, from acute mesenteric circulatory catastrophes, from renal colic, from cerebrovascular accidents, from mechanical obstruction of large or small intestine, from painful anal lesions, from certain drugs, or from fecal impaction. Of these, the last is the most embarrassing to overlook, since the puttylike mass filling the rectum makes the patient try to move his bowels and often results in frequent calls for a bedpan or visits to the toilet; such fruitless attempts at defecations may be called diarrhea, and the poor patient may receive anti-diarrheal medications! Rapid but complete physical examination including a digital examination of the rectum and proctoscopy is called for in all cases of constipation of acute onset; if no other physical signs to explain the sudden constipation are elicited, a low-pressure barium enema should be given to establish the site of obstruction if present and appropriate measures taken.

A long history of intermittent bouts of constipation, accompanied by abdominal distress relieved by defecation and by passage of hard stools of small caliber, with or without much mucus, is characteristic of the "irritable colon" syndrome, one of the commonest forms of anxiety met by the physician. The abuse of laxatives over many years is frequently added to the underlying emotional disturbance to aggravate the clinical picture. The symptoms are essentially exaggerations of normal physiologic activity of the colon, and in mild degrees have probably been experienced by most healthy people as, for example, the constipation associated with travel. Extensive studies of sigmoid motility in patients with this syndrome have verified the clinical impression that disturbed motor function correlates closely with emotional conflicts. Proctoscopic examination of these patients demonstrates an unremarkable rectum and a rectosigmoid which is often spastic, the lumen smaller than normal, the veins prominent, and the mucus more abundant than usual. The stools are negative for blood, parasites, and pathogenic bacteria; the x-ray examination is usually not abnormal.

Another common form of constipation is also chronic and is not characterized by the triad of symptoms of the irritable colon syndrome. Whether as the result of childhood training or of a perverse understanding of the necessity for bowel movements occurring with chronometric precision, these patients have equated general health with "regu-larity." This leads to a dependence on laxatives or enemas to hasten the overdue evacuation, so that over the years they lose the sensitivity of the rectal defecatory reflexes. Consequently, they do not have a regular schedule for moving their bowels, which for most normal people is most easily accomplished after breakfast and, if needed, after the heaviest meal of the day; over the years they no longer demonstrate any rhythmicity in defecation, take laxatives whenever they feel "run down," and have stools which may be alternately voluminous and watery or small and hard. Lax abdominal muscles and a pelvic floor weakened by multiple deliveries may contribute to poor defecatory performance. On physical examination these patients often have a palpable colon filled with feces, and on rectal examination feces fill the ampulla, the patient being unaware of this. Such types of rectal insensitivity have been called *atonic constipation, dyschezia,* and *rectal constipation.*

In both the above types of constipation, it is obvious that a thorough analysis by the physician of dietary habits, defecatory habits, use of laxatives, mode of living, and emotional problems must be made before proper therapy can be instituted. At the same time it must be stressed that such patients are not immune to the development of neoplasms of the large bowel, and it is a most difficult task for the physician to decide how often complete studies should be carried out on patients with long-standing, apparently static, complaints. The simplest solution is to do repeated stool examinations for occult blood and digital and proctoscopic examinations, remembering also that in patients who have difficulty with evacuation, anal diseases—fissures, ulcers, and hemorrhoids—are more common than in the general population.

A lifelong history of obstinate constipation may be associated with the enormous dilatation of the large bowel seen in idiopathic or acquired megacolon. In the former condition, the rectosigmoid is contracted and obstructing, because of its lack of the ganglionic cells necessary to pass on the propulsive waves of the proximal colon; in the latter condition, severe contraction of the voluntary anal sphincter produces enormous dilatation of the rectal ampulla and colon. Radiologic studies are usually very helpful in differentiating these two conditions.

When constipation is of recent onset and progressive, the investigation should be thorough and extremely comprehensive. This is the optimal time to detect a neoplasm of the large bowel. General physical and psychiatric examination may reveal a systemic disorder: hypothyroidism, hyperparathyroidism, tuberculosis, urinary tract disease, congestive heart failure; a major psychosis, profound depression, parkinsonism, or recent cerebrovascular accident may be responsible for progressive constipation. A careful history of drug ingestion may reveal that the patient received ganglionic-blocking agents or opiates prior to onset of symptoms or large amounts of sedation. A marked change in dietary regimen, particularly in combination with sedative drugs, may produce a marked decrease in frequency of bowel movements.

If the digital and proctoscopic findings fail to explain the constipation, a barium enema and upper gastrointestinal x-rays are indicated. Tumors of the gastrointestinal tract comprise nearly half of all cancer, and patients with colonic cancers have a better prognosis for survival after surgery than do those with gastric and esophageal lesions. A high index of suspicion for a neoplastic origin of changes in bowel habits, repeated tests for occult blood in the stools, and careful proctoscopy and x-ray studies will usually justify in salvaged lives the money and time spent.

REFERENCES

Mendeloff, A. I.: Chronic Diarrhea, Am. J. Digest. Diseases, 3:801, 1958.

Portis, S. A. (Ed.): "Diseases of the Digestive System," 3d ed., chap. 7, The Physiology of the Small and the Large Intestine; chap. 34, Diseases of the Small Intestine; chap. 37, Functional Disturbances of the Colon, Philadelphia, Lea & Febiger, 1953.

18 HEMATEMESIS AND MELENA

William H. Resnik

Hematemesis (vomiting of gross blood) and melena (passage of tarry stools) are with rare exceptions manifestations of hemorrhage in the upper digestive tract—esophagus, stomach, duodenum. In this discussion hematemesis may be used alone for the sake of brevity, although it is to be understood that both symptoms may occur as a result of the same hemorrhage, or either may appear alone. Whether hematemesis or melena takes place will depend on whether vomiting is aroused when the stomach or duodenum contains gross blood and how much blood gains access to the small intestine: melena may be the only symptom, even though the site is in the esophagus or the stomach; hematemesis may be the prominent symptom even though the bleeding originates in the duodenum. It has been demonstrated experimentally that at least 50 to 60 ml of blood is necessary to give the stool a tarry appearance.

There are no symptoms or signs that reveal accurately the size of the hemorrhage immediately after the event takes place. The statement of the patient regarding the amount of blood vomited is usually unreliable, and, in any case, a variable amount of blood has passed into the intestine. Blood counts and hematocrit determinations made shortly after the hemorrhage are of little value. Obviously, when signs of shock are clearly evident (pallor, cool moist skin, rapid thready pulse, hypotension, restlessness, cyanosis of finger tips, etc.), a serious loss of blood volume (40 per cent or more) has taken place. When the signs of shock are less apparent or absent, a fairly large hemorrhage may nevertheless have occurred and the patient may be in a compensated state. Despite the theoretic objections to the use of the Evans blue dye (T-1824) as a precise measure of plasma volume, for clinical purposes it can serve as a simple and rapid method of estimating the extent of the blood loss. After a number of hours has elapsed and time has been allowed for compensatory restoration of blood volume, the estimation of hemoglobin by an accurate method or, better still, of hematocrit levels, frequently repeated, affords additional information regarding the amount of blood lost and may indicate whether bleeding is continuous or recurrent. A well-marked decline in blood pressure in the sitting position may occur when the recumbent blood pressure is still normal. Decline in urine volume despite adequate fluid intake may also be a clue to onset of shock.

The severity of shock depends not only on the magnitude of the hemorrhage but also on the abruptness with which it takes place. Hemorrhage into the upper digestive tract is frequently associated with an elevation of the nonprotein nitrogen content of the blood, owing primarily to absorption of the digestion products of blood and enhanced in cases of extensive hemorrhage by the depression of renal function resulting from shock. The increase in urea nitrogen content of the blood usually reaches a peak in about 24 hr following a single hemorrhage, and its level serves as a measure of the severity of the hemorrhage. Preexisting renal disease leads to greater and more prolonged rises in urea nitrogen, so that one must include urinary findings in analyzing the situation. Elevation of temperature to 100°F is often manifest within 24 hr of the onset of the bleeding, and this may be due to the bleeding alone. Temperatures above 100°F and those lasting beyond the first 24 hr are usually due to the administered transfusions.

CAUSES OF HEMATEMESIS AND MELENA

Peptic Ulcer. This is the most common cause of hematemesis, accounting for about 50 per cent of the cases. Hemorrhage from duodenal ulcer comprises about 75 per cent of all bleeding ulcer cases. In most instances there is a history characteristic of ulcer, or the ulcer has been demonstrated by x-ray study. In a small percentage, hematemesis or melena may be the initial symptom. Bleeding usually results from the rupture of a small vessel in the ulcer or from an adjacent area of gastritis. More uncommonly, bleeding follows the erosion of a large sclerotic artery; it is in these latter cases that fatal hemorrhage is likely to ensue.

Gastritis and Esophagitis. These must constitute a large group, although an accurate estimation is rarely possible, for the diagnosis is often a wastebasket for unexplained hematemesis. Not infrequently hemorrhage due to gastritis appears to be unquestionably related to excessive intake of alcohol and frequently of aspirin. Even when a peptic ulcer is known to be present, a gastritis at some distance from the ulcer may harbor the bleeding point.

Carcinoma of the Stomach. About 3 per cent of the cases of hematemesis are accounted for by carcinoma of the stomach. Although this is often responsible for a moderate or severe anemia, usually the loss of blood takes place as a persistent ooze; only relatively uncommonly is there eroded a blood vessel large enough to cause a brisk hemorrhage.

Portal Hypertension. This is responsible for about 10 per cent of the cases, bleeding usually being due to an esophageal varix, but occasionally to a gastric varix. Of this group, cirrhosis of the liver (usually the Laennec type, and in certain regions liver disease due to schistosomiasis) is the most frequent cause. In the remainder, congestive splenomegaly without cirrhosis (splenic anemia or Banti's syndrome) is found.

Miscellaneous Causes. In the miscellaneous group fall the rarer causes of hematemesis and melena: benign polyps and other uncommon tumors of the stomach, duodenum, and small intestine; hiatal hernia; tumors and inflammation of the biliary tract; hereditary hemorrhagic telangiectasia, which may cause bleeding from the esophagus as well as from the pharynx and stomach; other blood dyscrasias, etc.—in all, about 2 or 3 per cent of the total.

The figures regarding the frequency with which the various causes of hematemesis and melena occur are approximate and will vary widely in different reported series. They will depend partly upon the material studied by different observers. A population containing a large number of Puerto Ricans or persons originating in other areas of the Caribbean or South America or Africa where schistosomiasis is prevalent may show figures that are heavily weighted with cases due to cirrhosis caused by this disease. In part, the figures will depend on what criteria are used to define the extent of the hemor-

rhage. In the main, the variations can be attributed to the thoroughness with which the investigations were carried out. Formerly, and still in many institutions, careful study was instituted only after 2 or 3 weeks had elapsed after the bleeding had subsided. At this time careful study failed to reveal any adequate cause for the hemorrhage in a considerable number of cases. In some, a typical history of ulcer made it probable that the ulcer was healed before the diagnostic studies were carried out. When no lesion could be discovered by x-ray or gastroscopy, it was often assumed that an ulcer had already healed, even when there was no previous history to suggest ulcer. In others, when there was no suggestive history, it was assumed that the hemorrhage had been caused by an acute superficial ulceration or by gastritis. Nevertheless, careful follow-up studies of such cases of unexplained hematemesis have often subsequently revealed previously undetected lesions such as peptic ulcer, carcinoma of stomach, tumors of small intestine, etc. However, the recently more frequent employment of the esophagoscope and gastroscope within the first few days of bleeding has revealed sources of hemorrhage such as mucosal erosions, or ulceration due to esophagitis or gastritis, or uncommon lesions such as hereditary hemorrhagic telangiectasia that could not have been detected before. Moreover, even when peptic ulcer or cirrhosis was known to be present, a cause of bleeding unrelated to these disorders has not infrequently been uncovered. For example, peptic ulcer may be present in almost 20 per cent of patients with cirrhosis, and the ulcer, not the varices, may have caused the hemorrhage. Even now, when early and thorough diagnostic studies have been carried out, a small residual group of cases will almost invariably be present in every reported series in which no adequate cause for the bleeding has been revealed even at autopsy.

Hematemesis and melena may be due to a number of disorders. However, the problem of diagnosis is simplified if it is borne in mind that 90 per cent of all cases are due to primary intragastric or duodenal diseases such as peptic ulcer (including gastrojejunal ulcers), gastritis, superficial ulceration, and benign and malignant tumors of the stomach. Most of the remainder are due to bleeding from esophageal varices.

PROCEDURE

It should be mentioned that a red color in the toilet bowl does not necessarily signify blood; occasionally, a person who has eaten beets or has been given an injection of Bromsulphalein may exhibit a reddish discoloration in the stool. Moreover, bright red blood in the stool is not an invariable sign of lower-bowel bleeding. A hemorrhage from the upper gastrointestinal tract may be associated with the presence of relatively unaltered blood in the stool, if transit time is rapid. Finally, it is not always easy to distinguish between bleeding originating from the gastrointestinal tract and that from the respiratory tract.

If unmistakable evidences of shock are present, the first obligation is to replace the lost blood and then to exclude hemoptysis and bleeding from the nose and pharynx as possible sources of swallowed blood. If bleeding persists, gastric lavage with ice water, using a French 30 Ewald tube, is frequently effective in stopping the hemorrhage. If shock is not present, 500 to 1000 ml whole blood may be given, depending on one's estimation of the amount of blood lost. While these measures are being instituted, historical data regarding indigestion, alcoholism, previous episodes of bleeding or a familial bleeding tendency, recent medication with drugs, such as salicylates, cortisone, or phenylbutazone, or severe vomiting just prior to the hematemesis should be obtained from the patient or his family, and physical findings such as enlargement of the liver or spleen, jaundice, spider angiomas, a palpable supraclavicular node, Blumer's shelf, and telangiectases should be searched for. Hematologic studies should also be pursued if there is a suspicion that a blood dyscrasia is present.

What studies are then carried out, and when they are begun, vary with the facilities that are available. In some clinics early investigation within the first 24 to 48 hr is initiated—by esophagoscopy, gastroscopy, and x-ray examination. If these studies are carried out skillfully and with suitable caution, the reports thus far indicate that little or no additional risk is imposed on the patient, while the advantages of ascertaining the precise point of bleeding are obvious. It is generally believed that all such procedures should be deferred as long as shock persists, and most authorities prefer to delay these investigations until bleeding has probably ceased. Even when expert endoscopic examination is not at hand, pneumatic tamponade of the esophagus can be employed as a therapeutic test for esophageal bleeding. Early or late x-ray examination will depend on the experience of the roentgenologist in handling such cases. Liver function tests are not of great value. There is no necessary correlation between impaired hepatic function and the degree of portal hypertension which is the basic cause of the development of varices.

A diagnostic approach, entirely different from that mentioned above has also been advocated. In the vast majority of patients, the important problem hinges on whether the hemorrhage has been caused by an ulcerative lesion in the upper gastro-intestinal tract or by a ruptured varix. Examination of the patient under emergency conditions by esophagoscopy, gastroscopy, x-ray must impose handicaps that may interfere with the accuracy of interpretation even in the most expert hands. The Sengstaken-Blakemore tube as a therapeutic test is not always reliable since a bleeding gastric varix may be distal to the gastric balloon. Besides, there are risks in using pneumatic tamponade, and these should be avoided when the balloon can do no good. Extensive experience has indicated that splenic pulp manometry can be employed with minimal risk and that pressures obtained by this method correlate very closely with portal pressures secured at operation. When a splenic pulp pressure of less than 250 mm H_2O is obtained, one can be assured that varices are not present and that bleeding is due to some other lesion. When the pressure is 290 or above, it is practically certain that varices are present and the probable cause of the hemorrhage. Values between 250 and 290 are indeterminate but still valuable. If the hemorrhage is caused by varices, the chances are good that tamponade will be effective. If active and persistent bleeding continues with the pulp pressure in the indeterminate range, it is then highly probable that the bleeding is caused by some other lesion than varices. Moreover, when it is important to resolve the doubt, portography will be decisive.

There is no unanimity regarding the criteria that determine when surgical intervention should be employed for bleeding not due to an esophageal lesion or a blood dyscrasia. Hematemesis should first be managed as a medical problem, and in any case, the patient should not be subjected to operation until he represents a good operative risk, which means restoration of the blood volume to near-normal levels. A full discussion of this matter should be consulted in Chaps. 271 and 279.

REFERENCES

Brick, I. B., and H. J. Jeghers: Gastrointestinal Hemorrhage (Excluding Peptic Ulcer and Esophageal Varices), New Engl. J. Med., 253:458, 511, 555, 1955.

Conn, H. O.: Hazards Attending the Use of Esophageal Tamponade, New Engl. J. Med., 259:701, 1958.

Jones, F. A., A. E. Read, and J. L. Stubbe: Alimentary Bleeding of Obscure Origin. A Follow-up Study and Commentary, Brit. Med. J., 1:1138, 1959.

Mackay, A. G., and H. G. Page: Hematemesis Associated with Hemobilia, New Engl. J. Med., 260:468, 1959.

Panke, W. F., L. M. Rousselot, and A. H. Moreno: Splenic Pulp Manometry in Differential Diagnosis, Surg., Gynecol. Obstet., 109:270, 1959.

19 JAUNDICE AND OTHER MANIFESTATIONS OF LIVER DISEASE (Including Tests and Diagnostic Features)

Gerald Klatskin

JAUNDICE

Normally the bilirubin derived from the breakdown of hemoglobin in the reticuloendothelial system is discharged into the blood and excreted by the liver. When the rate of excretion fails to match that of pigment production, bilirubin accumulates in the serum and ultimately stains the tissues, giving rise to the characteristic yellow pigmentation known as *jaundice* or *icterus.*

Although any tissue may become bile stained, those rich in elastic fibers have a special affinity for bilirubin, which accounts for the earlier appearance and greater intensity of the jaundice in the scleras and the skin of the face and upper trunk. It should be noted that jaundice is the consequence of bilirubin deposition in the tissue fibers and cells; it is not due to mere reflection of yellow light through the skin from the underlying interstitial fluid and plasma. For reasons not entirely clear, the tissues stain more readily with the direct- than with the indirect-reacting type of pigment (see below) and fail to stain in areas of edema and vitiligo.

Normal concentrations of serum bilirubin range from 0.5 to 1.2 mg per 100 ml. The precise level at which icterus becomes clinically evident varies; it depends, in part at least, on the type of bilirubin present in the serum and on the skill of the examiner. Usually when a high proportion of the pigment is of the direct-reacting type, as in obstructive and hepatocellular jaundice, icterus is detectable at levels of 2 to 3 mg per 100 ml, while in hemolytic states accompanied by predominantly indirect-reacting serum bilirubin, the concentration may rise to 3 or 4 mg per 100 ml before overt jaundice appears. Elevations of serum bilirubin unaccompanied by clinically detectable icterus are classified as *latent* or *subclinical jaundice.*

Early in the course of jaundice virtually all the pigment found in the serum is bilirubin. Later, however, small amounts of other unidentified pigments appear. Presumably these are bilirubin derivatives that arise in the bile-stained tissues, but their composition and origin are still uncertain. Not infrequently in deep jaundice the skin and scleras take on a greenish hue because of the presence of biliverdin, an oxidation product of bilirubin which may be detectable in the serum also.

Pigment Metabolism

Degradation of Hemoglobin to Bilirubin. When a circulating erythrocyte reaches the end of its normal life span of approximately 120 days, it is taken up by the reticuloendothelial system and destroyed, the end products being bilirubin, iron, and globin. The bilirubin is discharged into the plasma, ultimately to be excreted by the liver. In contrast, the

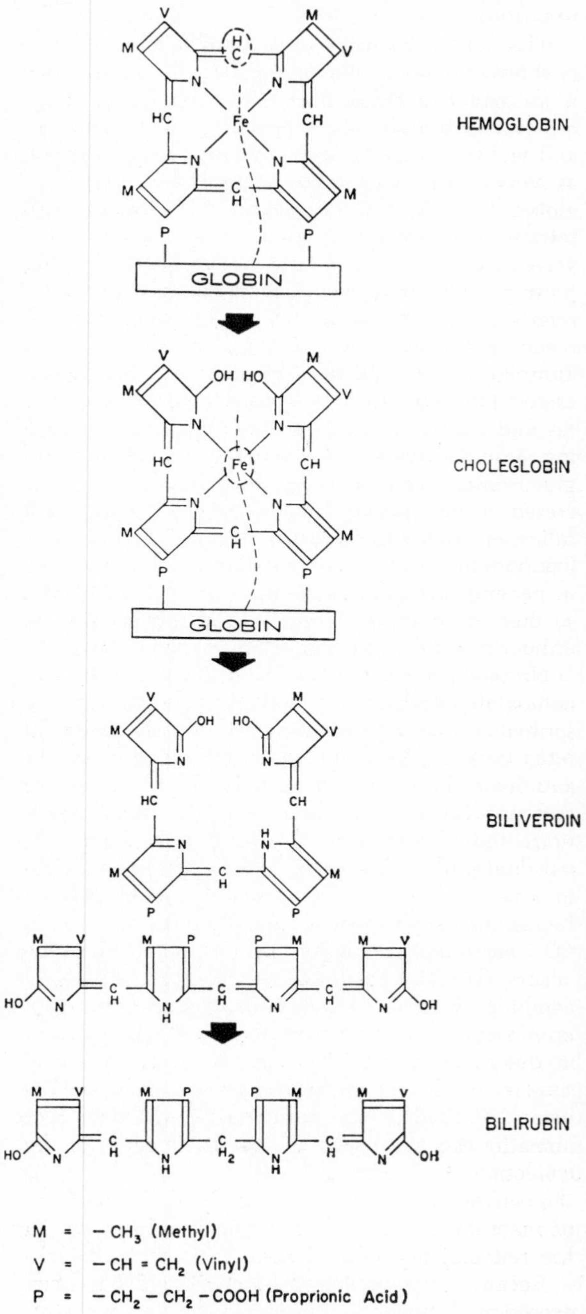

M = — CH₃ (Methyl)

V = — CH = CH₂ (Vinyl)

P = — CH₂ — CH₂ — COOH (Proprionic Acid)

FIG. 19-1. Degradation of hemoglobin to bilirubin.

iron is conserved for further use. Some is stored locally in the form of hemosiderin, a ferric hydroxide polymer, while the remainder is returned to the plasma where it is carried by a β_1-globulin, siderophilin, to other depots to be stored either as hemosiderin or as ferritin, a ferrous iron-protein complex. The fate of the globin is unknown, but recent studies do not support the widely held theory that it leaves the reticuloendothelium bound to bilirubin.

The normal pathway of hemoglobin degradation is shown schematically in Fig. 19-1. The first step is an oxidative removal of the carbon atom in the α-methene bridge, which opens the porphyrin ring and yields a green protein-pigment complex known as *choleglobin*. Subsequent removal of the iron and globin leads to the formation of a straight-chain tetrapyrrole, biliverdin, which on reduction is converted to bilirubin. The latter is discharged into the plasma where it combines with albumin to form a relatively stable protein-pigment complex. On reaching the liver the bilirubin is separated from albumin, conjugated with glucuronic acid, and excreted into the bile in the form of its protein-free di- and monoglucuronides, the former predominating. In obstructive and hepatocellular jaundice the glucuronides gain access to the blood and are excreted in the urine. As in the case of the free bilirubin discharged into the blood from the reticuloendothelium, they too combine with albumin, but in passing through the kidney the complex is split, so that the pigment is excreted in the urine in an unbound state, as in bile.

Normally most of the bilirubin derived from hemoglobin appears to follow the pathway described, the principal sites of formation being the reticuloendothelium of the bone marrow, spleen, and liver. However, under pathologic conditions, and possibly to some extent under normal conditions, bilirubin may be derived from hematin, the trivalent iron hydroxide of protoporphyrin IX. Thus, in severe hemolytic states, such as erythroblastosis fetalis, blackwater fever, and *Clostridium welchii* (*C. perfringens*) sepsis, *intravascular* hemolysis occurs, with the release of free hematin. The latter combines with serum albumin to form methemalbumin and then is converted to bilirubin, probably in the reticuloendothelial system by a mechanism similar to that involved in the degradation of heme. Similarly, the formation of bilirubin from hematin can be demonstrated in hematomas and collections of blood in the serosal cavities. Here, too, the conversion appears to occur under the influence of macrophages and endothelial cells belonging to the reticuloendothelial system.

Recent evidence, based on studies of stercobilin excretion following the administration of N[15]-labeled glycine, indicates that normally at least 10 per cent, and in diseases like pernicious anemia and congenital porphyria as much as 30 to 40 per cent, of the bile pigment produced is not derived from the degradation of hemoglobin in senescent erythrocytes. The source of this fraction of bilirubin has not been established, but the available evidence suggests that it probably arises in the bone marrow from heme or porphyrins produced in excess and not utilized in hemoglobin synthesis.

Bilirubin Conjugation and the van den Bergh Reaction. Since bilirubin is relatively insoluble at the pH of the body fluids, it must be solubilized for transport and excretion. Its linkage with serum albumin serves this purpose in the circulation, but in the liver the pigment-protein complex is split so that bilirubin must be conjugated with glucuronic acid before it can be excreted. This involves an active enzymatic process in which glucuronic acid is transferred from uridine diphosphoglucuronic acid to the carboxyl groups of bilirubin through the agency of glucuronyl transferase, an enzyme associated with the microsomes of the hepatic parenchymal cells. The freely soluble end products, bilirubin monoglucuronide (pigment I) and bilirubin diglucuronide (pigment II), are excreted in the bile, the latter predominating. Small amounts of other water-soluble bilirubin conjugates, and especially sulfate, are demonstrable in bile. These too are products of enzymatic action, although the reactions involved have not been worked out. There is suggestive evidence that under certain conditions a small fraction of bilirubin may undergo conjugation in the kidney to form pigment I.

One of the characteristic properties of bilirubin is its capacity to couple with diazotized sulfanilic acid to yield red azo compounds. This involves splitting of the bilirubin molecule, with the production of two molecules of azopigment A. Bilirubin diglucuronide behaves very similarly but gives rise to two molecules of azopigment B. The latter is identical with azopigment A except for the presence of a glucuronic acid side chain. The monoglucuronide yields one molecule each of azopigments A and B. The two azopigments are indistinguishable spectrophotometrically, but can be separated chromatographically.

Because of its relative insolubility at the low pH of the diazo reaction mixture, unconjugated bilirubin requires the addition of alcohol for solubilization before coupling. In contrast, its conjugates which are freely soluble can react in the absence of alcohol. These are known as the indirect and direct van den Bergh reactions, respectively.

By measuring the amount of pigment that diazotizes in the absence of alcohol (i.e., in the direct reaction), it is possible to estimate the approximate concentration of conjugated bilirubin in body fluids. Since free bilirubin can couple at a very slow rate in the absence of alcohol, while its conjugates react rapidly, it is customary to measure the direct-reacting pigment at the end of 1 min. This may underestimate the actual concentration of conjugated bilirubin, since there is some evidence to indicate that under favorable conditions it requires approximately 10 min for complete coupling.

The total bilirubin concentration is determined by carrying out the van den Bergh reaction in the presence of alcohol. On subtracting the amount of bilirubin found in the direct reaction, one obtains an estimate of the indirect-reacting or unconjugated fraction.

Normally the plasma contains up to 0.2 mg of direct-reacting bilirubin per 100 ml. Since it is not possible to identify such low concentrations of pigment chromatographically, it is still uncertain whether this fraction consists of conjugated bilirubin that has regurgitated into the circulation from the hepatic cells or the bile or represents the fraction of unconjugated bilirubin that is capable of diazotizing in the absence of alcohol. The fact that unconjugated bilirubin raises the concentration of direct-reacting pigment in serum to a higher level when it is infused in vivo than when it is added to serum in vitro favors the view that some degree of regurgitation occurs normally and that this may be enhanced when the excretion of conjugated bilirubin is accelerated. This probably accounts for the small but significant rise in direct-reacting serum bilirubin that often occurs in the course of hemolytic jaundice.

Fate of Bilirubin. On entering the intestinal tract bilirubin, as a consequence of bacterial action, undergoes a series of reductive reactions leading to the formation of two groups of compounds: (1) the colorless urobilinogens which characteristically react with Ehrlich's reagent to yield red aldehyde complexes and (2) their colored oxidation products, the urobilins, which on mixing with Schlesinger's solution (zinc acetate in alcohol) yield zinc complexes with an intense green fluorescence. Since all these compounds have the same physiologic significance and are measured together in quantitative analyses (following preliminary reduction of the urobilins), it is customary to consider them collectively as "urobilinogen," irrespective of their chemical structure or whether they are found in the urine, feces, or bile.

As shown in Fig. 19-2, bilirubin is reduced successively to mesobilirubin, dihydromesobilirubin, and finally to the two colorless urobilinogens, mesobilirubinogen and stercobilinogen. To a variable degree these are then oxidized to their respective urobilins, *i*-urobilin that is optically inactive and *l*-stercobilin that is levorotatory.

When the intestinal flora are suppressed by broad-spectrum antibiotics, unchanged bilirubin

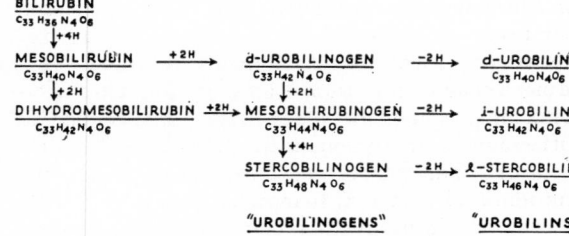

FIG. 19-2. Conversion of bilirubin to urobilinogen.

may be excreted in the feces. On reappearance of the organisms, *d*-urobilin, a strongly dextrotatory compound derived from *d*-urobilinogen, is excreted instead of *i*- or *l*-urobilinogen. Since *d*-urobilinogen is commonly found in the cecal contents of normal subjects, it may be a normal product that usually undergoes further reduction before appearing in the feces.

Normally a fraction of the urobilinogen formed in the intestine is reabsorbed and returned via the portal vein to the liver where it is reexcreted into the bile (the enterohepatic circulation). Under normal conditions a small amount escapes into the general circulation and is excreted by the kidneys in amounts not exceeding 4 mg per day. However, if the liver is diseased, or if the bilirubin output is greatly increased, as in hemolytic jaundice, so that the liver is no longer able to clear the blood of reabsorbed urobilinogen, the urinary excretion of urobilinogen increases.

The normal output of fecal urobilinogen ranges from 40 to 280 mg daily. If the excretion of bilirubin is decreased because of biliary obstruction or hepatocellular injury, or if the conversion of bilirubin to urobilinogen is interrupted by the administration of antibiotics that suppress the intestinal flora, fecal urobilinogen decreases.

In a normal individual with a blood volume of 5 liters and a hemoglobin concentration of 15 Gm per 100 ml, the total circulating hemoglobin is 750 Gm. Since approximately $\frac{1}{120}$ of the red cells are destroyed daily, 6.3 Gm of hemoglobin is released for degradation. Assuming quantitative conversion of heme to bilirubin and thence to urobilinogen, the expected daily output of urobilinogen would be approximately 250 mg plus an additional 15 to 30 mg derived from sources other than the hemoglobin of circulating erythrocytes. Often, however, the amount excreted is considerably less. The possibility that urobilinogen is further degraded to dipyrrolmethenes, such as mesobilifuscin, or is reabsorbed and reutilized in porphyrin synthesis appears unlikely in the light of recent studies with isotopically labeled pigments. The hypothesis that there is an alternative pathway for the degradation of hemoglobin that does not involve the formation of bilirubin is an attractive one, but as yet has not been established.

Urinary Excretion of Bilirubin. Normally the urine contains no bilirubin, although traces may be detectable by sensitive spectrophotometric methods. Often appreciable amounts are excreted in the presence of hepatocellular or obstructive jaundice, but bilirubinuria is rare in hemolytic jaundice unless it is complicated by liver damage.

Based on the observation that most of the bilirubin found in the urine is in the form of its glucuronides and on the assumption that, because such conjugates are more soluble than free bilirubin, they are more readily excreted, it is generally believed that the renal excretion of bilirubin is determined by the level of conjugated pigment in the plasma. However, the fact that the amount excreted is not closely correlated with the concentration of direct-reacting pigment in the serum suggests that other factors may be involved. Thus, at the onset of viral hepatitis, bilirubin often appears in the urine at minimally elevated serum levels of conjugated bilirubin, while during convalescence it may fail to do so at levels several times higher. Similarly, bilirubinuria is rare in hemolytic jaundice even when the concentration of direct-reacting serum bilirubin is significantly increased. One factor that may, in part at least, account for such discrepancies is that the renal clearance of the diglucuronide of bilirubin is greater than that of its monoglucuronide.

Since both bilirubin and its conjugates are firmly bound to albumin in the plasma, the excretion of pigment in the kidney cannot be a matter of simple glomerular filtration of a diffusible fraction. Although not conclusive, clearance studies point to the tubules as the probable site of excretion. Since almost all the pigment that appears in the urine is in the form of protein-free glucuronides, it must be assumed that the albumin is split off in the kidney and that the protein complex of conjugated bilirubin is more readily dissociated than that of free bilirubin.

PATHOGENESIS OF JAUNDICE

As previously noted, when bilirubin enters the circulation more rapidly than it is removed, it accumulates in the plasma and tissues, ultimately staining the latter to produce jaundice. Although this may occur under a wide variety of circumstances, only three basic mechanisms, either singly or in combination, are ever involved: (1) increased production of bilirubin, (2) impairment of the liver's capacity to take up, conjugate, or excrete bilirubin, and (3) regurgitation of bilirubin into the plasma from the bile or from the hepatic cells. As will be evident from the discussion to follow, multiple factors are implicated in most types of jaun-

dice, so that for clinical purposes it is customary to classify jaundice on the basis of pathogenesis rather than on the basis of the fundamental disturbances in pigment metabolism involved. Thus, most forms of jaundice are classified as being of obstructive, hepatocellular, or hemolytic origin. However, some cannot be categorized in this way and must be considered separately.

It is helpful diagnostically to subdivide the various forms of jaundice into those accompanied by predominantly conjugated, or direct-reacting, bilirubin in the serum and those with predominantly unconjugated, or indirect-reacting, bilirubin in the serum. At one time the terms "regurgitation" and "retention" jaundice, respectively, were applied to these two groups. However, these terms are objectionable in that they are too restrictive and imply that a single defect is involved in each group.

JAUNDICE WITH PREDOMINANTLY CONJUGATED BILIRUBIN IN THE SERUM

Obstructive Jaundice. The term *obstructive jaundice* should be limited to forms of jaundice in which an obstruction of the bile ducts can be demonstrated anatomically. Use of the term *intrahepatic obstructive jaundice* to describe atypical variants of hepatocellular jaundice in which an obstructive or regurgitative element is postulated solely on the basis of biochemical evidence is both inaccurate and misleading. These are more appropriately classified as forms of *cholestatic jaundice* (see below).

Complete obstruction of the *extrahepatic* bile ducts leads to an increase in serum bilirubin, particularly of the direct-reacting type, the appearance of bile in the urine, and the passage of clay-colored stools. As might be expected, the failure of bile to reach the intestine results in the virtual disappearance of urobilinogen from the urine and feces, except for traces derived from bilirubin that gains access to the intestinal lumen from the bile-stained mucosa. The concentration of bilirubin in the serum rises progressively and then stabilizes at a level that rarely exceeds 50 mg per 100 ml. Since the rate of hemoglobin breakdown is not diminished and the losses of bilirubin in the urine are negligible, it must be assumed that when a plateau is reached the daily increment of bilirubin is either diverted to the tissues or degraded to other compounds.

Partial obstruction of the extrahepatic bile ducts may also give rise to jaundice, but only if the intrabiliary pressure is greatly increased, since the excretion of bilirubin does not diminish until the intraductile pressure approaches the maximum secretory pressure of approximately 250 mm of bile. Jaundice may occur at very much lower pressures if the obstruction is complicated by infection of the ducts or hepatocellular injury. Bilirubinuria and clay-colored stools are inconstant findings in incomplete biliary obstruction, and the amount of urobilinogen varies with the degree of occlusion.

The functional reserve of the liver is so great that occlusion of the *intrahepatic* bile ducts does not give rise to jaundice unless the drainage of bile from a large segment of the parenchyma is interrupted. Thus, either of the two major hepatic ducts or a large number of secondary radicles may be occluded without producing jaundice. In experimental animals the ducts draining at least 75 per cent of the parenchyma must be occluded before jaundice appears.

Following occlusion of the bile ducts, conjugated bilirubin regurgitates into the circulation. The precise pathway involved is uncertain, but it has been suggested that bile escapes into the hepatic sinusoids or lymph spaces (1) from distended canaliculi that rupture, (2) through rents or functional leaks in the canals of Hering that connect the canaliculi with the terminal bile ducts, or (3) directly through the parenchymal cells from the canaliculi. As might be expected, the serum contains conjugated bilirubin predominantly, as in the bile. Early in the course of biliary obstruction the concentration of the diglucuronide (pigment II) may be higher than that of the monoglucuronide (pigment I), but later the reverse obtains. Invariably the serum contains abnormal amounts of unconjugated bilirubin also, which undoubtedly indicates impairment of hepatocellular function. On the basis of experimental studies it would appear that a defect in uptake and transport of bilirubin across the hepatic cells is involved. Although pigment I is found in bile, its concentration is lower than that of pigment II, so that its predominance in the serum late in obstructive jaundice cannot be due to regurgitation alone. It is generally believed that the accumulation of pigment I in the serum reflects a failure of the hepatic parenchymal cells to convert pigment I to pigment II. However, the alternative possibility that the excess of pigment I is due to conjugation of free bilirubin in extrahepatic sites, such as the kidney, or is only relative, as a consequence of the greater losses of pigment II in the urine, cannot be excluded.

Hepatocellular Jaundice. Theoretically it might be anticipated that the uptake, transport, and conjugation of bilirubin by the liver cells would be the dominant factors involved in hepatocellular jaundice and that retention of unconjugated bilirubin in the serum would result. Usually, however, the disturbance in pigment metabolism is almost identical with that of obstructive jaundice. Thus, the serum contains an excess not only of unconjugated bilirubin but also of both its glucuronides, pigments I and II, bilirubin is excreted in the urine, and fecal urobilinogen is reduced. In contrast to what happens in obstructive jaundice, urine urobilinogen may be increased, since the parenchyma no longer is capable of clearing the serum of urobilinogen entering from the intestinal tract. However, the excretion of bile may be suppressed to such an extent that virtually no bilirubin reaches the intestine. Under these conditions the stools are clay-colored, production and reabsorption of urobilinogen in the intestine are diminished, and the urine urobilinogen falls to a low level or disappears. Hepatocellular jaundice can seldom be differentiated from obstructive jaundice solely on the basis of changes in pigment metabolism, and, indeed, there are instances in which the two are indistinguishable on the basis of any biochemical criteria.

The retention of unconjugated bilirubin in the serum probably reflects the combined effects of impaired uptake, transport, and conjugation of bilirubin by injured hepatic cells. Since the serum invariably contains conjugated bilirubin, it must be assumed that some pigment regurgitates from either the bile or the hepatic cells. Several possible mechanisms have been postulated to account for this phenomenon: (1) rupture of the canaliculi as a consequence of necrosis of the hepatic cells that constitute their walls; (2) occlusion of the canaliculi by inspissated bile or their compression by edema in the surrounding parenchymal cells; (3) obstruction of the terminal intrahepatic bile ducts, the cholangioles, by inflammatory cells; (4) an increase in the permeability of the cholangioles; and (5) altered permeability of the parenchymal cells, permitting reflux of bile from the canaliculi. While the escape of bile through rents in the walls of canaliculi in areas of necrosis can be seen occasionally in histologic sections, and reflux of bile from the canaliculi into the sinusoids through injured but apparently viable cells has been demonstrated by fluorescent microscopy of the liver in rats injected with fluorescent dyes, the other mechanisms postulated to account for the regurgitation of bile in hepatocellular jaundice are purely speculative and open to question.

Since severe hepatocellular injury leads to a reduction in glucuronyl transferase activity, the question arises why high levels of conjugated bilirubin are found in the serum. Several explanations are possible: (1) injury to the hepatic cells impairs their capacity to excrete to a greater extent than their ability to conjugate bilirubin, so that the conjugate accumulates in the cells and ultimately diffuses out into the plasma; (2) even in severe hepatocellular injury some cells are spared and are capable of conjugating sufficient bilirubin to account for the amount found in the circulation; and (3) since glucuronyl transferase activity is demonstrable in the serum under conditions of severe hepatocellular necrosis, conjugation of bilirubin may occur outside the liver cells, in the hepatic lymph, the general circulation, or other tissues.

Cholestatic Jaundice. There is a form of jaundice of varied etiology in which the biochemical findings in the blood and many of the clinical features suggest obstruction of the bile ducts, but in which no anatomic defect in either the parenchymal cells or biliary tree can be demonstrated. It occurs (1) most commonly in *drug reactions* to such agents as chlorpromazine and methyl testosterone, (2) occasionally in *viral hepatitis,* (3) as a rare complication of *pregnancy,* (4) in the *Dubin-Johnson syndrome,* and (5) in the *Rotor syndrome.*

Characteristic of the group is the predominance in the serum of conjugated bilirubin. As in obstructive and hepatocellular jaundice, the serum contains bilirubin, pigment I, and pigment II, with a preponderance of pigment I. There is no defect in bilirubin conjugation. To account for this pattern it has been postulated that the basic defect involves the regurgitation of bile as a consequence of (1) increased permeability of the cholangioles, (2) compression of these ducts by inflammatory cells, or (3) obstruction of the canaliculi by thrombi of inspissated bile. This has led to use of such terms as "cholangiolitic" or "intrahepatic obstructive" jaundice. These appear to be inappropriate, since what evidence is available favors the view that the defect is in the hepatic cells, rather than in the cholangioles or canaliculi, and involves a functional disturbance in the transport mechanism and possibly the permeability of the cells.

JAUNDICE WITH PREDOMINANTLY UNCONJUGATED BILIRUBIN IN THE SERUM

Hemolytic Jaundice. The amount of bilirubin produced depends primarily upon the rate of red cell destruction. Normally the intact liver is capable of excreting all but a small fraction of this pigment, so that the concentration of bilirubin in the serum is maintained at a relatively constant low level. However, if bilirubin production is greatly increased as a consequence of abnormally rapid hemolysis, it may exceed the excretory capacity of the liver and give rise to hyperbilirubinemia and jaundice. It should be noted that the amount of bilirubin excreted by the normal liver is a function of the square of its concentration in the serum, so that as the rate of hemolysis is accelerated and the concentration of pigment in the serum rises the amount excreted by the liver increases. In addition, there is a limit to the amount of bilirubin that can be formed in the reticuloendothelium, approximately 1.5 Gm per day, irrespective of the amount of hemoglobin released for degradation. Because of

these two limitations, it takes a considerable degree of hemolysis to raise the serum bilirubin to abnormal levels, and even maximal hemolysis will rarely raise it above 3 to 5 mg per 100 ml unless it is complicated by some degree of hepatocellular dysfunction.

Unconjugated bilirubin is the principal pigment found in the serum of patients with hemolytic jaundice. Small amounts of direct-reacting pigment also are detectable, usually constituting less than 15 per cent of the total serum pigment. Although the presence of conjugated bilirubin has been confirmed chromatographically, its identity as a glucuronide has not been established. The significance of this fraction is still in doubt. According to some authorities it represents bilirubin that has been conjugated to pigment I in the kidney. Others regard it as a fraction of conjugated bilirubin that regurgitates from the bile when the amount of pigment excreted is increased by hemolysis.

In newborn infants with severe hemolysis and erythroblastosis due to isoimmunization, the concentration of direct-reacting bilirubin in the serum occasionally rises to the high levels seen in obstructive jaundice. This has been termed the "inspissated-bile syndrome" by those who attribute this type of jaundice to occlusion of the bile ducts by inspissated bile. However, the direct-reacting bilirubin under these conditions is in the form of pigment I exclusively, a finding that is more consistent with hepatocellular than obstructive jaundice. This interpretation is supported by postmortem evidence of hepatic necrosis in such cases.

The absence of bile in the urine is such a striking feature that hemolytic jaundice is known also as *acholuric jaundice.* As might be expected, the increase in pigment production gives rise to high levels of urobilinogen in the urine and feces. Other tests of hepatocellular function show no abnormalities, except when severe anemia or other complicating factors are present.

Neonatal Jaundice. With few exceptions, newborn infants develop a transient hyperbilirubinemia within the first few days of life. All but a small fraction of the serum bilirubin is unconjugated. This accumulation of pigment is due primarily to a relative deficiency of glucuronyl transferase activity in the liver which limits the excretion of bilirubin. In addition, the newborn infant may be further handicapped by a deficiency of uridine diphosphoglucose dehydrogenase, the enzyme required for the synthesis of uridine diphosphoglucuronic acid, the glucuronide donor essential for the conjugation of bilirubin. As the liver matures the activity of these two enzymes increases, ultimately attaining adult levels in a few weeks, which coincides with the return of the serum bilirubin level to normal.

The defect in bilirubin conjugation tends to be more severe in the premature infant, often resulting in inordinately high levels of serum bilirubin. Occasionally this gives rise to kernicterus, a serious neurologic disorder due to deposition of unconjugated bilirubin in the brain.

Congenital Familial Nonhemolytic Jaundice. Crigler and Najjar have described a rare form of hereditary jaundice in the newborn characterized by high levels of unconjugated bilirubin in the serum, the common occurrence of kernicterus, and a high mortality rate within the first year of life. Survivors remain deeply jaundiced throughout their lives. The basic defect involved is a genetically determined deficiency of glucuronyl transferase activity in the liver. Affected individuals are homozygous while both their parents are heterozygous for the mutant gene. Although the parents excrete bilirubin normally, they usually fail to conjugate other substances with glucuronic acid as effectively as normal individuals.

Nonhemolytic "Overproduction" Jaundice. Hyperbilirubinemia of the indirect-reacting type and increased fecal urobilinogen excretion are common findings in pernicious anemia. Since the life span of the red cell is reduced in this disorder, it is generally agreed that increased hemolysis is one of the factors involved in the retention of bilirubin. However, at least 40 per cent of the bile pigment excreted by affected individuals is derived from sources other than the hemoglobin of circulating erythrocytes. Accordingly it is quite possible that overproduction of bilirubin unrelated to hemolysis may contribute to the development of jaundice in pernicious anemia.

There is some evidence to indicate that the same mechanism may be responsible for the retention of unconjugated bilirubin in the serum and the increased urobilinogen excretion seen in the form of familial jaundice described by Israels and his associates and in the indirect-reacting type of hyperbilirubinemia that occasionally follows an attack of viral hepatitis.

Gilbert's Syndrome. There is a form of mild chronic jaundice seen in young individuals that is characterized by the presence in the serum of increased amounts of unconjugated bilirubin in the absence of overt hemolysis or hepatocellular disease. The disorder is ill-defined and includes a number of distinct etiologic entities, both hereditary and acquired, in which the basic mechanisms involved appear to differ. The latter include (1) a defect in the transport of bilirubin from the plasma to the site within the hepatic cells where it is conjugated, (2) a deficiency of glucuronyl transferase activity in the liver, and (3) nonhemolytic "overproduction" of bilirubin. A more detailed discussion of this group of disorders is given on p. 1699.

CLINICAL MANIFESTATIONS OF LIVER DISEASE

The functional reserve and regenerative capacity of the liver are so great that many lesions fail to produce overt signs of disease. This is particularly true of focal parenchymal lesions, localized obstructions of the intrahepatic blood vessels and ducts, and patchy fibrosis. However, diffuse hepatocellular injury, even when relatively minor in degree, usually results in significant impairment of function.

A number of ill-defined terms are used to describe the functional status of the diseased liver. In their broader sense the terms *hepatic decompensation* and *hepatocellular failure* imply any functional disturbance giving rise to symptoms. However, they are used more commonly to indicate a relatively severe degree of hepatocellular dysfunction, usually manifested by jaundice, ascites, edema, or coma. Liver disease is said to be *latent* when it is asymptomatic and unaccompanied by significant impairment of function.

Manifestations Referable to Extrahepatic Factors. Not all the symptoms in hepatic disease can be attributed to functional or structural changes in the liver. In many instances they are related to the extrahepatic effects of the underlying etiologic factor. As examples may be cited the diabetes in hemochromatosis and the malnutrition in Laennec's cirrhosis. Unfortunately, as in the case of the constitutional symptoms that often accompany liver disease, it is not always possible to distinguish between hepatic and extrahepatic manifestations.

Constitutional Symptoms. *Lassitude, weakness,* and *unusual fatigability* are seen in both acute and chronic liver disease. Their pathogenesis is not understood, although malnutrition, infection, and psychogenic factors may play a role in some instances.

Many patients with chronic liver disease exhibit a *low-grade fever.* Usually this is attributed to hepatic necrosis and inflammation, but on the basis of histologic studies the correlation does not appear to be very close. Spiking fever and chills, while rare in hepatocellular disease, occur with regularity in suppurative cholangitis, abscess, and pylephlebitis and undoubtedly are due to infection, often complicated by bacteremia.

Anorexia and *weight loss* are frequent in all forms of hepatic decompensation and are particularly striking in acute viral hepatitis. Fever, nausea, alcoholism, and ascites may be contributory factors but cannot be held accountable in all instances.

Abdominal Complaints. *Pain* in the region of the

liver is a common complaint in many types of hepatic disease and appears to be related to distention of Glisson's capsule and perihepatitis. Usually it is of a dull aching quality, but occasionally, for reasons that are not clear, may be colicky or lancinating in character.

Flatulence, nausea, and *vomiting* are relatively common. Gastroscopic studies suggest that they may be due to gastritis in viral hepatitis, but their pathogenesis in other forms of liver disease is obscure.

Changes in the Liver. *Hepatomegaly* is a frequent but not invariable finding in liver disease of all types. It may be due to (1) congestion, (2) infiltration with fat, glycogen, tumor, or amyloid, (3) inflammatory exudate, (4) regenerative activity, or (5) increase in water content. The largest livers are seen in malignant infiltration, biliary cirrhosis, and amyloidosis. A really *small liver* usually is indicative of cirrhosis, especially of the postnecrotic variety. *Tenderness* occurs in inflammatory disease and in conditions leading to rapid enlargement of the liver, and probably relates to distention and inflammation of Glisson's capsule. Often *induration* is indicative of cirrhosis or infiltrative disease, but occasionally it is the result of inflammation or congestion. *Palpable masses* in the liver may be due to tumor, the regenerating nodules of postnecrotic cirrhosis, cysts, or abscess. Only rarely can the fine nodules of other forms of cirrhosis be felt. A vascular *bruit* over the liver may be indicative of hemangioma or other types of intrahepatic tumor, but more often it is attributable to an extensive venous collateral circulation (Cruveilhier-Baumgarten syndrome). Occasionally a *friction rub* may be heard over the liver. Usually it is a sign of intrahepatic malignancy, but rarely it may be due to gonococcal perihepatitis or to the type of chronic peritonitis that follows repeated paracentesis. Frank *expansile pulsation* of the liver, which may be difficult to differentiate from a transmitted pulse from the aorta, is pathognomonic of tricuspid insufficiency.

In the presence of jaundice a *palpable gallbladder* usually indicates malignant obstruction of the extrahepatic bile ducts or carcinoma of the gallbladder itself. Only rarely is it found in patients with common duct stone, since the gallbladder usually is fibrotic and contracted because of associated chronic cholecystitis (Courvoisier's law). In the absence of jaundice, a palpable gallbladder usually signifies hydrops or carcinoma, but occasionally it is due to the presence of a large number of stones.

Jaundice. Since erythrocyte destruction, and hence bilirubin production, is a continuous process, any significant decrease in bilirubin excretion, whether due to hepatocellular injury or obstruction to the outflow of bile, will result in jaundice. It is noteworthy, however, that the functional capacity of the liver is so great that it may continue to clear the serum of bilirubin despite appreciable parenchymal damage or occlusion of numerous intrahepatic ducts. Also, the liver is capable of sustaining bile flow in the face of a significantly elevated intraductal pressure, so that partial obstruction of the common bile duct does not necessarily give rise to jaundice.

The differentiation between obstructive and hepatocellular jaundice depends more on collateral clinical and laboratory evidence than on any distinctive features of the jaundice per se. In both types the *urine* may be *dark* because of the presence of bilirubin, and if the suppression of bilirubin excretion is sufficiently great, the *stools* may become *clay-colored*. *Pruritus* is a frequent complaint in extrahepatic biliary obstruction and biliary cirrhosis, but it occurs also in viral and some forms of drug-induced hepatitis. Retention of bile salts is usually given as the reason for the pruritus, but the evidence for this is equivocal.

Not infrequently in chronic jaundice the skin shows a generalized increase in *melanin pigmentation,* and occasionally it has a greenish tinge owing to the presence of *biliverdin*. The latter is seen most commonly in malignant biliary obstruction but may occur in any form of prolonged deep jaundice. In biliary cirrhosis the jaundice may be accompanied by *xanthomatosis* of the skin. This is clearly due to intense and prolonged hypercholesteremia and is unrelated to the hyperbilirubinemia.

The course of the jaundice may be of diagnostic and prognostic significance. An abrupt onset and a rapid increase in intensity are more common in acute hepatocellular disease than in extrahepatic biliary obstruction. Characteristically in uncomplicated viral hepatitis the serum bilirubin level rises rapidly, reaching a peak in 1 to 2 weeks, and then falls progressively at a variable but somewhat slower rate. There is no plateau at the peak, and fluctuations are unusual, except during convalescence. In contrast, the jaundice of nonmalignant biliary obstruction deepens more slowly and tends to fluctuate, even if a plateau is reached, indicating that usually the obstruction is incomplete and subject to variation. In malignant obstruction the icterus often increases at a steady rate and then stabilizes when obstruction becomes complete. However, fluctuations, and even complete but temporary remission, may occur, particularly in carcinoma of the ampulla of Vater. The course of the jaundice in chronic hepatocellular disease, such as cirrhosis, varies considerably and may resemble that of either acute hepatitis or biliary obstruction.

Usually in acute hepatitis the depth of the jaundice is closely correlated with the extent of the hepatocellular injury, but there are notable exceptions. Similarly, in biliary obstruction the jaundice tends to vary with the completeness and duration of the obstruction, but marked discrepancies are not rare, particularly where the obstruction is complicated by biliary infection or hepatocellular injury. The occurrence of jaundice in cirrhosis usually indicates progressive hepatocellular failure.

Ascites and Edema. Abnormal fluid retention can be demonstrated in most forms of parenchymatous liver disease, and indeed, the ability to excrete a water load has been used as a test of hepatic function. However, the degree of retention is seldom sufficient to produce ascites and edema, except in the case of cirrhosis, hepatic vein obstruction (Chiari's syndrome), certain infiltrative diseases, and massive hepatic necrosis.

A number of interrelated factors are involved in the formation of ascites. These include (1) portal hypertension, (2) reduced plasma colloidal osmotic pressure, (3) increased hepatic lymph flow, and (4) retention of sodium and water secondary to alterations in renal and endocrine function.

Portal hypertension alone seldom gives rise to ascites, but in combination with a reduced plasma colloidal osmotic pressure it appears to be an important factor. Thus, while simple ligation of the portal vein has no effect, simultaneous lowering of the serum albumin level by means of plasmapheresis results in ascites formation. Also, reducing portal pressure by means of a portacaval shunt not infrequently leads to subsidence of the ascites in cirrhotic patients, despite the persistence of hypoalbuminemia.

In contrast to portal block, obstruction to the outflow of the hepatic veins almost invariably leads to ascites, even in the absence of hypoproteinemia. Experimental studies suggest that this is the consequence of a greatly increased hepatic lymph flow with leakage of lymph from the superficial lymphatic vessels of the liver capsule. However, since the protein content of the ascitic fluid under such circumstances is lower than that of hepatic lymph, it must be assumed that simple transudation of fluid from the peritoneal serosa also plays a role. Recent anatomic studies suggest that the occurrence of ascites in cirrhosis may be better correlated with a reduction in the size of the hepatic venous bed than with a decrease in the number and size of the intrahepatic portal channels, suggesting that intrasinusoidal hypertension may be of greater importance than portal hypertension in the pathogenesis of ascites.

The tendency for most patients with liver disease to retain water, even in the absence of portal hypertension and hypoproteinemia, and the frequent failure of ascites to appear when both are present make it clear that other mechanisms are involved. Retention of sodium appears to be one of these. Studies of renal function in individuals with cirrhosis and ascites indicate that tubular reabsorption of sodium is increased and that occasionally there is a slight reduction in glomerular filtration. Since there is no anatomic lesion in the kidney, and since the inability to excrete sodium is evident not only in the urine but also in the sweat, saliva, and intestinal secretions, it has been postulated that adrenal cortical activity is enhanced. In support of this theory it has been shown that the urinary excretion of aldosterone is increased. Although salt retention undoubtedly contributes to the formation of ascites, there is no evidence to indicate that it initiates the process. Rather, it appears to be a secondary phenomenon similar to that seen in other conditions accompanied by expansion of the extracellular fluid volume. The stimulus that initiates increased secretion of aldosterone and consequent sodium retention is not known, but in the case of liver disease at least, it may be related to the relative hypotonicity of the body fluids or to a relative reduction in effective circulating blood volume.

The cirrhotic patient with ascites tends to retain water in excess of the amount required to maintain the isotonicity of the body fluids, leading usually to a dilution type of hyponatremia. This may be an antidiuretic effect related to an increase in the secretion of antidiuretic hormone (ADH) by the posterior pituitary. Consistent with this interpretation is the frequent finding of increased antidiuretic activity in the urine. However, the level of ADH in the blood usually is normal, and there is some doubt about the origin of the antidiuretic substance in urine, so that it is by no means certain that the posterior pituitary is responsible for water retention.

Since there is rapid free exchange of water, protein, and electrolytes between the ascitic fluid and plasma compartments, and there is no obstruction to the outflow of ascitic fluid from the peritoneal cavity, it may be inferred that the accumulation of fluid is due to an increased rate of entry. The protein content of the ascitic fluid bears a direct relationship to that of the plasma but is usually significantly lower, ranging between 0.5 and 1.5 Gm per 100 ml. Rarely, the concentration may be as high as 4 or 5 Gm per 100 ml. The occurrence of blood-tinged or chylous ascites usually indicates the presence of malignancy or tuberculosis, but in rare instances may be seen in uncomplicated cirrhosis.

The disturbance in salt and water metabolism is closely correlated with the functional status of the liver. As hepatocellular function improves, there is a diuresis, and the ability to excrete sodium returns. Often this occurs despite the persistence of portal hypertension, and occasionally even before there is any change in the serum albumin level, suggesting further that the disturbance in salt and water metabolism is not merely a reflection of altered osmotic and hydrostatic relationships.

Edema may accompany the ascites or occur independently. Hypoproteinemia and sodium and water retention appear to be the principal factors involved. In patients with ascites the pressure in the inferior vena cava increases and may contribute to edema formation.

Small *pleural effusions*, chiefly right-sided, commonly occur in association with ascites. Since, in some instances, injected dye can be shown to pass freely from the abdominal cavity into the thorax but not in the reverse direction, it has been suggested that hydrothorax may be the consequence of ascitic fluid seepage through diaphragmatic lymphatic vessels. However, the forces leading to edema formation undoubtedly contribute to the accumulation of pleural fluid. Rarely, sudden *massive* hydrothorax is due to the passage of ascitic fluid through a rent in the diaphragm.

The *serum sodium level* tends to be low in advanced liver disease. In many instances, particularly in patients with ascites and edema, the hyponatremia is a dilution phenomenon related to excessive water retention and is accompanied by either normal or increased body stores of salt. As might be expected, therefore, it is not corrected by the administration of salt and does not give rise to symptoms. In contrast, cirrhotic patients occasionally exhibit a type of hyponatremia that is due to a deficit of salt related to an inadequate dietary intake or to excessive losses of salt following repeated paracentesis, prolonged mercurial diuresis, or vomiting and diarrhea. Often this form of hyponatremia is accompanied by the *salt depletion syndrome*, which is characterized by weakness, mental confusion, anorexia, nausea, vomiting, hypotension, muscle cramps, oliguria, azotemia, and hemoconcentration. Both the hyponatremia and the symptoms are promptly relieved by the administration of salt. However, it is still not clear whether it is the hyponatremia or the accompanying contraction of the plasma volume that is responsible for these clinical manifestations.

The *serum potassium* concentration may be decreased in advanced liver disease, although not so frequently as the sodium level. Often there are no associated symptoms, but occasionally clinical improvement follows correction of the hypopotassemia, suggesting that the latter may be of significance. Recent studies indicate that usually the body stores of potassium are diminished and that

repletion follows potassium administration. A poor dietary intake and losses of potassium in the urine, vomitus, and diarrheal stools probably account for the deficit.

Occasionally the *serum calcium* level is low, primarily because of a fall in serum albumin and a decrease in bound calcium. In patients with long-standing obstructive jaundice, hypocalcemia may be the consequence of steatorrhea and a disturbance in calcium absorption.

Portal Hypertension. Any obstruction to the outflow of portal blood from the main trunk of the portal vein to the right atrium may lead to an increase in portal pressure above the normal level of 100 to 200 mm H_2O. Often this is manifested clinically by the appearance of splenomegaly and by signs of an increased collateral circulation between the portal and systemic venous systems. In addition, as previously indicated, it may contribute to the development of ascites.

Cirrhosis is by far the most frequent cause of intrahepatic portal obstruction. Less common causes include intrahepatic tumors and cysts, certain granulomatous diseases, and hepatic vein thrombosis. Occasionally, the obstruction is both intra- and extrahepatic, as in the case of cirrhosis complicated by portal vein thrombosis.

The portal hypertension in cirrhosis is due, in part at least, to an increase in intrahepatic venous resistance related to partial obliteration and distortion of the vascular bed. Since occlusion of the hepatic artery causes a greater fall in portal pressure in the cirrhotic than in the normal person, there is reason to believe that abnormal arteriovenous shunts may play a role in the development of portal hypertension.

The *splenomegaly* of portal hypertension is due to congestion, fibrosis, and reticuloendothelial hyperplasia. Usually there are no accompanying symptoms, but occasionally the spleen is painful owing to perisplenitis or gives rise to a hematologic disorder characterized by anemia, leukopenia, thrombocytopenia, or pancytopenia ("hypersplenism"). Humoral mechanisms and increased stasis, sequestration, and phagocytosis have been postulated as the factors responsible for the increased rate of blood cell destruction in this syndrome. It should be noted that the same hematologic picture occurs in a wide variety of other diseases accompanied by splenomegaly. At present, the term *Banti's syndrome* is applied to any type of portal hypertension accompanied by splenomegaly and anemia. Almost always an obstruction to the outflow of portal blood can be demonstrated, either in the liver or in the portal vein itself, so that Banti's theory that the disease originated in the spleen and then gave rise to cirrhosis has been abandoned. However, there are occasional instances of Banti's syndrome in which no obstruction to portal flow can be demonstrated anatomically. It has been suggested that the portal hypertension and congestive splenomegaly in such cases may be due to increased blood flow, possibly through anomalous arteriovenous shunts, in the spleen, liver, or intestinal tract.

Not all forms of splenomegaly associated with liver disease are due to portal hypertension. In certain acute inflammatory diseases, such as viral hepatitis and infectious mononucleosis, hyperplasia of the reticuloendothelial lymphoid elements appears to be a response to infection. In other conditions, such as amyloidosis, sarcoidosis, and lymphoma, the spleen may be infiltrated with the same material found in the liver.

As a consequence of obstruction there are dilatation and congestion of the portal venous bed and shunting of blood through normal communications with the systemic veins found in (1) the submucosa of the esophagus, gastric cardia, lower rectum, and anus, (2) the falciform ligament of the liver, (3) the retroperitoneal bare area of the liver and mesentery, and (4) the splenorenal ligament. These collaterals tend to dilate and, in the relatively loose submucosa, give rise to *esophageal and gastric varices* and *hemorrhoids*. The former may rupture and often are an important source of massive gastrointestinal hemorrhage, resulting in either hematemesis or melena. The factors thought to be responsible for the rupture include mechanical trauma, peptic esophagitis, sudden increases in venous pressure produced by straining, and changes in the vessel walls and hemostatic mechanisms related to malnutrition and alterations in hepatic function. Hemorrhoids are a far less frequent cause of bleeding, and indeed, their relationship to portal hypertension has been questioned.

The increased collateral circulation through the periumbilical veins of the falciform ligament often results in the appearance of *dilated superficial veins* in the periumbilical area (*caput medusae*) and the anterior abdominal wall. These veins drain centrifugally from the umbilicus into branches of the superior and inferior vena cava. However, when the intraabdominal pressure is high, owing to ascites, all the drainage may be cephalad. A *venous hum* with systolic accentuation is heard occasionally below the xiphoid, around the umbilicus, or over the epigastric area of the liver (*Cruveilhier-Baumgarten syndrome*).

The extent of the collateral circulation in cirrhosis is variable and may be sufficiently great to overcome portal hypertension.

Arterial Spiders. Highly characteristic vascular skin lesions, known as *arterial spiders* or *spider nevi,* are seen in cirrhosis and, less commonly, in other forms of advanced liver disease. Although not pathognomonic of hepatic injury, since they occur in pregnancy, malnutrition, and occasionally in normal individuals, when large and numerous they almost invariably indicate the presence of liver disease. In general their number and size parallel the severity of the hepatocellular failure, and often they disappear following recovery.

The typical lesion, which measures 3 to 10 mm, consists of a bright or dusky-red, slightly elevated central arteriole with fine radiating branches on a background of normal skin. In large lesions the intervening skin may appear cyanotic. Compression of the central vessel with a fine point results in blanching of its branches; occasionally arterial pulsation can be demonstrated by palpation or gentle pressure with a glass slide. For reasons that are not clear, the lesions occur most frequently on the face, neck, and shoulders and are rare below the level of the costal margin.

The factors responsible for the occurrence of spider nevi in liver disease are not known. A high circulating estrogen level is thought to be important, but the evidence for this is far from convincing (see below).

Palmar Erythema (Liver Palms). Patients with advanced liver disease may exhibit a bright, sometimes mottled erythema of the thenar and hypothenar eminences and the finger tips. Not infrequently it is associated with spider nevi and is thought to be due to the same stimulus. However, it is far less diagnostic of liver disease, since it occurs in a variety of conditions and is especially common in rheumatoid arthritis and malnutrition.

Endocrine Disturbances. During the stage of hepatic decompensation, male cirrhotic patients often show *testicular atrophy,* a *decrease in libido and potentia,* and a *loss of axillary and pubic hair.* Less commonly they develop *gynecomastia.* These changes are usually ascribed to hyperestrogenemia resulting from a defect in the inactivation and excretion of estrogen by the liver. It is postulated that estrogen produces gynecomastia, loss of hair, and spider nevi by a direct action and that it induces testicular atrophy by suppressing the secretion of pituitary gonadotropin. This theory is supported by the evidence indicating that the normal liver is capable of inactivating and excreting estrogen and that in cirrhosis the urinary concentration of estrogen is high, while that of 17-ketosteroids, androgen, and gonadotropin is low. However, these abnormalities are inconstant findings and are poorly correlated with the occurrence of testicular atrophy, gynecomastia, spider nevi, or loss of hair, so that there is considerable doubt that estrogen plays a key role in the endocrine disturbances of liver disease.

The testicular atrophy and low androgen excretion may be due to malnutrition and wasting, as in many other diseases. Since the testicle usually shows atrophy of the germinal epithelium, thickening of the basement membrane, and intact Leydig and Sertoli cells, it is possible that the gynecomastia is a secondary phenomenon dependent on tubular atrophy, as in Klinefelter's syndrome and other related conditions. While gynecomastia usually appears during periods of hepatic decompensation, it may occur during the recovery phase when the patient is gaining weight at a rapid rate. This appears to be related to the type of gynecomastia that occurs in severely malnourished individuals following refeeding. It has been suggested that the loss of axillary and pubic hair, the low level of urinary 17-ketosteroids, and the tendency for patients with chronic liver disease to develop pigmentation are signs of relative adrenal cortical insufficiency. Indeed, the frequent finding of cortical atrophy at autopsy would appear to be consistent with this view. However, it is difficult to account on this basis for the paradoxic increase in urinary corticoids seen in some cirrhotic patients.

Premenopausal women with cirrhosis often exhibit amenorrhea and atrophy of the breasts. Whether these signs are manifestations of hepatic failure or the consequence of malnutrition and chronic illness is not certain. It is of interest that women with amenorrhea and low levels of urinary estrogen develop spider nevi and palmar erythema about as frequently as males. Loss of axillary and pubic hair is less striking than in the male. Rarely, young women with chronic liver disease exhibit hirsutism, acne, abdominal striae, obesity and moon facies, features reminiscent of Cushing's disease and suggestive of increased adrenal cortical activity.

Hepatic Coma. The changes in consciousness, behavior, and neurologic status that occur in advanced liver disease are known collectively as *hepatic coma*. Since similar manifestations are seen occasionally in the absence of liver disease, particularly in individuals with surgically induced portacaval anastomoses, there is reason to believe that the shunting of portal blood around the liver may be an important factor in the pathogenesis of hepatic coma. However, the symptoms associated with hepatocellular failure tend to be more severe and are less amenable to treatment, which suggests that they are due to a more complex metabolic derangement than occurs in the case of uncomplicated Eck fistula. The syndrome of hepatic coma, while still an ill-defined entity, must be differentiated from those forms of stupor due to hypoglycemia, hyponatremia, shock, and renal failure that occur occasionally in advanced liver disease.

Impending coma, the early phase of the syndrome, is characterized by mental confusion, difficulty in concentration, euphoria or apathy, drowsiness, inappropriate behavior, and untidiness. Often these signs are accompanied by a flapping tremor, other neurologic signs, electroencephalographic changes, and fetor hepaticus.

The *flapping tremor*, which is due to an inability to maintain postural tonus, is best demonstrated in the hands, although it may be seen also in the protruded tongue, the retracted lips, or the dorsiflexed feet. With the arms outstretched or resting on the bed, the wrists dorsiflexed, and the fingers spread apart, bursts of rapid, arrhythmic alternating flexion and extension movements occur at irregular intervals at the wrists, metacarpophalangeal joints, and less commonly, at the shoulders and elbows.

The *neurologic signs* are variable but often include fluctuating muscular rigidity, hyperreflexia, ankle clonus, and an extensor plantar response.

Characteristically, the *electroencephalogram* at this stage reveals paroxysms of bilaterally synchronous, slow waves of high voltage in the delta range ($1\frac{1}{2}$ to 3 per second) interspersed with or superimposed on a relatively normal alpha rhythm. These waves appear in the frontal region and then spread laterally and posteriorly until the entire record is one of slow activity.

Often the breath has a characteristic sweetish odor known as *fetor hepaticus*. Some authorities suggest that the odor may be due to methyl mercaptan (CH_3SH), a compound recovered from the urine and presumably derived from methionine [$CH_3 \cdot S \cdot CH_2 \cdot CH_2CH(NH_2) \cdot COOH$]. Others have tried to implicate a tertiary amine. The fact that broad-spectrum antibiotics sometimes eliminate the fetor suggests that these or other metabolites responsible for the odor may arise in the intestinal tract as a result of bacterial action.

As the precomatose state progresses to *frank coma*, drowsiness increases, culminating in deep stupor and unconsciousness. The muscles become flaccid, there is a tendency to areflexia, the flapping tremor ceases, and in some instances, muscle twitchings and convulsions appear. Often death ensues at this point, but it is not inevitable. Recovery may occur spontaneously or as a result of treatment but is rare once deep coma has been present for more than a few days.

The clinical course of hepatic coma varies, depending on the nature of the underlying disease and the precipitating factors involved. In general, the coma tends to be mild and reversible when portacaval shunting of blood and absorption of nitrogenous compounds from the intestinal tract are the principal factors. Often the neurologic signs do not progress to frank coma, and recovery may occur either spontaneously or as a result of treatment. The symptoms in this group vary in duration from a few hours to several months, and not infrequently they fluctuate in intensity. In contrast, coma that is due primarily to hepatocellular failure is likely to be severe, rapidly progressive, unresponsive to therapy, and fatal. In conditions like cirrhosis, where shunting and hepatocellular failure both play a role, the outcome is unpredictable.

The factors known to be important in precipitating hepatic coma include gastrointestinal hemorrhage, severe infection, prolonged episodes of alcoholism and malnutrition, surgical trauma, and the use of narcotics. Less commonly, coma appears following the administration of high protein diets, ammonium salts, urea, or methionine. In all instances the effects produced are due either to aggravation of the underlying hepatocellular failure or to the introduction into the gastrointestinal tract of nitrogenous compounds that exert a deleterious effect when absorbed (see below).

The nature of the cerebral disturbance in hepatic coma is poorly understood. While the brain usually shows diffuse proliferation and swelling of its protoplasmic astrocytes, and less commonly, regional degeneration of nerve cells, it is not known how these relate to the neurologic manifestations, nor how they are produced. At the present time it is generally believed that the encephalopathy of liver disease is due either to a disturbance in cerebral metabolic activity or to an intoxication with nitrogenous substances possibly derived from the intestinal tract. The old concept that coma was due to the retention of bile, which led to adoption of the now obsolete term *cholemia*, has been abandoned for lack of supporting evidence.

Often serum lactate, pyruvate, and alpha-ketoglutarate are increased in hepatic coma, suggesting a disturbance in carbohydrate metabolism involving the Krebs cycle. Similarly, alterations in the quantitative and qualitative pattern of the serum and urinary amino acids suggest a defect in protein metabolism. However, since these abnormalities may occur in liver disease in the absence of neurologic symptoms, it is doubtful that they are directly responsible for hepatic coma.

There is some evidence to indicate that ammonia intoxication may play a role in the pathogenesis of hepatic coma. It is believed that ammonia arising in the intestinal tract, as a result of bacterial action on nitrogenous compounds, may accumulate in the blood as a consequence of portacaval shunting or of a disturbance in the hepatic mechanism for the conversion of ammonia to urea. In support of this theory it has been shown that (1) intravenous ammonium salts are toxic for normal animals; (2) often the blood and spinal fluid levels of ammonia are elevated in both hepatocellular disease and uncomplicated portacaval shunt, and usually rise to higher levels when coma supervenes; (3) the administration of ammonium salts, urea, or large supplements

of protein or the occurrence of hemorrhage into the intestinal tract in such patients may raise the blood ammonia level and produce signs of impending or overt coma; (4) antibiotics that suppress bacterial growth in the intestine and glutamic acid, which combines with ammonia to form glutamine, tend to lower the blood ammonia level and occasionally induce clearing of the sensorium. Recent studies concerned with the metabolic activity of the brain during hepatic coma indicate that the cerebral uptake of ammonia is increased, while oxygen consumption is diminished. These observations have been interpreted as evidence that the fundamental disturbance in coma is a reduction in the oxidative metabolism of the brain related to diversion of alpha-ketoglutaric acid from the Krebs cycle as a result of its combination with ammonia to form glutamic acid. The increase in serum glutamine seen in hepatic coma is consistent with this hypothesis. However, the ammonia intoxication theory has by no means gone unchallenged. Indeed, it has been pointed out that (1) the ammonia measured in blood may represent a breakdown product of some other labile nitrogenous compound; (2) high levels of blood ammonia are not invariably accompanied by hepatic coma, and alterations in the level do not necessarily result in any change in the state of consciousness; (3) methionine is capable of producing impending hepatic coma without raising the blood ammonia level if it is administered to individuals with hepatocellular disease or portacaval shunt. Accordingly, it is now generally agreed that while ammonia intoxication may be a factor in the pathogenesis of coma in individuals with marked portacaval shunting of blood who experience gastrointestinal bleeding, or who ingest large amounts of other nitrogenous material, the type of hepatic coma associated with severe hepatocellular failure is a far more complex metabolic disturbance.

Manifestations of Renal Failure. There is no evidence to indicate that hepatic damage gives rise to a specific nephrotoxin that produces renal failure. Prolonged and severe jaundice may be associated with a mild form of tubular degeneration, known as *bile nephrosis*, but this rarely is accompanied by impairment of renal function unless other factors are involved. The oliguria and azotemia that occasionally complicate advanced hepatocellular disease are usually the result of salt and water retention, dehydration, or circulatory disturbances related to salt deprivation, hemorrhage, or shock. Not infrequently the latter give rise to acute tubular necrosis, in which case the renal failure may be severe. In some instances, as in carbon tetrachloride poisoning and leptospirosis, the liver and kidney are both injured simultaneously, so that renal failure is independent of hepatic damage.

The term *hepatorenal syndrome* was introduced by surgeons to describe a fatal form of coma, usually accompanied by hyperpyrexia, oliguria, and azotemia, that occasionally followed surgical manipulation of the biliary tract or trauma to the liver. Implied was the concept that the symptoms were of toxic origin and related to hepatic decompensation. At the present time, however, it is generally agreed that such symptoms are indicative of concomitant hepatic and renal failure and are due to infection, dehydration, hemorrhage, and shock. It is noteworthy that the syndrome has become far less common as better methods of managing these complications have become available. The term is still used by many clinicians to describe any form of renal failure that occurs in liver disease. This is an unfortunate practice, since it gives the erroneous impression that the hepatorenal syndrome is a specific clinical and pathologic entity, and tends to obscure the importance of extrahepatic factors in the genesis of renal failure in liver disease.

TESTS OF LIVER FUNCTION

A number of tests are available for estimating the functional status of the liver. These are useful in establishing the presence of liver disease and in gauging its severity and progress. Unfortunately, there are no tests that distinguish between the various forms of hepatocellular injury, and only a few that are helpful in discriminating between obstructive and hepatocellular jaundice.

The interpretation of liver function tests demands a sound knowledge of their physiologic basis and recognition of their limitations. The very term *liver function test* is misleading and, unless its implications are fully understood, may be the basis for misinterpretation. In the first place, many of the tests do not measure any of the normal physiologic activities of the liver. Thus, while the excretion of a foreign dye, such as Bromsulphalein, reflects the integrity of the parenchyma and the patency of the biliary tree, it is not a direct index of any known normal function. Secondly, some of the tests measure changes in the serum which reflect the presence of pathologic processes in the liver but do not necessarily indicate any impairment of function. The rise in serum globulin and the alterations in cephalin-cholesterol flocculation and thymol turbidity that accompany many forms of hepatocellular disease may be cited as examples. Finally, few, if any, of the chemical changes due to alterations in hepatic structure and function are pathognomonic of liver disease. Thus, hyperbilirubinemia may be indicative of increased hemolysis, Bromsulphalein retention a sign of circulatory collapse, hyperphosphatasemia an index of bone disease, and alterations in the serum globulin pattern an expression of extrahepatic infection. It is obvious, therefore, that the abnormalities disclosed by hepatic function tests do not necessarily indicate the presence of functional or structural changes in the liver.

Since hepatic damage does not necessarily affect all, or even any, of the multiple functions of the liver, it follows that no single test is capable of detecting all instances of disease. Similarly, no single test can be expected to distinguish between lesions in the parenchymal cells and the biliary tract under all conditions, since these two components of the liver are so intimately related anatomically that affections of one sooner or later lead to involvement of the other. For that reason there has been a growing tendency to use a battery of tests measuring not only alterations in a number of functions but also some of the biochemical changes that are related to specific lesions. While this trend is to be encouraged, it must be recognized that, as the number of tests multiply, they become increasingly difficult to interpret, especially since any increase in sensitivity is usually made at the expense of specificity. The value of any group of tests is enhanced as the clinician becomes more familiar with their biochemical and physiologic implications and as he has the opportunity of observing their behavior in the broad spectrum of disease.

The commonly used tests selected for discussion represent only a small fraction of the very large number that have been proposed. In the author's experience they provide about as much useful information as can be reasonably expected from this method of study and have the advantage that the technical methods required are reliable and can be carried out in any well-equipped clinical laboratory.

Serum Bilirubin. The direct-reacting bilirubin concentration may be estimated spectrophotometrically by measuring the amount of pigment diazotized in the absence of alcohol at the end of 1 min. Recent studies, based on the chromatographic isolation of the direct-reacting pigments in serum, indicate that a more accurate estimate is obtained at the end of 10 min of diazotization. However, the 1-min level is widely accepted in this country and has served as the basis for so many modern studies on jaundice that it has been retained in the following discussion as an index of direct-reacting bilirubin concentration, although, at best, it is only an approximation.

It is customary to add an equal volume of alcohol to the reaction mixture once the direct bilirubin level has been determined. At the end of 30 min the amount of diazotized pigment found represents the total bilirubin, consisting of both direct and indirect fractions.

Normal serum usually contains less than 0.2 mg of direct ("1-min") and 1.0 mg of total bilirubin per 100 ml. Values up to 0.3 and 1.3 mg, respectively, are of borderline significance.

The total serum bilirubin level is of diagnostic and prognostic significance in the detection of latent jaundice and in the recognition of fluctuations in the intensity of the jaundice not apparent to the eye. In hepatocellular disease and biliary obstruction the concentration may increase to 2 or 3 mg per 100 ml before icterus becomes evident, and in hemolytic disease the level may be even higher. Once jaundice appears, a great deal more can be learned about its course than is evident on inspection by carrying out serial determinations of the serum bilirubin concentration.

The percentage of total serum bilirubin that reacts directly has greater diagnostic significance than the absolute concentration of the direct-reacting fraction. In hepatocellular disease and biliary obstruction the latter usually constitutes 25 to 75 per cent of the total bilirubin, while in hemolytic disease the value is usually below 15 per cent. It must be emphasized that an increase in the percentage of direct-reacting pigment does not distinguish between hepatocellular and obstructive jaundice but may be helpful in excluding hemolytic disease. However, with mild hepatic injury the percentage may be low, while in severe hemolytic episodes, possibly because of associated liver damage, it may be high, so that the ratio of direct to total bilirubin is not always a reliable point of distinction. Even in uncomplicated hemolytic jaundice, the absolute concentration of the direct fraction often rises, but only in proportion to the total bilirubin, so that the ratio tends to remain within the normal range of 10 to 15 per cent. In contrast, in hepatocellular disease there may be an increase in the direct-reacting fraction without a concomitant rise in the total bilirubin level, a situation seen rather frequently in latent cirrhosis and early hepatitis.

In the absence of adequate laboratory facilities, the total bilirubin concentration may be crudely estimated from the *icterus index,* which measures the relative depth of color in serum as compared to a 1:10,000 aqueous solution of potassium dichromate. Normally serum has an index of 4 to 8 units, that is, a depth of color four to eight times that of the standard. The ratio between the bilirubin concentration and icterus index usually lies betwen 1:5 and 1:10, depending on the amount of interfering color present. Hemolysis, turbidity, carotenoids, and certain drugs introduce significant errors.

Urine Bilirubin. Bilirubinuria is a common finding in hepatocellular and obstructive jaundice but is rare in hemolytic disease, unless the jaundice is intense and accompanied by a marked increase in the percentage of the direct-reacting serum bilirubin. Occasionally bilirubin can be detected in the urine of individuals with liver disease who have a normal serum bilirubin level. However, the concentration of the direct-reacting fraction is usually, although not invariably, increased in such instances. It has been reported that with sufficiently sensitive methods it may be possible to detect traces of bilirubin in the urine of perfectly normal individuals. Often the urine contains bile salts when bilirubinuria is present, which accounts for the tendency of the urine to foam when it is shaken.

Tests for bilirubin in the urine are helpful in the differentiation of hemolytic from other types of jaundice. Also, since bilirubinuria may be present before overt jaundice appears, they are useful in detecting early hepatocellular and biliary obstructive disease. The reader is referred to p. 149 for a more complete discussion of the mechanisms governing the renal excretion of bilirubin.

Urine Urobilinogen. As indicated on p. 148, the bilirubin excreted into the intestinal tract is reduced by bacterial action to a group of compounds known collectively as *urobilinogen.* Most of the pigment is excreted in the feces, but a fraction is reabsorbed and returned by way of the portal vein to the liver, where it is reexcreted into the bile (the enterohepatic circulation of urobilinogen). A small amount of urobilinogen escapes into the general circulation and is excreted by the kidneys. Normally less than 4 mg is excreted in a 24-hr period. By the Watson method, which is simpler, but less specific, than the usual quantitative procedure, the value is less than 1.3 Ehrlich units in 2 hr. On simple qualitative test, urobilinogen may be detectable in dilutions up to 1:20.

The urinary excretion of urobilinogen increases when the pigment is not cleared from the serum. This may be a sign of hepatocellular injury or may be the consequence of abnormal hemolysis and excessive pigment production. If the amount of bile reaching the intestinal tract diminishes as a result of biliary obstruction or parenchymal disease, there is a corresponding decrease in urinary urobilinogen. Suppression of bacterial growth in the intestinal tract by means of antibiotics also reduces urobilinogen formation and excretion. It is essential, therefore, in interpreting the results of urine urobilinogen tests, to give due consideration to the amount of bilirubin reaching the intestine and the opportunity for its reduction to urobilinogen. Thus, while urine urobilinogen tends to be high in hepatocellular disease, it may be low if bile secretion is greatly diminished, or if antibiotics are administered. Similarly, in extrahepatic biliary obstruction urine urobilinogen usually is low, but it may be high if bacteria gain access to the ducts and convert bilirubin to urobilinogen.

The reader is referred to p. 148 for a more complete discussion of urobilinogen metabolism.

Fecal Urobilinogen. The urobilinogens derived from bilirubin are colorless but tend to oxidize in the intestinal tract to form urobilins, which impart a brown color to the feces. Other, as yet unidentified, pigments contribute to the color. Since the urobilins have the same significance as the urobilinogens, it is customary, as a matter of convenience, to speak of both groups of pigments as fecal urobilinogen, and indeed, both are measured together in quantitative procedures which entail a preliminary reduction of the urobilins to their corresponding urobilinogens. It is important to note that, in testing for the presence of pigment by qualitative methods, it is necessary to test for both urobilinogen and urobilin. Under normal conditions the feces contain no bilirubin, although the pigments present are often called bile. However, following the administration of broad-spectrum antibiotics that suppress the intestinal flora, bilirubin may appear.

Normally the amount of urobilinogen excreted in the feces ranges from 40 to 480 mg daily. In hemolytic disease it is increased, because of enhanced pigment production, while in hepatocellular and obstructive jaundice it is diminished, because of reduced bile flow into the intestine. With complete exclusion of bilirubin from the intestinal tract, urobilinogen excretion falls to less than 5 mg per day, the remaining traces being derived from bilirubin in the mucosa. This is seen in carcinomatous obstruction of the biliary tract but is rare in hepatocellular or nonmalignant obstructive jaundice, even when the stools are clay-colored, since the interruption of bile flow in these conditions is seldom complete or sustained.

Because the quantitative determination of fecal urobilinogen is time consuming, it is seldom employed as a routine procedure. However, it may be of diagnostic value in congenital atresia or malignant obstruction of the bile ducts by establishing the complete absence of bile in the feces and in hemolytic states by confirming the presence of increased hemolysis, particularly when jaundice is absent and other signs of hemolysis are equivocal. Ordinarily, simple inspection of the clay-colored stool suffices to establish cessation of bile flow. Qualitative tests are of very limited value and are seldom used.

Bromsulphalein (BSP) Excretion. Because intravenously injected BSP is eliminated almost exclusively by the liver, its rate of clearance from the plasma is a useful index of hepatocellular function. However, the excretion of this dye depends not only upon the functional capacity of the liver but also upon the state of the hepatic circulation and the integrity of the biliary tree, so that these factors must be taken into account in interpreting the results of this test.

Normally most of the dye is excreted in the bile, and less than 2 per cent in the urine. However, under conditions of abnormal dye retention, as in hepatocellular and obstructive jaundice, or when there is proteinuria, urinary losses of dye may be significantly greater. A small fraction may be destroyed extrahepatically. There is no convincing evidence that any of the dye is reabsorbed from the intestinal tract.

The removal of BSP from the plasma involves two steps: (1) passive uptake and concentration of dye in the liver and (2) active excretion of dye into the bile. Within limits the liver abstracts BSP from the plasma more rapidly than it is capable of excreting it. Under these conditions the liver removes a constant fraction of the dye reaching it per unit of time, so that the absolute amount cleared from the plasma is determined not only by the excretory capacity of the hepatic cells but also by the plasma concentration of BSP and the volume of hepatic blood flow.

In the liver some of the dye is conjugated with glutathione to form two BSP compounds which are excreted in the bile. Since more than half the dye is excreted in its free form, conjugation does not appear to be essential for excretion. In obstructive jaundice, and to a lesser extent in hepatocellular jaundice, the conjugates are demonstrable in the plasma, indicating that under these conditions the dye tends to regurgitate from either the hepatic cells or the bile. Although measurement of the conjugates by the cumbersome chromatographic method required gives some indication of the degree of regurgitation, it does not permit a quantitative estimate of the fraction of dye in the plasma attributable to regurgitation. Hence, the latter affects the apparent rate at which BSP is cleared from the plasma to an unpredictable degree, so that it is difficult in the face of obstructive or hepatocellular jaundice to interpret the results of the test in terms of hepatocellular function. The fraction of conjugated BSP in the plasma tends to be higher in obstructive than in hepatocellular jaundice. According to some investigators, the difference is sufficiently great to be of diagnostic value in distinguishing between these two forms of jaundice. On this basis they propose that the principal defect in hepatocellular jaundice involves the uptake and conjugation of dye, while that in obstructive jaundice is attributable to impaired excretion resulting in regurgitation of conjugated dye. Contradictory evidence has been reported by others indicating that in both forms of jaundice there is impairment of dye uptake and excretion and that the proportions of free and conjugated BSP in the plasma do not distinguish between them. Of interest is the fact that in the Dubin-Johnson syndrome, in contrast to other forms of hepatocellular jaundice, the uptake and conjugation of BSP appear to be normal, while excretion of dye is impaired and accompanied by reflux of BSP conjugates into the plasma.

Several methods of estimating BSP excretion are available. The one in most common use involves the intravenous injection of 5 mg dye per kg body weight and measurement of the percentage of dye retained in the serum at the end of 45 min. Normally there is less than 6 per cent retention, and in most individuals no dye can be detected.

In the absence of jaundice and circulatory disturbances, the degree of dye retention usually parallels the extent of hepatic parenchymal damage and, hence, is a highly valuable test of hepatocellular function. Although, as previously mentioned, the presence of jaundice complicates the interpretation of the BSP test, the latter may be of value in serial studies of patients whose jaundice is relatively stable. Moreover, when the jaundice is mild, the test may be helpful in distinguishing between obstructive and hepatocellular jaundice, since BSP retention tends to parallel the serum bilirubin level in the former and usually is proportionately greater in the latter. Since the rate of BSP clearance is in part determined by the volume of hepatic blood flow, some dye retention may be expected in shock, heart failure, and other conditions leading to disturbances in the hepatic circulation. No doubt this contributes to the dye retention in such intrahepatic diseases as cirrhosis.

Plasma Proteins. Often liver disease is accompanied by alterations in the composition of the plasma proteins. While these alterations are never pathognomonic, they may be of considerable diagnostic and prognostic value.

In hepatocellular disease there is a tendency for the *serum albumin* level to fall. Usually this is the result of a decrease in albumin synthesis in the liver, but malnutrition may be a factor in some instances. As a rule, the decline is slow, so that low concentrations of albumin are more common in chronic than in acute liver disease. However, the level may fall precipitously when parenchymal injury is extensive, as in acute massive necrosis of the liver. Since the albumin concentration tends to parallel the functional status of the parenchyma, it is a useful guide in following the progress of liver disease, especially when jaundice is present and other tests are difficult to interpret. Unfortunately, the albumin level may remain within normal limits when significant hepatic damage is present, so that it is a relatively insensitive index of liver function.

The *serum globulin* level tends to rise in both acute and chronic hepatocellular disease. Usually this is due to an increase in γ-globulin, but occasionally the α and β fractions also are increased. Not infrequently it is possible to detect these changes in the composition of the globulins electrophoretically

while the concentration of total globulin is still within the normal range. In obstructive jaundice, the β-globulins tend to rise and may be accompanied by hypergammaglobulinemia if the obstruction is complicated by infection or hepatocellular injury.

Since plasma cells and possibly other elements of the reticuloendothelial system are thought to be the source of γ-globulin, it is reasonable to suppose that the hypergammaglobulinemia of hepatic disease is related to inflammatory reactions in the liver. The questions of whether any of the γ-globulin increase is due to the occurrence of antibodies to autogenous antigens arising from the breakdown of liver tissue and whether the normal liver plays any role in the disposal or alteration of γ-globulin remain to be answered. It is important to recognize that an increase in γ-globulin is not diagnostic of liver disease and that it occurs in a wide variety of infections and in diseases affecting the reticuloendothelial system.

Usually the *total protein* content of the serum is low or normal in hepatocellular disease. However, occasionally, hyperglobulinemia is so marked that hyperproteinemia results. This is seen particularly in the chronic form of viral hepatitis and in posthepatitic cirrhosis.

The importance of the *albumin/globulin (A/G) ratio* has been overemphasized. While it often is reversed in hepatocellular disease, it should be emphasized that the albumin and globulin concentrations vary independently and that each has its own significance.

The *plasma prothrombin* level tends to fall in liver disease. Since the synthesis of prothrombin occurs in the liver and requires the presence of vitamin K, the decline in plasma prothrombin may be the result of hepatocellular injury or of failure to absorb vitamin K because of the absence of bile in the intestinal tract. Often both factors are operative. Theoretically the response to a parenteral injection of vitamin K should distinguish between hepatocellular and obstructive jaundice, but this has proved to be an unreliable diagnostic test. Several other plasma proteins concerned with blood coagulation may be reduced in advanced liver disease. These include fibrinogen, plasma *accelerator globulin* (factor V, labile factor), and *convertin* (factor VII, stable factor).

Flocculation and Turbidity Tests. A number of empirical tests have been devised to demonstrate subtle changes in the composition of the serum proteins in liver disease not apparent on routine fractionation by salting-out methods. While these tests often are useful in corroborating the presence of hepatocellular disease, it must be emphasized that they do not measure any specific function of the parenchymal cells, are not a direct index of hepatocellular dysfunction or injury, and may yield abnormal findings in any condition that alters the pattern of the serum proteins. Most of the tests reflect an increase or qualitative change in serum γ-globulin and/or a qualitative change in serum albumin. In addition, in the case of the thymol turbidity test, the phospholipids appear to be involved.

The two tests used most commonly are those of *cephalin-cholesterol flocculation* and *thymol turbidity*. These may be of value in confirming the presence of parenchymal disease and in differentiating between hepatocellular and obstructive jaundice. However, since they often remain abnormal for long periods following apparent recovery, they are unreliable guides in following the progress of established disease.

The results of these two tests overlap to a considerable extent but differ sufficiently to warrant their simultaneous use. Thus, the thymol turbidity test is somewhat more reliable in discriminating between hepatocellular and obstructive jaundice, since it is less likely to be affected by the hepatocellular changes and infection that often accompany obstruction of the biliary tree. The cephalin-cholesterol flocculation reaction, on the other hand, is more dependable in detecting cirrhosis. However, the thymol turbidity test may be of value in distinguishing between the various types of cirrhosis, since the values tend to be high in the posthepatitic variety and either normal or only slightly increased in the others. In general, extrahepatic infections affect cephalin-cholesterol flocculation to a greater degree than thymol turbidity, so that the former is more subject to errors in interpretation. A rise in the serum lipid level may increase thymol turbidity but does not affect cephalin-cholesterol flocculation.

It has been reported that the thymol flocculation test is more sensitive than the turbidity test in detecting hepatocellular injury, especially in chronic hepatitis. However, this has not been the experience of most investigators.

The range of values usually considered normal for the thymol turbidity test is 1 to 4 units, and for the cephalin-cholesterol flocculation test 0 to 1+ at 24 hr and 0 to 2+ at 48 hr.

Serum Lipids. The *total cholesterol* level of the serum tends to rise in obstructive jaundice but may fail to do so if the obstruction is minimal or of short duration. In contrast, the level usually remains within normal limits (150 to 250 mg per 100 ml) or falls when hepatocellular disease is present. However, if the parenchymal damage is not severe, and if it is accompanied by a high degree of bile retention, the cholesterol concentration may be high, as in primary biliary cirrhosis, cholestatic jaundice, and in the early stages of viral hepatitis. As hepatocellular function undergoes further deterioration or

bile flow is resumed in these conditions, the concentration tends to fall again, which explains why hypercholesteremia is relatively uncommon in hepatocellular jaundice. When the cholesterol concentration falls to subnormal levels, it usually indicates the presence of advanced parenchymal damage and is an ominous prognostic sign. Rarely such a fall is due to severe malnutrition.

The mechanisms responsible for the fluctuations in serum cholesterol are poorly understood, but there is some evidence to indicate that the tendency for the concentration to fall in hepatocellular damage is due to a decrease in cholesterol synthesis and that the rise that accompanies bile stasis, whether it be of parenchymal or of obstructive origin, may be due to an alteration in the physical properties of the serum proteins, possibly related to an increase in blood cholates, leading to interference with the normal removal of cholesterol from the blood.

The cholesterol in serum occurs in both free and esterified forms. In the absence of liver disease the *ratio of free to total cholesterol* remains remarkably constant within narrow limits (24 to 32 per cent), irrespective of the total cholesterol concentration. However, both in hepatocellular disease and biliary obstruction, there is a tendency for the ratio to increase. This apparent failure to esterify cholesterol is regarded usually as an index of hepatocellular dysfunction, but recent studies suggest that the percentage of free cholesterol may be more closely related to the severity of jaundice than to the degree of hepatocellular failure. Further studies are needed to validate these observations, since they are at variance with past experience.

The concentration of *serum phospholipid* in liver disease tends to parallel that of total cholesterol, although it often increases at a more rapid rate in conditions associated with hypercholesteremia. In contrast, the *triglyceride* content of the serum is little affected by liver disease, even when the other lipid fractions are increased. This probably accounts for the absence of turbidity in serums of high lipid content.

As compared with other tests, the serum lipid pattern is a relatively insensitive indicator of hepatocellular dysfunction. However, it may be useful in the differential diagnosis of jaundice and in estimating the severity of parenchymal damage.

Serum Alkaline Phosphatase. Often the serum alkaline phosphatase level is elevated in diseases of the liver and biliary tract. The mechanisms responsible for this increase are not fully understood. Since the enzyme occurs in a number of tissues, including the bones, intestinal mucosa, and liver, and is excreted in the bile, it is believed by some that the increase in serum phosphatase is a retention phenomenon reflecting a reduction in enzyme excretion due to either hepatocellular failure or biliary obstruction. While retention may be a factor in obstructive jaundice, it is difficult to see how it can account for the very much higher levels of alkaline phosphatase in obstructive than in hepatocellular jaundice or for the rise in alkaline phosphatase that occurs in nonicteric individuals with biliary fistula, cholangitis, or intrahepatic malignancy. According to another theory there is an increased production of enzyme in bone because of the development of osteomalacia secondary to the steatorrhea and vitamin D loss that occur in obstructive jaundice. Obviously this can hardly account for the hyperphosphatemia seen in nonicteric liver disease or for the prompt fall in the phosphatase level that follows relief of obstructive jaundice by external drainage of the common duct. Perhaps the most convincing case can be made for the theory that the alkaline phosphatase is due to overproduction of the enzyme by the liver in response to such diverse stimuli as hepatocellular injury, increased intraductile pressure, inflammatory disease of the ducts, and expanding lesions compressing parenchyma and ducts. A good many clinical and experimental observations may be cited as supporting evidence, but the two most impressive are the reports that (1) ligation of the pedicle of a single lobe of the liver raises the serum alkaline phosphatase level without producing jaundice, an effect that is prevented by excising the lobe at the time of ligation, and (2) creation of an external biliary fistula results in an increase in alkaline phosphatase concentration not only in the serum but also in the bile. However, this theory does not explain, any more than do the others, why the alkaline phosphatase level is higher in obstructive than in hepatocellular jaundice.

Several methods of measuring serum alkaline phosphatase activity are available. The normal range of values for the three in most common use are Bodansky 1 to 4 units, Shinowara-Jones-Reinhart (S-J-R) 2.2 to 8.6 units, and King-Armstrong (K-A) 3 to 13 units per 100 ml.

As previously indicated, the serum alkaline phosphatase tends to rise to a higher level in obstructive than in hepatocellular jaundice. Although there is some overlapping of values in the two groups, levels over 12 Bodansky, 15 S-J-R, or 30 K-A units usually indicate the presence of biliary obstruction, so that the test may be of value in the differential diagnosis of jaundice, particularly if serial determinations are carried out. Unfortunately, high values are not unusual in those forms of hepatocellular disease that present with signs suggesting obstructive jaundice so that the test is not always reliable.

The alkaline phosphatase level is a relatively insensitive index of hepatocellular function, so that it is of little value in detecting minimal changes in the liver. However, high values in the obstructive jaundice range may be seen in intrahepatic malignancy,

cholangitis, sarcoidosis, and other infiltrative lesions of the liver, even in the absence of jaundice or other overt signs of liver disease, so that the test may be of considerable help in establishing the presence of these diseases.

In interpreting the significance of changes in the serum alkaline phosphatase concentration, it is important to bear in mind that high values occur in a number of bone diseases accompanied by increased osteoblastic activity, such as Paget's disease, hyperparathyroidism, and osteogenic metastases. In fact, the very highest levels, 50 to 100 Bodansky units, are seen in this group. The only liver lesion that produces elevations of this magnitude is advanced intrahepatic malignancy with jaundice.

Serum Transaminases. Many tissues contain the enzyme *glutamic oxalacetic transaminase* (GOT), but the highest concentrations are found in the liver and myocardium. Normally, only low levels of activity (less than 40 Karmen units) are demonstrable in the serum. Tissue injury often raises the serum level, presumably by releasing intracellular GOT as a consequence of necrosis or altered permeability of cell membranes. This is seen most commonly in disorders of the liver and in myocardial infarction, but it may occur in a wide variety of other conditions including traumatic, inflammatory, and degenerative disorders of the muscles, acute pancreatitis, cerebral infarctions, trauma to the kidneys, leukemia and other forms of malignancy. Certain drugs, including aspirin, codeine, and the anticoagulants, bishydroxycoumarin (Dicumarol) and ethyl biscoumacetate (Tromexan), may also raise the serum GOT level; the underlying mechanism in this instance is not known.

The highest values of serum GOT are seen following acute hepatocellular injury due to the hepatitis virus, hepatotoxins, or drug sensitization reactions. Occasionally similarly high values are encountered in patients with congestive heart failure who develop acute pulmonary edema and/or shock, complications which result in extensive central hepatocellular necrosis. Chronic degenerative, inflammatory, and infiltrative disorders of the hepatic parenchyma, such as cirrhosis, fatty infiltration, granulomatous disease and tumors, and obstructive jaundice also increase serum GOT activity, but to a lesser extent. Values in excess of 500 units generally denote acute hepatocellular disease, but values below 500 units may be seen in both acute and chronic disorders of the liver and biliary tract. Thus, the serum GOT level may be helpful in distinguishing between acute hepatocellular and obstructive jaundice if it is very high, but is of no differential diagnostic value when it is only slightly or moderately elevated. In acute hepatocellular injury, serum GOT activity often rises sharply before the appearance of jaundice. This is an important point in connection with the early detection of viral hepatitis and drug reactions that affect the liver. Although the serum GOT level is a relatively nonspecific test of hepatocellular function, in that it is affected by so many other disorders, it does provide a relatively sensitive index of the integrity of the hepatic cells. In this way it is useful in following the recovery from hepatic damage.

Because the concentration of *glutamic pyruvic transaminase* (GPT) is higher in the liver than in the myocardium or any other tissue, it has been suggested that the serum level of GPT may be a more specific index of hepatocellular injury than that of GOT. Also it has been reported that the serum level of GPT is more sensitive than that of GOT is an index of acute hepatocellular injury. However, the two values are so closely correlated in most cases of liver disease that there does not appear to be any significant advantage in carrying out both determinations in the routine testing of hepatic function.

OTHER DIAGNOSTIC PROCEDURES

X-ray Studies. A *roentgenogram of the abdomen* may be helpful in estimating the size of the liver and spleen and may be of diagnostic value in demonstrating the presence of cholelithiasis, pancreatic calcification, the increased hepatic density of hemochromatosis, the localized tenting of the diaphragm over an underlying intrahepatic mass, or the intrahepatic calcification of a hemangioma, metastatic carcinoma, or hydatid cyst. Often a *gastrointestinal x-ray* study is useful in establishing the presence of esophageal and gastric varices, enlargement of the pancreatic head by carcinoma or cyst, or other intrinsic lesions that affect the hepatic parenchyma and bile ducts. The *cholecystogram* is of importance in the differential diagnosis of right upper quadrant pain, but its value in the investigation of jaundice is limited by the fact that the gallbladder usually fails to fill in the presence of jaundice. However, it may be possible to demonstrate stones when jaundice is minimal. With *intravenous cholangiography* it is possible to outline not only the gallbladder, but also the cystic, hepatic, and common ducts. This technique is particularly useful in demonstrating the presence of stones and dilatation of the ducts following cholecystectomy. Unfortunately, the lower end of the common duct is poorly visualized, and little or none of the dye is excreted when jaundice is present, so that often the test is valueless in situations where it may be needed most.

Esophagoscopy is far more reliable than the roentgenographic method of detecting esophageal varices, but it is not used as often because of its potential dangers. However, experience has shown that the procedure is relatively safe in the hands of an expert, even when bleeding is present.

Portal Pressure Measurements. A number of indirect methods have been devised for estimating the pressure in the portal vein. These include (1) measurement of the pressure within esophageal varices by means of a needle inserted through an esophagoscope; (2) measurement of the pressure in a small hepatic vein occluded by an open-ended cardiac catheter inserted through an antecubital vein and threaded through the right atrium and inferior vena cava into the liver; (3) measurement of the intrasplenic pressure through a fine needle inserted through the skin.

Transplenic Venography. By injecting radiopaque dyes such as Diodrast into the spleen by the percutaneous route, it is possible to outline the splenic and portal veins and thus demonstrate the presence and location of any obstruction to the outflow of blood. When obstruction is present, the vessels proximal to the block tend to dilate, collateral vessels are visualized, dye refluxes into the tributaries of the portal vein, and the emptying time of the dye-filled veins is increased. The procedure is particularly useful in differentiating between intra- and extrahepatic portal obstruction and thus may be of great assistance to the surgeon who is planning a remedial shunting operation. The objections to the method are that the injection of dye may provoke intraperitoneal bleeding and that the dye may fail to get into the spleen, particularly when the spleen is of normal size. Fortunately, however, there have been no reported fatalities from bleeding, and the accidental injection of dye into the peritoneum appears to be innocuous.

Duodenal Drainage. Occasionally microscopic examination of the spun sediment of aspirated duodenal contents is helpful in the differential diagnosis of jaundice. Calcium bilirubinate and cholesterol crystals usually indicate the presence of gallstones, while the demonstration of tumor cells by the Papanicolaou method may provide conclusive evidence of malignancy in the biliary tract or pancreas. Bacterial cultures are difficult to interpret, since contamination of the aspirating tube is inevitable. However, a heavy growth of enteric organisms may be indicative of infection in the biliary tract. The presence of a large number of polymorphonuclear leukocytes may have the same significance.

Needle Biopsy of the Liver. In many instances of overt or suspected liver disease, thorough clinical and laboratory investigation may fail to disclose the nature of the underlying lesion. Histologic examination of a liver biopsy specimen is often diagnostic in such cases. In addition, the procedure may be helpful in establishing the diagnosis in a number of diseases in which the liver is involved only secondarily. The chief advantages of securing the specimen by means of a needle, rather than by excision through a surgical wound, are that the procedure is simple, can be carried out at the bedside, does not require general anesthesia, and causes the patient little discomfort. Unfortunately, it may give rise to hemorrhage into the peritoneal or pleural cavity, to bile peritonitis, or to perforation of a viscus. The estimated morbidity rate is 1 per cent, and the estimated mortality rate 0.2 to 0.3 per cent, figures that are significantly lower than those for exploratory laparotomy. Certain precautionary measures and skillful technique appear to be important factors in keeping the number of accidents down to a minimum.

The situations in which needle biopsy of the liver have proved most useful include the following: (1) diagnosis of unexplained hepatomegaly, (2) differentiation between obstructive and hepatocellular jaundice, (3) confirmation of suspected cirrhosis, hepatitis, intrahepatic malignancy, hemochromatosis, amyloidosis, sarcoidosis, miliary tuberculosis, and brucellosis, (4) diagnosis of unexplained splenomegaly, (5) differentiation between intra- and extrahepatic portal obstruction, and (6) investigation of the pathogenesis and evolution of the hepatic lesions in viral hepatitis and cirrhosis.

REFERENCES

Billings, B. H., and G. H. Lathe: Bilirubin Metabolism in Jaundice, Am. J. Med., 24:111, 1958.

Dyrenfurth, I., C. H. Stacey, J. C. Beck, and E. H. Venning: Aldosterone Excretion in Patients with Cirrhosis of the Liver, Metabolism, 6:544, 1957.

Hyatt, R. E., and J. R. Smith: The Mechanism of Ascites: A Physiologic Appraisal, Am. J. Med., 16:434, 1954.

Laragh, J. H.: Mechanisms of Edema Formation and Principles of Management, Am. J. Med., 21:423, 1956.

Lloyd, C. W., and R. H. Williams: Endocrine Changes Associated with Laennec's Cirrhosis of the Liver, Am. J. Med., 4:315, 1948.

Nelson, W. P., III, and L. G. Welt: The Effects of Pitressin on the Metabolism and Excretion of Water and Electrolytes in Normal Subjects and Patients with Cirrhosis and Ascites, J. Clin. Invest., 31:392, 1952.

Sherlock, S.: Pathogenesis and Management of Hepatic Coma, Am. J. Med., 24:805, 1958.

Wahi, P. N., and S. Ramachandran: Adrenal Cortical Function in Portal Cirrhosis, A.M.A. Arch. Pathol., 66:482, 1958.

Zamcheck, N.: Needle Biopsy of the Liver: I. Its Use in Clinical and Investigative Medicine. II. The Risk of Needle Biopsy, New Engl. J. Med., 249: 1020, 1062, 1953.

Section 7: Polyuria, Oliguria, Uremia, and Edema

20 DISORDERED RENAL FUNCTION

Charles H. Burnett and Louis G. Welt

The kidneys provide the main channel for excretion, except for carbon dioxide, of metabolic end products and, in addition, selectively excrete normal body solutes and water in quantities sufficiently variable to permit maintenance within quite narrow limits of body fluid with a constant volume and composition. Although the mechanisms by which these functions of excretion and regulation are accomplished are in some instances only partially understood, most of them are ultimately related to the ability of the kidneys to vary widely both volume and solute concentration of the urine. Under appropriate stimuli, urine volume in the normal adult can vary from a few hundred milliliters to over 15 liters daily, and the total solute concentration from less than 50 mOsm to approximately 1,400 mOsm per liter. It should be recalled that

the osmolar concentration defines, the number of osmotically active units in a given volume, whereas the number of milliequivalents, or millimols, refers to concentration only from the standpoint of electrochemical reaction (see Chap. 50 for a full discussion of these points). Variability of excretory ability has also been demonstrated for essentially all urinary solutes. In the presence of normal renal function, maintenance of homeostasis may result in complete absence or marked diminution of some urinary solutes in the interest of conservation by the body; conversely, when required, great excesses are readily excreted. Similarly, urinary volume depends in general upon bodily requirements to reject or conserve water, except where there is a large solute load to be excreted. In the latter circumstance, osmotic diuresis or obligatory water excretion may occur despite inadequate body water (see below). The above considerations are of great importance for a basic understanding of the multiple factors involved in renal impairment and of the manifestations of disorders of the urinary tract.

ANATOMIC CONSIDERATIONS

The primary unit of the kidney is the nephron, of which there are approximately one million in each kidney. The nephron unit includes the glomerulus and its subjoined tubules. Subdivided renal arteries enter the glomerular tuft as the afferent arterioles, to form the glomerular capillaries, which branch and anastomose to emerge as the efferent arterioles, the latter branch again to form intertubular capillaries, which again unite to form finally the renal vein. The capillary endothelial cells of the glomerular vessels are probably separated by a single basement membrane from the endothelial cells of Bowman's capsule, which are continuous with those of the proximal convoluted tubules. Each of these consists of the pars convoluta and the pars recta. The latter forms the first portion of the descending limb of Henle, which changes to the thin limb and is of variable length. The long loops enter deep into the medulla and after making a sharp hairpin curve progress into the thin ascending limbs, which then change to the thick segment of the ascending limbs at the beginning of the area where cortex and medulla join. Short descending limbs have only a thick segment and hence do not enter into the medulla. In the human it is estimated that 85 to 90 per cent of the nephrons have short loops. All ascending loops return to the cortex where they touch their own glomerulus at the macula densa. The distal convolution begins at this point and continues until it joins to form collecting ducts. The latter are in close approximation with the long loops of Henle and with a dense network of intertubular blood vessels, the vasa rectae.

A clear visualization of the normal anatomic relationships is essential to an understanding of the mechanisms of renal function, especially those involved with concentration and dilution of the urine according to the countercurrent hypothesis (see below). Electron microscopy has provided information concerning the finer details of the nephron and vascular structure of the kidneys.

PHYSIOLOGIC CONSIDERATIONS

Urine formation begins with passage of an almost protein-free fluid across the glomerular membrane by a process of ultrafiltration effected by the hydrostatic pressure in the glomerular tuft. The various factors which influence the quantity of this filtrate—the capillary hydrostatic pressure, the oncotic pressure of the plasma, and the permeability of the glomerular membrane—are such that about 20 per cent of the plasma passing through the glomerular tufts is filtered. The ultrafiltrate then undergoes extensive alteration between the glomer-

ulus and the renal pelvis, as a result primarily of selective tubular reabsorption of solutes and water; a few solutes undergo active tubular secretion or transfer to the tubular fluid. Knowledge that the above phenomena do take place has come from a variety of sources but chiefly from micropuncture observations and from insights gained by use of clearance techniques.

Micropuncture Observations, Water Excretion, and Effect of Antidiuretic Hormone (ADH). From sampling of tubular fluids in rats and other mammals it is firmly established that at least two-thirds of the glomerular filtrate is reabsorbed in the proximal tubule. Throughout this process the fluid remaining in the tubule is isoosmotic with vena cava plasma (Fig. 20-1). All experimental data support the concept that active reabsorption of solutes with

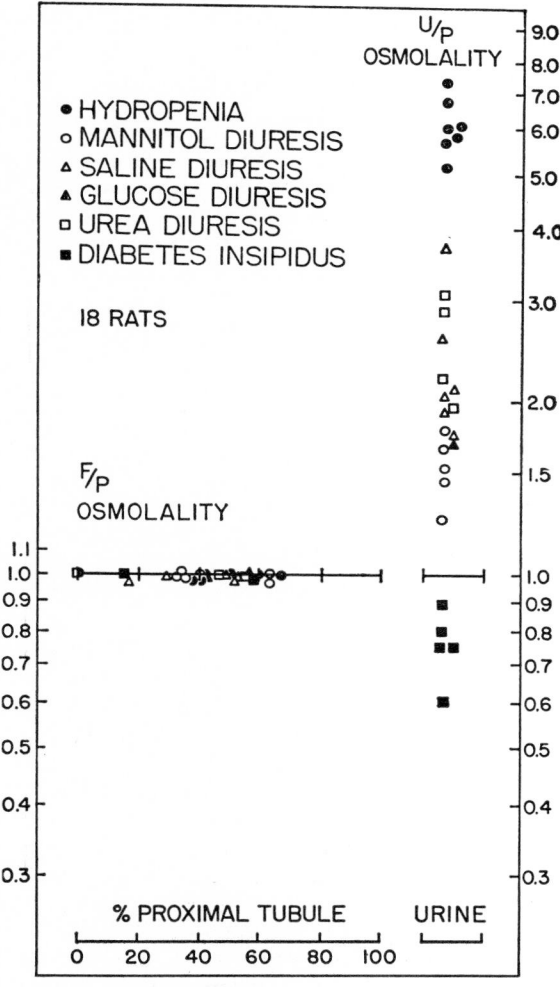

FIG. 20-1. Fluid to plasma osmolalities in proximal convolution under a variety of circumstances, concurrent with urine to plasma osmolalities. (*Carl W. Gottschalk and Margaret Mylle: Am. J. Physiol.,* 196:927, 1959.)

water following passively explains the proximal reabsorption.

Early distal tubular fluid, on the other hand, is hypoosmotic irrespective of final urine concentration. This dilution is an integral feature of the countercurrent multiplier system operating in the medulla. According to this important concept, a *gradual* concentration gradient increasing from cortex to the tip of the medulla is achieved by the following series of events: (1) active outward transport of solute, chiefly sodium and chloride, throughout the *ascending limb;* (2) delivery of hypoosmotic fluid to the distal tubule; (3) increased osmolality of medullary interstitial tissues, which results in (4) diffusion of water out of, and probably sodium, chloride, and urea into, the descending limb, bringing the intratubular fluid into os-

motic equilibrium with the interstitial tissues at any given level and (5) similar events such that adjacent vasa rectae and collecting tubules also come into osmotic equilibrium with the interstitium. Hence, at any given level the fluid in the medullary structures, excepting that in the ascending limb, is in osmotic equilibrium. The difference in osmolality between cortex and medulla is great; the difference between two closely adjacent levels in the medulla is small.

Subsequent alteration in the hypotonic early distal tubular fluid depends largely on the action, or lack of effect if absent, of the antidiuretic hormone (ADH). In the presence of ADH, two events contribute to a final urine which may exceed the osmolality of the plasma by a factor of 4. The presence of this hormone apparently permits diffusion outward of water so that the fluid at the end of the distal convolution is isoosmotic with plasma. It should be emphasized that reabsorption in the distal tubule involves both solutes and water. In this fashion, an isoosmotic fluid which is approximately 7 per cent of the volume of the original glomerular filtrate is presented to the collecting tubules. The latter in the presence of ADH are believed to be freely permeable to water. Since the collecting ducts pass through the hyperosmotic medullary interstitium, concentration of urine results by abstraction of water from collecting tubules (Fig. 20-2). In the absence of ADH the urine does undergo initial concentration in the loop of Henle, but the gradient is not so steep as that occurring in the presence of ADH. Tubular fluid is then diluted in the ascending limb and remains so as it passes through the distal convolution and collecting duct, apparently because these structures are more impermeable to water in the absence of ADH. The result is excretion of a dilute urine.

Glomerular Filtration Rate. Inulin is an example of a substance which permits estimation of glomerular filtration rate (GFR). Inulin is (1) freely filtered at the glomerulus, (2) neither reabsorbed nor secreted by the renal tubules, (3) unaltered by the kidneys, (4) readily analyzed in urine and plasma. Hence, the quantity of inulin which gains access to the urine is identical with the quantity that is filtered per minute. If one knows the quantity excreted per minute, as well as the concentration of inulin in the plasma from which it was filtered, one can calculate the volume of filtrate formed per minute. The following symbols are customarily employed for this calculation:

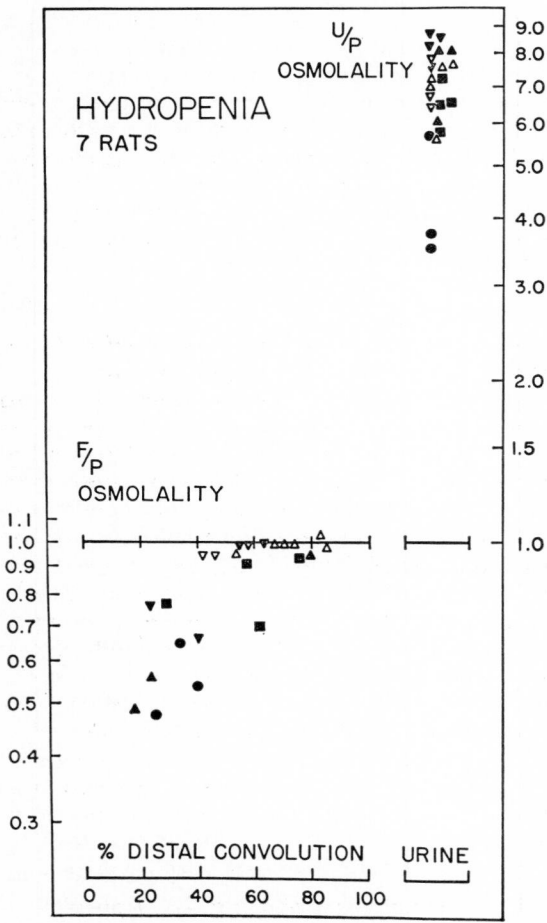

Fig. 20-2. Fluid to plasma osmolalities in distal convolution during maximum antidiuretic hormone activity, as well as concurrent urine to plasma osmolalities. (*Carl W. Gottschalk and Margaret Mylle: Am. J. Physiol.,* 196:927, 1959.)

U_{In} = concentration of inulin per ml of urine

V = rate of excretion of urine in ml/min

P_{In} = concentration of inulin per ml of plasma

Thus, if $U_{In} = 12.5$ mg/ml

$$V = 2 \text{ ml/min}$$

$$P_{In} = 0.25 \text{ mg/ml}$$

then,

$$\text{GFR} = \frac{U_{In}V}{P_{In}} = \frac{12.5 \times 2}{0.25} = 100 \text{ ml/min}$$

This calculation states that 100 ml of plasma water containing 25 mg of inulin was filtered in 1 min and excreted in 2 ml of urine. This formula is also known as the clearance formula and would be designated in this instance as C_{In}. It is an expression used to state the volume of plasma "cleared" of a substance per minute. It can be used only to estimate filtration rate when the test substance has the qualities listed above.

Renal Blood Flow and Tubular Maxima. From the above considerations the general concept of clearance can be stated as follows: clearance represents the smallest quantity of plasma from which the amount of urinary solute (UV) *could* be obtained in unit time. With any substance which is filtered and reabsorbed or filtered and also secreted by the tubules, UV/P becomes in a sense an abstraction unless considered in conjunction with the glomerular filtration rate. The clearance of a substance which is reabsorbed after filtration is less than the glomerular filtration rate, and that of a substance which is filtered and further secreted is greater. If a substance is filtered, reabsorbed, and *also* secreted, the clearance in relation to the glomerular filtration rate may be more or less than the glomerular filtration rate.

One group of foreign substances is very actively and rapidly secreted unchanged by the renal tubules, if administered at rates permitting *low* plasma concentrations. These substances, which include para-aminohippurate (PAH) and Diodrast, are virtually totally removed from the plasma and excreted into the urine during a single circulation through the kidney. The clearance of PAH or Diodrast, then, may be employed to estimate the rate of renal plasma flow. Because some of the plasma traversing the kidney does not come in contact with the tubular excretory system, about 90 per cent rather than 100 per cent is removed, and the clearance is referred to as *effective renal plasma flow*. About 650 ml plasma, or about 1,200 ml whole blood per minute, is estimated (from these methods) to pass through the kidneys.

Complete clearance is no longer effected if the plasma level of the above substances (e.g., PAH) is increased; clearance then no longer represents renal plasma flow. Progressive increments in plasma level eventually result in a saturation point which reflects the *maximal tubular secretory capacity*

(T_m) of that particular substance, and this is usually constant and reproducible for a given individual. Further, average values have been established for normal individuals corrected to a constant body surface area. This value can be readily calculated by the formula:

$$T_{m_{PAH}}\% = U_{PAH}V - fP_{PAH}C_{In}$$

where $U_{PAH}V$ is the urinary excretion of PAH in unit time, fP_{PAH} is that fraction of the plasma concentration which is filtrable at the glomerulus, and C_{In} is the simultaneous glomerular filtration rate. The quantity excreted minus the filtered load is the amount *secreted* and at a maximal level is the $T_{m_{PAH}}$.

The majority of solutes filtered at the glomerulus undergo partial to complete reabsorption. Some, such as glucose, are almost completely reabsorbed under normal conditions and hence are not present in the urine. Others, such as phosphates, undergo reabsorption in varying quantities according to the needs of the organism to conserve or reject them. Complete reabsorption will remove the solute from the urine. The rate of reabsorption of a given solute (T_x) may be estimated by determining the concentrations in the plasma (P_x) and the urine (U_x) of the solute and the simultaneous glomerular filtration rate:

$$T_x = P_xC_{In} - U_xV$$

The quantity reabsorbed is therefore equal to the filtered load minus the quantity excreted.

Maximal tubular reabsorptive capacities can be demonstrated for plasma constituents of low molecular weight which are completely filtered at the glomerulus and undergo partial or complete tubular reabsorption. Glucose, essentially absent from the urine under normal circumstances, is excreted when the amount filtered is increased to the degree that the capacity of proximal convoluted tubules for complete reabsorption is exceeded. The maximal capacity of some tubules to reabsorb glucose is reached earlier than others, which is a reflection of the fact that nephrons represent a varied population and are not all identical one with every other. When the filtered load of glucose is high enough, the capacity to reabsorb glucose is exceeded in all tubules, and a constant maximum quantity is reabsorbed per minute. This is referred to as the T_{m_G}.

A similar maximal transfer or reabsorptive capacity has been demonstrated for a number of other urinary solutes—phosphates, amino acids, and uric acid. For others, especially electrolytes, a maximal transfer has not been clearly defined. It seems clear that, with substances such as sodium and chloride, the quantity reabsorbed varies with the amount filtered and with other more poorly defined factors, such as the volume of body fluid, the amount of other solutes in the tubular fluid, and in some instances hormonal factors.

Solute or Osmotic Diuresis. In addition to the direct influence of ADH on the volume and osmolality of the urine, these parameters are also modified by the quality and the total quantity of solutes excreted. An understanding of the phenomenon of solute or osmotic diuresis is imperative to the interpretation of both normal and disordered renal function and of many clinical problems unassociated with primary renal disorders. The most important solutes normally in body water which affect urine flow and osmolality are urea, sodium chloride, glucose, and occasionally others; any of these substances may produce a solute diuresis. The sequence of events following the administration of a foreign substance such as mannitol which is osmotically active but almost totally unreabsorbable by the renal tubule provides some insight into the mechanism of such a diuresis. Mannitol is confined to the extracellular space, and when administered it will contribute more or less to the total osmolality of the extracellular fluid, depending on the concentration of the solution and the speed with which it is administered. Since mannitol cannot be reabsorbed by renal tubular cells and since the fluid throughout the proximal convolution is isoosmotic with plasma, it is implicit that mannitol must preempt a volume of water, diminish the fraction of filtered water that is reabsorbed, and promote the accession of a larger volume of fluid to that portion of the nephron beyond the proximal convolution. An increase in the rate of flow of fluid through the loop of Henle must diminish the efficiency of the countercurrent multiplier system so that even if the collecting tubular membrane was freely permeable to water (as would be the case in the presence of ADH) the interstitial osmolality would be less hypertonic and the final urine would likewise be less concentrated above the level that is isoosmotic with plasma. As the rate of excretion of mannitol increases (in the presence of ADH) the urine osmolality decreases and approaches that of plasma in an asymptotic fashion.

Furthermore, as mannitol becomes an increasingly prominent urinary solute (and, hence, Na and Cl must be present in ever-decreasing concentrations), the ability to free tubular fluid of solute and, hence, make the urine dilute becomes more and more difficult because the mannitol cannot be reabsorbed. Therefore, even in the *absence* of ADH the urine osmolality will rise from the characteristically low values to those which approach the osmolality of the plasma.

The use of mannitol to explain the phenomenon of solute diuresis is helpful and may be reasonably accepted as similar to the augmented flow of urine which accompanies glycosuria. However, the reader should be cautioned that certain qualities of the solute have importance. For example, reabsorbable solutes such as sodium and chloride behave similarly to mannitol in the presence of ADH, but may be associated with a lower urinary osmolality in the absence of ADH because these ions can be abstracted from tubular fluid. Urea as the loading solute is probably somewhere between glucose and NaCl since it at least is diffusible (and may even be actively transported).

All solutes which can promote an osmotic diuresis (including NaCl) are likely to increase the rate of excretion of salt. This is probably due to the rapid flow of fluid which may diminish the time available for active transport. It may be that this is more relevant at sites beyond the early distal convolution, since Gottschalk and Mylle have noted that the most dilute early distal tubular fluids were obtained when NaCl was the loading solute, suggesting that the increased rate and bulk of flow in the proximal tubule and Henle's loop did not diminish the ability to transport NaCl from the ascending limb of Henle.

Control of Acid-Base Equilibrium. The role of the kidney in maintenance of acid-base equilibrium and the factors influencing pH of the urine are discussed in Chap. 51.

PATHOPHYSIOLOGIC MANIFESTATIONS AND CAUSES OF RENAL INSUFFICIENCY AND RENAL FAILURE

The causes of alterations of renal function may be categorized according to different schemes and points of view. Such classifications include:

1. With respect to discrete alteration of:
   a. Renal blood flow.
   b. Glomerular filtration rate.
   c. Specific tubular excretory and secretory function.
2. From the viewpoints of severity, duration of disease, and prognosis:
   a. Acute renal failure, which may be reversible.
   b. Chronic renal *insufficiency*, which although not reversible may follow a prolonged and essentially benign course before progression to the next stage.
   c. Sudden deterioration of chronic renal insufficiency associated with acute insults such as dehydration, accelerated catabolic reaction, trauma, surgery, etc. Restoration to previous level of renal insufficiency may be possible.
   d. Chronic progressive renal *failure*, which ultimately ends in a fatal outcome.
3. From the viewpoint of specific pathogenesis—glomerulonephritis, pyelonephritis, etc.
4. From a morphologic point of view alone.
5. From the viewpoint which attempts, in the present state of our knowledge, to combine all the above factors into a unitary scheme.

An attempt will be made to follow the last approach in the subsequent discussion. Additional note will be made of some important manifestations of disease which are referable to the urinary tract but which do not reflect primary or intrinsic kidney disease. In patients with impaired renal function, many phases of the clinical state and most of the physiologic and biochemical abnormalities may partially be explained by consideration of the effects of absolute loss of nephrons. Experimental removal of three-quarters or more of renal tissue from an animal results in a state which closely resembles that seen in the human with advanced renal failure. Anatomic evidence suggests that loss of renal mass may be an important factor in humans dying of chronic renal disease. The events occurring in acute but reversible renal failure (e.g., acute tubular necrosis) could be the result of transient but complete inactivation of a large population of nephrons. It is equally possible that essentially all nephrons severely damaged by an acute insult are functioning inadequately in reversible renal failure. From a practical clinical standpoint, it should be recognized that acute reversible renal failure and chronic renal failure ending in a fatal outcome may be so similar that discrimination between the two states is not possible. Loss of renal tissue provides a rational explanation for many of the multiple and apparently bewildering and unrelated abnormalities occurring in renal failure. In addition, many of the observed anatomic and physiologic abnormalities should be interpreted as representing chiefly *compensatory* changes. Hence intelligent treatment of an individual with impaired renal function would include consideration of the possibility that clinical and physiologic deviations from normal may represent for that patient compensatory and, in a sense, desirable circumstances.

The classic dissections of Oliver have provided three-dimensional understanding of the true structural abnormalities in both acute and chronic renal failure. His work suggests the proposal that the physiologic abnormalities in renal failure may be the consequence of nephron destruction. In chronic Bright's disease, the nephrons that do remain undergo tremendous changes. Some are completely atrophied, and some discontinuous; some, however, show hypertrophy and hyperplasia. Only these latter few nephrons can be assumed to be elaborating urine, no matter how inadequate that urine may be in terms of maintaining homeostasis. Many of the abnormal functions of the kidney currently subject to measurement and most of the abnormalities of body water in renal impairment can be explained at least partially by these anatomic findings. Because the degree of destruction of nephrons and the compensatory changes in surviving nephrons

is uneven in respect to glomeruli and to various portions of the tubules, it is to be anticipated that the normal relationships between glomerular filtration and tubular function will be disrupted; this circumstance has been referred to as glomerulotubular imbalance.

It must be emphasized that intrinsic dysfunction of glomerular or tubular function apparently explains certain renal disorders (e.g., nephrotic syndrome, tubular acidosis).

In this discussion the biochemical and physiologic abnormalities of impaired renal function will be described first and subsequently correlated in so far as possible with clinical signs and symptoms of the syndrome commonly referred to as uremia.

Osmolality of Urine. Limitation of capacity to vary the volume and total concentration of the urine, despite variations in solute and water intake, is an almost invariable consequence of any disease of the kidneys which damages or inactivates a significant proportion of nephrons. Experimentally the same phenomenon rapidly occurs after removal of approximately three-quarters of rat kidney tissue.

The explanation for this important phenomenon is not clear. Probably multiple factors are responsible, and the role of specific factors in individual patients must vary. An elevated blood urea, if present, could provide a stimulus for a constant solute diuresis. It has also been proposed that, because relatively few nephrons are functional in renal insufficiency, these remaining nephrons are constantly presented with an unusually large volume of filtrate. The tubules of such nephrons presumably would be unable, despite compensatory changes, to reabsorb sufficient filtrate proximally to prevent delivery of excess fluid distally. The experimental work cited above supports this concept. In such an event a continuing solute diuresis would certainly impose limitations on the ability to concentrate the urine. The ability to elaborate a dilute urine might be preserved a little longer to the extent that distal elements of the nephron could still transport salt from lumenal fluid.

From the knowledge obtained in normal animals from micropuncture studies, it is reasonable to hypothesize that the normal concentrating mechanisms already described are injured by damage to the medullary structures. Potassium deficient uropathies, "water-losing nephritis" associated with multiple myeloma, and obstructive uropathies would almost surely fall into this group.

The widespread anatomic involvement of most chronic nephritides, however, will probably eventually demonstrate that the inability to concentrate the urine is due in varying degrees to all the factors mentioned above and others not yet disclosed.

The relationship of specific gravity to osmolality must be realized. The former is the measurement by which ability to concentrate the urine is routinely made in clinical settings. In most instances it reflects osmolality fairly well. However, since specific gravity is a function of the density or weight of urine per milliliter, and osmolality reflects the number of osmotically active substances in a similar quantity, there may be considerable differences in the two measurements in a given urine. Therefore, the specific gravity may inadequately reflect considerable changes in osmolality. However, from a practical standpoint, careful determination of the urinary specific gravity constitutes one of the most important methods of assessing renal function. Clearly, the finding of a high specific gravity is strong evidence against the presence of renal insufficiency. Conversely, a low specific gravity reflects renal disease only when prior sufficient stimulus for increased concentration has been produced.

Sodium Excretion. The urine of patients with isosthenuria (an inability to either concentrate or dilute the urine) contains sodium in significant quantities. Obligatory excretion of sodium proceeds in renal failure despite extracellular deficits of that cation. In addition to sodium excretion resulting from continuous solute diuresis or from damage to medullary structures, this cation may also be excreted in the urine as a result of impairment of hydrogen ion secretion and other factors contributing to the acidosis of renal insufficiency (see below and Chaps. 51 and 257).

Hyponatremia occurs eventually in practically all patients dying in uremia. Whether the lowered serum sodium concentration results from loss of urinary sodium in excess of water, dilution by retention of water, or whether it represents an asymptomatic hyponatremia is often difficult to assess. Many patients with uremia have heart failure; hyponatremia in patients with heart failure alone is most commonly agreed to result from chronic dilutional hyponatremia. Despite heart failure, however, most patients with uremia can be shown to be excreting significant quantities of sodium in the urine, presumably because of the abnormal renal mechanisms discussed above. The wasting and debilitation so frequently present terminally in uremia may in some patients provoke "asymptomatic" hyponatremia; in the latter, a lowered level of intracellular osmotic activity is suggested (see Chap. 258).

Despite the clear evidence for failure of the kidney in advanced renal failure to conserve salt, it is also well recognized that in renal insufficiency concentration of extracellular sodium may be remarkably well guarded for a long period of time. The fortuitous fact that the average American diet contains abundant salt may protect many patients who on a salt-free diet would develop evidence of sodium deficit.

Water Excretion. Sustained excretion of water per se is a mandatory compensatory phenomenon of renal *insufficiency.* When oliguria or anuria develops, the outcome is inevitably fatal unless urine flow can be restored. The mechanism of anuria or oliguria of acute or chronic renal failure is unclear. Immediately following acute contraction of plasma or interstitial volume, renal blood flow and filtration rate undergo severe reduction. After circulatory dynamics are partially or completely restored, continued oliguria or anuria may be due both to inactivation of large numbers of nephrons and to excessive back diffusion of glomerular filtrate through damaged tubular cells. The latter phenomenon may be the sole cause of oliguria in acute renal failure due to nephrotoxic agents. In chronic renal failure, both progressive destruction or inactivation of nephrons and back diffusion through existing nephrons may eventually terminate urine flow. The renal response to contraction of extracellular fluid volume in the presence of chronic kidney failure is probably even more sensitive than in the normal kidney. Internal renal vasoconstriction promptly decreases an already dangerously low filtration rate.

Renal excretion of large quantities of administered water (and probably also sodium) is, however, also limited as compared with the normal; many hours may be required to excrete a water load, most of which would be rejected within 2 hr by a normal person. This latter phenomenon is probably due to the fact that those nephrons which are forming urine are already doing so to a maximal degree in terms of filtration, reabsorption, and excretion.

Clinical and Therapeutic Implications. There are a number of therapeutic and clinical implications of inability to concentrate the urine and of the defects related to it. Because ability to adjust constant extracellular volume and osmolality is severely compromised, homeostasis is constantly threatened. Renal water and salt excretion proceed despite incipient dehydration. The patient with renal failure in whom urinary specific gravity is most often found to be 1.007 to 1.010 (about 300 mOsm per kg) obligates about four times as much water to excrete a given quantity of solutes as does a normal person, in whom a maximal concentration of 1,400 mOsm per kg is possible. This abnormal urine may contain significant quantities of sodium, despite a sodium deficit in the extracellular compartment. The common clinical observation that a patient with chronic renal insufficiency may deteriorate quickly following an episode of gastroenteritis, fever (and associated accelerated catabolic response), or a surgical procedure is readily understandable on consideration of pathophysiologic facts. Conversely, administration of excessive quantities of salt and water may result in edema, even in the absence of heart failure. Water alone can produce dilutional hyponatremia. The physician is confronted in such a patient with the problem of preventing dehydration on the one hand and edema on the other. Unless gastrointestinal disturbances prevent intake of food and water by mouth, *voluntary ingestion of water which is provoked by the patient's thirst mechanism is usually a far more sensitive indicator than the doctor's judgment.* When parenteral administration of fluid does become necessary, it is probably preferable to err on the side of slight overhydration. Decision as to whether hyponatremia should be corrected should be made by the same criteria that would be applied to any patient with a low serum sodium (see Chap. 50). If the proper criteria are met, no deleterious effects from parenteral hypertonic saline administration need be anticipated; in many instances it may be very beneficial. Salt restriction is considered by some advisable at certain stages in the course of renal insufficiency, chiefly for treatment of concomitant hypertension. In such instances it can be easily determined whether a salt-poor regimen will have adverse effects by comparing the rate of excretion of sodium or chloride to the intake and by remaining constantly alert for clinical evidence of salt depletion. The first evidence of the latter may be development or increase of azotemia.

Proteinuria and Hypoproteinemia. The presence of protein in the urine is an almost constant feature of renal impairment. It was originally noted by Richard Bright, however, that proteinuria is not invariably present. Except in occasional and unusual instances, such as multiple myeloma, the urinary proteins are those normally present in the plasma; albumin, however, predominates. Normally, small quantities of protein are thought to be filtered at the glomerulus and reabsorbed by the renal tubules. Interference with this reabsorptive process could result in significant proteinuria in view of the quantity of the glomerular filtrate without increased permeability of the glomerulus. The bulk of evidence, however, suggests that proteinuria originates from passage of protein into the capsular fluid as a result of changes in the glomerular membrane. Whether changes in the capacity of the tubules to reabsorb this increased quantity of filtered protein modify the total amount of protein excreted in the urine cannot be ascertained by present methods. The causes of the increased glomerular permeability are multiple. Actual glomerular injury due to disease can logically explain pro-

tein in the urine in many instances. Experimental ablation of from two-thirds to three-quarters of renal tissues results in significant and prompt proteinuria; nephron loss or reduction in renal mass alone therefore results in proteinuria. The predominance of albumin is explained by the fact that it is a smaller molecule than globulin.

From a pathophysiologic standpoint, proteinuria assumes importance as it relates to hypoalbuminemia resulting from depletion of body protein and formation of edema (Chaps. 21 and 50). From a diagnostic standpoint the importance of proteinuria can hardly be overestimated, for it is detectable by such simple methods. Proteinuria, on the other hand, is not always indicative of intrinsic renal disease; small amounts may be observed in normal individuals who have remained in an upright position for a considerable period. Such proteinuria may be quite intense in some individuals (orthostatic albuminuria). In normal persons following vigorous exercise some protein appears in the urine. Many febrile states are accompanied by proteinuria; and it is regularly present during congestive heart failure. Large numbers of leukocytes or erythrocytes may be interpreted as true proteinuria, unless the supernatant is tested after centrifuging the urine. The absence of casts in such urines also helps to exclude intrinsic renal disease. All the above conditions should be excluded before concluding that the presence of proteinuria reflects a significant renal lesion. The absolute quantity of protein lost in the urine varies from less than a gram daily to as much as 50 Gm. Quantities in excess of 2 to 3 Gm daily are rarely seen except in the nephrotic syndrome. The origin of urinary protein in this baffling syndrome is discussed elsewhere (Chap. 258).

Formed Elements in the Urine. Urinary cast formation (cylindruria) results from precipitation of protein in the tubular lumina. Hyaline casts reflect simply coagulated protein, which is present in small amounts in the normal glomerular filtrate; these casts therefore are seen in urine from normal persons. Desquamated tubular epithelium, leukocytes, and erythrocytes combine with tubular protein to form epithelial, white cell, or red cell casts. Combinations of all the above types may appear in a single cast; secondary changes produce granular, fatty, and waxy casts. Assessment of the significance of cylindruria must take into consideration (1) the total number and types of casts present and (2) the pH of the urine. Since the isoelectric point of proteins forming the matrix of casts is well on the acid side, they may be dissolved by an alkaline urine. The latter may be present on voiding; more frequently, urine becomes rapidly alkaline on standing, because of bacterial contamination which converts urea to ammonia. *A fresh urine is the only urine which regularly provides accurate information regarding cylindruria.* Hematuria, or free red cells in the urine, results from either passage of erythrocytes through the glomerular membrane or bleeding in any portion of the urinary tract. Hemoglobinuria should always be distinguished from hematuria. In the former, no erythrocytes are present in the urine. Hemoglobinuria originates from glomerular filtration of increased quantities of this substance in the blood stream; hemolysis of red blood cells may also occur in the bladder if the urine is extremely hypotonic. Leukocytes and bacteria may originate in any portion of the urinary tract, as a result of inflammation and infection. If a lower urinary tract source can be excluded, leukocytes and bacteria may be the chief or only clue to the presence of pyelonephritis, and the presence of white cell casts would provide further discrimination from other types of kidney disease. Caution should be exercised in interpreting the urine of a female, unless it is a catheterized specimen, or unless special care has been taken to provide a voided specimen uncontaminated by vaginal secretions.

Azotemia and Excretion of Urea. Historically, the first blood abnormality to be demonstrated in patients with renal failure was an increased concentration of urea. Hence the term *uremia* has, by usage, come to represent the entire clinical and pathophysiologic syndrome resulting from failure of kidney function. It has yet to be proved that elevation of blood urea concentration per se has any immediate harmful effects, although there is some evidence that such is the case. Urea is freely diffusible across most cell membranes and is therefore freely filtered at the glomerulus. Since a variable proportion diffuses back through tubular cells, urea clearance is less than that of inulin. There is good evidence that urea is in some way involved in the concentrating process in that it increases in concentration in the medulla. Former concepts of passive back-diffusion of urea must be reassessed in the light of newer knowledge. There is some inconclusive evidence that urea may undergo active transport in some portions of the nephron.

From a clinical standpoint, however, excretion of urea is determined largely by the rate of glomerular filtration. The renal capacity for urea excretion is such that approximately 50 per cent of the normal total number of functioning nephrons must be inactivated, and hence filtration rate must be reduced by 50 per cent, before significant increase in blood urea nitrogen (BUN) occurs.

If one assumes that a constant percentage of the filtered urea is excreted, then the rate of excretion of urea is determined by the plasma urea concentration and the glomerular filtration rate. The above relationship has a number of clinical and physiologic implications. (1) In the presence of severe diminution of glomerular filtration rate, elevation of the concentration of urea in the blood provides the adjustment by which total urea from body catabolism can be excreted. As filtration rate progressively falls with progression of disease, blood urea concentration correspondingly rises. Azotemia therefore is inevitable in renal failure and is compensatory in the sense that it provides a means for excreting the same daily load of urea despite the handicap of an inadequate filtration rate. (2) If the filtration rate is normal, increased excretion of urea can be accomplished by modest increments of plasma urea, whereas in the presence of marked diminution in filtration rate a comparable increase in urea excretion may require a very large increase in plasma urea concentration. (3) A physiologic implication of renal excretion of urea may be demonstrated as follows: a patient with kidney disease and a filtration rate one-third of normal— 60 liters per day—may have no azotemia. The BUN could be normal in such a patient if a small load of urea was presented for filtration, because endogenous intake of protein and catabolism were minimal. An increase in either of the latter factors could promptly result in azotemia but would not necessarily reflect deterioration of renal function. Similarly, drastic curtailment of protein intake in the presence of severe azotemia can effect significant decreases in blood urea nitrogen without improvement in the primary renal impairment. (4) A final implication is that any significant degree of azotemia may contribute to production of solute diuresis. Consequently, urine flow may be presumed to be maximal, a circumstance which in normal persons also results in maximal excretion of urea. If the above statement is true, it follows that urea excretion in renal failure is probably accomplished in the most efficient manner possible under the liability of severe reduction of glomerular filtration rate.

Excretion of some of the other nitrogenous end products, which are included in the total nonprotein nitrogen of the blood, follows the same general patterns as does excretion of urea. The mechanism of excretion of creatinine differs in that endogenous creatinine, in health, is not reabsorbed nor does it back-diffuse; further, catabolism of it proceeds at a relatively constant rate. Consequently, the level of serum creatinine varies more directly with filtration rate and is not influenced by protein intake. Uric acid, unlike urea and creatinine, undergoes tubular reabsorption; hyperuricemia nevertheless frequently occurs in uremia.

Abnormalities of Excretion of Phosphate, Sulfate, and Calcium, and Effects on the Extracellular Fluid. Serum concentration of phosphate and sulfate in most instances of renal failure increases as progressive decrements of glomerular filtration rate occur. Elevation of these anions in the extracellular fluid, in addition to possible deleterious effects from increased serum levels per se, initiates a number of pathophysiologic adjustments.

Acidosis. As is true of azotemia, hyperphosphatemia is directly related to a low glomerular filtration rate. Normally, phosphate is reabsorbed by the renal tubules, and maximal reabsorptive capacities can be defined. There is good evidence that, below a critical level of filtration rate of about 25 ml per min, reabsorption of phosphate is limited or absent. At even lower filtration rates, phosphate filtered is quantitatively transferred to urine, but extracellular phosphate increases. The same general relationships discussed above probably apply to sulfate excretion. Increased concentrations of plasma phosphate and sulfate in persons with uremia and severe renal failure usually accompany metabolic acidosis. The implications of this phenomenon are discussed in Chap. 51. In rare types of kidney disease hypophosphatemia may occur; such disorders represent specific tubular functional or anatomic defects as opposed to over-all reduction of or damage to total renal mass. (See Chap. 51 for further discussion of metabolic acidosis and calcium and phosphate metabolism in renal insufficiency.)

Calcium. The well-known but poorly understood reciprocal relationship between serum calcium and phosphorus concentration explains the characteristic *hypocalcemia* of renal failure. As serum phosphorus rises, serum calcium falls. The secondary effects of the above changes on the parathyroid glands and bone are discussed elsewhere (Chap. 77). Hypercalcemia rarely occurs in renal failure unless extrarenal factors are responsible, at least initially, for increased concentration of this cation in the extracellular fluid. The possible effects of hypercalcemia and hypercalcuria on the kidneys are discussed below.

Abnormalities of Potassium. Abnormalities in urinary potassium excretion and consequently in body potassium in impaired renal function are common. The serum potassium level may be high, low, or normal. Hyperpotassemia is most important and most frequent. It is almost always present at some time during the terminal stages of chronic Bright's disease (see also Chap. 50). In general, accumulation of this cation is associated with severe oliguria or anuria, but the former view that it cannot occur with an adequate urine flow is incorrect. The dangers and the therapeutic management of this feature of renal failure are well recognized (see Chap. 258). Hypopotassemia is most likely to occur in renal failure when intake of the cation is curtailed, extrarenal losses occur, and parenteral fluids containing glucose and sodium are administered. The abnormal renal mechanisms producing

hyper- or hypopotassemia are unclear. Ability to vary the urinary concentration of potassium appears quite clearly to be limited in renal failure. Hyperpotassemia would be expected where an excessive load was presented to a kidney in which ability to vary both concentration of potassium and volume of urine was limited. Similarly, potassium deficits would be anticipated in the presence of inadequate potassium intake because of limited renal conservation. Increased excretion of sodium by either a normal or an impaired kidney increases that of potassium, presumably by augmenting exchange with the latter by the renal tubule. Potassium depletion per se has been demonstrated to have both functional and anatomic renal effects in normal persons. Concentrating power of the urine is diminished, and the kidney is less responsive to ADH; a renal lesion is demonstrable which appears to be chiefly in the collecting tubule (in the rat).

ALTERATIONS IN THE VOLUME OR DIURNAL FLOW OF URINE

Polyuria. The wide variation possible in daily volume of urine and the mechanisms controlling the rate of urine flow have been discussed. In a person with normal renal function, polyuria may result either from inhibition of secretion of ADH or as a result of the necessity to excrete large quantities of solutes. In diabetes insipidus, lesions in the supraoptic and neurohypophyseal areas result in partial or total failure to produce ADH. Excessive volumes—as much as 20 liters daily—of a highly dilute urine are excreted, because of failure of the tubules selectively to abstract water. A hereditary nephrogenic diabetes insipidus has been described in which renal tubular cells fail to respond to ADH. In a normal person, ingestion of large quantities of water suppresses secretion of ADH; polyuria of a degree approaching that seen in true diabetes insipidus ensues. Prolonged and persistent excessive drinking of water may be ascribed to psychogenic factors; this condition has somewhat inappropriately been referred to as *psychogenic diabetes insipidus*. In addition, there are centers in the central nervous system which determine or modify the sense of thirst. Lesions in these areas could result in a condition in which primacy would be assigned to polydipsia and which should be differentiated from diabetes insipidus and from excessive water intake caused by psychogenic factors.

The necessity to excrete large quantities of urine in solute diuresis has been discussed; it is the cause of polyuria in diabetes mellitus. Patients receiving parenteral hypertonic solutions or tube feedings which produce a high solute excretion may develop similar polyuria, which if misinterpreted may result in serious consequences to the patients.

The polyuria of renal insufficiency has been discussed.

Oliguria and Anuria. Diminished urine volume most commonly is due to increased renal tubular reabsorption of water resulting from action of ADH; urine concentration is maximal. This type of oliguria permits compensatory conservation of water subsequent to water deficits from either decreased intake or increased loss through the skin, gastrointestinal tract, lungs, or urine. Oliguria also regularly occurs following contraction of extracellular volume from any cause; edema states are included in this group (see Chaps. 21 and 50). Multiple renal adjustments—decreased blood flow, decreased glomerular filtration rate, and increased tubular reabsorption of salt and water—all participate in the production of oliguria associated with dehydration or hypovolemia. The oliguria and anuria occurring in renal failure have been discussed. *Obstruction of any portion of the urinary tract must be excluded in any patient in whom oliguria or anuria is present.* The causes of such obstruction are discussed elsewhere (Chap. 258). The importance of prompt recognition of the causes of obstruction needs reemphasis, since most causes are remediable if recognized early enough.

Nocturia. Diurnal rhythm in renal function results in elaboration of sufficiently small quantities of urine at night so that healthy persons are not usually awakened to void. Any circumstances which oppose this normal adjustment, including all the causes of polyuria enumerated above, may produce nocturia. In the presence of renal insufficiency, the total daily urine volume is not necessarily excessive. Maximal concentration of urine in such a patient, however, is impossible, and rejection of excess water is delayed. Daily excretion of total water and solutes can be accomplished only by maintaining essentially the same minute volume and concentration throughout the 24 hr. Diurnal rhythm may actually be reversed in many diseases associated with generalized edema (Chap. 21); it is also reversed in adrenal insufficiency. Dysuria causes nocturia, because irritative stimuli arouse the patient often many times nightly to void small amounts of urine. The nocturia of renal insufficiency usually awakens the patient only once or twice, to void relatively copious quantities of urine.

DISORDERS OF URINATION

Dysuria. Difficult or painful urination is a common symptom; it is almost always associated with inflammation resulting from infectious or mechanical irritation of the lower ureters, bladder, or urethra. Infection or inflammation in the kidneys alone does not cause dysuria. However, since cystitis is frequently associated with intrarenal in-fection, the presence of dysuria may provide the clue leading to the important diagnosis of pyelonephritis. Dysuria frequently accompanies obstructive lesions in any portion of the lower urinary tract.

Frequency of Urination. Dysuria usually includes frequent urination. Recurrent passage of urine at short intervals is common in anxiety. Clear discrimination should be made between frequency where only small amounts of urine are voided and that due to polyuria and production of large quantities of urine.

Hesitancy. Difficulty in initiating and terminating urination, and subsequent dribbling of urine, commonly accompany dysuria. Obstructive lesions, especially those due to benign prostatic hypertrophy, are the most important causes of these symptoms. Difficulty in starting urination may be psychologic in origin.

Urinary Incontinence. Involuntary passage of urine in adults is seen most commonly associated with widespread spinal cord disease, in obstructive lesions of the lower urinary tract, in prolapse of the bladder in the female, during senility, during generalized seizures, and in coma. It is normal in infants but may persist for many years, manifested by enuresis. Severe fright may produce incontinence.

OTHER MANIFESTATIONS OF DISORDERS OF THE KIDNEY AND URINARY TRACT

Other important manifestations associated in varying degree with impaired renal function are discussed elsewhere:

1. Hypertension (Chap. 245)
2. Edema (Chap. 21)
3. Alterations in fluid and electrolyte balance (Chap. 50)
4. Alterations in acid-base equilibrium (Chap. 51)
5. Alterations in hematopoietic system (Chaps. 235 and 244)

MANIFESTATIONS OF ALTERATIONS IN THE COLLOIDAL STATE AND SOLUTE SATURATION IN THE URINE

The urine of healthy persons is usually a highly saturated complex solution, containing various organic constituents (urea, uric acid and its salts, etc.) and electrolytes. The reasons why these solutes remain in solution at a much higher concentration than would be predicted from individual solubilities of each in water are multiple and only partially understood. Some reasons which have been proposed include:

1. Protective colloids are present in the urine of normal persons. These colloids by forming a gel

keep crystalloids capable of stone formation in solution.

2. Urinary citrate decreases the degree of supersaturation of calcium in urine by forming undissociated calcium complexes. Citrate excretion increases as urinary pH rises, following administration of vitamin D and parathyroid extract and in other conditions associated with hypercalcemia. Thus, in the presence of cation excess, especially of calcium, citrates may provide a buffer mechanism analogous to titratable acidity and ammonia formation in acidosis.

3. The absence of contact of urine in the urinary passages with a nidus which initiates and acts as a focus for precipitation may also prevent crystallization.

Causes of Stone Formation and Nephrocalcinosis. Despite the above-mentioned mechanisms permitting excretion of a supersaturated urine, crystallization does frequently occur. Such precipitation results usually only in excretion of finely dispersed particles in the urine which may, in most instances, be readily identified in the sediment. Of those solutes for which the urine of average composition may be supersaturated, those in Table 20-1 are most important.

Presence of precipitated solutes in the urinary passages may, however, result in stone formation. Explanation for calculus formation is highly controversial. There is growing evidence that diminution or absence of colloids which increase ability to maintain supersaturated urinary crystalloids in solution is an important factor in calculus formation. The increase in the colloid state of the urine following administration of hyaluronidase is the basis for use of this substance as a means of preventing nephrolithiasis.

Hypercalcuria unquestionably contributes to stone formation; urinary calcium excretion varies with the dietary intake; hypercalcuria accompanies vitamin D administration, usually accompanies hypercalcemia from any cause, and is present in circumstances where calcium is mobilized rapidly from bone without production of hypercalcemia (e.g., acute osteoporosis resulting from immobilization, and Cushing's syndrome). On the other hand, it must be conceded (1) that of the total number of calcium stones encountered clinically, a significant,

and perhaps major, proportion are not accompanied by hypercalcuria, and (2) that many patients may have prolonged hypercalcuria without stone formation. However, the importance of defining the reasons for the fact that calcium is the primary component of the great majority of urinary calculi cannot be dismissed.

Decrease in urinary citrate excretion also predisposes to precipitation of calcium. Such a decrease has been reported in patients with renal tubular acidosis, a syndrome usually accompanied by nephrocalcinosis or nephrolithiasis. Experimental and clinical evidence indicates that intratubular precipitation of calcium under such circumstances may start in the distal portions of the proximal convoluted tubule and the first portion of the straight segment; the calcium casts may be demonstrated in the corticomedullary areas of the kidney. Carbonic anhydrase inhibitors decrease citrate and therefore increase excretion of ionized calcium, despite the fact that they increase urinary pH. The relationship of this latter effect to that already described for sodium, hydrogen, and potassium (see also Chap. 51) is conjectural. It should be further emphasized that the paucity of knowledge concerning normal mechanisms of calcium excretion renders accurate pathophysiologic correlations impossible.

In addition to the influence of hypercalcuria on calculus formation, there is considerable evidence, part of which has been cited above, that prolonged hypercalcuria associated with both intratubular and intrarenal calcification (nephrocalcinosis) results ultimately in renal failure. This type of uremia should be sharply separated or distinguished from other types of renal failure already discussed, including pyelonephritis, which is an almost inevitable sequel to persistent nephrolithiasis.

Infection in the urinary tract is commonly cited as a means for providing a primary nidus which permits precipitation, but in many instances of nephrolithiasis urine is initially sterile. Possibly of more importance than the primary nidus theory, if previous infection has occurred, is the evidence that certain species of bacteria may destroy urinary glucuronides. The latter substances markedly increase solubility of calcium and phosphate; they are excreted following salicylate administration. This latter fact provides a rationale for prolonged administration of salicylates for prevention of recurrence of calculus formation. Any condition leading to stasis and obstruction of urine flow favors infection and quite probably allows time for excessive precipitation on foci where crystallization has already started.

The pH of the urine influences stone formation. Mixed phosphate and calcium carbonate stones are more readily formed in an alkaline environment. Infection with bacteria which split urea to ammonia,

Table 20-1

Solute	Urine is supersaturated
Calcium acid phosphate	Above pH 5.3
Magnesium ammonium phosphate	Above pH 6.2
Uric acid	Below pH 6.0
Sodium or ammonium urate	From pH 4.6 to pH 9.0
Calcium oxalate	Above pH 4.0

forming a highly alkaline urine, is important in this respect. One of the most common types of stone encountered, calcium oxalate, is not affected by pH. Uric acid and cysteine stones are more readily formed in an acid urine. The latter are readily diagnosed and are probably much more frequent than appreciated (see Chap. 88).

A dilute urine is less likely to undergo precipitation. However, in some complex solutions, dilution may actually decrease the solubility of some of its components.

Calcium oxalate stones occasionally occur in patients with a disorder of metabolism in which large amounts of oxalates are formed—oxaluria. Usually, there is no oxaluria. Excretion of excessive quantities of phosphate favors calcium lithiasis; phosphaturia usually accompanies hypercalcuria and is influenced by diet and numerous other factors which alter bone and protein metabolism.

On the basis of the foregoing considerations, some general principles of management of nephrolithiasis can be stated: (1) Causes for stone formation should be vigorously investigated. Although too frequently the etiology of nephrolithiasis cannot be elucidated, the occasional gratifying cures in disorders such as hyperparathyroidism warrant extensive investigation. A corollary of the principle is that the composition of the stones should ideally always be determined. Knowledge of the type of stone provides clues to diagnosis, prognosis, and therapy. (2) The vast majority of calculi will result eventually in infection and pyelonephritis. Surgical removal, therefore, remains the first line of defense. (3) Attempts at dissolution of renal stones by retrograde solutions, although extensively tried, have not been successful. Dissolution of calcium stones by acidifying agents, such as ammonium chloride, is not warranted. (4) If infection exists with a ureasplitting organism (e.g., *Proteus vulgaris*), the urine is likely to be continuously more alkaline, owing to the production of ammonia from urea by the infecting organism. The constantly alkaline medium surrounding the stone promotes further deposition of calcium salts. (5) Very encouraging results, on the other hand, have been observed following large fluid intake and sufficient alkali to alkalinize the urine continuously in cysteine and uric acid stones. (6) Attempts should be made to prevent recurrence, if the stone can be removed surgically, or to minimize further stone formation if surgical management is impossible. Measures directed toward this aim include a large water intake, in the hope of increasing solubility in the urine and tubular fluid; a low calcium intake if the stone contains this cation; alkalinization for uric acid and cysteine stones. (7) Substances which increase the colloid state of the urine (hyaluronidase and salicylates) may be of value, though this is still unproved. (8) Vigorous treatment of any concomitant infection should be instituted. (9) Any obstruction present in any part of the urinary tract should be relieved.

CLINICAL MANIFESTATIONS OF IMPAIRED RENAL FUNCTION— UREMIA

The term *uremia* is commonly applied to the syndrome resulting from failure of kidney function; the manifestations are protean. Many clinical characteristics can be correlated readily with the profound changes, already discussed, in body water known to result from damage to the kidneys. Explanation for other well-recognized signs and symptoms remains undefined.

A sharper definition of uremia is possible if a separation is made between some features previously considered as integral and invariable accompaniments of uremia. The most important differentiation concerns the manifestations of vascular disease. These include hypertensive encephalopathy and other central nervous system sequelae of hypertension, retinitis, and heart failure. The vascular components, rather than renal failure, are presumably the major factors in eclampsia and acute glomerulonephritis. In terminal Bright's disease a clear separation of vascular factors from other manifestations of deteriorating renal functions may be extremely difficult. Whether a primary renal disorder may be responsible for hypertension is not germane to this discussion (see Chap. 245). Uremia may include any manifestations of hypertension, whether the latter preceded renal impairment, or whether a kidney disorder presumably initiated hypertension. The well-documented fact that patients with renal disease occasionally succumb without ever developing hypertension and vascular disease provides strong evidence that hypertension is not a prerequisite for uremia.

Circulatory insufficiency resulting from impaired cardiac function or decreased intravascular volume from hemorrhage, dehydration, or other causes produces prompt and extensive hemodynamic changes including decrease in renal blood flow and glomerular filtration rate (see Chap. 50). Azotemia ensues but is readily reversed if prompt correction of factors producing the hemodynamic changes is achieved. Although by strict definition such circumstances produce uremia, sharp separation from the syndrome under discussion should be made. If the hemodynamic factors persist long enough, they produce tubular necrosis and acute renal failure (see Chap. 257). Azotemia resulting from circulatory changes of the type mentioned above may occur under any circumstances which produces dehydration, from hemorrhage, in severe infections with circulatory failure, and during the course of congestive heart failure. Actual renal disease may accompany any of the above disorders, in which case demonstration of underlying renal disease may be difficult; it is usually possible by making appropriate clinical and laboratory observations.

It has been stated that it may be difficult to correlate known pathophysiologic events which occur in renal failure with many of the clinical features encountered in the patient with uremia. On the other hand, consideration of the probable effects on the patient of the biochemical and physiologic changes accompanying renal failure provides a rational explanation for many clinical features and therefore for a therapeutic approach. Thus the inability to concentrate the urine and to regulate the excretion of sodium and potassium partially explains the frequent occurrence of dehydration and of sodium and potassium abnormalities in the plasma and of the clinical manifestations of these abnormalities. Inability to excrete water or salt loads rapidly may also be responsible for some instances of edema in the absence of heart failure or hypoproteinemia. The retention of phosphorus contributes to the hypocalcemia, with its usual consequences. The impairment of hydrogen ion secretion, with deficit of titratable acidity and ammonia excretion, further accentuates the acidosis. Limitation of potassium secretion presumably results in hyperpotassemia; the latter is further accentuated by hyponatremia, possibly because exchange of sodium and potassium is compromised by the sodium deficit. Hypocalcemia subsequent chiefly to hyperphosphatemia plays a part in central nervous system manifestations. Disorders of bones, when present, are related to both the acidosis and to abnormalities of calcium and phosphorus metabolism. Abnormalities of potassium, sodium, and calcium all contribute to cardiotoxic disturbances which often constitute the greatest single threat to the patient's life. The anemia (Chap. 23) is frequently responsible for the majority of symptoms, especially during the early stages of chronic renal disease. Symptoms and signs deriving from the concomitant vascular disease have been mentioned.

The above considerations assume practical therapeutic importance. Treatment of renal insufficiency or renal failure implies thoughtful consideration of several interrelated questions: (1) Should demonstrable deficiencies be corrected (e.g., hyponatremia, hypocalcemia, lowered CO_2 content of the plasma, anemia)? (2) Should attempts be made to reverse or prevent further accumulations of substances present in excessive quantities in the plasma (e.g., azotemia, hyperpotassemia, hyperphosphatemia)? (3) How is any one individual abnormality related to others (e.g., hypocalcemia and hyper-phosphatemia, hyperpotassemia and hyponatremia)? (4) To what extent will therapeutically induced changes of one abnormality or a group of them interfere with compensatory mechanisms which have resulted from renal damage or destruction? Such treatment could have a deleterious effect (e.g., production of tetany by overenthusiastic correction of acidosis in the presence of hypocalcemia).

From a clinical and therapeutic standpoint, acute and chronic renal failure must be distinguished as causes of uremia. The specific diseases and disorders leading to both types are discussed elsewhere (Chap. 258). Acute and chronic renal failure may on occasion be very difficult to distinguish, for the pathophysiology and clinical characteristics are quite similar; nevertheless this important differentiation can usually be made. One important difference between the two types is exemplified by the severity of symptoms in acute renal failure; the entire response of the patient may be more dramatic and the prognosis poorer than in the patient with a comparable degree of impairment which has developed slowly. An individual with acute tubular necrosis may die with an aggregate of abnormalities (azotemia, acidosis, anemia, etc.), while an individual with the same laboratory findings in whom renal failure has slowly developed may be active and working. It should be clear, however, that the severity of the disease in acute renal failure may also be conditioned by the disorder primarily responsible for renal failure.

Although it is desirable to ascertain the nature of the primary kidney disorder which has ultimately resulted in renal failure, such discrimination is often of doubtful validity even on postmortem examination. The most common precursors of chronic renal failure are probably pyelonephritis, glomerulonephritis and nephrosclerosis, and obstructive uropathies in which pyelonephritis almost always is concomitantly present (see also Chap. 258).

Despite the frequency of renal disease and the predictability of features which in combination are highly suggestive of renal failure or impairment, the primacy of kidney disease may initially not be recognized; one of the protean manifestations of the syndrome may be misinterpreted and treated as an entity. For example, it is not uncommon for patients with uremia to be diagnosed as having primarily gastrointestinal disease.

The diverse manifestations of uremia were first clearly described by Richard Bright in 1827. Despite correlations mentioned above, many features of renal failure remain inexplicable.

Skin. The skin of patients with chronic and advanced renal failure may show a yellowish-brown discoloration (*café au lait*). The cause of this pigment is not positively known. Extreme pallor resulting from anemia accentuates this discoloration.

Pruritus of a severe degree is common. The itching and resultant scratching frequently cause excoriations. Furunculosis and infection of the skin are common. Purpura is quite prevalent in uremia; increased capillary permeability has been postulated but not proved as the cause. Eventually, after prolonged and severe azotemia, crystals, presumably of urea and called *urea frost,* may be visible on the skin.

Hematopoietic System. Severe normochromic and normocytic anemia is an almost invariable feature of uremia. Both depression of erythropoiesis and an intracorpuscular hemolytic component are thought to be responsible (Chap. 23).

Circulatory System. Although heart failure is common in renal failure, it can usually be ascribed to hypertension; as already discussed, the latter is not an invariable feature of uremia. Vascular retinopathy is usually absent in those patients who have no hypertension. Directly related to renal failure is the frequency of cardiac disorders resulting from abnormalities of extracellular or intracellular concentrations of potassium, calcium, and sodium. Calcium, sodium, and digitalis antagonize the cardiotoxic effects of hyperpotassemia. Conversely, in hypopotassemia, susceptibility to digitalis is increased. Since calcium and digitalis are additive in this respect, simultaneous administration of these substances can be quite dangerous in the patient who is simultaneously hypocalcemic and hypopotassemic.

Pericarditis occurs with great frequency in terminal renal failure; its appearance, therefore, is of grave import. Although it is usually painless, an occasional patient may suffer pain of such severity that coronary infarction or dissecting aneurysm must be considered. The mechanism of the pericarditis is entirely unknown.

Respiratory System. Kussmaul breathing (deep sighing respirations with only slight tachypnea) is frequently present, associated with the metabolic acidosis. Cheyne-Stokes respirations are not uncommon; slow, stertorous respirations coexist with increased intracranial pressure which is the consequence of hypertension. The rapid, labored breathing of heart failure, which is frequently present, is often seen in combination with the above types of respiratory abnormality. Roentgenographically, extensive fluffy shadows extending out for a short distance from the hilus of each lung have been demonstrated in patients with uremia but with few pulmonary symptoms. It is highly questionable whether this picture is specific for uremia and more likely that it is not any different from the usual findings in pulmonary edema.

Gastrointestinal Symptoms. Complaints referable to the gastrointestinal tract are among the most prominent and, to the patient, often the most dis-

tressing features of uremia. They vary from moderate anorexia to intractable nausea and vomiting. Diarrhea may be a troublesome feature. Hiccups are common. Ulcerative lesions of all portions of the gastrointestinal tract, especially in the mouth, add to the patient's discomfort and to the therapeutic problem. An apparent achlorhydria may actually be due to neutralization of hydrochloric acid by ammonia which has been converted from excessive amounts of urea in the gastric secretions. Excessive bleeding from the mucous membranes of the nasopharynx, the stomach, and the small or large bowel is a common terminal complication. At postmortem examination, ecchymosis or frank necrosis and ulceration may be demonstrated ("uremic colitis"). Dehydration and acidosis seem to accentuate many of the gastrointestinal symptoms, because correction of these abnormalities may provide temporary relief. It is nonetheless unfortunately true that understanding of the cause of the gastrointestinal symptoms and lesions is completely inadequate. Treatment of them is palliative and symptomatic at best.

Nervous System. Renal failure is associated with profound symptoms referable to both the peripheral and the central nervous systems; manifestations of both irritation and depression may coexist. Peripheral nerve involvement is intimated by complaints of tenderness and pain suggesting peripheral neuritis; yet objective evidence of the latter is usually absent. Central nervous symptoms usually first express themselves in the form of mental irritability; in time muscular twitchings appear. Although irritable, the patient is obtunded and tends to become drowsy; at this stage, however, he can be roused easily and he sleeps poorly. A variety of neurologic signs suggesting local lesions may be observed. The twitchings increase, generalized seizures appear, and coma sets in. Frequently, in this manner and indeed with little change since Richard Bright made his original observations, "the painful history of the disease is closed."

Localized brain lesions resulting from vascular disease may be demonstrated at necropsy, if hypertension was concomitant, but as often no anatomic lesions can be demonstrated which could explain the widespread nature of the neurologic signs during life. Some of the known pathophysiologic features of uremia can partially explain the nervous manifestations. The irritative phenomena can in part be ascribed to hypocalcemia and tetany. Dehydration and acidosis have profound effects on the central nervous system, although the nature of these effects is not clear. The majority of manifestations of renal failure on the nervous system at the present time can be given only the unsatisfactory explanation that they must in some unknown manner be the results of the multiple chemical abnormalities resulting from failure of kidney function.

CONCLUSIONS

Understanding of disorders of the kidney and urinary tract is greatly enhanced by consideration of current views of pathophysiologic mechanisms and of compensatory changes resulting from renal disease and destruction of large numbers of nephrons; such an approach is helpful in planning rational therapy. On the other hand, as Oliver has pointed out, the anatomic changes in patients dying of chronic renal insufficiency are incredibly extensive; inadequate attempts at compensation have resulted in a structure which can no longer be viewed as a kidney. Further, great as have been the advances in knowledge of normal renal physiology, great gaps still exist. It is clear that successful therapy of renal failure must await methods for early prevention or modification of changes brought about by glomerulonephritis, pyelonephritis, and nephrosclerosis, to name the most important. At the moment, the practical importance of differentiating those few conditions which may be reversible, for example, acute tubular necrosis and obstructive uropathies, is clear. Further, the importance of preventing if possible by active and persistent antibiotic therapy the one disease which accounts for a large percentage of patients with chronic renal failure, namely, chronic recurrent pyelonephritis, can hardly be overemphasized.

REFERENCES

Addis, T.: "Glomerular Nephritis: Diagnosis and Treatment," New York, The Macmillan Company, 1948.

Bricker, N. S., P. A. F. Morrin, and S. W. Kime: The Pathologic Physiology of Chronic Bright's Disease, Am. J. Med., 28:77, 1960.

Bright, Richard: Cases and Observations, Illustrative of Renal Disease Accompanied with the Secretion of Albuminous Urine, Guy's Hosp. Reps., 1:338, 1836.

Ciba Foundation Symposium: "The Kidney," Boston, Little, Brown & Company, 1954.

Gottschalk, C. W.: Micropuncture Studies of Tubular Function in the Mammalian Kidney (Bowditch Lectures), The Physiologist, 4:35, 1961.

Kleeman, C. R., H. W. L. Hew, and L. B. Guze: Pyelonephritis, Medicine, 39:3, 1960.

Merrill, J. P.: "The Treatment of Renal Failure," New York, Grune & Stratton, Inc., 1955.

Oliver, J.: "Architecture of the Kidney in Chronic Bright's Disease," New York, Paul B. Hoeber, Inc., 1939.

———: When Is the Kidney Not a Kidney? J. Urol., 63:373, 1950.

Smith, H. W.: "The Kidney: Structure and Function in Health and Disease," New York, Oxford University Press, 1951.

Strauss, M. B., and L. G. Raisz: "Clinical Management of Renal Failure," Springfield, Ill., Charles C Thomas, Publisher, 1956.

21 EDEMA

Charles H. Burnett and Louis G. Welt

Edema is a symptom or manifestation, not a cause, of many diseased states. Strictly defined, edema means simply "swelling"; in clinical medicine it signifies an increased volume of the extravascular component of the extracellular fluid—the interstitial fluid. Although an increase in interstitial fluid volume may be caused by shifts of intracellular fluid to an extracellular position (e.g., owing to hyperglycemia or to the infusion of hypertonic fluids whose solutes are restricted to an extracellular position), the edema encountered clinically can result from two or more processes: (1) Local redistribution of fluid in specific areas. Total extracellular volume may vary from no change to significant increases (e.g., edema associated with thrombophlebitis). (2) Redistribution of fluid, producing increment of fluid, in all portions of the interstitial compartment; eventually, total body water is also increased. Plasma and blood volume may or may not be changed. To the former of the above states, the term *localized* edema is applied and to the latter, *generalized* edema. The physical signs of edema vary from "pitting," or persistence of indentation of the skin following pressure (in particular against a bony eminence such as the tibia), to visually obvious generalized swelling. Edema, especially in obese individuals, may amount to several liters of fluid, with a corresponding gain in body weight, before retention of fluid can be appreciated on examination. *Ascites* and *hydrothorax* refer to accumulation of excess fluid in the peritoneal and pleural cavities, respectively. *Anasarca*, or "dropsy," implies generalized edema.

PATHOGENESIS

The primary (and qualitative) forces favoring extravascular transudation of fluid to the interstitial space were first proposed by Starling. A more complete explanation of generalized edema has required demonstration of secondary (and quantitative) factors which induce retention, chiefly in the kidneys, of salt and water in the body. Recently, sound evidence has been presented that hormonal factors are closely associated with, and probably requisite to, maintenance of these secondary factors. Hence edema should be viewed as the result of alterations in basic physiologic mechanisms operating similarly in a variety of diseased states. For generalized or extensive localized edema to develop, at least two conditions must be met: (1) Primary forces must be such that fluid enters the interstitial space faster than it is removed. (2) Secondary forces must induce circumstances which result in a total fluid output from the body that falls short of total fluid intake.

Primary Factors Favoring Increment of Interstitial Compartment. The basic physiologic mechanisms conditioning exchanges between plasma and interstitial tissues as originally proposed by Starling are now well accepted (see Chap. 13). A balance between the two compartments of the extracellular fluid is maintained normally by a combination of interacting forces, which include (1) capillary hydrostatic pressure, (2) tissue tension or interstitial hydrostatic pressure, (3) effective osmotic pressure of the plasma (It must be reemphasized that concentrations of sodium salts and other solutes of small molecular weight do not influence effective *plasma osmotic pressure*. The latter is determined chiefly by the large molecules, mainly the plasma proteins, which do not pass through to the capillary endothelium.), (4) effective osmotic pressure of the tissue fluids, and (5) lymphatic drainage.

According to the above principles, intravascular factors which favor transudation to the interstitial space include increased capillary hydrostatic pressure, due to localized or generalized increase of venous pressure, or decreased effective plasma osmotic pressure due to hypoproteinemia. If both the above features coexist, edema formation is greatly enhanced. The rate of transudation from capillaries to interstitial space is also affected by the tension of the tissues; as pressure builds up in the interstitial spaces, the rate of movement from capillaries diminishes. Hence the inherent ability of tissues to swell influences the sites of major accumulation of edema. For example, in certain circumstances edema around the eyes is prominent because expansibility of tissues in these areas is great. If the rate of removal of interstitial fluid by the lymphatic vessels is impaired, edema formation is further augmented. An increased rate of transudation from the capillaries may be compensated completely by a corresponding increased flow of lymph returning fluid from the interstitial space to the plasma, thus counteracting a tendency to edema formation. Conversely, elevation of lymphatic pressure in the absence of increased venous pressure may cause edema (chronic lymphangitis, etc.). In addition, small quantities of protein that do gain access to the interstitial fluid normally are removed by the lymphatic vessels. In the presence of obstruction of these channels, optimal rate of removal of fluid is impaired; the protein content of the interstitial fluid also increases. The latter circumstance promotes further edema formation because colloid osmotic pressure of the interstitial fluid is increased. The importance of the lymphatic vessels is frequently overlooked in assessing edema.

Damage to the capillary endothelium increases permeability of these vessels, permitting transfer of a protein-rich fluid to the interstitial compartment. Injury to capillary walls may be the result of chemical, bacterial, thermal, or mechanical agents. Edema that is a manifestation of hypersensitivity (angioneurotic edema) must also result from increased capillary permeability (see Chap. 232). Damage to capillary endothelium is primarily responsible for inflammatory edema, which is easily recognizable by the presence of other signs of inflammation—redness, heat, and tenderness. The high protein content of the fluid escaping into the tissues clearly favors further transudation. Capillary damage may be very severe and widespread; for example, in Rocky Mountain spotted fever, the amount of protein escaping into the tissues is sufficiently great to produce hypoproteinemia. Lymphatic reabsorption is of especial importance in the resolution of inflammatory edema.

Krogh showed that, even in the absence of inflammation and injury, simple dilatation of the capillaries favors edema formation. Theoretically, the increased rate of movement might be expected to operate equally in both directions, but actually dilatation of capillaries favors outward movement of fluid more than inward. This phenomenon may perhaps be explained by increased filtration alone subsequent to increased capillary hydrostatic pressure resulting from relaxation of arteriolar and precapillary sphincters during vasodilatation. However, according to one theory of capillary permeability, the entire endothelial surface is available for passage of small molecules soluble in water and lipids. Molecules insoluble in water and lipids, including proteins, probably pass only through intercellular pores. Increased capillary permeability resulting only from dilatations of these vessels appears to be of minor importance in edema formation. Nevertheless, vasodilatation increases the total area for filtration if the other primary factors for edema are coexistent. Further, in thyrotoxicosis and beriberi heart disease, in which vasodilatation is concomitant with the disease, the factors just mentioned are probably important in whatever edema formation occurs.

Secondary Factors Which May Be Associated with Generalized Edema. The primary factors discussed above initiate a redistribution of fluid among the several components of the extracellular compartment. In terms of specific major disease states, these factors may be listed as follows: (1) in the nephrotic syndrome a decrease in the plasma colloid osmotic pressure promotes a redistribution of fluid between the vascular and extravascular spaces in favor of the latter; (2) in cirrhosis with ascites, the portal hypertension, diminished colloid osmotic pressure and, probably, interference with lymphatic drainage of the ascitic sac favor accumulation of fluid in the peritoneal cavity and, in addition, in the pleural and interstitial spaces; (3) in congestive heart failure the sequence is more complicated but may be tentatively expressed as follows: defective systolic emptying redistributes blood from the arterial system to the chambers of the heart and to the venous system; the diminished arterial volume may then be responsible for retention of salt and water which, because of the failure of the heart as a pump, is sequestered on the venous side of the circulation; and, finally, there is an increase in interstitial fluid because the venous hypervolemia is accompanied by increased intravascular hydrostatic pressure, leading to an increased rate of transudation from capillaries.

The primary components of edema are salt and water, and the significance of the development and maintenance of the edematous state is that there has been a net positive balance of salt and water. Since the ingestion of these materials appears not to be affected in a primary sense, the problem is largely one of understanding the response of the kidneys in promoting this net positive balance. Of the two major components of edema, the retention of sodium appears to be primary to the retention of water. This is attested to by (1) the usual failure to accumulate edema if sodium is not available in the diet and (2) the success that accompanies the employment of pharmacologic agents and other measures which promote the excretion of sodium in the urine. In most circumstances the mechanisms that are responsible for the maintenance of a normal effective osmolality of the body fluids continue to operate efficiently so that the retention of sodium promotes thirst and the secretion of the antidiuretic hormone which, in turn, lead to the ingestion and retention of approximately 1 liter of water for each 140 mM of sodium retained. Similarly, measures which promote the loss of sodium into the urine are accompanied by antithetical responses leading to the net loss of an equivalent volume of water from the body.

Renal Factors. HEMODYNAMIC. The problem then is to define the manner in which the excretion of sodium is diminished in the various edema states. There are at least three ways in which the elimination of sodium in the urine might be diminished in states of edema by alterations of renal hemodynamics. These are:

1. Decreased filtered load (FL) of sodium

$$FL = GFR \times [Na_s^+]$$

2. Change in filtration among the population of nephrons

3. Increased filtration fraction (FF)

$$FF = \frac{GFR}{\text{renal plasma flow}}$$

The first and most securely established of these is the influence of a decrease in filtered load. There are innumerable examples of a direct correlation between a decrease in filtered load of sodium and a diminished rate of excretion of salt in the urine; furthermore, a depressed glomerular filtration rate is very common in congestive heart failure and may be a feature of the several other edema states. In fact, this may be the most important although not the only factor responsible for salt retention in congestive heart failure.

Another hemodynamic influence concerns the alteration of filtration rate among the population of nephrons. It has been recently emphasized that each of the 2 million nephrons cannot be considered identical, one with every other, and that they must be viewed as varying not only in certain anatomic characteristics but in functional terms as well. For example, some tubules might reabsorb a greater fraction of filtered sodium than others. This, in turn, could provide circumstances wherein the over-all rate of filtration from all 2 million glomeruli was unchanged but where the fraction of the total filtration which takes place in one group of nephrons decreases and in another increases in such a fashion as to change the rate of excretion of salt with no change in the total filtered load of sodium. The factors which would promote such a redistribution of filtration are unknown, but pressure changes in both the arterial and venous systems might very well be responsible.

A third hemodynamic alteration that may influence sodium excretion to some degree is the influence of a change in the filtration fraction. Since the hydrostatic pressure in the lumens of tubules and peritubular vessels is identical, the colloid osmotic pressure of the latter might promote a redistribution of water between the tubular lumen and vessel. This, in turn, would create a favorable diffusion gradient for solutes, including sodium and chloride and, hence, promote the reabsorption of both water and salt. The greater the filtration fraction, the higher the concentration of protein in the postglomerular plasma which perfuses the tubules, and to the extent that colloid osmotic pressure could influence reabsorption of water and salt this would be enhanced. Although there is undoubted active transport of solutes from tubular lumens, the influence referred to here could at least facilitate reabsorption. Thus, a decrease in renal plasma flow, even with no change in glomerular filtration rate, might in itself be responsible in some measure for the diminished excretion of salt and water.

REABSORPTIVE MECHANISMS. Although there is a considerable body of evidence to implicate one or more of these mechanisms discussed above in many states of edema, there are reasons to believe that these influences need not be operative or, at least, need not be the only factors which contribute to salt retention. It is pertinent, therefore, to examine the other major set of regulations which influence sodium excretion, namely, renal tubular reabsorption activity. The efferent arcs of reflexes responsible for implementing increased renal tubular absorption of salt would most likely be neural or humoral. There is no convincing evidence that renal tubular activity is influenced *directly* by neurogenic impulses.

Humoral Factors. There is, on the other hand, abundant evidence for the influence of humoral factors. Barger and his group suggested that a humoral agent from the autonomic nervous system may influence salt excretion. They noted that the injection of norepinephrine into one renal artery promoted a diminished rate of excretion and that this effect could be blocked by phenoxybenzamine (Dibenzyline). Furthermore, they noted that Dibenzyline alone had no effect on the excretion of salt by normal dogs, but its administration was followed by a natriuresis in dogs with experimental congestive heart failure. They suggest that a decrease in pressure in the carotid sinus sets in motion a series of responses, one of which is the secretion of a vasopressor material that somehow influences salt excretion.

The role of aldosterone in the renal response to heart failure and other states of edema is incompletely understood. This salt-retaining hormone is excreted in increased amounts in most instances of the several types of edema states in which the estimation has been made. The increased excretion of aldosterone by the adrenal cortex is presumably a response to the diminished arterial or *effective* plasma volume referred to earlier. (See Chap. 68 for a complete discussion of the regulation of aldosterone secretion.) However, increased quantities of aldosterone do not always promote the accumulation of edema as witnessed by the lack of striking fluid retention in most instances of primary aldosteronism. Furthermore, although normal subjects will retain some salt and water under the influence of a potent mineralocorticoid such as DOCA or 9-alpha-fluorohydrocortisone, this accumulation appears to be self-terminative despite continued exposure to the steroid and to salt and water. It is probable that the failure by normal subjects to accumulate fluid indefinitely is reflective of an increase in glomerular filtration rate (or other hemodynamic influences) which results from the increase in volume of the extracellular fluid compartments. The role of such a hormone in the accumulation of fluid in congestive heart failure may be more effective because these patients are unable to improve filtration rate owing to the failure of the heart; the

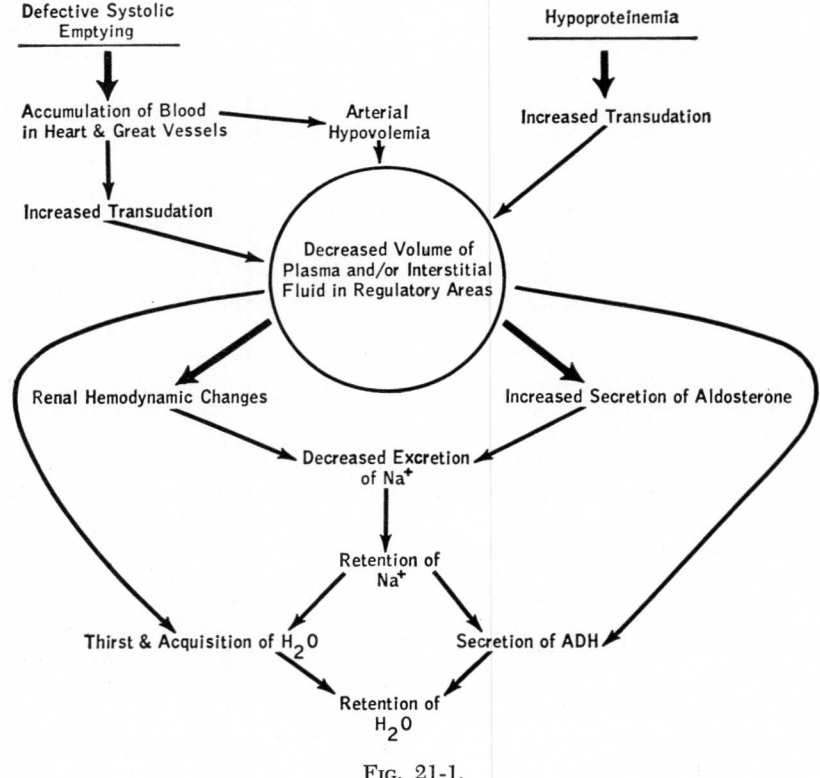

FIG. 21-1.

same is also true in nephrotic and cirrhotic patients because the increased volume of fluid does not repair the deficit of effective circulating blood volume but instead is sequestered in the interstitial, pleural, and peritoneal spaces owing to the basic distortion in the Starling forces inherent in the primary disorder.

A summary statement of the pathogenesis of edema is presented in Fig. 21-1. The basic assumption of this tentative description is that the primary disorder somehow promotes a set of circumstances wherein stimuli are aroused that reflect a diminution in plasma volume. There may be a decrease in the total plasma volume, or it may be diminution in the volume of some key segment, with little change or with an actual increase in the *total* volume. The diminished plasma volume is then represented as influencing the renal excretion of salt and water both by direct hemodynamic influences and by promoting the secretion of humoral agents which accelerate the processes. It is readily conceded that this proposal leaves many questions unanswered; hence, it represents at best an unsatisfactory hypothesis.

DIFFERENTIAL DIAGNOSIS

Despite numerous inconsistencies encountered in explanation of the various factors and mechanisms concerned in edema formation, the primary cause can usually be determined. As a rule, localized edema can be readily differentiated from generalized edema. The great majority of patients with noninflammatory generalized edema of significant degree suffer from cardiac, renal, hepatic, or nutritional disorders. Consequently, the differential diagnosis of generalized edema should be directed toward implication or exclusion of these several conditions. The considerations listed below should suffice to differentiate the common causes of edema.

Localized Edema. Edema originating from inflammation or hypersensitivity is usually readily identified; the characteristics of this type of edema have already been discussed. Localized edema due to venous or lymphatic obstruction (thrombophlebitis, chronic lymphangitis, resection of regional lymph nodes, filariasis, etc.) may demonstrate in a local area all the characteristics of edema occurring from generalized retention of salt and water. It should be reemphasized that lymphedema is peculiarly intractable, because restriction of lymphatic flow results in increased protein concentration in interstitial fluid, a circumstance which severely impedes removal of retained fluid.

Edema of Heart Failure. Evidence of heart disease as manifested by cardiac enlargement, diastolic murmurs, and gallop rhythm plus evidence of cardiac failure, such as dyspnea, basilar rales, diminished vital capacity, prolonged circulation time, venous distention, *increased venous pressure*, and hepatomegaly, usually provides abundant evidence of the pathogenesis of edema resulting from heart failure (Chap. 13).

Edema of the Nephrotic Syndrome. The classic triad—massive proteinuria, hypoproteinemia, and hypercholesterolemia—is usually present. This syndrome may occur during the course of a variety of kidney diseases (e.g., glomerulonephritis, diabetes and intercapillary glomerulosclerosis, and renal amyloidosis). A history of previous renal disease may or may not be elicited; more commonly it is not (see Chap. 258).

Edema of Acute Glomerulonephritis. The edema occurring during the acute phases of glomerulonephritis is characteristically associated with hematuria, proteinuria, and hypertension. Some evidence supports the view that the fluid retention is due to increased capillary permeability; but probably in most instances the edema in this disease is the result of heart failure or of primary retention of sodium by the kidneys.

Edema of Cirrhosis. Ascites plus evidence of hepatic disease (collateral venous channels, hepatomegaly, spider angiomas, and jaundice) characterize edema of hepatic origin. The ascites is frequently extremely refractory to treatment; the lack of therapeutic response can be ascribed to the fact that intraabdominal fluid collects as a result of the combination of portal hypertension, hypoalbuminemia, and frequently, a relatively high protein content of the ascitic fluid. The latter may be due to escape of a protein-containing fluid through the lymphatic vessels of the liver capsule or through the portal vessels, the lymphatic drainage of which is impeded. Edema may also occur in other parts of the body in patients with cirrhosis as a result of hypoalbuminemia.

Edema of Nutritional Origin. An inadequate diet over a prolonged period may produce hypoproteinemia and edema. In some instances of extreme malnutrition the degree of transudation appears to be disproportionately great for the degree of serum protein deficit observed. Coexisting beriberi heart disease may augment edema of this origin. In the latter condition, increased cardiac output and blood flow, in addition to those factors usually present in heart failure, and capillary dilatation may further favor edema formation.

General Differential Criteria. Aside from the criteria already mentioned, certain other points may be helpful in eliciting the cause of edema.

The *distribution of edema* is an important guide to the cause. Thus edema of one leg or of one or both arms is usually the result of vascular or lymphatic obstruction. Edema resulting from hypoproteinemia characteristically is generalized but is especially evident in the eyelids and face and tends to be most pronounced in the morning because of the recumbent posture assumed during the night. Edema associated with heart failure, on the other hand, tends to be more extensive in the legs and to be accentuated in the evening, a feature also determined largely by posture. In the rare types of cardiac disease, such as tricuspid stenosis and constrictive pericarditis, in which orthopnea is absent and the patient prefers the recumbent posture, the gravity factor may be equalized and facial edema observed. Less common causes of facial edema include trichinosis, allergic reactions, and myxedema. Unilateral edema occasionally results from cerebral lesions affecting the vasomotor fibers on one side of the body; paralysis also reduces lymphatic and venous drainage on the affected side.

The color, thickness, and sensitivity of the skin are important. Local tenderness and increase in temperature suggest inflammation. Local cyanosis may signify venous obstruction. Generalized but usually slight cyanosis is generally indicative of congestive heart failure. In individuals who have had repeated episodes of prolonged edema, the skin over the involved areas is thickened, hard, and often red.

The *venous pressure* is of great importance in evaluating edema. Elevation of this measurement in an isolated part of the body usually reflects venous obstruction. Generalized elevation of venous pressure is almost pathognomonic of congestive heart failure.

Ordinarily, significant increase in venous pressure can be recognized by the level at which cervical veins collapse; in doubtful cases, and for accurate recording, the venous pressure should be measured.

Determination of the concentration of serum proteins, and especially of the serum albumin, clearly differentiates those patients in whom the edema is due entirely or in part to diminished intravascular colloid osmotic pressure.

The presence of proteinuria affords useful clues. The complete absence of protein in the urine is evidence against either cardiac or renal disease as a cause of edema. In a patient with edema without proteinuria, the presence of a palpable liver constitutes strong evidence that hepatic disease may be the cause of the edema. Slight to moderate proteinuria is the rule in patients with heart failure, while persistent massive proteinuria usually reflects the presence of the nephrotic syndrome. Since the liver may be palpable in subjects with heart failure of hepatic disease, the presence of proteinuria in a patient who does not have a palpable liver would implicate the possibility of the nephrotic syndrome. Aside from the points mentioned, which bear directly on the question of the type of edema, much valuable information can be obtained from other features of the examination. Some of these are the presence or absence of heart disease, the character of the urinary sediment, the dietary history, and a history of alcoholism.

It should be emphasized that edema may originate from a variety of abnormal states; it is not therefore necessarily a consequence of only one of the disorders enumerated above. For example, in a diabetic patient with edema, hypoalbuminemia associated with the nephrotic syndrome of intercapillary glomerulosclerosis, the increased venous pressure associated with congestive heart failure due to atherosclerotic and hypertensive heart disease, and the anemia consequent to uremia may all contribute to edema formation.

SUMMARY

Edema limited to a local area suggests either obstruction or local capillary damage. The obstruction may be lymphatic or venous and the local capillary damage due either to inflammation or to allergy. Significant generalized edema may accumulate before it can be appreciated clinically. It appears first in tissues which are expansible and may be demonstrable only by pressure against a bony eminence such as the tibia. The presence of generalized edema requires investigation especially for evidence of cardiac, renal, or hepatic disease and occasionally for manifestations of nutritional deficiency.

The primary factors promoting transfer of fluid from the intravascular to the extravascular compartment of the extracellular fluid space are reasonably clear. The secondary factors which induce retention of salt and water include a variety of hemodynamic and hormonal mechanisms, the nature of which, although clarified by recent investigations, can still not be explained by any single hypothesis.

REFERENCES

Peters, J. P.: The Problem of Cardiac Edema, Am. J. Med., 12:66, 1952.

Starling, E. H.: The Fluids of the Body, in "The Herter Lectures," New York, W. T. Keener & Company, 1909.

Warren, J. V., and Eugene A. Stead, Jr.: Fluid Dynamics in Chronic Congestive Heart Failure: An Interpretation of the Mechanisms Producing Edema, Increased Plasma Volume and Venous Pressure in Certain Patients with Prolonged Congestive Failure, Arch. Internal Med., 73:138, 1946.

Welt, L. G.: Volume Receptors, Circulation, 21:1002, 1960.

Section 8: Alterations in Weight

22 GAIN AND LOSS OF WEIGHT

George W. Thorn and
Philip K. Bondy

Changes in body weight are of importance in diagnosis and in following the progress of treatment. Although single determinations may reveal deviations from normal, serial observations which show trends are of greater value. The interpretation of weight fluctuations requires an understanding of the factors whose interplay is reflected in changes of body mass—fluid exchange, assimilation of food, energy production, accumulation or breakdown of energy depots, and formation or destruction of functioning protoplasma—i.e., the ebb and flow of all metabolic processes. Since various influences acting simultaneously may increase the weight of certain body components while decreasing the weight of others, the changes observed clinically represent the resultant of several metabolic vectors.

What is meant by "normal" weight? The standard to which we usually refer is merely a series of tables representing the average weights of a large number of healthy people. Such tables usually correlate the weight with height, age, and sex (Table 22-1). These averages are not applicable to any particular individual; for example, tall, thin people with light bones and small muscles, those with a so-called "asthenic" habitus, have relatively low weights as compared with the "normal." On the other hand the heavily built, muscular "pyknic" type usually appears overweight by reference to the standard weight charts. Nevertheless both individuals may be within normal limits for their own body builds. Recognition of this fact has led to attempts to measure separately the skeletal mass, lean body mass (i.e., mass of fat-free, non-skeletal tissue), and the adipose tissue. Although such studies have not yet produced methods applicable to ordinary clinical practice, it seems likely that the standards of "normal" weight will ultimately be defined in terms of body composition. Until such scientific standards become available, the physician should determine the normal weight for an individual by observing his habitus as well as by reference to a standard of average weights.

GENERAL PRINCIPLES

In considering changes of weight, we can conveniently separate the body into two components:

Table 22-1. WEIGHT TABLES
Weight in Pounds According to Frame
(in Indoor Clothing)

Desirable Weights for Men, Ages 25 and over

Height (with shoes on) 1-in. heels ft	in.	Small frame	Medium frame	Large frame
5	2	112–120	118–129	126–141
5	3	115–123	121–133	129–144
5	4	118–126	124–136	132–148
5	5	121–129	127–139	135–152
5	6	124–133	130–143	138–156
5	7	128–137	134–147	142–161
5	8	132–141	138–152	147–166
5	9	136–145	142–156	151–170
5	10	140–150	146–160	155–174
5	11	144–154	150–165	159–179
6	0	148–158	154–170	164–184
6	1	152–162	158–175	168–189
6	2	156–167	162–180	173–194
6	3	160–171	167–185	178–199
6	4	164–175	172–190	182–204

Desirable Weights for Women, Ages 25 and over

Height (with shoes on) 2-in. heels ft	in.	Small frame	Medium frame	Large frame
4	10	92– 98	96–107	104–119
4	11	94–101	98–110	106–122
5	0	96–104	101–113	109–125
5	1	99–107	104–116	112–128
5	2	102–110	107–119	115–131
5	3	105–113	110–122	118–134
5	4	108–116	113–126	121–138
5	5	111–119	116–130	125–142
5	6	114–123	120–135	129–146
5	7	118–127	124–139	133–150
5	8	122–131	128–143	137–154
5	9	126–135	132–147	141–158
5	10	130–140	136–151	145–163
5	11	134–144	140–155	149–168
6	0	138–148	144–159	153–173

For girls between 18 and 25, subtract 1 lb for each year under 25.

SOURCE: Metropolitan Life Insurance Company, 1959.

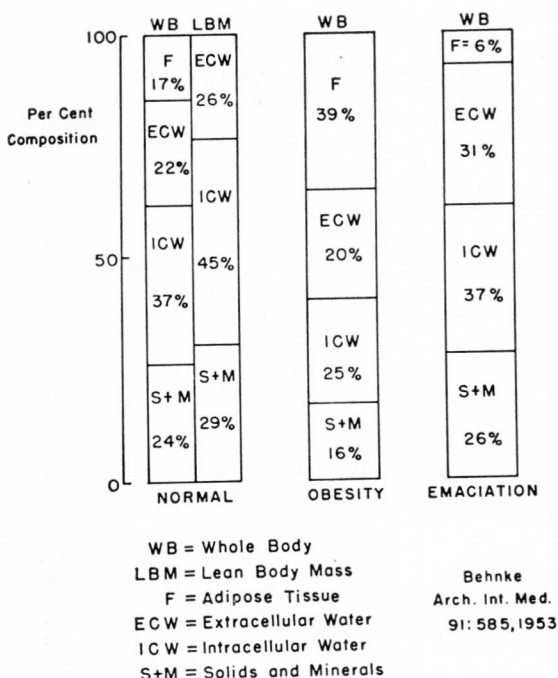

WB = Whole Body
LBM = Lean Body Mass
F = Adipose Tissue
ECW = Extracellular Water
ICW = Intracellular Water
S+M = Solids and Minerals

Behnke
Arch. Int. Med.
91: 585, 1953

FIG. 22-1: Changes in body composition associated with obesity and emaciation.

liquids and solids (Fig. 22-1). Body water comprises about 60 per cent of the total body weight, or about 70 per cent of the fat-free body mass. Extracellular fluid represents approximately 17 per cent of the total body weight, or 28 per cent of the total body water. The rest of the water is confined within the cells. The extracellular fluid includes the plasma, lymph, cerebrospinal fluid, and intercellular fluids. Under pathologic conditions there may be appreciable collections of fluid in the subcutaneous tissues or in the peritoneal, pleural, and pericardial cavities. All extracellular fluid contains sodium as its major cation, and the movement of water outside the cells is intimately concerned with the movement of sodium. Extracellular fluid is not ordinarily retained unless sodium is retained, and extracellular water is lost with increased sodium excretion. Since the excretion of sodium is influenced by many factors, changes of extracellular fluid volume commonly cause alterations of body weight.

Intracellular fluid is a component of the intracellular protoplasm. As a part of a complicated colloid system, it is intimately bound with cellular protein. Changes of intracellular water are, therefore, usually secondary to changes of tissue protein. The intracellular water is, however, in osmotic equilibrium with the extracellular fluid. In dehydrated individuals, intracellular fluid may therefore be released to the extracellular compartment; but such

shifts affect only a minor portion of the intracellular fluid volume.

Four solid components of the body must be considered: minerals, carbohydrates, proteins, and fats. Most of the weight of the minerals is found in the bones. Carbohydrate does not ordinarily make up much of the total body weight, since it can be stored only in small amounts as glycogen. Much of the dietary carbohydrate prior to oxidation is converted to fat and when excessive quantities are assimilated it is stored in this form. The body fat consists of the complex lipids, which represent only a small part of the total body fat and are found in all cells of the body, and the neutral fat, which is stored in the fat depots. These depots consist of actively metabolizing tissue including clumps of cells surrounded by supporting tissue and blood vessels. The composition of adipose tissue is approximately 14 per cent water, 63 per cent neutral fat, 22 per cent "sarcoplasm," and 1 per cent carbohydrate. It contains about 6 Cal per Gm. The term *depot* may be misleading, since it implies that the depot fat is withdrawn from the body's metabolism, whereas in actuality it is constantly being mobilized and replaced. Since the net result of this turnover is to maintain a total quantity of fat in the depots which changes only very slowly, it is sufficiently accurate for our purposes to consider that adipose tissue is a site of inactive storage.

Protein, the major solid component of the cellular protoplasm, is not stored in any type of inactive depot. A portion of the ingested protein is incorporated into functioning tissue; the rest is converted either to fat or carbohydrate and metabolized as such. Approximately 4 Gm water is needed for each gram of tissue protein. For this reason, the retention of 250 Gm protein, equivalent to 1000 Cal, causes a weight gain of 1,250 Gm, whereas the formation of fat deposits containing 1000 Cal (approximately 110 Gm) causes a weight gain of approximately 148 Gm. Consequently considerable alterations of body composition may occur without changes of total body weight. The flabby Easterner who spends a summer on a Western ranch may thus maintain a constant weight while losing 4 in. of girth. The laborer who is promoted to the ease of a desk job may, on the other hand, degenerate to paunchy obesity without putting on a pound of extra weight.

The caloric intake necessary to maintain body weight depends upon the basal metabolic rate and upon the person's activity (Table 22-2). If sufficient food is assimilated to permit an individual to carry on his activities, no change in weight occurs. The food requirement is increased if new protoplasm is being formed, e.g., in the fetus, the growing child, and the adult engaged in sufficiently

Table 22-2. FOOD AND NUTRITION BOARD, NATIONAL RESEARCH COUNCIL
RECOMMENDED DAILY DIETARY ALLOWANCES,* REVISED 1958
Designed for the Maintenance of Good Nutrition of Healthy Persons in the United States
(Allowances are intended for persons normally active in a temperate climate)

	Age, years	Weight, kg (lb)	Height, cm (in.)	Calories	Protein, Gm	Calcium, Gm	Iron, mg	Vitamin A, IU	Thiamine, mg	Riboflavin, mg	Niacin,† mg equiv	Ascorbic acid, mg	Vitamin D, IU
Men......	25	70 (154)	175 (69)	3200 ‡	70	0.8	10	5,000	1.6	1.8	21	75	
	45	70 (154)	175 (69)	3000	70	0.8	10	5,000	1.5	1.8	20	75	
	65	70 (154)	175 (69)	2550	70	0.8	10	5,000	1.3	1.8	18	75	
Women...	25	58 (128)	163 (64)	2300	58	0.8	12	5,000	1.2	1.5	17	70	
	45	58 (128)	163 (64)	2200	58	0.8	12	5,000	1.1	1.5	17	70	
	65	58 (128)	163 (64)	1800	58	0.8	12	5,000	1.0	1.5	17	70	
	Pregnant (second half)			+300	+20	1.5	15	6,000	1.3	2.0	+3	100	400
	Lactating (850 ml daily)			+1000	+40	2.0	15	8,000	1.7	2.5	+2	150	400
Infants §..	0–1/12 §				§	0.6	5	1,500	0.4	0.5	6	30	400
	2/12–6/12	6 (13)	60 (24)	Kg × 120									
	7/12–12/12	9 (20)	70 (28)	Kg × 100		0.8	7	1,500	0.5	0.8	7	30	400
Children...	1– 3	12 (27)	87 (34)	1300	40	1.0	7	2,000	0.7	1.0	8	35	400
	4– 6	18 (40)	109 (43)	1700	50	1.0	8	2,500	0.9	1.3	11	50	400
	7– 9	27 (60)	129 (51)	2100	60	1.0	10	3,500	1.1	1.5	14	60	400
	10–12	36 (79)	144 (57)	2500	70	1.2	12	4,500	1.3	1.8	17	75	400
Boys......	13–15	49 (108)	163 (64)	3100	85	1.4	15	5,000	1.6	2.1	21	90	400
	16–19	63 (139)	175 (69)	3600	100	1.4	15	5,000	1.8	2.5	25	100	400
Girls......	13–15	49 (108)	160 (63)	2600	80	1.3	15	5,000	1.3	2.0	17	80	400
	16–19	54 (120)	162 (64)	2400	75	1.3	15	5,000	1.2	1.9	16	80	400

* The allowance levels are intended to cover individual variations among most normal persons as they live in the United States under usual environmental stresses. The recommended allowances can be attained with a variety of common foods, providing other nutrients for which human requirements have been less well defined. See text for more detailed discussion of allowances and of nutrients not tabulated.

† Niacin equivalents include dietary sources of the preformed vitamin and the precursor, tryptophan. 60 mg tryptophan equals 1 mg niacin.

‡ Calorie allowances apply to individuals usually engaged in moderate physical activity. For office workers or others in sedentary occupations they are excessive. Adjustments must be made for variations in body size, age, physical activity, and environmental temperature.

§ The Board recognizes that human milk is the natural food for infants and feels that breast feeding is the best and desired procedure for meeting nutrient requirements in the first months of life. No allowances are stated for the first month of life. Breast feeding is particularly indicated during the first month when infants show handicaps in homeostasis due to different rates of maturation of digestive, excretory, and endocrine functions. Recommendations as listed pertain to nutrient intake as afforded by cow's milk formulas and supplementary foods given the infant when breast feeding is terminated. Allowances are not given for protein during infancy.

SOURCE: A Report of the Food and Nutrition Board, Publication No. 589, National Academy of Sciences—National Research Council, Washington, D.C.

arduous work to induce an increase in muscle mass. In each of these circumstances weight is gained. The energy required for the growth of protoplasm is greater than the equivalent caloric content of the deposited tissue, since the formation of protein is an energy-requiring process. If more calories are assimilated than are needed for growth and energy requirements, the extra energy is stored as fat.

When inadequate amounts of food are eaten, the individual must supply the caloric deficit from his tissues. Since the major source of stored energy is neutral fat, a considerable change in the metabolic pattern is necessary in order to achieve optimal conservation of body structure and prevent excessively rapid depletion of proteins and carbohydrates. Starvation therefore initiates a complex series of metabolic adjustments. These include rapid mobilization of fat from the depots to the liver and thence to the tissues, where it is burned for energy. Simultaneously there is a reduction in the ability of certain tissues to oxidize glucose, so that the respiratory quotient falls close to 0.7 and the metabolic pattern resembles somewhat that seen in diabetes. The metabolic rate falls, and the caloric requirement is consequently reduced. The rate of protein breakdown and nitrogen excretion is reduced below that normally present. If the rate of fat metabolism is too high, some degree of ketosis may develop, as the liver may produce ketone bodies more rapidly than they can be used in the periphery. Many of these adjustments can be facilitated if a small amount of carbohydrate—about 100 Gm daily—is made available. This small amount of carbohydrate reduces the nitrogen excretion to a still lower level and minimizes ketosis. If exogenous sources of carbohydrate are not available, endogenous carbohydrate must be used. The stores of carbohydrate are small and are rapidly exhausted; when this occurs, gluconeogenesis from protein must be accelerated, to supply the necessary carbohydrate. Since no stores of protein are known to exist, the catabolism of protein causes breakdown of functioning protoplasm and ultimately loss of cells. The protein breakdown proceeds, regardless of the amount of fat available for metabolism, as long as the carbohydrate intake remains inadequate. When fat stores are totally exhausted, the body must depend on protein for its entire energy requirement, and as a consequence there is rapid destruction of tissue terminally.

From this discussion of general principles of alterations of weight we shall proceed to discuss specific factors controlling the direction of weight changes in various physiologic and pathologic conditions.

BODY WEIGHT IN RELATION TO FLUID METABOLISM

Fluid Retention. Wide and rapid alterations of body weight may occur in association with the accumulation and loss of edema fluid and serous effusions. Dehydration may also reduce the body weight, although rarely by as much as 10 per cent of the total body weight. Detailed consideration of the factors affecting fluid balance will be found in Chaps. 50 and 21.

An interesting type of weight fluctuation is sometimes seen during the course of the menstrual cycle. During the latter part of the month, just before the onset of menstrual flow, some women gain a small amount of weight because they retain water. At the onset of menstruation a diuresis occurs and the weight returns to the normal level. Although these fluctuations are not usually noticeable clinically, the tendency to retain water in the premenstrual phase of the cycle may cause clinical edema in patients with underlying renal, cardiac, or hepatic disease.

Diuresis. In a patient who has retained salt and water, procedures causing a release of water cause a loss of weight. Diuresis may be produced by rest and digitalization in patients with heart disease, or it may occur spontaneously in recovery from acute glomerulonephritis. In patients with the nephrotic syndrome, diuretic crises occasionally occur without obvious cause, and large amounts of weight may be lost rapidly. An increase of water excretion may also occur after the administration of diuretic drugs. It is possible to cause a loss of weight by the restriction of salt intake, a measure particularly useful in the treatment of patients with congestive failure and early toxemia of pregnancy.

When edema has occurred as a result of reduced plasma albumin levels, restoration of the protein levels produces a diuresis and loss of weight.

In addition to loss of weight as a result of the excretion of abnormally accumulated water, weight loss may result from dehydration of a previously normal patient. For example, in cholera and other severe diarrheas, weight may be lost as a result of the water which is passed through the bowel. Excessive sweating may cause loss of weight.

The severe polyuria characteristic of uncontrolled diabetes mellitus may cause dehydration and weight loss, especially if acidosis supervenes and vomiting reduces the fluid intake. Patients with Addison's disease are subject to severe crises of dehydration as a result of vomiting, diarrhea, and the uncontrolled sodium diuresis characteristic of adrenocortical insufficiency. In both these diseases, however, the loss of weight attendant upon loss of water is acute and is usually complicated by loss of weight due to destruction of tissues.

BODY WEIGHT IN RELATION TO METABOLISM OF SOLIDS

In order to maintain its weight, the organism must assimilate sufficient calories to satisfy the requirements of its basal metabolic rate plus its activities. The basal metabolic rate is determined by many factors. Of these, the thyroid hormone is the most important. Hyperactivity of the thyroid increases the rate of activity of body processes, and reduction of thyroid activity reduces them. Fever also increases the metabolic rate, as do certain tumors, especially the lymphomas and leukemias, even in the absence of an elevation in temperature.

The requirement of energy in excess of that needed to satisfy the basal metabolism is determined by the activity of the organism. Sedentary workers require much less food to maintain their body weight than do laborers, while growing bodies need extra food to supply the materials for building protoplasm.

Gain in Weight. The total weight of the body solids increases when the caloric intake exceeds the energy demands of the body. The nature of the increase in weight depends somewhat on the need for functioning tissue. During periods of growth, or when strenuous exercise is causing an increase in muscle and bone mass, the excess of calories may be devoted entirely to the production of an increasing bulk of functioning tissue. If no such demand for tissue growth exists, the extra energy is stored in fat depots.

Growth. The processes leading to growth are complex and poorly understood. At least three factors are of importance: age, endocrine and other chemical environment of the growing cells, and physical activity. Thus, the rapid growth of the infant cannot be reproduced at any other time of life. This growth, however, does not occur unless appropriate amounts of pituitary, thyroid, adrenal, pancreatic, and gonadal hormones are present, together with the necessary nutritional elements. Replacement therapy at a later time will not produce normal growth in an infant who has been deprived of some essential hormone or nutriment at a critical point in his development. A normal growth curve is therefore a good indication of normal endocrine and nutritional status in infancy and childhood. Growth need not stop with maturity, however. Some of the weight gain during pregnancy must be considered to be growth, both of the fetus and of the maternal reproductive organs. True growth may also occur in individuals who, by active exercise, produce massive muscular and bony development.

Pathologic Growth Due to Endocrine Disease. Increase in the bulk of functioning tissue may result from hyperactivity of the acidophilic cells of the anterior hypophysis, producing the pituitary growth hormone, which causes either acromegaly or gigantism. In these diseases there is an increase in size of all functioning tissue. The bones become thicker and may grow longer if the epiphyses are not fused. The liver, spleen, kidneys, heart, tongue, and other organs also become enlarged. The increased weight is the result of a larger amount of functioning tissue. A similar mechanism accounts for the weight gain and exaggerated muscular development found in children or females having an excess of androgenic hormone. Adrenocortical tumors, or pathologic hyperplasia, arrhenoblastomas of the ovary, and rare testicular neoplasms can produce this masculinizing syndrome.

OBESITY

Obesity occurs when the caloric intake exceeds the energy requirements of the body both for physical activity and for growth. As a result there is an accumulation of fat which is stored in the adipose tissue. The excessive tissue may be distributed generally over the body, or it may be localized. The factors controlling the location of the fat are not all known, but such endocrine secretions as the estrogens and the adrenal hormones play some part. Obesity is a serious and common disease in those countries where a combination of generous food supplies and sedentary occupations readily permits the assimilation of more food than is necessary. The excessive deposition of fat is associated with an increased tendency to the development of the serious degenerative diseases such as atherosclerosis, diabetes, degenerative arthritis, hypertension, and even cancer; indeed the only common cause of death which does not strike earlier in the obese than in the lean population is suicide! The ill effects of obesity can be prevented and, to some extent, repaired by weight reduction.

The treatment of obesity is one of the most serious problems in preventive medicine in the United States today.

Etiology. Under normal circumstances there is a very exact adjustment of food intake to body requirements. Unfortunately, in certain individuals this adjustment is deranged, and the intake becomes excessive. The cause of the derangement is not clearly understood, because, at present, understanding of the mechanism of appetite control is inadequate. Several factors are clearly important, however.

Familial and cultural eating habits are firmly implanted at an early age. In groups in which great emphasis is placed on food, there is a tendency to overeat. Sometimes the cultural pattern equates success with obesity (as witness the common caricature of the obese banker) and thus encourages the ambitious person to achieve a comfortable corpulence. Moreover, when activity patterns change, eating habits may remain constant, so that the man who has previously been physically active may fail to reduce his caloric intake when he suddenly changes to a sedentary occupation. His habitual appetite causes him to overeat and tends to produce obesity; at the same time, disuse of his muscle mass causes atrophy. The result may be a conversion of active muscle tissue to flabby adipose deposits without change of total body weight. This tendency may be reinforced by the gradual decline of metabolic rate and of muscle activity which ordinarily accompanies aging.

Certain individuals have increased appetites for psychologic reasons. Such persons use food as a substitute for the satisfaction they should obtain from other emotional sources. In this respect, they are similar to alcoholics, who use alcohol as a substitute for such normal sources of satisfaction as their friends, their families, or success in their work.

It has been known for years that lesions involving the hypothalamus may lead to obesity. Experimental damage to the ventromedian nuclei of the hypothalamus, or of adjacent tracts, produces an increase in body weight of as much as 400 per cent. This increase is a result chiefly of increased caloric intake, but reduced physical activity may also play a part. When calories are restricted, hypothalamic-obese animals lose weight in a normal fashion. If unlimited calories are made available, the rapid weight gain lasts for only a short time; the animals then reach a plateau of weight at which they remain indefinitely. Lesions placed more laterally than those producing obesity may cause complete loss of interest in food, with resulting starvation. Hypothalamic lesions may rarely cause obesity in human beings, after trauma or infectious involvement of the hypothalamus. In view of the experimental relationship of the hypothalamus to hyperphagic obesity, it is commonly believed that control of appetite resides in the hypothalamus.

It is therefore clear that the basic cause of obesity is a derangement of the appetite-controlling mechanisms, permitting the assimilation of more food than is needed. It has been claimed that certain individuals are more efficient than others in their ability to digest, absorb, and utilize food, and therefore that they become obese at lower caloric intakes than might be expected. Extensive balance studies on such patients have never substantiated this explanation; at equivalent levels of physical activity and basal metabolism, there seems to be little variation in the required caloric intake. Recently it has been shown that young obese patients when tilted rapidly to the vertical position exhibit an impaired rise in serum unesterified fatty acids, in contrast to controls of normal weight.

Adipose tissue imposes a double load on the organism—a physical increase in the work which must be done in order to move about, and a metabolic increase in the amount of nutriment, oxygen, and blood needed to maintain the metabolism of the adipose tissue cells. Consequently, the addition of a given caloric increment to the diet of a person previously in equilibrium does not produce a continuous and infinite increase in body weight. After an appropriate amount of adipose tissue has been deposited, the additional caloric requirement imposed by the new tissue balances the added calories and the weight once again stabilizes at a higher level. This fact may explain in part the fact that weight gain tends to be rapid at first and later reaches equilibrium.

Pathology. The only pathologic lesion directly attributable to obesity is the presence of excessive amounts of adipose tissue. This tissue occurs chiefly in the subcutaneous areas, omentum, mesentery, and in the fat pads normally present around the kidneys and in the epicardium. The composition of the adipose tissue in obesity is identical with that found normally in smaller quantities in the same areas. It consists of clumps of fat cells, a special type of connective tissue cell which contains a relatively huge droplet of neutral fat displacing all other cell structures, together with supporting tissue such as blood vessels, lymphatic vessels, and fibrous tissue. Thus, although adipose tissue has a very high content of neutral fat, it also contains water, protein, and even small amounts of glycogen. A number of secondary pathologic changes are often seen in obese patients. These include premature atherosclerosis, fatty infiltration of the liver, and traumatic skeletal changes such as hypertrophic arthritis.

Clinical Picture. Obesity itself produces no symptoms, but the mechanical load of the excessive adipose tissue causes a series of secondary difficulties which may cause symptoms. These include postural adjustments which ultimately may cause backache and painful knees and feet, and also circulatory embarrassment, with dyspnea, easy fatigability, and orthopnea. Severe obesity is also frequently associated with menstrual disorders and infertility.

Diagnosis. No arbitrary aids to diagnosis are comparable to the information that can be obtained by simple inspection of the patient. From the standpoint of longevity, the ideal weight is one at which the patient is sparingly covered with a thin layer of adipose tissue. As soon as he accumulates enough subcutaneous adipose tissue to present a roll of redundant subcutaneous fat, he must be considered obese.

Treatment. The only effective method of treating obesity is restriction of caloric intake below the energy requirement; this can usually be accomplished without reducing the intake of essential minerals, vitamins, and amino acids below the danger point.

Motivation. In no disorder is the prescription so simple and the possibility of cure so high as in the treatment of obesity. Why, then, is there so much discussion concerning the "best diet," such concerted effort to seek the "magic pill," such quackery and chicanery surrounding attempts to restore weight to normal? The answer is readily apparent: caloric restriction maintained over any appreciable length of time requires courage and self-discipline of the highest order. To attain success a patient must possess sufficient motivation to enable him to carry through a prolonged uncomfortable program of relative starvation. If the ingestion of large quantities of food has provided essential emotional and psychologic satisfactions, caloric restriction may be accomplished only by substituting other sources of satisfaction or by increasing understanding of the nature of the emotional disturbances and subconscious conflicts which form a basis for the patient's present situation. In all these considerations the physician's patience and understanding are important determining factors in the success of the program. There are a few patients whose obesity has resulted from long-continued, modest excess of intake of calories, without deep underlying emotional conflict or overt disturbances in metabolism as the cause. For such as these it is simple to provide nutritional education and guidance. The number of such cases is diminishing rapidly as the appreciation of the dangers and difficulties which confront the obese individual becomes more widespread.

In general, motivation sufficient to sustain a patient in following the diet prescription arises from one or more of the following factors:

1. Pride in personal appearance
2. Symptoms of disordered physical function (shortness of breath, painful knees)
3. Fear of future disease (diabetes, arteriosclerosis)
4. An attempt to avoid the antagonistic reaction or "pressure" manifested by friends, relatives, or business associates

Obviously the last factor is the least satisfactory and, if at all potent, almost invariably leads to resentment. The danger in this instance is intensified by the probability that disturbed interpersonal relationships with mother, father, sister, or employer may have played an important role originally in the genesis of obesity. The submission to authority under these circumstances, while occasionally successful in accomplishing the immediate end (weight loss), may ultimately result in the development of much more serious emotional conflicts.

Although the presence of organic disease or the fear of its development may provide strong motivation for weight reduction, the fact that patients may have used the satisfaction derived from food as an important aid in meeting life's problems may create a serious conflict. On the one hand, there is fear of the physical consequences if weight is not reduced; on the other, the patient must face the loss of a necessary source of satisfaction. In some individuals who are incapable of making a reasonable, healthy adjustment to this predicament, the long-range effect of diet restriction may exert a detrimental effect on the underlying disease despite immediate benefits associated with weight loss.

Obese patients vary greatly in the ease with which dietary restriction enables them to lose weight. In instances in which only moderate restriction is necessary, success is almost certain with reasonable motivation, whereas patients requiring severe caloric restriction for prolonged periods need the strongest motivation. The skill with which the physician is able, on the one hand, to estimate the degree of dietary restriction which will be necessary and, on the other, to encourage the forces conspiring to motivate the patient will determine his success or failure in a therapeutic program.

It is helpful for a physician to determine whether it is possible for a given patient to continue on an unbroken restricted program for a prolonged period, whether he will do better with more rigid general restriction of calories than is necessary, thereby permitting a few special items of particular desirability to be included, or whether a certain patient is unable to maintain rigid restriction for a prolonged period but is able to maintain rigid restriction for a definite period followed by a short period of "relapse" or "relief." Over a period of months the same end may be attained by several pathways.

It must be apparent at this point that the "aura" which surrounds many diet fads and programs is an attempt to fortify the patient's motivation. One of the important aspects of the "cults" and "spas" is the reinforcement of resolution associated with constant supervision in a setting of group enterprise. Interest, pride, and cooperation are stimulated by the discussions which occur in conjunction with "classes" of patients on a similar regimen. The discussion of personal problems which may have arisen in conjunction with the application of the dietary program is helpful. For ultimate and permanent success, however, the individual must not become too dependent on the group. A physician in private practice may strengthen motivation by having certain of his patients on weight-reducing programs meet in his office in a group. This also offers the possibility of providing dietary instruction more efficiently. It is not, however, a substitute for individual attention. Since the emotional support supplied by the physician is most important during the early days of the diet, patients should be seen very frequently at first—probably once a week. Only when secure patterns of dietary restriction have been well established can visits become less frequent. Even when a normal weight level has been established, patients require continuing observation and support. It is depressingly common to have a patient return some months after having achieved a reasonable weight, once again obese and repentant. Constant support from the physician may prevent some lapses of this sort.

Dietary Prescription. In order to lose weight, the patient must assimilate fewer calories than he burns. The physician, in prescribing the diet, must have some concept of the total caloric requirement of the patient; and, in addition, he must know both the minimum nutritional requirements which the restricted diet must meet and the patient's dietary habits and prejudices. The use of a "standard" reducing diet is, therefore, not wise. In calculating the diet, at least 1 Gm protein per kilogram ideal weight should be included. Fats and carbohydrate should then be used to achieve the desired caloric level. The dietary habits of the patient should be consulted and the diet designed to resemble the patient's normal food preferencs as closely as possible.

The caloric prescription depends on many factors—height, weight, level of physical exertion, basal metabolic rate, and rate of desired weight loss. Although in some instances weight reduction can occur at intakes as high as 2500 Cal per day, the usual prescription is for 1800 Cal or less. The psychologic advantages of highly restricted diets with rest periods and of moderately restricted diets without interruption have already been discussed.

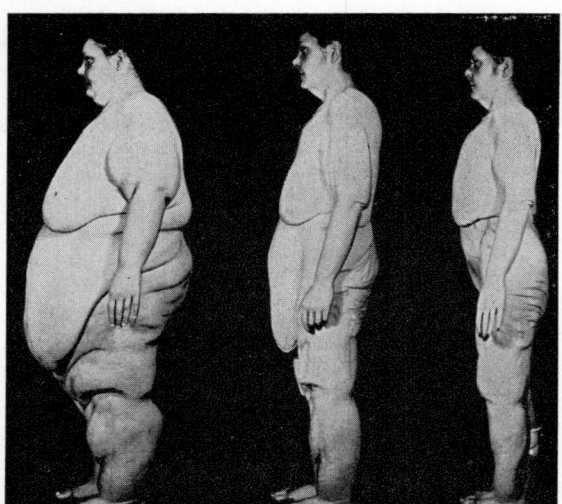

FIG. 22-2. Gradual weight reduction by diet alone in a 28-year-old woman with obesity due to overeating. Excess subcutaneous and connective tissue had to be removed surgically after a loss of 120 lb.

In deciding the proper caloric intake the physician must be empiric. Every patient is anxious to attain his ideal weight at the earliest possible moment. It is essential for the physician to decide the rate of weight loss which is most desirable for an individual patient. He must not be influenced unduly by his patient's demands. He must explain the advantages of a relatively slow rate of weight loss; he must point out that great weight loss may be accomplished over a prolonged period by moderate methods and that undue dietary restriction may be fraught with real dangers to health.

In most instances it is best to lose weight gradually rather than suddenly. A slow rate of weight loss allows better adjustment of the body and is a protection against nutritional deficiencies. There is opportunity for tissue to regain some of its elasticity, and the psychic and physical disturbances which occur with redundant folds of skin may be prevented (Fig. 22-2). Weight reduction should certainly proceed at a slow rate in the elderly, in the very young, and in pregnant and lactating women. Weight loss on a given caloric-deficient diet proceeds more rapidly in the first weeks than later. This is in part because of the compensatory fall in basal metabolic level which develops as dietary restriction is prolonged, and in part because of the early loss of relatively large quantities of minerals and water.

Total caloric intake should therefore be adjusted to produce a weight loss of 1 to 2 lb per week after the first 2 weeks. It should be remembered that very obese individuals may lose safely at a greater

rate than this, that growing children should lose more slowly than this, and that patients with cardiac insufficiency may lose large quantities of salt and water which should not be interpreted as tissue loss.

Most patients with moderate activity will lose satisfactorily on a 1200- to 1500-Cal intake. Some patients may have to be restricted to 1000 Cal or less. There is no real justification for diets under 800 Cal for ambulatory patients. Failure to lose weight on a diet prescription of 800 to 1000 Cal almost invariably means that the diet formula has been misunderstood or is not being followed. For short periods of time a diet of 500 to 600 Cal may be given, but the potential dangers of such rigid restriction should be appreciated.

Many excellent articles have been written with a view toward helping the physician and patient attain this end. In these discussions the advantages of bulk, the satiation value of foods high in protein, and the preparation of tasty foods of low caloric value are discussed at length. The means by which the diet is manipulated should not be confused with the end, which is only caloric restriction with the preservation of optimum essential food constituents.

Of great help to physician and patient during the early period of dietary regulation is the maintenance of a diary in which the patient writes down each article of food which he eats along with the approximate quantity. This should be checked over carefully by physician and patient together. Such a record is invaluable in suggesting necessary changes in diet, in rearranging meals and feedings, and in providing a simple means of detecting errors of omission as well as commission.

There is universal agreement that, in addition to caloric restriction, it is desirable to maintain a relatively high protein intake. Such a regimen reduces the negative nitrogen balance and prevents specific amino acid deficiencies which are more likely to occur in the presence of calorie-deficient diets. A high protein diet takes advantage of the specific dynamic action of protein, preventing to some extent the fall in metabolic rate which follows restriction of caloric intake. An adequate protein intake assists in maintaining a more constant blood sugar level, thus avoiding the relative hyperglycemia immediately after a predominantly carbohydrate meal and the relative "hypoglycemia" 2 to 3 hr later. Protein foods have increased "satiety" value. This, no doubt, is due, in part at least, to the increased specific dynamic action of proteins and the facilitation of gluconeogenesis.

Shifts in salt and water metabolism often induce relatively wide fluctuations in body weight from day to day. It is therefore preferable for patients to weigh themselves once weekly. This minimizes the effects of daily fluctuations and gives a true picture of the actual over-all effect of the dietary regimen. The fact that rapid shifts in body weight usually reflect alterations in salt and water intake or loss is taken advantage of by unscrupulous individuals who advertise "how to lose 12 lb in 12 days!" Physicians may take advantage of the effect of salt restriction in encouraging patients temporarily, since this will, of course, greatly increase the rate of weight loss. However, the disappointment which follows the slower rate of loss after a week or so on this regimen usually offsets its psychologic advantages. Physiologically, there is little advantage, and indeed some danger, in restricting unnecessarily the intake of sodium chloride on a weight-reduction program, unless edema or excess fluid retention is present. *Under no circumstances should water intake be restricted,* since dehydration is undesirable in a prolonged dietary regimen, and since edema is not effectively controlled by water restriction.

In female patients with active ovarian function, it is helpful to point out that weight gain normally occurs during the 10 days prior to the onset of menstruation, since patients who maintain their diet carefully may be disappointed to observe no weight loss during the premenstrual period. This periodic retention of salt and water adjusts itself automatically by a subsequent diuresis and increased rate of weight loss at the end of the cycle.

Exercise. Increased physical exercise is excellent for improving general health and body "tone" in individuals without serious organic disease. Patients should be informed, however, that it requires a great deal of exercise to assist appreciably in weight loss. Thus, if food intake is held constant (and this may present difficulties with increased exercise), playing 18 holes of golf may utilize 800 to 1000 extra calories. Exercise is helpful, and its value should not be underestimated, but the quantitative aspects should be carefully discussed with each patient. The dangers of excessive exercise by patients on a diet with rigidly restricted caloric intake have already been mentioned.

Vitamin and Mineral Supplements. Emphasis should be placed on a well-rounded, nutritious diet, since there may be essential factors of which we are not now cognizant. In addition, it is wise to provide an adequate supplement of the known vitamins. This is most easily accomplished by giving daily one or two of the readily available multivitamin tablets. Patients should know that it is vital for their good health that they abide by the restrictions imposed but that they also eat *all* the diet which they are permitted.

Only two mineral replacements need to be considered—calcium and iron. The indication for these is greatest during periods of growth and pregnancy.

Because skimmed milk is permissible in large amounts on most weight-reduction diets, it is usually unnecessary to prescribe additional calcium unless the patient cannot drink milk. Under these circumstances, calcium lactate in a dose of 0.3 Gm three times a day will supply ample calcium. Iron supplementation is necessary only in pregnancy, in growing children, and in patients suffering from iron-deficiency anemia.

Appetite Depressants. Depression of appetite by a pharmacologic agent can facilitate weight loss although it is apparent that as soon as the pharmacologic effect wears off, or the medication is discontinued, appetite will return and weight gain will recur unless the patient's inherent capacity to control his food intake has been altered fundamentally. That the pharmacologic agent used for these purposes be devoid of serious toxic side effects is axiomatic.

CENTRAL DEPRESSION OF APPETITE. Unfortunately there is no pharmacologic agent available at this time which acts primarily by depressing the "appetite center." This type of depression is seen regularly in disease states such as hepatitis and uremia and as a toxic manifestation of drugs such as digitalis. It will be of considerable clinical interest to observe whether or not it is possible to develop a pharmacologic agent which will effectively reduce appetite through its centrally mediated action without at the same time inducing some degree of nausea or general feeling of ill health.

SUBSTANCES WHICH DEPRESS APPETITE BY INDUCING A SENSE OF WELL-BEING. Amphetamine and its derivatives are the prototype of this group of substances. These agents are commonly referred to as "anorexigenic" or "anorectic." There is no evidence to show, however, that their action results from a depression of the "appetite center." As a result of stimulation, or a "lift," the patient's drive toward overeating may be significantly modified and as far as he is concerned the over-all effect of the drug is "appetite-depressing." Obviously, drugs which create such a state of euphoria may lead to habituation in certain individuals.

Amphetamine and its derivatives have been shown to depress food intake in man as well as in experimental animals. Patients experience a sense of well being after the ingestion of these drugs, and it is thought that the reduction in appetite is a consequence of distraction. At least in the hyperphagia which follows frontal lobotomy, no depression of appetite is induced by amphetamine or its congeners.

At present there is a large number of derivatives of amphetamine sulfate (Benzedrine) and closely related compounds available for clinical use, for example, dextroamphetamine sulfate (Dexedrine), levoamphetamine sulfate and phosphate, levoamphetamine alginate (Levonor), methamphetamine hydrochloride (Amphodroxyn, Desoxyephedrine, Desoxyn, Desyphed, Dexoval, Desoxyfed, Drinalfa, Efroxine, Methedrine, Norodin, Semoxydrine, Syndrox), phenylpropanolamine (Propadrine), phenmetrazine (Preludin), phenyl-tertbutylamine resin (Ionamin), and diethylpropion (Tenuate and Tepanil).

Although it is unfortunate that manufacturers avoid or disclaim the relationship of many of these substances with amphetamine, the fact is that the structural formulas differ very little (Fig. 22-3). The dextro form of amphetamine differs in its pharmacologic action from the levo form in that the cephalotropic effect is enhanced and the cardiovascular actions are less intense. However, this fact suggests that the dextro form might be expected to cause anxiety, restlessness or sleeplessness at the same dose level. The action of methamphetamine differs little from dextroamphetamine except in its somewhat enhanced cardiovascular effects. Since phenylpropanolamine may be sold without prescription, it has become a common ingredient of many weight-reducing tablets (Regimen, Didol, Rx 1121). Although if given in adequate dosage phenylpropanolamine may reduce appetite, in the usual dosage found in most weight-reducing tablets (25 mg or less) it is no more effective than a placebo. Phenmetrazine, although subjected to intensive study and claimed to be quite different, is a typical congener of amphetamine with the effectiveness of dextroamphetamine. Phenyl-tert-butylamine resin is advertised as not being an amphetamine drug although it clearly belongs to the amphetamine series as a study of its structural formula indicates (Fig. 22-3).

The usual dosage of amphetamine sulfate (Benzedrine) or dextroamphetamine sulfate (Dexedrine) is 5 mg given 30 to 60 min prior to meals. It may be necessary in some patients to omit the evening dose because of increased nervousness or sleeplessness.

Long-acting preparations which can be given in a single dose of 10 to 15 mg each morning are also useful. These substances may prove helpful for some patients during the early weeks of restricted food intake.

Although serious reactions are rarely encountered with amphetamine and its congeners, the physician must be alert to the sympathomimetic effect of these agents in causing a rise in blood pressure, increased cardiac rate and work, and the possible development of cardiac arrhythmias. Since tolerance to these drugs develops relatively rapidly, their usefulness is short-lived unless the dosage is increased. As noted above, habituation has been reported for some of these substances.

BULK PRODUCERS. Repeated attempts have been made to satiate the appetite by means of bulk of low caloric content. Leafy vegetables such as cabbage, spinach, lettuce, etc., are helpful in many patients and constitute an important element in most low-caloric diets. Methyl-cellulose has been advocated for its bulk and no-caloric content. For most patients, however, this has not proved satisfactory.

Metabolic Stimulants Including Hormones. Repeated efforts have been made to discover a nontoxic agent which would maintain a normal metabolic level in the face of weight loss. Dinitrophenol has had the widest use. The consensus today is that its undesirable toxic side reactions make its use unjustified.

In most instances, substances of this type are being employed by physicians or patients in an attempt to induce *weight loss without caloric restriction.* To do this, it is obviously necessary to raise basal metabolic level *above normal.* There is no known substance which can be used safely to increase metabolic level above normal for prolonged periods of time without danger of toxicity.

In the mind of the lay public, "hormones" are the most important cause of obesity and are hopefully considered to be its cure. The well-informed physician recognizes to what a small extent disturbances in hormone secretion are primarily responsible for obesity and how futile most types of hormone therapy are as cures of obesity.

No pituitary preparation now available is useful in weight reduction. Male and female gonadal hormones and adrenal cortical hormones have no place in therapy unless specific deficiency of these hormones exists. Thyroid therapy has received wide application and merits special discussion.

Thyroid therapy is effective substitution therapy in patients with hypothyroidism. Unfortunately, however, the number of patients with hypothyroidism among the obese is relatively small. Thyroid therapy has a definite and sustained effect on the metabolism of the hypothyroid case. Complete

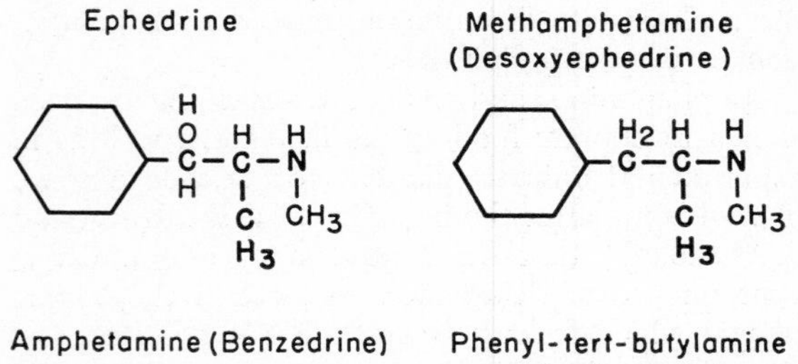

Fig. 22-3. Amphetamine and congeners.

thyroid deficiency may require 0.2 Gm thyroid (USP) daily; 0.1 Gm thyroid (USP) daily should be adequate for milder cases. A given dose of thyroid will produce a predictable rise in basal metabolic rate in a patient with hypothyroidism, and a daily dose of thyroid will maintain the increase in basal metabolic rate indefinitely. Unfortunately, in the minds of many physicians as well as patients, the term *hypometabolism* is synonymous with *hypothyroidism*. This readily leads to confusion and to the unwise and unwarranted administration of desiccated thyroid. In fact, it might be stated conservatively that at least 75 per cent of patients now taking thyroid extract do not need it.

When desiccated thyroid is used to increase the metabolic rate of a patient with hypometabolism rather than hypothyroidism, it is being used as a pharmacologic agent. With the initial dose of thyroid, some increase in basal metabolic rate will occur, since the total circulating thyroid present in the body will be increased temporarily. Since the thyroid gland is functioning in this patient, however, the continued administration of thyroid extract will exert a depressing effect on the gland, and before long the patient will have returned to the same level of circulating thyroid as he had prior to medication, the only difference being that he is now ingesting one-half or two-thirds of his thyroid hormone. Since the patient was stimulated by the first increment and since that effect appears to have worn off, the physician and the patient agree to increase the dose again, and the same cycle ensues. With each increment there is temporary stimulation of metabolism with a subsequent fall, until the total dose of thyroid exceeds that which the gland normally puts out, and persistent signs of hyperthyroidism become evident.

If such a patient on thyroid extract is seen by a skeptical physician, it is extremely difficult to persuade the patient that he does not need thyroid. First of all, he states that *he did feel better when thyroid was first given!* Second, if the thyroid medication is discontinued, the patient will almost certainly experience a marked fall in basal metabolic rate and will develop signs and symptoms of hypothyroidism which may be expected to persist for several weeks or months, until the thyroid gland is again normally stimulated to activity. It requires the utmost cooperation for a patient to undergo such a procedure, as he will most certainly tend to gain weight during the period of temporary hypothyroidism. It is easy to see why patients once started on thyroid extract may continue it unnecessarily for years.

Maintenance of Ideal Weight. Patients should understand thoroughly when they undertake a reduction diet that, in all probability, some degree of dietary restriction or discretion will be necessary permanently after ideal weight has been attained. The degree of dietary restriction is best attained by establishing the custom of weighing in each morning and adjusting the day's intake of food to the changes in body weight. It may be necessary at this time for the physician to review the comparative caloric content of certain foods which may have been withheld during the diet regimen. It is usually desirable to discuss in detail the calories contained in alcoholic beverages.

Once ideal weight has been attained, a patient should be encouraged to visit his physician every 3 to 6 months for examination and advice. The continued interest of the physician is of paramount importance to the health and happiness of his patient.

LOSS OF WEIGHT

Weight loss as a result of decreased body tissue may also be separated into loss of storage tissue and loss of functioning tissue. In this case, however, the separation is somewhat more arbitrary. It has already been pointed out that loss of fat stores cannot be separated entirely from protein and carbohydrate breakdown.

Starvation. When no appreciable intake of food occurs, the organism is completely dependent on its own tissues for the energy necessary to maintain life. Under these circumstances, protein breakdown is decreased, carbohydrate utilization is minimized, and fat becomes the chief substrate. The destruction of body tissues releases protein of high biologic value, and also minerals, vitamins, etc., which prevent the development of specific deficiency syndromes. Consequently, although the starved individual is greatly undernourished calorically, he does not develop malnutrition except as regards calories. In our civilization, complete starvation is not likely to occur except as a result of unusual accident, such as shipwreck; however, in certain postoperative patients where intake is restricted for prolonged periods to parenteral feeding and in emotionally disturbed patients with anorexia nervosa, a close approximation of starvation may appear. In contrast, patients receiving an inadequate caloric intake may develop deficiencies of various types, because the food supplied them is not complete in regard to vitamins, minerals, or amino acids. These deficiencies are discussed under manifestations of undernutrition.

Undernutrition. Nutritional inadequacies may occur when the total caloric intake is inadequate or when specific factors in the diet are lacking. Inadequate total caloric intake sometimes affects whole populations as a result of economic or political problems of food supply; however, in the United States it is usually the result either of neglect or of some disease process, such as gastrointestinal cancer, which interferes with the patient's ability to ingest adequate amounts of food. Lesions which interfere with digestion and absorption of food, such as chronic pancreatitis, gastritis, intestinal lipodystrophy, regional enteritis, sprue, etc., may cause a defect of caloric assimilation because undigested food is excreted. If a large segment of the intestine is removed as a result of surgery or is inoperative because a fistula short-circuits the fecal stream, inadequate absorption of food may result in malnutrition; however, since as little as 18 in. of normal small intestine may be enough to permit the maintenance of adequate nutrition, this type of malnutrition is rare. Undernutrition may also involve deficiencies of specific materials such as minerals, amino acids, vitamins, or essential fatty acids. The general problem of undernutrition will be considered under the following headings:

1. Total caloric and protein deficiency
2. Amino acid deficiency
3. Vitamin deficiency (see also Chaps. 58 through 61)
4. Mineral deficiency

Total Caloric and Protein Deficiency. When the caloric intake is insufficient to supply the energy requirement, weight is lost. Maintenance of body weight is, therefore, the simplest criterion of the caloric adequacy of the diet. The fact that the accumulation of edema may conceal the loss of tissue has been discussed above. The initial loss of weight occurs chiefly by sacrifice of the fat depots, especially if moderate amounts of carbohydrate are being supplied. Unless a low calorie diet is specifically planned to include a high proportion of protein, it is likely to be deficient in this material. Protein is the most expensive moiety of the diet and therefore is likely to be restricted first when economic limitations on food intake produce an inadequate nutrition. Moreover, protein absorption is readily deranged by disease of the pancreas, intestines, or stomach. Consequently, caloric inadequacy is commonly associated with an inadequate protein intake. In spite of this, the body protein can be conserved quite efficiently as long as the fat stores offer a ready source of calories to make up the deficit and as long as 50 to 100 Gm carbohydrate is included in the diet. Under these circumstances, caloric restriction produces a series of adjustments which tend to conserve the essential body constituents. Thus, carbohydrate utilization is reduced to a minimum, and a state of "starvation diabetes" ensues. Synthesis of fat from protein and carbohydrate ceases. Fat is mobilized and becomes the major energy-producing substrate. The basal metabolic rate is lowered and the caloric requirement is reduced as a result. As undernutrition becomes more severe, the secretion of pituitary gonado-

tropic hormones is greatly reduced, and reproductive function ceases, thus closing off another potential avenue for the loss of protein. The patient becomes somewhat more sluggish and moves about less actively; ultimately even mild exertion becomes impossible. As a result the caloric requirement is cut still further. By these mechanisms, the functioning portions of the body are preserved as long as possible, while less important fat depots and carbohydrate reserves are burned.

Whenever caloric intake becomes inadequate for energy requirements, a negative nitrogen balance develops. This is because of the fact that body protein is called upon to supply, in part, the calories required for energy. Under these circumstances, the quality of the dietary protein becomes of paramount importance. Protein intake is capable of maintaining nitrogen balance only in so far as *all essential amino acids are ingested and absorbed in adequate quantity*. With a daily intake of 100 Gm protein, one is practically assured of an adequate supply of the various essential amino acids. However, with a protein intake reduced to 50 Gm or less, it is necessary for the diet to contain an adequate quantity of all essential amino acids (Table 22-3) if nitrogen balance is to be preserved, even though adequate calories in fat and carbohydrate are supplemented. The smaller the total daily protein intake, the higher the relative "biologic value" or completeness of that protein must be in order to maintain a satisfactory nutritional state. Thus, it is readily possible for individuals on a high carbohydrate diet to develop protein deficiency because of inadequate protein intake or the ingestion of protein of low biologic value. In many instances in urban areas in the United States, deficiencies of this type are the result of "diet fads" or poorly supervised medical care. An ill-advised attempt to restrict the protein intake in kidney disease, for example, may result in the development of protein deficiency in addition to the renal difficulty.

Protein deficiency may also become manifest not primarily because of reduced intake but rather be-

Table 22-3. AMINO ACIDS

Essential	Nonessential
Arginine	Alanine
Histidine	Aspartic acid
Isoleucine	Citrulline
Leucine	Cystine
Lysine	Glutamic acid
Methionine	Glycine
Phenylalanine	Hydroxyglutamic acid
Threonine	Hydroxyproline
Tryptophan	Norleucine
Valine	Proline
	Serine
	Tyrosine

cause of increased needs. Infants and children during periods of rapid growth require much larger quantities of protein per kilogram of body weight than adults. Pregnancy and lactation impose a tremendous increase in requirement of both calories and protein. This is also true of men carrying on hard physical labor. The protein requirement also is increased with febrile illnesses and following operations and infections.

Despite a normal protein intake, a negative nitrogen balance may develop in certain gastrointestinal diseases, such as pancreatic deficiency, regional enteritis, or ulcerative colitis, because of increased intestinal motility or deficient intestinal enzymes and secretions. Patients entirely dependent on parenteral therapy for their nutrition may fail to maintain nitrogen balance, despite the administration of relatively large quantities of whole blood, plasma, human albumin, or amino acid solutions, since these preparations cannot ordinarily be given in sufficient quantities to supply an *adequate total caloric* intake. Fat emulsions suitable for intravenous administration can often be used to make up the caloric deficit. One such experimental preparation supplies 810 Cal in 600 ml of solution. In many instances, a positive nitrogen balance can be attained by intravenous feeding when protein solutions are supplemented with appropriate amounts of fat emulsions and carbohydrate is added in sufficient quantity to minimize ketosis.

In patients with prolonged or profuse bleeding from any source, one may encounter clinical evidence of protein deficiency. Under these circumstances, inadequacy in dietary protein intake will almost certainly precipitate a negative nitrogen balance and clinical symptoms of protein deficiency.

Amino Acid Deficiency. Although specific amino acid deficiencies may complicate the picture of severe nutritional deficiency, the multiple deficiencies present under most circumstances make it impossible to distinguish syndromes due to particular amino acid deficiencies. With diseases such as hepatitis or cirrhosis, chronic nephritis, or thyrotoxicosis, abnormal metabolism of one or more of the essential amino acids may take place, or the requirement of one or more may be specifically increased. For example, in severe thyrotoxicosis large quantities of creatine escape from the muscles and are excreted in the urine. It is known that arginine and glycine unite in the kidney to form glycocyamine, which, in turn, is methylated in the liver (methionine and choline) to form creatine. Thus, thyrotoxicosis necessitates an increased supply of at least three amino acids, i.e., arginine, glycine, and methionine, of which only glycine is synthesized within the body in quantities adequate for normal needs. In acute or chronic nephritis, large quantities of albumin, a protein of very high biologic value, may be excreted,

and in certain inborn errors of metabolism, such as alkaptonuria or phenylpyruvic oligophrenia, essential amino acids or their intermediate degradation products may be excreted in the urine in large quantities.

Deficiency of sulfur-containing amino acids shows up readily, with abnormalities in the growth of the skin, nails, and hair, all of which contain proteins with high sulfur-amino acid content. Methionine is also important, along with choline, as a source of "methyl groups" for many important liver functions. Deficiency of these groups is associated with fatty degeneration and infiltration of the liver. Other amino acids cause less striking individual manifestations but usually induce negative nitrogen balance with loss of muscular strength, osteoporosis, hypoproteinemia with edema, and deterioration of the organism. The most striking constitutional symptoms are lassitude and weakness. It is difficult to differentiate between deficiency symptoms due to amino acid inadequacy and those resulting from hypovitaminosis or avitaminosis.

Essential amino acid deficit will not occur in individuals provided with 1 Gm protein per kilogram of body weight and adequate caloric intake, unless some chronic organic disease is present. With reduction in protein intake below 0.5 Gm per kg per day, the biologic value of the protein must be excellent and the total caloric intake must be increased if deficiency is to be prevented. Low protein intake combined with low caloric intake will almost certainly lead to chronic amino acid deficiency.

Vitamin Deficiency. Specific vitamin deficiencies may color the clinical picture of more generalized nutritional inadequacy. There are also numerous instances in which total caloric and protein intake are adequate but in which a deficiency of one or more vitamins occurs. A good example of this is the difficulty which developed because of lack of an adequate supply of vitamin C during the long ocean voyages of the past century. The distribution of vitamin C among green vegetables and fresh fruits made this deficiency particularly likely to appear among sailors. Vitamin D deficiency is likely to occur among children, particularly in cold climates with little sunshine, or in warm climates where custom encourages the complete covering of the body with clothing, thus depriving the child of the natural means of supplying himself with adequate D from solar radiation. Pellagra in the Southern United States may occur in the presence of an adequate intake of total calories associated with an inadequate intake of nicotinic acid and the essential amino acid tryptophan. It seems probable that the vitamin requirement may vary considerably with the type of diet ingested.

Specific vitamin deficiencies are discussed in

Chaps. 58 to 61. It is well to point out here that there may be an increased need for certain vitamins in patients who are being fed for any prolonged period a relatively synthetic diet (intravenous glucose); also, patients with disturbed carbohydrate metabolism such as accompanies diabetic acidosis may require large quantities of the B-complex vitamins when the rate of glucose utilization is suddenly and tremendously increased, as occurs with the institution of insulin therapy.

The most certain method of preventing vitamin deficiency is to ingest a well-rounded diet. Although foods from various parts of the country may differ widely in their mineral and vitamin content, if food is prepared properly and if a diversified diet is ingested, little opportunity exists for the development of vitamin deficiency except in the presence of organic disease.

With the present custom of *massive* vitamin supplementation on the part of the American public, most individuals will exceed by several fold their daily needs. In some instances this may lead to carelessness in the selection of foods, with resultant amino acid or mineral deficiencies, although caloric and vitamin intake may continue to be optimal.

Mineral Deficiencies. Mineral deficiencies may arise in a number of different clinical situations; however these defects are seldom a result of undernutrition but rather a secondary effect of the disease itself. Thus it is impossible to produce sodium depletion in a normal individual by dietary restriction; but in a patient with Addison's disease, chronic diarrhea, or renal tubular insufficiency, the deficiency can easily be produced. Potassium also is supplied in large quantities by any sort of food, and potassium deficiency is unlikely to occur, therefore, unless an unusual avenue for potassium depletion has opened up, e.g., chronic diarrhea or the renal tubular defect associated with hypersecretion of aldosterone or comparable adrenal steroids. These defects are discussed in Chap. 52. Deficiencies of calcium, magnesium, and phosphate may occur rarely as a result of dietary deficiency; they are discussed in Chap. 57.

ANOREXIA NERVOSA

It is unusual for severe undernutrition to occur in the United States unless some severe organic disease is present. Psychogenic undernutrition does, however, occur in a small number of patients, chiefly young women. These individuals usually have a history of having previously been slightly overnourished. In an attempt to return their body weight to the level they consider esthetic, they begin to restrict calories, only to discover after a few weeks that they are unable to eat and consequently cannot stop their weight reduction. As a result, extreme loss of fat and atrophy of muscle may occur, with body weights becoming as low as 50 lb.

Etiology. The patients are usually severely emotionally disturbed. Often a history of incompatibility with parents can be obtained. There is frequently a story of some sort of sexual difficulty—either obsessive rejection of normal social sexual patterns or an unfortunate early experience with sex. Rejection of food represents a sort of suicidal tendency, and many of these patients attempt suicide by less indirect methods at some time in their disease. The physiologic disorders associated with the disease are caused by the lack of intake of calories and essential elements, as discussed above.

Pathology. The chief pathologic alteration is more or less complete disappearance of the normal fat depots. Although the normal feminine contours are lost as fat pads shrink, there is no atrophy of the breasts. In fatal cases, nonspecific changes in many organs may be demonstrated, probably chiefly as a result of lack of adequate protein and vitamin intake. Although a good deal of attention has been paid to the endocrine system, the only anatomic changes which are uniformly found are atrophy of the ovaries and endometrium.

Clinical Picture. The patient is very thin (Fig. 22-4) but usually maintains her strength and activities at a normal level; many such patients are able to carry out normal business and social activities. They are characteristically unconcerned with their undernourished state and are often brought under protest to the physician by worried relatives. The

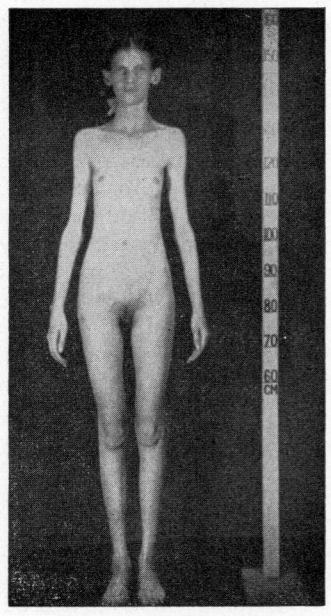

Fig. 22-4. A patient showing signs of marked undernutrition due to anorexia nervosa.

only characteristic alteration of function of which they complain is amenorrhea, which usually does not begin until after weight loss has been well established. On physical examination the blood pressure may be somewhat low, but there is no change of pigmentation, no loss of axillary or pubic hair, and the breasts are well developed. The examination is otherwise normal. Urinary 17-ketosteroid excretion may be somewhat depressed, the basal metabolic rate is depressed, but the serum protein-bound iodine is normal, and urinary gonadotropin excretion is low; other laboratory test results are within normal limits.

Diagnosis. The usual causes of emaciation must be considered in differential diagnosis, but such diseases as disseminated cancer, diabetes, or intestinal malabsorption syndromes are usually easily discarded because of the patient's subjective feeling of good health. Much has been said in the past about the differentiation of anorexia nervosa from hypopituitarism. Actually, the only similarity between these diseases is the fact that menstruation ceases in both. Otherwise, the persistence of normal body hair, normal breast tissue, normal thyroid and adrenal function, and good subjective strength and health should serve to eliminate pituitary dysfunction from consideration. This problem is discussed at greater length in Chap. 64.

Treatment. The patient will be completely cured if she can be persuaded to eat a normal diet. Since the emotional disorder precipitating this disease is usually severe and potentially self-destructive, these patients should be treated with the full cooperation of a psychiatrist. In some instances, complete recovery occurs spontaneously; however, many such patients remain maladjusted, and a considerable number die despite all attempts to maintain their nutrition. Tube feedings may be necessary to prevent the patient from starving to death during psychotherapy, but even forced feeding is not always successful. The use of high calorie, high vitamin foods of low satiety value may be advisable. Supplementary vitamins are often prescribed, but since the difficulty is usually with the quantity rather than with the balance of foods eaten, this type of therapy is not very successful. Numerous appetite stimulants have been suggested, including vitamins, "tonics," wine, and even cortisone. While any of these items may sometimes help, they do not improve the basic disorder and should therefore be used as adjuncts to treatment rather than as substitutes for more fundamental therapeutic approaches.

REFERENCES

Berkman, J. M.: Anorexia Nervosa: The Diagnosis and Treatment of the Inanition Resulting from Functional Disorders, Ann. Internal Med., 22:679, 1945.

Kekwick, A.: On Adiposity, Brit. Med. J., Aug. 6, 407, 1960.

Modell, Walter: Status and Prospect of Drugs for Overeating, J.A.M.A., 173:1131, 1960.

Rosenbeg, B. A.: A Double-blind Study of Diethylpropion in Obesity, Am. J. Med. Sci., 242:201, 1961.

Thorn, G. W.: Physiologic Considerations in the Treatment of Nephritis, New Engl. J. Med., 29:33, 1943.

Section 9: Anemia, Bleeding, and Lymphadenopathy

23 PALLOR AND ANEMIA
M. M. Wintrobe

Significance of Pallor. The color of the skin depends on many factors, which include the thickness of the epidermis, the quantity and type of pigment contained therein, and the number and degree of patency of the blood vessels, as well as the quantity and nature of the hemoglobin carried within them. Even the nature and fluid content of the subcutaneous tissue are significant factors. It is obvious, therefore, that pallor does not necessarily indicate that anemia is present.

A sallow complexion is present in certain individuals, as it was in their forebears before them, and may exist in the absence of any true anemia; the flush of excitement, on the other hand, or constant exposure to the sun and wind may produce an appearance which masks an underlying anemia. Physicians, at the turn of the present century, spoke of "rosy" chlorotics, as well as of green and pale ones. The number and pattern of distribution of the finer blood vessels vary in different individuals, and in the same person vasoconstriction may produce the appearance of pallor, whereas other factors, such as exercise, for example, may lead to the appearance of a "healthier" color. Certain disorders may affect

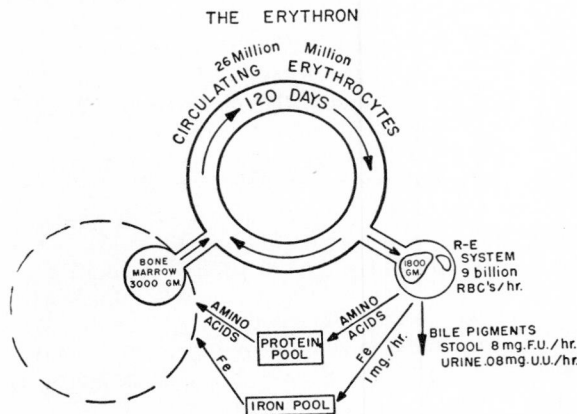

FIG. 23-1. The amount of blood in circulation represents the balance between production and destruction. In a 70-kg man the circulating red corpuscles carry approximately 770 Gm hemoglobin. Since the average life span of the red corpuscles normally is 120 days, the turnover rate per day is the total in the circulation divided by 120. In the average man this comes to approximately 2.16×10^{11} red corpuscles per day, or 9 billion per hour, and 6.4 Gm hemoglobin per day. From this are derived approximately 21 mg iron per day, 250 mg protoporphyrin, and 6.2 Gm globin. The iron and globin are reutilized. Of the protoporphyrin derived from the destroyed red corpuscles, somewhat less than 250 mg appears as fecal urobilinogen, since there are great variations in completeness of evacuation and also because of variations in the extent to which pigments giving this reaction are produced. Under normal conditions, through increased production and transformation of yellow marrow to red, the bone marrow is capable of approximately a seven- or eightfold increase in production capacity. Consequently, other things being equal, anemia will not develop as the result of increased blood destruction until the life span of the red corpuscles has been reduced to less than about 15 to 17 days.

the skin in such a way that a pallid appearance is produced, even though anemia is absent. These disorders include scleroderma, the various nephrotic states, and myxedema. The last two, however, may be accompanied by actual anemia.

ANEMIA

Definition

The Erythron. The *erythron* refers to the circulating red corpuscles as well as to that part of the hematopoietic system which is concerned with their production and destruction. As represented in Fig. 23-1, in the normal individual production is in equilibrium with destruction. Average wear and tear result in a "life span" of the red corpuscles which is approximately 120 days.

Hemoglobin, a compound of 67,000 mol wt, forms approximately 90 per cent of the red corpuscle (dry weight). It is made up of a colorless protein, globin, on the surface of which are four small prosthetic groups of heme molecules. Heme, which imparts the red color to the hemoglobin molecule, is a metal complex consisting of an iron atom in the center of a porphyrin structure (Fig. 23-2). The porphyrin has been designated protoporphyrin 9, type III. Like other porphyrin rings, it consists of four pyrrole nuclei connected to one another by methene $\left(\begin{smallmatrix} H \\ =C- \end{smallmatrix}\right)$ bridges. The iron, which has the capacity of binding oxygen reversibly, is linked to the nitrogen atom in each of the pyrrole groups and also to the imidazole nitrogen of the histidine in globin.

The structure of heme is identical in all mammals, but the properties of hemoglobin with respect to electrophoretic mobility, solubility, and resistance to denaturation by alkali vary in different species, apparently because of subtle differences in the composition of globin. In addition, in man a number of different types of hemoglobin, dependent on genetically determined differences in globin struc-

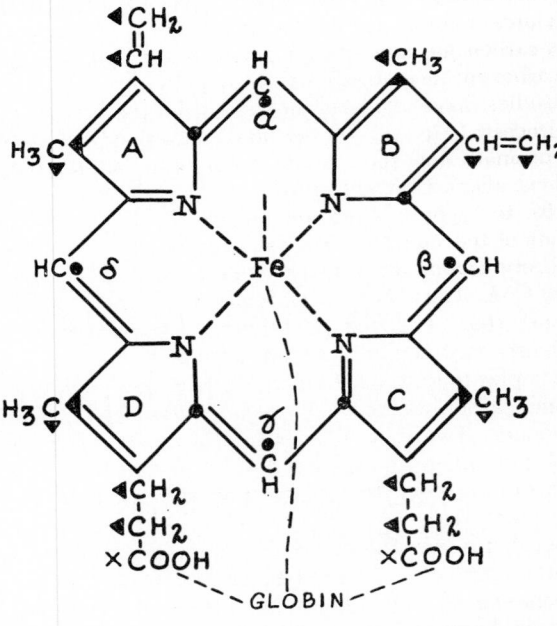

FIG. 23-2. Chemical structure of heme and its manner of union with globin to form hemoglobin. The carbon atoms derived from the alpha-carbon of glycine are represented by ●, those supplied from the methyl carbon of acetate by ▼, those derived from the carboxyl group of acetate by ✕. The unmarked carbons are those derived either from the methyl carbon atom of acetate or from the carboxyl atom. (*Prepared by Dr. G. E. Cartwright.*)

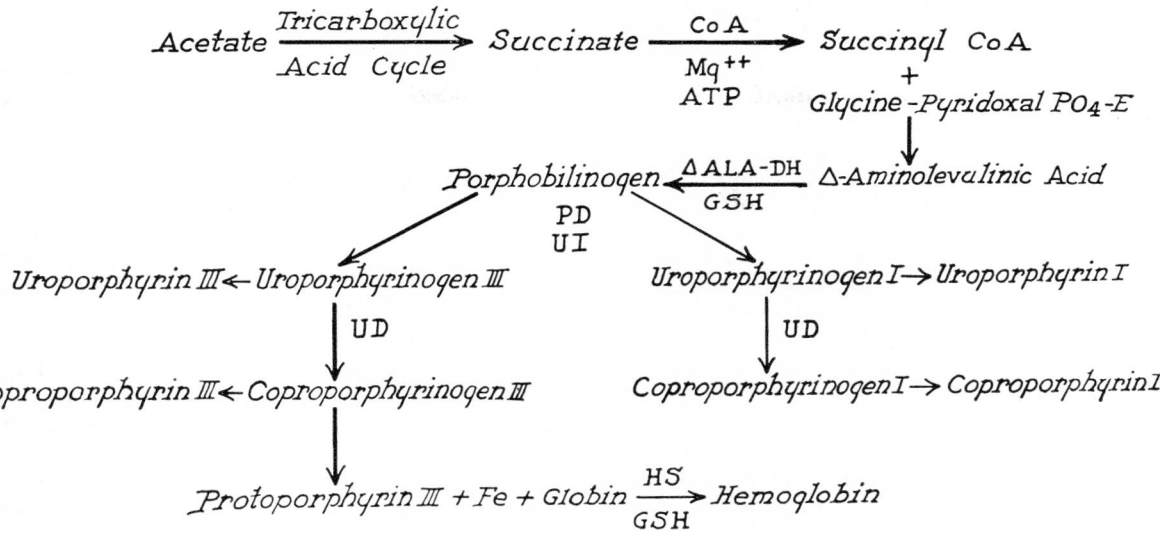

FIG. 23-3. The biosynthesis of hemoglobin and the by-products which are formed. (*Prepared by Dr. G. E. Cartwright.*) (*M. M. Wintrobe: "Clinical Hematology," 5th ed., Philadelphia, Lea & Febiger, 1961.*)

ture, have been discovered which in some instances govern the development of hematologic abnormalities and certain clinical manifestations (p. 1297).

Formation and Destruction of Hemoglobin. The source material for the formation of porphyrin is a 4-carbon asymmetric compound arising in the tricarboxylic acid cycle. In vitro as well as in vivo studies have clarified the steps in the synthetic process (Fig. 23-3). Acetate is transformed into succinate and this, in the presence of magnesium ions, adenosine triphosphate, and coenzyme A, gives rise to "active" succinate (succinyl CoA). This is one of the sites at which pantothenic acid functions in erythropoiesis, since this vitamin is a component of CoA. The vitamin pyridoxine is involved in the next step. The activated form of succinate condenses with a pyridoxal phosphate-glycine-enzyme complex to form delta-aminolevulinic acid (Δ-ALA) and carbon dioxide via several intermediate compounds. Two molecules of Δ-ALA in the presence of glutathione and an appropriate enzyme condense to form a monopyrrole, porphobilinogen. The subsequent steps leading to the formation of protoporphyrin are shown in the diagram. Ultimately protoporphyrin is converted to hemoglobin in the presence of iron, glutathione, globin, and an enzyme, heme synthetase. Amino acids are the source materials for the independent process which results in the formation of globin.

In the breakdown of hemoglobin, the protoporphyrin ring is opened by an oxidative removal of the α-methene bridge, the iron remaining and the union with globin persisting to form a green iron-protein compound, choleglobin or verdohemoglobin. How the cleavage is achieved is not clear, nor is

it understood how iron is ultimately split off and globin liberated to yield the bile pigment, biliverdin, a straight chain tetrapyrrole. It is known, however, that this takes place in the reticuloendothelial system and that the liberated iron is bound to protein in the tissues and then is transported as "plasma iron" via special transport proteins of the plasma (transferrins, siderophilins) either to the bone marrow, where it is used in the synthesis of new hemoglobin, or to the storage depots where it is deposited as ferritin, a ferrous iron-protein complex, or as hemosiderin, a ferric hydroxide polymer. The liberated globin is degraded and is returned to the body pool of amino acids. Biliverdin, as discussed earlier (p. 147), is rapidly reduced to bilirubin, which is then transported from the site of hemoglobin breakdown to the liver via the blood plasma, where it is carried with albumin as a relatively stable protein-pigment complex. On reaching the liver, bilirubin is separated from albumin, conjugated with glucuronic acid, and excreted via the bile canaliculi and the bile ducts in the form of protein-free di- and monoglucuronides, the former predominating.

Under pathologic conditions, free hemoglobin may escape into the circulation. This occurs in severe hemolytic states when there is intravascular hemolysis, as in erythroblastosis fetalis, blackwater fever, and *Clostridium welchii* (*C. perfringens*) sepsis. Such hemoglobin is promptly bound by certain α_2-globulins with affinity for hemoglobin, the *haptoglobins,* and is carried to the reticuloendothelial system for breakdown there and conversion to bilirubin. There are, in addition, two other serum proteins capable of carrying appreciable amounts of hemoglobin or its naturally occurring heme-containing metabolites. These are a heme-binding globulin and albumin which, by union with the ferric complex of protoporphyrin, form methemoglobin and methemalbumin. Free hemoglobin is demonstrable in plasma only when the hemoglobin-binding capacity of the plasma is exceeded. The so-called renal threshold for hemoglobin is probably not a true renal barrier but depends on the capacity of the binding proteins of the plasma and the reabsorptive capacity of the tubules. It is the free, unbound hemoglobin which appears in the urine. Then, in addition to hemoglobinuria, methemoglobinuria and methemalbuminuria may develop.

It has been held that bilirubin also can be derived from hematin, the trivalent iron complex of protoporphyrin 9. This may be formed in hematomas and collections of blood in serosal cavities.

It should be mentioned also that not all the bile pigment is derived from senescent erythrocytes. Studies of stercobilin excretion following the administration of N^{15}-labeled glycine indicate that normally at least 10 per cent, and in diseases like pernicious anemia and congenital porphyria as much as 30 to 40 per cent, is probably derived from heme or porphyrins produced in excess and not utilized in hemoglobin synthesis.

In the intestine, probably through the activity of the bacterial flora, bilirubin is converted to urobilinogen. *Urobilinogen* consists of three colorless chromogens, all of which are characterized by a strong Ehrlich aldehyde reaction, as well as by instability and ease of oxidation to three corresponding orange-yellow pigments which compose the urobilin group. The transition to urobilin can be hastened by mild oxidizing agents, such as iodine, and this is the basis of the Schlesinger (alcoholic zinc acetate) qualitative test for urobilin. Of the urobilinogen group, stercobilinogen is normally preponderant in the feces and urine. The remaining two substances are mesobilirubinogen and *d*-urobilinogen. Mesobilirubinogen is converted to stercobilinogen. *d*-Urobilinogen may be a precursor of mesobilirubinogen.

Although some investigators have maintained that the urobilinogens in urine come directly from bilirubin in the plasma, it is more generally held that they are derived from pigments absorbed from the colon into the portal circulation, most of which are returned to the liver and reexcreted in the bile but a small proportion of which escape into the general circulation and are excreted by the kidney.

The amount of urobilinogen excreted in the urine in 24 hr (UU) by the normal adult is 0 to 3.5 mg, most frequently 0.5 to 1.5 mg. The normal range for fecal urobilinogen (FU) as calculated from a 4-day period of collection is 40 to 280 mg per day, usually 100 to 200 mg. Lower values are found in young children. Mean values have been found to increase with age. The oral administration of chlortetracycline (Aureomycin) causes a marked decrease in the concentration of fecal urobilinogen, but this can be counteracted by the administration of aluminum hydroxide gel.

When the balance between the production and destruction of red corpuscles is altered in such a way that less than the normal quantity of red corpuscles is found in the circulation, anemia results. Anemia occurs, in other words, when production fails to keep up with demand. The latter may be normal, and yet anemia may develop because of (1) deficiency of materials required for the construction of the red corpuscles or (2) some defect in the metabolic processes concerned in erythropoiesis. On the other hand, anemia may occur in spite of vigorous production (3) because of blood loss or (4) as the result of excessive blood destruction (Table 23-1).

Pathogenesis

The simplest mechanism by which anemia develops is blood loss. Anemia due to blood loss may be acute or chronic. In the former the cause of the anemia is usually obvious, although sometimes a large hemorrhage may have occurred under conditions which do not reveal themselves readily. Hemorrhage in the gastrointestinal tract, as from a peptic ulcer, may be dramatic in its symptomatology and may be so severe as to cause shock; at other times it may be insidious in character and may occur without the development of pain or of symptoms pointing clearly to the gastrointestinal tract. Hemorrhage into one of the serous cavities can cause puzzling symptoms and signs: profound anemia may develop suddenly and icterus may even eventually appear as the result of absorption of blood from a serous cavity.

Chronic loss of blood occurs most commonly from the pelvic organs in females and from the gastrointestinal tract in the male. A common cause of chronic posthemorrhagic anemia in certain parts of the world is infestation with the hookworm.

For the construction of red corpuscles, as already stated, amino acids and protein, iron, and the precursors of porphyrin, are required. Certain minerals such as copper and cobalt are concerned in erythropoiesis, and under experimental conditions in animals it can be shown that anemia will develop when they are lacking. Perhaps still other minerals are involved. Certain of the B vitamins are important in erythropoiesis. These include pantothenic acid, pyridoxine, folic acid (pteroylglutamic acid), and vitamin B_{12}; riboflavin and nicotinic acid are possibly concerned as well.

Without doubt, protein deficiency results in anemia in man, but since there exists in the body a

Table 23-1. ETIOLOGIC CLASSIFICATION OF ANEMIA

I. Loss of blood
   A. Acute posthemorrhagic anemia
   B. Chronic posthemorrhagic anemia
II. Deficiency of factors concerned in erythropoiesis
   A. Iron deficiency
      Experimentally, also copper and cobalt deficiencies
   B. Deficiency of various B vitamins
      Clinically B_{12} and folic acid deficiencies (pernicious anemia and related macrocytic, megaloblastic anemias) and "pyridoxine-responsive" anemia
      Experimentally pyridoxine, folic acid, B_{12}, and nicotinic acid deficiencies; possibly also riboflavin, pantothenic acid, and thiamine deficiencies
   C. Protein deficiency
   D. Possibly ascorbic acid deficiency
III. Excessive destruction of red corpuscles resulting from
   A. Extracorpuscular causes
   B. Intracorpuscular defects, congenital (see IV, A below) and acquired
IV. Faulty construction of red corpuscles
   A. Congenital or hereditary
      1. Sickle-cell anemia and related disorders (hemoglobin C disease, etc.)
      2. Thalassemia
      3. Hereditary spherocytosis and nonspherocytic hemolytic anemias
   B. Acquired
      1. Anemia associated with infection
      2. Anemia associated with various chronic diseases (renal, etc.)
      3. Anemia in plumbism; following irradiation; in drug sensitivity (aplastic anemia)
      4. Anemia in myxedema and in other endocrine deficiencies
      5. Myelophthisic anemias (leukemia, Hodgkin's disease, myelofibrosis, malignancy with metastases, etc.)
      6. Anemia associated with splenic disorders ("hypersplenism")
   C. Unknown miscellaneous hypersideremic anemias
(For additional details see Tables 235-1, 235-2, 235-4, pp. 1281, 1289, and 1300, respectively.)

"dynamic equilibrium" of the proteins, the deficiency of protein must be very great before hemoglobin production suffers. The role of the specific amino acids in erythropoiesis in man remains to be worked out.

It is clear that in man anemia can occur as the result of iron deficiency. Cobalt deficiency has never been demonstrated in man, but a form of copper deficiency associated with hypoproteinemia and microcytic hypochromic anemia has been described in infants. Of the B vitamins, deficiency in man has been demonstrated only in the case of folic acid and vitamin B_{12}. Deficiency of these substances is characterized by macrocytic anemia and megaloblastic bone marrow. Quite possibly the other B vitamins are available in sufficient amounts, even under the extraordinary circumstances under which man sometimes finds himself, so that anemia clearly attributable solely to lack of nicotinic acid, riboflavin, or pantothenic acid has not been demonstrated. Pyridoxine-deficiency anemia has only once been produced experimentally in the human infant, but anemia responding to the administration of pyridoxine has been reported in several adults in whom it may have developed as the consequence of some metabolic defect.

More frequently deficiencies which result in anemia in man are not due to lack of the substance in the diet but are "conditioned" by special circumstances. Thus lack of vitamin B_{12} in pernicious anemia results from an inability to absorb this vitamin because of lack of a gastric "intrinsic factor." Again, in sprue, vitamin B_{12} or folic acid deficiency may develop, presumably as the consequence of inadequate absorption. The same condition is occasionally encountered following extensive resection of the small bowel or in the case of a gastrocolic fistula. Excessive demands in pregnancy and greater needs for growth in childhood and adolescence may "condition" the development of various types of deficiency, and anemia will then ensue. (See Table 235-1, p. 1281.)

The role of ascorbic acid in relation to anemia has not been established clearly; while anemia is seen in scurvy, it has not been shown that this is due directly to lack of vitamin C (see p. 540).

As already indicated, the whole red cell mass is replaced approximately every 4 months. Destruction at a more rapid rate is met by increased production of red corpuscles by the bone marrow, which is capable of approximately a sevenfold increase in activity. When destruction exceeds production, anemia develops. Such hemolytic anemias may be due to a large variety of causes which injure the red corpuscles (for extracorpuscular causes, see Table 235-2, p. 1289), or they may be associated with intrinsic defects in the erythrocytes. The latter condition will be considered in brief below.

A number of anemias cannot be attributed to blood loss, impaired production as the consequence of deficiency of essential building stones, or increased blood destruction as the result of the action of injurious agents. It is plausible to consider that a fourth mechanism by which anemia may develop is impairment of the synthetic processes which normally result in the production of the red corpuscles. The fault may be qualitative or quantitative, or both. In the last case, less than the normal quantity of cells would be made, but those formed might conceivably be entirely normal or abnormal to only an insignificant degree. If the defect is qualitative, defective red corpuscles may be produced which are destroyed more readily than is usual. As already indicated, increased production may be expected to make up for losses resulting from increased destruction unless the latter exceeds the productive capacity of the hematopoietic system. If the metabolic defect is both qualitative and quantitative, anemia will develop. Its manifestations may be expected to be those of impaired production or of increased destruction or both, in different degrees, depending on the nature of the fault in erythropoiesis.

Considerable evidence is now accumulating which gives support to this concept. First in this category are several types of anemia which are hereditary in nature and hemolytic in their manifestations. These anemias are usually classified as hemolytic anemias due to intracorpuscular defects (Table 235-2, p. 1289). It appears that they also belong in the category under discussion. Studies of the pathogenesis of sickle-cell anemia and certain related disorders have revealed that several different types of hemoglobin can be distinguished electrophoretically and that the production of an abnormal hemoglobin is the fundamental defect in these conditions. Thus it appears that a molecular abnormality in a simple protein may cause the sequence of events that characterize a single disease. There is evidence that a similar concept may apply to thalassemia. So far there is nothing to indicate that such a concept explains the pathogenesis of hereditary spherocytosis, but such an explanation seems plausible, since the abnormality in that disease has been shown to reside primarily in the red corpuscles. The pathogenesis of these disorders will be considered in more detail elsewhere (Chap. 235).

It seems likely that a fault in the construction of red corpuscles not only may be inherited but can also be acquired. It is possible that by one means or another, as will be mentioned below, the synthetic mechanisms by which red corpuscles are normally produced may become impaired. By interfering with erythropoiesis the metabolic disturbance may result in the production of fewer cells; or defective red corpuscles may be made which are destroyed more readily than is normal. Although the classical manifestations of hemolytic anemia are unusual in the types of anemia to be considered, it is conceivable that the rate of destruction, or perhaps even the manner of destruction, may be such that the classical manifestations of hemolytic anemia will be absent. In some instances, and even perhaps in all the types of anemia coming under this category, it is possible that both these mechanisms are involved; namely, fewer cells are produced, and many of those which are made are poorly constructed. The evidence to support this concept of the pathogenesis

of the anemias, which will be mentioned below, is still only suggestive. However, it is a useful one for the present.

Thus, it has been observed that infection is associated with a profound disturbance in iron metabolism. This is manifested by a low plasma iron, reduced plasma iron–binding capacity, and decreased incorporation of iron into hemoglobin. The defect cannot be altered by iron administration, even if iron is given parenterally in large quantities. An increase in free erythrocyte protoporphyrin and in serum copper occurs at the same time. Whether the anemia associated with infection is due directly to these changes or is related to them more remotely is unknown. In any event, the profound metabolic defect caused by infection, of which these are presumably some of the manifestations, can be overcome by appropriate treatment of the infection. As this is accomplished, the anemia is also relieved. Various other forms of therapy directed toward relief of anemia, such as the administration of iron, are of no value.

The pathogenesis of the anemia associated with chronic renal disease is an enigma. Unlike the anemia associated with infection, anemia of renal insufficiency does not have hypoferremia as a constant feature. Like the anemia of infection, however, it is closely tied with the underlying disease and is uninfluenced by measures other than those which affect renal function. An exception to this statement is the influence of cobalt on both the anemia of renal disease and that associated with infection (p. 491). The nature of this effect is obscure, but it is probably not concerned with the fundamental cause of the anemia.

In association with renal insufficiency, erythropoiesis becomes depressed. Two patterns have been described, namely, one in which the arrest of erythropoiesis is almost complete and the red cell mass falls rapidly, and another in which moderate or considerable depression of red cell mass is present and persists over long periods of time. Only the second variety is related to the degree of uremia. In general severe anemia is observed when the creatinine rises above 2 mg per 100 ml and the blood urea nitrogen becomes greater than 70 mg per 100 ml. Concurrently with either form of depressed erythropoiesis, red cell survival is decreased, in part at least, as the consequence of an extracorpuscular factor. The nature of this factor is obscure; there is no evidence of an autoimmune mechanism, nor is there a clear relation with any of the products which are retained in renal insufficiency. The relationship of the anemia associated with renal insufficiency to the erythropoietic serum factors which may be produced in the kidney is obscure.

Inhibition of hemoglobin synthesis by toxic action on porphyrin-forming mechanisms appears to be a factor in the pathogenesis of the anemia of plumbism. Many of the red corpuscles that are formed are imperfect, and their accelerated removal from the circulation, as compared with the life span of normally formed cells, is probably another factor in the pathogenesis of this form of anemia. The anemia which follows exposure to irradiation is related to the inhibition of nucleic acid synthesis, but depending on such factors as dose and duration of exposure, other mechanisms may be involved as well, namely, accelerated breakdown, perhaps due to injury of the circulating red corpuscles, damage to capillary walls with resulting diversion of erythrocytes into tissue spaces and lymphatics, and hemorrhage. Individual susceptibility, perhaps based on an underlying abnormality in a detoxifying mechanism, or other unrecognized factors seem to be involved in the anemia which follows ingestion of certain drugs.

The pathogenesis of the anemia observed in myxedema is obscure. Defective absorption of vitamin B_{12}, uninfluenced by intrinsic factor, has been demonstrated in some cases. The anemia disappears gradually as desiccated thyroid is given, but it seems unlikely that it is attributable directly to deficiency of the hormone. It has been suggested that it is brought about indirectly through the effect of the thyroid on the consumption of oxygen by the tissues. Moderate anemia is encountered in association with adrenal cortical insufficiency and in cases of hypopituitarism. The pathogenic mechanisms are not understood, but in view of what is now known concerning the functions of the hormones secreted by the adrenal glands and the pituitary gland, it is at least plausible that the anemia is the consequence of some metabolic disturbance resulting from deficiency of these hormones.

The pathogenesis of the anemia in leukemia, Hodgkin's disease, malignancy with metastases to bone marrow, myelofibrosis, and other similar conditions is as yet quite obscure. Such anemia has been classified as *myelophthisic*. The term myelophthisic implies wasting away of the marrow, but it is usually used to refer to encroachment on or replacement of the bone marrow by leukemia or metastases. There is little or no evidence, however, that the erythropoietic tissue is crowded out in these myelophthisic anemias. Measurements of red cell production rates have yielded normal or increased values. It has been suggested that in some cases erythrophagocytosis contributes to the anemia. A number of studies have shown the "life span" of the red corpuscles to be reduced, and occasionally frank hemolytic anemia develops. It is possible that no single explanation for the anemia associated with these diseases will be found, but it is plausible, at least, that a metabolic fault related to the underlying disease is an important factor.

The anemia accompanying certain disorders involving the spleen has been attributed to an exaggeration of the normal functional activities of this organ ("hypersplenism"), which include the removal of worn-out red corpuscles. Such anemia might therefore be regarded as hemolytic and resulting from extracorpuscular causes. That this is the sole cause of anemia accompanying various disorders of the spleen may be questioned, however. (See p. 1336.)

It should not be overlooked that, in any given patient with a chronic ailment accompanied by anemia, more than one factor may play a role. Thus, in any long-standing illness there may be nutritional deficiency because of reduced intake and sometimes also because of faulty absorption from the gastrointestinal tract. Blood loss may be an added factor. In addition, as already discussed, a metabolic disturbance, like that which accompanies infection, may play a role as well. As noted already, in some instances excessive blood destruction complicates the picture still further.

Symptomatology

Hemoglobin is the vehicle and the cardiovascular system the means of supply of oxygen to the tissues. Nevertheless, anemia may be present in severe degree and yet may be associated with few or no symptoms; on the other hand, mild grades of anemia may be found, and yet symptoms may be prominent. The development of symptoms in association with anemia depends on (1) the causative disorder; (2) the rapidity with which anemia has developed; (3) the degree of reduction in the oxygen-carrying power of the blood, as well as the extent of changes in total blood volume; and (4) the preexisting status of the cardiovascular system. The last factor is important because a defective

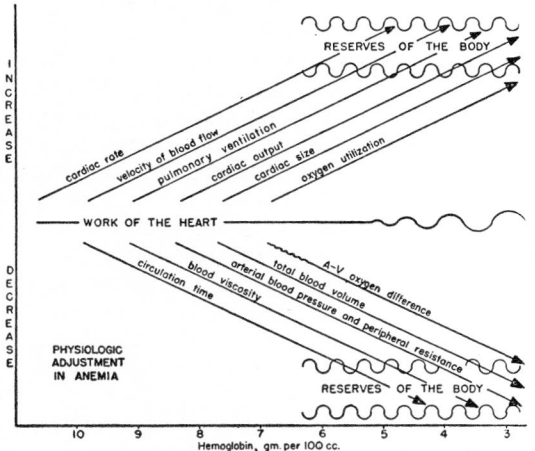

FIG. 23-4. Schematic diagram of physiologic adjustments to anemia. (*M. M. Wintrobe: Blood,* 1:121, 1946.)

cardiovascular system is less capable of adjustment to anemia than a normal one. The physiologic adjustments to anemia are represented diagrammatically in Fig. 23-4 and will be discussed shortly.

The nature of the condition which has led to the development of anemia is important, since disorders leading to anemia may—of themselves—cause pronounced symptoms which attract attention early; whereas other conditions are of such a nature that they are not likely to be detected until the effect of oxygen want, due to reduced oxygen-carrying power, becomes a factor. If anemia has developed so rapidly that there has been little or no time for physiologic adjustment, symptoms of oxygen want are likely to be prominent and to appear comparatively early; on the other hand, if the anemia has been insidious in onset, the adjustment may be so good that the red cell count may be even as low as 2 million cells per cu mm, or the hemoglobin as low as 6 Gm per 100 ml, without sufficient functional embarrassment occurring for the patient to appreciate his true condition.

When anemia is caused by the sudden loss of blood, the most prominent symptoms are those resulting from the reduction of the total blood volume, and they are relieved in large measure when the loss of blood is replaced by absorption of fluid from the tissues or by the artificial introduction of fluid or red cells. When there is rapid destruction of blood, the chief symptoms are those connected with the disposal of the products of blood destruction—namely, hemoglobinuria and jaundice. There may also be fever and even abdominal pain. When the anemia is caused by faulty formation of blood, its onset is much more insidious than in the above circumstances, and the symptoms are referred chiefly to the respiratory, circulatory, neuromuscular, and gastrointestinal systems.

Respiratory System. Respiratory symptoms in patients suffering from anemia are often noticeable only following exertion or excitement, although when the anemia is profound there may be dyspnea and rapid breathing even at rest in bed. Respiratory complaints are also dependent on associated myocardial changes and alterations in the cardiovascular system in general.

Cardiovascular System. Manifestations referable to the cardiovascular system depend on the severity of the anemia, the age of the patient, the rapidity of onset of the anemia, and the capacity of the cardiovascular system for adjustment. Anemia is one of the commonest causes of palpitation, shortness of breath, and pallor. If very severe, shock may develop. In chronic anemia, moderate dyspnea and palpitation may be the only symptoms related to the cardiovascular system, but, in certain cases, symptoms of congestive failure, angina pectoris, or intermittent claudication may be found as well.

Clinical evidences of an adjusting circulation in cases of anemia include a rapid heart rate, increased arterial pulsation, and increased pulse pressure; even capillary pulsation in the finger tips may be found, and still other signs of the "hyperkinetic syndrome" may be observed (p. 99). The heart may be dilated. These signs are due to increased venous return to the heart, with resulting increase in cardiac output. Thus the circulation time is shortened, and there may be a slight rise in right auricular pressure. Otherwise central venous and intracardiac pressures are not altered. The total circulating blood volume may decrease, although this is not always the case. Peripheral vascular resistance is lowered, and the oxygen dissociation curve is displaced to the right; that is, there is a reduction in the affinity of hemoglobin for oxygen. Extraction of oxygen by the tissues is therefore facilitated, and by this means tissue oxygen utilization can be maintained in spite of the narowed arteriovenous oxygen difference and the rapid circulation time.

Coincidentally with the cardiovascular changes, the rate and depth of respiration often are increased and the vital capacity together with the reserve and complemental air volumes are lowered. The residual air is somewhat increased, and minute ventilation is increased.

These and other changes which have been demonstrated to occur in association with anemia may not take place in an orderly manner and naturally become more pronounced as the anemia becomes more severe. The deviations from the normal values vary from patient to patient but generally are definite when the hemoglobin is less than 7.5 Gm per 100 ml blood and are greatest at the lowest levels of hemoglobin concentration. However, even at low levels of hemoglobin, anemic individuals at rest are able to compensate satisfactorily in the delivery of oxygen and the transport of carbon dioxide. On the other hand, during exercise, depending on the degree of anemia, the various hemodynamic adjustments become insufficient.

Severe anemia may produce a systolic murmur, which is usually most marked at the pulmonic area but may be heard elsewhere over the precordium, especially at the apex. Very rarely, diastolic blows are heard at the base. Over the vessels of the neck a curious humming sound, the *bruit de diable*, may be heard.

When compensatory adjustments become imperfect or fail, the clinical picture of cardiac failure ensues. Lateral displacement of the left cardiac border, basal rales in the dependent portions of the lungs, downward extension of the liver edge and liver tenderness develop. Edema is a frequent accompaniment of anemia. This may be the consequence of lowered renal blood flow but also is favored by such factors as hypoproteinemia and diminished tissue oxygen tension leading to increased capillary permeability. The reduction in the number of circulating red corpuscles is, of itself, of little importance in altering the osmotic pressure of the blood.

Neuromuscular System. Headache, vertigo, faintness, increased sensitivity to cold, tinnitus or roaring in the ears, black spots before the eyes, muscular weakness, and easy fatigability and irritability are common symptoms associated with anemia. Restlessness is an important symptom of rapidly developing anemia. Drowsiness develops in severe anemia. Headache due to anemia may be so severe as to simulate that of meningitis. Delirium is seldom seen except in pernicious anemia and in the terminal stage of leukemia. Retinal hemorrhage is by no means infrequent.

Paresthesias are common in pernicious anemia, and they may be accompanied by signs and symptoms of extensive peripheral nerve and spinal cord degeneration. They may also be encountered in chronic hypochromic anemia, but in the latter, spinal cord degeneration is very rare. In leukemia, involvement of cranial and peripheral somatic nerves occurs, but it is then almost always due to pressure or infiltration.

Alimentary System. Loss of appetite is not unusual as an accompaniment of anemia. Nausea, flatulence, abdominal discomfort, constipation, diarrhea, vomiting, or abnormal appetite may also be found. In pernicious anemia and, less often, in chronic hypochromic anemia, glossitis and atrophy of the tongue and papillae are common. In the latter condition, in particular, dysphagia may be found. Necrotic lesions in the mouth and pharynx may develop in patients with aplastic anemia, in granulocytopenia, and in acute leukemia.

Genitourinary System. Menstrual disturbances, most often amenorrhea, in the female and loss of libido in the male are frequently encountered in severe anemia. In other instances, excessive menstrual bleeding accompanies anemia. Slight proteinuria and even evidence of distinct renal function impairment may be seen in association with anemia.

Nutritional State. If the quantity of superficial fat is the criterion, the nutritional state may appear to be moderately or well preserved, in spite of the presence of anemia. When nutritional deficiency is present, the mucous membranes may be shiny and red, the tongue red and atrophic. Rarely there may also be fissures at the corners of the mouth, seborrheic accumulations about the nose, and erythematous lesions on the hands, face, neck, and elbows.

In severe anemia the basal metabolic rate may be moderately increased. Fever of mild degree is common when anemia is severe. A well-marked febrile reaction is characteristically found when there is rapid blood destruction.

Spleen. Enlargement of the spleen is rather frequent in various anemias of long standing. It is seen, in particular, in pernicious anemia, in chronic hypochromic anemia, and in the various hemolytic anemias, as well as in such conditions as leukemia, in which the spleen is specifically involved in the disease process. Moderate enlargement of the *liver* may be observed as well.

Integumentary System. The pallor which accompanies anemia has been discussed already. In addition, loss of normal skin elasticity and tone, thinning of the hair, and purpura and ecchymoses may develop in the chronic forms of anemia. When there is iron deficiency, the nails lose their luster, become brittle and break easily, and may become concave instead of convex (koilonychia).

So striking are its manifestations, and in certain parts of the country so common is the disorder, that special mention needs to be made of sickle-cell anemia. This condition exemplifies more than any other how varied the symptoms of anemia can be. The cardiac manifestations of sickle-cell anemia may be so pronounced as to be indistinguishable from those of rheumatic heart disease. Pain in the extremities may add to the confusion with rheumatic fever. Crises of abdominal pain have led to unnecessary operations many times, and the effects of thrombosis in the central nervous system have often raised the question of some neurologic disorder. Yet all these and still other bizarre symptoms and signs which are encountered in this disorder can be attributed to sickle-cell anemia alone.

Detection

The presence or absence of anemia is determined by the examination of the blood, but its existence may nevertheless be suspected and its degree even estimated with fair accuracy by proper examination of the patient. The skin itself, as already indicated, is an unreliable index of anemia; the mucous membranes (if not inflamed), the nail beds, and the palms of the hands are more dependable. The color of the conjunctiva may be very helpful, but one should not be misled by a coexistent conjunctivitis. The gums are not so useful as would be expected, for they may contain pigment or may be inflamed; furthermore, the pressure of the upper lip on the gums may produce some blanching if constriction of vessels results as the lip is retracted. Unless the hand has been held in an awkward position or has been exposed to cold or excessive heat, the nail beds and the palms of the hands will reveal anemia if much exists. In the palms the color of the creases is especially noteworthy, for they retain their red color even after the intervening skin of the palms has become definitely pale; when their color is lost, the hemoglobin may be judged as being below 7 Gm per 100 ml.

The presence or absence of anemia can be determined from the red cell count, the hemoglobin, or the volume of packed red cells as measured in the hematocrit. Of these procedures, the measurement of hemoglobin is the simplest but, unfortunately, hemoglobinometers are often imperfectly calibrated. Almost as simple, technically, and much more accurate as an index of anemia (or polycythemia) is the measurement of the volume of packed red cells. When this is measured in the hematocrit, additional information becomes available which is extremely useful in the routine survey of a patient. This includes the sedimentation rate of the red corpuscles, the volume of packed white cells and platelets, and the icterus index. If 5 ml blood is collected from a vein in a mixture of ammonium and potassium oxalate (6 mg of the former and 4 mg of the latter per 5 ml blood), or in ethylenediamine tetracetate (Versene), blood is available for a number of quantitative determinations. The white cell count can be determined without the necessity of obtaining more blood from the patient. A clue as to their number can be gained from the thickness of the layer of white cells above the layer of packed red cells. If the volume of packed red cells is abnormal, red cell counts and hemoglobin can be determined and the average volume and hemoglobin content of the red cells calculated. If the volume of packed platelets is abnormal, they can be enumerated, and if the color of the plasma appears unusual, the icterus index can be measured or a clue is obtained which suggests the need for other chemical determinations. Blood smears must be made directly from the finger. They should be examined in all instances of suspected anemia, for the morphology of the cells can serve as a valuable clue to the nature of the anemia and may be used to check the calculated mean corpuscular constants.

The normal values of red corpuscles for people at various ages are presented in the Appendix. These data are for persons living at sea level. At higher altitudes, higher values are found, roughly in proportion to the elevation above sea level. In general, the blood of normal persons tends to approach the mean for the sex. Provided the measurements are accurate, a deviation below the mean of more than 10 per cent should be looked upon with suspicion as representing mild anemia.

Study of a Patient with Anemia

Since anemia is a symptom, it is evident that the patient with anemia requires thorough examination. The *history* must be complete and must, in particular, give attention to the following details:

1. The possible occurrence of blood loss, either acute and in large amounts or chronic and long continued.

2. The diet, particularly with reference to the intake of foods rich in protein, vitamins, and minerals.

3. The presence or absence of symptoms suggesting an underlying disease such as chronic renal disease, chronic infection, or malignancy.

4. In the case of a child or adolescent, the rate of growth.

5. In the case of a woman, the nature of the catamenia (amount of flow, duration, and frequency); the number of pregnancies and abortions; the occurrence of excessive post-partum hemorrhage and the duration of lactation.

6. In certain cases, the possibility of exposure to poisons of various types should be investigated. In this last regard, attention must be given not only to the patient's occupation and its possible hazards but also to hobbies which may result in exposure to poisons, to possible exposure to insecticides, and to the taking of drugs which may be harmful (chloramphenicol, sulfonamides, gold, etc.).

7. The family history is sometimes of great importance in the study of anemia. A history of splenectomy in some member of the family may be a valuable clue to the diagnosis. If a familial or hereditary disorder is suspected, other members of the family should be examined if possible, since the family may be unaware of the existence of any detectable abnormality.

The *physical examination* must likewise be thorough. The examination of the skin and mucous membranes has been referred to already. The fundi of the eyes should be examined, for they may reveal hemorrhages or the exudates characteristic of chronic renal disease or of leukemia. The tongue may be atrophic, and the mucous membranes may reveal purpuric spots. A thorough check needs to be made for evidence of glandular enlargement, and it is good practice to palpate the bones. If done systematically such palpation may reveal tenderness in the sternum or nodules or tenderness in the ribs. In any condition leading to bone marrow hyperplasia, localized tenderness over the sternum is usually encountered if systematically sought out. In cases of multiple myeloma one may find nodules or tenderness in the ribs. The heart cannot be ignored, for it may give evidence of hemic murmurs or may yield the first clue to the existence of a subacute bacterial endocarditis. The liver and spleen must also be examined carefully, and the kidneys must be given attention, for it is not unusual for hypernephroma to cause an obscure anemia. Neither the pelvic nor the rectal examination can be neglected, for they may yield the first indication as to the nature and cause of the anemia. The nervous system, particularly in cases of macrocytic anemia, is likely to reveal abnormalities of significance.

The physical examination may need to be supplemented by roentgenography. A roentgenographic film of the chest may reveal unsuspected mediastinal enlargement, while roentgenograms of the bones may lead to the discovery of tumors or of periosteal elevations suggesting leukemia.

The *laboratory examination* may well commence with the collection of 5 ml of blood from a vein, as described already, together with a few blood smears. The discovery of anemia, as indicated by a reduced volume of packed red cells, should be followed by red cell counts and a hemoglobin determination; from them can be calculated the mean corpuscular volume, mean corpuscular hemoglobin, and mean corpuscular hemoglobin concentration. These findings should be checked by examination of the blood smear. In the latter may be found evidences of exaggerated erythropoiesis such as polychromatophilic red corpuscles, macrocytes, and even nucleated red cells. Evidences of disturbed red cell formation, such as poikilocytes, Cabot rings, and Howell-Jolly bodies, may also be found, or the smear may reveal an unsuspected protozoal parasite (e.g., that of malaria). An increased reticulocyte count gives evidence of physiologically stimulated red cell formation.

The fact should not be overlooked that the hematopoietic system functions as a physiologic unit. Consequently, when red cell formation is stimulated, it is found as a rule that there is, in addition, increased leukopoiesis and an increase in the quantity of platelets. Thus, following acute blood loss, there may be not only reticulocytosis but also moderate or even marked leukocytosis accompanied by an increase in the younger forms of leukocytes not ordinarily seen in such numbers in the blood ("shift to the left"). The quantity of platelets also is likely to be increased.

When erythropoiesis is impaired, owing to iron or to vitamin B_{12} deficiency or in aplastic anemia, one finds evidence of disturbed leukocyte and platelet formation as well. Thus, in pernicious anemia, leukopenia is a common accompaniment of the anemia and is usually associated with relative lymphocytosis and the presence of multisegmented polymorphonuclear leukocytes. Thrombocytopenia often exists as well.

Evidence of increased red cell destruction must also be sought out. The clue to this is generally given by the appearance of the plasma which, in cases of increased blood destruction, is distinctly icteric. The van den Bergh reaction reveals this to be of the "indirect" type, and examination of the urine in such cases reveals an increased quantity of urobilinogen (see p. 148). It is useful, where the facilities exist, to measure the quantity of uro-

bilinogen excreted in the stool as well. In relation to increased blood destruction, it is again important to look upon the hematopoietic system as a physiologic unit. Increased blood destruction, except in certain types of chronic hemolytic anemia, is accompanied not only by the chemical evidence just mentioned but also by reticulocytosis, leukocytosis, and thrombocytosis (see p. 1288). If there is reason to believe that one is dealing with a hemolytic anemia, special procedures will aid in the differential diagnosis, such as a test of the osmotic fragility of the red corpuscles, the Coombs test, and the presumptive test for warm, cold, and acid hemolysins (see Chap. 235).

The anemia associated with chronic infection or with chronic renal disease, like aplastic anemia due to the action of a poison, is differentiated from the anemias due to nutritional deficiency and the anemias due to exaggerated blood destruction by the lack of evidence of hematopoietic activity. Thus the anemia is usually normocytic and is accompanied by relatively little poikilocytosis or anisocytosis; reticulocytes are normal in number, and nucleated red cells are not found in the blood smear; the leukocytes are not altered in number from the normal except in so far as they may represent a reaction to the underlying disorder.

Knowledge of the chemical processes concerned in erythropoiesis has not yet reached the point where chemical examination is of great practical value in the recognition and differentiation of the various types of anemia. Nevertheless, interesting changes can be demonstrated. Thus the *plasma iron* content is reduced below the normal in cases of iron deficiency, in association with the anemia of chronic infection, and in various types of anemia in which blood regeneration is active. An interesting difference between the findings in cases of iron deficiency and in those caused by infection is the fact that the iron-binding capacity of the plasma is greatly increased above normal when the hypoferremia is due to iron deficiency, whereas it is less than normal when the hypoferremia is associated with the anemia of chronic infection. The plasma iron content is increased in pernicious anemia in relapse and in hemolytic anemias. However, the increased plasma iron of pernicious anemia in relapse falls to values below normal during the time when blood regeneration is occurring as the result of specific therapy. In certain circumstances, particularly in the anemia of chronic infection, the content of *free protoporphyrin in the erythrocytes* is increased. In this type of anemia the *serum copper* content is also in excess of the normal.

When the patient has been studied thoroughly in the manner indicated above, the number of instances in which *examination of the bone marrow* will be required is small. In Table 23-2 various

Table 23-2. CONDITIONS IN WHICH VARIOUS TYPES OF REACTION MAY BE OBSERVED, AS DEMONSTRATED BY BONE MARROW ASPIRATION

M/E (myeloid/erythroid) ratio increased	Nonmyeloid cells increased
Myeloid forms of leukemia	Other forms of leukemia
The majority of infections	Multiple myeloma
Leukemoid reaction	Metastases from carcinoma, etc.
Decrease in nucleated red cells	Gaucher's disease, Niemann-Pick disease
	Aplastic anemia (usually relative increase only)
	Infectious mononucleosis

Normoblastic hyperplasia	Megaloblastic hyperplasia
Hemorrhagic anemias	Pernicious anemia
Iron-deficiency anemia	Sprue, idiopathic steatorrhea, resection of small intestine (certain cases)
Hemolytic anemias	
Thalassemia	Tropical macrocytic anemia
Cirrhosis of the liver	
Polycythemia vera	Nontropical nutritional macrocytic anemia
Plumbism	
Anemia of chronic renal disease	Macrocytic anemia with diphyllobothrium infestation
	Megaloblastic anemia of infancy
	Megaloblastic anemia of pregnancy
	"Refractory megaloblastic" or "achrestic" anemia

types of reaction are listed which may be observed if differential counts on aspirated bone marrow are made. In the study of bone marrow as obtained by sternal, iliac crest, spinous process, or rib puncture, consideration should be given to the following:

1. What is the myeloid/erythroid (M/E) ratio? By this is meant the proportion of leukocytes of the myeloid series to nucleated red cells of all types.

2. If the M/E ratio is decreased—that is, if the proportion of nucleated red cells is greater than normal—this may be because of a decrease in the number of myeloid cells, as occurs in agranulocytosis, or it may be the consequence of an increase in erythroid cells. In the latter event, one must differentiate between normoblastic and megaloblastic hyperplasia.

3. Is there an increased number of cells other than those of the myeloid or erythroid series? These include lymphocytes, plasma cells, reticulum cells, and other forms (myeloma cells, carcinoma cells, Gaucher cells, etc.).

4. Since megakaryocytes form so small a proportion of the cells of the bone marrow, specific attention should be given them and a number of preparations of marrow should be examined. Do they appear to be increased or greatly decreased in number? Is their morphology normal?

5. If little material has been obtained by puncture, is the bone marrow aplastic, fibrotic, or otherwise abnormal, the material obtained being essentially only blood? In such a case, surgical biopsy may be necessary.

In Table 23-3 are given normal values for the differential nucleated cell count of bone marrow obtained by puncture, and representative findings in a number of conditions are presented. These must be regarded only as examples of findings in typical cases and do not give the range of variation in disease. The latter obviously depends on the stage of the disease and the presence or absence of modifying factors and is difficult to present in tabular form.

Although in all cases the material obtained by sternal puncture is of interest, bone marrow examination is an essential aid in diagnosis only in a limited number of conditions. These include aleukemic leukemia, multiple myeloma, Gaucher's and Niemann-Pick diseases, and unusual cases of macrocytic anemia. In the last-mentioned condition the demonstration of megaloblasts is very useful, since it suggests vitamin B_{12} or folic acid deficiency. In "aleukemic" leukemia, the bone marrow reveals numerous immature forms, thus dispelling the doubt raised by their absence or scarcity in the blood. In addition to these disorders, it may be added that, in cases of parasitic diseases such as kala-azar, the causative organisms may be discovered in the bone marrow when they cannot be found in any other way. Again, the cells of metastatic lesions may be demonstrated by sternal puncture.

In aplastic anemia it is the negative character of the marrow material which may be helpful. In cases suspected of being instances of "atypical leukemia," "agnogenic myeloid metaplasia," or "hypersplenism," sternal puncture followed by surgical biopsy may support one of these diagnoses or, instead, may reveal myelosclerosis or myelofibrosis.

It is customary to think of the blood in relation to a unit of volume. It is not unusual to forget that the sample examined is only a portion of the whole mass of blood. Fortunately, the unit obtained by venipuncture or from the finger is reasonably representative, and it is rarely necessary to measure the total blood volume; nor is it often practicable to perform the latter determination. It is necessary, nevertheless, to bear in mind the concept of total blood volume and to recall that an increase in the fluid portion of the blood—that is, an increase in the total plasma volume—may give a false impression of anemia, the total red cell mass having been reduced little or not at all. Of even greater importance is the fact that extracellular fluid deficit (dehydration) may mask an underlying anemia.

Table 23-3. REPRESENTATIVE DIFFERENTIAL COUNTS OF BONE MARROW OBTAINED BY PUNCTURE

Types of cells	Normal * average and range	Leukemia, acute †,‡	Leukemia,‡ chronic myelocytic	Leukemia,‡ chronic lymphocytic	Multiple myeloma §	Pernicious anemia	Hemolytic anemias	Irondeficiency anemia	Purpura hemorrhagica
Myeloblasts........	2.0 (0.3–5.0)	50.0–95.0 ‖	4.0	..	0.5	0.8	0.8	0.5	
Promyelocytes......	5.0 (1.0–8.0)	..	10.0	0.8	1.8	2.7	3.0	2.0	1.5
Myelocytes									
Neutrophilic.....	12.0 (5.0–19.0)	..	26.0	1.5	1.8	7.7	8.0	9.0	8.0
Eosinophilic......	1.5 (0.5–3.0)	..	2.0	0.7	..	0.8	2.0	0.8	
Basophilic.......	0.3 (0.0–0.5)	..	0.4	0.2	..	0.3			
Metamyelocytes....	22.0 (13.0–32.0)	..	22.0	8.0	3.3	14.5	18.0	15.0	15.3
Polymorphonuclear neutrophils.....	20.0 (7.0–30.0)	..	29.0	8.5	62.0	14.5	9.0	28.0	31.0
Polymorphonuclear eosinophils.......	2.0 (0.5–4.0)	..	0.8	1.0	3.5	0.5	0.6	0.2	0.5
Polymorphonuclear basophils........	0.2 (0.0–0.7)	..	0.4	3.0	1.2	0.2	..	..	0.2
Lymphocytes.......	10.0 (3.0–17.0)	..	1.4	60.0	13.0	9.5	10.0	1.0	2.5
Plasma cells........	0.4 (0.0–2.0)	..	..	..	4.5 §	0.2	0.4	0.7	0.8
Monocytes.........	2.0 (0.5–5.0)	..	0.2	..	0.2	0.3			
Reticulum cells.....	0.2 (0.1–2.0)	..	1.2	1.5	1.0	2.0	2.6	0.8	
Mitotic figures......	0	..	0.2	0.3	..	2.7	1.0		
Abnormal cells.....	0								
Megakaryocytes....	0.4 (0.03–3.0)	..	..	..	..	..	..	..	0.2 ¶
Megaloblasts.......	0	..	..	..	..	40.0			
Pronormoblasts.....	4.0 (1.0–8.0)	..	..	0.2	..	..	5.0	..	4.0
Normoblasts.......	18.0 (7.0–32.0)	..	2.4	14.3	9.0	3.0	43.0	40.0	36.0
M/E ratio.........	4:1 (3–5:1)	..	40:1	1.5:1	8:1	1:1.5	1:1	1.4:1	1.5:1

* Adapted from M. M. Wintrobe: "Clinical Hematology," 5th ed., Philadelphia, Lea & Febiger, 1961.

† The immature forms are listed in the table as myeloblasts merely as a matter of convenience. In acute lymphoblastic leukemia the cells are lymphoblasts, not myeloblasts. Often it is difficult to distinguish the various immature leukocytic cells seen in acute leukemia. The essential point is the great preponderance of very young forms.

‡ The bone marrow picture in *aleukemic leukemia* is similar to that of leukemia of the various types, whether or not changes can be demonstrated in the blood.

§ The characteristic cells in multiple myeloma differ somewhat from typical plasma cells in that the nuclear chromatin is relatively fine and the wheel-spoke arrangement of the chromatin is not present; the cytoplasm is basophilic and bright blue, not blue-green as in the plasma cell. A perinuclear clear zone is unusual.

‖ The most significant changes are shown in *italics.*

¶ Although the number of megakaryocytes may not appear to be increased, in typical purpura hemorrhagica the majority (64 per cent in the case cited) have no platelets about them and most of the remainder (32 per cent) have very few.

Erythrokinetics. The introduction of radioisotopes into the methodology of clinical medicine has made it possible to carry out quantitative measurements of hemoglobin production and destruction which have been helpful in gaining an understanding of the pathogenesis of various types of anemia. Thus, by tagging red corpuscles with Cr^{51} it is comparatively easy to measure their life span, and with the same isotope, an estimate of red cell mass can be made. Again, by incubating Fe^{59} with the subject's plasma for 20 min to allow it to combine with the iron-binding globulin and then injecting the plasma intravenously, the plasma iron turnover rate can be measured. The rate of incorporation of the iron into new red cells can also be measured. Furthermore, by the use of a scintillation counter, the sites of red cell production and destruction can be determined. When such data are available in addition to the reticulocyte count, the myeloid erythroid ratio of the bone marrow, and the fecal urobilinogen, a rough quantitative estimate of erythrocyte production and destruction can be made.

In diagnosis and for the successful treatment of the great majority of patients with anemia, such elaborate studies are unnecessary. Investigations by such methods, however, have provided two important concepts which are useful for the clinician. One concerns the balance between production and destruction. Reference has already been made to this, and the concept is illustrated in Fig. 23-1. It is conceivable that blood destruction might be greatly accelerated and yet no anemia would result, provided production is accelerated to an equal degree. This is known as "compensated hemolytic disease." Again, destruction may be accelerated only slightly above the normal, and yet anemia may ensue if production fails to keep pace with even this moderate acceleration. However, production could not be reduced below the normal rate and yet anemia fail to develop, since there is a normal wear and tear for which production must make up if anemia is not to occur.

It is also important to distinguish between *total* erythropoiesis and *effective* erythropoiesis. The application of quantitative methods has revealed that in certain disease states a large gap exists between the effort of the marrow and the red cells which reach the circulation. Red cell proliferation and hemoglobin synthesis can take place which do not result in the production of viable circulating erythrocytes. Such "shunts" have been observed in thalassemia, in pernicious anemia, and in patients with bone marrow failure. It is now recognized that qualitatively defective red cells can be formed in the marrow and destroyed there without reaching the circulation. This knowledge has proved helpful in understanding the manifestations of certain types of anemia.

Classification

Anemia, since it is a symptom, may be classified in various ways. It can be differentiated on the basis of etiology or pathogenesis as outlined in Table 23-1, and it can be classified on morphologic grounds. From one point of view the etiologic classification of anemia would be the most satisfactory. However, the incompleteness of our knowledge restricts the usefulness of the etiologic classification of anemia; furthermore, certain anemias can be classified on this basis under more than one heading. Since anemia must be classified after the patient's history has been taken and the physical examination as well as the blood examination have been made, there are certain advantages to be gained from a classification of anemia centering about morphology. On this basis anemias may be divided into three or four groups: (1) the macrocytic anemias, (2) the normocytic anemias, and (3) the microcytic anemias. These last anemias include a well-defined group, the hypochromic microcytic anemias, and another referred to as "simple microcytic," because in this anemia the reduction in the hemoglobin content of the cells corresponds to the reduction in red cell size, with the result that the mean corpuscular hemoglobin concentration is not significantly reduced. This morphologic classification is outlined in Table 23-4.

Macrocytic anemias are characterized by an increase in the average volume (MCV) and weight of hemoglobin (MCH) in the red corpuscles. The concentration of hemoglobin in the red cells (MCHC) remains normal. The macrocytic anemias, in general, are of two types. The megaloblastic macrocytic anemias are characterized by the presence of megaloblasts in the bone marrow and are related to a lack of vitamin B_{12}, pteroylglutamic (folic) acid, and related substances, as will be outlined fully later (p. 1280). To be distinguished from these are the nonmegaloblastic macrocytic anemias, which do not respond to administration of vitamin B_{12} or folic acid. These include cases of macrocytic anemia associated with hypothyroidism and with liver disease, as well as some cases of aplastic anemia. The nonmegaloblastic macrocytic anemias also include a number of conditions which ordinarily produce normocytic anemia. The macrocytosis depends on the fact that immature red cells, in general, are larger than their fellow mature corpuscles. Consequently, in conditions which ordinarily produce normocytic anemia, when there is an accompanying very intense activity of the bone marrow with liberation into the circulation of many immature cells, a temporarily macrocytic anemia develops.

The normocytic anemias are those characterized by red cells of normal average size and hemoglobin content. Theoretically and actually, they are due to (1) the sudden loss of blood; (2) the destruction of blood, acute or chronic; (3) lack of blood formation; or (4) hydremia, in which event there may be no true anemia (Table 23-5).

The simple microcytic anemias, as already mentioned, are characterized by a reduction in the size of the cells without a significant reduction in their hemoglobin content. This is the least well-defined of the morphologic groups of anemia and is found in association with subacute and chronic noninflammatory disease and in various chronic inflammatory conditions.

The hypochromic microcytic anemias are characterized by a reduction below normal in the average volume of the red cells, together with a marked reduction in the concentration of hemoglobin. Excepting a congenital and hereditary disorder known as *thalassemia* and combinations of thalassemia with certain abnormal hemoglobinopathies, and rare conditions such as *pyridoxine-responsive anemia*, a *hypocupremic syndrome* in infants, and a variety of uncommon *hypersideremic anemias*, the hypochromic microcytic anemias are due to iron deficiency. This deficiency may be the result of a lack

Table 23-4. MORPHOLOGIC CLASSIFICATION OF ANEMIAS

Class and severity	Number of red corpuscles	Mean corpuscular volume, vol/RBC	Mean corpuscular hemoglobin, Hb/RBC	Mean corpuscular hemoglobin concentration, Hb/vol	Summary
Macrocytic					Red cells increased in volume; *mean corpuscular hemoglobin proportionately increased;* increase in size and hemoglobin content of red cells roughly inversely proportional to number of cells; mean corpuscular hemoglobin concentration remains normal throughout or may be slightly reduced
Slight...............	−	+	+	0	
Moderate............	− −	+ +	+ +	0 −	
Severe..............	− − −	+ + +	+ + +	0 −	
Normocytic					Reduction in the number of red cells without any, or at most only slight, increase in mean corpuscular volume and mean corpuscular hemoglobin; mean corpuscular hemoglobin concentration normal throughout
Slight...............	−	0	0	0	
Moderate............	− −	+0	+0	0	
Severe..............	− − −	+0	+0	0	
Simple microcytic					Reduction in volume and hemoglobin content characteristically less marked than reduction in number of red cells; mean corpuscular hemoglobin concentration normal or only slightly reduced
Slight...............	−	0	0	0	
Moderate............	− −	−	−	0 −	
Severe..............	− − −	− −	− −	0 −	
Hypochromic microcytic					*Reduction in volume and hemoglobin content characteristically more marked than reduction in number of red cells;* mean corpuscular hemoglobin concentration characteristically reduced
Slight...............	0	−	− −	−	
Moderate............	−	− −	− − −	− −	
Severe..............	− −	− − −	− − − −	− − −	

Hb indicates the quantity of hemoglobin in grams per 1,000 ml blood; vol = volume of packed red cells in milliliters per 1,000 ml blood; RBC, the number of red cells in millions per cubic millimeter; +, increase; −, decrease; 0, no change from the normal; 0 −, no, or only slight, decrease; +0, slight or no increase. The amount of increase or decrease is indicated by the number of plus or minus signs, respectively.

of iron in the diet, defective absorption, chronic loss of blood, or excessive demands for iron (growth, repeated pregnancies), but it is most often produced by chronic blood loss (gastrointestinal tract, uterus), aggravated by several of the other factors operating in various degrees and combinations. These anemias respond to the administration of iron.

Management

In the sense that by their administration a specific deficiency is corrected, vitamin B_{12}, folic acid, and iron may be considered to be specific agents for the treatment of certain types of anemia. In macrocytic anemias characterized by megaloblastic bone marrow, of which pernicious anemia is the most common example, the administration of vitamin B_{12} corrects the deficiency and the anemia is relieved. In certain rare instances of macrocytic megaloblastic anemia, folic acid rather than vitamin B_{12} or purified liver extract relieves the anemia. Examples are the megaloblastic anemia of infancy, "refractory megaloblastic" or "achrestic" anemia, many cases of "pernicious anemia of pregnancy," and some cases of sprue. These agents are valueless in anemias other than those in which the bone marrow is megaloblastic.

Likewise iron therapy is effective in iron-deficiency anemias and is useless in all other types of anemia. Such therapy is almost always effective by mouth, and only in the rare instances of severe gastrointestinal intolerance and in cases of chronic

Table 23-5. MORPHOLOGIC AND CLINICAL CLASSIFICATION
OF ANEMIA

I. Macrocytic anemias (MCV * 94–160 cu μ, MCH †
32–50 $\gamma\gamma$, MCHC ‡ 32–36%)
   A. Those related to deficiency of vitamin B_{12} and
folic acid (*megaloblastic macrocytic anemias*)
     1. Pernicious anemia
     2. Sprue and other conditions in which intestinal
absorption is impaired
     3. Megaloblastic anemia of infancy
     4. Megaloblastic anemia of pregnancy
     5. Nutritional macrocytic anemias, refractory
megaloblastic anemia, etc.
     6. Antimetabolites and increased demands for
hematopoietic factors
   B. Where there is intense activity of the bone marrow and in other circumstances (*nonmegaloblastic
macrocytic anemias*)
     1. Reticulocytosis (acute posthemorrhagic ane-
mia, hemolytic anemias, and other conditions
usually associated with normocytic anemia)
     2. Some cases of hypothyroidism, liver disease,
aplastic anemia
     (For details, see Table 235-1, p. 1281)
II. Normocytic anemias (MCV 82–92 cu μ, MCH 28–32
$\gamma\gamma$, MCHC 32–36%)
   A. Sudden loss of blood
   B. Destruction of blood—acute and chronic hemo-
lytic anemias
   C. Lack of blood formation—hypoplastic and aplas-
tic or refractory anemias due to poisons, infec-
tion, metastases, etc.
   D. Hydremia—not a true anemia
III. Simple microcytic anemias (MCV 72–82 cu μ, MCH
21–27 $\gamma\gamma$, MCHC 30–36%)
   Anemia associated with chronic infection, chronic
renal disease, etc.
IV. Hypochromic microcytic anemias (MCV 50–82 cu μ,
MCH 12–27 $\gamma\gamma$, MCHC 24–32%)
   A. Iron deficiency due to
     1. Chronic blood loss
     2. Inadequate intake of iron together with
     3. Faulty absorption (achlorhydria, sprue, etc.)
and
     4. Excessive demands for iron (growth, menstru-
ation, pregnancies)
   B. Thalassemia and combinations with abnormal
hemoglobinopathies
   C. Rare miscellaneous causes [pyridoxine-respon-
sive anemia, hypocupremic syndrome of infants,
miscellaneous hypersideremic anemias]

* MCV refers to mean corpuscular volume.
† MCH refers to mean corpuscular hemoglobin.
‡ MCHC refers to mean corpuscular hemoglobin con-
centration.

ulcerative colitis with iron deficiency is it justifiable
to give iron parenterally. The parenteral administration of iron may be associated with a sense of
warmth and palpitation, nausea, vomiting, hyperpnea, and even precordial pressure.

Whether or not desiccated thyroid and ascorbic
acid should be classed as specific therapeutic
agents, as they are in Table 23-6, is debatable. It
is clear that the anemia accompanying hypothyroidism is relieved only by the administration of
thyroid, but whether this is the direct consequence
of the relief of a deficiency is less certain. The relationship of ascorbic acid therapy to the anemia
of scurvy is even less apparent, as already discussed
in this chapter.

Anemias which are neither due to deficiency of
iron nor caused by lack of vitamin B_{12} or folic acid
are most difficult to manage. Iron or liver therapy,
vitamins, or combinations of these, given orally or
parenterally, are useless and wasteful of the patient's funds and the physician's time. These anemias cannot, in the present state of our knowledge,
be relieved without the elimination of the underlying cause. Thus, the anemia of chronic renal disease
is difficult to treat because the renal disease itself
is usually so unremittent in character. Likewise, the
anemia of chronic infection persists as long as the
underlying infection continues. Aplastic anemias in
which the bone marrow has been damaged in general carry a very poor prognosis. In some instances
the destruction of hematopoietic tissue may not be
complete, and in such cases the maintenance of
life by transfusion may ultimately be followed by
some, or even occasionally by complete, regeneration of bone marrow. The anemia of leukemia is
relieved if the leukemic process can be checked by
the use of irradiation or chemotherapy. The same
is true of the anemia of Hodgkin's disease and other
disorders of the lymphoid tissue. In all these conditions the administration of iron, vitamin B_{12}, and
folic acid or liver is valueless, and the giving of
transfusions is but a temporary measure of limited
value.

Except in the management of the circulatory
collapse which may be associated with acute blood
loss or acute blood destruction, or when blood is
given to supply the antihemophilic substances or
prothrombin, *blood transfusion* must be regarded
as a nonspecific method of treatment. Yet it may
be of great value. As specific methods of treatment
are discovered, the need for blood transfusion is
reduced. Thus this measure is scarcely ever needed

Table 23-6. THERAPEUTIC AGENTS FOR ANEMIA

I. Specific: liver extract, vitamin B_{12}
   A. Folic acid
   B. Iron
   C. Desiccated thyroid(?)
   D. Ascorbic acid(?)
II. Nonspecific: blood transfusions
   A. Irradiation and chemotherapy (in leukemia, etc.)
   B. ACTH and adrenocorticosteroids
   C. Splenectomy

in pernicious anemia or in iron-deficiency anemia, even if the anemia is severe, for the patient has had time to become adjusted to the hemoglobin deficiency and can wait for physiologic regeneration following specific therapy. In other conditions, transfusion is useful in tiding the patient over until other measures may be decided upon or become effective, or until spontaneous recovery occurs. This is true in certain cases of hemolytic anemia, in leukemia, and in purpura hemorrhagica. In matching blood for transfusion in hematopoietic disorders, special care must be taken, for the repeated administration of transfusions may lead to the production of antibodies in such titers that serious reactions may occur. Again, the danger of producing pulmonary edema by overloading the vascular bed must not be overlooked. Where this is a possibility, the transfusion of washed red cells or of blood from which much of the plasma has been removed tends to reduce the volume and salt content of the transfused blood. In cases of aplastic anemia, where the number of transfusions used may become very great, actual hemosiderosis may be produced, since the iron from the introduced red corpuscles is not excreted. It is a good principle, therefore, to err somewhat on the side of giving fewer rather than too many transfusions, since this is but a palliative form of therapy.

Adrenocorticotropic hormone (ACTH) and adrenocorticosteroids are sometimes very useful in the management of acquired hemolytic anemias, and indirectly, when they affect the leukemic process, they serve to relieve anemia temporarily in acute lymphoblastic leukemia. These, too, must be classed as nonspecific agents in the treatment of anemia.

Splenectomy produces permanent relief of the anemia of hereditary spherocytosis and may be valuable in some cases of hemolytic anemia of the acquired type. This is especially true in the more chronic cases and when leukopenia and thrombocytopenia are also present. This operation is the most effective measure for the treatment of purpura hemorrhagica, and it can be helpful, together with venous shunt operations, in the management of the Banti syndrome. It is also valuable in certain cases characterized by "hypersplenism" (p. 1335). As in the case of other therapeutic measures which are known to be useful in the management of certain hematopoietic disorders, however, splenectomy should not be undertaken without a thorough diagnostic study and full knowledge of the risks involved—the operative mortality, the possibility of postoperative atelectasis or other complications, such as thromboses in association with the marked thrombocytosis which may develop after operation, and the likelihood of failure to achieve the result desired by this operation.

Details of the management of anemia will be discussed in later chapters in connection with the various types of anemia. In dealing with cases of anemia, the value of a diet containing food factors especially useful in blood regeneration, such as animal protein, the B vitamins, and iron, should not be overlooked. Such a diet offers much more than can be gained from vitamin capsules. The diet should also include all other nutritional essentials, such as ascorbic acid. In addition, the physician should assure a reasonable balance between rest and activity, and attention should be given to the need for reassurance and understanding concerning the patient's illness. Palliative measures may also be required for various complaints as they arise.

It should be apparent from what has been said already that adequate management of anemia is impossible without a thorough study of the patient and discovery of the nature and cause of the anemia.

REFERENCES

Laurell, C. B., and M. Nyman: Studies on the Serum Haptoglobin Level in Hemoglobinemia and Its Influence on Renal Excretion of Hemoglobin, Blood, 12:493, 1957.

Sproule, B. J., J. H. Mitchell, and W. F. Miller: Cardiopulmonary Physiological Responses to Heavy Exercise in Patients with Anemia, J. Clin. Invest., 39:378, 1960.

Wintrobe, M. M.: "Clinical Hematology," 5th ed., Philadelphia, Lea & Febiger, 1961.

24 BLEEDING
M. M. Wintrobe

Except for that which occurs during menstruation, the loss of blood is abnormal, and this symptom, therefore, is a definite indication for a search for disease. As indicated in Table 24-1, bleeding may arise from a great variety of causes, and these may involve any of the systems of the body. This table represents a systematic and logical classification rather than one based primarily on frequency.

The most common cause of hemorrhage is that resulting from injury of large vessels by trauma or by erosion from pathologic processes. Less common is that which is attributable to some form of generalized vascular disorder. Very rare are instances of hemorrhage which occur as a result of fragility of the skin and its blood vessels. Defects in the factors concerned in blood coagulation represented a comparatively infrequent cause of bleeding until bishydroxycoumarin (Dicumarol) and heparin were introduced as therapeutic agents.

Table 24-1. CLASSIFICATION OF CAUSES OF HEMORRHAGE

  I. Vascular abnormalities
   A. Injury of large vessels by trauma or by erosion from pathologic processes
   B. Hereditary hemorrhagic telangiectasia
   C. Nonthrombocytopenic purpuras
    1. Allergic purpuras (Henoch-Schönlein)
    2. Symptomatic nonthrombocytopenic purpuras (infections, chemical and animal agents, avitaminosis, certain chronic diseases)
    3. Hereditary familial purpura simplex
    4. Miscellaneous: mechanical purpura, orthostatic purpura, purpura senilis, purpura cachectica
 II. Extravascular and miscellaneous abnormalities
   A. Atrophy of subcutaneous tissues (purpura senilis, purpura cachectica)
   B. Fragility and hyperlaxity of skin (Cushing's syndrome, Ehlers-Danlos syndrome, epidermolysis bullosa)
   C. Purpura fulminans
   D. Purpura hyperglobulinemia
   E. Purpura simplex, vicarious bleeding, "autoerythrocyte sensitization"
III. Intravascular abnormalities
   A. Platelet abnormalities
    1. Quantitative deficiencies: symptomatic thrombocytopenic purpuras and idiopathic (Table 238-1)
    2. Qualitative abnormalities:
     a. With prolonged bleeding time: von Willebrand's disease, vascular hemophilia
     b. Other thrombocytopathies, congenital and acquired
     c. With defective clot retraction: Glanzmann's thrombasthenia
     d. Hemorrhagic thrombocythemia
   B. Coagulation defects
    1. Deficiency of factor VIII (AHG, AHF, hemophilia A)
    2. Deficiency of factor IX (PTC, Christmas disease, hemophilia B)
    3. Deficiency of PTA
    4. Congenital "hypoprothrombinemias"
     a. Congenital hypoprothrombinemia
     b. Congenital factor V deficiency (parahemophilia)
     c. Congenital factor VII (SPCA) deficiency (hypoproconvertinemia)
     d. Congenital factor X (Stuart-Prower) deficiency
    5. Acquired "hypoprothrombinemias"
     a. Newborn (hemorrhagic disease of the newborn)
     b. Vitamin K deficiency (obstructive jaundice, biliary fistula, impaired intestinal absorption, impaired bacterial growth in bowel)
     c. Miscellaneous diseases (liver disease, leukemia, etc.)

Table 24-1. CLASSIFICATION OF CAUSES OF HEMORRHAGE *(Continued)*

     d. Anticoagulant drugs (coumarin compounds, etc.)
    6. Hypofibrinogenemias
     a. Congenital
     b. Acquired. Fibrinolytic purpuras [complications of pregnancy (abruptio placentae, retention of dead fetus, amniotic fluid emboli), pulmonary manipulation, neoplastic diseases, disorders of bone marrow, severe liver damage, shock]
    7. Circulating anticoagulants
     a. Drug therapy (coumarin and related compounds, heparin)
     b. In association with coagulation defects (factors VIII and IX)
     c. Idiopathic and in association with pregnancy and various diseases

COAGULATION AND HEMOSTASIS

Before discussing the causes of hemorrhage it will be useful to consider first what is known about the process of coagulation and the mechanisms for hemostasis.

Hemostasis is the arrest of the flow of blood from a vessel and is effected through the combined actions of three fundamental groups of factors: (1) *extravascular,* such as subcutaneous tissue, muscle, and skin, which qualitatively depend upon age, mass, tonicity, tautness, and resiliency; (2) *vascular,* comprising the blood vessels, which vary as to age, type, size, tone, location, and nutritional state; and (3) *intravascular,* which includes all the factors concerned with coagulation, including the blood platelets.

When bleeding from a vessel occurs, these factors normally function in a coordinated manner. Although many details of the hemostatic mechanism have yet to be clarified, the course of events may be pictured as follows. Following injury, prompt vasoconstriction and retraction of the vessel occur. Egress of blood from the vessel into the surrounding tissues results in increased hydrostatic pressure in the tissues, while that in the vessel falls. These adjustments, in combination with normal tissue tone, tend to halt the escape of blood temporarily. Initial vasoconstriction is maintained for 3 to 4 min, during which time blood platelets agglutinate and adhere to the area of broken intima. Disintegrating platelets release a vasoconstrictor substance and other factors, while fibrin is deposited about them to form a plug at the interface of the open blood vessel and its tissue milieu. Coagulation of the escaped blood, markedly enhanced by tissue thromboplastin, extends to include the platelet plug. Vasoconstriction of vascular origin ceases, but narrowing of the vessel is maintained through the cohesive and vasoconstrictor properties of the platelet plug and its interlacing network of fibrin. Initiated at the time of bleeding, blood coagulation within the vessel continues, and fibrin reinforces the vascular side of the plug. Although intravascular coagulation soon ceases, permanent hemostasis occurs as the result of contraction and organization of the clot.

Theory of Coagulation. The classic theory of Morawitz which regarded coagulation as involving four essential components—thromboplastin, calcium, prothrombin, and fibrinogen—reacting in two stages now appears to have been an oversimplification. Although there is disagreement concerning details, the newer observations indicate clearly that the activation of thromboplastin is a separate, preliminary phase and that blood coagulation is a three-step process consisting of (1) activation of thromboplastin, (2) conversion of prothrombin to thrombin, and (3) formation of fibrin. Furthermore, blood clotting is thought of as a dynamic process in which positive forces leading to coagulation are antagonized by negative contrary forces, the latter including natural anticoagulants and agents which remove the formed clot.

For all students and physicians other than those who are continuously dealing with problems of coagulation, the process of coagulation and the disorders associated therewith represent one of the most difficult and confusing areas of clinical medicine. This is in part due to the limitations of knowledge and the fact that it has been necessary to study reactions without the aid of pure substances. Confusion arises also from the fact that a great variety of names has been used for essentially the same substances or reactions. Fortunately an internationally acceptable nomenclature now has been adopted. This, together with some of the synonyms which have been used, is presented in Table 24-2.

Figure 24-1 presents the essential features of the coagulation process as understood at the present time. Although the final stages of coagulation are comparatively clear, the initial steps are still obscure. Intra- and extravascular mechanisms differ somewhat from one another and may be considered separately. It is the intravascular process which has been particularly difficult to elucidate.

It is well known that coagulation is initiated by contact of blood with a foreign surface. The nature of the events which take place at this point has been the subject of much speculation, but it now appears that a coagulation activity known as *Hageman factor* (HF) is activated by contact with a surface. This factor was discovered in a family of that name in whom coagulation time was found to be greatly prolonged although no hemorrhagic tendency resulted. Activated HF reacts with *plasma thromboplastin antecedent* (PTA) to produce an

Table 24-2. SYNONYMS FOR VARIOUS COAGULATION FACTORS

International nomenclature	Synonyms
Factor I	Fibrinogen
Factor II	Prothrombin
Factor III	Thromboplastin
Factor IV	Calcium
Factor V	Proaccelerin, labile factor, accelerator globulin (AcG), thrombogen
(Factor VI	Accelerin)
Factor VII	Proconvertin (→ convertin), stable factor, serum prothrombin conversion accelerator (SPCA), autoprothrombin I
Factor VIII	Antihemophilic factor (AHF), antihemophilic globulin (AHG), thromboplastinogen, platelet cofactor I, plasma thromboplastic factor A, facteur antihémophilique A
Factor IX	Plasma thromboplastin component (PTC), Christmas factor, platelet cofactor II, autoprothrombin II, plasma thromboplastic factor B, facteur antihémophilique **B**
Factor X	Stuart-Prower factor
PTA	Plasma thromboplastin antecedent
Hageman factor	

active prothromboplastic factor. The remaining reactions are obscure, but it is known that factors IX, VIII, and X, as well as calcium, are required and that a platelet substance, the lipoprotein factor 3, or certain lipid constituents (phosphatidyl ethanolamine and phosphatidyl serine) are needed. Still another factor (V) is required in the ultimate development of the substance which promotes the conversion of prothrombin to thrombin.

As already mentioned, platelets are important in hemostasis because, by their adhesiveness and agglutination, they serve directly in sealing an injured blood vessel, and by liberation of the vasoconstrictor, serotonin, they play a part in the vasoconstrictive response observed when vessels are injured. Their adhesiveness is associated with another phenomenon, namely, viscous metamorphosis. This consists first in clumping of the platelets, then swelling of the mass, and finally release of granular material, possibly phospholipids, into the surrounding plasma. At the same time a change in permeability occurs so that the platelet plug, at first permeable to blood, soon becomes impermeable and bleeding ceases.

The extravascular process of coagulation is simpler. The substance, tissue thromboplastin, is a high molecular lipoprotein which is derived from tissues directly following injury and is widely distributed in the body as an intracellular compound. It is found in highest concentration in the brain, lungs,

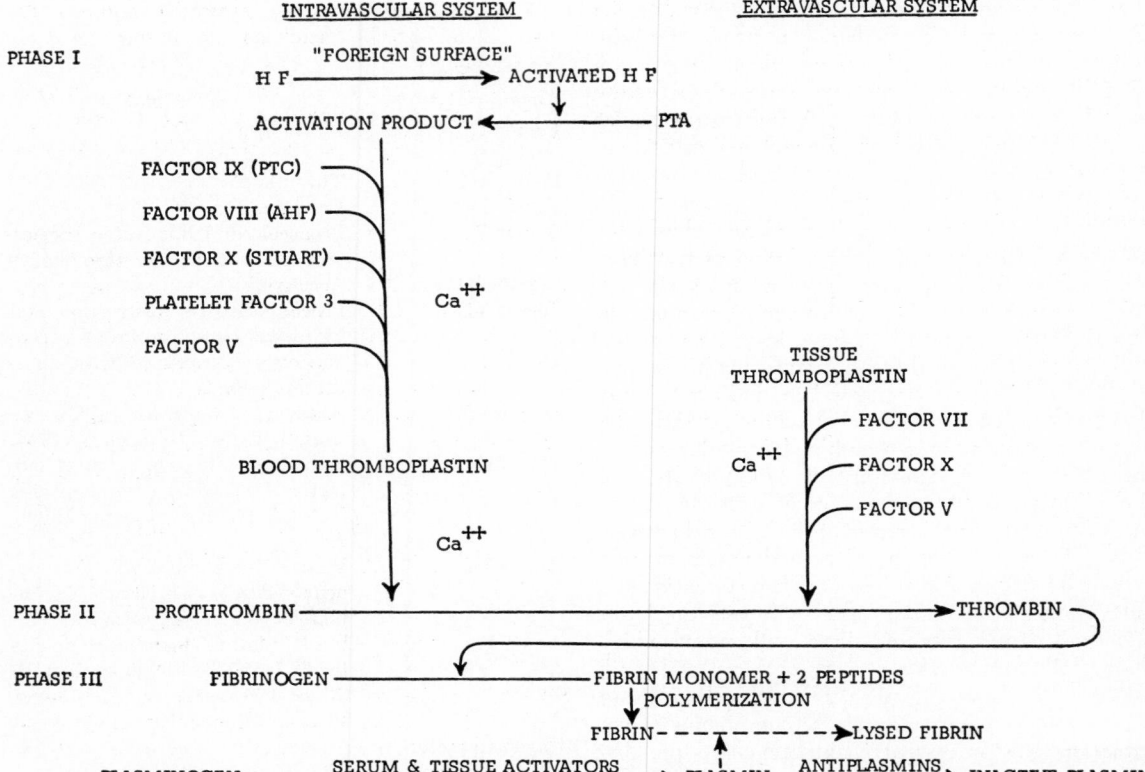

INTRAVASCULAR SYSTEM   EXTRAVASCULAR SYSTEM

FIG. 24-1. Outline of coagulation. The factors involved in the first phase of coagulation are shown more or less in the order in which they are thought to participate in the process. The counter forces are also indicated. (*M. M. Wintrobe: "Clinical Hematology," 5th ed., Philadelphia, Lea & Febiger, 1961.*)

placenta, thymus, and testes. Factors X and V and calcium are concerned in the extravascular process of coagulation, as well as in the intravascular, and an additional factor (VII) is also required to form, with tissue thromboplastin, a product which causes prothrombin to be converted to thrombin.

Factors VIII and V disappear during the normal clotting process, whereas factors IX, X, and VII, HF and PTA are not consumed. The action of the latter, therefore, would seem to be enzymatic, whereas factors VIII and V may serve as substrates. All these factors were discovered through the study of patients and families in whom they were deficient. The hemorrhagic disorders associated with such deficiencies will be discussed shortly, as well as in a later chapter (p. 1318).

All the events which have been described have the purpose of causing prothrombin to be converted to thrombin. Whether prothrombin, a glycoprotein, is converted to thrombin by an enzymatic or an autocatalytic process is unsettled, but it appears that a carbohydrate fragment is lost and that thrombin is a compound of half the molecular weight of prothrombin, or less. The activity of

thrombin is that of a proteolytic enzyme. It leads to polymerization of fibrinogen, a protein of large molecular weight, with the result that needle-shaped crystallike protofibrils are ultimately produced. These then become aligned into fiber strands by lateral association, and insoluble fibrin is formed.

The formation of fibrin, the end point of the process of clotting, is followed by clot retraction, a process which makes the seal firm and strong. Here, again, the platelets are involved. Soon after fibrin has been laid down, *intact* platelets in the interior of the mass converge toward the fibrin needles, adhere to them, and form large knots at their intersections. As the knots are being formed, the fibrin becomes bent, twisted, and shortened. Retraction of the clot is more complete, the higher the number of platelets, and the greater the concentration of thrombin in relation to the quantity of fibrinogen. In this process an actomyosin-like protein present in platelets is involved, and ATP is consumed. By these steps the *thrombus* is formed.

Coagulation is conceived to be like a chain reaction which develops at an ever-accelerating pace. The first phase is a relatively slow reaction, particularly the intravascular process. Once a small amount of thrombin has been formed, the velocity accelerates. To some extent the process of coagulation is such that it may compensate for a limited deficiency of the individual coagulation factors; only when severe deficiencies exist do clinical manifestations develop.

Negative forces exist which serve to oppose the solidification of the blood and favor the fluid state. One of the safeguards is the slowness of thrombin production. Another is the unbroken continuity of the vascular endothelium. In addition, certain lytic factors exist in the circulating blood, namely, antithrombin, heparin, and antithromboplastin. Furthermore, thrombin has an affinity for fibrin surface, which makes for a ready means whereby dangerous extension of a thrombus is prevented. There is also a mechanism for dissolution of the blood clot. This is achieved by proteolytic enzymes derived from the tissues and by the action of leukocytes, as well as by means of a specific proteolytic enzyme, plasmin. The last is derived from a precursor, plasminogen, which is carried in the globulin fraction of the plasma. Plasminogen activation occurs spontaneously or as a result of contact with activators of tissue, body fluid, or bacterial origin.

HEMORRHAGE AS THE RESULT OF INJURY OF LARGE VESSELS BY TRAUMA OR BY EROSION FROM PATHOLOGIC PROCESSES

Trauma is one of the chief causes of this type of bleeding. This may lead to external bleeding, in which event the cause and source are usually apparent. When the bleeding is internal, the true nature of the condition may not be discovered so readily. Different systems of the body may be affected. Intracranial hemorrhage is not uncommon following injury. The symptoms depend on the location of the hemorrhage. Injury to the chest may lead to the fracture of ribs, and this, in turn, by damaging the pleura, may lead to hemothorax. Abdominal injury may lead to rupture of viscera, with which some blood loss is associated. The rupture of the spleen in particular is accompanied by great loss of blood, since this is so vascular an organ. In fracture of the pelvis, severe retroperitoneal hemorrhage may occur.

Hemorrhage in the absence of trauma or of a disorder in the process of coagulation suggests the existence of some pathologic process or of a congenital abnormality as the cause of the bleeding. Occasionally, trauma is the precipitating factor, inducing hemorrhage from vessels which are congenitally abnormal or are already damaged by disease.

To list all the possible causes of hemorrhage resulting from pathologic processes is unnecessary,

but a number of the most important ones may be mentioned. In the *nervous system*, hemorrhage may be associated with hypertension or arteriosclerosis. In younger persons bleeding in the nervous system suggests rupture of a thin-walled and saccular congenital aneurysm in the circle of Willis. Inflammatory disease of the nervous system is rarely a cause of significant hemorrhage. Tumors, likewise, are not commonly associated with hemorrhage, although bleeding into a tumor is by no means unusual.

Hemorrhage from the *nose* is a common symptom. This may be the result of external trauma, but not rarely it is the consequence of local irritation and damage to the mucous membrane. Inflammatory processes involving the nasal mucous membrane (e.g., diphtheria, streptococcal infections) may cause such engorgement of Kesselbach's (Little's) area that a varix may develop which is readily made to bleed by mechanical factors. Epistaxis due to increased hydrostatic pressure is not unusual in hypertension. This symptom frequently is the initial and even the sole complaint in cases of multiple hereditary telangiectasia.

Bloody mucus, rather than free bleeding, is associated with perforation of the cartilaginous portion of the nasal septum, which may be produced by syphilis or by chromium poisoning or may be encountered in typhoid fever. Tuberculous perforation of the bony portion of the septum is not associated with bleeding. Only one type of nasal polyp leads to epistaxis. This is a fibroepithelioma which possesses a wide base and is situated on the septum.

Diseases of the nasal passages and sinuses other than those mentioned above are rarely a cause of hemorrhage. Trauma and severe streptococcal in-

Table 24-3. COMMON CAUSES OF HEMORRHAGE

I. Trauma to any part of the body
II. Congenital abnormalities or pathologic processes
    A. Nervous system: hypertension, arteriosclerosis, aneurysm in circle of Willis
    B. Nose, ears, and throat: local irritation, hypertension, skull fracture
    C. Lungs: mitral stenosis, tuberculosis, lung abscess, bronchiectasis, tumor
    D. Gastrointestinal tract: peptic ulcer, esophageal varices, carcinoma of the stomach, ulcerative colitis, hemorrhoids
    E. Urinary tract: glomerulonephritis, stone, tumor
    F. Genital apparatus: uterine fibroids, ruptured ectopic gestation
III. Generalized vascular disorders
    A. Hereditary hemorrhagic telangiectasia
    B. Allergic purpuras
    C. Symptomatic purpuras
IV. Defects in the factors concerned in coagulation
    A. Thrombocytopenic purpuras
    B. Hemophilia and PTC deficiency
    C. Induced hypoprothrombinemia

fections are the most common causes of bleeding from the *throat*. Hemorrhage from the *ear*, if not due to a direct blow, suggests fracture of the skull.

Hemorrhage from the *lungs* may arise in association with inflammatory, neoplastic, and vascular processes in the respiratory tract. Common causes of hemoptysis include tuberculosis, bronchiectasis, bronchogenic carcinoma, mitral stenosis, pulmonary infarction, and lung abscess. In pulmonary tuberculosis, arteriobronchial fistula may cause alarming hemorrhage from the lung which at times stops as abruptly as it begins, without the characteristic "tailing off" seen in bleeding from polyps and bronchial adenomas. When there is consolidation of the lung, as in pneumonia, the sputum may contain blood, but rarely is there much blood. Less common causes of bleeding from the respiratory passages include atypical pneumonia, coccidioidomycosis, broncholithiasis, and erosion of the respiratory passages by conditions affecting the mediastinum, such as aneurysm of the aorta and disease of the lymph nodes.

It is not always easy to determine whether the patient has coughed up or vomited the blood which has been expelled. Blood coming from the lungs is usually bright red in color and is often frothy, since it has been mixed with air. However, blood coming from the respiratory tract does not always present this classic appearance. Thus, if it comes from an area which is inflamed or congested, aeration may not be good and the blood may be somewhat dark, suggesting material obtained from the stomach. Furthermore, blood from the respiratory passages may be swallowed first and then vomited, with the result that it has all the characteristics of blood coming from the stomach. Blood arising in the stomach is generally dark because of the formation of acid hematin by mixture of hemoglobin with hydrochloric acid. It may be mixed with stomach contents.

By far the most common cause of massive *gastrointestinal bleeding* is peptic ulcer. Ruptured esophageal varices and carcinoma of the stomach cause less than 10 per cent of such bleeding. A hemorrhagic diathesis is the cause of gastric hemorrhage less than once in 100 cases.

Hematemesis and melena are discussed in a separate chapter (Chap. 18) and will not be considered in detail here. It should be mentioned, however, that a cause of hemorrhage hitherto little recognized is hiatus or diaphragmatic hernia. Massive bleeding may also be due to gastric polyps. Although malignant neoplasms of the stomach of the usual type rather infrequently cause severe hemorrhage, rhabdoleiomyomas have a definite tendency to cause free bleeding, but these are exceedingly rare. A phytobezoar in the stomach may cause ulceration of this origin and so lead to hemorrhage.

Meckel's diverticulum may cause massive hemorrhage from the intestinal tract. Benign polyps of the intestine may lead to blood loss, but this is rarely dramatic or large in amount. Ulcerative malignant processes will likewise cause hemorrhage, but this again is usually of a chronic character. The blood loss associated with inflammatory processes, except in the case of nonspecific ulcerative colitis or typhoid fever, is rarely of significant amount. When intussusception, volvulus, or mesenteric thrombosis is present, a bloody discharge rather than true hemorrhage is found. The rarer forms of tumor of the intestine, such as lymphosarcoma, sometimes cause bleeding. Hemorrhoids, of course, are an important source of blood loss. Large hemorrhages are rare in tuberculosis of the colon, but they do occur and then are likely to prove fatal. Of the parasites which may be found in the intestine, the hookworm, *Ancylostoma duodenale*, is an important cause of chronic blood loss. Hemorrhage from the alimentary tract may also be encountered in uremia.

Bleeding from the *urinary tract* (hematuria) is seen in glomerulonephritis or with stones or tumors in the bladder or kidney pelvis, such as benign or malignant papilloma of the bladder and hypernephroma of the kidney. A polycystic kidney sometimes produces this symptom. Severe bleeding, even with the production of clots in the bladder, may occur when only prostatic hypertrophy is present, perhaps because of the rupture of a varicose vein on the middle lobe. Of inflammatory processes, tuberculosis is the most common cause of hemorrhage from the urinary tract.

When cystitis is severe, much bleeding may occur. The urinary tract is the commonest site of bleeding complicating coumarin therapy.

Uterine fibroids are a common cause of abnormal bleeding from the *female genital tract*, while ruptured ectopic gestation is a common cause of internal bleeding. Much rarer is hemorrhage due to the rupture of an ovarian cyst.

BLEEDING DUE TO GENERALIZED VASCULAR DISORDERS

These include some well-defined, as well as certain vaguely differentiated, conditions associated with bleeding. The condition *hereditary hemorrhagic telangiectasia* is a vascular anomaly characterized clinically by hemorrhage and anatomically by multiple dilatations of capillaries and venules which are found in the skin and mucous membranes (Chap. 239). Trivial trauma sustained by these abnormal, relatively exposed vessels results in unusual bleeding. Although these telangiectases are usually quite evident when attention is called to them, not infrequently they are overlooked.

The so-called "nonthrombocytopenic purpuras" comprise a much less well-defined group of conditions associated with bleeding. They can be classified under four headings: (1) allergic purpuras, (2) symptomatic purpuras, (3) hereditary familial purpura simplex, (4) miscellaneous forms of purpura. In these different types of purpura, bleeding is due to direct alteration of the vessel wall, such as may occur in heart failure and shock (possibly on the basis of hypoxia), ascorbic acid deficiency, senility, allergic states or collagen diseases, or from the effects of toxins of bacterial, chemical, vegetable, or animal origin.

Allergic purpuras (Chap. 238) include a wide variety of conditions which are characterized clinically by bleeding into the skin, joints, and viscera and are associated with one or more of the common manifestations of allergy such as erythema, urticaria, or effusion of serum into subcutaneous tissues or viscera.

Purpura accompanying a large variety of disorders is termed *symptomatic*. Thus *infectious processes* too numerous to list may result in increased capillary permeability, with bleeding presumably on the basis of capillary damage produced by toxins. Important examples includes meningococcemia, staphylococcemia, rheumatic fever, subacute bacterial endocarditis, scarlet fever, smallpox, measles, diphtheria, and certain chronic infectious states. The purpuric manifestations of capillary permeability in these disorders are to be sharply distinguished from the embolic phenomena which also occur in some of these conditions. A multiplicity of *drugs* have been cited in isolated instances as causing purpura of a vascular nature. Although considered the result of idiosyncrasy, the mechanism of production of increased capillary permeability in such cases is not clear. It may be that endothelial cellular enzymes, necessary for the growth and integrity of the vessel wall, are actually inhibited by the antigen-antibody reaction or specific toxic substances. Certainly the hemorrhagic effects of certain snake venoms appear to be due to direct toxic injury of the endothelial lining of the capillaries and small veins.

Advanced *renal disease* and acute glomerulonephritis are sometimes associated with purpura. In chronic renal disease with azotemia, purpura of the skin and mucous membranes as well as large subcutaneous extravasations or hemorrhages into the internal organs may be found. Purpura in acute glomerulonephritis, on the other hand, is usually discrete and petechial and is likely to involve only the skin of dependent portions of the body. Purpura of the skin and mucous membranes and large subcutaneous extravasations or hemorrhages into the internal organs may be found when there has been acute destruction of the *liver*. This is because of lack of prothrombin and, sometimes, lack of fibrinogen as well. Hemorrhagic manifestations have been noted also in a number of cases of hemochromatosis, multiple myeloma, primary amyloidosis, and polycythemia.

These and certain rare hemorrhagic disorders such as *von Willebrand's disease* and *Glanzmann's thrombasthenia* will be discussed later (Chap. 238, p. 1317).

Of the miscellaneous forms of purpura not associated with abnormalities in the blood, there may be included the following:

Purpura simplex, a term generally applied to instances of mild purpuric skin manifestations unassociated with well-defined abnormalities in the blood. A hereditary, familial form has also been described.

Purpura fulminans, a term applied to a very rare form of nonthrombocytopenic purpura which has been observed in association with infections, such as scarlet fever, and with pregnancy and is characterized by sudden onset, fever, symmetric ecchymoses in the skin without hemorrhage from the mucous membranes and often a fatal course of 1 to 4 days. The same term has been used in relation to an extreme state of vascular collapse in meningococcemia (Waterhouse-Friderichsen syndrome). In most instances no abnormality in coagulation has been demonstrated, but factor V deficiency, excess antithrombin, and hypofibrinogenemia have been reported.

Mechanical purpura, which refers to purpuric manifestations associated with violent muscular contractions such as occur in whooping cough or convulsions, with the result that capillaries are ruptured.

Orthostatic purpura, a term describing purpura which develops in some persons in the lower extremities after prolonged standing. This purpura is presumably due to capillary weakness.

Prolonged *deficiency of vitamin C* may result in unusual hemorrhage which characteristically is perifollicular, gingival, and subperiosteal in location but also occurs in the skin, subcutaneous tissues, and muscles. The bleeding may be extensive and is attributed to increased capillary permeability due to lack of intercellular cement or ground substance. Bleeding ceases following the administration of lemon juice and similar antiscorbutic substances (ascorbic acid).

BLEEDING DUE TO ALTERATION OF EXTRAVASCULAR FACTORS OF HEMOSTASIS

Occasionally hemorrhage may be the result of fragility and hyperlaxity of the skin or atrophy of the subcutaneous tissue. This is seen most commonly in purpura senilis and purpura cachectica, where it is characterized by purplish ecchymoses of varying size appearing in the skin following trauma. The hemorrhagic manifestations seen in Cushing's syndrome are attributed to fragility of the skin, while those in the very rare Ehlers-Danlos syndrome are attributed to hyperlaxity of the skin. Occasionally hemorrhage, especially from the mucous membranes, is seen in epidermolysis bullosa. Other diseases associated with cutaneous hemorrhagic manifestations include annular telangiectatic purpura (Majocchi disease), angioma serpiginosum, Schamberg's disease, and pigmented purpuric lichenoid dermatitis.

Various forms of *dysglobulinemia,* whatever their cause, may be associated with purpura. These forms include the purpura sometimes encountered in multiple myeloma and in association with other instances of hyperglobulinemia and cryoglobulinemia (p. 1344). Under the title *purpura hyperglobulinemia* a miscellaneous group of cases have been described which are characterized by innumerable acute episodes of purpura, especially after unusual exertion, prolonged standing, or excessive pressure from garments. In these cases a considerable increase in γ-globulin and in the 7-component in the ultracentrifuge was observed. This probably does not constitute a diagnostic entity.

BLEEDING DUE TO ALTERATIONS OF INTRAVASCULAR FACTORS OF HEMOSTASIS

As outlined in Table 24-1, bleeding due to disturbances of blood coagulation may be related to (1) platelet abnormalities or (2) a defect in one of the factors concerned in coagulation.

Platelet abnormalities may be of two kinds: (1) quantitative deficiencies of platelets or (2) qualitative abnormalities. The latter are rare, the former relatively common. Thrombocytopenic purpura, which will be discussed in detail later (p. 1313), may be associated with and symptomatic of a large variety of disorders and can be produced by a number of chemical, physical, animal, and vegetable agents, but an "idiopathic" form of unknown etiology is also well recognized. Disorders associated with qualitative platelet abnormalities, the "thrombocytopathies," are becoming more clearly defined than they once were and will also be discussed later.

The number of recognized coagulation defects has increased as knowledge concerning the various factors involved in the clotting mechanism has been extended. Thus, instead of the single entity hemophilia, a number of bleeding disorders are now recognized, one of which resembles the classical disease even in its mode of inheritance, while others present a very similar clinical picture which can be differentiated only by more sensitive techniques than those which once served as the sole criteria, namely, the coagulation time and the bleeding time. It is also clear that disorders such as hemophilia may be inherited as comparatively mild defects which can be quite troublesome under certain circumstances but which cannot be recognized as being due to a defect in coagulation by such crude procedures as the measurement of coagulation time. Again, the measurement of prothrombin time, when used by itself, is not a sufficiently sensitive or specific technique for the study of hemorrhagic diatheses. The term *hypoprothrombinemia* was originally used to refer to a delayed reaction in certain tests which were assumed to measure prothrombin. These now are recognized as being influenced by a number of factors in addition to prothrombin, including factors V, VII, and X. Prothrombin has been isolated from plasma in highly purified form, and it appears that true hypoprothrombinemia is a very rare condition. However, hypoprothrombinemia, as demonstrated by the commonly used Quick test or by one of its modifications, is encountered frequently, both as an acquired condition and, much less often, as one of a number of congenital disorders.

Hemophilia and certain very closely related conditions will be discussed in a later chapter (p. 1318), but the hypoprothrombinemias and various other forms of bleeding due to alterations of intravascular factors of hemostasis may be considered here.

Diminution of the "Prothrombin" Content of the Blood. If the "prothrombin" content of blood is reduced to 10 per cent or below, hemorrhage may occur, since the blood will not clot properly. Such hypoprothrombinemia may arise in various ways.

Toxins. The toxic principle in spoiled sweetclover hay, which produces a hemorrhagic disease when fed to cattle, was found to be a coumarin compound. This, under the trade name Dicumarol, has become a widely used anticoagulant. Hypoprothrombinemia develops whenever this drug or a related compound, such as ethyl biscoumacetate (Tromexan), is administered. These agents produce low levels of true prothrombin and of factor VII, as well as somewhat lesser decreases of factor V. The levels of factors IX and X also fall but more slowly than that of factor VII. Bleeding due to Dicumarol- or Tromexan-induced hypoprothrombinemia usually occurs into the genitourinary and gastrointestinal tracts as well as in localized areas of the skin and subcutaneous tissue.

Administration of Salicylates. When salicylates are given in very large quantities, the prothrombin content of the blood plasma may be reduced. The mechanism of this action is not clear. Even when large doses are used therapeutically, however, salicylates are rarely a cause of bleeding.

Lack of Vitamin K. The liver is concerned in the formation of true prothrombin and probably is involved in some manner in the production of other coagulation factors. The fat-soluble vitamin K, a naphthoquinone, is related to this activity and may serve as the prosthetic group for an essential enzyme. It is found abundantly in alfalfa, spinach, cauliflower, cabbage, and kale. Since it is fat-soluble, bile salts are required for its absorption. Consequently, vitamin K deficiency may be found when there is complete obstruction of the flow of bile into the intestinal tract or when a biliary fistula exists. Deficiency may also develop where there is impaired absorption from the bowel as in sprue, the steatorrheas, gastrocolic fistulas, or following extensive surgical removal of much of the intestinal tract. Vitamin K is produced in abundance by bacteria growing in the intestinal tract, and for this reason lack of vitamin K in the diet is an extremely rare cause of vitamin K deficiency. However, in cases where prolonged use of drugs inhibits the growth of organisms in the gastrointestinal tract, vitamin K deficiency may ensue.

By the more refined techniques of the present day it has been shown that, when vitamin K is deficient, factors VII and X, and in some cases even factor IX, are depressed, in addition to true prothrombin. These defects can all be corrected by the intravenous administration of vitamin K.

Hemorrhagic Disease of the Newborn. The fetus and the newborn infant receive their store of prothrombin from the mother. After food has been taken by the infant and bacteria begin to grow in the intestinal tract, these serve to provide vitamin K. In occasional instances an infant may be born with a poor supply of prothrombin and may suffer severe hemorrhage before it has had an opportunity to produce vitamin K for itself. It is thought that this is the result of an accentuation of the hypoprothrombinemia which is normally observed in the newborn, perhaps as a consequence of functional immaturity of the liver. In some instances, trauma to the child at birth with hemorrhage and loss of coagulation factors may also play a role.

Liver Disease. Multiple serious plasma clotting-factor defects develop in the patient with decompensated hepatocellular disease. These include major deficiencies of prothrombin, factor VII, and factor V, and possibly also factor X and factor IX are deficient as well. These defects are not corrected by the administration of vitamin K. The treatment of the hemorrhagic state associated with severe liver disease requires the administration of blood and this must be fresh, or at least less than a week old.

Congenital and Idiopathic Hypoprothrombinemias. A hemorrhagic diathesis is encountered occasionally which is characterized by hypoprothrombinemia and yet cannot be attributed to the recognized causes, mentioned above. The clinical manifestations in such patients resemble those of hemophilia. The most common symptom is epistaxis. Other frequent symptoms are bleeding from the gums, spontaneous bruising, menorrhagia, and severe bleeding from injuries. Hematuria is moderately common, and hemarthroses have been recorded. Prothrombin time as measured by the one-stage method is prolonged, and when the defect is sufficiently severe, coagulation time is lengthened as well. Several forms have been differentiated.

True congenital hypoprothrombinemia is exceedingly rare, only three cases being known. Less rare is congenital *factor V deficiency* (parahemophilia) which appears to be inherited as an autosomal recessive (see p. 430) and has been observed in both sexes. The condition varies greatly in severity as does the degree of prolongation of prothrombin time and coagulation time and the decrease in prothrombin consumption. Congenital *factor VII (SPCA) deficiency* probably is the most common of the congenital hypoprothrombinemias and is thought to be inherited as an incompletely recessive autosomal characteristic with variable penetrance. By means of the prothrombin consumption and thromboplastin generation tests, factor VII deficiency has been distinguished from *factor X* (Stuart-Prower) *deficiency*, a condition which is thought to be inherited as a highly penetrant but incompletely recessive autosomal characteristic.

Recognition of the various types of congenital hypoprothrombinemia has been important because it has led to a better understanding of the clotting process through identification of the various factors involved. From a clinical standpoint, the idiopathic hypoprothrombinemias need to be differentiated from the much more common disorder hemophilia and from the various forms of purpura. Their treatment depends on supplying the missing factor. Vitamin K does not correct the prolonged prothrombin time. Fresh whole blood or plasma is necessary to correct factor V deficiency and serum or plasma to correct factor VII deficiency.

Decreased Fibrinogen. Afibrinogenemia and fibrinogenopenia are extremely rare causes of bleeding. A *congenital* disorder has been described in which hemorrhagic manifestations begin in infancy. This appears to be due to an inborn error of fibrinogen formation. *Acquired hypofibrinogenemia* develops under a variety of circumstances and as the effect of different mechanisms. Since it is formed in the liver, plasma fibrinogen may be reduced when severe destructive changes occur in this organ, as in acute yellow atrophy. Severe liver damage, however, produces impairment of prothrombin production before fibrinogen deficiency occurs, the latter being essentially a terminal event. In clinical practice, hypofibrinogenemia is more often the consequence of a pathologic fibrinolytic state than the result of fibrinogen deficiency.

In certain pathologic states, abnormal amounts of plasminogen activator may be released from the tissues into the circulation. In others, thromboplastic material may gain access to the circulation and, by bringing about intravascular clotting, consume fibrinogen and other clotting factors and set up a secondary fibrinolytic response. The clinical problem is usually complex, however, and a complete analysis of the events which take place is not yet available. The end result, in any event, is fibrinogenopenia. Other plasma coagulation factors, such as prothrombin and factors V and VIII, are often depleted as well, and thrombocytopenia may be found also, but these usually are not the primary factors involved in the development of the bleeding diathesis. In occasional instances, evidence of a circulating anticoagulant has been obtained, but this appears to be an unusual cause for fibrinogenopenia.

Clinically, fibrinolysis has been observed in five main conditions: (1) under conditions of stress and in association with severe and extensive physical trauma and following extensive burns; (2) following surgery, particularly pulmonary surgery; (3) as a result of obstetric complications of abruptio placentae, intrauterine retention of a dead fetus, and amniotic fluid embolism; (4) during the course of neoplastic disease, especially if the prostate or, less often, the lung, pancreas, or stomach is involved; and (5) in a variety of miscellaneous disorders, such as polycythemia vera, leukemia, sarcoidosis, and hepatic cirrhosis. The clinical picture may develop with great suddenness and be characterized by the appearance of extensive ecchymoses and severe bleeding from mucous membranes; or the symptoms may be of lesser severity and magnitude (*purpura thrombolytica, fibrinolytic purpura*).

The bleeding in cases of acquired fibrinogenopenia is often of extreme gravity and requires the prompt administration of whole, preferably fresh, blood and fibrinogen (4 to 10 Gm, occasionally even 15 to 20 Gm).

Circulating Anticoagulants. A hemorrhagic diathesis may occur as the result of the action of inhibitors of any of the factors concerned with coagulation, since they prevent clot formation. Heparin and Dicumarol are used therapeutically as anticoagulants in the management of thrombosis, and in clinical practice this is the most common manner in which excess anticoagulant produces hemorrhage. Heparin is normally found in blood in a concentration of 0.5 mg per 100 ml. The hypocoagulability of the blood of dogs in peptone or anaphylactoid shock is probably attributable to heparin, but the anticoagulant described in the blood following heavy exposure to irradiation or nitrogen mustards is not identical with heparin, as was once thought.

In addition to the anticoagulants which may be given deliberately or those which appear in various circumstances as described above, there are circulating anticoagulants that may cause hemorrhagic disorders. These may interfere with any phase of coagulation and can be classified in accordance with their mechanism of action. The type of anticoagulant most frequently encountered has been antithromboplastic in action. A significant number of the reported cases in this category represent cases of hemophilia in which an anticoagulant opposing the action of antihemophilic globulin developed following repeated transfusions. Other cases have occurred in women, usually in the childbearing period, the hemorrhagic manifestations developing some time after delivery. In a few cases a circulating antithromboplastin has been observed in association with some disease, especially disseminated lupus erythematosus, while in others the hemorrhagic disorder was of entirely obscure etiology.

SYMPTOMS PRODUCED BY HEMORRHAGE

The symptoms associated with blood loss differ according to whether the loss is large and rapid or relatively slow and long continued. They also depend on the site of the hemorrhage and on whether the bleeding occurs into a relatively nonexpansile space, such as a synovial joint, or in loose connective tissue. Acute and severe blood loss occurring within a matter of a few minutes results in syncope, but when the loss occurs over a period of hours the picture of shock is induced. The classic examples are seen in hemorrhage from peptic ulcer or ruptured ectopic pregnancy. The clinical picture and the pathogenesis of peripheral circulatory failure are discussed on pp. 92 to 103.

The acute loss of blood stimulates the hematopoietic system, with the result that the reticulocytes are increased in number, and if the hemorrhage is very severe, even occasional nucleated red cells of the normoblastic type may be found in the circulating blood. At the same time, the leukopoietic tissues are stimulated and a marked leukocytosis occurs. This leukocytosis is due to the liberation of cells formed in the bone marrow, with the result that the juvenile neutrophils are increased and even some myelocytes may appear. There is at the same time an augmentation in the number of blood platelets. Their number may be increased twofold, or even more. When the hemorrhage is entirely within the body, the absorption of the blood may produce hyperbilirubinemia. This, in turn, may result in an increase in the quantity of urobilinogen in the urine and may even be accompanied by noticeable jaundice.

Slow *chronic blood loss* ultimately produces anemia and the symptoms characteristic of anemia which have been described elsewhere (Chaps. 23, 235). The anemia eventually becomes hypochromic and microcytic in type, and instead of leukocytosis and thrombocytosis, one finds leukopenia with relative lymphocytosis, often accompanied by the presence of multisegmented polymorphonuclear neutrophile. At the same time there may be a somewhat reduced number of platelets. However, in spite of this "hypoplastic" blood picture, if the anemia is severe, occasional small nucleated red cells ("microblasts") will be found.

STUDY OF A PATIENT WITH HEMORRHAGE

Hemorrhage, if severe, first requires treatment by replacement of the blood which has been lost. Rational treatment beyond this, however, depends on a clear understanding of the cause of the hemorrhage. This entails recognition of whether or not the bleeding is the result of a fault in the process of coagulation, the consequence of dysfunction of the blood vessels, or the effect of trauma or pathologic processes unrelated to disorders of the blood. As is always the case, there is no short cut to the taking of an accurate history and the performance of a complete and thorough physical examination. The differential diagnosis of the causes of hemorrhage other than those concerned with disorders of the blood is beyond the scope of this section, for it entails consideration of disorders which include all the systems of the body. These are dealt with in other sections.

The history may reveal a story of trauma or the symptoms of some disorder of which the hemorrhage may be a manifestation; or one may learn about exposure to agents associated with the patient's occupation or hobby which may have caused bleeding, or the ingestion of drugs which the patient may have been taking from time to time for a number of years. A family history of bleeding should arouse suspicion of such conditions as hemophilia or of the various disorders which resemble classical hemophilia, or purpura hemorrhagica, or hereditary hemorrhagic telangiectasia (see pp. 1317 and 1321). The physical examination may reveal vascular anomalies, as in the case of hereditary telangiectasia, and may indicate the site of hemorrhage.

The examination of the blood should include the determination by reliable methods of coagulation time, clot retraction, prothrombin time, bleeding time, and the platelet count. A tourniquet test should be done as well. Some of these procedures are relatively crude, but if carefully performed they are useful, nevertheless. In special cases, other laboratory procedures are needed, as will be outlined below. Circumstances in which changes in these tests take place are summarized in Table 24-4.

The *coagulation time* is a measure of the capacity of the blood to clot after it has been removed from the body and, thus, in the absence of tissue factors. It can be carried out in siliconized as well as in uncoated test tubes. The latter measure the coagulation of blood after it has come into contact with a surface which can initiate the process. The coagulation time should be measured in test tubes of uniform size, and a control determination on the blood of a normal person should be made at the same time. In the determination of *prothrombin time,* it is important that a potent thromboplastin be used and that a determination be made on normal persons at the same time. It is important to recognize that by the one-stage technique a prolonged prothrombin time does not specifically indicate reduction of prothrombin, since prolongation also occurs with deficiencies of factor V, factor VII, and fibrinogen, these being vital to the speed and amount of clot formed, the end point of this method. Differentiation of these conditions from true hypoprothrombinemia is accomplished by means of certain special tests, which depend on the use of fresh and stored plasma, normal serum, and aluminum hydroxide–treated plasma.

The test for *bleeding time* is simple but crude, and unless it is done carefully a false normal result may be obtained. The test depends on the effect of a skin puncture in producing bleeding and is a measure of the hemostatic integrity of vascular and extravascular factors as well as the strength of the platelet plug. The bleeding time is characteristically prolonged in the thrombocytopenic purpuras because there is inadequate platelet activity. As arbitrarily defined the bleeding time is normal in hemophilia, but subsequent oozing after the initial factors of hemostasis have ceased to function may occur for days because of imperfect coagulation. Bleeding-time measurements, therefore, should be avoided in hemophiliac patients.

Platelet counts are notoriously difficult to perform with accuracy and should always be verified by examination of the blood smear, which should reveal gross discrepancies if they exist. Since *clot retraction* depends chiefly on an adequate supply of platelets, delayed retraction suggests thrombocytopenia, but it has also been observed in some cases of "thrombasthenia."

The *tourniquet test* is useful in demonstrating decreased capacity of the capillaries to withstand the effects of increased pressure. It depends primarily on the integrity of the capillary endothelial

Table 24-4. CAUSES OF ALTERATIONS IN MOST COMMON MEASURES OF COAGULATION

Laboratory finding	Condition	Mechanism
I. *Coagulation time* prolonged	A. Hemophilia	Deficiency of factor VIII (AHF)
	B. Factor IX deficiency	Deficiency of factor IX (PTC)
	C. PTA deficiency	Deficiency of PTA
	D. Hageman trait	Deficiency of Hageman factor
	E. "Hypoprothrombinemia"	When prothrombin time is greatly prolonged, deficiency of prothrombin or of factor V, VII, or X
	F. Afibrinogenemia or hypofibrinogenemia	Deficiency, rapid utilization, or destruction of fibrinogen
	G. Hyperheparinemia	Excess heparin or heparinoid substances (heparin therapy, anaphylactic and peptone shock)
	H. Circulating anticoagulants	Anti-VIII, anti-IX, anti-V, etc.
II. *Prothrombin time* (one-stage) prolonged	A. Excess Dicumarol or related therapeutic anticoagulant	Deficiency of prothrombin, factors VII and X
	B. "Parahemophilia"	Factor V deficiency
	C. "SPCA" deficiency	Factor VII deficiency
	D. Vitamin K deficiency	In newborn (hemorrhagic disease of newborn) and whenever absorption of vitamin K is impaired
	E. Liver disease	Reduction in prothrombin, factors V, VII, X and fibrinogen
	F. Circulating anticoagulants	Antiprothrombin, antithromboplastin
III. *Prothrombin consumption* or *thromboplastin generation* reduced	A. Thrombocytopenia	Impaired thromboplastin formation
	B. Thrombocytopathia	Diminished platelet factor 3
	C. Hemophilias	Deficiency of factor VIII, IX, or PTA
	D. Other deficiencies	Deficiency of factor V, X or Hageman factor
	E. Circulating antithromboplastin	Anti-VIII, anti-IX, anti-V, etc.
IV. *Bleeding time* prolonged	A. Thrombocytopenic purpura	Lack of platelets
	B. Any of the causes under I or II if sufficiently severe	Extreme deficiency of blood coagulation factors
	C. Vascular hemophilia (angiohemophilia, von Willebrand's disease)	Deficiency of plasma factor necessary for normal bleeding time
	D. Thrombocytopathia	Diminished platelet factor 3
V. *Tourniquet test* positive	A. Nonthrombocytopenic purpuras	Damage to capillary endothelium
	B. Thrombocytopenic purpuras	Platelets too few to support capillaries under pressure
	C. Scurvy	Deficiency of intercellular cement substance
	D. Thrombocytopathia	Diminished platelet factor 3
VI. *Thrombocytopenia*	Thrombocytopenic purpuras, primary and secondary	Platelet antibodies, megakaryocyte damage, etc.
VII. *Clot retraction* poor	A. Thrombocytopenias of various types	Insufficient platelets to induce fibrin contraction
	B. Thrombasthenia	Impaired platelet aggregation

SOURCE: From M. M. Wintrobe: "Clinical Hematology," 5th ed., Philadelphia, Lea & Febiger, 1961.

cells, the availability of intercellular cement substances, and the quantity of platelets. The tourniquet test is usually positive whenever there is severe thrombocytopenia and also, for a different reason, in many instances of nonthrombocytopenic purpura. It is negative as a rule in hemophilia and in other nonthrombocytopenic conditions involving the coagulation mechanism. It is noteworthy that a positive test result is encountered also in a high proportion of patients with diabetes complicated by vascular disease and in hypertension, in scurvy, in Weil's disease and other infections, and occasionally in apparently normal individuals.

It is important that all five determinations—bleeding time, platelet count, coagulation time, clot retraction time, and tourniquet test—be carried out. In a classic case of thrombocytopenic purpura the bleeding time is prolonged, the platelet count is reduced, coagulation time is normal but clot retraction is delayed, and the tourniquet test is positive. When these are the findings, one has confidence in the results of each of the tests. When there is a discrepancy between them, one should repeat these determinations and seek out possible sources of error.

Of the more specialized procedures employed in the study of bleeding disorders, the *prothrombin consumption test* is a relatively simple one. This test is based on the principle that, by determining the prothrombin before and after coagulation is complete, a measure of the plasma thromboplastin that reacts with prothrombin is obtained. The same reagents are required as in Quick's method for determining prothrombin. Another simple procedure which can be employed when there is a demonstrable defect in coagulation is to attempt to correct the defect in coagulation by the addition of blood or plasma of known composition; for example, stored plasma is deficient in factor V, serum contains factors VII and IX but no factor V, etc. When the bloods of patients with hemorrhagic disorders are available, they can be tested for their ability to correct the defect in the unanalyzed sample.

Simple screening tests for abnormal coagulation of blood are available, and there are special tests for circulating anticoagulants. Another valuable procedure is the *thromboplastin generation test*, a most useful method for differentiating abnormalities in coagulation in which there is impaired formation of blood thromboplastin, such as hemophilia and factor IX deficiency, and conditions in which there is abnormal platelet function. The procedure, however, requires training and some technical skill and, therefore, is not available in the average laboratory.

In any case of bleeding it is desirable to study the morphology of the red cells and the leukocytes and to determine the reticulocyte count. An increase of reticulocytes is the response of a normal bone marrow to hemorrhage, and its degree gives a rough index of the severity of the hemorrhage. The lack of reticulocytosis would mean either an inability on the part of the bone marrow to respond, as would be the case in aplastic anemia, or a less severe hemorrhage than other indications had suggested. The degree of leukocytosis, likewise, is an index of the severity of the hemorrhage and the capacity of the bone marrow to react. A low leukocyte count, in the face of a severe hemorrhage, would suggest some abnormality of the marrow, as might be the case in "aleukemic" leukemia or in aplastic anemia. The presence of very immature leukocytes suggests "aleukemic" leukemia, but it must be borne in mind that a few myelocytes form part of the picture of a vigorous response to hemorrhage.

REFERENCES

Biggs, Rosemary, and R. G. Macfarlane: "Human Blood Coagulation," 2d ed., Springfield, Ill., Charles C Thomas, 1957.

Macfarlane, R. G.: Blood Coagulation, Physiol. Revs., 36:479, 1956.

Quick, A. J.: "Hemorrhagic Diseases," Philadelphia, Lea & Febiger, 1957.

Wintrobe, M. M.: "Clinical Hematology," 5th ed., Philadelphia, Lea & Febiger, 1961.

25 ENLARGEMENT OF LYMPH NODES AND SPLEEN
M. M. Wintrobe

There are some 500 to 600 lymph nodes in the body, varying from less than 1 mm to 1 to 2 cm in size. These structures afford mechanical filtration for the lymph stream, removing cellular debris, foreign particles, and bacteria which may have gained access to the lymph from the various structures drained by the lymph channels. In the normal individual very few lymph nodes are palpable, even on careful physical examination. However, the access of disease-producing bacteria and certain viruses sets up an inflammatory reaction in the nodes, and various types of malignant cells can proliferate there. It has been aptly stated that in the exercise of their function the lymph nodes may sacrifice their own integrity for the welfare of the organism as a whole. One may wonder whether they do not mistakenly also nourish neoplastic tissue at their own expense.

These structures are also the site of formation of lymphocytes and of antibodies. Furthermore, the cells of the reticuloendothelial system contained within the nodes can revert to the task of blood formation. This is known as *myeloid metaplasia* and is a reflection of embryonal hematopoietic potentialities. This reaction is also accompanied by lymph node enlargement.

CAUSES OF LYMPH NODE ENLARGEMENT

Enlargement of the lymph nodes may be purely local, or it may be widespread. Such enlargement may be accompanied by all the signs of acute inflammation, such as heat, reddening of overlying skin, and tenderness; and the glands, instead of remaining discrete, may fuse with one another as the result of the perilymphangitis which occurs. Necrosis may even ensue and may be followed by rupture of the nodes and the formation of a sinus. On the other hand, very great enlargement of the lymph nodes may take place in the absence of any signs of inflammation whatever, and the glands may remain discrete at the same time. Enlarged lymph nodes may be extremely hard, or only moderately so, or may even be soft or feel cystic. When mediastinal, abdominal, or other deeply placed lymph nodes are affected, their enlargement may be first discovered as the result of the pressure such enlargement may produce. Thus acute mediastinal lymphadenitis in young children may lead to stridor, cyanosis, and dysphagia. Noninflammatory enlargement of the nodes in this region may lead to one or more of these signs. Again, if the condition is inflammatory in character, fever and leukocytosis and other signs of systemic involvement may be the first evidences of disease. When it is not due to infection, the glandular enlargement may be huge and evidences of systemic involvement may be wholly lacking; or, instead, wasting, anemia, and even fever may be more prominent than the glandular swelling.

The chief causes of lymph node enlargement are listed in Table 25-1. The strategic location of lymph

Table 25-1. CHIEF CAUSES OF LYMPH NODE ENLARGEMENT

I. Infections
   A. Acute, regional: etiologic agents include streptococcus, staphylococcus, Ducrey's bacillus, *Pasteurella tularensis, Treponema pallidum,* virus of lymphogranuloma venereum, *Pasteurella pestis* (plague)
   B. Acute, systemic: infectious mononucleosis, measles, rubella, chickenpox, etc.
   C. Chronic: tuberculosis, syphilis, fungous infections
II. Allergic reactions: serum sickness
III. Congenital abnormalities (lymphangiomas)
IV. Primary lymph node diseases: Hodgkin's disease, lymphosarcoma, reticulum cell sarcoma, etc.
V. Leukemia
VI. Metastases from malignant disease in breast, stomach, etc.

nodes along the lymph channels makes them likely to be involved in a variety of infections, both acute and chronic. The enlargement of the anterior cervical nodes in association with streptococcal sore throat, and enlargement of the epitrochlear node draining a digit which is infected are well-known examples of a regional reaction to local infection. The satellite node of tularemia is another example, as are the buboes of lymphogranuloma venereum and of plague. Many types of acute generalized infection are accompanied by lymphadenopathy which may be local or widespread. Lymph node enlargement frequently accompanies measles, rubella, mumps, and chickenpox. This is usually most prominent in the anterior cervical chain. In infectious mononucleosis, generalized lymph node enlargement is characteristic, but cervical glandular enlargement is often more striking than that found elsewhere in the body. Lymphadenopathy may be encountered in acute anterior poliomyelitis, especially in infants and children, in whom, in particular, the development of an acute infection of almost any variety is frequently accompanied by some degree of lymph node enlargement. Other acute infections are accompanied by adenopathy, but this may not be easily discernible (for example, the mesenteric lymph node enlargement which is seen in typhoid fever).

Of the chronic infections, tuberculosis and syphilis are the most common causes of lymphadenopathy. In tuberculosis the cervical, mediastinal, or mesenteric glands are most often involved. The enlargement usually is slowly progressive and is easily confused with that caused by Hodgkin's disease. However, tuberculous glands frequently are tender and firm and adhere to one another. Sometimes breakdown of the overlying skin occurs, leading to the production of a stubborn draining sinus. Rarely the lymph node enlargement is acute and rapidly developing, and in such cases the glands may remain discrete and freely movable. In relation to syphilis, mention may be made of the firm, painless swelling in the regional lymph nodes draining the primary lesions; the generalized, firm, shotty, nontender nodes which accompany the secondary stage; and the glandular swelling of various degrees which may accompany the late stages or the congenital form. Other chronic infections in which glandular swelling may be prominent include fungous infections and filariasis. Sarcoidosis, a rare disorder which in many ways resembles tuberculosis and Hodgkin's disease and which by some is regarded as a form of tuberculosis, often must also be considered. In sarcoidosis the pre- and postauricular lymph nodes, the submaxillary, submental, epitrochlear, and paratracheal glands are more often affected than in Hodgkin's disease. A history of involvement of the eyes and of the parotid glands (uveoparotid fever) suggests sarcoid, and punched-out areas in the small bones of the hands and feet may be demonstrable by roentgenography (see Chap. 228).

Serum sickness should not be overlooked as a cause of lymphadenopathy, particularly since it is usually accompanied by fever. Again, it may be noted that trauma, caused by running and jumping, has been known to lead to painful swelling of the inguinal and femoral lymph nodes. Of congenital abnormalities which may lead to lymphoid enlargement, simple or capillary lymphangiomas, cavernous lymphangiomas, and the cystic form (cystic hygroma) may be mentioned.

Hodgkin's disease, lymphosarcoma, reticulum cell sarcoma, and giant follicular lymphoma are frequently classed under the single heading of primary lymph node diseases or lymphomas because, clinically, they are usually indistinguishable. In these conditions the lymph node enlargement is characteristically localized at first; only as the disease progresses does wide dissemination occur. The glandular enlargement usually is discrete and firm and ranges greatly in degree. When the adenopathy becomes widespread, nodes may be discovered in locations where the presence of lymphoid tissue may not have been suspected. Such cases of lymph node enlargement are distinguished from those due to leukemia chiefly by the changes in the blood characteristically seen in the latter condition, but also by the asymmetry of the swellings which is often seen in the "lymphomas." In leukemia, lymph node enlargement is usually generalized and symmetric, although, especially in acute leukemia, adenopathy may be much more prominent in the neck than elsewhere.

Metastatic enlargement of lymph nodes, as a rule, is distinctly localized, and the glandular swelling ordinarily is very hard. Such enlargement may involve nodes which are easily discovered, such as those of the axilla in cases of carcinoma of the breast. It may be more often heard about than seen, such as Virchow's sentinel node above the clavicle in cases of carcinoma of the stomach or other abdominal organs. Or the adenopathy may exist in some region of the body inaccessible to physical examination but discoverable only by roentgenography or through the indirect effects of pressure produced by enlargement of the nodes. A very useful procedure for the differential diagnosis of certain diseases involving the lungs, such as sarcoidosis, is the biopsy of lymph nodes which are not palpable because they are situated deeply in the lower neck and upper mediastinum but which can be found by adequate exploration of the scalenus fat pad. This lies between the clavicle and the scalenus anticus and sternocleidomastoid muscles. It is easily removed under local anesthesia through a small incision in the supraclavicular fossa.

Lymph node hyperplasia is encountered in Addison's disease, hyperthyroidism, and hypopituitarism, in which conditions the adenopathy is noteworthy since it contrasts with the tendency for lymph node atrophy found in association with inanition due to other causes.

DIFFERENTIAL DIAGNOSIS OF LYMPH NODE ENLARGEMENT

It should be evident, from this discussion, that the discovery of the cause of glandular enlargement requires a thorough examination of the patient. It is important, of course, to determine the extent of the adenopathy. The systematic examination should especially include careful palpation of the cervical regions, the epitrochlear regions, the arms (for swelling of brachial nodes), the axillas, the lateral borders of the chest, the inguinal and femoral regions, and the popliteal spaces. Tenderness of lymph nodes suggests infection rather than one of the lymphomas, leukemia, or metastatic involvement. However, some degree of tenderness, as well as pain, may be encountered when the glands have enlarged rapidly, especially in Hodgkin's disease. A resilient firmness, somewhat like that of uncured gum rubber, is characteristic of lymphosarcoma and reticulum cell sarcoma and may be found in Hodgkin's disease. In the last condition, the presence of connective and fibrous tissue in the nodes may cause them to be harder than usual; they may have the consistency of cartilage. In carcinoma the glands are usually stony hard.

The location of the glandular enlargement may suggest the site of origin of the disease and sometimes may give some clue as to its nature. Acute cervical adenitis should direct attention to the mouth and pharynx, mastoid adenitis to scalp infections, axillary adenitis to the upper extremity and the breast, epitrochlear enlargement to involvement of the ulnar side of the hand or forearm, and inguinal swelling to the lower extremities and genitalia. Supraclavicular gland enlargement, it may be noted, may result from infection in the thumb and index finger as well as in the neck. If the gland is hard and not tender, it may be the seat of tumor. Lymph drainage to this node is such that, if the right node is enlarged, some primary process in the chest should be suspected; whereas enlargement of the left supraclavicular node should direct attention to the abdomen. Enlargement of the inferior deep cervical glands in the posterior triangle of the neck is more often due to Hodgkin's disease, or secondary to malignancy, than due to an infection arising in the throat. The occipital glands are not infrequently affected in rubella and in secondary syphilis. The finding of discrete, nontender nodes in regions where lymph nodes are rarely palpated, as along the brachial artery or in the femoral (as distinguished from the inguinal) region, should arouse suspicion of the existence of a systemic disorder involving the lymphatic system, such as leukemia.

The general examination of the patient must also be painstaking, for sometimes secondary glandular enlargement may be much more prominent than the primary cause. Thus, for example, cervical metastases from a nasopharyngeal tumor usually overshadow the primary growth, which is characteristically small and easily overlooked unless a careful nasopharyngoscopic examination is made. The study of the patient should include careful palpation of the sternum for tenderness and of the abdomen for splenic enlargement, as well as examination of the chest for evidence of mediastinal tumor. Rectal and pelvic examination must not be overlooked.

Important laboratory procedures include the serologic test for syphilis, examination of the blood for agglutination reactions, blood culture and culture of the throat, sputum, and other possible sources which might reveal infection, as well as examination of the blood and sometimes of the bone marrow for morphologic evidences of disease. Skin tests, such as tuberculin, histoplasmin, and coccidioidin, may also need to be performed; culture of the lymph nodes may be helpful occasionally; and roentgenograms may have to be taken of the lungs, the gastrointestinal system, the kidneys, or other structures. In chronic forms of lymph node enlargement, biopsy of a node is often necessary, especially when it is a matter of differentiating the various types of primary lymph node disease.

THE SPLEEN

It is very rare that one can palpate the spleen in a person who is entirely normal, although it must be admitted that very occasionally a person is encountered in whom the spleen is palpable and in whom even prolonged observation fails to reveal any evidence of disease. How often this may occur is difficult to state.

The pulp of the spleen is composed of (1) anastomosing strands of lymphoid tissue, (2) a reticular network and branching multipolar cells which are placed about blood sinuses and intermingle with the strands of lymphoid tissue, and (3) lymphocytes, granulocytes, and erythrocytes. The spleen is a very vascular organ and is capable of changing substantially in size, depending on its content of blood.

Functions of the Spleen. The spleen serves as a reservoir for blood and is concerned with blood destruction. There is good evidence that the spleen is the chief graveyard of the red cell. In man, in contrast to certain other mammalian species, the reservoir function does not seem to be very important. However, sequestration of red corpuscles takes place in the spleen, and this probably plays a role in the detection and removal of effete worn-out corpuscles and undoubtedly is important in the blood destruction which occurs in certain disorders of the blood (p. 1287). This organ, in contrast to the lungs and the kidneys, is able to dispose of the iron derived from red cell destruction and makes it available for the formation of new cells.

During embryonic life the spleen plays an important part in blood formation, and the potentialities of this organ for blood formation persist even in adult life. Lymphocytes are normally produced in the mature animal by the malpighian corpuscles of the spleen, and monocytes may also arise in that organ. In certain circumstances, foci of extramedullary blood formation can be found in the spleen; thus, when the functional activity of the bone marrow is impaired, the hematopoietic potentiality of the spleen may become an important asset. In this connection the interesting observation was made that the recovery of hematopoietic tissue following whole body radiation was significantly hastened by lead shielding of the exteriorized spleen. Other tissues have a similar though less striking influence. The protective factor was at first thought to be noncellular in nature, but it is now believed that recovery depends on the seeding or colonization of cells from the spleen.

Following splenectomy, certain characteristic alterations in the blood occur. Nucleated red cells appear, as well as corpuscles with Howell-Jolly bodies, and diffusely basophilic cells, target cells, and siderocytes are found, while the percentage of reticulocytes is increased. Leukocytosis occurs, and the number of platelets increases. These changes have been cited as evidence that the spleen exerts an inhibitory action on the bone marrow. In so far as the red cell changes are concerned, there is experimental evidence to support the view that the spleen normally *removes* the forms which are not usually seen in the blood in the absence of splenectomy or of hematopoietic disorders such as pernicious anemia or thalassemia. No evidence has been provided that the spleen exercises control over erythropoiesis in any other way. In relation to the leukocytes and platelets, however, there is at least some evidence to support the possibility that their production and liberation from the marrow may be influenced by the spleen. In addition, in certain situations the spleen appears to destroy these structures, especially the platelets, as, for example, when they are coated with antibodies.

In view of the large collection of reticuloendothelial cells and lymphoid tissue in the spleen, and for other reasons, it seems likely that the spleen plays a role in the defense mechanism of the body, perhaps through antibody production. In certain species, such as the dog and the rat, the spleen is important in maintaining natural resistance to certain bacterial, protozoal, and hematozoic infections. However, in man, at least, the spleen does not appear to be essential for these purposes, and no support has been found for the suggestion that the predisposition to infection is greater in splenectomized persons, even in young children, than in otherwise normal individuals.

Enlargement of the Spleen. This may occur under a great variety of circumstances. The chief ones are listed in Table 25-2.

Of greatest frequency is the enlargement of the spleen which occurs in association with infections. The "acute splenic tumor" accompanying various systemic infections such as typhoid fever and septicemia are examples. Like lymph node enlargement, splenic enlargement is frequently encountered in various contagious diseases and is often seen in infectious mononucleosis. Likewise, various subacute infections, notably bacterial endocarditis, are characteristically accompanied by enlargement of the spleen. Abscess of the spleen is rare.

Malaria is, perhaps, the most common cause of splenic enlargement when the world population is considered. Infection with other parasites which leads to splenic enlargement includes leishmaniasis,

Table 25-2. CHIEF CAUSES OF ENLARGEMENT OF THE SPLEEN

I. Inflammatory splenomegaly
  A. Acute splenic tumor of various systemic infections (typhoid, septicemia, infectious mononucleosis, various contagious diseases, etc.); abscess of spleen
  B. Subacute infections such as subacute bacterial endocarditis
  C. Malaria
  D. Other parasitic infections (leishmaniasis, trypanosomiasis, schistosomiasis, etc.)
  E. Chronic diseases such as tuberculosis, syphilis (especially congenital), chronic "infectious" arthritis, histoplasmosis, etc.
  F. Lupus erythematosus
II. Congestive splenomegaly ("Banti's disease," etc.)
III. "Hyperplastic" splenomegaly
  A. Acute and chronic, frankly hemolytic anemias
  B. Chronic anemias of various types (pernicious anemia, chronic hypochromic anemia, myelophthisic anemia, myelosclerosis, thalassemia, hemoglobin-C disease, etc.)
  C. Leukemia
  D. Polycythemia vera
  E. Thrombocytopenic purpura
IV. "Infiltrative" splenomegaly (Gaucher's disease, Niemann-Pick disease, amyloidosis, etc.)
V. Neoplasms and cysts
  A. Benign neoplasms and cysts (hemangioma, parasitic cysts, etc.)
  B. Lymphosarcoma, Hodgkin's disease, etc.

trypanosomiasis, and schistosomiasis. In kala-azar the spleen may be huge.

Primary tuberculous splenomegaly is extremely rare, but slight enlargement of the spleen accompanying a widespread tuberculous infection is by no means unusual. Splenomegaly may occur in connection with syphilis, especially congenital syphilis. Enlargement of this organ may also accompany the late stages of syphilis in association with gummas or amyloidosis. Chronic "infectious" arthritis, brucellosis, and sarcoidosis are other chronic diseases which may be accompanied by splenic enlargement. Splenic enlargement has been observed in about 25 per cent of cases of disseminated lupus erythematosus.

The vascularity of the spleen and its location in the portal bed make this organ liable to swelling as the result of increased venous pressure in that region. Such types of enlargement of the spleen can be classed under the general heading of "congestive splenomegaly," and include the syndromes known as "Banti's disease" and "splenic anemia," as well as the splenic enlargement which accompanies cirrhosis of the liver and thrombosis of the splenic or portal vein, and that which may be associated with cardiac failure.

The functions of the spleen in relation to the hematopoietic system result in enlargement of this organ when there is increased blood destruction (acute and chronic hemolytic anemias) or in the presence of chronic anemia of various types such as pernicious anemia, chronic hypochromic anemia, myelophthisic anemia, thalassemia, hemoglobin-C disease, and other hemoglobinopathies. Again, the spleen is enlarged, as a rule, in leukemia. In polycythemia vera splenomegaly is often encountered, and this finding helps to distinguish the primary disorder from secondary forms of polycythemia, where splenic enlargement is rare. The lymphatic hyperplasia which is associated with hyperthyroidism may be accompanied by splenomegaly. The spleen is also enlarged in conditions described under the names *primary splenic neutropenia* (p. 1323) and *primary splenic panhematopenia* (p. 1325).

Certain rare diseases such as Gaucher's disease and Niemann-Pick disease are characterized by splenic enlargement. In these conditions the swelling of the organ is probably due to the excessive storage of normal and abnormal metabolic products in the cells of the spleen.

Like other organs, the spleen may be enlarged as the consequence of the presence of neoplasms of various types. Hodgkin's disease, lymphosarcoma, reticulum cell sarcoma, and giant follicular lymphoma, however, are far more common causes of splenomegaly than other types of new growth. Carcinoma is the most frequent type of metastatic tumor, but even this is extremely rare. Benign tumors which may involve the spleen include lymphangiomas and hemangiomas. Cysts of the spleen may be of parasitic origin or nonparasitic. Of the latter, those containing serous or hemorrhagic fluid and due to trauma are the most common. They can sometimes be identified roentgenographically because of calcification of the wall.

DIFFERENTIAL DIAGNOSIS OF SPLENOMEGALY

A thorough physical examination, together with the history and examination of the blood, will serve to differentiate many of the causes of splenomegaly which have been outlined. Sometimes additional procedures may be required, such as blood culture, sternal puncture, a roentgenogram of the chest, serologic tests including those for syphilis, liver function tests, and spleen or lymph node biopsy.

The absence of fever is more helpful in differential diagnosis here than is its presence, since most of the conditions which have been mentioned may be accompanied by fever. However, at times, as in malaria and in undulant fever, the characteristic temperature curve is very helpful in making the diagnosis. In the septicemias the splenic enlargement is, as a rule, obviously only a minor feature of the whole clinical picture. The exanthemas are recognized by the respective characteristic changes in the skin. In their absence the skin should be inspected carefully for evidence of the petechiae which may accompany acute leukemia, thrombocytopenic purpura, or other hematopoietic disorders; the red petechiae occurring in crops together with the larger, slightly nodular and tender Osler nodes so characteristic of subacute bacterial endocarditis; or the spider telangiectases which accompany long-standing liver diseases. The plum-red "cyanosis" of polycythemia vera can hardly be overlooked.

Moderate lymph node enlargement accompanying splenomegaly is seen in many infectious diseases as well as in leukemia, but an asymmetric enlargement should arouse suspicion of Hodgkin's disease or lymphosarcoma. Great enlargement of the lymph nodes is seen in the last-named conditions as well as in chronic leukemia, especially in the lymphocytic form. The discovery of icterus suggests hemolytic anemia as a cause or, if there is little or no anemia and the splenic enlargement is only slight, infectious hepatitis. The splenomegaly associated with the Banti syndrome (congestive splenomegaly) and with cirrhosis of the liver is usually substantial in degree, and jaundice is not the rule under these circumstances. Malaria must be kept in mind among the causes of hemolytic anemia.

Lesions in the mucous membranes accompanying splenic enlargement are seen in measles (Koplik's spots), secondary syphilis (mucous patches), infectious mononucleosis (infection of the throat, tonsillar enlargement, sometimes signs of Vincent's angina), and acute leukemia (swollen, thickened gums which may be bleeding or purplish in color). In the leukemias, sternal tenderness may be quite pronounced.

The discovery of very great enlargement of the spleen tends to rule out the acute splenic tumor of various systemic infections, although sometimes the spleen may extend 4 to 6 cm below the costal margin in septicemia and in subacute bacterial endocarditis. Huge spleens are encountered in the chronic leukemias, in the Banti syndrome, in kala-azar, in schistosomiasis, in Gaucher's disease, in Hodgkin's disease and lymphosarcoma, in myelofibrosis, and in many instances of chronic hemolytic anemia.

Examination of the blood may indicate at once the nature of the disorder, as in malaria, the frank leukemias, or infectious mononucleosis. The discovery of icterus will lead to a reticulocyte count, examination of the stools and urine for the products of blood destruction, an erythrocyte fragility test, and other studies (see p. 1292) to rule out the various hemolytic anemias. The discovery of leukopenia should lead to the consideration of malaria, "aleukemic" leukemia, the Banti syndrome, typhoid fever, histoplasmosis, and leishmaniasis, but it must be kept in mind that the white cell count may sometimes be low also in infectious mononucleosis and in some cases of chronic hemolytic anemia. The demonstration of thrombocytopenia, as well as prolonged bleeding time, poor clot retraction, and positive tourniquet test, is an important finding, for it suggests acute leukemia. In that condition immature leukocytes will be found in the blood. In the "aleukemic" form, immature cells are absent from the blood or very scarce, but they are readily demonstrated by sternal puncture. In idiopathic thrombocytopenic purpura, the spleen is barely palpable in about 33 per cent of cases, but it is never very large. Thrombocytopenia only very rarely accompanies infectious mononucleosis and, while present in other conditions such as pernicious anemia, chronic hypochromic anemia, chronic hemolytic anemias, myelophthisic anemia, the Banti syndrome, Hodgkin's disease, and the related lymph node disorders, it is rarely severe in these diseases.

Sternal puncture may be very helpful if "aleukemic" leukemia, leishmaniasis, or Gaucher's disease is being considered seriously, for the characteristic cells or causative organisms may be demonstrated in this way. Sternal puncture does not often reveal malaria when the parasites have eluded careful study of the blood, but sometimes positive blood cultures for bacteria are obtained by this means when the usual method has failed. Splenic puncture is helpful when parasites, storage cells, signs of myeloid metaplasia, or granulomas are found, but this procedure should not be undertaken when hemorrhagic manifestations are present or in the absence of evidence of distinct splenic enlargement.

REFERENCE

Wintrobe, M. M.: "Clinical Hematology," 5th ed., Philadelphia, Lea & Febiger, 1961.

Section 10: Disorders of Nervous Function

INTRODUCTION

Raymond D. Adams

The symptoms and signs of nervous disease, which comprise the subject material of this section, are probably the most frequent and at the same time the most complex in all of medicine. Naturally they interest students of neurology and psychiatry, but they are so often found in patients who do not have classifiable diseases of the nervous system that they inevitably become the concern of every practitioner of medicine.

A lucid exposition of the diverse and complex manifestations of nervous disease is difficult to achieve, and a certain bias, which will become apparent at once to specialists in this field, is almost unavoidable. The method chosen in this discussion is somewhat unconventional and requires a few words of explanation. The aim has been to bring together all the expressions of disordered nervous function. They are described in some detail, and the most generally accepted explanations in terms of anatomy, biochemistry, physiology, and psychology are offered. No distinction is drawn between relatively simple phenomena such as motor and sensory paralysis, which are usually based on an easily demonstrated structural change, and the most complex ones such as anxiety, depression, or paranoia, to which at present no gross or microscopic pathologic changes can be assigned.

An attempt has been made, wherever indicated, to present both the neurologic and the psychologic conceptions of these phenomena, but the emphasis is on the neurologic, for it is more understandable to physicians and surgeons, the approach being the same as that to all other medical diseases.

NEUROLOGIC AND PSYCHOLOGIC CONCEPTIONS OF NERVOUS DISEASE

An understanding of these two conceptions of nervous disease is necessary in order to appreciate current trends in neurology and psychiatry. At the very beginning of this brief exposition of methodology and clinical approach, it should be stated that in the following pages the terms *neurologic* and *psychologic* do not denote the respective activities of neurologists and psychiatrists. By neurologic is meant the methods of medicine as applied to the study of nervous disease. They may be and are used by physicians, psychiatrists, and neurologists. By psychologic is meant another set of methods, largely nonmedical and used by many psychiatrists as well as by some neurologists and physicians. In other words the conception, the method, or the subject matter is not strictly within the province of any one discipline.

The *neurologic conception* has as its main tenet that all the phenomena of nervous disease are related to a pathologic process within the nervous system. This process may be obvious, like a cerebral infarct or tumor; or it may be impossible to see even with an ordinary light microscope, like the encephalopathy of delirium tremens. In all instances the pathologic process is the result of some physical or chemical change, and the visible lesion represents only its most advanced and often irreversible stage. The symptoms and clinical signs of nervous disease are the expressions of the activity of the pathologically altered nervous system. These clinical manifestations vary widely and include on the one hand the relatively simple, easily elicited, stereotyped objective signs, such as motor paralysis or ataxia, and on the other, the most complex, difficult to evoke, highly individualized, subjective signs, such as a hallucination, a delusion, or an obsessive thought. This is perhaps the most difficult idea for the student to grasp—that there is no necessary difference between "physical" and "mental" or "organic" and "functional" symptoms. To the neurologist, as to other physicians, all these symptoms have their objective as well as their "conscious" or subjective aspects, and the prominence of one or the other should not change our way of looking at them. In the paralyzed as well as the delirious patient, something of normal behavior has been lost as a consequence of his nervous disease, and something new in his behavior has emerged, presumably because of the unrestrained action of the undamaged parts of the brain. Some symptoms, like the dementia of general paresis, are understandable largely in terms of the structural alteration of the brain and the effects of the immediate stimulus of the environment upon the intact parts of it. No doubt previous personality structure, educational level, etc., modify the clinical picture. Other symptoms, such as a paranoid idea, though believed to be based on a neuropathologic process, are more difficult to analyze for we cannot identify the primary defect and the reaction of the patient to the defect. Such symptoms become more comprehensible when viewed against the background of all previous life experiences of which they may be a part. The previous life experiences thus become part of the present illness; but though possibly explaining the content of the nervous symptom and its mode of evolution, they do not explain its occurrence. The neurologic examination becomes merely a device which permits one to sample systematically the activities of the altered nervous system at one moment; and special techniques, especially refined psychologic methods may be needed to supplement it. Also, special laboratory procedures, such as biochemical tests of the blood, the electroencephalogram (EEG), the examination of the cerebrospinal fluid, x-rays, etc., provide additional objective data that cannot be obtained by observation. Pathologic study provides the final confirmation of the disease. The goal of the neurologic method or of neuropathology (the laboratory study of nervous disease) is to define the essential pathologic processes underlying disease and to determine their cause and mechanism. A complete theory of a nervous disease should embrace *all* aspects of it, the anatomic, biochemical, and physiologic, as well as the psychologic. The method is that of the medical sciences and of medicine itself.

The *psychologic conception of disease* makes many of the same assumptions as the neurologic concept. For example, it assumes that in many patients psychologic difficulties are caused by structural changes at the molecular, chemical, or tissue level. They may be due to a genetic or a developmental defect, and a lesion may be visualized. The main premise, however, is that the conscious processes of the mind are determined within broad limits by previous life experiences. Certain features of personality, the degree of emotional maturity, and the capacity to adjust adequately to a social situation are thought to depend to a considerable extent on learned patterns of reaction. Similarly, many of the aberrations of mental function are regarded as immature and unstable reactions to environmental circumstances, derived, it is believed, from an inadequacy of personality or traceable to a series of unfortunate experiences in early life. Some of these experiences are easily remembered, i.e., "con-

scious"; others are forgotten, i.e., "unconscious," and can be recalled with difficulty and sometimes only through the free association method of psychoanalysis. In either case the principal method of approach is to review the autobiography of the patient and to determine the relationship of the present symptoms to past experiences. The symptoms and signs of mental disease, whether the grandiose delusion of the general paretic or a phobia, are regarded as responses to a number of stimulus situations acting upon individuals who differ from normal mainly in that they have learned to think and to react emotionally in an abnormal way. Their symptoms are often traced in this way to psychic conflicts that have arisen in their personal life and are in this sense psychogenic. By interview and frank discussion, the physician endeavors to demonstrate these relationships to the patient and thereby to assist him to an understanding of his problems; and, if an untreatable medical disease is present, to help him make a satisfactory adjustment to it. The ultimate aim of the psychologic study of disease or of psychopathology, which is the scientific study of the psychologic origins of symptoms, is to discover abnormal mental processes and to find their psychologic cause and mechanism. Examples of some of the established mechanisms are conflict, projection, repression, conditioning, and arrest of libido. It is held, particularly by some of the more narrowly trained psychoanalysts, that all psychologic theories of mental disorder must be in psychologic terms and that anatomic, biochemical, physiologic, and pathologic terms have no place in such a formulation. The method is that of psychology, the conception is in line with rationalistic philosophy.

It seems to this editor that each method and each conception of disease has its place in medicine. The two methods operate at entirely different levels. In the *diagnosis* of nervous disease one's first responsibility is to record accurately all the symptoms and signs obtained in a single examination or a series of them. Here the neurologic method provides the only sound system. It permits one to approach the problem of nervous disease as one does any other medical problem. The psychologic method is not of great diagnostic value, because eliciting the patient's biography and finding psychologic explanations for his symptoms is a time-consuming procedure and commits one prematurely to a formula of the present illness which may be totally erroneous. In *therapy* and in the *management* of many diseases, including those for which there is no known treatment, a detailed knowledge of the patient's personality and his general reactions are, on the other hand, quite indispensable. One's whole success in all fields of medicine depends on the ability to deal with the patient as a troubled individual.

Here the psychologic method is of practical value, and the neurologic one often has relatively less to offer. This is a province of medicine where trained psychiatrists may function with great skill. In *theorizing* about disease and in doing *medical research*, however, the neurologic method and concept provide the soundest approach, for they embrace all the methods of medicine and the medical sciences, the anatomic, physiologic, biochemical, and neuropathologic, as well as the psychologic. Here the psychologic method has limited application and, though yielding useful data regarding the evolution of symptoms and their content or form, will probably never give us a complete explanation of a disease of the nervous system.

Thus we become confronted with one of the crucial problems of neurology—that of defining nervous diseases. Failure to do this has resulted in great confusion and has been an obstacle to research. The authors propose as a definition of nervous disease *one in which there is a lesion in the nervous tissue or in which there is reasonable evidence of an anatomic abnormality or a consistent physical or biochemical disturbance.* This should be distinguished from an abnormal psychologic reaction which is defined as *a disorder of behavior caused apparently by maladjustment in social relations.* Worry over the loss of a job or the ill health of a child, with all its potential visceral reverberations, would not be classified as a disease. These and countless other daily problems are better looked upon as natural physiologic reactions to social problems and dealt with at a psychologic level. A persistent anxiety state without obvious cause in a previously healthy young housewife, on the other hand, would be viewed differently. Most psychiatrists would consider it a reaction to some unconscious conflict, whereas many neurologists would consider the possibility that it is an unexplained, socially evoked disorder as mysterious as was hyperthyroidism a century ago. Anyone who essays to investigate it should do so with a completely open mind and be prepared to review critically any apparently satisfactory explanation, whether psychologic or neurologic. Mania, depression, paranoia, and the several varieties of schizophrenia, the major problems of psychiatry, have, unfortunately, an uncertain status. Many experienced psychiatrists would probably agree that they are diseases, rather than deviate ways of living or abnormal psychologic reactions, and that the more comprehensive methods of medicine and the medical sciences offer a more promising approach than does psychology. To the neurologist the major deficiencies in the study of nervous disease in the past few years have been the relative overemphasis on psychopathology and the relative neglect of neuropathology, using this term in its broadest connotation.

THE FIELDS OF NEUROLOGY AND PSYCHIATRY

All that has been said is by way of explaining the different ways in which neurologists and psychiatrists conceptualize the problems of nervous disease. Actually the fields of neurology and psychiatry are broad and ramify through all the medical and surgical specialties. They overlap in so far as both are concerned with disturbances of behavior, conduct, thinking, and emotional control due to diseases of the brain. They diverge in that neurology is concerned with many diseases of the nervous system which do not alter mind, and psychiatry is occupied with countless problems of adjustment in daily life which are sources of much unhappiness and disability, and yet cannot be defined as nervous diseases.

THE IMPORTANCE OF PSYCHOLOGIC MEDICINE

In planning this textbook the editors have undertaken to provide a comprehensive account of all the major psychiatric and neurologic diseases. Certain principles and problems of psychiatry are covered in the first half of the book. The reader will find that psychiatry has been introduced in Part One, Approach to the Patient. The cardinal manifestations and syndromes of psychiatric disease are discussed in the following pages, rather than in the second half of the book. This departure from the general plan of the book is a concession to contemporary psychiatric thought, which maintains that many of these conditions are but psychologic reactions and not diseases. The author believes that this position will probably be proved incorrect within the next decade.

The magnitude of the field of psychologic medicine can hardly be overestimated, and the emphasis here on the neurologic method does not indicate a wish to depreciate the importance of the psychologic approach. Every physician would agree that illness invariably creates problems for the patient and his family. Some, such as the temporary loss of employment or interruption of normal activities, are relatively minor. Others, such as fear of disability or death, may be so overwhelming as to demand the most thoughtful treatment. The need for an understanding of the patient and his reactions must be taken into account in every medical procedure, even in history taking, where the reliability and validity of symptoms must be evaluated against the background of the patient's personality and his cultural environment. The group of illnesses called the *psychoneuroses* or *neuroses* are manifested by a wide variety of symptoms which may be confused with those of medical disease.

Lastly there is a large category of diseases of unknown origin (peptic ulcer, mucous colitis, ulcerative colitis, bronchial asthma, atopic dermatitis, urticaria, angioneurotic edema, hay fever, Raynaud's disease, hypertension, hyperthyroidism, amenorrhea and other disturbances of menstruation, enuresis, dysuria, rheumatoid and other forms of arthritis, headache, syncope, and epilepsy) in which a stressful personal problem appears often to be associated with the initial development, exacerbation, or prolongation of symptoms. Three lines of evidence tend to set these latter so-called *psychosomatic diseases* apart from all others. (1) A large series of observations, made by Cannon, Wolff, Mittelman, Wolf, Cobb, Finesinger, White, Jones, have established the fact that the function of the offending organ is excited and deranged by one of the strong emotions and assuaged by feelings of security and relaxation. (2) A careful analysis of the biographies of patients with these diseases has shown what is believed to be an inordinately high incidence of resentment, hostility, dependence or independence, suppressed emotionality, inability to communicate matters of emotional concern or to differentiate between reality and subjective falsification (cf. studies of Lindemann, Dunbar, French, and Alexander). Preliminary studies of personality promised at first to show a special group of personality traits to be operating in each disease, but subsequent inquiry indicates that this is not the case. (3) A search through the biographic data of patients with these diseases has related exacerbations of symptoms with the occurrence of frustrating or disturbing incidents, and unsuccessful medical therapy has seemed to be due to a neglect of emotional factors.

In this latter field of psychosomatic disease, despite intensive investigation by psychiatrists in the last 20 years, the reports of which have led to the accumulation of an enormous literature, very few facts have been established. Surely it can be said that like the psychoneuroses they are "part disturbances" of the personality. But they differ from the psychoneuroses in that (1) they have different symptoms; (2) as a rule they are of longer duration; (3) they have in most instances a known and demonstrable pathologic basis and often a known cause, e.g., allergy in asthma and atopic dermatitis; (4) the treatment has been concerned more directly with the relief of symptoms and has tended to be directed by different groups of specialists; (5) the incidence of frank psychoneuroses in this group of patients is no greater than in the population at large, and these psychosomatic disorders are not more frequent in neurotic individuals. No complete proof has thus far been adduced that psychic factors are the primary cause of any of these psychosomatic diseases, any more than they are the cause of angina pectoris or exophthalmic goiter. To argue so from present data would be no more logical than to say that the war between the states was caused by the attack on Fort Sumter. Moreover, the concepts which have been formed about these diseases in recent years, although educationally useful, have not been of great value from the theoretical point of view. There is no evidence that the therapeutic results obtained by a thoughtful understanding physician, unsophisticated in psychologic theory, are less good than those of the most experienced psychiatrists.

The basic fault in the whole of this field of psychologic medicine, as it was in the "somatic medicine" which flourished in the days before and after the First World War, is that one aspect is stressed, with too little reference to the other. As pointed out by Wolff in his scholarly exposition of the mind-body relationship, the logical fallacy of such ideas as "psychogenic," "psychosomatic," and "emotional causes of disease" is that they imply a mind acting in opposition to a body.

The approach to this broad area of medicine which appeals to the editors is the ancient one, first suggested by Claude Bernard and ably espoused by Adolph Meyer. Man is regarded as a psychobiologic unit functioning in relationship to his physical and his uniquely social environment. Disease represents a faulty or inadequate adaptation of the organism to the environment. Sometimes the maladaptation can be traced to a single agent in the environment such as the tubercle bacillus without which the disease tuberculosis could not develop. In other instances, a recurrent infection is much more complex, being a manifestation of a primary physical defect in the individual, as in agammaglobulinemia. Again, exhaustion from a prolonged, stressful situation or malnutrition may render the patient susceptible to a given infectious agent. Seldom, however, even in a straightforward disease such as tuberculosis, can one reduce the problem to a single physical or psychic factor. Hence a rigid and narrow physical or psychologic approach must be supplanted by this broader, more biologic one which attempts to weigh each of the several factors entering the equation of disease. At present this is difficult, for all the factors, particularly in the so-called psychosomatic diseases, have not been isolated and studied. Until such time as new facts are obtained, the physician must attempt to cope with a huge population of patients, comprising as much as 50 per cent of his clientele, with inadequate methods of diagnosis and treatment. Fortunately, most of these patients suffer from relatively minor ailments which time and kindly reassurance alleviate or from psychoneuroses which do not result in a major derangement of life's activities. The physician and student must acquire a sensitivity to psychologic problems without, at the same time being so mindful of them that every illness is reduced to a naive psychologic formula. Above all, an open-minded attitude should be adopted—that will permit a critical review of all postulations in this field and an acceptance only of those based on the valid data of controlled clinical observation and scientific experiment.

REFERENCES

Cobb, S.: "Emotions and Clinical Medicine," New York, W. W. Norton & Company, 1950.

Finesinger, J. E.: Psychiatric Components in Medical Disease: Psychosomatic Medicine, New Engl. J. Med., 227:578, 1942.

Masserman, J. H.: "Behavior and Neurosis. An Experimental Psychoanalytic Approach to Psychobiologic Principles," Chicago, University of Chicago Press, 1943.

Wolf, S., and Wolff, H. G.: "Human Gastric Function. An Experimental Study of a Man and His Stomach," New York, Oxford University Press, 1947.

26 DISTURBANCES OF THE MOTOR SYSTEM
I. Motor Paralysis

Raymond D. Adams

The motor activities of man are commonly deranged by disease. Loss of power of voluntary movement probably surpasses all other neurologic symptoms in frequency and importance. Alterations of posture and involuntary movements represent another type of motor disorder, less frequent perhaps, but no less dramatic and disabling in their effects. The next two chapters present the main clinical features of these abnormalities of movement, along with such neuroanatomic and neuropathologic data as are necessary for their proper interpretation.

The motor functions constitute some of the most important aspects of human behavior. In a sense the greater part of man's nervous system is designed for the purpose of moving his body in space and the various parts of the body in relationship to one another. For this to be accomplished, the contraction of specific groups of muscles must be accompanied by the maintenance of certain postures which counteract gravity and other opposing forces. It should also be mentioned that many of man's thought processes are concerned with the planning of present and future motor activity.

Certain parts of the nervous system are known to be engaged primarily in the effectuation of movement: (1) The large motor nerve cells in the anterior horns of the spinal cord and the motor nuclei of the brain stem, with axones extending into the cranial nerves and into the anterior spinal roots and spinal nerves en route to the skeletal muscles, are called the *lower* or *primary motor neurones*. They are the "final common path" by which all nervous impulses subserving motor activity are transmitted to muscle. (2) The large motor cells of Betz in the cerebral cortex near the Rolandic fissure are connected with the spinal motor neurones by a system of fibers known, because of its shape in transverse sections through the medulla, as the *pyramidal* (corticospinal) *tract*. They represent the second or *upper motor neurones*. (3) Many other parts of the cerebral cortex, viz., those concerned with tactile, visual, and auditory sensation and the more anterior parts of the frontal lobes, are connected by fiber tracts with the motor cortex. They provide for the sensory regulation of motor function and are the means of coordinating thought and action. This is the highest level of motor function. (4) Several nuclear masses in the center of the brain, such as the caudate and lenticular nuclei, parts of the thalamus, the subthalamic and red nuclei, the substantia nigra, and the reticular formation in the brain stem, and also the pontine nuclei and the cerebellum, which subserve the neural mechanisms for posture and movement, are connected with one another and with the cerebral cortex and spinal cord by short relay neurones, all of which are entirely separate from the pyramidal tract. For this reason these latter structures are called *extrapyramidal*.

The motor activities of man may be analyzed physiologically, without regard to the morphology of the nervous system. The simplest, most stereotyped and most predictable are reflexes, such as the withdrawal of a limb from a painful stimulus (nociceptive or flexion reflex), the contraction of a muscle when its tendon is suddenly stretched (myotactic, stretch, or tendon reflex), or the constriction of the pupil in a bright light (pupillary reflex). These reflexes, based on inherited neural mechanisms, are centered in the spinal cord or brain stem. In simplest form they consist of an afferent or sensory neurone and an efferent motor neurone. There are, in addition, more complex reflexes, such as those subserving postural and righting reactions. These basic reactions, also unlearned, owe their integrity to the midbrain structures, but the nuclei on which they depend have not been ascertained. They are manifest in the decerebrate animal (one with a complete transverse lesion between the red nuclei and the pontine nuclei) which stands with all four limbs rigidly extended, with opisthotonos of cervical and other spinal muscles, and in the decorticate animal (an animal without cerebral cortex and white matter) which is capable of standing, righting itself, walking, and avoiding obstacles. In man comparable states may be observed.

At the other end of the physiologic scale are the most complex and variable and the less predictable movements, which in man are under voluntary control and can occur only when some degree of consciousness is retained. They are mediated by the motor cortices and the pyramidal tracts acting in relation to sensory cortical mechanisms. Although to some extent innate, these patterns of movement are largely learned and are perfected by training. Their execution, in the beginning at least, requires concentration, and once established, the patterns are retained as memories or engrams, arousable under proper stimulus conditions. With practice many of these movement patterns become automatic and no longer require close attention. Examples of this type of movement are the many habitual skills of craftsmen.

In human development the simple spinal and brain stem reflexes are already established at birth, and the more complex postural and righting reflexes appear in the first weeks of life. The various automatic movements organized in connection with cortical sensory functions (cortical automatisms, e.g., grasping and groping reactions), volitional movements, and the more refined motor skills await the maturation of the cerebrum, particularly the frontal lobes. The same systematization of simple and complex reflex patterns and instinctual reactions can be traced through the animal scale. Only the higher primates achieve a fine degree of manual precision, i.e., have the cerebral organization required for the use of tools. The motor neurones in the spinal cord, brain stem, cerebellum, and basal ganglions which are the basis of the motor activity in the newborn child become subjugated to cortical mechanisms as the nervous system matures. This evolution of motor functions is usually conceived as a synthesis of simple reflexes into more complex patterns of movement, but some of the more intricate, specialized movements may be better explained as differentiations, occurring during infancy and childhood, from crude, diffuse, or generalized motor activities.

The motor system may undergo dissolution in several ways during the course of disease. In diffuse disorders of the cerebrum there may be a disintegration first of the highest nervous integrations and then of the lower ones. Concepts or memories of specialized movement patterns may be lost while less complicated volitional and automatic movements are retained. Later there may be a paralysis of all volitional movements, without change or even with exaggeration of reflex activities. In lesions of the spinal cord all movements, both volitional and reflex, may be abolished. Other diseases damage particular parts of the motor system. The resulting impairments may be subdivided into (1) paralysis due to affection of lower motor neurones,

(2) paralysis due to a disorder of upper motor neurones, (3) apraxic or nonparalytic disturbances of purposive movement, and (4) abnormalities of movement and posture due to disease of the extrapyramidal motor systems. The first three types of motor disorder will be discussed briefly here, and the fourth type will be explained in the following chapter.

MOTOR PARALYSIS

Definitions. The term *paralysis* is derived from two Greek words: *para*, beside, and *lysis*, a loosening. In medicine it has come to refer to an abolition of function, either sensory or motor. When applied to voluntary muscles, paralysis means a loss of contraction due to interruption of some part of the pathway from the cerebrum to the muscle fiber. Lesser degrees of paralysis are sometimes spoken of as *paresis*, but in everyday medical parlance motor paralysis usually stands for either partial or complete loss of function. The word *plegia* comes from the Greek word meaning stroke; and the word *palsy*, from an old French word, has the same meaning as paralysis. All these words tend to be used interchangeably in medical practice, though it is preferable to use paresis for slight and paralysis or plegia for severe loss of motor function.

Paralysis Due to Disease of the Lower Motor Neurones

The essential facts concerning the anatomy and physiology of this system of motor nerve cells are well known. A few points, however, deserve brief comment because they provide an explanation for important clinical phenomena.

Each motor nerve cell through the extensive arborization of the terminal part of its fiber comes into contact with 100 or 200 or more muscle fibers; altogether they constitute "the motor unit." All the variations in force, range, and type of movement are determined by differences in the number and size of motor units called into activity and the frequency of their action. Feeble movements involve only a few small motor units; powerful movements recruit many more units of increasing size. When a motor neurone becomes diseased, as in progressive muscular atrophy, it may manifest increased irritability and all the muscle fibers that it controls may discharge sporadically in isolation from other units. The result of the contraction of one or several such units is a visible twitch, or *fasciculation*, which can be recorded in the electromyogram as a large diphasic or multiphasic action potential. If the motor neurone is destroyed, all the muscle fibers to which it is attached undergo a profound atrophy, viz., denervation atrophy. For some unknown reason the individual denervated muscle fibers now begin to contract spontaneously, though they can no longer do so in response to a nerve impulse or as part of a motor unit. This isolated activity of individual muscle fibers is called *fibrillation* and is so fine that it cannot be seen through the intact skin, but can be recorded only as a repetitive short-duration spike potential in the electromyogram. (See Chap. 56.)

The motor nerve fibers of each ventral root intermingle as the roots join to form plexuses; and although the innervation of the muscles is roughly metameric, or according to segments of the spinal cord, each large muscle comes to be supplied by two or more roots. For this reason the distribution of paralysis due to disease of the anterior horn cells or anterior roots differs from that which follows a lesion of a peripheral nerve.

All motor activity, even of the most elementary reflex type, requires the cooperation of several muscles. The analysis of a relatively simple movement such as the clenching of the fist affords some idea of the complexity of the underlying neural arrangements. In this act the primary movement consists of a contraction of the flexor muscles of the fingers, the flexor digitorum sublimis and profundus, the flexor pollicis longus and brevis, and the abductor pollicis brevis. In the terminology of Beevor, these muscles act as *agonists* or prime movers in this act. In order that flexion may be smooth and forceful the extensor muscles (*antagonists*) must relax at the same rate as the flexors contract. The muscles which flex the fingers also flex the wrist; and since it is desired that only the fingers flex, the muscles which extend the wrist must be brought into play to prevent its flexion. The action of the wrist extensors is *synergic,* and these muscles are called *synergists* in this particular act. Lastly the wrist, elbow, and shoulder must be stabilized by appropriate flexor and extensor muscles, which serve as *fixators.* The coordination of agonists, antagonists, synergists, and fixators involves reciprocal innervation and is managed by segmental spinal reflexes under the guidance of proprioceptive sensory stimuli. Only the agonist movement in a voluntary act is believed to be initiated at a cortical level.

If all or practically all peripheral motor nerves supplying a muscle are destroyed, both voluntary and reflex movements are abolished. The muscle becomes soft and yields to passive stretching, a condition known as *flaccidity.* Muscle tone—the slight resistance that normal relaxed muscle offers to passive movement—is reduced (hypotonia or atonia). The denervated muscles undergo extreme atrophy, usually being reduced to 20 or 30 per cent of their original bulk within 3 months. The reaction of the muscle to sudden stretch, as by tapping its tendon, is lost. And finally, it may be demonstrated that the muscle will no longer respond to electrical

stimuli of short duration, i.e., faradic stimuli, but still does respond to currents of long duration, galvanic stimuli. This alteration of electrical response is known as *Erb's reaction of degeneration.* If only a part of the motor units in the muscles is affected, only partial paralysis or paresis will ensue. The atrophy will be less, the tendon reflexes weakened instead of lost, and the reaction of degeneration may not be obtained. Quantitative testing by the determination of strength-duration curves is a means of showing partial denervation, but there may also be electromyographic evidence of fibrillations and fasciculations.

The tonus of muscle and the tendon reflexes are now known to depend on the muscle spindles and the afferent fibers to which they give origin and on the small anterior horn cells whose axones terminate on the small muscle fibers within the spindles. These small spinal motor neurones are called gamma neurones in contrast to the large alpha neurones. A tap on a tendon by stretching the spindle muscle fibers activates afferent neurones which terminate in alpha motor neurones. The result is the familiar muscle contraction or tendon reflex. The spindle muscle fibers are relaxed by an inhibitory mechanism, which is the means of terminating the reflex. Thus the setting of the spindle fibers and state of excitability of the gamma neurones (normally inhibited by the corticospinal fibers and other supranuclear neurones) determines the level of activity of the tendon reflexes and the responsiveness of muscle to stretch.

The signs and symptoms of a lower motor neurone lesion vary according to the location of the lesion. Probably the most important question for clinical purposes is whether sensory changes coexist. The combination of flaccid, areflexic paralysis and sensory changes indicates involvement of a mixed motor and sensory nerve or affection of both anterior and posterior roots. If sensory changes are absent, the lesion must be situated in the gray matter of the spinal cord, in the anterior roots, or in a purely motor branch of a peripheral nerve. The distinction between nuclear (spinal) and anterior root (radicular) lesions may at times be impossible to make. The coexistence of spastic weakness in muscles innervated by segments situated below the level of the lesion points to intraspinal disease.

Paralysis Due to Disease of the Upper Motor Neurones

There are several anatomic and physiologic facts concerning the upper motor neurones that are worthy of note. It was formerly believed that the corticospinal tract originated from the large motor cells of Betz in the fifth layer of the precentral convolution. However, there are only about 25,000 to 30,000 Betz cells, whereas the pyramidal tract at the level of the medulla contains approximately one million axons. This tract must, therefore, contain many fibers which do not arise from the Betz cells of the motor cortex (area 4 of Brodmann) but rather from the smaller cells of area 4 and the cells of the adjacent precentral (area 6) and postcentral cortex (areas 1, 3, 5). Furthermore, since about half the fibers in the pyramid remain intact after removal of the precentral and postcentral convolutions (i.e., hemispherectomy), these must originate in subcortical structures and descend to the spinal cord or ascend from spinal levels, as recently shown by Brodal and his associates. The pyramidal tract is the only long fiber connection between the cerebrum and the spinal cord. At the level of the internal capsule these corticospinal fibers are intermingled with many others destined to end in the globus pallidus, substantia nigra, and reticular substance. The fibers to the cranial nerve nuclei become separated at about the level of the midbrain and cross the midline to the contralateral cranial nerve nuclei (Fig. 26-1). These fibers form the corticopontine and corticobulbar tracts. The decussation of the pyramidal tract at the lower end of the medulla is variable in different individuals. A small number of fibers, 10 to 20 per cent, do not cross but descend ipsilaterally as the uncrossed pyramidal tract. The termination of the corticospinal tract is

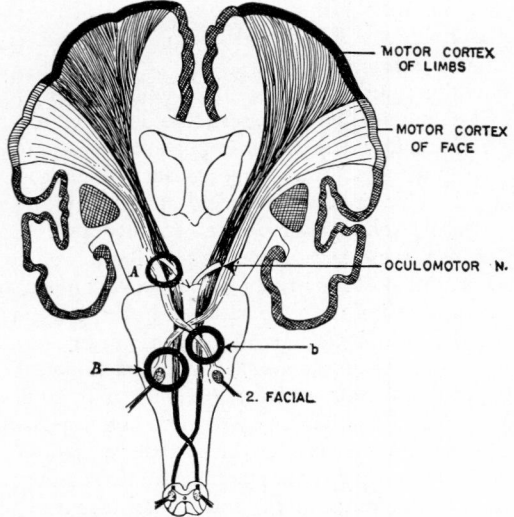

FIG. 26-1. Diagram of the corticospinal and corticobulbar tracts. Lesion at (*A*) produces ipsilateral oculomotor palsy and contralateral paralysis involving face, arm, and leg. Lesion at (*B*) causes ipsilateral facial paralysis of peripheral type and contralateral paralysis of arm and leg. Lesion at (*b*) results in ipsilateral facial weakness of upper motor neurone of central type and contralateral paralysis of arm and leg. (*Bergmann and Staeheln: "Krankheiten des Nervensystems," Berlin, Springer-Verlag, 1939.*)

in relation to nerve cells in the intermediate zone of gray matter, and not more than 10 to 15 per cent establish direct synaptic connection with anterior horn cells. These facts must of necessity modify current views of the anatomy of the pyramidal tract and suggest new interpretations of symptoms that result from the interruption of this tract.

The motor area of the cerebral cortex is difficult to define. It includes that part of the precentral convolution which contains Betz cells, but as already mentioned it probably extends both anteriorly into area 6 and posteriorly into the parietal lobe, where it overlaps the sensory areas. Physiologically it is defined as the region of the cortex from which isolated movements can be evoked by stimuli of minimal intensity. The muscle groups of the contralateral face, arm, trunk, and leg are represented in the motor cortex, those of the face being at the lower end of the precentral convolution and those of the leg in the paracentral lobule on the medial surface of the cerebral hemisphere. These motor points are not fixed but vary somewhat with the conditions of previous stimulation. The parts of the body capable of the most delicate movements have, in general, the largest cortical representation. Area 6, the premotor area, is also electrically excitable but requires more intense stimuli to evoke movements, and the movements produced are more complex than those evoked from area 4. Very strong stimuli elicit movements from a wide area of premotor frontal and parietal cortex, and the same movements may be obtained from several points. From this it may be assumed that one of the functions of the motor cortex is to synthesize simple movements into an infinite variety of finely graded, highly differentiated patterns.

Paralysis due to a lesion of the upper motor neurones always involves a group of muscles, never individual muscles, and the proper relationships between agonists, antagonists, synergists, and fixators are always preserved. The paralysis never involves all the muscles on one side of the body. Those movements which are invariably bilateral, such as movements of eyes, jaw, pharynx, larynx, neck, thorax, and abdomen, are little affected if at all. The hand and arm muscles suffer most severely, the leg muscles next, and of the cranial musculature only the muscles of the lower face and tongue are involved to any significant degree. Broadbent was the first to call attention to this distribution of paralysis, and this predilection of certain muscles to paralysis with pyramidal tract disease is referred to as *Broadbent's law*. Paralysis of pyramidal type is rarely complete for any long period of time and in this respect it differs from the total and absolute paralysis due to a lesion of the lower motor neurones. The paralyzed arm may suddenly move during yawning and stretching, and various reflex activities can be elicited at all times. However, acute disorders may abolish function in parts of the nervous system distant from the site of the lesion. For example, a sudden lesion of the pyramidal tract not only may cause a paralysis of voluntary movements but may abolish spinal reflexes as well. This is known as *spinal shock*. It usually lasts but a few days or weeks and is replaced by spasticity of the paralyzed muscles. This phenomenon of spasticity is another characteristic of lesions of the upper motor neurones and is due to a release of spinal reflex mechanisms or the release of a "normal component in movement from its natural competitor" (Denny-Brown). Spasticity does not set in immediately after the onset of a sudden lesion but develops gradually in the course of a few months. In exceptional cases the paralyzed limbs remain flaccid. The spasticity affects some muscle groups more than others. The arm is usually held in a flexed position, and any attempts to extend it encounter resistance, which is maximal at the beginning and then yields (clasp-knife phenomenon). The leg is maintained in an extended position, and passive flexion is resisted. If the limbs are moved to a new position, either flexion or extension, that position is maintained (lengthening and shortening reaction). If patients have suffered a paresis due to a lesion of the pyramidal tract, they not infrequently display associated movements upon attempting to carry out a voluntary movement with the weak limb. Attempts to flex the arm may result in involuntary pronation (the pronation phenomenon); or when the hemiplegic leg is flexed, the foot automatically dorsiflexes and everts (Strümpell's tibialis phenomenon). When the patient is asked to alternately pronate and supinate the paretic limb, the healthy limb may mimic these movements (i.e., *mirror movements*).

Table 26-1, modified from Stewart, shows the main differences between paralyses of the lower and those of the upper motor neurones.

APRAXIC OR NONPARALYTIC DISORDERS OF MOTOR FUNCTION

Aside from upper and lower motor neurone paralysis there may be a loss of purposive movement without paralysis or loss of movement. This is called *apraxia* and may be explained as follows. Many simple actions are acquired by learning or practice. Movement patterns, particularly those which involve manufacture, i.e., the use of tools and instruments, as well as gestures, once established, are remembered and may be reproduced under the proper circumstances. Any purposive act may be conceived as occurring in several stages. First, the idea of an act must be aroused by an appropriate stimulus situation, and then there is a mental representation

Table 26-1. DIFFERENCES BETWEEN PARALYSIS OF UPPER AND LOWER NEURONE TYPES

Upper, supranuclear, or corticospinal (pyramidal) paralysis	Lower, spinomuscular, or infranuclear paralysis
1. Muscle groups affected diffusely; never individual muscles	1. Individual muscles may be affected
2. Atrophy slight and due to disuse	2. Atrophy pronounced, 70 to 80 per cent of total bulk
3. Spasticity with hyperactivity of the tendon reflexes	3. Flaccidity and hypotonia of affected muscles with loss of tendon reflexes
4. Babinski sign +	4. Plantar reflex, if present, is of normal flexor type
5. Fascicular twitches never present	5. Fascicular twitches may be present
6. Normal reactions to galvanic and faradic current	6. Loss of reaction to faradic and retention of galvanic reaction—reaction of degeneration

of it as a whole. This idea or concept is then translated into action by the excitation of the motor cortex and the corticospinal tracts, which not only initiate particular movements of individual muscle groups but also modify or suppress the subcortical mechanisms that control the basic attitudes and postures of the body. In right-handed and most left-handed individuals the neural mechanisms for the formulation of an idea of an act and its reproduction are believed to be centered in the posterior and inferior part of the left parietal lobe, near the angular gyrus, and are connected with the motor areas of the right cerebral hemisphere.

A failure to execute certain acts in the correct context while retaining the individual movements upon which such acts depend is the main feature of *apraxia*. The most adequate clinical tests of motor deficits of this type are a series of verbal requests to perform a series of actions such as using a comb, a razor, a toothbrush, or a common tool, or as gesturing, i.e., to wave good-bye, to salute, to shake the fist as though angry, or to blow a kiss. Of course failure may be due to an aphasia which prevents understanding of the spoken or written word or an agnosia which makes recognition of a tool or object impossible. But aside from these sources of difficulty there remains a peculiar motor deficit in which the patient appears to have lost his memory of how to perform a given act, especially if called upon to perform it in an unnatural, artificial setting. The maximal degree of it is called *ideomotor apraxia* and implies an inability to translate the idea of the movement into a precise well-executed movement. The failure may be evident both upon spoken command and when asked to imitate a movement made by the examiner. The least degree of it, bordering upon paralysis of willed movement, is sometimes called motor apraxia, a state which is poorly defined. The maximum degree is often observed in confused or demented patients who may fail entirely to understand what the examiner requests and are unable to perform certain acts. Only if this deficit is out of proportion to all others, thus reflecting a specific loss of certain learned patterns of movement (a specific amnesia so to speak, analogous to the amnesia of words in aphasia), can one recognize the condition in such patients. This latter state is called *ideational apraxia*. Probably all three conditions, ideational, ideomotor, and motor apraxia, are but varying degrees of a single memory deficit of learned patterns of movement, most clearly in evidence when there is no motor paralysis or incoordination and mental function is clear. An added element of mental confusion imparts to it the form of ideational apraxia, a disorder which is bilateral; and an added element of voluntary motor paralysis converts it to a motor apraxia. Apraxia becomes manifest only with cortical lesions and is most frequent with parietal lesions. If the lesion is in the left dominant cerebral hemisphere the apraxia is usually bilateral; if in the right hemisphere the apraxia is in the left arm and leg.

Lesions of areas 6 and 8 which leave the more posterior part of the motor and the sensory cortex intact may produce a curious syndrome in which many voluntary movements are retained but are slow and awkward. Moreover, grasping and sucking reflexes are manifest. The tendon reflexes are lively, and the plantar reflexes are flexor. In some cases there is a persistence of hand and foot flexion on tactile stimulation of the palmar and plantar surfaces, so that the patient is unable to release his grip or dorsiflex his foot (tonic innervation) voluntarily as long as the stimulus is present. In lesions of the parietal lobe a whole series of aversion or avoidance reactions to sensory stimuli become manifest. For a more complete discussion of the several types of apraxia, see Chap. 37.

EXAMINATION SCHEME FOR MOTOR PARALYSIS AND APRAXIA

The first step is to inspect the paralyzed limb, taking note first of its posture and of the presence or absence of muscle atrophy, hypertrophy, and fascicular twitchings. The patient should then be called upon to move each muscle group, and the power and facility of movement are graded and recorded. The range of passive movement is then determined by moving all the joints. This provides information concerning alterations of muscle tone, i.e., hypotonia, spasticity, and rigidity. Dislocations, disease of joints, and ankyloses may also be revealed by these same maneuvers. Enlargement of muscles with increased strength denotes true hypertrophy, which may be either physiologic or a manifestation of myotonia congenita. Slight atrophy may be due to disuse from any cause, i.e., pain, fixation as the result of a cast, or any type of paralysis. However, a pronounced atrophy usually occurs only with denervation of several weeks or months standing.

The tendon reflexes should then be tested. The usual routine is to try to elicit the jaw jerk (increased in pseudobulbar palsy), the supinator, biceps, triceps, quadriceps, and Achilles tendon reflexes. Two cutaneous reflexes are then tested, the abdominal and the plantar reflexes. (The extensor plantar reflex is the Babinski sign.)

If there is no evidence of upper or lower neurone disease but certain acts are nonetheless imperfectly performed, one should look for a disorder of postural sensibility or of cerebellar coordination or rigidity with abnormality of posture and movement due to disease of the basal ganglions. In the absence of these disorders, the possibility of a hysterical disorder of motor function should be investigated.

Hysterical paralysis is easily distinguished from chronic lower motor neurone disease by the areflexia and severe atrophy that are so characteristic of the latter condition. It is only in certain acute cases of upper motor neurone disease lacking all the usual changes in reflexes and muscle tone that diagnostic difficulty may arise. In hysterical paralysis one arm or one leg or all of one side of the body may be affected. The hysterical gait is sometimes diagnostic in itself (see Chap. 43). Often there is loss of sensation in the paralyzed parts and sometimes loss of sight in the eye, of hearing in the ear, and of smell in the nostril on the paralyzed side, a group of sensory changes that is never seen in organic brain disease. The patient should be asked to move the affected limbs, and as he does so, the movement is seen to be slow and jerky, often with contraction of both agonist and antagonist muscles simultaneously or intermittently. Hoover's sign and Babinski's combined leg flexion test are helpful in distinguishing hysterical from organic hemiplegia. To elicit Hoover's sign the patient, lying on his back, is asked to raise one leg from the bed; in a normal individual the back of the heel of the contralateral leg is pressed firmly down, and the same is true when the patient with organic hemiplegia attempts to lift the paralyzed leg. To carry out Babinski's combined leg flexion test, a patient with an organic hemiplegia is asked to sit up without using his arms; when he does so, the paralyzed or weak leg flexes at the hip, and the heel is lifted from the bed while the heel of the sound leg is pressed into the bed. Both these signs are absent in hysterical hemiplegia.

If there is no definite paralysis except in the

performance of certain specific acts, then the possibility of apraxia must be considered. This defect is best demonstrated by asking the patient to carry out certain commands such as to make a fist, to put out his tongue, to stamp his foot, to touch his nose, to place one heel on the opposite knee, to brush his hair, to light a cigarette, or to drink a glass of water. One must also take note of the state of mentation and of the speed of comprehension. Confusion and aphasia interfere with the understanding of spoken commands.

DIFFERENTIAL DIAGNOSIS OF PARALYSIS

The diagnostic consideration of paralysis may be simplified by the following subdivisions which relate to the location and distribution of the weakness.

1. *Monoplegia.* This term refers to a weakness or paralysis of all the muscles in one limb, whether leg or arm. It should not be used for paralysis of isolated muscles or groups of muscles supplied by a single nerve or motor root.

2. *Hemiplegia.* This is the most common distribution of paralysis—loss of strength in arm, leg, and sometimes the face on one side of the body.

3. *Paraplegia.* Paraplegia indicates a weakness or paralysis of both legs. It is most commonly found in spinal cord disease.

4. *Quadriplegia.* This indicates weakness of all four extremities. It may result from lesions involving peripheral nerves, gray matter of the spinal cord, or the corticospinal tracts bilaterally in the cervical cord, upper brain stem, or cerebrum. Diplegia is a special form of quadriplegia in which the legs are affected more than the arms.

5. *Isolated paralyses.* This term refers to weakness localized to one or more muscle groups.

Monoplegia

The physical examination of patients complaining of weakness of one extremity often discloses an unnoticed weakness in another limb, and the condition is actually one of hemiplegia or paraplegia. Or, instead of weakness of all the muscles in a limb, only isolated groups are found to be affected. Ataxia, sensory disturbances, or pain in an extremity will often be interpreted by the patient as weakness, as will the mechanical limitation resulting from arthritis or the rigidity of parkinsonism.

In general the presence or absence of atrophy of muscles in a monoplegic limb can be of diagnostic help.

Paralysis without Muscular Atrophy. Long-continued disuse of a limb may lead to atrophy, but this is usually not so marked as in diseases which denervate muscles; the tendon reflexes are normal, and the response of the muscles to electrical stimulation and the electromyogram are unaltered.

The most frequent cause of monoplegia without muscular wasting is a lesion of the cerebral cortex. Only occasionally does it occur in diseases which interrupt the corticospinal tract at the level of the internal capsule, brain stem, or spinal cord. A vascular lesion (thrombosis or embolus) is most common, but of course a tumor or abscess may have the same effect. Multiple sclerosis and spinal cord tumor, early in their course, may cause weakness of one extremity, usually the leg. As indicated above, weakness due to damage to the corticospinal system is usually accompanied by spasticity, increased reflexes, and an extensor plantar reflex (Babinski sign), and the electrical reactions and electromyogram are normal. However, acute diseases which destroy the motor areas of the cerebrum may at first (for several days) reduce or leave unaltered the tendon reflexes and cause hypotonia (the condition known as spinal shock). This does not occur in partial or slowly evolving lesions. In acute diseases affecting the lower motor neurones the tendon reflexes are always reduced or abolished, but atrophy may not appear for several weeks. Hence one must take into account the mode of onset and the duration of the disease in evaluating the tendon reflexes, muscle tone, and degree of atrophy, prior to reaching an anatomic diagnosis.

Paralysis with Muscular Atrophy. This condition is more frequent than paralysis without muscular atrophy. In addition to the paralysis and reduced or abolished tendon reflexes there may be visible fasciculations. If completely paralyzed, the muscles exhibit an electrical reaction of degeneration and the electromyogram shows reduced numbers of motor units (often of large size), fasciculations at rest and fibrillations. The lesion may be in the spinal cord, the spinal roots or peripheral nerves. Its location can usually be decided by the distribution of the palsied muscles (whether the pattern is one of nerve, spinal root or spinal cord involvement), and by the associated neurological symptoms and signs and special tests (cerebrospinal fluid examination, x-ray of spine and myelogram).

The many diseases which may cause an atrophic monoplegia need only to be listed here. Acute anterior poliomyelitis, amyotrophic lateral sclerosis and progressive muscular atrophy, syringomyelia, spinal cord tumor, and spinal cord trauma are the most frequent diseases of the spinal cord. Injuries of the brachial plexus and nerves, neoplastic involvement of spinal roots and plexus are well recognized causes of this syndrome. It should be noted that multiple sclerosis almost never causes atrophy, and that ruptured intervertebral disk and the many varieties of neuritis rarely paralyze all or most of the muscles of a limb. Muscle dystrophy may begin in one limb, but by the time the patient is seen the typical more or less symmetrical pattern of proximal limb and trunk involvement is in evidence.

Hemiplegia

This is the most frequent distribution of paralysis in man. With rare exceptions (a few unusual cases of poliomyelitis or motor system disease) this pattern of paralysis is due to involvement of the corticospinal tract.

Location of Lesion Producing Hemiplegia. The site or level of the lesion, i.e., cerebral, capsular, brain stem, spinal cord, can usually be deduced from the associated neurologic findings. Diseases localized in the cerebral cortex, cerebral white matter (corona radiata), and internal capsule usually evoke a weakness or paralysis of the face, arm, and leg on the opposite side. The occurrence of convulsive seizures or the presence of a defect in speech (aphasia), a cortical type of sensory loss (astereognosis, loss of two-point discrimination, etc.), anosognosia, or defects in the visual fields suggest a cortical or subcortical location.

Damage to the corticospinal tract in the upper portion of the brain stem (see Fig. 26-1) may cause a paralysis of the face, arm, and leg on the opposite side. The lesion in such cases is localized by the presence of a paralysis of the muscles supplied by the oculomotor nerve on the same side as the lesion (Weber's syndrome) or other neurologic findings. With low pontine lesions a unilateral abducens or facial palsy is combined with a contralateral weakness or paralysis of the arm and leg (Millard-Gubler syndrome). Lesions of the lowermost part of the brain stem, i.e., in the medulla, affect the tongue and sometimes the pharynx and larynx on one side and arm and leg on the other side. These "crossed paralyses," so common in brain stem diseases, are described in Chap. 31.

Rarely, a homolateral hemiplegia may be caused by a lesion in the lateral column of the cervical spinal cord. At this level, however, the pathologic process more often induces bilateral signs, with resulting quadriparesis or quadriplegia. If one side of the spinal cord is extensively damaged, the homolateral paralysis is combined with a loss of vibratory and position sense on the same side and a contralateral loss of pain and temperature (Brown-Séquard syndrome).

Muscle atrophy of minor degree often follows lesions of the corticospinal system but never reaches the proportions seen in diseases of the lower motor neurones. The atrophy is due to disuse. When the motor cortex and adjacent parts of the parietal lobe are damaged in infancy or childhood, the normal development of the muscles and the skeletal system in the affected limbs is retarded. The palsied limbs and even the trunk on one side are small. This does not occur if the paralysis begins after skeletal growth is attained. In the hemiplegia due to spinal cord injury there is often an atrophy of muscles at the level of the lesion as a result of damage to anterior horn cells or ventral roots.

Causes of Hemiplegia. In this condition vascular diseases of the cerebrum and brain stem exceed all others in frequency. Trauma (brain contusion, epidural and subdural hemorrhage) ranks second, and other diseases such as brain tumor, brain abscess and encephalitis, demyelinative diseases, complications of meningitis, tuberculosis, and syphilis are of decreasing order of importance. Most of these diseases can be diagnosed by the mode of evolution and the conjoined clinical and laboratory data which are presented in the chapters on neurologic diseases.

Paraplegia

Paralysis of both lower extremities may occur in diseases of the spinal cord and the spinal roots or of the peripheral nerves. If the onset is acute, it may be difficult to distinguish spinal from neural paralysis, for in any acute myelopathy spinal shock may result in abolition of reflexes and flaccidity. As a rule in acute spinal cord diseases with involvement of the corticospinal tracts, the paralysis affects all muscles below a given level; and often, if the white matter is extensively damaged, sensory loss below a particular level (loss of pain and temperature with lateral spinothalamic tracts and loss of vibratory and position sense with posterior columns) is conjoined. Also, in bilateral disease of the spinal cord, the bladder and bowel sphincters are paralyzed. Alterations of cerebrospinal fluid (dynamic block, increase in protein or cells) are frequent. In peripheral nerve diseases both the sensory and motor loss tend to involve the distal muscles of the legs more than the proximal ones (an exception is acute idiopathic polyneuritis), and the sphincters are often spared or only briefly deranged in function. Sensory loss, if present, is more likely to consist of a distal impairment of touch, vibration, and position sense, with pain and temperature spared in many instances. The cerebrospinal fluid protein may be normal or elevated.

For clinical purposes it is helpful to consider separately the acute and the chronic paraplegias and to divide the chronic ones into two groups, those which occur in infancy and those which begin in adult life.

Acute paraplegia, beginning at any age, is relatively infrequent. Fracture dislocation of the spine with traumatic necrosis of the spinal cord, spontaneous hematomyelia with bleeding from a vascular malformation (angioma, telangiectasis), thrombosis of a spinal artery with infarction (myelomalacia), and dissecting aortic aneurysm or atherosclerotic occlusion of nutrient spinal arteries arising from the aorta with resulting infarction (myelomalacia) are the most common varieties of sudden paraplegia (or quadriplegia if the cervical cord is involved). Postinfectious or postvaccinial myelitis, acute demyelinative myelitis (Devic's syndrome if the optic nerves are also affected), necrotizing myelitis, and epidural abscess or tumor with spinal cord compression tend to develop somewhat more slowly, over a period of hours or days, or may have a subacute onset. Poliomyelitis and acute idiopathic polyneuritis, the former a purely motor disorder with meningitis, the latter predominantly motor but often with minimal sensory disturbances (paresthesias or objectively demonstrated impairment), must be distinguished from the other acute myelopathies and from one another.

In pediatric practice, delay in starting to walk and difficulty in walking are also common problems. These conditions may be associated with a systemic disease such as rickets or may be indicative of mental deficiency or, more commonly, of some muscular or neurologic disease. Congenital cerebral disease accounts for a majority of cases of infantile diplegia (weakness predominant in the legs, with the arms minimally affected). Present at birth or manifest in the first months of life, it may appear to progress, but actually it is stationary and only becomes apparent as the motor system develops. Later there may seem to be slow improvement as a result of the normal maturation processes of childhood. Congenital malformation of the spinal cord or birth injury of the spinal cord are other possibilities. Friedreich's ataxia and familial paraplegia, progressive muscular dystrophy and the chronic varieties of polyneuritis tend to appear later during childhood and adolescence and are slowly progressive.

In adult life multiple sclerosis, subacute combined degeneration, spinal cord tumor, ruptured cervical disk and cervical spondylosis, syphilitic meningomyelitis, chronic epidural infections (fungous and other granulomatous diseases), Erb's spastic paraplegia and motor system disease, and syringomyelia represent the most frequently encountered forms of spinal cord disease. The several varieties of polyneuritis and polymyositis must be considered in their differential diagnosis for they, too, may cause a paraplegia.

Quadriplegia

All that has been written about the common causes of paraplegia applies to quadriplegia. The lesion is usually in the cervical rather than the thoracic or lumbar segments of the spinal cord. If situated in the low cervical segments and involving the anterior half of the spinal cord, as in occlusion of the anterior spinal artery, the arm paralysis may be flaccid and areflexic and the leg paralysis spastic (anterior spinal syndrome). There are only a few points of difference between the common paraplegic and quadriplegic syndromes. In infants, aside

from developmental abnormalities and anoxia of birth, an inherited cerebral disease (Schilder's disease, metachromatic leukoencephalopathy, lipid storage disease) may be responsible for a quadriparesis or quadriplegia. Congenital forms of muscle dystrophy may be recognized soon after birth and also infantile muscular atrophy (Werdnig-Hoffmann's disease).

In adults repeated cerebral vascular accidents may lead to bilateral hemiplegia, usually accompanied by pseudobulbar palsy.

Isolated Paralysis

Paralysis of isolated muscle groups usually indicates a lesion of one or more peripheral nerves. The diagnosis of a lesion of an individual peripheral nerve is made on the presence of weakness or paralysis of the muscle or group of muscles and an impairment or loss of sensation in the distribution of the nerve in question. Complete transection or severe injury to a peripheral nerve is usually followed by atrophy of the muscles which it innervates and loss of their tendon reflexes. Trophic changes in the skin, nails, and subcutaneous tissue may also occur.

A knowledge of the muscular and sensory function of each individual nerve is needed for a satisfactory diagnosis. Since lesions of the peripheral nerves are relatively uncommon in civil life, it is not practical for the general physician to keep all these facts in his memory, and a textbook of anatomy or a compendium on nerve injury should be consulted. It is, however, of considerable importance to decide whether the lesion is a temporary one of conduction only (neuropraxia) or whether there has been a pathologic dissolution of continuity, requiring nerve regeneration for recovery. Electromyography may be of great value.

All the diseases mentioned in the differential diagnosis of monoplegia, hemiplegia, paraplegia, and quadriplegia will be discussed in the neurologic section of the book.

MUSCULAR PARALYSIS AND SPASM UNATTENDED BY VISIBLE CHANGE IN NERVE OR MUSCLE

A discussion of motor paralysis would not be complete without some reference to a group of diseases which appear to have no basis in terms of visible structural change in motor nerve cells, nerve fibers, motor end-plates, and muscular fibers. This group is comprised of myasthenia gravis, myotonia congenita (Thomsen's disease), familial periodic paralysis, disorders of potassium, sodium, calcium, and magnesium metabolism, tetany, tetanus, botulinus poisoning, black widow spider bite, and the thyroid myopathies. In these diseases, each of which possesses a fairly distinctive clinical picture, the abnormality is purely biochemical, and even if the patient survives for a long time, no visible microscopic change develops. An understanding of these diseases requires a knowledge of the processes involved in nerve and muscle excitation and in the contraction of muscle.

Excitation of Nerve and Muscle Fiber

All nerve and muscle fibers in their resting state have an electric charge, i.e., there is an electrical difference between the surface and the interior. This is readily demonstrated by recording from a fine electrode inserted into the substance of the fiber and applying another to its surface. When the two are connected to a voltmeter, the inside is found to be negative in relation to the surface, which is therefore positive. The difference, i.e., the electrical potential, is of the order of 90 μv; it has been shown to depend on the difference in concentration of potassium ions between the inside and outside of the fiber, the inside being rich in potassium, the outside being poor. The membrane of the fiber with this electrical charge is said to be *polarized*. Upon injury, or application of an electrical or chemical stimulus to the fiber, the electrical charge, or *resting potential*, is reversed and the surface or fiber membrane becomes negative to the interior. Potassium ions leave the fiber and sodium ions enter. The fiber is said now to be *depolarized*, though actually it is now polarized in the opposite direction. This surface negativity spreads along the axone of the nerve fiber as a wave of electrical charge, being accompanied always by this flux of K and Na ions. This is the nerve or muscle action potential, which by convention is recorded in an oscillograph as an upward deflection—a sharp wave at the usual speeds of recording. The excited fiber, if it reacts at all, does so maximally (all-or-none law). As would be expected, the threshold of excitability of the nerve and muscle fiber is influenced by the concentration of K and Na ions in the extracellular fluids, and there is good evidence that Ca and Mg are also influential.

The point at which the nerve fiber comes in contact with the muscle fiber, i.e., the neuromuscular junction (Doyère's hillock or motor end-plate), is of special importance. As the branching axone of a single anterior horn cell comes to rest on several hundred muscle fibers, one slip of nerve ends on each muscle fiber, the total ensemble comprising the motor unit. This nerve terminal, usually made up of several filaments, more or less indents the surface of the fiber but is always separated from its interior by the true neurilemma and sarcolemma. There is good evidence that acetylcholine is formed at the terminal nerve filaments and is the means whereby the nerve impulse is transmitted to the muscle cell. Acetylcholine is in itself capable of depolarizing the muscle cell. It has been found that a small amount of it is liberated constantly at the motor end-plate, enough to keep it electrically negative but yet insufficient to discharge the adjacent parts of the sarcolemmal membrane. This is called the *end-plate potential*. Upon the arrival of a nerve impulse, more acetylcholine is formed, and the action potential of the end-plate quickly passes the length of the muscle fiber along the sarcolemmal membrane. This action potential is followed within a millisecond by a contraction of the entire fiber. The action potential is separate from the contractile response. The former is measured as a wave of negative polarity which is very brief, the latter as a mechanical change, a shortening of the fiber which lasts longer. It is possible therefore for a second nerve and muscle action potential to arrive before the contractile process of the first is finished, i.e., before the fiber has relaxed. If the frequency of nerve impulse is between 25 and 50 per second, there is a complete fusion or prolongation of the contractile process. This mechanical response of the muscle is called a *tetanus*.

In order for the muscle fiber to respond to any succeeding nerve impulse, the end-plate must be repolarized, and this is possible only if the acetylcholine is removed or destroyed. This is done by a special enzyme called *cholinesterase*, which hydrolyzes acetylcholine into acetate and choline. The latter also has some depolarizing effect and is more slowly removed. If an excess of acetylcholine is formed, or if cholinesterase fails to destroy it (the latter may be insufficient or may be inhibited), the motor end-plate remains depolarized and is then incapable of responding to nerve impulses. Compounds such as neostigmine (Prostigmine), pyridostigmine (Mestinon), edrophonium (Tensilon), physostigmine (eserine), diisopropyl fluorophosphate (DFP), tetraethylpyrophosphate (TEPP), and several of the "nerve gases" act in this way to paralyze muscle, i.e., as anticholinesterases. Several other chemical substances, such as decamethonium and succinylcholine, have an action similar to that of acetylcholine and produce a depolarizing type of block of neuromuscular transmission. They are called *depolarizing blocking agents*. If their action is prolonged, this continuous depolarization results in paralysis. Curare and *d*-tubocurarine are believed to act in a different way. They compete with acetylcholine for the receptor site in the end-plate and thus prevent acetylcholine from acting. They have been called *competitive blocking agents*. This is also the mode of action of some of the quaternary ammonium ions.

A disturbance of the biochemical mechanism in nerve and muscle and at their junction may account not only for the impairment of the contractile process but also for its enhancement. There may be an excessive irritability, under which circumstance "spontaneous" discharges may occur; or a single nerve impulse may set off a train of action potentials in nerve or muscle. The common cramps in the calf muscles and small muscles of the feet (painful, sustained involuntary contractions with motor unit discharges up to 300 per second) are apparently due to increased excitability of the peripheral parts of the motor nerve. They may occur in hypocalcemic or hyponatremic states or after unaccustomed use of a muscle. Quinine and warmth tend to prevent them.

The manner in which the muscle action potential initiates the contractile response has not been fully determined. The energy for this process is derived from the action of adenosinetriphosphate (ATP) on the special muscle proteins, actin and myosin, and the change in the shape of these protein molecules results in shortening of the muscle fiber. The high-energy phosphate bonds of ATP must be replenished constantly, a reaction which involves interchanges with phosphocreatine. Myoglobin, another important muscle protein, plays a part in the transfer of oxygen, and a series of enzymes are involved in this exchange.

Biochemical Basis of Special Neuromuscular Diseases

From this brief account it is evident that the muscle fiber, which is totally dependent on nerve for its stimulus to normal contraction, may be paralyzed in a number of ways. This may be accomplished by any agent which blocks the transmission of the nerve impulse; it may be due to a failure of the nerve to conduct the impulse, an insufficiency of acetylcholine to depolarize the muscle cell, an inaccessibility of the motor end-plate to normally released acetylcholine due to a competing substance such as tubocurarine, excessive quantities of acetylcholine or some other depolarizing substance which impair neuromuscular conduction by keeping the end-plate depolarized, or a failure of the membrane of the muscle fiber to transmit the impulse to all the fiber or to initiate the contractile process. Similarly, fascicular twitching, cramps, and muscle spasm may be due to excessive activity at a number of points in the neuromuscular apparatus.

Power of muscle contraction is impaired in a number of conditions which alter the concentration of certain electrolytes in extracellular fluids. If the plasma level of *potassium is below 2.5 mEq per liter or above 7 mEq per liter*, weakness of the extremities usually occurs; and when the concentration reaches 2 mEq or 9 mEq, there is flaccid paralysis of the extremities and later of respiratory muscles, with relative sparing of the cranial muscles. In addition the tendon reflexes are diminished, and the electrocardiogram is altered. The contraction of muscle to percussion is also reduced, which suggests an impairment not only of transmission in nerve and at neuromuscular junction but also of the reactivity of the muscle fibers themselves. Hypocalcemia at levels of 7 mg per 100 ml or below, as in rickets and hypoparathyroidism (or at times only a reduction in ionized calcium as in hyperventilation), causes an increased irritability and spontaneous discharge of sensory and motor nerve fibers and muscle fibers. The sensory manifestations are tingling and tightness in fingers, lips, tongue, and feet; the motor manifestations consist of spasms of distal musculature (tetany) in the hands, forearms, feet, and face, laryngospasm, and occasionally convulsions. In latent tetany the nerve irritability can be evoked by percussing the nerve, as in the Chvostek test (tapping the facial nerve to induce facial spasm), or compressing the nerve with a tourniquet (Trousseau's sign). Also there is a decrease in faradic excitability of nerve fibers, with frequent repetitive and finally spontaneous discharges. *Hypercalcemia*, above 12 mg per 100 ml (as in vitamin D intoxication, hyperparathyroidism), causes a reduction in excitability of nerve and muscle fibers and also an increase in the release of acetylcholine. *Reduction in the plasma concentration of magnesium* results in muscle spasm and convulsions; and an *increase in magnesium levels* leads to muscle weakness, depression of central nervous system, and vasodilatation with fall in blood pressure. The weakness of muscle is said to be due mainly to a reduction in release of acetylcholine as well as an inhibition of the depolarizing action of acetylcholine on the motor end-plate. A *rise or fall in the plasma concentration of sodium* causes a generalized lassitude and muscular weakness, due presumably to the depolarizing action of the sodium in nerve and muscle. Sodium loss may result in muscle cramps, as do hypocalcemia and hypoxia.

In *myasthenia gravis* (described more fully on pp. 736 to 739), with its characteristic weakness of ocular, bulbar, and, to a lesser extent, limb and trunk musculature, which is worsened by activity and improved by anticholinesterase compounds, there is no evidence of abnormality in the central or peripheral nervous system. Moreover, the muscle responds normally to direct stimulation. The principal defect is at the neuromuscular junction. This is shown by the steady decline of the contractile response to repeated nerve stimulation and the enhancement of weakness by small doses of curare or similarly acting compounds. The nature of the block is unknown. The possibility of a defect in acetylcholine or an excessive production of cholinesterase has been considered, but the failure of injected acetylcholine to correct the abnormality or of anticholinesterase drugs completely to restore muscular power argues against these explanations. Also a competitive blocking agent, possibly elaborated by the thymus gland, has been suggested but has never been substantiated. Grob, Johns, and Harvey now believe the disorder may be one of a "competitive block produced by the choline that is released in a normal manner during neuromuscular transmission."

In *myotonia congenita* or *dystrophica* (see pp. 734 and 741), in which every strong contraction persists for many seconds despite all attempts to relax, at least part of the abnormality must reside in the muscle fiber itself. This phenomenon, called *myotonia,* persists after muscle has been denervated or paralyzed by the action of curare and can be initiated in a single muscle fiber by the application of an electrical stimulus to the muscle fiber itself. Moreover, percussion which acts directly on the muscle fibers induces myotonia. Acetylcholine and potassium have a more prolonged action than in normal muscle. Quinine suppresses myotonia, but its mode of action is not known, nor is it understood how repeated muscle contraction, calcium, and ephedrine diminish it. Myotonia is certainly not the antithesis of myasthenia.

In *familial periodic paralysis* there is also a neuromuscular block and defective propagation of the action potential along the muscle fiber. Patients with this condition are sensitive to factors which modify the concentration of extracellular potassium, e.g., epinephrine and the administration of glucose. More recently it has been shown, however, that retention of sodium and high levels of aldosterone precede and accompany the attacks of paralysis. The administration of KCl relieves or aborts attacks in some cases, but there are also recorded examples of the disease in which levels of serum K remains normal at all times. Hence we are not justified in assuming that familial periodic paralysis is due simply to an alteration of K metabolism. Other factors must operate.

In *tetanus poisoning* the characteristic rigidity of jaw muscles (trismus), facial muscles (risus sardonicus), extensors of the neck and trunk (opisthotonos), and convulsions are due to the presence of a toxin which acts to impair the spinal inhibitory mechanism of the motor nerve cells. The spasm can be abolished by the administration of curare. In *botulinus poisoning,* with its characteristic weakness of ocular, jaw, facial, tongue, limb, and trunk musculature, the toxin appears also to act on the motor nerve endings, there being a reduction in the formation of acetylcholine at the motor end-plate. Little is known of the site or mode of action of the toxin of the *black widow spider,* which also heightens the excitability of the neuromuscular apparatus.

In several endocrine diseases, the speed, strength, and duration of the contractile process of the muscle fiber are altered. In some instances, this may be traced to a change in electrolytes, whereas in others, such as hypo- or hyperthyroidism, the abnormality has not been defined. In the latter the most striking biochemical change has been in creatine tolerance, discussed on pp. 727 to 728.

Methods of Clinical Study

In all these diseases of the neuromuscular apparatus, the weakness and paralysis, the fasciculation or spasm, cramps or myotonia usually occur without coincident atrophy or reflex loss. Helpful in diagnosis are a number of procedures, some clinical, others pharmacologic, which systematically test the state of different parts of nerve and muscle.

Table 26-2. SOME HELPFUL DIAGNOSTIC PROCEDURES

I. Tests of general nerve hyperexcitability (suspected when tingling, cramps, spasms, tetany, and seizures are observed).
   A. Elicitation of muscle twitching by gently percussing the nerve trunk. Chvostek test of tetany (facial twitch on tapping the facial nerve) is the most practical.
   B. Erb's test: decreased threshold of electrical excitation, expressed in terms of rheobase, chronaxie or shown by strength-duration curves.
   C. Trousseau's test: the application of a tourniquet over the proximal part of the nerve, with the production of tetany.
      (N.B. As a rule with nerve hyperexcitability, sensory and motor nerve fibers are both affected, sensory > motor.)

II. Tests of general nerve hypoexcitability (suspected when there is decrease in strength and tone of muscle).
   A. Elevated threshold of electrical excitability, high rheobase and chronaxie, and altered strength-duration curves.
      (N.B. Smooth muscle is often affected simultaneously with resulting anorexia, nausea, vomiting, and constipation.)

III. Tests of failure of neuromuscular conduction.
   A. Neostigmine test. For children 0.5 mg and for adults 1 mg neostigmine methylsulfate is injected intramuscularly. If weakness is due to myasthenia gravis, an unmistakable improvement in strength will occur within 30 min. Marked fasciculation occurs with large doses, particularly in the nonmyasthenic patient. Atropine sulfate 0.65 mg may be given to allay the muscarine effects, i.e., nausea, vomiting, and abdominal cramps. Edrophonium (Tensilon) may be used instead of neostigmine. The dose is 2 to 10 mg, given intravenously. The action occurs within 20 to 60 sec and lasts only 1 or 2 min.

IV. Tests of failure of or excessive excitability of neuromuscular junction.
   A. Curare test. This test has been used extensively at the Mayo Clinic; their method is to inject tubocurarine chloride. In testing the myasthenic

Table 26-2. SOME HELPFUL DIAGNOSTIC PROCEDURES
(*Continued*)

patient, who is sensitive to extremely small doses, a solution containing 3 mg per ml is used. For each 40 lb body weight, 0.1 mg solution is drawn into the syringe and diluted by sufficient sterile water to make 4 ml. Each 4 ml then contains about $\frac{1}{10}$ the effective curarizing dose for the normal person. First, 0.5 ml of this dilute solution ($\frac{1}{80}$ the curarizing dose) is given intravenously, and the patient is tested for increasing weakness. If none is present after 2 min, another 0.5 ml is given. Only the myasthenic patient develops weakness of eyelids, diplopia, and weakness of the neck on $\frac{1}{20}$, $\frac{1}{40}$, or $\frac{1}{80}$ of the curarizing dose. The full curarizing dose may be given cautiously to the patient with tetanus, and spasms should disappear. Caution should be exercised in using curare because of the risk of respiratory paralysis. The test should be performed only in a hospital with a respirator close by.

V. Tests of excessive or altered responsiveness of muscle.
  A. Response to tapping. Local spasm which spreads slowly to adjacent fibers is the positive sign. Excessive idiomuscular irritability may also occur in denervation, e.g., in anterior horn cell diseases.
  B. Percussion myotonia. A strong tap causes a contraction of a muscle fascicle, which remains contracted for a minute or more.
  C. Quinine test for myotonia. Quinine sulfate 0.6 Gm is given by mouth every 2 hr for three doses. A positive test will depend on the loss or diminution of the myotonic reaction.
  D. Prolongation of tendon reflex. The duration of a tendon reflex contraction may last two or three times as long as normal in hypothyroidism.
VI. Tests of reduced responsiveness of muscle tissue.
  A. Reaction of degeneration—Erb's test. Galvanic stimulus is more effective than faradic (the reverse of normal). Strength-duration curves are also altered. A greater strength of stimulus (voltage) is required to evoke a response within a short period of time, 1 msec or less, than in the normal person. These latter are the familiar tests of denervation and may be supplemented by electromyograms, which may show fibrillations and fasciculations.

27 DISTURBANCES OF THE MOTOR SYSTEM
II. Abnormalities of Posture; Involuntary Movements
Raymond D. Adams

The phasic, modifiable activities of the cortico-spinal motor system (phylogenetically, the "new motor system") and the disturbances of these activities by disease were discussed in the preceding chapter. This chapter discusses automatic, static, and less modifiable postural activities of the human nervous system. These are believed, on good evidence, to be an expression of the activity of the "older motor system," meaning, according to S. A. K. Wilson, who introduced this term, the extrapyramidal motor structures in the basal ganglions and brain stem.

In health the activities of both the old and the new motor system are blended. The static postural activities are indispensable to voluntary, or willed, movement. According to Wilson:

The apparatus for the autoregulation of attitude must be in being if cortical excitations are to effect movements and acts. With each displacement of the head a given attitude of the whole body is determined and it follows that for each intended "voluntary" movement the body finds itself, reflexly or automatically, in such a position as to enable the appropriate contraction of the muscles to be attained at the moment of production of that voluntary movement.

This close association of the pyramidal and extra-pyramidal or the new and old motor systems is best shown by disease of the human nervous system. Lesions of the pyramidal tract result not only in a paralysis of volitional movements of the contralateral half of the body but in the appearance of a fixed posture or attitude in which the arm is maintained in flexion and the leg in extension (predilection type of Wernicke-Mann). Similarly, decerebration from a lesion in the upper pons or midbrain releases another posture in which all four extremities are extended and the cervical and thoracolumbar spine dorsiflexed. In these released action patterns one has evidence of the postural and righting reflexes which are mediated through bulbospinal and other brain stem structures.

If an oversimplification may be permitted for clarity of exposition, the extrapyramidal motor system may be subdivided into two parts: (1) the striatopallidonigral and (2) the cerebellar. Disease in either of these parts will result in disturbances of movement and posture without significant paralysis. These two major systems and the symptoms which result when they are diseased are reviewed on the following pages.

EXTRAPYRAMIDAL MOTOR DISTURBANCES DUE PRIMARILY TO DISEASES OF THE BASAL GANGLIONS

Probably no field of neuroanatomy and neurophysiology has been developed more rapidly in the past 50 years than that of the basal ganglions; but despite immense research activity and a rapidly accumulating literature, it is not possible to write on this subject with any degree of finality.

According to anatomists the basal ganglions consist of the caudate and lenticular nuclei, the claustrum, and the amygdaloid nucleus. These are the primitive parts of the forebrain that lie between the cerebrum and the thalamus. Physiologists, analyzing the function of the nervous system have regrouped these structures and have added others whose activities appear to be related. The caudate nucleus and putamen, alike in development and in histology, are grouped together as the neostriatum or simply the striatum. The globus pallidus or the pallidum, as it is called, is the inner part of the lenticular nucleus but is anatomically different from the putamen. Other nuclei usually included in the basal ganglion complex are the subthalamic body of Luys, the red nucleus, and the substantia nigra. The connections between the basal ganglions are intricate. They receive fibers from the cerebral cortex

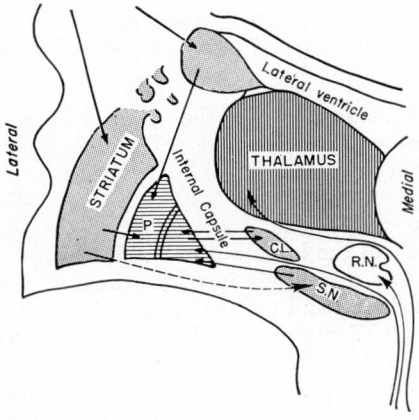

Posterior

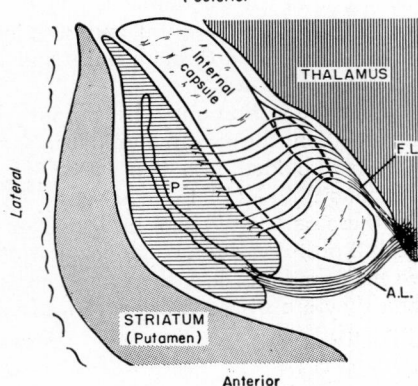

Anterior

FIG. 27-1. Frontal (coronal) section of the brain through the basal ganglia showing relationships of the cortex to the striatum (putamen and caudate nucleus), of the globus pallidus (*P*) to the corpus Luysi (*CL*), of the striatum to the substantia nigra (*SN*), and of the red nucleus (*RN*) to the thalamus and the pallidum. (*Modified from J. P. Martin: Remarks on the Functions of the Basal Ganglia, Lancet* I:999, *May,* 1959.)

and from the thalamus. The main projection of the striatum is to the pallidum, and the latter is connected with the subthalamic nucleus of Luys, the thalamus, the red nucleus, and by systems of fibers known as the *ansa lenticularis* and *stria lenticularis.*

Another anatomic system of great importance is the cerebellum and brachium conjunctivum, which consists of fibers arising in the dentate nucleus, passing through the superior cerebellar peduncle, and then dividing, some fibers descending to the lower brain stem, others ascending, decussating, and continuing as a ventral and a dorsal dentatorubrothalamic and dentatorubropallidal tract. These ascending fibers from the cerebellum, together with ascending fibers from the substantia nigra which in turn project to the cerebral cortex, constitute a system of great importance in the primate and in man. Thus it can be seen that the ventrolateral nucleus of the thalamus, the pallidum, and other related parts of the reticular formation represent crossroads of a major mesencephalic and cerebellar ascending and a corticostriatal descending pathway. All these structures come to bear on the reticular nuclei of the brain stem and finally upon the spinal cord (striorubrospinal and reticulospinal systems).

The functions of the basal ganglions have been peculiarly elusive. Stimulation experiments in monkeys have shown both the putamen and globus pallidus to be completely inexcitable. Occasional fleeting movements were induced when the stimulating electrode passed through the striate nucleus or pallidum, but they were never constant and could have been due to spread of electric current to the adjacent pyramidal tract. In decorticate cats and dogs with both pyramidal tracts degenerated, a variety of responses were recorded, including swallowing, sniffing, chop-licking, and salivation. No phasic movements were observed, but if an extremity happened to be maintaining a posture, stimulation of the caudate nucleus promptly inhibited the posture. It has also been found that cortically induced movements were inhibited by stimulation of the caudate nucleus. These same inhibitory effects have been obtained from the suppressor areas in the cerebral cortex. Stimulation of the pallidum in the intact animal during cortically induced movement provokes a tonic contraction of the contralateral limb which persists after the cortical stimulus is removed. When the nucleus of Luys is stimulated, there is a contraction of the contralateral dorsal trunk muscles. Stimulation of the red nucleus induces contraction of the ipsilateral dorsal trunk muscles, a flexion of the ipsilateral forelimb, and extension of the contralateral hind limb. Stimulation of the substantia nigra causes an increase in extensor posture, mainly on the opposite side.

Experimental lesions in the basal ganglions of animals have resulted in three types of motor disorder: (1) Lesions placed in the subthalamus of primates by the Horsley-Clarke stereotoxic instrument have induced unequivocal, abnormal, involuntary movements on the opposite side of the body which have been likened to the choreoathetosis and hemiballismus of human beings (Whittier and Mettler). These abnormal movements were said to have been abolished by operative destruction of the medial segment of the globus pallidus, the lenticular fasciculus, or the ventrolateral nucleus of the thalamus. (2) Lesions in the reticular formation in the tegmentum of the midbrain and upper pons have been followed by a static tremor (Magoun and associates). (3) Lesions in the inferior olivary nucleus have resulted in palatal myoclonus (Bender and associates). However, clinicians who have examined these animals are not agreed as to how these abnormalities of movement should be designated, for they are not perfect replicas of chorea, athetosis, and dystonia.

Many other experiments have been performed, with inconclusive results. Circumscribed striate lesions have caused little or no disturbance of function. Even with large lesions in the striatum bilaterally there is only slight impairment of skilled movement. A slight but persistent hypertonia in the contralateral limbs has been observed after the production of a combined lesion in the striatum and pallidum. Decortication, leaving the basal ganglions intact, has a somewhat different effect on the experimental monkey than does decerebration, which removes them along with the cortex. The latter abolishes leaping and movements of progression, defense, and emotional display, all of which are retained in the decorticate animal. Some of these functions are undoubtedly mediated by the thalamus and hypothalamus.

From these physiologic studies it is difficult to form any conception of the role of the basal ganglions. It appears that the striatum is closely related to the premotor cortex and forms with it a functional unit. Similarly the dentato-rubral-thalamic and pallidal system appears to form another functional unit; and it may be that ascending fibers from the substantia nigra represent a third one, but this is still a matter of speculation. Denny-Brown's statement, that "no single functional pattern of motor response is identified with any of these nuclei," still seems to be valid. He has concluded that "the physiological evidence indicates that the basal ganglia and the subthalamic nuclei are essential for the motor integration of stereotyped behavior. It is only the means by which this is accomplished that eludes us." Much research is being done in this field.

Human clinicopathologic studies have yielded some of the most significant facts concerning the role of the basal ganglions in behavior. In 1912 S. A. K. Wilson delineated the syndrome of chronic lenticular degeneration, and in 1920 Oskar and

Cécile Vogt described a number of other motor disturbances associated with lesions limited to the striatum. Lewy was one of the first to describe the pathology of paralysis agitans, and Tretiakoff (in postencephalitic forms) and Hassler (in paralysis agitans) have established the localization in the substantia nigra. A long series of observations, the most recent ones being those of J. Purdon Martin, have demonstrated the relationship between a hemiballismus and hemichorea and lesions in the subthalamic nucleus of Luys. Unfortunately many of the classic cases left much to be desired. In some instances the disease process was of diffuse type, and many other parts of the brain were affected, as in Wilson's hepatolenticular degeneration; even now the topography of the pathologic findings in several of these diseases (e.g. dystonia musculorum deformans) has not been fully determined.

Table 27-1 presents clinicopathologic correlations accepted by many neurologists; however, there is still much uncertainty as to finer details.

The symptoms that lend themselves best to clinical analysis are rigidity, chorea, athetosis, dystonia, and tremor.

Table 27-1. CLINICOPATHOLOGIC CORRELATIONS

Symptoms	Principal location of morbid anatomy
Unilateral plastic rigidity with static tremor (Parkinson's syndrome)	Contralateral substantia nigra
Unilateral hemiballismus and hemichorea	Contralateral subthalamic nucleus of Luys, prerubral area, and Forel's fields
Chronic chorea (Huntington's chorea)	Caudate nucleus, putamen, pallidum(?), and corpus Luysi
Athetosis and dystonia...	Striatum and pallidum(?), thalami(?)
Cerebellar ataxia, i.e., intention tremor, slowness in starting and stopping, alternating, voluntary movements, hypotonia, rebound phenomenon	Homolateral cerebellar hemisphere or middle and inferior cerebellar peduncles, superior brachium conjunctivum (ipsilateral if below, contralateral if above the decussation)
Decerebrate rigidity, i.e., opisthotonos, extension of arms and legs, modification of these postures by turning of head and neck—increased extensor and decreased flexor tone on side toward which head is turned	Lesion usually bilateral in tegmentum involving red nuclei or structures between red nuclei and vestibular nuclei
Palatal and facial myoclonus (rhythmic)	Lesion in the central tegmental tract, inferior olivary nucleus, and olivodentate connections

*Rigidity, Spasticity, and Alterations
of Muscle Tone in Athetosis*

Already it has been pointed out that muscle tone (the small resistance to muscle stretch offered by healthy muscle) is enhanced in the many conditions which cause a paralysis of voluntary movement by interrupting the corticospinal tract. The special distribution of the increased tone, i.e., greater in antigravity muscles (extensors of leg and flexors of the arm, in man), the sudden augmentation of tone with gradual yielding (the lengthening reaction or clasp-knife phenomenon) upon quick movement and the absence of resistance upon slow movement, its disappearance in relaxed muscle with "electromyographic silence," and exaggerated tendon reflexes are the identifying characteristics of this spasticity. This type of hypertonus is believed in some instances to be due to hyperactivity of the small gamma motor neurones with increase in the sensitivity of the spindle muscle fibers to stretch; in other instances it seems related to an excessive activity of the larger alpha motor neurones. The "gamma spasticity" is abolished by procaine injection of the motor nerve (procaine paralyzes the small motor and sensory fibers, leaving the large ones intact) without weakening the willed contractions of the muscle, whereas the "alpha spasticity" is not affected.

In the state known as rigidity the muscles are continuously or intermittently firm, tense, and prominent; and the resistance to passive movement is slow and even like that noted in bending a lead pipe or in stretching a strand of toffee. Although present in all muscle groups, both flexor and extensor, on the whole it tends to be more prominent in those which maintain a flexed posture, i.e., flexor muscles of trunk and limbs. It appears to be somewhat greater in the large muscle groups, but probably this may be merely a question of muscle mass. The smaller muscles of the face and tongue and even those of the larynx are often affected. The tendon reflexes are not enhanced. Nevertheless, like the "gamma spasticity" this rigidity is said to be abolished by procaine (Rushworth), and Walshe, and later Foerster, had demonstrated that it is reduced by this means or eradicated by posterior root section. In the electromyographic tracing, motor unit activity is more continuous than in spasticity, persisting even after relaxation.

A special type of rigidity, first noted by Negro in 1901, is the cogwheel phenomenon. When the hypertonic muscle is passively stretched, the resistance may be jerky, as though the limb were pulled over a ratchet. A number of different explanations of this phenomenon have been suggested. Wilson postulated that it might be due to a minor form of the lengthening-shortening reaction, but it seems to the author that a more likely explanation is an associated static tremor which has been masked by the rigidity during an attitude of repose but emerges faintly during the manipulation.

Rigidity is prominent in paralysis agitans, postencephalitic Parkinson's syndrome, hepatolenticular degeneration, and some cases of dystonia musculorum deformans.

The "tension hypertonus of athetosis" differs from both spasticity and rigidity. Strictly speaking it takes two forms, one which occurs during the involuntary athetotic movement, the other which appears in the absence of any involuntary motion. Clinically these forms of hypertonus are variable from one moment to the next and are paradoxic in sometimes disappearing during a rapid passive movement or when the limb is passively shaken. The tendon reflexes may be normal or brisk. The lengthening and shortening reactions are absent. This form of variable hypertonus is found in cases of "double" athetosis, choreoathetosis, and in some cases of dystonia musculorum deformans. Usually in Sydenham's and Huntington's chorea there is hypotonia.

Involuntary Movements

Chorea. From the Greek word meaning "dance," chorea refers to widespread arrhythmic movements of forcible, rapid, jerky type. These movements are involuntary and are noted for their irregularity, variability, speed, and brief duration. They are quite elaborate and of variable distribution. In some respects they resemble a voluntary movement; yet they never combine into a coordinated act. The patient may, however, incorporate them into a deliberate movement, as if to make them less noticeable. They may be limited to a limb or to an arm and leg on one side (hemichorea), or they may involve all parts of the body. They may cause grimacing or peculiar respiratory sounds and may be superimposed on voluntary movements, giving to these a grotesque and exaggerated character. Usually they are discrete, but if very numerous may flow into one another; the resultant picture resembles athetosis. Normal volitional movements are of course possible, for there is usually no paralysis, but they, too, may be excessively quick and poorly sustained. The limbs are often unusually slack or hypotonic. A choreic movement may be superimposed on a tendon reflex, giving the "hung-up reflex." The tendon reflexes tend to be pendular (i.e., when the knee jerk is elicited with the patient sitting, the leg swings back and forth four or five times, like a pendulum).

Chorea appears in typical form in Sydenham's chorea, and was noted also in the acute stages of epidemic encephalitis lethargica. In Huntington's chorea (chronic chorea), the movements are more typically choreoathetotic. Vascular lesions in the subthalamus, particularly those in and near the subthalamic nucleus of Luys, may result in wild flinging movements of the opposite arm and leg (hemiballismus). As these subside they become indistinguishable from chorea.

Athetosis. This term is from a Greek word meaning "unfixed" or "changeable." The condition is characterized by an inability to sustain the fingers and toes in any one position in which they are placed and by continuous, slow, sinuous, purposeless movements. They are most pronounced in the digits and the hands, but often involve the tongue, throat, and face. Basic patterns of movement, such as extension and pronation of the arm, alternating with flexion and supination, and an alternate flexion and extension of the fingers, are evident in most cases. They may be unilateral, especially in children who have suffered a hemiplegia at some previous date (posthemiplegic athetosis). The movements are slower than those of chorea, but in many cases gradations between the two (*choreoathetosis*) are seen. Most athetotic patients exhibit variable degrees of motor deficit owing in some instances to associated pyramidal tract disease. Discrete individual movements of the tongue, lips, and hand are often impossible, and attempts to perform such voluntary movements result in a contraction of all the muscles in the limb—an intention spasm. Variable degrees of rigidity are generally associated, and these may account for the slow quality of athetosis in contrast to chorea. It must be admitted, however, that in some cases it is almost impossible to distinguish between chorea and athetosis.

Athetosis or choreoathetosis of all four limbs is a cardinal feature of a curious state known as *double athetosis,* which begins in childhood or adolescence. Athetosis appearing in the first months of life usually represents a congenital or postnatal condition such as hypoxia, kernicterus, or birth injury. Postmortem examination in some of the cases has disclosed a peculiar pathologic change of unknown etiology, a status marmoratus in the striatum; in others there has been a loss of medullated fibers, a status dysmyelinisatus, in the same regions.

Torsion Spasm, or Dystonia. This is closely allied to athetosis, and the two may coexist. Dystonia is chiefly distinguished by the fact that it preponderantly affects the trunk musculature and proximal segments of the limbs. It results in retraction of the head, excessive lordosis, twisting of the trunk, and a variety of contortions. If it is mild, the dystonic movements cease at rest, and the limbs are then quite flaccid. Involuntary spasm may return upon the initiation of voluntary movement.

Dystonia may be seen in the condition of double athetosis after hypoxic damage to the brain, in kernicterus, and even in Wilson's hepatolenticular degeneration. It is most characteristic in the syndrome designated *dystonia musculorum deformans.* The etiology of this disorder is unknown.

Chorea, athetosis, and dystonia are all closely related. The movements are elaborate and depend for their expression on cortical mechanisms. Paralytic lesions involving the pyramidal tract abolish the involuntary movements. The hypotonia in chorea and some cases of athetosis, the pendular reflexes, and some degree of incoordination of movement are reminiscent of the syndrome which follows disease of the cerebellum.

Tremor. This consists of a more or less regular rhythmic oscillation of a part of the body around a fixed point, owing to alternate contractions of agonist and antagonist muscles. The rate is usually 4 to 6 beats per second and in any one individual is fairly constant in all affected parts, regardless of the size of the involved muscle mass. It is generally most pronounced in the distal parts of the limb but may involve the head, tongue, face, and trunk.

There are many different types of tremor, and only a few varieties are recognized as related to disease of the extrapyramidal motor system; but since tremors have not been discussed elsewhere, all the different types will be considered here.

Tremors can be classified in several ways. They may be subdivided according to their distribution, amplitude, regularity, and relationship to volitional movement. The following tremors should be familiar to every physician.

Static (Parkinsonian) Tremor. This is a coarse rhythmic tremor, with an average rate of 4 to 5 beats per second, most often localized to one or both hands, the feet, or occasionally the jaw or tongue. Its most characteristic feature is that it occurs when the limb is held in an attitude of repose and is at least temporarily suppressed by willed movement. If the tremulous limb is completely relaxed, the tremor usually disappears, but the average patient rarely achieves this degree of relaxation. In some cases the tremor is constant; in others it varies from time to time and may move from one group of muscles to another. It may be rather gentle and more or less limited to the distal muscles, as in paralysis agitans, or may be of wider range and involve proximal muscles as in postencephalitic Parkinson's disease and hepatolenticular degeneration. In many cases there is an associated rigidity of plastic type. The tremor interferes with voluntary movements surprisingly little; it is not uncommon to see a patient who has been trembling violently raise a full glass of water to his lips and drain the contents without spilling a drop. The handwriting of these patients is often small and cramped (micrographia). The gait may be of a festinating type. (Disturbances of Gait, Chap. 30.) The combination of static tremor, slowness of movement, rigidity, and flexed postures, without true paralysis, constitutes Parkinson's syndrome. The exact pathologic anatomy of static tremor is unknown. In paralysis agitans and postencephalitic Parkinson's syndrome, the lesions are predominantly in the substantia nigra. A similar tremor, without rigidity or slowness of movement, is seen in senile individuals and in some cases of hepatolenticular degeneration.

Action Tremor. This term refers to a tremor present when the limbs are actively maintained in a certain position, as when outstretched, and throughout voluntary movement. It may increase slightly as the action of the limbs becomes more precise, but never approaches the degree of intention tremor. It disappears completely when the limbs are relaxed. Probably the term *action tremor* embraces two different types of tremor:

1. A fine 8 to 10 per second tremor, somewhat irregular and involving the outstretched fingers and head, less often the lips and tongue, interferes little with voluntary movements such as handwriting and speech. This type of tremor is seen in numerous medical, neurologic, and psychiatric diseases and is therefore more difficult to interpret than static tremor. It may occur as the only neurologic abnormality in several members of a family and is then known as *familial* or *hereditary tremor.* Familial tremor persists throughout adult life, being worse when the patient is under observation. It is a source of embarrassment because it suggests to the onlooker that the patient is nervous. A curious fact about familial tremors is that one or two drinks of an alcoholic beverage may abolish them, and they may become worse after the effects of the alcohol have worn off. Similar tremors are seen in delirious states such as delirium tremens, in the chronic alcoholic patient as an isolated symptom, and in general paretics. An action tremor usually more rapid than the above is also characteristic of hyperthyroidism and other toxic states, while a similar tremor is frequently observed in patients suffering from intense anxiety.

2. The other type of action, or postural, tremor is much slower (4 to 6 per second) and coarser, involving most often an arm or the head and neck. It has the same frequency as the tremor of Parkinson's disease. An example of this type of tremor is the typical "wing beating" of Wilson's disease but it may be seen with other types of disease which involve the ascending fibers of the brachium conjunctivum above the level of the red nucleus. In the experimental animal (monkey) this tremor was never obtained by placing lesions within the striatum, substantia nigra, or "reticular substance" (see Carrera and Mettler).

Intention Tremor. The word *intention* is ambiguous in this context because the tremor itself is not intentional. The tremor requires for its full expression the performance of a deliberate, willed movement. Perhaps a better term is *ataxic tremor,* as suggested by Mettler, for it is always combined with cerebellar ataxia. The tremor is absent when the limbs are in repose and during the first part of a voluntary movement, but as the action continues and greater precision of movement is demanded (e.g., in touching a target such as one's nose or the examiner's finger), a jerky, more or less rhythmic interruption of forward progression, with a side-to-side oscillation, appears. It continues for a second or two after the act is completed. The tremor may seriously interfere with the patient's performance of skilled acts. Sometimes the head is involved (titubation). This type of tremor is invariably indicative of disease of the cerebellum and of its connections.

Hysterical Tremor. Hysterical tremors may simulate any of the aforementioned varieties and are difficult to diagnose. One notable feature is that they usually do not correspond to any of the better known types of organic tremor. Most often they are restricted to a limb and are seldom as regular as the static tremors of paralysis agitans. If the affected limb is restrained by the examiner, the tremor may move to another part of the body. It persists during movement and at rest and is less subject to the modifying influences of posture and willed movement than are organic tremors. In the author's experience this manifestation of hysteria is exceedingly rare.

Other Involuntary Movements. There is a variety of other abnormalities of movement, but limitation of space permits no more than a few words about each. They vary from simple irritative phenomena to complex psychologic phenomena such as compulsions. Many have no particular relation to the extrapyramidal motor system but may be conveniently discussed here. The reader should consult one of the standard books on neurology for further details.

Fascicular Twitchings. These coarse twitchings of individual fascicles of muscle, i.e., motor units, were mentioned under atrophic paralysis. As isolated phenomena they may occur in healthy individuals and in the absence of muscle weakness, atrophy, and reflex change probably have no clinical significance. The laity refers to them as "live flesh"; a generalized form of this disorder is sometimes seen and is called by the medical profession *benign fasciculations,* or *myokymia.* Except for being more localized, of longer duration, and more repetitious in a single fascicle, they are almost indistinguishable from the fasciculations of anterior horn cell disease, which are observed in completely relaxed muscles but nearly always in association with other signs of motor disease. During voluntary muscular contractions fasciculations may be seen in tremulous individuals and in patients with cachexia or partially atrophic muscles. In the latter instance —the so-called "action fasciculation"—an uneven recruitment of motor units appears to account for the phenomenon.

Hemifacial Spasm. This is a curious condition in which all or part of the muscles supplied by the facial nerve on one side contract intermittently. It may follow Bell's palsy or occur without previous disease of the facial nerve. Grouped motor unit potentials, typical of nerve irritation, may be seen in the electromyogram. The current view of this condition is that it is due to a constriction of the facial nerve in the fallopian canal. The treatment is said to be decompression of the nerve, but this operation has had limited success.

Blepharospasm. Elderly individuals occasionally develop an involuntary spasm of the orbicularis oculi muscles, often accompanied by photophobia. The cause is unknown. It is not a neurotic symptom, and there is no known treatment except crushing the branches of the facial nerves to the orbicularis oculi muscles, which is justifiable only in severe cases.

Spasmodic Torticollis. This is an intermittent or continuous spasm of sternomastoid, trapezius, and other neck muscles, usually on one side, with turning or tipping of the head. It is involuntary and cannot be inhibited and differs from habit spasm or tic. The writer is of the opinion that this condition should be considered a form of dystonia. It is worse when the patient sits, stands, or walks, and contactual stimulation of the chin or of the back of head partially alleviates the muscle imbalance. Psychiatric treatment is ineffectual. In severe cases muscle sectioning, neurectomy, or section of the anterior cervical roots has given the best results.

Tics and Habit Spasms. Many individuals throughout life are prone to habitual movements such as sniffing, clearing the throat, protruding the chin, blinking, etc., whenever tense. The patient will admit that the movements are voluntary and that he feels compelled to make them in order to relieve tension; they can be inhibited by effort of will. In certain cases they become so ingrained that the person is unaware of them and unable to control them. Children between five and ten years of age are especially liable to habit spasms. The movements are often purposive, coordinated acts, originally provoked by some physical or emotional stimulus and continued as a habit. They are arrhythmic and stereotyped. Multiple convulsive tics (Gilles de la Tourette's disease) is a more severe form of the same condition. In children it is best to ignore the habit spasm and at the same time to arrange for more rest and a calmer environment. In adults relief of nervous tension by tranquilizing drugs and psychotherapy is helpful, but the disposition to tic formation persists.

Spasmus Nutans. This is a peculiar involuntary rotatory, nodding, or side-to-side tremor of the head seen in children with congenital nystagmus. It ceases when the eyes are closed. Usually it disappears after a few weeks to months. *Head rolling* and *head banging* are other varieties of movement exhibited by many small children from six to eighteen months of age. The rhythmic movement seems to provide some sort of physiologic satisfaction; it is unaccompanied by nystagmus and disappears when the child begins to walk. The significance of these movements is unknown, but they are particularly common in children confined to institutions. Some pediatricians believe that they are expressions of the loss of parental affection. This may be a factor, but the movements are so common that some other explanation should be sought.

Myoclonus. Several different motor phenomena are included under this term. Some neurologists use it to denote a brief contraction of a single muscle or part of a muscle. Again, it has been applied to a sudden abrupt contraction of a group of muscles, regardless of their functional state. The latter contractions may be arrhythmic and diffuse or rhythmic and confined to one part of the body. An example of the latter phenomenon is "nystagmus of the palate," or palatal myoclonus—rhythmic contractions of the soft palate and pharyngeal muscles and sometimes of the vocal cords, diaphragm, or facial muscles, at the rate of 10 to 50 or more per minute. The lesions producing this sign, whether vascular, neoplastic, or encephalitic, have been situated in all instances in the central tegmental tract, in the inferior olivary nucleus, or in the olivocerebellar tracts. Diffuse arrhythmic myoclonus is sometimes associated with dementia and epilepsy and has been referred to as the *familial myoclonic epilepsy of Unverricht and Lundborg.* In the author's opinion, this myoclonus is a form of epilepsy, a disseminate form of epilepsia partialis continua. Nonfamilial forms in childhood are due to "inclusion body encephalitis" or lipoid-storage diseases, and in adults, to a degenerative cerebral disease of unknown etiology, associated with dementia, i.e., Jakob-Creutzfeld's disease, and as a sequel to hypoxic encephalopathy. Isolated myoclonic jerks occur in epileptic patients, particularly in children with petit mal. This is the most frequent form of arrhythmic myoclonus.

One of the most remarkable discoveries of recent years, to be credited largely to the pioneering efforts of Meyer and Cooper, has been the abolition of tremors, rigidity, and involuntary movements of the limbs by the induction of a surgical lesion in the medial segment of the globus pallidus or the ventrolateral nucleus of the thalamus. The effects are contralateral. Usually the lesion has been made by the injection first of procaine (Novocain) and then alcohol (Cooper), by electrocoagulation (White and Sweet and Leksell), by ultrasound (Meyer), or by a proton beam (Leksell). The operation has been successful in a high percentage of cases of unilateral paralysis agitans, dystonia musculorum deformans, double athetosis, and violent intention tremor. It has been perfected to the point where the mortality is relatively low, 3 to 4 per cent, and the risk of hemiplegia or some other sequel is less than 10 per cent. This therapeutic effect indicates that the pallidum and ventrolateral nucleus, possibly through their connections with the cerebral cortex (motor cortex and its pyramidal pathway), are essential for the expression of these extrapyramidal syndromes. The indications for these surgical procedures will be discussed in Chap. 290.

EXTRAPYRAMIDAL MOTOR DISTURBANCES DUE PRIMARILY TO DISEASES OF THE CEREBELLUM

In recent years the comparative anatomic studies of Larsell and his associates have made possible a satisfactory subdivision of the cerebellum into three main parts, the vestibular portion, known as the *flocculonodular lobe*, a spinocerebellar part, and the cerebellar hemisphere, sometimes called the *neocerebellum*.

Isolated lesions in the midline flocculonodular lobe result in grave disturbances of equilibrium. Often the symptoms are exhibited only when the patient attempts to stand and walk. He sways, staggers, titubates, and reels (see the Cerebellar Gait in Chap. 30). There may be no disturbance in coordination and no intention tremor of the limbs. A midline tumor of the cerebellum, such as a medulloblastoma, usually produces this syndrome.

Extensive lesions of one cerebellar hemisphere, especially the anterior lobe, cause disturbances of volitional movements of the ipsilateral arm and leg. This is known as *ataxia*. The movements "are characterized by an inappropriate range, rate and strength of each of the various components of the motor act and by an improper sequence of those components." Electromyographic analysis has shown that ataxia is manifested as a decomposition of movement consisting of abnormal duration and sequences of bursts of contraction and relaxation of agonists and antagonists of a joint, usually a large joint (Carrera and Mettler). This incoordination is also called an *asynergia*. The defects are particularly noticeable in acts requiring rapid alternation of movements. A slowness in acceleration and deceleration, which is almost invariably present, impedes the performance. The direction of purposive movement is frequently inaccurate. Ow-

ing to delay in arresting the movement, it may overshoot its mark. The antagonist muscles do not come into play at the proper time, possibly because of the hypotonia that is almost always present. This may be demonstrated by having the patient flex his arm against a resistance which is suddenly released. The patient with cerebellar disease will sometimes strike his face because he fails to check the flexion movement (rebound phenomenon). In movements requiring accurate direction, as the limb approaches its destination it may stop short and then advance by a more or less rhythmic series of jerks. In addition to hypotonia there may be, in acute cerebellar lesions, some slight weakness. Bilateral lesions of the cerebellar hemispheres and midline flocculonodular lobe lead to such a severe disturbance in all movements that the patient may be unable to stand or walk or use his limbs effectively. In addition, there are ocular and speech disturbances, viz., nystagmus, skew deviation of the eyes, and dysarthria. Lesions of the cerebellar peduncles have the same effect as extensive hemispheral lesions. This syndrome of one cerebellar hemisphere (neocerebellum) may be observed in a tumor or abscess of the cerebellar hemisphere, or in vascular lesions of the brain stem and cerebellar peduncles. It tends to be bilateral and symmetrical in primary atrophy or degeneration of the cerebellum.

Lesions of the dentate nuclei and the parts of the brachium conjunctivum which project to brain stem segmental structures also produce ataxia in the primate. If the ventral component of the crossed ascending limb to the red nucleus, globus pallidus, and thalamus is also interrupted, tremor will be added. Tremor and ataxia are effects of injury of efferent cerebellar tracts, according to Mettler, who has reproduced these disorders in the monkey.

EXAMINATION AND DIFFERENTIAL DIAGNOSIS

In Chap. 26 the methods of examining the motor system were described at some length, so that only a few additional remarks concerning extrapyramidal disorders need be made here. These abnormalities are demonstrated best by seeing the patient in action. If he complains of a limp after walking a distance or of difficulty in climbing stairs, he should be observed under these conditions. Tests of rate, regularity, and coordination of voluntary movement must be sufficiently varied and demanding of the patient's motor coordination to bring out his defect. The physician must cultivate the habit of accurately observing and describing abnormalities of movement, and should not be content merely to give the condition a name or force it into some category such as chorea or tic or myoclonus. The main postures of the body in all common acts should be noted. Aside from the assessment of muscle power and of gait, the usual test applied to the upper limb is to ask the patient to touch the examiner's finger tip and then the tip of his own nose repeatedly (finger-to-nose test). In testing the leg the patient is asked to place his heel on one knee and then to run it down his shin and back to the knee (heel-to-knee-to-shin test). Finer movements of the hand may be tested by having the patient successively touch each finger to his thumb or pat his thigh rapidly, or by observing him as he uses tools or handles objects. The performance of rapidly alternating movements such as pronation and supination of the hands is another valuable test.

The fully developed extrapyramidal motor syndromes can be recognized without difficulty once the physician has become familiar with the typical pictures. He should form a mental picture of Parkinson's syndrome with its slowness of movement, poverty of facial expression, static tremor and rigidity, and absence of true paralysis or reflex changes. Similarly the gross distortions and postural abnormalities of dystonia, whether widespread in trunk muscles or involving only neck muscles, as in spasmodic torticollis, should be familiar. Athetosis, with its instability of postures, ceaseless movements of fingers and hands, intention spasm, and chorea, with its abrupt and complicated movements which flit over the body, are other standard syndromes. Characteristic of all is the lack of pyramidal tract signs (i.e., motor paralysis, spasticity, increased tendon reflexes, and Babinski signs), the effects of emotional stimuli which invariably exaggerate the symptoms, the quieting effect of relaxation and sleep, and the presence of a mild defect in voluntary movement.

The clinical differences between pyramidal and extrapyramidal disorders are summarized in Table 27-2.

Early or mild forms of these conditions, like all medical diseases, may offer special difficulties in diagnosis. Cases of paralysis agitans, seen before the appearance of tremor, are often overlooked. The patient may complain of being nervous and restless or may have experienced an indescribable stiffness and aching in certain parts of the body. Because of the absence of weakness or of reflex changes, the case may be considered psychogenic or rheumatic. It is well to remember that Parkinson's syndrome often begins in a hemiplegic distribution, and the case may be misdiagnosed as cerebral thrombosis. A slight masking of the face, a suggestion of a limp, blepharoclonus, or uninhibited blinking of eyes when the bridge of the nose is tapped, a mild rigidity, failure of an arm to swing naturally in walking, or loss of certain movements of cooperation will be of assistance at this time. Every case pre-

Table 27-2. CLINICAL DIFFERENCES BETWEEN PYRAMIDAL AND EXTRAPYRAMIDAL SYNDROMES

	Pyramidal	Extrapyramidal
Character of rigidity	Clasp-knife effect	Plastic, equal throughout; passive movement or intermittent (cogwheel rigidity)
Distribution of rigidity	Flexors of arms, extensors of leg	Flexors of all four limbs and trunk
Shortening and lengthening reaction	Present	Absent
Involuntary movements	Absent	Presence of tremors, chorea, athetosis, dystonia
Tendon reflexes...	Increased	Normal or slightly increased
Babinski sign.....	Present	Absent
Paralysis of voluntary movement	Present	Absent or slight

senting the syndrome of Parkinson or other abnormality of movement and posture in adolescence or early adult life should be surveyed for hepatolenticular degeneration by tests of liver function, slit-lamp examination for corneal pigmentation (Kayser-Fleischer ring), and if facilities are available, urinary amino-nitrogen excretion and copper excretion.

Mild or early chorea is often mistaken for simple nervousness. If one sits for a time and watches the patient, the diagnosis will often become evident. There are cases, nonetheless, in which it is impossible to distinguish simple nervousness from early Sydenham's chorea, especially in children, and there is no laboratory test that one can depend upon. The first postural manifestation of dystonia may suggest hysteria, and it is only later, when the fixity of the postural abnormality, the lack of the usual psychologic picture of hysteria, and the relentlessly progressive character of the illness become evident, that accurate diagnosis is reached. Another common error, which the writer has made more than once, is to assume that a patient, at present bedfast, who has complained of dizziness, staggering, and headache and exhibits no other neurologic abnormality, is suffering from hysteria. The flocculonodular cerebellar syndrome is demonstrable only when the patient attempts to stand and walk.

REFERENCES

Carrera, R. M. E., and F. A. Mettler: Function of the Primate Brachium Conjunctivum and Related Structures, J. Comp. Neurol., 102:151, 1955.

Denny-Brown, D.: "Diseases of the Basal Ganglia and Subthalamic Nuclei," New York, Oxford University Press, 1945.

Martin, J. Purdon, and Ian R. McCaul: Acute Hemiballismus Treated by Ventrolateral Thalamolysis, Brain, 82:104, 1959.

28 DISORDERS OF SENSATION

Maurice Victor and
Raymond D. Adams

Under normal conditions sensory function and motility are interdependent, as was dramatically illustrated by the early animal experiments of Claude Bernard and Sherrington, in which practically all movement of a limb was abolished by sectioning only the posterior roots or some other part of the sensory pathway. Also, as indicated below in Chap. 37, man's orientation in space depends on a constant influx of sensory impulses and the motor adaptations to these impulses. At every level of the nervous system from the spinal cord to the cerebrum, sensory and motor neurones are closely connected. The Rolandic fissure, for example, does not form an absolute division between motor and sensory areas; the parietal lobe is nearly as essential as the frontal lobe for regulated movement. In a sense, "movement is sensation."

By common practice, however, sensory functions have come to be considered separately from movement. Since the major anatomic pathways of the sensory system are distinct from those of the motor system, and may be selectively disturbed by disease, tests of the functional state of the sensory apparatus often provide important clues to diagnosis. It is from this point of view that disorders of sensory function are considered here. Since the special senses—vision, hearing, taste, and smell—are dealt with in connection with the cranial nerves, only exteroceptive cutaneous and proprioceptive sensory function are taken up in this chapter.

ANATOMIC AND PHYSIOLOGIC CONSIDERATIONS

An understanding of sensory disorders depends on a knowledge of physiology and applied anatomy. These subjects were introduced in Chap. 3, General Considerations of Pain, and other aspects of the physiology of sensation are taken up at appropriate points in the discussion of the clinical syndromes; only some general anatomic features are reviewed here. Charts showing segmental sensory topography and the distribution of cutaneous sen-

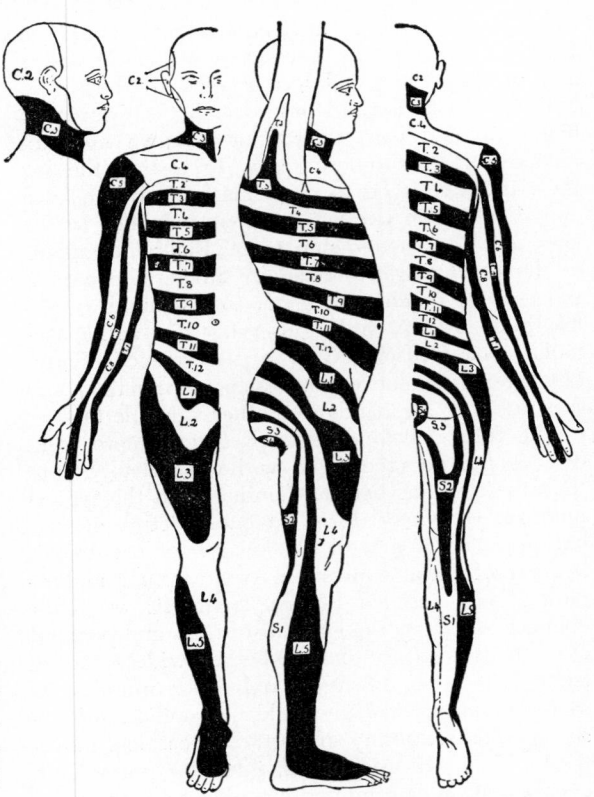

FIG. 28-1. Distribution of the sensory spinal roots on the surface of the body. (*Holmes: "Introduction to Clinical Neurology,"* Edinburgh, E. & S. Livingstone, Ltd., 1946.)

sory nerves are included (Figs. 28-1 and 28-2), and these subjects will not be discussed further.

Ordinarily every sensation depends on impulses excited by the adequate stimulation of receptors and conveyed to the central nervous system by afferent or sensory fibers. Sensory receptors are of two main types—the exteroceptors, which relate us to "the world about," and the proprioceptors, which inform us of changes going on within our body. Practically all structures contain receptors. Those in the skin are particularly numerous and give rise to four types of sensory experience—warmth, cold, touch, and pain. Deeper structures are supplied with proprioceptors, which inform us of the position of our body in space, of the force, direction, and range of movement of the muscles, and of pressure, both painful and painless.

For many years it has been taught that each of the primary modalities of cutaneous sensation is subserved by a morphologically distinct end organ with separate peripheral nerve fibers. Histologically, a large number of complex end organs were described. According to this hypothesis, usually associated with the names of von Frey and Gold-

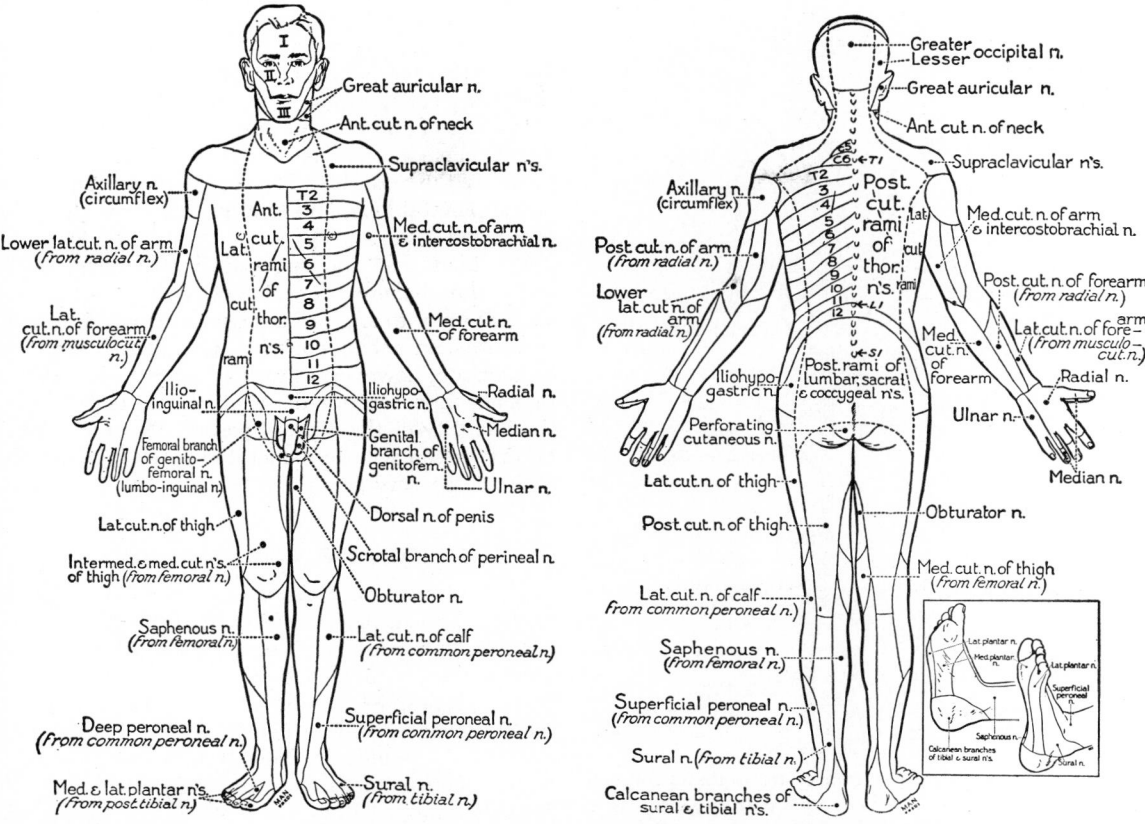

FIG. 28-2. The cutaneous fields of peripheral nerves. (*Haymaker and Woodhall: "Peripheral Nerve Injuries,"* *Philadelphia, W. B. Saunders Company, 1945.*)

scheider, each type of end organ responds only to a particular sensory stimulus and gives rise to a specific modality of sensation. This concept of specific sensory endings has been seriously discredited, largely as a result of the observations of Weddell and his colleagues. They admit that some of the previously described end organs exist, but deny that they are essential for the appreciation of cutaneous sensibility. With the appropriate stimulation of the cornea, for example, each of the four primary modalities of common sensibility (touch, warmth, cold, pain) can be recognized, despite the fact that it contains only fine freely ending nerve filaments. Of interest also are the recent observations of Kibler and Nathan in regard to warm and cold spots, i.e., those small areas of skin which most consistently respond to thermal stimuli with a sensation of warmth or cold. They found that a cold stimulus applied to a warm spot gave rise to a sensation of cold, and vice versa; that painful stimulation of a warm or cold spot gave rise only to a painful sensation; and that mechanical stimulation of these spots gave rise to a sensation of touch or pressure. A current hypothesis of cutaneous sensibility proposes that any given nerve fiber

and its ending may convey impulses; that different stimuli set up different spatial and temporal patterns of impulses; and that the recognition of the nature of the stimulus (the psychical state called sensation) depends on the particular pattern of impulses reaching the brain.

The proprioceptive fibers run mainly in the motor nerves, while the cutaneous fibers are carried in sensory or mixed sensory and motor nerves. All the sensory neurones have their cell bodies in the dorsal root ganglions; the central projections of these cells enter the spinal cord via the dorsal or posterior roots where they are first rearranged according to function. A medial group made up of large fibers enters the dorsal column of the same side and runs uninterrupted to the medulla, terminating in the gracile and cuneate nuclei. In this column are contained the fibers subserving proprioceptive sensation and a portion of those for touch. The nerve cells of the nucleus gracilis and cuneatus give rise to a secondary afferent path, which crosses the midline in the medulla and ascends in the brain stem to the thalamus as the medial lemniscus (Fig. 28-3).

The lateral bundle in the posterior root consists

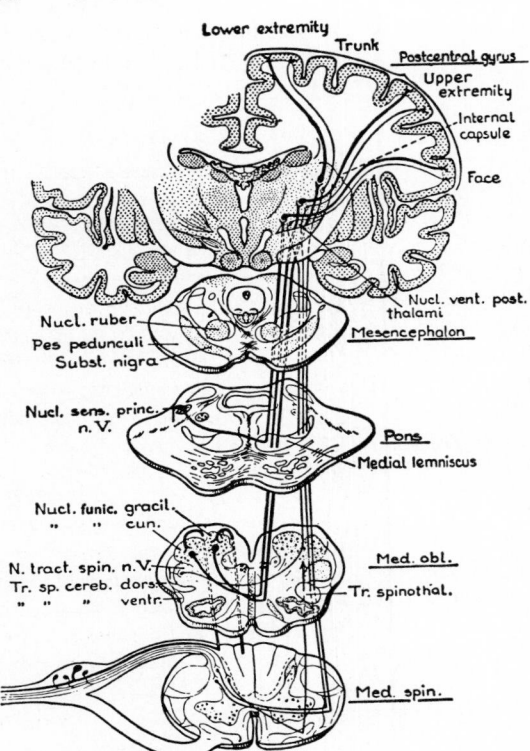

FIG. 28-3. A composite diagram of the somatic sensory tracts. Redrawn and slightly modified from Rasmussen (1932). (*Brodal: "Neurological Anatomy in Relation to Clinical Medicine,"* New York, Oxford University Press, 1948.)

of fine fibers which synapse around the cells of the dorsal horn of the spinal cord within a few segments of their point of entry. The dorsal horn cells in turn give rise to secondary tracts, which cross to the opposite side of the spinal cord; one tract, carrying pain and thermal impulses, ascends in the ventral part of the lateral column as the lateral spinothalamic tract. The other tract, in the anterior column, known as the anterior spinothalamic tract, conveys those tactile impulses not carried in the posterior column. The dorsal and ventral spinocerebellar tracts are secondary pathways for unconscious proprioception.

The pathways of cutaneous sensation from the face and head, especially those of touch, pain, and temperature, are important clinically. Impulses are conveyed to the brain stem mainly by the trigeminal nerve; after entering the pons, the pain and temperature fibers run caudally as the descending trigeminal root and terminate in a long vertical nucleus which lies beside it and extends to the upper cervical segments of the cord. Fibers from this nucleus then cross the midline and join the most medial portion of the spinothalamic tract.

In the midbrain the medial lemniscus and spinothalamic tract merge and ascend to the nucleus ventralis posterolateralis of the thalamus. Below the thalamus, collaterals are given off to the reticular formation of the entire brain stem. From the thalamus, fibers project to the sensory cortex, which includes the postcentral gyrus, the adjacent parts of the parietal lobe, and to a much lesser extent the precentral gyrus.

Provided that the subcortical structures, especially the thalamus, are intact, certain sensations such as pain, touch, pressure, and extremes of temperature can reach consciousness. Their accurate localization, however, as well as the patient's ability to make fine sensory discriminations, depends on the integrity of the sensory cortex. This fundamental distinction will be elaborated further in dealing with the sensory syndromes.

EXAMINATION OF SENSATION

The examination of sensation is the most difficult part of the neurologic examination. For one thing, test procedures are relatively crude and inadequate, and at times no objective sensory loss can be demonstrated despite symptoms that clearly indicate the presence of such a deficit. Also, a response to a sensory stimulus is difficult to evaluate objectively, the examiner's conclusions depending on the patient's interpretation and editing of sensory stimuli. This in turn will depend on his general awareness and responsiveness, his desire to cooperate, and his fatigability, as well as his intelligence, education, and suggestibility. At times, children and relatively uneducated persons, by virtue of their simple and direct responses, are better witnesses than more sophisticated individuals who are likely to analyze their feelings minutely and report small differences.

Before proceeding to sensory testing, the physician should question the patient about his symptoms, attaching special importance to such complaints as "pins and needles," tingling, coldness, burning, or pain. The term *numbness*, frequently employed by patients, may have a variety of meanings; careful questioning may be required to determine whether it actually signifies a lack of sensation.

The degree of detail in which sensation is tested will be governed by the clinical situation. If the patient has no sensory complaints, it is sufficient to examine vibration and position sense in the fingers and toes, to test the appreciation of pain over the face, trunk, and extremities, and to determine whether this sensation is the same in symmetrical parts of the body. A rough survey of this sort may detect sensory defects of which the patient is unaware. On the other hand, more thorough testing is in order if the patient has complaints referable to the sensory system, or if there is a localized atrophy or weakness, an ataxia, trophic changes of joints, or painless ulcers.

A few other general principles should be mentioned. One should not press the sensory examination in the presence of fatigue, for an inattentive patient is a poor witness. When first dealing with a patient, sensory testing is of necessity preceded by a history and often by a general examination; under these circumstances it is best to aim for a quick orientation regarding the whole sensory system, and to return to the details when the patient is rested. The examiner must also avoid suggesting symptoms to the patient. After having explained in the simplest terms what is required, he should interpose as few questions and remarks as possible. Consequently the patient must not be asked "Do you feel that?" each time he is touched, but simply to say "Yes" or "Sharp" every time he has been touched or feels pain. The patient should not be permitted to see the part under examination. For short tests it is sufficient that he close his eyes; during more detailed testing it is preferable to interpose a screen between his eyes and the part examined. Finally, all the findings of the sensory examination should be accurately recorded on a chart.

Sensation is frequently classified as superficial (cutaneous, exteroceptive) and deep (proprioceptive); these are convenient terms for examination and reporting. The former comprises the modalities of light touch, pain, and temperature; the latter includes the sense of position, passive motion, vibration, and deep pain.

Sense of Touch. This is usually tested with a wisp of cotton. The patient is first acquainted with the nature of the stimulus by applying it to a normal part of the body. Then he is asked to say "Yes" each time he is touched in various other parts. A patient simulating sensory loss may say "No" in response to a tactile stimulus. Cornified areas of skin, such as the soles and palms, will require a heavier stimulus, whereas the hair-clad parts are sensitive to a lighter stimulus because of the numerous nerve endings around the follicle. A moving stimulus of any kind is more effective than a stationary one. The application of the examiner's or preferably the patient's finger tips is a useful method of testing, particularly, as Trotter originally showed, in mapping out an area of tactile loss following peripheral nerve injury.

More precise testing is possible by using a von Frey hair. By this method a stimulus of constant strength can be applied and the threshold for touch sensation determined.

Sense of Pain. This is most efficiently estimated by pinprick, although it can be evoked by a great diversity of noxious stimuli. The patient must understand that he is to report the degree of sharpness of the pinprick and not simply the feeling of contact or pressure of the point or even a special sensation due to penetration of the skin. A few other simple rules should be kept in mind. If the pinpricks are applied rapidly, their effects may be summated, and excessive pain may result; therefore they should be delivered not too rapidly, about one per second, and not over the same spot.

It is almost impossible, using an ordinary pin or needle, to apply each stimulus with equal intensity. This difficulty can be largely overcome by the use of an algesimeter, which enables one not only to give constant stimuli but to grade their intensity and determine threshold values. Even when the pinpricks are of equal intensity, an isolated stimulus may be reported as excessively sharp, apparently because of direct contact with a pain spot.

If an area of diminished or absent sensation is encountered, its boundaries should be demarcated, to determine whether it has a segmental or peripheral nerve distribution, or whether sensation is lost below a certain level. Such areas are best delineated by proceeding from the region of impaired sensation toward the normal, and the changes may be confirmed by dragging a pin lightly over the skin.

Deep Pressure Sense. One can estimate this sense simply by pinching or pressing deeply on the tendons and muscles; no special virtue is attached to the traditional and somewhat sadistic use of the testicle for this test. Pain can often be elicited by heavy pressure even when superficial sensation is diminished; conversely, in some diseases such as tabetic neurosyphilis the loss of deep pressure sense may be more prominent.

Thermal Sense. The proper evaluation of this sensation requires attention to certain details of procedure. One may fail consistently to evoke thermal stimuli if small test objects are used. The perception of heat and cold is relatively delayed, especially if the test objects are applied only lightly and momentarily against the skin. At a temperature below 10°C or above 50°C, sensations of cold or warmth become confused with pain. As the temperature of the test object approaches that of the skin, the patient's response will be modified by the temperature of the skin itself.

The following procedure for testing thermal sensation is therefore suggested. The areas of skin to be tested should be exposed for some time before the examination. The test objects should be large, preferably Erlenmeyer flasks containing hot and cold water. Thermometers, which extend into the water through the flask stoppers, indicate the temperature of the water at the moment of testing. At first, extreme degrees of heat and cold (e.g., 5 and 50°C) may be employed, to delineate roughly an area of thermal sensory disturbance; over such an area the patient will report that the flask feels "less hot" or "less cold" than over a normal part. If areas of deficit are found, the borders may be more accurately determined by moving the flask along the skin from the insensitive region to the normal one than by applying the flask at intervals. The qualitative change should then be quantitated as far as possible by estimating the *differences in temperature* which the patient is capable of recognizing, the patient reporting whether one stimulus is *warmer or colder* than another. The patient should not simply be asked whether a given stimulus is warm or cold, since the cooler of two stimuli may be interpreted as warm. The range of temperature difference between the two flasks is gradually narrowed by mixing their contents. A normal person is capable of detecting 1° of difference when the temperature of the flasks is in the range of 28 to 32°C. In the warm range he should readily recognize differences between 35 and 40°C, and in the cold range between 10 and 20°C. In many older people and in others with poor peripheral circulation (especially in cold weather), the responses may be modified in an otherwise normal patient.

The sensation of heat or cold depends not only on the temperature of the stimulus, but also on the time and area over which it is applied. This principle may be employed to detect slight impairment of sensation; the patient may be able to distinguish small differences in temperature when the bottom of the flask is applied for 3 sec and be unable to do so if only the side of the flask is applied for 1 sec. Throughout the test procedure, especially when dealing with small temperature differences, the area of sensory disturbance should be continually checked against perception in normal parts.

Postural Sense and the Appreciation of Passive Movement. These modalities are usually lost together, although in any particular case one may be disproportionately affected.

Abnormalities of postural sensation may be revealed in any of several ways. With the upper limbs extended in front of the patient, his eyes being closed, the affected arm will wander from its original position, and if the fingers are spread apart they may undergo a series of slow changing postures ("piano-playing" movements or pseudoathetosis).

The lack of position sense in a lower limb may be demonstrated by displacing the limb from its original position, and asking the patient to point to his large toe. If postural sensation is defective in both lower limbs, then the patient will be unable to maintain his balance with feet together and eyes closed (Romberg's sign). This sign should be interpreted with caution. Even a normal person in the Romberg position will sway slightly more with his eyes closed than open. It follows that a patient with a lack of balance due to motor weakness or cerebellar disease will also sway more if visual cues are removed. Only if there is a marked discrepancy between the state of balance with eyes open and closed can one confidently state that the patient has a Romberg's sign, i.e., a loss of proprioceptive sensation. Mild degrees of unsteadiness in nervous or suggestible patients may be overcome by diverting their attention, as by having them alternately touch the index finger of each hand to their nose while standing with their eyes closed.

The appreciation of passive movement is first tested in the fingers and toes, and the defect, when present, is reflected maximally in these parts. It is important to grasp the digit firmly at the sides opposite the plane of movement, for otherwise the patient may judge the direction of movement from the source of pressure of the examiner's fingers. This applies as well to the testing of the more proximal segments of the limb. The patient should be instructed to report each movement as "up" or "down" in relation to the previous stationary position, and not in relation to the neutral position. It is useful to demonstrate the test with a large and easily identified movement, but once the idea is clear to the patient, the smallest detectable changes in position should be tested. The range of movement normally appreciated in the digits is said to be as little as 1°. Clinically, however, defective appreciation of passive movement is judged by comparison with a normal limb, or if bilaterally defective, on the basis of what the examiner has through experience learned to regard as normal. Slight impairment may be disclosed by a slow response or, if the digit is displaced very slowly, by a relative unawareness that movement has occurred; or after the digit has been displaced in the same direction several times, the patient may misjudge only the first movement in the opposite direction; or after the examiner has moved the toe, he may detect that the patient is trying to determine the position of the part by making small voluntary movements of the digit, a sign probably of uncertainty.

The Sense of Vibration. This is a composite sensation comprising touch and rapid alterations of deep pressure sense. It depends for its conduction on both cutaneous and deep afferent fibers, which ascend in the dorsal columns of the cord. It is therefore rarely affected in lesions of single nerves but will be disturbed in polyneuritis and disease of the dorsal columns, medial lemniscus, and thalamus. Except in cases of cortical lesions, vibration and position sense are usually lost together. There are exceptions to this statement, however, for in some instances the loss of vibration sense is more severe than loss of position sense (e.g., combined system disease). With advancing age, vibration sense may be diminished at the toes and ankles.

Vibration sense is tested by using a tuning fork with a low rate of vibration (128 d.v.) placed over the bony prominences. The examiner must make sure that the patient responds to the vibration and not to just the contact stimulus. Although there are mechanical devices to quantitate the intensity of vibration sense, it is sufficient for clinical purposes to compare the point tested with a normal part of the patient or of the examiner. A 256-d.v. fork can be used for finer testing. The level of vibration-sense loss due to spinal lesions can be estimated by placing the fork over successive vertebral spines.

Discriminative Sensory Functions. Damage to the sensory cortex or to the sensory projections from thalamus to cortex results in a special type of disturbance affecting mainly the patient's ability to make sensory discriminations. Lesions in these structures may disturb postural sense but leave the primary modalities (touch, pain and temperature, and vibration sense) relatively little affected. In such a situation, or if a cerebral lesion is suspected on other grounds, discriminative function should be tested further by the following tests.

Two-point Discrimination. The ability to distinguish two points from one point is tested by using a compass, the points of which should be blunt and applied simultaneously and painlessly. The distance at which such a stimulus can be recognized as double varies greatly, being 1 mm at the tip of the tongue, 3 to 6 mm at the finger tips, 1.5 to 2 cm on the palms and soles, 3 cm on the dorsa of the hands and feet, and 4 to 7 cm on the body surface. It is characteristic of the patient with a lesion of the sensory cortex to mistake two points for one, although occasionally the opposite is true.

Cutaneous Localization and Number Writing. Cutaneous localization is tested by touching various parts of the patient's body and asking him to point to the part touched or to a corresponding part of the examiner's limb. Recognition of *number writing* or of the direction of lines drawn on the skin also depends on the localization of tactile stimuli.

Appreciation of Texture, Size, and Shape. Appreciation of *texture* depends mainly on cutaneous impressions, but the *recognition of shape and size* of objects is based on impressions from deeper receptors as well. The lack of recognition of shape and form, therefore, though frequently found with cortical lesions, may also be present with lesions of the spinal cord and brain stem, due to interruption of the tracts transmitting postural and tactile sensation. Such a sensory defect, called *stereoanesthesia*, should be distinguished from astereognosis which connotes an inability to identify an object by palpation, the primary sense data being intact. The latter defect is essentially a tactile agnosia and is associated with lesions lying posterior to the postcentral gyrus. In practice, a pure astereognosis is rarely encountered, and the term is employed where the impairment of tactile and joint sense is of such slight degree that it could not account for the difficulty.

Extinction of Sensory Stimuli and Cortical Inattention. In response to bilateral simultaneous testing of symmetrical parts, the patient may acknowledge only the stimulus on the sound side, or he may improperly localize the stimulus on the affected side, whereas those applied individually are properly appreciated. This phenomenon of *extinction* or cortical *inattention* is characteristic of parietal lobe lesions, the symptomatology of which is considered in pp. 348 and 349.

A few other terms require definition, since they may be encountered in reading about sensation. Most of them are pedantic, and it is recommended that the simplest terms possible be used. *Anesthesia* refers to a loss and *hypesthesia* to a diminution of all forms of sensation. Loss or impairment of specific cutaneous sensations is indicated by an appropriate prefix or suffix, e.g., *thermoanesthesia* or *thermohypesthesia*, *analgesia* (loss of pain) or *hypalgesia*, *tactile anesthesia* (loss of sense of touch), and *pallanesthesia* (loss of vibratory sense). An alteration or perversion of sensation such as burning, prickling, or formication, is referred to as *paresthesia* or *dysesthesia*. The term *hyperesthesia* requires special mention; although it implies a heightened receptiveness of the nervous system, careful testing will usually demonstrate an underlying sensory defect, i.e., an elevated threshold to tactile, painful, or thermal stimuli; once the stimulus is perceived, however, it may have a severely painful or unpleasant quality (hyperpathia).

SENSORY SYNDROMES

Sensory Changes Due to Interruption of a Single Peripheral Nerve. These changes will vary with the composition of the nerve involved, depending on whether it is predominantly muscular, cutaneous, or mixed. Since proprioceptive fibers run for a time at least with the muscular (mainly motor) nerves, and cutaneous sensibility is carried in sensory nerves, each of these sensory systems may be affected separately. In lesions of cutaneous nerves, it is said that the area of tactile anesthesia is more extensive than the one for pain, but there is no universal agreement on this point.

Because of the overlap from adjacent nerves, the area of sensory loss following division of a cutaneous nerve is always less than its anatomic distribution. If a large area of skin is involved, the sensory impairment characteristically consists of a central portion, in which all forms of cutaneous sensation are lost, surrounded by a zone of partial loss, which becomes less marked as one proceeds from the center to the periphery. The sense of deep pressure and passive movement is intact, being carried by muscular nerves.

In lesions involving the brachial and lumbosacral plexuses, the sensory disturbance is no longer confined to the territory of a single nerve and is accompanied by muscle weakness and reflex changes.

Sensory Changes Due to Multiple Nerve Involvement (Polyneuropathy). In most instances of polyneuropathy the sensory changes are accompanied by varying degrees of motor and reflex loss. Usually the sensory impairment is symmetrical, notable exceptions being some instances of diabetic and periarteritic neuropathy. Since the longest and largest fibers are most often affected, the sensory loss is most severe over the feet and legs, and less over the hands. The abdomen, thorax, and face are spared except in the most severe cases. The sensory loss usually involves all the modalities, and although it is manifestly difficult to equate the degrees of impairment of pain, touch, temperature, vibration, and position sense, one of these may seemingly be impaired out of proportion to the others. One cannot accurately predict, from the patient's symptoms, which mode of sensation may be disproportionately affected. The term *glove and stocking anesthesia* is frequently employed to describe the sensory loss of polyneuropathy. Although this term draws attention to the predominantly distal pattern of sensory involvement, it is incorrect in that no sharp border exists between normal and impaired sensation. The sensory loss shades off gradually, the transition to normal sensation occurring over a variable vertical extent of the limb. In hysteria, by contrast, the border between normal and very absent sensation is usually sharp.

Sensory Changes Due to Involvement of Multiple Spinal Nerve Roots. Because of considerable overlap from adjacent roots, division of a single spinal sensory root does not produce complete loss of sensation in any area of skin. Compression of a single sensory cervical or lumbar root (in herniated intervertebral disks, for example) causes varying degrees of impairment of cutaneous sensation. When two or more roots have been completely divided, a segmental zone of sensory loss can be found, with reduction of touch and pain being about equal in extent. A narrow zone of partial loss surrounds the area of anesthesia in which a raised threshold may or may not be present and accompanied by overreaction ("hyperesthesia"). The presence of muscle paralysis, atrophy, and reflex loss indicates involvement of ventral roots as well.

The Tabetic Syndrome. This results from damage to the large proprioceptive fibers of the posterior lumbosacral roots. It is usually caused by neuro-

syphilis, less often by diabetic or other types of neuritis. Numbness or paresthesias and lightning pains are frequent complaints, and areflexia, atonicity of the bladder, abnormalities of gait (Chap. 30), and hypotonia without muscle weakness are found on examination. The sensory loss may consist only of loss of vibration and position sense in the lower extremities, but in severe cases some loss or impairment of superficial or deep pain sense or of touch may be added. The feet and legs are most affected, less often the arms and trunk.

Complete Spinal Sensory Syndromes. In a complete transverse lesion of the spinal cord, all forms of sensation are abolished below a level which corresponds with the lesion. There may be a narrow zone of "hyperesthesia" at the upper margin of the anesthetic zone. It is important to remember that during the evolution of such a lesion there may be a discrepancy between the level of the lesion and the level of the sensory loss, the latter ascending as the lesion progresses. This can be understood if one conceives of a lesion evolving from the periphery to the center of the cord, affecting first the outermost fibers carrying pain and temperature sensation from the legs. Conversely, a lesion advancing from the center of the cord may affect these modalities in the reverse order.

Partial Spinal Sensory Syndromes. *Hemisection of the Spinal Cord (Brown-Séquard Syndrome).* In rare instances disease is confined to one side of the spinal cord. Provided that the lesion is above the level where pain and temperature fibers have completely decussated (about the tenth thoracic segment), there will result a loss of pain and temperature sensation on the opposite side and of proprioceptive sensation on the same side as the lesion. The loss of pain and temperature sensation begins two or three segments below the lesion. An associated motor paralysis on the side of the lesion completes the syndrome. Touch is not affected, since the fibers from one side of the body are distributed in tracts (posterior columns and anterior spinothalamic) on both sides of the cord.

Lesions of the Central Gray Matter (Syringomyelic Syndrome). Since fibers conducting pain and temperature cross the cord in the anterior commissure, a lesion in this location will characteristically abolish these modalities on one or both sides, tactile sensation being spared. The commonest cause of such a lesion is syringomyelia, less often tumor and hemorrhage. The sensory loss usually occurs in a segmental distribution, and since the lesion frequently involves other parts of the gray matter, varying degrees of amyotrophy, loss of reflexes and of touch sensation may be added.

Posterior Column Syndrome (e.g., Subacute Combined Degeneration of the Cord). There is loss of vibratory and position sense below the lesion, with relatively little affection of the sense of pain, temperature, and touch. This may be difficult to distinguish from the tabetic syndrome. In some diseases, as mentioned earlier, vibratory sensation may be selectively involved, while in others position sense is more affected. It is important to remember that a lack of proprioceptive impulses may interfere with discriminative sensory function such as two-point discrimination and recognition of size, shape, and weight, and that impairment of this function may occur solely with posterior column disease. Paresthesias are a common complaint with posterior column disease, and pain stimuli may produce unpleasant sensations.

The Anterior and Lateral Column Syndrome. With occlusion of the anterior spinal artery or other destructive lesions that predominantly affect the ventral portion of the cord, there is relative or absolute sparing of proprioceptive sensation and loss of pain and temperature sensation below the level of the lesion. Since the corticospinal tracts and the ventral gray matter also fall within the area of distribution of the anterior spinal artery, paralysis of motor function forms a prominent part of this syndrome.

Disturbances of Sensation Due to Lesions of the Brain Stem. A characteristic feature of lesions of the medulla and lower pons is that in many instances the sensory disturbance is crossed; i.e., there is loss of pain and temperature sensation of one side of the face and of the opposite side of the body. This is accounted for by involvement of the trigeminal tract or nucleus and the lateral spinothalamic tract on one side of the brain stem. In the upper pons and midbrain, where the spinothalamic tracts and the medial lemniscus become confluent, an appropriately placed lesion may cause a loss of all superficial and deep sensation over the contralateral side of the body. Cranial nerve palsies, cerebellar ataxia, or motor paralysis is often associated, as indicated in Chap. 31, Disturbances of Cranial Nerve Function.

Sensory Loss Due to a Lesion of the Optic Thalamus (Syndrome of Déjerine-Roussy). Involvement of the nucleus ventralis posterolateralis of the thalamus, usually due to a vascular lesion or tumor, causes loss or diminution of all forms of sensation on the opposite side of the body. Position sense is affected more frequently than any other sensory function, and deep sensory loss is usually, but not always, more profound than cutaneous loss. There may be spontaneous pain or discomfort ("thalamic pain") on the affected side, and any form of stimulus may have a diffuse, unpleasant, lingering quality. Interestingly, this overresponse is usually associated with an elevated threshold; i.e., a stronger stimulus is necessary to produce a sensation, in spite of the greater discomfort experienced by the patient once the sensation had been evoked.

Sensory Loss Due to Lesions in the Parietal Lobe. There is a disturbance mainly of discriminative sensory functions on the opposite side of the body, particularly the face, arm, and leg. Astereognosis, loss of position sense, impaired tactile localization, elevation of two-point threshold, and a general inattentiveness to sensory stimuli on one side of the body are the most prominent findings. Although pain and temperature, touch, and vibratory sense are stated to be intact in cortical lesions, this is only relatively true, and the impairment of these latter modalities may take a form other than an elevation of threshold. Thus, on one examination, sensation may appear almost normal, while on a second examination the patient's responses may be inconstant and irregular. This type of response is often attributed to hysteria. Other features of parietal lobe symptomatology and the differences between dominant and nondominant parietal lobe syndromes will be considered in Chap. 37.

Sensory Loss Due to Suggestion and Hysteria. The possibility of suggesting sensory loss to a patient has already been mentioned. In fact, hysterical patients almost never complain spontaneously of cutaneous sensory loss, although they may use the term *numbness* to indicate a paralysis of a limb. Complete hemianesthesia, often with reduced hearing, sight, smell, and taste, as well as impaired vibration sense over only half the skull, is a common finding in hysteria. Anesthesia of one entire limb or a sharply defined sensory loss over part of a limb, not conforming to the distribution of root or cutaneous nerve, is also frequently observed. Postural sensation is rarely affected. The diagnosis of hysterical hemianesthesia is best made by eliciting the other relevant symptoms of hysteria, or if this is not possible, by noting the discrepancies between this type of sensory loss and that which occurs as part of the usual sensory syndromes.

REFERENCES

Holmes, Gordon: "Introduction to Clinical Neurology," 2d ed., chaps. 8, 9, Baltimore, The Williams & Wilkins Company, 1952.

Kibler, R. F., and P. W. Nathan: A Note on Warm and Cold Spots, Neurology, 10:874, 1960.

Mayo Clinic: "Clinical Examinations in Neurology," Philadelphia, W. B. Saunders Company, 1956.

Oppenheimer, D. R., E. Palmer, and G. Weddell: Nerve Endings in the Conjunctiva, J. Anat., 92:322, 1958.

Walshe, F. M. R.: "Critical Essays in Neurology," Baltimore, The Williams & Wilkins Company, 1948.

29 DISTURBANCES OF AUTONOMIC FUNCTION

Raymond D. Adams

The visceral activities of man are regulated to a large extent by the autonomic, or vegetative, nervous system. These functions are essential to life and at the same time are unconscious and involuntary. Why nature has divorced the vegetative functions from volition is not known. One would like to think that the mind, being occupied continuously with the discriminative and aesthetic activities of life, could not very well turn aside to regulate the heartbeat. Claude Bernard expressed the same idea in less laudatory terms when he wrote that, "Nature thought it prudent to remove these important phenomena from the caprice of an ignorant will."

Diseases that exert their morbid effects directly and exclusively on the autonomic nervous system are few and hardly require more than passing comment. On the other hand, the number of diseases the symptoms of which are expressed by some derangement of vegetative function is large, and even more important is the fact that this part of the nervous system is the neural effector apparatus for all emotional and affective experience, which will figure prominently in later chapters. In order to understand some of these phenomena of disease, the physician must have his anatomic and physiologic facts well in hand.

ANATOMIC AND PHYSIOLOGIC CONSIDERATIONS

Probably the most remarkable feature of this part of the nervous system is its location, outside the cerebrospinal axis and near the structures which it innervates. This position alone would seem to symbolize its relative independence from the cerebrospinal system. The autonomic nervous system consists essentially of aggregates of motor neurones whose cell bodies are collected into two large ganglionated chains, or cords, in the thoracic region, one on each side of the vertebral column, and in isolated ganglions elsewhere. The axones of these ganglion cells pass via the gray communicating rami to the spinal nerves and supply the blood vessels, sweat glands, and pilomotor structures in the various segments of the body; they also form plexuses of fibers which are distributed to the viscera. These autonomic motor neurones are called the *postganglionic neurones*. The autonomic ganglions are under the influence of the motor nerve cells of the lateral horns of the spinal cord and of the special visceral nuclei in the brain stem. The axones of these craniospinal nuclei traverse the anterior roots and then enter the autonomic ganglions via the

white (medullated) communicating rami. They are the preganglionic neurones and, together with the postganglionic neurones, they comprise the lower motor neurones of the autonomic nervous system.

From the anatomic viewpoint the autonomic nervous system is divided into the thoracolumbar (sympathetic) and the craniosacral (parasympathetic) divisions (see Fig. 29-1). The parasympathetic division consists of the special visceral nuclei in the brain stem, i.e., the nucleus of Edinger-Westphal, the superior and inferior salivary nuclei, and the dorsal motor nucleus of the vagus, the axones (preganglionic fibers) of which are important components of the oculomotor, facial, glossopharyngeal, and vagus nerves. The vagus is the most important of these nerves. The axones of the nucleus of Edinger-Westphal course through the oculomotor nerves and synapse in the ciliary ganglions in the orbits. The postganglionic neurones extend via the short ciliary nerves to the ciliary and pupillary constrictor muscles. Preganglionic fibers of the superior salivatory nucleus enter the facial nerve, and at a point near the geniculate ganglion they form the great superficial petrosal nerve, by which they reach the sphenopalatine ganglion. The cells of this ganglion innervate the lacrimal gland. Other of these fibers pass along the seventh nerve

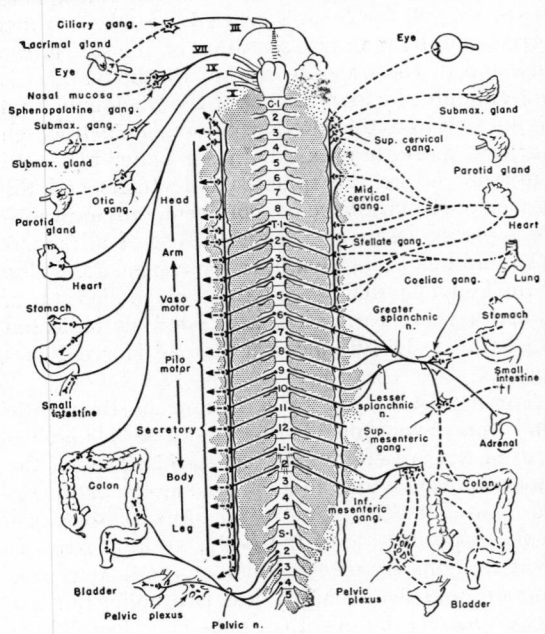

Fig. 29-1. Diagram of the spinal cord and brain stem with thoracolumbar or sympathetic nerves and ganglions on the right and craniosacral nerves and ganglions on the left. This shows the dual autonomic nerve supply of the viscera. (*Courtesy, Dr. L. M. Eaton and W. B. Saunders Company, Philadelphia.*)

to the chorda tympani and eventually join with the submaxillary ganglion; thus cells of this ganglion innervate the submaxillary and sublingual glands. The axones of the nerve cells of the inferior salivary nucleus enter the glossopharyngeal nerve and reach the otic ganglion through the tympanic plexus and lesser superficial petrosal nerve. The otic ganglion sends fibers to the parotid gland. The preganglionic neurones of the dorsal motor nucleus of the vagus enter the vagus nerve and terminate in ganglions situated in the walls of the many thoracic and abdominal viscera which it supplies.

The sacral part of the parasympathetic system is largely made up of preganglionic neurones in the lateral horns of the second, third, and fourth sacral segments. Their axones traverse the sacral nerves and synapse with ganglions which lie within the walls of the colon, bladder, and other pelvic organs. These sacral autonomic neurones, like the cranial ones, have long preganglionic and short postganglionic fibers, which would be expected from the peripheral location of the ganglion cells.

The cell bodies of the thoracolumbar preganglionic neurones are situated in the lateral horns of the gray matter of spinal cord from the first thoracic to the third lumbar segments. They enter the paravertebral chain of ganglions which extend from the base of the skull to the coccyx via the white communicating rami. There are three cervical (superior, middle, and inferior, the latter also called *stellate*), eleven thoracic, and four to six lumbar ganglions. The postganglionic neurones enter the splanchnic, mesenteric, and hypogastric plexuses and are distributed to all organs which receive sympathetic innervation. The cranium receives its sympathetic supply from the eighth cervical and first two thoracic cord segments, the fibers of which pass through the inferior and middle cervical and synapse with the nerve cells of the superior cervical. Postganglionic fibers from these cells follow the internal and external carotid arteries and innervate the blood vessels, smooth muscle, sweat, sebaceous, lacrimal, and salivary glands of the cranium. The upper extremity receives its postganglionic innervation from the upper four or five thoracic segments via the stellate ganglion. The cardiac plexus and other thoracic sympathetic nerves are derived from the upper thoracic ganglions, and the abdominal visceral plexuses from the fifth to the ninth or tenth thoracic ganglions. The lower three lumbar and first sacral ganglions have no visceral connections, however. They supply only the lower extremities.

Somewhat arbitrarily, anatomists have declared the autonomic nervous system to be purely motor in function. This, however, overlooks the fact that all the visceral nerves contain afferent fibers which convey sensory impulses from the viscera. The cell bodies of these sensory neurones lie in the posterior root ganglions; some of their central axones synapse with the lateral horn cells of the spinal cord, subserving visceral reflexes, and others carry sensory impulses to the thalamus via the lateral spinothalamic tract.

Within the autonomic nervous system there are arrangements for both excitation and inhibition of visceral function; this appears to be accomplished through the release of adrenergic and cholinergic substances. For the most part the sympathetic postganglionic fibers liberate sympathin and act in opposition to the parasympathetic ones, which release acetylcholine. There are exceptions to this generalization, however. For example, the blood vessels, piloerector muscles, and sweat glands receive only a sympathetic nerve supply; yet the sudomotor system reacts only to cholinergic drugs.

Stimulation of the sympathetic nerve fibers causes dilatation of the pupil, sweating, piloerection, acceleration of the heart, dilatation of bronchi, inhibition of intestinal peristalsis, and closure of bladder and bowel sphincters. Stimulation of the cranial part of the parasympathetic nerve fibers results in slowing of the heart, peristalsis, relaxation of sphincters, and secretion of digestive juices. Stimulation of the sacral part of the parasympathetic nerve leads to contraction of the detrusor muscles of the bladder and relaxation of the vesical sphincter, contraction of the colon and rectum, with relaxation of the anal sphincter. Reproduction is served by both the parasympathetic and the sympathetic systems; the latter causes contraction of prostatic muscle and ejaculation of sperm but when fully activated will inhibit erection of the penis.

The two divisions of the autonomic nervous system, acting in conjunction with the endocrine glands, with which they are closely related, maintain the homeostasis of the organism. Cannon has expounded this theory in admirable fashion. The sympathetic nervous system serves to marshal the energy reserves of the body during strong emotion and provides the mechanism for the emergency reactions to acute or prolonged stress. Man (or animal) may survive if deprived of his sympathetic nervous system but only if he is kept in a sheltered environment.

CENTRAL NERVOUS REGULATION OF VISCERAL FUNCTION
(The Visceral Brain)

Among the most important advances in knowledge of neuroanatomy has been the relatively recent discovery of autonomic regulating mechanisms in the brain. Small insignificant-appearing nuclei in the walls of the third ventricle beneath the thalami (hypothalamus), and in buried parts of the cerebral cortex, formerly judged to have purely olfactory functions, are now known to control the autonomic nervous system. This is accomplished in two ways—through direct descending nervous pathways to the spinal cord and through the pituitary and other endocrine glands.

This supranuclear regulatory apparatus of the autonomic nervous system consists of three main groups of structures: (1) the hypothalamus, (2) the mesial transitional cortex and archicortex (the rhinencephalon or smell brain, the hippocampus, amygdaloid nuclei, olfactory cortex, and cingulate gyri), and (3) the frontal lobe cortex.

The *frontal lobe cortex*—the least understood and most uniquely human arrangement—appears to be the highest level of integration of autonomic function. Stimulation of one frontal lobe may evoke changes in temperature and sweating in the contralateral arm and leg, and massive lesions here, which usually cause a hemiplegia, may modify these functions in the direction of either inhibition or facilita-

tion. Bilateral lesions in the paracentral lobules in man result in loss of voluntary control of the bladder; unilateral lesions have no effect. The descending pathways subserving bowel and bladder function are believed to be close to the corticospinal fibers, but their exact course is not known. Most likely a large contingent of these fibers terminate in the medial transitional and archicortex and the hypothalamus, which in turn sends fibers on to the brain stem and spinal cord.

The *transitional mesocortex and archicortex* have now been identified as important parts of the so-called "cerebral autonomic centers." Together they have been called the *visceral brain*. Lesions here in animals have given variable results. A remarkable placidity and lack of fear was observed in macaques and sham rage in cats. Sham rage, in which the animal automatically reacts by rage to every stimulus, had formerly been associated with removal of cerebral hemispheres, leaving the hypothalamus and brain stem intact, but the more recent work of Bard and his associates has demonstrated that the removal of the meso- and archicortex is essential to the development of this condition. These facts are of great importance to students of behavior, for it would appear that there are cortical mechanisms here for both the facilitation and the inhibition of affective or emotional reactions. The manner in which these emotional reactions are integrated with nervous activity in general has yet to be learned.

The *hypothalamus* has been the subject of intensive study. It is comprised of three main groups of nuclei: (1) the *anterior group* includes the supraoptic and paraventricular nuclei; (2) the *middle group* includes the ventrimedian, dorsomedian, and tuberal nuclei; and (3) the *posterior group* includes the mammillary bodies and posterior hypothalamic nuclei (see Fig. 29-2). The supraoptic and paraventricular nuclei send fibers into the posterior lobe of the pituitary gland, i.e., the *supraopticohypophyseal* tract. The tuberal nuclei project onto the infundibulum and the pars intermedia, and together compose the tuberoinfundibular system. The mammillary bodies send fibers to the thalamus and the mesocortex (cingulate gyri). Afferent sensory fibers, largely pain fibers, enter the reticular formation of the upper brain stem and hypothalamus. Descending cortical fibers, including the medial forebrain bundle, partly terminate here. Also the archicortex is connected with the mammillary bodies via the fornix. Descending fiber systems from the hypothalamus have also been demonstrated; they extend to the medulla and spinal cord. Physiologically it appears that the anterior portion of the hypothalamus is related to the parasympathetic nervous system and the posterior part to the sympathetic system.

The hypothalamus is a part of the diencephalon

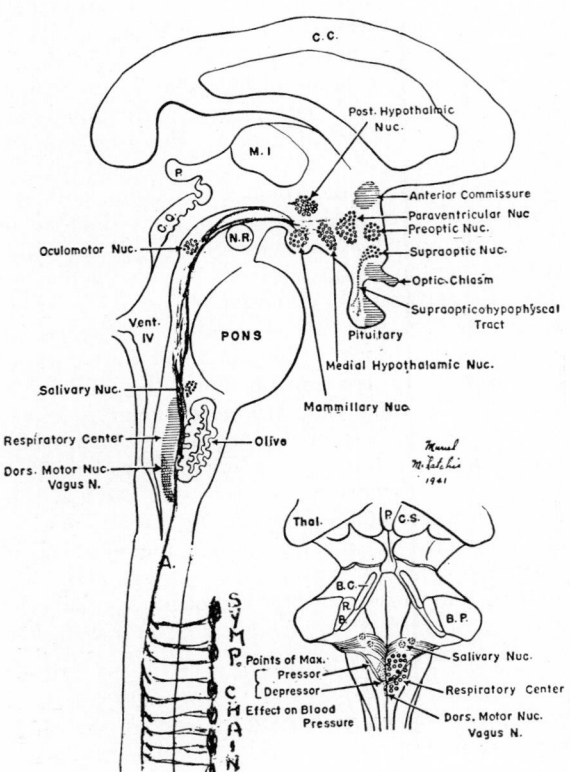

FIG. 29-2. (*Left.*) Sagittal section of corpus callosum (*CC*), brain stem, and spinal cord to show the central autonomic connections. Note hypothalamic nuclei and descending fiber system (*A*) to lateral horn cells in thoracic cord which give rise to preganglionic fibers. (*Right.*) Dorsal view of brain stem and upper spinal cord. (*Courtesy, Dr. J. C. White.*)

and, being situated just above the pituitary gland, is the crossroad between the cerebrospinal and the endocrine systems. There is now substantial evidence that it is involved in some of the most fundamental reactions, including emotion, sleep, temperature and water regulation, sexual activity, sugar and fat metabolism.

AUTONOMIC SYNDROMES

Emergency and Alarm Reactions

Inasmuch as the central and peripheral autonomic nervous apparatus and the endocrine glands, particularly the adrenals, have been accepted for many years as the neural and humoral basis of all instinctive and emotional behavior, it is remarkable how little sound information has been acquired about the role of this apparatus in disease. In chronic anxiety, acute panic reactions, the altered emotionality of depressive psychosis, mania, and schizophrenia, and the many so-called "psychosomatic" diseases, some of which have an alluring similarity to primitive emotional reactions, no consistent autonomic or endocrine dysfunction has been demonstrated. This has been disappointing, since Cannon, with his attractive emergency theory of sympathoadrenal action, had given us such a promising new conception of the neurophysiology of acute emotion and Selye had extended this theory so plausibly to explain all the reactions of the human and animal organism to chronic stressful situations. According to this theory strong emotion, such as anger or fear, excites the sympathetic nervous system and also the medulla of the adrenal glands, which is under both direct nervous and hormonal control. These sympathoadrenal reactions are brief and capable of sustaining the animal in flight or fight; but they are likely to prove fatal if continued for more than a few minutes. Prolonged stressful situations stimulate the anterior pituitary, probably through the hypothalamus, and an excess of ACTH is produced. This in turn stimulates the adrenal cortex, which elaborates a number of hormones, referred to collectively as *steroids*. These more prolonged defensive and adaptive reactions develop, according to Selye, in three stages. The first stage is the *alarm reaction*, i.e., the initial calling forth of the body's defensive forces. The second is the *stage of resistance*, which develops if the stress is not too strong and if the adaptation is effective. The final stage is *exhaustion and death*. Animals deprived of adrenal cortex or human beings with Addison's disease cannot tolerate stress because they are incapable of mobilizing either the adrenal medulla or the adrenocortex. Exercise, cold, oxygen lack, and surgical injury all are said to evoke

the same defensive reactions in animals. Some of the latter are accompanied by adrenal enlargement, thymic and lymphatic hyperplasia, and gastric ulceration, irreversible tissue changes which have been regarded as experimental products of psychosomatic disease. This extension of the theory, although attractive, has received little or no support. Critics have pointed out that the conditions to which the experimental animal has been subjected and those of human disease are not sufficiently close to permit conclusions as to their identity. More critical studies of the anatomy and physiology of the hypothalamus, pituitary and adrenal glands, and autonomic nervous system are needed before many of these problems can be settled.

Special Autonomic Syndromes

The disorders of autonomic nervous function may be divided into three groups, involving the peripheral autonomic, spinal autonomic, and cerebral autonomic apparatus.

Peripheral Autonomic Disorders. *Horner's Syndrome and Stellate Ganglion Syndrome.* Section of the cervical sympathetic fibers in the neck or at any point along the internal carotid arteries (postganglionic fibers) or the removal of the superior cervical ganglions results in myosis of the pupil, drooping of the eyelid, enophthalmos, and abolition of sweating over one side of the face. The same syndrome may be caused by interruption of the preganglionic fibers from the eighth cervical and first through third thoracic spinal segments or the descending uncrossed hypothalamospinal pathway in the lateral tegmentum of the medulla or cervical cord. The common causes of the syndrome are tumorous or inflammatory involvement of cervical lymph nodes, surgical trauma in operations on cervical structures, neoplastic invasion of the proximal part of the brachial plexus, basal skull fractures, tumor, syringomyelia, or traumatic lesions of the first and second thoracic spinal segments, and infarcts or other lesions of the lateral part of the medulla (Wallenberg's syndrome). There is also an idiopathic variety which may at times be hereditary. If Horner's syndrome develops early in life, the iris on the side of the lesion fails to become pigmented and remains blue or mottled gray-brown and blue. A lesion of the stellate ganglion, e.g., a tumor arising from the superior sulcus of the lung or compression by cervical rib, produces the interesting combination of Horner's syndrome and paralysis of sympathetic reflexes in the arm (the hand is warm and dry).

Other Pupillary and Salivary Disturbances. A disorder of the oculomotor nerve, in addition to paralyzing four of the extraocular muscles and the levator muscle of the eyelid, causes a dilatation of the pupil, with an abolition of the constriction which normally occurs as a reaction to light; also there is a loss of accommodation, i.e., of near vision, owing to paralysis of the ciliary muscle. Diseases which involve the facial, glossopharyngeal, and vagus nerves seldom induce recognizable parasympathetic changes. However, a severe facial palsy (Bell's palsy) may be followed by imperfect regeneration and misdirection of nerve fibers. For example, fibers which should innervate the salivary glands may reach either the lacrimal or the sweat glands in the preauricular and temporal regions. Eating, with its attendant reflex salivation, then provokes lacrimation (*syndrome of crocodile tears*) or temporal sweating (*auriculotemporal syndrome*).

Disturbances of Bladder and Bowel Function. As already stated, the bladder receives a dual nerve supply, the sacral parasympathetic via sacral nerves (second through fourth sacral segments) and the sympathetic via the hypogastric plexus (first and second lumbar segments). The afferent fibers for pain and feelings of distention course through the pelvic as well as the hypogastric nerves, and those from the urethra and external sphincter pass through the pudendal nerves to the third and fourth sacral spinal segments. Bladder evacuation is effected by the detrusor muscles, which also form the internal sphincter in such a way that when they contract the internal sphincter relaxes and vice versa. The action of the detrusor and internal sphincter muscles is both reflex and voluntary. Their spinal connections are through the pelvic afferents, second and third sacral spinal segments, and their pre- and postganglionic parasympathetic motor neurones. The sympathetic nervous system has relatively little influence on bladder function. It supplies mainly the blood vessels in the wall of the bladder.

The act of micturition is complex. When the normal person is asked to empty his bladder, there is first a relaxation of the perineum, then an increased tension of the abdominal wall, a slow contraction of the vesical muscle itself (the detrusor) with an associated opening of the internal sphincter, and finally a relaxation of the external sphincter. From the studies of Denny-Brown and Robertson it appears that the vesical orifice opens only after the voluntary contraction of the detrusor. When the external sphincter is voluntarily closed, the vesical contraction subsides. The abdominal muscles have no power to initiate micturition except when the detrusor muscle is abnormal. This voluntary control of the bladder is a cortical affair, motor fibers arising in the paracentral lobules and descending in the spinal cord just anterior to the corticospinal tracts, so close that a lesion which affects the latter will often interfere with the voluntary control of micturition. There are also said

to be other suprasegmental mechanisms in the upper brain stem, but their exact location and action are not known.

Cerebral lesions which lead to mental confusion are often accompanied by urinary and fecal incontinence (so-called "frontal lobe incontinence"). The patient does not appear to appreciate his immediate circumstances and voids in inappropriate places. Usually he is unaware of having soiled his clothes or the bed linen, and when his attention is called to it he may deny any responsibility for it or offer an excuse. In addition there may be a bilateral affection of the paracentral lobules which will abolish voluntary control of the bladder. Often one or both legs will also be weakened or paralyzed. Unilateral lesions of the paracentral lobule or of the corticospinal tract at any level from cortex to sacral cord result at most in only transitory loss of voluntary control of bladder and bowel. Transection of the spinal cord, regardless of the nature of the disease, causes a flaccid paralysis of the bladder and bowel, just as it does of the leg muscles. The bladder rapidly becomes distended, and overflow incontinence follows. Later, as spasticity and heightened spinal reflex activity of the legs develop, the bladder, too, becomes spastic and contracted, its stretch reflex being now exaggerated. The distention produced by urine then provokes reflex contraction, and relatively complete micturition results. This is the *automatic* or *reflex bladder*. If the cord lesion is incomplete and weak voluntary control remains, the patient reports urgency and precipitancy of urination and difficulty in both initiating and inhibiting bladder action. Sensation of bladder filling and distention may or may not be present, according to whether or not sensory tracts are interrupted. Posterior root lesions, e.g., tabes dorsalis, impair sensation and also the reflex tone of the detrusor muscle; the bladder is then both insensitive and hypotonic. It overfills without the patient being aware of it, and with a rise in intraabdominal pressure during strain, turning in bed, or stooping, there will be overflowing and dribbling. The urinary stream is feeble. Sacral cord lesions (spina bifida or tumor) or anterior root lesions also leave the bladder partially paralyzed and hypotonic, but in this case (unlike a denervated skeletal muscle) even though completely isolated from spinal control, the bladder does regain tone and becomes capable of some functional activity. However, the isolated bladder does not empty itself completely, and infection of the residual urine always remains a serious hazard.

The colon, rectum, and anal sphincters have an innervation similar to that of the bladder, and their function is disturbed in the same way with central and peripheral lesions. The colon may be hypotonic and distended and the anal sphincters lax. The anal and, in the male, the bulbocavernosus reflex may be abolished. Or defecation may be urgent and precipitant in higher spinal lesions. Since the same spinal segments and nearly the same spinal tracts subserve bladder and bowel function, so-called "double incontinence" is often manifest. However, since the bowel is less often filled and its content is solid, fecal incontinence is usually less troublesome than urinary incontinence.

Disturbances of Sexual Function. Sexual function in the male, which is not infrequently affected in neurologic disease, is another highly complex act; it is conveniently divided into several parts: (1) sexual impulse, drive, or desire, often referred to as *libido;* (2) penile erection, whereby the act of sexual intercourse can be effected (potencia); (3) ejaculation of semen by the prostate through the urethra, whereby impregnation of the female may be accomplished. These different parts of the sexual act may be affected separately. Loss of libido may depend on both psychic and somatic factors. It may be complete, as in old age or in medical and endocrine diseases, or it may occur only in a certain circumstance or in relationship to a certain person. In the latter case, which is usually due to psychologic factors, penile erection and even emission of semen may occur nocturnally and effective sexual intercourse with another person is possible. Sexual desire can on occasion be altered in the opposite direction; i.e., it may be excessive as a sign of neurologic disease. This has been observed in encephalitis and tumors affecting the diencephalon and temporal lobes. Sexual desire on the other hand may be present but penile erection may be impossible to attain or sustain, a condition called *impotence.* This happens often in patients who suffer disease of the sacral cord segments and their afferent and efferent connections (e.g., cord tumor, tabes, diabetic polyneuritis). The parasympathetic nerves cannot then be activated to cause tumescence of the corpora cavernosa. Diseases of the spinal cord may be accompanied by penile erection, reflexly induced and sustained for long periods of time. This is called *priapism;* it is a reminder that all the neural apparatus for the control of sexual function is organized through the lower spinal segments and that it may function effectively even when completely removed from voluntary control by the spinal cord lesions. Another sexual difficulty may be the premature ejaculation of semen, a common complaint in neurotic individuals, though by no means peculiar to them. After lumbar sympathectomy the semen may be ejected back into the bladder because of paralysis of the periurethral muscle (prostate) at the verumontanum. Finally, as will be pointed out later, diseases of the testes accompa-

nied by insufficient spermatogenesis or diseases of the seminal vesicles which prevent emission of sperm result in sterility. In these cases libido and potencia may or may not be normal.

Aberrations of sexual function also occur in the female but are more difficult to analyze. Lack of sexual desire or failure to attain orgasm (frigidity) is much more frequent in the female than in the male, occurring in a significant percentage of neurotic women and in others who exhibit no further signs of psychic disorder. States of excessive sexual excitability are known in psychopathic individuals and, rarely, in those who suffer disease of the brain. Fecundity and sterility are often unrelated to the other aspects of sexuality, being the result of diseases of the ovaries, fallopian tubes, and uterus, as well as of other less clearly defined factors discussed later.

The genesis of sexual perversions remains obscure. Endocrine, biochemical, and psychologic studies have failed to clarify the cause and mechanism.

The Effects of Thoracolumbar Sympathectomy in Man. Operative removal of the sympathetic ganglions has provided the clinician with the only clear-cut example of extensive injury to the peripheral autonomic nervous system, although in orthostatic hypotension a fundamental or similar defect in the peripheral autonomic nervous system has long been suspected (cf. Chap. 33). In general it may be said that total sympathectomy results in surprisingly few physiologic changes. Aside from loss of sweating over the denervated areas of the body, the most pronounced abnormality in these individuals is an impairment of vasomotor reflexes. In the upright posture, syncope is frequent because of the pooling of blood in the splanchnic bed and lower extremities. There is a steady fall in blood pressure to shock levels and little or no pallor, nausea, vomiting, or sweating, the usual accompaniments of syncope. Bladder, bowel, and sexual function are preserved, though in some males the semen is ejaculated into the posterior urethra and bladder. No consistent abnormalities of renal or hepatic function are found.

Other Disturbances of the Peripheral Autonomic Nervous System. Hirschsprung's disease is presently ascribed to a failure of development or a loss of the parasympathetic ganglion cells in the enteric plexus. Some cases of megaloureter are also attributed to similar defects.

Excessive sweating, a sympathetically mediated disorder, may be a troublesome complaint in some patients. Its cause is not known. One variety, presumably of congenital origin, may affect the palms. The social embarrassment of a "dripping paw," as lay people term it, is often intolerable. It is taken to be a sign of nervousness, though many persons with this condition disclaim all other neurotic symptoms. It is likely that this type of sweating is related to nervousness, for cold, clammy hands are common in individuals with anxiety neurosis and hysteria, and indeed this has been a useful sign in distinguishing an anxiety state from hyperthyroidism, in which the hands tend to be warm and moist. Cervical sympathectomy will relieve the more severe cases of palmar sweating. Excessive perspiration is also observed in some cases of peripheral neuropathy, i.e., causalgia and the "burning foot syndrome," in which burning and painful paresthesias and hyperhydrosis are combined.

Anhydrosis in restricted skin areas may be a frequent and useful finding in peripheral nerve disease. The loss of sweat corresponds to the area of sensory loss. In contrast, spinal root disease does not affect sweating.

Autonomic Disturbances with Lesions of the Spinal Cord and Brain Stem

That the somatic afferent and efferent nerves join the cord at all levels from the cervical to the sacral, whereas the sympathetic efferents all leave the cord from the first thoracic to the third lumbar, explains the lack of correspondence in the distribution of the sympathetic and somatic sensorimotor functions after lesions of the spinal cord. An acute cervical lesion may cause a disturbance of sympathetic function over the entire body including the head, whereas the sensorimotor paralysis is limited to those parts below the level of the lesion. A lumbar lesion, on the other hand, will have no effect upon sympathetic function, and yet it will impair sensation and motor power. Only in the thoracic lesion is there a rough concordance between the distributions of somatic and autonomic motor deficits.

If the spinal cord is transected in the cervical or thoracic levels, interrupting the descending cerebrospinal sympathetic fibers, several autonomic disturbances may be observed. Below the level of the lesion the skin is warm and dry; cold stimuli have less vasoconstrictive effect than normally; and if the patient is tilted upright, there may be a postural hypotension. Dermographia is slightly increased at the level of the lesion and decreased below. There is loss of the pilomotor reaction to skin pinching in the denervated segments of the body. If the cervical cord is hemisected, hypohydrosis or anhydrosis occurs ipsilaterally. After "spinal shock" subsides, the skin below the level of the lesion becomes warm and moist and paroxysms of excessive sweating may occur. These episodes may be combined with other manifestations of spinal "mass" reflexes, such as flexor or extensor spasms and involuntary micturition. Pinching of the skin above the spinal cord lesion will induce a pilomotor reaction—goose flesh—which will not extend to skin areas below the level of the lesion. Nevertheless, the pilomotor reflex is still excitable from the denervated areas. With partial cord lesions, autonomic dysfunction is relatively rare, except in syringomyelia, in which destruction of the lateral horn cells may be responsible for anhydrosis.

With lesions of any type in the lateral tegmentum of the pons and medulla there may be an ipsilateral paralysis of autonomic function in the arm, trunk, and leg. These parts are warm and dry. In addition a Horner's syndrome may occur.

Hypothalamic Syndromes

Within comparatively recent times the following syndromes referable to the hypothalamus have been delineated.

Diabetes Insipidus. This condition is due to involvement of the supraoptic nuclei or supraopticohypophyseal tract. It is discussed in Part Four, Section 2.

Disturbances of Temperature Regulation. Lesions in the more anterior parts of the hypothalamus may result in hyperthermia. The heat-dissipating mechanisms of the body are impaired. This often follows operations in the region of the floor of the third ventricle. The temperature rises to 106°F or higher and remains elevated until death some hours or days later. Icy coldness of the extremities, dry skin, tachycardia, and tachypnea are also present. Acetylsalicylic acid has rather little effect on central hyperthermia; the temperature may, however, be reduced by sodium phenobarbital and chlorpromazine and by cooling the body. Lesions in the more posterior parts of the hypothalamus are sometimes attended by hypothermia or poikilothermia. The latter often passes unnoticed unless the patient's temperature is taken after lowering and raising the room temperature. Somnolence and hypotension are often associated.

Adiposogenital Dystrophy—Froehlich's Syndrome. Destruction of the tuberal nuclei and the tuberoinfundibular tracts results in a delay or an arrest of sexual development. This is often combined with obesity and will be described in detail in Part Four, Section 2. Many cases are idiopathic; craniopharyngioma is the most frequently demonstrated cause. In the *Laurence-Moon-Biedl* syndrome, obesity and hypogenitalism are combined with mental retardation, polydactyly, and retinal pigmentation. In several instances this syndrome has been familial. *Sexual precocity* as a clinical phenomenon is rare and has in several autopsied cases been traced to an anomalous overdevelopment of tuberal nuclei. The author has observed this in cases with von Recklinghausen's disease and tuberous sclerosis. Both sexes may be affected; this type of *pubertas praecox* evidently has a basis different from that of the sexual precocity in pinealoma, which is limited to males. In *Albright's syndrome* sexual precocity in the female is combined with bone cysts and spots of cutaneous pigmentation.

Gastric Hemorrhage and Other Disorders. Lesions in or near the tuberal nuclei also are accompanied by superficial erosions, ulcerations, and hemorrhages from the gastric mucosa (Cushing's ulcer). Massive gastrointestinal hemorrhage may occur with any type of acute brain disease. In experimental animals this has been most consistently produced by lesions in or near the tuberal nuclei. However, in human cases coming to autopsy lesions usually have not been found in the hypothalamus.

Disturbances in sugar metabolism have been produced by experimental lesions in the hypothalamus but are of infrequent occurrence in man. The transitory hyperglycemia and glycosuria observed in some cases of stroke can rarely be traced to a lesion in the hypothalamus. The author has not encountered hypoglycemia with brain disease; if it occurs it must be extremely rare.

Hypersomnia, pathologic appetite for food (hyperbulimia) with or without confusion may follow head-injury, encephalitis, etc. (*Kleine-Levin syndrome*).

Emotional and Personality Disorders

At some time or other almost every conceivable disorder of personality and emotional control has been ascribed to disease of the cerebrum or hypothalamus. Alpers in 1939 pointed out in a review of published work on the hypothalamus how uncritical some of these clinicopathologic correlations have been. The author's own studies of the hypothalamic lesions in Wernicke's disease have suggested that mental confusion and severe learning and memory defects of the type described as *Korsakoff's psychosis* may in fact be due to lesions in the walls of the third ventricles. This idea has received support from the observations of Cobb and White and others that similar mental symptoms accompany pituitary adenomas and craniopharyngiomas. Apathy, disinterest, and drowsiness are noted in many of these patients. Immobility and speechlessness, amounting at times to a veritable *akinetic mutism,* characterize some of them. Other patients with more anteriorly placed lesions have exhibited excitement and maniacal behavior. Visual hallucinations with relatively clear mentation and good insight have been reported in cases with disease of regions adjacent to the hypothalamus, the "peduncular hallucinosis" of Lhermitte, the exact anatomy of which is unsettled. *Sham rage* has been observed in human beings with disease of the basal forebrain. As mentioned above, this is a remarkable state in which every stimulus evokes a violent outburst of wild rage resembling that of an infuriated

individual. The patient will spit, strike, bite, or scratch every person or object with which he comes in contact; he can be cared for only by confining him to a room or restraining him and giving heavy sedation. Finally, so-called "epileptic attacks with autonomic discharges," mainly of sympathetic type, the so-called "diencephalic autonomic epilepsy of Penfield," have been ascribed to a lesion of this part of the brain. Only one case was reported, however, and it was so complicated (a diencephalic tumor with hydrocephalus) that the epileptic nature of the syndrome and its hypothalamic localization are uncertain.

Remarkable changes in emotional control, character, and personality in patients with lesions in the medial parts of the temporal lobes have only recently been brought to the attention of the medical profession. Most of the cases studied were subject to psychomotor or temporal lobe epilepsy and may also have had disease in other parts of the nervous system. Nevertheless, new arrangements for the nervous control of autonomic and visceral function and for the regulation of emotion are suggested and will surely be scrutinized with great care.

The peculiar syndrome described in Chap. 283, under Anhydrotic Ectodermal Dysplasia, probably represents a central disturbance of autonomic regulation.

TESTS FOR ABNORMALITIES OF THE AUTONOMIC NERVOUS SYSTEM

With few exceptions, such as Horner's syndrome, it is relatively difficult to demonstrate and to evaluate dysfunction of the autonomic nervous system. Many experienced neurologists tend to rely entirely on palpation and inspection of the skin. Nonetheless, several special laboratory techniques can be used to confirm clinical impressions.

Tests of Vasomotor Reactions. Measurement of the skin temperature is a useful index of vasomotor function. Vasomotor paralysis results in vasodilatation of skin vessels and a rise in temperature; vasoconstriction lowers the temperature. With a skin thermometer one may compare the affected with the normal areas under standard conditions. The normal skin temperature is usually 31 to 33°C when the room temperature is 26 to 27°C. Vasoconstrictor tone may also be tested by measuring the temperature of the area in question before and after immersing the hands in cold water.

Tests of Sudomotor Activity. Of these there are several. The neatest and generally most satisfactory is the galvanic skin resistance test. This consists of a string galvanometer which indicates the resistance offered by the skin to the passage of a weak galvanic current through the skin. Increase in sweating lowers the resistance; anhydrosis raises it. Sweat can also be weighed after it is absorbed by small squares of filter paper. Powdered charcoal dusted on the skin will cling to moist areas and not to dry ones. The starch test or a color indicator such as chinizarin 2-6 disulfonic acid may be used. If the amount of sweating is not sufficient to show by these tests, the patient should be warmed up with blankets and given a diaphoretic such as hot tea or a dose of pilocarpine.

Bladder function is best demonstrated by the cystometrogram, i.e., by measuring intravesicular pressure while sterile saline solution is permitted to flow by gravity into the bladder. Relatively simple apparatus is available for this purpose. The rise of pressure as 500 ml sterile saline flows into the bladder and emptying contractions may be recorded by a manometer. The size and motility of the colon can be tested in similar fashion.

REFERENCES

Association for Research in Nervous and Mental Disease, "The Hypothalamus," Research Publications, vol. XX, Baltimore, The Williams & Wilkins Company, 1939.

Kuntz, A.: "The Autonomic Nervous System," Philadelphia, Lea & Febiger, 1929.

White, J. C., and R. H. Smithwick: "The Autonomic Nervous System," New York, The Macmillan Company, 1941.

30 VERTIGO AND DISORDERS OF EQUILIBRIUM AND GAIT

Maurice Victor and Raymond D. Adams

States of disordered equilibrium occur in the course of many medical and neurologic diseases. The terms used to describe the sensation of unbalance are rather ambiguous. *Dizziness* is used by the patient to indicate not only a sense of rotation but also such vague sensory experiences as uncertainty, insecurity, unsteadiness, weakness, faintness, a swimming sensation in the head, and lightheadedness. *Giddiness* has almost the same significance, with perhaps more implication of altered consciousness, blurred vision, and swaying sensation. *Vertigo* literally means "sense of turning," either of one's body or of the surroundings, a definition which, with a few important qualifications to be mentioned, is used throughout this chapter. *Equilib-*

rium refers simply to a state of balance or equipoise in which opposing forces such as gravity and postural reflexes exactly counteract each other.

Disorders of equilibrium are suitably considered in connection with dizziness and vertigo because these states so frequently go together (vertiginous ataxia). However, there are other disorders of equilibrium quite independent of vertigo, e.g., those due to a loss of joint and muscle sense (sensory ataxia) or cerebellar disease (cerebellar ataxia). These are also considered briefly in this chapter.

ANATOMIC, PHYSIOLOGIC, AND PSYCHOLOGIC CONSIDERATIONS

The mechanisms which are responsible for the maintenance of a balanced posture and make us aware of the body's position in relation to its surroundings must be understood before considering the clinical aspects of this subject.

Afferent impulses from the eyes, labyrinths, muscles, and joints inform us of the position of the body in space. In response to these impulses the many fine and rapid adjustments necessary to maintain equilibrium are carried out. Normally we are unaware of these adaptive movements, since they operate for the most part at a reflex level. The most important of the afferent impulses are the following:

1. Visual impulses from the retina and possibly proprioceptive impulses from the ocular muscles. By such impulses we judge the distance of objects from the body, and are enabled to produce a sharply focused image on the retina.

2. Impulses from the labyrinths, which are highly specialized spatial proprioceptors. The primary function of the semicircular canals and the vestibule is to register changes in direction of motion (either acceleration or deceleration) and in the position of the body. The semicircular canals respond to movement and angular momentum, while the otoliths—the sense organs of the utricle and saccule—are mainly concerned with the orientation of the organism with reference to gravity.

3. Impulses which arise from the proprioceptors of the joints and muscles. Those from the neck are of special importance in relating the position of the head to the rest of the body. Impulses from the lower limbs and the trunk are concerned with the position of the body in relation to sitting, standing, and walking.

The afferent nerve fibers from these sense organs are connected with the cerebellum, the vestibular nuclei, the medial longitudinal fasciculi, and the red nuclei. These are the central structures concerned with regulation of posture. Experimental transection of the brain stem of an animal above the level of the red nuclei does not interfere with the maintenance of upright posture, even if this posture is forcibly altered. The role of the cerebral hemispheres is to coordinate impulses conveyed by the afferent paths with the activity of the efferent paths which, through voluntary and involuntary movements, modify the position of the body in space. The three great efferent paths are (1) the pyramidal tract, linking the precentral cortex with the anterior horn cells; (2) the frontopontine, temporopontine, and pontocerebellar fibers connecting the cerebral cortex with the cerebellum and, hence, indirectly with the other postural reflex centers of the midbrain; (3) the several tracts which descend from the basal ganglions to the reticular formation and thence by way of the reticulospinal and vestibulospinal tracts to the spinal cord.

Important psychologic phenomena are also involved in the maintenance of equilibrium, viz., those which deal with the relationship between ourselves and the external world. A lucid exposition of this subject is to be found in the article by Brain, and the following statements are a summary of his views. We perceive that portion of space occupied by our body and construct from sensory data a general concept called the *body schema*. The space around our body, i.e., the external world, is represented by another schema. These two schemata are neither static nor independent; they are constantly being modified and adapted to one another; their interdependence is ascribed to the fact that the various sense organs which supply the information on which the two schemata are based are usually simultaneously activated by any movement of our bodies. By a process of learning we see objects as having motion when we are either moving or stationary. Motion of an individual in space is always relative. At times, especially when our own sensory experience is incomplete, we mistake movement of our surroundings for movements of our own body as, for example, the feeling of movement which is experienced in a stationary train when a neighboring train is moving. Hence in this frame of reference, orientation of the body in space is possible only by the maintenance of an orderly relationship between the bodily schema and the schema of the external world; as a corollary, disorientation in space, or disequilibrium, occurs when this relationship is upset.

Disorders of equilibrium may thus have widely differing origins. They may be part of a syndrome which currently is regarded as psychogenic (anxiety neurosis); or there may be an abnormality of the proprioceptive mechanisms, the postural reflex centers, or the motor pathways. On clinical grounds, disorders of equilibrium may be divided into three groups: (1) true vertigo, (2) pseudovertigo, or giddiness, and (3) abnormalities of equilibrium without either vertigo or giddiness.

VERTIGO

Characteristics. In disorders in which vertigo is a leading symptom, the patient's history assumes special importance in diagnosis, for this symptom may be accompanied by no objective signs. The diagnosis of vertigo is an easy matter when the patient reports that objects in his environment spun around, or his body was turning, or his head was spinning. Very often, however, he is not so explicit. He may state that there was a feeling of to-and-fro or up-and-down movement of the body, usually the head; or he may relate that objects in his environment suddenly sank or rose up toward him or that he was pulled strongly to one side or to the ground. The feeling of impulsion is particularly characteristic of vertigo; the patient feels as though impelled or moved by some force acting outside his body. In walking he may have felt unsteady, tending to veer to one side. In exceptionally severe attacks the patient may without warning be thrown violently to the ground and only then experience vertigo, nausea, and vomiting. If vertigo is at all severe, equilibrium is almost invariably affected and the patient usually notes that his symptoms are especially troublesome when he attempts to sit, stand, and walk. With intense vertigo it may be impossible for him to do so. This type of gait disturbance, which depends on an abnormality of labyrinthine or vestibular function, may be called *vertiginous ataxia*. It is noteworthy that under these circumstances the coordination of individual movements of the limbs is never impaired. With milder degrees of vertigo, the patient may have difficulty in describing his symptoms. It may be of help to ask him whether his present symptoms are similar to the feelings of movement one experiences when coming to a halt after being rapidly rotated.

The symptoms of vertigo are usually paroxysmal and of short duration, but at times they may linger for weeks or even months. The chronic state may or may not follow an acute attack; in this latter instance the patient complains of a continuous state of imbalance, swaying, or a vague sense of movement in the environment. Characteristically the vertigo is made worse or may only become manifest on assuming the erect posture or on movement, so that the patient has to walk carefully and may become nervous about descending stairs or crossing a road.

Distinction between True and False Vertigo. It is important to distinguish clearly between true vertigo and a second group of symptoms which do not have the same significance (*pseudovertigo*). Some patients may describe a feeling of uncertainty, lightheadedness, or a swimming sensation; others may feel as though they were going to fall or were walking on air. These sensory phenomena are particularly common in psychoneurotic states, in introspective individuals with an overawareness of various parts of their body. They may complain of other peculiar aberrations as, for example, great lengthening of their legs or a sensation as if the ground were receding from beneath them. A feeling of lightheadedness is frequently brought about by hyperventilation, and similar symptoms often occur in patients with anemia, hypertension, and pulmonary disease, particularly emphysema. In anemia, mild hypoxia is the probable mechanism, and the same is probably true of emphysematous patients, in whom an attack of coughing may cause dizziness or even fainting, owing to impaired venous return to the heart (tussive syncope). The dizziness which so often accompanies hypertension is more difficult to evaluate. In some cases it may be due to an associated psychoneurosis; in others, one cannot be sure that it does not depend upon transient changes in the intracranial vasculature. A similar complaint is that of *postural* dizziness. Poorly conditioned individuals and many elderly people upon arising from a recumbent position or after stooping are troubled with a momentary giddiness or a swaying type of dizziness with dimming of vision or spots before the eyes. This is probably due to a momentary failure of reflex vasoconstriction in overcoming the "pooling" effect of gravity upon the circulating blood. This type of dizziness may occur in normal individuals on arising from a hot bath and is frequent in patients convalescing from debilitating illness. A mild syncopal reaction of any type may give rise to similar symptoms and be described by the patient as "dizziness." Finally, petit mal epilepsy may be referred to as a "dizzy spell."

In practice it is not difficult to separate these symptoms from true vertigo; there is not the feeling of rotation and impulsion so characteristic of the latter symptom. In addition, a number of ancillary symptoms accompany true vertigo, including varying degrees of nausea, vomiting, headache, pallor, and sweating. Actual loss of consciousness may occur as part of a vertiginous attack, but it is very rare and usually signifies another category of disorder such as syncope or convulsion. Both the vertigo and the nausea and vomiting are made worse by movement, so that characteristically the vertiginous patient remains immobile during an attack.

Neurologic Significance. A disorder of any of the following structures may give rise to vertigo:

1. Cerebral cortex
2. Ocular muscles
3. Cerebellum
4. Labyrinthine-vestibular apparatus
5. Brain stem

That vertigo may constitute the aura of an epileptic seizure gives support to the view that a *cortical lesion* can produce vertigo. This usually occurs with lesions of the temporal lobe, mainly on the lateral aspect of the middle and posterior portions or at the parietotemporal junction. The patients experience a sensation of movement, either of their body away from the side of stimulation or of the environment in the opposite direction. This observation also supports the concept that the sensation of vertigo depends largely on the perception of relative movement between the body and the external world. Vertiginous seizures may occur very rarely as a reflex phenomenon, the result of vestibular (e.g., caloric) stimulation.

Ocular disturbances may give rise to vertigo and may even be accompanied by staggering and nausea; this occurs most frequently at the outset of an ocular muscle paralysis when the patient looks in the direction of action of the paralyzed muscle. The vertigo is apparently due to a faulty projection of the visual field, the patient being presented with two conflicting images. Some people experience a type of giddiness or uncertainty when wearing bifocal lenses for the first time. The necessity of adapting to an unusual visual environment, as in looking down from a height, may result in a similar sensation.

Whether *lesions of the cerebellum* are capable of producing vertigo seems to depend on what portion of this structure is involved. Thus vertigo may be absent despite large lesions of the cerebellar hemispheres but may be present if the vestibulocerebellar connections are damaged.

Although cortical, ocular, and cerebellar causes should all be considered in the differential diagnosis of vertigo, they are clinically uncommon. Usually the problem resolves itself into deciding whether vertigo has its origin in the labyrinth, in the vestibular division of the eighth cranial nerve, or in the vestibular nuclei and their immediate connections with other structures in the brain stem. A number of features, especially the form of the attack and the associated symptoms, help one to make this decision.

Vertigo of labyrinthine origin (aural vertigo) tends to occur in paroxysmal attacks. It has an abrupt onset, is maximal at the beginning, and subsides in a matter of minutes or in an hour or two. Similarly the nausea, vomiting, pallor, immobility, and ataxia associated with the attack are short-lived. The accompanying nystagmus tends also to be transient and characteristically is rather fine, rotatory, and most pronounced when the eyes are turned away from the offending labyrinth. Occasionally, patients with labyrinthine disease may have a more chronic form of vertigo. However, it seldom continues for more than a few days or weeks, the central mechanisms apparently compensating for the peripheral lesion. Labyrinthine vertigo is frequently associated with deafness and tinnitus, since the pathologic process in the inner ear encroaches on the cochlear apparatus.

Ménière's syndrome is the name applied to recurrent aural vertigo, accompanied by tinnitus and deafness. The latter symptoms are usually, but not always, present before the onset of vertigo and are increased in severity during an acute attack. With milder forms of the syndrome the patient may complain more of head discomfort and of difficulty in concentration than of vertigo and may be thought to be neurotic. Provided that deafness is not complete, the recruitment phenomena can be demonstrated (p. 294). Ménière's syndrome has its onset most frequently in the fifth decade of life, though young adults and the elderly are not spared. The pathologic changes in Ménière's syndrome consist of a distention of the membranous labyrinth and a degeneration of the organ of Corti, although the relation of these changes to paroxysmal disorder of labyrinthine function is unknown. During an acute attack, rest in bed is the most effective treatment, since the patient can usually find a position in which no vertigo is present. Dimenhydrinate (Dramamine) in doses of 25 to 50 mg t.i.d. is useful in the more protracted cases. A low-salt diet is still a generally accepted treatment, but its usefulness is difficult to judge. Usually the deafness is progressive, and when it is complete the vertiginous attacks cease. However, the course is variable, and where the attacks persist in a severe manner, permanent relief can be obtained by surgical destruction of the labyrinth or section of the vestibular portion of the eighth nerve intracranially.

Another disorder of labyrinthine function is characterized by the occurrence of paroxysmal vertigo and nystagmus, with the assumption of certain critical positions of the head. This is the *positional vertigo of Bárány,* or the so-called "benign paroxysmal type." A highly diagnostic feature of this disorder is the development of transient vertigo and rotary nystagmus when the patient rapidly assumes a supine position. The optimal position in which to bring out this disorder is to tip the patient backward with the head 30° below the level of the bed and rotated 30 to 45° to one side. On repetition of the test, the response is characteristically reduced or entirely absent. Deafness only rarely accompanies this disorder, and the presence of mild ear infections or other labyrinthine disease can be detected in only a small proportion of cases. It is thought that positional nystagmus of the benign paroxysmal type is due to a lesion of the otolith apparatus which results in a qualitatively abnormal response to the positional stimulus.

There are many other causes of aural vertigo, such as purulent labyrinthitis complicating meningitis, serous labyrinthitis due to infection of the middle ear, "toxic labyrinthitis" due to drug intoxication (e.g., from alcohol, quinine, streptomycin, and salicylates), motion sickness, trauma and hemorrhage into the internal ear. In these instances the attacks of vertigo tend to last longer than in the recurrent form, but in other respects the symptomatology is similar. The causative role of occlusive vascular disease in the genesis of aural vertigo has not been pathologically settled, but has been postulated on clinical grounds. There are patients who suffer the abrupt onset of severe vertigo, nausea, and vomiting without tinnitus or deafness, in whom the vertigo tends to persist for several weeks and labyrinthine function is permanently ablated. Occlusion of the labyrinthine division of the internal auditory artery would logically explain this syndrome.

Vertigo of vestibular nerve origin may occur with diseases that involve the nerve in the petrous bone or the cerebellopontine angle. Except that it is less severe and is less frequently paroxysmal, it has many of the characteristics of labyrinthine vertigo. The adjacent auditory division of the eighth cranial nerve may also be affected, which explains the frequent coincidence of tinnitus and deafness. The function of the eighth cranial nerve may be disturbed by tumors of the lateral recess (especially acoustic neuroma), as well as by meningeal inflammation in this region or, very rarely, by compression from an abnormal vessel.

Under the titles of *vestibular neuronitis* and *epidemic vertigo,* there has been described a clinical state, occurring mainly in young adults, and characterized by the abrupt onset of vertigo, nausea, and vomiting, without impairment of hearing. Otoscopic examination and tests of cochlear function disclose no abnormality, but the caloric responses are reduced, usually on both sides. The symptoms are benign, subsiding, as a rule, in 2 to 3 weeks. Although many of the reported cases have been associated with signs of systemic disease, and a few with signs of polyarteritis nodosa, the exact cause remains unknown. Similarly, the precise site of the lesion is not known, although it has been the subject of considerable speculation.

Cogan has described a peculiar syndrome in young adults, in which a nonsyphilitic interstitial keratitis is associated with vertigo, tinnitus, nystagmus, and rapidly progressive deafness. The prognosis for life and vision is good, but the deafness is usually permanent. The etiology of this disease is not understood, although several cases later developed periarteritis nodosa.

The vertigo of brain stem origin usually lasts much longer than aural vertigo and may disorganize the patient's equilibrium for several weeks or even longer. In these cases, auditory function is usually spared, since vestibular and cochlear fibers become separated soon after entering the brain stem. It is a fairly reliable clinical rule that the combination of auditory and vestibular symptoms occurs only in diseases that involve the inner ear or eighth cranial nerve. The nystagmus accompanying central lesions tends to be coarse and protracted, is more marked on lateral gaze to one side than the other, and may have a vertical component, particularly on upward gaze. Vertical nystagmus nearly always indicates disease of the brain stem. A small plaque of multiple sclerosis may affect vestibular connections, and this diagnosis should always be considered when a young person has a severe and protracted attack of vertigo without auditory symptoms. Vascular and neoplastic lesions may also give rise to vertigo through involvement of the vestibular nuclei and their immediate connections. In addition, there may be signs of interference with the long sensory and motor tracts which pass through the brain stem. This feature clearly points to a brain stem location of the lesion and is, in the final analysis, the most important point in differentiation from aural vertigo.

DIAGNOSIS

When the patient's complaint is dizziness, it is first necessary to obtain a clear description of the symptoms. The element of rotation or a similar sensation, the sense of impulsion, and the accompanying nausea and vomiting, if present, usually distinguish the case of true vertigo from one of giddiness. The latter has no element of rotation or impulsion, and nausea, vomiting, tinnitus, and deafness are absent. Although fearful of falling or swooning, the patient can nonetheless walk without difficulty if forced to do so. Blurred vision, smothering and choking feelings, palpitation, trembling, sweating, and a sense of fear or apprehension complete the usual clinical picture of neurotic dizziness. Frequently in cases of recurrent aural vertigo or Ménière's syndrome, the symptoms of anxiety and depression may be added to the total clinical picture, which adds to the difficulty of interpretation.

If the physician is uncertain as to whether the patient has vertigo or giddiness, it is sometimes helpful to induce these sensations in order that the patient may compare them with his usual attacks. This can be done by having the patient breathe deeply for 3 min (which causes giddiness in most people), stoop over for a minute and then straighten up (postural giddiness), and while standing, turn rapidly in one direction ten times in order to provoke vertigo. If the patient fails to distinguish these sensations, his history is probably inaccurate, and he should be asked to take careful note of his sensations during his next spontaneous attack.

In some cases the attack may be so abrupt and severe that the patient falls immediately to the ground without loss of consciousness. Here the diagnosis may be clarified by the nausea, vomiting, and dizziness which almost invariably follow such a fall. If the vertigo has been very mild in degree, it is helpful to elicit a history of disinclination to walk during the attack, a tendency to list to one side, discomfort in sitting or riding in a vehicle, and a preference for maintaining one position fixedly.

A neurologic examination, including tests of ocular movements and nystagmus, cranial nerve function, gait, and coordination of limbs, should be carried out on all patients with dizziness as the presenting complaint. The eardrums should be inspected and hearing tested by the methods indicated in Chap. 31, Disturbances of Cranial Nerve Function. Vestibular function should also be tested. This is usually done by irrigating the ear with 5 ml ice water, the head being tilted back 30° from the vertical, since in this position the horizontal canal is stimulated maximally. The normal labyrinthine responses consist of falling to the side of the vestibular lesion, past pointing to that side, and rotary nystagmus on gaze to the opposite side. The nystagmus begins about 20 sec after the irrigation and persists for 90 to 120 sec. The duration of these periods is variable, however, and more important is the comparison of the affected and normal labyrinths.

DISTURBANCES OF GAIT

Probably no aspect of neurology is more interesting or affords greater opportunity for brilliant diagnosis than the study and analysis of gait.

The normal gait seldom attracts attention. The body is erect, the head straight, and the arms hang loosely and gracefully at the sides, each moving rhythmically forward with the opposite leg. The feet are slightly everted, and the steps are of moderate length and approximately equal. With each step there is a coordinated flexion of hip and knee and dorsiflexion of foot and a barely perceptible elevation of the hip so that the foot clears the ground. The heel strikes the ground first, and inspection of shoes will show that this is the part most subject to wear. In the erect posture, the muscles of greatest importance in the maintenance of equilibrium are the erector spinae and the extensors of the hips and knees.

There are many individual variations of gait, and it is a commonplace observation that the sound of an individual's footsteps, notably his pace and heaviness of tread, may permit his identification. The manner of walking and the carriage of the body provide clues to the character and personality of a person and sometimes indicate his occupation. Furthermore, the gaits of the male and the female differ, the steps of the latter being quicker and the movement of the trunk and hips more graceful and delicate. Certain female characteristics of gait, if observed in the male, immediately impart an impression of femininity; or male characteristics in the female, one of masculinity.

When confronted with a disorder of gait, the examiner must observe the patient's natural stance and the attitude and dominant positions of the legs, trunk, and arms. It is good practice to watch the patient as he walks into the examining room, because he is apt to walk more naturally then than during special tests. He should be asked to stand with his feet together, head erect, and eyes first open and then closed. Swaying due to nervousness may be overcome by asking that he touch the finger first of one hand, then of the other, to the tip of his nose. Next the patient should be asked to walk forward and backward, first with his eyes open and then with them closed. Any tendency to reel to one side, as in cerebellar disease, can be checked by having him walk around a chair. When the affected side is toward the chair, the patient tends to walk into it; and when it is away from the chair, he veers outward in ever-widening circles. More delicate tests of gait are walking a straight line heel-to-toe (Frankel's test) or having the patient arise quickly from a chair and walk briskly, and then stop or turn suddenly (Fournier's tests). If all these tests are successfully executed, it may be assumed that any difficulty in locomotion is not due to disease of the proprioceptive mechanisms or cerebellum. Detailed neurologic examination is then necessary in order to determine which of the many other possible diseases is responsible for the patient's disorder of gait.

The following abnormal gaits are so distinctive that with a little practice they can be recognized at a glance.

Cerebellar Gait. In the cerebellum the proprioceptive impulses from the body musculature are integrated with the cerebral impulses concerned with motion. By its efferent connections the cerebellum exerts a coordinating influence upon the action of voluntary muscles. The main features of cerebellar disease in regard to gait are *wide base* (separation of legs), *unsteadiness, irregularity,* and *lateral reeling.* Steps are short and uncertain, with sudden lurching to one side or the other. The unsteadiness is more prominent on quickly arising from a chair and walking, on stopping suddenly while walking, or on turning abruptly. If the ataxia is severe, the patient cannot stand without assistance. Standing with feet together and head erect, with eyes either open or closed, may be difficult. In its mildest form the ataxia is best demonstrated by having the patient walk a line heel-to-toe. After two or three steps he loses his balance and must step to one side

to avoid falling. The Romberg sign, i.e., marked swaying or falling with the eyes closed but not with the eyes open, is not a feature of cerebellar disease. The abnormality of gait may or may not be accompanied by other signs of cerebellar incoordination and intention tremor of the arms and legs. The presence of the latter signs depends on involvement of the cerebellar hemispheres as distinct from midline structures; if the lesion is unilateral they are always on the same side. Cerebellar gait is most commonly seen in multiple sclerosis, medulloblastoma of the cerebellar vermis, and the cerebellar atrophies.

Gait of Sensory Ataxia. This is due to an impairment of kinesthetic sensation resulting from interruption of afferent nerve fibers in the peripheral nerves, posterior roots, posterior columns of the spinal cord, or medial lemnisci; it may also be produced by a lesion of both parietal lobes. Whatever the location of the lesion, the patient is deprived of knowledge of the position of his limbs. The principal features of the resulting gait disorder are the *uncertainty,* the *irregularity,* and the *stamp* of the feet. Hunt characterized this type of gait very well when he said that the ataxic patient is recognized by "his stamp and his stick." There is great difficulty in standing and walking, and in advanced cases there is a complete failure of locomotion, although muscular power is retained. The legs are kept far apart to correct the instability, and the patient carefully watches the ground and his legs. As he steps out the legs are flung brusquely forward and outward, often being lifted higher than necessary. The steps are of variable length, and many are attended by an audible stamp as the feet are banged down on the floor. The body is held in a slightly flexed position, and the weight may be supported on the cane which the severely ataxic patient so often carries. The incoordination is greatly exaggerated when the patient is deprived of visual cues, as in walking in the dark. If asked to stand with feet together and eyes closed, he shows increased swaying or actual falling (Romberg's sign). It has been said that a lame man whose shoes are not worn in any one place is probably suffering from sensory ataxia. There is almost invariably a loss of vibratory and position sense in the feet and legs. Gaits of this type are observed in tabes dorsalis, Friedreich's ataxia, subacute combined degeneration, syphilitic meningomyelitis, chronic polyneuritis, and those cases of multiple sclerosis in which posterior column disease predominates.

Hemiplegic and Paraplegic (Spastic) Gaits. In hemiplegia the leg is held rigidly and does not swing freely and gracefully at the knee and hip. It tends to rotate outward and describes a semicircle, first away from and then toward the trunk (circumduction). The foot scrapes along the floor, and the outer side of the sole of the shoe is worn. One can diagnose the hemiplegic gait by hearing the slow rhythmic scuff of the foot along the floor. The other muscles of the body on the affected side are weak and stiff to a variable degree, particularly the arm, which is carried in a flexed position and does not swing naturally. This type of gait disorder is most frequent after vascular disease of the brain.

The spastic paraplegic gait is entirely different from the gait of sensory ataxia, though the two may be combined. Each leg is advanced slowly and stiffly with restricted motion at the knee and hip. The patient looks as though he were wading in water or walking in thick mud. The legs are extended or slightly bent at the knees and may be strongly adducted at the hips, tending almost to cross ("scissors gait"). The steps are regular and short. The forepart of the shoe becomes worn because there is a tendency for the advancing foot not to clear the ground. Movements are generally slow and the patient may be able to advance only with great effort. The laity have referred to this state as "creeping palsy." An easy way to remember the main features of this gait is by the letter S, which begins each of its descriptive adjectives—spastic, slow, scuffing. Multiple sclerosis, cerebral spastic diplegia, syringomyelia, spinal syphilis, combined system disease, and spinal cord compression are the common causes of spastic paraparesis.

Festinating Gait. This term comes from the Latin word *festinatio* meaning "haste" and is appropriate for the gait disorder of both paralysis agitans and postencephalitic Parkinson's syndrome. The general attitude is one of flexion. Rigidity or immobility of the body is another conspicuous feature. The trunk is bent forward, and the arms are carried ahead of the body. There is a paucity of the automatic movements made in sitting, standing, and walking. The arms do not swing; the head does not turn on looking to one side; the arms are never folded, nor the legs crossed. The hands are held stiffly as though in preparation for writing, and the facial expression is unblinking and masklike. The legs are stiff and bent at knee and hip. The steps are short, and the feet barely clear the ground as the patient shuffles along. Once forward or backward locomotion is started, the upper part of the body advances ahead of the lower part, as though the patient were chasing his center of gravity. His steps become more and more rapid, and he may fall if not given assistance. This is the festination, and it may occur when the patient is walking forward or backward, taking the form of either propulsion or retropulsion. *Rigidity, shuffling,* and *festination* are the cardinal features of this gait; when they are joined to the typical tremors, generalized rigidity, and slowness of movement there can be no doubt as to the diagnosis. Other unusual gaits are sometimes observed in the postencephalitic

patient. For example, he may be unable to take his first step forward until he hops or takes one step backward; or walking may be initiated by a series of short steps which give way to a more normal gait; occasionally such a patient may run better than he walks.

Athetotic, Dystonic, and Choreic Gaits. These are less common than the preceding gait disorders. The athetotic patient is rigid, and his body often assumes the most grotesque postures. One arm may be held aloft and the other one behind the body with wrist and fingers alternately undergoing slow flexion, extension, and rotation. The head may be inclined in one direction, the lips alternately retract and then purse, and the tongue intermittently protrudes from the mouth. The legs advance slowly and awkwardly. Sometimes the foot is plantar flexed at the ankle, and the weight is carried on the toes; or it may be dorsiflexed or inverted. This type of gait is typical of congenital athetosis.

In dystonia musculorum deformans the first symptom may be a limp due to inversion or plantar flexion of the foot or a distortion of the pelvis. The patient stands with one leg rigidly extended or one shoulder elevated. The trunk may be in a position of exaggerated lordosis, and the hips are partly flexed, with a tilting forward of the pelvis. Because of the muscle spasms which deform the body in this manner, the patient must walk with knees flexed. The gait may seem normal as the first steps are taken, but as the patient walks, one or both legs become flexed, giving rise to the "dromedary gait." In the more advanced stages walking becomes impossible, owing to torsion of the trunk or the continuous flexion of one leg.

In *chorea* the gait is often bizarre. As the patient stands or walks there is a continuous play of irregular "choreic" movements affecting the face, neck, and hands, and in the advanced stages the large proximal joints and trunk. The positions of the trunk and upper parts of the body vary with each step. There are jerks of the head, grimacing, squirming, and twisting movements of the trunk and limbs, and peculiar respiratory noises. The general features of these conditions are described more fully in Chaps. 27 and 290.

Steppage, Drop-foot, or Equine Gait. This is caused by paralysis of the pretibial and peroneal muscles. The legs must be lifted abnormally high in order to clear the ground. There is a flapping noise as the foot strikes the floor. The anterior and lateral border of the sole becomes worn. The steps are regular and even; otherwise walking is not remarkable. The steppage gait may be unilateral or bilateral and occurs in diseases which affect the peripheral nerves of the legs or motor neurones in the spinal cord, such as poliomyelitis, progressive muscular atrophy, and Charcot-Marie-Tooth disease (peroneal muscular atrophy). It is also observed in patients with peripheral types of muscular dystrophy.

Waddling Gait. This gait is characteristic of progressive muscular dystrophy. The attitude of the body may be straight, but more often there is accentuation of the lumbar lordosis. The steps are regular but a little uncertain. With each step there is an exaggerated elevation of the hip, and once the weight is put on this hip, it yields to an abnormal degree so that the upper trunk then inclines to that side. This alternation of lateral trunk movements results in the rolling gait or *waddle*, a term suggested by Oppenheim. The gluteal musculature is weak and inefficient, although leg muscles may appear well developed. Muscular contractures may lead to an equinovarus position of the foot, particularly in childhood cases, so that the waddle is combined with circumduction of the legs and "walking on the toes."

Staggering or Drunken Gait. In the drunken gait the patient totters, reels, tips forward and then backward, threatening each moment to lose his balance and fall. Control over trunk and legs is greatly impaired. The steps are irregular and uncertain. There is a wide diversity of excursions of all parts of the body. The reeling is in many different directions, unlike the cerebellar gait, and no effort is made to correct it by watching the legs or the ground, as in sensory ataxia. The patient appears stupefied and indifferent to the quality of his performances, but under certain circumstances he can momentarily correct his defect. A staggering gait is characteristic of alcoholic and barbiturate intoxication. The gait in severe disease of the cerebellum may be similar, but it is not so irregular and bizarre.

Hysterical Gait. This may take any one of several forms. The patient may have a hysterical monoplegia, paraplegia, or hemiplegia; the muscles may be rigid with contracture or may be flaccid. The paralysis is usually of sudden onset and complete, though under unexpected stress the patient may move the affected part. The monoplegic or hemiplegic patient does not lift the foot from the floor while walking; instead he drags it as a useless member or pushes it ahead of him as though it were a skate. The characteristic circumduction is absent in hysterical hemiplegia, and the typical hemiplegic posture, the hyperactive tendon reflexes, and Babinski signs are missing. The hysterical paraplegic cannot very well drag both legs, and usually he depends on a crutch or remains helpless in bed, sometimes with severe contractures. The hysterical paraplegic gait may be quite dramatic. Some patients look as though they were walking on stilts, and others lurch wildly in all directions, actually demonstrating by their gyrations the most remarkable ability to make rapid postural adjustments.

Astasia-abasia, in which the patient, though unable to either stand or walk, retains normal use of his legs while in bed, is nearly always hysterical. When such a patient is placed on his feet, he takes a few normal steps then becomes unable to advance his feet; he lurches wildly and crumples to the floor if not given assistance.

Senile Gait. Elderly people often complain of difficulty in walking, and examination may disclose no abnormality other than the slightly flexed posture of the "senile" and the short uncertain steps, *marche à petits pas.* At times the patient halts to advance without great effort, but with a little assistance he does much better. Speed, balance, and all the graceful, adaptive movements are lost.

Frontal Lobe Ataxia. Equilibrium and the capacity to stand and walk may be severely disturbed by diseases which affect the frontal lobes, particularly their medial parts. Although this disorder is spoken of as an ataxia, it really represents an apraxia of gait, since the difficulty in walking cannot be accounted for by weakness or loss of sensation alone. The movements become slow, hesitant, and poorly directed, and at the same time dementia may develop. Grasping, groping, hyperactive tendon reflexes, and bilateral Babinski signs may or may not be present. One of the unique features of this disorder is a failure to perform certain skilled movements, even though the capacity for crude movement is retained. In some of the reported examples of this disorder, however, all movements of the legs are slow, hesitant, and awkward, and the limbs when passively moved offer variable resistance (gegenhalten). Such cases have characteristics of both extrapyramidal (Parkinsonian) and premotor cortical disorder (magnetic apraxia of Denny-Brown). Pronounced degrees of this difficulty interfere with locomotion. There is difficulty in standing and walking and even of turning in bed. The end result is a "cerebral paraplegia in flexion." If one frontal lobe is affected, an awkwardness of movement appears in the opposite arm and leg, simulating cerebellar ataxia at times, except for the absence of intention tremor, pendular reflexes, Holmes' rebound sign, etc. This apractic motor defect is discussed further in Chap. 26.

REFERENCES

Alpers, B. J.: "Vertigo and Dizziness." Modern Medical Monographs, New York, Grune & Stratton, Inc., 1958.

Brain, W. R.: Vertigo, Brit. Med. J., p. 605, Sept. 17, 1938.

Citron, L., and C. S. Hallpike: Observations upon the Mechanism of Positional Nystagmus of the So-called "Benign Paroxysmal Type," J. Laryngol. and Otol., 70:253, 1956.

Symonds, C.: The Significance of Vertigo in Neurological Diagnosis, J. Laryngol. and Otol., 66:295, 1952.

31 DISTURBANCES OF CRANIAL NERVE FUNCTION

Maurice Victor and Raymond D. Adams

The cranial nerves subserve the special senses—vision, hearing, taste, and smell—and govern the movements of the eyes, jaws, face, larynx, pharynx, tongue, and respiratory muscles. A knowledge of the anatomy of the cranial nerves is particularly important. In the case of intramedullary lesions, it enables us to localize accurately the segment of brain stem involved, and in extramedullary lesions to recognize a variety of neurologic syndromes involving single cranial nerves or several nerves as they lie in relationship to one another and to the brain.

In this chapter each of the cranial nerves will be considered in turn. In relation to each nerve certain anatomic features will first be discussed, but only those which have an immediate clinical application; then the methods of examination and the disorders of function will be described.

THE FIRST, OR OLFACTORY, NERVE

Olfactory nerve fibers have their cells of origin in the mucous membrane of the superior part of the nasal cavity. They pass as fine filaments through the cribriform plate of the ethmoid bone and synapse with cells in the olfactory bulb. The axones of these cells form the olfactory tract, which courses along the olfactory groove of the frontal bone and terminates mainly in the anterior (ventral) part of the uncus and to a lesser extent in the posterior part of the orbital cortex (the prepiriform area) and the anterior perforated space. The further central connections of the olfactory impulses are not fully known.

The first nerve is generally not tested unless the patient complains of loss of smell or is suspected of having disease at the base of the brain. The patient may not always realize that his principal difficulty is one of olfactory anesthesia. Instead he may complain of loss of taste (ageusia), because taste depends largely on the volatile substances in foods and beverages, and the sensation of flavor is a combination of smell and taste.

To test the sense of smell the patient is asked to close his eyes and, with first one nostril blocked and then the other, to sniff several test odors. Coffee, peppermint, cloves, and tobacco are satisfactory stimuli. Ammonia and similar pungent substances should not be used because they stimulate the trigeminal nerves. If the patient can detect odors in each nostril, even if he cannot name them, it may be assumed that the olfactory nerves are intact.

Anosmia, or loss of the sense of smell, may occur after fractures through the anterior cranial fossa, with severe head injuries, with meningiomas or gliomas in the inferior part of the frontal lobes, or in tabes dorsalis. However, the diagnostic value of this finding is lessened by the fact that upper respiratory infections may produce a similar effect by obstructing the nasal passages or injuring the olfactory mucosa and nerve filaments.

Parosmia, or perversion of the sense of smell, may occur with local nasal conditions such as empyema of the paranasal sinuses. Minor degrees of this phenomenon are not necessarily abnormal for unpleasant odors have a way of lingering and being reawakened by other olfactory stimuli for several hours.

Olfactory hallucinations are always of central origin. As described on pp. 333 and 334, a disagreeable odor may be the aura of a seizure. The evocative lesion is usually in the inferior and medial part of one or the other temporal lobe, in or near the uncus, and the seizure it produces is therefore called *uncinate.* Also, schizophrenic patients sometimes complain of disagreeable odors emanating from their bodies and causing other people to shun them. These olfactory experiences rarely have the objectivity of a hallucination but are rather in the nature of a delusion. The sense of smell is demonstrably intact.

THE SECOND, OR OPTIC, NERVE

The first neuronal elements in the visual pathway are the rod and cone cells situated in the deepest layer of the retina. The cones are responsible for sharp vision and color discrimination, and they alone are present in the fovea. The rods, which are more sensitive to low intensities of light, predominate in the rest of the retina. The visual impulses are then transmitted through the second system of neurones, the bipolar cells, to the ganglion cells, whose axones form the optic nerve by perforating the sclera at the optic disk, creating a sievelike structure, the lamina cribrosa. The absence of visual end organs at this point accounts for the blind spot in the field of vision. Thus, the optic nerve is actually a part of the central nervous system, with glial cells between its fibers but no Schwann cells as in the other cranial and spinal nerves. The optic nerves extend from the disk to the optic chiasm, where their fibers undergo partial decussation (Fig. 31-1). The rearranged optic fibers continue as the optic tract, which partially encircles the cerebral peduncles and synapses with cells in the lateral geniculate body. From these cells arises the fourth system of neurones, the final visual pathway, comprising the geniculocalcarine tract and the optic radiations. These fibers lie close to the wall of the temporal horn of the lateral ventricle. The upper ones take a direct course posteriorly, the lower ones loop forward over the temporal horn of the lateral ventricle into the temporal lobe (Meyer's loop) before they pass posteriorly and join the upper fibers on their way to the calcarine cortex.

In the assessment of any patient complaining of impaired vision, it is first necessary to exclude primary ocular disease (e.g., glaucoma, refractive errors) before assuming that the defect is one of the nervous pathways. Examination of the optic nerve includes tests of visual acuity, plotting of visual fields, and inspection of the fundi. Distant vision may be accurately tested by means of a Snellen chart. The capacity to read ordinary newsprint indicates that central vision is approximately normal. The visual fields can be plotted at the bedside by the confrontation test. With one of the patient's eyes covered and the other looking into the corresponding eye of the examiner (patient's right eye and examiner's left), a moving target, such as a finger or a white pinhead, is brought from outside toward the center of the visual field. With the target placed equally distant between the examiner's and patient's eyes, the patient's fields are compared with those of the examiner. In young children or uncooperative patients the integrity of the fields may be roughly estimated by observing whether the patient is attracted to objects in his peripheral field, or whether he blinks in response to sudden threatening gestures in one-half the visual field. In every case of suspected visual field defect, perimetric tests should be done, and the Bjerrum tangent screen should be used for finding and outlining scotomas. Fundoscopic examination completes the examination of the second nerve. Since the retinas and optic nerves are direct outpouchings of the brain, they represent in a sense small windows to the intracranial structures. Thus an increase in intracranial pressure is manifested by a swelling of the optic disks ("choked disk," or papilledema), and in cases of hypertension the retinal arterioles reflect more or less accurately the state of the arterioles of the brain.

The types of visual field defect resulting from lesions in different parts of the visual pathways are shown in Fig. 31-1. A prechiasmal lesion causes

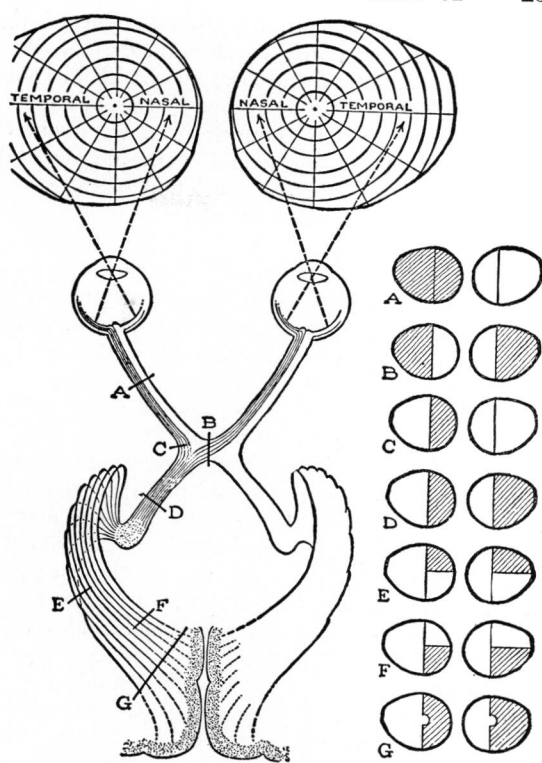

Fig. 31-1. Diagram showing the effects on the fields of vision produced by lesions at various points along the optic pathway. *A,* complete blindness in left eye; *B,* bitemporal hemianopsia; *C,* nasal hemianopsia of left eye; *D,* right homonymous hemianopsia; *E* and *F,* right upper and lower quadrant hemianopsias; *G,* right homonymous hemianopsia with preservation of central vision. (*Homans: "A Textbook of Surgery,"* Springfield, Ill., *Charles C Thomas, Publisher,* 1945.)

either a *scotoma* (an island of impaired vision within the visual field) or a cut in the peripheral part of the visual field. A small scotoma in the macular part of the visual field may seriously impair visual acuity. Demyelinative diseases, toxic (methyl alcohol, quinine) or nutritional disorders, and vascular disease involving the papillomacular bundle in the optic nerve are the usual causes of central scotomas. The toxic and nutritional states cause bilateral and more or less symmetrical scotomas; the vascular lesions cause unilateral scotomas, while demyelinative diseases give unilateral or asymmetrical bilateral scotomas. If the lesion is near the optic disk, there may be swelling of the optic nerve head, i.e., papillitis, which can usually be distinguished from papilledema by the marked impairment of vision which it produces.

Another common defect encountered on visual field examination is concentric constriction. This may be due to papilledema, in which case it is usually accompanied by an enlargement of the blind spot. A concentric constriction of the visual field, at first unilateral and later bilateral, and pallor of the optic disks (optic atrophy) should suggest chronic syphilitic optic neuritis. The treatment of neurosyphilis with tryparsamide frequently produced an acute bilateral constriction of the visual fields. Glaucoma is another cause of this type of field defect. Tubular vision, i.e., a constriction of the visual field to the same degree regardless of the distance of the visual test stimulus from the eye, is a sign of hysteria. In organic disease the area of the constricted visual field enlarges as the distance between the patient and the stimulus increases.

Hemianopsia means blindness in one-half the visual field. *Bitemporal hemianopsia,* indicating a lesion of the decussating fibers of the optic chiasm, is usually due to tumors of the pituitary gland, of the infundibulum or third ventricle, to a meningioma of the diaphragm of the sella, or occasionally to a large suprasellar aneurysm of the circle of Willis. *Homonymous hemianopsia* (a loss of vision in corresponding halves of the visual fields) indicates a lesion of the visual pathway behind the chiasm and, if *complete,* gives no more information than that. An *incomplete homonymous hemianopsia,* however, has more localizing value: if the field defects in the two eyes are similar (congruous), the lesion is in the calcarine cortex; if incongruous, the visual fibers in the parietal or temporal lobe are implicated. Since the fibers from the peripheral lower quadrants of the retina extend for a variable distance into the temporal lobe, lesions of this lobe may be accompanied by a homonymous upper quadrantic field defect. Parietal lobe lesions may affect the lower quadrants more than the upper.

If the entire optic tract or calcarine cortex on one side is destroyed, there is a complete homonymous hemianopsia, including half the field which represents the macula. Incomplete lesions of the optic tract and radiation, as well as lesions of the anterior part of the calcarine cortex, may spare the central (macular) vision. It must be kept in mind that apparent macular sparing is frequently due to imperfect fixation of gaze. A lesion of the tip of one occipital lobe produces a central homonymous hemianopsia, because half the macular fibers of both eyes terminate there. Lesions of both occipital poles result in bilateral central scotomas; and if all the calcarine cortex on each side is destroyed, there is complete "cortical" blindness. Altitudinal or horizontal hemianopsias are nearly always due to lesions of the occipital lobes below or above the calcarine cortex.

In addition to blindness, i.e., visual anesthesia, there is another category of visual impairment, which consists of a defect of visual perception, i.e., *visual agnosia.* The patient can see but cannot recognize objects unless he hears, smells, tastes, or palpates the object in question. The failure of visual recognition of words is called *alexia.* Lesions producing visual object agnosia are usually bilateral in the parietooccipital regions and the white matter beneath the angular gyri; those producing alexia are in the region of the major angular gyrus.

The optic nerves also contain the afferent fibers for the pupillary reflexes. These fibers leave the optic tract and terminate in the superior colliculi. A lesion of the optic nerve or tract may abolish the pupillary light reflex; the pupil is dilated and unreactive. Cerebral lesions, on the other hand, leave the pupillary light reflex unaltered. The lack of direct reflex in the blind eye and of consensual reflex in the sound one means that the afferent limb of the reflex arc (optic nerve) is the site of the lesion. A lack of direct light reflex with retention of the consensual reflex places the lesion in the efferent limb of the reflex arc (the homolateral oculomotor nucleus or nerve).

Amaurosis refers to blindness from any cause. *Amblyopia* refers to a dimness of vision not due to an error of refraction or some other disease of the eye. *Nyctalopia,* or night blindness, means poor twilight or night vision and is associated with vitamin A deficiency and retinitis pigmentosa.

THE THIRD, FOURTH, AND SIXTH NERVES

The oculomotor, trochlear, and abducens nerves innervate the extrinsic and intrinsic musculature of the eye. Their function is similar, and many diseases tend to involve all of them at once. It is customary, therefore, to discuss them together.

The oculomotor nucleus consists of several groups of nerve cells ventral to the aqueduct of Sylvius, at the level of the superior colliculi. The nerve cells which innervate the iris and ciliary body are situated anteriorly in the so-called "Edinger-Westphal nucleus." Below this nucleus are the cells for the superior rectus, inferior oblique, internal rectus, and inferior rectus, in that order from above downwards. Convergence is under the control of the medial groups of cells, the nuclei of Perlia. The cells of origin of the trochlear nerves are just inferior to those of the oculomotor nerves. The sixth nerve arises at a considerably lower level, from a paired group of cells in the floor of the fourth ventricle at the level of the lower pons. The intrapontine portion of the facial nerve loops around the sixth nerve nucleus before it turns anterolaterally to make its exit; a lesion in this locality usually causes a homolateral paralysis of both the lateral rectus and facial muscles.

All three nerves, after leaving the brain stem, course anteriorly and pass through the cavernous sinus, where they come into close proximity with the ophthalmic division of the fifth nerve, and together they enter the orbit through the superior orbital fissure. The oculomotor nerve supplies all the extrinsic ocular muscles except two—the superior oblique and the external rectus—which are innervated by the trochlear and abducens nerves, respectively. The voluntary part of the levator palpebrae muscle is also supplied by the oculomotor nerve, the involuntary part being under the control of autonomic fibers which also supply the sphincter pupillae and the ciliary muscles (muscles of accommodation).

Although all the extraocular muscles probably participate in every movement of the eyes, particular muscles are especially effective in moving the eye in certain fields. The lateral rectus rotates the eye outward; the medial rectus inward. The function of the vertical recti and the obliques varies according to the position of the eye. When the eye is turned outward, the elevators and depressors of the eye are the superior and inferior recti; when the eye is turned inward, they are the inferior and superior obliques, respectively. In contrast, torsion of the eyeball is effected by the oblique muscles when the eye is turned outward, and by the recti when it is turned inward.

Accurate binocular vision is achieved by the associated action of the ocular muscles, which allows a visual stimulus to fall on exactly corresponding parts of the two retinas. Conjugate movement of the eyes is controlled by centers in the cerebral cortex and brain stem. Area 8 in the frontal lobe is the center for voluntary conjugate movements of the eyes to the opposite side. In addition there is a center in the occipital lobe concerned with contralateral following movements. Fibers from these centers pass to the opposite sides of the brain stem, where they connect with lower centers for conjugate movements: those for right lateral gaze are in the proximity of the right abducens nucleus, those for left lateral gaze are near the left abducens. Simultaneous innervation of one internal rectus with the other external rectus during lateral gaze is a function of the medial longitudinal fasciculus. The arrangements of nerve cells and fibers for vertical gaze and convergence are situated in the superior colliculi and tegmental parts of the midbrain, respectively.

Pupil size is determined by the balance of innervation between the dilator and constrictor fibers. The pupillodilator fibers arise in the posterior part of the hypothalamus, descend in the lateral tegmentum of the midbrain, pons, medulla, and cervical spinal cord to the eighth cervical and first thoracic segments, where they synapse with the lateral horn cells. The latter give rise to preganglionic fibers which synapse in the superior cervical ganglion; the postganglionic fibers course along the internal carotid artery and traverse the cavernous

sinus to join the first division of the trigeminal nerve, finally reaching the eyes as the long ciliary nerves. The pupilloconstrictor fibers arise in the nucleus of Edinger-Westphal, join the oculomotor nerve, and synapse in the ciliary ganglion with the postganglionic neurones which innervate the iris and ciliary body.

The pupils are usually equal in size, though if the eyes are turned to one side the pupil of the abducting eye dilates slightly. Pupil size varies with light intensity; as one pupil constricts under a bright light (direct reflex), the other unexposed pupil does likewise (consensual reflex). Pupillary constriction is also a part of the act of convergence and accommodation for near objects.

Interruption of the sympathetic fibers either centrally, between the hypothalamus and their point of exit from the spinal cord, or peripherally, in the neck or along the carotid artery, results in miosis and ptosis (due to paralysis of the levator palpebrae), with loss of sweating of the face, and occasionally enophthalmos (*Bernard-Horner syndrome*). Stimulation or irritation of the pupillodilator fibers has the opposite effect, i.e., lid retraction, slight proptosis, and dilatation of the pupil. The ciliospinal pupillary reflex, evoked by pinching the neck, is effected through these efferent sympathetic fibers. Abnormal dilatation of the pupils (mydriasis), often with loss of pupillary light reflexes, may result from midbrain lesions and is a frequent finding in cases of deep coma. Extreme constriction of the pupils (miosis) is commonly observed in pontine hemorrhage, presumably because of bilateral interruption of the pupillodilator fibers.

The functional integrity of the sympathetic and parasympathetic nerve endings in the iris may be determined by the use of certain drugs. Atropine and homatropine dilate the pupils by paralyzing the parasympathetic nerve endings, while physostigmine and pilocarpine constrict them, the former by inhibiting cholinesterase activity and the latter by direct stimulation of the sphincter muscle of the iris. Cocaine dilates the pupils by stimulating the sympathetic nerve endings. Morphine acts centrally to constrict the pupils.

In chronic syphilitic meningitis and other forms of late syphilis, particularly tabes dorsalis, the pupils are usually small, irregular, and unequal, do not dilate properly in response to mydriatic drugs and fail to react to light, although they do constrict on accommodation. This is known as the *Argyll Robertson pupil*. The exact locality of the lesion is not known; it is generally believed to be in the tectum of the midbrain proximal to the oculomotor nuclei, where the descending pupillodilator fibers are in close proximity to the light-reflex fibers. The possibility of a partial third nerve lesion or a lesion of the ciliary ganglion has not been excluded. A

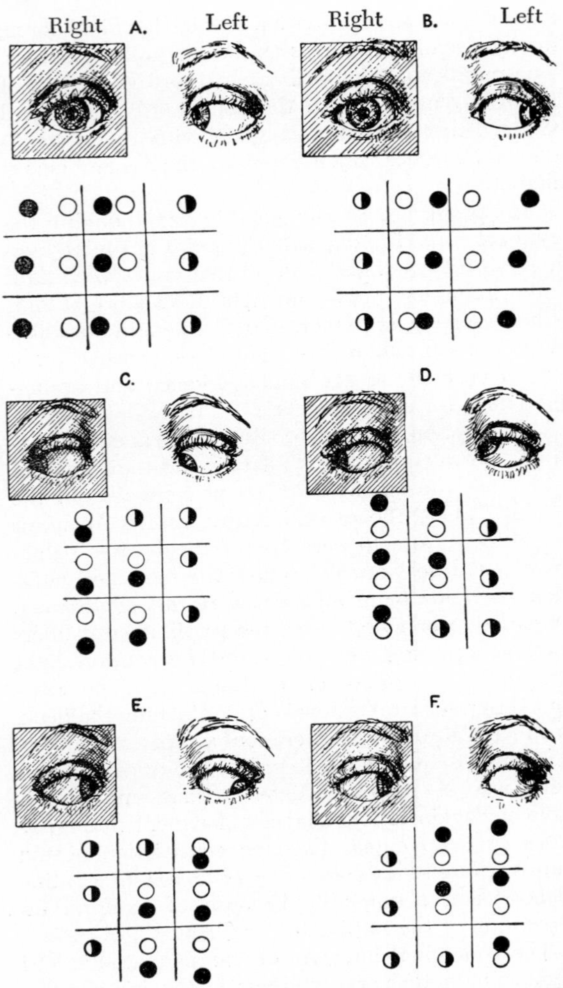

FIG. 31-2. Diplopia fields with individual muscle paralyses. The dark glass is in front of the right eye, and the fields are projected as the patient sees the images. A. Paralysis of right external rectus. Characteristic: right eye does not move to the right. Field: horizontal homonymous diplopia increasing on looking to the right. B. Paralysis of right internal rectus. Characteristic: right eye does not move to the left. Field: horizontal crossed diplopia increasing on looking to the left. C. Paralysis of right inferior rectus. Characteristic: right eye does not move downward when eyes are turned to the right. Field: vertical diplopia (image of right eye lowermost) increasing on looking to the right and down. D. Paralysis of right superior rectus. Characteristic: right eye does not move upward when eyes are turned to the right. Field: vertical diplopia (image of right eye uppermost) increasing on looking to the right and up. E. Paralysis of right superior oblique. Characteristic: right eye does not move downward when eyes are turned to the left. Field: vertical diplopia (image of right eye lowermost) increasing on looking to left and down. F. Paralysis of right inferior oblique. Characteristic: right eye does not move upward when eyes are

dissociation of the light reflex from the accommodation-convergence reaction is sometimes observed in other midbrain lesions, e.g., pinealoma and multiple sclerosis, and also in diabetes mellitus. In these diseases miosis, irregularity of pupils, and failure to respond to a mydriatic are not constantly present. Another interesting pupillary abnormality is the myotonic reaction, sometimes referred to as *Adie's pupil*. The patient may complain of blurring of vision or may have suddenly noticed that one pupil is larger than the other. The reaction to light and convergence are absent if tested in the customary manner, although the size of the pupil will change slowly on prolonged stimulation. Once contracted or dilated, the pupils remain in that state for some minutes. The affected pupil reacts promptly to the usual mydriatic and miotic drugs but is unusually sensitive to 2.5 per cent solution of mecholyl, a strength which will not affect a normal pupil. The myotonic pupil usually makes its appearance during the third or fourth decade and may be associated with absence of knee jerks, and hence be mistaken for tabes dorsalis.

There are three types of paralysis of extraocular muscles: (1) paralysis of isolated ocular muscles, (2) paralysis of conjugate movements (gaze), and (3) syndromes of mixed gaze and ocular muscle paralysis.

Ocular Muscle Palsies. These are among the most common neurologic signs. If an individual ocular muscle is weak or paralyzed, there is a deficiency of movement of the affected eye in the direction of traction of the paretic muscle. The perfect alignment of the two eyes is lost, with a resulting strabismus (squint) and diplopia, since the visual image now falls on disparate parts of the two retinas. The affected eye is often displaced by the unopposed antagonists in the direction opposite to that of the paretic muscle. The head may be tilted or turned in the direction of action of the weak muscle.

Characteristic clinical disturbances result from lesions of the third, fourth, and sixth cranial nerves. A complete third nerve lesion causes ptosis (since the levator palpebrae is supplied both by the third nerve and sympathetic fibers), an inability to rotate the eye upward, downward, or inward, a divergent strabismus due to unopposed action of the lateral rectus muscle, a dilated nonreactive pupil (iridoplegia), and paralysis of accommodation (cycloplegia). When only the muscles of the iris and ciliary body are paralyzed, the condition is termed *internal ophthalmoplegia*. Fourth nerve lesions result in an extorsion of the eye and a weakness of

turned to the left. Field: vertical diplopia (image of right eye uppermost) increasing on looking to left and up. (*Cogan: "Neurology of the Ocular Muscles," 2d ed., Springfield, Ill., Charles C Thomas, Publisher, 1956.*)

downward gaze, so that patients commonly complain of special difficulty in going downstairs. Head tilting, to the opposite shoulder, is especially characteristic of fourth nerve lesions. This maneuver causes a compensatory intorsion of the lower eye, enabling the patient to obtain binocular vision. Lesions of the sixth nerve result in paralysis of abduction and a convergent strabismus owing to the unopposed action of the internal rectus muscles. With incomplete sixth nerve palsies, turning the head toward the side of the paretic muscle may overcome diplopia. The foregoing signs may occur in various degrees of completeness, depending on the site of the lesion or lesions.

Ocular palsies may be central, i.e., due to a lesion of the nucleus or the intramedullary portion of the cranial nerve, or peripheral. Ophthalmoplegia due to lesions in the brain stem is usually accompanied by involvement of other cranial nerves or long tracts. Peripheral lesions, which may or may not be solitary, have a great variety of causes; the most common are aneurysm of the circle of Willis, tumors of the base of the brain, carcinomatosis of the meninges, herpes zoster, and syphilitic meningitis. The third nerve palsy which occurs with diabetes is probably due to infarction of the third nerve, and the prognosis for recovery in such cases, as with other nonprogressive diseases of the peripheral nerve, is usually excellent. The points of difference between lesions within and outside the brain stem are tabulated in Table 31-1, and the various intramedullary and extramedullary cranial nerve syndromes are described in Tables 31-2 and 31-3.

When the ocular palsy is slight, there may be no obvious squint or defect in ocular movement; yet the patient experiences diplopia. The study of the relative positions of the images of the two eyes then becomes the most accurate way of determining which muscle is involved. The image seen by the affected eye is usually less distinct, but the most reliable way of distinguishing the two images is by the red glass test. *A red glass is placed in front of the patient's right eye.* He is then asked to look at a flashlight, held at a distance of a meter, in various segments of his visual fields and to state the position of the red (right) and white (left) images. The relative positions of the two images are plotted as indicated in Fig. 31-2.

Three rules aid in the analysis of ocular movements by the red glass test: (1) The direction in which the distance between the images is at a maximum is the direction of action of the paretic muscle. For example, if the greatest separation is in looking to the right, either the right abductor or the left adductor muscle is weak. (2) The image projected farther to the side belongs to the paretic eye. If the patient looks to the right and the red image is farther to the right, then the right abducens mus-

cle is weak. If the white image is to the right of the red, then the left internal rectus muscle is weak. (3) In testing vertical movements, again the image of the eye with the paretic muscle is the one projected most peripherally in the direction of eye movement. One ignores lateral separation at this time. It must be remembered that there are two elevator and two depressor muscles. The responsible muscle may be either one of the obliques or vertical recti muscles. For example, if the maximum separation of images occurs on looking downward and to the left, and the white image is projected farther down than the red, the paretic muscle is the left inferior rectus. If the maximum separation occurs on looking down and to the right, with the white image being lower than the red, the paretic muscle is the left superior oblique. Separation of images on looking up and to the right or left will similarly distinguish paresis of the inferior oblique and superior rectus muscles.

If the defect in ocular rotation is due to a weakness or paralysis of an ocular muscle, it is termed *paralytic strabismus*. If the defect is one of ocular muscle imbalance, it is referred to as *concomitant strabismus*. It differs from the paralytic variety in that there is no diplopia and each eye exhibits a full range of motion when tested separately.

Monocular diplopia may occur and is related to diseases of the lens and refractive media of the eye. Another nonparetic form of diplopia is that which accompanies heteronymous visual field defects (e.g., bitemporal hemianopia with pituitary adenomas). Also paresis of accommodation may produce diplopia for near vision; its cause is unknown.

Paralysis of Conjugate Movement (Gaze). The term *conjugate gaze*, or *conjugate movement*, refers to the simultaneous movement of the two eyes in the same direction. An acute lesion in one frontal lobe may cause a paralysis of lateral gaze. The eyes turn toward the side of the lesion, and the patient seems disinclined to look toward or sustain his gaze to the contralateral side. The ocular disorder is temporary, and after several days the range of eye movement is again full. In bilateral frontal lesions the patient may be unable to turn his eyes voluntarily (*oculomotor apraxia*) in any direction—up, down, or to the side—but retains fixation and following movements, which are occipital lobe functions. Gaze paralysis of cerebral origin is not attended by strabismus or diplopia. The usual causes are vascular occlusion with infarction, hemorrhage, and abscess or tumor of the frontal lobe. With diseases of the basal ganglia, e.g., postencephalitic parkinsonism, Huntington's chorea, etc., there may be a limitation of ocular movements in all directions, especially upward. Lesions of the superior colliculus, near the posterior commissure, interfere with voluntary and reflex upward gaze, and often movements of convergence as well as the pupillary light reflexes are abolished (Parinaud's syndrome). There also exists a pontine center for conjugate lateral gaze, probably in the vicinity of the abducens nuclei. A lesion here causes the eyes to turn to the opposite side. The palsy tends to last longer than with cerebral lesions and is frequently accompanied by other signs of pontine disease. Fully developed forms of gaze paralysis are readily discerned, but lesser degrees may be overlooked unless one pays special attention to the predominant position of the eyes and tests the ability to sustain conjugate movement.

Skew deviation is a poorly understood disorder of gaze, characterized by a maintained deviation of one eye above the other. The deviation differs from peripheral muscle palsy in being constant in all fields of gaze. It may occur with any lesion of the posterior fossa but particularly with a lesion of the cerebellum.

Mixed Gaze and Ocular Paralyses. These are always a sign of intrapontine or mesencephalic disease. With a lesion of the lower pons in or near the sixth nerve nucleus, there is a homolateral paralysis of the lateral rectus muscle and a failure of adduction of the opposite eye, i.e., a combined paralysis of the sixth nerve and of conjugate lateral gaze. Lesions of the medial longitudinal fasciculi interfere with lateral conjugate gaze in another way. On looking to the right, the left eye fails to adduct; on looking to the left, the right eye fails to adduct. The abducting eye shows nystagmus. This condition is referred to as *internuclear ophthalmoplegia* and should always be suspected when the medial recti alone are affected. If the lesion is in the lower part of the medial longitudinal fasciculi, convergence is intact; if the lesion is in the higher part, i.e., near the ocular motor nuclei, convergence may be lost.

Nystagmus. This refers to involuntary rhythmic movements of the eyes and may be divided into an oscillating or pendular type and a rhythmic or jerk type. In jerk nystagmus, the movements are distinctly faster in one direction than the other; in pendular nystagmus, the oscillations are roughly equal in rate for the two directions, although on conjugate lateral gaze, the pendular type may become converted to a jerk type with the fast component to the side of gaze.

In testing for nystagmus, the eyes should first be examined in the central position and then during upward, downward, and lateral movements. If nystagmus is monocular (as in the "ataxic" nystagmus described below), each eye should be tested separately, with the other one covered. Labyrinthine nystagmus is most obvious when visual fixation is prevented by shielding the eyes; brain stem and cerebellar nystagmus are brought out best by having the patient fixate on a finger. Labyrinthine nystagmus may vary with the position of the head; hence these various tests should be performed with the head in several different positions. In particular, the postural nystagmus of Bárány is evoked by hyperextension of the neck, with the patient in the supine position. Opticokinetic nystagmus should be tested by asking the patient to look at a rotating cylinder on which several stripes have been painted.

A few irregular jerks are observed in many normal individuals when the eyes are turned far to the side. These so-called "nystagmoid movements" are probably similar to the tremulousness of a muscle that is contracted maximally. Occasionally a fine rhythmic nystagmus can be obtained in extreme lateral gaze, but if it is bilateral and disappears as the eyes move a few degrees toward the midline, it usually has no clinical significance.

Pendular nystagmus is found in a variety of conditions in which central vision is lost early in life, such as albinism and in various other diseases of the retina and refractive mediums. The syndrome of *miners' nystagmus,* formerly a common cause of industrial disability, occurs after many years of work in comparative darkness. The oscillations of the eyes are very rapid, increase on upward gaze, and are often associated with vertigo, head tremor, and intolerance of light. *Spasmus nutans* is a specific type of pendular nystagmus of infancy and is accompanied by head nodding and occasionally by wry positions of the neck. The prognosis is good, most cases recovering within a few months.

Jerk nystagmus is the more common type. It may be lateral or vertical, particularly on ocular movement in these planes, or it may be rotary. By custom, the direction of the nystagmus is named according to the direction of the fast component. There are several varieties of jerk nystagmus. When one is watching a moving object—e.g., the passing landscape from a train window or a rotating drum with vertical stripes—a rhythmic jerk nystagmus called *opticokinetic nystagmus* normally appears. The slow phase is a result of visual fixation; the quick phase is compensatory. With unilateral cerebral lesions, particularly in the parietooccipital region, there is loss of opticokinetic nystagmus when the moving visual stimulus, e.g., the drum, moves toward the side of the lesion.

Aside from opticokinetic nystagmus, jerk nystagmus usually signifies disease of the labyrinthine-vestibular apparatus. Labyrinthine stimulation or irritation produces a nystagmus with the fast phase to the opposite side. The slow component reflects the effect of impulses derived from the semicircular canals, while the fast component is a corrective movement. Vestibular-labyrinthine nystagmus may be horizontal, vertical, or, most characteristically, rotary. Vertigo, nausea, vomiting, and staggering are the usual accompaniments, as in Ménière's syndrome or labyrinthitis (see Chap. 30). Brain stem lesions often cause a coarse unidirectional nystagmus, which may be horizontal or vertical; the latter is usually brought out on upward gaze, and rarely on downward gaze. The presence of a vertical nystagmus is pathognomonic of disease in the tegmentum of the brain stem. Vertigo is inconstant, and signs of disease of other nuclear structures and tracts in the brain stem are frequent. Jerk nystagmus of this type is frequent in demyelinative or vascular disease, in tumors, syringobulbia, and the Arnold-Chiari malformation. Cerebellopontine-angle tumors cause a coarse, horizontal nystagmus with the fast component to the side of the lesion. Nystagmus probably does not occur with cerebellar disease unless the fastigial nuclei and their connections with the vestibular nuclei are involved. The so-called "ataxic" nystagmus which occurs only in the abducting eye and is said to be a pathognomonic sign of multiple sclerosis probably represents an incompletely developed form of internuclear ophthalmoplegia. The movement of the adducting eye (which does not show nystagmus) is impaired.

Convergence nystagmus is a rhythmic oscillation, in which a slow abduction of the eyes in respect to each other is followed by a quick movement of adduction. It is usually accompanied by other types of nystagmus and by one or more features of Parinaud's syndrome. Occasionally there is also a jerky retraction movement of the eyes (nystagmus retractorius), or a maintained spasm of convergence, best brought out on attempted elevation of the eyes to command. These unusual phenomena all point to a lesion of the upper midbrain tegmentum and are usually manifestations of vascular disease or of pinealoma.

Oscillopsia refers to illusory movement of the environment, which may or may not occur with turning of the eyes and consequent displacement of the image on the retina. When the eyes are turned voluntarily, the environment is interpreted as being stationary, whereas passive displacement of the eye or nystagmus from stimulation of the labyrinth results in oscillopsia during the slow phase of movement.

THE FIFTH, OR TRIGEMINAL, NERVE

This is a mixed sensory and motor nerve. It conducts sensory impulses from the greater part of the face and head, from the mucous membranes of the nose and mouth, and from the cornea and conjunctiva. The cell bodies of the sensory part of the nerve lie in the Gasserian or semilunar ganglion. The proximal branches of the axones of these cells form the sensory root. On entering the pons they divide into short ascending and long descending branches. The former are concerned mainly with touch and deep sensation and terminate in the principal and mesencephalic nuclei, respectively. The long descending branches form the spinal trigeminal tract and convey impulses for pain and temperature. The spinal trigeminal tract, together with its nucleus, extends from the junction of the pons and medulla to the uppermost segments of the spinal cord. From the nucleus, fibers of the second order cross to the opposite side and ascend to the thalamus in the most medial part of the spinothalamic tract.

The peripheral branches of the Gasserian ganglion form the three sensory divisions of the nerve. The first division (ophthalmic) passes through the superior orbital fissure; the second (maxillary) leaves the middle fossa through the foramen rotundum; the third (mandibular) leaves the skull through the foramen ovale.

The motor portion of the fifth nerve, which supplies the masseter and pterygoid muscles, has its origin in the midpons; the fibers pass underneath the Gasserian ganglion and become incorporated into the mandibular nerve.

The masseter muscles are tested by asking the patient to clamp his jaws while the examiner palpates the muscles and attempts to separate the jaws by pressing down on the chin. Only major degrees of weakness can be detected in this way. Weakness of the pterygoids is demonstrated by failure to open the mouth against resistance. With unilateral weakness of the pterygoid muscle, the jaw deviates to the side of the weakened muscle. Testing of the sensory part of the fifth nerve has been described in Chap. 28, Disorders of Sensation.

Because of their wide anatomic distribution, complete interruption of both the motor and sensory fibers of the trigeminal nerve is rarely observed. On the other hand, partial affection of the trigeminal nerve, particularly of the sensory part, is common. The various brain stem and cranial nerve syndromes in which the fifth nerve is involved are tabulated in Tables 31-2 and 31-3.

The sensory portions of the trigeminal nerve, especially the maxillary and mandibular divisions, are subject to a paroxysmal disturbance known as *trigeminal neuralgia* or *tic douloureux*. This occurs in middle-aged and elderly individuals and consists of excruciating paroxysms of pain in the lips, gums, or chin. The pain seldom lasts more than a few seconds or a minute or two but is so intense that the patient winces; hence the term *tic*. It recurs frequently, both day and night, for several weeks at a time. Another characteristic feature is the initiation of pain by obvious stimuli to certain areas on the face, lips, or tongue, so-called "trigger zones." Sensory loss cannot be demonstrated in these cases. Kugelberg and Lindblom have studied the relationship between stimuli applied to the trigger zone and the pain paroxysm. They found that the adequate stimulus for precipitating an attack is touch and possibly tickle, rather than pain or temperature. Usually a spatial and temporal summation of impulses was necessary to trigger an attack, which was followed by a refractory period of up to 2 or 3 min. They suggest that the mechanism for the paroxysmal pain is situated in relation to the nucleus of the spinal tract of the fifth nerve.

The diagnosis of this disorder must rest upon these strict clinical criteria, and the condition must be distinguished from other forms of facial and cephalic neuralgia and pain arising from diseases of the jaw, teeth, or sinuses. Tic douloureux is usually without assignable cause, although occasionally it is a manifestation of multiple sclerosis or of herpes zoster. Very rarely a tumor in the posterior fossa which has caused only an early irritative lesion in the nerve or its root may produce pain clinically indistinguishable from that of tic douloureux. Usually, however, space-occupying lesions, such as aneurysms, neurofibromas, meningiomas, etc., produce a loss of sensation.

The conventional treatment for tic douloureux is alcohol injection of the affected nerve at the foramen ovale and rotundum or section of the root of the trigeminal nerve between the ganglion and the brain stem. Antiepileptic drugs such as diphenylhydantoin (Dilantin) have been found by some authors to shorten the duration of the attacks. Temporizing and using chlorpromazine, inhalations of trichlorethylene, or injections of vitamin B_1 or vitamin B_{12} may permit a spontaneous remission to occur.

Tonic spasm of the masticatory muscles, known as *trismus,* is symptomatic of tetanus, although it may occur in hysteria, and lesser degrees may be associated with disease of the temporomaxillary joint or of the teeth and gums.

THE SEVENTH, OR FACIAL, NERVE

The seventh cranial nerve is mainly a motor nerve supplying all the muscles concerned with facial expression on one side. The sensory component is small (the nervus intermedius of Wrisberg); it conveys taste sensation from the anterior two-thirds of the tongue and probably cutaneous sensation from the anterior wall of the external auditory canal. The taste fibers originally traverse the lingual nerve (a branch of the mandibular) but then leave this nerve to join the chorda tympani. Visceral motor fibers innervate the lacrimal gland through the greater superficial petrosal nerve, and secretomotor fibers travel to the sublingual and submaxillary glands via the chorda tympani.

Several other anatomic facts are worth remembering. The motor nucleus of the seventh nerve is anterior and lateral to the abducens nucleus, and in their intrapontine course the facial nerve fibers hook around the abducens nucleus before they emerge from the pons at a point just lateral to the corticospinal tract. After leaving the pons they enter the internal auditory meatus with the acoustic nerve. The facial nerve then bends sharply forward and downward around the anterior boundary of the vestibule of the inner ear. At this angle lies the sensory ganglion (named *geniculate* because of its close proximity to the genu). The nerve continues its course in its own bony channel, the facial canal, and makes its exit from the skull at the stylomastoid foramen. It then passes through the parotid gland and subdivides to supply the facial muscles, the stylomastoid, and the posterior belly of the digastric muscle. Within the facial canal, just distal to the geniculate ganglion, it gives off the branch to the sphenopalatine ganglion, i.e., the greater superficial petrosal nerve, and somewhat more distally it gives off a small branch to the stapedius and is joined by the chorda tympani.

A complete interruption of the facial nerve at the stylomastoid foramen paralyzes all muscles of facial expression. The corner of the mouth droops, the creases and skin folds are effaced, the forehead is unfurrowed, the palpebral fissure is widened, and the eyelids will not close. Upon attempted closure of the lids, the eye on the paralyzed side rolls upward (Bell's phenomenon). The lower lid sags also, and if the punctum falls away from contact with the conjunctiva, tears spill over the cheek. Food collects between the teeth and lips, and saliva may dribble from the corner of the mouth. The patient complains of a heaviness or numbness in the face, but no sensory loss is demonstrable and taste is intact.

If the lesion is in the facial canal above the junction with the chorda tympani but below the geniculate ganglion, all the above symptoms occur and, in addition, there is loss of taste over the anterior two-thirds of the tongue on the same side. If the nerve to the stapedius is paralyzed, there is hyperacusis (painful sensitiveness to loud sounds) and the sound produced by moving the jaw and facial muscles is no longer present in the ear on the affected side. If the geniculate ganglion or the motor root proximal to it is involved, lacrimation may be reduced. Lesions at this point may also affect the adjacent auditory nerve, causing deafness, tinnitus, or dizziness. Intrapontine lesions that paralyze the face usually affect the abducens nucleus and often the corticospinal tract.

If the peripheral facial paralysis has existed for some time before the return of motor function, a contracture of muscles may develop. The palpebral fissure becomes narrowed and the nasolabial fold deeper. Attempts to move one group of facial muscles result in contraction of all of them (associated movements or synkinesis). Facial spasm may be present. Anomalous regeneration of the seventh nerve fibers may result in curious disorders. If fibers originally connected with the orbicularis oculi become connected with the orbicularis oris, closure of the lids may cause a retraction of the mouth; or if fibers originally connected with muscles of the face later come to innervate the lacrimal gland, anomalous tearing (crocodile tears) may occur with any activity of the facial muscles, such as eating (Bogorad's syndrome). With the passage of time, the face and even the tip of the nose become pulled to the unaffected side.

The commonest disease affecting the facial nerve is Bell's palsy, presumably due to an inflammatory reaction in or around the nerve near the stylomastoid foramen. The onset is acute, and the paralysis may evolve over a few hours, although pain behind the ear may have been present for a day or two. Occasionally taste sensation is lost, and more rarely hyperacusis is present. In some cases there is mild pleocytosis in the cerebrospinal fluid. Fully 80 per cent of cases recover within a few weeks. A reaction of degeneration at the end of 10 days indicates long delay in recovery until regeneration occurs. Electromyography may be of value in distinguishing temporary conduction defects from a pathologic interruption in continuity of nerve fibers. Protection of the eye during sleep, massage of the weakened muscles, a splint to prevent drooping of the lower face are the measures which one generally employs in the management of such cases.

Tumors which invade the temporal bone may produce a facial palsy, but the onset is insidious and the course progressive. Herpes zoster of the geniculate ganglion (Ramsay-Hunt's syndrome), which gives a severe facial palsy, is associated with a vesicular eruption in the external auditory canal and other parts of the cranial integument, and often the eighth cranial nerve is affected. Acoustic neuromas frequently involve the facial nerve. Vascular lesions or tumors are the common forms of pontine disease which may cause facial palsy. Bilateral facial paralysis (facial diplegia) occurs in acute infectious polyneuritis and in a variety of sarcoidosis known as *uveoparotid fever* (*Heerfordt's syndrome*). *Melkersson's syndrome* refers to a rarely encountered triad of recurrent facial paralysis, recurrent—and eventually permanent—facial (particularly labial) edema, and less constantly, plication of the tongue. The etiology is unknown.

All these forms of nuclear or peripheral facial palsy must be distinguished from the supranuclear type. In the latter the frontalis and orbicularis oculi muscles are involved less than those of the lower face, since the upper facial muscles receive upper motor neurone innervation from both sides of the cortex. In supranuclear lesions there may be a dissociation of emotional and voluntary facial movements, and often some degree of paralysis of the arm and leg or an aphasia (in dominant hemisphere lesions) is conjoined.

A curious disorder is the facial hemiatrophy of Romberg. This occurs mainly in females and is characterized by a disappearance of fat in the dermal and subcutaneous tissues on one side of the face. It usually begins in adolescence or early adult years and is slowly progressive. In its advanced form the face is gaunt and the skin is thin, wrinkled, and rather dark. The hair may turn white and fall out, and the sebaceous glands become atrophic. The muscles and bones are as a rule not involved. The condition is probably a form of lipodystrophy, and the restricted localization within a dermatome indicates the operation of some neural factor, of unknown nature.

The facial muscles on one side may be affected by irregular clonic contractions of varying degree (facial hemispasm). This may be due to an irritative lesion of the facial nerve (e.g. an acoustic neuroma) or may represent a transient or permanent sequel to a Bell's palsy. In the most common form, however, the cause and pathology are unknown. Allied to the latter form is an involuntary recurrent spasm of the eyelids (blepharospasm) which may occur as an isolated phenomenon or with varying degrees of spasm of the facial muscles.

THE EIGHTH, OR VESTIBULOCOCHLEAR, NERVE

This cranial nerve has two separate divisions, the cochlear, subserving the sense of hearing, and the vestibular, subserving the sense of balance.

The vestibular division has its cell bodies in Scarpa's ganglion, which lies in the internal auditory meatus. The ganglion is composed of bipolar cells, the peripheral processes of which terminate in the ampullae of the semicircular canals and the otoliths of the saccule and utricle. The cochlear division arises from biopolar cells in the spiral ganglion of the cochlea. The peripheral processes of these cells convey auditory impulses from the specialized neuroepithelium of the inner ear, the spiral organ of Corti. The central fibers from both these ganglions lie in close proximity; they enter the cranial cavity through the internal auditory meatus and course together toward the brain stem, which they penetrate at the junction of the pons and medulla. Here the cochlear and vestibular fibers become separated, the former terminating almost at once in the cochlear nuclei, the latter penetrating the brain stem for some distance and terminating in the vestibular nuclei. Each cochlear nucleus is connected with the cortex of both temporal lobes, so that hearing is unaffected by unilateral cerebral lesions.

The central connections of the vestibular nuclei, the methods of testing, and the disordered function of this nerve are considered in Chap. 30.

The principal symptoms of disease of the auditory nerve are tinnitus and deafness. Tinnitus, or ringing in the ears, is a purely subjective phenomenon and may also be reported as a buzzing, whistling, hissing, or roaring sound. It is a very common symptom in adults and may be of no significance, as for example the hissing sound due to wax in the external auditory canal or a blocked eustachian tube. On the other hand, it is regularly associated with disease of the eighth nerve, inner ear, or ossicles, and tinnitus in the presence of normal hearing is very rare. If tinnitus is localized to one ear and is described as having a tonal character, such as ringing or a bell-like tone, and particularly if the recruitment phenomenon (see below) is present, it is probably cochlear in origin. Noises described as rushing water or escaping steam point to disease of the nerve or even the brain stem. Clicking sounds are caused by intermittent contraction of the tensor tympani. A pulsating tinnitus synchronous with the pulse may be related to an intracranial vascular malformation; however, this symptom must be carefully judged, since introspective individuals often report hearing their pulse when lying down. Certain drugs such as salicylates and quinine produce tinnitus and transient deafness. Nervous individuals are less tolerant of tinnitus than are more stable persons; depressed or anxious patients may demand relief from a tinnitus that has existed for years.

The examination of hearing should always begin with an inspection of the external auditory canal and the tympanic membrane. A watch or whispered words are suitable means of testing hearing at the bedside, the opposite ear being closed by the finger. If there is any suspicion of deafness or a complaint of tinnitus or vertigo, or if the patient is a child with a speech defect, then hearing must be tested further. This can be done with the use of tuning forks of different frequencies, but the most accurate results are obtained by the use of an electric audiometer and the construction of an audiogram, which reveals the entire range of hearing at a glance. An auditory recruitment test may also be helpful: the difference in hearing between the two ears is estimated, and the loudness of the stimulus delivered to each ear is then increased by increments. In nonrecruiting deafness (characteristic of a nerve trunk lesion) the original difference in hearing persists in comparisons above threshold. In recruiting deafness (as occurs in Ménière's disease)

the bad ear gains in loudness and finally is equal to the good ear.

Deafness is of two types: (1) nerve deafness, due to interruption of cochlear fibers, and (2) conduction deafness, due to disease of the middle ear (or occlusion of the external auditory canal or eustachian tube). In differentiating these two types, the tuning fork tests are of value. When the vibrating fork is held several inches from the ear (the test for air conduction), sound waves can be appreciated only as they are transmitted through the middle ear and will be reduced with disease in this location. When the fork is applied to the skull (test for bone conduction), the sound waves are conveyed directly to the cochlea, without the intervention of the middle ear apparatus, and will therefore not be reduced when the disease is confined to the middle ear. With affection of the cochlea or eighth nerve, both air and bone conduction will be reduced or lost. Normally air conduction is better than bone conduction. These principles form the basis for several tests of auditory function.

In *Weber's test,* the vibrating fork is applied to the forehead in the midline. In middle ear deafness the sound is localized in the affected ear, in nerve deafness in the normal ear. In *Rinné's test,* the fork is applied to the mastoid process, the ear being closed by the observer's finger. At the moment the sound ceases, the fork is held at the auditory meatus. In middle ear deafness the sound cannot be heard by air conduction after bone conduction has ceased (abnormal or negative Rinné test). In nerve deafness the reverse is true (normal or positive Rinné test), although both air and bone conduction may be quantitatively decreased. In *Schwabach's test,* the patient's bone conduction is compared with that of a normal observer. In general, high-pitched tones are lost in nerve deafness and low-pitched ones in middle ear deafness, but there are frequent exceptions to this rule.

The common causes of middle ear deafness are otitis media, otosclerosis, and rupture of the eardrum. Nerve deafness has many causes. The internal ear may be aplastic from birth (hereditary deaf mutism), or it may be damaged by rubella in the pregnant mother. Acute purulent meningitides or chronic infections spreading from the middle ear are common causes of nerve deafness in childhood. The auditory nerve may be involved by tumors of the cerebellopontine angle or by syphilis. Deafness may also result from a demyelinative plaque in the brain stem. Hysterical deafness may be difficult to distinguish from organic disease. In the case of bilateral deafness, the distinction can be made by observing a blink (cochleoorbicular reflex) or an alteration in skin sweating (psychogalvanic skin reflex) in response to a loud sound. Unilateral hysterical deafness may be detected by an audiometer, with both ears connected, or by whispering into the bell of a stethoscope attached to the patient's ears, closing first one and then the other tube without the patient's knowledge.

THE NINTH, OR GLOSSOPHARYNGEAL, NERVE

This nerve arises from the lateral surface of the medulla by a series of small roots which lie just rostral to those of the vagus nerve. The glossopharyngeal, vagus, and accessory nerves leave the skull together through the jugular foramen and are then distributed peripherally. This nerve has a sensory component with cell bodies in the petrosal ganglion and the small superior ganglion, the central fibers of which end in the tractus solitarius. It also receives the nerve of Hering from the carotid body. The somatic efferent fibers of the ninth nerve are derived from the nucleus ambiguus, the visceral efferent (secretory) fibers from the inferior salivatory nucleus. These fibers contribute to the motor innervation of the striated musculature of the pharynx and the glands in the mucosa.

The sensory functions of this nerve are not entirely clear. It is commonly stated that with complete interruption of the ninth nerve sensation is blunted on the faucial tonsil, posterior wall of the pharynx, and part of the soft palate, taste sensation is abolished on the posterior third of the tongue, and the pharyngeal or gag reflex is diminished on one side. However, cases with unilateral or bilateral section of the nerve have been reported in which no sensory loss was observed, suggesting that the tenth nerve may be responsible for this function in some individuals. There is also evidence that the ninth nerve, through its innervation of the carotid sinus, plays a part in the reflex control of circulation.

One may occasionally observe a glossopharyngeal palsy in conjunction with vagus and accessory nerve involvement due to a tumor in the posterior fossa or an aneurysm of the vertebral artery that extends into the jugular foramen. Hoarseness due to vocal cord paralysis, some difficulty in swallowing, deviation of the soft palate to the sound side, anesthesia of the posterior wall of the pharynx, and weakness of the upper trapezius and sternomastoid muscles comprise the total clinical picture.

Glossopharyngeal neuralgia is a syndrome which in many respects resembles trigeminal neuralgia. The pain is intense and paroxysmal; it originates in the throat, approximately in the tonsillar fossa. In some cases the pain is localized in the ear or may radiate from the throat to the ear, because of implication of the tympanic branch (Jacobson's nerve). Spasms of pain may be initiated by swallowing. There is no demonstrable sensory or motor deficit. Division of the nerve near the medulla is the treatment of choice. Very rarely, herpes zoster may involve the glossopharyngeal nerve.

THE TENTH, OR VAGUS, NERVE

This nerve has an extensive sensory and motor distribution. It has two ganglions, the jugular, which contains the cell bodies of the somatic sensory nerves, and the nodose, which contains the cell bodies of the afferent fibers from the pharynx, larynx, trachea, esophagus, and the thoracic and abdominal viscera. The central processes of these ganglions terminate in relation to the nucleus of the spinal trigeminal tract and the tractus solitarius, respectively. The motor fibers of the vagus are derived from two nuclei in the medulla, the nucleus ambiguus and the dorsal motor nucleus. The former supplies somatic motor fibers to the striate muscles of the larynx, pharynx, and the palate, and the latter supplies visceral motor fibers to the heart and other thoracic and abdominal organs.

Complete interruption of the intracranial portion of one vagus nerve results in a characteristic paralysis. The soft palate droops and does not rise in phonation. There is loss of the gag reflex on the affected side, as well as of the "curtain movement" of the lateral wall of the pharynx, whereby the faucial pillars move medially as the palate rises in saying "Ah." The voice is hoarse, often nasal, and the vocal cord lies immobile in an abducted or cadaveric position. There may also be loss of sen-

Table 31-1. COMPARISON OF LESIONS WITHIN AND OUTSIDE THE BRAIN STEM

Effect	Lesions within the brain stem	Lesions external to the brain stem
Involvement of multiple contiguous nerves	±	+
Involvement of sensorimotor tracts	+, often "alternating" or crossed sensory or motor palsies	±
Disturbance of consciousness	+	0 (+late)
Evidence of other segmental disturbances of the brain stem such as decerebrate rigidity, tonic neck reflexes, pseudobulbar palsy	+	0 (+late)
X-ray evidence of erosion of cranial bones or enlargement of foramens	0	+

sibility at the external auditory meatus and back of the pinna. Usually no change in visceral function can be demonstrated.

Complete bilateral paralysis is said to be incompatible with life, and this is probably true if the nuclei are involved in the medulla by poliomyelitis or some other disease. However, in the cervical region both vagi have been blocked with procaine (Novocain) for the treatment of intractable asthma,

without mishap. The pharyngeal branches of both vagi may be affected, as in diphtheria; the voice has a nasal quality, and regurgitation of liquids through the nose occurs during the act of swallowing.

The vagus nerves, especially the left, are most often damaged as a result of thoracic disease. Aneurysm of the aortic arch, an enlarged left atrium tumors of the mediastinum and bronchi

Table 31-2. BRAIN STEM SYNDROMES WHICH INVOLVE CRANIAL NERVES

Eponym	Site	Cranial nerves involved	Tracts and nuclei involved	Signs	Usual cause
Weber's syndrome	Base of midbrain	III	Corticospinal tract	Oculomotor palsy with crossed hemiplegia	Vascular occlusion; tumor; aneurysm
Claude's syndrome	Tegmentum of midbrain	III	Red nucleus	Oculomotor palsy with contralateral cerebellar ataxia and tremor	Vascular occlusion; tumor; aneurysm
Benedikt's syndrome	Tegmentum of midbrain	III	Red nucleus and corticospinal tract	Oculomotor palsy with contralateral cerebellar ataxia, tremor and pyramidal signs	Softening; hemorrhage; tuberculoma; tumor
Nothnagel's syndrome	Tectum of midbrain	Unilateral or bilateral III	Superior cerebellar peduncles	Ocular palsies, paralysis of gaze, and cerebellar ataxia	Tumor
Parinaud's syndrome	Tectum of midbrain	Supranuclear coordinating mechanism for upward gaze	Superior colliculi	Paralysis of upward and sometimes downward gaze; fixed pupils; divergence of eyes	Pinealoma
Millard-Gubler syndrome and Raymond-Foville syndrome	Base of pons	VII and often VI	Corticospinal tract	Facial and abducens palsy and contralateral hemiplegia, sometimes palsy of gaze to side of lesion	Softening or tumor
Avellis' syndrome	Tegmentum of medulla	X	Corticospinal tract Sometimes descending pupillary fibers, with Bernard-Horner syndrome	Paralysis of soft palate and vocal cord and contralateral hemiplegia	Softening or tumor
Jackson's syndrome	Tegmentum of medulla	X, XII	Corticospinal tract	Avellis' syndrome plus ipsilateral tongue paralysis	Softening or tumor
Wallenberg's syndrome	Tegmentum of medulla	Spinal V, IX, X, XI	Lateral spinothalamic tract Descending pupillodilator fibers Spinocerebellar and olivocerebellar tracts	Ipsilateral V, IX, X, XI palsy, Bernard-Horner syndrome, and cerebellar ataxia Contralateral loss of pain and temperature	Occlusion of posterior-inferior cerebellar artery

are much more frequent causes of an isolated vagus palsy than intracranial disorders. The nerve may be implicated at the meningeal level by tumors and infectious processes and within the medulla by vascular lesions and tumors, e.g., the lateral medullary syndrome of Wallenberg, and by motor system disease. Herpes zoster may attack this nerve. Polymyositis and dermatomyositis, which cause hoarseness and dysphagia owing to direct involvement of laryngeal and pharyngeal muscles, may be confused with disease of the vagus nerves.

When confronted with a case of laryngeal palsy, the physician must attempt to determine the site of the lesion. If it is intramedullary, there are usually other signs such as ipsilateral cerebellar signs, loss of pain and temperature sensation over the ipsilateral face and contralateral arm and leg, and ipsilateral Bernard-Horner syndrome. If the lesion is extramedullary, the glossopharyngeal and spinal accessory are frequently involved (jugular foramen syndrome). If it is extracranial in the posterior laterocondylar or retroparotid space, there may be a combination of ninth, tenth, eleventh, and twelfth cranial nerve palsies and Bernard-Horner syndrome. Combinations of these lower cranial nerve palsies are sometimes called the *syndrome of Collet-Sicard* and *syndrome of Villaret* (see Table 31-3), respectively. If there is no sensory loss in the palate and pharynx, or no palatal weakness, the lesion is below the origin of the pharyngeal branches, which leave the vagus nerve high in the cervical region. The usual site of disease is then the mediastinum.

THE ELEVENTH, OR ACCESSORY, NERVE

The accessory is a purely motor nerve. Its fibers arise from the anterior horn cells of the upper five cervical cord segments and enter the skull through the foramen magnum. Intracranially, the accessory nerve travels for a short distance with that part of the tenth nerve which is derived from the most caudal cells of the nucleus ambiguus (referred to as the vagal accessory nerve or the cranial root of the accessory nerve). Together, the two roots leave the skull through the jugular foramen. The aberrant vagus fibers then rejoin the main trunk of the vagus, and the purely spinal fibers continue as the external ramus to innervate the sterno-cleidomastoids and trapezii muscles. Only the latter fibers constitute the accessory nerve in the strict sense.

A complete lesion of the accessory nerve results in a partial paralysis of the trapezius and sterno-mastoid muscles. This can be demonstrated first by asking the patient to shrug his shoulders; the affected shoulder will be found to be weaker, and there will often be evident atrophy and some degree of rotation of the scapula. Second, when the patient turns his head forcibly against the examiner's hand, the sternomastoid of the opposite side does not contract firmly beneath the fingers. This muscle

Table 31-3. CRANIAL NERVE SYNDROMES

Site	Cranial nerves involved	Eponym	Usual cause
Sphenoidal fissure.......	III, IV, ophthalmic V, VI, sometimes II	. . . .	Invasive tumors of sphenoid bone, aneurysms
Lateral wall of cavernous sinus	III, IV, ophthalmic V, VI, often with proptosis Maxillary V sometimes involved	Foix's syndrome	Aneurysms of cavernous sinus, cavernous sinus thrombosis, invasive tumors from sinuses and sella turcica
Petrosphenoidal space...	II, III, IV, V, VI	Jacob's syndrome	Large tumors of middle cranial fossa
Apex of petrous bone....	V, VI	Gradenigo's syndrome	Petrositis, tumors of petrous bone fossa
Internal auditory meatus	VII, VIII	. . . .	Tumors of petrous bone (dermoids, etc.), infectious processes
Pontocerebellar angle...	V, VII, VIII, and sometimes IX	. . . .	Acoustic neuromas, meningiomas
Jugular foramen........	IX, X, XI	Vernet's syndrome	Tumors and aneurysms
Posterior laterocondylar space	IX, X, XI, XII	Collet-Sicard syndrome	Tumors of parotid gland, carotid body, and secondary tumor
Posterior retroparotid space	IX, X, XI, XII, and Bernard-Horner syndrome	Villaret's syndrome	Tumors of parotid gland, carotid body, secondary tumor, lymph node tumors, tuberculous adenitis

can be further tested by having the patient press his head forward against resistance or raise his head from the pillow. Double sternomastoid and trapezius palsy which occurs with primary disease of muscles, e.g., polymyositis and muscular dystrophy, may be difficult to distinguish from a lesion of both accessory nerves.

HYPOGLOSSAL NERVE

Arising as a series of rootlets from the medulla, this nerve issues from the skull at the hypoglossal foramen and supplies the genioglossus muscle, which acts to protrude the tongue, the styloglossus, which retracts and elevates its root, and the hypoglossus, which causes the upper surface to become convex. Complete interruption of the nerve results in paralysis of one side of the tongue. The tongue curves slightly to the healthy side as it lies in the mouth, but on protrusion it deviates to the affected side owing to the unopposed push of the healthy genioglossus muscle. In the mouth the tongue cannot be moved with natural facility. The denervated side becomes wrinkled and atrophied, and "fibrillary" twitches are seen.

Lesions of the hypoglossal nerve roots or ansa hypoglossi are rare. Occasionally an intramedullary lesion damages the emergent fibers of the hypoglossal nerve, the corticospinal tract, and medial lemniscus. Paralysis and atrophy of one side of the tongue, together with spastic paralysis and loss of vibration and position sense in the opposite arm and leg, result. Poliomyelitis and motor system disease may destroy the hypoglossal nuclei. Lesions of the basal meninges and the sphenoid and occipital bones may involve the nerve in its extramedullary course, and it is sometimes damaged in operations on the neck.

MULTIPLE CRANIAL NERVE PALSIES

As will be readily understood, several cranial nerves may be affected by the same disease process. One of the clinical problems that arise is whether the disease is within or outside the brain stem. Table 33-1 calls attention to the main differentiating features of these two classes of disease. Many eponyms have been attached to the intramedullary syndromes in which cranial nerve palsies are combined with signs of sensory and motor tract disease. The latter are always contralateral to the cranial nerve disturbance, a finding which localizes the disease to the brain stem. It is hardly to be expected that the medical student or physician will remember the names of these many syndromes, but they are listed in Table 31-2 for his convenience.

Involvement of multiple cranial nerves outside the brain stem is frequently the result of a meningeal carcinomatosis, sarcoma, chordoma, or other type of tumor. Owing to special anatomic arrangements, particularly at the points of exit of the nerves from the cranial cavity, a number of rather distinctive syndromes can be identified. They are listed in Table 31-3. Polyneuritis cranialis refers to an asymmetrical affection of multiple cranial nerves analogous to the variety which affects spinal roots and nerves, having no known cause but a good prognosis. Garcin has described unilateral cranial nerve disorder with Schmincke tumor, i.e., transitional cell carcinoma of the nasopharynx. This combination of findings has been called Garcin's syndrome. It may also occur with chordomas of the clivus.

REFERENCES

Brodal, A.: "The Cranial Nerves," Springfield, Ill., Charles C Thomas, Publisher, 1959.

Cogan, D. G.: "Neurology of the Ocular Muscles," 2d ed., Springfield, Ill., Charles C Thomas, Publisher, 1956.

Staff of Mayo Clinic: "Clinical Examinations in Neurology," Philadelphia, W. B. Saunders Company, 1956.

Wilson, S. A. K.: "Neurology," 2d ed., Baltimore, The Williams & Wilkins Company, 1955.

32 CEREBROSPINAL FLUID, HYDROCEPHALUS, AND MENINGEAL IRRITATION
Raymond D. Adams

The information yielded by examination of the cerebrospinal fluid (CSF) provides the most important aids to neurologic diagnosis. Every physician, therefore, must be familiar with the technique of lumbar puncture and the methods of examining the CSF. Many of the latter are relatively simple and can be performed at the time of lumbar puncture.

It must be supposed that the reader possesses a certain general knowledge of the anatomy and physiology of the CSF and of the routine tests done on it. No attempt at a thorough review of this subject is made here. Some of the results of recent research which have modified ideas about the CSF are reviewed, and certain common sources of error in CSF examination are mentioned.

One can hardly think about the CSF without also considering the choroid plexuses and arachnoid villi and pia-arachnoid, in the meshes of which much of the CSF is contained. Therefore a few brief comments are also made on the anatomy of the meninges. The symptoms and signs of diseases of the meninges, particularly meningitis and hydrocephalus, although not strictly cardinal manifestations of nervous disease, are reviewed briefly.

FORMATION, CIRCULATION, AND ABSORPTION OF CEREBROSPINAL FLUID

The general notion of CSF which has been taught for years is that it is formed from the choroid plexuses by secretion and by dialysis of blood plasma; and that it flows successively from the lateral ventricles via the foramen of Monro, to the third ventricle, aqueduct of Sylvius, fourth ventricle, basal foramens of Magendie and Luschka to the subarachnoid space, from which it is absorbed into the cerebral and spinal veins through the arachnoid villi. Although this is a useful way of thinking about the formation, flow, and resorption of CSF, recent studies by Sweet and his associates and others show that it is not altogether correct. When stable and radioactive isotopes of Na, Cl, K, and deuterium and radioactive albumin are injected intravenously into human beings and animals and the time of their appearance in the lateral ventricle, cisterna magna, and lumbar subarachnoid space is calculated minute by minute, they are found to enter the CSF both in the ventricle and in the subarachnoid space at rates which vary with "the site of formation and the substance used." Also water, electrolytes, and albumin leave the ventricles and subarachnoid space, again at dissimilar rates. It appears that the rate of exchange at any one site varies inversely with the molecular size of the material studied; in decreasing order of the velocity of exchange, the substances are water, electrolytes, and albumin. Water in particular is found to move back and forth between blood vessels and ventricles and subarachnoid space very rapidly, probably more rapidly through the pia-arachnoid vessels than through ependymal ones. The electrolytes enter the ventricles more rapidly than they do the subarachnoid space, suggesting a special secretory activity of the choroid plexuses. Protein, on the other hand, enters the subarachnoid space more rapidly than the ventricles. It is concluded from these studies that the CSF is both a secretion and an ultrafiltrate. The rate of formation and the volume of fluid in any one part of the ventricular system and subarachnoid spaces are said to be determined by the diffusion rates and concentration of electrolytes and albumin. This concept of CSF circulation, which emphasizes the diffusion of electrolytes and proteins and their osmotic pressures rather than the flow of water, is still not altogether satisfactory, for it does not completely explain the high pressures that occur in the lateral ventricles when the ventricular system is blocked at one point (obstructive hydrocephalus).

Most histologic and embryologic studies have shown that the pia and arachnoid develop as a single membrane and cover the whole of the brain and spinal cord. The CSF lies between these two membranes in the subarachnoid space. The pia is tightly adherent to the spinal cord and brain, and there is no space beneath it. The pia and arachnoid are connected by trabeculae except over the cauda equina and in the cisterns of the brain. Here they are widely separated, and large pools of CSF collect; this fluid may be safely aspirated from the lumbar subarachnoid space and the cisterna magna. There are, in addition, spinal subdural and epidural spaces and a cerebral subdural space; these have no connection whatsoever with the subarachnoid spaces and CSF. The subdural space is only a potential one and contains very small amounts of fluid. It is of interest to clinicians when it harbors blood or pus.

The amount of CSF is estimated to be 125 to 200 ml. The rate at which it is formed has been determined only by highly artificial methods, which suggest a turnover of the total volume several times a day. Nothing new has been learned in recent years about the absorption. Presumably it takes place through the arachnoidal villi along the cerebral veins and dural sinuses and to a small extent in the lateral recesses of the spinal subarachnoid space along the posterior roots.

The only known function of the CSF is that of protection. It serves as a water jacket to guard the brain and spinal cord against everyday knocks and blows. Although reflecting some of the metabolic activities of the brain, there is no evidence that the CSF participates in any of them.

INDICATIONS FOR LUMBAR AND CISTERNAL PUNCTURE

Lumbar puncture is necessary under the following conditions: to obtain pressure measurements and at times to relieve elevated intracranial pressure; to secure a sample of fluid for cellular, chemical, or bacteriologic examination; to administer therapeutic substances such as streptomycin or other antibiotics; to perform spinal anesthesia; and to inject for diagnostic purposes radiopaque materials such as Pantopaque (myelography) and air (pneumoencephalography). Lumbar puncture is contraindicated if the cerebrospinal fluid pressure is high, as shown by headache and papilledema, for it increases the possibility of a fatal cerebellar and tentorial pressure cone. However, if it seems important, in a given case of suspected increased intracranial pressure, to have the information yielded by CSF examination, the lumbar puncture may be performed with a fine-bore needle (No. 22 or 24) as the last part of the clinical study. Cisternal puncture, although safe in the hands of experts, is too risky a procedure to entrust to inexperienced house officers and students. The lumbar puncture is always to be preferred. The cisternal puncture should be done only when a spinal subarachnoid block exists and it is necessary to have a sample of fluid from above the block, to introduce an antibiotic above a spinal subarachnoid block so that it may reach the more superior recesses of the subarachnoid space, or to inject Pantopaque in order to demonstrate the upper level of the spinal lesion.

Experience with diagnostic neurologic problems teaches the importance of meticulous technique. If done carefully with procaine anesthesia and under sterile conditions, the procedure should be harmless and painless; and if it is accomplished by a single clean puncture, using a fine needle, not more than one of five patients will have a postpuncture headache from the continuous leakage of CSF. The "dry tap" is more often due to an improperly placed needle than to a compressive lesion of the spinal cord or chronic adhesive arachnoiditis. A "bloody tap" due to the transfixion of a meningeal vessel may result in hopeless confusion as regards diagnosis, if it is erroneously interpreted as a subarachnoid hemorrhage. The improper testing of CSF dynamics or of pressure may lead to unnecessary pneumoencephalography, myelography, or even a useless operative procedure.

ROUTINE METHODS OF EXAMINATION

Pressure and "Dynamics." (See Appendix for normal values of CSF.)

The normal pressure is less than 180 mm H_2O with the patient in the lateral decubitus position with the spine strictly horizontal. The pressure is elevated in many cases of brain tumor, brain abscess, brain hemorrhage, subarachnoid hemorrhage, meningitis, hydrocephalus, intracranial sinus thrombosis, and heart failure. Common sources of error are permitting fluid to escape before the manometer is applied and thereby obtaining a lower pressure than originally existed; the failure to note that the patient is tense and unrelaxed and that by holding abdomen and thorax taut he has raised the pressure; or failure to position properly an obese patient whose heavy thighs, pressed against the paunchy abdomen, raise the intraabdominal and thence the intraspinal pressure. In these latter two circumstances straightening out the patient's legs, calming him, or asking him to take several deep breaths and then to relax will lower the pressure to a normal level within a few minutes. The most fre-

quent causes of subnormal pressures are imperfect placement of the needle in the subarachnoid space or a previous lumbar puncture; rarely, it is due to a spinal block.

The Queckenstedt test is performed by manually compressing both jugular veins in the side of the neck. This results in an immediate congestion of intracranial veins and sinuses and a rapid rise in intracranial pressure, usually to over 300 mm H_2O. If the spinal subarachnoid space is unobstructed, this pressure is transmitted to the lumbar puncture needle. If there is a spinal block, the pressure in the lumbar region will either rise and fall slowly or not at all, or once risen, will require longer than 20 sec to return to its previous level. Holding a deep breath and straining down with the abdominal muscles will cause congestion of the thoracic and lumbar spinal veins and raise the pressure in the lumbar needle with or without a spinal block. The common causes of a spinal block are tumor, fracture-dislocation, epidural abscess, purulent or tuberculous meningitis, and chronic adhesive arachnoiditis. Usually the CSF protein is then high, and the fluid may be yellow and may clot spontaneously (Froin's syndrome). The Queckenstedt test is often incorrectly performed, the usual sources of error being failure to compress the jugular veins (checked by wrapping a blood pressure cuff around the neck and inflating it to 40 mm Hg for 20 to 40 sec) or improper placement of the needle, i.e., touching the meninges (checked by observing whether or not a prompt rise and fall are obtained by abdominal compression and straining and by the presence of good pulse and respiratory waves). Refinements of spinal dynamics, such as charting the CSF pressures at varying intervals of time after different degrees of jugular vein occlusion, have no real advantage over the above method. Compression of each jugular vein separately gives useful information only in some suspected cases of lateral sinus thrombosis. The Queckenstedt test is indicated only in suspected spinal lesions; it should not be done in cases of intracranial tumor, abscess, or subarachnoid or cerebral hemorrhage.

The gross appearance of the CSF is also informative. Normally clear and colorless, indistinguishable from water, it becomes cloudy, white, or some slight off-tone of white when there is a purulent meningeal exudate; and pink or red with red blood cells and oxyhemoglobin with hemorrhage; xanthochromic from bilirubin with subarachnoid hemorrhage, jaundice, and in conditions which elevate the total protein; and brown or black from the methemoglobin with massive hemorrhage. In most diseases which cause only a lymphocytosis of a few hundred cells the CSF remains clear. Pus may be seen at the bottom of the tube in purulent meningitis. A delicate white coagulum often forms in tuberculous and other types of meningitis because of the presence of fibrin in the subarachnoid exudate. The cobweb-like clot of tuberculous meningitis may take several hours to form but should be watched for and examined under the microscope because it often harbors tubercle bacilli. A few red blood cells (10 to 100 or more) may be found in any specimen, even when the puncture appeared to be perfect and the CSF entirely clear. A common error is to misidentify them as lymphocytes in a counting chamber. This is easily avoided by adding a few drops of acetic acid to the CSF, which will hemolyze the red blood cells, or by preparing a smear and staining with Wright's stain. Larger amounts of blood, 500 red blood cells or more, raise the question of subarachnoid hemorrhage versus "bloody tap"—an accidental injury to a subarachnoid vein by the lumbar puncture needle. Usually the bloody tap can be recognized by the fact that the first fluid to escape (the first tube) usually contains more blood than that in later tubes. Furthermore, if the fluid is grossly bloody, a clot will form, which does not happen with subarachnoid hemorrhage where the blood appears to have been defibrinated in the subarachnoid space. Xanthochromia is a sign of subarachnoid hemorrhage of one or several days' standing, unless the hemorrhage is massive (usually a million or more red blood cells per cu mm), in which instance enough serum bilirubin is present to color the CSF almost at once. Crenation of red blood cells is not a reliable indication of subarachnoid hemorrhage. Subarachnoid hemorrhage is usually due to head injury, ruptured aneurysm, brain hemorrhage, angioma, venous thrombosis, or arterial embolism with, hemorrhagic infarction, and rarely to a malignant tumor. Xanthochromia becomes evident in 12 to 24 hr and deepens during the following week as the red blood cells disappear. The fluid usually becomes clear in 2 to 3 weeks unless further bleeding occurs.

Cytologic Changes. The normal CSF usually contains no cells or at most not more than five. Lymphocytes, neutrophilic leukocytes, rarely monocytes or plasma cells which may appear in abnormal CSF arise from the meninges. Tumor cells are occasionally seen in cases of metastatic tumor or glioma. Low cell counts, less than 200 per cu mm, are usually predominantly mononuclear or a mixture of lymphocytes and neutrophilic leukocytes. A predominantly neutrophilic leukocytic pleocytosis indicates a bacterial infection, and a predominantly lymphocytic pleocytosis, a viral or spirochetal infection. In poliomyelitis, during the "meningitic" phase, and in tuberculous meningitis there is usually a mixture of neutrophilic leukocytes and lymphocytes. White cells in the CSF may always be taken as a sign of meningeal irritation, owing to infection in or near the meninges. However, they may also be found in cases of recent subarachnoid hemorrhage or tumor (glioma, metastatic carcinoma, lymphocytoma).

The protein content of the CSF should normally not exceed 45 to 50 mg per ml, and of this 2.5 to 5.0 mg is globulin and the rest albumin. Pandy's reaction gives a rough indication of the presence of an excess of albumin and globulin. The content of protein can be judged with semiquantitative accuracy by adding 5 per cent sulfosalicylic acid to the fluid and comparing it to a standard which contains 50, 100, and 200 mg protein. The globulin can be measured with approximate accuracy by the $ZnSO_4$ precipitation test and by the Lange first zone colloidal gold reaction, which indicate in the first dilutions a relative increase in globulin in relation to albumin. The Ross-Jones test using ammonium sulfate permits bedside detection of a globulin excess. The protein content is increased in all inflammatory diseases, in pyogenic more than in virus infections (though it may be normal in viral infections), and in tumors, abscesses of brain, all types of subarachnoid and ventricular bleeding, hypertensive encephalopathy, myxedema, and certain types of multiple neuropathy. A high globulin content, out of proportion to albumin, is most often found in neurosyphilis and multiple sclerosis.

The sugar content of the CSF is important only with infections of the meninges, although it may be depressed or elevated in states of hypoglycemia and hyperglycemia. Intravenous glucose will also increase the amount of sugar in the CSF. Bacterial or fungous infections and, rarely, extensive involvement by tumor (carcinomatosis or lymphomatosis of the meninges) will lower the sugar below 40 mg per 100 ml. Virus infections do not consistently alter it either by increasing or decreasing it. A useful roughly quantitative test of sugar content is to add 1, 2, 3, 4, and 5 drops of CSF to five tubes, each containing Fehling's solution, and heat them. Usually a plus reaction will be obtained in the tubes with 4 and 5 drops; if it does not occur the sugar is probably less than 40 mg. The chloride content of the CSF is reduced in all forms of meningitis but more in the tuberculous variety than in others.

Smears of CSF, stained by methylene blue or Wright's stain, and cultures are essential in all cases of suspected meningeal infection. The Wassermann reaction and an appropriate precipitation reaction should be routine; in nonsyphilitic forms of meningitis which increase the permeability of vessels, syphilitic antigen may reach CSF from the blood stream in cases of latent syphilis and give a false positive reaction.

THE SYNDROME OF MENINGEAL IRRITATION

This is most frequently manifested in two conditions—meningitis and subarachnoid hemorrhage. Headache, stiffness of the neck on forward bending, some degree of alteration of consciousness ranging from slight drowsiness and confusion to coma, and an absence of other neurologic signs compose the clinical picture. Convulsions, more frequent in infants and children than adults, ocular palsies, and minor neurologic signs may appear in some cases.

Headache is present in nearly every case, though of course it is not a complaint in infants and small children. It is generalized, often extends into the neck and as far down as the interscapular area, but is really not in any way distinctive. The cause of the headache is probably the irritation of the meninges, quite possibly augmented by increased intracranial pressure.

The *stiff neck* on forward bending (detected by placing the hand under the occiput and passively flexing the neck) is a manifestation of heightened activity of flexor reflexes, presumably due to inflammation of the meninges and spinal roots. J. F. Fulton's explanation of the phenomenon seems most plausible, that the activation of flexor or protective reflexes immobilizes the inflamed meningeal and radicular tissues. Shortening of the spinal axis, accomplished by extension of the neck and back and flexion of the hips and knees, diminishes tension on these inflamed structures. Flexion of the neck as well as the trunk and straight leg, i.e., the Kernig and Brudzinski signs, tend to lengthen the spine and stretch the spinal roots. These maneuvers not only are countered by the muscles engaged in these flexor reflexes but are also painful. *Back retraction* and *opisthotonos* represent the extreme degree of this spinal splinting. Of these several signs, the stiff neck is the most reliable. Nonetheless it may be absent in infants, in whom a bulging fontanel is said to be a more dependable sign of meningitis, and occasionally in the aged patient. Other types of stiff neck, in no way related to meningeal irritation, may be confused with it. Stiffness of neck in all directions of movement or in some direction other than flexion is usually due to disease of the cervical spine or to rigidity of neck muscles which may be a part of generalized rigidity in extrapyramidal diseases or tetanus. The Kernig and Brudzinski signs are likely to be present only in the more advanced and severe cases of meningeal inflammation.

The alteration of consciousness, which tends to be mild in many cases, may take numerous forms such as drowsiness, confusion, delirium, stupor, and coma. In the beginning stages of disease it must be distinguished from the mental changes which may accompany any systemic infection. Its greater prominence in both meningitis and subarachnoid hemorrhage should always alert the physician to the possibility of meningeal disease. Its cause and mechanism are not clear. Presumably it represents an encephalopathy due to the presence of bacteria or blood in the pia-arachnoid next to the cortex. The factor of increased intracranial pressure may be of importance in some cases. Convulsions, which are frequent in meningitis, may have the same explanation. In subarachnoid hemorrhage, coma usually occurs only with massive bleeding in the meninges or with a meningocerebral clot. The CSF pressure is high.

In any widespread meningeal disease, either neoplastic, chemical, i.e., "post spinal anesthesia arachnoiditis," or bacterial, an unusual *meningoradicular syndrome* may develop. Single or multiple cranial and spinal roots may be involved, and even the spinal cord may be compressed or constricted. To this may be added cerebral symptoms and at times hydrocephalus. The abducens, oculomotor, and facial nerves are the ones most often affected intracranially. The lumbosacral roots are most susceptible intraspinally. The resulting clinical syndrome may show multiple variations of meningeal, radicular, spinal cord and hydrocephalic symptoms. Some cases have resembled an acute infectious or other type of polyneuropathy because of the widespread sensory and motor paralysis. The CSF pleocytosis, rarely observed in peripheral neuropathy, is helpful in diagnosis.

HYDROCEPHALUS

This term refers to an increase in the quantity of ventricular fluid, i.e., an increase in the size of the ventricles and consequently in the volume of CSF which they contain. This may result from an atrophy or destruction of brain tissues, a compensatory hydrocephalus (hydrocephalus *ex vacuo*), in which instances the ventricular and the lumbar pressures are normal. Or it may be due to an excessive formation, an obstructed circulation, or a faulty absorption of CSF, in which instances the intraventricular and lumbar pressures are elevated (obstructive hydrocephalus).

Obstructive hydrocephalus obviously has many causes, but they all relate to disease of the choroid plexuses, walls of the ventricles, or meninges. Little is known about diseases of the choroid plexuses except that an occasional example of hyperplasia or hypertrophy has been reported as the sole cause of a hydrocephalus. Apparently the formation of CSF then exceeds the capacity of the drainage or absorptive channels. Even less is known about defects in the absorption of CSF back into the venous blood. Thrombosis of the superior sagittal sinus, which should be the best example of this, does not in fact result in ventricular enlargement, and the high intracranial pressure and papilledema which follow are probably the result of venous congestion. An obstruction to the flow of CSF may occur at any point between the lateral ventricles and cerebral subarachnoid space. Frequent sites are the third ventricle and foramen of Monro, the aqueduct of Sylvius, the fourth ventricle, the basal foramens of Magendie and Luschka, and the subarachnoid space around the midbrain and pons. Usually the obstruction is incomplete, and the ventricles above the block slowly dilate. (Complete obstruction is said to have caused death in 24 to 48 hr.) If the sutures have not closed, the head enlarges; if they have closed, the skull bones become unevenly thin (the convolutional markings or hammered silver appearance seen in the x-ray), but the head does not alter in size and shape. The enlargement of ventricles is mainly at the expense of white matter. The cause of the obstruction may be a tumor, a developmental atresia of the aqueduct of Sylvius or the basal meninges (foramens of Luschka and Magendie), or an Arnold-Chiari malformation with spinal meningomyelocele, tumor, chronic ependymitis, purulent meningitis, or postmeningitic fibrosis. Julien Marie has ascribed hydrocephalus in infants to hypervitaminosis D (*Julien Marie syndrome*).

The symptomatology depends on the age of the patient, the nature of the lesion, and the speed of development of the obstructive process. In congenital hydrocephalus, enlargement of the head is the most prominent symptom, being present at birth or developing rapidly in the first weeks of postnatal life. Because of this easy expansibility of the infant's skull, the intracranial pressure may remain only slightly elevated. Convulsions, progressive blindness with optic atrophy, and bilateral pyramidal tract signs, particularly in the legs, occur later; and the mental state varies from relatively normal to severe impairment.

Headache, vomiting, and papilledema are the common signs of rapidly acquired hydrocephalus in the older child or adult. The headache at first is severe, generalized with nuchal radiation and sometimes head retraction; later it is nearly continuous. *Crises of hydrocephalus* due to intermittent block may be manifested by severe headache, slow mental reactions, episodic impairment of vision, numbness of the face or extremities, and weakness and buckling of the knees, with sudden falls. The blood pressure may rise, pulse may become slow, and respirations may be slow and irregular. Acquired hydrocephalus of more gradual evolution in the older child or adult is more difficult to recognize. Headache, vomiting, and papilledema are not at all prominent. Failing mental function, i.e., psychomotor retardation, inattention, poor emo-

tional control, and other aberrations of behavior, cranial nerve palsies especially bilateral abducens palsy, hypopituitarism with obesity and genital hypoplasia in adolescents, bilateral pyramidal tract signs, and sometimes a mild ataxia of the limbs compose the picture. This chronic hydrocephalic syndrome simulates a dementia and is difficult to differentiate from intracranial tumor and other expanding lesions, except by ventriculography. The dementia, moreover, may obscure the symptoms and signs of the causative lesion, e.g., acoustic neuroma, a dermoid cyst of the cerebellum, a craniopharyngioma, or a cysticercosis of the fourth and third ventricles. These problems will be discussed in further detail in Chap. 283, Developmental Abnormalities of the Nervous System, and Chap. 286, Tumors of the Brain and Spinal Cord.

REFERENCES

Association for Research in Nervous and Mental Diseases: Research Publication XXXIV, chap. VIII, The Formation, Flow and Absorption of CSF: Newer Concepts Based on Studies with Isotopes, Baltimore, 1954.

Fulton, J. F.: "Physiology of the Nervous System," 2d ed., chap. 6, New York, Oxford University Press, 1943.

Merritt, H. H., and F. Fremont-Smith: "The Cerebrospinal Fluid," Philadelphia, W. B. Saunders Company, 1938.

33 FAINTNESS, SYNCOPE, AND EPISODIC WEAKNESS

Raymond D. Adams and T. R. Harrison

Episodic faintness, lightheadedness or giddiness, and reduced alertness are frequent and vexatious symptoms. The patient may refer to these symptoms as "weak spells" when he actually means loss of vigor, a weakness of limbs, or an impaired alertness. Any difference, then, between faintness and syncope would appear to be only quantitative. Since syncope, though less common, is more definite, it will be considered in greater detail. Those types of episodic weakness, such as myasthenia gravis and familial periodic paralysis, which are associated with striking reduction of muscular strength but are unaccompanied by impairment of consciousness, are discussed in other chapters. Epilepsy, which is also associated with episodic unconsciousness, differs from syncope in most other respects. It is discussed in Chap. 36.

CARDINAL FEATURES OF SYNCOPE

The term *syncope* literally means a "cutting short," "cessation," or "pause" and is synonymous with *swoon* or *faint*. Syncope comprises a generalized weakness of muscles, with an inability to stand upright and an impairment of consciousness. Abrupt onset, brief duration, and complete recovery within a few minutes are other distinguishing features. Faintness, in contrast, refers to a lack of strength, with a sensation of impending faint. It is an incomplete faint. Both faintness and syncope vary somewhat according to their mechanism, but both conform roughly to the following pattern.

The syncopal attack develops rapidly, but it is doubtful whether consciousness is ever terminated with the absolute suddenness of a seizure, even when there is an arrest of cardiac action. At the beginning of the attack, the patient is nearly always in the upright position, either sitting or standing. Usually the warning of the impending faint is a sense of "feeling badly." He is assailed by giddiness, the floor seems to move, and surrounding objects begin to sway or spin around. His senses become confused, he yawns or gapes, there are spots before the eyes, or vision may dim and the ears ring. Nausea and sometimes actual vomiting accompany these symptoms. If the patient can lie down promptly, the attack may be averted without complete loss of consciousness. If he cannot, there is "loss of senses" and falling to the ground. What is most noticeable, even at the beginning of the attack, is a striking pallor or ashen-gray color of the face, and very often the face and body are bathed in a cold perspiration. As a rule the deliberate onset enables the patient to lie down or at least to protect himself as he slumps. A hurtful fall is exceptional.

The depth and duration of the unconsciousness vary. Sometimes the patient is not completely oblivious of his surroundings. His senses are confused, but he may still be able to hear the voices or see the blurred outlines of people around him. Again, coma may be profound, and there may be complete lack of awareness and of capacity to respond. The patient may remain in this state for seconds to minutes or even as long as half an hour.

Shortly after the beginning of unconsciousness, convulsive movements occur in some cases. These usually consist of several clonic jerks of the arms and twitchings of the face. Rarely is there a generalized tonic-clonic convulsion. Usually the person who has fainted lies motionless, with skeletal muscles completely relaxed. Sphincter control is maintained in nearly all cases. The pulse is thin or cannot be felt; the blood pressure is low and breathing is almost imperceptible. This reduction in vital functions, the striking pallor, and unconsciousness simulate death.

Once the patient is in the horizontal position, perhaps from having fallen, gravitation no longer hinders the flow of blood to the brain. The strength of the pulse improves, and color begins to return to the face. Breathing becomes quicker and deeper. Then the eyelids flutter, and consciousness is quickly regained. There is from this moment onward a correct perception of the environment. The patient is nevertheless keenly aware of physical weakness; and if he rises too soon, another faint may be precipitated. Headache and drowsiness, which, with mental confusion, are the usual sequelae of a convulsion, do not follow a syncopal attack.

CLASSIFICATION OF CAUSES OF RECURRENT WEAKNESS, FAINTNESS, AND DISTURBANCES OF CONSCIOUSNESS

The following list is based on established or assumed physiologic mechanisms. Some of the disorders frequently cause episodic weakness but rarely cause syncope. A few are especially apt to cause syncope associated with convulsions. These features are indicated in accompanying parentheses. Unless this specific notation is made, it may be assumed that the disorder in question is likely to cause faintness (when mild) and syncope (when severe).

I. CIRCULATORY (deficient *quantity* of blood to the brain—common causes of either faintness or syncope)

  A. Peripheral circulatory failure (defective venous return to the heart) (Chap. 13)

    1. Psychogenic (vasovagal) syncope

    2. Postural hypotension

    3. Increased intrathoracic pressure, e.g., tussive syncope

    4. Other causes of peripheral circulatory failure (Chap. 13)

  B. Cardiac (acute cardiac failure, see Chap. 13)

    1. Alterations in rate or rhythm

      a. Ectopic tachycardias (Chap. 250)

      b. Bradycardia

        (1) *Myogenic* (heart block, see Chap. 250, convulsions frequently occur)

        (2) Neurogenic (reflex bradycardia)

          (*a*) *Hypersensitive carotid sinus*

          (*b*) Rarer causes of reflex bradycardia

    2. *Acute myocardial injury* (especially infarction, see Chap. 3)

    3. Mechanical hindrance

      a. Aortic stenosis

      b. Disorders of pulmonary vessels, e.g., embolism

II. OTHER CAUSES OF WEAKNESS AND EPI-
SODIC DISTURBANCES OF CONSCIOUSNESS

   A. Chemical (defective *quality* of blood to the
      brain)
      1. *Hyperventilation* (faintness common; syncope
         seldom occurs)
      2. *Hypoglycemia* (episodic weakness common,
         faintness occasional, syncope rare)
   B. Cerebral
      1. *Epilepsy* (akinetic, see Chap. 36, other con-
         vulsive disorders common)
      2. Cerebral vascular disturbances (cerebral is-
         chemic attacks)
      3. Hypertensive encephalopathy
      4. Emotional disturbances (hysterical seizures)

This list of the conditions which cause weakness, faintness, and disturbances of consciousness is deceptively long and involved. Closer study, however, reveals that the more common types of faint are reducible to a few simple mechanisms. In order not to obscure the central problem of fainting by too many details, only a few of the more common varieties likely to be encountered in clinical practice are discussed below.

COMMON TYPES OF SYNCOPE

Vasovagal, Vasodepressor (Psychogenic) Syncope. This is the ordinary faint, and the description already given applies most perfectly to this form of it. The loss of consciousness usually takes place when the systolic pressure falls to 70 mm Hg or below. The pulse is weak or imperceptible, and its rate may be either slowed or slightly increased. Sudden vasodilatation, particularly of intramuscular vessels, is responsible for the fainting. It has been thought to represent a response to an emotional or physical stimulus which would ordinarily call for immediate strenuous physical activity. In the absence of such activity, there is sudden pooling of blood in the muscles, with inadequate venous return, decline in cerebral blood flow, and loss of consciousness. These considerations explain the rarity of vasovagal syncope in the recumbent position or during active muscular exercise, which increases the venous return. However, this explanation is somewhat speculative, and there are surprisingly few studies of this type of syncope.

Vasovagal or vasodepressor faints occur (1) in normal health as a consequence of a strong emotional experience or in conditions which favor vasodilatation, e.g., hot crowded rooms, especially if the person is tired, hungry, or ill; (2) in anxiety states and neurocirculatory asthenia; (3) during pain; (4) after injury to tissues as a consequence of shock, pain, and psychologic factors.

Postural Hypotension with Syncope. This type of syncope affects persons who have a chronic defect in or a variable instability of vasomotor reflexes. The character of the syncopal attack differs little from that of the vasovagal or vasodepressor type. The effect of posture is the cardinal feature of it. Sudden arising from a recumbent position or standing still is the condition under which it usually occurs.

Nature has provided man with several mechanisms by which his circulation adjusts to the upright posture. The pooling of blood in the lower parts of the body is prevented by (1) pressor reflexes which induce constriction of peripheral arteries and arterioles; (2) reflex acceleration of the heart by means of aortic and carotid reflexes; (3) improvement of venous return to the heart by activity of the muscles of the limbs and by increased rate of respiration. A normal individual placed on a tilt table to relax his muscles and tilted upright has a slightly diminished cardiac output, and blood accumulates in the legs to a slight degree. This is followed by a slight transitory fall in systolic blood pressure and then, within a few seconds, by a compensatory rise. Some normal individuals if tilted on a table will faint. In them it has been found that at first the blood pressure falls slightly and then stabilizes at a *lower* level. Shortly thereafter these compensatory reflexes suddenly fail, and the blood pressure falls precipitously. This also happens in some of the conditions listed below. In others, e.g., after surgical sympathectomy and in the unusual condition of chronic orthostatic hypotension, the blood pressure never stabilizes after tilting but falls steadily to a level at which cerebral circulation cannot be maintained.

Postural syncope tends to occur under the following conditions: (1) in otherwise normal individuals who for some unknown reason have defective postural reflexes (chronic orthostatic hypotension); (2) rarely as part of a syndrome which comprises orthostatic hypertension and symptoms and signs of pyramidal and extrapyramidal nervous disorder; (3) after prolonged illness with recumbency, especially in elderly individuals with flabby muscles; (4) after a sympathectomy which abolishes vasopressor reflexes; (5) in diabetic neuropathy, tabes dorsalis, and other diseases of the nervous system which cause flabby, weak muscles and paralysis of vasopressor reflexes; (6) in persons with varicose veins because of pooling of blood in the abnormal venous channels.

In chronic orthostatic hypotension, a special form of this type of syncope and a relatively rare condition, the postural hypotension differs from that already described in that the systolic and diastolic blood pressures fall rapidly as soon as the patient assumes an upright position but without compensatory tachycardia, pallor, sweating, nausea, or other symptoms. The loss of consciousness is usually abrupt and may be attended by confusion. Recumbency restores the circulation of the brain, with a prompt return of consciousness. The pooling of blood in the abdomen and legs does not excite vasoconstriction of peripheral vessels. This is apparently because of an abnormality in the autonomic nervous system. There is also evidence that patients with this type of postural hypotension have deficiency in release of norepinephrine and epinephrine. Repeated attacks may result in mental confusion, slurred speech, and other neurologic signs.

Syncope of Cardiac Origin (Cardiac Syncope). The occurrence of fainting in patients with a permanently slow pulse was first described by Morgagni and subsequently by Adams and by Stokes. It is today known as the *Adams-Stokes syndrome*. The pulse is usually under 40, and the electrocardiogram shows a transient or permanent atrioventricular block. Usually without more than a momentary sense of weakness, the patient suddenly loses consciousness. This may occur at any time of day or night regardless of the position of the body. In the upright position the unconsciousness will develop after a briefer period of asystole than in the recumbent position. According to Engel, 4 to 8 sec of asystole produces coma in the erect position, and 12 to 15 sec is required in recumbency. If cardiac standstill is more than 12 sec, the patient turns pale, falls unconscious, and may exhibit a few clonic jerks. The blood pressure falls rapidly during the period of asystole. With the resumption of the heartbeat the face and neck become flushed. Longer periods of asystole, up to 5 min, result in coma, ashen-gray pallor giving way to cyanosis, stertorous breathing, fixed pupils, incontinence, and bilateral Babinski signs. Prolonged confusion and neurologic signs due to the relative ischemia of parts of the brain supplied by narrowed, arteriosclerotic arteries may persist in some cases, and permanent impairment of mental function is not unknown. Cardiac faints of this type may recur several times a day. Occasionally the heart block is transitory, and the electrocardiogram taken later shows only evidence of myocardial disease. Another form is that in which the heart block is reflex and due to irritation of the vagus nerves. Examples of this phenomenon have been observed with esophageal diverticula, mediastinal tumors, carotid sinus disease, glossopharyngeal neuralgia, pleural and pulmonary irritation. However, reflex bradycardia is more commonly of the sinoatrial type than of the atrioventricular type.

Aortic stenosis and, less often, insufficiency dispose to fainting attacks. The mechanism is not well understood. In some cases it appears to be due to

heart block, but not all cases can be explained in this way. A characteristic clinical feature is that the faint occurs during or immediately after exertion. There may be an initial pallor, weakness, or lightheadedness, or no warning whatsoever. Unconsciousness may last as long as half an hour, and convulsions sometimes occur.

Paroxysmal atrial and ventricular tachycardia cause unconsciousness by interfering with cardiac filling and output. A series of ventricular asystoles may have the same effect. Most patients who faint because of paroxysmal ectopic tachycardia are aware of the preliminary rapid heart action. Otherwise, the syncopal attack does not differ from the aforementioned types.

A cardiac faint, sometimes fatal, may occur in patients with disease of the coronary arteries. No explanation for death is found at autopsy. Also fainting is not infrequent in myocardial infarction. During acute coronary occlusion several factors—pain, ventricular tachycardia, momentary ventricular fibrillation, and heart block—are probably of importance.

Carotid Sinus Syncope. The carotid sinus is normally sensitive to stretch and gives rise to sensory impulses which are carried via the intercarotid nerve of Hering (branch of the glossopharyngeal nerve) to the medulla oblongata. Massage of one or both carotid sinuses, particularly in elderly people, causes a reflex slowing of the heart or even heart block, a fall of blood pressure without cardiac slowing, or an interference with the circulation of the ipsilateral cerebral hemisphere.

Syncope due to carotid sinus sensitivity may be initiated by turning the head to one side, by a tight collar, or as in one reported case, by shaving over the region of the sinus. The absence of such stimuli is of no aid in diagnosis, since spontaneous attacks may occur. The attack nearly always begins when the patient is in the upright position, usually when he is standing. The onset is sudden, often with falling. Clonic convulsive movements are not infrequent in the vagal and depressor type of carotid sinus syncope. Unilateral paresthesias or convulsions have been reported in the central type. The period of unconsciousness seldom lasts longer than a few minutes. The sensorium is immediately clear when consciousness is regained. The majority of the reported cases have been in males.

In a patient displaying faintness on compression of one carotid sinus, it is important to distinguish between the benign disorder, hypersensitivity of one carotid sinus, and a much more serious condition, atheromatous narrowing of the opposite carotid or of the basilar artery (see Chap. 284).

Tussive Syncope ("Laryngeal Vertigo"). This condition is rare but should be mentioned because it illustrates another mechanism of fainting—that resulting from a paroxysm of coughing. The few patients that the authors have observed have been men with chronic bronchitis. After hard coughing the patient suddenly becomes weak and loses consciousness momentarily. The unconsciousness that results from breath holding in infants is probably similar. Not all the underlying physiologic changes are known. It is said that the intrathoracic pressure becomes elevated and interferes with the venous return to the heart. The Valsalva maneuver of trying to exhale against the closed glottis is believed to produce an identical effect. Episodes of faintness and lightheadedness are not infrequent in pertussis and chronic laryngitis.

CONDITIONS OFTEN ASSOCIATED WITH EPISODIC WEAKNESS AND FAINTNESS BUT NOT WITH SYNCOPE

Anxiety Attacks and the Hyperventilation Syndrome. This condition is discussed in detail in Chap. 42, and it is necessary here only to state that this disorder is one of the commonest causes of recurrent faintness without actual loss of consciousness, the symptoms *are not relieved by recumbency,* and the diagnosis depends in large measure on reproducing the symptoms by hyperventilation. Two mechanisms are involved in the attacks: loss of carbon dioxide as the result of hyperventilation and release of epinephrine. Both these mechanisms are said to be initiated by anxiety or allied emotional disturbances.

Of aid in diagnosis, as well as in therapy, is the demonstration to the patient of many of the symptoms of the anxiety attack by voluntary hyperventilation for a period of 2 to 3 min and the intramuscular injection of 1.0 cc of a 1:1,000 solution of epinephrine. However, it must be admitted that the initial symptoms of the attack are not reproduced and that in some cases such measures are entirely without demonstrable effect.

Hypoglycemia. Another frequent cause of obscure episodic weakness is spontaneous hypoglycemia. When severe, the condition is likely to be due to a serious disease such as a tumor of the islets of Langerhans or advanced adrenal, pituitary, or hepatic disease, in which instances there may be a confusion or even a loss of consciousness. When mild, as is usually the case, hypoglycemia is of the reactive type (Chap. 71) and occurs 2 to 5 hr after eating. The fasting blood glucose is normal. The diagnosis depends largely upon the reproduction by the injection of insulin of a symptom complex exactly similar to that occurring in the spontaneous attacks.

Acute Internal Hemorrhage. This condition, usually within the gastrointestinal tract, is an occasional cause of syncope. Peptic ulcer is the most common source of the hemorrhage. When pain is absent, as it not infrequently is, and when there is no hematemesis, the cause of the weakness, faintness, or even unconsciousness may remain obscure until the passage of a black stool.

Cerebral Ischemic Attacks. Some patients with arteriosclerotic narrowing or occlusion of the major arteries of the brain may have repeated attacks, all of identical pattern, in which there is a temporary focal deficit in cerebral function. The main symptoms vary from patient to patient and include dim vision, hemiparesis, numbness of one side of the body, dizziness, and thick speech; and to these may be added an impairment of consciousness. The mechanism of this vascular syndrome has not been fully elucidated. Some physicians hold that localized vasospasm is responsible; others ascribe the attacks to small focal vascular lesions. The authors' own investigations suggest some other mechanism than either of these. The condition is discussed more fully in Chap. 284.

Hysterical Fainting. This subject is discussed more fully in Chap. 43. Fainting, which is rather frequent, usually occurs under dramatic circumstances. Unconsciousness may begin at any time, regardless of the position of the patient, and a surprising number of attacks occur when the patient is with friends at the theater or is engaged in some social activity. During the attack, there may be no motion whatsoever, but struggling, mumbling, and even well-directed movements of resistance of the limbs are sometimes observed. Bizarre postures may be seen. The patient usually recovers within a few minutes but may remain in this condition for hours or days. The spell then has the aspect of a trance rather than a faint. This fainting is unattended by any outward display of anxiety. The evident lack of change in pulse and blood pressure or color of the skin and mucous membranes requires that it be distinguished from the vasodepressor faint induced by a shocking emotional experience.

It is doubtful whether the patient in a hysterical faint is unconscious at all. Certainly the electroencephalograms are normal, and by amobarbital (Sodium Amytal) interviews the patient may be able to recall events that took place during the faint—recall which would be impossible with a real faint. The diagnosis is based on the bizarre nature of the attacks in a person who exhibits the general personality and behavior characteristics of hysteria (see Chap. 43).

PATHOPHYSIOLOGY OF SYNCOPE

In the final analysis the loss of consciousness in these different types of syncope must be caused by a change in the nervous elements in those parts of the brain which subserve consciousness. Syncope resembles epilepsy in this respect; yet there is an important difference. In epilepsy, whether major or minor, the arrest in mental function is almost instantaneous and, as revealed by the electroencephalogram, is accompanied by a paroxysm of activity in certain groups of cerebral neurones. Syncope, on the other hand, is probably never so sudden; even when due to cardiac arrest there is often a brief warning. This difference relates to the essential pathophysiology—a sudden spread of an electrical discharge in epilepsy, and the more gradual failure of cerebral circulation in syncope.

During syncopal attacks, measurements of cerebral circulation (Schmidt-Kety and Gibbs's methods) demonstrate a significant degree of reduction in cerebral blood flow and of cerebral oxygen utilization (cerebral metabolism). Cerebral vascular resistance is decreased. The electroencephalogram reveals high voltage, slow waves of 2 to 5 per second coincident with the loss of consciousness. Hyperventilation results in hypocapnia, alkalosis, increased cerebrovascular resistance, and decreased cerebral blood flow.

DIFFERENTIAL DIAGNOSIS

Of Syncope from Other Transitory Nervous Disorders. The recognition of the more typical varieties of syncope is of importance in clinical medicine, and they must be distinguished from other disturbances of cerebral function, the most frequent of which is the epileptic seizure. It is now believed that some epileptic patients, especially those subject to typical or atypical forms of petit mal, may lose consciousness and fall to the ground without a quiver. In these latter attacks, sometimes called *akinetic epilepsy*, there may be complete loss or only slight impairment of consciousness. In the more pronounced form of each condition—akinetic or minor epilepsy and syncope—there are nonetheless clinical differences that often make for clear distinction between them. Epilepsy may occur day or night, regardless of the position of the patient; syncope appears only under special conditions when the patient is awake and in an erect position, the only exception being some types of cardiac syncope. The patient's color does not change in epilepsy; pallor is usually an early and invariable finding in all types of syncope, except chronic orthostatic hypotension and hysteria, and precedes unconsciousness. Epilepsy is sudden in onset, and if an aura is present it rarely lasts longer than a few seconds before consciousness is abolished.

The onset of syncope is usually more deliberate. Even in the cardiac types in which there is asystole, the oxygen supply of the brain will maintain consciousness for several seconds. There are exceptions to this rule, however, for in some cases of Adams-Stokes syndrome consciousness may be lost without any warning whatsoever. Injury from falling is frequent in epilepsy and rare in syncope for the reason that only in the former are protective reflexes instantaneously abolished. Tonic convulsive movements with upturning eyes are frequent in epilepsy in contrast to syncope, though the same cannot be said of clonic movements of the arms. The period of unconsciousness tends to be longer in epilepsy than in syncope. Urinary incontinence is frequent in epilepsy and rare in syncope; but since it may be observed in syncope, it cannot be used as a means of excluding syncope. The return of consciousness is prompt in syncope and slow in epilepsy. Mental confusion, headache, and drowsiness are the common sequelae of epilepsy, whereas physical weakness with clear sensorium characterizes the postsyncopal state. Repeated spells of unconsciousness in a young person at a rate of several per day or month are much more suggestive of epilepsy than syncope. It should be emphasized that no one of these points will absolutely differentiate epilepsy from syncope, but taken as a group they provide a means of distinguishing the two conditions.

Of the Different Types of Syncope. The differentiation of the several conditions which cause a diminution in cerebral blood flow is discussed in some detail in Chap. 34, and only a few points need to be repeated here.

When faintness is related to a reduced cerebral blood flow resulting directly from a disorder of cardiac function, there is likely to be a combination of pallor and cyanosis, pronounced dyspnea, and distention of the veins. When on the other hand the peripheral circulation is at fault, pallor is usually striking but is not accompanied by cyanosis or respiratory disturbances, and the veins are collapsed. When the primary disturbance lies in the cerebral circulation, the face is likely to be florid and the breathing slow and stertorous. During the attack a heart rate faster than 150 per minute indicates an ectopic cardiac rhythm, while a striking bradycardia (rate less than 40) suggests the presence of complete heart block. In a patient with faintness or syncope attended by bradycardia, one has to distinguish between the neurogenic reflex and the myogenic (Adams-Stokes) types. Occasionally electrocardiographic tracings will be needed, but as a rule the Adams-Stokes seizures can be recognized by their longer duration, by the greater constancy of the heart rate, by the presence of audible sounds synchronous with atrial contraction, and by the marked variation in intensity of the first sound, despite the regular rhythm (Chap.

250). Clinical diagnosis may at times be difficult or impossible.

The color of the skin, the character of the breathing, the appearance of the veins, and the rate of the heart are therefore valuable data in diagnosis *if the patient is seen during an attack.* Unfortunately the physician does not have the opportunity to see most of the patients during their "spells" of weakness. Hence he must obtain the proper clues from the patient's story. It is therefore of primary importance that the physician be familiar with the *circumstances* and the *precipitating* and *alleviating* factors in a given episode of weakness or fainting.

Type of Onset. When the attack begins with relative suddenness, i.e., over the period of a few seconds, carotid sinus syncope or postural hypotension is likely. When the symptoms develop gradually during a period of several minutes, hyperventilation or hypoglycemia (spontaneous or induced by insulin) is to be considered. Onset of syncope during or immediately after exertion is suggestive of aortic stenosis, and in elderly subjects, of postural hypotension. Exertional syncope is likewise occasionally seen in persons with aortic insufficiency.

Position at Onset of Attack. Attacks which are due to hypoglycemia, hyperventilation, hypertensive encephalopathy, or heart block are likely to be independent of posture. Faintness associated with a decline in blood pressure (including carotid sinus attacks) and with ectopic tachycardia usually occurs only in the sitting or standing position, while faintness resulting from orthostatic hypotension or orthostatic tachycardia is apt to set in shortly after the change from the recumbent to the standing position.

Associated Symptoms. The associated symptoms during the attack are important, for palpitation is likely to be present when the attack is due to anxiety or hyperventilation, to ectopic tachycardia, or to hypoglycemia. Numbness and tingling in the hands and face are frequent accompaniments of hyperventilation. Irregular jerking movements and generalized spasms without loss of consciousness or change in the electroencephalogram are typical of the hysterical faint. Genuine convulsions during the attack, although characteristic of epilepsy, may occasionally occur with heart block and with hypertensive encephalopathy.

Duration of Attack. When the duration of the seizure is very brief, i.e., a few seconds to a few minutes, one thinks particularly of carotid sinus syncope, vasodepressor syncope, or one of the several forms of postural hypotension. A duration of more than a few minutes, but less than an hour, is particularly suggestive of hypoglycemia or hyperventilation.

SPECIAL METHODS OF EXAMINATION

In many patients who complain of recurrent weakness or syncope but do not have a spontaneous attack while under the observation of the physician, an attempt to *reproduce* attacks is of a great assistance in diagnosis. In order to avoid the effects of suggestion, rigid controls must be adopted. Thus if one wishes to determine whether the attacks in a given subject are hypoglycemic in type and may be reproduced by insulin injection, it is necessary to control the observations by injecting other drugs such as atropine, nitroglycerin, or histamine which evoke subjective symptoms of a different type. When properly controlled, the insulin test is of great value in the diagnosis of spontaneous hypoglycemia. Without such controls the procedure is useless.

When hyperventilation is accompanied by faintness, the pattern of symptoms can be reproduced readily by having the subject breathe rapidly and deeply for 2 or 3 min. This test is often of therapeutic value also, because the underlying anxiety tends to be lessened when the patient learns that he can produce and alleviate the symptoms at will simply by controlling his breathing.

Among the other conditions in which the diagnosis is commonly clarified by reproducing the attacks are carotid sinus hypersensitivity (massage of one or the other carotid sinus), orthostatic hypotension, and orthostatic tachycardia (observations of pulse rate, blood pressure, and symptoms in the recumbent and standing positions). In all such instances one should remember that *the crucial point is not whether symptoms are produced* (the procedures mentioned frequently induce symptoms in healthy persons) but whether the exact pattern of symptoms which occurs in the spontaneous attacks is reproduced in the artificial seizures.

Multiple mechanisms of syncope frequently coexist. Combinations of hypoglycemia, hyperventilation, and postural hypotension, or any two of them, are frequent. In order to reproduce exactly the spontaneous symptoms, it may be necessary to have the patient stand and hyperventilate at a time when the blood sugar has been reduced by insulin administration. When tremor, palpitation, and fright are present in the spontaneous attacks, it may be necessary to carry out these procedures in association with the administration of epinephrine. There is great psychotherapeutic value to the patient in *knowing* that the physician can turn his "spells" on and off at will, and, therefore, is not guessing about their cause and significance.

Lastly, the electroencephalogram is also helpful in diagnosis. In the interval between epileptic seizures it may show some degree of abnormality in 40 to 80 per cent of cases. In the interval between syncopal attacks it should be normal.

TREATMENT

Fainting in most instances is due to a relatively innocent cause. In dealing with patients who have fainted the physician should think first of those causes of fainting which constitute a therapeutic emergency. Among them are massive internal hemorrhage and myocardial infarction, which may be painless. In an elderly person a sudden faint, without obvious cause, should arouse the suspicion of complete heart block, even though all findings are negative when the physician sees the patient. When this suspicion is strong, it may be wise to institute appropriate therapy (Chap. 250), even before further episodes have confirmed the diagnosis.

If the patient is seen during the preliminary stages of fainting or after he has lost consciousness, one should make sure that he is in a position which permits maximal cerebral blood flow, i.e., with head lowered between the knees, if sitting, or lying supine. All tight clothing and other constrictions should be loosened and the head turned so that the tongue does not fall back into the throat, blocking the airway. Peripheral irritation such as sprinkling or dashing cold water on the face and neck or the application of cold towels is helpful. If the temperature is subnormal, the body should be covered with a warm blanket. If available, aromatic spirit of ammonia may be given cautiously by inhalation. Epinephrine, 0.5 ml of a 1:1,000 solution, or phenylephrine hydrochloride (Neo-synephrine), 0.5 mg intravenously or 5.0 mg subcutaneously, may be administered. One should be prepared for a possible emesis. Nothing should be given by mouth until the patient has regained consciousness. Then 1/2 tsp aromatic spirit of ammonia in a half glass of cold water or a sip of brandy or whisky may be given. The patient should not be permitted to arise until his sense of physical weakness has passed, and he should be watched carefully for a few minutes after rising.

As a rule the physician sees the patient after the faint has occurred, and he is asked to explain why it happened and how it can be prevented in the future. The prevention of fainting depends on the mechanism involved. In the usual vasovagal faint of adolescents, which tends to occur in periods of emotional excitement, fatigue, hunger, etc., it is enough to advise the patient to avoid such circumstances. If the patient is sickly, measures to improve general health and circulatory efficiency are useful. In postural hypotension the patient should be cautioned against arising suddenly from bed. Instead he should first exercise the legs for a few seconds, then sit on the edge of the bed and make

sure he is not lightheaded or dizzy before starting to walk. He should sleep with the headposts of the bed elevated on wooden blocks 8 to 12 in. high. A snug elastic abdominal binder and elastic stockings are often helpful. Drugs of the ephedrine group (ephedrine sulfate, 0.025 Gm t.i.d.) may be useful if they do not cause insomnia. If there are no contraindications, a high intake of sodium chloride, which expands the extracellular fluid volume, may be beneficial.

In the syndrome of chronic orthostatic hypotension, oxytocin (Pitocin) has recently been found to give dramatic relief in some cases.

The treatment of carotid sinus syncope involves first of all the instruction of the patient in those measures which minimize the hazards of a fall (see below). Loose collars should be worn, and the patient should learn to turn the whole body, rather than the head alone, when looking to one side. Atropine or the ephedrine group of drugs should be used, respectively, in patients with pronounced bradycardia or hypotension during the attacks. Radiation or surgical denervation of the carotid sinus has apparently yielded favorable results in some patients but is rarely necessary. Once the possibility that the attacks are due to a narrowing of major cerebral arteries has been excluded, emphatic reassurance is essential for such patients, the majority of whom are under the mistaken impression that strokes or cardiac disease are responsible for the episodes.

The treatment of the various cardiac arrhythmias which may induce syncope is discussed on pp. 1394 to 1405. The treatment of hypoglycemia will be found on p. 662, and of the hyperventilation syndrome and hysterical fainting on pp. 403 and 404.

The chief hazard of a faint in most elderly persons is not the underlying disease but rather of fracture or other trauma due to the fall. Therefore, patients subject to recurrent syncope should cover the bathroom floor and bathtub with rubber mats and should have as much of the home carpeted as is feasible. Especially important is the floor space between the bed and the bathroom, because faints are common in elderly persons when walking from bed to toilet. Outdoor walking should be on soft ground rather than hard surfaces, when possible, and the patient should avoid standing still, which is much more likely than walking to induce an attack.

SUMMARY

In conclusion it should be emphasized that the majority of conditions which produce recurrent weakness and syncope are not serious. When the less frequent conditions, such as heart block, ventricular arrhythmias, myocardial infarction, aortic stenosis, internal hemorrhage, hypertensive encephalopathy, and organic lesions of the brain, have been excluded, the assumption of a relatively benign disorder is usually justified. The same may be said of the chemical disorders which usually induce episodic weakness rather than syncope.

Attacks of both types are likely to be interpreted by the patient, and occasionally by the physician, as being due to serious disease of the circulatory apparatus or of the nervous system. Many of these patients are therefore worried and anxious, often out of all proportion to the seriousness of the condition. Once the mystery has been solved by careful study, and its exact significance has been explained to the patient, his fears are usually allayed.

A number of the topics considered in this chapter are discussed elsewhere in the book. The mechanisms of the circulatory disorders which may cause syncope are considered in Chap. 34. Epilepsy as a cause of recurrent unconsciousness is discussed in Chap. 36. The hyperventilation syndrome is considered in Chap. 42.

REFERENCES

Bradbury, S., and C. Eggleston: Postural Hypotension, Am. Heart J., 1:73, 1925.

Chapman, E. M., and E. Asmussen: On the Occurrence of Dyspnea, Dizziness, and Precordial Distress Occasioned by the Pooling of Blood in Varicose Veins, J. Clin. Invest., 21:393, 1942.

Ellis, L. B., and F. W. Haynes: Postural Hypotension, Arch. Internal Med., 58:773, 1936.

Engel, G. L.: "Fainting," Springfield, Ill., Charles C Thomas, Publisher, 1950.

Ferris, E. B., Jr., R. B. Capps, and S. Weiss: Carotid Sinus Syncope and Its Bearing on the Mechanism of the Unconscious State and Convulsions, Medicine, 14:377, 1935.

Gowers, W. R.: "The Borderland of Epilepsy," London, J. A. Churchill, 1907.

Harris, Seale: Hyperinsulinism and Dysinsulinism, J.A.M.A., 83:729, 1924.

Harrison, T. R.: Clinical Syndromes Produced by Temporary Disturbances of the Cerebral Circulation, J. Mt. Sinai Hosp., 8:612, 1942.

—— and R. M. Finks: Glucose Deficiency as a Factor in the Production of Symptoms Referable to the Cardiovascular System, Am. Heart J., 26:147, 1943.

Luft, Rolf, and Ulf S. von Euler: Two Cases of Postural Hypotension Showing a Deficiency in Release of Nor-epinephrine and Epinephrine, J. Clin. Invest., 22:1065, 1953.

Stead, E. A., Jr.: Fainting, Am. J. Med., 13:387, 1952.

Weiss, S.: in "The Oxford Loose-leaf Medicine," vol. 2, p. 250, H. A. Christian (Ed.), New York, Oxford University Press, 1949.

Wolf, L.: The Cardinal Manifestations of Paroxysmal Tachycardias. II. Vascular Collapse, New Engl. J. Med., 232:527, 1945.

34 COMA AND RELATED DISTURBANCES OF CONSCIOUSNESS

Raymond D. Adams

The practitioner of medicine is frequently called upon to treat patients whose principal abnormality is an impairment of consciousness which varies from simple confusion to coma. In large municipal hospitals it is estimated that as many as 3 per cent of total admissions are due to diseases which have caused coma, and although this figure seems high, it serves to emphasize the importance of this class of neurologic diseases and the necessity for every student of medicine to acquire a theoretic as well as a practical knowledge of them.

The terms *consciousness, confusion, stupor, unconsciousness,* and *coma* have been endowed with so many different meanings that it is almost impossible to avoid ambiguity in their usage. This arises from the fact that they are not strictly medical terms, but literary, philosophic, and psychologic ones as well. The word *consciousness* is the most difficult of all. William James once remarked that everyone knew what consciousness was until he attempted to define it. To the psychologist consciousness denotes a state of awareness of one's self and one's environment. Knowledge of one's self, of course, includes all "feeling attitudes and emotions, impulses, volitions, and the active or striving aspects of conduct" (English)—in short, an awareness of all of one's own mental functioning, particularly the cognitive processes. These can be judged only by a verbal account of the patient's introspections and indirectly by his actions. Physicians, being practical men for the most part, have learned to place greater confidence in their observations of the patient's general behavior and his reactions to overt stimuli than to what he says. For this reason when they employ the term *consciousness* they usually do so in its commonest and simplest signification, viz., a state of awareness of the environment. This narrow definition has another advantage in that the word *unconsciousness* is its exact opposite—a state of unawareness of environment or a suspension of those mental activities by which man is made aware of his environment. However, it must be pointed out that in psychoanalysis the word *unconscious* has a different meaning, standing for that repository of memories of previous experiences that cannot be immediately recalled to the conscious mind.

DESCRIPTION OF STATES OF NORMAL AND IMPAIRED CONSCIOUSNESS

The following definitions, while admittedly unacceptable to most psychologists, are of service to medicine, and the student will find that they provide him with a convenient grammar for describing the mental states of his patients.

Normal Consciousness. The condition of the normal individual when fully awake, in which he is responsive to psychologic stimuli and "indicates by his behavior and speech that he has the same awareness of himself and his environment as ourselves." This normal state may fluctuate during the course of the day from keen alertness or deep concentration with a marked constriction of the field of attention to general inattentiveness and drowsiness.

Sleep. A state of physical and mental inactivity from which the patient may be aroused to resume normal consciousness. A person in sleep gives little evidence of being aware of himself or his environment, and in this respect he is unconscious. Yet he differs from the comatose patient in that he may still respond to unaccustomed stimuli and at times is capable of some mental activity in the form of dreams which leave their traces in memory. And, of course, he can be recalled to a state of normal consciousness when stimulated.

Coma. A state in which the patient appears to be asleep but is at the same time incapable of sensing or responding adequately to either external stimuli or inner needs. Coma may vary in degree, and in its deepest stages no reaction of any kind is obtainable. Corneal, pupillary, pharyngeal, tendon, and plantar reflexes are all absent. There may or may not be extensor rigidity of the limbs and opisthotonos, signs which, Sherrington showed, indicate decerebration. Respirations are often slow and may be periodic, i.e., Cheyne-Stokes breathing. In lighter stages, referred to as *semicoma,* most of the above reflexes can be elicited, and the plantar reflexes may be either flexor or extensor (Babinski sign). Moreover, pricking or pinching the skin, shaking and shouting at the patient, or an uncomfortable distention of the bladder may cause the patient to stir or moan and his respirations to quicken.

Stupor. A state in which mental and physical activity are reduced to a minimum. Although inaccessible to many stimuli, the patient opens his eyes, looks at the examiner, and does not appear to be unconscious. Response to spoken commands is either absent or slow and inadequate. As a rule there are no alterations of tendon or plantar reflexes. On the other hand, tremulousness of movement, coarse twitching of muscles, restless or stereotyped motor activity, grasping and sucking reflexes are not infrequent. It should be pointed out that in psychiatry the term *stupor* has a special meaning —a state in which impressions of the external world are normally received, but activity is marked by negativism, e.g., catatonic schizophrenia.

Confusion. A state in which the patient is incapable of thinking with customary rapidity and coherence. A severely confused person is usually unable to do more than carry out a few simple commands. His capacity for speech is limited to a few words or phrases. He is unaware of much that goes on around him and does not grasp his immediate situation. A moderately confused individual can carry on a simple conversation for short periods of time, but his thinking is slow and incoherent, and disorientation for time and place is evident. In mild degrees of confusion the disorder of thinking may be so slight that it is overlooked unless the examiner is objective in his analysis of the patient's behavior and conversation. The patient may be roughly oriented as to time and place and able to speak freely on almost any subject. Only occasional irrelevant remarks betray an incoherence of thinking. Patients with mild or moderately severe confusion may be submitted to psychologic testing. The degree of confusion often varies from one time of day to another, tending to be least pronounced in the early morning. Severe confusion or stupor may resemble semicoma during periods when the patient is drowsy or asleep. Many events which happen to the confused patient leave no trace in memory; in fact, capacity to recall later events that transpired in any given period is one of the most delicate tests of mental clarity.

Some neurologists regard *delirium* as a state of confusion combined with excitement and hyperactivity, and in some medical writings delirium and confusion are used interchangeably. It is undoubtedly true that the delirious patient is nearly always confused. However, the vivid hallucinations which characterize delirious states, the relative inaccessibility of the patient to other events than those to which he is reacting at any one moment, his extreme agitation and tremulousness, and the tendency to convulse suggest a cerebral disorder of a different type from that under consideration here. The clearest evidence of the relationship of confusion, stupor, and coma is that the patient may pass through all three states as he becomes comatose or emerges from coma. The present author has not observed any such relationship between coma and delirium, and for that reason would prefer to discuss the latter as a separate entity (cf. Chaps. 37 and 38).

At times a patient with certain types of aphasia, especially jargon aphasia, may create the impression of confusion, but close observation will reveal that the disorder is confined to the sphere of language and that behavior is otherwise natural.

THE ELECTROENCEPHALOGRAM AND DISTURBANCES OF CONSCIOUSNESS

One of the most delicate confirmations of the fact that these states of altered consciousness are expressions of neurophysiologic changes is the electroencephalogram. In the normal waking state the electrical potentials of the cortical neurones are integrated into regular waves of two frequency ranges, from 8 to 15 (alpha rhythm) and 16 to 25 (beta rhythm). These wave forms are established by adolescence, but certain individual differences as to the general pattern and dominance of alpha waves are maintained throughout adult life. With sleep there is a slowing of these cortical potentials and an increase in amplitude (voltage) of the individual waves. At one stage in light sleep characteristic bursts of 14 to 16 per second waves appear, the so-called "sleep spindles," and in deep sleep all the waves of normal frequency and amplitude are replaced by slow ones of high voltage ($1\frac{1}{2}$ to 3 per second). Similarly, some alteration in brain waves occurs in all disturbances of consciousness except the milder degrees of confusion. This alteration usually consists of a disorganization of the electroencephalographic pattern with random, slow waves of high voltage in stages of confusion; more regular, slow, 2 to 3 per second waves of high voltage in stupor and semicoma; and slow waves or even a suppression of all organized electrical activity in deep coma (see Chap. 55). The electroencephalograms of deep sleep and light coma resemble one another. Not all diseases which cause confusion and coma have the same effect on the electroencephalogram. Some, such as barbiturate intoxication, may cause an increase in frequency and amplitude of the brain waves. In epilepsy the disturbance of consciousness is usually attended by paroxysms of "spikes"—fast waves of high amplitude—or by the characteristic alternating slow waves and spikes of petit mal. Other diseases such as hepatic coma characteristically cause a slowing in frequency and an increasing amplitude of "brain waves," and special triphasic waves. Whether all metabolic diseases of the brain induce similar changes in the electroencephalogram has not been determined. Probably there are differences between them, some of which may be significant.

MORBID ANATOMY OF COMA

For a long time it has been known to neuropathologists that lesions situated in the upper midbrain and diencephalon are most likely to be accompanied by prolonged disturbances of consciousness. This was anticipated by Herbert Spencer in his "Principles of Psychology" when he suggested that the seat of consciousness would be found to reside where there is a confluence of sensory pathways. His idea was based on sound psychologic reasoning and not on mystical speculations, as was Galen's localization of consciousness in the lateral ventricles or Descartes', in the pineal gland.

Since the time of Hughlings Jackson it has been suggested that both the cerebral cortex and diencephalon provide the anatomic substratum of consciousness. Following the observation of pathologic coma in some cases of pituitary tumor and the hypersomnia of encephalitis lethargica, attention turned to the hypothalamus. Research on this part of the brain has done much to elucidate the neural mechanisms of wakefulness and sleep. More recently it was discovered that the reticular nuclei of the midbrain and the intralaminar and anterior nuclei of the thalami are part of a diffuse recruiting or activating system that influences large parts of the cerebral cortex. Lesions in this system of neurones diffusely alter the electrical activity of the cortex and produce coma. Collaterals from the medial and lateral lemnisci, i.e., the main sensory afferents, terminate in this region. Thus it would appear that stimulation of sensory neurones has a double effect, conveying to the body information of the outside world and also providing the energy for activating those parts of the nervous system on which consciousness depends. The nervous system, in the opinion of Martin, is like a radio set. The electricity must be turned on and the set warmed up before it is ready to receive radio waves; the human nervous system must be activated and the individual must be conscious before he can become aware of stimuli impinging upon his body. The analogy is not a good one, however, because it would appear that sensory stimulation provides the energy for both the background of consciousness and its content.

MECHANISMS WHEREBY CONSCIOUSNESS IS DISTURBED IN DISEASE

Knowledge of diseases of the nervous system is so limited that it is not possible to identify all the different mechanisms by means of which consciousness is disturbed. Already several ways are known in which the mesencephalic-diencephalic-cortical systems are deranged, and there are probably many others.

In a number of disease processes there is a direct interference with the metabolic activities of the nerve cells in the cerebral cortex and the cerebral nuclear masses of the brain. Hypoxia, hypoglycemia, and deficiencies of thiamine, nicotinic acid, vitamin B_{12}, pantothenic acid, and pyridoxine are well-known examples. The intimate details of these underlying biochemical changes have not as yet been fully elucidated, but methods are becoming available for their study. The rate of cerebral blood flow can now be determined in human beings with considerable accuracy (Schmidt-Kety method) by measuring the rate of diffusion of inert gases such as N_2O or krypton into the brain, viz., the time required for the gas to reach the same degree of concentration in the jugular venous blood as in arterial blood after 10 min of inhalation of the gas. The normal value of cerebral blood flow (CBF) is 750 ml per min. The cerebral metabolic rate (CMR-oxygen consumption per minute) is determined at the same time by measuring the oxygen difference between arterial and jugular blood and multiplying this difference by the rate of cerebral blood flow. The normal value of the cerebral metabolic rate is 46 ml per min. In hypoglycemia the cerebral blood flow is normal or above normal, whereas the cerebral metabolic rate is diminished owing to deficiency of substrate. In thiamine and vitamin B_{12} deficiency the cerebral blood flow is normal or slightly diminished, and the cerebral metabolic rate is diminished, presumably because of insufficiency of coenzymes. Extremes of body temperature, either hyperthermia (temperature over 106°F) or hypothermia (temperature below 97°F), probably induce coma by exerting a nonspecific effect on the metabolic activity of neurones.

Diabetic acidosis, uremia, hepatic coma, and the coma of systemic infections are examples of endogenous intoxications. The identity of the toxic agents is not known. In diabetes acetone bodies (acetoacetic acid, β-hydroxybutyric acid, and acetone) are present in high concentration, and in uremia there is probably accumulation of phenolic derivatives of the aromatic amino acids. In both conditions "dehydration" and acidosis may also play an important role. In hepatic coma an elevation of blood NH_3 to levels of five to six times normal has been found in many cases. The mode of action of bacterial toxins is unknown. In all these conditions the cerebral metabolic rate is reduced, whereas cerebral blood flow remains normal.

In toxic and metabolic diseases the patient usually approaches coma through a state of drowsiness, confusion, and stupor, and the reverse sequence occurs as he emerges from it. Each disease probably manifests itself by a characteristic clinical picture which will be described in the appropriate chapter in a later section of the book.

A critical decline in blood pressure, usually to a systolic level below 70 mm Hg, affects neural structures by causing a decrease in cerebral blood flow and, secondarily, a diminution in cerebral metabolic rate. If decline in blood pressure is episodic, the corresponding clinical picture is syncope (see Chap. 33). Here the clinical feature is one of physical weakness usually preceding and following the loss of consciousness, the whole process being acute and promptly reversible.

The sudden, violent, and excessive discharge of epilepsy is another mechanism. Usually a Jacksonian convulsion has little effect on consciousness until it spreads from one side of the body to the other. There is then immediate onset of coma, presumably because the spreading of the seizure discharge to central neuronal structures paralyzes their function. Other types of seizure in which consciousness is interrupted from the very beginning are believed to take origin in the diencephalon. Concussion exemplifies still another special pathophysiologic mechanism. In "blunt" head injury it has been shown that there is an enormous increase in intracranial pressure of the order of 200 to 700 lb per sq in., lasting a few thousandths of a second. Either the vibration set up in the skull and transmitted to the brain or this sudden high intracranial pressure is believed to be the basis of the sudden paralysis of the nervous system which follows head injury. That the increased pressure itself may be the main factor has been suggested by experiments in which raising the intraventricular pressure to a level approaching diastolic blood pressure has abolished all vital functions.

Large, destructive, and space-consuming lesions of the brain such as hemorrhage, tumor, or abscess interfere with consciousness in two ways. One is by direct destruction of the midbrain and diencephalon; the other, far more frequent, is by producing a herniation of the medial part of the temporal lobe through the opening of the tentorium and crushing the upper midbrain against the opposite free edge of the tentorium. The latter, usually referred to as the "tentorial pressure cone" is responsible for the dilated (Hutchinson's) pupil on the side of a large cerebral lesion or bilaterally, the ipsilateral hemiparesis and bilateral Babinski signs, the coma, and slowing or irregularity of respirations.

CLINICAL APPROACH TO THE COMATOSE PATIENT

Coma is not an independent disease entity but is always a symptomatic expression of disease. Sometimes the underlying disease is perfectly obvious, as when a healthy individual is struck on the head and rendered unconscious. All too often, however, the patient is brought to the hospital in a state of coma, and little or no information about him is immediately available. The physician is then required to subject the clinical problem to careful scrutiny from many directions. To do this efficiently he must have a broad knowledge of disease and a methodical approach to the problem that leaves none of the common and treatable causes of coma unexplored.

It should be pointed out that when the comatose patient is seen for the first time certain simple therapeutic measures take precedence over diagnostic procedures. A quick survey must be made to make sure that the comatose patient has a clear airway and is not in shock (circulatory collapse) or, if trauma has occurred, is not bleeding from a wound. In patients who have suffered a head injury there may be a fracture of the cervical vertebras, and therefore one must be cautious about moving the head and neck lest the spinal cord be inadvertently crushed. There must be an immediate inquiry as to the previous health of the patient: whether the coma was of sudden or gradual onset, whether the patient had suffered a head injury or had been seen in a convulsion, and the circumstances in which he was found. The persons who accompany the comatose patient to the hospital should not be permitted to leave until they have been questioned.

Diagnostic Procedures. The temperature, pulse, respiratory rate, and blood pressure are of aid in diagnosis. Fever suggests a severe systemic infection such as pneumonia, bacterial meningitis, or a brain lesion that has disturbed the temperature-regulating centers. An excessively high body temperature, 107 to 110°F, associated with dry skin should arouse the suspicion of heat stroke. Hypothermia is frequently observed in alcoholic or barbiturate intoxication, extracellular fluid deficit, or peripheral circulatory failure. Slow breathing points to morphine or barbiturate intoxication, while deep rapid breathing (Kussmaul's respiration) suggests diabetic or uremic acidosis, but may also occur in intracranial diseases. Rapid breathing accompanied by an expiratory grunt and associated with fever is a frequent finding in lobar pneumonia. Diseases which elevate the intracranial pressure or damage the brain, especially the brain stem, often cause slow, irregular, or periodic (Cheyne-Stokes) breathing. The pulse rate is less helpful, but if exceptionally slow it should suggest heart block or, if combined with periodic breathing and hypertension, an increase in intracranial pressure. A tachycardia of 160 or above calls attention to the possibility of an ectopic cardiac rhythm with insufficiency of cerebral circulation. Marked hypertension occurs in patients with cerebral hemorrhage and hypertensive encephalopathy and, at times, with increased intracranial

pressure; whereas hypotension is the usual finding in the coma of diabetes, alcohol or barbiturate intoxication, or internal hemorrhage.

Inspection of the skin may also be a source of valuable information. Multiple bruises, and in particular a bruise or boggy area in the scalp, favor cranial trauma. Bleeding from an ear or nose or orbital hemorrhage also raises the possibility of trauma. Puffiness and hyperemia of face and conjunctivas and telangiectasia are the usual stigmas of alcoholism, while marked pallor leads to a suspicion of internal hemorrhage. The presence of a maculohemorrhagic rash indicates the possibility of meningococcal infection, staphylococcus endocarditis, typhus, or Rocky Mountain spotted fever. Pellagra may be diagnosed from the typical skin lesions on face and hands.

The odor of the breath may provide clues to the nature of a disease causing coma. The odor of alcohol is easily recognized. The spoiled-fruit odor of diabetic coma, the uriniferous odor of uremia, and the musty fetor of hepatic coma are distinctive enough to be identified by physicians who possess a keen sense of smell.

Physical Examination. The next step is a careful physical examination with special attention to the neurologic function. Although limited in many ways, careful observation of the stuporous or comatose patient may yield considerable information concerning the function of different parts of the nervous system. One of the most helpful procedures is to sit at the patient's bedside for 5 to 10 min and observe what he does. The predominant postures of the body, the position of the head and eyes, the rate, depth, and rhythm of respiration, and the pulse should be noted. The state of responsiveness should then be estimated by noting the patient's reaction when his name is called, his capacity to execute a simple command, or to respond to painful stimuli.

Usually it is possible to determine whether or not the coma is accompanied by meningeal irritation or focal disease in the cerebrum or brain stem. With meningeal irritation from either bacterial meningitis or subarachnoid hemorrhage, there is resistance to active and passive flexion of the neck, but not to extension, turning, or tipping the head. Resistance to movement of the neck in all directions indicates disease of the cervical spine or is part of generalized rigidity. In infants, bulging of the anterior fontanel is at times a more reliable sign of meningeal irritation than stiff neck. A cerebellar pressure cone or decerebrate rigidity may also cause limitation in passive flexion of the neck and may be confused with meningeal irritation.

Evidence of disease of midbrain, pons, or medulla can be obtained even though the patient is comatose by noting the prevailing posture of the body and by examination of the cranial nerves. Decerebrate rigidity is indicated by extension of all four extremities and opisthotonos, and may be continuous or intermittent; if intermittent, it is sometimes referred to as a tonic cerebellar fit. Tonic neck reflexes, i.e., extension of the right arm and leg and flexion of left arm and leg upon turning of the head to the right, and the opposite movements when the head is turned to the left, may be demonstrated in some cases of decerebration. These attitudes and postures signify a disorder of upper pons and midbrain, and although it may be due to a functional derangement, as in a toxic or metabolic disorder, more often it points to a gross structural lesion such as a hemorrhage, basilar artery occlusion, or temporal lobe pressure cone. In contrast, the "decorticate" patient lies with arms rigidly flexed and legs extended, or at times with diagonal postures, i.e., one arm and the opposite leg flexed and other limbs extended. By "decorticate" is usually meant a lesion not of the cerebral cortex but of the motor parts of the cerebral hemispheres or the internal capsules.

Lesions of the oculomotor and abducens nerves can be detected by pupillary inequality, unequal width of palpebral fissures, or strabismus. It must be remembered that in coma the eyes tend to diverge slightly owing to relaxation of the effort of accommodation. In light coma the eyes can often be induced to move to either side by turning the head: e.g., when the head is turned to the right, the eyes move conjugately to the left, and when the head is turned to the left, the eyes move to the right. A sustained conjugate deviation of both eyes in one direction indicates either a paralysis of gaze in the opposite direction or a contralateral homonymous hemianopia. Loss of the pupillary light reflex on one side means either blindness of that eye or a lesion in midbrain or oculomotor nerve and its nucleus. A loss of consensual reflex as well as direct light reflex places the lesion in the efferent limb of the reflex arc (i.e., oculomotor nucleus or nerve). Bilateral constriction of the pupils may occur in pontine hemorrhage or in opiate intoxication. Absent corneal reflex on one side implicates the trigeminal nerve or its spinal nucleus in the pons or medulla. The same may be said of failure to wince or avert the head when one side of the face is pricked. Hemianesthesia of cerebral origin may also weaken or abolish the corneal and pharyngeal reflexes on one side. Severe facial paralysis can be demonstrated by pressure upon the supraorbital ridges to make the patient grimace, and by drooping and flaccidity of one side of the face when in repose. Also the cheek on the paralyzed side may puff out with each expiration.

Integrity of the auditory nerve is sometimes shown by blinking of the eyes at a loud sound.

Persistent nystagmus, especially when unidirectional, is suggestive of disease of vestibular nuclei. Nystagmus in all directions of eye movement in a drowsy or confused patient should suggest barbiturate intoxication. Swallowing movements can be observed, and a few drops of water in the mouth will test their adequacy. They may be abolished in deep coma or in diseases which cause lesions in both cerebral hemispheres or upper brain stem. Gag reflexes are evoked by stimulating each side of the pharyngeal wall. Facility of movement of the tongue may be determined by stroking the lips and observing spontaneous licking, vocalizing, and masticatory movements. In stupor or coma the patient may be unable to inhibit closing the eyes when in a bright light or closing the mouth and clenching the jaw when an object such as a throat stick is placed in the mouth. This may be mistaken for negativism or voluntary resistance.

Paralysis of the arms and legs can be discovered if the patient is restless, by the lack of movement in certain parts. Another useful maneuver is to lift the limbs from the bed, feeling the muscle tone on passive movement, and permitting them to fall. Paralyzed limbs fall more heavily, remain in uncomfortable positions, and flatten out on the bed more than nonparalyzed ones. Pinprick may provoke movements of the limbs. Failure to heed a painful stimulus on one side, and a response such as quickening of respirations and groaning or grimacing or restless movement on the other, suggest hemianesthesia. If sensation is intact but one arm and leg are paralyzed, a grimace, a groan, and restless movements may occur when a painful stimulus is applied to either side. Of course the withdrawal of one arm and leg from the stimulus is prevented by the hemiplegia. The tendon reflexes are often unequal on the two sides, tending to be diminished on the side of a recent acute hemiplegia and increased on the side of a chronic hemiplegia. The plantar reflexes may be bilaterally extensor but may be absent or more definitely extensor on the paralyzed side.

A history of headache before or at the onset of coma, recurrent vomiting and papilledema afford the best clues to increased intracranial pressure. This can be confirmed by lumbar puncture, which is usually safe unless there is a herniation of the temporal lobe through the tentorium or of the cerebellum through the foramen magnum. In the latter instance the cerebrospinal fluid pressure may not reflect intracranial pressure. Papilledema may develop within 12 to 24 hr in brain trauma and brain hemorrhage, but if pronounced, usually signifies brain tumor or abscess of longer duration. Multiple retinal or large subhyaloid hemorrhages are usually associated with ruptured saccular aneurysm or hemorrhage from an angioma. Papilledema, with widespread retinal exudates, hemorrhages, and arteriolar changes, is an almost invariable accompaniment of hypertensive encephalopathy. In patients with evidence of increased intracranial pressure, lumbar puncture, although admittedly dangerous because it may promote further herniation, is nevertheless necessary in some instances. See Chap. 45 for further discussion of retinal changes.

Laboratory Procedures. Unless the diagnosis is established at once by history and physical examination, it is necessary to carry out a number of laboratory procedures. If poisoning is suspected, the gastric contents must be aspirated and saved for later chemical analysis. A catheter is passed into the urinary bladder, and a specimen of urine is obtained for specific gravity, sugar, acetone, and albumin content. Urine of low specific gravity and high protein content is nearly always found in uremia, but proteinuria may also occur for 2 or 3 days after a subarachnoid hemorrhage or with fever. Urine of high specific gravity, glycosuria, and acetonuria are almost invariable in diabetic coma; but again glycosuria and hyperglycemia may result from a massive cerebral lesion. If bromide or barbiturate intoxication is suspected, it can be verified by special tests for these substances. A blood count is made, and in malarial districts a blood smear is examined for malarial parasites. Neutrophilic leukocytosis occurs in bacterial infections and also with brain hemorrhage and softening. Venous blood should be examined for glucose, nonprotein nitrogen, CO_2, sodium, potassium, and chlorides. The cerebrospinal fluid must be drawn, and the pressure, presence of blood, white cell count, and results of Pandy's test should be recorded. Bloody cerebrospinal fluid occurs in cerebral contusion, subarachnoid hemorrhage, brain hemorrhage, and occasionally with hemorrhagic infarcts due to thrombophlebitis or embolism. If there is a pleocytosis, a stained smear of the sediment should be searched for bacteria, and a rough quantitative sugar determination should be done. The standard cerebrospinal fluid formula in bacterial meningitis is elevated pressure, high white cell count (10,000 to 20,000), elevated protein, and subnormal sugar values. The fluid should be saved for quantitative tests for sugar and protein, and a bacterial culture and Wassermann reaction should be performed. If the pressure is suspected of being elevated, a No. 20 needle should be used. A very high pressure must be slowly reduced by removal of 10 to 15 ml over a period of 15 to 20 min. Afterward the foot of the bed should be elevated. Jugular compression tests are obviously contraindicated. X-rays of the skull should be obtained as soon as possible after these procedures, preferably on the way from the emergency ward to the hospital room.

CLASSIFICATION OF COMA AND DIFFERENTIAL DIAGNOSIS

The demonstration of focal brain disease or meningeal irritation, with cerebrospinal fluid abnormality, is of aid in the differential diagnosis. The diseases which frequently cause coma can be conveniently divided into three classes, as follows:

CLASSIFICATION OF COMA

I. Diseases which cause no focal or lateralizing neurologic signs or alterations of the cellular content of the cerebrospinal fluid
  A. Intoxications (alcohol, barbiturates, opiates, etc.)
  B. Metabolic disturbances (diabetic acidosis, uremia, Addisonian crisis, hepatic coma, hypoglycemia, hypoxia)
  C. Severe systemic infections (pneumonia, typhoid fever, malaria, Waterhouse-Friderichsen syndrome)
  D. Circulatory collapse (shock) from any cause, cardiac decompensation in the aged
  E. Epilepsy
  F. Hypertensive encephalopathy and eclampsia
  G. Hyperthermia or hypothermia
II. Diseases which cause meningeal irritation, with either blood or an excess of white cells in the cerebrospinal fluid, usually without focal or lateralizing signs
  A. Subarachnoid hemorrhage from ruptured aneurysm, occasionally trauma
  B. Acute bacterial meningitis
  C. Some forms of virus encephalitis
  D. Neurosyphilis
III. Diseases which cause focal or lateralizing neurologic signs, with or without changes in the cerebrospinal fluid
  A. Brain hemorrhage (Chap. 284)
  B. Brain softening due to thrombosis or embolism (Chap. 284)
  C. Brain abscess (Chap. 152)
  D. Epidural and subdural hemorrhage and brain contusion (Chap. 285)
  E. Brain tumor (Chap. 286)
  F. Miscellaneous, i.e., thrombophlebitis, some forms of virus encephalomyelitis

If the history and the examination of the comatose patient and the accessory laboratory procedures enable the physician to decide which of these three classes of neurologic disease his patient has, the differential diagnosis is greatly simplified. Class I includes essentially the toxic and metabolic encephalopathies, and usually any definite sign of localized lesion in one cerebral hemisphere, the brain stem, or cerebellum, or a cellular change in the cerebrospinal fluid, is sufficient to exclude these diseases.

It must be conceded that clinical cases are complex and that even the most careful analysis will not always yield the correct diagnosis. If the patient has had a focal brain lesion before the onset of his present illness, the signs of it could become more pronounced during coma from toxic or metabolic diseases, and this may at times be a source of error. Or a difficult lumbar puncture resulting in a "bloody tap" may also cause an erroneous diagnosis. Finally, certain rare diseases like lead encephalopathy in infants may induce a mild pleocytosis and elevation in the protein content of the cerebrospinal fluid. Another difficulty sometimes encountered in dealing with the comatose patient is that the level of unconsciousness is so deep that it is impossible to detect focal or lateralizing signs. Often, however, such an illness is so completely beyond the control of the physician that diagnosis becomes unimportant.

It must be remembered that diagnosis has as its prime purpose the direction of therapy, and it matters little to the patient whether or not we diagnose a disease for which we have no treatment. The treatable forms of coma are drug intoxications, toxemia from systemic infections, epidural and subdural hematoma, brain abscess, bacterial and tuberculous meningitis, diabetic acidosis, and hypoglycemia.

INCIDENCE OF DISEASES WHICH CAUSE COMA

There have been only a few attempts to determine the relative incidence of diseases which lead to coma. A report from the Boston City Hospital includes the largest series of clinical cases, but the material was heavily weighted by the large local alcoholic population. The cases at Cook County Hospital have also been summarized, but only the figures on the fatal cases were presented. These statistics are combined in Tables 34-1.

It can be seen at once that trauma and vascular disease of the brain are two leading causes of coma in municipal hospitals and that the mortality rate from these diseases is extremely high. Alcoholism and drug intoxication are also frequent but are seldom fatal. In the cases studied at Cook County Hospital accuracy of diagnosis, when checked by postmortem examination, was not more than about 50 per cent and did not improve with the increasing length of survival. More than half the fatal cases had died in the first 24 hr, and two-thirds within the first 48 hr.

The differential diagnosis of the diseases which cause focal or lateralizing neurologic signs and meningitis will be taken up under the discussions of traumatic, neoplastic, vascular, and infectious diseases of the brain.

CARE OF THE COMATOSE PATIENT

Impaired states of consciousness, regardless of their cause, are often fatal because they represent not only an advanced stage of many diseases but also add their own characteristic burden to the primary disease. The main objective of therapy is, of course, to find the cause of the coma—according

Table 34-1. RELATIVE INCIDENCE OF DISEASES WHICH CAUSE COMA*

Disease	Boston City Hospital series † (clinical cases)			Cook County series ‡ (autopsied cases)	
	No.	Per cent	Mortality, %	No.	Per cent
Alcoholism	690	59.1	2	16	4.6
Trauma	152	13.0	31.5	94	27.5
Cerebral vascular disease	118	10.0	77.0	120	35.0
Poisoning	33	3.0	9.0		
Epilepsy	28	2.4	0		
Diabetes	20	1.7	55	8	2.3
Bacterial meningitis*	20	1.7	100	29	8.5
Pneumonia	20	1.7	90	18	5.4
Cardiac decompensation	17	1.4	70		
Neurosyphilis	7	0.6	0	4	1.2
Uremia	7	0.6	100	37	10.9
Eclampsia	7	0.6	68.4		
Miscellaneous	48	4.1	75.0	16	4.6
Total	1,167	100		342	100

* These figures were collected in 1933 before the introduction of most of the sulfonamide drugs or antibiotics.
† Reported by Solomon and Aring.
‡ Reported by Holcomb.

Table 34-2. IMPORTANT POINTS IN THE DIFFERENTIAL DIAGNOSIS OF SOME OF THE MORE COMMON CAUSES OF COMA

General group	Specific disorder	Important clinical findings	Important laboratory findings	Remarks
Coma with focal or lateralizing signs of brain disease	Brain tumor	Stertorous breathing, neurologic signs dependent on location, papilledema	CSF pressure elevated Protein often > 100 mg	Steady progression of signs and symptoms
	Cerebral hemorrage	Stertorous breathing, hypertension, flushed skin, hemiplegia	CSF grossly bloody and under increased pressure	Sudden onset, elderly patients
	Cerebral thrombosis	Unilateral and bilateral paralysis of abrupt onset	CSF normal	Stupor or coma
	Cerebral embolism	Sudden onset of paralysis	CSF normal	Evidence of heart disease
	Hypertensive encephalopathy	Convulsions, headache, severe hypertension, hypertensive retinopathy	CSF pressure normal or increased Protein 50–200 mg	Confusion, stupor, or coma Acute or sudden onset Duration several days
	Fracture or concussion	Signs of skin trauma	Skull fracture in x-ray CSF bloody and under increased pressure	Bleeding from nose or ears History of trauma
	Subdural hematoma	Slow respiration, rising blood pressure	Normal or increased fluid pressure	History of trauma
Coma without focal or lateralizing signs but with evidence of meningeal irritation	Meningitis	Stiff neck, positive Kernig, fever	Changes in spinal fluid	Subacute onset
	Subarachnoid hemorrhage	Fever, stertorous breathing, hypertension, stiff neck, positive Kernig	Bloody or xanthochromic CSF under increased pressure	Sudden onset after headache
Coma without focal neurologic signs or evidence of meningeal irritation	Alcohol intoxication	Hypothermia, hypotension, flushed skin, alcohol breath	Elevated blood alcohol	
	Barbiturate intoxication	Hypothermia, hypotension	Barbiturate in urine	
	Opium intoxication	Slow respiration, cyanosis, constricted pupils		History of intake of intoxicating substance
	Bromide intoxication	Hyperthermia, delirium	Blood bromides ++	
	Carbon monoxide intoxication	Cherry-red skin	Carboxyhemoglobin	
	Diabetic coma	Signs of extracellular fluid deficit, deep respiration, "fruity" breath	Glycosuria, hyperglycemia, reduced CO_2 Acetone bodies in urine	History of polyuria, polyidpsia, weight loss, or diabetes
	Uremia	Hypertension, yellowish-brown skin, uriniferous breath	Proteinuria, blood urea ++	Vascular retinopathy

Table 34-2. IMPORTANT POINTS IN THE DIFFERENTIAL DIAGNOSIS OF SOME OF THE MORE COMMON CAUSES OF COMA
(*Continued*)

General group	Specific disorder	Important clinical findings	Important laboratory findings	Remarks
Coma without focal neurologic signs or evidence of meningeal irritation	Hepatic coma	Jaundice, ascites, flapping movement of outstretched arms	Elevated blood NH₃ levels CSF yellow with normal protein	Onset over a few days or after hemorrhage from varices or paracentesis
	Severe infections Heat stroke	Extreme hyperthermia, rapid respiration	Vary according to cause	Evidence of a specific infection, of heat stroke, or intracranial disease
	Idiopathic epilepsy	Episodic disturbance of behavior or convulsive movements	Characteristic electroencephalogram	History of previous attacks

to the procedures already outlined—and to remove it. It often happens, however, that the disease process is one for which there is no specific therapy; or as in hypoxia or hypoglycemia, the disease process may already have expended itself before the patient comes to the attention of the physician. Again the problem may be infinitely complex, for the disturbance of cerebral function may not be attributable to a single cause but rather to several possible factors acting in unison, no one of which could account for the total clinical picture. In lieu of direct therapy, supportive measures must be used, and indeed it may be said that the patient's chances of surviving the original disease often depend in large measure on their effectiveness.

The physician must give attention to every vital function in the insensate patient. The following is a brief outline of the more important procedures. In order for them to be carried out successfully a well-coordinated team of nurses under the constant guidance of a physician is needed.

1. If the patient is in shock, this demands precedence over all other abnormalities. The treatment of shock is discussed in Chap. 13.

2. Shallow and irregular respirations and cyanosis require the establishment of a clear airway and oxygen. The patient should be placed in a semiprone position so that secretions and vomitus do not enter the tracheobronchial tree. Pharyngeal reflexes are usually suppressed, and therefore an endotracheal tube can be inserted without difficulty. Stagnant secretions should be removed with a suction apparatus as soon as they accumulate, since they will lead to atelectasis and bronchopneumonia. Oxygen can be administered by mask in a 100 per cent concentration for 6 to 12 hr, alternating with 50 per cent concentration for 4 hr. The depth of respiration can be increased by the use of 5 to 10 per cent carbon dioxide for periods of 3 to 5 min every hour. Atropine should not be given; edema

of the lungs and fluid in the tracheobronchial passages are not glandular secretions. Furthermore, atropine thickens this fluid and also may disturb temperature regulation of the body. Aminophylline is helpful in controlling Cheyne-Stokes breathing. Respiratory paralysis dictates the use of a tank-type respirator or electrophrenic stimulator, but in the author's experience neither has been effective in comatose states in which there is disorganization of respiratory centers.

3. The temperature-regulating mechanisms may be disturbed, and extreme hypothermia, hyperthermia, or an unrecognized poikilothermia may occur. In hyperthermia, removal of blankets and use of alcohol sponges and cooling solutions are indicated.

4. The bladder should not be permitted to become distended. If the patient does not void, a retention catheter should be inserted. If more than 500 ml of urine is found in the bladder, decompression must be carried out slowly over a period of hours. Urine excretion should be kept above 800 to 1,000 ml per day. The patient should not be permitted to lie in a wet or soiled bed.

5. Diseases of the central nervous system may upset the control of water, glucose, and salt. The unconscious patient can no longer adjust his intake of food and fluids by hunger and thirst. Salt-losing and salt-retaining syndromes have both been described with brain disease. Water intoxication, severe hypopotassemia or hyperpotassemia, or hyponatremia may of themselves prove fatal. The maintenance of water and electrolytes will be discussed in Chap. 50. If coma is prolonged, the insertion of a stomach tube will make the problem of feeding the patient and maintaining fluid and electrolyte balance much easier.

6. One should attempt to forestall the development of bronchopneumonia by the prophylactic use of penicillin and streptomycin or some other broad-spectrum antibiotic. The legs should be ex-

amined each day for signs of phlebothrombosis.

7. If the patient is capable of moving, suitable restraints should be used to prevent a possible fall out of bed.

8. Convulsions should be controlled by measures outlined in Chap. 36.

REFERENCES

Holcomb, B.: Causes and Diagnosis of Various Forms of Coma, J.A.M.A., 77:2112, 1921.

Munro, D.: "Craniocerebral Injuries, Their Diagnosis and Treatment," New York, Oxford University Press, 1938.

Purdon-Martin, G.: Consciousness and Its Disturbances, Lancet, 1946, I:1, 48.

Solomon, P., and C. D. Aring: The Causes of Coma in Patients Entering a General Hospital, Am. J. Med. Sci., 188:805, 1938.

—— and ——: Differential Diagnosis in Patients Entering a General Hospital in Coma, J.A.M.A., 105:7, 1935.

35 SLEEP AND ITS ABNORMALITIES

Raymond D. Adams

Sleep, that familiar yet inexplicable condition of repose in which consciousness is in abeyance, is obviously not abnormal; yet there is no absurdity in the consideration of it in connection with abnormal phenomena. There are no doubt irregularities of sleep which approach serious extremes, just as there are unnatural forms of waking consciousness.

Everyone has had much personal experience of sleep, or the lack of it, and has observed others in sleep; so it requires no special knowledge of medicine to know something about this condition or to appreciate its importance to health and well-being. Nearly all the great writers of the past have expressed their views on the psychologic and physical benefits of sleep but probably none with more feeling than Sterne, who has Tristram Shandy remark:

'Tis the refuge of the unfortunate—the enfranchisement of the prisoner—the downy lap of the hopeless, the weary, the broken-hearted; of all the soft, delicious functions of nature this is the chiefest; what a happiness it is to man, when the anxieties and passions of the day are over. . . .

Physicians are often sought out by individuals who suffer an illness caused by or accompanied by some derangement of sleep. Most often the problem is one of sleeplessness, but sometimes it concerns peculiar phenomena occurring in connection with sleep. As these disorders cannot be satisfactorily treated without a clear conception of the sleeping-waking mechanism, this chapter reviews briefly certain points concerning its physiology that will assist in understanding the pathology of sleep.

NORMAL SLEEP

Sleep is ordinarily preceded by a period of drowsiness during which sustained attention is difficult. Warmth, mental and physical inactivity, monotony of environmental stimuli, and the ingestion of a large and satisfying meal are all conducive to drowsiness. The awareness of physical fatigue becomes increasingly insistent at this time. Eventually the individual gives in to it and either falls asleep where he is or retires to bed. Often, however, a person goes to bed and promptly falls asleep without any awareness of fatigue or of preliminary drowsiness. Sleep automatically follows upon completion of all the usual arrangements for the night. Such instances as these remind us of the nature of sleep as a reaction to a definite and regular set of stimuli.

During sleep the individual looks as though he were comatose, with the important difference that strong stimulation will arouse him to a normal waking state (see Chap. 34). The eyelids are usually closed, although there are exceptions to this, the eyeballs rolled up, and the pupils constricted. The pulse is decreased 10 to 20 beats per minute. The blood pressure is lowered, and breathing becomes slower, deeper, and more audible. In normal elderly adults Cheyne-Stokes respirations may occur, without any special significance. The body temperature undergoes modification during sleep, both in children and adults, falling 0.5 to 2.0°F, chiefly for 2 to 3 hr after midnight. It falls similarly during the day in those who work by night and sleep by day. Helmholtz found that the average person gives off 40 cal of heat per hour by night and 112 cal in the same time by day. The skeletal muscles are relaxed, but this is variable, because individuals are known to sleep in sitting positions or while standing, in which postures complete relaxation would be impossible. During sleep all sensory thresholds are raised. Reflex movements can be evoked quite readily. Often a sleeping person will respond to commands or requests which call forth only a simple movement or response. Urine is formed in smaller quantity by night, the amount being a fourth of that excreted by the kidneys during the waking day. Sweating is normally decreased during sound sleep, as shown by increased resistance of the skin to the passage of electric current.

An intermediate state between sleeping and waking can be detected as the individual goes to sleep and awakens. This is usually brief, a matter of seconds to minutes, but may rarely be prolonged. Several different terms have been suggested, but most psychologists refer to it as the *hypnagogic state.* Falling to sleep requires a progressive relaxation of voluntary musculature; as this is being achieved, stimulation may cause a sudden start, with movement of the entire body or a limb. Thought processes, too, must gradually cease, but may emerge several times as the sleep state is attained. In waking from sleep there is a rapid readjustment of sensory thresholds to those of the waking state and a resumption of all cognitive and affective processes. Muscle tension increases, the eyes open, and normal consciousness returns. Individuals vary in the rapidity with which this is achieved. Some, even after being up and moving about for some time, are still in a condition comparable to the drowsiness which precedes sleep, whereas others become fully alert quite promptly. This difference between individuals may be related to the character of their work curves, i.e, whether they work most efficiently early or late in the day.

The amount of sleep required by any one person is variable within rather narrow limits. Apparently the majority of people sleep about 8 hr a night. In addition some adults who are normal in every respect sleep for a short time after the large meal of the day, either at noon or in the evening. Exceptional individuals can function well on a few hours of sleep a day, and others need 10 hr. Women usually require more sleep than men. A cheerful interest in the activities of the day, strong motivation, and purpose in life will overcome fatigue and enable an individual to work efficiently with small amounts of sleep.

The time of sleep during the day and night and the depth or intensity of sleep have been observed by a number of psychologists. The newborn sleeps much of the time, day and night, awakening only when in need of nourishment. His sleep curve is called polyphasic. Infants and small children sleep throughout the night and in the late morning as well as in the afternoon. The amount of sleep declines up to adolescence, and as it does so the nocturnal monophasic pattern of the adult is established. Adults also vary in their sleep requirement and pattern according to their activities and the demands placed upon them. If idle they may doze after lunch and especially after their dinner. The intensity or depth of sleep at any given moment has been measured in terms of the strength of stimulus necessary to awaken the subject. Kohlschütter found that the depth of sleep in normal persons is greatest at the end of the first hour, and from the second to third hour onward it lightens rapidly to the point of waking. However, the curve is far from smooth, showing much irregular oscillation. Another period of increased depth occurs in the latter part of the sleep curve, about the fifth to sixth hours. It has been suggested that this second drop is more frequent in children. An analysis of the sleep curves of a large number of individuals has shown variations. While the striking feature of all the curves is the sharp increase in intensity shortly after falling asleep, Michelson obtained evidence of two classes of individuals, in this respect. There are those with morning dispositions who exhibit a maximum of mental efficiency in the early part of the day and upon going to bed sleep most deeply by the end of the first hour (type A); and those with evening dispositions whose maximum efficiency comes later in the day and whose curve for sleep reaches the maximum of intensity with relative slowness, 1¾ to 3½ hr after falling asleep (type B).

ANATOMY AND PHYSIOLOGY OF THE SLEEP-WAKING STATE

The condition of the sleeping man or animal was formerly likened to that of an individual deprived of cerebral hemispheres and capable only of the most elementary sensorimotor acts. This is now known to be inaccurate because the "decorticate" animal exhibits a sleep-wake rhythm. Moreover, there is evidence that many parts of the nervous system are quiescent in sleep, and those functions which persist are carried on in a modified manner.

Do certain parts of the nervous system regulate the sleep-waking rhythm, or does the nervous system as a whole merely respond to the effect of some outside influence such as a toxin or reduced blood flow? Physiology now provides the answer to this question—there are neural structures in the tegmentum of the midbrain which maintain a state of wakefulness. Somnolence of several weeks' duration has been produced in monkeys by making lesions between the posterior hypothalamus and midbrain. As pointed out in Chap. 34, the structures in the tegmentum of the midbrain are activated by the collaterals of afferent sensory neurones, and in turn exert a widespread effect on the cerebral cortex. In addition there is probably a corticifugal influence on the midbrain by which afferent volleys of nerve impulses may be prevented from having their influence on the cortex.

Assuming that this or a neighboring part of the nervous system is essential to the maintenance of the sleep-waking rhythm, by what means does it periodically subside into tranquillity? No satisfactory answer has been found to this question, as may be surmised from the many theories of sleep now entertained. The available evidence provides increasing support for the view put forth long ago by Purkinje —that sleep represents "a physiological interruption of afferent pathways at a central point."

The electroencephalogram reveals a number of stages of progression from waking to sleeping. First, as the person becomes drowsy, there is a regularization of the 8 to 10 per second normal alpha rhythm and, in light sleep, an increase in frequency and amplitude of waves, with the formation of "spindles." Delta waves appear, and the spindles are no longer seen in deep sleep. A sensory stimulus at any time makes the alpha waves return suddenly over the whole cortex, and the same restoration of the normal electroencephalographic pattern occurs during natural awakening. During light sleep the proportion of alpha to delta (waves of less than 4 per second frequency) activity increases. Movements during sleep are nearly always preceded by a return of alpha waves. The ratio of alpha/delta activity reflects the trend toward wakefulness or sleep.

The total cerebral blood flow and cerebral metabolism do not appear to be reduced during sleep, an observation which refutes the idea that sleep is the consequence of a general cerebral ischemia.

THE EFFECTS OF LOSS OF SLEEP

Of the conditions making for human efficiency sleep is one of the most important. Sleep is absolutely essential to normal body metabolism. Experimental animals deprived of sleep will die within a few days, no matter how well they may be fed, watered, and housed.

Despite the many studies of the effect of sleeplessness on human beings and animals, we still do not know as much as we should about it. Experiments on human beings have taken the form of enforced abstention from sleep for several days, with tests administered before, during, and after. One group of psychologists succeeded in keeping their subjects going in a state of apparent wakefulness for 90 hr. The surprising result was that on tests such as tapping, aiming at targets, reading letters, and calculation there was no failure of performance even after the loss of two nights of sleep. The sleepless subjects did fail, however, in tasks requiring sustained attention. They could do as well as they normally would on short tests, but on longer ones of the same degree of difficulty they became slow and inaccurate. Another characteristic was sluggishness of attention in shifting from one task or one test item to another. It was difficult for the subjects to redirect their activity; once started on a given line they could hardly be diverted from it. Whatever their achievement on the tests, all subjects reported numerous symptoms such as burning eyes, headache, dazed feeling, nervousness, emotional instability, loss of motor power and coordination, and distressing visual hallucinations. In general deportment they were alternately irritable and silly, tending to laugh at anything said to them.

The reason for the relatively good test performance in the face of these bodily sensations is the ability of the normal individual to compensate. He can "shake himself out of it" and apply himself with an effort that overcomes his deficiencies. This extra effort put forth in keeping oriented to the task cannot be maintained without cost. The energy consumed during an arithmetic task, as measured by the metabolic rate, is about three times greater in persons who have lost sleep.

Another surprising finding was that subjects recovered on less than 35 per cent of the sleep that had been lost. In other words the amount of sleep required after the experiment is not equal to the number of hours that they were kept awake. Probably the explanation is that the subjects were not fully awake at all times, and in the latter part of the experiment they may have been half asleep.

A corollary of this hypothesis would be that persons who sleep for long periods do not necessarily obtain the maximum benefits from sleep. Sleep may be sound and restful, or light and fitful. In sound sleep the psychogalvanic test of skin resistance of the palm is raised, and in poor sleep it remains the same as in the waking state. It has also been found that only in sound sleep does the blood pressure fall. From these fragmentary studies it must be concluded that the value of sleep to the metabolism of the human organism is a function of its depth multiplied by its length and that long hours spent in bed are no substitute for sound sleep.

DERANGEMENTS OF SLEEP

The essential facts concerning the abnormalities and abnormal relationships of sleep are set forth on the following pages under separate topics.

Insomnia. The word *insomnia* signifies the want of sleep and is used popularly to indicate any interference with the duration or depth of sleep. As every physician knows from practical experience this is not a disease but a symptom of many diseases, which differ widely in their nature and gravity. It is associated equally with trivial ailments and with conditions which jeopardize life. The persistence and severity of it are no guide to the diagnosis of the condition on which it depends.

Since insomnia is often a symptom of a minor illness, there is a tendency for the physician to make light of it. Yet there are few common conditions which cause more misery and discomfort to the patient. When deprived of the nightly restoration of his energies, he grows weary and his whole mental and physical vigor is impaired. He seems to exhaust his fund of reserve force. His tolerance of pain, noise, and the countless irritations of every-day life is reduced. This in turn reflects itself in his psychologic reaction to all the ordinary symptoms of disease. Also, the capacity for effective work is intimately related to the ability to sleep; in fact this is one of the most reliable measures of sound health.

In former times there was a tendency to formulate elaborate classifications of insomnia according to the nature of the diseases in each of the different organ systems of the body. This approach has little to offer, because in the final analysis the factors operating in all these diseases are relatively few. Most instances of unyielding insomnia are due to (1) the presence of pain and discomfort or (2) anxiety and other nervous disorders.

Several types of sensory disorder may cause abnormal wakefulness. The pain of spine and root or peripheral nerve disease may be particularly troublesome at night, and the same is true of abdominal discomfort in a number of gastrointestinal diseases such as pancreatic carcinoma. Tired, aching, restless legs, which has been described as the "restless leg syndrome" (anxietas tibialis) may regularly delay the onset of natural sleep. Excessive fatigue may give rise to many abnormal muscular sensations of a similar nature. Acroparesthesias, that peculiar nocturnal tingling numbness of the hands which is so common in women, may awaken the patient nightly.

Insomnia is a frequent complaint of patients suffering from psychiatric disease. Its simplest form is that of a reactive nervous state in which domestic and business worries keep the patient in a turmoil. Also, vigorous mental activity late at night or excitement counteracts drowsiness and sleep. Under these circumstances there is difficulty in falling asleep and a tendency to sleep late in the morning. Sleeplessness is also commonly recorded in the histories of patients suffering from psychoneuroses and psychoses. In a valuable study of the character of sleep in psychiatric patients Muncie informs us that in illnesses in which anxiety and fear are prominent symptoms there is usually difficulty in falling asleep and light, fitful, or intermittent sleep. Also, disturbing dreams, so common in such conditions, may awaken the patient, and he may even try to stay awake in order to avoid them. In contrast the depressive illnesses, particularly manic-depressive or involutional depression, cause early morning waking and inability to return to sleep. If anxiety is combined with depression, both the above patterns are observed. In states of mania all types of sleep disorder are known to occur. The sleep rhythm may be totally deranged in acute confusional states and delirium. In the latter the patient may only doze for short periods both day and night. The total amount and depth of sleep in a 24-hr period is reduced. Frightening hallucinations may prevent sleep. The senile and arteriosclerotic patient tends to catnap during the day and then refuse to go to bed at night; his nocturnal sleep is intermittent, and the total amount may be either increased or decreased.

Finally there are occasionally patients who are convinced of the absolute necessity of obtaining sleep of a certain ideal quantity and quality. These are the "sleep pedants" and the "sleep hypochondriacs" of Laudenheimer. They become obsessed with the importance of sleep. Every night they are in a panic lest they remain awake; they cannot sleep because of their anxiety over it. They demonstrate the truth of William McDougall's statement that "peace of mind is an essential preliminary to sleep." Especially interesting is that group for whom insomnia becomes the excuse for all inadequacies and failures in adjustment to the everyday problems of living. Such individuals, although they want to sleep, worry about the loss, and their mental agitation actually opposes sleep.

Whatever the cause may be, the physician should always be on his guard when listening to reports of the amount of sleep lost by sufferers from insomnia because they are usually exaggerated. Every individual who has lain awake at night will recall how much longer the time seemed than it actually was. This is an example of illusion in the perception of unfilled time.

Disturbances in the Transitional Period of Sleep (Somnolescent Starts, Sensory Paroxysms, and Nocturnal Paralysis). As sleep comes on it would appear that certain nervous centers may be excited to a burst of insubordinate activity. The result is a sudden start that rouses the incipient sleeper. It may involve one or both legs or the trunk; less often, the arms. If the start occurs repeatedly during the process of falling to sleep and is a nightly event, it may become a matter of grave concern to the patient. These starts are more apt to occur in individuals in whom the sleep process develops slowly, and it has been observed that they are especially frequent in tense, nervous individuals. It is probable that some relationship exists between these nocturnal starts and the sudden isolated jerk of a leg, or arm and leg, which may occur in healthy, fully conscious individuals. It does not appear to be related to epilepsy despite certain superficial resemblances. Disturbances of this nature may be the stimulus for night terrors. These somnolescent starts must be distinguished from flexor spasms of the legs, which occur in individuals who have suffered disease of the pyramidal tracts and from a rare condition known as nocturnal myoclonus.

Sensory centers may be disturbed in a similar way, either as an isolated phenomenon or in association with those phenomena inducing motion. As the patient drops off to sleep he may be roused by a sensation that darts through his body. It may or may not be followed by a start. Such sensory symptoms are often in the domain of one of the special senses, especially hearing. A sudden clang or crashing sound disturbs commencing sleep. Sometimes a sudden flash of light occurs as sleep is coming on. A sensation of being lifted and dashed to earth or of being turned is probably a similar sensory paroxysm involving the labyrinthine mechanism.

Curious paralytic phenomena, so distressing to a patient as to cause him to seek medical advice, may also occur in that transition from the sleeping to the waking state. Nocturnal paresis or paralysis was the subject of an interesting study by Weir Mitchell. Sometimes in an otherwise healthy individual a state supervenes in the morning in which, although awake, conscious, and fully oriented, he is unable to innervate a single muscle. He lies as though still asleep with eyes closed and is all the while engaged in a struggle for movement. He has the impression that if he could but move a single muscle, the spell would instantly vanish and he would regain full power. It has been reported that the slightest cutaneous stimulus such as the touch of a hand may abolish the paralysis. Such attacks are usually transient and of no special significance. They have also been reported to occur during the development of sleep. They may be related to narcolepsy.

Nightmares and Night Terrors. Awakening in a state of terror has happened to nearly everyone. Children and nervous young adults are especially prone to it. Fevers dispose to it, and it has been said that any upsetting condition of the body, such as a disturbance of digestion, may have a similar effect. Bad dreams, stimulated directly by the recent memory of bloodcurdling television programs before going to bed, may account for night terrors in children. Some psychologists have drawn a distinction between the nightmare which is merely a terrifying dream and the night terror in which there are visual hallucinations and motor activity. Considering the predominantly visual nature of dreams, it is doubtful if such a separation is valid. Probably any difference is only one of degree.

A night terror is probably always connected with an alarming dream. The victim sits up or jumps out of bed, shouts or rushes frantically from his room. He is at first unconscious of his surroundings, but usually the intensity of the emotional disturbance and the physical activity awaken him. The following morning he may have only a hazy recollection of the experience.

Such phenomena are of little clinical significance as isolated events in childhood but require to be distinguished from nocturnal epilepsy. They seldom persist beyond early adult life. If they occur with excessive frequency and continue very long, a relationship to other disturbances such as a psychoneurosis usually exists.

Somnambulism and Sleep Automatism. Examples of sleepwalking come to the attention of the practicing physician not infrequently. This condition likewise occurs more often in children than in adults. After being asleep for a time the patient arises from his bed and walks about the house. He may turn on a light or perform some other familiar act. There is no outward sign of emotion; the eyes are open and the sleeper is guided by vision, thus avoiding familiar objects. The sight of an unfamiliar object may awaken him. If spoken to, he makes no response; if told to return to bed, he may do so but more often must be led back to it. The following morning he usually has no memory of the episode.

Most psychiatrists hold that these are dissociated mental states similar to the hysterical trance and fugue, except that they begin during sleep. Undoubtedly this is true and sleepwalking may be accepted as evidence of a nervous disorder, probably of the psychoneurotic variety. There are nonetheless examples of this in adults who have no other signs of mental illness. One can only regard such a case as an isolated disorder of sleep-waking mechanism. It is probably allied to talking in one's sleep, though the two conditions seldom occur together.

Half-waking somnambulism, or sleep automatism, is a state in which an adult patient, half-aroused from sleep, goes through a fairly complex routine such as going to a window, opening it, and looking out, but afterward retains a recollection of only a part of the episode. The patient may injure himself during sleepwalking.

Nocturnal Epilepsy. Paroxysmal abnormalities of the brain waves of the type seen in epilepsy tend to occur in epileptic patients during or shortly after the onset of sleep. This characteristic electroencephalographic pattern has been found so frequently in the epileptic patient that the practice of artificially inducing sleep in order to obtain confirmation of epilepsy has been adopted in many laboratories. Of course it has long been known that epilepsy occurs during sleep.

The sleeping epileptic patient attracts attention by a cry, violent motor activity, or labored breathing. As in the diurnal seizure, after the tonic-clonic phase the patient becomes quiet and falls into a state resembling sleep but from which he cannot be aroused. His appearance depends on the phase of the seizure he happens to be in when first observed. Seizures of this type may occur at any time during the night, and some patients may have all their seizures at night. If the seizure during the night is unobserved, the only indication of it may be a few drops of blood on the pillow, wet bed linen from urinary incontinence, a bitten tongue, or sore muscles. Rarely, a patient may die in an epileptic seizure during sleep, presumably from being smothered by bedclothes.

Other less well-defined types of seizure occur at night. The patient may arise as though in a night terror and perform complex acts. He may be excited and overactive and if restrained becomes combative. After some minutes he is subdued and returns to sleep. The following morning he disclaims all memory of the episode. Whether this represents a psychomotor seizure or a night terror is difficult to decide. An electroencephalographic study is helpful in such cases.

Nocturnal jerks of the legs, also called nocturnal myoclonus, is another troublesome symptom for it interferes with sleep night after night. Only recently has it been classified as a form of myoclonic epilepsy. It is unaccompanied by all other epileptic manifestations. Anticonvulsant drugs are said to control the condition, though in two cases the author has had better success with an occasional dose of Pantopon. It differs from the restless leg syndrome in that involuntary movements occur.

Epilepsy may occur in conjunction with both night terrors and somnambulism, and the question then arises whether the latter are of the nature of a postepileptic automatism. Usually no such relationship is established.

Prolonged States of Sleep and Reversal of Sleep-Waking Rhythm. Encephalitis lethargica or "epidemic encephalitis," that remarkable illness which appeared on the medical horizon during the great pandemic of influenza following the First World War, has provided some of the most dramatic instances of prolonged somnolence. In fact, protracted sleep lasting days to weeks was such a prominent symptom that the disease was called the "sleeping sickness." The patient appeared to be in a state of continuous sleep, or "somnosis," and remained awake only while stimulated. Although the infective agent was never isolated, the pathologic anatomy was fully divulged by many excellent studies, all of which demonstrated a destruction of neurones in the midbrain, subthalamus, and hypothalamus. Patients surviving the acute phases of the illness often had difficulty in reestablishing the normal sleep-waking rhythm. As the somnolence disappeared, some patients exhibited a reversal of sleep rhythm, tending to sleep by day and stay awake at night.

Other diseases localized to the floor and walls of the third ventricle are known to produce continuous somnolence. Small tumors in the posterior hypothalamus and midbrain have been associated with arterial hypotension, diabetes insipidus, and

a somnolence lasting many weeks. Such patients can be aroused but if left alone immediately fall asleep. Traumatic brain lesions and other diseases have been found to produce similar clinical pictures.

Narcolepsy and Cataplexy. The term *narcolepsy* has been used rather loosely. According to most authorities it should refer to peculiar brief recurrent attacks of sleep, and not to prolonged or continuous sleep. Although a few of the reported cases are doubtless examples of hysteria, there is unquestionably a well-defined clinical entity which bears no relationship to neurosis or any other known psychiatric condition.

Typical narcolepsy occurs in males and females equally and often has its onset during adolescent or adult years. Brief episodes of natural sleep recur throughout the day with a variable periodicity. A sudden yawning and heaviness of the eyes assails the patient, and the desire for sleep becomes so imperative that he gives way to it within a few minutes regardless of where he is. If the subject is spoken to or touched, the sleep is immediately interrupted, and if left alone he arouses himself within a few minutes and often feels refreshed. An impressive feature of the condition is that sleep may come on while the person is standing or engaged in conversation or some other activity. He can prevent it by effort of will for a time, but must in the end give way to it. In exceptional cases there may be no preliminary drowsiness, or the patient may feel as if he were in a trance rather than asleep. The sleep attacks come more frequently at some times of day than others. Nocturnal sleep is usually normal.

Another component of the narcoleptic attack is its relation to strong emotion. Instances have been cited of the induction of attacks of sleep by hearty laughter resulting from amusement or joy, or by anger, compassion, and anxiety. Far more frequent is the phenomenon of *cataplexy*, i.e., attacks in which there is loss of muscle tone and power (*Tonusverlust*) after emotional excitation. The usual sequence is for irresistible laughter to culminate in a transitory paralysis of all parts of the body. The patient's knees give way and he sinks to the ground helpless to move for a few moments, yet fully conscious. Less complete attacks amount to only a weakness of the knees, a dropping of the jaw, or inability to speak. Objective examination may show the limbs to be slack, with temporary loss of the tendon reflexes. The total duration of the attack is not longer than a few seconds as a rule, and normal muscle power is then restored.

Wilson lists many transitional states and combinations of narcolepsy and cataplexy. In some, sleep was associated with the cataplectic state; or if sleep was resisted, cataplexy took its place; or cataplexy developed spontaneously without antecedent emotional excitation. Even *catalepsy*, which is a condition of sustained immobility with or without clouding of the sensorium, and flexibilitas cerea, i.e., the holding of whatever attitudes and postures the limbs are placed in, have been observed in brief attacks. The term *flexibilitas cerea* is not well chosen for this condition, however, since it has been used to designate a number of dissimilar syndromes, usually hysterical or schizophrenic.

The search for possible causes of the narcoleptic and cataplectic state so far has been unrewarding. Most cases have had no other neurologic abnormality. There have been no other signs of hypothalamic disease, and the sella turcica is of normal size. A very few cases have accompanied multiple sclerosis or have followed encephalitis or trauma. A rapid gain in weight has occurred in some cases and raises the question of an endocrine disturbance. The condition is never fatal, and no complete postmortem examination of a typical case of idiopathic narcolepsy has been conducted.

Sleep Palsies and Acroparesthesias. There are curious and at times distressing paresthetic disturbances which develop during sleep. Everyone is familiar with the phenomenon of a limb falling asleep. The immobility of the limbs and the maintenance of uncomfortable postures without being aware of them permits pressure to be applied to exposed nerves. The ulnar, radial, and peroneal nerves are quite superficial in places; pressure of the nerve against an underlying bone may interfere with intraneural circulation of the compressed segment. If this lasts for half an hour or longer, a sensory and motor paralysis sometimes referred to as *sleep palsy* may develop. This condition usually lasts only a few hours or days, but if the compression is prolonged, the nerve may be severely damaged so that functional recovery awaits regeneration. Unusually deep sleep, as in alcoholic intoxication, or anesthesia renders the patient especially liable to sleep palsies merely because he does not heed the discomfort of an unnatural posture.

Acroparesthesias are frequent in adult women and are not unknown in men. The patient will say that after being asleep for a few hours she is awakened by an intense numbness, tingling, prickling, or "pins and needles" feeling in fingers and hands. There are also aching, burning pains, or tightness and other unpleasant sensations. At first there is a suspicion of having slept on the arm, but the usual bilaterality and the occurrence regardless of the position of the arms dispel this notion. Usually the paresthesias are in the distribution of the median nerves. Vigorous rubbing of the hands restores normal sensation and the paresthesias subside within a few minutes, only to return later or upon first awakening in the morning. The condition never

occurs during the daytime unless the patient is lying down or sitting with the arms and hands in one position. It may be unilateral but is more often bilateral. It never occurs in the feet. When acroparesthesias are frequent, the hands may at all times feel swollen, stiff, clumsy, and slightly numb. Careful examination discloses little or no objective sensory loss, though in some cases touch and pain sensation have been slightly altered in parts supplied by the median nerves. Slight atrophy and weakness of the abductor pollicis brevis and opponens pollicis have been noted. The use of the hands for heavy manual work during the day seems to aggravate the condition, and a holiday or a period of hospitalization may relieve it. It often occurs in young housewives with a new baby or in factory workers who perform a routine skill. Recently it has been demonstrated that there is a compression of the median nerves in the carpal tunnel at the wrist. The injection of 50 mg of hydrocortisone beneath the carpal ligament or the sectioning of the flexor retinaculum has given immediate relief in a respectable number of cases.

DIAGNOSIS OF DISORDERS OF SLEEP

The diagnosis of the cause of insomnia may be troublesome. The difficulty is usually not with the acute case of insomnia as much as with the chronic one. A common source of error is to fail to recognize an underlying psychiatric illness such as an anxiety neurosis or depressive psychosis. This failure can be avoided only by having the main symptoms of these illnesses clearly in mind and making particular inquiry concerning them in every case.

Somnolescent starts, somnolescent sensory paroxysms, and night terrors may all be confused with nocturnal epilepsy, but actually the only real problem here is to distinguish between night terrors and epilepsy. This may at times be difficult if not impossible. The occurrence of other types of seizures, especially if they occur during the daytime, the lack of any display of terrifying emotion, the presence of urinary incontinence and tongue biting are all points indicative of epilepsy. Often electroencephalographic confirmation can be obtained.

In the diagnosis of diseases which cause protracted somnolence, a thorough neurologic study with x-rays of skull, electroencephalogram, and lumbar puncture must be employed. Diabetes insipidus, signs of pituitary insufficiency, blindness in parts of visual fields, ophthalmoplegia, and sometimes extrapyramidal motor disturbances are helpful in that they indicate disease in areas adjacent to the posterior hypothalamus and midbrain.

Narcolepsy may be confused with normal states of somnolence in healthy individuals and with states of excess fatigue and lethargy in neurotic persons. The businessman who invariably falls asleep after lunch or during an evening bridge game, or the bored housewife who feels drowsy in the presence of her friends, is doing little more than showing the usual response to sleep-inducing stimuli. The intrusion of sleep in uncomfortable and unnatural circumstances is a point in favor of narcolepsy, and the coincidence of cataplexy—a much more easily recognized condition—is confirmatory. Increasing drowsiness may also be an early symptom in brain tumor, chronic subdural hematoma, and other neurologic diseases.

Sleep palsies must be distinguished from other diseases affecting the peripheral nerves. The onset during sleep, the maximum functional disturbance immediately afterwards, and steady improvement are the main characteristics. A delay in the appearance of muscular atrophy may be perplexing unless it is remembered that it takes 2 to 3 months for denervation atrophy to develop fully. The syndrome of acroparesthesias is often mistaken for ruptured cervical disk, anterior scalene and cervical rib syndrome, peripheral neuritis, or multiple sclerosis. The nocturnal incidence, the localization to the fingers and hands in the median nerve distribution, and the lack of other neurologic signs are diagnostic. A tourniquet around the arm just above the elbow may reproduce the acroparesthetic syndrome.

TREATMENT

In general, there are three varieties of wakefulness. For best management, treatment should be based on the type exhibited by the patient. In younger patients the most frequently observed type of insomnia is the inability to fall asleep. These individuals have developed more and more tenseness during the day and are unable to relax. This type of insomnia usually lasts from 1 to 3 hr, and then the individual sinks into an exhausted, deep sleep which continues through the night. For these patients a quick-acting, fairly rapidly destroyed hypnotic such as secobarbital (Seconal)—0.1 Gm given 15 to 20 min before going to bed—is desirable.

The second group consists of patients who are able to go to sleep but who awaken in 1 or 2 hr and lose sleep in the middle of the night. Some are alternately awake and asleep all night. Often these are sick individuals with a debilitating or painful illness who develop more pain and restlessness as muscles relax, leaving painful areas unsplinted. In others, fever, sweats, dyspnea, or other distressful symptoms develop and demand attention. Frequently, these patients secure good relief from 0.1 Gm pentobarbital (Nembutal) given at bedtime. In cardiac patients who have Cheyne-Stokes respiration or moderate orthopnea, a rectal suppository of aminophylline, 0.5 Gm given at bedtime, will frequently relieve the respiratory distress and promote sleep. When pain is a factor in insomnia, acetylsalicylic acid (0.3 to 0.6 Gm) should be given with the sedative. Occasionally codeine phosphate (30 mg) may be required when pain is severe.

The third group of insomnia patients consists of those who go to sleep promptly and sleep well most of the night only to awaken too early in the morning. Most of these individuals are older people who turn night into day. They go to bed and get up earlier and earlier so that soon they are sleeping during the day and are alert during the night. Into this category also fall those individuals who are under great tension, worry, or anxiety, or are overworked and exhausted. These people sink into bed and sleep through sheer exhaustion but around 4 or 5 A.M. awake with their worries and are unable to get back to sleep. Most of these patients are benefited by barbital (0.3 Gm) given with fruit juice or milk at bedtime. For debilitated patients the compressed tablets of insoluble material should be crushed to ensure proper absorption, or sodium barbital should be substituted. Chloral hydrate (1.0 Gm) given with fruit juice at bedtime is also effective and may be substituted for the barbital if desired.

Patients with serious mental agitation, delirium, or excitement who require prompt, easily controlled, relatively safe sedation should receive paraldehyde, 15 to 30 ml by mouth in iced fruit juice, or the same dose by rectum but diluted with 200 ml physiologic saline solution or 120 ml olive oil. Generally it is wise to avoid the use of barbiturates in highly agitated patients, since occasionally they may precipitate serious mental confusion, excitement, or even manic tendencies. Chloral hydrate, 1.0 to 2.0 Gm by mouth or rectum, is useful in the management of these individuals and frequently proves more satisfactory than the barbiturates.

A word of caution about oversedation is wise in any discussion of sedative drugs. All too frequently they are abused in that they are given when not needed, the dose is too great, or the wrong preparation is used. These drugs are a common source of constipation, lead to fatigue and lack of energy and strength, and interfere with the patient's recovery from his illness.

When large doses of quicker-acting barbiturates, 0.4 to 0.6 Gm daily, are given for more than a week or two, there is real danger of habituation which, once it has developed, is pernicious in character. Withdrawal, unless done skillfully and in graded steps, may cause serious mental disturbance or precipitate convulsions. The patient should not be encouraged to use sedative drugs as a crutch on which to limp through life. One should search out and correct the underlying difficulty, using sedation when necessary, as a temporary helpful tool.

Barbiturate sedatives may be of value in the treatment of night terrors, and if their differentiation from nocturnal epilepsy is impossible, a trial on Dilantin Sodium and phenobarbital is indicated. (See Chap. 36 for further information concerning anticonvulsant medication.)

Amphetamine sulfate and other sympathomimetic drugs are effective in controlling narcolepsy. The dose should be regulated so that diurnal sleep attacks are reduced to a minimum (usually not all of them can be prevented) and nocturnal sleep is normal. Doses of 10 to 20 mg amphetamine sulfate three to five times daily are usually sufficient. Interspersed naps are also helpful and make sleep attacks less frequent. Another drug which has proved to be useful is pipradol (Meratran) in a dose of 2.5 mg morning and noon.

REFERENCES

Gilbert, J. A., and G. I. W. Patrick: On the Effects of Loss of Sleep, Psychol. Rev., 3:469, 1896.

Kremer, M., R. W. Gilliatt, J. S. R. Golding, and T. G. Wilson: Acroparesthesiae in the Carpal-tunnel Syndrome, Lancet, 1953, II:590.

Miller, H. R.: "Central Autonomic Regulations in Health and Disease," p. 260, New York, Grune & Stratton, Inc., 1942.

Muncie, W.: "Psychobiology and Psychiatry," p. 104, Sleep, St. Louis, The C. V. Mosby Company, 1939.

Wilson, S. A.: "Modern Problems in Neurology," Chap. 5, London, Edward Arnold & Co., 1928.

36   RECURRENT CONVULSIONS
Raymond D. Adams

The magnitude of the problem of epilepsy and its importance in our society can hardly be overstated. The statistics of Lennox show that there are at least 500,000 persons in this country who are or have been subject to seizures. Epilepsy follows apoplexy in being the most frequent neurologic disorder. Therefore, it is desirable for the physician, if he is to achieve some measure of precision in diagnosis and treatment, to know something of the nature and etiology of this common disorder and of the mechanism of production of its symptoms.

Epilepsy is an intermittent disorder of the nervous system due presumably to a sudden, excessive, disorderly discharge of cerebral neurones. This was the postulation of Hughlings Jackson, the eminent British neurologist of the nineteenth century, and modern electrophysiology offers no evi-

dence to the contrary. This discharge results in an almost instantaneous disturbance of sensation, loss of consciousness, convulsive movements, or some combination thereof. A terminologic difficulty arises from the diversity of the clinical manifestations. It seems improper to call a condition a convulsion when only an alteration of sensation or of consciousness takes place. The word *seizure* is preferable as a generic term and also lends itself to qualification. Motor or convulsive seizure is therefore not tautologic, and one may speak also of sensory seizures. The word *epilepsy*, which in the days of our forefathers meant the "falling evil," has many unpleasant connotations and, although a useful medical term, probably is best avoided in open discussions until such time as the general public becomes more enlightened.

Epilepsy may begin at any age. It may occur once in the lifetime of an individual or several times a day. Sometimes it is an obvious symptom of a brain disease which also manifests itself in other ways, sometimes it is the solitary expression of deranged cerebral function in an individual who otherwise maintains perfect health. The latter is the more frequent circumstance and explains why the convulsive state has for so long been looked upon as a disease entity. However, the illogicality of the concept that a convulsion occurring by itself represents a disease whereas one occurring in combination with other symptoms is but a manifestation of a disease should be apparent to all. The convulsive state must always be looked upon as symptomatic. Resort to such epithets as "genuine" or "essential" or "idiopathic" in no sense changes its status.

THE COMMON TYPES OF CONVULSIVE DISORDERS

In a statistical survey of nearly 2,000 patients it was reported that 51 per cent of all epileptic patients had had generalized convulsions; 8 per cent, minor seizures referred to as petit mal; 1 per cent, psychic or psychomotor seizures; and the remaining 40 per cent, two or even all three types, the most prominent form being psychomotor. Thus psychomotor epilepsy, as pointed out by Singh, is probably as frequent as grand mal. Although the total number of seizures having a focal onset was not determined, these data give some notion of the principal forms of the convulsive state in the majority of patients and provide a starting point for the ensuing discussion.

The Generalized Convulsion (Grand Mal, Major Epilepsy)

The term *convulsion* is most applicable to this form of seizure. The patient may sense its possible approach by any one of several subjective sensations. For some hours he may feel apathetic, depressed, irritable, or the opposite—unusually alert or even ecstatic. Flatulence, constipation, headache are other prodromal symptoms, and myoclonic twitches, i.e., sudden movements affecting one or another limb or the trunk, may precede the convulsion by some hours. In approximately half the cases there is some type of sensation or movement of one part of the body before the loss of consciousness or the generalized convulsion. This is called the *aura*, and as will develop later it provides the most reliable clue to the location of the underlying disease. The most frequent aura is an epigastric sensation, a sinking or gripping feeling, a strangulation or palpitation. A tingling numbness of the fingers or lips or some other part of the body, a flashing light or panorama, a disagreeable taste or odor are other well-known sensory auras. Clonic twitches, tonic contraction of the muscles of a limb, and turning of the head and eyes constitute somatic motor auras. These latter may spread from one part of the body to another in an orderly, predictable sequence. Usually by the time all of one side of the body is affected there is a loss of consciousness. The aura, though truly a warning of the oncoming seizure, is actually the first part of the seizure and not a prodrome. It seldom lasts for more than a few seconds.

The generalized convulsion, or fit, as it is often called, begins with a sudden loss of consciousness and falling to the ground. The whole musculature is seized in a violent spasm. The contraction of the diaphragm and chest muscles produces a characteristic cry. The eyes turn up or to one side, the face is contorted, the jaw is set, often with biting of the tongue and oozing of saliva or blood from the lips, and the limbs may assume any one of several positions. With continued spasm of the respiratory muscles breathing is impossible, and the color of the skin and mucous membranes becomes dusky or cyanotic. After a fraction of a minute the rigid or tonic state of the muscles gives way to a series of clonic jerking movements. Air begins to enter the lungs in short convulsive gasps, and a bloody froth, a mixture of saliva and blood from a bitten tongue or cheek, forms on the lips. The arms, legs, face, and head jerk violently. After a minute or two the movements become slower, then irregular, and finally cease. The patient then lies relaxed, breathing rather deeply and sweating profusely. There may have been loss of control of urine and occasionally of feces. The state is now one of deep coma, and even the most intense pain fails to evoke a response. After a few minutes the patient stirs and then opens his eyes. His first remarks or questions usually betray mental confusion. For the next several minutes or even hours

there is a tendency toward incoherence of thought and drowsiness. Often the patient falls into a deep sleep. Headache is another frequent postseizure or postictal symptom. The patient himself is completely unaware of what has happened or at most remembers only the aura. He may come to his senses in a hospital or other strange place, and his only way of telling that something has happened is by the hiatus in his memory, his disheveled appearance, the sore tongue, and a soreness of the vigorously exercised muscles. Injury may be sustained during the fall, and as a consequence of violent muscular contraction, a vertebra may be crushed.

Convulsions of this type ordinarily come singly or in groups of two or three and may occur when the patient is awake or when he is asleep. About 5 to 8 per cent of patients at some time have a series of seizures without regaining consciousness between times. This is known as *status epilepticus* and demands urgent treatment. Or instead of the whole sequence of changes described above, only one part of the seizure may occur. For example, there may be only the aura without loss of consciousness, or the entire spell may consist of a brief loss of consciousness and momentary spasm of the limbs.

Petit Mal (*Minor Epilepsy, the Small Illness, l'Absence*)

In contrast to the generalized seizure these attacks are so brief that they are often overlooked. In fact many patients may have them for years before their true nature is recognized.

The attack comes without warning and consists of sudden loss of consciousness. The person is motionless, and a staring expression of the face and a failure to speak or to respond to commands are the only signs of abnormality. In contrast to grand mal, motor disturbances are conspicuously absent, and at most only a few flickering contractions of the eyelids and facial muscles and jerking of the arms at a rate of three contractions per second are seen. The patient does not fall, as a rule, and may continue such complex acts as walking or even riding a bicycle during an attack. After 2 to 15 or more seconds consciousness is regained abruptly and fully, and the patient promptly resumes whatever action was taking place before the seizure. To the patient there is only a blank place, "an absence" in his stream of consciousness.

Closely related to petit mal are the akinetic seizures, in which the patient suddenly loses consciousness and falls motionless to the ground, and the myoclonic seizure, which consists of a sudden violent contraction of some part or all of the body, often with falling and loss of consciousness of a few seconds' duration (generalized myoclonus).

Because of frequent association with petit mal and the similarity of the electroencephalographic pattern, Lennox groups petit mal, the akinetic seizure, and myoclonic seizure into a single entity called the *petit mal triad*.

Episodes of this type are much more frequent in childhood and adolescence. Another characteristic is their great frequency. As many as several hundred may occur in one day. Although benign, they may, if frequent, derange the mental processes so that the patient does poorly in school. Rarely, a series of them in close succession will interrupt consciousness for a longer period of time. This is known as *petit mal status*. Pyknolepsy is an almost obsolete term for frequent petit mal during childhood, terminating at puberty. When present as the only type of seizure during childhood, petit mal may, as the patient grows older, give way to or be combined with grand mal.

Psychomotor Epilepsy (*Epileptic Equivalents, Psychic Variants, Epileptic Mania or Delirium, Epilepsia Procursiva*)

This differs in several ways from the two types of seizure discussed above. (1) The aura, if it occurs, is often of the nature of a complex hallucination or perceptual illusion. There may be an unpleasant smell or taste or the revival of a complicated visual scene involving people, dwellings, etc., usually taken from past experiences and resembling a dream. Furthermore, the patient's perception of what is seen and heard and his relationship to the outside world are altered. Objects appear to be far away or unreal (*jamais vu*); or strange objects or people may seem familiar (*déjà vu phenomenon*). Hughlings Jackson applied the term *dreamy state* to these psychic disturbances. (2) Instead of losing all control of his thoughts and actions the patient behaves as though he were partially conscious during the attack. He may get up and walk about, unbutton or remove his clothes, attempt to speak, or even continue such habitual acts as driving a car. If he is asked a specific question or given a command it is evident that he is out of contact with the examiner and does not understand. When restrained he may resist with great energy and at times can be violent. This type of behavior is said to be *automatic*, presumably because the patient behaves like an automaton. (3) Convulsive movements when present are likely to consist of chewing, smacking and licking of the lips, and less often, tonic spasms of the limbs or turning of the head and eyes to one side.

In any given case one or several of these phenomena may be observed. In the series studied by Lennox, which numbered 414 cases, 43 per cent displayed some of these motor or psychomotor phenomena, 32 per cent the automatic state, and 25 per cent the psychic changes. Because of the concurrence of these three symptom complexes he has referred to the whole group as the *psychomotor triad*. These types of seizure vary in frequency and duration. Some are very brief, lasting only for seconds, and others continue for hours or days. This fact calls to mind that the duration of the seizure is an unsatisfactory criterion for classification. Two-thirds of the cases have generalized convulsions at some time in their life.

In addition to these three major types the clinicians of the nineteenth century recognized many other special forms of epilepsy, some of which were given descriptive names. The term *tonic seizure* referred to tonic muscle contractions, to the exclusion of phasic qualities. *Epilepsia partialis continua* specified a repetitive clonic contraction of one group of muscles. The terms *focal motor* or *focal sensory* epilepsy were applied to a tonic or clonic movement or a sensation restricted to one portion of the body. Myoclonic epilepsy referred to a syndrome of epilepsy and isolated twitches of a muscle or group of muscles, called *myoclonus* (see Chap. 27). Random, arrhythmic myoclonus in a sense might be designated as *epilepsia partialis discontinua et disseminata*. It is usually caused by a more or less diffuse disease of the cerebral and cerebellar cortex and possibly other parts of the nervous system such as the thalamus.

It is obvious that the traditional division of seizures into three general types leaves much to be desired. Petit mal is a more or less homogeneous type, whereas grand mal represents a phase of generalization of the seizure discharge, regardless of its origin or the initial symptoms of the seizure. Psychomotor epilepsy, as will become evident upon further analysis, is not a uniform syndrome, but encompasses a diversity of clinical phenomena. Moreover, careful study of the first symptoms of the seizure and the use of the electroencephalogram have given us a new means of subdividing seizures according to other more significant attributes. The seizure pattern provides information that not only is of great value in determining the topography of the disease causing the convulsive disorder but affords a new basis of classification that will serve until such time as the etiology is discovered.

COMMON SEIZURE PATTERNS

A number of seizure patterns have been identified; they are so helpful in the localization of cerebral lesions that every student of medicine should be familiar with them. These types of epilepsy are often termed *focal* because they can be traced to a circumscript lesion of the brain. Many cases of this type come under the surveillance of neurosurgeons, and their contributions to this field have been of great value.

Motor Seizures (Generalized, Contraversive, Focal Motor, and Jacksonian Motor Seizures)

A lesion in one or other frontal lobe may give rise to a generalized or major convulsive seizure of the type described above, without introductory sensory aura. In some cases there is a turning movement of head and eyes to one side, simultaneous with loss of consciousness, and in others there are no turning or versive movements. It has been postulated that in both types of seizure, the one with and the one without contraversive movements, there is an immediate spread of the discharge from the frontal lobe into an integrating center such as the thalamus, with immediate loss of consciousness. In cases with head and eye turning, the discharge is believed to reach area 8 (area for contralateral turning of head and eyes), although it has been found that contralateral turning of the head and eyes can be induced in the experimental animal by stimulation of temporal or occipital as well as of the premotor cortex.

Do most cases of generalized motor seizures (grand mal) of idiopathic type have a frontal lobe focus? Unfortunately this question cannot be answered at the moment. Actually such a focus has been found in only a small number of such cases, and these may not be representative of the whole group.

The characteristics of the Jacksonian motor seizure are well known. It begins usually with a twitching of the fingers of one hand, the face on one side, or one foot. The movements are clonic and rhythmical; their speed varies. They may occur in bursts or paroxysms. The disorder then spreads or marches from the part first affected to other muscles on the same side of the body—from the face to the neck, hand, forearm, arm, trunk, and leg; or if the first movement is in the foot, the order is reversed. The high incidence of onset in the lips, fingers, and toes probably is related to the greater cortical representation of these parts of the body. The disease process or focus of excitation is usually in the Rolandic cortex, area 4 (Fig. 37-1) on the opposite side; in a few cases it has been found in the post-Rolandic convolution. Lesions confined to the premotor cortex (area 6) are said to induce tonic contractions of an arm, face, neck, or all of one side of the body. Perspiration and piloerection, sometimes of the parts of the body involved in a focal motor seizure, suggest that these autonomic functions have a cortical representation in the Rolandic area. Some neurologists distinguish focal motor and Jacksonian motor seizures by the absence of a characteristic march in

the former, but both have essentially the same localizing significance.

There is another type of focal motor epilepsy, designated as *epilepsia partialis continua*, which consists of rhythmic clonic movements of one group of muscles, usually in the face, arm, or leg. These may continue for a variable period of time, minutes to weeks or months. The seizure usually does not march to other parts of the body. Its localizing value has not been settled. Some cases have a lesion in the opposite sensorimotor areas of the cerebral cortex.

Somatic, Visual, and Other Sensory Seizures

Somatic sensory seizures, either focal or "marching" to other parts of the body on one side, nearly always indicate a parietal lobe lesion. The usual sensory disorder is described as a numbness or a tingling or "pins and needles" feeling. Other variations are sensations of crawling (formication), buzzing, electricity, or vibration. Pain and thermal sensations are infrequent. The onset is in the lips, fingers, and toes in the majority of cases, and the spread to adjacent parts of the body follows a pattern determined by sensory arrangements in the postcentral (post-Rolandic) convolution of the parietal lobe. In Kristiansen and Penfield's series the seizure focus was found in the postcentral convolution in 24 of 55 cases. In the others it was central, either pre-Rolandic or post-Rolandic in 18, and precentral in 7. One may conclude that this type of sensory phenomenon is always indicative of a focus in or near the post-Rolandic convolution of the opposite cerebral hemisphere; if localized in the head, the locus is in the lowest part of the convolution, near the Sylvian fissure; and if in the foot or leg, the upper part near the superior sagittal sinus is involved.

Visual seizures are also of localizing significance. Lesions in or near the striate cortex of the occipital lobe usually produce a sensation of lights, of darkness, or of color. According to Gowers, red is the most frequent color, followed by blue, green, and yellow. The patient may tell of seeing stars or moving lights in the visual field on the side opposite the lesion. Sometimes they appear to be straight ahead of the patient. Often, if they occur on only one side of the visual field, he believes only one eye to be affected, the one opposite the lesion, probably because the average person is unaware that he has two corresponding visual fields. It is curious that a lesion arising in one occipital lobe may cause momentary blindness in both eyes. It has been noted that lesions on the lateral surface of the occipital lobes (Brodmann's areas 18 and 19) are more likely to cause twinkling or pulsating lights. Complex visual hallucinations are usually due to a focus in the posterior part of the temporal lobe, near its junction with the parietal, and may be associated with auditory hallucinations. Often the visual images, either those of the hallucination or of objects seen, are distorted, being too small (micropsia) or unnaturally arranged.

Auditory hallucinations are rather infrequent as an initial manifestation of a seizure. Occasionally a patient with a focus in the superior temporal convolution on one side will report a buzzing or a roaring in his ears. A human voice sometimes repeating recognizable words has been noted a few times in patients with lesions in the more posterior part of one temporal lobe.

Vertiginous sensations of a type suggesting vestibular stimulation may be the first symptom of a seizure. The lesion is usually localized in the superior, posterior temporal region or at the junction between parietal and temporal lobes. Foerster is said to have evoked a sensation of vertigo by stimulating the parietal lobe, and one of Penfield's cases had a lesion here. Occasionally with a temporal focus the vertigo is followed by an auditory sensation. Giddiness is also a frequent prelude to a seizure, but this has so many different meanings that it is of little diagnostic import.

Olfactory hallucinations are often associated with disease of the inferior and medial parts of the temporal lobe, usually in the region of the hippocampal convolution or the uncus (hence the term *uncinate seizures,* after Jackson). Usually the smell is exteriorized, i.e., projected to someplace in the environment, and is of a disagreeable nature. Gustatory hallucinations have also been recorded in proved cases of temporal lobe disease. Sensations of thirst and salivation may be associated. Stimulation of the upper surface of the temporal lobe in the depths of the Sylvian fissure during neurosurgical operations has reproduced peculiar sensations of taste.

Visceral sensations arising in the thorax, epigastrium, and abdomen are among the most frequent of auras. They are described as a vague, indefinable feeling, a sinking sensation in the pit of the stomach, a weakness in the epigastrium or substernal area which rises to the throat and head. In several such cases the seizure discharge has been localized to the upper bank of the Sylvian fissure, but a few cases had lesions in the upper intermediate or medial frontal areas near the cingulate gyrus. Palpitation and acceleration of pulse at the beginning of the attack have also been related to a temporal lobe focus.

Psychic Phenomena

The studies of many neurologists have served to establish the close relationship between psychic changes and the temporal lobe. Disease of either temporal lobe may be accompanied by seizures that have many of the characteristics outlined in the section on psychomotor epilepsy. In addition to olfactory and gustatory hallucinations, there are often others of more complex visual and auditory type, resembling dreams. Curious illusions of perception and feelings of unreality and partial or complete interruption of consciousness may be observed. Compulsive thoughts or actions may recur in a fixed pattern during each seizure. Automatic behavior or even frank psychoses of many different types, lasting for hours or days, may be induced by seizure discharges or electrical stimulation of the temporal lobe. Masticatory movements are also frequent.

Loss of Consciousness

A lapse of consciousness is the initial event in petit mal, which is believed now to represent a disorder of the diencephalon, the so-called "centrencephalic epilepsy." Lesions in the prefrontal regions have been observed to abolish consciousness at the very beginning of the seizure, presumably through their effects on the diencephalon and midbrain structures.

The various motor, sensory, or psychic phenomena may be combined in many different sequences. These presumably indicate the spread of a seizure discharge from one cortical area to another. A flash of light followed by tingling of one side of the body suggests that the epileptic discharge began in the occipital lobe and extended to the somatic sensory areas in the parietal lobe. A smell of something burning, followed by chewing and smacking movements and then loss of speech, would be interpreted as a spread of the seizure discharge from the region of the uncus to the upper parts of the temporal and the inferior frontal lobe. A focal motor seizure followed by a tonic contraction of one side of the body and then turning of the head and eyes contralaterally would indicate a successive involvement of the motor, premotor, and contraversive cortical field for head and eyes. Little is known about the factors which facilitate or inhibit the spread of seizure discharges from one part of the brain to another.

The various clinical types of seizure patterns and their localizing significance are summarized in Table 36-1.

THE EVOCATION OF SEIZURES
(Reflex Epilepsy)

For a long time it has been known that seizures could be evoked in certain epileptic individuals by a physiologic or psychologic stimulus. Approximately 1 in every 15 patients will have remarked that their seizures occur under special circumstances, such as being exposed to flickering light,

Table 36-1. COMMON SEIZURE PATTERNS

Clinical type	Localization
1. Somatic motor:	
Generalized (grand mal)	Complete motor
Jacksonian (local motor)	Pre-Rolandic gyrus
Masticatory	Lower Rolandic
Simple contraversive	Frontal
Tonic postural (decerebrate, opisthotonic)	Brain stem
2. Somatic and special sensory (auras):	
Somatosensory	Post-Rolandic
Visual	Occipital, or temporal
Auditory	Temporal
Vertiginous	Temporal
Olfactory	Infratemporal
Gustatory	Sylvian-temporal
3. Visceral:	
Autonomic	Diencephalic
4. Psychic:	
Dreamy state	Temporal
Automatism (ictal and postictal)	
Psychotic states (primary or secondary)	Temporal
5. Petit mal	Diencephalon(?)

SOURCE: Modified from Penfield and Erickson, "Epilepsy and Cerebral Localization," Springfield, Ill., Charles C Thomas, Publisher, 1941.

passing from darkness to light or the reverse, being startled by a loud noise, hearing a series of monotonous sounds or music, touching, rubbing, or hurting a particular part of the body, making certain movements, eating a large meal or experiencing digestive changes, or being subjected to a fright or other strong emotion. The evoked seizure may be focal (beginning often in the part of the body which has been stimulated) or generalized and may take the form of one or a series of myoclonic jerks, a petit mal or grand mal. In a few instances such reflex epilepsy, as it is called, has been due to a focal cerebral disease, such as tumor, but more often its cause cannot be ascertained. W. Watson has discovered a strong tendency to familial incidence in a variety of myoclonic jerking elicited by photic stimulation, and some patients in whom this phenomenon had been noted were unaware of ever having had a seizure. Also of interest in these cases of evoked seizure has been the phenomenon of willfully averting the seizure by undertaking some mental task, e.g., thinking about some distracting subject, counting, etc., or by initiating some physical activity.

Patients of this type suggest to us that epilepsy is a natural state, a physiologic event resulting from the excitation and subsequent inhibition of an injured part of the cerebrum.

PATHOPHYSIOLOGY AND BIOCHEMISTRY OF EPILEPSY

From what has been said about epilepsy it is obvious that a satisfactory theory must account for the following clinical and pathologic data. (1) The majority of demonstrable epileptogenic lesions are situated in or near the cerebral cortex, which suggests that some property of the neural organization of the cortex disposes to this condition. (2) The foci induced by any given disease may or may not give rise to epilepsy; some peculiarity of the lesion must, therefore, determine this phenomenon. (3) The epileptic focus once present is known to become active, i.e., to discharge, only on occasion, or at least the electrical discharge which attends it may be detected in the electroencephalogram and the seizure occurs only from time to time. (4) Several events appear to activate the focus, some of physiologic or psychologic nature and others, biochemical. The former include photic and other sensory stimuli; the latter pentylenetetrazol (Metrazol), picrotoxin, acetylcholine. (5) The seizure discharges upon reaching a certain magnitude spread along preformed pathways from their site of origin to other cortical areas and to the diencephalon. (6) Some inhibitory process counteracts and ultimately terminates the seizure discharge. (7) In many human cases no cortical lesion has been demonstrated by current neuropathologic methods, and in this group there may be a genetic factor. The evidence on this latter point is not altogether convincing. Certainly epilepsy and paroxysmal disturbances in the electroencephalogram have been observed in a large series of identical twins. However, the incidence of convulsions in the blood relatives of epileptic patients is only two or three times that in the public at large.

Much experimental work has been done to obtain explanations of these phenomena, but limitations of space permit no more than a condensed review of it here. Investigators have centered their attention on human cases of focal epilepsy and on focal epileptic lesions in the mammalian cortex. In both man and animal the neurophysiologic analogue to the human convulsive seizure has been the repetitive, self-sustained discharge of electrical activity which continues after a stimulus to a circumscript cortical area has terminated. The neurosurgeon has found this so consistently in or near epileptic foci and has observed so frequently a seizure discharge to accompany it that he has accepted it as the electrical sign of the epileptic lesion. As pointed out by Symonds in his Hughlings Jackson Lecture, the afterdischarge, once started, continues at a regular frequency of 10 to 14 per second. Within a short time (seconds to minutes), the intervals between spikes increase, they tend then to be grouped and their voltage rises. When the pauses between bursts reach ½ sec or more, the afterdischarge ceases altogether and the area of cortex becomes electrically inactive and inexcitable. Adrian in his study of this state interprets its cessation as indicative of a rivalry between two opposing processes, the initial one excitatory, the final one inhibitory. A possible physiologic basis of these two processes has been demonstrated by Eccles. Each motor anterior horn cell, when activated, stimulates through a collateral branch another cell, the Renshaw cell, which is inhibitory in its action and imposes this inhibition on the anterior horn cell itself. Similarly, Phillips has noted an arrangement between the Betz cells in the cerebral cortex and other interneurones which inhibit the Betz cells. Thus both the anterior horn cells and Betz cells initiate excitation to another cell via their main axone and an inhibition of their own activity by means of an adjacent inhibitory nerve cell. Moreover, on the afferent side of nervous activity all recent physiologic work has shown that each sensory neurone from the end organ to the cerebral cortex is monitored by a central, descending inhibitory system.

A convulsive seizure could be conceived, therefore, as an excessive excitation resulting from a narrowly focused afferent stimulation on the injured cerebral cortex or a deficiency of suppressive influences either from the afferent neurones or the special inhibitory neurones of the cortex. It is of interest that strychnine, one of the most potent agents for discharging neurones and producing seizures, does not facilitate the excitatory postsynaptic potential of motor neurones but rather diminishes their inhibitory postsynaptic potentials. Furthermore it has been shown that solutions of strychnine, by themselves too weak to have any effect on the cortex, would condition it in such a fashion that sensory stimuli conveyed to it could discharge the altered neurones and thus produce convulsive activity. This state of affairs resembles that which prevails in human epilepsy, where a silent, subliminal epileptic focus is discharged by a particular type of sensory stimulus and is restored to its quiescent state by inhibitory neurones.

Since electrical activity is believed to depend on chemical changes (flux of Na, K, Ca, Mg), it is rather to be expected that a search would have been made for special excitatory and inhibitory substances in the brain. Acetylcholine is known to be an effective convulsive agent when applied to the animal cortex, and cholinesterase inhibitors such as isopropylfluorophosphate also produce seizures. Human epileptic cortical lesions have been found to contain an increased amount of acetylcholinesterase and in a test tube are unable to "bind acetylcholine." After a seizure there are increased amounts of acetylcholine in human cerebrospinal fluid. Barbiturates and diphenylhydantoin (Dilantin) are said to act as anticonvulsants because they enhance the acetylcholine-binding power of the cerebral cortex.

With respect to inhibitory substances Florey found that cerebral and spinal cord tissue contain an agent identified as gamma aminobutyric acid (GABA) which, if applied to the cortex, blocks excitation of the superficial layer and augments inhibition—an action opposite that of strychnine. It is formed from glutamic acid, and one of the coenzymes which catalyzes its synthesis is pyridoxine (vitamin B_6), a lack of which is known to produce seizures in animals and man. Metrazol and picrotoxin prevent the inhibitory effect of GABA. The action of GABA as an intrinsic anticonvulsant has not been fully explored. Given intravenously it is said to protect animals against chemically induced seizures. There is disagreement on this point, however, for others have found it to be ineffective when given by this route and have noted that it fails to cross the blood-brain endothelial barrier. If true, only a lesion which destroys this barrier would be expected to permit the entrance of GABA into the discharging focus. This subject is still under investigation.

Whatever the basic chemistry of the process it is reasonably well established that changes in the blood such as oxygen supply, acid-base equilibrium, calcium, magnesium, glucose, chloride, and fluid balance alter the seizure threshold. Lennox has depicted the relationship of these many factors to epilepsy by drawing an analogy to a reservoir. Water enters this reservoir from various underground springs, each of which represents one cause of the seizures. As the reservoir fills it periodically overflows the restraining dam, the overflow representing the seizure. The height of the restraining dam indicates the seizure threshold and the amount of water in the reservoir, the force of the influences which cause seizures. The restraining dam is lowered by alkalosis, decreased oxygenation, hydration, hypoglycemia, and elevation of intracranial pressure, and raised by the opposite conditions. This metaphorical reservoir stresses the importance of the factors which operate to prevent seizures in any given patient.

Although high-amplitude activity of a group of neurones represents the "functional unit of epilepsy," it is the spread of this electrical potential to other parts of the nervous system that characterizes the whole convulsive seizure both clinically and electroencephalographically. The spread of these discharges proceeds along preformed pathways, i.e., via the uncinate fibers to adjacent cortical fields, via the corpus callosum to corresponding parts of the contralateral cerebral hemisphere, or along corticothalamic and thalamocortical pathways to the diencephalon and reticular formation. Little is known about factors which interfere with the spread of the seizure discharge. The corpus callosum has been sectioned in animals and human beings for this purpose, and although the results were not conclusive, the seizures usually remained unilateral. The anticonvulsant activity of phenobarbital and diphenylhydantoin is believed to be mainly in preventing the spread of seizure discharges, and these drugs are said to have rather little suppressive action on the epileptic focus.

These many investigations raise more new questions than they answer, but one fact is certain—scientists are now searching out the basic facts concerning the epileptic discharge and are coming to view it in both its biochemical and neurophysiologic aspects. Approximate explanations are no longer acceptable. The observation that a lesion in the motor cortex causes focal or Jacksonian seizures does no more than center attention on one link in a chain of causal events. It enables us to say only that such a lesion provides suitable conditions for the development of a convulsion.

Certain occurrences in the seizure, such as the cry, the motor activity, the sensory experience, may be regarded as the direct manifestation of the seizure discharge in the brain. Some of these immediate effects when regarded from the more general neurophysiologic point of view are excitatory, and others, like the lapse of consciousness of petit mal, are inhibitory. Electrical stimulation of the brain through the intact skull, as in electroshock convulsions for the treatment of depression, or by the application of electrodes on the surface of the brain is observed to produce the same changes. This initial outburst lasts for only a brief period of time and is often followed by a total or subtotal paralysis or inhibition of cerebral function. A focal motor seizure, for example, may result in suppression of activity in motor areas and a temporary paralysis of the involved muscles (Todd's postepileptic or exhaustion paralysis). The loss of consciousness which follows a generalized motor seizure, in contradistinction to that of petit mal, is probably due to a postexcitatory paralysis of either diencephalic or midbrain structures. Vital functions may also be arrested, but usually for only a few seconds. In rare instances, however, death may occur owing to a cessation of respiration, derangement of cardiac action, or some unknown cause. The automatic behavior so characteristic of psychomotor epilepsy appears in some instances to be a direct stimulatory effect in the temporal lobe and in others is a postexcitatory, inhibitory, or paralytic effect.

The electroencephalogram provides a delicate proof of Hughlings Jackson's theory of epilepsy—that it is an excessive, disorderly discharge of cortical neurones. At the onset of the focal seizure this is registered in or near the focus as a series of spikes or sharp waves interrupting the normal alpha and beta waves. The clinical spread of the seizure has its electroencephalographic equivalent in the extension of the abnormal electrical waves; and with generalization of the seizure (grand mal) the entire electroencephalographic recording surface of the brain exhibits spikes of high voltage. Petit mal is accompanied by a characteristic slow wave—spike complex occurring simultaneously in all cortical leads and presumably taking origin from a diencephalic focus. At first it was thought that there was a characteristic electroencephalographic picture for psychomotor epilepsy, but further studies have not confirmed this. The postseizure state, sometimes called postictal disturbance of cerebral function, also has its electroencephalographic correlate in random, generalized slow waves; with recovery the electroencephalogram returns to normal. If the electroencephalographic tracing is obtained during the interval between seizures, it is abnormal to some degree in approximately 40 per cent of fully conscious and 75 per cent of sleeping patients.

The electroencephalographic changes are discussed in Chap. 55.

CLASSIFICATION OF CONVULSIVE DISORDERS

The classification of McNaughton, presented in Table 36-2, combines the best features of older descriptions with present concepts of focal cerebral and diencephalic seizures. Furthermore, it has the merit of subdividing seizures according to their main clinical attributes, which can be ascertained by a detailed history and careful observation of the patient.

DISEASES CAUSING SYMPTOMATIC EPILEPSY

In the list of diseases of the nervous system with which every physician must be familiar, a few stand apart by reason of their tendency to produce recurrent convulsions. The seizures are said to be symptomatic in contrast to the large majority of cases in which epilepsy is idiopathic. The physician must distinguish by the usual clinical and laboratory methods the different diseases that may cause, accompany, or precipitate convulsions.

Diseases Localized in the Cerebral Hemispheres

Almost any type of cerebral lesion may cause seizures; on the other hand, no cerebral lesion is invariably accompanied by them. In patients with cerebral lesions the seizures are usually focal, lead-

Table 36-2. A CLASSIFICATION OF CONVULSIVE DISORDERS

Group	Attack pattern	Electroencephalographic findings	Radiographic findings	Pathologic findings
1. Focal epilepsy (cortical or subcortical)	Focal attack pattern usual; may be major or minor in degree. This includes focal temporal seizures with automatism	Focal spikes, sharp waves, etc.	Cranial asymmetry may be present. Pneumogram may show focal changes	Clinical examination may show focal neurologic changes due to agenesis (and other congenital causes), scar, neoplasm, abscess, etc., or to unknown cause
2. Central or "centrencephalic" epilepsy	Focal attack pattern unusual. Major or minor (petit mal). Myoclonic jerks common	3 per sec wave and spike, bilateral synchronization	Cranium usually normal. Pneumogram normal or may show symmetrical enlargement	Cause usually unknown. Birth trauma and hypoxia possible factors
3. Epilepsy, unlocalized, due to known causes	Focal attack pattern unusual. Major or minor	Generalized multiform (including slow spike and wave)	Pneumogram normal, or showing diffuse changes, usually atrophic	May be due to: *a.* Diffuse cerebral lesions, e.g., syphilis, lead, parasites, encephalitis, trauma, degenerative diseases, diffuse cerebral vascular disease *b.* Causes acting generally, e.g., fever, hypoglycemia, cerebral anemia, hypoxia
4. Epilepsy, unlocalized, due to unknown causes	Focal attack pattern unusual. Major or minor	Normal or indefinite	Normal or indefinite	Unknown or indefinite. Further investigation may lead to classification under 1, 2, or 3

SOURCE: McNaughton, F. M.: The Classification of the Epilepsies, Epilepsia, Series III, 1:7, 1952.

ing in most instances to a generalized convulsion of grand mal type; less commonly they are of the psychomotor and only rarely of the petit mal type.

Cerebral Tumors. They give rise to seizures in 35 to 60 per cent of cases, and in approximately 10 per cent of all cases of tumor the seizure is the initial symptom. The nearer the tumor is to the excitable motor cortex, the greater is the likelihood of seizures. Tumors of the cerebellum and brain stem are seldom associated with any of the types of seizures described above, but may cause episodes of decerebrate rigidity, i.e., opisthotonos and extension of all four extremities, sometimes called *tonic cerebellar fits.*

Cerebral Trauma. It may cause seizures immediately after the injury, i.e., within hours or days, or after an interval of several months or years. The former are rare; the latter vary in incidence, being more frequent in the more severe grades of head injury. Uncomplicated concussion results in epilepsy in only about 0.5 per cent of cases, which is about the expected frequency in the population at large, while with penetrating injuries, the incidence rises to approximately 20 per cent, some figures having been as high as 40 per cent. The average interval between the head injury and the first seizure is about 9 months, with a range of 6 months to 2 years or longer.

Cerebrovascular Diseases. It has been said that although seizures occur at the time of hemorrhage or infarction in a small percentage of cases, vascular disease is rarely responsible for recurrent convulsions. Recently, however, analysis of our own material showed that cases of vascular disease of the cerebral cortex, particularly of infarction due to embolism, had recurrent convulsions in about the same frequency as traumatic disease of the cerebral cortex. Hypertensive encephalopathy is often attended by convulsions. Venous thrombosis and infarction are a notable cause of focal epilepsy, and the same is true of vascular lesions in infancy and childhood, which may be either arterial or venous in nature. Seizures are also a frequent manifestation of vascular malformations.

Cerebral Infections. All types of cerebral infection may lead to epilepsy. Brain abscess is accompanied by seizures in about 50 per cent of cases, and they may continue after the abscess has been drained or removed surgically. The seizures that accompany dementia paralytica and other inflammatory diseases of the brain are related to cortical lesions. Inclusion-body encephalitis and subacute sclerosing encephalitis give rise to arrhythmic myoclonus which is often combined with progressive dementia. In those diseases which do not involve the cerebral cortex, such as encephalitis lethargica, there is little or no disposition to epilepsy.

Degenerative Diseases. All types of degenerative diseases, if they affect the cerebral cortex, may be associated with recurrent seizures. Lipid-storage diseases and Jakob-Creutzfeldt disease must be added to the list of myoclonic dementias. Tuberous sclerosis almost invariably gives rise to seizures. They occur but are infrequent in Alzheimer's disease and Pick's disease. About 5 per cent of cases of multiple sclerosis have convulsions in some phase of their illness.

Congenital Maldevelopment of the Brain. This is frequently associated with epilepsy. The latter may be part of the syndrome of mental retardation, spastic diplegia, and other disturbances of motor function. The seizures usually develop in the first weeks or months of life. Special types of infantile and childhood seizures are discussed later in Chap. 283.

PHYSIOLOGIC DISTURBANCES

Conditions which disturb the metabolism of the brain may induce recurrent seizures. With hypoxia of whatever cause which damages the cerebral cortex, a series of seizures may begin within a few hours to days and continue intermittently for a variable period of time, usually a few days. The author's surviving cases usually have not been subject to epilepsy. Cerebral edema, resulting from excess ingestion of water or large infusions of glucose and water, may be attended by one or several generalized convulsions followed by headache and mental confusion. Uremia is accompanied by muscular twitching and occasionally one or more terminal convulsions. Low blood calcium due to rickets or hypoparathyroidism often results in both tetany and seizures. Hypoglycemia caused by an overdose of insulin or an insulin-secreting islet cell

tumor often induces seizures, but they invariably follow an initial period of mental confusion, stupor, or coma. The usual history is for the attack to occur several hours after a meal or following a period of fasting. Seizures occur frequently in alcoholic patients and in those who have become addicted to barbiturates, particularly after the withdrawal of these substances.

Drug Intoxications. The classic examples of direct seizure evocation by drugs are camphor, Metrazol, and picrotoxin. Withdrawal from barbiturates and alcohol in addicted individuals also gives rise to generalized convulsions.

APPROACH TO THE CLINICAL PROBLEM OF RECURRENT SEIZURES

A history of recurrent attacks of loss of consciousness or awareness associated with abnormal movements or confusion is usually sufficient to establish a diagnosis of epilepsy. In such patients a very thorough history, a complete physical and neurologic examination, examination of the visual fields, and laboratory study, including x-ray examination of the skull and an electroencephalogram, should be done. The results of these essential procedures will determine to which of the categories in the above classification the case belongs and whether or not it should be labeled idiopathic epilepsy.

The history should be particularly searching in regard to epilepsy in the family history, occurrence of head trauma or infections in the past; and careful description of the seizure itself, including prodromas, aura, manifestations during the seizure, and the postictal period must be obtained. The report of seizures in the family history is a point in favor of the diagnosis of idiopathic epilepsy. Signs of pulmonary or ear infection or of congenital heart disease with a right-to-left shunt should suggest, in a patient with recently acquired seizures, the possibility of a brain abscess. The presence of a heart murmur and fever or of atrial fibrillation favor embolism. Head trauma of a serious nature, followed by seizures at an interval of several weeks to 2 years, indicates that an injury may have given rise to the convulsions. A regularly recurring aura, especially of a focal nature, may indicate the presence of a localized lesion in the brain. Similarly, the description of a focal convulsive movement at the onset of the seizure indicates the high probability of a localized cerebral lesion. A transient monoplegia or hemiplegia (Todd's paralysis) in the postictal period also has considerable significance as to localization of a lesion. In fact its presence may provide the best clue to a focal brain lesion. A history of other neurologic symptoms such as headache, localized paralysis, or mental changes often indicates that special diagnostic studies should be conducted.

A complete physical examination, including a careful survey of nervous function, is mandatory in each case of epilepsy. The findings can act as clues to the legion of conditions associated with epilepsy. The presence of protuberances over the skull may suggest an underlying pathologic condition. Vascular nevi over the body, especially over the face and in the retina, may be associated with vascular abnormalities within the skull. Small tumors, often pedunculated, distributed over the body surface bring to mind the diagnosis of von Recklinghausen's disease, and when associated with seizures may indicate an intracranial glioma or neurofibroma. Sebaceous adenomas of the face in the typical butterfly distribution point to the diagnosis of tuberous sclerosis. The presence of cranial nerve disturbances is also helpful in diagnosis; thus a sixth nerve paralysis is often associated with increased intracranial pressure. Localized weakness, difference in reflexes, or the presence of abnormal reflexes such as a Babinski response are all of potential localizing value. Coupled with the history, such findings in the examination will often yield a localizing as well as an etiologic diagnosis.

The question of what laboratory procedures should be done in cases of epilepsy can be answered only on the basis of the clinical findings. X-rays of the skull should be taken in all cases. Findings of significance in regard to increased intracranial pressure include erosion of the clinoid processes, increase in the cortical markings, and, in infants and children, separation of the sutures. Hyperostoses, erosions of the skull, abnormal vascular markings, and intracranial calcifications are other findings of importance that may appear in skull x-rays. Because of the frequency of cerebral metastases from primary carcinoma of the lung, films of the chest should be made in all patients suspected of having intracranial neoplasm.

Lumbar puncture can be of considerable value in the elucidation of the causes of epilepsy. If the history, neurologic examination, or skull x-rays show any abnormality, especially if it is suggestive of a focal lesion in the brain, then a lumbar puncture is mandatory. Of special importance is the determination of the pressure, cell count, total protein, and serologic tests. An increased pressure points to an expanding intracranial lesion. An abnormal cell count is often indicative of an infectious process. An elevation in total protein (greater than 100 mg per 100 ml) favors the diagnosis of a tumor. If the pressure is normal, but other symptoms or signs point to a recently acquired, localized brain lesion, a pneumoencephalogram may be done. If, in addition to localizing signs, the patient shows signs of increased intracranial pressure, whether by papil-

ledema or high cerebrospinal fluid pressure, then a ventriculogram is preferred to a pneumoencephalogram. The visualization of the cerebral ventricles by these procedures may be of particular help to the neurosurgeon in localizing the lesion and in planning a surgical approach to it.

The electroencephalogram, although now routinely employed in the definitive diagnosis of cases with epilepsy, is not absolutely conclusive, since it may be normal in some patients, particularly if the seizures are relatively infrequent, or is abnormal in diseases which do not cause epilepsy. The test is of particular value in diagnosis of petit mal, for here clinical or subclinical attacks are apt to be frequent enough to register during the electroencephalographic test. Abnormal electric waves may manifest themselves in other types of epilepsy as well, and the electroencephalogram may be abnormal during the interseizure period, demonstrating either focal or generalized abnormalities of cortical activity. Activation of the electroencephalogram by photic stimulation, drug-induced sleep, or Metrazol injection is now standard procedure in many laboratories.

Other laboratory tests that should be used routinely include examination of the urine and fasting blood sugar. The determination of the blood calcium and a glucose-tolerance test are indicated in some cases.

The type of clinical study in any given case is dictated to some extent by the age of the patient. Up until early adulthood the plan should be outlined as above. Most cases in this age group turn out to have idiopathic epilepsy. As one approaches the older age groups, the incidence of idiopathic epilepsy becomes less and the occurrence of symptomatic epilepsy increases. Thus the appearance of convulsions for the first time at a period past middle age should be presumptive evidence of a diagnosis of brain tumor until every effort has been made to rule it out. However, in the last analysis

Table 36-3. CAUSES OF RECURRENT CONVULSIONS IN DIFFERENT AGE GROUPS

Age of onset, years	Probable cause
Infancy, 0–2	Congenital maldevelopment, birth injury; metabolic (hypocalcemia), B$_6$ deficiency
Childhood, 2–10	Birth injury, trauma, infections, thrombosis of cerebral arteries or veins, idiopathic
Adolescence, 10–18	Idiopathic, trauma, congenital defects
Early adulthood, 18–35	Trauma, neoplasm, idiopathic, alcoholism, drug addiction
Middle age, 35–60	Neoplasm, trauma, vascular disease, alcoholism, drug addiction
Late life, over 60	Vascular, degenerative, tumor

each case must be dealt with on an individual basis, subsequent procedures depending on the previous findings.

The most frequent causes of recurrent convulsions in different age groups are presented in Table 36-3.

DIFFERENTIAL DIAGNOSIS

The clinical differences between a seizure and syncopal attack were presented in Chap. 33 and need not be repeated here. It must be emphasized once again that there is no single criterion for distinguishing between them. The author has erred in calling akinetic seizures a simple faint and in mistaking cardiac or carotid sinus faints for seizures. Petit mal may be difficult to identify because of the brevity of attacks. One helpful maneuver is to have the patient count for 5 to 10 min. If he is having petit mal he will blink or stare, pause in counting, or skip one or two numbers. Psychomotor seizures are the most difficult of all to diagnose. These attacks are so variable in character and so likely to induce minor disturbances in conduct rather than obvious interruptions of consciousness that they may be diagnosed as temper tantrums, hysteria, psychopathic behavior, or an acute psychosis.

A special problem in diagnosis is offered by states of mental dullness and confusion. Epileptic patients as seen in hospital and office practice usually show no mental deterioration, regardless of the type of seizure. Therefore the appearance of dementia, confusion, or some other derangement of mental function should suggest the possibility of recurrent subclinical seizures which have not been controlled by medication, drug intoxication, postseizure psychosis, or a brain disease which has caused both dementia and seizures. To distinguish these clinical states may require careful observation, along the lines suggested in Chap. 37, and electroencephalography.

TREATMENT

The treatment of epilepsy can be divided into three parts: the removal of causative and precipitating factors, the regulation of physical and mental hygiene, and the use of anticonvulsant drugs.

The Removal of Causative and Precipitating Factors. Infections of the central nervous system, such as the meningitides and syphilis, which may give rise to convulsive seizures should be treated by the antibiotics and the sulfonamide drugs. Disturbances of the endocrine system resulting from adenomas of the pancreas or hypoparathyroidism require surgery and appropriate replacement therapy, respectively.

Whenever convulsive seizures are associated with a surgically removable lesion of the brain, such as tumor or abscess, removal of such a lesion is indicated. It must be remembered, however, that the relief of convulsive seizures will occur in only about 50 per cent of cases of meningioma of the brain and in a much smaller percentage of cases of glioma or abscess of the brain. In such cases, further treatment with drugs is necessary.

Surgery has also been advocated for the removal of cortical scars secondary to cerebral trauma, vascular lesions, and birth injuries, on the assumption that such scars produce an irritation of neighboring cortex, which acts as a trigger mechanism for the seizures. Reduction in the frequency of seizures has been reported as a sequel to these operations by a number of neurosurgeons. This treatment should be limited to the group of patients with focal attacks which do not respond to medical therapy. In addition, the excision of such lesions should be performed only by neurosurgeons who have facilities for the adequate localization of the lesion. Medical treatment must also be used in these patients after operation.

Patients with infantile hemiplegia and convulsive seizures that have not responded to anticonvulsant therapy have been subjected to a radical neurosurgical procedure, the complete removal of the cerebral hemisphere involved. Good results have been reported in some of these cases, but it is still too early to evaluate the long-range effect of such an operation.

The anterior tip of the temporal lobe has been removed in many patients with psychomotor seizures who failed to respond to medical therapy and in whom it was possible to demonstrate a temporal lobe focus by electroencephalography. Favorable results have been reported for this procedure by some neurosurgeons. On the other hand, an almost intractable type of grand mal attack has occurred following this operation in some of the patients.

Physical and Mental Hygiene. The epileptic patient should have a wholesome, regular diet consisting of simple foods with an abundance of vegetables and fresh fruits. Alcoholic beverages of any sort are strictly forbidden. Constipation can be a troublesome symptom and should be avoided by the establishment of regular bowel habits. This can be developed by training and the use of mild laxatives when necessary.

The patient should be encouraged to maintain regular hours of sleep. Physical activity is desirable and a moderate amount of physical exercise should be recommended. With proper safeguards, even the more dangerous sports, such as horseback riding and swimming, may be permitted. The uncontrolled epileptic patient, however, should not be allowed to drive an automobile or operate unguarded machinery.

Simple, superficial psychotherapy will frequently prevent or help overcome the feelings of inferiority and self-consciousness present in many epileptic patients. Both the patient and his family will benefit from such therapy, and a proper family attitude should be established. Oversolicitude and overprotection should be discouraged. It is important to emphasize that the patient be allowed to live as normal a life as possible.

Every effort should be made to keep children in school and adults should be encouraged to work. Many communities have vocational rehabilitation centers, and advantage should be taken of such facilities. Patients should be encouraged to participate in available recreational activities, such as movies, dancing, and parties.

The Use of Anticonvulsant Drugs. Success in the management of patients with epilepsy depends upon the ability of the physician to prevent the occurrence of seizures. Approximately 75 per cent of patients with convulsive seizures can have their attacks controlled or reduced in frequency by the use of anticonvulsant drugs. Although these drugs are not a cure for epilepsy, their use is the most important step in the treatment of patients with convulsive disorders.

For a long time the bromides and phenobarbital were the only two drugs available for the medical treatment of epilepsy. Recently, however, many new compounds have appeared. The search for a more effective anticonvulsant is constantly going on, and new compounds are being given therapeutic trials in many clinics.

The drugs commonly used at present in the treatment of patients with convulsive seizures are the barbiturates, hydantoins, oxazolidinediones, and, to a lesser extent, the acetylureas and bromides. The available products which have been given a thorough clinical trial and their daily dosages are given below:

1. Barbiturates:
   a. Phenobarbital (0.1 to 0.3 Gm)
   b. Mebaral (0.2 to 0.6 Gm)
2. Hydantoins:
   a. Dilantin (0.2 to 0.6 Gm)
   b. Mesantoin (0.2 to 0.8 Gm)
3. Oxazolidinediones:
   a. Tridione (0.6 to 3.0 Gm)
   b. Paradione (0.6 to 3.0 Gm)
4. Bromides (1.0 to 3.0 Gm)
5. Mysoline (1.0 to 3.0 Gm)
6. Milontin (1.0 to 3.0 Gm)

General Principles. Certain drugs are more effective in one type of seizure than in another, and it is necessary to use the proper drugs in the optimum dosages for the different types of seizures. If satisfactory results are not obtained with one of the drugs, the others should be tried, but frequent shifting of drugs is not advisable, and each should be given an adequate trial before another is substituted. In some patients a combination of two or more drugs will produce better results than one alone.

The author has obtained the best therapeutic results by having the patients chart daily their medication and the number, time, and circumstances of their seizures. Ideally such a base line should be established before medication is begun, but often this is impractical. Changes in medication should be made only when a given program is shown to be inadequate. As shown by Buchthal and his associates, frequent measurements of blood levels of diphenylhydantoin and barbiturate are useful. For Dilantin, the therapeutic level is about 15 μg per ml. Clinical and electroencephalographic improvement were not noted below 10 μg per ml, and one-half of patients have side effects at 30 μg per ml. The therapeutic level for phenobarbital is probably about 15 to 20 μg per ml, though the range has not yet been exactly determined. Side effects appear in patients on long-term treatment at 25 μg per ml.

When changing medication, the dosage of the new drug should be gradually increased to an optimum level, and then the dosage of the old drug should be decreased gradually. The sudden withdrawal of a drug may lead to status epilepticus, even though a new drug is substituted. Once an anticonvulsant or a combination of anticonvulsants is found to be effective, its use should be maintained for a period of years.

The therapeutic dose for any patient must be determined by trial and error. Not uncommonly a drug is discarded as being ineffective, whereas in reality a slightly increased dosage would have led to a complete disappearance of all the attacks. It is, however, inadvisable to administer a drug to the point where the patient is so dull and stupid that he is more incapacitated by the toxic effects of the drug than by the seizures. It is highly doubtful whether the prolonged administration of anticonvulsant medication is a factor in the development of the mental deterioration that occurs in a small percentage of the patients with convulsive seizures. The evidence at present indicates that with rare exceptions the mentality of the patient is unchanged by medical treatment, unless the drugs are given to the point of intoxication. It is not uncommon to note an improvement in the mental faculties of some patients following control of the seizures by the use of anticonvulsant drugs. The recent claim of pulmonary fibrosis after prolonged Dilantin therapy seems to be unfounded.

Indications for Use of Specific Drugs. GRAND MAL SEIZURES. For those patients with infrequent grand mal seizures (from one to four per year) phenobarbital can be tried first because of its high therapeutic index and its relatively low toxicity. When the seizures are more frequent, diphenylhydantoin sodium (Dilantin Sodium) is the drug of choice. A combination of diphenylhydantoin sodium (0.3 to 0.4 Gm) and phenobarbital (0.1 to 0.2 Gm) is often more effective than either of the drugs used alone. When these drugs are used in combination, a full therapeutic dose of each drug must be given. Occasionally, methylphenylethyl hydantoin (Mesantoin), a combination of this drug with the diphenylhydantoin sodium, or primidone (Mysoline) will give the best results. Rarely, the bromides or a combination of bromides and phenobarbital or diphenylhydantoin sodium will be most effective.

The toxic effects of phenobarbital are drowsiness and mental dullness, nystagmus, staggering, and skin eruptions. Only the latter is a contraindication to its further use; otherwise these symptoms can be controlled by reducing the dose. Dilantin causes ataxia of gait, nystagmus, hypertrophy of gums and, in large doses, stupor or coma. Skin rashes may also occur which require discontinuation of the medication. Reduction of dose controls the other symptoms. Rare complications of therapy are hirsutism and psychotic behavior.

PSYCHOMOTOR ATTACKS. Drugs effective in the treatment of grand mal seizures are effective in the treatment of patients with psychomotor attacks. Larger doses are required, and the results on the whole are not so good as in patients with grand mal seizures.

PETIT MAL ATTACKS. As a rule drugs effective in the treatment of grand mal and psychomotor seizures are not effective in the treatment of patients with petit mal attacks. Trimethadione (Tridione), paramethadione (Paradione), and phensuximide (Milontin) are the drugs of choice in patients with frequent petit mal attacks.

The dose of trimethadione and paramethadione is 0.9 to 1.5 Gm per day in children over 6 years of age. The beginning dose is 0.3 Gm thrice daily; for infants 0.3 Gm per day, and small children 0.6 Gm per day may be given. Toxic symptoms are skin eruptions and photophobia. Aplastic anemia has been reported, hence monthly blood counts during the first year are indicated. The dose of methyl phenylsuccinamide is 0.6 to 1.8 Gm per day for children and 0.9 to 3 Gm per day for adults. Although less effective than the diones, it is also less toxic. Methyl-methylphenylsuccinamide (Celontin), adult dose 0.3 Gm three or four times a day, and acetazolamide (Diamox), adult dose 0.25 to 0.75 Gm per day, have been useful in controlling difficult cases of petit mal and massive myoclonus in children.

MINOR SEIZURES AND FOCAL ATTACKS. The same drugs effective in the treatment of grand mal and psychomotor seizures are effective against minor seizures and focal attacks. Minor seizures, which appear in patients whose grand mal attacks have been controlled, can occasionally be checked by simply increasing the dose of the drug or drugs that the patient is already taking. If the minor attacks are very infrequent and nonincapacitating, no great effort need be made to treat them.

PETIT MAL PLUS OTHER TYPES. When patients are subject to petit mal seizures as well as grand mal or psychomotor seizures, they should receive Tridione or Paradione plus diphenylhydantoin sodium, phenobarbital, or Mesantoin. The treatment of the special types of convulsions in infancy and childhood is discussed in Chap. 283.

Myoclonic Epilepsy. Mysoline (1.0 to 3.0 Gm) and phenobarbital (0.1 to 0.2 Gm) have been the most effective agents in this type of seizure. The treatment of massive myoclonus in infants is discussed in Chap. 283.

STATUS EPILEPTICUS. Recurrent convulsions at a frequency which does not allow consciousness to be regained in the interval between seizures (status epilepticus) probably constitute the most serious therapeutic problem. Most patients who die of epilepsy do so because of uncontrolled recurrent seizures or an injury sustained as a result of seizure. Rising temperature, circulatory collapse, and lower nephron nephrosis is a sequence of events which the author has encountered in a number of fatal cases.

It must be conceded that at present no known drug will safely control all recurrent convulsions. This is not surprising, for there are many causes of convulsions and not all cases are alike. Clinical experience teaches that in some patients the convulsive tendency is so overwhelming that no amount of anticonvulsant medication, even deep ether anesthesia, will prevent recurrence of seizures. In others the liability to recurrent convulsions lasts only a few hours or at most a few days, regardless of whether anticonvulsant medication is given. The real hazard in treating resistant recurrent convulsions is that consciousness and vital functions may be suppressed to a degree incompatible with life. The risk of deep coma without convulsions is greater than semicoma or stupor with an occasional convulsion.

The following medications have been recommended for recurrent convulsions with brain disease and for status epilepticus.

1. Sodium phenobarbital in doses of 0.2 to 0.3 Gm intramuscularly, repeated every 1 to 2 hr up to a maximum of 0.8 to 1.0 Gm per 24 hr.

2. Diphenylhydantoin sodium (Dilantin) in doses of 0.4 to 0.5 Gm per day orally (through stomach tube) or intravenously. This is usually given morning, noon, late afternoon, and evening.

3. Trimethadione (Tridione) in doses of 1.0 to 2.0 Gm intravenously.

4. Paraldehyde intravenously in doses of 1.0 to 8.0 ml. It may also be given by rectum, 1 part paraldehyde to 2 parts vegetable oil in doses of 5.0 ml paraldehyde per 15 lb body weight. Some physicians inject it intramuscularly in doses of 10.0 to 15.0 ml, but there is danger of sensory and motor paralysis if the drug is injected in the vicinity of a peripheral nerve.

5. Thiopental (Sodium Pentothal) in doses of 0.3 to 0.6 Gm intravenously or intramuscularly.

6. Tribromoethanol (Avertin) by rectum in doses of 25 mg per kg body weight and followed by 10 to 15 mg per kg body weight at 15- to 30-min intervals as indicated by the response of the patient.

7. Ether by inhalation.

These many treatments attest to the fact that no one of them is altogether satisfactory. The author has had greatest success with the following program. When an adult patient is first seen, an intramuscular injection of 0.3 Gm sodium phenobarbital is given. Diphenylhydantoin sodium, 0.1 to 0.2 Gm, is then administered intravenously or through a stomach tube and additional amounts later to a total of 0.5 Gm per day. If seizures continue for the next hour, 0.2 Gm sodium phenobarbital is again injected. If the seizures cease for an hour or two and then recur, this amount of barbiturate may be given in repeated doses up to a total amount of 1.0 Gm per 24 hr. If the seizures are not controlled by the diphenylhydantoin and the first two injections of sodium phenobarbital, 1.0 Gm Tridione may be injected intravenously. If seizures continue, all medication except diphenylhydantoin sodium should be discontinued, and either a light ether anesthesia or a light Pentothal anesthesia, up to 0.5 Gm intravenously, should be tried. Should the seizures continue despite all these medications, one is justified in the assumption that the convulsive tendency is so strong that it cannot be checked by reasonable quantities of anticonvulsants. One then depends entirely on diphenylhydantoin sodium 0.5 Gm and sodium phenobarbital 0.4 Gm per day. For infants and children, correspondingly smaller doses should be administered.

Hyperthermia, which occurs in most cases of severe status epilepticus, must be controlled by the measures outlined in Chap. 104.

REFERENCES

Lennox, W. G., and S. Cobb: The Relation of Certain Physicochemical Processes to Epileptiform Seizures, Am. J. Psychiat., 8:839, 1929.

McNaughton, F. M.: The Classification of the Epilepsies, Epilepsia, Series III, 1:7, 1952.

Penfield, W., and T. C. Erickson: "Epilepsy and Cerebral Localization," Springfield, Ill., Charles C Thomas, Publisher, 1941.

—— and K. Kristiansen: "Epileptic Seizure Patterns," Springfield, Ill., Charles C Thomas, Publisher, 1951.

Symonds, C.: Excitation and Inhibition in Epilepsy, Brain, 82:133, 1959.

Tower, D. B.: Mechanisms of Seizures Investigated by Experimental Production and Control of a Biochemical Lesion Present in the Epileptogenic Cortex, Epilepsia, Series III, 1:9, 1952.

37 THE CLINICAL SIGNS OF FOCAL CEREBRAL DISEASE AND THE SYNDROME OF DEMENTIA

Raymond D. Adams

Every physician sooner or later discovers through clinical experience the necessity of acquiring a special competence in assessing the mental faculties of his patients. He must become capable of observing with detachment and complete objectivity their character, intelligence, mood, memory, judgment, and other attributes of personality in much the same fashion as he observes the nutritional state and the color of the mucous membranes. The systematic examination of these affective and cognitive functions permits him to reach certain conclusions regarding the mental status, and this is of value in understanding the patient and his illness. Without accurate knowledge of the mental status, errors will be committed in evaluating the reliability of the patient's history, in diagnosing the neurologic or psychiatric disease from which he suffers, and in conducting any proposed therapeutic program.

Perhaps the purpose of this and the next two chapters will be more clearly understood if a few introductory remarks are made. In Chap. 34, Coma and Related Disturbances of Consciousness, there was brief reference to states of confusion and stupor, which are of course abnormalities of human behavior. However, the main emphasis was on coma, or abolition of consciousness, as a clinical state, and confusion was mentioned only as a lesser degree of the same condition. This chapter and the two following are concerned more particularly with other disturbances of behavior that result from brain diseases. These disturbances are discussed under three headings, *dementia, the acute confusional states,* and *schizophrenia.*

Definition of Terms. Again a preliminary definition of terms is inescapable. Defining terms which refer to normal and abnormal states of mind is always troublesome because they have been given so many meanings in literature and in textbooks of psychology and medicine. English in his useful little "Dictionary of Psychological Terms" reminds us that Alice was puzzled by this problem of the meaning of words in her journeys through Wonderland but learned its solution.

"The question is," said Alice, "whether you *can* make words mean so many different things."
"The question is," said Humpty Dumpty, "which is to be master—that's all."

If we are ever to be the masters of these complex psychologic disorders and the derangements of the higher integrations of nervous function on which they depend, we must strive for a precise and uniform terminology. The following nomenclature, though tentative, is useful and will be employed throughout this textbook.

The term *dementia* means loss of one's reason, or more particularly a deterioration of intellect. Implied in this word is the idea of a general enfeeblement of mental powers in a person who formerly possessed a normal mind. *Amentia*, by contrast, indicates a congenital feeblemindedness. *Confusion* is a more general term denoting a state in which the patient cannot think with customary speed and efficiency. This may depend on any one of several factors. In the discussion of coma it was pointed out that drowsiness and reduced awareness may interfere with clarity of thinking. Inability to assimilate and retain new impressions seems to be responsible for the disturbed mentation in certain of the organic psychoses, and in delirium there is a fluctuation of attention and the intrusion of hallucinatory experiences. The phrase *organic reaction type* comprehends both dementia and acute confusional psychosis. *Delirium*, from the Latin word *delirare* (to rave) has a rather uncertain nosologic position. Some writers use this term to designate all types of confusion of thinking or disturbance of behavior. The author, however, prefers to let it represent a special disorder, nearly always transitory and characterized by psychomotor and autonomic overactivity, sleeplessness, and aberrations of sense perception in the form of illusions and hallucinations. Mental confusion is unquestionably present, but delirium is distinguished from the simple confusional psychoses by the presence of hallucinations and frenzied excitement and overactivity.

OBSERVABLE ASPECTS OF BEHAVIOR

The components of behavior which may be subjected to scrutiny at the bedside in the diagnosis of mental disease are temperament and mood, the capacity for coherent thinking and the quality of ideational and associative processes, the accuracy of perception and distortions of the perceptual process, impulse and drive, and insight.

The emotional life of the patient, so important to all who deal with the sick, may be manifested in a variety of ways. There are in the first place rather marked individual differences in basic temperament, some persons being throughout their life cheerful, gregarious, optimistic, and free from worry, and others being just the opposite. It is believed that there is an association between temperament and particular psychiatric diseases. For example, the volatile, cyclothymic individual appears to be liable to manic depressive psychosis, and the suspicious, introverted person to schizophrenia and paranoia. Certain overwhelming emotions such as love, fear, anger, and worry may cause physiologic changes, and the student soon learns that they may be the basis of or add to certain clinical syndromes. The degree of responsiveness to emotional stimuli, another variable quality of personality, may undergo alteration in disease; it may be excessive, labile, and uninhibited, as in the syndrome of pathologic laughter and crying that often accompanies *pseudobulbar palsy*, or it may be reduced and overinhibited or lacking altogether, as in apathetic states or depressions. Again, the emotional response may be inappropriate to the stimulus, as in schizophrenia.

Since there are relatively few overt manifestations of temperament, mood, and emotional experience, the physician must learn of these conditions largely through conversation, in which the individual is encouraged to verbalize his feelings. This requires that the physician establish rapport with the patient and attempt at the same time an objective appraisal of the affective responses.

For purposes of examination, the emotional experiences are arbitrarily divided into mood, feeling, and affect. By *mood* is meant the prevailing emotional state of the individual, unconditioned by the stimuli immediately impinging upon him. For example, a person awakens and finds himself in a pleasant state of emotion. The world about him appears serene; he feels optimistic and cheerful as he meditates on the tasks which lie ahead. Conversely, he may be dejected, melancholy, and pessimistic, dreading the prospects of the day's activities. Mood is thus a state of emotion not evidently related to the immediate environmental situation. In observing the emotional state of the patient much reliance is placed on his language, i.e., the adjectives he uses, e.g., happy, elated, exhilarated, and ecstatic or depressed, morbid, unhappy, melancholy; and usually the attitude and facial expression are also of value.

By contrast, feeling and affect are emotional experiences evoked by environmental stimuli. *Feel-*

ing is the subjective component; *affect* the overt manifestation. Feeling and affect may modify mood. Illustratively, a person awakening in the morning in a happy frame of mind, upon hearing a disparaging remark is provoked to anger, or upon being told of a threatening danger, may be overcome by fear or anxiety. The patient will tell of his feeling of anxiety, and the affect will be manifested by the facial expression, pallor, trembling, sweating, and rapid pulse.

The difference between mood as a prevailing emotional state and feeling and affect as emotional reactions to stimuli may seem rather tenuous, but nevertheless these distinctions are of practical value. Mood is probably the resultant of both the basic temperament of the individual and reactions to a series of emotional stimuli, many of which pass unnoticed. Feeling and affect, which if deranged may represent the patient's main complaint, may be understood only through a knowledge of environmental circumstances and the basic mood.

Another important part of mentation is the *content of thought* and the *quality of the ideational and associative processes*. For purposes of examination one may consider thinking from the point of view of ideational content, the coherence and logical relationship of ideas, the quality and quantity of associations to any given idea, and the propriety of feeling and affect engendered by an idea or content of thought at any one moment.

Information concerning the thought processes and associative functions is best obtained by analyzing the patient's spontaneous verbal productions. If he is taciturn or mute, one must then depend on his responses to direct questions, or upon written material, i.e., letters, etc. One must note whether the patient's ideas are unreasonable, vague, circumstantial, tangential, and irrelevant or whether they are to the point, direct, and concise. Is the patient excessively critical, rationalizing, obsessive, or hairsplitting? Are his thought processes shallow and completely fragmented? Do certain ideas dominate the mind to the exclusion of all others? Are judgments reached and held tenaciously even though illogical?

It may be found that the patient flits nimbly from one idea to another and that his associations are numerous and haphazard, a veritable *flight of ideas*, so common in mania; or there may be a *poverty of ideas* and associations, as in depression. The patient's own subjective analysis of his thought processes is of importance. He may state that his mind is inadequate, a remark which always suggests a depressive mood, or that it is impossible to escape from certain thoughts which recur with all the force of an obsession or a delusion. Thinking may be distorted and the patient may fail to check his ideas against reality. When a false belief

persists in spite of normally convincing contradictory evidence the patient is said to have a *delusion*. Ideas may seem to be implanted in the mind by some outside agency such as radio, telepathy, or atomic energy. These are referred to as *passivity feelings*.

Perception, i.e., the process of acquiring through the senses a knowledge of the "world about" or of one's own body, may also be deranged in certain ways. The capacity to focus attention or to concentrate for prolonged periods on one stimulus may be impaired. Disturbances of this type, designated by the words *inattentiveness, fluctuations of attention,* and *distractibility,* are important signs of neurologic disease. In delirium and confusional psychoses certain stimulus objects may be incorrectly perceived, with the patient fully conscious of the aberration, as in *illusory experiences;* or objects, people, and situations may be misinterpreted without the patient knowing of his mistake, i.e., *sensory misinterpretations*. Nonexistent objects or people may be perceived as though real in *hallucinatory experiences*, with or without full insight on the part of the patient. And finally, there may be an inability to perceive simultaneously all the elements of a given situation, a *failure of subjective reorganization*.

Insight, by which is meant an accurate appraisal of functional deficits and more particularly the awareness of symptoms and their degree of severity, is another common index of neurologic and psychiatric status. Full insight presupposes an alert, attentive mind as well as adequate functioning of language mechanisms by which such observations may be reported. Often the patient is totally unaware of being ill or ignores or denies the existence of obvious sensory, motor, or psychic deficits. The degree of lack of insight may be estimated by comparing the patient's statement of his disability with the objective findings on examination.

Lastly, observations concerning physique, impulse, intelligence, and ego are of relevance in evaluating patients with psychiatric diseases. Certain of these qualities are sources of maladjustment in everyday life and are also believed to dispose the patient to particular forms of mental illness. Much has been made of body habitus. The short, stocky *pyknic body type* is likely to be associated with *cyclothymic temperament;* the slender, nonathletic, *leptosomal body type* tends to be accompanied by a withdrawn, *schizoid personality. Impulse,* that basic biologic urge, driving force, or energy potential, varies in strength from person to person. Probably the most conspicuous deviation here is weakness of impulse in certain neurotic individuals or complete lack of it in cases of bilateral frontal lobe disease (*akinetic mutism*). The capacity to learn and to reason abstractly, the essential features of intelligence, are other variable qualities of personality. Here there is an observed range from idiocy through imbecility, to normalcy and genius, and each level of intelligence tends to be related to particular types of psychologic problems and a liability to certain psychiatric illnesses. Finally, there is the vague category of personality known as *ego*. This term refers to the strength and direction of self-regard. Again there are evident variations in what has been called "ego strength" in different personalities, ranging from domineering egocentricity to meekness, timidity, and depreciation.

In this and the following two chapters it will be seen that these various components of personality and behavior are subject to particular types of derangement and that the diagnosis of these states requires a systematic and objective appraisal of these qualities of mental function.

FUNCTIONS OF DIFFERENT PARTS OF THE CEREBRUM

Symptoms and signs of disease of one part of the cerebrum may occur singly or in combination with dementia and these provide important information as to the locality of a disease process and at times to its nature. This is an appropriate place, therefore, to review briefly the known effects of disease of different parts of the cerebrum. Agnosia, apraxia, and aphasia will be only mentioned, since they are treated more extensively in Chaps. 26 and 40.

Frontal Lobes. The frontal lobes have long been recognized as having an important role in intellectual processes. The first direct evidence of this was obtained in Harlow's famous crowbar case, reported in 1868. The patient, Phineas Gage, survived an injury in which a crowbar penetrated the left frontal lobe. He was changed as a result of the accident from a competent, pious foreman of a crew of laborers and head of a household to an irresponsible, irreverent man, incapable of intelligent, planned activity. Numerous studies of other patients have since been made. In recent years the widespread use of lobotomy (sectioning the central white matter of both frontal lobes), lobectomy (excision of both frontal lobes), and gyrectomy (removal of certain convolutions of frontal lobes) for the treatment of schizophrenia and other psychiatric conditions have provided an almost unique opportunity to study frontal lobe function in man.

In Fig. 37-1, it may be seen that the frontal lobes lie anterior to the central, or Rolandic, sulcus and superior to the Sylvian fissure. They consist of several functionally different parts which are conventionally designated in the neurologic literature by numbers (according to a scheme devised by

Brodmann) and by letters (in the scheme of von Economo and Koskinas).

The posterior parts, areas 4 and 6 of Brodmann, are specifically related to motor function. Voluntary movement in man depends on the integrity of these areas, and lesions in them produce a spastic paralysis of the contralateral face, arm, and leg. This is discussed in Chap. 26, Disturbances of the Motor System—I. Motor Paralysis. In areas 8 and 24 of Brodmann are localized the mechanism concerned with turning the head and eyes contralaterally. Areas 44 and 45 subserve vocalization, deglutition, and chewing. Lesions in area 44 of the dominant cerebral hemisphere, usually the left one, have often resulted in loss of verbal expression, the aphasia of Broca. In the medial limbic, or piriform, cortex (areas 23 and 24) are localized the mechanisms controlling respiration, circulation, and micturition.

The remainder of the frontal lobes (areas 9, 10, 11, 12, and 13 of Brodmann), sometimes called the prefrontal areas, have less specific and measurable functions. The following groups of symptoms have been observed in patients with diseases limited to one or both frontal lobes or to the central white matter and anterior part of the corpus callosum by which they are joined.

1. Change of personality, usually expressed as lack of concern over the consequences of any action, which may take the form of a childish excitement (*moria* of Jastrowitz), an inappropriate joking and punning (*Witzelsucht* of Oppenheim), or an instability and superficiality of emotion, or irritability.

2. Slight impairment of intelligence usually referred to as lack of concentration, vacillation of attention, inability to carry out planned activity, difficulty in changing from one activity to another, loss of recent memory, lack of initiative and spontaneity.

3. Motor abnormalities such as decomposition of gait and upright stance, trunk ataxia of Brun, abnormal postures, reflex grasping or sucking, and incontinence of sphincters.

In many of the reported cases the exact localization of the disease was not known, and it probably encroached upon the posterior parts of the frontal lobes concerned with motor and speech function.

The most pronounced changes have been observed in cases with bilateral disease of frontal lobes, and there has been much doubt as to the effect of a lesion involving only one frontal lobe. Nevertheless, the most careful psychologic tests on patients with lesions of either frontal lobe demonstrate a slight elevation of mood with increased talkativeness and tendency to joke, a lack of tact, inability to adapt to a new situation, and loss of initiative.

Several careful studies of lobotomized patients

have now been published. Of course very few of these patients were normal before the operation, so that the base-line measurements of mental ability are not obtainable. However, some patients of normal intellect have received this treatment for a severe neurosis or intractable pain. They are said to have shown little or no loss of ability in their performance on intelligence tests, depending on the extent of the procedure; and if worry, fears, compulsions, and suffering from pain were incapacitating, the loss of these traits resulted in test scores actually higher than before the operation. However, careful examination usually will disclose a slight lowering of general intelligence, a decrease in drive or energy, a definite change of personality in the form of shallow emotional life, a lack of tact, and inability to direct and sustain activity towards future goals. Also traits related to neuroticism such as suggestibility, rigidity of character, self-criticism, and introversion decrease.

The function of the frontal lobes cannot be determined simply by the study of human beings who have suffered injury or disease of this part of the brain. Symptoms from lesions of a part of the nervous system are not identical with the functions of that part. The symptoms of frontal lobe deficit must depend both on a loss of certain parts of the cerebrum and on the functional activity of the remaining portions of the nervous system. There is no doubt that the human mind is changed by disease of the frontal lobes, but it is difficult to say in what way it is changed. Intelligence, emotional feeling and expression, memory, visual fixation, postural control, regulation of respiration and blood pressure—all are intact in animals and human beings without frontal lobes. Perhaps at present it is best to regard the frontal lobes as that part of the brain which orientates the individual, with all his percepts and concepts formed from past life experiences, towards action that is projected into the future.

Temporal Lobes. The boundaries of the temporal lobes may be seen in Fig. 37-1. The Sylvian fissure separates the superior surface of each temporal lobe from the frontal and anterior parts of the parietal lobes. There is no definite anatomic boundary between the temporal and occipital lobes either inferiorly or laterally or between temporal and parietal lobes. The temporal lobe includes the superior, middle, and inferior temporal, fusiform, and hippocampal convolutions, and the transverse convolutions of Heschl, which is the auditory receptive area present on the superior surface within the Sylvian fissure. The hippocampal convolution was once believed to be related indirectly to the olfactory bulb, but now it is known that lesions here do not cause anosmia. The fibers from the homolateral lower quadrant of each retina course

through the central white matter en route to the occipital lobes, and lesions which interrupt them characteristically produce a contralateral homonymous upper quadrant defect of visual fields. Hearing and labyrinthine function, also localized in the temporal lobes, are bilaterally represented, which accounts for the fact that unless both temporal lobes are affected, there is no demonstrable loss of hearing. Loss of equilibrium has not been observed with temporal lobe lesions. Extensive disease in the superior and middle convolutions of the left temporal lobe, in right-handed individuals, results in Wernicke's aphasia. This syndrome, discussed in Chap. 40, Affections of Speech, consists of jargon aphasia, inability to read, to write, or to understand the meaning of spoken words. Probably the basic defect in all these is the loss of memory for words.

Between the auditory and olfactory projection areas there is a large expanse of temporal lobe which has no assignable function. This is the temporal association area. Patients with tumors and vascular lesions of this part of the brain have been examined on numerous occasions, but usually

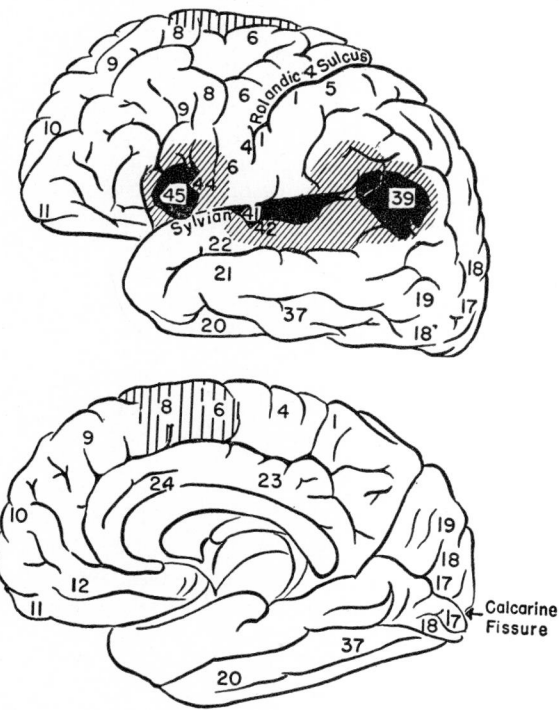

Fig. 37-1. Diagram to show cortical areas, numbered according to the scheme of Brodmann. The speech areas are in black, the three main ones being 39, 41, and 45. The zone marked by vertical stripes in the superior frontal convolution is the secondary motor area which like the Broca's area 45 if stimulated causes vocal arrest. (*Redrawn from "Handbuch der Inneren Medizin," Berlin, Springer-Verlag, 1939.*)

the full extent of the disease has not been determined. Cases of temporal lobectomy for tumor have provided more valuable material, but again it has seldom been possible to be certain that other parts of the brain were not involved. The most careful psychologic studies have shown a difference between cases with loss of the dominant and the nondominant temporal lobe. With lesions of the dominant side there is impairment in learning verbal material presented auditorially and in nondominant lesions a similar failure in tests with visually presented material (e.g., poor score in a visual anomalies test). In addition about 20 per cent of such cases have shown a syndrome similar to that described for the prefrontal parts of the brain; but more significant is the fact that the other cases have exhibited little or no defect in personality. The study of cases of uncinate epilepsy, with the characteristic dreamy state, olfactory or gustatory hallucinations, and masticatory movements, suggests that all these functions are organized through the temporal lobes. Similarly, stimulation of the posterior parts of the temporal lobes of epileptic patients during surgical procedures has brought to light the interesting fact that complex memories and visual and auditory images, some with strong emotional content, can be aroused in fully conscious human beings. Recent studies of the effect of stimulation of the amygdaloid nucleus, which is in the anterior and medial part of the temporal lobe, have shed additional light on this subject. There are remarkable autonomic effects. Blood pressure rises, pulse increases, respirations are increased in frequency and depth, and the patient looks frightened. Complex emotional experiences that have occurred previously may be revived. These effects have been discussed in Chap. 36, Recurrent Convulsions. Ablation of the hippocampal convolutions bilaterally has been carried out recently, with a disastrous loss of ability to learn new experiences or to establish new memories (Korsakoff's psychosis). All this would suggest the important role of the temporal lobes in auditory and visual perception and imagery, in learning and memory, and in the emotional life of the individual.

Bilateral ablations of temporal lobes, so far studied only in monkeys, have resulted in an animal that displays a curious tendency to react to every visual stimulus without seeming to recognize it (psychic blindness) and to examine every object in its environment by oral and manual contact. Placidity, with lack of the usual emotional response to stimuli, was another prominent feature.

To summarize, in man the temporal lobe syndromes include the following:

I. Effects of unilateral disease of the dominant temporal lobe
  A. Quadrantic homonymous anopia

  B. Wernicke's aphasia
  C. Impairment in verbal tests of material presented through the auditory sense
II. Effects of unilateral disease of nondominant temporal lobe
  A. Quadrantic homonymous anopia
  B. Impairment· of mental function with inability to judge spatial relationships in some cases
  C. Impairment in nonverbal tests of visually presented material

Parietal Lobes. This part of the human nervous system is the subject of one of the most interesting discussions of cerebral function that has occurred in this century—that of its role in the formation of the body image or body schema.

It has long been known that the postcentral convolution is the terminus of somatic sensory pathways from the opposite half of the body. It has also been learned that destructive lesions here did not abolish cutaneous sensation but instead caused mainly a defect in sensory discrimination with variable impairment of sensation. In other words pain, touch, and thermal and vibratory sensation are largely retained, whereas stereognosis, sense of position, distinction between single and double contacts (two-point threshold), and the localization of sensory stimuli are lost. This type of sensory disturbance, sometimes called "cortical sensory defect" is discussed in Chap. 28, Disorders of Sensation. Also it was discovered long ago that lesions deep in the white matter of the parietal lobes produce a contralateral homonymous hemianopia, and lesions in the angular gyrus of the dominant hemisphere produce an inability to read.

More recent investigations have centered about the function of the parietal lobes in the perception of one's position in space and of the relationship of the various parts of the body to one another. Since the time of Babinski it has been known that patients with a large lesion of the minor parietal lobe are often unaware of their hemiplegia and hemianesthesia. Babinski called this condition *anosognosia*. Related psychologic disorders are lack of recognition of the left arm and leg when seen or felt by the other hand, neglect of the left side of the body in dressing, an imperception of external space on the left side, and constructional apraxia, an inability to perform the movements of constructing simple figures. The terms *agnosia* and *apraxia* are discussed in Chaps. 26 and 40.

Another frequent constellation of symptoms, usually referred to as *Gerstmann's syndrome*, occurs with lesions of the dominant parietal lobe. This consists of inability to write (agraphia), inability to calculate (acalculia), failure to distinguish right from left, and loss of recognition of various parts of the body. An ideomotor apraxia may or may not be conjoined.

The effects of disease of the parietal lobes differ then according to whether the dominant (left hemisphere in a right-handed person) or nondominant lobe is involved. These may be tabulated as follows:

I. Effects of unilateral disease of parietal lobe, right or left
   A. Cortical sensory syndrome
   B. Mild hemiparesis, unilateral muscular atrophy in children
   C. Homonymous hemianopia or visual inattention, and sometimes neglect of one-half of external space
   D. Abolition of opticokinetic nystagmus
II. Effects of unilateral disease of dominant parietal lobe—left hemisphere in right-handed patients: Additional phenomena
   A. Disorders of language (especially alexia)
   B. Gerstmann's syndrome
   C. Bimanual astereognosis (tactile agnosia)
   D. Bilateral apraxia of ideomotor type
III. Effects of unilateral disease of minor parietal lobe—right hemisphere in right-handed patients: Additional phenomena
   A. Anosognosia
   B. Neglect of left side of body
   C. Neglect of visual space to the left of the midline

In all these lesions if the disease is sufficiently extensive there may be a reduction in the capacity to think clearly, inattentiveness, and impairment of memory.

It is impossible at present to enunciate a formula of parietal lobe function in general. It does seem reasonably certain that the parietal and occipital lobes both participate in sensory functions, especially in those which provide for consciousness of one's surroundings, of the relationship of objects in the environment to one another, and of the position of the body in space. In this respect, as C. M. Fisher has recently suggested, the parietal lobe may be regarded as a suprasensory mechanism.

Occipital Lobes. The occipital lobes are the terminus of the visual pathways and are essential for visual sensation and perception. Lesions in one occipital lobe result in homonymous defects in the contralateral visual fields. Bilateral lesions cause cortical blindness, a state of blindness without change in optic fundi or pupillary reflexes. If areas 18 and 19 of Brodmann are affected (Fig. 37-1), there is a loss of visual recognition with retention of some degree of visual acuity, a state termed *visual agnosia* or *mind-blindness*. In the classical form of this blindness an individual with intact mental powers is unable to recognize objects even though by tests of visual acuity and perimetry he appears to see sufficiently well to do so. Psychologists have demonstrated several special types of visual agnosia. In the simultagnosia of Wolpert, the patient, though capable of seeing the individual parts of a picture, is unable to gather the meaning of the whole. Similarly in prosopagnosia the patient is unable to recognize a human face even though he sees all the individual details of it. Alexia, or inability to read, and visual spatial agnosia, or inability to recognize actual or abstract space, with resulting disorientation, are other special types of agnosia. Often the patient with bilateral lesions of the occipital lobes (cerebral cortical blindness) is unaware of his visual difficulty, i.e., has an agnosia for it. This state is known as *Anton's syndrome*. In *Holmes syndrome* visual disorientation may be combined with a homonymous hemianopia.

This whole problem of both visual and tactile agnosia has recently been reexamined. In most of the reported cases tests of primary visual sensation or visual acuity have been inadequate. By controlling the time factor in visual perception and the adaptation time, and by testing the simultaneous perception of multiple points in the visual field, it is possible to show that the visual function is more often impaired than was at first suspected. The division of the visual process into sensation and perception becomes highly artificial.

Visual function is discussed further in Chap. 31.

Diagnosis of Focal Cerebral Disease. In summarizing the special effects of disease of different parts of the cerebral hemispheres several points should be made. Extensive lesions in one or both frontal lobes often encroach on motor areas and in doing so cause a weakness of muscle groups on the opposite side of the body. This is especially noticeable in the face and is sometimes more pronounced during emotional expression than on voluntary movement. It may affect the arm and leg as well. In some instances the weakness may be rather slight, and a slowness and stiffness of movement with grasp reflex, slightly increased tendon reflexes, and Babinski sign on the contralateral side are observed. A rather "absent-minded" type of urinary and fecal incontinence is also frequent. Expressive aphasia—an inability to speak—indicates involvement of the inferior frontal convolution of the dominant frontal lobe. Anosmia and blindness are neighborhood symptoms, resulting from an extension of a lesion on the orbital surfaces of the frontal lobes to the olfactory bulbs and optic nerves.

An upper quadrantic homonymous anopia is the most reliable sign of disease of either the right or left temporal lobes; this localization should always be considered if dementia and this visual disturbance are conjoined. Uncinate or psychic seizures also establish a temporal lobe lesion but do not indicate the laterality. Bizarre disturbances of thinking and affect, often indistinguishable from schizophrenia, may follow temporal lobe seizures. In lesions of the dominant temporal lobe, Wernicke's aphasia is the most characteristic feature.

Cortical sensory deficit is the common neurologic abnormality in disease of either parietal lobe and is often combined with hemiplegia. With left-sided lesions in the inferior parietal lobule there is alexia and a contralateral homonymous hemianopia. Gerstmann's syndrome localizes a lesion in the more posterior parts of the parietal and the lateral occipital lobes of the dominant hemisphere. The curious disturbances of body awareness or body scheme and of the visuotactile appreciation of space on the left of the midline are usually found with lesions of the nondominant parietal lobe. Focal seizures arising in the parietal lobe usually consist of a focal or Jacksonian sensory disturbance.

Occipital lesions are distinguished by the almost exclusive affection of visual functions, a circumstance which rarely occurs in pure form with temporal or parietal lesions. The affection may take the form of a homonymous hemianopia or of one of the more complex disorders of visual recognition.

Obviously deterioration of intellect cannot at present be assigned to lesions in any one territory of the brain, and certainly not to any conventional division of the cerebrum. Stated in another way, the effects of disease of any of the known anatomic structures are not equivalent to dementia. Nevertheless a disorder of personality and in thinking and memory does occur with a large lesion of any part of the cerebrum, particularly the frontal and temporal association areas.

Probably the most satisfactory formula that can be offered is the one which postulates all cerebral function in terms of sensorimotor mechanisms. Sensation is the beginning and movement the end of this function. But action at a cortical level is not necessarily the immediate consequence of sensory stimulation; instead there may be a long delay. This temporal factor is one of the most striking perquisites of the human brain—that present action can be modified in the light of past experience and that present sensory data, endowed with appropriate emotional tone, can influence action that will not be consummated until some future time.

Widespread destruction of the cerebral cortex in many lobes of both hemispheres deprives the patient of all the aforementioned functions and in addition removes all capacity for rational behavior (dementia) and reduces general awareness or consciousness. Such states may occur in anoxic encephalopathy or Jakob-Crentzfeldt's disease. Lesser degrees of *decortication* are more common and their clinical manifestations are discussed in the next section.

CLINICAL SYNDROME OF DEMENTIA

In current neurologic parlance the term *dementia* usually denotes a clinical state comprising a failing memory and loss of intellectual functions due to a chronic progressive degenerative disease of the brain. It may or may not be associated with signs of disease in one or more of the so-called projection areas of the cerebrum. The chronicity of the process is ordinarily emphasized, but the illogicality of setting apart any one constellation of cerebral symptoms on the basis of their speed of onset or duration is obvious.

The earliest signs of dementia may be so subtle as to escape the notice of even the most discerning physician. Often an observant relative of the patient or an employer is the first to become aware of a certain lack of initiative, of irritability, of loss of interest, and of inability to perform up to the usual standard. Later there is distractibility of attention, inability to think with accustomed clarity, a reduction in general comprehension, perserveration in speech, action, and thought, and defective memory, especially for recent events. Frequently a change in mood becomes apparent, deviating more often toward depression than elation. The direction of this deviation is said to depend on the previous personality of the patient rather than upon the character of the disease. Excessive lability of mood may also be observed, i.e., an easy fluctuation from laughter to tears on slight provocation. Moral and ethical standards are lost, early in some cases and late in others. Paranoid ideas and delusions may develop. As a rule the patient has little or no realization of these changes in himself; i.e., he lacks insight. As the condition progresses there is loss of almost all intellectual faculties, with mental retardation and extreme incoherence and irrationality. Mutism, unresponsiveness, dysarthria, aphasia, and sphincteric incontinence may be added to the clinical picture. In a late state a secondary physical deterioration also takes place. Food intake, which may be increased in the beginning of the illness, is in the end usually limited, with resulting emaciation. Finally the patient remains in bed most of the time and dies of pneumonia or some other intercurrent infection. This whole process may evolve over a period of months or years.

Many of these alterations of behavior are the direct result of disease of the nervous system; or, expressed in another way, the symptoms are the primary manifestations of neurologic disease. Others are secondary, in the sense of being reactions to the catastrophe of losing one's mind. For example, the dement is said to seek solitude to hide his affliction and may thus appear asocial or apathetic. Again, excessive orderliness may be an attempt to compensate for failing memory; or apprehension, gloom, or irritability may be the expressions of general dissatisfaction with a necessarily restricted life. Even in a state of fairly advanced deterioration the patient is still capable of reacting to his illness and to the individuals who care for him.

Attempts to relate loss of memory and failing intellectual function to lesions in certain parts of the brain have been eminently unsuccessful. Two types of difficulty have obstructed progress in this field. (1) There is the problem of defining, analyzing, and determining the significance of the so-called "intellectual" functions. (2) The morbid anatomy of these diseases is so complex that it cannot be fully defined and quantitated.

In the most careful analyses of the intellectual functions, certain general and certain specific factors have been isolated. The general factors are not localized at the moment to any one area of the brain, whereas the specific ones do have at least a regional localization in the cerebrum. Spearman, Thurstone, and others have been able to single out a number of specific factors such as verbal capacity, ability to appreciate spatial relationships, ability to learn and to reason inductively and deductively, facility in the use of numbers and in numerical calculation, and retentive memory. All these qualities are tested in standard intelligence and achievement tests. Memory correlates poorly with all the other factors and seems to be an independent factor. There is an intercorrelation between all the other factors. In other words a person who performs well in tests of verbal capacity tends to do well on tests of spatial orientation, numerical relationships, learning, and reasoning tests. Some general factor, ? G factor of Spearman, is being measured by each test and determines in part the level of performance. In addition there are special aptitudes or factors, S factors of Spearman, that account for individual superiorities or (in disease) inferiorities in one or another test.

In dementia the memory impairment which is a constant feature may occur with extensive disease in any part of the cerebrum. Yet it is interesting to note that the function of the diencephalon may be more fundamental to retentive memory than integrity of cortex, and, as will be pointed out below, it may be the thalamotemporal connections that are particularly concerned with this function. Failure in tests of verbal function (the most advanced degree is aphasia) is closely associated with disease of the dominant cerebral hemisphere, and particularly the speech areas in the frontal, temporal, and parietal lobes, and insula. Loss of capacity for arithmetic reasoning and numerical calculation (acalculia) is related to lesions in the posterior part of the left (dominant) cerebral hemisphere. Impairment in drawing or constructing simple and complex figures with blocks, sticks, picture arrangement, etc., as shown by tests of visual construction, is most pronounced in right (nondominant) parietal lobe lesions, as was pointed out above.

Thus the clinical picture which results from cerebral disease depends in part on the extent of the lesion, i.e., the amount of cerebral tissue destroyed, and on the specific locality of the lesion.

MORBID ANATOMY AND PATHOLOGIC PHYSIOLOGY OF DEMENTIA

Dementia is related usually to obvious structural disease of the cerebrum and the diencephalon. Knowledge of the detailed anatomy of the diencephalic nuclei and their connections with one another and with the various parts of the cerebral cortex is so limited that it has thus far been impossible to define either the topography of many of the diseases with which we are concerned or the nature of the lesion. In some diseases, such as Alzheimer's and Pick's presenile or senile dementia, the main process appears to be a degeneration of nerve cells in the association areas, with secondary changes in the cerebral white matter. In others, such as Huntington's chorea, Jakob-Creutzfeldt pseudosclerosis, and the cerebrocerebellar degenerations, loss of neurones in the cerebral cortex is accompanied by a similar degeneration of neurones in the putamen and caudate nuclei, the lenticular and subthalamic nuclei, and the cerebellum, respectively. Arteriosclerotic vascular disease results in multiple foci of infarction all through the thalami, basal ganglions, brain stem, and cerebrum and in the latter in the motor, sensory, or visual projection areas as well as the association areas. Severe trauma may cause contusions of cerebral convolutions and degeneration of the central white matter (Strich) with resulting protracted stupor or dementia (rare). Most of the diseases which produce dementia are quite extensive, and the frontal lobes are affected more often than other parts of the cerebrum.

Other mechanisms than the destruction of brain tissue may operate in some cases. Chronic increased intracranial pressure or chronic hydrocephalus, regardless of cause, is often associated with a general impairment of mental function. The compression of one or both cerebral hemispheres by chronic subdural hematomas may cause a widespread disturbance of cortical function. A diffuse inflammatory process is at least in part the basis for dementia in syphilis and in neurotropic virus infections. Lastly, several of the toxic and metabolic diseases discussed in Chap. 34 may interfere with nervous function over a long period of time and create a clinical picture similar to, if not identical with, that of dementia.

APPROACH TO THE CLINICAL PROBLEM OF DEMENTIA

The physician presented with a patient suffering from a diffuse brain disease must adopt an examination technique designed to expose fully the intellectual defect. Abnormalities of posture, movement, sensation, and reflexes cannot be relied upon, for it must be remembered that the association areas of the brain may be severely damaged without demonstrable neurologic signs of this type.

Three categories of data are required for the recognition and differential diagnosis of dementing brain disease:

1. A reliable history of the illness
2. Findings on mental examination, i.e., so-called "mental status," as well as on the rest of the neurologic examination
3. Special laboratory procedures, lumbar puncture, x-rays of the skull, electroencephalogram, and sometimes pneumoencephalogram

The history should always be supplemented by information obtained from a person other than the patient, because, through lack of insight, he is often unaware of his illness; and indeed he may be ignorant even of his chief complaint. Special inquiry should be made about the patient's general behavior, capacity for work, personal habits, and such faculties as memory and judgment.

This performance of an examination of the mental status must be systematic. At a minimum it should include:

I. Insight (patient's replies to questions about his chief symptoms): What is your difficulty? Are you ill? When did your illness begin?
II. Orientation (knowledge of personal identity and present situation):
   Person: What is your name? What is your occupation? Where do you live? Are you married?
   Place: What is the name of the place where you are now? How did you get there? What floor is it on? Where is the bathroom? What are you doing now?
   Time: What is the date today? What time of day is it? What meals have you had? When was the last holiday?
III. Memory:
   Remote: Tell me the names of your children and their birth dates. When were you married? What was your mother's maiden name? What was the name of your first schoolteacher?
   Recent past: Tell me about your recent illness. (Compare with previous statements.) What did you have for breakfast today? What is my name or the nurse's name? When did you see me for the first time? What were the headlines in the newspaper today?
   Retention: Repeat these numbers after me. (Give series of 3, 4, 5, 6, 7, 8 digits at speed of 1 per second.) Now when I give a series of numbers, repeat them in reverse order.
   Visual span: Show the patient a picture of several objects and then ask him to name what he has seen and to note any anomalies.

IV. General information: Ask about names of presidents, well-known historic dates, the names of large rivers, of large cities, etc.
V. Capacity for sustained mental activity:
   Calculation: Test ability to add, subtract, multiply, and divide. Subtraction of serial 7s from 100 is a good test of calculation as well as attention.
   Abstract thinking: See if the patient can detect similarities and differences between classes of objects, or explain a proverb or a fable.
VI. General behavior: Attitudes, general bearing, stream of thought, attentiveness, mood, manner of dress, etc.

In order to enlist the patient's full cooperation he must be prepared for questions of this type. Otherwise, the first reaction will be one of embarrassment or anger because of the implication that his mind is not sound. It should be pointed out to the patient that some individuals are rather forgetful and that it is often necessary to ask specific questions in order to form some impression about their degree of nervousness when being examined. Reassurance that these are not tests of intelligence or of sanity is helpful.

A more formal and reliable method of examining the mental capacity of adults is the Wechsler-Bellevue test. This can be given by a psychologist or by the physician if he carefully reads the instructions for administering and scoring the test. The "Mental Examiners' Handbook," by F. L. Wells and J. Ruesch, published by the Psychological Corporation, is of help to those not familiar with this type of examination. Tests of retention of verbal material and the recall of a series of learned digits or of visually presented objects are of value in estimating the degree of deterioration. In the Wechsler test the discrepancy between the vocabulary, picture completion, information, and object assembly tests as a group (these correlate well with premorbid intelligence and are relatively insensitive to dementing brain disease) and arithmetic, block design, digit span, and digit-symbol tests provides an index of deterioration.

Although the form of the dementia is not indicative of a particular disease, certain combinations of symptoms and neurologic signs are more or less characteristic and may be of aid in diagnosis. The mode of onset, the clinical course, the associated neurologic signs, and the accessory laboratory data constitute the basis of differential diagnosis. It must be admitted, however, that some of the rarer types of "degenerative" brain disease are at present recognized only by pathologic examination. The correct diagnosis of treatable forms of senile (over sixty years of age) or presenile (forty to sixty years) dementias, such as general paresis, subdural hematoma, brain tumor, bromide or other chronic drug intoxication, pellagra and related deficiency states, and hypothyroidism, is of greater practical importance than the diagnosis of any of the untreatable ones.

BEDSIDE CLASSIFICATION OF DEMENTING DISEASES OF THE BRAIN

The conventional classification of dementing diseases of the brain is usually according to etiology, if known, or pathology. Another more practical approach that follows logically from the method by which the whole subject has been presented in this book is to subdivide the diseases into three categories on the basis of the associated clinical and laboratory signs of medical disease and the accompanying neurologic signs. Once the physician has determined that the patient suffers a dementing illness, he must then decide into which category the case fits by the medical, neurologic, and laboratory data. This classification may at first seem somewhat artificial. However, it is likely to be more useful to the student or physician who is not conversant with the many diseases which cause dementia than a classification based on pathology.

CLASSIFICATION

I. Diseases in which dementia is usually associated with other clinical and laboratory signs of medical disease
  A. Hypothyroidism
  B. Cushing's disease
  C. Nutritional deficiency states such as pellagra, Wernicke's disease and Korsakoff's syndrome, pernicious anemia, and subacute degeneration of spinal cord and brain
  D. Neurosyphilis—general paresis and meningovascular syphilis
  E. Hepatolenticular degeneration
  F. Cerebral arteriosclerosis
  G. Bromidism
II. Diseases in which dementia is associated with other neurologic signs but not with other obvious medical disease
  A. Invariably associated with other neurologic signs:
    1. Huntington's chorea
    2. Schilder's disease and related demyelinative diseases
    3. Amaurotic family idiocy and other lipid-storage diseases
    4. Myoclonic epilepsy
    5. Jakob-Creutzfeldt disease
    6. Cerebrocerebellar degeneration
    7. Dementia with spastic paraplegia
  B. Often associated with other neurologic signs:
    1. Cerebral arteriosclerosis
    2. Brain tumor
    3. Brain trauma, such as cerebral contusion and midbrain hemorrhage, chronic subdural hematoma

III. Diseases in which dementia is usually the only evidence of neurologic or medical disease
  A. Alzheimer's disease and senile dementia
  B. Pick's disease
  C. Marchiafava-Bignami disease
  D. Some cases of brain tumor of frontal lobes and corpus callosum

Many of these diseases are discussed more fully in other sections of this book. The special features of the dementia which accompanies arteriosclerotic, senile, syphilitic, traumatic, nutritional, and degenerative diseases are discussed in the appropriate chapters.

DIFFERENTIAL DIAGNOSIS

The first difficulty in dealing with this class of patients is to make sure of deterioration of intellect and personality change. It may be necessary to examine the patient several times before one is confident of the clinical findings.

There is always a tendency to assume that mental function is normal if patients complain only of nervousness, fatigue, insomnia, or vague somatic symptoms, and to label the patients psychoneurotic. *This will be avoided if one keeps in mind that psychoneuroses rarely begin in middle or late adult life.* A practical rule is to assume that all mental illnesses beginning during this period are due either to a structural disease of the brain or to a depressive psychosis.

A mild dysphasia must not be mistaken for dementia. The aphasic patient appears uncertain of himself, and his speech may be incoherent. Furthermore he may be anxious and depressed over his ineptitude. Careful attention to the patient's language performance will lead to the correct diagnosis in most instances. Further observation will disclose the fact that the patient's behavior, except for speech, is within normal limits.

The depressed patient presents another type of problem. He may remark that his mental function is poor or that he is forgetful and cannot concentrate. Scrutiny of his conversation will show, however, that he actually remembers all the details of his illness and that no qualitative change in mental ability has taken place. His difficulty is one either of lack of energy and interest or of anxiety which prevents focusing of attention on anything except his own problems. Even during mental tests his performance may be impaired by his emotions, in much the same way as that of the worried student during his examinations. This condition of emotional blocking is called "experiential confusion." When the patient is calmed by reassurance, his mental function is normal, a proof that intellectual deterioration has not occurred. The hypomanic patient fails in tests of intellectual function because of his restlessness and distractibility. It is helpful to remember that the demented patient rarely has sufficient insight to complain of mental deterioration; and if he admits to poor memory, seldom realizes the degree of his disability. The physician must never rely on the patient's statements as to the efficiency of mental function and must always evaluate a poor performance on tests in the light of the emotional state and the motivation at the time the test is given.

The neurologic syndrome associated with metabolic or endocrine disorders, i.e., ACTH therapy, hyperthyroidism, Cushing's disease, Addison's disease, or the post-partum state, may be difficult to diagnose because of the wide variety of clinical pictures which may be shown. As stated above, some patients appear to be suffering from a dementia, others from an acute confusional psychosis; or if mood change or negativism predominates, a manic-depressive psychosis or schizophrenia is suggested. In these conditions some degree of clouding of sensorium and impairment of intellectual function can usually be recognized, and these findings alone should be enough to exclude schizophrenia and manic-depressive psychosis. It is well to remember that an acute onset of mental symptoms is always suggestive of a confusional psychosis or delirium. In as much as many of these conditions are completely reversible, they must be distinguished from dementia.

Once the decision that the patient suffers a dementing disease is made, the next step is to decide by careful physical examination whether there are signs of a medical or of a focal neurologic disease. This enables the physician to place the case in one of the three categories in the bedside classification. X-rays of skull, electroencephalogram, and lumbar puncture should be carried out in most cases. Usually these procedures necessitate admission to a hospital. The final step is to determine by the total clinical picture which disease within any one category the patient has. Table 39-2 shows the major points in differential diagnosis.

Care of the Demented Patient

Dementia is a clinical state of the most serious nature, and usually it is worthwhile to admit the patient to a hospital for a period of observation. The physician then has an opportunity to see the patient several times in a new and fairly constant hospital environment, and certain special procedures such as x-rays of the skull, lumbar puncture, analysis for blood bromides, basal metabolic rate, and an electroencephalogram can be carried out at this time. The management of the demented patient in the hospital may be relatively simple if he is quiet and cooperative. If the disordered mental function is severe, a nurse, attendant, or member of the family must stay with him at all times. Provision must be made for adequate food and fluid intake and control of infection, using the same measures outlined for the delirious patient.

Once it is established that the patient has an untreatable dementing brain disease, a responsible member of the family should be apprised of the medical facts. The patient should be told that he has a nervous condition for which he is to be given rest and treatment. Nothing is accomplished by telling him more. The family should be given the prognosis, if the diagnosis is sufficiently certain for this to be possible. If the dementia is slight and circumstances are suitable, the patient may remain at home, continuing activities of which he is capable. He should be spared responsibility and be guarded against injury which might result from imprudent action. If he is still at work, plans for occupational retirement should be carried out. If the home situation is unsuitable, or when, in the more advanced stages of the disease, mental and physical enfeeblement become pronounced, institutional care should be advised. Seizures should be treated symptomatically. Nerve tonics, vitamins, and hormones are of no value in checking the course of the illness or in regenerating decayed tissue. They may, however, offer moral support for the patient and the family.

38 THE ACUTE CONFUSIONAL STATES

Maurice Victor and
Raymond D. Adams

The singular event in which a patient with a previously intact mentality becomes acutely psychotic is observed almost daily on the medical and surgical wards of a general hospital. Occurring as it does during an infective fever, in the course of another illness such as cardiac failure, or following an injury, operation, or the excessive use of alcohol, it never fails to create grave problems for the physician, the nursing personnel, and the family. The physician has to cope with the problem of diagnosis without the advantage of a lucid history, and his program of treatment may constantly be threatened by the agitation, sleeplessness, and uncooperative attitude of the patient. The nursing personnel is often sorely taxed by the necessity of providing a satisfactory environment for the convalescence of the patient and, at the same time, of maintaining a tranquil atmosphere for the other patients on the ward. And the family is appalled by the sudden specter of insanity and all that it entails.

Under such circumstances it is a great temptation to rid oneself of the clinical problem by transferring the patient to a psychiatric hospital. This, in the authors' opinion, is an unwise action for it may result in the inexpert management of the underlying medical disease and may even jeopardize the patient's life. It is far better for the physician to assume full responsibility for the care of such patients and to familiarize himself with this group of nervous disorders.

TERMINOLOGY

The term *confusional states* used in the title of this chapter finds no universal acceptance, and the authors have had to be somewhat arbitrary in denoting a group of syndromes by one common attribute—that of *thinking with less than accustomed clarity and coherence*. It is their impression that this term conveniently designates a broad group of mental disorders and includes at least three syndromes:

1. A confusional state associated with an increase in psychomotor and autonomic activity, i.e., delirium
2. A confusional state associated with reduced psychomotor activity, i.e., primary mental confusion
3. Senile or other dementing brain disease aggravated by fever or some other medical state, i.e., beclouded dementia

The subdivision of the confusional states in this manner seems justified in that each of these syndromes appears to be separable on clinical grounds, to have particular relationships to other medical diseases, and to depend on relatively specific mechanisms.

The term *delirium* [from *delirare* to rave; literal derivation, "to wander from the *lira* (furrow)," i.e., "to go off the track,"] denotes a transient illness characterized by overalertness and vigilance, excitation of autonomic nervous functions, psychomotor overactivity, talkativeness, disorders of perception with prominent hallucinations, a low seizure threshold, and a relatively normal electroencephalographic pattern. Delirium is generally related to the excessive ingestion of alcohol or other drug.

The second type of confusional psychosis has as its cardinal feature a *reduced state of alertness and responsiveness*. This type also is transitory in nature, but in contrast to delirium is characterized by mental dullness, reduced attentiveness, drowsiness, faulty perception, psychomotor underactivity, a comparatively slight tendency to hallucinate and convulse, and a disordered electroencephalogram pattern.

The third syndrome, the beclouded dementia, consists of mental dullness, drowsiness, impairment of perception, and clouding of consciousness superimposed on the syndrome of dementia (see Chap. 37).

Finally, it should be pointed out that schizophrenia and manic-depressive psychosis may at times coincide with some other medical illness and may simulate the other conditions described in this chapter.

In this chapter only the three types of confusional psychosis are described in detail; the other forms of psychosis are considered in Chaps. 39 and 44.

The terminology which the authors have chosen is at variance with that found in many medical writings. For example, Bonhoeffer, in his authoritative exposition of the confusional and delirious states, referred to both of them as the *exogenous reaction type* or *symptomatic psychosis*, implying that they are induced by acute infections and other medical diseases. Other writers, noting their association with infective fevers, designate them as the *toxic psychoses*, the *infective-exhaustion psychoses*, *fever delirium*, and *acute delirious mania and stupor*. Adolf Meyer introduced the term *dysergastic reaction*, which in his nomenclature included all mental disturbances "due to disorders of the nutrition and circulatory support of the brain."

SYNDROMES OF WHICH MENTAL CONFUSION IS A MAJOR COMPONENT

Delirium

Clinical Features. These are most perfectly depicted in the alcoholic patient. The symptoms usually develop over a period of 2 or 3 days. The first indications of the approaching attack are restless irritability, tremulousness, insomnia, and poor appetite. The patient's rest becomes troubled by unpleasant and terrifying dreams. There may be momentary disorientation or an occasional irrational remark. These initial symptoms rapidly give way to a clinical picture which, in severe cases, is one of the most colorful and dramatic in medicine. He talks incessantly and incoherently, and looks distressed or perplexed, an expression which is in keeping with his vague notions of being pursued by someone seeking to injure him. From his manner and from the content of his speech it is evident that he misinterprets the meaning of ordinary objects and sounds around him and has vivid visual, auditory, and tactile hallucinations, often of a most unpleasant type. At first he can be brought into touch with reality and may in fact answer questions correctly; but almost at once he relapses into his preoccupied confused state. Before long he is unable to shake off his hallucinations even for a second and does not recognize his family or his physician. Tremor and restless movements are usually present and may be violent. The countenance is flushed and the conjunctivas are injected, the pulse is rapid and soft, and the temperature may be raised. There is much sweating, and the urine is scanty and of high specific gravity. The symptoms abate, either suddenly or gradually, after 2 or 3 days, although, in exceptional cases, they may persist for several weeks. The most certain indication of the end of the attack is the occurrence of sound sleep and of lucid intervals. Recovery is usually complete.

Delirium is subject to all degrees of variability, not only from patient to patient but in the same patient from day to day and hour to hour. The entire syndrome may be observed in one patient and only one or two symptoms in another. In its mildest form, as so often occurs in febrile diseases, it consists of an occasional wandering of the mind and incoherence of expression interrupted by periods of lucidity. This form, shorn of motor and autonomic overactivity, is sometimes referred to as a *quiet delirium,* and is difficult to distinguish from other confusional states. The more severe form, sometimes called *active delirium* and best exemplified by delirium tremens, is characterized by a great excess of motor activity and marked confusion which may progress to a "muttering stupor" and in about 10 per cent of patients ends fatally.

The dominant clinical manifestations of delirium are:

1. Disturbances of attention and concentration and disorders of perception (clouding of the sensorium)

2. Illusions and hallucinations

3. Delusions

4. Excessive motor activity, i.e., tremulousness, restlessness, overtalkativeness

5. Disorders of mood and affect

6. Overactivity of autonomic nervous functions, i.e., rapid pulse, sweating, fever

Disturbances of Attention and Concentration and Disorders of Perception. There is also an impairment of those faculties of attention and perception which enable the patient to place himself properly in time and space. This appears to account for his disorientation and inability to grasp the meaning of his surroundings. Thus he may be unaware of the most obvious features of his immediate situation, such as whether he is standing or lying, what clothing he is wearing, and whether he is indoors or on the street.

There is always in the delirious state a *diminished power of attention and concentration,* and an inability properly to perceive environmental stimuli (*clouding of the sensorium*). The patient has difficulty understanding what is said to him, and his answers are diffuse and rambling. Even if sporadic responses are to the point, he cannot sustain a coherent and rational conversation for long. In fact, compelling him to concentrate on a given task is one of the best ways of revealing minor sensorial defects.

As this attention defect becomes more severe, formal mental testing becomes impossible. At times the patient cannot be distracted by any means from a persistent preoccupation with some abnormal activity or thought process. Paradoxically, despite his inaccessibility when preoccupied, the patient at all times is vigilant and may respond to the slightest change in his environment. Any new stimulus may make only a momentary impression or, on the other hand, it may become the focal point for a new thought process, from which it is again difficult to turn the patient's attention. If one can but attract the patient's attention for a brief period, momentary flashes of clear insight and accurate responses are obtained. He may recall material which he was asked to remember at a previous examination and which left him seemingly unimpressed at that time. These observations would indicate that the confusion is largely due to a sensorial defect—inattention and inaccurate interpretation of sensory experiences. Other aspects of intellectual function, particularly the loss of memory of newly formed impressions, are, in this respect, secondary phenomena.

Illusions and Hallucinations. The disorder of the perceptual process is more dramatically illustrated by the occurrence of illusions and hallucinations. The content of the abnormal percept may or may not be based on objective reality. Thus in many instances the patient may falsely interpret sensory impressions (*illusions*). He *misidentifies* people or *misinterprets* the meaning of sounds and shadows; or some familiar object may become distorted as he looks at it. The disorder in perception may be further illustrated by the patient's ready response to suggestion. He can, for example, be provoked to go through the motions of opening and drinking down a bottle of beer or lighting a cigar, by suggestively handing him such imaginary objects.

On the other hand, the patient may have a disorder of perception quite unfounded in reality, i.e., *hallucinations.* Actually it is impossible to draw a sharp line between his hallucinations and illusions, because one can never be certain that some sense impression is not involved in the genesis of the hallucination. In practice one speaks of illusions when the sensory stimulus is obvious to the bystander and of hallucinations when it is not so. The hallucinations may be visual, auditory, less commonly tactile, and rarely olfactory or gustatory; or there may be a mixture of these forms. Unlike the schizophrenic hallucinations, they are usually projected into space; i.e., they are said to be coming from a certain place. While actively hallucinating the patient usually has no appreciation of the unreality of his new sensory experiences. His reaction to them is quite appropriate; he may cower when faced with a menacing visual image; on hearing threatening voices he may call on the police for protection or barricade and arm himself against intruders; and even more dramatically he may perform suicidal acts in an attempt to avoid what the voices threaten.

Delusions. These are false beliefs which cannot be rectified by reason. Usually the abnormal ideas are closely interwoven with misinterpretations, illusions, and other perceptual disorders. However, in some cases, they are the most prominent part of the clinical picture. The delusional ideas are not as a rule well-systematized and are not retold with any consistency. Frequently they have a paranoid coloring—the patient believes that he is being stalked or pursued, and that he is in imminent danger of being injured. He may recount tales of being robbed and tortured, or of taking part in pitched battles.

Excessive Motor Activity. Several forms of *excessive motor activity* are discernible in the majority of cases. *Restlessness* is an invariable feature. The patient is unable to sleep naturally throughout the delirious period. In the more violent forms, he is constantly moving, looking suspiciously about him, arranging the bedclothes, wandering about the room, or tugging at his restraints. More complex restless movements are also common; they are usually in relation to some delusion or hallucination. Especially characteristic are the turning of the head and eyes to engage in an imaginary conversation, the persistent searching movements in which the patient ransacks his bedclothes for some object which he supposes to be concealed there, the reenacting of complex habitual acts, such as driving a car, or of some part of the patient's occupational activities. Some of his incessant activity may be explained by the common misbelief that he is imprisoned in some building from which he is attempting to escape and return home. He strives to get out of bed and out of doors, and although momentarily persuaded to return to his bed, is soon attempting to get up again. Other characteristic motor abnormalities include picking and fumbling movements. It is also noteworthy that the patient startles easily, and voluntary movements are jerky and uneven.

The excessive motor activity is reflected in the patient's *speech.* Not only is it increased in amount, but much of it is slurred, garbled, and unintelligible. The patient may shout and scream for hours on end; or when he is seriously ill, speech may be reduced to an almost inaudible muttering. At times he falters over words as though he had forgotten what he wished to say, or he may speak in neologisms. A close analysis of these faults of speech indicates both a disturbance of articulation and a mild dysphasia.

The *tremor* which usually affects the extremities, face, and tongue is added to the restless movements. It is present as long as the limbs are activated and fluctuates in severity, increasing markedly with any sustained action or emotional upset. The tremor, particularly in delirium tremens, may be so coarse and violent as to render the simplest tasks such as walking, eating, or talking quite impossible.

Disorders of Mood and of Affect. The patient's *mood* and his outward display of emotion (*affect*) show no constancy in delirium; in fact they are marked by their lability and changing character. The mood may be one of either depression or elation. Or an attitude of complete detachment may be preserved with only minor tendencies toward facetiousness, quizzicality, or perplexity. At any moment these attitudes may be transformed to suspicion, truculence, or fear. Vague apprehension and fear, a response appropriate to the patient's belief of impending calamity, are the rule; and when threatened by imaginary danger the patient may react not only with visible concern or terror but with all the physiologic concomitants of fear as well.

Overactivity of Autonomic Nervous Functions. Dilated pupils, tachycardia, and an elevated temperature, often attributable to no cause other than the delirium, are common findings. Excessive sweating is frequent and may result in severe dehydration. There may also be excessive pilomotor responses, pallor or flushing, nausea, constipation, and diarrhea.

Morbid Anatomy and Pathophysiology. The brains of patients who have died in delirium, especially delirium tremens, are said to show many pathologic changes, including edema, swelling of the nerve cells with vacuolization, pigmentation, and chromatolysis, and also degeneration of nerve fibers. Not all authors report such changes, however, and those who do, fail to agree on a uniform pathologic picture. The authors' own observations lead them to believe that no definite pathologic changes in the brain in fatal cases of delirium have yet been discovered and that most if not all those reported are in the nature of artefacts or are expressions of agonal processes. There are, however, a number of diseases which may cause delirium and also give rise to focal lesions in the brain, such as focal embolic encephalitis, virus encephalitis, Wernicke's disease, trauma, etc. The topography of these lesions is of particular interest. They tend to be localized in certain parts of the brain, particularly in the midbrain and subthalamus and in the temporal lobes. Hallucinations have been observed with focal lesions in these parts. Penfield's studies of the human cortex during surgical exploration clearly indicate the importance of the temporal lobe in the production of visual, auditory, and olfactory hallucinations. With subthalamic and midbrain lesions, there may occur visual hallucinations of a pleasurable type accompanied by good insight, viz., the peduncular hallucinosis of Lhermitte.

The value of the electroencephalogram in studying delirium has largely been limited by the difficulty of obtaining records free of movement artefact. There is some evidence that the electroencephalogram in severe delirium shows nonfocal slow activity in the range of 5 to 7 per second, a state which rapidly returns to normal as the delirium clears. However, in others only activity in the fast beta frequency is seen and in milder degrees of delirium there is usually no abnormality at all.

An analysis of the several conditions inducive to delirium suggests at least two different physiologic mechanisms. In alcoholism and barbiturate intoxication the clinical manifestations appear after the withdrawal of drugs which are known to have a strong inhibitory effect on the central nervous system. In the case of bacterial infections and poisoning by certain drugs such as atropine and scopolamine the delirious state probably results from the direct action of the toxin or chemical.

Psychophysiologic mechanisms have also been postulated, but they rest on only random observations, and the hypotheses formulated are based largely on analogies to other types of mental disturbance. It has long been suggested that some individuals are much more liable to delirium than others. There is much reason to doubt this hypothesis, for it has been shown that all of a group of randomly selected persons would develop delirium if the causative mechanisms were operative. This is to be expected, for any healthy person under certain circumstances may experience phenomena akin to those found in delirium. Thus after repeated auditory and visual stimulation the same impressions may continue to be perceived even though the stimuli are no longer present. A soldier, for example, may hear the sound of shells long after he has left the battlefield. Moreover, it has been shown that a healthy individual can be induced to hallucinate by placing him in an environment as free as possible of sensory stimulation. The similarity between hallucinations which form the aura of a convulsive seizure and those of delirium, already mentioned, suggests that an irritative lesion in certain parts of the cerebral cortex may be at work in a hallucinatory state. A relation between delirium and dream states has been postulated because in both there is a loss of appreciation

of time, a richness of visual imagery, and indifference to inconsistencies. Moreover, patients may refer to some of their delirious symptoms as a "bad dream"; normal persons may hallucinate in the so-called "hypnagogic state," the short period between sleeping and waking. "The emergence into awareness of imagery belonging to subconscious thought" and other formulations in the field of dynamic psychology seem more reasonably to account for the topical content of delirium rather than to explain its occurrence. Wolff and Curran, having observed the same content in repeated attacks of delirium due to different causes, concluded that the content depends more on the age, sex, intellectual endowment, occupation, personality traits, and past experiences of the patient than on the cause or mechanism of the delirium.

The main difficulty in understanding delirium arises from the fact that it has not been possible from clinical studies to ascertain which of the many symptoms have physiologic significance. What is the basis of this lack of harmony between actual sensory impressions of the present and memory of those in the past? Obviously there is something missing from total behavior, something that leaves the patient at the mercy of certain sensory stimuli and unable to attend to others and at the same time incapable of discriminating between sense impression and fantasy. There appears to be some lack of inhibition of sensory processes which may also be the basis of the sleep disturbance (insomnia) and the convulsive tendency.

Confusional States Associated with Reduced Alertness and Responsiveness (*Primary Mental Confusion*)

Clinical Features. In the most typical examples of this type of confusion all mental functions are reduced to some degree, but alertness, attentiveness, and the ability to grasp all elements of the immediate situation suffer most. In its mildest form the patient may pass for normal and only a failure to recollect and reproduce happenings of the past few hours or days reveals the inadequacy of mental function. The more obviously confused patient spends much of his time in idleness. Only the more automatic acts and verbal responses are properly performed, but these may permit the examiner to obtain from the patient a number of relevant and accurate replies to questions about age, occupation, and residence. Reactions are slow and indecisive, and it is difficult to sustain a conversation. The patient dozes during the interview and is observed to sleep more hours each day than is natural. Responses tend to be rather abrupt, brief, and mechanical. Perceptual difficulties are frequent, and voices, common objects, and the actions of people are frequently misinterpreted. Often one cannot discern whether the patient hears voices and sees things that do not exist, i.e., whether he is actively hallucinating, or is merely misinterpreting stimuli in the environment. This inadequacy of perception and forgetfulness results in a constant state of bewilderment. Failing to recognize his surroundings and having lost all sense of time, he repeats the same questions and makes the same remarks over and over again.

As the confusion deepens, conversation becomes more difficult, and at a certain stage the patient no longer notices or responds to much of what is going on around him. Replies to questions may be with a single word or a short phrase, in a soft tremulous voice or whisper. Or the patient may be mute. Irritability may or may not be present. Some patients are extremely suspicious; in fact a paranoid trend may be the most pronounced and troublesome feature of the illness.

In its most advanced stages confusion gives way to stupor, and finally the stupor to coma. As the patient improves he may pass again through the stage of stupor and confusion in the reverse order. All this informs us that at least this category of confusion is but a manifestation of the same disease processes which in their most severe form cause coma.

In some instances the mental aberration never exceeds that of confusion with stupor; in others, with more than the usual degree of irritability and restlessness, one cannot fail to notice the striking resemblance to delirium. In both there is a clouding of consciousness and impairment of attention, a slowness and disordered perception and association of ideas. Indeed, if the delirious state were shorn of its tremor, vivid hallucinations, vigilant excited attitude, insomnia, and the low convulsive threshold, the differentiation would be impossible. Actually typical cases showing one or other of these two syndromes are easily distinguished, but it must also be admitted that in numerous patients with an acute confusional state the differentiation is impossible.

Morbid Anatomy and Pathophysiology. All that has been said on this subject in Chap. 34 is applicable to at least one subgroup of the confusional states. In the others no consistent pathologic change has been found. The electroencephalogram is of interest because it is almost invariably abnormal in the more severe forms of this syndrome, in contrast to delirium, where the changes are relatively minor. High-voltage slow waves in the 2 to 3 per second (delta) range or the 5 to 7 per second (theta) range are the usual finding.

Senile and Other Dementing Brain Diseases Complicated by Medical Diseases (Beclouded Dementia)

Many elderly patients who enter the hospital with a medical or surgical illness are mentally confused. Presumably the liability to this state is determined by preexisting brain disease, in this instance senile dementia, which may or may not have been obvious to the family before the onset of the complicating illness.

All the clinical features of confusion described in the previous sections may be present. The severity may vary greatly. The confusion may be reflected only in the patient's inability to relate sequentially the history of his illness, or it may be so severe that he is virtually *non compos mentis*.

Although almost any complicating illness may bring out this confusion, it is particularly frequent in infectious disease, especially in those cases which resist the effects of antibiotic medication; in posttraumatic and postoperative states, notably after concussive brain injuries and removal of cataracts (in which case the confusion is probably related to being temporarily deprived of vision); in congestive heart failure, chronic respiratory disease, and severe anemia, especially pernicious anemia. Often it is difficult to determine which of several possible factors is responsible for the confusion in this heterogeneous group of illnesses. There may be more than one factor. A cardiac patient with a confusional psychosis may be febrile, have marginally reduced cerebral blood flow, be intoxicated by one or more drugs, or be in electrolyte imbalance. The same is true of postoperative confusional states, where a number of factors such as fever and infection, dehydration, and drug intoxication may be incriminated. The presence of alcoholism may further complicate the matter.

With recovery from the recently acquired medical or surgical illness, the patient usually returns to his premorbid state, though his shortcomings, now drawn to the attention of the family and physician, may be more obvious than before.

Coincidental Development of Schizophrenia or Manic-depressive Psychosis during a Medical or Surgical Illness

A certain proportion of psychoses of the schizophrenic or manic-depressive type first become manifest during an acute medical illness or following an operation or parturition. A causal relationship between the two is usually sought but cannot be established. Usually the psychosis had its onset long before but was not recognized. The diagnosis of the psychiatric illness must proceed along the lines suggested in Chaps. 39 and 44. Close observation will usually reveal a clear sensorium and relatively intact memory which permit differentiation from the acute confusional states.

The Residual Mental States Following Delirium and Confusion, Korsakoff's Psychosis (Amnestic-Confabulatory Syndrome)

The majority of patients suffering from delirium and confusion recover completely after a few days or weeks. Afterwards one can detect no evidence of damage to the nervous system. In contrast, in cases of beclouded dementia as the sensorial disturbance subsides the patient is left with the same mental weakness that existed before the onset of the confusional state. Sometimes the dementia seems more pronounced afterward, and the family will later remark that the patient's mind failed at the time of the acute illness. However, one has the impression that they merely became aware of the insidiously developing dementia at this time.

There is another group of cases, by no means small or insignificant, in which the acutely delirious or confused patient is left with a severe deficit. The inattentiveness, hallucinations, and sleep disorder disappear. The patient is alert, easily engaged in conversation, and quite proper in his general deportment. Nevertheless he is incompetent to look after himself. A careful evaluation of his mental status will reveal a severe memory deficit of the type found in Korsakoff's psychosis. The distinguishing feature of this latter illness is not memory loss alone but the disproportionate affection of memory in relation to the patient's alertness and the integrity of other faculties. It is further characterized by the inability to learn new facts and, in its early stages, by confabulation. This state, once fully developed, may be permanent, though often there is some improvement in learning capacity and memory as the months pass. It represents a special type of dementia.

The clinical features of Korsakoff's psychosis are presented in detail in Chap. 288. Although frequently observed in patients who suffer from alcoholism and malnutrition, the same clinical picture may occur with other diseases, such as ruptured saccular aneurysm and subarachnoid hemorrhage, tuberculous meningitis, tumors in the walls of the third ventricle, etc.

Other residual states may occur, as would be expected with diseases which may exert a variable effect on the brain. The authors have several times seen a severe and permanent dementia combined with cerebellar ataxia and pyramidal tract signs following an infectious disease with hyperpyrexia.

CLASSIFICATION OF THE ACUTE CONFUSIONAL STATES

The only satisfactory basis for classification is the syndrome itself and its main clinical relationships, until such time as the actual cause and pathophysiology are discovered. The tendency in the past to subdivide the syndromes according to their most prominent symptom or the degree of severity, e.g., "picking delirium," "microptic delirium," "acute delirious mania," "muttering delirium," has no fundamental value.

I. Delirium
  A. In a medical or surgical illness (no focal or lateralizing neurologic signs and cerebrospinal fluid usually clear)
     1. Typhoid fever
     2. Pneumonia
     3. Septicemia, particularly erysipelas and other streptococcal infections
     4. Rheumatic fever
     5. Thyrotoxicosis and ACTH intoxication (rare)
     6. Postoperative and posttraumatic states
  B. In neurologic disease that causes focal or lateralizing signs or changes in the cerebrospinal fluid
     1. Vascular, neoplastic, or other diseases, particularly those involving the temporal lobes and upper brain stem
     2. Cerebral contusion and laceration (traumatic delirium)
     3. Acute purulent and tuberculous meningitis
     4. Subarachnoid hemorrhage
     5. Encephalitis due to viral causes and to unknown causes, e.g., infectious mononucleosis
  C. The abstinence states (after drug intoxications) or postconvulsive states or intoxications—signs of other medical, surgical, and neurologic illnesses being absent or coincidental
     1. Delirium tremens and chronic barbiturate intoxication
     2. Drug intoxications—camphor, caffeine, ergot, bromides, scopolamine, atropine, amphetamine
     3. Postconvulsive delirium
II. Confusion associated with psychomotor underactivity
  A. Associated with a medical or surgical disease (no focal or lateralizing neurologic signs and cerebrospinal fluid clear)
     1. Metabolic disorders: hepatic stupor, uremia, hypoxia, hypercapnia, hypoglycemia, porphyria
     2. Infective fevers—especially typhoid
     3. Congestive heart failure
     4. Postoperative, posttraumatic, and puerperal psychoses
  B. Associated with drug intoxication (no focal or lateralizing signs and cerebrospinal fluid clear) —opiates, barbiturates, bromides, Artane, etc.

C. Associated with diseases of the nervous system (the focal or lateralizing neurologic signs and cerebrospinal fluid changes of this condition are more common than in delirium)
   1. Cerebral vascular disease, tumor, abscess
   2. Subdural hematoma
   3. Meningitis
   4. Encephalitis
   5. Preexisting neurologic disease (e.g., senile dementia) complicated by a medical or surgical disease
III. Beclouded dementia (see Chap. 37 for subdivisions)

DIAGNOSIS AND MANAGEMENT

The first step in diagnosis is to recognize that the patient is confused. This is obvious in most cases, but, as pointed out above, the mildest form of confusion, particularly when some other acute alteration of personality is prominent, may be overlooked. In these mild forms a careful analysis of the patient's thinking as he gives the history of his illness and the details of his personal life will usually reveal an incoherence. The serial subtraction of 7s from 100 is a useful bedside test of the patient's capacity for sustained mental activity. Memory of recent events is one of the most delicate tests of adequate mental function, and may be brought out by having the patient relate all the details of his entry to the hospital, laboratory tests, etc.

Once it is established that the patient is confused, the differential diagnosis must be made between delirium, simple or primary mental confusion, Korsakoff's psychosis, and a beclouded dementia. This can be done usually by careful attention to the patient's degree of alertness and wakefulness, his capacity to solve new problems, his memory, the accuracy of perception, and hallucinations. The presence of Korsakoff's psychosis may not become evident until the patient's general state improves. The distinction between confusional states and dementia is also difficult at times. It has been said that the patient with the acute confusional psychosis has a clouded sensorium; i.e., he is inattentive, and inclined to inaccurate perceptions and hallucinations, whereas the patient with dementia has a clear sensorium. However, it is the authors' impression that many severely demented patients are as beclouded as those with confusional psychoses and that the two conditions are at times indistinguishable, except for their different time courses. All this suggests that the parts of the nervous system affected may be the same in both conditions. When the physician is faced with this problem, the history of the mode of onset becomes of great value. The confusional psychosis has an acute or subacute onset and is usually reversible, whereas dementia is always chronic and tends to be more or less irreversible.

Once a case has been classified as a delirium, a primary mental confusion, or Korsakoff's psychosis, it is important to determine its clinical associations. A thorough medical and neurologic examination and often a lumbar puncture should be done. The other medical and neurologic findings are of great value in indicating the underlying disease which must be treated, and they also give information concerning the prognosis. In the neurologic examination particular attention should be given to language functions, visual fields and visual-spatial discriminations, cortical sensory functions, calculation and other test performances requiring normal functioning of the temporal-parietal-occipital lobes. Confusional states are frequent with diseases of these parts of the brain. Moreover, some of the signs of disease of these parts of the brain are often mistaken for a confusional psychosis.

Schizophrenia and manic-depressive psychosis can usually be separated from the confusional states by the presence of a clear sensorium and good memory.

The treatment is directed to the underlying disease process.

Care of the Delirious Patient. There is an advantage to treating the delirious patient in a general hospital, because he often suffers from a medical disease which can be dealt with more adequately there than in a psychiatric hospital. Furthermore, a delirium seldom lasts more than a few days, and if the patient can be kept on a medical ward, the social stigma which attaches to incarceration in a mental institution is avoided. In the authors' experience only a few delirious patients are so agitated and noisy as to annoy others; if this does happen, many general hospitals now have some facilities for isolating the mentally disturbed patient. Delirium of this severity is rare in infectious diseases but is of course not infrequent in alcoholism (delirium tremens), drug intoxication, and other medical diseases.

The first objectives are to quiet the patient and protect him against injury. A private nurse, an attendant, or a member of the family should be with the patient at all times, if this can be arranged. Depending on how active and confused the patient is, various types of restraint must be employed. If he is extremely active and vigorous, a locked room, screened windows that cannot be opened by the patient, and a low bed or mattress on the floor should be arranged. It is often better to let the patient walk about the room than to tie him into bed which may excite or frighten him so that he struggles to the point of complete exhaustion and collapse. If he is less active, the patient can usually be kept in bed by leather wrist restraints, a restraining sheet, or a net thrown over the bed. Unless contraindicated by the primary disease, the patient should be permitted to sit up or walk about the room part of the day.

All drugs that could possibly be responsible for delirium—particularly opiates, barbiturates, bromides, atropine, hyoscine, cortisone, adrenocorticotropic hormone (ACTH), and salicylates in large doses—should be discontinued. Paraldehyde and chloral hydrate are the only sedatives that can be trusted under these circumstances. Paraldehyde, which is preferred, may be given orally or rectally in doses of 10 to 12 ml. For oral administration, mixing it with fruit juices makes it more palatable, though alcoholic patients will take it in any form and seem to enjoy it. One must be cautious in attempting to suppress the agitation completely. To accomplish this may require the use of very large doses of drugs, and vital functions may be dangerously impaired. The purpose of sedation is to assure rest and sleep so that the patient does not exhaust himself. Continuous warm baths or warm packs are also effective in quieting the delirious patient, but very few general hospitals have proper facilities for this valuable method of treatment.

A fluid intake and output chart should be kept, and any fluid and electrolyte deficit should be corrected according to the methods outlined in Chap. 50. The pulse and blood pressure should be recorded at intervals of 2 hr in anticipation of circulatory collapse, which is sometimes the cause of death, particularly in delirium tremens. In the event of circulatory collapse, transfusions of whole blood and vasopressor drugs may be lifesaving.

Finally, the physician should be aware of many small therapeutic measures which may allay fear and suspicion and reduce the tendency to hallucinations. The room should be kept well lighted, and if possible the patient should not be moved from one room to another. Every procedure should be explained in detail, even such simple ones as the taking of blood pressure or temperature. The presence of a member of the family may be a means of enabling the patient to maintain contact with reality.

It may be some consolation and also a source of professional satisfaction to remember that most delirious patients tend to recover if placed in good hygienic surroundings and competently nursed. The family should be reassured on this point. They must also understand that the abnormal behavior and irrational actions of the patient are not willful but rather are symptomatic of a brain disease.

39 SCHIZOPHRENIA, PARANOIA, PUERPERAL AND ENDOCRINE PSYCHOSES

Justin M. Hope, Dean M. Laird, and Raymond D. Adams

SCHIZOPHRENIA (Dementia Praecox)

The schizophrenic patient, as remarked earlier, often has the appearance of being demented. This is partly because of his bizarre behavior and relative inaccessibility to interview and psychologic test, and also because of an obscure and relatively permanent "mental weakness" which afflicts him in the late stages of the illness.

The differential diagnosis of the dementing brain diseases, as well as of delirium and the confusional psychoses, must therefore always include schizophrenia. Schizophrenia is the most serious unsolved disease in American society, according to "Medical Research: A Midcentury Survey," and merits the thoughtful consideration of all practitioners of medicine.

Definition. Schizophrenia is a disease or group of diseases in which there is a slow, steady deterioration of the personality, beginning usually during adolescence and early adult life and involving particularly the affective life, thinking, conduct, and the depth of insight. The cause is unknown, and no definable neuropathologic changes have been established. A hereditary factor operates in a certain proportion of cases.

Historical Background. Morel, Kahlbaum, Hecker, and Kraepelin wrote the earliest descriptions of the disease. Kraepelin not only separated the disorder from manic-depressive psychosis but also observed that the several different syndromes of hebephrenia, catatonia, and paranoid psychosis were but varieties of this one pathologic process. Bleuler considered the disease misnamed because many cases instead of being "precocious" had their onset later in life and the term dementia did not adequately characterize the fundamental disorder. He considered the main abnormality to be a dissociation of emotional experience and overt behavior, for which the term schizophrenia was proposed.

Cause and Mechanism. Any statement on this subject should begin with the role of heredity. Kallman pointed out in 1952 that "no analysis of a statistically representative group of blood relatives of schizophrenic and manic-depressive patients has so far been completed in any country without showing a significant increase in the expectancy rate for either psychosis." The expectancy rate for schizophrenia in the general population is between 0.7 and 0.9 per cent. The genetic data may be summarized as follows: 11 per cent of 5,000 siblings of schizophrenic patients were found to be suffering from the same disease; in 90 sets of fraternal twins, one of whom had schizophrenia, the disease occurred in the second twin in 11 per cent of cases—the same incidence as in non-twin siblings; in 62 sets of identical, or monozygotic, twins, however, the disease occurred in the second twin in 68 per cent of cases.

The manner in which a genetic factor can operate an interval of time after birth to produce this disease has never been determined. Obviously a genetic mechanism cannot transmit mental experience but only the capacity for having mental experiences. A variety of hypotheses have been advanced but all are as yet unproved. Autointoxication, a metabolic abnormality, an endocrine disorder, an aplasia or hypoplasia of the circulatory system have all had their exponents. Concerning the existence of a metabolic abnormality it may be said that the metabolic rate of cerebral tissue (oxygen uptake) and the total cerebral blood flow are within normal limits. Suggestive evidence of an anti-insulin factor in the blood and urine for schizophrenic patients has been obtained, and at least one investigator is cited as having found a "general cellular difference in carbohydrate metabolism in schizophrenics as compared to normals." So far, however, no convincing data have been forthcoming, and this hypothesis of carbohydrate lack serves only to indicate a possible line of research. A claim was made by Swedish neuropathologists for an insufficiency in the formation of nucleoproteins by the nerve cells in schizophrenic patients, but this too has not been confirmed. In biopsies of the cerebral cortex of schizophrenic patients, analyzed for enzymatic activity, no consistent abnormality has been found. The possibility of an endocrine disorder in schizophrenia has attracted attention. It has been noted that approximately two-thirds of hospitalized schizophrenic patients give an inadequate adrenocortical response to stress, as compared with normal persons. Furthermore, they do not respond by enhanced adrenal cortical secretion to the administration of ACTH. Replacement therapy has not relieved the symptoms, however, and it is not known whether or not the lack of response to ACTH is the result of prolonged inactivity and hospitalization.

The intensified interest in the effects of tranquilizing drugs such as reserpine and chlorpromazine, which have had such remarkable effects in quieting the schizophrenic patient, has led to the suggestion that the parts of the brain upon which these drugs act may be the site of disease in schizophrenia. So far no information of practical value has come from the investigation of this thesis. Nor has the unusual tolerance of the schizophrenic patient for lysergic acid, which produces a peculiar schizoid psychosis in many normal individuals, led to new understanding of the schizophrenic process. Recently reported is a blood factor in schizophrenic patients that will produce a psychotic reaction in normal individuals, but this has not been confirmed. More recently a small molecular substance which is dialyzable and combines loosely with proteins has been isolated from the blood of normal and schizophrenic patients by Hoagland and his associates. This substance when injected into rats previously conditioned to rope climbing abolishes this conditioned response. At present these investigators are working on a method of measurement to ascertain whether this substance is present in greater quantity in schizophrenic than in normal subjects. Many of these studies are open to the criticism that they were done on chronically ill, hospitalized patients. The effects of inactivity, inanition, etc., have not been controlled. At the moment one is forced to accept the conclusion of Kety that it appears to require as much glucose and oxygen "to think an irrational thought as a rational one."

The psychopathologic approach has also been pursued with vigor and with equally unrewarding results. Meyer's psychobiologic formulation of the disease has had wide appeal in this country. The essence of his views was that schizophrenia is due to a progressive maladaptation of the individual to his environment. It is not a disease, therefore, but a number of "reaction types," all with certain common features. Inheritance, physical factors, endocrine disorders, intellectual inadequacy, and other factors, any one or a combination of which may be operative in a given case, interfere with successful adaptation. A "shut-in," "withdrawn," or excessively introverted personality is the consequence of this maladaptation. Early signs of the schizoid personality, as it is called, are an excessive concern about health (hypochondriasis) or other unreasonable fears, a tendency to solitary activities, undue sensitiveness, bashfulness, precocious mental development and occupation with bookish pursuits, persistent juvenile attitudes, prudishness, and selfishness. Personalities of this type are said to be especially liable to schizophrenia, but it would be as reasonable to say that these are the earliest signs of the disease. Various other psychopathologic formulations have been offered by members of the Freudian school, but they merely stress one or other aspect of this abnormal personality development. The reader should refer to textbooks of psychiatry for further information concerning these hypotheses. Needless to say none of them, the psychologic or chemical, has been validated, nor have they been particularly useful in the prevention or treatment of this disease. Most physicians and neurologists have come to regard schizophrenia as a series of clinical syndromes caused by an inherited biochemical disorder of unknown type, affected to varying degrees by environmental circumstance and little influenced by formal psychotherapy.

Neuropathology. Much has been written on the neuropathology of schizophrenia, and a wide variety of abnormalities have been described. They are reviewed in the "Proceedings of the First International Congress of Neuropathology." It is fair to say that no convincing nerve cell loss or neuroglial or other cellular reactions have been demonstrated.

Incidence. Strecker estimated that at least 30,000 individuals develop this disease each year in the United States alone, an occurrence rate of about 25 per 100,000, which is not too different from that of tuberculosis.

Clinical Manifestations. The illness declares itself largely by certain abnormalities of affectivity and thinking which are most clearly demonstrated by an examination of the mental functions of the patient. The medical history has not always been helpful in the authors' experience. It is true, as stated above, that in some cases the family will report a long-standing inability to form warm and satisfactory contacts with people, and a tendency to shun activities of an "outgoing" nature, especially with members of the opposite sex, a disposition to indulge largely in solitary pursuits and daydreaming, all of which are special behavioral abnormalities of the introverted, schizoid, or dystonic type. However, other patients have shown no prepsychotic behavioral abnormality whatsoever.

Primary Signs. The specific and characteristic signs unique to schizophrenia are (1) disturbances in affect, (2) disturbances in thought processes and associations, (3) disturbances in attention.

INAPPROPRIATE OR INADEQUATE AFFECT. In many though not all patients with schizophrenia the affect, or outward expression of emotion, is bland, rigid, inappropriate, or ambivalent. Personal events of serious importance are discussed in a casual manner without any outward show of emotional concern, i.e., *inadequate or bland affect.* The patient may discuss the death of a near relative, the dinner menu, and his admission to the hospital with the same apparent feeling and affect; i.e., the affect is rigid. He may relate that he has been pursued by his enemies or is at the moment about to be killed by a secret machine and, instead of expressing fear and anxiety, he appears faintly amused; i.e., emotional response is inappropriate. A friendly or unfriendly act on the part of a member of the family may fail to excite any response. He appears to be neither pleased nor displeased. As one patient expressed it, "Doctor, when you have had as much experience as I, you will find that strong feelings for and against balance each other, and you do not feel strongly about anything." This emotional response is termed *ambivalent.*

DISTURBANCES IN THINKING AND IDEATIONAL ASSOCIATION. In the patient's spontaneous utterances and in his replies to questions one finds that his thinking about any given topic is apt to be illogical, tangential, and irrelevant. When asked why he came to the hospital the patient may reply, "My brother brought me"; "The doctor suggested it"; "The ambulance brought me"; or "It was the hospital nearest my house." All these statements may have been true, but in each instance there had been a conspicuous behavioral change which had caused the family great concern and had led to the patient's commitment. The reason for admission offered by the patient must thus be considered clearly "peripheral" or tangential. Inappropriate explanations may be offered. A patient seen tearing his shirt to shreds said that he was doing it because it was raining outside—an example of *illogical association.* In conversation, seemingly unrelated and impertinent items may be brought up and even given as answers to direct questions. Such disturbances in thinking are called *associational irrelevancies.*

Not infrequently ideas that would at first appear illogical or irrelevant are actually quite sensible on further analysis. The lack of coherence is often, and may be in nearly all such instances, the result of *associational gaps* or *associational condensation.* In the former the patient makes a series of statements without supplying the connecting details, which he appears to consider unnecessary. One of the authors' patients stated that her present trouble was due to "speech and financial matters"; only after careful questioning was it learned that there had been a heavy financial loss because of poor crops on the farm and that she believed the neighbors to be speaking disparagingly of her and her family. These beliefs were reported to the sheriff who, upon finding them completely fallacious, sent her to a hospital for examination. Another patient said he came to the hospital because "First come best." This proved on further inquiry to indicate a series of ideas that an older brother whom he believed to be persecuting him was always favored by his family. The problem finally came to medical attention when he assaulted the brother with a knife because he had borrowed one of the patient's neckties. Probably this process of associational condensation accounts for some of the neologisms that appear in the speech and writing of schizophrenic patients.

The essence of the thinking disorder in schizophrenia is that the usual cause and effect relationships and the usual method of drawing conclusions from factual evidence are not respected. The thinking is not rambling, incoherent, and chaotic, as in confusional psychoses, but instead appears to be directed inexplicably into certain devious channels. One often has the impression that with time and patient questioning some logical thread could eventually be followed through the disconnected, irrelevant, and distorted ideas; but, communication being limited, this is usually not possible.

DISTURBANCES IN ATTENTION. Often there are lapses in attention or preoccupation with other ideas, and at these times the patient may ignore the questions of the examiner. Later he may respond alertly and focus his attention on the problem at hand and in fact may indicate that he heard the examiner's earlier questions even though he did not reply to them. In the later stages of the illness he appears continuously preoccupied and it is impossible to attract or to hold his attention even momentarily.

Secondary Signs. The term *secondary* denotes those signs which appear to derive from the aforementioned disorders of thinking, emotion, and attention. The most important of these are delusions, hallucinations, rigidity, resistiveness, negativism, and mannerisms. Although not unique to schizophrenia, they occur with sufficient frequency to be of importance, and at times they appear to dominate the clinical picture.

DELUSIONS. These false beliefs in schizophrenic patients are frequently of the *paranoid type.* The paranoid delusion has two components, a grandiose idea of one's own importance and an "idea of persecution." The patient may rationalize his delusion in several ways. Believing himself to be an important person and observing his signal lack of success in competitive life, he assumes that he suffers the fate of many prominent people, that of being persecuted by jealous rivals. Or, conscious of his own inadequacies, he continuously projects the blame on others. In addition, the schizophrenic patient suffers *somatic delusions,* usually beliefs that some part of his body is deteriorating or diseased, and *nihilistic delusions,* in which he denies the existence of himself and of everyone and everything around him. These delusions are related to the primary disorders of thinking but may at times be the most striking feature of the illness.

HALLUCINATIONS. Hallucinations are also a prominent symptom in schizophrenia. They may be auditory, visual, olfactory, or tactile. Unlike the hallu-cinations of delirium, they are usually rather ambiguous psychic phenomena, not always well enough described so that one can be sure of the sensory modality involved; and seldom are they projected into extracorporeal space. The patient admits to hearing voices but often does not state whence they come. In addition, sensory *misinterpretations* also occur. If two individuals are seen talking together, the patient assumes that he is the subject of their conversation and that they are making derogatory remarks about him. A casual gesture, a peculiar odor, an unusual sound are all interpreted as being intended to annoy him. These are called *ideas of reference.* Another unusual and closely related symptom is that in which the patient feels that his thoughts and actions are being controlled by some person or outside agency; these are called *ideas of influence,* or "passivity feelings."

CATATONIA, RESISTIVENESS, AND NEGATIVISM. These are closely related phenomena. The catatonic patient lies immobile and is mute. He may permit himself to be dressed and led about or will sit or stand in one position for hours or days. No effort is made to eat or drink or even to empty the bladder and bowels for long periods of time. There may be incontinence and utter neglect of toilet and dress. This state of speechlessness and motionlessness suggests the possibility of aphasia or anarthria with paralysis, but it is ordinarily recognized for what it is by the lack of pathologic reflexes and the occasional normal movement or speech. Although the limbs may be supple, often attempts at passive movement demonstrate rigidity, which on closer observation suggests a deliberate or willed *resistiveness.* An extreme degree of resistiveness is *negativism,* in which the patient makes an action opposite to the one requested. When asked to open the eyes, he closes them tightly; if requested to protrude the tongue he clenches his jaw; and if told to sit down, he will stand up. These phenomena of immobility, rigidity, resistiveness, and negativism are known collectively as catatonia. The term *stupor* is often added, even though there is no important disorder of consciousness and the patient is able to recount accurately all that transpired during the period of unresponsiveness.

STEREOTYPY OF UTTERANCE AND MOVEMENT, BIZARRE MANNERISMS, GRIMACES. The schizophrenic patient may utter certain words or expressions over and over again. This is termed *echolalia.* Certain movements may be repeated incessantly. The face may be set in a silly expression. Stereotyped, relatively automatic rituals may be reproduced again and again, seemingly dictated by some impulse and without regard as to their appropriateness.

Frequency of the So-called "Primary" and "Secondary" Signs. In order to obtain some notion of the relative incidence of these signs in schizo-phrenia, 30 cases in whom the diagnosis was veri-fied by several psychiatrists were tabulated. Each case was evaluated on the basis of 22 specific points, the ones usually used in mental status ex-aminations. This sample of schizophrenic cases is obviously heavily weighted with those who were suffering from severe and relatively irreversible forms of the disease. Nevertheless, the data are informative. For purposes of comparison the same rating scheme was applied to 30 cases which had been diagnosed as psychosis with cerebral arterio-sclerosis. Most of the latter were probably suffering from senile dementia. Table 39-1 shows the signs which significantly differentiate the two psychoses.

Other Physical Findings. In contrast to these im-portant behavioral abnormalities, other objective neurologic signs are conspicuously absent. Certain difficulties in the interpretation of neurologic find-ings are encountered when contractures have de-veloped in limbs that have been held in one posi-tion for a long time. The extremities then may be edematous and cyanotic, and the tendon reflexes are difficult to elicit. Pinprick or painful stimulation may fail to evoke response from certain areas of the body. Blood pressure is low and the heart small. The circulation time may be reduced. One is also impressed, when a group of these patients are gath-ered together, with the peculiar appearance and dysplastic physique of many of them. However, these abnormalities do not compose a recognizable clinical syndrome.

The Composite Clinical Picture and Natural Course of Schizophrenia. In a large proportion of cases the disease develops slowly and insidiously over a period of months and years during late childhood and adolescence. If the patient is exam-ined at this stage it may be difficult to ascertain the nature of the illness. One may observe only

Table 39-1. SIGNS IN 30 SCHIZOPHRENIC PATIENTS
(N = 30) *

Abnormal signs in sphere of:	No. of patients	Per cent	Standard error of per cent
Affect.................	30	100	0.0
Associations............	28	93.3	−4.57
Thought processes.......	27	90.0	−5.48
Feeling................	25	83.3	−6.81
Perception.............	24	80.0	−7.30
Subjective reorganization	18	60.0	−8.94
Speech................	13	43.3	−9.65
Awareness.............	8	26.7	−8.08
Memory..............	3	10.0	−5.48

* All values are significant at the 0.001 level of con-fidence.

that the patient is vague, suggestible, rather apa-thetic, and uninterested in his daily affairs. In reply to questions, he says repeatedly that he does not know the answer or does not care. He may be excessively preoccupied with his health, a rather unnatural state in adolescents. Often there is an appearance of mild depression. The physician who first examines the patient is apt to make a diagnosis of "nervousness," psychoneurosis, or some obscure medical disease.

The psychiatric nature of the illness becomes evident, as a rule, when the patient expresses overtly some delusional idea or becomes excited and begins to hallucinate. This may be precipitated by an infectious disease or an operation, or may seemingly result from worry or guilt over some problem that has arisen in the home or at school. A scene follows in which the patient attempts to escape, to seclude himself, or to assault someone whom he blames for his predicament. Exception-ally, and this is particularly true of the catatonic syndrome, the illness develops acutely, no ante-cedent symptoms having been known. This clinical state is recognized at once as being the result of a psychiatric illness. Once a diagnosis of schizo-phrenia is reached, it is usually not difficult to distinguish the special form of the disease.

Formerly it was asserted that schizophrenia was a hopeless and incurable disease, but now it is viewed with less pessimism. Some patients make a fairly prompt recovery within a few weeks and remain well thereafter. Of course, one never knows whether the diagnosis was correct, but at least the patient had shown all the usual clinical signs. The remission rate is estimated to be 11 to 20 per cent, but this figure is not applicable to all cases, since it was obtained from a study of discharge rates from psychiatric hospitals and was therefore based on the more severe cases, all of which were treated in some way, even if the treatment amounted to no more than hospitalization. The remissions may be complete or partial. In the latter state the patient leaves the hospital and returns to work but carries on at a reduced level of efficiency and continues to have minor symptoms. Factors said to influence the outcome favorably are early age of onset, a cata-tonic form of illness, acute development of symp-toms, and retention of relatively normal affectivity. The temporary improvement seen in some cases following an intravenous injection of Sodium Amy-tal is said to favor the possibility of a good progno-sis. Of those patients who recover some will later relapse.

Ordinarily the mental illness, once it has devel-oped, progresses for a time and then becomes more or less stationary. Many of the active symptoms of the progressive period subside, and the patient settles down to a custodial existence for the remainder of his life. In this fixed, chronic stage he is often classed as demented or deteriorated. However, the dementia, even in the most advanced stages, differs from that of general paresis and certain other organic brain diseases. If one can allow sufficient time to observe and to interview the patient, he may say or do something which indicates that he is and has been aware of what is going on around him and can also remember recent happenings. Other patients will remain mute, and of course there is no way of judging the quality of their mental activity. Another difference from degenerative brain disease is the potential reversibility of the process, with resumption of adequate psychic function. This phenomenon, admittedly rare in the late stages of the illness, is one of the reasons for calling schizophrenia a "functional psychosis."

Death may rarely occur during a period of intense excitement and excessive psychomotor activity which has lasted several days, and usually no explanation for it is found at autopsy. As a rule, however, the schizophrenic patient lives for many years and eventually dies of some other disease. As he is neglectful of health and nutrition, his age at death is apt to be younger than that of the general population. The coincidence of schizophrenia and of tuberculosis is high.

Special Types of Schizophrenia. The following subtypes are recognized: (1) simple, (2) hebephrenic, (3) catatonic, (4) paranoid, (5) acute undifferentiated, (6) chronic undifferentiated, (7) schizoaffective, (8) childhood, (9) pseudoneurotic. Of these, the physician should be familiar with the paranoid and catatonic varieties since they may have an acute onset at times while the patient is in the hospital for some other illness. The simple and hebephrenic forms are usually seen in the population of patients found in a mental hospital. The essential features of each type are listed below.

Simple. This form, the most difficult to diagnose, is manifested chiefly by a reduction in interests and by impoverishment of social relationships. Often the patient appears simply to have adjusted at a lower psychobiologic level. Apathy and indifference mark all his behavior and are rarely accompanied by delusions or hallucinations. The onset is often so insidious that one hardly can decide when the patient who is regarded as eccentric began to be psychotic. Once the symptoms develop, they may gradually increase in severity over long periods, usually ending with apparent mental deterioration. This condition must be distinguished from the schizoid personality, in which abnormal character traits seem not to interfere with education and work.

Hebephrenic. This is characterized by shallow, inappropriate affect, unpredictable giggling, silly behavior and mannerisms, delusions that are often of a somatic nature, hallucinations, and regressive behavior.

Catatonic. Motor abnormalities such as stupor, mutism, negativism, and waxy flexibility or excessive activity and excitement are characteristic. The patient may improve or regress to a more or less vegetative state in which he remains for long periods of time.

Paranoid. Here autistic, unrealistic thinking, delusions of persecution and grandeur, ideas of reference, and often hallucinations are the leading clinical findings. Often behavior is unpredictable, with a prevailing attitude of hostility and aggression. There may be excessive concern over religion, with or without delusions of persecution, and expansive delusions of omnipotence, genius, or special ability.

Acute Undifferentiated. This category includes cases exhibiting a wide variety of schizophrenic symptomatology such as confusion of thinking and turmoil of emotion, ideas of reference, fear and dream states, and dissociative phenomena. Like catatonia, these symptoms appear acutely, often without apparent precipitating stress. There may have been prodromal symptoms of similar type. Very often the reaction is accompanied by a pronounced deviation of mood, either excitement or depression. The symptoms may subside in a few weeks but may later recur. If the reaction subsequently progresses, it ordinarily crystallizes into one of the other definable reaction types.

Chronic Undifferentiated. In this syndrome, which is one of the most frequent, there is a mixed symptomatology that does not conform to any of the more clearly defined types of schizophrenia. The so-called "late," "incipient," "prepsychotic" schizophrenic reactions usually fall in this category.

Schizoaffective. This category is intended for those cases showing significant admixtures of schizophrenic and manic-depressive reactions. The mental content may be predominantly schizophrenic, with pronounced elation or depression; or predominantly affective changes may be complicated by schizophrenic-like thinking or bizarre behavior. The "prepsychotic personality" may be at variance with the predominant trend of the illness. On prolonged observation, such cases usually prove to be schizophrenic.

Childhood. The schizophrenic reactions occurring before puberty are placed in this category. The clinical picture may differ from schizophrenic reactions occurring in other age periods because of the immaturity and plasticity of the patient at the time of onset of the reaction. Psychotic reactions in

Table 39-2. DIFFERENTIAL DIAGNOSIS OF MAJOR PSYCHIATRIC SYNDROMES

Syndrome	Mental status examination	Physical examination
Anxiety neuroses	Restless Tense Anxious Sighing respirations Voluble	Few abnormal physical findings, including: High resting pulse rate Respiratory rate over 20 Tremor of fingers Hyperactive tendon reflexes
Hysteria	Overtalkative Friendly, ingratiating manner Emotional response—casual, objective, indifferent, or anxious Chief complaint—nonspecific, multiple, or irrelevant Symptoms described in dramatic, histrionic fashion	Weakness or paralysis of arm and leg or both legs Hemianesthesia, aphonia, blindness No objective physical findings
Psychasthenia	Affect appropriate Motor activity—restless, tense, and anxious Vasomotor overactivity—blushing and sweating Associations—direct and to the point Mental content—obsessions, compulsions, and phobias No formal thought disorder Evidence of concern or depression of mood in relation to symptoms	Facial and respiratory or other tics but usually no other abnormal physical findings
Depression	Facial expression—plaintive, troubled, or anguished Mood—depressed, discouraged, "blue," "unhappy," "low in spirits," "glum," "morbid" Speech—retarded to point of mutism or push of speech with restricted content Motor activity—decreased to point of stupor or accelerated to point of agitation Content—pessimistic thoughts; fear of cancer or other serious disease, self-depreciation, self-accusation, feeling of inferiority or guilt, somatic delusions, e.g., "rotting," "blood dried up" Suicidal preoccupation or attempts Abstract judgment colored by depressed mood Personal judgment present or absent Nihilistic delusions and hallucinations consistent with morbid mood in severe cases Thought processes, mood, and affect parallel	Signs of neglect and dehydration may be present in cases of severe depression Weight loss, severe constipation
Mania	Mood—happy, elated, exalted—"feel good," "best ever" Stream of speech—rapid, digressible, with flight of ideas Motor activity—increased, great activity, may be increased to point of incessant activity Affect—mercurial, rapidly changing through euphoria, exaltation, irritability, and violent anger Content—consistent with elevated mood and may embrace overconfidence, exaggerated self-esteem, and delusions of grandeur Unsystematized paranoid delusions may occur Impairment of judgment or insight	Signs of dehydration may be present
Dementia	Change in personality (by history) Intellectual impairment Disturbances in orientation Defective intellectual capacity and grasp Disturbance in clarity of thinking Memory impairment, particularly for recent events Distractibility of attention Perseveration in speech, actions, and thoughts Blunting of moral and ethical standards (by history) Lability of emotional response, vacillating from depression, elation, or irritability to violent anger	Signs consistent with basic disease process Dysarthria Aphasic disturbances Sphincter disturbances Signs of focal brain disease are evidenced by pyramidal, extrapyramidal, or cranial nerve disturbance

Table 39-2. DIFFERENTIAL DIAGNOSIS OF MAJOR PSYCHIATRIC SYNDROMES (*Continued*)

Syndrome	Mental status examination	Physical examination

Delirium	Facial expression perplexed, bewildered
	Clouding of sensorium
	Attention—distractible and poorly sustained; span increased (increased vigil)
	Perceptual disturbance—illusions, hallucinations (visual, auditory, or olfactory)
	Delusions—dictated by perceptual impairment
	Affect parallels perceptual content and is usually apprehensive, anxious, or fearful
	Upon recovery there is amnesia for the illness
		Autonomic overactivity
		  Flushed face
		  Rapid pulse
		  Fever
		  Sweating
		  Dilated pupils
		Usually no focal neurologic signs
		Tremor of extremities

Primary mental confusion	Facial expression—perplexed Confusion in relationship to external stimuli Attention—detached, preoccupied—span restricted (decreased vigil) Perceptual disturbance—illusions and hallucinations Delusions—consistent with perceptual disturbance Affect—concerned or fearful Motor activity usually slowed—may be retarded to point of stupor	Consistent with disease process, or exogenous, noxious agent responsible for condition
Schizophrenia	Disturbance in affect—bland, rigid, or inappropriate Disturbance in associations—vague, tangential, irrelevant, or neologistic Impairment of insight—nil Thought processes—shallow, illogical, or fragmented Feeling—occasionally tense and anxious but usually phlegmatic, dull, or apathetic Delusions—paranoid, somatic, nihilistic, ideas of influence and reference Hallucinations—visual, auditory, olfactory—usually not vivid Emotional response does not parallel thought processes	There are no physical signs directly related to the disease process
Psychopathic personality	History of poor social adjustment, poor work record, civilian arrests, suicidal attempts, proved theft, chronic alcoholism, and failure to advance in army or civilian life Usual reason for referral—behavioral disturbances and/or multiple somatic complaints Examination—voluble, plausible, friendly, and oversolicitous—tendency to explain away difficulties in terms of misfortune or a fault of others Longitudinal history reveals conspicuous inability to profit by experience	There are no physical signs directly related to the disease process
Post-partum psychosis	Onset 4 to 10 days following delivery Facial expression—somber, dejected, puzzled, or bewildered Emotional reaction—depressed Attention—preoccupied Awareness—restricted or perplexed. Depersonalization or derealization may be present Motor activity—increased to point of agitation or decreased to point of stupor Speech stream shows blocking and paucity of ideas Hallucinations and delusions Retrograde, amnesia may be present Insight lacking Confusion	Physical signs present are those of the normal post-partum state, viz., breast engorgement, subinvolution of the uterus, and lochia. In many cases there is evidence of dehydration, shown by dryness of lips, mucous membranes, and skin

children manifesting primarily autism (tendency to preoccupation with dreams, fantasies, and ruminations) are classified here. Cases of this type are at present often classified as *Heller's syndrome.*

Pseudoneurotic. The presence of numerous neurotic symptoms including anxiety attacks, gross hysterical symptoms, somatic preoccupation, phobias, obsessions, and compulsions occurring in a patient with few cardinal symptoms of schizophrenia distinguishes the condition as the pseudoneurotic form of the disease.

Patients with any of the above conditions may improve sufficiently to be able to get along in the community, yet continue to show recognizable residual symptoms in thinking and affectivity. Such cases are classed as *schizophrenia, residual type.*

Differential Diagnosis. Already it has been pointed out that the schizoid or mildly schizophrenic individual is often considered nervous, eccentric, or psychoneurotic. At this early stage the disturbances in thinking and affect so characteristic of schizophrenia are not recognized. The illness presented by the acutely excited or "stuporous" schizophrenic must be distinguished from mania, severe depression, acute confusional psychoses and delirium, and some of the endocrine psychoses. Here a common source of error in the very disturbed, speechless patient is to misdiagnose a rapidly advancing brain disease as schizophrenia. The authors have seen hypoxic encephalopathy, encephalitis, lipoid-storage disease, Schilder's disease, brain tumor, and epileptic psychoses all mistaken for schizophrenia. The usual source of error has been that the patient was mute and resistive and, because of muteness, it had been impossible to evaluate thinking and emotional reactions. Chronic alcoholic hallucinosis and paranoid schizophrenia are easily confused. In fact the authors have not been able to separate them except by the knowledge of their mode of onset and the history of prolonged alcoholism before the illness. The deteriorated schizophrenic must be distinguished from the patient with true dementia. Schizophrenic patients who exhibit rigid attitudes and postures must be differentiated from those who suffer basal ganglion diseases. (See Table 39-2 for differential diagnosis.)

Many of the above errors can be avoided if one insists that at least three of the following mental signs—disturbance of affect, disturbance of insight, disturbance in ideational association, perceptual disorders, and abnormality in subject-object differentiation—be present. If these signs alone are manifested, a diagnosis of *simple schizophrenia* is justified. If in addition the patient has persecutory delusions, grandiose ideas, and hallucinations, a more specific diagnosis of paranoid schizophrenia is assured. The addition of negativism, resistiveness, rigidity, and apparent "stupor" categorizes the case as one of catatonic schizophrenia; while the conjunction of mannerisms, inappropriate laughter, giggling, immature emotional development places it in the group of hebephrenic schizophrenia. Finally, it is only proper to say that until such time as some reliable and incontrovertible test for schizophrenia is developed, diagnosis will always be uncertain in many cases.

Treatment and Management. The management of the schizophrenic patient is difficult, and in most instances it is best to refer him to a psychiatrist. Mild cases may be cared for by a general physician and undoubtedly many of them are under a mistaken diagnosis. However, once the patient has had a frankly psychotic episode, hospitalization is usually necessary, and some advantage to the patient and his family accrues from establishing a relationship with a psychiatrist who has had experience with this type of case.

Several new methods of therapy have been introduced in recent years. They have been difficult to evaluate because of uncertainty as to the natural course of the illness. The most important have been custodial treatment and psychotherapy, insulin coma, electric or Metrazol therapy, lobotomy, chlorpromazine, and reserpine, and other new drugs collectively termed "tranquilizers." The results obtained by these methods are summarized in Table 39-3.

From these data it is obvious that schizophrenia is a serious disease and one for which there is no specific therapy. The older methods of prolonged institutional or custodial care have resulted in fewer remissions than vigorous supportive treatment in a more natural hospital environment. The tranquilizing drugs are opening a new field of therapy and may provide fresh insight into the nature of the basic process.

Table 39-3. EFFECTS OF VARIOUS TYPES OF THERAPY EMPLOYED IN SCHIZOPHRENIA

Type of therapy	No. of patients	Complete remission and social remission, per cent
Custodial and supportive treatment	11,080	19
Convulsive therapy	7,357	29
Insulin coma	9,433	43
Lobotomy	1,211	18
Chlorpromazine	1,517	34
Reserpine	897	22

PARANOIA AND PARANOID REACTIONS

Already it has been pointed out that suspiciousness and distrustfulness are distortions of thinking which may occur as symptoms of several clinical syndromes, particularly depressive psychosis and schizophrenia, and sometimes in dementing diseases. More important from the viewpoint of the general physician is the not infrequent occurrence of an acute paranoid syndrome during the course of a focal or systemic infection, or following an operation. This condition has also been observed in military personnel who suffer extreme fatigue (combat psychosis). Only upon the closest examination will it be noted that these patients are not perfectly oriented as to their present surroundings, are unable to recollect the details of all that has happened in the preceding days, are disorganized in their activities, and sleep relatively little. These facts, once established, enable one to recognize the illness as an example of either an acute confusional psychosis or a mild delirium, and proper use of sedation and careful nursing usually result in a gratifying recovery within a few weeks. Certainly these several different conditions should always come to mind whenever ideas of self-reference and delusions of persecution are observed.

There is, however, another group of illnesses, relatively rare to be sure, in which an elaborate, systematized delusion of persecution develops insidiously in middle or late adult life and is not accompanied by any other psychical abnormality. Such individuals are said to be suffering from a strange malady called *paranoia*. Limitations of space do not permit further discussion of this condition. The interested reader should refer to one of the textbooks of psychiatry.

PUERPERAL OR POST-PARTUM PSYCHOSIS

This psychosis is difficult to classify. It resembles in some respects either schizophrenia or manic-depressive psychosis but also has features peculiar to delirium and the acute confusional psychoses. It is mentioned here with schizophrenia because this is the condition with which it is most likely to be confused in clinical medicine.

THE ENDOCRINE PSYCHOSES

One of the most provocative discoveries in the field of psychiatry in contemporary times is that relatively normal individuals may become psychotic when they develop hyper- or hypothyroidism, Cushing's disease, or adrenal insufficiency, or receive therapeutic doses of ACTH. If these conditions were no more than examples of drug-induced psychosis, they would be interesting enough. The fact is, however, that they differ considerably from the usual toxic delirium or confusional state. The syndrome, reminiscent of puerperal psychosis and some cases of "combat psychosis" seen during the Second World War, comprises features that are suggestive of a manic-depressive psychosis or schizophrenia on the one hand and of the confusional psychoses on the other. These endocrine psychoses have far-reaching medical significance, for they provide experimental models of psychoses that can be created by the manipulation of metabolic factors.

ACTH and Cortisone Psychoses. This psychiatric syndrome is now occurring far less frequently than when these hormones were first introduced into medicine. Presumably the products are now more refined and there are more reliable data as to safe dosage. The psychosis usually develops over a period of a few days after the patient has received the hormone for one or more weeks. The features are extremely variable. Some of the patients become elated, euphoric, excited, and talkative, as though under pressure to speak while others are mute. Thinking may be confused, illogical, tangential, and incoherent. Hallucinations and sensory misinterpretations may appear. The prevailing emotional response varies from apathy to anxiety and panic, depression, or elation. Although mental confusion is not prominent, the state of awareness is not altogether normal, and at times the patient is frankly bewildered. In the motor sphere there may be incessant activity or immobility, resistiveness, and even negativism verging on catatonia. Clouding of the sensorium, disorientation, and confusion, the hallmarks of deliria and the confusional psychoses, have not been prominent in the ACTH and cortisone psychoses. Once established, these psychoses have lasted for several weeks and recovery has been complete. Usually the hormone was stopped as soon as the diagnosis was established.

The mechanism of this psychosis is not known. From the few available studies it has been learned that the occurrence of the psychosis is not related to the premorbid personality. Although the dosage of ACTH or cortisone has usually been high, there has been no exact correlation between dose level and the occurrence, severity, and duration of the psychosis. The mental disturbance appears unrelated to the rapidity and intensity of the therapeutic response to ACTH and cortisone.

Thyroid Psychoses. A great deal has been said and written about the pervasive effects of abnormal thyroid function on all organs including the neuromuscular apparatus and central nervous system. These effects are discussed in the chapters on endocrine disease.

The hyperthyroid patient often shows minor changes in his emotions and mentation. Restlessness, irritability, apprehension, emotional lability, and even at times agitation may occur. Either of two trends may be observed in the relatively rare psychotic thyroid patient. There may be mania with its characteristic increase in psychomotor activity, overtalkativeness, flight of ideas; or depression with its somber mood, weeping, and agitation. Visual and auditory hallucinations are present in both groups of cases. The clinical picture is seldom clear. Usually the psychiatrist finds something more than simple mania or agitated depression, usually some clouding of the sensorium with perplexity and confusion suggestive of delirium. The condition is said to be related to the premorbid personality, some personality types being more vulnerable, but this point is disputed. The condition is not directly related to the level of the basal metabolic rate. Careful studies of cerebral blood flow and cerebral metabolism during and after the psychosis have not been done. Treatment of hyperthyroidism does not result in prompt arrest of the psychic disorder, but usually recovery takes place over a period of months. One must distinguish this illness from other types of recurrent psychosis which happen to coincide with or be precipitated by hyperthyroidism.

With myxedema there is also a characteristic slowness and thickness of speech, mental dullness, listlessness and apathy, irritability, and sometimes suspiciousness. This can usually be distinguished from depression by the lack of definite melancholia and the presence of a memory disturbance particularly for recent events. The cerebrospinal fluid total protein is usually elevated. Reduced cerebral blood flow and cerebral metabolism have been found, and with improvement on therapy these functions are restored to normal.

Other Endocrine Psychoses. Mental aberrations have been observed in Cushing's disease and Addison's disease. They are rare, and because of limitations of space the reader is referred to the current medical literature for references on the subject.

REFERENCES

American Foundation: "Medical Research: A Midcentury Survey," Boston, Little, Brown & Company, 1956.

Bleuler, E.: "Textbook of Psychiatry," English ed. by A. A. Brill, New York, The Macmillan Company, 1934.

Kraepelin, E.: Dementia Praecox, translated from "Textbook of Psychiatry," 8th German ed., Edinburgh, E. J. Livingstone, 1918.

40 AFFECTIONS OF SPEECH
Raymond D. Adams

Language or speech functions are of fundamental significance to man, both in his social intercourse and in his private intellectual life; and when disordered as a consequence of developmental anomaly or disease of the brain, the resultant physiologic loss exceeds all others in gravity—even blindness, deafness, and lameness.

The physician is concerned with all derangements of language function, including those of reading and writing, because they are the source of much unhappiness and disability and are almost invariably the manifestations of disease of the brain. Furthermore, language is the means whereby the patient communicates his complaints and his feelings to his physician and, at the same time, the medium for that interpersonal transaction between physician and patient which we call psychotherapy. Any disease process which interferes with speech or the understanding of spoken words touches the very core of the patient-doctor relationship. Finally, the clinical study of language disorders serves to illuminate the abstruse relationship between psychologic functions and the anatomy and physiology of the cerebrum. Language mechanisms fall halfway between the well-localized sensorimotor functions and the complex mental functions, such as imagination and thinking, which cannot be localized.

GENERAL CONSIDERATIONS

It has often been remarked that man's commanding position in the world rests on the possession of two faculties: (1) his ability to employ verbal symbols as a "background for his own ideation" and as a means of transmitting his thoughts to others of his kind and (2) the remarkable facility for the use of his hands. One curious and provocative fact is that the evolution of both speech and manual dexterity occurs in relationship to neurophysiologic pathways located in one cerebral hemisphere. This is a departure from nearly all other localizable neurophysiologic patterns, which are organized according to a bilateral and symmetrical plan. This dominance of one cerebral hemisphere, usually the left, emerges with speech and the preference for the right hand, especially in writing; and a lack of development or loss of cerebral dominance as a result of disease entails a disturbance of both these traits.

There is abundant evidence that higher animals are able to communicate with each other by vocalization and gestures. However, the content of their communication is their feeling tone of the moment.

This emotional language, as it is called, was studied by Charles Darwin, who noted that it underwent increasing differentiation in the animal kingdom. Similar instinctual patterns of emotional expression are observed in man. In fact they are the earliest type of speech to appear (in infancy) and may have been the first to develop in primitive man. Moreover, the language we use to express joy, anger, and fear is retained even after destructive lesions of the dominant cerebral hemisphere. The neural arrangements which subserve emotional expression are bilateral and symmetrical and do not depend on the cerebrum. The experiments of Cannon and Bard have amply demonstrated that emotional expression is possible in animals after the removal of both cerebral hemispheres, provided the diencephalon, and particularly the hypothalamus and lower parts of the neuraxis, remain undamaged. In the human infant emotional expression is well developed at a time when the cerebral cortex is still immature.

Propositional or symbolic speech differs from emotional speech in several ways. Instead of communicating feeling it is a means of transferring ideas from one person to another and requires in its development the substitution of a series of sounds or marks for objects or concepts. This type of speech is not found in animals nor in the human infant. It is not instinctive but learned, and is therefore subject to all the modifying influences of social and cultural environments. However, the learning process becomes possible only after the nervous system has reached a certain degree of development. Facility in symbolic language, which is acquired over a period of 15 to 20 years, depends, then, on both maturation of the nervous system and education.

THE DEVELOPMENT OF LANGUAGE

The acquisition of symbolic language by the infant and child has been observed methodically by a number of eminent scientists, and their findings provide a basis for understanding the various derangements of speech.

First there is the *babbling* or *lalling stage* during which the infant a few weeks of age emits a variety of sounds in combinations of vowel and labial or nasoguttural consonants. This predominantly motor speech activity is no doubt stimulated and reinforced by auditory sensations which become linked to the kinesthetic ones arising from the speech musculature. It is not clear whether the capacity to hear and understand the spoken word precedes or follows the first motor speech. Possibly it varies from one infant to another, and certainly both speaking and auditory reception of words develop

very early in life. Soon babbling gives way to *echo speech*, in which the infant repeats parrot-like whatever he hears. Thereafter auditory, visual, and kinesthetic sensations are gradually combined, and a sound comes to stand for or symbolize an object. Nouns are learned first, then verbs and other parts of speech. Single words and groups of words are used meaningfully in thinking and talking. They form propositions which, according to Hughlings Jackson, are the very essence of speech. By the age of eighteen to twenty-four months the average infant can construct a phrase; in the months and years which follow, he learns to speak in full sentences. A six-year-old child has a speaking vocabulary of several thousand words and an even larger understanding vocabulary.

The child is now ready for the next stage, reading. This involves the association of graphic symbols with the auditory, visual, and kinesthetic images of words that have already been acquired. Writing is learned soon after reading, and word symbols must become linked to cursive movements of the hand. Only those destined to become literate learn to read and write; and to be a complete master of the art of writing is an attainment of only a few select members of our society.

Language development proceeds in an orderly manner, but there are individual variations in the actual time at which each successive stage is reached, and to a limited extent in the order of the different stages. The pattern appears to be set by the neurologic equipment of the individual at any given age. Psychologic factors are of minor importance, at least in the beginning. There is, therefore, good reason why educators have found it unprofitable to teach reading and writing before the sixth year.

Anthropologists have suggested that the individual merely recapitulates the language development of his race. It is supposed that gestures and the utterance of simple meaningful sounds first occurred in primitive man as a differentiation of emotional speech. Gradually these movements and sounds became the conventional signs and verbal symbols of concrete objects, then of the abstract qualities of objects. Signs and spoken language were the first means of human communication; graphic records appeared much later. The American Indian, for instance, never reached the stage of a written language. Writing commenced as pictorial representation, and only much later were alphabets devised. The reading and writing of words and propositions have been relatively recent developments.

The increasing importance of language in contemporary society may be overlooked unless we reflect on the proportion of man's time devoted to purely verbal pursuits. *External speech*, by which we mean the expression of thoughts by spoken and written words and reception of the thoughts of others, is an almost continuous activity when human beings are gathered together; and *internal speech*, or the formation in our minds of unuttered words on which it depends, is the "coin of mental commerce." The latter goes on even during man's preoccupation, when he is apt to think in words and may, in doing so, subconsciously utter words.

THE ANATOMY OF THE LANGUAGE FUNCTIONS

The conventional teaching is that there are four language areas, situated, in the majority of individuals, in the left cerebral hemisphere (Fig. 37-1). Two are receptive and two are executive. One of the former, an area where the neural mechanisms for auditory memory images of words are said to be located, is situated in the posterior part of the first and second temporal convolutions (areas 41 and 42) near the auditory receptive area in Heschl's convolution; the other is for the visual memory, i.e., images of words, and occupies the angular convolution (area 39) in the inferior parietal lobule, near the areas concerned with vision. The intervening area between auditory and visual word centers (area 37), the posterior part of the temporal lobe and the supramarginal convolution, is believed also to be concerned with language formulation. Of the executive areas, one at the posterior end of the third frontal convolution (usually referred to as Broca's convolution or area 44) is for motor speech, and the other, situated at the foot of the second frontal convolution above Broca's area, is for writing. These sensory and motor areas are connected by nerve fibers which pass through the subcortical white matter, the isthmus of the temporal lobe, and the external capsule of the lenticular nucleus. They are also connected with the thalamus and to corresponding areas in the minor cerebral hemisphere through the corpus callosum and anterior commissure.

There has been much difference of opinion concerning these cortical areas, and objection has been made to calling them centers, for they do not represent circumscribed neural structures of constant function and fixed localization. Actually there is almost no exact information concerning the anatomy and physiology of these areas. A competent neuroanatomist could not distinguish under the microscope the cortical speech areas from other parts of the cerebral cortex. Electrical stimulation of the parts of the cortex concerned with speech while the patient is alert and talking (during craniotomy under local anesthesia) causes only an arrest of speech. Knowledge of the location of speech functions has come almost exclusively from the study of human beings who have succumbed to focal brain diseases. From the available information it seems almost certain that the whole language mechanism is not divisible into a number of parts, each depending on a certain fixed group of neurones. Instead, speech must be regarded as a sensorimotor process roughly localized in the opercular region of the left cerebral hemisphere, and the more complex elaborations of speech probably depend on the entire cerebrum.

Henschen, in a monograph consisting of three large volumes, collected the clinical and pathologic findings in all the 1,500 cases of aphasia in the literature published prior to 1920, and included 60 of his own. These and other concepts of speech have recently been reviewed by Brain in "Neurology," by Wilson and Bruce. Some of the more crucial pieces of anatomic evidence have been summarized in the valuable monograph of Nielsen and are of such fundamental importance that they have been itemized below.

1. Hemispherectomy, i.e., ablation or destruction of all the speech areas in the left cerebral hemisphere, was recorded in 18 cases. There was complete or almost complete inability to speak in 14 cases, and in only 1 was this function preserved. Reading and writing were lost in every case. Comprehension of spoken language was abolished in 10 cases and was fair to excellent in the other 8.

2. Destruction of Broca's area and, to a variable extent, of the adjacent cortex and the subcortical white matter was recorded in 43 cases. There was loss of the power to speak in 25; in the other 18, although this power was reduced at first, recovery was fair to complete. Approximately half these cases were unable to write (agraphia). Comprehension of spoken and written language was affected only slightly in most cases.

3. Temporal lobectomy, either surgical for tumor or pathologic (due to occlusive vascular disease), was recorded in 10 cases. Comprehension of spoken language was lost in all except 1 case. Spontaneous speech was poor in 6 and fair in 4 cases. Only 2 of the 10 were able to read after the lesion had developed. Paraphasia (the substitution of an inappropriate word for the intended word in speech) was present in 8 of the 10 cases, in contrast to the cases with hemispherectomy, where it was not observed.

4. Bilateral destruction of the superior and middle temporal convolution was recorded in 4 cases. There was retention of hearing because the transverse convolution of Heschl was preserved on one or both sides. All subjects were unable to comprehend spoken words (word deafness). There was agraphia in 2 cases, without disturbance of

reading. Spontaneous speech was only slightly impaired.

5. Destruction of the inferior parietal lobe involving the supramarginal and adjacent parts of the superior temporal convolution was recorded in 7 cases. All patients except 1 lost the ability to read, and all were unable to write. Spontaneous speech was fair. Understanding of spoken words was impaired in some cases, and paraphasia was noted in several.

6. Lesions of the isthmus of the temporal lobe, according to Nielsen's own studies, have abolished spontaneous speech and writing and have also produced an inability to comprehend spoken or written words. There was a homonymous hemianopia in nearly every case.

7. Lesions in the insular cortex, external capsule, and putamen were recorded in 12 cases. In all there was a loss of spontaneous speech, an inability to write, and paraphasia. Reading ability was reduced in some cases; spoken language was understood fairly well.

From these clinical and pathologic data it may be concluded that the locus of the anatomic lesion is more significant than the extent of brain damage. However, localization is not specific. Several cases with lesions in Broca's area did not suffer the same disturbance of speech. This lack of consistency in the anatomy of any given speech disorder has engaged the attention of many students of aphasia and several different hypotheses have been proposed for its explanation. The "classic" one has been that the net effect of any lesion depends on the degree of cerebral dominance. If cerebral dominance is poorly established, a left-sided lesion has less effect on speech than if dominance is strong. Unfortunately, handedness and cerebral dominance were not recorded in many of Henschen's cases.

CEREBRAL DOMINANCE AND ITS RELATIONSHIP TO SPEECH AND HANDEDNESS

The functional supremacy of one cerebral hemisphere is so crucial to language function that it must be considered in greater detail. There are three ways of determining that the left side of the brain is dominant: (1) the loss of speech when disease occurs in the left hemisphere and its preservation in diseases involving the right hemisphere; (2) the greater facility in the use of the right hand, foot, and eye; (3) the arrest of speech immediately after the injection of amobarbital (Sodium Amytal) or some other drug in one of the internal carotid arteries. Only (2) and (3) are of use in deciding the cerebral dominance of a living and healthy patient.

Of the general population approximately 90 to 95 per cent are right-handed; the remainder prefer the left hand. A person is said to be right-handed if he chooses the right hand for intricate, skilled acts and is more skillful with it. The preference is more complete in some than others. Most individuals are neither completely right-handed nor completely left-handed, but use one hand for most complicated tasks and the other for other tasks. Orton refers to this as *intergrading*. The manner in which dextrality and sinistrality are acquired is of interest. Most infants and small children are ambidextrous in their first actions. Writing may be carried out with either hand at first, and "mirror writing" at this stage is frequent. Between the ages of two and six years one hand and one foot are selected for throwing and kicking a ball, sawing a board, cutting bread, etc. By middle childhood there is usually no doubt as to the dominant side. The reason for hand preference is still controversial. There is strong evidence of a hereditary factor, but the mode of inheritance is uncertain. Learning is also a factor; many children are shifted at an early age from left to right (shifted sinistrals) because it is a handicap to be left-handed in a right-handed world. Many right-handed people sight with the right eye, and it has been said that eye preference determines hand preference. Even if true this still does not account for eye dominance. It is noteworthy that handedness develops simultaneously with language, and the most that can be said at present is that speech localization and the preference for one eye, one hand, and one foot are both manifestations of some fundamental and inherited tendency not yet defined. There is no observable anatomic difference between the dominant and the minor cerebral hemispheres except that the occipital horn of the left lateral ventricle is usually larger than the right, and the left sulcus lunatus more prominent. No consistent differences in the electroencephalogram between the two hemispheres has been found.

Left-handedness may result from disease of the left cerebral hemisphere in early life, and this probably accounts for its higher incidence amongst the feebleminded and brain-injured. Presumably the neural mechanisms for language become centered in the right cerebral hemisphere. Handedness and cerebral dominance may fail to develop in some individuals, and this is particularly true in certain families. Developmental defects in speech and reading, stuttering, "mirror writing," and general clumsiness are much more frequent in these families.

Differences in degree of cerebral dominance do unquestionably account for some of the inconsistency in the cerebral localization of speech in different individuals.

TYPES OF LANGUAGE DISORDER ENCOUNTERED IN MEDICINE

These can be divided into four categories. (1) Disturbances of speech which occur with diseases which affect the higher nervous integrations, viz., delirium and dementia. Speech is seldom lost in these conditions, but is instead merely deranged as part of a general impairment of intellectual functions. *Palilalia* and *echolalia*, in which the patient repeats, parrot-like, the syllables and words which he hears, are special abnormalities usually observed in states of dementia with extrapyramidal signs. (2) The loss or disturbance of speech due to a cerebral lesion that does not deprive a man of his reason or paralyze other motor or sensory functions. This condition has been termed *aphasia;* milder degrees of it have been called *dysphasia.* (3) A defect in articulation with intact mental functions and normal comprehension and memory of words. This is a pure motor disorder of the muscles of articulation and may be due to flaccid or spastic paralysis, rigidity, repetitive spasms (stuttering), or ataxia. The term *anarthria* or *dysarthria* has been applied to these conditions. (4) A loss of voice due to disease of the larynx or its innervation, with resulting *aphonia* or *dysphonia.* Articulation and internal language are unaffected.

In the practice of medicine the most frequent and troublesome disorders of speech are aphasia, stuttering, dysarthria, and aphonia. The remainder of this chapter will be devoted to these clinical problems and their diagnostic significance.

Types of Aphasia

The following tests will usually make it possible to decide whether the patient has a *global aphasia* (with loss of all or nearly all speech functions), an *expressive* or *motor aphasia* (sometimes called verbal, or executive, or Broca's aphasia), or a receptive aphasia (Wernicke's aphasia) predominantly of either auditory or visual type. Writing is disturbed to some extent in the majority of cases of aphasia and is not separately deranged.

Global (Central) Aphasia. This is due to a lesion which destroys a large part of the speech areas of the major cerebral hemisphere. It is most commonly due to occlusion of the left internal carotid or middle cerebral artery, but an infiltrative tumor or other lesion may also cause this syndrome. The middle cerebral artery nourishes all the speech areas, and nearly all aphasic disorders due to vascular occlusion are caused by involvement of this artery or its branches. The only exceptions are (1) Heubner's recurrent branch of the left anterior cerebral artery, which supplies the subcortical white matter of the frontal lobe; occlusion of it is said to cause subcortical motor aphasia; and (2) the temporal branch of the posterior cerebral artery, which supplies part of area 37; occlusion of this may rarely cause a difficulty in the visual recognition of words and amnesic aphasia, i.e., an inability to name objects seen. In many cases of global aphasia the patient is unable to say more than a few words, cannot read or write, and can at most understand a few simple spoken words and phrases. Recovery depends on the nature and extent of the disease and whether or not the right cerebral hemisphere had previously engaged in language formulation and expression. If the left hemisphere was strongly dominant there will usually be no recovery, a fact which casts doubt on the popular notion that the right hemisphere can take over speech function.

Expressive Aphasia. This condition is due to a lesion in the posterior part of the inferior or third frontal convolution, the subcortical white matter of the insula, or the external capsule of the lenticular nucleus. Softening due to occlusion of branches of the middle cerebral artery is a more frequent cause than neoplasm or trauma. The patient loses the power of expressing himself by spoken words. He is unable to speak spontaneously, to read aloud, or to repeat what he hears. And yet he is not dumb. He can usually say "Yes" and "No" and a few other words previously habitual with him. One may mistake this difficulty for an anarthria until it is observed that the patient has no difficulty in other acts such as chewing and swallowing which require movement of the tongue, lips, palate, and larynx. For a time there may be an inability to purse the lips properly to blow out a candle, or to make other purposeful lip movements. This motor incapacity for certain acts in the absence of paralysis of the necessary muscles or groups of muscles is called *apraxia,* and it has been contended that expressive aphasia is actually a verbal apraxia. The patient repeats his few words over and over again as if compelled to do so. Words in a well-known song may be sung and others uttered as expletives when the patient is angered or excited, illustrating the point that the patient, though "speechless" under ordinary conditions, has not become "wordless." Usually he can recognize some of his own mistakes and may express exasperation or despair over them. Most patients are unable to write, and even though hemiplegic and so denied the use of their right hand, they are unable to write recognizable words with the left hand. An occasional patient with Broca's aphasia has been observed to be able to repeat some words spoken by the examiner, to read aloud, and to copy words; this condition is called *transcortical motor aphasia.* Sometimes the ability to write is retained in the face of a severe Broca's aphasia, and the ability to read and understand spoken language is faultless, showing that inner language is undisturbed. This is called *subcortical motor aphasia*. Alajouanine has traced the regression of expressive aphasia along two lines: (1) through stereotyped, obligatory verbal utterance to agrammatism, in which only a skeleton of nouns and verbs is spoken; (2) from anarthria through dysarthria with various degrees of phonetic disintegration.

Receptive or Sensory Aphasia. Sensory aphasia is more difficult to define than expressive aphasia. It usually appears as a rather complex syndrome consisting essentially of a loss of comprehension of spoken language and of written words and an inability to write. The patient is able to speak, often volubly, but misuses words. According to present terminology the defects are, respectively, auditory verbal agnosia; visual verbal agnosia, or alexia; agraphia; and paraphasia. The term *agnosia* was first introduced by Sigmund Freud and means a disturbance of recognition or identification with relatively intact sensation. In word deafness, hearing is not reduced but there is an agnosia for spoken words (an inability to comprehend words, or word deafness with intact hearing). All these elements were noted by Wernicke, and it is now customary when the entire syndrome is present, to refer to it as *Wernicke's aphasia*. The lesion is variable in its extent but usually involves the posterior part of upper temporal convolutions and the supramarginal convolution and white matter beneath it. Special interest attaches to the patient's manner of speech. His articulation is normal, unless there is an associated expressive aphasia. He often pauses or gropes for a word, substitutes an incorrect word, omits words, and is unable at times to construct a sentence. When he begins to speak, the first sentence or two is well composed, but as he continues, the difficulty becomes increasingly evident. When the speech is severely disorganized it gives way to *jargon aphasia*, also called *choreatic aphasia* (Kussmaul) and *syntactical aphasia* (Head). During recovery one may observe progress from an undifferentiated through an asemantic and then paraphasic jargon. The patient does not seem to notice his own errors and is not much disturbed by them.

The basic disorder in paraphasia has been disputed. Some investigators believe that the patient has merely lost the ability to understand his own spoken words, i.e., has an auditory verbal agnosia. This simple explanation does not seem to account for all the facts. Head's explanation is more likely the correct one, that internal language mechanisms are deranged, i.e., the mental processes by which visual and auditory word memories are evoked in response to certain ideas are disordered.

Many aphasic patients present only part of the syndrome. The term *transcortical sensory aphasia* is applied to the state in which the patient can repeat what he hears but without comprehension; he also reads aloud without understanding the words. *Amnesic* or *nominal aphasia* may also be present in Wernicke's aphasia but may occur as a solitary symptom. The patient is unable to affix a name to many common objects when they are visually presented. He tells instead the use of the object, and if the auditory receptive centers are intact he can immediately recognize the name when it is spoken by the examiner. The question of location of the responsible lesion is still debated. Nielsen believes it to be in area 37 or near the isthmus of the temporal lobe and has observed this type of aphasia in cases with temporal lobe abscess, tumors, or vascular lesions. *Visual aphasia, word blindness,* or *alexia* may also occur in relatively pure form, but usually the patient displays some degree of *agraphia* because there is also loss of memories of written or printed words. If capacity to write is conserved, the defect is called *subcortical* visual aphasia, and the lesion is believed to be in the subcortical white matter deep to the inferior parietal lobe. As pointed out by Osler, it is often associated with a contralateral homonymous hemianopia.

Pure agraphia, i.e., inability to write with preservation of all other elements of speech and good strength and sensation in the hand, has not been reported. This is one of the reasons for doubting the existence of a writing center.

Approach to the Clinical Problem of Aphasia. In investigating a case of aphasia it is first necessary to inquire into the patient's native language, his handedness, and his previous education. Many naturally left-handed children are trained to use their right hand for writing; therefore in determining this point we must ask which hand is used for throwing a ball, threading a needle, or using a spoon or common tools such as hammer, saw, or bread knife. Next, one should quickly ascertain whether the patient has other signs of a gross cerebral lesion such as hemiplegia, facial weakness, homonymous hemianopia, or cortical sensory loss.

It is important before beginning the examination to determine whether the patient is alert and mentally clear or is suffering from confusion, because this may prevent accurate assessment of language. One must also avoid as far as possible the effects of fatigue by making the interview short. Explanation of the purpose of the tests, sympathy, and encouragement are often necessary to assure full cooperation.

Many elaborate examination schemes have been devised for testing the language functions, and some of them lead to refinements that are of little physiologic or clinical significance. The following procedure will yield sufficient data for diagnosis.

1. Can the patient spontaneously utter intelligible words in proper sequence and well-constructed phrases and sentences? The fluency of speech, the extent of vocabulary, the grammatical construction of sentences, the accuracy of word usage, and clarity of enunciation should all be observed and examples incorporated into the record of the interview. Wrong choice of words, misplacement of words or syllables, omission of essential words, and use of disjointed phrases may be slight in degree and take the form of paraphasia, or if severe may result in an unintelligible jabbering or jargon.

2. Can the patient understand what he hears? If he is unable to speak, give him a series of commands of increasing complexity. Ask him to close his eyes, open his mouth, hold up his left hand, place the index finger of the left hand to the right ear, etc. Often the patient will execute the first one or two simple commands correctly and will fail on all others, sometimes repeating the first act over and over (perseveration).

3. Can the patient read? Written questions or commands should be presented and the responses observed.

4. Can the patient write spontaneously? If his right hand is paralyzed, he should be encouraged to try his left. It must also be determined whether or not he can write from dictation or can copy words or sentences.

5. If he is able to speak, can he name common objects shown visually, such as a penny, button, pencil, fountain pen, handkerchief, the various parts of a wrist watch, safety pin, key, flashlight, matches? If not, does he recognize the correct name when he hears it? Can he repeat the words that he hears? Can he read aloud from a newspaper or magazine? Are his gestures appropriate?

Disorders in the Development of Language in Children

A close parallelism exists between the symptoms observed in adults who have suffered a loss in language as a result of brain injury and those to be seen during the development of the language faculty. This reminds us that there may be a faulty development of language and of cerebral dominance. It has been found that a high percentage of these patients have a strong family background of speech disorders and that strong preference for the right or the left hand is not present.

Developmental disorders of language and congenital deafness are far more frequent than aphasia. The latter includes developmental alexia (special reading disability, congenital word blindness), developmental agraphia (special writing disability), developmental word deafness, developmental motor aphasia (motor speech delay), and developmental apraxia (abnormal clumsiness of the limbs). The development of language, instead of proceeding in the manner outlined in the early part of this chapter, becomes arrested or is delayed. These conditions are often misunderstood by parents, teachers, and physicians. Sometimes the unfortunate child is judged to be feebleminded or lazy. Another frequent error is to assume the condition to be due to psychologic factors. Space does not permit a description of each of these syndromes.

Congenital Word Deafness. If an individual is born deaf, he never learns to talk without special training; he is "deaf and dumb." Should deafness develop within the first few years of life, after speech has been acquired, he gradually loses speech but can be retaught by the lip-reading method. His speech is harsh, poorly modulated, and unpleasant, and he is apt to make many peculiar throat noises of a snorting or grunting kind. Such patients are bright and alert and clever at pantomime and gesturing. They are inattentive to household noises and do not appear to understand what is said to them. The deafness can be demonstrated at an early age by careful observation of the child's responses to sounds, but cannot be accurately tested before the age of three to four years. The psychogalvanic reflex technique for testing reaction to sounds and tests of the labyrinths, which are usually unresponsive in the deaf-mute, may be helpful. In contrast the idiot or moron is stupid in all his actions and talks little because he has no ideas. Developmental word deafness may be difficult to distinguish from true deafness. Usually the parents have noted that the word-deaf child responds to loud noises and music, though obviously this does not assure perfect hearing, particularly for high tones. The word-deaf child does not understand what is said, and there is a delay and distortion of speech. These children are alert, active, and inquisitive and may chatter incessantly. They adopt a language of their own design, and attentive parents come to understand it. This peculiar type of speech is known as *idioglossia*. It is also observed in children who have marked difficulty in the articulation of certain consonants. They learn to lip-read very quickly and are clever at acting out their ideas.

Congenital Word Blindness (Alexia). In this unusual condition the patient has good eyesight, is able to see the word, but is unable to grasp its meaning. There is no loss of the ability to recognize the meaning of objects, pictures, and diagrams. Usually with assiduous training, the patient, who is otherwise bright and intelligent, can learn to read individual letters and a few simple words. Spelling is impossible. Often the patient cannot write anything of his own composition but can copy skillfully. Lesser degrees of congenital alexia are more common than the severe forms and pose serious problems in the classroom. A few of the severely handicapped children have a right homonymous hemianopia or a right-sided sensory loss; but most of them show no other abnormality.

Abnormalities of Articulation and Phonation (Lisping, Dyslalia). A number of other odd varieties of deficient articulation may come to the notice of the physician. One is *lisping,* in which the *s* sound is replaced by *th,* e.g., "thister" for "sister." Another condition, called *lallation* or *dyslalia,* a common speech disorder observed in early childhood, is characterized by multiple substitutions or omissions of consonants. In severe forms, speech may be almost unintelligible. These children are unaware that their speech differs from that of other people and are distressed at not being understood. Milder degrees consist of the failure to pronounce only one or two consonants. For example, there may be imperfect enunciation of the sound *r* so that it sounds like *w.* "Running a race" becomes "wunning a wace." The nature of this disorder is not known. It has been suggested that the development of language in some children is so rapid that there is a partial failure of both perceptive and imitative speech. The patient usually recovers spontaneously from this disorder, or if not, responds promptly to speech therapy, which is best carried out at about the age of five years. These abnormalities are more frequent amongst feebleminded than normal children, and mental defect should always be suspected if numerous consonants are mispronounced and the condition persists beyond the age of twelve or thirteen years. The speech disorder resulting from *cleft palate* is easily recognized. Many of these patients also have a harelip, and the two abnormalities together interfere with suckling, and later in life with the enunciation of labial and guttural consonants. The voice has an unpleasant nasality and often, if the defect is severe, there is an audible escape of air through the nose.

Stammering and Stuttering. *Stammering* and *stuttering* are difficult to classify. In some respects they belong to the developmental disorders but differ from them in being largely centered in articulation. They consist of a spasm of the muscles of articulation upon attempting to speak. The spasm may be tonic and result in a complete block of speech, sometimes called stammering, or a repetitive spasm which leads to repeated utterance of the first syllable, a stutter. Certain syllables offer greater

difficulty than others. The patient falters on an initial consonant or syllable, which he repeats over and over again before he finally succeeds in enunciating the rest of the word, e.g., *p-p-p-paper, b-b-b-boy.* The severity of the stutter is increased by excitement, as in speaking before strangers or a group of people. The spasms may overflow into other muscle groups not directly concerned with speech. Males are affected three times as often as females. The time of onset may be when the child first begins to talk, that is at two or three years of age, or between the ages of six and eight years. These are the two critical periods of language development. Many of these children also have some degree of reading and writing disability. Slowness in developing hand preference or enforced change from left- to right-handedness are noted in many cases. If mild, the condition tends to be present only during periods of emotional distress; and it may disappear spontaneously during adolescent or early adult years. If severe, it persists all through life, regardless of treatment, but tends to improve as the patient grows older.

The essential character of stuttering is difficult to define. There is no detectable paralysis or incoordination of the speech musculature, which seems to function normally in other commonplace acts and when the patient is alone and relaxed or singing. Stuttering differs from apraxia in that the muscles, when called upon to perform the specific act, go into a voluntary spasm, but since the spasm does not occur during other movements in which these muscles are involved, it differs from the intention spasm of athetosis. It appears to represent a special category of movement disorder and is much like writer's cramp, another motor disorder of unknown etiology.

Everyone who has studied this condition has been impressed with the high incidence of similar disabilities in other members of the same family, sometimes going back several generations. This and the preponderance in males suggest a sex-linked characteristic, but the inheritance does not follow a simple pattern.

Many of the patients, probably as a natural result of this impediment to free social intercourse, become increasingly fearful of speaking and have feelings of inferiority after a few years. By the time adolescent and adult age are reached emotional factors are so prominent that many physicians have mistaken stuttering for a neurosis. Usually there is no evidence of any personality deviation before the onset of stuttering, and psychotherapy by competent psychiatrists, though unquestionably helpful in relieving emotional tension and assisting a satisfactory adjustment to the condition, has not significantly modified the underlying defect.

Occasionally stuttering will develop during adult life as a consequence of brain disease.

Disorders of Articulation and Phonation

Lastly it is necessary to consider disorders of articulation. In simple dysarthria there is no abnormality of the cortical centers. The dysarthric patient is able to understand perfectly what he hears, and if literate reads and has no difficulty in writing, even though unable to utter a single intelligible word. This is the strict meaning of being inarticulate.

The act of speaking is a highly coordinated sequence of contractions of the larynx, pharynx, palate, tongue, lips, and respiratory musculature. These are innervated by the hypoglossal, vagal, facial, and phrenic nerves. The nuclei of these nerves are controlled through the corticobulbar tracts by both motor cortices. As with all movements, there is also an extrapyramidal influence from the cerebellum and basal ganglions. A current of air is produced by expiration and the force of it is finely regulated and coordinated with the activity of other muscles engaged in speech. Phonation, or the production of vocal sounds, is a function of the larynx. Changes in the size and shape of the glottis and in the length and tension of the vocal cords are effected by the action of the laryngeal muscles. Vibrations are set up and transmitted to the column of air passing over the vocal cords. Sounds thus formed are modified as they pass through the nasopharynx and mouth, which act as resonators. Articulation consists of contractions of the tongue, lips, pharynx, and palate which interrupt or alter the vocal sounds. Vowels are of laryngeal origin, as are some consonants; but the latter are formed for the most part during articulation. For instance, the consonants *m*, *b*, and *p* are labial, *l* and *t* are lingual, and *nk* and *ng* are nasoguttural.

Defection of the articulatory process and phonation is best demonstrated by listening to the patient during ordinary conversation or reading aloud from a newspaper or a book. Test phrases or the rapid repetition of lingual, labial, and guttural consonants may bring out the particular abnormality. Disorders of phonation call for an examination of the apparatus of voice. The movements of the vocal cords should be inspected with the aid of a hand mirror or, even better, a laryngoscope, and those of the tongue, palate, and pharynx by direct observation.

Defects in articulation may be subdivided into several types: paralytic dysarthria, spastic and rigid dysarthria, and ataxic dysarthria.

Paralytic Dysarthria. This is due to a neural or bulbar (medullary) paralysis of the articulatory muscles (lower motor neurone paralysis). Bulbar poliomyelitis and "progressive bulbar palsy" are examples of diseases which may produce a partial or complete anarthria. In the latter the shriveled tongue lies inert in the floor of the mouth, and the lips are relaxed and trembling. Saliva constantly collects in the mouth because of dysphagia, and drooling is troublesome. Speech becomes less and less distinct. There is special difficulty in the correct utterance of vibratives such as *r*; and as the paralysis becomes more complete, lingual and labial consonants are finally not pronounced at all. Lesser degrees of this abnormality are observed in myasthenia gravis. Bilateral paralysis of the palate, which may occur with diphtheria, poliomyelitis, or involvement of the tenth cranial nerve by tumor, produces a disorder of articulation similar to that of cleft palate. The voice has a nasal quality, since the posterior nares are not closed during phonation, and certain consonants such as *n*, *b*, and *k* are altered. The abnormality is sometimes less pronounced in recumbency and increased when the head is thrown forward. Bilateral paralysis of the lips interferes with enunciation of labial consonants; *p* and *b* are slurred and sound more like *f* and *v*.

Spastic and Rigid Dysarthria. These are more frequent than the paralytic variety. Diseases which involve the corticobulbar tracts, usually vascular disease or motor system disease, result in the "syndrome of pseudobulbar palsy." The patient may have had a minor stroke some time in the past affecting the corticobulbar fibers on one side; but since the bulbar muscles are probably represented in both motor cortices there is no impairment in speech or swallowing from a unilateral lesion. Another stroke occurs with involvement of the other corticobulbar tract and possibly the corticospinal tract at the pontine, midbrain, or capsular level; immediately the patient becomes anarthric or dysarthric and dysphagic. Unlike bulbar paralysis due to lower motor neurone involvement, there is no atrophy or fasciculation of the paralyzed muscles, the jaw jerk is exaggerated, the palatal reflexes are retained, emotional control is poor (pathologic laughter and crying), and sometimes breathing becomes periodic (Cheyne-Stokes). The patient may be anarthric and aphonic for a time, but as he improves, or in lesser degrees of the same condition, speech is thick and indistinct, much like that of partial bulbar paralysis.

In paralysis agitans, or postencephalitic Parkinson's syndrome, one observes an extrapyramidal disturbance of articulation. The patient speaks slowly and articulates poorly, slurring over many syllables and trailing off the ends of the sentences. The voice is low-pitched, monotonous, and lacking inflection. The words are pronounced hastily. In advanced cases speech is almost unintelligible. It may happen that the patient finds it impossible to talk while walking but is able to resume speech upon sitting or lying down. In chorea and athetosis, speech may also be severely affected, and the defect is difficult to distinguish from the speech of pseudobulbar palsy or paralysis agitans, being slow and slurred in all. Grimacing and the other characteristic motor signs must be depended upon for diagnosis. Pyramidal and extrapyramidal disturbances of speech may be combined in generalized cerebral diseases such as general paresis, in which slurred speech is one of the cardinal signs.

In many cases of "capsular hemiplegia" or partially recovered Broca's aphasia the patient is left with a dysarthria which may be difficult to distinguish from a pure articulatory defect. Careful testing of other language functions, especially writing, may bring out the aphasic quality.

Ataxic Dysarthria. This is characteristic of acute and chronic cerebellar lesions. It may be observed in multiple sclerosis, Friedreich's ataxia, cerebellar atrophy, and heat stroke. The principal abnormality of the speech is slowness; imprecise enunciation, monotony, an unnatural separation of the syllables of words (scanning) are other features. Coordination of speech and respiration is poor. There may not be enough breath to utter certain words, and others may be ejaculated explosively. *Scanning dysarthria* is distinctive, but in some cases, especially if there is some possibility of spastic weakness of the tongue from corticobulbar tract involvement, it is impossible to predict the anatomy of the disease from analysis of speech alone. Myoclonic jerks involving the speech musculature may be superimposed on the cerebellar ataxia in a number of diseases.

Aphonia and Dysphonia. Lastly, a few points should be made concerning disturbances of voice. In adolescence and early adult life there may be a persistence of the unstable "change of voice" normally seen in males soon after puberty. As though by habit the patient speaks part of the time in a falsetto voice. This can usually be overcome by training.

Paresis of the respiratory movements, as in poliomyelitis and acute infectious polyneuritis, may affect voice because insufficient air is provided for phonation and speech. Also, disturbances in the rhythm of respiration may interfere with the fluency of speech. This is particularly noticeable in so-called extrapyramidal diseases, and one may note that the patient tries to talk upon inspiration. Reduced volume of speech due to limited excursion of the breathing muscles is another common feature; the patient is unable to speak loudly or to shout.

Paresis of both vocal cords causes complete aphonia. There is no voice, and it is possible for the patient to speak only in whispers. Since the vocal cords normally separate during inspiration, their failure to do so when paralyzed may result in an inspiratory stridor. If one vocal cord is paralyzed the voice becomes hoarse, low-pitched, and rasping.

Another curious condition about which little is known is spastic dysphonia. The author has seen several cases, all middle-aged or elderly males and otherwise healthy, who gradually lost the ability to speak quietly and fluently. Any effort to speak resulted in contraction of all the speech musculature so that the patient's voice was strained and articulation was labored. Apparently this is a neurologic disorder of undetermined kind. The patients are not neurotic, and psychotherapy has been ineffective.

DIAGNOSIS

There are so many facets of the complex act of speech that it has not been possible to present all of them. Nothing, for example, has been written in this chapter about the changes in speech during various psychiatric illnesses. This does not mean that the present author considers the psychiatric syndromes unimportant, for there is no doubt that hysterical aphonia, the various tics that interrupt the speech of tense individuals, and the altered rate, fluency, and content of speech in the psychoses pose formidable problems.

In the diagnosis of disorders of speech the physician must attempt in every case to decide first whether the problem is one of aphasia, dysarthria, or dysphonia. The examination procedure outlined above will, if carried out systematically, permit this first and important step to be made. If the patient is aphasic, it should be determined whether his aphasia is global, expressive, or sensory in type. Global aphasia signifies a disease involving the posterior frontal, the superior temporal, or inferior parietal and intervening insula and external capsular parts of the left cerebral hemisphere in a right-handed person, or rarely the right cerebral hemisphere in a left-handed person. Expressive aphasia indicates a lesion in the insular region and frontal lobe; sensory aphasia points to disease more posteriorly, in the temporoparietal region. Contralateral hemiplegia, hemianesthesia, and hemianopia with sensory aphasia are frequently associated with motor aphasia.

The general physician is frequently called upon to examine children who show some disorder of speech or delay in language development. From the above remarks it will be seen that these disorders fall into several broad categories, of which stuttering, delay in the onset of speech, dyslalia, partial or complete deafness, word deafness, cleft palate, lisping, and word blindness are the most frequent. When faced with problems of this type, the physician must ask several questions. Is the child partially or completely deaf? Does he have a more generalized mental or neuromuscular defect —is he feebleminded or suffering from an infantile hemiplegia or spastic diplegia? Does he stammer, stutter, or show dyslalia? In attempting to answer these questions, the parents' account of the child's development and his behavior at home is most helpful. Failure to respond to noise of any kind suggests deafness. An interest in sounds and music but not in stories or conversation, together with slowness in development of understanding for and use of speech are points indicative of high-tone deafness or word deafness (auditory verbal agnosia). Delay in the onset of suckling, head control, sitting, standing, walking, etc., should lead to a neurologic examination; one should look particularly for spastic weakness or rigidity of the limbs and poor motor control of the tongue, as well as mental retardation. The latter can be assessed at an early age by special intelligence tests such as the performance part of the Stanford-Binet test. If the child is otherwise normal, the recitation of a nursery rhyme will disclose a stammering, stuttering lallation or cleft-palate speech. Disturbances of articulation point to involvement of a different set of neural structures, such as the motor cortices, the corticobulbar pathways, the VII, IX, X nuclei, the brain stem, and extrapyramidal nuclei and tracts. Often it is necessary to use other neurologic findings to decide which of these are implicated in any given case. The important distinction between the pseudobulbar or supranuclear palsies and the bulbar palsies, is grasped only with difficulty by the average student. The information obtained by the localization of these two major types of dysarthria is extremely helpful in differential diagnosis. Dysphonia should lead to an investigation of laryngeal disease either primary or secondary to an abnormality of innervation.

TREATMENT

The sudden loss of speech would be expected to cause great apprehension, but, except for almost pure motor defects, most patients show remarkably little concern. It would appear that the very lesion that deprives them of speech also causes at least a partial loss of insight into their own disability. This reaches almost a ludicrous extreme in cases of Wernicke's aphasia, in which the patient will become indignant when others cannot understand his jargon. Nonetheless, as improvement occurs many patients do become discouraged. Reassurance and a positive program of speech rehabilitation are the best ways of helping the patient at this stage.

The contemporary methods of training and re-education in overcoming an aphasic defect have never been critically evaluated. Most aphasic difficulty is due to vascular disease of the brain, and this nearly always is accompanied by some degree of spontaneous improvement in the days, weeks, and months which follow the stroke. Sometimes recovery is complete within hours or days; again not more than a few words are regained after a year or two of assiduous speech training. Nevertheless it is the opinion of many experts in the field that speech training is worthwhile.

One must decide about each patient whether speech training is needed and when it should be started. As a rule, therapy is not advisable in the first few days of an aphasic illness, because one does not know how lasting it will be. Also, if the patient suffers a severe global aphasia and can neither speak nor understand spoken and written words, the speech therapist is helpless. Under such circumstances, one does well to wait a few weeks until some one of the language functions has begun to return. Then the physician may begin to encourage and help the patient to use that function to a maximum degree. In milder aphasic disorders the patient may be sent to the speech therapist as soon as the illness has stabilized.

The methods of speech training are specialized, and it is advisable to call in a person who has been trained in this field. However, inasmuch as the benefit is largely psychologic, an interested member of the family or a schoolteacher can be used if a speech therapist is not available in the community.

The language problems of children, if serious, demand skillful diagnosis and treatment, and often excellent results can be obtained. Most of the well-organized urban school systems have remedial reading teachers who will take over the problem once it has been evaluated medically. The emotional problems that often cause these developmental disturbances of language and of cerebral dominance to become manifest must be dealt with gently and firmly.

The physician should by wise counseling assist the patient to an understanding of the nature of his problem and try to avoid some of the secondary emotional problems that the speech disorder creates. Prolonged psychotherapy helps with the emotional problems but has not, in the author's experience, corrected the underlying speech defect. Fortunately the natural course of mild stuttering is toward improvement during adolescence, and many recover spontaneously by adult life. The severe cases have a life-long problem to face and none of the present methods of therapy, including psychoanalysis, have corrected the defect.

There is no special treatment for the dysarthric disturbances of speech.

REFERENCES

Alajouanine, T.: Verbal Realization in Aphasia, Brain, 79:1–29, 1956.

Brain, R.: Aphasia, Apraxia, Agnosia, chap. 83 in "Neurology," 2d ed., vol. 3, S. A. K. Wilson and N. Bruce (Eds.), Baltimore, The Williams & Wilkins Company, 1955.

Nielsen, J. M.: "Agnosia, Aphasia, Apraxia: Their Value in Cerebral Localization," New York, Paul B. Hoeber, Inc., Medical Department of Harper & Brothers, 1948.

Orton, S. T.: "Reading, Writing and Speech Problems in Children," New York, W. W. Norton & Company, Inc., 1937.

41 LASSITUDE (INCLUDING NEURASTHENIA) AND WEAKNESS (with Remarks on the Psychoneuroses)

Raymond D. Adams

From a simple descriptive point of view the psychoneuroses include seven clinical syndromes as follows: (1) fatigue or neurasthenia, as it was formerly called, (2) simple nervousness, anxiety neurosis or neurocirculatory asthenia, (3) phobic neurosis, (4) obsessive compulsive neurosis (also called psychasthenia), (5) hysteria, (6) hypochondriasis, and (7) reactive depression. Although they are easily identifiable and separable, if presenting in pure form, experience shows that many patients exhibit symptoms which belong to more than one of these categories, and hence must be classed as having "mixed psychoneuroses."

The causes and the exact mechanisms of symptom production in these many syndromes are unknown. It is a generally accepted proposition that all involve maladjustment in interpersonal (social) relations, in other words they may be psychogenic. But the more penetrating students of psychiatry do not dismiss lightly genetic or obscure biochemical factors. Even Freud, the most emphatic exponent of the psychogenic etiology, underscored the importance of heredity, constitution, and endocrine abnormalities. There is also general acceptance of the idea that the psychoneuroses need not be and usually are not disabling; i.e., they are "partial reactions" in an otherwise healthy person, not "total reactions," as in the psychoses.

According to Finesinger and Cobb, patients with psychoneuroses may be studied advantageously from the following points of view. (1) *Verbal accounts* given by the patient. Here reference is made to the patient's statements concerning his feelings, fantasies, and ideas. These are believed to provide the best clues to diagnosis. Supplementary data concerning the emerging patterns of thought may be secured by the free association of ideas, a methodology widely employed in psychoanalysis. Unfortunately information of this type although of great theoretical interest has not been used for the critical testing of the original postulates of the psychoanalytical school. (2) *Motor behavior* (besides the verbal accounts) such as visible facial expressions and other acts which denote worry, tension, restlessness, excitement, or their opposites. These activities involve the cerebrospinal nervous system. (3) *Visceral reactions.* These involve the autonomic nervous system, which controls the activities of smooth muscle and glands. Derangements in this sphere express themselves during emotion as combinations of rapid heartbeat, accelerated respiration, intestinal and bladder contractions, pupillary dilatation, sweating, flushing, pallor, etc. Four major emotional states—rage, fear, love, and sorrow—may thus be differentiated. (4) *Reactions to environmental stimuli*, past or present. The patient's symptoms are examined in relation to stimulus situation. Here the remarkable feature is that in the psychoneuroses the emotional reaction is not consonant with the manifest external or professed internal stimuli. Anxiety under the circumstances of a potentially threatening situation is of course an understandably normal reaction, but in the neurotic a similar reaction occurs without evident cause. It is the contention of many experienced psychiatrists that the stimulus situation is there and may be discovered only by the free association of psychoanalysis or by the exploration of biographical details, i.e., remembered (conscious) and forgotten (subconscious) experiences. Or in the language of the behaviorist or reflexologist, the inexplicable emotion may be regarded as a conditioned response to an inapparent or forgotten fragment of an emotionally charged experience. Therapy in either instance logically consists of making these connections known to the patient or of interrupting the conditioned reaction. The symptoms then become natural, meaningful, and tolerable. Unfortunately there are no accurate data as to the efficacy of these modes of therapy.

Each of the major types of psychoneuroses will be found in the following chapters. In the remainder of this chapter lassitude and asthenia, symptoms common to many psychiatric and medical diseases, will be discussed in detail.

LASSITUDE AND ASTHENIA

The term *weakness* is used by patients to describe a variety of subjective complaints which vary in their import and prognostic significance. Most of the subjective disorders embraced by this term will be found, upon careful questioning, to fall within the following classification.

I. Lassitude, fatigue, lack of energy, listlessness, and languor. These terms, while not synonymous, shade into each other; all refer to weariness and a loss of that sense of well-being typically found in persons who are healthy in body and mind. Symptoms of this type are present in a large majority of all patients and have little diagnostic significance. For the sake of brevity this group of complaints will be considered together under the heading Lassitude and Fatigue.

II. Weakness, loss of muscular strength, and asthenia. These may be either persistent or episodic:
  A. Persistent weakness: This may be (1) restricted to certain muscles or groups of muscles (palsy, paresis, paralysis) or (2) general, involving the entire musculature, in which instance the term *asthenia* or *myasthenia* is used. Paralysis is discussed as a separate topic in pp. 240 to 244. The generalized type of muscular weakness will be considered below, under the title Asthenia. It is far less common than lassitude and more likely to indicate serious disease.
  B. Recurrent weakness: Many patients complain of "attacks of weakness," and careful questioning reveals that a diminished sense of alertness, a feeling of lightheadedness, or a sensation of faintness is the actual symptom. Since these complaints are subjectively different from lassitude and asthenia, and since the causes are likewise different, such recurrent attacks of weakness are discussed in Chap. 33.

It should be restated that the unqualified term weakness is so vague as to be almost useless, and that a sound clinical approach to this problem entails, as the initial step, an analysis of what the patient himself means when he uses this and similar terms.

LASSITUDE AND FATIGUE (Lack of Energy, Languor, Listlessness, Weariness, Neurasthenia)

Of all symptoms these are amongst the most frequent and at the same time the most abstruse. More than half of all patients make direct complaint of this group of symptoms or admit of their presence when questioned. During the Second World War they figured so prominently in military medicine that the term *combat fatigue* was applied to all acute psychiatric illnesses on the battlefield. Therefore, it behooves every student of medicine to learn as much as possible about these symptoms

and their physiologic and psychologic antecedents.

Our understanding of the nature and mechanisms of lassitude and fatigue and their full significance in practice remains peculiarly limited. This is not from want of interest in them, for they have been objects of clinical study for more than a century by some of the most eminent physicians, including Beard, DaCosta, Weir Mitchell, Mosso, and Freud. There are, however, several new facts concerning chronic fatigue that have come to light in recent years and many old ones that deserve consideration.

Lassitude or fatigue most commonly refers to a feeling of weariness or tiredness. Patients who complain of this symptom have a more or less characteristic way of describing it. They speak of being "all in," "without pep," having "no ambition," "no interest," or "being fed up." They are inclined to lie down. On close analysis this is a difficulty in initiating activity, and also in sustaining it.

This condition is the familiar aftermath of prolonged labor or great physical exertion, and under these circumstances is accepted as a physiologic reaction. When, however, the same symptoms or similar ones appear in the abence of vigorous exercise they are recognized as being unnatural, and the patient rightly suspects some recently acquired disease.

The physician's first task then is to determine whether or not his patient is merely suffering from the physical and mental effects of overwork without realizing it. Overworked and overwrought people are everywhere observable in our society. Their actions are both instructive and pathetic. They seem to be impelled by notions of duty and refuse to think of themselves. Or, as is often the case, some personal inadequacy prevents them from deriving pleasure from any activity except their work, in which they indulge as a defense mechanism. Such individuals often experience a variety of symptoms such as weariness, irritability, nervousness, and sleeplessness. The behavior of these individuals and their varied symptomatology are best understood by referring to psychologic studies of the effect of fatigue on normal individuals.

The Effect of Fatigue on the Normal Person. According to the most authoritative sources, fatigue has several effects, some explicit, others implicit. These are (1) a series of physiologic changes in many organs of the body, (2) an overt disorder of behavior in the form of reduced output of work, known as work decrement, and (3) an expression of dissatisfaction and a subjective feeling of tiredness or weariness in association with a variety of psychologic changes.

Fatigue indicates the presence of changes in the

physiologic balance of the body. Continuous muscular work results in a depletion of muscle glycogen and the accumulation of lactic acid and probably other metabolites which handicap the prolonged contractility and the recovery of active muscle. It is said that the injection of the blood of a fatigued animal into a rested one will produce the overt manifestations of fatigue in the latter. During fatigue states muscle action is tremulous, and movements become clumsy and cannot be sustained for long without increasing effort. The rate of breathing increases; the pulse quickens; the blood pressure is raised and the pulse pressure widens; and the white blood count and the metabolic rate are increased. These reactions bear out the hypothesis that fatigue is in part a manifestation of altered metabolism.

The decreased capacity for work or productivity which is the direct consequence of fatigue has been investigated by industrial psychologists. Their findings show clearly the importance of the motivational factor on work output, whether it be in the operation of an ergograph or the performance of heavy manual labor. Also it appears that there are individual differences in the energy potential of human beings, just as there are differences in physique and temperament. Some people are strong and vigorous from birth, whereas others are weak and lacking in energy.

The subjective feelings of fatigue have been carefully recorded. Aside from weariness the tired person complains of nervousness, restlessness, inability to deal effectively with complex problems, and a tendency to be upset by trivialities. The number and quality of his associations in tests of mental function are reduced. Behavior tends to be less rational than normal, and the capacity to deliberate and to reach sound judgments is impaired. The worker physically exhausted after a long, hard day is unable to perform adequately his duties as head of a household, and the example of the tired businessman who becomes the proverbial tyrant of the family circle is well known. A disinclination to try, and the appearance of ideas of inferiority, are other characteristics of the fatigued mind.

Instances of fatigue and lassitude resulting from overwork are not difficult to recognize. A description of the patient's daily routine will usually suffice; and if he can be persuaded to live at a more reasonable pace, his symptoms promptly subside. Errors in diagnosis are usually in the direction of ascribing fatigue to overwork, chronic infection, or anemia when in fact it is a manifestation of a psychoneurosis.

Fatigue as a Manifestation of a Psychiatric Disorder. The great majority of patients who suffer from unexplained chronic fatigue and lassitude have been found to have some type of psychiatric illness. In former times the term *neurasthenia* was applied to this group of patients, but since fatigue rarely exists as an isolated phenomenon, the current practice is to label such cases according to the total clinical picture. The usual associated symptoms are nervousness, anxiety, irritability, depression, insomnia, palpitation, headaches, breathlessness, inability to concentrate, sexual disorders, and disturbances of appetite. In one series of cases of severe fatigue in a general hospital, 75 per cent were diagnosed as anxiety neurosis or tension state. Depression and "psychosomatic disease" accounted for another 10 per cent, and the remainder had miscellaneous illnesses with hysterical, obsessive, or phobic symptoms.

Several features are common to the psychiatric group. The fatigue is frequently worse in the morning. The patient is often aware of a desire to lie down but finds himself unable to sleep when he does. The feeling of fatigue relates more to some activities than to others; at times certain affairs are prosecuted with great vigor; while even the thought of others completely exhausts the patient. A careful inquiry into the circumstances under which the fatigue occurred the first time or recurs often reveals a specific relationship to certain events. Instances of an acute episode of fatigue coming on during an unpleasant emotional experience, in connection with a grief reaction, or after a surgical operation have been noted. And finally the feeling of tiredness extends to mental as well as physical activities. The individual's capacity for sustained mental effort, as in solving problems or carrying on a difficult conversation, is impaired.

Depressing emotion, whether grief from bereavement, or a phase of manic-depressive psychosis or involutional psychosis, has its characteristic effect on the impulse life and energy of the individual. The initiation of activity is difficult, and the capacity for work is reduced. Lassitude and fatigue are a more prominent feature in many mild depressive illnesses than is the depression of mood. Patients typically complain that everything they do, whether mental or physical, requires great effort, and all their accustomed activities no longer give the usual satisfaction and enjoyment. Sleep is poor, with a tendency to early morning waking. Such individuals are at their worst, both in spirit and in energy output, in the morning and tend to improve as the day wears on. It is difficult to decide whether their fatigue is a primary effect of disease or is secondary to a lack of interest.

Many physicians may question whether all patients with chronic fatigue as seen in everyday practice deviate far enough from normal to justify a diagnosis of psychoneurosis or depressive psychosis. There are some people who because of circumstances beyond their control have no purpose in life and much idle time. They become bored with the monotony of their daily routine. Such conditions are conducive to fatigue, just as optimism or enthusiasm for a new enterprise dispels fatigue. There are other patients who, as far as one can tell, were reasonably healthy and well-adjusted until they met some adversity which aroused fear and worry. They then develop a state which may be classified as simple nervousness or reactive anxiety with the usual lassitude and fatigue, sleeplessness, and difficulty in concentration. Reactions such as these are understandable to everyone who has had stage fright or buck fever. The sense of physical weakness, the utter incapacity to act, the sudden transformation of a normally well-ordered mind into intellectual chaos, and the exhaustion which follows the episode are indelible experiences in the minds of most of us.

Psychologic Theories. The significance of lassitude and fatigue in these different life situations and psychiatric illnesses has been the subject of much speculation. Physiologists have remarked on the enervating effect of strong emotion and have argued that a simple prolongation of the emotional experience would provide a rational explanation for all the symptoms of chronic anxiety. This, however, only takes the explanation one step further back and does not account for the patient's being emotionally aroused at a time when there is no overt stimulus to emotion.

The dynamic schools of psychiatry, particularly the psychoanalytic, have postulated that chronic fatigue, like the anxiety from which it derives, is a danger signal that something is wrong; some activity or attitude has been persisted in too intensely or too long. The purpose of fatigue may be regarded as self-preservation, not merely as a protection against physical injury but also to preserve the individual's self-esteem, his concept of himself. Another hypothesis is that the fatigue is the result of the exhaustion of one's store of energy by the demands of repression. The characteristic situation in which the fatigued patient finds himself is said to be one in which effective behavior is of a type forbidden by the patient's own idea of what is permissible to him as a member of society. Fatigue then is not a negative quality, a lack of energy, but an unconscious desire for inactivity. A reciprocal relationship is believed to exist between fatigue and anxiety. Both are believed to be protective devices, but anxiety is the more imperative. It calls the individual to take some positive action to extricate himself from a predicament, whereas fatigue calls for inactivity. Both fatigue and anxiety operate blindly. The individual does not perceive what it

is that must be done or stopped. All this happens at an unconscious level.

Other psychiatrists are not satisfied with the psychoanalytic hypothesis, especially for cases of lifelong weakness and fatigability. They point out that individuals differ basically in energy potential. Certain persons, it is believed, seem endowed with a limited store of energy. The physiologic or psychologic basis for this deficiency is unknown. Eugene Kahn regards it as a constitutional inadequacy and states that at present it cannot be decided whether this is inborn or acquired. Under the heading "Psychopath Weak in Impulse," he describes the individual who has an evident physical inferiority. He is a weakling; his vitality is low. He is unusually susceptible to disease and requires longer to convalesce than the average. Such a person may spend half his life recuperating from illnesses that would not bother a normal person. Vigorous games tire him, and his performance is usually so poor that he takes no interest in sports. Unless born in favorable economic circumstances he earns a meager livelihood. He seeks and accepts subordinate positions and usually cannot establish an independent social position of his own. He gives the impression of weakness of will, dullness, or nervousness, though many such individuals possess an average or superior intellectual endowment. His success is limited by his lack of drive and industry. Sexual impulse is also weak and he may find marriage impossible. He requires medical attention throughout life and whenever subjected to any unusual stress is apt to break down and complain of nervousness, lassitude, insomnia, and many other vague symptoms. The physical inferiority and lack of sexual impulse bring to mind that dwarfs of endocrine origin often show this same deficiency in impulse life. This weakness in impulse is found in the chronic invalid seen in everyday practice.

It is perfectly obvious that these various psychologic theories are not mutually exclusive. Undoubtedly there are certain individuals whose impulse to activity is weak throughout life, and this deficiency probably is largely, if not exclusively, determined by genetic factors. It is equally clear that boredom, lack of interest, depression of mood, and strong emotion, regardless of the conditions under which they arise, are usually accompanied by fatigue and lassitude. The more chronic varieties of fatigue are probably in most instances related to psychiatric illnesses, and here the proposition that fatigue, like anxiety, is part of a psychologic defense mechanism seems most applicable.

Lassitude and Fatigue in Chronic Infection and Endocrine Diseases. Chronic infection is another cause of chronic fatigue, though a much less frequent one. Everyone has at some time or other sensed the abrupt onset of a tired ache in all the muscles of the body as an acute infection develops, or the listlessness that accompanies an afternoon fever. In chronic infections the patient has lassitude, fatigue, mental depression, and vague aches and pains. Also, there is often a period of easy fatigability, irritability, inability to work effectively, after a protracted febrile illness. Some diseases, e.g., influenza and hepatitis, are more likely to be followed by these convalescent symptoms than others. If symptoms of this type are prolonged, it is often difficult if not impossible to decide whether they are due to the disease in question or to the presence of chronic anxiety or depression. In many chronic diseases such as infectious hepatitis and brucellosis, neurotic symptoms are often added to those of the original disease.

Metabolic and *endocrine disturbances* (see pp. 249 and 371) of various types may produce lassitude or fatigue. The symptom is likely to be extremely marked and to be associated with true muscular weakness. In Addison's disease and Simmonds's disease it dominates the clinical picture. In persons with hypothyroidism with or without frank myxedema, lassitude is usually pronounced. It is also present in many patients with hyperthyroidism, although often less troublesome than the associated nervousness. Uncontrolled diabetes may be accompanied by excessive fatigability. Hyperparathyroidism, Cushing's disease, and hypogonadism are other instances of endocrine diseases in which lassitude may be prominent. Any type of nutritional deficiency may, when severe, cause lassitude, and in the early stages of the disease this may be the only complaint. Weight loss and the dietary history may be the only objective clues as to the nature of the illness.

Differential Diagnosis. Since a large variety of physical and emotional disorders may be accompanied by lassitude, the following discussion is limited to causes likely to be obscure.

When chronic fatigue and lassitude are the presenting symptoms, the most common cause is a psychoneurosis or depressive psychosis. The basis of diagnosis is the nature of the symptom and its pervasive effect on both mental and physical function, the associated psychiatric symptoms, usually of anxiety or depression, and the absence of signs of somatic disease. However, since psychic and somatic disorders frequently coexist, it is wise to search for organic disease before concluding that the illness is entirely psychogenic. The clinical examination should be thorough and prompt; unnecessary prolongation of the procedure may aggravate an anxiety state, if present. A careful inquiry should be made for situational factors in the patient's life which could possibly be related to the psychiatric symptoms. If found, measures should be taken to assist the patient to an understanding of how these factors are affecting him. If reassurance that no somatic disease is present and discussion of the patient's problems do not afford relief, a psychiatric consultation is desirable. If the diagnosis is obscure, psychiatric appraisal should be part of the initial examination. Common errors are to mistake a depressive illness in which the leading symptom is chronic fatigue for a psychoneurosis; to fail to recognize the basic energy lack in an "asthenic psychopath" and to attempt to treat him as an individual with a chronic somatic disease or a recently acquired neurotic illness; and to misjudge the relative importance of psychic and somatic factors in a chronic medical disease.

Obscure infections and surgical operations may cause symptoms which closely resemble those of psychoneurosis. Indeed, individuals who have suffered from all three conditions report that the "nuclear" emotional state is similar. As a rule aches and pains, weight loss, and low-grade fever are more prominent in chronic infection, and anxiety is in the foreground of the neurotic illness. In the United States tuberculosis, subacute bacterial endocarditis, chronic brucellosis, chronic pyelonephritis, subacute infectious hepatitis, or certain parasitic infections such as malaria and hookworm should be considered as a cause of an illness of this type. The status of chronic brucellosis has been especially difficult to evaluate. Unfortunately there is no reliable method (other than blood culture, which is rarely positive in chronic cases) of diagnosing this condition.

Anemia (Chap. 23) when moderate to severe, and regardless of the cause, is likewise frequently responsible for lassitude. The severity of the symptom is more likely to parallel the hemoglobin level of the blood than the number of erythrocytes. It is the author's impression that mild grades of anemia are usually asymptomatic and that lassitude is ascribed to anemia much too often. *Nutritional deficiency* in many parts of the world is a source of lassitude and fatigability; it is often combined with anemia.

The diagnosis of the fatigue and lassitude which accompany endocrine diseases may be difficult. These conditions are relatively rare in comparison to the psychiatric diseases which cause chronic fatigue. One of the most helpful points to keep in mind is that many of these patients are actually experiencing some degree of asthenia as well as fatigue. Details as to the most reliable methods of diagnosis of these rare diseases will be found in later chapters of the book.

Almost any type of chronic *exogenous* or *endogenous intoxication* is likely to be associated with lassitude, which, however, is only rarely the chief complaint. Among the more common examples are alcoholism, bromism, prolonged ingestion of barbiturates, morphine addiction, and uremia. In these the clue to diagnosis is usually provided by the more troublesome complaints. In persons with acute infections, in patients with malignant tumors, and in many individuals with almost any type of serious disease, the other symptoms are in the foreground and are much more likely to have diagnostic significance than the associated lassitude.

Lassitude of sudden onset is likely to be due to (1) an acute infection, (2) a disturbance of fluid balance, especially one producing extracellular fluid deficit, or (3) rapidly developing circulatory failure of either peripheral or cardiac origin. In these various disorders, discussed in detail in later chapters, the subjective manifestation—lassitude—is likely to be accompanied by outspoken objective phenomena, i.e., fever, tachycardia, etc.

Generalized Muscular Weakness, Debility, Asthenia

This symptom is relatively uncommon, as compared with the great frequency of lassitude. True asthenia is probably never due to psychogenic disorders alone and is not likely to result from anemia or from the chronic infections, except in their advanced stages. It is observed in the terminal phases of most wasting diseases and throughout the course of severe acute fevers. Its most common causes are senility and prolonged confinement to bed, regardless of the underlying disease process. When asthenia is the presenting symptom in a patient who is not senile and has not been at bed rest, one should think of the severe forms of the common anemias, of nutritional deficiencies, of the diffuse disorders of the motor system, and of the diseases of the pituitary, adrenal, thyroid, and parathyroid glands, such as Addison's disease and Simmonds's disease, which may give rise to both fatigability and asthenia.

The distinction between lassitude and asthenia is not a sharp one; the former symptom shades into the latter. All patients with asthenia also have lassitude, but most patients with lassitude do not have genuine asthenia. Before concluding that a person has true loss of strength rather than the more common and less serious loss of energy, one either should be able to demonstrate the muscular weakness objectively, or should obtain a story from the patient that he is no longer able to perform specific muscular acts which previously could be done readily.

One not extremely rare cause of asthenia merits special attention—namely, myasthenia gravis. In this remarkable disorder the patient may have nearly normal muscular strength following prolonged rest, but quickly develops weakness of the affected muscles following repeated contraction. The muscles supplied by the cranial nerves, ocular movement, swallowing, and speech are especially involved (see pp. 736 and 738).

When more than one member of the family is subject to recurrent attacks of weakness proceeding to the point of actual paralysis, but without loss of consciousness, and when such seizures are separated by intervals of good health, one should be suspicious of a rare disorder—familial periodic paralysis (see pp. 250 and 739). Recurrent and persistent weakness and aching of muscles after exercise should suggest McArdle's disease (see pp. 729 and 743). Persistent weakness is a common feature of polymyositis and cortisone myopathy (see pp. 725 and 728).

There are probably several mechanisms of asthenia, but only a few are known. In myasthenia gravis it has been said that a toxic substance with an action very similar to that of curare interferes with the neuromuscular transmission of nerve impulses. It can be inhibited by cholinergic drugs such as neostigmine, which are of great therapeutic value. (See p. 249 for other theories.) Familial periodic paralysis is believed to be intimately linked to potassium metabolism; and low serum potassium levels, found in some but not all cases at the time of the paralysis, interfere with the contractility of muscle fibers. McArdle's syndrome was recently shown to be due to a deficiency of an enzyme phosphorylase which is normally present in the striated muscle fibers. Thyrotoxic myopathy is associated with a reduced creatine tolerance and an impairment of muscle metabolism. Probably the asthenia of senility, cachexia, and other metabolic diseases will ultimately be traced to metabolic changes in muscle.

Differential Diagnosis. *Procedure in a Patient with Obscure Persistent Weakness as the Presenting Symptom.* Some of the more important points in differential diagnosis are indicated in Table 41-1.

The decision as to whether an obscure but active chronic infection exists is made largely on the basis of measurements of *temperature* (preferably taken at 2-hr intervals and under conditions of activity if the resting temperatures are normal), *leukocyte count,* and *sedimentation rate.* If any of these are persistently elevated, there is strong likelihood that the patient has either an infection or some other process such as neoplasm, thrombosis with infarction, arteritis, etc., which is causing tissue injury. These tests are not infallible, for individuals, otherwise healthy, may have a slight elevation of temperature or an elevated sedimentation rate. (The procedures utilized in differentiating these various

Table *41-1*. IMPORTANT POINTS IN DIFFERENTIAL DIAGNOSIS OF SOME OF THE MORE COMMON CAUSES OF OBSCURE PERSISTENT WEAKNESS

General group of causes	More specific causes	Commonly associated symptoms	Likely physical findings	Remarks
Obscure chronic infection	Any chronic infection	Aches and pains Fatigue Anorexia Weight loss	Slight fever Tachycardia	Rapid sedimentation rate
	Tuberculosis	Weight loss and cough	Incipient: none Advanced: rales, etc., fever, sweating	X-ray, positive tuberculin test * Tubercle bacilli in sputum
	Chronic brucellosis	Fatigue Malaise Fever	None	History of ingestion of raw milk Positive brucellergin test * Brucella agglutination, blood culture positive
	Subacute rheumatic fever	Weight loss, cough, and palpitation	Early signs of valvular disease Disproportionate tachycardia	History of joint pain, chorea, or epistaxis Response to salicylates Electrocardiogram
Anemia	. . . .	Palpitation Fatigue Anorexia	Pallor	Reduction of hemoglobin, cell volume, etc.
Endocrine and metabolic disorders	Hypothyroidism	Coldness Drowsiness Loss of hair Slow speech Deep voice	Puffy facies Dry skin Delayed relaxation of tendon reflexes	Basal metabolic rate decreased Blood cholesterol increased
	Hyperthyroidism	Nervousness Palpitation Polyphagia Weight loss	Tachycardia Goiter; tremor Exophthalmos Warm, moist skin	Basal metabolic rate increased
	Diabetes	Polyphagia Weight loss Polyuria Polydipsia	None	Urine sugar Fasting blood sugar Glucose tolerance test
	Simmonds' disease	Extreme anorexia Loss of libido Smooth skin	Hypothermia Hypotension	Fasting hypoglycemia Flat glucose tolerance curve
	Addison's disease	Nausea Vomiting Diarrhea	Hypotension Cutaneous and oral pigmentation	Low blood sodium (during crises) Water load (Kepler test) Eosinophil test
Muscle diseases: Myasthenia gravis	Neuromuscular block	Rapid fatigue with effort (especially of eyelids)	Involvement of cranial muscles > limbs	Prostigmine test EMG change
Polymyositis. . .	Muscle fiber degeneration	Proximal muscle weakness	↓ or 0 reflexes Dermatitis (50%) Other connective tissue disease	↑ transaminase ↑ creatine excretion, ↓ creatinine excretion EMG

* The presence of a positive skin test does not constitute adequate grounds for the assumption that tuberculosis or brucellosis is the cause of the symptoms.

conditions are discussed in pp. 60 to 64.) The presence of persistently normal values for these functions makes it unlikely that a bacterial infection exists at a sufficiently active level to cause weakness, but does not exclude parasitic and other infections which may produce weakness by causing anemia or by interfering with nutrition.

The presence of a persistent tachycardia (greater than can be accounted for by the level of the temperature) is suggestive of thyrotoxicosis, subacute rheumatic fever, or a psychogenic disorder. In the last condition, unlike the other two, the *sleeping pulse rate* is likely to be normal, and the hands, though moist, are usually cold.

The decision as to whether anemia, from whatever cause, is of sufficient severity to cause weakness can be made readily by measurement of the hematocrit. Measurements of the number of red blood corpuscles and the quantity of hemoglobin are often inaccurate, so that whenever these values are low they must be checked in order to determine their accuracy. There is no absolute level of anemia at which weakness may be expected. Its rate of development is important; acute blood loss has a much greater effect than chronic. Minor degrees of anemia are usually not the correct explanation of weakness. Once anemia of significant degree has been demonstrated, the problem becomes one of determining its nature and cause (Chap. 23).

In deciding whether advanced nutritional deficiency is responsible for weakness, one can rely on objective methods; but *in the earlier states of the deficiency diseases reliance has to be placed on the dietary history,* supplemented, in certain instances, by vitamin saturation tests, etc. (see Chap. 57).

Concerning the possible causative role of the more common endocrine and metabolic factors, a few simple clinical observations and laboratory tests will usually suffice. The rarer types require more elaborate tests for diagnosis. These are discussed in the chapters on endocrinology.

The history as regards habits (alcohol), *occupation* (lead, etc.), and *drugs* offers the main clue for the diagnosis of exogenous intoxication as the cause of weakness.

The social history as regards the patient's adjustment to his family and friends, his happiness, and the existence of personal problems in relation to his home and work is helpful in deciding whether or not lassitude and possible weakness are of emotional origin.

The considerations mentioned will lead to an accurate evaluation of the cause of weakness in many patients. Even so, there will remain a group of subjects (unfortunately, not rare) in whom the most exhaustive investigation fails to uncover the cause. In some such individuals time will furnish the answer, but in others recovery will eventually occur without the cause being known.

REFERENCES

See Chap. 44.

42 THE ANXIETY STATE AND PSYCHASTHENIA

Raymond D. Adams and Justin M. Hope

THE ANXIETY STATE

Psychologists, psychiatrists, philosophers, and social historians have been increasingly preoccupied with the subject of anxiety for the past century. In the opinion of the psychologist and psychiatrist it is "the fundamental phenomenon and the central problem of neurosis; . . . a nodal point, linking up all kinds of most important questions; a riddle of which the solution must cast a flood of light upon our whole mental life" (Freud). From the viewpoint of the social historian, anxiety is said to be the "most prominent mental characteristic of Occidental civilization" (Willoughby).

In these contexts anxiety has a broad meaning, more or less the equivalent of social and psychologic unrest. Its more strictly medical meaning, and the one under consideration in this chapter, is an "emotional state arising when a continuing strong desire seems likely to miss its goal" (McDougall), a state of fearful apprehension with many of the physiologic accompaniments of fear.

Incidence of the Anxiety States and Other Psychiatric Syndromes in a General Hospital. As a clinical syndrome the anxiety state outranks all other diagnostic problems in general medicine, as shown in Table 42-1, compiled by one of the authors (Hope). For these reasons a chapter has been devoted to anxiety and its medical implications.

Definition. The anxiety state is characterized by a subjective feeling of fear and uneasy anticipation (apprehension), usually with a definite topical content, associated with the physiologic concomitants of fear, i.e., breathlessness, palpitation, restlessness, increased muscular tension, tightness in the chest, giddiness, trembling, sweating, flushing, choking, and broken sleep. By *topical content* is meant the idea, the person, or the object about which the patient is anxious. The several vasomotor, visceral, and chemical changes which underlie many of the symptoms and signs are mediated by the autonomic nervous system, particularly the sympathetic part of it.

Anxiety manifests itself in acute episodes, lasting a few minutes, or in a protracted state continuing for several weeks, months, or even years. In the acute attacks, called "anxiety attacks" or "panics," breathlessness, palpitation, choking, sweating, and trembling tend to dominate the clinical picture. In the states of chronic anxiety, sometimes called *neurocirculatory asthenia,* nervousness, restlessness, irritability, excitability, headache, fatigue, and insomnia are the major symptoms. Discrete anxiety attacks and protracted states of anxiety are by no means mutually exclusive, though they often occur separately.

Syndromes in Which Anxiety Is a Prominent Feature. The anxiety state is not a disease *sui generis* or the manifestation of a single psychiatric illness. Instead it is a syndrome which may occur in relatively pure and uncomplicated form, as in anxiety neurosis; or it may accompany hysteria, psychasthenia, depression, schizophrenia, and various organic brain diseases.

CLASSIFICATION OF SYNDROMES IN WHICH ANXIETY IS A PROMINENT FEATURE

I. Acute anxiety attacks (panics, vasovagal attacks of Gowers)
   A. Anxiety neurosis
   B. Agitated depression
   C. Hysteria
   D. Psychasthenia
   E. Delirium tremens
   F. Early schizophrenia
II. Protracted anxiety states
   A. Chronic anxiety neurosis—chronic neurocirculatory asthenia
   B. Agitated depression
   C. Hysteria
   D. Psychasthenia
   E. Schizophrenia
   F. Dementing and other brain diseases

The Acute Anxiety Attack. This attack is a common feature of all these diseases, but as a solitary recurrent symptom it is most often observed in an acute anxiety neurosis. The attack usually begins with a distressing presentiment of fear or sense of imminent dissolution. The patient feels as though he will die (angor animi) or lose his mind. This is followed within a few seconds or minutes by palpitation, difficulty in breathing, tightness in the throat, a feeling of smothering or suffocating; trembling, sweating, and giddiness. Hyperventilation may be pronounced, and as a consequence paresthesias of the lips and fingers and even carpopedal spasms may occur. Angor animi is manifested by such expressions as "I am dying," "This is the end," "Oh, my God, I am going." Sometimes there is a sense of unreality or feeling that one cannot move or is in a trance. The symptoms point to a disorder of function, mostly in organs supplied by the vagus nerves. Indeed Gowers was so impressed with this fact that he called spells of this type *vasovagal attacks,* and Nothnagel referred to them as *angina pectoris vasomotoria.*

Such attacks come on most often when the pa-

Table 42-1. INCIDENCE OF PSYCHIATRIC SYNDROMES IN A DIAGNOSTIC HOSPITAL*

Anxiety state †		223
Depression		520
Hysteria		65
Other psychiatric syndromes		110
"Mixed psychoneuroses"	20	
Obsessive compulsive syndrome (psychasthenia)	13	
Anorexia nervosa	4	
Traumatic neuroses (compensation neuroses)	4	
Hypochondriasis	5	
Psychopathic personality	7	
Cyclothymic personality	7	
Schizoid personality	6	
Paranoia	1	
Schizophrenia	11	
Manic-depressive psychoses—manic phase	0	
Chronic alcoholism	4	
Toxic psychoses	3	
Delirium tremens	4	
Drug addiction	1	
Psychoses with organic brain disease	10	
Cerebral arteriosclerosis	3	
Senile dementia	5	
Presenile dementia	2	
Alzheimer's disease 2		
Pick's disease 0		
General paresis	0	
Other (feebleminded, behavior disorder, etc.)		1
Undiagnosed		61
No psychiatric disease		65
Total		1,045

* All patients were studied during the year 1955–1956 at the New England Center Hospital, Boston, Mass. There were 4,660 admissions to the Medical Service during this period. This hospital is primarily a diagnostic clinic

† The diagnosis indicates the dominant syndrome. In some cases classified as depression, hysteria, schizophrenia, etc., there were also symptoms of anxiety.

tient is in a crowd. He feels pent-up, oppressed, unable to breathe, and tries to leave as quickly as possible. Other provocative situations are small, closed rooms, elevators, tunnels, and subway cars. Some attacks begin when the patient is alone in his own home or walking down the street. They may occur at night and awaken him from a sound sleep. At times they appear to be induced by a troublesome dream. A particular situation may invariably provoke an anxiety attack.

Except in minor details, all the attacks are alike in any one individual. Their duration varies from a few minutes to an hour. Immediately following an attack, distressing weakness to the point of exhaustion may become apparent and persist for several hours or days. Between attacks, except for being upset over such an alarming experience, the patient may feel well, though often he complains of being tired, "nervous," and preoccupied with a fear of further attacks. Attacks of this type may occur once or several times a day. Many patients believe that they are having a heart attack and call their physician, regardless of the hour. Some physicians have reported that anxiety attacks are the most frequent cause of emergency calls at night.

Overwhelming anxiety or panic may also occur in an acute psychosis of either the schizophrenic or manic-depressive type. Faulty insight, distortions of logical thinking, delusions, hallucinations, associational disturbances, inappropriateness of affect, or depression of mood are then in the foreground of the clinical picture of these psychoses. Nevertheless acute anxiety attacks may also occur in pure form in anxiety neurosis or neurocirculatory asthenia.

The Protracted Anxiety States. An individual who develops this syndrome may have been healthy before the onset of symptoms, or he may have been anxious in the past and may have had acute attacks of anxiety. From the history alone, two general categories of patients may be differentiated: those who give convincing evidence of good health, nervous stability, and ability to do muscular work and to engage actively in athletics without fatigue prior to the onset of illness; and those who have had a lifelong illness with symptoms of poor exercise tolerance, inability ever to do hard work, tenseness, "nervousness," and intolerance to crowds. The former group of patients suffer from a chronic anxiety neurosis; the latter group have chronic neurocirculatory asthenia.

Chronic Anxiety. The onset of this syndrome is rare before the age of eighteen or after thirty-five to forty; the mean age of onset in Cohen's series was twenty-five. The illness is twice as frequent in women as men. The course is variable. Most often there are periods of several weeks' duration when the symptoms are so severe as to interrupt the patient's activities. These may be separated by periods of partial or complete remission. There is a high familial incidence of this syndrome, but the explanation of this is not known.

In addition to one or many typical anxiety attacks, the patient usually complains of fatigue, restlessness, tenseness, apprehension, and "nervousness" developing over a period of weeks. Pressure headaches, often described as a bandlike sensation encircling the head, and palpitation are other prominent and troublesome symptoms. The physician, finding little or nothing by objective examination, often attributes the fatigue and other symptoms to low blood pressure or anemia, and prescribes a tonic or vitamins. The patient, upon learning that no evidence of structural disease was found on examination, may be reassured for a few days, but as his symptoms return he is again assailed by doubts concerning his health. Anxiety attacks are usually the reason for the patient seeking medical aid for the first time.

The relative frequency of 20 different symptoms that comprise the syndrome of acute anxiety neurosis has been tabulated by Cohen and by Miles and Cobb. Nervousness, apprehension, palpitation, and breathlessness head the list; while trembling, fatigue on effort, chest pain, dizziness, sweating, and headache occurred in more than 50 per cent of cases. Paresthesias, sighing, smothering, vascular throbbing, nightmares, anorexia, pain radiating to the left arm, fatigue on minor exertion, depression, and syncope were less frequent. Concerning the smothering, the patient usually remarks, "I can't get enough air," "I have to fight for my breath." The chest pain consists of a feeling of pressure or aching, usually in the precordium, and rarely of darting or stabbing pains. The dizziness is of the type referred to as giddiness (see Chap. 30). Faintness is frequent; actual syncope is uncommon. Nevertheless, the patient's fear of fainting may cause him to seek the quiet of his own home and shun people. The appetite is poor, and digestive complaints, e.g., nausea, epigastric pressure, a sensation of abdominal fluttering, are not infrequent.

The physical examination usually yields relatively little of positive value. Cohen, in one of the most thorough and objective reports on this condition, has noted only (1) slight and inconstant tachycardia, (2) slight tachypnea, (3) sighing respirations, (4) flushed face and neck, (5) tremor of the outstretched fingers, and (6) brisk tendon reflexes. The results of standard clinical laboratory procedures—i.e., blood cell counts, urine, blood sugar, nonprotein nitrogen values, basal metabolic rate, electrocardiogram, and electroencephalogram—are within normal limits.

CHRONIC NEUROCIRCULATORY ASTHENIA. A chronic, perhaps lifelong illness, chronic neurocirculatory asthenia (effort syndrome, irritable heart, soldier's heart, DaCosta's syndrome, nervous heart, vasomotor neurosis, chronic vasomotor instability, cardiac neurosis,) manifests itself by excessive fatigability, palpitation, and dyspnea on slight exertion. It usually becomes apparent during adolescence and interferes with the physical activity of the patient, particularly his participation in vigorous games. Nervousness, tenseness, and the other symptoms listed under the "acute anxiety state," including frank anxiety attacks, also occur in chronic neurocirculatory asthenia.

Patients with neurocirculatory asthenia frequently consult cardiologists because of the suspicion that they suffer from heart disease, and indeed many such cases are mistakenly diagnosed as mild rheumatic heart disease because of the chance finding of a systolic murmur or an unexplained tachycardia.

Many of these individuals make a satisfactory adjustment to their illness by limiting their activities. In times of war, when they are inducted into the army, their nervous instability and cardiopulmonary symptoms are so prominent as to render them unfit for active duty. All the more important studies of neurocirculatory asthenia were begun during or after a war.

The physical findings are the same as those of the chronic anxiety state. Occasionally there is a slight systolic murmur and the T waves may be flattened in leads I and II. Approximately half the children of patients with neurocirculatory asthenia have been found to suffer from the same syndrome. A 20-year follow-up on 173 cases by Wheeler, White, Reed, and Cohen showed that the symptoms were still present in 88 per cent but only 15 per cent had had moderate to severe disability from them. Most of the patients were able to work and enjoy a normal family and social life. Psychosomatic illnesses or other types of psychoneurosis had not developed.

Anxiety in Hysteria and Other Psychoneuroses. The occurrence of anxiety in hysteria and psychasthenia, or obsessive-compulsive neurosis, is discussed on pp. 395 and 399.

Agitated Depression, Dementing Diseases, and Delirium. These are discussed in Chaps. 44, 37, and 38, respectively.

Cause, Mechanism, and Biologic Significance of the Anxiety States. There has been much speculation as to the cause of anxiety. The psychologist has come to regard it as anticipatory behavior, i.e., a state of uneasiness concerning something, which the individual believes may happen or will happen in the future. It is believed to be based on an inherited instinctual pattern (fear), and the occurrence of this emotional state without an obvious and natural provocation is explained as an example of a conditioned or learned response.

The only well-systematized psychiatric theory is that put forth by the psychoanalysts, who look upon anxiety as a response to a situation which in some manner threatens the security of the individual. Anxiety is a response to danger, either actual or symbolic. It is pointed out that the somatic symptoms of anxiety are similar to those of fear. The postulated danger is internal rather than external; some primitive drive that is not compatible with one's conscience has been aroused and could be satisfied only at risk to the individual.

Most psychiatrists accept this theory and believe that, through psychotherapeutic interviews, an anxiety-provoking stimulus of which the patient is not aware can usually be found. Once the patient gains insight into the psychodynamic mechanism his anxiety symptoms are said to subside.

A search for physiologic or pathologic changes in cases of anxiety has been unrewarding thus far. The patient with neurocirculatory asthenia has a limited capacity for physical work, and effort uncovers a defect in aerobic metabolism as evidenced by increased oxygen consumption and blood lactate concentration. He is unable to tolerate the physiologic and biochemical effects of work as well as the average person. Whether these differences are of primary significance or are due to a lack of training or poor physical condition has not been settled.

A number of endocrinologic studies have been done and have yielded interesting data. In some patients with neurocirculatory asthenia, the urinary excretion of epinephrine has been found to be elevated; in others, an increase in the urinary excretion of norepinephrine was found; while in still a third group, normal values for both epinephrine and norepinephrine were obtained. Recently Elmadjian and his associates have found that the aldosterone excretion of anxiety-neurotic patients is two to three times that of normal control persons. This work has been in part corroborated by Venning, who demonstrated an increase in aldosterone excretion in medical students experiencing worry and overt anxiety while preparing for examinations. The significance of these observations is not immediately apparent.

Diagnosis. The clinical diagnosis of anxiety state depends upon recognition of the implicit or subjective disturbance, i.e., the uneasiness and apprehension, and the more objective vasomotor and visceral changes. The presence of diffuse or more or less circumscribed attacks of autonomic excitation without the psychic counterpart, i.e., the feeling of nervousness and apprehension, does not establish the clinical diagnosis of anxiety, but only suggests anxiety as a diagnostic possibility. Similar autonomic disturbances in acute attacks may occur as a manifestation of diencephalic, autonomic epilepsy as described by Penfield, in cases of pheochromocytoma, of thyrotoxicosis, and of hypoglycemia. These conditions are discussed elsewhere in this book. They can usually be distinguished from anxiety attacks if one makes a careful analysis of the history and findings. A disturbance in the function of somatic structures or of viscera that are not under the control of the autonomic nervous system is, on the other hand, sufficient grounds for excluding an anxiety state, at least as the full explanation for the clinical picture. (See Table 39-2 for differential diagnosis.)

Once the diagnosis of the anxiety state, with or without anxiety attacks, has been established with reasonable certainty, the next problem is to determine its significance. Is it merely one manifestation of schizophrenia or of a depressive psychosis? Is it combined with other neurotic symptoms which dominate the clinical picture such as phobic obsessive-compulsive psychoneurosis or hysteria? Is it merely fear due to some event that has recently upset the life of the patient, or is it a chronic lifelong illness? Is it a symptom of a reactive state in a patient with organic brain disease?

In order to answer these questions the physician must make pointed inquiry as to the presence of mood depression, distortion of logical thinking and inappropriateness of affect, hysterical symptoms, obsessions, compulsions, phobias, and dementia. A useful practical rule is that any anxiety state that develops for the first time after the thirty-fifth year of life almost invariably proves to be an agitated or involutional depression or an organic disease of the brain.

Anxiety states are frequently misdiagnosed. When cardiac and pulmonary symptoms are prominent, coronary or chronic rheumatic heart disease is assumed; trembling and sweating suggest hyperthyroidism; excessive fatigue raises the possibility of anemia or Addison's disease; and headache, blurred vision, dizziness, and peculiar spells raise the question of a neurologic disease. Cohen has summarized a number of crucial points which are of aid in the differential diagnosis.

Anxiety neurosis and neurocirculatory asthenia differ from coronary heart disease in the following respects: The onset of anxiety neurosis is before the age of thirty-five years; coronary heart disease usually begins after the age of forty years. Anxiety neurosis is more frequent in women; coronary heart disease is more frequent in men. The pain of coronary heart disease or angina pectoris is usually midline, substernal with radiation to the arms, and of constricting quality; the pain of anxiety neurosis is usually on the left side, precordial or epigastric, is aching or stabbing in type, and seldom radiates to the arms. The electrocardiogram is essentially normal in anxiety neurosis or neurocirculatory asthenia except for minor S-T and T-wave changes in an occasional case. Anginal attacks are more likely to be precipitated by muscular exertion, especially in cold weather or after eating; they last a minute or two and cause the patient to stop what he is doing. Anxiety attacks come on in a warm, crowded place or while the patient is at rest or even in bed; they are of longer duration and the patient may get up and walk about during the attack. It should be remembered, however, that the patient who has had a coronary occlusion may also walk while in pain. Cardiac asthma or attacks of paroxysmal nocturnal dyspnea differ from anxiety attacks in that there is evidence of left-sided heart failure, cough, rales, and squeaks in the chest. Fear and acute dyspnea are common to both conditions. Congestive heart failure and anxiety neurosis may sometimes occur together, but this can be recognized if one is mindful that cough, edema, exertional dyspnea, low vital capacity, cyanosis, rales in the lungs, enlarged liver, and evident heart disease are characteristic of the former, while sighing respirations and dyspnea at rest, palpitation, fear and apprehension, and giddiness are typical of the latter. Paroxysmal auricular tachycardia differs from anxiety attacks in that the beginning and the end of the attack is abrupt, the pulse is 160 beats per minute or higher, and the rhythm is regular. There may be other symptoms but they are more in the nature of weakness or faintness.

Thyrotoxicosis can usually be distinguished from anxiety neurosis by its onset, usually in middle or late life, and the presence of eye signs, marked weight loss, radioactive iodine uptake of more than 50, protein-bound iodine values greater than 8 mg per 100 ml, and increased basal metabolic rate, none of which occurs in anxiety neurosis. Cold hands, nervous chills, dizzy spells, headaches, smothering and sighing respirations, so common in anxiety neurosis, are not symptoms of thyrotoxicosis. The basal metabolism test is not always a reliable means of distinguishing between these two conditions. Patients with anxiety neurosis are seldom at basal conditions and some of them, especially if sighing respirations are frequent, have an elevated metabolic rate. A normal value is therefore more meaningful than an elevated one. The nervousness of thyrotoxicosis is in the nature of restlessness, awareness of trembling, and easy excitability; that of anxiety neurosis is fear and apprehension. Probably this condition is more often confused with anxiety than any other illness. In some clinics as many as half the patients who have had thyroidectomy for hyperthyroidism are suffering instead from anxiety neurosis. The elderly patients with "masked hyperthyroidism" may be particularly difficult to diagnose.

Bronchial asthma is readily identified by audible wheezing respirations, and by chronic cough, squeaks, and wheezes in the chest. Dyspnea and tightness in the chest are common to both conditions.

Anxiety neurosis may be distinguished from the menopausal syndrome with some difficulty because typical anxiety attacks are not too infrequent at this age. "Hot flashes," labile emotionality, irritability, and change in the menstrual cycle in a middle-aged woman are characteristic of the menopause. When the typical anxiety symptoms are added, the case usually proves to be one of involutional melancholia. Only the vasomotor symptoms of menopause respond at all to the administration of estrogens.

Most experienced physicians are able to recognize the anxiety state and to distinguish it from the aforementioned syndromes. Frequently, however, anxiety is combined with some other disease such as bronchial asthma or cardiac decompensation. To separate the effects of the two diseases and to manage them properly requires much clinical skill. The mistake often made is to expect the anxiety symptoms to respond to the treatment of the associated disease.

Management and Treatment. There is rather little available information as to the effectiveness of different methods of treatment in anxiety neurosis and neurocirculatory asthenia. The few published reports suggest that supportive medical care, simple psychotherapy, deep psychotherapy such as psychoanalysis and institutional psychiatric therapy, all give results that are roughly comparable, i.e., improvement in about 50 to 70 per cent of cases. Many psychiatrists are of the opinion that frequent psychotherapeutic interviews have produced the highest percentage of cures, but this conclusion cannot be drawn from the published data.

Adequate examination and detailed case study as performed in a hospital are an important part of therapy. The patient should be reassured that there is no serious medical disease. He should be told firmly and convincingly that he is suffering from a nervous disorder from which he will recover. His illness should not be passed off as imaginary. Many physicians encourage their patients to give up smoking because this tends to aggravate the pulmonary and vasomotor symptoms; but if smoking appears to relieve their tension, they probably should not be deprived of this support. If the patient is extremely irritable and upset, a trial of sedatives is indicated. Barbital in doses of 0.3 Gm b.i.d. or phenobarbital 0.032 Gm t.i.d. should be given for 2 or 3 weeks. During the past few years encouraging results have been obtained by the authors in allaying anxiety with the use of meprobamate in doses of 200 to 400 mg or methaminodiazepoxide (Librium), 5 to 10 mg, four times a day. Tonics and vitamins are sometimes of value as supportive measures. However, since there is no serious medical disease, and in order to be consistent, it is well to avoid the use of all medication and encourage the patient to resume his activities. If anxiety symptoms recur he should be as tolerant of them as possible. Obvious sources of anxiety should be avoided. The hyperventilation symptoms which occur in the last part of the anxiety attack can to some degree be voluntarily controlled and this is often reassuring to the patient, for he then knows that he is the master of at least part of his attacks.

These few simple measures will relieve symptoms in about half or more of the cases, particularly the more acute ones in which fear of disease is paramount. Chronic and severe cases should be referred to a psychiatrist, if one is available. Psychotherapy should probably not be prolonged. Some of the more experienced psychoanalysts, including Freud, have stated that psychoanalysis is not indicated for this condition.

Chronic neurocirculatory asthenia is best managed as any other chronic incurable medical ailment. The patient is given every possible assistance in adjusting to his disability.

PSYCHASTHENIA (Obsessive-Compulsive Neurosis, Phobic Neurosis, Obsessive-Compulsive-Ruminative State)

The terms *psychasthenia* and *neurasthenia* have quite different meanings in psychiatry. The former refers to an illness characterized by obsessions, morbid fears, and doubts. It is discussed in some detail below. The latter term had wide popularity in the nineteenth century and is now obsolete. It referred to a state in which the major symptoms were chronic fatigability, lack of endurance, backache, and headache. Upon further study most patients of this type proved to be suffering from anxiety neurosis, neurocirculatory asthenia, a depressive psychosis or hysteria. There seems now to be no need for this diagnostic category.

Psychasthenia in its fully developed form is a relatively rare condition, probably occurring in not more than 0.5 per cent of the population for whom psychiatric consultation is sought in a diagnostic clinic. Lesser degrees of it, manifest as excessive hand washing and other irrational habits or rigid, obsessional thinking is much more frequent, and it may interfere with the therapy and management of medical disease.

Psychasthenia is discussed in the chapter on anxiety because anxiety is a prominent feature in the majority of patients.

Clinical Description. This type of neurosis, like many others, usually develops during adolescence or early adult years, and females and males are both affected, the former somewhat more frequently. The beginning of the illness is gradual in most cases and no date can be assigned to it, but in others its onset may be precipitated by some unusual event in the personal life of the patient with which he is unable to cope.

The outstanding characteristics of the illness are *obsessions, phobias, compulsions,* and *anxiety.* Westphal, who was the first to make a study of obsessions, concluded that anxiety is always secondary to the obsession, but this opinion appears to be too absolute, for in some cases anxiety precedes the obsession. Rosanoff and others are inclined to the view that obsessions and anxiety are "two manifestations of the same fundamental psychic disorder."

An *obsession* may be defined as an imperative idea which persists in the patient's mind despite his desire to be rid of it. It is like a tune "running in the head," which every normal person has experienced from time to time. Often these thoughts are unpleasant, and some are frightening. Obsessions are of various forms. The most common are the *intellectual obsessions*, in which the mind of the patient is occupied either by some abstract or concrete idea—a word, an object, or image of a scene; *impulsive obsessions*, in which the mind is dominated by an impulse to kill oneself, to stab one's children, or to perform some other objectionable act; *inhibiting obsessions*, in which every act must be ruminated upon and analyzed before it is carried out—a "doubting mania." Every effort of will or deliberate attempt at distraction fails to rid the patient of the obsessive thought. It engulfs his mind; it renders him miserable and inefficient. Probably the most disturbing of these are the impulsive obsessions, in which the patient is constantly struggling with the fear that he will put his terrible thought into execution. Even as he tells of his obsession he seeks reassurance that he will not yield to it. Fortunately, such patients rarely obey their fatal impulses.

Phobias are similar to obsessions. In fact they are really obsessive fears. The most common phobias are those of open places, closed places, high places, dirt, traveling, syphilis or other venereal disease, cancer, insanity, or death.

Compulsions are the third feature of the illness. These are single acts or series of acts which the patient feels he must carry out in order to put his mind at ease or to relieve his nervousness. Examples are repeatedly checking the locks on the doors or the gas jets, adjusting articles of clothing, repeated hand washing, wiping with a clean handkerchief objects which have been touched, etc. An illustration of the complexity of some of these compulsive acts was provided by one of the author's patients who went through a time-consuming ritual each night before retiring. This consisted of arranging all removed garments in an orderly fashion on a chair in his room, then taking a bath and, after washing scrupulously, standing on a mat and permitting the air to dry him completely, returning to his room by opening and closing the doors with his elbows, putting on clean pajamas, turning out the light with his elbow, going to the chair where his clothes were, turning his head in the opposite direction and picking up the articles of clothing at random and throwing them piece by piece in the air and letting them fall where they would. This was repeated twice a day, consuming several hours of his time.

Certain motor disturbances of an apparently less meaningful nature are also present in many cases. Usually they involve a small group of muscles and are of limited extent. They consist of repetitious movements of the shoulders, arms, hands, and certain of the facial muscles, i.e., habit spasms, also called *tics*. Their outstanding feature, unlike other involuntary movements, is that they take place only with accompanying consciousness. The person thinks of the movement which he dislikes and knows he can't control and then feels compelled to make the movement. Often a phobia dictates the compulsive act, e.g., hand washing may be the result of a fear of dirt and germs.

In all these phobias, obsessions, compulsions, and motor agitations the patient recognizes the absurdity of his behavior, yet is incapable of controlling himself, much as he desires to do so. He suffers a curious feeling of insufficiency or incompetency in being unable to expel these troublesome thoughts.

The majority of these patients are tense, nervous, and apprehensive. They may complain of typical anxiety attacks. After the condition has persisted for a time they may become discouraged or depressed over their helplessness in escaping from their obsessions and compulsions. This distraught emotional state is usually inconstant and is often related to the fear that an idea may eventuate in reality. Fatigue, anorexia, and general lack of interest, which are often present, are probably related to the anxiety and depression. In other respects the patients do not deviate from normal. There are no disturbances in formal thinking, no illusions, hallucinations, or delusions. Insight is intact; the patient realizes fully that his fears are irrational and groundless. The facial expression is usually appropriately animated. There is a tendency to be restless, and excessive vasomotor activity such as blushing and sweating are often in evidence. Once the patient feels confident in his physician, there is usually no reluctance to tell of his upsetting symptoms, for most individuals afflicted in this way are desperately seeking help.

Cause and Mechanism. Phenomena such as obsessions, phobias, and compulsions have attracted the attention of all who would interpret behavior in psychologic terms. Theories are legion. Ribot was of the notion that obsessions and phobias are the more or less permanent effects of some exceptionally intense and profound emotional experience, particularly fear, that may have occurred in the highly impressionable period of childhood. Janet expounded the theory that the very domination of the mind by these disturbing thoughts indicates a defect in what is commonly called will power. It was his impression that such individuals really differ from the normal person in that they have less power of mental inhibition and that the processes of attention do not function normally, which is why distracting and irrelevant thoughts cannot be eliminated. Indecisiveness is believed to be another common manifestation of this weakness. For all these fundamental defects Janet has suggested the term *psychasthenia*, and by this he vaguely implies a genetic origin but offers no further evidence on this point.

The psychoanalysts have offered a theory in terms of their familiar postulates concerning the human psyche. To them the psychasthenic behavior is the result of the imperfect repression of some disagreeable wish. They conceive of this wish as having an ideational content and an emotional, or affective content. The latter is the attached libido. If the whole of the disagreeable wish is completely repressed, the energy of the affect may be converted into a physical symptom such as hysterical paralysis or anesthesia (conversion hysteria). If repression is imperfect or incomplete so that only the ideational content is thrust out of the mind, the energy of the affect may then be converted into fear with a resultant phobia, or displaced to another idea which then becomes an obsession or compulsion. The puzzling persistence of the idea or fear is, for them, due to the emotional energy of another idea which cannot be recalled except by the aid of free association.

Janet's and Freud's theories are not incompatible. Janet has described the condition of the psychasthenic mental state and Freud, the conditions which bring about each specific psychasthenic phenomenon. To the neurologist, however, both theories appear to be only partial explanations. One rather expects that some more basic defect, as yet unexplained, must allow these irrational ideas or compulsions to dominate the mind.

Diagnosis. Since the prevailing emotional state in patients with psychasthenia is one of anxiety and depression, it is necessary to distinguish this condition, anxiety neurosis, and depressive psychosis. There are important differences between them, and they can be distinguished rather easily in most instances. In psychasthenia the depression tends to be evanescent and closely related to the obsessive thinking. As the latter improves the depression lightens. In uncomplicated anxiety states, although baseless fears are not uncommon, they are never so persistent or so disabling as in psychasthenia; and the indecisiveness, compulsive actions, and habit spasms are lacking. Schizophrenia must be considered when an adolescent or young adult begins to harbor peculiar ideas, but then the mental status almost invariably reveals the other disturbances in affectivity, thought, and attention, which are described in Chap. 39.

Treatment. The treatment of these rare forms of psychoneurosis is probably best left to psychiatrists, or at least there should be a trial of psychotherapy in most cases. Whereas a few spectacular improvements are said to have been accomplished by psychoanalysis, for the most part the results which have been obtained in a series of patients have never been reported. Presumably the outlook for recovery is poor. In exceptionally severe cases electroconvulsive and insulin shock therapy has been undertaken as a last resort, with some degree of success. The former has proved effective when a strong depressive element colors the clinical picture. Tranquilizing drugs are just now being tried, but it is too soon to draw any conclusions as to their efficacy.

REFERENCES

See Chap. 44.

43 HYSTERIA AND THE PSYCHOPATHIC PERSONALITY (with Remarks on Malingering)

Justin M. Hope and
Raymond D. Adams

Up to this point in the discussions in this book of cardinal manifestations it has been assumed that the patient's symptoms always represent the objective or subjective manifestations of serious disease. But the student soon must learn that symptoms may have other meanings as well. They may, for example, actually express only some trivial disorder of normal body function and, if a source of much concern, may then be indicative of depression, worry, fear, or some related mental state rather than of visceral disease. Symptoms may continue long after their cause has ceased, or may actually be feigned, in order that the patient may continue his role as an invalid or gain some other desired objective.

In order to comprehend the significance of symptoms in all these varied circumstances the physician must be alert to the several possibilities whenever he undertakes to analyze a clinical problem. In making this evaluation it is necessary to maintain a calm, objective, realistic attitude toward the patient and his problem. Both excessive gullibility and excessive skepticism must be avoided. The physician's manner at all times should be one of friendliness and sympathy, and he must show neither surprise nor annoyance when the symptoms appear trivial or spurious. The suspicion that sometimes permeates the medical atmosphere in military hospitals and the medical departments of insurance agencies, where many of the patients tend to make exaggerated claims, is particularly deplorable for it serves only to antagonize the patient and to prevent the formation of a proper patient-doctor relationship.

The circumstance in which a patient believes or pretends that he has a disease which does not exist is not too uncommon in medicine. In many instances the reason for this unusual behavior is rather obvious, such as fear of a disease which has affected another member of his family or a friend, the evasion of work or military duty, or the gaining of compensation for a real or fancied injury. There are other instances, and this is especially true of female hysterics, in which the reason for the illness may not be evident, though the physician may readily enough imagine a plausible explanation.

The diagnosis of hysteria may be difficult. Errors of two types are likely to be committed. The condition may be mistaken for some other medical or neurologic disease, and not until a series of expensive, and at times dangerous, diagnostic procedures have been completed or several unnecessary operations performed will the hysterical nature of the illness finally be ascertained. Or an obscure medical or surgical disease, not sufficiently advanced to permit diagnosis, may erroneously be called hysteria. These errors emphasize the fact that there is no certain means of arriving at a correct diagnosis in every case, or of confirming the diagnosis once it has been made. The physician must therefore become familiar with the major clinical manifestations of this illness and must know the background upon which this unusual behavior is usually engrafted. Clinical diagnosis will depend, then, not on the mere exclusion of other diseases, i.e., the negative approach, which is always hazardous, but rather on the fulfillment of positive diagnostic criteria.

There are two clinical syndromes, not completely separable, in which a patient may dissemble an obvious physical symptom or an illness: hysteria and psychopathy, sometimes called *constitutional psychopathic state*.

HYSTERIA

Clinical Description. The so-called "classic" form of hysteria without doubt predominates in women, as confirmed in all contemporary clinical studies. One of the authors (Hope) has not observed a typical case of hysteria in a man during the past 10 years. During this period, in which several thousand psychiatric cases were seen in consultation, the diagnosis of female hysteria was made 813 times. There were, however, eight male cases with an illness that bore some resemblance to the classic form of hysteria, but they differed in one important respect—a tangible, material compensation factor was present in each. From this, however, it must not be assumed that a neurosis in which compensation factors are prominent is limited to men, for one sees it in many women as well. One must conclude that classical hysteria is exceedingly rare in males and that women are as likely to develop an illness in which a tangible financial gain is a factor as are men.

Because of this and other important differences between the classic form, which is predominantly a female disease, and the forms of the disease which involve compensation factors and which occur in both men and women, each is presented separately on the following pages. Under the heading Hysteria is described the classic form of the disease, as the authors have observed it in women and as it has been described in the literature, while that variety of compensation neurosis so often observed in the male segment of the population is introduced in a special section under the heading Hysteria with an Important Factor of Compensation.

"Classic" Hysteria. By a careful review of the history of any given case it can usually be learned that the disease had its onset at the time of puberty or adolescent years. A few cases may appear to begin before puberty, at the age of eight or nine up to fourteen years, but before this period of life it is so rare that it should seldom be considered as a diagnostic possibility. Once established, hysteria often appears to be a lifelong illness or type of reaction, and symptoms continue to occur intermittently, though with lessening frequency, throughout adult years even to an advanced age. There are, no doubt, cases of lesser severity which exhibit symptoms only once or a few times, just as there are lesser degrees of all conditions. The patient may be seen for the first time during the middle period of life or later, and the earlier history may not at first be obtained. Careful probing, however, will almost invariably reveal that the earliest manifestations of this illness had appeared before the age of twenty-five years.

Other interesting and valuable data are also brought to light by a careful past history. During late childhood and adolescence the normal activities of the patient, including education, have usually been interrupted by periods of illness. Sometimes diseases such as rheumatic fever, tuberculosis, or other obscure diseases were suspected. Later in life, problems in work adjustment and marriage are frequent. There is a notably high incidence of marital incompatibility, separation, and divorce. The patient's life history is punctuated with symptoms and illnesses which do not conform to recognizable patterns of medical and surgical disease. For these, many forms of therapy, including surgical operations, have been performed. Rarely has adult life been reached without at least one abdominal operation, usually done because of pain, persistent nausea, and vomiting, or generalized weakness. The indications for the surgical procedure have usually been unclear, and further, the same symptoms or others have recurred to complicate the convalescence. The biographies of these patients are also replete with difficulties which center about menstrual, sexual, and procreative functions. Menstrual periods may be painfully prostrating, irregular, or excessive. Sexual intercourse may be painful, unpleasant, or unsatisfactory. Pregnancies may be difficult: the usual vomiting of the first trimester may persist all through the gestational period, with weight loss and prostration; labor may be severe and prolonged, and all manner of unpredictable complications are said to occur during and after parturition.

Hysteria is, then, rarely a monosymptomatic disease. Expressed another way, the only forms which can be diagnosed with any degree of assurance are polysymptomatic, involving almost every organ system. The only limit to their variation and pleomorphism is the limit of the patient's ability to produce them by an effort of will (conscious or unconscious). Accordingly, symptoms and signs which are beyond volitional control cannot be accepted as manifestations of hysteria. A list of the most frequent symptoms, all statistically significant, which were elicited during a study of 50 unmistakable cases of female hysteria and compared with a control group of 50 healthy women of the same age who were working regularly in a factory and who appeared to have no recognizable psychiatric illness (Cohen, Robins, et al.) include the following: headache, blurred vision, lump in the throat, loss of voice, dyspnea, palpitation, anxiety attacks, anorexia, nausea and vomiting, abdominal pain, food dyscrasia, sexual indifference, painful intercourse, paresthesias, dizzy spells, nervousness, and easy crying.

The examination of the female hysteric patient demonstrates a number of useful findings, mostly in the sphere of mental status. One becomes suspicious of the possibility of a psychiatric illness almost at once by the patient's response to questions regarding the chief complaint. Usually a vague reply or the narration of a series of symptoms or problems, many of which prove to have little or no relevance to the obvious disability is obtained. However, unlike a psychotic illness insight is intact, and there is no evidence of hallucinations, delusions, disturbance in logical thinking, or loss of appreciation of the reality of the situation. The manner of the patient is often amiable and even ingratiating. The description of symptoms tends to be dramatic and exaggerated and does not necessarily accord with the facts as elicited from other members of the family; yet at the same time a rather casual emotional reaction is manifested. The patient may insist that everything in her life is quite natural and serene, which is obviously not true. This calm attitude toward a turbulent illness is so common that it has been singled out as an important characteristic and has been given the name *la belle indifférence*. Other patients, however, are obviously tense and anxious, and frank anxiety attacks are reported by many of them. Also, "any attempt at disproving the somatic nature of the complaints meets with anxiety and dramatic protest." Memory defects are usually demonstrated while taking the history; the patient appears to have forgotten important segments of the history, particularly those which relate to the development of her symptoms (Lindemann).

There are no characteristic physical findings. Although many writers have commented on the rather youthful, girlish appearance and coquettish manner of many of the patients, this by no means characterizes all of them. The so-called stigmas of hysteria, i.e., corneal anesthesia, absence of gag reflex, spots of pain and tenderness over the scalp, sternum, breasts, lower ribs, and ovaries, are often suggested by the examiner and are too inconsistent to be of much help in diagnosis.

Special Hysterical Syndromes. A few hysterical syndromes recur with great regularity, and every physician may expect to encounter them. They constitute some of the most puzzling diagnostic problems in medicine.

HYSTERICAL PAIN. This may involve any part of the body; generalized or localized headache, "atypical facial neuralgia," abdominal pain, back pain with camptocormia are the most frequent and most troublesome to the clinician. Here the greatest source of error is to mistake the pain of osteomyelitis, metastatic carcinoma, or brain tumor, before other symptoms have developed, for a manifestation of hysteria. In many of these patients the response to analgesic drugs has been unusual, and not a few of them are suspected of or may be suffering from drug addiction. They may respond to a placebo as though it were a potent drug, but it should be pointed out that this is a notoriously unreliable means of distinguishing hysterical pain from that of other diseases. The most helpful diagnostic features are inability of the patient to give a clear, concise description of the type of pain, its location, and other features; the dramatic elaborations of its intensity and effects; its persistence, either continuous or intermittent, for long periods of time; the lack of conformation to other pain syndromes; the absence of other diseases which could account for pain; the assumption of bizarre attitudes and postures; the coexistence of other hysterical symptoms.

HYSTERICAL VOMITING. This is often combined with pain and tenderness in the lower abdominal quadrants and results in many unnecessary appendectomies and the removal of pelvic organs in adolescent girls and young women. The vomiting is somewhat unusual, in that it often occurs after a meal, leaving the patient hungry and ready to eat again; it may be induced by unpleasant circumstances. Some of these patients can vomit on command, regurgitating food from the stomach like a ruminant animal. Vomiting may persist for weeks with no cause being found. Weight loss may occur but seldom to the degree anticipated. The usual first trimester vomiting of pregnancy may continue throughout the entire 9 months, and occasionally pregnancy will be interrupted because of it. Anorexia may be another prominent symptom.

HYSTERICAL SEIZURES AND OTHER PHYSICAL STATES, E.G., TRANCES AND FUGUES. These conditions seem to be less frequent than in the days of Charcot when *la grande attaque d'hystérie* was often exhibited before medical audiences. Nevertheless they do occur and must be distinguished from convulsive seizures and catalepsy. To witness an attack is of great assistance in diagnosis. The lack of aura, initiating cry, hurtful fall, and incontinence, the presence of peculiar movements such as grimacing, squirming, biting, striking at or resisting those who offer assistance, the retention of consciousness during a motor seizure which involves both sides of the body, the long duration of the seizure and abrupt termination by strong sensory stimulation are all typical of the hysterical attack. Sometimes hyperventilation will initiate an attack and is therefore a useful maneuver in the hospital or clinic. Both epilepsy and hysteria may be combined in the same patient, in which instance the resulting illness invariably causes difficulty in diagnosis. Hysterical trances or fugues, in which the patient wanders about for hours or days and carries out complex acts, may also simulate temporal lobe epilepsy, epilepsy equivalent, or any of the conditions which lead to confusional psychosis or stupor. Here the most reliable point of differentiation comes from observation of the patient, who, if hysterical, is likely to indicate a degree of alertness and promptness of response not seen in confusional states. After the episode is past, an interview with the patient under the influence of hypnosis, strong suggestion, Pentothal, or scopolamine will often bring to light memories of what happened during the episode. This will exclude the possibility of an epileptic fugue.

HYSTERICAL PARALYSES AND TREMORS. Hysterical palsies usually involve an arm, leg, one side of the body, or both legs. If the affected limb can be moved at all, muscle action is weak, and often the strength of voluntary movement is in proportion to the resistance offered. Movements are characteristically slow, tentative, and poorly sustained. One can feel agonist and antagonist muscles contracting simultaneously. When the resistance is suddenly withdrawn, there is no follow-through, as with normal movements. The muscular tone in the affected limbs is usually normal, but rigidity may sometimes be found. Walking may be impossible, there may be a veritable astasia-abasia, or the gait may be bizarre (see Chap. 30). This discrepancy between the ability to walk and to move the legs is, of course, not unique to hysteria; it also occurs in frontal lobe apraxia and in ataxia from midline cerebellar lesions. If the limb has been held in a rigid posture for a long time, contractures may set in. The features of hysterical tremor are described in Chap. 27 and need not be repeated here. The tendon reflexes are always normal, but with hysterical anesthesia of one-half the body, the abdominal and plantar reflexes may be suppressed on the affected side. Anesthesia or hypesthesia is almost always inadvertently induced by the examining physician. Seldom is sensory loss a spontaneous complaint of the patient, though the complaints of "numbness" and paresthesias are not uncommon. The sensory loss may involve one or more limbs below a sharp line (stocking and glove distribution) or may involve one-half the body. Touch, pain, taste, smell, vision, and hearing may all be affected on that side, which is an anatomic impossibility from a single lesion.

HYSTERICAL AMNESIA, SOMNAMBULISM, AND PSEUDODEMENTIA (GANSER'S SYNDROME). Patients brought to a hospital in a state of amnesia are usually hysterics or psychopaths. Usually after a few hours or days, with encouragement they divulge their whole life history. The epileptic patient or the victim of a concussion or acute confusional psychosis does not come to a hospital asking for help in establishing his identity. Moreover, the complete loss of memory for all previous life experiences by a patient who is otherwise able to comport himself normally is not observed in any other conditions.

In Ganser's syndrome, which usually occurs in psychopathic males involved in a crime, the patient pretends to have lost his mind or to have become insane. He acts in the way he believes an insane or feebleminded person should act. He may babble and give silly and obviously incorrect answers to every question asked of him. Usually his behavior is obviously an act.

UNEXPLAINED HYPERPYREXIA. Among the sporadic cases of unexplained fever which turn up in every diagnostic clinic, there are always a few hysterical patients. Although our clinical material is not large, the authors have been impressed with the number of student nurses, nurses, and nursing aides among them. Some of these patients will be found to have no fever if the nurse or doctor checks the temperature. Others have oral temperatures of 99 to 100°F, which must be regarded as normal for some individuals. Finally, there are a few well-documented cases of verified hyperpyrexia, said to be of psychogenic origin. In these the possibility of some obscure hypothalamic disorder cannot be excluded. Diagnosis is assisted by a longitudinal history and the elicitation of the other symptoms of hysteria.

DERMATITIS FACTITIA (HYSTERICAL DERMATONEUROSIS). This condition is seen more often in the psychopathic than in the hysteric patient. The skin eruptions induced by the patient are characterized by erythema, ulcerations, gangrene, and variable degrees of dermatitis. Usually a caustic or irritant chemical or a sharp instrument such as a nail file has been used. The lesions are most commonly observed on parts of the body accessible to the right hand, i.e., right side of the face, neck, anterior trunk, anterior surface of left arm. They are multiple, sharply outlined, appear at variable intervals of time, and do not conform to any of the standard dermatologic diseases. They resist all treatment until protected from the continued manipulations of the patient and then they heal promptly.

Hysteria with an Important Factor of Compensation. As stated before, hysteria in men is most often encountered in patients who serve the military, veterans' hospitals, and in places where injured civilian workers are treated. As in the classic form of hysteria described above, multiple symptoms are noted in the majority of cases, certainly in all eight cases which one of the authors (Hope) examined. Furthermore, many of the symptoms are the same as those listed under female hysteria, i.e., headache, nervousness, irritability, pain in the back and extremities, dizziness, dyspnea, palpitation, nausea, vomiting, paresthesias, blurred vision, anxiety attacks, depression, faints, amnesia, loss of libido, and trance states. A tangible gain from the illness may easily be discovered by simple questioning. This is usually in the form of monetary compensation, which, surprisingly enough, is often less than the patient could earn if he returned to work. Another interesting feature is the frequency with which the patient expresses extreme dissatisfaction with the medical care given him; he is often

frankly hostile toward the physicians and nurses. Descriptions of symptoms tend to be lengthy and circumstantial and fail to give details which are so useful in diagnosis. Many of these patients have already been subjected to an excessive number of hospitalizations when first seen, and rather dramatic mishaps may have occurred in carrying out diagnostic and therapeutic procedures. The majority have been suspected of and many accused of malingering by at least one physician in the past, which may be responsible for the aggressive behavior and uncooperative attitude of some of the patients. In fact compensation hysteria, as pointed out below, is at times almost indistinguishable from malingering. The diagnosis of hysteria in the male probably should be made with great caution unless some obvious compensation factor is present.

Women who suffer injury while at work or are involved in auto accidents may exhibit these same symptoms and signs. Both men and women with hysterical personalities may also be excessively disposed to accidents. This is one of the causes of the *accident-prone syndrome.*

Cause and Pathogenesis. In speculating upon the cause or causes of hysteria one must call attention to a number of factors. Age and sex have already been mentioned. Native endowment is commonly believed to be important; intellectual capacity is usually only average or below average, but it would be a mistake to conclude that hysteria affects only the illiterate and the feebleminded. The number of psychotic, psychoneurotic, and psychopathic relatives seems always to exceed that found in a more normal segment of the population. However, in the present state of knowledge, the influence of heredity cannot be separated from that of environment. Social and economic conditions also may contribute to hysteria. There seems to be ample evidence that the majority of cases come from what is called the "better and poorer classes," from the "froth and dregs of society," where lack of discipline, instability, impulsiveness, and violent conflicts between the individual and his social environment come particularly to the fore. Prolonged illness during early life also tends to breed neurotic character, perhaps by arousing fear and preventing the realization of ambition. And finally the aggravating effect of a major social disturbance may evoke a hysterical reaction in that segment of society which is unstable, nervous, worried, weak, poorly educated, artistic, disappointed, and maladjusted. Indeed many persons with incipient mental disease have gotten along without a serious outbreak until some major catastrophe occurs.

Over the years, from the time when hysteria was first recognized, many theories and hypotheses have been advanced purporting to explain its cause and mechanism. It is safe to say that, up to the present, none of these theories or hypotheses has been validated. However, of the many theoretic explanations of the psychopathology of hysterical phenomena, three are most deserving of attention, those of Babinski, Janet, and Freud. Charcot had presented a rigid conception of hysteria as a disease and had described all the stages of it in the typical seizure. It was Babinski who pointed out that the salient characteristic of the illness was hypersuggestibility, and that the seizures, paralyses, and anesthesias were the result of this mental trait. By hypersuggestibility he meant the acceptance of or the realization of an idea which was manifestly irrational. He insisted, moreover, that all the manifestations of hysteria could be removed by persuasion, i.e., the presentation of an idea which was reasonable.

Pierre Janet accepted the notion of hypersuggestibility but went further in attempting to account for the particular forms of hysteria. He postulated the existence of a peculiar hysterical personality characterized first of all by what he termed a weak or imperfect synthesis. This functional synthesis, well integrated in the normal individual, never develops in the hysteric patient, because of some inherent or adventitious condition. If this synthesis is marginally weak, fatigue, an emotional crisis, or ill health may further weaken it and cause an outbreak of symptoms. A second feature of the hysterical personality is "chronic retraction of the field of consciousness," which is probably the basis of the heightened suggestibility. Other qualities are the puzzling and changeable character of the hysteric and the weakness of will power which results in his impulsive behavior. Hysterical paralysis represents a dissociation from the normal synthesis of the affected parts of the body. The hysteric cannot feel or move a part because all that pertains to it is dissociated from his mind; and for the same reason he can maintain a spasm or contracture indefinitely without fatigue. Janet's theory is far more detailed and systematic than Babinski's theory but does not explain adequately how the individual symptom arises.

The psychoanalytic theory, as expounded by Freud and his early students, has undergone so many variations that a single statement of their views is difficult. They, too, recognize the existence of a defective personality due presumably to genetic and environmental forces. The personality make-up is one of psychic infantilism, i.e., immaturity of sexual development. A series of unfortunate experiences in such a person is believed to lead to an arrest or a misdirection of sex instincts, which include not only the instinct for reproduction proper but all allied impulses. In the infant these instincts embrace all pleasure-giving impulses. No longer is the process of maturation of the sexual impulses from undifferentiated sexuality through the stage of narcissism, homosexuality, and finally heterosexuality, continued to completion. In the language of the psychoanalysts, the libido becomes "fixated" at an infantile level. The neurotic personality is thus defined as one in which heterosexuality has not properly developed, though the individual himself is not aware of it. This abnormality is ordinarily prevented from becoming manifest by inhibitions and defense mechanisms in the form of ideals and self-discipline which everyone acquires. Fantasies and complexes of ideas arising from these powerful misdirected sexual impulses are in conflict with the patient's ideals, and this is said to explain his peculiarities of conduct, nervousness, and weakness. These complexes of ideas are repressed, but the energy of the emotion attached to them constantly seeks expression. Although these ideas and their affective or emotional content may not express themselves directly during waking hours, they may during sleep, when inhibiting mechanisms are relaxed. Meaningful dreams and somnambulism are the result. Or they may declare themselves indirectly, either through consciousness or through a motor pathway. If the emotional affect is displaced or transferred to some associated ideas, these will then persist in consciousness as an obsession. If the affective energy finds expression through a motor pathway, a conversion hysteria occurs, by which is meant a conversion of a psychic conflict into a state of physical distress or dysfunction. This mechanism of conversion is believed to be central to the whole problem of hysterical symptomatology. Indeed the capacity for conversion is probably present in everyone under conditions of great emotional strain (fright, trauma) and comes to light in civilian life when injury offers a substantial financial gain. This is the situation in the compensation hysteric. However, in classic hysteria there is always "an inner conflict which is linked to the patient's sexual development and secondary gain is of minor importance" (Lindemann).

Another important part of the psychoanalytical theory is that the symptoms and signs are a symbolic expression of the repressed complex. Thus hysterical vomiting stands for a desire to be rid of something repugnant; an hysterical paralysis, a desire to remain ill and to maintain an infantile state of dependency. By this theory the psychoanalysts attempt to explain both the pathogenesis of the hysterical personality and the form of the neurotic symptom. The chief criticism has been the emphasis on misdirected sexuality as the basis of this and all psychoneuroses. Although it is alluringly systematic and accounts plausibly for many of the symptoms, many physicians believe still, as did Janet and others, that it is incomplete, explaining only the content or character of the symptoms and not the basic process. There must still be a basic constitutional defect, not as yet defined, in cases of classic hysteria.

Diagnosis. The method of diagnosis subject to the least error is that employed in medicine generally, i.e., an informative history (obtained from the patient himself as well as from sources other than the patient) and a physical and mental status examination (see Table 39-2). The elicitation of the attributes of a neurotic character by interview and special so-called "projective" tests (Rorschach and Thematic Apperception Tests), methods popular with dynamic psychiatrists, may be helpful but are by no means infallible. Even evidence of extreme suggestibility and the tendency to dramatize symptoms cannot be taken as absolute criteria of the disease, for they may appear under certain conditions in nonhysterical individuals. The psychiatrist obtains help from an analysis of the character of the patient, but this is not likely to be of use to physicians who are not versed in special psychiatric techniques. A longitudinal history, the manner and attitude of the patient, and the absence of symptoms and signs of other medical and surgical disease probably will permit the accurate diagnosis of the majority of cases.

Treatment. The treatment of hysteria may be considered from two aspects: the correction of the long-standing basic personality defect, and the removal of the recently acquired physical symptoms.

Since the main defect in thinking and in character development in the hysteric patient may be quite profound, little or nothing can be done about it at present in the most severe cases. Psychoanalysts have attempted to modify it by long-term reeducation, but their results are unavailable and there are no control studies for the few reports of therapeutic success. One has the impression that in many cases the underlying illness is so pervasive that nothing can be accomplished except to grant that the patient is inadequate in certain respects and requires medical support. Many psychiatrists, for this reason, are inclined to regard the female hysteric with a life-long history of ill health as having a severe psychopathy. In other less severe cases and especially in those in whom the hysterical symptoms have appeared under the pressure of a major crisis, psychotherapy appears to have been helpful and the patients have been able thereafter to resume their places in society.

The acute outbreak of symptoms can usually be controlled by persuasion. Here the best tactic is to treat the patient as though he has had an illness and is now in the process of recovering. The earlier this is done after the development of symptoms, the more likely they are to be eradicated. In chronic cases strong pressure to get out of bed and resume function must be applied. Compensation neuroses are often quite difficult to treat, and a settlement of claims may be necessary before the symptoms are relieved.

The following therapeutic principles should be observed in the average case of hysteria where expert psychiatric opinion is not available or in severe cases where previous psychiatric treatment has failed.

1. Hysteria must be treated as a tangible, definite illness. The patient should never be told, "There is nothing wrong with you," or "It's just your imagination." This at once alienates the patient, and he almost invariably terminates his relations with the physician. The patient should not be dismissed as a malingerer or a faker of illness.

2. Simple understandable language should be employed in interviews with these patients; abstruse psychologic terms should be avoided. It is unnecessary to employ the term *hysteria* in discussions with these patients or their families, since it conveys a derogatory connotation which the physician should not imply.

3. The care of the patient should be entrusted to one physician.

4. All indicated examinations and laboratory procedures for the investigation of the chief complaints should be conducted before actual treatment is begun. Once the treatment is started, one should avoid, if possible, rechecking or repeating laboratory or examination procedures.

5. Persuasion and suggestion, both direct and indirect, should be employed in the treatment of patients. Illustratively, the patients should be encouraged, told that they are better, urged to resume work or household duties and to continue participation in routine activities. Symptoms should be ignored and medication should be withheld.

6. There should be several personal interviews in which the patient is permitted to direct the discussion. He should be assured of the privacy of the interview, of the impersonal, "morally neutral" position of the physician, and of the advantages of "thinking things out more thoroughly." Any questions which the patient asks should be answered truthfully in accordance with the physician's knowledge, in simple, direct terms.

7. Every illness in such patients should be evaluated as a possible manifestation of hysteria. The possibility of other diseases must not be overlooked. Surgical procedures should be used only if strict criteria of surgical disease are satisfied.

How successful this program will be over a long period of time is not known. The eradication of some recently acquired hysterical symptom is relatively easy. The real test of therapy is, however, whether it assists the patient to a satisfactory adjustment to family and to daily activities, prevents unnecessary medical treatments and operations, and makes possible the prompt diagnosis of any medical or surgical disease which may strike a hysteric patient just as it does any other person.

PSYCHOPATHIC PERSONALITY
(Constitutional Psychopathic Inferiority, C.P.I.)

Aside from those patients who suffer from psychoneuroses, epilepsy, psychoses, and feeblemindedness, there still remains a large number who do not fit any of these categories but are still incapable of making a satisfactory adjustment to civilized society. This group is rather heterogeneous and includes drug addicts, many habitual criminals, the chronically unemployed, and those who are more or less constantly under the care of social welfare agencies. Only a small segment of this group, those who develop symptoms and signs suggestive of disease, ever come to the attention of the medical profession. However, all these cases, with as well as without symptoms, seem in some manner to be lacking an essential trait which permits a normal, stable adjustment to life. As a consequence, they remain social misfits all their lives.

The group of these patients which displays behavioral disturbances for which medical advice is sought in general hospitals is not large. Only 33 were found among 10,039 patients examined by the Psychiatric Service of the New England Center Hospital over an 8-year period (see also Table 42-1). However, in large municipal hospitals and in service and veterans' hospitals the number of cases is much greater.

Clinical Description. This disorder becomes manifest early in life, and both sexes are equally susceptible. However, recognition before the age of twenty-one is difficult because one depends for diagnosis largely on evidence of protracted behavioral disturbances over many years. The common turbulent emotional outbreaks during adolescence are particularly difficult to assess in this respect. Experienced physicians know that many boys and girls who appear destined for a life-long psychopathy settle down and become stable citizens, once adulthood is reached.

The most distinctive feature of the constitutional psychopath is his *impulsivity*. He seems unable to control his impulse to any act which provides immediate gratification of his urges and instinctual drives. Without any apparent concern he will withdraw from a team, quit a job, abandon his family, seek financial gain regardless of the means, drink excessively, or be sexually promiscuous. When brought to task for his misdemeanor he appears sorry and may persuade others that he will reform, only to repeat the same act or some other one equally irresponsible when the occasion arises. This *inability to profit from experience* despite adequate intelligence and a proved capacity to learn in school is another noteworthy feature. These defects result in an apparent inability to conform to the moral and ethical standards of his social group; hence he is classed as a "moral imbecile."

The complaints and somatic symptoms which bring these individuals to a general hospital are multiple and varied. Like the hysteric, they have amnesias, trances, fits, paralyses, gait disturbances, unexplained prostration, alleged hemorrhage, unexplained fever, etc. Psychotic episodes may also occur but are remarkably brief as a rule. They tend to develop at the time of some crisis or during an episode of heavy drinking or drug addiction and consist of outbursts of uncontrollable temper, fits of depression with feeble attempts at suicide, and unsystematized delusions and hallucinations. Often they clear up within 2 or 3 days after entering a mental hospital. Their reckless impulsivity predisposes some of these patients to accidents (accident-prone syndrome).

At the time of examination the manner and attitude of the patient are especially informative. He is engaging, talkative, and very persuasive, often convincing the physician and family of the correctness of his position and arousing their sympathy. He may be courteous, ingratiating, and flattering to those around him. On the other hand some such patients are irritable and irascible and may be provoked to anger by some triviality. Only when his story is checked against that of the family does one begin to realize that the present episode has followed a pattern of behavior which has created endless problems over a period of years. Furthermore it is then apparent that the patient himself has no real insight into his condition and is inclined to blame his plight on ill luck, various injustices perpetrated by others, or destiny. Even when caught rubbing his thermometer on the bed sheet to feign the fever of some infectious disease, or when found picking his gums to produce obscure gastrointestinal bleeding, he appears totally uninterested and leaves the hospital saying he is sorry that the doctors did not believe him.

In recent years it has been discovered that a number of these patients have minor electroencephalographic abnormalities, some of clearly paroxysmal type compatible with epilepsy, and others, nonspecific and diffuse. Also psychologic tests may in some instances reveal findings of the type seen in patients with brain disease.

Cause and Pathogenesis. For such a heterogeneous group of behavioral disorders as this represents, one would hardly expect to find a common etiologic factor or mechanism. The word *constitutional* is deplorably ambiguous, for it refers both to genetic factors and to those which result from unfavorable environmental influence. All diseases, in this sense, are constitutional. Yet the term will probably continue to be used until it is possible to separate the particular entities which it presently embraces and to find their cause or mechanism.

Two general theories have been elaborated to account for these aberrations in behavior: (1) character neurosis, (2) structural disease of the nervous system. According to the theory of character neurosis, the abnormal nervous and mental processes are due to psychogenic factors which operated in early life. Here one is on treacherous ground, for little evidence has been forthcoming in favor of this idea, and critics of the theory maintain that the adverse effects of psychologic factors is the result of an intrinsic brain disease rather than the cause of the illness. Adherents of the concept of neurologic disease refer to the remarkable variety of behavioral changes, often limited to emotional control and character structure, which followed in the wake of the great epidemic of lethargic encephalitis after the First World War, and also to the rather high incidence of electro-encephalographic abnormalities. Here again evidence is wanting, for no thorough neuropathologic studies have been made. A final opinion on this matter cannot be expressed at this time. One can only say that the problems involved in such cases are at present beyond the realm of scientific knowledge.

Diagnosis. The key to diagnosis is the evidence by well-documented history of a long-enduring behavior disturbance in which impulsive actions, inadequate self-discipline, weak inhibition, faulty judgment, and the failure to learn by experience have led to a series of immoral and unethical actions (see Table 39-2). In addition, there are the physical symptoms of the type seen in the malingerer and hysteric. Finally the mercurial affective response, varying from a nonchalant, persuasive manner or boastfulness to open hostility, and the utter lack of insight complete the picture.

Alcoholic psychoses, schizophrenia, and manic-depressive psychosis must at times be differentiated, and this is usually possible when all the data of the history and mental examination are at hand. Needless to say, however, some of these individuals do develop frank alcoholic psychoses or have epilepsy, particularly of the temporal lobe type. Such cases can easily be confused with hysteria because of their multiple spurious somatic symptoms. The differentiation is usually not difficult if it is remembered that the number of symptoms is much greater in the hysteric than in the psychopath and, in the cases of male hysteria, the possibility of material gain is more obvious. Hysterical stigmas are not prominent and are certainly less impressive than their tendency to "put on an act." The defect in the psychopath shows most clearly in his inability to make a satisfactory adjustment to school, to work, and to marriage. Lastly, unethical or immoral conduct is peculiar to the psychopath. When alcoholism is added to a psychopathic personality state, the resulting psychoses differ in no way from those occurring in other individuals.

Treatment. The early recognition of psychopathic personality with proper instruction of the family as to the serious nature of the illness may save much expense and embarrassment. Unfortunately many of these individuals are so nearly normal that the possibility of mental disease may not be considered. As yet no treatment has emerged which has modified the behavior of these patients. Reeducation, superficial or "deep" psychotherapy is of little value because of the inability of these patients to profit by experience.

MALINGERING

This problem frequently arises in connection with both hysteria and psychopathic personality, and the physician should know how to deal with it. It is rarely a medical diagnosis, except under the rare circumstances in which a patient is caught in the act of producing a sign of disease or confesses to have done so. The term *malingering* means to consciously and deliberately feign an illness or disability in order to attain a desired goal. It would be correct to say that it does not occur as an isolated phenomenon and that whenever it occurs it must be interpreted as a sign of a serious personality disturbance, often one which prevents effective work or military combat, though noteworthy exceptions to this statement can be found.

The relationship between hysteria and malingering is nebulous to say the least. Certainly there is a close similarity in the two conditions and there may be great difficulty in establishing a clinical differentiation. Jones and Llewellyn have observed:

Nothing . . . resembles malingering more than hysteria; nothing hysteria more than malingering. In both alike we are confronted with the same discrepancy between fact and statement, objective sign and subjective symptom—the outward aspect of health seemingly giving the lie to all the alleged functional disabilities. We may examine the hysterical person and the malingerer, using the same tests, and get precisely the same results in one case as the other.

The main points of difference between the two conditions which are cited by most authors are (1) the conscious or unconscious quality of the motivation, being always more or less unconscious in the hysteric and more or less conscious in the malingerer; (2) the influence of persuasion, which is usually effective in hysteria and not in the malingerer; (3) the attitude of the patient, the hysteric appearing more genuinely ill and inviting examination, the malingerer not.

The tendency of the psychopath to malinger has already been mentioned. Most of the more obvious cases of malingering which the authors have seen have been psychopaths, and for this reason comment on this phenomenon is made in relationship to this disease.

One observes in the malinger pain, hyperesthesia, anesthesia, limping gait, tremor, contracture, paralysis, amaurosis, deafness, stuttering, mutism, amnesia, epileptiform seizures and fugues, unexplained gastrointestinal bleeding, pains and unexplained skin lesions, in short, almost the same array of symptoms and signs as in the psychopath and the compensation hysteric. Indeed the line between the two, especially between the malingerer and the "compensation hysteric," is too ambiguous to be of clinical value. Probably the medical profession has placed too great a reliance on degree of conscious awareness of deception. In such "weak-minded," unstable, and morally defective individuals, the words *conscious, unconscious,* and *deception* are too vague and subjective to serve as useful guides in practical work.

REFERENCES

See Chap. 44.

44 DEPRESSION, MANIA, INVOLUTIONAL MELANCHOLIA, AND HYPOCHONDRIASIS

Justin M. Hope, Jean N. Angelo, and Raymond D. Adams

Each term in the title of this chapter stands for a highly distinctive clinical state which receives separate description in the following pages. Nevertheless they are often linked in regular combinations, which is the justification for considering them as a related group of diseases. Depression is the most important member of the group and in fact is one of the most frequent of all major psychiatric illnesses. The statistics in Table 42-1 show that depression was the main symptom in 520 patients, nearly 50 per cent of 1,045 psychiatric consultations that had been requested among a total of 4,660 medical admissions to a diagnostic clinic. Some illnesses of this type take the form of relatively pure and uncomplicated *depression.*

Others are mixed with anxiety and agitation and, because of their tendency to occur for the first time during the middle and late years of life, have been called *involutional melancholia.* Some are clearly reactive states and if persistent are regarded by some psychiatrists as neuroses. *Mania* is less frequent than depression and may develop as a relatively pure clinical state or may be preceded or followed by episodes of depression, in which instance the illness is called manic-depressive psychosis. Lastly there are not a few mild depressions which masquerade as *hypochondriasis;* although this psychiatric syndrome may rarely occur as manifestation of a protracted and obstinate neurosis, it will not prove misleading to think of it always in relationship to depression.

For several reasons, aside from the prevalence of depression, mania, and hypochondriasis, physicians and medical students should be acquainted with these symptom complexes. One of the paramount dangers is suicide, which may at times be attempted and successfully executed even before the depressive symptoms are recognized, i.e., while the patient is being treated for low blood pressure, "nerves," anemia, and chronic infection. Prompt diagnosis may therefore prevent a tragedy in a family. Furthermore, the syndrome of depression can often be treated successfully, and the patient may thus be spared a prolonged and disagreeable illness.

DEPRESSION

Symptoms and Signs. Knowledge of the depressive reaction, like knowledge of all other psychiatric syndromes, is gained from three sources: the history as obtained from the patient himself, the history as obtained from a relative or friend in close contact with the patient, and the findings on examination. From these sources it is learned that the patient has several of the following symptoms.

Mood Depression. This is the cardinal symptom, and the patient may describe it in any of several ways. Usually he complains of "not feeling well," of being vaguely aware that his emotional reactions have changed. He may speak of feeling depressed, dejected, or melancholy and express these feelings in terms such as being "blue," "low in spirits," "unhappy," "glum," or "morbid."

Lassitude, Fatigue, Lack of Energy. A decrease in energy output is another common symptom. There is a complaint of being continuously without energy and of tiring without reference to the amount of work done. The appetite is usually poor; the patient derives no real enjoyment from eating and may comment, "I only eat to live," "I only eat because I have to." Weight loss is common and probably due to the decrease in food intake; and the majority of severely depressed patients are constipated.

Loss of Interest and Incapacity for Enjoyment. These are noted by both the patient and his family. Where formerly the patient found pleasure in his work and was quite capable of doing it well, even the simplest tasks now demand great effort. He feels that he lacks his former efficiency in his work and often ascribes this to forgetfulness. However, when one questions his employer, one learns that there has been no impairment of memory or judgment but only a lack of the usual interest in and enthusiasm for work. Also when one systematically tests his memory, one finds that the deficit in memory of which he complains is a difficulty in concentration rather than a true memory deficit. This lack of interest and enthusiasm extends also to other activities. Absorbing recreational pursuits now give no pleasure. Cherished friendships are abandoned simply because it is too much of an effort to see people. Waning of libidinal interests or complete loss of libido is common. Irritability is also frequent, and patients who by nature were quite placid and imperturbable find themselves easily irritated by trivial happenings. The noises of children playing about the house are intolerable. However, if the patient is overcritical or harsh with them, he feels guilty and reproaches himself.

Worry and Diffuse Concern. These symptoms are prominent in most cases of depression. Patients find themselves worrying about things that have not happened or feeling apprehensive and fearful about the outcome of some ordinary activity. Incidents that occurred years before may be the objects of concern. For example, the patient may become very much upset and unhappy and may cry about the death of a relative which occurred many years before. He is assailed by pessimistic thoughts and by feelings of inadequacy and unworthiness, and is often preoccupied with the possibility of suicide.

Insomnia. Almost always present, insomnia manifests itself in several ways. The patient may find it difficult to fall asleep; or when he retires sleep may come quickly, but soon he awakens and is unable to return to sleep. Some patients state that they do not awaken during the night but their sleep is restless and unsatisfactory. Usually when unable to sleep they cannot remain quietly in bed. Plagued by pessimistic thoughts, they arise, walk about the house, smoke a cigarette, get something to eat, and resort to various measures to induce sleep. Bad dreams or nightmares are common. Occasionally there is excessive sleep, the patient finding relief from his worries in slumber.

A closely related complaint is that of not feeling rested upon awakening in the morning. Patients frequently state, "I feel more tired upon awakening than I did before I went to sleep." A diurnal variation in mood swing is characteristic of this illness. In most patients all the symptoms are worse in the morning and improve as the day progresses. Occasionally the reverse is true, the symptoms being worse in the afternoon or evening than in the morning.

Anxiety. A large proportion of depressed patients experience anxiety. There may be anxiety attacks in which the patient becomes tense and apprehensive, perspires freely, and experiences palpitation and labored respiration. These symptoms may occur in discrete attacks or may continue in milder form over a longer period of time. There may be crying spells in association with attacks of tenseness and palpitation for reasons not apparent to the patient or an observer.

Nervousness. This is another common symptom. Very often depressed patients and psychoneurotic patients state that nervousness is their chief complaint. Inquiry as to what they mean by this term may reveal only that it denotes a vague, ineffable psychologic state. Or it may denote a feeling of uneasy expectancy or of impending doom, the precise nature of which they are uncertain. Again, the word "nervousness" may refer to tenseness, inner tremulousness, or a diffuse uneasiness. Depressed patients also employ the term "nervousness" to express a feeling of sadness, with outbreaks of spontaneous weeping.

Pain. Though not generally appreciated, pain may occasionally be one of the earliest, if not the first, manifestation of a depression, occurring before other obvious depressive symptoms put in their appearance. The pain is often described as "tearing," "pulling," "twisting," "burning," "clamping" and may be localized or migratory. In one of the authors' patients it appeared first in the right external auditory canal and then successively in the right chest and shoulder, the left pudendal region, and in both lower extremities, starting in the left instep and radiating upward to the left groin, then in the right instep and radiating to the right groin. The pain is usually constant from the time of onset. There may, however, be fluctuations in severity with exacerbations which the patient associates with fatigue and emotional disturbances.

Signs of Depression. Before considering the objective signs on examination, it should be pointed out that the chief abnormalities occur in three domains of psychic function: emotion, ideation, and psychomotor activity. Abnormalities in these three spheres are designated by some psychiatrists as the cardinal signs or "unit symptoms" of the disorder.

The *facial expression* is often plaintive, troubled, pained, or anguished. The patient's attitude and manner betray the prevailing mood of depression, discouragement, and despondency. In other words the affective response, which is the outward expression of feeling, is consistent with the depressed mood. The patient's eyes during the course of the interview may become lacrimose or he may burst into tears.

The stream of speech, from which the ideational content is determined, is slow. At times the patient is mute and speaks neither spontaneously nor in response to questions. Again, he may speak very slowly with a long latent period between his various spontaneous utterances, or there may be a long delay between the questions posed by the examiner and the answers given by the patient. The retardation is present regardless of the topic of conversation and is not restricted to certain subjects as it is in the case of emotional blocking (selective retardation) seen in other psychiatric illnesses. At times the flow of speech is accelerated rather than retarded, but still the topical content tends to be restricted to a few subjects such as the patient's symptoms and his personal problems.

The *motor activity may be decreased* in varying degrees from slowness and deliberateness of movement to complete suppression even to the point of stupor. Frequently the patient will sit for hours in one place without moving; the slightest movement appears to require great effort. Again, the motor activity may be increased to the point of restlessness and agitation, the patient pacing the floor, wringing his hands, and loudly bemoaning his fate.

The *content of speech* varies and is largely conditioned by the past experiences of the patient. Conversation is replete with pessimistic thoughts and fears of cancer or other serious diseases. Ideas of self-depreciation, self-accusation, feelings of unworthiness, inferiority, and guilt, a belief that life is not worthwhile, and suicidal preoccupations are frequent. Although systematized ideas of persecution are not common in depressions, the patient often believes he is not liked by his relatives or friends. The patient's reaction to these ideas is usually one of agreement, since he himself feels unworthy and sees no reason for people wanting him around or enjoying his company. In severe depressions some of the ideas expressed by the patient are bizarre and assume the form of somatic and nihilistic delusions. Various parts of the body are said to be "rotting"; there have been "no normal bowel movements for weeks or months"; "all my blood is dried up," "I am dead," etc. In severe depressions auditory, visual, tactile, or olfactory hallucinations occur, and as a rule the salient features of their content are consistent with the depressed mood.

Personal and abstract judgment is often pessimistically tinged by the depressed mood. The patient evaluates his illness as a hopeless one and

his business as destined for certain failure. His outlook toward the future is pessimistic and hopeless. Insight may be entirely lacking, the patient feeling that he is suffering from malignancy or some incurable disease despite repeated reassurance to the contrary. However, some patients do realize that they are depressed and that their feelings are for the most part dictated by this depression.

Etiology and Mechanism. Psychiatrists are not in complete agreement concerning the cause of the depressive syndrome. There are two schools of thought, one of which contends that the depressive reaction has its genesis in hereditary factors; the other, based largely on psychoanalytic theory, considers it to be a psychogenic disturbance brought about by the inability of a rigid personality to adjust its instinctual drives to the demands of the environment. The latter theory, while interesting, has not been substantiated and has not resulted in the development of effective psychotherapeutic measures.

Classification. The chief merit of the following classification lies in the fact that it is simple and subdivides the syndrome according to the major clinical settings in which it is likely to occur.

  I. Reactive depressions
     A. In association with medical disease
     B. In association with emotional problems
 II. Depression as a transitory symptom in the psychoneuroses
III. Depression as a concomitant of demonstrable neurologic disease (depression plus neurologic disease), e.g., general paresis, senile brain disease, arteriosclerotic brain disease, brain tumor, Alzheimer's disease, Pick's disease
IV. True or uncomplicated depression
     A. Manic-depressive psychosis—depressed phase
     B. Involutional melancholia

(In subdividing the true or uncomplicated depressions into manic-depressive psychosis—depressed phase—and involutional melancholia, the authors do not intend to imply that they represent distinct disease entities. They may indeed represent the same disease occurring at different periods of life. They are separated in this classification out of deference to time-honored psychiatric teaching, and because such a separation appears to be of aid to the physician in diagnosis.)

Reactive Depression. This term is used to denote a depressive syndrome precipitated by physical or emotional factors which in themselves could conceivably sadden the average person. Though some authorities, viz., Kraepelin, Kretschmer, and Bleuler, tend to minimize the importance of reactive features in the production of depression, it is certain that one encounters the depressive reaction after a physical or emotional disturbance in individuals whose basic temperament does not conform to that of the manic-depressive group.

IN ASSOCIATION WITH MEDICAL DISEASE. Depression in patients with serious medical disease does not appear to differ markedly from idiopathic depression. The patients exhibit the same depressed mood, pessimistic ideational content, and agitation or slowing of psychomotor activity. Their thought content centers on the physical disease from which they suffer and the incapacity induced by it. Great concern is expressed because of the change in life pattern imposed by the disease. Chronic, debilitating, incapacitating illnesses such as tinnitus, Ménière's disease, paralysis agitans, arthritis, diabetes mellitus, pernicious anemia, tuberculosis, and malignancy are the ones upon which the depressive reaction is most frequently engrafted. Physical examination and appropriate laboratory studies demonstrate the typical findings of these diseases. A careful history may reveal that the symptoms of the physical disease may have antedated the depressive reaction by many months. The prognosis for recovery from the depressive syndrome is largely determined by the prognosis of the physical disease with which it is associated. If the latter can be successfully treated and the patient's normal life pattern restored, there may be a concomitant disappearance of the depressive symptomatology. In many cases, however, the depression outlasts the medical disease and must be treated as a separate illness. Conversely, if the medical disease is incurable, the likelihood of the depression responding to treatment is poor.

IN ASSOCIATION WITH EMOTIONAL PROBLEMS. Depression as a reaction to various emotional disturbances such as the death of relatives or loved ones, serious financial reverses, marital problems, unrequited love, or a series of stressful environmental impacts is qualitatively identical with that encountered in the previously described circumstances. However, quantitatively it is often less severe than the depression of manic-depressive psychosis or involutional melancholia. The discussion of the particular emotional factor with which the depressive reaction is associated brings forth an outburst of sadness and weeping. Conversely, when the conversation is diverted from the patient's emotional problems to neutral topics, a surprising elevation of the mood with a lightening of the depression becomes almost immediately apparent. Usually these patients do not have hallucinations or delusions. Weight loss is infrequent. Suicide is not so common in this group as in the true depressions. From the history it is clearly evident that the existence of the emotional problem antedated the appearance of the depressive reaction. Recovery from the depression usually occurs. The length of time that the depressive reaction exists before recovery ensues is determined largely by the patient's ability to resolve the emotional problem with which it is associated.

Psychoneurotic Depression. Depressive symptoms in psychoneurotic individuals unquestionably do occur. It may be difficult to decide whether they are a part of the psychoneurosis with a particular psychodynamic mechanism or an independent illness. In anxiety neurosis, hysteria, and psychasthenia, saddening or depression of mood is usually transitory, lasting only a few minutes or a few hours and rarely longer than a day or two. It bears direct temporal relationship to the incapacity induced by the psychoneurosis or to the exacerbations of symptoms of the psychoneurosis. On the other hand the authors have encountered clear-cut depressive episodes of varying duration occurring in patients who have had the symptoms of chronic neurocirculatory asthenia or hysteria for many years preceding the onset of the depression. The occurrence of a typical involutional depression late in life in patients who have had anxiety neurosis or hysteria for many years has also been witnessed. In each of these circumstances the previous existence of the psychoneurosis in no way altered the natural course of the depression. The authors are inclined to believe that such patients have two illnesses, i.e., psychoneurosis and depression.

Depression as a Concomitant of Demonstrable Neurologic Disease. Depression as one of the early manifestations of organic disease of the brain is readily recognized by the cardinal symptoms of depressed mood and pessimistic ideational content associated with psychomotor retardation or agitation, in conjunction with dementia and other neurologic abnormalities. At times the depressive reaction may be so marked as to obscure the basic neurologic aspects of the clinical picture. A careful history of change in established behavior patterns, defective judgment, and moral lapses, and the observation of marked lability of affect, distractibility of attention, impairment of memory (especially for recent events), defects in retention and recall, disorientation in time and space, a depleted fund of knowledge, a reduction in general comprehension, and perseveration in speech, action, and thought are the usual distinguishing features. Positive neurologic findings, as described in Chap. 37, are demonstrable in many cases. The occurrence of the depressive reaction in these disorders is considered by most authorities to represent an exaggeration of the previous personality pattern; i.e., the depressed patient is said to have had a premorbid temperament of the cyclothymic type. The outlook for recovery from the depression in these cases is to a large extent dependent upon the prognosis of the coexistent neurologic disease. In general it is unfavorable.

True or Uncomplicated Depression. MANIC-
DEPRESSIVE PSYCHOSIS. True depression occurs most
often in individuals who suffer a curious illness
known as *manic-depressive psychosis*. This disease
has been known to the medical profession since the
appearance of the first article on the subject by
Falret in 1854. Later Baillarger, Kahlbaum, and
Kraepelin described the disease more fully. Its
cause is unknown. Many observers have remarked
that it occurs more often in those of pyknic physique
and cyclothymic temperament, i.e., in those who
are disposed to wide mood swings, from depression
to elation. A hereditary predisposition has been
found in 60 to 80 per cent of cases. Other members
of the family may have been subject to recurrent
depressions or manic attacks, and it is not too
unusual to learn that several members over two or
three generations had ended their lives by suicide.
Other types of mental illness, often not classifiable
either as neurosis or psychosis, are frequently recorded. Otherwise the mental make-up of these
individuals is noteworthy only in so far as they
are likely to be somewhat unstable, bright, frankly
optimistic, and overly aggressive.

Manic-depressive psychosis, as the name implies,
consists of episodes of mania or depression or both.
Mania, which has not been described in previous
sections of this book, is undoubtedly one of the
most dramatic of all psychiatric illnesses. Within
days or weeks a reasonably well-balanced individual
may become uncontrollably maniacal in the true
sense of the word. In *hypomania,* the mildest form
of the illness, it is not always easy to decide whether
the patient is mentally sick or merely acting peculiarly because of some change in the circumstances of his work or family life; often some unusual event may appear to have affected him
unduly. First it may be noticed that the patient is
attracting more attention than ordinarily. The
routine of daily living is suddenly broken. Facial
expression is more gay and animated; dress is less
restrained or eccentric in some way. All actions and
reactions are more brisk. Conversation is louder,
and there is a tendency to talk excessively and to
be argumentative. The handwriting is larger and
suggestive of haste and impatience. The mind is
more active, and ideas come more freely, sometimes
with the result that the patient is more witty and
socially more agreeable than usual. New theories
which solve the most abstruse problems come to
mind; new enterprises may be enthusiastically
undertaken without due deliberation and then
abandoned a few days later, only to be replaced by
others. The patient is physically more active. He
is restless, paces the floor, moves from one place to
another, sleeps rather little, and has an almost in-
exhaustible energy. Friends or members of the
family, realizing that something may be wrong and

that the patient needs supervision, soon become
weary and perplexed with his noisy, changeable
ways. Another disturbing symptom is a loss of inhibitions and deviation from customary standards
of conduct. The patient may be less discreet than
formerly; he thinks nothing of discussing personal
or family problems before strangers. If opposed,
he may be irritable and argumentative.

As these symptoms become more prominent, the
family may seek medical help; often this is
prompted by some act which upsets the family or
the community. It may be an assault upon someone
who has criticized or disagreed with the patient, to
or some deviation from moral standards, such as
excessive sexual indulgence or alcoholism. The patient has relatively little insight, as a rule, and may
resist attempts at treatment or hospitalization. To
make matters more difficult, he is plausible at this
stage and has a ready and often coherent explanation for his actions. There is no clouding of consciousness or forgetfulness. The physician seeing
the patient for a short time may note only the
extreme restlessness and overactivity as being at
all peculiar.

Acute mania is a more severe degree of hypomania. At this stage the abnormality of the patient's
behavior is abnormal beyond question. Ideas now
flow rapidly, one suggesting another and another,
the connecting threads being very loose. This is
termed *flight of ideas*. The associations are usually
obvious and the coherence superficial, unlike those
of the schizophrenic. Motor activity likewise increases until finally there is at times almost a frenzy
of excitement. The stream of thought and activity
may be difficult to interrupt; yet at any time there
may be a pause, and momentarily the patient is able
to recognize his physician and his whereabouts and
to make a sensible remark. Hallucinations may
occur but are transitory, and delusions, if present,
are usually changeable and poorly elaborated. The
mood is merry, gay, but interrupted by periods of
irritability and anger. Memory and intellectual
functions are impossible to examine accurately, but
there is nothing to suggest that they are disordered.
Judgment and insight are limited or absent.

In *hyperacute* or *delirious mania* the patient is
completely uncontrollable. He paces the floor and
if restrained constantly struggles and tosses about.
Speech is completely incoherent and his utterances
make no sense at all. The patient gives no thought
to his actions, exposes himself unabashedly, is
careless in his habits and totally uncooperative.
There are auditory and visual hallucinations, suspicions, and delusions.

Manic illnesses of this type may last for weeks or
months, but in the majority of instances the symptoms gradually subside. A few patients pass into
a stage of chronic mania which may persist indefi-

nitely. After an acute or hyperacute mania termi- nates, there is usually little or no memory for the details of what has happened.

At all stages of mania *the elated mood* and *in- crease in psychomotor activity* are the evident and characteristic qualities of the illness. In the hypo- manic state the clarity of the sensorium distin- guishes it from a mild delirium. Acute and hyper- acute mania, however, in which orientation, think- ing, and judgment are deranged, are at times almost impossible to distinguish from delirium or from an excited schizophrenic state unless one knows the background of the illness and the early symptoms.

Transitional phases between pure manic excite- ment and pure depression are not too infrequent. Here the rather difficult diagnosis is usually estab- lished by the fact that the patient is known to have manic-depressive psychosis and then begins to ex- hibit a mixture of the symptoms of both phases of the illness. These "mixed states," as originally de- scribed by Kraepelin, may take the form of a maniacal stupor, agitated depression, nonproduc- tive mania, depression with flight of ideas, and akinetic mania.

In the depressed phase the clinical picture is the converse of mania. There is simple retardation with slowing of both mental and physical functions and depression of mood. The milder forms may masquerade as hypochondriasis, but the more severe ones are easily recognized. *Depressive stu- por,* in which the patient remains in bed, refuses to speak, has to be fed and urged to attend to blad- der and bowels is the most severe grade of depres- sion. The patient's thoughts are pessimistic, and he has no interest in anything. Delusions are usually present. Mental retardation is so marked that the patient may take no notice of objects and people around him. Consciousness appears befogged. For- tunately depressive stupor and maniacal delirium are rare and are not likely to be encountered by the physician in general practice.

The different phases of manic-depressive psy- chosis may succeed each other in the same in- dividual; or a patient may be subject only to recurrent attacks of depression and mania separated by periods of normalcy. An attack of depression may be replaced by one of mania, or a manic epi- sode may be followed by a depressive episode. The duration of these episodes is subject to extraordinary variation; they may last from a few weeks to a year or more. As a rule, however, depressive pa- tients are more subject to recurring depressions than to mania, and the same may be said for the manic patient.

In manic-depressive insanity the prognosis is relatively good. A young person nearly always re- covers from an individual attack. There is no evidence to suggest that repeated attacks ever lead to dementia. For this we have the authority of Kraepelin, who wrote, "Usually all morbid mani- festations completely disappear but where that is not the case, only a rather slight, peculiar psychic weakness develops, which is just as common to the types here taken together as it is different from dementias in diseases of other kinds." (See Table 39-2 for differential diagnosis.)

INVOLUTIONAL MELANCHOLIA. This is likely to occur in individuals whose temperaments are char- acterized by rigidity, overscrupulousness, overcon- scientiousness, meticulousness, and high ethical standards. They have usually been very active, busy, and hard-working and may have performed a dull, uninteresting job in a methodical fashion. Shortly before the actual onset of the illness, there is usually a precipitating or exciting factor such as an illness which temporarily changes the patient's life pattern, the breaking up of his home, a change in family relationships, business problems, or the death of a relative.

Involutional melancholia is more common in women than in men, the ratio being about 3:2. The age range of onset is stated arbitrarily in the literature as being between forty and fifty-five years in women and between fifty and sixty-five years in men. However, we have encountered involutional depression in classic form occurring as early as thirty-two years of age in women and forty-two years of age in men, and as late as sixty-eight years in women and eighty-one years in men. Because of the occurrence of these depressions in the age epoch picturesquely referred to as the "involutional period," and because of their association with the symptoms of the menopause in women, attempts have been made to relate them to the endocrino- logic change of the climacterium. However, the most careful workers in this field have failed to establish this mechanism, and attempts at therapy with varying doses of androgenic, estrogenic, and progestational substances both orally and paren- terally have failed to effect any change in the nat- ural course of the illness.

In its fully developed form the clinical picture of involutional melancholia is that of an agitated depression. The mood is anxious, apprehensive, despondent, and dejected, and there is often an undercurrent of irritability. Instead of exhibiting a paucity of ideas and retardation of speech, many of these patients are communicative and talk a great deal. The content of their utterances is repe- titious and monotonous. Moreover, if the patient's speech is interrupted by a question, it is usually answered tersely and to the point, following which there is immediately a return to his complaints, with much rumination and a repetition of the same phrases again and again. The patient's state of dependence is evidenced by his frequent visits to the physician for reassurance. Ideas with a depressive coloring, self-recrimination and self-depreciation, somatic preoccupations with fears regarding the existence of incurable disease, nihilistic delusions, suicidal preoccupations, fatigue, anorexia, and insomnia sum up the clinical picture. In their motor excitement the patients walk about wringing their hands, plucking at their wearing apparel, and generally tormenting themselves and those about them by continually lamenting their fate. These patients are mentally clear as to their surroundings, perceive accurately, and are well oriented. In its mildest form the clinical picture is characterized by tenseness, anxiety, apprehension, uneasiness, self-concern, fatigue, insomnia, and anxiousness with or without prominent delusion formation and lesser degrees of depression.

Often patients with an agitated depression have any one or several of the cardiovascular, genitourinary, or other diseases common to this age group. These associated diseases, strangely enough, may be ignored by the patient and are only discovered on routine physical examination. A common mistake is to confuse the symptoms of depression with those of some other organic disease and to expect the depressive symptoms to disappear when the latter is treated.

The prognosis was poor before the advent of modern therapy.

Treatment. In the management of the true depressions, i.e., manic-depressive psychosis (depressed phase) and involutional depression, the first question to be considered by the physician is whether to treat the patient himself or refer him to a psychiatrist. Mild or moderately severe depressions can, in many instances, be safely managed by competent general practitioners who are aware of the dangers inherent in the disease. The chief risk is suicide, particularly in the early stages of the depression, sometimes before the symptoms are fully recognized, and in the late stages, just as the symptoms are subsiding. The patient may commit suicide after having denied even the thought of such action. His relatives must therefore understand the nature of the illness and guard against such an eventuality by constant supervision. However, the maintenance of this supervision must be tactful and unobtrusive so that the patient does not get the idea that he is being "spied upon," "watched," or "policed" and thus have the suicidal impulse accentuated by inadvertent harmful suggestion. Failing to secure such cooperation from the relatives, the physician should refuse to accept responsibility for the management of the patient.

The treatment should consist of psychotherapy and pharmacotherapy. The psychotherapy employed should consist of reassurance, education as to the nature and course of the illness, and the employment of favorable suggestion. The patient should be told that his illness is not a serious one, and the self-limited quality of the illness should be emphasized. In patients who have had a previous depressive illness, the recovery from that episode should be dwelt upon and used as a point of reassurance in the present illness. The physician should not say, "There is nothing wrong with you," or that the symptoms are imaginary. Instead he should state that though real and distressing, the symptoms do not have their basis in demonstrable structural disease. The expressed belief of the patient or his relatives that he "should fight this thing off," or "It's up to me, I'll just have to snap myself out of it," should not be encouraged. He should be told not to force himself into activities which are repellent but to resume them as he improves in spirits. A helpful point in management is to work out a daily program which includes mild exercise, physical therapy, rest, simple diet, and a few activities which the patient is likely to enjoy. This gives him and his family a tangible approach to the problem. At the outset, interviews in which these psychotherapeutic principles are employed should be conducted once or twice weekly. As the patient improves he should be urged, at first cautiously and within the limits of symptomatic tolerance, to increase the range of his activities until his normal routine is reestablished.

Along with psychotherapy, drugs should be employed. It was shown by Lindemann in 1931 and later by other workers that Sodium Amytal, employed in nonhypnotic doses is an effective antidepressant and produces at least temporary amelioration of depressive symptoms. When it is employed in conjunction with amphetamine, a synergistic effect occurs. The dose found to be effective in mildly and moderately depressed patients is Sodium Amytal, 0.12 to 0.20 Gm, in conjunction with Dexedrine sulfate, 5 to 10 mg twice daily. As a synergist for Sodium Amytal, Benzedrine sulfate works equally as well as Dexedrine sulfate. However, the latter drug is preferable because it does not elevate the blood pressure. Since the depressive reaction is characteristically worse in the morning, the medication is given upon arising and after the midday meal. In patients in whom anorexia and weight loss are prominent, it is better to prescribe the medicine after breakfast as well as after the midday meal, since the Dexedrine sulfate may increase the anorexia. If the beneficial effects produced by the medicine wane late in the afternoon, a third dose can be given. However, it is inadvisable to give Dexedrine after 6 P.M., unless a strong sedative is prescribed upon retiring, because it may interfere with sleep. There is considerable individual variation, and the dose here prescribed may have to be adjusted to secure optimal benefit. If the patient becomes torpid, drowsy, or somnolent 20 to 30 min after taking the medicine, the Dexedrine sulfate should be increased to 12.5 mg. On the other hand, if apprehension, tenseness, or palpitation supervenes 20 to 30 min after the medicine has been taken, the Dexedrine sulfate should be reduced to 5 mg. At times it is not necessary to employ nocturnal sedation, since the patient may sleep well on the regimen outlined. If nocturnal sedation is necessary because of insomnia, a barbiturate preparation should not be used since additional amounts of barbiturates decrease the patient's tolerance to the beneficial effects of Sodium Amytal. Chloral hydrate, 1 to 2 Gm, or paraldehyde, 8 to 10 ml, is usually efficacious.

In the past several years a great many drugs collectively known as "tranquilizers" have been employed in the treatment of various psychiatric illnesses. In the authors' experience few of these drugs, when employed alone, has been effective in controlling the depressive syndrome. In some instances, however, when slight to moderate improvement has occurred on the drug regimen described in the preceding paragraph, a greater amelioration of symptoms has been obtained when chlorpromazine, in doses of 10 to 25 mg, meprobamate, in doses of 200 to 400 mg, or Librium, 5 to 10 mg at 10 A.M., 2 P.M., and 6 P.M. has been added. In some depressed patients failing to respond to these drug regimens, the authors have obtained good results with imipramine (Tofranil) 5 to 10 mg two to four times daily. When Tofranil is prescribed, the blood pressure should be carefully recorded since severe postural hypotension may occur in some patients. Dryness of the mouth, dysuria, and urinary retention, other side effects of Tofranil administration, can be combated with pyridoxine hydrochloride, 25 mg two to four times a day. Great caution must be exercised in the use of these drugs, particularly of chlorpromazine, since jaundice, resulting from interstitial hepatitis, and leukopenia may develop. Another complication observed by Campbell is a blood picture resembling chronic granulocytic leukemia or myeloid metaplasia. In most instances, however, these complications disappear when chlorpromazine is discontinued. Hypotension is another troublesome symptom but is not apt to occur unless oral doses of chlorpromazine exceed 20 to 50 mg daily.

Reserpine should not be employed in the treatment of the depressive syndrome for it may produce depressive symptoms in patients who have shown no evidence of depression preceding its usage. Because of the tendency of reserpine to produce depressive symptoms, it occurred to the authors to employ it in the treatment of the manic phase of manic-depressive psychosis. Although controlled data have not been secured, it is their clinical impression that the manic phase of this illness may respond to oral doses of 0.5 to 1.0 mg three to four times a day or parenterally in a dose of 2.5 mg twice a day.

Whenever possible the custody and administration of the medicine should be consigned to a responsible member of the family. When this cannot be done, the total amount of medicine prescribed at a given time should be small so as to avoid the tragedy of self-inflicted harm should the patient, in a suicidal attempt, take all the medicine in his possession.

If the mild or moderately depressed patient fails to show signs of improvement after a satisfactory trial period of 2 to 3 weeks on this combined conservative regimen, he should then be referred to a psychiatrist for treatment. The delay imposed by trial of conservative treatment, though it be unsuccessful, does not prevent the patient from responding favorably to treatment carried out by a psychiatrist.

All severe depressions, as soon as the diagnosis is reasonably certain, should be referred to the psychiatrist for treatment. In most instances severely depressed patients should be admitted to a psychiatric hospital where electric shock therapy and appropriate medical measures to ensure adequate nutrition and elimination can be provided. There must be facilities for the prevention of self-inflicted injury. These measures are augmented by appropriate occupational, recreational, and physical therapy. Electric shock therapy appears to have had its greatest success in the treatment of involutional depression and the depressed phase of manic-depressive psychosis. Although carefully controlled experiments cast some doubt upon the efficacy of electric shock therapy in terminating an individual depressive episode or preventing recurrences, nevertheless it is the authors' clinical impression that it does indeed favorably influence the course of the individual depressive episode. This type of treatment should be given by a psychiatrist.

Neurosurgical treatment in the form of prefrontal lobotomy has been introduced in recent years. If it is to be used at all it should be reserved only for those severe and chronic cases which have failed over a period of many years to improve on other methods of therapy.

Patients with reactive depressions in association with emotional problems require psychotherapy, which is often quite time-consuming and beyond the scope of the average general practitioner. In a patient with long-standing psychoneurosis and a complicating depression, the latter should be treated by the measures outlined for uncomplicated depressions.

HYPOCHONDRIASIS

The status of hypochondriasis as a psychiatric illness has changed over the years. Originally it was believed to be a particular form of mental illness of the same general category as hysteria; current psychiatric opinion now favors the view presented by Bleuler that it is a symptom complex which may occur in psychoneuroses, schizophrenia, manic-depressive psychosis, or involutional depression.

The authors' experience has led them to believe that hypochondriasis is usually a manifestation of a mild depression, and for this reason they have classified it with the depressions. However, there are a few patients in every medical clinic, quite rare to be sure, in whom hypochondriasis appears to have persisted for long periods of time without other attendant psychiatric symptoms. This illness should probably then be classified as a psychoneurosis.

Hypochondriasis (so-named because the symptomatology usually relates to the subcostal viscera) *is a condition in which the patient is unjustifiably preoccupied with the functions of his own body and with matters of health.* The main clinical characteristics of this illness are (1) the great number and variety of symptoms and complaints, all seemingly without foundation, and (2) the patient's peculiar attitude and reaction to his symptoms. There may be some complaints referable to every organ of the body, but those which occur most frequently are referable to the abdominal and pelvic viscera. Rectal pain, dryness or mucus and other abnormalities of the stool, difficulty in swallowing, epigastric distress, bloating, belching, abdominal cramps, fullness and pressure in the genital organs, frequency of urination and dysuria, nasal discomfort, difficulty in breathing, fatigue, backache, chest pains, and insomnia are some of the complaints. As regards the patient's attitude and reaction to the symptoms, it is to be noted that in his mind they represent manifestations of disease. Often no amount of argument or of negative examinations and laboratory tests will persuade him that he is wrong. The pervasive influence of these symptoms is revealed by the patient's manner of discussing them. He is overtalkative and dominates the interview with an endless description of his ailments. The pressure of speech may be so great that the examiner finds it difficult to interrupt its flow in his quest for specific information. The descriptions may be vague and the language rather bizarre, but in many instances they are meticulous, detailed, and repetitious. The patient speaks of his symptoms

with great familiarity, as though they have been subjects of careful study, and it is evident that he has been so much engrossed with them that they have interfered with his work and social activities. It is impossible usually to divert the patient's conversation to any other topic. Physical examination may disclose no abnormality or only a number of relatively unimportant signs of unrelated diseases. The same may be said of the neurologic examination.

The nature of the illness of which hypochondriasis is a part is revealed by other psychiatric symptoms. In the few cases of relatively pure uncomplicated hypochondriasis which the authors have seen, the habit of self-observation and worry about health can often be traced to childhood or adolescence and may have begun during some protracted period of ill health, such as rheumatic fever, tuberculosis, or osteomyelitis, at this time. Sometimes the parents had evinced a similar concern over health problems. Rigid habits of eating, dress, elimination, and elaborate measures to avoid infections were established early and have continued throughout life. Other neurotic symptoms may have appeared during adult years. The patient shows no evidence of depression, distortion of "reality appreciation," delusions, or hallucinations.

Far more common than the above picture is that in which the hypochondriasis has developed in the middle or late years of adult life in a setting of mild depression. The latter may be obscured by the hypochondriasis unless one makes pointed inquiry about the patient's mood, affect, energy output, interests, and capacity for work and enjoyment.

The appearance of bizarre somatic symptoms in adolescence should always raise in the physician's mind the possibility of schizophrenia, the diagnosis of which is made by obtaining evidence of the typical disorder of affect, thinking, and attention described in Chap. 39.

The cause of hypochondriasis must be as varied and uncertain as that of the neuroses and psychoses of which it is a part. Current theories of the rare lifelong forms of hypochondriasis are for the most part psychologic. It has been proposed that the patient is merely imitating the patterns observed in his parents, or that he uses the symptoms unconsciously in order to obtain indefinitely the privileges of being ill and receiving attention and affection. Feelings of insecurity, parental oversolicitude, fear of punishment, unhappiness in the home or school are emphasized in some formulations of the psychologic problem.

The treatment of uncomplicated hypochondriasis is extremely difficult. If it is part of a disabling neurotic state the problem is best managed by a psychiatrist. For the innumerable elderly adults with mild hypochondriacal symptoms who are among the most faithful attendants of every outpatient clinic, the management should be by general physicians. Reassurance, sympathetic evaluation of symptoms, a program which includes symptomatic measures, regularly scheduled periods of work and rest, encouragement to carry on normal activities despite symptoms enable many of these patients to carry on with reasonable comfort. Sodium Amytal, Dexedrine, and similar drugs as outlined above should be used if depressive symptoms coexist.

REFERENCES

Carter, A. B.: The Prognoses of Certain Hysterical Symptoms, Brit. Med. J., 1:1076, 1949.

Cohen, M. E.: Neurocirculatory Asthenia: Anxiety, Neurosis, Neurasthenia, Effort Syndrome, Cardiac Neuroses, Med. Clin. N. Amer., 33:1343, 1949.

Cohen, M. E., E. Robins, J. J. Purtell, M. W. Altmann, and D. E. Reid: Excessive Surgery in Hysteria, J.A.M.A., 151:977, 1953.

Freud, S.: "Selected Papers on Hysteria and Other Psychoneuroses," translated by A. A. Brill, Nervous and Mental Disease Monograph Series No. 4, 1920.

Huston, P. E., and L. M. Locher: Involutional Psychosis: Course When Untreated and When Treated with Electric Shock, Arch. Neurol. Psychiat., 59: 385, 1948.

Janet, P.: "The Major Symptoms of Hysteria," New York, The Macmillan Company, 1907.

Jones, A. B., and L. J. Llewellyn: "Malingering," New York, McGraw-Hill Book Company, Inc., Blakiston Division, 1917.

Kahn, E.: "Psychopathic Personalities," New Haven, Yale University Press, 1931.

Lamson, E. T., F. Elmadjian, J. M. Hope, P. Pincus, and D. Jorjorian: Aldosterone Excretion of Normal, Schizophrenic and Psychoneurotic Subjects, abstracted in J. Clin. Endocrinol. and Metabolism, 16:954, 1956.

Lindemann, E.: Psychological Changes in Normal and Abnormal Individuals under the Influence of Sodium Amytal, Am. J. Psychiat., 11:1080, 1932.

———.: Hysteria as a Problem in a General Hospital, Med. Clin. N. Am., 22:591, 1938.

Purtell, J. J., E. Robins, and M. E. Cohen: Observations in Clinical Aspects of Hysteria, J.A.M.A., 146:902, 1951.

Robins, E., J. J. Purtell, and M. E. Cohen: Hysteria in Men, New Engl. J. Med., 246:677, 1942.

Rosanoff, A. J.: "Manual of Psychiatry," New York, John Wiley & Sons, Inc., 1920.

Shands, H. C., J. E. Finesinger, and A. L. Watkins: Clinical Studies of Fatigue States, Arch. Neurol. Psychiat., 60:210, 1949.

Venning, E. H., I. Dyrenfurth, and J. C. Beck: Effect of Anxiety upon Aldosterone Excretion in Man, J. Clin. Endocrinol. and Metabolism, 17:1005, 1957.

Wheeler, E. O., P. D. White, E. W. Reed, and M. E. Cohen: Neurocirculatory Asthenia, J.A.M.A., 142: 878, 1950.

Section 11: Disorders of the Eye

45   OCULAR MANIFESTATIONS OF SYSTEMIC DISEASE

J. Lawton Smith and Frank B. Walsh

The importance of the eye in diagnosis is evidenced by the fact that 38 per cent of all the fibers in the central nervous system are concerned with this organ and its function, that one-half of the cranial nerves subserve it, and that it is the only place in the body where both blood vessels and nervous tissue may be observed directly by the clinician. This chapter considers certain disorders of the eye likely to be encountered by the general physician, emphasizing their recognition and pointing out indications for ophthalmologic consultation.

A thorough examination of the eyes by the internist is easily carried out with the simple equipment and supplies illustrated in Fig. 45-1. Such an examination should include *history*, determination of *visual acuity, external examination,* and *ophthalmoscopy.*

HISTORY

The ease of direct visualization of virtually every structure in the eye often leads to negligence in taking a history. The structure and function of the eye are such that lesions of any type can produce a limited variety of symptoms. These usually fall into two categories: *disturbances of vision* (as blurred vision, diplopia, halo vision, night blindness) and *discomfort* (ranging from "tiredness" and pruritus of the lids to photophobia and trigeminal neuralgia). Within these two groups, many symptoms are sufficiently characteristic to be of great help in diagnosis.

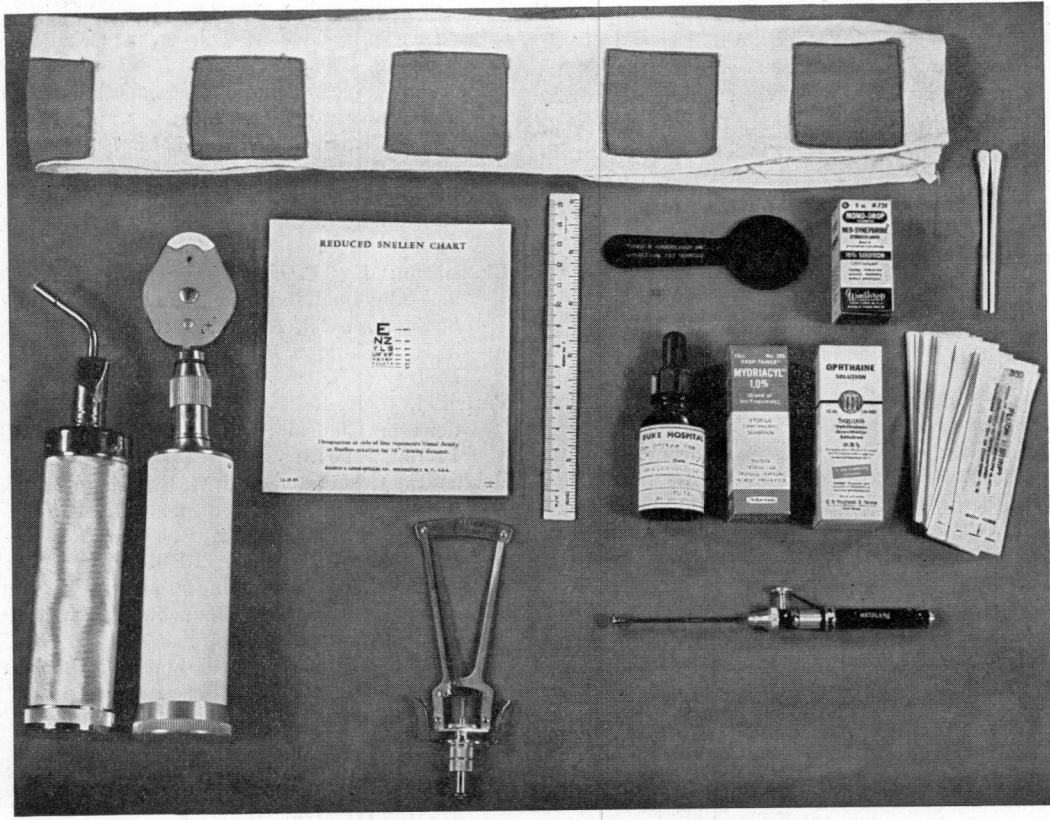

FIG. 45-1. Equipment and supplies for ophthalmologic examination.

Visual Disturbances. The *duration* is important. The *amaurosis fugax* (transient blindness) of cerebrovascular insufficiency usually persists for 5 to 15 min, as opposed to the *transient obscurations* of papilledema, which almost invariably last less than 15 sec. *Scintillating scotomas*, suggestive of migraine or occipital lobe disease, are often described as fire, ripples on water, or zigzags in the visual fields. A *diurnal variation* in acuity can occur in retinal detachment, better vision being noted after retinal settling during the night and visual deterioration occurring during the day. *Halo vision* is characteristic of glaucoma or corneal disease. These spectral "rainbows" may be confused with the scattering of light by early lens opacities, and slit-lamp examination is necessary in patients with this complaint. *Binocular diplopia* has been discussed elsewhere (p. 288). *Uniocular diplopia* should not be assumed to be functional or hysterical in origin without ophthalmologic consultation; true uniocular diplopia may occur in early cataract, irregular astigmia, and the Marfan syndrome (p. 1884), or other forms of lens displacement. *Teleopsia, micropsia,* and *macropsia* may occur with temporal lobe lesions, but distortions of objects (as *metamorphopsia*) are most commonly seen with macular disease, the changes of which are sometimes so slight that they can be missed on routine ophthalmoscopy.

A common error in taking histories occurs when a patient with a right-sided *visual field* defect complains of difficulty with the right *eye,* or similarly on the left. It is also surprising how often individuals who are blind in one eye are not aware of this and discover "sudden" blindness only after a foreign body or target practice causes them to close the normal eye for the first time.

Headache. Many patients who complain of headache are referred to an ophthalmologist. It is of interest that significant refractive errors are uncommon in this group of patients. Aneurysms and neurologic lesions often present as pain in and behind the eye, and the authors, therefore, consider *perimetry* a more important examination in the patient with headache than *refraction.* Symptoms related to refractive errors or ocular muscle imbalances are broadly described as "asthenopia." Such patients usually note a relationship between use of the eyes and symptoms such as blurring or a tired feeling after reading, going to the movies, or watching television. Patients with *glaucoma* not infrequently complain of recurrent mild headaches.

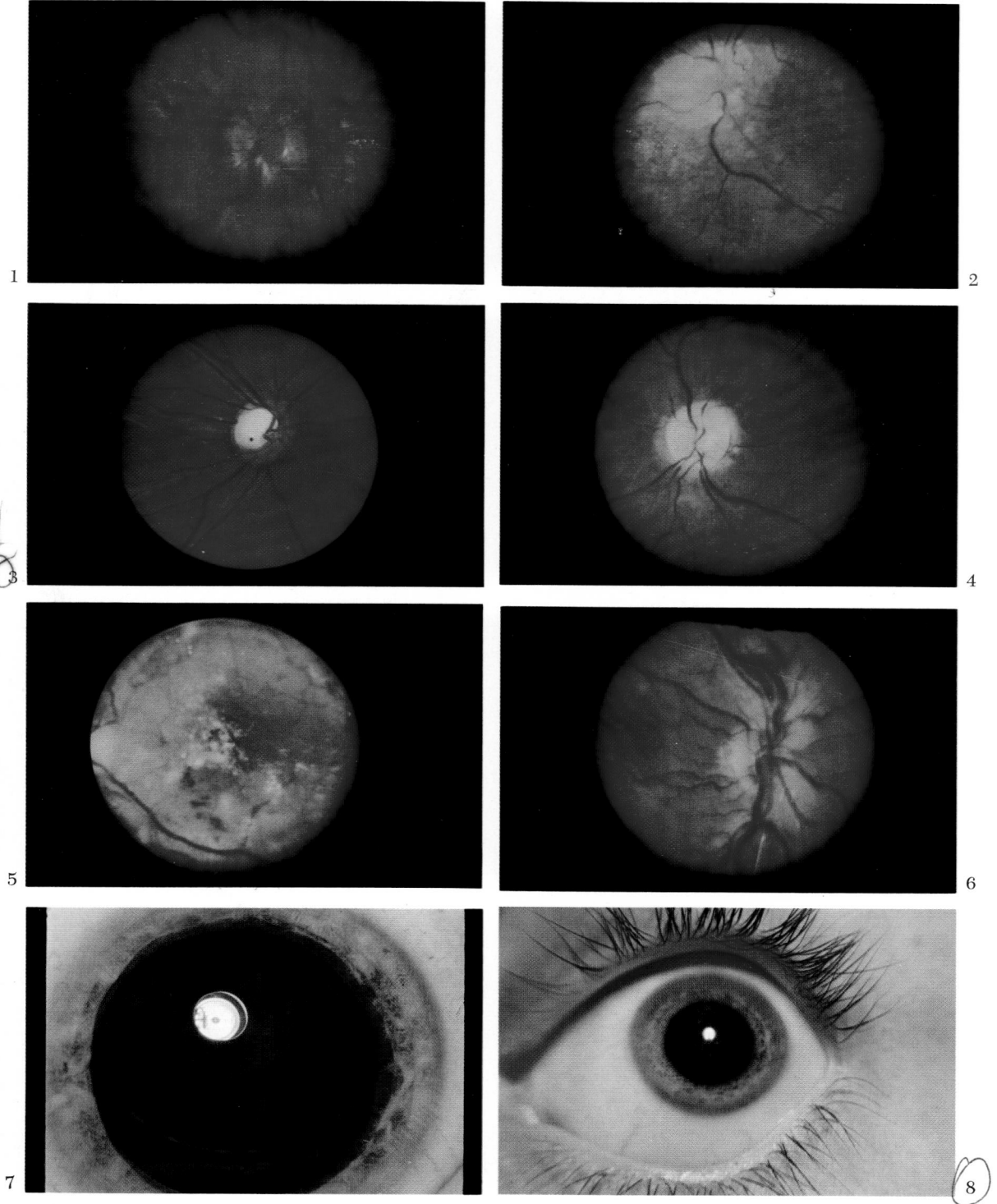

1. Papilledema. 2. Unusually extensive drusen of optic nerve in a patient with retinitis pigmentosa. 3. Glaucoma. 4. Arteriosclerosis of the retinal vessels with optic atrophy. 5. Advanced diabetic retinopathy. 6. Polycythemia vera. 7. Displacement of crystalline lens. 8. Kayser-Fleischer ring of Wilson's disease.

Becoming sleepy with near work is a classic symptom of *convergence insufficiency,* one of the commonest disorders of optic function in young adults. Because these patients can often be relieved by base-out prism exercises, they should be referred to an ophthalmologist.

Severe ocular pain is most common with acute lesions: foreign bodies, recurrent erosion or corneal abrasion, exposure to intense light such as a welding arc (photophthalmia), acute iridocyclitis, or acute glaucoma of the angle closure type.

Pain on motion of the globe is characteristic of optic neuritis, although it occurs in only about one-fifth of patients with this disorder.

Tearing. *Epiphora* is tearing due to blockage of normal channels of flow, whereas *lacrimation* is excessive production of tears. Common causes of epiphora include malposition or stenosis of the lower punctum, previous lid lacerations involving the canaliculus, fractures, prolonged use of irritating drops, chronic dacryocystitis, and nasal disease. A complaint of *unilateral* epiphora and ill-fitting dentures should raise the possibility of a neoplasm of the antrum.

Other Points in History. In uveitis, a complete review of systems, including exposure to animals (toxoplasmosis) and raw milk (brucellosis), and visits to foreign lands (trypanosomiasis, parasitic disease) is indicated. In *strabismus,* the birth weight, obstetric history, age of onset, whether the deviation is monocular or alternating, and frequency of deviation should be noted. Diabetes and syphilis so commonly produce eye disease that the past history should always be investigated for these. A family history is not uncommon in diabetes, glaucoma, strabismus, congenital cataract, and high myopia (with related retinal detachment).

Ingestion of drugs must be evaluated in any patient with optic neuritis (see Table 45-1). The most common cause of *oculogyric crises* at the present appears to be a reaction to prochlorperazine (Compazine). Diplopia and sixth nerve palsies have been attributed to furaltadone (Altafur). The commonest cause of vertical nystagmus is barbiturate or diphenylhydantoin (Dilantin) administration, and this point should always be remembered in evaluating this otherwise ominous sign of posterior fossa disease. The three commonest causes of pin-point pupils are morphine, miotics, and pontine lesions; a hypodermic mark or a bottle of drops in the pocket may provide a prompt explanation of miosis in an unconscious patient.

EXAMINATION

Visual Acuity. The reduced Snellen near card (seen in Fig. 45-1) is a convenient method of

Table 45-1. CAUSES OF TOXIC AMBLYOPIA

Analine	Marihuana
Anoxia	Mescaline
Arsenic	Methyl alcohol
Aspidium	Methyl bromide
Barbital	Mushroom poisoning
Benzene	Para-aminosalicylic acid
Bromides	Plasmocide
Carbon disulfide	Prestone
Carbon monoxide	Quinacrine (Atabrine)
Carbon tetrachloride	Quinine
Chloramphenicol	Salicylates
(Chloromycetin)	Santonin
Digitalis	Sodium iodoacetate
Dinitrobenzene	Snake bite
Diphenylhydantoin	Spinal anesthesia
(Dilantin)	Stramonium
Diphtheria toxoid	Streptomycin
Disulfiram (Antabuse)	Sulfonamides
Ergot	Tansy
Ethyl alcohol	Thallium
Ethylhydrocupreine	Tobacco
(Optochin)	Toluene
Ethyl pyridine	Trichlorethylene
Finger cherries	Trimethadione
Hair dye (coal tar)	(Tridione)
Hexamethonium	Tryparsamide
Iodine	
Lead	

determining visual acuity for the general physician. The patient should wear his reading glasses; a tissue placed under one lens provides rapid occlusion for monocular testing. The card must be placed at the specified distance (usually 16 in.), and if a tape measure is employed and a good light source used, the visual acuity obtained will be interchangeable with that obtained at a 20-ft range. If a visual acuity less than 20/20 (equivalent) is obtained by this method, the *stenopeic disk (multi-pinhole)* is a rapid means of determining whether or not the reduced visual acuity is due to refractive error or to some other lesion. As all rays of light passing through a lens are deviated except those passing through the optical axis, the stenopeic disk functions simply by excluding all but the latter (or paraxial) rays. Thus, the patient with even a profound refractive error possesses normal visual acuity with a pinhole aperture. The failure to improve reduced acuity with this method indicates a nonrefractive disease. Likewise, *reduction* of visual acuity with the pinhole is a significant finding, as this points to an opacity in the media or a central scotoma.

External Examination. Inspection of the patient's face is first performed to note facial asymmetry or flattening of the nasolabial fold. This is followed by examination with a good hand light of the brows, lashes, lids, and lacrimal apparatus. Ever-sion of the upper lid allows inspection of the lacrimal gland. The commonest causes of acute dacryoadenitis are infectious mononucleosis and mumps; chronic involvement occurs in sarcoidosis, lymphoma, and Sjögren's syndrome (p. 1917). The Schirmer test is useful in assessing lacrimal function. Strips of filter paper (30 by 5 mm), Floristrips, or litmus paper strips may be used for this purpose. One end is folded over and inserted into the lower conjunctival cul-de-sac. In 5 min, the paper is normally moistened 15 to 20 mm. Less than 10 mm is indicative of slight, and less than 5 mm of definite, deficiency in lacrimal secretion. A simple test for patency of the lacrimal passages is to instill 3 drops of sterile fluorescein into the lower cul-de-sac and have the patient blow his nose 1 min later. Inspection of the gauze or tissue will reveal the presence of the dye if the nasolacrimal system is normally patent. In chronic dacryocystitis, pressure over the lacrimal sac produces regurgitation of mucopurulent material from the puncta.

The cornea, conjunctiva, and sclera should be examined with oblique illumination. The widest dimensions of the palpebral aperture, and the pupils as well, should be measured with a millimeter rule if neurologic disease is suspected. Horner's syndrome not uncommonly presents only 1 to 1.5 mm ptosis and 0.5 to 1.0 mm miosis on the affected side, and can be easily missed without measurements. Old photographs of the patient are helpful in excluding small degrees of congenital ptosis and facial asymmetry. If an oculosympathetic paresis is suspected, pupillary size should be measured before and 30 to 45 min after instilling 3 drops of 4 per cent cocaine into each eye. Failure or lag of dilatation of the affected pupil corrobo-

rates the diagnosis. Other pharmacologic pupillary tests of value include Scheie's (Mecholyl) test (p. 288). The 2 per cent Mecholyl test is not specific, however, as responses to this drug have been encountered in paresis, tabes, and familial amyloidosis as well. The *misdirection in regeneration phenomenon* is common following oculomotor nerve palsies due to aneurysm or trauma (p. 271), is rare in syphilis and neoplasm, and does not occur in diabetic ophthalmoplegia. Three types of pupil may be seen following a third nerve palsy—the pupil may remain dilated and fixed, it may return to normal, or it may become a pseudo-Argyll Robertson pupil (i.e., contracts on adduction but not to light).

Adequate examination of the cornea and lens requires slit-lamp biomicroscopy (Table 45-2). *Iridodonesis* (tremulousness of the iris) indicates dislocation or absence of the lens. The commonest cause is surgical aphakia. In the Marfan syndrome (p. 1884), subluxation of the lens is always bilateral. If only unilateral subluxation is found with careful slit-lamp examination, syphilis and trauma are the most common causative factors.

Ophthalmoscopy. With the pupils well dilated (Mydriacyl is excellent for this purpose), and the direct ophthalmoscope set at +8 or +10, the *media* are evaluated. *Asteroid hyalitis* has a striking appearance, with myriads of whitish round mobile deposits like snowballs in the vitreous. It is monocular in 75 per cent of cases and is usually asymptomatic. Diabetes mellitus should be excluded in patients with this disorder. *Vitreous veils* are seen on slit-lamp or ophthalmoscopic examination in familial amyloidosis. A common finding in elderly patients is the syndrome of *vitreous detachment*. These patients often note a sudden, slight blurring of vision in one eye, perhaps associated with flashes of light and, at times, slight pain on motion of the globe. This may come on without apparent cause, or it may follow coughing, straining, or bending. Characteristically, the symptoms subside in a few weeks, but slit-lamp examination thereafter reveals a characteristic appearance. Such patients merit ophthalmologic examination to exclude the onset of retinal holes, precursors of retinal detachment.

Ophthalmoscopic examination also includes the optic nerve, vessels, macula, and retinal periphery. The characteristic findings have been described elsewhere in *hypertension* (p. 1354), *diabetic retinopathy* (p. 655), and *collagen disease* (p. 1893). There have been described fundus changes in *mucoviscidosis,* consisting of papilledema, retinal vein distention, retinal edema, and macular changes. In *macroglobulinemia* of Waldenström (p. 1344), there is sometimes a striking ophthalmoscopic picture, consisting of dilated tortuous retinal vessels, along with small newly formed vessels in the periphery.

Table 45-2. INDICATIONS FOR SLIT-LAMP BIOMICROSCOPY

Corneal Lesions

Chloroquine keratitis (in patients on this medicine for chronic discoid lupus or other reasons)
Hurler syndrome
Groenouw's dystrophy in ectodermal dysplasia
Cystine crystals in Fanconi syndrome
Phlyctenular keratitis and monilial keratitis in hypoparathyroidism
Band keratopathy in Still's disease
Keratitis sicca in Sjögren's syndrome
Heavy metal deposits in the cornea (Kayser-Fleischer ring of copper in Wilson's disease; gold, silver, calcium)

Lens Lesions

Diabetes mellitus	Rothmund's syndrome
Hypoparathyroidism	Marfan syndrome
Myotonic dystrophy	Marchesani syndrome
Galactosemia	Posterior subcapsular lens
Hereditary nephritis	Opacities are reported in
Werner's syndrome	chronic steroid administration

A *rete mirabile* of minute aneurysms and new-formed vessels is typical in the fundus in *pulseless disease* (p. 1367). Ophthalmodynamometry reveals extremely low ophthalmic artery pressures in this condition. Angioid streaks are seen in the Groenblad-Strandberg syndrome (p. 1887), occur in about 3 per cent of patients with Paget's disease, and have been reported in 6 per cent of patients with sickle-cell disease. Angioid streaks can be difficult to differentiate from sclerotic choroidal vessels, and ophthalmologic consultation is advisable to evaluate these lesions. The characteristic small arteriovenous aneurysmal lesions of *sickle-cell hemoglobin C* disease are virtually diagnostic. Woods and Wahlen have noted an association between macular lesions and *histoplasmosis*. The "cherry red spot" at the macula, classically seen in central retinal artery occlusion and Tay-Sachs disease (p. 1859), may be black in Negroes with amaurotic family idiocy.

Characteristic ophthalmoscopic features of *retinitis pigmentosa* include waxy pallor of the disk, marked arteriolar attenuation, and "bone corpuscle" pigmentation in the retinal periphery. The ophthalmoscopic differential diagnosis of these findings consists of eight entities: (1) retinitis pigmentosa, (2) syphilitic chorioretinitis, (3) choroidal sclerosis, (4) trauma, (5) nematode endophthalmitis, (6) dislocated, cataractous lens in the vitreous, (7) Vogt-Spielmeyer disease, and (8) rubella retinitis. Fortunately, the differentiation of these rather similar lesions of the fundus is easy on clinical grounds in all but the first two conditions. Trauma and *nematode* endophthalmitis are almost invariably uniocular. The latter occurs almost entirely in children, and ophthalmologic examination usually suffices to make the diagnosis, although these lesions have been confused with retinoblastoma. Intrauterine rubella (p. 1160) produces associated and characteristic defects other than retinitis. A history of seizures and progressive deterioration is present in the child with Vogt-Spielmeyer disease (p. 1860). Choroidal sclerosis occurs with other fundus changes of vascular disease in the elderly. The two conditions, therefore, that are difficult to differentiate in the adult are true retinitis pigmentosa and syphilitic chorioretinitis. Because of the poor prognosis in retinitis pigmentosa, and the not-infrequent finding of seronegativity in long-standing cases of ocular syphilis, particularly with antibiotic therapy, the authors feel that every patient with the fundus picture suggesting retinitis pigmentosa merits a treponemal immobilization test. True unilateral retinitis pigmentosa is a great rarity.

The *optic disk* should be examined for size, shape, color, and cupping. The temporal margin is normally more distinct, and the nasal half is normally pinker—points to be remembered in assessing temporal pallor and papilledema. The differentiation of true papilledema from pseudopapilledema may be difficult. The findings of retinal striae, hemorrhages on the disk margin, and significant enlargement of the blind spot are absolute criteria of papilledema. Pseudopapilledema is sometimes a result of high hypermetropic or astigmatic distortion of the papilla, and may be seen with congenital tortuosity of the vessels. Ophthalmologic consultation should be obtained in such patients prior to consideration of lumbar puncture. An important feature is the presence or absence of a normal spontaneous *venous pulse* on the disk. This is seen in most normal patients if looked for assiduously. Loss of this normal pulse assumes great significance as the earliest sign of papilledema. *Pseudotumor cerebri* (p. 1820) may produce such choking of the disks as to resemble bilateral central vein occlusion; however, the simultaneous occurrence of venous occlusion in both eyes has never been observed by the authors.

Another anomaly of the optic disk which may be confused with papilledema is *drusen* (hyaline bodies) *of the optic nerve*. These should not be confused with the whitish, round, discrete drusen (colloid excrescences of Bruch's membrane) seen elsewhere in the fundus. Drusen of the nerve may be striking, resembling clear transparent grapelike bodies on the disk, but in other cases may require special ophthalmologic techniques (Hruby lens) for detection. Drusen of the nerve may be spontaneous or familial and are seen in optic atrophy, tuberous sclerosis (p. 1733), and retinitis pigmentosa. They usually do not interfere with vision.

Ischemic optic neuritis includes a large group of vascular lesions of the optic nerve. With an infarct in the retrobulbar portion of the optic nerve, the papilla may show no ophthalmoscopic change, but there is usually slight swelling of the nerve, with a small linear hemorrhage or two at the disk margin. A sudden visual drop in one eye in an elderly individual with a wedge-shaped visual field defect extending into the fixation point is common. A normal sedimentation rate allows the exclusion of active temporal arteritis (p. 1899) in such cases.

Ophthalmodynamometry. A simple test helpful in the diagnosis of internal carotid arterial insufficiency is measurement of the ophthalmic artery pressures with the Bailliart ophthalmodynamometer. This test is performed with widely dilated pupils (Mydriacyl) and after instillation of a topical anesthetic (Ophthaine). It is more easily performed with indirect ophthalmoscopy and an assistant, but may be done alone and with the ordinary direct ophthalmoscope. As the observer watches the disk, pressure is gradually applied to the temporal portion of sclera. The onset of a striking arterial pulse in the papilla is recorded as diastolic

Table 45-3

Indications for ophthalmodynamometry
  1. Any person with amaurosis fugax
  2. Aortic arch syndrome
  3. Pulseless disease (Takayasu)
  4. Any person with visual claudication
  5. To assess effectiveness of Matas test
  6. To follow several stage carotid ligation and effectiveness of carotid artery clamping or ligation
  7. Evaluating transfacial collaterals in carotid-cavernous fistulas

Indications for the ophthalmodynamometric posture test
  1. Any person with amaurosis fugax or symptoms of carotid disease in which diagnostic differences in pressure are not noted in one position
  2. Study of postural hypotension
  3. Symptoms related to change of posture
  4. Study of cerebrovascular disease

pressure (in the units of the instrument). Three checks may be made without removing the footplate. Pressure is then increased until the arteries collapse and the disk blanches. The pressure is then gradually lowered until the arteries will suddenly fill with blood; the reading at this point is recorded as systole. The procedure is then repeated as promptly as possible in the other eye. Average values will be in the range of $8\%_0$. These cannot be correlated exactly with brachial blood pressure, although the diastolic reading obtained will be in the range of two-thirds and the systolic about three-fourths of those obtained in the arm. The highest reading on the instrument is 150; in hypertensive patients, the ophthalmic artery pressure may be recorded as, for example, 150+/75. Once this technique is mastered, a reproducible difference of over 10 units, systolic or diastolic (with pressure in the normal range), is indicative of carotid insufficiency on the side of the lower pressure. The test is simple, painless, rapid, and safe. It is *not reliable* in the presence of a *cardiac arrhythmia*. It is of interest that one may differentiate the fundus picture of optic atrophy and narrowed arterioles due to a central retinal artery occlusion from that secondary to internal carotid artery thrombosis by this technique. After recanalization of the central ophthalmic artery, pressures are normal. See Table 45-3 for other uses of ophthalmodynamometry.

DISORDERS OF THE CONJUNCTIVA

The mucous membrane of the eye is divided into the tarsal conjunctiva, which lines the lids and extends into the fornices, and the bulbar conjunctiva, which covers the globe and whose epithelium becomes continuous with that of the cornea at the limbus. Differences between conjunctiva and other mucous membranes are of interest. The scantiness of normal conjunctival flora is due to excellent drainage through the nasolacrimal duct and the presence of lysozyme in tears. Its susceptibility to infectious agents differs markedly from that of the adjoining nasal mucosa. The conjunctiva is relatively immune to the common cold viruses, and the nasal mucous membrane is not affected by the trachoma virus or the gonococcus despite direct contact with these organisms. The conjunctiva also shows differences in susceptibility which are of help in diagnosis. Trachoma (p. 1175) and vernal conjunctivitis (p. 1259) involve predominantly the upper tarsal conjunctiva; folliculosis and inclusion conjunctivitis (p. 1175) the lower tarsal conjunctiva, while phlyctenular conjunctivitis (p. 421) involves predominantly the bulbar conjunctiva.

The common lesions of the conjunctiva are foreign body, inflammation, hyperemia, hemorrhage, trauma, and pterygium.

Hyperemia of the conjunctiva without exudation is extremely common. Frequent causes are irritants, refractive errors, muscle imbalances (convergence insufficiency is the most common), blepharitis, rhinitis, and mild infections.

Subconjunctival hemorrhage alarms the patient because of its appearance, but is not indicative of hypertension or other general disease. Usually all that is needed is reassurance that the blood will resorb in about 2 weeks.

Foreign bodies frequently are overlooked in the upper retrotarsal sulcus, unless the upper lid is everted, when they are easily removed with a cotton applicator. *Trauma* may be mechanical, chemical, or thermal. An acute keratoconjunctivitis frequently follows exposure to *ultraviolet light* (as welder's arcs, sun lamps, operating rooms, and reflection from snow at high altitudes). A latent period of 6 to 12 hr is the rule after such exposure, so that the patients usually are seen in the early morning hours complaining that they were awakened with extreme ocular pain and photophobia. A drop of Ophthaine or other topical anesthetic brings instantaneous relief. Simply covering the eyes for several hours will relieve this condition.

Pterygium is a wing-shaped membrane extending from the limbus onto the cornea, usually on the nasal side. If it is enlarging or interfering with vision, an ophthalmologist may advise removal. A *pingueculum* is a small, yellowish nodule of fatty tissue at the limbus, usually preceding the formation of a pterygium.

Conjunctivitis is conjunctival inflammation, and unlike hyperemia, is characterized by cellular infiltration and exudation. Many forms exist, but the cause can usually be determined by clinical, bacteriologic, and pathologic examination. In all forms of conjunctivitis, the usual symptoms are those of inflammation: hyperemia, pain, exudation, secretion, and foreign body sensation. Conjunctivitis may be classified into *acute catarrhal, purulent, pseudomembranous, follicular, allergic,* and *chronic* forms. In every case of severe or stubborn conjunctivitis, smears, scrapings, and cultures of both the conjunctiva and lid margin should be made. Smears are more often helpful than cultures in routine practice. A predominantly polymorphonuclear reaction suggests the pyogenic cocci; eosinophils, allergy; a monocular reaction, adenovirus infection (p. 1116) or epidermic keratoconjunctivitis (p. 1176), and numerous large macrophages are highly suggestive of trachoma (p. 1175). Biopsy is rarely indicated except in the granulomatous diseases and in the diagnosis of tumors. Hyperacute or purulent forms of conjunctivitis are usually due to gonococci (p. 927), meningococci (p. 924), or Koch-Weeks organisms (p. 955). As corneal involvement and ulceration may lead to early loss of the eye in such forms, prompt antibiotic therapy is important. Because of the universal use of Credé prophylaxis at birth, the gonococcus has been almost excluded in the differential diagnosis of ophthalmia neonatorum, and the present-day causes in order of frequency are: (1) staphylococcus, (2) inclusion conjunctivitis, (3) pneumococcus, and (4) *Hemophilus influenza.* The common "pink eye" is usually a catarrhal conjunctivitis, with the pneumococcus, Koch-Weeks influenza group, and *Staphylococcus aureus* as the most common causes. Beta streptococci, *Neisseria catarrhalis,* and gram-negative bacilli are less common etiologic agents. Chloramphenicol 0.5 per cent ophthalmic solution, a drop to the affected eye every hour or two by day, will usually clear this condition, but the medication should be continued four to five times per day for a few days after exudation subsides to prevent recurrence. In a recurrent *unilateral* conjunctivitis, one should recall the possibility of nasolacrimal duct obstruction. Three common causes of lacrimal conjunctivitis are (1) streptothrix canaliculitis, (2) congenital nasolacrimal duct stenosis in the newborn, and (3) chronic dacryocystitis in the adult. The 1-min fluorescein test (p. 418) is helpful in evaluating nasolacrimal duct obstruction. *Phlyctenular* conjunctivitis consists of a small, hard, reddish lesion at the limbus associated with marked photophobia. It usually occurs in poorly nourished children, and at times is indicative of tuberculosis. In many cases it has been seen in association with hypoparathyroidism (p. 601); these patients have a tendency also to develop *Candida albicans* keratitis. A child with severe photophobia and limbal lesions merits a serum calcium determination. Vernal conjunctivitis is an allergic condition with giant papillae on the upper tarsal conjunctiva "like a cobblestone street,"

and with a mucoid, stringy, ropy secretion. It is common in children, and recurs in spring and fall. Itching is the chief complaint. This condition usually responds to topical steroids.

Other conjunctival lesions are of medical interest. The oculoglandular syndrome of Parinaud (p. 1179), consists of conjunctival granuloma formation, with preauricular lymphadenopathy and fever. The differential diagnosis includes tuberculosis (p. 146), syphilis (p. 1068), lymphogranuloma venereum (p. 1177), tularemia (p. 963), fungi (p. 1051), and cat-scratch disease (p. 1178). Characteristic lesions of the conjunctiva occur in ataxia-telangiectasia (p. 1734). These may be mistaken for conjunctivitis, and this should be sought for in the ataxic child. It has been pointed out that the sickling phenomenon may be noted in conjunctival vessels on slit-lamp examination. Conjunctival manifestations are common in acne rosacea (p. 76), benign mucous membrane pemphigoid (p. 1928), erythema multiforme (p. 1924), dermatitis herpetiformis (p. 75), molluscum contagiosum (p. 1174), and erythema nodosum (p. 1924).

DISORDERS OF THE CORNEA

The cornea functions as a shield, a window, and a strong magnifying glass. Its efficiency as a shield is remarkable considering that it is just over half a millimeter thick. Transparency imposes limitations upon the thickness of a medium and necessitates both anatomic regularity of structure and avascularity. A flat cornea could serve as a window or shield, but the curvature of the normal cornea renders it an even more powerful refracting instrument than the crystalline lens. Scars from corneal lesions may interfere with vision not only by creating an opacity but by distorting this normal curvature.

Corneal symptoms occur in four main groups: (1) pain, (2) impaired vision, (3) lacrimation, and (4) photophobia. Severe pain in corneal disease is, interestingly enough, usually of good prognostic import, as it suggests the likelihood of a superficial lesion. Deep corneal lesions may be attended by little pain. Absence of pain in spite of epithelial destruction occurs in neuroparalytic keratopathy or severe vitamin A deficiency.

A *corneal ulcer* is most often associated with direct implantation of organisms by trauma. *Hypopyon,* a collection of pus in the anterior chamber forming a yellowish-white fluid level in the lower part of the anterior segment, is an ocular emergency, and such patients should be promptly sent to an ophthalmologist. Adequate examination of the cornea requires the use of a slit-lamp biomicroscope (see Table 45-2) so that the broad field of corneal disease can be but touched upon here.

The most common form of keratitis in the United States today is dendritic keratitis due to *Herpes simplex* virus (p. 1170). This has a characteristic morphology when stained with fluorescein, with branching arborites or arms radiating from a central lesion. *The use of local steroids is contraindicated in this condition.* Perforation of the globe has occurred in several instances after topical steroids. For this reason, *combinations of antibiotics and steroids should be avoided in inflammatory eye disease when the diagnosis is not well established.* A rising incidence of other corneal fungous infections has also followed widespread use of topical steroids, and these lesions have a very poor visual prognosis.

A slit-lamp examination may help in general diagnosis in many patients who have no ocular symptoms at all. Examples are: corneal cystine crystals in Fanconi syndrome, band keratopathy in hypercalcemia and Still's disease, sarcoidosis, Riley-Day syndrome, chloroquine keratitis, keratoconus in mongolism, corneal changes in the Hurler syndrome, and Groenouw's dystrophy in ectodermal dysplasia. A disk-shaped keratitis may be produced by herpes simplex, herpes zoster, vaccinia, or varicella. It is of interest that systemic steroids have been reported to be quite successful in herpes zoster ophthalmicus (p. 1169), whereas, as mentioned, topical steroids are strongly contraindicated in herpes simplex keratitis.

GLAUCOMA

Glaucoma may be defined as a pathologic state in which the intraocular pressure is elevated, intermittently or constantly, to a level which the eye cannot withstand without damage to structure or impairment of function. More simply stated, glaucoma is *ocular hypertension.* Normal intraocular pressure is 13 to 23 mm Hg. Most ophthalmologists consider an intraocular pressure of 24 to 29 mm as suspicious, and 30 mm or over as diagnostic of glaucoma.

It is of interest that, normally, the intraocular pressure is the highest extravascular tissue tension in the body. Comparative figures are: eye 20 mm Hg, cerebrospinal fluid pressure 7 mm Hg, and peripheral tissue tension 2 mm Hg. This high intraocular pressure must be rather constantly maintained for optical purposes. Critical in this function is the aqueous humor. In contrast to the vitreous, which, once lost, is never replaced, the aqueous normally maintains a constant circulation, so much so that the anterior chamber evacuated at surgery usually refills spontaneously within a few minutes. The aqueous is secreted by the ciliary processes into the posterior chamber, passes through the pupil to the trabecular meshwork in the angle of the anterior chamber, and thence via the canal of Schlemm and episcleral veins, through the ophthalmic veins to the cavernous sinus. Two variables in aqueous circulation can increase intraocular pressure—excessive secretion or impaired outflow. It is well established that in glaucoma, impaired outflow is virtually always the cause.

Glaucoma is one of the commonest causes of blindness. It affects 2 per cent of the population over forty years of age. Because there are many possible causes of increased intraocular pressure, glaucoma is divided into primary and secondary types. In the latter, the elevated pressure occurs as a consequence of another eye disease, such as blockage of the anterior chamber angle from inflammatory debris or adhesions (uveitis), red blood cells (hyphema), pupillary block from an intumescent or subluxated lens, and many others.

The most common form, however, is *primary glaucoma,* in which the elevation of intraocular pressure and its sequelae constitute the sole recognizable ocular abnormality. Primary glaucoma is subdivided into two types: open angle glaucoma (glaucoma simplex) and angle closure glaucoma. These are differentiated by a technique utilizing a contact lens and the slit lamp (gonioscopy). This differentiation is of fundamental importance (Table 45-4).

The *virtual absence of symptoms* in the majority of patients with glaucoma cannot be too strongly emphasized. As visual field loss in this disease cannot be restored, all therapy is directed toward maintaining the vision existing at the time of diagnosis. Because of the rarity of symptoms in the most common type (open angle glaucoma), we are dependent upon routine *tonometry* for diagnosis. Ophthalmologists customarily measure the intraocular pressure with the tonometer in all persons over the

Table 45-4. GLAUCOMA

	Open angle glaucoma	Angle closure glaucoma
Symptoms...	Usually none	May have pain, halos, blurring
Sex.........	Slightly more common in men	Slightly more common in women
Mydriasis and use of atropine-like drugs	Safe	Not safe
Therapy.....	Medical	Surgical
Indication for surgery	Loss of visual field on maximum medical therapy	Making the diagnosis

age of forty, and whenever indicated in younger persons. The procedure is brief, painless, and simple. The symptoms of an acute congestive attack of angle closure glaucoma (pain, nausea, vomiting) have been overemphasized in the past. Such symptoms are uncommon, and many more patients will simply note tired eyes, rainbow or halo vision, and occasional headaches after watching movies or television.

Several other points about glaucoma are of interest. The patient who complains that he has had several changes of glasses in the past year or two without relief should alert the physician to the fact that the three most common causes of frequent changes of refraction are *glaucoma, diabetes,* and *incipient cataract.* Many physicians are aware of the relationship between central retinal venous occlusion and diabetes mellitus, yet do not realize that the relationship between central retinal venous occlusion and glaucoma is even more frequent. The incidence of open angle glaucoma is 48 to 72 per cent in the fellow eye in central vein occlusion, and 10 per cent in the fellow eye in branch vein occlusion. A point to stress is that some patients with hypertensive vascular disease and controlled chronic simple glaucoma, when placed on antihypertensive drugs (as ganglionic blocking agents), will experience a loss of visual field from an intraocular pressure which was previously tolerated. *In patients with hypertension and glaucoma, when commencing antihypertensive therapy, the internist should alert the ophthalmologist in order that the glaucoma may be more closely followed.* Likewise, ophthalmologists should notify the general physician when placing a patient with glaucoma on one of the potent new miotics (Humorsol and Phospholine iodide) because cramping abdominal pain and diarrhea may follow the use of these drugs in some patients. When a diagnosis of chronic simple glaucoma is made, the patient must be followed regularly for life. Good practice is to check the intraocular pressure, visual fields, and vision every 3 months.

Congenital glaucoma is worthy of comment. The usual symptoms are photophobia, tearing, and clouding and enlargement of the corneas in a child. It has been seen in association with the Pierre Robin syndrome (micrognathia, cleft palate, and glossoptosis) and in Lowe's syndrome (mental deficiency, loss of muscle tone, congenital glaucoma, cataract, and aminoaciduria). In the Sturge-Weber syndrome, a helpful clinical point is the fact that, when the naevus flammeus involves the upper lid, congenital glaucoma is usually present in the ipsilateral eye, whereas glaucoma is usually not seen if the upper lid is spared. The therapy of congenital glaucoma is surgical. In the great majority of all types of glaucoma, the disease can be controlled and blindness prevented with good management if the diagnosis is made in time.

UVEITIS

The uveal tract (*uva,* grape) consists of the iris, ciliary body, and choroid. Because of a common blood supply, the iris and ciliary body are usually involved together in disease processes, as are the retina and choroid. *Anterior uveitis* is thus iridocyclitis, and retinochoroiditis is often termed *posterior uveitis.* The ophthalmologist often differentiates a case of uveitis into one of two large groups—granulomatous and nongranulomatous—on the basis of the criteria in Table 45-5.

This clinical differentiation is of definite help in outlining the diagnostic procedures to be carried out. If the internist has been told that the patient has granulomatous disease, his attention is directed to the common causes listed in the table. Pertinent laboratory studies would then include: chest x-ray, lymph node biopsy, tuberculin skin tests, toxoplasma skin test (p. 1208), Sabin dye titer (p. 1209), and serologic test for syphilis (if negative, TPI). Likewise, if the patient has nongranulomatous disease, laboratory studies should include x-rays of the sacroiliac joints, sedimentation rate, LE preparation, urological examination, etc.

The patient with uveitis complains of blurring of vision, redness, and injection of the eye, tearing, photophobia, and ocular pain. Examination reveals a ciliary flush, perhaps focal tenderness of the

Table 45-5. UVEITIS

	Granulomatous	Nongranulomatous
Onset......	Insidious	Acute
Course.....	Chronic	Intermittent
Inflammation	Less	More
Keratitic precipitates	Mutton fat (epithelioid) cells	Small, pin-point cells (lymphocytes)
Iris.........	Thickening of stroma and nodule formation	No iris nodules; hyperemia
Fundus......	Chorioretinitis	Posterior segment *not* involved (only at times some neuroretinal edema)
Common causes	Sarcoidosis, toxoplasmosis, syphilis, cytomegalic inclusion disease	Rheumatoid spondylitis, "bacterial" allergy
Uncommon causes	Tuberculosis, Behcet's disease, Harada's disease, sympathetic ophthalmia	Serum sickness, systemic lupus erythematosus

ciliary body on palpation around the limbus, sluggish pupil at times, and later an irregular pupil fixed by posterior synechias. Such patients should be promptly referred to an ophthalmologist.

PROPTOSIS

The diagnostic possibilities in the patient presenting with *unilateral* exophthalmos are many. The three most common causes of unilateral proptosis are thyroid disease, pseudotumor of the orbit, and primary orbital neoplasm. The commonest cause of pulsating exophthalmos with a bruit is carotid-cavernous fistula. The commonest cause of pulsating exophthalmos without a bruit is neurofibromatosis (p. 1732), with a bony defect in the orbital roof. The commonest primary neoplasms of the orbit include hemangioma, lymphoma, lacrimal gland tumor, neurofibroma and neurilemmoma, dermoid, meningioma, and glioma of the optic nerve. Evaluation of such a patient should include a complete ophthalmologic, medical, and neurological examination. X-rays of orbit and optic foramens are indicated. The authors' practice is to obtain thyroid function tests (including protein bound iodine and radioiodine uptake), and then to give 100 μg. of triiodothyronine three times daily along with large doses of systemic steroids for the next 2 weeks. The radioiodine uptake is then repeated.

The commonest source of orbital cellulitis in adults is ethmoiditis; in infants a tooth bud eroding into the antrum may cause an orbital cellulitis. The commonest metastatic tumor to the eye and the orbit is carcinoma of the breast. The commonest cause of proptosis under the age of two years is metastatic neuroblastoma of the adrenal; scurvy with subperiosteal hematoma formation should also be remembered as a possible cause for proptosis in an infant. Unilateral proptosis with partial ophthalmoplegia in a diabetic, simulating cavernous sinus thrombosis, may be rhinomucormycosis (p. 1063).

LEGAL BLINDNESS

Data provided through the courtesy of the National Society for the Prevention of Blindness reveal that in the United States there are 350,000 legally blind persons, 1,400,000 others are blind in one eye only, and there are 1,860,000 partially sighted persons (visual acuity 20/70 to 20/200 after refraction). Furthermore, an estimated 29,500 additional persons are becoming blind each year. Industrial or legal blindness is defined as follows: (1) best corrected visual acuity in the better eye of 20/200 or less, or (2) total diameter of the visual field in the better eye of 20 degrees or less. Such patients are often unaware of the blind benefits to which they are entitled. The major ones include: (1) *double income tax deduction.* A simple note signed by a physician stating the individual's name, date, and visual acuity will allow such patients a $1,200 per annum personal deduction. This is applied only to the patient or his spouse and not to other dependents under current law. (2) *Transportation pass.* A statement by the physician attesting the patient's visual acuity as meeting the above definitions of legal blindness, sent along with two small photographs of the patient, to the American Foundation for the Blind, 15 West 16th Street, New York 11, N.Y., will provide, at no cost, a small passport which will allow such a patient to travel on any train or bus with a companion, the two at one fare. Airlines do not reciprocate with this. This point is often of benefit to patients with poor vision who must return to a clinic for regular follow-ups. (3) *Talking books.* The Library of Congress, Washington, D.C., provides phonograph records of many books in many languages for low vision patients at no expense. If the patient does not own a phonograph, the American Foundation for the Blind will provide one at cost. This organization has many other services available at cost to these patients—such as special insulin syringes for blind diabetics, braille watches, magnifiers and visual aids, and lists of recommended schools for the blind. A simple inquiry by the low vision patient about these benefits often brings the comfort that something is being done for him despite the fact that perhaps his vision cannot be restored.

PART THREE
Biologic Considerations

Section 1: Inheritance and Aging

46 GENETICS AND DISEASE
Victor A. McKusick

Increasingly in recent years the importance of genetics to medicine has come to be appreciated. The relative importance of those conditions in which genetic factors play a leading role has increased as some other etiologic categories of disease, e.g., infectious and nutritional, have become better understood and better treated.

The mutant gene should be considered an etiologic agent. The variability, yet predictability, of the clinical picture in a genetic disorder in which the etiologic agent, a gene, operates from within is very similar to that of an infectious disease in which the etiologic agent invades from the environment. In studying progressive muscular dystrophy of the pseudohypertrophic type, one is not searching for its cause. The cause, a sex-linked recessive gene, is known. It is the mechanism by which the mutant gene produces the clinical manifestations, and methods for interrupting that mechanism, that are sought by research in muscular dystrophy.

In addition to those conditions for which a single mutant gene in single or double dose is quite directly responsible, and in addition to those disorders which result from chromosomal aberrations, there are many disorders, including some of the commonest affections of man, e.g., atherosclerosis, hypertension, and rheumatoid arthritis, in which genetic factors and environmental factors collaborate in a complex manner. For a majority of the diseases of man, causation must not be viewed in the rigid sense of a single etiologic agent—a pattern of thinking engendered by the bacteriologic era of medicine—but rather as a nexus, a network of multiple interacting factors among which the genetic factor or factors are always likely to be important. In coronary artery disease, for example, one cannot say that heredity, high-fat diet, cigarette smoking, particular forms of stress, or any other of many postulated factors is *the* cause. The controversy between genetics and environment, nature and nurture, of an early day has now subsided since it is appreciated that both types of factors are important.

The collaboration of heredity and environment is well illustrated by primaquine sensitivity (glucose 6-phosphate dehydrogenase deficiency) in which hemolytic anemia usually occurs only if the genetically predisposed person is exposed to a chemical of a particular type (p. 1291); and by suxamethonium (succinylcholine) sensitivity (pseudocholinesterase deficiency) in which the genetically predisposed person suffers no obvious ill effects of his defect unless given the agent mentioned as a muscle relaxant in anesthesia.

Definitions. *Congenital* means "present at birth" and is not synonymous with genetic. Genetic factors may or may not be of importance in the cause of individual congenital malformations. On the other hand, hereditary conditions are not necessarily congenital; at least, clinical manifestations may not appear until much later in life. *Hereditary, genetic,* and *heritable* are roughly synonymous. *Familial* and *heredofamilial* were used previously to designate conditions inherited as recessives, i.e., conditions which often occur in multiple siblings with both parents normal. Since a recessive disorder is as genuinely inherited as a dominant one, these terms have little justification. Possibly the only use for the term *familial* is in connection with disorders with a familial aggregation not yet proved to be genetic in basis.

The word *genotype* refers to the genetic constitution of the individual; *phenotype* refers to the outward expression. The phenotype is, of course, that which the physician observes and from which he makes deductions about the genotype. The difference is comparable to that between character and reputation—"genotype" and "character" refer to the true nature of the individual, "phenotype" and "reputation" to the apparent nature.

Abiotrophy is a term introduced by Gowers (1902) to describe the behavior of genetic disorders, such as Huntington's chorea and the spinocerebellar ataxias, in which a system functions normally and may be histologically normal up to a stage more or less late in life. The term refers to an inborn defect which leads to premature deterioration of a particular tissue, organ, or system.

Syndromes. Many hereditary disorders have manifold manifestations, the combination of which is referred to as a syndrome ("running together"). (Of course, conditions predominantly nongenetic may also occur as syndromes.) Hereditary syndromes, excluding those like mongoloid idiocy which are due to a chromosomal aberration, appear to be produced by a single mutant gene which has multiple expressions in the phenotype because the protein, enzymatic, or other, which is specified by the gene, has wide implications, at least multiple implications, in the economy of the organism.

427

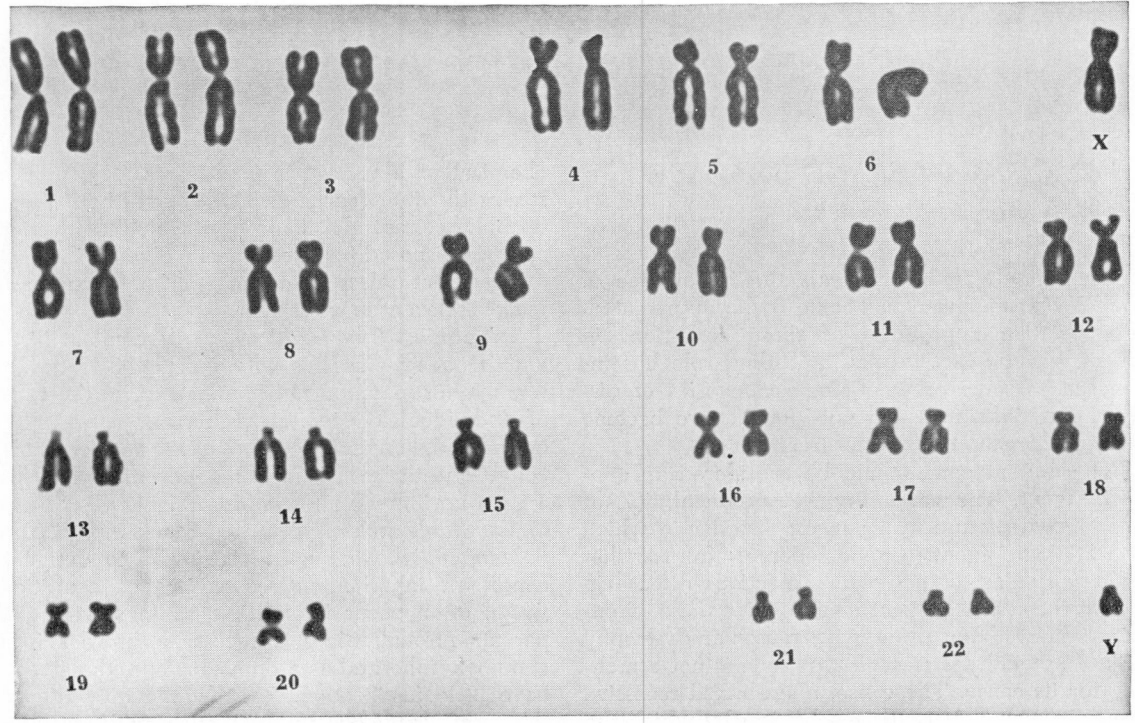

FIG. 46-1. The chromosomes of a normal male. The photographic images of the chromosomes of a single cell in a squash preparation have been cut out and arranged according to descending length and varying arm ratio. It will be noted that the X chromosome is shown in the upper right hand portion of the photograph in close association with chromosomes 4, 5, and 6 to which it has morphologic resemblance. The Y chromosome, on the other hand, is shown in the lower right hand portion of the photograph in close association with chromosomes 21 and 22 which it resembles. Note the XY sex chromosome constitution of the male and contrast with the XX constitution of the female, as shown in Fig. 46-2.

Genetic linkage—the location on the same chromosome of separate genes for each aspect of the syndrome—cannot account for the syndromal relationships observed in clinical medicine.

The investigation of members of a family with regard to a particular disease trait usually begins from a *proband,* or *propositus (-a).* The proband is the affected person through whom the family is ascertained. The proband is comparable to the *index* case of epidemiologic studies. Often in family studies it is desirable to compare the frequency of a discontinuous trait on the mean level of a biometric trait in the relatives of probands and in the relatives of controls. Data are almost meaningless unless the degree of relationship of the relatives studied is indicated. It means little, for example, to state that 5 per cent of the relatives of patients with rheumatoid arthritis have rheumatoid arthritis, but more significance can be attached to the statement that 5 per cent of first degree relatives have rheumatoid arthritis. *First degree relatives* are parents, siblings, and offspring; on the average their genetic resemblance to the proband is 0.50,

if genetic identity is 1.0. *Second degree relatives* are grandparents, aunts and uncles, and grandchildren of the proband; on the average their genetic resemblance to the proband is 0.25.

The aspects of genetics which are of particular significance to clinical medicine are at least three: (1) cytogenetics, i.e., the study of the chromosomes; (2) pedigree patterns, i.e., the behavior of genetic disease in families; and (3) biochemical genetics. Each of these three aspects is discussed separately in the following sections.

CYTOGENICS IN MAN

It was not until 1956 that the correct chromosome number in man (46) was known and not until 1959 that a microscopically identifiable chromosomal aberration was reported to be the cause of disease in man. These advances were made possible by the introduction of two modifications of technique: (1) the use of colchicine in cell cultures to cause an accumulation of cells in metaphase of mitosis, the stage most favorable for counting the chromosomes;

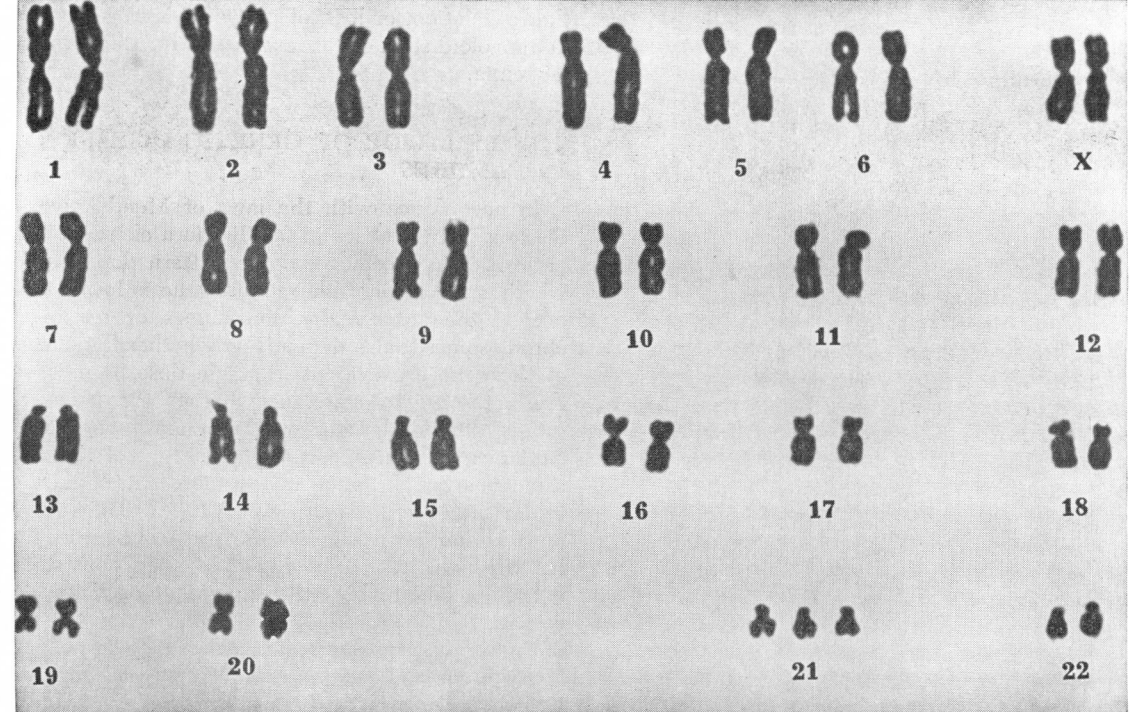

Fɪɢ. 46-2. The chromosomes in mongolism. The chromosomal constitution (karyotype) is that of the normal female except for the presence of an extra chromosome in the set numbered 21.

and (2) the use of hypotonic solutions to produce swelling of the nucleus and separation of the chromosomes. The cells studied have been derived from the bone marrow by the usual aspiration technique or from explants of skin or other tissue. Cells grown from the peripheral blood in short-term culture have been particularly useful for family studies and surveys. The chromosomes are studied by light microscopy after appropriate fixing and staining (Fig. 46-1).

Mongolism (mongoloid idiocy) was found to be characterized by 47 chromosomes, the extra one being one of the smallest autosomes, or nonsex chromosomes (Fig. 46-2). In the *Klinefelter syndrome* it was found that there are 47 chromosomes and a sex chromosome constitution XXY (Fig. 46-3). In the *Turner syndrome* (gonadal aplasia) it was found that there are 45 chromosomes, there being only one sex chromosome, the so-called XO sex chromosome constitution (Fig. 46-4). In both of the latter two cases an abnormality of the sex chromosomes had been suspected because of paradoxic findings on Barr's test of nuclear sex. In the Klinefelter syndrome the subject is ostensibly male but shows the "chromatin-positive" pattern of the normal female; in the Turner syndrome the phenotypic female shows in a majority of cases the

"chromatin-negative" pattern of the normal male (Fig. 46-5).

The three conditions above appear to arise through the accident of nondisjunction occurring either during meiosis in one parent (that is, in spermatogenesis or oogenesis) or in the first mitotic cleavage of the zygote. In meiotic nondisjunction both chromosomes of a given pair pass into one cell product rather than separating. Abnormal cells of two types are produced: one with one chromosome too many and one with one chromosome too few. In mongolism the strikingly higher frequency in the offspring of older mothers appears to be due to a higher risk of nondisjunction in older females.

Many other chromosomal aberrations have been discovered. Those which affect the sex chromosomes include XXX, XXXY, XXXXY, XXYY, and XXXX constitutions. Trisomic states (conditions in which, as in mongolism, three chromosomes rather than two of a particular set are present) have been described in which the chromosomes involved are different ones than in mongolism. Deletions and translocations have also been discovered and correlated with phenotypic changes.

The relationship of demonstrable changes in the chromosomes to neoplastic disease is under active investigation. In many cases of chronic myeloid

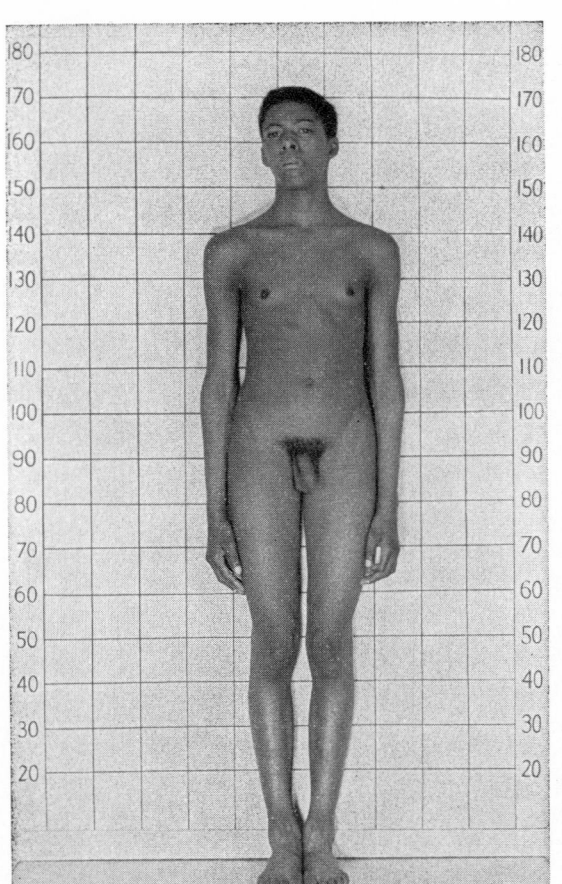

leukemia a consistent change in one of the four smallest autosomes has been observed. It is possible that a deletion, or loss, of part of this chromosome in a myeloid stem cell is responsible for this form of leukemia.

THE BEHAVIOR OF GENETIC DISEASE IN FAMILIES

In accordance with the laws of Mendel, many diseases in man occur in families in a characteristic pattern. The specific pedigree pattern depends on whether the responsible mutant gene is located on one of the autosomal chromosomes or on an X chromosome. It also depends on whether the effects of the gene are evident in single dose, that is, in the heterozygous state, or whether the gene requires double dosage, or the homozygous state, for its expression. According to the type of chromosome bearing the gene in question, a trait is said to be either *autosomal* or *sex-linked*. Depending on whether expression of the gene occurs in the heterozygous state or only in the homozygous state, a trait is said to be either *dominant* or *recessive*, respectively.

Figure 46-6 presents an idealized pedigree pattern of an *autosomal dominant trait*. Within the limits of chance, half the sons and half the daughters of an affected person are affected. This follows directly from the fact that the mutant gene is carried by one of a pair of autosomes and that there is a 50 per cent chance of the affected

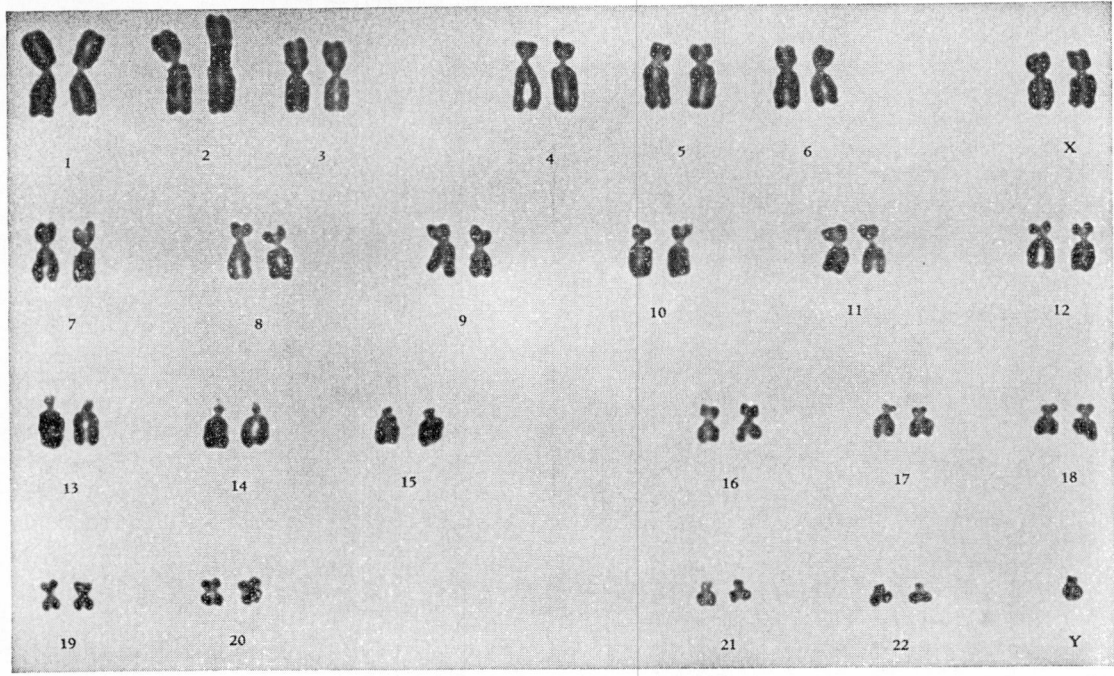

FIG. 46-3. (*Above*) A patient with the Klinefelter syndrome. Note the long legs, gynecomastia, and sparse body hair. (*Below*) The chromosomes in the Klinefelter syndrome. The karyotype is abnormal in the presence of three sex chromosomes (XXY).

430

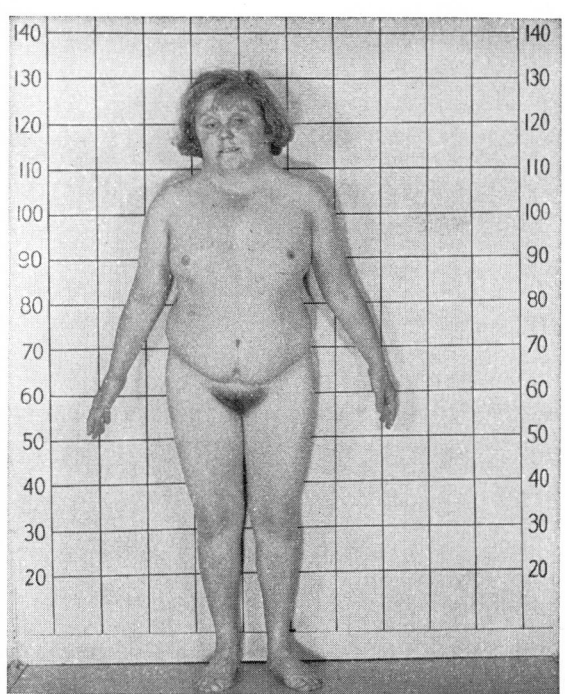

parent contributing that chromosome to any given offspring.

As a generalization, dominant traits are less severe than recessive traits. In part an evolutionary or selective reason for this observation can be offered. A dominant mutation which determines a grave disorder making reproduction impossible will promptly disappear. On the other hand, even though in the homozygous condition a recessive mutation precludes reproduction, it can gain wide dissemination in heterozygous carriers, if it endows these carriers with a selective advantage.

A biochemical explanation is also possible for the greater severity of recessive traits. One might anticipate a greater derangement when both genes specifying a particular protein, let us say an enzyme, is of mutant type than if only one is mutant.

Another characteristic of dominant characters is wide variability in severity. The degree of severity is referred to as the *expressivity*. Sometimes the expressivity is so much reduced that the presence of the gene cannot be recognized at all, at least by the methods at one's disposal. When this is the case, the trait is said to be *nonpenetrant*. Sometimes in pedigrees of families with a dominant trait, so-

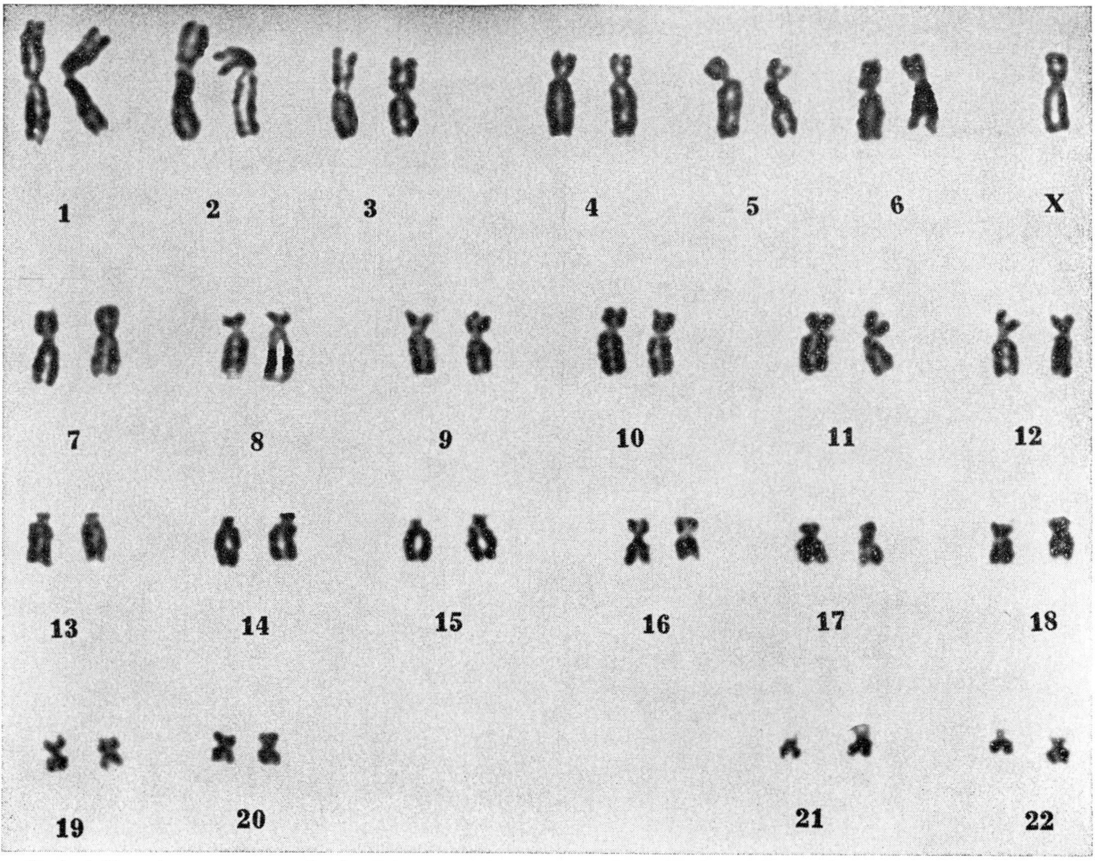

FIG. 46-4. (*Above*) A patient with the Turner syndrome. Note the short stature, broad shieldlike chest with wide intermammary distance, hypoplastic mandible, low-set ears, and webbed neck. Note the scar of the operation for resection of coarctation of the aorta. (*Below*) The chromosomes in the Turner syndrome. The karotype is abnormal in the absence of one sex chromosome.

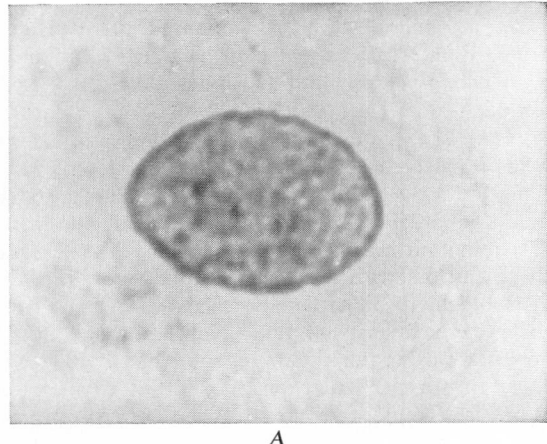

A

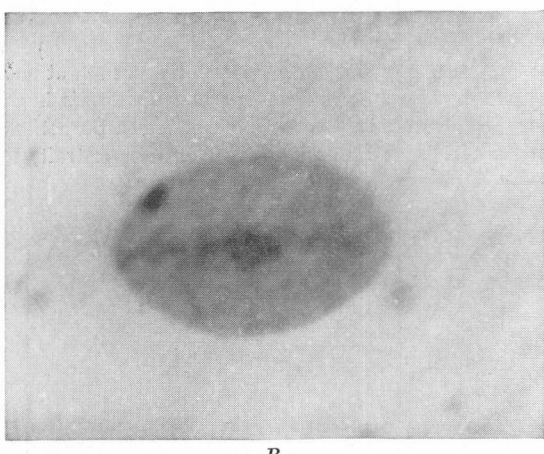

B

FIG. 46-5. *A.* Cell in buccal smear from normal male. No sex chromatin mass is seen in this "chromatin-negative" pattern which is shown also by most patients with the Turner syndrome. *B.* Cell in buccal smear from normal female, showing a sex chromatin mass adjacent to the nuclear membrane. This "chromatin-positive" pattern is also shown by patients with the Klinefelter syndrome.

called skipped generations occur. In the "skipped" individual, expressivity is so low that the presence of the gene is not recognizable, i.e, the trait is non-penetrant in that person. The variability results from differences in the environment and in the rest of the genetic make-up, the genome. At least in part the variability of dominant traits may be the result of differences in the "normal" allele which accompanies the mutant allele in the heterozygous affected individual. Evidence of the last is provided when one can demonstrate that sib-sib correlations for behavior of the given disease are stronger than the parent-sibling correlations.

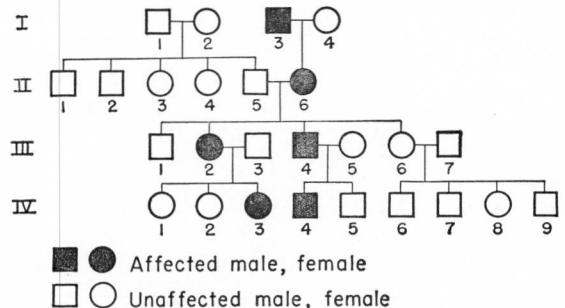

FIG. 46-6. Pedigree pattern of an autosomal dominant trait.

Autosomal recessive traits (Fig. 46-7) likewise occur equally often in males and females, as a rule. The affected individuals usually have normal parents, but both parents are heterozygous carriers of the gene in question. Since related individuals are more likely to be heterozygous for the same mutant gene, consanguineous mating, of first cousins for example, are more likely to result in offspring affected by a recessive trait. Viewed in another way, a greater proportion of the parental matings in families affected by recessive traits are likely to be consanguineous than is true generally. The rarer the recessive trait, the higher is the proportion of consanguineous parental matings.

On the average, among the offspring of two heterozygous parents one-fourth of males and females are expected to be homozygous-affected. One-half will be heterozygous carriers for the trait, and one-fourth will be homozygous for the normal allele.

Affected sibships can usually be ascertained only through the appearance of one or more affected members. Since there is no way to recognize those matings of two appropriately heterozygous parents who are so fortunate as to have no affected children, a collection of sibships containing at least one affected child is a biased sample. More than

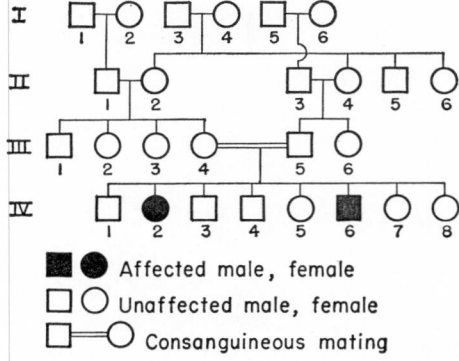

FIG. 46-7. Pedigree pattern of an autosomal recessive trait.

the expected one-fourth will be affected. Methods for correcting for the so-called "bias of ascertainment" are available.

If an individual affected by a recessive trait marries a homozygous normal person, none of the children will be affected, but all will be heterozygous carriers. If an individual affected by a recessive trait marries a heterozygous carrier, one-half of the offspring are likely to be affected. A pedigree pattern superficially resembling that of a dominant trait can result. It was previously thought that two genetic forms of alkaptonuria (p. 746) exist—one inherited as an autosomal recessive and one as an autosomal dominant. Closer investigation reveals that the apparently dominant form was the same disease as the clearly recessive one. Because of much inbreeding, homozygous affected individuals frequently mated with heterozygous carriers and a quasi-dominant pedigree pattern resulted.

When two individuals affected by the same recessive disease mate, all their offspring are likely to be affected. However, an exception to this generalization occurs if the recessive trait which phenotypically is identical in two parents is in fact determined by genes at different loci. The exception illustrates the genetic axiom: The phenotype is no necessary indication of the genotype. Different genotypes can result in the same phenotype (so-called "genetic mimics" or "genocopies"). Or an environmental insult can result in a phenotype indistinguishable from that produced by a mutant gene (a so-called "phenocopy").

Dominant and *recessive* are somewhat arbitrary concepts. When our methods are sufficiently acute, the effect of a recessive gene in heterozygous state can be recognized. Furthermore a gene which has

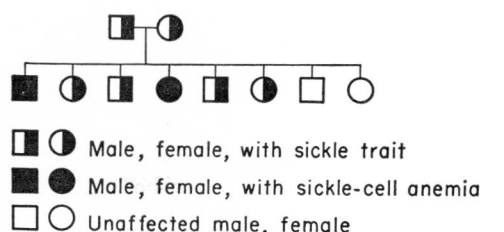

Male, female, with sickle trait

Male, female, with sickle-cell anemia

Unaffected male, female

Fig. 46-8. Pedigree pattern of an autosomal intermediate trait as illustrated by sickle state.

obvious expression in the heterozygous individual and is therefore considered dominant may have a different effect, quantitatively and even qualitatively, in the homozygous state. The gene for sickle hemoglobin and the states referred to as sickle-cell anemia and sickle-cell trait illustrate the arbitrary nature of the distinction. If sickle-cell anemia is considered as the phenotype, then the condition is recessive, since a homozygous state of the gene is required. The phenotype sickling, however, is dominant since the gene in heterozygous state is expressed. *Intermediate inheritance* is the term sometimes applied to this type of pedigree pattern (Fig. 46-8).

Codominance is the term used for characters which are both expressed in the heterozygote. For example, persons with the blood group AB demonstrate the effects of both the gene for antigen A and the gene for antigen B. Neither is recessive to the other. Similarly the genes for different hemoglobins are both expressed, for example, in the person with both hemoglobin S and hemoglobin C. These examples of codominance again indicate that whether we view the phenotype as recessive

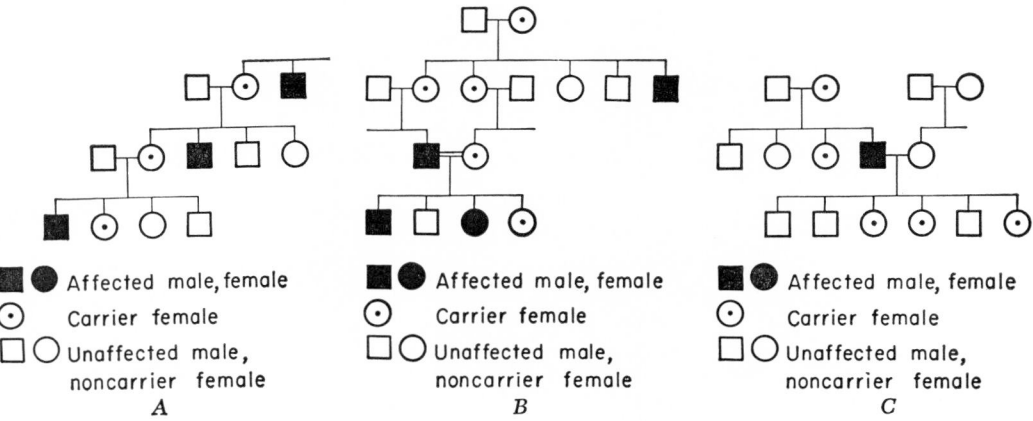

Affected male, female

Carrier female

Unaffected male, noncarrier female

A

Affected male, female

Carrier female

Unaffected male, noncarrier female

B

Affected male, female

Carrier female

Unaffected male, noncarrier female

C

Fig. 46-9. Pedigree patterns of a sex-linked recessive trait. *A.* Note the "oblique" pattern. *B.* An affected female can result from the mating of an affected male and a carrier female, as in the case of a consanguineous marriage shown here. *C.* An affected male mating with a normal, noncarrier female has all normal sons, all carrier daughters.

or dominant is dependent largely on the acuteness of our methods for recognizing the products of gene action.

In traits determined by genes on the X chromosome, either dominance or recessiveness may be observed, just as in autosomal traits. The female with two X chromosomes may be either heterozygous or homozygous for a given mutant gene, and the trait can demonstrate either recessive or dominant behavior. On the other hand, the male with one X chromosome can have only one genetic constitution, namely, hemizygous. Regardless of the behavior of the mutant gene in the female, whether recessive or dominant, the mutant gene, if present in the male, is always expressed.

An important characteristic of sex-linked inheritance, both dominant and recessive, is the absence of male-to-male (that is, father-to-son) transmission of the disease. This is a necessary result of the fact that the male contributes his X chromosome to all his daughters but to none of his sons.

Sex-linked (X-linked) recessive inheritance (Fig. 46-9) is illustrated in a classical manner by hemophilia. The pedigree pattern of an autosomal dominant trait is a horizontal one, with affected persons in successive generations. The pedigree pattern of an autosomal recessive trait tends to be a vertical one, with affected persons confined to a single generation. The pedigree pattern of a sex-linked recessive character tends to be an oblique one because of transmission to the sons of normal carrier sisters of affected males. Bateson compared this pattern to the knight's move in chess. Tracing of sex-linked recessive characters through many generations is often difficult because the patronymic of affected persons tends to change with each generation.

To have hemophilia a female must be homozygous for this recessive gene. She must have received a gene for hemophilia from each parent. Such can occur, and has been observed, when a hemophiliac male marries a carrier female (Fig. 46-4B). As with other recessive traits this homozygous state is more likely to result from consanguineous matings. A hemophilic female may also occur if a carrier mother is impregnated by a mutant sperm from a normal father, or if the phenotypic female has in fact an XO sex chromosome constitution (the Turner syndrome) or an XY constitution (the syndrome of testicular feminization). (In these comments reference is, of course, made to sex-linked recessive hemophilia A and B and not to other hemophilioid states which occur equally frequently in males and females.)

A hemophilic male can have gotten the hemophilia gene *only* from his mother and can transmit it only to his daughters but to none of his sons. *All* daughters of a hemophilic male are carriers (Fig. 46-9C).

In man one can enumerate two dozen or more other diseases which are inherited as sex-linked recessives, including such significant entities as primaquine sensitivity (p. 1291), the Duchenne type of progressive muscular dystrophy (p. 730), and agammaglobulinemia (p. 752). In some, for example, primaquine sensitivity and nephrogenic diabetes insipidus, a partial defect can be demonstrated in the heterozygous female carrier, and one might prefer to call the inheritance sex-linked intermediate. In another condition, choroideremia, hemizygous males, but only the males, have severe impairment of vision, and from this point of view the disease is a sex-linked recessive; but the heterozygous female carriers show striking changes in the fundus oculi on ophthalmoscopy, even though vision is unaffected.

At least one common trait, colorblindness, is inherited as a sex-linked recessive. It is sufficiently frequent (about 8 per cent of white males are colorblind) that the occurrence of homozygous colorblind females is no great rarity—0.08^2, or 0.6 per cent.

In sex-linked (X-linked) dominant inheritance both females and males are affected and both males and females transmit the disorder to their offspring, just as in autosomal dominant inheritance. Superficially the pedigree patterns in the two types of inheritance are similar, but there is a critical difference (Fig. 46-10). In sex-linked dominant inheritance, although the affected female transmits the trait to half her sons and half her daughters, the affected male transmits it to *none* of his sons and to *all* his daughters. Furthermore, in a series of cases females are expected to occur twice as often as males. One of the best studied sex-linked dominant traits is vitamin D–resistant rickets, or hypophosphatemic rickets (p. 713). In this condi-

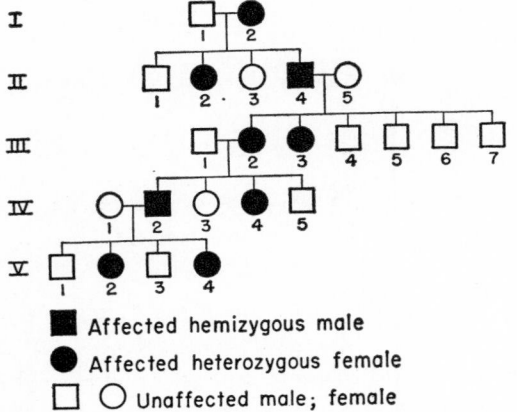

■ Affected hemizygous male

● Affected heterozygous female

□ ○ Unaffected male; female

FIG. 46-10. Pedigree pattern of a sex-linked dominant trait.

tion the hemizygous affected male tends to have more severe clinical involvement than does the heterozygous affected female.

Occurrence of the following types of inheritance in man is uncertain: (1) *holandric (all-male) inheritance,* resulting from the possible location of a gene on the Y chromosome, and (2) *partial sex-linkage,* resulting from the location of a gene on possibly homologous parts of the X and Y chromosomes between which crossing over might occur.

Before leaving sex-linked inheritance, one should note the distribution between sex-linked inheritance and sex-influenced (or sex-limited) autosomal inheritance. Baldness appears to be such a sex-influenced autosomal trait. In man baldness is inherited as an autosomal dominant, but in women for baldness to occur the gene must be in homozygous state, that is, in women baldness behaves like a recessive. In women who develop masculinizing tumors of the ovary, baldness can occur if the genotype is proper. As another example, one can imagine a mutant gene whose sole effect was that of preventing lactation in the female. Even though it were located on an autosomal chromosome, it would not have expression in the male. Idiopathic hemochromatosis (p. 785) results from the pathologic effects of excessive accumulations of iron within the body, probably as a result of a hereditary defect in the intestinal mechanism regulating iron absorption. Although the inheritance seems to be autosomal dominant, females are rather rarely affected because they have a safety valve on excessive iron accumulation—menstruation and pregnancy.

Note the difficulties in distinguishing sex-linked recessive inheritance from sex-limited autosomal dominant inheritance, if the nature of the disease is such that reproduction of affected males does not occur. The syndrome of testicular feminization (p. 665) is an example. The affected individuals are genetic males but, because of the production of female hormones by the testis, female external genitalia and all the secondary sex characters of the female develop. The affected male does not reproduce and normal females are carriers. The pedigree pattern is precisely that of a sex-linked recessive trait. However, the inheritance can equally well be sex-linked autosomal dominant. In diseases too severe to permit reproduction of affected males—the Pelizaeus-Merzbacher disease (a form of cerebral degeneration), the Duchenne variety of muscular dystrophy (p. 730), one variety of gargoylism (p. 1742)—there is on the basis of pedigree patterns no way to distinguish sex-linked and sex-limited inheritance.

Genetic Counseling. Familiarity with the patterns of disease is useful in diagnosis; if the pedigree pattern is consistent with the mode of inheritance usual for a suspected entity, the diagnosis of that entity is thereby strengthened. Knowing what individuals in a kindred are at risk, one can watch for the earliest signs of hereditary disease.

Furthermore, familiarity with pedigree patterns is essential to genetic counseling. The risk of having an affected child can be stated as 1 in 2 for a person affected by a dominant trait and as 1 in 4 for a couple which has already had a child affected by a recessive disease. For the sister of a male affected by a sex-linked recessive trait the risk of being a carrier is (unless the affected brother represents a new mutation) 1 in 2, of having an affected son one-half of that, or 1 in 4, and the risk of any affected child (considering both sexes) one-half of that, or 1 in 8.

Other genetic considerations such as the severity of the disease in question, including its severity in the specific family, must be included in the evaluation. Only the risks should be stated to the persons seeking counsel. The decision as to what action they should follow must be theirs and must take account of factors such as economic status and emotional fortitude. Socially valuable traits partially determined by genetic constitution may be present in the family and outweigh the disadvantage of a mutant gene. Counseling will be strengthened when methods for detecting heterozygous carriers, for example the female carrier of sex-linked recessive traits, are available.

Often the statement of risks is a relief to the persons involved and is not disturbing. For example, a young man with pseudoxanthoma elasticum (p. 1887), an autosomal recessive trait, was relieved to learn that the likelihood that his children by an unrelated wife would be affected by the severe eye involvement and tendency to hemorrhage is essentially nil. In families affected by a clear-cut, nearly fully penetrant autosomal dominant trait normal persons are sometimes surprised to learn, and considerably relieved, that there is virtually no risk of their offspring being affected.

PRINCIPLES OF BIOCHEMICAL GENETICS IN MAN

Biochemical genetics had its origin in the early part of this century, with a physician, Archibald Garrod, and his "inborn errors of metabolism." The disorders he considered were defects in intermediary metabolism resulting from an inherited abnormality of particular enzymes. In its broader implications, biochemical genetics is concerned with the chemical nature of the genetic code and with all the biochemical steps by which that code is translated into an observed characteristic, for example, an inherited disease.

The genetic information passed from generation

to generation is coded in some manner in the sequence of purine and pyrimidine bases in the deoxyribonucleic acid (DNA) of the chromosomes. The primary action of any given gene is to specify the amino acid sequence of a particular protein or of one polypeptide component of a protein. There is some rather direct relationship between the base sequence of DNA and the amino acid sequence of the protein specified. Ribonucleic acid (RNA) appears to be involved in transferring the code from its place of storage in the nucleus to the site of primary gene action, that is, protein formation, in the ribosomes of the cytoplasm.

In accordance with the current views, all properties of a protein are a consequence of its amino acid sequence. Probably the proteins specified by genes are not only enzyme proteins but also may be structural proteins, e.g., collagen, or proteins with other functions and properties, such as hemoglobin or erythrocyte antigens. The useful concept of "one-gene-one-enzyme" requires modification to "one-gene-one-polypeptide," or (see below) "one-cistron-one-polypeptide."

In the schema outlined above mutation represents a change in the code, that is, a change in the base sequence of DNA. Mutations may be of two types. In "mis-sense" mutations a different amino acid is substituted at a given site in the particular protein, for example, valine for glutamic acid, changing "normal" hemoglobin to sickle hemoglobin. In "non-sense" mutations the change in the base sequence of DNA is such that there is no corresponding amino acid and none of a given protein, e.g., an enzyme, may be found.

The limits of the gene have become clearer. As a functional unit, called by Benzer the *cistron*, the gene is that portion of DNA responsible for specification of a single polypeptide and a *locus* is physically that portion of the linearly arranged genetic material (DNA) occupied by the cistron or gene. The alternative forms of the gene which occur at the same locus are called *alleles*. For example, the genes for A, B, and O blood types are multiple alleles at one locus. Within a locus there are many mutable sites. Obviously if the gene at a locus is responsible for specifying all the many amino acids in a complex protein, there are many base pairs which are vulnerable to mutation. This much smaller unit is called by Benzer the *muton*. In the third place the genetic unit as revealed by recombination is referred to as the *recon*.

As stated above, the mutant gene can result in the formation of a different protein or of no protein at all of a given type. If the protein in question is an enzyme, none at all may be formed or an enzyme may be formed which is so impaired in its function that the net effect is the same. In intermediary metabolism such a change can have

pathogenetic consequences through any of several mechanisms or through some combination of these. We can represent a hypothetical metabolic process as follows:

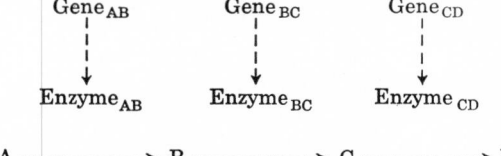

$$A \longrightarrow B \longrightarrow C \longrightarrow D$$

If a mutant form of gene$_{CD}$ results in no formation of enzyme$_{CD}$ or in the formation of functionally defective enzyme, then the effects may be of several types:

1. The disease characteristic may reflect the deficiency of product D:

$$A \longrightarrow B \longrightarrow C \longrightarrow\!\!/\!\!\longrightarrow (D)$$

Albinism (p. 788) might be cited as an example; melanin is not formed because of a block in tyrosine metabolism. In several forms of genetic cretinism (p. 585), thyroid hormone is not formed because of blocks of this type; in the adrenogenital syndrome (p. 623), hydrocortisone is not found.

2. A metabolite just proximal to the block may accumulate in toxic amounts.

$$A \longrightarrow B \longrightarrow \begin{matrix}C\\C\\C\end{matrix} \longrightarrow\!\!/\!\!\longrightarrow (D)$$

An example is alkaptonuria. Homogentisic acid is not metabolized normally. It is excreted in the urine in large amounts. Furthermore its increase in the body in some way leads to a form of degenerative arthritis.

3. If the reactions in question are reversible, there may be an accumulation of precursors farther back from the site of block.

$$\begin{matrix}A\\A\\A\end{matrix} \rightleftharpoons \begin{matrix}B\\B\end{matrix} \rightleftharpoons C \longrightarrow (D)$$

An example is the accumulation of glycogen in the form of glycogen storage disease (von Gierke's disease) in which the primary defect involves glucose 6-phosphatase (p. 772).

Glycogen ⇌ glucose 1-phosphate ⇌ glucose 6-phosphate

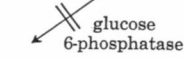

glucose
6-phosphatase

4. There may be production of products through an accessory pathway which is normally of minor significance.

$$A \longrightarrow B \longrightarrow C \longrightarrow\!\!/\!\!\longrightarrow (D)$$
$$\downarrow$$
$$X \longrightarrow Y \longrightarrow Z$$

In phenylketonuria, phenylketone products are produced in unusual amounts from phenylalanine which is not properly metabolized. In hyperoxaluria, an excess production of oxalate may be the result of a defect in the normal metabolism of glyoxylate:

$$\text{Glycine} \rightleftarrows \text{glyoxylate} \longrightarrow \text{formic acid} + CO_2$$
$$\searrow \searrow$$
$$\text{oxalic acid}$$

Undoubtedly these do not exhaust the possible mechanisms of a pathogenetic effect from a mutation in a gene controlling an enzyme.

Metabolic processes are in most instances chains, indeed often networks. A mutation in the genes controlling any of several metabolic steps may lead to the same phenotypic result. Thus, the phenotoype is not an indication of the specific genotype. Identical diseases may be produced by mutation of different genes; "genetic mimics," they are called.

Another type of process, not strictly enzymatic, by which mutations have pathogenetic effects involves changes in active transport mechanisms in the kidney and elsewhere. Cystinuria (p. 747) is an example. Other active transport systems can be cited, such as those involved in the movement of substances such as amino acids across the intestinal mucosa, of substances like bilirubin into and out of the liver cell, and of electrolytes across the muscle cell membrane. All these mechanisms are vulnerable to the effects of mutation in the determinant genes, and diseases for which such mutation is probably responsible can be cited.

REFERENCES

Ferguson-Smith, M.A.: Cytogenetics in Man, A.M.A. Arch. Internal Med., 105:627, 1960. Also, Chromosomes and Human Disease, in "Progress in Medical Genetics," A. G. Steinberg and D. Adlersberg (Eds.), New York, Grune & Stratton, Inc., 1961.

Stanbury, J. B., J. B. Wyngaarden, and D. S. Fredrickson (Eds.): "The Metabolic Basis of Inherited Disease," New York, McGraw-Hill Book Company, Inc., Blakiston Division, 1960.

Stern, C.: "Principles of Human Genetics," 2d ed., San Francisco, W. H. Freeman and Co., 1960.

47 BLOOD GROUPS
M. M. Wintrobe

VARIETY OF BLOOD GROUP SYSTEMS AND FACTORS

In 1900 Karl Landsteiner studied the clumping which occurs when blood from one person is mixed with that of certain others and showed that this is due to completely normal properties in the cells and serum of the blood. These observations not only laid the ground for practical transfusion therapy but opened a field of knowledge which has not yet been exhausted. In addition to the A-B-O system with which Landsteiner first became engrossed, at least ten other "systems" of blood factors have been discovered (Table 47-1). The ramifications of these discoveries are of the utmost importance in human genetics and anthropology as well as in relation to disease and in the medicolegal field.

The number of different known blood factors is continuously enlarging. Thus it was found that there are qualitative differences in agglutinogen A. There are two main varieties, A_1 and A_2, thereby making two subgroups of A and two of AB (A_1B, A_2B). Still other variants of agglutinogen A exist, designated as A_x, A_m, and A_g. It appears, furthermore, that group O is not the negative character (i.e., no A, no B) which was once assumed. Anti-O serums have been found to be of two kinds, namely, one which is inhibited by the addition of saliva of secretors of any group ("anti-H") and one which is not ("anti-O"). The H antigen may represent a positive characteristic of group O.

The discovery of a blood factor S related to the long-known M-N system, and the finding of still another blood factor, s, reciprocal to S, made it possible to distinguish nine M-N-S-s types. This, however, does not appear to be the end. There is evidence for a third allele at the Ss locus, Ss or S^u. There appear to be three alleles, M_1, M_2, and N, and perhaps still another, M^g. On the same chromosome but not allelic are Hu, He, Mi^a, Vw (Gr), and Vr. The P system, discovered at the same time as M and N and thought at first to be of little clinical or medicolegal significance, may prove to be of more importance than was thought at first.

As is well known, the Rh system, which came next in the expanding catalogue of blood groups, has proved to be of major importance and also of great complexity. The discovery of anti-f made it necessary to postulate a fourth series of allelic antigens in the Rh system, f and a still hypothetical F, supplementing Dd, Cc, and Ee. The newest of the Rh antibodies is anti-V, which may represent another pair, Vv, and there may be still another factor, G. In addition, a number of alleles of these Rh antigens have been discovered, such as C^w, C^x, c^v, C^u, D^u, E^u, and E^w. The differences between the Fisher-Race and the Wiener systems of terminology and the genetic theories on which they are based cannot be considered here, but it should be mentioned that Wiener makes a distinction between an agglutinogen, a substance present on the surface of red blood cells that is identified by certain agglutination reactions with diagnostic reagents, and blood *factors*, which are attributes of the agglutinogen molecule that enable it to combine with antibodies. These have been named Rh^A, Rh^B, Rh^C, and Rh^D. Unfortunately, the inherent complexities of the subject are not being made easier by disagreement concerning nomenclature.

Other blood group systems listed in Table 47-1 include the reciprocal factors, Kell-Cellano (K, k) and several related alleles; antibodies for K have been found in occasional serums from mothers of erythroblastotic babies and not infrequently in serums from persons who have had hemolytic transfusion reactions; Duffy (Fy^a, Fy^b), which has been responsible for a number of serious intragroup hemolytic transfusion reactions; and Kidd (Jk^a). The Lewis (Le^a, Le^b) and Lutheran (Lu^a, Lu^b) systems have not been thought to be of much importance antigenically in man, but anti-Le^a has been encountered in a few instances in which there was a history of transfusion. The Lewis system may be primarily an antigen system of the saliva and serum and only secondarily an antigen system of the red cells.

There is increasing evidence that the antigen *Diego* defines another locus controlling antigens of the red cells and saliva. This antigen is generally presumed to be a Mongolian character. It has been found in the blood of South American Indians, Japanese, and Chinese and only as an extreme rarity in the blood of Europeans and West Africans.

Still another well-established blood group system is Sutter and, besides this, a number of "*private*" *blood groups* have been discovered (Be^a, By, Rm, Wr^a, Levay, and others) which are of such infrequent occurrence that they appear to be almost the private property of particular families. "*Public*" antigens, that is, those possessed by the vast majority of people, include Vel, Yt^a, and I.

MEDICOLEGAL AND ANTHROPOLOGIC IMPORTANCE

The three genes, A, B, and O, can occupy the same locus on a certain chromosome; that is, they are allelic. Each person inherits one of these genes from each of his parents. As a result six different combinations are possible, AA, BB, OO, AO, BO, AB. However, the factor O seems to be recessive to both A and B. Consequently the heterozygotes AO and BO cannot be differentiated by the usual typing techniques from the homozygotes AA and BB, respectively. For this reason only four blood groups are distinguishable out of the six possible combinations.

The genes for the other blood group systems are thought to be present on different chromosome pairs, and there is no evidence that any of the groups are inherited together, or linked. Consequently the usefulness of serologic examinations in medicolegal and anthropologic work becomes apparent. It has been calculated that, with the ABO system and the two subgroups of A, the MNSs blood groups, P, the Rh system, Lutheran, Lewis, and Kell, the total number of possible different combinations of serologic recognizable phenotypes is 23,616 and the number of genotypes is 972,000. Because of technical and other difficulties, the P, Lewis, Kell, Duffy, and Kidd systems are not recommended for use in problems of parentage or identity, but even without them, when blood of the mother, the child, and the alleged father is available, it is possible to exonerate 51 per cent of all men wrongfully accused of paternity.

Of additional medicolegal importance is the fact that the antigens A, B, and H are present in saliva. The ability to secrete them is inherited as a mendelian dominant character which is not linked to the ABO genes. Persons whose red cells are Le^a positive are salivary nonsecretors of A, B, or H substance, whereas those who are Le^b are secretors. There are two distinct forms of the antigens: (1) a water-soluble form not present in the red cells or serum but present in most of the body fluids and organs of a secretor; and (2) an alcohol-soluble form, not influenced by the secretor gene, which is present in all tissues (except the brain) and in the red cells, but not present in the secretions. In secretors, blood group substances can be extracted with aqueous solutions from tissues and organs, especially salivary glands and gastric mucosa, and can be found in high concentration in secretions such as saliva, gastric juice, and semen.

Table 47-1. BLOOD GROUP FACTORS

Name of system	Factors of clinical importance	Other identifiable factors
ABO	A, B	O, H
MNSs	S, s, Ss, Mi^a, Vw	M_1, M_2, N, Hu, He, M^g
P		P_1, P_2, p, P^k
Rh	D, D^u C, C^w, C^x, c^v, C^u, c E, e, E^u	E^w f, V, G
Kell	K	k, Kp^a, Kp^b, K_o
Duffy	Fy^a	Fy^b
Kidd	Jk^a	Jk^b, Jk
Lewis	Le^a	Le^b
Lutheran		Lu^a, Lu^b
Diego		Di^a
Sutter		Js^a

Table 47-2. DISTRIBUTION OF A-B-O, M-N, AND RH SYSTEMS

	A-B-O				M-N			Rh-Hr						
	O	A	B	AB	M	MN	N	cde	CDe	cDE	CDe/cDE	cDe	Cde	cdE
American Indians (Utah)............	*97.4*	2.6	0	0	*58.7*	34.6	6.7	0	33.7	*28.8*	*37.5*	0	0	0
Australian aborigines..	48.1	*51.9*	0	0	2.4	30.4	*67.2*	0	58.2	8.5	30.4	1.3	1.7	0
Basques.............	57.2	41.7	1.1	0	23.1	*51.6*	25.3	*28.8*	55.1	7.8	6.0	0.6	1.8	
English..............	47.9	42.4	8.3	1.4	28.7	47.4	23.9	15.3	54.8	14.7	11.6	2.3	0.6	*0.7*
Negroes (U.S.A.).....	51.5	29.5	15.5	3.5	23.0	51.5	25.5	8.1	20.2	22.4	5.4	*41.2*	*2.7*	0.5
White (U.S.A.).......	42.2	39.2	13.5	5.1	29.9	50.2	19.9	13.5	33.5	13.0	13.8	2.5	0.5	0.5
Chinese.............	30.7	25.1	34.2	*10.0*	33.2	48.6	18.2	1.5	60.6	3.0	34.1	0.9	0	0
Asiatic Indians.......	32.5	20.0	*39.4*	8.1	.....	.....	.....	7.1	*70.5*	5.1	12.8	1.9	2.6	0

Italic figures—highest value in column; ..... —no information.

As a consequence it is possible to apply blood grouping to the examination of dried stains of saliva or semen and to saline extracts of muscle tissue.

In human genetics and anthropology the blood groups are of the utmost value for a number of reasons. The first is that they are sharply distinguishable "all-or-none" characteristics which do not grade into each other. Then again, they are simple, genetically speaking, and are inherited in a known way according to mendelian principles. Furthermore, they owe nothing to environment in their inheritance, nor are they subject to variations because of natural selection as is the case, for example, with skin color. Hence the blood groups are especially fitted to throw light on the moderately remote as well as the recent origins of mankind. Wide differences in frequency in different races have been observed. Consequently the blood groups provide the most valuable anthropometric measurements available.

Considerable and interesting data are being accumulated concerning the ethnologic distribution of the blood groups. Thus the incidence of B has been found highest in certain parts of Asia and declines in all directions from central Asia except for a subsidiary high center in Africa. In the Old World the lowest figures have been found in the Scandinavian countries, while in Australia the gene seems to have been absent until very recent times. A similar complete absence has been found in the living aborigines of North America as well as in the Basques. Group O reaches levels of practically 100 per cent among certain Indian tribes in the United States. In the aborigines of America the gene for N is relatively rare, while in those of Australia it is very common. The factor P is much more common in the blood of American Negroes than in that of American whites. The Rh-negative gene (cde) has

been found in 13 to 17 per cent of modern inhabitants of Europe and in white inhabitants of America. In the Basques it reaches very high levels (28.8 per cent); in contrast, in a study of Eskimos only 1 out of 2,522 was found to be Rh-negative. Some representative figures are given in Table 47-2.

CLINICAL IMPORTANCE

Before discussing the relation of blood groups and blood transfusion, several other aspects may be considered briefly. It is well established that blood group incompatibility is responsible for at least one disease, hemolytic disease of the newborn (p. 1289). From the standpoint of the pathogenesis of other acquired hemolytic anemias, the finding of anti-e in a patient with acquired hemolytic anemia whose red cells were of a genotype containing ee and other similar observations bring up the possibility that autosensitization may occur under special circumstances (p. 1290).

It is possible that blood groups may be of clinical importance in other ways. It has been postulated that blood groups are examples of balanced polymorphism and that different combinations of genotypes may have different survival values. Unfortunately, information on this topic is as yet inadequate. Reports concerning an association between ABO blood groups and fertility are conflicting and difficult to interpret. It is also hard to evaluate the significance of reports concerning the relationship of these blood groups and prematurity and stillbirth or blood group "conflicts" and aberrant salivary secretion in spontaneous abortion.

Much has been written concerning the association of blood groups and various diseases. Thus, it has been reported that there is a close association between blood group A and gastric cancer and pernicious anemia. Some regard the evidence indicating a high incidence of duodenal ulcer in people of group O as "overwhelming." Similar studies have been carried out with reference to many other conditions, but less strong support has been uncovered concerning the association of blood groups and these diseases. Nevertheless, the studies are of great interest and importance. However, investigations of this kind must be interpreted with great caution as the sources of error and chances for misinterpretation are very great.

As indicated in Table 235-5, blood transfusion reactions are of great variety. Those related to the blood groups are among the most serious and, unfortunately, though preventable, are all too frequent. The blood groups A and B or D (Rh) are involved in by far the great majority, perhaps 95 per cent of cases. This is because anti-A and anti-B antibodies occur naturally, and D is, like A and B, a strong antigen to which antibodies are produced readily. The first exposure to A or B of a person who does not possess the factor results in a hemolytic reaction if such blood is introduced. The transfusion of D blood to a person who is Rh-negative usually only sensitizes him; a second such transfusion may result in a hemolytic reaction. The Kell system (Kk) is also important because many K-negative persons can be sensitized to K by transfusion. The same holds true for E and c, but the danger is smaller. The remaining blood group factors are of still less importance. Nevertheless, it has been estimated that over 80 per cent of all transfusions given are possibly sensitizing ones. Scarcity of serums and the labor involved make it impractical to type routinely for all the known factors. The use of a sensitive cross-match test together with the Coombs test for "incomplete" antibodies is a helpful safeguard.

REFERENCES

Boyd, W. C.: "Genetics and the Races of Man," Boston, Little, Brown & Company, 1950.

Clarke, C. A., D. A. P. Evans, R. B. McConnell, and P. M. Sheppard: Secretion of Blood Group Antigens and Peptic Ulcer, Brit. Med. J., 1:603, 1959.

Owen, R. D., C. Stormont, I. B. Wexler, and A. S. Wiener: Medicolegal Applications of Blood Grouping Tests, J.A.M.A., 164:2036, 1957.

Plotkin, S. A.: The A-B-O Blood Groups in Relation to Prematurity and Stillbirth, J. Pediat., 52:42, 1958.

Race, R. R., and Ruth Sanger: "Blood Groups in Man," 3d ed., Oxford, Blackwell Scientific Publications, 1958.

Sussman, L. N.: Pitfalls of Paternity Blood Grouping Tests, Am. J. Clin. Pathol., 33:406, 1960.

Wintrobe, M. M.: "Clinical Hematology," 5th ed., Philadelphia, Lea & Febiger, 1961.

48 AGING AND INVOLUTION
William Dock

DEFINITION AND GENERAL CONSIDERATIONS

Aging includes the acquired changes which require time for their development, and also involutional changes which are as much a part of mammalian life as the autumnal involution of the leaves of deciduous trees. Accumulations of fat, of cholesterol in the arteries or gallbladder, of chalk in the cartilages, all require time; hence, they are more advanced in the aged than in the young. Changes in the subdeltoid tendon sheath or about the vertebral bodies occur from stress—the oftener the stress is repeated, the more marked the changes. Hence old people show more change than younger ones. Involution probably also plays a part in altering the composition of the tissue in all these cases, but age and repeated exposure to a noxious influence are also necessary to evoke clinical evidence of impaired function.

Aging, then, may be defined as the sum of the losses of function and structure and of the callosities, scars, and nodular hyperplasias due to "wear and tear" and to involution. Wear and tear includes trauma; infection; overstimulation by emotional, dietary, or other abuses; dietary inadequacies; exposure to inclement weather; exhausting activity; etc. Changes in metabolism not due to such abuses or overstimulation must be ascribed to involution, if it occurs in a large proportion of members of certain families after the age of maturity. The effects of such involution may not become apparent under ideal conditions. Thus diabetes may not become manifest so frequently in those obliged to live on a low-calorie diet. One interpretation of this would be that diabetes is due to dietary excess, even though it never develops in most of those who live on faulty diets. We accept the other view, that pernicious anemia, gout, and diabetes developing after maturity are due to innate involutional faults.

The boundary between what one chooses to classify as involutional and abiotrophic is arbitrary. If *involutional* designates "the usual or expected change occurring with age," and *abiotrophic* "the exceptional progressive anatomic and functional loss which may occur at any time during development or senescence," then gout and diabetes, idiopathic Parkinson's disease, and pernicious anemia are all abiotrophies, along with, perhaps, amyotrophic lateral sclerosis, Alzheimer's psychosis, and progressive muscular atrophy. In the future we may expect to learn more about the genetics and the external factors which control these disorders. Then we may include in aging many cases of Paget's disease, Graves's disease, myxedema, etc., which are now called idiopathic, or we may narrow aging to those disorders which are inevitably present in all men or women who reach the age of seventy, or ninety. Thus baldness and even graying of hair would be classified as abiotrophies, because they do not invariably manifest themselves before ninety.

AGING AND THE VASCULAR SYSTEM

Even in the aged, the vascular bed is able to grow and to adapt itself to circulatory needs. Tumors in the aged become well vascularized, and arteries leading to them enlarge strikingly. Only when the arterial lumen is severely encroached on by clots or atheromas does the vascular supply fail in the organs and brain of the aged. Inflammatory disease also may lead to vascular inadequacy at any age; and in the coronary arteries of the heart, atheromas may cause trouble soon after puberty in patients with very high blood cholesterol levels. The vessels of the legs also may suffer soon after maturity in such patients, and in severe hypertension, bilaterally symmetric and diffuse lesions of small arteries may become evident in the brain, retina, and kidneys, even before maturity. In the absence of initial unilateral lesions in the normotensive person, and in the absence of retinal lesions in the hypertensive one, it is never wise to ascribe changes in memory, judgment, and originality to cerebral arteriosclerosis. In the absence of angina or evidence of a myocardial infarct, it is equally unwise to ascribe cardiac failure to arteriosclerosis. In the heart there is only coronary atheromatosis involving the large epicardial branches; even in hypertension the arterioles in the myocardium usually remain unaltered.

The most vigorous objection must be registered to the notion that men are "as old as their arteries." Men may die of coronary atherosclerosis before they are old enough to vote; these arteries are diseased and not "old." Temporal arteries may stand out as large, tortuous vessels in men under thirty, yet at ninety the same men may be alert and in good health. This is due to fibrosis with ectasia, a clinically unimportant vascular involution. Men are as old as their skins, their scalps, their cerebral cortices, and all their other tissues. Since aging shows up most strikingly in the skin and brain, even when these have excellent vasculature, a man might be said to be no older than his ectoderm. He is vulnerable to death from a congenital weakness in 5 mm of his circle of Willis, or from an atheroma in 1 cm of one coronary artery.

MANIFESTATIONS OF INVOLUTION

The tissues of the body undergo aging at very different rates in different organs, species, and individuals. To some degree the rates are influenced by environment, nutrition, infection, trauma, or abuse, but even these influences are minimal—great variations in aging of specific tissues are obvious in individuals and in families as well as in species. Grizzly bears and gorillas have graying of the hair on reaching maturity; other bears and primates have none at advanced ages; some families turn white in the thirties, others not until after seventy. Wrinkling of the face and neck may occur early in members of families who become neither bald nor gray until old age. Pulmonary elastic fibers may age and emphysema become troublesome in men whose elastica ages slowly in the skin or the arteries.

The pattern of graying, baldness, and coarsening of the hair of the face, nostrils, and ears shows clearly how atrophy may proceed in one area while hypertrophy is occurring in another. Focal hyperplasia in the presence of atrophy is a commonplace of aging of the skin, breast, prostate, and thyroid, and in the gastric mucosa. Symmetric degeneration of neurones may occur in certain parts of the cerebral cortex, or the cerebellum, or the substantia nigra, while preservation of neurones in adjacent regions is still excellent. This is often incorrectly ascribed to vascular disease; in the scalp no loss of vascularity is necessary to cause baldness or graying, and in the brain no local ischemia precedes the symmetrical loss of neurones. In many organs, involutional atrophy of the parenchyma precedes disuse atrophy of the vascular bed, which then undergoes secondary degenerative changes.

Physiologic involution, such as that in the lens and uveal tract which causes loss of near vision (presbyopia, or the "elder's eye"), may be associated with minimal histologic change. Anatomic involution, such as disseminated cortical atrophy of the frontoparietal regions, may be grossly striking, with almost no functional loss. In the former type, chemical systems age and wear out, but cell structure is little altered; in the latter, cells disappear but the effect is minimal because vital activity is carried on in adequate fashion by the remaining tissue. The aging heart recovers less rapidly during diastole than does the young heart; consequently, heart failure occurs under conditions which a few decades earlier did not even cause transient dilatation. In all such cases, the diagnosis of involution is made from two sets of facts. The mature patient may become senile in certain tissues at almost any age, and, therefore, maturity is one essential datum. The other is the demonstrated absence of infections or metabolic or vascular disorders capable of accounting for the phenomenon in question. Thus pellagra may simulate involution of the brain, beriberi simulate involution of the heart, and syphilitic aortitis simulate senile dilatation and elongation of the aorta. Much the most convincing evidence for involutional causation is a familial similarity in age of onset and distribution, and the widespread occurrence of similar disorders in aging mammals of various species.

Fortunately, many involutional losses are readily corrected—the hair can be dyed, the long hairs in the ears and nostrils clipped, the bald scalp can be wigged with a toupee. Others are turned to assets: the faulty memory of the aged and their deafness excuse much and spare effort and annoyance. Finally, some chemical involutions can be corrected. Those which cause pernicious anemia and combined cord lesions are effectively treated with vitamin B_{12}; senile heart failure is usually responsive to digitalis; presbyopia is easily corrected by eyeglasses, etc. Some physicians hesitate to diagnose disease as due to involution until after threescore years and ten, or avoid this diagnosis altogether because it suggests an incurable disorder. Both these reasons are incorrect. Many involutions, like presbyopia, can be demonstrated in larval stages in the twenties in nearly everyone; others, like baldness and the disorders of urate metabolism called gout, are manifest before forty, in a very appreciable percentage of all those finally recognized; and many involutions, after rapid progress for a few years, become arrested and often compensated.

The involution of greatest importance to society and to the physician is that of the central nervous system. Anatomically, this is characterized by loss of neurones, which is demonstrable in the spinal cords and brains of mice, rats, and men. Loss of motor neurones decreases the fiber count of the spinal nerves and probably contributes to the loss of agility and athletic prowess, with sustained capacity for prolonged heavy loads of work, which is typical of middle and old age. Loss of neurones in the basal ganglions accounts for tremor, rigidity, and even full-blown clinical disorders such as idiopathic parkinsonism.

But most important of all is the loss of cortical neurones which diminishes the acuteness of observation, and when severe leads to the apathy, irritability, stolidity and garrulousness, overly great concern for minutiae, and loss of concern about essentials which are characteristics of senile psychoses and of many older people merely regarded as eccentric or bureaucratic. Older patients' histories are notoriously undependable. For every man or woman in whom "old experience do attain to something like prophetic strain," there are half a dozen in the asylums and several score who "ain't what they used to be." It is the physician's function to detect the remediable disorders, such as brain tumor, pellagra, pernicious anemia, or myxedema, which masquerade as senile behavior, and

to do what is possible to secure maximum comfort and effectiveness from the waning powers of aging men and women. Nothing is gained by refusal to recognize the fact that all men age and die and that involution of many tissues sets in with maturity, not in old age.

One of the great tragedies of urban civilization is the treatment of elderly people slipping into second childhood or second infancy (with loss of concern for cleanliness, bowel or bladder function) as if they were insane. In rural or primitive cultures, such people are cared for by their relatives in the familiar environment of their homes. This can become impossible in small apartments, and there should be orphan asylums and foundling homes to provide for unwanted people in second childhood and infancy. They are not helped by psychiatric treatment, are upset by the strange environment of hospital or asylum, and deteriorate rapidly under sedative therapy.

This problem will grow as science brings arterial disease and neoplasia under control. These disorders, by removing aging people, serve an important biologic purpose, creating opportunity and removing burdens from those in the child-rearing age. During the nineteenth century when pneumonia killed more people, Sir William Osler called it "the old man's friend" for, like Ecclesiasticus, he considered death kind to the old and feeble. Inheritance of resistance to involution, arterial disease, and cancer is evident in many families, but this biologic blessing is often paid for by the necessity to live with or support aged relatives. In an urban society, such obligations favor late marriage and few or no children. Success in eradicating arteriosclerosis, cancer, and rapid aging will tend to be frustrated by natural selection, and the survival of more grandchildren in families with few living grandparents. Atherosclerosis and neoplasia are now the chief factors in determining that we do not decline into second childhood, do not overstay our biologically allotted span of life too long.

REFERENCES

Andrews, W.: The Reality of Age Difference in Nervous Tissue, J. Gerontol., 14:259, 1959.

Birren, J. E.: "Handbook of Aging and the Individual," Chicago, University of Chicago Press, 1959.

Strehler, B. L., et al.: Rate and Magnitude of Age Pigment Accumulation in Human Myocardium, J. Gerontol., 14:430, 1959.

Wolff, K.: "The Biological, Sociological, and Psychological Aspects of Aging," Springfield, Ill., Charles C Thomas, Publisher, 1959.

Section 2: Neoplastic Diseases

49 PRINCIPLES OF NEOPLASIA

Ivan L. Bennett, Jr., and
Sumner Wood, Jr.

DEFINITIONS

A *neoplasm* is a proliferation of new cells that may progress, become quiescent, or regress. Although *tumor* literally signifies swelling of any etiology, the terms neoplasm and tumor are often used synonymously in clinical parlance. While the initiating factor in human tumors is usually unknown, it is clear that progressive, uncontrolled, and autonomous growth can continue after cessation of the provocative stimulus, indicating an heritable disorder of cellular multiplication.

A *benign* neoplasm is composed of normal or nearly normal cells whose growth is local, demarcated, or encapsulated. *Malignant* tumors or *cancers* are characterized by uncoordinated growth, usually without sharp delimitation of borders; as cellular multiplication progresses and becomes autonomous, morphology frequently becomes atypical or undifferentiated ("anaplastic"), infiltration and invasion of adjacent tissues follow, and dissemination to remote sites can result in secondary growths, or *metastases*.

It is important to recognize that the term *cancer* designates disorders of many etiologies; biologically, physically, and chemically, its meaning is no more specific than *inflammation, degeneration,* or *infection.* Consequently, it is extremely difficult to generalize about many aspects of neoplastic disease; for detailed discussions, the reader should refer to the monographs listed at the end of the chapter.

Biochemical differences between neoplastic and normal tissues have been investigated extensively, but no universal specific or distinctive alteration has been found.

Even a consistent morphologic classification of tumors is lacking. While malignant tumors usually show significant aberrations in growth pattern and cytologic features, the histology of a malignant, metastasizing tumor, such as follicular carcinoma of the thyroid gland, can be identical with that of the normal tissue from which it arises. The recognition that many neoplasms are malignant has come only from careful correlation of the histologic patterns observed by the pathologist with the biologic behavior and clinical course of the tumors in man. It is obvious that the distinction between benign and malignant neoplastic disease is of fundamental importance in therapy and prognosis.

A malignant tumor derived from ectodermal or entodermal structures is a *carcinoma,* and one derived from *mesoderm* is a *sarcoma.* Even this basic distinction is not always clear-cut, an example being the melanoma or melanosarcoma, whose cellular origin is uncertain although its morphology and clinical behavior are well established. Tumors of the central nervous system (see p. 1811) are classified separately, and tumors arising from lymph nodes or related structures are often referred to as *lymphomas.*

A *teratoma* is a neoplasm arising from both mesodermal and ectodermal (or entodermal) tissues. Most are benign but one or more components may be malignant; the recognition of the malignancy of a teratoma sometimes poses great difficulty for the pathologist.

A *hamartoma* is a focal proliferation of cells normally present in an organ and is probably best regarded as a congenital malformation rather than a true neoplasm.

ETIOLOGY

No precise causes are known for the majority of human tumors. It can only be hoped that accumulating knowledge of agents that will elicit cancer in experimental animals and of the many factors such as heredity, diet, and occupational exposure that seem to influence the incidence of neoplastic diseases in different ethnic groups and geographic areas will eventually clarify the situation.

Genetic Factors. Experimentally, the role of heredity is easily demonstrable by the inbreeding of animals with the production of strains which show a very low or very high incidence of spontaneous tumors. Isolated examples of human families in which tumors of several types have occurred with extraordinary frequency in as many as four generations are also well documented. Among the neoplastic diseases of man with known familial occurrence are von Recklinghausen's neurofibromatosis (p. 1732), polyposis coli, retinoblastoma, osteochondroma, and pheochromocytoma. Other new growths such as nevi, hemangiomas, chondromas, neurofibromas, teratomas, neuroblastomas, and Wilms's tumors of the kidney are often congenital, being present at birth. The high incidence of leukemia in patients with mongolism, now established as a chromosomal disorder (see p. 429), implies an association between chromosomal aberrations and neoplasms; this is further suggested by the occurrence of the so-called "Philadelphia chromosome" in chronic myeloid leukemia.

Viruses. Viral etiology has been established for tumors in many experimental animals, including the chicken, frog, rabbit, mouse, and hamster. In man, present evidence indicates that a virus causes warts. However, it must be emphasized that the absolute identification of a virus as the causative agent of a human cancer would not be an indication for reclassifying the tumor. The lesion would still be a neoplasm—a neoplasm of known etiology similar to malignant growths induced by chemicals or ionizing radiation.

Physical Agents. The major physical agent known to produce both animal and human neoplasms is *ionizing radiation*. Examples in man include osteogenic sarcoma ("phossy jaw") after occupational exposure to radium, cutaneous carcinomas after x-ray exposure, and the high incidence of leukemia among those who were survivors of the atomic blast at Hiroshima. Thymic or pharyngeal irradiation during infancy has been associated with an increased frequency of thyroid carcinoma in young individuals, and therapeutic irradiation of benign giant-cell tumors of bone has resulted in osteogenic sarcoma. The so-called "Schneeberg carcinomas" of the lung in cobalt miners in Saxony are the result of the inhalation of radon. There is an increase in cutaneous cancer among individuals exposed chronically to the sun's actinic rays, noted especially in sailors, farmers, and fair-skinned races. Carcinoma of the skin is forty-five times as frequent in Caucasians living in Hawaii as it is among Orientals and Hawaiians. The congenital disorder *xeroderma pigmentosum,* characterized by unusual sensitivity to sunlight, is well known to predispose to cutaneous carcinoma at an early age.

Mechanical trauma is virtually never a primary or contributory cause of cancer.

Chemical Agents. More than 500 different compounds of diverse chemical structure will produce experimental neoplasms. In man, the scrotal carcinoma of chimney sweepers was the first-recognized "occupational tumor." Others include cancer of the lip in Scottish fishermen who customarily held the tarred twine used in mending nets between the teeth, carcinoma of the lung in chromate workers (and possibly in nickel workers), and carcinoma of the bladder among aniline-dye workers exposed to *beta-naphthylamine.* There is a strong statistical correlation between cigarette smoking and lung cancer; the controversy over the etiologic significance of this will continue for a long time. Two

examples of the role of chemical (or thermal) irritation in human tumorigenesis are observed in South Asia: the so-called "Andhra carcinoma" of the hard palate in South Indian women who smoke *chottas,* native cigars, "hotside in," and the well-documented increase in oral cancer among chewers of betel (areca) nut.

Hormones. A variety of hormones, especially the sex steroids, are capable of inducing malignant tumors in animals. While no direct causal relationship is known between hormones and tumors in man, striking alterations in the course of prostatic or breast cancer have been produced by giving sex hormones, by castration, by hypophysectomy, or by adrenalectomy. That these substances sometimes play a contributory or permissive role in human neoplasms seems beyond doubt.

Miscellaneous Factors. A variety of studies illustrate the multiplicity of potential carcinogens or cocarcinogens. Laryngeal and esophageal cancer are more frequent in alcoholics. Hepatic cancer is associated with nutritional imbalance in Bantus and in the United States; more than 50 per cent of these tumors occur in adults with cirrhosis of the liver. Studies among different ethnic groups in Hawaii have shown that gastric cancer is two and one-half times as common in Japanese males as it is in Caucasian men, that prostatic cancer is nine times as common in Caucasians as it is in Japanese, that the incidence of mammary carcinoma in Japanese women is less than one-fourth of that in Caucasian women, and that although Chinese compose only 6 per cent of the population, 76 per cent of nasopharyngeal carcinomas occur in Chinese patients.

The presence of neoplastic disease predisposes to cancer, as evidenced by the observation that a patient with one malignant tumor is two to six times more likely than others to develop a second primary cancer.

There are, obviously, many "statistically significant" differences in the incidence of neoplasms among ethnic and racial groups, but the interpretation of these data is complicated by many differences in diet, climate, occupation, and coexisting endemic diseases. Presently, the usefulness of epidemiologic studies of human cancer is sharply limited by the problem of multiple factors that cannot yet be isolated from one another. While findings in surveys often suggest excellent subjects for experimental testing, they rarely suffice for any new etiologic conclusions.

INCIDENCE

With increase in life expectancy and lowering of the number of deaths from infectious agents, incidence of and mortality from cancer have risen. As a cause of death in the United States, cancer is second only to circulatory disease in adults and to accidental trauma in children. About half the childhood deaths from malignant disease are caused by leukemia.

In the United States, the most frequent cancer in males is cutaneous, and mammary carcinoma is the commonest in women. The pattern varies enormously in other countries and geographic areas and generalizations cannot be made.

PROPERTIES OF MALIGNANT NEOPLASMS

There are endless variations in the growth rate of different tumors, in their local invasiveness, and in their routes and sites of metastasis. While multiplication of neoplastic cells usually proceeds more rapidly than that of many normal cells, this property alone does not imply malignancy of a tissue; indeed, the generation time of cells during embryogenesis, regeneration of liver, or the normal replacement of intestinal mucosa is shorter than that of most tumors.

Basal cell carcinoma of the skin is locally invasive but metastasis is exceedingly rare. Epidermoid carcinoma of the skin metastasizes by way of lymphatics rather frequently, but melanomas can spread to regional nodes and also disseminate widely by the blood stream while the primary lesion is still minute and inconspicuous.

Progressive growth, ulceration with bleeding, or pressure upon adjacent structures resulting in pain or obstructive phenomena may call attention to the primary tumor. Generally, cancer cells are less cohesive than normal cells, a property which may be of great importance in their detachment from the main growth, making possible their detection by the methods of exfoliative cytology.

Precancerous Lesions, *in Situ* Carcinoma, and Malignant Transformation. Generally, it is very rare for a benign tumor to become a cancer. However, on a purely empirical basis, it has come to be recognized that certain lesions that are themselves benign are so often associated with later development of cancer that excision or other treatment is indicated. Leukoplakia of the oral cavity or female genitalia, senile keratosis of the skin, arsenical keratosis (p. 812), intestinal polyps (p. 1642), and cutaneous nevi showing "junctional activity" (p. 1932) fall into this group. Other lesions that may be complicated by cancer are cirrhosis of the liver (p. 1696), thermal burn scars, and the atrophic gastritis of pernicious anemia (p. 1285). Benign chondromas are often difficult to excise completely, and serial recurrences and removals for many years may lead to the development of chondrosarcoma at the local site. Whether this is the natural course of the tumor or malignant transfor-

mation resulting from repeated surgical trauma is not known. However, in the absence of repeated specimens indicating that a tumor was benign, the criticism can always be raised that it was malignant from the first and that no transformation was involved.

The terms *intraepithelial carcinoma* and *carcinoma in situ* are used interchangeably to describe foci of cytologically abnormal cells in which there is also disruption of normal arrangement or sequence of cell types without invasion of adjacent tissue. They are used most often in connection with lesions of the uterine cervix and breast but are also applied to skin, stomach, bladder, bronchus, etc. The very names imply the malignant potential of the lesion, and it is customary to manage such foci as though they were indeed malignant. However, the true incidence of invasive carcinomas that arise in such lesions if they are undisturbed is not known. Indeed, to determine their existence requires excision and, consequently, those who prefer to believe that the lesion is premalignant can account for failure of cancer to appear in a patient with *carcinoma in situ* by claiming that the original biopsy also constituted surgical excision. Valuable as the definitive information would be, it seems unlikely that long-term studies in untreated patients will ever now be completed under conditions that will yield reliable answers.

Metastasis. The occurrence of metastasis is the most decisive factor determining the choice of treatment and the success of therapy. Wound contamination by tumor cells can result in local *implant metastases*, largely preventable by meticulous surgical technique.

Invasion of lymphatics and spread to regional nodes is usually managed by excision of the tumor with dissection and removal of the nodes or postoperative irradiation of them.

The frequency of direct venous invasion and hematogenous transport of tumor cells has been emphasized in recent studies. Venous invasion is demonstrable in about 40 per cent of resected carcinomas of the rectosigmoid, 70 per cent of lung cancers, and 80 per cent of gastric cancers. Manipulation or operative trauma increases the number of cells released from the primary lesion into lymphatics and blood vessels. The presence of large numbers of tumor cells in the blood is a poor prognostic sign. However, *tumor cell embolism* is not *metastasis;* many patients with venous invasion and circulating tumor cells have survived for many years after surgical excision of the primary growth. Experimental studies have revealed that an enormous number of cells must be injected into the blood stream to produce a single metastasis.

The mechanisms responsible for the *organ selectivity* of metastasis are unknown.

Grading and Staging. For uniform evaluation of the natural behavior and response to therapy, methods of grading and staging have been proposed for specific tumors. *Grading* refers to the degree of histologic differentiation. Low-grade neoplasms (grade I) consist of well-differentiated, nearly normal-appearing cells, whereas grades III and IV neoplasms are pleomorphic or anaplastic. *Staging* refers to extent; in the colon, stages include involvement of mucosa, of muscularis, of local lymph nodes, or of distant sites.

SYSTEMIC EFFECTS

Nutritional. Weight loss and eventual inanition are frequent in extensive malignant neoplastic disease. This is usually attributable to a combination of anorexia, blood loss, diarrhea, fever, etc., rather than to any specific property of the tumor.

Specific Metabolic Changes. The tissue concentrations of enzymes such as catalase and lactic acid dehydrogenase are nonspecifically lowered. Serum acid phosphatase level is elevated in disseminated prostatic cancer, and serum alkaline phosphatase level often rises when the liver or bones contain metastatic tumor. Hypercalcemia can accompany bronchogenic or other carcinomas (see p. 607), and hypoglycemia is a rare manifestation of mediastinal neoplasms and fairly common with hepatic cancers. Peculiar neuropathy or myopathy (p. 1560) and clubbing of the fingers (p. 1920) are often reversed by removal of a small bronchogenic carcinoma. The systemic effects of serotonin elaborated by malignant carcinoid (p. 755), intractable peptic ulceration (Zollinger-Ellison syndrome, p. 1594) accompanying tumors of the pancreatic islets or duodenum, and the hormonal effects of gonadal (pp. 669 and 677), hypophyseal (p. 568), adrenal (p. 619), pancreatic islet (p. 661), or pineal (p. 688) neoplasms are other systemic effects. *Thrombophlebitis* sometimes precedes other symptoms of pancreatic, bronchogenic or gastric tumor by months, and intractable *pruritus* is the first manifestation of Hodgkin's disease in some patients.

Elevation of blood uric acid level or of basal metabolic rate is seen in Hodgkin's disease and leukemia. Some tumors are apparently capable of elaborating humoral substances with hormone-like action. While none of these has been identified, there is much to indicate that the hypercalcemia accompanying occasional bronchogenic tumors and the hypoglycemia which is produced by other tumors involve such a mechanism. Finally, the often-noted association between Cushing's disease and malignant tumors is now believed to represent, in many cases, secondary stimulation of the adrenal glands by an ACTH-like substance rather than suscepti-

bility of patients with hypercorticism to neoplastic disease.

Fever, the mechanism of which is not understood, accompanies many tumors, especially lymphoma, renal carcinoma, and hepatic metastases.

Psychologic Effects. The patient with cancer requires sympathetic, diligent, and optimistic care. There are no rules that the physician can learn, but experience, an awareness of the terror that the words "tumor," or "growth," and especially "cancer" hold for most patients, and above all, a combination of professional skill, common sense, and compassion will usually suffice (as they will in the care of patients with almost any serious chronic disease).

CANCER AND OTHER DISORDERS

The clinical association between benign or malignant tumors and other diseases is poorly understood in most instances. A partial list of tumors and diseases with which they seem to be clinically associated includes pernicious anemia (gastric carcinoma), cirrhosis or hemachromatosis (hepatoma), congenital cystic disease (bronchogenic carcinoma), polyposis coli (colonic carcinoma), chronic ulcerative colitis (colonic carcinoma), Paget's disease of the nipple (mammary duct carcinoma), Paget's disease of bone (osteogenic sarcoma), myasthenia gravis (thymoma), mongolism (leukemia), xeroderma pigmentosum (skin cancer), Peutz-Jeghers syndrome (colonic carcinoma), acanthosis nigricans (visceral carcinoma), and dermatomyositis (several types).

DIAGNOSIS

Other sections of this book describe the clinical manifestations of specific tumors and the use of laboratory tests, endoscopy, and x-ray studies in diagnosis. The discussion that follows is confined to the problem of the definitive diagnosis of tumors by microscopic examination of biopsy specimens or of smears of exfoliated cells.

In the examination of excised tissue, accurate diagnosis depends upon the skill and experience of the pathologist. The clinician should remember that the interpretation of histologic findings in terms of the individual patient is not an "objective" exercise in exact morphology but can vary importantly with the patient's age, sex, medication, and x-ray findings (especially in bone tumors). All pertinent data should be made available to the pathologist, tissue specimens should be adequate in size, and the occasional need for additional biopsies should be recognized. It is not unusual, for instance, to find nonspecific and nondiagnostic changes in the structure of one or two excised lymph nodes, only to discover the characteristic lesion of Hodgkin's disease in a third specimen from the same patient.

The common practice of having histologic sections and x-rays reviewed and reinterpreted by another pathologist and radiologist when a patient comes under the care of another clinician illustrates the importance of individual skill and experience. This practice does not signify any innate unreliability of the methods employed or a distrust of the professional opinions of others; it is no more difficult to understand than the insistence of a clinician on taking his own history and performing his own physical examination on a patient, no matter how frequently others may have carried out the same procedures.

Clinically benign lesions that may be mistakenly identified as histologically malignant include pseudoepitheliomatous hyperplasia secondary to insect bites (p. 1243) or a benign tumor called granular cell myoblastoma, juvenile fibromatosis, fibroxanthomas, intraductal hyperplasia or papillomas of the breast, oral lichen planus (p. 76), myositis ossificans, and a poorly understood entity known as pseudosarcomatous fasciitis.

Lesions that may be histologically benign in appearance but can behave as malignant tumors include smooth-muscle neoplasms of the stomach, villous polyps of the colon, mixed salivary gland tumors, follicular thyroid tumors, and cartilaginous tumors. These can pose serious problems in clinical management because of the difficulty of accurate histologic distinction between malignant and benign forms.

Exfoliative Cytology. The examination of exfoliated cells in vaginal secretions by the method of Papanicolaou is extremely accurate in detecting early carcinoma of the uterine cervix. The so-called "Pap smear" for this tumor is actually the only screening technique that is simple and sensitive enough to be applied in a practical way to mass examination of the population.

Accurate cytologic diagnosis is also possible for carcinoma of the larynx (sputum), lung (sputum, bronchial washings), kidney and bladder (urine), gastrointestinal tract (saline washings), biliary tract (duodenal washings), and breast (nipple secretions). Furthermore, the certain identification of cancer cells in cerebrospinal fluid, peripheral blood, and effusions into pleural, pericardial, peritoneal, or synovial cavities is feasible. However, for all these other tumors, the preparation of the patient, the collection and processing of specimens before cells degenerate, the concentration of cells, and the thorough examination of numerous smears require meticulous technique and many expensive hours of the time of professional personnel. Simplification of

tedious methodology without sacrificing sensitivity and accuracy are needed before cytopathology can be made available on a large scale for these diseases.

The use of exfoliative cytology for the detection of cervical cancer in totally *asymptomatic* women is well established, and the Pap smear is becoming almost as routine as the blood count in physical checkups. However, no comparable test of the accuracy of cytologic methods for detecting *unsuspected* and *asymptomatic* tumors of other types has yet been possible. Most experience has been limited to patients with symptoms or signs of disease in a specific organ system, and it is highly unlikely that methods will ever be simplified to an extent that will permit general "screening" of the population for malignant disease.

Presently, exfoliative cytology is a valuable diagnostic method in selected cases and supplements without eliminating the need for other diagnostic methods.

THERAPY AND THE EVALUATION OF THERAPEUTIC RESULTS

As in other chronic, disabling illnesses, attention to nutrition, judicious use of blood replacement, relief of pain, and maintenance of morale are of utmost importance.

The major avenues of attack upon the neoplastic process are surgery, irradiation, and chemotherapy.

Total excision of tumors is obviously desirable whenever possible. Advances in anesthesiology, general supportive care, and plastic surgery have made possible many radical and supraradical operations, but these have largely reached the limits imposed by anatomy. Evaluation of the results in terms of cure and palliation balanced against immediate operative mortality and patient disability remains to be completed for many of these procedures. It is not surprising that there is considerable controversy over specific surgical techniques among different clinics and that the relative merits of surgery, irradiation, and chemotherapy in management of certain tumors are hotly debated.

Irradiation, including supervoltage x-rays, cobalt "bombs," and the systemic or local use of radioactive isotopes, is curative for certain tumors and is, generally speaking, preferable to surgery for palliation or suppression in patients with systemic spread of tumors. The evaluation of results of treatment of "deep" tumors (lung, esophagus) using high-voltage beams awaits careful follow-up studies. Ionizing radiation should be avoided for benign or banal lesions except under very rare circumstances. A combination of radiation and surgery or radiation and chemotherapy sometimes offers advantages; the judicious application of the available methods in the individual patient can increase survival in many incurable tumors and prolong active, pain-free, and useful life for months or years.

With rare exceptions, chemotherapy is palliative or suppressive rather than curative. Of the two general classes of anti-tumor drugs in wide use, the antimetabolites and the alkylating (sometimes called radiomimetic) drugs, all are toxic to normal tissues; this limits sharply their dosage and raises many problems because of undesirable, uncomfortable, and dangerous side reactions. It is unlikely that any chemical agent that injures neoplastic cells will be totally without action on other tissues. Furthermore, the wide differences in tumors themselves make it just as unlikely that any single universal "cure" for cancer will be discovered as it is that any antibiotic will be found that can cure all bacterial, rickettsial, and viral infections.

The use of hormones and castration can produce striking remissions in prostatic or mammary carcinoma, and adrenal steroids often ameliorate symptoms of neoplastic disease without modifying its course. In certain cases of leukemia and lymphoma, corticosteroids may also exert some direct, though transient action upon the tumor itself.

Agents such as stilbamidine, urethan, bacterial toxins, venoms, and viruses are occasionally effective; all have their advocates and many are under continuing investigation, but the usefulness of all is limited.

Techniques such as intraarterial injection or isolated perfusion of a diseased organ to allow delivery of larger doses of a drug to the tumor without systemic toxicity are very useful in special cases.

An enormous program for discovery of new chemotherapeutic agents and generous support of cooperative clinical trials of their effectiveness and toxicity is sponsored on a continuing basis by the United States Public Health Service; eventually, improved agents may become available.

For many types of cancer, knowledge of the natural history of the disease and of the variations that can occur in the absence of treatment is incomplete, a fact which obviously makes the evaluation of therapeutic regimens difficult. For most tumors, the results of therapy can also be expected to depend upon the extent of the lesion at the time treatment is initiated. It is in the attempt to standardize this variable that techniques of *staging* and *grading* have been developed for several common cancers. Of most importance is the fact that it is virtually impossible to conduct "double-blind" or placebo-controlled investigations of human cancer and that no study can be conclusive without continued observations of patients for many years. When this attempt to carry out long-term observations is coupled with attempts to evaluate not only *cures* but also extent of relief of symptoms, etc., in palliation and suppression, the difficulties are almost insurmountable.

The results of therapy are often recorded as 5- and 10-year disease-free survival rates. For cervical, pulmonary, and gastric carcinomas, patients who live for 5 years without residual or recurrent disease can generally look forward to many more years of survival. However, recurrence or metastasis of carcinoma of the breast or thyroid is a threat for so many years after initial recognition and treatment of a tumor that the relative merits of therapeutic regimens are difficult to assess with certainty.

In most clinics, the operative mortality rates are higher and the 5-year survival rates lower for charity than for private patients. Survival figures are generally better for asymptomatic than for symptomatic tumors, regardless of grade or stage. Finally, the 5-year survival rates tend to be higher for females than for males treated in the same fashion for carcinoma of the lung, stomach, thyroid, esophagus, salivary glands, and tongue, and for melanoma and Hodgkin's disease.

REFERENCES

Ackerman, L. V., and J. A. Regato: "Cancer: Diagnosis, Treatment and Prognosis," 3d ed., St. Louis, The C. V. Mosby Company, 1961.

Cole, W. H., H. W. Southwick, S. Roberts, and G. O. McDonald: "Dissemination of Cancer: Prevention and Therapy," New York, Appleton-Century-Crofts, Inc., 1961.

Everson, T. C., and W. H. Cole: Spontaneous Regression of Cancer. Preliminary Report, Ann. Surg., 144:366, 1956.

Ewing, J.: "Neoplastic Diseases," 4th ed., Philadelphia, W. B. Saunders Company, 1940.

"Fourth National Cancer Conference Proceedings," Philadelphia, J. B. Lippincott Company, 1961.

Greenstein, J. P.: "Biochemistry of Cancer," 2d ed., New York, Academic Press, Inc., 1954.

Hills, A. G., and K. A. Woeber: The Syndrome of Intrathoracic Neoplasia and Bilateral Hyperfunction of the Adrenal Cortex, Ann. Int. Med., 54:1295, 1961.

Papanicolaou, G. N.: "Atlas of Exfoliative Cytology," Cambridge, Harvard University Press, 1954.

Quisenberry, W. B.: Sociocultural Factors in Cancer in Hawaii, Ann. N.Y. Acad. Sci., 84:795, 1960.

Warren, S.: Criteria for Traumatic or Occupational Causation of Cancer, Ann. Surg., 117:585, 1943.

Wood, S., Jr., E. D. Holyoke, and J. H. Yardley: Mechanisms of Metastasis Production by Blood-borne Cancer Cells, Canadian Cancer Conference, 4:167, 1961.

Section 3: Fluids, Electrolytes, and Acid-Base Balance

50 FLUIDS AND ELECTROLYTES
Louis G. Welt and
Charles H. Burnett

PHYSIOLOGIC CONSIDERATIONS

Volumes of Body Fluid

The total volume of body fluid is equivalent to 50 to 70 per cent of the body weight. Since adipose tissue is relatively free of water, the figure is closer to 50 per cent in the obese and approximates 70 per cent in lean individuals. This fluid is compartmented into two major phases: the intracellular and the extracellular, and several subdivisions thereof. Approximately two-thirds of the total water is within the cells. The extracellular fluid (one-third of the total and approximately equivalent to 16 to 20 per cent of the body weight) is further partitioned among the plasma, interstitial fluid, and several smaller but specialized units such as the cerebrospinal fluid, the aqueous humor of the eye, and the lymph.

The volume of several of these major compartments can be estimated. The technique entails the administration of some material whose distribution is considered to be uniform throughout the compartment in question. If a known amount of the test material is administered, and the amount lost from the body during the time necessary for complete mixing can be determined, and the concentration per liter at the time of equilibration can be estimated, the volume of distribution of the test substance can be calculated. The volume of total body water can be estimated by using water labeled with deuterium or tritium. A variety of substances, such as inulin, sucrose, sulfate, etc., has been used to define the volume of the extracellular fluid. The volume of the intracellular fluid cannot be estimated directly but may be inferred from the difference between the total volume of body water and the volume of the extracellular fluid. Plasma volume (approximately 5 per cent of the body weight) has been calculated from the volume of distribution of protein-bound dyes, such as T-1824, and of albumin tagged with I^{131}. However, since the proteins, particularly albumin, are not wholly confined to the vascular compartment and gain access to the interstitial spaces and the lymph, the volume of distribution of tagged albumin is likely to be in excess of the plasma volume itself. This extravascular distribution of labeled albumin may be exaggerated in many states of edema, and its use in these circumstances is thought by many to provide spuriously high values for the plasma volume. The volume of the red cell mass is considered to be more reliable and may be estimated utilizing erythrocytes tagged with an isotope of iron, phosphorus, or chromium.

Each of these measurements has been of value in the investigation of both the normal and pathologic exchanges of water and electrolytes. There is no doubt that such measurements would provide considerable aid in the management of patients whose illness is complicated by a disorder of hydration and of electrolyte imbalance. Unfortunately these techniques are not as yet applicable as routine clinical tools. Nevertheless, the background of information gained from their use in the careful study of small series of patients, plus the less precise qualitative data that the clinician may gather from the history, physical examination, and the intelligent use of the laboratory techniques that are readily available usually allow a fairly shrewd appraisal of the quantitative character of deficits and excesses of fluid volume.

Composition of Body Fluids

There are major differences in the composition of the intra- and extracellular fluids, and minor differences among the several components of the latter. The composition of the extracellular fluid is better understood and more precisely defined, both because it is a more simple fluid and because it is available for analysis in the form of serum and transudates into the serous cavities. The only cells that can be obtained in relatively pure form in any bulk are the erythrocytes. Generalizations from the characteristics of this unique and highly specialized cell to all cells would, of course, be most hazardous.

The *interstitial fluid* of the extracellular compartment is an ultrafiltrate of serum and differs from the latter in that it contains very low concentrations of large molecular species such as proteins and lipids. The usually accepted normal range of values for the concentrations of electrolytes in serum is as follows:

Cations, mEq/L	Anions, mEq/L	
Sodium..... 132–142	Chloride.....	98–106
Potassium .. 3.5–5.0	Total CO$_2$....	26–30 (mM/L)
Calcium.... 4.5–6.0	Phosphate and	
Magnesium . 1.5–3.0	sulfate.....	2–5
	Organic anions	3–6
	Proteins......	15–2.5

The average total cation concentration approximates 150 mEq per liter and this is considered to be identical with the total anion concentration. Although these concentrations are conventionally expressed in relation to a unit volume of serum, it is understood that these ions are for all intents and purposes distributed in the aqueous phase of the serum. The average water content of serum is about 93 per cent, and, hence, to express these concentrations in terms of serum water, they should each be divided by 0.93. The concentrations in the water of serum can then be translated to the concentrations in the interstitial fluid by applying a correction factor to account for the asymmetric distribution of ions across the capillary membrane. This latter is related to the presence in the serum of nondiffusible ions, the proteins. The Donnan ratio that describes the relative concentrations between serum and an ultrafiltrate thereof is approximately 1.05 for the univalent cations and 0.95 for the univalent anions.

The compositions of joint fluid, aqueous humor of the eye, and the cerebrospinal fluid are all similar to an ultrafiltrate of serum, but there are enough differences in the aqueous humor and spinal fluid to suggest that these are not pure dialysates but are, in part at least, formed by an active process of secretion.

The composition of the intracellular fluids cannot be examined directly, and, hence, the characteristics of cell fluid are inferred from analyses of whole tissue and the use of certain "reasonable" calculations. The total tissue water can be readily estimated from the difference in weight between the fresh wet tissue and the weight after it has been dried at 100°C for 72 hr. The volume of this water which is to be ascribed to the extracellular phase is calculated from knowledge of the concentration of chloride in the tissue and serum and with the assumption that the chloride is in an extracellular position. The values for the volume of the extracellular fluid and the concentrations of sodium and potassium in this fluid (as derived from their values in serum) are used to calculate the quantity of these two ions in the noncellular phase. The difference between the total tissue sodium and potassium and the quantity in the extracellular phase represents the amount in cells. The difference between the total water and the extracellular volume is the intracellular water. The concentration of sodium

and potassium in the intracellular fluid can then be calculated. These details have been recited to emphasize the indirectness with which cell composition is defined.

The average data, derived largely from muscle analyses, obtained in this inferential manner are as follows:

Cations, mEq/L	Anions, mEq/L	
Sodium......... 10	Bicarbonate...	10 (mM/L)
Potassium...... 150	Phosphate and	
Magnesium...... 40	sulfate......	150
	Proteins.......	40

Granting validity to the calculations, there is still much that is unknown about the physicochemical state of these materials. For example, the characteristics of the phosphate, sulfate, and proteins in terms of valence are unknown. It is not certain that all the potassium and magnesium is in a free and ionized state. Furthermore, it is probably unrealistic to speak of intracellular fluid as an entity, since diverse tissue cells have major differences in composition. Lastly, the intracellular fluid of a single cell type is probably not an entity, since it, in turn, is compartmented at least into an extra- and intra-mitochondrial fluid.

The most complicated characteristics of cell composition and the marked differences between it and the environment of the cells serve to emphasize the highly specialized functions of cells, the complex mechanisms that must be available to maintain these compositional differences, and the possibilities for alterations in metabolic pathways that may result from even subtle alterations in composition.

In contrast to the marked differences in the composition of these two major phases, it is believed that the total solute concentration in these fluids is identical. This, in turn, is due to the presumed free permeability of most of the cell membranes to water. This concept has been challenged in recent years, and although a categorical statement is not appropriate, the preponderance of evidence continues to support the concept that the cellular fluids are, in fact, isotonic with respect to their environmental fluid. This may not apply for those cells which secrete a hypotonic fluid such as the sweat and salivary glands, and for the renal tubular cells that tolerate fluids of markedly different osmolalities on each surface.

Internal Exchanges of Water

When two aqueous solutions are separated by a membrane that is freely permeable to water, molecules of water will move from one compartment to the other. There will be an equilibrium with respect to water when the same number of water molecules pass in each direction per unit of time. At such a time there is no *net* alteration in volume in either of the compartments separated by the membrane. The tendency for the molecules of water to pass from one compartment to the other is spoken of as an "escaping tendency" and is referred to as the *chemical potential* of the water. Whenever the chemical potentials of the water of two contiguous solutions differ, there will be a net movement of water from the phase with the higher chemical potential to that with the lower, until equilibrium is reached. The chemical potential of water is reduced when solutes are added, and the reduction is proportional to the concentration of solutes. In contrast the chemical potential of water molecules is enhanced by increases in hydrostatic pressure and temperature.

Thus the addition of a solute that can traverse a membrane with freedom will result in its uniform distribution throughout the volumes of fluid separated by that membrane. The addition of this solute will diminish the chemical potential of the water molecules, but since the water in both compartments is influenced to the same degree, there is no *net* change in the volume of water on either side of the membrane. The only effect is that fewer molecules of water, but an equal number of them, move in each direction per unit of time. In contrast, if the added solute were unable to permeate the membrane in question, it would be confined to the side to which it was added and would diminish the chemical potential of the molecules of water on that side alone. Under this circumstance molecules of water would continue to *enter* this phase at the rate which obtained prior to the addition of the solute, but water molecules would *escape from* this compartment at a slower rate, and there would be a net change in volume, such that there would be an accumulation of water in the compartment to which the solute had been added. The redistribution of water would continue until a new state of equilibrium was established.

Ordinarily these problems are discussed in terms of osmotic pressure. In this context the addition of a solute that can permeate membranes freely, such as urea, contributes to the total osmotic pressure, but it is not effective in terms of promoting a redistribution of water. Glucose which is not free to enter cells by passive diffusion not only contributes to the total osmotic pressure of a solution to which it is added, but it contributes what is referred to as an *effective osmotic pressure* (as opposed to *total* osmotic pressure) and does condition a redistribution of water.

With respect to biologic fluids and membranes, it may be said that an increase in the concentration of those solutes that permeate membranes freely augments the total osmotic pressure (decreases the chemical potential of the water molecules) in all compartments of the body fluids. However, an increase in the concentration of a solute that cannot penetrate a membrane freely will increase the *effective* osmotic pressure as well as the total (diminish the chemical potential of the molecules of water) in the fluid in which the concentration has been altered. If this fluid is separated by a membrane that is freely permeable to water, there will be a net alteration in volume in favor of the compartment to which the solute has been added. Despite long usage and familiarity, the terms total and effective osmotic pressure will be replaced in the rest of this discussion with the terms total and effective *osmolality*. This should serve to recall that it is the activity of the molecules of water that is under discussion, and not the technique (utilizing hydrostatic pressure) which may be used to estimate these activities. However, since hydrostatic pressure increases the chemical potential of molecules of water, a change in hydrostatic pressure may counterbalance the influence of solutes so that a *difference* in total solute concentration across a membrane may be unassociated with net transfers of water.

Sodium salts represent almost all the solutes that usually contribute to the effective osmolality of the extracellular fluid. Hence in most instances an increase or a decrease in the concentration of sodium in the serum may be equated with an increase or decrease in the effective osmolality of the extracellular fluid and, in turn, will promote a movement of water from or into the cellular compartment.

There are two circumstances when a depressed concentration of sodium in serum may not necessarily represent a diminished effective osmolality of the serum water. It will be recalled that it would be more precise to speak of the concentration of an ion such as sodium in terms of its concentration in the water of serum. Since the determination is actually performed on a diluted aliquot of serum, and since the per cent of serum that is water is so commonly between 90 and 93 per cent, the convention is to refer the concentration to a unit (usually a liter) of serum. In circumstances characterized by hyperlipemia, the lipids may occupy a significant volume of the serum, and the per cent of serum that is water may be drastically reduced, to as low as 70 to 80 per cent. An average concentration of sodium of 138 mEq per liter in a serum whose water content was 93 per cent would represent a concentration of 148.3 mEq *per liter* of serum *water* (138/0.93). If this same concentration obtained in the water of a *lipemic* serum where the water content was only 75 per cent, the concentration per liter of *serum* would be 111.2 mEq (148.3 × 0.75). Thus a striking hyponatremia in this instance would not mean a diminished effective osmotic pressure of the water of the serum.

Although glucose contributes to the effective osmolality of the extracellular fluid, the magnitude is usually small. At a concentration of 100 mg per 100 ml (1,000 mg per liter) this would amount to 5.5 mOsm per liter. However, if hyperglycemia supervenes, the corresponding increase in the effective osmolality will promote a movement of water from the cells. This will dilute the concentration of sodium and may depress the level to the point of frank hyponatremia. In this instance the interpretation that the hyponatremia signifies a decrease in effective osmolality would be in error. For these reasons the concentration of sodium in a patient with diabetes mellitus should be interpreted with knowledge of the simultaneous concentration of glucose in the serum.

Significance of Hyponatremia. Hyponatremia is observed frequently in hospital practice. Not all instances of hyponatremia have the same pathogenesis; many are poorly understood, and a decision as to their management may be difficult. This discussion excludes those instances in which hyponatremia is not equivalent to a decrease in the effective osmolality of the body fluid, such as those cited in relation to hyperlipemia and hyperglycemia.

The most common situations in which hyponatremia is observed are those cases of dehydration or edema in which salt has been lost in excess of water, or water has been retained in excess of salt. A modest deficit of sodium is frequently accompanied by an equivalent loss of water. The sequence of events may be something as follows: (1) the loss of sodium induces a mild reduction of the concentration of this cation in the extracellular fluids, (2) this, in turn, suppresses the secretion of the antidiuretic hormone (ADH), and (3) the excretion of water is increased until the concentration of sodium has been restored. This is frequently referred to as a "sacrifice of volume in the interests of tonicity of the body fluids." However, as the volume deficit assumes more significant proportions, equivalent losses of water no longer follow further deficits of sodium salts, and a hyponatremia is established. It may be that the deficit in volume, or some expression thereof, is a stimulus for the secretion of ADH despite hyponatremia; or the volume deficit may influence renal function, in some fashion independent of ADH, to conserve water. It is clear from this sequence that one very important implication of a state of dehydration accompanied by hyponatremia is that the intensity of the dehydration is probably severe. In addition, the decrease in effective osmolality of the extracellular water will have promoted a movement of water into the cellular compartment. Thus the deficit in volume of the extracellular phase is greater than the total external loss. Lastly, the dilution of the intracellular fluid may be expected to have untoward consequences with respect to cell functions. These latter are most clearly expressed on a clinical level by a clouded sensorium, which may progress to frank coma and may be accompanied by seizures.

In patients who have a disturbance characterized by the development of edema, it seems clear that the retention of sodium salts is primary to the retention of water. This is attested to by the limitation placed on the accumulation of edema that may be imposed by a rigid regimen of salt restriction, and the success of those measures designed to relieve edema by promoting a loss of salt in the urine. Here, as is the case with the early phases of dehydration, the interrelationships between the effective osmolality of the body fluid, ADH, and the kidneys serve to maintain the concentration of sodium within normal limits. However, as the disorder responsible for the edema becomes more profound, a retention of water (despite the lack of ingestion of salt and in the absence of its excretion in the urine) proceeds, with the establishment of a *chronic dilutional hyponatremia*. The precise mechanisms responsible for this situation are not clear. It is not clear, for example, why these patients continue to ingest water. The stimulus for thirst must be other than an increase in the effective osmolality and may be the result of some consequence of the pathophysiology of the disease, or, simply, habit. Once again, as in dehydration, an important implication of the hyponatremia with edema concerns the severity of the disorder and suggests a very grave prognosis. Moreover, if this has occurred in the natural progression of the disease, it is most unlikely that restoration of the concentration of sodium is desirable; it is usually followed by increased thirst, the administration or ingestion of water, the retention of water, and consequent redilution.

Patients with edema may develop an *acute* dilutional hyponatremia. There are limits to the maximal rate of excretion of water which are imposed by such factors as the glomerular filtration rate, the volume of fluid gaining access to the distal segments of the nephron, and the intensity of antidiuretic hormone activity. In the absence of the antidiuretic hormone the flow of urine is conditioned largely by the rate of excretion of solutes. The edematous patient whose renal tubules reabsorb most or all of the filtered salt, and whose excretion of urea is diminished owing to less nitrogen turnover or depressed filtration rate or both, has serious limitations on the maximum rate at which he can excrete water. This limitation ordinarily conditions less thirst; hence, a normal concentration of sodium in serum is easily maintained. However, on occasion these patients are urged to drink beyond the dictates of thirst, or if they are unconscious and the decision concerning the volumes to be administered are ill-advised and too large, they will retain water and develop *acute dilutional hyponatremia.* This intoxication with water promotes an unphysiologic state whose serious consequences include a disturbed sensorium, coma, convulsions, and death. It is, therefore, desirable to restore the concentration of sodium to normal. This can be accomplished by the restriction of water, the administration of some solute such as urea which may promote a diuresis of water, or the administration of a hypertonic solution of sodium salts. In the patient who is already edematous, the first two measures have obvious advantages. In only the rare instance when the water intoxication appeared to be life-threatening would it be reasonable to include the last measure.

There are *rare* instances wherein acute dilutional hyponatremia has some of the features of dehydration with hyponatremia and may be expected to be benefited by correction. These acute episodes may occur following the removal of large volumes of ascitic or pleural fluid or after an unusually brisk response to a diuretic agent. In the case of the withdrawal of segregated collections of fluid such as ascites, there is good evidence that the procedure is followed by an increased rate of transudation from the plasma, leading to a reduction in plasma volume. This is accompanied by thirst and oliguria. Water ingested at this time is retained, and an acute dilution of the body fluids is induced. Such patients may have the signs and symptoms associated with impaired peripheral blood flow and water intoxication. This complication may be prevented, or at least modified, by the support of blood volume at the time of the procedure. At any rate, to the extent that the signs, symptoms, and disability which accompany this event can be ascribed to the acute reduction in volume (presumably plasma volume), the hyponatremia, and the consequent transfer of water to the cells, they may be benefited by the administration of a hypertonic solution of sodium salts.

A new interpretation of certain instances of hyponatremia suggests that some patients have an *inappropriate secretion of antidiuretic hormone* owing to some consequence of an intrathoracic or intracerebral lesion. Usual quantities of water are ingested, but because of the antidiuretic hormone secretion the urine is more concentrated than it would otherwise be. Water is retained and the patients become hyponatremic. In addition, the rate of excretion of salt may be augmented owing to the expansion of body fluid volume (and consequent suppression of aldosterone secretion and increase of glomerular filtration rate), and the pic-

ture then is one of hyponatremia coincident with considerable salt in the urine. Since the expansion of body fluid volume need not be great, edema may not be clinically evident, which adds further difficulties to the interpretation of the syndrome. However, the association of hyponatremia and salt in the urine in the absence of dehydration, with normal or even low levels of blood urea nitrogen, and urine osmolalities (or specific gravities) which are higher than anticipated under the circumstances should suggest the diagnosis of *inappropriate ADH secretion.* The management of this problem is limitation of the intake of water so that the positive balance of water can be dissipated and its recurrence prevented. This will serve to restore the level of serum sodium to normal, diminish the excretion of salt in the urine, and to the extent that there are symptoms of water intoxication, these will abate.

There is at least one other group of patients with hyponatremia who may have neither dehydration nor edema. They are found among patients with severe, usually chronic, debilitating diseases such as advanced tuberculosis, metastatic carcinoma, etc. These patients appear to have no signs, symptoms, or physiologic abnormalities that can be ascribed to the hyponatremia per se. They respond to salt restriction in a normal fashion by excreting a urine virtually free of sodium in 3 to 5 days. They seem to differ only in that their "normal" concentration of sodium in the serum is significantly lower than the usual range of 132 to 142 mEq per liter. These patients have been referred to as having "asymptomatic" hyponatremia. The mechanism is not clear, but it has been suggested that these patients may have sustained a primary decrease in the effective osmolality of the intracellular fluids, thus establishing a new level for the osmolality of the body fluids. As in the other conditions cited above, the hyponatremia is the hallmark of a severe disorder and the prognosis for these patients is poor. It is, of course, quite possible that some patients with edema have a similar disorder. In this instance, however, they would achieve a reduction in the osmotic activity of body water commensurate with the assumed primary change in the cells by the ingestion and retention of water, since the disturbance associated with the edema conditions a retention of salt by the kidney. Although it would be impossible to discriminate between such patients and those with chronic dilutional hyponatremia cited initially, the implications and the management would be the same in either instance.

Another way that hyponatremia might develop is by virtue of a movement of sodium from the extracellular compartment to cells or to bone. There is some evidence that such an intercompartmental shift of sodium may occur in adrenal cortical insufficiency. Sodium may accumulate in cells deficient in potassium, and some investigators have considered that certain instances of hyponatremia are related to this transfer from the extracellular compartment.

An assessment of the pathogenesis of hyponatremia can usually be made on the basis of the above discussion, and hence the therapeutic implications can usually be arrived at according to the above criteria. It must be conceded, however, that the best opinion on this subject is confused.

Significance of Hypernatremia. In contrast to hyponatremia, an increase in the concentration of sodium in the serum is a reflection of a loss of water in excess of salt, or of the administration (or ingestion) of salt in excess of water. The hypernatremia, which is the chemical expression of a deficit of water, in turn incites the following responses, which result in the acquisition of more water, the most efficient conservation of same, and the most desirable distribution of the available water, viz.:

1. Thirst
2. Secretion of the ADH which promotes the excretion of a concentrated urine
3. A movement of water from the cells to the extracellular space, thus mitigating the deficit of volume in this latter compartment
4. Diminution in the loss of insensible perspiration
5. A decrease in the rate of secretion of sweat

Comments on Correction of Hypo- and Hypernatremia. One other implication of the free permeability of cell membranes to water and a uniform osmolality throughout the body fluids concerns the manner in which the concentration of sodium in the serum is restored to normal from both hypo- and hypernatremic levels.

If hyponatremia complicates an illness and it is considered advisable to correct this abnormality, the amount of sodium that is required is equivalent to the deficit in concentration per liter multiplied by the estimated number of liters of *total body water*. If there is to be osmotic equality throughout the body fluids, it is implicit that the concentration of sodium in the extracellular phase cannot be increased without an equivalent increase in solute concentration in the cellular fluid. The administered sodium will increase the osmotic activity of intracellular fluid, not by entering the cells, but by promoting a movement of water from the cells to the extracellular compartment as the osmolality of the latter is increased. If it is desired to restore the concentration of sodium reasonably promptly, or if it is to be accomplished with a small volume of fluid, the sodium salts must be administered in a hypertonic solution. The amount of sodium that must be administered to restore the concentration to normal is equal to the normal concentration of

Na_s (138 mEq/liter) minus the current concentration of Na_s multiplied by the total volume of body water. For example: In a 70-kg adult with an assumed body water content of 60 per cent (42 liters) and a concentration of sodium in the serum of 128 mEq per liter,

$$(138 - 128) \times 42$$

$$= 420 \text{ mM deficit of sodium chloride}$$

Since there are 17.1 mM per Gm of NaCl, 420/17.1, or 24.56 Gm NaCl, would be necessary to restore the sodium to 138 mEq per liter. This could be supplied in 500 ml of 5 per cent NaCl solution.

The same principles apply to the estimation of the volume of water that may be necessary to reduce the concentration of sodium in the serum from hypernatremic to normal levels. Since the intensity of the hypernatremia (due to the loss of water in excess of or without salt) is proportionate to the deficit of total body water, the following relationship obtains:

$$\frac{\text{Normal concentration } Na_s}{\text{Elevated concentration } Na_s}$$

$$= \frac{\text{current vol total body H}_2\text{O}}{\text{assumed normal vol total body H}_2\text{O}}$$

The value for the current volume of total body water can be calculated, and the difference between it and the assumed normal volume for total body water represents the deficit of water. For example, in the same adult mentioned above but with a concentration of sodium in the serum of 160 mEq per liter:

$$\text{Current vol total body H}_2\text{O} = \frac{138}{160} \times 42 = 36.2 \text{ liters}$$

The deficit would be $42 - 36.2 = 5.8$ liters of water.

Exchanges between Plasma and Interstitial Fluid. The net exchange of fluid between the plasma and interstitial space is conditioned by a series of forces. Some of these forces favor transudation from the vascular system, such as the hydrostatic pressure within the vessels and the colloid osmotic pressure of the tissue fluids. The tissue tension and the colloid osmotic pressure of the plasma favor the reabsorption of fluid from the interstitium. It should be emphasized that, unlike the cell membranes, the capillary endothelial membrane is freely permeable not only to water but to all the solutes of the plasma except the large molecular species such as the proteins and the lipids. Thus, the concentration of sodium and its salts does not influence the distribution of water between these two major components of the extracellular compartment. Although the proteins do not contribute a large osmolality, they alone contribute to the effective osmolality since they are unable to permeate the endothelial membrane except in very small quantity. Thus, hypoalbuminemia may promote an expansion of the interstitial fluid, with diminution in plasma volume and hemoconcentration, with normal values for the concentration of sodium.

A change in the forces governing the net exchange between the plasma and the interstitial fluid need not necessarily condition a redistribution of volume between these two compartments. A net increase in transudation could be largely compensated by the return of this increment of fluid to the vascular system by way of the lymphatics. Lymphatic flow is frequently increased when the interstitial fluid volume is expanded, and this influence must be carefully considered when analyzing the forces that govern the disposition of fluid within the extracellular compartment.

Internal Exchanges of Electrolytes

Although it is apparent that ions such as sodium, potassium, magnesium, etc., move in and out of cells, it is equally apparent that their net movements are not a consequence of free passive diffusion. Large concentration gradients are established and maintained between the two major fluids, and the responsible mechanisms, the sources of energy, the nature of the carrier systems that may implement the active transport of materials across cell membranes are poorly understood.

One example of the transport of ions from one compartment to the other is referred to as an *ion exchange*. This implies a reciprocal and, presumably, a virtually simultaneous transfer of one ion, e.g., potassium, from the cell to the extracellular fluid and the movement of one other ion of similar charge, e.g., sodium, from the extracellular fluid to the cell. It has been postulated that an ion exchange mechanism operates between the luminal fluid and the renal tubular cells. In this context the reabsorption of sodium is thought to be accompanied by an exchange for hydrogen or potassium ions.

The change in composition of the cellular fluid with potassium deficiency illustrates some aspects of an exchange mechanism. Analyses of muscle tissues in many investigations of potassium depletion have shown an accumulation of sodium in the cell fluid. This exchange of sodium for potassium is not invariable, but when it does occur there is evidence under some experimental conditions that it is in a ratio of 2 mM sodium gained for each 3 mM potassium lost by the cells. Under these same conditions evidence has been presented which suggests that 1 mM hydrogen ion may have been exchanged for the third millimole of potassium. Furthermore, this substitution of hydrogen ion for potassium may be viewed as a transfer of the hydrogen ion from the extracellular fluid to the cell. This, in turn, may be at least partially responsible for the extracellular alkalosis seen so often in potassium depletion.

To the extent that the renal tubular cells share in a general deficit of potassium, a limitation may be imposed on the exchange of potassium in the process of sodium reabsorption. It has been suggested that this circumstance conditions a greater exchange of hydrogen and ammonium ions for reabsorbed sodium. This might promote an augmented excretion of hydrogen ions and add to other factors that tend to establish an extracellular alkalosis in potassium depletion.

Bone as a reservoir of ions other than calcium has attracted increased attention recently. Approximately a third of the total body sodium is in bone, and only 15 per cent of this can be ascribed to the extracellular phase. About one-half of the total body content of magnesium is in bone. Potassium is present in much smaller amounts. Deficits of sodium, potassium, and magnesium are shared by bone, and this tissue participates in exchanges which articulate with alterations in acid-base relationships. (See also Chap. 51, Acid-Base Equilibrium.)

External Exchanges of Electrolytes and Water

Thirst. In considering the net exchange of water between the individual and his environment it seems reasonable to begin with a discussion of thirst. This is the sensory impression that motivates the ingestion of water. There are several stimuli which may give rise to the sensation of thirst, and the most important of these is an increase in the effective osmolality of the body fluids. This appears to hold true whether the hypertonicity is promoted by a loss of water in excess of salt or the administration of salt in excess of water. These two circumstances differ in that in the first instance the volume of the extracellular fluid is decreased, and in the second this volume is expanded. However, in each circumstance the volume of the cells is diminished by virtue of a shift of water to the extracellular phase. A secondary stimulus is related somehow to a deficit of volume (or some expression of such a deficit) in some key portion of the extracellular space. Other factors which condition and modify the sensation of thirst include exposure of the oropharyngeal and esophageal tissues to water, the fullness of the stomach, and emotional as well as social factors. The central nervous system is responsible for the appreciation of and the response to thirst in both a specific and a nonspecific manner. There is now abundant evidence that lesions in key portions of the central nervous system—predominantly in the hypothalamus—may induce hypodipsia or polydipsia. The latter need not be accompanied by diabetes insipidus. The polydipsic center can be stimulated by exposing it to tiny volumes of hypertonic, but not isotonic, solutions of saline. It can also be aroused by electrical stimulation.

In a less specific sense the central nervous system conditions the reception and response to stimuli provoking thirst in relation to the level of the state of consciousness. The frequency with which patients with a clouded sensorium or coma are allowed to develop significant deficits of water is sufficient justification for emphasizing the obvious fact that such patients can neither appreciate nor respond to their own thirst mechanism.

Potassium depletion may be accompanied by thirst and polydipsia. This may reflect, in part, the inability of the kidneys to conserve water appropriately in this condition. However, it is also possible that there may be a primary influence on some aspect of the stimulus-response pathways concerned with thirst.

Insensible Perspiration. Water is continuously lost from the body in the expired air and from the skin. The sum of these losses is spoken of as "insensible loss" of water and is equivalent to about 600 to 1,000 ml per day in the average adult. This loss is augmented with increase in metabolic activity (fever, exercise, hyperthyroidism) and respiratory exchange. The catabolism of tissues produces 200 to 300 ml of water per day; hence, the *net* loss of insensible water may be considered as 400 to 700 ml per day. Since this loss is water without solutes, it should be replaced as water without salt (e.g., 5 per cent glucose in water when fluid balance is being maintained by parenteral techniques).

Sweat. The production of sweat is primarily responsive to heat. The latter presumably excites afferent impulses to centers that regulate the motor activities that promote the loss of heat. The important centers in the central nervous system are in the anterolateral portions of the hypothalamus. Sweat is not a simple fluid, and the details of its secretion are not well understood. It is always a hypotonic solution except in adrenal cortical insufficiency and in patients with fibrocystic disease (mucoviscidosis) of the pancreas. Among other influences, the rate of sweating is diminished by an increase in the effective osmolality of the body fluids. An average composition for sweat, in millimoles per liter, is as follows: sodium 48.0, potassium 5.9, chloride 40.0, ammonia 3.5, and urea 8.6. The characteristics of this fluid dictate the replacement of losses incurred as sweat by a solution which is one-third to one-half isotonic saline. This is readily satisfied for intravenous administration with 1 part isotonic saline to 1 or 2 parts of 5 per cent glucose in water.

Gastrointestinal Tract. The exchange of water and solutes between the body fluids and the lumen of the gastrointestinal tract is large. It is contrib-

uted to by the saliva, and the secretions of the stomach, liver, pancreas, and the intestinal mucosa. The volume of these secretions may exceed 8 liters a day under ordinary circumstances, but the net loss from the body is negligible. However, when there are losses through vomitus, diarrhea, or drainage from enterostomies, colostomies, or fistulas the deficits of water and electrolytes may be prodigious. Loss of fluid through these routes probably represents the most common pathogenesis of significant dehydration in clinical practice.

Aside from saliva, which is a hypotonic solution, the secretions mentioned are close to isotonicity with the extracellular fluids. However, they differ from the latter in composition. For example, the gastric secretion, if it contains free HCl, has a much lower pH, less sodium and bicarbonate, and more chloride than the extracellular fluid. In contrast, the pancreatic secretion has a higher pH and more bicarbonate. Most of the gastrointestinal secretions have more potassium than the extracellular fluid. Thus, although losses of gastrointestinal secretions per se represent isotonic deficits, the derangements that accompany the dehydration will be conditioned by the particular portion of the gastrointestinal tract from which the lost fluid derived. In many instances, however, these losses can be successfully replaced by equal volumes of isotonic saline solution. The potassium lost with the loss of these secretions and the consequences thereof must also be adequately replaced.

Renal Exchanges of Electrolytes and Water. The kidneys represent the major organs of conservation as well as of excretion in terms of the net balance of water and electrolytes. The kidneys are capable of excreting large volumes of excess water and large quantities of unwanted ions and other solutes. In addition, they respond to the need for the conservation of water by the excretion of small volumes of highly concentrated urine. Their response to a deficit of sodium is the excretion of a urine virtually free of salt. The conservation of magnesium is also good and subjects subsisting on a diet deficient in magnesium may excrete as little as 1 mEq of this ion per day. Although the excretion of potassium is very much diminished when there is a deficit of this cation, the efficiency with which the kidneys conserve potassium is not quite so great as it is with sodium, chloride, or magnesium.

The excretion of sodium is markedly reduced when there is primarily a deficit of water, despite the fact that this is accompanied by hypernatremia. This has the advantage of eliminating a major solute from the urine and, by reducing urine flow, furthers the conservation of water.

The kidneys display other exquisitely sensitive responses to most of the alterations in the composition, volume, tonicity, and pH of the body fluids. Details of these responses and the mechanisms involved therein are discussed in Chap. 257.

CLINICAL CONSIDERATIONS

An understanding of the pathogenesis and management of disorders of fluid and electrolyte balance is dependent on an appreciation of the approximate net exchanges of water and the several ions that have occurred during the course of a patient's illness. In essence, many of the problems concerning clinical disorders of hydration are resolved by the simple expediency of setting up a balance sheet in which the total estimated losses are accumulated, the total intake is summated, and the net differences are calculated. Although not quantitatively precise, this practice usually defines the qualitative nature of the alterations and provides an approximation of the quantitative characteristics. Many of these data can be obtained from the carefully taken history or the well-documented hospital chart. In addition, the physical examination, the chemical analyses of serum and urine, and other laboratory data provide additional insights. The management of the problem then becomes largely one of providing those materials which will restore the normal state of hydration. It is not an oversimplification to state that the majority of these problems are easily resolved with simple arithmetic.

In many instances a disordered state of hydration could have been avoided by the provision of adequate replacement of certain predictable and mandatory losses. It is desirable, therefore, to define the characteristics of the basal requirements for water and electrolytes, and to describe how these are modified by a variety of conditioning circumstances.

Basal Requirements

For the purposes of this discussion it will be assumed that the patient must receive the necessary water, electrolytes, and other materials by parenteral routes, that he has accumulated no antecedent deficits, that he is not sustaining any unusual losses, and that he has normal renal function. One other qualification is that the problem is one of short duration and that the need for calories and protein is not a major consideration. The task then is to prescribe a regimen which will maintain a normal state of hydration, avoid depletion of the major essential minerals, and minimize the most immediate threats of starvation.

The volume of water recommended per day is the sum of (1) the probable net insensible loss, 500 ml, (2) a reasonable volume for urine, 1,000 ml, and (3) perhaps a small additional volume, 300 ml, which is provided to anticipate other losses such as sweat, etc., but which, if not lost by extrarenal routes, can be readily excreted in the urine. These total 1,800 ml.

If a patient has been previously ingesting an average diet, he has probably been receiving about 8 to 10 Gm (135 to 170 mM) NaCl per day. If the intake of salt is suddenly eliminated, the patient will probably be able to excrete a urine essentially free of sodium in about 5 days. During this interval of 5 days a negative balance of sodium is allowed to develop. This is likely to be accompanied by an equivalent loss of water in the interests of maintaining a normal concentration of sodium in the extracellular fluid. This deficit in volume is probably not harmful in itself, but it prejudices the patient's ability to withstand other losses that may occur during the course of his illness. Therefore, unless there is some specific contraindication, it is recommended that the patient receive 4 to 5 Gm (70 to 85 mM) NaCl each day.

As noted earlier, the conservation of potassium is not quite so efficient as that of salt, and, unless the urinary excretion of this cation is replaced, a deficit of potassium will be ultimately achieved. From 40 to 60 mM potassium per day should be adequate to avoid a negative balance of this cation.

It has been stated that approximately 100 Gm carbohydrate is necessary for the operation of the Krebs cycle. Unless this is made available from preformed endogenous or exogenous carbohydrate, the catabolism of protein and fat will be accelerated and 4-carbon ketones will be formed faster than they can be utilized. The acid products of protein catabolism and the excess ketones must be excreted to avoid a metabolic acidosis; they are excreted in part as sodium salts, which adds another drain to the body's store of sodium. Each of these complications can be avoided by the provision of an adequate quantity, 150 to 200 Gm, of glucose per day.

The total basal requirements can now be listed as follows:

Water............	1,800 ml
NaCl.............	70–85 mM (4–5 Gm)
KCl.............	40–60 mM (3–4.5 Gm)
Glucose...........	150–200 Gm

An appropriate fluid prescription to meet these requirements is:

1,300 ml........	10% glucose in water
500 ml........	5% glucose in isotonic saline solution
4 Gm.......	KCl (added to the total water to be administered)

It should be reemphasized that this prescription is appropriate for the patient with qualifications set forth in the initial paragraph of this discussion on Basal Requirements.[1]

Additional Requirements. There are many circumstances which would require revision of the above prescription. Fever, restlessness, and increased respiratory activity will augment the loss of water as insensible perspiration. A hot environment and fever will promote sweating. Water loss in urine will be accelerated during an osmotic diuresis due to glycosuria or unusual amounts of urea. The latter situation is observed when unnecessarily large amounts of protein are administered to patients who are experiencing a reaction to injury and, hence, are limited in the ability to store nitrogen. Additional amounts of salt may be lost with glycosuria. Impaired renal function will demand an increased volume of urine, and the conservation of sodium may be less efficient than in patients with normal kidneys.

Fluids Available for Parenteral Administration. There is available a number of specially prepared solutions, such as "gastric replacement fluid," "intestinal replacement fluid," etc., aimed at meeting the requirements of particular types of loss. Their use should be discouraged. The basic tenet of the individualization of therapy applies here, as it does elsewhere in clinical practice. The proper management of disorders in fluid and electrolyte balance demands an analysis of the specific characteristics of the distortion in the particular patient at hand. The routine use of a special solution tends to diminish the diligence with which this analysis is made in the false sense of security provided by the claims of the value of the particular solution. This is not to imply that solutions other than glucose in water and isotonic saline are not frequently needed. However, when the need arises, the appropriate fluid should be designed for the particular patient and his problem. A great variety of special problems can be met by the preparation of a special solution from the following list of raw materials:

1. 5%, 10%, 50% glucose in water
2. 0.9% NaCl (154 mM/liter)
3. 5.0% NaCl (855 mM/liter)
4. 7.5% $NaHCO_3$ (900 mM/liter)
5. 14.9% KCl[2] (2,000 mM/liter or 2 mM/ml)

[1] Some suggest that small amounts of magnesium should be provided as maintenance as well. The recommended dose is 1 to 2 Gm $MgSO_4$ (8 to 16 mM) per day. There is much still to be learned about magnesium metabolism before sound recommendations can be made.

[2] This is a highly concentrated solution of potassium chloride and should never be administered unless it is diluted.

Lastly it should be emphasized that the most appropriate replacement fluid for lost blood is whole blood; and where the particular need is to expand plasma volume, the use of whole blood, plasma, or a plasma expander is recommended.

Techniques of Administration of Fluids

Fluids may be given by vein, by hypodermoclysis, or by gavage into the stomach. The latter method has many advantages, especially where the problem is likely to last for some time and where the considerations of calories, proteins, and other essential foodstuffs merit attention. The intravenous route is convenient, and the use of plastic tubing threaded into larger veins has eliminated some of the technical problems. The rate of administration of fluid deserves some attention, and in patients with cardiovascular disease the patient should be observed carefully and frequently to ensure the earliest recognition of an untoward response. The potential hazard of a cardiovascular complication may serve to modify the fluid prescription and the speed with which the fluids are administered. However, it should certainly not interfere with the proper management of dehydration.

The subcutaneous route may have some advantages in patients with heart disease. The access of fluid from the subcutaneous tissue to the blood stream is obviously slower than when fluid is introduced directly into the vein, but, in addition, its absorption may be even further delayed if there is a rise in venous pressure. In this fashion there is an added factor of safety. If fluids are administered by hypodermoclysis, two precautions must be borne in mind:

1. The fluid should be isotonic with the plasma. If it is hypertonic, there will be a tendency initially for water to leave the plasma and enter the clysis pool. This will cause an initial decrease in plasma volume, which is undesirable, especially if the patient is already dehydrated. Moreover, a hypertonic solution may be quite irritating to the subcutaneous tissue and result in a bad slough of tissue.

2. A solution of 5 per cent glucose in water should not be administered by clysis if the patient is dehydrated. When glucose is administered in this fashion, concentration gradients are established for the diffusion of glucose from clysis pool to plasma and for diffusion of sodium from plasma to clysis pool. Sodium diffuses more rapidly than glucose, the fluid in the pool, therefore, becomes hypertonic, and this, in turn, promotes a movement of water from the plasma. This reduction in plasma volume superimposed on the antecedent deficit may be sufficient to induce a state of peripheral vascular collapse.

Dehydration

The term *dehydration* continues to mislead, since it implies to many physicians the loss of water alone. Clinical dehydration is rarely represented by a pure deficit of water. Dehydration is usually associated with losses of both salt and water (in proportionate or disproportionate quantities), with deficits of other ions such as potassium, and with the frequent complication of a disturbance in acid-base equilibrium. All these factors must be considered in planning appropriate management. For purposes of orientation and discussion, clinical dehydration may be classified into three major groups as follows:

1. Loss of water in excess of sodium
2. Loss of sodium in excess of water
3. Isotonic losses of sodium and water

Loss of Water in Excess of Sodium. The failure to drink is the most common cause of a deficit of water. This is observed most frequently in severely debilitated patients with clouding of consciousness or coma. Not only are these patients too weak and ill to respond to thirst, but they are even unable to communicate the fact that they are thirsty to their family or to their physicians. The size of the water deficit, though it may increase each day, may be small and, hence, easily overlooked. However, this deficit can achieve significant proportions and contribute greatly to the severity of the patient's illness.

Solute diureses due to glycosuria are usually characterized by a loss of water in excess of salt. This is the situation, for example, in almost all patients with significant degrees of diabetic acidosis.

In recent years another type of solute diuresis has been found to be responsible for a deficit of water. Many physicians have become impressed with the therapeutic value of feeding large quantities of protein. There are many situations in which this is desirable. However, in the early stages of the reaction to an injury, the ability to store nitrogen may be very seriously impaired, and large amounts of protein (usually administered by gavage) will find its way to urea, demanding excretion in the urine. If the patient is able, he may complain of thirst if the urine flow is large enough to induce a deficit of water. The unconscious patient cannot provide this help. Delay in recognition is due, in great measure, to the misinterpretation of the significance of a large flow of urine, especially when the latter is not concentrated. This is equated with an appropriate state of hydration, whereas, in fact, the large volume of unconcentrated urine may be causing the deficit of water (see Chap. 258).

Diabetes insipidus may be responsible for large deficits of water. Unfortunately acute diabetes insipidus is commonly associated with trauma or infection in the central nervous system, and hence a clouded or comatose state is not unusual. Major deficits of water may occur in a matter of hours. A large volume of very dilute urine should alert the clinician to this possibility. The defect in the tubular reabsorption of water is easily corrected by the administration of pitressin (see Chap. 258).

The loss of sweat contributes to a deficit of water in excess of salt loss. To the extent that water alone is ingested and retained to replace the volume of lost sweat, a dehydration characterized by a loss of water in excess of salt loss is readily converted to one characterized by a loss of salt in excess of water loss. This serves to emphasize the point that the characteristics of the net deficit are conditioned not only by the quantity and quality of the fluid lost, but also by the characteristics of the fluid used as replacement.

The hallmark of a dehydration characterized by a loss of water in excess of salt loss is an increase in the effective osmolality of the extracellular fluids. In most instances this is reflected in an increase in the concentration of sodium in the serum, and the intensity of the hypernatremia may be used as a gauge to calculate the relative deficit of water (see earlier discussion).

Deficit of Salt in Excess of Water Deficit. *Adrenal cortical insufficiency* is probably the classic example of this type of dehydration. Although the loss of sodium may be the primary event in the pathogenesis of the dehydration in this disorder, it does not necessarily follow that the concentration of sodium will be depressed in the early phase (see prior discussion, Significance of Hyponatremia). However, as the contraction of volume becomes more significant, further deficits of sodium salts are not accompanied by equivalent deficits of water, and hyponatremia supervenes. The dehydration is severe, the cells are overhydrated, and the contracted volume of the plasma may compromise the renal blood flow and glomerular filtration rate, leading to azotemia and some degree of acidosis. The excretion of potassium is diminished. This is owing, according to most of the evidence, to the failure to reabsorb sodium at a site in the renal tubule where potassium secretion is coupled with sodium reabsorption. Hyperpotassemia out of proportion to the azotemia and hyponatremia is characteristic of this disorder. Peripheral vascular collapse is common, as are hypoglycemia, restlessness, and an altered sensorium (see Chap. 68).

Patients with chronic renal insufficiency may exhibit an inability to conserve salt properly. This may be of striking proportions and has been known to mimic and be misdiagnosed as adrenal cortical insufficiency. More commonly, the defect is much less intense and may be unmasked only when such patients are advised to restrict the use of dietary salt.

The loss of salt each day may not be great, but in the course of time a significant deficit may develop, accompanied by hyponatremia. The dehydration is associated with alterations in renal hemodynamics, and further reduction of an already deficient renal function is a common and dangerous complication. The hazard of a salt-poor regimen in patients with chronic renal disease should be recognized, and it is the responsibility of the physician who prescribes the program to make certain that the patient can tolerate the treatment. Careful evaluation of daily weights, observations with respect to changes in concentration of blood urea nitrogen and the concentration of sodium in serum, and an estimation of the total 24-hr excretion of salt in the urine are helpful in evaluating the response (see Chap. 258).

Some patients with lesions in the central nervous system may excrete large quantities of salt in the urine. Most of these may well represent instances of *inappropriate secretion of ADH* described in an earlier section. A few patients, however, have appeared to be dehydrated and were found to have azotemia. The question remains open as to whether a lesion in the central nervous system can induce a loss of salt by way of the urine that may lead to true salt depletion dehydration.

Isotonic Deficits of Salt and Water. In general, these deficits are primarily incurred by losses of fluid from the gastrointestinal tract. The ultimate character of the net deficit will be determined in part by the quality and quantity of fluids that the patient may receive. If the patient refrains from the ingestion of fluids and none have been administered by a parenteral route, the continued loss of insensible perspiration, sweat, and urine will determine a net deficit characterized by the loss of water in excess of salt loss. If the patient drinks water and vomits, the net deficit will be a loss of salt in excess of water loss.

Analysis of the Characteristics of Dehydration. The discussion presented above concerns the pathogenesis of dehydration in rather isolated terms, and in the hope of achieving clarity the price of oversimplification has been paid. Most patients have experienced a variety of insults of different magnitudes and for shorter or longer periods of time. The essence of the analysis of the characteristics of the dehydration is an assessment of all the data, in both quantitative and qualitative terms. These data are derived from the history, the physical examination, and the laboratory.

History. A careful review of the sequence of events during the course of the illness provides most important information concerning the quality and magnitude of the deficits of electrolytes and water. These data should actually be tabulated, and it is most desirable to develop the habit of preparing a balance sheet to use in the analysis. A sheet with the simple headings indicated below will usually suffice:

Intake:	Output:
Date/time	Diarrhea
Weight	Vomitus
Character of fluid	Urine
Volume	Insensible loss
	Sweat
	Blood

The systematic analysis of these data should provide a fair estimate of deficits in terms of volume, salt, potassium balance, and acid-base equilibrium. In an illness of short duration, information relating to the patient's usual and current weight may be helpful in estimating the volume of fluid that has been lost. The presence or absence of fever and sweating is relevant, as are data concerning the possibility of renal insufficiency or diabetes mellitus. Information concerning the usual level of blood pressure is helpful, since a "normal" blood pressure may be hypotensive for a patient whose blood pressure is usually in the hypertensive range. The symptom of thirst is most significant and can be most helpful in calling the physician's attention to a disorder of hydration which might otherwise be neglected. Thirst is most often due to a primary deficit of water, although it may also reflect a contracted volume, even when salt has been lost in excess of water.

A disorder of hydration may develop during the course of hospitalization. The data referred to above should certainly be available in a precise fashion in the hospital chart. The administration of parenteral fluids should be recorded with as much attention to detail as the record of drug therapy. It might even be anticipated that the very process of recording the data with respect to output and the administration of fluids would help to prevent serious disorders of hydration by focusing attention, if even for a brief period each day, on the quality and quantity of fluids that must be administered to replace the daily losses.

Physical Examination. The physical signs may provide important information concerning the analysis of the deficits of electrolytes and water. The appearance of the skin, its elasticity, texture, temperature, and color, the appearance of the mucous membranes, the tension of the eyeballs, the blood pressure, and the pulse rate all contribute to an estimation of the magnitude of the deficit. The state of consciousness may be related to the magnitude of the deficit. Muscle weakness and diminished-to-absent deep tendon reflexes may suggest potassium depletion.

The character of respiratory activity may suggest a disequilibrium in acid-base relationships. The respirations in metabolic acidosis, with dehydration as an almost invariable concomitant feature, are deep and eventually accelerated, and one can usually detect an effort toward the end of expiration. A systemic alkalosis is suggested by a positive Chvostek reflex; this may also be present if the patient has hypocalcemia despite a concurrent acidosis. Clinically detectable changes in respiration in alkalosis can rarely if ever be appreciated. The odor of acetone on the breath implies a ketonemia.

Laboratory Data. The value of the *packed cell* (hematocrit), the concentration of *hemoglobin,* and the concentrations of *total proteins* in the serum can be helpful in evaluating the degree of contraction (or expansion) of the plasma volume. Since this inference is dependent on *changes* in the concentrations, these data are of help primarily in evaluating those disorders that develop while the patient is under observation, and in following the progress of a patient whose dehydration is undergoing correction.

The significance of the concentration of sodium in the serum has been discussed earlier in this chapter. It is, however, worthwhile to reemphasize that the concentration of sodium per se cannot possibly be equated with the presence or absence of a state of dehydration. The *concentration* of sodium is merely a statement of the amount of sodium in a liter (or any other unit of volume) of extracellular fluid. The patient with a normal concentration of sodium in the serum may have no disorder of hydration, he may have gained many liters of fluid, or lost a large volume of fluid. The significance of the normal concentration of sodium is simply that if the patient gained or lost fluid, the gain or loss of water was accompanied by a gain or loss of sodium approximately equal to 140 mM per liter of the water that was gained or lost. Similarly, a variety of states of hydration may be accompanied by hypo- and hypernatremia. Hyponatremia signifies a gain of water in excess of salt gain or a loss of salt in excess of water loss; and hypernatremia implies a gain of salt in excess of water gain or a loss of water in excess of salt loss. A dehydration associated with a normal concentration of sodium implies that the total deficit of volume derives from the extracellular compartment. Dehydration associated with hypernatremia implies a loss of volume from both compartments. Dehydration with hyponatremia implies a loss of volume from the extracellular compartment and a *gain* of water by the cells.

The concentrations of potassium and total CO_2 content of the serum may be altered, and these deviations are frequently accompanied by disturbances in acid-base equilibrium. These matters are discussed in more detail in Chap. 51. Hypo- or hypermagnesemia may be present. The former is not uncommon in the same situations that are characterized by deficits of potassium such as diabetic acidosis, gastrointestinal disturbances including the malabsorption syndrome, and in the postoperative period.

The excretion of urea is related to the amount filtered less the amount reabsorbed through the renal tubules. This latter process is considered to be passive and, hence, is favored by high concentration gradients between renal tubular and interstitial fluid. Therefore it is clear that a diminished rate of filtration at the glomerulus, or a highly concentrated urine, or both will favor a diminished rate of excretion and an increase in urea concentration in the body fluids. To the extent that dehydration is responsible for these alterations in renal function, the concentration of urea in blood may serve as a gross index of the severity of the dehydration.

The urinalysis contributes considerable information. In the first place it provides information concerning the probability of renal disease. A urine of high specific gravity, in the absence of glucose or protein, suggests good renal function and an antidiuretic response. This, in turn, carries certain implications with respect to alterations in the internal environment. The excretion of salt despite hyponatremia may indicate one of the salt-wasting disorders.

Principles of Management of Dehydration. The initial goals of the management of a state of dehydration are simple and include the restoration of the body fluids to normal in terms of volume, effective osmolality, composition, and acid-base relations. The quality and quantity of fluids required to satisfy these goals are dependent on the analysis of the characteristics of the dehydration. On the basis of this analysis it should be possible to outline a course of action. Since the analysis cannot be expected to be precise, it is wise to include in the outline a plan to interrupt therapy at an appropriate point to allow a reevaluation of the status of the patient. This reevaluation should employ all the available clinical and laboratory data relevant to the problem. The initial plan of management may then be modified in accord with this second analysis. Like the management of many other clinical problems, management of dehydration requires a combination of information, logic, and empiricism. In many instances the restoration of a normal volume and tonicity of the body fluids, and the repair of a deficit of potassium, if present, will be accompanied by the coincidental correction of a complicating disturbance in acid-base balance. The administration of insulin and, at an appropriate time, of glucose and potassium is obviously necessary in a patient with diabetic acidosis. Since the alleviation of the acid-base disturbance is dependent on normal renal and respiratory function, these problems are more complex in patients with renal and pulmonary disease (see Chap. 51). The basic principles of the management of adrenal cortical insufficiency do not differ from those presented above; however, the administration of cortisone or hydrocortisone and of 9-α-fluorohydrocortisone is added to the regimen. The management of the water deficit in diabetes insipidus differs from that of other deficits of water only in so far as the patient with diabetes insipidus should be given a preparation of the posterior pituitary gland to replace the deficiency of the ADH.

When these first goals have been realized, plans must be made to maintain the normal state of hydration. The fluid prescription must be developed in relation to the usual basal requirements and their possible alterations in this particular patient, and to the need to replace losses other than those included in the former category.

No attempt will be made to discuss the problems of management in any further detail. In fact the very essence of the goal of this discussion is to emphasize that the details of management must be defined in relation to the particular patient. Therapy must be designed to meet the problems of the individual patient in terms not only of the quality and quantity of the fluids to be administered, but also of the route and speed of administration. These details can be appreciated only when the specific requirements for repair of the dehydration are evaluated within the context of the patient's total disease picture.

REFERENCES

Elkinton, J. R., and T. S. Danowski: "The Body Fluids, Basic Physiology and Practical Therapeutics," Baltimore, The Williams & Wilkins Company, 1955.

Strauss, M. B.: "Body Water in Man," Boston, Little, Brown & Company, 1957.

Water and Electrolyte Metabolism. A Symposium, J. Chronic Diseases, II, 187, 1960.

Welt, L. G.: "Clinical Disorders of Hydration and Acid-Base Equilibrium," 2d ed., Boston, Little, Brown & Company, 1959.

51 ACID-BASE EQUILIBRIUM
Louis G. Welt and
Charles H. Burnett

PHYSIOLOGIC CONSIDERATIONS

An understanding of the physiologic regulation and the clinical disorders of acid-base balance is often needlessly difficult because of the multiple uses and misuses of the terms *acid* and *base*. In the past these terms have been applied to anions and cations. This is not now acceptable, although the respectability of long usage has tended to perpetu-

ate the error. Moreover, this is not a semantic quibble, since the use of these inadequate and misleading definitions creates a major handicap in the efforts to appreciate the very nature of the problem. In this discussion the term *acid* will refer to any substance that can donate a hydrogen ion (H^+), and a *base* will refer to any substance that can accept a hydrogen ion. This statement may be rewritten as follows:

$$\text{Acid} \rightleftharpoons \text{base} + H^+$$

Some substances may serve as an acid *or* a base. For example, $H_2PO_4^-$ can dissociate to H^+ and HPO_4^{--}, or it can accept a hydrogen ion to form H_3PO_4. In the first instance it serves as an acid, and in the second, as a base. These definitions serve to focus attention on the hydrogen ion as the significant item in acid-base balance. The manner in which the concentration of hydrogen ions may be expressed and the inferences which may be drawn from this expression therefore become a highly relevant issue.

The dissociation of an acid, HA, may be expressed in the following manner:

$$HA \rightleftharpoons H^+ + A^- \tag{1}$$

The rate at which this reaction proceeds to the right is proportional to the molar concentration of the acid and may be said to be equivalent to $k_1[HA]$. Likewise, the rate at which the reaction proceeds to the left is proportional to the product of the molar concentrations of H^+ and A^- and may be described as equivalent to $k_2[H^+][A^-]$. At equilibrium the two rates are equal, and, therefore:

$$k_1[HA] = k_2[H^+][A^-] \tag{2}$$

This equation can be rearranged to

$$\frac{k_1}{k_2} = \frac{[H^+][A^-]}{[HA]} \tag{3}$$

The ratio of the two constants can be included in one new constant, K, and the statement can be rearranged to function as an expression of the concentration of hydrogen ions:

$$[H^+] = K \frac{[HA]}{[A^-]} \tag{4}$$

Sorenson introduced the alternative method of expressing the concentration of hydrogen ions as the negative logarithm. The latter is denoted as pH, and the following statement emerges:

$$pH = pK + \log \frac{[A^-]}{[HA]} \tag{5}$$

This may be stated in the more general form:

$$pH = pK + \log \frac{[\text{base}]}{[\text{acid}]} \tag{6}$$

which is referred to as the *Henderson-Hasselbalch equation*. The logarithm of 1.0 is zero, and therefore when the concentrations of the base (the hydrogen ion acceptor) and the acid (the hydrogen ion donor) are equal to each other, the pH is equal to pK.

Buffers

A buffered solution is one that is able to minimize the deviation of pH by the addition to that solution of a strong acid or a strong base. A buffer pair is composed of a weakly dissociated acid or base and a highly dissociated salt. Such a pair might be designated as HA and NaA. The addition of a strong acid, such as HCl, to this solution would promote the following reaction:

$$HA + NaA + HCl \rightarrow 2HA + NaCl$$

In this fashion a weak acid is substituted for the strong acid. The concentration of hydrogen ions will be increased to the extent that the increment of weak acid dissociates. This increase is clearly considerably less than that which would have occurred had the HCl been added to pure water.

The pH of a buffered solution will be defined by the ratio of the molar concentrations of the members of the buffer pair:

$$pH = pK + \log \frac{[NaA]}{[HA]}$$

Several characteristics of buffer activity are implicit in this equation. The deviation in pH consequent to the addition of an acid stronger than HA will be equated with a decrease in the concentration of A$^-$ (represented by the numerator of the ratio) and an increase in the concentration of HA. This implies that, for a given increment of acid, the least change in pH will occur when the buffer ratio has a value of 1. Another implication is that, at *any* specific ratio of the concentrations of the pair, the addition of a given quantity of acid will alter the ratio less if the concentrations of the members of the pair are high rather than low. Finally, it is apparent that the capacity to buffer is lost when there is no hydrogen ion acceptor (base) left.

A solution may contain several buffers. The ratio of the concentrations of the components of each buffer pair is determined by the pH and, in turn, determines the pH. The ratios of each pair will be different at a specific pH in accordance with the individual dissociation constant for the system. Therefore, in a solution with several buffers a change in one component of any pair will dictate a change in the ratio for every other pair.

As mentioned in the preceding chapter, the body fluid most accessible for analysis is the plasma, and the pH of the extracellular fluid can be defined by the relationship between NaHCO$_3$ and H$_2$CO$_3$, or,

more precisely, the tension of CO$_2$(P_{CO_2}).[1] This is expressed by the equation:

$$pH = 6.1 + \log \frac{NaHCO_3}{H_2CO_3 + \text{dissolved } CO_2}$$
$$\updownarrow$$
$$CO_2 + H_2O$$

The ratio of the concentrations of sodium bicarbonate and the carbonic acid plus dissolved CO$_2$ is 20:1 at the pH of serum 7.40. This is far removed from the more efficient ratio of 1:1, and in a closed system this would be a poor buffer system at that pH. However, the buffer is unique in that its acid component is a gas whose excretion can be rapidly accelerated or diminished by variations in respiratory exchange, and it is ubiquitous in that it is constantly being formed as a metabolic end product.

Although much of the buffer activity within the body is reflected and mirrored in the bicarbonate–carbonic acid system, this is by no means the only important buffer system in the body's fluids. The proteins of the plasma, the hemoglobin of the red blood cells, and the bicarbonate, phosphate, and proteins of the intracellular fluids all play a significant role in buffer activity. The sum total of the anions of the buffer salts which are capable of accepting hydrogen ions (i.e., the sum total of *base*) represents the first line of defense in absorbing the insult of the accession of an acid load in the body. The total of all body buffers (including those contributed by cations from cells and bones) cannot be estimated readily; some indication of their magnitude and a reflection of changes therein may be obtained from a consideration, as developed by Singer and Hastings, of the buffers present in whole blood alone.

The buffers in whole blood include the bicarbonate, proteins, and phosphate of the plasma, and the hemoglobin, bicarbonate, and phosphate salts in the red blood cells. In addition, since the anionic properties of hemoglobin vary between the reduced and oxygenated state, the degree of saturation of hemoglobin with oxygen must be stipulated. The sum of these buffers has been referred to as *buffer base*. Initially this term was used to mean the cation equivalents of the buffer anion. It is now more proper to use the term interchangeably with buffer anion itself. The range of normal values for the sum of the buffer base is 46 to 52 mM per liter. The values for buffer base and P_{CO_2} can be read from a nomogram prepared by Singer and Hastings if the pH of the blood, the hematocrit, and the total CO$_2$ content of whole blood or plasma are known. Since the anionic properties of the proteins vary directly with pH, the primary retention

[1] The term P_{CO_2} refers to the partial pressure of carbon dioxide and is usually close to 40 mm Hg.

or loss of carbon dioxide and bicarbonate, as in respiratory disturbances, is accompanied by reciprocal changes in the buffer base value for the proteins. Hence the characteristic of respiratory acidosis and alkalosis will be the lack of deviation from normal in the value for buffer base. In contrast, the value for buffer base will be diminished in metabolic acidosis and increased in metabolic alkalosis.

Acidosis and Alkalosis

It should be clear from the above that the status of the acid-base relationship cannot be evaluated solely from knowledge of the total CO_2 content of the serum. This latter represents the sum of the members of the buffer pair and includes bicarbonate as well as carbonic acid and CO_2 gas. The total provides no information with respect to the relative proportions of the components of the buffer pair. In fact a high or low concentration of total CO_2 is compatible with either an acidosis or an alkalosis. The pH of arterial blood (or blood obtained from a limb vein after warming the part at 45°C for about 10 min) is ultimately necessary to define the acid-base relationship. The pH, however, may be found to be disturbed more or less than the deviation in total CO_2 content of the serum. This depends, in part, on the sequence of events, the speed with which the distortion has supervened, and the success or failure of the compensatory mechanisms. Furthermore, in more complicated circumstances, the estimation of both P_{CO_2} and whole blood buffer base may be necessary to unravel the nature of the disturbance in acid-base relationships.

Calculation of P_{CO_2} and Partition of Total CO_2 Content

The quantity of carbon dioxide dissolved in a liquid is proportional to the P_{CO_2} and can be expressed in millimoles per liter as equal to alpha P_{CO_2}. The term *alpha* is equal to 0.0301 (millimole/liter/mm Hg) for plasma at a temperature of 38°C. At different body temperatures an appropriate correction must be made. In turn, dissolved CO_2 is in equilibrium with H_2CO_3, and therefore the sum of dissolved CO_2 and carbonic acid can be said to be proportional to P_{CO_2}. Since the quantity of dissolved CO_2 is so much greater than the concentration of carbonic acid, the denominator of the ratio in the Henderson-Hasselbalch equation will be taken as our value.

In the sample calculation to follow, it will be assumed that the pH is 7.40, the total CO_2 content is 26 mM per liter, and the pK for the bicarbonate-CO_2 system is 6.10. The Henderson-Hasselbalch equation may be written as follows:

$$pH = 6.10 + \log \frac{(HCO_3^-)}{(\alpha P_{CO_2})}$$

Since the concentration of bicarbonate in plasma is equal to the difference between the total CO_2 content and P_{CO_2}, the equation may be rewritten:

$$pH = 6.10 + \log \frac{(\text{total } CO_2) - (\alpha P_{CO_2})}{(\alpha P_{CO_2})}$$

$$7.40 = 6.10 + \log \frac{(26) - (.0301\, P_{CO_2})}{(.0301\, P_{CO_2})}$$

$$7.40 - 6.10 = 1.3 = \log \frac{(26) - (.0301\, P_{CO_2})}{(.0301\, P_{CO_2})}$$

$$\text{Antilog } 1.3 = \frac{(26) - (.0301\, P_{CO_2})}{(.0301\, P_{CO_2})}$$

Antilog $1.3 = 19.95$, therefore:

$$19.95\,(.0301\, P_{CO_2}) = (26) - (.0301\, P_{CO_2})$$

$$19.95\,(.0301\, P_{CO_2}) + (.0301\, P_{CO_2}) = 26$$

$$P_{CO_2} = 41.2 \text{ mm Hg}$$

The sum of the concentrations of dissolved CO_2 and H_2CO_3 is equal to:

$$.0301\, P_{CO_2} = .0301 \times 41.2 = 1.24 \text{ mM/L}$$

Since the concentration of bicarbonate ion is the difference between total CO_2 content and the value for dissolved CO_2 and H_2CO_3,

$$(HCO_3^-) = 26 - 1.24 = 24.76 \text{ mM/L}$$

Regulation of Acid-Base Equilibrium

In general, the problem of the regulation of acid-base balance in health is that of protecting the pH from alterations that may be induced by the continuous formation of acid end products of metabolism. In health the pH of the extracellular fluids is maintained at a level between 7.35 and 7.45. This is accomplished by buffer activity (discussed earlier), by exchange of ions between the two major fluid compartments, and by adaptations of respiratory and renal function.

Regulation by Ion Exchange. The exchange of *anions* across membranes appears to be restricted to the red cells and, probably, the renal tubular cells. Chloride and bicarbonate ions can diffuse across the erythrocytic membrane, and their distribution between the red cell and plasma water is responsive to changes in their concentrations and pH. For example, an increase in the P_{CO_2} of the plasma due to the addition of carbon dioxide is followed by diffusion of the gas into the red cell, where part of it is hydrated to H_2CO_3. The dissociation of this acid increases the concentration of bicarbonate ions, and these diffuse from the cell. This, in turn, is accompanied by a movement of chloride into the red cells. The net effect of this redistribution of anions in terms of the acid-base relationships of the extracellular fluid is to increase the concentration of bicarbonate in this compartment. This increase in the concentration of HCO_3^- tends to offset the effect of the initial increase in P_{CO_2} on the buffer ratio of the Henderson-Hasselbalch equation.

The exchange of *cations* such as sodium, potassium, and, perhaps, calcium as well, from muscle cells and bone for hydrogen ions in the extracellular fluid (and vice versa) plays a significant role in modifying the alterations in pH of the extracellular fluids. It has been estimated, for example, that approximately 50 per cent of an acid load administered to dogs was neutralized by such an exchange of sodium and potassium for hydrogen ions. In another study it was suggested that 25 per cent of the "neutralization" of an infusion of $NaHCO_3$ had been achieved by the exchange of extracellular sodium for intracellular hydrogen ions. Similar exchanges are reported in studies of both respiratory acidosis and respiratory alkalosis.

Respiratory Regulation. The lungs play a major role in the excretion of acid as carbon dioxide. Moreover, the centers that regulate the rate and depth of ventilation are exquisitely sensitive to subtle changes in the composition of the blood and extravascular fluids. The central chemoreceptors located in the medullary respiratory centers are responsive to the P_{CO_2} and pH of their environment in such a way that an increase in P_{CO_2} or hydrogen ion concentration promotes an increase in pulmonary ventilation. In contrast, a decrease in CO_2 tension or increase in pH tends to inhibit ventilation. In either case it is clear that the alteration in respiratory activity tends to correct the primary deviation in P_{CO_2} or pH. The P_{CO_2} appears to be the more potent stimulus of the two. In addition, there are peripheral chemoreceptors located in the carotid and aortic bodies. These are relatively insensitive to pH and P_{CO_2}, but are responsive to the arterial oxygen tension (P_{O_2}).

An interesting aspect of the chemoregulation of pulmonary ventilation concerns the phenomenon of a change in the "sensitivity" of the central respiratory centers to a specific P_{CO_2}. It appears as though a period of hypercapnia diminishes "sensitivity," and hypocapnia enhances the intensity of the response to a given tension of CO_2. The precise nature of this altered response is not clear. An appreciation of this adaptation is helpful in understanding certain complications of acid-base disorders which will be discussed in more detail later (see Chap. 260 for a more complete discussion of respiratory regulation).

Renal Regulation. The kidneys contribute to the regulation of acid-base balance by varying the net rate of excretion of hydrogen ions and by processes of selective reabsorption and rejection of cations and anions. These two processes are interdependent to the extent that the reabsorption of sodium is closely related to the secretion of hydrogen ions and potassium. The total rate of *secretion* of hydrogen ions by the tubular cells may be calculated from the sum of the titratable acid, ammonium ion, and a fraction which is equivalent to the difference between the filtered and excreted bicarbonate. The part each of the above phenomena plays in the urinary *excretion* of acid or alkaline loads is discussed below.

The titratable acid is equivalent to the quantity of NaOH that must be added to the urine to change its pH to that of the plasma. It represents the hydrogen ions present in free acid compounds and incorporated in the buffer components of the urine. Caution must be exercised to avoid the error of necessarily equating a low urinary pH with a high rate of excretion of acid. A small quantity of a dissociated acid in a poorly buffered urine will lower the pH considerably. This same quantity of titratable acid in a buffered solution might be accommodated with very little depression of pH.

Pitts and his collaborators are responsible for the demonstration that the urinary excretion of acid may be in excess of that which can be accounted for by filtration and preferential reabsorption. They developed the hypothesis that hydrogen ions are secreted into the tubular fluid in exchange for sodium. The source of the hydrogen ions for this secretory process is not known for certain, although it is usually represented as having been derived from carbonic acid. The latter, in turn, is believed to be formed from the hydration of carbon dioxide:

$$H_2O + CO_2$$
$$\updownarrow$$
$$H_2CO_3$$
$$\updownarrow$$
$$H^+ + HCO_3^-$$

This reaction accelerated by the enzyme carbonic anhydrase.

The rate of tubular *secretion* of hydrogen ions is probably conditioned by many factors, some of which include the pH of the renal tubular cell fluid, the P_{CO_2} (rather than the pH) of the extracellular fluid, the availability of buffers in the tubular fluid, the intensity of the stimuli primarily responsible for the reabsorption of sodium, and the status of the stores of potassium in the tubular cells. A decreased pH in the cell fluid, hypercapnia, and a diminished content of potassium in the renal tubular cells tend to favor the secretion of hydrogen ions. These ions cannot be secreted against a concentration gradient in excess of approximately 800:1. A diminished tubular content of buffer will therefore impose a restriction on the rate of secretion of hydrogen ions by failing to resist the decrease in pH consequent to this secretion.

The rate of excretion of ammonia does not change as acutely as is the case with titratable acid, but in

The reactions involved in the acidification of the urine may be expressed as follows:

I. *Interstitial fluid*	*Tubular cell*	*Tubular fluid*	*Urine*

$$
\begin{array}{lll}
\text{I. } \textit{Interstitial fluid} & \textit{Tubular cell} & \textit{Tubular fluid} & \textit{Urine} \\
 & \overset{\longleftarrow}{\text{H}^+ \quad \text{HCO}_3^-} & \text{Na}^+ \quad \text{HCO}_3^- & \\
 & \quad\quad\quad\downarrow & \quad\quad\downarrow & \\
\text{NaHCO}_3 \longleftarrow & \text{Na}^+ \quad \text{HCO}_3^- & \text{H}_2\text{CO}_3 & \\
 & & \quad\quad\downarrow & \\
\text{CO}_2 \longleftarrow & \longleftarrow\! & \text{CO}_2 + \text{H}_2\text{O} \longrightarrow & \text{H}_2\text{O}
\end{array}
$$

appropriate circumstances the excretion of ammonia may make a greater contribution in quantitative terms. Ammonia is formed in the renal tubular cells, and the largest fraction (about 80 per cent) is derived from glutamine. The deamidation of glutamine is accelerated by the enzyme glutaminase, which is present in the kidneys. The specific factors that regulate the rate of excretion of ammonia are not well understood but include those which influence the activity of enzymes, such as glutaminase, the availability of ammonia precursors, and the pH of the luminal fluid. It is not clear whether ammonia diffuses into the tubular fluid and becomes NH_4^+ by reacting with hydrogen ion, or whether NH_4^+ is actively secreted as such. Within the context of the first of these two views, the accession of NH_3 to the

It will be noted that the reabsorption of the filtered bicarbonate is somewhat indirect. The sodium which is reabsorbed by exchange with hydrogen ion is then transported from the cell to the interstitial fluid of the kidney along with the bicarbonate remnant of the carbonic acid which had donated the hydrogen ion. The carbonic acid left behind in the tubular fluid is then dehydrated to CO_2 and H_2O, and the carbon dioxide diffuses back to the body fluids.

The exchange of sodium for hydrogen ion may also involve the sodium associated with the salt of phosphate. This operation converts the disodium phosphate salt to the monosodium salt and promotes the reabsorption of sodium bicarbonate. This sequence of events may be depicted as follows:

$$
\begin{array}{lll}
\text{II. } \textit{Interstitial fluid} & \textit{Tubular cell} & \textit{Tubular fluid} & \textit{Urine} \\
 & \overset{\longleftarrow}{\text{H}^+ \quad \text{HCO}_3^-} & \text{Na}^+ \ \text{Na}^+ \ \text{HPO}_4^{--} & \\
 & \quad\quad\downarrow & \quad\quad\downarrow & \\
\text{NaHCO}_3 \longleftarrow & \text{Na}^+ \ \text{HCO}_3^- & \text{NaH}_2\text{PO}_4 \longrightarrow & \text{NaH}_2\text{PO}_4
\end{array}
$$

luminal fluid and its reaction with hydrogen ions can be looked upon simply as a buffering action. To the extent that this activity reduces the gradient for hydrogen ion concentration between tubular cell and luminal fluid, secretion of hydrogen ions will be favored. Thus, the secondary factors that might be considered to condition an increase in the rate of excretion of ammonia would include a diminution in the amount of buffer (bicarbonate, phosphate) in the tubular fluid, an intense stimulus for the reabsorption of sodium (without its associated anion), and a limited ability to secrete potassium.

The utility of the transfer of sodium and hydrogen ion with both bicarbonate and phosphate in aiding the compensation of disturbances in acid-base equilibrium will be illustrated later. This type of reaction may proceed as long as there is adequate buffer in the tubular fluid to prevent the concentration of hydrogen ions from achieving a value which represents a prohibitive gradient for secretion of these ions by the tubular cell. It may be that the excretion of ammonia is provoked by such a situation as that just suggested. This sequence is portrayed in the next panel:

$$
\begin{array}{lll}
\text{III. } \textit{Interstitial fluid} & \textit{Tubular cell} & \textit{Tubular fluid} & \textit{Urine} \\
 & \overset{\longleftarrow}{\text{H}^+ \quad \text{HCO}_3^-} & \text{Na}^+ \quad \text{Cl}^- & \\
 & \quad\quad\downarrow & \quad\quad\downarrow & \\
\text{NaHCO}_3 \longleftarrow & \text{Na}^+ \ \text{HCO}_3^- & \text{H}^+ \quad \text{Cl}^- & \\
 & \text{Glutamine} \rightarrow \text{NH}_3 \longrightarrow & & \\
 & & \quad\quad\downarrow & \\
 & & \text{NH}_4 \quad \text{Cl} \longrightarrow & \text{NH}_4\text{Cl}
\end{array}
$$

It is suggested that the diminished pH of the tubular fluid traps the ammonia. This would tend to drive the reaction: glutamine → NH_3, and the faster the ammonia diffused away, the faster it would be formed (provided there was adequate precursor). In the process, the pH of the tubular fluid is modified to allow the continued secretion of hydrogen ion.

Consideration of all three of the above reactions illustrates a very important implication in the mechanisms of acidification: more bicarbonate may be returned to the interstitial fluid than is filtered at the glomerulus. This circumstance is a corollary of Pitts' observation that more hydrogen ion may be excreted in the urine than is filtered.

The reabsorption of sodium may be associated with an exchange for potassium in lieu of hydrogen ion. These alternatives are frequently pictured as competing one with the other. It has already been noted that potassium depletion and intracellular acidosis would be expected to favor the secretion of hydrogen ions. In contrast, potassium excess (as may occur with the administration of potassium) and an intracellular alkalosis would be expected to promote the secretion of potassium rather than of hydrogen ions. These interrelationships may explain, in part, the aciduria which may accompany potassium depletion despite an extracellular alkalosis; and this may also explain why the administration of $NaHCO_3$ is accompanied by an augmented excretion of potassium.

The administration of a carbonic anhydrase inhibitor suppresses all these reactions, which are dependent on a readily available source of hydrogen ions. Such an agent promotes an increased excretion of sodium, bicarbonate, and potassium and decreases the rate of excretion of titratable acid and ammonia. Some of these alterations are observed in patients with renal disease characterized by tubular dysfunction. The defect in these instances is also associated with an impaired ability to secrete hydrogen ions properly and is, in part at least, responsible for the acidosis noted in renal insufficiency.

The role of the kidneys in acid-base regulation will be further discussed later in this chapter. The nature of the specific responses in each type of acid-base disturbance will serve to illustrate the particular contributions of the kidneys.

A comment is in order concerning the significance of *compensation*. The responses which have just been described are initiated by a distortion of one or more of the physicochemical characteristics of the body fluids. If the response were such as to efface the distortion, the stimulus for the response would be removed and the distortion would reappear. Thus, it is unlikely that compensation can ever

be perfect since it would automatically be self-destructive so long as the initial basis for the disturbance persisted. Hence, if a patient with an obvious acid-base disturbance has a normal value for pH, or P_{CO_2}, or total CO_2 content, the implication is that this is almost certainly an instance of a *mixed* acid-base disturbance.

CLINICAL CONSIDERATIONS

There are four major disturbances in acid-base equilibrium, and it is convenient to discuss them individually and as separate entities. Nevertheless it should be remembered that mixed disturbances occur fairly frequently. In this discussion the aim is to present an analysis of each of these disorders in terms of the primary alteration, the impact of this insult and the compensatory respiratory and renal responses on the Henderson-Hasselbalch equation, the nature of the compositional changes, and the approach to the management of the disorder. The Henderson-Hasselbalch equation is re-presented here with respect to the bicarbonate–carbonic acid buffer system. Reference to this equation, which defines the pH, is most helpful in visualizing the sequence and consequence of primary and secondary events in the pathogenesis of acidosis and alkalosis:

$$pH = 6.1 + \log \frac{NaHCO_3}{\underset{\underset{CO_2 + H_2O}{\Updownarrow}}{H_2CO_3 + \text{dissolved } CO_2}}$$

The ratio of the concentrations of the buffer pair is 20:1.

Respiratory Acidosis

A respiratory acidosis is due to an inadequate elimination of CO_2 by the lungs because of hypoventilation or because of uneven ventilation in relation to blood flow. It is unlikely to be associated solely with impaired diffusion across the alveolar capillary membranes, since the diffusion of CO_2 is so rapid. Respiratory acidoses are found commonly in patients with conditions such as emphysema, pulmonary fibrosis, and cardiopulmonary disease.

The retention of CO_2 will increase the P_{CO_2} and the concentration of carbonic acid. The increase in the value for the denominator of the buffer ratio will change this to something less than 20:1 and will define a decrease in the pH. The CO_2 can penetrate cell membranes freely, and in this fashion a considerable quantity of acid can be buffered in the intracellular fluids. In addition there is evidence that hydrogen ions from the extracellular fluids exchange for potassium and sodium from cells and bone.

The increase in P_{CO_2} and the decrease in pH both serve to stimulate ventilation, and further accumulation of CO_2 may be prevented or, at least, retarded thereby. The renal response is characterized by an increased excretion of titratable acid, ammonium, and chloride with a diminished excretion of bicarbonate. The above-mentioned response clearly implies a net increase in the total rate of *secretion* of hydrogen ions by the renal tubule, a circumstance which is not necessarily the case in metabolic acidosis (see below). In this manner the kidneys help to eliminate acid, but, in addition, they alter electrolyte composition so that the concentration of bicarbonate in the extracellular fluid increases at the expense of chloride. To the extent that this increase in the concentration of bicarbonate restores the buffer ratio toward 20:1, the deviation of the pH is minimized. The ability to tolerate a high P_{CO_2} has an additional advantage in that a greater quantity of CO_2 is excreted per unit of ventilation. This increment may be sufficiently large to allow the excretion of CO_2 to equal its production. In this circumstance no further increase in P_{CO_2} will occur unless the primary disease worsens.

It was stated earlier that the increase in CO_2 tension stimulated respiratory activity, but as the hypercapnia is maintained the respiratory centers appear to develop a decrease in sensitivity to this stimulus. A diminution in the respiratory response to the next increment of P_{CO_2} will promote a more intense hypercapnia. This new level of P_{CO_2} serves to maintain some increase in ventilation until a new level of desensitization develops and the vicious cycle is repeated. Ultimately the hypercapnia becomes extreme and the increased P_{CO_2} no longer serves as an appropriate stimulus to increase ventilation. At this time the most important stimulus for respiratory activity is the accompanying hypoxia. It has been said that if patients with respiratory acidosis were left to their own devices they would probably succumb to hypoxia rather than to the hypercapnia or acidosis. The slower diffusion of oxygen would be expected to promote an incapacitating hypoxia prior to the development of a CO_2 narcosis or a pH incompatible with life. However, if such patients are treated by exposure to a breathing mixture with a high content of oxygen in an effort to relieve the hypoxemia, they may quickly become confused, lapse into coma, and die. The improvement in the hypoxia may remove the last effective stimulus for respiratory activity. As a result of the diminished ventilation, there is a further decline in the excretion of CO_2, leading to the grave consequences of extreme hypercapnia. This should not be interpreted to suggest that such patients should never be treated with oxygen; but it should serve to emphasize the need for close observation when oxygen therapy is used to detect the earliest evidences of this complication. If morphine is used in these patients, it should be administered with caution, since this drug may affect the respiratory center in such a manner as to induce hypoventilation. This, in turn, will promote a sharp increase in the P_{CO_2}, the intensity of the acidosis, and the degree of hypoxia.

The management of these patients includes all those measures which may be expected to improve the basic disease condition responsible for pulmonary insufficiency, as discussed in Part Eight, Sec. 4, Introduction and Chap. 268. However, these measures may fail, and the extreme hypoxia and hypercapnia may require immediate attention. In this situation the use of artificial respiration (employing a mechanical respirator) may offer a valueble therapeutic approach. The increase in ventilatory exchange induced by the respirator improves the hypoxia and promotes an increased excretion of CO_2. In the course of a few days this may be successful in reducing the P_{CO_2} to more normal levels. This, in turn, may restore the sensitivity of the respiratory center to lower levels of CO_2, and a rising P_{CO_2} may again serve as a proper stimulus to respiratory activity.

The use of the carbonic anhydrase inhibitor Diamox has been recommended in the management of this problem. Although it has not been uniformly successful, some patients appear to have improved as a result of its use. Furthermore, the observed data are not sufficiently consistent to permit certainty as to the precise sequence of events by which it has been effective. A reasonable working hypothesis suggests that the first event is an augmented excretion of bicarbonate in the urine, leading to a decrease in the concentration of bicarbonate in the extracellular fluids. This change should dictate a decrease in pH. If this latter were successful in stimulating an increase in respiratory activity with an augmented excretion of CO_2, the pH would be restored toward normal and the P_{CO_2} would be diminished. The decrease in the hypercapnia would be expected to restore the sensitivity of the respiratory centers to lower tensions of CO_2, and this would have the same beneficial effect as that described above with respect to the use of artificial respiration. However, the data do not always support this hypothesis, and some suggest that Diamox has an effect on the respiratory center itself which may serve to improve ventilation. Another agent that may be useful is salicylate, which may be ingested as aspirin or administered intravenously as the sodium salt. This drug definitely increases the sensitivity of the respiratory center to carbon dioxide and may be helpful in patients with chronic hypercapnia. Progesterone is one other agent which has been reported to influence the sensitivity of the respiratory center to carbon dioxide.

The compositional changes in the serum have been mentioned; a fairly typical pattern of concentrations of electrolytes in a patient with respiratory acidosis is:

Na............... 137 mEq/L
K................ 4.5 mEq/L
Total CO_2........ 40 mM/L
Cl............... 90 mEq/L
pH............... 7.31
P_{CO_2}............ 79 mm Hg

The pattern neglecting pH and P_{CO_2} would also be compatible with a metabolic alkalosis. The gross characteristics of the underlying clinical problem will usually dictate the appropriate selection between these two alternatives. The normal concentration of potassium suggests that this is not a metabolic alkalosis. The arterial pH clearly resolves the problem in the above instance. It is not usually necessary to make this determination to make the necessary clinical differentiation.

Metabolic Acidosis

Metabolic acidosis is due to either an accumulation of acids or a primary loss of bicarbonate. An accumulation of acids is observed classically in diabetic acidosis and in renal insufficiency, and a primary loss of bicarbonate may be observed in renal disease as well. In diabetes the offenders are the four carbon ketones, and if these may be represented by the expression HK, the consequences of their accession to the extracellular fluid may be visualized as follows:

$$HK + NaHCO_3 \rightleftharpoons NaK + H_2CO_3$$

If this buffering of the ketone acid is related to the effect on the Henderson-Hasselbalch equation, it is readily observed that the reduction in bicarbonate and increase in carbonic acid will decrease the ratio to something less than 20:1 and will define a decrease in the pH. The latter as well as the presumed initial increase in P_{CO_2} both serve as stimuli to increase pulmonary ventilation, the excretion of CO_2 will be accelerated, P_{CO_2} will fall, the buffer ratio will be restored toward 20:1, and the deviation in pH is minimized. The violent respiratory response to the acidosis characterized by an increase first in depth and later in frequency of respirations is referred to as *Kussmaul breathing*. If one observes the characteristics of this respiratory activity closely, it is usually noted that the effort appears to be on the expiratory phase in contrast to the inspiratory effort noted in patients with oxygen lack.

Since the P_{CO_2} is depressed along with the decrease in pH, the inference is either that the latter is now solely responsible for the increased respiratory activity, or that the hypocapnia has induced a state of increased sensitivity of the respiratory cen-

ters to low tensions of CO_2. The latter appears quite likely, and it has recently been pointed out that during the recovery phase of several types of metabolic acidosis, the pH reaches normal values while the P_{CO_2} is still depressed. This would be an unlikely event unless the respiratory center was responsive to these lower levels of P_{CO_2}.

The renal response to this metabolic acidosis includes virtual total reabsorption of filtered bicarbonate and an increase in the net *urinary excretion* of acid as titratable acid and ammonia. The increase in net excretion of acid does not necessarily imply an increase in the net *secretion* of hydrogen ions. This will be apparent if it is recalled that the secretion of hydrogen ions to effect total reabsorption of a small filtered load of bicarbonate may be considerably less than that needed for incomplete reabsorption of bicarbonate when there is a much higher filtered load, as is the case normally or in respiratory acidosis. The net rates of excretion of acid may be similar in respiratory and metabolic acidosis, although presumably more hydrogen ion is secreted in the former to effect the larger bicarbonate reabsorption. Thus, although higher levels of P_{CO_2} favor the secretion of hydrogen ions, the renal response, in terms of the *net excretion* of acid, is not jeopardized by the hypocapnia of a metabolic acidosis.

A fairly typical pattern of the concentrations of electrolytes in the serum in diabetic acidosis is:

Na............... 125 mEq/L
K................ 3.5 mEq/L
Total CO_2........ 5 mM/L
Cl............... 90 mEq/L
Glucose.......... 800 mg per 100 ml
pH............... 7.01
P_{CO_2}............ 19 mm Hg

It will be noted that the sum of the concentrations of CO_2 and chloride is 95 mEq per liter. The difference between this sum and the concentration of sodium is 30 mEq per liter, which is significantly higher than the usual difference of 5 to 10 mEq per liter and implies an unusual concentration of some anion other than CO_2 and chloride. In diabetic acidosis this is likely to be almost all represented by ketones. (Although the concentration of sodium is depressed, the effective osmolality of the extracellular fluids will be found to be increased if one calculates the osmolar contribution of the elevated concentration of glucose.)[2]

The management of the acid-base disturbance in diabetic patients is not usually a primary concern. The administration of adequate amounts of insulin can be expected to promote the utilization of glucose and to decrease the production of ketones.

[2] 180 mg per cent of glucose is approximately equivalent to 10 mOsm per liter.

Under these circumstances the ketonemia is soon dissipated by utilization and excretion, and as the ketonemia subsides, the concentration of bicarbonate increases and the pH is soon restored to more nearly normal levels.

A metabolic acidosis due to the loss of bicarbonate in the urine is not uncommon in chronic renal insufficiency. It is due, presumably, to an inadequate reabsorption of bicarbonate by the renal tubular cells. This may, in turn, be due to one of several steps that must precede the actual secretion of hydrogen ions in the process of exchange with sodium. Since this is primarily a reflection of tubular dysfunction, it has been stated that it is seen more commonly in chronic pyelonephritis than in glomerulonephritis or other forms of chronic Bright's disease; it may occur, however, in all types of chronic renal failure. In one rather rare form of renal disease there is relatively little functional evidence of glomerular disease. In some of these disorders, the tubular defect may be congenital in origin. The net effect of the defect is a reduction in the concentration of bicarbonate in the extracellular fluids, accompanied by a reciprocal increase in the concentration of chloride. The diminution in concentration of bicarbonate defines a decrease in the pH of the extracellular fluid. This latter serves as a stimulus to respiratory activity, the increased excretion of CO_2 promotes a decrease in P_{CO_2}, and pH approaches a normal value as the ratio of the buffer pair approaches a value of 20:1. Since the ability to secrete hydrogen ions is not totally defunct, the excretion of bicarbonate diminishes only to the point where the filtered load of bicarbonate reaches a value no longer in excess of the residual capacity to secrete hydrogen ions. This disorder may also be associated with an increased excretion of calcium and potassium. The latter is not unexpected in virtue of the competitive relationship between hydrogen ions and potassium for exchange with sodium. The reason for the augmented excretion of calcium is less clear. It may be due, in part, to the effect of the systemic acidosis in mobilizing calcium from bone. It may also represent some specific renal response of an adaptive nature.

A characteristic set of concentrations of electrolytes in the serum is:

Na................	134 mEq/L
K.................	3.5 mEq/L
Total CO_2.........	12 mM/L
Cl................	115 mEq/L
PO_4..............	2 mEq/L
pH...............	7.25
P_{CO_2}.............	26 mm Hg

It should be noted that the sum of the concentrations of CO_2 and chloride, 127 mEq per liter, dif-

fers only by 7 mEq per liter from the concentration of sodium, and that the phosphate concentration is normal. This makes it clear that the depression of CO_2 cannot be ascribed to the accumulation of anions other than chloride. This same pattern might be observed in a patient who had received large doses of NH_4Cl or Diamox, or who had a respiratory alkalosis. The determination of the pH readily resolves the directional deviation in this instance. In clinical situations the history alone should reveal whether this pattern had resulted from a renal lesion or from the administration of ammonium chloride or a drug.

In instances of renal insufficiency accompanied by a significant decrease in filtration rate, there is an accumulation of acidic metabolic end products. These are represented, in part, by the acids of phosphate and sulfate. Since these acids are more highly dissociated than carbonic acid, they are buffered in a fashion similar to that described for the ketone acids in the discussion of diabetic acidosis. The accumulation of these products in addition to an impaired ability to secrete hydrogen ions accounts for most instances of metabolic acidosis associated with renal insufficiency. The sum of the concentrations of total CO_2 and chloride subtracted from the concentration of sodium in the serum will usually equal a value in excess of 5 to 10 mEq per liter. This type of acidosis is the one most commonly encountered in chronic renal failure. A characteristic set of concentrations is:

Na..............	130 mEq/L
K...............	5 mEq/L
Total CO_2........	12 mM/L
Cl..............	93 mEq/L
PO_4.............	7 mEq/L
pH..............	7.25
P_{CO_2}............	26 mm Hg

Note that the total CO_2 plus chloride subtracted from the sodium equals 25 mEq per liter. The hyperphosphatemia accounts for part of this excess, and sulfates would, if measured, probably be equally increased. Note also the slight hyperpotassemia (see Chap. 258).

The correction of a metabolic acidosis due to renal insufficiency can be achieved by the administration of sodium bicarbonate. In this fashion the concentration of bicarbonate can be increased, and the buffer ratio may be restored to a normal value. This correction can be made effectively in many instances simply by prescribing the ingestion of sodium bicarbonate either in addition to or in lieu of table salt. The reduction in the intake of NaCl is particularly desirable where there is some reason to avoid an excessive intake of sodium, or the substitution of sodium bicarbonate for sodium chloride is indicated where the acidosis is due to a primary loss of bicarbonate and the concentration of chloride is already high. The amount of sodium bicarbonate necessary as a daily supplement must be gauged in an empirical manner by correlating the dose with the response. The use of 2 to 4 Gm NaHCO₃ per day is safe to start with. Two complications may mar the success of this treatment. Since these patients have lost the capacity for proper discriminatory function on the part of the kidneys, it is possible to overcorrect the acidosis. The possibility of such overcorrection may be increased by the maintenance of a low P_{CO_2} due to an increased sensitivity of the respiratory center to CO_2 as a stimulus. The second complication deals with the possible development of tetany. Many of these patients have hyperphosphatemia and hypocalcemia. The acidosis may serve to protect against tetany from the hypocalcemia, and this protection may be lost as the pH is corrected with NaHCO₃. The ingestion of several grams of calcium gluconate or lactate may be adequate to prevent this complication. In addition, the daily ingestion of aluminum hydroxide may promote an increased excretion of phosphate in the bowel. This may contribute to a diminution in the hyperphosphatemia and, hence, may modify both the intensity of the acidosis and the hypocalcemia. The obvious advantages of the correction of the metabolic acidosis include the elimination of the hyperpnea which may be a troublesome symptom, in most cases some relief from subjective discomfort, and the maintenance of an internal environment that is better able to buffer sudden increments of acid. The increase in excretion of calcium and potassium that may accompany the acidosis may be diminished as well.

So far this discussion has concerned management in a noncritical chronic phase of the disease. When patients with renal insufficiency experience an episode of dehydration with further decompensation in renal function, they may develop acute and more intense disturbances in acid-base balance. However, it is frequently in these very circumstances that the physician may be most effective in the correction of a disabling acidosis. The efficient correction of the acidosis is dependent on increasing the concentration of bicarbonate in the extracellular fluid. This can be accomplished most dramatically when hyponatremia accompanies the disorder, since the concentration of sodium can be raised together with the bicarbonate by administering a hypertonic solution of NaHCO₃. The quantity of sodium to administer is calculated as discussed in Chap. 52. This should represent too much bicarbonate but, in fact, it rarely does. The second most dramatic correction may be accomplished when the patient with acidosis has a normal concentration of sodium but is dehydrated. The administration of an isotonic solution of a sodium salt will expand the volume of the extracellular fluid and repair the dehydration. If the salt is the bicarbonate, the concentration of this anion will be increased.

The possibility of provoking hypocalcemic tetany must always be considered when sodium bicarbonate is administered in these circumstances. It is recommended that prior to the infusion of NaHCO₃ the patient should receive at least 10 ml of a 10 per cent solution of calcium gluconate intravenously. In addition, the presence of the Chvostek reflex should be checked during the administration of the bicarbonate and more calcium administered if the reflex is elicited. The solution of calcium should not be mixed with bicarbonate, since this will result in the precipitation of calcium carbonate.

Respiratory Alkalosis

A respiratory alkalosis is due to hyperventilation and results from the excretion of carbon dioxide in excess of its production. This reduces the tension of CO_2, increases the value for the ratio of the buffer pair, and defines an increase in the pH. This disorder may be observed in the early phases of pulmonary and cardiopulmonary disease when hyperventilation is induced by hypoxia. It is more commonly observed as a manifestation of anxiety and tension, and it may be due to a lesion in the area of the central nervous system responsible for respiratory regulation. This last is the least common variety, but it is the circumstance in which one may see the most significant deviations from normal.

The anxious and tense patient, usually a woman, who hyperventilates in response to emotional stimuli, may develop an acute, although transient, alkalosis accompanied by a variety of symptoms which include giddiness and lightheadedness, circumoral and peripheral paresthesias, muscle tremors, and frank carpopedal spasm. Since these episodes are shortlived, there is insufficient time for a significant renal response in the nature of a compensatory effort. For the same reasons the only compositional changes are the increase in pH and decrease in P_{CO_2}.

In those instances of a relatively sustained hyperventilation, as in an irritative lesion in the reticular formation of the medulla, compensatory responses and compositional changes may be prominent. The renal responses are characterized by an increased excretion of bicarbonate, a decreased excretion of chloride, and an augmented excretion of potassium and sodium. The diminution in renal tubular reabsorption of bicarbonate is due, presumably, to a decrease in the secretion of hydrogen ions for the exchange with sodium. This may be due to the hypocapnia. The lessened secretion of hydrogen ions may be responsible for an increase in the secretion and excretion of potassium. The most significant consequence of these renal responses is a decrease in the concentration of bicarbonate in the extracellular fluids. This alteration tends to reduce the value for the ratio of the buffer pair toward 20:1 and, hence, minimizes the deviation in pH. The other alterations in composition include an increase in the concentration of chloride in the serum, along with a tendency to a lowered concentration of sodium and potassium.

These alterations in the electrolyte pattern may mimic those of a metabolic acidosis. It is important to recognize a respiratory alkalosis as distinct from a metabolic acidosis, since the administration of bicarbonate, which may be desirable in the acidosis, may be detrimental to the patient who is already alkalotic.

The management of patients with hyperventilation as a manifestation of anxiety and tension is primarily directed toward helping the patient to understand the pathogenesis of the disorder. It is frequently helpful to have the patient induce an episode by voluntary hyperventilation and then to demonstrate how this may be modified by rebreathing into a paper bag or by holding the nose and covering the mouth. This demonstration is usually quite convincing and helps to furnish the motivation for the patient to train herself to discontinue this habit. In those instances where the hyperventilation has provoked carpopedal spasm, the immediate need is to use some technique to increase the P_{CO_2} of the body fluids. This is most easily accomplished by having the patient rebreathe into a paper bag.

Metabolic Alkalosis

A metabolic alkalosis is characterized by an increase in the concentration of bicarbonate unattended by an equivalent increase in the P_{CO_2}, so that the ratio of the concentrations of the buffer pair is in excess of 20:1 and the pH is elevated. This condition may arise as a consequence of (1) the administration of sodium bicarbonate (or sodium salts of organic acids such as citrate or lactate); (2) the loss of chloride as HCl, as in vomiting or gastric suction; (3) the loss of chloride with sodium in a ratio in excess of that which characterizes their relative concentrations in the extracellular fluid; (4) an excessive excretion of acid in the urine; (5) the movement of hydrogen ions from the extracellular fluid to the cells in consequence of a deficit of potassium. The interrelationships among these possible primary events are intimate, and each of them provokes responses of an interdependent character, so that it is rare to find a metabolic alkalosis that is not multicausal. The interplay of primary events and subsequent responses can be illustrated by examining the sequence that may follow each of the major initiating events.

Throughout the discussion it will be well to visualize the effects of compensatory mechanisms that would tend to mitigate the deviation in pH as these may be surmised from the Henderson-Hasselbalch equation. These include an increase in the CO_2 tension, which may be induced by hypoventilation, and a reduction in the concentration of bicarbonate in the extracellular fluid. Hypoventilation would, presumably, be favored by the increase in pH. However, this path of compensation is not usually of great quantitative significance. There are limiting influences on the hypoventilation, which include the development of hypoxia and hypercapnia. These are both stimuli to increased respiratory activity. The reduction in the high concentration of bicarbonate may be achieved to some extent by the accelerated excretion of $NaHCO_3$ in the urine. To the extent that an increase in P_{CO_2} tends to enhance the reabsorption of bicarbonate, it may be said that a more successful hypoventilatory response would impose serious limitations on the efficiency of the renal response. Other limitations imposed on the compensating mechanisms will be illustrated in the discussions to follow. Furthermore, there may be specific deleterious effects on renal function and anatomic integrity as a consequence of certain features of a metabolic alkalosis. One of these effects is potassium depletion, and another may be the alkalosis per se, although this is not so firmly established.

Alkalosis Induced with Sodium Bicarbonate. The administration of $NaHCO_3$ will induce a metabolic alkalosis, which is dependent, in part, on the magnitude and rapidity with which a particular load of this salt is administered. However, the ability to accelerate the excretion of $NaHCO_3$ in the urine is so great that it is difficult to maintain any serious degree of alkalosis in this fashion in the absence of other conditioning influences. The ingestion or administration of $NaHCO_3$ is accompanied by an augmented excretion of potassium. If the ingestion or administration of potassium is inadequate to match the accelerated urinary loss, a deficit of potassium develops. The depletion of potassium has several consequences that tend to intensify rather than mitigate the alkalosis:

1. A deficit of potassium tends to diminish the secretion of potassium and enhances the exchange of hydrogen ions for sodium in the renal tubular reabsorptive mechanism. The augmented secretion of hydrogen ions promotes an increased reabsorption of sodium as bicarbonate, which imposes a limit on the efficiency with which bicarbonate may be excreted.

2. A large experimental literature dealing with the production of potassium depletion by the utili-

zation of diets essentially free of this cation and by the administration of $NaHCO_3$ describes an increase in the quantity of sodium in tissue cells. However, in most instances the quantitative relationship is such as to suggest that some other cation has gained access to the cell along with sodium. In some instances, at least, this appears to be hydrogen ion. To the extent that this transfer of hydrogen ions from the extracellular fluids to cells is operative, the intensity of the extracellular alkalosis will be augmented.

As long as potassium depletion is avoided, large amounts of administered bicarbonate may fail to induce a significant alkalosis.

Metabolic Alkalosis Due to Loss of Gastric Secretion by Vomiting or Suction. The primary cause of the alkalosis in this instance is the loss of HCl with the consequent increase in the concentration of bicarbonate, and a decrease in the concentration of chloride in the extracellular fluids. The renal response to this alkalosis is similar to that just described and is characterized by an accelerated excretion of sodium and potassium bicarbonate in the urine. The loss of potassium in the urine added to the loss of this ion in the gastric fluid represents an early potassium deficit. The nature of the primary event precludes the retention of ingested food or fluid, and if potassium is not administered parenterally and the gastric losses continue, the intensity of the potassium depletion increases. Furthermore, the loss of sodium in the gastric fluid and in the urine, if unreplaced, induces a deficit of this ion as well. The deficits of potassium and sodium both impose limitations on the mechanisms that tend to compensate the alkalosis. Those related to potassium depletion have just been described. The limits imposed by the depletion of sodium may operate as follows: As the deficit of sodium develops there is a loss of fluid. If no water is ingested or administered, the net deficit tends toward a loss of water in excess of sodium loss. If water is ingested and promptly vomited, or if water without salt (e.g., glucose in water) is administered by vein, the net deficit will be of sodium in excess of water. In either event, there will be a contraction of the extracellular volume. This, in turn, will promote a decreased rate of excretion of sodium. To the extent that the renal tubular reabsorption of sodium is increased, a serious limitation is imposed on the excretion of bicarbonate. Moreover, if sodium reabsorption is virtually complete and that fraction of sodium reabsorption which transpires by cation exchange is achieved with exchange for hydrogen and ammonium ions in lieu of potassium (because of deficit of the latter), the urine may no longer be alkaline but acid. This implies an increase in the *net* excretion of acid despite the extracellular alkalosis. These conditioning factors are, presuma-

bly, the genesis of the paradoxical aciduria that may be noted in clinical disorders associated with metabolic alkalosis. It is probable that the aciduria is conditioned not only by the deficit of potassium but also by a condition which demands virtually total reabsorption of sodium.

These considerations have very important therapeutic implications and serve to emphasize the need for an over-all evaluation of the problem in management. For example, the administration of ammonium chloride to such a patient could correct the alkalosis by virtue of adding the complications of a metabolic acidosis, but it would probably enhance the loss of potassium and sodium and serve very poorly to improve the patient's status. In contrast, the therapeutic measures that are clearly indicated include the following:

1. The dehydration should be corrected by the administration of salt and water. The proportion in which they should be administered is dependent on the net character of the deficits. If there is hypernatremia, the patient needs more water than salt, and if he is hyponatremic the need is for more salt than water. If one is in doubt, isotonic saline solution will usually be adequate. The amount to administer must be judged by an evaluation of the quantity of the deficit, made on the basis of history, physical examination, laboratory data, and the observed response to therapy (see Chap. 50).

2. The deficit of potassium must be corrected. The manner in which this may safely be accomplished will be discussed in the section on potassium depletion that follows later in this chapter.

3. Sufficient carbohydrate should be administered to minimize protein catabolism and ketonemia.

Once the antecedent deficits are restored, care must be taken to ensure appropriate replacement of current losses so that a new state of depletion will not obtain.

Altered Urinary Composition Due to Organic Mercurial Diuretic and Steroid Therapy. The administration of an organic mercurial compound promotes an increased excretion of sodium, chloride, titratable acid, ammonia, and potassium. The ratio of Na:Cl in the extracellular fluid is approximately 1.25:1.0, whereas the ratio of Na:Cl in the urine following the successful administration of an organic mercurial compound is 1:1 or less. This loss of sodium in relation to chloride will promote a contraction of the extracellular compartment (the successful goal of this therapy), with an accompanying increase in the concentration of bicarbonate. This, alone, would be sufficient to establish a metabolic alkalosis. However, in addition, the augmented excretion of hydrogen and ammonium ions and of potassium would each tend to enhance the extracellular alkalosis. The development of this disturbance inhibits the response to a mercurial diuretic, and, hence, this complication should be recognized and corrected. It can be successfully treated with NH_4Cl, and with KCl if there is an element of potassium depletion. Most patients who receive mercurials are digitalized, and one other complication of the development of a deficit of potassium is evidence of digitalis intoxication. This may be dramatically improved by the administration of a potassium salt.

The enhanced excretion of hydrogen ions, ammonia, and potassium is also observed when the reabsorption of sodium is increased by the administration of a salt-retaining steroid. These compounds presumably accelerate the reabsorption of sodium in an ion exchange operation, leading to the accelerated excretion of acid and potassium. A negative balance of potassium can be avoided by increasing the intake of a potassium salt or by diminishing the ingestion of sodium salts. If a rigid regimen of salt restriction is practiced, the loss of potassium is not observed.

Deficit of Potassium. The manner in which a deficit of potassium interrelates with a state of metabolic alkalosis has already been described. There are many causes of a deficit of this ion, including prolonged periods of parenteral alimentation without adding potassium, excessive losses in gastrointestinal fluid, diarrhea due to disease or induced with cathartics, excessive losses in the urine, as with the use of organic mercurial diuretics, chlorothiazide, and steroid hormones, potassium-losing renal disease, Cushing's syndrome, and primary aldosteronism.

Potassium is the major intracellular cation, and depletion is accompanied by disorders of structure and function in various tissues. These tissues include skeletal muscle, the smooth muscle of the gastrointestinal tract, the myocardium, cartilage, the kidneys, and gastric mucosa. Weakness of the muscles and hyporeflexia are common, alterations in the electrocardiogram are well established, and abnormalities in the motor and secretory activity of the gastrointestinal tract are well documented. An inability to concentrate the urine appropriately, a decrease in the rate of filtration at the glomerulus, and a defect in the transport of para-aminohippurate have all been reported.

Although a deficit of potassium may have serious consequences, judgment must be exercised in the technique of repletion to avoid the complications of therapy. The most significant hazard is the possibility of administering a potassium salt in too great a quantity or too rapidly so that cardiotoxic levels are reached in the serum.

In the course of the development of a deficit of potassium, the patient may become sufficiently dehydrated or acidotic so that the depletion is not mirrored in a hypopotassemia. This is seen quite often, for example, in diabetic acidosis. It would appear to be safer under these circumstances to refrain from the administration of potassium until partial correction of the dehydration and utilization of the carbohydrate have induced a decrease in the concentration of potassium in the serum and there is clear evidence of satisfactory flows of urine. Potassium salts may be administered more safely by mouth than by a parenteral route. There is sufficient delay in absorption from the gastrointestinal tract to provide some assurance that a sudden increase in the concentration of potassium in the serum will not obtain.

These precautionary comments should not be interpreted to mean that potassium salts cannot be safely administered by the intravenous route. There are many circumstances where for obvious reasons the salt cannot be administered orally and potassium repletion is clearly indicated. However, some control should be exercised with respect to the rate of administration. It is reasonably safe to administer potassium at a rate of about 20 mEq per hr, but it would be desirable to limit the first replacement to 50 to 100 mEq. After this first phase of replacement has been completed, the level of potassium in the serum should be determined. A change in the pattern of the electrocardiogram can also be used as a guide. The change in concentration will provide some guide as to the safe dose to administer in the next phase of therapy. Unfortunately there is no way to estimate the magnitude of the deficit with any precision from knowledge of the concentration of potassium in the serum. There is, of course, a gross correlation, but this is an inadequate premise on which to base a safe prediction.

Since the rate of an infusion may vary with change of position of the needle, it is always possible that the plan of administration may fail. An additional safeguard is provided by limiting the concentration of potassium in the infusate to approximately 50 mEq per liter. Under this circumstance an accidental increase in the rate of administration of the infusion will have less effect on the rate of administration of potassium.

Once again it must be emphasized that, although this discussion has presented the disturbances of acid-base equilibrium as four distinct and separate entities, mixed clinical pictures are common. However, these should not be too difficult to analyze if the principles described are recalled. In addition, it must be remembered that a disturbance in acid-base equilibrium may be only one aspect (and not necessarily the most important) of the patient's total disease picture. In fact, in some instances attention to the primary disorder may improve the disturbance in acid-base equilibrium so that no therapy for the disequilibrium per se is necessary. Moreover, there are circumstances in which a correction of abnormal chemical values may be undesirable in that it may destroy an adequate compensation.

REFERENCES

Clark, W. M.: "Topics in Physical Chemistry," 2d ed., chap. 8, Baltimore, The Williams & Wilkins Company, 1952.

Davenport, H. W.: "The ABC of Acid-Base Chemistry," Ann Arbor, Mich., Edwards Bros., Inc., 1947.

Orloff, J.: The Role of the Kidney in the Regulation of Acid-Base Balance, Yale J. Biol. and Med., 29:211, 1956.

Singer, R. B., and A. B. Hastings: An Improved Clinical Method for the Estimation of Disturbances of the Acid-Base Balance of Human Blood, Medicine, 27:223, 1948.

Section 4: Intermediary Metabolism

52 SOME PATHWAYS OF INTERMEDIARY METABOLISM

Albert E. Renold and
George W. Thorn

The metabolic activities of living cells may be arbitrarily divided into (1) reactions serving to support growth and differentiation and (2) reactions serving to produce useful energy. It need hardly be stressed that these two groups of reactions are not mutually exclusive. The first set of reactions is mainly concerned with the elaboration and the maintenance of the complex and highly specific structural elements which distinguish one cell type from another, among which proteins and nucleic acids are predominant; the second set of reactions serves to provide the energy necessary for the maintenance of cellular functional integrity and for the interactions of the cell with its environment. This energy derives from the alteration of suitable metabolic "fuels" and, in the mammalian organism, is mainly the result of the stepwise oxidation of carbohydrate and fat, and, to a lesser degree, of protein.

Between the entrance of metabolic fuels into the cell on the one hand, and the disposal of the oxidized end products on the other hand, a number of intermediary reactions occur. Some of these are peculiar to the metabolism of one class of fuels only (e.g., carbohydrate), while others represent a metabolic system common to all. These intermediary reactions have been grouped together under the designation *intermediary metabolism*. Although certain elements of intermediary metabolism may be peculiar to a given tissue, the over-all plan is similar in most tissues and can be discussed in general terms. It should be clearly stated, however, that many of these reactions (or the enzymes catalyzing them) have not as yet been individually established in human tissues, and that the evidence relating to their participation in human metabolism is as yet frequently inferential.

The energy requirements of a given organism or tissue vary widely with varying conditions, such as the quantity of mechanical work to be performed or the temperature gradient to be maintained. To satisfy these changing requirements, adjustments have to be made in the consumption of metabolic fuels and therefore in the rate of some or all of the reactions of intermediary metabolism. These adjustments are controlled in part by changes in the concentrations of available fuel and in part by a system of physical and chemical agents, among which hormones play an important part.

Derangements of intermediary metabolism may occur either as a result of direct interference with intermediary reactions (e.g., cyanide intoxication), or as a result of an abnormality in the regulatory system (e.g., thyrotoxicosis). Indeed, most if not all disease processes are accompanied by derangements in rate or coordination of intermediary reactions in one tissue or several. Although most of these alterations of intermediary metabolism in disease have not as yet been clearly defined, it has become evident that even their partial elucidation in any given instance adds significantly to understanding of the disease process involved and to the ability to cope with it therapeutically. A general understanding of intermediary metabolism is therefore not only of theoretic but also of great practical importance.

Detailed descriptions and analyses of the individual reactions of intermediary metabolism are available in biochemical texts. In this chapter an attempt is made to recall the general outline of intermediary metabolism, giving emphasis to those aspects of physiologic regulation and pathologic derangements which have improved understanding of disease.

OVER-ALL PLAN OF INTERMEDIARY METABOLISM

The over-all purpose of intermediary metabolism is to make available to the organism the energy stored in organic compounds. The latter is derived originally from the energy of light in photosynthetic processes. Photosynthesis results in the incorporation of carbon dioxide and water into hydrocarbons; intermediary metabolism results in an ordered and gradual reversal of the energetics of the photosynthetic processes within living cells and in the return of the photosynthetic energy to the organism in usable form.

In mammalian tissues it is convenient to consider separately the following steps:

1. The uptake of glucose into cells and its metabolic activation to glucose 6-phosphate
2. The storage of activated glucose as glycogen, and the mobilization of glycogen
3. The metabolism of glucose 6-phosphate to pyruvic or lactic acid
4. The synthesis of glycogen and glucose from pyruvic or lactic acid
5. Alternate metabolic pathways for glucose 6-phosphate
6. The metabolism of pyruvate to acetyl coenzyme A and to oxaloacetate
7. The oxidation of acetyl in the tricarboxylic acid cycle
8. The synthesis of fatty acids from acetyl coenzyme A, their storage as glycerol esters, and their mobilization and oxidation
9. The metabolism of acetoacetate
10. Other metabolic fates of acetyl coenzyme A
11. The metabolism of amino acids and proteins
12. The transport of electrons from substrate to oxygen and the liberation of useful energy

Uptake of Glucose into Cells and Its Metabolic Activation to Glucose 6-Phosphate. Glucose is highly soluble in water but poorly soluble in less polar solvents. The surface of certain body cells has the physicochemical characteristics of a lipid. In order to be available for intracellular metabolism, glucose first must pass through the cell membrane, and it is well established that the membrane (or surface) of many cells is a highly effective diffusion barrier for glucose. To account for the rapidity of its uptake into most cells it is necessary to postulate in the cell membrane a catalytic transport system for glucose; the existence of such a system in certain cells such as muscle or erythrocytes appears quite probable. It should simply be remembered at this point that the transport of glucose into cells is a complex process.

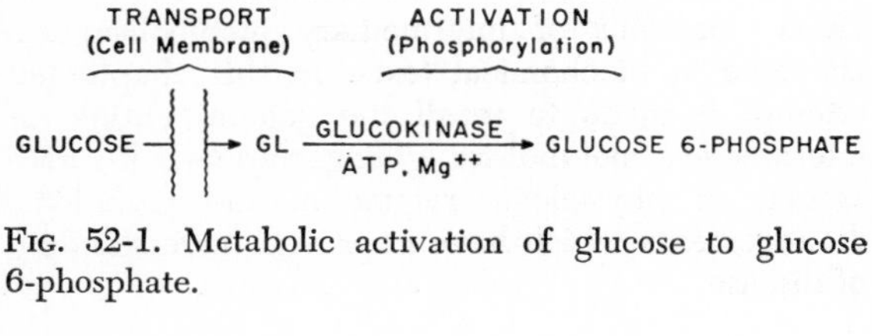

Glucose per se is a stable substance in the mammalian organism. Prior to its utilization it has to be "activated" by its phosphorylation to glucose 6-phosphate. Glucose 6-phosphate contains more energy than glucose, and the reaction requires the presence of adenosinetriphosphate (ATP) as well as that of an enzyme (*glucokinase* or *hexokinase*) and of magnesium ions. In the course of the reaction the terminal phosphate of ATP is transferred to glucose and the energy provided by the splitting of the "high-energy" terminal phosphate bond of ATP is thus transferred in part to the newly formed glucose 6-phosphate.

It should be understood that the phosphorylation of glucose has two distinct effects. First it increases the total energy associated with the glucose molecule. Second, the molecule so produced is more labile, more reactive, and hence better suited for further metabolism. Its kinetic stability is less than that of glucose. This latter result is the more important one and accomplishes the *activation* of the glucose molecule. Kinetic stability has been lucidly described in simple terms by Stetten.

The reactions considered so far are summarized in Fig. 52-1.

Storage of Activated Glucose as Glycogen and the Mobilization of Glycogen. Glucose 6-phosphate, once formed, can be stored as glycogen, a glucose polymer. The reactions involved result in the transfer of the activation energy present in the ester bond of glucose 6-phosphate and glucose 1-phosphate to glucosidic bonds between glucose molecules.

It is now recognized that glycogen synthesis and glycogen breakdown are controlled by two separate series of reactions. Glycogen *synthesis* probably results primarily from the reaction of glucose 1-phosphate with uridine triphosphate (UTP), with formation of uridine diphosphoglucose (UDPG). Glucose is then transferred from uridine diphosphate to the free (nonreducing) end of a glycogen chain, resulting in a new glucosidic 1,4 link, with elongation of the chain by one glucose unit. After a given elongation of each glycogen chain, branching points are established in the presence of branching enzyme (amylo-1,4-1,6 transglycosidase) by the formation of 1,6 links, thereby originating new chains of 1,4 links. Glycogen *breakdown,* on the other hand, is catalyzed by the enzyme phosphorylase, resulting in cleavage (phosphorolysis) of successive 1,4 links, with formation of glucose 1-phosphate, until a 1,6 link is encountered. To rupture this bond, amylo-1,6 glucosidase is required, with formation of free

TRANSPORT (Cell Membrane)	ACTIVATION (Phosphorylation)

GLUCOSE ⟶ ⊢ ⟶ GL $\xrightarrow[\text{ATP, Mg}^{++}]{\text{GLUCOKINASE}}$ GLUCOSE 6-PHOSPHATE

FIG. 52-1. Metabolic activation of glucose to glucose 6-phosphate.

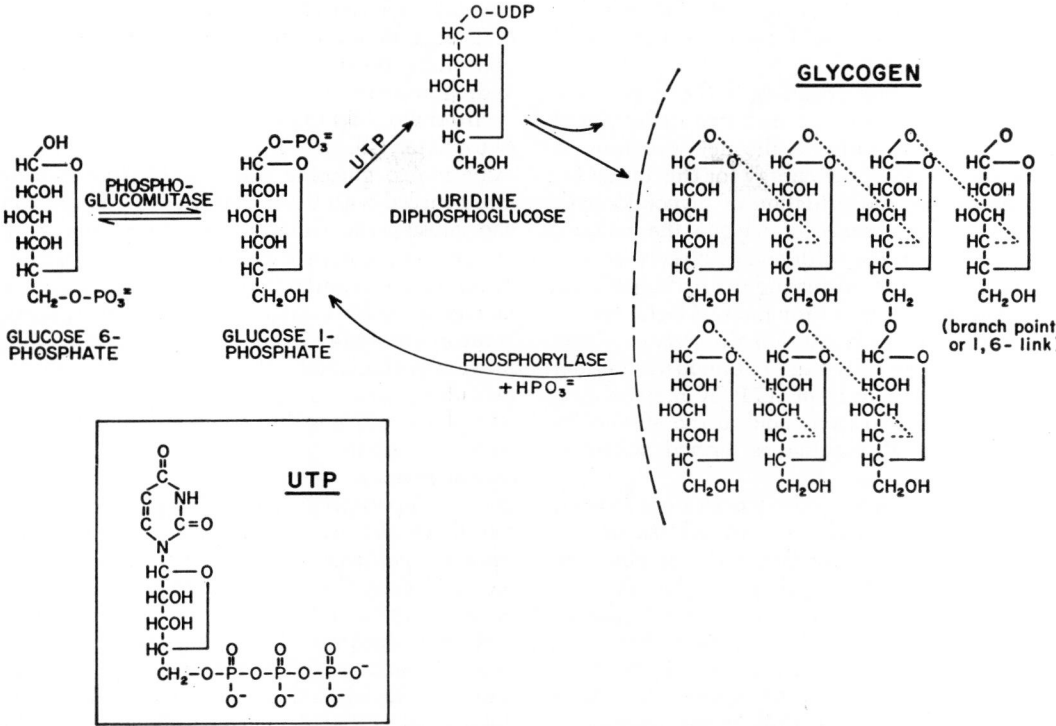

FIG. 52-2. Pathway of glycogen synthesis and breakdown.

glucose. The ratio of 1,4 links to 1,6 links in glycogen averages 8 to 1. Although the existence of a separate synthetic pathway of glycogen metabolism was established only in 1957, and although its presence has not as yet been demonstrated in a large number of tissues from different species, its acceptance makes it possible to resolve many previously existing contradictions in terms of metabolic control, as will be outlined further on. The reactions which have been mentioned are summarized in Fig. 52-2.

It is important to understand that the glucose molecules stored as glycogen are already activated and can therefore be transformed into glucose 6-phosphate without the expenditure of energy necessary for the transformation of glucose into glucose 6-phosphate.

Metabolism of Glucose 6-Phosphate to Pyruvic or Lactic Acid. This series of reactions is also known as "glycolysis" or "the Embden-Meyerhof pathway." It is schematized in Fig. 52-3. Essentially it consists in isomerization of glucose 6-phosphate to fructose 6-phosphate, the addition of a second phosphate radical in position 1 (again at the expense of one molecule of ATP), resulting in the formation of fructose 1-6-diphosphate, which is then reversibly split in the presence of aldolase into two phosphorylated 3-carbon fragments, glyceraldehyde

phosphate and dihydroxyacetone phosphate. These two 3-carbon compounds are interconvertible, and further metabolism occurs by way of glyceraldehyde phosphate, which is oxidized in the presence of diphosphopyridine nucleotide (DPN) and inorganic phosphate to diphosphoglyceric acid. In this reaction the energy necessary for the addition of a second phosphate radical to glyceraldehyde phosphate is provided not by the splitting of ATP but by the simultaneous oxidation of the 3-carbon compound. Diphosphoglyceric acid is then dephosphorylated in a series of reactions resulting in the

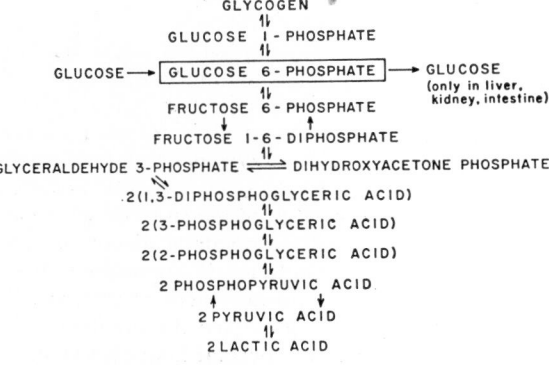

FIG. 52-3. Pathways of glycolysis.

formation of pyruvic acid along with the regeneration of two molecules of ATP for each molecule of pyruvic acid formed.

The over-all reaction, resulting in the transformation of one glucose molecule into two molecules of pyruvic acid, thus results in the net formation of two molecules of ATP, the energy for this formation being provided by the oxidation of glyceraldehyde phosphate. In the absence of oxygen the reduced DPN resulting from the oxidation of glyceraldehyde can be reoxidized by transferring the hydrogen from DPNH$_2$ to pyruvate with formation of lactic acid, a reaction catalyzed by lactic dehydrogenase. Under these circumstances cells can continuously produce useful energy in the form of ATP by metabolizing glycogen or glucose to lactic acid in the absence of oxygen. This over-all reaction is termed *anaerobic glycolysis.*

Synthesis of Glycogen and Glucose from Pyruvic or Lactic Acid. Although the over-all reaction of anaerobic glycolysis is reversible under aerobic conditions, it is important to understand that the synthetic sequence of reactions (i.e., toward glucose 6-phosphate) differs in three points from the catabolic sequence (i.e., toward pyruvic or lactic acid). First, the reaction *phosphopyruvic acid →* *pyruvic acid,* although reversible in the presence of ATP, apparently does not proceed in the reverse direction to any quantitatively significant degree, at least in liver cells. Instead pyruvic acid reacts with CO$_2$ in the presence of TPNH$_2$ to form malic acid which in turn forms oxaloacetic acid and DPNH$_2$. In the presence of inosine or guanosine triphosphate, oxaloacetic acid then may be directly metabolized to phosphopyruvic acid and CO$_2$. Second, whereas fructose 6-phosphate is phosphorylated to fructose 1,6-diphosphate in the presence of ATP and the enzyme *phosphofructokinase,* the reverse reaction is catalyzed by *fructose diphosphatase* and results in the formation of inorganic phosphate. Finally, while glucose is phosphorylated to glucose 6-phosphate in the presence of ATP and of *hexokinase,* the dephosphorylation of glucose occurs in the presence of *glucose 6-phosphatase* and again results in the formation of inorganic phosphate. This last enzyme, glucose 6-phosphatase, is present only in liver, kidney, and intestinal mucosa, thus providing a ready explanation for the fact that only liver and kidney (and, to a lesser degree, intestinal mucosa) can contribute endogenous glucose to the blood stream. The presence of separate reactions for synthesis or catabolism of glucose and glycogen, provided at three separate points of glycolysis, may well be of major importance in permitting directional control of the over-all reactions toward synthesis or toward catabolism (see the discussions by Krebs, 1957). It is also important to understand that the synthesis of one molecule of glucose from two

molecules of pyruvic acid results in the expenditure of energy at least equivalent to four high-energy phosphate bonds as well as in the utilization of hydrogen in the form of DPNH$_2$ and TPNH$_2$.

Alternate Metabolic Pathways for Glucose 6-Phosphate. Glucose 6-phosphate can also undergo oxidation to gluconic acid 6-phosphate (an oxidation coupled with the reduction of TPN to TPNH$_2$) and subsequent oxidative decarboxylation (an oxidation again coupled with the reduction of TPN to TPNH$_2$) to ribulose 5-phosphate. The further metabolic transformation of this phosphorylated pentose eventually results in its reentrance into the previously discussed pathways of glycolysis, thereby permitting continuing regeneration of glucose 6-phosphate and possibly complete oxidation of glucose to carbon dioxide and water by repeated rearrangements and recycling. This pathway of glucose 6-phosphate metabolism has been termed the direct oxidative pathway, the *phosphogluconate oxidative pathway,* the pentose phosphate pathway, the Lipmann-Dickens pathway, or finally the "shunt." Its biologic importance probably results in part from the formation of important intermediary products such as pentoses necessary for the synthesis of nucleic acids and in part from the production of TPNH$_2$ which becomes available for reductive synthetic steps such as the biosynthesis of fatty acids and other lipids. It is not surprising, therefore, to find that the enzymes of the direct oxidative pathway for glucose 6-phosphate are present in highest concentration in those tissues which specialize in the synthesis of fatty acids and sterols, e.g., adipose tissue and the adrenal cortex.

Glucose 6-phosphate can also be metabolized, through glucose 1-phosphate and uridine diphosphoglucose (as in Fig. 52-2), to uridine diphosphoglucuronate and glucuronic acid. This pathway, the *glucuronic acid pathway,* thus results in oxidation of the other end of the glucose molecule. The glucuronic acid formed may be of importance as a constituent of many mucopolysaccharides, or as a compound frequently used in the conjugation of substances such as bilirubin, phenols, or sterols. The quantitative importance of this pathway, whose existence has been established beyond reasonable doubt by Horecker and Hiatt, has not as yet been clearly defined.

The metabolic pathways open to glucose 6-phosphate have been summarized in Fig. 52-4.

Metabolism of Pyruvic Acid to Acetyl Coenzyme A and to Oxaloacetic Acid. Whereas in plants pyruvic acid is mainly decarboxylated to acetaldehyde, this reaction has not been observed in animal tissues. Oxidative decarboxylation is probably the major fate of pyruvic acid in mammalian cells and results in the formation of CO$_2$ and of acetyl coenzyme A, though other metabolic pathways have

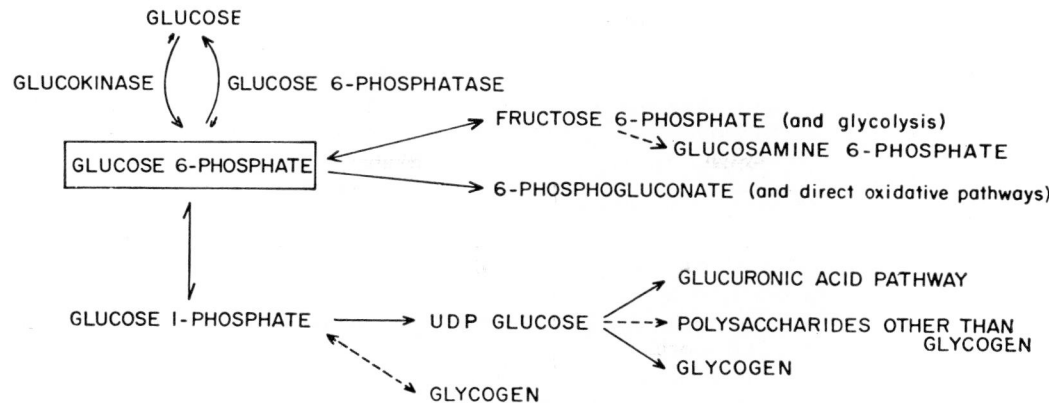

FIG. 52-4. Metabolic pathways of glucose 6-phosphate.

been described. This important and complex reaction requires the presence of *at least* two enzyme fractions, of four coenzymes (DPN, thiamine pyrophosphate, coenzyme A, and alpha-lipoic acid), and of Mg^{++} ions or Mn^{++} ions. It results in the formation not of free acetic acid but of the ester of acetic acid and the free thiol ending of coenzyme A, i.e., acetyl coenzyme A. Acetyl coenzyme A bears a relationship to acetic acid similar to that of glucose 6-phosphate to glucose; it is an *activated* acetic acid which participates readily in further enzymatic reactions (required by further intracellular metabolism), whereas acetic acid itself is unreactive. The

$$R\overset{\overset{\textstyle O}{\|}}{C}\text{—SCoA}$$ bond is a high-energy bond comparable to the terminal phosphate bond of ATP. The oxidative decarboxylation of pyruvate is not reversible.

In the presence of biotin, ATP, Mn^{++} and $TPNH_2$ pyruvic acid can also react with CO_2 to yield malic acid first, then oxaloacetic acid, as already discussed. These reactions are the principal source of the oxaloacetic acid needed to "spark" the tricarboxylic acid cycle and to keep it from "running down," thereby lending to pyruvate probably one of its important metabolic characteristics. Compounds which can be metabolized to pyruvate can also give rise to a net oxaloacetate production and thus provide for continued operation of the tricarboxylic acid cycle.

Acetyl CoA has several pathways open to it, of which four are of major quantitative importance: oxidation in the tricarboxylic acid cycle, synthesis of fatty acids, synthesis of cholesterol, and metabolism to acetoacetate and beta-hydroxybutyrate.

Oxidation of Acetyl in the Tricarboxylic Acid Cycle. The acetyl residue from acetyl coenzyme A reacts with oxaloacetic acid in the presence of condensing enzyme to form citric acid. Citric acid is then further metabolized, as shown in Fig. 52-5, and regenerates one molecule of oxaloacetic acid. In

each revolution of this cycle one acetyl residue is consumed, two molecules of CO_2 are evolved, and eight hydrogen atoms are transferred to their appropriate acceptors and ultimately to oxygen with the formation of water. It is not necessary to discuss here the details of these reactions, but it is important to understand (1) that these reactions are of great quantitative importance, since they account for the major portion of oxidative metabolism in mammalian tissues and as a consequence for the major part of energy formation during life; and (2) that oxaloacetate, although regenerated at the end of each revolution of the cycle, apparently does undergo some utilization in the process (for example, transamination, decarboxylation by metal ions, metabolism to phosphopyruvic acid and thence synthesis of glucose or glycogen), thus making the periodic supply of oxaloacetate from other sources mandatory for continued operation of the tricarboxylic cycle. Finally it should be pointed out that the oxidative decarboxylation of alpha-ketoglutaric acid to succinate results in the formation of suc-

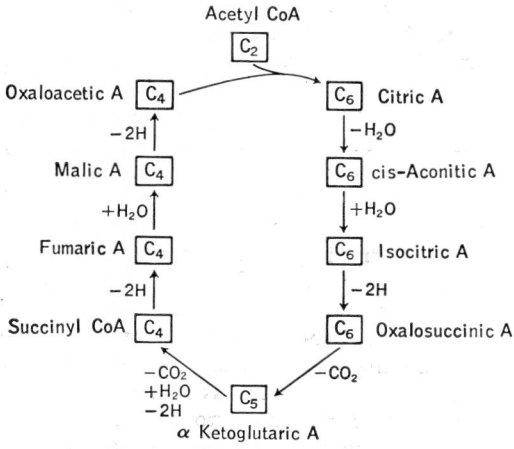

FIG. 52-5. The tricarboxylic acid cycle.

cinyl coenzyme A in a manner similar to the formation of acetyl coenzyme A during the oxidative decarboxylation of pyruvate.

The Synthesis of Fatty Acids from Acetyl Coenzyme A, Their Storage as Glycerol Esters, and Their Mobilization and Oxidation. When acetyl CoA is present in excess of immediate oxidative needs, it is primarily stored as long-chain fatty acids esterified with glycerol. The synthesis of long-chain fatty acids from acetyl CoA is a *reductive* synthesis, two molecules of hydrogen being required for the incorporation of each acetyl residue into a saturated fatty acid chain. After elongation of each chain to 16 or 18 carbons, while still attached to coenzyme A, the acyl residue can be transferred from the sulfhydryl group of coenzyme A to a hydroxyl group of alpha-glycerophosphate, finally resulting in glycerol esters of the fatty acids. At this writing, many uncertainties as to the exact mechanism of fatty acid synthesis remain, and presentation of a detailed schema does not seem warranted here. The following generalizations, however, are relevant to the working scheme of intermediary metabolism which we are developing in this introduction.

Contrary to the view generally accepted until recently, *fatty acid synthesis is likely to proceed by pathways separate from fatty acid catabolism.* Not only are the enzymes involved different, but different intermediates are probably formed (in particular the intermediate malonyl CoA), and the hydrogen needed for synthesis has to be provided as $TPNH_2$, whereas the dehydrogenation occurring during catabolism results in the formation of $DPNH_2$ as well as reduced flavine-adenine dinucleotide (FAD). Thus, control over synthesis and catabolism is likely to be exerted separately, and the availability of appropriate oxidized or reduced cofactors is likely to be of particular importance in exerting this control. For details, the reviews by Wakil and by Green should be consulted (the latter in the volume edited by Greenberg).

Storage of fatty acids in large quantities requires the formation of neutral glycerol esters. The synthesis of glycerides requires the presence of both fatty acids (as acyl CoA) and glycerol (as glycerolphosphate) in activated form. Hydrolysis of glycerides, however, probably results primarily in the formation of free fatty acids and free glycerol. It is likely that here, again, metabolic regulation may be exerted by controlling separately the availability of activated precursors and of lipolytic activity.

It is important to understand clearly that before any fatty acid can react in intermediary metabolism, either in the direction of further synthesis or in the direction of catabolism, it has to be activated by esterification with the thiol group of coenzyme A, a process requiring the expenditure of ATP and quite comparable to the initial phosphorylation of glucose to glucose 6-phosphate. A masterful presentation of this newly developed and important field was given early by Lynen in his Harvey Lecture of 1953; his conclusion follows.

The role of coenzyme A in fatty acid metabolism may be compared to the role of inorganic phosphate in carbohydrate metabolism. The sugar molecule is introduced into the chain of degradations and transformations by conversion into a phosphorylated derivative. Quite analogous to this, fatty acids are linked in the first step to the sulfur of coenzyme A, and only then can the enzymatic oxidation within the cell proceed. For medicine, the recent developments in the field of fatty acid metabolism are significant because now the chemical transformations are known and the individual enzymatic steps can be tested separately. Biochemistry thus supplies medicine with facts and with methods for recognizing metabolic failures.

Metabolism of Acetoacetate. Acetoacetyl CoA is formed primarily as a result of the condensation of two acetyl CoA molecules, with or without the intermediate formation of malonyl CoA. Whenever acetyl CoA is formed in large quantities in the course of cellular metabolism, acetoacetyl CoA accumulates. In certain tissues, predominantly the liver, free acetoacetate may be produced under these conditions. Whereas it was thought until recently that CoA is split off directly in the presence of a specific deacylase, it appears more likely from the recent work of Lynen that the reaction is a more complex one, involving the intermediary formation of beta-OH, beta-methyl glutaryl CoA, as shown in Fig. 52-6, which further points out that this metabolite also represents an intermediate in the course of the synthesis of cholesterol.

Once acetoacetate has been formed in the liver, it readily appears in the blood stream and can then be reactivated and used by all tissues either by direct reaction with coenzyme A in the presence of ATP or by transfer of coenzyme A to acetoacetate from succinyl coenzyme A formed in the oxidation of citric acid; the latter, more economic transfer reaction is catalyzed by a specific enzyme which is not present in liver but is present in muscle and other tissues, thus establishing a useful transport system, acetoacetate being produced in the liver and utilized in the periphery. Acetoacetate is also easily reduced to beta-hydroxybutyric acid, which can be activated by reaction with coenzyme A in the presence of ATP. Finally acetoacetate can be decarboxylated to acetone—probably a reaction of small biologic significance. However, some evidence indicates that acetone can undergo oxidation to pyruvate and thus represents a possible pathway for carbohydrate synthesis from acetoacetate and therefore from fatty acids. The reaction, although possible, probably does not occur to a degree that would be quantitatively significant.

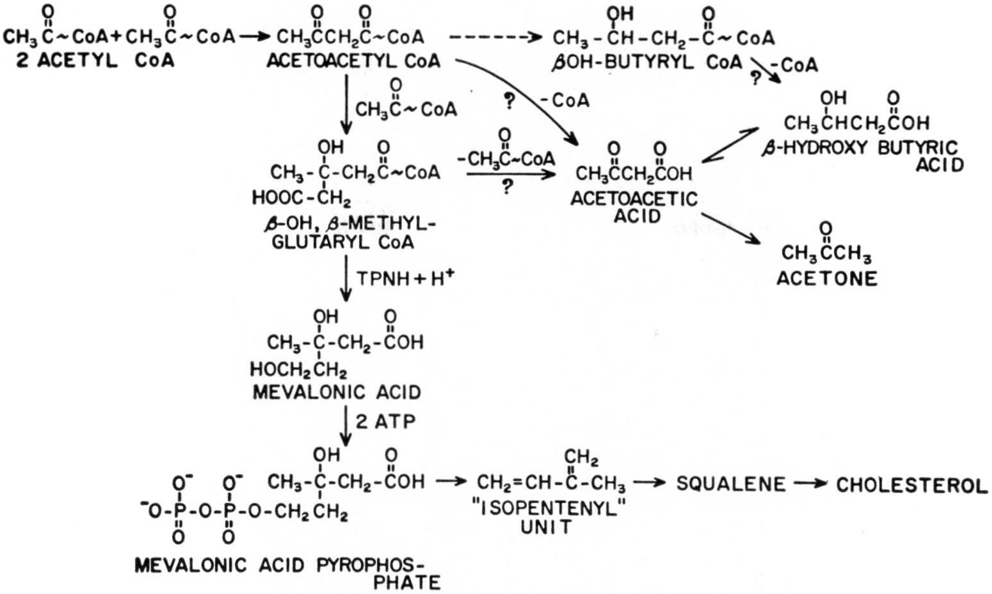

$$CH_3\overset{O}{\overset{\|}{C}}\sim CoA + CH_3\overset{O}{\overset{\|}{C}}\sim CoA \longrightarrow CH_3\overset{O}{\overset{\|}{C}}CH_2\overset{O}{\overset{\|}{C}}\sim CoA \dashrightarrow CH_3-\overset{OH}{\overset{|}{C}}H-CH_2-\overset{O}{\overset{\|}{C}}\sim CoA$$

2 ACETYL CoA   ACETOACETYL CoA   βOH-BUTYRYL CoA

$$\downarrow CH_3\overset{O}{\overset{\|}{C}}\sim CoA$$

? - CoA

$$CH_3-\overset{OH}{\overset{|}{C}}-CH_2\overset{O}{\overset{\|}{C}}\sim CoA$$
$$\overset{|}{HOOC-CH_2}$$
β-OH, β-METHYL-GLUTARYL CoA

$$\xrightarrow[?]{-CH_3\overset{O}{\overset{\|}{C}}-CoA} CH_3\overset{O}{\overset{\|}{C}}CH_2\overset{O}{\overset{\|}{C}}OH$$
ACETOACETIC ACID

$$CH_3\overset{OH}{\overset{|}{C}}HCH_2\overset{O}{\overset{\|}{C}}OH$$
β-HYDROXY BUTYRIC ACID

$$CH_3\overset{O}{\overset{\|}{C}}CH_3$$
ACETONE

$$\downarrow TPNH + H^+$$

$$CH_3-\overset{OH}{\overset{|}{C}}-CH_2-\overset{O}{\overset{\|}{C}}OH$$
$$\overset{|}{HOCH_2CH_2}$$
MEVALONIC ACID

$$\downarrow 2\ ATP$$

$$\overset{O^-}{\underset{O}{\overset{\|}{P}}}\overset{O^-}{\underset{O}{\overset{\|}{P}}}\ CH_3-\overset{OH}{\overset{|}{C}}-CH_2-\overset{O}{\overset{\|}{C}}OH$$
$$^-O-P-O-P-O-CH_2CH_2$$
MEVALONIC ACID PYROPHOS-PHATE

$$\longrightarrow CH_2=CH-\overset{CH_2}{\overset{\|}{C}}-CH_3 \longrightarrow$$ SQUALENE $\longrightarrow$ CHOLESTEROL
"ISOPENTENYL" UNIT

FIG. 52-6. Pathways of cholesterol synthesis and ketogenesis.

Other Metabolic Fates of Acetyl Coenzyme A. It has already been pointed out that acetyl CoA is also the precursor of cholesterol (and other steroids) through a complicated synthetic sequence very briefly sketched in Fig. 52-6, and recently reviewed by Bloch, Popjak, and Tchen (see Ciba Symposium on steroids and the pertinent chapter in the volume edited by Greenberg). Relatively less hydrogen is required for the synthesis of cholesterol than for the synthesis of long-chain fatty acids. Acetyl CoA also links the metabolism of carbohydrates and fats to that of certain amino acids, carotenoids, and acetylated compounds such as acetylcholine. It represents a true "crossroad of metabolism" which has been schematized in Fig. 52-7.

Metabolism of Amino Acids and Proteins. Much has been learned in recent years with regard to the synthesis of proteins from amino acid, and it is of particular interest that, again, activated amino acid

intermediates have to be formed prior to their utilization in synthesis. Reference is made to the recent Harvey Lecture of Zamecnik. In this chapter, however, and with relation to the working plan of intermediary metabolism being developed, it is necessary to mention only that amino acids, in addition to their structural significance as building units of proteins, may participate significantly in intermediary metabolism and energy production. Under certain conditions this participation is a major one. Most amino acids appear to enter the metabolic pool by means of transamination reactions. Their metabolites then enter previously described pathways, principally by preliminary transformation to pyruvic acid, acetyl coenzyme A, alpha-ketoglutaric acid, or oxaloacetate. Alpha-ketoglutaric acid is probably a particularly important meeting point of amino acid metabolism and the metabolism of carbohydrate and fat, since it arises from deamination and oxidation of glutamic acid.

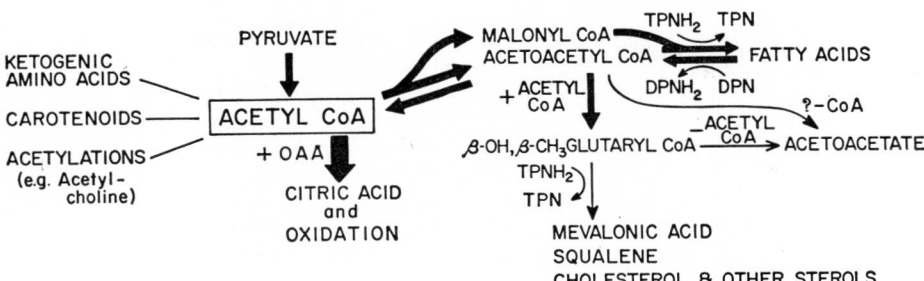

FIG. 52-7. Fates of acetyl CoA.

At this crossroads of the metabolic pathways of amino acids and other metabolic fuels, ammonia may be conveniently disposed of by condensation with other compounds.

In many cells amino acids are found in concentrations many times higher than their concentrations in plasma, thereby suggesting the presence of an active transport mechanism which may play an important role in the regulation of tissue growth and more generally in intracellular amino acid and protein metabolism (Noall, Riggs, Walter, and Christensen).

Transport of Electrons from Substrate to Oxygen and the Liberation of Useful Energy. The over-all purpose of intermediary metabolism is that of generating useful energy as a result of substrate oxidation. At the substrate level this oxidation usually is a dehydrogenation with transfer of the hydrogen to DPN or TPN, resulting in the formation of reduced DPN or TPN. Reduced DPN or TPN is usually then reoxidized by appropriate electron acceptors, and this process of coupled oxidation and reduction is repeated several times as electrons are transported from acceptor to acceptor (flavine-adenine dinucleotides and cytochromes). Finally, under aerobic conditions, oxygen reacts with the hydrogen released from the last acceptor, usually cytochrome oxidase, thus completing the "respiratory chain." In the course of this electron transfer,

energy is liberated and is fixed, to a considerable extent, as chemically useful energy in the form of high-energy bonds, of which the high-energy phosphate bond is the most frequently used example. It is important to realize, however, that high-energy bonds other than phosphate bonds are also generated and used, such as the carbon-sulfur bond in acetyl coenzyme A. These high-energy bonds are then available for transformation of their energy, in the presence of appropriate systems, into useful thermal or mechanical work. The exact mechanism of these energy transfers is as yet unknown. The coupling of electron transfer in the respiratory chain with the generation of high-energy bonds—more specifically high-energy phosphate bonds—is usually termed *oxidative phosphorylation*. In living cells this complex aggregate of serial and simultaneous reactions is to a large extent localized anatomically to mitochondria (see Green and Goldberger).

Simplified Working Scheme of Intermediary Metabolism. It is highly desirable and indeed essential for the student of disease to have at his disposal a working scheme of intermediary metabolism sufficiently simple for daily use. It is evident that such working schemes will vary from individual to individual according to special interests and needs. However, as an example, a simplified working scheme which has been found useful by the authors of this chapter is presented in Fig. 52-8.

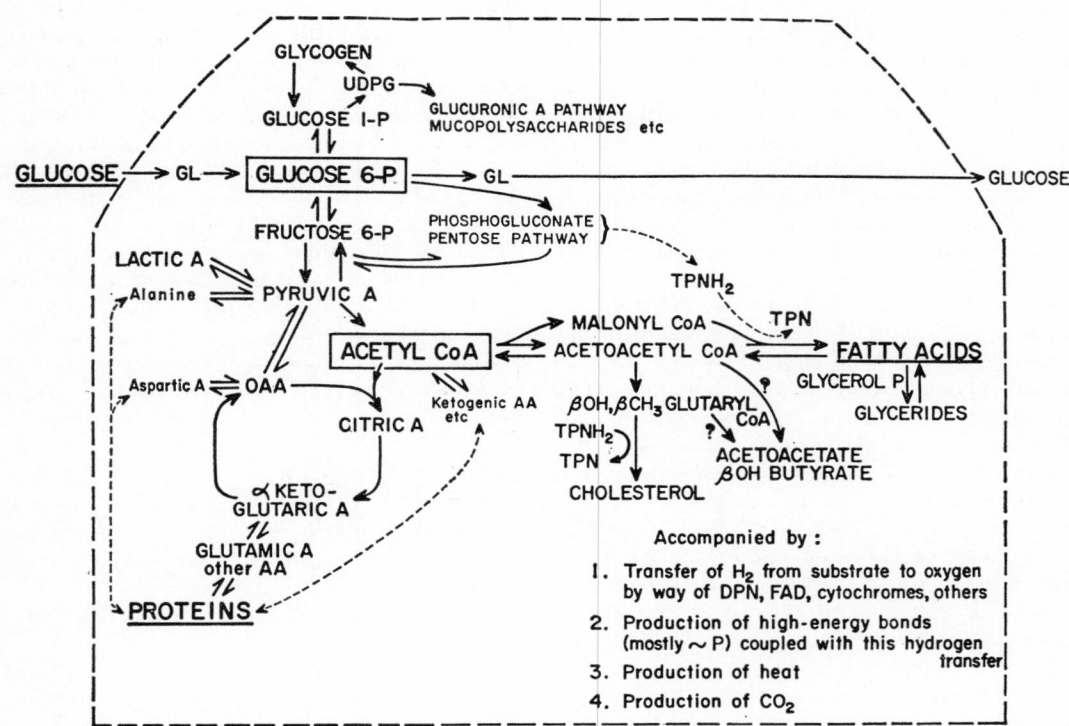

FIG. 52-8. Simplified working scheme of intermediary metabolism.

REGULATION OF INTERMEDIARY METABOLISM

Having briefly recalled the major features of intermediary metabolism, we shall next recall some of the regulating factors which affect it. *It is important to remember that the biologic effect of any metabolic regulator results from its chemical or physical nature and from the specific responsiveness of individual tissues.* The importance of the specific responsiveness of individual tissues has often been neglected, although no true understanding of the biologic effectiveness of a regulator such as a hormone will be achieved before its site and mode of action *and* the relative responsiveness of each tissue to the hormone are known.

The regulating factors which affect intermediary metabolism may be grouped into (1) *nutritional factors,* both nonspecific (e.g., fasting) and specific (e.g., vitamins or essential amino acids); (2) *hormonal factors;* (3) *other environmental factors* such as the absolute and relative concentrations of ions, the presence of certain "trace elements"; and (4) *neural factors,* although these are at present but poorly understood with respect to intermediary metabolism. Most of what is presently known concerns nutritional and hormonal regulation. The plan of intermediary metabolism previously outlined will be followed in considering its regulation. It should be clearly appreciated that this area of knowledge is at present a particularly fluid one.

Regulation of Glucose Entrance into Cells and of Its Metabolic Activation to Glucose 6-Phosphate. The accelerating effect of insulin upon glucose transport and/or phosphorylation by skeletal and heart muscle, adipose tissue, and lens is the best-documented regulation of this sector of intermediary metabolism. At present it would seem more likely that insulin exerts this effect upon glucose transport into the cell rather than upon its subsequent phosphorylation. An attractive suggestion is that made recently by Barnett and Ball, i.e., that insulin accelerates pinocytosis (accelerated cellular drinking by a process akin to phagocytosis) at least in some insulin-sensitive tissues. This regulatory action of insulin affords an excellent example of varying responsiveness of individual tissues. Whereas insulin increases glucose uptake by muscle and adipose tissue within minutes of its administration, this effect upon liver is delayed, and glucose transport and phosphorylation of brain, kidney, and intestinal mucosa remain unaffected by the administration of even larger insulin doses. Although some evidence suggests that insulin does, under certain circumstances, affect glucose balance across the liver within minutes of its administration, this is likely to be primarily due to decreased hepatic *output* of glucose. Muscular activity by as yet unknown mechanisms also facilitates glucose uptake by skeletal muscle.

Prolonged fasting or a diet low in carbohydrate, administration of large doses of pituitary growth hormone, and epinephrine administration have been shown to result under certain conditions in decreased glucose uptake and phosphorylation by tissues such as muscle. Furthermore the glucokinase reaction is markedly affected by the presence or absence of ions such as Mn^{++} or K^+ and requires the presence of adequate supplies of ATP. It is evident that this region of intermediary metabolism is highly sensitive and is also well suited for regulatory influences, since it controls the over-all supply to individual cells of a major metabolic fuel, glucose.

Regulation of Glycogen Synthesis and Breakdown. Muscle and liver represent the two major sites of glycogen storage. Quite generally conditions associated with an abundant supply of glucose, such as high carbohydrate diet, result in a facilitation of glycogen synthesis by mechanisms not as yet completely understood, although acceleration of the transglycosidase reaction from UDPG to glycogen may be involved (Larner). Glycogen breakdown is mainly controlled by two hormonal factors: epinephrine and glucagon. *Epinephrine* action results in rapid breakdown of both muscle and liver glycogen, the former process resulting in accumulation of pyruvate and lactate, the latter in accumulation of glucose. Epinephrine is generally released under emergency conditions, and the effects just described are appropriate; they result in the facilitation of anaerobic glycolysis in muscle and in the supply of additional glucose to the blood stream for use by essential tissues such as brain. Even the previously mentioned inhibitory effect of epinephrine upon glucose utilization by muscle fits well into this scheme, since in the presence of increased muscular activity glucose uptake by muscle might otherwise exceed the blood glucose supply and result in a highly dangerous curtailment of glucose available for use in the central nervous system.

Glucagon, in contrast, affects only hepatic glycogen. Both hormones appear at present to exert their effect by maintaining a larger proportion of phosphorylase than usual in its active form, thus increasing the effective concentration of the enzyme mainly responsible for glycogen breakdown. The effect of both glucagon and epinephrine upon glycogen metabolism is mediated by the initial formation of cyclic adenylic acid (adenine-ribose 3',5'-phosphate).

The increased hepatic glycogen content which results from the administration of certain adrenal corticosteroids probably reflects increased gluconeogenesis and therefore increased intrahepatic concentrations of glucose 6-phosphate and glucose 1-phosphate, conditions which result in facilitation of glycogen synthesis. Again this region of intermediary metabolism is highly sensitive to environmental factors, such as absolute and relative concentration of ions, and maintains a delicate balance frequently affected by disease.

Regulation of Glucose 6-Phosphate Metabolism to Pyruvic Acid and Vice Versa. There can be little doubt that a number of factors regulating the metabolism of glucose 6-phosphate to pyruvic acid will in time be demonstrated, particularly since the presence of an alternate pathway of glucose 6-phosphate metabolism (i.e., the phosphogluconate–pentose phosphate pathway) provides many regulatory possibilities. However, at present the established facts are few and mostly concern ionic environment and the presence of certain cofactors. On the other hand considerable information has accumulated with regard to the conditions which favor the operation of glycolysis *in reverse,* leading to the accumulation of glycogen and glucose, a process usually referred to as *gluconeogenesis.* Gluconeogenesis occurs principally, of course, in those tissues which can liberate glucose from glucose 6-phosphate, i.e., liver and, to a lesser degree, kidney. Gluconeogenesis necessitates the expenditure of energy in order to accomplish the necessary phosphorylations and the reduction of diphosphoglyceric acid to phosphoglyceraldehyde. Furthermore in the course of gluconeogenesis, two enzymes—fructose 1,6-diphosphatase and glucose 6-phosphatase—catalyze essentially irreversible reactions and thus provide potential directional flow valves. It would appear at present that insulin inhibits and that certain *adrenal corticosteroids* markedly stimulate gluconeogenesis. Prolonged fasting or a diet high in protein similarly appear to stimulate gluconeogenesis. Although the exact mechanism of these effects is unknown, it is interesting to note that the activity of the two essentially unidirectional enzymes mentioned above has been found to be increased in conditions associated with increased gluconeogenesis; hepatic glucose 6-phosphatase activity markedly increases in the absence of insulin and in the presence of excess glucocorticoid activity, and fructose 1,6-diphosphatase activity also increases after glucocorticoid administration.

Regulation of Oxidative Pyruvate Decarboxylation to Acetyl Coenzyme A. This important and highly complex reaction is dependent on the presence of four cofactors—DPN, thiamine pyrophosphate, coenzyme A, and alpha-lipoic acid—and of Mn^{++} or Mg^{++} ions. Since pantothenic acid is necessary for coenzyme A synthesis, this and other coenzyme A–dependent reactions may be expected to be interfered with in pantothenic acid deficiency. Nicotinamide is necessary for DPN synthesis and thiamine for the synthesis of *thiamine pyrophosphate.* The importance of pyruvate decarboxylation

is well illustrated by the thiamine-deficiency syndrome (beriberi), characterized by severe cardiovascular and neurologic disturbances. It is quite likely that the syndrome represents the direct and indirect result of inadequate oxidative decarboxylation of pyruvate and of other alpha-keto acids such as alpha-ketoglutaric acid, and it would appear therefore that both heart muscle and nervous tissue are particularly dependent on the proper functioning of these reactions. Further elaboration of cofactor-deficiency syndromes appears superfluous in this chapter since they are fully described in Chap. 61. An endocrine regulation of the oxidative decarboxylation of pyruvate has not as yet been established, although it has been suggested that adrenal corticosteroids exert an inhibitory effect.

Regulation of Acetyl Coenzyme A Metabolism. Figure 52-7 presents a summary of the possible metabolic fates of acetyl coenzyme A. A number of regulating influences have been demonstrated at this level. *Insulin* administration or a diet high in carbohydrate favor the synthesis of long-chain fatty acids by liver and adipose tissue. Insulin and carbohydrate feeding also favor the hepatic condensation of acetyl coenzyme A with oxaloacetate to form citric acid but inhibit the accumulation and release of acetoacetate and tend to decrease the synthesis of cholesterol. Fasting, diets low in carbohydrate and protein, epinephrine, and certain *adrenal corticosteroids* as well as certain *anterior pituitary preparations* inhibit the synthesis of long-chain fatty acids by liver and adipose tissue, favor the catabolism of stored fatty acids, and favor the hepatic synthesis and release of acetoacetate. These observations have been coordinated into the following working hypothesis: (1) Factors which tend to increase the availability of glucose 6-phosphate from exogenous glucose or from glycogen favor the condensation of acetyl CoA with oxaloacetate, the synthesis of long-chain fatty acids, and the storage of fatty acids as glycerides. These effects might be explained as brought about by (*a*) increased availability of malate and oxaloacetate from pyruvate, as a result of active glycolysis; (*b*) increased availability of the appropriate reduced coenzyme ($TPNH_2$) and of acetyl CoA as a result of active glycolysis *and* active metabolism of glucose 6-phosphate in the phosphogluconate-oxidative pathway; (*c*) increased availability of α-glycerophosphate as glycerol donor in the synthesis of glycerides, as a result of active glycolysis with formation of α-glycerophosphate from dihydroxyacetone phosphate. (2) Factors which tend to increase gluconeogenesis (reverse glycolysis) inhibit the synthesis of long-chain fatty acids and favor the accumulation of acetoacetate and perhaps the synthesis of cholesterol. Although the mechanism of these effects is not established, it would seem reasonable that reverse glycolysis would (a) decrease the amount of pyruvate available for keeping the tricarboxylic acid cycle from "running down," and (b) accelerate the oxidation of fatty acids to acetyl CoA (by requiring $DPNH_2$ and $TPNH_2$) while simultaneously decreasing the synthesis of long-chain fatty acids (because of the limited activity of the phosphogluconate-oxidative pathway and therefore limited $TPNH_2$ formation). Both these factors would reasonably tend to increase the accumulation of acetoacetyl CoA with overflow formation of acetoacetate. If, furthermore, acetoacetate is primarily formed through alpha-hydroxy, beta-methyl glutaric acid (Fig. 52-6), then acetoacetate and cholesterol production, having one additional precursor in common, might reasonably vary in roughly parallel fashion. It has also been suggested that, since the reductive synthesis of cholesterol from acetyl CoA requires less $TPNH_2$ than the reductive synthesis of long-chain fatty acids (since cholesterol is less completely reduced than, for instance, palmitic acid), it is reasonable to expect that it would remain relatively unaffected even in the presence of severe curtailment of fatty acid synthesis.

The important possible sequence of events underlying the regulation of cholesterol synthesis, especially as related to dietary intake, have been discussed by Siperstein.

Regulation of Amino Acid and Protein Metabolism. With regard to intermediary metabolism, knowledge concerning protein and amino acid metabolism is fragmentary. A diet rich in carbohydrate, *insulin, male and female sex hormones,* and, under certain conditions, *growth hormone* favor protein synthesis from amino acids (or inhibit protein hydrolysis to amino acids), whereas fasting, *adrenal glucocorticoids, thyroid hormones,* and certain pituitary fractions favor protein catabolism to amino acids (or inhibit protein synthesis from amino acids). The mechanism of these effects is as yet unclear, although it would again appear to be related in part to the activity and direction of glycolysis as well as to the activity of the phosphogluconate oxidative pathway. Direct hormonal effects on protein synthesis probably also exist. Amino acids, once present in excess in the blood stream, are metabolized at a more rapid rate. However, no clear evidence has yet been obtained to indicate that the rate of oxidative deamination of amino acids is hormonally controlled.

The effects of male and female sex hormones on the growth of such tissues as the male accessory glands or the uterus are so marked and may occur so rapidly that careful analysis of these processes is likely to contribute greatly to the elucidation of the regulatory mechanisms involved in tissue growth and protein synthesis. Christensen and coworkers have suggested that the regulation of amino acid transport into the cells may be of major importance.

Regulation of Electron Transport and Formation of Useful Energy. The stepwise, enzyme-linked transfer of electrons (and hydrogen) from substrate molecule to oxygen is performed by the mitochondria of living cells. The electron transport apparatus has been shown to consist of enzymes, many of which are metalloenzymes: zinc in the dehydrogenases, copper in many oxidases, iron in the heme enzymes. The cofactors required by some of the oxidative enzymes contain vitamins: nicotinamide in DPN and TPN, riboflavin in the flavin nucleotides, and possibly vitamin K and vitamin E in as yet unknown sites. The vital role of these tissue components is exerted even though their concentrations are very low; metals and vitamins thus offer sensitive target systems through which extraneous control mechanisms can be exerted. The effects of such extraneous agents, or of deficiencies leading to clinical manifestations, are not always attributable simply to the oxidative functions in tissues. Thus, pellagra is a disease complex not obviously related to the deficiency of a dehydrogenation cofactor. On the other hand, the chemical reactivity of iron to cyanide or to carbon monoxide makes the symptoms of cyanide or carbon monoxide toxicity predictable: There is a generalized interference with tissue respiration which may lead to sudden suspension of life.

The electron transport systems are the main route by which the *energy* derived from the oxidation of a complex molecule is transferred to the metabolic patterns of the cell *in useful form.* The medium of energy transmission is usually a reactive chemical bonding, and its energy is further transmitted when the bond is broken or transferred. The chief "high-energy" bond is a phosphate link, as in ATP. The production of high-energy bonds via oxidations, *oxidative phosphorylation* (see above), is a mechanism not yet known in detail, but it is very sensitive to external physical or chemical agents, and here again is a crucial target system for external controls. Experimental evidence from animal tissues indicates that excessive levels of *thyroid hormones* increase the rate of oxidations but simultaneously diminish the production of high-energy phosphate; this suggests that hyperthyroidism may be viewed as *inefficient hyperoxidation,* rather than as hypermetabolism. However, the thyroid hormones have also been shown to inhibit certain dehydrogenating enzymes, malic dehydrogenase in particular.

METABOLIC AND ENZYMATIC ADAPTATION

The repeated or prolonged exposure of an organism to unusual and unfavorable environmental conditions frequently results in gradually improved tolerance for these conditions. This improved tolerance is frequently termed *adaptation,* more specifically *metabolic adaptation.* The exact nature of metabolic adaptation in any given instance is usually unknown and probably highly complex, comprising nutritional, endocrine, and neural regulation. In certain instances, however, it has been shown that among the factors contributing to the metabolic adaptation is a change in the enzymatic architecture of certain cells, resulting in increased or decreased concentrations of certain enzymes and, on occasion, in the appearance of new enzymes. This phenomenon, *enzymatic adaptation,* has been most frequently encountered and studied in microorganisms (e.g., adaptation of bacteria which ordinarily utilize glucose to other sugars such as galactose), but recent studies suggest that the induction of enzymes may play an important role in the adaptation of mammals to environmental changes. An excellent review of this field has been published by Knox, Auerbach, and Lin.

INTERMEDIARY METABOLISM IN DISEASE

It is likely that medical textbooks published 20 years hence will devote most of the available space to the consideration of metabolism in disease and of the means available to influence it. Already metabolic considerations form an important part of many of the chapters concerned with specific disease processes; the discussion here will be limited to pointing out briefly some of the areas where specific information concerning intermediary metabolism is presently available. It may be useful to consider three arbitrarily selected groups:

1. Diseases associated with a specific, demonstrated metabolic lesion which may be reasonably considered as causative.

2. Diseases whose primary metabolic nature is highly likely, although the specific metabolic lesion has not as yet been demonstrated

3. Diseases which may not be primarily metabolic but which result in metabolic anomalies which may become predominant and which may be remediable

The first group includes diseases determined by genetic factors (e.g., *galactosemia,* see Chap. 94; *glycogen-storage diseases,* see Chap. 94) or nutritional factors (e.g., *beriberi,* see Chap. 60). This group, as yet, is relatively small.

The second group is a large one and includes diseases about which a great deal of metabolic information is available, as well as diseases which have as yet been considered from a mainly descriptive point of view. *Many endocrine disorders* fall into this general category, as well as most nutritional disorders. Whereas in the case of *diabetes mellitus* it is almost possible to reconstitute the major features of the syndrome by starting from a single metabolic lesion (i.e., decreased glucose transport into *or* activation within certain tissues, see Chap. 70), it is as yet difficult to differentiate primary and secondary anomalies in endocrine disorders such as *Cushing's syndrome* (Chap. 68), *acromegaly* (Chap. 64), *thyrotoxicosis* (Chap. 66), *pellagra* (Chap. 59), or *potassium depletion.* It is of interest that several endocrine disorders can now be assigned to the first group, as in the case of several types of adrenogenital syndromes associated with inherited anomalies of steroidogenesis (Chap. 68), and several types of thyroid dysfunction are associated with anomalies of thyroidal iodine metabolism (Chap. 66).

The third group is best represented by the syndromes resulting from failure of specific organ systems, such as *renal, hepatic,* or *cardiac failure.* Some progress has been made in the study of the metabolic derangements involved, but much remains to be done. Questions may be raised with regard to the potential usefulness of this search, since these syndromes are *secondary* to failure of the organ system involved; however, it may be reasonable to point out that the defect presumably responsible for at least the juvenile form of diabetes mellitus is inadequate insulin *synthesis* (absolute or relative), a defect which we are as yet unable to correct; yet, by supplying the finished product, insulin, considerable therapeutic success can be achieved. Further disorders in this group include those associated with normal and neoplastic growth as well as those associated with aging.

REFERENCES

Barnett, R. J., and E. G. Ball: The Effect of Insulin on Adipose Tissue, Am. J. Clin. Nutrition, 8:666, 1960.

Cahill, G. F., Jr., B. Leboeuf, and A. E. Renold: Factors Concerned with the Regulation of Fatty Acid Metabolism by Adipose Tissue, Am. J. Clin. Nutrition, 8:733, 1960.

Chaikoff, I. L.: Metabolic Blocks in Carbohydrate Metabolism in Diabetes, Harvey Lectures, 47:99, 1951–1952.

"Ciba Symposium on Terpenes and Sterols," Boston, Little, Brown & Company, 1958.

Fredrickson, D. S., and R. S. Gordon: Transport of Fatty Acids, Physiol. Revs., 38:585, 1958.

Greenberg, D. M. (Ed.): "Metabolic Pathways," vols. 1 and 2, New York, Academic Press, 1960.

Green, D. E., and R. F. Goldberger: Pathways of Metabolism in Heart Muscle, Am. J. Med. 30:666, 1961.

Horecker, B. L., and H. H. Hiatt: Pathways of Carbohydrate Metabolism in Normal and Neoplastic Cells, New Engl. J. Med., 258:177, 1958.

Knox, W. E., V. H. Auerbach, and E. C. C. Lin: Enzymatic and Metabolic Adaptation in Animals, Physiol. Revs., 36:164, 1956.

Krebs, H. A., and H. L. Kornberg: A Survey of the Energy Transformations in Living Matter, Ergeb. Physiol., biol. Chem. u. exp. Pharmakol., 49:212, 1957.

Lynen, F.: Acetylcoenzyme A and the Fatty Acid Cycle, Harvey Lectures, 48:210, 1952–1953.

——, O. Henning, C. Bublitz, B. Sörbo, and L. Kröplin-Rueff: Der chemische Mechanismus der Acetessigsaurebildung in der Leber, Biochem. Z., 330, 269, 1958.

Noall, M. W., T. R. Riggs, L. M. Walker, and H. N. Christensen: Endocrine Control of Amino Acid Transfer, Science, 126:1002, 1957.

Park, C. R., H. E. Morgan, M. J. Henderson, D. M. Regen, E. Cadenas, and R. L. Post: The Regulation of Glucose Uptake in Muscle as Studied in the Perfused Rat Heart. Recent Progr. in Hormone Research, 17:493, 1961.

Renold, A. E., J. Ashmore, and A. B. Hastings: Regulation of Carbohydrate Metabolism in Isolated Tissues, Vitamins and Hormones, 14:139, 1958.

Ross, E. J.: The "Permeability" Hypothesis of the Action of Insulin, Medicine, 35:355, 1956.

Siperstein, M. D.: Inter-relationships of Glucose and Lipid Metabolism, Am. J. Med., 26:685, 1959.

——: The Homeostatic Control of Cholesterol Synthesis in Liver, Am. J. Clin. Nutrition, 8:645, 1960.

Stanbury, J. B., J. B. Wyngaarden, and D. S. Fredrickson: "The Metabolic Basis of Inherited Diseases," New York, McGraw-Hill Book Company, Inc., Blakiston Division, 1960.

Stetten, DeW., Jr.: Thermodynamic, Kinetic and Biologic Stability, Am. J. Med., 13:251, 1952.

—— and M. R. Stetten: Glycogen Metabolism, Physiol. Rev., 40:505, 1960.

Villar-Palasi, C., and J. Larner: Insulin-mediated Effect on the Activity of UDPG Glycogen Transglucosylase of Muscle, Biochim. Biophys. Acta, 39: 171, 1960.

Wakil, S. J.: The Mechanism of Fatty Acid Synthesis, Am. J. Clin. Nutrition, 8:630, 1960.

Wertheimer, E., and E. Shafrir: Influence of Hormones on Adipose Tissue as a Center of Fat Metabolism, Recent Progr. in Hormone Research, 16:467, 1960.

Zamecnik, P.: Historical and Current Aspects of the Problems of Protein Synthesis, Harvey Lectures, 65:256, 1960.

53 METALS AND METABOLISM
Bert L. Vallee

The role of inorganic constituents, other than the so-called electrolytes, in the physiology, intermediary metabolism, and pathology of man merits attention. More than 60 elements have been discovered in bacteria, fungi, higher plants, animals, and man. Few of these elements have been studied intensively. Investigation has necessarily been restricted to those occurring in amounts large enough to be measurable, even if not always precisely, by available techniques: calcium, carbon, chlorine, hydrogen, iodine, iron, nitrogen, oxygen, phosphorus, potassium, sodium, sulfur, and magnesium (although the last has presented difficulties in analysis).

Trace elements, micronutrients, microelements, minor elements, and *oligelements* are terms applied to the remaining elements occurring in biologic systems in minute quantities.

The following are generally included among the trace elements: aluminum, antimony, arsenic, barium, boron, bromine, cadmium, chromium, cobalt, copper, fluorine, gallium, lead, lithium, manganese, mercury, molybdenum, nickel, rubidium, silver, strontium, tin, titanium, vanadium, and zinc. These elements have been grouped together quite arbitrarily. They have in common (1) the difficulty of measurement in biologic fluids because of low concentration, which varies from 1×10^{-6} to less than 1×10^{-12} Gm per Gm wet organ, and (2) a resistance to definitive appraisal as to physiologic function.

Determination of the concentration of trace elements, like that of other metabolites, in tissues, cells, subcellular particles, and fluids is a corollary to the elucidation of their role in disease. This knowledge has awaited the development of techniques and methods permitting the determination of minute concentrations of elements with precision. Through advances in chemical and physical knowledge, gained as recently as the past decade, great strides have been made in the design of techniques and methods which make possible precise determination of minute concentrations of elements. More important yet, these technical advances have permitted the formulation and testing of hypotheses not previously susceptible to experimentation.

BIOCHEMISTRY AND PHYSICAL CHEMISTRY

The search for an explanation of the physiologic role of the trace elements has emphasized their association with enzyme systems in living cells. For operational purposes the enzymes which are affected by metals can be considered in two groups: *metalloenzymes* and *metal-enzyme complexes.*

A *metalloenzyme* contains a metal as an integral part of the molecule (Table 53-1). There is a fixed amount of metal per molecule of protein. The metal cannot be separated from the protein by mild procedures. When the element is split from the protein residue by more vigorous manipulation, all measur-

Table 53-1. METALLOPROTEINS ISOLATED FROM HUMAN AND OTHER SOURCES

Protein	Metal	μg metal per Gm protein	Source	Year isolated
Hemoglobin	Iron	3,350	Equine erythrocyte	1886
Myoglobin	Iron	3,450	Equine myocardium	1932
Chlorocruorin	Iron	12,000	*Spirographis spallansanii*	1933
Catalase	Iron	900	Equine liver	1938
Cytochrome C	Iron	4,300	Bovine myocardium	1939
Verdoperoxidase	Iron	1,000	Human leukocytes	1941
Peroxidase	Iron	1,200	*Armoracia rusticana*	1942
Lactoperoxidase	Iron	900	Bovine milk	1944
Hemocyanin (sycotypin)	Copper	2,450	*Helix pomatia*	1933
		2,450	*Busycon canaliculatum*	
		2,500	*Octopus vulgaris*	
		2,600	*Loligo peali*	
		1,730	*Limulus polyphemus*	
		1,870	*Homarus americanus*	
Hemocuprein	Copper	3,400	Bovine erythrocyte	1938
Hepatocuprein	Copper	2,500	Bovine liver	1938
Tyrosinase	Copper	3,000	Psalliota	1938
Ascorbic acid oxidase	Copper	2,500	*Cucumis sativus*	1940
Laccase	Copper	2,500	*Rhus vernicifera*	1940
Milkcuproprotein	Copper	1,900	Bovine milk	1942
Ceruloplasmin	Copper	3,200	Human serum	1948
Hepatocuprein	Copper	2,350	Equine liver	1954
Erythrocuprein	Copper	3,400	Human erythrocytes	1959
Cerebrocuprein I	Copper	2,900	Human brain	1959
Carbonic anhydrase	Zinc	2,100	Bovine erythrocyte	1940
Leukocyte Zn protein	Zinc	3,000	Human leukocytes	1954
Carboxypeptidase A	Zinc	2,000	Bovine pancreatic juice	1954
Alcohol dehydrogenase	Zinc	1,800	Yeast	1955
Alcohol dehydrogenase	Zinc	1,820	Equine liver	1956
Glutamic dehydrogenase	Zinc	260	Bovine liver	1955
Lactic dehydrogenase	Zinc	700	Rabbit muscle	1956
Alkaline phosphatase	Zinc	1,500	Porcine kidney	1959
Alkaline phosphatase	Zinc	1,800–2,400	*Escherichia coli*	1960
Carboxypeptidase B	Zinc	1,900	Porcine pancreas	1960
Metallothionein	Cadmium	50,000	Equine kidney cortex	1960
	Zinc	10,000		

able biologic activity is lost and is not readily restored by readdition of this or any other metal. Some metals are parts of prosthetic groups, as found in hemoglobin, catalase, or peroxidase. Table 53-1 summarizes the small group of known metalloproteins, with and without known enzymatic function, which are sufficiently characterized to be considered "pure." Though only a few of these metalloproteins, which may be considered as a class of biochemical substances, have been obtained from human sources, their significance with respect to the biochemistry, physiology, and pathology of man is becoming increasingly clearer, since their action in different species constitutes a common biologic denominator.

If hemovanadin, a vanadium-containing protein of ascidian blood, as yet incompletely characterized, is also included, it is seen that these metalloproteins incorporate transition elements between atomic numbers 23 to 30. Only these metals have thus far been found to be joined to proteins by bonds sufficiently strong to allow their isolation as metalloproteins. Proteins containing the elements 24 (Cr), 27 (Co), and 28 (Ni) are missing from Table 53-1; they have now been found in substantial concentrations in ribonucleic acids. Thus these elements may play an important though as yet undetermined role in protein synthesis, a presumable function of some ribonucleic acids. Similarly, cadmium, very similar to zinc in many respects, has been found in concentrations of 5 per cent in a protein of the renal cortex, suggesting a biologic role for this element. The biologic significance of cobalt has already been amply demonstrated, though no cobalt-containing protein has thus far been isolated; instead, it has been found to be an essential component of the vitamin B_{12} group, the cobalamins. Structurally, chemically, and biologically similar metalloenzymes are found in a variety of phyla, demonstrating that these enzymes are significant in the biochemical processes of species of widely diversified evolutionary histories, and thereby indicating their general metabolic importance.

Most of these metalloproteins have been shown to have specific enzymatic functions. Study of their enzymatic properties has usually preceded demonstration of their metal content, probably because until very recently methods for enzyme activities have been more sensitive than the methods for the small quantities of metals involved. Moreover, the purification and isolation of enzymes and other proteins from complex tissues has reached a high degree of perfection only quite recently. In certain cases, however, this course of events has been reversed. Thus, cytochromes and ceruloplasmin were isolated on the basis of their physical-chemical properties, were found to contain a metal, and subsequently were shown to have important implications for metabolic processes. The oxygen-transporting agents contain a metal, and some metalloproteins act as storage or transport agents for metals, or perhaps as hormones.

This group of metalloenzymes may be contrasted with metal-enzyme complexes.

Metal-enzyme complexes compose a far larger group of enzymes that are very loosely associated with a metal, the criterion of association being the *activation* of catalysis. In this group, the specificity of the association is lacking. The metals may be removed, and different ones may substitute for one another in many instances. The metal ion is not an integral part of the molecule, and in most instances the enzyme is apparently active in the absence of the metal ion. These facts increase the difficulties of assessing the *biologic* significance of these in vitro findings. Some investigators have considered the difference between these two groups of metal-enzyme systems to be a matter only of degree and not of kind; a continuous spectrum of the firmness of association between metal and protein has been postulated, with metalloenzymes at one end, and metal-enzyme complexes at the other, but both having similar biochemical function. Other workers

have emphasized the dissimilarities. Whatever the hypotheses, operationally the metalloenzyme group lends itself more readily to a definitive assessment of the physiologic role of metal-enzyme systems at this time, since experimentally, the element and the enzyme may be studied jointly in vitro and in vivo, the inherent specificity of their association lending biologic significance to the results.

Even though there are great difficulties in physiologic interpretation of work with the enzyme-metal complexes, great advances may be expected once a satisfactory experimental procedure for the further elucidation of their mechanism of action is evolved. Their importance in the understanding of catalytic phenomena cannot be stressed sufficiently.

MEDICAL IMPLICATIONS

In the minds of many investigators, iron, iodine, and fluorine have virtually been removed from the group considered as trace elements, and their medical significance is no longer questioned. In a 70-kg individual there are a total of 4 to 5 Gm iron and 30 to 60 mg iodine. This may be contrasted with about 20 Gm magnesium, 2 Gm zinc, and about 100 to 150 mg copper in the same individual; these latter are considered trace elements at present. It is clear that concentration of an element in biologic matter is *not* the sole criterion of either its importance in health and disease, or the extent of knowledge concerning it.

Unlike the highly colored iron and copper complexes and proteins and the violet iodine fumes, compounds of zinc, cadmium, or magnesium are colorless and do not attract attention, complicating the identification or recognition of these elements in biologic materials. Since these last elements, and others, have become measurable by adequate analytic, chemical means quite recently, knowledge of their significance to medical problems is of similarly recent origin.

The identification of a number of zinc enzymes during the last few years, for example, has brought about unexpected fundamental knowledge to serve as the basis for clinical exploration, replacing the empiricism previously necessary. The relationship of iron to anemia, iodine to thyroid disease, cobalt to pernicious anemia, and copper to Wilson's disease is too obvious to require emphasis, except to point out that we can soon expect much new knowledge of similar significance concerning other metals and diseases.

The subsequent discussion is concerned with cadmium, cobalt, copper, fluorine, magnesium, and zinc. Neither their toxicology nor data from mammalian physiology are considered.

COBALT

Physiology. The study of the function of cobalt in human physiology is an excellent example of the anomalous state of trace element research. A great deal of information has been accumulated concerning the *effect* of this element on health and disease of animals and man, particularly in erythropoiesis, while knowledge of the element's natural *occurrence* is quite fragmentary.

All attempts to show that cobalt has physiologic significance in animals other than ruminants and man have at best yielded equivocal answers. The discovery in 1948 that the anti-pernicious anemia factor contains 4 per cent of cobalt stimulated investigation of the function of cobalt as part of this vitamin.

The daily requirement of cobalt in man is unknown, though about 0.1 μg cobalt per day would be sufficient to supply the amount needed to synthesize an adequate amount of vitamin B_{12}. A normal diet supplies about 5 to 8 μg per day. In view of the small quantities of cobalt present, its quantification has been a major problem, and many data that have been presented are of dubious value. In animals, orally ingested or intravenously administered cobalt is excreted primarily in the urine. The greater part of ingested cobalt is not absorbed, but is excreted in the stool, and the fraction retained is concentrated mostly in the liver and kidneys. The

mode of storage is, however, uncertain. Much of this work has been done by studying the distribution of radioactive Co^{58} or Co^{60} rather than by chemical analysis.

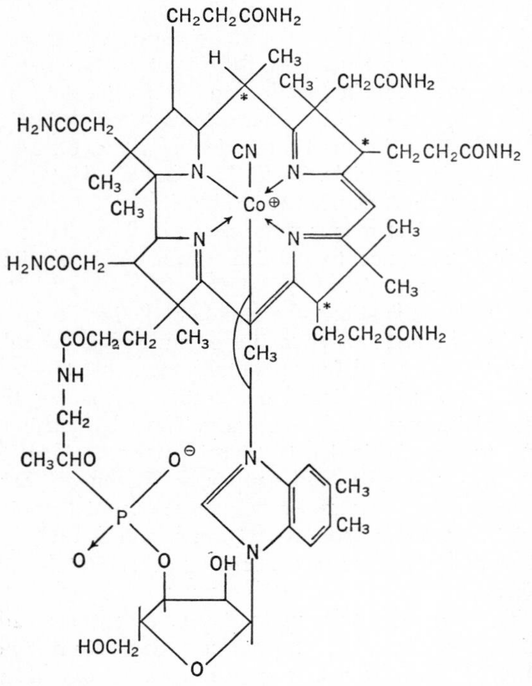

The cobalt concentration of human plasma is about 60 to 80 $\mu\mu$g per ml and that of whole blood 80 to 300 $\mu\mu$g per ml. While the determination of cobalt itself at these concentrations is a difficult analytic problem, its estimation by bioassay, when it is part of vitamin B_{12}, has become a clinical test in recent years (see Chap. 235).

Biochemistry. Vitamin B_{12} and Related Compounds. Vitamin B_{12} and vitamins $B_{12a\text{-}d}$ contain about 4 per cent cobalt and are termed *cobalamins;* derivatives are named according to the cobalt coordination complex present, e.g., cyanocobalamins, hydroxycobalamins, etc. No distinction will be made between the effect of vitamin B_{12} and its closely related compounds. The chemical structure of this vitamin was elucidated in 1955 and is shown in Fig. 53-1. The porphyrin ring differs from those typical of the hemes. The side chains are structurally similar to those of several coenzymes. Vitamin B_{12} is now known to function as a coenzyme in the synthesis of the methyl group of methionine from formaldehyde, the decomposition of glutamate by way of β-methylaspartate, and in the exchange of succinate and propionate in the presence of biotin. Coenzyme B_{12} can be isolated from bacteria, particularly *Proprioni bacterium shermanii,* and from the livers of various animals. The structure of coenzyme B_{12} is similar to that of the vitamin except that the cyano group, linked to cobalt, is replaced by an adenine nucleoside. Several hypotheses have been formulated to explain the pharmacologic action of vitamin B_{12} and its interrelation with folic acid.

Vitamin B_{12} causes a remission of pernicious anemia when administered parenterally in microgram quantities. In pernicious anemia, iron, zinc, and copper metabolism are disturbed, and it is of some, if at present only philosophical, interest to note that their metabolism is restored to normality by a cobalt-containing substance (see Chap. 235).

The vitamin B_{12} content of normal human serum has been stated to vary from 100 to 900 $\mu\mu$g per ml, whereas patients with pernicious anemia have levels from less than 10 to 110 $\mu\mu$g per ml, i.e., a hypocobaltemia.

Cobalt and Polycythemia. Very small quantities of cobalt in metallic or ionic form, when ingested, will produce a true polycythemia in rats, mice, guinea pigs, rabbits, dogs, pigs, chickens, ducks, and frogs. The development of this polycythemia is apparently independent of other metals but is inhibited or prevented by cystine, methionine, cysteine, histidine, choline, nicotinamide, and ascorbic

FIG. 53-1. The structure of the vitamin B_{12} molecule.

acid. The administration of cobalt has been reported to lower the ascorbic acid, sugar, and glutathione levels of blood serum.

The mechanism of this polycythemia and its relationship to polycythemia vera is unexplained.

While a true polycythemia of the magnitude observed in polycythemia vera, or following the administration of cobalt in animals, has not been observed in man, an increase in *erythrocyte mass* and hemoglobin of normal individuals has been described by several observers. It has been speculated that the erythrocyte changes represent adaptations to a relative hypoxia induced in the bone marrow because of oxygen-binding complexes of cobalt with histidine and cysteine. However, no chemical evidence for this or other theoretic propositions has been brought forth. Current evidence favors the view that the polycythemia is produced by a circulating erythropoietic factor.

The use of cobalt in certain anemias of man is, at present, almost entirely restricted to investigative efforts. Beneficial effects have been reported in the anemia of infection and in anemia associated with chronic nephritis and azotemia, while the administration of inorganic cobalt salts has no effect on pernicious or other macrocytic anemias. Cobalt has been claimed, however, to cause thyroid enlargement, though this has been doubted by others. Caution in its indiscriminate use as a pharmacologic agent seems indicated at this time.

COPPER

Physiology. The normal copper intake of man is estimated at 2.5 to 5 mg per day, an amount adequate for the maintenance of positive copper balance. Normally, a very small amount, 0 to 100 μg, of copper is excreted in the urine per 24-hr volume, independently of the intake. The balance is excreted through the bile and stool. The total amount of copper in the body is about 100 to 150 mg. Copper is found in all human tissues, varying from about 3 to 45 μg per Gm dry weight. Spleen, lung, bone, adrenal, kidney, spinal cord, voluntary and heart muscle, and intestine vary between 3 and 18 μg per Gm, while various areas of the brain contain between about 20 and 30 μg of copper per Gm dry weight of tissue. Adult liver contains about 45 μg per Gm, though fetal liver may contain as much as five to ten times as much. On a normal diet copper is not accumulated preferentially by any tissue.

Human whole blood contains about 100 μg per 100 ml copper, distributed about equally between cells and plasma. The copper content of leukocytes is insignificant when compared to that of erythro-cytes and plasma. The serum copper level in normal individuals is very constant, varying by no more than 5 per cent over periods of a month; it is independent of age, sex, the menstrual cycle, food intake, diurnal or seasonal influences, and tissue stores.

The serum copper level rises slowly during the first trimester of pregnancy and increases at an accelerated rate until parturition. Serum copper levels of 250 to 300 μg per 100 ml and above are reached. Following parturition, the serum copper level returns to normal within 2 to 3 weeks.

The serum copper concentration of human infants at birth is low compared with that of adults and has been reported to vary between 50 and 75 μg per 100 ml. The copper content of erythrocytes in the newborn is normal.

The relationship of copper to iron metabolism has long been a subject of great interest but has recently received renewed emphasis. Copper influences heme synthesis, and its deficiency apparently reduces iron absorption. The copper level in tissues seems to be a more important factor in this relationship than the copper level in the diet. The deficiency of copper apparently results in a failure to utilize iron for hemoglobin synthesis and in the production of red cells with shortened survival time. The significance of these investigative efforts to the physiology and pathology of man has not yet been scrutinized adequately. A relationship between molybdenum and copper metabolism in ruminants has also aroused interest but has not been studied in man.

Biochemistry. Copper Proteins and Copper-protein Complexes. *Ceruloplasmin.* It has been shown that well over 90 per cent of all copper in human serum is associated with ceruloplasmin, a specific copper protein isolated and named by Holmberg and Laurell. The protein has a molecular weight of 151,000 and contains 8 atoms of copper per molecule, equivalent to 0.32 per cent copper per gram dry weight of protein. The copper atoms of ceruloplasmin can be removed in the presence of ascorbic acid. The copper-free, colorless apoceruloplasmin recombines with cuprous ions to form ceruloplasmin. The metalloprotein has a characteristic spectrophotometric absorption and oxidizes paraphenylenediamine, benzidine, and other phenols including catecholamines. A good correlation between the copper content of serum and its capacity to oxidize these substances has been shown.

Six distinct ceruloplasmins have been demonstrated on the basis of chromatography and electrophoresis. The remainder of the serum copper has been described as "loosely bound," and its possible interaction with serum proteins is the subject of active investigation.

Hemocuprein. This blue copper protein of molecular weight 35,000, containing 0.34 per cent of copper per gram dry weight of protein (Table 53-1), has been isolated by Keilin and Mann from erythrocytes of the ox, sheep, and horse. It is probably closely related to, if not identical with, a protein from human erythrocytes, erythrocuprein.

Erythrocuprein. This faintly greenish-blue protein of human erythrocytes was isolated by Markowitz, Cartwright, and Wintrobe in 1958. The molecular weight is about 33,000, and it contains 0.32 to 0.36 per cent copper per gram dry weight protein. It is distinctly different from ceruloplasmin and accounts for virtually all the copper of erythrocytes. The function of this protein is presently unknown, and alterations in disease have not yet been reported.

Hepatocuprein. Hepatocuprein, another metalloprotein (Table 53-1), has been obtained from bovine and equine liver; it is colorless. Though hemocuprein and hepatocuprein are thought to be intimately related substances, they are differentiated because of their difference in color. No enzymatic activity or physiologic function is known for hepatocuprein, but, like hemocuprein, it is thought to represent an important step in copper metabolism.

Cerebrocuprein I. This bluish-green protein from human and bovine brain was isolated by Porter and Folch in 1957. The molecular weight is between 30,000 and 40,000; it contains 0.25 to 0.3 per cent copper. Extracts of brains from patients with hepatolenticular degeneration (see Chap. 93) contain an abnormal copper-protein compound which is isolated together with cerebrocuprein I. A protein with high copper affinity has also been demonstrated in the liver of such patients by Uzman.

Tyrosinase. Tyrosinase or phenoloxidase activity has been found in the melanocytes of human skin and melanoma tissue. The enzymatic activity is associated with the mitochondrial elements of this cell and is responsible for melanin pigment formation. A pure preparation of the enzyme has been obtained from mushrooms; it has a molecular weight of about 34,000 and contains 0.2 per cent copper. The skin of albino human beings possesses no detectable tyrosinase activity, indicating that a deficiency of this enzyme is responsible for the absence of pigment found in the skin and the uveal tract.

Other Cuproproteins. Copper was suggested to be a component of cytochrome oxidase as long as 20 years ago. The definitive demonstration has been a subject of continuing controversy, though recent evidence would seem to confirm the presence of both 1 Gm atom of copper and of iron per mole of enzyme. This is of some interest in view of the decrease in cytochrome oxidase activities in copper deficiency.

A variety of copper enzymes (most of them oxidases) found in plants and animals is suspected to play a role in human biochemistry. Though enzymatic activity for some of them has been found in man, the structural presence of the enzyme has not always been unequivocally identified.

Beta Metal-combining Globulin (Fraction IV-7). This protein, identified as the iron-binding protein of human serum, has been shown to form complexes with copper in vitro. However, at physiologic pH, the protein has a higher affinity for iron, which readily displaces copper. The physiologic significance of this observation is questionable.

Chemical Pathology. Changes in blood copper concentrations are generally due to changes in the *serum* or *plasma* content, the erythrocyte content remaining stable.

INCREASE OF COPPER. The copper level is increased in acute, as well as chronic, infectious disease: the common cold, tonsillitis, pharyngitis, pneumonia, scarlet fever, diphtheria, rheumatic fever, rheumatoid arthritis, acute nephritis, infectious hepatitis, septicemia, subacute bacterial endocarditis, lung abscess, tuberculosis, and brucellosis. Copper levels of 200 μg per 100 ml and above are not unusual, and they return to normal upon recovery. Marked elevations of the serum copper level have been noted in myocardial infarction and acute leukemia, and less dramatic ones in hyperthyroidism, chronic leukemia, and Laennec's cirrhosis. Elevations of the serum copper level of lesser magnitude have been noted in pernicious anemia, aplastic anemia, thalassemia, sickle-cell anemia, iron-deficiency anemia, and hemochromatosis. Hypercupremia has been observed in hepatitis, cirrhosis, chronic alcoholism, pellagra, carcinoma of the lung, pancreas, uterus, rectum, liver, stomach, esophagus, in Hodgkin's disease, and lymphosarcoma.

The suggestion, first advanced in 1941, that schizophrenia is accompanied by hypercupremia has since been repeatedly confirmed and denied. In 1957, Ackerfeldt reported that an increase of ceruloplasmin in the serums of schizophrenic patients could serve as an aid in the diagnosis of schizophrenia and other mental diseases. Many workers have now shown this conclusion to be incorrect and to be based on inadequate selection of patients and controls.

Correlation between hypercupremia and increase in the erythrocyte sedimentation rate has been claimed. Though coexistence can undoubtedly be observed, efforts at correlation, symptomatically or etiologically, are quite unconvincing.

Though androgens and estrogens cause hypercupremia and increase the ceruloplasmin concentrations of serum, a precise hormonal control mechanism is not as yet known, however. Thyroid and pituitary hormone—melanotropin and corticotropin—also seem to exert a regulatory effect.

The significance of hypercupremia has been subjected to close scrutiny but without marked success. Serum copper level is remarkably stable in healthy individuals, and thus deviations in certain physiologic and many pathologic states take on special interest.

Such findings as have been reported are of empirical value. No physiologic function in copper metabolism has been found thus far for the β_1-metal-combining globulin. The mode of binding of "loosely bound" copper and its possible relation to this protein are not clear.

DECREASE OF SERUM COPPER. Decrease of ceruloplasmin and, usually, hypocupremia seem to be characteristic of Wilson's disease, as is the deposition of copper in the cornea (Kayser-Fleischer ring). The physiologic role of copper in relation to this process is discussed elsewhere in Chap. 93. Decrease of serum copper concentrations has also been reported in dysproteinemia of infants. This uncommon malady of infants is characterized by edema, hypoproteinemia, anemia, hypoferremia, hypocupremia, and reduction of ceruloplasmin concentrations. Two types are observed which are thought to differ in their etiology. The depression in serum proteins in one group is thought to be due to a decreased concentration of albumin, while in the second, both albumin and globulins are diminished. Decreased concentrations of ceruloplasmin are also seen in kwashiorkor, celiac disease, tropical and nontropical sprue, the nephrotic syndrome, idiopathic hypoproteinemia, and intestinal scleroderma. Though hypoferremia was present, normal serum copper levels were found in prisoners of war on grossly inadequate diets.

CHANGES IN ERYTHROCYTE COPPER. Red cell copper may decrease in hyperthyroidism and increase as a result of intravenous injection of copper salts. Mean corpuscular copper increases in pernicious anemia while the copper concentration per cell remains normal.

Changes in copper concentrations of tissues, particularly liver and brain, have been observed in a variety of clinical conditions, but these findings have not explained the disease process or the physiologic role of copper.

URINE. Hypercupruria accompanied by aminoaciduria has been found in Wilson's disease (see Chap. 93). Hypercupruria due to urinary excretion of as much as 5 per cent of the total, normal ceruloplasmin is seen in the nephrotic syndrome, which is also accompanied by increased urinary elimination of iron. Ceruloplasmin accounts for 60 to 80 per cent of the copper excreted by these patients. Ceruloplasmin is not detected in the urine of normal individuals.

FLUORINE

Physiology. Fluorides occur in small amounts in all foods and most mineral water. The "normal" fluorine intake from water and food ranges from 0.5 to 4.0 mg fluorine per day. The level of intake is dependent upon the source of the water and the make-up of the diet. Sea food, fish, and tea are sources of exceptionally high amounts of fluorine. No measurable storage of fluorine occurs on an intake of 0.6 mg per day. Fluorine is excreted primarily through the urine. A 24-hr specimen of urine closely reflects the fluorine content of the ingested fluoride. Perspiration may account for an appreciable part of fluorine excretion. The blood fluoride concentration varies from 10 to 40 mμg per ml.

The element is taken up preferentially by osseous and dental tissues, the amount deposited being a function of the chemical mode of occurrence of fluorine and the quantities ingested. The amount laid down in bone increases with age. Bones take up fluoride throughout life, and considerable quantities may be deposited on a high fluorine intake by the time advanced age is reached. However, on lowering the intake the element is readily mobilized. The normal average bone content is stated to be 0.5 to 2.1 μg per Gm. The fluorine content of the enamel of normal teeth is about 100 μg per Gm, while that of dentine has been estimated at about 330 μg per Gm. Fluorides are not readily transferred across the placenta. The debate on the *essentiality* of fluorine to human physiology has been caused by studies relating it to *dental caries, dental fluorosis* (mottled enamel), and *fluorotic osteosclerosis*.

Chemical Pathology. Dental Caries. The development of dental caries has been shown to bear a definite inverse relationship to the fluorine intake during the formative period of tooth development. Teeth take up fluorine only during their formative period (up to twelve to fourteen years of age), though recent evidence indicates that the outermost, superficial layers of the enamel may contain as much as five- to tenfold as much fluorine as the innermost layers. This suggests that only a small amount of fluoride is laid down in the inner bulk of the enamel during its formation but that the surface of the unerupted tooth continues to accumulate the element, serving as a protective coating. Dental integrity for adult life seems to be ensured during this early period, and increasing the fluorine intake thereafter protects the teeth against decay in only 15 per cent of cases studied; some fluoride still continues to accumulate but only in the outermost layers and at an exceedingly slow rate. Thus fluoride seems to prevent caries as a surface protective agent.

One part per million of fluorine in water seems

to ensure an optimal daily fluorine intake to safeguard the integrity of teeth. The intake of the element will vary somewhat depending upon local geologic conditions, water intake, diet, and climate. The fluorine intake will reflect itself in the fluorine content of dentine and enamel.

Extensive epidemiologic investigations have positively established the relationship between fluorine and dental caries, and the partial prevention of caries by this element. The findings are resulting in the addition of fluorides to many communal water supplies, similar to the addition of iodides to table salt. A level of 1 ppm fluorine in drinking water is generally considered safe in Northern temperate regions: "*eufluorosis*," the point of maximum health with maximum safety. Many doubtful objections to this valuable public health measure have, however, been raised because of the suspected toxicity of the element.

Dental Fluorosis (*Mottled Enamel*) *and Fluorotic Osteosclerosis.* In the case of high fluoride intake from water supplies with 2 to 8 ppm, or foods exceptionally high in fluorine content, dental fluorosis develops in growing teeth. This affliction is the most delicate index of fluoride toxicity. Its signs are opaque white spots or bands distributed irregularly over the surface of the teeth; they occur at sustained levels of fluorine intake of 2 ppm. The opacities turn brown at prolonged fluoride ingestion of 4 ppm or more. At higher intakes, hypoplasia of the enamel over all surfaces is seen; surfaces subject to attrition show marked wear, with prominent, discrete, or confluent pitting. There is a direct relationship between magnitude of exposure to fluoride and severity of response. Mottled enamel due to high fluorine ingestion can be produced only during the period of tooth development.

Prolonged high fluorine intake in adults results in skeletal abnormalities, which begin as thickening of the trabeculae and eventually manifest themselves as osteosclerosis, osteopetrosis, and exostosis of the long bones, vertebras, pelvis, jaw, and flat bones. The condition eventually leads to calcification of tendons and ligaments and almost complete synostosis of various joints. There follow restriction of motion, "stiff back," pain, embarrassment of thoracic respiration, cachexia, and anorexia. The condition is eventually fatal. Changes in the dermal appendages may be attributable to the same process, but their etiologic relationship to it needs to be sustained.

Since fluorine is an effective inhibitor of a large number of enzymes, the explanation of its physiologic and pathologic effects is very likely to be expected from studies of its role in regulating enzyme action.

Public Health Measure. It cannot be stated with certainty that fluorine is *directly* related to the integrity of human teeth. The mechanisms which induce dental caries *may* be only indirectly connected with fluorine metabolism. However, the adjustment of drinking water to 1 ppm of fluorine is doubtless the soundest and most effective preventive measure known at present and should be instituted wherever possible. There is no convincing evidence that this course of action causes any deleterious systemic effects.

ZINC

Physiology. The normal human zinc intake of 10 to 15 mg per day is excreted mainly through the stool which contains about 10 mg per day, while the urine contains 0.4 mg per day.

The total amount of zinc in the body has been estimated at 2 to 3 Gm. Zinc is found in all human tissues, varying from 10 to 200 μg per Gm wet weight. Most organs, including the pancreas, contain 20 to 30 μg. Liver, voluntary muscle, and bone contain 60 to 180 μg. Large quantities of zinc have been found in corneal epithelium, the iris, retina, and lens. Zinc is not accumulated preferentially by any tissue, though the prostate, prostatic secretions, and spermatozoa are remarkably high in their content of zinc, which is not accounted for by their content of either carbonic anhydrase or phosphatase.

Human whole blood contains about 900 μg zinc per 100 ml. Normal serum zinc levels range from about 80 to 160 μg per 100 ml and average 121 μg per 100 ml. Normal erythrocytes contain 1.44 mg per cc of packed red blood cells. Three per cent of all blood zinc is found in human leukocytes, which contain 3.2×10^{-2} μg zinc per million cells, about twenty-five times more than is found in comparable numbers of erythrocytes. Blood zinc concentrations do not exhibit seasonal or diurnal variations, and there is no difference in concentration between the sexes. Claims for changes in blood zinc concentrations of pregnant women do not appear justified.

The zinc content of erythrocytes of newborn infants is only about 25 per cent of that found in adults; zinc has been shown to be transferred across the placenta.

Biochemistry. Zinc is closely associated with various proteins. Since several different zinc proteins may be present in most organs, total zinc content of tissues is no guide to functions of the metal, which may be manifold. A considerable number of zinc enzymes and two complexes of proteins with zinc have been shown to be of importance in human metabolism.

Zinc Proteins and Zinc-protein Complexes. *Carbonic Anhydrase.* This enzyme catalyzes the reaction $CO_2 + H_2O \rightleftharpoons H_2CO_3$. It is present in erythrocytes in high concentration, and many tissues exhibit activity to catalyze this reaction. Without this enzyme, carbon dioxide elimination could not take place with sufficient rapidity to sustain life; it is as important to carbon dioxide transport as is hemoglobin to oxygen transport. Carbonic anhydrase is a metalloenzyme and contains a fixed amount of zinc per gram dry weight of protein. When purified from ox erythrocytes, it contains 0.21 per cent zinc, which does not exchange freely against ionic zinc. The zinc content of human carbonic anhydrase is not known. In blood, all carbonic anhydrase activity is found in erythrocytes; none has been found in serum or leukocytes, though such activity has been detected in many other tissues. Close correlation has been obtained between the zinc content and enzyme activity in red blood cells under both normal and pathologic conditions.

Zinc-containing Protein of Human Leukocytes. A protein from human leukocytes contains 0.3 per cent of zinc per gram dry weight of protein. It is responsible for 80 per cent of all zinc found in human leukocytes and has been differentiated clearly from carbonic anhydrase. A zinc-containing alkaline phosphatase, recently isolated from leukocytes, may well be identical with this protein.

Carboxypeptidase. Carboxypeptidase A and B of bovine pancreatic juice have recently been shown to be zinc enzymes. The enzymes contain 1 atom of zinc per molecule of protein. Zinc is firmly bound to the proteins and is apparently indispensable for their enzymatic activities, thus constituting a prosthetic group. In carboxypeptidase A, zinc has been shown to be bound to sulfur and nitrogen. These findings seem to explain previous observations demonstrating that about 6.5 per cent of a dose of radioactive zinc administered to dogs was found in their pancreatic juice within 5 days. Zinc, at least in part, is eliminated into the gastrointestinal tract as carboxypeptidase; it is thus implicated in proteolysis.

Zinc-containing Dehydrogenases. Four enzymes responsible for dehydrogenation reactions have been shown to contain zinc that is essential for their action. All four enzymes are dependent upon diphosphopyridine nucleotide (DPN) for their activity: alcohol dehydrogenase of yeast, alcohol dehydrogenase of horse liver, glutamic dehydrogenase of beef liver, and lactic dehydrogenase of rabbit skeletal muscle. Yeast alcohol dehydrogenase contains 4 atoms of zinc per molecule of protein; alcohol dehydrogenase of horse liver contains 2; and glutamic dehydrogenase of beef liver contains 2 to 4 zinc atoms. The molecular weight of lactic dehydrogenase of rabbit skeletal muscle is not known; thus, no figure for the molar ratio of zinc to protein can be given. All four enzymes have been crystallized. The zinc is firmly bound and is essential to the action of these enzymes.

The detection of zinc in these enzymes may explain the high concentrations of this element in the liver and the retina, since it has been shown that alcohol dehydrogenase of horse liver oxidizes vitamin A_1 and reduces retinene, probably being identical with retinene reductase. Thus far, no other metals have been identified with certainty in similar dehydrogenases. These findings were the first indication that zinc is in any way associated with their catalytic action, thus implicating this metal for the first time in cellular oxidation. There is presumptive evidence that many other pyridine nucleotide dependent dehydrogenases may contain zinc or another metal.

Alkaline Phosphatase. Both the alkaline phosphatase of porcine kidney and that of *Escherichia coli* have been demonstrated to contain stoichiometric quantities of zinc which is essential to their activity. A decrease in the activity of this enzyme had long been noted in zinc-deficient experimental animals, a change which may now be attributed to a failure of synthesis of the active holoenzyme.

Zinc-protein Complexes. In blood serum, zinc exists in at least two fractions: firmly bound zinc, amounting to about 34 per cent, and loosely bound zinc, amounting to 66 per cent of the total zinc content. The firmly bound zinc protein, a globulin, satisfies the criteria of metalloproteins, whereas the loosely bound zinc protein should be defined as a metal-protein complex. The firmly bound zinc protein has not been purified adequately to state the percentage of zinc that it contains. Neither substance has been shown to exhibit enzymatic properties. The loosely bound complex appears to be concerned primarily with zinc transport. The ubiquitous occurrence of zinc and its participation in cellular and gaseous respiration as well as in proteolysis point to its cardinal role in metabolism. These discoveries foreshadow a recognition of its significance in pathologic processes.

Zinc Insulin. The crystallization of insulin as a zinc salt has led to general confusion concerning the chemical structure of this hormone in vivo. Active insulin may be obtained as an amorphous material, free of zinc below pH 4. It can be crystallized with zinc, nickel, cobalt, or cadmium. There is no evidence substantiating the contention that zinc is necessary for the action of insulin or that insulin occurs in the body as a metalloprotein or a metal-protein complex. Cobalt-containing insulin is as active as the zinc-free or zinc-containing material. Glucagon does not contain zinc.

Chemical Pathology. *Changes in Serum Zinc Concentration.* DECREASE OF ZINC. In pneumonia, bronchitis, erysipelas, and pyelonephritis, serum zinc has been shown to decrease significantly: the higher the body temperature, the greater the decrease. This correlation has been found to be statistically significant. At the height of fever the serum zinc concentration is lowest (60 to 80 μg per 100 ml); upon recovery, normal serum zinc levels are restored (120 to 140 μg per 100 ml).

In untreated pernicious anemia, serum zinc levels are about 80 to 90 μg per 100 ml. Twenty-four hours following institution of therapy, the zinc level rises, reaching a maximal value during the first week, with a concomitant increase in the number of reticulocytes.

In all other anemias studied thus far the data either indicate normal serum zinc levels or are so sketchy that no definitive conclusions may be drawn.

Decreased zinc serum levels in patients with a variety of primary tumors have been reported, but no uniform pattern exists. Normal serum zinc values have been observed in acute rheumatic fever, ulcerative colitis, diabetes, acute nephritis, and peptic or duodenal ulcers.

Recent observations demonstrate that the serum zinc concentrations in patients with myocardial infarction are markedly lowered. The concentrations in myocardial infarction were reported as 73 $\pm$ 20 μg zinc per 100 ml.

INCREASE OF ZINC. No increases in serum zinc values have been observed and substantiated. Variations in serum zinc levels are attributed to fluctuations in the "loosely bound" fraction, the "firmly bound" zinc remaining constant. The physiology of control of zinc in serum is not understood. No plausible explanations for pathologic changes have been offered.

Changes in Erythrocyte Content. INCREASE OF ZINC. The zinc content and carbonic anhydrase activity of red cells parallel each other and are significantly correlated. In normal individuals as well as in those afflicted with anemia, polycythemia vera, secondary polycythemia, leukemia, and congestive failure, both parameters vary directly with the hematocrit level and the hemoglobin concentration.

In untreated pernicious anemia, however, the erythrocyte zinc concentration and carbonic anhydrase activity are close to normal, though the hematocrit, erythrocyte count, and hemoglobin levels are markedly decreased. The mean corpuscular zinc concentration and carbonic anhydrase activity are increased several times more than the high mean corpuscular hemoglobin, and out of all proportion to the increase in cell size. Upon remission, zinc concentration and carbonic anhydrase activity return to normal values. Erythrocyte zinc concentration and carbonic anhydrase activity have also been found increased in sickle-cell anemia and acute intermittent porphyria.

DECREASE OF ZINC. The zinc content and carbonic anhydrase of erythrocytes of normal infants at birth is only 25 per cent of the adult value, and it is even lower in premature infants. Both values gradually rise to normal levels, doubling at age one, and reaching adult values at ages ten to twelve. Certain intractable types of cyanosis and dyspnea of infants at birth have been thought to be benefited by transfusion of adult red cells, with their higher carbonic anhydrase content.

A decrease of 50 per cent in the concentration of zinc in whole blood of Chinese suffering from protein deficiency, acute and chronic beriberi, and pellagra has been reported. No separate values for erythrocytes and serum were obtained, and no hematologic data are given.

Change in Leukocyte Content. INCREASE OF ZINC. Marked increases of leukocyte zinc have been observed in patients with anemias "refractory" to all therapy and accompanied by leukocyte counts below 2,000 per cu mm.

DECREASE OF ZINC. The zinc concentration of leukocytes in acute and chronic lymphatic and myelogenous leukemia is decreased to 10 per cent of the normal value. With successful therapy the zinc concentration returns to normal values. Administration of zinc salts intravenously fails to raise the leukocyte zinc concentration or influence the course of the disease. The phenomenon is apparently independent of the stage of maturation of the cells.

Zincuria. The normal zinc content of urine, 0.3 to 0.4 mg per 24-hr volume, has been found to rise sevenfold, to 2.1 mg per 24-hr volume, in patients with albuminuria.

Zinc and Postalcoholic Cirrhosis. A marked abnormality of zinc metabolism in patients with postalcoholic cirrhosis of the liver has been demonstrated. The serum concentrations in "severe" disease are lowered to 66.7 $\pm$ 19.2 μg per 100 ml. The lowest serum zinc concentrations are seen in hepatic coma, and values below 30 μg per 100 ml are a poor prognostic finding. Simultaneously, these patients excrete abnormally large quantities of zinc in their urine; this zinc excretion may become subnormal terminally, however. The zinc excretion was found to be 1016 $\pm$ 196 μg per 24 hr in patients with cirrhosis, compared to 457 $\pm$ 120 μg per 24 hr in a normal group. The zinc and iron concentrations are decreased significantly in the livers of patients dying with the disease, while the concentration of other metals does not change.

These studies were prompted by the discovery of the zinc-containing dehydrogenases (see above), which are cardinally involved in intermediary carbohydrate and protein metabolism. It has been suggested that the low serum zinc concentration in cirrhosis reflects a change in the synthesis, degradation, metal content, or specific activity of these enzymes. It cannot be stated at this time whether these abnormalities of zinc metabolism constitute primary or secondary manifestations of the disease, though they emphasize the significance of the metal to this nosologic entity.

Zinc and Porphyria. A zinc-uroporphyrin complex occurring in liver and urine is characteristic of intermittent acute porphyria and differentiates this type of porphyria from the congenital type. A zinc-coproporphyrin complex has been identified in the urine in lead poisoning and in acute rheumatic fever. The origin and metabolism of these complexes is not known.

Zinc and Diabetes. No significant difference in the zinc content of the pancreas in normal persons and diabetic patients has been detected. Most of the studies concerning this subject were motivated by erroneous notions concerning zinc insulin referred to above. Zinc blood levels of diabetic individuals are normal.

CADMIUM

Cadmium has been detected in most human organs, though the concentrations are of the order of 1 μg per Gm wet tissue. The kidney (sheep, hog, cow, horse, and human) contains amounts varying from 10 to 70 μg per Gm wet tissue.

The physiologic function of cadmium is unknown; it has been suggested, however, without documentation, that it is a "toxic" element and an etiologic factor in essential hypertension. Analyses of kidney cortex, containing the major fraction of the renal cadmium content, reveal no differences between normal material and that obtained from individuals succumbing from hypertension or a variety of renal disorders. Physiologic studies in rabbits show cadmium salts to exhibit a *hypotensive* action.

A protein containing 5 per cent of cadmium has been isolated from the cortex of horse kidney; it has a molecular weight of 10,000 and contains 9.3 per cent of sulfur and 2 per cent of zinc in addition to cadmium. The metals are bound to sulfur atoms, hence the name metallothionein. This is the first instance of the demonstration of a natural product containing cadmium, implying a biochemical and physiologic role which is yet to be discovered.

MAGNESIUM

Though the total body magnesium content of 25 Gm should remove this element from consideration as a trace element, the paucity of knowledge concerning its role in biology, physiology, and pathology is comparable to that of the trace elements here discussed.

Physiology. The daily intake of magnesium on an average diet is about 300 mg per day. There is no known factor which controls the absorption of magnesium in a manner similar to that of vitamin D in calcium absorption.

The stool magnesium represents that portion of the ingested ion which is not absorbed; it varies, therefore, with the magnesium intake. The bowel does not represent a major excretory pathway for absorbed magnesium in man.

In normal adults, about 60 to 200 mg a day is excreted in the urine. The factors which regulate the urinary excretion of magnesium are not known. Nor is it known whether adrenal steroids have any effect on renal magnesium excretion, although alterations of the metabolism of this element do occur in both adrenal insufficiency and hyperfunction.

Magnesium is filtered by the glomerulus and is reabsorbed by the tubules; it may in fact, like potassium, be excreted by a tubular mechanism.

The adult body contains 21 to 28 Gm magnesium, or about 43 mg per kg fat-free tissue. About half the total body content is present in bone, the ash containing 0.5 to 0.7 per cent magnesium.

Magnesium is similar to potassium in its distribution, being relatively concentrated in the intracellular space. The liver and striated muscle have the highest concentrations of about 20 mEq per liter. The brain and kidney contain about 17 and 13 mEq per liter, and the red cell concentration is about 6 mEq per liter. The normal serum content ranges from 1.6 to 2.4 mEq per liter, with a mean of 2 mEq per liter. It does not vary with age.

A portion of the serum magnesium is bound to protein. In the physiologic pH range, about 35 per cent of the total magnesium is protein-bound, a percentage which is almost identical to that of calcium over a wide range of hydrogen ion concentrations. The magnesium content of the cerebrospinal fluid is considerably higher than that of serum, the mean ranging from 2.4 to 3.0 mEq per liter.

Next to potassium, magnesium is the major intracellular cation. The mechanism governing the exchange between the intracellular, extracellular, protein-bound, and free moieties is not understood. There is an apparent reciprocal relationship between serum calcium and magnesium; at least under some circumstances, an increase of one results in the lowering of the other.

Biochemistry, Magnesium Proteins and Magnesium-protein Complexes. Though its precise mode of action is not known, even a cursory perusal of the literature implicates magnesium in a larger and more diverse number of biochemical reactions than almost any other metal. Most of this in vitro work has been carried out on material derived from other than human sources, so that implications to in vivo phenomena of man can only be speculated upon. These enzymes fall into the group of metal-enzyme complexes. The majority of the reactions involving adenosine triphosphate (ATP) are activated by magnesium ions; in their absence activity is either very much reduced or absent. The individual systems in which the metal participates are too numerous to detail here. Suffice it to say that this ion usually participates in group-transfer reactions: the transfers of phosphate, pyrophosphate, sulfate, methyl, formyl, acetyl, alkyl, and the glycol aldehyde groups utilize magnesium for activation. Thus it is involved in virtually all important metabolic processes, such as oxidative phosphorylation, protein, fat, carbohydrate, and nucleic acid anabolism and catabolism, muscle contraction, and glucose utilization. None of the purified enzymes involved has been shown to contain magnesium as part of the molecule, though methodology has curtailed decisive studies. It may be of more than passing interest that many "magnesium enzymes" also require thiamine pyrophosphate as a coenzyme. Finally, certain peptidases require the ion for activity.

Chemical Pathology. Symptomatic magnesium deficiency was first observed to occur in the rat almost 30 years ago. In this, as well as in all other mammalian species in which magnesium deficiency has been produced, it manifests itself as tetany. In cattle, in addition to the experimental varieties of magnesium deficiencies, a spontaneous type occurs. These observations have long suggested that a symptomatic magnesium deficiency would also be found to occur in man, but a discrete clinical syndrome comparable to that observed in animals has been described only recently.

Human Magnesium-deficiency Tetany. Clinically the human magnesium-deficiency syndrome is indistinguishable from hypocalcemic tetany. It is manifested by the presence of either a Chvostek's or Trousseau's sign when tetany is latent, or frank carpopedal spasms when tetany is active. As in hypocalcemic tetany, the neuromuscular irritability is aggravated by mechanical, auditory, or visual stimulation. The similarity is further increased by the presence of a lowered threshold response to galvanic stimulation.

The manifestations of human magnesium deficiency are virtually identical with those which occur spontaneously or which may be induced experimentally in numerous animal species. In all these instances, tetany is the primary sign of lack of magnesium and, like the human syndrome, it is indistinguishable from hypocalcemic tetany except by the measurement of the serum concentration of the two ions. The magnesium-deficiency tetany syndrome is therefore one of the rare illnesses of man which mimic a corresponding disorder of animals almost exactly.

Dietary restriction alone does not produce tetany nor does prolonged debilitation. Malnutrition has been a factor in all the patients afflicted, and a reduced dietary intake of the element occurs in most of them. In each instance that the syndrome has been observed it was brought about or intensified by some other factor which either prevented the absorption or increased the excretion of magnesium: a "conditioned deficiency," failure to absorb a metabolite, inability to synthesize it into a biologically active intermediate, and excessive excretion are the simplest examples of conditioning factors. Severe debilitating disease, prolonged acute infections, severe alcoholism accompanied by malnutrition, prolonged intestinal malabsorption, or drainage of gastrointestinal contents, continued parenteral treatment with magnesium-free fluids provide the setting in which this syndrome may be observed.

Conclusive proof that the syndrome is due to an alteration of magnesium metabolism is afforded by the correlation of symptoms and signs with chemical changes in the serum. The serum magnesium concentrations are markedly depressed, varying from 0.6 to 1.3 mEq per liter, while calcium concentrations are normal. Restoration of normal magnesium concentrations in serum through the parenteral administration of magnesium sulfate promptly and completely reverses the symptoms and signs.

Hypomagnesemia Accompanying Other Conditions. A lowered magnesium concentration has been observed in idiopathic epilepsy, cirrhosis, congestive heart failure, chronic nephritis, eclampsia, diabetic acidosis, pancreatitis, hyperparathyroidism, and hyperaldosteronism, though a causal relation of magnesium deficiency to these conditions has not been demonstrated. Among these, delirium tremens has received particular attention because of the similarity of the symptoms of patients afflicted with this condition to those of magnesium deficient animals. While delirium tremens is often accompanied by hypomagnesemia, the existent data do not support the hypothesis that there is a unique causal relationship between magnesium deficiency and this disease.

Hypermagnesemia. An increase in serum magnesium concentrations has been noticed in some patients with chronic and acute renal failure and in Addison's disease. The administration of magnesium sulfate to patients with severe renal disease is contraindicated.

Somnolence, loss of reflexes, general anesthesia, prolonged AV and intraventricular conduction time, similar to the effects of hyperpotassemia, accompany hypermagnesemia, simulating symptoms observed in the uremic state; some of these manifestations may well be attributable to the abnormalities of magnesium metabolism.

OTHER TRACE ELEMENTS

Although much information on other trace elements has been gathered in plants and animals, no unequivocal data on their role in human health and disease exist.

REFERENCES

GENERAL

Lamb, C. A., O. G. Bently, and J. M. Beattie (Eds.): "Trace Elements," New York, Academic Press, Inc., 1958.

Underwood, E. J.: "Trace Elements in Human and Animal Nutrition," New York, Academic Press, Inc., 1956.

Vallee, B. L.: Metal and Enzyme Interactions: Correlation of Composition, Function and Structure, p. 225, in "The Enzymes," 2d ed., vol. 3, part B, P. D. Boyer, H. Lardy, and K. Myrbäck (Eds.), New York, Academic Press, Inc., 1960.

Williams, R. J. P.: Coordination, Chelation and Catalysis, p. 391, in "The Enzymes," 2d ed., vol. 1, P. D. Boyer, H. Lardy, and K. Myrbäck (Eds.), New York, Academic Press, Inc., 1959.

CADMIUM

Kägi, J. H. R., and B. L. Vallee: Metallothionein; a Cadmium- and Zinc-containing Protein from Equine Renal Cortex, J. Biol. Chem., 235: 3460, 1960 and 236: 2435, 1961.

COBALT

Arnstein, H. R. V.: The Metabolic Function of Vitamin B_{12}, in Proceedings of the Fourth International Congress of Biochemistry, Vienna, 1958, W. Umbreit and H. Molitor (Eds.), vol. XI, p. 286, New York, Pergamon Press, 1960.

Biochemical Society Symposia No. 13: "The Biochemistry of Vitamin B_{12}," New York, Cambridge University Press, 1955.

COPPER

Adelstein, S. J., and B. L. Vallee: Copper Metabolism, in "Mineral Metabolism," vol. II, C. Comar and F. Buonner (Eds.), New York, Academic Press, Inc., 1961.

Scheinberg, I. H., and I. Sternlieb: Copper Metabolism, Pharmacol. Revs., 12:355, 1960.

FLUORINE

Moulton, F. R. (Ed.): "Dental Caries and Fluorine," American Association for the Advancement of Science, Washington, D.C., 1946.

Shaw, J. A. (Ed.): "Fluoridation as a Public Health Measure," American Association for the Advancement of Science, Washington, D.C., 1954.

Sognnaes, R. F. (Ed.): "Advances in Experimental Caries Research," American Association for the Advancement of Science, Washington, D.C., 1955.

MAGNESIUM

Vallee, B. L., W. E. C. Wacker, and D. D. Ulmer: The Magnesium Deficiency Tetany Syndrome in Man, New Engl. J. Med., 262:155, 1960.

Wacker, W. E. C., and B. L. Vallee: Magnesium Metabolism, New Engl. J. Med., 259:431, 475, 1958.

ZINC

Vallee, B. L.: Biochemistry, Physiology and Pathology of Zinc, Physiol. Revs., 39:443, 1959.

Section 5: Electrophysiology

54 PRINCIPLES OF ELECTROCARDIOGRAPHY

Elliot V. Newman

The purpose of this chapter is to present logically the basic principles concerning the origin and formation of the electrocardiogram. It is necessary to understand the principles while learning to use the electrocardiogram for clinical practice. No attempt will be made to cover the entire range of abnormalities. Enough illustrations of application of the method will be given to show how the principles apply when interpreting disorders. Emphasis is placed on ventricular muscle and conduction.

The heart and the body form a three-dimensional spatial system. The electrical events are therefore also three-dimensional. The fourth dimension is time. A single electrocardiographic tracing is unidimensional electrically. We must develop a three-dimensional sense from multiple unidimensional pictures. The fifth dimension of electrocardiography is the correlative knowledge of simultaneous clinical, pathologic, and physiologic events.

The electrocardiogram as used by the physician is a partially summated distant picture of multiple electrical events in the heart. The surface recording is a composite result of a series of processes. In the millions of individual muscle fibers the electrical events arise from changes in the energetic mechanisms in the cell, which are dependent ultimately on chemical or metabolic transactions in the cell protoplasm. The intracellular biochemical processes are in turn dependent on adequate supplies of fuel, of oxygen, and on adequate perfusion by blood of the proper chemical composition.

The electrical events of the cells reach the surface of the body through a series of boundaries and pathways. The first boundary of prime importance is the individual cell membrane. Each cell may be considered a small battery, with one pole inside the cell and the other outside the membrane. Discharge and recharge of the cell are accompanied by transfer of charges and salts across the membrane. The second boundary of importance is the anatomic configuration of the whole cardiac muscle, the syncytium of cells. Not all cells discharge and recharge simultaneously. Thus the pathway, or the sequential order in which the cells discharge and recharge, governs greatly the configuration of the distant picture. This order is determined usually by the special conduction apparatus of the heart. However, while the anatomic arrangement of cardiac muscle to a certain extent governs the electrical configuration at a distant observation point, the pathways of discharge and recharge may have varied arrangements as the masses of cells vary their quantity and sequence of electrical activity. In this way, an organ of constant anatomic structure or configuration can produce manifold electrical configurations by varying the time order, the numbers, and the pathways of cellular electrical events. Added to this there may be variations due to alterations in the intracellular metabolism of individual cells and in the condition of the cell membranes. "Electrical shape" of the heart's picture is only partly governed by the anatomic shape.

Once the electrical forces are liberated by the cells, they are conducted through tissue to the surface of the body. These myriads of forces have varying magnitudes and directions. The conduction through tissues is governed again by anatomic configuration, but it also obeys the laws of flow of electricity through volumes of liquids of varying electrical properties. It is interesting that the heart muscle itself, while it is the source of the electrical forces, is also part of the volume of tissues which conducts to the surface. An electrical force liberated in one part of the muscle is conducted from one part of the heart to another as it travels through tissue. Also, the blood in the heart chambers conducts. These myriads of electrical forces compete with each other, so that equal and opposite forces in different parts of the heart may cancel each other, with the net result that the surface force may be much smaller than the sum of the individual forces in the muscle. As with any kind of force, the magnitude will vary with the distance it must travel.

Also, forces will not be recorded from leads (electrodes) unless the orientation of the forces are in the direction of the flow of current between the observation posts (lead axis). Because of the distance factor, and the internal cancellation of forces, and the direction factor, localized potentials may be recorded clearly only at the surface of the structure within which the events have occurred. It is for this reason that the intimate details of cardiac electrical events can be finally determined only by electrodes placed within the cardiac cavities or in the muscle itself.

Finally, the appearance of the record called the electrocardiogram will be governed to some extent by the properties of the instruments used for detecting and depicting the forces in some visible and measurable form. The visible form of the final record of these events will also depend in part on some rather arbitrary choices of conventions for visible representation. The choice of surface "leads" gives only special views of the whole electrical process. An understanding of the underlying processes and form of the whole picture gives a sound basis for the interpretation of abnormalities.

THE SINGLE CELL

If one electrode is placed inside a resting cell and another outside, there will be found a high electrical potential difference between the two terminals, or poles. In other words, a current will flow if the terminals are externally conducted. The cell is therefore *polarized*. The direction of flow will be from the outside to the inside. The inside of the cell is therefore said to be negative, and the outside surface positive. As much as 80 to 100 millivolts (mv) potential difference exists across the cell boundary. The spontaneous discharge of this potential is called *depolarization*. This process of discharge of potential, or depolarization, may occur in a wave proceeding across the cell membrane and from cell to cell. The spread of depolarization is called the *excitation*, or *accession*, *wave* or process.

Following depolarization there is a recovery or *repolarization* so that the cell is ready again for excitation. Depolarization is a rapid process in cardiac muscle, occurring in a few hundredths of a second. The excitation wave can spread through the heart at a velocity of about 3 ft per sec. In contrast, repolarization is a slower process and may occupy two- or three-tenths of a second.

The storage of energy in the cell depends on the metabolic processes which keep a marked difference of concentration of ions between the inside and the field outside the cell membrane. Potassium is present in a concentration inside which is roughly twenty times that of the outside fluid. The reverse is true of sodium concentration. During depolarization, there is an exchange of ions, with sodium entering the cell and potassium leaving. During recovery, the reverse takes place. Thus the flow of electric potentials depends on ionic flow. The maintenance of the stored energy depends on active metabolic processes which build these charges by the arrangement of ionic concentrations. It is at this cellular level of activity that drugs, electrolyte concentrations, and disease affect the electrical properties by modifying the depolarization and repolarization process of the cell.

THE VENTRICULAR MUSCLE

The electrical anatomy of the cardiac ventricular muscle begins with the atrioventricular node (AV node), which receives its excitation stimulus from the descending wave from the atria. The AV node is situated at the top of the interventricular septum, at the junction of the atria and the interatrial septum. The AV node and the bundle of His lie closer to the left ventricular cavity surface just under the right aortic cusp and are in the muscular ring of the aortic orifice. The bundle branches into right and left pathways, which then spread in the Purkinje network throughout the endocardial surfaces of each ventricle. Conduction of the electrical excitation wave proceeds more rapidly through the special network than through the muscle itself.

The *excitation,* or *depolarization,* wave of the muscle mass begins on the left side of the interventricular septum and proceeds from left to right and upward, initially. Then follows a rapid excitation of the endocardial walls with the wave proceeding from inside outward. Because the excitation wave starts on the left side of the septum, the progression of depolarization to the right side of the heart is a little later. The last part of the heart muscle to be depolarized may be at the base. As the wave proceeds from the endocardial to the epicardial muscle it arrives at the surface of the heart. There is some disagreement among students of electrocardiography regarding the exact order of depolarization in various parts of the heart. However, there is general agreement that there is first a movement from left to right in the septum; secondly, a progression from endocardium to epicardium; and, lastly, a wave at the base.

There is evidence that the Purkinje fibers which activate the left ventricle are divided into an anterolateral and a posterobasal group. These groups occasionally respond as units and have a characteristic response to injury.

As the front of the depolarization wave proceeds through the muscle, it defines a continuously changing electrical anatomic boundary. Each muscle fiber, in its turn, contributes its share of electrical force in a direction determined by the conduction pathway. These myriads of forces are added together according to well-known principles of the behavior of electrical forces in a fluid medium.

The Addition of the Ventricular Muscle Depolarization Forces. The heart muscle itself and the blood in the ventricular chambers are conductors of the electrical forces liberated by depolarization. The muscle and the blood inside form a so-called "volume conductor" of electricity, in contradistinction to a linear conductor such as a metal wire. This volume, being made of two types of tissue, namely, blood and muscle, is inhomogeneous, electrically speaking. The conductivity of blood is roughly ten times that of muscle. Thus we have, in essence, a hollow, roughly spherical shell of muscle filled with relatively highly conductive fluid.

The simplest principle of electrical addition of forces is that equal and opposite forces will cancel each other. An electrical force can be represented as a line or an arrow, like this:

The origin of the arrow represents the location of the origin, or source, of the electrical force. The length of the arrow represents the magnitude of the force. The direction of the force is defined by the facts that (1) it is drawn on a flat surface (the *plane* of the paper); (2) it has a direction which can conveniently be defined by the angle it subtends on the *coordinates,* or sides, of the paper. The coordinates used to define the direction of the force are sometimes called the *reference frame.* The reference frame for this purpose is selected on the basis of convenience. The plane of this paper at the moment is convenient, but it is apparent that there are other planes and that the force (the arrow) can point in any direction when one is dealing with a volume conduction system (three-dimensional) rather than with a single-plane system like the paper surface (two-dimensional). The many arrows will be pointing in all directions toward the observer and away from him, as well as along the surface of the plane represented on this thin piece of paper, which can reflect only the forces manifest along its own surface, or plane.

Equal and opposite forces cancel each other, e.g.,

$$\longleftarrow + \longrightarrow = 0$$

This really comprises a special case of a general principle of addition. These forces, called *vectors,* have the properties of *magnitude, direction,* and *sense*. Magnitude and direction have already been defined, respectively, by the length of the line and by the direction as revealed by its position with reference to a convenient reference frame, or coordinate system.

The property of *sense* is described by the adjectives "positive" and "negative." In the case of the single cell, previously described, the outside of the cell is said to be positive and the inside negative. This is based on the convention that in a battery electricity flows from the positive to the negative pole. When the outside of the cell is connected to the inside of a single muscle cell, the current flows inward. With a mass of cells having a depolarization wave proceeding through it, the front of the wave is positive and the tail is negative. Thus in ventricular muscle, as the excitation wave proceeds from the endocardium toward the epicardium, a vector pointing outward is produced. In this instance, if one electrode, or pole, were placed inside the heart and the other outside, the outside would be positive and the inside negative. Or, in other words, there would be a vector pointing outward and in the general direction of the pathway of the front of the depolarization wave. If all the myriads of forces in all directions at any instant are added together, the net result, or addition of forces, can be represented as one single *mean vector*.

There is one more general principle of addition of vector forces to be considered before this summation of all forces at any instant into one *mean manifest vector* can be accomplished. The special case of addition of equal and opposite vectors has been considered, e.g.,

$$\overleftarrow{\bullet} \overset{+}{\bullet} \overrightarrow{} = 0$$

But what if the vectors are not equal and not exactly opposite in direction? The forces are then added by this rule:

If two forces act on a point and if two lines be drawn from that point representing the forces in magnitude and direction, and a parallelogram be constructed on these lines as their sides, their resultant will be represented in magnitude and direction by that diagonal which passes through the point.

For example:

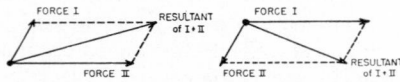

With these principles of electrical conduction and resolution of forces, one can turn to the problem of the resolution of the multitudinous forces liberated by the excitation wave proceeding through the fibers of the hollow muscle mass of the heart. In order to elucidate further the mechanism of addi-

tion of electrical forces in such a three-dimensional system, it is helpful to consider first a simplified model which resembles the heart. The model consists of a perfectly spherical hollow shell of muscle filled with highly conductive fluid such as blood. The depolarization, or excitation, is represented as starting on the endocardial spherical surface at all points simultaneously and proceeding in a perfectly uniform and symmetrical wave to the surface. At each instant in time after the beginning of depolarization the electrical boundary of the wave forms a perfect sphere (Fig. 54-1).

It is immediately apparent that every force will be perfectly balanced by an equal and opposite force and the resultant force of the whole process will be always zero. Each segment of muscle will have an equal and opposite in the sphere. This will result in complete *cancellation of forces*. The presence of highly conductive blood in the cavity allows transference, or short circuiting, of the forces liberated by depolarization in divergent directions.

In the human heart the excitation wave proceeds, as in the above model, in divergent directions and there is much cancellation. Actually, roughly 90 per cent of the forces of depolarization are canceled, and only about 10 per cent of the total is the net force which can be detected outside the organ. The heart will manifest a vector force only if the resultant of all forces proceeding in some direction is greater than the forces in divergent directions. Thus the heart's vector at any time will represent only the unbalanced or uncanceled portion of all the forces. This means that a change in the contour of the pathway of the excitation wave in a relatively small area of muscle can greatly affect the size and direction of the heart's vector. To illustrate this, one can make slight changes in the shape of the perfectly hollow sphere by adding some muscle on one side. As before, the depolarization starts everywhere simultaneously on the inner surface and proceeds in an orderly sequence of spherical waves toward the surface. However, in this example, the wave continues through the additional muscle after it has penetrated the surface in all other parts of the sphere. As soon as this oc-

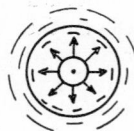

FIG. 54-1. The forces of depolarization are symmetrically oriented so that the net force of the whole process is zero, which is represented by the dot in the center of the sphere. There is complete cancellation of all forces because of the perfect symmetry of the electrical events proceeding uniformly through the mass.

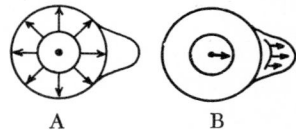

FIG. 54-2. *A*. The net force of the depolarization process is zero (dot in center) as long as it is proceeding through the symmetrical part of the spherical mass. *B*. As soon as the wave proceeds through the additional asymmetrical part of the mass, the forces are unopposed and a vector force appears, represented by the arrow, having its origin in the center and its direction toward the extra muscle.

curs there is an isolated uncanceled wave proceeding in one direction unopposed by any wave in the opposite direction. A vector force will then appear. This summated force can be represented by the arrow arising in the center of the circle and pointing in the direction of the wave. This is an example of a vector produced by additional muscle, or ventricular *preponderance* (Fig. 54-2).

Another model example of unbalancing of the forces is produced by distorting the muscle by removing a segment or rendering a part incapable of depolarization. The depolarization wave proceeds outward to the perimeter of normal muscle with complete cancellation. As soon as the perimeter of the wave reaches the "dead" area, the normal muscle in a comparable opposite position is no longer canceled. There is an unbalancing of the forces, producing a vector pointing toward the normal opposite area. This illustrates the important principle that an *electrically dead area of muscle causes the heart vector to point away from that area and in the direction of the depolarization wave through normal muscle* (Fig. 54-3).

Regardless of the alterations in shape of the depolarization wave or the shape of the muscle, one can represent the sum of the forces at any instant as a single vector having its origin from a *point source* in the electrical center of the heart.

So far, only consideration of the behavior of normal depolarization of muscle has been presented. The normal ventricular muscle exhibits a net force of zero when it is resting, or not excited. Injured muscle, however, may have a chronic discharge of potential. This is called *injury current*. The "injured" area creates a force which is in the direction of the normal tissue. Thus, in the resting state of the ventricle if there is an injured area, this injured part is actually not resting, electrically speaking. One might call this a state of local chronic depolarization. In the model, the vector force can again be added and represented as before by a single arrow from a point source in the center. Now an interesting phenomenon occurs if this muscle model is depolarized in the same fashion as before, viz., from the inside surface outward in a symmetrical spherical wave of progression. The injured part is still capable of acute depolarization as the excitation wave passes through it. The depolarization of the injured area temporarily disposes of the injury potential, so that the vector of injury disappears. Actually, the usual methods of recording potentials do not reveal whether there is a constant injury current present in the muscle when it is in the resting state. The injury current is "unmasked" by the depolarization of the whole muscle (Fig. 54-4).

Ventricular Muscle Repolarization and the Addition of Forces. Repolarization of the muscle fiber is the process of electrical recovery which replaces the electrical potentials lost during depolarization. Repolarization also proceeds through the muscle in a wave pattern, but the sequence in various parts of the muscle has been less well defined than for depolarization waves. If a repolarization wave proceeds throughout the muscle mass in exactly the same direction, the total force produced will be exactly equal and opposite in direction to the forces of depolarization. Again, the principle of cancellation of forces holds. Thus in the symmetrical spherical model shell of muscle, the net total force will be zero. However, if the pathway is asymmetrical, there will be imbalancing of forces and a vector of depolarization will appear. Since the repolariza-

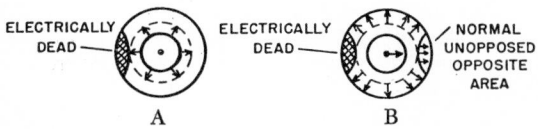

FIG. 54-3. *A*. As long as the depolarization wave proceeds through the symmetrical part of the muscle the force will be zero, all forces being canceled by equal and opposite forces. *B*. As soon as the wave reaches the electrically "dead" area, there is a vector force pointing away from the dead area because of the unbalanced forces of the opposite normal muscle. This vector is represented as an arrow arising in the center pointing toward the normal unopposed area.

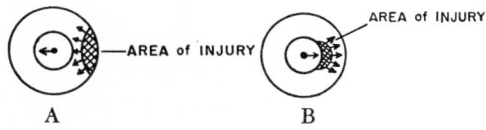

FIG. 54-4. *A*. This injured area results in a continuous potential across the boundary to the normal area, resulting in a steady force represented by the vector arrow pointing away from the injured area. In this case, the injured area is in the epicardial region. *B*. When the injured area is in the endocardial region on the same side, the vector force points in the opposite direction but still toward the normal (muscle) area boundary.

tion process may not occur in the same order as depolarization, neither the direction nor the magnitudes of force of each may be the same. It is true that each single cell may have discharged and regained the same total electrical energy, but the variable amount of cancellation of forces of some parts of the muscle mass by other parts may make the summation of the whole process a very small and variably directed quantity.

One striking and important difference between depolarization and repolarization is the speed. Repolarization is relatively a very slow process. Depolarization, being rapid, produces a large force which lasts a short time, and repolarization a smaller force which lasts a longer time. This is analogous to discharging a storage battery by using a large current for a short time and then replacing the same amount of energy, or recharging the battery, with a small current for a long time.

Another very important feature of the repolarization, or recovery, process is its marked variability under the influence of mechanical, chemical, and physiologic factors. Heat, cold, drugs, electrolyte concentrations, oxygen tension, blood pressure may change the course of repolarization without changing the pattern of depolarization. Under normal circumstances the distribution of the forces of repolarization are quite constant and reproducible. While it is a different pattern from that of depolarization, yet the repolarization process ordinarily follows an order which has been determined by the preceding order of depolarization. For example, if the wave of depolarization were started at an odd place (ectopic focus) in the muscle, and followed a different course from the normal, then one could expect that the repolarization wave would also follow a different pattern.

The differences in pathway of depolarization and repolarization can be summarized by comparing the magnitude and direction of forces of the two processes. This is of great importance in the detection of abnormalities of the repolarization process. In other words, one cannot tell if repolarization is abnormal in its direction and timing unless the direction and timing of the depolarization are known. This concept will be further elaborated later under discussion of quantitative expressions of the differences in the two processes and their relationships.

THE CONDUCTION OF FORCES FROM THE HEART TO THE SURFACE OF THE BODY

The tissues of the body are conductors of electrical forces in all directions. As already mentioned, this type of conductor is called a *volume conductor,* in contrast to a linear conductor such as a metal wire; the heart muscle itself and the blood in the cavities conduct the electrical forces liberated in one part to all other parts. From the confines of the heart, these forces are conducted through the tissues to the surface. Since the tissues of the body are seemingly quite different in their composition, one might expect that the forces would be conducted through devious pathways of least resistance. If this were the case, the body would be an *electrically inhomogeneous volume conductor.* Blood, for example, has a conductivity roughly ten times that of muscle. However, a rather remarkable constancy of conductivity of tissues exists outside the heart. In effect, the body is a remarkably *homogeneous volume conductor.* It seems odd that tissue like the lungs has approximately the same conductivity as muscle, when lungs contain so much air. It happens that the lungs are a mixture of air, which has very low conductivity, and blood, which has high conductivity, in such proportions that the total effect is like that of muscle. Thus the conduction of forces in this apparently heterogeneous mass of tissue, the body, turns out to follow quite accurately the principles of conduction in a homogeneous volume conductor. The behavior of electrical forces produced by a small electrical generator ("point source") and conducted through a homogeneous volume follows well-defined laws. Actual measurements in the human body show that the *heart behaves like a point source generator and the body like a homogeneous volume conductor with an accuracy of roughly 90 per cent.* While there are discrepancies between the ideal behavior and the actual result, one must proceed in practice on generalizations which best fit all the evidence in hand. Corrections for those errors which are known will be necessary when it is shown that the errors interfere with the practical applicability of methods based upon the generalized ideal.

This behavior of the heart and surrounding tissues means that forces measured in or on the surface of the body are the sums of all the forces liberated in the heart added together as though the resultant arises from a point somewhere near the center of the whole volume. Stated in another way, this means that forces measured at a distance from the heart do not represent selectivity, or preferential areas, in the heart muscle closer to the site of measurement. Proximity of the site of measurement to the heart gives no exclusive information about the muscle which anatomically is closer to the site. Distance of the point of measurement from the source only modifies the force in its magnitude, following the familiar rule that *magnitude varies inversely as the square of the distance from the source.*

Other changes in magnitude of the forces measured at a distance from the heart are due to variation in orientation of the site of measurement with respect to the direction of the summated source vector. Differences in the appearance of the changes of force throughout the time course of the cardiac cycle are due to the variable position of the observer who places his observation points. This means that all views of the cardiac electrical forces are related to one another, in that they are special views of the same process. The simplest example of this is the equal and opposite view. For every site within the system there is another directly opposite view which will give a mirror image of the forces. Another special case is the observation line in the system which will detect no record of force because the line of observation is oriented exactly at right angles to the direction of the force. In other words, to the observer there will be no force measurable unless it has some motion referable to the direction of the line of observation.

THE PRINCIPLES AND TECHNIQUES OF REPRESENTING AND RECORDING FORCES

The application of two metal electrodes to the surface of the body establishes a pathway between the two points for the flow of electricity. The electric potential between the two electrodes can be measured by leading wires from the electrodes to a suitable meter. The changing potential will cause movements of the meter, or galvanometer. These changes can be continuously recorded by making the meter inscribe its motion on a moving strip of paper. The inscription can be made directly or by a photographic process.

For purposes of analysis, the electrodes can be considered as defining a reference line drawn between the two poles. This is commonly called a *bipolar lead.* One of the terminals, or poles, of a lead is designated as positive and the other negative. By convention, a positive potential is represented on the record paper by an upward inscription and conversely a negative potential by a downward inscription. The position of the pen or writing mechanism of the meter in the resting state is called the zero potential or *isoelectric line* on the record.

Having established a reference line by applying a bipolar lead system to the body, the problem is to determine what part of the central cardiac force will be recorded in this distant lead. The force, or potential, which will be recorded by the lead will depend on the magnitude and direction of the cardiac vector and its orientation with respect to the lead line. For example, it is common practice to place an electrode on the left arm and right arm, forming "lead I," with the left designated positive and the right negative. A simple geometric calculation can be made of the component of the cardiac vector translated to the lead I reference line. The magnitude of the component on the lead line is the

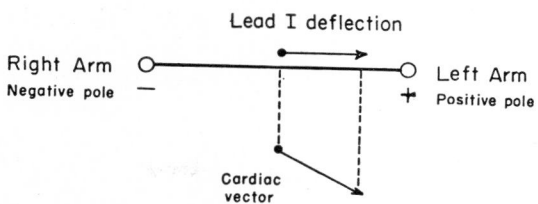

FIG. 54-5. The geometric representation of the component on a lead axis of a vector force (arrow) which arises from a point equidistant from the two poles of the lead. The lines drawn perpendicularly from the origin and terminus of the arrow to the lead axis line define the magnitude and direction of the component on the lead line.

distance between the two points at which perpendicular lines drawn from the origin and end of the cardiac vector intersect. Since the component in the lead I reference line points toward the designated positive pole, the deflection produced and recorded will, by definition, be positive and upward on the record (Fig. 54-5). In this illustration, the assumption has been made that the point of origin of the cardiac vector lies opposite the center of the lead line and that this point is equidistant from the two poles (see Einthoven hypothesis, below). The important special case in which lead I alone will give no information about the cardiac vector is when the vector itself is perpendicular to the lead line. In this instance, there will be no component of this force translated to the reference lead line. In other words, the reference lead will record only forces which have *components in the axis of the lead.* Forces having direction perpendicular to this axis will have no components, and therefore other leads are necessary to establish accurately the magnitude and direction of the cardiac vector. Another special case is when the lead line is parallel to the cardiac vector. This will give the maximal representation on the lead line (Fig. 54-6).

The most familiar and longest-used reference

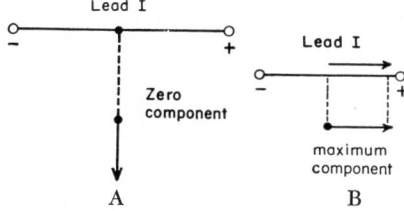

FIG. 54-6. A. When the vector force is perpendicular to the lead axis line, there will be no component on the lead line. This lead alone, therefore, will give no information about the magnitude and direction of forces perpendicular to it. B. When the vector is parallel to the lead line, the component on the lead line will be maximum.

frame for recording the components of the cardiac vector is the *triangular system of Einthoven*. This is based on the essentially accurate hypothesis that the electrical center of the heart, or the point source of the cardiac vector, lies in the center of an equilateral triangle formed by the three bipolar leads between, first, the right arm and left arm; second, the right arm and left leg; and third, the left arm and left leg. In this system, the components of the cardiac vector are recorded on the three so-called "standard leads." The designated polarity of the electrodes and waves of the leads are those which were first arbitrarily selected by Einthoven and subsequently established by conventional use. This triangular system with the polarities arranged in this fashion results in the interesting geometric fact that the component in lead II is equal to the sum of the components in leads I and III. Actually, therefore, it is necessary to have only any two leads to define the magnitude and direction of the cardiac vector in this one plane (Fig. 54-7).

Another type of reference system is formed by leads placed on the body so that the lines of the leads are theoretically at right angles to each other. This is called an *orthogonal system*. For example, electrodes placed on the upper back from side to side can form one axis (X axis), and the vertical axis (Y axis) can be formed by a lead between the electrode on the right upper back and another directly below. The components of the cardiac vector are then measured along these axes. Or conversely, the magnitude and direction of the cardiac vector can be determined as the resultant of the two com-

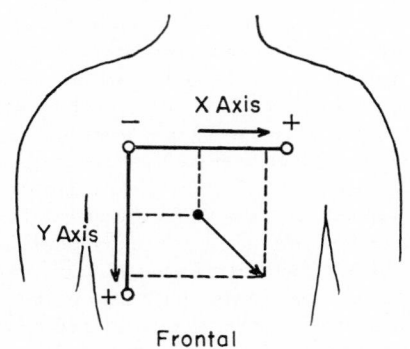

FIG. 54-8. An orthogonal reference frame for the frontal plane formed by leads placed along axes at right angles to each other. Many other types of reference frames can be used.

ponents on these axes (or any other axes of known spatial orientation). (Fig. 54-8.)

So far, the reference frames considered have been restricted to one plane of the body. *Any two axes or leads define a plane.* The Einthoven lead system and the orthogonal axes above are in the *frontal plane* of the body. The forces of the heart, however, are not restricted to one plane. The cardiac vector has components in all directions. A plane is a two-dimensional representation, the cardiac vector is three-dimensional (Fig. 54-9). Just as a lead will show no detectable components of forces directed at right angles to it, so also leads in one plane will not show components directed at right angles to, or perpendicular to, the plane of these leads. Thus leads in the frontal plane will not give information about the magnitude and direction of the cardiac forces in the sagittal and transverse

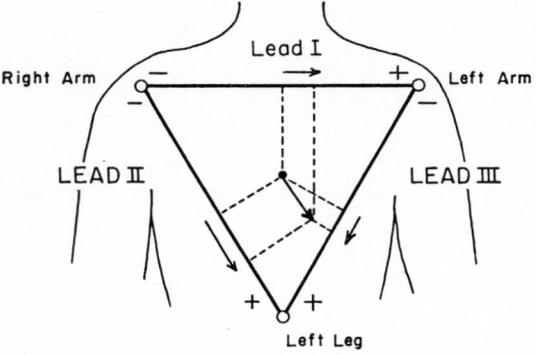

FIG. 54-7. The conventional reference frame of the Einthoven Standard Lead System, representing the cardiac vector as arising from a point in the center of an equilateral triangle formed by the leads between the electrodes on three extremities of the body. The components of each axis are represented for the cardiac vector. In this particular example, the three lead components will all have a positive sense because the arrows point toward the designated positive poles of the leads. These leads are one way of showing the forces in the frontal plane of the body.

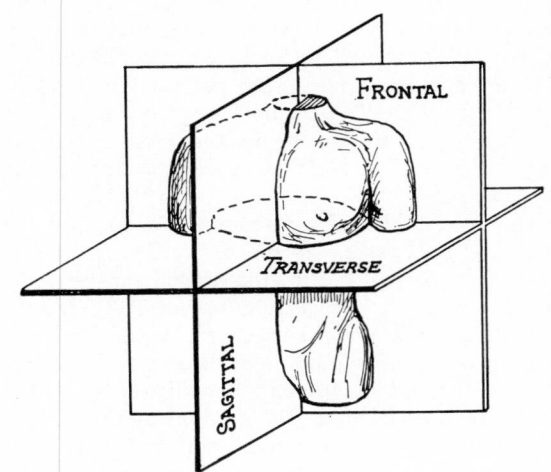

FIG. 54-9. Illustrating the three planes of the body which form a convenient conceptual framework in which to describe the spatial orientation of electrocardiographic forces.

planes. The sagittal plane components can be determined by a lead system which records the components along a vertical axis (Y axis) and a horizontal axis (Z axis) (Fig. 54-10). The transverse plane components can be determined by a lead system which records the components along the X axis and the Z axis (Fig. 54-11). There are other types of lead systems and reference frames for measuring the components of the cardiac forces. While these systems are not perfectly accurate, they are based on essentially sound facts and assumptions. It is a general truth that the magnitude of the component of the cardiac force which is represented in any lead is governed by the spatial orientation of the lead with respect to the cardiac forces. Differences in the components in different leads depend, therefore, on differences in orientation. They are merely different views of the same forces and do not represent different forces or separate parts of the total force.

Discussion so far has been of recording systems which employ the *bipolar leads*. Another type of lead is that devised by Wilson and called the *unipolar lead*. The term unipolar is perhaps confusing because, in reality, no lead system can record a potential unless there are two poles to complete the circuit. The unique feature of the unipolar system is that one of the terminals, or poles, is a combination of electrodes connected together. Wilson took advantage of the fact that in a triangular reference system the sum of the potentials at the corners of the triangle is always zero. This is known as *Kirchhoff's law*. This law holds for any triangle, equilateral or not. For an equilateral triangle, however, such as the Einthoven system, the pole formed by connecting the electrodes at the corners of the tri-

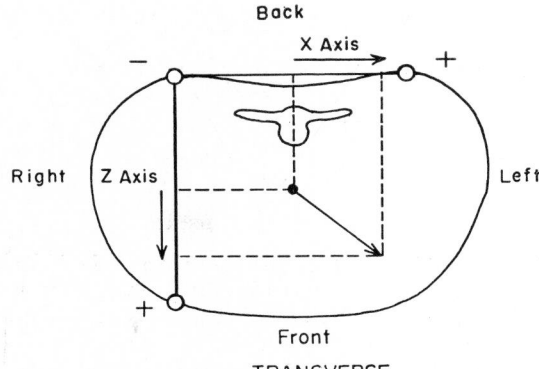

FIG. 54-11. A lead system which can be used to represent the forces in the transverse plane of the body.

angle may be represented as lying in the center of the triangle and at the electrical center of the heart. This common or *central terminal* (sometimes called the "indifferent electrode") is designated as the negative pole, and another electrode placed anywhere else on the body is designated the positive pole. The positive pole is frequently referred to as the *exploring electrode*. In effect, the unipolar lead is a bipolar lead formed by the central terminal and the exploring electrode. Such leads are generally called *V leads* or *Wilson leads* (Fig. 54-12).

The axis of the V lead may be represented by a line drawn from the location of the exploring electrode to the electrical center of the heart. In the Einthoven system this is the center of the triangle. For example, the application of the exploring electrode to the right arm (VR), left arm (VL), and left leg (VF) form lead axes from the corners of the triangle to the center. The components of the cardiac vector will then be measured along these axes, and the cardiac vector has its origin, or source, at the electrical center. When the cardiac vector points toward the exploring electrode, the component potential is positive (as illustrated in VF and VL in Fig. 54-13), and when away, it is negative (as illustrated in VR).

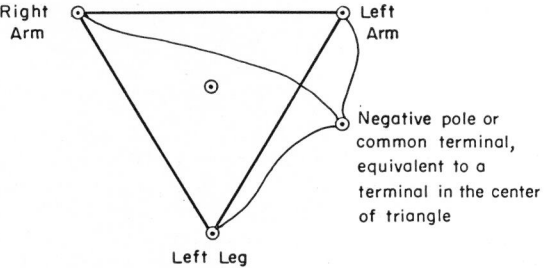

FIG. 54-12. Illustrating the arrangement for producing an "indifferent" or "control terminal" negative pole for the Wilson V leads, which theoretically should have zero potential.

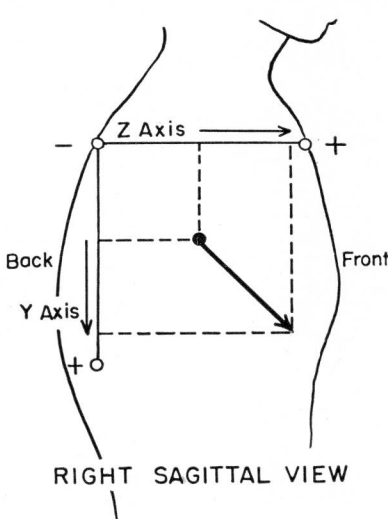

RIGHT SAGITTAL VIEW

FIG. 54-10. Two leads which define the sagittal plane in an orthogonal system of recording.

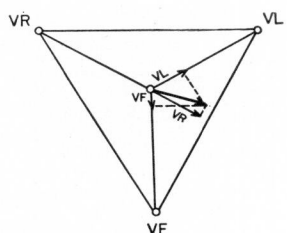

FIG. 54-13. Showing the reference frame of the V limb leads and the components of a cardiac vector on the lead axes. The negative side of all V leads is, by definition, the control terminal, which we can represent as lying in the electrical center of the heart at the origin of the cardiac vector.

In the case of V leads from the limbs, the potential measured is small because the electrode on the limb is connected to the negative central terminal, as well as being the exploring electrode. Goldberger introduced a modification of the V limb leads which "augments" the potential by disconnecting the exploring electrode from the central terminal. These augmented unipolar limb leads are referred to by the symbols AVR, AVL, and AVF.

It is common practice to use the Wilson or V lead by placing the exploring, or positive, electrode at various points on the front surface of the chest. Each position of the electrode connects with the electrical center somewhere in or near the center of the heart. For the sake of uniformity in practice, electrocardiographers have agreed upon six positions on the chest wall for recording V leads. These six positions are defined arbitrarily by surface anatomic geography as follows: V_1 is at the right border of the sternum in the fourth interspace; V_2 is at the left border of the sternum in the fourth interspace; V_3 is halfway between the left midclavicular line and the V_2 position and over the fifth rib; V_4 is at the left midclavicular line in the fifth interspace; V_5 is at the left anterior axillary line on a line drawn horizontally from V_4; V_6 is at the midaxillary line at the same level as V_4 and V_5 (Fig. 54-14).

Each position of the V lead defines its own axis, represented by a line drawn from the electrical center of the heart to the exploring electrode. None of these axes lies exactly in one of the three standard reference planes of the body. Therefore, in order to depict the orientation of the lead axes of the conventional chest V leads, one must examine the projection of the axes on two planes. In the transverse plane, the V lead axes are spread out over an arc of roughly 110°. While the V lead axes are usually represented as lying in the transverse plane, and while some do represent most transverse plane forces, it is apparent that the axes of the V_4, V_5, and V_6 are pointed downward toward the foot and very much to the left. Perhaps V_1, V_2, and V_3 are more nearly truly transverse plane axes than any of the others. They are more parallel to the Z axis of the body and have less tilt downward than V_4, V_5, and V_6. Actually, V_5 and, particularly, V_6 are really more in the frontal plane than in the transverse plane. Since they point to the left and downward, they are apt to be opposite in view to the axis of VR, which points to the right and upward. In other words, a component in VR which is positive is likely to be found simultaneously in V_5 or V_6 as a negative potential. The magnitude of components varies considerably in the V chest leads because of the great variation in distance of the electrode from the center, due to the contour of the chest cage. The fact that V_5 and, particularly, V_6 really form frontal plane lead axes results in the interesting relationship between the components measured in V_6 and those in AVF and AVL. When the cardiac vector points footward ("vertical"

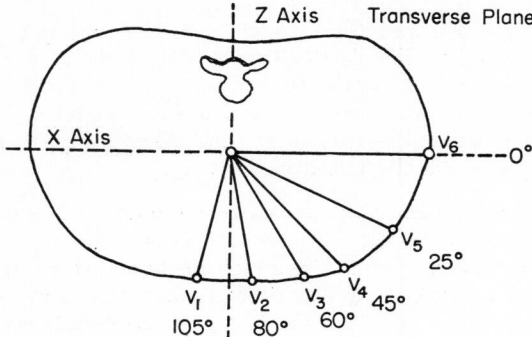

FIG. 54-14. The projection of the chest V lead axes on the transverse plane showing the approximate orientation of the lead axes with respect to the X and Z axes of the body. The actual lead axes, however, do not lie exactly in this plane, but have a variable tilt footward. This figure also shows that the distance of the electrode from the heart varies considerably. Much of this depends on the contour of the chest and position and size of the heart.

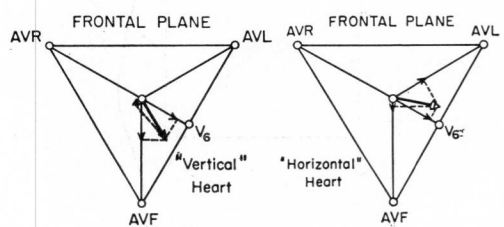

FIG. 54-15. Showing the relationship of the "unipolar" extremity leads to the chest lead V_6. The component in V_6 is likely to be exactly opposite to that of AVR and will resemble that of AVL or AVF, depending on whether the cardiac vector is vertically or horizontally directed.

heart), the components in AVF and V_6 are similar, with a small or negative component in AVL. When the cardiac vector points upward and to the left ("horizontal" heart), the components in AVL and V_6 are similar, with a small or negative component in AVF (Fig. 54-15).

THE ERRORS IN LEAD SYSTEMS FOR REPRESENTING THE CARDIAC VECTOR

In the discussion so far the assumption has been made that two electrodes constitute two poles between which a straight line, called the axis of the lead, can be drawn. Then it is assumed that all electrical forces arising anywhere in the heart will have components on this lead axis which can be calculated by simple geometric rules for the resolution of forces. Implicit in these assumptions is the condition that any other lead axis parallel to the same plane will give the same result (Fig. 54-16).

In actuality, the forces are not conducted along straight lines between the two electrodes. For example, the flow of electricity between two poles such as in lead I follows curved lines. These lines of flow are called the *lead* field. The lead field of lead I is not a series of straight lines but is like what one would expect from the flow of fluid through the body into one arm and out the other (Fig. 54-17).

Thus, in actuality, the reference lines representing lead axes are not all straight. Vector forces which have the same direction and magnitude in different parts of the heart may not have exactly the same components in the lead axis because of a curving linear reference line in one part. According to ideal theory, a force which in the heart is perpendicular to the theoretical lead axis should not have a component on the lead; but, in actuality, it may have a component on this lead because of conduction from the heart to the electrode along curved rather than straight lines. This accounts for the fact that Einthoven's law is not completely ac-

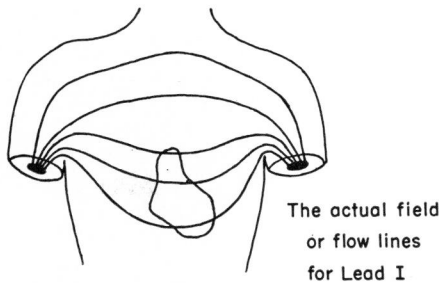

The actual field or flow lines for Lead I

FIG. 54-17. The flow lines through the region of the heart which are established by lead I are only approximately parallel to a line which conventionally represents the lead I axis (Fig. 54-16). This means that forces from some parts of the heart have a vertical direction and may influence lead I potentials, which would not be the case if the flow lines were perfectly parallel.

curate, that the heart does not behave exactly like a point source of electrical force, that the electrical center of the heart is not exactly in the center of an equilateral triangle, and that the central terminal of the V leads is not exactly at zero potential at all times.

In spite of these errors, the idealization of the facts which is made by using the vector theory is useful and practical because it is 80 to 90 per cent correct. The deviations from ideal behavior do not detract from the usefulness of the concepts.

Our present leads are not perfect. They need to be straightened out. Much of modern research is directed toward improving the leads. It is important for the student of medicine (from the first year of medical school to the end of his career) to know the basis of the electrocardiogram so that he will be prepared to understand the advances which are certain to occur.

THE TIME COURSE OF THE CARDIAC VECTOR AND ITS RELATIONSHIP TO AXIAL COMPONENT RECORDS

While there is considerable variation in the direction of the cardiac vectors due to variations in the position of the heart in the chest, there are general features of the time course which may be outlined. The time course of the magnitude and direction of the cardiac forces and their components can be illustrated best by a consideration of them as projected on the simple framework of the three planes of the body: viz., *frontal* (X against Y axis) (Fig. 54-18), *sagittal* (Y against Z axis) (Fig. 54-19), and *transverse* (X against Z axis) (Fig. 54-20). The illustrations are made from an actual record of a normal patient. Each numbered dot represents the end of an instantaneous vector

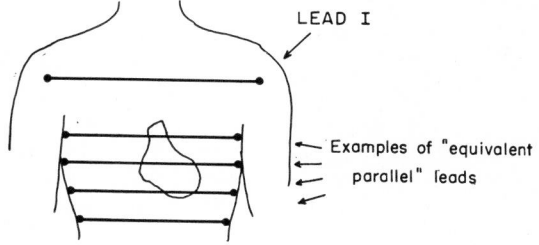

LEAD I

Examples of "equivalent parallel" leads

FIG. 54-16. If lead I records only forces which have components in the direction of the lead axis, then the lines of flow, or the "lead field," can be represented as a series of parallel lines. Under these conditions, one might expect any lead oriented parallel to the X axis in the same plane to give the equivalent results.

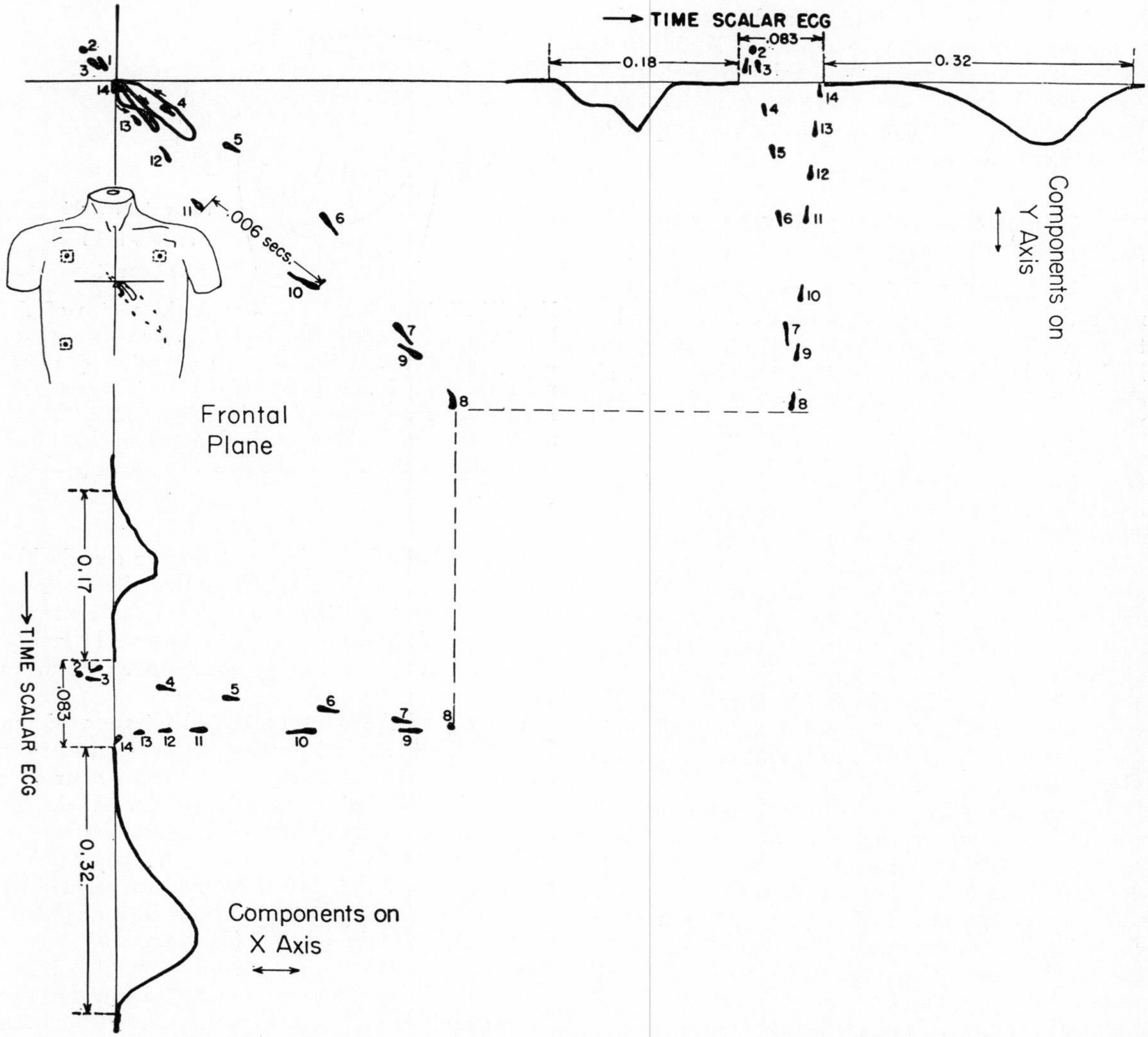

FIG. 54-18. In the upper left-hand corner is a frontal plane vectorcardiograph recorded from electrodes located on the back of a person in the positions illustrated. There are three loops: the smallest (solid line), which doubles on itself, is caused by atrial depolarization, and the larger solid-line loop is caused by ventricular repolarization. The largest (interrupted numbered dots) is due to ventricular depolarization. They are sometimes referred to as the "P," "T," and "QRS" loops, because their components on the lead axes describe deflections having these designations (see Fig. 54-22). It is better to call them the "atrial" and "ventricular" loops. See text for further explanation. The durations, in seconds, of the major intervals of the cycle are given on scalar records.

arrow. The time course is indicated by the distance between dots, which is 0.006 sec, or 6 msec. The direction in which the vector is moving is revealed by the tapered end which points in the direction of motion. For each position of the vector on the planar surface, there is a simultaneous axial component for both axes of the plane. These axial components are taken simultaneously and are the electrocardiographic time-based or *scalar tracings* of the potentials along each axis. They are arranged in the proper spatial relationship as components of the cardiac vector on each axis.

A line drawn from the center of the vector figure to any of the dots gives the magnitude and direction of the vector at that time. From the illustration one sees that in the first few milliseconds the forces of ventricular depolarization are small (short distance from center) and point frontward to the right and very slightly upward. Remembering the pathway of the depolarization wave of the ventricular muscle, one can correlate the magnitude and direction of the vector with it. The first event is a wave in the septal region from left to right. Thus the initial forces are normally small and directed from

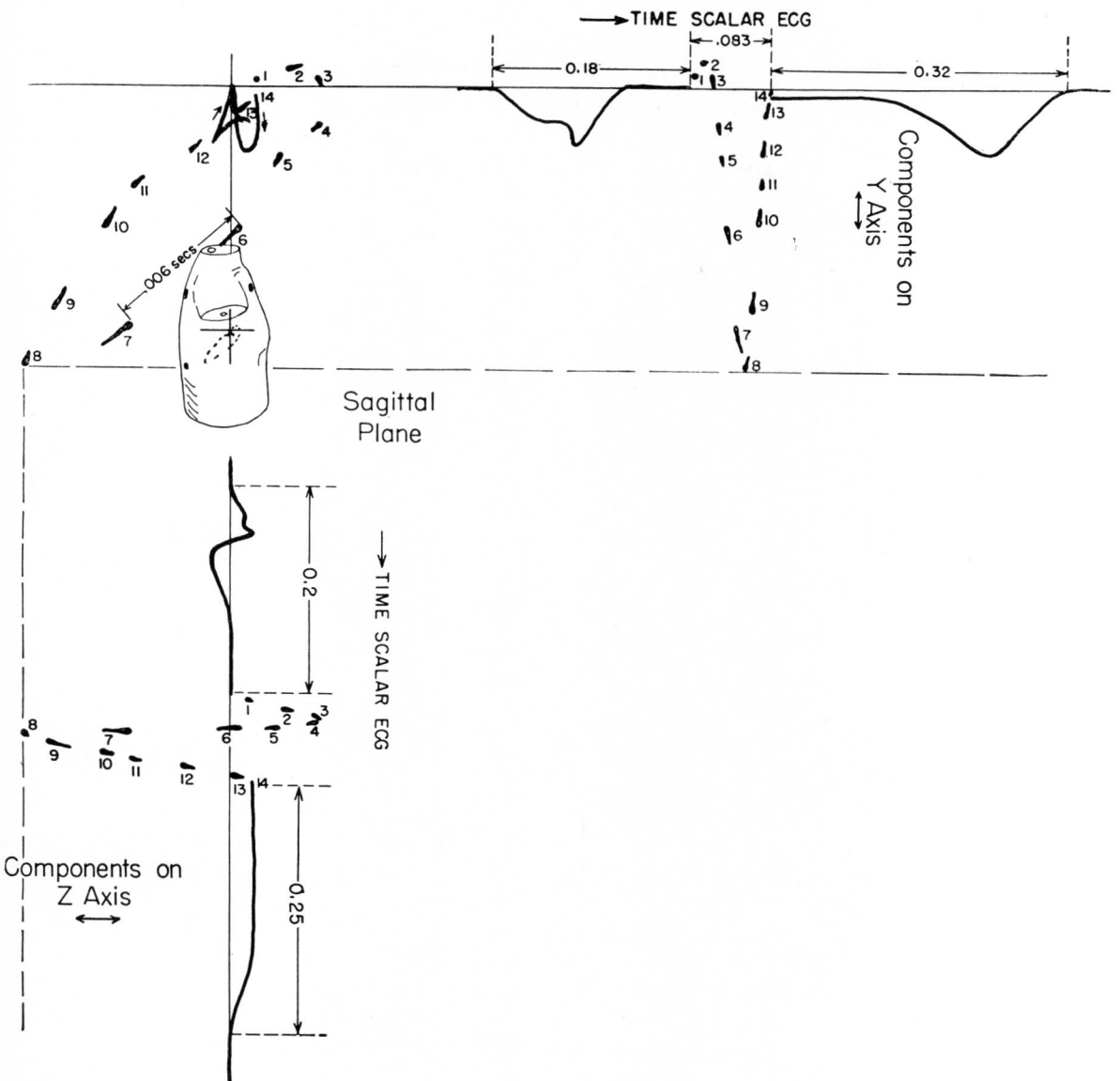

FIG. 54-19. A normal sagittal plane vectorcardiograph with the time scalar components on each axis. (Same person as in Figs. 54-18 and 54-20.)

left to right, and frontward and upward (vector dots 1, 2, and 3). Next, the wave spreads to the inner surfaces of both right and left ventricles and begins to move through from inside outward. The net effect is a balancing of left and right ventricular forces, which moves the cardiac vector to the left and downward (vector dots 4, 5, and 6). Finally, the left ventricular mass predominates and the vector is larger and is pointed to the left, backward and downward (vector dots 7, 8, 9, and 10). The final smaller portion to be depolarized results in a diminution of the vector magnitude and a re-

turn to the center, or null point (vector dots 11, 12, 13, and 14). Sometimes the terminal vector will be directed slightly to the right and upward as well as backward, correlating with the last wave of depolarization upward toward the base of the heart.

If the ends of the cardiac vectors are connected with a continuous line, the result is what is called a *vector loop*. Sometimes these records are made with a continuous line or loop. A three-dimensional model can be made with flexible wire to make a "spatial vector loop."

The forces of ventricular depolarization are large

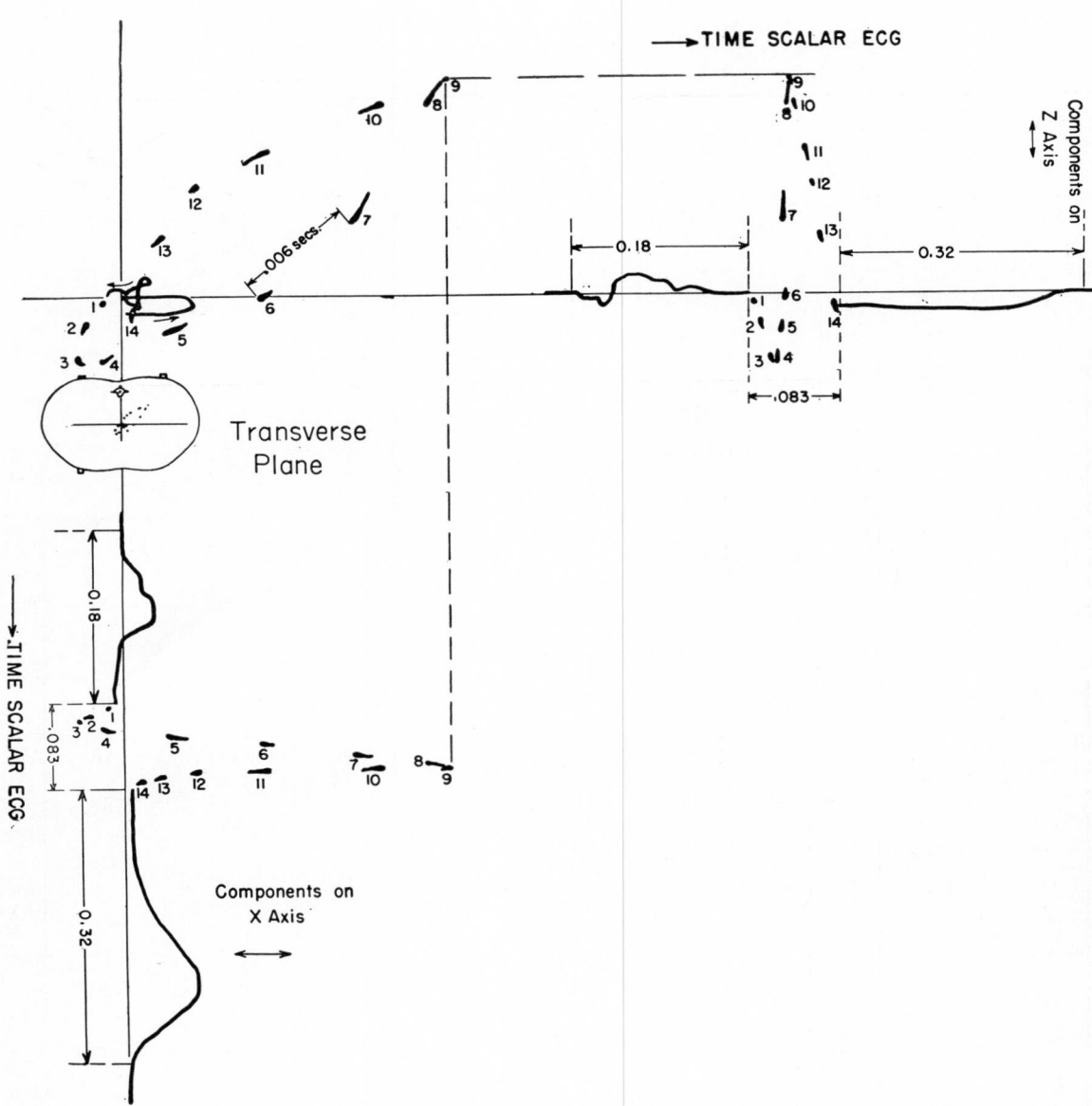

FIG. 54-20. A normal transverse plane vectorcardiograph with the time scalar components on each axis. (Same person as in Figs. 54-18 and 54-19.)

and rapid, as revealed by the larger distance between the equal time dots. The forces of repolarization are smaller and slower to move. Thus the vector loop of the repolarization forces is represented as a smaller, slower-moving loop. It is noteworthy that the general direction in space of the depolarization forces is normally the same as that of repolarization. The small loop is inside the large one. However, there is a normally slight difference in general direction of the repolarization forces, so that on some reference axes or in some leads the components of the two processes may not be pro-

portional or may result in opposite scalar direction (above or below the base line of the axis). An example of this may be seen in the Z axis electrocardiographic scalar components, where the depolarization forces are mostly on one side of the center of the axis and the repolarization forces are on the other. This explains the result that in certain leads in the normal person the sum of the depolarization forces may be opposite in sense to the repolarization process. In this case, it would occur in leads similar to the Z axis, such as in the chest leads, V_1 and V_2.

THE ATRIA

From the illustration of the frontal, sagittal, and transverse components of the atrial depolarization, one can see that the direction of the wave is to the left, downward and slightly backward (see Figs. 54-18, 54-19, and 54-20). These findings are correlated with the anatomic knowledge that the beginning of the electrical depolarization wave is at the sinoatrial node and that the wave spreads over the walls of atria which lie in the chest, mainly to the left and downward from the sinoatrial (SA) node.

The general direction of the atrial forces ensures that the components in lead I and lead II are always positive in the normal, and VR is negative, since the wave direction is away from the VR positive pole. In lead III, the component is quite variable, since the general direction of the forces is nearly perpendicular to this reference axis. In the chest leads, the components of the atrial forces may be small or negative in the leads to the front (V_1 and V_2), since the vector points to the left and sometimes a little backward (Fig. 54-21).

The repolarization of the atria, like that of the ventricles, is a much slower process than depolarization, but unlike the ventricles, the forces of atrial repolarization are directed generally opposite to those of depolarization. Usually in the scalar electrocardiogram, or time-based record of the axial components, the repolarization forces are not recognizable because they occur simultaneously with the much larger ventricular depolarization forces. However, if the interval between atrial depolarization and ventricular depolarization is prolonged, it may be revealed as a small component opposite in sense to the atrial depolarization component.

CONVENTIONAL ELECTROCARDIOGRAPHIC TERMINOLOGY AND METHODS

The usual electrocardiographic method is to record the potentials in one lead at a time. As already

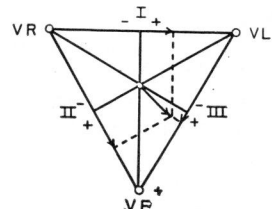

FIG. 54-21. Showing why the normal atrial depolarization forces always give a positive deflection in the frontal plane in lead I and lead II but a deflection in lead III which varies considerably in magnitude and sense.

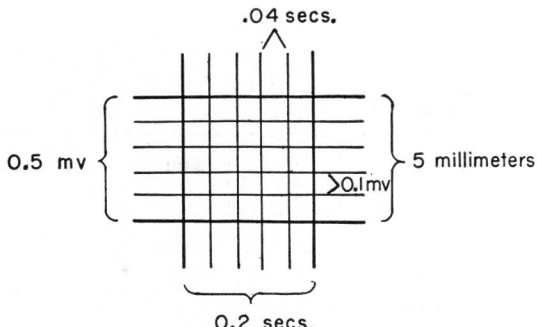

FIG. 54-22. The conventional time and amplitude markings of electrocardiographic record paper.

mentioned, the position of the galvanometer when there is no cardiac electrical activity is described by a line called the *isoelectric line*.

Any deflection above the isoelectric line is called positive, and any below negative. The polarity of the leads is arbitrarily chosen by convention. It is perhaps sometimes confusing when the cardiac muscle depolarization wave direction is spoken of as being positive but ends up on the conventional electrocardiograph tracing as a negative deflection. This is because the depolarization wave may be advancing toward the designated negative pole of the lead axis. At any rate, it is necessary to get into the habit of thinking of positive, or upward, deflections as representing forces having components in the direction of the designated positive pole of the lead axis, and of negative, or downward, deflections as representing forces which have components in the direction of the designated negative pole along the lead axis.

The time and the amplitude markings on the paper are agreed upon by convention (Fig. 54-22). Each small space on the time axis is 0.04 sec, the heavier lines representing 0.20 sec. On the amplitude axis each small space is 0.1 mv and the heavier lines are 0.5 mv apart. In some of the figures in this chapter, time and voltage lines have been omitted when they are not necessary for the purpose of the illustration.

The light lines are 1.0 mm apart.

The first deflection in the normal cycle (Fig. 54-23) is the atrial wave, or *P wave* (it may be positive, negative, or biphasic).

The first obvious negative deflection after the P wave is called the *Q wave*.

The first obvious positive deflection after the P wave is called the *R wave* (whether there is a Q wave or not).

A negative deflection following the R wave is called an *S wave*.

A second positive deflection following an R wave is called an *R'*.

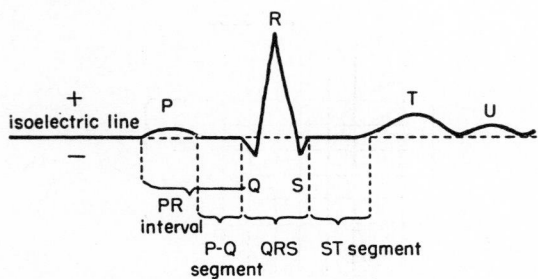

Fig. 54-23. The terminology of the scalar electrocardiogram.

A second negative deflection after the R wave is called an S'.

The whole series which represents the ventricular depolarization process is called the QRS *complex.*

It is apparent that the terminology may result in labeling the same cardiac forces with different symbols in different leads. For example, a Q wave in one lead may be a component of the identical cardiac forces which produce an R wave in a lead having a differently oriented axis. It would be better, perhaps, to think of all lead deflections due to ventricular depolarization as occurring in three time groups: viz., initial forces, middle forces, and late forces, rather than labeling some deflections arbitrarily with different letters regardless of identical origin.

The deflection coincident with and due to ventricular repolarization is called the *T wave.* That part of the tracing which immediately follows ventricular depolarization is called the *S-T segment.* (Even if there is no S wave, it is called the S-T segment.)

From the beginning of ventricular depolarization to the end of repolarization (marked by the end of the T wave) is called the *Q-T interval.*

Following the T wave there may be evident another small deflection called the *U wave.* This component is considered to be related to a repolarization process which is very late and slow to occur and is associated with readjustment of electrolyte concentration within the muscle cells. It will be remembered that depolarization is associated with loss of potassium and gain of sodium ions within the cells. It may be that readjustment of these ions is not completely accomplished by the end of the T wave but is completed coincident with the U wave. Good evidence for this relationship is the finding that clinical disease with electrolyte derangements involving potassium and sodium may cause marked deviations in the form and size of the U waves as well as in the T waves.

The time from the beginning of atrial depolarization to the beginning of ventricular depolarization is called the *P-R interval.* Actually, the purpose is to measure the atrioventricular conduction time. In some leads it turns out to be not the P-R interval but the P-Q interval. This is because in some leads the initial forces may have no component on the lead axes, so that the P-R segment includes some of the depolarization time. The lead which has a clearly visible, early deflection of the P wave which gives the shortest "P-R" interval is the correct one.

The time from the beginning of the Q wave and the end of the S wave is called the QRS *duration* and represents an important measurement of the duration of depolarization. The duration may seem to be shorter in some leads because of the absence of one of the components of the initial or late depolarization forces. In this case, the longest interval is the correct one.

INTERPRETATION OF THE ELECTROCARDIOGRAM

The process of interpretation of the electrocardiogram is carried out by the physician in stages. In the first place, he inspects the records to be certain that they are technically satisfactory and accurate. It is always wise to check the markings of the tracings to be sure that they represent correctly placed leads and that they belong to the right patient.

Certain quantitative measurements are noted, such as the duration of the various intervals previously mentioned. The rest of the process involves quite a remarkable mental accomplishment. It involves an estimate of the magnitudes and directions of the QRS deflections relative to those of the T waves, and then a comparison of these estimates with normal experience. One of the most difficult parts of the process of interpretation is to define the limits of normal variation and separate the normal from the abnormal.

Finally, the abnormalities found must be interpreted on the basis of physiologic principles and on the basis of correlative information obtained from the clinical history and physical examination, from histologic, biochemical, and other special observations. The electrocardiographic instrument is a very accurate tool. It reveals accurate electrical information. However, the electrocardiographic examination of the patient is only as accurate as the physician who interprets the records. The interpreter's success depends on his knowledge and understanding of the physical and physiologic principles combined with long and careful correlative clinical study. There are many unsolved problems and much still to be learned about the basis of the electrocardiogram.

One of the most frequent errors of electrocardiographic interpretation is to attach too much significance to minor variations in one part of the process (commonly the T wave) without consideration of the relationships of this part to the whole picture, that is, the whole electrocardiographic as well as the whole clinical picture.

RELATION OF MAGNITUDE AND DIRECTION OF DEPOLARIZATION (QRS) FORCES TO THOSE OF REPOLARIZATION (T)

The problem of assessing the relationship of QRS to T is susceptible to quantitative methods based on sound physiologic principles. To illustrate this fact, a simplified model of a segment of muscle can be used again. If the depolarization wave proceeds from endocardium to epicardium, the result can be represented as a positive deflection in the lead along this axis. Now, if repolarization starts on the endocardial surface and follows *exactly the same pathway* (although more slowly), the result will be an exactly *oposite deflection* (Fig. 54-24). (It should be noted that although the direction of the movement of the process is the same, one is a discharge and the other is a recharge, giving opposite electrical force directions.) In addition, the total area enclosed by the deflections and the isoelectric line should be equal, because the net energy change (force × time) of the two processes is zero. Now, if one examines the case where repolarization follows a *pathway exactly opposite* to that of depolarization, it is found that both deflections in the lead are in the *same direction* still with *equal areas* (Fig. 54-25).

Transferring this concept to the whole heart in the body, one can say that if repolarization follows exactly the same pathway through the muscle, it can be expected that every electrocardiographic lead on the surface of the body will show the QRS area to be opposite in electrical sense to the T area. (If the QRS area is positive, the T area will be negative and vice versa.)

To represent this concept in a quantitative and spatial way, the *areas* of the QRS and T can be plotted as *vectors*. This is reasonable because the

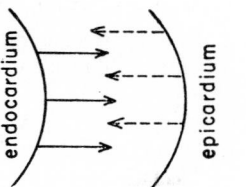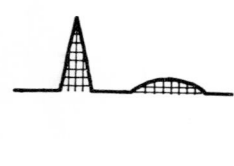

Fig. 54-25. When the direction of repolarization (dotted arrows) is opposite to that of depolarization (solid arrows), the sense of the QRS and T areas will be the same.

areas do have direction as well as magnitude. Areas have direction for the same reason that instantaneous vectors have direction, namely, that the direction of the depolarization and repolarization is spatially oriented within the body. The *area*, when used as a vector, is an expression of the *mean direction* of forces. This can be examined spatially by seeing how the *area vector manifests* itself on each body plane (Fig. 54-26).

From this illustration it is apparent that any lead axis from the center to the surface which lies anywhere in the shaded zone will give a positive area QRS and a negative T (vice versa on the other side of the sphere). The line drawn at right angles to the area vectors is the lead axis where the net area of the QRS and T are zero. Thus while different leads will give varying magnitude of the areas of the QRS and T, the *relative* magnitude of the areas will always be the same in this example.

A method for determining these area vectors is as follows: The net area in each lead for each process can easily be estimated by counting the number of small boxes enclosed by the QRS and T deflections, taking into account that if the QRS or T is biphasic (partly positive and partly negative), the areas of each process are added algebraically; the areas of the QRS on each lead axis are treated as components of the spatial QRS area vector; the two area components (AQRS on the X axis and AQRS

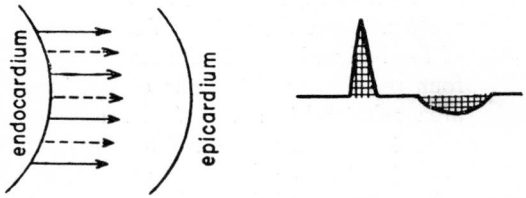

Fig. 54-24. When the directions of the depolarization (solid arrows) and repolarization (dotted arrows) pathways are identical, the scalar deflections will show the QRS area to be equal and opposite in sense to the T area.

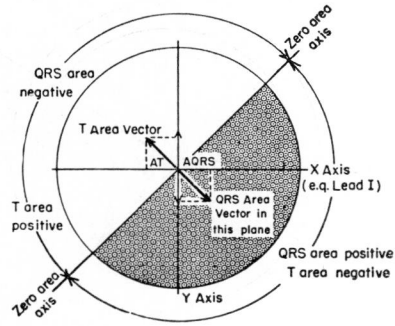

Fig. 54-26. The use of the QRS and T areas as vectors in one plane to define the relationship of QRS and T deflections to be expected from any lead in that plane.

on the Y axis) are added vectorwise to obtain the resultant which is the *resultant manifest vector for the plane defined by the two leads*. The same is done for the T waves.

All is not so simple and orderly, however, when one examines the behavior of the human heart with respect to depolarization-repolarization pathways. But if the principles just outlined are followed, reasonable order is found in the deviations of behavior or in what may seem like a disorderly array of lead patterns. For most of these concepts medicine is indebted to Dr. Frank Wilson, who stands together with Waller and Einthoven, the great scientists in electrocardiography.

In the human heart, the repolarization process does not follow the same pathway as depolarization. There is a different order. Indeed, it may start in different parts of the muscle at different times and be quite inhomogeneous in its progress. The result is that the QRS and T areas have different relative magnitudes and directions in various leads.

In spite of the difference in pathway of repolarization, the relationship to the depolarization pathway shows a reliable regularity which is predictable and quantifiable. In other words, in the normal heart there are fairly regularly predictable interdependent pathways for both processes.

In Fig. 54-27, the circle is divided into segments by the lines drawn at right angles to the QRS and T area vectors. These lines are the T area = zero line, and the QRS area = zero line.

Plotting the mean direction and magnitude of both the QRS and T areas as vectors manifest on the frontal plane of the body for a normal person gives the diagram which immediately reveals what will be the relationship of the QRS to T area in any electrocardiographic lead in the frontal plane.

There are two important conclusions to be drawn from this. First, it is obvious that the manifest direction of the repolarization pathway is not the same as that of depolarization (not as in Fig. 54-26), but is almost opposite.

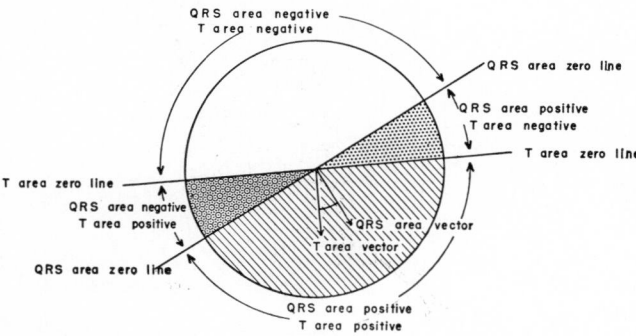

FIG. 54-27. The relationships of QRS and T areas in the leads in a plane similar to the relationships found in the frontal plane of a normal human being.

Secondly, the angle between the QRS and T area vectors is small, which means that only in leads in a small segment of the surface of the body will the QRS and T deflections have opposite areas. From the diagram it is readily seen that this angle between the QRS and T area vectors, when rotated 90° in either direction, is the same angle which determines the size of the segments of the sphere where leads will give QRS opposite to T areas in the tracings.

Thus it is seen that in the normal heart depolarization proceeds generally from inside outwards, and repolarization mainly from outside inward (see Fig. 54-25). The slower repolarization of the inner layers of myocardium is due supposedly to a poorer blood supply and higher tension in the inner layer during ventricular systole. Repolarization occurs during ventricular systole while the ventricular muscle is ejecting blood. The second heart sounds which mark the end of mechanical systole are nearly simultaneous with the end of "electrical systole," which is marked by the end of the T wave.

The angle between the QRS and T area vectors is perhaps one of the best single indications of normality. It is quite constant in normal hearts. One of the reasons why the angle between the two vectors is valuable is that it is quite independent of the position of the heart in the body. Different body configurations may make the general direction of both the QRS and T areas quite variable from one person to another. However, these "positional" variations will not change the fundamental spatial relationship between QRS and T areas, which is expressed by the angle between the two area vectors. This angle depends on the normality of the pathways of depolarization and repolarization in the heart muscle, and not upon the position of the heart in the body.

While the QRS and T area vectors have been represented diagrammatically as manifest in one plane, the spatial QRS and T area vectors do not necessarily lie in this plane. When considered three-dimensionally, the QRS and T area vectors divide the body into four pieces. These pieces are obtained by slicing the body along planes which are at right angles to the two vectors. These four pieces define the parts of the body wherein lead axes will give the four possible combinations of QRS and T area relationships: viz. (QRS area +, T area +), (QRS area −, T area −), (QRS area +, T area −), (QRS area −, T area +). Examples of the exploded sliced pieces of the body representing the four zones are given for a normal person (Fig. 54-28) and for a person with left ventricular hypertrophy due to hypertension (Fig. 54-29).

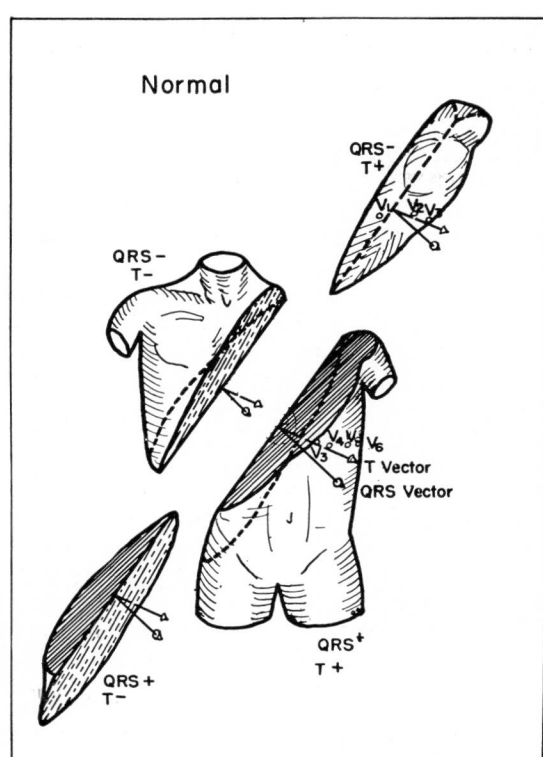

FIG. 54-28. The three-dimensional segments of a body "exploded" to show a normal example of the zones where various relationships between QRS and T areas exist. When put together, the upper right piece fits on front, the lower left piece fits on back. The planes of the two slices are identified by the continuous lines and the interrupted lines on the surfaces of the slices. (Same person as in Fig. 54-32.)

In the latter case, not only is the mean QRS direction altered because of the preponderance of the left ventricular muscle mass, but also the mean direction of the T is markedly different from that of the QRS. The disease has caused a marked change in the general direction of repolarization. In contrast to the normal, in the hypertensive heart a reversal of the relationships of QRS and T directions is found.

INJURY, INFARCT, AND ISCHEMIA

When the blood supply to an area of cardiac muscle is insufficient to maintain the life of the muscle and to support its function, there appear in the electrocardiogram usually three distinct deviations from the normal which correlate with the anatomic-pathologic picture (Fig. 54-30). The word *infarct* is used electrocardiographically to describe the area of muscle which is completely dead and has no more electrical activity. In and around the

area of dead muscle there is usually a zone of muscle which is still electrically active, but whose function has been severely disturbed. This area is called *injured* because it produces the injury current in the electrocardiogram (Fig. 54-31). A third area of muscle associated with an infarct is called *ischemic*, which implies that the muscle is functioning but under the stress of poor blood supply. Electrocardiographically, the ischemic area of muscle produces abnormalities in the time course and pathway of repolarization, the process which is so sensitive to interference with cellular metabolism and chemical environment. Thus when a patient who has had a myocardial infarction is examined, there may be evidence of the three anatomic and electrical stages of severity of disease: infarct, injury, and ischemia.

In the usual case, the three abnormal zones of muscle produce their own characteristic vector abnormalities. In Fig. 54-30, the three areas in a segment of ventricular muscle wall are illustrated diagrammatically. The vector arrows of each process are placed opposite outside the heart as though these vectors were being recorded from a lead parallel to the arrows, with the positive pole to the

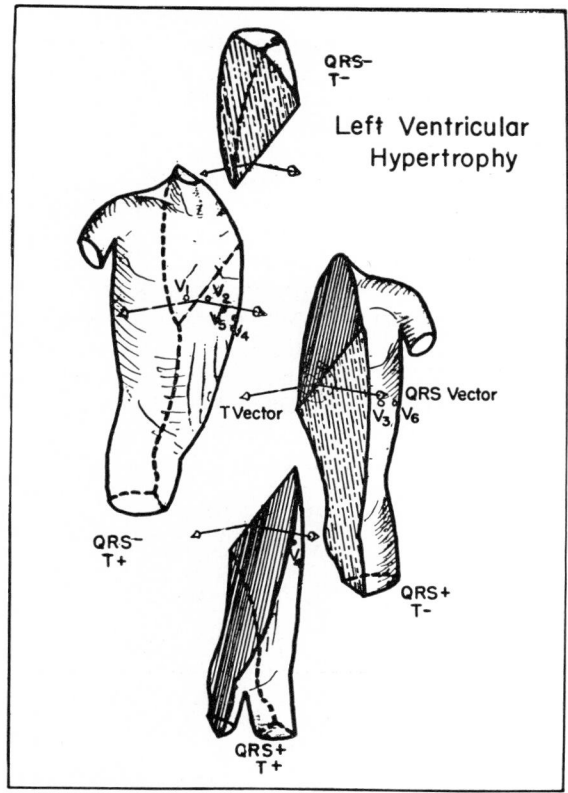

FIG. 54-29. The four segments of the body defined according to relationships of QRS- and T-area directions in a patient with left ventricular hypertrophy.

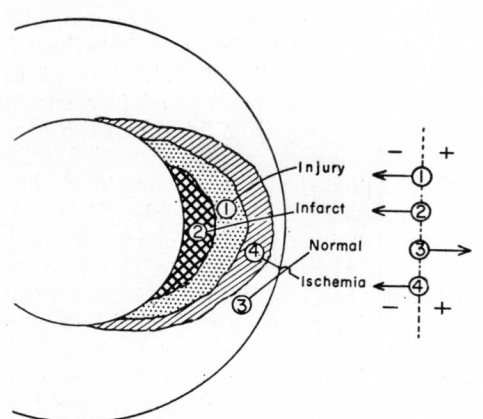

FIG. 54-30. The three anatomic-electrical zones of abnormality associated with a myocardial infarction represented diagrammatically.

right and the negative pole on the other side to the left. A diagrammatic scalar electrocardiogram which represents for one cardiac cycle the time sequence of the electrical events on this lead is given in Fig. 54-31.

First, it can be seen that the injury current has caused the "base line," or isoelectric line, to be shifted downward because of the negative vector of the injury current. Secondly, the beginning of the depolarization process results in a negative deflection (Q wave in this lead) because of the unbalancing effect of the dead muscle. In other words, if the dead area were alive the initial deflection would have been upright or positive. Thirdly, there is the upright deflection (R wave) due to the depolarization of the normal muscle.

At the end of depolarization (the beginning of the S-T segment), the deflection has not returned to the base line as in the normal, but shows an elevation. This S-T segment elevation is actually caused by the disappearance of the injury current during depolarization. Gradually, the injury current reappears, causing the S-T segment to return to the original level. At the same time the fourth event takes place, viz., the abnormal inversion of the T

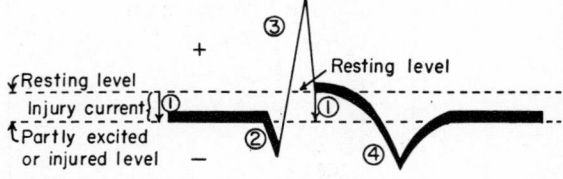

FIG. 54-31. A diagrammatic scalar electrocardiogram showing the effects upon its components of the three zones or processes associated with a myocardial infarction. The numbers refer to the zones and vectors illustrated in Fig. 54-30.

wave due to the abnormal forces of repolarization arising in the ischemic area. Normally the T wave would be positive, or upright.

CORRELATION OF ELECTROCARDIOGRAPHIC WITH CLINICAL AND PATHOLOGIC EVIDENCE OF ABNORMALITY

One of the most important principles of correlation is to *make repeated or serial observations* of change in the picture. This is particularly important in cases where coronary insufficiency, ischemia, injury, and infarction are suspected. This is the fifth dimension of electrocardiographic interpretation, namely, the correlation of the repeated electrocardiographic observation with the time course of the disease as revealed by repeated clinical, pathologic, and physiologic observations. The initial insult caused by a coronary occlusion or by pericarditis may produce characteristic changes which are different in type and degree from the later effects of the insult. Thus in the very early stage of an eventual myocardial infarction, the changes of injury may predominate. The changes of muscle death or infarction may appear a few hours later, with variable degrees of ischemia. As one might expect from the high degree of variation of size and location of the disorders in the coronary vessels and in the muscle, the serial changes in the electrocardiogram are quite variable.

Sometimes the electrocardiographic changes may seem "extensive," while the clinical pathologic picture shows only evidence of mild injury to the myocardium. This seeming lack of correlation together with some experimental evidence has led some students of electrocardiography to the theory that the electrocardiogram is more influenced by some parts of the myocardium than by others. One must remember, however, that the electrocardiogram represents a small part of the total forces produced because of the cancellation of forces (see p. 502 and Figs. 54-3A and 54-3B). This makes the picture sensitive to localized disorders which may not be extensive but which can unbalance markedly the canceled portion of the forces. To illustrate by a crude calculation, since the electrocardiogram represents roughly only 10 per cent of the forces produced, a small change in the 90 per cent canceled fraction can upset the observed 10 per cent dramatically. One single muscle cell has as much as 80 to 100 mv potential difference across its membrane! The surface electrocardiogram reveals only a few millivolts.

An excellent example of extensive change in the electrocardiogram with small localized change in the myocardium occurs in *pericarditis*. In acute pericarditis there may be in all leads a large injury current, manifested by a shift in the S-T segment. From the physiologic point of view, the heart may function perfectly well as a pump. From the standpoint of pathology, there can be found only a slight cloudy swelling of the myocardium limited to the

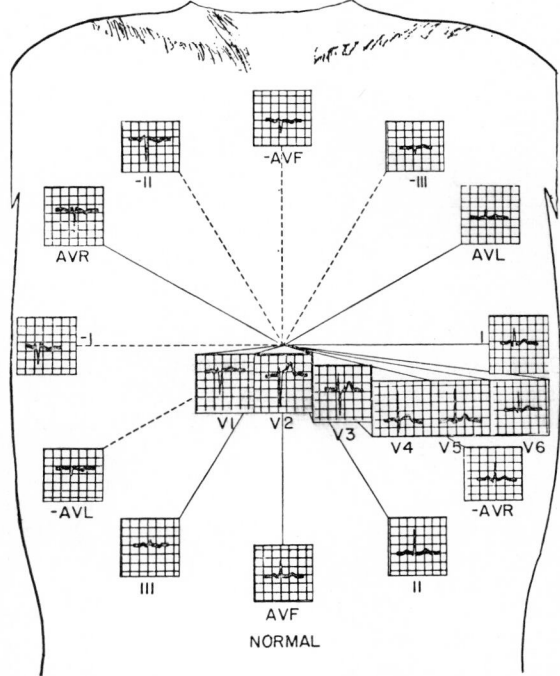

Fig. 54-32. The conventional scalar electrocardiographic tracings of a normal person (same person as in Fig. 54-28). One cardiac cycle for each lead is shown. The time lines are 0.2 sec. The smaller time lines of 0.04 sec which are usually shown on scalar tracing paper have been omitted for the sake of clarity. The tracings are arranged on a body figure according to the orientation of the lead axes with respect to the ideal theoretical electrical center of the heart. The chest leads V_1 to V_6 are placed in their approximate spatial relationship, showing their axes projected inward to the center. The standard leads I, II, III and the unipolar leads AVR, AVL, and AVF are placed at both the positive and negative poles of their axes. The negative axes are dotted lines.

As one inspects the tracings, proceeding around the periphery of the frontal plane, the relationship of one lead to another is readily apparent. Cne can also readily see that the lateral chest leads (V_5 and V_6) are very similar to the frontal plane leads (AVR and I). The amplitude of the chest leads is larger when the electrodes are closer to the heart, but diminished at a distance, as in V_6. Thus the relative amplitude of one part (QRS) to the other (T) is more important than the relation of amplitude from lead to lead. These scalar tracings should be inspected in relation to the body segments shown in Fig. 54-28 of the same person.

layer of the epicardium, measuring only a fraction of a millimeter. In other words, one does not think of pericarditis as an extensive myocardial disease, but the electrocardiogram may show "extensive" changes. After the pericarditis is healed, there may be a permanent residual abnormality in the electrocardiogram consisting of several inverted T waves, because of residual distortion of the repolarization pathway through this thin layer of muscle. This does not necessarily mean, however, that the clinical electrocardiogram is more sensitive to the outer layer than any other layer of myocardium.

A good example of unbalancing of the electrical forces occurs with *ventricular ectopic beats* (ventricular premature contractions or ventricular extrasystoles). The complex produced by an ectopic focus in the ventricle reveals a much larger voltage and is of longer duration than the normal. This larger voltage in the electrocardiogram is the result of less cancellation of forces, and the longer duration is due to the longer, slower spread of the depolarization wave from the ectopic focus through the muscle than would occur through the normal rapid pathway of the special conduction system (Purkinje system and bundles).

Defects in the ventricular conduction system such as *right or left bundle branch block* produce characteristic abnormalities in the electrocardiogram because of delay in the depolarization wave reaching and spreading through either the right or left muscles. In both cases the total depolarization time (QRS duration) is prolonged (greater than 0.10 sec). With *right bundle branch block*, the depolarization wave proceeds normally through the septum (see pp. 510–511) and the left ventricle, but the spread through the right ventricular wall is delayed. This produces late vector forces pointing to the right, upward and forward. Thus in leads AVR and V_1, there appears a late wide R wave. A similar picture can be produced by *right ventricular hypertrophy*. The greater thickness and mass of muscle in the right ventricle causes a longer and larger "right ventricle vector." With *left bundle branch block* the septum depolarizes mainly from right to left. The wave through the left ventricle is delayed and produces a late vector force pointing to the left and slightly backward. A normal electrocardiogram illustrating the tracings obtained from the conventional leads is illustrated in Fig. 54-32.

REFERENCES

Burch, G. E., and Travis Winsor: "A Primer of Electrocardiography," Philadelphia, W. B. Saunders Company, 1955.

Craib, W. H.: The Electrocardiogram, Med. Research Council (Brit.) Spec. Rept. Ser. No. 147, 1930.

Grant, R. P.: Clinical Electrocardiography: The Spatial Vector Approach, New York, McGraw-Hill Book Company, Inc., Blakiston Division, 1957.

Hecht, Hans H. (Ed.): The Electrophysiology of the Heart, Ann. N.Y. Acad. Sci., 65:653, 1957.

McFee, R., and F. D. Johnston: Electrocardiographic Leads: I. Introduction, Circulation, 8:554, 1953.

——, and ——: Electrocardiographic Leads: II. Analysis, III. Synthesis, Circulation, 9:255, 868, 1954.

Shedlovsky, Theodore: "Electrochemistry in Biology and Medicine," New York, John Wiley & Sons, Inc., 1955.

Wilson, F. N., A. G. Macleod, and P. S. Barker: "The Distribution of the Currents of Action and of Injury Displayed by Heart Muscle and Other Excitable Tissues," Ann Arbor, University of Michigan Press, 1933.

Wolff, Louis: "Electrocardiography," Philadelphia, W. B. Saunders Company, 1956.

55 PRINCIPLES OF ELECTROENCEPHALOGRAPHY

Robert S. Schwab

The electroencephalographic examination is a part of the complete clinical study of a neurologic patient, but it may also be used in the evaluation of the nervous effects of a number of medical diseases. This chapter in no sense attempts to describe the details of the electroencephalographic interpretation nor the technique of making the examination. Adequate manuals are available for this and are mentioned in the bibliography.

History. Electroencephalography had its roots in neurophysiology and neuroanatomy. In 1875 Caton in England, using a sensitive coil galvanometer coupled to an optical "multiplier," recorded electrical potentials from the exposed brains of rabbits. In 1895 Einthoven made a still more sensitive galvanometer, placing a quartz thread in the strong magnetic field of a horseshoe magnet, and then connecting each end of this string to one of the pair of electrodes. These were moist pads tied to silver plates; each was fastened to a wrist of the subject. There was sufficient voltage from the beating heart to twist or displace this thread a few degrees, and the tiny mirror on the thread could then reflect a focused beam of light onto a moving film and register by such *enlargement* the wave form of this electrical discharge of the electrocardiogram. It should be noted that there is no amplification of the electrical heart wave but only enlargement, but the technique was not adequate to record the feeble ($\frac{1}{10}$ the voltage) electric discharge from the bone-enclosed brain. In 1928 Hans Berger in Germany added a vacuum-tube amplifier to a string galvanometer. He was then able to record the electrical waves from the brain through electrodes on the scalp. His first subject was his son. Berger coined the word *electroencephalogram* to describe these *rhythms* and wrote 16 different papers, all in German.

Verification of these findings came from the laboratory of E. D. Adrian at Cambridge University in 1933, and in his reports, the first published in English, he referred to these recordings of the electrical activity of the brain as the EEG or the Berger rhythm. For this work and other pioneer investigations he received the Nobel prize. He was the first to use an ink-writing oscillograph to record the waves. From this time on the practice of using electronic amplifiers and various types of ink-writing recorders spread all over the world.

The Origin of the Electrical Activity of the Cerebrum. The electrical activity of the brain is essentially a specialized form of the general phenomenon of electricity in living cells. To the neurophysiologist the brain appears as a superbly organized and very complicated network of many billions of cells, each of which consists of a rhomboid-shaped (0.05 to 0.1 mm in diameter) perikaryon, a single transmitting filament called the *axone* which may be as short as 0.5 mm or as long as 2 m, and multiple short processes called *dendrites* which are the receiving elements of the nerve cell. The nucleus has about a millivolt negative charge of direct current in reference to the positively charged surface membrane. It builds up and maintains this electrical potential much as does the muscle cell of the heart (cf. p. 501), by the entrance of potassium ions and the exodus of sodium ions. The living cell membrane and the nucleus are integral factors in this ionic exchange, a process which consumes energy and requires oxygen and glucose. A nerve cell in this state is polarized.

Both the inside of the dendrites and the axone, like the cell body, are negative to their surface membrane, i.e., are polarized. A stimulus of adequate electrical or chemical strength received at one of the dendrites will destroy this chemical equilibrium and depolarize the membrane. Sodium now enters, potassium leaves, and for a brief period of time (0.5 to 1 msec) a current flows toward the cell body and thence along the axone to its branching tip. It moves, however, by a series of depolarizing chemical changes identical to that initiated by the original stimulus in the dendrite. It does not flow as an electric current in a wire. Its speed becomes less as the diameter of the fiber becomes smaller. Many stimuli from the axones of other cells are too weak to set off this depolarization but nevertheless do reduce its charge and prepare it for the next stimulus, which may then activate the cell and start the nerve impulse on its way.

The origin of the rhythmic electrical activity recorded from the surface of the brain has been disputed. It used to be thought that the brain waves were conglomerates or envelopes of many action spikes from activated cells, waxing and waning together in some kind of sinusoidal rhythm; but recent evidence points to the receiving dendrites in the outer layers of the cerebral cortex as the source. The electrical potentials in this dendritic network build up and partially discharge as subliminal stimuli of neighboring cortical and thalamic axons converge on it. The 10-per-second rhythm fits the properties of this dendritic network. Rhythmic activity has not been obtained from the deepest layers of the cortex; and the white matter, where one might find axone spikes, is singularly silent when reached by depth electrodes.

These basic 8 to 10 per second alpha rhythms, which are dependent upon thalamocorticothalamic circuits, might well serve as a scanning mechanism. Whether they are autonomous or derive their energy from a minuscule portion of the huge sensory inflow that is present at all times is not known. It has been postulated that the reverberations of the 10 per second brain rhythm could maintain the activity of cell networks involved with previous sensations, memories, or emotional feelings. Certain appropriate stimuli would selectively enhance these circuits and other sensory impulses, having no effect, would pass unnoticed. According to this hypothesis the brain rhythm acts as a filter or gate to exclude from mind many of the useless details provided by our sensory apparatus.

EEG Laboratory. The modern laboratory uses commercially built apparatus capable of recording from several areas over the scalp at the same time. The usual console model electroencephalograph has from 8 to as many as 16 separate amplifying and recording units. The amplified brain rhythms are strong enough to move an ink-writing pen which reproduces the wave form of the brain discharges on paper moving at a standard speed of 3 cm (1¼ in.) per sec. [Cf. standard EKG paper speed of 2.5 cm (1 in.) per sec.] The resulting electroencephalogram appears as a number of parallel, wavy lines, as many as there are units, or "channels." Electrodes, which are solder or silver disks 0.5 cm in diameter, are placed over the scalp by means of adhesive material such as bentonite or collodion, using ordinary cardiographic paste under the electrode to make contact with the scalp. Patients are usually examined while seated with their eyes closed and relaxed in a comfortable chair or lying on a bed. The procedure is entirely painless and takes ½ to 1¼ hr.

In addition to the resting record, a number of so-called "activating" procedures are usually carried out:

1. The patient is requested to breathe deeply twenty times a minute for 3 min. The resulting alkalosis may uncover or activate characteristic seizure patterns or other abnormalities.

2. A very powerful flashing light such as a stroboscope is placed over the patient's eyes and flashed at frequencies from 1 per second to 16 per second. This is done with the patient's eyes opened and closed. The occipital visual system may then show abnormal or localizing discharges.

3. The patient is allowed to fall into natural sleep or is given sedative drugs by mouth or by vein, and the pattern is recorded during the sleep period.

4. Small amounts of Metrazol (100 mg per min) may be given intravenously alone or during the flashing of the light to see if the threshold for Metrazol-activating discharges is lower than normal. Other methods of activation such as sounds, insulin, etc., are not so useful as those mentioned. The purpose of these procedures is to produce diagnostically useful abnormalities without inducing convulsions.

The EEG record (electroencephalogram) consists of 50 to 100 pages, each 12 in. long and representing 10 sec of time. These are studied in the same careful manner as in the interpretations of x-rays or electrocardiograms. Competent analysis requires knowledge of the limitations and artefacts produced by the technique, the apparatus, or the movements of the patient.

Types of Normal Recordings. The normal electroencephalographic record in adults is usually easy to identify. The pattern shows symmetrical 10 per second, 50 μv sinusoidal waves in both the occipital and the parietal regions. These wax and wane spontaneously and disappear promptly when the patient opens his eyes or fixes his attention on some object (Fig. 55-1A). The frontal part of the normal record shows waves of lower amplitude, 10 to 20 μv, and faster rhythm, 18 to 24 per second, which are called *beta waves* and are also symmetrical on both sides. Slow waves or sharp spikes or other unusual patterns are absent in a normal record. When the normal subject falls asleep, the rhythm slows in a symmetrical and regular way, and if the sleep is induced by barbiturates an increase in the fast frontal frequencies is characteristic and is considered to be a normal change (Fig. 55-1B).

The record of the normal adult is not activated by the flashing light, although it is quite usual to see an occipital response to each flash of light. This is called the *normal evoked response*, or photic "driving." The arrival of the visual stimulus in the calcarine part of the occipital lobe (just under the midoccipital protuberance in man) occurs about 19

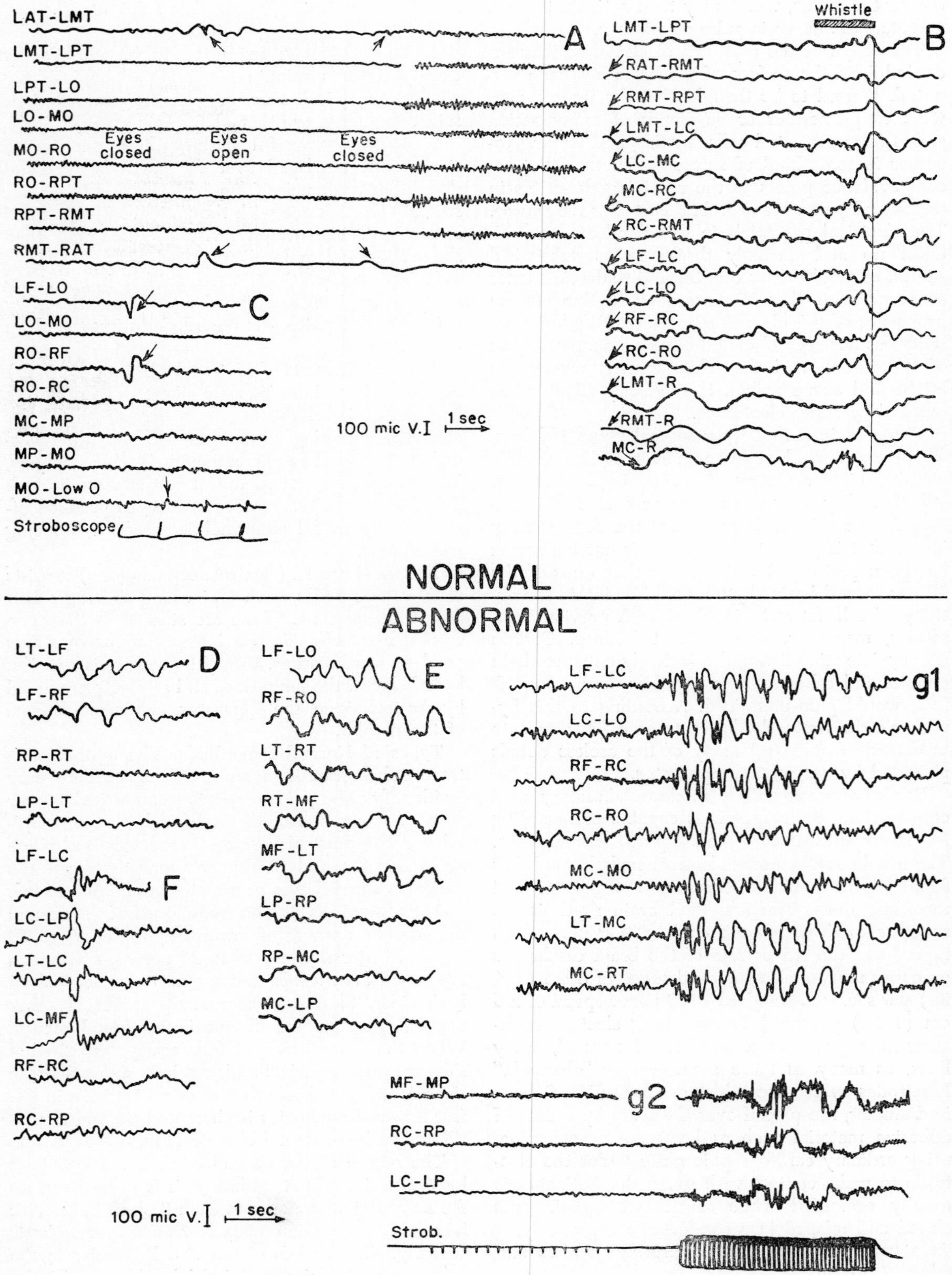

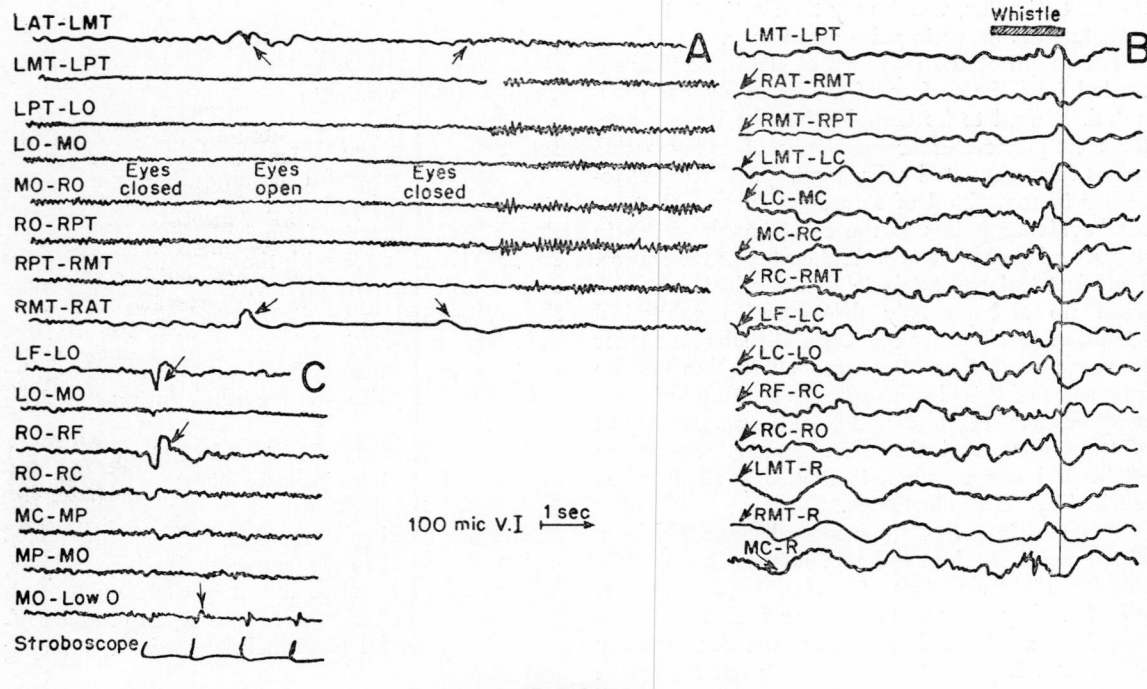

NORMAL

ABNORMAL

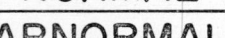

FIG. 55-1. (Caption on next page.)

msec after the flash of light. In animals it has been shown that this event produces in the cortex an extremely brief spike discharge, only a few milliseconds long and only 50 μv in amplitude. With the scalp electrodes 1 to 2 cm away from the brain and with the ink-writing oscillograph which cannot follow or record such brief duration discharges, this primary evoked response is not seen in the EEG. The primary response, however, secondarily activates a great many more neurones which communicate with cells in the thalamus, with other areas in the cortex, and the reticular cells in the midbrain, which in turn reverberate their electrical activity back to the occipital cortex. Now the discharge is some 60 to 80 msec long and 200 or more μv in amplitude. This is called the *secondary evoked response* and can be seen in 90 per cent of all subjects, even in the presence of the background of the regular brain waves. It takes some 50 or 60 msec after the primary response for the secondary one to appear, the total latency between the flash and the secondary evoked response (Fig. 55-1C) being 70 to 90 msec.

The clinical usefulness of this evoked occipital response has increased the scope of electroencephalography in several ways. First of all, one can be reasonably sure that a person with such a response can see or at least can perceive the light. Therefore a patient with such a response who claims he is totally blind is suffering from hysteria or is malingering. In situations where this evoked response is absent on one side of the head but present on the other, there is physiologic evidence of a lesion interfering with normal transmission between the optic decussation and the occipital lobe on this side and can imply the presence of a hemianopsia. Finally when the flashing light causes the occipital response to spread all over the cortex and activate abnormal waves, there is evidence of a very hypersensitive cortex. This will produce seizure patterns in the EEG if the activation procedure is continued, or if still more sensitive, frank, myoclonic jerks of face or arms, or rarely major convulsions.

Overbreathing usually does not change the record in the normal adult. Metrazol has little effect on normal persons when less than 500 mg (in patients who weigh 150 lb) is injected at the rate of 100 mg per min. Children and adolescents are more sensitive to all the activating agents mentioned, and a different set of standards has to be applied. It is customary for children to develop slow activity of between 3 and 4 waves per second during the middle and latter part of overbreathing. This promptly disappears within a minute after the hyperventilation has stopped. Here it is to be noted that the frequency of the occipital rhythms in newborn infants is normally less than 3 per second and very irregular. There is a gradual steady increase in frequency of these occipital rhythms with maturation, and so by the age of twelve to fourteen years the normal 9 to 10 per second alpha is the dominant pattern. It is agreed among electroencephalographers that children's and infants' records are the most difficult to interpret, since the wide range of normal values makes sharp separation impossible. Nevertheless asymmetrical records or records with seizure patterns are clearly abnormal in children of any age.

Types of Abnormal Recordings. The most pathologic finding of all is the disappearance of the EEG pattern and its replacement by a flat line. This means that the electrical activity of the entire cortical mantle is in abeyance. When it persists all over the head for more than 10 sec, it is unlikely that any brain activity exists, and in such cases the damage is often irreversible.

Localized areas of such flattening may also occur in cases where there is a large area of softening or an extensive surface tumor or clot lying between the cerebral cortex and the electrodes. With such

---

FIG. 55-1. Abbreviations used in illustrations: R—right; L—left; F—frontal; C—central (motor area); T—temporal; P—parietal; O—occipital; A—anterior; M—mid; R—reference or inactive lead (such as nose, both ears, or midpost neck); mic V.—microvolt; sec—second; Strob.—stroboscope.

A. 8-channel record; normal subject with eyes open and closed. Note symmetry on the two sides and disappearance of alpha when eyes are open. Arrows show artefact in anterior temporal region from the eye movement.

B. A strip of 15-channel recording; subject asleep. Note slow waves, absence of normal alpha, and symmetry on the two sides. Block on first line shows whistle and evoked response in all leads at line. The small arrows indicate the channel for each electrode pair.

C. Normal subject, showing flash in eye and the evoked response in occipital area. It is seen only in low occipital lead. Arrows show eye movement in frontal leads.

D. Abnormal; brain tumor. Left frontal region showing slow delta waves.

E. Abnormal; head injury. Showing slow data 3 per second, and 5 per second theta both sides.

F. Abnormal; epilepsy (seizure pattern). Focal type with spike and slow-wave focus left temporal region occurring spontaneously.

G. Abnormal; epilepsy (seizure pattern). (1) Petit mal type, showing 3 per second spike and wave (activated by overbreathing). (2) Myoclonic jerk, short seizure activated by 15 per second stroboscope flash, but not by 5 per second flash.

a finding, the localization of the abnormality is precise, but of course the nature of the lesion cannot be ascertained. Abnormal waves arise in the borders of the lesion.

The abnormal waves that have been alluded to are best defined as *slower* and of higher amplitude than normal. Those which are 3 per second with amplitude from 50 to 350 μv are called *delta waves* (Fig. 55-1*D,E*), and the higher-voltage, faster waves are known as *spikes* or *sharp waves* (Fig. 55-1*F*). These fast and slow waves may be combined, and when a series of them suddenly interrupts relatively normal EEG patterns they are highly suggestive of epilepsy. The one associated with the lapses of petit mal spells is a 3 per second spike and wave that characteristically appears in all leads of the electroencephalogram at the same time and disappears equally suddenly at the end of the seizure (Fig. 55-1*G*). This has led to a theoretic localization of at least part of the petit mal discharge in the thalamus or some deep central structures, and there is some experimental evidence that confirms this.

Certain preparations are necessary if electroencephalography is to be done under optimal conditions. The patient should not be sedated and should not have been for a long time without food, for both sedative drugs and relative hypoglycemia modify the normal EEG pattern. The same may be said of mental concentration, extreme nervousness, or anxiety which tend to suppress the normal alpha rhythm. For those suspected of having epilepsy, if the referring physician and the electroencephalographer agree, the test should be done 24 hr after withdrawal of the anticonvulsant drug. It is unusual for seizures to begin in this short time after withdrawal of anticonvulsants, though it may happen. Longer periods without drugs are hazardous. Some physicians prefer to have the first examination made while the patient is receiving drugs, and to withdraw anticonvulsants only if the EEG is normal. In some patients with proved epilepsy a normal-interval record may be found when the patient is receiving anticonvulsant medicines. The type of activation procedure can usually be worked out in advance by contacting the electroencephalographer. In patients with suspected tumors it is helpful to request a definite localization study and to indicate the suspected side.

Neurologic Conditions with Abnormal EEGs. In the following groups of neurologic disorders the EEG may be of considerable help in reaching the correct diagnosis. In others, as will be mentioned, it is of little or of questionable value.

Epilepsy. It may be said that all types of epileptic seizures are associated with some abnormality in the electroencephalogram provided the record-ing is made at the time of the seizure. The only exception is in some deep temporal lobe foci where the discharge never reaches the scalp in sufficient amplitude to be seen against the background activity of the normal scalp EEG, particularly if there is a strong alpha rhythm. In these exceptional cases an anterior temporal electrode, which is most free of occipital alpha frequencies, is most likely to show such a discharge from the depths. A nasopharyngeal lead will usually pick it up. In perhaps 2 to 5 per cent of cases the only way in which this deep activity can be sampled is by opening the skull and inserting an electrode into the substance of the brain. Some electroencephalographers have become enthusiastic over the possible uses of the depth electrode and feel a great deal of information about temporal lobe epilepsy can be obtained by this technique. Whereas it is true that a rare case with temporal lobe epilepsy and a normal EEG at the time of a seizure may be erroneously labeled as hysterical from the EEG alone, the clinical state itself is of help. Certainly most neurologists would be unwilling to allow depth electrode recordings to be made on any of their patients except the few who are having an operation on the brain.

Some of the different types of convulsive seizure patterns are shown in Fig. 55-1*D,E,F*. The petit mal, atypical petit mal, the myoclonic jerk, and the grand mal patterns correlate closely with the clinical seizure type. A fact of importance is that between seizures approximately 20 per cent of all epileptic patients show a normal pattern, and it is for this reason that activation procedures are necessary. Moreover, the records of many epileptic patients are abnormal during and between seizures, but the abnormality is nonspecific, and therefore the diagnosis of epilepsy can be made only by the correct interpretation of the EEG abnormality in relation to the clinical data.

Brain Tumor, Abscess, and Subdural Hematoma. Space-occupying intracranial lesions are associated with abnormalities in the EEG in 9 out of 10 patients. Tumors and abscesses which are above the tentorium and subdural hematomas have correct lateralization in the EEG in 8 out of 10 and more precise localization in 7 out of 10. Conversely, with a normal EEG in patients suspected of having one of the above conditions there are 9 chances to 1 against its presence. Both the positive and the negative values of the EEG in such situations may be helpful in the clinical study, particularly when integrated with the other laboratory and clinical findings.

Cerebrovascular Diseases. Cerebral infarcts and intracranial bleeding usually produce diffuse as well as localized slowing of the EEG during the first 2 or 3 days. There is, however, a disappearance of the diffuse abnormality during the ensuing week. If large arteries are thrombosed with extensive infarction there is a partial improvement in the focal slow activity, but the record remains abnormal. By the use of serial EEGs at regular intervals a considerable amount of useful clinical knowledge about prognosis and progression in such cases can be elicited. Furthermore the differential diagnosis between the cerebral infarct and a tumor becomes nicely clarified by such serial electroencephalographic studies. The usefulness of the EEG in the differential diagnosis of the different forms of vascular disease has not been determined as yet, however.

Brain Injury. Cerebral concussion is accompanied by a transitory disturbance in brain waves, but this is usually over before a recording can be made. Cerebral contusion or hemorrhage on the lateral or superior surfaces of the brain produces a lasting, focal slow-wave abnormality which usually disappears over a period of weeks or months. The EEG is useful in following the rate of recovery and changes in the type of electrical activity. Often sharp waves or spikes appear in the focus and may precede the occurrence of posttraumatic epilepsy (Fig. 55-1F). Serial EEGs, then, are of value in estimating prognosis.

Other Diseases of the Cerebrum. There are many disorders of nervous function that cause little or no alteration in the EEG. Some of the demyelinating diseases, such as multiple sclerosis, are examples, though many advanced cases will have an abnormal record. The different types of encephalitis produce variable alterations, and in general exacting clinical and electroencephalographic correlations are not possible. Neuroses and psychoses, such as manic-depressive disturbances or schizophrenia, either do not modify the normal record or create only nonspecific abnormalities. Little is to be gained by investigating them in a routine manner.

Senility. In senility the normal 10 per second alpha rhythm begins to slow slightly to 9 and 8 per second, particularly after the seventieth year. In the absence of cerebrovascular lesions, a normal 8 per second alpha is to be expected in the eighth and ninth decades. In the presenile dementias, e.g., Alzheimer's disease, the wave frequencies are often reduced to 5 and 6 per second (theta waves). This abnormality is diffuse and mostly over frontal and temporal areas. However, the agreement between the EEG change and intellectual loss as measured by the IQ or cortical atrophy as seen in the air encephalogram is far from perfect. In some demented patients the EEG is relatively normal. The effect of aging on the EEG is illustrated by the author's cases of Parkinson's disease, which in its early form causes no EEG abnormality. In 37 such

cases (1938) with an age range of forty to fifty-five, only one had an abnormal record. In a recent 1959 series of 100 patients averaging sixty-five years of age, 45 per cent had abnormal records (usually 5 to 7 per second theta waves and rare 3 per second delta waves).

Diseases Which Cause Coma and States of Impaired Consciousness. The EEG is abnormal in all conditions in which there is some impairment of consciousness. In general, the more profound the loss of consciousness, the more abnormal the EEG recording. In such situations the slow waves are bilateral, of high amplitude, and tend to be more conspicuous over the frontal regions (see Fig. 55-1E). In hepatic coma the degree of abnormality in the EEG corresponds with the degree of confusion, stupor, or coma. Moreover, paroxysms of bilaterally synchronous wave and spike or "triphasic waves" are characteristic. Uremic and diabetic coma produce slow delta waves in both frontal areas which spread over the rest of the head to a less extent. Diffuse degenerations of the brain that involve the cortex are accompanied by various degrees of diffuse nonspecific EEG abnormality. In all these situations, the diffuse abnormal EEG is useful in emphasizing the presence of structural or biochemical abnormalities of the brain. A normal EEG in a patient who is apathetic, slow, depressed, or forgetful is a point in favor of the diagnosis of an affective disorder or schizophrenia.

Special Applications of the EEG. The EEG can be of value in the diagnosis of hysterical blindness, as stated above. Similarly, the auditory evoked response, seen only in light sleep, can be of help in confirming the presence of hearing in a patient who feigns total deafness (see Fig. 55-1B).

The EEG provides information concerning the status of the cerebral cortex in hypoxic encephalopathy. In the regular operating room the EEG machine can be used to monitor the presence of a living cerebral cortex while the new cardiac and vascular surgical procedures are undertaken. Apparatus has been available for some time now that indicates to the anesthetist the level of anesthesia. It is expected that a simple EEG apparatus may be used to monitor both the cardiac and cerebral status of all patients being subjected to surgical anesthesia.

In the neurosurgical operating room the EEG can be recorded from the exposed brain (electrocorticogram) and seizure patterns localized more precisely than from the regular scalp recording. Resections of such abnormal tissue have helped about 50 per cent of the epileptic patients who have undergone such procedures.

The Clinical Value of Minor EEG Abnormalities. Certain findings in the EEG tracing are of value only if they are correlated with some clinical phenomenon. Borderline deviations in an entirely normal person have no clinical weight whatsoever. These same findings, when associated with certain neurologic signs, even though they too are of minimal clinical significance, acquire diagnostic import. For example: a 34-year-old woman with a history of tension headaches since the age of 14 is under neurologic study because of insomnia, weight loss, and an increase in the frequency of her headaches. The neurologic examination, spinal fluid, and x-rays of skull are all within normal limits. The EEG shows a clear-cut reduction of voltage in the left occipital parietal area and less of the 10 per second alpha, as contrasted to the same area on the right side. This finding of an asymmetry in the brain wave has no clinical significance in this case and should be disregarded. On the other hand, this same finding in a 32-year-old man who was rendered unconscious in an automobile accident 9 days before, and who shows slight awkwardness in his right hand and a continuous dull headache with a lack of his usual alertness, now carries considerable diagnostic meaning. It points to the left hemisphere, which might show contusion or the presence of a subdural hematoma.

In Table 55-1 the relative value of EEG findings is summarized in relation to clinical neurologic examination (NE). The weights run from 0 to 2, with 0 meaning no value and 2 a maximum value.

In conclusion, the electroencephalogram, like the electrocardiogram, is part of the clinical examination and is meaningful only in relation to the clinical status of the patient at the time it was taken.

Table 55-1

EEG findings	Weight* with normal NE	Weight with positive minimal findings on NE	Weight with positive findings on NE
Borderline EEG			
Voltage asymmetry.......	0	1	2
Scattered 6 per sec rhythm	0	1	2
Early or severe breakdown to slow waves on hyperventilation that disappears promptly........	0	1	2
Abnormal EEG			
Seizure discharge; definite slow waves in a focus or absence of normal rhythms..............	2	2	2

* 0 = no value; 2 = maximum value.

REFERENCES

Adrian, E. D., and B. H. C. Matthews: The Berger Rhythm: Potential Changes from the Occipital Lobes in Man, Brain, 57:355, 1934.

Berger, H.: Über das Elektrenkephalogramm des Menschen, Arch. f. Psychiat., 87:527, 1929.

Caton, R.: "Researches on Electrical Phenomena of Cerebral Gray Matter," Trans. Intern. Med. Congr., 9th Session, Section VIII (Physiology), vol. 3, pp. 246–249, Washington, 1887.

Cohn, R.: "Clinical Electroencephalography," New York, McGraw-Hill Book Company, Inc., 1949.

Gibbs, F. A., and E. L. Gibbs: "Atlas of Electroencephalography," 3d ed., Cambridge, Mass., Addison-Wesley Publishing Company, 1953.

Hill, D., and G. Parr (Eds.): "Electroencephalography: A Symposium on Its Various Aspects," London, Macdonald & Co., Ltd., 1950.

Schwab, R. S.: "Electroencephalography in Clinical Practice," Philadelphia, W. B. Saunders Company, 1951.

Strauss, H., and M. Ostow: "Diagnostic Electroencephalography," New York, Grune & Stratton, Inc., 1952.

56 ELECTROMYOGRAPHY
Leonard W. Jarcho

The earliest demonstration of the existence of electric currents in the vertebrate body was the work of Galvani (1794). Striated muscle was the tissue in which the discovery was made; yet electromyography, the study of electrical events in striated muscle, has lagged behind other electrical techniques in attaining clinical usefulness. The reasons are largely two, one anatomic, the other technical. The heart and the brain, though exceedingly complex, are single organs, and their total electrical output can be sampled effectively for clinical purposes from a limited number of standard electrode positions. The voluntary muscles, on the other hand, are numerous and scattered. In some areas they are coarse and bulky, being modified for crude mechanical labor. Elsewhere, they are delicate and finely structured, as befits more accurate tasks. As a result, no small series of leads will give an average picture of their electric activity. They must be tested laboriously one at a time. In addition, disease tends to affect skeletal muscle in a spotty fashion, subdividing the tissue in such a way that normal findings in one area do not guarantee against pathologic events close by. These anatomic difficulties pose the technical problem of finding suitable electrode systems for electromyography. External plate electrodes, such as those used in electrocardiography and electroencephalography, will pick up potentials representing the chance summation of activity in a group of fibers or muscles of uncertain boundaries. Such recordings may be useful in assessing the average function of the group. A more intimate physiologic dissection is possible by means of needle electrodes, which register the activity of smaller numbers of fibers.

Three types of needle electrodes are in general use: unipolar, bipolar, and concentric. All three are made of fine wire or hypodermic needle tubing coated with insulating material so as to leave at the tip only a few microns of bare, conducting metal. In the unipolar application, a single needle is used, the other electrode being a diffuse skin lead. Bipolar electrodes consist of two needles, separated by a distance of 2 mm or less for most uses. A concentric electrode may be made from a hypodermic needle by inserting a shellacked wire in the lumen, so that one lead encircles the other. The potential forms seen with these three types are not identical. Most satisfactorily explained according to current theory are the records obtained with bipolar needles.

Such electrodes pick up the action potentials of those few muscle fibers which lie in the immediate vicinity of their bare tips. If the needles are oriented in the long axis of the muscle fibers, the action potential reaches first one, then the other. The electrode on the active, or depolarized, portion of the fiber becomes negative to its mate, and the recording instrument is deflected from the base line. By convention, the negative potential is recorded as an upward deflection (Fig. 56-1). As the potential propagates further along the muscle fiber, it reaches a point equidistant from the two electrodes, and the record returns to base line. When the action potential reaches the second electrode, a deflection opposite to the first is inscribed. Thus a diphasic potential is recorded. Because of the extreme rapidity of these events, the inertia-free cathode-ray oscillograph (CRO) is the preferred recording instrument for electromyography.

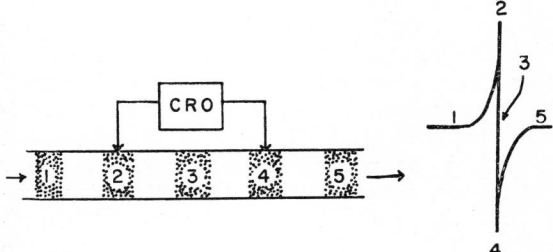

FIG. 56-1. The active (shaded) area is negative to all other points on the fiber surface. It is shown at five points in its course (from left to right) along the fiber. At each point, the correspondingly numbered portion of the diphasic potential is inscribed on the face of the cathode-ray oscillograph (CRO).

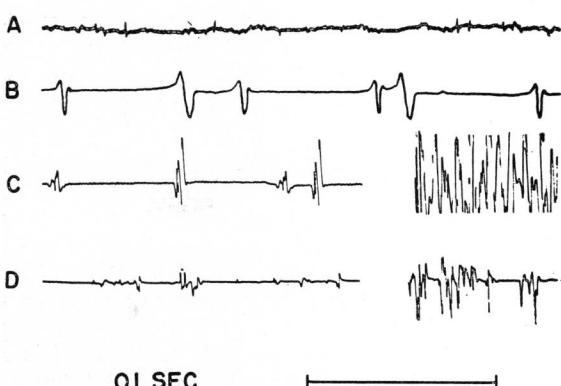

0.1 SEC |⎯⎯⎯⎯⎯⎯⎯⎯⎯⎯⎯⎯⎯|

FIG. 56-2. Electromyographic patterns. *A.* Fibrillation. Tibialis anterior, 11 years after gunshot wound of nerve. Totally random potentials of 1 to 2 msec in duration and maximum amplitude of about 0.1 mv. *B.* Fasciculation. Amyotrophic lateral sclerosis. Potentials of two units, each firing with its own fairly regular rhythm. Maximum amplitude of about 3 mv. *C.* Normal muscle. Contraction starts gently with two motor units (amplitudes of about 1 and 3 mv). Right-hand record shows "interference activity." *D.* Muscular dystrophy. Contraction starts with several units of abnormally low voltage (maximum of about 0.3 mv) and bizarre form. Maximal effort is insufficient to maintain "interference" pattern.

The Motor Unit. The simple diphasic potential discussed above should theoretically result from the activity of a single muscle fiber. In healthy muscle, single fibers do not act alone. Normally, excitation arrives via the motor nerves. A single motor axone branches, and its subdivisions may innervate a few fibers (as in the facial muscles) or several hundred (in the large leg muscles), and in either case the whole group is termed a *motor unit,* as was described in Chap. 26. Within a motor unit, the fibers are not necessarily of uniform diameter, length, or shape, and their spatial orientation with regard to the electrodes will vary. Normal muscle activated through its nerve therefore produces rather complex potentials, presumably the result of summation of single-fiber potentials of varying characteristics. Some of the factors involved in producing the wave forms seen in normal muscle have been demonstrated in animal experiments, but the limits of normal variation are not yet well defined.

Fibrillation. The two phenomena of fibrillation and fasciculation have often been confused with each other. Fasciculation, defined in detail in the next paragraph, consists of synchronous contraction of *groups of muscle fibers* tied together by a single axone into a motor unit. Fibrillation is the contraction of *single muscle fibers* when death of their axone has dissolved their association in a motor unit.

When a motor neurone is killed by disease, or when its axone is severed, the axone degenerates, a process which takes several days. The muscle fibers formerly innervated by the branches of the dead axone (a motor unit) are no longer held together as a functional unit. For reasons which are still obscure, 8 to 12 days after death of the axone the denervated fibers develop spontaneous activity, that is, even while no effort is being made to contract the muscle, action potentials restlessly flow along the denervated muscle fibers. Each fiber fires at its own rate and without relation to the activity of its fellows. There results a totally random conglomeration of diphasic potentials (Fig. 56-2A), among which it is occasionally possible to pick out by some unusual characteristic the repeated firing of a particular fiber. This activity is termed *fibrillation*. Fibrillary potentials have a duration of 1 to 2 milliseconds (msec). They rarely exceed 200 μv in amplitude, but much smaller ones will be recorded from fibers relatively distant from the electrodes. When potentials of this sort are observed in resting muscle, it may be concluded that some of the fibers are denervated. Diseases such as poliomyelitis, which produce death of motor axones or injuries of peripheral nerves or anterior spinal roots, frequently produce only partial denervation of the involved muscles. In such muscles, one electrode placement may pick up fibrillation at rest in denervated fibers and normal potentials during activity from nearby healthy fibers. Fibrillation continues until the muscle fiber is reinnervated by the outgrowth of new axones from the central nervous system, or until the fiber is replaced by connective tissue. The phenomenon has been observed as late as several years after poliomyelitis.

Since the action potential normally accompanies contraction in muscle, it is not surprising to find that fibrillating muscle is mechanically as well as electrically active. In the tongue, where the epithelium is thin and wet, faint shimmering motions may be seen as the fibers contract. Elsewhere in the body the isolated contraction of single fibers is ordinarily not of sufficient strength to be visible through the skin. Visible twitchings, sometimes loosely called fibrillation in the clinic, are usually fasciculation.

Fasciculation. Fasciculation is the spontaneous, involuntary contraction of motor units, singly or in groups. Since a relatively large number of muscle fibers contracts in synchrony, visible dimpling or twitching of the skin occurs, though ordinarily not enough power is exerted to move a joint. The form of the accompanying potential varies, presumably because it is made up of the summed activity of variable numbers of fibers of slightly differing characteristics. Commonly, it will have three to five phases, a duration of 8 to 10 msec (somewhat less in the facial muscles) and an amplitude of several millivolts (Fig. 56-2B). The pattern tends to repeat at a fairly regular rate, indicating a rhythmic activation of the fibers by the responsible axones.

Traditionally, fasciculation occurs in chronic, slowly advancing, destructive disease of the anterior horn cells such as amyotrophic lateral sclerosis and progressive spinal muscular atrophy. It has been reported in the early stages of poliomyelitis, less commonly than in the chronic diseases mentioned, perhaps because the affected cells die too rapidly. In all these cases, the damaged neurone seems to be "irritated" by the disease process. It fires repetitively and beyond the patient's control and, in so doing, trips off activity in all the muscle fibers that it innervates. It has been shown, however, that fasciculation may also follow peripheral nerve lesions, giving way to fibrillation upon death of the axone. More important is the fact that fasciculation occurs occasionally in many normal people, constantly in some, so that it need not be evidence of disease at all. Shivering and the twitchings associated with depressed serum calcium are also forms of fasciculation. Finally, when needle electrodes are inserted into normal muscles, the mechanical irritation which they produce may cause the activation of a few fibers. Brief bursts of fibrillary potentials result, called *insertion activity*. This usually subsides within a few minutes after insertion of the electrodes.

The Normal Electromyogram (EMG). Normal muscle is electrically silent when it is at rest. Once insertion activity following placement of the needles has died down, the electrodes record no propagated action potentials. In very tense individuals, it may take considerable training to reach this point of complete relaxation, for properly placed electrodes will record minimal activity of which the person is not conscious. If now the muscle is voluntarily contracted, action potentials appear on the CRO screen. Slowly graded contraction allows one to observe the manner in which force is normally accumulated (Fig. 56-2C). As contraction begins, the potentials of one or a few motor units appear. Each will usually be relatively constant in the form characteristic for its own motor unit, and it will differ slightly from the potentials of other units in number of phases, shape, duration, amplitude, and rate of repetition. If contraction is maintained at this minimal level, the record is indistinguishable from that of fasciculation, which is also the activity of a few motor units, except that here the activity is voluntary and disappears at rest. As the strength of contraction is increased, more motor units enter the picture and their potentials begin to overlie each other. There results a disorderly tangle of violent oscillation of the CRO beam, which now never comes to rest at the base line. Individual potentials of motor units can no longer be distinguished. The total amplitude of oscillation is many millivolts. Obviously, a weak muscle with few contracting fibers will produce a smaller total potential than normal. However, unless reduction in output is sufficient to destroy the "interference" pattern just described, so that individual motor unit potentials become identifiable, we have no certain evidence of abnormality. As long as a muscle is held actively contracted, the interference pattern continues. Gradual relaxation will show a gradual dropping out of motor units, until only a few are left firing, then one, then none.

Skeletal muscle may also be artificially stimulated to contract. In man the usual method is the application of electric shocks to the skin overlying a motor nerve. With proper stimulating conditions, there will be one response for each shock. The form of this response will depend upon the number of motor units activated and the number sampled by the recording electrodes. If repeated shocks are given, each response will have the same form and amplitude, until fatigue supervenes. Normal muscle will follow rates of stimulation as high as 25 per sec for periods of at least 60 sec before decrement of the action potential indicates the failure of some fibers to respond. The ability of muscle to follow repetitive stimulation is altered in certain diseases (see below).

Muscular Dystrophy and Myositis. Clinically, the muscular dystrophies are not a uniform group (see Chap. 85). Electromyography, however, is not yet sufficiently refined to allow clear differentiation among them. They share with various forms of myositis certain features which are responsible for the electric picture they present. They are all primary diseases of muscle, that is, they do not appear to result primarily from damage to nervous tissue. In the course of these diseases, single muscle fibers are destroyed while their neighbors remain whole. This type of injury gradually produces loss of motor units, and eventually whole muscles may be replaced by noncontractile tissues which can no longer transmit the propagated action potential. Early in the course of such a disease the total force which an affected muscle can exert may be markedly diminished; but as long as enough motor units are active to produce the interference pattern discussed above, it is difficult to detect electric abnormality. At the beginning or end of voluntary contraction, isolated motor unit potentials may be seen, and they may be abnormal (Fig. 56-2D). Duration may remain in the normal range (8 to 10 msec), while amplitude is lost, indicating dropping out of fibers from the unit. As more and more fibers are affected and the motor unit comes to consist of only straggling survivors, motor unit potentials may resemble groups of fibrillary potentials, differing from the latter only in that they do not occur spontaneously when the muscle is at rest. When destruction

is completed, no potentials appear, no matter how hard the patient may try to contract his muscle. Neither fibrillation nor fasciculation is a part of the picture of muscular dystrophy, since neurones are not primarily affected. As in normal muscles, there is "electrical silence" when the affected muscle is at rest. In some cases of myositis, however, fibrillary potentials may be recorded from the resting muscle. It is presumed that these signify the denervation of occasional fibers as a result of implication of terminal motor nerve twigs in a destructive inflammatory process.

Myotonia. In myotonic muscle, contraction persists despite voluntary attempts at relaxation. The symptom occurs in two hereditary diseases, myotonia congenita (Thomsen) and dystrophia myotonica (Steinert), appearing in the latter in combination with a definite pattern of muscle wasting and certain other stigmas (see Chap. 85). Minor forms occur sporadically under other circumstances. The characteristic electrical picture occurs after voluntary contraction or direct stimulation of the muscle, either electrically or by a blow. The motor unit potential appears entirely normal, but it is not followed by the silence which normally occurs on relaxation. Instead there is a burst of rapid activity, which may take as long as several minutes to subside (Fig. 56-3A). Some of the potentials of this prolonged discharge have the duration, amplitude, and form of single-fiber activity, while others appear to have the characteristics of motor unit potentials. Interestingly enough, if the muscle is activated repeatedly at short intervals, either voluntarily or by a series of taps, this late discharge becomes more and more brief and eventually disappears (Fig. 56-3A). Simultaneously the patient finds that he can relax the exercised muscle at will. This phenomenon has been called *warm-up*. Although there is evidence of abnormal reflex patterns in myotonia, the characteristic repetitive discharge does not arise in the nervous system, for it is not blocked by curare. Apparently, then, myotonic muscle responds to excitation with a normal contraction followed by persistent involuntary twitching of single fibers.

Myasthenia Gravis. The typical symptom of myasthenia gravis is not so much weakness as abnormal fatigability. The affected muscles tire after repeated use, and a similar phenomenon is seen in the EMG (Fig. 56-3D). The original motor unit potentials evoked by stimulating the motor nerve appear normal. After a few shocks at rates as low as 10 to 12 per sec (or less in some cases), the amplitude of the potentials falls off and may reach zero, if stimulation is continued, while normal muscles follow the stimulus without decrement at rates as high as 40 to 50 per sec for brief periods. This defect is remarkably similar to the partial block produced at the neuromuscular junction by curare, and like it,

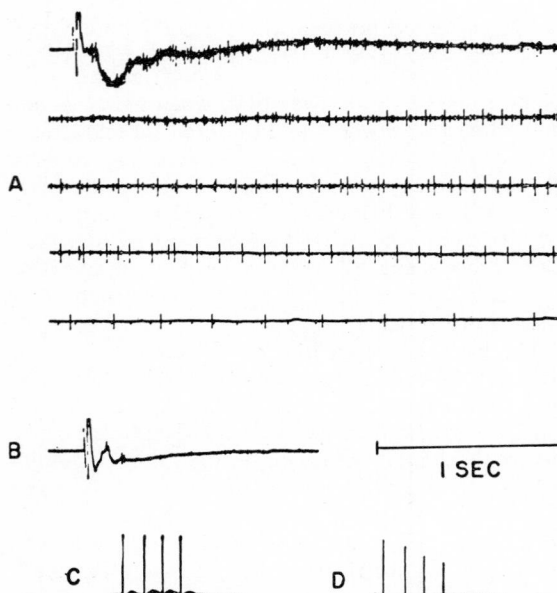

FIG. 56-3. Myotonia and myasthenia. *A.* Myotonia congenita (Thomsen's disease). The five lines are a continuous record of activity in the biceps brachii following a tap on the tendon. The initial response is within normal limits, but it is followed by a prolonged burst of rapid activity, gradually subsiding over a period of many seconds or minutes. *B.* Same electrode placement as in (*A*). Response to the fifth of a series of tendon taps. "Warm-up" has occurred, and the characteristic prolonged myotonic activity is no longer evident. *C.* Response of normal muscle to shocks applied to the motor nerve at a rate of approximately 3 per sec. At this rate of stimulation the amplitude of the first response is maintained throughout the series of four shocks. *D.* Myasthenia gravis. Same conditions as in (*C*). The first potential is of normal amplitude, but as stimulation continues, the response falls off and may eventually reach zero if stimulation continues. (*Records C and D courtesy of Dr. David Grob, Department of Medicine, Johns Hopkins Hospital.*)

may be relieved by neostigmine. The abnormality is thus apparently located at the neuromuscular junction, but its nature is obscure. Similar decline of the action potential with repetitive stimulation may occur in poliomyelitis, raising the question of whether there may be damage elsewhere than in nerve cells in this disease.

Peripheral Neuropathies. Laboratory evidence of disease of the peripheral nervous system may be obtained by electromyographic study or by the measurement of the conduction velocity of the nerve itself.

The electromyogram in lesions of the nerve, whatever the type of disease, is much the same. As stated above, if the nerve is completely interrupted, the paralyzed, flaccid, areflexic muscle is at first electrically silent, and after 1 to 2 weeks, fibrillations appear. As often happens, however, the nerve is less severely damaged, leaving many intact axones or motor units and a muscle which contracts with less than normal force. The intact motor units, during voluntary contraction, are then observed to be abnormally large, i.e., the amplitude or voltage is excessive (? due to collateral regeneration of intramuscular motor nerves and reinnervation by adjacent nerves of some of the denervated muscle fibers from previously destroyed axones). The interference pattern, then, is abnormal because of the reduction of the number of active units in proportion to the strength of contraction, but also with respect to their high amplitude. This picture contrasts to that of myopathic disease (dystrophy or myositis) where the interference pattern may be normally rich in motor units but abnormal because of their brevity and low voltage.

Conduction Velocity of Nerve. Data of considerable clinical interest may be obtained by determining conduction velocity in peripheral nerve. Any accessible nerve is stimulated through the skin while the resulting muscle action potential is recorded with needle electrodes. Conduction time is measured from the shock artefact to the onset of the response. A second stimulus is then applied to another point along the nerve and the new conduction time is measured. The distance between the two points of stimulation divided by the difference in conduction times gives a measure of velocity of propagation of the nerve action potential. When studies are carried out in this manner, the calculated velocities are those of the largest motor fibers. In normal adults the range is between 45 and 75 meters per sec. Lower values are recorded in infants and in the aged.

Conduction velocity measured in this manner may be markedly reduced in acute or chronic peripheral neuropathies of whatever etiology. The technique has been found clinically useful in differentiating lesions of peripheral nerve from central lesions and from primary muscle disease. It may give objective evidence at an early stage of disorders otherwise manifested only by indefinite sensory findings.

Statistical Analysis. In electrocardiography, it is frequently possible to decide that a single complex is abnormal because its measurements lie outside of well-established limits for the lead under consideration. For reasons discussed above, it is often difficult to make this decision in the case of an individual motor unit potential in skeletal muscle. As a result, attempts have been made to establish curves of frequency distribution for various parameters, such as duration and amplitude of potentials. It has been found that duration varies in different normal muscles and that it tends to increase with age. In the dystrophies, a normal distribution of durations occurs, while some types of myositis show a shift of the curve toward shorter durations. Muscles weakened as a result of disease of neurones tend to produce prolonged potentials. In poliomyelitis there is evidence that more pronounced prolongations forebode poor functional recovery. The meaning of all these findings is still obscure. Further research is necessary before electrical abnormalities can be correlated with other pathologic findings.

REFERENCES

Buchthal, F., and P. Pinelli: Analysis of Muscle Action Potentials as a Diagnostic Aid in Neuromuscular Disorders, Acta Med. Scand., 142(Suppl.):315, 1952.

Denny-Brown, D., and J. B. Pennybacker: Fibrillation and Fasciculation in Voluntary Muscle, Brain, 61:311, 1938.

Hodes, R., M. G. Larabee, and W. German: The Human Electromyogram in Response to Nerve Stimulation and the Conduction Velocity of Motor Axons, Arch. Neurol. Psychiat., 60:340, 1948.

Jarcho, L. W., C. L. Vera, C. G. McCarthy and P. M. Williams: The Form of Motor-unit and Fibrillation Potentials, Electroencephalog. and Clin. Neurophysiol., 10:527, 1958.

Licht, S.: "Electrodiagnosis and Electromyography," New Haven, Elizabeth Licht, Publisher, 1956.

Mayo Clinic Staff: "Clinical Examinations in Neurology," chap. XV, Philadelphia, W. B. Saunders Company, 1956.

Petersen, I., and E. Kugelberg: Duration and Form of Action Potential in the Normal Human Muscle, J. Neurol. Neurosurg. Psychiat., 12:124, 1949.

Thomas, P. K., T. A. Sears, and R. W. Gilliatt: The Range of Conduction Velocity in Normal Motor Nerve Fibers to the Small Muscles of the Hand and Foot, J. Neurol. Neurosurg. Psychiat., 22:175, 1959.

Weddell, G., B. Feinstein, and R. E. Pattle: The Electrical Activity of Voluntary Muscle in Man under Normal and Pathological Conditions, Brain, 67:178, 1944.

PART FOUR
Metabolic and Endocrine Disorders

Section 1: Nutritional Deficiencies

57 GENERAL CONSIDERATIONS AND MISCELLANEOUS DEFICIENCIES

William J. Darby

The human being has a dietary requirement for calories, protein, vitamins, minerals, and perhaps fat.[1] Obviously, inorganic nutrients must be derived from exogenous sources. Of the organic nutrients, some can be synthesized by the body from various precursors (carbohydrates, fats, or protein); the nonessential amino acids may be built up within the organism so that they do not have to be supplied in the diet. On the other hand, some organic materials cannot be made by the organism, and since they play an essential metabolic role, the organism must obtain them from food. This latter group includes the vitamins, the essential amino acids, and the essential fatty acids. The body may have a limited capacity to make a given metabolite, but under certain conditions the need may exceed this capacity, in which case there appears a dietary requirement for the nutrient.

There is a great adaptive capacity in the use of nutrients, even of the essential nutrients. This capacity varies with the storage reservoirs and metabolic characteristics of the nutrient, but for most essentials there is a wide range between the intake level that barely prevents clinically evident deficiency disease and the level of maximally filled stores of the nutrient. In other words, there is a wide spectrum of nutriture, or "condition as to nourishment," between maximally nourished and deficient states. In the case of a few nutrients, e.g., calories, vitamin A, carotene, and vitamin D, the capacity to store—or, perhaps, the limited ability to destroy, metabolize, or excrete—may be overwhelmed by an excessive intake, which, accordingly, may lead to undesirable states of excess (obesity or hypervitaminosis). These states may result from overeating, i.e., taking in excess calories or carotene, or from overdosing with supplements (vitamins A or D).

Clinically, two zones of nutriture may be considered deficiency states: (1) Latent deficiency disease (for example, latent scurvy) is characterized by vague, indefinite, nonspecific symptoms which are suggestive of a deficiency but which alone do not permit a diagnosis. The diagnosis may be established by the judicious appraisal of the history and findings, by therapeutic trial, or by biochemical tests. (2) Clinically manifest deficiency disease, both mild and severe, is the zone in which signs characteristic of deficiency diseases are evident. These signs may be mild and require careful examination to detect (angular cheilosis, dermatitis of mild pellagra, mild gingival lesions of scurvy, etc.), or they may be severe and evident. Biochemically, one may estimate the body stores of certain essential nutrients (for example, vitamin A, ascorbic acid, thiamine, riboflavin, or iron) and thereby determine whether the customary intake has been adequate to permit accumulation of the nutrient above the minimum level required to prevent clinical deficiencies.

A lower nutriture, and thereby a deficiency disease, results from a decreased dietary intake of a nutrient or from a conditioning factor (disease or physiologic state) which increases the demand for the nutritive essential. Such conditioning factors include states with impaired absorption (e.g., sprue syndrome, pernicious anemia), or those which result from certain operative procedures on the gastrointestinal tract (gastrectomy or short-circuiting operations), and conditions in which there is excessive loss (iron loss in chronic bleeding) or increased requirement (hyperthyroidism, growth, pregnancy, or lactation).

Dietary deficiencies develop as a result of factors which unduly restrict the variety of foods consumed. These include economic limitations, ignorance, self-imposed dietary restrictions, and ill-advised therapeutic regimes. The displacement of food by the chronic overindulgence in alcohol may result in the development of deficiency manifestations because of the decreased intake of protein, thiamine, nicotinic acid, etc. Because of metabolic interrelationships, the requirement of some nutrients may be higher when one type of diet is consumed than in the case of another. Thus, thiamine requirement is higher on a high carbohydrate, low fat, rice dietary than on the usual Western diet.

The most common form of malnutrition in the United States is caloric excess, or obesity. Florid deficiency states of dietary origin, more prevalent in the past, are now encountered infrequently.

Dietary deficiencies are met more often among the economically underprivileged groups, and hence are more prevalent in wards of charity hospitals

---

[1] Quantitative changes in nutrition, that is gain and loss of weight, are discussed in Chap. 22.

than in private institutions. As already mentioned, in some areas it is not unusual to see cases of deficiencies arising from the displacement of food with alcohol. Although food faddists, alcoholics, and persons who receive greatly restricted therapeutic diets may develop deficiency diseases regardless of their economic position, among the middle and upper economic groups the most frequently encountered deficiency diseases are of the "conditioned" type.

In any consideration of vitamin deficiency states it is useful to make certain generalizations. The absorption, storage, and excretion of vitamins seem to follow two broad patterns. Water-soluble vitamins (ascorbic acid, vitamins of the B-complex group) are diffusible, and examples of their impaired absorption (except for vitamin B_{12} in pernicious anemia) are not common; these vitamins may be stored in amounts sufficient to prevent the development of clinically manifest deficiency states over a period of deprivation of 4 months to a year or so; also, they (or their metabolic products) are excreted in the urine, and, hence, the accumulation of toxic quantities from excessive doses does not easily occur. The fat-soluble factors (carotene, vitamins A, D, E, and K) are absorbed along with lipids, and derangements of their absorption are seen in steatorrheas and biliary obstruction; the body has great storage capacity for these factors, and it often requires upward of a year of deprivation in the adult to obtain evidence of clinically manifest deficiency; they are not excreted in the urine of healthy subjects and may accumulate to toxic levels if grossly excessive quantities are given repeatedly. Representatives of both classes may be synthesized by the intestinal flora of man.

The signs of mild clinically manifest deficiency disease are nonspecific and are often simulated by nonnutritional causes. Only those signs due to deficiency will respond to nutritional therapy, and their response is usually quite rapid. Failure to understand these principles has resulted in much useless supplementation of patients with a great variety of preparations containing vitamins. False reliance on vitamin therapy has sometimes resulted in delayed institution of effective treatment.

To date the therapeutic effectiveness in man of the following vitamins has been clearly demonstrated: vitamin A and carotene, vitamin D, vitamin K, ascorbic acid, thiamine, riboflavin, nicotinic acid, folic acid (pteroylglutamates), vitamin B_6, and vitamin B_{12}.

There has been no convincing demonstration of clinically recognizable syndromes due to a spontaneously occurring deficiency of pantothenic acid, biotin, tocopherols, or other vitamins required by lower species. Despite the numerous claims of spectacular therapeutic results from administration of large doses of *tocopherols* in a variety of obscure

clinical conditions, there has been no critically designed study which substantiates them. It can be admitted, however, that tocopherol administration has been followed by reproducible metabolic changes in premature and newborn infants and in cases of steatorrhea. The changes include effects on in vitro hemolysis of erythrocytes in hydrogen peroxide and on the urinary excretion of creatine and of a pentose. As regards *pantothenic acid*, a symptom complex of lethargy, weakness, burning paresthesia of the feet, cramps, and mild tetany has been produced in adults by feeding a purified, pantothenic acid–deficient diet plus α-methylpantothenic acid (an antivitamin). Thus, the evidence is increasing for the essential role of these factors in human metabolism. Failure, to date, to recognize spontaneously occurring clinical syndromes attributable to a lack of these (and other) vitamins may be due to an exceedingly small human requirement which is met by the quantity contained in even the most limited diet, to the absorption of requisite amounts from the gut following intestinal synthesis of the vitamins, or, less likely, to a slight synthetic ability by the human organism. The limitations of knowledge do not allow us to deny that these several factors may serve essential metabolic roles in man; they do permit the conclusion that to date there has been no demonstration of their usefulness in treating deficiencies.

Exact quantitative statements of daily minimal requirements of nutrients cannot be made. A useful "objective toward which to aim in the planning of practical dietaries" is provided by the Recommended Daily Dietary Allowances compiled by the Food and Nutrition Board of the National Research Council (Table 22-2, p. 189). Allowances are recommended for adults in terms of a hypothetical standard 65-kg man and are purposely sufficiently generous to maintain normal individuals in the zone of saturation or of unsaturation without functional impairment. The allowances can be met by ingestion of a variety of readily available foods *without supplementation*. They serve as useful standards for the planning of adequate therapeutic diets. Indeed, any therapeutic diet which fails to provide the quantity of nutrients recommended by these standards should be carefully considered before it is used for prolonged periods: it is important that any therapeutic diet meet the criteria of nutritional adequacy as well as possess the particular attribute for which it is designed.

The question of the proper use of supplementary vitamins frequently arises. An appropriately varied diet as usually consumed in the United States provides a sufficient quantity of these nutrients to meet requirements except under extraordinary circumstances. Conditioning factors may increase the requirement and justify a protective supplementation.

Specific supplementation with vitamins C, D, and in some instances, A is indicated during periods of infancy. During pregnancy vitamin D supplementation may be desirable. The therapeutic use of supplements in treatment of true deficiency states is clearly of value. Despite uncritically considered claims, the nonspecific general toniclike influence often attributed to vitamins is but a placebo effect. The indiscriminate or "routine" prescription of vitamin preparations is indefensible, it is poor medical practice and may substitute for a proper diagnosis or delay institution of effective therapy, and it is costly to the patient.

When multivitamin preparations are indicated, it is important to distinguish between the categories of multivitamin preparations available: (1) those containing approximately one-half the Recommended Dietary Allowances and suitable as dietary supplements where such are indicated, (2) those containing one to one and one-half times the Recommended Allowances and which are useful as supplements to therapeutic regimes likely to induce prolonged deprivation, (3) those which contain five times as much as the Recommended Allowances. These should be reserved for use as therapeutic agents for the treatment of demonstrable deficiency states.

Ariboflavinosis. A deficiency of riboflavin (vitamin B_2) results in a syndrome (ariboflavinosis) of angular oral fissures, corneal vascularization, photophobia, and lingual and skin changes. Ariboflavinosis may result from an intake of less than approximately 0.6 mg riboflavin daily. This syndrome is often associated with evidences of a lack of other members (especially nicotinic acid) of the B complex. Although not common in the United States at the present time, it was frequently associated with pellagra during the 1930s and has been described as occurring in Newfoundland, China, India, Malaya, Africa, and England. The oral lesions develop as a pallor of the labial mucosa at the angles of the mouth, followed within a few days by maceration and the appearance of transverse fissures. The active lesions may become covered with a honey-colored crust; redness and swelling of the mucosa of the lip may develop at the height of the process. Upon healing, the site of the fissures is marked by barely visible pinkish scars. The lingual papillae may become shorter, and the filiform papillae assume a mushroom appearance. The typical glossitis of riboflavin deficiency is described as magenta colored.

The nasolabial area and the butterfly region of the face are often covered with fine, scaly, slightly greasy desquamation. Fissures and maceration at the nasolabial junction sometimes resemble in appearance the local lesions which may accompany an upper respiratory infection. Maceration of the external palpebral junction may be seen. Scrotal dermatitis has been described.

The corneal involvement in ariboflavinosis is first manifest as circumcorneal injection and may be evident grossly. Invisible but preexisting subepithelial capillaries, best seen with the slit lamp, are thought to open up under conditions of hypoxia, as they respond to irritation from any cause.

The clinical picture of ariboflavinosis varies, depending upon the predominant lesion. When ocular manifestations are prominent, the patient complains of photophobia and dimness of vision, a burning sensation of the eyes, roughness or a "sandpapery" feeling of the eyelids, and blurring of vision. Conjunctival injection is especially marked in the pericorneal region. Corneal vascularity is observed with either the slit lamp or the ophthalmoscope. Opacities of the cornea may be present.

Angular fissures, cheilosis, and glossitis may be present and are frequently associated with the dermatitis described above. Oral or ocular lesions may occur alone or in combination. Manifestations of ariboflavinosis may be the sole deficiency sign, or changes characteristic of pellagra may be associated.

Careful inquiry into the dietary history of the patient reveals a diet devoid of those foods rich in riboflavin—milk, liver, lean meat, green leafy vegetables, etc.

There are no characteristic laboratory findings in ariboflavinosis. Riboflavin excretion in the urine is decreased, whether measured in a timed specimen or following a load test. It is not possible at this time to state that a given urinary excretion level will necessarily be associated with clinically manifest disease. Excretion of less than 10 μg of riboflavin in the urine in 6 hr may be regarded as consistent with ariboflavinosis. On the other hand, a urinary excretion value above 30 to 50 μg per 6 hr makes unlikely the diagnosis of ariboflavinosis. The concentration of riboflavin in erythrocytes may be of confirmatory usefulness.

The clinical picture, the dietary history, and an associated low urinary excretion of riboflavin should lead to the consideration of ariboflavinosis as a possible diagnosis. The rapid specific response to riboflavin aids in the establishment of the diagnosis.

The ocular lesions of riboflavin deficiency must be differentiated from conjunctivitis of various origins, from traumatic keratitis, syphilis, and other causes. Examination with the slit lamp of the cornea of healthy individuals reveals an occasional healthy person with one or more asymptomatic vascular "streamers" in the cornea. Such findings are not to be confused with those of ariboflavinosis. The angular fissures and glossitis of ariboflavinosis must be distinguished from lesions due to deficiency of nicotinic acid or of iron or those caused by the irritation produced by ultraviolet light or by the drooling of saliva. A careful dietary history is of value in making this distinction. The patient with nicotinic acid deficiency usually gives a history of considerable intake of corn, while ariboflavinosis has not been so closely related to an intake of maize. Milk is rich in riboflavin, and an intake of a pint per day almost eliminates the possibility of riboflavin deficiency. The finding of a hypochromic microcytic anemia is helpful in differentiating iron deficiency and ariboflavinosis. Angular fissures resistant to riboflavin therapy are often noted in older patients with ill-fitting dentures. These lesions, presumably due to the distortion of the labial angles, have been termed *pseudoariboflavinosis*. Some patients with angular fissures have been reported to respond to treatment with other members of the B complex, particularly pyridoxine and pantothenic acid.

Ariboflavinosis is prevented by the ingestion of 1 mg or more of riboflavin in the diet daily. The daily recommended allowance (Table 22-2, p. 189) is a somewhat higher level. This quantity may easily be obtained by including daily portions of milk, lean meat, green leafy vegetables, and occasional servings of organ meats in the diet. Specific curative therapy consists of the oral administration of 5 to 15 mg riboflavin daily. In addition, an effort should be directed toward correction of the patient's dietary pattern to assure the regular inclusion of good sources of this vitamin.

Vitamin B_6 Deficiency. Hyperirritability, increased "startle" responses, convulsive seizures associated with nondiagnostic electroencephalographic changes, and sometimes gastrointestinal distress appeared among infants fed a prepared formula containing 60 μg vitamin B_6 per liter. This clinical picture developed as a result of a 2- to 5-month period of deprivation on such a dietary regimen and presumably is the result of a dietary lack of vitamin B_6 (pyridoxine). Biochemical evidences of pyridoxine deficiency included the urinary excretion of xanthurenic acid after the administration of tryptophan and diminished excretion of N-methylnicotinamide in the urine after administration of tryptophan. Treatment with daily doses of 5 to 10 mg pyridoxine orally arrested the convulsions, and if vitamin B_6 intake was continued, the manifestations did not recur.

Although an identical syndrome has not been observed in adults, there are reports of clinical response of muscular weakness and cheilosis to pyridoxine. These observations are of more credence since it has been found that the antivitamin, 4-desoxypyridoxine, plus a vitamin B_6–deficient diet will produce irritability, depression, seborrheic dermatitis of the nasolabial folds and about the eyes, cheilosis, angular stomatitis, glossitis, and peripheral neuritis—again accompanied by the above-noted biochemical defects and responding to pyridoxine. Pyridoxine-responsive microcytic anemia has been reported (p. 205). During pregnancy elevated urinary excretion of xanthurenic acid has been reported which can be reduced by giving pyridoxine. However, despite these and other metabolic changes which can be influenced by pyridoxine administration during the course of normal and pathologic pregnancy, there is no conclusive evidence that these findings indicate a relative vitamin B_6 deficiency in pregnancy or that such a postulated lack is causative in the human being of complications of pregnancy such as toxemia, vomiting of pregnancy, preeclampsia, or eclampsia.

A neuritis occurs in some patients receiving antituberculosis therapy with isoniazide (INH) in large doses. The administration of INH enhances the urinary loss of pyridoxal, presumably through the formation of a pyridoxal-INH compound. It lowers whole blood glutamic oxalacetic transaminase (GOT). Fifty milligrams daily of pyridoxine prevents this "conditioned deficiency."

The manifestations and mode of development of vitamin B_{12} and folic acid deficiencies are discussed elsewhere (Chaps. 23, 235).

REFERENCES

Aykroyd, W. R., and B. G. Krishnan: Stomatitis Due to Vitamin B_2 Deficiency, Indian J. Med. Research, 24:411, 1936.

Bessey, O. A., M. K. Horwitt, and R. M. Love: Dietary Deprivation of Riboflavin and Blood Riboflavin Levels in Man, J. Nutrition, 58:367, 1956.

Council on Foods and Nutrition: Vitamin Preparations as Dietary Supplements and as Therapeutic Agents, J.A.M.A., 169:109, 1959.

Coursin, D. B.: Effects of Vitamin B_6 on the Central Nervous Activity in Childhood, Am. J. Clin. Nutrition, 4:354, 1956.

Darby, W. J.: Some Considerations Pertaining to the Proper Use of Supplementary Vitamins, J. Chronic Diseases, 6:178, 1957.

Food and Nutrition Board, National Research Council: "Recommended Dietary Allowances," revised 1958, National Academy of Sciences—National Research Council Publication 589, Washington, D.C.

Gordon, H. H., and H. M. Nitowsky: Some Studies of Tocopherol in Infants and Children, Am. J. Clin. Nutrition, 4:391, 1956. See Discussion by C. W. Woodruff, *ibid.*, p. 405.

Lubin, R., K. A. Daum, and W. B. Bean: Studies of Pantothenic Acid Metabolism, Am. J. Clin. Nutrition, 4:420, 1956.

Sebrell, W. H., and R. E. Butler: Riboflavin Deficiency in Man, Public Health Repts. U.S., 53:2282, 1938.

Strauss, M. B.: The Role of the Gastrointestinal Tract in Conditioning Deficiency Disease, J.A.M.A., 103:1, 1934.

Sydenstricker, V. P., W. H. Sebrell, H. M. Cleckley, and H. D. Kruse: The Ocular Manifestations of Ariboflavinosis, J.A.M.A., 114:2437, 1940.

Vilter, R. W.: The Metabolism of Vitamin B₆ in Human Beings, Am. J. Clin. Nutrition, 4:378, 1956.

58 ASCORBIC ACID DEFICIENCY (Scurvy)

Richard W. Vilter

Definition and History. Scurvy, a disease due to deficiency of vitamin C, has been recognized since ancient times. Clinical descriptions are found in the Ebers papyrus, dating from about 1500 B.C., and in the works of Hippocrates. Scurvy was a factor in the failure of the crusades and assumed considerable importance when long sea voyages for discovery and conquest became popular in the 1500s. In 1753 James Lind, a ship's surgeon, wrote an excellent treatise on scurvy and recognized the preventive qualities of oranges and lemons. Sir Thomas Barlow differentiated infantile scurvy from rickets in 1883, but not until 1907 was scurvy reproduced in the guinea pig by Holst and Frolich. This achievement paved the way for studies on pathology and pathologic physiology by Zilva, Wolbach and Howe, Farmer and Abt, and many others. Finally in 1928, vitamin C was isolated from natural sources by Szent Gyorgyi and by Waugh and King. Synthesis of the vitamin was accomplished by Reichstein, but as yet its exact mode of action remains to be discovered, though many of its chemical functions are known.

Physiology. Although scurvy is now a rare disease, it is still encountered in infants who are fed only unsupplemented milk formulas. It occurs also in recluses, usually males and often bachelors, and in food faddists who avoid vegetables and fruits, particularly of the citrus varieties. Most animals are able to synthesize vitamin C from glucose by the following reactions:

$$\text{D-glucuronate} \underset{}{\overset{\text{TPNH}}{\rightleftharpoons}} \text{L-gulonate} \overset{\text{DPN}}{\rightleftharpoons}$$

$$(\text{3-keto-L-gulonate}) \rightarrow \text{L-ascorbate}$$

Primates, including man, and guinea pigs are dependent on exogenous sources for the vitamin because they lack the enzyme system necessary for the conversion of 3-keto-L-gulonate to L-ascorbate. Citrus fruits and tomatoes are the most reliable sources of this heat-labile vitamin. Many other vegetables are rich in vitamin C but lose it in preparation and cooking. Raw milk contains some vitamin C, most of which is destroyed by pasteurization, evaporation, or drying.

When tissues of human beings have acquired all the vitamin C they can hold, they are said to be saturated. Under these conditions, the tissues of an adult person contain about 4 Gm of the vitamin, and the levels in the plasma, whole blood, and buffy coat (white cells and platelets) are, respectively, 0.8 to 1.0 mg per 100 ml, 1 to 1.2 mg per 100 ml, and 25 to 38 mg per 100 ml. Any additional vitamin C absorbed will exceed the renal threshold (1.4 mg per 100 ml) and will be excreted in the urine. Since vitamin C is almost completely absorbed from the gastroenteric tract, little will appear in the stool, and about 50 per cent of the intake of a well-saturated person will appear in the urine. A dietary intake of 75 mg daily for the adult person and 30 mg for the infant will more than maintain this satisfactory state.

Should all dietary sources of vitamin C be cut off, the level in the plasma will fall to zero in 6 weeks, and little or none of the vitamin will appear in the urine. The whole-blood concentration will reach levels too low to measure in 3 months, and the buffy coat level will fall under 4 mg per 100 ml in 4 to 5 months. By this time, most of the body stores of vitamin C will have been depleted. After 6 months, clinical scurvy may appear. Pregnancy, lactation, and thyrotoxicosis, which increase demands for vitamin C, and diarrheal states, which increase losses of the vitamin, shorten these time intervals and increase a person's susceptibility to scurvy.

Symptomatology. Prodromal complaints are weakness, fatigue, and aching in the muscles, bones, and joints. The skin becomes dry, and the hair follicles, particularly on the legs and buttocks, become hyperkeratotic. The hairs coil, crack, and break off or become buried in the follicle. Erythema and then hemorrhages occur in these abnormal hair follicles, producing the first distinctive manifestation of scurvy, the perifollicular hemorrhage. Later hemorrhages appear on the lower and then the upper extremities, especially about joints, along scratch marks, or in traumatized areas. They may become confluent, and ultimately an entire extremity may be involved in purpuric discoloration. Palisades of splinter hemorrhages appear under the nails. Deep hemorrhages occur in muscles, causing painful lumps, or into joints, causing hemarthroses. Less frequently hemorrhages occur in the viscera, and blood may appear in the urine and stool. Rarely there is bloody pericardial effusion, and petechiae may occur in the brain, causing convulsions and coma.

Only when teeth or tooth remnants are present may one see the typical gum lesions of scurvy. Infected pyorrheic gums are more prone to this lesion than previously healthy ones. Hemorrhages occur at the tips of the interdental papillae, which ultimately become boggy, friable blue-red masses of blood and are sometimes so swollen that they extend beyond the edges of the teeth. Infarcts of the papillae occur, and ultimately the necrotic gum tissue becomes gangrenous and falls away from the teeth.

Bones become osteoporotic, fractures previously incurred fail to heal, and teeth become loose and fall out. In the adult person, however, one does not find the bone lesions typical of scurvy in the growing infant or child which are described below.

Wounds fail to heal or, if recently healed, may break down. The skin becomes pigmented with melanin and hemosiderin, pallor due to anemia and jaundice due to breakdown of blood in large hematomas appear, and the temperature may be elevated to 101 to 102°F. Blood pressure falls, confusion and somnolence supervene, and convulsions, coma, and death will ensue if treatment is not instituted.

In the infant, scurvy usually does not occur before the fourth month of life. Loss of appetite, irritability, fretfulness, and a disinclination to be touched or lifted usually make up the initial manifestations. The baby lies with legs drawn up and abducted, and the lower ends of the femora or the upper ends of the humeri, where subperiosteal hemorrhages most frequently occur, are the sites of exquisite tenderness. Ecchymoses in the skin and muscles are less common than in the adult person, and gum lesions occur only after the teeth have erupted. Costochondral separation may occur and, as a result, the sternum may sink inward, leaving a sharp elevation, the "scorbutic rosary," on the rib side of the junction.

Pathologic Physiology. The cause of all the clinical manifestations is a defect of mesenchymal tissue characterized by failure of formation of intracellular cement substance. In connective tissue this material is known as *ground substance,* an amorphous mucopolysaccharide product, presumably, of the fibroblast, which cements together the fibrils into bands of collagen. When ground substance is defective, as in scurvy, wounds fail to heal properly.

In bone, this material is called *matrix* or *osteoid,* and this is ultimately ossified to form new bone. In growing bones of infants and children with scurvy, osteoid is not normal and cannot be ossified. At the epiphyseal end of the diaphysis and in the epiphysis, the provisional zone of calcification of cartilage appears, and because of slow growth of cartilage, this area becomes more compact than

usual. Osteoblasts, which should invade the cartilaginous columns and lay down osteoid, revert to fibroblasts and form a meshwork of loose connective tissue just shaftward from the provisional zone of calcification. This, of course, does not ossify. It is called the *zone of rarefaction.* In fact, since bone resorption continues, osteoporosis occurs throughout the shaft and epiphysis. Minute fractures appear just beneath the zone of provisional calcification. Periosteal osteoblasts fail to lay down normal matrix but proliferate much like fibroblasts, producing a layer of cells which separates the periosteum from the cortex of the shaft. Hemorrhages, which begin in the minute fractures at the zone of rarefaction, break out into this area of loose connective tissue and spread up and down the shaft but do not pass the periosteal attachments. These are the subperiosteal hemorrhages. As a result of these anatomic changes, the characteristic x-ray signs of infantile scurvy appear—the white line (the dense zone of provisional calcification and the surrounding osteoporosis) and the "corner sign" (the minute fractures into the zone of rarefaction, visualized best at the ankle and wrist).

A similar pathologic process affects the teeth. Odontoblasts become inactive, and the matrix between pulp and dentine is abnormal. Alveolar bone is resorbed, and the teeth become loose and fall out.

Defectiveness of the intracellular cement substance accounts for poor wound healing. Under normal circumstances, vitamin C accumulates in the new connective tissue of healing wounds, but when, because of vitamin deficiency, this cannot occur, scanty and abnormal collagen is laid down. The tensile strength of such a scar is poor. A similar defect in intracellular cement substance of capillaries accounts for greatly increased fragility of these vessels and for the petechiae, ecchymoses, and bleeding swollen blue-red gums that are so characteristic of the scorbutic state.

The anemia which occurs in the scorbutic infant is usually microcytic and hypochromic when iron deficiency also is a problem. Otherwise it is normocytic or slightly macrocytic. Occasionally, at any age, severe macrocytic megaloblastic anemia may be found. Many factors are responsible for the anemia. Infection, iron deficiency, blood loss, and folic acid deficiency are probably most important in infants. In adult scorbutic patients, there is considerable blood lost into tissues in areas of large ecchymoses, and folic acid metabolism frequently is abnormal. Whether vitamin C deficiency interferes directly with blood formation or causes intravascular hemolysis are points still debated.

The specific derangements of body chemistry which must be responsible for these pathologic changes have not been discovered. Vitamin C, in general, governs oxidation-reduction potentials within the cells. The conversion of dehydroascorbic acid to ascorbic acid is facilitated in animals and plants by reduced triphosphopyridine nucleotides (TPNH) and related enzyme systems by way of reduced glutathione (GSH) and other compounds containing SH groups. For instance,

$$\left(\begin{matrix} \text{TPNH} \\ \text{TPN} \end{matrix}\right) \left(\begin{matrix} \text{GSH} \\ \text{GSSG} \end{matrix}\right) \left(\begin{matrix} \text{Ascorbic acid} \\ \text{Dehydroascorbic acid} \end{matrix}\right) \left(\begin{matrix} \text{H}_2\text{O} \\ \tfrac{1}{2}\text{O}_2 \end{matrix}\right)$$

is a reaction which is said to be irreversible to the right, but it is possible that quinones may act as hydrogen acceptors during an oxidation phase, and triose phosphate, malate, and isocitrate may act as hydrogen donors during the reduction phase. In this way, ascorbic acid may be involved in an important hydrogen transfer system and regulate cellular oxidation-reduction potentials.

Folinic acid, a reduction product of folic acid, will not remain in the reduced state without vitamin C or some similar reducing agent, and it is likely that vitamin C is required for other steps in the reaction which forms the folic acid coenzymes from folic acid conjugates found in food. This is probably the explanation for the megaloblastic anemia that occurs in association with scurvy, since a marginal amount of folic acid is quite inadequate when vitamin C is deficient also.

The oxidation of tyrosine and phenylalanine is dependent upon an adequate supply of ascorbic acid. Scorbutic persons, given a load test of tyrosine, excrete large amounts of intermediate products of tyrosine metabolism in the urine.

Ascorbic acid has a protective action also on vitamin A and the tocopherols and is depleted from the adrenal cortex, a region very rich in ascorbic acid, under the stimulating influence of ACTH. There is no definite evidence, however, that ascorbic acid is necessary for the synthesis of the adrenal steroids, nor that any of the manifestations of scurvy are due to adrenocortical insufficiency. In spite of all the knowledge that is available, it is not yet possible to translate the morphologic changes of scurvy into chemical terms.

Diagnosis. Scurvy is a clinical state and cannot be diagnosed with assurance by any chemical test. The best that the laboratory can do is to confirm or deny a degree of deficiency of vitamin C compatible with scurvy. A serum vitamin C level of 0 mg per 100 ml merely indicates that the patient has not eaten foods containing vitamin C for about 6 weeks. A level of less than 4 mg per 100 ml in the buffy coat of the blood indicates severe tissue depletion and is compatible with a diagnosis of scurvy or a prescorbutic state. Various load tests have been proposed to determine the degree of tissue unsaturation. The one most commonly used involves the oral administration of 15 mg vitamin C per kilogram body weight to the fasting adult patient or 200 mg intramuscularly to the infant. Blood and urine specimens are collected before and at hourly intervals for 4 or 5 hr after this dose. In the infant, a 4-hr specimen is sufficient. Persons whose tissues are completely desaturated will excrete little or no ascorbic acid in the urine during this period, and the blood level will rise to 0.4 mg per 100 ml at the highest and then rapidly fall back to zero. Such a result is also compatible with a diagnosis of scurvy. The clinical features already described and, in the infant, the appearance of the bones in the x-ray, make the diagnosis. The skin and mucous membrane lesions may be confused with those of other types of purpura, particularly the thrombocytopenic and vascular types. Petechiae associated with various forms of sepsis may be confused with perifollicular hemorrhages, and the gum lesions of acute, especially monocytic, leukemia and those of diphenylhydantoin (Dilantin) hypersensitivity may be confused with scorbutic gums, though the blue-red color of the scorbutic gum lesion is usually quite distinctive.

Prevention and Treatment. A diet rich in citrus fruits, tomatoes, and vegetables will keep the tissues normally saturated with vitamin C. A marginal diet containing as little as 25 mg vitamin C per day will prevent scurvy but will not keep the tissues well saturated. Infants who are given orange juice regularly are adequately protected; those who are reared primarily on unsupplemented milk formulas run the risk of the disease.

One orange (equivalent to 50 mg vitamin C) will temporarily relieve the manifestations of scurvy. Usually, however, one prescribes 100 mg ascorbic acid five times daily by mouth, or if the patient is unable to take oral medication, an equal amount of sodium ascorbate is given in divided doses by the intravenous or intramuscular routes. As soon as the patient can eat, a diet rich in vitamin C and in all other essential nutrients should be prescribed. Under such a regimen, gum lesions begin to clear in 2 or 3 days and subperiosteal hemorrhages in the infant begin to calcify in 7 to 10 days. Even massive ecchymoses will have disappeared in 3 weeks.

REFERENCES

Crandon, J. H., C. C. Lund, and D. B. Dill: Experimental Human Scurvy, New Engl. J. Med., 223: 353, 1940.

Ralli, E. P., and S. Sherry: Adult Scurvy and Metabolism of Vitamin C, Medicine, 20:251, 1941.

Sebrell, W. H., Jr., and R. S. Harris: Ascorbic Acid, pp. 177–391, in "The Vitamins," vol. 1, New York, Academic Press, Inc., 1954.

59 NICOTINIC ACID DEFICIENCY (Pellagra)

William J. Darby

Definition. Pellagra is a deficiency syndrome characterized by dermatitis (usually symmetric lesions of exposed surfaces), glossitis and stomatitis, diarrhea, and in later stages, dementia.

Etiology and Pathogenesis. Pellagra may occur as the result of a dietary deficiency or may be conditioned by other diseases, particularly those of the gastrointestinal tract. The typical pellagragenic diet derives 60 per cent or more of its calories from maize (corn), is monotonously restricted, includes almost no green leafy vegetables, and is very poor in sources of animal protein (meat, eggs, milk, cheese). Such diets are relatively low in, but not devoid of, nicotinic acid. The nicotinic acid present is mostly in the bound form. They provide scanty quantities of tryptophan, the amino acid precursor of nicotinic acid. Approximately 60 mg of tryptophan are equivalent to 1 mg of nicotinic acid. The protein of corn is of poor biologic quality, with an imbalanced pattern of amino acids—low in tryptophan and excessive in leucine. The relationship of this imbalance to the development of pellagra is not yet clear, but it is possible that it accounts for the long-postulated pellagragenic activity of maize. It is not essential under all circumstances that corn be included in the diet in order that pellagra occur. For example, pellagra was noted in prisoners of war in the Philippines during the Second World War despite the absence of corn from the diet. Under these circumstances nutritional edema was universal.

Pellagra is a seasonal disease. When it was epidemic in the Southern United States, the peak of the season occurred in May, June, and July, and the incidence decreased during the latter part of the summer to reach the lowest point during the winter. The incidence of pellagra parallels remarkably the seasonal variation in intensity of the sunlight. It has been established that the dermatitis of exposed surfaces may be precipitated in pellagrins by exposure to the sun, as it may be by any other type of trauma.

In summary, then, pellagra may be thought of as the syndrome which results from exposure to the sun of the person depleted of nicotinic acid and protein (tryptophan). Manifestations of a deficiency of other B vitamins may frequently coexist.

Secondary or conditioned pellagra has been related to a multitude of associated diseases and conditions, including diseases of the alimentary canal, hepatic disease, surgical procedures, infections, pregnancy and lactation, and neoplastic disease. Alcoholic pellagra is similar to the endemic disease except that, etiologically, alcohol has displaced other foods to such an extent that the person becomes depleted of the pellagra-preventive factor(s).

Incidence and Epidemiology. Sporadic cases of pellagra occur throughout the world. Areas in which epidemics have occurred include the Southern United States, Transcaucasia, Bulgaria, Rumania, Spain, Italy, Africa, Yucatán, Chile, Egypt, Yugoslavia, and India. In the last two decades the florid disease has disappeared almost completely from the Southern United States. For example, in 1928, 6,969 deaths were reported from the registration area, while in 1946 only 804 deaths were attributed to pellagra. This decrease has been continuous since the early 1930s and is most logically attributable to many factors, including educational efforts directed toward improvement of agricultural practices, food preparation, conservation, and dietary habits; improved economic position of the poorer groups in the population; increased availability of a wide variety of nutritious processed foods; the decrease in area isolation as a result of better systems of communication and travel; the gradual change from the one-crop system of farming; and the industrialization of many regions.

Pathologic Findings. The pathologic findings in pellagra are not specific. The tissues involved include skin, mucosal surfaces, gastrointestinal tract, and nervous system, and in some instances, the blood is involved.

The initial skin change ascribable to nicotinic acid deficiency is rarefaction of the corium and dilatation of the blood vessels. Simultaneously occurring epithelial changes include hyperkeratosis, parakeratosis, and acanthosis. Bullae are attributed to separation of the epidermis due to the changes in the corium. Later the superficial layers of the epidermis and the sebaceous glands become atrophic.

The mucosal surfaces—mouth, esophagus, vagina—exhibit similar dilatation of blood vessels and epithelial atrophy. Ulcerations of the mucosa may develop. The epithelium of the colon may be atrophic, and the walls thickened and inflamed, exhibiting cysts or ulcerations. The relationship of these colonic lesions to nicotinic acid deficiency is not clearly established, and it has been noted that they are quite similar to the changes observed in pantothenic acid–deficient swine.

Anemia is inconstantly associated with pellagra. It may be microcytic, normocytic, or macrocytic in character. Indeed, contrary to former impressions, microcytic iron-deficiency anemia appears now to be more commonly associated with pellagra than does macrocytic anemia. When macrocytic, the anemia responds to administration of folic acid or vitamin B_{12}. Nicotinic acid lack does not per se appear to result in anemia; the role of protein deficiency cannot yet be defined.

The angular fissures and "magenta tongue" may, on occasion, be signs of ariboflavinosis. Ocular lesions of ariboflavinosis may also be present at times.

Fatty infiltration of the liver has been described in pellagra and is emphasized particularly in the disease as seen in Africa. This finding is most likely a manifestation of a deficiency of lipotropic substances rather than of nicotinic acid. Furthermore, the term *pellagra* has often been wrongly applied to protein deficiency (kwashiorkor) in Africa; it is not certain, therefore, that the fatty liver is ascribable to nicotinic acid deficiency.

The lesions described as occurring in the nervous system are quite variable and nonspecific.

It is obvious that the syndrome of pellagra represents, in the main, a deficiency of nicotinic acid which may be associated with the findings of any of a number of other deficiency states. This view readily explains the variable pathologic and clinical picture of the disease.

Clinical Findings. It is rare to find a "typical pellagrin" who exhibits all the manifestations of the disease. However, the pellagrin usually experiences for some weeks lassitude, anorexia, rather vague digestive symptoms, and emotional instability described by the patient as "nervousness." Following a few days of work in the field (exposure to sun), the patient notes some burning and stinging of the hands, face, and neck, and within a day or so there appears a fiery red erythema, which may be interpreted as sunburn. Vesiculation, progressing to bullous lesions, appears on the backs of the hands and sometimes on the face and neck. When seen by the physician the bullae may have been opened or may have ruptured spontaneously. In some instances they become secondarily infected. Soreness of the tongue and mouth and symptoms of vaginitis often develop in association with the erythematous changes. The acute phase of the disease is accompanied by diarrhea and increased anorexia.

The initial relatively mild nervous manifestations of headache, irritability, insomnia, and burning of the hands and feet give way in the acute pellagrin to definite personality changes. These patients react slowly, are uninterested, may become mildly to completely disoriented, and exhibit hallucinations and delusions. The mental symptoms at times so dominate the picture that pellagrins have been referred to mental institutions before the correct diagnosis became apparent. Nevertheless, severe mental symptoms occured in but a small percentage of the cases of endemic pellagra.

On occasion the history may disclose that the patient has experienced in previous years one or more somewhat similar episodes. The dietary history reveals a monotonous intake of the pattern already described.

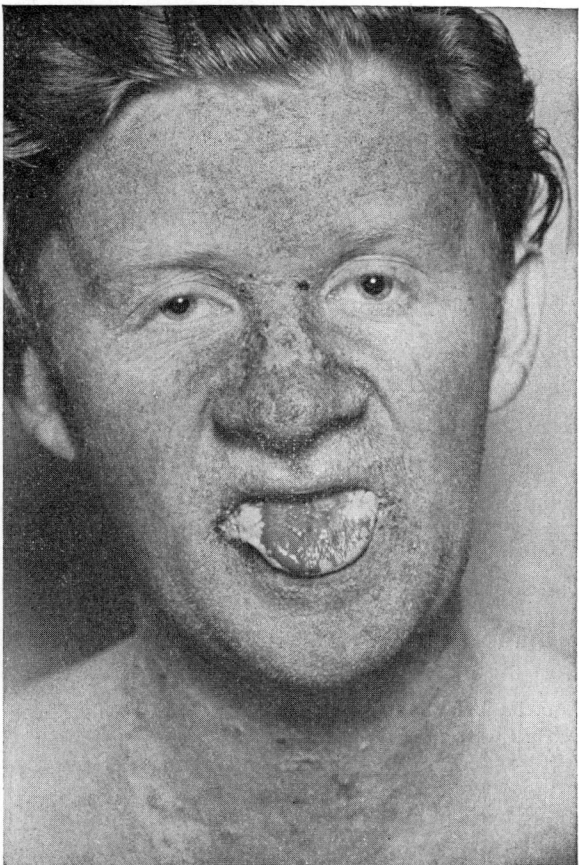

Fig. 59-1. Photograph of a pellagrin, on admission, showing marked dermatitis over face and neck, and extensive and severe glossitis with membranes on the margins of the tongue. There were plugs in the orifices of the sebaceous glands and fissures at the corners of the mouth. (*Smith and Ruffin: Intern. Clinics,* 2:103, 1940.)

Upon physical examination, the pellagrin may be somewhat underweight, with varying degrees of dehydration, depending upon the severity of the gastrointestinal disturbance. The characteristic skin lesions (Figs. 59-1, 59-2) are the symmetric changes of the exposed surfaces, especially over the wrists and tops of the feet. In addition, one may find the so-called "dyssebacia" around the nose, mouth, and forehead—i.e., the plugging of sebaceous glands with dry, yellowish material. These lesions are often termed *shark skin*. Over bony prominences, such as the knees and elbows, hyperkeratotic areas associated with increased pigmentation are frequent. Such lesions occur most often in those pellagrins who have been bedridden for a period of time. Excoriations are common in the genital region, especially in the female. A bright red, sore tongue, sometimes described as "beefy"

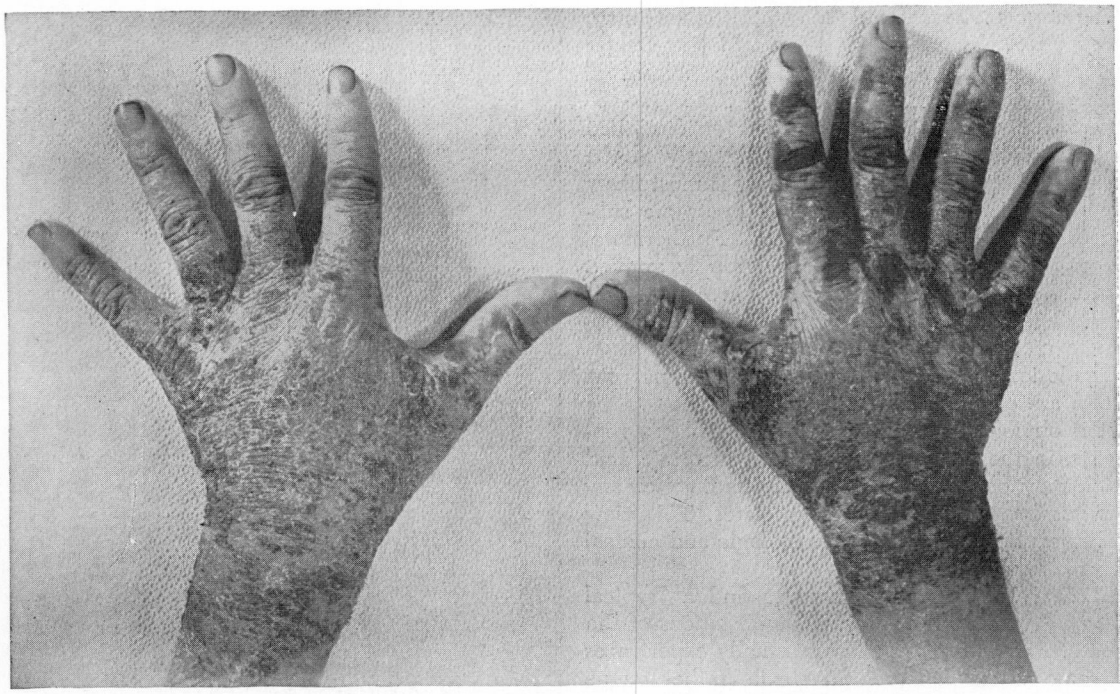

FIG. 59-2. Photograph of the hands of the same patient as in Fig. 59-1, on admission. Similar but less extensive lesions were present on the feet. (*Smith and Ruffin: Intern. Clinics,* 2:103, 1940.)

in appearance, is usual. Finally, cheilosis and angular oral fissures may be encountered. In many instances, the cheilosis and angular fissures respond to nicotinic acid therapy; but in others, they do not heal until riboflavin is administered. Dyssebacia may follow similar therapeutic patterns.

Laboratory Findings. No decisive chemical tests exist for the detection of pellagra. The occurrence of abnormal urinary pigments has been reported in this disease, but much confusion exists concerning the identity and significance of these substances. The nicotinic acid metabolite, N^1-methylnicotinamide, may be rendered fluorescent and, hence, is conveniently measured. The urinary excretion of this metabolite is decreased in clinically manifest nicotinic acid deficiency. This decrease is apparent in either 24-hr urinary specimens or in timed specimens following a standardized test dose of nicotinamide. Because of the very great overlapping of values between those found in deficient patients and those showing no evidence of nicotinic acid deficiency, this test is of little value in establishing the diagnosis in an individual case. Blood and tissue coenzyme concentrations have not proved of clinical value to date.

As previously indicated, the pellagrin may or may not exhibit anemia. This when present ranges from microcytic to macrocytic in character. Serum protein values are not usually altered.

Diagnosis. The diagnosis of pellagra rests upon the clinical and dietary history, the clinical findings, and the response to specific therapy. Evaluation of therapeutic response is rendered difficult unless the patient is carefully controlled in order to prevent the occurrence of spontaneous remissions due to bed rest and improved dietary intake.

The distinction between sprue and pellagra is sometimes a problem but can usually be made upon consideration of the following points: (1) A more severe macrocytic anemia and megaloblastic bone marrow are usually found in sprue. (2) Pellagrous dermatitis is not seen in sprue, unless the two diseases coexist. (3) Although diarrhea is present in both diseases, steatorrhea and its concomitant findings are not usually encountered in pellagra. (4) The oral glucose tolerance test result is not significantly abnormal in pellagra. (5) The response to specific therapy differs.

Mild clinically manifest nicotinic acid deficiency may be characterized entirely by the vague symptoms of early pellagra as well as glossitis and, in some cases, angular fissures. In such instances, the condition must be differentiated from ariboflavinosis, chronic iron deficiency, pernicious anemia, pseudoariboflavinosis, allergic glossitis, and even lingual neoplasms. If mental symptoms predominate, the disease may be confused with psychoses of various origins.

Treatment. The symptoms of pellagra are relieved by administration of nicotinic acid in doses of 50 mg two or three times a day orally. If the patient's condition contraindicates oral administration, nicotinamide (100 mg daily) may be given parenterally. Such specific therapy should be accompanied by an adequate diet of relatively high protein, high vitamin content.

Additional dietary supplements may be given as indicated by evidence of specific deficiencies. Crude liver extracts given orally have proved of particular benefit in the restoration of many pellagrins.

General supportive measures should be instituted. In the presence of dehydration, prompt administration of saline and glucose is necessary. Bed rest, good nursing care, and sympathetic encouragement to consume a liberal diet should be part of the treatment of all such patients.

Continuous maintenance therapy with nicotinic acid is unnecessary after subsidence of the disease. It is essential, however, that the patient's eating habits be altered in order to allow for the consumption of an adequate diet.

Prognosis. The prognosis in pellagra depends upon the severity of the disease. In the usual mild or moderately severe cases, mortality should approach zero, unless the disease is complicated by some more serious disturbance. In severely ill patients, death may occur despite the most skillful handling. For example, at Duke University a mortality of 3.7 per cent was reported for the group of patients who were treated shortly after the introduction of nicotinic acid therapy.

Vigorous early treatment of patients with mental changes results in recovery. If the dementia has been of long standing, however, permanent residua may remain.

REFERENCES

Bean, W. B., T. D. Spies, and M. A. Blankenhorn: Secondary Pellagra, Medicine, 23:1, 1944.

Chick, H.: The Causation of Pellagra, Nutrition Abstr. & Revs., 20:523, 1950–1951.

Food and Agriculture Organization of the United Nations: "Maize and Maize Diets," p. 94, Rome, 1953.

Goldberger, J., and G. A. Wheeler: The Experimental Production of Pellagra in Human Subjects by Means of Diet, U.S. Public Health Serv., Hyg. Lab. Bull. 120, 1920.

Goldsmith, G. A.: Niacin-Tryptophane Relationships in Man and Niacin Requirements, Am. J. Clin. Nutrition, 6:479, 1958.

Lewis, C. F., and M. M. Musselman: Observations on Pellagra in American Prisoners of War in the Philippines, J. Nutrition, 32:549, 1946.

Smith, D. T., and J. M. Ruffin: Effect of Sunlight on the Clinical Manifestations of Pellagra, Arch. Internal Med., 59:631, 1937.

—— and ——: Pellagra Therapy, Intern. Clinics, 2:103, 1940.

Sydenstricker, V. P.: The History of Pellagra, Its Recognition as a Disorder of Nutrition and Its Conquest, Am. J. Clin. Nutrition, 6:409, 1958.

60 THIAMINE DEFICIENCY (Beriberi)

William J. Darby

Definition. Beriberi is a deficiency disease characterized by multiple neuritis, changes in the cardiovascular system, and, frequently, edema. The primary manifestations are attributable to thiamine lack.

Etiology. Thiamine is a water-soluble, heat-labile vitamin, the principal food sources of which are whole cereals, legumes, lean meats (especially organ meats), nuts, and yeast. Highly refined foodstuffs, such as polished (white) rice, low-extraction flour, and refined sugar, are practically devoid of the vitamin. The dietary requirement of thiamine is related directly to the intake of nonfat calories. Fat and, to a lesser extent, protein exert so-called "thiamine-sparing action."

The typical diet associated with the development of beriberi is a monotonous low protein, low fat, high carbohydrate diet in which a highly milled cereal such as rice is the chief source of calories. The existence of this food pattern accounts for the distribution of beriberi in the Orient, in many of the islands of the Pacific, in sections of the West Indies, South America, and Africa, and in circumscribed regions of North America (the rice-growing area of southern Louisiana and, formerly, Newfoundland). The sporadic case of beriberi in the United States is commonly associated with alcoholism. This association was formerly thought to be due to an increased use of thiamine in the metabolism of alcohol but is now known to be due to the displacement of thiamine-containing foodstuffs by alcohol. Alcohol, surprisingly enough, has a thiamine-sparing action.

Beriberi is seen in both sexes and at all ages. In the United States the majority of reports indicate a predominance in men. In the Orient and the Philippines, however, the disease not infrequently complicates pregnancy or lactation. It may occur in the breast-fed infant or, in rare cases, as a congenital disease of the newborn. Infantile beriberi most characteristically occurs in the one- to four-month age group.

There is no doubt that beriberi is a deficiency

disease. In addition, there is an opinion that its development is at times attributable to consumption of dirty or spoiled rice which, presumably, contains a hypothetic beriberi-producing factor. Thiaminase, an enzyme occurring in certain fish, destroys the vitamin and, hence, may render a food deficient in thiamine. Synthetic antimetabolites for thiamine have been produced; none, however, has been isolated from foodstuffs. Live yeast, when introduced into the gastrointestinal tract, "soaks up" thiamine, converts it to a phosphate derivative, and renders it unabsorbable. Whether there are other microorganisms with similar activities has not been ascertained. A beriberi-like syndrome attributed to microbiologic thiaminase activity has been reported from Japan. Bacteria with potent thiaminases have been isolated from the feces of patients with this "thiaminase disease."

Pathologic Findings. The pathologic findings in beriberi are marked by their nonspecificity and lack of constancy. The most important lesions are noted in the heart and peripheral nerves. The heart may be enlarged, particularly to the right. This enlargement is usually due to cardiac dilatation, although hypertrophy has been described. Microscopically, degenerative changes in the cardiac muscle, interstitial edema, and hydropic degeneration of the myocardial fibers may be seen.

Degenerative changes involving the central, peripheral, and autonomic nervous systems may exist. Degeneration of the myelin sheath and fragmentation of the axis cylinder comprise the most frequently described lesions of the peripheral nerve. Swelling and chromatolysis of the sympathetic chain and degeneration of the vagus nerve are found in some cases.

It is not possible to ascribe these pathologic changes specifically to thiamine deficiency. In experimental studies in which only thiamine deficiency was produced, neurologic changes were not observed. Some of the findings may be due to concomitant deficiencies of one or another dietary factor other than thiamine.

Clinical Picture. The clinical picture of beriberi may for convenience be divided into three types: (1) wet beriberi, in which the finding of edema and serous effusions predominates; (2) dry beriberi, in which the predominant picture is referable to the nervous system and edema is minimal or absent; and (3) acute cardiac beriberi, in which the cardiac symptoms predominate and in which sudden death may occur.

At least 3 months on a grossly deficient diet are required for the development of beriberi. The onset is seldom acute but rather is marked by gradually increasing fatigability, irritability, cardiac palpitation, muscle tenderness (especially of the calf muscles), and leg pains exacerbated by assuming a squatting position. The appearance of paresthesias, superficial hyperesthesia, loss of superficial cutaneous sensation, and diminution of deep reflexes mark the development of the peripheral neuritis. Flaccid paresis, foot drop, and muscular wasting may follow. The peripheral neuritis first appears in the lower extremities and may later develop in the upper extremity.

During the initial phases of the peripheral neuritis, edema may appear in the wet type of beriberi. The edema is first noted around the ankles, and initially it disappears after a few hours in bed. It may progress, however, to generalized anasarca with pleural, peritoneal, and pericardial effusions. In the absence of cardiac failure, the cause of this edema is unknown.

Clinicians working in China have described two types of cardiac beriberi: (1) the acute fulminating disease, which appears suddenly and, if untreated, results in death within a few hours; and (2) the less acute beriberi heart disease with congestive failure. The patient with beriberi heart complains of excessive fatigue, palpitation on exertion, and shortness of breath. In the congestive type, edema is always present, the pulse rate may or may not be increased, and the blood pressure may be normal or elevated. The heart is dilated, the circulation time is decreased, venous pressure may be elevated or normal, and less difference than normal exists between the oxygen content of arterial and venous blood. The characteristic picture of high-output failure (Chap. 13), with exaggeration of the heart sounds, systolic murmurs, and a full bounding pulse, is usually seen. Thus the precordial phenomena may mimic those of mitral insufficiency, while the peripheral signs resemble those of aortic insufficiency. Electrocardiographic changes are variable and nonspecific. Dramatic recovery may follow specific therapy with thiamine. The recovery is marked by relief of general symptoms, diuresis, and a progressive decrease in cardiac size over a period of a few weeks.

Some clinicians believe that less rigid criteria for the diagnosis of beriberi heart disease should be accepted, and the following have been proposed: (1) insufficient evidence for other cause of the failure, (2) 3 months or more on a thiamine-deficient diet, (3) signs of neuritis or pellagra, (4) enlarged heart with sinus rhythm, (5) dependent edema, (6) elevated venous pressure, (7) minor electrocardiographic changes, and (8) recovery with decrease in heart size or autopsy consistent with beriberi heart disease.

Other deficiency diseases, such as avitaminosis A and pellagra, or anemia, may be associated with the beriberi syndrome.

Laboratory Findings. Many laboratory procedures have been used for the investigation of thiamine metabolism in man. Among them are the determination of thiamine in the blood, in the white cell–platelet layer, and in 24-hr urinary excretion, as well as various load tests in which the urinary loss of thiamine is estimated following standardized doses of the vitamin. Unfortunately, none is dependable clinically for the establishment of the diagnosis of beriberi.

Probably the most promising test for the diagnosis of the thiamine deficiency state is determination of the carbohydrate metabolism index (CMI). In the absence of thiamine, the metabolism of pyruvic acid is impaired. Slightly elevated basal pyruvic acid concentrations (above 1.2 mg per 100 ml) occur in severe beriberi. Except in severe thiamine deficiency, the determination of fasting pyruvic acid levels in the blood is not a reliable indicator of thiamine deficiency. The rate of disposal (and, hence, the blood concentration) of pyruvic acid depends partly upon the metabolic load of glucose and lactic acid. Accordingly, the simultaneous determination of these three constituents under proper conditions seems to provide more useful information concerning thiamine status than does a measure of one alone. The procedure is as follows: 9 ml of 20 per cent glucose per kilogram is administered orally after withdrawing a fasting basal blood sample. Sixty minutes later a mild exercise test is applied. This consists of walking down and up and down and up again a flight of 21 steps 19 cm high in a period of 60 sec. Five minutes later, blood is again sampled. The CMI, as was empirically developed, is calculated by the formula:

$$CMI = \frac{L - \dfrac{G}{10} + 15P - \dfrac{G}{10}}{2}$$

G, L, and P, respectively, are levels of glucose, lactic acid, and pyruvic acid in milligrams per 100 ml blood. On the basis of studies of induced thiamine deficiency in man, 15 has been set as the upper limit of normal CMI.

Diagnosis. The diagnosis of beriberi is made from the history, physical findings, and controlled response to specific therapy. Determination of pyruvic acid levels or of CMI may be useful diagnostic procedures. The measurement of cardiac size by x-ray is especially valuable as a means of evaluating the effect of specific therapy. Two procedures of value in examining for peripheral neuritis of beriberi are to (1) have the patient squat on his heels and determine whether this produces leg pain and whether he is able to rise without using his hands; (2) squeeze the calf muscles to test for tenderness.

Peripheral neuritis, when present, must be differentiated from the neuritis of lead poisoning or arsenic. The history, the absence of edema in toxic neuritis, the presence of a lead line on the gums, or the presence of stippled cells in the blood smear serves to distinguish these.

Treatment. Preventive therapy consists in the establishment of proper dietary habits which will ensure sufficient intake of the vitamin (see Table 22-2). Curative treatment consists of the administration of thiamine orally or parenterally. Oral doses of 3 to 5 mg may be given two or three times a day. The evidence indicates that oral doses larger than 5 mg are no more efficient than this amount, because of limitation of absorption. From 5 to 25 mg thiamine hydrochloride parenterally per day may be given. The oral route is to be preferred except in critical cases, and once response has begun in these critical cases, oral administration may safely be substituted. Along with the specific therapy, every effort should be made to correct faulty dietary habits responsible for development of the deficiency. Provision of a liberally adequate diet is of added value in many cases because of the accompanying deficiencies.

Prognosis. The prognosis in beriberi depends upon the stage of the disease and the time which elapses before proper therapy is instituted. Properly instituted therapy is followed by rapid remission in most uncomplicated cases. On the other hand, a death rate as high as 50 per cent has been reported for "occidental beriberi heart disease" in recent years. This has been attributed to the establishment of an irreversible process.

REFERENCES

Blankenhorn, M. A., C. F. Vilter, I. M. Scheinker, and R. S. Austin: Occidental Beriberi Heart Disease, J.A.M.A., 131:717, 1946.

Burgess, R. C., et al.: Beriberi, Federation Proc., 17: Suppl. 2, p. 3, 1958.

Hayoshi, R.: Bacterial Synthesis and Destruction of Thiamine, Nutrition Revs., 15:65, 1957.

Horwitt, M. K., and O. Kreisler: The Determination of Early Thiamine-deficient States by Estimation of Blood Lactic and Pyruvic Acids after Glucose Administration and Exercise, J. Nutrition, 37:411, 1949.

Keefer, C. S.: The Beriberi Heart, Arch. Internal Med., 45:1, 1930.

Platt, B. S., and G. D. Lu: Chemical and Clinical Findings in Beri-beri with Special Reference to Vitamin B₁ Deficiency, Quart. J. Med., 5(n.s.):355, 1936.

Wintrobe, M. M., et al.: A Study of Thiamine Deficiency in Swine, Bull. Johns Hopkins Hosp., 71: 141, 1942; 73:169, 1943.

61 THE LIPID-SOLUBLE VITAMINS

William J. Darby

The lipid-soluble vitamins which are clearly of importance for man include vitamin A and carotene, vitamin D, and vitamin K. The status of the tocopherols is discussed in Chap. 57. Physiologically it is convenient to consider these nutrients together, since all are soluble in fats and are associated with lipids in the process of absorption. Indeed, conditioned deficiencies of all these fat-soluble vitamins may occur in disease states in which defective lipid absorption is present. These nutrients, in contrast to the water-soluble factors, are not excreted in appreciable amounts in the urine. Accordingly, they may accumulate in relatively large amounts in the body as a result of excessive intake.

VITAMIN A

The absorption of vitamin A is dependent upon normal absorption of fats. It appears in the lymphatics following ingestion. In those conditions in which fat absorption is impaired, water-dispersible or emulsified preparations of vitamin A are better absorbed than the oily preparations. Vitamin A is stored in the liver of the well-fed adult in quantities sufficient to meet estimated requirements for a period of 200 to 400 days or longer. Only negligible quantities are normally excreted in the urine, although there is increased excretion in some renal diseases and infections.

Carotenes serve as precursors of vitamin A, the site of conversion being either the liver or the intestinal wall. Carotene is less efficiently absorbed than vitamin A; and if the total vitamin A requirement is met from carotene alone, the minimal requirement is greater than if the dietary source is preformed vitamin A.

It is well established that vitamin A enters into the constitution of visual purple (rhodopsin). When light falls on the retina, visual purple is broken down. Accordingly, there is a constant cycle of breakdown and resynthesis of this derivative of vitamin A. In the absence of vitamin A, the resynthesis is retarded and night blindness (nyctalopia) occurs.

Avitaminosis A

Vitamin A–deficiency syndrome is termed *avitaminosis A*. It may be manifested by an impaired capacity for dark adaptation, night blindness, xerophthalmia, and keratomalacia. The occurrence of Bitot spots and hyperkeratotic lesions of the extensor surfaces of the skin may be associated lesions.

Avitaminosis A results from a dietary lack of vitamin A or its precursors (carotenes) or from failure to absorb these lipid-soluble substances because of alterations in absorption of fat. Conditioned deficiencies may be found in sprue, celiac disease, fibrocystic disease of the pancreas, intestinal lipodystrophy, and other steatorrheas. Long-continued ingestion of mineral oil with meals may render carotene or vitamin A unabsorbable and thereby lower significantly the nutriture of the individual, particularly when the dietary contains borderline amounts of vitamin activity largely derived from carotene. In hepatitis and cirrhosis of the liver, decreased blood levels of vitamin A may be encountered. The impairment of dark adaptation in hepatic cirrhosis may reflect a defect in the metabolism of vitamin A.

Avitaminosis A is uncommon in the United States, but dietary deficiencies have been reported frequently from the Orient, India, Indonesia, southeast Asia, Africa, and, formerly, northern Europe. The reports from northern Europe were chiefly of institutionalized children. The rare instances of severe avitaminosis A reported from the United States have usually been conditioned.

This deficiency disease is more likely to be encountered in infants than in adults for two reasons: (1) The requirement for the vitamin is higher during growth than for simple maintenance. (2) The newborn infant has relatively small stores of the vitamin, which, therefore, are more easily depleted by a deficient diet.

Pathologic Findings. Vitamin A is concerned with the maintenance of normal integrity of certain epithelial tissues and the orderly development of bones and teeth. Epithelial lesions of avitaminosis A are characterized by atrophy and proliferation of the basal cells, with metaplasia into stratified keratinizing epithelium. It is sometimes difficult to separate the epithelial changes seen at autopsy into those due to vitamin A lack and those attributable to associated conditions, such as fibrocystic disease. Corneal lesions may be especially noteworthy, with keratinization of the epithelium, followed by infiltration, vascularization, and sometimes, ulceration. Alterations in the lacrimal glands may result in atrophy and fibrosis, and these processes may account for the ocular xerosis. There is no general agreement on this point, however. Skin lesions attributed to vitamin A deficiency are follicular, somewhat pigmented papules with a central core consisting of a keratinized epithelial plug. Histologic study shows hyperkeratinization and hyperplasia of the epithelium with associated degeneration of the sweat glands. To these changes is attributed the dryness of the skin. The specificity of these lesions has recently been questioned, and some workers hold that the skin lesions are due to associated B-complex deficiencies or lack of unsaturated fatty acids. The important pathologic changes which occur in the skeleton, nervous system, teeth, retina, and other structures in experimental deficiencies in lower animals have not been clearly identified in man.

Clinical Picture. The clinical picture of avitaminosis A varies with the age of the person. In infants, night blindness, xerophthalmia, and keratomalacia are the most frequent manifestations. The nutritional history of the infant indicates a diet lacking in vitamin A or carotene, or else there is an associated disease, such as cystic fibrosis of the pancreas or biliary obstruction, which would lead to defective absorption of vitamin A. The syndrome is not infrequently associated with kwashiorkor. In the adult, xerophthalmia occurs but rarely and then only in the more advanced cases. The earliest clinical manifestation of vitamin A depletion in the adult is decreased dark adaptation, detectable by one of the several adaptometers. Some time later, clinical night blindness develops.

Skin changes consist of generalized dryness of the skin, or xeroderma, followed by the appearance of localized papular eruptions on the anterolateral aspect of the thighs and posterolateral surfaces of the upper arms. These lesions (phrynoderma) may involve extensor surfaces of both upper and lower extremities and then extend over the buttocks, shoulders, abdomen, and neck. The distribution is symmetric, and the skin over the involved sites generally appears darker than normal. The lesions are seen to be horny plugs projecting from the hair follicles. They are described with increasing frequency after puberty but are rare before that age. Prior to the onset of puberty, skin changes of avitaminosis A are primarily those of dryness without the associated hyperkeratosis. Failure to recognize this point has led to much confusion. The common childhood lesion of keratosis pilaris has often been mistakenly attributed to avitaminosis A, despite the fact that it is not associated with any of the other findings of A deficiency, is associated with satisfactory blood levels of vitamin A, and does not respond to administration of the vitamin. On the other hand, much evidence from India attributes phrynoderma to a deficiency of essential fatty acids rather than to avitaminosis A.

Bitot spots are characteristic grayish-white, foam-like, superficial lesions of the bulbar conjunctiva. The lesion is usually seen in both eyes. It occurs most frequently on the lateral aspect. These changes are widely held to be manifestations of avitaminosis A. They may disappear upon the administration of the vitamin, but this is by no means a constant finding. Evidence is unconvincing that these signs are in fact due to vitamin A lack. Bitot spots are easily differentiated from the thickened, gelatinous-appearing, triangular pinguecula which are so common in adults and which are not manifestations of vitamin A deficiency.

Within 3 months after the start of a vitamin A- and carotene-free diet, the plasma level falls to a stable concentration of 10 to 40 IU per 100 ml (6 to 24 μg per 100 ml). Total carotene content of plasma of well-nourished individuals usually ranges upward from 120 to 300 IU per 100 ml (72 to 180 μg per 100 ml). In states of deprivation, the very low carotene values may not actually represent biologically active precursors of vitamin A but, instead, other carotenoid pigments. Concentrations of carotene less than 80 IU, or 50 μg, per 100 ml are presumptive evidence of low dietary intake or of some impairment of absorption.

Under conditions leading to a deficiency of vitamin A, the blood concentration of the vitamin itself falls much more slowly than does the concentration of carotene. No appreciable fall in vitamin A concentration occurs in adults until after about 8 months on a diet totally devoid of the vitamin or its precursor. It is widely accepted that values of vitamin A as low as 70 IU per 100 ml are consistent with health. Concentrations as low as 50 IU per 100 ml are not infrequently encountered in otherwise healthy individuals. Deterioration of dark adaptation does not occur until the plasma level has fallen below 50 IU per 100 ml. Concentrations below 40 or 50 IU per 100 ml may be associated with defective night vision or other clinical manifestations of avitaminosis A. On the other hand, such levels may be encountered in apparently healthy adults. Clinical findings due to vitamin A deficiency are consistently accompanied by plasma levels below 40 or 50 IU.

Blood levels of vitamin A are normally lower in infants, the newborn, and in the latter part of pregnancy. Infant blood is usually low or devoid of carotene.

The diagnosis of avitaminosis A may be made upon finding the suitable combination of signs and a history of a diet low in vitamin A and carotene over a long period of time or of some defect in absorption which might effectively decrease the absorption of vitamin A and carotene, coupled with consistently low blood levels. Measurement of dark adaptation by leading to the detection of a definitely abnormal final rod threshold and lengthening of the cone-rod transition time is of value in establishing the diagnosis of avitaminosis A. The subsequent response of these abnormalities of adaptation to administered vitamin A or carotene is further evidence in support of such diagnosis.

The treatment of avitaminosis A should be preventive and curative. Preventive therapy consists of the establishment of proper dietary habits in order to ensure a sufficient intake of the vitamin (Table 22-2).

Curative treatment consists of administration of 5,000 to 25,000 IU of vitamin A or an equivalent amount of carotene daily for a period of some 6 weeks or until the lesions have cleared. If the avitaminosis is conditioned by faulty absorption, one of the water-dispersible preparations of vitamin A may be more effective. Complete therapy involves correction of the dietary defect and of the conditioning abnormality underlying the development of the disease syndrome.

The prognosis in cases of avitaminosis A is good except where corneal involvement is sufficiently extensive to result in permanent scarring. In these instances, permanent blindness may result despite the clearing of the xerophthalmia.

Hypervitaminosis A

Hypervitaminosis A results from a greatly excessive intake of vitamin A, usually in the form of concentrates or high-potency fish-liver oils. Because of the large margin of safety between active therapeutic dose and toxic quantities of the vitamin, the condition is relatively rare. Nevertheless, on occasions the ingestion of amounts of vitamin A of 160,-000 to 180,000 IU or more per day over a sufficient period of time has resulted in a picture of toxicity.

The usual syndrome of hypervitaminosis A is characterized by hepatomegaly, splenomegaly, leukopenia, anemia, periosteal changes, sparse, coarse hair, increased serum vitamin A levels, and increased serum lipids. The serum vitamin A values may range from 600 to 1,000 IU per 100 ml. An increased bleeding tendency, probably due to hypoprothrombinemia, may be observed.

The toxicity of polar bear and seal liver has been attributed to the tremendously high vitamin A content of these tissues. It is held that the acute symptoms of drowsiness, irritability, severe headache and vomiting, and "peeling of the skin" which may occur after ingestion of polar bear liver may be attributed to acute hypervitaminosis A.

Upon withholding of vitamin A, the hypervitaminosis subsides gradually over a 2- or 3-month period. Specific therapy is unnecessary unless hypoprothrombinemia occurs, in which event administration of vitamin K may be of use.

VITAMIN D

Vitamin D may be ingested in foods or formed within the skin by the ultraviolet irradiation of 7-dehydrocholesterol. The irradiation of this sterol produces the vitamin. For the maintenance of a normal healthy state, the recommended minimal daily intake of vitamin D in human beings is 400 IU per day in term infants, growing children, adults, and pregnant or lactating women; and 600 to 800 IU per day in premature infants. For avitaminosis D to develop, it is necessary that the diet be deficient in the preformed vitamin and that the person not be exposed to ultraviolet light of the wavelength which will convert 7-dehydrocholesterol into the active vitamin.

Only ultraviolet light of the wavelength within the range of approximately 250 to 310 mμ is active in the conversion of precursors of vitamin D to vitamin D (hence, possesses antirachitic potency). The wavelengths of solar radiation range upward from approximately 290 mμ. Accordingly, sunlight possesses antirachitic properties, and where the solar radiation is intense and not obstructed by fog, clouds, smoke, or other atmospheric conditions, it provides some protection against rickets. For this property of sunlight to be effective, the shorter ultraviolet rays must contact an appreciable portion of the skin surfaces. Heavy clothing or ordinary window glass will obstruct active ultraviolet irradiation from the sun. Furthermore, it is commonly stated that the pigmented skin of the darker races serves to "filter out" the antirachitic rays and that the greater frequency of rickets in the Negro in the United States may be attributed to this phenomenon. Economic and dietary factors are most likely of considerable importance also in this difference in incidence.

Avitaminosis D (see also Chap. 79, Osteomalacia and Rickets)

Definition. Deficient systemic levels of vitamin D [calciferol (vitamin D$_2$) or activated 7-dehydrocholesterol (vitamin D$_3$)] result in the nutritional disorder avitaminosis D. This is characterized by insufficient calcium absorption from the gastrointestinal tract and inadequate saturation of body fluids with the ion product of calcium and phosphate. As a result there is decreased formation of bone because of defective calcification of the protein osseous matrix. In patients with an inadequate systemic response to physiologic doses of vitamin D (vitamin D–resistant rickets), there also is insufficient renal tubular reabsorption of phosphate. This contributes to the subnormal ion product of plasma calcium and phosphate. The metabolic bone disorder that results from this defect in bone formation is called *rickets* in infants and young children and *osteomalacia* in adults. Although avitaminosis D is only one of the causes of rickets or osteomalacia, the term rickets often is employed as if it were synonymous with rickets resulting from vitamin D deficiency. The other causes of these bone disorders are discussed in Chap. 79.

Etiology. Avitaminosis D may result from (1) an insufficient content of preformed vitamin D in the diet; (2) poor absorption of fat-soluble vitamin D because of disturbed gastrointestinal function (as in nontropical sprue, celiac disease, chronic pancreatitis, cystic fibrosis of the pancreas, congenital atresia of the bile ducts, and prolonged obstructive jaundice from intra- or extrahepatic biliary tract disease); (3) resistance to the action of vitamin D so that three to ten times the usual amount is required to induce normal physiologic responses; and (4) inadequate formation of activated 7-dehydrocholesterol (vitamin D_3) from ergosterol within the skin by the ultraviolet irradiation of sunlight because of insufficient exposure to the sun.

Incidence. Rickets from avitaminosis D occurs primarily in the Temperate Zone, in large towns, and in thickly populated industrial areas. Because diagnostic criteria vary, the exact incidence in the United States is not known, although the disease is less prevalent than it was several decades ago. Osteomalacia from avitaminosis D in adults is rare in the United States. The low incidence of vitamin D deficiency in this country is related to the fact that the large majority of the population eats an adequate diet, including foods fortified with vitamin D, and is exposed liberally to sunlight. Osteomalacia from vitamin D lack is found occasionally in women of certain religious orders who are continuously protected from the sun by their robes and who are living on a suboptimal diet. Avitaminosis D, with its osseous manifestations, is common in children and adults (especially pregnant women) in northern China and Japan and in the Balkans and the Middle East.

Pathology. In the normally growing child, the long bones increase in length by a process which involves (1) continuous proliferation and maturation of the cartilage cells of the epiphysis, (2) the alignment of the older cartilage cells during maturation into parallel rows at the junction of ossification, (3) deposition of calcium salts in the cartilaginous matrix lying between the rows of cartilage cells, (4) disintegration of the oldest cartilage cells nearest the area of bone formation, (5) invasion of the lacunas by proliferating blood vessels accompanied by osteoblasts, (6) laying down of osteoid by osteoblasts, (7) deposition of calcium and phosphate as hydroxyapatite in the osteoid to form new bone, and (8) resorption of some of the newly formed bone to facilitate remodeling and molding. In rickets, this normal process is interrupted; osteoblastic activity proceeds with the laying down of osteoid, but the deposition of calcium and phosphate to produce ossification does not occur. In addition, the destruction of the older cartilage cells, the invasion of the blood vessels, and the calcification of the cartilaginous matrix fail to take place. The normal costochondral junction presents a narrow, sharp, well-demarcated union between cartilage and bone; the rachitic junction shows a broad, disorganized band with a wide zone of proliferating cartilage cells and considerable irregularity in calcification. The costochondral junction of rickets appears grossly as an enlarged, softened, irregular lesion which produces such clinical manifestations as beading of the ribs or enlarged wrists. The osseous lesions of children with rickets due to avitaminosis D also include the defects in endosteal bone formation that occur in the osteomalacia of adults (see Chap. 79).

The failure to absorb adequate amounts of calcium and phosphate from the gastrointestinal tract results in a lowered plasma calcium, and this, in turn, leads to secondary parathyroid hyperplasia. Hence, evidence of osteitis fibrosa may be superimposed on the lesions of rickets or osteomalacia. The administration of vitamin D with the consequent improved calcium absorption permits restoration of the plasma calcium level to normal and results in the correction of both the pathologic process associated with vitamin D deficiency and the changes resulting from secondary hyperparathyroidism.

Clinical Features, Laboratory Findings, and Diagnostic Criteria. In general, these are the same as those for rickets and osteomalacia due to other factors. The diagnosis of avitaminosis D is suggested by a history of circumstances which would lead to deprivation of vitamin D, such as an inadequate intake of the vitamin, gastrointestinal disease, and lack of exposure to sunlight. In the mildest cases of rickets, the child is irritable, restless during sleep, and may present almost no physical signs other than slightly exaggerated beading of the ribs (rachitic rosary). The latter may be confused with the costochondral beading of scurvy, but the presence of bone tenderness in scurvy facilitates the differentiation. The response to therapeutic doses of vitamin D may aid in establishing the diagnosis in mild obscure cases. The severe disease is characterized by widespread bony deformities, and the child is fretful, pale, and ill.

The bony deformities are the most characteristic findings. Enlargement of the costochondral junctions, while not pathognomonic of rickets, is one of the earliest of detectable signs. The most severe beading, which accompanies long-continued rickets, may be associated with flaring of the lower ribs and a depression along the line of attachment of the diaphragm (Harrison's groove). Retraction of the sternum to form the so-called "funnel chest" may or may not occur. In the moderate or more severe cases of rickets, the head appears large, with prominent frontal bosses, there may be flattening of the crown, and areas of softening of the cranial bones may be detected upon palpation. The presence of these softened areas is termed *craniotabes*. Delayed closure of the sutures may be noted.

In cases of some duration, the long bones exhibit enlargement of the metaphyses, especially noticeable at the wrists, knees, and ankles. Varying degrees of deformities, such as bowing of the legs, knock-knees, and pelvic deformities, may occur, depending upon the duration of the process and the amount of stress to which the skeleton has been subjected.

The musculature generally is lax, and this, in association with the rachitic bone changes, gives rise to the protuberant abdomen aptly termed *potbelly*.

Any one or a combination of the above signs may be present in varying degrees. On the other hand, the signs may occur in the absence of a rachitic process. Accordingly, diagnosis cannot be made on the basis of the physical findings alone. Roentgenologic examination of moderate to advanced cases of rickets reveals cupping of the ends of the bones, especially of the ulna, a frayed margin of the epiphyseal end of the shaft, and diminished calcification of the shafts. X-ray examination is less helpful in efforts to establish the diagnosis of mild rickets, since many of the normal changes in growing bone may easily be confused with slight alterations in structure sometimes attributed to rachitic processes. Laboratory evidence of avitaminosis D consists of increased serum alkaline phosphatase and normal to low serum calcium and/or inorganic phosphorus.

Prognosis. The prognosis for patients with avitaminosis D is good provided that adequate treatment is instituted and as long as associated skeletal deformities are compatible with life. An initial response is observed in days to weeks, and the alleviation of the bone disease with restoration of normal growth (where the epiphyses are not yet closed) is apparent in weeks to months. Patients who have recovered from avitaminosis D should thereafter be given preventive amounts of vitamin D.

Prevention. Although avitaminosis D can be prevented by exposure to ultraviolet light (from natural or artificial sources), the most practical measure for preventing vitamin D deficiency is the daily administration of 400 IU of the vitamin. Evaporated and dehydrated milk preparations are fortified with vitamin D in amounts calculated to provide this amount of vitamin activity in the reconstituted fluid milk. Breast feeding of infants helps to prevent avitaminosis D. When there is doubt concerning the adequacy in children of the vitamin D intake from natural or fortified food sources, a preventive dose of a vitamin D–containing preparation should be administered (see p. 189). This

may be given as cod-liver oil, high-potency fish-liver oil, fish-liver oil concentrates, calciferol (vitamin D_2), viosterol, or activated 7-dehydrocholesterol (vitamin D_3). In equivalent doses, these preparations have equal efficacy in the human being in preventing rickets, in facilitating growth, and when given in excess, in producing hypercalcemia. Hypervitaminosis D from excessive doses of the vitamin may result from overenthusiastic efforts to provide an abundant nutritional intake in growing children. The calcium intake should be supplemented if the supply from natural sources is not adequate. In adults, as compared with children, the use of supplemental medication containing preventive amounts of vitamin D and calcium usually is not necessary because of the lowered requirements for the vitamin and for calcium, the widespread use of milk and other vitamin D and calcium-containing foods, and the adequate exposure to sunlight. Such supplements are recommended, however, for women during pregnancy and lactation and for some elderly individuals.

Treatment. The measures for treating avitaminosis D in children include (1) administration of 5,000 to 10,000 IU per day of a concentrated vitamin D preparation such as calciferol in cases resulting from "simple" vitamin D lack and 10,000 to 50,000 IU per day in cases associated with gastrointestinal disorders; (2) use of a diet high in calcium and supplemented (if necessary) with calcium gluconate or lactate, so that the total intake is 1.5 to 2.0 Gm calcium per day in cases resulting from "simple" vitamin D lack and 15 Gm calcium per day in cases associated with gastrointestinal diseases; (3) adherence to the daily allowances recommended by the Food and Nutrition Board of the National Research Council (see Table 22-2) for protein, ascorbic acid, B-complex vitamins, and vitamin D in all cases except those associated with insufficient absorption because of gastrointestinal diseases. The latter require a low fat, high protein diet, large amounts of all the fat-soluble vitamins (A, D, E, and K) as well as of ascorbic acid and B-complex vitamins, and special therapy for the gastrointestinal disease; (4) therapy with iron preparations if iron deficiency is present; (5) appropriate orthopedic measures to avoid deformities; and (6) intravenous administration of calcium (a *very slow* drip of 5 to 20 ml 10 per cent calcium gluconate four times a day and repeated as long as necessary) to control tetany or laryngeal spasm if these manifestations are present. In children with rickets associated with gastrointestinal diseases, the administration of small doses of corticoid steroids (50 mg cortisone or equivalent per day) may improve gastrointestinal function and thus increase vitamin and mineral absorption. The treatment of avitaminosis D in adults is essentially the same in principle as that employed in children. The therapeutic measures are discussed in detail elsewhere (see p. 710).

Once the avitaminosis D has been cured, *continuation of vitamin D therapy in large doses not only is unnecessary but may lead to hypervitaminosis D.* The danger point occurs when the plasma alkaline phosphatase level drops to normal and the urinary calcium excretion rises. When these indices appear, the vitamin D intake should be reduced to an amount just sufficient to maintain a normal plasma calcium level.

Results of Treatment. The response of patients with avitaminosis D to treatment is dramatic. With proper doses of vitamin D, attacks of tetany disappear within a few days, the plasma calcium and phosphate concentrations are restored to normal levels within a week to 10 days, and normal growth of ununited epiphyses occurs again within a month. The plasma alkaline phosphatase level usually returns to normal in 2 to 3 months, and at that time no evidence remains of lack of calcification of the endochondral and endosteal osseous tissues. Residual evidences of bone involvement may be found, however, for example, the deformities which cannot be eliminated by orthopedic measures and the bone areas which have become osteosclerotic from excessive compensatory repair.

Vitamin D Resistance

After a period of continuous administration of the vitamin D sterols in the treatment of hypoparathyroidism and in the management of the various forms of "resistant" rickets or, particularly, in the treatment of osteomalacia associated with renal failure or steatorrhea, the patient may become insensitive or "resistant" to the actions of the vitamin even though previously it had been effective in ameliorating the disease. When "resistance" has developed, increasing the dose of the particular sterol usually fails to produce an effect upon the pathologic condition. In this situation, a therapeutic response may be obtained either (1) by stopping the particular agent for a time and then reinstituting therapy with it, or (2) by changing from this agent to another vitamin D sterol (e.g., from vitamin D_2 to dihydrotachysterol).

Hypervitaminosis D

Hypervitaminosis D results from a greatly excessive intake of vitamin D. In adults, vitamin D poisoning has been associated with the ingestion of approximately 100,000 IU or more of vitamin D preparations daily for a prolonged period of time; in infants, with the administration of 20,000 to 40,000 IU of vitamin D per day although early symptoms of toxicity may be apparent at much lower doses (1,800 to 5,000 IU daily). A series of cases of hypercalcemia in infants which occurred in England was attributed to ingestion of vitamin D at levels of some 2,500 IU daily. The syndrome of hypervitaminosis D is similar in infants and adults. The symptoms, all attributable to hypercalcemia, include anorexia, lassitude, constipation, nausea, vomiting, muscular weakness, headache, polyuria, and polydipsia.

Laboratory examinations reveal an increased plasma calcium level, essentially normal plasma alkaline phosphatase values, and mild anemia. Plasma phosphate levels may be high, normal, or low, depending upon the intake of phosphates. The electrocardiogram may show characteristic changes of hypercalcemia, i.e., a shortened Q-T, a depressed S-T segment, and flat to inverted T waves. The biochemical picture is reminiscent of the syndrome of hypophosphatasia (p. 720); it has been suggested by some investigators that the hypophosphatasia syndrome is a disorder resulting from hypersensitivity to vitamin D. Others have proposed that hypersensitivity to vitamin D may be an important factor in the hypercalcemia of sarcoidosis (p. 1246) and of idiopathic hypercalcemia in infancy (p. 607). Renal damage is indicated by proteinuria, the finding of casts on microscopic study, an elevated nonprotein nitrogen, and impaired renal function as measured by the phenolsulfonphthalein and concentration tests. The characteristic x-ray finding is calcification of the periarticular structures. The bones themselves may show osteoporosis. Metastatic calcification of other soft tissues occurs, for example, calcification of the prostate or kidney. In some of the fatal cases, extensive calcification of the inner portion of the media of arteries and of the heart valves has been described. Renal calcification has been reported in the lumen of collecting tubules, in the tubular cells, and in the arterioles.

Because of the widespread misuse of highly potent vitamin D preparations, hypervitaminosis D should be suspected in all cases of hypercalcemia. Careful questioning of the patient should reveal whether massive vitamin D ingestion has occurred. The absence of elevated serum alkaline phosphatase levels is useful in differentiating the condition from the hypercalcemia of hyperparathyroidism. The hypercalcemias associated with multiple myeloma and skeletal neoplasms may be differentiated by the roentgenologic findings, history, and blood chemical findings, including plasma protein changes.

The outcome of the toxicity may be fatal unless administration of vitamin D is interdicted. When administration of vitamin D is stopped, relatively prompt relief of the acute symptoms may be obtained. The correction of the hypercalcemia may be greatly facilitated by the prompt administration of glucocorticoids. A suggested dose schedule is 100 to 200 mg cortisone daily until the plasma calcium is normal (roughly 10 days to 2 weeks). Unless renal damage has become too severe, a gradual fall in nonprotein nitrogen will occur in association with other evidence of improved renal function, as indicated by the phenolsulfonphthalein test and renal concentration tests. In some cases, permanent renal damage may persist.

VITAMIN K

Vitamin K is a lipid-soluble factor necessary for the formation of prothrombin and convertin, or factor VII. Pronounced deficiency results in the familiar bleeding tendency associated with hypo-prothrombinemia. Whether the human being is dependent on a dietary source of this vitamin, which is synthesized by microorganisms of the gastrointestinal tract, has not been determined. Deficiency states are invariably of the conditioned type and result from absorptive defects (biliary obstruction, sprue, fibrocystic disease of the pancreas, intestinal lipodystrophy, or other steatorrheas, or chronic diarrhea). This deficiency is discussed in Chap. 24 and under the associated conditioning diseases.

REFERENCES

Adlersberg, D., H. Sobotka, and B. Bogatin: Effect of Liver Disease on Vitamin A Metabolism, Gastroenterol., 4:164, 1945.

Aykroyd, W. R., et al.: Hypovitaminosis A, Federation Proc., 17: Suppl. 2, 103, 1958.

Bagchi, K., K. Halder, and S. R. Chowdhury: The Etiology of Phrynoderma, Am. J. Clin. Nutrition, 7:251, 1959.

Blegvad, O.: Xerophthalmia, Keratomalacia, and Xerosis Conjunctivae, Am. J. Ophthalmol., 7:89, 1924.

Clausen, S. W.: The Absorption of Vitamin A and Its Storage in the Tissues, Harvey Lectures, 38:199, 1942–1943.

Danowki, T. S., A. W. Winkler, and J. P. Peters: Tissue Calcification and Renal Failure Produced by Massive Dose Vitamin D Therapy of Arthritis, Ann. Internal Med., 23:22, 1945.

Donegan, C. K., A. L. Messer, and E. S. Orgain: Vitamin D Intoxication Due to Ertron: Report of Two Cases, Ann. Internal Med., 30:429, 1949.

Frazier, C. N., and C. K. Hu: Cutaneous Lesions Associated with a Deficiency in Vitamin A in Man, Arch. Internal Med., 48:507, 1931; Arch. Dermatol. Syphilol., 33:825, 1936.

Gopalan, C.: The Aetiology of "Phrynoderma," Indian Med. Gaz., 82:16, 1947.

Isler, O., and O. Wiss: Chemistry and Biochemistry of the K Vitamins, Vitamins and Hormones, 17:53, 1959.

Jeghers, H., and H. Marraro: Hypervitaminosis A: Its Broadening Spectrum, Am. J. Clin. Nutrition, 6: 335, 1958.

Mellanby, Sir Edward: "A Story of Nutritional Research," Baltimore, The Williams & Wilkins Company, 1950.

Oomen, H. A. P. C.: Xerophthalmia in the Presence of Kwashiorkor, Brit. J. Nutrition, 8:307, 1954.

Spence, J. C.: A Clinical Study of Nutritional Xerophthalmia and Night Blindness, Arch. Disease Childhood, 6:17, 1931.

Vitamin A Sub-Committee of the Accessory Food Factors Committee: "Vitamin A Requirements of Human Adults: An Experimental Study of Vitamin A Deprivation in Man," Medical Research Council, Special Report Series, No. 264, London, His Majesty's Stationery Office, 1949.

62 SPRUE AND OTHER MALABSORPTION SYNDROMES

Frank H. Gardner

Definition. Sprue is an inclusive term applied to a malabsorption syndrome characterized by impaired absorption of foods, minerals, and water by the small bowel. The majority of the clinical symptoms are a reflection of nutritional deficiencies which result from impaired absorption or from altered intestinal activity.

Classification. The early clinical observations of recurrent diarrhea among Europeans living in tropical areas of the Far East initiated interest in malabsorption of the small bowel. This disorder was called tropical sprue. For many years the disease was thought to be limited to hot, humid climates. However, in 1932, Thaysen aroused interest in such a malabsorption syndrome in the Temperate Zone, and thus the term *nontropical sprue* was introduced. During the last few decades, clinical observations have emphasized the similarity of the gastrointestinal dysfunction in children with celiac disease and that seen in sprue, and it is now recognized that numerous adult patients with nontropical sprue represent the continuing manifestations of the childhood disorder.

For convenience, sprue may be classified as *acute* or *chronic*. The acute form may be self-limited and is observed only in tropical climates. Most cases of nontropical sprue are observed during a chronic phase of the disease. The adult form of celiac disease is considered to be a chronic form of nontropical sprue.

The secondary forms of sprue listed in Table 62-1 represent a wide range of malabsorption states. Patients with intrinsic bowel wall disease or obstruction of lymphatics are rarely seen. More frequently, surgical alterations of the stomach (sub-

Table 62-1. CLASSIFICATION OF SPRUE

Primary sprue	*Secondary sprue*

Primary sprue

1. *Acute:* May be self-limited; usually observed in tropical climate
2. *Chronic*
   a. Tropical sprue
   b. Nontropical sprue
   c. Adult celiac disease

Secondary sprue

1. *Intrinsic bowel wall alterations*
   a. Intestinal tuberculosis
   b. Regional enteritis
   c. Amyloid disease
   d. Lymphoma
2. *Obstruction of intestinal lymphatics*
   a. Intestinal lipodystrophy (Whipple's disease)
   b. Lymphoma
3. *Anatomic alterations*
   a. Diverticula of jejunum and ileum
   b. Enteroenteric fistula
   c. Postgastrectomy syndrome

total gastrectomy) and blind loops ("bypass" surgery of the ileum) cause impaired absorption.

Etiology. *Primary Sprue.* The cause of tropical sprue is not known. Efforts have been made in the past to associate the disorder with various bacteria or an imbalance of the bacterial flora of the bowel. However, no proposed cause has withstood critical evaluation. It may be of significance, nevertheless, that despite failure to isolate a specific bacterial agent tropical sprue has responded to sulfonamide (sulfaguanidine) and antibiotic (chloramphenicol and tetracyclines) therapy. In the presence of generalized malnutrition and dietary deficiencies, folic acid has been cited as a specific nutritional defect in tropical sprue in areas where malnutrition is common. However, by the methodology available, a systemic folic acid depletion has not been observed in such cases. It is difficult to explain why so few cases of tropical sprue are observed in the geographic areas where nutritional deficits are widespread. It is noteworthy that the symptoms of sprue may develop after 1 or 2 months' residence in tropical areas where the disease is endemic, or they may appear years later after return to nontropical areas. Such observations should encourage further investigations of infectious agents. The infrequency of sprue in Africa as compared to that in the Far East may reflect racial, dietary, and constitutional factors.

NONTROPICAL SPRUE (ADULT CELIAC DISEASE). Studies in Holland and England have demonstrated that most children with celiac disease respond dramatically when wheat, barley, and rye flour are excluded from the diet. Similar results have been observed in the majority of adult patients with nontropical sprue, especially if dietary

control is rigid and is followed for at least 6 months. More specifically, the offending agent appears to reside in the protein fraction of the flour (gluten). The exact mechanism by which gluten may interfere with absorption by the small bowel mucosa is not known. Two widely held views favor an antibody immune response or an enzymatic defect in the epithelium. The possibility cannot be excluded that other nutritional agents may act in a fashion similar to that of gluten.

Secondary Sprue. The invasion of the bowel epithelium or submucosal area by tumor (lymphoma) or the development of lymphatic obstruction (Whipple's disease) impairs absorption or transport of foodstuffs. Diverticula or blind loops allow stagnation of chyme, with resultant profuse bacterial overgrowth. It has been suggested that the competitive demands of such bacterial flora could utilize vitamins and nutrients or that the metabolic products of the bacteria could irritate the bowel mucosa (jejunitis). Normally, there is no resident bacterial population in the small bowel as far down as the terminal ileum.

Alterations in motility of the small bowel produced by the absence of pylorus (subtotal gastrectomy) or the ileocecal valve (ileocolostomy) decrease transit time and lessen absorption. Inadequate mixing of stomach contents with pancreatic enzymes probably is the most important defect to account for malabsorption after subtotal gastrectomy.

Pathologic Findings. Observations are scanty concerning morphologic changes in the acute phase of primary sprue. However, biopsy material obtained from the jejunum within 2 months after the onset of symptoms has revealed alterations similar to the changes described for the more chronic forms of primary sprue. Although repeated observations are not available, one assumes that the alterations are reversible or that compensatory changes allow normal bowel function since this phase responds quickly to therapy. In all types of chronic sprue, the mucosal changes are more frequent in the jejunum than in the ileum. Jejunal biopsy specimens show short, blunted villi, and the width of the crypts of Lieberkühn is increased. These changes are associated with abnormal columnar cells and cellular infiltration of the lamina propria (Fig. 62-1). The enzyme functions of the columnar cells in patients with nontropical sprue have been shown by histochemical measurements to be altered. The microvilli (brush border) are sparse, blunted, and fused. Similarly, the mitochondria are enlarged and vacuolated, in contrast to those of the normal columnar cell. These mitochondrial changes have also been observed in tropical sprue, but the microvilli have not been found to be as distorted. The shortened villi and decreased abnormal microvilli re-

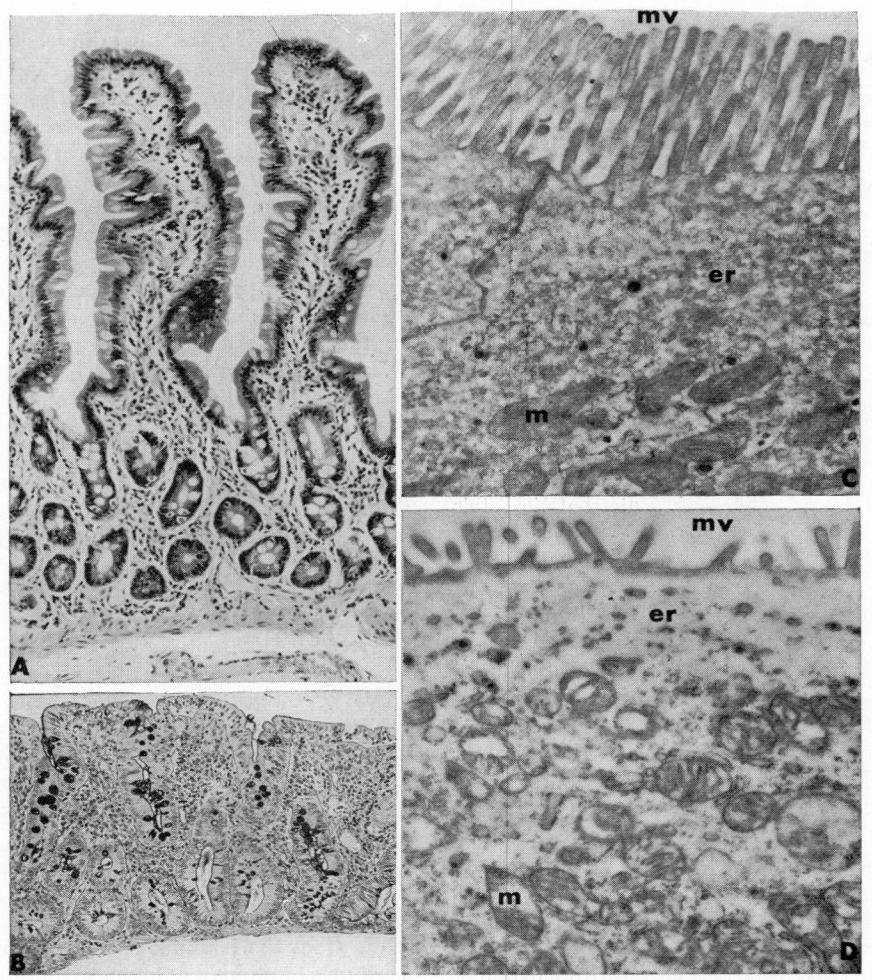

FIG. 62-1. A. Biopsy specimen of normal jejunum. The villi are prominent, slender, erect, and the columnar cells are arranged in an orderly palisade. (H and E approximately ×100.)

B. Biopsy specimen of jejunum in nontropical sprue. Villi are virtually absent; when present they are severely blunted. The epithelial surface is diminished considerably, whereas, proportionately, the area of the crypts of Lieberkuhn appears to be increased. (P.A.S. and H. approximately ×100.)

C. Electronmicrograph of a portion of a normal jejunal columnar villous cell. A distinct border of microvilli (mv) faces the intestinal lumen. Under this border is a region of five cytoplasmic tubules of the endoplasmic reticulum (er), beneath which are an abundance of normal-appearing mitochondria (m). (Approximately ×20,000.)

D. Electronmicrograph of a portion of an absorptive columnar cell of jejunum in nontropical sprue. The microvilli (mv) are shorter, fewer, and relatively irregular (in many samples, they appear normal). The cytoplasmic tubules of the endosplasmic reticulum (er) appear to be reduced in number and compactness. Mitochondria (m) exhibit abnormalities of form and internal structure. Histochemically, these mitochondria show a deficiency in succinic dehydrogenese. (Approximately ×20,000.) (*Kindly prepared by Dr. John J. Ladman.*)

flect a major loss of the bowel absorptive area. These morphologic alterations are found in the absence of starvation and may be observed in patients manifesting a clinical remission of their disease. Treatment of tropical sprue with folic acid and vitamin B_{12} has not reversed mucosal changes, but the prolonged use of a gluten-free diet in non-tropical sprue has been associated with villous alterations toward the normal pattern. Instillation of wheat flour into the ileum of patients with non-tropical sprue when there are minimal epithelial changes causes mucosal alterations of the villi like those described above within a few days and is associated with the onset of diarrhea. Degeneration of the myenteric and submucosal plexus, with vacuolization and neurolysis, has also been noted in the small intestine. Such neurogenic changes may contribute to motor dysfunction and defective propulsive activity of the bowel.

Secondary sprue disorders usually do not involve the epithelium. In instances of diverticula or fistula, the bacteria may cause an inflammatory reaction (jejunitis) with cellular infiltration of the lamina propria. Such changes are reversible when the bacterial contamination is removed.

The availability of small bowel (jejunal) biopsy specimens by the use of various intraluminal instruments passed into the bowel by mouth has allowed a more definitive diagnosis of the bowel lesion. For complete understanding of these disorders, microscopic study of the mucosa should be done to facilitate classification and therapy.

With prolonged folic acid and vitamin B_{12} depletion, there is megaloblastic erythroid hyperplasia of the bone marrow. In early descriptions of sprue, aplastic fatty marrow was reported in untreated patients as a terminal manifestation in the cachectic patient, and depleted fat depots and marked atrophy of the liver and spleen were described. At the present time such degrees of malnutrition are not seen, and death is rarely attributable to malabsorption.

Physiology. The term *idiopathic steatorrhea* has been applied by many to the malabsorption syndromes since the impaired absorption of fats alters the character of the feces in a striking fashion. However, the morphologic changes of the mucosa in reality impair absorption of all foodstuffs. In primary sprue, usually fat intolerance is observed early in the disorder, and more extensive deficiencies of absorption appear later. It is not known whether the impaired absorption by the small bowel represents a primary alteration of intracellular enzymatic function or a mucosal response with changes in secretion that impair absorption. Alterations in the mucoprotein secretion and increased viscosity of the succus entericus have been demonstrated. These changes may reflect a mucous barrier overlying the epithelial surface which prevents absorption. Increased leakage of plasma proteins into the bowel lumen has been observed in nontropical sprue as well as regional enteritis. This transudation is the major mechanism accounting for the decreased plasma protein levels (hypercatabolic hypoproteinemia) and increased fecal nitrogen wastage. The immense loss of bowel wall epithelial area caused by blunted villi and poor propulsive motor activity are the major alterations that impair absorption.

Analysis of the duodenal secretions reveals normal values for pancreatic enzymes and bile salts. In the jejunum there is adequate emulsification of fats and digestion of proteins. No defective function of the succus entericus has been described. It appears that food products are prepared properly for absorption by the digestive ferments but are unable to pass through the abnormal small bowel mucosa. Malabsorption of fats related to pancreatic insufficiency, however, does allow normal absorption of other substances noted below. Ulcerogenic tumors of the pancreas (Zollinger-Ellison syndrome) often are associated with pancreatic steatorrhea because the hypersecretion of stomach acidity inactivates the pancreatic enzymes in the duodenal juice.

Decreased absorption of simple molecular substances (D_2O, KI^{131}, Fe^{59}, SO_4, and $Na^{29}Cl$) may be detected with isotope labeling procedures. The absorption of more complex foodstuffs such as fats, amino acids, sugars, and vitamins can be measured by dietary balance studies. Not all substances are associated with the same degree of impaired transfer across the mucosa. The presence of an abnormal bacterial flora in diverticula and blind loops is especially prone to impair absorption of vitamin B_{12}. This defect is noted when there is ileal involvement (regional enteritis) since, in human beings, vitamin B_{12} absorption is restricted to this area of the bowel. The abnormal mucosa also impairs the reabsorption of the vitamin B_{12} and cholesterol which are excreted in the bile.

Impaired absorption of vitamin K often produces hypoprothrombinemia. Secondary physiologic alterations are associated with deficiency of electrolytes. Hypomotility of the small bowel may be enhanced by hypopotassemia. Hypocalcemia and demineralization of the skeleton are observed with the negative calcium balance occurring in sprue, both primary and secondary.

Clinical Picture. The syndromes in primary and secondary sprue are characterized in most instances by a slow insidious onset. A history of intermittent diarrhea for months or years may be elicited. Some patients may have a normal stool habit, but the volume is great. About one-third of the patients with nontropical sprue have a past history of intestinal disorders in infancy or childhood. During the episodes of diarrhea, the stools may be mushy, light-colored, frothy, foul smelling, and associated with explosive flatus. At the onset, the diarrhea may be limited to two or three bulky stools in the morning without additional stools during the day. Intermittent constipation often is present between bouts of diarrhea. Associated with the diarrhea there is severe lassitude and fatigue, possibly because of excessive loss of electrolytes in the feces. Moderate to severe weight loss is noted in all patients, depending on the duration of the disorder. Often patients become accustomed to an altered bowel habit and do not seek medical advice until secondary deficiencies become prominent. Severe emotional or physical stress may convert intermittent diarrhea to a constant condition, which in turn is associated with more generalized clinical manifestations of other deficiencies. When there is more active diarrhea, nausea and vomiting may be noted as well as epigastric pain. In rare instances, the abdominal distress may simulate intestinal obstruction. Progressive abdominal distention during the day, which disappears at night, is a frequent observation. A nocturnal diuresis often is observed in the adult patient with nontropical sprue, and such a symptom may be helpful to orient the physician to a more detailed study of the bowel.

As malabsorption becomes chronic, clinical signs and symptoms of nutritional deficiencies develop. Muscle cramps occur at some time in all patients, while a few may have tetany. Hypoprothrombinemia is associated with widespread hemorrhagic lesions. Glossitis is seen at some time in all patients with chronic malabsorption. The lesions may be limited to mild atrophic changes at the tip of the tongue or may be associated with widespread denudation of the papillary surface, with numerous small aphthous lesions. Tongue changes may appear within a few days but cannot be distinguished from those of other states of nutritional deficiency. With severe glossitis dysphagia contributes to further weight loss. Progression of secondary deficiencies results in inadequate reserves of iron, folic acid, and vitamin B_{12}. All the symptoms of anemia may therefore be present. Clubbing of the fingers and toes rarely may be seen. Edema and ascites may result from hypoproteinemia and anemia. Fractures, especially of the long bones, are associated with osteomalacia. Hypocalcemia with tetany is seen in nontropical sprue but is rare in tropical sprue, possibly because of the greater exposure to sunlight in the latter.

Laboratory Findings. Stools are not consistently altered; in mild cases their appearance may be normal. In more severe disease the stools are light tan (almost acholic in appearance), frothy, greasy, foul smelling, and tend to float on water. These changes are associated primarily with the content of fat and will not be detected if the patient has avoided fat. Fat particles and fatty acid crystals may be detected by microscopic examination of the stool.

EXAMINATION FOR FAT. A small 5-mm sample of stool is emulsified with a few drops of water and an aliquot placed on two glass slides. To the first slide is added two drops of 95 per cent ethanol followed by three drops of a saturated 95 per cent ethanol solution of Sudan III. A cover slip is applied, and the preparation is examined microscopically for yellow, pale orange refractile globules of fat with a high dry lens ($430\times$). The edge of the cover slip should be examined especially carefully.

These globules represent neutral fat and may be seen in patients with pancreatic insufficiency or following the ingestion of oily laxatives. The majority of patients with steatorrhea have adequate lipolytic enzymes to break down fat to fatty acids.

EXAMINATION FOR FATTY ACIDS. On the second prepared slide, the aliquot of stool is mixed with three drops of 36 per cent acetic acid followed by three drops of the saturated solution of Sudan III. A cover slip is applied after mixing, and the slide is heated gently over a low flame until bubbling is noted under the cover slip. The heating allows hydrolysis of the fatty acid in the presence of acetic acid. After cooling, the slide is examined as noted above. With cooling, the fatty acids may crystallize as colorless, needlelike sheaves.

The normal stool usually contains as many as 100 globules of fatty acid per high dry field, usually less than 4 μ in diameter. With increased fatty acids the globules are larger, varying from 10 to 75 μ in diameter, and the relationship to fecal material in the background varies with the degree of steatorrhea. With profound steatorrhea only fatty acid globules may be observed. These fecal examinations are of no value without adequate fat intake in the diet (more than 60 Gm daily). The examiner must train his visual interpretation by repeated examinations of normal stools.

The bulk is increased (normal 100 to 200 ml; sprue 500 to 1,000 ml) and reflects increased liquid volume. No consistent bacterial flora are observed, although the absolute number of bacteria is increased, probably reflecting the utilization of unabsorbed nutrients from the small bowel.

Absorption Studies. Dietary balance studies reveal increased fecal loss of nitrogen and fats. Normal subjects excrete 5 Gm or less of fecal fat when consuming the average 50 to 100 Gm daily of dietary fats. Usually, in severe malabsorption 15 to 30 Gm or more of fat will be excreted daily. In most instances 6- to 12-day serial determinations are needed for careful evaluation, inasmuch as wide fluctuations in daily excretion occur.

The chronic deficiency state is reflected in low fasting serum levels of neutral fats, cholesterol, phospholipids, vitamin A, carotene, vitamin B_{12}, folic acid, vitamin C, iron, copper, total proteins, calcium, potassium, and prothrombin. However, the various nutritional components are not depressed uniformly in a particular patient. The fasting carotene and vitamin A levels have been the most useful laboratory measurements. Serum mucoprotein levels are elevated in malabsorption states associated with mucosal invasion (primary sprue, Whipple's disease and regional enteritis).

A variety of "tolerance" tests has been used to evaluate impaired bowel function. The absorption of glucose has been measured most frequently.

About one-third of normal subjects have a "flat tolerance curve," however, making the test of doubtful value. Two screening procedures can be used with ease to estimate sugar and fat absorption.

Absorption of D-Xylose. The fasting patient ingests 25 Gm of D-xylose with several glasses of water. The urine is collected for a 5-hr period thereafter, and the amount of the pentose excreted is determined (normal persons excrete 5 to 8 Gm; sprue patients excrete 3 Gm or less).

Postprandial Lipemia. Lipemia curves can be standardized by semiquantitative measurements of serum optical density (O.D.) changes. The fasting patient receives a standardized breakfast meal of 30 Gm of butter, two slices of bread with jelly, 100 ml of fruit juice, and sweetened tea or coffee. A fasting serum sample as well as collections at 2, 3, 4 and 5 hr is measured in a colorimeter at 540 $m\mu$ for optical density changes with the fasting sample as a control. The normal subject has a peak lipemia in the second to fourth hour, with an optical density above 0.1. The sprue patient usually has values below 0.05 and gives no evidence of a postprandial lipemia in this short interval. Other tolerance tests are more difficult to perform and add little diagnostic information.

Hematology. About two-thirds of the patients with primary sprue demonstrate mild to severe macrocytic anemia. Morphologic changes of the peripheral blood and bone marrow are indistinguishable from those of Addisonian pernicious anemia. With impaired iron absorption, the anemia may be normocytic or hypochromic. At that time a double red cell population may be present; such changes are referred to as *dimorphic* anemia. Urinary and fecal excretion studies of folic acid, Fe^{59} salts, and Co^{60} vitamin B_{12} have demonstrated impaired absorption of these erythropoietic agents. Diverticula and blind loops, especially, show impaired absorption of vitamin B_{12}, possibly by competitive bacterial utilization of the vitamin or binding of intrinsic factor.

Roentgenologic Observations. Ingestion of a barium sulfate suspension normally reveals a fine feathery pattern of the jejunal and ileal mucosa. In cases of primary sprue, segmentation and clumping of the barium meal and emphasis of the haustral marking are found instead (Fig. 62-2). Such "puddling" of the barium meal may be absent in the early phase of the disorder, but in chronic disease some alterations of the bowel pattern are always observed. The flocculation of the barium suspension has been attributed to excess mucus in the small bowel, but aspiration studies have not demonstrated increased secretion. Transit time of the barium meal is delayed in the small bowel. Dilatation of the colon may be noted. Secondary sprue associated with intrinsic bowel wall alterations or

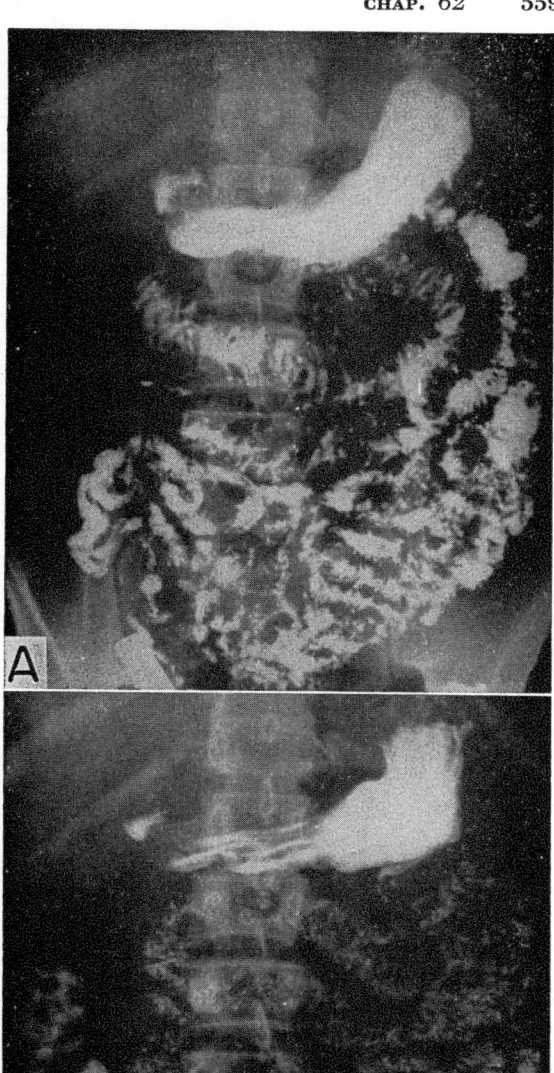

FIG. 62-2. *A.* Small bowel x-ray studies in tropical sprue. The barium suspension is segmented (puddled) in the small bowel. *B.* Tropical sprue (same patient) during folic acid therapy. A normal feathery appearance is observed throughout the jejunum and upper ileum.

obstruction of lymphatics shows a similar pattern with the barium suspension. Radiologic examination is the only method by which anatomic lesions (blind loops, diverticula, fistulas) can be detected and separated from primary sprue. While absorption tests may be similar, the x-ray studies and biopsy specimens of small bowel are necessary for complete classification. With prolonged impaired calcium absorption, demineralization of the skeleton is seen and alteration in the growth of the long bones may be noted if the adult patient represents a recrudescence of a childhood celiac disease.

The general appearance of these patients, as well as the association of weight loss, anemia, and weakness, has often suggested the diagnosis of postpubertal panhypopituitarism. However, endocrine functions are normal as measured by the response of target glands to pituitary hormones.

Treatment. The acute primary sprue seen in the tropics responds well to numerous forms of treatment. Bland diets (milk, bananas, liver soups, and puréed meats) have been successful. Physical and emotional rest in the acute phase of the disease hasten recovery. Oral folic acid (5 mg twice daily) appears to be the most efficacious therapy for acute and chronic tropical sprue. Such treatment relieves lassitude, diarrhea, and weight loss even in the absence of anemia or clinical evidence of secondary nutritional deficiencies. Maintenance therapy of 5 mg daily should be given for a 4- to 6-month period. Return to temperate zones usually is associated with remission of the disorder. Tropical sprue does not respond to elimination of wheat gluten from the diet. Some patients have responded to sulfonamides and antibiotics (chloramphenicol), an observation which suggests that overgrowth of bacterial flora may be a contributing feature of the illness. Possibly the success of various dietary programs is attributable to the alteration of bacterial growth which is associated with a high protein diet. The secondary nutritional deficiencies and megaloblastic anemia likewise respond to folic acid. Usually, oral or parenteral iron salts are necessary for a complete hematologic remission. However, some patients continue to manifest some degree of impaired absorption of all foodstuffs. In such instances dietary limitation of fats and starches may be necessary for control of intermittent diarrhea. Parenteral vitamin B_{12} likewise has been successful in amelioration of anemia, but the ease of oral folic acid administration for patient care has made it the treatment of choice.

Adults with celiac disease (nontropical sprue) must be given a gluten-free diet. The patient may use any food that does not contain wheat, barley, or rye gluten. The absorption defect is altered slowly, and the dietary restriction must be continued for at least 6 months before the physician can conclude that it is not helpful. Such patients need folic acid, vitamin B_{12}, and other vitamins only if anemia and nutritional deficiencies are pres-

ent. The use of vitamins and hematinics may correct anemia and initiate clinical improvement, but this is not comparable to the more spectacular responses noted in tropical sprue. One may anticipate that the majority of patients with chronic sprue in nontropical areas have adult celiac disease. In the absence of a childhood history of intestinal complaints, a gluten-free diet may be tried empirically. Instructions for careful dietary restriction of fats and starches should be given and a high protein diet provided. In patients with malnutrition, therapy may be initiated with adrenocortical hormones (cortisone acetate or prednisone at dosage levels of 200 mg and 40 mg, respectively), but prolonged therapy is not advised. Hormonal therapy is dramatic, with improved absorption and relief of diarrhea noted in 2 to 3 days. Some patients have been given corticosteroids when the gluten-free diet is started, anticipating that the hormone therapy will be discontinued in 4 to 8 weeks. If the drug is used alone, most patients require 50 to 75 mg cortisone acetate or 10 to 15 mg prednisone daily to control bowel symptoms. Improved absorption of foodstuffs is noted within 1 week and is maintained for the duration of hormone therapy. Initially, corticosteroids often accentuate tetany (possibly by increased fecal calcium loss), and oral calcium salts should be given. Tetany from hypocalcemia can be controlled rapidly with intravenous 10 per cent calcium gluconate. Special attention to electrolyte replacement, especially potassium salts, is of great importance in the relief of lassitude and weakness. Usually potassium chloride is given in amounts of 2 to 3 Gm daily. Hemorrhagic complications (hypoprothrombinemia) respond to intramuscular menadione (10 mg daily).

Secondary sprue associated with specific defects in the small bowel can be treated only after recognition of the cause. Diverticula, intestinal strictures, and blind loops may improve dramatically with antibacterial therapy. However, relapse follows when the bacterial flora is allowed to regrow. Antibacterial therapy is a helpful adjunct to prepare the patient for surgical correction of the anatomic defect. Jejunal biopsies are helpful to plan proper chemotherapy for lymphosarcoma and Hodgkin's disease. Intestinal lipodystrophy may respond to adrenocortical hormones, but further experience has emphasized that the results are not so promising as initially claimed. Some patients have had partial or complete remissions with antibiotic (chloramphenicol, tetracyclines) treatment without an adequate explanation for the response.

The treatment of the postgastrectomy patient has been difficult. Weight gain has been associated with (1) frequent small feedings to assure adequate pancreatic secretions from the proximal loop of the anastomosis, (2) addition of pancreatin to the diet,

(3) androgens for their anabolic effects. In many patients, the malabsorption defect lessens over a period of years. These patients absorb iron poorly, and an iron deficiency anemia is observed frequently within 5 years after surgery. Symptoms of the "dumping syndrome" may be associated with hypoferremia and are relieved in part by parenteral iron therapy.

Prognosis. Diagnostic procedures are now available to define the various types of malabsorption. With such information, therapy can be planned with anticipation of improved bowel function. Information is still sparse regarding the mechanisms of absorption across the bowel mucosa. The accumulated evidence relating nontropical sprue to a similar defect found in celiac disease has emphasized the long duration (lifetime) and points to a probable epithelial enzyme deficiency. Additional studies are needed to determine if the bowel manifestations in primary sprue are related to systemic metabolic abnormalities.

REFERENCES

Castle, W. B., C. P. Rhoads, H. A. Lawson, and G. C. Payne: Etiology and Treatment of Sprue; Observations on Patients in Puerto Rico and Subsequent Experiments on Animals, Arch. Internal Med., 56:627, 1935.

Crosby, W. H. (Ed.): Tropical Sprue: Studies of the U.S. Army's Sprue Team in Puerto Rico, U.S. Walter Reed Army Institute of Research, Med. Sci. Pub. No. 5, 1959.

Drummey, G. D., J. A. Benson, Jr., and C. M. Jones: Microscopical Examination of the Stool for Steatorrhea, New Engl. J. Med., 264:85, 1961.

French, J. M., C. F. Hawkins, and N. Smith: The Effect of a Wheat-gluten-free Diet in Adult Idiopathic Steatorrhoea, Quart. J. Med., 26:481, 1957.

Gardner, F. H., and E. W. Strauss: Disorders Related to Disturbed Absorption of the Small Bowel, Advances Internal Med., 10:137, 1960.

Thaysen, Th. E. H.: "Non-Tropical Sprue: A Study in Idiopathic Steatorrhoea," Copenhagen and London, Levin & Munksgaard, 1932.

Section 2: Hormonal Disturbances

63 GENERAL CONSIDERATIONS
George W. Thorn

Isolation, purification, identification, and synthesis of new hormones continue to proceed at a rapid rate, and it is reasonable to assume that within the near future those few remaining unidentified principles will also succumb to the technical advances of chemistry and biophysics. Noteworthy among recorded achievements are the determination of the structure and amino acid sequence of adrenocorticotropin, melanocyte-stimulating hormone, and insulin, the synthesis of posterior pituitary hormone and a host of adrenal and gonadal steroid hormones, and the identification and isolation of several new thyroid substances. Coupled with these chemical advances there has also occurred a rapidly expanding body of knowledge concerning the regulation of hormonal secretion and the precise locus of hormonal action. Although this latter field has barely been opened, the effect of insulin on cell permeability to certain sugars, the mechanism whereby estrogens provide energy for the growth of their target organs, and the physical modification of mitochondrial particles by thyroxin illustrate the type of information which rapidly is becoming available.

It is now generally agreed that hormones do not initiate new events in the complicated biochemistry of metabolic processes, but rather produce their effects by regulating enzymatic and other chemical reactions already present. In view of the relatively large number of hormones, their diverse chemical structures, and their multiple sites of action, it can be assumed that scarcely a single important metabolic event can escape the effect of their primary or secondary action. From this one may conclude that a true understanding of any disease process or physiologic disorder must encompass an appreciation of the possible etiologic role of hormones and the factors which regulate their synthesis, release, and degradation. In this regard, one can point to such widely diverse actions as the effect of catechol amines (adrenal medulla) on brain metabolism and psychologic behavior, the effect of adrenal steroids on the inflammatory reaction associated with infection, trauma, surgery, or burns, the effect of insulin on adipose tissue metabolism, and the importance of growth hormone on the fabrication of body proteins.

Primary endocrine disorders may mimic the clinical picture of epilepsy as a consequence of hypoglycemia (insulinoma, hypopituitarism, or adrenal cortical insufficiency); primary neuromyopathy because of hypo- or hyperpotassemia due to an excess or deficiency of hydrocortisone or aldosterone; primary visual difficulty as a consequence of diabetic retinopathy or optic nerve compression from a pituitary tumor; a fracture in which the important etiological factor is an unrecognized generalized osteoporosis (hyperparathyroidism, hyperthyroidism, or Cushing's syndrome); heart disease in which fatigue and cardiac irregularity are due primarily to hyperthyroidism; hypertension resulting from a functioning pheochromocytoma or aldosteroma, unregulated diabetes mellitus with nephropathy, and renal disease secondary to hypercalcemia and hypercalcuria (hyperparathyroidism); or psychologic disturbances requiring institutionalization as a consequence of undetected abnormal adrenal (medullary as well as cortical), thyroid, or parathyroid secretion.

In addition to the wide spectrum of syndromes presented by patients with primary endocrinopathies, one must be cognizant of the importance of secondary abnormalities in hormonal secretion or metabolism in nonendocrine disease, for example, the detrimental influence of secondary hyperaldosteronism in edema of cardiac, hepatic, or renal origin; of estrogenic hormones on the course of certain breast tumors; of androgens on prostatic cancer; of secondary hyperparathyroidism in late stage renal disease and the accentuation of gastric secretion and peptic ulcer with cyclical increase in corticosteroid secretion. In many of the foregoing situations, correction of the secondary endocrine abnormality may offer an important and practical approach to clinical improvement.

MECHANISMS FOR ENDOCRINOPATHIES

1. Increased or decreased liberation of normal hormones
2. Secretion of abnormal hormones
3. Aberrations in hormone conjugation and degradation
4. Abnormalities inherent in local tissue responsiveness
5. Continued, rather than cyclical, elaboration of hormones

Characteristically, endocrine abnormalities arise as a consequence of increased or decreased hormone secretion. In the majority of patients, the clinical manifestations derive from an excess of or deficiency of the *normally* secreted hormone. However, in certain syndromes, such as some cases of adrenal virilism, the endocrinopathy may result from the secretion of an abnormal hormone. In addition, hormonal disorders may result from aberrations in the metabolism or degradation of hormones. For example, a deficiency of plasma proteins may decrease the quantity of hormone-carrying protein in the blood and hence modify significantly the balance between "free" and "bound" thyroid hormone; liver disease may alter the conjugation or degradation of steroid hormones, giving rise to abnormal blood and tissue hormone levels. In such types of abnormalities, however, serious endocrine disorders will result only if the "servo-regulating" mechanism or "feedback" response fails to stimulate the appropriate reaction in the target gland. Endocrine abnormalities may also develop as a consequence of inability of local tissues to respond to a normal hormonal level. For example, localized myxedema over the tibia may occur in the presence of thyrotoxicosis or euthyroidism; in cases of pseudohypoparathyroidism, the abnormalities observed in hypoparathyroidism occur despite the presence of normal parathyroid glands. In some endocrinopathies, a heightened tissue susceptibility to hormone action is the determining factor in the genesis of the syndrome, for example, hirsutism in young women with a minimal abnormality in androgenic steroid secretion, Cushing's syndrome with cortical hyperplasia, or extreme degrees of hyperpigmentation as observed in patients with early adrenal insufficiency and increased melanin pigmentation on a racial basis.

Hormonal secretions in general show wide fluctuations throughout the 24-hr period, periods of high activity often alternating with those of reduced secretion, for example, the early morning high level of adrenal cortical secretory activity. Evidence is accumulating that endocrinopathy may result not only from a total daily increase in over-all secretion but also from a loss of cyclical diurnal pattern due to a more or less constant hormonal elaboration throughout the day and night, resulting in only a slight increase, if any, in total secretion. Two important considerations have been derived from these observations: (1) Interpretation of single determinations of hormone content—of blood, tissues, or urine—reflecting instantaneous or relatively short collection periods may be unreliable; for final evaluation, repeated determinations, longer collection periods, or isotopic "turnover" studies may be required. (2) Clinical application of the cyclic method of hormone administration has been quite successful in minimizing undesirable hormone side effects while maintaining control of the underlying disease process.

The suspicion that an endocrine abnormality may play a role in a patient's illness will often derive initially from the gross physical appearance of the patient as in myxedema, hyperthyroidism, pituitary dwarfism or gigantism, acromegaly, hypogonadism, carotenemia (diabetes mellitus or hypothyroidism), Addison's disease, Cushing's syndrome, and the adrenogenital syndrome. Although a careful history and physical examination will in most instances provide presumptive evidence of an underlying endocrine disorder, the definitive diagnosis will almost invariably depend upon the values obtained from laboratory examinations. Here, accuracy in diagnosis will depend upon the specificity of the laboratory test, its precision and its reproducibility, the care and understanding with which specimens are collected, and the reliability of the laboratory which carries out the procedures. In the past, endocrine abnormalities were established for the most part on the basis of nonspecific laboratory examinations such as the basal metabolic rate, roentgenograms, glucose tolerance test, and blood sugar, calcium, sodium, and potassium determinations. Today, tests of endocrine dysfunction are employing more and more frequently measurement of the specific hormones under consideration, for example, protein bound iodine level, blood and urinary steroid values, urinary gonadotropins, and blood ACTH or insulin levels. It is essential for the practicing physician to realize, however, that a single determination of a specific hormone (in blood, urine, or tissue) does not necessarily establish or exclude an endocrine abnormality. The addition of hormonal "turnover" or "secretory" measurements by means of isotopic techniques represents a great step forward. The use of stressful situations or specific substances such as ACTH (adrenocorticotropin) for the adrenal, thyroid-stimulating hormone (TSH) for the thyroid, and glucose for the detection of early diabetes permits one to test the functional reserve of these endocrine systems and thereby facilitates the diagnosis of potential endocrine deficiency at a time when prophylactic measures may prove effective. In the succeeding chapters, particular attention will be devoted to indicating the usefulness and limitations of diagnostic methods and the degree of specificity which may be attached to the procedure. Because of its great practical importance, the source of common errors related to these determinations will also be emphasized.

With the general use of the corticosteroids, thyroid, and the sex hormones as nonspecific therapeutic agents, new and difficult problems present themselves to the internist and endocrinologist. One may be faced on the one hand with iatrogenic Cushing's syndrome, hyperthyroidism, or virilism— or severe adrenal insufficiency or hypothyroidism if hormone therapy is discontinued rapidly or completely. The special problems relating to these phenomena as they present themselves in general practice will, because of their seriousness, be discussed at length in relation to each of the specific hormones so implicated. The use of hormones as nonspecific therapeutic agents, while offering great promise in many serious and often fatal diseases, is fraught with difficulties and requires, in addition to a thorough knowledge of the endocrine preparations, a comprehension of their physiologic and pharmacologic effects, the exercise of sound judgment on the part of the physician, and complete cooperation on the part of the patient. Without these the end result accompanying endocrine pharmacotherapeutics may be more disabling than the untreated cause of the primary disease.

64 DISEASES OF THE ANTERIOR AND INTERMEDIATE LOBES OF THE PITUITARY GLAND

Don H. Nelson and
George W. Thorn

DISEASES OF THE ANTERIOR PITUITARY GLAND

Diseases of the anterior pituitary gland may be simply divided into those due to excess production of one of the hormones secreted by this gland or the syndrome of deficiency of pituitary secretion. Because of the many different hormones produced by this small organ, no other tissue in the body of similar size exerts a more widespread direct effect on the function of such widely different tissues than does the anterior pituitary. Thus, adrenocorticotropin (ACTH) acts particularly on the adrenal gland, thyrotropin (TSH) stimulates thyroid function, follicle-stimulating hormone and luteinizing hormone (FSH and LH) exert their effect on the gonads. Growth hormone has specific effects on growth and intermediary metabolism, and the lactogenic hormone or luteotropic hormone (LTH) is effective in maintaining the corpus luteum of pregnancy, and may be important in the stimulation of progesterone secretion, as well as having effects on the mammary gland and lactation. Melanocyte-stimulating hormone (MSH) is produced by the anterior or intermediate lobes of the pituitary gland and has widespread effects on pigmentation.

In addition to these hormones, the existence of which is well demonstrated, it is possible that other substances produced by the anterior pituitary gland may have important physiologic effects. For instance, the "adrenal weight factor" which has been demonstrated to have effects on adrenal growth but not on corticosteroid secretion may be separated from ACTH which produces an increase in secretion of the adrenal cortical steroids from the adrenal gland. Another hormone which may be produced by the pituitary gland is an exophthalmus-producing substance (EPS). It has been shown, chiefly in animals, that a pituitary substance separate from TSH may be responsible for exophthalmus in Graves's disease. Also suggested as pituitary

Table 64-1. ANTERIOR PITUITARY HORMONES

Hormone	Approximate molecular weight	Probable nature	Availability for therapy
Adrenocorticotropic (ACTH).....	3,800	Polypeptide	Intravenous and long- and short-acting intramuscular preparations available
Growth (GH).... S.T.H..........	44,000	Protein	Hormone obtained from primate pituitary glands appears to be effective but is not generally available
Follicle-stimulating (FSH).......	69,000	Protein	Available preparations are likely to promote antihormone formation. No pure preparations of either hormone are available for clinical use, but substances obtained from pregnant subjects' urine and pregnant horse serum have biologic activity of this type
Luteinizing (LH)..............	40,000–90,000	Protein	
Luteotropic (LTH).............	32,000	Protein	Doubtful clinical usefulness at present
Thyroid-stimulating (TSH)......	10,000	Protein	Used for distinguishing between primary and secondary hypothyroidism. Not therapeutic
Melanocyte-stimulating (MSH) ..	2,177	Polypeptide	For investigation only, at present

hormones are a fat-mobilizing factor (adipokinin) and an erythropoietic factor.

Of additional interest is the fact that although these various hormones, whether they are proteins or polypeptides (Table 64-1), have a primary function in most cases of stimulating secretion of specific hormones from their target gland, they may also have general metabolic effects as does growth hormone. Although it is not certain whether such effects are truly physiologic, ACTH, for example, does have fat-mobilizing activity.

In addition, hormones not produced by the pituitary act on the endocrine glands. There is clear evidence of an aldosterone-stimulating hormone which is not produced by the anterior pituitary gland but which has considerable effect on aldosterone secretion from the adrenal gland. In addition to these widespread effects which, as mentioned, are of as yet unproved physiologic significance, are the cross activities enjoyed by some of these hormones. All preparations of ACTH appear to have some melanocyte-stimulating activity and large, nonphysiologic, doses of pitressin will stimulate adrenal cortical secretion.

Because of the multiple secretions of a relatively small amount of tissue characteristic of the pituitary gland, it is uncommon for only one organ system to be involved in any destructive process acting on the gland, and in cases of hypopituitarism, the most common finding by far is a general loss of anterior pituitary secretions. With hyperfunction of the gland, however, the opposite case appears to be true, and it is rather rare for more than one pituitary hormone to be produced in excess in a single individual. Tumors of this gland are either nonsecretory or secrete large quantities of a specific hormone. Examples of the latter are the eosinophilic tumors which produce excess growth hormone and the basophilic or chromophobic tumors of the pituitary gland which produce excess ACTH. Notable by their absence are pituitary tumors which secrete specifically gonadotropins in large quantities.

Histology. The classic histology of the anterior pituitary gland divides the cells into chromophobe cells, eosinophils, and basophils, with the respective division of these various cells in the adult being 52, 37, and 11 per cent. It has generally been believed that the chromophobe cells do not secrete tropic hormones, and the eosinophilic cells secrete all but ACTH, TSH, and FSH, which are said to be secreted by the basophilic cells. Recent evidence, however, suggests that chromophobe cells, as in pituitary tumors associated with Cushing's syndrome, may secrete ACTH, and other methods of classification of cells have been devised. There is no good correlation between cell type and hormonal secretion at the present time.

Physiology. The physiologic effects of most of the anterior pituitary hormones have been extensively studied. Growth hormone increases the rate of skeletal growth and produces a gain in body weight. Adrenocorticotropin is the chief stimulus to adrenal steroid secretion, with the exception of aldosterone. Thyrotropin induces hyperplasia of the thyroid gland, stimulates the synthesis of thyroid hormone, and accelerates its release into the circulation. Follicle-stimulating hormone stimulates the growth of graafian follicles and aids in estrogen production. It is also essential for spermatogenesis, stimulating the seminiferous tubules of the testes. The luteinizing hormone (LH) is necessary for ovulation and corpus luteum formation in the ovary and stimulates the production of estrogens and progesterone. In the male, LH (sometimes called interstitial cell–stimulating hormone, or ICSH) stimulates the testicular Leydig cells and leads to the secretion of testosterone and other androgens. Lactogenic hormone, or luteotropin (LTH), maintains the corpus luteum of pregnancy, stimulates progesterone formation, and is essential for mammary gland development and lactation.

The secretion of anterior pituitary hormones appears in some cases to be regulated by the amount of specific hormone either secreted by the endocrine glands or administered exogenously. For example, the administration of large doses of corticosteroids depresses ACTH secretion. It has been suggested that an increased blood level of a hormone suppresses secretion of its specific pituitary tropic hormone. It is also true, however, that if there is sufficient stimulus to secretion from the gland as in conditions of stress, increased secretion of ACTH may occur while corticosteroids in the circulation are considerably elevated. An intact hypothalamus appears to be a necessary part of the normal response to stress. In addition, there is evidence that dietary intake and nutritional status may modify the secretion of the anterior hormones. Thus with starvation one may observe a decrease in gonadotropic hormones and a reduction in 17-ketosteroid and 17-hydroxycorticosteroid excretion.

The protein nature of the majority of the preparations presently available and their capacity for inducing an antibody response limit their use, in many instances, to diagnostic procedures. Thus, in practice, a deficiency of one of the anterior pituitary hormones is generally corrected by replacing the hormone or hormones liberated by the target gland. Even in those cases where antihormones are not a problem, as with the adrenocorticotropic hormone, it is much more satisfactory to administer cortisone or one of its analogues to a patient with adrenocorticotropic deficiency than to attempt continuous therapy with the tropic hormone.

Decreased Anterior Pituitary Secretion

Panhypopituitarism

Prepuberal. Prepuberal panhypopituitarism, which was first described in 1871 by Lorrain, is a rare condition usually associated with suprasellar cyst or craniopharyngioma. The disease is characterized by dwarfism and subnormal sexual development. Mentality is usually normal. The impairment of growth is symmetric, and the body proportions

are normal. As in other cases of hypopituitarism, the skin often is described as having a pale yellowish appearance and increased wrinkling. Sexual maturation is delayed, and in rare cases there may be obesity from hypothalamic involvement. If the tumor is of sufficient size to affect the optic chiasm, there may be bitemporal or complete blindness. X-ray studies reveal delayed fusion of the epiphyses, and destruction of the sella turcica is frequently noted. The condition may be distinguished from genetic dwarfism and from hypothyroidism by subnormal sexual development, failure to mature, normal mentality, and the normal body proportions which are generally present. Treatment should be similar to that described below, with thyroid and cortisone doses scaled to age and size. In addition the administration of human or monkey growth hormone in doses of 1 to 3 mg weekly has had considerable success in producing growth in these patients. Because of the psychologic-sociologic importance of reaching normal stature, every attempt should be made to obtain such therapy for these patients if the epiphyses have not closed.

Postpuberal. In 1914 Simmonds described a case of post-partum necrosis of the pituitary gland with marked cachexia. He correlated his clinical-pathologic findings with Paulesco's experimental observations on the profound effects of hypophysectomy, and the term *Simmond's disease* has since been applied to patients who have marked insufficiency of the target glands and profound cachexia. The term *Sheehan's syndrome* is more commonly used to refer to those cases in which there is post-partum pituitary insufficiency but no significant weight loss. A careful history usually reveals increased blood loss at time of delivery. Following delivery, these patients may fail to lactate or may have some function for a period of a few months followed by gradual loss of pituitary secretion. The most common symptomatology in hypopituitarism consists of asthenia, lethargy, loss of libido, impotence, amenorrhea, and intolerance to cold. Failure of lactation and of menses following difficult labor should always suggest this diagnosis. Common physical signs consist of pallor, loss of axillary and pubic hair, wrinkling of the skin, and general loss of secondary sex characteristics with atrophy of the genitalia and breasts.

Etiology. Post-partum pituitary necrosis due to thrombosis is the most common cause of panhypopituitarism. Chromophobe adenomas and craniopharyngiomas may cause atrophy by pressure on normal tissue. Tumors which lead to specific types of hyperpituitarism (e.g., eosinophilic adenomas with acromegaly) may be associated with hypopituitarism because of replacement of normal tissue or following surgical removal of the gland. Other less common etiologies are gliomas which invade the pituitary, brain injuries, various granulomatous processes such as sarcoid or Hand-Schüller-Christian disease, injuries which affect blood supply to the gland, and rarely, infectious processes.

Craniopharyngiomas are the most common cause of hypopituitarism before the age of puberty and represent a secretory vestige of Rathke's pouch, which has been cut off from its origin in the roof of the pharynx. The viscous, cholesterol-containing fluid of such suprasellar cysts is prone to calcification and may give a clue as to the etiology of the process on x-ray examination. Although much more common in the younger age group, such tumors are occasionally found in adult life.

Chromophobe adenomas of the anterior pituitary deserve special mention because of their relative frequency as a cause of hypopituitarism. About two-thirds of all pituitary adenomas and one-fifth of all intracranial tumors are chromophobe adenomas of the pituitary gland. They are usually nonsecretory and produce symptoms only through pressure on neighboring organs and replacement of normal pituitary tissue. Thus in addition to the classical symptomatology of hypopituitarism, there may be increased intracranial pressure, destruction of the sella turcica, involvement of the optic chiasm with bitemporal hemianopsia, and the signs and symptoms of diabetes insipidus, usually mild. An important complication of these tumors is progressive involvement of the optic nerves which may lead to blindness if proper therapy is not instituted.

Pathology. Irrespective of the etiology of the pituitary destruction leading to panhypopituitarism, the secondary pathologic effects on the endocrine organs of the body are similar. Thus there is marked atrophy of the thyroid, adrenals, and gonads. Interference in growth occurs if the lesion appears prior to puberty. Of interest from the point of view of pituitary secretion is the relatively large amount of the pituitary gland which may be destroyed or replaced by various pathologic processes with continued secretion of the hormones in physiologic amounts by the gland. Various studies carried out in animals have suggested that destructive processes of the anterior pituitary are likely to interfere first with gonadotropic function, secondly, thyroid function, and lastly, adrenal function as a progressively larger part of the gland is destroyed.

Incidence. Although the incidence of panhypopituitarism is not great, it cannot be classed as a rare disease as considerable numbers of these patients are found. In 1942 Escamilla was able to collect 595 cases from the literature.

Laboratory Findings. Laboratory findings are generally those which reflect decreased function of the endocrine organs which are involved. Thus plasma protein-bound iodine (PBI) is low as is the radioactive iodine (RAI) uptake, and there is a decrease in metabolic rate. Unlike primary myxedema, the level of plasma cholesterol is rarely elevated despite very low thyroid function. Urinary 17-ketosteroids and 17-hydroxycorticosteroids or 17-ketogenic steroids are low, as are urinary gonadotropins. Blood levels of ACTH are said to be low, but these are not generally available or useful for the diagnosis of the condition. A normochromic anemia is frequently present. Hypoglycemia of a mild variety may be present, and more importantly these patients are extremely sensitive to insulin.

Differential Diagnosis and Physiologic Tests of Function. The chief problem in the differential diagnosis of panhypopituitarism is differentiation from failure of an individual target organ or from some general debilitating process which may simulate hypopituitarism. Primary failure of the thyroid or the adrenal cortex can generally be differentiated from secondary failure by the administration of TSH or ACTH to the patient. Thus a patient with hypopituitarism, although starting at the same low levels of plasma protein-bound iodine and radioactive iodine uptake as a patient with primary myxedema, will respond to the administration of TSH with an increase in both these values (see p. 587). Likewise the patient with adrenal failure, secondary to pituitary disturbance, will respond to ACTH administration by an increase in the 24-hr excretion of urinary 17-ketosteroids and 17-hydroxycorticosteroids or 17-ketogenic steroids. Such patients often fail to respond to a single day's infusion of ACTH, but administration of 50 units intravenously over an 8-hr period on 3 or 4 successive days is characterized by lack of response early and an increasing response on the second to the fourth day of administration. No such test is readily available for the estimation of response to gonadotropins, but the presence or absence of urinary gonadotropins is an important diagnostic test in the diagnosis of hypopituitarism. Unfortunately, many patients who are chronically debilitated, either from illness or from undernutrition due to anexoria nervosa, may have low gonadotropin excretions. The response to ACTH is generally of more diagnostic significance in this group of patients without pituitary involvement but in whom target organ responses are definitely decreased, the cause may be pituitary suppression due to long-term malnutrition.

The disease most commonly confused with panhypopituitarism is anorexia nervosa. Such patients commonly give a history of amenorrhea, but careful investigation may reveal anorexia preceding this change. In young adult nulliparous women, panhypopituitarism is very rare, whereas anorexia nervosa occurs predominantly in younger women. The differentiation of psychologic disturbance from endocrine abnormality is, however, difficult, particularly as patients with panhypopituitarism may have major psychologic difficulties, related either to brain tumor or hypoglycemia. A most helpful differential diagnostic test in these patients is the presence of a normal or near normal urinary corticosteroid values and a positive response to substances such as 2-methyl-1,2 bis-(3-pyridyl)-1-propanone (SU 4885), a stimulator of endogenous pituitary function. This substance inhibits the 11-hydroxylation on the steroid molecule, and following its administration, there are increased quantities of 11-deoxy-17-hydroxycorticosterone secreted and decreased amounts of 17-hydroxycorticosterone (hydrocortisone). This results in increased ACTH secretion from the anterior pituitary gland and a marked increase in adrenal secretion and thereby urinary excretion of 17-hydroxycorticosteroids. Thus patients with normal adrenal-pituitary function, when given this substance, will have an increase in urinary corticoids. Patients with either primary or secondary adrenal insufficiency will fail to demonstrate such an increase in urinary 17-hydroxycorticosteroids. It is important in performing the test to be certain that the adrenal is capable of responding to ACTH. This is usually established by carrying out the standard ACTH test referred to above, and then carrying out the test with the SU 4885. Such a test has particular use in evaluation of the patient who produces fairly normal quantities of corticosteroids during the unstressed state but appears unable to increase secretion following a stress. This test simulates a response to stress.

Other tests which are sometimes employed are insulin tolerance and response to a water load. Patients with hypopituitarism are very sensitive to insulin administration. This test should, therefore, be carried out only under close supervision of the patient. These patients also excrete a water load poorly, but this test may be falsely positive in the presence of primary adrenal or renal disease, and thus more specific tests of hormonal secretion are preferred. In addition, water intoxication may be produced in patients who are not carefully observed throughout the test.

Treatment. When the lesion is found to be a chromophobe adenoma or a craniopharyngioma, x-ray therapy is recommended. Unfortunately, the result of x-ray treatment in craniopharyngioma is often unsatisfactory. In the presence of compression of the optic chiasm, surgical intervention followed by irradiation is required. It is to be emphasized that patients with panhypopituitarism respond poorly to operation unless proper hormonal replacement therapy is given because of the lack of normal secretion of adrenocorticotropic hormone. In those cases coming to operation or subjected to a variety of stresses, corticosteroid replacement therapy is definitely required. In most cases it should be as-

sumed that the adrenal glands are unresponsive, and full therapeutic doses of cortisone, not ACTH, such as are described for carrying the Addisonian patient through a stressful situation, should be administered (see Chap. 68).

In the endocrine management of panhypopituitarism, multiple pituitary tropic hormones would be true replacement therapy. Unfortunately, however, TSH and ACTH must be given by daily injection, and pituitary gonadotropins cannot be used successfully for any prolonged period because of the tendency to form antibodies. In practice, the physician must rely on replacement therapy with the target gland hormones. USP thyroid should be started at a dose of 15 mg a day and gradually increased to 90 to 120 mg over a period of several weeks. Cortisone acetate should be started at a level of approximately 5 to 10 mg per day and increased to 15 to 30 mg as is needed. Deoxycorticosterone or other salt-retaining corticosteroid is generally not required, as these patients continue to secrete aldosterone in the absence of ACTH. Although hyponatremia is not a general part of the picture, these patients like the Addisonian patients are unable to excrete excess fluids normally, and may become hyponatremic following a water load. Particular care should be taken that thyroid is not given prior to the administration of corticosteroid replacement therapy, as this may precipitate an Addisonian crisis which may be fatal. Testosterone cyclopentylpropionate in a dose of 100 to 200 mg intramuscularly every 3 to 4 weeks is beneficial in some patients. In a few cases, estrogens may be given to women patients. Treatment with these hormones is aimed at only normal physiologic replacement, and thus the harmful effects of corticosteroid administration in large doses are not seen, but psychic disturbances of various kinds may be noted if the patient is changed suddenly from no steroid or thyroid medication to full replacement doses. Another problem often noted is that of excessive appetite in the patient who has not received steroids, perhaps for some years, and who is then placed on cortisone therapy. This must be regulated by diet and in some cases a decrease in cortisone dosage.

Specific Deficiencies of Pituitary Secretion

Specific deficiencies of secretion of anterior pituitary hormones with normal secretion of the other secretory products of this gland, although reported in a number of instances, are very rare. The diagnosis can be made only after careful study of all parameters of pituitary function and certainly should never be made without such studies. Thus, in the postulated specific deficiency of ACTH, it is necessary to demonstrate that adrenal secretion is very low, that it responds poorly but in the characteristic stepwise manner to intravenous infusion of ACTH, and that aldosterone function is present in the absence of normal corticosteroid secretion. It is then necessary to demonstrate that gonadotropins are present and that the thyroid function is normal as indicated by plasma protein-bound iodine and radioactive iodine uptake. Similar functional studies are necessary prior to making a diagnosis of specific TSH or gonadotropin insufficiency. Present diagnostic techniques certainly do not allow the diagnosis of relative ACTH, TSH, or gonadotropin insufficiency to be made. It may be that, in some cases, patients who have been considered to have specific deficiencies of pituitary secretion actually have lesions of the hypothalamus in the areas which control secretion of these specific hormones, but as stated previously, such diagnoses should be made cautiously. A patient mistakenly diagnosed as having pituitary deficiency of only TSH when ACTH was also deficient might be treated with thyroid hormone and no corticosteroids. Such a patient may develop acute adrenal insufficiency.

Increased Secretion from the Anterior Pituitary Gland

Increased pituitary secretion is generally associated with a tumor of the gland. There is, in the authors' opinion, no clear-cut syndrome of general pituitary hyperfunction, with the exception of those cases of acromegaly or gigantism that have evidence of multiple endocrine gland hyperactivity.

Growth Hormone (Increased Secretion)

In addition to its effects on growth, this hormone has been shown to have a wide influence on a variety of metabolic processes. In the young animal there is an increase in growth, storage of protein, phosphorus, calcium, and an elevation of serum inorganic phosphorus and alkaline phosphatase. In addition, growth hormone has an anti-insulin or diabetogenic effect which leads to glucosuria, impaired glucose tolerance, and increased insulin resistance. There is a species specificity of growth hormone preparations. Only primate hormone has been shown to have significant physiologic effects in man and be capable of inducing growth.

Gigantism. The characteristic picture of increased growth hormone secretion during the prepubertal period is excessive growth with resulting gigantism. With this condition there is generalized symmetric overgrowth of the skeleton and soft tissues so that a well-proportioned giant results. At the onset these individuals are usually physically strong, alert, and intelligent. Later in the disease, however, pituitary insufficiency may develop, and they may progress to a point of weakness and easy fatigability although maintaining their gigantic size. The underlying lesion is generally an eosinophilic or mixed

cell adenoma of the anterior lobe which may or may not be visible radiologically. The condition is extremely rare, and generally little difficulty is encountered in making the diagnosis. The only other endocrine abnormality contributing to excessive growth to be considered in differential diagnosis is the increased height sometimes obtained by the eunuch. These patients have the abnormalities of proportion which are characteristic of the eunuchoid habitus and gonadal failure. Such patients, unlike the patient with typical gigantism, may continue to grow into late life, with failure to close their epiphyses. Treatment of the pituitary giant is similar to that described below for acromegaly.

Acromegaly. The same pituitary tumor producing excess growth hormone which results in the production of a giant when it occurs during the prepubertal period will produce acromegaly in the adult.

Clinical Findings. The condition is first noted by change in facial features, size of head, hands, and feet which may necessitate increases in hat, glove, or shoe size. Other patients first note signs and symptoms of an intercranial tumor which may produce headache or visual disturbances. The fully developed syndrome is unmistakable. The hands and feet are greatly enlarged, the ends of the digits are square, there is prognathism which may be so marked as to interfere with mastication. These patients may have symptoms of arthritis and show osteoarthritic-like bone changes. The features are coarse, in part because of thickening of the skin; the malar and supraorbital ridges are prominent; the tongue is much enlarged, and the lips are thickened. The speech may be thick and hoarse, and there is general visceromegaly. These patients are particularly subject to psychiatric disturbances and may have emotional instability (Fig. 64-1).

Among the associated endocrine disturbances, enlargement of the thyroid and an increased basal metabolic rate are of frequent occurrence. Frank hyperthyroidism, however, occurs in only a small percentage of cases. Diabetes mellitus is present in 10 to 15 per cent of these patients. It is typically mild but may be relatively resistant to insulin therapy. Libido may be increased at the onset, but is lost subsequently, and gonadal atrophy may occur late in the disease. The course of the disease is usually one of benign chronicity, but fatalities may occur as a result of cardiac failure, local complications of the tumor, or unrecognized hypopituitarism.

Diagnosis. Diagnosis is made by the typical changes in body configuration, demonstration of pituitary tumor by x-ray or visual field defects, and particularly a recent change in facial features or growth of hands and feet. A high level of serum inorganic phosphorus is characteristic of the active disease and may be helpful in deciding whether a

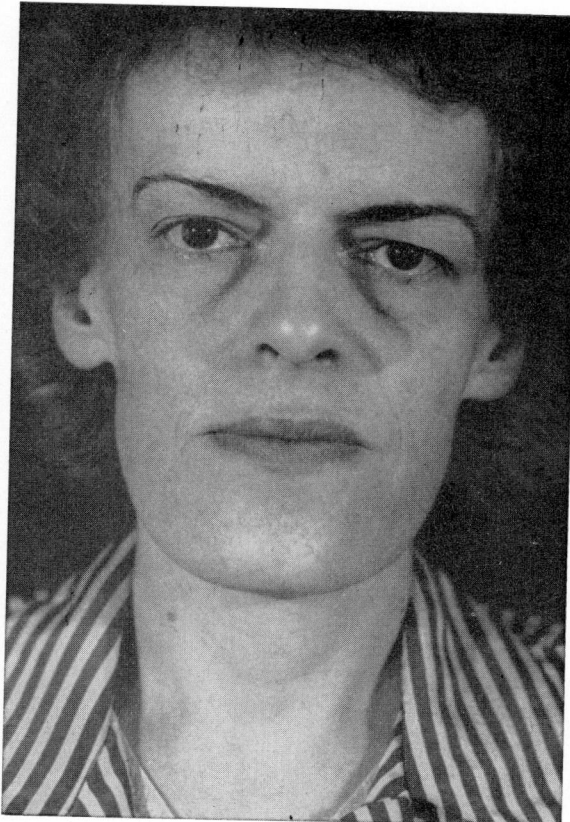

FIG. 64-1. Photograph of a 44-year-old woman with acromegaly, arrested. Onset of the disease occurred 20 years before, at which time a moderately enlarged sella turcica was demonstrated by x-ray. Following x-ray therapy of the pituitary she has shown no further progression of the disease.

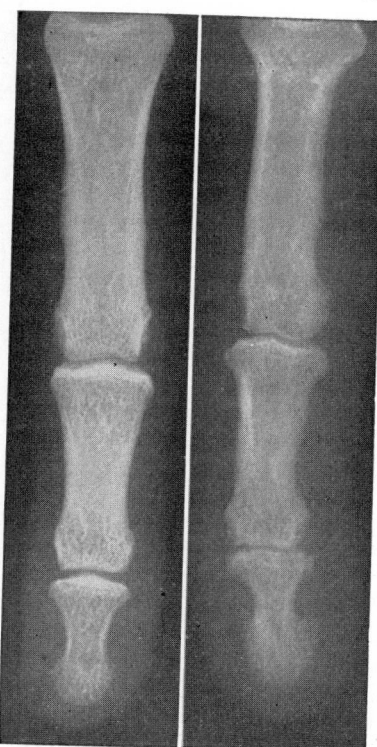

FIG. 64-2. Characteristic tufting or "arrowhead" appearance of the terminal phalanx in acromegaly (*right*). Normal phalanx for comparison (*left*). Note also the thickness of the acromegalic finger.

course of irradiation to the pituitary gland has been successful. Patients should also be followed carefully for changes in bony growth (Fig. 64-2).

Because of the difficulty in objectively demonstrating changes in skeletal size, particularly over a short interval of time, and because of the wide variation in levels of plasma inorganic phosphate, it is frequently problematical to determine the presence or absence of growth activity in patients with acromegaly. Determination of growth hormone in plasma using immunochemical methods has been somewhat successful, but the assay is technically extremely difficult. The presence or absence of growth activity can also be determined using the patients own tissues, for example, the relative cellularity of costochondral cartilage, indicating endochondral bone formation.

Treatment. Eosinophilic adenomas are generally sensitive to irradiation, but in some cases hypophysectomy may be required, particularly in the patient who has pressure on the optic chiasm from a tumor of sufficient size to threaten the eyesight of the individual. If hypopituitarism develops, diagnosis and therapy may be made as previously described. There is an additional reason for urgency in the therapy of this condition in order to reduce the disfigurement which the disease often produces.

ACTH (*Increased Secretion*)

Increased secretion of ACTH from the pituitary gland is a normal accompaniment of stressful situations. Thus, it has been demonstrated that with severe trauma, such as abdominal operation, there is an increased circulating level of ACTH. Such secretion of ACTH can be suppressed by the administration of corticosteroids if the stress is relatively mild, but in conditions of severe trauma, very high levels of plasma corticosteroids may be associated with markedly elevated plasma ACTH levels. Response to stress is mediated through the hypothalamus, and lesions of this area will prevent the normal increase in ACTH and corticosteroid secretion which is associated with trauma. The exact mechanism by which control over ACTH secretion is maintained is unclear, and experimental evidence suggests that there are other central nervous system areas which may act to inhibit or stimulate the se-

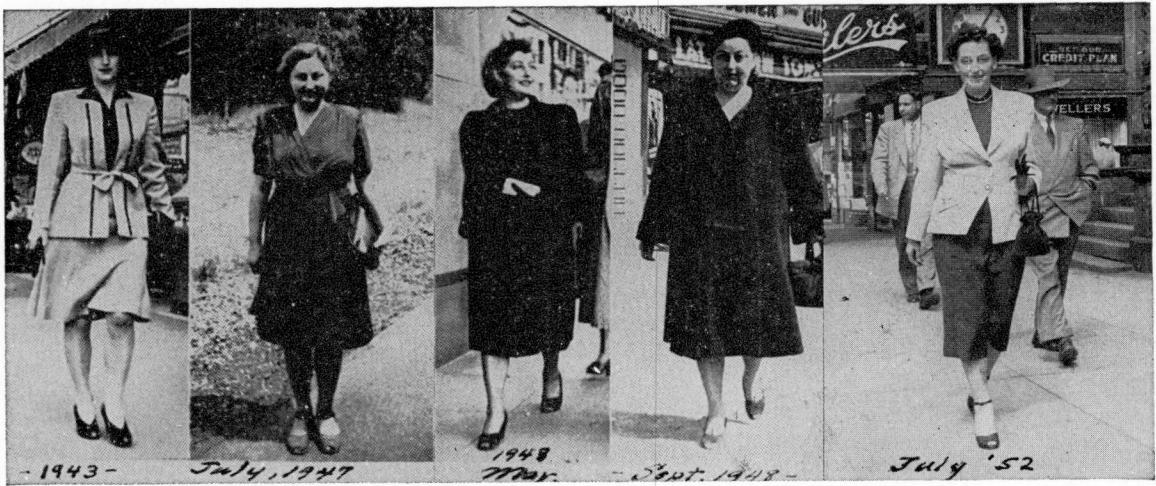

FIG. 64-3. Photographs of a 38-year-old woman with Cushing's disease. (1) Patient before the onset of the disease, age 33. (2) Patient 5 to 6 months after the onset of symptoms, age 37. (3) Improvement following x-ray treatment to the pituitary (2,800 roentgen units) and to the adrenal region (600 roentgen units). (4) Return of the full-blown disease, just prior to admission to the Peter Bent Brigham Hospital. (5) Remission following bilateral adrenalectomy.

cretion of ACTH. Increased production of ACTH results in the secretion of hydrocortisone and, to a lesser extent, corticosterone from the adrenal cortex. In addition to this, compounds possessing androgenic activity are also stimulated by ACTH. Although ACTH affects aldosterone secretion to some extent, it is not the chief controlling factor in the secretion of this hormone.

Cushing's Syndrome. This syndrome, which is described more fully in Chap. 68, p. 617, may be of adrenal or pituitary etiology. When the anterior pituitary gland is responsible, the effect is mediated by increased secretion of ACTH from this gland. A relatively small percentage of these cases may be demonstrated to have tumors of the anterior pituitary gland which produce excess quantities of ACTH. A larger group, however, have hyperplasia of the adrenal cortex with little or no demonstrable change in the pituitary. Although attempts to demonstrate increased secretion of ACTH in these patients are not conclusive, it is believed that Cushing's syndrome with adrenal hyperplasia is produced by increased secretion of ACTH. The mechanism by which such ACTH production is increased is not clear. Pituitary tumors, when present, have generally been described as being of a basophilic type; although, as noted below, chromophobe tumors of the pituitary gland seen following adrenalectomy for Cushing's syndrome may also produce ACTH.

The clinical characteristics of Cushing's syndrome are described more fully in Chap. 68, p. 618. The most important changes are obesity, rounding of the face, abdominal striae, hypertension, diabetes, osteoporosis, and elevated corticosteroid excretion. The primary diagnostic points in the laboratory examination of such patients are: high resting levels of 17-hydroxycorticosteroids or 17-ketogenic steroids, and in the case of adrenal hyperplasia, increased or hyperactive secretion following the administration of intravenous ACTH. The increment of urinary corticosteroid excretion over control day is greater in the patient receiving intravenous ACTH who has Cushing's syndrome and adrenal hyperplasia than it is in the normal subject. Patients with primary adrenal disease such as adrenal adenoma or carcinoma are less likely to show a hyperactive response to intravenous ACTH. Following the administration of corticosteroid, such as dexamethasone, in quantities of 2 mg per 24 hr (0.5 mg every 6 hr), corticosteroid excretion is usually suppressed in the normal individual. In patients with Cushing's syndrome and adrenal hyperplasia it is not suppressed by this quantity of dexamethasone but may be if doses in the neighborhood of 8 mg per day (2 mg every 6 hr) are given. Many patients with adrenal tumors will fail to suppress adrenal secretion when even larger amounts of corticosteroids are given. The extent to which other laboratory findings such as hyperglycemia and diabetic glucose tolerance test, hypopotassemia, and alkalosis are present is dependent upon the severity and the duration of the disease. Patients with tumors of the anterior pituitary gland of this type should be treated with irradiation of the pituitary gland as described below, and if this fails to reduce adrenal secretion satisfactorily, surgery is indicated.

Pituitary Tumors Occurring Following Adrenalectomy for Cushing's Syndrome. A number of patients have developed pituitary tumors following bilateral adrenalectomy for Cushing's syndrome. It is not possible to say at the present time whether a small tumor was present prior to operation, and continued to grow, or whether the adrenalectomy stimulated the production of the pituitary tumor. Most of these patients have, however, been examined prior to adrenalectomy with no evidence of such tumor being present. The tumors are associated with intense pigmentation of the skin, which is generally much more pronounced than the pigmentation seen in Addison's disease. These patients often have exceedingly high levels of ACTH in their plasma. The tumor, in a few cases, has been demonstrated to be of a chromophobe type. It is unclear whether the tumor produces melanocyte-stimulating hormone in addition to ACTH. ACTH in the quantities present would have some melanocyte-stimulating effect. Therapy for this condition, as other pituitary tumors, is first, irradiation, which if unsuccessful should be followed by hypophysectomy. These patients may in addition exhibit the symptomatology of local pituitary destruction or pressure on related areas, as previously described. It is not felt that the finding of this type of tumors of the anterior pituitary gland, following adrenalectomy for Cushing's syndrome, should be taken as a reason for partial rather than total adrenalectomy in Cushing's syndrome. A few pituitary tumors of this type have also been noted in patients who were partially adrenalectomized and who later were found to have increased secretion of corticosteroids from their remaining adrenal tissue and increased levels of ACTH in their peripheral plasma.

Increased Plasma ACTH in Adrenal Insufficiency and Congenital Adrenal Hyperplasia. There is increased production of ACTH in patients who have adrenal insufficiency of a primary type. Thus, most patients with Addison's disease have elevated levels of plasma ACTH when not receiving corticosteroids or prior to receiving a dose of cortisone. This excess production of ACTH is not pathologic and has not been associated with pituitary tumors, but may be a factor responsible for the pigmentation which occurs in this disease. Patients with congenital adrenal hyperplasia also have elevated levels of ACTH in their plasma as a result of their deficient production of hydrocortisone. The primary pathologic change is not, however, in the pituitary gland but in the adrenal gland, and the excess production of ACTH may be easily suppressed by the administration of normal quantities of corticosteroids (see Chap. 68).

Thyrotropin

The relationship between hyperthyroidism and secretion of thyroid-stimulating hormone is not clear. Although some investigators have claimed to find elevated levels of TSH in the blood of patients with hyperthyroidism, such assays have not been consistently reproducible by different techniques, and the role which this pituitary hormone may play is unproved. It does appear, however, that certain pituitary tumors may produce excess TSH and be associated with thyroid hyperplasia and increased secretion of thyroid hormones from this gland. TSH secretion may be increased by stimuli arising in the hypothalamus, and it is thought that a mechanism acting through higher central nervous system centers may be related to the not infrequent appearance of thyrotoxic symptoms following major emotional or psychic trauma. It is also probable that an increase in TSH secretion is involved in cases of hyperthyroidism associated with acromegaly.

Gonadotropins

There are no definite clinical syndromes associated with increased secretion of gonadotropins from the anterior pituitary gland. There are, however, cases of sexual precosity due usually to lesions of the hypothalamus, in which it is probable that hypersecretion of gonadotropic hormones does occur. Such patients are characterized by virilization and increased androgen production and are usually seen in infancy or childhood.

Other Syndromes Related to Pituitary Function

There are two syndromes, the etiology of which are as yet poorly defined, which may have some pituitary or hypothalamic origin. They are Froehlich's syndrome and the Laurence-Moon-Biedl syndrome, both associated with failure of gonadal development. No constant lesions are observed in the anterior pituitary, however, and if the gonadotropic abnormality is produced by a diminution of gonadotropic secretion, it must be secondary to hypothalamic disturbance.

Froehlich's Syndrome

The clinical picture described for Froehlich's syndrome is a combination of adiposity and genital atrophy. There is underdevelopment of the gonads and secondary sex characteristics and a white, delicate skin. Also sometimes associated are mental retardation, visual disturbances, diabetes insipidus, and disturbances in skeletal growth. It is important to differentiate between cases of Froehlich's type of habitus (obesity and apparent delayed genital development) and true Froehlich's syndrome. Patients with the former condition actually may have normal sex organs which are hidden in the adipose tissue. Restoration of weight to normal and patient observation is usually sufficient to correct the condition. Most such boys at the time of puberty develop normally without treatment. In true Froehlich's syndrome, associated with a tumor of the hypothalamic-pituitary origin, treatment should be directed at the tumor.

Laurence-Moon-Biedl Syndrome

The Laurence-Moon-Biedl syndrome is a hereditary disease characterized by adiposity, genital atrophy, mental retardation, skull deformities, and associated congenital malformations such as polydactyly and retinitis pigmentosa. Less than 100 cases have been reported, and there is no evidence of pituitary lesions in these patients. The adiposity and genital atrophy are assumed to be caused by a dysfunction of the hypothalamic-pituitary region.

Tumors of the Pituitary

Pituitary adenomas, often microscopic in size, are found in approximately 10 per cent of human pituitary glands. They may be classified, according to the predominant cell type, as chromophobic, eosinophilic, and basophilic adenomas. Eosinophilic adenomas are usually limited in location to the anterior pituitary, whereas basophilic adenomas not infrequently are located within the pars nervosa.

Other types of pituitary tumors include carcinomas, cysts lined with ciliated epithelium, and craniopharyngiomas.

Pituitary adenomas of the eosinophilic or basophilic type may be accompanied by excessive hormone secretion (see Acromegaly, p. 568, and Cushing's syndrome, Chap. 68). In all types of tumors of the pituitary, decreased function is likely to occur late in the disease as a result of increased pressure and necrosis. In addition, because of the proximity of the numerous vegetative centers in the hypothalamic region, expansion of cysts or tumors very frequently induce not only changes in vision because of pressure on the optic chiasm but also changes in many of the more primitive vegetative functions (see Panhypopituitarism, p. 565). Normal pituitary tissue is particularly insensitive to irradiation, so that normal pituitary function may be seen following destruction of tumor tissue which is sensitive to the therapy. Once hypopituitarism has developed, it is uncommon to see return to normal endocrine function following therapy. Whereas, improvement in visual fields is common.

DISEASES OF THE INTERMEDIATE LOBE OF THE PITUITARY GLAND
(Melanocyte-stimulating Hormone)

The intermediate lobe of the pituitary gland is the probable site of production of the melanocyte-stimulating hormone (MSH). The hormone is a polypeptide composed of the same 13 amino acids which form the first 13 amino acids of ACTH. Thus, ACTH preparations always have melanocyte-stimulating effects, but the converse is not true and MSH does not cause adrenal cortical secretion. It is of interest that cortisone administration may suppress MSH as well as ACTH secretion from the pituitary gland.

Rarely do tumors of the pituitary gland occur which are primarily MSH producing. These appear to be even less common than the tumors previously described which are seen in patients who have been adrenalectomized for Cushing's syndrome and which appear to produce increased quantities of MSH and ACTH. The hyperpigmentation which is seen in patients with Addison's disease may also be influenced by increased production of MSH. The ability of ACTH to produce similar effects on pigmentation to those seen with MSH have confused our understanding as to whether ACTH alone produces such pigmentation or whether MSH is also produced in excess quantity. Variations in MSH production may also be related to the increased pigmentation seen in patients with hyperthyroidism, biliary cirrhosis, sprue, and other chronic diseases, and it is likely that decreased production of MSH is associated with the decreased pigmentation often seen in patients with panhypopituitarism. The relationship of secretion of this hormone to various types of pigmentation will be better understood as better methods for the estimation of the hormone become available.

REFERENCES

Antoniades, Harry N. (Ed.): "Hormones in Human Plasma," Boston, Little, Brown & Company, 1960.

Daughaday, W. H., W. D. Salmon, and F. Alexander: The Measurement of Serum Sulfation Factor as an Index of Somatotrophin Activity in Man, J. Clin. Invest., 37:888, 1958. Proc. Endocrinol. Soc., 1958.

Henneman, P. H., A. P. Forbes, M. Moldawer, E. F. Dempsey, and E. L. Carroll: Effects of Human Growth Hormone in Man, J. Clin. Invest., 39:1223, 1960.

Jailer, J. W., and D. A. Holub: Remission of Graves's Disease Following Radiotherapy of a Pituitary Neoplasm, Am. J. Med., 28:497, 1960.

Lerner, A. B.: Hormonal Control of Pigmentation, Ann. Rev. Med., 11:187, 1960.

Liddle, G. W., H. L. Estep, J. W. Kendall, W. C. Williams, and A. S. Townes: Clinical Application of a New Test of Pituitary Reserve, J. Clin. Endocrinol., 19:875, 1959.

Nelson, D. H., J. W. Meakin, and G. W. Thorn: ACTH-producing Pituitary Tumors Following Adrenalectomy for Cushing's Syndrome, Ann. Internal Med., 52:560, 1960.

Raben, M. S.: Treatment of a Pituitary Dwarf with Human Growth Hormone, J. Clin. Endocrinol., 18:901, 1958.

Schwartz, Drew: Patterns in the Amino-Acid Sequences of the Corticotropins, Nature, 183:464, 1959.

Wolstenholme, G. E. W., and C. M. O'Connor: "Human Pituitary Hormones," vol. 13, Ciba Foundation Colloquia on Endocrinology, Boston, Little Brown & Company, 1960.

65 DISEASES OF THE NEUROHYPOPHYSIS

Joseph F. Dingman and George W. Thorn

Oliver and Schäfer in 1894 demonstrated a pressor effect of pituitary extracts, and in 1897 Howell showed that the pressor principle resided in the posterior lobe. The oxytocic action of posterior pituitary extracts was described by Dale in 1909, and the antidiuretic action by von den Velden in 1913. Fisher, Ingram, and Ranson in 1938 demonstrated a functional relationship between certain hypothalamic nuclei and the posterior pituitary. The studies of Scharrer and Scharrer since 1928 concerning the secretory activity of nerve cells (neurosecretion), the demonstration by Bargmann in 1949 of secretory granules in the neurones of the supraoptic and paraventricular nuclei of the hypothalamus, and the recent successful synthesis of oxytocin and vasopressin by du Vigneaud and co-workers represent important advances in current understanding of the endocrine function of the neurohypophysis.

GENERAL CONSIDERATIONS

The principal effects of posterior pituitary extracts are to enhance the reabsorption of water by the renal tubules (antidiuretic effect); stimulate uterine contraction (oxytocic effect); promote the secretion of milk from the lactating breast (milk-ejecting effect); and only in *anesthetized* mammals, produce a rise in blood pressure (vasopressor effect). The neurohypophyseal hormones are vasopressin (antidiuretic hormone, ADH) and oxytocin. The former is predominantly responsible for pressor and antidiuretic actions, whereas the latter is most potent in uterine stimulation and milk ejection. The neuroendocrine unit responsible for production and secretion of these hormones has been designated the *neurohypophysis* (Fig. 65-1), which includes the neurones of the supraoptic and paraventricular nuclei of the anterior hypothalamus, the axones which form the supraopticohypophyseal tract traversing the pituitary stalk, and the posterior lobe of the pituitary gland, the pars nervosa, throughout which the axone endings ramify.

Classic concepts of the endocrine function of the neurohypophysis ascribed the role of hormone production to parenchymatous secretory cells in the posterior lobe; however, an impressive body of evidence has been accumulated recently to show

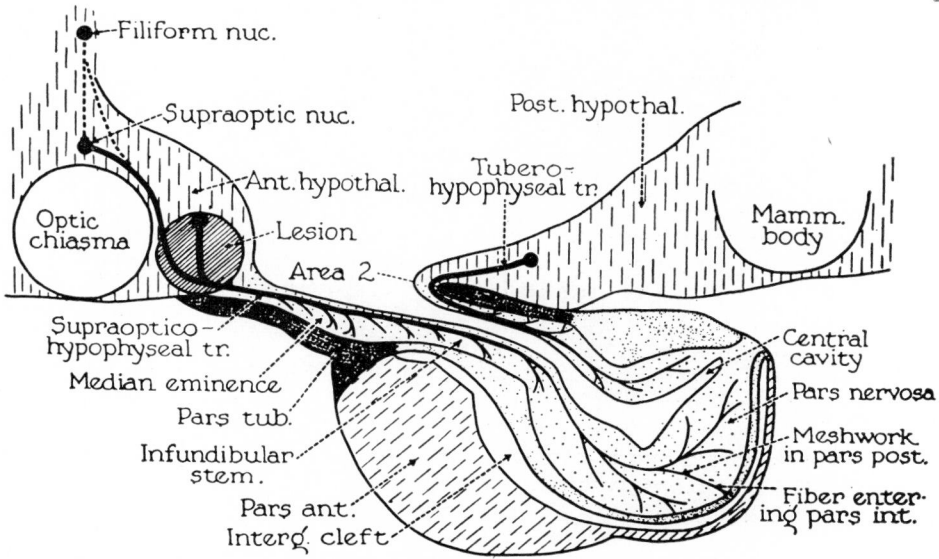

Fig. 65-1. Diagram of a midsagittal section through the hypothalamus and hypophysis. The broken lines indicate proposed filiform-supraoptic connections and the tractus paraventricularis. The obliquely striped circle indicates the position of a typical lesion designed to produce diabetes insipidus. (*Fisher, Ingram, and Ranson: "Diabetes Insipidus and the Neuro-Hormonal Control of Water Balance," Fig. 2, Ann Arbor, Mich., Edwards Brothers, Inc., 1938.*)

that the hormones are actually secreted by the neurones of the supraoptic and paraventricular nuclei. Gomori's chromalum hematoxylin stain for the beta cells of the pancreatic islets has been used to demonstrate secretory granules within the cytoplasm of these neurones which migrate along the axones into the posterior pituitary, accumulating in axone end-plates in close proximity to blood vessels. The bulk of neurohypophyseal hormone is contained in the posterior lobe; the tuber cinereum, stalk, and hypothalamic nuclei accounting for a small fraction of total activity. The posterior lobe, then, may serve mainly as a reservoir of hormone available for rapid secretion into the systemic circulation.

Removal of the posterior lobe will lead to hormonal deficiency only if most of the axones of the supraoptical hypophyseal tract are severed, which results in retrograde degeneration of the cell bodies in the hypothalamus. With severance of the stalk close to the posterior pituitary, short axones terminating at a higher level may escape injury and the remaining viable neurosecretory cells apparently can maintain secretion and release of hormones, probably into the vessels of the stalk and the hypothalamus.

The physiologic significance of the peculiar anatomic location of this neurosecretory organ, in which hypothalamic neurones extend their processes over relatively great distances into the posterior pituitary,

is obscure. Such an arrangement may have been necessary, teleologically, in order to provide rapid access of the hormones into the systemic circulation through the highly vascularized posterior pituitary. However, there is good evidence that the neurohypophysis produces a neurohormone, identical with or closely related to vasopressin, which regulates the release of ACTH from the anterior pituitary (corticotropin-releasing factor, CRF), and additional evidence that oxytocin regulates the secretion of prolactin or lactogenic hormone by the anterior lobe. Thus, the secretions of the neurohypophysis may provide an important link between the central nervous system and the secretion of anterior pituitary tropic hormones which so profoundly influence the body economy.

In view of this evidence, consideration of the posterior pituitary as an endocrine gland warrants revision, and reference should be made to the neurohypophysis when discussing this endocrine system. However, the terms posterior pituitary gland and posterior lobe hormone are still in common usage at the present time.

NATURE OF NEUROHYPOPHYSEAL HORMONES

Extracts of the neurohypophysis are assayed biologically with reference to oxytocic, vasopressor and antidiuretic activity. One international USP or BP unit is defined as the activity of 0.5 mg of an international standard posterior pituitary powder. In

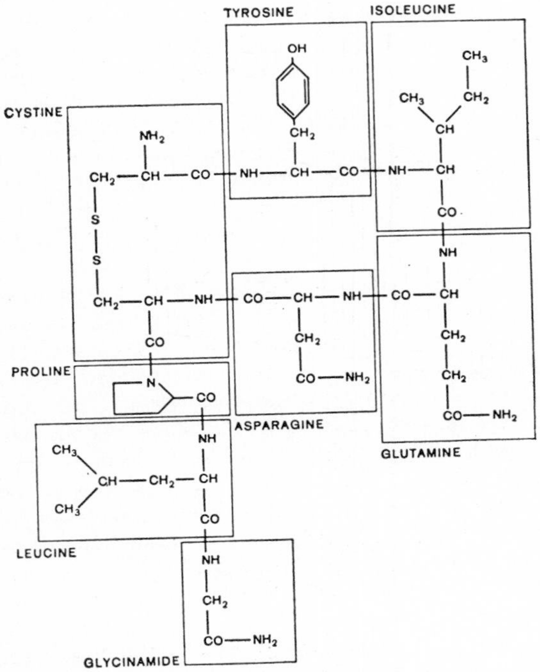

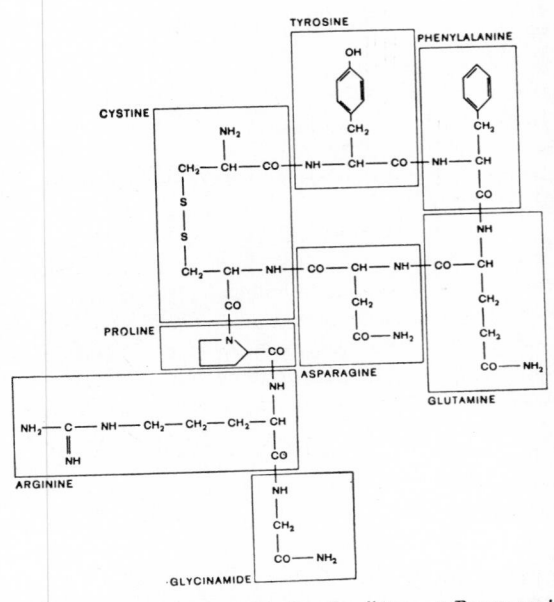

FIG. 65-2. Oxytocin. (B. Berde: "Recent Progress in Oxytocin Research," Fig. 1, Springfield, Ill., Charles C Thomas, 1959.)

FIG. 65-3. Vasopressin. (B. Berde: "Recent Progress in Oxytocin Research," Fig. 2, Springfield, Ill., Charles C Thomas, 1959.)

crude extracts of the posterior lobe the biologic activity appears to reside in a homogeneous protein or polypeptide fraction having a molecular weight of the order of 30,000 and an isoelectric point of pH 4.8. Such fractions show approximately equal vasopressor and oxytocic activities in terms of the reference powder, of the order of 16.6 IU per mg. It has not been conclusively established whether this protein represents the natural secretion of the neurohypophysis or whether vasopressin and oxytocin, which are loosely bound to the protein by electrostatic forces, are released in a free form into the circulation.

Using modern technics of ion exchange chromatography and countercurrent distribution, highly purified preparations of vasopressin (600 IU per mg) and oxytocin (500 IU per mg) have been obtained from posterior lobe extracts.

Both vasopressin and oxytocin have been shown to contain eight amino acids and 3 moles of ammonia. The peptide structure of each hormone has been determined, and both hormones have been successfully synthesized by du Vigneaud and his coworkers, representing a milestone in protein chemistry and hormone research. Both hormones are composed of five amino acids arranged in the form of a ring closed by the disulfide linkage of cystine, with a side chain of three amino acids. Oxytocin contains cystine, tyrosine, isoleucine, glutamic acid, and aspartic acid in the ring, with proline, leucine, and glycine in the side chain (Fig. 65-2). Vasopressin differs from oxytocin by only two amino acids. Phenylalanine replaces isoleucine in the ring, and leucine in the side chain is replaced by arginine (human, beef vasopressin, Fig. 65-3) or lysine (hog vasopressin). The molecular weight of oxytocin is 1,007 and that of arginine vasopressin 1,084. Both are ampholytes, oxytocin having an isoelectric point (IP) of pH 7.7, and arginine vasopressin being considerably more basic, with an IP of pH 10.9.

Oxytocin has been shown to possess slight but definite pressor and antidiuretic effects, whereas vasopressin contains not only equal pressor and antidiuretic activities, but also significant intrinsic oxytocic and milk-ejecting properties. Partially purified posterior pituitary preparations available commercially include Pitocin (oxytocin) and Pitressin (vasopressin), each fraction being slightly contaminated by the other in pharmaceutic preparations. Synthetic oxytocin is also available for clinical use under the trade name of Syntocinon.

REGULATION OF SECRETION OF NEUROHYPOPHYSEAL HORMONES

The neurohypophysis responds to a wide variety of physiologic and pharmacologic stimuli, generally by secretion of both hormones irrespective of the nature of the stimulus. Since the kidney is exquisitely sensitive to the antidiuretic action, a decrease in urine flow is most easily demonstrable following neurohypophyseal stimulation. The effects of oxytocin on the uterus and breast are less obvious, except in special experimental situations, because of the relatively large doses required to elicit a detectable response. Elaboration of vasopressin (ADH) can be induced by a rise in the osmotic pressure of the extracellular fluid, by circulatory changes and by direct nervous system stimulation. The first mechanism is probably of major significance in the daily control of water balance and is mediated principally by changes in the concentration of sodium in the extracellular fluid. The locus of response to osmotic stimulation is somewhere within the distribution of the internal carotid arteries and may reside within the neurohypophysis. The osmotic response may be absent in some patients with posterior pituitary destruction or vascular insufficiency or following surgical extirpation. Secretion of vasopressin with hypothalamic (neural) stimulation may be maintained, however, indicating preservation of hypothalamic centers for vasopressin production. These findings suggest that the osmotic regulation of vasopressin secretion may depend on the presence of posterior pituitary tissue or an intact hypophyseal circulation although they may also be explained on quantitative differences in vasopressin release with osmotic and neurogenic stimuli.

A decrease in plasma osmotic pressure (osmolality) such as occurs with water administration inhibits the secretion of vasopressin and allows a diuresis of water to ensue; secretion is restored when plasma osmolality returns to normal. This very sensitive osmoregulatory mechanism normally protects and maintains an optimal state of body hydration.

An auxiliary mechanism regulating vasopressin secretion, which may be of more importance than osmotic pressure, especially in pathologic conditions, is the influence of the state of intravascular volume on neurohypophyseal function. Thus, the antidiuresis of quiet standing, hemorrhage, venous congestion, etc., is probably mediated either through an alteration of the volume of blood flowing to the neurohypophysis or by an over-all contraction of effective blood volume leading to stimulation of the hypothalamic nuclei by ill-defined afferent nervous pathways. There is some evidence that stretch receptors in the wall of the right atrium sensitive to volume or pressure changes may initiate afferent nervous impulses to the hypothalamus, regulating vasopressin release.

Of the two vascular modalities, osmolality and volume, the former apparently operates effectively in most normal situations by retaining or releasing body water to suit the needs of the body. However, in pathologic conditions characterized by a decrease in intravascular volume or in cardiac output, volume regulation supersedes osmoregulation. In this situation, vasopressin secretion may persist despite the simultaneous occurrence of hypotonicity. A primary decrease in osmolality, such as seen in the hyponatremia of Addison's disease, salt-losing nephritis, long-standing congestive heart failure, etc., would result in severe depletion of body water if osmolality were the only factor governing vasopressin secretion. A regulator of secretion sensitive to the volume of the body water or the fullness of the vascular compartment or both would protect against desiccation and vascular collapse in these situations, the body giving up an optimal osmotic state for the vital requirements of the tissues for water. This antidiuretic mechanism, although protective in nature, may lead to serious complications, particularly in disorders already characterized by fluid retention and edema, since constant water retention in salt-restricted subjects may lead to severe hyponatremia, water intoxication, and further compromise of circulation and renal function.

There are similar regulatory mechanisms for sodium conservation, mediated at least in part through the secretion of salt-retaining adrenal steroids, of which aldosterone is the most potent. Aldosterone secretion is influenced by the plasma concentrations of sodium and potassium as well as by the intravascular or extracellular volume. Aldosterone secretion may be inhibited by volume expansion despite the presence of hyponatremia. In this respect regulation of aldosterone secretion resembles that of vasopressin secretion, the influence of fluid volume having precedence over ionic concentration. It is probable that an intimate relationship exists between the adrenal steroid, aldosterone, governing sodium metabolism, and vasopressin controlling water metabolism.

Current studies into the hypothalamic regulation of ACTH secretion have shown that neurohypophyseal substances resembling but not identical to vasopressin may be mediators of ACTH release. The secretion of aldosterone is regulated in part by ACTH as well as by the hypothalamus and other areas of the central nervous system. The hypothalamus, then, may influence water and sodium metabolism by regulating both vasopressin and adrenal steroid secretion. The rapid effect of intravascular volume changes on the secretion of these hormones may reflect a first line of defense whereby hormone secretion is governed by the quantity of blood perfusing the glands or some critical intravascular receptor area. The hypothalamic-pituitary mechanism may serve to augment secretion under conditions that would require more prolonged hormonal effects.

In view of the fact that the neurohypophyseal hormones represent secretions of the nervous system, further studies of the neural control of the neurohypophysis have assumed great importance in neuroendocrine physiology. There is little doubt that the central nervous system exerts a dominant role in the control of neurohypophyseal secretion, neural stimuli easily superseding the relatively weak effect of fluid volume and osmolality on vasopressin release. Secretion of vasopressin has been produced in man and monkeys by electrical stimulation of the subcortical "limbic system," including the hippocampal gyrus, the amygdoloid nucleus, and the septal region, as well as by electrical stimulation of the hypothalamus. Electrical stimulation of various areas of the cerebral cortex, however, has been shown not to evoke vasopressin release, suggesting that neural reflexes regulating the neurohypophysis may be transmitted primarily via the more primitive areas of the brain rather than through cortical pathways.

Numerous centrally acting substances influence the neurohypophysis. Some of these include emotional stresses such as fright, noise, and pain; fainting, which may also act through volume regulators; coitus, suckling, changes in environmental temperature, etc.; and numerous drugs such as nicotine, acetylcholine, and many hypnotics and sedatives. Alcohol inhibits vasopressin secretion. Of the various hormones and endogenous substances, small doses of epinephrine inhibit and large doses stimulate the release of vasopressin, at least in animals. Ferritin, the iron-containing hepatic vasodepressor substance, is antidiuretic by virtue of stimulating the neurohypophysis, and the hydrocortisone-like adrenal steroids have been shown to inhibit vasopressin secretion (see below).

Thus, it is readily apparent that the neurohypophyseal hormones are secreted in diverse situations. Their importance in the body economy and in the pathogenesis or the complications of disease is poorly defined. With the availability of synthetic preparations, specific assay methods, and greater knowledge of the mechanisms of hormone production and secretion, significant advances in neurohypophyseal physiology may be anticipated in the not-too-distant future.

PHYSIOLOGIC ACTIONS OF NEUROHYPOPHYSEAL HORMONES

Vasopressin (ADH). The pressor and antidiuretic activities of vasopressin are properties of a single molecule. The antidiuretic action is of profound importance in the regulation of water balance. The current hypothesis as to the mechanism of action of vasopressin on water reabsorption by the kidney, based upon experiments with various biologic membranes such as frog skin and toad bladder, is that it renders the cells of the distal convoluted tubules and perhaps the collecting tubules permeable to water, permitting passive diffusion of tubular water along an osmotic gradient across the cell and into the peritubular vessels. The antidiuretic action of vasopressin is best demonstrated during excess hydration and water diuresis; *this effect represents the true physiologic role of the hormone on water metabolism, which is to prevent the bulk of the filtered water entering the distal tubular segment from escaping into the urine.* The effect of vasopressin during hypertonic urine flow is extremely variable and limited by a maximum rate of water reabsorption which the concentrating mechanism of the collecting tubules can achieve.

An interesting aspect of the studies of the action of vasopressin on biologic membranes has been the demonstration that this hormone has a pronounced effect on transport of sodium as well as water across cell boundaries. The effect of vasopressin on sodium excretion by the kidneys is, however, extremely variable and dependent upon the experimental design. It is probable that vasopressin does not have a direct effect on salt excretion and that any observed change in sodium or chloride balance is secondary to the modifying influence of this hormone on the total volume and the distribution of body water.

Vasopressin has been shown to exert a pressor effect in persons with postural hypotension, and large intravenous doses may also produce transient increases in blood pressure even in normal man. The significance of this observation in relationship to blood pressure regulation in normal persons is unknown. Generally, posterior lobe preparations as used therapeutically in man have no consistent effect on blood pressure, probably because of compensatory adjustments elsewhere in the circulation.

Oxytocin. Studies with purified and synthetic oxytocin have significantly advanced understanding of the role of this hormone in uterine function and milk secretion. Oxytocin has been shown to be the hormonal substance of posterior lobe extracts responsible for release of milk from the lactating breast, as little as 0.5 unit, or 1 μg, of synthetic hormone producing a copious flow of milk within 30 sec after intravenous injection. Synthetic oxytocin has also been used successfully in the initiation of labor, and as previously mentioned, there is good evidence that oxytocin stimulates or sustains the secretion of prolactin by the anterior pituitary. Oxytocin therefore appears to play a very important and fundamental role in reproduction. Vasopressin also possesses oxytocic and milk-ejecting properties but is much less potent than oxytocin in this regard.

Other effects of oxytocin which warrant consideration include its marked but evanescent and unsustained vasodepressor action demonstrable both in human beings and in experimental animals and its effects on water excretion and renal function. In appropriate experimental situations, oxytocin has been shown to antagonize the antidiuretic action of vasopressin and to increase renal plasma flow and the excretion of sodium, the latter effect currently attributable to an action of the hormone on the brain which is abolished by hypophysectomy or the induction of diabetes insipidus. The demonstration that some of the actions of oxytocin are directly opposed to those of vasopressin imply a physiologic system for regulation of the volume and composition of the body fluids as well as the arterial pressure under the control of the central nervous system and the hypothalamus which, although obscure at this time, may prove to be of clinical significance in the future.

ADRENOCORTICAL-NEUROHYPOPHYSEAL RELATIONSHIPS

Ever since crude adrenal cortical extracts were found to protect against water intoxication and enhance the diuretic response to water administration, the interaction of adrenal steroids and ADH on water metabolism has been studied extensively. Hydrocortisone, the principal glucocorticoid secreted by the human adrenal cortex, has been shown to inhibit the release of vasopressin from the neurohypophysis. This inhibition appears to act selectively on the hypothalamic (neural) control of vasopressin release, since secretion with osmotic stimulation of the neurohypophysis is not similarly affected.

Steroids may induce a transient water diuresis in normal subjects, but the loss of body water and the induction of hypertonicity will activate the osmoregulatory control of vasopressin secretion. In patients with neurohypophyseal insufficiency, a more complete state of diabetes insipidus can be induced with hydrocortisone administration, and a greater loss of solute-free water from the kidney occurs. The physiologic importance of this effect of hydrocortisone on secretion of the hormone governing water metabolism has not been fully delineated, but it may represent a hormonal mechanism for independent regulation of the body content of sodium and water. Thus, the diuretic effect of adrenal steroids may be mediated not through primary effects on water metabolism, but indirectly by alteration of the secretory activity of the neurohypophysis.

Patients with complete absence of vasopressin secretion do not have a true water diuresis with adrenal hormone administration. However, since these hormones, at times, increase solute excretion by the kidney, there may be a concomitant increase in water excretion because of an inability of the kidney, in the absence of vasopressin, to increase adequately the solute concentration of the urine. This diuresis may be termed "an obligatory excretion of solute-free water" and cannot be regarded as being hormonally mediated.

An additional effect of adrenal steroids on water metabolism, which may be related to their action on the neural control of the neurohypophysis, is the occasional production of polydipsia with steroid therapy. A steroid effect on thirst-regulating centers of the hypothalamus which are in close proximity anatomically to the supraoptic nuclei may be responsible for the polydipsia. A similar mechanism may account for the experimental production of a polydipsic syndrome in animals receiving large doses of adrenal steroids. The polydipsia is quickly relieved by withdrawal of hormone treatment.

Although demonstrable in animals, an antagonistic effect of adrenal steroids on the antidiuretic action of vasopressin has not been observed in man. The adrenal steroids appear to influence water metabolism in three ways in man: (1) by inhibition of the neural control of vasopressin secretion and diuresis of water subsequent to a decrease in vasopressin action on the kidney; (2) by occasionally increasing the obligatory excretion of water, in the absence of vasopressin, secondary to a solute diuresis; (3) by production of the sensation of thirst, possibly by influencing hypothalamic thirst centers which may be sensitive to alterations in autonomic activity in the region of the supraoptic nuclei.

VASOPRESSIN DEFICIENCY— DIABETES INSIPIDUS

Diabetes insipidus is a chronic symptom complex characterized by the passage of large quantities of pale, dilute urine, with secondary polydipsia. It results from a defect in the chain of events by which vasopressin is released from the neurohypophysis and acts on the cells of the renal tubules. The classic anatomic and physiologic studies of Fisher, Ingram, and Ranson revealed that the disease may be caused by interference with the functional integrity of the neurohormonal unit comprising the supraoptic and paraventricular nuclei of the hypothalamus, the supraopticohypophyseal tract, and the posterior lobe of the hypophysis. The full-blown disease occurs only with interruption of the tract close enough to the hypothalamus to cause degeneration of at least 85 per cent of the supraoptic and paraventricular

neurones. There is also a relatively rare disorder of nephrogenic diabetes insipidus which exhibits a familial distribution. This disorder may be due to a hereditary refractoriness of the renal tubules to vasopressin, and it is presumed that there is no neurohypophyseal disease in this group.

The incidence of classical diabetes insipidus following hypophysectomy may be significantly diminished if damage to the supraoptic neurones is minimized by careful severance of the pituitary stalk as close to the pituitary gland as possible. The polyuria of hypophysectomized persons has been shown to vary with the magnitude of vasopressin deficiency, those patients devoid of this secretion demonstrating persistent polyuria despite withdrawal of adrenocortical replacement therapy. These observations illustrate the important role of vasopressin in determining the rate of water excretion and corroborate the concept that the diuretic effect of adrenal steroids is mediated indirectly through an effect on vasopressin secretion. The adrenal steroids may increase urine volume in such patients, however, by increasing solute excretion.

The thyrotropic and growth hormones of the anterior pituitary are necessary for maintenance of polyuria, probably by influencing the nutritional state and solute turnover as well as by sustaining renal function. A peripheral antagonism of vasopressin action by thyroid hormone has been demonstrated, but this effect may not be a direct one.

Incidence. Diabetes insipidus is a rare disease, having a slightly greater incidence in youth and in males. In 1924 Rowntree reported 10 and 16 cases, respectively, in two series of 100,000 admissions to the Mayo Clinic. With the advent of hypophysectomy in recent years for the treatment of far-advanced breast carcinoma and other serious disorders, the disease is becoming much more frequent in the general hospital population.

Etiology. As shown by Fink's pathologic studies in 107 cases, the great majority of instances of this disease are due to anatomic lesions involving the hypothalamic-hypophyseal system and hence, presumably, interfering with the production of vasopressin. In clinical practice, it will often be impossible to elicit any other evidence of such a lesion; while the label *idiopathic* may be justifiable for such cases ante mortem, the finding of an anatomic lesion at autopsy generally may be predicted.

Pathology. The primary pathologic processes associated most frequently with the syndrome have been tumors of the diencephalopituitary region, basilar meningitis, and, in children, xanthochromatosis (Hand-Schüller-Christian syndrome). Transitory and occasionally permanent polyuria frequently follows severe cranial injuries. Pathologic changes consist of those due to the primary disorder, such as tumor, brain injury, inflammation, etc.; and secondary changes in the urogenital tract, such as dilatation and hypertrophy of the bladder with megaloureter.

Clinical Picture. The chief symptoms of diabetes insipidus are polyuria and polydipsia. The loss of large amounts of pale urine of low specific gravity (1.001 to 1.005), often as much as 15 to 29 liters per day, results in dehydration and, consequently, in such related symptoms and signs as dry skin, constipation, and an intense, almost insatiable thirst. Water deprivation to the limit of tolerance does *not* prevent polyuria, nor does it lead to a significant increase in urinary specific gravity. Thus, in this disease, polydipsia is secondary to polyuria, in contrast to patients with psychogenic polydipsia, who pass large quantities of urine as an aftermath of a large fluid intake. In patients with diabetes insipidus, no consistent physical or chemical changes are noted other than those of dehydration. However, there may be symptoms referable to the localized disease process causing the syndrome.

The role of trauma in the production of diabetes insipidus deserves special comment, since the polyuria which sometimes follows head injury is not infrequently transient, as contrasted with the chronicity of most other forms of the disease. A similar syndrome may develop subsequent to cerebrovascular accidents or intracranial surgery, and in association with other forms of cerebral disease. When the full-blown syndrome develops under these conditions, serious dehydration may occur before the diagnosis is suspected, particularly in the incontinent patient or in the patient with clouded sensorium who is unable to request or partake of an adequate volume of fluids. The dehydration, which is due principally to water loss, may be accentuated by the administration of isotonic saline or solutions containing large amounts of protein. Such large solute loads will aggravate the renal loss of water in these patients because of a failure to increase adequately the solute concentration of the urine.

Diagnosis. The symptoms plus the large urine volume with specific gravity below 1.010, unassociated with a history of other findings of diabetes mellitus or of chronic renal disease, will quickly suggest diabetes insipidus. Since, however, this diagnosis commits the patient to a regimen of daily injections for an indefinite period, it is not to be made lightly, and the clinical impression should be supported by careful studies made under hospital conditions. All cases of diabetes insipidus, moreover, should be studied carefully for active intracranial lesions, which should be presumed present until proved otherwise. Thus, examination should include, in addition to the differential tests of water

excretion outlined below, a study of the spinal fluid, roentgenograms of the skull and chest (metastatic disease), electroencephalogram, serologic test (syphilis), the serum protein level, sternal marrow aspiration (multiple myeloma), and visual fields.

Differential Diagnosis. The syndrome must be differentiated from psychogenic polydipsia, chronic nephritis, diabetes mellitus and the polydipsia and polyuria so characteristically associated with the hypochloremic alkalotic syndrome, and the hypercalcemic syndrome associated with such conditions as hyperparathyroidism and vitamin D intoxication. Chronic nephritis may be excluded by the absence of protein or formed elements in the urine, a normal blood nonprotein nitrogen level, and normal kidney function tests. Often the most difficult differential diagnosis is that between diabetes insipidus and psychogenic polydipsia. Other procedures which are helpful in making a differential diagnosis may be described as follows:

1. Dehydration for 8 to 12 hr should be performed cautiously during the day, with close observation of the patient for signs of vasomotor collapse, which can occur with sudden severe dehydration. An inability to increase the specific gravity of the urine to hypertonic levels is characteristic of diabetes insipidus and serves to differentiate this syndrome from psychogenic polydipsia but not from chronic nephritis. Great care must be taken in suspected psychogenic cases to be certain that the patient does not have access to water or other fluids.

2. Alleviation of symptoms will follow repeated small doses of Pitressin, i.e., 0.2 ml every 3 to 4 hr. This differentiates diabetes insipidus from chronic nephritis but not from psychogenic polydipsia. The possibility of Pitressin-resistant diabetes insipidus must always be kept in mind, since 5 to 15 per cent of cases of diabetes insipidus fall into this category.

3. Tests of secretory function. Since the secretion of vasopressin can be initiated by either neurogenic or osmotic stimuli, both the hypothalamic neurones and the osmoregulators must be stimulated in turn for proper evaluation of the integrity of this neurohormonal unit. In addition, the adequacy of renal tubular responsiveness to vasopressin must also be measured to understand fully the nature of the polyuria. The functional integrity of the neurohypophyseal-renal system may be fairly completely evaluated within a period of a few hours by serial intravenous injections of nicotine, hypertonic saline solution, and Pitressin under constant water-loading conditions. Acute changes in solute-free water clearance (C_{H_2O}) during a water diuresis reflect the action of vasopressin on the renal tubular reabsorption of water and may be regarded as a useful index

of the secretory capacity of the neurohypophysis.[1]

Technique. The patient is hydrated with 20 ml water per kg body weight over a 30- to 60-min period. Preliminary dehydration is unnecessary and may be dangerous. Urine is collected by spontaneous voiding if at all possible or else through an indwelling catheter at 15- to 30-min intervals, and a constant state of hydration is maintained by oral or intravenous administration of a volume of fluid equal to that excreted during the preceding collection period. When a sustained high rate of urine flow is reached (over 5 ml per min), a nicotine solution is injected intravenously over a period of 1 to 3 min—1 mg nicotine base to nonsmokers and as much as 3 mg to smokers. As an alternative, the subject may smoke 1 to 3 cigarettes rapidly and with deep inhalation. The dose of nicotine is gradually increased by 0.5 to 1.0 mg at intervals of 30 min until a clear-cut antidiuretic response ensues or the occurrence of symptoms of nicotine intoxication (i.e., vertigo, nausea, vomiting) precludes further administration.

The normal response to nicotine which occurs within 15 to 30 min after injection is associated with a fall in urine flow and free water clearance and a rise in urinary creatinine, chloride, and total solute (Fig. 65-4). Patients with diabetes insipidus usually do not evidence a fall in water excretion with normal doses of nicotine; however, many of them will have an antidiuresis of some degree with much larger amounts (5 to 6 mg nicotine base), suggesting residual neurohypophyseal activity insufficient to influence water balance significantly. When urine flow returns to control levels, 15 to 25 milliunits

[1] The urine volume (V) is equal to the algebraic sum of the osmolal clearance (C_{osm}) and solute-free water clearance (C_{H_2O}).

$$C_{H_2O} = V - C_{osm}$$

$$C_{osm} = V \frac{\text{total solute conc. urine}}{\text{total solute conc. plasma}}$$

C_{osm} represents the volume of water required to contain the urinary solutes in a solution isosmotic with plasma. C_{H_2O} represents the net excess or deficit of water beyond the osmolal clearance; it will be positive during a water diuresis and negative when urine is concentrated by the abstraction of solute-free water, as in antidiuresis. C_{H_2O} usually parallels urine flow during water diuresis studies, since osmolal clearance remains relatively constant. This index is particularly useful in determining the changes in water excretion occurring during the solute diuresis usually observed with hypertonic saline administration. Not infrequently, a large increase in C_{osm} may mask a concomitant decrease in C_{H_2O}. In this instance, urinary flow may fall only slightly or may actually increase even though an increase in water reabsorption may be under way, under the influence of released vasopressin.

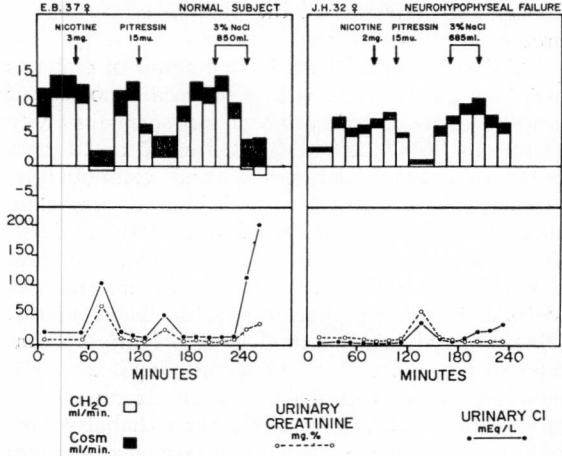

EFFECT OF INTRAVENOUS NICOTINE, HYPERTONIC SALINE AND PITRESSIN IN A NORMAL SUBJECT AND IN A PATIENT WITH DIABETES INSIPIDUS

FIG. 65-4. See text and footnote. Patient J.H., a nonsmoker, was given twice the usual dose of nicotine.

aqueous Pitressin is injected intravenously. The response to Pitressin differentiates renal disease from true diabetes insipidus.

The administration of water is discontinued with the Pitressin injection to decrease the volume of retained water in preparation for the administration of hypertonic saline solution, since excessive hydration may abolish the osmotic response by diluting the hypertonic saline as it enters the circulation. When the antidiuresis to Pitressin is completed, 3 per cent saline (10 ml per kg) is infused rapidly intravenously over a 30- to 45-min period. In normal persons a marked reduction in water excretion will occur during the infusion or within the following 30 min. In patients with diabetes insipidus, this antidiuresis does not occur and a rise in free water clearance is frequently observed (Fig. 65-4). Patients with psychogenic polydipsia demonstrate a normal antidiuresis to the hypertonic saline infusion but, curiously, many do not respond normally to nicotine, suggesting some derangement in hypothalamic function and neural regulation of vasopressin release in this disorder.

The response to nicotine, to hypertonic saline solution, and to Pitressin may be used to differentiate the locus of the functional disturbance which is responsible for the polyuria, i.e., hypothalamus, osmoregulators, and renal tubules.

By the serial use of these techniques, it has been possible to demonstrate that certain patients with diabetes insipidus apparently have secreting neurohypophyseal tissue which is responsive to normal doses of nicotine but not to hypertonic saline solution. Postmortem studies on one such patient with metastatic breast carcinoma demonstrated an abundance of secretory granules within the neurones of the intact supraoptic nuclei, but the posterior pituitary and stalk were devoid of hormone and completely destroyed by tumor. This phenomenon suggests that a selective failure of osmoregulatory function may be responsible for the syndrome of diabetes insipidus in certain patients with posterior pituitary disease in whom significant neurohypophyseal function may still be demonstrable.

Treatment. Treatment of diabetes insipidus may be divided into two phases: (1) correction of the underlying intracranial difficulty, if present, and (2) replacement therapy with vasopressin.

Usually the hormone must be continued throughout life. It may be given as subcutaneous injections of aqueous Pitressin, as nasal insufflation of posterior pituitary powder, or preferably as Pitressin tannate in oil by subcutaneous or intramuscular injection.

Pitressin is a brand of vasopressin or beta-hypophamine; it is supplied in 0.5- and 1-ml ampuls with a strength of 20 IU pressor activity per milliliter. The quantity of Pitressin required to ameliorate the symptoms is very small (0.1 to 0.2 ml), but the evanescent action of the aqueous preparation necessitates repeated injections at 3- to 4-hr intervals, making this form of treatment impractical for prolonged periods.

Nasal insufflations of dried posterior pituitary powder (supplied in 5- and 30-Gm bottles) every 3 to 6 hr, depending upon the amount insufflated, accomplish the same purpose and are more easily administered, but some patients develop a chronic rhinopharyngitis and even gastritis from powder which is swallowed.

Pitressin tannate in oil is supplied in 1-ml ampuls with a strength of 5 IU per ml. This preparation provides relatively long action of the hormone with a single injection administered every 24 to 72 hr. A test dose of 0.3 to 0.5 ml (1.5 to 2.5 units) should be given initially to determine the effectiveness of treatment and to guard against the serious, but fortunately rare, occurrence of excess fluid retention and water intoxication in particularly sensitive individuals. For practical purposes of economy, chronic treatment with 1.0-ml doses of hormone should be tried and the frequency of injection gauged by the recurrence of symptoms. Most patients will retain 1 to 2 kg water following an injection, and the dissipation of effective hormone levels will be attended with a sudden polyuria and loss of body weight prior to the onset of polydipsia. In general, injections should be timed to coincide with the onset of polyuria in order to prevent marked fluctuations in body water content and fluid compartmental shifts. The hormone is preferably given in the evening to ensure a restful night. *Great care should be employed to caution patients to warm the vial of Pitressin tannate and to shake it repeatedly and thoroughly, since the active material has a tendency to precipitate out in the vial.*

Occasionally, patients with vasopressin-sensitive diabetes insipidus may develop resistance to the action of the hormone, in some cases accompanied by allergy either to the hormone or to the oily menstruum. Allergy to the latter may be easily corrected by use of a different medium, and hormone allergy may be overcome by desensitization. Vasopressin resistance is also observed in patients with hypercalcemia or hypercalcuria, and disorders of calcium metabolism should be investigated and treated in all such instances.

Both chlorothiazide and hydrochlorothiazide have been shown to increase free water reabsorption in diabetes insipidus. These drugs, however, will decrease urine flow by no more than about 30 to 50 per cent, and patients usually will continue to require vasopressin therapy as well to prevent abnormally large urine volumes. The thiazide derivatives may have their greatest usefulness in lessening polyuria in the rare form of vasopressin-resistant diabetes insipidus. The average daily dose of chlorothiazide is 0.5 to 1.0 Gm and of hydrochlorothiazide 0.05 to 0.1 Gm given in divided doses.

The prognosis of this chronic deficiency syndrome if adequate replacement therapy is given is that of the initiating disease process.

EXCESS OF ANTIDIURETIC HORMONE

Abnormally elevated levels of antidiuretic substances in blood and urine have been reported in a variety of disease states associated with edema or defects in water diuresis, including cardiac failure, cirrhosis with ascites, nephrosis, and Addison's disease. While the hypothesis that excessive antidiuretic activity may be responsible for the water retention observed in edematous patients is quite attractive, proof has not been clearly established. It is generally agreed that patients with these disorders do not show excessive sensitivity to or a delayed inactivation of exogenously administered Pitressin. Some studies with nicotine stimulation of endogenous vasopressin secretion in patients with edema have yielded normal results, but some patients whose disease is associated with severe hyponatremia have shown enhanced neurohypophyseal response to nicotine and other stimuli. Many of the studies which minimize the role of vasopressin in edema formation are based upon data obtained from patients in equilibrium with their fluid retention who are capable of excreting water loads, although at a somewhat depressed rate. It is obvious that vasopressin release mechanisms should be evaluated during the active phase of edema formation, but studies in such patients have been hampered by the fact that they frequently cannot excrete administered water, which automatically vitiates the biologic end point of vasopressin action, i.e., antidiuresis. Further advancement in this field will depend upon the development and application of precise and reliable methods for measurement of vasopressin levels in the plasma.

The level of vasopressin in the body fluids need not necessarily be increased to account for water retention, since even physiologic amounts effectively halt a water diuresis. The abnormality in water metabolism may be primarily related to a *persistence* of vasopressin secretion despite the presence of an excess body water or of hypotonicity, situations which normally should invoke a water diuresis. It appears that the distribution rather than the total quantity of body water may determine the secretory activity of the neurohypophysis, and more extensive studies of the precedence of volume versus osmoregulation of vasopressin secretion should shed more light on the nature of fluid retention in these disorders.

The interrelationships between the neurohypophyseal secretion and the adrenal secretion of aldosterone are not well defined. Patients with aldosterone-secreting adrenal tumors do not usually develop edema, and normal subjects treated with aldosterone have been shown to escape readily from sodium and water retention. Furthermore, patients with diabetes insipidus will retain sodium with aldosterone therapy but will not retain water unless they simultaneously receive vasopressin. It is probable that both vasopressin and aldosterone are necessary for the retention of edema fluid and that their secretion is sustained in patients with fundamental derangements in circulation.

REFERENCES

Arimura, A., and J. F. Dingman: Specific and Sensitive Assay Method for Vasopressin and Oxytocin Using Glass Paper Chromatography, Nature, 184:1878, 1959.

Berde, B.: "Recent Progress in Oxytocin Research," Springfield, Ill., Charles C Thomas, 1959.

Dingman, J. F.: Hypothalamus and the Endocrine Control of Sodium and Water Metabolism in Man, Am. J. Med. Sci., 235:79, 1958.

——, K. Benirschke, and G. W. Thorn: Studies of Neurohypophyseal Function in Man: I. Diabetes Insipidus and Psychogenic Polydipsia, Am. J. Med., 23:226, 1957.

—— and R. H. Despointes: Adrenal Steroid Inhibition of Vasopressin Release from the Neurohypophysis of Normal Subjects and Patients with Addison's Disease, J. Clin. Invest., 39:1851, 1960.

Du Vigneaud, V.: Trail of Sulfur Research: From Insulin to Oxytocin, Science, 123:967, 1956.

Fink, E. B.: Diabetes Insipidus: A Clinical Review and Analysis of Autopsy Reports, Arch. Pathol., 6:102, 1928.

Fisher, D., W. R. Ingram, and S. W. Ranson: "Diabetes Insipidus," Ann Arbor, Mich., Edwards Bros., Inc., 1938.

Lewis, A. A. G., and T. M. Chalmers: A Nicotine Test for the Investigation of Diabetes Insipidus, Clin. Sci., 10:137, 1951.

Scharrer, E., and B. Scharrer: Hormones Produced by Neurosecretory Cells, Recent Progr. Hormone Research, 10:183, 1954.

Van Dyke, H. B., K. Adamsons, Jr., and S. L. Engel: Aspects of the Biochemistry and Physiology of the Neurohypophyseal Hormones, Recent Progr. Hormone Research, 11:1, 1955.

Verney, E. B.: Absorption and Excretion of Water, Lancet, II:739, 1946.

Williams, R. H., and H. Cole: Nephrogenic Diabetes Insipidus: Transmitted by Females and Appearing during Infancy in Males, Ann. Internal Med., 27:84, 1947.

66 DISEASES OF THE THYROID GLAND

S. Richardson Hill, Jr., and Herbert A. Selenkow

Diseases of the thyroid gland result as a consequence of either increases in gland size (goiter, neoplasm) or alterations in its hormonal secretions. Changes in gland size and weight (normally 16 to 35 Gm) are associated with toxic or nontoxic goiter, adenomas, thyroiditis, or malignancies. Symptoms may arise from local compression in the neck and superior mediastinum, from disturbances in hormonogenesis producing hypothyroidism or hyperthyroidism, or from malignancy. With abnormalities in the secretion of hormone, far-reaching metabolic disturbances occur. The thyroid hormones normally regulate the rate of cellular oxidative processes throughout the body, but the exact mechanism by which they act is not completely understood. An excess of thyroid hormones induces a significant rise in basal oxygen consumption of tissues (hypermetabolism). Insufficiency of thyroid hormones is followed by a reduction in the rate of oxidative reactions (hypometabolism).

In 1891 Murray, an English physician, administered thyroid substance to a myxedematous patient, who subsequently improved remarkably. The material employed was a glycerine extract obtained from sheep thyroids. Magnus-Levy, in 1895, observed that thyroid medication was followed by an increase in basal metabolic rate in patients with hypothyroidism. In 1896 Baumann obtained an acid hydrolysate of thyroid tissue in powder form which contained 10 per cent of iodine, thus establishing the high iodine content of thyroid. Oswald, 8 years later, prepared iodothyroglobulin, thus suggesting that the thyroid hormone was a protein substance. Thyroxin was first isolated by Kendall in 1915 and subsequently synthesized by Harington and Barger in 1927. 3,5,3′-Triiodothyronine was isolated chromatographically from plasma and thyroid tissue and identified in 1952 by Gross and Pitt-Rivers and by Roche, Lissitsky, and Michel.

The activity of the thyroid gland is controlled by the anterior pituitary thyrotropic or thyroid-stimulating hormone (TSH) (see p. 571). Reduction in the quantity of circulating thyroid hormones stimulates the output of TSH, which in turn increases the secretory activity of the thyroid gland. Conversely, increased levels of circulating thyroid hormones in normal persons tend to depress the secretion of TSH and so in turn reduce thyroid activity. It is thought that thyrotropic hormone is inactivated by thyroid tissue and possibly also by lymphoid and thymic tissue.

The intrathyroidal pathways of iodine metabolism (Fig. 66-1) may be divided into four basic interdependent synthetic processes. In the biosynthesis of thyroid hormones, iodide which has been absorbed into the plasma from the gastrointestinal tract is specifically concentrated or "trapped" by thyroid cells (step I). This arbitrarily designated "trap" maintains an iodide gradient across the cellular membrane between plasma and thyroid. Such a mechanism permits the thyroid gland to concentrate iodide 10 to 1,000 times above plasma levels. The gradient is increased by TSH directly, or indirectly via low thyroidal iodide stores. Inorganic anions such as perchlorate or thiocyanate inhibit the mechanism responsible for maintenance of the gradient and thus either prevent the cells from concentrating iodide or release stored iodide into the circulation. This latter phenomenon can best be demonstrated in subjects with hyperthyroidism in whom organic binding (step II) is blocked. An analogous situation has now been shown to exist in congenital goitrous cretins who exhibit the inborn error of inability to iodinate tyrosine (binding defect). These children have increased rates of trapping, as evidenced by elevated I^{131} uptakes, but release their trapped iodide upon administration of perchlorate or thiocyanate.

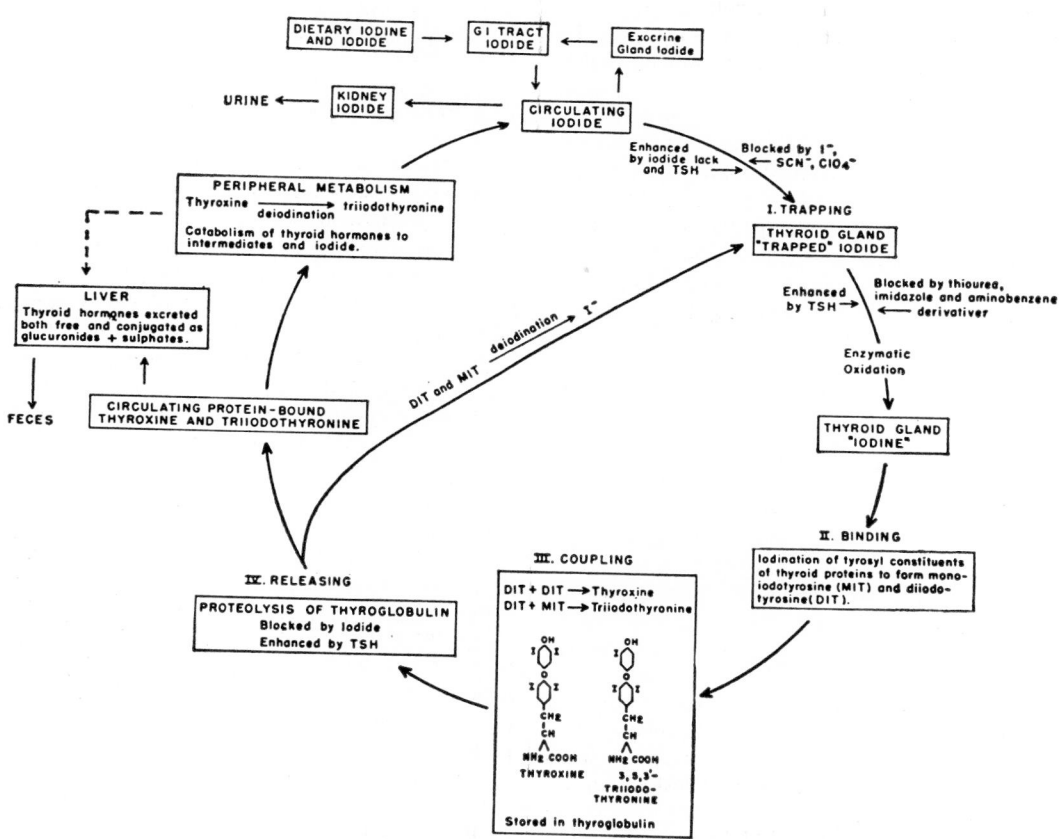

FIG. 66-1. Simplified representation of the chemical pathways of thyroid hormonogenesis.

Under physiologic conditions the trapped iodide is oxidized to a higher valance form, possibly iodine or hypoiodite, which exists only momentarily (step II). This oxidative process which apparently is enzymatically controlled, can be blocked by organic

I. TRAPPING: Plasma I^- $\xrightarrow{\text{gradient}}$ Thyroid I^-

II. BINDING : I^- $\xrightarrow{\text{oxidation}}$ $[I]$ $\longrightarrow$ Monoiodotyrosine (MIT)

             MIT + $[I]$ $\longrightarrow$ Diiodotyrosine (DIT)

III. COUPLING: DIT + DIT $\longrightarrow$ Thyroxin (T4)

             DIT + MIT $\longrightarrow$ Triiodothyronine (T3)

IV. RELEASING: Thyroglobulin $\xrightarrow{\text{proteolysis}}$ MIT + DIT + T3 + T4

             T3 + T4 $\longrightarrow$ Plasma T3 + T4

             MIT + DIT $\xrightarrow{\text{deiodination}}$ Tyrosine + Thyroid I^-

antithyroid compounds such as thiourea, mercaptoimidazole, or aniline derivatives. The iodine then rapidly combines with the tyrosine contained in thyroidal proteins to form monoiodotyrosine and diiodotyrosine. Two diiodotyrosine molecules or one each of monoiodotyrosine and diiodotyrosine are coupled in a second oxidative reaction to form thyroxin or 3,5,3'-triiodothyronine (step III). This synthesis of the thyroid hormones probably occurs while the iodotyrosine moieties are in polypeptide or protein form. Triiodothyronine may also be formed in nonthyroidal tissues by the deiodination of thyroxin. Thyroxin and 3,5,3'-triiodothyronine are stored in the thyroid follicles as thyroglobulin. Under physiologic conditions, thyroglobulin does not enter the circulation. Proteolytic enzymes in the thyroid gland hydrolyze thyroglobulin into its constituent amino acids (step IV). This hydrolysis is enhanced by TSH and decreased by iodide.

During proteolysis of thyroglobulin, the iodinated compounds released include mono- and diiodotyrosine as well as the active hormones thyroxin and triiodothyronine. However, neither mono- or diiodotyrosine enters the circulation under physiologic conditions. Tyrosine desiodinase present in normal thyroid glands removes iodide from the mono- and diiodotyrosine released by proteolysis but not from thyroxin or triiodothyronine. Thus, mono- and diiodotyrosine are prevented from entering the circulation and their iodide is conserved by being permitted to reenter the cycle. Another group of goitrous cretins appears to exemplify a defect in this enzymatic deiodination. These children release mono- and diiodotyrosine into the circulation in addition to small quantities of active thyroid hormones. Other tissues of these goitrous cretins are incapable of deiodinating iodotyrosines, thus also permitting mono- and diiodotyrosines to be excreted in their urine.

In the circulation, the thyroid hormones are al-

most entirely bound to plasma proteins, the major portion of serum thyroxin electrophoretically migrating between α_1- and α_2-globulins. The small, but probably metabolically significant remainder appears to exist unbound or "free." The inter-α-globulin which binds thyroid hormone is apparently a specific glycoprotein and is generally referred to as thyroxin-binding protein, or TBP. Some degree of thyroxin binding also occurs in both the albumin and prealbumin fractions of plasma. During pregnancy, there is an increase in the plasma protein-bound iodine level of approximately 4 μg per 100 ml which appears to be due to an absolute increase in thyroxin-binding protein. Such an increase has been reproduced in normal men and women by the administration of estrogens. In contrast, there may be a decrease in the plasma protein-bound iodine level in patients with the nephrotic syndrome which is due to an absolute decrease in TBP. The "available" or free thyroxin in both of these conditions may be entirely normal. Whereas 3,5,3'-triiodothyronine is weakly bound to plasma proteins and diffuses freely into the body cells, thyroxin is more firmly bound, dissociates slowly, and penetrates cells more slowly. This difference in binding may, in part, explain the quantitative differences in physiologic activity of these two hormones. For practical purposes, the level of endogenous organic iodine in the blood is a measure of the amount of circulating thyroxin. This is estimated as butanol-extractable iodine (BEI) or as protein-bound iodine (PBI). Serum protein-bound iodine levels following the administration of triiodothyronine to athyreotic subjects are disproportionately low when compared to the metabolic status of the patient; contrariwise, the serum protein-bound iodine levels following the administration of thyroxin tend to be somewhat elevated compared to the metabolic status of the patient.

Triiodothyronine has metabolic activity approximately fourfold that of an equimolecular quantity of thyroxin. Since various tissues have been shown to form small amounts of triiodothyronine from thyroxin, it is interesting to speculate that the rate of this transformation within the cells might constitute an autoregulatory mechanism whereby tissues may control their metabolic activity. Both hormones given orally or parenterally will simulate all the known actions of endogenous thyroid hormone. Triiodothyronine not only is more potent but also acts more rapidly than thyroxin, but for a correspondingly shorter period of time. The exact physiologic roles of the naturally occurring structural isomers of triiodothyronine, other partially iodinated thyronines, and the pyruvic and acetic acid metabolites of these hormones have not been determined.

HYPOTHYROIDISM

History. The concept that sporadic cretinism was due to the absence of the thyroid gland was first expressed by Dr. C. H. Fagge at Guy's Hospital in 1871. In 1874 Gull described adult myxedema, stating that it resembled cretinism but occurred in adult life. The term myxedema, or mucous edema, must be credited to Ord (1878). During the subsequent 4 to 5 years, the Reverdin brothers of Geneva and Kocher of Berne observed that following thyroidectomy for goiter there appeared what they termed postoperative myxedema, or cachexia strumipriva.

Incidence. Cretinism is rare in this country. The incidence of myxedema (juvenile and adult) is estimated to be 1 in every 1,500 hospital admissions. Adult myxedema occurs five times as frequently in women as in men and most frequently between the ages of thirty and sixty years.

Etiology. Hypothyroidism may be either primary (thyroid gland failure) or secondary (anterior pituitary failure). Primary hypothyroidism dating from birth results in a clinical picture characteristic of cretinism. It may occur either sporadically, as a result of athyreosis or failure of the thyroid to develop normally, or endemically, as a result of maternal iodine deficiency or genetic factors. In the endemic variety there is generally an associated goiter, whereas no thyroid tissue is palpable in the usual sporadic type. Several varieties of a familial type of sporadic goitrous cretinism have been described in which inborn errors of thyroid hormonogenesis are responsible for the inability to secrete thyroid hormones. The occurrence of primary thyroid deficiency later in life gives rise to the syndromes of juvenile and adult myxedema. Under these circumstances, inadequate production of thyroid hormones results from destruction of the thyroid gland by disease, atrophy, or ablative procedures (thyroidectomy, radioactive iodine therapy, or external radiation). Secondary hypothyroidism results from a deficiency of pituitary thyrotropin (TSH) and may occur at any age as a consequence of anterior pituitary failure (Chap. 64). Several examples of hypothyroidism following long-term iodide ingestion have also been reported.

Physiopathology. The most frequent cause of spontaneous hypothyroidism is idiopathic atrophy of the thyroid gland. Such atrophy may possibly represent the end result of an autoimmune response to thyroglobulin or other thyroid antigens and, therefore, be related to one form of chronic thyroiditis, struma lymphomatosa (Hashimoto's struma). The finding of thyroid autoantibodies in over 80 per cent of patients with spontaneous hypothyroidism does not in itself prove that preexist-

ent lymphoid thyroiditis was etiologically responsible. Low titers of similar antibodies have been found in approximately 60 per cent of patients with thyrotoxicosis and 30 per cent of patients with nontoxic colloid goiter and thyroid cancer. Excessive iodine intake over long periods of time may also produce hypothyroidism in susceptible individuals. Goiter formation may result from substances in the diet such as are present in the Brassica vegetables (turnips, rutabaga, kale, rape), from calcium in large amounts in the presence of suboptimal iodine intake, and occasionally from medications containing thiocyanate, p-amino salicylic acid, phenylbutazone, or cobalt. This form of goitrogenesis occasionally may be associated with some degree of hypothyroidism. Endemic cretinism is frequently found among the children of goitrous mothers in whom prenatal iodine deficiency, rather than genetic factors, appears to be the predominant cause. Under such circumstances, thyroid hormone administered within the first few months of life should correct most of the abnormalities. This type of endemic cretinism may be associated with deaf-mutism. In sporadic cretinism, athyreosis may be accompanied by other defects, particularly in the central nervous system. Under these circumstances early thyroid replacement therapy may not correct all existing defects. Four major groups of patients with sporadic, familial cretinism and nodular goiter have been delineated on the basis of biochemical anomalies. These anomalies include: (1) failure to bind iodide into an organic form despite normal trapping, (2) failure of intrathyroidal conservation of iodide due to an inability to deiodinate iodotyrosines, (3) failure to couple iodotyrosines to form iodothyronines, and (4) production and secretion of abnormal iodoproteins.

Postthyroidectomy and postirradiation myxedema occur frequently as compared with the spontaneous variety. Hypothyroidism secondary to anterior pituitary failure may result from atrophy, necrosis, or tumor (pituitary myxedema) and is often complicated by adrenal and gonadal deficiencies as well.

Clinical Picture. The general appearance of children with hypothyroidism varies considerably, depending on the age at which the deficiency begins and the promptness of replacement therapy. Signs and symptoms of cretinism may be clinically evident at birth, or more commonly within the first several neonatal months, depending upon the completeness of thyroid failure. The children are dwarfed, stocky, and somewhat overweight, with a broad, flat nose; eyes set apart because of failure of nasorbital development; coarse features with thick lips, protruding tongue, and pale, mottled skin; poor muscular tone and intestinal activity; spadelike, stubby hands with x-ray evidence of retarded bone age and epiphyseal dysgenesis; delayed eruption of the teeth, and malocclusion resulting from the macroglossia. In infancy the characteristic facies, the hoarse cry, the large tongue, the "potbelly," and the presence of an umbilical hernia should call attention to the diagnosis of severe degrees of thyroid deficiency. Diagnosis and treatment at the earliest possible date in infancy are important since the extent of mental retardation may be related to the age at which treatment is instituted. Good results are obtained only when the diagnosis is established early and adequate therapy is instituted at once. If therapy is delayed, most of the clinical features of cretinism may still be reversed, but some degree of mental retardation usually persists.

The adult and older child with myxedema have a typical facies characterized by a dull, uninterested expression and puffy eyelids, often with an alopecia of the outer third of the eyebrows. The skin of the face exhibits creamy pallor and occasionally a peach coloring over the malar prominences. The changes in coloring result from anemia combined with carotenemia. The skin elsewhere on the body is dry and rough. The subcutaneous tissue is indurated and doughy, because of interstitial fluid of high protein content. The hair is brittle, and dry, and there is frequent premature graying. There is swelling of the tongue and larynx and a halting, slurred, hoarse speech, with slowing of mental and physical activity. Anemia, constipation, and increased sensitivity to cold are present as well as increased capillary fragility, as evidenced by susceptibility to bruising. Women with myxedema during the active ovarian cycle usually note prolonged menstrual bleeding. Some patients with hypothyroidism complain of constant rhinorrhea, coryza, or deafness. There may also be arthralgia, symptoms indistinguishable from peripheral neuropathy, signs and symptoms of cerebellar disturbance, muscular weakness, or myotonia.

The cardiac silhouette is usually larger than normal, partially because of dilatation but mostly from pericardial effusion. Rarely, the cardiac silhouette may be small; if so, pituitary myxedema should be considered. Thyroid tissue is rarely palpable except in the presence of chronic thyroiditis, endemic goiter, or goitrous cretinism. Skeletal growth is usually normal in the adult patient with myxedema, but in children or adolescents may be significantly retarded. The relaxation time of the deep tendon reflexes is characteristically slowed in patients with myxedema. Severe ileus with a picture of megacolon is also seen. Psychoses (myxedema madness) may dominate the clinical picture in some patients with myxedema. Untreated patients with profound degrees of myxedema may exhibit hypothermic coma (myxedema coma), a serious and usually fatal complication. Some of the features of myxedema coma are related to respiratory depression and consequent CO_2 narcosis.

Laboratory examinations reveal a low basal metabolic rate, elevated serum cholesterol level, low plasma protein-bound iodine level, depressed red blood cell uptake of radioactively tagged triiodothyronine, and decreased radioiodine uptake in the region of the thyroid. The extraneous factors which may modify the plasma protein-bound iodine level or the radioiodine uptake of the gland are enumerated in Table 66-1. In some varieties of goitrous cretins, the thyroid uptake of radioactive iodine may be increased. In those in whom I^{131} remains unbound, it may be discharged from the gland following the administration of potassium thiocyanate or perchlorate.

It is noteworthy that the spinal fluid protein concentration may be elevated in patients with profound myxedema. There may be a significant normocytic or slightly macrocytic anemia, as well as gastric achlorhydria. The electrocardiograph may reveal a marked decrease in voltage with flattened or inverted T waves.

The diagnosis of myxedema will almost always be suggested by the facial appearance and voice of the patient.

The signs and symptoms in hypothyroidism without the classical syndrome of myxedema are less striking. Palpable thyroid tissue may be absent, or there may occasionally be a goiter. Patients with mild hypothyroidism may complain of easy fatigability, disturbed emotional control, vague aches and pains, menstrual disturbances, and pallor. The laboratory findings, however, should reflect decreased thyroid function as evidenced by a basal metabolic rate below −20 per cent, a serum protein-bound iodine level below 4.0 μg per 100 ml, and a 24-hr radioactive iodine uptake below 15 per cent.

Hypothyroidism secondary to anterior pituitary deficiency may present a picture indistinguishable from that of primary myxedema. However, the accumulation of subcutaneous fluid (myxedema fluid) is usually not so pronounced in patients with pituitary myxedema as in those with primary myxedema. Careful investigation will usually reveal associated gonadal and adrenocortical deficiency out of proportion to that seen in primary myxedema. In general, the serum cholesterol level is within, or close to, normal limits in patients with hypothyroidism secondary to anterior pituitary failure, whereas it is usually elevated in primary myxedema. In contrast to patients with primary myxedema, who respond readily and satisfactorily to thyroid replacement therapy, administration of this hormone to patients with pituitary myxedema may be less effective and may precipitate adrenal crisis. The administration of pituitary thyrotropic hormone

Table 66-1. COMPARATIVE VALUES FOR TESTS OF THYROID FUNCTION IN COMMON CLINICAL SITUATIONS

Diagnostic and clinical status	24 hr I^131 uptake, %	Serum PBI,* µg/100 ml	Serum BEI,* µg/100 ml	BMR, % normal standard	RBC uptake, %
Euthyroidism:					
Normal values..............	15 to 50	4 to 8	3 to 7	−15 to +15	11.5 to 19 (male) / 11 to 17 (female)
Pregnancy.................	Normal/increase	Increase	Increase	+20 to +25	Decrease (<11)
Iodide deficiency...........	Increase	Normal/decrease	Normal/decrease	Normal/decrease	Normal/decrease
Iodide Rx (>3.0 mg/day)....	Decrease	Increase	Normal	Normal	Normal
Thyroid, USP (>120 mg/day)	Decrease	Normal/increase	Normal/increase	Normal/increase	Normal/increase
L-Thyroxin (>0.4 mg/day)...	Decrease	Normal/increase	Normal/increase	Normal/increase	Normal/increase
L-Triiodothyronine (>0.1 mg/day)	Decrease	Decrease	Decrease	Normal/increase	Normal/increase
Antithyroid drug Rx (during).	Decrease	Normal	Normal	Normal	Normal
Antithyroid drug Rx (shortly after).................	Increase	Normal	Normal	Normal	Normal
Congestive heart failure......	Variable	Normal	Normal	Variable	Normal
Hyperthyroidism:					
Untreated.................	50 to 100	7 to 20	5 to 15	Increase	>19 (male) / >17 (female)
Pregnancy.................	Increase	Increase	Increase	Increase	
Iodide therapy (>2.0 mg/day)...........	Normal/decrease	>20	5 to 15	Increase	Increase
Thyroid, USP†.............	>20	Increase	Increase	Increase	Increase
L-Thyroxin (0.4 mg/day)†....	>20	Increase	Increase	Increase	Increase
L-Triiodothyronine (0.1 mg/day)†............	>20	Increase	Increase	Increase	Increase
Antithyroid drug Rx (euthyroid)..............	Normal/decrease	Normal	Normal	Normal	Normal
Thyroiditis (acute)..........	Decrease	Increase	Increase	Increase	Increase
Myxedema (primary):					
Untreated.................	0 to 15	0 to 4	0 to 3	−20 to −50	<11.5 (male) / <11.0 (female)
Thyroid USP (120 mg/day-euthyroid)....	Decrease	Normal	Normal	Normal	Normal
L-Thyroxin (0.4 mg/day-euthyroid).....	Decrease	Normal	Normal	Normal	Normal
L-Triiodothyronine (0.1 mg/day-euthyroid).....	Decrease	Decrease	Normal	Normal	Normal

* The presence of trace amounts of mercury in serum will render the values for the PBI and BEI factitiously low.
† Suppression test.

(TSH), 10 to 30 USP units over a 24- to 72-hr period, to patients with pituitary hypothyroidism is usually followed in 24 to 48 hr by a rise in the thyroidal uptake of radioactive iodine and in serum protein-bound iodine.

Differential Diagnosis. Little difficulty will be experienced in the diagnosis of classic cretinism, juvenile or adult myxedema. Occasionally a mongoloid infant may be confused with a cretin. However, the characteristic mongoloid eyes, the hyperextensibility of the finger joints, and the normal skin and hair texture distinguish the mongoloid imbecile from the hypothyroid cretin. Chronic nephritis and especially nephrosis may simulate juvenile myxedema. This is particularly true of the chronic uremic patient with retarded mental acuity and characteristic facial expression. The difficulty in diagnosis is made more confusing because hypothyroidism may coexist in nephrotic patients. In nephrosis, the basal metabolic rate is usually below normal, as is the level of the serum protein-bound iodine. Since the nephrotic patient may also exhibit anemia, hypercholesterolemia, and anasarca (simulating myxedema fluid), the differential diagnosis may be confusing. However, the uptake of radioactive iodine is usually normal in nephrotic patients, and the low level of serum protein-bound iodine is due to a decrease in thyroid-binding protein secondary to proteinuria. The hyperactive deep tendon reflexes of the uremic patient, as contrasted with the slowed relaxation phase of the reflexes in patients with myxedema may be of clinical aid in distinguishing the two conditions. Not infrequently patients with hypothyroidism exhibit severe anemia and clinically resemble patients with pernicious anemia. The anemia of uncomplicated hypothyroidism is most often normocytic or occasionally macrocytic, but not megaloblastic. It responds rather slowly to thyroid medication. Patients with Addison's disease and hypometabolism may be distinguished by the pigmentary changes in the former. The 17-ketosteroid and 17-hydroxycorticoid excretion may be reduced in both conditions but will be markedly reduced only in the case of Addison's disease. A differential diagnosis may be established with the use of the 48-hr pituitary adrenocorticotropin test (p. 566) and by the radioactive iodine uptake.

The most serious problem in differential diagnosis is that presented by patients with a moderate reduction in basal metabolic rate. Unfortunately, in the minds of many physicians, hypometabolism and hypothyroidism are synonymous. The greatest help in differential diagnosis under these circumstances will be obtained by studying the uptake of radioactive iodine by the thyroid gland or from a determination of the butanol-extractable or protein-bound iodine level of the serum. One may also follow the clinical course carefully during the administration of small doses of thyroid hormone (30 to 60 mg thyroid, USP, daily). Patients with primary hypothyroidism show progressive objective and subjective improvement on adequate thyroid substitution therapy until euthyroidism is attained. Patients whose basal metabolic rates are subnormal owing to causes other than thyroid hormone insufficiency will not exhibit this response to thyroid therapy.

Table 66-2. APPROXIMATE EQUIVALENT DOSES OF VARIOUS THYROID PREPARATIONS

Preparation	*Average daily oral maintenance dose, mg*
Desiccated thyroid USP	120.0
L-Thyroxin	0.3
3,5,3'-L-Triiodothyronine	0.1
3,5,3'-Triiodothyroacetic acid	6.0
Tetraiodothyroacetic acid	9.0
3,5,3'-Triiodothyropropionic acid	6.0
Tetraiodothyropropionic acid	12.0

Treatment. Desiccated thyroid substance (thyroid, USP) is usually administered as 30-, 60-, and 120-mg tablets. Sodium L-thyroxin is available as 0.05-, 0.1-, and 0.2-mg tablets, showing approximately 300 times the activity of USP thyroid. The rapidly acting thyroid hormone, 3,5,3'-triiodothyronine, is available in 5.0- and 25-μg tablets; 1 μg L-triiodothyronine is roughly equivalent to 1 mg desiccated thyroid (Table 66-2). These substances constitute the therapeutic choice for all types of hypothyroidism except in cases due to a specific iodine lack. In all instances, except perhaps in myxedema coma, it is desirable to institute therapy with a relatively small dose of thyroid substance, since a sudden change in metabolic level may induce undesirable psychologic or cardiovascular disturbances, especially in the older age group of patients. The occurrence of angina pectoris or congestive heart failure during therapy for myxedema is an indication to proceed with caution, since rapid changes in metabolic rate may precipitate, as well as increase, the severity of these conditions. In many patients, generalized muscular aching follows initiation of therapy regardless of the dosage of thyroid hormone, and occasionally coryza is noted. It is essential in patients with cretinism or juvenile myxedema to maintain therapy at close to toxic levels in order to ensure the desired growth re-

Table 66-3. AVERAGE DOSE OF DESICCATED THYROID FOR VARIOUS AGE GROUPS

Age	*Daily maintenance dose, mg*
Infant <1 year	60*
2–6 years	90*
Adults	90–120

* In infants and children, the therapeutic maintenance dose should be kept at the maximum nontoxic level. The initial dose should be approximately one-fourth the maintenance dose and may be increased in a stepwise fashion until the desired state of euthyroidism is clinically achieved.

sponse. The requirement for optimum bone growth appears to be higher than that usually needed for satisfactory maintenance of the over-all clinical picture. Children need somewhat more thyroid in proportion to their size than do adults. Dosage usually must be adjusted according to clinical evaluation of the effects obtained, at the same time avoiding symptoms of overdosage such as tachycardia, irritability, continuous weight loss, diarrhea, or sweating. In panhypopituitarism, thyroid hormone therapy should not be instituted until after adrenocortical replacement therapy has been initiated, and the initial dose of desiccated thyroid should be small and increased gradually by 15 mg increments at 3-week intervals. In adults one may begin with a dose of 15 mg per day, gradually increasing the dose at weekly or biweekly intervals. In patients over forty to fifty years of age, thyroid therapy should be given cautiously, with longer intervals between the increments in dosage. The usual maintenance dose of desiccated thyroid necessary to maintain an athyreotic patient in euthyroidism is 90 to 120 mg. In the presence of any evidence of cardiovascular disease, the total dosage should not exceed 30 to 60 mg daily until the patient has been followed for several weeks at this dosage level. The maximum effect from a given dosage level will not be obtained for at least 7 to 10 days, and thyroid hormone action will persist for several weeks after the last dose. It is not necessary to give desiccated thyroid more than once daily. Because of its relatively more rapid onset and shorter duration of action, triiodothyronine may be given in divided doses. Equivalent therapeutic quantities of various thyroid preparations are given in Table 66-2. It should be noted that patients with myxedema, like patients with Addison's disease, are extremely sensitive to many drugs, such as morphine, and to most stressful situations, such as operations. Patients with myxedema coma should be treated with parenteral triiodothyronine and, in addition, artificial respiration should be used if CO_2 narcosis exists.

Some workers have advocated the use of thyroid hormone analogs such as D-thyroxin, 3,3′-diiodothyroacetic acid, and 3,3′,5′-triiodothyronine as serum cholesterol–lowering agents in euthyroid subjects. However, their ultimate therapeutic role has not been determined. It is of interest that some dissociation of the cholesterol-lowering and metabolic rate responses may be obtained with most thyroactive compounds when small doses are used.

HYPERTHYROIDISM

History. Dr. Caleb Parry described a disease characterized by thyroid enlargement, dilatation of the heart, palpitation, exophthalmos, and nervous as well as menstrual symptoms in 1786. Graves and Basedow, between the years 1835 and 1843, independently published treatises on the syndrome which now bears their names. That hyperthyroidism was the fundamental disorder in Graves's disease was formulated by Möbius in Germany in 1887. The use of iodine in the treatment of thyrotoxicosis was popularized by Plummer. Recent advances in the medical therapy of hyperthyroidism include the use of antithyroid substances such as thiourea and imidazole derivatives as well as potassium perchlorate and other goitrogenic agents. Radioactive iodine now occupies a prominent position as a therapeutic agent in the treatment of thyrotoxicosis.

Incidence. Hyperthyroidism is a relatively common disorder which may occur at any age, especially during puberty and the menopause. The disease is much more frequent in females than in males. In nongoitrous areas the ratio of predominance in females may be as high as 8:1. In endemic goitrous areas, the ratio is smaller. Hyperthyroidism is comparatively rare in children. When it occurs there is usually a diffuse goiter free of nodules.

Etiology. At present the cause of thyrotoxicosis is poorly understood. It has been assumed that, in patients with exophthalmic goiter with diffuse enlargement of the thyroid gland (Graves's disease), excessive thyrotropic hormone might be responsible for the initiation of the syndrome. Convincing proof of this is lacking in most patients. However, in a large number of cases there is a clue in the correlation between episodes of psychic trauma, infections, injury, or other types of stress and the onset of thyrotoxicosis. An abnormal thyroid stimulator which differs from thyroid-stimulating hormone (TSH) in its prolonged action on the thyroid of the guinea pig and in its prolonged intravascular half-life in the rat has been detected in the blood of some patients with Graves's disease. The observation that the thyroid gland of patients with hyperthyroidism is not inhibited following thyroid hormone administration and is stimulated following TSH administration has suggested to some that this disease is not due to excessive endogenous TSH secretion. Thyrotoxicosis associated with nodular goiter (Plummer's disease) may represent a phase in the natural history of nodular colloid goiter. In the hyperfunctioning single adenoma it is evident that the adenoma is occasionally the autonomous source of excess thyroid hormone. In some patients hyperthyroidism occurs without clinical evidence of goiter, and in very rare instances the hyperplastic thyroid tissue may be ectopic, for example, in the ovary (struma ovarii). The exophthalmos present in many patients with Graves's disease may be due to effects of both excessive thyroid hormone and a specific anterior pituitary factor.

Pathology. In typical Graves's disease the thyroid gland is bilaterally diffusely enlarged, soft, and vascular. The essential pathologic picture is that of parenchymatous hypertrophy and hyperplasia, characterized by increased height of the epithelium and redundancy of the follicular wall, giving the picture of papillary infoldings and cytologic evidence of increased activity. Such hyperplasia may involve the entire parenchyma of the thyroid, or it may be limited to certain areas. In hyperthyroidism associated with nodular goiters, the major part of the thyroid tissue shows colloid involutional changes with hyperplastic paranodular areas which exhibit the functional changes responsible for the hyperthyroidism. This type of gland is thought to represent the end stage of an involuted nodular goiter and is erroneously termed "toxic adenoma." True thyroid tumors (adenomas) which produce hyperfunction occur only rarely, and in these the paranodular tissue is inactive.

Following iodine medication in patients with hyperthyroidism, there is intense colloid storage, which sometimes causes enlargement and increased firmness of the gland. Long-continued thyrotoxicosis leads to characteristic lymphocytic infiltration of the thyroid and other tissues and degeneration of the skeletal muscle fibers, enlargement of the heart, fatty infiltration or diffuse fibrosis of the liver, decalcification of the skeleton, loss of body tissue (including fat depots, osteoid, and muscle), and thymic and lymphatic hypertrophy.

Clinical Picture. Classic manifestations of thyrotoxicosis include exophthalmos, goiter, fine tremor especially of the extended fingers and tongue, increased nervousness, irritability and emotional instability, sweating, and hyperkinesis. Loss of weight and of strength usually exist without loss of appetite, although occasionally anorexia, nausea, vomiting, and diarrhea occur. There may be intolerance to heat, dyspnea, palpitations, paroxysmal arrhythmias, and not infrequently in individuals over the age of forty, cardiac failure. Oligomenorrhea and amenorrhea are more common than menorrhagia. In general, nervous symptoms dominate the clinical picture in younger individuals, whereas cardiovascular symptoms predominate in older subjects with thyrotoxicosis.

Significant physical findings are related to skin changes, eye signs, cardiac signs, and local changes in the thyroid gland. The skin is warm and moist, with a velvety texture, and the hair is fine and silky. Occasionally, increased loss of hair from the temporal aspects of the scalp and in the axillas may be noted. Excessive melanin pigmentation is frequently observed. Ocular signs include infrequent blinking (Stellwag), lid lag (von Graefe), failure of convergence (Möbius), and failure to wrinkle the brow on upward gaze (Joffroy).

Local changes in the thyroid gland consist chiefly of diffuse or nodular enlargement, a bruit best heard directly over the gland, and rarely, signs of tracheal or substernal obstruction. A hyperplastic pyramidal lobe of the thyroid may often be palpable if carefully sought.

Cardiovascular findings include a wide pulse pressure, sinus tachycardia or atrial fibrillation, frequent systolic murmurs, increased intensity of apical first sound, cardiac enlargement, overt heart failure, and usually a poor response to digitalization. A to-and-fro high-pitched sound may be audible in the pulmonic area and may simulate a pericardial friction rub (Means-Lerman scratch).

Childhood hyperthyroidism is relatively uncommon. It is usually benign, and a portion of the cases appear to recover spontaneously. In nearly all instances there is a diffuse goiter and marked nervousness, with striking tachycardia. Depending upon the severity and duration of the disease and the caloric intake, growth and development may be greater or less than normal. Precocious eruption of the teeth may be a helpful diagnostic finding in juvenile hyperthyroidism.

Diagnosis. Most cases of thyrotoxicosis are so striking that diagnosis presents little difficulty. In these there are goiter, eye signs, loss of weight despite good appetite, tachycardia, sweating, psychic instability, tremor, increased basal metabolic rate, a high serum protein-bound iodine and butanol-extractable iodine, an increased red blood cell uptake of radioactive triiodothyronine, and a rapid and increased thyroidal uptake of radioiodine (Table 66-1).

In a few patients the clinical picture may be one of apathy rather than of hyperactivity, and the basal metabolic rate elevation may be relatively slight. In such instances the clinical detection of underlying thyrotoxicosis is difficult, but the thyroidal uptake of radioactive iodine, the red blood cell or resin uptake of radioactive triiodothyronine, and the serum protein-bound iodine levels are usually diagnostic. A barium swallow may be helpful in demonstrating displacement of the esophagus or trachea by substernal enlargement of the thyroid. All patients with unexplained cardiac failure or irregularities in rhythm, especially supraventricular tachycardias, should be surveyed carefully for underlying thyrotoxicosis. In patients with preexistent cardiac disease, even mild thyrotoxicosis may induce severe disability. The circulation time may be rapid or normal in the presence of an elevated venous pressure, and the response to digitalis is usually poor.

Although eye signs are important, it should be recognized that exophthalmic ophthalmoplegia may occur antecedent to, or in the absence of, the metabolic abnormalities of thyrotoxicosis and that, in certain nationalities and in certain families, prominent eyes and wide palpebral fissures occur normally. Prominence of the eyes is occasionally seen in advanced uremia with normal thyroid function. Exophthalmos and an elevated thyroidal uptake of radioiodine may occur in some patients with nonthyroidal disorders, but in these patients the elevated uptake can be suppressed with triiodothyronine (see below).

Differential Diagnosis. Since the basal metabolic rate measures over-all oxygen consumption and not specifically thyroid function, extrathyroidal disturbances such as unrecognized infections, leukemia, neoplasms, hypertensive cardiovascular disease, congestive heart failure, aortic stenosis, diabetes, pheochromocytoma, chronic pulmonary insufficiency, and polycythemia may lead to hypermetabolism not consequent to hyperthyroidism. The presence of perforated eardrums may also lead to a spuriously high basal metabolic rate through oxygen leakage. In all the aforementioned circumstances, the plasma protein-bound iodine and radioiodine uptake are of considerable diagnostic value. It is to be noted, however, that the ingestion of thyroid substances or iodine-containing compounds may interfere with the correct values of many of these tests, in so far as determining the actual functional capacity of the thyroid gland is concerned (Table 66-1). The administration of iodine in any form (cough sirup, radiopaque dyes, salt substitutes, or Lugol's solution) will invalidate the radioiodine uptake, as well as the serum protein-bound iodine but not the red blood cell or resin uptake of radioactively tagged triiodothyronine. The butanol-extractable iodine determination is usually valid in the presence of moderate excesses of iodide but is spuriously elevated by organic iodine compounds. Considerable aid may be obtained from a study of the daily temperature and pulse records. Thyrotoxicosis frequently induces a mild hyperthermia with a very narrow diurnal swing in comparison to the wider changes in temperature from morning to night associated with most infections. The response of the clinical manifestations, basal metabolic rate, and serum protein-bound iodine levels, under controlled conditions, to antithyroid medication may constitute a helpful clinical therapeutic trial.

A suppression test for hyperthyroidism has proved helpful in delineating patients whose clinical status is equivocal and whose radioactive iodine uptake and serum protein-bound iodine are in the "high normal" range. The daily administration of 100 to 150 μg of L-triiodothyronine by mouth for 8 days causes a fall in the 24-hr I^{131} uptake to below 20 per cent in patients with normal thyroid function. On the other hand, patients with hyperthyroidism or euthyroid patients with the ocular manifestations of this disorder fail to suppress below 20 per cent.

Anxiety states may simulate thyrotoxicosis, and an associated tachycardia and weight loss may be quite pronounced. In patients with anxiety, however, there is often marked vasomotor instability, with cold rather than warm extremities. It is essential to detect underlying thyrotoxicosis in patients with emotional and psychic instability, since correction of the underlying thyrotoxicosis may result in improvement of the emotional difficulties. In patients with anxiety states, basal metabolic rate determinations are both difficult and unreliable unless they are done under anesthesia or sedation; a more direct determination of thyroid hyperfunction, such as the level of serum protein-bound iodine or the percentage uptake of radioiodine following a tracer dose (Table 66-1), is the most expedient diagnostic approach.

Treatment. Hyperthyroidism is characteristically a disorder with cyclic phases of exacerbation and remission; occasionally patients with mild forms of the disorder may recover spontaneously. In most instances, however, medical or surgical therapy is required and must be directed toward decreasing the thyroidal production of excessive quantities of its hormones.

There are three major approaches to the treatment of hyperthyroidism: drug, surgical, and radiation. Each has its advantages and disadvantages. Selection of a particular program must be predicated not only upon the clinical circumstances, but also upon social and economic factors, emotional stability, and the patient's reliability. The use of iodide solutions alone in the medical management of patients with hyperthyroidism is usually unsatisfactory. Although some improvement from iodide therapy may be evident within a week or so after institution, complete control of the disorder is seldom satisfactorily accomplished solely by this means. Except in anticipation of subtotal thyroidectomy, the use of iodides, either alone or in combination with antithyroid therapy, interferes with the practical employment of most laboratory tests of thyroid function and with the use of therapeutic amounts of radioactive iodine.

In general, the long-term use of antithyroid drugs is reserved for children, adolescents and young adults, and for pregnancies complicated by hyperthyroidism. Subtotal thyroidectomy is elected in those under the age of forty years in whom a definitive ablative procedure is required. Indications for subtotal thyroidectomy include relapse following drug therapy, a large or enlarging goiter, toxic reactions, failure of the patient to follow a medical regimen or to return for periodic examinations. Radioactive iodide is employed in all patients over the age of forty years and in patients with complicating systemic disorders contradicting safe elective surgery and those with severe heart disease.

Satisfactory regulation of thyrotoxicosis may be obtained with propylthiouracil or methimazole (Tapazole) in appropriately selected cases. Patients with small diffuse thyroid enlargement do better in general than those with nodular goiter. Since the agents employed are inhibitors of thyroid activity, it is essential that an effective level of the therapeutic agent be maintained throughout the 24-hr period. In the medical management of thyrotoxicosis, antithyroid drugs may be given for an 18- to 24-month course in an initial dosage of 100 mg propylthiouracil or 10 mg methimazole every 6 to 8 hr, until euthyroidism is achieved. In nodular goiter with hyperthyroidism it is occasionally necessary to increase the initial daily dose of propylthiouracil to 600 to 1,000 mg or equivalent doses of methimazole for satisfactory control.

Once euthyroidism is achieved, the daily dose of propylthiouracil may be maintained at 300 mg or that of methimazole at 30 mg, in three divided doses, and to this should be added 120 mg desiccated thyroid daily. By this regimen, the thyroid gland can be maximally suppressed by the antithyroid medication and hypothyroidism prevented by the concomitant administration of thyroid replacement therapy. Such combination therapy provides several further advantages, such as a beneficial effect on the ophthalmopathy, some tendency to reduction in the size of the goiter, and a more stabilized clinical course. It also has the added advantage in that it can be used as a prognostic device when the course of drug therapy is completed. By continuing the 120 mg of thyroid daily for 3 months following discontinuance of the antithyroid compound, a thyroid suppression test can be easily performed. If the uptake of radioactive iodine is less than 20 per cent in 24 hr at this time, a favorable prognosis for a permanent remission is indicated.

Leukopenia is the principal undesirable side effect of antithyroid drugs. Mild transient leukopenia may occur in approximately 10 per cent of patients treated and is not necessarily an indication for discontinuing therapy. When the absolute number of polymorphonuclear leukocytes reaches 1,500 or less, antithyroid medication should be discontinued. Drug rashes and sensitivity develop in approximately 3 to 5 per cent of patients. On rare occasions (in less than 0.2 per cent) agranulocytosis may occur suddenly.

Prolonged remission or permanent cure of the thyrotoxicosis by this method may be anticipated in approximately 50 per cent of the patients on long-term therapy. If prolonged drug therapy is impractical, a more definitive therapeutic approach such as subtotal thyroidectomy or radioiodine ther-

apy should be undertaken. Preparation for the former can be accomplished readily by the addition of iodine, 15 to 30 drops of Lugol's solution daily by mouth, to the therapeutic program of propylthiouracil or methimazole 10 to 14 days prior to surgery. Thyroidectomy should be an elective procedure and performed only when the patient is euthyroid.

During the treatment of hyperthyroidism occurring with pregnancy, the basal metabolic rate should not be maintained at a lower value than is physiologic for that particular trimester in order to assure a normal thyroid status in the fetus. During the last trimester of pregnancy the basal metabolic rate should usually be maintained between plus 25 and plus 30 per cent, and the plasma protein-bound iodine level will usually remain around 8 to 11 μg per 100 ml. The use of thyroid replacement therapy is especially efficacious when antithyroid compounds are employed in the treatment of hyperthyroidism during pregnancy.

The rapid, but rarely massive, enlargement of the thyroid gland which occasionally occurs following therapy with antithyroid drugs usually abates with continuation of therapy. Some embarrassment of respiration or deglutition may occasionally occur in patients with appreciable gland enlargement in the retrosternal space. The use of thyroid in conjunction with an antithyroid drug may reduce the thyroid enlargement as well as the vascularity of the gland, making thyroid surgery less difficult. Although some authorities use iodine routinely in conjunction with antithyroid drugs, the combination of iodine and antithyroid drugs is usually reserved for patients with hyperthyroidism who are being prepared for surgery. Recently, the inorganic compound potassium perchlorate has been found to be quite effective in the control of hyperthyroidism in doses of 250 mg three to four times daily. This compound may be more toxic than the organic goitrogens, but sufficient experience with it has not been available for comparison.

Effective reduction of thyroid activity may be accomplished by subtotal thyroidectomy following medical preparation. In skilled hands there is a high rate of cure and a low incidence of serious complications (see Table 66-4). Careful preparation of a patient with propylthiouracil or methimazole for a minimum of several months followed by iodine administration (5 to 10 drops of Lugol's solution three times daily for 10 days or 2 weeks prior to operation) usually ensures excellent preoperative control of thyrotoxicosis. Potassium perchlorate may be employed successfully to control hyperthyroidism. However, it may not be employed in the preoperative period, since its effects are antagonized by the simultaneous administration of iodide.

Radioactive iodine (I^{131}) affords a relatively

Table 66-4. COMPLICATIONS FOLLOWING THYROIDECTOMY
AND RADIOACTIVE IODINE THERAPY FOR HYPERTHYROIDISM
(REPRESENTATIVE ORDER OF MAGNITUDE)

Complication	Surgery, per cent	Radioactive iodine, per cent
Hypothyroidism.............	3–5	8–10
Recurrent hyperthyroidism.....	3–10	2
Vocal cord paresis...........	5	0
Vocal cord paralysis..........	3	0
Hypoparathyroidism (permanent)...................	0.5–1.0	0
Mortality...................	<0.4	0

simple and effective medical means of treating thyrotoxicosis. Radiation of the thyroid can be readily accomplished by the administration of this isotope orally. With appropriate doses and sufficient thyroid uptake of radioiodine, cure of the thyrotoxicosis is almost certain and complications are minimal (Table 66-4).

The undesirable late effects of radioisotopic therapy remain to be evaluated, but current evidence suggests that for the most part serious complications will not be significant. Many physicians prefer to reserve radioiodine therapy for patients over forty years of age, feeling that one is not justified in administering an agent of undetermined radiation potentialities to younger persons. Patients with recurrent thyrotoxicosis following surgery, those who refuse surgery, or those who have complicating illnesses contraindicating surgery are excellent candidates for radioiodine therapy. The usual therapeutic dose for diffusely enlarged thyroid glands ranges between 120 to 140 μc per estimated gram of thyroid tissue (approximately 4 to 8 mc total dose). Nodular goiters require somewhat larger doses, usually 8 to 12 mc. Repeated doses are sometimes required, and these may be given at intervals of 3 to 6 months until euthyroidism is achieved.

Radiation thyroiditis from radioiodine may contraindicate its use in patients with large substernal goiters likely to induce respiratory embarrassment upon swelling. Patients exhibiting severe hyperthyroidism, heart failure, or progressive ophthalmopathy may first be rendered euthyroid by the use of methimazole or propylthiouracil; by discontinuing antithyroid treatment for 2 to 3 days or longer and then administering radioactive iodine, a good therapeutic response may be obtained.

In the presence of intractable cardiac failure or angina, one may deliberately attempt to induce hypothyroidism. In administering doses of radioactive iodine to cardiac patients, caution should be observed around the fifth to the seventh day following therapy, since the occasional occurrence of radiation thyroiditis with liberation of increased amounts of metabolically active thyroid hormones into the circulation may exacerbate underlying cardiac disease. Radioactive iodine therapy is contraindicated during pregnancy and is usually limited to patients outside the childbearing age. Under extenuating circumstances, complicating systemic conditions justify the use of radioactive iodine therapy at any age. Outstanding examples include severe forms of cardiac, renal, hepatic, or pulmonary disease, diabetes, psychoses, and conditions which hinder the proper preparation of patients for surgery (such as severe drug reactions to antithyroid medications).

In all instances, the over-all status of the patient, including his environmental, social, and economic aspects, forms an important basis for evaluating the type of therapy to be employed. A diet of high caloric and vitamin content, rich in carbohydrate, protein, and calcium, and adequate rest and sedation are indicated in both the medical and surgical management of all patients with hyperthyroidism.

THYROTOXIC CRISIS

The clinical picture of thyrotoxic crisis or "storm" is that of a fulminating increase in all the signs and symptoms of thyrotoxicosis. This disturbance is most often observed postoperatively in poorly prepared patients. There is usually extreme irritability, delirium or coma, hyperpyrexia to 106°F or more, tachycardia up to 200, hypotension, vomiting, and diarrhea. Rarely, the clinical picture may be more subtle, with apathy, myopathy, prostration, and coma predominating and accompanied by only slight elevation of temperature. It is thought that in certain patients thyrotoxic crisis is associated with or precipitated by adrenocortical insufficiency. The possibility of this complication gains support from evidence indicating greatly increased adrenocortical hormone requirements in experimentally induced thyrotoxicosis and from the indication of markedly reduced adrenal reserves in this disorder.

It is extremely rare to observe thyrotoxic crisis in patients properly prepared for thyroidectomy. With the preoperative use of antithyroid drugs and iodine and the capacity to control the metabolic rate, body weight, and nutritional status, postoperative thyrotoxic crisis should not occur. If such an event does occur, however, treatment should consist of the intravenous administration of large quantities of hypertonic glucose, 100 to 200 mg hydrocortisone, and iodide; the intramuscular administration of large doses of reserpine and thiamine; and the continuation of large doses of antithyroid drugs. The patient should be placed in an oxygen tent, and hyperpyrexia should be treated, as indicated. Sedation with barbiturates may be necessary, and intravenous doses of Pentothal sodium may occasionally be necessary. Full digitalization should be employed only in the presence of cardiac failure. If shock exists, intravenous pressor agents such as levarterenol may be employed, but with extreme caution, since patients with hyperthyroidism are particularly sensitive to pressor amines.

EXOPHTHALMOS

When exophthalmos progresses rapidly and becomes the major concern in Graves's disease, the clinical condition is usually referred to as "malignant exophthalmos." The term "exophthalmic ophthalmoplegia" refers to the ocular muscle weakness causing strabismus usually accompanied by diplopia, and the description "hyperophthalmopathic Graves's disease," refers to the ophthalmopathy which is occasionally seen without the associated metabolic abnormalities of hyperthyroidism. Clinically, exophthalmos is accompanied by marked proptosis, lid retraction, and the classic eye signs already described (p. 590). In addition, there are chemosis of the conjunctiva, edema of the eyelids, limitation of ocular movements, and diplopia. The appearance of these latter signs during the course of Graves's disease may be a more reliable forewarning of future serious ophthalmopathy than is exophthalmos alone. Exophthalmos may occur with a high, normal, or low metabolic rate and is usually accompanied by edema, fat, and round-cell deposits within the orbital tissues. Occasionally, these changes are severe enough to interfere with the orbital circulation.

It is probable that the ophthalmopathy of Graves's disease results from some factor or factors of the anterior pituitary gland or the hypothalamus, although the genesis of this disorder is not definitely known. The exophthalmos may stabilize or decrease following treatment of the hyperthyroidism, but usually follows a course independent of the therapeutic metabolic response. Rapid progression of exophthalmos with marked chemosis and edema is generally a grave prognostic sign and should serve as a warning that progressive eye changes may be anticipated. In the treatment of this type of exophthalmos it is important to bring the thyrotoxicosis under control gradually and to prevent the development of hypothyroidism. Subtotal thyroidectomy or radioactive iodine therapy may occasionally enhance the progression of exophthalmos. Propylthiouracil or other antithyroid drugs may be more gradual than thyroidectomy or radioactive iodine in their effects on reducing thyroid function. Although there appears to be little difference in the incidence of progressive eye changes following the various forms of therapy of hyperthyroidism, antithyroid drug therapy seems to be the least provocative of severe or "malignant exophthalmos." The long-continued administration of thyroid to maintain euthyroidism may favor the regression of the exophthalmic changes.

Application of ophthalmic hydrocortisone, 5 mg per ml, locally every 2 hr may produce symptomatic improvement and slight regression of the chemosis. Use of tinted glasses and methylcellulose eye drops may afford some protection against irritation from dust or wind. Hydrocortisone, cortisone, or ACTH given systemically in high dosage may be helpful temporarily, but should be used only in selected cases. Elevation of the head of the bed during sleep, a low sodium diet with added diuretic therapy, and cold compresses or pressure dressings applied to the eyes may occasionally be beneficial. X-ray irradiation to the orbit or pituitary has been successful in some instances. Tarsorrhaphy may be beneficial in protecting the cornea during sleep and in helping contain the exophthalmos. Corneal ulcerations must be vigorously treated. In cases which appear to progress despite all therapy, orbital decompression by surgery may be ultimately necessary to preserve the vision of the patient.

LOCALIZED PRETIBIAL MYXEDEMA

Localized myxedema, a circumscribed deposition of mucinous material in the deeper layers of the skin over the lower portions of the legs or dorsa of the feet, occurs in patients with past or present Graves's disease and is in no way related to hypothyroidism. The affected area of skin may be pruritic, with increased pigmentation, hirsutism, and a *peaux d'orange* appearance which is sharply delineated from the normal skin. The clinical course resembles that of exophthalmos, with which it is frequently associated. It may also be associated with clubbing of the fingers. About half of the cases occur during the active stage of thyrotoxicosis, and in the remainder the lesions develop following treatment of the thyrotoxicosis. The activity of the disorder is usually self-limited. No form of therapy is entirely satisfactory, although the local injection of hyaluronidase or triiodothyronine has been transiently beneficial in some cases.

THYROTOXIC HEART DISEASE

The cardiac manifestations of hyperthyroidism have been described (p. 590). Many elderly patients may exhibit manifestations of obvious cardiac disease but without the usual clinical appearance of hyperthyroidism. These thyrocardiac patients have been called "apathetic" or "masked." They occasionally represent difficult diagnostic problems, but if one maintains a constant awareness of thyrotoxicosis in patients with heart disease, the correct diagnosis is almost always suspected. In these patients hyperthyroidism is usually associated with a toxic nodular goiter. Although the basal metabolic rate is not consistently elevated, the plasma protein-bound iodine, the erythrocyte or resin uptake of radioactive triiodothyronine, and the radioactive iodine uptake of the thyroid are often specifically diagnostic.

In patients with cardiac decompensation and thyrotoxicosis, the cardiac output is frequently above normal, with a rapid or normal circulation time in spite of an elevated venous pressure. This condition is one of several which is responsible for so-called "high-output failure." Even though elevated above normal, the cardiac output is unable to satisfy the high metabolic requirements of the body, and thus heart failure occurs. It is probably wise to obtain such thyroid studies as the protein-bound iodine and the radioactive iodine uptake in all patients with atrial fibrillation or congestive heart failure of undetermined etiology, since the finding of thyrotoxicosis affords a remediable form of cardiac disease.

There is evidence to suggest that the production of hypothyroidism, and consequently hypometabolism, is beneficial in appropriately selected euthyroid patients with congestive heart failure from any cause, or in those with angina pectoris or intractable supraventricular tachycardias. This hypothyroidism may be effectively accomplished by the administration of radioactive iodine.

THYROTOXIC MYOPATHY

Weakness and impairment of muscular function of varying severity often accompany thyrotoxicosis. Certain patients, however, exhibit these symptoms entirely out of proportion to the degree of thyrotoxicosis. Occasionally the myopathic picture is complicated by lymphocytosis simulating a leukemoid reaction. In patients presenting signs and symptoms of myopathy, an intensive search for excessive thyroid activity should be made (see Chap. 84, pp. 727 to 728).

THYROTOXIC BONE DISEASE

Urinary excretion of excessive amounts of calcium and phosphorus in hyperthyroidism produces a prolonged state of negative balance. Despite this, serum levels of calcium and phosphorus are usually within normal limits and the levels of alkaline phosphatase are usually normal or only slightly elevated. Clinically, significant degrees of skeletal demineralization are rarely seen in hyperthyroidism except in elderly individuals; in these, preexistent osteoporosis upon which is superimposed a high rate of skeletal demineralization may occasionally result in vertebral wedging or collapse. (See Chap. 77, p. 699 and Chap. 78, p. 707.)

TUMORS OF THE THYROID GLAND

Simple Goiter

History. Simple goiter has been recognized since antiquity, being described as early as the fifteenth century B.C. and later by the Greeks and Romans. Burnt sponge and seaweed, which are rich in iodine, were used against goiter in the Middle Ages. It was not, however, until the classic experiment of Marine and Kimball was carried out on school girls in Akron, Ohio, in 1916 that iodine was shown clearly to prevent goiter.

Incidence. Simple goiter may arise endemically in geographic areas deficient in iodine in soil and water. Endemic areas in the United States are located principally in the Great Lakes Basin. Sporadic goiter is most common at puberty, during pregnancy and lactation, or following the menopause. It is ten times more frequent in females than in males.

Etiology. In the presence of an absolute iodine deficiency, as in endemic goiter or with the ingestion of goitrogenic agents, such as cabbage, thiocyanates, or milk from cows fed on plants containing goitrogens (see p. 585), the secretion of thyroid hormones may decrease. Such a change may also occur with relative iodine deficiency during periods of increased body demand, such as may occur at puberty. In response to a lowered circulating thyroid hormone level, the pituitary output of thyroid-stimulating hormone (TSH) is increased and hyperplasia of thyroid cells occurs. Some workers feel that an abnormal inactive thyroglobulin may be formed and the colloid is therefore of "poor quality" (basophilic staining and poor in iodine content). Later, colloid disappears and further cellular hyperplasia occurs. On iodine administration, thyroid hormone is again formed and liberated. The rising blood level of protein-bound iodine inhibits thyrotropic hormone production, and there is restoration of active, acidophilic, iodine-rich colloid surrounded by flattened acinar epithelium. From this it may be seen that early in simple iodine-deficiency goiter the histologic appearance may be that of a colloid goiter; whereas later the histologic appearance might be described as a parenchymatous goiter. There seems to be little doubt that hereditary factors play a prominent but poorly understood role in the pathogenesis of simple goiter, especially sporadic varieties.

Pathology. Pathologically, one may observe diffuse enlargement (simple or adolescent goiter) with an increase in the number of cells (paren-chymatous goiter) or increase in colloid content (colloid goiter); or the abnormality may be manifest in the development of one (uninodular) or usually many nodules (multinodular).

Clinical Picture. In early simple goiter there is symmetric diffuse enlargement of the thyroid (adolescent goiter), usually associated with no disturbance of function, although in some instances mild hypothyroidism may occur. In areas of endemic goiter, the diffuse enlargement of the thyroid that occurs in adolescence usually disappears, but if it persists, it almost always eventually becomes nodular. The chief clinical findings include evidence of tracheal or esophageal compression, occasionally with severe obstructive symptoms if the goiter becomes large enough. Compression of the recurrent laryngeal nerve is rare but is noted to produce hoarseness in a few cases of benign goiter. In addition, superior mediastinal compression may occur with large intrathoracic goiters. These multinodular goiters will often lead to hyperthyroidism between the ages of fifty and sixty. One form of familial sporadic goiter associated with deaf-mutism (Penrod's syndrome) has been shown to be due to a partial defect in the binding of trapped iodide by the thyroid.

Treatment. The incidence of endemic goiter can be greatly reduced by the use of iodized salt in iodine deficient areas. Mild and early forms of goiter in these areas can be treated by iodine in the form of Lugol's solution, 10 drops three times daily for 2 to 3 months followed by smaller amounts such as are contained in iodized salt for an indefinite period. The majority of patients with well-established endemic goiter and almost all those with sporadic goiter do not respond to iodine therapy; they do, however, usually respond to the administration of desiccated thyroid, in doses of 120 to 180 mg a day given for a period of 12 months or longer. In many of these patients, treatment should be continued indefinitely. Surgical removal is indicated only if obstructive symptoms arise rapidly (as following hemorrhage into the gland) or persist after an adequate course of suppression by thyroid medication. Thyroid (USP), 120 to 180 mg daily, should also be given postoperatively for an indefinite period of time, if well tolerated, in an effort to prevent compensatory hypertrophy or nodular development in the remaining thyroid tissue.

Thyroid Neoplasms

Adenomas. Adenomas of the thyroid may arise at any location from the base of the tongue (thyroglossal duct) to the diaphragm, most commonly within the thyroid itself. They may vary greatly in size and may contain a solitary adenoma or, more commonly, multiple nodules.

Thyroid Carcinoma. Cancers of the thyroid gland are pathologically plemorphic and seldom of a pure type. Definitive pathologic classification is difficult, and the degree of malignancy as determined histologically is not necessarily consistent with the clinical course of the disease. A modification of Warren's classification is given below:

Table 66-5. CLASSIFICATION OF THYROID TUMORS

I. Tumors of low malignancy
    A. Adenomas with blood vessel invasion
    B. "Histologic carcinoma" (small tumors found incidentally at operation; without symptoms, recurrence, or metastases)
    C. Papillary adenocarcinoma (occurs in young age group; lymphangioinvasive)
II. Tumors of moderate malignancy
    A. Nonpapillary, solid or alveolar, adenocarcinoma (occurs in older age group; hemangioinvasive; histologically the metastases may appear benign —"benign metastasizing struma")
    B. Hurthle cell adenocarcinoma (occurs in middle age group; usually locally invasive, occasional skeletal or pulmonary metastases)
III. Tumors of high malignancy (rare)
    A. Small-cell carcinoma (simplex)
    B. Giant-cell carcinoma
    C. Epidermoid carcinoma
    D. Fibrosarcoma
    E. Lymphoma

From a clinical point of view, primary thyroid carcinomas are of three major types: (1) A small number are highly anaplastic and histologically undifferentiated. These are often quite malignant and for the most part are not surgically removable nor radiosensitive. (2) A similarly uncommon type is the so-called benign metastasizing thyroid carcinoma. This variety has a predilection for metastases to bone and is often first discovered when a metastatic lesion is biopsied. (3) The largest number of thyroid cancers present with varying degrees of differentiation. The commonest of these is papillary adenocarcinoma. This latter group is generally of low virulence, metastasizes to regional lymph nodes, and is the most amenable to both medical or surgical therapy. Determination of the degree of functional differentiation may be accomplished by use of the scintogram obtained after administration of radioactive iodine. The degree of I^{131} uptake in the nodule may thus be determined and compared to the normal tissue present. In this manner, thyroid nodules may be arbitrarily divided into "hot" or "cold" nodules, depending upon whether or not they take up more or less I^{131} than the normal portions of the gland. Generally speaking, the "cold" nodules have a greater likelihood of being malignant because of their lesser function, but it must be remembered that many benign nodules and cysts are likewise "cold" and that this test should not be used as the sole determinant of malignancy or operability.

Diagnosis and Treatment. The diagnosis and management of malignancies of the thyroid gland present several problems, each of which must be taken in proper perspective. In the past, statistical analyses of the incidence of thyroid cancer in surgical specimens led to a concept upon which was based the rationale for surgical removal of thyroid nodules in the prophylaxis or therapy of thyroid cancer. This concept proposes that goiters be surgically removed to prevent cancer and is predicated upon the finding of a high incidence of cancer in goiters containing either a single nodule or multiple nodules. Recent reappraisal of the basic tenets of this concept has shown that, although the incidence of thyroid cancer in surgical specimens appears to be increasing, the actual incidence of thyroid cancer in the general population is quite low, somewhere in the range of 2.5 cases per 100,000 population per year. The death rate from thyroid cancer is probably below 0.6 per 100,000 population per year. The low death rate from this disease has suggested that the pathologic diagnosis of thyroid cancer upon which most statistics are based may be misleading and that thyroid malignancy is indeed quite rare.

Signs and symptoms most suggestive of thyroid cancer are rapid and progressive growth of the thyroid (not to be confused with overnight enlargement of a nodule which is usually due to hemorrhage or infarction), hoarseness due to recurrent laryngeal nerve paralysis, presence of lymph node enlargement in the neck or supraclavicular area, or fixation of the thyroid gland to contiguous structures. Hyperthyroidism or hypothyroidism is rarely associated with thyroid cancer. Needle biopsy of the thyroid is contraindicated in the diagnosis of thyroid malignancy because of the tendency of these neoplasms to "seed" in the incised area.

Conservatism in the treatment of most thyroid malignancies is currently the most realistic approach to this problem. Thyroid cancer of high degrees of malignancy usually progresses so rapidly that it is frequently beyond any form of treatment by the time diagnosis is established. External radiation therapy is the only rational therapeutic measure available and usually is of little benefit. Because of the extremely low degree of malignancy of most differentiated forms of thyroid cancer, current trends are directed toward avoidance or limitation of surgical procedures in the prophylaxis or therapy of thyroid cancer. This trend includes both solitary nodules and multinodular goiter and is especially pertinent in individuals over the age of forty. However, for solitary nodules in individuals under forty years and especially in children, it is currently justifiable to recommend as the treatment of choice simple excision of the nodule with a large band of surrounding normal tissue. Individuals with nodular goiters or those over the age of forty should be treated with suppressive doses of USP thyroid, in the range of 120 to 180 mg daily. This dose usually does not cause any untoward symptoms in most patients.

Following surgery of the thyroid, all patients should be kept on 120 to 180 mg of thyroid daily. The dose of thyroid used should be the minimum dose which completely inhibits the uptake of I^{131} in the thyroid, this being an indirect measure of inhibition of the TSH effect on the gland.

THYROIDITIS

Thyroiditis is a comparatively rare disease. It may be specific (suppurative or nonsuppurative), acute or subacute nonspecific, or chronic (Hashimoto's or Riedel's struma).

Specific Thyroiditis. This condition may be due to almost any known pathogenic organism, pyogenic or nonpyogenic, and is relatively rare compared to the nonspecific varieties. It may occur after infection of the mouth, pharynx, upper respiratory tract, or cervical lymph nodes. Very rarely tuberculosis, actinomycosis, syphilis, or infection with pyogenic organisms may result in single or multiple abcesses or in suppuration. Classically there are redness, swelling, and tenderness of the skin over the thyroid, together with fever and other signs of systemic infection. There may be hyperthyroidism and, rarely, thyrotoxic crisis. Therapy consists for the most part of specific chemotherapeutic or antibiotic agents along with surgical drainage where indicated.

Acute or Subacute Nonspecific Thyroiditis. This type of thyroiditis is of unknown etiology. It occurs predominantly in middle-aged women and is characterized by rapid, painful swelling of the neck, with systemic manifestations of inflammation. An elevated sedimentation rate and a low radioiodine uptake (which responds to TSH administration) are characteristic. The basal metabolic rate and serum protein-bound iodine levels may be elevated, and there may be mild symptoms of hyperthyroidism. A needle biopsy may be helpful in the diagnosis. Therapy is conservative, since spontaneous recovery is the rule. Treatment with ACTH gel (80 units intramuscularly once a day) or cortisone (50 mg every 6 hr by mouth) for up to 1 week greatly reduces the symptoms. Usually, codeine and aspirin suffice. X-ray therapy has also been found to be therapeutically effective in subacute forms of this disease.

Chronic Thyroiditis. There are two varieties of chronic thyroiditis of undetermined etiology which may be diagnosed histologically, *Hashimoto's struma* (struma lymphomatosa, lymphadenoid goiter) and *Riedel's struma*. Struma lymphomatosa, the commoner of the two, occurs predominantly in middle-aged women. It is characterized by a firm, rubbery, lobular swelling of the thyroid, simulating multinodular goiter. The serum of patients with this disorder may contain increased amounts of γ-globulin and the thymol turbidity, cephalin flocculation tests may be abnormal. The hypothyroidism commonly found in this disorder results from replacement of the functional thyroid structures by lymphoid or fibrous tissue. The serum protein-bound iodine and the 24-hr radioactive iodine uptake may be low, and there is often no response in these indices to TSH administration. Occasionally, there are abnormal, noncalorigenic, iodinated proteins circulating which raise the serum protein-bound iodine but not the butanol-extractable iodine.

Of particular interest in this disorder is the detection of circulating autoantibodies to thyroglobulin. These are precipitating as well as complement-fixing antibodies and may be measured by gel diffusion technics or quantitatively by the tanned erythrocyte hemagglutination assay. It has been postulated that Hashimoto's struma is an example of an autoimmune disease in which the damaging effects of the antigen-antibody combination in the thyroid gland lead to destruction of functional thyroid tissue. Detection of circulating antibodies to thyroglobulin is not specifically diagnostic of Hashimoto's struma, however, since they may be found in other thyroidal disorders. In addition, cytotoxic effects on human thyroid cells have been obtained with serums from patients with Hashimoto's struma; the factor responsible for these effects is apparently distinct from the autoantibodies.

Diagnosis of Hashimoto's struma is suspected on clinical grounds when nodular goiter is present with hypothyroidism. Definitive diagnosis depends upon histologic confirmation, which may be obtained by needle biopsy and by the presence of high titers of thyroglobulin antibody. Treatment consists of replacement doses of 120 to 180 mg USP thyroid daily to correct or avoid hypothyroidism and to reduce the size of the goiter. When Hashimoto's disease is first diagnosed following subtotal thyroidectomy, it is particularly important to institute thyroid substitution therapy to avoid the common postoperative consequence of hypothyroidism.

Riedel's struma produces a firm, ligneous swelling of the thyroid which may involve surrounding neck structures. This disorder is quite rare and must be differentiated from thyroid neoplasia. Needle biopsy should not be employed in the diagnosis of any thyroid disorders if malignancy is suspected. In those instances where histologic diagnosis is required to exclude malignancy, open biopsy is preferred.

REFERENCES

Astwood, E. B. (Ed.): "Clinical Endocrinology," vol. I, New York, Grune & Stratton, Inc., 1960.

Brunton, C.: Exophthalmos, Physiol. Revs., 29:260, 1949.

Chapman, E. M., and F. Maloof: The Use of Radioactive Iodine in the Diagnosis and Treatment of Hyperthyroidism: Ten Years' Experience, Medicine, 34:261, 1955.

Ciba Foundation Colloquia on Endocrinology, vol. 10, Regulation and Mode of Action on Thyroid Hormones, London, 1957.

Crile, C., Jr., and J. B. Hazard: Classification of Thyroiditis: Use of Needle Biopsy, J. Clin. Endocrinol. and Metabolism, 11:1123, 1951.

Folis, R. H.: Skeletal Changes Associated with Hyperthyroidism, Bull. Johns Hopkins Hosp., 92:405, 1953.

Hamilton, H. E., R. O. Schultz, and E. L. DeGowin: The Endocrine Eye Lesion in Hyperthyroidism, A.M.A. Arch. Internal Med., 105:676, 1960.

Hill, S. R., Jr., S. B. Barker, J. H. McNeil, J. O. Tingley, and L. L. Hibitt: The Metabolic Effects of the Acetic and Propionic Acid Analogs of Thyroxine and Triiodothyronine, J. Clin. Invest., 39:523, 1960.

Means, J. M.: "The Thyroid and Its Diseases," 2d ed., Philadelphia, J. B. Lippincott Company, 1948.

Modern Concepts of Thyroid Physiology, Ann. N.Y. Acad. Sci., 86:311, 1960.

Nickerson, J. F., S. R. Hill, Jr., J. H. McNeil, and S. B. Barker: Fatal Myxedema with and without Coma, Ann. Internal Med., 53:475, 1960.

Pitt-Rivers, R., and J. R. Tata: "The Thyroid Hormones," New York, Pergamon Press, Inc., 1959.

Quinby, E. H., S. Feitelberg, and S. Silver: "Radioactive Isotopes in Clinical Practice," Philadelphia, Lea & Febiger, 1958.

Rawson, R. W., J. E. Rall, and M. Sonnenberg: The Chemistry and Physiology of the Thyroid, in "The Hormones," New York, Academic Press, Inc., 1955.

Selenkow, H. A., and S. P. Asper, Jr.: The Effectiveness of Triiodothyronine and Thyroxine Administered Orally in the Treatment of Myxedema, J. Clin. Endocrinol. and Metabolism, 15:285, 1955.

—— and F. Colaço: Clinical Pharmacology of Antithyroid Drugs, Clin. Pharmacol. and Therap., 2:191, 1961.

—— and F. J. Marcus: Masked Hyperthyroidism and

Heart Disease, Med. Clinics N. Am., 44:1305, 1960.

Stanbury, J. B.: Familial Goiter, in "The Metabolic Basis of Inherited Disease," J. B. Stanbury, J. B. Wyngaarden, and D. S. Frederickson (Eds.), New York, McGraw-Hill Book Company, Inc., Blakiston Division, 1960.

Symposium on the Pathologic Physiology of Thyroid Disease, Am. J. Med., 20:651, 1956.

Symposium—The Thyroid Gland, Brit. Med. Bull., 16: 89, 169, 1960.

Thorn, G. W., and H. A. Eder: Studies on Chronic Thyrotoxic Myopathy, Am. J. Med., 1:583, 1946.

Warren, S.: Classification of Tumors of the Thyroid, Am. J. Roentgenol., 46:447, 1941.

Werner, S. D.: "The Thyroid," New York, Paul B. Hoeber, Inc., Medical Department of Harper & Brothers, 1955.

67 DISEASES OF THE PARATHYROID GLANDS

Daniel S. Bernstein, Alan Goldfien, and George W. Thorn

The parathyroid glands were first recognized as separate structures and described by Sandstrom in 1880. Shortly thereafter Gley (1881) and others performed extirpation experiments demonstrating that tetany was caused by the removal of the parathyroids rather than the thyroid, as had been suggested on the basis of earlier observations. The classic experiments of McCallum and Voegtlin in 1908 showed that hypoparathyroid tetany was due to a lowered plasma calcium and that tetany ceased with the intravenous injection of calcium. Further proof of the endocrine nature of these glands followed the preparation of parathyroid extracts by Collip in Canada, by Hanson and Berman in the United States, and by the demonstration that these extracts were capable of inducing an elevation of plasma calcium.

ANATOMY AND PHYSIOLOGY OF THE PARATHYROID GLANDS

Anatomy. The parathyroid glands originate from the posterior halves of the third and fourth pairs of pharyngeal pouches. Therefore, like the thyroid, the parathyroids are entodermal in origin. In man the parathyroids are reddish or yellowish brown and are flattened, ovate, or pyriform bodies located on the posterior surfaces of the lateral lobes of the thyroid. There are normally four glands. The number may vary from two to ten, and their location is extremely variable. They have been found within the thyroid gland, in the mediastinum, and in scattered regions of the neck. The average size of a human parathyroid gland is 5 by 3 by 3 mm, and the combined weight of four glands averages about 120 mg.

In the adult, the parathyroid gland contains chief cells and oxyphil cells. The chief cells are more numerous and are probably the source of the parathyroid hormone. These cells are 6 to 8 μ in diameter and contain glycogen. The oxyphil cells appear in the human gland at about the tenth year of life. They contain no glycogen, and their nuclei are somewhat pycnotic. They may represent a more mature or inactive chief cell. Another cell, the large water-clear cell (*wasserhelle* cell) derived from the chief cell, is the commonest cell type observed in hypertrophy and hyperplasia of the parathyroids.

Function. The parathyroid glands exert a regulatory effect on calcium, phosphate, and bone metabolism. Parathyroid hormone has been shown to increase urinary phosphate excretion, decrease plasma inorganic phosphate level, increase plasma calcium level, and increase the urinary excretion of calcium. These changes are effected by the regulation of the tubular reabsorption of phosphorus and increased mobilization of calcium and phosphate from bone. This hormone has also been shown to influence bone matrix resorption directly, although the mechanism whereby this occurs is as yet unclear. Discussion of the mechanism of parathyroid hormone action can be found in Chap. 77.

The role of parathyroid hormone in the homeostatic regulation of calcium and phosphate concentration in body fluids can be summarized as follows: (1) if the component processes (absorption, storage, utilization, release, and excretion) of mineral metabolism result in a fall in the plasma calcium concentration, the parathyroid glands are stimulated to secrete more hormone; (2) if the dietary intake is high in calcium, there is less of a negative calcium balance and the bone depot may be spared; otherwise bone resorption occurs.

There is no conclusive evidence that a calcium-phosphorus solubility product exists in the plasma, and likewise it has not been shown conclusively that a high plasma phosphate level stimulates the parathyroid glands to produce more hormone. Recently it has been shown that parathyroid hormone causes an increased absorption of calcium from the gastrointestinal tract and this, along with the prevalence of high calcium intake in the diet, might help to explain the numerous cases of hyperparathyroidism where there is no evidence of bone resorption. At the present time there is no unanimity of opinion regarding the actions of parathyroid hormone among investigators in the field, but most believe that parathyroid hormone has a direct action on bone, resulting in dissolution of the mineral phase of the bone.

Parathyroid Hormone. In recent years major progress has been made in the purification of parathyroid hormone. While no one investigator has been able to crystallize the hormone, it is apparent that the parathyroid hormone is a protein containing some 20 or more amino acids. There has not been any separation of fractions, and it appears that the active portion contains both calcium mobilizing and renal tubular phosphate blocking properties. The molecular weight of the hormone is about 9,000. It is not available for commercial use at present. Parathyroid extract, USP, is standardized by biologic assay so that 1 ml contains 100 to 120 USP units. The USP unit is defined as one-hundredth of the amount required to raise the plasma calcium level of a normal male dog weighing 10 to 12 kg by 1.0 mg per 100 ml within 16 to 18 hr after a single subcutaneous injection.

Regulation of Parathyroid Activity. The parathyroid glands do not appear to be under the direct control of a tropic hormone elaborated by the anterior pituitary, nor is there evidence of nervous control of their secretory activity. However, a number of observations point to an indirect relationship to other endocrine organs. Parathyroid hyperplasia has been reported in cases of acromegaly, Cushing's syndrome, Addison's disease, and pancreatic islet cell adenomas. Experimentally, hypophysectomy in animals causes some involution of the parathyroids, whereas growth hormone, adrenocorticotropin, crude anterior pituitary extracts, and adrenal steroids cause hyperplasia. It is possible that these changes are secondary to the alteration in serum mineral levels mediated by the pituitary, thyroid, adrenal, gonadal, and islet cell hormones. A number of cases of multiple tumors involving the anterior pituitary, pancreatic islet tissue, and the parathyroids have been reported. Since tumors of these glands are quite rare, their association can scarcely be explained as a matter of chance. Also the familial occurrence of multiple tumors of this type has been noted. Although unexplained, the association of these tumors is of clinical importance.

The parathyroid glands alter their production of hormone in response to changes in the plasma level of ionized calcium. It is generally agreed that hormone production is stimulated by hypocalcemia and decreased by hypercalcemia. Hyperplasia of the parathyroids is found in those conditions in which there is a tendency toward a low plasma calcium level, viz., rickets (or osteomalacia), calcium deprivation, and renal insufficiency with acidosis. There is conflicting evidence concerning an increase in parathyroid hormone production in patients with hyperphosphatemia in the absence of hypocalcemia.

It is not possible to measure satisfactorily parathyroid hormone levels in blood or urine. For this reason assessment of endogenous parathyroid secretion must depend on the evaluation of the changes in metabolic processes known to be influenced by the parathyroid glands. Changes in the plasma calcium, phosphate, and alkaline phosphatase levels are the most important indicators of the state of parathyroid function (see Chap. 77).

HYPOPARATHYROIDISM

History. One of the causes of tetany is total or extensive parathyroidectomy. Tetany received its name from Corvisart in 1852. MacCallum and Voegtlin in 1908 showed that the mechanism of this type of tetany was dependent upon hypocalcemia. The Swiss surgeons Reverdin and Kocher in 1882 described postoperative tetany after a complete thyroidectomy for goiter without realizing that the condition was due to parathyroid deficiency.

Etiology and Pathology. Primary parathyroid deficiency is extremely rare, usually occurring in patients under the age of sixteen, but often persisting throughout adult life. In most instances, clinical evidence of parathyroid deficiency is secondary to thyroidectomy. During the past decade increased knowledge and experience in surgical techniques have decreased the incidence of permanent parathyroid deficiency secondary to thyroidectomy. Transient deficiency is not unusual and is attributed to trauma, edema, hemorrhage, and temporary interference with the blood supply to the remaining parathyroid glands. There have been no documented cases of hypoparathyroidism secondary to the administration of radioactive iodine in the treatment of thyrotoxicosis.

Pathologic Physiology. There is a pronounced disturbance of calcium and phosphate metabolism as reflected by plasma calcium levels as low as 2.5 mEq per liter (5 mg per 100 ml) and plasma inorganic phosphate levels as high as 3 to 4 millimoles per liter (9.3 to 12.4 mg per 100 ml) and phosphorus levels of 1.0 millimole per liter (3.1 mg per 100 ml). The decrease in calcium facilitates the transmission of impulses across the myoneural junction, which is responsible for much of the clinical picture.

Clinical Picture. The most striking symptom is an increased neuromuscular excitability resulting from a decrease in the plasma ionized calcium. The presenting complaint in most (70 per cent) of these patients is tetany or tetanic equivalents. Tetany is manifested by carpopedal spasm in which the stiff, hollowed hand with rigid fingers is flexed at the metacarpal-phalangeal, wrist, and elbow joints, and the legs and feet are extended. The tetanic equivalents include tonic and clonic convulsions, laryngeal stridor (spasm) which may be fatal, paresthesias, numbness, muscle cramps, dysphagia, dysarthria, muscular palsies, and cardiac irregularities. Spasm may involve the smooth muscle of the eye, gastrointestinal tract, bladder, and blood vessels. About 40 per cent of these patients are seen because of epileptic seizures. The electroencephalographic findings in these patients suggest that occasionally underlying factors unrelated to plasma calcium levels play an important part in lowering the threshold for convulsive seizures. Mental changes are frequent and include anxiety, depression, increased irritability, and psychoses. Acute symptoms may be precipitated by infection, undue fatigue, menstruation, and emotional upsets and by an increase in the phosphate content of the diet. In some cases, the symptoms may be quite mild, varied, and even vague. Patients have manifested fatigue, muscular weakness, palpitations, numbness and tingling of the extremities, and other signs of latent tetany for as long as 30 years before a diagnosis of chronic hypoparathyroidism was established.

On examination, increased neuromuscular excitability may be demonstrated by contraction of the facial muscles in response to a light tap over the facial nerve in front of the ear (Chvostek's sign). This test is almost always positive in untreated hypoparathyroidism; however, it does occur occasionally in normal individuals. Dorsal flexion and abduction of the foot may be elicited by tapping the lateral surface of the fibula just below its head (peroneal sign). If the circulation to the arm is occluded by inflation of a blood pressure cuff above the level of systolic pressure, the hand may assume the typical position seen in carpopedal spasm within 3 min (Trousseau's sign). This sign is sometimes negative in marked hypoparathyroidism. Extensive tropic changes of the ectoderm may be seen. The hair is likely to be sparse, prematurely gray, and is occasionally absent in the axillary and pubic regions. Generalized or patchy erythema may be found. The skin is rough, dry, and scaling, and there may be papules, vesicles, or bullae. A number of skin diseases have been described in association with hypoparathyroidism, including moniliasis of the skin, nails, tongue, and mouth. However, no etiologic relationship has been established. The nails are deformed and brittle, showing transverse ridging. In children one finds evidence of faulty dentition, including pitting and ridging of the enamel. Cataracts are frequently present, their extent being related to the duration and severity of the hypocalcemia. Early lens changes, not apparent on ophthalmoscopic examination, can usually be found with the aid of a slit lamp. Papilledema has been observed. The electrocardiogram usually shows a prolongation of the Q-T interval. The density of the bone may appear normal or increased. Abnormalities of dentition, such as deformed or absent roots, may be helpful in determining the age of onset of the disease. The pronounced disturbance of calcium and phosphate metabolism is reflected by lowered plasma calcium and elevated plasma inorganic phosphate levels. The alkaline phosphatase is normal or low. Hypocalcuria may be present, as shown by a negative Sulkowitch test (see p. 603). The spinal fluid may be under increased pressure without other abnormalities. When this occurs in the presence of papilledema, the diagnosis of a brain tumor may be made incorrectly. In primary hypoparathyroidism, bilateral symmetrical calcification of the basal ganglia is commonly seen on the skull film. Other areas, such as the cerebellum and choroid plexus, are occasionally calcified.

Differential Diagnosis. The principal causes of tetany are hypocalcemia and alkalosis. Of the nonparathyroid causes of hypocalcemia, rickets, osteomalacia, steatorrhea, and renal insufficiency are the most common. Recently, there has been described a new syndrome of "decreased tissue calcium with tetany." This condition is manifested by severe tetany with normal plasma levels of calcium, magnesium, potassium, and carbon dioxide content. It has been demonstrated by radioactive calcium studies that the tissue calcium pool is lower than normal and that treatment with vitamin D will tend to bring the level of calcium in this pool toward normal. Extreme caution must be employed since the difference between the therapeutic and toxic dose of vitamin D is narrow.

In rickets, osteomalacia, and steatorrhea, a low value for plasma calcium is almost invariably associated with a normal or low value for plasma phosphate. In late-stage renal insufficiency with hypocalcemic tetany, the elevation in plasma phosphate level is disproportionately higher than that which occurs with a given level of hypocalcemia in parathyroid tetany. Nitrogen retention, as evidenced by an elevated blood urea nitrogen or nonprotein nitrogen, is nearly always present and differentiates the two conditions. A lowered plasma magnesium can also produce tetany. Magnesium salts have been used to eliminate hypocalcemic tetany. Furthermore, the level of plasma potassium plays an important part in the clinical manifestation of hypocalcemic tetany. The relationship of these three ions in the serum as regards tetany can be formulated as follows: calcium $\times$ magnesium/potassium. This is especially important in the treatment of renal failure where all three of these ions are drastically altered.

In addition to general renal insufficiency, there are two specific tubular lesions to be considered.

The first is a failure of reabsorption of certain amino acids (Fanconi syndrome, Chap. 88 and p. 748) in which there is increased excretion of phosphate and low phosphate rickets, and the second is a rare selective failure of calcium reabsorption accompanied by metabolic acidosis and often by renal calcinosis.

Alkalosis causes tetany with no demonstrable change in the concentration of calcium in the plasma. Alkalosis may be due to hyperventilation, to prolonged vomiting of acid gastric contents, or to excessive alkali ingestion. With hyperventilation, the carbon dioxide *content* of the plasma is reduced; whereas with vomiting, and alkali ingestion, the carbon dioxide combining power of the plasma may be increased greatly (see Chap. 51). Alkalotic tetany occurs most frequently in association with acute infection, particularly in children.

Treatment. The object of treatment is to increase and maintain the plasma calcium at an approximately normal level.

Management of Acute Hypoparathyroidism. Immediate correction of hypocalcemia may be accomplished by intravenous injections of calcium gluconate (10 ml of a 10 per cent solution) or calcium chloride (10 ml of a 5 per cent solution or an intravenous drip of 500 ml of 0.2 per cent solution over a 1-hr period) (see Table 67-1). The effect is transitory, lasting only a few hours, and additional calcium may have to be administered. Caution should be exercised with patients on digitalis, since rapid infusion of calcium may cause cardiac arrest.

Parathyroid extract injection may be instituted along with the infusion of calcium and will give more prolonged action (12 to 24 hr). Parathyroid extract is available in injectable form containing 80 to 120 USP units per milliliter. From 100 to 200 units should be administered intravenously. Administration should proceed slowly initially since anaphylactoid reaction may occur and necessitate discontinuance. From 25 to 50 units of parathyroid extract may be given every 6 to 12 hr during the acute phase of hypoparathyroidism.

Dihydrotachysterol should be administered in doses of 1 to 3 ml (1.25 to 3.75 mg) one to three times daily by mouth until calcium appears in the urine, as indicated by the Sulkowitch test. The dose is then adjusted to maintain a normal serum calcium level. Treatment may be continued with this preparation or with a cheaper but just as adequate preparation of calciferol (vitamin D_2). Supplementary calcium preparations should be given orally as soon as possible. Calcium chloride is most effective, since it forms an acid solution which favors calcium absorption and also contains a higher percentage of available calcium. It may be administered in doses of 10 ml of a 30 per cent solution, well diluted, three times a day after meals (see Table 67-1). A licorice sirup medium will conceal the taste of calcium chloride solution.

Management of Chronic Hypoparathyroidism. The objective of therapy in chronic hypoparathyroidism is to reduce the plasma phosphate and raise the plasma calcium levels. This is best accom-

Table 67-1. CALCIUM-REGULATING COMPOUNDS

Type	Route of administration	Dosage	Effect on plasma calcium
Calcium gluconate (USP)....	Intravenous Intramuscular	5 to 20 ml of 10% aqueous solution (i.v.) 10 ml of 5% solution (1 to 2 times daily i.m.)	Immediate but of only short duration
	Oral	10 to 25 Gm daily	
Calcium chloride (USP).....	Intravenous	55 ml of 0.2% over 1 hr (i.v.) or 10 ml of 5% aqueous solution slowly (i.v.)	Immediate but of only short duration
	Oral	10 ml of 30% aqueous (2 to 3 times daily)	
Calcium lactate...........	Oral	10 to 15 Gm daily (as a clear solution)	Immediate but of only short duration
Dihydrotachysterol (AT 10)..	Oral	3 to 4 ml (1.25 mg per ml) daily initially; 1 ml (3 to 5 times weekly) as maintenance	Delayed, with a maximum in 48-96 hr. Prolonged effect
Calciferol (vitamin D_2)......	Oral	50,000 to 200,000 units daily (1.25 to 5 mg)	Delayed. Prolonged effect
Parathyroid..............	Subcutaneous or intramuscular	100 to 200 units in severe tetany and then 25 to 50 units every 6 to 12 hr. Not recommended maintenance	Moderately rapid, with maximum in 8 to 18 hr

plished by a combination of dietary and drug therapy. The diet should include as much calcium as tolerated, but there is nothing to be gained by reducing the amounts of phosphate in the diet unless it is eaten in excess. From 4 to 8 Gm of the various calcium salts shown in Table 67-1 should be given.

Parathyroid hormone is rarely used except in critical situations since it must be given daily and may be associated with local reactions. There is no evidence that antibodies will develop to chronically administered parathyroid hormone. It is almost always advantageous to administer vitamin D_2 (calciferol) in ranges of 50,000 to 150,000 units daily, in order to enhance plasma calcium levels. Dihydrotachysterol, a synthetic derivative of ergosterol, may also be used, but while its action is similar to vitamin D_2 in all respects, it is much more expensive and rarely must be resorted to in favor of vitamin D_2. When vitamin D_2 or AT 10 (dihydrotachysterol) is used in therapy, the plasma calcium should be determined at frequent intervals, because persistent hypercalcemia and hypercalcuria may lead to deleterious effects. Since vitamin D_2 or AT 10 will cause an increase in the urine calcium before affecting a rise in blood calcium levels, it is important to check the urine level of calcium often as well as the plasma calcium, either by total 24-hr calcium excretion or by the Sulkowitch test. The Sulkowitch solution has the following composition:

Oxalic acid	2.5 Gm
Ammonium oxalate	2.5 Gm
Glacial acetic acid	5.0 ml
Distilled water q.s. ad	150.0 ml

The test is performed by adding 5 ml of the reagent to 5 ml urine in a test tube, noting the speed of appearance and the density of the precipitate. The result is graded 0, 1, 2, 3, or 4 plus. Routine use of the test for a short time enables one to become familiar with a normal response. The calcium intake (e.g., quantity of milk) as well as marked concentration or dilution of the urine should be taken into account. A negative test after a week on a diet free of milk and cheese suggests hypocalcemia— less than 3.5 mEq per liter (7.0 mg per 100 ml)— and a 3 to 4 plus test suggests hypercalcemia— more than 5.2 mEq per liter (10.4 mg per 100 ml). While this test can be run by the patient it is important to check plasma levels from time to time. A 2 plus Sulkowitch reaction is the most desirable.

An adjunctive mode of therapy is the use of probenecid (Benemid) by mouth in doses ranging from 0.5 to 1.5 Gm (daily). This agent is most useful in treating the tetany seen directly after inadvertent surgical removal of the parathyroids but is of little help in the chronic treatment of hypoparathyroidism. Rarely can Benemid be used alone.

Its action is on the kidney blocking the reabsorption of phosphate by the renal tubule in a similar manner to the way it blocks the tubular reabsorption of uric acid. If epilepsy is evident, Dilantin or other antiepileptic drugs should be employed.

PSEUDOHYPOPARATHYROIDISM

The first description of this rare condition was given by Albright and his coworkers in 1942. This disease presents the same clinical and chemical features as hypoparathyroidism, except that these patients have round faces and short, thick figures. Subcutaneous centers of ossification are seen. There is a characteristic shortening of some of the metacarpal and metatarsal bones as a result of early epiphyseal closure, so that a dimple rather than a knuckle shows upon clenching of the fist. Most of the patients show some degree of mental deficiency. Not all these characteristics are necessarily present; any one or a combination of them may be found. The apparent parathyroid deficiency in these patients appears to be due to a lack of end organ response. This is supported by the failure to respond to parathyroid extract, the finding of normal or hyperplastic glands where biopsy specimens have been obtained, and the failure to demonstrate antibodies to parathyroid hormone in the serum of patients in whom studies were done. The failure of these patients to respond to parathyroid extract need not be complete, and there are cases which have almost normal response to injected hormone.

It was suggested that the abnormalities seen in pseudo-pseudohypoparathyroidism and which are also found in pseudohypoparathyroidism are probably due to separate genetic factors, which may penetrate independently. Subsequent reports support this concept. Albright and his group have reported a case of a young woman with a rounded face, thickset figure, characteristic smile, shortened fingers and toes, and subcutaneous calcium deposits. However, the plasma calcium and phosphate levels were normal, and the Chvostek and Trousseau signs were absent.

Diagnosis. Because of the frequent history of convulsions, the condition may be incorrectly labeled epilepsy. The symptomatology, chemical findings, and physical signs are those of hypoparathyroidism. The relative resistance to parathyroid extract as measured by failure to produce a phosphate diuresis (Ellsworth-Howard test) serves to distinguish it from hypoparathyroidism.

The Ellsworth-Howard Test. The test is performed as follows: The patient, in the fasting state, is given 2 ml (200 units) of parathyroid extract intravenously, and the urinary phosphate content is determined hourly for 3 hr prior to, and for 3 to 5 hr following, the injection. Occasional anaphylactoid reactions to the extract demand slow and careful administration. Parathyroid extracts are assayed by their effect on the plasma calcium level, and recent preparations have not been so effective in producing an increased phosphate excretion as those previously available. It is best to compare the response of the patient to that of a normal control given the same amount of hormone. The degree of phosphate diuresis induced by parathyroid hormone is dependent upon both the level of endogenous parathyroid secretion and the responsiveness of the phosphorus reabsorbing mechanism of the renal tubules. Following the injection of a standard amount of parathyroid extract, there is a five- to sixfold increase in urine phosphate in normal persons, a tenfold or greater increase in patients with hypoparathyroidism, and at the most a twofold increase in patients with pseudohypoparathyroidism (parathyroid hormone resistance). Patients with hyperparathyroidism show a variable response to the extract.

Treatment. The therapy is the same as that outlined under chronic hypoparathyroidism.

PRIMARY HYPERPARATHYROIDISM

History. Generalized osteitis fibrosa cystica, a generalized disease of bones, was described in 1891 by von Recklinghausen. Askanazy associated this condition with a parathyroid tumor in 1904, and in 1925 Mandl removed a parathyroid adenoma from a patient suffering from this disease, noting a remarkable improvement. The occurrence of hyperparathyroidism without bone disease was pointed out by Albright in 1934. The clinical and metabolic studies subsequently carried out by Albright, Bauer, Aub, and Cope are classic.

Incidence. The exact incidence of the disease is unknown, but thanks to the work of Albright and his colleagues there has been a deliberate search for the disease, with a consequent increase in the frequency of diagnosis. The disease occurs most often in middle life, and about 70 per cent of the reported cases are women. It has been shown that hyperparathyroidism can exist without evident disease of bone and that skeletal involvement represents a relatively late development. Involvement of the urinary tract is much more common than bone disease in the United States, presumably because of the high calcium intake, and in several series of cases more than 5 per cent of all kidney stones have been associated with hyperfunction of these glands. Many cases of hyperparathyroidism in the United States are "masked" by insignificant or atypical alterations in plasma calcium and phosphate levels resulting from a high phosphate intake.

Etiology. Hypersecretion of the parathyroid glands may be caused by adenoma, hyperplasia, or carcinoma. The most common cause of primary hyperparathyroidism is an adenoma (90 per cent of cases), hyperplasia is rather infrequent, and carcinoma is rare.

Pathology. Adenomas are usually limited to one gland. Norris collected from the literature 322 cases of parathyroid adenoma, with only 20 cases (6.2 per cent) having multiple tumors. The pathologic overactivity of these tumors is not closely associated with their size. The adenomas are encapsulated, soft, orange-brown masses embedded in fat. They are occasionally lobular. The appearance, grossly, differs from that of the hyperplastic gland, which is irregular in shape and a darker, mahogany brown in color. The adenoma usually involves the entire gland but may involve only part of it. Adenomas are found in all the locations of the normal parathyroid glands. In one large series, 75 per cent were found in the mediastinum. All cell types may be present, forming cords, glands, and solid masses. Cyst formation is common.

In primary diffuse hypertrophy and hyperplasia all the glands are involved but not necessarily to the same extent. The glands show a uniformity of structure, with a predominance of very large *wasserhelle* cells and a tendency to gland formation. There is a good correlation of size to the degree of overactivity.

Carcinoma of the parathyroid gland is extremely rare, accounting for 1 per cent of functioning parathyroid tumors. They are generally larger than adenomas and in most cases have been clinically palpable. All these tumors have been associated with severe hyperparathyroidism with bone disease. They are generally slow growing, tending to recur locally when excised, and are very resistant to x-ray therapy. Metastases to the regional lymph nodes, lungs, and liver may occur. There is evidence indicating that carcinoma may develop from an adenoma.

The skeletal lesions observed in conjunction with long-standing hyperparathyroidism are discussed in Chap. 79, Osteomalacia and Rickets. Degenerative changes occur in the renal tubular epithelium, heart muscle, and gastric mucosa and are often followed by calcification. About 80 per cent of the cases show some evidence of renal damage such as nephrolithiasis, pyelonephritis, and calcium deposits in and around the tubules.

Mineral Levels. Characteristically, the plasma calcium is elevated and may attain values as high as 10 mEq per liter (20 mg per 100 ml). The plasma inorganic phosphate level is reduced below 1 millimole per liter (3.1 mg per 100 ml) unless renal damage has resulted in secondary phosphate retention. In the presence of a high phosphate intake, many patients with hyperparathyroidism have plasma phosphate levels which fall within normal limits, with minimal elevation in plasma calcium levels. The excretion of calcium and phosphate in the urine is increased. With extensive bone involvement, the alkaline phosphatase may reach levels as high as 20 to 30 Bodansky units.

Clinical Picture. The earliest symptoms rarely lead to a diagnosis. They may be recognized in retrospect as an accompaniment of hypercalcemia. The symptoms include muscular weakness, anorexia, nausea, and constipation. Polyuria and polydipsia accompany the excessive calcium, phosphate, sodium, and potassium excretion as well as the renal lesions, which cause a loss of the ability of the kidney to concentrate urine even before structural changes have occurred. Often the first indication of hyperparathyroidism is renal colic or a spontaneous fracture. Deafness, paresthesias, and bone pain have been observed, and weight loss may be marked. On examination one may find hypotonia, muscular weakness, calcific keratitis (band keratitis), skeletal deformities, fractures, and tumor masses, especially in the jaw (epulis). When bone disease is present, x-ray studies may show a generalized decrease in bone density, cysts, tumors, fractures, and deformities, which are most marked in the hands, long bones, vertebras, pelvis, skull, and jaw. Bone marrow depression is common, with anemia, leukopenia, and occasionally thrombocytopenia. Peptic ulcer occurs in many patients with this disorder.

Diagnosis. Classic cases of chemical hyperparathyroidism with von Recklinghausen's disease (osteitis fibrosa generalisata or osteitis fibrosa cystica) are diagnosed easily from the clinical picture and the chemical findings of hypercalcemia, hypophosphatemia, hypercalcuria, and an increased plasma alkaline phosphatase (Table 67-2). It is important to carry out simultaneous calcium and total protein determinations, as marked hypoproteinemia (with accompanying decrease in calcium proteinate) may mask an increase in diffusible ionized calcium, the fraction of importance in this disease. It is also important to obtain plasma calcium levels on several occasions, particularly if the first determination is not elevated. While neither the protein nor the ionic fraction can be measured with ease directly, both can be estimated from the concentration of total calcium and total protein by use of the readily available nomogram of McLean and Hastings. Bone lesions may be absent or minimal when calcium and protein intake have been high or when the disease is relatively mild or of short duration. In such cases the plasma alkaline phosphatase level may not be elevated. The diagnosis of hyperparathyroidism should be carefully ruled out in all patients with renal stones. Lithiasis often occurs in mild cases in which no other symptoms are present and plasma mineral levels show minimal changes.

Table 67-2. SUMMARY OF CHEMICAL FEATURES OF DISEASES WITH DISTURBED PLASMA CALCIUM AND PHOSPHATE

Disease	Serum			Urine		Feces*	
	Calcium	Phosphate	Alkaline phosphatase	Calcium	Phosphate	Calcium	Phosphate
Hyperparathyroidism . .	Increased	Decreased	Normal or increased	Increased	Increased	Normal	Normal
Paget's disease.	Normal	Normal	Increased	Normal	Normal	Normal	Normal
Hypoparathyroidism. . .	Decreased	Increased	Normal	Decreased	Decreased	Normal	Normal
Renal insufficiency.	Decreased	Increased	Normal or increased	Decreased	Decreased	Normal	Increased
Osteomalacia.	Decreased or normal	Decreased	Increased	Decreased	Decreased	Normal or increased	Decreased
Senile osteoporosis.	Normal	Normal	Normal	Normal	Normal	Normal	Normal
Multiple myeloma.	Normal to increased	Normal	Normal	Normal to increased	Normal to decreased	Normal	Normal
Milk-alkali syndrome. . .	Increased	Normal to increased	Normal	Normal to decreased	Normal to decreased		
Vitamin D intoxication.	Increased	Increased	Normal	Increased	Decreased		
Metastatic carcinoma . .	Normal to increased	Normal	Normal to increased	Increased	Normal	Decreased	Decreased
Sarcoidosis.	Increased	Normal to increased	Normal to increased	Increased	Decreased	Decreased	Decreased
Hyperventilation (alkalosis).	Normal	Normal	Normal	Normal	Normal		

* On low calcium diet.

Although hypercalcuria occurs in the absence of hyperparathyroidism, particularly in patients with nephrolithiasis, it is helpful in establishing the diagnosis from other causes. If after 7 to 14 days on a diet of 200 mg calcium the patient excretes more than 200 mg calcium in the urine in 24 hr, hypercalcuria is present. In the presence of avitaminosis D or renal insufficiency, hypercalcuria may not be found in hyperparathyroidism. An approximation of the urinary calcium concentration may be made with the Sulkowitch test.

The early diagnosis of hyperparathyroidism in the absence of renal and skeletal lesions may be extremely difficult, and several procedures have been devised to facilitate diagnosis.

Intravenous Calcium Test. When a calcium load is administered intravenously, the normal individual responds with a rise in the plasma phosphate level and a fall in the urinary phosphate excretion. This is due to the fact that calcium will "shut off" the parathyroids if the plasma level is high enough. Theoretically, patients with hyperparathyroidism should not show the decrease in urinary excretion of phosphate, but the results are often inconclusive. Patients with hypoparathyroidism show a marked phosphate diuresis, and this test is probably most useful in diagnosing true hypoparathyroidism.

Tubular Reabsorption of Phosphate. Parathyroid hormone decreases the tubular reabsorption of phosphate in the renal tubules, and it has been found that patients with hyperparathyroidism have a tubular reabsorption of phosphate which is distinctly lower than normal. This can be best demonstrated by giving these patients an oral phosphate load and calculating the tubular maximal transport of phosphate. It can be shown that, when there is a normal inulin clearance, this type of determination is valid and is further evidence for the tubular blocking action for phosphate by parathyroid hormone.

Cortisone Test. The action of cortisone on the normal patient is to decrease the absorption of calcium from the gastrointestinal tract and to increase the urinary output of calcium. In those patients with sarcoidosis and hypercalcemia, multiple myeloma, vitamin D intoxication, infantile hypercalcemia with failure to thrive, and metastatic carcinoma with hypercalcemia, cortisone has been shown to lower the plasma calcium within a matter of a few days to 2 weeks. When the diagnosis of hyperparathyroidism is uncertain, this test can often help make the correct diagnosis since cortisone does not affect the hypercalcemia due to a parathyroid adenoma.

Differential Diagnosis. Careful observation may be required to differentiate less typical cases from the following skeletal disorders:

Osteoporosis. In this disease there is a negative calcium balance and a decreased bone mass. Calcium, phosphate, and alkaline phosphatase are normal. This is frequently seen in women after the menopause and involves the spine and pelvis, very rarely the skull. The negative calcium balance can be reversed by the administration of estrogens or androgens, and recent work has shown that the balance can be made positive by the administration of large doses of calcium in the diet alone.

Osteomalacia. This implies failure to mineralize an otherwise normal matrix, seen especially in steatorrhea, vitamin D deficiency, and primary renal acidosis. Both plasma calcium and phosphate are decreased, while plasma alkaline phosphatase is increased. The urinary calcium excretion is decreased in the first two disorders and increased in the last.

Multiple Myeloma. This condition may show sharp demarcation of bone lesions by x-ray, with increased plasma and urine calcium, possible stones, a variable phosphate level, increased globulin, Bence-Jones protein (50 per cent), and plasma cells in the bone marrow. Even though massive bone disease may be seen by x-ray, the alkaline phosphatase usually remains within normal limits.

Metastatic Malignancies. These may present a variable x-ray picture, depending on whether the origin of the primary tumor is the breast, prostate, kidney, bronchus, or thyroid. Plasma calcium and alkaline phosphatase may be increased. An increase in the prostatic fraction of the total acid phosphatase is presumptive evidence for carcinoma of the prostate. The acid phosphatase may be elevated in other types of metastatic cancer to bone.

Renal Osteitis Fibrosa. In this condition there exists a history of onset of renal difficulties prior to skeletal changes. However, this differentiation is often extraordinarily difficult to ascertain. It should be stated that if an elevated plasma calcium is found with severe long-standing renal disease this is most likely due to primary hyperparathyroidism.

Sarcoidosis. While it once was believed that the bone lesions seen as punched out lesions in the hands and feet were responsible for the cases of hypercalcemia in association with sarcoid, this has been shown not to be the case. Indeed, the association of hypercalcemia in sarcoidosis is rarely seen in those cases where the bones are involved. There is little doubt at present that the hypercalcemia is secondary to an increased sensitivity to vitamin D and that moderate exposure to bright sunlight is enough to induce hypercalcemia in the 20 to 30 per cent of those afflicted with sarcoid who have this sensitivity. The hypercalcemia responds rapidly to cortisone administration and serves to distinguish this disease from hyperparathyroidism in most instances. An increased globulin, pulmonary fibrosis, splenomegaly, hepatomegaly, and a positive Kveim test help to establish the diagnosis.

Other Skeletal Diseases. Gaucher's disease, Niemann-Pick disease, Hand-Schüller-Christian syndrome, Hodgkin's disease, osteogenesis imperfecta, osteomyelitis, xanthomatosis, chronic radium poisoning, polycythemia vera, erythroblastosis, etc., may have to be considered in the differential diagnosis. A more complete discussion of these individual skeletal disorders is given in Part Four, Sec. 3.

Hypercalcemia Associated with Renal Insufficiency and Prolonged Milk or Alkali Ingestion. Burnett and his coworkers (1949) described a syndrome with many features common to primary hyperparathyroidism and secondary renal damage. The characteristic features in patients with this syndrome were a history of prolonged and excessive intake of milk and absorbable alkali, hypercalcemia without hypercalcuria or hypophosphatemia, marked renal insufficiency, calcinosis, and mild alkalosis. The differentiation of this syndrome from primary hyperparathyroidism may be very difficult because of the high incidence of ulcer symptoms in hyperparathyroidism. Treatment consists of a low milk, low alkali diet and a high fluid intake. The azotemia and hypercalcemia may diminish and the chemical imbalance may be restored to normal, but residual renal damage may persist.

Vitamin D Intoxication. Excessive vitamin D administration induces a clinical and pathologic picture similar to hyperparathyroidism. The symptoms of intoxication are those secondary to hypercalcemia and hypercalcuria already described. Recovery depends upon prompt diagnosis and upon the severity of the toxicity. Cortisone is the treatment of choice, as well as complete elimination of all sources of vitamin D, in moderate to severe cases of poisoning. The dose of cortisone should range from 75 to 150 mg per day and should be maintained at this level until a normal plasma calcium is attained. The severe manifestations of the hypercalcemia will recede in a week to 10 days under such treatment, but other minor side effects, such as lassitude, weakness, loss of appetite, etc., may take anywhere from weeks to months before disappearing.

Hypercalcemia in Carcinoma without Metastases. Recently there have been numerous instances in which a picture resembling hyperparathyroidism was abolished by removing a cancer locally. These cases were not associated with any demonstrable bony metastases. The cause of the hypercalcemia is not evident, although it has been presumed that these tumors have secreted a substance with plasma calcium raising properties. The cortisone test is often a useful tool in differentiating this cause of hypercalcemia from hyperparathyroidism.

Immobilization. Any patient with diffuse skeletal disease or chronic disease, if immobilized, can develop hypercalcemia and hypercalcuria, unless appropriate measures to prevent its occurrence are taken. No patient with Paget's disease should be put to bed for any long interval since such a patient is especially prone to develop hypercalcuria.

Idiopathic Hypercalcemia of Infancy with Failure to Thrive. This is a new syndrome first described in Great Britain by Lightwood and his associates. These infants often have mental retardation, elfin facies, elevated cholesterol levels in the plasma, and hypercalcemia with all its secondary effects on the kidney and elsewhere. They will respond to cortisone or a diet devoid of vitamin D and calcium. It has been postulated that these children have an abnormal sensitivity to vitamin D similar to that found in sarcoidosis.

Idiopathic Hypercalcuria. There is a large group of stone formers who characteristically have hypercalcuria, low plasma phosphate, and a normal plasma calcium. They may or may not have a lowered tubular reabsorptive rate for phosphate. Bone lesions and elevation of the alkaline phosphatase are absent. While the etiology of this syndrome is not clear at the present time, it is possible that these patients have a variant of hyperparathyroidism and should be followed carefully. Should they develop hypercalcemia at any time in their clinical course, neck exploration for an adenoma should be considered seriously.

Other Causes of Hypercalcemia. Thyrotoxicosis has been described in association with hypercalcemia, although this is a rare phenomenon.

Treatment. Once the diagnosis of primary hyperparathyroidism is established, fluids should be forced, intake of calcium restricted, and surgical consultation obtained with a view toward neck exploration. Difficulty in locating the offending gland or glands because of inconstant anatomic positions, and because the noninvolved glands show compensatory atrophy, may necessitate not only extensive but also repeated surgical exploration. Careful x-ray studies of the neck, including the esophagus and the mediastinum, may be helpful in attempting to locate the tumor before exploration, but are often misleading. Removal of an adenoma or removal of all except a portion of one gland in case of hypertrophy and hyperplasia may be expected to cure the condition. When plasma alkaline phosphatase is markedly elevated, large quantities of calcium may be required postoperatively to prevent recurrent tetany since the bone will avidly remove calcium from the plasma in order to recalcify the bone lesions. The treatment of postoperative tetany is similar to that described in the treatment of hypoparathyroidism except that more vigorous treatment may have to be continued for some time to control the acute manifestations. A diet high in calcium and phosphate should be given post-operatively, but there is no need for increased doses of vitamin D over the normal intake unless there is a problem of chronic tetany. Under normal circumstances great improvement may be noted in the skeletal lesions as well as the renal function.

Acute Parathyroid Intoxication. Acute parathyroid intoxication occurs occasionally as an acute complication of hyperparathyroidism and is characterized by weakness, lethargy, and intractable nausea and vomiting, an extreme elevation of the plasma calcium level, gradual elevation of plasma phosphate, and finally coma and sudden death. The patient should be given intravenous dextrose, in saline solution, and often supplements of potassium in order to replace lost electrolytes and help maintain renal function. Chelating agents such as sodium ethylenediaminetetraacetic acid may help when given intravenously, but great care should be taken during their administration. Dialysis on an artificial kidney is of little benefit since the plasma calcium will rise rapidly to predialysis levels following such a procedure. The discovery and removal of a hyperfunctioning parathyroid tumor offers the only chance of survival in most instances.

SECONDARY HYPERPARATHYROIDISM

History. The existence of enlargement of the parathyroid glands secondary to another disease process in the body was first noted in 1905 by MacCallum in a case of nephritis. One year later, Erdheim noted similar findings in rickets, and since that time the syndrome of secondary hyperfunction of the parathyroids has been recognized.

Incidence. As a complication of advanced renal disease, hyperfunction of the parathyroids is relatively common. In 1933 Pappenheimer and Wilens reported that in a series of 21 cases of nephritis the mean parathyroid weight was 50 per cent greater than that in a control group.

Etiology. The most common cause of this condition is chronic, long-standing renal disease, as in glomerulonephritis and pyelonephritis. The term "renal rickets" does not apply to cases of secondary hyperparathyroidism and should be reserved for those cases seen most often in children where true rickets is secondary to prolonged and chronic renal disease and the supervening acidosis. Both secondary hyperparathyroidism and rickets have been described in the same patient as a complication of chronic renal disease. Reports of secondary hyperparathyroidism have been noted in a variety of diseases, such as osteogenesis imperfecta, Paget's disease, multiple myeloma, carcinoma with bone metastases, and pituitary basophilism.

Pathology. The parathyroid glands are enlarged diffusely and are hyperplastic. No single adenomas are visible. The cells are normal in size and easily differentiated from those seen in primary hyperparathyroidism. The former are principally chief cells with some increase in oxyphil cells, as opposed to the huge, water-clear cells of primary hyperparathyroidism due to hypertrophy and hyperplasia. The bone lesions are entirely similar to those seen in primary hyperparathyroidism, viz., generalized decalcification and bone cysts, with or without outright fracture.

Pathologic Physiology. It is unclear at the present time what the precise mechanisms for the development of parathyroid hyperplasia are in renal disease. It was believed that the presence of long-standing phosphate retention was the *sine qua non* for the development of the syndrome. It has been suggested by many that the metabolic acidosis secondary to renal disease may be the important factor in the development of a low plasma calcium. The parathyroid glands respond to this lowering of the plasma calcium in a uniform manner by increasing their output of hormone in order to maintain a normal plasma calcium. If the acidosis persists, then parathyroid hyperplasia is induced. While this may not be the true explanation for the development of parathyroid hyperplasia secondary to renal disease, it is a more plausible one since it correlates very closely with the types of bone disease seen in response to primary renal disease.

Clinical Picture. The symptoms are usually those of the primary disease process before any evidence of hyperparathyroidism is noted. Classic glomerulonephritis or pyelonephritis, uremia, and evidence of renal insufficiency dominate the clinical picture. In children, dwarfism and pathologic fractures may be the presenting complaints.

Diagnosis. The chemical findings of a normal or low normal plasma calcium with hyperphosphatemia and a high alkaline phosphatase, with the classic skeletal x-rays of bone cysts and generalized demineralization, lead to the diagnosis of parathyroid hyperfunction with renal disease. The history of early renal disease is often the only differential diagnostic point, since the primary cases are often complicated late in the disease by renal failure secondary to long-standing hyperparathyroidism. It is important to remember that an elevated plasma calcium in the face of uremia indicates primary hyperparathyroidism.

Treatment. Of greatest importance is the establishment of the correct diagnosis. Once this is accomplished, all therapy is directed at the primary disease and an attempt is made to correct the acidosis and to diminish the intake of phosphate by oral administration of aluminum hydroxide gel. The acidosis can be aided by administration of alkaline salts, such as sodium citrate. In rare cases the parathyroids have been surgically removed with little benefit, the patient ultimately dying of the primary renal disease.

NONFUNCTIONING TUMORS OF THE PARATHYROID GLANDS

Nonfunctioning carcinoma of the parathyroids has been reported, but these cases have not been generally accepted because of the difficulty in establishing the origin of the tumor. Other nonfunctioning tumors include oxyphil adenomas (which may be burned out primary adenomas), metastatic carcinoma, and cysts. Microscopic cysts are common in hyperplastic and adenomatous glands, whereas gross cysts are quite rare. Symptoms, when present, are due to pressure on local structures, including the recurrent laryngeal nerve. Most tumors have been found in the lower glands.

REFERENCES

Albright, F., and E. C. Reifenstein, Jr.: "Parathyroid Glands and Metabolic Bone Diseases," Baltimore, The Williams & Wilkins Company, 1948.

Baker, W. H.: Abnormalities in Calcium Metabolism in Malignancy: Effects of Hormones, Am. J. Med., 21:714, 1956.

Bergstrand, C. G., K. Ekengren, R. Filipsson, and A. Huggert: Pseudohypoparathyroidism: Familial Incidence and Comparison with Idiopathic Hypoparathyroidism, Acta Endocrinol., 29:201, 1958.

Bogdonoff, M. D., A. H. Woods, J. E. White, and F. L. Engel: Hyperparathyroidism, Am. J. Med., 21:583, 1956.

Bourne, G. H.: "The Biochemistry and Physiology of Bone," New York, Academic Press, Inc., 1956.

Bronsky, D., D. S. Kushner, A. Dubin, and I. Snapper: Idiopathic Hypoparathyroidism and Pseudohypoparathyroidism, Medicine, 37:317, 1958.

Calcium and Phosphorus Metabolism in Man and Animals with Special Reference to Pregnancy and Lactation, Ann. N.Y. Acad. Sci., vol. 64, art. 3, 1956.

Castleman, B.: Tumors of the Parathyroid Gland, in "Atlas of Tumor Pathology," sec. 4, fasc. 15, Washington, D.C., Armed Forces Institute of Pathology, 1952.

Chambers, E. L., G. S. Gordan, L. Goldman, and E. C. Reifenstein, Jr.: Tests for Hyperparathyroidism: Tubular Reabsorption of Phosphate, Phosphate Deprivation, and Calcium Infusion, J. Clin. Endocrinol. and Metabolism, 16:1507, 1956.

Ciba Foundation Symposium, Bone Structure and Metabolism: Boston, Little, Brown & Company, 1956.

Cope, O.: Surgery of Hyperparathyroidism: The Occurrence of Parathyroids in the Anterior Mediastinum and the Division of the Operation into Two Stages, Ann. Surg., 114:706, 1941.

Fanconi, A., and G. A. Rose: The Ionized, Complexed, and Protein-bound Fractions of Calcium in Plasma, Quart. J. Med., 27:463, 1958.

Heaney, R. P., and G. O. Whedon: Radiocalcium Studies of Bone Formation Rate in Human Metabolic Bone Disease, J. Clin. Endocrinol. and Metabolism, 18:1246, 1958.

Howard, J. E., T. R. Hopkins, and T. B. Connor: On Certain Physiologic Responses to Intravenous Injection of Calcium Salts into Normal, Hyperparathyroid, and Hypoparathyroid Persons, J. Clin. Endocrinol. and Metabolism, 13:1, 1953.

Rasmussen, H.: Purification of Parathyroid Polypeptides, J. Biol. Chem., 235:3442, 1960.

Recent Advances in the Study of the Structure, Composition, and Growth of Mineralized Tissues, Ann. N.Y. Acad. Sci., vol. 60, art. 5, 1955.

Rodahl, K., J. T. Nicholson, and E. M. Brown, Jr.: "Bone as a Tissue," New York, McGraw-Hill Book Company, Inc., Blakiston Division, 1960.

Underdahl, L., L. B. Woolner, and B. M. Black: Multiple Endocrine Adenomas: Eight Cases Involving Parathyroids, Pituitary, and Pancreatic Islets, J. Clin. Endocrinol. and Metabolism, 13:20, 1953.

68 DISEASES OF THE ADRENAL CORTEX

*George F. Cahill, Jr.,
Dalton Jenkins, and
George W. Thorn*

Thomas Addison's description in 1849 of a clinical syndrome which resulted from destruction of the adrenal glands first attracted attention to these organs. Seven years later Brown-Séquard demonstrated that removal of both adrenals from experimental animals caused death soon after operation, while sham-operated controls survived. Subsequent investigations established that the life-maintaining hormone was elaborated by cells in the cortex, since destruction of all medullary tissue was not accompanied by the classical signs and symptoms of adrenal insufficiency noted after complete removal of the glands.

Between 1927 and 1930, Hartman and his associates, Rogoff and Stewart, and Pfiffner and Swingle all independently described methods for preparing potent adrenal cortical extracts. During the following decade, crystalline steroid substances were isolated from these extracts by Kendall, by Grollman, and by Reichstein. In 1937, Steiger and Reichstein synthesized the first natural corticosteroid, 11-deoxycorticosterone, a year before it was identified in adrenal extracts. From 1940 to 1950, a synthesis of several 11-oxygenated compounds was achieved, including both cortisone and hydrocortisone, the contributions of Reichstein and his group and Kendall and his associates being outstanding. In 1954, aldosterone, the principal salt-retaining hormone was identified by Simpson and Tait in collaboration with the Swiss group under Reichstein, and the chemical synthesis of pure D-aldosterone was achieved several years later.

NORMAL FUNCTION OF THE ADRENAL CORTEX

For clinical and physiologic purposes, it is sufficient to consider that the gland secretes three general classes of hormones. These are: (1) glucocorticoids (hormones involved with the intermediary metabolism of organic compounds—to be specifically defined later), (2) mineralocorticoids (hormones involved with the regulation of sodium and potassium metabolism), and (3) hormones possessing androgenic or estrogenic activities. A given steroid, whether natural or synthetic, may exhibit various potencies between classes, i.e., aldosterone which has an extremely potent mineralocorticoid action compared to its glucocorticoid effects, deoxycorticosterone which is a potent mineralocorticoid but lacks glucocorticoid activity, or hydrocortisone,

which is relatively a more potent glucocorticoid than mineralocorticoid.

Although numerous steroids have been isolated from the adrenal cortex, only a few appear to be of major metabolic significance. These are illustrated in Fig. 68-1 and include hydrocortisone, cortisone, corticosterone, and aldosterone. Other important natural steroids with metabolic activity are 11-dehydrocorticosterone; 11-deoxycorticosterone; 17-hydroxy, 11-deoxycorticosterone; and steroids with androgenic effects including androstenedione, dehydroepiandrosterone, and 11-hydroxyandrostenedione. In addition, small quantities of estrogens are secreted by the adrenal. Hydrocortisone and aldosterone are the steroids of predominant importance in the metabolism of normal man. In other species, corticosterone may replace hydrocortisone.

Approximately 25 mg hydrocortisone and 0.1 to 0.2 mg aldosterone are secreted by the adrenals daily. Hydrocortisone is normally present in plasma in a concentration of 5 to 20 μg per 100 ml and is bound to a specific globulin with a high affinity but limited capacity for hydrocortisone, becoming saturated at a plasma hydrocortisone concentration of

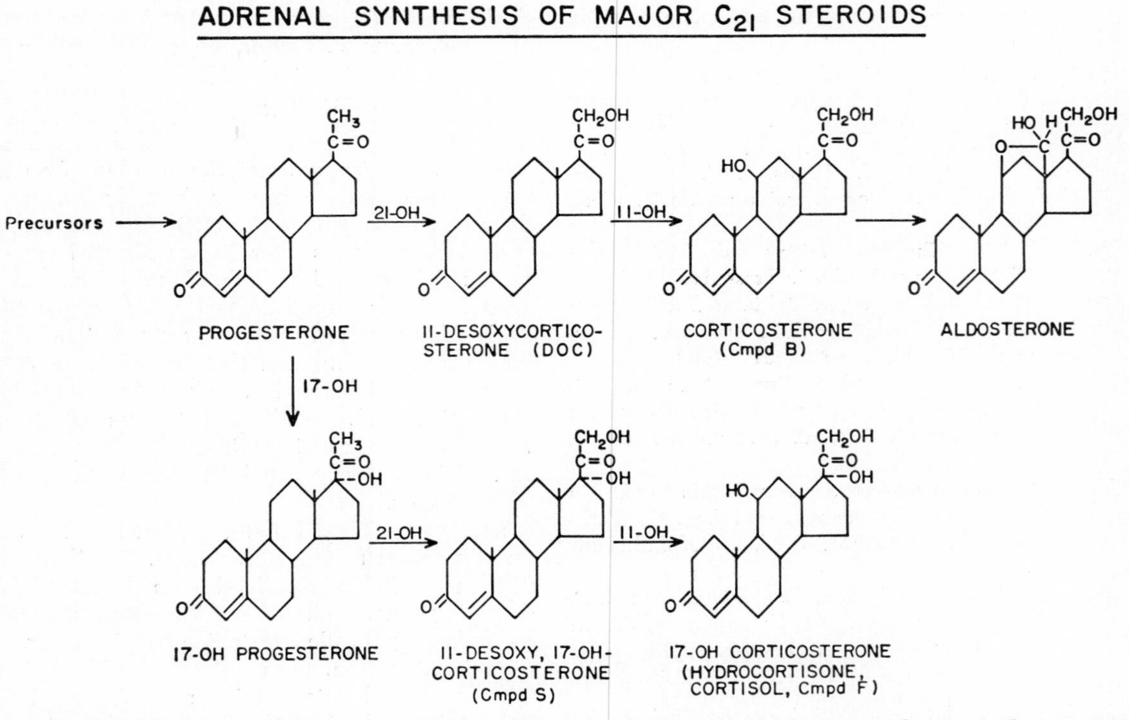

ADRENAL SYNTHESIS OF MAJOR C_{21} STEROIDS

FIG. 68-1. Simplified scheme of synthesis of principal C_{21} steroids showing the two general groups, those with a hydroxyl on carbon-17 and those without. The two hydroxylating enzymes for carbon-21 and carbon-11 are depicted for each series, and a deficiency of either of these enzymes is easily visualized with respective accumulation of 17-OH progesterone and progesterone and their metabolites such as pregnanediol and pregnanetriol in the case of carbon-21 hydroxylase deficiency, and DOC and compound S in the case of deficiency of hydroxylation at carbon-11.

20 μg per 100 ml. The plasma half-life of hydrocortisone is between 60 and 90 min. It is primarily removed from the circulation by the liver which reduces the double bond in ring A and the keto group at the 3-position followed by conjugation with glucuronic acid. In addition, a large quantity is also reduced in carbon-20. Lastly, a small proportion of the steroid is cleaved between carbons 17 and 20 to form one or more 17-ketosteroids (Fig. 68-2).

One of the most popular assays for the clinical determination of glucocorticoids was described by Porter and Silber and involves a colorimetric reaction with steroids bearing a 17,21-dihydroxy, 20-keto side chain. Of the hydrocortisone secreted by the adrenals, about 25 per cent is excreted in the urine as conjugated-reduced Porter-Silber chromogens (e.g., tetrahydrocortisol). About 35 per cent more is excreted reduced also in the 20 position and is thus not measured by the Porter-Silber reaction, but is measured in conjunction with Porter-Silber positive compounds as 17-ketogenic steroids after oxidation. A very small quantity of free, unchanged hydrocortisone, namely, 0.1 mg or less, may be normally excreted in the urine daily. Excretion and secretion of aldosterone and androgenic hormones will be discussed in subsequent sections.

Hormone Action

Glucocorticoid. The glucocorticoid "characteristics" of a hormone encompass a wide variety of metabolic effects. These include the ability to increase hepatic glucose synthesis, resulting in an increase in hepatic glycogen, hepatic glucose production, and subsequently a rise in blood glucose. Associated with these effects and possibly the primary site of action of the hormone are an increase in the mobilization of peripheral supporting structures, including the matrix of bone and connective tissue, as well as an increase in release of amino acids into the blood stream from muscle and probably other tissues. These amino acids are then trapped by the liver, deaminated, and utilized in glucose synthesis followed by increased glycogen deposition and hepatic glucose production, the nitrogen being disposed in the form of urea. In addition, intracellular electrolytes such as potassium and phosphorus are also lost, probably as a passive or secondary phenomenon in this over-all catabolic process. The metabolic effects of glucocorticoids include the ability to inhibit inflammatory and fibroplastic processes, including antigen-antibody reactions, together with the ability to cause suppression and dissolution of certain reticuloendothelial elements such as lymphatic and thymic tissue. The latter effect may be evidenced clinically in lowered circulating eosinophil concentrations and possibly in the involution of certain malignancies arising from reticuloendo-

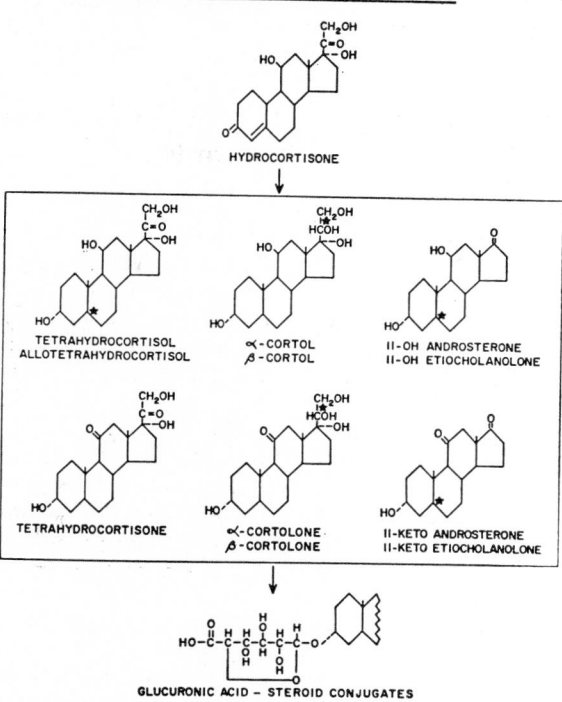

METABOLISM OF HYDROCORTISONE

Fig. 68-2. Principal metabolites of hydrocortisone. Since reduction at carbon-5 or carbon-20 introduces a new point of asymmetry, as marked by the asterisk, two new compounds may arise, such as the androstane series in which the hydrogen atom is in the α-position or below the plane of the molecule or in the etiocholane series in which the hydrogen atom is in the β-position.

thelial elements. Among other glucocorticoid effects is the capacity to raise the glomerular filtration rate, to permit a rapid urinary excretion of a water load, to allow vascular tissue to constrict in response to adrenergic stimulation, and to permit the release of free fatty acids from adipose tissue during fasting or adrenergic stimulation. Lastly, and obviously of prime significance in the maintenance of adrenal function, is the glucocorticoid capacity to suppress pituitary elaboration of adrenocorticotropic hormone (ACTH).

Mineralocorticoid. The mineralocorticoid effects are largely limited to excretory tissues and, therefore, the kidney is the most significant site of action. Mineralocorticoids promote sodium retention and the secretion of potassium, possibly by augmenting the exchange of potassium for sodium in the distal tubule. In addition, these hormones control the loss of sodium by sweat and salivary glands and probably also, but of less physiologic importance, exert effects on sodium and potassium metabolism in the gut. Also, a primary effect on ionic shifts and secondarily on the contractility of heart and vascular smooth muscle have been postulated.

Androgens and Estrogens. Adrenal androgens and estrogens appear to exert their physiologic effects in a manner similar to hormones secreted by the gonads. The possibility of differences in action cannot be excluded until adrenal androgenic and estrogenic steroids can be given in pure form to human beings.

Control of Adrenal Function

Several factors seem to be involved in the regulation of adrenal cortical function. By far the most significant is pituitary ACTH which apparently stimulates production of all hormones elaborated by the cortical portion of the gland. Of these, hydrocortisone is the most important, since as the principal glucocorticoid in man, its level serves to regulate pituitary secretion of ACTH, possibly by acting on a center in the hypothalamus which, in turn, governs pituitary elaboration of ACTH via a humoral mechanism. Thus, as circulating effective hydrocortisone falls, ACTH is elaborated to stimulate the adrenal until the level of hydrocortisone is sufficient again to inhibit the hypothalamic–anterior pituitary axis. Although the synthesis and secretion of adrenal androgens are under the control of ACTH, there is no evidence that their level serves to regulate pituitary ACTH secretion.

On the other hand, ACTH produces only a small and transient increase in aldosterone secretion; and following hypophysectomy, aldosterone secretion may continue at normal or even increased rates. Aldosterone secretion appears ordinarily to be stimulated by a decrease in effective circulating volume. Thus, sodium deprivation, hemorrhage, and diuretic agents all appear to be stimuli to aldosterone secretion. Receptors are located probably in major vessels and the heart, and by afferent nerves, signals are sent to higher centers in the diencephalic area to secrete a humoral factor which in turn stimulates aldosterone secretion. Some evidence implicates centers located along branches of the carotid arteries as the site of "volume" reception; other evidence suggests the kidney as a site of another tropic factor stimulating aldosterone secretion.

HYPOFUNCTION OF THE ADRENAL CORTEX

Adrenal cortical hypofunction includes all conditions in which the secretion of adrenal steroid hormones falls below the metabolic and functional requirements of the body. Various types of adrenal insufficiency are encountered and may be divided into two general categories: (1) those associated with primary inability of the adrenal to elaborate sufficient quantities of hormone and (2) those as-

Table 68-1. CLASSIFICATION OF ADRENAL INSUFFICIENCY

I. Primary adrenal insufficiency
  A. Anatomic destruction of the gland (chronic and acute)
    1. Infection or metastatic invasion
    2. Hemorrhage
    3. "Idiopathic" atrophy
    4. Surgical removal
  B. Metabolic failure in hormone production
    1. Congenital as in certain types of virilizing hyperplasia
    2. Specific enzyme inhibitors (i.e., 11-hydroxylase inhibitor)
    3. Nonspecific inhibitors (i.e., amphenone)
II. Secondary adrenal insufficiency
  A. Atrophy of gland due to lack of tropic hormone
    1. Hypopituitarism due to pituitary disease
    2. Suppression of hypothalamic-pituitary axis
      a. Exogenous steroid
      b. Endogenous steroid from tumors after removal of the tumor
      c. Pharmacologic agents

sociated with a secondary failure due to a primary failure in the elaboration of ACTH.

Addison's Disease (Chronic Adrenal Cortical Deficiency)

Addison's classical description of primary adrenal insufficiency in 1855, namely, "general languor and debility, remarkable feebleness of the heart's action, irritability of the stomach, and a peculiar change of the color of the skin," summarizes the dominant clinical features of the disease. Advanced cases usually cause little difficulty in diagnosis, but recognition of the disease in its earlier phases may present a real challenge. Since the disease, when unrecognized and untreated, carries an almost uniformly poor and frequently fatal prognosis, early diagnosis is important since present-day therapy may provide a complete correction of the metabolic derangement.

Incidence. Adrenocortical insufficiency is relatively rare; the admission rate in general hospitals appears to be approximately 1 in 5,000 cases. It may occur at any age in life and affects both sexes with equal frequency.

Clinical Signs and Symptoms. Adrenocortical insufficiency is most frequently characterized by an insidious onset with slowly progressive fatigability, weakness, anorexia, nausea and vomiting, weight loss, cutaneous and mucosal pigmentation, hypotension, and occasionally hypoglycemia. These signs and symptoms compose the classical syndrome of Addison's disease; however, the spectrum may vary, depending on the duration and degree of adrenal hypofunction, from a complaint of mild chronic fatigue to the fulminating shock associated with acute massive destruction of the glands in the type

Table 68-2. INCIDENCE OF SYMPTOMS AND SIGNS IN 125 CASES OF ADDISON'S DISEASE, PER CENT

Weakness	99	Hypotension (below	
Pigmentation of skin	98	110/70)	87
Pigmentation of mu-		Abdominal pain	34
cous membranes	82	Salt craving	22
		Diarrhea	20
Weight loss	97	Constipation	19
Anorexia, nausea, and		Syncope	16
vomiting	90	Vitiligo	9

of syndrome described by Waterhouse and Friderichsen. Table 68-2 lists the incidence of symptoms and signs noted in classical cases of Addison's disease.

Asthenia is the cardinal symptom of Addison's disease. Early it may be sporadic, usually most evident at times of stress; as adrenal function becomes more impaired, the weakness progresses until the patient is continuously fatigued, necessitating bed rest. Even the voice may fail, so that speech finally becomes listless and indistinct.

Pigmentation is the most striking sign of the disease. It commonly appears as a diffuse brown, tan, or bronze darkening of both exposed and unexposed parts of the body, with accentuation over pressure points such as elbows or creases of the hand and in areas normally pigmented such as the areolas about the nipples. In many patients, bluish-black patches appear on the mucous membranes. Some patients develop dark freckles, and occasionally irregular areas of vitiligo may paradoxically appear. As an early sign, patients may notice an unusually persistent tanning following exposure to the sun.

Arterial hypotension is also extremely frequent and in severe cases may be extreme, with blood pressures in the range of 80/50 or less. Postural accentuation is common, and syncope may occur. Abnormalities of gastrointestinal function are not only extremely frequent but often are the presenting complaint. Symptoms may vary from mild anorexia with weight loss to fulminating nausea, vomiting, diarrhea, and various types of ill-defined abdominal pain which at times may be so severe as to be confused with an acute "surgical abdomen." Rarely a Landry's type of ascending paralysis with flaccid quadriplegia and mixed sensory defects accompanied by ascending muscular weakness has been noted in conjunction with a high serum potassium. In these instances, the electrocardiogram may reflect the hyperpotassemia. In addition, patients with adrenal insufficiency frequently have marked personality changes, usually in the form of excessive irritability and restlessness.

Laboratory Findings. In the milder forms, sometimes called "partial" or "incomplete" Addison's disease, there may be no demonstrable abnormalities in any of the parameters measured in the rou-

tine laboratory, and even plasma and urinary steroid determinations may indicate values relatively low but yet within normal range. However, definitive studies of adrenal stimulation with ACTH show abnormalities even in this stage of the disease. In the more advanced stages, levels of serum sodium chloride and bicarbonate are reduced while serum potassium is elevated. These patients may show a marked reduction in heart size, and in about one-quarter of the patients suprarenal calcification is seen but is, unfortunately, not pathognomonic. The electrocardiogram may show nonspecific changes and the electroencephalogram a striking reduction and slowing of the predominant activity. The basal metabolic rate may be low, but other thyroid indices are ordinarily normal. There may be a normocytic anemia, a relative lymphocytosis, and usually a moderate eosinophilia.

Diagnosis. The definitive diagnosis of adrenocortical insufficiency requires demonstration of a failure of the gland to respond to adrenocorticotropic hormone (ACTH). The degree of response is best evaluated by serial determinations of urine or plasma 17-hydroxycorticoids. One frequently employed method involves the collection of two consecutive 24-hr urine samples followed by intravenous infusion of 25 to 50 USP units of ACTH in saline over each first 8-hr period of two succeeding days. By one method of assay, normal persons excrete 1 to 10 mg 17-hydroxycorticoid per 24 hr, and with ACTH excrete 5 to 25 mg more on the first day and 15 to 40 mg on the second. Patients

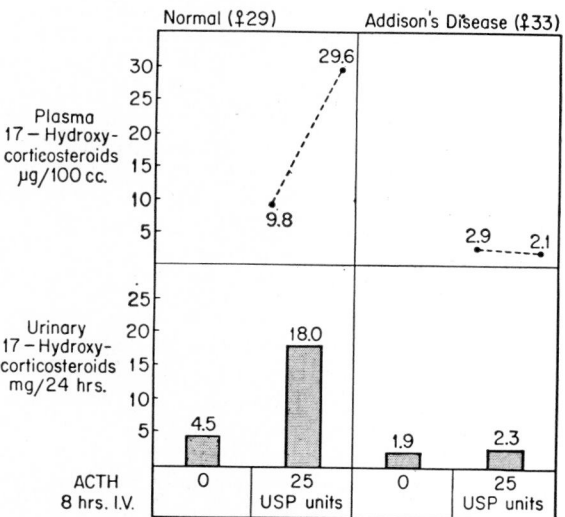

FIG. 68-3. Response of plasma and urinary 17-hydroxycorticosteroids to ACTH in a normal person and in a patient with Addison's disease. Urinary measurements were obtained from 24-hr urine collections; plasma measurements were obtained on samples drawn immediately before and after 6 hr of ACTH infusion.

with Addison's disease may show either no response or a very slight response on the first day. If no response is observed by the second day, the infusions should be continued for two more days, since patients with adrenal atrophy due to a prolonged decrease in pituitary elaboration of adrenocorticotropic hormone (pituitary disease or suppression by exogenous steroid) may not show a response until the second or third day. In the patient with Addison's disease, the 17-ketosteroids also fail to show any response. In addition, plasma levels of hydrocortisone show no increase following the infusion of ACTH, when compared to the control level before the infusion.

Emphasis is placed on the utilization of saline as diluent for ACTH, since patients with inadequate adrenal reserve may experience an acute febrile episode while or shortly after receiving glucose in water. In addition, since ACTH preparations are essentially foreign proteins, an allergic or anaphylactic response may occur following its administration, particularly in patients with diminished adrenal reserve. This danger may be minimized by previous administration of 1 mg of a potent steroid such as dexamethasone or fluorohydrocortisone. The excretory products of these compounds do not add appreciably to the amount of 17-hydroxycorticoids measured in the urine and, therefore, do not interfere with the test.

An alternative to the intravenous infusion of ACTH in saline is twice daily injections of 40 to 80 units of ACTH; however, due to variations in its absorption, the response is not as dependable. As an initial screening procedure or in those instances where definitive steroid analyses are unobtainable, the response of the adrenal may be assessed by following circulating eosinophils after intramuscular injection of ACTH. In normal persons, eosinophils measured 4 hr after the injection of 25 USP units are 30 per cent or less of the initial concentration. If this test is suggestive of Addison's disease, steroid analyses must nevertheless be performed for definitive diagnosis.

Indirect tests of adrenal cortical function include: (1) a delay in water excretion following an acute water load; (2) defective renal conservation of sodium when a low sodium, high potassium diet is imposed; (3) a tendency toward hypoglycemia during fasting and hypoglycemic unresponsiveness following the intravenous administration of insulin. Since ACTH has become generally available for direct evaluation of adrenal cortical function, the use of these procedures is rarely indicated, and furthermore, in a patient with adrenal cortical insufficiency, water intoxication, sodium deprivation, or hypoglycemia may all be life-threatening situations.

Differential Diagnosis. Since weakness and fatigue are such common complaints, clinical diagnosis of early adrenal cortical insufficiency is frequently difficult. However, mild gastrointestinal distress with weight loss, anorexia, and a suggestion of increased pigmentation make mandatory ACTH stimulation to rule in or out adrenal insufficiency, particularly before treatment with steroid is begun. Racial pigmentation in Negroes, Orientals, Indians, Spanish Americans, and Latins and other diseases with hyperpigmentation form a major problem. These include hemochromatosis, acanthosis nigricans, porphyria, thyrotoxicosis, polyostotic fibrous dysplasia, chronic metal poisoning (bismuth, lead, arsenic, silver), chronic malnutrition (starvation, anorexia nervosa, sprue syndrome, pellagra), progressive malignancy, chronic anemia, salt-losing nephritis with hypotension, renal tubular acidosis, and hepatic cirrhosis. In most cases, differentiation from Addison's disease is not difficult, but when doubt exists, ACTH administration ordinarily provides clear-cut differentiation.

Etiology and Pathogenesis. Addison's disease results from progressive adrenal cortical destruction. The adrenal is a frequent site for chronic infectious diseases of the granulomatous variety, predominately tuberculosis but also including fungal infections such as histoplasmosis, coccidioidomycosis, and cryptococcosis. In previous years, tuberculosis was found at post mortem in 70 to 90 per cent of cases; however, the most frequent finding at present is "idiopathic" atrophy, and it has been suggested that an autoimmune mechanism may be responsible for this process. Rarely other lesions are encountered, such as bilateral tumor metastases, amyloidosis, or sarcoidosis.

Treatment. All patients with Addison's disease should receive specific hormone replacement therapy. Similar to the treatment of patients with diabetes, proper care also requires careful and persistent education in regard to the disease. Since the adrenal elaborates three general classes of hormone, of which two, glucocorticoids and mineralocorticoids, are of primary clinical importance, replacement therapy should correct both deficiencies. Cortisone (or hydrocortisone) is the mainstay of treatment; however, its mineralocorticoid effect, when given in sufficient dosage to replace the endogenous hydrocortisone deficiency, is inadequate for complete electrolyte balance, and therefore the patient usually requires other supplementary hormone. Cortisone dosage varies from 12.5 to 50 mg daily, with the majority of patients taking 25 to 37.5 mg in divided doses. Because of its direct local effect on gastric mucosa, patients are advised to take their cortisone with meals, or if this is impractical, with milk or an antacid preparation. In addition, the larger proportion of the dose is taken in the morning, i.e., 25 mg, and the remainder, 12.5 mg, in the late afternoon, to simulate somewhat the diurnal adrenal rhythm of the normal. Some patients may exhibit insomnia, irritability, mental excitement, and even frank psychosis soon after initiation of therapy; in these the dosage should obviously be reduced. Other indications for maintaining the patient on smaller amounts are the presence of hypertension, diabetes, or active tuberculosis.

Since, as mentioned earlier, this amount of cortisone or hydrocortisone fails to replace the mineralocorticoid component of the adrenal gland, supplementary hormone is usually needed. The simplest means is daily oral administration of 0.1 to 0.2 mg of 9α-fluorohydrocortisone. If parenteral administration is indicated, 2.0 to 5.0 mg of deoxycorticosterone acetate in oil can be given every day intramuscularly. An alternative method of therapy is an injection of 25 to 50 mg of deoxycorticosterone trimethylacetate in oil intramuscularly every 3 to 4 weeks, but similar to the previous use of subcutaneous implantation of pellets of deoxycorticosterone which lasted for 8 to 10 months, most patients prefer the simplicity of daily oral administration of the 9α-fluorohydrocortisone.

Complications of cortisone therapy, with the exception of peptic disease, particularly ulcer or gastritis, are extremely rare in the doses used in the treatment of Addison's disease. However, overtreatment with deoxycorticosterone preparations or 9α-fluorohydrocortisone is more frequent and may present as edema, hypertension, cardiac enlargement, or even congestive failure due to sodium retention. Overtreatment may also present as weakness, progressing to total paralysis due to hypopotassemia. In the management of patients with Addison's disease, regular measurement of body weight, serum potassium, heart size, and blood pressure and serial electrocardiograms are useful.

Special Therapeutic Problems. During periods of intercurrent illness, the dose of cortisone or hydrocortisone should be increased to levels of 75 to 150 mg per day. When oral administration is not possible, parenteral routes should be employed. Likewise, prior to surgery or dental extractions, excess steroid should be administered. The patients should all be advised of these facts in addition to carrying an identification card bearing detailed instructions for the administration of steroid in case of acute illness or injury. Patients should also be advised to increase the dose of 9α-fluorohydrocortisone and should add excess salt to their otherwise normal diet during periods of excessive exercise with sweating, during extremely hot weather, or during periods of gastrointestinal upsets. In spite of animal

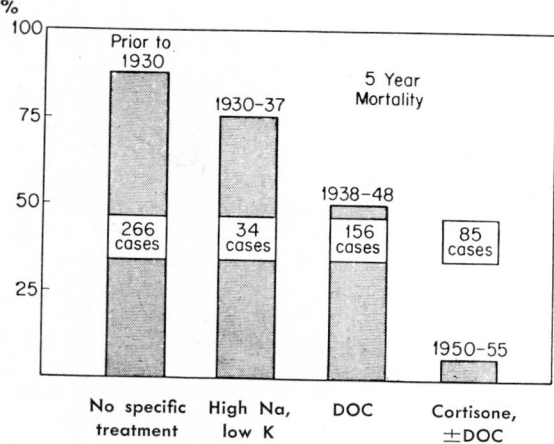

Fig. 68-4. The effect of hormone therapy on the 5-year mortality rate in Addison's disease.

studies demonstrating an increased susceptibility to tubercular spread associated with excess steroid administration, patients with Addison's disease and tuberculosis may be maintained safely on 12.5 to 25 mg cortisone daily.

Course and Prognosis. Untreated Addison's disease characteristically runs a chronic and relentless course. In some patients, its advance is relatively slow, but in all patients, the disease may rapidly deteriorate into adrenal crisis. With treatment, the prognosis of the disease is extremely favorable. In fact, some of the degenerative vascular problems such as hypertension or congestive failure are more easily handled in an Addisonian compared to a patient with intact adrenals. In Fig. 68-4 are plotted the 5-year mortality statistics during the historic development of treatment.

Acute Adrenocortical Insufficiency

Acute adrenocortical insufficiency may result from several processes. One of these, usually termed "adrenal crisis," is a rapid and overwhelming intensification of chronic adrenal insufficiency. Another process involves an acute hemorrhagic destruction of both adrenal glands, usually associated with an overwhelming septicemia. A third, and probably the most frequent cause of acute insufficiency, results from the rapid withdrawal of steroids from patients with adrenal atrophy secondary to chronic steroid administration.

Adrenal Crisis

The long-term survival of patients with Addison's disease largely depends upon the prevention and treatment of adrenal crisis. Consequently, the occurrence of infection, trauma (including surgery), gastrointestinal upsets, or other forms of stress requires an immediate increase in hormone. In previously untreated patients, preexisting symptoms are intensified. Nausea, vomiting, and abdominal pain may become intractable. Fever is frequently severe, but may be absent. Lethargy deepens into somnolence, and the blood pressure and pulse fail as hypovolemic vascular shock ensues. In contrast, patients previously maintained on hormone therapy may not exhibit severe dehydration or hypotension until preterminally, at which time there is an extremely rapid decline.

Treatment is primarily directed toward the rapid elevation of circulating adrenal cortical hormone in addition to the replacement of the sodium and water deficit. Hence, an intravenous infusion of 1,000 ml of 5 per cent glucose in normal saline containing 100 to 200 mg of any of several soluble hydrocortisone preparations is begun rapidly, with the first 250 ml infused in the first ½ to 1 hr and the remainder over the ensuing 4 to 8 hr. If the condition is extreme, immediate intravenous infusion of 100 mg hydrocortisone in the first few minutes is suggested, followed by a rapid infusion as described above. Epinephrine 0.2 mg intravenously may also be indicated. In any case, it is also advisable to administer 100 mg cortisone acetate intramuscularly in case the infusion becomes infiltrated or inadvertently stopped. If the crisis was preceded by prolonged nausea, vomiting, and dehydration, several liters replacement are indicated. With large doses of steroid, the patient receives a maximal mineralocorticoid effect, and supplementary deoxycorticosterone is superfluous. After the initial infusion, depending on the patient's condition a second similar infusion may be given or if there has been marked improvement, the patient may be offered oral fluids and be given 50 mg cortisone acetate intramuscularly every 12 hr until gastrointestinal absorption is guaranteed, at which time the steroid can be given orally. Steroid dosage is then tapered over the next few days to maintenance levels, with reinstitution of supplementary mineralocorticoid, if needed.

Adrenal Hemorrhage

Adrenal hemorrhage (adrenal apoplexy) is usually associated with overwhelming septicemia (Waterhouse-Friderichsen syndrome); however, it may also occur in the absence of sepsis. Occasionally, massive bilateral adrenal hemorrhage results from birth trauma. The infant may be either stillborn or die soon thereafter, with shock and hyperpyrexia. Adrenal hemorrhage also occurs in patients with advanced hypertension and arteriosclerosis, during pregnancy, following idiopathic adrenal vein thrombosis, during convulsions in epilepsy or during electroconvulsive therapy, with excessive anticoagulant therapy, and after trauma or surgery. Pain in the flank and epigastrium is frequent, and if the hemorrhagic process ruptures into the abdomen, signs of peritoneal inflammation are present.

The adrenal hemorrhage associated with septicemia is most frequent with meningococcemia but is also seen with overwhelming infections due to the pneumococcus, staphylococcus, or *Hemophilus influenzae*. The onset is often explosive, with a shaking chill, violent headache, vertigo, vomiting, and prostration. A petechial rash appears on the skin and mucous membranes and progresses rapidly to a confluent, extensive purpura. Large areas of skin may become grossly hemorrhagic. Body temperature may be subnormal, but is usually markedly elevated. Circulatory collapse rapidly ensues, and death may occur within 6 to 48 hr. Specific diagnosis requires immediate identification of the organism. Frequently, the septicemia is so massive that organisms may be seen in peripheral blood smears or petechial scrapings. Time is not sufficient for determination of adrenal function; however, a plasma sample for later determination of 17-hydroxysteroid may be of academic interest.

Treatment must be immediate and intensive. Control of the infection by vigorous administration of parenteral, preferably intravenous, antibiotics is indicated in addition to the steroid schedule delineated for adrenal crisis. Intravenous norepinephrine (4 to 8 mg per liter) may also be required for maintenance of vascular tone. Since shock may also be associated with massive septicemia without adrenal hemorrhage, one is never completely certain whether adrenal insufficiency is contributing to the patient's decompensation; however, the authors feel that because of the increasing frequency of survival of patients treated with steroid, some degree of adrenal insufficiency, whether relative or absolute, is present, and steroid treatment is therefore indicated in all patients in whom there is a fulminating septicemia associated with shock.

Adrenal Insufficiency Due to Metabolic Failure in Hormone Production

This group of patients includes those with congenital adrenal hyperplasia (to be discussed in detail later) and those receiving one of several pharmacologic agents which are capable of inhibiting hormone synthesis in the gland. These include 3,3 di-(*p*-aminophenyl) butanone-2-hydrochloride (Amphenone), which appears to inhibit synthesis of all hormones early in the sequence of reactions from cholesterol, and concomitantly results in hypertrophy of the gland; various derivatives of diphenyl dichloroethane, of which the *o,p*-dichloro derivative is the most active (*o,p*-DDD or Perthane) and causes atrophy and even necrosis of adrenal cortical tissue; and lastly, 2-methyl-1,2-bis-(3-pyridyl)-1-propanone (SU 4885), a compound similar to the other two but more specific in that it selectively inhibits hydroxylation of the steroid nucleus at the 11-position. Amphenone and *o,p*-DDD have been used in the treatment of adrenocortical carcinoma, and SU 4885 has been used as a laboratory test for pituitary reserve (see Chap. 64).

Adrenal Insufficiency Due to Peripheral Inhibition of Steroid Action

This theoretical possibility presents itself in two situations. The presence of a salt-losing steroid in certain patients with congenital adrenal hyperplasia has been suggested; however its isolation and identification have so far not been certain. The other situation is the use of aldosterone antagonists such as the spirolactones as diuretic agents, to inhibit the sodium-potassium exchange and thereby increase urinary sodium excretion. In patients with normal adrenal reserve, they induce a temporary sodium diuresis, but in patients with insufficient adrenocortical reserve, their use (similar to other diuretic agents) may result in excessive sodium and water loss and potential vascular collapse. The occasional use of progestational agents as diuretics also probably serves to inhibit peripherally the metabolic effects of aldosterone.

Secondary Adrenal Insufficiency

Secondary adrenal cortical insufficiency results from inadequate production of ACTH. Patients with pituitary disease due to any number of causes such as tumor, cysts, infection, infarction, etc., may have secondary adrenal cortical insufficiency, but since ACTH is usually one of the last functions to be lost, other insufficiencies, such as gonadotropic and thyrotropic, are usually more apparent. Cases with a pure deficiency in ACTH elaboration have been described but are exceedingly rare. In contrast to patients with Addison's disease, pigmentation is nearly always absent, and in fact, patients with hypopituitarism usually present with marked pallor. In addition, hypoglycemic episodes are much more prominent in patients with hypopituitarism than in those with primary adrenocortical insufficiency.

Differentiation between primary and secondary adrenal cortical failure is easily made by the ACTH-stimulation test, the patients with pituitary disease showing a progressively increasing response to ACTH stimulation compared to lack of response in patients with Addison's disease. The diagnosis of secondary adrenal insufficiency is suggested by low baseline values for 24-hr urinary 17-ketosteroids and hydroxysteroids, with a return to or toward normal values with ACTH stimulation. However, a definitive diagnosis of pituitary insufficiency can be established only with the use of agents such as 2-methyl-1,2-bis-(3-pyridyl)-1-propanone (SU 4485)

which in the normal individual results in increased ACTH release as a consequence of the decrease in blood hydrocortisone level. The increase in endogenous ACTH secretion may be measured directly by ACTH assays in the blood or indirectly by an increase in compound S excretion in the urine, which can be detected by methods which measure either total 17-hydroxy or 17-ketogenic steroids (see Chap. 64).

Another form of secondary adrenal insufficiency is seen in patients who have received prolonged therapy with steroids capable of suppressing pituitary secretion of ACTH. These include cortisone and hydrocortisone, prednisone, and any other of the synthetic anti-inflammatory steroids. As a result, the adrenal cortex undergoes atrophy. Consequently, exogenous stress may induce adrenal crisis. Susceptibility is greatest following hormone withdrawal, but acute adrenal insufficiency may also occur during continued hormone administration when stress is severe and hormone dosage not increased. These patients should therefore be handled as an Addisonian on maintenance therapy, requiring additional steroid during episodes of stress and increased parenteral steroids during surgery, gastrointestinal upsets, etc. Lastly, newer pharmacologic agents capable of suppressing the hypothalamic-pituitary axis and thereby the secretion of ACTH are available, but as yet they have not proved to have sufficient potency to induce failure in man.

HYPERFUNCTION OF THE ADRENAL CORTEX

Since the adrenal cortex secretes three general classes of hormone, glucocorticoids, mineralocorticoids, and hormones with androgenic or estrogenic potencies, disordered hypersecretion, whether resulting from hyperplasia or neoplasia, may result in several separate clinical syndromes and in several other interpolated or mixed syndromes resulting from various degrees of hyper- or hyposecretion. The "pure" syndromes are:

1. Glucocorticoid—Cushing's syndrome
2. Mineralocorticoid—hyperaldosteronism (Conn's syndrome)
3. *a.* Androgenic—virilization
   b. Estrogenic—feminization

For the sake of simplicity, each of these "pure" syndromes will be discussed separately, with full knowledge that clinical states may also involve excessive secretion of two or more types of hormone.

Cushing's Syndrome

With a collation of the clinical and pathologic findings in a collected series of 12 patients, Harvey Cushing in 1932 established a syndrome charac-

Table 68-3. INCIDENCE OF SIGNS AND SYMPTOMS IN
35 CASES OF CUSHING'S SYNDROME, PER CENT

Typical habitus	97	Amenorrhea	77
Increased body weight	94	Cutaneous striae	67
Fatigability and weakness	87	Personality changes	66
		Ecchymoses	65
Hypertension (above 150/90)	82	Edema	62
		Polyuria, polydipsia	23
Hirsutism	80	Hypertrophy of clitoris	19

terized by "a peculiarly disposed adiposity," hypertension, fatigability and weakness, amenorrhea or impotence, hirsutism, "purplish lineae atrophicae," purpura-like ecchymoses, edema, glucosuria, osteoporosis, and increased susceptibility to infection.

Incidence. The disease is relatively rare; however, as steroid analyses are becoming more a part in the medical workup of persons with osteoporosis, diabetes, hypertension, etc., many more patients with mild degrees of adrenal hyperfunction are discovered. Its frequency in females is three to five times that in males. Although cases have been encountered at all ages, the onset usually occurs during the third or fourth decade.

Clinical Signs and Symptoms. The frequency of clinical findings are listed in Table 68-3. From knowledge of the physiologic effects of glucocorticoids, many of the signs and symptoms logically follow. As a result of mobilization of peripheral supportive tissue, there is muscle weakness and fatigability, osteoporosis, and cutaneous striae (weakening and rupturing of collagenous fibers in the dermis, thereby exposing the heavily vascularized subcutaneous tissues). Likewise, because of weakening of vascular tissue, there is easy bruisability, and ecchymoses often appear at sites of mild trauma. The osteoporosis may be so severe that collapse of vertebral bodies and pathologic fractures of other bones are frequently encountered. As a reflection of increased hepatic gluconeogenesis from these mobilized precursors, there may be frank diabetes with polydipsia and polyuria due to severe glucosuria; or more frequently, in the presence of an adequate reserve of insulin, there is metabolism of this excess glucose into fat in certain depots, most notably the upper face (the classical "moon" facies), the interscapular area (the "buffalo" hump), and the mesenteric bed (producing the classical "truncal" obesity). The reason for this peculiar distribution of lipid is not known. The face also appears "plethoric," even in the absence of any increase in red cell concentration. Hypertension is most always present, and frequently there are profound emotional changes ranging from irritability or emotional lability to severe depression, confusion, or even frank psychosis. Even in the absence of any secretion of androgenic hormone,

hirsutism in women patients is frequent and often appears as a fine "downy" coat over the face, forehead, and upper trunk. Likewise, in women patients, olig- or amenorrhea is a frequent disturbance.

Laboratory Findings. With rare exceptions, plasma and urinary 17-hydroxycorticoid levels are elevated. Circulating eosinophils are below 100 cells per cu mm in 90 per cent of the cases, and some patients may show a mild neutrophilic leukocytosis. In spite of markedly plethoric facies, the hematocrit is usually within the normal range, but occasionally erythemia with higher hematocrits are encountered, particularly when associated with excessive production of 17-ketosteroids in the mixed syndromes. Serum sodium concentration is usually normal; however, depending on the degree of secretion of hormones with mineralocorticoid potency, there may be hypopotassemia, hypochloremia, and metabolic alkalosis with an elevated concentration of serum bicarbonate. More than three-fourths of patients exhibit intermittent glucosuria, and all have a decreased rate of disappearance of infused glucose from the circulation. Some patients may

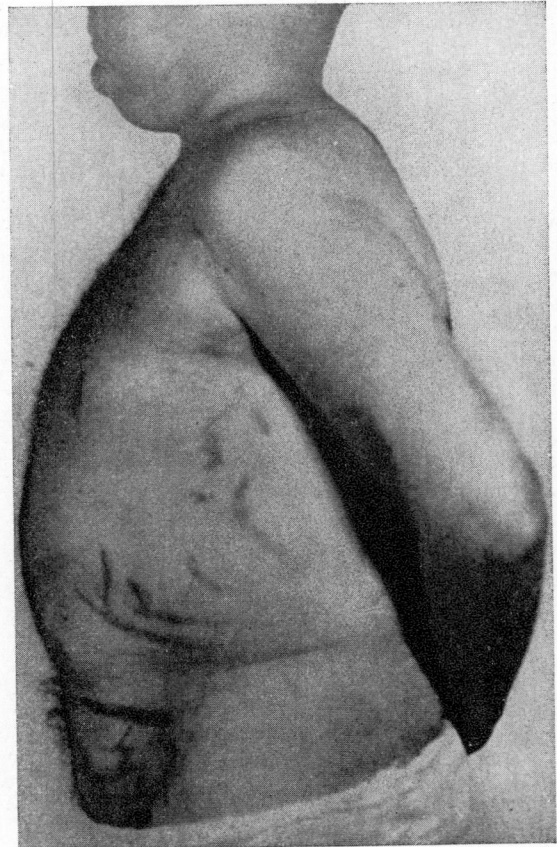

FIG. 68-5. A 26-year-old male with typical Cushing's syndrome. Note the bison neck and the deep red striae.

have frank diabetes necessitating insulin therapy. X-ray studies usually reveal generalized osteoporosis, most marked in the spine and pelvis, but also frequently including the skull with disappearance of the lamina dura, and fractures are often seen in the vertebras. Intravenous pyelography and laminograms with or without retroperitoneal insufflation of gaseous material (to provide contrast to soft tissues) may demonstrate adrenal enlargement, particularly when an adenoma or carcinoma is the pathologic cause of the disease. Frequently, however, the truncal obesity makes radiologic interpretation difficult.

Diagnosis. The specific criterion for the diagnosis of Cushing's syndrome can best be defined as an inappropriate hypersecretion of glucocorticoid hormone. Since hydrocortisone is the predominant glucocorticoid in man, demonstration of an unexplained elevated plasma level of 17-hydroxycorticoid or of an increased urinary excretion of 17-hydroxycorticoid at a time when the patient is not under acute exogenous stress is strongly in favor of the diagnosis. Using the radioactive dilution technique, an increased secretion of hydrocortisone by the gland may be directly determined. Other ancillary tests include the determination of the "free" unbound and unreduced hydrocortisone in the urine, which is probably a reflection of the level of free, unbound hormone in plasma, and in normal persons is less than 100 μg in 24 hr. In patients with Cushing's syndrome, urinary free hydrocortisone may be more than ten times this amount. In addition, the diurnal pattern of adrenal secretion may be absent, again demonstrating the "inappropriateness" of steroid secretion. In normal persons, twice as much 17-hydroxycorticoids appear in the urine between 7:00 A.M. and 7:00 P.M. In patients with even early or mild Cushing's syndrome, equal quantities may appear in both 12-hr periods, or occasionally this normal pattern may even be reversed. In addition, administration of amounts of synthetic steroids with marked glucocorticoid activity (i.e., 0.5 mg dexamethasone or 9α-fluorohydrocortisone every 6 hr for 3 to 4 days) which in the normal person suppresses adrenal secretion of hydrocortisone by suppressing pituitary elaboration of ACTH (the "suppression" test) fails to do so or does so only very minimally in patients with Cushing's syndrome.

Differential Diagnosis. Exogenous obesity, essential hypertension, and diabetes mellitus, occurring singly, or particularly in combination, may be mistaken for Cushing's syndrome. However, in these conditions adiposity is usually generalized, skin changes are usually absent, and most significant, 17-hydroxycorticoid values are normal. Osteoporosis not due to Cushing's syndrome rarely involves the skull or lamina propria. The bone changes associated with hyperparathyroidism are easily separable by the altered serum calcium and phosphorus levels and the normal 17-hydroxycorticoid values. Rarely, patients with impaired metabolism of steroids due to hepatic disease may exhibit some manifestation of Cushing's syndrome associated with increased levels of circulating steroid. In addition, patients with excessive thyroid hormone or patients with high levels of estrogen, either exogenously administered or endogenously produced, may have elevated levels of circulating 17-hydroxycorticoid, but in these the increase is due to an increment in the "bound" fraction secondary to an elevation in protein binding.

Etiology and Pathogenesis. The immediate cause of Cushing's syndrome is adrenal cortical hypersecretion. While Cushing conceded that the same clinical findings could occur in association with adrenal tumors, he believed "the fact that the syndrome may accompany a basophil adenoma in the absence of any apparent alteration of the adrenal cortex other than a possible secondary hyperplasia" indicated that the pituitary gland probably played a dominant etiologic role.

In the rare cases occurring in childhood, an adrenal tumor is nearly always present, and is most frequently a carcinoma. In adults, approximately 60 per cent have bilateral adrenal cortical hyperplasia, while 35 per cent have adrenal tumor, of which one-half are malignant. Approximately 10 per cent may show no discernible anatomic abnormality. Some cases may have hyperplastic glands without an increase in total adrenal weight; however, there is frequently a thickened cortex with accentuated convolutions and nodulation.

The etiology of bilateral hyperplasia continues to remain obscure. During Cushing's era, attention was focused on the pituitary as the primary site of the pathologic changes, and indeed all patients show cytologic hyalinization of the pituitary basophils (Crooke's changes). These changes, however, are now considered to be a result rather than a cause of adrenal overproduction of glucocorticoid, since similar changes are noted in patients who have received exogenous glucocorticoids for prolonged periods of time. Nevertheless, a small basophilic adenoma was present in approximately one-third of the early cases; and less commonly, other types of pituitary adenomas were found at necropsy.

Since the surgical approach to the treatment of Cushing's syndrome by adrenalectomy has become practical and, more important, since the availability of cortisone and related compounds for adequate postoperative and chronic maintenance, prolonged follow-up of patients who previously had bilateral adrenal hyperplasia with Cushing's syndrome has revealed, in about one-sixth of the cases, a progressive increase in pigmentation in spite of adequate steroid maintenance therapy. In some of these, enlargement of the sella turcica and signs and symptoms of pituitary tumor have appeared. When optic nerve encroachment or pituitary hemorrhage necessitate surgical intervention, these tumors are found, surprisingly, to be chromophobe adenomas. Indeed, some patients with active Cushing's syndrome may already have evidence of expansion of the sella turcica prior to removal of their hyperplastic adrenals. The question is therefore raised whether, as Cushing suggested, all patients with hyperplasia and excessive production of glucocorticoid have primary pituitary disease, with inability to inhibit elaboration of ACTH in the face of excessive circulating levels of 17-hydroxycorticoids, or whether some of these patients may have a primary ACTH-producing chromophobe adenoma as the original cause of their Cushing's syndrome.

When the pathogenic agent of Cushing's syndrome is an adrenal adenoma or carcinoma, the surrounding normal tissue and the contralateral gland undergo atrophy. Carcinomas may be highly malignant, with early metastases to the liver or lungs or with direct invasion into the kidney and local tissues. Other pathologic changes with Cushing's syndrome may include not only all the changes of vascular deterioration associated with hypertension, but also renal calcinosis, fatty necrosis of the pancreas, osteoporosis, and ovarian fibrosis. Rarely, malignant tumor of the lung may be associated with Cushing's syndrome, and likewise, patients with adenomas of other endocrine tissues (Werner's syndrome) may have associated Cushing's syndrome with an adenoma of the adrenal cortex.

Further Comments on Diagnosis and Treatment. Once the presence of excessive secretion of glucocorticoid has been demonstrated by any of the previously mentioned tests, it is of importance to try specifically to define the type of lesion, since initial treatment involves either direct adrenal excision or a more conservative approach with pituitary irradiation. In general, adrenal carcinomas secrete high levels of both 17-hydroxy and 17-ketosteroids and fail to be stimulated by ACTH or suppressed by administration of exogenous steroid. Cortical adenomas producing Cushing's syndrome, on the other hand, may secrete almost solely 17-hydroxycorticoids and may or may not be stimulated or suppressed. When an adenoma or carcinoma is suspected, adrenal exploration is performed, with excision of the tumor. Because of probable atrophy of the contralateral adrenal, the patient is prepared and treated pre- and postoperatively for total adrenalectomy even when a solitary lesion is suspected, the routine being similar to that for an Addisonian patient undergoing elective surgery.

In the presence of high base-line 17-hydroxy and 17-ketosteroids, a hyperactive response to ACTH and failure to suppress adequately on 2 mg per day of dexamethasone or 9α-fluorohydrocortisone for a period of several days, the diagnosis is most likely bilateral adrenocortical hyperplasia. This is particularly substantiated if large doses of this highly potent synthetic glucocorticoid, such as 8 mg per day, do suppress the patient's steroid values. Several forms of treatment may then be considered.

In the absence of severe hypertension, overt diabetes, psychosis, osteoporosis with pathologic fractures, or any other of the more serious sequelae of Cushing's syndrome, pituitary irradiation of not less than 3,000 r may be given. One-half of these patients with a milder degree of the disease may undergo complete or partial remission following irradiation, but in only one-half of this group does the remission remain permanent. It is also extremely difficult to evaluate the efficacy of this form of treatment since remissions are not rare without treatment, and the disease itself, although usually progressive, may wax and wane spontaneously.

If the patient has a more advanced degree of Cushing's syndrome, or if the patient has received a course of pituitary irradiation without remission, therapy is directed toward removal of adrenal tissue. In order to avoid recurrence, the total gland is removed from the right and 85 per cent of the gland removed from the left. It should be pointed out that, in advanced Cushing's syndrome associated with bilateral adrenal dysfunction, the adrenals at operation grossly may appear completely normal. However, even in subtotally adrenalectomized patients, recurrences are not infrequent; on the other hand, it is not infrequent for the patient to require replacement hormone because of inadequate functioning capacity of the remaining tissue. It is therefore felt by many that total bilateral adrenalectomy is the treatment of choice, followed by institution of standard total replacement therapy, thus avoiding both the risk of a recurrence or of relying on an adrenal remnant with borderline maximal secretory capacity. Reversal of the changes produced by Cushing's syndrome occurs slowly and may require a year or more. Radiologic improvement of the osteoporosis is difficult to demonstrate; however, pain and pathologic fractures cease. Hypertension, if of long-standing duration, may occasionally also not be relieved.

As mentioned earlier, approximately one-sixth of patients adrenalectomized for Cushing's syndrome develop signs and symptoms of pituitary tumor, with marked skin pigmentation, high levels of circulating ACTH by assay, and occasionally symptoms of anatomic expansion of the tumor such as optic nerve compression. As more and more patients are adrenalectomized for Cushing's syndrome and followed for longer periods of time, the incidence of these tumors is increasing. It is therefore felt advisable to irradiate prophylactically the pituitary of any patient undergoing bilateral adrenalectomy for Cushing's syndrome if there is any suspicion of a change in the sella turcica or a suggestion of abnormal pigmentation. Likewise, if, in the face of adequate glucocorticoid replacement, pigmentation becomes marked after adrenalectomy, or if there is any change in the sella turcica, pituitary irradiation is indicated in an attempt to halt further development of the suspected pituitary tumor.

Hyperaldosteronism

Aldosterone is the primary mineralocorticoid secreted by the adrenal. Excessive secretion can be attributed either to primary adrenal disease or to some other extraadrenal pathologic process which, in turn, induces secondary secretion of the hormone. The primary form of the disease was first summarized by Conn in 1956 and is characterized by muscular weakness, tetany, paresthesias, polyuria, polydipsia, hypopotassemia and alkalosis, and demonstration of inappropriate excessive secretion of aldosterone. Classically, the disease results from an aldosterone-producing adrenal adenoma (or carcinoma); however, cases with bilateral adrenal hyperplasia and cases with histologically normal adrenals without any other pathologic process have been described and may be included as primary hyperaldosteronism until an etiologic agent is described.

Incidence. In 75 per cent of patients with hyperaldosteronism, an adrenal adenoma is found at surgery. This form of the disease is twice as common in females as in males. The peak incidence is in the fifth decade. However, the other 25 per cent of patients (those without adenomas) do not have this increased incidence in the female; indeed, those under the age of twenty are predominantly males. Hyperaldosteronism due to carcinoma is rare.

Classical Signs and Symptoms. Symptoms may be subdivided into two separate groups, one related to hypopotassemia and alkalosis and the other related to hypertension. Muscle weakness is frequent and may be marked by periodic episodes often progressing to paralysis. Muscles innervated by cranial nerves are usually spared except in the most severe episodes. Typical tetany may occur with accompanying paresthesias, pain, and a positive Chvostek sign. Because of the inadequate concentrating ability of the kidney associated with potassium deficiency, polyuria and polydipsia may be marked. Hypertension is usually present but except in the juvenile cases is rarely severe; however, it may be associated with headache, cardiac enlargement, electrocardiographic changes, and hypertensive retinopathy. Edema is usually absent or

minimal, unless there is associated congestive failure or severe renal vascular changes or preexisting abnormalities such as thrombophlebitis.

Laboratory Findings. Serum electrolytes are consistent with hypopotassemic alkalosis, with a serum potassium concentration frequently below 3.0 and occasionally below 2.0 mEq per liter and an elevated serum bicarbonate. Serum sodium may be normal or slightly elevated, and chloride low. Serum pH is high. The urine is neutral or alkaline with a low, fixed specific gravity with little, if any, response to administration of pituitary antidiuretic hormone. Urinary 17-hydroxy and 17-ketosteroids are usually within normal limits and respond normally to ACTH stimulation. Electrocardiographic and electroencephalographic tracings frequently show changes consistent with hypopotassemia. The markedly decreased concentration of sodium in sweat and saliva provides additional laboratory evidence.

Diagnosis. The specific diagnosis of primary hyperaldosteronism is made by the demonstration of excess secretion of aldosterone by the adrenals under physiologic conditions designed not to stimulate hypersecretion, in other words, in patients with an adequate effective circulating volume, not depleted of sodium and maintained on a liberal sodium intake. This can be done most accurately by calculation of aldosterone secretion following administration of radioactive aldosterone and measurement of the specific activity and quantity of one or more urinary metabolites. Using this method, aldosterone secretion rates in normal subjects are approximately 50 to 150 μg per 24 hr, as long as the subjects are on an adequate sodium intake. In normal subjects on sodium restriction, secretion may rise to 1,000 μg per 24 hr or more. Urinary aldosterone may be determined and accounts for only a small percentage of that secreted, and in normal persons is less than 10 μg per 24 hr. Since the methods for the demonstration of excess aldosterone production, whether by the secretion rate or by urinary metabolites, require special techniques and equipment, a simpler method is the demonstration of an inappropriate secretion of mineralocorticoid as reflected by its physiologic effects. This is best done by placing the subject on a liberal sodium intake and finding high levels of urinary potassium in the presence of abnormally low serum potassium concentrations. In accord with this, but not as reliable, is the demonstration of low levels of sodium in samples of sweat and saliva.

Emphasis is placed on adequate sodium intake during diagnostic studies, since sodium restriction not only increases aldosterone secretion and recovery of urinary aldosterone and its metabolites in normals but also may correct all the metabolic changes noted with primary hyperaldosteronism, including the hypopotassemic alkalosis, the symptoms of tetany and muscle weakness, and the polydipsia and polyuria even in patients with hyperaldosteronism due to tumor.

In some cases, an adrenal cortical tumor can be demonstrated by pyelograms, tomograms, or radiography after retroperitoneal injection of carbon dioxide, but usually the tumor is of such small size that localization is difficult.

Differential Diagnosis. The most frequent problem in the differential diagnosis of primary hyperaldosteronism is hypertension due to other causes. If placed on restricted sodium, as mentioned previously, increased aldosterone levels are found in all subjects, and on the other hand, the patient with primary hyperaldosteronism may lose all the classical associated metabolic changes of the disease. If the hypertensive patient has been given diuretic agents, particularly the chlorothiazide derivatives, hypopotassemia may be induced, complicating the picture even further. Definitive differentiation is again made by providing a liberal sodium intake and demonstration of an inappropriately increased secretion of aldosterone, either directly by chemical determination or indirectly by electrolyte balance studies in the face of this adequate sodium intake. Another diagnostic problem is the patient with hypopotassemia due to other causes, such as gastrointestinal disease or following excessive use of laxatives and other agents producing diarrhea. These patients may present with polydipsia, polyuria, muscle weakness, tetany, etc., but urinary potassium is extremely low because of the kidney's effort to conserve potassium in contrast to the high urinary potassium concentration in patients with primary hyperaldosteronism.

Other problems in the differential diagnosis include various forms of potassium-losing renal disease. In these, there is usually an associated loss of sodium and calcium and a metabolic acidosis; and in Fanconi's syndrome and its variants, there may also be aminoaciduria and phosphaturia. Lastly, patients with familial periodic paralysis with transitory episodes of paralysis and hypopotassemia usually have a marked family history; in addition they are most frequently seen in the first or second decades.

Etiology and Pathogenesis. Approximately three-fourths of patients with primary hyperaldosteronism have a solitary adrenal adenoma. These may be several centimeters in diameter; however, cases have been reported with functioning tumors less than 1 cm in size, found only on sectioning the adrenal after its removal. Hyperaldosteronism due to carcinoma is extremely rare. The remaining cases may show generalized adrenal hypertrophy and nodulation, particularly of the subcapsular zone (zona glomerulosa), or else no demonstrable histologic abnormality. The duration of symptoms of the disease may vary from several months to many years.

Treatment. Treatment is directed to surgical excision of the hyperfunctioning tissue. Preferably, both adrenals are exposed, and if an adenoma is found, it is excised. If no adenoma is detected, or if small adenomas not apparent until the gland is sectioned are found, both adrenals are excised to remove all potential aldosterone-secreting tissue. Obviously, the patient, prior to surgery, should be prepared for eventual total adrenalectomy, with both repository and intravenous steroid. All patients should receive large supplements of potassium chloride postoperatively to replete the body stores.

Course and Prognosis. Without treatment, patients with this disorder progress into irreversible uremia or hypertensive-cardiovascular disease. Sodium restriction and administration of potassium chloride may alleviate the progression of the disease to a certain extent. With removal of the hyperfunctioning adrenal tissue, a marked improvement is usually noted; however, depending on the duration and severity of the disease, the hypertension and renal changes may not be completely reversed. In addition, there is frequently mild to severe chronic pyelonephritis which also may result in irreversible renal damage.

Secondary Aldosteronism

Secondary hyperaldosteronism describes the condition of increased adrenal secretion of aldosterone associated with other pathologic states; almost invariably it is associated with low urinary sodium output on a normal diet in contrast to the normal or relatively high levels of sodium output in patients with primary hyperaldosteronism. Patients with congestive heart failure usually secrete amounts of aldosterone similar to normal persons; however, once digitalization or a low sodium diet or diuretic therapy is instituted, there is a marked increase in adrenal aldosterone production. Similarly, patients with hepatic cirrhosis, nephrosis, inferior vena caval obstruction, and other edematous states usually have some degree of secondary hyperaldosteronism, particularly when placed on sodium restriction and diuretic agents. Increased secretion of aldosterone has also been associated with malignant hypertension; its role, however, in the pathogenesis of this disease is at present difficult to evaluate.

Aldosterone and Edema

Patients with primary aldosteronism rarely have more than a trace of ankle edema. When aldosterone (or any other mineralocorticoid) is given in excess to a normal person, sodium retention occurs until extracellular fluid volume is expanded approximately 3 liters. Any further intake of sodium and water is rapidly excreted by the kidney, even in the presence of continued excessive mineralocorticoid. This phenomenon has been described as the "escape mechanism" and has been related to an increase in renal hemodynamics. It is the threshold for this escape mechanism which is apparently altered in the various edematous states usually associated with secondary hyperaldosteronism, and it is not the aldosterone itself which is producing the edema as a primary phenomenon.

Adrenal Virilism

Adrenal virilism results from excessive production of adrenal hormones with androgenic activity. Similar to other states of adrenal hyperfunction, the disease may result from adenoma, carcinoma, or hyperplasia. In addition, it may be associated with secretions of greater or lesser amounts of other adrenal hormones and may, therefore, present as either a "pure" syndrome of virilization or a "mixed" syndrome associated with excessive production of glucocorticoid and some of the characteristics of Cushing's syndrome. In the congenital forms it may be associated with either excessive or decreased secretion of mineralocorticoid or decreased production of glucocorticoid.

The enzymatic composition of the adrenal as determined by heredity (and perhaps other factors as well) determines the relative synthesis of hormones with glucocorticoid activity and of hormones with androgenic activity. Since in man hydrocortisone is the principal adrenal steroid suppressing pituitary elaboration of ACTH, and since ACTH stimulates production of both hydrocortisone and adrenal androgen, this enzymatic structure of the adrenal may markedly influence the hormonal milieu. On one hand, the adrenal may produce primarily hydrocortisone with only insignificant amounts of androgen. On the other hand, the adrenal with its enzymatic machinery more geared to androgen production may induce minor degrees of virilization in order to produce sufficient hydrocortisone to suppress pituitary ACTH. In extreme situations, such as the patient with a marked degree of congenital virilizing hyperplasia, the adrenal may be incapable of producing adequate hydrocortisone, in which case the virilization may be associated with clinical adrenal "insufficiency," even in the face of anatomic adrenal hyperplasia.

From Fig. 68-1, the steps in the synthesis of hydrocortisone from 17-hydroxyprogesterone involve first hydroxylation in position-21 and then in position-11. One group of patients with "congenital adrenal hyperplasia" associated with virilism, have been shown to be deficient in hydroxylation of carbon-21. These patients therefore, stimulated by their own pituitary ACTH, produce excessive quantities of adrenal androgen. Their urine contains not only excessive metabolites of the androgens as 17-ketosteroids but also metabolites of 17-hydroxyprogesterone (the steroid accumulating before the block) such as pregnanetriol or pregnanetriolone. If the deficiency to hydroxylate at position-21 is more or less complete, the patient may suffer in addition to virilization, adrenal insufficiency due to failure in the synthesis of hydrocortisone, and possibly also the synthesis of aldosterone. The degree of insufficiency in these patients may be so extreme that secretion of a "salt-losing" steroid has been postulated in some of these more severe cases.

Insufficiency in the enzyme hydroxylating carbon-11 results in adrenal virilization and synthesis of not only adrenal androgens, but also certain 11-deoxysteroids such as compound S and deoxycorticosterone which have mineralocorticoid effects (Fig. 68-1). Thus, these patients may exhibit symptoms from an increased secretion of mineralocorticoid such as hypertension, hypopotassemia, and alkalosis, in addition to their virilization. These patients have been referred to as the "hypertensive" form of congenital virilizing hyperplasia.

Incidence. Congenital bilateral adrenocortical hyperplasia is by far the most common adrenal disorder of infancy and childhood. It has also been described to occur later in life, predominantly in women. Its appearance in postpuberal men would obviously not be as clinically apparent; nevertheless, it has been reported. The most common form of significant "noncongenital" adrenal virilization is that seen with bilateral adrenocortical hyperplasia and is most frequently associated with various degrees of excessive production of glucocorticoid and the clinical signs and symptoms of Cushing's syndrome.

Clinical Signs and Symptoms. *The Congenital Form.* In females there may be various degrees of pseudohermaphroditism with hypertrophy of the clitoris. The labia majora are large, usually fused in the midline and may resemble a scrotum. The labia minora are atrophic. At the base of the clitoris, there is frequently a common urogenital sinus simulating hypospadias. Pubic hair usually appears by the age of three years. In males the condition may not be recognized until this age, at which time the phallus enlarges and sexual hair and acne appear. The testes, unlike those of patients with congenital precocious puberty, remain small and atrophic. In both sexes, somatic growth is accelerated and body growth and skeletal development are advanced relative to age. If untreated, early closure of the epiphyses may result, and the child, although larger than his contemporaries during childhood, usually ends below average in size as an adult.

If the disease is due to inability to hydroxylate carbon-11 effectively, there may be hypertension and its associated symptoms. If the disease is due to a relative inability to hydroxylate carbon-21 and the degree of enzyme deficiency is marked, the patient may suffer all the signs and symptoms of classical adrenocortical insufficiency with hypotension, anorexia, etc., frequently resulting in death if not diagnosed. This condition is most striking in male infants in whom the symptoms of adrenal insufficiency may precede any noticeable objective degree of virilization.

The Postnatal Form. If the disease occurs prepuberally, accelerated adolescence may be noted in males. In females, heterosexual precocity occurs with acne, pubic and axillary hair, hypertrophy of the clitoris, and failure of the menarche and breast development. In adult women, the clinical picture includes amenorrhea, hirsutism of masculine distribution, enlargement of the clitoris, acne, deepening of the voice, increased muscularity, and development of a male habitus. As mentioned earlier, pure virilism in adults is relatively rare; more often, features of Cushing's syndrome are also present and the anatomic cause is bilateral hyperplasia, not of the classical "congenital" variety due to a specific enzyme deficiency.

Laboratory Findings. Since adrenal androgens are relatively less potent than testosterone, an increased level of urinary 17-ketosteroids is present in all cases of virilization due to adrenal disease. By one commonly used assay, women excrete approximately 10 to 15 mg urinary 17-ketosteroids per 24 hr and men 15 to 20 mg per 24 hr; however, there is a fairly wide individual variation. Children obviously excrete much smaller amounts, and newborn infants less than 1 mg per 24 hr. Likewise, 17-ketosteroid secretion falls slightly in old age.

Diagnosis. The diagnosis of adrenal virilization requires demonstration of increased adrenal production of androgenic hormone. Usually, abnormally elevated levels of urinary 17-ketosteroids are sufficient. When associated with elevated levels of 17-hydroxycorticoids and some clinical signs and symptoms of glucocorticoid activity as mentioned before, one is dealing with a "mixed syndrome." If there is a markedly hyperactive response of 17-ketosteroid and 17-hydroxycorticoid excretion to ACTH stimulation and suppression by only large amounts of dexamethasone or 9α-fluorohydrocortisone, the pathogenic cause is probably bilateral cortical hyperplasia. Failure to stimulate or to suppress is again suggestive of carcinoma.

On the other hand, virilization with elevated urinary 17-ketosteroids and normal or low 17-hydroxycorticoids is suggestive of the congenital types of adrenal disorders and not simple bilateral cortical hyperplasia. In these, suppression of ketosteroid excretion to normal levels by administration of amounts of glucocorticoid equal to that amount expected to be secreted by the patient's own

adrenals supports the diagnosis, and confirmation is secured by demonstration of abnormal quantities of blocked hydrocortisone "precursors" such as pregnanetriol. Lastly, virilization with elevated 17-ketosteroids which fails to respond to ACTH or suppress with exogenous glucocorticoid is indicative of an adrenal adenoma or carcinoma, more frequently the latter.

Differential Diagnosis. The most common problem in the differential diagnosis of adrenal virilism is the young woman with abnormal hirsutism and either irregular or absent menstrual periods. Contributing to the problem, many of these patients excrete 17-ketosteroids either in the high normal or slightly higher than normal range. However, they do not excrete markedly abnormal quantities of pregnanetriol as expected with patients with one of the types of congenital virilizing adrenal hyperplasia, and their response to exogenous ACTH may not be hyperactive. Culdoscopy or laparotomy frequently reveals normal ovaries, or the classical polycystic ovary as described by Stein and Leventhal, or a less markedly abnormal ovary with various degrees of thickening of the capsule. Whether these patients have a primary disturbance of the ovary with production of androgen or whether their disease primarily arises from the adrenal as a case of "partial" congenital virilizing hyperplasia is controversial. However, many seem to improve with administration of small suppressive doses of glucocorticoid in order to inhibit secretion of endogenous ACTH and thereby adrenal androgen production. These patients possibly form a link between normal women and those with the classical form of congenital adrenal virilization. This concept is supported by the fact that in some families one sibling may have the former and another sibling the latter syndrome. In essence, both are probably congenital virilizing adrenal hyperplasia with different degrees of penetrance.

Another problem in differential diagnosis is virilization in the absence of elevated urinary 17-ketosteroids, suggesting production of highly potent androgen, such as testosterone. In boys this may be due to a Leydig cell tumor of the testis or in girls to an ovarian tumor such as an arrhenoblastoma. Likewise, children with various degrees of hermaphroditism may be confused with congenital virilizing hyperplasia, but in these urinary 17-ketosteroid excretion is within normal limits, and determination of sexual chromatin or direct chromosomal counts may aid in the true diagnosis.

Treatment. Treatment of adrenal virilism is dependent on the type of suspected pathologic changes. In the classical forms of congenital hyperplasia, with elevated urinary 17-ketosteroids and a hyperactive response to ACTH, and (in the more common variety with deficient 21-hydroxylating capacity) demonstrable abnormal levels of pregnanetriol, treatment is simply administration of maintenance doses of glucocorticoid (dexamethasone, prednisone, cortisone, etc.) to suppress pituitary ACTH secretion. In children, this results not only in suppression of urinary ketosteroid excretion but also in cessation of virilization and the associated problems of hyperandrogenicity. Some children (the "salt wasters") may also require mineralocorticoid, most easily satisfied (similar to the Addisonian) by small doses of 9α-fluorohydrocortisone. In addition, markedly altered genitalia may require isosexual surgical correction, such as clitoral amputation. If the adrenal virilism is associated with excessive quantities of glucocorticoid secretion resulting in a mixed syndrome and is associated with an excessive response to ACTH, treatment is similar to that for "pure" Cushing's syndrome due to adrenal hyperplasia, namely, pituitary irradiation for the milder and adrenalectomy for the more advanced cases. Virilization with high urinary ketosteroids unresponsive to ACTH or to suppressive doses of glucocorticoid is suggestive of adrenal adenoma or carcinoma and is thus treated surgically.

In the borderline cases with mild hirsutism, high normal or minimally abnormal urinary 17-ketosteroid excretion, and menstrual irregularities, a trial on suppressive doses of glucocorticoid is indicated and may frequently result in return not only of normal menses and suppression of hair growth, but occasionally in ovulation and pregnancy.

Prognosis. Children with congenital virilizing hyperplasia, when treated with adequate suppressive doses of glucocorticoid, develop normally and many females followed from childhood have married and borne children. However, virilization if of long duration may result in certain irreversible changes. In particular hirsutism, once established, may take many years to decrease after the source of the androgen has been removed. In some cases, there may be a substantial improvement in hirsutism but never a total return to the previrilized state.

Adrenal Feminization

Adrenal feminization is an extremely rare entity and is most frequently due to adrenal carcinoma. In one or two instances, feminization has been described associated with bilateral adrenal hyperplasia.

NONSPECIFIC USE OF ACTH AND ADRENAL STEROIDS IN CLINICAL PRACTICE

The widespread application of ACTH and adrenal steroid therapy in many branches of medicine and surgery emphasizes the need of a thorough understanding of the metabolic effects of these agents if clinical use is to be most effective and if undesirable side reactions are to be minimized. Prior to instituting adrenal hormone therapy, a physician should weigh carefully the gains that can reasonably be expected versus the potentially undesirable metabolic actions of the particular hormone. Accurate appraisal will require familiarity with the reports of others in similar instances, a critical evaluation of the statistical significance of such reports, as well as a clear understanding of the chemical, physiologic, and psychologic changes which hormone preparations of this type are known to induce.

Perhaps an approach to the problem presented by a particular patient may be facilitated by reviewing the specific considerations outlined in Table 68-4.

1. *How serious is the underlying disorder?* The use of any nonspecific or "symptomatic" pharmacologic agent must be weighed against the seriousness of the underlying disorder. Each pharmacologic agent has a "price tag" which must be evaluated carefully prior to the institution of a therapeutic program. With the antibiotic agents this price tag may consist of the possibility of inducing drug-sensitivity reactions or the development of antibiotic-resistant strains of pathogenic organisms; with the agents employed for hypertensive-cardiovascular disease the price tag may consist of disturbing side effects referable to the autonomic nervous system. With the corticosteroids, effective therapy may be purchased at the risk of inducing

Table 68-4. CONSIDERATIONS PRIOR TO THE USE OF CORTICOSTEROIDS AS PHARMACOLOGIC AGENTS

1. How serious is this disorder?
2. How long will therapy be required?
3. What is the usual dosage required for this disorder?
   a. To achieve improvement.
   b. To suppress effectively the signs and symptoms of the disorder.
4. Is the patient predisposed to any of the known hazards of corticosteroid therapy by virtue of:
   a. Cardiovascular-renal disease.
   b. Gastric hypersecretion.
   c. Osteoporosis.
   d. Diabetes.
   e. Tuberculosis or other infections.
   f. Psychologic abnormalities.
5. Which adrenal preparation is preferable?
   a. ACTH—long-acting (intramuscular) or intravenous administration.
   b. Cortisone or hydrocortisone—oral, intramuscular, local, or intravenous.
   c. Derivatives of cortisone such as prednisone, triamcinolone, and dexamethasone.
6. Supplementary adjuvants employed to minimize metabolic abnormalities.

undesirable side reactions such as peptic ulceration, osteoporosis, or psychologic abnormalities. Clearly in a patient whose life is threatened by unexplained shock or in one in whom other measures have failed to modify the course of disseminated lupus erythematosus, the physician need not hesitate to employ massive steroid therapy. On the other hand, one should exercise restraint in administering suppressive steroid therapy to a patient with early rheumatoid arthritis who as yet has not received the possible benefits of physiotherapy and a well-organized program of general medical care.

2. *How long will therapy be required?* The problems which arise in connection with evaluating the seriousness of the underlying disorder naturally involve the expected or anticipated duration of therapy. Thus the use of intravenous hydrocortisone for 24 to 48 hr in the treatment of severe status asthmaticus or acute serum sickness or a drug reaction does not present the problems which arise in considering steroid therapy in the treatment of chronic, lifelong asthma or psoriasis. In general, contraindications to steroids for severe, short-lived disorders will be few, whereas in suppressive therapy for chronic, persistent disorders one must envisage the serious problem presented by Cushing's syndrome which results from prolonged ingestion of exogenous glucocorticoid.

3. *What is the usual dosage required for this disorder?* Hormone therapy may be employed in a relatively low schedule calculated to achieve clinical improvement but not necessarily to achieve complete or almost complete suppression of all signs and symptoms of the disorder. In the former case 50 to 75 mg cortisone or hydrocortisone (or the equivalent amount of one of its derivatives) may be required to attain worthwhile clinical improvement, whereas 150 to 300 mg cortisone or hydrocortisone may be needed to suppress all evidences of activity of the disease. At the 50- to 75-mg level of cortisone or hydrocortisone, it might be feasible to embark on long-term therapy with minimal risk of serious complications resembling Cushing's disease, whereas at the 150-mg dose level, relief of one disease may be attained only at the risk of inducing another (Cushing's syndrome). In general, doses of hydrocortisone or cortisone of 75 mg or less may be tolerated by most patients for prolonged periods of time with a minimum of underlying metabolic disabilities, whereas doses of cortisone or hydrocortisone of 100 mg or more will usually be associated with progressive metabolic aberrations. Dosages of cortisone or hydrocortisone in the range of 25 to 50 mg daily can, in all probability, be tolerated by most patients for life.

4. *Is the patient predisposed to any of the known complications of corticosteroid therapy?*

a. Cardiovascular-renal disease. In general the so-dium-retaining propensity of most adrenal steroid preparations requires that caution be used when they are employed in the presence of cardiovascular disease. The availability of preparations in which sodium-retaining activity is minimal (triamcinolone and dexamethasone), restriction of dietary sodium intake, the use of resins, diuretic agents, and particularly of supplementary potassium salts will permit the safe use of steroid therapy where important indications exist. Of course in congestive failure or pericardial effusion associated with acute rheumatic activity, or in patients with nephrotic edema, steroid hormone preparations may act as effective diuretic agents.

All patients in whom prolonged steroid therapy is contemplated should have careful evaluation of their cardiovascular-renal status, which should include a chest film for *heart size*. The chest film is essential also in excluding pulmonary tuberculosis.

b. Peptic ulcer, perforation, and bleeding. It appears evident that patients with a history of gastric hypersecretion or peptic ulcer are likely to experience an aggravation of their symptoms during adrenal hormone therapy. It is not known for certain whether the aggravation of peptic ulceration and complicating gastrointestinal hemorrhage reflect the increased gastric secretory activity so frequently associated with adrenal hormone therapy, or whether the nitrogen-depleting effect of these hormones accelerates the process of ulceration and perforation. Antacid therapy and an ulcer diet are useful precautions in susceptible patients. *The development of anemia in a patient on ACTH or cortisone therapy should immediately suggest gastrointestinal bleeding*, and patients should be cautioned to note black or tarry stools. A clear-cut history of peptic ulcer is a contraindication to ACTH and cortisone therapy unless extreme precautions are taken.

c. Osteoporosis. All patients on prolonged cortisone-like steroid therapy are likely to develop some degree of osteoporosis. Obviously a considerable change in bone structure must occur before it is radiologically demonstrable. For this reason patients should have standard films of the spine and pelvis in order to establish the status of the bony framework prior to therapy and for comparative purposes later. Postmenopausal women patients and men and women of advanced age will be predisposed to the earlier development of serious changes of this type. The skin also participates in the depletion of body protein, becoming thin and atrophic, with easy bruisability. It is possible that ACTH may cause less osteoporosis for a given level of steroid therapy because of a concomitant increase in adrenal androgen secretion. This possible advantage of ACTH over crystalline steroids is offset by the increased difficulty with which an exact pharmacologic dosage of endogenous steroid is maintained with the tropic hormone. Supplementary calcium therapy in the form of calcium lactate, 1 Gm three times daily, and estrogen and androgen therapy should be considered in those patients known to be susceptible to the catabolic action of adrenal steroids. Of course the presence of any degree of osteoporosis *a priori* would constitute strong evidence against the desirability of embarking upon prolonged high-dosage adrenal hormone therapy.

d. Diabetes mellitus. Prolonged ACTH or cortisone-like steroid therapy may unmask latent diabetes mellitus and aggravate preexisting disease. For this reason a careful history to exclude familial incidence of diabetes is important, as well as an examination of the blood and urine for excess glucose levels. It is more valuable to carry out these examinations following a test load of carbohydrate. A convenient method consists in measuring blood and urinary glucose 2 to 3 hr following the ingestion of a breakfast containing approximately 100 Gm carbohydrate (see Chap. 70). Obviously the presence of frank diabetes mellitus or the demonstration of impaired glucose tolerance will affect the physician's decision regarding the desirability of instituting adrenal hormone therapy. However, if such therapy appears necessary or desirable in the presence of latent diabetes, the judicious use of supplementary insulin should be seriously considered. The insulin requirement of known diabetics will usually need to be increased with ACTH or cortisone-like therapy except in those rare instances in which the diabetic patient is suffering from some degree of insulin-protein reaction in which the "anti-inflammatory" or "antiallergic" effect of cortisone enhances the metabolic effectiveness of the insulin sufficiently to "balance off" its diabetogenic action.

e. Tuberculosis or other infections. Before prolonged steroid therapy is seriously entertained, it is imperative to exclude the presence of tuberculosis and other infections. Continued steroid therapy, without a specific antibiotic agent, can lead to serious spread of infection. A chest film is essential prior to prolonged steroid therapy, and the desirability of cultures from the nose and throat, and of the urine and feces, if symptoms point to any disturbances, is evident.

f. Psychologic abnormalities. From time to time steroid therapy may be complicated by severe psychologic disturbances, and of course less severe abnormalities are relatively frequent. In general, serious psychologic disturbances are more closely related to the patient's personality structure than to the actual dose of hormone, although, as might be anticipated, the larger doses of hormone will be associated with more serious reactions. At present

there is no reliable method of determining beforehand a patient's psychologic reaction to steroid therapy. Patients with known psychologic difficulties undoubtedly experience more frequent and more severe disturbances. Further difficulty arises because previous tolerance of steroids does not necessarily ensure immunity from subsequent courses of therapy, and outward psychologic reactions on one occasion does not invariably mean that the patient will respond unfavorably to a second course of treatment. This is one area in which the physician must follow his patient carefully during the early period of steroid therapy, and one in which he must take a responsible member of the family into his confidence.

The foregoing considerations constitute important data on which the physician's ultimate decision for or against hormone therapy will rest.

5. *Which adrenal preparation is preferable?* For practical purposes there is no clearly demonstrable qualitative difference among cortisone, hydrocortisone, prednisone, triamcinolone, and dexamethasone; the latter three groups of substances, however, have much less sodium retaining effect in relation to their anti-inflammatory activity. Excluding the mineralocorticoid effect, the formulas and therapeutic potencies per milligram of these and similar substances are illustrated in Fig. 68-6 and Table 68-5.

In most cases, the only decision of major consequence will revolve around the possible use of ACTH rather than one of the adrenal steroid preparations. In general, it can be stated that adrenal steroid therapy is effective by mouth and can be regulated more accurately than ACTH therapy. The latter will fluctuate considerably in the amount of steroid produced from day to day, depending on the rate and extent of absorption of ACTH and on the state of the adrenal cortex. ACTH therapy does involve the secretion of adrenal androgens as well as hydroxysteroids. The former may have advantages in certain diseases, such as dermatomyositis

HYDROCORTISONE AND NATURAL AND SYNTHETIC ANALOGUES

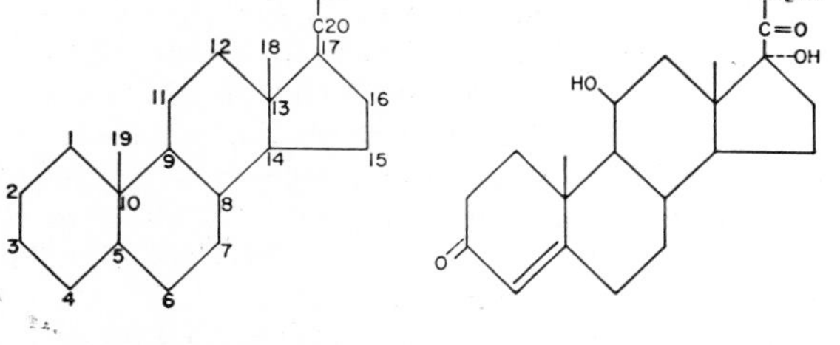

PREGNANE NUCLEUS

HYDROCORTISONE
(PREGN-4-ene-11β,17α,21-triol-3,20-dione)

FIG. 68-6

Table 68-5. ADRENAL PREPARATIONS

Commonly used name	Other names	Estimated potencies	
		Gluco-corticoid	Mineralo-corticoid
Hydrocortisone............	Cortisol, Hydrocortone Compound F, 17-hydroxycorticosterone PREGN-4-ene-11β,17α,21-triol-3,20-dione	1	1
Cortisone.................	Cortone, compound E 11-Dehydro-17-hydroxycorticosterone PREGN-4-ene-17α,21-diol-3,11,20-trione	0.8	0.8
DOC.....................	Percorten, cortexone, 11-deoxycorticosterone PREGN-4-ene-21-ol-3,20-dione	0	25
Aldosterone..............	Electrocortin PREGN-4-ene-11β,21-diol-18-al-3,20-dione	? 0.5	200–400
Prednisolone.............	Meticortelone, Δ¹-hydrocortisone PREGN-1,4-diene-11β,17α,21-triol-3,20-dione	5	0.5
Prednisone...............	Meticorten, Δ¹-cortisone PREGN-1,4-diene-17α,21-diol-3,11,20-trione	4	0.5
Methyl prednisolone.......	Medrol, 6-methyl-Δ¹-hydrocortisone	8–10	? ±
Triamcinolone.............	Aristocort, Kenacort 16α-Hydroxy-9 α-fluoro-Δ¹-hydrocortisone	6–8	? ±
Dexamethasone...........	Decadron, Deronil 16α-Methyl-9 α-fluoro-Δ¹-hydrocortisone	25–50	? ±
Fluorohydrocortisone.......	Florinef, Fluoro-F 9α-Fluorohydrocortisone	10–25	100

in which the adrenal androgens may prove helpful in maintaining the muscle mass, while the inflammatory reaction is being suppressed by the 17-hydroxycorticosteroids. Combined androgen and corticoid therapy may, of course, attain the same objective. Sodium retention with ACTH has often been more marked than with cortisone or, particularly, with prednisone therapy. It is not probable that ACTH stimulates aldosterone secretion to any significant degree.

There is little support for the belief that ACTH stimulates the production of naturally useful steroids—not available commercially. Of course the use of ACTH presupposes a normally responsive adrenal cortex, an assumption which cannot always be verified in serious and prolonged disorders. Obviously both ACTH and steroid administration will induce pituitary inhibition, and in addition steroid therapy will induce adrenal suppression. For practical purposes the use of ACTH is largely confined to initiating a therapeutic response and to actuating the adrenal cortex prior to discontinuing steroid therapy. It, of course, has a very important use in the diagnostic approach to disorders of adrenal function.

6. *Supplementary adjuvants employed to minimize metabolic disabilities.* Since the continued use of ACTH or adrenal steroids induces a hypopotassemic, hypochloremic metabolic alkalosis, supplementary potassium therapy should be given daily to patients receiving these hormone preparations. Enteric-coated tablets of potassium chloride (1 Gm) are usually well tolerated if given with meals in a dose of 3 to 9 Gm (40 to 120 mEq of potassium) daily. In addition the authors have found a solution of "triplex" potassium salts[1] to be an effective and often well-tolerated means of administering potassium. Each teaspoonful (5 ml) contains 15 mEq of potassium. Renal insufficiency is the only contraindication to continued potassium therapy.

Antacid therapy and an ulcer diet may be required in patients with evidence of marked gastric acidity or a previous history of peptic ulceration. Testicular androgen therapy (testosterone) must be considered, particularly in female patients on long-continued corticoid therapy. This is not necessary in male patients or in patients on ACTH. Restriction of sodium chloride intake is essential, and the excessive intake of food can be safely restricted only if adequate consideration is given to the problem of related increased gastric secretion. Adrenal steroid therapy in diabetes or prediabetic patients must be accompanied by increased insulin adminis-

[1] Formula: potassium acetate, 100 Gm; potassium bicarbonate, 100 Gm; potassium citrate, 100 Gm; sugar-free vehicle: saccharin sodium, 0.6 Gm; solution of amaranth, 3 ml; glycerin, 200 ml; water, *ad* 1,000 ml.

tration. Adrenal cortical hormones have been given safely to patients with infections in whom a highly specific antibiotic was being administered simultaneously. The possible usefulness of the new "tranquilizing" drugs in minimizing psychologic difficulties encountered in steroid treatment has yet to be determined.

Summary. Several general facts should be considered in the management of patients receiving prolonged steroid therapy.

1. There is real danger of inducing acute adrenal failure if steroid therapy is suddenly withdrawn. Furthermore, inadequate adrenal reserve may be present for a prolonged period following the cessation of steroid therapy. Under these circumstances, patients must be warned regarding the additional risk of acute stress reactions such as injuries, operations, and infections. Both the patient and his doctor should be aware of this problem, and supplementary corticoid therapy should be readily available at all times.

2. Patients who are being maintained on a constant dose of steroid over a prolonged period should be protected by the provision of an increase in their hormone therapy during a period of surgery or endocrine stress. It may be necessary to increase the basic dose of cortisone or its equivalent 17-hydroxy-corticoid by as much as 100 mg daily.

3. When using steroids such as prednisone which usually do not invoke appreciable sodium retention or edema, one must be on the alert for more subtle evidences of overdosage during a prolonged therapeutic program. Special attention should be given to disturbance in the gastrointestinal tract, as indicated by the appearance of digestive symptoms or occult blood in the stool. One should also watch carefully for signs suggestive of bone pain due to the development of underlying osteoporosis.

4. All patients on prolonged steroid therapy should have periodic checks, which should include body weight, blood pressure, urine sugar, and appraisal of the cardiovascular, digestive, and skeletal systems; and the possibility of the development of posterior subcapsular cataracts must be considered.

Adrenal hormone therapy constitutes a potent pharmacologic agent in the armamentarium of every practicing physician. As with all potent medicaments, a physician's responsibility must include an adequate knowledge of the pharmacologic actions of these agents as well as of the indications and contraindications for their use.

REACTIONS TO INJURY AND STRESS

A febrile response, leukocytic changes, and alterations in the erythrocyte sedimentation rate are well recognized indexes of injury and the body's reaction to it. More gradually it has been recognized that the reaction to injury involves the whole organism. A series of integrated responses occurs, which includes important changes in the circulation as well as psychologic and neuromuscular changes and a whole group of chemical and metabolic reactions initiated by neurohormonal mediators and chemical substances which arise from the injured tissues. These reactions entail the participation at least of the pituitary and the adrenal glands, the liver, the kidneys, and the hematopoietic tissues. They result in alterations in circulation and in protein, carbohydrate, and fat metabolism, as well as in various electrolytes. At the same time, important psychologic reactions take place.

Selye has applied the descriptive title of "the alarm reaction" to the series of events which may be initiated by such varied stresses as emotional disturbances, infection, hemorrhage, trauma, or undue exposure to heat and cold. Injury such as occurs with full-thickness burns gives rise to the most intense pattern of reaction.

In the original hypothesis it was assumed that the increased liberation of adrenal hormones, both medullary and cortical, was largely responsible for initiating the widespread metabolic changes characteristic of this syndrome. It was postulated by Long and others that the release of epinephrine provided the trigger mechanism which initiated the hypothalamic-pituitary release of adrenocorticotropin (ACTH). This in turn stimulated the release and formation of greatly increased quantities of adrenal cortical steroids, which in turn were responsible for the chemical and metabolic changes observed.

By the use of highly purified ACTH preparations or synthetic adrenal steroids, it has been possible to reproduce many of the changes characteristic of this general response of the organism to stress. Thus increased excretion of nitrogen, potassium, and phosphorus, retention of sodium chloride and water, reduction in circulating eosinophils and lymphocytes, increase in polymorphonuclears, elevation of blood sugar level with decreased glucose tolerance, changes in important plasma constituents such as cholesterol and globulin, and alterations in gastrointestinal secretions, as well as fundamental changes in psychologic behavior and neuromuscular function, have all been observed in patients and in normal persons given large quantities of ACTH, cortisone, or hydrocortisone (compound F) (see Chap. 64).

Although widespread changes of this type can be induced by stimulating the intact adrenal gland of man with purified ACTH preparations, or by the administration of the appropriate adrenal steroids, recent studies indicate that mechanisms other than those related to activation of the pituitary-adrenal axis are capable of inducing similar metabolic and chemical effects. Indeed, only in severe stress or tissue injury does a measurable increase in blood or urine adrenal steroid level occur. Thus it appears more correct to interpret the total response of the organism to stress as representing (1) adrenal cortical activation, (2) other as yet undisclosed mechanisms, (3) varying combinations of both. Although the importance of adrenal cortical participation in the stress response appears to be well substantiated, the theory that increased adrenal cortical secretions dominate the reaction needs important modification.

A valuable contribution to the understanding of the problem has come from the studies of Ingle, who has shown that the provision of a constant level of adrenal cortical hormone during the application of stress permits survival over a wide range of stressful situations. It is well known that adrenalectomized animals exhibit a very limited response to noxious agents. Thus the concept of the "permissive" action of the adrenal steroids has been proposed. In this theory it is suggested that a basic level of adrenal steroids permits a satisfactory total metabolic response of the organism over a relatively wide range of adverse conditions. Of course, under very severe stress the level of adrenal steroids must be greatly increased. According to this view, the stresses of everyday life can be met by chemical and psychologic responses which require the presence of adrenal cortical steroids but not necessarily an *increased* secretion of them. This explanation is consistent with the known difficulty of demonstrating a significant increase in the blood or urine steroid level under any type of stress short of those which threaten life.

Regarding the theory that epinephrine constitutes a key substance in initiating the hypothalamic-pituitary adrenal cortical activation, it is of some interest to note that, to date, no increase in the blood or urine level of ACTH or adrenal steroids has been observed in man following the administration of epinephrine either subcutaneously or intravenously, in single or in repeated doses, or following continuous intravenous infusion. Thus although the participation of the adrenal medullary hormones is essential in man's successful response to stress (Cannon), there is no evidence that epinephrine or norepinephrine in physiologic doses is capable of initiating increased secretion of ACTH or adrenal steroids. Under special circumstances in experimental animals, an increase in the adrenal steroid content of adrenal venous blood has been observed following epinephrine administration in sympathectomized dogs. It is important to note, however, that in man epinephrine itself has been demonstrated to be capable of inducing eosinopenia in the absence of demonstrable functioning adrenal cortical tissue.

REFERENCES

Albright, F.: Cushing's Syndrome, Harvey Lectures, 38:123, 1942–43.

Brown, J. H. U.: Specific Inhibitors of the Adrenal Cortex, Nature, 4272:985, 1960.

Conn, J. W., and I. H. Louis: Primary Aldosteronism, a New Clinical Entity, Ann. Internal Med., 44:1, 1956.

Cushing, H.: The Basophil Adenomas of the Pituitary Body and Their Clinical Manifestations (Pituitary Basophilism), Bull. Johns Hopkins Hosp., 50:137, 1932.

Laidlaw, J. C., W. J. Reddy, D. Jenkins, N. A. Haydar, A. E. Renold, and G. W. Thorn: Advances in the Diagnosis of Altered States of Adrenocortical Function, New Engl. J. Med., 253:747, 1955.

Nelson, D. H., J. W. Meakin, and G. W. Thorn: ACTH-producing Pituitary Tumors following Adrenalectomy for Cushing's Syndrome, Ann. Internal Med., 52:560, 1960.

Selye, H.: "Physiology and Pathology of Exposure to Stress," Montreal, ACTA, Inc., 1950.

Soffer, L. J., A. Iannaccone, and J. L. Gabrilove: Cushing's Syndrome: A Study of 50 Patients, Am. J. Med., 30:129, 1961.

Tomkins, G. M., and J. S. McGuire, Jr.: The Adrenogenital Syndrome in "The Metabolic Basis of Inherited Disease," J. B. Stanbury, J. B. Wyngaarden, and D. S. Fredrickson (Eds.), New York, McGraw-Hill Book Company, Inc., 1960.

69 DISEASES OF THE ADRENAL MEDULLA

George W. Thorn and Alan Goldfien

The cells of the adrenal medulla arise from the ectoderm of the primitive neural crest. The common stem cell is the sympathogonia, which may develop along two possible pathways: (1) It may differentiate to form a sympathoblast or neuroblast and later a mature ganglion cell, or (2) it may give rise to a chromaffin cell.

The recognized diseases of the adrenal medulla are the result of neoplasms of these cell types. Since these cells are present not only in the adrenal medulla, but wherever there is sympathetic nervous tissue, similar tumors may arise in the sympathetic nerve ganglions and plexuses and in the organ of Zuckerkändl at the lower end of the aorta.

Physiology. The cells of the adrenal medulla synthesize, store, and secrete norepinephrine and epinephrine. The biosynthesis of these hormones proceeds by the sequential conversion of phenylalanine to tyrosine, dihydroxyphenylalanine (dopa), dihydroxyphenylethylamine (dopamine), norepinephrine, and finally to epinephrine. Therefore, norepinephrine, in addition to its role as a hormone of the adrenal medulla, serves as the immediate precursor of epinephrine. Epinephrine constitutes 80 per cent of the amines stored in the human adrenal medulla, whereas norepinephrine appears to be the important neurohumor released at adrenergic nerve endings.

The physiologic activities of these two hormones differ in several respects. Norepinephrine produces marked peripheral vasoconstriction leading to a rise in systolic and diastolic pressures, and this increase in blood pressure usually results in a reflex bradycardia. Small doses of epinephrine cause a net vasodilatation, although the vessels of the skin are constricted. Epinephrine increases the pulse pressure and heart rate, thereby augmenting cardiac output. These latter changes are associated with increased muscle, cerebral, and visceral blood flow. Epinephrine also causes relaxation of bronchiolar smooth muscle. Epinephrine and norepinephrine both increase myocardial contractility and excitability in the isolated heart.

Epinephrine has prominent metabolic effects shared only to a slight degree by norepinephrine. It increases oxygen consumption and body temperature. It also raises the blood glucose level by stimulating the formation of adenosine 3',5'-(cyclic) phosphate. This substance activates the enzyme phosphokinase, which catalyzes the regeneration of active phosphorylase required for breakdown of glycogen and the release of glucose from liver and lactic acid from muscle (see Chap. 52). In contrast to these actions, the mobilization of fatty acids from adipose tissue is stimulated to a similar extent by both epinephrine and norepinephrine.

The metabolic degradation of the adrenal medullary hormones is rapid, more than half of the active amines being removed from the circulation within a minute after their entry. Only a small percentage of these are excreted unchanged into the urine, with the remainder metabolized through the pathways illustrated in Fig. 69-1. When either isotopically labeled epinephrine or norepinephrine is administered to man, 30 to 40 per cent of the label is recovered as metanephrine or normetanephrine and their conjugates, and a similar amount is recovered as 3-methoxy-4-hydroxymandelic acid (vanillo-mandelic acid, VMA).

Although the adrenal medulla is not necessary to maintain life, it is an adjunct to the adrenal cortex in aiding the organism to cope with acute stress. In contrast to other parts of the sympathetic nervous

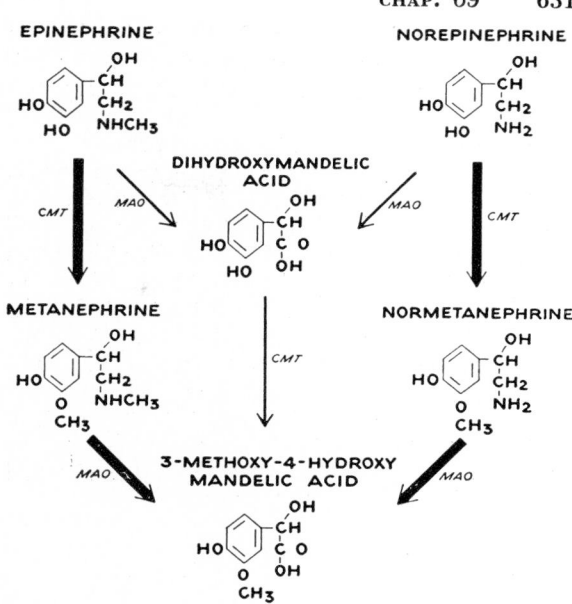

Fig. 69-1. The degradation of epinephrine and norepinephrine by catechol O-methyl transferase (CMT) and monamine oxidase (MAO). All the above compounds appear in the urine in the free form or conjugated to glucuronide or sulfate. The heavier arrows indicate the major pathways. 3-Methoxy-4-hydroxymandelic acid is derived from epinephrine and norepinephrine.

system, which appear to have tonic activity, the adrenal medulla has a low basal secretion but does respond readily to a variety of stimuli of reflex or central origin, such as hemorrhage, hypoxia, hypoglycemia, exercise, fear, and rage. Hypofunction of the adrenal medulla has been demonstrated in children with spontaneous idiopathic hypoglycemia. These individuals show no increase in urinary epinephrine excretion during spontaneous or insulin-induced hypoglycemia.

FUNCTIONING TUMORS

Pheochromocytoma

This relatively uncommon functioning tumor arises in the chromaffin tissue of the sympathetic nervous system. The association of a pheochromocytoma (chromaffinoma) and paroxysmal hypertension was first reported by Labbé in 1922. In 1927, C. H. Mayo removed such a tumor in the retroperitoneal tissues, with resultant complete relief of the associated hypertension. Pheochromocytomas may occur in all age groups but more often in adults. There is no predilection for male or female, but a familial occurrence has been noted. Although usually found in the adrenal, pheochromocytomas may also arise from chromaffin tissue elsewhere in the body. Cutaneous neurofibromatosis is a coincidental finding in about 5 per cent of the cases. The over-all incidence of multiple tumors in patients with pheochromocytomas is 10 to 20 per cent; however, the incidence is higher in younger age groups.

Pathology. The tumors vary in size but often are small and are usually lobulated, vascular, and well encapsulated. The cut surface is yellowish brown in color and frequently shows evidence of hemorrhage and cystic degeneration. Microscopically, the tumor cells appear large, irregular, and polyhedral, with granular cytoplasm. The tumors contain many thin-walled blood vessels, and there is a fine connective tissue stroma. Histologically it is very difficult to distinguish between benign and malignant tumors since many show invasion of the capsule and blood vessels, yet are clinically benign. However, metastases to the liver, lymph nodes, and bone have been found in 7 to 10 per cent of cases.

Clinical Picture. In addition to individual differences which lead to variation in the clinical manifestations of any disorder, the syndrome produced by pheochromocytoma will depend upon whether the tumor releases its amines continuously or intermittently, and upon whether the tumor secretes predominately norepinephrine or epinephrine. In those patients where the tumor releases norepinephrine predominantly, the evidence of hypermetabolism may be less prominent or, on rare occasions, absent.

The presence of pheochromocytoma is usually characterized by hypertension, either paroxysmal or sustained. The classical syndrome of paroxysmal hypertension occurs in approximately 50 per cent of the patients, while about a third of the patients with persistent hypertension have superimposed paroxysmal attacks. During an episode, hypertension, headache, and sweating are found, often associated with anxiety, palpitations, dizziness, and peripheral vasoconstriction. Nausea, vomiting, and precordial pain may be present. Bradycardia is found in approximately 20 per cent of cases. Paroxysms are occasionally precipitated by changes in posture, physical exertion, or emotional upsets. Early in the disease, the attacks tend to occur infrequently, but with time the frequency characteristically increases and the episodes may become more severe. The blood pressure may rise to levels of 150 to 300 mm Hg systolic and 150 to 175 mm Hg diastolic. Hyperglycemia, glucosuria, and albuminuria may accompany the attacks, and death may occur from pulmonary edema, ventricular fibrillation, or cerebral hemorrhage.

In patients with sustained hypertension, one may find an elevated basal metabolic rate, heat intolerance, and excessive sweating, hyperglycemia, glucosuria, polydipsia, and polyuria. Postural hypotension is often present. These patients are usually thin and have a history of recent weight loss.

Diagnosis. If the physician maintains a high index of suspicion, the classical syndrome is not difficult to diagnose. In less typical cases, the clinical picture may closely mimic that of essential hypertension, diabetes mellitus, thyrotoxicosis, anxiety neurosis, or impending myocardial infarction. Diencephalic hypertensive attacks and hypertensive crises in patients with lead poisoning, tabes dorsalis, porphyria, or spinal cord injury also may simulate paroxysms due to pheochromocytoma.

Since the finding of elevated blood pressure is very common and the incidence of pheochromocytoma is low, extensive studies to rule out the disease cannot be carried out in every hypertensive individual. However, particular attention should be given to patients with hypertension under the age of thirty in the absence of a family history of hypertension; to those with malignant hypertension, hypermetabolism without hyperthyroidism, spells of headache and sweating, severe hypertension and diabetes mellitus; and to those with severe hypertension of short duration plus a history of weight loss. The presence of a pheochromocytoma also should be considered in those patients who develop marked blood pressure elevations during the induction of an anesthetic and in patients exhibiting paradoxic responses to ganglionic blocking agents administered for the treatment of their hypertension. It becomes apparent, then, that one is more often faced with the problem of excluding the presence of a pheochromocytoma than with confirming a clinical diagnosis.

Investigation of these patients has been facilitated by the availability of blood and/or urine assays for epinephrine, norepinephrine, or products of their metabolism (Fig. 69-1). In the normal subject at rest, plasma and urine epinephrine levels reflect adrenal medullary activity and are quite low. Plasma levels range from 0 to 1.0 μg per liter, and the urinary excretion rate is about 5 μg per 24 hr. Plasma and urine levels of norepinephrine and normetanephrine primarily reflect peripheral sympathetic activity. 3-Methoxy-4-hydroxymandelic acid is derived from both hormones, and in the resting state reflects norepinephrine secreted at adrenergic nerve endings. When elevated in amount, however, its hormonal origin cannot be defined. At rest, plasma norepinephrine levels are 1.0 to 2.0 μg per liter or less, depending on the analytic methods used. The excretion rate for norepinephrine is 20 to 40 ug per 24 hr and that for 3-methoxy-4-hydroxymandelic acid 1 to 3 mg per 24 hr.

In patients with pheochromocytomas, the level of the catechol amines in plasma and urine will depend on the magnitude of the secretion of the tumor, as well as of the duration of its activity. In patients with persistent hypertension one usually finds a markedly elevated urinary excretion of the catechol amines and their metabolites. In a small percentage of patients, particularly those with intermittently secreting tumors, the total urinary secretion of epinephrine and norepinephrine is less than 200 μg and may be as low as 75 to 100 μg per 24 hr. Although this is above the normal resting level, one must take into account the fact that the 24-hr urinary excretion of catechol amines may be considerably increased following severe exercise, surgical procedures or other forms of trauma, myocardial infarction, and febrile illnesses.

A small percentage of patients with paroxysmal hypertension have tumors which secrete significant amounts of the amines only at intervals. In these patients, more information can be obtained by the use of plasma catechol amine estimations, which reflect the level at a given moment rather than integrating the secretion over a 24-hr period. Here the diagnosis can best be made by obtaining plasma during an attack, either spontaneous or induced with histamine. Since the life of the amines in plasma is so short, in order to be definitive the specimen must be obtained at the height of symptoms (Fig. 69-2). The collection of timed urine specimens may also be of use. However, the time required for excretion of epinephrine and norepinephrine and their metabolites is important. That portion of the amines excreted unchanged rapidly appears in the urine, whereas the methylated metabolites appear slowly over a period of hours. It has been reported from some clinics that, in this particular group of patients, the elevations in excretion rates of 3-methoxy-4-hydroxymandelic acid may be more marked than those found for the catechol amines.

Care must be taken to withhold medications which interfere with any of the above assays, particularly fluorescence measurements. Also bananas, which contain large amounts of norepinephrine, must be avoided.

Pharmacologic Aids to Diagnosis. Pharmacologic agents can be used either to stimulate the secretion of a tumor in a patient in whom the blood pressure has been normal, or to induce a fall in blood pressure by the use of an adrenolytic compound in a patient whose blood pressure is elevated. Provocative tests are employed when the blood pressure is below 170/110 mm Hg. Of these, the histamine test is most widely used. In the normal person, histamine, when given quickly intravenously in a dose of 0.01 to 0.025 mg, causes flushing, headache, and a slight blood pressure fall, with a return to normal within 1 to 2 min. A rise in blood pressure significantly greater than the cold pressor response

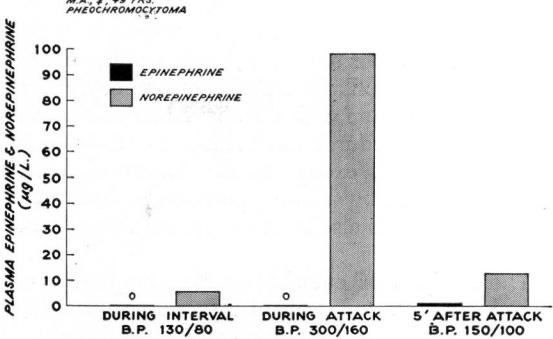

FIG. 69-2. The plasma epinephrine and norepinephrine levels before, during, and after a spontaneous paroxysm. The change in levels illustrates the intermittent secretory activity shown by some tumors and underlines the importance of obtaining samples for diagnostic purposes *at the height* of a spontaneous or induced attack.

within 2 min of injection is considered a positive result. The cold pressor test must be performed as part of this procedure. A typical response occurs in most but by no means all cases of pheochromocytoma. False positive results also occur. When alarming rises in blood pressure result, they usually can be controlled by the injection of 5 mg phentolamine intravenously. The severity of spontaneous attacks is a useful guide to ill effects to be anticipated in an induced paroxysm.

Blocking agents are used when the blood pressure is elevated. Here the preferred drug is phentolamine (Regitine) because of low incidence of untoward effects and ease of administration. Phentolamine administered intravenously in a dose of 5 mg to a patient with pheochromocytoma produces a rapid fall in blood pressure lasting 10 min or longer. In the absence of uremia or sedatives or other medications, a fall of 35 mm or more systolic and 25 mm diastolic is considered to be a positive response. False positive tests are frequently encountered, but false negative results are rare. Phentolamine may also be administered intramuscularly but is not as reliable by this route.

The inconvenience, risks, and not infrequent false positive or false negative results restrict the diagnostic value of the pharmacologic agents. They are primarily of value when hormonal measurements cannot be made, or when used in conjunction with them as noted above.

Localization of Tumors. Localization of the tumor is highly desirable before operation. In a few patients, a mass or displaced kidney may be palpated in the flank and a rise in arterial blood pressure may occur when the suspected site is palpated. In the majority of patients, however, the tumor is small and additional examinations will be required.

A tumor mass or displacement of the kidney may be detected by urologic x-ray procedures, including a film of the upper abdomen, pyelography, or presacral oxygen insufflation. Tomography may also be used in combination with the above procedures. Gas insufflation procedures are subject to errors in interpretation and, except in the hands of an experienced radiologist, are potentially hazardous. Arteriography has also been found useful in selected patients.

The analysis of catechol amines in plasma obtained from selected parts of the venous system has proved useful. A radiopaque catheter is introduced under fluoroscopic control, and samples are obtained at various levels of the venous drainage.

Since the proportion of epinephrine and norepinephrine in plasma and urine has been found to be similar to that contained by the tumor, suggestive information may be obtained through these analyses. Tumors containing epinephrine as well as norepinephrine are usually located in the adrenals. Tumors producing only norepinephrine, although sometimes found in the adrenal glands, may be situated at some distance from them.

Treatment. The symptoms of a pheochromocytoma can be controlled for a limited period of time by the use of oral phentolamine or longeracting adrenergic blocking agents. Although these agents are useful adjuncts in the preoperative management, definitive treatment requires surgical removal of the tumor. A transperitoneal approach allows satisfactory exploration of all possible tumor sites in the abdomen. However, large adrenal tumors are more easily removed through a flank or transthoracic incision. The choice of proper anesthetic and premedication is important. Adequate preoperative sedation is necessary. Agents, such as cyclopropane, which may cause serious arrhythmias in the presence of increased levels of epinephrine, should be avoided. Extremes of hypertension often occur during the induction of anesthesia and with manipulation of the tumor but can be controlled by the use of intravenous phentolamine. Later, with ligation of the tumor vessels, a precipitous fall in pressure usually occurs. This may be corrected by the use of intravenous norepinephrine. In the postoperative period intramuscular pressor agents such as Neo-Synephrine and mephentermine may be given subcutaneously to correct mild hypotension. Although in these patients there is a normal hematocrit before surgery, isotope dilution studies indicate that their blood volume may be significantly reduced. Removal of the tumor is followed by vasodilatation and expansion of the vascular bed. The disparity between the circulating blood volume and the enlarged vascular bed may play an important role in the persistent hypotension observed in many of these patients. In these cases, replacement of blood in amounts sufficient to restore a normal blood volume is an important part of the management and may reduce or eliminate the need for pressor agents following removal of a tumor.

If the blood pressure remains elevated following the removal of a pheochromocytoma, the possibility of residual tumor tissue should be excluded. After the initial drop, the blood pressure of the majority of patients will stabilize at normal levels. In some patients, however, the pressure will return to hypertensive levels and then return to normal over a period of months. In a few, the pressure will remain elevated on the basis of a preexisting essential hypertension or because of a renal vascular disease, secondary to the pheochromocytoma.

Other Functioning Tumors of Sympathetic Origin

The syndrome of paroxysmal hypertension associated with the release of large quantities of epinephrine and norepinephrine has also been described in connection with histologically malignant neuroblastoma.

In children, the association of ganglioneuromas and ganglioneuroblastomas with a clinical picture resembling the celiac syndrome has been observed. Chronic diarrhea, wasting, and abdominal distention are the most prominent symptoms, but hypertension may also be present. These children excrete excessive amounts of the pressor amines and their metabolites. Removal of the tumor is associated with remission of the hypertension and gastrointestinal symptoms.

NONFUNCTIONING TUMORS OF THE ADRENAL MEDULLA

Tumors may develop from any of the primitive or mature cell types which make up the sympathetic nervous system and the adrenal medulla.

The *sympathogonioma* is an uncommon, highly malignant tumor which appears in early infancy or intrauterine life. It metastasizes early to retroperitoneal lymph nodes, liver, and bone. It is a large, soft, cellular growth which often shows evidence of hemorrhage and necrosis. The prognosis is poor.

The *ganglioneuroma*, on the other hand, is a small, well-encapsulated, slow-growing tumor which occurs in adults and is usually an incidental finding at post mortem. It contains many mature ganglion cells separated by a network of myelinated or nonmyelinated nerve fibers.

The *neuroblastoma* is one of the commonest malignant tumors of early childhood. It grows rapidly, forming a bulky mass in the flank and often displacing the kidney. It metastasizes early to regional lymph nodes, liver, bones, and orbit.

The presenting symptoms may be those of a local tumor mass, with abdominal enlargement, vomiting, and perhaps pain; or they may be those of malignancy in general, with weakness, pallor, loss of weight, and fever. In one-quarter of cases there is generalized lymphadenopathy. Metastases introduce the disease in some cases. The child may suffer from bony skull swellings, proptosis, discoloration of the eyelids, or blindness, with optic neuritis or profound anemia.

Other possible diagnoses which must be considered are Wilms's tumor, lymphosarcoma, chloroma, Hand-Schüller-Christian syndrome, and Ewing's sarcoma of bone.

Pathologically the tumors are large and cellular. The cut surface is firm, pink, and gritty, with many areas of hemorrhage and necrosis. The cells are oval, with dark, round nuclei and thin rims of cytoplasm. They are often arranged in rosettes and are separated by fine fibrils.

The prognosis is poor. Radical surgery followed by deep x-ray therapy may provide some cures. Farber reported 10 cures in 40 cases treated in this manner and followed over a 10-year period. It should be noted that in some of these children complete surgical removal of the tumor had not been possible.

REFERENCES

Axelrod, J.: Metabolism of Epinephrine and Other Sympathomimetic Amines, Physiol. Revs., 39:751, 1959.

de Bodo, R. C., and N. Altszuler: Insulin Hypersensitivity and Physiological Insulin Antagonists, Phys. Revs., 38:389, 1958.

von Euler, U. S.: "Noradrenaline," Springfield, Ill., Charles C Thomas, Publisher, 1956.

—— and Ström, G.: Present Status of Diagnosis and Treatment of Pheochromocytoma, Circulation, 15:5, 1957.

Green, M., R. E. Cook, and W. Matanzy: Occurrence of Chronic Diarrhea in Three Patients with Ganglioneuromas, Pediatrics, 23:951, 1959.

Kvale, W. F., G. M. Roth, W. M. Manger, and J. T. Priestley: Present Day Diagnosis and Treatment of Pheochromocytoma, J.A.M.A., 164:854, 1957.

Pack, G. T., E. D. Horning, and I. M. Ariel: Neuroblastoma (Sympathicoblastoma), J. Neuropathol. Exptl. Neurol., 11:235, 1952.

Sjoerdsma, A., L. C. Leeper, L. L. Terry, and S. Udenfriend: Studies on the Biogenesis and Metabolism of Norepinephrine in Patients with Pheochromocytoma, J. Clin. Invest., 38:31, 1959.

Smithwick, R. H., W. E. Greer, C. W. Robertson, and R. W. Wilkins: Pheochromocytoma, New Engl. J. Med., 242:252, 1950.

Symposium on Catecholamines, Pharmacol. Rev., 11: part 2, 1959.

70 DIABETES MELLITUS

Peter H. Forsham, Albert E. Renold, and George W. Thorn

Definition. Diabetes mellitus is a chronic disorder of carbohydrate metabolism which is characterized by hyperglycemia. The resulting glucosuria as well as the alterations, probably secondary, of protein and fat metabolism lead to polyuria and in severe cases to ketoacidosis, dehydration, coma, and death. It is generally accepted that this metabolic disorder results from relative or absolute insulin deficiency. The predisposition to the disorder is inherited, although the nature of the inherited anomaly is as yet unknown.

History. Diabetes has been recognized from antiquity. Aretaeus described the disease and gave it its name, meaning in Greek, "to run through a siphon." Chinese medical writings as early as the seventh century mentioned polyphagia, polydipsia, and polyuria. In the sixteenth century Paracelsus noticed that diabetic urine produced an unusually abundant residue on drying, but he mistook the sugar for salt. In the seventeenth century Willis described sweetness of the diabetic urine "as if imbued with honey or sugar," and Helmont noted the presence of lipemia in a diabetic patient.

In 1850 Claude Bernard clearly demonstrated the increased glucose content of diabetic blood and recognized hyperglycemia as the cardinal sign of the disease. The careful work by clinicians such as Bouchardat, Kussmaul, Naunyn, Allen, and Joslin led to a significant measure of therapeutic success with diet. In 1869 Langerhans described the islet-cell formations in the pancreas which now bear his name. Von Mering and Minkowski carried out their classic experiments in 1889, in which they demonstrated that diabetes mellitus could be induced in dogs by extirpating the pancreas. In 1921, Banting, Best, and Macleod prepared an extract of pancreas from dogs who had previously undergone ligation of the pancreatic duct and found it capable of inducing a reduction in blood glucose level. Elimination of toxic substances and concentration of the active principle, insulin, were accomplished by Collip working with this group. Improvement in the regulation of diabetic patients followed Hagedorn's discovery in 1936 that the action of insulin could be prolonged by combining it with protamine. In 1953 Sanger established the chemical structure of beef insulin; Smith and Sanger reported the complete structure of human insulin in 1960. The accidental discovery of the hypoglycemic action of carbutamide by Franke and Fuchs in 1955 and the earlier experimental work of Loubatieres initiated the use of "oral hypoglycemic agents."

Incidence and Inheritance. The importance of

diabetes mellitus to public health is great because of its high incidence throughout the world and the long period during which patients require medical supervision. One and one-half million individuals with recognized diabetes in the United States alone may be expected to live an average of 20 years with their disease. Quite common among all races, the incidence of diabetes is perhaps higher among Jews. It appears to be less frequent among Chinese, Japanese, and East Indians, and is also mild as long as they remain on their native low caloric diets. Communities with a high degree of obesity have a high incidence of diabetes.

The trait for diabetes is recessive, and genetic carriers, estimated at 20 million in the United States at present, are increasing in number. The carrier does not necessarily develop diabetes during his lifetime but may transmit the recessive trait to his offspring. Depending upon the family history of the mate and whether he or she is a carrier of the same trait, some of the offspring may develop clinical diabetes during their lifetime. Among diabetic patients fewer than 10 per cent develop the disease before reaching maturity (prematurity onset), and more than 90 per cent develop it during or after middle life (postmaturity or adult type). More than 50 per cent of patients develop diabetes prior to the age of 50, although 75 to 90 per cent of all diabetic deaths occur between the sixth and ninth decades. Diabetes occurs more frequently in women than in men and particularly in women who have borne children.

Etiology

Although the exact mechanism underlying the development of diabetes is obscure, it is generally accepted that the common etiologic denominator in all cases is a relative or absolute insulin deficiency. This is based primarily on studies on the experimental production of diabetes. *Permanent* diabetes may be produced experimentally by (1) surgical removal of at least 90 per cent of the pancreas, (2) chemical destruction of the insulin-producing beta cells of the islets of Langerhans by administration of compounds such as alloxan, (3) injection of anterior pituitary extracts, including purified growth hormone, (4) prolonged administration of large quantities of glucose parenterally. *Transient* diabetes has been produced by the administration of purified pituitary adrenocorticotropic hormone and species-specific antibodies to insulin. It is thought that growth hormone affects carbohydrate metabolism chiefly by decreasing the peripheral utilization of glucose, that pituitary adrenocorticotropin and adrenal steroids affect it mostly by increasing hepatic gluconeogenesis, and that excessive thyroid hormone does so by producing an increased food intake and a generally

ACTH

heightened level of metabolic activity. It has been postulated that all these experimental conditions have one common denominator: the creation of a continued demand for increased insulin production, with resulting strain on the insulin-producing cells and consequent reduction of available insulin. In all instances in which permanent diabetes mellitus has been produced experimentally, degenerative changes in the *beta cells* of the islet tissue have been observed.

In man diabetes mellitus has been produced by pancreatectomy incidental to removal of malignant tumors and has been noted during and after severe pancreatitis, including that due to mumps. In addition, hemochromatosis (p. 785), although rare, is a well-established cause of diabetes mellitus. Following the deposition of iron pigment in the pancreas and in other tissues, secondary fibrosis and loss of functioning tissue occur. The disease affects males predominantly. Seventy-five per cent of patients with hemochromatosis ultimately develop diabetes. Whereas in these instances, all rare, a clear correlation exists between the development of diabetes in man and destruction of the pancreatic islets, poor correlation is seen between morphologic damage to the islets and the severity of the disease (see also Pathology).

Although insulin is virtually absent in the pancreas of young diabetic patients at postmortem examination, this is not true in elderly, obese diabetics. Factors other than impaired insulin secretion appear to play important roles in the genesis of the disease. This is best illustrated by the cases of clinical diabetic syndrome associated with overactivity of the adrenal cortex (Cushing's syndrome, see p. 617) or of the anterior pituitary (Acromegaly, see p. 568); in these cases the diabetic syndrome improves markedly or often disappears when the overactive tissue is removed surgically or destroyed by roentgen therapy. The common denominator of the etiologic factors leading to diabetes, excluding primary lack of insulin, is the production of conditions increasing insulin requirement which leads to relative insulin deficiency, either temporary or permanent. During the early stages of the disease, insulin reserve may be normal, but insulin *release* in response to elevation of blood glucose levels may be sluggish or delayed (Yalow and Berson).

Three important etiologic factors appear to be *heredity, obesity,* and possibly *hormonal disturbances* (other than insulin deficiency). It is now well established that the diabetic *trait is inherited.* In the past the importance of hereditary factors has been somewhat obscured by the failure to appreciate the fact that diabetes may develop in the offspring before it becomes manifest in the parent. Hence, in history taking, it is important to note that at the onset of diabetes 20 per cent of children have diabetic relatives, whereas 20 years later the incidence of diabetic relatives among the same group has risen to 55 per cent. Obviously parents who succumb to other diseases early in life may have masked their potentialities for developing diabetes. It appears probable that the diabetic trait is mainly inherited according to the mendelian ratio for recessive characteristics (see Chap. 46).

Although cases of diabetes mellitus present at birth or shortly thereafter have been described, the inherited trait is as a rule a *predisposition*, and the disease itself appears later in life. One of the most important unsolved problems in the study of the disease is the nature of the process which diminishes a previously adequate insulin reserve.

The exact relationship between *obesity* and diabetes is not known, but the high coincidence of the two disorders is unquestioned. It should not be inferred that all obese individuals become diabetic, but the fact remains that in the elderly adult group diabetes selects 9 out of 10 of its victims from among the ranks of the obese. Leanness among adults confers a decreased susceptibility to the disease. Two provisional conclusions appear justified in relation to diabetes and obesity: (1) Relative insulin deficiency may be shown in many obese individuals and may be reversed by dieting to normal weight. (2) The continued high demand for insulin in the obese individual may well be an important factor in precipitating clinical manifestations of the disease in those who carry the diabetic trait.

Hormonal disturbances other than insulin deficiency have frequently been postulated, but only rarely demonstrated, as etiologic factors in the genesis of diabetes mellitus. The pituitary, the adrenal cortex, the thyroid, and the gonads have been implicated. The postulated mechanisms of action, none of which has been proved, include a direct effect on insulin secretion, competition with or inhibition of insulin action, or the creation of conditions necessitating the secretion of more insulin than normal. It has been recently shown that the maternal environment during pregnancy influences the incidence of early diabetes in the child and may well explain the reported higher incidence of diabetes in children of diabetic mothers than diabetic fathers.

Infections are common in patients with diabetes mellitus. However, except in rare instances of extensive involvement of the pancreas with pancreatitis, it appears that the etiologic role of acute infections in the genesis of diabetes is confined to unmasking potential diabetes, thereby precipitating the clinical manifestations of the disease. Infections may decrease glucose tolerance by (1) increased insulin "antagonism" resulting from increased elaboration of adrenal cortical hormone in response to the stress; (2) decreased efficiency of insulin re-

sulting from fever, heightened metabolic level, dehydration, and acidosis; (3) possible decreased insulin production following toxic parenchymatous changes in islet tissue.

Pathology

The earliest *change in the islets of Langerhans* consists of "hydropic degeneration," shown by Toreson to represent reversible intracytoplasmic infiltration of beta cells with glycogen. The most common finding is that first described by Opie in 1901 of "hyalinization" of the islets in patients who died of diabetes. Such changes occur in less than half of patients with diabetes mellitus, but this phenomenon is only rarely observed in patients who are not diabetic. *Fibrosis* and *lymphocytic infiltration* of the pancreas are found more rarely, the latter especially in patients who die within a few weeks of the onset of the disorder. Extensive quantitative studies of the total mass of the beta cells of the islets of Langerhans in diabetic patients have demonstrated some decrease in all patients with the juvenile, severe form of the disorder and in more than 80 per cent of elderly, obese, nonketotic diabetics (Ogilvie, Gepts). Application of electron microscopic techniques to the study of pancreatic islets promises to reveal changes in nearly every case of diabetes mellitus, and already more specific perivascular and perigranular lesions are being established (Hartroft, Lacy).

Extrapancreatic lesions observed post mortem in diabetics are varied and are presumably secondary to the long-continued metabolic disturbance evidenced by hyperglycemia, lipemia, and ketosis. The *deposition* and *distribution of glycogen* are frequently abnormal. While it may be depleted in the liver in the terminal phases of acidosis, it is abnormally deposited within the nuclei. Except in this terminal phase of the disease, glycogen levels in diabetic patients appear to be equal to or higher than those in nondiabetic persons, particularly in the fasting state. In the kidney an accumulation of glycogen is commonly found in the renal epithelium, especially in the loops of Henle. Other tissues such as heart muscle, iris and ciliary bodies of the eye, and skin are frequently found to contain an accumulation of glycogen. *Fatty infiltration* and enlargement of the liver are common findings in untreated diabetics and especially in diabetic children.

Vascular lesions comprising morphologic changes in the intima of venules, capillaries, arterioles, and smaller muscular arteries occur in addition to ordinary atheromatous and arteriosclerotic lesions in the larger vessels of all diabetics. Whereas the former are confined practically exclusively to the diabetic, the latter are found in all patients coming to autopsy, but appear to occur some 10 years earlier and with greater severity in the diabetics.

The capillary lesion is easily demonstrable in retinal and renal glomerular vessels, with increasing frequency as the duration of the diabetes increases, particularly after 13 years or more. The typical lesion of *diabetic retinopathy* consists of a saccular microaneurysm, most commonly at the level of the venule, with a halolike hemorrhage around it, making it visible on ophthalmoscopic examination. Dilatation and beading of the larger retinal veins, due to weakening of the basement membrane, are seen earlier. Later stages comprise white exudates, retinal hemorrhages extending into the vitreous with subsequent organization leading to development of retinitis proliferans, and sooner or later retinal detachment. Diabetic retinopathy is frequently but not always associated with a characteristic lesion of the small vessels of the kidney. The basal membrane of kidney capillaries and venules, made up of mucopolysaccharide bound to protein, undergoes swelling, reduplication, and proliferation toward the lumen. This intramural material becomes impregnated with certain components of the plasma, forming hyalin, which eventually obstructs the lumen in the form of a hyaline nodule. Whereas the characteristic nodular distribution of the hyalin is practically pathognomonic of the diabetic state and is known as *intercapillary glomerulosclerosis*, the diffuse lesion may occasionally be found in nondiabetic renal disease. Either may be associated with the Kimmelstiel-Wilson syndrome, viz., diabetes, hypertension, proteinuria, and edema. At autopsy one frequently finds the combination of three distinct renal pathologic processes which have been termed *diabetic nephropathy*, consisting of nephrosclerosis, chronic pyelonephritis, and intercapillary glomerulosclerosis. The greater frequency of urinary infections in diabetic patients predisposes to the serious complication of necrotizing papillitis in some. With advanced vascular disease, interruption of blood supply to the papillae leads to the desquamation of their tips and to mechanical blockage of urine flow.

Probably specific lesions known as *diabetic angiopathy* have more recently been recognized in the arterial trunk, consisting of an obliterating endarteritis with marked proliferation of swollen endothelial cells, quite distinct from the fibrosis and hyalinization seen in arteriosclerosis.

Atherosclerosis of major arteries appears to occur more frequently in diabetics, and at an earlier age. At postmortem examination coronary occlusions are four times as frequent and vascular insufficiency of the lower extremities is found some 65 times as often in diabetes as in nondiabetics of similar age groups. In the medium-sized muscular arteries medial calcifications of the Mönckeberg type frequently accompany the atheromatous type of lesion; in fact, fibrotic changes are more common than fatty ones early in the disease. It has recently been suggested that the small vessel disease in diabetes may be a greater culprit in complications such as patchy gangrene, arteriosclerotic heart disease, neuropathy, and skin lesions such as necrobiosis lipoidica diabeticorum than the somewhat accelerated process of arteriosclerosis. It is of interest that arteriosclerosis of the *cerebral* vessels does *not* appear to be more frequent in diabetics than in nondiabetics.

Pathologic Physiology

Endocrine Defect in Diabetes. As discussed above, evidence to date would indicate that, in all likelihood, diabetes mellitus develops as a consequence of a disturbance in the balance between insulin production, on the one hand, and factors modifying the requirement for it, on the other. The success with which most diabetic patients are treated with insulin or insulin substitutes, irrespective of cause or type of diabetes, indicates the important role which relative or absolute insulin deficiency plays in the pathogenesis of the disease. Greater weight is presently given to the evidence suggesting initial regulatory dysfunction of insulin release (Yalow and Berson) or of insulin effectiveness (Bornstein, Taylor, Steinke, et al.) than to that indicating a primarily depressed synthesis of insulin.

Pathogenesis of the Syndrome Associated with Severe Insulin Deficiency. According to present concepts, insulin deficiency first limits carbohydrate utilization at normal blood glucose levels. This is compensated for in part by a rise in blood sugar, by means of increased carbohydrate formation (gluconeogenesis) and increased liberation of glucose from liver glycogen (glycogenolysis). In most patients, unfortunately, the elevation in blood sugar exceeds renal reabsorptive capacity and the benefit derived from increased utilization of carbohydrate at the higher blood sugar levels is offset by loss of carbohydrate in the urine. Inadequate glucose utilization despite hyperglycemia stimulates mobilization of fat in the form of fatty acids and their breakdown to ketone bodies in the liver. The latter substances comprise a normal source of energy but, in the presence of impaired glucose utilization, may be formed in excess of the capacity of the tissues to utilize them, leading to a rising blood ketone level and ketonuria. Because of the acidic nature of the ketone bodies and the limited renal ability to excrete an acid urine, it is necessary for the kidney to excrete cations with the ketone acids, leading to both sodium and potassium loss.

In unregulated diabetes the body loses glucose, ketone bodies, cations, and water. Dehydration and acidosis resulting from the loss of cations and water, as well as from the excess of circulating anions, further impair the utilization of glucose and increase the insulin requirement, thus aggravating the already serious insulin deficit. Transitory antagonists of insulin action appear in the blood. With increasing ketosis and dehydration, coma may supervene. Since insulin is not believed to exert a direct effect upon carbohydrate utilization by nervous tissue, coma is probably due to the direct effect of acidosis, ketosis, and dehydration on the central nervous system.

That primary lack of available carbohydrate may lead to the syndrome of diabetic coma is well illustrated by the similar syndrome of ketonemia in lactating cows. In the latter case excessive milk production results in a negative carbohydrate balance, and ketosis and coma supervene in the presence of *hypoglycemia;* the syndrome can be dramatically reversed by a single large intravenous administration of glucose.

The many pathogenetic factors involved in the production of late diabetic complications, mainly vascular, remain to be clarified.

Metabolic Defects in Diabetes. A working analysis of intermediary metabolism has been presented in Chap. 52, as well as the necessity for separate consideration of hepatic (mainly carbohydrate-producing) and peripheral (mainly carbohydrate-utilizing) tissues. Figure 70-1 summarizes the chief known metabolic defects in diabetic tissues. Peripheral tissues in this instance mainly include muscle (including heart) and adipose tissue. The importance of adipose tissue as an actively metabolizing tissue highly sensitive to hormone action has only recently become fully apparent. Sites of abnormal metabolic slowing (bars) and acceleration (heavy arrows) have been indicated by superimposing the appropriate symbols upon the previously discussed working schemes. Diabetic metabolism is mainly characterized by (1) decreased glucose utilization by both periphery and liver, (2) decreased incorporation of acetyl coenzyme A into fatty acids, (3) accelerated release of free fatty acids from adipose tissue, (4) increased catabolism of protein (to amino acids) and fat (to ketone bodies), and (5) increased hepatic release of glucose, as a result of both accelerated glycogenolysis and accelerated gluconeogenesis from pyruvate, lactate, and amino acids. It is important to understand that *all* these metabolic defects can be corrected by the administration of insulin. While some defects are corrected within minutes of the beginning of insulin therapy, others may not be fully corrected until 24 hr later.

Mechanism of Insulin Action. The exact mechanism by which insulin acts remains unknown, although much work has been carried out in many laboratories during the last 40 years. Most investigators agree that in insulin-responsive tissues, *insulin primarily facilitates the conversion of extra-cellular glucose to intracellular glucose 6-phosphate and thus increases the metabolic availability of glucose.* Some 15 years ago, Cori and his collaborators postulated that insulin directly alters hexokinase activity in the presence of inhibitory pituitary or adrenal components. This has not been adequately confirmed. However, Levine and his collaborators, as well as Ross, and Park and his collaborators, have since obtained conclusive evidence that insulin acts directly on the cell membrane and facilitates the entry of glucose and similar substances into insulin-responsive cells. Under certain circumstances, the presence of insulin in muscle (Morgan and Park, Kipnis and Cori) may result both in increased penetration of glucose *and* in correction of the decreased phosphorylation in diabetes, suggesting that glucose transport into cells and activity of phosphorylation within cells may have components in common. Liver has no demonstrable permeability barrier to glucose; yet the diabetic state in liver is characterized by inability to phosphorylate glucose, suggesting a direct effect of insulin on the phosphorylating mechanism in this tissue.

Whatever the exact mechanism by which insulin accelerates glucose metabolism in insulin-sensitive tissues, it is generally agreed that many of the metabolic effects of insulin in vivo and in vitro can be related directly or indirectly to the primary effect of the hormone on glucose utilization. In addition, however, there are some well-documented effects of insulin which cannot readily be explained on this basis alone, such as the accelerating effect of the hormone on amino acid incorporation into protein by skeletal muscle. *It is necessary, therefore, to remain open-minded not only as to the exact mechanism of insulin action on glucose transport and utilization, but also as to the possible existence of physiologically important actions of insulin which are not related to the initial metabolism of glucose.*

Tissues vary markedly in their responsiveness and sensitivity to insulin. At present, skeletal muscle, heart muscle, and especially adipose tissue appear to be the most sensitive to physiologic concentrations of the hormone and are the most likely major sites of insulin action. In addition, insulin probably alters directly the release of glucose by the liver, particularly when glucose is being released as a result of glycogenolysis. Although some tissues, such as brain, are usually classified as nonresponsive to insulin, specific structures of small bulk within these tissues, for example, hypothalamic areas concerned with the regulation of food intake, may evidently be affected.

Clinical Picture

Three general types of diabetes are now clearly distinguished. The *prematurity onset* juvenile dia-

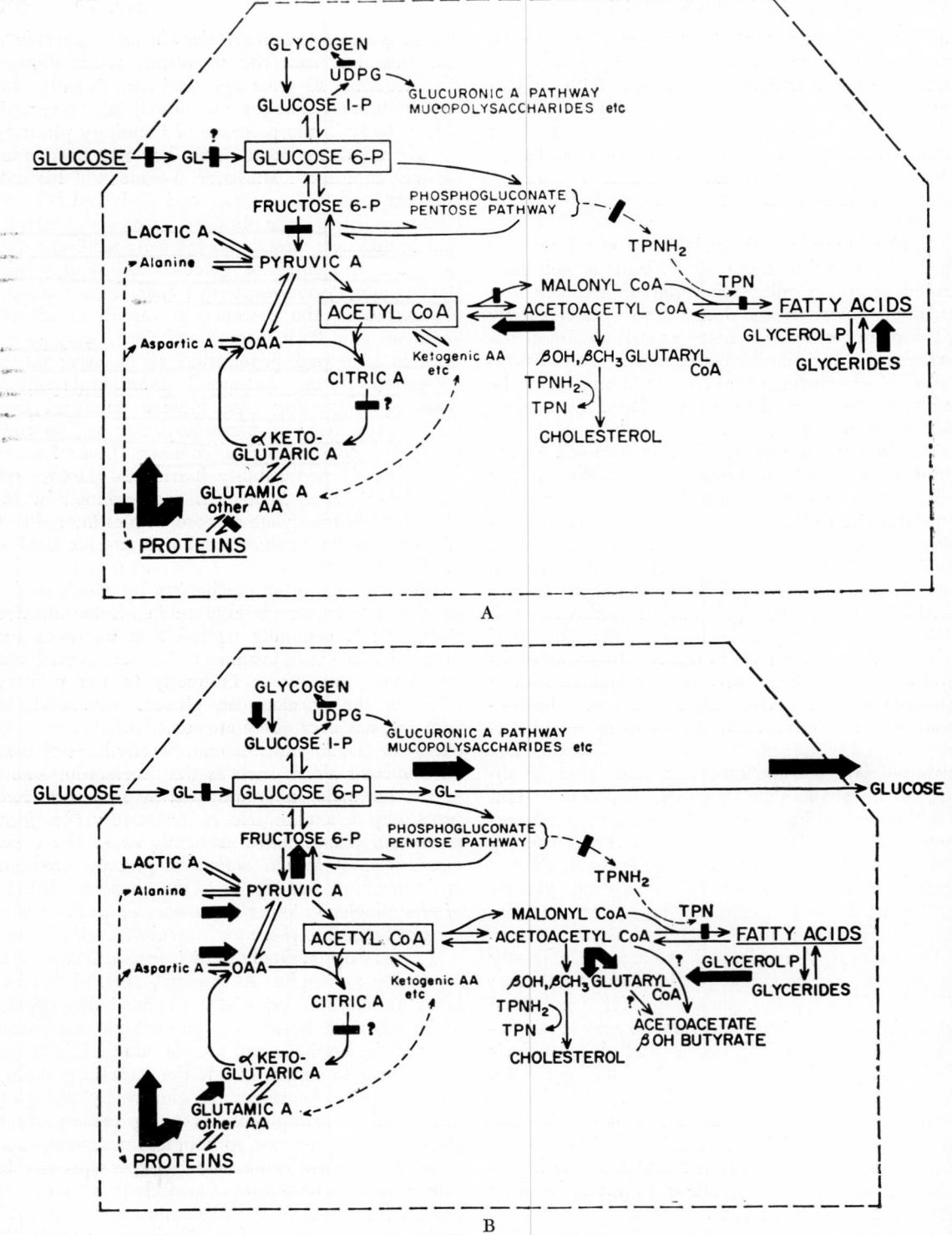

Fig. 70-1. Metabolic defects in diabetes, as applied to the working scheme of intermediary metabolism presented in Chap. 52. Abnormal metabolic slowing is indicated by heavy bars, acceleration by heavy arrows. *A.* Adipose tissue and muscle. In addition adipose tissue accumulates free fatty acids from glycerides and releases them; muscle accumulates and releases amino acids from protein. *B.* Liver. In addition there is increased availability to hepatic metabolism of free fatty acids and amino acids transported from adipose tissue and muscle.

betes, with onset under age twenty-five, is characterized by insulin deficiency, unresponsiveness to sulfonylurea, and proneness to ketoacidosis. These patients are thin, although a brief period of weight gain may precede the onset of the disease. When treated with insulin they show marked fluctuations in blood glucose, e.g., plus or minus 100 mg per 100 ml, and their control is characterized as "brittle." Although this type of diabetes is most frequent in the younger age group, as indicated by its name, it does also occur in some adults, albeit rarely.

The *maturity onset* adult diabetes usually occurs after age twenty-five. These patients are frequently obese, respond to sulfonylureas, may show normal or high circulating insulin levels, and have an easily controllable blood sugar level. They are sometimes known as "stable" diabetics.

Miscellaneous diabetic syndromes include states in which insulin antagonists are produced in excess. Temporary diabetes eventually leads to permanent or metadiabetes, presumably because of continued hyperglycemia leading to exhaustion of the beta cells. The diabetes of acromegaly (excess growth hormone), Cushing's syndrome (excess hydrocortisone), thyrotoxicosis (excess thyroxin), and the rare pheochromocytoma (excess epinephrine) fall into this category. Another syndrome is the *lipoatrophic type of diabetes* in which absence of subcutaneous fat tissue, usually in young females, may lead first to an insulin-resistant hyperglycemia due to a block in the major pathway for glucose disposal, viz., its incorporation into fat, and eventually to an insulin-deficient type of diabetes. Since children with lipoatrophic diabetes exhibit accelerated growth, metabolic hyperpituitarism may also be involved.

All types of the diabetic syndrome may have an unrecognized onset during which underutilization of carbohydrate is compensated for by a gradual rise in blood glucose levels. This compensatory hyperglycemia eventually results in glucosuria (above 160 to 200 mg glucose per 100 ml blood), leading to polyuria, polydipsia, and polyphagia, as well as general weakness and loss of body weight.

The *acute* manifestation of diabetes is *diabetic coma*, usually precipitated by infection. The cheeks are flushed and the clinical signs of dehydration, ketoacidosis, and eventually coma are present, such as dry skin and mucous membrane, low blood pressure, hypothermia, rapid pulse, air hunger or Kussmaul respiration, abdominal tenderness, and varying degrees of disorientation and unresponsiveness (Table 70-1). A critical differential diagnosis presents itself in patients with glucosuria and coma. With a *cerebrovascular accident* and glucosuria, it is unusual to observe ketonuria unless the patient has not eaten for a considerable period. The carbon dioxide–combining power is usually normal, and dehydration may be absent. The reflexes may be asymmetric and the blood pressure normal or elevated.

In the *subacute* stage of diabetes, skin changes such as pruritus, pyodermia, perigenital moniliasis, blurred vision from disturbances in accommodation, constipation due to dehydration, and dizziness due to loss of circulating blood volume may represent suspicious symptoms and signs.

In the *chronic* state of diabetes, after many years of unrecognized mild disease, the degenerative complications make their appearance as recognizable symptoms and signs. This is particularly true in the older age group, in which one may see, as the first overt indication, large fatty livers, early cataracts,

Table 70-1. DIFFERENTIAL DIAGNOSIS

	Hypoglycemia	Diabetic coma
History...............	Insufficient food; excess insulin; excess exercise	Insufficient insulin; infection; gastrointestinal upset
Onset................	Following *short-acting insulin:* Suddenly, a few hours after injection	Gradually, over many hours
	Following *long-acting insulin:* Relatively slower, many hours after injection	
Course...............	Anxiety; sweating; hunger; headache; diplopia; incoordination; twitching; convulsions; coma (headache, nausea and haziness especially following long-acting insulin)	Polyuria; polydipsia; anorexia; nausea; vomiting; labored deep breathing; weakness; drowsiness; possibly fever and abdominal pain; coma
Physical findings........	Pale, moist skin; full, rapid pulse; dilated pupils; normal breathing; B.P. normal or elevated; overactive reflexes; positive Babinski sign	Florid, dry skin; Kussmaul breathing with acetone odor; decreased B.P.; weak, rapid pulse; soft eyeballs
Laboratory findings.....	Second urine specimen sugar- and ketone-free; low blood sugar; normal serum CO_2	Urine contains sugar and ketone bodies; high blood sugar; low serum CO_2

advanced diabetic retinopathy, diabetic nephropathy, or gangrene of the feet or toes. Diabetic neuropathy may include isolated motor nerve defects, deficits of the autonomous nervous system such as poor bladder control, impotence, amenorrhea, nocturnal diarrhea and constipation, and general loss of sensation in the extremities together with painless destruction of joints (Charcot joint). Frequently diabetes mellitus is revealed by the patient seeking medical care for one of the complications, and the underlying metabolic disorder is then discovered. Common complaints are: poor wound healing, skin infections, angina in women, aches and pains, coldness of the extremities, and perialveolar bone resorption with caries. Whether the degenerative complications of diabetes are truly complications, or whether they represent a basic part of the inherited disease itself is as yet open to question.

Diagnosis

The diagnosis of diabetes mellitus is frequently suggested by the history. More often, however, the discovery of glucose in a routine urine specimen will initiate a careful search for other evidence of the disease. Glucosuria is most likely to be present immediately following a meal. Glucosuria alone is not conclusive evidence of the presence of diabetes mellitus. *Glucosuria associated with ketonuria is almost always pathognomonic of diabetes mellitus.* The final diagnosis, however, should be made only after demonstrating a high fasting blood glucose level or impaired glucose tolerance.

Fasting Blood Glucose. The range of normal for the "true" blood glucose level taken in the fasting postabsorptive state is approximately 70 to 110 mg per 100 ml whole blood. With a value above 130 mg per 100 ml under fasting conditions, a presumptive diagnosis of diabetes mellitus may be made. It is essential, however, to confirm this observation by repeated analyses.

Table 70-2. 100-GM CARBOHYDRATE BREAKFAST

Food	Quantity	Carbohydrate, Gm
Orange juice.........	8 oz	24
Cooked cereal.......	4 oz	
or		16
Dry cereal..........	1 oz	
Bread..............	2 slices	32
Egg...............	1	
Butter.............	2 pats	
Milk..............	6 oz	9
Cream.............	3 oz	4
Sugar.............	3 tsp	15
Coffee or tea........	ad lib.	
		100

A simple but effective "screening test" consists in the determination of the blood glucose level on a single sample of blood taken 2 hr after the ingestion of a breakfast containing approximately 100 Gm carbohydrate, as detailed in Table 70-2. A value within normal limits at this time makes the diagnosis of diabetes mellitus unlikely.

Glucose Tolerance Tests. A patient should be properly prepared for a glucose tolerance test by the administration of at least 300 Gm carbohydrate daily for 2 to 3 days prior to the test. This prevents abnormalities in the tolerance curve which might occur as a consequence of a decreased carbohydrate tolerance due to starvation or to a diet of low carbohydrate content. In the test, blood glucose levels are determined in conjunction with the administration of a measured quantity of glucose. At appropriate intervals during the test, the urine is examined for the presence of sugar.

Oral Glucose Tolerance Test. A sample of urine and one of whole blood are obtained from the patient in the fasting state. The patient is then given 100 Gm glucose dissolved in 500 ml water and flavored with lemon juice. Samples of urine and whole blood are taken for determination of glucose ½, 1, 2, and 3 hr after the ingestion of the glucose.

The fasting level for glucose is normally below 100 mg per 100 ml. The maximum level in normal persons properly prepared in advance is 150 mg per 100 ml, and this usually occurs in a specimen taken at the end of the first hour. The blood glucose level should return to or below the normal fasting level within 3 hr (Fig. 70-2A). Abnormally high levels of blood glucose attained during the first hour of the test with a rapid fall to normal values (characteristic of hyperthyroidism) or flat curves with no appreciable rise (hypothyroidism or sprue) most frequently reflect primary alterations in the rate of intestinal glucose absorption. However, flat curves are frequently seen in normal individuals as well.

Intravenous Glucose Tolerance Test. Under certain circumstances it is desirable to study glucose utilization without reference to gastrointestinal absorption. Glucose may be given intravenously in a dose of 0.5 Gm per kg body weight in an aqueous solution containing approximately 20 Gm glucose per 100 ml pyrogen-free distilled water. It is administered by intravenous infusion, regulated to a constant rate, such that the total volume is given in ½ hr. Samples of urine and whole blood are collected 30, 60, 90, and 150 min after the intravenous infusion is begun. The fasting blood sugar level is normally reestablished in 90 min.

Whereas the intravenous administration of 0.5 Gm glucose per kg body weight over ½ hr approximates the maximal normal rate of intestinal glucose absorption, and thus allows for comparative evalua-

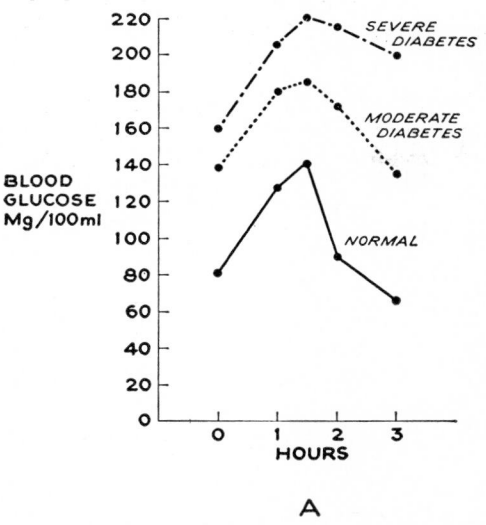

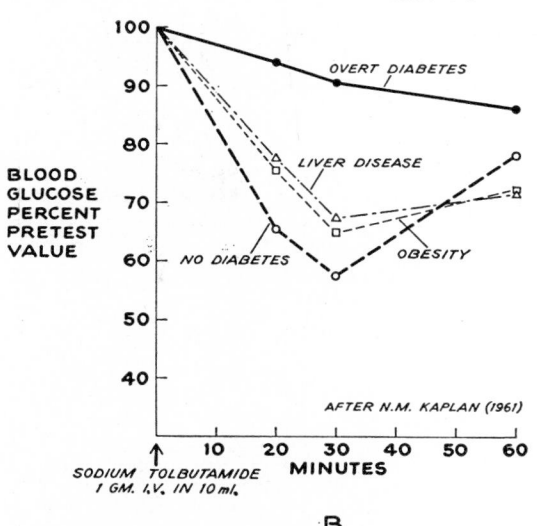

FIG. 70-2. *A.* The characteristic oral glucose tolerance test following administration of 100 Gm of glucose or its equivalent by mouth at zero hour. *B.* Characteristic curves of the intravenous sodium tolbutamide test. Note that although there is a gradual fall of blood sugar up to about 15 to 20 per cent in a postmaturity onset diabetic (shown in the figure), no fall whatever is observed in prematurity onset cases (not shown). Patients with liver disease and obesity closely approach the nondiabetics, which is not always so in the oral glucose tolerance tests.

tion of oral and intravenous glucose tolerance, the *rapid intravenous glucose tolerance test* is being increasingly used today. In this test, 0.5 Gm glucose per kg body weight is administered over 2 min or less, and blood samples are obtained at intervals of 10 min for at least 60 min. Under these conditions the rate of blood glucose decrease is an exponential one, and a glucose disappearance constant may be calculated. In normal individuals, glucose disappearance usually exceeds 1.5 per cent of the administered dose per minute, while values below 1 per cent are clearly diabetic.

Intravenous Tolbutamide Test. This, the latest in the available tests based on blood glucose measurements, depends specifically on the ability of the patient to respond to tolbutamide by a prompt rise in insulin secretion. The patient is given 1 Gm sodium tolbutamide intravenously in 10 ml distilled water in the fasting state. Blood glucose levels are obtained before the injection and after 20 and 30 min (Fig. 70-2*B*). The intravenous tolbutamide test clearly differentiates between insulinopenic diabetics of the prematurity type, who show no response whatever, the adult type diabetics who show a fair but delayed decrease in blood glucose, and individuals with normal pancreatic reserve who exhibit a brisk and prompt response. This test differentiates well between diabetes and liver disease or hyperthyroidism, since tolbutamide-induced hypoglycemia is more severe in these instances. The test promises to be of value since it is simple to perform, rapidly concluded, and critical in terms of the

therapeutically important question: Is there an available insulin reserve in the patient tested?

Provocative Tests with Cortisone. Fajans and Conn have proposed a glucose tolerance test after priming with cortisone as an attempt to establish susceptibility to diabetes in presently nondiabetic homozygous relatives of diabetic patients. This test therefore attempts to uncover the presence of *pre-diabetes*. Oral glucose tolerance tests are carried out before and after a standard cortisone acetate dosage (50 mg by mouth 8 and 2 hr before the second glucose tolerance test for patients under 70 kg, and 65 mg, similarly, for patients above 70 kg). Whereas all but one of the 100 normal subjects without a diabetic family history showed an abnormal elevation after the administration of cortisone, approximately 25 per cent of patients with diabetic relatives, but with normal initial glucose tolerance, showed abnormal glucose tolerance after cortisone administration. As a technical instrument for early detection and characterization of the diabetic trait, this test and an increasing number of modifications of it should yield valuable information in the future.

Differential Diagnosis

Persistent melituria will most often be found to be glucosuria and a manifestation of diabetes mellitus. Persistent glucosuria also occurs in the presence of a lowered renal threshold. This may be present in otherwise normal persons, in pregnant women, and in patients with chronic renal disease.

In all these situations glucose disappears from the urine as the blood sugar level approaches 100 mg per 100 ml. True renal glucosuria (see Chap. 94) is a rare familial abnormality *in which glucose is present in all specimens of urine,* including those passed after an overnight fast. The condition is not prediabetic. *Transient glucosuria* may occur occasionally in nondiabetic persons under conditions of stress or following the ingestion of a high carbohydrate meal (alimentary glucosuria). Under such conditions, the fasting blood sugar and the glucose tolerance values will be normal. This condition may be prediabetic.

Melituria Other than Glucosuria. (See also Chap. 94.) Lactose is found in the urine of lactating women but not, as a rule, in appreciable quantities before the third trimester of pregnancy. Sugars other than glucose may be found in the urine following the ingestion of large quantities of fruit (fructosuria). Pentosuria and fructosuria also occur as inborn errors of metabolism. Characterization of a urinary reducing substance as glucose has become simple since the specific enzyme glucose oxidase has become commercially available in the form of impregnated indicator strips (Testape or Clinistix).

Increased intracranial pressure due to cerebral tumor, brain trauma, or arterial hypertension may on occasion give rise to glucosuria and hyperglycemia. It is often difficult to differentiate the hyperglycemia and glucosuria associated with these conditions from true diabetes mellitus. The presence of ketonuria with an adequate dietary intake strongly points to diabetes mellitus. Signs and symptoms of intracranial disease usually suggest the true diagnosis. In most instances of this type, the disturbance in carbohydrate metabolism disappears with improvement in the cerebral disorder. In elderly diabetic patients with advanced cerebral vascular disease, one may, of course, encounter a combination of both conditions. A negative history of diabetes prior to the onset of the intracranial disease is extremely helpful. Occasionally hyperglycemia and glucosuria will be noted with the glucose tolerance test in patients with liver disease. Presumably the ability to store glucose as glycogen is impaired.

Treatment

The aims of diabetic management are (1) the correction of the underlying metabolic abnormalities by insulin therapy or oral hypoglycemic agents and dietary management, (2) the attainment and maintenance of ideal body weight, (3) the prevention of complications commonly associated with the disease. In the treatment of a patient with diabetes mellitus, the physician has an excellent opportunity to accomplish and maintain complete rehabilitation. Successful therapy will depend upon the thorough-

ness with which the physician understands the particular problems in each individual case and upon how conscientiously the patient cooperates.

In approaching the treatment of a patient with diabetes mellitus, it is essential to be certain at the onset that there is no active focus of infection anywhere in the body. Infections of the urinary tract, gallbladder, teeth, and sinuses should be looked for particularly, and a chest x-ray is a requisite. It is also desirable to obtain a careful evaluation of the state of the cardiovascular and renal system to serve as a subsequent point of reference.

Insulin Therapy. Whereas practically all diabetic patients with prematurity onset require insulin, many obese adult diabetics respond to dietary management and weight reduction alone. However, failure to maintain a normal fasting blood sugar level under prolonged dietary management calls for use of supplementary insulin therapy or of oral hypoglycemic agents. When ketonemia or ketonuria is also present, the use of insulin is clearly indicated.

The insulin preparations available for clinical use consist of two principal types: soluble or unmodified insulin acting rapidly, as opposed to modified preparations that act more slowly.

Crystalline insulin consists of an aqueous solution of the crystalline preparation of the antidiabetic principle of the pancreas. It has a relatively short period of action (6 to 8 hr) which demands relatively frequent administration for adequate control. The *modified insulin* preparations may be divided into two types: combinations with basic proteins or insulin zinc suspensions.

Protamine zinc insulin consists of a solution of crystalline insulin to which an excess of protamine has been added. This preparation has a long period of action. The excess of protamine combining with fibrinogen forms small emboli. This accounts in part for its rather irregular rate of absorption from day to day. With a period of action of up to 30 hr, the release of soluble insulin over a given period of time is slow, and thus the preparation does not control elementary hyperglycemia. This has led in the past to the use of "tailor-made" mixtures of crystalline insulin and protamine given in a single injection. One must note, however, that when mixing equal quantities of the two the effective preparation will show two-thirds the activity of protamine zinc insulin and only one-third that of crystalline insulin owing to the excess of protamine present in protamine zinc insulin.

Neutral protamine Hagedorn (NPH) insulin contains protamine in amounts exactly sufficient to combine chemically with the insulin present. The duration of action is shorter, amounting to approximately 24 hr. There being no excess of protamine, absorption from the injection sites is more predictable and mixtures with crystalline insulin show

Table 70-3. INSULIN ACTION CURVES

Type of insulin	Maximum action, hr after injection	Duration, hr	Time of maximal hypoglycemia
Crystalline zinc .	4–6	6–8	10 A.M. to 1 P.M.
Globin	6–10	12–18	3 P.M. to 6 P.M.
NPH	8–12	18–24	3 P.M. to 6 P.M.
Lente	8–12	18–30	3 P.M. to 6 P.M.
Protamine zinc..	14–20	24–36	6 to 8 A.M.
Ultra Lente	16–24	26–36	6 to 8 A.M.

rapid action to the extent that crystalline insulin was added to the NPH.

Globin insulin consisting of insulin bound to globin is practically identical to NPH in action.

Insulin zinc suspensions represent the latest class and consist of *ultra Lente, semi-Lente,* and a mixture of the two in the proportion of 7:3 known as *Lente insulin.* Their prolonged action is due to the use of acetate instead of phosphate buffer, as a result of which insulin and zinc keep in a state of suspension without the use of any protamine or other foreign substance. Ultra Lente closely resembles protamine zinc insulin in its action, whereas semi-Lente acts more like NPH with a small amount of crystalline insulin added. The most commonly used preparation in this series is Lente, which has an action curve practically identical with that of NPH (Table 70-3).

In the case of uncomplicated diabetes the patient should be put on an appropriate diet and insulin therapy at once. As a rule, middle-aged, mildly diabetic patients will do well on protamine zinc or NPH insulin alone, whereas younger patients and those with severe diabetes usually require combination of crystalline with one of the modified insulins with an intermediate period of action. Patients who require more than 40 units a day do better on two daily injections of NPH or Lente insulin, three-quarters of the dose before breakfast and one-fourth before supper; under these circumstances, it is important that a bedtime snack containing both carbohydrate and protein be taken.

The *insulin dosage* will be established in one of two ways: (1) In mildly diabetic patients one may start arbitrarily with 10 units of ultra Lente or NPH insulin daily and increase this dose by 5 units daily every third day until the urinary sugar has been reduced to zero after an overnight fast. It should be appreciated that the therapeutic effect of a standard dose of long-acting insulin is not attained until the second or third day of continued administration. In general, it is not wise to exceed a daily dose of 50 units of ultra Lente or protamine zinc insulin. If this is insufficient, two injections of

Lente should be given. (2) A second method of initiating insulin therapy is to estimate the 24-hr urine sugar on a standard diet and to administer 1 unit of insulin for every 2 Gm urine sugar found. While it is true that a clear quantitative relationship between glucose in the urine and insulin requirement does not exist, this rough approximation has been found to be helpful. This may be given as ultra Lente or protamine zinc insulin in a single dose, or as NPH insulin, or Lente, in one or two doses daily, or as crystalline insulin in divided doses throughout the day. Every other day the dosage is raised 5 to 10 units, depending on urine sugar.

Young diabetic patients require relatively large quantities of insulin for adequate control (30 to 100 units) in contrast to elderly persons with diabetes. Patients with complicating liver disease unable to store glucose satisfactorily as liver glycogen tend to display postprandial hyperglycemia and easily develop hypoglycemia with insulin therapy.

In initiating insulin therapy for diabetic management, it is essential for the patient to be able to test his urine for reducing substances and for ketone bodies. It is of great assistance in establishing the adequacy of diet and insulin therapy for a patient to keep a daily chart in which the urine is checked prior to breakfast, lunch, dinner, and retiring (Table 70-4). One should not use the "fractional" method, testing the total specimen obtained between meals, but rather the "spot" test obtained by discarding the first urine and then collecting for a 20-min period just prior to a meal. Consideration of the times during the 24 hr in which the patient displays glucosuria or ketonuria will permit accurate readjustment of the preceding insulin dosage and dietary intake.

Insulin Reactions. Patients must be instructed concerning insulin reactions. Crystalline insulin given in excess produces a rapid and characteristic reaction associated with hunger, anxiety, sweating, palpitation, confusion, weakness, and tachycardia (epinephrine effect). Patients are usually well aware of these early symptoms and are immediately and completely relieved by the ingestion of carbohydrate with rapid action such as orange juice.

Modified insulin, on the other hand, causes a gradual reduction in blood sugar which is more frequently associated with headache. In most instances reactions to ultra Lente or protamine zinc insulin occur during sleep or in the morning. Residual weakness, incoordination, and headache often follow a hypoglycemic attack (see Table 70-3). In elderly patients with hypertensive cerebral vascular disease, headaches associated with reaction to modified insulin may be mistaken for a slight cerebral vascular disturbance. Nocturnal hypoglycemia is often characterized by lethargy on awakening as well as bad dreams, restlessness, night sweats, and pal-

Table 70-4. ILLUSTRATIVE CASES IN DIABETIC MANAGEMENT

Case	Dietary prescription			Carbohydrate distribution				Insulin	Premeal urine sugar			Urinary ketone bodies		
	C, Gm	P, Gm	F, Gm	Brkf.	Lunch	Dinner	Bed-time		8 A.M.	12 N.	6 P.M.	8 A.M.	12 N.	6 P.M.
Severe diabetes in young men (weight 70 kg)	220	90	80	1/3	1/3	1/3	...	CI 40 U 8 A.M. 20 U 12 N.	++	+	0	+	+	+
				2/7	1/7	2/7	2/7	PZI 40 U 8 A.M.	+	++	0	0	0	0
				2/7	2/7	2/7	1/7	PZI 45 U 8 A.M. CI 20 U 8 A.M.	±	+	0	0	0	0
				2/7	2/7	2/7	1/7	NPH 60 U 8 A.M.	+	0	0	0	0	0
				2/7	2/7	2/7	1/7	Lente 45 U 8 A.M. Lente 15 U 6 P.M.	0	0	0	0	0	0
Mild diabetes in elderly women (weight 50 kg)	220	80	60	2/7	2/7	2/7	1/7	PZI 20 U 8 A.M.	±	+	0	+	0	0
	180	80	60	2/7	2/7	2/7	1/7	PZI 10 U 8 A.M.	0	0	0	0	0	0
	160	90	70	2/7	2/7	2/7	1/7	PZI 0 U 8 A.M.	±	±	0	0	0	0

pitations; yet by the time the patient rises there may be a considerable amount of glucose and acetone in the urine. In treating reactions to long-acting insulin preparations, one must be mindful of the possibility of recurrent bouts of hypoglycemia following glucose administration due to their continued effect. To counteract these, frequent carbohydrate feedings should be given throughout the remainder of the day or night.

Diabetics on insulin and especially those known to have recurrent hypoglycemic episodes should be given a *glucagon* emergency pack (1 mg as an amorphous powder with diluent). This can be injected subcutaneously by a relative whenever the patient is unable to swallow glucose containing material and will lead to a transient rise in blood sugar long enough for him to receive oral carbohydrate.

Recurrent hypoglycemic attacks, with their attendant anxiety, headache, confusion, and loss of concentration power, are a serious handicap to the diabetic patient. Repeated severe attacks of hypoglycemia may lead to marked intellectual deterioration as a result of irreversible damage to cortical neurones. The patient must be told about the prodromal symptoms, so as to prevent a full-blown insulin reaction. *Whenever exercise is anticipated, the patient should reduce the dose of insulin or take extra carbohydrate,* since exercise increases glucose utilization without relation to insulin action. Hypoglycemic attacks during the daytime call for a reduction of crystalline insulin, whereas those occurring in the afternoon, evening, and early morning hours are best prevented by reduction in the dose of modified insulin. If weight gain has not occurred, carbohydrate intake may be increased at the appropriate meal. A reduction in dietary fat will be necessary in patients who exceed ideal weight.

Other Complications of Insulin Therapy. Early in the treatment with insulin, *a local reaction*, char-acterized by redness, swelling, pain, and nodule formation, may occur at the site of insulin injections, particularly with protamine-containing modified insulins. These reactions persist for variable lengths of time and appear less and less frequently as the use of insulin continues (spontaneous desensitization). Where such local irritation is actually an *allergic manifestation*, itching is usually present also. *Hypersensitivity to insulin* may appear in the form of a generalized allergic reaction or, rarely, as an anaphylactic shock. Changing to an insulin derived from another animal species or to one prepared by a different manufacturer may be all that is necessary to prevent hypersensitivity reactions. Boiling crystalline or Lente insulin for 5 min in a water bath often reduces these sensitivity reactions. Patients who require prolonged insulin action and have become hypersensitive to protamine may do well on insulin zinc suspensions such as Lente. Occasionally desensitization is required. *Skin infections at the site of insulin injections* are distinct from the above reactions, are extremely rare, and call for appropriate treatment.

Insulin lipodystrophy is characterized by either hypertrophy or a complete atrophy of the subcutaneous fat at the site of insulin injection. In the latter case, localized deep hollows are produced in the subcutaneous tissue. This condition is more frequent in women and children and has no significance other than the obvious esthetic one. Over a period of time these defects will gradually disappear, especially when injecting insulin into the same sites after a rest period. When hypertrophy of the subcutaneous adipose tissue has occurred, injection at these sites is often preferred by the patient because of decreased sensation of pain. Preferential injections of these sites should be avoided, however, since decreased vascularity of the hypertrophic adipose tissue may lead to poor or unpredictable insulin absorption.

Insulin sensitivity is related to the rapidity of response of the blood sugar to an injection of insulin. In severe juvenile diabetes, insulin reactions may occur quite frequently. In contrast, patients with mild diabetes of late adult life may be relatively insensitive to insulin. A suddenly increased insulin sensitivity should bring the possibility of early adrenal or pituitary hypofunction to mind.

Insulin Resistance. Insulin resistance may be arbitrarily defined as the inability to obtain satisfactory regulation of diabetes with 200 units or more of insulin per day. This situation may arise because of inactivation of insulin at the site of injection or because of enhanced insulin destruction in the circulation or in tissues. Occasionally high titers of antibodies against insulin may be produced and have been shown to be related to the insulin resistant state. Insulin resistance may be observed in diabetic patients in severe acidosis, when neutralization of insulin by a plasma-borne anti-insulin factor has been demonstrated. Insulin resistance has also been observed in the presence of hepatic involvement, in patients with hemochromatosis, in patients with leukemia and other types of neoplasm.

In the case of insulin resistance associated with shock and severe acidosis, blood and plasma transfusions and sodium bicarbonate administered intravenously are indicated in order to improve circulation and reduce acidosis. With correction of shock and acidosis, increased responsiveness to insulin may be anticipated and depots of insulin may be abruptly mobilized. In acidosis associated with shock, one should not rely on sodium lactate as a ready source of available base, since the rate of lactate metabolism may be seriously impaired. The anti-insulin inactivation found in the plasma of acidotic diabetic patients will gradually disappear as the condition comes under control.

When insulin resistance is related to the presence in the patient's serum of increasing insulin-binding capacity (demonstrated by the fixation of added insulin labeled with I^{131} in the γ-globulin region), an immunologic basis for the resistant state may be assumed. Under these conditions, treatment with highly concentrated preparations of crystalline insulin (500 units) is preferable. Up to 10,000 units or more per day may be required during the most active resistance phase. When feasible, a change to an insulin preparation obtained from a single species may be attempted (pure beef and pure hog insulin are usually available, insulin from other preparations on occasion only; standard insulin preparations contain as a rule mixed beef and hog insulin). Cortisone may prove helpful, although its continued administration is undesirable. In adult diabetics, oral hypoglycemic agents of the sulfonylurea series may occasionally be substituted for insulin with beneficial effect. For reasons as yet unexplained, severe insulin resistance of the type just discussed characteristically follows a waxing and waning course and usually remits over a period of months.

During the course of severe infections, in Cushing's syndrome, acromegaly, and hyperthyroidism, and during the response to severe stress, one may observe temporary insulin resistance. Under these circumstances, 500 units or more of insulin per day may be required. With the amelioration of the underlying difficulty, normal responsiveness to insulin is usually restored.

Transient presbyopia occurs in an appreciable number of patients during the initial period of insulin therapy. This disturbance is related to a reduced elasticity of the lens dependent upon an alteration in osmotic equilibrium between the lens and ocular fluids. The change is bilateral and tends to disappear after 2 to 4 weeks of insulin therapy. It is wise to wait until the diabetes has been under satisfactory control for at least 6 weeks before obtaining prescription lenses, if they are needed.

Oral Hypoglycemic Agents. A number of compounds, ranging from salicylates to the clinically useful sulfonylureas and biguanides, are known to lower the blood sugar level. The latter have a definite use in the treatment of maturity onset diabetes once weight reduction by dietary restriction has been achieved without significant improvement in diabetic control. At present approximately 40 per cent of adult patients are on insulin, 35 per cent on oral hypoglycemic agents, and 20 per cent are managed on diet alone in the average diabetic clinic.

The sulfonylureas presently used clinically are tolbutamide and chlorpropamide. They primarily act by enhancing the secretion of insulin by the beta cells of the pancreas, while probably also exerting a limited direct effect on intermediary metabolism. Ideal candidates for their successful use should be over thirty years of age, should be using no more than 30 units of insulin daily, should have been on antidiabetic therapy for no more than 5 years, and should not reveal a tendency to ketosis or give a history of coma. Patients without insulin reserve, especially juvenile cases, do not respond. Only a portion of apparently suitable diabetics respond satisfactorily. If fasting blood sugar levels are above 250 mg per 100 ml, a lasting response is usually unlikely. This then limits an adequate response to the group of middle-aged diabetics with mild disease or of recent onset. If upon insulin withdrawal acetone appears in the urine together with glucosuria, the likelihood of tolbutamide responsiveness is small. However, in the absence of ketonuria one may proceed with the administration of the sulfonylurea by mouth.

Tolbutamide, acting much like crystalline insulin

with a biologic half-life of 6 hr, is given in 0.5 Gm doses before meals three to four times a day. Little is achieved by increasing the dose above 2.0 Gm.

Chlorpropamide is given in doses of 0.1 to 0.3 Gm before breakfast only once a day. With a half-life of 36 hr it acts more like the Lente insulins. Observation of a decrease in urine sugar and an approach to normal fasting blood sugar levels after 3 days of treatment heralds successful control with the oral sulfonylurea, but there are a few isolated instances in which the hypoglycemic effect does not become apparent for weeks. These cases require a longer therapeutic trial. As patients show a tendency to gain weight on these agents, continued dietary restriction is imperative. In making a choice between tolbutamide or chlorpropamide, the greater convenience of one single dose for the latter has to be weighed against the more insidious and more severe hypoglycemic episodes and the slightly greater toxicity.

Secondary failure in the hypoglycemic response to tolbutamide has been noted in as much as 30 per cent of groups treated for a number of years. The same holds true for chlorpropamide but to a lesser extent. Some cases with resistance to tolbutamide show a good response to chlorpropamide. If such a substitution fails, insulin therapy should be reinstituted.

Whereas chlorpropamide is not altered in the body, tolbutamide undergoes chemical change, and the excretory product in the urine may give rise to false positive tests for albumin, since it is precipitated by acidifying the urine.

Sulfonylureas have been in widespread clinical use for only 5 years, and little can be said about their long-range efficacy. Since they tend to enhance the secretion of insulin at a slow and continuous rate, most patients who show a good hypoglycemic response may actually do better in the long run than patients on insulin in whom the regulation is less smooth. Conversely, poor control under the mantle of seemingly adequate oral therapy, because of the high glucose threshold found in some older patients, may accelerate degenerative processes.

Side effects of tolbutamide occur in less than 5 per cent of patients. They include urticaria, erythematous rashes, epigastric pain and vomiting, exacerbation of duodenal ulcers, transient leukopenia, rarely purpura, and hypoplastic anemia. Fatal liver failure has not been reported. In contrast, the side effects of chlorpropamide have been more severe when the dose used was excessive, and some cases of fatal hepatitis have been reported.

The *biguanide* compounds, of which *phenformin* has had the greatest clinical use in this country, exert a direct action on intermediary metabolism and do not enhance insulin secretion. It has been claimed that, by increasing anaerobic glycolysis at the expense of the hexose monophosphate shunt, this compound raises utilization of glucose without inducing lipogenesis. Thus the limited application of phenformin might be in middle-aged or aged diabetics with a tendency to obesity. Subjects with highly labile blood sugar levels while on insulin have on occasion shown considerable stabilization of their blood sugar with the concomitant use of phenformin and insulin. The combined use of the latter with sulfonylureas is also under investigation. Phenformin has gastrointestinal side effects and leads to nausea of central origin. The recent introduction of a preparation which dissolves slowly has decreased this difficulty. In practice one should begin therapy with a dose of 25 mg four times a day or 100 mg of the long-acting preparation, and not exceed a 24-hr total of 150 mg. After 2 years of usage no acquired resistance has been noted. However, when a patient shows reduction of blood glucose to normal levels, and yet increasing ketonuria, the drug must be discontinued when weight loss has reached a level 10 per cent below that of the ideal weight. Children should *not* be treated exclusively with this essentially nonanabolic agent during their growth phase.

Although biguanide preparations are now generally available, it should be stressed that their usage is clearly still at the investigative stage and should be limited to individuals and institutions adequately equipped for metabolic evaluation and with adequately stable follow-up practices.

Diet. There is no diet therapy which has been influenced as greatly by new discoveries and differing viewpoints as that of diabetes. Principal considerations in the design of diabetic diets include: (1) caloric intake adequate to satisfy the activity requirement of the patient without excess weight gain, (2) sufficient protein intake for tissue anabolism, (3) optimum supply of vitamins and minerals, (4) adequate variety and palatability.

Protein. There is general agreement on the amount of protein necessary for diabetic patients. The requirement varies with age, weight, activity, and the ability of the kidneys to excrete nitrogenous waste products. Adult patients usually receive 1.0 to 1.5 Gm and children 2.0 to 3.0 Gm protein per kg of body weight. In the presence of azotemia it may be necessary to decrease the protein intake to minimal anabolic levels, i.e., 0.5 Gm protein per kg of body weight.

Carbohydrate. A minimum of approximately 2 Gm per kg per day of carbohydrate is necessary to prevent ketoacidosis. In general, diets containing 40 per cent of the caloric intake as carbohydrate are most practicable. Carbohydrate intake should be increased to meet caloric expenditure from growth and exercise.

Fat. Since derangement of serum lipids of the types frequently associated with atheromatous disease is found with an increased incidence in diabetic patients, an effort should be exerted to keep the serum lipids at a nearly normal pattern. A reduction in the higher density beta lipoproteins may be achieved by limitation of dietary saturated fatty acids. Supplantation of these by polyunsaturated fats, in general, may be expected to achieve a reduction in the higher density beta lipoprotein cholesterol. In patients presenting elevation in low density lipoproteins, limitation of total caloric intake is necessary to effect a reduction in serum triglyceride levels.

Example of dietary prescription follows:

Patient's actual weight........ 190 lb (86 kg)
Patient's ideal weight......... 150 lb (68 kg)

It is estimated that the patient should be restricted to 68 × 20, or 1360 Cal daily for weight reduction.

Protein = 68 × 1 = 68 Gm =	272 Cal
Carbohydrate = 40% of total Calories =	544 Cal
	816 Cal

Fat = 1360 − 816 = 544 Cal

Final diet: Carbohydrate...............	136 Gm
Protein....................	70 Gm
Fat.......................	60 Gm

In converting the above diet prescription to a satisfactory or convenient menu, it is necessary to indicate both the type of food and the distribution of the diet throughout the day. For practical purposes, this is done by first apportioning the carbohydrate. It is apparent that diabetic regulation will be simpler with a greater number of feedings involving small quantities of carbohydrate, rather than with infrequent meals containing large quantities of carbohydrate. Such dietary regulation minimizes peaks in the daily blood sugar curve.

The number of meals will depend upon a patient's habits and his opportunities for eating. It is desirable, in so far as is possible, to encourage a patient to lead a normal life. Most patients will experience no difficulty in arranging three regular meals and a late evening feeding. In the case of children or adults at home, it may be possible to provide supplementary nourishment at 10:30 A.M. and 4 P.M. The distribution of the quantity of food in the diet will also vary with the type of insulin employed (Table 70-3). The degree of cooperation and effectiveness obtained in dietary management will parallel the patient's understanding of basic dietary principles. Simplicity in apportioning the calories is essential. The diet should minimize unnatural concern for nonessential details. In Tables 70-5 and 70-6, food equivalents are presented in a simplified form. Utilizing these tables, it is relatively

simple for a patient to substitute one equivalent for another and thereby obtain variety as well as relative accuracy in dietary management. A diet adapted to the individual's food habits will have a much better chance of being followed. It is desirable to ingest a well-rounded diet to ensure an adequate intake of the essential vitamins and minerals. A vitamin supplement, particularly with vitamins of the B complex, is desirable for most diabetic patients and essential for those on a reduced caloric intake. Under the latter circumstance, the need for supplementary calcium and iron should also be considered.

Teaching and Training of Patient. It is a relatively simple matter to obtain good regulation, provided a patient's cooperation has been obtained. If the patient tests his urine for sugar and acetone in the morning on arising, just before lunch, in the evening before dinner, and at night before retiring, fluctuations in blood sugar level can be detected, and adjustment of diet and insulin therapy may be made as indicated. It is not necessary for patients to carry on this multiple type of testing for any

Table 70-5. FOOD EXCHANGES

LIST 1. MILK[1]
Carbohydrate 12 Gm, protein 8 Gm, fat 10 Gm per serving.

Food	Approximate measure 1 exchange	Weight, Gm
Milk.................	1 cup (8 oz)	240
Milk, evaporated......	½ cup	120
Milk, powder, skim[2]....	⅓ cup (5⅓ tbsp level)	48
Milk, powder, whole....	½ cup (8 tbsp level)	35
Buttermilk[2]..........	1 cup	240
Milk, skim[2]..........	1 cup	240

LIST 2. VEGETABLES[1]
One or more fat exchanges from the diet allowance may be used to season the vegetables.
Carbohydrate 7 Gm, protein 2 Gm, fat negligible.

Beets	Peas, green	Squash, winter[3]
Carrots[3]	Pumpkin	Turnip
Onions	Rutabagas	

[1] Modified from Meal Planning with Exchange Lists. Obtainable from the American Diabetes Association, Inc., 1 East 45th Street, New York 17, N.Y.

[2] Add 10 Gm fat (2 fat exchanges). Most commercial buttermilk is skimmed. Check local supplies.

[3] These vegetables have high vitamin A content; use at least one serving each day. All other vegetables, except those listed under Bread Exchanges, contain negligible carbohydrate, protein, and fat. They may be used as desired.

Table 70-5. FOOD EXCHANGES (*Continued*)

LIST 3. FRUITS

Fresh, cooked, canned, or frozen *unsweetened*. Carbohydrate 10 Gm per exchange, protein and fat are negligible.

Fruit	Approximate measure 1 exchange	Weight, Gm
Apple, 1 small........	2″ diameter	80
Applesauce..........	½ cup	100
Apricots, dry.........	4 halves	20
Apricots, fresh........	2 medium	100
Banana..............	½ small	50
Berries (blackberries, raspberries, and strawberries)........	1 cup	150
Blueberries..........	⅔ cup	100
Cantaloupe⁴.........	½ (6″ diameter)	200
Cherries.............	10 large or 15 small	75
Dates...............	2	15
Figs, dried..........	1 small	15
Figs, fresh..........	2 large	50
Grapefruit⁴..........	½ small	125
Grapefruit⁴..........	½ cup	100
Grapes..............	12	75
Grape juice..........	½ cup	60
Honeydew melon.....	⅛ (7″ diameter)	150
Mango..............	½ small	70
Nectarines..........	1 medium	100
Orange⁴.............	1 small	100
Orange juice⁴........	½ cup	100
Papaya.............	⅓ medium	100
Peach..............	1 medium	100
Pear...............	1 small	100
Pineapple..........	½ cup, cubed	80
Pineapple juice.......	⅓ cup	80
Plums..............	2 medium	100
Prunes, dried........	2 medium	25
Raisins.............	2 tbsp level	15
Tangerine⁴..........	1 large	100
Watermelon..........	1 cup diced 1 slice 3″ × 1½″	175

⁴ These fruits are rich sources of vitamin C; use at least one serving each day.

prolonged period unless regulation is extremely difficult. It is desirable for most severe diabetic patients to test the urine on arising. Simplified chemical outfits today allow the tests to be made with ease and rapidity.

The difficulty of obtaining satisfactory regulation in a diabetic person under emotional stress is well known and should be considered whenever unduly wide swings from hyperglycemia to hypoglycemia are encountered in a patient who is faithfully following his prescribed regimen. It is often impossible, under such circumstances, to obtain satisfactory

Table 70-5. FOOD EXCHANGES (*Continued*)

LIST 4. BREAD EXCHANGES

Carbohydrate 15 Gm, protein 2 Gm, fat is negligible.

Food	Approximate measure 1 exchange	Weight, Gm
Bread, baker's........	1 slice	25
Biscuit, roll..........	2″ diameter	35
Muffin..............	2″ diameter	35
Cornbread...........	1½″ cube	35
Cereals, cooked.......	½ cup, cooked	100
Cereals, dry (flakes, puffed, and shredded varieties)...........	¾ cup, scant	20
Rice, macaroni, noodles, spaghetti............	½ cup, cooked	100
Crackers:		
Graham.............	2 (2½ × 2¾″)	20
Oyster.............	20 (½ cup)	20
Saltines............	5 (2″ square)	20
Soda..............	3 (2½ × 2½″)	20
Round, thin varieties.	6–8 (1½″ diameter)	20
Vegetables:		
Beans, peas, dried (cooked) Includes limas, navy, kidney beans, black-eyed peas, cowpeas, split peas, etc..........	½ cup, scant	100
Corn..............	⅓ cup or ½ ear	80
Parsnips...........	½ cup	125
Potatoes:		
White, baked......	2″ diameter	100
White, boiled, mashed.........	½ cup	100
Sweet or yam......	¼ cup	50
Ice cream, vanilla⁵.....	⅛ qt	70
Sponge cake, no icing...	1½″ cube	25

⁵ Omit 2 fat exchanges.

regulation with any regimen until the psychologic and emotional difficulties have been dealt with.

General Hygiene Measures. The diabetic patient must ever keep in mind his propensity for infection. Keeping the number of infections at a minimum is largely dependent upon the individual's personal hygienic habits. Personal hygiene in the diabetic patient refers primarily to cleanliness. Careful and frequent cleansing of the skin should be emphasized. Immediate attention to all skin abrasions will often prevent serious sequelae. The nails should be kept clean, but the cuticle should not be cut. All areas of pruritus should be kept clean, dry, and free from irritation. Good oral hygiene is helpful in reducing tooth infection and in delaying the onset of tooth decay. The lower extremities with their at-

Table 70-5. FOOD EXCHANGES (*Continued*)

LIST 5. MEAT EXCHANGES

Carbohydrate negligible, protein 7 Gm, fat 5 Gm per serving. All items expressed in cooked weight. One or more fat exchanges from the diet may be used to cook or season these foods.

Food	Approximate measure 1 exchange	Weight, Gm
Meat: Beef, fowl, lamb, veal (medium fat), liver, pork, ham (lean).......	1 oz	30
Cold cuts: Salami, minced ham, bologna, cervelat, liver sausage, luncheon loaf	1 slice 4½" diam. × ⅛"	45
Frankfurters (8 to 9 per lb)	1	50
Fish:		
Cod, haddock, halibut, herring, etc..........	1 oz	30
Salmon, tuna, crabmeat, lobster.............	¼ cup	30
Shrimp, clams, oysters (medium)..........	5	45
Sardines.............	3 medium	30
Cheese:		
Cheddar type.........	1 oz	30
Cottage..............	3 tbsp level	45
Peanut butter[6]..........	2 tbsp scant	30
Egg.................	1	50

[6] Limit to one serving per day unless adjustment is made to balance carbohydrate content.

LIST 6. FAT EXCHANGES

Carbohydrate and protein negligible, fat 5 Gm per serving.

Food	Approximate measure 1 exchange	Weight, Gm
Avocado.................	⅛ (4" diam)	24
Butter or margarine......	1 tsp level	5
Bacon, crisp.............	1 slice	10
Cream, light, sweet, or sour—20%..........	2 tbsp level	30
Cream, heavy—40%.....	1 tbsp level	15
Cream cheese...........	1 tbsp level	15
French dressing.........	1 tbsp level	15
Mayonnaise.............	1 tsp level	5
Nuts...................	6 small	10
Oil or cooking fat.......	1 tsp level	5
Olives.................	5 small	50

SOURCE: Committee on Calculation of Diabetic Diets of the Diet Therapy Section of the American Dietetic Association.

Table 70-6. CONVERSION OF A DIET PRESCRIPTION TO DIETARY MENU: A DIABETIC DIET ORDER

	Amount	Carbohydrate, Gm	Protein, Gm	Fat, Gm
Milk (skim)*......	2 cups	24	16	0
Vegetables........	1 serving	7	2	0
Fruit exchanges....	3 servings	30	0	0
Bread exchanges...	5 servings	75	10	0
Meat exchanges....	6 servings	0	42	30
Fat exchanges.....	6 servings	0	0	30
Total..................		136	70	60

The servings may be divided into meals and between-meal feedings according to the habits of the patient and the type of insulin he is receiving.

* For every cup of whole milk substituted, two fat exchanges less are prescribed.

tendant vascular changes require a more special type of attention.

Care of Feet. In patients with diabetes mellitus, arterial changes progress more rapidly than in nondiabetic persons. Among the vessels frequently affected are those of the extremities. Care and attention to the feet may prevent long periods of disability. Every patient with diabetes should be given careful instruction in this matter. Simple rules include:

1. Cleanliness: Wash feet with warm, not hot or cold, water and a bland soap each evening. Dry thoroughly but gently between the toes. Then rub feet gently with rubbing alcohol. If the skin is dry, use lanolin or cocoa butter two or three times weekly.

2. Wear clean hose, loosely fitting and without seams or wrinkles.

3. Insert lamb's wool between overlapping toes.

4. Avoid injuries to the feet.

5. Cut toenails cleanly and straight across with scissors or nail clipper, never with a knife, and only after a foot bath.

6. In cold weather fleece-lined "stadium boots" are ideal footwear, being warm, nontraumatic, and inexpensive.

Pointed shoes and loose-fitting heels are dangerous and should be avoided. Corns are caused by ill-fitting shoes. Properly fitting shoes are most important, and protective pads are helpful. Corns should be treated only by an accredited chiropodist or surgeon. Epidermophytosis is best treated with cleanliness and appropriate medicated powder such as calcium propionate or undecylenic acid preparations. Special exercises and measures for improving the circulation of the feet are an invaluable adjunct in many elderly patients.

General Considerations in Treatment

Most authorities attempt to eliminate glucosuria in so far as is practicable and to restore the blood sugar to normal levels.

Adequate but not ideal diabetic control may be taken as the state in which the patient consistently excretes less than 10 per cent of the carbohydrate ingested. Whenever feasible, ideal control (no glucosuria and blood glucose levels consistently below 150 mg per 100 ml) should be attempted. Diabetic angiopathy, nephropathy, and neuropathy are often more severe and progress more rapidly in patients who have been poorly controlled. Whether their prevention can be attributed to the constant and adequate supply of insulin, to the fact that blood sugar levels are consistently kept below 150 mg per 100 ml, or to the consumption of a more balanced diet is not known. Those who believe that the insulin effect is more important than the diet advocate a free diet permitting the patient to choose his own food according to his appetite, spilling in the urine any excess sugar which cannot be taken care of by what is considered an adequate physiologic amount of insulin. This regimen may be justified in some children and certainly is the management of choice for older patients with coronary artery disease. The vast majority of patients fall into an intermediate class requiring moderate yet liberal control. It is best to acquaint patients with a dietary system at the onset of the disease so as to make them able to evaluate their food intake. This diet will then be liberalized by the patient's own inability to pursue a strict diet prescription in everyday life, but excessive variations in intake will not occur. Glucosuria—really just a barometer for the utilization of available carbohydrates—still remains the criterion of reasonable diabetic control, except in progressive renal impairment, when it no longer reveals the true level of the blood sugar because the renal threshold is elevated.

While there may be some disagreement as to the importance of maintaining normal blood sugar levels in diabetic regulation, all authorities agree that the preservation of normal lipid and cholesterol levels in the blood is of the utmost importance in decreasing the incidence of late-stage serious atherosclerotic vascular complications. Whether the serum cholesterol or the lipoprotein molecules of flotation constants above 20 is the more important factor in the genesis of arteriosclerosis is debatable. Determinations of either or both in the serum of diabetic patients, preferably at yearly intervals, are part of careful regulation. If either is elevated, attempts should be made to cut down dietary fats of animal origin, substituting vegetable fats containing a high percentage of polyunsaturated fatty acids, and to increase carbohydrate and protein. Unfortunately,

diet has relatively little effect once vascular disease has become established, and a low fat, high protein and adequate carbohydrate diet, combined with adequate control, represents the best prophylactic measures to date.

Physicians should have a clear understanding of the hardships of dietary restrictions and the special nursing problems involved in making up to children and sensitive adults the loss of the pleasure of an unrestricted diet. They should also appreciate the effect on a patient of the knowledge that he has an incurable disease, and the feeling of rejection which is aroused, especially in children, by the regimen imposed by the disease. The patient and his family should be aware of the nature and frequency of negativism and personality changes in diabetic patients which accompany excessively low blood sugar levels. They are likely to occur immediately prior to meals and on arising in the morning, if modified insulins are being used. Each patient is to be considered an individual problem. If the physician feels that in each instance he has helped the patient to achieve the best possible diabetic control without severe psychologic hardship, he is less likely later to question the wisdom of his management.

Patients with diabetes should understand clearly the risk incurred for their progeny if they marry a diabetic person or one with a family history of diabetes.

Pruritus. This is a common symptom among patients with poorly regulated diabetes. Skin infections often develop from scratching the itching areas. Pruritus vulvae may be very disturbing. Severe local skin irritation and infection are usually present. The pruritus usually vanishes within a few days after the disappearance of sugar from the urine.

Epidermophytosis. Although its occurrence is no more frequent among diabetic than among normal persons, epidermophytosis in a diabetic patient is much more serious, since it provides a portal of entry for bacterial infections.

Furuncles. Repeated bouts of furuncles also suggest the diagnosis of diabetes; they are observed with great frequency among persons with unregulated diabetes. Not infrequently, they may proceed to more extensive involvement, such as *carbuncle* formation.

Urinary Tract Infections. These are particularly likely to occur when diabetes is poorly regulated. Bowen has observed an incidence of approximately 50 per cent among female diabetic patients. Since pyuria does not always accompany a urinary tract infection, a urine culture is absolutely essential in the diabetic person suspected of having such a condition. The treatment of pyelonephritis and cystitis in diabetic patients is identical with that in nondiabetic persons except that prolonged chemotherapy is often necessary. It is essential to keep the urine free from sugar for successful therapy.

Occasionally one may encounter a fulminating and often fatal form of renal infection, *renal necrotizing papillitis*. It is characterized by the almost complete destruction of papillae, with an ascending involvement of renal parenchyma. In intravenous pyelograms, the papillary tips are often seen to be broken off.

Cholecystitis and Cholelithiasis. There is a high incidence of cholecystitis and cholelithiasis among diabetic patients. In addition to the obstructive symptoms which a stone may cause, a chronically diseased gallbladder may be a focus of infection, which makes regulation of diabetes more difficult. The possible relationship of chronic cholecystitis and cholelithiasis to pancreatitis must be given particular consideration in diabetic patients.

Pulmonary Tuberculosis. The presence of diabetes, particularly if poorly regulated, markedly increases the seriousness of pulmonary tuberculosis. A chest film should be taken once yearly as a routine prophylactic measure. In most instances, diabetes precedes the development of clinical tuberculosis, and tuberculosis is most likely to become manifest in the presence of weight loss and poor regulation of the underlying disease.

Whenever diabetic regulation becomes difficult or whenever there is an unexplained increase in insulin requirement, a hidden focus of infection should be suspected and searched for diligently

Diabetic Acidosis and Coma

The treatment of a patient in diabetic coma necessarily varies greatly from patient to patient, depending upon the degree of acidosis, age, vascular status, and presence of infection. The general principles of treatment in diabetic coma are as follows:

1. Immediate and adequate insulin therapy
2. Treatment of acidosis, dehydration, and shock by means of parenteral fluid and electrolytes and whole blood or plasma
3. Treatment of complicating infection with appropriate antibiotic therapy
4. Prevention of aspiration of vomitus by gastric suction
5. Institution of fluid therapy by mouth as soon as tolerated

Plan of Treatment. *Insulin Therapy.* The first and foremost necessity is to administer adequate insulin immediately. A justifiable criticism of the treatment of diabetic coma in most institutions is that insufficient insulin is used. Often a patient's life may be saved by the administration of 50 to 100 units of insulin by the attending physician prior to hospitalization or en route to the hospital. In 123 cases of

coma treated at the Joslin Clinic, the average dose of insulin was 216 units in the first 3 hr.

The dose of insulin to be administered every 1 to 2 hr may be gauged by one of the following rules of thumb: as soon as the diagnosis of diabetic coma is established, 100 units of crystalline insulin should be given intravenously or subcutaneously if the blood sugar exceeds 500 mg per 100 ml or if undiluted serum gives a strong (4 plus) reaction for acetone. It should be accompanied by the subcutaneous injection of an additional 100 units of crystalline insulin if the carbon dioxide–combining power is less than 10 millimoles per liter (22 vol per 100 ml). If the blood sugar level is between 300 and 500 mg per 100 ml, 50 to 100 units of insulin should be given intravenously and 50 units subcutaneously. When the blood sugar level is below 300 mg per 100 ml, an initial subcutaneous injection of 50 units of crystalline insulin may be adequate, provided severe acidosis is not present. Crystalline insulin should be given every 1 to 2 hr and thereafter in amounts appropriate to blood sugar levels as described above or according to the following plan. A 4 plus (red) reaction in the urinary sugar test calls for 50 units, and 1 plus (green) 10 units. A rapid drop in the blood or urine sugar indicates that insulin dosage should be reduced or omitted, if a hypoglycemic reaction is to be avoided. Perhaps the most logical method is that of Duncan, whereby a 4 plus reaction in the acetone test (Rothera's test) done on undiluted serum calls for 200 units of insulin, and the same reaction in serial dilutions of serum calls for proportionally larger amounts. In the presence of severe acidosis or persistently high blood sugar levels, it may be necessary to give as much as 100 to 200 units of crystalline insulin hourly. Once the blood sugar level approaches 200 mg per 100 ml, glucose and insulin or fruit juice, if tolerated, should be administered until the last trace of ketone bodies has disappeared from the urine.

Modified insulins with a delayed action are not recommended for initial use in diabetic coma, since they are too slow to intervene effectively in early treatment and may subject the patient to severe hypoglycemic reactions during the convalescent period. However, once hyperglycemia and ketosis have been corrected, modified insulin should be given as soon as possible, since the more sustained, somewhat smoother action of this type of insulin is of great advantage.

Fluid Therapy. Patients with diabetic acidosis and coma present a serious problem in fluid and electrolyte deficiency. The magnitude of the deficit depends upon the duration and intensity of the unregulated diabetic state. In the most severe cases the loss of water may be extreme, amounting to 10 per cent or more of body weight, and a total of 4 to

8 liters of fluid is usually required over the first 24-hr period.

The basic disturbances in the patient suffering from diabetic acidosis and coma are (1) severe dehydration, in which the cells have sustained a relatively greater loss of water than the extracellular space, (2) depletion of sodium and chloride, in the ratio in which they normally occur in extracellular fluid, viz., 3:2, and (3) depletion of potassium and phosphorus. The reader is referred to Chaps. 50 and 51 for fundamental concepts underlying fluid and electrolyte therapy.

Fluid therapy should be instituted immediately in conjunction with insulin administration. In the comatose or severely acidotic patient, the intravenous route of administration is to be preferred; in the less severe cases, or as improvement occurs, oral administration should be encouraged. As a rule, 1 to 2 liters of hypotonic saline solution, with added sodium bicarbonate, may be administered rapidly even to patients presenting evidence of circulatory impairment, since the latter is usually secondary to marked contraction in plasma volume and extracellular fluid, further replacement may proceed more slowly. In the presence of profound shock, plasma and whole-blood transfusions should be employed, and the output of urine should be followed carefully as a guide to the adequacy of therapy and the status of renal function.

The sequence of fluids employed most advantageously in replacement therapy is as follows: (1) Initially, hypotonic saline solution (0.45 or 0.5 per cent) to which sodium bicarbonate has been added: for example, 500 ml isotonic sodium chloride (approximately 72 mEq sodium and chloride) plus 500 ml distilled water, to which has been added 50 ml of a solution containing 44.6 mEq sodium bicarbonate (obtainable in a sterile ampul). Such a solution contains a total of approximately 117 mEq sodium and 72 mEq chloride per liter and in addition provides an excess of water for cellular rehydration and metabolic needs. (2) In the absence of severe ketoacidosis or circulatory failure 1,000 ml of $\frac{1}{6}$ M sodium lactate may be used to replenish plasma volume while reducing the acidosis gradually at the time. (3) With a fall in blood sugar level to 250 mg per 100 ml or less and a marked decrease in urinary glucose output, 5 per cent glucose in 0.5 N saline may be employed with advantage. The administration of glucose at this time will accelerate the control of acidosis and ketonuria.

Although the deficit of potassium may exceed 200 mEq in individual instances, a conservative rate of potassium replacement, viz., 20 to 25 mEq per hr, appears satisfactory for most patients. In general, it is best not to begin intravenous potassium administration until the urine output has increased to 50 to 75 ml per hr and 2 to 3 liters of intravenous fluid has been given. Since potassium deficiency is almost invariably associated with deficiency of phosphorus in diabetic patients, it is common practice to supply the potassium for intravenous use as a solution of potassium phosphate. A convenient preparation is an ampul containing 2.0 Gm dibasic potassium phosphate and 0.4 Gm monobasic potassium phosphate, in 5 ml water. This provides approximately 25 mEq potassium and 14 millimoles phosphate. The contents of this ampul can be added to the flask used for intravenous medication. In most instances, by the time 100 mEq potassium has been given, sufficient clinical improvement has occurred to permit cessation of intravenous administration of fluid and the patient is encouraged to drink fruit juices and broth, which contains relatively large quantities of potassium. It has been estimated that, for every 100 ml water retained by the patient in the correction of dehydration, at least 6 mEq sodium, 6 mEq potassium, and 4 mEq chloride will be required. During the first 24-hr period of therapy, 80 per cent of the total deficit of sodium chloride and water and 50 per cent of the total deficit of potassium, magnesium, and phosphorus can be replaced with advantage. Although hypopotassemia is rare before 3 to 4 hr of effective insulin and fluid therapy have elapsed, the presence of this complication must be considered whenever satisfactory progress fails to occur. To obtain routinely an electrocardiographic tracing within the first 2 hr is considered good practice.

Recently considerable interest has been expressed in the possibility of using fructose in the treatment of severe diabetic acidosis, since it has been shown that this sugar disappears from the blood of diabetic patients in the absence of insulin. However, careful reinvestigation of this problem has revealed the fact that fructose is to a large extent deposited in the liver as glycogen or converted by the liver to glucose, but is not used to any significant degree peripherally by such tissues as muscle and brain in the presence of circulating glucose. Thus, fructose could be added to glucose and insulin in an attempt to diminish ketone formation more effectively, but fructose should never replace glucose and insulin in the management of patients with severe acidosis and coma.

Accessory Procedures in Treatment of Diabetic Acidosis and Coma. Gastric lavage with diluted sodium bicarbonate, leaving a residue in the stomach, is useful in all patients. Patients in collapse should be treated with stimulants, and the general measures employed in the treatment of shock should be followed. Infections should be treated vigorously by the administration of antibiotics. It is the senior author's custom to administer immediately a mixture of intramuscular penicillin and dihydrostreptomycin in all cases of severe acidosis and coma after bacterial cultures have been obtained. Catheterization should be avoided, but if it must be done, an indwelling catheter should not be used, for fear of producing a urinary tract infection. Lumbar puncture should not be undertaken unless a cerebrovascular accident is seriously suspected, and then only a 22-gauge needle should be used. Fecal impactions of the rectum occur frequently and should be broken up.

Aftercare. The patient must be followed closely until he is completely responsive and the urine is free of acetone, with a glucosuria of 2 plus or less. At this point, the acute phase of the illness may be considered terminated. During the subsequent 12 hr, the patient should receive a soft diet, which should include foods such as orange juice and salty broth. It is essential to begin with small feedings at frequent intervals. Intravenous fluid administration may be discontinued as soon as the patient is able to retain adequate quantities of food and liquid by mouth. Within 48 hr, it is possible to reestablish most patients on their standard diabetic regimen, including long-acting insulin preparations.

Degenerative Changes

In spite of adequate clinical control of diabetes, as judged by prevailing criteria, an insidious progress of degenerative vascular changes takes place continuously. Two pathologically distinct processes occur in diabetes of long standing: *small vessel degenerative disease and atherosclerosis.* These processes, either singly or combined, lead to changes in the eyes, kidneys, heart, and nerves and, tragically, to great morbidity in the group of juvenile diabetic patients of 20 years standing or longer made worse by poor control.

Capillary Degenerative Disease. *Diabetic retinopathy* may be demonstrated in more than 90 per cent of diabetic patients after 15 years or more of the disease. Not infrequently it is most severe in the middle-aged, untreated, mildly diabetic person, although it may affect those with the brittle, juvenile type of diabetes just as much. Among those certified as legally blind, diabetics have recently become the most numerous.

The earliest recognizable lesions on routine funduscopic examination are dilatation and beading of retinal venules (Fig. 70-3) and punctate hemorrhages consisting of the aneurysms surrounded by a halo of extravasated blood. These lesions soon become organized and, unlike free hemorrhages, remain unchanged for many years. All are a consequence of proliferative changes in the basement membrane of the small vessels containing mucopolysaccharide, and the characteristic sludging of the blood in the conjunctival vessels of diabetic and prediabetic patients may well be based on similar alterations. Unless the aneurysms and hemorrhages

occur in the macula, there will be no impairment of vision. Transitory haziness, occurring early in the disease, is related to formation of reversible exudates. Sooner or later, however, these lipid exudates become organized and appear hard, circumscribed, and yellow. Occurring in the macular region they diminish visual acuity. As retinal hemorrhages increase throughout, they become organized and neovascularization takes place, emanating from the region of the optic disks (retinitis proliferans, Fig. 70-3). The same process in the vitreous leads to formation of fibrous tissue, which may shrink and lead to retinal detachment and complete blindness.

The clinical picture is made worse by associated atherosclerosis, hypertensive vascular disease, and renal insufficiency. This may account for a sudden, rapid progression of visual impairment after years of an asymptomatic presence of the typical lesions of diabetic retinopathy.

The progression of diabetic retinopathy may be slowed down considerably by *careful control.* A radical and as yet experimental approach in therapy consists in pituitary stalk section or pituitary destruction by surgery or proton irradiation. By abolishing anti-insulin factors, diabetic control may become better, and in addition some ill-defined, direct

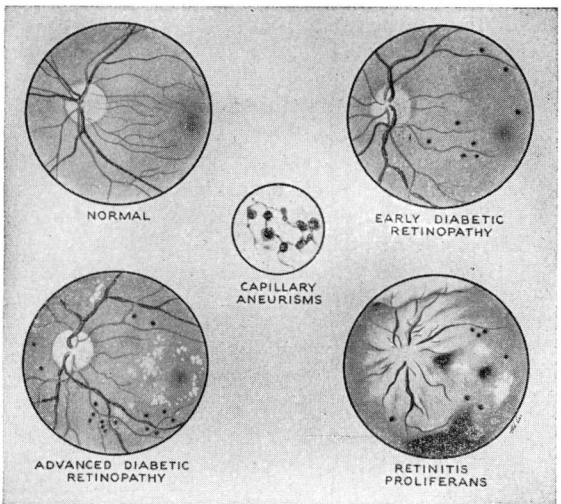

FIG. 70-3. Note the early dilatation of the venules and the punctate hemorrhages in *early diabetic retinopathy* actually representing capillary aneurysms surrounded by hemorrhages, as shown in a microscopic preparation of the retina (*center*). In *advanced diabetic retinopathy*, note in addition the typical hard, waxy exudates. In *retinitis proliferans* are seen papilledema and the spread of connective tissue, revealed as a white material emanating from the optic disk, together with endovascularization in the form of small irregular vessels. Note the detachment of the retina at the top of the figure, and the larger hemorrhages.

detrimental effects of these anti-insulin factors on the vasculature may be diminished. Although there is indirect evidence suggesting that certain anterior pituitary secretions, notably growth hormone, tend to favor the progression of capillary disease, it must be emphasized that direct proof for their etiologic role in diabetic retinopathy is lacking. Results with hypophysectomy have shown a 25 per cent improvement and a 25 per cent arrest of diabetic retinopathy.

In terms of degenerative changes in connective tissue, it is of interest that cataracts are more common in diabetic patients of all ages than in normal persons. *Diabetic nephropathy* has as its major component the hyalinization of glomerular capillaries, in addition to nephrosclerosis and scattered areas of pyelonephritis. The former is known as *intercapillary glomerulosclerosis* or as the *Kimmelstiel-Wilson syndrome.* Proliferative changes in the capillary basement membrane are quite similar to the changes in the retinal capillaries. While the pathologic changes are demonstrable in more than 65 per cent of diabetic patients coming to autopsy, only 15 per cent of these patients will have shown any clinical manifestations. Clinical signs consist first of albuminuria, which gradually increases. With a fall in serum albumin, anasarca develops and the serum cholesterol rises, producing a nephrotic syndrome in addition to the existing diabetes. An increasingly severe hypertension follows, and the patients eventually succumb to renal insufficiency with azotemia, cardiac failure, and thrombotic episodes involving the coronary or cerebral vessels. The course of the disease is variable, depending on the extent of the hypertension and infection associated with nephrosclerosis and pyelonephritis superimposed upon the lesions of intercapillary glomerulosclerosis.

The treatment of the diabetic nephropathy is that of diabetes and urinary tract infection, hypertension, the nephrotic syndrome, and eventually renal failure. Insulin requirements often fall off by 50 per cent or more as renal disease advances; the renal threshold for glucose rises, so that regulation by urine tests becomes difficult if not impossible, necessitating frequent blood glucose determinations for careful control. As a rule a more liberal regimen, with fasting blood glucose above 150 mg per 100 ml, must be followed. The renal disease has shown little improvement following hypophysectomy in patients with decreased renal clearances.

Atherosclerosis. Atherosclerotic changes in the medium-sized and large arteries are found frequently in the diabetic patient. This finding reflects in part the advanced age of diabetic persons as a group and in part the particular effect of diabetes in initiating or accelerating degenerative arterial changes. Even under optimal control, vascular changes appear in diabetic patients on an average of 10 years earlier than they do in nondiabetic persons.

The earliest change in the diabetic vasculature may be the depolymerization of a mucopolysaccharide which makes up the basement membrane of the smaller blood vessels, both arterioles and venules. The presence of an elevated blood lipid level in diabetic patients probably predisposes to increased deposition of cholesterol and fatty acid in the damaged vessel wall. Atheromatous and patchy thickening of the intima of the larger arteries predominate in diabetic patients. The first evidences of this process are usually seen in the vessels of the extremities and the heart. The roentgenologic appearance of the pelvic vessels has been shown to serve as a good index of the vascular state. Calcification of the vas deferens is more frequent in diabetic than in nondiabetic males.

Heart disease leads as a cause of death among diabetic patients. *Coronary artery disease* is approximately five times as frequent in males as in females among the nondiabetic population, whereas the incidence is equal among the sexes in the diabetic group. Those afflicted may do better if the blood glucose level is not regulated too closely, because of the danger of an epinephrine-induced coronary attack during hypoglycemia.

Cerebral vascular disease is of particular importance in diabetes because of the ease with which vascular accidents may be confused with coma on the one hand and with hypoglycemia secondary to excessive insulin on the other. Yet, the incidence is not increased over that in normal persons, in contrast to a fourfold excess of myocardial infarctions and a sixtyfold increase in gangrene of the lower extremities.

Gangrene. Gangrene of the lower extremities is a serious and relatively frequent complication of diabetes. Small vessel obliterative changes may make it more difficult to develop collateral circulation as occlusions of large vessels occur. A small gangrenous area on the foot may totally incapacitate an otherwise relatively healthy diabetic patient. Intermittent claudication is a frequent precursor of arteriosclerotic gangrene. Prophylaxis in the care of the feet and legs, the avoidance of infections in the extremities, and the use of exercises designed to maintain and increase circulation to the legs and feet, in conjunction with good diabetic regulation, comprise the principal methods of delaying the onset of this complication. It is essential to examine carefully the state of the circulation in the extremities of all diabetic patients. The use of the histamine flare test is often very helpful. Although occlusion of arterioles and more rarely segmental vascular occlusion is the principal pathologic change accounting for diminished blood flow, it is not unusual to observe varying degrees of associated arterial spasm. If such is the case, great improvement of an otherwise hopelessly slow-healing process may be obtained by lumbar sympathectomy.

Gangrene of the extremities may also follow severe neuropathic changes. One should suspect neuropathic gangrene, rather than primary vascular occlusion, in a patient who presents bilateral, symmetrical gangrenous areas. The improved prognosis for successful surgery in the presence of neuropathic gangrene indicates the importance of appreciating the etiologic factor.

Diabetic Neuropathy. Neuropathic changes are common in diabetic patients, particularly among the poorly nourished and poorly regulated and those over forty (Table 70-7). In the former it may represent an acute vitamin deficiency or a toxic insult to poorly protected nerves; this relatively acute form of diabetic neuropathy often responds satisfactorily to treatment, i.e., improved control of the diabetic state. Vitamin supplements are often used, although their usefulness is not clearly established. In the more chronic type of neuropathy found in the older age group with longer duration of the disease, an added damaging factor is the effect of occlusive vascular disease on peripheral nerves. In these instances treatment does not restore the patient to normal as a rule, although some improvement may be achieved. Neurogenic bladder, pseudotabes, postural hypotension, and nocturnal diarrhea occur in only the long-standing cases. It has been stated that diabetic neuropathy may mimic *any* neurologic syndrome. It is not generally appreciated that the protein content of the spinal fluid is frequently increased, usually without accompanying changes in cell count or dynamics.

Table 70-7. DIABETIC NEUROPATHIES

1. *Sensory changes:*
   Numbness, tingling, and paresthesias
2. *Neuromuscular dysfunction:*
   Muscular cramps, tenderness, aching, weakness, paralysis; occasional "shooting pains"; diminished or absent tendon reflexes
3. *Autonomic nerve disease:*
   Edema; decreased or absent sweating; intolerance to temperature extremes; night sweats; skin changes due to decreased function of sebaceous glands and vascular lability; miotic, occasionally irregular, pupils, reacting sluggishly to light
4. *Orthostatic hypotension or tachycardia:*
   Faintness, dizziness, syncope on standing
5. *Genitourinary and sphincter disturbances:*
   Sexual impotency; urinary and fecal incontinence; atony and paralysis of bladder
6. *Gastrointestinal dysfunction:*
   Severe constipation; chronic diarrhea (nocturnal); anorexia and nausea
7. *Bones and joints:*
   Degenerative joint disease (neuropathic foot)

Treatment consists essentially of careful diabetic regulation with a high protein intake. Supplementary vitamin therapy, especially large quantities of B complex and B_{12}, is usually recommended. Liver extract may be worthy of trial.

Reversal of early neuropathic changes may be anticipated following good regulation and a high protein and supplementary vitamin intake in those whose disease is not based on endarteritis primarily. With the more chronic and more serious neuropathic changes, it may take weeks or months to obtain maximum (still incomplete) improvement. Paradoxically, it should be noted that symptoms may be transiently aggravated following the institution of insulin therapy or improved diabetic regulation.

Surgery and Diabetes Mellitus

Diabetic patients may be affected by any disease, but there are certain surgical conditions, such as gangrene, cholecystitis, and cholelithiasis, to which they are more prone than the average person. The present average mortality rate in surgery in diabetics is practically the same as the over-all average for the general population. The surgical risk is increased in diabetics in the presence of poor regulation, obesity, arteriosclerosis, or cardiovascular disease. Certainly diabetes is not a contraindication to any necessary operation, and if the case is an emergency there is no need for delay.

Management of Surgery in the Diabetic. The extent to which special management is required will depend on whether there has to be much curtailment of food intake or changes in the usual hour of insulin administration. With minor surgical procedures under local anesthesia, where there is little interference with routine daily nourishment of the diabetic, there need be no special changes made. However, major surgery under general anesthesia in patients on insulin or on oral hypoglycemic agents requires a preoperative improvement in control, including all aspects such as glucosuria, hyperglycemia, dehydration, ketoacidosis, and restitution of depleted glycogen and vitamin stores. Except in emergencies, this calls for a delay of surgery to carry out this preparation. It includes a diet containing at least 200 Gm of carbohydrate for 3 days prior to surgery while keeping urine sugars between a negative and 2 plus by adequate insulin therapy. Preparation for and treatment during and after surgery should aim at allowing the patient to utilize about 1000 Cal derived from carbohydrate per day so as to prevent ketoacidosis. Patients on long-acting insulin receive one-half the usual dose the day before surgery in order to prevent hypoglycemia after a long preoperative fast. In patients receiving oral hypoglycemic agents, the evening dosage should be omitted and the patient should be changed to insulin on the day of surgery until able to take food by mouth again. On the morning of surgery, one-half the usual dose of insulin is administered subcutaneously and an infusion of 1,000 ml of 10 per cent dextrose in water at 20 to 30 drops per minute is begun. From 2,000 to 3,000 ml is given on the day of surgery and during subsequent days if there is inadequate food intake.

In the presence of an increased capillary fragility found so frequently in diabetics and a somewhat reduced ability for wound healing, preoperative supplementation of ascorbic acid (300 to 500 mg per day), pyridoxine (50 to 100 mg per day), and vitamin B_{12} (500 μg intramuscularly daily) must be considered, together with the possible administration of anabolic hormones. A preoperative check on prothrombin time should be carried out in all diabetics.

Anesthesia must be selected so as to minimize anoxia and acidosis and to disturb carbohydrate metabolism least. Local anesthesia is preferred; spinal anesthesia is satisfactory; cyclopropane, nitrous oxide, and ethylene are relatively safe. Intravenous Pentothal sodium should be used cautiously and only over short periods. Ether is undesirable because of the nausea that often follows its use. Chloroform and Avertin are definitely contraindicated because of the adverse action on liver glycogen storage.

During the first 6 hr in the operating room no attention need be paid to hyperglycemia or glucosuria since the long-acting insulin preparation or for that matter any crystalline insulin given prior to surgery should be more than covered by the slow infusion of glucose and the stress of surgery. It is after 6 hr that one must turn one's attention to maintaining the blood sugar and urine sugar within reasonable limits, viz., 150 ± 30 mg per 100 ml or a 1 to 2 urine reduction. Strict control should not be aimed at inasmuch as danger from hypoglycemia far outweighs that of a moderate hyperglycemia. If a patient is able to urinate spontaneously, urine sugars should be determined every 6 hr and crystalline insulin administered subcutaneously in minimum doses of 20 units for 4 plus reduction, 15 units for 3 plus reduction, and 10 units for 2 plus reduction. If at all possible catheterization of the diabetic patient should be avoided because of the real danger of starting intractable urinary infections. If no urine is passed, a blood sugar determination at 8:00 A.M. and 5:00 P.M. may be used to gauge the insulin requirements. A minimum of 10 units of crystalline insulin is administered every 8 hr for every 50 mg elevation of blood sugar above 150 mg per 100 ml. Not only is this management necessary in patients whose urine output is poor and irregular, but it may be preferable to using urine glucose determinations while the patient receives intra-venous glucose. The addition to the intravenous solutions of sodium and potassium chloride or sodium lactate will be governed by prevailing electrolyte losses and the presence or absence of ketoacidosis. This postoperative management must be carried on for as long as the patient is unable to take food by mouth. On the first postoperative day, again half the usual dose of long-acting insulin is given and glucosuria or blood sugars are controlled on the above-mentioned sliding scale with crystalline insulin. During the postoperative period, food by mouth should be commenced early with orange juice and clear soups. At that time either long-acting insulin preparations or oral hypoglycemic agents may be resumed in larger quantity and be then rapidly increased up to or beyond the preoperative level.

Amputation of a part of or a whole extremity is often necessary in diabetic patients and is usually indicated if gangrene or osteomyelitis is present. If the infection or gangrene is located in the toe, transmetatarsal amputation has proved successful if adequate circulation is present. If the condition extends higher than the toes, a low thigh amputation provides the best chance for subsequent healing.

The diagnosis of acute abdominal lesions occasionally presents some difficulty in the diabetic patient, since many of the signs and symptoms of diabetic acidosis are similar to those resulting from abdominal emergencies. An abdominal emergency will be suggested by a sharp localization of the pain and by the lack of improvement after several hours of adequate diabetic control.

Pregnancy and Diabetes Mellitus

The problem of management during pregnancy has assumed increasing importance during the past two decades, as young diabetic patients survive and are capable of procreation. Infertility in both male and female diabetic patients, common prior to insulin therapy, is rarely seen with good diabetic control. The increasing number of diabetic persons maintained in excellent health has, of course, increased the importance of considering the effect of the disease upon the mother and fetus.

The first problem which must be answered is one of genetic, social, and ethical significance. Diabetics should not be encouraged to procreate diabetics. Hence the family history of the nondiabetic partner is of great importance. A diabetic patient with a spouse possessing a positive family history of diabetes preferably should not bear children. A negative family history for diabetes in the nondiabetic parent permits the serious consideration of procreation without danger of overt diabetes occurring in the offspring.

Today pregnancy carries but slightly added risk

for the well-managed diabetic mother. In the pre-insulin era, maternal mortality among diabetic women often reached 25 to 30 per cent, whereas today less than 1 per cent of diabetic mothers succumb during pregnancy. In contrast, however, fetal mortality is still high. Stillbirths among diabetics are six times as common as among nondiabetics. White and Smith and Smith have reported chorionic gonadotropin and sex hormone imbalance to be associated with the increased fetal mortality rate among diabetics. In White's series 96 per cent of diabetic patients with normal sex hormone balance had surviving fetuses, whereas 50 per cent fetal mortality rate was observed in patients with marked hormonal imbalance. Correcting the sex hormonal imbalance with estrogens and progesterone resulted in a reduction to 15 per cent fetal mortality. However, these endocrine abnormalities are not the only cause for increased fetal mortality since equally good fetal survival has been obtained in the absence of estrogen therapy by merely assuring very careful diabetic control throughout pregnancy. The work of Hoet points to the great importance of adequate blood sugar control in the mother in order to prevent damage to the fetal pancreas and hence increase the chance of avoiding the development of diabetes in later life. Hoet has also suggested that abnormal carbohydrate metabolism during the early part of pregnancy may increase the incidence of fetal anomalies in general.

Diagnosis. In patients who are not known to be diabetic, the diagnosis of diabetes mellitus may offer some difficulty because of the frequency with which glucosuria is observed among nondiabetic pregnant women. In such cases a history of frequent miscarriages or a series of babies with increasing birth weight from 8 to 11 lb and a family history of diabetes should lead to a strong suspicion on the part of the attending physician that a prediabetic state is present.

The diagnosis may be established with certainty only by repeated analyses of the fasting blood sugar level and a glucose tolerance test (see Melituria, p. 715). By these means it is possible to distinguish between the glucosuria associated with lowered renal threshold during pregnancy and true diabetes mellitus. In the former the fasting blood sugar levels and the glucose tolerance curve will be normal.

Treatment. The treatment of pregnant diabetic patients entails the same general health measures as those recommended for nondiabetic pregnant women. It is desirable to maintain a high intake of protein (i.e., at least 2 Gm per kg body weight per day) and an adequate intake of calcium, iron, and iodine. The diabetes is regulated throughout pregnancy with tolbutamide or insulin. The patient usually requires two injections of NPH or Lente insulin a day; because of the lowered renal threshold

for glucose it is wise not to attempt to keep the urine sugar-free, but rather to give adequate carbohydrate and insulin to ensure the utilization of at least 200 Gm carbohydrate daily. Such a regimen will prevent acidosis despite mild glucosuria. It is often difficult to manipulate the diet satisfactorily so as to avoid hypoglycemia and excessive weight gain which appears to predispose to complications of the diabetic pregnancy such as toxemia and large babies.

Care of a diabetic woman through the first trimester is perhaps the most difficult, because of nausea and vomiting. It is essential to maintain an adequate caloric intake during this period, and if frequent small feedings are not well tolerated, intravenous glucose must be administered at regular intervals. Because of the unpredictability of the nausea and vomiting, it is preferable to use small doses of crystalline insulin several times daily, rather than to attempt to use a single injection of long-acting insulin, at the risk of possible hypoglycemic reaction if food is not retained. The second trimester offers less difficulty, and little change in carbohydrate or insulin requirement is noted. In the third trimester the insulin requirement usually increases, concurrently with a rise in adrenal cortical activity, and good control of the mother's diabetes prevents an undue load on the fetal pancreas. Spontaneous hypoglycemia in the newborn may be reduced by careful regulation of the mother's diabetes during the last trimester as will the dreaded hypoxia due to intrapulmonary membrane formation.

It is of utmost importance to detect preeclamptic toxemia, since treatment of this complication offers great opportunity to reduce infant mortality. The most successful management of the diabetic mother demands delivery from below by induction or, if difficult, cesarean section at the thirty-sixth week. This has the advantage of removing the fetus prior to its becoming too large and before the degeneration of the placental circulation, which is either the cause or effect of the tendency to toxemia. It also reduces the incidence of postnatal hypoglycemia and perhaps the development of diabetes in later life. The administration of 5 to 10 mg hydrocortisone intramuscularly during the first 2 to 5 days after delivery may greatly improve the state of the newborn.

Normal labor and cesarean section should be treated as a surgical procedure. A sudden decrease of the insulin requirement usually follows delivery.

Diabetes in Childhood

Diabetes in childhood with prematurity onset differs from that seen in the adult in being in general more severe and subject to more rapid and wider fluctuations in blood sugar. This is presumably due to the absolute lack of insulin. Diabetic children make up approximately 5 per cent of the diabetic population in this country. The age of incidence is approximately twelve for girls and fourteen for boys, thus corresponding to the most rapid periods of growth. These observations correlate well with the theory that overactivity of the anterior pituitary and its satellite glands plays an important role in unmasking the disease.

Of particular importance is the fact that the patient is first seen in most instances in acidosis or coma, and that protein depletion may be very great, necessitating the administration of at least 3 Gm per kg body weight for prolonged periods to make up for an accumulated deficit and to provide for adequate growth. Furthermore, the criteria of good management in the adult (i.e., normal blood sugar level and absence of glucosuria) are much less important in judging the effectiveness of treatment in children with diabetes than is the restoration of normal growth rate and freedom from acidosis.

Diabetic children, at the time the disease is diagnosed, are inclined to be above average in height but below average in weight. Hepatomegaly and splenomegaly are common. Hepatomegaly disappears rapidly on a good therapeutic regimen and is thought to be due to fatty infiltration.

Satisfactory criteria of management include the following:

1. Prevention of acidosis, coma, and insulin reactions
2. Maintenance of ideal weight and growth rate
3. Healthy psychologic development
4. Maintenance of normal serum cholesterol and lipoprotein levels

Diet calculations should be made on the basis of ideal weight, not actual weight, and should include supplementary minerals and vitamins, especially of the B-complex group containing pyridoxine and vitamin B_{12}. Intermediate nourishment should be arranged. The use of intermediate acting insulin such as Lente, NPH, or globin insulin preferably twice a day has greatly improved the management of diabetic children.

Of great importance in the management of diabetic children is the physician's attitude toward developing a healthy personality in the child. The presence of a chronic incurable disease, the necessity for daily injections of insulin, the occasional periods of hospitalization, and the constant necessity for diet regulation can be balanced effectively only by continued understanding and help on the part of both physician and parents. It is in this realm that the idea of greater latitude in diet is perhaps of much greater help in personality development than the small chemical advantage to be obtained by undue concern over matters of less importance. Combined with such a liberal attitude in respect to carbohydrate ingestion should be a serious appreciation of the need for continued good regulation if the complications which plague diabetic children are to be prevented or postponed.

In the fully established case of juvenile diabetes *insulin* is an *absolute necessity* for adequate control. However, recently Fajans and Conn have shown that the administration of 1.5 Gm tolbutamide to children with only a moderate elevation of blood sugar but a diabetic blood sugar curve may result in complete return to normal which suggests that the production of insulin by the residual beta cells of the pancreas is enhanced and stabilized by such treatment. This preliminary work affords a faint hope for the prevention of diabetes mellitus if the trend is discovered early.

REFERENCES

These references are collections of reviews and essays on specific aspects of diabetes pathophysiology and treatment:

Forsham, P. H. (Consulting Editor): Current Trends in the Management of Diabetes, Ann. N.Y. Acad. Sci., 82:191, 1959.

Joslin, E. P., H. F. Root, A. Marble, and P. White: "Treatment of Diabetes Mellitus," Philadelphia, Lea & Febiger, 1958.

Renold, A. E., and G. F. Cahill, Jr.: Diabetes Mellitus, in "The Metabolic Basis of Inherited Disease," J. Stanbury, J. Wyngaarden, and D. Fredrickson (Eds.), New York, McGraw-Hill Book Company, Inc., 1960.

Warren, S., and P. M. LeCompte: "The Pathology of Diabetes Mellitus," 2d ed., Philadelphia, Lea & Febiger, 1958.

William, R. H. (Ed.): "Diabetes," New York, Paul B. Hoeber, Inc., 1960.

Young, F. G. (Ed.): Insulin, Brit. Med. Bull., 16:175, 1960.

———: "The Mechanism of Insulin Action: A Symposium," Oxford, Blackwell Scientific Publications, 1960.

SPECIFIC REFERENCES

Cahill, G. F., Jr., J. Ashmore, A. E. Renold, and A. Baird Hastings: Blood Glucose and the Liver, Am. J. Med., 26:264, 1959.

Campbell, J., and C. H. Best: Physiologic Aspects of Ketosis, Metabolism, 5:95, 1956.

Colwell, A. R.: Histology of Small Blood Vessel Disease in Diabetes, Editorial, Diabetes, 9:503, 1961.

Fajans, S. S., and J. W. Conn: Comments on the Cortisone Glucose Tolerance Test, Diabetes, 10:151, 1961.

Field, R. A., W. A. Hall, J. S. Contreras, and W. H. Sweet: Hypophyseal-stalk Section in the Treatment of Advancing Diabetic Retinopathy, New Engl. J. Med., 264:689, 1961.

Foa, P. P., G. Galansino, and G. Pozza: Glucagon, a Second Pancreatic Hormone, Recent Progr. Hormone Research, 13:473, 1957.

Hoet, J. J.: Carbohydrate Metabolism during Pregnancy, Diabetes, 3:1, 1954.

Lawrence, R. D.: Three Types of Human Diabetes, Ann. Internal Med., 43:1199, 1955.

Lee, C. T., and G. G. Duncan: Diabetic Coma: The Value of a Single Test for Acetone in Plasma—An Aid to Diagnosis and Treatment, Metabolism, 5:144, 1956.

Renold, A. E., J. Ashmore, and A. B. Hastings: Regulation of Carbohydrate Metabolism in Isolated Tissues, Vitamins and Hormones, 14:139, 1956.

Ross, E. J.: The "Permeability" Hypothesis of the Action of Insulin, Medicine, 35:355, 1956.

Schwartz, Robert, Irwin A. Schafer, and Albert E. Renold: Generalized Lipoatrophy, Hepatic Cirrhosis, Disturbed Carbohydrate Metabolism and Accelerated Growth (Lipoatrophic Diabetes), Am. J. Med., 28:973, 1960.

Stadie, W. C.: Current Concepts of the Action of Insulin, Physiol. Revs., 34:52, 1954.

———: Recent Advances in Insulin Research, Diabetes, 5:263, 1956.

Thorn, G. W., A. E. Renold, and G. F. Cahill, Jr.: The Adrenal and Diabetes: Some Interactions and Interrelations, Diabetes, 8, 337, 1959.

Van Eck, W. F.: The Effect of a Low Fat Diet on the Serum Lipids in Diabetes and Its Significance in Diabetic Retinopathy, Am. J. Med., 27:196, 1959.

White, P.: Childhood Diabetes: Its Course and Influence on the Second and Third Generations, Diabetes, 9:345, 1960.

Yalow, R. S., and S. A. Berson: Plasma Insulin Concentrations in Nondiabetic and Early Diabetic Subjects, Diabetes, 9:254, 1960.

71 HYPERINSULINISM
Albert E. Renold and George W. Thorn

The maintenance of a constant blood glucose level is an essential part of homeostasis. Reduction in blood glucose levels to low or lower than normal values, regardless of the mechanism, initiates first a derangement in cerebral function and second a marked autonomic reaction accompanied by a wide variety of symptoms. Clinically, the latter may be noted first. The symptoms associated with any given reduction in blood glucose vary with the rate at which blood glucose falls and with the variable and individual susceptibility of the underlying state of the central nervous system.

The blood glucose level at any given time reflects the balance of two groups of physiologic processes: (1) those which add glucose to the blood, viz., (a) absorption of ingested carbohydrate, (b) formation of carbohydrate from nonglucose sources (gluco- neogenesis), and (c) mobilization of glucose from glycogen stores; and (2) those which remove glucose from the blood, viz., utilization of glucose by muscle, adipose tissue, liver, brain, and other organs. Persistent excessive secretion of insulin by the pancreatic islet cells induces hypoglycemia, with its characteristic attendant signs and symptoms. The increased secretion of insulin may arise from normal, adenomatous, or malignant islet cell tissue.

FUNCTIONAL ISLET CELL TUMORS

History. In 1924, Harris, having observed the syndrome of insulin-induced hypoglycemia in a diabetic patient, postulated the existence of spontaneous hypoglycemia due to endogenous overproduction of insulin. Wilder, in 1927, reported a case of spontaneous hypoglycemia caused by cancer of the islets of Langerhans. Two years later Graham successfully removed a benign adenoma of the islet cells and cured a patient of recurrent bouts of hypoglycemia.

Pathology. In a series of 149 cases of islet cell tumor, 106 (71 per cent) were found to be benign adenomas; 15 (10 per cent) were definitely malignant with identified metastases; and in 28 (19 per cent) the tumors were described as malignant under microscopic examination, but grossly and clinically they appeared benign. In 11 of the 149 cases, diffuse hyperplasia was also present. The diagnosis of hyperplasia is based upon the number and size of the islets judged by an increase from the normal diameter. The age range was ten to seventy-three years, with a majority of cases occurring between thirty and fifty years. Benign islet cell adenomas varying in size from 0.14 to 15 cm in diameter have been described, the majority being between 0.5 and 2 cm. They are usually encapsulated, purplish in color, highly vascular, and firmer than the normal pancreas. They tend to be distributed throughout the body and tail of the pancreas, with a slightly higher incidence in the head. In approximately 12 per cent of the cases multiple adenomas are found. Rarely, benign adenomas of islet cell tissue may occur outside the pancreas. Malignant adenocarcinomas usually metastasize to the regional lymph nodes and the liver. Both benign and malignant tumors have been found to contain insulin. The association of multiple adenomas of the islet cells with adenomas of the parathyroid and of other endocrine glands has been recently emphasized by Underdahl, Woolner, and Black.

Severe hypoglycemia has also been found in conjunction with *large* extrapancreatic tumors, most frequently retroperitoneal or mediastinal, with the histologic appearance of *sarcomas* or *fibromas*. It has been suggested that these tumors are modified islet cell tumors or that their hypoglycemic action is exerted through an excessive rate of utilization of glucose by the tumor itself. Neither theory has as yet been verified. In rare instances, malignant tumors involving the adrenal cortex have been associated with both clinical features of Cushing's syndrome (see Chap. 68) and hypoglycemia. A review of 20 cases of extrapancreatic tumors associated with severe hypoglycemia has been published by Frantz.

Clinical Picture. Hyperinsulinism due to islet cell adenoma may develop insidiously. It may be characterized by periodic hypoglycemic attacks, which gradually become more frequent and more severe, or by sudden convulsive seizures with loss of consciousness. Factors predisposing to attacks are fasting and exercise. Since the longest daily fasting period is the overnight fast, early morning hypoglycemia is particularly frequent. Symptoms include weakness and excessive fatigue, nervousness, anxiety, tremulousness, faintness, nausea, sweating, syncope, circumoral numbness, epigastric pain, and palpitation. More severe manifestations of central nervous system disturbance include irritability, confusion, diplopia, nystagmus, aphasia, mania, convulsions, unconsciousness, and coma. Once the attack pattern has developed, it usually persists in any given patient. Between attacks there may be no signs or symptoms. Patients may show profound personality changes and often become obese from frequent ingestions of food in an effort to prevent an attack. Chronic hypoglycemia may also result in damage to the anterior horn cells of the spinal cord, with progressive muscular atrophy.

Diagnosis. In the presence of hyperinsulinism, symptoms rarely develop unless the level of blood glucose has fallen below 30 to 40 mg per 100 ml (Nelson-Somogyi or enzymatic methods). Attacks characteristically occur while fasting and respond immediately to the administration of glucose. Whipple has emphasized that unless these three conditions are met the diagnosis of true hyperinsulinism is unlikely. Patients with hyperinsulinism may sometimes show decreased sensitivity to insulin, but glucose tolerance tests are not diagnostic. In contrast to true hyperinsulinism, functional or reactive, hypoglycemia occurs characteristically 2 to 5 hr after a meal of high carbohydrate content and usually is not associated with low blood sugar levels in the morning prior to breakfast or following a 24-hr fast. In infants and children, however, spontaneous idiopathic hypoglycemia not associated with known anomalies of the insulin-producing cells is relatively frequent and is a fasting, not a reactive, type of hypoglycemia. Patients with tumors of the islets of Langerhans have been misdiagnosed as representing hysteria, neurosis, psychotic state, alcoholic intoxication, brain tumor, epilepsy, encephalitis, duodenal ulcer, and hypoparathyroidism. The

presence of severe hypoglycemia after an overnight fast is not observed in any of these conditions but does occur in disorders of glycogen storage, Addison's disease, pituitary insufficiency, hypothyroidism high-grade hepatic failure, including congestive heart failure, and severe primary renal glycosuria.

The most helpful procedure in doubtful instances is prolonged fasting for up to 72 hr, with or without a subsequent exercise test as suggested by Conn. The usefulness of this procedure has been well documented in the large series of patients reported by Scholtz and coworkers. Total fasting may be replaced by a 1200 Cal diet of low carbohydrate content (50 Gm). Fajans and Conn have also suggested the diagnostic usefulness of a provocative test with tolbutamide. They have reported that *failure to recover within 3 hr* from tolbutamide-induced hypoglycemia is characteristic of insulin-producing tumors. This failure of hypoglycemia to recover spontaneously (hypoglycemia unresponsiveness) can also be demonstrated where hypoglycemia is induced by other means, such as insulin administration, and is a characteristic finding in these patients. In general, however, it should be understood that the diagnosis made is usually that of "fasting hypoglycemia" and that the diagnosis of insulin-producing tumor is arrived at by exclusion of the other possible causes of fasting hypoglycemia mentioned above. The possibility of *factitious hyperinsulinism,* as a result of self-administration of insulin, should always be considered, particularly in nurses and other medical personnel.

Although insulin in plasma can be estimated either by measuring the biologic insulin-like activity of plasma or by immunochemical means, the diagnostic usefulness of these measurements has yet to be established. The finding of elevated serum insulin-like activity or elevated immunologically reactive insulin *in the presence of hypoglycemia* (when low levels of circulating insulin are to be expected) supports, but does not establish, the diagnosis of hyperinsulinism. The final diagnosis of true hyperinsulinism is made at surgical exploration, with identification of the small, firm adenoma by palpation of the pancreas.

Treatment. Following the diagnosis of hyperinsulinism, surgery should not be delayed. Early surgery is indicated because of the possibilities of malignant change with metastases, of further irreversible damage to the central nervous system due to hypoglycemic episodes, of the deleterious effect of reactive sympathetic discharge on the heart of older patients with coronary insufficiency, and of increased obesity which will make surgical management more difficult. The administration of alloxan has not proved satisfactory because of the narrow margin between toxicity in general and selective destruction of the beta cells. After excision of the adenoma or subtotal pancreatectomy the patient is usually cured, except for rare cases of islet cell hyperplasia or of multiple tumors, which are usually located in the head of the pancreas. In approximately 20 per cent of the cases diagnosed histologically as carcinoma, follow-up observations have failed to reveal a recurrence of symptoms or tumor for several years.

REACTIVE HYPOGLYCEMIA

Reactive hypoglycemia is a common physiologic disorder in which one assumes excessive insulin secretion in response to an elevation of the blood glucose following meals or periods of excitement. This condition occurs almost uniformly in conjunction with anxiety and increased nervous tension. Following a meal the patient complains of weakness, faintness, and symptoms of adrenergic overactivity such as tachycardia, headache, trembling, and palpitation. Ingestion of carbohydrate usually ameliorates the symptoms but initiates a vicious cycle (see diagram).

CYCLE OF REACTIVE HYPOGLYCEMIA

Anxiety state
↓
Excessive carbohydrate intake and accelerated gastric emptying
↓
Elevated blood sugar levels
↓
Reactive hypoglycemia
↓
Excessive autonomic and adrenal activity

Diagnosis. The diagnosis of reactive hypoglycemia is indicated by the clinical picture of weakness and faintness 2 to 5 hr following the ingestion of carbohydrate. This is associated with some lowering of the blood sugar level. In contrast, the fasting morning blood glucose level is normal. An intravenous glucose tolerance test may show a rapid rise and a precipitous fall in blood sugar. Patients exhibit normal sensitivity to injected insulin. Intravenous injection of 0.1 unit per kg body weight leads to a 50 per cent fall in fasting blood sugar within ½ hr. A rise in fasting blood sugar of 30 to 100 mg within 20 min following injection of epinephrine (0.3 mg intramuscularly) or glucagon (1.0 mg intramuscularly) indicates normal liver glycogen storage. In severe hepatic disease, glycogen storage may be impaired, and consequently one may observe reactive hypoglycemia, although fasting hypoglycemia and increased insulin sensitivity are more common.

The majority of patients suspected of organic hyperinsulinism usually are discovered to have reactive hypoglycemia associated with evidence of emotional and psychologic disturbances. Hypoglycemia of the reactive type also occurs with the "dumping syndrome" seen most frequently after extensive gastric surgery. When the hypoglycemic symptoms appear to be associated with meals of a high protein content, the *possibility of hypoglycemia precipitated by leucine should be considered.* This syndrome has been described by Cochrane, Payne, Simpkiss, and Woolf and has since been reported in a number of families both in England and in this country. Present evidence reviewed by DiGeorge and Auerbach suggests that in these individuals leucine administration results in accelerated insulin release, or at least in elevated blood levels of insulin-like material. Hypoglycemia of the reactive type also may be an early symptom of diabetes mellitus.

Treatment. The weight should be restored to normal in the frequent cases in which obesity is present. In general the patients do well on a high protein, high fat, low carbohydrate diet and with the strict avoidance of large quantities of concentrated carbohydrate at any one time. Administration of parasympathicolytic agents, such as tincture of belladonna every 6 to 8 hr, using two less than the number of drops found to induce poor vision in the particular patient, is suggested as of possible benefit in decreasing insulin secretion. In rare instances stabilization of blood sugar in such patients may be improved by cortisone therapy in a dosage of 12.5 mg of the acetate orally on arising, at bedtime, and, if necessary, once during the day. The fundamental approach requires improvement in the psychologic and emotional status of the hypoglycemic patient.

REFERENCES

Conn, J. W., and H. S. Seltzer: Spontaneous Hypoglycemia, Am. J. Med., 19:460, 1955.

Crain, E. L., Jr., and G. W. Thorn: Functional Pancreatic Islet Cell Adenomas, Medicine, 28:427, 1949.

DiGeorge, A. M., and V. H. Auerbach: Leucine-induced Hypoglycemia, Am. J. Med. Sci., 240:792, 1960.

Fajans, S. S., et al.: The Diagnostic Value of Sodium Tolbutamide in Hypoglycemic States, J. Clin. Endocrinol. and Metabolism, 21:371, 1961.

Frantz, V. K.: Tumors of Pancreas, fasc. 27 and 28 of Section VII of Atlas of Tumor Pathology, Washington, D.C., Armed Forces Institute of Pathology, 1959, F 27-79 to 141 and F 27-142 to 149.

Garland, H.: Endogenous Hypoglycemia, Proc. Royal Soc. Med., 51:979, 1958.

McQuarrie, I.: Idiopathic Spontaneously Occurring Hypoglycemia in Infants, J.A.M.A., 83:729, 1924.

Renold, A. E.: Insulin in Blood, p. 663 in "Clinical Endocrinology," vol. I, E. B. Astwood (Ed.), New York, Grune & Stratton, Inc., 1960.

Scholtz, D. A., W. H. ReMine, and J. T. Priestley: Hyperinsulinism: Review of 95 Cases of Functioning Pancreatic Islet Cell Tumors, Proc. Staff Meetings Mayo Clinic, 35:545, 1960; also Am. J. Surgery, 99:413, 1960.

Whipple, A. O.: Islet Cell Tumors of the Pancreas, Can. Med. Assoc. J., 66:334, 1952.

72 DISEASES OF THE TESTES

George F. Cahill, Jr., S. Richardson Hill, Jr., and George W. Thorn

Androgen deficiency resulting from loss of testicular tissue was undoubtedly recognized by prehistoric man, as was the associated sterility; indeed, testicular tissue was recommended for impotence over 30 centuries ago. This dual function of the testes, as both the site of spermatogenesis and as the primary site of male hormone production, was clearly defined in the middle of the nineteenth century when Berthold returned to the capon the characteristics, both physical and behavioral, of the cockerel by testicular grafts and when his contemporaries, the anatomists von Kolliker, Leydig, Sertoli, and Schweigger-Seidel, defined the morphology of the gland. They recognized the spermatogonia, spermatids, the Sertoli (or sustentacular) cells, and cells located interstitially between the tubules (the Leydig or interstitial cells).

The tropic role played by the anterior pituitary gland in the development and maintenance of testicular function was demonstrated by Smith and Engle in 1927, and several years later, Butenandt isolated androsterone from male urine. By 1935, testosterone had been both chemically synthesized from cholesterol and isolated in crystalline form from bull testes. In addition, it was conclusively shown to be the most significant natural androgenic material.

DEVELOPMENT

Embryogenic. In the fourth to sixth week of fetal development, the primitive genital ridge differentiates into cortical and medullary components. If the sperm bares a Y chromosome, the embryo is a genotypic male (XY), and its destiny is to be a phenotypic male. Normally, in the presence of this genotypic pattern, the primitive interstitial cells direct somatic development along masculine lines, the cortical component of the gonad atrophies, and the medullary component develops into fetal seminiferous tubules. If the sperm bares an X chromosome, the embryo is genotypically female (XX), the medullary component of the gonad atrophies, and the cortical component persists as the future ovary. More important, in the absence of the masculinizing effects caused by the primitive interstitial cells and evoked by the presence of the Y chromosome, somatic development proceeds along feminine characteristics.

Aberrations in Embryonic Development. If the interstitial cells in the genotypic male (XY) fail to develop or function, fetal organs then differentiate according to the female pattern and may result in an infant with complete external female genitalia (syndrome of testicular feminization). Indeed, this condition may be so extensive as to be completely unrecognized, only to be discovered later in life as primary amenorrhea in an otherwise apparent female. Examination of these patients reveals absence of uterus and fallopian tubes and the presence of rudimentary testes, usually located intra-abdominally. Partial failure in the elaboration of fetal masculinizing hormone may result in varying degrees of feminization, encompassing slight hypospadias, through failure of fusion of the labioscrotal folds, to complete feminization as described above. Animal experiments have demonstrated that many of the effects of fetal masculinizing hormone occur locally to the gland, probably by direct diffusion of hormone into the tissues. Thus, unilateral damage or developmental failure of one fetal testis may produce feminization on one side and masculinization on the other, resulting in a true "unilateral" hermaphrodite. In an analogous fashion, since development proceeds along female lines unless directed by the masculinizing hormone, administration of androgenic or potentially androgenic agents to a pregnant female may induce in a genotypic female fetus various degrees of irreversible masculinization.

Aberrations in Fetal Development. Assuming a normal male chromosomal content (22 pairs of autosomes and a single X and Y chromosome) and normal production of fetal masculinizing hormone, the male infant develops a normal infantile male soma with persistence of the Wolffian system, atrophy of the Müllerian system, and complete closure of the urogenital sulcus except for the urinary meatus at the end of the phallus. Further sexual alterations do not occur until the time of puberty; however, the testes may change in location, at any time, from the abdominal cavity into the scrotum. The age at which this descent takes place is highly variable, occurring as early as the latter months of intrauterine life or as late as 15 or 16 years after birth. At birth, the testes are approximately 1 cm in length and weigh but $\frac{1}{2}$ Gm each. During adolescence each gland increases to 4 cm in length and weighs 15 to 20 Gm, but again, there is much variability, normal function and fertility being present in glands far less than half the size of the mean.

PHYSIOLOGY

Production of androgenic hormone by the interstitial cells under the influence of pituitary gonadotropins at the time of puberty effects the numerous somatic changes noted in the adolescent male. These include enlargement and increased pigmentation of the external genitalia, hypertrophy of the larynx with lowering of the voice, a generalized increase in hirsutism with growth of a beard and a typical masculine pelvic escutcheon and forehead hair line, enlargement of the prostate and seminal vesicles, and an over-all increase in muscle development. Metabolic balance studies demonstrate a retention of electrolytes, nitrogen, and phosphorus, and radiologic examination shows acceleration of osseous development.

The testes in the normal male elaborate between 6 and 10 mg of testosterone daily. Approximately half of this amount appears in the urine as measurable 17-ketosteroids, primarily androsterone and etiocholanolone (Fig. 72-1). The total 17-ketosteroid daily excretion for males, which includes the steroid derivatives from the testes and adrenal cortex, amounts to approximately 13 to 20 mg, of which approximately 5 mg is derived from the testes and the remainder from the adrenal. Assay of testosterone in the plasma suggests that males possess approximately 0.2 μg per 100 ml and females approximately one-quarter of this amount. With increasing age, 17-ketosteroid secretion in the normal male gradually diminishes, but whether there ever naturally occurs a sudden cessation in gonadal function analogous to the female menopause is dubious.

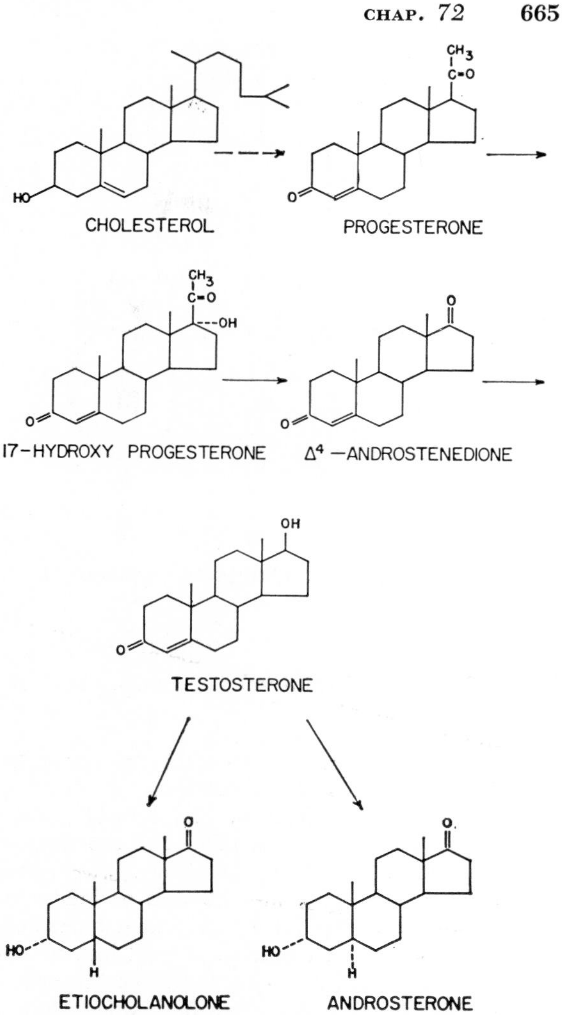

HYPOGONADISM

The clinical term *hypogonadism* refers to failure in interstitial cell function, resulting in decreased or absent production of androgenic hormone. (It should be qualified, however, that states of androgen-estrogen "imbalance" not directly attributable to interstitial cell function may also present as the clinical state of hypogonadism.) Interstitial cell function either may be decreased by a primary defect in the number or function of cells or may be secondarily decreased because of lack of pituitary tropic hormone. The hormone elaborated by the anterior pituitary gland which induces development and then functional maintenance of the testicular interstitial cell has been appropriately labeled interstitial cell–stimulating hormone (ICSH) and reportedly is identical to the luteinizing hormone (LH) in the female.

The precise interrelationships of the elaboration of testicular hormone and pituitary function are not completely defined. It is generally accepted that

FIG. 72-1. Synthesis and metabolism of testosterone. The broken arrow between cholesterol and progesterone signifies a series of reactions, all of which, including the conversion to 17-hydroxyprogesterone to Δ^4-androstenedione and then to testosterone, occur in the testis. The further metabolism of testosterone to etiocholanolone and androsterone occurs mainly in liver, and these products are then conjugated with glucuronic acid and secreted in the urine as the principal urinary metabolites of testosterone.

the Leydig cell is the site of testosterone synthesis and is stimulated by ICSH and that the seminiferous tubules are stimulated by the follicle-stimulating hormone (FSH) (Fig. 72-2). Production of estrogen by the testes has been demonstrated, and it has been suggested that it may arise from the Sertoli cells and may serve to inhibit pituitary production of gonadotropins. The role of the Leydig cell and possibly that of ICSH has been suggested by the observation of patients with absent Leydig cells, a lack of many of the masculine secondary

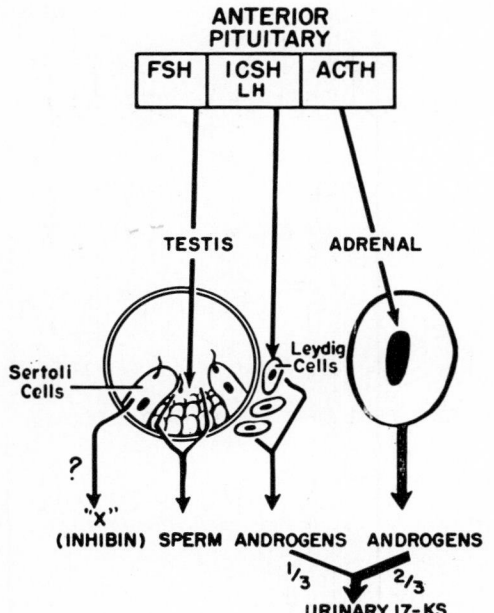

FIG. 72-2. Scheme showing anterior pituitary–testis relationship.

sexual changes and yet the presence of spermatogenesis, the so-called "fertile eunuchs."

Prepuberal Hypogonadism. The clinical picture of hypogonadism is directly related to the time of development of androgen deficiency. Prepuberal deficiency results in varying degrees of failure to develop the expected secondary sexual characteristics associated with maturity. A total lack of androgen production by the testes results in persistence of infantile morphology, a high voice, partial or total lack of facial, axillary, and pubic hair, infantile genitalia, and a barely palpable prostate. Because of lack of osseous maturation, epiphyseal closure is delayed, resulting in a tall "eunuchoid" habitus with long graceful arms and legs and wide hips. Gynecomastia and girdle obesity may also be present. The skin is pale and delicate and may show early "wrinkling" of age. Acne is absent.

Prepuberal hypogonadism remains obviously inapparent (unless there are gross physical anomalies of the testes which may signal pathologic changes at an earlier age) until the expected time of puberty. A total absence of any of the usual changes of adolescence at approximately age fourteen or fifteen suggests that interstitial cell function may be abnormal. However, as in other developmental states, there is a wide range of normal variation, just as complete sexual maturity (see Hypergonadism) may be present in the seventh or eighth year without demonstrable testicular or adrenal pathologic changes. Likewise, puberal changes may not be noticeable in certain other and yet normal boys

until the sixteenth year when voice, genital, and hirsutic changes may only then begin to become apparent. This latter phenomenon causes much concern to patient, family, and physician, and most frequently receives some form of hormonal therapy followed by somatic changes which undoubtedly would have occurred without the therapy.

Postpuberal Hypogonadism. Postpuberal hypogonadal changes decrease or are minimized when the hypogonadal state develops late in adult life; thus, castration of elderly men may result in none of the alterations seen in younger individauls. In the latter, there is usually a diminution in beard growth and a thinning of axillary and other body hair. The skin becomes smoother, the prostate atrophies to the point of being barely palpable, and sexual desire and performance wane. The genitalia lose pigmentation and may decrease somewhat in size. The voice does not change, but gynecomastia may appear. In older men, none of the changes may be noted; beard and body hair growth usually persist, and there may be no noticeable change in libido or sexual function.

Etiology of Hypogonadism. Primary hypogonadism (not secondary to failure of elaboration of pituitary tropic hormone) may be the result of numerous causes. It may be present at birth as either a genetic or embryologic defect or may occur any time later in life as a result of either testicular infections such as mumps, tuberculosis, brucellosis, leprosy, or syphilis or following trauma, irradiation, neoplasm, or castration, either surgical or accidental. In this group, besides the obvious physical characteristics of hypogonadism, the patient may excrete excessive quantities of pituitary gonadotropins in the urine as measured by any of a number of bioassay procedures, such as the routine measurement of follicle-stimulating hormone (FSH). In addition, because of lack of testosterone synthesis, there will be a slightly lower excretion of total urinary 17-ketosteroids and a more marked decrease in the excretion of androsterone and etiocholanolone. More significant, there are low or absent urinary androgens as bioassayed by growth of the cockerel's comb or some other similar androgen-sensitive bioassay. It should be stated here and cannot be overemphasized, however, that the most significant bioassay is the patient's own tissues, as seen clinically.

Secondary hypogonadism results from failure of pituitary elaboration of the necessary tropic hormones, specifically interstitial cell–stimulating hormone. In most cases there is an associated loss of other pituitary tropic hormones resulting in decreased thyroid and adrenal function as well as decreased gonadal function. However, when there is a progressive destruction of pituitary tissue from either granulomatous processes such as sarcoid or neoplasm (i.e., craniopharyngeoma or chromophobe adenoma) or cysts, the first deficiency is usually in the secretion of gonadotropic hormones, and the patient may therefore appear in the clinic as a case of isolated hypogonadism. In addition, idiopathic deficiency of gonadotropic hormones without demonstrable loss of other hormones occurs not infrequently.

Laboratory tests may demonstrate an absence of pituitary gonadotropins, and skull x-ray may reveal enlargement of the sella turcica or erosion of the clinoids. Thyroid and adrenal studies may also reveal clinically unsuspected hypofunction, and visual field examination may show an early involvement of the optic nerves.

Klinefelter's Syndrome (Seminiferous Tubule Dysgenesis). Klinefelter, Reifenstein, and Albright described in 1942 a clinical syndrome of hypogonadism which includes gynecomastia, eunuchoidism, elevated urinary gonadotropins, and decreased testicular size associated with hyalinization of the tubules. Barr demonstrated that many of these were "chromatin-positive," exhibiting nuclei similar to the nuclei seen in females (see Chap. 46). Culture of marrow cells in vitro in the presence of colchicine has permitted direct chromosomal counting and classification, as shown in Fig. 72-3, and indeed, many patients with the triad described by Klinefelter et al. have been shown to contain an extra sex chromosome, resulting in a karyotypic classification of 22 autosomes plus two X chromosomes and one Y chromosome (see Chap. 46). Thus, they have 47 instead of 46 chromosomes, and it is therefore not surprising that many of these patients also have various degrees of mental deficiency (similar to mongolism where the extra chromosome may be autosomal). Some patients with Klinefelter's syndrome, however, lack the clinical findings of gynecomastia, hypoplastic testes, and eunuchoidism and may be discovered only when they appear in the fertility clinic with a finding of oligospermia or aspermia; thus, the spectrum of Klinefelter's syndrome is quite broad, including obviously feminized males on one end and on the other, grossly normal, virilized men with only abnormal microscopic testicular anatomy.

Froelich's Syndrome and the Laurence-Moon-Biedl Syndrome. In 1901 Froelich described an obese, hypogonadal boy with signs of a tumor in the hypothalamic area. Since then, his name has been inappropriately applied to a large group of overweight boys with slightly retarded maturation but without demonstration of any hypothalamic lesion and, therefore, without any real clinical significance. On the other hand, the Laurence-Moon-Biedl syndrome engrosses a group of congenital malformations (the trait being inherited as a recessive characteristic) including hypogonadism, dwarfism, mental retardation, polydactyly, syndac-

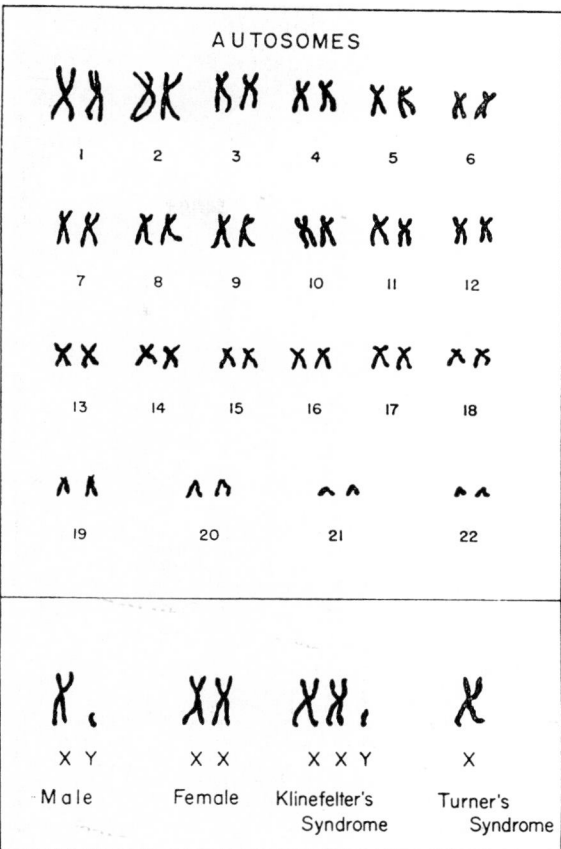

FIG. 72-3. Schematic drawing of 22 pairs of autosomes and aberrations in the number of sex chromosomes as seen in patients with Klinefelter's or Turner's syndrome.

tyly, obesity, retinitis pigmentosa, and diabetes insipidus.

Androgen-Estrogen Imbalance. This ill-defined group of diseases includes hepatic decompensation with supposed failure in the removal of circulating estrogens, as exemplified by Laennec's cirrhosis, various feminizing tumors of the testes and adrenals with excessive production of estrogens and, lastly, intentional or unintentional intake of exogenous estrogen. The result of all these is again decreased sexual function and desire, decreased testicular size, gynecomastia, and loss of hair. The changes, however, are highly variable, depending on the duration and intensity of female hormone exposure, the age of the patient, and most important, a wide degree of variation from individual to individual.

Treatment of Hypogonadism. In general, hypogonadal states, when treatment is indicated, are treated by direct administration of preparations of testosterone. Most commonly used are any one of the long-acting depot injections listed in Table 72-1. The usual method of therapy is to start with rela-

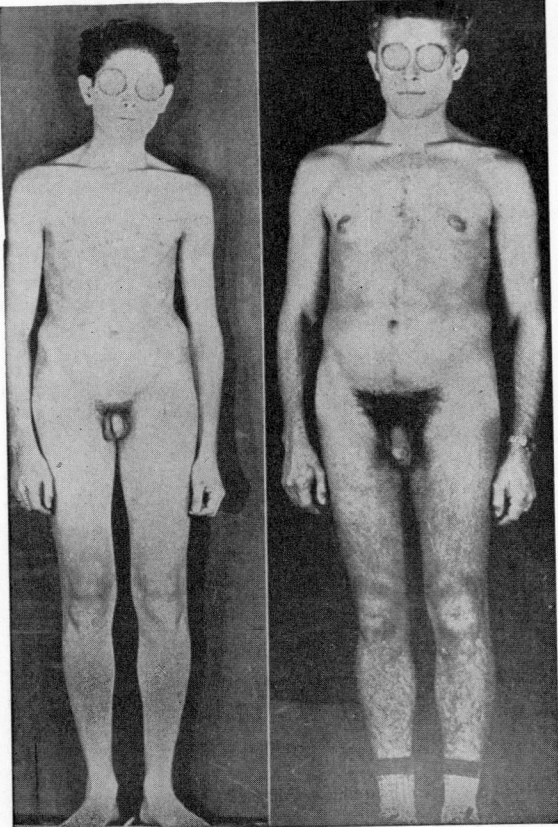

FIG. 72-4. (*Left*) Male, age 25 years, with eunuchoidism untreated. (*Right*) The same patient, age 30 years, after male hormone therapy for 5 years (*Werner: Am. J. Med.*, 3:52, 1947.)

suggested for the treatment of undescended testes in the adolescent.

STERILITY, IMPOTENCE, AND LIBIDO

Sterility, impotence, and loss of libido (or sexual desire) are frequently confused. Sterility in the male implies the continuous failure of the ejaculate to fertilize an ovum in a normal female. Since the average ejaculate contains 60 to 120 million sperm of which 60 to 80 per cent are active in approximately 4 ml of seminal fluid, sterility may be due to inadequate volume, inadequate concentration of sperm, or an abnormal proportion of immobile sperm. These factors may be due to a structural process, such as occluded ducts due to active or old infection (frequently gonorrhea), testicular disease, or occasionally to a total lack or destruction of seminiferous tubules, to an idiopathic dysgenesis of the tubules (del Castillo syndrome), or to Klinefelter's syndrome. Diagnosis of sterility in a male requires a microscopic examination of semen, or if unobtainable (or if obtained and an obvious deficiency is observed) by testicular biopsy.

Impotence, on the other hand, is usually not of endocrine origin and most frequently reflects a psychiatric and occasionally a neurologic disturbance. Loss of libido is more difficult to assess and may reflect a psychiatric disturbance, a true endocrine imbalance, or may be due to many other factors. Loss of libido is frequently the first sign of incipient hypogonadism due to either primary gonadal disease or to loss of gonadotropins; for example, the earliest sign of hypopituitarism in a previously normal male may be a waning of sexual desire. Likewise, loss of libido may be associated with any chronic disease, including infection and malignancy.

The treatment of impotence is obviously through psychiatric support, or if neurologic in origin such as secondary to tabes or diabetes, by treatment of the underlying process. The treatment of sterility due to production of inadequate semen is essentially supportive. If there is oligospermia or decreased motility, the various maneuvers discussed in the chapter on infertility (Chap. 75) may be employed to facilitate contact of sperm with the cervical os. If aspermia is present, the patient should be informed of the fact in order that continuous emotional distress of repeated attempted conception be avoided. The treatment of decreased libido, if associated with diagnosed hypogonadism, is the administration of androgen (Table 72-1). If not associated with hypogonadism, treatment of decreased libido by androgen should be considered with caution, since the underlying process is prob-

tively small doses, such as 150 mg of a depot preparation intramuscularly every 3 to 4 weeks, gradually increasing the dose to 250 or 300 mg for the same period of time. Excessive acne formation, retention of sodium resulting in edema, and excessive personality changes are all indications of overtreatment, and the dose should therefore be diminished.

In patients with hypogonadism in the puberal or prepuberal age group, testosterone administration has been reported to cause pathologic changes in the seminiferous tubules, resulting in azoospermia and sterility. Hence, caution must be exercised in its use in this group. If the hypogonadism is secondary to failure of gonadotropin secretion by the pituitary, a trial on chorionic or pituitary gonadotropins may be indicated, starting with injections of 500 to 1,000 units two or three times weekly, increasing the dose over a period of several weeks to see if changes occur. A similar schedule has been

Table 72-1. TESTOSTERONE PREPARATIONS
COMMONLY USED

Short acting	Dosage
Testosterone proprionate in oil...............	10–25 mg intramuscularly 3 to 5 times per week
Methyltestosterone tablets	10–100 mg by mouth
Long acting	
Testosterone cyclopentyl-proprionate in oil......	100–300 mg intramuscularly every 3 to 4 weeks
Testosterone enanthate in oil................	100–300 mg intramuscularly every 3 to 4 weeks
Testosterone phenylace-tate, aqueous suspension	100–300 mg intramuscularly every 3 to 4 weeks

Table 72-2. CAUSES OF MALE SEX PRECOCITY

Type of precocity	Cause	Per-centage
Complete genital pre-cocity, true preco-cious puberty	Idiopathic	55
	Pineal neoplasm	12
	Cerebral (hypotha-lamic disease)	13
Incomplete genital pre-cocity, precocious pseudopuberty, dis-sociated virilization (failure of testes to mature)	Adrenal cortical lesion	16
	Interstitial cell tumor of testis	4

SOURCE: Seckel, and Dorfman and Shipley.

ably some other systemic disease or a reflection of an emotional disturbance.

HYPERGONADISM

The production of excessive quantities of andro-genic hormone in the adult male results in little, if any, morphologic or functional change. However, in the child, the somatic changes associated with puberty may be induced at an early age and there-fore become clinically apparent (precocious pu-berty).

Hypergonadism may be due to excessive andro-gen production from a functioning testicular tumor, the Leydig or interstitial cell carcinoma. Children with these tumors show all the changes associated with puberty, such as increased hair growth and phallic enlargement, and usually have a palpable testicular tumor. However, the presence of the tu-mor may be difficult to determine if the testes are undescended or if the tumor is extremely active in producing hormone but still very small in size. The urine may contain excessive quantities of biologi-cally active androgen. Because of the marked po-tency of testosterone, the total 17-ketosteroids may be normal or only slightly increased in the presence of marked androgenicity. Pituitary gonadotropins are absent.

Hypergonadism may also appear in the presence of excessive quantities of adrenal androgen. These boys, often called "infant Hercules" because of their precocious puberty and muscle development, also show all the changes of sexual maturity in addition to accelerated growth and muscle development. The testes remain, however, infantile and atrophic, and gonadotropins are absent. The diagnosis is made on the basis of markedly elevated urinary 17-ketosteroids. For further discussion see Chap. 68.

A third variety of hypergonadism is that associ-ated with an early onset of what appears to be a normal puberty. These boys may have pubic hair, deepening of the voice, increased size of phallus and scrotum at age four or five, and occasionally

earlier. The testes are enlarged for the patient's age but are in accord with the size expected for that degree of maturity exhibited by the remainder of his somatic development. More important, gona-dotropins are present in the urine, and 17-ketoster-oids are also elevated for his chronologic age, but like the testicular and other secondary sexual changes, the ketosteroids are in the range of an adolescent. This trait of precocious puberty seems to run in families and, similar to that seen with excessive production of adrenal androgen, results in relatively excessive growth during childhood, fol-lowed by early closure of the epiphyses, ending in an adult who frequently is smaller than his con-temporaries. In certain instances, precocious pu-berty has been associated with cysts and tumors located in the pineal body or hypothalamic area (Table 72-2).

NEOPLASMS OF THE TESTES

Neoplasms of the testis are relatively uncommon. It is generally believed that they occur more com-monly in the cryptorchid testis (1 in 2,000) than in the normal testis (1 in 100,000). They may be classified as follows, in their relative order of fre-quency:

1. Seminoma (germinoma)
2. Teratocarcinoma
3. Embryonal carcinoma
   a. Chorioepithelioma
4. Teratoma
5. Interstitial cell tumor
6. Fibroma, lipoma, adenoma, myxoma
7. Unclassified varieties

The incidence of teratocarcinoma is roughly con-stant throughout life, whereas the incidence of seminoma tends to rise with age. One-year survival is rare for embryonal carcinomas and chorioepitheliomas, not uncommon for teratocarcinomas and teratomas, and the rule for seminomas.

Endocrine changes such as gynecomastia and increased secretion of gonadotropins giving a positive Aschheim-Zondek test result are occasionally seen in chorioepitheliomas as well as in embryonal carcinomas and teratocarcinomas. The endocrine effects of interstitial cell tumors have been discussed.

Diagnosis. The diagnosis is made by palpating a mass, usually firm, smooth, and painless. Neoplasms must be distinguished from tuberculosis or old gonorrheal epididymitis (usually hard and nodular), from syphilis (usually accompanied by a positive serologic test and a response to specific therapy), and from the various fluid-containing cysts (hydrocele, spermatocele), which may be transilluminated. The diagnosis may be aided also by finding an increased urinary excretion of 17-ketosteroids, estrogens, or gonadotropins, the latter giving a positive Aschheim-Zondek test. Rarely, tumor cells may be identified in the semen.

Treatment. Surgical removal is always indicated in any tumor of the testis and will usually effect a cure in the benign varieties. If the tumor is malignant, a radical operation followed by irradiation should be employed. X-ray therapy has been shown to effect a cure in the majority of cases of seminoma. Results of therapy may be followed by repeated determinations of the 17-ketosteroids or estrogens, or by the Aschheim-Zondek test, if originally positive. Certain testicular tumors, particularly the chorioepitheliomas, have been shown to be exquisitely sensitive to certain antimetabolic agents such as 4-amino-N^{10}-methylpteroylglutamic acid (Methotrexate).

DISEASES OF THE PROSTATE

Adenocarcinoma of the prostate is one of the most common tumors of men. It is rare before the age of forty, and the incidence rises rapidly with advancing age, occurring microscopically in 10 to 15 per cent of men in the fifth decade and as high as 40 per cent in those in the eighth decade. However, only one-fourth may become clinically apparent prior to death. Three-fourths of these tumors arise in the posterior lobe. The largest majority are easily palpable; hence routine frequent rectal examinations are indicated as a means of demonstrating early and operable tumors. Although the whole gland need not be enlarged, the presence of stony, hard, and indurated nodules or masses strongly suggests the presence of an adenocarcinoma. Frequently there may be an elevation in the "prostatic" fraction of serum acid phosphatase while the tumor is still localized within the prostatic capsule, and elevation of this enzyme may serve to differentiate a benign hypertrophic nodule from a malignancy.

Once the tumor has spread locally from the gland and particularly after it has metastasized, total serum acid and alkaline phosphatase may be greatly elevated.

Therapy consists of radical prostatectomy; irradiation by x-ray, radium, or radioactive isotopes (colloidal gold); and hormonal treatment (especially when metastatic disease develops) to decrease the androgen and increase the estrogen levels. Androgens are decreased by orchidectomy and by adrenalectomy or adrenal cortical suppression following cortisone administration (50 to 100 mg cortisone given orally in divided doses); estrogen levels are increased by administering diethylstilbestrol, 10 to 15 mg daily, or the equivalent doses of other estrogenic products.

REFERENCES

Albert, A., L. O. Underdahl, L. F. Greene, and N. Lorenz: Male Hypogonadism: I, II, III, IV, V, VI, VII, Proc. Staff Meetings Mayo Clinic, 28: 409, 557, 698, 1953; 29:131, 317, 368, 1954; 30: 31, 1955.

Dorfman, R. I., and R. A. Shipley: "Androgens—Biochemistry, Physiology and Clinical Significance," New York, John Wiley & Sons, Inc., 1956.

Ferguson-Smith, M. A., and A. W. Johnston: Chromosome Abnormalities in Certain Diseases of Man, Ann. Internal Med., 53:359, 1960.

Howard, R. P., R. C. Sniffen, F. A. Simmons, and F. Albright: Testicular Deficiency: A Clinical and Pathological Study, J. Clin. Endocrinol., 10:121, 1950.

Leadbetter, W. F.: Treatment of Testis Tumors Based on Their Pathological Behavior, J.A.M.A., 151:275, 1953.

McCullagh, E. P., J. C. Beck, and C. A. Schaffenburg: A Syndrome of Eunuchoidism with Spermatogenesis, Normal Urinary FSH and Low or Normal ICSH ("Fertile Eunuchs"), J. Clin. Endocrinol. and Metabolism, 13:489, 1953.

Seckel, H. P. G.: Precocious Sexual Development in Children, Med. Clin. N. Am., 30:183, 1946.

73 DISEASES OF THE OVARIES
John C. Laidlaw, Kendall Emerson, Jr., and George W. Thorn

History. The ovulatory function of the ovaries was first described by a Dutch physician, Reinier de Graaf, in 1673. He recognized small fluid blisters, now known as graafian follicles, which had succeeded in reaching the surface of the ovaries prior to ovulation. The hormonal function of the ovaries was first demonstrated in 1896 by the German biologist Knauer, who showed that ovarian grafts in the dog would prevent the uterine atrophy which follows castration. It was next observed by Marshall and Jolly that the ovarian secretion which produced estrus differed from that which was formed by the corpus luteum. The presence of estrogens in the follicles was proved by R. T. Frank, and their occurrence in urine was established by Allen and Doisy, who demonstrated the effectiveness of potent urinary extracts in producing estrus in the vaginal mucosa of rodents. This relatively simple biological assay method became of incomparable help in the isolation and synthesis of estrogenic compounds. In 1929 Butenandt and Doisy and associates isolated estrone in a crystalline form from human pregnancy urine. In 1930 estriol was identified by Browne in human placenta, and in 1936 MacCorquodale obtained estradiol, the most potent natural estrogen, from ovarian follicular fluid. The progestational activity of the corpus luteum hormone was first demonstrated by Corner and Allen in 1929. Five years later progesterone was isolated and identified, simultaneously and independently, by Butenandt, Allen, Slotta, and Hartmann.

Physiology. The human ovaries possess three closely interrelated functions: (1) as a result of secretion of estrogenic hormone the ovaries are responsible for the maturation and maintenance of the genitalia and secondary sexual characteristics; (2) they produce ova which are capable of fertilization by the spermatozoa of the male; (3) the ovaries form the corpus luteum, a highly specialized structure which appears after ovulation and secretes the second ovarian hormone, progesterone. It is this hormone which, along with estrogen, periodically prepares the endometrium for the reception and nourishment of a fertilized ovum. In the event that fertilization takes place, the ovarian secretion loses its cyclic character and becomes continuous. Thereby the endometrium is maintained in a state suitable for nourishment of the ovum until the latter has developed to the point where the trophoblast itself begins to secrete estrogen and progesterone. All three functions of the ovary are dependent upon a delicately maintained balance between the hypothalamus, the gonadotropins of the anterior pituitary, and the hormones of the ovaries.

The manifestations of ovarian estrogen secretion first make their appearance about the age of ten with the development of budding of the nipples and breasts and growth of the bony pelvis. There follows in gradual fashion the growth of pubic hair, thickening and cornification of the vaginal epithelium, and growth of the external and internal genitalia. Pigmentation of the nipples and axillary hair growth are next to appear, and finally, about the

age of thirteen, menstruation begins. The menstrual flow consists of endometrial cells, secretions, and blood. It lasts 3 to 7 days, occurs approximately every 4 weeks, and brings to a conclusion a regularly occurring series of changes in the uterine mucosa. These changes are the reflections of cyclic fluctuations in ovarian estrogen and progesterone secretion. At first the menstrual periods are irregular and anovulatory, but by the middle teens, when full sexual maturation has taken place, ovulation and menstruation are occurring at regular intervals. All these signs of sexual maturation are maintained through the reproductive period into the forties, when estrogen production diminishes, ovulation and progesterone production cease, and menstruation, after a period of irregularity, gradually disappears. This is the menopause. Thereafter, regressive changes in the breasts and genitalia slowly evolve.

Of the large number of follicles present at puberty, the vast majority degenerate either as primitive follicles or at various stages of development (atretic follicles). With each menstrual cycle many follicles begin to mature, but only one "favored follicle" reaches full maturity, penetrates the surface of the ovary, and discharges its ovum into the peritoneal cavity. This phenomenon, ovulation, occurs approximately 2 weeks prior to the onset of menstrual flow. The ovum then finds its way into the fallopian tube and thence is carried to the uterine cavity. There, within a few days, it disintegrates unless it has been fertilized in transit, in which case it implants itself within the uterine mucosa. Following ovulation the ruptured follicle is transformed into the corpus luteum, a richly vascularized body composed of progesterone- and estrogen-secreting cells. This body reaches maturity about 1 week before the next menstrual period, then, over the course of weeks to months, gradually involutes to a tiny scar (the corpus albicans). If the previously discharged ovum has been fertilized and pregnancy has occurred, the corpus luteum does not regress but becomes larger. This "corpus luteum of pregnancy" continues to secrete progesterone and estrogen until the second half of gestation, when involution occurs in the usual way.

The maturation of the graafian follicle is dependent upon the anterior pituitary follicle-stimulating hormone (FSH) (Fig. 73-1). This hormone stimulates the growth of the granulosa cells and the production of follicular fluid which surrounds the ovum. Along with the luteinizing hormone (LH or ICSH) FSH induces the cells of the theca interna to secrete estrogens. Estrogen secretion increases rapidly during the week prior to ovulation, maintains a plateau over the ensuing 2 weeks, and diminishes rapidly just before menstruation. The increased estrogen secretion is responsible for the proliferative changes which occur in the endome-

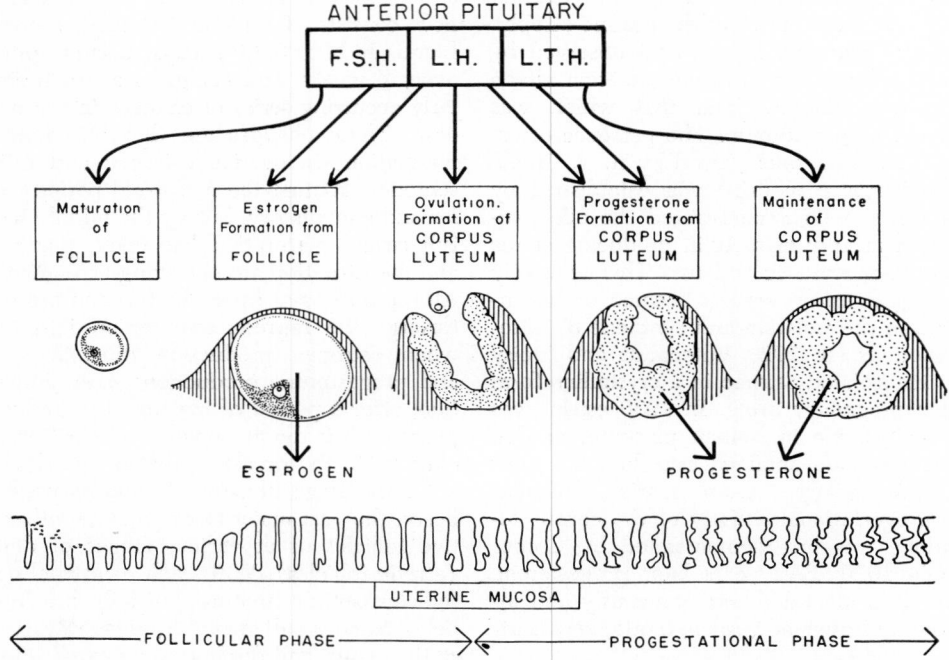

ANTERIOR PITUITARY

| F.S.H. | L.H. | L.T.H. |

| Maturation of FOLLICLE | Estrogen Formation from FOLLICLE | Ovulation. Formation of CORPUS LUTEUM | Progesterone Formation from CORPUS LUTEUM | Maintenance of CORPUS LUTEUM |

ESTROGEN   PROGESTERONE

UTERINE MUCOSA

←————FOLLICULAR PHASE————→|←————PROGESTATIONAL PHASE————→

FIG. 73-1. Semidiagrammatic representation of the relation of anterior pituitary gonadotropic hormones to ovarian and uterine changes during the menstrual cycle in normal women.

trium during the first half of the menstrual cycle. The phenomena of ovulation and transformation of the remaining follicular cells into the corpus luteum are dependent upon the secretion of luteinizing hormone alone. In conjunction with LH, a third anterior pituitary hormone, LTH (luteotropin or prolactin), stimulates the corpus luteum to secrete progesterone. Progesterone secretion reaches a peak about the middle of the luteal phase, then gradually falls to low levels just prior to menstruation. The increased progesterone secretion is reflected in secretory changes which take place in the endometrium during the last half of the menstrual cycle. If fertilization occurs and pregnancy ensues, luteotropin continues to maintain the corpus luteum through the first few months of the gestation period. In this action LTH is aided by the placental secretion of chorionic gonadotropin.

OVARIAN HORMONES

Ovarian hormones are steroids. The *estrogens* (Fig. 73-2) are characterized chemically by the presence of a benzene ring and a phenolic hydroxyl group which makes them soluble in alkali, a property used in their chemical separation from the adrenal cortical steroids. Estradiol is the principal and most potent estrogen secreted by the human ovary. In the liver it is in part transformed to the less potent estrogens, estrone and estriol. All three

steroids circulate in the blood and are excreted in the bile and urine largely as conjugates with glucuronic and sulfuric acids. The process of conjugation takes place in the liver. Estriol is the principal estrogen found in urine. It should be emphasized, however, that only a small proportion of the estradiol secreted by the human ovary has been accounted for by the metabolites described. Some 11 different urinary metabolites of estradiol have now been isolated from human urine, mostly in small quantities. The estrogenic effects involved in the process of sexual maturation have already been discussed. In addition, small doses of estrogen will stimulate pituitary gonadotropin, principally LH, secretion. Large doses of estrogen inhibit pituitary gonadotropins and cause sodium, calcium, phosphorus, nitrogen, and water retention. Undesirable side effects of estrogen administration include painful breasts, uterine bleeding, nausea, and vomiting. The salt and water retention observed with large doses of estrogens may precipitate or aggravate cardiac failure. The potential carcinogenic effect of these substances requires that one be alert to the development of cancer in the breasts and genital tracts of women on long-term estrogen therapy.

Progesterone (Fig. 73-3) bears a striking chemical resemblance to the adrenal cortical steroids. It is largely degraded in the liver, and a small fraction appears in the urine as the inactive pregnanediol glucuronide. The major metabolites of proges-

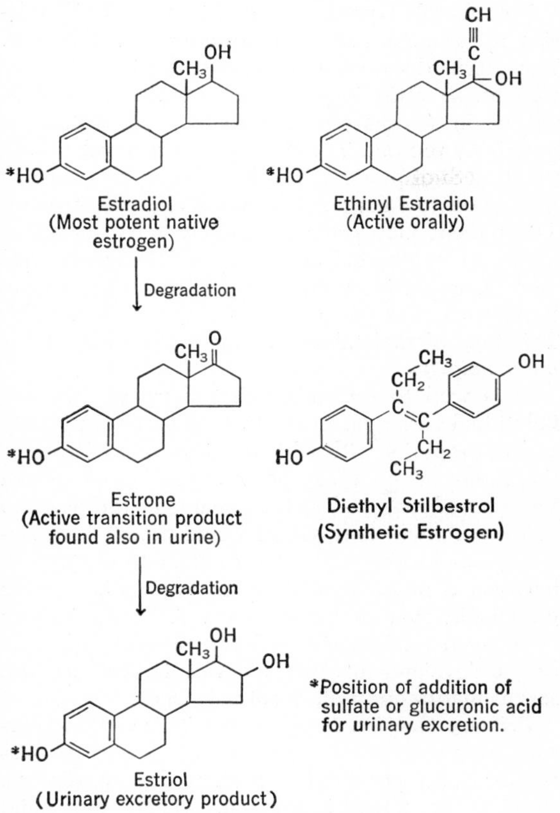

FIG. 73-2. Common estrogens.

terone are unknown. In addition to its effect on the endometrium, progesterone decreases uterine motility and activates the secretory tissue of the breast. No undesirable side effects accompany progesterone administration. Such is not the case, however, for the synthetic progestational compounds 17α-ethynyl-19-nortestosterone (Norlutin) and its $\Delta^{5(10)}$ isomer, norethynodrel (Enovid). The administration of these substances during pregnancy may result in masculinization of the female fetus.

MEASUREMENT OF PITUITARY-OVARIAN ENDOCRINE FUNCTION

Estrogens. The chemical and biological methods presently available for the assay of urinary estrogens are hampered by the relatively small quantities present in the urine of the nonpregnant female. A gross and indirect estimate of estrogen secretion may be obtained from examination of an endometrial biopsy or vaginal smear. The absence of cornification in the latter specimen indicates marked diminution of estrogen production.

Progesterone. Once progesterone secretion has been detected by any procedure, it may be assumed that ovulation has occurred and a corpus

luteum has formed. Adequate progesterone production is indicated by the presence of 5 to 10 mg pregnanediol glucuronide in a 24-hr urine collection during the second half of the menstrual cycle. A further indication of progesterone activity is the finding of secretory changes in an endometrial biopsy, which is preferably taken a few days prior to the expected onset of menstruation or soon after the beginning of uterine bleeding. A daily basal temperature record which reveals an abrupt rise of approximately 1°F in the middle of the menstrual cycle suggests the presence of a functioning corpus luteum. Vaginal smears are not reliable for the detection of progesterone secretion.

Gonadotropins. An estimate of the follicle-stimulating hormone (FSH) activity in urine may be made by the measurement of the ability of urine extracts to produce uterine growth in mice. Normal values in women during the reproductive period range from 10 to 50 mouse units. High levels are found in primary ovarian insufficiency and diminished levels in secondary ovarian insufficiency. No clinically feasible methods for the determination of blood or urinary LH and LTH activity are currently available. The male frog test and the Aschheim-Zondek and Friedman tests for pregnancy are based on the ability of urinary chorionic gonadotropin to produce spermatozoa in the frog and hemorrhagic ovarian follicles in the mouse and rabbit, respectively.

OVARIAN PREPARATIONS FOR CLINICAL USE

Four types of *estrogenic substances* are available (Fig. 73-2):

1. The naturally occurring estrogens related to estradiol. These include estrone, estradiol, and its long-acting esters, estradiol benzoate and dipropionate. These substances are less active by mouth than by injection. They may be used as solutions in oil for intramuscular use. Estrone sulfate isolated from pregnant mare's urine may be given orally and does not induce gastric irritation. This prepa-

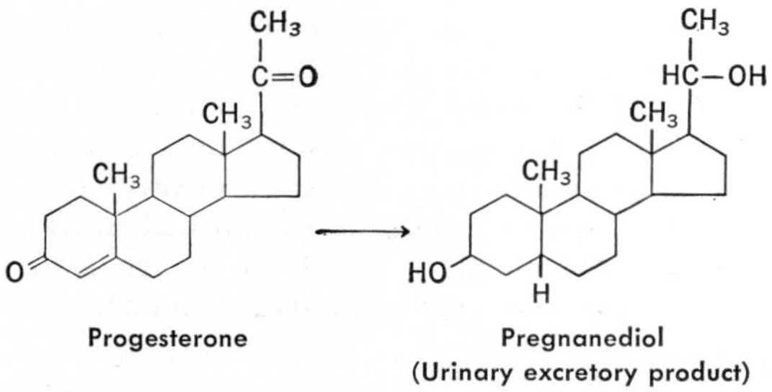

FIG. 73-3. Progesterone and its principal urinary metabolite.

ration is administered in doses ranging from 0.625 to 5 mg per day.

2. The synthetic ethynyl derivative of estradiol may be given by mouth. It may occasionally produce nausea. The dose of this compound is 0.05 to 0.2 mg per day.

3. Synthetic estrogens made up of two aromatic rings joined by a short aliphatic chain are also available. The most commonly used preparation is diethylstilbestrol. This is potent by mouth, but occasionally it causes nausea. The dose ranges from 0.5 to 2.0 mg per day.

4. A synthetic compound having a prolonged action, tri-para-anisylchloro-ethylene (TACE), may be given by mouth in daily doses of 12 to 24 mg.

Progesterone may be given by intramuscular injection in oil in doses ranging from 5 to 50 mg per day. An oral preparation, anhydrohydroxyprogesterone, is administered in doses of 20 to 100 mg per day. Two synthetic progestational compounds, 17-α-ethynyl-19-nortestosterone (Norlutin) and its $\Delta^{5(10)}$ isomer norethynodrel (Enovid) which also contains ethynyl estradiol, may be given orally in doses of 5 to 20 mg per day. As previously noted, some of the synthetic progestational compounds, if given during pregnancy, may bring about masculinization of the female fetus.

DISEASES OF THE OVARY

The diseases discussed in this section are associated with disturbances in the secretion of ovarian hormones. Such disturbances may occur as the result of disease in the ovaries themselves or may be due to hypothalamic or pituitary disorders which alter gonadotropin secretion. Such hypothalamic or pituitary conditions lead to changes in ovarian hormone secretion because both ovaries are secondarily involved. In contrast, not all forms of primary ovarian disease are accompanied by an endocrine disturbance. A number of congenital, inflammatory, cystic, degenerative, and neoplastic diseases of the ovary may cause no endocrine disorder when the lesion is confined to one ovary and the uninvolved gonad is capable of maintaining adequate hormone secretion. In certain instances, however, unilateral ovarian disease does lead to endocrine disturbances, as in the case of the hormone-producing tumors. These disorders are characterized by increased, rather than decreased, hormone production.

Conditions which cause disturbances in ovarian hormone secretion may be conveniently divided into those which result in diminished secretion (ovarian hypofunction) and those which lead to excessive secretion (ovarian hyperfunction).

Ovarian Hypofunction

The manifestations of this state differ according to whether it is present before or after puberty.

Prepuberal Hypofunction. In prepuberal ovarian hypofunction sexual maturation fails to occur. The uterus does not enlarge, and the infantile cervicouterine ratio is preserved. Menstruation does not begin (primary amenorrhea), and sterility is invariably present. The breasts do not develop, and the growth of pubic and axillary hair is sparse. The pelvis fails to enlarge. Osteoporosis may be present. The patient may grow excessively tall because of failure of epiphyseal union. In addition there may be a disproportion between the extremities and the trunk such that the arm span exceeds the height. This type of skeletal development is referred to as *eunuchoidism.*

It is well to remember that there are marked individual variations in the time of onset of puberty and the rapidity with which it develops. Menstruation in normal girls may begin at any time between the ages of nine and sixteen years. In the absence of menstruation and sexual development in a sixteen-year-old girl, it is often difficult to distinguish between a physiologic delay in maturation and a pathologic ovarian insufficiency. A family history of delayed adolescence and the presence of some breast development are favorable indications that sexual maturation will eventually occur.

Primary Ovarian Insufficiency. This condition results from congenital hypoplasia or absence of ovaries or from postnatal castration due to disease, surgery, or x-ray irradiation. When the child reaches the age of puberty, pituitary gonadotropins are released but there is little or no ovarian tissue to respond. Consequently estrogen and progesterone secretion is diminished to absent, and, from the time of puberty onward, urinary gonadotropin excretion is high.

GONADAL DYSGENESIS (TURNER'S SYNDROME) (See Chap. 46). In this condition the "ovaries" consist of a fibrotic streak or chord in each broad ligament. Examination of nuclei in skin biopsies, smears of buccal mucosa, and leukocytes has shown that approximately 80 per cent of cases have chromatin-negative (male pattern) nuclear sex. Furthermore, such cases have an XO sex-chromosome constitution with no Y chromosome and a diploid number of 45. Patients with gonadal dysgenesis show signs of estrogen deficiency: infantile female genitalia, primary amenorrhea, lack of breast development, and osteoporosis. Axillary and pubic hair usually develop normally though their appearance may be somewhat delayed. Rarely androgenic manifestations such as hirsutism and clitoral enlargement may be present; these findings have been attributed to the presence of androgen-secreting hilus cells in the ovarian anlagen. The condition of gonadal dysgenesis is usually associated with shortness of stature and multiple congenital abnormalities. The commonest of these are short metacarpals, cubitus valgus, eye disorders, webbing of the neck, shield-like chest, coarctation of the aorta, and lymphedema of the extremities. The appearance of the patient is often sufficient to suggest the diagnosis.

These patients should receive continuous estrogen replacement therapy from the chronologic age of puberty. Estrogen may be given as diethylstilbestrol in doses of 0.5 to 2 mg daily. The therapy should be administered cyclically, with 3 weeks of treatment followed by 1 week of rest, whether or not withdrawal bleeding occurs. On this therapy sexual maturation is achieved, but sterility, of course, remains.

CASTRATION. This condition may occur as the result of surgery, x-ray sterilization, and tuberculosis, or in rare instances, it may be a sequela of brucellosis or mumps. Individuals with this condition are of normal or increased height. Some exhibit normal body proportions, while others are eunuchoid. The signs of estrogen deficiency are present. Treatment is as described for gonadal dysgenesis.

Secondary Ovarian Insufficiency. This condition results from diseases which directly or indirectly affect the hypothalamus or anterior pituitary in a manner which interferes with gonadotropin secretion. Thus, in contrast to patients with the primary type of ovarian insufficiency, patients with the secondary type show low rather than high urinary gonadotropin excretion.

HYPOTHALAMIC INFANTILISM. Ovarian insufficiency occurring in association with destructive lesions of the hypothalamus and with congenital conditions such as the Laurence-Moon-Biedl syndrome has been described previously (see Chap. 64, Diseases of the Anterior and Intermediate Lobes of the Pituitary Gland).

GENERAL METABOLIC DISTURBANCES ASSOCIATED WITH OVARIAN INSUFFICIENCY. Conditions such as obesity, chronic malnutrition, diabetes mellitus, nephrosis, and chronic renal failure may be associated with a failure of sexual maturation presumably because of interference with hypothalamic or anterior pituitary function. Successful treatment of the primary condition is usually followed by normal sexual development.

HYPOPITUITARISM. Hypopituitarism occurring in the prepuberal period is most commonly due to the presence of a craniopharyngioma. Rarely the condition may result from trauma or inflammatory disease. Under these conditions there may be a selective deficiency of gonadotropin secretion or varying degrees of the full picture of panhypopituitarism with thyroid, adrenal, ovarian, and growth hormone insufficiency (see Chap. 64).

THE ADRENOGENITAL SYNDROME. The most common adrenal disease of childhood is congenital adrenal cortical hyperplasia with increased androgen secretion. In females this condition leads to pseudo-hermaphroditism and failure of sexual maturation. The ovarian insufficiency is believed to be due to the inhibitory effect of the adrenal androgens on gonadotropin secretion. Cortisone therapy usually induces normal sexual maturation (see Chap. 68, Diseases of the Adrenal Cortex).

Postpuberal Hypofunction. The characteristic symptoms of ovarian insufficiency which is due to a condition arising after puberty are amenorrhea (secondary amenorrhea) and sterility. These may be the *only* clinical manifestations. Gradually the ovarian hormone deficiency leads to hypoplasia of the sex organs and loss of secondary sex characteristics without, however, a regression to the immature state. Eunuchoidism does not occur if normal skeletal development has preceded the onset of the ovarian insufficiency. Osteoporosis will appear only when the condition has been of long duration.

Primary Ovarian Insufficiency. FEMALE CLIMACTERIC OR MENOPAUSE. This state has its onset, in the majority of instances, between the ages of forty-five and fifty-five years. Commonly there is a progressive irregularity in the frequency, duration, and amount of menstrual flow until finally amenorrhea ensues. Persistent metrorrhagia, or a recurrence of bleeding after a period of amenorrhea, in a woman of menopausal age requires careful investigation and must be considered to be due to uterine or ovarian neoplasm until proved otherwise. Along with the disappearance of menstruation at the climacteric a more gradual regressive change in the uterus, vagina, and breasts occurs. Pubic and axillary hair tend to become sparse, and after some time osteoporosis may become evident. Mild hirsutism, usually confined to the face, is not infrequent. In keeping with the view that the menopausal state is a type of primary ovarian insufficiency, one finds a high urinary gonadotropin excretion.

Certain vasomotor and nervous symptoms may accompany the menopausal changes just described. These include periodic feelings of warmth in the face, neck, and upper thorax ("hot flushes"). Less frequently, sudden surges of heat involve the whole body and are accompanied by drenching sweats ("hot flashes"). There may be nervousness and irritability, fatigability, and lassitude. While these symptoms appear in many women at the climacteric, in only a small proportion are they of a marked degree or more than a few months in duration. Most patients with climacteric symptoms respond well to simple psychotherapy and the administration of mild sedatives. These measures should always be employed first before hormonal substitution therapy is considered. Estrogen treatment is reserved for a relatively small group of patients whose distress is not relieved by the simple measures described. Diethylstilbestrol, in an initial dose of 0.5 mg per day, or equivalent doses of other estrogen preparations may be given cyclically, with 3 weeks of treatment followed by 1 week of rest. Once benefit is achieved, the hormone dose may be lowered to that which maintains relief. Estrogen should not be used indefinitely, however, in these patients. It is suggested that after a period of 3 to 6 months the hormone be gradually withdrawn. The treatment of postmenopausal osteoporosis is discussed in Chap. 78.

PREMATURE CLIMACTERIC. The spontaneous onset of the climacteric before the age of forty is regarded as premature. Treatment is as described for the normal climacteric, except that estrogens are more frequently required and in somewhat larger doses (initial dose of diethylstilbestrol, 1 to 2 mg per day). The estrogen therapy is usually maintained until the early forties, when it is gradually withdrawn. It is important to continue cyclic estrogen therapy up to the normal menopausal age in order to prevent premature onset of degenerative disease.

CASTRATION. Postpuberal castration may result from surgery, x-ray sterilization, or inflammatory disease. Treatment is as prescribed for premature climacteric.

Secondary Ovarian Insufficiency. In postpuberal ovarian insufficiency which is secondary to disturbances of the hypothalamus and anterior pituitary, the clinical picture is virtually the same as that seen in primary ovarian hypofunction. In two important respects, however, the two states differ. In the secondary type of the disease the vasomotor symptoms of the menopause do not occur, and there is a diminished rather than an excessive urinary gonadotropin excretion.

PSYCHOGENIC AMENORRHEA. Emotional disturbances are one of the most common causes of amenorrhea and sterility. Other signs of ovarian insufficiency, however, are usually absent. It is believed that emotional disorders induce amenorrhea through their influence on hypothalamic centers which control gonadotropin secretion. In these patients successful psychotherapy is usually followed by restoration of normal menstrual function.

GENERAL METABOLIC DISTURBANCES ASSOCIATED WITH OVARIAN INSUFFICIENCY. A number of metabolic disturbances may be accompanied by amenorrhea and sterility but rarely by any of the other signs of ovarian hypofunction. Such disorders include obesity, chronic malnutrition, diabetes mellitus, hyperthyroidism, and chronic renal disease. It is believed that the amenorrhea is due to a disturbance of hypothalamic or pituitary function. Successful treatment of the primary condition usually results in the reappearance of normal menstruation in these patients.

HYPOPITUITARISM. Hypopituitarism occurring in the postpuberal female is often due to pituitary necrosis associated with post-partum hemorrhage (Sheehan's syndrome). Less commonly the condition may be the result of pressure atrophy due to the presence of a pituitary tumor (chromophobe or eosinophil adenoma). Under these conditions there may be selective deficiency of gonadotropin secretion or the full picture of panhypopituitarism with thyroid, adrenal, and ovarian hypofunction (see Chap. 64, Diseases of the Anterior and Intermediate Lobes of the Pituitary Gland).

VIRILIZING SYNDROME. Bilateral hyperplasia or tumor of the adrenal cortex and such ovarian lesions as arrhenoblastoma and hilus cell tumor may produce masculinization and ovarian insufficiency as the result of excessive secretion of androgenic hormones. The ovarian hypofunction is believed to be the result of the inhibitory effect of androgens on gonadotropin secretion (see Chap. 68, Diseases of the Adrenal Cortex).

STEIN-LEVENTHAL SYNDROME. Another ovarian condition which may be associated with gonadal hypofunction is the *polycystic ovary syndrome* described by Stein and Leventhal. The etiology of this syndrome is obscure. It usually appears within the first 10 to 15 years after the menarche and is characterized clinically by amenorrhea and sterility, frequently by hirsutism, and occasionally by obesity. Pathologically there is enlargement of the ovaries (except in early cases) with a thick tunica albuginea, many follicular cysts and hyperplasia, and not infrequently luteinization, of the theca interna. Urinary 17-ketosteroid excretion is normal. Bilateral ovarian wedge resection frequently results in restoration of normal menstrual function. The hirsutism, however, is rarely ameliorated by this procedure. It should be noted that some patients with amenorrhea and "Stein-Leventhal ovaries" also have bilateral adrenal hyperplasia and increased 17-ketosteroid excretion. In this group of patients the menses may be restored and conception may occur following suppression of the adrenals with small doses of a glucocorticoid such as Prednisone, 2.5 mg three times a day.

Ovarian Hyperfunction

As with hypofunction, a state of hyperfunction in the ovary may be due to primary gonadal changes or may be secondary to alterations in hypothalamic or pituitary function. Ovarian hyperfunction may be said to be present when there is a premature appearance of ovarian hormone secretion (prepuberal hyperfunction) or when there is an excessive hormone secretion in adult life (postpuberal hyperfunction).

Prepuberal Hyperfunction. The early onset of *normal* (adult) ovarian hormone secretion leads to precocious puberty. In this syndrome there are the premature appearance of pubic and axillary hair, enlargement of the genitalia and breasts, periodic uterine bleeding, and rapid skeletal growth, but also premature closure of the epiphyses. Ovulation is present, and conception is possible. Precocious puberty is usually associated with hypothalamic disorders which prematurely initiate gonadotropin secretion.

The appearance of an *abnormal* quantity of ovarian hormone secretion in the prepuberal period leads to the syndrome of precocious pseudopuberty. In this syndrome, which is produced by granulosa cell tumors of the ovary, ovulation does not occur and only the signs of estrogen hypersecretion are present.

Constitutional Precocious Puberty. Precocious puberty which develops in the absence of demonstrable disease is said to be constitutional. This condition has been attributed to early maturation of the hypothalamic sex center.

Hypothalamic Precocious Puberty. Precocious puberty may develop in infants in whom there is involvement of the hypothalamus by tumors or cysts or by lesions which follow meningitis or encephalitis.

Albright's Disease. This congenital condition is a special form of polyostotic fibrous dysplasia. It is characterized by scattered fibrous bone cysts, brown pigmentation ("coast-of-Maine-shaped" *café au lait* spots) and precocious puberty in the female. The etiology of the condition is unknown (see Chap. 78).

Granulosa Cell Tumor of the Ovary. While the majority of granulosa cell tumors occur during the reproductive period and after the menopause, they may occasionally appear before puberty and, owing to their ability to form estrogens, they may give rise to the syndrome of precocious pseudopuberty (see below).

Choriocarcinoma (Chorionepithelioma) of the Ovary. This is an extremely rare type of teratoma which occurs in childhood. Its ability to secrete chorionic gonadotropin leads to stimulation of the normal ovarian tissue. The tumor itself may produce both estrogen and progesterone. The increased ovarian hormone secretion leads to a syndrome of precocious pseudopuberty (see below).

Postpuberal Hyperfunction—Abnormal Uterine Bleeding. The prime manifestation of postpuberal ovarian hyperfunction is abnormal uterine bleeding. No overt changes in the external genitalia or secondary sexual characteristics occur. The abnormal uterine bleeding may be represented by a reappearance of bleeding following a normal menopause or by changes in the menstrual cycle during the childbearing period. In the latter instance there may be metrorrhagia (frequent bleeding), menorrhagia (excessive bleeding), or both. There may be periods of amenorrhea irregularly interrupted by periods of uterine hemorrhage (metropathia hemorrhagica).

Table 73-1. CAUSES OF ABNORMAL UTERINE BLEEDING

General
    Abnormalities in blood coagulation
    Hypothyroidism
    Estrogen therapy

Local
    Pregnancy states—abortion, ectopic pregnancy
    Tumors of cervix and body of uterus
    Feminizing ovarian tumors
    Infections of uterus and adnexa
    Endometriosis
    Functional uterine bleeding

It is important to emphasize that abnormal uterine bleeding may be caused by a multitude of conditions, only a few of which are associated with ovarian hyperfunction (see Table 73-1). It is evident that abnormal menstrual flow during the active reproductive period or the reappearance of uterine bleeding following the menopause requires extremely thorough investigation. The causes of abnormal uterine bleeding which are associated with ovarian hyperfunction include the feminizing ovarian tumors, choriocarcinoma (chorionepithelioma) of the uterus, and "functional uterine bleeding." The *feminizing ovarian tumors* will be discussed below. *Choriocarcinoma of the uterus* may produce bleeding partly through its local effect, partly by virtue of its secretion of estrogen and progesterone, and also because of its elaboration of chorionic gonadotropin which stimulates ovarian estrogen secretion. The urinary excretion of this tropic hormone will give rise to a positive pregnancy test.

Three common gynecologic conditions with an endocrine background which must be considered in the differential diagnosis of abnormal uterine bleeding are midcycle bleeding, endometriosis, and leiomyoma of the uterus. *Midcycle bleeding* may occur at the time of ovulation. It is painful at times (mittelschmerz) and associated with light staining. No treatment is necessary. *Leiomyomas of the uterus* ("fibroids") develop during the childbearing period. Their growth is stimulated by estrogen. Further growth of these tumors ceases at the time of the menopause. Bleeding associated with leiomyomas occurs when the tumor involves the endometrium. Treatment is by myomectomy or hysterectomy, depending on the age of the patient.

Endometriosis is a disease of young women in which uterine mucosa may be found around the large bowel, the adnexa, and most commonly, the ovaries. The ectopic or metastatic endometrium frequently participates in the cyclic changes induced by ovarian hormones. Chocolate cysts are the characteristic lesions. Local irritation, intraabdominal hemorrhages, and adhesions may occur. In many patients there are no symptoms. When the latter occur, they include abdominal pain, dysmenorrhea, irregular menses, and infertility. Treatment is aimed at suppression of the cyclic changes in the mucosal implants or at removal of the ectopic endometrium. The former may be achieved with gradually increasing doses of norethynodrel and ethynyl estradiol (Enovid) to a limit of 50 mg per day over a period of 6 months. Such treatment suppresses ovarian function and leads to degeneration of the ectopic endometrial tissue. On withdrawal of therapy, prolonged palliation frequently results. Surgical treatment of endometriosis involves removal of implants, presacral neurectomy for relief of pain, and uterine suspension if retroversion is present. Sterilization by ovariectomy should be reserved for the most intractable cases.

Functional Uterine Bleeding. This condition is common but often transitory during the active reproductive period. It is physiologic at the extremes of this period, that is, for a short time following the menarche and just before the cessation of menstruation. Its exact etiology is not known. Whatever the cause may be, an anovulatory state frequently exists and there is a deficiency of progesterone in the presence of normal or elevated estrogen production. The abnormal pattern of hormone secretion may lead to menorrhagia, metrorrhagia, or metropathia hemorrhagica. The diagnosis of functional uterine bleeding should be made only after the other causes of abnormal uterine bleeding have been carefully eliminated (see Table 73-1). There are two aims in the treatment of functional uterine bleeding. Of first importance is the control of excessive blood loss. Secondly, it is hoped, particularly in the young adult female, to restore normal menstrual function and fertility. Functional uterine bleeding which is mild in degree and of short duration requires no therapy; the condition is frequently temporary, and normal menstrual periods may soon be resumed. When bleeding is more severe or prolonged, the curettage, which is carried out to exclude other causes of uterine bleeding, is not infrequently followed by restoration of normal menstrual function. When this procedure fails, medical therapy should first be tried. Progestational agents alone may be administered as progesterone in oil, 50 mg in a single intramuscular injection, or as Norlutin or Enovid, 10 mg by mouth daily for 7 days. The course of progesterone is repeated every 4 weeks for a period of 3 to 4 months. Occasionally following such a regimen, normal menstrual periods are resumed. When progesterone alone is unsuccessful in controlling the excessive bleeding, the patient may be given cyclical estrogen and progesterone therapy. The estrogen may be administered as diethylstilbestrol, 0.5 to 1 mg by mouth per day for a 3-week period, followed by a course of progesterone as described above. At the end of the period of withdrawal bleeding, the course of treatment is resumed and repeated cyclically over a period of 3 to 4 months. Prolonged functional uterine bleeding results in iron deficiency, not always demonstrable by hematocrit or red cell count alone, and may be cured in some cases by restoration of normal body stores of iron. Only when medical treatment has failed to control a prolonged and excessive blood loss should surgical treatment be considered. The surgical procedure of choice is hysterectomy without removal of the ovaries. This operation is preferable to simple sterilization by ovariectomy since the chief focus of symptoms may be removed without the loss of secondary sexual characteristics or the appearance of menopausal symptoms.

Functional Neoplasms of the Ovary

A list of ovarian tumors which may be useful in the differential diagnosis of ovarian masses is shown in Table 73-2. Relatively few of these tumors secrete hormones. They may produce androgens or estrogens, occasionally progesterone, and very rarely chorionic gonadotropin. The uncommon struma ovarii may secrete thyroid hormone.

Feminizing Tumors. Feminizing ovarian tumors when they occur in the prepuberal period give rise to the syndrome of precocious pseudopuberty. In the adult female little change in secondary sexual characteristics results. When the tumors develop prior to the menopause there is commonly excessive uterine bleeding, though occasionally amenor-

Table 73-2. NEOPLASMS OF THE OVARY

Tumors arising from coelomic epithelium (vaginal, endocervical, endometrial, endosalpingial)	Tumors arising because of continuity
Cystadenoma (endometrioma, endosalpingioma, adenoma, fibroadenoma)	Adrenal cell* Kidney cell (hypernephroma) Mesonephroma Brenner (renal pelvis, ureter, or urethra)
Papillary cystadenoma Malignant papillary cystadenoma Solid carcinoma	*Tumors arising from ova*
Tumors arising from primitive mesenchyme	Teratoma, chorionepithelioma,* struma* Dermoid cyst
Arrhenoblastoma* Granulosa cell, theca cell* Hilus cell* Luteoma* Dysgerminoma Fibroma Sarcoma	*Metastatic tumors* From uterus (endometrial) From stomach (Krukenberg) From intestine (small or large), eye, rectum, breast, bile duct, etc.

* Only these seven are endocrinologically active.
SOURCE: Modified from J. V. Meigs: New Engl. J. Med., 228:53, 1943.

rhea is observed. Sterility is present. In the post-menopausal female, feminizing ovarian tumors are associated with a reappearance of uterine bleeding. Surgical removal of these tumors leads to disappearance of the signs of feminization.

Granulosa Cell Tumor. These are the most common hormone-producing tumors, comprising about 10 per cent of all solid ovarian neoplasms. They are usually unilateral, often cystic, and not infrequently malignant. The uninvolved ovary is atrophied, presumably because of pituitary inhibition, by the high level of circulating estrogen arising from this type of tumor. The incidence of uterine leiomyoma and adenocarcinoma is increased. While pure granulosa cell tumors have been occasionally encountered, commonly a mixture of granulosa and theca cells is found. These cells may rarely secrete progesterone as well as estrogen. The majority of the tumors are found after the menopause, but they may appear during the reproductive period and before puberty. The clinical picture has been described above. Biopsy of the uterine mucosa usually reveals a proliferative endometrium, though occasionally secretory changes are observed. Urinary assays show increased estrogen but decreased gonadotropin excretion. Surgical therapy is the treatment of choice. In premenopausal patients with a well-encapsulated unilateral tumor, the affected ovary is removed but the uterus and opposite ovary may be left intact. If there is evidence of malignancy, a radical pelvic dissection is performed. The latter procedure is recommended for the postmenopausal patient because of the higher incidence of recurrence and of associated uterine cancer. Postoperative radiotherapy should be used when the tumor is malignant.

Theca Cell Tumor (Thecoma). Pure theca cell tumors are rare. They are almost always unilateral, usually solid, and seldom malignant. The average age incidence is similar to that of granulosa cell tumors. Theca cell tumors, however, are uncommon during the reproductive period and extremely rare in infancy. The clinical picture, laboratory findings, and therapy are as described for granulosa cell tumors.

Luteoma. When all or the greater portion of an ovarian tumor is transformed into luteal tissue, the tumor is known as a *luteoma.* Luteomas which are accompanied by a syndrome of feminization are believed to represent luteinization in a granulosa cell or theca cell tumor. Treatment, therefore, is as described for these tumors.

Choriocarcinoma (Chorionepithelioma) of the Ovary. This is an extremely rare tumor, a type of teratoma, which may be found in the ovaries of prepuberal females. It is highly malignant. Its ability to secrete chorionic gonadotropin, estrogen, and progesterone leads to the syndrome of preco-cious pseudopuberty. An ovarian mass in conjunction with a positive pregnancy test in a prepuberal female may suggest the diagnosis. Treatment consists of radical pelvic surgery followed by chemotherapy, methotrexate or vincoleucoblastin. It should be noted that in the adult female choriocarcinoma of the uterus frequently metastasizes to the ovaries.

Masculinizing Tumors. The manifestations of masculinizing ovarian tumors may vary from a mild increase of facial hair to a full picture of virilization with generalized hirsutism, loss of scalp hair, acne, muscularity, deepening of the voice, atrophy of breasts and uterus, amenorrhea, and sterility. The urinary 17-ketosteroid excretion is often normal and only rarely very high. Hence, the finding of normal urinary 17-ketosteroids in a patient with masculinization does not exclude the presence of an ovarian tumor. Surgical removal of such tumors is followed by the disappearance of most of the clinical manifestations. Not infrequently, however, the hirsutism is unaffected or only slightly diminished. It is important to emphasize that virilization in the adult female is only rarely due to a functioning ovarian tumor. The differential diagnosis and management of the syndrome of masculinization have been discussed previously (see Chap. 68, Diseases of the Adrenal Cortex).

Arrhenoblastoma. This uncommon tumor is believed to arise from male-directed embryonic rests in the ovary. It is usually unilateral and only rarely malignant. The tumor is commonly solid, though occasionally cystic degeneration may be observed. The uninvolved ovary is often atrophied, presumably because of inhibition, by high circulating androgen levels of pituitary gonadotropin secretion. Microscopically there are strands of primitive cells arranged in adenomatous formation, in cords or in tubules. Interstitial cells resembling testicular Leydig cells can often be identified. The arrhenoblastoma is found predominantly during the reproductive period. It occasionally occurs beyond the menopause. No patient under sixteen years of age has been known to develop this tumor. Signs of masculinization are found in association with a pelvic mass and a normal or slightly elevated urinary 17-ketosteroid excretion. In younger patients simple removal of the ovary and tube on the affected side is sufficient. In older women, particularly if they are past the menopause, hysterectomy and removal of the adnexa on both sides are advised because of the greater incidence of malignancy at this later age.

Hilus Cell (Leydig Cell) Hyperplasia or Adenoma. Characteristic cells, indistinguishable from testicular Leydig cells, have been found in the hilus of the normal ovary. On very rare occasions these cells may show hyperplasia or adenomatous formation and give rise to a syndrome of virilization. The hyperplastic tissue may be bilateral and large in size; the tumors are usually small and confined to one ovary. The urinary 17-ketosteroid excretion may be normal or slightly increased. Treatment is surgical removal.

Miscellaneous Masculinizing Tumors. Rare tumors, variously described as adrenal-like tumors, luteomas, masculinovoblastomas, and virilizing lipoid cell tumors have been described in association with a syndrome of virilization. The confusion regarding the cellular origin of these tumors arises from difficulty of distinguishing between proliferating adrenocortical and luteal cells. These tumors may be highly malignant. Urinary 17-ketosteroid levels are usually increased. Treatment consists of surgical removal.

Struma Ovarii. Struma ovarii is an extremely rare type of ovarian teratoma in which the predominant tissue is thyroid. These tumors are unilateral and usually benign. Hyperthyroidism may be present as a result of excessive production of thyroid hormone. Treatment is surgical removal.

REFERENCES

Ferguson-Smith, M. A.: Cytogenetics in Man, A.M.A. Arch. Internal Med., 105:159, 1960.

Grumbach, M. M., and M. L. Barr: Cytological Tests of Chromosomal Sex in Relation to Sexual Abnormalities in Man, Recent Progr. Hormone Research, 14:255, 1958.

Katzman, P.: Metabolism of Steroids, Ann. Rev. Biochem., 28:257, 1959.

Morris, J. Mc., and R. E. Scully: "Endocrine Pathology of the Ovary," St. Louis, The C. V. Mosby Company, 1958.

Pincus, G.: The Physiology of Ovarian and Testis Hormones, vol. III in "Hormones: Physiology, Chemistry and Applications," G. Pincus and K. V. Thimann (Eds.), New York, Academic Press, Inc., 1955.

Sohval, A. R.: Physiology of the Ovary, in "Diseases of the Endocrine Glands," 2d ed., L. J. Soffer (Ed.), Philadelphia, Lea & Febiger, 1956.

Wilkins, L.: "The Diagnosis and Treatment of Endocrine Disorders in Childhood and Adolescence," 2d ed., Springfield, Ill., Charles C Thomas, Publisher, 1957.

74 DISEASES OF THE BREAST
Kendall Emerson, Jr.

History. The earliest description of cancer of the breast, and probably of cancer in any form, is credited to the Egyptian physician Imhotep in 3000 B.C. and is recorded in the Edwin Smith Surgical Papyrus under Case number 39, "Bulging Tumor of the Breast." The gross anatomy of the lactating breast must have been familiar to the author of the Song of Solomon in the year 1014 B.C., who likened it to "a cluster of grapes." Aside from its obvious function of lactation, however, little was known about the mammary gland, and interest in it throughout the ages has been more esthetic and symbolic than scientific until the studies of Sir Astley Cooper in 1845 provided us with an adequate morphologic description of this organ and the first suggestion of its possible relationship to menstrual dysfunction. In the latter half of the nineteenth century the German investigators discovered that normal breast development in animals depended upon intact ovarian function, and in 1896 Sir George Beatson first demonstrated the inhibition of the growth of mammary cancer by oophorectomy in human beings. The role of the corpus luteum and pituitary in the development of the breasts has been brought to light during the present century by the works of L. Loeb, Gardner, Riddle, Corner, Turner, and many others.

CONGENITAL ANOMALIES

The occurrence of aberrant breast tissue (polymastia) and supernumerary nipples (polythelia) situated along the so-called milk line extending from the mid-clavicle to the inguinal ligament has been noted in art and legend since recorded time. One wonders if these anomalies may not have been more common when man was closer in evolution to his multiparous animal forebears, since the number of breasts allotted to each member of the animal kingdom is in proportion to the average size of its litter. Absence of one or both breasts (amastia) occurs very rarely but was recorded long ago by the aforementioned author of the Song of Solomon.

ENDOCRINE RELATIONSHIPS

The most comprehensive recent studies of the endocrine factors determining the growth and function of the mammary glands in rats are those of Lyons which are very briefly summarized here because they seem to support most of the observations in human beings. The development of the normal nonlactating breast is directly dependent upon the synergistic action of three major hormones: estrogens, pituitary growth hormone, and adrenal cortical steroids. Growth hormone alone will cause some growth of mammary ducts, whereas estrogens and adrenal hormones have no effect by themselves. Prolactin (luteotropic hormone, LTH) and progesterone are essential for the functional development of the alveolar lobules and the secretion of milk, whereas in the adult gland estrogens inhibit lactation by suppressing LTH activity. Prolactin with adrenal steroids is capable of inducing lactation in the absence of progesterone.

Following section of the pituitary stalk in patients with cancer of the breast, lactation has been observed to occur while at the same time the growth of cancer is suppressed. Stalk section has been shown to destroy at least 80 per cent of the cells of the anterior lobe of the pituitary (Ehni and Eckles, 1959). The effects of this procedure are interpreted, therefore, as indicating that the cells producing growth, adrenocortical and follicle stimulating hormones are destroyed and estrogen secretion is inhibited, all of which results in inhibition of the cancer growth. The cells secreting prolactin, however, are preserved and become activated following removal of inhibition by estrogen. Since these patients are provided with hydrocortisone replacement therapy, the stage is set for lactation to occur just as it does following removal of the placental source of estrogen at the termination of pregnancy. These considerations are of practical importance because it has been shown that the growth of breast cancer in man may be stimulated by estrogens and in some instances by human growth hormone (Pearson and Ray, 1959), although there is conflicting evidence on this point (Lipsett and Bergenstal, 1960). Such growth stimulation by progesterone, however, has not been demonstrated in human beings although it may occur under certain circumstances in strains of mice with a high hereditary tendency to develop cancer. It is also apparent that prolactin is not ordinarily a stimulant to the growth of human mammary cancer, but our knowledge is still too incomplete to say that this may never be so. The hormones of greatest clinical importance in relation to the breast in man are the estrogens.

Painful engorgement of the breasts may be seen as a transient phenomenon in newborn infants due to the high level of circulating estrogens of placental origin. The normal development of the female breast at puberty, which is sometimes accompanied by intermittent tenderness and edema, results from the rising level of circulating estrogens secreted by the maturing ovarian follicles just prior to the menarche. Precocious breast development may occur as a result of inherited or constitutional factors, of abnormal pituitary, ovarian, or adrenal activity associated with functional tumors or hyperplasia of these organs, or of locally irritating lesions such as tumors of the pineal or fourth ventricle, fibrous dysplasia of the bones of the base of the skull, as occurs in Albright's disease (polyostotic fibrous dysplasia), or rarely following viral encephalitis.

Gynecomastia occurs physiologically in normal males at puberty and may persist through adolescence. (In some animals such as the bat, the func-

tion of lactation is retained by the male who may assist his partner in suckling their young.) This breast enlargement usually subsides spontaneously, but if it presents a sufficiently serious psychologic problem simple mastectomy with preservation of the nipples is justified since any hormonal treatment is ineffective. Gynecomastia should always raise the suspicion of seminiferous tubule dysgenesis with fibrosis, a variant of Klinefelter's syndrome, in which there is usually an elevated urinary excretion of follicle-stimulating hormone and a female pattern of sex chromatin (see Chap. 72).

Marked degrees of breast development in adolescent males or the onset of gynecomastia in later life may indicate the presence of an estrogen secreting tumor of the adrenal. These tumors are usually associated with an elevation of the urinary 17-ketosteroids, the excretion of which is not further stimulated by ACTH or suppressed by adrenal steroids. Every effort should be made to locate such tumors by radiographic means and to remove them surgically because, though rare, a high percentage, if not all, are malignant.

Choriogenic tumors and more rarely interstitial cell, and granulosa cell tumors of the testes may produce gynecomastia. This condition is also seen in males with cirrhosis of the liver and in states of severe malnutrition, presumably in both instances due to failure of inactivation of circulating estrogens. It regularly follows iatrogenic administration of estrogenic compounds in the treatment of carcinoma of the prostate and even occasionally occurs during testosterone therapy in eunuchoidism. Transient gynecomastia occurs as a normal physiologic phenomenon in elderly men.

INFECTIOUS DISEASES

Acute pyogenic infections of the breast are largely confined to the first 2 months of lactation and usually involve the staphylococcus, less often a beta streptococcus. They should be prevented by proper hygiene and treated with appropriate antibiotics. Very rarely an acute mastitis may occur during the course of paratyphoid or typhoid fever, brucellosis, or mumps, unassociated with lactation.

Chronic tuberculous mastitis is a rarity today. It usually results from the extension of tuberculosis of the underlying bone into the breast tissue and should be suspected from the presence of multiple sinus tracts and the finding of active tuberculosis elsewhere.

INFLAMMATORY LESIONS

Mammary duct ectasia (Haagensen) is a benign condition usually seen in elderly women with atrophic breasts wherein the mammary ducts in or just beneath the nipple become dilated and filled with cellular debris and lipid-containing material. Intermittent pain and local inflammatory changes may be present, and because a discharge, at times bloody, and retraction of the nipple may occur, this condition must be differentiated from carcinoma. Excision of the nipple is usually indicated.

Fat necrosis is a common occurrence following trauma, which may be so slight as not to have been noticed. It presents as a painful lump usually associated with some ecchymosis and may be followed by local atrophy and dimpling of the skin, at which stage biopsy must be performed to distinguish it from carcinoma.

Sarcoid may very rarely involve the skin of the chest. Eosinophilic granuloma may occur in the submammary folds.

It must not be forgotten that carcinoma of the breast may rarely present as a subacute red, warm, indurated mass, resembling a bacterial cellulitis, the so-called "inflammatory carcinoma." This lesion may be suspected when the skin over it presents the characteristic *peau d'orange* appearance.

FIBROCYSTIC DISEASE

With each menstrual cycle there is a recurring biphasic stimulation first of proliferation of breast tissue by estrogens, then of alveolar secretory activity by progesterone, followed by a period of involution. In most women these changes are of such slight degree as to cause few if any clinical symptoms. Not infrequently, however, well-marked inflammatory changes may occur preceding each menses, with tenderness, engorgement, and increasing nodularity of the breasts. This is more often seen in nulliparous women and may subside after childbearing and lactation. Methyl testosterone 5 mg daily for 7 to 10 days before each menstrual period will often provide relief.

In the later years of reproductive life the continued recurrent stimulation and involution of the breasts in the course of each menstrual cycle may result in diffuse and nodular fibrosis and the formation of cysts of varying sizes, so-called chronic cystic mastitis. This condition can simulate carcinoma but is usually distinguishable by the fact that it is intermittently painful and may subside to some extent following menstruation. Nevertheless carcinoma may coexist and be masked by the diffuse nodularity of the cystic disease. Moreover, the incidence of mammary carcinoma is greater in patients with fibrocystic disease of the breasts, and it is unwise to delay biopsy of suspicious areas in the hope that they may subside by the end of the next menstrual cycle. In severe cases simple mastectomy is fully justified.

TUMORS OF THE BREAST

Benign fibroadenomas of the breast may occur at any age but are more common in women under the age of thirty. They may be distinguished from carcinomas by their mobility and well-defined margins, but biopsy is nonetheless imperative.

Benign intraductal papillomas may occur and cause a bloody discharge from the nipple. They are usually small and difficult to feel but may be located by noting that area of the breast on which pressure causes the bleeding. Excision is always advisable.

Sarcomas of all types make up less than 3 per cent of all breast tumors. Fibrosarcomas are the most frequent; lymphosarcomas occasionally originate in the breast. Liposarcomas and hemangiosarcomas have been reported rarely. Cystosarcoma phyllodes is a curious, very large, relatively rapidly appearing tumor arising usually from a preexisting fibroadenoma. It presents as a tender, warm, cystic mass often replacing the whole breast. The skin over it is thinned, and the superficial veins are dilated. The tumor consists of fibrous cords covered with epithelium arising from the duct system. The cords are separated by cystic areas which becomes filled with leaflike (phyllodes) projections of epithelial tissue. Although usually benign, blood-borne metastases have been reported, and surgical removal of the tumor is always indicated.

Carcinoma. Carcinoma of the breast is the most frequent malignant tumor to which the human female is subject and accounts for a greater number of deaths than any other single form of cancer in women. It occurs with increasing frequency from the age of twenty-five or thirty up to the menopause, when its incidence levels off until a second rise in frequency occurs after the age of sixty-five.

Etiology. In common with most forms of malignant disease, the etiology of breast cancer is not known. A few factors affecting its incidence are, however, reasonably well established. The very strong hereditary influence seen in mice can be carried over, though in a much smaller degree, to human beings. A two- to sevenfold increase in the familial incidence of the disease is reported. There is good evidence that the frequency of mammary cancer is inversely related to the number of children nursed, a fact which many modern pediatricians fail to realize. The role of the estrogenic hormones in the genesis of breast cancer in human beings has not yet been settled. The view most widely accepted at the present time is that estrogens do not initiate the cancer but may, nevertheless, hasten its development in genitically susceptible individuals. The prolonged use of these hormones, especially at or beyond the menopause, or in patients with a family history of cancer, should be discouraged.

Pathology. The primary site is usually in the ducts, less often in the alveoli. Multicentric origins are a frequent occurrence, and all gradations of differentiation may be observed. It is common to see a marked proliferation of dense connective tissue surrounding groups of malignant cells, whether primary or metastatic, the so-called scirrhous carcinoma. Unfortunately all degrees of differentiation may be found in different portions of the same tumor, and little prognostic value can be attached to the histologic appearance of any one area of such a malignancy.

Mammary carcinoma is prone to metastasize relatively early to the regional lymph nodes—axillary and supraclavicular if the primary site is in the outer half of the breast, the internal mammary chain if the disease arises in the inner quadrants of breast tissue. From thence spread occurs primarily to bone, lungs, liver, skin, and subcutaneous tissues generally, less frequently to the brain. Blood-borne metastases may occur even before lymphatic spread is clinically evident. It is interesting that there is a predilection for metastases to occur in the ovaries, adrenals, and pituitary—areas rich in the hormones stimulating the growth of this type of epithelial cell.

Diagnosis. The diagnosis of breast cancer is facilitated by the fact that it is possible to palpate directly this type of neoplasm, a procedure which should be done gently because of the possibility of spreading the disease. Unfortunately, the diffuse nodularity of the adult female breast makes it difficult to detect early lesions. As a rule the physician must depend on such evidence as hardness, fixation to underlying structures, or dimpling of the overlying skin to distinguish a malignant mass from a benign nodule of breast tissue, and by the time these distinguishing signs have become apparent the cancer has all too often metastasized. The majority of patients with breast cancer suggest the diagnosis themselves because of their ready detection of abnormal lumps or masses during self-examination. Although the procedure of periodic self-examination of the breasts may be decried as tending to encourage neuroticism and cancerphobia, it is the only practical way by which we can succeed in reducing the death rate from cancer of the breast until a final cure for cancer has been found.

Treatment. Total surgical excision provides the only permanent cure for carcinoma of the breast and x-ray therapy the best palliation for localized disease. The technical details of the surgical and radiologic treatment of breast cancer are beyond the scope of this chapter as is the controversy over radical versus simple mastectomy and extensive local irradiation, as advocated by McWhirter and others. Because of the susceptibility of breast cancer to changes in its endocrine environment, how-

ever, every physician should be cognizant of the remarkable palliative effect which can be achieved in inoperable mammary cancer by intelligent hormonal manipulations.

In considering appropriate therapy for metastatic breast cancer, it is convenient to divide the patients into four age groups which may be termed premenopausal, intramenopausal, postmenopausal, and senescent. The primary growth stimulant for the malignant mammary cell in the premenopausal and the majority of intramenopausal patients is the estrogens; it follows, therefore, that in these patients every effort should be made to remove all sources of these hormones. Oophorectomy or adequate x-ray castration will induce subjective and/or objective remissions in approximately 40 per cent of such patients, lasting from 4 months to more than 2 years. The addition of small doses of adrenal cortical hormones, such as prednisone 5 mg twice daily, has been advocated in order to prolong this remission by suppressing the compensatory synthesis of adrenal estrogens which follows ovarian ablation. There is increasing evidence that prophylactic castration and prednisone suppression at the time of mastectomy may significantly prolong the survival of those patients with metastases ostensibly confined to axillary lymph nodes.

When the regression following oophorectomy has ended, or if it fails to occur, prednisone in doses of 15 to 20 mg per day, or the equivalent amounts of other synthetic adrenal cortical steroids, may induce a very satisfactory remission in a significant number of cases. At this point bilateral adrenalectomy, as advocated by Huggins, or hypophysectomy, as first carried out by Olivacrona, should be seriously considered whenever adequate facilities are available. These procedures provide objective remissions in 40 to 50 per cent of patients in the early postmenopausal period and are more likely to be successful in patients who have previously responded favorably to oophorectomy or adrenal cortical hormones. Similarly successful results have been reported following hypophyseal stalk section or the transnasal implantation of yttrium 91 and other radioactive substances, as well as by proton beam bombardment of the pituitary. The usefulness of these procedures is obviously limited by the requirement of a cooperative team of skilled surgeons to carry out the procedures and conscientious internists to handle the subsequent hormone replacement problems of adrenal or pituitary insufficiency. When these facilities are not available, further benefit may be obtained from the use of androgens or pharmacologic doses of estrogens, as will be described below.

As ovarian activity wanes during the course of the menopause, the estrogens come to play a lesser role and other factors, some at least of pituitary origin, a more important one in stimulating the growth of breast cancer. There appears to be a small group of patients in this age group who may actually be adversely affected by oophorectomy perhaps because the secretion and stimulating activity of growth hormone or other pituitary factors on the cancer cell is enhanced by removal of estrogen inhibition. There is no way of predicting such a result in the present state of our knowledge, but fortunately it is a rare occurrence. Such patients may well be the ideal candidates for hypophyseal ablation, or sex hormone administration.

In the postmenopausal group, treatment must be individualized. Some patients may show continued ovarian activity even up to the age of seventy; a very high incidence of ovarian stromal hyperplasia, which is considered to be evidence of persistence of estrogen synthesis beyond the period of ovulation, has been observed among postmenopausal patients with mammary cancer. Such estrogen activity may be most easily detected by demonstrating the presence of more than 10 per cent of cornified cells in the vaginal smear stained by the Papanicolaou method. When present, oophorectomy is indicated and may produce dramatic remissions even in patients over the age of seventy years.

In the younger group of patients, less than 8 to 10 years postmenopausal, who show no such evidence of persistence of ovarian activity, as well as in those who have shown a remission following oophorectomy, hypophysectomy should be seriously considered if their disease is not too far advanced and the proper facilities for their management are available. Otherwise the use of androgens and estrogens may achieve a successful remission.

In the older postmenopausal patients and the senescent group, 15 years or more past the menopause, large doses of estrogens may provide remarkable palliation and is the treatment of choice. This paradoxic effect of estrogens, first clearly described by Nathanson, has never been fully explained.

The place of androgens and estrogens in the treatment of metastatic breast cancer has been well defined by the recent report of the American Medical Association's Council on Drugs, based on a 10-year nationwide cooperative study. In summary, androgens produced objective remissions in approximately 20 per cent of patients both before and after the menopause. Estrogens, which should not be used before the menopause, will induce remissions in about 36 per cent of patients during the first 8 postmenopausal years and in more than 38 per cent in later years. Estrogens have a greater relative effect on soft tissue and visceral metastases than on bone, but equal or exceed the effect of androgens on all types of tissue. It should be emphasized that estrogens must be employed in large doses to achieve these results, such as stilbestrol 15 mg or ethinyl estradiol 3 mg daily. Smaller amounts may adversely affect the tumor. Nausea and vomiting may occur at the onset of treatment but can be controlled by antiemetic agents and will disappear in time. Uterine bleeding may be troublesome but can usually be controlled by the cyclic administration of progesterone or methyl testosterone.

The optimum dose of androgens has been found to be equivalent to 100 mg of testosterone propionate given intramuscularly three times weekly. Recent experience indicates that the newer anabolic androgens such as fluoxymestrone in oral doses of 20 mg daily may be equally effective with much less tendency to produce the undesirable masculinizing side effects of testosterone.

All patients, but especially those within the first 8 postmenopausal years, should be observed carefully during the first few days and weeks of treatment because both androgens and estrogens may cause an exacerbation of their disease, estrogens by a direct stimulating effect and androgens presumably by being converted in small but effective amounts to estrogens. One of the most serious complications which can be produced by administration of these hormones in patients who exhibit extensive skeletal metastases is calcium intoxication. This is presumed to result from the sudden stimulation of growth of the bony metastases by the hormone, with correspondingly rapid destruction of bone and flooding of the circulation with calcium. There is a marked increase in urine calcium excretion, and the serum calcium level may rise to as high as 15 to 20 mg per 100 ml, and drowsiness, coma, convulsions, and death from renal failure may ensue. It is important to distinguish this condition from cerebral or liver metastases or the terminal effects of widespread cancer because it can be reversed by forcing fluids, withdrawal of the offending hormone, and administration of large amounts of hydrocortisone, 200 mg daily by slow intravenous drip or in divided oral doses daily, until symptoms subside.

Currently, extensive studies are being made of the value of carcinolytic chemical agents as adjuncts to other forms of therapy for mammary cancer. To date, definite and repeated regression of cutaneous and subcutaneous metastases have been observed following the use of thio-triethylene phosphoramid and 5-fluoro-uracil. Unfortunately, these effects are transient and the value of these agents is limited at present by their bone marrow toxicity.

Carcinoma occurs in the male breast at least 100 times less frequently than in the female. Otherwise it behaves in exactly the same manner. The treatment is the same except that orchiectomy replaces oophorectomy. Prednisone and hypophysectomy have both been shown to induce remissions when the primary disease has metastasized.

REFERENCES

Lyons, W. R., C. H. Li, and R. E. Johnson: Hormonal Control of Mammary Growth and Lactation, Recent Progr. Hormone Research, 14:219, 1958.

Haagensen, C. D.: "Diseases of the Breast," Philadelphia, W. B. Saunders Company, 1956.

Pincus, Gregory (Ed.): "Recent Progress in Hormone Research," New York, Academic Press, Inc., 1958.

Segaloff, Albert (Ed.): "Breast Cancer," The Second Biennial Louisiana Cancer Conference, St. Louis, The C. V. Mosby Company, 1958.

75 INFERTILITY
Melvin L. Taymor

Definition. Infertility may be defined as the inability to conceive during the course of normal sexual activity. It is generally held that a marriage should not be considered infertile until a year of unprotected coitus has been allowed to pass. However, each couple's problems should be judged individually, and diagnosis and treatment instituted at an earlier or later date as indicated.

Etiology. The two fundamental concepts to be kept in mind are (1) the multiplicity of etiologic factors and (2) the equal responsibility of male and female partners. To delineate these possible factors working either singly or in concert, one need only review the pathways of conception in male and female and the disorders of these pathways that may ensue.

Deficiency of sperm production in quantity and quality accounts for the majority of the *male*'s contribution to the problem of infertility. Sperm production may be adversely affected by congenital influences such as germinal aplasia or cryptorchidism, by hormonal deficiencies of the pituitary or thyroid glands, by infection such as mumps orchitis, and by environmental factors such as nutritional deficiencies, noxious chemicals and drugs, radiation, excess local heat, and altitude. Often the cause is not ascertainable by diagnostic methods available at present. Sperm transport is affected by congenital malformations, surgical trauma, and infections. Impotency, an important factor in many cases, is commonly on a psychologic basis, although local infection or general systemic disorders may play a contributory role.

Defects in the *female* are related to production of ova and interference with their union with spermatozoa. Vaginal causes are organic or functional.

Although organic changes such as congenital malformation and infection may cause interference with the ascent of the sperm by preventing normal coitus, dyspareunia on a functional basis is more frequent. Often a deep-seated emotional conflict lies at the root of this complaint. The ascent of the spermatozoa may be halted at the level of the cervix by chronic endocervicitis or an endocrine deficiency, both of which may result in inadequate or unsatisfactory cervical mucus production during the preovulatory phase. Occasionally retroversion of the uterus prevents adequate contact of the external os with the seminal pool, particularly if the volume of the ejaculate is inadequate. Uterine disorders such as malformation or tumors more commonly result in repeated abortion but occasionally may contribute to inability to conceive. The fallopian tubes may be obstructed, completely or partially, by congenital narrowing, postinflammatory states, or adnexal tumors. The tubes may be patent, but the ova may not reach the tube due to peritubal adhesions or fixation of the ovary by postinflammatory adhesions or endometriosis. Anovulation may be due to genetic absence or incomplete development of the follicular apparatus, but is more commonly the result of a relative inadequacy of pituitary function, particularly in the production of luteinizing hormone. Such changes in pituitary function may be caused by constitutional, nutritional, or emotional factors, excess adrenal production, hypo- or hyperthyroidism, chronic disease, or debilitating states. Ovulation may occur, but there may be a relative deficiency of estrogen or progesterone or both due to any of the above causes. A relative deficiency of these hormones may interfere with endometrial implantation of the fertilized egg.

Emotional factors, in addition to producing dyspareunia and interference with ovarian function, may possibly cause tubal spasm and interference with functions as yet undelineated. In the male, emotional factors interfere with coital function and possibly with sperm production via hormonal pathways or direct nervous inhibition.

Diagnosis. A complete history and examination of both partners, together with sufficient laboratory procedures needed to rule out congenital, infectious, or metabolic diseases, should be an integral part of every infertility investigation. In addition, the physician should take this opportunity to investigate the marital relationship of the couple for the purpose of uncovering both superficial sexual maladjustments and deep-seated emotional disturbances.

Each couple should then undergo a series of minimum tests with further special studies indicated in individual cases.

Treatment. As in diagnosis the two general principles of "the couple as a unit" and the multiplicity

Table 75-1. TESTS FOR INFERTILITY

I. In the male.
  A. Routine.
    1. Semen analysis. The semen is delivered into a clean glass container by withdrawal or masturbation. The following characteristics are considered normal:
      a. Volume—3 to 5 ml.
      b. Sperm count—above 60 million per ml is unquestionably normal, below 30 million per ml unquestionably indicates reduced fertility. The significance of counts between 30 million and 60 million depends upon the quality of motility and the degree of fertility in the female partner. A highly fertile female would be more susceptible to a count of borderline fertility.
      c. Motility—40 per cent or more still actively motile 4 to 5 hr after collection.
      d. Morphology—at least 60 per cent of the spermatozoa should be of normal size and shape.
    2. Examination of prostatic smear—excess leukocytes indicates that an infection may play a contributory role.
  B. Special tests—for the male with reduced fertility as indicated by semen analysis.
    1. Evaluation of thyroid function by basal metabolic rate, protein-bound iodine, or radioactive iodine uptake.
    2. Testicular biopsy—in most cases this will result in a definitive diagnosis. In only a few cases, however, will it demonstrate a remediable defect.
    3. Urinary gonadotropins—these may be low in pituitary deficiency. Excretion is high in primary gonadal failure.
    4. Sex chromatin determination.
II. In the female.
  A. Routine.
    1. Postcoital test—examination of the cervical mucus for its preovulatory qualities of clarity, spinnbarkeit (ability of the mucus to form a thread 5 to 10 cm in length when stretched between slide and cover slip), ferning (ability of the mucus to form fernlike pattern when dried and examined under low power of microscope), and for the number of viable spermatozoa 8 to 12 hr after coitus.
      a. Good test—more than 20 active spermatozoa per high-power field.
      b. Fair test—5 to 20 spermatozoa per high-power field.
      c. Poor test—less than 5 spermatozoa per high-power field. A poor postcoital test in the presence of good preovulatory mucus suggests a semen deficiency, a deficiency of the coital method, or malposition of the cervix. A poor postcoital test combined with poor mucus in the preovulatory phase and a normal semen analysis indicates a hostile

Table 75-1. TESTS FOR INFERTILITY (*Continued*)

      cervix either on an inflammatory or an endocrine basis.
    2. The evaluation of tubal patency—initially by insufflation with carbon dioxide (Rubin test) and followed at a later date by hysterosalpingography in those cases which show failure of carbon dioxide to pass or who fail to conceive after an interval of time despite a normal Rubin test.
    3. Evaluation of ovulation and hormonal factors by:
      a. Measurement of basal body temperature, which characteristically show a sustained rise after ovulation. Studies have shown that actual ovulation may occur as long as 2 days before or 2 days after the beginning of the temperature rise. The value of the temperature chart as an exact indicator of ovulation timing for purposes of timing of coitus or insemination treatments can be overestimated.
      b. Endometrial biopsy with the demonstration of secretory changes in the endometrium is valid evidence that ovulation has occurred. The presence of endometrium out of phase with the time of biopsy is evidence of a progestational deficiency.
  B. Special tests should be carried out when indicated.
    1. Evaluation of thyroid function.
    2. Endocrine assays, such as urinary gonadotropin and 17-ketosteroid determination, in cases of anovulation or inadequate luteal function.
    3. Further studies of ovulation timing utilizing vaginal or urinary smears and studies of cervical mucus.
    4. Culdoscopy to detect early endometriosis, pelvic adhesions interfering with tube-ovarian function, or polycystic ovaries.

of etiologic factors should be constantly considered in the therapy of the infertile couple. Treatment of any defects, either minor or major, in both the husband or the wife should be carried out concomitantly so that the total fertility potential of the couple will be raised to an optimum level.

In the *male* with azoospermia, in whom spermatogenesis is normal as shown by testicular biopsy, and in whom a block has been demonstrated, epididymovasostomy can result in return of fertility in 10 to 20 per cent of cases. When hormonal studies reveal a deficiency of pituitary gonadotropin, treatment with human chorionic gonadotropin (5,000 units APL intramuscularly twice weekly for 2 to 6 months) is indicated. However, sperm deficiencies not associated with specific pituitary defects will not respond to pituitary or pituitary-like extract. Azoospermia or severe oligospermia will not respond in any significant degree to the administration of hormones, vitamins, thyroid preparations, or diet unless a specific deficiency can be demonstrated. In the present state of knowledge, little can be offered in the vast majority of cases of azoospermia or severe oligospermia.

This degree of pessimism should not be carried over to the infertile male with moderate degree of oligospermia (10 to 30 million per ml) or to the male partner of an infertile couple with only a moderately lowered sperm count (30 to 60 million per ml), particularly if one considers the "couple as a unit" concept of infertility. A modest improvement in the sperm count or motility combined with attention to the factors in the female partner may raise the fertility of the couple above a critical level. Avoidance of excess alcohol and tobacco, sufficient sleep and exercise, an optimum diet, adjustment of local excesses of heat, administration of thyroid preparations in minor degrees of hypofunction—all these singly or together may prove of definite benefit.

In the *female* specific attention should be directed to the cervical factor by correction of unfavorable coital habits, correction of retroversion of the uterus by a pessary, improvement in quality and quantity of preovulatory mucus by the daily administration of small dosages of estrogen (0.1 mg diethylstilbestrol daily for three or four cycles), by the use of a plastic cervical cap, and by the correction of cervicitis by systemic and local antibiotics or by cervical cauterization. Cauterization must be conservative lest more harm than good be produced by cervical stenosis or obliteration of mucus secreting glands. When cervical stenosis is found, dilatation under anesthesia is of definite value.

Attempts to overcome tubal occlusion by repeated insufflations, diathermy, and high dosage of estrogen occasionally meet with success. Plastic repair of tubes or cornual implantation is followed by success in only 10 to 20 per cent of cases. Surgery for tube-ovarian blockade, due to ovaries fixed by endometriosis, peritubal or periovarian adhesions, but associated with essentially normal tubes, results in a higher percentage of success. Infrequent ovulation accompanied by gross irregularity will respond to thyroid preparations when specifically indicated and to the correction of a specific dietary or vitamin deficiency. Ovulation accompanied by an inadequate luteal phase should be treated with progesterone preparations (17-ethynyl-19-nortestosterone, 2.5 mg daily for 10 days) or injections of human chorionic gonadotropin (HCG, 1,000 units intramuscularly every other day for five doses). Treatment should begin on the fifth or sixth day after the mid-cycle rise in the basal body temperature. Absence of ovulation is rarely corrected by pituitary hormone preparations.

When caused by a specific defect in thyroid function, nutrition, adrenal activity, or the psyche, correction of these defects will improve the condition. Wedge resection of polycystic ovaries, if bilaterally enlarged, is accompanied by 60 to 80 per cent resumption of ovulatory cycles.

Psychotherapy is of value in improving the coital habits of the couple, in reducing tubal spasm, and in the correction of some deficiencies of hormonal nature. Finally, the manner and attitude of the physician plays a role in the outcome by preventing undue feelings of guilt and depression from gaining the upper hand, and by instilling sufficient hope and fortitude to allow the couple to carry through with the tedious and sometimes painful diagnostic testing and therapeutic maneuvers.

REFERENCES

Buxton, C. L., and A. L. Southam: "Human Infertility," New York: Paul B. Hoeber, Inc., Medical Department of Harper & Brothers, 1958.

MacLeod, J., R. Z. Gold, and C. M. McLane: Correlation of Male and Female Factors in Human Infertility, Fertility and Sterility, 6:112, 1955.

Meeker, S. R.: "Human Sterility, Causation, Diagnosis and Treatment: A Practical Manual of Clinical Procedures," Baltimore, The Williams & Wilkins Company, 1933.

Nelson, W. O.: The Klinefelter Syndrome, Fertility and Sterility, 8:527, 1957.

Stone, A., and M. E. Ward: Factors Responsible for Pregnancy in 500 Infertility Cases, Fertility and Sterility, 7:1, 1956.

76 DISEASES OF THE PINEAL AND THYMUS GLANDS

Julian I. Kitay

DISEASES OF THE PINEAL GLAND

It appears that the pineal gland is not a functionless vestige, as has been commonly believed. Histochemical studies of the gland in monkeys, rats, and other animals have shown the presence of ribonucleoprotein, deoxyribonucleoprotein, glycogen, acid and alkaline phosphatase, and succinic dehydrogenase in the parenchymal cells. Radioisotope experiments in rats have demonstrated that the uptake of P^{32} per 100 mg fresh tissue is greater in the pineal gland than in any other organ studied. Hypophysectomy in rats results in an even greater pineal uptake of P^{32}, whereas corticotropin administration decreases the uptake to prehypophysectomy levels. Pinealectomy in chicks, mice, rabbits, or rats is associated with gonadal hypertrophy and acceleration of vaginal opening in immature animals and with prolongation of estrus and shortening of diestrus in mature animals. On the other hand, pineal extract administration in these animals consistently reversed these changes. Constant exposure to light has been shown to result in pineal atrophy. Other studies have implicated the pineal region with regulation of aldosterone secretion. Recently, a methoxyindole compound, N-acetyl-5-methoxy-tryptamine, has been isolated from pineal gland extracts which is extremely potent in lightening frog skin in vitro (Lerner and Case). Another pineal extract has been described as beneficial in the therapy of psychosis (Altschule; Eldred, et al.). Injection of pineal extracts in man has been observed to decrease urinary 17-ketosteroid excretion and to increase both blood glutathione concentration and the number of circulating eosinophils. These studies suggest that the pineal gland is a functioning endocrine organ. Further research must be carried out, however, before its function can be defined.

Anatomy and Pathology. The human pineal gland is a small conical organ, gray in color, that lies deep in the brain along the quadrigeminate groove between the superior colliculi. It is attached anteriorly to the posterior wall of the third ventricle by the pineal stalk, which is continuous with the superior habenular and posterior commissures. Histologic descriptions of the gland are varied and controversial; however, most authorities agree that it contains at least two types of cells—pineal parenchymal cells and neuroglia. The normal human pineal gland weighs between 140 and 200 mg. Pineal weight does not decrease at puberty or in senescence.

Calcification in the pineal gland is seen in about 50 per cent of routine skull roentgenograms. The incidence of such calcification is negligible in the first decade of life; it approximates 25 per cent in the second decade; and it increases gradually from the third to the eighth decades. The visible calcium deposits in the gland are frequently used as an anatomic landmark in roentgenographic localization of brain tumors. It should be noted that similar deposits occurring in the habenular region may often be confused with pineal calcification.

Many pineal lesions have been described, including tumors, fibrosis, infarction, atrophy, agenesis, and a variety of histopathologic changes that occur in association with diseases elsewhere in the body. With the exception of tumors, none of these lesions has demonstrable clinical significance.

Pineal Tumors. Neoplasms are the most common pineal lesions; however, their incidence is low in most series of intracranial tumors. Only 583 cases have been reported in any detail; 189 additional cases are briefly mentioned in reports on series of brain tumors. Over 50 per cent of the total have been reported in patients twenty years of age or younger. The incidence is three times as frequent in men as in women. Histopathologic descriptions are varied and confusing, and more than 25 types of tumor have been described. All these types may be generally classified as either tumors of parenchymal origin (e.g., pinealomas) or tumors of nonparenchymal origin (e.g., teratomas, gliomas, and cysts). However, such classification may be difficult because pinealomatous and teratomatous tissues have frequently been noted to coexist in the same lesion.

Clinical Features. The neurologic signs most frequently associated with pineal tumors include hydrocephalus, papilledema, and paralysis of upward gaze (Parinaud's syndrome) with weakened convergence and decreased pupillary reaction to light. Diabetes insipidus is occasionally seen, usually in association with tumors of parenchymal origin.

Precocious puberty (Pellizzi's syndrome) has been observed in 53 patients with verified pineal tumors. All these patients were boys whose ages at autopsy (or operation) were under seventeen years. The total number of pineal tumors reported in children one to sixteen years old is 214; 176 of these were found in boys. Accordingly, the over-all incidence of sexual precocity associated with pineal tumors is 25 per cent, and its incidence in boys with pineal tumors is 30 per cent. The current explanation of the mechanism whereby a pineal tumor causes precocious puberty is that the expanding lesion indirectly stimulates the pituitary gland by compressing or destroying hypothalamic areas that regulate anterior pituitary function. This trauma presumedly increases the secretion of gonadotropins, with consequent development of precocity. Proponents of this theory believe that the histologic composition of the tumor is of no importance and that only its location is significant. It should be noted, however, that this hypothesis was formulated because sexual precocity occurs in connection with both pineal and other intracranial lesions, and some workers wished to explain all sexual precocity due to intracranial disease on the basis of a single mechanism.

Although the above-mentioned theory has been widely held, recent reexamination of the available data has called attention to certain findings that tend to controvert it. Pineal tumors of parenchymal origin and those of nonparenchymal origin are equally distributed in children one to sixteen years of age. However, sexual precocity is associated with nonparenchymal tumors four times as often as with parenchymal tumors—a statistically significant disproportion. Moreover, hypogenitalism also has been reported in association with pineal tumors, and in these cases parenchymal tumors predominate by a ratio of 2.5:1. The "pressure" hypothesis outlined above is incompatible with these findings. A better explanation must await more definitive experimental studies.

Treatment. Surgical removal offers the only hope of cure; cerebral decompression and irradiation merely provide palliation. The possibility that parenchymal tumors can be destroyed by uptake of administered radioactive phosphorus warrants investigation.

DISEASES OF THE THYMUS GLAND

It is thought by some that the thymus should be classified as one of the glands of internal secretion. However, classic extirpation experiments in a variety of animals have given no conclusive proof of its endocrine nature, and certainly thymectomy in the human being causes no recognizable clinical syndrome. There is no doubt that the thymus is a storehouse of essential body constituents which may be readily mobilized in times of stress. Thymus hyperplasia and atrophy are characteristically associated with a wide variety of clinical conditions.

Anatomy and Pathology. The normal thymus of infants consists of a well-defined cortex composed of closely packed masses of lymphocytes and a medulla. During the process of differentiation into cortex and medulla, Hassall's corpuscles, or concentric masses of cells, appear in the sheets of epithelial cells of the medulla. The gland is a thick, solid structure which in infants may occupy most of the anterior mediastinum. Later in life its size decreases, relatively. Involution is accompanied by replacement with adipose tissue. There exists an inverse relation between the size of the thymus and adrenal cortical activity—hyperactivity induces thymic and generalized lymphoid atrophy, whereas adrenal cortical insufficiency is characteristically associated with thymic hypertrophy and generalized lymphadenopathy. It is probable that the so-called "accidental involution of the thymus" so characteristic of severe illness is mediated by the increased adrenal activity in response to stress.

Tumors of the Thymus. Tumors of the thymus, or thymomas, are difficult to classify. They are usually encapsulated, and a single tumor may contain many different states of histologic differentiation. Tumors of the thymus may be adherent to surrounding organs, but distant metastases are rare.

"Status Thymicolymphaticus." It is possible that some cases of sudden death formerly attributed to "status thymicolymphaticus" were in reality deaths due to acute adrenal insufficiency. Recent studies also indicate that many of the sudden deaths previously attributed to thymic obstruction or status thymicolymphaticus were actually explained by congenital obstructive anomalies or inflammatory lesions of the trachea and larynx. It is also probable that unrecognized cases of overwhelming infections complicated by shock have in the past been classified as deaths due to status thymicolymphaticus.

Relation of the Thymus Gland to Myasthenia Gravis. In 1941 Blalock reported on the improvement of patients with myasthenia gravis following removal of the thymus. Since that time a number of studies have been made relating to the efficacy of thymectomy or irradiation of the thymus as a method of treatment of myasthenia gravis. Reports vary widely as to the efficacy of these procedures. Eaton and Clagett have reported a long-term survey of 472 patients with myasthenia gravis including 77 with thymoma and have evaluated the effects of thymectomy compared to medical therapy alone. A total of 121 patients received thymic surgery of whom 51 were shown to have thymoma. The results demonstrated that thymectomy is of value in the treatment of female patients with myasthenia gravis who are less than fifty years of age and in whom there is no evident thymoma. Beneficial effects of surgery are less evident if the disease has been present 10 years or more. The value of thymectomy in male patients is less conclusive but should be considered in light of the surgical risk involved. Prognosis is generally poorer in patients with thymoma, but thymic surgery perhaps should be undertaken provided there is no evidence of inoperability. In any event, the selection of therapy should depend upon careful evaluation of all the data available concerning each patient.

REFERENCES

PINEAL GLAND

Altschule, M. D.: Some Effects of Aqueous Extracts of Acetone-dried Beef-pineal Substance in Chronic Schizophrenia, New Engl. J. Med., 257:919, 1957.

Case Records, Massachusetts General Hospital, New Engl. J. Med., 263:965, 1960.

Eldred, S. H., N. W. Bell, and L. J. Sherman: A Pilot Study Comparing the Effects of Pineal Extract and a Placebo in Patients with Chronic Schizophrenia, New Engl. J. Med., 263:1330, 1960.

Kitay, J. I., and M. D. Altschule: "The Pineal Gland: A Review of the Physiologic Literature," Cambridge, Mass., Harvard University Press, 1954.

Lerner, A. B., and J. D. Case: Melatonin, Federation Proc., 19:590, 1960.

Posner, M., and G. Horrax: Eye Signs in Pineal Tumors, J. Neurosurg., 3:15, 1946.

THYMUS GLAND

Eaton, L. M., and O. T. Clagett: Present Status of Thymectomy in Treatment of Myasthenia Gravis, Am. J. Med., 19:703, 1955.

Section 3: Metabolic Disorders of Bone

77 GENERAL CONSIDERATIONS

Edward C. Reifenstein, Jr.

CALCIUM AND PHOSPHATE METABOLISM

Calcium in Body Fluids. The normal level of the total calcium in the plasma for adults and for children is 10.0 ± 0.5 mg per 100 ml (5.0 ± 0.25 mEq per liter or 2.5 ± 0.125 mM), depending upon the laboratory and the method employed. The total plasma calcium can be divided into three fractions: (1) the nondiffusible or protein-bound calcium (0.85 mM), which is bound primarily to albumin (0.67 mM) and to a lesser extent to globulin (0.18 mM), with the amount proportional to the total concentration of the proteins (when the total plasma protein level is 7 Gm per 100 ml, the protein-bound fraction is approximately 3.4 mg calcium per 100 ml); (2) the complexed calcium (0.32 mM), which is complexed to phosphate (0.07 mM), bicarbonate (0.17 mM), or citrate (0.08 mM); and (3) the remaining portion of the calcium, 5.4 mg per 100 ml, is present as the ionized calcium (1.35 mM), which is the physiologically active form. Both these latter fractions (total 1.65 mM) are diffusible. Thus, approximately 67 per cent of the plasma calcium is diffusible, and approximately 33 per cent is bound to protein. Of the diffusible component, approximately 80 per cent is ionized. The ionized fraction is concerned with the various functions of calcium and in physiologic states is maintained within a constant range by homeostatic mechanisms. The concentration of calcium in the extracellular fluid is approximately 70 per cent of that in the plasma; the concentration in the cerebrospinal fluid is 4.5 to 6 mg per 100 ml. The current laboratory methods for measuring the plasma concentration of calcium determine the total calcium content. Since the ionized fraction is important physiologically, measurements of the total calcium level are of limited value unless the total protein content of the plasma is measured at the same time. The measurement of the diffusible calcium concentration may be of value, particularly if the temperature and the pH of the procedure are controlled, but the currently available methods require a great deal of skill and care to give reproducible results.

Phosphate in Body Fluids. The normal level of inorganic phosphate in the plasma for adults is 3.5 ± 0.5 mg per 100 ml (2.0 ± 0.3 mEq per liter), and for children is higher by 1 to 2 mg per 100 ml (0.5 to 1 mEq per liter). The total phosphate in the plasma is divided into three fractions: (1) the lipid phosphate (about 8 mg per 100 ml), (2) the ester phosphate (about 1 mg per 100 ml), and (3) the inorganic phosphate (about 3.5 mg per 100 ml). Thus the total phosphate content of the plasma is approximately 12.5 mg per 100 ml. The inorganic phosphate fraction of the plasma is influenced by the parathyroid hormone, the gonadal hormones, the adrenal cortical glucogenic hormone, the anterior pituitary growth hormone, and insulin. The plasma inorganic phosphate level normally fluctuates directly with the blood sugar concentration. For this reason the plasma phosphate level can be evaluated more adequately when the blood sample for the determination is taken in the morning under standard fasting conditions. The cerebrospinal fluid normally contains about 1.3 to 2.0 mg inorganic phosphate per 100 ml.

Plasma Calcium-Phosphate Relationship. Under normal physiologic conditions, the calcium ion activity and the phosphate ion activity can be considered to exist in the extracellular fluid in a state of equilibrium with the exchangeable hydroxyapatite crystals in bone, with the ion product at any given time (under constant metabolic conditions) equal to a constant. Thus, if the calcium ion activity is increased, the phosphate ion activity falls, and vice versa. Such a concept is an idealization, because the moment there is a change in the concentration of either ion compensatory physiologic adjustments occur. Actually, in many pathologic states there is a reciprocity between the concentration of calcium and that of phosphate in the plasma which suggests that under a variety of circumstances the relationship between the exchangeable bone mineral and the circulating ions can be considered for practical purposes to be that of a simple solubility relationship. However, even if the extraosseous physiologic conditions are assumed to be constant, the possibility exists that the bulk of the process of ion-exchange between the circulating ions and the ions of the exchangeable bone compartment is mediated by the cellular activity of the osteoblasts.

The maintenance of an approximately constant ion product in the plasma during a variety of changing physiologic or metabolic conditions is achieved by adjustments in four major processes: (1) resorption (and to a lesser extent, formation) of bone, (2) absorption of calcium by the gastrointestinal tract, (3) excretion of phosphate by the kidney, and (4) excretion of calcium by the kidney. Of paramount importance in the regulation and the coordination of these processes are the D vitamins; this is indicated by the fact that the ion product falls in states of vitamin D deficiency. The parathyroid hormone does not appear to be necessary for the maintenance of a constant ion product in the plasma; furthermore, the product is maintained in the constant range independently of the status of the parathyroid gland activity. The parathyroid hormone increases the calcium ion activity of the plasma and maintains it at a level higher than that achieved with physiologic amounts of vitamin D; the hormone also lowers the phosphate ion activity of the plasma. The growth hormone of the anterior pituitary gland has an important influence on the value of the ion product in the plasma; the product is higher in growing children and in patients with acromegaly. The nutritional status and the activities of the adrenal gland and the gonads also have an effect upon the value of the ion product.

The concentrations of calcium and phosphate in the plasma normally are such that they form a metastable solution with respect to the formation of apatite crystals. This means that the plasma may be stored in vitro indefinitely without any apatite crystals being formed. However, if the plasma is exposed to bone mineral, calcium and phosphate separate from the plasma and form more solid. Furthermore, if collagen is placed in metastable calcium phosphate solutions, hydroxyapatite crystals form within the collagen fibrils. The initial process of crystal deposition is known as nucleation. Since either bone mineral or collagen can act in the plasma as a nucleating agent, the body fluids are considered to be *supersaturated* with calcium and phosphate in relation to bone. This state is maintained by cellular activity through a complex regulatory system which involves the control of the calcium and phosphate ion exchange in the kidney, in the gastrointestinal tract, and in the bone. When the ion product falls in the extracellular fluid, ions leave the exchangeable compartment of bone and enter the extracellular fluid so that the ion product returns to or toward its normal value; in this respect, the exchangeable area of bone can be considered to serve a buffering function. This mechanism alone usually is not sufficient for the complete restoration of the ion product, and some other active process such as increased absorption of calcium from the gastrointestinal tract, increased reabsorption of calcium by the renal tubules, or increased resorption of nonexchangeable bone must take place to restore the ion product to its physiologic value. Active resorption of bone (osteoclastic or otherwise) results in the removal of calcium and phosphate from the nonexchangeable osseous compartment and the return of these ions (after solubilization) to the extracellular fluid; this increases the ion product (calcium activity times phosphate activity).

The assumption that the product of the calcium ion activity *times* the phosphate ion activity in the plasma is maintained in an approximately constant range during a variety of changing physiologic or metabolic conditions is a useful concept in the diagnosis and the therapeutic management of various metabolic disorders. For practical purposes, the product of the total calcium level in milligrams per 100 ml *times* the inorganic phosphate level in milligrams per 100 ml in the plasma is a convenient index of this relationship. Under normal physiologic conditions, the product thus calculated is about 30 to 40 for adults, and about 40 to 55 for growing children.

PHYSIOLOGY OF ADULT BONE

Protein Composition. From a metabolic point of view, adult human bone consists of a mass of protein tissue in which has been deposited a calcium phosphate salt. The protein matrix is primarily collagen, a coiled helix of fibrous protein with 27 amino acids, which is rich in glycine, proline, and hydroxyproline and which contains as well small amounts of methionine, lysine, hydroxylysine, and tyrosine. The bone collagen appears to be similar structurally to that found in other connective tissues although it may be more highly crosslinked. Chemically, it does not differ significantly from collagen of other sources (tendon, and so forth). In fact, collagen from many different connective tissues can be dissolved in weak acids, following which they can be reconstituted into fibrils relatively free of "ground substances." The reconstituted fibrils assume various fibrillar forms depending upon the conditions employed. Of these reconstituted collagen fibrils, only those having the so-called "native-type structure" with a 640-Å axial repeating pattern (as observed in the electron microscope or by low-angle x-ray diffraction) are able to initiate the nucleation of an apatite crystal from solutions of calcium-phosphate which are metastable with respect to the formation of apatite crystals. The hydroxyapatite crystals form at specific sites within the hollow collagen fibrils. The collagen, therefore, induces the nucleation, the orientation, and the growth limitation of these crystals. The specific sites within the collagen molecule where nucleation occurs are not known, but the charged groups of lysine and hydroxylysine have been suggested. Since the apatites are primarily phosphate salts, it may be the interaction of the phosphate ions in solution with the positively charged groups in the collagen (epsilon-amino groups of lysine) which is the primary event in the process of nucleation.

The other components of the organic matrix include a number of poorly defined proteins and a group of acid mucopolysaccharides and mucoproteins. These constituents comprise the so-called "ground substance." The polysaccharide components, such as chondroitin sulfate, probably are formed in the bone through the pathways of carbohydrate metabolism involving the uridine nucleotides. It has been postulated that the ground substance of bone holds the collagen fibers together and may be important in regulating the supply of salts to the calcifiable collagen substrate. This regulation could take place through changes in the concentration or in the degree of polymerization of the ground substance, since it is known that the more highly polymerized mucopolysaccharides have a greater cation-binding capacity than that of their precursor or depolymerized forms. The matrix also contains small amounts of lipids, enzymes, glycogen, and minerals (in addition to the bone salt crystals). These organic constituents are synthesized and organized structurally through the activity of the osteoblasts and their enzymes so that the matrix as it is laid down is calcifiable. However, some workers believe that vitamin D must act on bone matrix before it can be calcified.

Mineral Composition. The calcium phosphate salt of bone appears to be hydroxyapatite, with the formula $Ca_{10}(PO_4)_6(OH)_2$. The growth of a crystal of this salt requires energy and involves the symmetric repetition of calcium, phosphorus, oxygen, and hydrogen atoms in the proportions of hydroxyapatite until a unit of structure is achieved. This unit, with a continuous slight spiral dislocation, is translationally repeated until the lattice of the hydroxyapatite crystal is formed. The best estimates are that the crystals are no larger than $500 \times 250 \times 100$ angstroms. It is postulated that, because of the large surface area of the crystals, they absorb excess phosphate thereby lowering the calcium/phosphorus ratio. This chemisorption in turn leads to the binding of water, which produces a so-called "hydration shell" of water on the crystal surface. Throughout the life of the crystal, all its reactions involve the transfer of ions across this crystal solution interface. In addition, it seems likely that certain ions, such as the sodium ion, can replace the calcium ion on the surface of the crystal but not in the interior of the crystal. Such a phenomenon could account for the sodium content of bone. In the living organism, the crystals are exposed to a solution of many different ions. Some of these can penetrate to the ion layer on the crystal surface, and others can replace ions in the interior of the crystal. These ion-exchange reactions

account for the observed variability in the composition of the bone mineral and explain the rapid exchange of such isotopes as Ca^{45} with bone mineral. These reactions provide an explanation for the fact that changes in the concentration of the hydrogen ions, the bicarbonate ions, or the sodium ions in the extracellular fluid are buffered by exchanges with the bone crystals.

The biologic fluids of the living organism contain many substances which apparently are not wanted in the lattice of the growing hydroxyapatite crystal. These materials are excluded from the internal structure and deposited on the surface of the lattice. These adventitious substances include carbonate, citrate, magnesium hydroxide, sodium, fluoride, and either excess phosphate or excess calcium as the case may be. The composition of the surface mixture reflects that of the surrounding biologic fluid and, therefore, varies both qualitatively and quantitatively throughout life. The ions of potassium, chloride, and sulfate of the surrounding fluid do not appear to be deposited on the lattice surface in any appreciable quantity.

The growth of the bone salt is continued by the development of a new hydroxyapatite crystal lattice on top of an old one; thereby, the extraneous surface substances of the moment are entrapped within the enlarging mass. Certain atoms (such as strontium, barium, and lead), which usually are not present in significant quantities in human biologic fluids, can replace the calcium atoms within the crystal lattice. Thus the chemical composition of the bone salt as it develops in nature differs from person to person, and also from time to time and from location to location in the same individual. As the hydroxyapatite crystals are deposited and grow, they displace water from the fixed amount of collagen in bone. Growth ceases when the crystals have displaced so much water that the ions no longer can diffuse into or out of the area at appreciable rates.

Calcium stored in the body is located almost exclusively in the skeleton. Average figures for a 70-kg adult indicate that of a total of 1,160 Gm of calcium in the whole body, 1,150 Gm is present in bone. The small fraction of calcium not in the skeleton or teeth is found chiefly in the extracellular fluid, where it has a number of important functions.

About 36 per cent of the ash of bones is calcium, of which 85 per cent is in the form of calcium phosphate (hydroxyapatite) and 12 per cent as calcium carbonate. Regardless of the form of the calcium complex or of the variations in the total mineral content of bone, the calcium-phosphorus ratio is approximately 2.2:1 wherever bone is being laid down or resorbed. In the normal adult, the amount of calcium that enters the skeleton is offset by an equal amount released from it; thus bone maintains a state of dynamic equilibrium, and there is no net change in the total calcium content.

There is no similar turnover of calcium in the teeth. If calcium metabolism is faulty in early childhood, the teeth may fail to calcify. However, if calcium metabolism is defective after the teeth are formed, there is no decalcification. Around the teeth there is a condensation of alveolar bone called the *lamina dura*. This structure is present at all ages, is easily discerned in dental roentgenograms, and is a convenient index of osseous calcification because of the unchanging contrast of the adjacent teeth.

Metabolic Processes in Normal Bone. The calcified mass of adult bone can be considered to have three types of surfaces: (1) one on which nothing appears to be happening (this type includes about 90 per cent of bone surfaces), (2) one on which bone is being formed, and (3) one on which bone is being resorbed.

Bone resorption is a biologic process which consists of two events: (1) the removal of the matrix (*matrix resorption*) and (2) the release of the calcium phosphate salt, which involves the breakdown and solubilization of hydroxyapatite crystals from the fully calcified nonexchangeable stable bone. Usually, these events appear to take place simultaneously; however, the matrix actually may be the first to be removed. In addition, bone mineral may leave the partially calcified exchangeable compartment of bone by the process of ion-exchange (*mineral mobilization*), a process which appears to be predominantly physicochemical in nature. Minor adjustments can be made in the mineral levels of the body fluids by mineral mobilization without involving the other processes.

The continual growth and dissolution of bone are dynamic processes which are under cellular control. Although the nature of the cell type involved in bone resorption is still debated, some role is played by large multinuclear cells called *osteoclasts*, in contrast to the single-nuclear cells called *osteoblasts* which are concerned with bone formation. These two cells may have a common origin and be converted from one type to the other under the influence of the environment and of various agents. The actual gross dimensions of an individual bone normally are determined not only by the rate of bone collagen deposition, but also by the rate of bone resorption because of the necessity of maintaining the calcium ion activity of the extracellular fluid relatively constant in the presence of increased requirements of minerals for bone growth.

The fully calcified nonexchangeable stable bone represents more than 99 per cent of the mass of compact bone. The progressive mineralization leading to nonreactive bone does not result in an entire skeleton of stable mineral because of the constant remodeling process of the Haversian systems; this is demonstrated by the continual redistribution of radiocalcium or radiophosphorus deposited in the skeleton. Each day, Haversian remodeling accounts for 500 mg of calcium removed from the extracellular fluid and deposited as new bone (accretion), and for 500 mg of calcium removed from bone (resorption) and returned to the extracellular fluid. There are two possible sites from which calcium in bone can be returned to the body fluids: (1) from the mineral in the fully calcified nonexchangeable stable portion of bone and (2) from the mineral in the partially calcified exchangeable portion of bone.

If the calcium returned to the extracellular fluid comes from a nonexchangeable area of bone, an active cellular process in some manner must break down the bone and solubilize it. The present evidence supports the view that active resorption of bone (osteoclastic or otherwise) involves the removal of both the matrix and the mineral, and there is some evidence that the matrix actually may be the first to be removed. This active cellular process is probably controlled by agents such as the parathyroid hormone, thyroxine, and the D vitamins. The calcium and phosphate thus removed from a nonexchangeable area of bone, solubilized, and returned to the extracellular fluid will increase the calcium times phosphate ion product.

If the calcium returned to the extracellular fluid comes from an exchangeable area of bone, there must be a net removal of calcium ions from the partially calcified bone before there can be a net increase in the calcium ion concentration of the extracellular fluid. This process, therefore, must be clearly differentiated from the continuously occurring process of exchange between two calcium ions, in which a calcium ion in the extracellular fluid changes places with a calcium ion in the lattice of the hydroxyapatite crystal, and there is no net change in the total number of calcium ions in either the extracellular fluid or the crystal lattice. A net increase in the calcium ion concentration of the extracellular fluid as a result of the removal of calcium from the exchangeable portion of bone can be brought about by: (1) a fall in the calcium-phosphate ion product in the extracellular fluid, (2) the replacement of calcium ions in the bone crystal lattice by cations other than calcium, and (3) a modification in the effective product of the ions bathing the bone crystal induced by cellular activity which changes the pH, the organic acid concentration, and so forth. The first of these is the important mechanism in most conditions. The exchange of other cations for calcium occurs to a limited extent in certain disorders, but the mobilization from bone of calcium alone without matrix as a result of cellular activity is not clearly established.

It appears, therefore, that calcium and phosphate leave the exchangeable compartment of bone only when there is a fall in the concentration of these ions in the extracellular fluid, and leave the nonexchangeable compartment of bone only when there is cellular activity resulting in osteolysis. This latter process is of major importance in: (1) maintaining the calcium-phosphate ion product of the extracellular fluid in a constant range and (2) altering the macroscopic structure of the bone in response to external demands.

Bone formation consists of two steps: (1) the laying down of the matrix (*matrix formation*) and (2) the deposition therein of the calcium-phosphate salt (calcification), a physicochemical process which involves: (*a*) the nucleation and growth of hydroxyapatite crystals (*apatite formation*) and (*b*) ion-exchange reactions between the hydration shell, the crystal surface, and the crystal interior and additional mineral ions (*mineral accumulation*). Usually these steps appear to take place simultaneously. However, minor adjustments can be made in the mineral levels of the extracellular fluid and the plasma by mineral accumulation without involving the other processes.

The continual growth and dissolution of bone are dynamic processes under cellular control, as previously discussed. The role of the osteoblast is confined to the laying down of a calcifiable collagen fibril in a suitable ground substance. This function probably is achieved through the activities of enzymes, such as *alkaline phosphatase*, which apparently are elaborated by the osteoblasts. Thus, in the absence of liver disease, the alkaline phosphatase level in the plasma is an index of osteoblastic activity, and hence of matrix formation. The normal level of the alkaline phosphatase in the plasma for adults is 3 to 5 Bodansky units (3 to 10 King-Armstrong units), and for children is higher, up to 12 Bodansky units (20 King-Armstrong units). At present, the factors controlling the activity of the osteoblasts are poorly understood. One of these factors is mechanical stress upon the bone; the manner in which this influence is translated into a biochemical stimulus is completely unknown. The actual gross dimensions of an individual bone normally are determined by the rate of bone collagen deposition and by the rate of bone resorption. Adequate amounts of protein, ascorbic acid, vitamin A, growth hormone, and gonadal hormones are required for normal osteoblastic activity.

Another factor which regulates the rate and degree of calcification in bone matrix is the availability of water as the process proceeds. Because the process of the initiation of calcification (nucleation) and the rate of the deposition of mineral are dependent upon the degree of saturation of the extracellular fluids, the living organism maintains a fairly constant level of the calcium and the phosphate ions in order to ensure a continuing orderly calcification of the organic matrix. The maintenance of these levels is under the control of cellular factors, thus providing biologic regulation of a predominantly physicochemical process. The major factor which determines the net transfer of calcium from the extracellular fluid into bone is the amount of new osseous matrix which recently has been deposited and calcified (completely or partially).

A net decrease in the calcium ion concentration of the extracellular fluid as a result of the accretion of calcium in the exchangeable portion of bone can be brought about by: (1) an increase in the rate of deposition of new matrix as a result of cellular activity, (2) a rise in the calcium-phosphate ion product in the extracellular fluid, and (3) the replacement of cations other than calcium of the bone crystal lattice by calcium ions. An increase in the rate of matrix formation and a rise in the extracellular fluid calcium-phosphate ion product are the most important mechanisms. The exchange of other cations for calcium in the crystal lattice occurs to only a limited extent.

It appears, therefore, that calcium and phosphate enter the exchangeable compartment of bone when there is cellular activity resulting in osteogenesis and a simultaneous rise in the concentration of these ions in the extracellular fluid. Calcium and phosphate are deposited as hydroxyapatite crystals in a small area of the exchangeable compartment of bone. This area grows and becomes maximally mineralized at which time it is converted to a nonexchangeable compartment of bone through the displacement of water by the growing crystals. A point is reached when so much water has left the nonexchangeable compartment of bone that calcium and phosphate ions can no longer readily diffuse in or out of this area at any appreciable rate.

Types of Bone Formation. Three types of bone formation are found: (1) endochondral, (2) membranous, and (3) endosteal. In the first, bone formation takes place after a preliminary formation of cartilage; in the second, bone formation occurs in specialized mesenchymal tissues in the embryo without a preliminary cartilaginous phase; in the third, bone is formed by apposition to the cortex and trabeculae as part of the constant remodeling of bone. In the final analysis, all three types of bone formation involve essentially the same process—the laying down of the extracellular matrix (osteoid) and the deposition into this osteoid of a calcium phosphate salt.

BONE AND MINERAL HOMEOSTASIS

Dynamic Equilibrium of Normal Bone. In the normal individual, simultaneous bone resorption and bone formation maintain the calcified mass of bone in a state of dynamic equilibrium, as previously discussed.

Adjustments to Physical Activity. Since the normal stimulus to osteoblastic activity appears to be the stress and strain of weight bearing, the skeleton tends to be heavier in persons who lead physically active lives and lighter in those who have sedentary habits. For example, lumberjacks have bones which are seen in roentgenograms to be more dense than those of accountants. Some individuals subject their skeletons to wide seasonal variations in stress. This group is exemplified by sedentary workers who engage in strenuous activity on vacation and athletes engaging in seasonal sports. During the period of strenuous physical exercise, osteoblastic activity is greatly accelerated and the calcified bone mass is considerably increased. Fractures suffered by individuals undertaking strenuous physical exercise and athletic training tend to occur early in this period of adjustment. The cessation of strenuous activity, at the end of this period, eliminates the stimulus to new bone formation. Furthermore, since at this point the mass of calcified bone is greater than that needed by the less active skeleton, there is a compensatory increase in the osteolytic activity of the osteoclasts and consequently in the rate of bone resorption until the mass of calcified bone is restored to a new state of equilibrium. The decrease in bone formation and the increase in bone resorption lead to an augmented excretion of calcium in the urine. If fluid intake is inadequate during this period, renal calculi may complicate the return to normal bone equilibrium. The physiologic adjustments of the "intermittent exerciser" illustrate the mechanisms involved in the more serious situation (acute osteoporosis of disuse) that arises when a very active adult or child is immobilized by a fracture or by some other acute illness (see Chap. 78).

Changes in the direction in which physical forces are applied to a bone alter the osteoblastic activity in that bone. This is best illustrated in the case of fractures which have healed with a poor alignment of bone fragments. The different stresses involved cause new bone to be laid down where it will be of the greatest mechanical advantage to the bone; at the same time, bone is resorbed from the area of decreased stress. As a result, the deformed bone ultimately develops a strength that is adequate for all normal stresses, and the angulation from imperfect alignment becomes less conspicuous.

The shifts in the quantity of calcified bone mass which result from excessive stress or from immobilization can bring out detectable changes in the size and the density of bones in roentgenograms and in the urinary excretion of calcium. However, these adjustments usually do not produce observable alterations in the plasma levels of calcium, phosphate, or alkaline phosphatase (except when acute osteoporosis of disuse and its sequelae are induced). Whether excessive stress in itself can create a pathologic situation is open to question, since the human physiologic mechanisms for adaptation to increased stress have a capacity that can be exceeded with difficulty, if at all.

Differences in Rates of Bone and Mineral Homeostatic Processes. The cellular activities involved in bone formation or bone resorption are biologic processes which do not accelerate or decelerate abruptly. It appears that the saturation of calcium and phosphate ions can deviate from the normal range for some time before there are recognizable adjustments in the rates of the cellular activities of bone metabolism. Similarly, the mineral constituents of the body fluids can be restored to the normal range for a considerable period before the cellular processes return to a physiologic level of activity. In osteomalacia (rickets in the child) the body fluids have inadequate saturation of the calcium and phosphate ions for optimum calcification of the matrix (see Chap. 79). Since bone resorption is continuing at a normal rate, the mass of calcified bone gradually decreases in amount. As a consequence of this weakening of the skeleton, osteoblastic activity is stimulated. In the healing phase of osteomalacia, the saturation of calcium and phosphate ions in the body fluids apparently can be restored to normal and maintained in this state for some time without appreciable reduction in osteoblastic activity. During this period the previously formed matrix is quickly calcified and additional osteoid with its deposits of minerals accumulates at a diminishing rate on the endosteal surfaces. The end result of this response is a greater than normal bone mass (hyperosteogenesis), which by roentgenogram appears as abnormally dense bone. The index of increased osteoblastic activity is the level of the plasma alkaline phosphatase, and the concentration of this enzyme also drops very slowly to the normal range. The alkaline phosphatase level provides a useful means of following the effect of therapy in osteomalacia and rickets. Bones which have become dense from compensatory repair eventually may be restored to a normal bone mass; but if the amount of repair has been extensive, the dense bone appears to persist almost indefinitely.

In osteitis fibrosa generalisata the mechanisms involved in stimulating compensatory bone repair are the same as those in osteomalacia. However, in osteitis fibrosa generalisata the total mass of calcified bone is decreased in amount and rendered more susceptible to stresses by increased bone destruction instead of by decreased bone formation (see Chap. 67).

Adjustments to Acute Changes in Mineral Concentrations of Body Fluids. In conditions with acute changes in the concentrations of calcium and phosphate in the body fluids, the previously described ion-exchange mechanism, between the ions in the exchangeable bone mineral compartment and those in the fluids, plays a buffering role. For example, following the infusion of calcium, the product of the calcium ion and phosphate ion activities increases, which leads in turn to a net movement of ions into the bone crystals; in contrast, the infusion of a chelating agent such as sodium versenate leads to a fall in the ion product and to a net movement of ions into the fluids. However, as soon as the compensatory physiologic adjustments take place and the product returns to its normal value, the ions move back from the fluids into the exchangeable compartment of the bone mineral.

Adjustments to Chronic Changes in Mineral Concentrations of Body Fluids. An imbalance between the rate of bone deposition and the rate of bone resorption will soon lead to changes in the concentrations of the calcium and phosphate in the body fluids. If the imbalance is small, changes in the function of the kidney and of the gastrointestinal tract may be able to bring about compensatory adjustments. A major imbalance invariably leads to a disordered metabolism of calcium and phosphate such as is present in the various metabolic bone diseases. Abnormalities in the mineral concentrations of the body fluids, such as a lack of calcium, may be corrected by alterations in the function of the kidney, in the function of the gastrointestinal tract, or in the function of the bone. In the case of bone, additional calcium is made available to the body fluids by the development of an imbalance in which the rate of bone resorption exceeds the rate of bone formation, either because resorption is increased or because deposition is decreased. The ability of both the kidney and the gastrointestinal tract to make such compensatory adjustments is limited; furthermore, frequently it is an impairment in the function of one of these two organs which causes the abnormality in the mineral concentration (such as the lack of calcium) in the body fluids. Consequently, the major system responsible for maintaining the constancy of the plasma calcium concentration is the regulation of the balance between the rate of resorption and the rate of deposition of bone.

Role of Bone in Mineral Homeostasis. In mineral homeostasis, therefore, bone acts in two capacities: (1) the exchangeable compartment of the bone mineral serves a buffering function by rapidly compensating for acute changes in the plasma concentrations of calcium and phosphate; and (2) the cellular regulation of the dynamic processes of bone remodeling serves a homeostatic function by adjusting the balance between the rate of bone formation and the rate of bone resorption so that it compensates for chronic changes in the plasma concentrations of calcium and phosphate.

ACTION OF PARATHYROID HORMONE ON CALCIUM, PHOSPHATE, AND BONE METABOLISM

Action on Bone. As a result of direct parathyroid hormone action on bone, potentially osteogenic cells are converted into osteolytic-type cells which are either multinucleated giant cells (osteoclasts) or osteolytic fibroblasts. Osteoblastic activity initially is decreased, and the active osteolysis leads to increased bone resorption with simultaneous release of both matrix and mineral components from bone, raising the plasma calcium and phosphate concentrations. As well, the hormone causes a net loss in phosphate by either blocking tubular reabsorption of phosphate or increasing distal tubular secretion of phosphate. The loss of phosphate results in a fall in the calcium-phosphate ion product which is buffered by further dissolution of the mineral components from the exchangeable compartment of bone. However, as bone resorption is increased by the hormone and the ion product is returned to the normal range, calcium and phosphate leave the extracellular fluid and return to the exchangeable compartment of bone mineral. Thus, this compartment serves as a buffer which may be controlled in part by osteoblastic activity. Since the increase in bone resorption impairs the weight-bearing capacity of bone, this leads to increased mechanical stress and compensatory activation of resting osteogenic cells into active osteoblasts, thereby inducing an increase in the rate of bone growth and mineral accretion.

Integrated Concept of Mechanism of Action. When one considers the points in the living organism at which the regulation of the calcium metabolism could be achieved, four sites come to mind: the bone, the kidney, the gastrointestinal tract, and the lactating mammary gland. There is experimental evidence that the parathyroid hormone influences the exchange of calcium at each of these sites. It must be emphasized that calcium reabsorption by the renal tubule, calcium absorption from and secretion into the gastrointestinal tract, calcium deposition into and resorption from bone, and calcium secretion into milk continue in the complete absence of the parathyroid glands. The parathyroid hormone, in common with all other mammalian hormones, does not initiate any process *de novo,* but exerts a regulatory influence by controlling the rates of one or more of the metabolic reactions involved in the process. The net effect of these actions is to increase the calcium ion activity of the plasma.

Dependence of Parathyroid Hormone Actions on the Presence of Adequate Vitamin D. From a physiologic point of view, the function of the D vitamins appears to be that of maintaining the concentration of calcium and of phosphate in the plasma at levels sufficient to ensure calcification of the bone matrix (i.e., to maintain the product of the calcium ion and phosphate ion activities above a certain critical level), whereas the actions of the parathyroid hormone are superimposed upon this basic system to control the level of the calcium ion activity in the plasma.

ACTION OF STEROLS ON CALCIUM, PHOSPHATE, AND BONE METABOLISM

Sterols with Vitamin D Activity. In the group of the D vitamins, there are three main sterols with physiologic activity. *Calciferol, or vitamin D_2,* is the major biologically active product obtained from the irradiation of ergosterol, a sterol derived from fungi and yeast. Calciferol has a potency per milligram of 40,000 International Units. *Vitamin D_3, or activated 7-dehydrocholesterol,* is the D vitamin obtained from a variety of natural animal sources, such as fish oils, and is thought to be the active form of the vitamin produced by the irradiation of the human skin with ultraviolet light. *Dihydrotachysterol,* more commonly known as A.T.10, is the third sterol of biologic importance. This substance is a derivative of one of the major components of the mixture of sterols formed by the irradiation of ergosterol. This compound was developed in 1933 by Holtz. It should be noted that *vitamin D* is the generic name for this group of substances, and that there is no preparation called vitamin D_1.

Effects of Vitamin D. The complete elimination of vitamin D induces the following effects: (1) a decrease in the absorption of calcium from the gastrointestinal tract, apparently through a direct effect upon the calcium transport mechanism; (2) a decrease in the excretion of calcium in the urine, possibly as a result of an increase in the tubular reabsorption of calcium; (3) hypocalcemia; (4) an increase in the excretion of phosphate in the urine, probably as a result of a decrease in the proximal tubular reabsorption of phosphate; (5) either normophosphatemia or hypophosphatemia; (6) an increase in the excretion of amino acids in the urine, most likely as a result of a decrease in the proximal tubular reabsorption of amino acids; (7) a decrease in the resorption of bone; (8) hypocitremia; (9) hypocitruria; (10) a decrease in the content of citrate in the bone; and (11) a decrease in the content of citrate in the kidney.

The development of these abnormalities can be prevented in man by the administration of as little as 40 to 400 IU of vitamin D per day. In the treatment of the well-defined clinical entity of vitamin D deficiency, higher doses of vitamin D are recommended (see Chap. 79).

Differences in Effects of Sterols with D Vitamin Activity. In the past, dihydrotachysterol was considered to be a sterol with predominantly calcium-mobilizing activity but with little or no antirachitic activity. This assumption now has been shown to be incorrect. All three agents, vitamin D_2, vitamin D_3, and dihydrotachysterol, possess an antirachitic effect in man. These agents apparently differ only in their speed of action—dihydrotachysterol being the more rapidly acting sterol and calciferol or vitamin D_2 the least rapid.

Comparative Effects of D Vitamins and Effects of Parathyroid Hormone. The important differences in activity are: (1) the D vitamins in physiologic and pharmacologic doses are more effective in increasing the gastrointestinal absorption of calcium than the parathyroid hormone; (2) the parathyroid hormone is a more potent phosphaturic agent than the D vitamins and is a more potent bone-resorbing agent; and (3) the parathyroid hormone also has a more rapid onset of action than the D vitamins.

ACTION OF OTHER HORMONES ON CALCIUM AND PHOSPHATE METABOLISM AND ON BONE

The hormones of certain other endocrine glands alter the metabolism of calcium and phosphate, and thus have an influence upon the actions of the parathyroid hormone and of the sterols with vitamin D activity. Similarly, the parathyroid hormone and the D vitamins alter the metabolism of calcium and phosphate and, hence, have an influence upon the actions of the hormones of these other glands.

Gonadal Hormones. The physiology of the gonads and their hormones are presented elsewhere (Chaps. 72 and 73). The gonadal hormones, androgen and estrogen, have important effects on calcium and phosphate metabolism and on bone. Androgenic substances have a protein anabolic action and induce the retention of nitrogen, phosphate, potassium, sulfur, and water in the proportions that exist in protoplasm. Thus, androgens stimulate the growth of all tissues, including the matrix of cartilage and the matrix of bone. In addition, androgens induce the retention of calcium and additional phosphate in the proportions that exist in bone probably as a secondary consequence of the matrix formation and calcification. Estrogenic substances likewise have a general protein anabolic action,

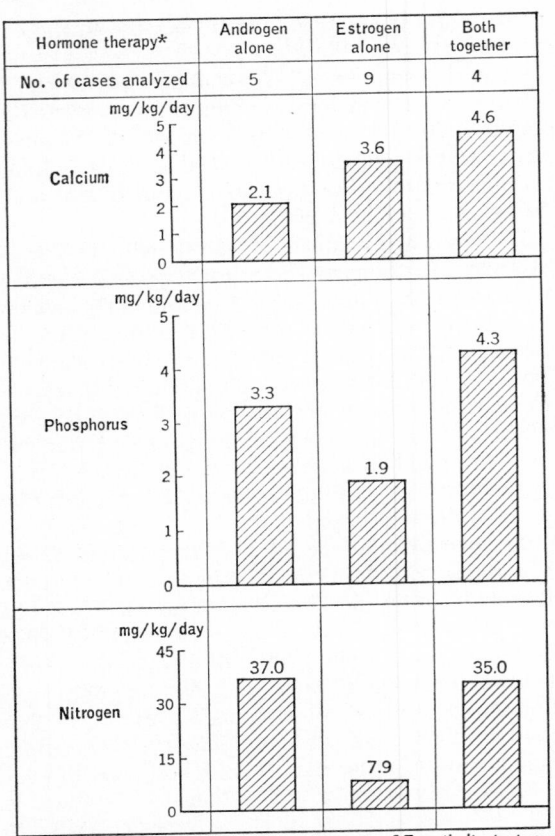

Hormone therapy*	Androgen alone	Estrogen alone	Both together
No. of cases analyzed	5	9	4
Calcium (mg/kg/day)	2.1	3.6	4.6
Phosphorus (mg/kg/day)	3.3	1.9	4.3
Nitrogen (mg/kg/day)	37.0	7.9	35.0

*Androgens: testosterone, testosterone propionate, 17-methyltestosterone
Estrogens: estradiol benzoate, diethylstilbestrol

Fig. 77-1. Chart to illustrate the average net retention of calcium, phosphorus, and nitrogen with prolonged androgenic and estrogenic therapy alone and in combination in patients with postmenopausal and/or senile osteoporosis during metabolic balance studies. The periods of analysis during therapy varied from 15 to 48 days. Note that when estrogen is given alone, there is a greater retention of calcium and a lesser retention of nitrogen than when androgen is given alone. Note further that, although the combination of both gonadal hormones does not result in more nitrogen retention than is obtained with androgen alone, the combination results in a greater calcium retention than with either estrogen or androgen alone.

which is considerably less marked than that of the androgens. However, estrogen is thought to have a specific stimulating effect on the osteoblasts, and thereby causes an increase in their activity, with matrix formation and, secondarily, calcium and phosphate deposition as part of the process of bone formation. Estrogen causes more calcium retention than androgen, but the combination of these hormones induces a greater effect than either agent alone (Fig. 77-1). Both hormones reduce the urinary and fecal calcium content as part of their

action in stimulating osteogenesis. Adequate quantities of protein foodstuffs, ascorbic acid, and growth hormone (in the child), as well as a physiologic amount of estrogen and androgen (in the adult), are necessary for the full function of the osteoblasts in bone formation.

The gonadal hormones exert an effect upon the plasma inorganic phosphate level. The onset of adolescence is accompanied by a fall in this level, and the administration of androgens or estrogens results in a decrease in plasma phosphate level in patients with acromegaly, in excessively tall children, in postmenopausal women, and in castrate individuals. The mechanism of this action is not clear, although it has been postulated that suppression of pituitary growth hormone by the gonadal hormones in part may be responsible.

In most clinical conditions, the administration of androgenic or estrogenic hormones alone or in combination does not induce an alteration in the concentration of the calcium in the plasma. However, in patients with osseous involvement due to metastatic neoplasm, administration of gonadal hormones may be followed by hypercalcemia, particularly when the bone lesions are of the osteolytic type. The hypercalcemia appears to be related only indirectly to the actions of the gonadal hormones. It is believed that the hormones stimulate the tumor cells to grow more rapidly, and this leads to increased osteolysis; the amount of calcium released by the bone that is being destroyed by the tumor frequently exceeds the maximum excretory capacity of the kidney and thus causes an increase in the plasma calcium concentration. Furthermore, prolonged hypercalcuria (which commonly occurs with osteolytic lesions) may impair the calcium excretory mechanism so that the maximum filtration capacity is reduced.

Adrenal Cortical Hormones. The physiology of the adrenal cortex and its steroid hormones is presented elsewhere (Chap. 68). One of the major actions of the glucogenic steroids, hydrocortisone (cortisol) and cortisone, is to increase the rate of gluconeogenesis. This results in the depletion of body protein, particularly the protein moiety of connective tissue of which the matrix of cartilage and bone is a major constituent. Excessive glucocorticoids induce a negative calcium balance which is an important factor in the production of osteoporosis. A negative calcium balance is brought about by the reduction of calcium absorption in the intestine and the facilitation of calcium excretion in the urine. In bone, the manifestations of the antianabolic action of the glucocorticoid agents is a reduction in the rate of activity of the osteoblasts and, consequently, a decrease in the rate of formation of bone. This leads to the development of osteoporosis. In contrast to the effect of cortisol, there is at least experimental evidence that the mineralo-corticoids facilitate calcification of cartilage (see Addison's disease, Chap. 68). In man, hypercalcuria following cortisol administration is not accompanied by hypercalcemia.

In addition to the glucogenic steroids, the adrenal cortex synthesizes other hormones, including substances with androgenic and with estrogenic actions whose effects mimic those of gonadal origin. In children with the adrenogenital syndrome, there is an acceleration in the rate of osseous growth and also in the rate at which the epiphyses close, the net result being normal or slightly decreased height and thickened bones.

Thyroid Hormone. The physiology of the thyroid gland and its hormonal substances are discussed elsewhere (Chap. 66). One of the chief actions of the thyroid hormone is to increase the basal energy metabolism of all living cells. For example, in the absence of the thyroid hormone, there is a marked retardation in endochondral bone formation (growth) and in maturation of the epiphyseal cartilage. In addition, there is a decrease in the rate of activity of all the biologic processes concerned with the absorption, metabolism, and excretion of minerals and the formation and resorption of bone. In contrast, an excess of thyroid hormone accelerates the rates of all these biologic processes and creates a need for increase in the quantity of all the materials that participate in these systems. As a consequence of this, the rate of calcium absorption is increased in the gastrointestinal tract and there is an over-all increased requirement for calcium and vitamin D intake.

Patients with hyperthyroidism frequently have hypercalcuria, which is associated usually with normocalcemia, and rarely with hypercalcemia and an accelerated rate of bone turnover as indicated by an increased rate of turnover of injected radiocalcium (Ca^{45}). It is suggested that the sequence of events in the action of the thyroid hormone on bone and mineral metabolism may be: (1) an initial effect of increasing the rate of bone resorption, (2) hypercalcemia as a result of the accelerated resorption of bone, (3) a decrease in the production of the parathyroid hormone as a result of the elevated plasma calcium concentration, (4) a compensatory decrease in the rate of bone resorption as a result of the decreased amount of parathyroid hormone, (5) a compensatory decrease in the tubular reabsorption of calcium as a result of the decreased amount of parathyroid hormone, and (6) hypercalcuria as a result of the decreased tubular reabsorption of calcium. These postulated compensatory adjustments usually are sufficient to maintain the plasma concentration of calcium in the physiologic range. However, in severe hyperthyroidism, the excessive amount of bone resorption leads to hypercalcemia in spite of the compensatory underproduction of parathyroid hormone. In the patient with hyperthyroidism, biopsy of bone often reveals evidence of an increase in osteolytic activity with osteitis fibrosa generalisata. In addition, severe hyperthyroidism may lead to disturbances in protein metabolism with a negative nitrogen balance and osteoporosis.

Growth Hormone. The somatotropic or growth hormone of the anterior pituitary gland has a primary action of stimulating the basal energy metabolism of all living cells. Therefore, some of the effects of this hormone on mineral and bone metabolism may result from the same mechanisms which were suggested for the thyroid hormone (see above). For example, lack of growth hormone leads to a retardation of endochondral bone growth and of epiphyseal maturation. An excess of growth hormone, like an excess of thyroid hormone, leads to osteoporosis in many patients with acromegaly. In addition, however, growth hormone has a direct stimulating effect on membranous bone formation; the manifestations of this action are readily apparent in patients with acromegaly. When an increased amount of growth hormone is present (as in growing children or acromegalic patients), the plasma phosphate level is greater than the physiologic range of the mature young adult.

Other Anterior Pituitary Tropic Hormones. It is generally believed that there is no tropic hormone from the anterior pituitary gland which regulates the secretion of the parathyroid hormone by the parathyroid glands. Although other tropic hormones of the anterior pituitary gland (such as adrenocorticotropin, thyrotropin, and gonadotropin) have complex effects upon the growth and the turnover of bone, these effects appear to be mediated by the actions of these tropic hormones upon their respective target glands.

Insulin. The hormone of the pancreatic islet cells, insulin, is essential for normal carbohydrate metabolism. Patients with diabetes mellitus (Chap. 70) characteristically exhibit increased gluconeogenesis and a negative nitrogen balance. In addition, in the presence of ketoacidosis, increased quantities of calcium may be eliminated in the urine. However, today, with insulin therapy, diabetes mellitus alone rarely is the cause of severe osteoporosis. The plasma phosphate level usually is increased in diabetes mellitus and decreased in hyperinsulinism.

RELATION OF CERTAIN METALLIC AND NONMETALLIC ELEMENTS TO BONE METABOLISM

Mineral elements are involved in many of the processes concerned with the chemistry and physiology of normal bone. It is to be expected, therefore, that at times these processes may be affected by abnormal concentrations of certain elements which usually either are absent from the body fluids of the normal individual or are present only in trace amounts.

These extraneous elements can participate in bone metabolism at several points: they may (1) replace atoms within the hydroxyapatite crystal structure; (2) deposit as surface adherents on the hydroxyapatite crystals; (3) combine with or replace constituents of the protein components of the osteoid, thus altering its characteristics and ability to become calcified; (4) alter the activity of osteoblasts or osteoclasts by exerting on them stimulating or inhibiting effects; (5) modify enzyme activity involved in bone metabolism; (6) modify the manner in which plasma and other biologic fluids handle calcium and phosphate; (7) affect the activity of the parathyroid glands, the other endocrine glands, the intestinal tract, the kidneys, or the other organs concerned with the processes of calcium and phosphate metabolism; or (8) exert other systemic effects which indirectly affect bone and its normal mineral constituents. A common sequence which apparently follows the introduction of a foreign element into the osteoblasts, the osteocytes, or the osteoclasts is: (1) stimulation of activity with a small concentration, (2) inhibition of activity with a larger concentration, (3) secondary necrosis and fibrosis from the irritation and/or radiation produced by the element, and (4) secondary bacterial invasion of the involved cells.

The following is a partial list of chemical elements which may become involved in bone metabolism: arsenic, bismuth, cadmium, gold, lead, and silver (see Chap. 102); barium, fluoride, magnesium, and phosphorus (see Chap. 103); radium (see Chap. 108); americium, beryllium, cerium, curium, lanthanum, manganese, plutonium, strontium, and yttrium. The effects of certain of these elements on bone are entirely innocuous; the effects of others are as yet inadequately described. The manifestations induced by these substances on bone are discussed in other sections of the book (see above). Certain recent observations deserve mention. Beryllium has a marked stimulating effect on osteoblasts, and intoxication with this substance in animals has resulted in neoplastic lesions resembling osteogenic sarcoma. Alkaline earth metals such as strontium, barium, and radium are localized predominantly in the skeleton and generally are affected by the same conditions which affect calcium metabolism. Metals such as yttrium and plutonium have some distribution in soft tissues (such as the uncalcified osteoid matrix) but are localized chiefly in bone, particularly in the areas where resorption is occurring. Metals such as cerium,

lanthanum, americium, and curium are taken up in large amounts initially by the liver as well as by bone. These metals disappear from the liver in a few months but remain rather firmly fixed in the skeleton.

DEFINITION AND CLASSIFICATION OF METABOLIC BONE DISORDERS

A metabolic disorder of bone may be defined as a disease of bone arising from a disturbance in the general metabolism of the body. Metabolic bone diseases, therefore, are generalized or systemic bone diseases which influence all the bones of the body. However, it is not uncommon for some parts of the skeleton to respond with a more pronounced degree of disorder than others. For example, there may be generalized decalcification as part of the bone disease with hyperparathyroidism, and in addition there may be localized cysts and tumors. Similarly, all the bones of the body may be affected by the loss of stresses and strains which leads to atrophy (osteoporosis) of disuse; however, the patient immobilized in bed who develops osteoporosis of his limbs still uses his skull and mandibles as much as when he is up and about, and hence these bones do not manifest the bone disease. Likewise, estrogen deficiency affects all the tissues of the body, including the bones; in spite of this, the vertebras show the most marked osteoporosis, and the skull is rarely involved.

To be contrasted with the metabolic diseases of bone are the localized diseases of bone. The one essential feature in establishing that a bone disorder is localized is the finding of an uninvolved area with normal bone. At the same time it should be pointed out that localized bone disease may be very widespread. For example, Paget's disease of bone may involve 95 per cent of the skeleton, but a careful roentgenographic survey will disclose normal bone in some areas with a sharp line of demarcation between it and the involved bone.

The metabolic bone disorders can be divided into two main groups in terms of the total amount of calcified bone present in the body: there can be either too little calcified bone or too much calcified bone. Since the mass of bone in the body is in a state of dynamic equilibrium, an alteration in the total mass of calcified bone can be brought about in two ways: either by changes in the amount of bone formation or by changes in the amount of bone resorption.

In Table 77-1, metabolic bone diseases are classified according to this scheme. It will be noted that a further subdivision is necessary, since bone formation consists of two steps: (1) the laying down of the matrix by the osteoblasts and (2) the deposition of the calcium salts into this matrix.

Table 77-1. CLASSIFICATION OF METABOLIC BONE DISORDERS

I. Too little calcified bone
  A. Too little bone formation
    1. Defect in matrix formation: osteoporosis
    2. Defect in matrix calcification: osteomalacia or rickets
  B. Too much bone resorption: osteitis fibrosa generalisata
II. Too much calcified bone
  A. Too much bone formation
    1. Increased matrix formation: hyperosteogenesis
    2. Increased matrix calcification: nonexistent
  B. Too little bone resorption: osteosclerosis

Thus, there may be a defect in the formation of the matrix or a defect in the calcification of the matrix, both of which would lead to too little bone formation. When the defect is in matrix formation, the condition is spoken of as *osteoporosis;* when the defect is in the calcification of the matrix, the defect is spoken of as *osteomalacia* (adult rickets). Too much bone resorption produces the condition called *osteitis fibrosa generalisata.*

Increased matrix formation leads to too great bone formation and, hence, to too much calcified bone; this condition is called *hyperosteogenesis.* The evidence indicates that the matrix is either calcified or not calcified and that it cannot become supercalcified; hence, there is no heading under "too much calcified bone" which corresponds to osteomalacia under "too little calcified bone." Too much calcified bone also results from too little bone resorption; this condition is called *osteosclerosis.*

In Table 77-2, metabolic bone disorders are classified according to the pathologic mechanisms which lead to the osseous condition into two main groups: (1) disturbances in bone turnover and (2) disturbances in bone calcification. The conditions with alterations in bone turnover involve disorders in which there are: (1) disturbances in the equilibrium between bone formation and bone resorption and (2) disturbances in the amount of bone turnover. Since increased calcification of the matrix does not occur (see Table 77-1), the disturbances in bone calcification include only conditions in which there is an insufficient amount of hydroxyapatite deposited for the amount of matrix that is formed.

Disturbances in the equilibrium between the rate of the cellular process (osteoblastic activity) involved in the formation of bone and the rate of the cellular process (osteolytic activity) involved in the resorption of bone result in osseous disorders in which the density of the bone may be either decreased or increased. Conditions with decreased bone density result either from decreased osteoblastic activity or from increased osteolytic activity;

Table 77-2. CLASSIFICATION OF PATHOLOGIC MECHANISMS LEADING TO METABOLIC BONE DISORDERS

I. Disturbances in bone turnover
  A. Disturbances in equilibrium between bone formation and bone resorption (abnormal bone density)
    1. Decreased bone density
      a. Decreased osteoblastic activity: osteoporosis
      b. Increased osteolytic activity: osteitis fibrosa generalisata
    2. Increased bone density
      a. Increased osteoblastic activity: hyperosteogenesis
      b. Decreased osteolytic activity: osteosclerosis
  B. Disturbances in amount of bone turnover (normal bone density)
    1. Increased bone turnover
      a. Increased osteoblastic and osteolytic activity
        i. Hyperparathyroidism*
        ii. Hyperthyroidism*
    2. Decreased bone turnover
      a. Decreased osteoblastic and osteolytic activity
        i. Hypoparathyroidism†
        ii. Hypothyroidism†
II. Disturbances in bone calcification
  A. Disturbances in equilibrium between matrix production and hydroxyapatite deposition (decreased bone density)
    1. Normal plasma product of calcium and phosphate ion activities
      a. Increased rate of matrix production with normal rate of hydroxyapatite deposition: osteomalacia or rickets
    2. Decreased plasma product of calcium and phosphate ion activities
      a. Normal rate of matrix production with decreased rate of hydroxyapatite deposition: osteomalacia or rickets

* Initial or mild stage with a compensatory increase in osteoblastic activity sufficient to restore the equilibrium between the rate of bone resorption and the rate of bone formation.

† Late or severe stage with a compensatory decrease in osteoblastic activity sufficient to restore the equilibrium between the rate of bone resorption and the rate of bone formation.

SOURCE: Modified from a classification by R. H. Follis, Jr., Am. J. Med., 22:469, 1957

those with increased bone density result either from increased osteoblastic activity or from decreased osteolytic activity. It should be noted that conditions in which there is a decrease in the amount of calcification of the matrix also result in osseous disorders in which the density of the bone is decreased.

A decrease in osteoblastic activity leads to a decrease in the number and the thickness of the normally calcified bone trabeculae and to a decrease in the width of the bone cortex. This osseous condition is called *osteoporosis*. An increase in osteolytic activity is characterized by an increase in osteoclastic activity. This osseous condition is called *osteitis fibrosa generalisata,* a name derived from the fact that, in addition to the increased number of osteoclastic cells, increased osteolysis also is accompanied by a proliferation of the fibrous connective tissue at the sites of bone resorption. Furthermore, there usually is a compensatory increase in osteoblastic activity in prolonged or severe osteitis fibrosa generalisata.

An increase in the density of bone is characterized by an increase in the number and the size of the bone trabeculae and by an increase in the width of the bone cortex. This condition may result either from an increase in osteoblastic activity (*hyperosteogenesis*) or from a decrease in osteolytic activity (*osteosclerosis*). Some disorders, such as hypoparathyroidism, which are characterized by a decrease in osteolytic activity, usually exhibit only a minimal increase in bone density because there is a compensatory decrease in osteoblastic activity which eliminates the imbalance between osteogenesis and osteolysis in spite of the decrease in the rate of turnover of bone. Similarly, in the initial phase or in a mild degree of hyperparathyroidism, there may be an increase in both the osteogenesis and the osteolysis without a change in the balance between these two types of activity. Similar alterations in the rates of the processes involved in the turnover of bone without a disturbance in the dynamic equilibrium between these rates probably occur as well in hypothyroidism and in hyperthyroidism. In such conditions, the bone appears to be normal by radiologic and histologic examination; hence, in the classic sense, no disorder of bone exists. However, by the use of radioisotope technics, it is possible to demonstrate a definite change in the rate of turnover of bone in these various endocrine states.

Disturbances in the rate and the degree of calcification of the matrix of cartilage and/or bone with a decrease in the amount of calcification result in osseous disorders in which the density of bone is decreased. It should be noted that conditions in which there is a disturbance in the equilibrium between the rate of the cellular activities concerned with bone formation and/or bone resorption characterized by either decreased osteoblastic activity or increased osteolytic activity also result in osseous disorders in which the density of bone is decreased. In some conditions, the amount of deposition of hydroxyapatite in cartilage or bone matrix is not sufficient for the amount of matrix that is formed by the osteoblastic activity. This

osseous disorder is called *rickets* (in the child) or *osteomalacia* (in the adult).

Diagnostic Significance of Bone Roentgenograms. In this discussion, the terms *osteoporosis* and *osteomalacia* are used to indicate specific disease conditions and not to describe any state of bone in which too little density is seen by x-ray. There is a tendency on the part of roentgenologists to call any bone which appears to have less than the normal amount of density, osteoporotic or osteomalacic. It is apparent from the previous discussion, however, that it is impossible to determine *just from the amount of density present* whether the patient has osteoporosis, osteomalacia, or osteitis fibrosa generalisata. Furthermore, the early stages of bone disease of any of these three types escape recognition in the x-rays because it is impossible to detect with accuracy changes in density until approximately 30 to 50 per cent of the calcium has been lost. Similarly it is very difficult to detect recalcification by x-ray (in osteomalacia or osteitis fibrosa generalisata) because a considerable amount of calcium must be regained before an increase in density can be observed in the x-ray films. Attention is called also to the tendency to use the terms "*de*calcification" (*de*calcified) or "*de*mineralization" when the terms "*a*calcification" (*un*calcified) or "*a*mineralization" are meant.

It should be pointed out that any bone which contains too little calcified mass may exhibit deformity. For example, deformities of the vertebra (codfish vertebra, wedged vertebra, crushed vertebra, and herniation of the nuclei pulposi into the end-plate of the vertebra) occur in osteoporosis, osteomalacia, and osteitis fibrosa generalisata, although they may be somewhat more common in osteoporosis. In differentiating these three osseous disorders by x-ray, however, those experienced in interpreting x-ray films usually arrive at the correct diagnosis by evaluating simultaneously: (1) the type of osseous deformity (for example, there is a greater tendency for bones to bend in osteomalacia, while spontaneous fractures are more likely to occur in osteoporosis and in osteitis fibrosa generalisata); (2) the location of the overt osseous lesions (for example, osteoporosis commonly involves the spine and pelvis but rarely the skull and extremities, osteomalacia frequently involves the extremities, and osteitis fibrosa generalisata frequently involves the skull); (3) the degree of osseous involvement (for example, the degree of involvement usually is greater in osteitis fibrosa generalisata and leads more often to an absence of the lamina dura); (4) the structure of the bone density (for example, the absence of transverse but not vertical trabeculation in osteoporosis); and (5) the predilection of certain osseous lesions for a specific location in a particular bone disorder (for example, the codfish vertebras in osteoporosis or the "rugger jersey" spine in osteomalacia). The occurrence of bone cysts, "brown tumors," and lesions of the hands in osteitis fibrosa generalisata and of pseudofractures in osteomalacia is of considerable diagnostic assistance. It must be emphasized, however, that generalized decreased density *in itself usually has no particular* diagnostic significance except to indicate that a metabolic bone disorder is present.

REFERENCES

Albright, F.: The Effect of Hormones on Osteogenesis in Man, Recent Progr. in Hormone Research, 1: 293, 1947.

—— and E. C. Reifenstein, Jr.: "The Parathyroid Glands and Metabolic Bone Disease: Selected Studies," Baltimore, The Williams & Wilkins Company, 1948.

——, F. C. Bartter, E. F. Dempsey, A. P. Forbes, P. H. Henneman, and E. C. Reifenstein, Jr.: Serum Albumin and Bone Matrix, Trans. Macy Conf. on Metabolism Interrelations (with Special Reference to Calcium), 5:227, 1954.

Armstrong, W. D.: Phosphorus Metabolism in the Skeleton, in "A Symposium on Phosphorus Metabolism," E. C. McElroy and B. Glass (Eds.), vol. 2, chap. VII, pp. 698–731, Baltimore, Johns Hopkins University Press, 1952.

Follis, R. H., Jr.: A Survey of Bone Disease, Am. J. Med., 22:469, 1957.

Glimcher, M. J.: Molecular Biology of Mineralized Tissues with Particular Reference to Bone, Rev. Mod. Phys., 31:359, 1959.

Harrison, M., and R. Fraser: Bone Metabolism in Rats, Studied with Stable Strontium, J. Endocrinol., 21:191, 1960.

——: Bone Structure and Metabolism in Calcium-deficient Rats, J. Endocrinol., 21:197, 1960.

——: The Parathyroid Glands and Calcium Deficiency in the Rat, J. Endocrinol., 21:207, 1960.

Harrison, M., R. Fraser, and B. Mullan: Calcium Metabolism in Osteoporosis, Lancet, May, 1961, p. 1015.

Henneman, P. H.: Effects of High Calcium Intakes on Renal Function, Federation Proc., 18:1093, 1959.

Howard, J. E.: Calcium Metabolism, Bones and Calcium Homeostasis: A Review of Certain Current Concepts, J. Clin. Endocrinol. and Metabolism, 17: 1105, 1957.

Jackson, W. P. U., and C. Dancaster: A Consideration of the Hypercalciuria in Sarcoidosis, Idiopathic Hypercalciuria, and That Produced by Vitamin D: A New Suggestion Regarding Calcium Metabolism, J. Clin. Endocrinol. and Metabolism, 19:658, 1959.

Krane, S. M., G. L. Brownell, J. B. Stanbury, and H. Corrigan: The Effect of Thyroid Disease on Calcium Metabolism in Man, J. Clin. Invest., 35:874, 1956.

Malm, O. J.: "Calcium Requirement and Adaptation in Adult Men," Oslo (Norway), Oslo University Press, 1958.

McLean, F. C., and M. R. Urist: "Bone: An Introduction to the Physiology of Skeletal Tissue," Chicago, The University of Chicago Press, 1955.

Neuman, W. F., B. J. Mulryan, and G. R. Martin: A Chemical View of Osteoclasis Based on Studies with Yttrium, Clin. Orthopaedics, 17:124, 1960.

Nordin, B. E. C.: The Pathogenesis of Osteoporosis, Lancet, May, 1961, p. 1011.

Rasmussen, H.: Parathyroid Hormone: Nature and Mechanism of Action, Am. J. Med., 30:112, 1961.

Reifenstein, E. C., Jr. (Ed.): Transactions of Macy Foundation Conferences on Metabolic Interrelations (with Special Reference to Calcium), New York, The Josiah Macy, Jr. Foundation; vol. 3, 1951; vol. 4, 1952; and vol. 5, 1953.

——: The Relationship of Steroid Hormones to the Development and the Management of Osteoporosis in Aging People, Clin. Orthopaedics, 10:206, 1957.

Rodahl, K., J. T. Nicholson, and E. M. Brown, Jr. (Eds.): "Bone as a Tissue," New York, McGraw-Hill Book Company, Inc., Blakiston Division, 1960.

Snapper, I., and A. Kahn: Tubular Reabsorption of Phosphorus in Avitaminosis D, Clin. Orthopaedics, 17:297, 1960.

Stanbury, J. B., J. B. Wyngaarden, and D. S. Fredrickson (Eds.): "The Metabolic Basis of Inherited Disease," pp. 1177–1221, 1222–1245, and 1367–1378, New York, McGraw-Hill Book Company, Inc., Blakiston Division, 1960.

Urist, M. R. (Ed.): Symposium on the Clinical Physiology and Pathology of Bone, Clin. Orthopaedics, 17:3, 1960.

Whedon, G. D.: Effects of High Calcium Intakes on Bone, Blood and Soft Tissues; Relationship of Calcium Intake to Balance in Osteoporosis, Federation Proc., 18:1112, 1959.

——: Expansion of the Concept of Altered Bone Metabolism in Osteoporosis: Importance of Nutritional Factors, Acta Endocrinologica, 35:Suppl. 51:519, 1960.

Wolstenholme, G. E. W., and C. M. O'Connor (Eds.): "Ciba Foundation Symposium on Bone Structure and Metabolism," Boston, Little Brown & Company, 1956.

78 OSTEOPOROSIS

Edward C. Reifenstein, Jr.

Osteoporosis is the result, primarily, of insufficient production of bone matrix by osteoblasts to maintain the rate of bone formation in equilibrium with the rate of bone resorption, and therefore belongs to that category of "too little calcified bone" in which the decrease of calcified bone tissue is due to inadequate bone formation. There is evidence to suggest that a simple deficiency of calcium is sufficient to produce the disease. In man, whatever matrix is formed is normally calcified and the bone formation rate is normal as measured with the isotope Ca^{45}. The plasma calcium, phosphate, and alkaline phosphatase levels are normal.

Osteoporosis may develop rapidly with disuse, since under these circumstances immobilization reduces the stress of weight bearing and hence reduces the stimulation to osteoblastic activity. Thus with the reduced stress of weight bearing there occurs a compensatory increase in the osteolytic activity with a consequent rapid increase in bone resorption.

CLINICAL TYPES (See Table 78-1)

Postmenopausal and/or Senile Osteoporosis. *Incidence.* The exact incidence of senile osteoporosis cannot be determined at present because of the technical difficulties inherent in estimating a decrease in bone mass—a decrease of approximately 50 per cent in bone density being required before a significant change can be detected with certainty in the roentgenogram. Surveys indicate that more than half of men and women over the age of sixty have a degree of osteoporosis sufficient to be detected in roentgenograms of the vertebras. In aging women, osteoporosis occurs much more frequently and at an earlier age than in men, and tends to be more severe. The incidence of osteoporosis in elderly women appears to be approximately five times that seen in men of comparable age. In women over fifty, half will show roentgenographic evidence of decreased bone mass, about 30 per cent will exhibit a previously unrecognized fractured vertebra, although only 10 per cent will complain of symptoms directly referable to osteoporosis. The occurrence and severity of symptoms frequently show no correlation with the degree of osteoporosis as recorded by roentgenograms.

Etiology. It is recognized that all tissues atrophy with age, and bone is no exception. Skeletal atrophy is termed osteoporosis.

It is necessary at this point to define postmenopausal osteoporosis in women and senile osteoporosis in men and women. Those women who develop clinical osteoporosis after menopause at any time up to the age of sixty-five are said to have postmenopausal osteoporosis. Those women and men who first develop clinical osteoporosis after the age of sixty-five are said to have senile osteoporosis. The evidence suggests that the pathologic process underlying the development of postmenopausal osteoporosis does not differ significantly from that which develops at a later age in men and women (senile osteoporosis).

Table 78-1. PROVISIONAL CLASSIFICATION OF CAUSES OF OSTEOPOROSIS

I. Insufficient osteogenic activity of osteoblasts: osteoporosis
   A. Calcium deficiency
      1. Dietary
      2. Sprue
   B. Decrease in physiologic stimulus to osteoblasts: loss of stress and strain
      1. Sedentary physical activities
      2. Atrophy (osteoporosis) of disuse or immobilization
   C. Damage to osteoblasts by external agents
      1. Radiation
      2. Poisoning from certain chemicals
   D. Genetic defect in osteoblasts or matrix structures
      1. Osteogenesis imperfecta
      2. Ehlers-Danlos syndrome
   E. Insufficient nutrition of osteoblasts
      1. Protein deficiency and general malnutrition
      2. Scurvy (hypovitaminosis C; ascorbic acid deficiency)
      3. Deficiency of other nutrients essential for activity of osteoblasts or for formation of osteoid matrix
      4. Hyperthyroidism with insufficient protein intake
      5. Diabetes mellitus with insufficient protein intake
   F. Endocrine imbalance: hormonal inhibition greater than hormonal stimulation of osteoblasts
      1. Absolute increase in antianabolic (inhibiting) hormones over anabolic (stimulating) hormones: corticosteroid excess with normal androgen and/or estrogen levels
        a. Cushing's syndrome
        b. Hyperadrenocorticism from chronic corticosteroid medication
        c. Prolonged stress
      2. Relative increase in antianabolic (inhibiting) hormones over anabolic (stimulating) hormones: androgen and/or estrogen deficiency with normal corticosteroid levels
        a. Hypogonadism in individuals with preadolescent development
        b. Gonadal dysgenesis and Turner's syndrome
        c. Hypogonadism in individuals with postadolescent development
        d. Postmenopausal and senile individuals with osteoporosis
   G. Mechanism unknown
      1. Acromegaly
      2. Idiopathic osteoporosis
      3. Tumor cells in bone marrow

SOURCE: Modified from a classification by R. H. Follis, Jr., Am. J. Med., 22: 469, 1957.

There appear to be at least two major factors in the etiology of postmenopausal or senile osteoporosis: (1) a reduction in the amount of gonadal hormones without a concomitant decrease in adrenal glucogenic hormones and (2) an inadequate intake of calcium. Hormone production by the gonads decreases more abruptly and at an earlier age in women than in men, and this may be an important predisposing factor. These hormonal alterations increase the amount of calcium required to maintain the calcium balance in equilibrium. In addition, the possible effects of pregnancy, lactation, physical activity, and genetically determined factors must be considered.

Pathology. Bone sections from patients with acute osteoporosis may show a decrease in the calcified mass with very few osteoclasts and rare osteoblasts; in these cases the trabeculae are few and narrow. In the long-standing cases, a small number of osteoid seams of normal width are seen. In many of these cases it may be impossible to tell from any given section of a bone biopsy that the total mass of calcified bone is reduced in amount.

Pathologic Physiology. The rate of bone formation is not adequate to maintain an equilibrium with the rate of bone resorption. As bone resorption continues, the amount of calcified bone is gradually decreased until symptoms arise. The decreased bone mass becomes increasingly susceptible to the stresses and strains of weight bearing, and eventually these stresses stimulate osteoblastic activity sufficiently to restore the equilibrium. However, by the time that this occurs, a considerable reduction in calcified bone mass will have taken place.

Clinical Manifestations. Patients with symptomatic postmenopausal or senile osteoporosis complain of pain in the bones, particularly in the back. They show deformities resulting from spontaneous fractures and may exhibit symptoms from renal calculi which have developed during the acute manifestations of the disease. They have thin skin and may exhibit weakness, anorexia, and manifestations of estrogen deficiency. Osteoporosis tends to involve the spine and pelvis and, rarely, the skull and extremities. There is a greater tendency to spontaneous fractures than to bending of the bones. It should be emphasized that there can be a great deal of deformity without any symptoms. This is particularly true of wedged and collapsed vertebras which may be less serious clinically than appears by x-ray. In spite of collapsed vertebras, patients very rarely show damage to the spinal cord. The tendency is to exaggerate the seriousness of these collapsed vertebras and to immobilize the patient in a plaster cast for a long period of time, thus inducing atrophy of disuse which will increase the amount of osteoporosis.

Laboratory Findings. In the typical case of long-standing postmenopausal or senile osteoporosis with symptoms, the plasma calcium, inorganic phosphate, and alkaline phosphatase levels are in the normal range. The plasma protein concentration may be normal or slightly low. The urinary calcium excretion is either within the normal range or rarely increased. When acute osteoporosis of disuse is superimposed on senile osteoporosis, there may be a transient hypercalcuria and a tendency toward hypercalcemia.

Diagnosis. In postmenopausal or senile osteoporosis, one finds characteristically a middle-aged or elderly patient with: (1) pain in the back, (2) x-ray changes which indicate a decreased calcified bone mass, (3) normal plasma chemistry, (4) possibly a history or evidence of renal calculi, (5) no other apparent cause for the osteoporosis, and (6) a favorable response to therapy with calcium, estrogens, and or androgens.

Differential Diagnosis. It has been pointed out that generalized demineralization involving the spine and the long bones occurs predominantly in osteoporosis, but it may be found occasionally in osteomalacia and in osteitis fibrosa generalisata. Both of the latter conditions may be excluded in the presence of normal values for plasma calcium, inorganic phosphate, and alkaline phosphatase. A picture similar by x-ray to osteoporosis may be found in multiple myeloma. In these cases the plasma calcium may be normal or elevated, and the plasma phosphate and alkaline phosphatase levels are usually normal as in the case of senile osteoporosis. The presence of an elevated plasma globulin level, plasma cells in the peripheral blood or on bone marrow biopsy, Bence-Jones protein in the urine, and punched-out radiologic lesions in the skull and long bones help to confirm the diagnosis of multiple myeloma. Osteogenesis imperfecta occurs in young individuals with blue scleras, nerve deafness, and a family history of bone pathology. Metastatic malignancy, sarcoidosis, xanthomatosis, neurofibromatosis, Paget's disease of bone, polyostotic fibrous dysplasia (osteitis fibrosa disseminata, Albright's syndrome) usually present characteristic localized x-ray changes, abnormal plasma chemistry values, or other distinguishing features. Since tumor metastases may be present in bone without overt manifestations, the patient with demonstrated osteoporosis should be examined carefully for primary neoplastic lesions.

Prognosis. The prognosis for most patients with postmenopausal or senile osteoporosis is relatively good; however, the condition requires prolonged treatment. By the time the diagnosis is established, the disease will have been present for some years and the bone involvement is marked. Furthermore, by this time, osteoblastic activity will have been accelerated by the abnormal responsiveness of the thin skeleton to the stress and strain of weight bearing so that an equilibrium between bone formation and bone resorption will have been approximated.

Treatment. Therapy is designed to eliminate pain and to prevent further vertebral fractures. Since the majority of patients with postmenopausal or senile osteoporosis exhibit a negative calcium balance, a cardinal factor in treatment is the induction of a positive balance. This can be accomplished in most instances by giving calcium orally at a dose level of 2 to 3 Gm daily. The preparations of calcium for oral use are enumerated in Table 67-1. In addition, hormonal therapy may be expected to benefit most patients since such therapy decreases the amount of calcium required to induce a positive balance. In female patients with osteoporosis, estrogen is recommended in doses sufficient to produce cyclic menstrual bleeding, i.e., 21 days on medication and 7 days off. It is believed that a dose of estrogen sufficient to produce withdrawal bleeding is adequate to induce a positive calcium balance. In the absence of the uterus, cyclic therapy is not necessary and estrogen can be administered without interruption. In this instance, the level of estrogen needed must be empirical since there is no objective end point, i.e., uterine withdrawal bleeding. It is important to be certain that stenosis of the uterine cervix does not exist and that there is no carcinomatous change in the cervix or breast. Table 78-2 lists some of the available estrogenic preparations. There is some evidence that there may be advantages in administering a combination of androgen-estrogen therapy in conjunction with supplementary calcium for both men and women. Preparations which have been employed for this purpose are also listed in Table 78-2. Although the combined hormone preparations rarely give rise to undesirable androgenic side effects in women when properly administered, this fact must be weighed in the over-all utilization of such preparations. In men patients with osteoporosis, androgenic hormone therapy alone or combined hormone preparations may be used to supplement oral calcium medication. When androgens are used in this age group,

Table 78-2. GONADAL HORMONE PREPARATIONS

	Usual dose
Diethylstilbestrol	0.5–3 mg/day
Ethynyl estradiol	0.02–0.05 mg/day
Equine conjugated estrogens	1.25–5.0 mg/day
Estradiol valerate	20 mg IM/2 weeks
Testosterone propionate	50 mg IM/week
Testosterone enanthate	200 mg IM/month
Combined therapy: ethynyl estradiol with methyltestosterone	0.02–0.04 mg with 5–10 mg/day
Combined therapy: estradiol valerate with testosterone enanthate	8 mg with 180 mg IM/month

careful examination of the prostate for both benign prostatic hypertrophy or neoplasm should be carried out. This study should also include measurement of prostatic acid phosphatase.

Contrary to what might be anticipated, supplementary vitamin D administration is not indicated in the treatment of postmenopausal or senile osteoporosis as this frequently leads to the overabsorption of calcium with its inherent dangers of hypercalcemia, hypercalcuria, renal calculi, and renal calcinosis. A diet which provides adequate calories and a protein intake of high biologic value is desirable. In the presence of malabsorption, serious consideration must be given to the type of food, the frequency of feeding, and the advantage of supplementary medication (see Sprue and Other Malabsorption Syndromes, Chap. 62).

Prolonged or excessive immobilization must be avoided to minimize the atrophy of disuse. It is essential, however, to provide support for collapsed vertebras, and the use of a corset or brace should be considered. Because of the rather wide-spread distribution of senile osteoporosis, it is wise for physicians to consider this possibility during their examination and evaluation of elderly patients. With x-ray evidence of mineralization of bones, a prophylactic therapeutic program of 2 to 3 Gm of calcium salts daily is recommended. It is thought by some that the gonadal hormones can be used prophylactically with advantage under these circumstances. Gastrointestinal malabsorption as a possible etiologic factor should be excluded in all instances.

Atrophy of Disuse. Osteoporosis associated with immobilization of a previously active portion of the skeleton represents one of the most frequent causes of osteoporosis. Metabolic studies on normal young adults indicate that immobilization produces a loss of 1 to 2 per cent of the total body calcium in a period of 5 or 6 weeks. Thus, each day, 100 to 200 mg that normally would be added to the bone mass is lost from the body by the cessation of bone formation. Atrophy of disuse frequently complicates other types of osteoporosis, particularly those which occur in the older age group. Immobilized patients should receive a liberal fluid intake, and in addition the urinary calcium excretion should be determined at frequent intervals to minimize the incidence of hypercalcuria and its attendant renal damage.

Malnutrition. The role of diet in osteoporosis is not clear. If the diet is inadequate in protein, insufficient amounts of protein tissue are formed in the body, and thus the organic matrix of bone will not be formed in adequate amounts, and osteoporosis may result. However, a frequent accompaniment of an insufficient diet is a reduction in calcium intake, and this can be a very important factor in the production of osteoporosis.

Hypogonadism. In preadolescent hypogonadism (in either males or females), gonadal dysgenesis, or Turner's syndrome, and in postadolescent hypogonadal individuals, there is a hormonal imbalance similar to that observed in postmenopausal women and elderly men. This imbalance is characterized by a decrease in the production of anabolic steroids (androgens and estrogens) and by a maintenance of the normal production (and hence a relative excess) of antianabolic steroids (corticosteroids) by the adrenal cortex. In patients with Turner's syndrome, there is as well an inherent disease of the connective tissue which in many instances contributes to the often seen osteoporosis. Many individuals in the adolescent age exhibit as an early manifestation of the gonadal hormone deficiency, a delayed union of the epiphyses which has been called *epiphysitis*. Long-standing, untreated eunuchoids may present with osteoporosis which is clinically indistinguishable from that observed in elderly men and women; however, eunuchoid males who have been adequately and continuously treated with androgen from the chronologic age of puberty do not develop osteoporosis. In general, the same principles apply to the treatment of the osteoporosis associated with hypogonadism as to the management of postmenopausal and senile osteoporosis.

Acromegaly. Patients with acromegaly show hypercalcuria and a decrease in the density of bone, an increased plasma inorganic phosphate level, and plasma calcium and alkaline phosphatase values in the normal range. The bone disease, therefore, is consistent with osteoporosis and inconsistent with almost all other metabolic bone disorders. This decrease in the density of bone occurs in spite of the fact that certain portions of the skeleton of acromegalic patients are growing. The cause of the demineralization of bone is obscure.

Cushing's Syndrome. A discussion of Cushing's syndrome and its relation to osteoporosis will be found in Chap. 68. It is sufficient at this point to indicate that Cushing's syndrome is the result of overproduction of hydrocortisone or the long-term administration of glucocorticoids. One of the fundamental actions of a glucocorticoid appears to be the stimulation of glucose formation from known carbohydrate precursors as, for example, the glucogenic amino acids. The conversion of glucogenic amino acids to carbohydrate (gluconeogenesis) diverts these building blocks from protein synthesis. Thus an excess of the glucocorticoids, through their antianabolic effect, leads to an insufficiency of amino acids for protein synthesis and interferes with the building up of protein matrix and the formation of bone. It is of interest to note that local tissue factors must exert a regulatory effect on this process; it is not uncommon to observe extensive demineral-ization of the vertebral bodies with normal appearing density of the adjacent long bones. The osteoporosis associated with Cushing's syndrome may present in a severe and malignant form.

The treatment of osteoporosis in patients with Cushing's syndrome requires the elimination of excess production of glucocorticoids. A small proportion of patients will respond to pituitary irradiation; the majority will require removal of adrenal or pituitary tissue. The subsequent restoration of a positive calcium balance in such patients will be facilitated by a high calcium intake and the use of gonadal hormone preparations.

Patients with iatrogenic Cushing's syndrome in whom steroid therapy must be continued should receive supplementary calcium and, in most instances, gonadal hormones as well. Of prime importance, of course, is the reassessment at regular intervals in order to reduce the glucocorticoid dosage if at all possible.

Prolonged Stress. The concepts involved in a consideration of the osteoporosis resulting from prolonged stress can be summarized briefly as follows: When an individual is subjected to any kind of noxious stimulus such as a fracture, an operation, an injection, an exposure to heat or cold, or a toxic reaction to a drug, he reacts to the stimulus by setting in motion a series of adaptive mechanisms. One of the integral parts of this adaptation is a change in the production of adrenal cortical hormones, which results, for a temporary period, in an increased production of cortisol. This initial or "catabolic" phase resembles, from the hormone imbalance point of view, Cushing's syndrome. A few patients have been observed in whom this catabolic phase has persisted much longer than one normally would have expected it to, and in whom, as a result, there has been interference with the anabolism of all tissues and, in particular, with bone formation. Supplementary calcium and gonadal hormone therapy should prove helpful in minimizing the changes exhibited in these circumstances.

Hyperthyroidism. Osteoporosis does occur in some patients with prolonged hyperthyroidism. This probably is a negative nitrogen and/or calcium balance associated with the hypermetabolic condition. It is essential to correct the hyperthyroid state as rapidly as possible, and the therapy outlined for patients with senile osteoporosis may be used advantageously as a supplement.

Idiopathic Osteoporosis. When all the other types of osteoporosis have been eliminated, there are still a few individuals in whom the cause of the osteoporosis cannot be determined. These include young women with normal ovarian function, as well as young adult men. Many types of therapy have been tried on these cases without benefit, including vitamins A, C, and D; estrogenic and androgenic hormones; sodium fluoride; and a high protein intake. The use of pooled plasma albumin infusions has proved of benefit in some cases.

It is not uncommon for two or more factors to be present in the same individual. For example, a woman past the menopause who develops osteoporosis from hormonal imbalance frequently is immobilized and then may develop a superimposed osteoporosis of disuse. Similarly, a patient who has undergone an immobilizing operation may show osteoporosis from the combination of atrophy of disuse and the metabolic response to surgery.

REFERENCES

See Chap. 77.

79 OSTEOMALACIA AND RICKETS

Edward C. Reifenstein, Jr.

Definition. Osteomalacia or rickets falls in that category of "too little calcified bone" in which the decrease in calcified bone tissue is the result of inadequate bone formation because of insufficient saturation of the body fluids with calcium and phosphate. When the ion product of the plasma calcium:phosphate is reduced below normal because of too little calcium or inorganic phosphate, precipitation of the calcium phosphate salt into the bone matrix will not occur. In osteomalacia and rickets, one finds the plasma calcium level normal or low and the plasma phosphate level low or normal; thus the product of the plasma calcium and the plasma phosphate concentrations in milligrams is lower than the normal range, i.e., 30 to 40 for adults and 40 to 55 for growing children (see Chap. 77).

Because of the lack of calcification in osteomalacia and rickets, the bones become weak and more responsive to stress and strain; this leads to increased osteoblastic activity, elevated plasma alkaline phosphatase level, and deposition of wide osteoid seams, which are uncalcified. When osteomalacia occurs in infants and young children, it is called *rickets;* the pathologic physiology is the same, but there are additional defects in the growing epiphyseal cartilage, particularly faulty calcification of the zone of provisional calcification. In other words, rickets is "childhood osteomalacia," and conversely, osteomalacia is "adult rickets" (see Chap. 61).

Etiology. Throughout the world, the principal cause of osteomalacia is a deficiency of vitamin D,

which results in a deficiency of calcium and phosphate in the plasma. The main causes of osteomalacia in the United States are steatorrhea and renal acidosis.

Pathology. Bone sections from osteomalacia in the adult patient show a decrease in the calcified mass, with very few osteoclasts and large numbers of osteoblasts. Most of the trabeculae are covered with osteoid seams which are considerably wider than normal. The marrow spaces are enlarged, but the amount of fibrous tissue is not increased.

Clinical Types. Osteomalacia or rickets may be classified as follows: (1) chemical osteomalacia with high plasma phosphatase level, in which there are no pseudofractures and acalcification of bone is not apparent; (2) Milkman's syndrome, in which the plasma alkaline phosphatase level is high, pseudofractures are present, and acalcification of bone is not apparent; and (3) "advanced osteomalacia," in which the plasma alkaline phosphatase level is high, pseudofractures are present, and acalcification of bone is readily detected.

Milkman's Syndrome. Milkman's syndrome is an x-ray diagnosis which calls attention to the fact that osteomalacia or rickets may present as ribbon-like zones of acalcification. These zones of acalcification or pseudofractures, first described by Milkman, tend to occur in symmetric locations and in areas where arteries parallel the surface of the bone. Presumably they are caused by stress at the weak points in the skeleton. The mechanism is probably: (1) partial fracture, (2) filling of the defect with matrix through the activity of the osteoblasts, and (3) failure of the matrix to calcify because of the underlying osteomalacia. The pseudofractures tend to occur particularly in the neck of the femurs, the rami of the pubic and ischial bones, and the ribs. The underlying osteomalacia in these cases frequently is so mild that it escapes detection. However, plasma alkaline phosphatase level may be elevated, indicating that systemic bone disease is present. Since at least 30 to 50 per cent of the density of the bone must be lost before recognizable changes can be detected in the x-ray films, it is not surprising that a number of early cases are observed in which osteomalacia is present, but in which the degree of general bone involvement is not sufficient to give detectable changes in the roentgenograms.

Clinical Manifestations. Clinically, adult patients with osteomalacia exhibit anorexia, loss of weight, pain in the bones, deformity of the bones, muscular weakness, renal calculi, chronic pyelonephritis, and urinary tract infections. The number of symptoms is related to the severity of the bone disease. The bone pain is of an aching nature, and the bones are tender to pressure. Because of the frequent involvement of the long bones and the tendency of the

Table 79-1. CHEMICAL FINDINGS IN VARIOUS TYPES OF OSTEOMALACIA OR RICKETS

Alterations in calcium and/or phosphate and cause	Plasma					Urine			Other findings (footnote)
	Alkaline phosphatase	Ca	P	CO_2	Cl	Ca	NH_4	Titratable acidity	
Insufficient absorption:									
Dietary factors (calcium, phosphate, vitamin D)	H	N or L	L	N	N	L	N	N	1
Gastrointestinal disease (steatorrhea; pancreatic and biliary tract disease)	H	N or L	L	N	N	L	N	N	2
Excessive excretion:									
Renal tubular acidosis	H	N or L	L	L	H	H	L	L	3
Renal tubular phosphate reabsorption defect (vitamin D–resistant rickets; phosphate diabetes)	H	N	L	N	N	N	N	N	4
Renal tubular phosphate and organic acid reabsorption defects (vitamin D–resistant rickets; Fanconi syndrome)	H	N or L	L	L	N	H	H	H	5
Loss from breast or placenta	H	L	N	N	N	L	N	N	
Excessive utilization:									
Healing phase of osteitis fibrosa generalisata (after removal of parathyroid tumor)	H	L	L	N	N	L	N	N	

[1] Plasma carotenoids normal; vitamin A and K tests normal.
[2] Plasma carotenoids low; vitamin A and K tests low.
[3] Plasma sodium or potassium may be low.
[4] Urinary phosphate high.
[5] Urinary phosphate high; plasma potassium low; glucosuria +; aminaciduria +; cystinosis +.
H = high; L = low; N = normal; + = present.

bones to bend, a waddling gait is common. Tetany occurs particularly in those patients in whom the causative factor is insufficient absorption of calcium. It is seen much less commonly in cases due to excessive calcium excretion, since the latter usually is accompanied by an acidosis which tends to minimize tetany. The signs and symptoms of tetany are discussed elsewhere (Chap. 67).

Laboratory Findings. The laboratory findings in the different types of osteomalacia are summarized in Table 79-1. Attention is called to the fact that in the group labeled "renal tubular acidosis" one may also encounter a low plasma sodium or low plasma potassium level. In the Fanconi syndrome, the blood level of amino acids is not elevated, but the renal threshold for amino acids is lowered. As a result, excessive amounts of amino acids appear in the urine, and there is a high ratio of amino acid nitrogen to total nitrogen in the urine. Glucosuria and phosphaturia also occur in this syndrome, and cystinuria may be present. In these patients, calcium excretion in the urine will be elevated. The excretion of calcium in the urine will be decreased in patients with osteomalacia or rickets caused by avitaminosis D.

When steatorrhea is the cause of osteomalacia or rickets, one often finds the plasma carotenoid and vitamin A levels low and the prothrombin time increased.

The x-ray findings in osteomalacia depend to some extent upon the degree of severity of the disease. Osteomalacia commonly involves the extremities and the pelvis, less frequently the spine and skull. Spontaneous ununited fractures, or pseudofractures, which are typical of Milkman's syndrome, have been mentioned. The bones are soft and more prone to deformity by bending than they are to fracture. In more advanced cases, the demineralization is readily apparent. The lamina dura will be absent in the long-standing cases. The roentgenograms may reveal renal calculi or, more commonly, nephrocalcinosis (multiple deposits of calcium in the collecting tubules).

Diagnosis. To make the diagnosis of osteomalacia and rickets, one relies chiefly on the plasma calcium and phosphate values. The severity of the disease is determined by the plasma alkaline phosphatase level, cupping and irregular enlargement of long-bone metaphyses (in children), and x-ray evidence of pseudofractures and generalized amineralization. In establishing the etiologic factor, one considers the history of calcium and vitamin D intake, the exposure to sunlight, the presence of gastrointestinal disease or acidosis and renal disease, the amount of calcium in the urine, and the history of frequent pregnancies and prolonged lactation. The special diagnostic signs should be employed to uncover latent tetany. The amount of calcium in the plasma should be measured to differentiate tetany due to hypocalcemia from that of alkalosis or hypomagnesemia. The response to therapeutic doses of vitamin D may aid in establishing the diagnosis of rickets due to avitaminosis D in patients with mild obscure manifestations.

Differential Diagnosis. The differentiation of osteomalacia and rickets from other metabolic bone diseases depends largely upon the chemical findings. Tetany does occur, of course, in conditions other than osteomalacia. It is found in hypoparathyroidism. The differential diagnostic point, in essence, is the fact that the plasma inorganic phosphate level is high in hypoparathyroidism, whereas it is practically always normal or low in patients with osteomalacia. Tetany also occurs as a result of alkalosis. The commonest cause of this is hyperventilation in individuals who are emotionally unstable. Tetany arising from this cause is readily recognized by the fact that the plasma calcium and the plasma inorganic phosphate levels are normal. Furthermore, there is calcium in the urine in this type, whereas in the tetany resulting from hypoparathyroidism and in many of the cases arising from osteomalacia, the urinary calcium is practically absent. In the tetany caused by alkalosis, the plasma total base value will be found to be absolutely or relatively increased, with an increase in plasma carbon dioxide–combining power and a decrease in plasma chloride values.

Three renal conditions which give rise to metabolic bone diseases are renal osteitis fibrosa generalisata ("renal rickets"), renal acidosis with osteomalacia, and the Fanconi syndrome with osteomalacia. It is interesting to note that renal rickets is really renal osteitis fibrosa generalisata with increased bone resorption resulting from the persistence of the acidosis and the secondary hyperparathyroidism. All three of the above-mentioned conditions are accompanied by hypercalcuria and plasma acidosis. Renal rickets is recognized readily by the elevated plasma phosphate level, in contrast to the other two conditions which have normal or low plasma phosphate levels. The Fanconi syndrome can be differentiated by the increase of titratable acidity and of ammonia in the urine, in contrast to the decrease of these two "base sparers" in the urine of patients with osteomalacia due to other types of renal acidosis. The osteonephropathies are discussed in detail elsewhere (see p. 712).

Prognosis. The prognosis for patients with rickets or osteomalacia is good provided the underlying cause can be corrected, the treatment is adequate, and the residual skeletal deformities are compatible with life. The clinical and chemical manifestations respond in days to weeks, the osseous involvement in weeks to months. Patients who have recovered from avitaminosis D should receive thereafter preventive amounts of vitamin D. In cases resulting from renal acidosis, therapy to overcome the acidosis usually must be continued as long as the patient lives.

Treatment. The treatment of osteomalacia and rickets depends upon the etiology. In those cases in which insufficient absorption is the major factor, the primary objective in treating the osseous disorder is to give calcium and vitamin D. In adults, 1 to 3 glasses of milk a day will supply a high intake of calcium, and this can be supplemented by giving 5 Gm calcium gluconate, or calcium lactate, dissolved in water, three times a day. Since acidosis tends to alleviate tetany, it is helpful in some instances to make the patient slightly acidotic. Calcium chloride administered by mouth produces a slight acidosis because more chloride is absorbed than calcium. A favorite prescription in the past has been 10 ml of a 30 per cent solution of calcium chloride diluted in water three times daily after meals. In addition, calciferol (vitamin D_2) is administered in a dosage of 25,000 to 100,000 units a day. Patients with osteomalacia associated with resistance to vitamin D may require as much as 600,000 units of vitamin D daily. Although calciferol usually is administered orally, intramuscular and intravenous preparations of vitamin D are available commercially; occasionally these may be tolerated better than the oral medication. In children with rickets arising from avitaminosis D, the same principles of therapy apply as in adults, although smaller amounts of vitamin D and calcium are required; the therapeutic measures are discussed in detail elsewhere (Chap. 61, p. 550). Once the osteomalacia or rickets has been cured, continuation of the vitamin D therapy in large doses not only is unnecessary but may lead to *hypervitaminosis*. The danger point can be determined by following the plasma alkaline phosphatase level; when it drops to normal, the vitamin D intake should be reduced to an amount just sufficient to maintain a normal plasma calcium level. During the administration of vitamin D to patients with osteomalacia or rickets arising from insufficient absorption of calcium, the plasma calcium level should be followed at frequent intervals in order to detect promptly the development of hypercalcemia and, hence, the necessity for reducing the dosage of vitamin D. The Sulkowitch test has not proved to be a reliable method for estimating the amount of the urinary calcium excretion or for determining the need for adjustment in the dosage of the calcium-regulating therapy; the test may be very misleading.

The cases of osteomalacia or rickets resulting from insufficient absorption because of gastrointestinal disease require the additional therapeutic agents which are indicated for the control of the particular gastrointestinal disorder. In general the administration of corticosteroids may improve gastrointestinal function and thus increase vitamin and mineral absorption. A low fat, high protein diet should be prescribed, and the fat-soluble vitamins should be given in large amounts between meals. It is important to give *all* the fat-soluble vitamins, including vitamins A, K, and E.

In those forms of osteomalacia or rickets arising from excessive excretion of calcium (base) through the kidney, there are two important principles of therapy: (1) to control the acidosis and (2) to replace the calcium. Inasmuch as the initial disturbance is a deficiency of base, the first item of treatment is the administration of base. This is best given in the form of a salt of a mineral base with an organic acid, for example, sodium citrate, sodium lactate, or calcium gluconate. If low plasma potassium or low plasma sodium levels are factors, a combination of sodium citrate and potassium citrate should be given. The organic acid is metabolized after absorption, leaving the base free to help in the excretion of acid in the urine. An organic acid, such as citric acid, which will be largely metabolized after absorption, can be given in addition in order to increase the gastrointestinal acidity and hence favor calcium absorption. A useful prescription for adults consists of 140 Gm citric acid and 98 Gm sodium citrate dissolved in 1 liter of water; the patient takes 50 to 100 ml of this mixture, depending upon the amount needed to overcome the acidosis. The second step in therapy is the administration of agents which will increase calcium absorption in the gastrointestinal tract, namely, calcium salts and vitamin D. These are used in larger amounts than in osteomalacia or rickets arising from insufficient absorption. Supplementary calcium should be given during pregnancy and lactation as a preventive measure.

The osteomalacia resulting from excessive utilization of calcium and phosphate in compensatory bone formation following the removal of a parathyroid tumor requires prolonged and continuous treatment of offset the tetany (pp. 607 to 608).

Results of Treatment. The response of patients with osteomalacia or rickets to treatment is most spectacular. In a relatively short time, the pseudofractures disappear, the bones become much stronger, and normal growth occurs in patients in whom the epiphyses have not yet united. The plasma alkaline phosphatase level usually returns to normal within 2 to 6 months, and at that time the manifestations of acalcification of the endochondral and endosteal osseous tissues will have disappeared and the osteomalacia or rickets is cured. The deformities which are not amenable to orthopedic measures and the areas of osteosclerosis from excessive compensatory bone repair are the residual evidence of osseous involvement.

The elimination of rickets or osteomalacia per se has no effect upon the underlying disease which originally lead to the osseous disorder. In the cases resulting from the dietary factors (see below), the therapy that cures the bone disease also corrects the underlying disease. In some of the gastrointestinal disorders resulting in bone disease, additional specific therapeutic measures permanently may eliminate the tendency to develop rickets or osteomalacia; however in most of these disorders, the underlying disease will recur when the specific therapy is discontinued and with it the potential for a recurrence of the metabolic bone disorder if the calcium-regulating therapy also is discontinued. In cases with renal disease, the combined therapy with alkali, vitamin D, and calcium gluconate does not effect appreciably the impaired renal function, with its serious prognosis in terms of renal failure, or the anemia if this is present. In such patients, also, rickets or osteomalacia will tend to recur when the therapy is discontinued. The cause of the osseous condition which leads to the osteomalacia complicating the healing phase of the osteitis fibrosa generalisata of hyperparathyroidism already has been eliminated by the removal of the parathyroid tumor.

OTHER CONDITIONS ASSOCIATED WITH OSTEOMALACIA OR RICKETS

Insufficient Gastrointestinal Absorption of Calcium and/or Phosphate. This may result from: (1) dietary factors, (2) gastrointestinal disease, and (3) vitamin D disturbances.

Dietary Factors. An insufficient absorption of calcium may be the result of an inadequate calcium intake. In the United States, because of the widespread use of milk as a food, the diet generally is adequate in calcium, so that a low intake is rarely a cause of osteomalacia in adults and only occasionally a cause of rickets in children. However, low calcium intake appears to be the common cause of osteomalacia or rickets in China where vitamin D insufficiency also is a contributing factor. An inadequate intake of phosphate is very rare. A change in the pH of the gastrointestinal contents affects the absorption of calcium; acidity facilitates while alkalinity inhibits the calcium uptake. Many acidic radicals form insoluble complexes with calcium and thus decrease its absorption; among these are included oxalate (spinach) and phytate (present in large quantities in certain cereal grains). Aluminum salts form insoluble complexes with phosphate and decrease its absorption. A high protein diet facilitates calcium absorption, and vice versa. However, a high protein diet often is also a high phosphate diet, and excessive amounts of phosphate may decrease the absorption of calcium.

Gastrointestinal Disease. Disease of the gastrointestinal tract, especially when associated with steatorrhea or removal of large portions of the gastrointestinal tract, may result in the inability to absorb calcium. The chief causes of steatorrhea in the United States are (1) idiopathic steatorrhea or nontropical sprue or, in children, celiac disease (juvenile sprue) and (2) chronic pancreatitis. In these conditions a large amount of fat is retained within gastrointestinal tract, and the calcium combines with it to form an insoluble soap so that the calcium is not absorbed. Furthermore, vitamin D, which is fat-soluble, also is not absorbed, nor are the other fat-soluble vitamins. A similar mechanism is responsible for osteomalacia and fat-soluble vitamin deficiencies in patients who have had considerable portions of the gastrointestinal tract removed so that insufficient absorption takes place. Gastrointestinal disease as the cause of osteomalacia or rickets and fat-soluble vitamin deficiencies is frequently overlooked; similarly, osteomalacia or rickets and fat-soluble vitamin deficiencies as complications of gastrointestinal disease frequently are not recognized. Since bile and pancreatic secretions also are of importance in the absorption of calcium and vitamin D, rickets is found in children with congenital atresia of the bile ducts or with cystic fibrosis of the pancreas, and osteomalacia in adults with prolonged obstructive jaundice from intra- or extrahepatic biliary tract disease (where osteoporosis may be present as well because of the chronic protein depletion). Surgical procedures involving the gastrointestinal tract which result in a chronic excessive absorption of chlorides, such as the transplantation of the ureters into the sigmoid or other portions of the colon, also may result after some years in osteomalacia or rickets; in these cases, the mechanism leading to the osseous disorder is not insufficient gastrointestinal absorption of calcium but excessive excretion of the mineral in the urine as a consequence of the chronic acidosis.

Excessive Excretion of Calcium and/or Phosphate. Calcium can be excreted from the body in excessive amounts from four portals: (1) the kidney, (2) the gastrointestinal tract, (3) the breast, and (4) the placenta. There are four different types of renal disease that result in an excessive excretion

of calcium and/or phosphate in the urine and, hence, in the development of osseous disorders: (1) renal rickets; (2) renal tubular acidosis with rickets or osteomalacia, (3) renal tubular phosphate reabsorption defect with rickets or osteomalacia (vitamin D–resistant rickets), and (4) renal tubular phosphate and organic acid reabsorption defects with rickets or osteomalacia (vitamin D–resistant rickets, Fanconi syndrome). These conditions are spoken of, therefore, as osteonephropathies. It is to be noted that only the last three conditions lead to a clinically significant degree of rickets or osteomalacia; however, for the sake of clarity the pathologic physiology of all four disorders will be described at this point.

Renal Rickets. In the first type of osteonephropathy there is renal disease with glomerular insufficiency as well as tubular insufficiency. Renal rickets is often confused with renal osteitis fibrosa generalisata (secondary hyperparathyroidism). True renal rickets is usually seen in prepuberal children with chronic renal disease, for example, chronic glomerulonephritis or chronic pyelonephritis. The mechanism by which osteomalacia develops in these children is not clear.

Renal Tubular Acidosis with Rickets or Osteomalacia. In the second type of osteonephropathy, glomerular insufficiency is minimal or absent, and the pathologic state results from a distal tubular insufficiency with a decreased ability to secrete hydrogen ions and to excrete an acid urine. This leads to the utilization of fixed base for excretion in the urine with the acid radicals; this may result in a loss of sodium, potassium, and calcium. With depletion of sodium, the patient may present symptoms suggestive of adrenal cortical insufficiency with hyponatremia; with loss of potassium, the patient may present symptoms similar to those seen in familial periodic paralysis and other disorders associated with hypopotassemia; with depletion of calcium, the patient may present symptoms of tetany and exhibit chemical osteomalacia with hypocalcemia. As a result of the low plasma calcium level, the activity of the parathyroid glands is increased and secondary hyperparathyroidism results. The acidosis and the secondary hyperparathyroidism lead to an increased excretion of phosphate in the urine and then to a lowering of the phosphate concentration in the plasma. This produces an increase in the requirement for calcium in the plasma, which is met by calcium that is absorbed from the gastrointestinal tract or, failing this, by calcium that is mobilized from bone by the action of the parathyroid hormone. This mechanism brings about a rise in the plasma calcium level which tends to offset the previously low concentration. The net result, however, is a low plasma phosphate level and either a normal or a low plasma calcium level;

since the concentrations of these mineral ions are below the normal range of the ion product (see Chap. 77), mineral deposition in newly formed matrix fails to occur. The plasma chemical changes and the bone histologic picture, therefore, are those of osteomalacia, although on careful histologic examination there usually is some evidence of osteitis fibrosa generalisata as well. The plasma alkaline phosphatase activity of these patients usually is high. Because of the difficulty in excreting acid radicals, the plasma carbon dioxide level usually is lowered and the plasma chloride level usually is increased. Furthermore, the hypercalcemia may lead to kidney stones and nephrocalcinosis. This disease is often described in females and is believed by many to be hereditary.

Renal Tubular Phosphate Reabsorption Defect with Rickets or Osteomalacia (Vitamin D–resistant Rickets). In the third type of osteonephropathy, glomerular insufficiency is minimal or absent, and the primary defect is an insufficiency in the proximal convoluted tubules with a decreased ability to reabsorb a sufficient quantity of phosphate. This leads to a low plasma phosphate level with a normal plasma calcium level and, thus, to a lowering of the calcium: phosphate ion product to a level below normal range (see Chap. 61). As a result, deposition of minerals in newly formed matrix fails to occur, and the patient develops rickets or osteomalacia. The plasma alkaline phosphatase level of these individuals usually is high. There is no acidosis and no abnormality of other constituents of the plasma. This disorder is resistant to ordinary doses of vitamin D and frequently is classified as a case of "vitamin D–resistant" rickets. The disease tends to occur in families and may be genetically determined. This third type of osteonephropathy is very similar to the fourth type (see below) except that the latter disorder has one or more additional defects in tubular function.

Renal Tubular Phosphate and Organic Acid Reabsorption Defects with Rickets or Osteomalacia (Vitamin D–resistant Rickets, Fanconi Syndrome). In the fourth type of osteonephropathy, glomerular insufficiency is minimal or absent, and the pathologic disturbance results from defects in the proximal convoluted tubules with not only a decreased ability to reabsorb a sufficient quantity of phosphate (as in the third type), but also one or more additional defects in tubular function which result in glucosuria, aminoaciduria, and the excretion of excessive amounts of other organic acids. The defect in the tubular reabsorption of phosphate leads to a low plasma phosphate level; the defects in the tubular reabsorption of the organic acids result in an increased urinary excretion of base (particularly calcium) in combination with these acids which may lead to hypercalcuria. There is a marked lower-

ing of the plasma product of the calcium and phosphate ion activities. As a result, deposition of minerals in newly formed matrix fails to occur, and the patient develops rickets or osteomalacia with hypophosphatemia and a low plasma calcium level. The low concentration of phosphate in the plasma produces an increase in the requirement for calcium in the plasma, which is met by calcium that is absorbed from the gastrointestinal tract, or failing this, by calcium that is mobilized from bone. As a result of the low plasma calcium level, the activity of the parathyroid glands is increased and secondary hyperparathyroidism occurs. The acidosis and the secondary hyperparathyroidism also lead to an increase in bone resorption. The bones in cases of this disorder, therefore, tend to have some histologic evidence of osteitis fibrosa generalisata as well as the predominant picture of rickets or osteomalacia. The plasma alkaline phosphatase level of these patients usually is high. As a result of the shortage of base, the plasma carbon dioxide level is lowered, although the plasma chloride level usually is normal. Furthermore, the large amount of calcium that is excreted in the urine may lead to kidney stones. This disorder is resistant to ordinary doses of vitamin D, and occasionally is diagnosed as a case of vitamin D–resistant rickets; more commonly, it is classified as a case of the Fanconi syndrome. This disease occurs in families and appears to be genetically determined.

Nonrenal Chronic Acidosis. In some patients, chronic acidosis arises from conditions which are not renal disorders. For example, surgical procedures involving the gastrointestinal tract, such as the transplantation of the ureters into the sigmoid or other portions of the colon, may be followed by a chronic excessive absorption of chlorides, and after some years the hyperchloremic acidosis may lead to rickets or osteomalacia in these individuals. The pathologic physiology is similar to that described for the Fanconi syndrome except that the excess of acids in the plasma is not the result of renal tubular disease but of some other nonrenal disturbance. In these cases, the renal mechanisms to combat the acidosis, although normal, are unable to eliminate all the acid radicals even when functioning at maximal capacity; hence, there is increased urinary excretion of base (particularly calcium) with these excess acids. This leads to hypercalcuria, to a low plasma calcium level, and to a reduced plasma product of the calcium and phosphate ion activities. As a result, deposition of minerals in newly formed matrix fails to occur, and the patient develops rickets or osteomalacia. Furthermore, the low plasma calcium level induces an increased activity of the parathyroid glands and secondary hyperparathyroidism. The acidosis and the secondary hyperparathyroidism also lead to an increase in bone resorption. The bones in these cases, therefore, also tend to show some histologic evidence of osteitis fibrosa generalisata as well as the predominant picture of rickets or osteomalacia. The treatment of these various renal osteonephropathies is directed toward the restoration of a normal acid-base balance and the utilization of vitamin D as outlined on p. 602.

Frequent Pregnancies and Prolonged Lactation. Pregnancy per se is a relatively unimportant cause of calcium depletion in the mother. The placenta becomes a source of appreciable calcium loss only during the last 2 months of pregnancy. The total depletion of a normal 70-kg woman during pregnancy is approximately only 1.8 per cent of her calcium content, two-thirds of which is lost during the last 60 days. Therefore, the average pregnant woman who eats an adequate diet has little need for supplemental calcium medication. The calcium should be supplemented in women who are malnourished, who are not maintaining an adequate intake, or who are having a pregnancy shortly after a previous one. In China and Japan, the tendency toward osteomalacia that results from the suboptimal intake of calcium and vitamin D is aggravated by the additional calcium loss during pregnancy, and fetal rickets is common in the newborn infants of osteomalacic mothers.

In contrast to pregnancy, lactation causes a far greater drain of calcium from the mother. One quart of human milk contains about 400 mg calcium. More than four times as much calcium is lost during 9 months of lactation as is lost during pregnancy. The total depletion of a normal 70-kg woman during 9 months of lactation is approximately 7.2 per cent of her calcium content. Therefore, supplemental calcium medication supplying at least 0.5 Gm calcium per day as an addition to the complement of an otherwise adequate diet should be administered during lactation.

Excessive Utilization of Calcium and/or Phosphate. In patients who have osseous disease with increased bone formation, the utilization of calcium and phosphate in bone formation under certain conditions may be so excessive that there is a fall in the plasma calcium and phosphate ion product, with the development of osteomalacia.

Osseous Disease with Increased Bone Formation. Osteomalacia or rickets may occur during the healing phase of overt osteitis fibrosa generalisata associated with primary hyperparathyroidism. In such cases, the removal of the entire quantity of pathologic parathyroid tissue at one surgical operation usually results in a fall in the plasma calcium concentration to the level of tetany. The significant factors that contribute to the development of hypocalcemia following the decrease in the amount of parathyroid hormone are the decrease in the rate of

absorption of calcium from the gastrointestinal tract and, particularly, the decrease in the rate of bone resorption. Furthermore, following the surgical procedure, the plasma phosphate level instead of rising frequently falls and does not rise for some time after the plasma calcium concentration has decreased.

Insufficient Mobilization of Calcium and/or Phosphate. When an insufficient amount of calcium is available from the gastrointestinal tract to maintain the mineral homeostasis of the body fluids, calcium is withdrawn from the skeleton by the processes of bone apatite and bone matrix resorption (see Chap. 77). In patients who have osseous disease with decreased bone resorption, the mobilization of insufficient calcium from bone in the presence of a reduced calcium intake may result in a fall in the plasma calcium and phosphate ion product, with the development of osteomalacia.

Osseous Disease with Decreased Bone Resorption. Osteomalacia or rickets may occur in patients with osteopetrosis (see Chap. 80) who have an inadequate calcium intake. These individuals have difficulty in obtaining mineral from the skeleton by resorbing bone, and hence they have difficulty in maintaining the calcium concentration of the body fluids when the calcium intake is moderately reduced.

Excessively Rapid Formation of Matrix. In certain conditions, there is a disturbance in the equilibrium between matrix production and hydroxyapatite deposition, because there is an increased rate of matrix production associated with a normal plasma product of calcium and phosphate ion activities and hence a normal rate of matrix calcification. These conditions include: (1) rapid matrix formation, particularly in premature infants and very rapidly growing children, (2) healing fractures, and (3) healing scurvy.

Rapid Osseous Growth. During the period of very rapid bone growth in young infants and children, the formation of bone osteoid may proceed so rapidly that calcification of the matrix lags behind. This gives rise to histologic and sometimes radiologic evidence of rickets. There are no clinical manifestations, however, and the babies or youngsters appear in every other respect to be healthy, rapidly growing children. As the child grows older and the rate of growth slows down, the process of ossification catches up with the laying down of the matrix, and the microscopic and x-ray evidence of rickets disappears. The relatively common occurrence of this disparity between the rate of osteoid formation and the rate of matrix calcification should be recognized in interpreting the roentgenograms of rapidly growing children.

Defect in Calcification Process. A disturbance in the equilibrium between matrix production and hydroxyapatite deposition can occur because there is a defect in the calcification process which is not associated with a decrease in the normal plasma product of calcium and phosphate ion activities or a decrease in the rate of matrix production. This appears to be the mechanism in hypophosphatasia.

Hypophosphatasia. See Chap. 81, p. 720.

OSTEOMALACIA OR RICKETS AND SECONDARY HYPERPARATHYROIDISM

Almost all cases of osteomalacia are accompanied by hypertrophy and hyperplasia of the parathyroid glands, and as a consequence, it generally is believed that there is hyperfunction of the parathyroid glands (secondary hyperparathyroidism) in this disorder. The sequence of events appears to be this: (1) the calcium level in the plasma is reduced, because of insufficient absorption, excessive excretion, or excessive utilization of calcium; (2) the low plasma calcium level leads to parathyroid hyperplasia; (3) the increased amount of circulating parathyroid hormone results in hyperphosphaturia, hypophosphatemia, increased plasma calcium requirement, and finally an increase in the low plasma calcium concentration to either a normal or a minimally depressed level.

REFERENCES

See Chap. 77.

80 OSTEOSCLEROSIS AND HYPEROSTEOGENESIS

Edward C. Reifenstein, Jr.

Definition. Osteosclerosis is in that category of "too much calcified bone" in which the mechanism of the osseous disturbance is "too little bone resorption" (see Table, 77-1).

Clinical Types. A provisional classification of the causes of osteosclerosis is given in Table 80-1. These include: (1) a genetic defect in the osteoclasts with decreased osteolytic activity [osteopetrosis (see below)]; (2) a decrease in the hormone stimulus to osteoclastic activity [hypoparathyroidism (see below) or hypothyroidism]; and (3) various miscellaneous conditions such as the deposition of heavy metals (lead, Chap. 102, p. 813, bismuth, Chap. 102, p. 813).

OSTEOPETROSIS

Osteopetrosis (marble bones, Albers-Schönberg disease) is a rare hereditary disease in which decreased resorption of bone leads to a marked in-

Table 80-1. PROVISIONAL CLASSIFICATION OF CAUSES OF OSTEOSCLEROSIS

I. Decreased osteolytic activity of osteoclasts: osteosclerosis
   A. Genetic defect in osteoclasts
      1. Osteopetrosis
   B. Endocrine disturbance: decrease in hormone stimulation of osteoclasts
      1. Hypoparathyroidism*
      2. Hypothyroidism*
   C. Miscellaneous
      1. Erythroblastosis fetalis
      2. Deposition of heavy metals
         a. Lead (plumbism)
         b. Bismuth and other heavy metals

* Initial or mild stage without a compensatory decrease in osteoblastic activity to restore the equilibrium between the rate of bone resorption and the rate of bone formation.

SOURCE: Modified from a classification by R. H. Follis, Jr., Am. J. Med., 22:469, 1957.

crease in the density of the skeleton. There is a decreased remodeling of bones, in which the primary trabeculae fail to be resorbed and are replaced by criss-cross secondary trabeculae. This results in a peculiar "celery" appearance of metaphyseal bone. In some instances, islands of cartilage can be seen within the long bones. The cortex of the bone, as well as the trabeculae, is thickened. The bone marrow is decreased or absent in the denser portions of bone and is often compressed into layers which appear as bands of decreased density in roentgenograms. There may be constriction of the cranial nerve foramina of the skull. In spite of increased density, the bones are brittle and tend to fracture readily.

The manifestations of this disease usually appear in childhood, although individuals have been known to remain asymptomatic throughout life. Growth may be retarded, the head is square and enlarged, and deformities of the chest and spine may be present. Fractures are frequent and may give rise to deformities. Bone healing, however, is usually satisfactory. Teeth are abnormal and tend to decay. Involvement of the skull leads to visual disturbances (optic atrophy) and deafness. Cataracts may be present. As the marrow space is reduced, a myelophthisic anemia may develop accompanied by enlargement of the liver, spleen, and lymph nodes. Osteomyelitis is a frequent complication.

The diagnosis is usually established by roentgenograms which demonstrate the generalized increase in bone density with clubbing at the ends of the long bones. Plasma calcium, phosphate, and alkaline phosphatase values are normal. Because patients with osteopetrosis have difficulty in obtaining minerals from the skeleton by resorbing bone, they have difficulty in maintaining the calcium concentration of the body fluids. Thus, on a moderately reduced calcium intake, they tend to develop osteomalacia (or rickets) and tetany. There is no treatment, and the prognosis is, in general, unfavorable. Death usually results from anemia and/or intercurrent infection.

HYPOPARATHYROIDISM

In parathyroid insufficiency, decreased osteoclastic stimulation leads to inadequate resorption of bone. Since bone formation continues at a normal rate, the bones may, over a long period, increase in density. Thus one may observe osteosclerosis as a complication of long-continued hypoparathyroidism. However, most cases of hypoparathyroidism usually exhibit only a minimal increase in bone density because there is a compensatory decrease in osteoblastic activity which eliminates the imbalance between osteogenesis and osteolysis in spite of the decrease in the rate of turnover of bone. It is to be noted, however, that in patients with markedly reduced plasma calcium levels osteomalacia and acalcification of the teeth may be seen. Other aspects of hypoparathyroidism are considered in Chap. 67.

HYPEROSTEOGENESIS

Definition. Hyperosteogenesis is in that category of "too much calcified bone" in which the mechanism of the osseous disturbance is "too much bone formation" because of increased matrix formation.

Table 80-2. PROVISIONAL CLASSIFICATION OF CAUSES
OF HYPEROSTEOGENESIS

I. Increased osteogenic activity of osteoblasts: hyperosteogenesis
   A. Increase in physiologic stimulus to osteoblasts: excessive stress
      1. Strenuous physical activities
      2. Compensatory bone repair
         a. Healing phase of osteomalacia
         b. Healing phase of osteitis fibrosa generalisata
   B. Stimulus to osteoblasts by external agents
      1. Radiation
      2. Poisoning from certain chemicals
         a. Fluorosis
         b. Elemental phosphorus
         c. Beryllium and other elements
         d. Vitamin A intoxication
   C. Miscellaneous
      1. Hypertrophic osteoarthropathy
      2. Progressive diaphyseal dysplasia
      3. Melorheostosis
      4. Metastatic tumors

SOURCE: Modified from a classification by R. H. Follis, Jr., Am. J. Med., 22:469, 1957.

Clinical Types. A provisional classification of the causes of hyperosteogenesis is given in Table 80-2. These include: (1) an increase in the physiologic stimulus to the osteoblasts from excessive stress (strenuous physical activities, compensatory bone repair), (2) a stimulus to the osteoblasts by external agents (radiation, poisoning with certain chemicals), and (3) various miscellaneous conditions. The adjustments of the biologic processes of bone metabolism to variations in physical activity and the differences that can develop between the rates of the bone and the mineral homeostatic processes during compensatory adjustments such as bone repair are discussed elsewhere (Chap. 77). Excessive stress will result in a skeleton that is heavier than average, but one cannot properly classify this as a pathologic state with "too much" bone for the requirement. Matrix formation may be increased to a pathologic degree, however, with radiation (Chap. 108) or with poisoning from certain chemicals such as fluoride, elemental phosphorus, beryllium (see Chap. 103), or vitamin A in toxic doses.

REFERENCES

See Chap. 77.

81 UNCLASSIFIED DISORDERS OF BONE

Edward C. Reifenstein, Jr.

POLYOSTOTIC FIBROUS DYSPLASIA

Polyostotic fibrous dysplasia is a disease which in its complete form shows: (1) a disseminated osteitis fibrosa of both the hyperostotic and the hypoostotic type, with a segmental distribution which suggests a neurologic or embryologic relationship; (2) areas of brown (*café au lait*) cutaneous pigmentation with a segmental distribution suggesting some connection between them and the bone lesions; and (3) sexual and somatic precocity in females, but probably not in males (several atypical cases in males have been reported as polyostotic fibrous dysplasia with sexual precocity). Incomplete forms of the syndrome occur with either one or a combination of any two of the triad of typical manifestations.

Polyostotic fibrous dysplasia (osteitis fibrosa disseminata, Albright's syndrome) is a localized bone disease which frequently is mistaken for hyperparathyroidism with bone disease. The condition can be differentiated from hyperparathyroidism because the bone lesions are not generalized and the plasma calcium is normal. Furthermore the bone lesions are hyperostotic as well as hypoostotic, which is most unusual in hyperparathyroidism. In addition, pigmentation and sexual precocity are not manifestations of hyperparathyroidism. In 15 cases of polyostotic fibrous dysplasia the parathyroid glands were explored and found to be normal. Patients with cystic bone lesions should be carefully investigated for polyostotic fibrous dysplasia, especially if four apparently normal parathyroid glands have been demonstrated by surgical exploration.

The skull abnormalities are spotty in distribution and consist of multiple localized lesions with normal bone elsewhere. The lesions will involve the multiple bones of one extremity or of one digit and entirely miss the other extremity or the other digits. The occiput, the metatarsals and metacarpals, the phalanges, the upper ends of the femurs, and the tibias are the sites of predilection. The epiphyses of the phalanges, metatarsals, and metacarpals usually, but not always, escape involvement. The base of the skull is especially likely to be very dense and hyperostotic (platybasia); this may lead to proptosis of one or both eyes. There may be a marked prominence in the region of the occiput. Pathologic fractures are common but usually heal well. The upper ends of the femur, when involved, usually show outward bowing, which produces the "shepherd-crook deformity." On histologic examination the involved bone shows the characteristic findings of osteitis fibrosa except that occasionally there are islands of cartilege. By roentgenogram the lesions sometimes show a "torn-paper" appearance. The bone age is usually advanced in those females who develop precocious puberty.

The brown cutaneous pigmentation exhibits a very irregular outline (coast-of-Maine) in contrast to the relatively regular outline (coast-of-California) observed in neurofibromatosis, although the color is similar. The mucous membranes of the mouth may be involved. In several cases the pigmentation was discovered only by a careful examination of the scalp. The pigment is melanin. The cutaneous pigmentation usually shows a segmental distribution; it tends to stop at the midline. Although the bone and the skin lesions are often on the same side of the body, they may occur predominantly on opposite sides. Polyostotic fibrous dysplasia should be differentiated from neurofibromatosis.

The sexual precosity in females is a true precocity, since the pituitary and ovarian glands function in a normal manner. A case has been observed in which catamenia was established before the age of one, the woman bore several normal children, and finally developed menopause at the age of fifty-four after 53 years of normal ovarian function! The patients grow rapidly and are large for their chronologic ages; however, because of early closure of the epiphyses, they usually are rather short at maturity. No consistent abnormality in gonadal function has been found in male patients. It is believed that the precocity results from the premature release of the follicle-stimulating hormone of the anterior pituitary gland as a consequence of some hypothalamic disturbance, resulting in the production of estrogen in the female but not of androgen in the male. The precocious puberty of polyostotic fibrous dysplasia must be differentiated from the other types of true precocity, such as those associated with (1) tumors of the walls or floor of the third ventricle (with or without internal hydrocephalus), (2) tuberous sclerosis with a tumor in the region of the corpora mammillaria, and (3) diffuse encephalitis or infectious process in the wall of the third ventricle. True precocity must be differentiated also from pseudoprecocious puberty in which the genital organs are without function, as in patients with granulosa and theca cell tumors of the ovary, with Leydig cell tumors of the testis, or with tumors or hyperplasia of the adrenal cortex.

The blood chemistry is normal in polyostotic fibrous dysplasia, although there may be some elevation of the plasma alkaline phosphatase, particularly if there is extensive involvement of bone (see Table 67-2). The bone lesions show only a slight tendency to progress, never clear up spontaneously, and are not radiosensitive. Hyperthyroidism has been observed in a number of the cases. No abnormality has been found in the urinary excretion of hormone metabolites. Some patients have had mental retardation. Albright feels that the primary disturbance is in the central nervous system, possibly in the hypothalamus, because the bone cysts and the cutaneous pigmentation have a segmental distribution corresponding to the spinal nerves. The only known treatment is orthopedic therapy for the skeletal deformities and fractures. Pain in the bones, which is commonly present, is sometimes relieved by x-ray treatment of the involved area.

PAGET'S DISEASE OF BONE
(Osteitis Deformans)

Paget's disease of bone (osteitis deformans) is a localized bone disease in which the primary lesion results in bone destruction. The etiology of the primary lesion is not known. The parathyroid glands have been found to be normal in patients with Paget's disease. The possibility that the disease is caused by a vascular disorder has also been considered. Evidence consistent with this hypothesis arises from the observation that the disease is frequently associated with generalized arteriosclerosis, is intensified with age, and exhibits evidence of excessive circulation of blood in the area of the lesions. The lesion simulates an arteriovenous shunt because of the pooling of blood in large venous lakes with increased total blood flow. Several cases of cardiac failure arising from this cause have been reported. Paget's disease of bone appears to be related to skeletal stress and strain. The bones most frequently involved are those subjected to the greatest stress. For example, the sacrum is involved more often than the lumbar vertebras, the lumbar more often than the thoracic, the thoracic more often than the cervical vertebras, and the lower extremities more often than the upper. The skull is frequently involved also, and apparently the pull of the temporal muscles has some influence on this site of the lesions.

Paget's disease of bone is a fairly common disease, occurring in 3 per cent of all persons over forty years of age. Cases have been observed in patients in their twenties. Pathologically the lesions are characterized by marked vascularity and fibrosis. About half the surfaces exhibit osteoclastic activity and bone resorption, the rest show osteoblasts and bone repair. Calcification is normal since the osteoid seams are normal in width. Osteoblastomas and brown tumors are rare in Paget's disease. The arrangement of trabeculae is poor in Paget's disease, so that the bone has a very poor architectural value. Because bone destruction and bone repair occur over and over again in the same area, there is a bizarre and patternless mosaic of cement lines.

If one accepts that the initial lesion results in bone destruction, one can explain all the other findings in Paget's disease. The destruction, which leads to hypercalcuria and renal calculi, also causes weakened bones which have a tendency to fracture and which respond more markedly than normal to stress and strain. This leads to an increase in osteoblastic activity with an elevation of the plasma alkaline phosphatase level, an increase in bone repair, and an overgrowth of bone which is compensatory and which results in deformity. However, the bone destruction continues, and areas that have just been repaired are destroyed again.

Evidence that the initial lesion results in bone destruction is obtained from the following sources. (1) The histology of the advancing edge shows definite bone destruction. (2) In certain situations, particularly in the skulls of women after menopause, one can find normal bone, then bone destruction, and then bone repair at three adjacent zones which are visible by x-ray. Furthermore, these zones progress with time in the same relationship to each other. (3) In some patients the initial involvement of bone is an osteolytic lesion (often called *osteoporosis circumscripta*) which precedes by some years the appearance of the osteoblastic manifestations of the disease. During this interval the plasma

alkaline phosphatase level is not elevated. In roentgenograms this initial lesion may resemble a punched-out area in the skull or a cortical cyst in the long bones.

The onset of the disease is insidious, and the course is slowly progressive. Many cases are asymptomatic, and the disorder is discovered inadvertently because: (1) characteristic changes in bone structure are detected in roentgenograms obtained for other reasons, (2) the plasma alkaline phosphatase level is found to be elevated in the absence of liver disease, or (3) the patient becomes aware of a bony deformity. Several patients have presented themselves with the following sequence: (1) the pain in one knee joint proves to be involved with hypertrophic arthritis; (2) then it is discovered that the patient has Paget's disease in the opposite tibia or femur with trivial symptoms; (3) the history reveals that the Paget's disease has been present for some time and that the patient has been favoring the leg with the Paget's involvement; and (4) it becomes apparent that the cartilages of the opposite knee have worn out from overuse, with the development of hypertrophic arthritis and sufficiently severe symptoms to bring the patient to the physician. The presence of this disorder should be considered in patients with high output cardiac failure.

Pain may be the first symptom of Paget's disease. It is primarily dull, deep, constant, and aching in character, increasing in intensity with time. The other clinical manifestations are headache, deformities of the legs and the arms, enlargement of the skull, progressive kyphosis with shortening in stature, and fractures. As the skull enlarges, the superficial blood vessels become tortuous and distended; those in the temporal region often are conspicuous. The patient with advanced Paget's disease presents a characteristic picture with a shortened stature, a pendulous abdomen, a large protruding head, bowed shin bones, and a waddling gait. The involved bones are very susceptible to fracture with slight trauma. As the long bones become involved, there are numerous partial fractures (infractions) in the cortex which are associated with the bowing of these bones; tripping on the stairs or turning in bed may be sufficient stress to cause a break of the femur. Fracture of the sternum may occur with the progression of kyphosis.

By x-ray one observes increased density of bones ("tufts of cotton") with coarse trabeculation, an increased size of the bone, bowing of the extremities with partial infractions, and finally the three zones at the advancing edge of the lesions. The bones most frequently involved are the skull, the tibias, the pelvis, the vertebras, the femora, and the humeri, but no bone is immune. The lesions may be limited to one or two bones, but many parts of the skeleton may be involved. However, it is always possible to find an area of normal, uninvolved bone; hence, the disorder is classified as a localized or nonmetabolic bone disorder.

The laboratory findings of Paget's disease include a normal plasma calcium level, a normal or slightly high plasma inorganic phosphate level, a high plasma alkaline phosphatase level, and frequently a high urinary calcium level.

Three complications occur in patients with Paget's disease: (1) renal calculi, (2) osteogenic sarcoma, and (3) hypercalcemia. Renal calculi result from the hypercalcuria. Osteogenic sarcoma occurs quite commonly in patients who have had a preexisting Paget's disease. It should be suspected in those patients who experience a marked increase in the intensity of their bone pain or other symptoms or a sudden marked increase in their plasma alkaline phosphatase level. Whenever a patient with Paget's disease is immobilized as a result of a fracture or some other illness, the amount of bone repair is sharply decreased, and osteoporosis of disuse occurs. Since bone destruction continues unabated, a large amount of calcium which before immobilization has been put back into bone must now be excreted into the urine. The quantity of calcium may exceed the ability of the kidney to excrete it. As a result, hypercalcemia will develop, with nausea, vomiting, dryness of the mouth, and even chemical death. The urinary calcium excretion of immobilized patients should be determined at frequent intervals in order to detect promptly any tendency toward the development of hypercalcuria and, hence, of hypercalcemia.

The treatment of Paget's disease in the ambulatory patient differs from the management of the immobilized patient. In the *ambulatory patient* there are three objectives: (1) to decrease bone resorption, (2) to increase bone repair, and (3) to decrease bone pain. The first of these, the decreasing of bone resorption, can be brought about by giving a high calcium phosphate intake, for example, two glasses of milk per day. In order to increase bone repair, one keeps the patient as active as possible and administers anabolic steroids to stimulate bone formation. Large doses of corticosteroids (such as 300 mg or more of cortisone orally per day) appear to reduce, at least temporarily, the initial bone destruction of the Paget's disease process, but when administered in these amounts as chronic therapy they have the undesirable actions of inducing osteoporosis (see Chap. 78) and other Cushingoid manifestations. Since the corticosteroid therapy rapidly decreases the elevated skeletal blood flow through the osseous lesions and reduces the cardiac output to the normal level, it is of particular benefit in patients with cardiac failure arising from Paget's disease. Bone pain at times can be decreased by giving large amounts of ascorbic acid, up to 1,000 mg per day. X-ray irradiation will alleviate the bone pain in some instances.

The objective of treatment in the *immobilized patient* with Paget's disease is to decrease the urinary calcium excretion. The patient is given a diet low in calcium and phosphate, milk and vitamin D are avoided, and the water intake is increased. If hypercalcemia occurs, dextrose and saline, citrate, or a chelating agent (such as ethylenediaminetetraacetic acid) are administered intravenously. The administration of inositol sodium hexaphosphate (sodium phytate) will produce insoluble and unabsorbable complexes with calcium and thus help to decrease the elevated serum calcium level. The administration of corticosteroids also may reduce the hypercalcemia. Therapy with anabolic steroids may help to maintain bone formation at a maximal rate.

OSTEITIS FIBROSA GENERALISATA

See Chap. 67.

OSTEITIS FIBROSA LOCALISATA

Osteitis fibrosa localisata (solitary bone cyst, benign giant-cell tumor) produces solitary cystic bone lesions which on biopsy are indistinguishable from those of osteitis fibrosa generalisata. These lesions are found particularly at the ends of long bones, where they occasionally lead to pathologic fractures. Solitary bone cysts usually appear before the second or third decade. Pain and swelling are not common. Benign giant-cell tumors usually appear after the second or third decade. Trauma appears to be a precipitating factor, and pain is the outstanding symptom. These tumors usually respond well to treatment with roentgen-ray irradiation. The fact that the plasma calcium, phosphate, and alkaline phosphatase levels are normal serves to indicate that these solitary lesions are not manifestations of an underlying metabolic bone disease.

Solitary cystic bone lesions with both hyperostotic and hypoostotic features are probably incomplete forms of polyostotic fibrous dysplasia. All patients with solitary bone lesions should be checked for the cutaneous pigmentation which occurs with polyostotic fibrous dysplasia and with neurofibromatosis. The presence of sexual and somatic precosity in females indicates that the bone cyst is associated with the syndrome of polyostotic fibrous dysplasia; the presence of cutaneous nodules indicates that the lesion is associated with the syndrome of neurofibromatosis.

HYPOPHOSPHATASIA

Osseous disturbances which simulate those of rickets occur in hypophosphatasia. This condition is a heritable (probably an autosomal recessive), generalized disorder with the cardinal pathologic feature of inadequate calcification of bone matrix. Although the condition usually is apparent in infancy or childhood, it may not induce manifestations until adult life. The characteristic features of the disorder are: (1) impaired mineralization of bone which appears radiologically and histologically indistinguishable from rickets (in infants and children) or osteomalacia (in adults), (2) decreased levels of tissue and plasma alkaline phosphatase activity, (3) the presence of phosphoethanolamine in the plasma and urine, (4) a normal plasma phosphate concentration, and (5) hypercalcemia and hypercalcuria in severe cases. There may be premature synostosis of the cranial vault (and its sequelae), nephrocalcinosis, premature loss of teeth, or pseudofractures (in adults). Heterozygotes may have a low plasma alkaline phosphatase concentration, the presence of phosphoethanolamine in the urine, or both without evidence of bone disease. The administration of vitamin D has not proved to be of value in the treatment of hypophosphatasia and may be hazardous to those patients with hypercalcemia; some data suggest that patients with this disorder have hypersensitivity to vitamin D. Some patients (but not all) appear to respond favorably to small doses of corticosteroid medication. The unusual feature of fundamental interest in hypophosphatasia is the presence of phosphoethanolamine (a normal constituent of brain tissue) in the plasma and in the urine. This substance has been found also in the urine in cases of celiac disease, hypothyroidism, scurvy, liver disease, and erythroblastosis fetalis. The role of this amine in bone metabolism and its relation to the decreased tissue and plasma alkaline phosphatase levels are not known. The chemical findings of value in the differential diagnosis of hypophosphatasia and certain bone and related disorders are given in Table 67-2.

REFERENCES

See Chap. 77.

82 NEOPLASMS OF BONE
Edward C. Reifenstein, Jr.

PRIMARY NEOPLASMS

Primary neoplasms of bone occasionally are accompanied by metabolic manifestations that may be confused with metabolic bone disorders. More than 60 per cent of these tumors are osteogenic sarcomas, and the remainder are other types of sarcomas. Those who consider multiple myeloma as a neoplasm include it in this group of tumors.

Osteogenic Sarcoma. This is a malignant degeneration of the osteoblasts, the bone-producing cells. It is likely to occur in the long bones, and in those conditions in which there is an accelerated rate of bone formation, as in Paget's disease (osteitis deformans). Bone formation and bone destruction occur simultaneously in the same tumor, and the ratio of formation to destruction may differ widely in different tumors.

When bone formation is predominant, the tumor is classed as osteoblastic; it is characterized by a very high alkaline phosphatase activity in the bone tissue (six to one hundred times that of normal bone tissue) and in the plasma (twenty to forty times that of normal plasma). The level of the plasma alkaline phosphatase activity parallels the course of the tumor, being reduced by excision or x-ray irradiation of the lesion and being increased by extension of the tumor or by metastasis to other tissues (lung, lymph nodes, or soft parts). Those tumors in which bone destruction is predominant are classed as osteolytic; they rarely show an increase in plasma or bone alkaline phosphatase activity.

The plasma levels of calcium and of phosphate usually are not abnormal in either the osteoblastic or the osteolytic type of osteogenic sarcoma. Pain is the predominant symptom. Amputation of the affected limb is the only effective therapy.

Other Primary Neoplasms. These rarely exhibit manifestations that suggest a metabolic bone disorder. The plasma alkaline phosphatase level may be markedly elevated in patients with chondrosarcoma, and moderately increased in those with malignant giant-cell tumor. The level usually is normal in patients with Ewing's tumor (sarcoma), fibrosarcoma, lymphosarcoma, or liposarcoma.

METASTATIC MALIGNANCY

Metastatic tumors to bone may be accompanied by bone destruction as well as bone formation although the ratio of destruction to formation varies with different tumors. When the rate of destruction exceeds that of formation, the tumor is classified as predominantly *osteolytic*. Typical examples of this type of lesion are metastases to bone from carcinoma of the lung, kidneys (hypernephroma), thyroid, breast, rectum, or from a neuroblastoma. Osteolytic lesions often result in hypercalcuria and the magnitude of the increased excretion depends on the rate of bone destruction which increases directly with the rate of growth of the tumor and the rate of compensatory bone formation. A pronounced increase in mineral excretion suggests an acceleration of the rate of tumor growth. In general, the plasma alkaline phosphatase level is either normal or only slightly to moderately increased in osteolytic lesions; but the acid phosphatase may be slightly elevated indicating the dissolution of bone.

In certain patients with osteolytic metastases to bone, hypercalcemia occurs spontaneously. This condition gives rise to symptoms of polyuria, polydipsia, dehydration, and anorexia. The excess calcium appears to arise largely from increased bone destruction by the tumor and occasionally from decreased bone reparation when the patient is immobilized. The hypercalcemia may result from an inability of the kidney to excrete the large amounts of calcium presented to it. In the later stage renal damage results from prolonged hypercalcemia and hypercalcuria and there may be an associated impairment of calcium excretory mechanisms with further aggravation of the hypercalcemia.

Therapeutic approaches to hypercalcemia should be directed toward retardation of osteolysis by appropriate hormonal treatment and radiation. The patient should be mobilized to stimulate bone formation and the calcium intake should be reduced. The volume of urine should be increased by forcing fluids and appropriate corrections of electrolyte loss and acid-base imbalance instigated. Corticoid steroids may reduce the hypercalcemia as discussed elsewhere (Chap. 67).

Osteoblastic neoplasms occur when the rate of bone formation exceeds that of bone destruction as exemplified in the metastatic bone lesions from carcinoma of the prostate. Osteoblastic lesions are often characterized by a low excretion of calcium in the urine and a normal plasma calcium level. The plasma alkaline phosphatase level is almost always elevated in patients with carcinoma of the prostate with bone formation around the lesions. Hypercalcemia occurs rarely in patients with predominating osteoblastic metastases.

The acid phosphatase which is often elevated in osteolytic lesions is also elevated in the metastatic lesions to bone from carcinoma of the prostate; however, this acid phosphatase elevation is derived from the secretion of the prostatic carcinoma cells and can be differentiated from bone acid phosphatase. The level of prostatic acid phosphatase is elevated by androgens and depressed by estrogens.

The most outstanding symptom of osseous metastases is pain, often dull in the beginning but becoming progressively more severe. Occasionally the onset of bony metastases may be associated with sharp, agonizing pain with disability. The x-ray appearance of bone lesions in metastatic malignancy usually is different from that of the bone lesions in hyperparathyroidism with bone disease, since in the former condition the areas involved usually show sharply demarcated lesions and areas of normal bone are found quite readily. The plasma calcium may be high; there may be hypercalcuria and azotemia and renal calculi. The plasma phosphate may be normal or high, but there are instances where the plasma phosphate is low. A primary focus should be sought in the breast, prostate, kidney, bronchus, thyroid, rectum, or in a neuroblastoma.

A consideration of the specific therapeutic procedures employed in the treatment for cancer are discussed in the following chapters: breast, Chap. 74; thyroid, Chap. 66; prostate, Chap. 72.

REFERENCES

See Chap. 77.

Section 4: Diseases of Striated Muscle

83 GENERAL CONSIDERATIONS
Frank H. Tyler and
Raymond D. Adams

The muscle fiber has been more thoroughly studied than any other cell of the human or animal body, but until comparatively recent times little had been learned of the diseases to which it is subject. However, clinicians and pathologists are concentrating on the conditions which impair its function and imperil its existence; and even in the period that has elapsed since the publication of the first edition of this book several monographs, devoted exclusively to muscle diseases, have appeared.

The muscle tissue is the principal organ of locomotion as well as a vast metabolic reservoir. Disposed in more than 450 separate muscles, this tissue comprises as much as 40 per cent of the weight of adult man. Intricacy of structure undoubtedly accounts for its diverse susceptibilities to disease, and for this reason reference should be made to the following anatomic characteristics.

A single muscle is composed of thousands of fibers which course for variable distances along its longitudinal axis. Each fiber is a multinucleated cell, itself of relatively large size and complexity. Although the fiber functions as an indivisible unit, disease may affect only a part of it, leaving the remainder to degenerate or regenerate according to the nature of the pathologic process. The nuclei of each cell, which may number into the hundreds, lie beneath the cytoplasmic membrane (sarcolemma), hence are called sarcolemmal. The cytoplasm (sarcoplasm) of the cell is abundant and contains the striated myofibrils and various other organelles such as microsomes, mitochondria, and endoplasmic reticulum. The myofibrils are composed of longitudinally oriented filaments (microfilaments) of contractile proteins (actin and myosin). Droplets of stored fat, glycogen, other proteins, and myoglobin, the latter imparting the red color to muscle, have been identified within the sarcoplasm.

The individual muscle fibers are supported by delicate strands of reticular connective tissue (endomysium) and blood vessels. A similar tissue and sheets of intercellular collagen (perimysium and epimysium) bind together groups of muscle fibers. These connective tissue tunics are richly vascularized, and many fat cells are embedded within their interstices. The muscle fibers are attached at their ends to tendon fibers, which in turn connect with the skeleton; it is by this means that contraction of muscle maintains posture and imparts movement.

Each fiber receives a nerve twig from a motor nerve cell in the anterior horn of spinal cord or brain stem nucleus which joins it at a point called the neuromuscular junction, and as was pointed out in Chap. 26, groups of muscle fibers with a common innervation from one anterior horn cell constitute the "motor unit" which is the basic physiologic unit in all reflex and voluntary activity. Acetylcholine and cholinesterase which play a special role in neuromuscular transmission are concentrated at this junction zone. In addition to the motor nerves there are two types of sensory receptors (proprioceptors), the muscle spindles and Golgi tendon organs which participate in the regulation of reflexes, and free nerve endings that subserve pain sensation.

CLASSIFICATION OF DISEASES OF MUSCLE

Examples of diseases which act on one or more of the aforementioned components of muscle have been identified; that is, pathologic processes are known which attack muscle through its nerve supply, nutrient arteries or veins, or connective tissue sheaths. Or, the muscle fibers themselves may

be affected by an agency which involves the whole cell or some substance, e.g., an enzyme within it. Finally, the muscle fiber, though itself intact, may be rendered powerless to contract by blockage or excited to continuous contraction by facilitation of the transmission of the nerve impulse across the neuromuscular junction or along the surface of the muscle fiber. The anatomy of these separable pathologic processes reflects various pathways of disease and could be the basis of a classification until such time as primary causation is established. However, the purposes of the physician with practical interests are probably better served by a classification which subdivides muscle diseases in accordance with the syndromes by which they most commonly manifest themselves. Recognition of the syndrome then provides the clinical approach to a given category of disease, the subtypes of which may thereafterward be differentiated.

CLINICAL MANIFESTATIONS OF PRIMARY DISEASES OF MUSCLE

It is at once obvious from the above classification that muscle diseases manifest themselves by relatively few symptoms, the most frequent of which are weakness or paralysis, atrophy, twitching, spasm, cramp, and pain. They may also affect the state of the blood and other organs by altering the metabolism of the body, but this is usually discovered only by means of special laboratory procedures and would not be discerned from clinical study.

Impairment of contractility is described by the patient as generalized or localized weakness. Fatigability may also be a symptom, but as was pointed out in Chap. 41, it is in no way characteristic of muscle disease. Special features of the weakness or paralysis may be demonstrated by appropriate tests of the speed, power, and endurance of muscular action. There are variations, first in the pattern of weakness in the major groups of cranial, trunk, and limb muscles during maximal contraction, and their recognition is useful in diagnosis. For example, the cranial and especially the ocular muscles are usually weakened in myasthenia gravis and certain forms of thyroid disease, all the limb and trunk muscles in periodic paralysis, and the proximal limb and trunk muscles in progressive muscular dystrophy and polymyositis. Then, too, the power of successive or sustained contractions may prove to be informative. The progressive weakness of continued movements and rapid recovery after rest are the most reliable index of myasthenia gravis, and useful confirmatory tests are the rapid restoration of power upon intravenous injection of Tensilon or neostigmine and the marked weakening

Table 83-1. SYNDROMIC CLASSIFICATION
OF MUSCLE DISEASES

I. Acute (days) or subacute (weeks) paralytic disorders of muscle (may cause weakness or paralysis)
   A. Acute spinal or peripheral nerve diseases (denervation paralysis) (paralysis often severe and widespread; atrophy may or may not be present)
      1. Poliomyelitis
      2. Acute idiopathic polyneuritis, or other forms of polyneuropathy (porphyria, beriberi, etc.)
   B. Primary diseases of muscle
      1. Rarely fulminant myasthenia gravis
      2. Polymyositis and dermatomyositis
      3. Cortisone myopathy
      4. Acute paroxysmal myoglobinuria
         (*Note:* first attack of episodic weakness may enter into differential diagnosis)
II. Chronic (i.e., months to years) paralytic disorders of muscle (weakness usually with severe atrophy)
   A. Progressive muscular dystrophy
      1. Duchenne type
      2. Facioscapulohumeral type (Landouzy-Déjerine)
      3. Limb girdle type (Erb)
      4. Distal type (Gowers, Welander)
      5. Myotonic dystrophy (Steinart's disease)
      6. Progressive ophthalmoplegic type
   B. Chronic polymyositis
   C. Progressive muscular atrophy and other forms of motor system disease (amyotrophic lateral sclerosis, progressive bulbar palsy) and infantile muscular atrophy (Werdnig-Hoffmann disease)
   D. Chronic neural muscular atrophy
      1. Peroneal muscular atrophy (Charcot-Marie-Tooth)
      2. Hypertrophic polyneuritis (Déjerine-Sottas)
      3. Amyloid polyneuropathy
      4. Chronic nutritional and arsenical polyneuropathy
   E. Chronic thyrotoxic myopathy
III. Episodic weakness of muscle
   A. Myasthenia gravis
   B. Familial periodic paralysis
   C. Hereditary adynamia (Gamstorp)
   D. Paramyotonia congenita (von Eulenberg)
   E. Hyper- and hypopotassemia
   F. Acute thyrotoxic myopathy (also thyrotoxic periodic paralysis)
IV. Stiffness, soreness, involuntary spasm, and cramp
   A. Congenital myotonia (Thomsen's disease) and paramyotonia congenita
   B. Tetanus
   C. Tetany
   D. Black widow spider bite
   E. Hypothyroidism and pseudomyotonia (Debré-Semelaigne and Hoffman syndromes)
   F. Myopathy resulting from phosphorylase defect (McArdle)
   G. Contracture with Addison's disease
V. Myalgic states
   A. Connective tissue diseases (rheumatoid arthritis,

Table 83-1. (*Continued*)

      lupus erythematosus, scleroderma, polymyositis)
   B. Localized fibrositis or fibromyositis
   C. Many forms of polyneuritis
   D. Trichinosis
   E. Myopathy of myoglobinuria and McArdle's syndrome
   F. Myopathy with hypoglycemia
VI. Localized muscle mass(es)
   A. Rupture of a muscle
   B. Muscle hemorrhage
   C. Muscle tumor
      1. Rhabdomyosarcoma
      2. Desmoid
      3. Angioma
   D. Localized and generalized myositis ossificans

effect by small doses of curare (described on p. 250). Slowness in relaxing a muscle or group of muscles after strong contraction is the mark of myotonia, and the same persistence of contraction upon tapping a muscle (percussion myotonia) is a confirmatory sign (easily distinguishable from the local bulge induced by a sharp tap in the muscle of a cachetic patient—myoedema). The effect of cold on muscle contraction is also informative; paresis and myotonia may be evoked or enhanced by cold in the paramyotonia of von Eulenberg. The repeated contraction of the forearm or leg muscles after the application of a tourniquet above arterial pressure to the proximal part of a limb will often elicit latent tetany, and a strong or repeated voluntary contraction of limb muscles in patients with mild or localized tetanus will often lead to the recruitment of a spreading involuntary spasm.

The volume of the muscular mass is another clinically demonstrable attribute but is less often the subject of comment by the patient. Setting apart innate differences in muscle development and the slight diminution of bulk and slackness which attend any chronic disabling illness, extreme degrees of enlargement or atrophy are usually of clinical significance. Increased volume is most commonly induced by exercise and conditioning but is also observed in patients with hypothyroidism, in congenital myotonia (the circus freaks with the phenomenal muscle development often have this disease), in congenital athetosis and feeble-mindedness (de Lange's syndrome), and occasionally in an early stage of a familial muscular dystrophy. Muscle enlargement in the latter condition is more often due to a pseudohypertrophy, with fat cells replacing muscle fibers; it is revealed by a progressive weakness of the enlarged muscle. Other muscles are usually atrophied in the same patient. Denervation due to lesions of peripheral nerve or spinal cord leads to a loss of bulk up to 75 per cent of the original volume within 3 months, and this becomes a useful sign in all the denervation diseases, provided that they have affected a sufficient number of all the motor fibers to a muscle and enough time has elapsed for the atrophy to occur. There is also a loss of bulk in the primary diseases of muscle, which progressively destroys its fibers.

The tendon reflexes are altered in the majority of muscle diseases, particularly those which involve their peripheral nerves. In muscle dystrophy and polymyositis they tend to be reduced in proportion to the reduction in muscle power. In the myopathy of hypothyroidism, in which the contractile process is slowed, there is a prolongation of the tendon reflex, and the opposite condition of quickening of the tendon reflex has been less reliably demonstrated in hyperthyroidism.

Fascicular twitchings during rest, if pronounced and combined with muscle weakness and atrophy, usually signify motor neurone disease. If pronounced they suggest amyotrophic lateral sclerosis and progressive muscular atrophy but may be seen in lesser degrees in other diseases of the gray matter of the spinal cord (e.g., syringomyelia), in lesions of anterior roots (e.g., ruptured disk), and in peripheral neuropathies. Benign fasciculations (myokymia), a common finding in otherwise normal individuals, can usually be distinguished by the lack of muscular weakness and atrophy.

Cramps at rest or with movement are frequently observed in motor system disease, but there is a benign form which may rarely be a source of disability in which no other neuromuscular disturbance exists. The condition tends to subside upon the administration of procaine amide. A particularly malignant and progressive form of painful spasm may occur in the "stiff man syndrome." Continuous spasm, intensified by action of muscles, is a common manifestation of tetanus and also follows shortly the bite of the black widow spider. Continuous, nonpainful contraction of the limbs with or without increased tendon reflexes and clonus is usually due to disease of the central nervous system (see Chap. 26, on Disturbances of the Motor System—spasticity and rigidity).

Pain localized to a group of muscles is extremely severe in wryneck, fibrositis and fibromyositis, acute brachial neuritis, radiculitis, Bornholm disease and pleurodynia, and the "stiff man syndrome," but little is known of the underlying pathology in any of them. In contrast, the established forms of muscle disease, even the more serious ones such as polymyositis, are usually painless. In the latter condition, if pain is present, it usually indicates a coincident involvement of connective tissues and joint structures. Tenderness of muscle is much more definite in polyneuritis and poliomyelitis than in polymyositis; and in the various forms of dys-

trophy and other myopathies there is no increase in the sensitivity of the muscle tissue.

Continuous shortening of a muscle when not due to spasm is called *contracture* and may develop in any condition that causes skeletal fixation with the limb remaining in one position for long periods of time. It is distinguished from ankylosis by the demonstration that tightness of the muscle during passive movement is the limiting factor. Contracture is prominent in progressive muscular dystrophy and polymyositis but may also occur in the denervation diseases.

REFERENCES

Adams, R. D., D. Denny-Brown, and C. Pearson: "Diseases of Muscle," 2d ed., New York, Paul B. Hoeber, Inc., Medical Department of Harper & Brothers, 1962.

84 SUBACUTE MYOPATHIC PARALYSIS

*Frank H. Tyler and
Raymond D. Adams*

As was remarked in Chap. 26 sudden paralysis of skeletal muscles in a limb or sector of the body, developing over a period of minutes or hours, can usually be traced to a vascular disorder of spinal cord or brain, and rarely to a myelitis or encephalitis. Acute paralysis, developing in the course of days (1 to 14), is usually due to poliomyelitis or acute idiopathic polyneuritis (Landry-Guillain-Barré syndrome) or other form of polyneuropathy (porphyria, beriberi). The primary diseases of muscle, by contrast, rarely cause a rapidly developing, widespread paralysis. Instead, their course is usually subacute (2 to several weeks) or chronic. The only exceptions that the authors have observed are rare cases of myasthenia gravis where the evolution of the disease to a severe and incapacitating paresis has been over 2 or 3 days and in some of the cases of acute thyrotoxic myopathy which we have suspected of being a combination of myasthenia gravis and hyperthyroidism. In some of the cases of paroxysmal myoglobinuria, a moderately severe weakness of the limbs has appeared within a few hours of physical exertion, but usually the clinical picture has been at once complicated by renal damage and anuria. A pronounced, rapidly developing paralysis of the limbs and respiratory and cranial musculature may occur after the bite of certain species of ticks (tick-bite paralysis); and botulism causes a fulminant paralysis of ocular and other cranial muscles, leading to respiratory failure and death in a few hours or days (cf. Chap. 144). The initial attack of periodic paralysis or of hyper- or hypopotassemia must also enter the differential diagnosis of the acute muscle paralysis. The clinical analysis of these acute syndromes is aided by certain laboratory data such as the electrocardiogram, serum potassium, sodium, and chloride values, protein-bound iodine measurement, and the cerebrospinal fluid may be of great help. The response to neostigmine or edrophonium (Tensilon) (Chap. 26) aids in the diagnosis of acute myasthenia gravis.

The two principal categories of subacute myopathy are dermatomyositis (polymyositis if no skin involvement) and polymyopathy due to metabolic diseases.

DERMATOMYOSITIS AND POLYMYOSITIS

Definition. These are relatively common diseases which affect primarily the striated muscle, skin, and other connective tissues of the body. The terminology varies according to the distribution of the pathologic process. If restricted clinically to the striated muscles the disease is called polymyositis; if the skin is involved it is designated as dermatomyositis; and if other connective tissues are implicated, the term of choice is dermatomyositis with rheumatoid arthritis, rheumatic fever, lupus erythematosis, or scleroderma.

History. Polymyositis has been known since the original descriptions by Wagner in 1863 and 1887, and the dermatomyositis form was first reported by Unverricht in 1887. The literature since that time and a general statement of present knowledge are found in the monograph of Walton and Adams in 1958.

Etiology. The cause of the disease is unknown. All attempts to isolate an infective agent have been unsuccessful. Its close association with diseases of connective tissue suggests a common etiology or pathogenesis, possibly an autoallergic inflammation. The clinical grouping of patients in this category is not overly precise and probably results in the inclusion of other diseases of noninflammatory type, viz., metabolic myopathies.

Pathology. The principal changes in muscle tissue consist of widespread destruction of muscle fibers, with all the expected cellular reaction thereto (myophages and fibroblastic proliferation), and infiltrates of inflammatory cells (lymphocytes, mononuclear leukocytes, plasma cells, and rare neutrophilic leukocytes). Evidences of regenerative activity in the form of proliferating sarcolemmal nuclei, basophilic (ribonucleic acid-rich sarcoplasm), and the development of new myofibrils are almost invariable. Many of the residual muscle fibers are small, with increased numbers of sarco-

lemmal nuclei. Either the degeneration of muscle fibers or the infiltrations of inflammatory cells may predominate in any given patient, especially if the pathologic sample was obtained by a biopsy. There are also inflammatory changes in the skin and other organs, but these will be discussed in Chaps. 301 and 302.

Clinical Manifestations. This type of muscle disease tends to appear in several clinical settings, as follows.

Polymyositis. A subacute symmetrical weakness of proximal limb and trunk muscles without dermatitis or with minimal skin lesions. The onset is usually insidious and the course slowly progressive over a period of several weeks or months. The disease may develop at almost any age (one to eighty years) and in either sex. The majority of the authors' cases have been middle-aged adults. A respiratory or obscure systemic infection may precede the muscle weakness, but in many patients the first symptoms develop during excellent health. The patient first becomes aware of a painless weakness of the proximal limb muscles, and acts such as arising from a squatting or kneeling position, climbing or descending stairs, walking, putting an object on a high shelf, or combing the hair become increasingly difficult. In restricted forms of the disease only the neck muscles or quadriceps may be involved. Pain of aching variety, in buttocks, joints, and calves, is experienced in only a few cases. The weakness progresses over a period of weeks and months. When the patient is first seen the facial, anterior and posterior neck muscles (head may loll), the pharyngeal and laryngeal muscles (dysphagia and dysphonia), all the trunk, the girdle muscles of shoulders and hips, upper arms and thighs are usually involved. Ocular muscles are almost never affected; the forearm, hand, leg, and foot muscles are usually spared but are found to be weakened in some patients. The muscles are usually not tender, and atrophy and reduction in tendon reflexes though present are not so pronounced as in denervation diseases. The skin and mucous membranes, joints, and heart are unchanged. As a rule, evidence of systemic infection is absent. Exceptionally there is low grade fever, especially if joint pain coexists, and one or a few spots of dermatitis may be present at one stage of the illness.

Dermatomyositis. The skin changes may precede or accompany the muscle syndrome and take the form of a localized or diffuse erythema, maculopapular eruption, scaling eczematoid dermatitis, or even an exfoliative dermatitis. Itching may be troublesome in some cases. The skin lesions are restricted and unimportant in some cases, consisting, as mentioned, of only one or more patches of dermatitis. Periorbital and perioral edema is frequent. Signs of other connective tissue diseases are more frequent than in the examples of pure polymyositis. The limb weakness is usually proximal but may be diffuse, i.e., distal and proximal.

Connective Tissue Diseases with Polymyositis or Dermatomyositis. This occurs in patients with rheumatic fever, rheumatoid arthritis, scleroderma, or lupus erythematosus who exhibit greater muscular weakness and atrophy than can be accounted for by the original disease. Inasmuch as pain in arthritis may also impair the power of voluntary movement, the diagnosis is not easy and sometimes reliance must be put on muscle biopsy, urinary excretion of creatine and creatinine, and measurements of muscle enzymes in the serum. Malaise, aches, and pains may be the only symptoms in the early stages of the disease (cf. Chap. 300, Miscellaneous and Rarer Diseases of Connective Tissue).

Carcinoma with Polymyositis or Dermatomyositis. This syndrome is placed in a separate category, although the muscle and skin changes are indistinguishable. Approximately 10 per cent of all adults, especially the elderly, who have polymyositis or dermatomyositis are found to have a carcinoma or some other tumor. Some cases of thymoma are accompanied by polymyositis. The incidence of this neoplastic syndrome is slightly higher in men than women. Over 500 examples have been reported in the literature being linked most often with bronchogenic carcinoma. The tumors, however, have occurred in every organ of the body. The muscle and skin tissues show no evidence of tumor cells. The polymyositis may antedate the clinical manifestations of the malignancy by 1 to 2 years. The relationship is not understood.

Laboratory Findings. Creatine excretion in the urine is moderately elevated in most cases, and creatinine excretion is low. The several types of transaminase and other tissue enzymes such as aldolase are more elevated in the blood serum than in any other type of muscle disease. Serum γ-globulin values are often elevated. Myoglobin is occasionally found in the urine in severe cases. The sedimentation rate is normal and elevated. LE preparations of blood smears are negative, as a rule. The electromyogram reveals a typical "myopathic pattern," i.e., many abnormally brief action potentials of low voltage and, in addition, numerous fibrillation potentials (cf. Chap. 26). The electrocardiogram has been normal in a few of the authors' cases. The muscle biopsy, if taken from an affected muscle, usually demonstrates the typical pathologic changes of the disease.

Diagnosis. Patients with a pure polymyositis are often suspected of having progressive muscular dystrophy because of the similar distribution of weakness (proximal and trunk muscles). Unlike dystrophy, however, the development is much more

rapid, individuals may be affected at all ages (one rarely sees a dystrophy begin after thirty years of age), and the laryngeal, pharyngeal, and neck muscles are usually involved (seldom observed in dystrophy). It must be conceded, however, that in some patients, especially children, it is virtually impossible to distinguish a chronic polymyositis from a rapidly advancing dystrophy.

A few of the patients with the myositis of carcinoma will exhibit a myasthenic type of reaction, first demonstrated by Eaton and Lambert, and this type of illness must be distinguished from myasthenia gravis. It differs in one respect in that the patient may experience a sense of stiffness like myotonia which diminishes during the course of successive voluntary contractions.

The painful varieties of the polymyositis must be separated from early connective tissue disease. If the latter is not established, it may be impossible to reach a correct diagnosis even after all the laboratory data have been obtained. Such patients may be classified as hysteric or neurotic or depressed or may be suspected of having some metabolic disease.

Trichinosis may be confused with idiopathic polymyositis, especially if the history of ingested pork is not obtained. The high eosinophil counts in the blood, the relatively slight weakness of limbs, the conjunctival edema, the ocular and lingual weakness, the symptoms of cerebral involvement (hemiplegia, aphasia, coma, etc.), the positive skin reaction to trichinae antigen, and the muscle biopsy establish the diagnosis in most cases.

Treatment. The various measures which have been suggested are of uncertain value. The most promising results have been obtained by a program which consists of (1) acetylsalicylic acid 0.9 Gm every 4 hr except during the night (blood levels of 20 to 30 mg per 100 ml), (2) prednisone 40 to 60 mg per day for a month and gradual reduction in steps of 5 mg and finally 1 mg every week over many months, (3) physiotherapy—gentle massage, passive movement and then resistance exercises as the evidences of activity (elevated sedimentation rate and high serum transaminase values) subside. Vitamin E or alpha-tocopherol has been used with doubtful benefit. Oral penicillin should be taken most of the year (200,000 units twice a day) to prevent streptococcal infections.

Every patient should be reexamined every few weeks for malignancy. If found, it should be excised, if possible, or treated by x-ray or chemical agents.

Prognosis. Only a few of the patients with an acute condition will die. The majority improve upon therapy, and in fact, the muscle weakness may lessen even in those patients with an advancing malignancy. A few patients recover completely, but more often some weakness of the shoulders and hips, usually not disabling, remains. Relapse may occur at any time up to 1 to 15 years or more. Corticosteroids should not be used longer than a few months unless there is continuous threat of relapse. Acetylsalicylic acid and penicillin may possibly reduce the relapse rate.

METABOLIC DISEASES OF MUSCLE

The boundaries of this category of disease cannot be sharply drawn at this time. With advance in knowledge it is probable that many diseases, presently classified as degenerative and possibly some labeled as polymyositic, will be linked to specific defects in enzymes within the muscle walls. Limitations in space permit the description of only a few representative forms of the better known metabolic myopathies.

The Thyroid Myopathies

During the past two decades several myopathic diseases related to alterations in thyroid function have been recognized. These are: (1) chronic thyrotoxic myopathy, (2) exophthalmic ophthalmoplegia (infiltrative ophthalmopathy), (3) myasthenia gravis associated with toxic diffuse goiter or with hypothyroidism, (4) periodic paralysis associated with toxic diffuse goiter, (5) muscle hypertrophy and slow muscle contraction and relaxation associated with myxedema and cretinism. Although not frequent, several examples of each of these diseases may be seen in a single year in any large general hospital.

Chronic thyrotoxic myopathy is a disease characterized by progressive weakness and atrophy of skeletal musculature, occurring in conjunction with overt or covert (masked) hyperthyroidism. The muscular disorder may reach proportions such as to suggest progressive muscular atrophy (motor system disease). It is estimated that the middle-aged patient is most likely to suffer from this complication of hyperthyroidism and that men are more susceptible than women. The onset is insidious, the weakness progresses over weeks and months, and exophthalmos need not be present. The pelvic girdle and thigh muscles are weakened more than others (Basedow's paraplegia), though all are affected to some extent, even bulbar and rarely ocular. However, the shoulder and hand muscles are the ones which show the most conspicuous atrophy. Tremor and coarse twitching during contraction may occur, but the authors have not seen fasciculations at rest or true fibrillations (in the electromyogram). The tendon reflexes are normal or lively. Creatine excretion in the urine is increased and tolerance to ingested creatine diminished, but the degree of it has not been correlated with the degree

of weakness. Electromyograms have disclosed no definite abnormality, and biopsies of muscle, except for slight volumetric reduction in fibers, have been normal. Injections of neostigmine have no effect. Muscle power and bulk are gradually restored when thyroid function is reduced to normal levels.

Exophthalmic ophthalmoplegia is a weakness of external ocular muscles (pupillary and ciliary muscles are always spared) which is conjoined with exophthalmos. The latter varies in degree, being sometimes absent at an early age of the disease, and is not in itself responsible for the weakness. Both the ocular weakness and exophthalmos may precede the hyperthyroidism or follow the effective treatment of it. The ocular palsy may occasionally be unilateral, especially in the beginning. Many of the fibers of the eye muscles in biopsies and in autopsy material have degenerated, and infiltrations of lymphocytes, mononuclear leukocytes, and lipocytes are present, hence the term infiltrative ophthalmopathy. All external eye muscles may be affected, often one more than others, accounting for strabismus and diplopia; upward movements are usually limited to the greatest degree. Prostigmine has no effect. The condition often runs a self-limited course like the exophthalmos itself, and therapy is difficult to evaluate. Lugol's solution, 1.0 cc three times daily, may be helpful, and certainly the maintenance of an euthyroid state is desirable (see Chap. 66 for treatment of hyperthyroidism). If the exophthalmos reaches a degree which threatens injury of the cornea, the operation of unroofing the orbits, introduced by Naffziger, is indicated.

Thyrotoxic periodic paralysis resembles the familial periodic paralysis (described below) and consists of attacks of mild to severe weakness of limb and trunk muscles, usually with sparing of those of the cranium, which develops in a few minutes or hours and lasts part of a day longer. In some series as many as half of the cases of periodic paralysis have been in individuals who suffered from hyperthyroidism. It is believed that the thyrotoxicosis evokes a muscle disease which had been latent. In some cases the serum potassium levels have been low during an attack and the administration of several grams of KCl terminates the attack. Treatment of the hyperthyroidism abolishes the symptomatic manifestations of the muscular disorder.

Myasthenia gravis in typical neostigmine-responsive form may accompany hyper- or hypothyroidism. In hyperthyroidism the typical weakness and poorly sustained contraction of the aforementioned chronic thyrotoxic myopathy are added to the myasthenia, without appearing to affect the response to or requirement for neostigmine. In contrast, hypothyroidism, even of mild degrees, seems to aggravate the myasthenia gravis, greatly increasing the need for neostigmine and at times inducing a myasthenic crisis. Thyroxin is beneficial and, with respect to myasthenia, restores the patient to his status before the onset of the thyroid insufficiency. The myasthenia gravis (described in Chap. 86) is independent of thyroid disease. Each disease must be treated separately.

Hypothyroidism, whether in the form of myxedema or cretinism, is often accompanied by a series of changes in skeletal muscle consisting of increased volume, stiffness and slowness of contraction, and prolonged tendon reflexes (see Chap. 87). These changes probably account for the large tongue and typical dysarthria of this disease. The clinical syndrome simulates hypertrophia musculorum vera and myotonia congenita. Cretinism manifesting these muscle symptoms is known as Debré-Semelaigne's syndrome, and myxedema with a similar muscle picture is called Hoffmann's syndrome. In either of these two syndromes there is no real evidence of myotonia by either clinical test or electromyogram, and muscle biopsies have revealed only large fibers. Creatine excretion is reduced, creatine tolerance is increased, and transaminase values in the serum are normal. The administration of thyroxin corrects the abnormality of muscle.

The effect of thyroid secretion on the muscle fiber in all these myopathies is still a matter of conjecture. Clinical data indicate that this hormone influences in some manner the contractile process without interfering in any way with the transmission of impulses in the peripheral nerves or across the myoneural junctions. In hyperthyroidism this functional disorder enhances the speed of the contractile process and reduces its duration, the net effect being a weakening, an excess fatigability, and a loss of endurance in muscle action. In hypothyroidism the converse of these changes occurs.

The thyroid hormone also acts on the central nervous system, and in some syndromes such as myxedema and the acute toxic encephalopathy and myopathy of hyperthyroidism, it is possible to observe the effects of both a neurologic and a muscular disorder.

Cortisone Myopathy

The widespread use of adrenal corticosteroids in recent years has brought to light a new muscle disease, probably not dissimilar to that which has been noted in rabbits receiving cortisone. The proximal limb and girdle musculature becomes extremely weak to the point where it is difficult to elevate the arms and to arise from a sitting, squatting, or kneeling position, and walking itself may be hampered. The electromyogram shows the myopathic pattern of small but abundant action poten-

tials and also fibrillations; in biopsies there is evidence of scattered degenerating and regenerating muscle fibers without infiltrates of inflammatory cells. The serum transaminase and aldolase levels are raised, and there is a creatinuria. Discontinuation of the corticosteroid administration leads to recovery within a few weeks. The dose levels of cortisone or prednisone have usually been high and sustained over a period of months, and improvement upon lowering the dose has been reported. Corticosteroid preparations containing fluorine are said to have been particularly culpable. A similar myopathy has been observed in patients who suffer from Cushing's syndrome. The mechanism of the muscle disease is unknown.

Myopathy and Myoglobinuria

In any disease that results in rapid destruction of striated muscle fibers, myoglobin and other muscle proteins may enter the blood stream and appear in the urine. The latter is a dark red or burgundy-colored, much like the urine in hemoglobinuria. The myoglobin can be identified and distinguished from hemoglobin by spectroscopic examination. If present in excess amounts, especially if the urine is acid, it may precipitate and form casts in the renal tubules; shock and renal obstruction damage the kidneys, with resulting anuria. The latter is often temporary but may persist and prove fatal. Alkalinization of the urine by the ingestion of sodium bicarbonate is said to protect the kidney by preventing the formation of myoglobin casts, but it is of doubtful value and the sodium may actually be harmful if anuria has occurred.

The following conditions may give rise to myoglobinuria:

1. Crush injury to a limb.

2. Strain or excessive use of muscles, especially the pretibial muscles which are confined in the tight pretibial compartment (pretibial syndrome).

3. Extensive infarction as in occlusion of the main artery of a limb or a subcutaneous infusion into the lower leg (with resultant swelling and probable ischemia).

4. Haff disease, which results from eating fish poisoned by toxic resinous acids derived from cellulose. This was first reported in the bay (Haff) of Königsberg, Germany.

5. Familial myoglobinuria, a disease which occurs in families with or without a diffuse chronic myopathy or dystrophy. The attack of myoglobinuria may be precipitated by strenuous exertion or possibly by an infection. Weakness, stiffness, and tenderness or swelling of muscles are the principal symptoms and vary in intensity. The muscle fibers are later found in various stages of degeneration and regeneration. The degree of renal injury

usually determines the outcome. No therapy is known except that of complete inactivity and measures which assist return of renal function. Since the patient often has a life-long disposition to attacks of myoglobinuria, physical activity must be curtailed and exertion avoided. Nothing is known of the precise mechanism by which the muscle fibers are damaged, but presumably an enzymatic defect of the muscle fibers reduces the tolerance of the muscle to maximal activity—? a fault in anaerobic metabolism.

Other Metabolic Myopathies

A progressive areflexic muscular atrophy giving rise to a syndrome of infantile muscular atrophy or slack child has been recorded in two of the five established forms of glycogen storage disease (see Chap. 94).

A syndrome of painful muscles and generalized weakness has been reported in hypoglycemia (see Chap. 71).

In hyperparathyroidism and osteomalacia resulting from renal tubular acidosis (a form of Milkman's syndrome), muscular weakness, fatigability, atrophy, and discomfort after exercise have been noted. The tendon reflexes are normal or hyperactive.

A contracture of hamstring muscles which prevents upright stance has been found several times in patients with Addison's disease. Biopsy has revealed normal muscle tissue; the electromyogram is normal; and the tendon reflexes are retained.

A primary defect of phosphorylase has been established as the cause of another condition known as McArdle's syndrome. This is a chronic familial myopathy with weakness, stiffness, and discomfort in the muscles following exercise. Therefore it is more likely to be considered in connection with the myalgic and muscle stiffness syndromes (Chap. 87).

REFERENCES

Walton, J. N., and R. D. Adams: "Polymyositis," Edinburgh, E. S. Livingstone, Ltd., 1958.

85 CHRONIC MUSCULAR WASTING AND PARALYSIS

Frank H. Tyler and Raymond D. Adams

As intimated in the clinical classification (Table 83-1, p. 723), one of the major causes of the syndrome of progressive weakness and wasting of the musculature of the limbs and trunk is muscular dystrophy. This category of disease can usually be differentiated from the familial or nonfamilial varieties of neuropathy by the pattern of the muscle involvement (usually proximal in the dystrophies and distal in most of the neuropathies), the absence of sensory disturbances, the less severe reduction of tendon reflexes, the cerebrospinal fluid examination (normal in dystrophies, protein often elevated in neuropathies), the characteristic electromyogram, and the findings in a muscle biopsy. It can usually be distinguished from spinal muscular atrophy, exemplified in the adult by motor system disease and in the infant by Werdnig-Hoffman's muscular atrophy, by the proximal pattern of muscle involvement (total lack of pattern in motor system disease and usually asymmetric, either forearms and hands or legs or proximal and girdle muscles), the lack of coarse fasciculations, and the characteristic electromyogram and biopsy changes. These two forms of chronic muscular atrophy are described in Chaps. 290 and 291 and will not be discussed further in this section.

THE MUSCULAR DYSTROPHIES

History and Terminology. Progressive muscular dystrophy (*dystrophia musculorum progressiva; primary myopathy*) was described by several prominent physicians in the latter half of the nineteenth century. The many names used since that time to designate these diseases have been a source of confusion. Duchenne reported a group of patients with muscular enlargement as well as atrophy, who have since been referred to as examples of *pseudohypertrophic* type of progressive muscular dystrophy. Leyden and Möbius called attention to a clinically similar group in which, however, muscular enlargement was lacking. Thus arose the name *simple atrophic* type. Landouzy and Déjerine described a form of muscular dystrophy in which the facial and pectoral girdle muscles were the first to be involved, which they called the *facioscapulohumeral* type. Erb reported a group of patients with little or no facial involvement which he described as having "juvenile dystrophy." Recently, Walton and others have distinguished Erb's case of "limb-girdle dystrophy" from facioscapulohumeral dystrophy by their earlier onset and lack of typical dominant inheritance in the pedigrees as well as the lack of facial involvement. A number of other syndromes have been described, but as they are rare and, in some cases, of doubtful relationship to the more typical disorders, they will not be considered here.

It is now generally agreed that all these groups represent only insignificant variations of a single disease process. From clinical and genetic evidence, at least six syndromes can be defined. They are childhood, facioscapulohumeral, limb-girdle, distal, ocular, and myotonic dystrophy. They are distinguished by mode of inheritance, age of onset, rate of progression, localization of initial involvement, and prognosis. Nearly all patients with typical muscle disease and other dystrophic features fit well into one of these syndromes. It should be emphasized that other much rarer types do exist, but description of their characteristics is beyond the scope of this discussion.

Pathologic Anatomy. The atrophic muscles appear white or fatty, a change frequently described as "fish flesh," and the diagnosis may be suspected from the gross appearance. Microscopically, the earliest change is an enlargement of the muscle fibers and a marked increase in the number of sarcolemmal nuclei, which may form chains and appear centrally in the muscle fiber. Other fibers within a microscopic field may appear entirely normal, and the distribution of involved muscle fibers is an entirely random affair within a given muscle. The damaged and atrophic fibers ultimately disappear and are progressively replaced by fibrous tissue and fat cells.

The lesions are similar in all types of dystrophy. In the very advanced cases, where all muscle fibers have disappeared, it may be difficult to recognize the tissue as muscle. The peripheral and central nervous system are unchanged, although in the late stages of the disease there may be a secondary loss of nerve cells and fibers.

Pathogenesis. The pathogenesis of progressive muscular dystrophy is obscure. There is convincing evidence that in the majority of patients a genetic mechanism underlies the disease process. Although in many instances a family history cannot be obtained by direct questioning of the patient, on careful examination of the members of the pedigree other affected individuals are frequently found. Other considerations lead to the conclusion that the disease may be caused either by a previously latent recessive trait or by the occurrence of a mutation. Although it is quite possible that the same clinical manifestations may occur occasionally as the result of a nongenetic mechanism, the occurrence of the genetic pattern in the majority of instances must be included in any concept of the mechanism of these disorders.

By analogy with the other known genetic disorders, it must be presumed that some abnormality in the intracellular metabolism is caused by the genetic abnormality. This could be a modified or absent enzyme system within the muscle cell or some defect in the muscle metabolism resulting from inability to absorb or to metabolize normally a substance vital to muscle function.

The occurrence of creatinuria in patients with muscular dystrophy has led to extensive study of creatine synthesis as a site of the metabolic anomaly. Although there is some evidence both of increased creatine synthesis and inability to control creatine synthesis normally, the significance of this to the fundamental anomaly is as yet unknown. Many other metabolic systems in the muscle are under investigation or have been investigated in the past. As yet, no clear-cut mechanism by which the observed chemical changes could lead to the muscular damage has been proposed.

The pattern of development of muscular atrophy is remarkably similar from one patient to another with the same type of dystrophy. Within a local group of muscles, it has been suggested that the affection bears a relationship to the order of development of the muscles in the embryo, those muscles which appear earliest manifesting the first and most severe weakness and atrophy. Even when one part of the muscle develops earlier than another, the atrophy follows this order. Thus, the upper fibers of the trapezius form very early at the same time as the muscles innervated by the cranial nerves, while the lower fibers are among the earliest of girdle muscles to develop; and the disease always involves the lower part of the muscle most severely. On the other hand, the variation in severity in different patients and variation in area of initial involvement in the various types make the possibility of this embryologic factor an incomplete explanation of the process.

As in other genetically determined metabolic disorders, it is probable that a single enzymic abnormality underlies the entire disease process and accounts for all its manifestations, even in such a disease as myotonic dystrophy in which many systems are involved. Only continued search at the basic level of metabolic processes will lead to an understanding of the pathogenesis of these disorders.

Childhood Type (Duchenne's Pseudohypertrophic Muscular Dystrophy)

Clinical Pattern. Progressive muscular dystrophy of childhood appears in boys usually before they reach the age of six. Some children manifest weakness or enlargement of the calf muscles before they learn to walk. In a few rare individuals, manifestations indistinguishable clinically from those of the childhood disorder develop in adult life. Occasionally a girl is seen whose clinical picture fits that of progressive muscular dystrophy of childhood better than any other well-defined neuromuscular disorder, although, more frequently than not, atypical features are found on close study.

Children with this disease are usually normal at birth, and their early muscular and other development is indistinguishable from that of a normal child. Prenatal forms have been described but are rare. The most frequent initial complaint is that the child falls frequently. On examination, easily demonstrable weakness and atrophy of the peroneal, tibial, thigh, pelvic girdle, spinal, and pectoral girdle muscles are found. These weaknesses usually have not been recognized by the patient or his family. The onset and progression are generally so insidious that it is nearly impossible to date the events accurately in the history. An occasional individual will relate the onset to an acute illness or injury. As far as can be determined, such illness or injury has no causal relation to the disease but does affect its course in a fashion which will be pointed out below.

There are rarely any symptoms other than those relating directly to the muscular disability. An occasional child will complain of aching or nagging pain in the legs or of muscular cramps. The disease is steadily progressive without striking remission or relapse, although the patients may claim to feel better and stronger on certain days. When these patients are confined to bed by acute illnesses or for other reasons, disproportionately rapid increase in the severity of the disease appears to have occurred during the period of inactivity. For this reason, confinement and body casts should be avoided, if possible.

As the disease becomes more severe, a characteristic pattern of muscular wasting—the best diagnostic criterion of the disease—becomes evident. Slight symmetric weakness of the entire group of facial muscles, usually most marked in the zygomaticus and orbicularis oris, occurs in some patients. These changes result in only minimal changes in facial expression, a transverse smile, and some pouting of the lips. The other muscles supplied by cranial nerves are essentially normal. The cervical muscles are rather diffusely affected, but all of them remain functional to a certain extent, with the extensors and sternocleidomastoids least seriously impaired. In contrast, certain of the muscles of the pectoral girdle may be entirely absent. Among the earliest to disappear are the middle and lower fibers of the trapezius, the rhomboids, the latissimi, and the sternal head of the pectoralis major. The serratus anterior usually is only moderately involved. This combination of changes results in elevation and slipping out and forward of the scapulas, which stand out behind the patient like wings when tension is placed on them by having the patient push against a wall or raise the arms. The anterior chest develops a flattened appearance which is sometimes complicated by depression of the sternum (pectus excavatum). The deltoid sometimes shows striking atrophy of its upper half in contrast to the relatively intact lower part.

The triceps and biceps brachii are moderately to severely involved. The brachioradialis becomes atrophic and even disappears at an early stage, but the other forearm muscles retain fair strength and mass until most of the central musculature is very atrophic. The intrinsic musculature of the hand is not severely involved until quite late in the disease.

Soon all the axial musculature becomes involved, and the changes progress rapidly. Severe lumbar lordosis and inability to extend the trunk on the pelvis without support are evident. This leads to the characteristic maneuver which these children develop, of literally climbing up their own legs with their hands in order to bring the trunk to its precarious vertical position. They fall whenever this carefully maintained balance is disturbed.

All the thigh muscles are involved, but the process is usually most severe in the quadriceps femoris. The lower leg shows a striking disproportion between the severely involved tibial and peroneal groups and the usually much less weak calf and foot muscles. Sometimes the tibial group shows a significantly more severe degree of atrophy than the peroneal, but in the average patient, the involvement is similar in the two groups. The muscular loss is relatively symmetric at all stages of its development, a fact which is useful diagnostically.

The gastrocnemius and soleus show a striking and diagnostically useful sign of enlargement in most of these patients. Indeed, the enlargement may be the very first sign, as has been noted already under the term *pseudohypertrophy*. It is symmetric when present, and is seen in other muscles as well, most frequently the deltoid and triceps. It occurs infrequently and irregularly in other diseases of muscle. Although the affected muscles are weaker than might be expected from their size, severe loss of strength is unusual. They do not become atrophic or weak so rapidly as the other involved muscles. The enlarged muscles feel firm and doughy in contrast to normal or atrophic muscles.

Neurologic examination shows only defects which are secondary to the muscular atrophy and loss of tone. The reaction to electric stimulation is normal except that increased current is required to produce contraction in the involved muscles. Deep tendon reflexes may be depressed or absent, depending on the amount of atrophy and loss of tone in the muscles tested. Sensation is intact in all modalities; coordination is markedly impaired by the muscular weakness, but no evidence of deficiency of cerebral or spinal motor centers is found in typical cases. Intellectual development is not hindered by the disease, although mental deficiency may be present as a separate hereditary or developmental anomaly and other neurologic abnormalities as well.

When the disease becomes severe, the patients are confined to bed or a wheelchair because of their inability to stand and walk without support.

Strength may still be fair in the hands and forearms. The facial involvement is not progressive. Normal facial movement is the rule even in the completely bedridden patient, with little evidence of functional voluntary muscle elsewhere.

Complications. As the activity of the patient is reduced by his disability, deforming contractures frequently develop. The Achilles tendons and hamstrings are involved most frequently. During this same period, marked scoliosis and kyphosis may develop because of the severity of the atrophy in the axial musculature. These may result in deformities, particularly of the chest, but seldom are they severe enough to produce symptoms of respiratory insufficiency.

Certain of these patients become quite obese when they are bedfast. There is often a high dietary intake, sometimes related to the emotional problems of invalidism. Obesity is a serious problem because of the manner in which it complicates nursing care and increases disability. Only by proper supervision of food intake can the obesity be controlled. Other patients become quite emaciated and have little muscle or subcutaneous tissue.

An unusual but apparently directly related complication is the development of *congestive heart failure* as the result of involvement of the myocardium by the dystrophic process. In the majority of patients in whom there are no other signs or symptoms of cardiac disease, sinus tachycardia is found. Symptoms of cardiac involvement might be much more frequent if the muscular disability did not limit activity. The congestive failure is often mild and responds to the usual management. Although it can be fatal, remissions frequently occur in which symptoms and signs of cardiac disease may no longer be detectable clinically, and they may not recur during the ensuing years of life. Electrocardiographic abnormalities are found in nearly all cases.

In general, the patients are normal in other respects, except for the occurrence of unrelated anomalies. Most of the patients die in adolescence or early adult life from infections, most frequently respiratory, which develop as a result of their disability. The most common lethal effect of the disease is myocardial insufficiency, which may often become manifest abruptly and may terminate fatally.

Laboratory Data. The electromyogram (EMG) exhibits a characteristic pattern of low voltage, abnormally brief action potentials, unlike those of denervation atrophy. Muscle biopsy demonstrates the loss and degeneration of muscle fibers, large and small fibers in haphazard distribution, fibrosis, and fat-cell infiltration.

The other laboratory findings are not highly specific and are not so helpful in diagnosis as the clinical findings. The blood is consistently normal in the absence of complications. The urine is negative. The spinal fluid shows no abnormalities. Determination of *creatine* and *creatinine* in the urine may be diagnostically useful. The best available evidence indicates that ingested or endogenous creatine is stored mainly in muscle. Amounts in excess of the quantity that can be stored lead to a marked increase in serum levels of creatine and result in excretion of creatine in the urine. Creatinine is the anhydride of creatine, and when formed it is excreted in the urine. Creatinine appears to be derived by a nonenzymatic change in creatine phosphate which occurs either in vivo or in vitro at a constant rate. For this reason it is thought that the 24-hr excretion of creatinine is an accurate measure of the total body store of creatine and thus of the functional muscle mass in the body.

Normal adult males excrete little or no creatine in the urine, but women and children may excrete small amounts of creatine even on a creatine-free diet.

The usual laboratory procedure for the determination of creatine and creatinine is to measure the creatinine and then to convert the creatine to creatinine by heating in acid solution and to redetermine the creatinine. The creatine can then be estimated from the difference multiplied by a factor (1.32) for conversion of creatinine to creatine hydrate.

The creatinine excretion is frequently expressed as an index which is derived by dividing the 24-hr creatinine excretion in milligrams by the body weight in kilograms. Normal values are usually between 14 and 25, depending on the muscular development of the individual.

More or less in proportion to the reduction in muscle mass, patients with childhood muscular dystrophy excrete much less than the normal amount of creatinine and greatly increased amounts of creatine in the urine. The average patient excretes between 200 and 300 mg creatinine and 400 to 600 mg creatine per day on a creatine-free diet. This much distortion of the creatinine-creatine excretion pattern is seldom seen in any other disorder except muscle dystrophy, polymyositis, or severe and long-standing thyrotoxicosis. It must be kept in mind, however, that other neuromuscular and metabolic diseases may lead to creatinuria, and care must be taken not to put undue reliance on this finding in differential diagnosis.

The concentration of a number of serum enzymes is elevated in the early stages of childhood dystrophy. Transaminases, lactic dehydrogenase, aldolase, and creatine phosphokinase all show abnormalities early and tend to become normal, more or less in that order, as the disease progresses. In the few instances in which they have been examined, they have been abnormal before the clinical manifestations of the disease were apparent, and thus may identify the trait earlier than any other procedure. The quantity of these enzymes is also elevated in the acute myopathies and active phases of polymyositis. Whether the enzymes are entirely derived from degenerating muscle cells or, at least in the dystrophies, reflect abnormal permeability of the membrane of the muscle fibers is uncertain. In the adult dystrophies, which are more chronic and less severe, there is little or no elevation of these enzymes.

Inheritance. This type of muscular dystrophy is frequently familial in character, and more than one male child of a family often manifests the disease. The parents are normal. In some families, male children of various members of the female line are affected. This fact, together with its nearly complete limitation to males and its frequent apparently sporadic occurrence, suggests that the condition depends usually on the transmission of a sex-linked recessive gene which arises by frequent mutation from the normal gene.

Families have been reported in which the dominant type of inheritance seemed to be present. It is possible that essentially the same abnormality is transmitted by different genes in different families, but extensive experience has failed to reveal any pedigrees of this type. The study of the problem is complicated by the probably fortunate fact that the patients only rarely have children and therefore the trait can be traced only in collaterals of involved individuals.

Treatment. See under Facioscapulohumeral Type below.

Facioscapulohumeral Type

Clinical Pattern. Facioscapulohumeral dystrophy is closely related to childhood dystrophy. The average age of onset is thirteen years but ranges between nine and twenty years. A few patients even beyond fifty years of age are found on close examination to have the disorder, although they have not recognized their disability. As this implies, the degree of involvement may be extremely slight; other patients, however, are significantly incapacitated before the age of twenty.

The pattern of muscular involvement differs from that of other dystrophies, as is indicated by the name. Weakness of facial muscles is nearly always present. All the facial muscles are involved in the process, but the orbicularis oris shows a patchy and often asymmetric atrophy which results in abnormal movements and inability to pucker the mouth or whistle normally. There is weakness of the orbicularis oculi and diffuse flattening of the face; and asymmetric movements, particularly about the mouth, are extremely characteristic. The

diagnosis may be suspected after watching the patient's face while he gives his history. The facial weakness may be the earliest change.

The muscles of the pectoral girdle are involved early in the course of the disease in almost the same pattern as in childhood dystrophy. Frequently there is complete atrophy of one muscle and its mate on the opposite side of the body, with no evident disease in a nearby pair of muscles. The patients cannot raise their arms above their heads because of the loss of muscles of the pectoral girdle, but they frequently maintain normal strength in the forearms and hands until an advanced age.

The axial and pelvic musculature is not involved extensively until late in the disease, but atrophy in the tibial and peroneal groups begins early.

These patients show the same complications and associated abnormalities as patients with childhood dystrophy, but there are fewer associated congenital anomalies; and heart disease due to the dystrophy and contractures is extremely rare. The average patient lives out a normal life span, becoming completely incapacitated only very late in life if at all.

Inheritance. The disease is inherited as an autosomal dominant, with complete penetrance. This, plus the fact that involved persons are not incapacitated during the childbearing period, accounts for high familial incidence in a single generation.

Laboratory Data. Laboratory examinations yield no abnormalities except creatinuria, which is usually not so marked as in childhood dystrophy, and creatinine excretion is not so greatly reduced as in childhood dystrophy. Some patients, particularly those with minimal involvement, may have relatively insignificant creatinuria.

Distal Type

Gowers many years ago and Welander more recently have called attention to patients with slowly progressive atrophy of the muscles of the hands and feet. In these patients muscle biopsy has shown the characteristic lesions of muscular dystrophy. The disorder apparently begins in youth and is slowly progressive but produces only moderate disability. Welander was able to establish the existence of an autosomal dominant transmission of the trait in some of the families which she studied. The disorder must be unusual for the authors have observed only two such patients in Salt Lake City and Boston over a period of years. It should be noted that the cardinal manifestation of this disorder, i.e., atrophy and weakness of the lower leg and hand muscles, is characteristic of peroneal muscular atrophy. This latter disease is also a genetically determined disorder of autosomal dominant inheritance in which the patients usually develop more severe atrophy and weakness in the lower leg, the forearm, and hand, in contrast to the distal type of dystrophy. This, and other features of neuropathy such as delayed conduction velocity of peripheral nerves, prove to be useful in differential diagnosis.

Progressive Ophthalmoplegia

Isolated dystrophic involvement of the extraocular muscles is another relatively rare form of muscle dystrophy. The disorder usually appears in adult life and must be differentiated from other causes of ophthalmoplegia. A progressive external ophthalmoplegia (sparing of pupils and muscles of accommodation), ptosis, and sometimes weakness of orbicularis oculi, extending over a period of years, represents the typical clinical syndrome. Isolated involvement of other cranial or spinal muscles may be conjoined. Affection of eye muscles is a relatively uncommon feature of the other forms of muscular dystrophy. Similarity of the histologic findings on biopsy to other varieties of dystrophy has been the means of establishing the myopathic character of this disorder.

Therapy. Treatment of these disorders is entirely unsatisfactory at the present time. *Vitamin E and inositol* and modified vitamin E preparations, pyridoxine, testosterone, and glycine, among others, have been proposed, but there is no well-documented, long-term evidence of satisfactory results.

Two factors are of definite importance in the management of these diseases—avoidance of prolonged bed rest and inactivity and encouragement of the patient to maintain as full and normal a life as possible. These measures are indicated to prevent the rapid progress associated with inactivity and to maintain a healthy attitude of mind. A diet which is adequate in all normal requirements but which will not result in progressive weight gain is desirable. No evidence is available that any type of dietary supplement beyond the normal level is of value.

MYOTONIC DYSTROPHY

Definition. Myotonic dystrophy (myotonia dystrophica, myotonia atrophica, Steinert's disease) is a hereditary disease characterized by myotonia, muscular wasting of a characteristic pattern, cataracts, testicular atrophy, and frontal baldness.

Clinical Pattern. Except for the myotonia, which frequently develops many years before the other manifestations, this disease usually begins in early adult life. Myotonia consists of an inability to relax a muscle normally after its contraction and is the result of repetitive discharge of the motor endplate. It is a symptom which may be seen in an occasional patient with any of several other neuromuscular disorders. It is seen most characteris-

tically in the adductors of the thumb. The patient's inability to let go after shaking hands may give the clue to the proper diagnosis. This difficulty disappears after repetitive motion. Contractions elicited by direct percussion of the muscle are also delayed in relaxation. This latter sign (percussion myotonia) may be present when the grasp response and other clinical evidence of myotonia are not found. The muscular atrophy which develops is in some respects similar to that in the disease described above. A different type of facial involvement occurs, however. In general the patient exhibits a rather dull, expressionless facies, with severe ptosis of the eyelids due to weakness of levator muscles. The forehead is furrowed as a compensatory effort on the part of the frontalis muscle to overcome the ptosis. This becomes so severe that the patient must tip his head back to see straight ahead. The "dystrophic" facial movements of facioscapulohumeral dystrophy do not occur. The voice becomes nasal and expressionless. Atrophy of the temporalis muscles is usually severe.

Loss of the sternocleidomastoids is disproportionately marked; the other muscles of the anterior part of the neck may be so atrophic that the trachea is seen immediately beneath the skin. There is extreme difficulty in flexing the neck, but extension is usually moderately good because of the preservation of the spinalis group of muscles.

The loss in other muscle groups is similar to that of childhood dystrophy, except that much earlier and more severe atrophy of the muscles of the leg, forearm, hands, and feet develops and may even exceed in severity that of the central musculature.

These patients, whether male or female, also develop progressive *alopecia,* usually frontal, at an early age. Testicular atrophy with androgenic deficiency usually develops in males. The latter are frequently sterile and sometimes impotent. In some patients, gynecomastia and elevated gonadotrophin excretion are found. Testicular biopsy may show peritubular fibrosis. Thus, all the clinical characteristics of Klinefelter's syndrome may be present. Rarely, the nuclei of skin or bone marrow cells may be shown to have "sex chromatin mass"; and at least one individual with myotonic dystrophy has had a sex chromosome complement of XXY. However, even in those individuals who develop severe testicular atrophy in early life, the nuclei usually do not show the "sex chromatin mass" and are presumably of the usual male XY sex chromosome constitution. Ovarian deficiency occasionally develops in females. This is seldom severe enough to interfere with the menstrual pattern or fertility. The lens opacities of myotonic dystrophy are of two types. The first consists of fine dustlike subcapsular deposits which frequently appear scintillating and colored under the slit lamp but often cannot be seen with the ordinary ophthalmoscope. This type of opacity is virtually always present in patients with other signs of the disorder. Their appearance is so characteristic as to be virtually diagnostic. The second type of cataract is like the usual senile cataract, and seldom appears except in elderly patients, being of little diagnostic usefulness. *Blepharoconjunctivitis* is an extremely common finding, even in patients with little weakness of facial muscles, and is universal in advanced cases.

Neurologic examination reveals no sensory or other motor abnormalities.

Dystrophic heart disease is common in this disorder, as it is in childhood dystrophy, in contrast to the facioscapulohumeral type. Because it usually occurs at an advanced age and presents no specific features, it is difficult to differentiate from other types of heart disease common in elderly persons.

Among the dystrophies the myotonic variety is the most variable. Rarely a patient may exhibit only one of the features, particularly myotonia or the characteristic cataracts; not uncommonly one or more of the dystrophic features may be missing. Nonetheless diagnosis is seldom difficult on physical examination alone if care is taken to look for the features described. The diagnosis is obvious in patients who have significant disability from their myotonic dystrophy.

Routine laboratory data are of no aid in making the diagnosis. Creatinuria is irregular and frequently absent. The characteristic after-potentials of myotonia can be demonstrated electromyographically and may be useful where clinical demonstration of myotonia is difficult. In addition, the electromyogram shows the usual myopathic pattern of many low voltage, brief action potentials of myopathy. In muscle biopsies one sees the usual findings of muscle dystrophy and in addition many rows of central nuclei, ring bundles of myofibrils encircling the muscle fibers, and curious sarcoplasmic masses.

Two rare but distinct diseases are closely related to myotonia dystrophica and need mention in order that they may not be confused with it, *myotonia congenita* (*Thomsen's disease*) a familial disorder of dominant inheritance in which there is lifelong myotonia, which is most severe following rest, excitement, or anxiety, but without the other manifestations of myotonia dystrophica; and *paramyotonia congenita,* an even more rare disorder, in which myotonia occurs only following exposure to cold. The latter is also familial, of dominant inheritance, of lifelong duration, and benign in character. It is genetically separate from both the other myotonias. Both these disorders respond to quinine, as described below.

Inheritance. Myotonia dystrophica is inherited as a typical mendelian dominant, but certain members of a given line may manifest only one or two of the usual group of findings. Myotonia is the most common finding on physical examination, while cataracts are often mentioned in family histories. Care must be used, however, in the evaluation of this evidence, because cataracts of other etiology may occur in the nondystrophic line and lead to confusion. Search by history and examination for other features of the syndrome in individuals with cataract will usually prevent such errors.

Treatment. *Quinine* has a mild curare-like action at the motor end-plate and thus relieves the myotonia. Although symptomatic relief of the myotonia is usually achieved, the drug has no effect on the progress of the muscle atrophy or other degenerative aspects of the disease. The usual dose is 0.3 to 0.6 Gm orally, repeated as needed about every 6 hr. Mild toxic symptoms such as tinnitus may develop before enough quinine has been given to obtain satisfactory relief of the myotonia. Some patients find these symptoms more distressing than the myotonia and prefer not to take quinine except on special occasions when the myotonia is troublesome in a particular activity.

Treatment with cortisone will also relieve the myotonia in some patients but may accelerate the progress of the muscular atrophy and should not be used. Procaine amide (0.25–0.50 Gm) will relieve the myotonia in some patients with fewer side effects than observed with quinine.

Surgical management of the cataracts when they are mature is indicated.

Administration of androgen therapy when deficiency is apparent may be given for symptomatic benefit, but a relation of the hormone to the pathogenesis of the disease is not established.

REFERENCES

CHILDHOOD TYPE

Benedict, Jean D., Helen J. Kalinsky, Louis A. Scarrone, Arthur R. Wertheim, and DeWitt Stetten, Jr.: The Origin of Urinary Creatine in Progressive Muscular Dystrophy, J. Clin. Invest., 34:141, 1955.

Bowden, R. E. M., and E. Gutman: Observations in a Case of Muscular Dystrophy with Reference to Diagnostic Significance, Arch. Neurol. Psychiat., 56:1, 1946.

Gowers, William Richard: "Pseudohypertrophic Muscular Paralysis," London, J. & A. Churchill, 1879.

Perkoff, G. T., and F. H. Tyler: Differential Diagnosis of Progressive Muscular Dystrophy, Med. Clin. N. Am., 37:545, 1953.

Tyler, F. H., and F. E. Stephens: Studies in Disorders of Muscle: IV. Clinical Manifestations and Inheritance of Childhood Progressive Muscular Dystrophy, Ann. Internal Med., 35:169, 1951.

Walton, John N., and F. J. Nattrass: On the Classification, Natural History and Treatment of the Myopathies, Brain, 77:169, 1954.

Wilson, S. A. Kinnier: "Neurology," Baltimore, The Williams & Wilkins Company, 1941.

FACIOSCAPULOHUMERAL TYPE

Landouzy, L., and J. Déjerine: De la myopathie atrophique progressive, Rev. méd. (Paris), 5:81, 1885.

Tyler, F. H., and F. E. Stephens: Studies in Disorders of Muscle: II. Clinical Manifestations and Inheritance in Facioscapulohumeral Dystrophy in a Large Family, Ann. Internal Med., 32:640, 1950.

MYOTONIC TYPE

Brown, G. I., and A. M. Harvey: Congenital Myotonia in the Goat, Brain, 62:341, 1939.

Thomasen, Eivind: "Myotonia (Thomsen's Disease), Paramyotonia and Dystrophia Myotonica," vol. 17 of "Opera ex Domo Biologiae Hereditariae Humanae Universitatis Hafniensis," translated by Finn Brink Carlson, Copenhagen, Ejnar Munksgaard, 1948. (A mine of valuable information about the myotonias.)

86 EPISODIC MUSCULAR WEAKNESS

Frank H. Tyler and Raymond D. Adams

Characteristic of most of the muscular diseases included in this chapter is the episodic nature of the weakness, the patient being normal or only slightly weak between attacks, and the evident disorder of neuromuscular transmission or of muscle membrane excitability (see Chap. 26).

The following diseases should be considered when a patient with an apparently intact nervous system and relatively normal appearing muscles complains of episodic or fluctuating weakness or paralysis. In myasthenia gravis and thyrotoxic myopathy with myasthenia or periodic paralysis, some degree of weakness is persistent at all times but is made worse by activity. Muscle weakness with drug intoxication (phenothiazine drugs, barbiturates, and bromides), neurasthenia, depression, and other states of excess fatigability can be separated as a rule on clinical grounds (see Chap. 33).

I. Myasthenia gravis
II. Episodic myasthenia of other types
    A. Familial periodic paralysis
    B. Adynamia episodica hereditaria (Gamstorp)
    C. Paramytonia congenita (von Eulenberg)
    D. Hypo- and hyperpotassemia and aldosteronism

MYASTHENIA GRAVIS

Definition. This disease is characterized by weakness and easy fatigability which most frequently affect the facial, oculomotor, laryngeal, pharyngeal, and respiratory muscles.

Clinical Pattern. Myasthenia gravis occurs at all ages and in both sexes. The disease most frequently appears, however, in the third or fourth decade. There is no significant familial incidence.

The onset may be in the facial or, more frequently, oculomotor muscles. The weakness of facial muscles and drooping of the eyelids, which may be unilateral at first, give rise to a smooth, relatively immobile face. The smile is frequently unnatural in that the lips elevate but do not retract; it resembles a snarl. Diplopia due to unequal weakness of the ocular muscles may appear early; it is often a transient and intermittent symptom but may persist to some degree and at times cause complete paresis of ocular movement. The pupils are never affected.

The laryngeal and pharyngeal muscles may be the first to manifest abnormalities. Choking and aspiration of food are common and obviously serious symptoms. Fluids may flow from the nose when swallowing is attempted, as a result of paresis of the palatal muscles. The involvement of tongue, laryngeal, and facial muscles results in abnormal speech of a rather feeble, nasal quality; if the patient continues to talk for a short time, the abnormality becomes more severe, and it is sometimes impossible to understand what the patient is saying. This is in striking contrast to the psychoneurotic patient, who also complains of weakness but can talk interminably without change in voice or enunciation.

A generalized weakness of skeletal muscles is also present in advanced cases of myasthenia gravis but seldom occurs in the absence of involvement of muscles innervated by cranial nerves. Easy *fatigability* and relatively prompt, partial recovery after rest are quite typical, and this history of it can be elicited in most cases. It is most characteristically demonstrated by having the patient perform a repetitive motion with some involved muscle. Sometimes no abnormality may be demonstrated in one muscle although it is easily evident on ordinary activity at other sites. As the process becomes more severe and of longer duration, it also tends to be more extensive. There are no other neurologic abnormalities in the average patient.

The disease process may be aggravated to a variable extent by a number of factors. The most frequent of these are upper respiratory infections, excitement, general fatigue, loss of sleep, menstruation, high carbohydrate meals, and the intake of alcohol. Medications which increase the neuromuscular block, such as curare, quinine, and quaternary ammonium compounds, should be avoided because they may produce severe paralysis in amounts which are quite ineffectual in normal individuals.

Muscular atrophy is not seen in the great majority of patients but may be present, particularly when the process has been of long duration. It most frequently involves the temporal, masseter, cervical, and proximal shoulder girdle muscles and is assumed to be due to disuse.

The illness usually develops over a few weeks (exceptionally in a few days), it may advance irregularly or remain at the same level of severity for a long time. Remissions are common and almost always occur after weeks or months of difficulty. They may be partial or complete. There may also be relapses, completely unpredictable as to time of occurrence or severity, but they usually reproduce the initial syndrome when they occur.

The life of the patient with severe myasthenia is endangered by intercurrent infections, particularly respiratory ones; and these are tolerated poorly. The sulfonamides and antibiotics are effective in controlling the serious effects of such infections when bacteria susceptible to the agents are responsible. Some female patients have a reduced fertility, but pregnancy does occur and may be followed by a normal delivery. Remissions and occasionally relapse have been reported to accompany pregnancy. The offspring may have mild or severe *myasthenia* at birth which may threaten their lives. This type of neonatal myasthenia lasts for a few weeks, and spontaneous recovery is the rule.

Respiratory insufficiency may develop quite abruptly or may be insidiously progressive. Of those complications which are the direct result of the disease, respiratory failure is the most common fatal one. Fatal accessions of profound weakness may be caused by an overdose of neostigmine.

Pathology. In some cases one or a few degenerating muscle fibers and frequent collections of small round cells, presumably lymphocytes, are seen among the muscle fibers and around the small blood vessels. Other organs may also show similar cellular infiltrations. Single muscle fibers or groups of fibers in a state of degeneration have been found in a few muscles in about half the fatal cases. There is no lack of cholinesterase at myoneural junctions, but two groups of investigators have noted that the motor ending on the surface of the muscle fiber was abnormally thin and unbranched. In as many as 20 per cent of certain series of cases, *tumors of the thymus* have been found. They may be either benign or malignant. In most of the remaining cases, there is persistence of an unusually large or a hyperplastic thymus.

Pathogenesis. This disease now appears to be the result of a specific functional abnormality at the *neuromyal junction.* Normally, acetylcholine is released at this junction, which facilitates the passage of impulses across it. Cholinesterase is normally present and hydrolyzes the acetylcholine (see Chap. 26). Physostigmine and neostigmine antagonize cholinesterase. Conduction of nerve impulses from the motor nerve to the muscle syncytium is impaired in myasthenia gravis (see Chap. 26). This may be shown in the electromyogram (Chap. 56) as a progressive decline in the voltage of action potentials. The exact nature of the defect is not clear. The administration of curare, quinine, or the quaternary ammonium compounds, which normally impair transmission across the neuromyal junction or over the surface of the muscle fiber, act in unusually small dosages to enhance the weakness in myasthenic patients. A circulating curare-like factor has never been demonstrated, and exchange transfusions have been of no value. A faulty catabolism of acetylcholine has also been postulated.

Diagnosis. The diagnosis usually is made without difficulty if one carefully evaluates the history and thinks of the disease. The characteristic pattern of *myasthenic fatigability* is easy to demonstrate by having the patient make some repetitive or sustained movement such as look up toward the ceiling for 2 to 3 min. The eyelids progressively droop until they cover the iris. Intramuscular injection of 0.5 to 2.0 mg neostigmine usually results in prompt relief of the muscular weakness, which is evident to the patient and physician. When the larger doses of neostigmine are used, it is important to administer about 1 mg atropine prior to the neostigmine in order to minimize the side effects of the neostigmine. Many times a patient who is unable to sit up, speak, or swallow will in the course of 5 min after neostigmine administration regain strength in a dramatic fashion. Occasionally patients with localized ocular palsies do not respond promptly to neostigmine, but the effect is nearly always obvious in other groups of muscles. Edrophonium chloride (Tensilon) is very similar in its action to neostigmine. For diagnostic testing it has the advantage that the response to an intravenous injection is almost instantaneous and the action is dissipated within a few minutes. The usual dose is 10 mg. Also severe side reactions are uncommon, making it unnecessary to administer atropine except in patients with asthma or cardiac disease. Although the short duration of action of this drug makes it unsatisfactory for maintenance therapy, in a myasthenic crisis it may be given by continuous intravenous drip. Another use is to determine if the weakness which develops in a myasthenic patient on neostigmine or similar therapy is the result of an exacerbation of the myasthenia gravis or of overtreatment with neostigmine or related compounds which of themselves may cause weakness. If due to the latter, 5 or 10 mg edrophonium administered intravenously, because of the short duration of action, may determine whether or not the profound weakness is due to a severe exacerbation of the disease or to overmedication. If, on the other hand, improvement ensues, higher doses of neostigmine or other longer-acting agent can be given safely. Curare must be used cautiously in patients with myasthenia and should be limited to the unusual circumstance in which the diagnosis seems improbable but needs to be more effectively ruled out (see Chap. 26). The weakness of thyrotoxic myopathy and motor system disease and the tiredness of neurasthenia which are sometimes confused with myasthenia gravis do not show the fluctuations of myasthenia gravis nor respond to neostigmine. Such patients develop large numbers of fasciculations after prostigmine, as do many normal persons. In thyrotoxicosis, however, a typical prostigmine myasthenia may occur and be added to the thyroid myopathy, and, as was stated above, hypothyroidism, if present, actually enhances myasthenic weakness (see Chap. 84).

Treatment. The management of these patients is divided into two parts: the treatment of acute episodes of severe paralysis and long-term management. Neostigmine is by far the most useful drug during acute attacks and should be given parenterally in doses of 1 mg and in multiples of this amount until the desired degree of improvement has been attained. The side reactions are gastrointestinal and uterine cramps, which may be partially controlled by the simultaneous administration of atropine.

Other problems which must be taken care of during the acute episode are to protect the patient from hypostatic pneumonia and other infections and to watch for impaired respiratory exchange with resulting cyanosis and respiratory acidosis due to failure of respiratory excretion of normal amounts of carbon dioxide. At times a Drinker respirator or other mechanical device for maintaining respiratory exchange may be lifesaving. If these complications are prevented, most patients experience a remission after a few weeks or months. Some recover completely. Others, as time goes on, relapse, and a slow general trend toward increasing severity of the disease may become apparent.

Mild cases may require no special medical attention except during relapse. In the slightly more severe case, neostigmine in oral doses of 15 mg every 2 or 3 hr, or multiples of this dose, as needed, is the most useful medication and may be quite effective. Over a period of months or years, the dosage may have to be increased progressively, and the cost becomes nearly prohibitive for some

families. The maximal effect of neostigmine given orally appears in half an hour and decreases rapidly after that time. If the patient becomes resistant to this medication, Mestinon bromide (60 mg is equivalent to 15 mg neostigmine) may be substituted, tablet for tablet. Mytelase chloride (5 to 7.5 mg is equivalent to 15 mg neostigmine) may also be tried, beginning always with a small dose of 5.0 mg every 2 hr and increasing to tolerance and to maximum therapeutic effect. All three of these drugs are available in syrup form (for tube feeding) and in delayed timespace tablets which have an effect for 3 to 12 hr.

Supplementing neostigmine with ephedrine (25 mg three times daily) and potassium salts (KCl, 25 per cent aqueous solution in doses of 4 to 6 cc t.i.d.) may be of therapeutic value in certain cases, particularly in relieving the weakness which occurs between doses of neostigmine. The possible usefulness of these agents must be investigated for each patient. Many anticholinesterase agents other than neostigmine have been investigated in an attempt to find an agent with more prolonged action and fewer side effects. Of these, pyridostigmine (Mestinon) is probably the best and does have a more prolonged period of activity. Ambenonium (Mysuran) is also said to be effective in some patients. The most severe and chronic forms of myasthenia gravis do not respond to any of these drugs, and the patient is forced to live a miserable existence in and out of a respirator. The mortality rate is high.

Variation in the intensity of the disease at different times makes evaluation of any type of management extremely difficult. This statement is nowhere better demonstrated than in attempting to assess the results of thymectomy and radiation of the thymus. Although a few dramatic and apparently permanent cures have been effected by these measures, particularly excision of the thymus, the majority of patients continue to have symptoms of myasthenia after thymectomy. Some proponents of the procedure believe that only early, chronically active but not too severe cases should be selected for operation. One authority has noted particularly beneficial effects of thymectomy in young women. However, it should be noted that these are the patients in whom spontaneous remissions are most frequent. The postoperative management of these patients is difficult (see books by Osserman and by Viets and Schwab if it is to be undertaken); it requires oxygen, a respirator, an aspirator, and excellent nursing. Parenterally administered neostigmine should be used in place of oral medication. Intravenous prostigmine (1 mg being equivalent to 15 mg of the oral dose) may be given during and after surgery in 1 liter of 5 per cent glucose and water or normal saline over a 4-hr period. The adequacy of treatment may be checked by the response to Tensilon. Because of the unpredictability of remissions, the relatively few examples of striking improvement, and the great danger to the patient, thymectomy cannot be recommended as a routine procedure.

EPISODIC MYASTHENIA OF OTHER TYPES

At least four different muscle syndromes of recurrent muscle weakness have now been identified. These are: (1) familial periodic paralysis, (2) hyperthyroidism with periodic paralysis; (3) congenital paramyotonia (von Eulenberg), and (4) hereditary periodic adynamia (Gamstorp). In each of these conditions the patient may develop over a period of a few hours a disorder of skeletal muscles which may vary from weakness to total paralysis and which subsides and disappears completely after a few hours or days. Differences between them are small, but the latter two appear to share, in some instances at least, a mild degree of restricted myotonia. The syndrome must be differentiated from cataplexy [always of seconds or a few minutes' duration, precipitated by strong emotion and conjoined with narcolepsy (see p. 326)], from syncope [the physical weakness is always combined with impairment of consciousness (see p. 305)], from hydrocephalic attacks with limb weakness [headache and signs of increased intracranial pressure (see p. 303)], and from "drop seizures," one of the varieties of epilepsy (see petit mal triad and myoclonus, p. 331).

Familial Periodic Paralysis

Clinical Pattern. Familial periodic paralysis is a very rare disorder which occurs in certain families, usually being inherited as a mendelian dominant trait. The clinical story is a striking one. The patients are normal except for well-demarcated episodes in which intense weakness or complete paralysis of limb and trunk muscles develops. The attacks begin in early life and may come at varying intervals throughout life, being more frequent in adolescence or early adult life.

A single attack may last from a few minutes to several days, the average duration being 12 to 48 hr. The attacks in many patients have a periodicity and duration characteristic for that individual or family. During the episode there is marked hypotonia of the affected muscles and hyperextensibility of the joints. The tendon reflexes are absent or greatly reduced but return to normal as strength and tone return. The muscles are refractory to electric stimulation. The facial, pharyngeal, thoracic, and diaphragmatic muscles are affected only in very severe cases, but respiratory embarrassment and death have been reported.

The attacks are precipitated by several factors, such as violent exercise or a large high carbohydrate meal. Many attacks occur during sleep or are present on awakening. Profuse diaphoresis may precede the attack. Usually no definite precipitating cause can be discovered.

In the average patient there is no evidence of progressive muscular disease, and physical examination of a patient between attacks frequently demonstrates no abnormality. Exceptionally some degree of weakness, usually mild, persists after the termination of the attack and is cumulative in successive attacks.

Pathogenesis. During the attack the *serum potassium level* drops sharply. This apparently results from the sudden passage of potassium into the cells of the body, because the urinary excretion of potassium falls at the same time. The intracellular potassium of muscle has been demonstrated to rise during attacks. The relation to excess carbohydrate intake has frequently been noticed; there· is a fall in serum potassium and rise in intracellular muscle and liver potassium during rapid glycogen storage. However, the timing of the two events is frequently not similar. The initial potassium changes are observed in all individuals during the first few hours after carbohydrate ingestion, while the paralysis in periodic paralysis is frequently delayed by 8 to 12 hr and is associated with a second series of changes in potassium levels. Thus the mechanism of the metabolic anomaly is not entirely clear. Biopsies of muscle taken during the attacks of paralysis reveal sarcoplasmic vacuolization.

Hyperthyroidism with Periodic Paralysis

(See Chap. 84)

Congenital Paramyotonia (von Eulenberg)

The principal feature of this disease is stiffness (myotonia), weakness, or paralysis which follows exposure to cold. At first only the myotonic features of this disease were described, and it was always regarded as a variant of congenital myotonia (Thomsen). Shy has called attention to the fact that in some cases there are also attacks of weakness similar to those of periodic paralysis. The latter need not be related to cold. It is of interest that serum potassium is reduced in attacks and that myotonia of the hands may persist in spite of the hypopotassemia.

The relationship between myotonia congenita, myotonica dystrophica, paramyotonia congenita, adynamia episodica hereditaria, and familial periodic paralysis is close but remains controversial.

Adynamia Episodica Hereditaria (Gamstorp)

This is a hereditary disease (mendelian dominant) characterized by periods of weakness or paralysis of skeletal muscle not unlike that described in familial periodic paralysis. The onset is between the ages of five and ten years. The attacks, which may last for one to many hours, tend to occur during rest after physical exertion, particularly if the patient is wet, cold, or hungry. Tingling of lips, fingers, and toes may occur at the onset of attacks. Weakness varies in degree. Respiratory embarrassment has not been noted. Between attacks the patient is symptom-free though in a few a mild weakness persists, as in the family of Tyler.

Serum potassium rises transiently during the attack, and in the electrocardiogram the T waves are high and peaked. Urinary potassium does not increase before or during attacks. Administration of 2 to 5 Gm of KCl induces an attack. Glucose tends to prevent this phenomenon.

Puberty is the worst age, and after this period the prognosis is good both for survival (no fatal cases) and effective work.

Hyperaldosteronism and Other Alterations of Potassium Metabolism

Another syndrome of potassium depletion recognized recently has been called primary *hyperaldosteronism, Conn's syndrome,* or potassium-losing nephritis. This disorder results in marked hypopotassemia, with episodes of paralysis similar to those of periodic paralysis. Tetany, polyuria, hypertension, and other manifestations not found in the hereditary cases are commonly present. Most of the patients appear to have adrenal tumors which secrete aldosterone and possibly other steroids. Care should be taken that these patients are not confused with those having familial periodic paralysis.

The same clinical picture may be observed in patients with other disorders when serum potassium is depleted, as in severe diarrhea or in overtreatment with deoxycorticosterone of a patient with Addison's disease, but the plasma potassium levels observed are usually lower than those found during attacks of periodic paralysis.

Extreme hyperpotassemia is also accompanied by muscular weakness or paralysis (see Chap. 26).

Treatment of Episodic Myasthenia. Episodes of familial periodic paralysis with hypopotassemia are treated by the oral administration of potassium salts in doses of 2 to 8 Gm until the attack is relieved. In the rare instance when acute respiratory or pharyngeal paralysis appears, it may be necessary to give potassium intravenously. Great care should be observed in its use, as it may be quite toxic if administered too rapidly. In the flaccid paralysis which results from adynamia episodica hereditaria with hyperpotassemia, potassium is contraindicated. Normal renal function, sufficient fluids to maintain a good urine volume, and slow

administration are the most important precautions which should be taken in giving potassium salts intravenously. In patients with periodic paralysis who have frequent episodes, attacks may be prevented by giving 4 to 8 Gm potassium chloride in divided doses per day by mouth.

REFERENCES

Grob, D.: Course and Management of Myasthenia Gravis, J.A.M.A., 153:529, 1953.
——— and A. McG. Harvey: Abnormalities in Neuromuscular Transmission, with Special Reference to Myasthenia Gravis, Am. J. Med., 15:695, 1953.
Osserman, K. E.: "Myasthenia Gravis," New York, Grune & Stratton, Inc., 1958.
Talbott, John H.: Periodic Paralysis: A Clinical Syndrome, Medicine, 20:85, 1941.
Viets, Henry R.: Myasthenia Gravis, New Engl. J. Med., 251:97, 141, 1954.
Viets, H., and R. S. Schwab: "Myasthenia Gravis," Grune & Stratton, Inc., 1958.

87 OTHER MAJOR MUSCLE SYNDROMES

Frank H. Tyler and Raymond D. Adams

These are the other syndromes by which diseases of muscle declare themselves clinically.

CONGENITAL DISEASES OF MUSCLE WITH STIFFNESS

In some of the primary diseases of muscle (in contrast to the neurologic diseases attended by spasticity and rigidity) passive movement may evoke no abnormality even though myotonia is present and hampers strong voluntary movements. If the myotonia is diffuse and lifelong, and if there is a family history of similar disease and no evidence of muscle wasting, the diagnosis of congenital myotonia or Thomsen's disease is the only likely possibility. On the other hand, if the stiffness and slowness of movement are acquired during childhood or adult life, are diffuse in distribution, and are not accompanied by reflex changes, or evidence of myotonia, three conditions suggest themselves—hypothyroidism, some form of congenital myopathy, and the "stiff-man syndrome." Hypothyroidism, McArdle's syndrome, and central core disease of Shy et al. have already been discussed. The stiff-man syndrome is a rare condition seen in only a few adults by Henry Woltman and others, and its cause has not been established. It may be attended by violent and painful spasms, sometimes localized to one muscle group but more often diffuse. Over a period of years, it progresses to involve all the skeletal muscles to the point where the patient is completely disabled. Spasms of pain, general stiffness, and slowness of movement, particularly in the legs may occasionally be observed in patients with osteoporosis and osteomalacia. The symptoms may improve on vitamin D therapy (see Chap. 80).

Tetanus and tetany, discussed in Chaps. 143 and 26, need only be mentioned in passing. In tetanus the spasm is of acute onset, beginning some days after a wound, may be generalized or localized, is increased by muscular activity and excitement, and lasts for several weeks to months. It is superimposed on a background of muscle stiffness especially in the masseter (trismus) and trunk muscles. In tetany the spasms are always intermittent and are localized principally in the hands and feet, viz., carpopedal spasms. They are accompanied by prickling and tingling, positive Chvostek's and Trousseau's signs, and a characteristic electromyogram change (see Chap. 26). Extreme spasm localized mainly to the trunk muscles which assume boardlike rigidity may arise as the consequence of the bite of the black widow spider. Several of the newer phenothiazine compounds acting on the brain may also produce an acute rigidity of muscles but usually with attendant tremors of the jaw and limbs, dystonic postures, weakness of muscles, and sometimes syncope or confusion, in various combinations. These latter phenomena should permit easy distinction from myotonia, tetanus, and tetany.

Congenital Myotonia (Thomsen's Disease)

Definition. This is a hereditary disease in which a difficulty in initiating movement is combined with slowness of relaxation. Originally described by Julius Thomsen who suffered from the disease himself, later descriptions by Strumpell, Erb, and Westphal served to establish its nosologic position as a lifelong, familial disease. Erb provided the first description of its pathology and called attention to two additional unique features, muscular excitability and hypertrophy.

Clinical Manifestations. The disease begins in the first years of life (usually by the age of six to eight years) and persists throughout its span. The disorder appears to be transmitted as an autosomal dominant trait. However, the patient frequently fails to give a family history, and myotonia may be difficult to demonstrate clinically in some individuals who nonetheless have typical electrical myotonia. It may be present in a milder subclinical degree early in life and interfere with learning to stand and walk. However its chief feature, myotonia, is seldom demonstrable before mid-child-

hood, and it becomes more intense at adolescence (in myotonia dystrophica, myotonia usually has a later onset). Muscular hypertrophy may also be noted during the early years of life. The typical slowness of contraction and persistence of contraction upon attempted relaxation is best provoked by strong voluntary movements after a period of inactivity, but it may be induced by electrical stimulation or by percussion. It is most prominent in the legs where the first movements of walking or running after a period of rest are slow and stiff. It is also present in the hands and arms and even the face and eye muscles. With repetition of the contraction, the movement characteristically becomes more facile and rapid and relaxation more prompt, until both are normal. Clinically this slowness of relaxation is most easily demonstrated in the forearm and hand muscles and in the orbicularis oculi during voluntary effort. Percussion myotonia, which may be evoked in any of these muscles and in the tongue, consists of a persistent contraction, for half a minute or more, of a segment of a muscle which has been tapped. Myotonia does not accompany the tendon reflex, but it may alter the abdominal and cremasteric reflexes. The muscles being repeatedly involved in these strong contractions are hypertrophied, though Patterson and Maas call attention to the development of a mild dystrophic change in some cases. Cataract, temporal baldness, testicular atrophy, and muscle weakness and wasting do not occur in Thomsen's disease. When present, they always signify myotonic dystrophy.

Laboratory Data. The only metabolic abnormality is a mild creatine intolerance and increased urinary excretion in some patients. The electromyogram is characteristic (see Chap. 56) in that upon voluntarily arresting muscle contraction there is a persistence of action potentials for several seconds. The biopsy of muscle reveals little or nothing of interest except large fibers with occasional rows or central displacement of sarcolemmal nuclei.

Treatment. Quinine sulfate 0.3 to 0.6 Gm three times daily reduces or relieves the myotonia, but often patients dislike it because of side effects (tinnitus, etc.). Procaine amide in doses of 250 to 500 mg orally three times daily is said to be superior to quinine.

Prognosis. The disease remains unchanged throughout the patient's life. The later development of dystrophy must be exceptional.

Paramyotonia Congenita (von Eulenberg)

This rare disease, already discussed as occasionally presenting as an episodic weakness, is one in which slowness and stiffness of movement are most clearly evoked by cold. The myotonia tends to be rather mild and is often restricted to the hands and tongue or facial muscles (eyelids). The aforementioned episodes of weakness may also be induced by cold but may occur spontaneously. The myotonia is seldom of sufficient intensity to require treatment.

Debré-Semelaigne and Hoffmann Syndromes in Hypothyroidism

These conditions were described in Chap. 84 on myopathy due to thyroid disease. The principal findings are relatively large muscles and slowness of movement. Myotonia and paramyotonia do not occur. The diagnosis of this muscular disorder usually offers no difficulty, for the other symptoms of deficient thyroid function (cretinism and myxedema) are fairly obvious, as a rule. The delayed tendon reflex, found in no other disease, is a useful clinical test.

Muscle Cramps

Everyone has experienced muscle cramps. They are common in the feet and legs especially at night when the limbs are cool, particularly after there has been some unusual exertion during the day. A strong movement tends to initiate the cramp; the muscle becomes hard and painful, and relief can be obtained only by massaging and stretching of the offending muscle. The electromyogram shows a continuous burst of action potentials of abnormally high frequency and voltage. Patients may also use the word cramp to describe other sensations, pains usually, but without spasm. A few questions in these instances should enable the examiner to ascertain that reference is being made to a different order of phenomena, a dysesthesia.

The most common variety of pathologic cramping is that which occurs during physical activity, e.g., in the legs while walking, so-called intermittent claudication, and it indicates a serious impairment of circulation in the extremity. It contrasts to cramps at rest which have not this meaning at all. A severe, persistent tendency to cramp in many of the muscles of the body may appear in the following conditions: (1) salt loss from excessive sweating or diarrhea, e.g., cholera; (2) tetany from whatever cause; (3) motor system diseases; (4) *a benign generalized cramp syndrome* in which painful spasms and fasciculations, both of obscure origin, are the only manifestations. The underlying pathophysiology of all varieties of cramp is hyperexcitability of the motor nerve fiber or the membrane of the muscle fiber. Typical of both levels of disorder is enhancement by ischemia. The treatment is to correct any existing alteration of electrolytes such as sodium chloride depletion from excess sweating. In the benign cramping syndrome, quinine sulfate 0.3 to 0.6 Gm t.i.d. by mouth has been beneficial in some cases, and procaine amide orally in a dose of 0.5 Gm one to three times a day has recently been introduced as a therapeutic agent.

MYALGIC STATES

Diffuse muscle pain, which merges with malaise, is a frequent expression of a large variety of systemic infections, e.g., influenza, brucellosis, dengue, Colorado tick fever, glanders, measles, malaria, relapsing fever, rheumatic fever (cf. growing pains), salmonellosis, toxoplasmosis, trichinosis, tularemia, and Weil's disease. When remarkably intense and especially if localized to one group of muscles, the most likely diagnostic possibility is epidemic myalgia (also designated as pleurodynia, devil's grip, painful neck, and Bornholm disease). Poliomyelitis also may be accompanied by intense pain at the onset of neurologic involvements, and later the paralyzed muscles may ache. Herpes zoster is another well-known cause of segmental pain. Nothing is known of the pathologic basis for the pains of either pleurodynia or poliomyelitis. The muscle tissue has been little studied by pathologists, and random biopsies have proved to be relatively uninformative.

Fibromyositis and myogelosis (see Chap. 300). One would suppose that by definition fibrositis or fibromyositis would represent an inflammation of the fibrous tissues of the muscles, fascia, aponeuroses, and probably nerves as well. Unfortunately, the pathologic changes remain obscure. Only the clinical facts are at hand: a muscle or group of muscles become painful and tender after exposure to cold, dampness, minor trauma, or for no reason that can be discerned. The neck and shoulders are the common sites. Firm, tender zones, sometimes several centimeters in diameter, are found within the muscles, and palpation and active contraction or passive stretching of them increases the pain— points of diagnostic value. In Europe, following the descriptions by Lange and Schade in 1921, the term "myogelosis" was applied to this condition, but it has never gained popularity in the United States. Usually the condition clears up in a few days, and local heat and massage are found to give comfort while symptoms are present. The condition is a "favorite" with physiotherapists and osteopaths who believe their maneuvers and adjustments to be helpful, as indeed they may. Rarely a similar syndrome is but the forerunner of what proves after some days, with the onset of neurologic signs, to be a radiculitis, brachial neuritis, or an outbreak of herpes zoster.

Diffuse muscular soreness and aching may at times be the initial symptoms in rheumatoid arthritis, preceding the signs of joint involvement by a period of weeks or months. The muscles are tender, but since this may be found in individuals, particularly otherwise normal individuals, particularly women, it is difficult to interpret. An increased sedimentation rate, a positive latex-fixation test, or other of the laboratory aids listed in Chap. 300 may clarify the diagnosis. Muscle biopsy may reveal a nonspecific interstitial nodular myositis. Occasionally a localized weakness of muscle, a slightly reduced tendon reflex, or a zone of impaired cutaneous sensation within the territory of a nerve will indicate the existence of a disease of the peripheral nervous system—an interstitial polyneuritis—which can sometimes be confirmed by the finding of infiltrates of lymphocytes, mononuclear leukocytes, and plasma cells in a nerve or muscle biopsy.

In thin, asthenic adults who exhibit this rather ambiguous symptomatology without other abnormalities, the authors have found it difficult to exclude hysteria or other psychoneurosis or depression. In every such individual it is well to search for evidence of rheumatic state and brucellosis as well as the metabolic myopathy which accompanies hyperparathyroidism and renal tubular acidosis, hypoglycemia, the intrinsic phosphorylase defect (McArdle's syndrome), and myoglobinuria before calling for a psychiatric consultant. Patients with these latter diseases often complain of soreness, stiffness, and lameness after any strenuous muscular effort.

The treatment for each of these conditions will be found in the appropriate section of the book.

LOCALIZED MUSCLE MASSES

This may happen in a variety of clinical settings, and the clinical findings in each one have a different significance.

Muscle rupture giving rise to a large bulge upon contraction is usually caused by a violent strain attended by an audible snap and then a bulge which appears when the muscle contracts. A weakening in contractile power and mild discomfort are usually noted by the patient. The biceps muscle is the one most often affected. Treatment is immediate surgical repair; if delayed, little can be done for the condition.

Hemorrhage into muscle may occur as a consequence of trauma, as a complication of the use of anticoagulants, in hematologic diseases, or after a minor trauma in a patient with Zenker's degeneration who is convalescing from typhoid fever or other infection.

Tumors include desmoid tumor (a benign massive growth of fibrous tissue in parturient women and after surgery), *rhabdomyosarcoma* (a highly malignant tumor with strong liability to local recurrence and metastasis), and *angioma.*

Thrombosis of arteries or, more often, of veins cause congestion and infarction of muscle.

Myositis ossificans refers to the deposit of bone within the substance of a muscle. Two types are recognized. One is a localized form which appears in a single muscle or group of muscles after trauma, and the other is a progressive, widespread ossifying process in many muscles of the body and entirely unrelated to trauma. In the localized traumatic form, after a single traumatic blow or the tear of a muscle or repeated minor trauma, a painful area, probably a herniation, develops in the muscles. It is gradually replaced by masses of solid cartilaginous consistency, and within 4 to 7 weeks' time a solid mass of bone can be felt and becomes visible in the x-ray. As would be expected, this most frequently happens in vigorous adult men, and the pectoralis major, biceps, brachii, or thigh muscles of militiamen, cavalrymen, and athletes are the usual sites of the abnormality. Symptoms tend to subside if the patient desists from the activity which produced the mass.

Generalized myositis ossificans is a disease of unknown origin and consists of bone formation within muscles of children or adolescents. Only this latter disease need be discussed in any further detail here.

Pathology. The first stage is believed to be as an interstitial myositis or fibrositis. Biopsies of early indurated swellings have revealed extensive proliferation of interstitial connective tissue in which little inflammatory cell reaction is found. The adjacent muscle fibers become compressed by the connective tissue which retracts and calcifies. Osteoid and cartilage formation occur at a later stage, developing in the connective tissue and enclosing intact muscle fibers.

Clinical Manifestations. Nearly 75 per cent of all reported cases have had congenital anomalies, the most frequent of which is a failure of development of the great toes or thumbs and less often other digits. The first symptom is often a firm swelling in a vertebral or cervical muscle. There is, in addition, a mild tenderness and a discomfort during muscle contraction, and the overlying skin may be reddened and slightly swollen. A trauma may have been recalled as the initiating factor, but as the months pass other muscles not injured in any recognizable way become similarly involved. At first x-rays reveal no important changes, but within 6 to 12 months calcium deposits are observed and one can feel stony-hard masses within the muscle. As the disease advances, limitation of movement, contractures, and deformities become increasingly evident, and occasionally the patient is converted into a virtual "stone man." Scoliosis, rigidity of spine, abnormal postures, and limited expansion of the thorax may ultimately occur.

Diagnosis. The principal problem in diagnosis is to differentiate this condition from calcinosis universalis, which usually occurs in relationship to scleroderma or polymyositis. It is not clear whether a sharp dividing line can be drawn between the two conditions. In calcinosis universalis there is said to be calcinosis (calcium deposit) in the skin, subcutaneous tissues, and connective tissue sheaths around the muscles, whereas in myositis ossificans there is bone formation within the muscles. Probably the pathologic data are too meager to justify this distinction at present. Vitamin D calcinosis, resulting from the prolonged ingestion of large doses of vitamin D, may also produce widespread deposition of masses of calcium around muscles, joints, and subcutaneous tissue.

Prognosis. The disease may undergo spontaneous remissions and exacerbations and may halt at a point where the patient is capable of adequate function, remaining in this state for years. If death is to occur, it is related to the enfeebled, debilitated, malnourished condition of the patient, the final illness often being a terminal pneumonia or other intercurrent infection.

Treatment. No medical treatment is of proved value. Excision of bony deposits may be undertaken if it is certain that they are causing particular trouble. Some of the calcium deposits in calcinosis universalis have disappeared under cortisone therapy, and because of the unclear relationship of this disease to generalized myositis ossificans, it is probably advisable to try this form of therapy, using the same plan as that described in the chapter on diseases of connective tissue (Chap. 300).

REFERENCES

Adams, R. D., D. Denny-Brown, and C. Pearson: "Diseases of Muscle," 2d ed., New York, Paul B. Hoeber, Inc., Medical Department of Harper & Brothers, 1962.

Adams, R. D., L. M. Eaton, G. M. Shy: Neuromuscular Disorders, Res. Pub. Assoc. for Research in Nervous and Mental Dis., vol. 38, Baltimore, Williams & Wilkins Co., 1961.

Section 5: Errors of Metabolism

INTRODUCTION

W. Eugene Knox

The errors of metabolism constitute a very large group of individually rare hereditary conditions, each distinguished by some striking biochemical departure from the usual. Far from being curiosities of no general importance, these conditions provided the conceptual schemes which linked the sciences of genetics and biochemistry to each other and to the science of medicine. The central idea emerged in 1902 in a paper by Sir Archibald Garrod entitled "The Incidence of Alkaptonuria, A Study in Chemical Individuality." To alkaptonuria he later added cystinuria, albinism, and pentosuria, calling them "inborn errors of metabolism." He realized that these conditions, biochemical peculiarities "which advertised their presence in some conspicuous way," were only prototypes of a potentially large number of differences between individuals of greater or less significance:

If it be, indeed, the case that in alkaptonuria and the other conditions mentioned, we are dealing with individuality in metabolism and not with the results of morbid processes, the thought naturally presents itself

that these are merely extreme examples of variations of chemical behavior which are probably everywhere present in minor degrees and that just as no two individuals of a species are ever absolutely identical in bodily structure neither are their chemical processes carried out on exactly the same lines. Such chemical differences will be obviously far more subtle than those of form, for whereas the latter are evident to any careful observer the former will only be revealed by elaborate chemical methods.

Since then, many further examples of the same kind of thing have been discovered, adding detail to Garrod's concept without altering his general principles.

The central idea of Garrod's concept was the relationship between gene, enzyme and disease. At a time when mendelian inheritance was not known in man, Garrod saw that the aggregation of cases of an inborn error of metabolism in particular families followed the law of recessive inheritance. At a time when the mysteries of metabolism were still unexplored, Garrod hypothesized that metabolism occurred in a series of chemical steps each catalyzed by a specific enzyme and with each enzyme produced by a specific genetic factor. The gene-determined inactivity of a single enzyme blocked that step in metabolism. Accumulation of the intermediate before the block, or deficiency of the intermediate coming after the block, produced the signs and symptoms of the associated disease. At a time when morbidity was being ascribed with great success to extraneous agents such as bacteria or poisons, Garrod perceived that morbid processes could also be inborn.

The idea of the relationship of gene, enzyme, and disease has flowered with time. The excretion of homogentisic acid in alkaptonuria and of L-xylulose in pentosuria and the signs and symptoms of these conditions can now be traced back to the gene-determined inactivity of the specific enzymes which normally metabolize these compounds. The same relationship in the form of the *one gene–one enzyme* hypothesis became the key for the study of intermediary metabolism in the lower forms of life by experimental genetics. The purview of Garrod's idea has also extended beyond the inborn abnormalities of intermediary metabolism. The cystine excretion of cystinuria results not from a block in metabolism, but from failure of a specific renal tubular reabsorption mechanism. Therefore genes play a role in the formation not only of the enzymes of metabolism but also of the specific enzyme-like transport systems. Still more recently it has been learned that genes determine the detailed structure of functional proteins such as the hemoglobins. There are still other subtle chemical differences among individuals such as the blood group antigens that are genetically determined. The present development of Garrod's concept envisages the primary equipment of the cell as a cadre of molecules, for the most part functional proteins, whose molecular structures and therefore functions are determined by the arrays of nucleotides of deoxyribonucleic acid in the genes. These molecules fashion the cell from its environment. The inborn structural variations of these molecules account for the inborn diversities in the biochemical make-up of human beings. When the physiologic consequences of a particular molecular alteration are sufficiently grave, the condition may appropriately be considered a hereditary molecular disease. The term "molecular disease," first introduced by Pauling to describe sickle-cell anemia, indicates both the modern chemical definition of the "error" first conceived by Garrod and our modern knowledge of the detailed pathologic consequences to the individual from such a molecular alteration.

The enduring fruitfulness of Garrod's concept results from the happy combination of its esthetic attractiveness and its wide applicability to biologic problems. The discrete alteration in a single type of functional molecule represents an experiment of nature whose subtlety has long captivated biologists. Through such errors we have gained insight about pathways and functions whose existence was unsuspected so long as they operated smoothly. The discovery of new examples of such errors has continued unabated since Garrod's time, and no decrease is to be expected. The possible number of such diseases is commensurate with the number of genes. All variant genes should produce variant molecules. Therefore, the molecular abnormalities are not restricted to the recessively inherited types that were first singled out. Individuals with abnormal genes inherited dominantly or recessively, and even individuals with one abnormal gene, the heterozygous carriers of a recessive gene, have a portion of abnormal molecules produced by that gene. Because heterozygous carriers of a gene for a rare recessive disease are so enormously more frequent than patients with the disease, it turns out that most individuals must possess some abnormal genes and some abnormal molecules.

The specifically medical interest in the inborn errors centers on the pathogenetic pathways by which a chemical abnormality of a molecule produces the signs and symptoms of disease. The pathologic consequences of the precise chemical disturbances in these conditions contributes fundamental information about disease mechanisms in general. Such information is equally applicable to the mechanisms of nonheritable diseases which share similar final common pathways. The inborn errors studied so far have inexorably produced certain pathologic consequences with little influence by ordinary environmental conditions. Now examples are being recognized in which the molecular abnormality does not lead inevitably to disease: environmental influences must interact in some essential way for a pathologic result. Such a hereditary abnormality that is a necessary but not sufficient cause for disease is the deficiency of glucose 6-phosphate dehydrogenase in red cells. In this condition the hemolytic anemia results only when there is exposure to certain substances like the fava bean. The participation of environmental influences in the pathogenesis of a disease promises to clarify the hereditary basis of many common diseases whose familial occurrence is too highly variable to be proved hereditary by simple mendelian expectations.

It is not to be anticipated that environmental influence can alter the primary defect either in a gene or in the functional molecule made by the gene. But the consequences of gene action are being continuously altered by environmental influences. Given knowledge of how a disease results from the fundamental chemical disturbance, the play of environment can often be altered by design to minimize or prevent the disease consequences which would otherwise result from an inborn error of metabolism.

88 DISORDERS OF AMINO ACID METABOLISM

W. Eugene Knox

ALKAPTONURIA

Definition. Alkaptonuria is the lifelong excretion in the urine of the strongly reducing compound, homogentisic acid (2,5-dihydroxyphenylacetic acid). Old or alkaline *urine turns dark,* and after middle life the darkened mesenchymal tissues (*ochronosis*) appear blue through the skin and *degenerative joint changes* occur.

History. The condition was named by Bödeker in 1859. He found in the urine of a patient with lumbar arthritis a substance which when alkalinized darkened the urine from the surface down and caused the urine to take up more than its own volume of oxygen: "I call it for this reason 'Alkapton' (admittedly a somewhat barbarous combination from the Greek participle of καπτεῖν, to suck up greedily, and the Arabic, *alkali*), after its outstanding behaviour toward oxygen in alkaline solution." Virchow in 1866 reported as a pathologic curiosity a patient with "arthritis deformans," the coal blackness of whose cartilages and tendons he called ochronosis. Albrecht in 1902 demonstrated the connection between ochronosis and alkaptonuria at the section of a patient with gray-blue ears "like dilated veins" and with residual bladder urine which darkened on standing. Sir William Osler (1904) was the first to diagnose ochronosis during life on the basis of the darkened scleras, ears, and nose of two alkaptonurics. He failed to connect the disabling arthritis in one of his patients with the alkaptonuria. This was done in 1913 by Umber on the basis of a family with five alkaptonurics, all five with arthritis.

Alkaptonuria was the prototype of the inborn errors of metabolism. It was the first of these diseases that Garrod studied, and the one to which he fitted the definition of the group.

Etiology. Alkaptonuria is inherited as a very rare autosomal recessive characteristic. The sexes are equally affected, but parents and offspring of a patient are usually unaffected. An average of one in four siblings is affected, and the parents are often related. The incidence is about 1 in 200,000 persons. The molecular basis is the complete hereditary inactivity of homogentisate oxidase which normally catalyzes a step in tyrosine metabolism. Approximately 4 Gm per day of homogentisic acid accumulates at this metabolic block to be rapidly excreted by the kidneys. The amount excreted can be decreased by a low protein diet (short of negative nitrogen balance) and increased by administration of extra protein or the amino acids, phenylala-

nine and tyrosine. At neutral pH or above, homogentisic acid is rapidly oxidized to the brown or black polymer which accounts for the darkening of the urine on standing and the staining of wetted linen. A slower accumulation in the body of a similar polymer bound to cartilages and related tissues produces the ochronosis and the degeneration of the stained structures seen by middle life.

Clinical Picture. Most patients have been found by an atypical positive test for reducing substances in the urine, raising the question of diabetes. More males than females are found because more males have urine tests. Less commonly the darkening of the urine leads to the diagnosis. Wet diapers turn black in hours. It is remarkable how often this phenomenon will go unnoticed throughout the life of an affected individual. The condition is completely benign until thirty or forty years of age when the degenerative joint changes begin in at least half the cases. The large joints and spine are affected with pain and stiffness, sometimes there are acute inflammatory episodes, and the process progresses in time to ankylosis. Degeneration of the intervertebral disks with subsequent calcification and vertebral osteophyte formation makes the spine appear radiologically like the ties and rails of a railroad track. The ochronosis can be seen in the transmitted blueness of cartilages of the ear, nose and costochondral junctions, and the superficial tendons, and brown areas in the scleras at the rectus insertions on both sides of the irides. The affected tissues when exposed present an arresting sight of coal blackness. Staining also occurs in the arterial intima, sclerotic plaques, and other elements of the cardiovascular system. Older patients often exhibit degenerative cardiovascular disease. The association may be one of chance.

Diagnosis. Chemical identification of homogentisic acid should be required even in the presence of the triad of arthritis, ochronosis, and darkening urine. Undarkened urine plus sodium hydroxide turns red brown, then blackens as it absorbs oxygen. The urine strongly reduces alkaline copper solutions, but since it turns black in the process the erroneous diagnosis of glucosuria can be avoided. It does not give a positive test with glucose oxidase test papers, nor does it reduce bismuth reagents for sugar (Nylander's test). Undeveloped photographic film exposed to the light will be immediately blackened by the urine just as it will be by the chemically similar hydroquinone developer. This is the clinical test of choice.

In carbolochronosis from the long-continued absorption of large amounts of phenol or its derivatives, the tissues are stained as in alkaptonuria, and the urine may be dark from hydroquinone formed metabolically. Acute phenol poisoning and rarely melanomas will also produce dark urines.

Treatment. A low but adequate protein diet for life should be instituted at an early age to avoid excessive homogentisate formation and possibly to delay the degenerative changes. "Wishful" treatments should be avoided, including insulin, liver extracts and cortisone, and ascorbic acid which merely keep homogentisate in the urine bleached.

CYSTINURIA

Definition. Cystinuria is the inborn and lifelong excretion in the urine of large amounts of the dibasic amino acids, cystine (about 1 Gm per day), lysine, arginine, and ornithine. It results from a hereditary defect in a specific reabsorptive process of the renal tubule. Recurrent cystine urinary calculi and their sequelae are the sole clinical manifestations.

History. The first amino acid available in relatively pure form was the cystine in the stones from cystinurics. The condition has been recognized by the stones or by the microscopic crystalluria since the early nineteenth century, but its critical definition dates from the medical thesis of Niemann in 1876. On the basis of 53 cases then known, he defined the disease, excluded age and environmental factors as causes, noted its familial occurrence, and suggested an arrest of cystine metabolism as the cause. Garrod's contribution, coming after the rediscovery of Mendel's laws of inheritance, was to recognize that most of the familial cases followed the pattern of recessive inheritance. The erroneous belief that intermediary cystine metabolism was defective persisted in the face of evidence to the contrary until recently. Then three other amino acids, previously unnoticed because of their high solubility in urine, were found to be excreted by cystinurics along with cystine. Dent and Harris thereupon promptly and completely explained the renal physiology and genetics of cystinuria.

Etiology. In two-thirds of the families so far studied, cystinuria was inherited as a recessive condition, with the parents of affected individuals having no abnormality of amino acid excretion. In the remaining third of the families the condition was incompletely recessive, with the heterozygous carriers of one abnormal gene showing raised excretions of cystine and lysine. The amount of cystine excreted is almost always less than 250 mg per Gm creatinine. Above this amount stone formation may occur. These heterozygotes account for the high incidence (1 in 250) of chemically detectable cystinuria without stones which is found in the population. Matings between the two types are needed to determine if the two kinds of genes are allelic.

The four amino acids excreted in cystinuria have two basic groups separated by four or five carbon atoms. Possibly this is the structural basis for their reaction with a single transport system that has an enzyme-like specificity. Because of the inactivity of this specific transport system in a cystinuric, the renal clearances of these amino acids closely approach the glomerular filtration rate. In the normal or heterozygous person an administered load of one of these amino acids will competitively inhibit the reabsorption of the others. The blood levels of the four amino acids are low in cystinuria rather than elevated as would be expected from a blocked metabolism with an overflow type of excretion.

The amount of cystine excreted depends directly upon its blood level. Methionine, and not cystine itself, is the component of dietary protein which elevates the blood cystine level and so increases cystine excretion. The amount excreted is usually 0.4 to 1.2 Gm per day or 0.3 to 0.8 mg per min, and this amount is primarily determined by body size and diet. The solubility of cystine in urine at body temperature is less than 0.4 mg per ml through the readily attainable range of urine pH. A urine flow above 2 ml per min (3 liters per day) may therefore be needed throughout the 24 hr to carry in solution the cystine which will be excreted. The decreased urine flow in the early morning hours is often responsible for the supersaturation of cystine, its crystallization, and the accretion into calculi unless washed away by the daytime diuresis. First stones appear randomly at all ages among cystinurics when this precarious equilibrium fails, as it eventually does in nearly all untreated cystinurics. Recurrent calculi and progressive renal damage then usually occur.

Diagnosis. The only clinical manifestations are those referable to recurrent urinary calculi of the kidney, ureters, bladder, or urethra, or to the passing of gravel. These are not clinically distinguishable from other urologic conditions of this type. With infection, the urine may develop a particularly foul odor from the decomposition of ornithine and lysine to putrescine and cadavarine. Because of the high atomic number of sulfur, the cystine stones are radiologically dense, more so than urate and comparable to the density of calcium oxalate. Because effective treatment is possible, every effort should be made to identify the 1 per cent of urinary calculi that are cystine, and when possible to diagnose the condition before calculi appear.

The microscopic appearance of cystine crystals in the sediment of the first morning urine is a sufficiently sensitive test to detect cystinuria, especially if combined with a urine concentration test and if the urine plus glacial acetic acid to pH 4.5 is chilled for a few hours before centrifuging. The crystals are hexagonal plates resembling the formula of a benzene ring. Crystalluria is nearly restricted to those cystinurics excreting more than 250 mg cystine per day who may develop stones and who occur with an incidence of perhaps 1 in 50,000 persons.

The nitroprusside tests for cystine in urine will detect the cystinurics and also the very much more frequent heterozygotes of the incompletely recessive form (1 in 250 persons). It will also detect some rarer conditions in which cystine excretion is part of a general aminoaciduria. Urinary cystine must first be reduced to cysteine with sodium cyanide to give this test.

The specific aminoaciduria consisting of the excretion of cystine, lysine, arginine, and ornithine in comparable amounts is diagnostic. The specific pattern can be demonstrated with paper chromatography. It distinguishes cystinuria from all other diseases, including cystinosis.

Treatment. Medical treatment can prevent formation and growth of stones. Over a long period it can sometimes also bring about stone dissolution, but usually the accepted urologic procedures for dealing with calculi should be followed. The progressive renal insufficiency that follows recurrent episodes of calculi complicates the medical treatment even while it produces a more dilute urine that diminishes the cystine precipitation.

The basis of the medical treatment is the quantitative estimation of the 24-hr cystine excretion. From this and the known solubility of cystine in urine, an adequate urine flow to carry the excreted cystine in soluble form can be calculated. The flow must be maintained throughout the 24 hr by nocturnal fluids. The total amount of cystine excreted can be minimized by a diet low in methionine, obtained by replacing animal protein with vegetable protein. The diet must be chosen for its long-term adequacy for the patient. The efficiency of the regimen is monitored by periodic checks to determine that cystine saturation is not exceeded in either the day or night urines. Occasionally it may be necessary to use in addition the small increase in cystine solubility obtainable by alkalinizing the urine.

CYSTINOSIS AND THE FANCONI SYNDROME

Definition. Two groups of cases will be distinguished from the tubular nephropathies that share some or all of the features of generalized aminoaciduria, renal glucosuria, hypophosphatemia, chronic acidosis, and defective mineralization of bone matrix (resistant rickets or osteomalacia). These are the features of the "adult Fanconi syndrome." Cystinosis is seen in infants and children. They have in addition cystine crystals deposited throughout most tissues.

History. In 1903 Abderhalden described the finding at autopsy of crystalline cystine deposits in the tissues of a twenty-one-month-old infant dead of "inanition." He called the disease *familial cystine diathesis* since two siblings died in a similar way, and moderate excretion of cystine occurred in adult members of the family. The next child, described in 1924 by Lignac-Leider, was unique in having in addition cystine urinary calculi. Nevertheless, there is no justification for confusing the condition with the quite different disease of cystinuria. Later cases in adults and children were described from different points of view under a variety of eponyms such as the Fanconi-Lignac-Debré–de Toni syndrome to refer to various combinations of signs. Central to all these is the renal tubular disorder.

Etiology. Cystinosis and adult Fanconi syndrome appear to be genetically distinct entities transmitted as recessive characters. In families with one of these conditions, it would be unusual to find the other (or cystinuria).

In both conditions there is a shortened and narrowed "swan-neck" deformity of the proximal renal tubule. This has been demonstrated by microdissection. It is probable that the morphologic and functional defects are related, since most of the findings can be attributed to failure of many reabsorptive and other functions of the (proximal) renal tubule. There is absence of alkaline phosphatase in the proximal tubule, probably a secondary effect of the disease.

Glucose reabsorption is certainly a proximal tubule function, and possibly so are the reabsorptions of amino acids, phosphate, bicarbonate, and potassium. Glucosuria, scant and intermittent or profuse and constant, occurs with a normal blood sugar level. The carbohydrate wastage is extreme enough to produce ketosis in about one-fourth of the patients. This may contribute to the acidosis. The generalized aminoaciduria occurs without an increased blood level of α-amino nitrogen. The pattern of amino acids excreted resembles that of plasma. The aminoaciduria is innocuous, amounting perhaps to a loss of as much as one-tenth of the dietary protein in the urine. This loss may contribute to the dwarfism and body wastage and may participate in calcium excretion by chelation. The phosphaturia produces hypophosphatemia and together with the acidosis results in osteomalacia. The loss of phosphate from bone counteracts acidosis because dissolution of bone converts $PO_4{}^{3-}$ to $HPO_4{}^=$ and so buffers one hydrogen ion. Low bicarbonate resorption results in bicarbonate excretion at a lower urine pH than normally and in depletion of body alkali stores. It also contributes to the defect in urinary acidification. Thus bicarbonate loss also contributes to the acidosis and to the hyperchloremia. The potassium wastage results in hypopotassemia and sometimes causes profound muscular weakness or paralysis. Potassium depletion may in turn produce renal tubular damage by positive feedback, resulting in polyuria and inability to concentrate urine and inability to excrete urine more acid than pH 6 to 7 despite the severe acidosis. Potassium depletion can by itself cause the vacuolation of proximal tubule cells seen in this condition and can predispose to the development of renal infection. Thus the proximal tubular anomaly can be considered to initiate a self-maintained renal injury with widespread metabolic consequences. The condition often produces glomerular damage with hyalinization, often pyelonephritis, and eventual death with hypertension and uremia.

Clinical Picture. In addition to the distinction between young and adult cases, each individual patient differs considerably from others in the particular combination and severity of his pathologic changes. In the adult Fanconi cases, at least, the renal tubular dysfunction precedes the development of the usual presenting complaints caused by osteomalacia. The typical urinary abnormalities have been found in relatives without bone disease who were followed until bone changes did develop. Such individuals also have hypophosphatemia and mild acidosis. Over a period of years, rheumatic type pains develop which restrict movement until the patient is bedridden. Severe osteomalacia is seen radiologically with its characteristic pseudofractures. These are bilateral, symmetrical lines of decalcification whose location can be predicted since they occur adjacent to the course of blood vessels curving round the bones.

The condition seen in children is more fulminating. Failure to thrive and severe resistant rickets with dwarfing develop in the first few months of life. In children death usually occurs by ten years of age, although treated cases have survived as long as 35 years. The intracellular deposition of considerable amounts of cystine (about 0.5 Gm per Gm tissue nitrogen) in most tissues (not only in the reticuloendothelial system) is a unique and puzzling feature in the young cases. An altered active transport of cystine and possibly of other amino acids into cells might be suggested, but such a mechanism cannot now be related to the renal abnormality which determines the main clinical features. The presence of these crystalline rods or plates in the cornea and conjunctivas demonstrable by a slit lamp is of diagnostic importance.

Usually there is no difficulty in assigning a patient to this general group, but classification within the group is seldom satisfactory because of the variations between patients and in the same patient at different stages of the disease. A closely related group of patients with renal tubular acidosis shares many of the defects of the Fanconi syndrome, including low reabsorption of bicarbonate. However, formation of renal calculi, nephrocalcinosis, and absence of aminoaciduria distinguish renal tubular acidosis from the Fanconi syndrome. The differential diagnosis may consider diabetes or even diabetic acidosis on the basis of the urine findings, but the normal blood glucose should prevent this error.

Treatment. Because patients vary widely in the severity of the several defects making up this syndrome, they will also vary in their response to the several therapeutic procedures available. These are merely replacement therapies and are not curative: alkali therapy with Shohl's solution (98 Gm sodium citrate and 140 Gm citric acid per liter) to correct acidosis when present; 50,000 to 400,000 units of vitamin D daily to improve the calcium balance by decreasing the fecal loss without expectation of reducing the urinary loss; supplementary neutral phosphate to improve the phosphate balance despite a continued or even increased urinary loss; correction of hypopotassemia, especially before any glucose tolerance tests which may precipitate a "dextrose shock" by further reduction of the serum potassium to a critical value. Potassium and calcium supplements should be given only when indicated by plasma measurements; otherwise the basic regimen should be continued indefinitely. Great symptomatic improvement is possible, but the treatment does not prevent the slow progression of renal impairment with ultimate glomerular failure and uremia. Because of this and the increased susceptibility of potassium deficient subjects to renal infection, urinary tract infections should be carefully sought and specifically treated.

PHENYLKETONURIA (Phenylpyruvic Oligophrenia)

Definition. Phenylketonuria is a recessively inherited failure to oxidize phenylalanine to tyrosine, characterized by the excretion of phenylpyruvic acid, mental deficiency, epileptic seizures, and mild pigmentation.

History. Følling in 1934 described 10 mentally deficient patients whose urine contained phenylpyruvic acid, identified by the blue-green color produced with $FeCl_3$. Surveys in the Western world based on this urine test revealed that about 0.7 per cent of the inmates in institutions for the mentally defective were so affected. Jervis proved that phenylketonuria was inherited through a single autosomal recessive gene. He also located the metabolic error by demonstrating a very large accumulation of phenylalanine in the body fluids and the absence of the normal rise in plasma tyrosine following a dose of phenylalanine. In 1953 Jervis demonstrated the inactivity of phenylalanine hydroxylase of the liver in these patients, thus completing for the first time a proof of the relationships between gene, enzyme, and disease postulated for the inborn errors of metabolism by Garrod.

Etiology. The parents of a phenylketonuric child each have one defective gene for phenylalanine hydroxylase, manifesting itself in a slightly reduced capacity to oxidize phenylalanine, but without any mental or clinical abnormalities. On the average, one in four children of such a union receive two defective genes and so have no active phenylalanine hydroxylase. This enzyme is restricted to liver, where it appears during the first few weeks after birth. The failure of active enzyme to appear in the phenylketonuric infant results in the gradual accumulation of phenylalanine from the diet to as much as thirty times the normal blood level after several weeks. It then overflows via transamination into the rapidly excreted phenylpyruvate. Several other related metabolites are also excreted in abnormal amounts. Among these phenylalanine and o-hydroxyphenylacetic acid may have diagnostic usefulness.

After six months of age, mental development is retarded, and seizures and other neurologic abnormalities suggesting extrapyramidal disease appear. Since the mental defect is stationary and not progressive in older children or adults, the brain injury appears to be limited to a particularly sensitive stage in brain development. Delayed myelination has been found at autopsy in the youngest children, but there are no other neuropathologic findings to account for the mental disease.

The mild pigmentation of hair, eyes, and skin results from the competitive inhibition by phenylalanine of the melanin formation by tyrosinase. Eczema has been commonly described, but it is not a specific sign.

Diagnosis. Chemical diagnosis is essential for successful treatment, since the neurologic abnormalities once established are largely irreversible. The FeCl₃ urine test is remarkably effective after one month of age: several drops of 5 per cent FeCl₃ in 5 ml of fresh urine produces first some precipitation of phosphates, then with several more drops a blue- or olive-green color slowly appears within 2 min and fades after 1 or 2 hr. Paper strips for the test are available. Confirmation is obtained by formation of a yellow precipitate on addition to the urine of a few drops of saturated 2,4-dinitrophenylhydrazine in 2 N HCl. Diagnosis before one month of age must depend upon the grossly elevated level of plasma phenylalanine, as should the final corroboration of the diagnosis before treatment is started.

Treatment. The biochemical abnormalities can be corrected by preventing the accumulation of phenylalanine. This is done by a special diet in which protein is replaced by an amino acid mixture low in phenylalanine (Ketonil, Merck; Lofenolac, Mead Johnson). Supplementary foods are given to supply only the amount of L-phenylalanine needed for body growth. An infant requires at least three times as much per kilogram body weight as an older child. Normal weight gain and near normal plasma phenylalanine levels should be maintained. Treatment should continue at least until four years of age. Normal development has been obtained in some patients treated from early infancy. Little permanent improvement can be achieved by treatment begun after the age of three years.

OTHER CONDITIONS

Albinism. The virtual absence of melanin pigment from skin, hair, and eyes is recessively inherited. The sole consequence is sensitivity to light: the skin sunburns easily and the pink-appearing eyes are affected with photophobia and nystagmus. The melanocytes, which are normally recognized by their pigment in mitochondria-like organelles, have not certainly been identified in human albino tissues. They are present as "clear" cells in the skin of certain albino mice. The known occurrence of (amelanotic) melanomas in two human albinos suggests that melanocytes are present and that the albino defect is subcellular. Possibly an enzyme is missing. The tyrosinase system which oxidizes tyrosine through dopa to melanin can normally be detected histochemically by the dopa oxidase reaction, but it is inactive in human albino skin. A sex-linked form of ocular albinism is also known in which the pigment defect is limited to the eye structures. Other localized absences of pigment occur commonly, often dominantly inherited as "white streaks," or as part of more serious congenital anomalies.

Argininosuccinic Aciduria. This ninhydrin-positive amino acid intermediate of the urea cycle was excreted in large amounts (1 to 2 Gm per day) by two siblings who were both seriously mentally retarded. Other siblings and the parents were normal. Presumably the condition represents a new inborn error of metabolism. Systemic urea formation was not abnormal as would be expected if the "splitting enzyme" normally acting on argininosuccinate was lacking in the liver. Some particular defect in the central nervous system is suggested by the fact that two to three times as much argininosuccinic acid has been noted in the cerebrospinal fluid as in the blood.

Hartnup Disease. This condition, also called *H disease,* was first detected in four of eight children from a first-cousin marriage. At least 13 cases are now known. It is characterized by intermittent attacks of a red, scaly pellagra-like rash appearing after exposure to sunlight, attacks of cerebellar ataxia, and occasionally psychiatric changes ranging from emotional instability to delirium. There is a massive aminoaciduria, renal in origin, with at least 12 amino acids excreted in a characteristic pattern. For example, the four amino acids excreted in cystinuria and the proline excreted in generalized aminoacidurias such as Fanconi syndrome are not abnormally excreted in Hartnup disease. There is also excretion of large amounts of indican and other indole derivatives formed from tryptophan by bacteria in the gut. It is possible that a specific active transport system for certain amino acids into cells is defective. In consequence renal reabsorption fails and produces the aminoaciduria, slowed intestinal absorption occurs and permits the bacterial action on tryptophan, and diversion of tryptophan from its normal route of degradation to nicotinic acid results in niacin deficiency. Oral doses of nicotinamide have markedly improved the pellagra-like dermatitis and the neurologic signs. A high protein diet is also recommended to offset the urinary amino acid loss.

Maple Syrup Urine Disease. Several familial cases of a disease uniformly fatal in the first years of life have been observed characterized by the onset of central nervous system symptoms soon after birth (muscular hypertonicity, poor feeding, vomiting, and mental retardation) and intermittently by the odor of maple syrup to the urine. The disease is analogous to phenylketonuria: there is an accumulation of ten times the normal plasma levels of methionine and the branched amino acids leucine, isoleucine, and valine; an overflow type of excretion of these amino acids in the urine; and the urinary excretion of α-keto acids, mainly those derived from isoleucine and leucine. Identification of the latter compounds by precipitation with a solution of 2,4-dinitrophenylhydrazine in 2 N HCl added to urine is diagnostically more reliable than the urine odor. The metabolic defect leading to accumulation of these amino acids is unknown. One patient has been successfully treated by restricted intake of the accumulated amino acids.

Primary Hyperoxaluria and Oxalosis. (See also Chap. 46.) This is a rare recessive condition with continuous high urinary oxalate excretion, progressive bilateral calcium oxalate urolithiasis and nephrocalcinosis beginning in childhood, and extrarenal crystalline calcium oxalate deposits or "oxalosis." It results in death from renal failure by early adult life. Oxalate is normally not further metabolized. The 0.02 mg per mg creatinine (< 50 mg per day) normally excreted comes from the few per cent of that in the diet which is absorbed plus that formed endogenously. In hyperoxaluria the excretion of oxalate is consistently several times the maximum normal value. The extra oxalate is formed endoge-

nously. Some ingested ascorbic acid is converted to oxalate, but the amount cannot account for the extra oxalate formed in hyperoxaluria. The other major route of oxalate formation involves the conversion of glycine (and serine through glycolic acid) to glyoxylic acid. Normally and in hyperoxaluria about half the oxalate excreted comes from glycine, representing a normal conversion of about 0.5 per cent of the daily glycine turnover. The metabolic defect in hyperoxaluria therefore probably consists of a failure to metabolize glyoxylic acid by some other route, leaving more to be oxidized to oxalate. The possible routes of glyoxylic acid metabolism which may be defective include its transamination to glycine, oxidation to formic acid, and reduction to glycolic acid. Administration of pyridoxine, necessary as a coenzyme of transamination, will decrease the normal excretion of oxalate. Attempts to decrease oxalate excretion in hyperoxaluria by a restricted protein diet or by administration of sodium benzoate to trap glycine produced only small or temporary changes. All three measures warrant further trial, in conjunction with the avoidance of oxalate-rich foods.

REFERENCES

Garrod, A. E.: The Incidence of Alkaptonuria, A Study in Chemical Individuality, Lancet, II:1616, 1902.

———: Inborn Errors of Metabolism, Lancet, II:1, 73, 142, 214, 1908.

Harris, H.: "Human Biochemical Genetics," London, Cambridge University Press, 1960.

Knox, W. E.: Sir Archibald Garrod's "Inborn Errors of Metabolism," Am. J. Human Genetics, 10:3, 95, 249, 385, 1958.

Schwartz, W. B.: Case 44341 (Fanconi Syndrome), New Engl. J. Med., 259:392, 1958.

Stanbury, J. B., J. B. Wyngaarden, and D. S. Fredrickson (Eds.): "The Metabolic Basis of Inherited Disease," New York, McGraw-Hill Book Company, Inc., 1960.

Stauffer, Martha: Oxalosis: Report of a Case, with a Review of the Literature and Discussion of the Pathogenesis, New Engl. J. Med., 263:386, 1960.

89 CONGENITAL DYSPROTEINEMIAS

Frederic L. Hoch

The congenital dysproteinemias are defined as genetic alterations in plasma protein synthesis. The genetic alteration or defect may affect protein synthesis directly, as when an apparently normal cell fails to synthesize a normal plasma protein, or indirectly, as when the cell itself is not developed into mature form, and secondarily, perhaps, demonstrates an altered pattern of synthesis of plasma proteins. Both defects may lead to a lack of synthesis of a normal protein, synthesis of too little or too much normal protein, or synthesis of abnormal proteins. Dependent on the function of the protein affected, major, minor, or no clinical findings may be associated with the abnormality.

The apparent incidence of these abnormalities depends on two factors: (1) the means used for their detection and (2) the known function of the protein affected. If the results of the genetic alteration change the function of a normal protein, as, for example, when protein factors in blood clotting are not synthesized, the defect is readily recognized through the occurrence of abnormalities in bleeding, etc. If the function of a normal plasma protein is not as yet recognized, the dysproteinemia may be detected only through examination of the physical or chemical characteristics of the plasma proteins.

The present usual means of detection of abnormal plasma proteins—as those of proteins in general—depend upon changes in their molecular mass, density, dimensions, charge distribution, reactive end groups, optical properties toward plane and polarized light, composition, amino acid sequence, and immunologic reactivity. Physical and chemical methods measuring one or more of these parameters increasingly have found clinical application, and more dysproteinemias, and perhaps normal genetic variants, have been recognized; many more may be expected to be detected. Once an abnormal protein, or the absence or excess of a normal one, has been identified, the recognition of similar defects in the family of the patient is required for diagnosis.

The congenital dysproteinemias should be differentiated from the numerous acquired changes in plasma protein concentrations and from those apparently acquired diseases involving syntheses of abnormal proteins which circulate in the plasma. Thus, hyperglobulinemia is frequently observed in many conditions, including transient infections where the β- and γ-globulins are increased, and in immune reactions, where γ-globulin increases. Diseases such as multiple myeloma and macroglobulinemia, which involve increased numbers of abnormal plasma cells synthesizing abnormal proteins, may be termed *paraproteinemias* (see p. 1342).

The congenital dysproteinemias may be classified on the basis of the protein which is the end product of the synthetic pathway modified by the genetic variation.

Albumin. Hyperalbuminemia rarely if ever occurs except adventitiously, as by hemoconcentration. Congenital defects of two types have been identified: *paralbuminemia* and *analbuminemia*. In paralbuminemia, an additional abnormal albumin circulates, the two albumins representing two autosomal alleles of equal dominance, giving rise to a definite genetic pattern of occurrence among the relatives of the propositus. The abnormal albumins have been shown to contain one or more tyrosine molecules substituted for carboxyl-containing amino acids; the change in charge alters the electrophoretic mobility. No known symptoms are associated with this change.

Analbuminemia is an exceedingly rare condition, in which the serum albumin component is apparently missing. An increase in total globulin concentrations, observed in the few cases studied, perhaps accounts for the maintenance of 50 per cent of the normal oncotic pressure. Only slight ankle edema occurs, and hypotension is noted.

Blood Coagulation Protein Factors. Defects in the synthesis of proteins concerned in clotting have long been recognized because of the obvious disturbance in coagulation. They may be due to decreased plasma concentrations of normal factors or to replacement of the normal proteins by nonfunctioning ones; little evidence is at hand to aid in such resolution.

The blood coagulation disorders may be considered as congenital dysproteinemias if they represent the latter phenomenon. For a discussion of afibrinogenemia and the thromboplastin deficiencies, see Chaps. 238 and 239.

γ-Globulin. A synthetic defect, probably due to a defect in the formation of plasma cells, results in *congenital agammaglobulinemia*. Synthesis may not be completely absent, as shown by the small amounts of reactive protein detected in these cases by very sensitive and selective immunologic techniques. This condition is a sex-linked recessive defect, appearing only in males. It is usually detected in children from infancy; they are subject to repeated infections, usually bacterial. A large proportion of these children exhibit a syndrome resembling rheumatoid arthritis; some exhibit other "collagen diseases." The failure of synthesis of antibodies is reflected by absence of the γ-globulin peak on examination by electrophoresis or other methods. Administration of normal plasma or immune proteins may be of transient therapeutic value. Even the natural isohemagglutinins involved in blood group characterization are absent in the majority of these patients. In some cases, two β-globulins are also absent, perhaps because they arise from the same cells as the γ-globulins.

Metal-binding Proteins. The genetic patterns of the iron-binding globulins or transferrins vary in normal individuals. A marked deficiency, a very rare occurrence, lays open the carrier to toxic reactions from free iron ions when the plasma iron-binding capacity is exceeded. Genetic defects occur in *haptoglobin* synthesis. These proteins, distinguished by their ability to bind hemoglobin, normally appear as seven or eight distinct fractions, the resultant of a rather complex genetic interplay, and so of questionable medicolegal value in disputes over parentage. Some normal individuals lack haptoglobins; their role in iron conservation and hemoglobin transport is therefore questionable.

Ceruloplasmin concentrations are lowered markedly through the genetic defects occurring in Wilson's disease (see p. 768), which are inherited as autosomal recessives. Serum copper is low; this is accounted for by the decrease in ceruloplasmin, the major copper-protein of plasma, to as low as 30 per cent of normal concentration. The defect is not in abnormally rapid breakdown of ceruloplasmin, since the turnover of administered ceruloplasmin is normal in these patients. The primary genetic target may be the defect in copper metabolism, so that ceruloplasmin synthesis fails secondarily.

Since hormones are components of the normal circulating plasma, it might be questioned whether such a disease as *diabetes mellitus* might be considered a dysproteinemia because of the defect in synthesis resulting in insufficient insulin to maintain homeostasis. Similar considerations hold for the newly discovered large group of circulating enzymes, some of which are carried in several serum fractions, but little information is as yet on hand as to genetic variations.

It should be pointed out that the term dysproteinemia is a descriptive and symptomatic one. The alterations of circulating proteins are due to genetic effects in cells synthesizing these proteins. As the pathways of plasma protein synthesis are elucidated, the dysproteinemia will likely be renamed, to fall into such groups as diseases of liver cells, plasma cells, lymphocytes, etc.

REFERENCE

Putnam, F. W. (Ed.): "The Plasma Proteins," vol. II, New York, Academic Press, Inc., 1960.

90 SEROTONIN METABOLISM AND THE CARCINOID SYNDROME

Seymour J. Gray

Although the presence of a vasopressor substance in clotted blood has been known since 1868, the responsible factor has been isolated only recently and identified as 5-hydroxytryptamine, a powerful smooth muscle stimulant and vasoconstrictor known as *serotonin*. This compound is formed predominantly in the argentaffin cells of the gastrointestinal tract. It is transported in the blood by the platelets and is present in the brain and other tissues.

Serotonin was discovered in considerable quantities in carcinoid tumors (argentaffinomas) by Lembeck in 1953. One year later Thorson, Biorck, Bjorkman, and Waldenström described the clinical picture of the "carcinoid syndrome" in patients with metastatic (malignant) carcinoids. The syndrome is characterized by episodic flushing of the skin, patchy cyanosis, telangiectasia, diarrhea, asthma, and valvular heart disease.

The excess secretion of serotonin by the endocrine tumors and a disturbance in tryptophan metabolism appear to be responsible for the various manifestations. The profound and dramatic effects of serotonin upon various organ systems have stimulated considerable investigation in the physiologic and pharmacologic properties of this hormone and related hydroxyindoles.

SEROTONIN METABOLISM

The metabolic pathway involved in the formation and breakdown of serotonin (5-HTA) is presented in Fig. 90-1. The amino acid, tryptophan, a constituent of many dietary proteins, is hydroxylated to form 5-hydroxytryptophan (5-HTP), or serotonin precursor. 5-HTP then undergoes rapid decarboxylation to form 5-hydroxytryptamine (5-HTA) or serotonin. The enzyme, monoamine oxidase, converts serotonin by oxidative deamination to 5-hydroxyindoleacetic acid (5-HIAA), which is excreted in the urine.

Hydroxylation of Tryptophan to 5-Hydroxytryptophan. Approximately 1 per cent of dietary tryptophan is normally metabolized by the 5-hydroxyindole pathway. Its relationship to the major catabolic pathway of tryptophan to kynurenine and nicotinic acid is depicted in Fig. 90-2. Patients with carcinoidosis can convert as much as 60 per cent of the dietary tryptophan to 5-hydroxyindole compounds. The excessive diversion of tryptophan in this direction may decrease the amount available for protein and nicotinic acid, resulting in a pellagra-like picture (Fig. 90-2).

Although the site of tryptophan hydroxylation is unknown, it may take place in the argentaffin cell. 5-Hydroxytryptophan has been identified chromatographically in the urine of patients with malignant carcinoidosis, and C^{14}-labeled tryptophan has been shown in the human to be converted to C^{14}-labeled 5-HTP, lending considerable support to the concept that 5-HTP is an intermediate in the biosynthesis of serotonin.

Decarboxylation of 5-Hydroxytryptophan to 5-Hydroxytryptamine. The enzymatic decarboxylation of 5-HTP to 5-HTA takes place in the liver,

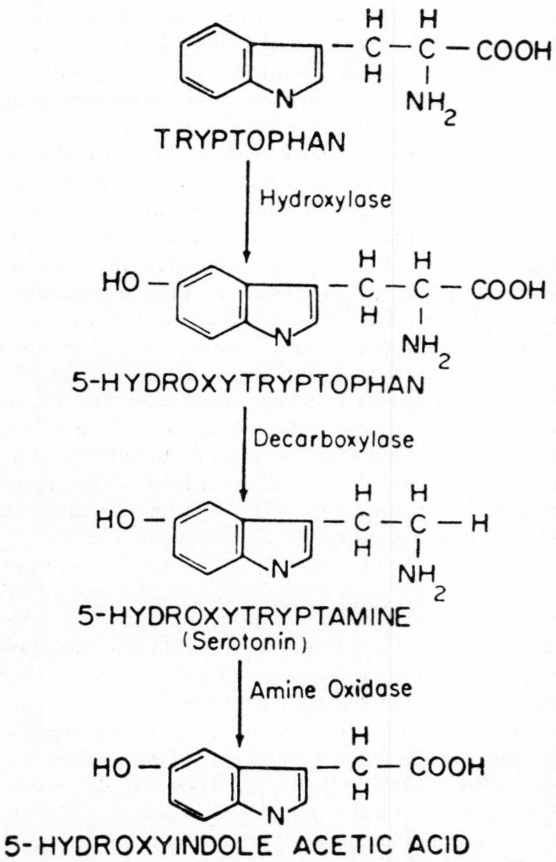

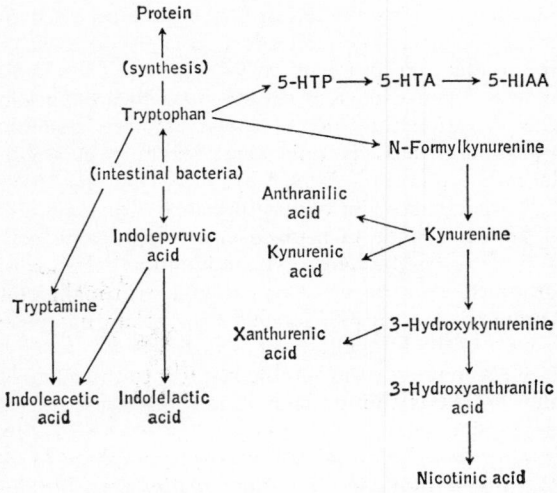

FIG. 90-1. Metabolic pathway of serotonin.

kidney, gastrointestinal mucosa, brain, lung, and carcinoid tumor. Only the L-form of 5-HTP is normally decarboxylated to serotonin. In the central nervous system the localization of the enzyme, 5-

hydroxytryptophan decarboxylase, in the hypothalamus and upper brain stem parallels the distribution of serotonin. The presence of a metal as well as pyridoxal phosphate (vitamin B_6) is required for its activity. Diminished formation of serotonin from 5-HTP has been demonstrated in pyridoxine deficient animals.

Serotonin. Serotonin is the biologically active compound resulting from tryptophan hydroxylation. The major depot in the body is the gastrointestinal tract. Serotonin is also found in blood platelets, brain, spleen, lungs, and other tissues. Postmortem examination of human brains for 5-HTA content has revealed the highest quantities in the mesencephalic and diencephalic structures. In nature serotonin may be found in bananas, tomatoes, certain mushrooms, insect venoms, and Crustacea.

Serotonin is active only in the free form. Biologic activity is apparently lost with binding to tissues or platelets. The mechanism of binding and release remains uncertain, although ATP may play a role. When 5-HTA is released from tissue stores into the blood, it is rapidly taken up by the platelets. There is no evidence that platelets synthesize or metabolize serotonin or that serotonin plays a role in platelet function or hemostasis. Normal human whole blood contains only 0.1 to 0.3 μg per ml of serotonin virtually all of which is bound to the platelets and released into the plasma when the platelets disintegrate.

5-Hydroxyindoleacetic Acid. In the presence of monoamine oxidase, free serotonin rapidly undergoes oxidative deamination to form 5-HIAA, the final major metabolic derivative of the 5-hydroxyindole pathway. Monoamine oxidase activity has been demonstrated in gastrointestinal mucosa, lung, kidney, brain, and liver. Very small amounts of serotonin may be degraded by mechanisms other than oxidative deamination.

Physiology and Pharmacology

Gastrointestinal Tract. Approximately 90 per cent of the total body serotonin is found in the argentaffin cells of the gastrointestinal tract. Small doses of serotonin or serotonin precursor administered intravenously to man produce marked intestinal contractions, increased intestinal tone, abdominal cramps, nausea, and vomiting. Although the intestinal response has been attributed to stimulation of postganglionic cholinergic fibers, recent experiments indicate that serotonin acts directly on autonomic ganglions at sites different from those of acetylcholine. In vitro studies suggest that serotonin may sensitize the mucosal stretch receptors for initiation of the peristaltic reflex, indicating an important function for 5-HTA in the regulation of normal gastrointestinal motility.

FIG. 90-2. Metabolic pathways of tryptophan.

Pathologic Physiology. Serotonin inhibits gastric secretion in animals. Adequate studies in human beings have not been reported. Achlorhydria is present in some patients with carcinoidosis, but there is no consistent abnormality of gastric acid secretion. An increased incidence of gastric and duodenal ulcerations has been noted in patients with metastatic carcinoid and in animals following the administration of 5-HTP or serotonin. The exact mechanism of ulcer production is unknown. Smooth muscle spasm, vasoconstriction, or histamine release may be implicated.

An increase in urinary 5-HIAA is observed in some patients with nontropical sprue, with a return to normal following the elimination of gluten or gliadan from the diet, suggesting a possible abnormality in serotonin metabolism.

Although a deficiency of serotonin has been postulated in the pathogenesis of hepatic coma, the urinary excretion of 5-HIAA is normal in patients with decompensated hepatic cirrhosis with and without encephalopathy. The urinary excretion of 5-HIAA, however, does not necessarily reflect the metabolism of 5-hydroxyindoles in the central nervous system. A greater than normal urinary excretion of 5-HIAA is observed following the intravenous administration of 5-HTP in patients with decompensated cirrhosis, suggesting altered metabolism in the cirrhotic liver in the presence of excess 5-HTP.

Central Nervous System. A physiologic role for serotonin in brain function as a chemical mediator of parasympathetic impulses has been proposed by Brodie and Shore. Serotonin, 5-hydroxytryptophan decarboxylase, and monamine oxidase are present in the brain, particularly in the hypothalamus and those areas where autonomic integration occurs. Although serotonin itself does not enter the brain from peripheral tissues, it can be synthesized within the brain from its precursor 5-HTP which is able to pass the blood-brain barrier.

The concept that 5-HTA may be of physiologic importance in cerebral function is based on the following: (1) the finding of serotonin in brain tissue, (2) the hallucinogenic effects of certain antagonists and analogues of serotonin, (3) the depressant effects of reserpine which liberates serotonin (and epinephrine) from the brain, (4) the stimulatory effects of the amine oxidase inhibitor, iproniazide, which blocks serotonin degradation, and (5) the pronounced central nervous system effects of exogenously administered 5-HTP. Further studies are necessary, however, to establish the importance of serotonin in brain function. There is no proof that serotonin metabolism is disturbed in mental disease. Evidence that 5-hydroxyindole metabolism may be altered in schizophrenia has not been confirmed, and abnormal mental function or striking emotional disorders are observed only rarely in patients with carcinoidosis. A significant increase in the total 5-hydroxyindoles of the cerebrospinal fluid in hydrocephalus and an increased serotonin level in tuberculous meningitis have been reported.

Anaphylaxis. In animals, both histamine and serotonin are released by anaphylaxis. Although mast cells of rats and mice contain serotonin as well as histamine, serotonin is not demonstrable in the mast cells of man. There is no conclusive evidence, furthermore, linking serotonin to allergic manifestations in man. Serotonin antimetabolites neither suppress anaphylactic reactions nor do they influence asthma in patients with malignant carcinoidosis.

Smooth Muscle. Serotonin is an extremely powerful smooth muscle constrictor, and the bioassay of serotonin utilizes the constrictor effects upon the guinea pig ileum, pulmonary artery of dogs, rat uterus, and clam heart. The actions of serotonin on smooth muscle may be responsible in part for the cutaneous vascular changes, the bronchoconstriction, and the abnormal intestinal motility observed in patients with malignant carcinoidosis. Aerosolized serotonin may induce bronchial constriction in some asthmatic patients.

Cardiovascular-Renal. Serotonin constricts arteries and veins and dilates capillaries. Infusion of the amine decreases blood flow, increases vascular volume, and produces flushing and cyanosis of the skin. It induces intense spasm of the infused vein. Serotonin has been reported to increase cardiac output in human beings and may elevate the pulmonary artery pressure in human beings and animals. Its effect on the systemic blood pressure is variable and inconsistent. Serotonin may act as a regulator of glomerular filtration by constricting the afferent renal arterioles. It can exert an antidiuretic effect in animals and human beings and may cause ischemic cortical necrosis of the kidneys in rats.

THE CARCINOID SYNDROME (Carcinoidosis)

The clinical aspects of the carcinoid syndrome reflect the effects of serotonin excess upon the cardiovascular and respiratory systems and the gastrointestinal tract. Abnormal tryptophan metabolism, malnutrition, and diarrhea may predispose the patient to protein deficiency or a pellagra-like state. The generalized signs and symptoms of the syndrome do not appear until the carcinoid metastasizes to the liver and high levels of blood serotonin are attained.

Carcinoids occur from adolescence to extreme old age. Metastasizing carcinoids are commoner in the older age group and are seen equally among the sexes. The symptoms may extend over many years in spite of metastases because of the slow growth of the tumor.

Clinical Features

Vasomotor. The most distinctive and often the earliest symptom of the carcinoid syndrome is the acute, reddish, cutaneous flush which starts in the face and neck and may extend to the chest, arms, and legs. Colors range from bright red to violaceous. The flush usually lasts only a few minutes but may persist longer and recur many times during the day, precipitated at times by emotional disturbances, physical exertion, manipulation of the tumor, food, alcohol intake, or the injection of histamine. Periorbital edema, hypotension, tachycardia, abdominal pain, diarrhea, and wheezing often accompany the flushing. The flush tends to be more frequent and severe as the disease progresses. Facial vascular congestion may become permanent, and some patients develop localized telangiectasia in the affected area or chronic cyanosis resembling polycythemia.

The flushing is probably caused by an increase in the blood serotonin level since the excretion of 5-HIAA in the urine may increase with the flush, and the infusion of serotonin into the brachial arteries of man produces a deep flush in the injected arm. Epinephrine or norepinephrine may play a role in the release of serotonin. Ballistocardiograms demonstrate involvement of the entire circulatory system during the flushing episode. Observation of the peritoneum during abdominal laparotomy reveals peritoneal flushing as well. Cardiac catheterization performed during flushing demonstrates an elevated pressure in the pulmonary vasculature—a well-described serotonin effect in animals.

Waldenström has noted an increased urinary excretion of histamine in some patients with malignant carcinoidosis. Since carcinoid tumors do not contain excess histamine it has been postulated that serotonin may release histamine from normal tissue stores, producing a peculiar bright red, patchy flush. Tumors secreting both 5-HTP and serotonin may be more potent in histamine release.

Gastrointestinal. Recurrent or chronic diarrhea is one of the most frequent manifestations of the disease and may be accompanied by borborygmi, colicky abdominal pain, and other signs of hyperperistalsis. Diarrhea is often the first symptom noted. An enlarged liver usually signifies metastatic involvement, although metastases may be present without hepatomegaly. An increased incidence of peptic ulcer has been reported.

Carcinoids of the appendix may obstruct the lumen, presenting the picture of acute appendicitis, or in the small bowel they may cause symptoms of intestinal obstruction. Rarely tumors obstructing the biliary system may produce jaundice or steatorrhea.

Cardiac Involvement. Right-sided cardiac involvement, primarily pulmonary stenosis, appears late in the disease and occurs in about 50 per cent of advanced cases. Although the tricuspid and pulmonic valves are most commonly involved either alone or in combination, all four valves may become sclerotic. Characteristically, the pulmonic and tricuspid valves present a pearly, gray fibrosis with sclerosis, thickening, and retraction of the chordae tendinae. Rigidity, thickening, and contractures may explain the physical findings of stenosis and regurgitation. Right-sided heart failure may develop. In some instances, the mural endocardium becomes markedly thickened. The cause of endocardial fibrosis is unknown. It has been attributed to chemical irritation from the high levels of blood serotonin. Hepatic metastases are invariably present when cardiac involvement appears.

The serotonin in the blood passing from the right to the left side of the heart may be rapidly oxidized by the monamine oxidase in the lungs, explaining the predominance of right-sided cardiac lesions. This concept is supported by the finding of valvular heart lesions involving both sides of the heart in a patient with carcinoidosis and a patent foramen ovale. However, the serotonin content of pulmonary artery blood is not consistently greater than that of the pulmonary vein. There is no significant change in systemic blood pressure.

Respiratory. Asthmatic wheezing attacks and dyspnea are noted in some patients, particularly during flushing episodes, presumably related to bronchiolar constriction produced by serotonin.

Other Symptoms. Other symptoms include abnormal pigmentation of the skin with pellagra-like lesions and hyperkeratosis in severe cases, arthritis with swelling and stiffness of the joints, sudden localized edema of the hands or face, dependent edema, and weight loss.

The Carcinoid Tumor

The term *carcinoid* was first proposed by Oberndorfer in 1907 to emphasize the malignant appearance but benign course of the tumor. Carcinoid tumors arise from the argentaffin cells (Kultschitzky cells) of the intestinal mucosa near the bases of the crypts of Lieberkuhn, and often contain cytoplasmic granules with an affinity for silver or chromium compounds. The fresh tumors are yellow firm, and consist of clumps or strands of epithelial cells with a tendency to tubular or acinar formation.

Site. These serotonin-producing tumors may be found anywhere from the stomach to the rectum, although 80 to 95 per cent are located in the region of the ileocecal valve, principally in the appendix and the terminal ileum. Carcinoids may also be present in the gallbladder, bile ducts, and ampulla of Vater and are multiple in 15 to 25 per cent of cases. Occasionally a carcinoid may arise from an ovarian or testicular teratoma. Bronchial adenomas of the carcinoid type may give rise to the syndrome, and although usually benign, metastasize to the liver occasionally. This type of bronchial adenoma does not always give an argentaffin staining reaction, although it frequently contains serotonin. In general, carcinoid tumors of all types vary considerably in their serotonin content and silver staining properties.

Metastasis. Appendiceal carcinoids metastasize rarely, if at all. Carcinoid tumors involving the ileum, cecum, colon, or stomach metastasize more frequently, usually to the liver and regional lymph nodes, and occasionally to the ovaries, lungs, and bones. Metastatic lesions may appear late, grow slowly, and assume massive proportions.

Relationship of Liver Metastases to the Clinical Syndrome. The clinical features of the carcinoid syndrome in most instances signify malignant carcinoidosis of the liver and a high blood level of serotonin. The serotonin formed by metastatic tumors in the liver escapes destruction and enters the hepatic vein and the general circulation. In the absence of liver metastases the serotonin secreted by the intestinal carcinoid is inactivated in the liver by monamine oxidase, resulting in an increased excretion of 5-HIAA in the urine without clinical manifestation of the carcinoid syndrome. Serotonin secreted by extraportal carcinoids, such as ovarian tumors, enters the systemic circulation directly through the vena cava and may produce the syndrome without metastasis to the liver.

Diagnosis and Management of the Carcinoid Syndrome

Laboratory Aspects and Diagnosis. The diagnosis can be established by measuring the level of 5-HIAA in the urine. Urinary levels of 50 to 1,000 mg per day are found in patients with the carcinoid syndrome compared to normal values of 2 to 10 mg. A simple screening test for 5-HIAA, consisting of a purple color when a nitrosonaphthol solution is added to urine, becomes positive when the daily excretion of 5-HIAA exceeds 40 mg. Marked increases do not occur except in carcinoidosis, although a slight elevation may be observed in some patients with nontropical sprue and transiently after the administration of reserpine. The ingestion of bananas, which contain significant amounts of serotonin (4 mg per banana), can also increase the urinary excretion of 5-HIAA. Decreased excretion has been noted in renal insufficiency and in some instances of phenylketonuria. Medications containing mephenesin carbamate and phenothiazines interfere with the determination.

The malignant carcinoid usually contains 1.0 to 3.0 mg of serotonin per Gm of tumor. The level of 5-HIAA in the urine is a measure of the extent of the functioning tumor mass and may be helpful in following the clinical course of the patient after surgery or other therapy. It returns to normal when the carcinoid is completely removed if no metastases are present.

The serotonin pool in the body of a carcinoid patient approximates 2,800 mg. The blood serotonin levels vary from 0.5 to 3.0 μg per ml (normal 0.1 to 0.3 μg per ml). Normally the serotonin in the urine is barely detectable compared to 0.5 to 12 mg daily in the carcinoid patient. Hypoalbuminemia and hypoproteinemia are seen in some instances.

Prognosis. Since carcinoids often grow very slowly, patients may live as long as 10 to 20 years after the symptoms have developed. The immediate prognosis is not necessarily poor with inoperable carcinoids or those which have already metastasized. Death is caused by heart failure, metastatic liver disease, malnutrition, or intercurrent infection.

Management. Surgery is indicated in spite of metastases, because of the remarkably slow progression of the carcinoid tumors. Surgical removal of the primary lesion and metastases when feasible may decrease, delay, or ameliorate symptoms by reducing serotonin production. Removal of the primary tumor is recommended to prevent local complications such as obstruction. Vitamin supplements, particularly niacin, are recommended.

The serotonin antagonists and antimetabolites including lysergic acid diethylamide (LSD), brominated LSD, and the benzyl analogue of serotonin (BAS) interfere somewhat with serotonin action but do not prevent its formation and have proved ineffective therapeutically. Phenylacetic acid diminishes 5-HIAA excretion in some patients probably by its action on renal excretory mechanisms but does not ameliorate the symptoms. Reserpine, which releases serotonin from tissue stores, is also of little value.

Chlorpromazine, 25 mg every 6 hr, may be effective in diminishing the diarrhea and the severity of the flush in some instances, although it does not decrease the urinary excretion of 5-HIAA. X-ray therapy and radioactive gold have been tried without success.

Recently α-methyl-dopa (α-methyl-3,4-dihydroxyphenylalanine) has been shown to block serotonin formation by inhibiting decarboxylase activity and to produce an increase in urinary 5-HTP with a decrease in 5-HIAA. Its final clinical evaluation in the treatment of the carcinoid syndrome awaits further study. This agent is also under consideration as an antihypertension drug, presumably related to its inhibitory effect upon epinephrine and nor-epinephrine.

REFERENCES

Page, I. H.: Serotonin (5-Hydroxytryptamine): The Last Four Years, Physiol. Revs., 38:277, 1958.

Resnick, R. H., and S. J. Gray: Serotonin Metabolism and the Carcinoid Syndrome, Med. Clin. N. Am., 44:1323, 1960.

Sjoerdsma, A., H. Weissbach, and S. Udenfriend: Clinical, Physiologic and Biochemical Study of Patients with Malignant Carcinoid (Argentaffinoma), Am. J. Med., 20:520, 1956.

Thorson, A. H.: Studies on Carcinoid Disease, Acta Med. Scand., 161:1, 1958 (Suppl. 334).

Waldenström, J.: Carcinoid Tumors, Clinical Aspects, pp. 92–100, in "Modern Trends in Gastroenterology," Series II, F. A. Jones (Ed.), New York, Paul B. Hoeber, Inc., Medical Department of Harper & Brothers, 1958.

91 DISORDERS OF PORPHYRIN METABOLISM

George E. Cartwright

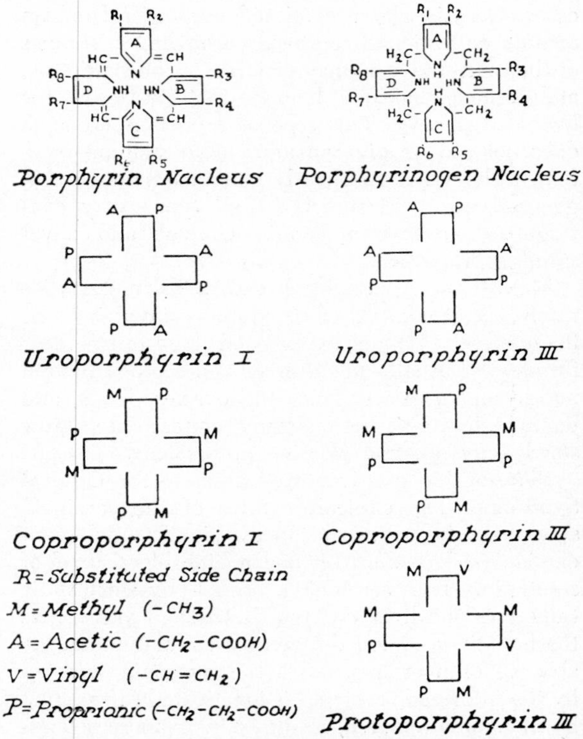

Definitions. The porphyrins are pigments possessing a basic structure of four pyrrole rings linked by methene bridges (Fig. 91-1). These pigments are widely distributed throughout the plant and animal worlds. The individual porphyrins differ from each other according to the nature of the eight possible side chains. In addition, each porphyrin has a number of stereoisomers. The basic pigment of chlorophyll is *actinoporphyrin* and that of hemoglobin is *protoporphyrin*. The porphyrins are also vital components of enzyme systems such as the cytochromes and catalases.

The term *porphyrinuria* refers to the excessive excretion of porphyrins in the urine. *Coproporphyrinuria*, the excretion of increased amounts of coproporphyrin, is not uncommon and occurs in a variety of conditions. The term *porphyria* embraces a group of diseases, each with unusual and characteristic clinical manifestations, which have in common the excessive excretion of uroporphyrin and coproporphyrin and/or porphyrin precursors (Δ-aminolevulinic acid and porphobilinogen) in the urine and/or feces.

History. To Hans Fischer and his school at Munich goes credit for much of the knowledge of the chemistry of the porphyrins. These workers in 1915 described, named, and isolated in crystalline form the uroporphyrins and coproporphyrins from

FIG. 91-1. The structural formulas of the porphyrin and porphyrinogen nuclei and diagrammatic formulas of the important naturally occurring porphyrins.

the urine of their now famous case of congenital porphyria (Petry). Shemin and his group in New York made substantial contributions to recent knowledge of the biosynthesis of the porphyrins. Congenital porphyria was first described by Günther in 1911, and contributions to the understanding of the manifestations of porphyria have come from Waldenström in Sweden, Barnes and Dean in South Africa, and Watson and Schwartz in this country.

Biosynthesis. The rather complex porphyrin molecule is synthesized in the body from two simple precursors, acetate and glycine (Fig. 91-2). Acetate enters the Krebs tricarboxylic acid cycle (Chap. 52, p. 479) and is converted into succinate. Succinyl CoA (active succinate) is then formed in the presence of Mg^{++} ion, adenosine triphosphate (ATP), and coenzyme A (CoA). The activated form of succinate condenses with a pyridoxal phosphate-glycine enzyme (glycine-PE) to form the 5-carbon compound, Δ-aminolevulinic acid (Δ-ALA), and carbon dioxide by the decarboxylation of glycine. This step is enzymatically controlled, and several intermediate compounds have been suggested. Two molecules of Δ-aminolevulinic acid, in the presence of glutathione (GSH) and an enzyme, Δ-aminolevulinic acid dehydrase (Δ-ALA DH), condense to form a substituted monopyrrole, porphobilinogen, which contains acetic acid (A) and proprionic acid (P) side chains. In the next step in heme synthesis, four molecules of porphobilinogen condense to form the reduced tetrapyrrolic structure, uroporphyrinogen. This step is catalyzed by at least two enzymes, porphobilinogen deaminase (PD) and uroporphyrin isomerase (UI). Details of the action of these enzymes and the sequence of reactions leading from porphobilinogen to uroporphyrinogen types I and III are not known. Uroporphyrin III is not in the direct pathway of heme synthesis as was formerly assumed but is a by-product. Uroporphyrinogen III (reduced uroporphyrin) is converted to coproporphyrinogen by the enzyme, uroporphyrinogen decarboxylase (UD). Coproporphyrinogen III is then converted to protoporphyrin III. Coproporphyrin III is a by-product, whereas the available evidence suggests that protoporphyrin III is in the direct pathway of heme synthesis. Protoporphyrin III is converted to hemoglobin in the presence of iron, glutathione, globin, and the enzyme, heme synthetase (HS). The intermediate steps between protoporphyrin and hemoglobin have not been identified. It is not known whether heme or a porphyrin-globin compound is an intermediate in this reaction, although the former possibility seems more likely.

Metabolism. The most important of the naturally occurring porphyrins are uroporphyrin (isomer types I and III), coproporphyrin (types I and III), and protoporphyrin (type III).

Protoporphyrin III is present in hemoglobin and is, therefore, the most important of the porphyrins from the physiologic standpoint. It is normally absent from urine. The concentration of fecal protoporphyrin is related to the amount of blood in the gastrointestinal tract and the rate of liberation of protoporphyrin from hemoglobin by fecal bacteria.

Coproporphyrin is the predominant porphyrin in urine and feces under normal circumstances. Coproporphyrinuria occurs in a variety of clinical conditions, such as lead poisoning, poliomyelitis, liver disease, acute alcoholism, hemolytic anemia, and Hodgkin's disease. In all these disorders the increased coproporphyrinuria accompanies the underlying disease, and it is unlikely that the abnormality in porphyrin metabolism contributes significantly to the clinical picture. Coproporphyrinuria is also found in patients with porphyria. Abnormally high fecal coproporphyrin values are found in patients with hemolytic anemia, and low values occur in patients with liver disease.

Uroporphyrin is normally excreted in urine in only trace amounts. The urinary excretion of this porphyrin is moderately increased in lead poisoning and is greatly increased in patients with porphyria.

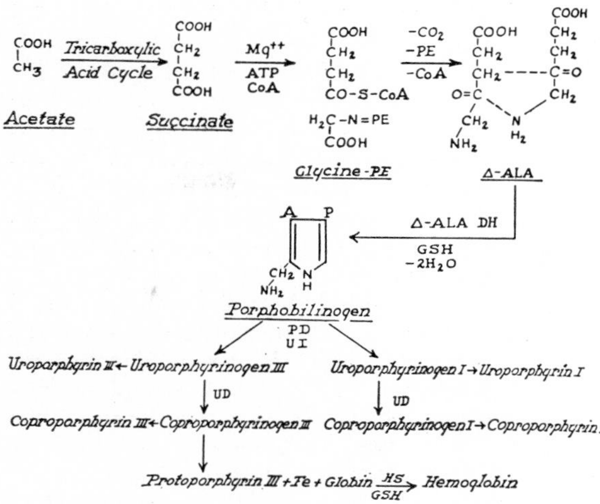

FIG. 91-2. The biosynthesis of the porphyrins from acetate and glycine and the biosynthetic pathway of hemoglobin. CoA, coenzyme A; ATP, adenosine triphosphate; PE, pyridoxal phosphate enzyme; Δ-ALA, delta-aminolevulinic acid; Δ-ALA DH, delta-aminolevulinic acid dehydrase; GSH, glutathione; PD, porphobilinogen deaminase; UI, uroporphyrin isomerase; UD, uroporphyrinogen decarboxylase; HS, heme synthetase; A, acetic; P, proprionic.

PORPHYRIA

Porphyria may be divided into two general groups (Table 91-1). In porphyria erythropoietica, excessive quantities of porphyrins are synthesized in the bone marrow. In porphyria hepatica, excessive porphyrin production occurs in the liver. Hepatic porphyria may be subdivided further into at least three different types: acute intermittent porphyria, porphyria cutanea tarda hereditaria, and porphyria cutanea tarda symptomatica. Not all patients with hepatic porphyria can be so classified, and it is entirely possible that more than a single entity is contained in each subtype of hepatic porphyria.

Porphyria Erythropoietica (Congenital Porphyria)

This is a very rare disease, inherited probably as a recessive mendelian characteristic. The clinical manifestations appear very early in life, sometimes

Table 91-1. CLASSIFICATION OF PORPHYRIA

I. Porphyria erythropoietica (congenital porphyria)
II. Porphyria hepatica
    A. Acute intermittent porphyria (pyrrolia)
    B. Porphyria cutanea tarda hereditaria (mixed porphyria, porphyria variegata, South African Caucasian porphyria, protocoproporphyria)
    C. Porphyria cutanea tarda symptomatica (South African Bantu porphyria)
    D. Unclassified

even a few days after birth, but often they are not observed until after an interval of a year or two. The disease is characterized by the excessive deposition of porphyrin in the tissues, leading to pronounced photosensitization. The early lesions of photodynamic origin are the blisters of hydroa estivale (hydroa vacciniforme) on skin surfaces exposed to light, especially of the face and hands. In time, scarring and mutilation occur. After years of continued photosensitivity, the mutilation becomes extensive, with loss of fingers, portions of the nose, ears, scarring of the cheeks and about the mouth, ectropion, or symblepharon. Skin not exposed to light remains unaffected. Hemolytic anemia and splenomegaly are an integral part of the disease. Erythrodontia may be observed in those cases in which sufficient porphyrin has been deposited in the teeth to make them grossly red or reddish brown. Teeth which do not show erythrodontia in ordinary light may exhibit red fluorescence in Wood's light. Red fluorescence may be seen in the phalangeal bones if a strong source of ultraviolet light is allowed to shine through the fingers. There is no marked disturbance of the nervous system, nor is there abdominal colic.

Because of the demonstration of large quantities of uroporphyrin and coproporphyrin in the normoblasts in the bone marrow, it has been suggested that in this type of porphyria the excessive quantities of porphyrin are formed in the marrow. It is for this reason that the disease has been called *erythropoietic porphyria* rather than congenital porphyria.

The color of the urine varies from pink to red. Uroporphyrin I and coproporphyrin I are the predominant porphyrins excreted. If the concentration of uroporphyrin is sufficiently great, the urine, on the addition of hydrochloric acid, exhibits an intense band at about 552 mμ and a weaker band at 596 mμ when viewed in a hand spectroscope. The excretion of porphyrin precursors, Δ-aminolevulinic acid and porphobilinogen, is not increased.

The disease is slowly progressive, and death is usually due to an intercurrent infection or severe hemolytic anemia. At autopsy there is extensive deposition of porphyrins in the skeleton and tissues. This may be so pronounced as to color the bones red. Erythroid hyperplasia of the bone marrow and splenomegaly are additional pathologic features.

Treatment. Exposure to sunlight should be avoided. The harmful and disfiguring effects of light may be ameliorated by the use of quinine cream. Splenectomy is indicated if there is evidence of increased erythrocyte destruction. Splenectomy may be associated not only with amelioration of the hemolytic anemia but also with a reduction in photosensitivity and porphyrin excretion.

Acute Intermittent Porphyria

This is an uncommon but not a rare disease which affects both sexes, with a slight predilection for the female. Young adults or the middle-aged are most frequently affected. Acute porphyria is extremely rare below the age of 15 and after the age of sixty. The familial occurrence of the disease is marked. It is probably transmitted as a mendelian dominant characteristic. The disease is characterized clinically by (1) periodic attacks of intense abdominal colic, usually accompanied by nausea and vomiting; (2) obstinate constipation; (3) neurotic or even psychotic behavior; and (4) neuromuscular disturbances. The mortality rate is high.

Abdominal pain is frequently the presenting complaint. The pain is usually colicky in nature and may be extremely severe and associated with spasm without localizing signs but with fever, tachycardia, and leukocytosis. The abdominal signs may be, and frequently are, mistaken for manifestations of renal colic, acute appendicitis, cholelithiasis, or pancreatitis. It is not uncommon for patients with porphyria to have multiple surgical scars on the abdomen. The neurologic manifestations are quite varied and may include neuritic pain in the extremities, areas of hypoesthesia and paraesthesia, and foot and wrist drop. Paraplegia or a complete flaccid quadriplegia may ensue and may be followed by bulbar paralysis and death. Except for pain in the extremities, sensory changes are usually not prominent and signs of upper motor neurone changes are usually absent. The neurologic manifestations may simulate a wide variety of conditions, including poliomyelitis, encephalitis, and arsenic or lead poisoning. A true ascending paralysis of the Landry type is not observed.

The patients frequently have many vague "neurotic" complaints, even when in remission from an attack. With an attack they may become confused or even psychotic. Hypertension may accompany an attack, there may be temporary loss of vision, and convulsions have been described.

The course of the disease is extraordinarily variable. Recurrent abdominal crises may be present for years, or the patient may die in the first attack. It is not at all uncommon to find in one parent or in several siblings of a patient with porphyria that porphobilinogen, the diagnostic feature of porphyria, is present in the urine even though they have never had active symptoms of the disease. This condition is called *latent porphyria*. In general, the neuromuscular and psychotic symptoms are late manifestations, and with their appearance the prognosis becomes more grave. Between attacks there may be no symptoms. The mechanism by which the latent disease is converted to manifest disease, i.e., an attack of acute porphyria, is unknown, but it is known quite definitely that attacks may be provoked by the administration of certain drugs, particularly barbiturates. Menstruation, pregnancy, infection, alcohol, or lead may be the precipitating factor in a few patients.

The freshly voided urine is frequently normal in color and on standing in the sunlight turns to a Burgundy wine color or even black. This color change can be hastened by adding a small amount of acid to the urine and boiling for 30 min. The explanation for these color changes is that porphobilinogen (colorless) and not uroporphyrin (red) is excreted in the urine. Heating of porphobilinogen in an acid medium results in the nonenzymatic formation of uroporphyrin, together with a dark-brown or reddish-brown nonporphyrin pigment.

In acute intermittent porphyria during relapse the presence of porphobilinogen is a constant feature. During remission the porphobilinogen reaction is usually positive, but a negative test does not exclude the diagnosis of this type of porphyria. The qualitative determination of porphobilinogen by the Watson-Schwartz modification of the Ehrlich reaction is, therefore, a simple and valuable screening procedure. In this test 5 ml freshly voided urine is mixed with 5 ml Ehrlich's reagent (0.7 Gm para-dimethylaminobenzaldehyde, 150 ml concentrated hydrochloric acid, and 100 ml water). After mixing, 10 ml aqueous saturated sodium acetate is added. The solution is then extracted with an equal volume of chloroform. Both porphobilinogen and urobilinogen form a red aldehyde compound with Ehrlich's reagent. However, porphobilinogen can be distinguished from urobilinogen by the fact that it remains in the aqueous (upper) layer, whereas urobilinogen is soluble in chloroform and is extracted into the lower chloroform layer. This test is quite specific for acute intermittent porphyria. The test is negative in erythropoietic porphyria and in porphyria cutanea tarda symptomatica. It is positive in patients with porphyria cutanea tarda hereditaria during acute attacks but is negative in the interval between such episodes.

In addition to porphobilinogen, patients with acute intermittent porphyria excrete excessive quantities of uroporphyrin (types I and III), coproporphyrin (types I and III), and other as yet unidentified porphyrins. As mentioned previously, the porphyrins are formed in the renal tubules by the nonenzymatic transformation of porphobilinogen into uroporphyrin at an acid pH. Examination of the tissues of such patients, in contrast to the findings in erythropoietic porphyria, has revealed that the porphyrin content of the bone marrow is normal. The liver, on the contrary, regularly exhibits increased quantities of porphyrin, especially porphyrin precursors. For this reason, acute intermittent porphyria is classified among the hepatic porphyrias.

Treatment. The use of barbiturates should be avoided completely at all times because of their known action in precipitating acute attacks. Chloral hydrate and paraldehyde may be used for sedation. Opiates, Demerol, or ganglioplegics such as tetraethylammonium may be used for relief of pain. Chloropromazine, in doses of 50 to 100 mg, is reported to effect rapid relief of acute symptoms but without change in the underlying disease process. The rauwolfia derivatives may have supplementary value as maintenance therapy. ACTH, corticosteroids, and chelating agents such as BAL (2,3-dimercaptopropanol) and EDTA (disodium ethylenediaminetetraacetate) have been reported to be effective in alleviating acute attacks. However, evaluation of drugs is made difficult by the intermittent nature of the disease.

Porphyria Cutanea Tarda Hereditaria

Porphyria cutanea tarda hereditaria is characterized clinically by cutaneous lesions or acute attacks of abdominal colic and not infrequently by both. The disease is inherited as a non-sex-linked mendelian dominant. The onset of symptoms is usually between the ages of 10 and 30 years. The outstanding biochemical feature of the disorder is the increased excretion of coproporphyrin and protoporphyrin in the feces *at all times* in the course of the disease.

During the latent phase of the disease the patients are entirely asymptomatic. Porphyrinuria is usually absent and the porphyrin precursors, Δ-aminolevulinic acid and porphobilinogen, are not excreted in increased amounts. The disease can be diagnosed only during the latent phase by examination of the stools for porphyrins. A simple screening test can be done by obtaining a small specimen of stool on a glove. The specimen is extracted with about 2 ml of solvent containing equal parts of glacial acetic acid, amyl alcohol, and ether. The supernatant solution is then decanted and viewed in a Wood's lamp. Negative specimens show a green or gray fluorescence, a positive specimen a brilliant pink. Excess chlorophyll may give rise to a false positive test.

In a number of patients, particularly males, the skin is unusually sensitive to light and blisters and abrades easily. Healed depigmented scars may be present over the exposed surfaces, particularly the hands. Hyperpigmentation of the skin may occur, and hirsutism has been observed in females. The photosensitivity and cutaneous deformities are not so great as in erythropoietic porphyria.

Acute attacks of jaundice and abdominal colic accompanied in some cases by psychotic manifestations and motor paralysis may intervene in the course of the disease. Indeed any or all of the manifestations of acute intermittent porphyria may make their appearance. As in acute intermittent porphyria, death or recovery may occur. During the acute attacks the excretion of porphyrins in the feces frequently decreases and the excretion of coproporphyrin and uroporphyrin in the urine increases. Both Δ-aminolevulinic acid and porphobilinogen are usually excreted in increased amounts in the urine during acute attacks. It has been suggested that the disease remains asymptomatic as long as the liver is capable of excreting the porphyrins in the bile (latent phase); when this capacity is impaired bilirubinemia, porphyrinemia, porphyrinuria, and cutaneous lesions appear (cutaneous phase); and finally when porphyrin metabolism is greatly disturbed Δ-aminolevulinic acid and porphobilinogen appear in the urine and all the manifestations of acute intermittent porphyria may develop (acute phase). Porphyria cutanea tarda hereditaria is not an entirely suitable name for this disorder since not all patients develop cutaneous lesions. It is for this reason that the designation *porphyria variegata* has been suggested.

Porphyria Cutanea Tarda Symptomatica

This type of porphyria is characterized clinically by cutaneous lesions, hyperpigmentation of the skin, evidences of liver disease, and hypertrichosis; and chemically, by the excretion of large amounts of uroporphyrin and lesser amounts of copropor-

phyrin in the urine. Abdominal pain and neurologic complications are conspicuously absent. The urine does not contain increased quantities of Δ-aminolevulinic acid or porphobilinogen. The excretion of protoporphyrin in the feces is normal; the excretion of coproporphyrin in the feces is usually within normal limits but in a few patients may be slightly increased.

The skin lesions are indistinguishable from those observed in porphyria cutanea tarda hereditaria. The skin is unusually sensitive both to light and to mechanical trauma. Blisters appear on the exposed skin areas, frequently ulcerate, and finally lead to scar formation. The photosensitivity is similar to that in erythropoietic porphyria but not as marked.

This disorder is probably acquired and has been described (1) in male subjects, forty to seventy years of age, with alcoholic cirrhosis of the liver; (2) in Bantu subjects in South Africa with nutritional cirrhosis of the liver; (3) in children and adults in Turkey who have ingested the fungicide, hexachlorobenzene; (4) in three elderly subjects with a tumor of the liver; and (5) in an occasional young adult without a history of alcoholism or drug exposure.

Experimental Porphyria

A condition resembling in many respects porphyria erythropoietica in human beings has been produced experimentally in rats, rabbits, and chickens by the administration of lead, phenylhydrazine, or the dye rose bengal, as well as by excessive exposure to sunlight. A bovine form of porphyria erythropoietica, inherited as a recessive trait, has been recognized and studied in some detail.

Table 91-2. DISTINGUISHING FEATURES OF THE SEVERAL TYPES OF PORPHYRIA

Characteristics	Erythropoietic porphyria	Hepatic porphyria				
		Acute intermittent		Cutanea tarda hereditaria		Cutanea tarda symptomatica
Inheritance	Recessive	Dominant		Dominant		Acquired
Sex	Both	Both		Both		Both
Age of onset	0–5 yr	15–40 yr		10–30 yr		Any age
Phase of disease	....	Latent	Acute	Latent	Acute	
Cutaneous lesions	++++	0	0	0	+ or 0	+
Abdominal colic, psychoses, and/or neurologic disease	0	0	+	0	+	0
Urine Δ-ALA	N	++	++++	N	++	N
Urine PBG	N	++	++++	N	++	N
Uroporphyrinuria	++++	++	++	N	+++	++++
Coproporphyrinuria	++	++	++	N	+++	++
Fecal porphyrins	++	N	+	++++	+++	N

0, absent; N, normal; +, increased; ++++, greatly increased.

Δ-ALA = Δ-aminolevulinic acid; PBG = porphobilinogen.

A condition resembling porphyria hepatica of the acute intermittent type has been produced in animals and in chick embryos by the administration of the sedative Sedormid (allyl-isopropyl-acetyl-carbamide).

REFERENCES

Barnes, H. D.: The Excretion of Porphyrins and Porphyrin Precursors by Bantu Cases of Porphyria, South African Med. J., 33:274, 1959.

Dean, G., and H. D. Barnes: Porphyria in Sweden and South Africa, South African Med. J., 33:246, 1959.

Vannotti, A.: "Porphyrins, Their Biological and Chemical Importance," London, Hilger & Watts, 1954.

Waldenström, J.: The Porphyrias as Inborn Errors of Metabolism, Am. J. Med., 22:758, 1957.

Watson, C. J.: Porphyria, vol. 5, p. 235, in "Advances in Internal Medicine," W. Dock and I. Snapper (Eds.), Chicago, Year Book Publishers, Inc., 1954.

Wolstenhölme, G. E. W., and E. C. P. Millar: "Ciba Foundation Symposium on Porphyrin Biosynthesis and Metabolism," Boston, Little, Brown & Company, 1955.

92 GOUT
Warren E. Wacker
and George W. Thorn

History. Gout is an inherited disturbance of uric acid metabolism characterized by acute arthritic episodes and the eventual deposition of uric acid crystals in various tissues. It has been recognized since ancient times, being mentioned in the writings of Hippocrates. The name is derived from the Latin *gutta*, a drop, signifying the presence of noxious drops (of uric acid) in the joints. Uric acid was first associated with gout by Scheele in 1776 through the demonstration of its presence in urine; Wollaston shortly thereafter identified it in a renal calculus obtained from a gouty patient. The hyperuricemia of gout was discovered by Garrod in 1848. Emil Fischer derived the structural formula of uric acid, while Folin developed the first adequate method for its measurement.

Incidence. Gout is not rare; in the United States almost a half a million persons are estimated to be afflicted with the disease. In careful genealogic studies the familial incidence is found to be as high as 75 per cent. In addition to clinical gout, however, the incidence of asymptomatic hyperuricemia is even higher in the families of gouty patients. The defect in uric acid metabolism is probably due to a single autosomal dominant gene, clinical gout occurring in a small percentage of

heterozygotes. Clinical gout occurs chiefly in males, only about 5 per cent of patients being females; the incidence of asymptomatic hyperuricemia is much more nearly the same in both sexes. In women clinical gout is rare before the menopause, while the most frequent age of onset for men is in the third and fourth decades. The infrequent occurrence in women probably represents an altered expression of the defect rather than a sex-linked genetic process. The common perception that gout is due to overindulgence in food and wine is without basis in fact.

Etiology. Gout represents the accumulation of large amounts of uric acid, identified by an increased concentration in serum, an increased total body uric acid pool, and in advanced gout by the precipitation of urates in various tissues.

In man uric acid is the end product of purine metabolism. The two purines, adenine and guanine, are present in the body chiefly as components of the nucleic acids, ribonucleic acid (RNA) and deoxyribonucleic acid (DNA). Normally two purine sources are responsible for uric acid production, purines obtained by the hydrolysis of ingested nucleic acids and those obtained by the hydrolysis of endogenous nucleic acids. Uric acid, 2-6-8 trioxypurine, is formed by the stepwise enzymatic oxidation of adenine and guanine. The further degradation of uric acid to allantoin appears not to occur in man though it does in most other mammalian species; however, there is evidence that limited uricolysis may occur in man, although the biochemical mechanism is currently unknown.

The accumulation of uric acid in patients with gout (Fig. 92-1) may come about through several possible mechanisms: simple overingestion of dietary nucleic acid has been excluded; a constantly increased degradation of endogenous nucleic acids, while occurring in patients with gout secondary to diseases associated with an excessive cell destruction, sufficient to provide this amount of nucleic acid, such as polycythemia vera, leukemia, or lymphoma, has been ruled out as a cause of primary gout; direct overproduction of uric acid from simple purine precursors or an impedance of the normal excretory process are the remaining possibilities.

The biochemical pathways of uric acid synthesis have been elucidated in detail; it is formed from several simple precursors, glycine, aspartic acid, CO_2, and glutamine. Uric acid is normally derived from the degradation of purines previously incorporated into nucleic acids; however, in some patients with primary gout there exists an alternate pathway for the direct synthesis of uric acid, which does not involve prior incorporation into nucleic acid. The rate and extent of incorporation of isotopically labeled glycine into urinary uric acid has

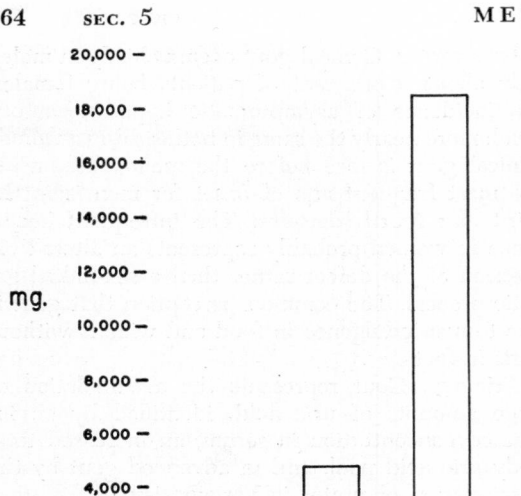

FIG. 92-1. Uric acid pool in normal and gouty persons.

been employed to demonstrate this abnormal mechanism. In some patients with gout fed isotopically labeled glycine a greater amount appears in urinary uric acid; the rapid rate of appearance of the isotope precludes the possibility that the labeled uric acid is derived from the normal degradation of nucleic acid purines. The accumulation of uric acid in these patients may thus be explained on the basis of an abnormal *increased synthesis*. The enzymatic defect(s) responsible for the shunt mechanism are not known; however, an abnormality in purine biosynthesis in patients with gout is revealed by an altered excretory pattern of several purine compounds, 8-hydroxy-7-methylguanine, and 6-succinoaminopurine.

Abnormal synthesis of uric acid, however, does not occur in all patients with primary gout; it appears to be limited to those who excrete an excessive amount of uric acid in the urine. In many patients, despite an elevated serum uric acid content, the urinary acid excretion does not exceed the normal range of 300 to 600 mg per 24 hr. In these patients it is not possible to demonstrate increased synthesis as measured by the incorporation of N^{15} labeled glycine into uric acid, suggesting instead an impairment of the excretory mechanism. The only significant mechanism for the excretion of uric acid is the renal pathway. It appears that uric acid is excreted largely by tubular secretion, most, if not all, of that filtered by the glomerulus being reabsorbed. The ability of chlorothiazide and pyrizinamide to cause hyperuricemia through an alteration of the renal excretory process strongly supports

the concept of tubular secretion. In a converse fashion so does the occurrence of hypouricemia in Wilson's disease and the de Toni–Fanconi syndrome, diseases characterized by other known renal tubular defects. Therefore in those patients with primary gout in whom it is impossible to demonstrate increased synthesis and the concomitant hyperexcretion of uric acid, an abnormality of the tubular secretory mechanism may represent the primary pathologic defect. This hypothesis is supported by the observation that the renal clearance of uric acid in these gouty patients is much lower than that achieved by normal persons in whom the plasma uric acid concentration has been raised artificially by the administration of urate precursors.

Thus there are at least two biochemical defects which can be responsible for the occurrence of primary gout: a defect in purine biosynthesis leading to a direct overproduction of uric acid, and an abnormal renal tubular secretory mechanism for uric acid. They may operate independently or jointly.

There is a simple relationship between the clinical manifestations of chronic tophaceous gout and the biochemical alterations leading to an increase in plasma uric acid and the total body uric acid pool. Uric acid is quite insoluble and therefore precipitates to form tophi in the joints, bones, cartilage, kidneys, and other soft tissue. In the pathogenesis of acute gouty arthritis, however, such a simple relationship does not exist. Acute gouty arthritis does not correlate with the degree of hyperuricemia, nor does it occur in normal persons whose plasma uric acid is raised artificially. This lack of correlation has led to the concept that acute gouty arthritis is caused by the evanescent presence of some as yet unidentified product of purine metabolism. The absence of gout in patients with renal failure having marked hyperuricemia is cited to support this hypothesis. It should be pointed out, however, that clinical gout appears to occur simply as a result of the hyperuricemia secondary to polycythemia or leukemia.

Pathology. The pathognomonic lesion of gout is the deposit of sodium urate crystals resulting in inflammatory and eventual degenerative changes. The lesions occur chiefly in joints, bones, bursae, and cartilaginous structures. The marked insolubility of urates at the acid pH characteristic of these tissues may account for the preferential precipitation at these sites. Any joint may be affected; however, those of the lower extremities, and chiefly those of the great toe, are favored. Urate deposits occur in the articular cartilage and periarticular structures, causing bone destruction, joint narrowing, degeneration of the synovium, bony ankylosis and exostoses. The precipitates in nonarticular tissues are called tophi, meaning "chalkstones." The cartilage of the ears, the tendons, the tarsal plates of the eyes, and the olecranon and patellar bursae are the most common locations. Urates also precipitate in the collecting tubules of the kidney, leading to obstruction and pyelonephritis. Glomerular fibrosis, arteriolar and arterial nephrosclerosis are invariably present to some extent in the kidneys of patients with gouty nephropathy. Arteriosclerosis, with its attendant hypertension and cardiac hypertrophy, occurs more frequently in patients with gout than in others of comparable age.

Clinical Picture. Gout is often unrecognized in its early stages before the obvious destructive changes of chronic tophaceous gout have appeared. Its onset is characterized by acute attacks of joint pain with intervals of complete well-being. Later, the intervals become progressively shorter until the final state of persistent, deforming arthritis is reached.

Acute Gout. Acute arthritis usually heralds the disease although occasionally renal colic, from urate stones, may be the initial manifestation. The metatarsophalangeal joint of the great toe is the primary site of attack in 60 per cent of cases, according to Scudamore (Fig. 92-2); frequently the arthritis is bilateral. Other common sites in the order of their frequency include the instep, ankle, heel, knee, and hand. Acute attacks are often preceded by a stressful or traumatic episode, i.e., mild physical trauma to the joint, acute infection, surgery, cold exposure, injection of foreign protein or drugs such as mercurials, epinephrine, ergotamine, or liver extract. The onset of acute joint pain in a male patient following surgery should immediately raise the possibility of an acute episode of gout. Attacks may also be associated with sudden changes in atmospheric pressure. The attack often occurs several hours before midnight, awakening the patient from sleep. Some patients are able to recognize that an attack is imminent by a mild sensation of burning, tingling, numbness, or warmth in the affected joint. Often, however, the attack begins suddenly, the joint becoming swollen, tender, violaceous in color, and excruciatingly painful. Lymphangitis and true cellulitis are rare complications. The involvement may be monarticular or of a migratory polyarticular type. General malaise, headache, tachycardia, and fever associated with an elevated leukocyte count and erythrocyte sedimentation rate and an elevated serum uric acid concentration complete the clinical picture. The duration of the attack is a function of the time before the initiation of therapy and of its effectiveness. Untreated, an acute episode may last 2 weeks.

Interval Gout. Early in the course of the disease symptom-free periods between acute attacks may vary from months to years. As the disease progresses, however, the asymptomatic periods become

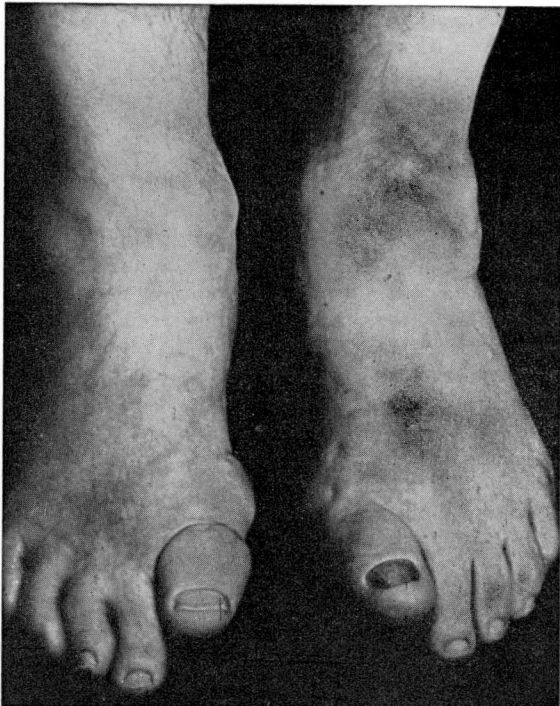

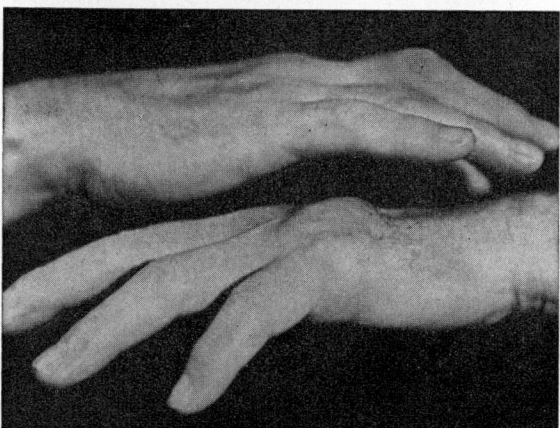

Fig. 92-2. (*Upper*) Appearance of feet in chronic gout. Note swelling of the great toes as well as subcutaneous deposits of uric acid opposite the first metatarsal joint. (*Lower*) Appearance of hands in chronic gout. Note joint enlargement due to deposits of uric acid.

shorter and shorter until finally persistent deforming arthritis appears.

Chronic Gout. This stage of the disease occurs after a variable period of time; it is characterized by irreversible, deforming changes in the joint spaces, capsules, tendons, and bursae. Tophi in the cartilaginous structures and subcutaneous tissues are usually present. Ankylosis, multiple draining sinus tracts, and complete crippling inactivation are the hallmarks of the final stages of untreated gout.

Complications. Renal disease, secondary to the deposition of urates in the kidney parenchyma, is the major, direct, serious complication of gout. Although autopsy studies indicate that renal damage is present to some degree in most patients with the disease, severe renal failure does not occur in more than 10 per cent of patients. Clinically the earliest manifestation of gouty renal disease is albuminuria, which may persist for several decades before nitrogen retention ensues. The terminal stage of gouty renal disease is the uremic syndrome with its attendant hypertension and anemia. Secondary pyelonephritis causing additional renal impairment is a frequent occurrence in gout.

About 20 per cent of patients with gout have a history of renal colic. Most frequently the stones are composed entirely of urate salts; however, they may have a mixed composition consisting of calcium phosphate or oxalate as well as urate. The passage of urate stones may be the first indication of the disease. The complete combustion of a urate stone in a flame allows its differentiation from a calcium stone which imparts a brick red color to the flame.

Hypertension and atherosclerosis occurring at an earlier age than in the normal population are quite common in patients with gout and are reflected in a high incidence of myocardial infarction in young males with the disease.

Diagnosis. Acute gouty arthritis is easily recognized by its explosive onset. The severe pain and exquisite tenderness of the affected joint, the elevated serum uric acid concentration (greater than 6 mg per 100 ml in males), and the rapid response to treatment with colchicine, a drug which fails to alter the course of other types of arthritis, confirms the diagnosis. The disease, however, is frequently overlooked in the interval phases. Specific interrogation of all patients who complain of arthritic symptoms will prevent misdiagnosis in most instances. Since gout is the only variety of chronic arthritis for which an effective form of therapy is known, it is important to recognize the disease as early as possible. The most valuable clues are a family history of gout (or rheumatism), a delayed onset of acute joint symptoms following mild trauma, or the passage of renal stones.

Chronic gout may be diagnosed by the presence of deposited urates, either as tophi in soft tissue or in the joints and bursae. Removal of the chalky contents of a tophus and the chemical identification of the material as sodium urate provide an absolute diagnosis of gout. Roentgenologic changes in affected joints are often lacking in the early stages of gout. The typical roentgenologic finding is a punched out, destructive lesion representing a urate deposit (Fig. 92-3). Narrowing and destruction of the joint spaces also occur. The extent of these processes depends, of course, on the stage of the disease.

Although an elevated serum uric acid concentration (6.0 mg per 100 ml in males; 5.0 mg per 100 ml in females) is a necessary accompaniment of gout, it is not pathognomonic. Hyperuricemia also occurs secondary to renal disease; for this reason the blood urea nitrogen should be determined simultaneously with the serum uric acid. In patients with renal disease hyperuricemia will corre-

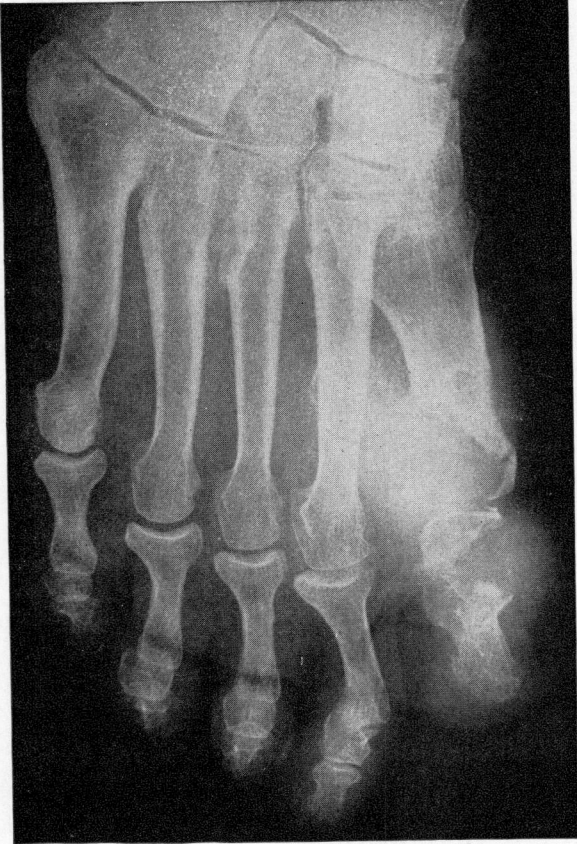

FIG. 92-3. X-ray of a foot in a case of chronic gout. Note marked destruction of the first and second metatarsal joints and adjacent punched-out areas of diminished density.

Table 92-1. SERUM URIC ACID AND BLOOD UREA NITROGEN LEVELS IN PATIENTS WITH GOUT AND NEPHRITIS

	Normal	Gout	Nephritis
Serum uric acid (mg per 100 ml).............	2–5	8	6
Blood urea nitrogen (mg per 100 ml)..........	8–15	15	45

late with the increased blood urea nitrogen (Table 92-1).

Differential Diagnosis. Acute gout must be differentiated from acute rheumatic fever, rheumatoid arthritis, infectious arthritis, osteoarthritis, cellulitis, bursitis, tendonitis, and thrombophlebitis. Palindromic arthritis in women, manifested by episodes of acute arthritis with periods of complete remission, is unusually similar to gout. All these conditions are excluded by the presence of hyperuricemia and the response to colchicine.

Secondary Gout. The accumulation of uric acid by a direct increase of nucleic acid catabolism occurs in patients with hematologic disorders chiefly polycythemia, leukemia, or lymphoma. Acute gout may actually represent the first clinical manifestation of the underlying disease.

Treatment. The knowledge that the metabolic abnormalities of gout result in an accumulation of uric acid provides the basis for the long-term therapy of this disease; the potentiation of uric acid excretion. Therapy, however, may be separated conveniently into the treatment of the acute attack, of chronic gout, of interval gout, and of the azotemia secondary to progressive renal involvement.

Acute Gouty Arthritis. Colchicine remains the best drug for the treatment of acute gout. To be maximally effective, treatment should be started as early in the course of an attack as is possible. The drug should be administered according to the following schedule: 0.5 to 0.6 mg every hour until the arthritis abates or gastrointestinal side effects, consisting of nausea, vomiting, or diarrhea, appear. The maximum tolerable dose ranges from 4 to 10 mg; since it varies from person to person it must be established empirically for each individual. The distressing diarrhea, if encountered, may be controlled with tincture of opium. To avoid therapeutic failure it is important to continue the hourly dosage schedule until the maximum dose has been given.

Phenylbutazone is also effective in treating acute gout, but its chief use is in the management of patients who have not responded to colchicine, often because of inadequate dosage. Following an initial dose of 0.4 Gm, 0.1 Gm four times a day should be given for 2 to 3 days. The serious toxicities of phenylbutazone are infrequent when it is given for this short period of time. The risk is not, however, entirely eliminated.

Adrenocorticotropic hormone (ACTH) as well as being a potent uricosuric agent is also effective in the treatment of acute gout; 100 mg ACTH gel should be administered daily until symptoms subside. The dose should then be decreased gradually over the next several days to prevent an exacerbation due to sudden withdrawal of adrenal stimulation. Cortisone and its analogues may also be employed, but are said to be less effective than ACTH. ACTH and cortisone may also be used to minimize undue gastrointestinal sensitivity to colchicine.

Supportive therapy consists of bed rest and immobilization of the affected joint. In contrast, however, to other forms of acute arthritis, mobilization may be allowed as soon as the joint is no longer painful. Codeine may be used if pain is severe. Sufficient fluids to correct dehydration should be given.

Chronic Gout. Since the precipitation of urate crystals is responsible for the deforming arthritis of chronic gout, the major therapeutic goal must be the mobilization and excretion of excess urate. The discovery of several potent uricosuric agents (probenecid, zoxazolamine, and sulfinpyrazone) has provided the means to achieve this goal. These drugs promote the excretion of uric acid by a direct effect on the kidney, preventing the reabsorption of uric acid from the glomerular filtrate.

Probenecid has been used extensively and is known to have a very low order of serious toxicity. On this basis it may be considered the optimal uricosuric agent. It should be given in amounts varying between 1.0 and 2.0 Gm a day in divided doses. Initially a dose of 1 Gm a day will prevent the precipitation of uric acid crystals in the renal tubules during the course of the initial excretion of large amounts of excess urate. For the same reason all patients, throughout the course of therapy, should maintain a high fluid intake (2.5 to 3 liters per day). Patients having a history of urate stones may be treated with sodium citrate to alkalinize the urine and render uric acid more soluble.

Probenecid prevents the extension of the disease, reducing the size of tophi and the deposits of urate in the joints. Since uricosuric drugs do not alter the deranged biochemical mechanisms responsible for primary gout, therapy, to be successful, must be continuous. Salicylates antagonize the uricosuric action of these agents; therefore the two drugs should not be given concomitantly.

Strict dietary limitations have not been beneficial in the management of gout; only those few foods containing a large amount of purine should be prohibited (Table 92-2).

Although uricosuric therapy ultimately diminishes the attack rate of acute gout, initially it is unaltered; therefore, therapy to prevent acute attacks is indicated. Colchicine, in doses of 0.5 to 2

Table 92-2. FOODS WITH HIGH PURINE CONTENT*

Sweetbreads	Liver
Anchovies	Kidneys
Sardines	Meat extracts

* Not allowed in diet of patients with gout.

mg a day, represents the optimal therapy for the prevention of acute gout. In this instance a modest dose of cortisone, i.e., 50 mg per day, may permit an effective therapeutic dose of colchicine to be given and will also enable patients to continue combined colchicine and Benemid prophylactic or interval therapy. The necessary dose should be established for each patient such that while it is therapeutically adequate it does not cause gastrointestinal side effects. Continuous combined therapy with a potent uricosuric agent and colchicine provides a simple, effective program which prevents the disabling consequences of gout.

Surgical treatment may occasionally be employed to remove large, painful subcutaneous tophi, discharging sinuses associated with a tophaceous deposit, and to repair the consequences of extensive osseous involvement of the fingers and toes.

Prophylaxis. Hyperuricemia occurs frequently in relatives of patients with gout; however, a relatively small number of these individuals develop symptomatic gout. It is accepted that those who develop clinical gout should be treated. There is, however, no universal agreement concerning the management of patients with asymptomatic hyperuricemia. The facts concerning the prophylactic treatment of affected relatives are as follows:

1. The incapacitating and potentially lethal effects of gout are *certainly* caused by the deposition of uric acid.

2. The accumulation of uric acid, reflected by *hyperuricemia,* can be prevented by a safe and simple program of drug therapy.

Therefore to prevent the disease, relatives of patients with gout having significant elevations of the concentration of uric acid in serum (above 8 mg per 100 ml) should be treated with a uricosuric drug. To be successful such a program of preventive medicine *requires* the full understanding and cooperation of the patient and the recognition by the physician of the absolute necessity for frequent, detailed, and continued close observation.

REFERENCES

Buchanan, J. M.: The Enzymatic Synthesis of the Purine Nucleotides, Harvey Lecture Series, 14:104, 1960.

Combined Staff Clinic: Metabolic and Clinical Aspects of Gout, Am. J. Med., 22:807, 1957.

Nugent, C. A., and F. H. Tyler: The Renal Excretion of Uric Acid in Patients with Gout and in Nongouty Subjects, J. Clin. Invest., 38:1890, 1959.

Seegmiller, J. E., and A. I. Grayzel: Use of the New Uricosuric Agents in the Management of Gout, J.A.M.A., 173:1076, 1960.

Stetten, D., Jr.: Recent Contributions to the Understanding of the Metabolic Defect in Gout, Geriatrics, 9:163, 1954.

Talbott, J. H.: "Gout," New York, Grune & Stratton, 1957.

—— and K. L. Terplan: The Kidney in Gout, Medicine, 39:405, 1960.

Weissmann, B., and A. B. Gutman: The Identification of 6-Succino-aminopurine and 8-Hydroxy-7-methylguanine as Normal Urinary Constituents, J. Biol. Chem., 229:239, 1958.

Yu, T. F., B. Weissmann, L. Sharney, S. Kupfer, and A. B. Gutman: On the Biosynthesis of Uric Acid from Glycine N^{15} in Primary and Secondary Polycythemia, Am. J. Med., 21:901, 1956.

93 HEPATOLENTICULAR DEGENERATION (Wilson's Disease)

George E. Cartwright

Definition. Hepatolenticular degeneration (progressive lenticular degeneration, Wilson's disease, pseudosclerosis of Westphal and Strümpell, tetanoid chorea of Gowers) is an uncommon, familial, progressive, fatal disease which becomes manifest usually in the first three decades of life and is characterized by the triad of basal ganglion degeneration, cirrhosis of the liver, and a ring of brown pigment at the corneal margins known as the Kayser-Fleischer ring.

History. Kinnier Wilson, in 1912, in his classic monograph, "Progressive Lenticular Degeneration," first clearly defined the disease entity to which his name is now affixed. A similar condition had previously been described in 1883 by Westphal and later by Strümpell. The symptoms resembled those of multiple sclerosis, but no demyelinative plaques were observed. For that reason it was called *pseudosclerosis.* The cirrhosis of the liver was overlooked until Spielmeyer reexamined the cases many years later. His studies and the clinical observations of Hall left little doubt that hepatolenticular degeneration and pseudosclerosis were the same disease. The corneal ring was described in 1902 by Kayser in a case diagnosed as "multiple sclerosis," but to Fleischer is due the credit for appreciating its significance in relation to the disease as it is now known.

A marked increase in the copper content of both the brain and the liver was demonstrated by Haurowitz in 1930 and was later confirmed by Glazebrook and Cummings. Mandelbrote and his associates in 1948 observed by chance that the urinary output of copper was high and that this output is increased by the administration of BAL. In the same year Uzman and Denny-Brown found that a persistent aminoaciduria is associated with the disease.

Inheritance. The condition is inherited as an autosomal recessive trait, the affected individuals inheriting the gene from both parents who, while phenotypically normal, are heterozygous for the abnormal allele. Since the frequency of the abnormal gene is low in the general population, affected individuals may be expected to be, most often, the products of consanguineous marriages. This has proved to be the case.

Pathogenesis. Two different types of metabolic disturbance have been described, viz., (1) abnormalities in the metabolism of copper and (2) impairment in renal tubular reabsorption.

A number of alterations in the metabolism of copper has been described (Table 93-1). The amount of copper in the tissues, particularly in the liver and brain, is increased about tenfold above the normal. The golden-brown pigment of the Kayser-Fleischer ring contains copper. The amount of copper excreted in the urine is increased. The specific copper protein of plasma, ceruloplasmin, is almost invariably decreased. On the other hand, the "direct-reacting" fraction of plasma copper, the copper which is probably loosely bound to albumin, is increased. Since there is a greater reduction in ceruloplasmin copper than there is increase in direct-reacting copper, the net effect on the total plasma copper is such that there is usually hypocupremia. In an occasional patient the total plasma copper may be as high as 100 μg per 100 ml. Patients with this disease retain more than the normal amount of copper in the body. This is apparently because of an increased rate of absorption of copper from the gastrointestinal tract. Whether or not copper is excreted by the liver into the bile at the normal rate has not yet been determined with certainty. There may be a normal copper content in the bile, but this is not normal when the total copper content of the liver is considered.

Renal dysfunction which is present in many, but not all, patients include abnormalities in tubular reabsorption manifested by aminoaciduria, peptiduria, proteinuria, glucosuria, uricosuria, or phosphaturia. The aminoaciduria involves most of the amino acids found in normal urine and, in addition, proline and citrulline. Taurine, aspartic acid, isoleucine, methyl histidine, and arginine are excreted in amounts close to the normal range. The urinary amino acid pattern and the severity of the aminoaciduria depend in part upon the amount and type of protein ingested and vary considerably from patient to patient without relation to the type, duration, or stage of disease. The aminoaciduria is not accompanied by any significant elevation in the blood α-amino nitrogen level. The uricosuria may be associated with a diminished level of uric acid in the serum. The phosphaturia may result in hypophosphatemia and eventually in osseous changes.

Table 93-1. BIOCHEMICAL ALTERATIONS IN WILSON'S DISEASE

Chemical findings	Normal subjects	Wilson's disease
Total plasma copper, μg/100 ml.	114 (79–149)	61 (19–103)
Direct-reacting plasma copper, μg/100 ml	7 (0–21)	26 (12–40)
Ceruloplasmin, mg/100 ml.	34 (23–44)	9 (0–19)
Urine copper, μg/24 hr	10 (0–23)	522 (95–1,300)*
Liver copper, μg/Gm wet tissue	5 (3–10)*	79 (53–100)*
Urine α-amino nitrogen, mg/day	164 (118–204)	337 (90–519)

The figures in parentheses refer to ± 2 standard deviations.

* Range.

The pathogenesis of the metabolic and pathologic changes is not fully understood. Because of the excessive deposition of copper in the tissues of patients with Wilson's disease, it has been suggested that the lesions in the liver and in the lenticular nuclei are the consequence of the excessive deposition of copper in these tissues and that the accumulation of copper in the kidney causes a functional impairment in the reabsorption of amino acids, peptides, and other substances. In support of this concept is the observation that excessive deposition of copper in the liver precedes the development of significant parenchymal damage. In at least some patients with the disease, the mobilization of copper from the body is apparently associated with dramatic improvement in the clinical state of the patient.

Copper absorbed from the gastrointestinal tract enters first into the direct-reacting fraction of plasma copper. Therefore, the increase in this fraction reflects the increased turnover of copper between the gastrointestinal tract, the tissues, and the excretory routes. The copper in this fraction is easily dissociable from the albumin, and the increase in the direct-reacting fraction probably accounts for the increased excretion of copper by the kidneys.

The most widely held concept of the disease is that the inherited defect is an inability to synthesize ceruloplasmin. However, some individuals heterozygous for the gene may have as low a ceruloplasmin concentration as some patients with the disease. Furthermore, there is a poor correlation between the ceruloplasmin level and the severity or duration of the disease. An additional difficulty with this theory is that a mechanism whereby a deficiency of ceruloplasmin can lead to excessive tissue deposits of copper is not known.

Another theory which has been proposed is that the genetically determined abnormality in protein metabolism results in the formation of abnormal tissue proteins which have a high avidity for copper. The difficulty with this theory is that it does not explain the low concentrations of the plasma copper protein, ceruloplasmin.

Pathology. The characteristic pathologic findings are in the liver and the brain. The liver is usually small, firm, and coarsely nodular. It may or may not be bile stained. Nodules of regenerating liver cells are separated by trabeculae of fibrous connective tissue. The picture is that of healed subacute yellow atrophy or the nonalcoholic variety of Laennec's cirrhosis. The most striking gross finding in the brain is cavitation of the putamen on each side and rarely of cerebral cortex and white matter. In many cases, probably more than half, the putamen and caudate nuclei are atrophic and of light, grayish-brown color, and there is no evidence of cavitation. Microscopic examination almost invariably reveals a remarkable hyperplasia of protoplasmic astrocytes in the cerebral cortex, lenticular and caudate nuclei, subthalamic nuclei of Luys, substantia nigra, dentate and red nuclei. Nerve cell loss is widespread but is most pronounced in the lenticular and dentate nuclei and cerebral cortex. The protoplasmic astrocytosis does not differ from that observed in cases of hepatic coma. Splenomegaly is a common finding.

Clinical Manifestations. The disease usually begins in adolescence, but it may appear as early as the age of four or as late as age forty. The mode of onset is somewhat variable. In a few cases the first manifestation is related to liver insufficiency, i.e., jaundice, ascites, or splenomegaly. More often the initial symptom is related to the neurologic system: tremor, dysarthria, ataxia, incoordination, or personality change. The disease may run an acute course of several months' duration associated with fever, rapid emaciation, and mental deterioration, or an extremely chronic afebrile course of 30 or 40 years' duration. The usual course is 5 to 10 years.

The clinical picture of a well-developed case is quite characteristic. *Tremor* of one or both of the upper extremities is an outstanding as well as an early manifestation. The tremor consists of regular, rhythmic, alternating contractions and may occur in the earliest stages only on movement of the extremity. Later it is also present when the arm is maintained in an attitude of repose. It is accentuated by excitement or by attention being drawn to it. One of the most certain ways of demonstrating the tremor is by having the patient extend the arms in front of the body. In this position "flapping" or "wing-beating" may be noted. The tremor may also increase during fine volitional movements, taking a form that resembles intention tremor. Indeed, in some cases cerebellar ataxia and tremor are the principal neurologic manifestations. In severe cases a tremor of the mandible or even of the entire head is present. *Abnormal movements* of choreic or choreoathetoid type are present in some patients but are not frequent. *Rigidity* of the skeletal muscles, often reaching an extreme degree, is another characteristic. The rigidity may be intermittent or constant, and the resulting clinical state may vary from transient spasms in the acute cases to permanent *contractures* and *deformities* in the chronic. In the late stages of the disease the facial muscles become set in a stiff, vacuous smile, the neck and trunk become rigid, the upper extremities are held rigidly in flexion at the elbow, wrist, and metacarpal joints, and the lower extremities are held in a position of extension. *Dysarthria* or even anarthria in advanced cases is an almost constant finding. *Cachexia* and muscular wasting may be extreme. Some form of *mental disturbance* is common, and in severely affected patients changes in character and personality and terminally marked mental deterioration may be present. The sensory system is intact and the reflexes are essentially normal. Pyramidal signs are usually absent.

The clinical course of the liver disease is extremely variable. In many patients signs of liver insufficiency are completely lacking, even though the liver function tests are abnormal and cirrhosis can be demonstrated by needle biopsy. In other patients the signs of liver insufficiency, such as splenomegaly, ascites, jaundice, hepatomegaly, hematemesis, and spider angiomas, dominate the clinical picture. When liver function is markedly impaired, anemia, leukopenia, and thrombocytopenia may be found to accompany the splenomegaly.

The most remarkable, unique and consistent feature of the disease is the Kayser-Fleischer ring (Plate I, facing p. 416), a golden-brown or greenish-brown ring of pigment located at the periphery of the cornea in Descemet's membrane. The pigment usually goes completely around the cornea; occasionally there may be only a crescent-shaped distribution. Although the rings are frequently visible in ordinary light, in the early stages of the disease or in patients in whom the color of the iris is brown, it may be necessary to use a slit lamp to visualize the rings. Under slit-lamp examination, the ring is seen to be composed of a multitude of granular specks. When present the rings are pathognomonic of the disease. Since the metabolic changes in Wilson's disease have been recognized, there has not been a single patient with the disease reported without Kayser-Fleischer rings. The presence of the rings is a more reliable and consistent feature of the disease than any single one of the biochemical alterations.

Skeletal abnormality, manifested by roentgenographic evidences of osteomalacia, cartilage injury, or bone fragmentation, is a frequent finding in the disease. Azure lunulas, bluish crescent areas at the nail bases, have been observed in several patients.

Diagnosis. The triad of Kayser-Fleischer rings, cirrhosis of the liver, and signs of basal ganglion disease is pathognomonic of this condition.

The various clinical findings combine to form several different clinical pictures, the most frequent of which is Parkinson's syndrome. Occasionally cerebellar ataxia, chorea, choreoathetosis, or dystonia predominates. If signs of liver insufficiency are not evident from physical examination, liver function studies or needle biopsy of the liver will demonstrate the presence of liver disease. Rubeanic acid stain may be used to demonstrate the excessive deposition of copper. In young patients in whom neurologic disease is not manifest and the signs of liver disease are marked, the condition has been confused with "juvenile" or "familial" cirrhosis.

The presence of hypocupremia, hypoceruloplasminemia, hypercupruria, and hyperaminoaciduria confirms the diagnosis, although it is rarely necessary to perform the difficult laboratory examinations in order to establish the diagnosis. In a rare patient with the disease, hypocupremia and hypoceruloplasminemia may not be present. Hypocupremia and hypoceruloplasminemia may be present in some normal individuals who are heterozygous for the gene. These two biochemical alterations are also present in all normal newborn infants and in at least some patients with kwashiorkor, sprue, celiac disease, and the nephrotic syndrome. Hypercupruria may be present only in the last condition mentioned. Hypercupruria may be present in patients with alcoholic cirrhosis of the liver, but the copper excreted rarely exceeds 200 μg per day; in this condition the concentration of copper and ceruloplasmin in the plasma is either normal or increased.

Prognosis. The disease is progressive and invariably fatal if untreated. It is still too early to know for certain if death can be prevented or delayed by the early continuous and energetic therapy outlined below. Death results from intercurrent infection or hepatic failure.

Treatment. The therapy of Wilson's disease is directed toward (1) the prevention of the continued accumulation of copper in the body and (2) the removal of copper already deposited. Potassium sulfide (potash sulfurated technical, 20 mg three times daily with meals) prevents the absorption of copper by the formation of insoluble, unabsorbable copper sulfide in the gut. No undesirable side effects have been observed when such therapy has been given continuously for periods up to 5 years. The administration of copper-chelating agents such as BAL (2,3-dimercaptopropanol), amino acids, Versenate (calcium disodium salt of ethylenediaminetetraacetic acid), or penicillamine (β,β-dimethyl cysteine), results in the mobilization of copper from the tissues and an increase in its excretion in the urine. Of the chelating agents, penicillamine is the most effective. D-Penicillamine, 1 to 4 Gm daily in four divided doses, on an empty stomach, should be given continuously for the lifetime of the patient. Fever, skin rashes, leukopenia, and thrombocytopenia may result from penicillamine therapy but are rarely sufficiently severe to require more than temporary cessation of therapy and gradual desensitization by the administration of increasing amounts of the agent. The L-form of penicillamine is a pyridoxine antagonist and theoretically could produce manifestation of pyridoxine deficiency. Such complications have not yet been observed in patients on long-term therapy. A diet high in protein promotes the urinary excretion of copper and may be of value in the treatment of the liver disease.

Therapy as outlined above has resulted in some degree of improvement in the clinical manifestations in about 1-month's time in some but not all patients. If mental changes are present they may revert toward normal, while the tremors and rigidity become less pronounced, sometimes to a remarkable degree. Improvement in liver function or in plasma copper aberrations are not observed with therapy. The partial remissions may last for months to years.

REFERENCES

Bearn, A. G., and H. G. Kunkel: Abnormalities of Cooper Metabolism in Wilson's Disease and Their Relationship to the Aminoaciduria, J. Clin. Invest., 33:400, 1954.

Bush, J. A., J. P. Mahoney, H. Markowitz, C. J. Gubler, G. E. Cartwright, and M. M. Wintrobe: Studies on Copper Metabolism: XVI. Radioactive Copper Studies in Normal Subjects and in Patients with Hepatolenticular Degeneration, J. Clin. Invest., 34:1766, 1955.

Cartwright, G. E., H. Markowitz, G. S. Shields, and M. M. Wintrobe: Studies on Copper Metabolism: XXIX. A Critical Analysis of Serum Copper and Ceruloplasmin Concentrations in Normal Subjects, Patients with Wilson's Disease and Relatives of Patients with Wilson's Disease, Am. J. Med., 28:555, 1960.

Scheinberg, I. H., and I. Sternlieb: The Pathogenesis and Clinical Significance of the Liver Disease in Hepatolenticular Degeneration (Wilson's Disease), Med. Clinics of N. Am., 44:665, 1960.

—— and ——: Environmental Treatment of an Hereditary Illness: Wilson's Disease, Ann. Internal Med.,
53:1151, 1960.

Wilson, S. A. K.: Progressive Lenticular Degeneration:
A Familial Nervous Disease Associated with Cirrhosis of the Liver, Brain, 34:395, 1912.

94 DISORDERS OF CARBOHYDRATE METABOLISM (Other than Diabetes Mellitus)

Albert E. Renold

A working scheme of intermediary metabolism
has been developed in Chap. 52, and its application to the interrelations of carbohydrate, fat, and
protein metabolism has been illustrated during the
discussion of diabetes mellitus (Chap. 70). In this
chapter, errors of carbohydrate metabolism other
than those occurring in diabetes will be briefly discussed and similarly related to the plan of intermediary metabolism. Since most of the defects to
be discussed concern the region between glucose
6-phosphate and glycogen, a region only briefly
outlined in Figs. 52-2 and 52-8, a somewhat more
detailed, still abbreviated, working scheme is presented in Fig. 94-1, which should serve as both
introduction and summary.

In the practice of medicine, most of the abnormalities to be discussed in this chapter present
either as problems of glycogen storage with hepatomegaly or hypoglycemia, or as problems in the
differential diagnosis of melituria. Accordingly, the
material will be grouped under these headings.

DISORDERS OF GLYCOGEN STORAGE AND MOBILIZATION

With continuing elucidation of the details of the
reactions involved in the synthesis and breakdown
of glycogen, biochemical as well as clinical characterization of several distinct disorders of glycogen
storage and mobilization has become possible. We
shall follow here the classification proposed by
Field as an extension of that previously introduced
by G. Cori, as summarized in Table 94-1.

The numbering system used can be directly
transferred to the localization of the defects in Fig.
94-1.

**Hepatorenal Glycogen Storage Disease with Hy-
poglycemia.** Von Gierke, in 1929, described a condition in children, characterized by enlargement of
the liver and kidneys, with excessive glycogen
deposition in the cells of these organs. The disorder is congenital, frequently familial, and appears to be transmitted as a mendelian recessive
characteristic. This is probably the most frequent
form of glycogen storage disease.

Pathology. The organs most severely involved are
the liver and kidneys. The liver is markedly enlarged, smooth, firm, and brownish in color. The
liver cells, which are enlarged up to three times
the normal size, are filled with glycogen and, frequently, fat. The kidneys may be increased to
twice the normal size, with excess glycogen in the
proximal tubules. Characteristically, glycogen may
be found in all these organs long after death, suggesting a greatly impaired rate of glycogenolysis.

Pathologic Physiology. Glucose is converted to
liver glycogen during and shortly after the ingestion of carbohydrate foods; in the fasting state,
liver glycogen is reconverted to glucose by a process known as glycogenolysis. The final step of

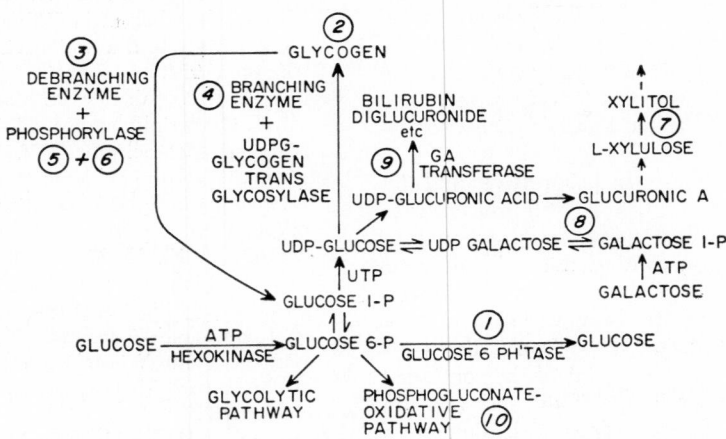

FIG. 94-1. Summary of metabolic pathways and metabolic lesions of carbohydrate metabolism, other than diabetes mellitus. The numbers are referred to in the text, excepting number 2 which indicates that, in cardiomegalic glycogen storage disease, glycogen is present in excessive amounts although no metabolic lesion has as
yet been detected.

hepatic glucose release is the hydrolysis of glucose 6-phosphate, a process catalyzed by the enzyme glucose 6-phosphatase (Fig. 94-1). In hepatorenal glycogen storage disease, glycogenolysis is abnormally slow, and *hepatic glucose 6-phosphatase activity* is absent or very low. In contrast *glycogen structure is normal.* Abnormally low glucose 6-phosphatase activity could account for most of the metabolic abnormalities which can be demonstrated in these patients. Thus, little or no elevation of blood glucose is observed following the injection of epinephrine or glucagon, and in the fasting state, *hypoglycemia* develops readily because of decreased rate of hepatic glucose release. Intravenously administered fructose or galactose, which for all intents and purposes is solely metabolized by the liver and is for the most part converted to blood glucose via glucose 6-phosphate, in the absence of glucose 6-phosphatase cannot appear in the blood as glucose. Ketonemia, lipemia, and ketonuria are frequent because of the relative unavailability of glycogen stores and the resultant tendency to hypoglycemia, which places an increased demand on the mobilization and utilization of fat for energy requirements. Marked lactacidosis occurs.

Clinical Picture. The patient with hepatorenal glycogen storage disease usually comes to medical attention during infancy or early childhood because of a markedly distended abdomen and delayed growth and development. Subjective complaints are infrequent despite severe hypoglycemia. Occasionally epileptiform seizures or vomiting occurs. The child is usually pale and undersized, with a fat face and neck, but with thin buttocks. The abdomen is markedly distended, with a huge liver. Ascites and splenomegaly are absent. Laboratory investigation reveals fasting hypoglycemia, ketonuria, anemia, and at times lipemia. The blood and white blood cell glycogen level may be elevated. After glucose ingestion or intravenous glucose infusion, the fall in blood glucose level is slower than normal. This pseudodiabetic curve is probably due to impaired storage of glucose as glycogen rather than to failure to utilize glucose normally in the periphery. Severe prolonged hypoglycemia may be induced by small doses of insulin. The liver function tests are usually normal. Final diagnosis is made by biochemical analysis of hepatic specimens obtained at biopsy.

In the past, most patients with this disorder have died during infancy or early childhood as a result of either hypoglycemia or intercurrent infections. However, earlier recognition, the availability of chemotherapy, and the possible effectiveness of dietary measures, together with administration of thyroxin, glucocorticoids, or glucagon in facilitating the stabilization of blood glucose levels, may well lead to considerably improved life expectancy. It is possible also that the disease tends to become less severe in those patients who survive beyond the first 5 years. Survival to thirty-two and thirty-eight years of two cases first reported in 1929 and 1932 has recently been recorded (Van Creveld), although one of these patients may have suffered from type 3 (Table 94-1) glycogen storage disease.

Cardiomegalic or Neuromuscular Glycogen Storage Disease (Pompe). In this disorder the outstanding pathologic finding is cardiomegaly, with marked infiltration of the myocardium by glycogen.

Table 94-1. DISORDERS OF GLYCOGEN STORAGE AND MOBILIZATION*

Cori type	Enzyme defect	Organ	Glycogen structure	Eponymic name	Suggested clinical name
1	Glucose 6-phosphatase	Liver, kidney	Normal	Von Gierke's disease	Glucose 6-phosphatase deficiency hepatorenal glycogenosis
2	?	Generalized	Normal	Pompe's disease	Idiopathic generalized glycogenosis
3	Amylo-1,6-glucosidase	Liver, heart, muscle	Abnormal: missing or very short	Forbes' disease	Debrancher deficiency limit dextrinosis
4	Amylo-(1,4 → 1,6)-transglucosidase (brancher)	Liver, probably other organs	Abnormal: long inner and outer branches	Andersen's disease	Brancher deficiency amylopectinosis
5	Muscle phosphorylase	Muscle	Normal	McArdle-Schmid-Pearson disease	Myophosphorylase deficiency glycogenosis
6	Liver phosphorylase	Liver	Normal	Hers' disease	Hepatophosphorylase deficiency glycogenosis

* From R. A. Field: "The Metabolic Basis of Inherited Diseases," p. 175, 1960.

Sometimes excessive deposition of glycogen also occurs in skeletal muscle, particularly the tongue, and in brain. When looked for, glycogen accumulation is also found in white blood cells. Functional tests of carbohydrate metabolism (response to fasting, epinephrine, glucagon, etc.) are normal, as is glycogen structure. An enzymatic defect has not as yet been found.

Clinical Picture. The onset of the disease is early in infancy and is marked by progressive symptoms of cardiac failure with, on occasion, muscular weakness and neurologic abnormalities. The course is short, with death resulting from heart failure or infection, usually within the first year.

Glycogen Storage Disease with Cirrhosis. In this disorder glycogen structure is abnormal, as a result of either abnormal debranching enzyme (3, Fig. 94-1) or abnormal branching enzyme (4, Fig. 94-1) activity. The debranching enzyme anomaly is more common. Abnormal glycogen structure is found both in liver and in muscle. Increase in periportal connective tissue is characteristic and may represent a tissue reaction to the deposits of abnormally structured glycogen.

Clinical Picture. Symptoms appear in late infancy or early childhood. Complaints are most frequently referable to hepatomegaly with, at later stages, hepatic dysfunction and splenomegaly. Hypoglycemia is not so characteristic of this form of the disease as of the hepatorenal form, since glucose formed during gluconeogenesis can be liberated into the blood stream, glucose 6-phosphatase activity being preserved. There is, however, decreased tolerance to fasting and increased tendency to fasting ketonuria, since a major portion of the glycogen stores of liver and muscle is not available to metabolism.

The course is variable and as yet ill defined, since specific diagnosis has been made only in recent years. A high protein, relatively low fat diet, with frequent feedings, seems logical. Intercurrent infections must be treated promptly, and the probability of myocardial involvement may warrant prohibition of strenuous exercise and caution in the use of cardiodepressant drugs or anesthetics.

Glycogen Storage Disease with Abnormal Phosphorylase Activity. Phosphorylase (5, Fig. 94-1) catalyzes glycogen breakdown to glucose 1-phosphate and is thus the enzyme primarily concerned with making glycogen available to cellular metabolism. Although liver and muscle phosphorylase catalyze the same reaction, present evidence indicates that they are distinct chemical entities. Recently, a syndrome associated with deficient muscle phosphorylase has been described, and defective hepatic phosphorylase has been added to the possible causes of anomalous hepatic glycogen storage.

Defective or absent muscle phosphorylase (McArdle, Schmid, Pearson) has been described in patients with unexplained episodic muscular weakness brought on by short but strenuous exercise, particularly as a result of ischemic muscle work. During anaerobic contraction, glycogenolysis followed by anaerobic glycolysis to lactate probably represents the major source of energy available to the contracting muscle, beyond the immediate emergency reserve of ATP and creatine phosphate. In individuals without muscle phosphorylase, the normal rise in blood lactate which follows violent exercise does not occur, and muscular atrophy with myoglobinuria is sometimes noted. Although glycogen synthesis is normal, excess glycogen storage is not seen. Hepatic glycogen phosphorylase activity appears to be maintained. A single recessive mode of inheritance appears most likely (Schmid), although only few instances of the disorder have as yet been recorded. The syndrome was first described by McArdle, although it was not related by him to defective phosphorylase activity.

Defective hepatic phosphorylase has been suggested as one of the causes of excessive accumulation of structurally normal hepatic glycogen by Hers. As yet, the resulting syndrome has not been clearly defined, and the diagnosis is based on enzymic analysis of liver biopsy material. Additional possible enzymatic anomalies, including low glucose 6-phosphate dehydrogenase activity, have recently been suggested by Weber.

NONDIABETIC MELITURIA

Definition. Nondiabetic melituria may be defined as excessive excretion of sugar in the urine in the absence of underlying diabetes mellitus. Excessive dietary intake of unusual sugars should always be ruled out.

Physiology. Normally, the renal tubules (mostly the proximal part of the proximal tubule) absorb all except traces of glucose filtered through the glomeruli. There is a maximum tubular reabsorption capacity, however, even in the normal adult (approximately 350 mg glucose per minute), which may be exceeded by a large increase in the glucose filtered per unit of time through the glomeruli. In most instances the increased glucose level presented for tubular reabsorption is the result of an increased blood glucose concentration. However, the so-called "renal threshold" is not defined by the blood glucose level alone, but rather reflects the relationship between the total quantity of glucose filtered per unit of time (glomerular filtration rate X concentration) and the tubular capacity to reabsorb glucose. When the latter is decreased, true renal glucosuria results.

Table 94-2. CLASSIFICATION OF NONDIABETIC MELITURIA

I. Glucosuric melituria
   A. True, permanent renal glucosuria
      1. Isolated
      2. Associated with other renal tubular defects
   B. Transient renal glucosuria
      1. Pregnancy
      2. Nephritis
   C. Alimentary glucosuria
   D. Transient hyperglycemic nondiabetic glucosuria
II. Nonglucosuric melituria
   A. Pentosuria
   B. Fructosuria
   C. Galactosuria
   D. Lactosuria
   E. Other

In *true renal glucosuria,* transient or permanent, the glucosuria is due to a decreased tubular capacity to reabsorb glucose. In general this results in the presence of glucose in the urine at all times, even in the fasting state. It is important to distinguish true renal glucosuria from patients with mild intermittent glucosuria in whom a clear-cut decrease in the tubular reabsorptive capacity for glucose *cannot* be demonstrated. Whereas in the former group diabetes rarely develops, in the latter group the development of diabetes is more frequent than in the general population; this latter condition has sometimes been termed *pseudorenal glucosuria.*

Incidence. Among 22,000 cases of melituria collected at the Mayo Clinic and in Montreal and 50,000 cases of melituria classified at the Joslin Clinic, only two or three per thousand appeared to have true renal glucosuria. Transient nondiabetic glucosuria has been observed in 0.3 per cent of army inductees. *Nonglucose* melituria, other than lactosuria, is rare. Among 50,000 patients with melituria, only 10 patients with pentosuria and 4 with fructosuria have been observed in the Joslin Clinic.

GLUCOSURIC MELITURIA

True, Permanent Renal Glucosuria. *Isolated.* Glucosuria which persists in the fasting state and with blood glucose levels below 100 mg per 100 ml is considered true renal glucosuria. The incidence is small, only 16 cases being observed among a group of 9,000 patients with glucosuria. The condition is thought to be hereditary and persists throughout life. The importance of its recognition derives from its harmlessness and the fact that patients with this disease rarely develop diabetes; it is important that the patient and his family or employers be made to recognize the benign nature of the anomaly. The diagnosis of true renal glucosuria is best established by precise measurement of renal glucose clearance under specified conditions (measurement during gradually increasing glucose administration). The anomaly found is either that of a fixed lowered maximal reabsorptive tubular capacity for glucose (below 200 mg per min) or that of significantly increased urinary glucose loss well before maximal reabsorptive capacity is reached. Since these measurements are not always available, the following clinical criteria can also be used in establishing the diagnosis:

  1. Fasting blood glucose within normal limits or lower than normal
  2. Glucose tolerance curve normal or flat
  3. Glucose present in every specimen, whether voided in the fasting state or after a meal

Acetonuria after an overnight fast is often noted in true renal glucosuria and should not be interpreted as suggesting the presence of diabetes mellitus.

Associated with Other Renal Tubular Defects. Decreased tubular reabsorptive capacity for glucose may be part of a more extensive tubular dysfunction, as in the Fanconi syndrome (see p. 748). In these cases glucosuria is frequently accompanied by aminoaciduria and renal loss of phosphate and calcium. Clinically, nephrolithiasis, failure to grow, and osteoporosis, in addition to glucosuria, suggest the presence of this syndrome.

Transient Renal Glucosuria. From 10 to 15 per cent of normal pregnant women may show glucosuria. The usual explanation is increased blood volume, increased renal blood flow, and hence glucosuria at correspondingly lower blood sugar levels. It is probable that the mechanism is more complex than this, involving altered threshold for glucose, amino acids, and other substances. The condition is benign and disappears after parturition.

Glucosuria may be observed at times in patients with nephritis and particularly in the early stage of toxic nephrosis due to mercury, uranium salts, or cyanide. Glucosuria under these circumstances results from impaired tubular absorption of glucose.

Alimentary Glucosuria. This term is employed to designate the urinary excretion of glucose by certain apparently normal individuals after the ingestion of large quantities of cane sugar, glucose, or starch. The incidence of alimentary glucosuria is increased with impairment of hepatic function because of impaired glycogen storage; with thyrotoxicosis, because of an increased rate of intestinal absorption; with amputation of extremities, because of greatly decreased muscle mass; with gastrectomy and other gastrointestinal operations, because of altered absorption rate.

Transient Hyperglycemic Glucosuria. A variety of disturbances may cause temporary elevation of the blood sugar level and, hence, in the presence of normal or increased glomerular filtration rate, induce glucosuria. Frequently this is the result of permanent or transient exacerbation of hitherto latent diabetes mellitus, but often the disorder cannot be so classified because decreased glucose tolerance cannot be demonstrated by standard tests. In most instances a "stress" is present. Among the more frequent causes of transient hyperglycemic glucosuria are cerebrovascular accidents and brain injuries, particularly in the presence of increased intracranial pressure, acute coronary occlusion, thyrotoxicosis, and asphyxia. Pheochromocytoma, although rare, frequently is associated with glucosuria.

This group of glucosurics undoubtedly includes individuals who harbor the diabetic *trait* but in whom decreased glucose tolerance has not as yet reached the stage at which it can be detected by the usual procedures. This probably explains the observation that diabetes develops subsequently more frequently in this group than in the population at large and has led to the use of the term "pseudorenal glucosuria," which we consider imprecise and undesirable.

NONGLUCOSURIC MELITURIA

When urine contains substances which reduce Benedict's solution and which are carbohydrate in nature, *the presence of nonglucosuric melituria can be specifically established by showing that the substance is not affected by the enzyme glucose oxidase.* Glucose oxidase is available commercially and has been conveniently prepared for semiquantitative (Clinistix, Tes-tape) as well as quantitative analysis. *Alimentary nonglucosuric melituria* due to excessive ingestion of foods containing the suspect sugar should always be considered and ruled out.

Pentosuria. *Essential pentosuria* is a benign inborn error of metabolism in which the pentose L-xylulose is excreted in the urine in amounts varying between 1 and 4 Gm daily. The anomaly is almost exclusively limited to individuals of Jewish descent and is in no way related to diabetes mellitus. The enzymatic defect is almost certainly related to the metabolism of glucuronic acid and probably concerns specifically the reduction of L-xylulose to xylitol (7, Fig. 94-1). As a result, L-xylulose accumulates and is excreted in the urine. A specific renal lesion does not appear to be present. The anomaly is inherited as an autosomal recessive trait. The condition is entirely benign and requires no treatment. Its presence should be suspected when a nonglucose reducing substance is consistently found in the urine of an individual, particularly of the Jewish race. Identification of the pentose is best carried out by *paper chromatography*. In addition, since L-xylulose is a stronger

reducing substance than glucose, it reduces Benedict's solution at relatively lower temperatures (10 min at 55°C or 3 hr at 25°C); it is not fermented by yeast.

Fructosuria. *Essential fructosuria* is a rare, benign inborn error of metabolism reported so far only in Jews and probably inherited as a recessive trait. The origin of the urinary fructose is dietary, and the excessive urinary excretion appears to be the result of decreased fructose utilization, with resultant increased levels of fructose in blood and, hence, fructosuria. Since fructose is primarily utilized in the liver, under normal circumstances, and since its initial hepatic metabolism is its phosphorylation to fructose 1-phosphate, a reaction catalyzed by the enzyme fructokinase, it is likely that the enzymatic defect involved in this anomaly is inadequate or absent hepatic fructokinase activity. However, this hypothesis still lacks direct enzymatic confirmation. The condition is entirely benign, requires no treatment, and is not related to diabetes mellitus. The presence of fructose in the urine is best established by paper chromatography or by the formation of a salmon red color with resorcinol (Seliwanoff reaction). Fructose is fermentable by yeast and levorotatory; in the presence of fructose, Benedict's solution is reduced at relatively low temperatures as described above for xylulose; the urine specimen tested should be fresh since fructose may be formed from glucose in alkaline urine.

Fructosuria with Hypoglycemia. In at least two families reported from Switzerland (Froesch and Prader), and at least one additional patient, fructosuria was associated with tendency to severe hypoglycemia, hepatomegaly, and retarded growth and intellectual development. In these individuals, hypoglycemia with somnolence and vomiting is regularly brought on by the feeding of cane sugar or fruits and is accompanied by elevated blood levels of fructose and fructosuria. Although the exact nature of the enzymatic defect involved is not known, indirect evidence has been presented which indicates that fructose 1-phosphate accumulation occurs and that subsequent events might be the result of the intracellular accumulation of fructose 1-phosphate (as also postulated for galactose 1-phosphate in galactosuria, discussed below). The disorder should be thought of when the characteristic association of somnolence, vomiting, and sweating is associated with feeding of cane sugar or fruits. When fructose-containing foods are avoided, symptoms and signs gradually disappear.

Galactosuria. Galactose tolerance is sometimes used as a test in hepatic disease and in hyperthyroidism. In these two conditions, the ingestion of galactose is said to be followed by significant galactosuria. Large quantities must be ingested by normal persons to induce appreciable galactosuria.

Congenital Galactosemia. Congenital galactosemia is an inborn error of metabolism characterized by inability to utilize ingested galactose. Galactose tolerance is decreased, and the ingestion of galactose or lactose is associated with galactosemia and galactosuria. The inability to utilize galactose is the result of defective or absent galactose 1-phosphate uridyl transferase (8, Fig. 94-1) and results not only in accumulation of galactose but also in accumulation of galactose 1-phosphate. There is evidence to suggest that this intracellular accumulation of galactose 1-phosphate is responsible for the cellular damage associated with galactose feeding in afflicted individuals. Particularly affected are nervous tissue, liver, kidney, and lens. The enzymatic defect can be directly demonstrated in erythrocytes and thus allows for biochemical diagnosis in each instance. The anomaly is probably inherited as an autosomal recessive trait. The heterozygous (carrier) state may be characterized in some instances by subnormal (but not absent) activity of the enzyme, as measured in red blood cells.

Clinical Picture. Clinical signs and symptoms are dependent upon galactose feeding, a nearly universal occurrence since milk sugar, lactose, is a galactose and glucose disaccharide. Accordingly, clinical signs and symptoms usually appear shortly after birth. They include nutritional failure, with mental retardation, hepatosplenomegaly, and formation of cataracts. The affected infants usually appear normal at birth, but after some days or weeks of milk ingestion develop vomiting, diarrhea, impaired nutrition and growth and after a few weeks, jaundice and evidence of cataract formation. Depression of blood glucose levels during milk ingestion is frequently seen and may lead to clinical evidence of hypoglycemia.

In some instances, the clinical picture may be less characteristic, particularly when milk intake is early limited because of "milk intolerance." In these individuals, diagnosis may be delayed for several months or even years, as clearly suggested by the detection of previously unrecognized adult patients with galactosemia in mental institutions.

Diagnosis is usually suggested by the clinical findings and should be considered in each instance of nutritional failure with early postnatal onset. It is supported by finding a non-glucose-reducing substance in the urine, which can then be identified as galactose. Galactosuria may be accompanied by glucosuria and aminoaciduria which appear to be secondary toxic effects of the accumulation of galactose metabolites in the renal tubule. Although galactose tolerance is decreased, this should not be specifically tested for because of the risk involved. Blood galactose is elevated, while blood glucose may be lowered. The definitive diagnostic procedure of choice is the measurement of erythrocyte galactose 1-phosphate uridyl transferase activity, for which a convenient test has been described. The accumulation of galactose 1-phosphate in erythrocytes can also be measured, but the procedure is more time-consuming and less convenient.

Treatment and Course. Early diagnosis is essential since mental retardation, once present, is permanent. Treatment should be initiated whenever the diagnosis is suspected, prior to definitive substantiation. When galactosemia is considered prior to birth, on genetic grounds, a sample of umbilical cord blood should be obtained at birth and assayed for erythrocyte galactose 1-phosphate uridyl transferase. The treatment consists of avoidance of galactose in the diet by using essentially lactose-free milk substitutes such as Nutramigen, Dextri-Maltose, or soybean preparations. It is probable that traces of galactose present in some of these commercially available substitutes are not harmful. When treatment is initiated at birth or within a few weeks, subsequent development is normal. Furthermore, with aging, galactose intolerance probably decreases somewhat, as the result of increasing ability of the organism to metabolize galactose 1-phosphate to UDP galactose in the presence of UTP by a reaction similar to that involved in the formation of UDP glucose from glucose 1-phosphate (Fig. 94-1). Hepatosplenomegaly and cataracts, when present, gradually improve on the galactose-free regimen. Aminoaciduria disappears within a few days.

Lactosuria. Lactosuria occurs in a considerable proportion of women during the second half of pregnancy and during lactation. It is sometimes observed in men when milk is an important component of the diet. It must be regarded as of no clinical importance. Lactose is a non-glucose-reducing disaccharide, best identified by paper chromatography. Also, it leads to gas production when incubated with *Escherichia coli*, but not with *Salmonella paratyphi*.

Additional Instances of Melituria. Maltosuria has been reported, as well as sucrosuria. In the latter instance, sucrose apparently passes the intestinal barrier without prior hydrolysis and leads to polyuria with high specific gravity. Benedict's solution is not reduced prior to hydrolysis of the sucrose molecule. Mannoheptulosuria occurs in some, but not all, individuals after the ingestion of avocado.

OTHER ANOMALIES

Disorders of glucuronide formation and of reactions of the phosphogluconate oxidative pathway are discussed elsewhere but are mentioned here in order to complete the survey of known metabolic errors associated with this portion of the metabolic scheme. Disorders of glucuronide formation (9, Fig. 94-1) occur in certain types of jaundice associated with decreased ability to conjugate bilirubin and thus to prepare it for biliary excretion as the diglucuronide (see Chap. 280). Disorders of the enzymes concerned with the oxidation of glucose 6-phosphate in the phosphogluconic oxidative pathway (10, Fig. 94-1) appear to be associated with several anomalies of red blood cells, leading to alteration of their survival characteristics (see Chap. 235).

SUMMARY

When considering the summary presented in Fig. 94-1, perhaps the most striking feature is the following. As the details of this small area of intermediary metabolism have been uncovered, the occasional occurrence of anomalies at almost every step has been encountered. Some of these anomalies are purely incidental findings and of no importance to the affected individuals, except inasmuch as their presence may lead to erroneous diagnosis (e.g., essential pentosuria or fructosuria misdiagnosed as diabetes). Others are accompanied by minor or major functional defects which result in definite pathologic syndromes compatible with limited or unlimited survival. Undoubtedly still others are not compatible with survival and present as lethal factors at some stage of embryonic development. If this segment of intermediary metabolism is representative of intermediary metabolism in general, then it is evident that an almost endless variety of inborn variants of metabolism are yet to be discovered and may well in time significantly contribute to our understanding of the nature and variability of disease, as well as to the detailed analysis of alternate pathways of intermediary metabolism and of their relative survival value.

REFERENCES

Cori, G. T.: Glycogen Structure and Enzyme Deficiencies in Glycogen Storage Disease, Harvey Lectures, 48:145, 1952–53.

Diseases of Glycogen Storage, Editorial, Lancet, I:206, 1961.

Marble, A.: Non-diabetic Melituria, p. 717, in E. P. Joslin, "The Treatment of Diabetes Mellitus," Philadelphia, Lea & Febiger, 1959.

Mudge, G. H.: Disorders of Renal Tubular Function, Combined Staff Clinics, Am. J. Med., 20:448, 1956.

Stanbury, J. B., J. B. Wyngaarden, and D. S. Fredrickson: "The Metabolic Basis of Inherited Disease," McGraw-Hill Book Company, Inc., New York 1960. In particular the chapters by R. A. Field, p. 156, Glycogen Deposition Diseases; H. H. Hiatt, p. 121, Pentosuria; S. M. Krane, p. 144, Fructosuria, and p. 1246, Renal Glycosuria; and K. J. Isselbacher, p. 208, Galactosuria.

Symposium on Biochemical Lesions of Carbohydrate Metabolism, Federation Proc., 19:971, 1960.

Van Creveld, S.: Glycogen Disease, Arch. Disease Childhood, 34:298, 1959.

Weber, G., and E. R. Harpur: Liver Enzymes in Glycogen Storage Disease, Metabolism, 9:880, 1960.

95 XANTHOMATOSIS AND LIPIDOSIS

Donald S. Fredrickson and George W. Thorn

Lipidosis is a general term applied to disorders characterized by abnormal concentrations of lipids in tissues or in extracellular fluid. *Xanthomatosis* is often employed in the same sense, although it more specifically refers to certain morphologic changes in tissues associated with lipid accumulation. It is convenient to consider the lipidoses as either *primary*, due to some initiating metabolic defect in lipid metabolism, or *secondary*, arising from another disease process. The known primary lipidoses include at least four familial syndromes. The most common is *essential hyperlipidemia*, in which elevated concentrations of plasma lipids are the basic manifestation. Three others are characterized by intracellular accumulation of lipid, mainly sphingolipids. These are *Gaucher's disease, Niemann-Pick disease*, and *amaurotic family idiocy*, the characteristic lipid involved in each being cerebrosides, sphingomyelin, and gangliosides, respectively. There is at least one other familial neurolipidosis—*metachromatic leukodystrophy*—a condition in which abnormal sphingolipid metabolism is present.

The etiologies of these diseases are not understood, and the primary biochemical abnormalities may involve the metabolism of substances other than lipid.

A recently discovered rare inheritable disorder, *a-beta-lipoproteinemia*, in which hypocholesterolemia is associated with the absence of one of the major plasma lipoprotein groups, illustrates that deficiency of a protein can be manifested by striking changes in lipid metabolism. This syndrome also emphasizes that a "lipidosis" may involve a decrease rather than increase in lipid concentrations in the affected tissue.

Among the secondary lipidoses are included the *Hand-Schüller-Christian* syndrome and a group of similar disorders in which characteristic xanthomas may develop, probably as a result of proliferative disease of reticuloendothelial (RE) cells. Secondary accumulation of lipid may occur in tissues or blood in many other diseases, such as diabetes, hypothyroidism, biliary cirrhosis, the nephrotic syndrome, and within the localized lesions of many granulomatous processes.

ESSENTIAL HYPERLIPIDEMIA

Definition. Increased concentrations of plasma lipids persisting throughout life and not explained by other primary disease are not rare findings in clinical medicine. Perhaps the majority of such patients have hypercholesterolemia and represent a heritable disorder, usually called *essential familial hypercholesterolemia,* even though plasma phospholipids are always, and triglycerides occasionally, elevated as well. Significant hyperglyceridemia, producing lactescence in plasma (hyperlipemia), is less common. Usually called *essential hyperlipemia,* this syndrome probably does not represent a single genetically determined disease. Inheritable defects in removal of dietary fat from the blood are definitely involved in some cases. Biochemical tests are lacking for clear separation of the hyperlipidemic syndromes, and the generic term, essential (familial) hyperlipidemia, is frequently useful in classification. Essential hyperlipidemia is commonly associated with xanthomatosis and accelerated development of atherosclerosis.

History. An inheritable tendency toward hypercholesterolemia, frequently associated with xanthomatosis and atherosclerosis, has been recognized for many years. Among the first to describe xanthomas were Addison and Gull in 1851. Associated atheromatous involvement of the heart and great vessels was soon recognized and observed to be familial. In recent years it has been accepted that hypercholesterolemia is the common manifestation and that development of xanthomatosis depends upon genotype and possibly other factors determining the duration and severity of the elevated plasma lipids. The first case of essential hyperlipemia was reported in a child by Bürger and Grütz in 1932 and the first familial incidence by Holt, Aylward, and Timbres shortly thereafter. Both of these patients demonstrated a dependence of hyperlipemia upon dietary fat intake.

Etiology. The biochemical abnormalities underlying the several essential hyperlipidemic syndromes remain unknown. In essential familial hypercholesterolemia the homeostasis of plasma cholesterol is apparently altered. Significant abnormalities have not been demonstrated in either hepatic cholesterol synthesis or in removal of cholesterol by the two major pathways, excretion into the gut or conversion to bile acids. Since all cholesterol is transported in plasma associated with other lipids and protein as lipoprotein molecules, abnormalities in the metabolism of the other lipoprotein constituents, phospholipid, triglyceride, or protein, may have an etiologic role.

In essential hyperlipemia it has often been observed that the elevated triglycerides are predominantly in the form of chylomicrons and that the severity of hyperlipemia is directly related to the dietary intake of fat. Defective removal of chylomicrons has been clearly demonstrated in some patients. The amount of lipolytic activity appearing in plasma after administration of heparin, due mainly to release or activation of an enzyme, lipoprotein lipase, may be low in such cases. An essential role of this enzyme in chylomicron removal has not been proved, however. Some cases do not respond to low fat diets and may have post-heparin lipolytic activity which is greater than normal. Abnormalities in endogenous fatty acid metabolism remain a distinct etiologic possibility in such types of essential hyperlipemia. There is also a definite linkage to abnormal carbohydrate metabolism in many instances of severe essential hyperlipemia since associated hyperglycemia, abnormal glucose tolerance tests, and family history of diabetes are common.

Clinical Picture. Hyperlipidemia is frequently the only manifestation in these syndromes. It is always accompanied by elevated concentrations of *low density* lipoproteins of one or more flotation (S_f) classes. In *essential familial hypercholesterolemia,* the S_f 0 to 20 (beta) lipoproteins are most frequently elevated, and their high cholesterol/phospholipid ratio becomes a characteristic feature of the total serum lipids. The triglyceride-rich lipoproteins of higher flotation rate may also be elevated; hyperlipemia may be present in some, but not necessarily all, hypercholesterolemic members of the same pedigree. Xanthomas may or may not be present in skin and tendons. The various types which are seen include xanthelasma, tendon, plane, tuberous and eruptive xanthomas, in this order of frequency. The latter type is always associated with hypertriglyceridemia. Evidence of atherosclerosis, especially coronary artery disease, is very common, and death from myocardial infarction may occur in early adulthood. Corneal arcus occurs in about 50 per cent of patients. The hypercholesterolemic trait is inherited as a mendelian dominant. There is evidence that homozygotes for the trait may develop greater hyperlipidemia and earlier and more severe xanthomatosis.

Essential hyperlipemia is currently defined as hypertriglyceridemia with proportionately much less associated increase in other lipids. Several biochemical disorders are doubtless included. "Classical" essential familial hyperlipemia is due to an unknown defect in clearing exogenous fat from the blood. Postabsorptive chylomicronemia is present; other low density and high density (alpha) lipoproteins may actually be decreased. The hyperlipemia is quickly reduced by an intake of only 5 to 10 Gm of fat per day.

In contrast, marked hyperlipemia observed in another group of patients may be unresponsive to fat intake. Such "endogenous" cases are often seen in obese adults with poor carbohydrate tolerance. Low fat, high carbohydrate diets may actually cause triglycerides to rise in some. In addition, many mild cases of hyperlipemia are seen with triglyceride levels of 200 to 400 mg per 100 ml (normal 150). It is possible that these patients may represent lesser expression of one of the disorders mentioned above. The genetic determination of essential hyperlipemia is uncertain, however, because any responsible traits have not been clearly defined.

Regardless of origin, severe hyperlipemia is frequently accompanied by hepatosplenomegaly, eruptive xanthomas, foam cells in reticuloendothelial tissues, and lipemia retinalis. Bouts of severe abdominal pain, frequently associated with nausea, vomiting, and signs of peritoneal irritation, may recur and last for several days. Infrequently this is accompanied by clinical signs of acute pancreatitis. Rarely, febrile episodes associated with clearing of hyperlipemia may occur. About half the patients with essential hyperlipemia have diabetic-type intravenous glucose tolerance tests. An occasional patient may have marked hyperlipemia, hyperglycemia, and glucosuria for years without significant ketosis. Insulin has no significant effect in clearing essential hyperlipemia.

Diagnosis. Essential hypercholesterolemia developing before the age of thirty or accompanied by xanthomatosis is almost invariably familial. Uncomplicated hypercholesterolemia in adults, especially in the range of 250 to 350 mg per 100 ml, cannot be assumed to be genetically determined. In every case proof should always be obtained by examination of other family members. Full-blown cases of essential familial hyperlipemia of the exogenous type have triglyceride concentrations of 1,000 to 10,000 mg per 100 ml on a free fat intake. Their response to a low fat diet should be dramatic, and this constitutes the most practical diagnostic test. Some have a lower than normal lipolytic response in plasma after injection of sodium heparin, 0.1 mg per kg; however, this test is not generally available. Insulin-responsive diabetes and myxedema must be excluded by appropriate tests and trial of specific therapy. It may be impossible to determine the antecedent condition in patients who have both hyperlipemia and evidence of chronic pancreatitis.

Treatment. The only widely accepted therapy is dietary. Patients with exogenous hyperlipemia should receive the lowest practical fat intake based on measurements of response of plasma triglycerides. Dietary recommendations for other hyperlipidemics based on current concepts include (1) maintenance of ideal weight; (2) reduced intake of saturated fat, including substitution of skim for whole milk products, and use of more fish and chicken than meats of higher saturated fat content; (3) liberal use of unsaturated oils for salads, cooking, and baking. Very low fat, high carbohydrate diets are to be avoided.

Absence of Beta-Lipoprotein. This is a rare familial syndrome characterized by hypocholesterolemia, erythrocytes having a crenated appearance (acanthocytosis), retinopathy, and ataxic neuropathy. There may be associated steatorrhea or fat intolerance. The full-blown syndrome is characterized by almost complete absence of beta-lipoprotein when measured by sensitive immunochemical tests.

GAUCHER'S DISEASE

The clinical manifestations of this disease are discussed in Chap. 242. The characteristic cells contain abnormally large amounts of cerebrosides, lipids containing equimolar amounts of sphingosine, fatty acid, and hexose. In the visceral lesions of Gaucher's disease, the cerebrosides also contain predominantly glucose instead of the normal galactose moiety. In infants, ganglion cell destruction, glial proliferation, and demyelination may be found in the brain, although abnormal cerebroside content has not been demonstrated. The nature of the defect in cerebroside metabolism presumably responsible for this disorder has not yet been elucidated.

In practically every case, plasma acid phosphatase activity is increased when measured with phenylphosphate as substrate. In contrast to the prostatic enzyme, the acid phosphatase activity is not inhibited by *l-tartrate*. Plasma cerebroside levels may be elevated in splenectomized patients with Gaucher's disease.

NIEMANN-PICK DISEASE

Definition. This is a rare familial disorder, first described in 1914, in which lipid, mainly sphingomyelin, accumulates in reticuloendothelial cells throughout the body. There is associated destruction of ganglion cells in both the central and autonomic nervous systems. Hepatosplenomegaly and retarded nervous and physical development are usually observed within the first 6 months of life, and death from inanition or intercurrent infection usually occurs within 1 to 3 years. The disease may progress more slowly, and the typical tissue changes have been unsuspectingly found at autopsy in adults.

Etiology and Morbid Anatomy. The biochemical basis for the accumulation of sphingomyelin and lesser amounts of other phospholipids and cholesterol is unknown. The disease is apparently inherited as a simple mendelian recessive, both sexes being equally involved. The disease has not been observed in more than one generation in a single pedigree. Over half the reported cases have been in Jews, but many other ethnic groups have been involved. Foam cells (20 to 90 μ in diameter), filled with vacuoles and having a "mulberry" appearance may be found everywhere, but are especially prominent in spleen, liver, lymph nodes, and bone marrow. Throughout the nervous system the ganglion cells undergo swelling, vacuolation, and degeneration of Nissl substance. There is also demyelination, scarring and fibrosis, and proliferation of glial cells which become converted to foam cells. In the retina, destruction of ganglion cells in the surrounding area may leave a grayish background against which the macula stands out as a "cherry-red spot." Although the anatomic changes in the nervous system resemble closely those in Tay-Sachs disease, these two diseases are distinctly separate entities.

Clinical Manifestations. In addition to hepatosplenomegaly, there may be generalized lymphadenopathy, infiltrative lesions in the lung visible by x-ray, and xanthomatous or infiltrative lesions of the skin. The earliest sign usually is poor feeding patterns in infants. A relentless and widely varied pattern of neurologic disturbances follows until a nearly vegetative state may be reached before death. Visceral changes may be present for years in the absence of neurologic signs. The cherry-red spot is seen in only about one-half the cases.

Diagnosis. There are no characteristic laboratory tests. Slight hyperlipemia is common, but plasma sphingomyelin levels are normal. Vacuolation of lymphocytes and monocytes is commonly seen in blood smears. The appearance of the foam cells, usually obtained by marrow aspiration, affords a tentative diagnosis. Biopsy of rectal mucosa showing changes in the ganglion cells of the myenteric plexus may also be helpful. A positive Smith-Dietrich stain is usually obtained, but specific histochemical tests for sphingomyelin are not available. Similar clinical and morphologic findings have been obtained in one family in which the stored lipid was inosamine phosphatide rather than sphingomyelin. Diagnosis should, therefore, always be confirmed by lipid analysis of involved tissues.

Treatment. There is no specific therapy.

AMAUROTIC FAMILY IDIOCY

Definition. This is a general term for several closely related familial neurologic disorders which are characterized by varying degrees of blindness and dementia. Other terms, such as "cerebromacular" or "retinocerebral" degeneration are sometimes employed to describe this group. They are considered as a lipidosis because, at least in one of the special clinical types within the group, the characteristic lesions in the nervous system have been shown to be associated with an increase in gangliosides.

Special Clinical Types. Amaurotic family idiocy can be further subdivided into varieties which differ from one another in age of onset and extent and location of the pathologic process. Thus, the following are recognized:

Tay-Sachs Disease (see Chap. 290). This classic form occurs in infants. Involvement is extremely widespread, including prominent retinal changes (macular cherry-red spot) and a rapid progression of impaired motor control of trunk and limbs, hypotonia with retained reflexes or mild spasticity, seizures, and impaired vision. The average age at onset is six months, and the average age of death is about twenty-four months.

Late Infantile Form (Bielschowsky). This disease has a more chronic course and results in optic atrophy rather than macular cherry-red spot, spastic or hypotonic weakness of the limbs, cerebellar ataxia, tremor and other abnormalities of posture and movement, seizures, and mental deterioration. Death usually occurs by the tenth or twelfth year.

Juvenile Form (Spielmeyer-Vogt). Here the onset is still later, and the course is prolonged (6 to 7 years or more), with a tendency to pigmentary degeneration of the retina (a form of retinitis pigmentosa). Blindness, imbecility, cerebellar ataxia, myoclonic epilepsy, and pyramidal tract signs comprise the picture.

Adult Form (Kufs, Hallervorden). This is considerably rarer than the childhood varieties. The nervous system changes tend to be less widespread than at earlier ages, with corresponding differences in the clinical manifestations, and blindness is not nearly so constant a feature. Dementia, seizures, and athetosis have characterized some of the cases. The course is prolonged, some patients having lived for 10 years or even longer after the onset of the illness.

Etiology. The ganglioside content of the brain is greatly increased in Tay-Sachs disease. Smaller increases have also been reported in a few juvenile and adult cases, but these observations await confirmation. These lipids, characterized by their high content of sialic acid are an important normal constituent of ganglion cells and, hence, of gray matter of the brain. It is assumed that, because of an inheritable metabolic defect in ganglioside metabolism, these lipids accumulate and eventually cause the death of the ganglion cells. The same defect may not be responsible for all forms of amaurotic family idiocy. Tay-Sachs disease occurs primarily in Jewish families, while the juvenile form rarely does. The latter has been seen most frequently in Scandinavia.

Pathology. Abnormality is limited to the nervous system. The characteristic pathologic change is engorgement and distention of nerve cell bodies. In infantile or childhood cases, this is so extensive that all nerve cells in every location, including those in peripheral ganglions, show this alteration. In relation to this destruction, prominent reactive glial changes occur. In infantile cases, surviving beyond fifteen months, this glial reaction is associated with an actual increase in the size of the brain, and the cranial measurements concomitantly become larger than normal. The classic cherry-red spot is due to destruction of ganglion cells in the macular area of the retina, leaving a gray zone against which the macula stands out as a red spot. In juvenile cases with atrophy and pigmentary deposits, the deeper layers of the retina as well as nerve cells degenerate and the pigment epithelium proliferates.

In severe cases, the white matter is abnormal also. This can often be accounted for by the destruction of nerve cell bodies, with consequent degeneration of their axonal processes. The occasional finding of large regions of white matter which are totally necrotic, however, suggests a primary disorder of the structure of white matter as well. It is possible that the metabolism of the myelin-typical lipids such as cerebrosides and sphingomyelin, which have certain structural similarities to gangliosides, are also affected by the disease process.

In general, the older the individual, or the more chronic the course, the less widespread are the neuronal changes. In infants it has been repeatedly observed that the ontogenetically most recent areas of the brain seem most susceptible to the disease process. In others there is no constant localization, but in juvenile cases the cerebellum is nearly always affected. In some cases the alterations in the basal ganglions have been particularly prominent.

The morphologic features of the neuronal alterations of amaurotic family idiocy are indistinguishable from certain other diseases. In gargoylism, gangliosides and mucopolysaccharides of similar composition accumulate in both the brain and other tissues (Chap. 296). In Niemann-Pick disease, discussed above, sphingomyelin accumulates in reticuloendothelial cells throughout the body. The

changes in the white matter are also reminiscent of the leukodystrophies (Chap. 290, p. 1861), which may also eventually prove to be primary disorders of lipid metabolism.

Clinical Features. In infants and children, the combination of rapidly progressive dementia, blindness, retinal changes, and generalized convulsive seizures, often with widespread myoclonic jerks, forms a consistent picture. Frequently the earliest sign is a neuroirritative one, such as hyperacusis. As already noted, the characteristic appearance of the macula in infantile cases yields place in older children and young adults to optic atrophy, possibly with pigment accumulations in the retina. In juvenile cases, striking vacuolation of the agranulocytes is frequently noted on examination of the peripheral blood smear. This may also be seen in asymptomatic family members, presumably heterozygous for the trait.

In the rarer adult cases there is no single characteristic feature. Dementia, myoclonic jerks, and variable degrees of rigidity, spasticity, weakness, ataxia, and involuntary movements may be encountered, with a slowly progressive course measured in years. At present, there is no generally useful biochemical determination which will assure the diagnosis of amaurotic family idiocy during life.

Differential Diagnosis. In typical infantile or childhood cases, there is usually no difficulty in recognizing this condition. In older children and adults, the diagnosis may be suspected only after other diffuse disorders—neoplastic, infectious, nutritional, or toxic—have been eliminated by the various currently used diagnostic measures. It should always be considered in myoclonic epilepsy, with mental deterioration, progressive cerebellar ataxia, and progressive dementia with seizures and athetosis.

EOSINOPHILIC XANTHOMATOUS GRANULOMA (Hand-Schüller-Christian Syndrome)

Frequently considered among the lipidoses are several disorders which belong to a large group of closely related diseases of the reticuloendothelial system. In each, the pathologic lesions contain common features, present in variable degrees. Those include, in the usual order of progression, proliferation of reticuloendothelial tissues, accompanying granulomatous changes, featuring eosinophils and giant cells, conversion of the reticulum and histiocytic cells to foam cells or xanthomas, and, finally, fibrosis.

The sites of involvement and the stage of tissue reaction predominating are quite variable. A rapidly progressing and usually fatal proliferative reaction in infants and children is represented by the

Letter-Siwe syndrome. Eosinophilic granuloma refers to usually solitary, granulomatous or xanthomatous bone lesions. When skeletal lesions are combined with others in the orbit, and in the dura or brain, such that function of the posterior pituitary is affected, the resulting triad of exophthalmos, diabetes insipidus, and the bone defects describe the classical *Hand-Schüller-Christian syndrome.* These conditions are discussed in Chap. 242. The typical pathologic changes may be found in widely distributed lesions of the skin and mucous membranes (*xanthoma disseminatum*). Fibrotic lesions associated with extracellular lipid deposits located under the tongue and in the pharynx and larynx, so-called *lipid proteinosis,* may also represent an end stage of xanthoma disseminatum.

The xanthomatous lesions associated with these disorders are characterized by a great increase in tissue lipids, primarily cholesterol. There is no associated hyperlipidemia, and it has been proposed that abnormal cholesterol metabolism might be the primary cause of xanthoma formation. It is more widely held that lipid accumulation is a secondary and inconstant feature of a more generalized process, the etiology of which is unknown.

There is no tendency for familial involvement as in the inheritable lipidoses discussed above.

Xanthoma Disseminata. The characteristic skin lesion is a mahogany-colored papular eruption, most commonly in the axillas, antecubital fossas, and on the sides of the neck. The mucous membranes of the mouth and vulva are other sites of predilection. Widespread chronic ulcerations with secondary infection may be present.

CEROID STORAGE DISEASE

Extensive tissue storage of ceroid, a pigmented lipid of unknown chemical composition, has been reported in several rare instances. This may be associated with cirrhosis of the liver and intestinal malabsorption. Organ involvement may be sufficiently widespread to produce a clinical picture similar to severe Niemann-Pick disease. Ceroid may be identified histochemically by the combination of red periodic acid-Schiff stain, acid-fastness, and fluorescence. Deposition of this material has also been seen in aorta, liver, intestinal musculature, and other tissues in a variety of conditions, including tocopherol deficiency. The biochemical basis for ceroid formation and storage is not known.

REFERENCES

Fredrickson, D. S.: The Lipidoses, in "The Metabolic Basis of Inherited Disease," J. B. Stanbury, J. B. Wyngaarden, and D. S. Fredrickson (Eds.), New York, McGraw-Hill Book Company, Inc., Blakiston Division, 1960.

Oppenheimer, E. H., and Edward C. Andrews, Jr.: Ceroid Storage Disease in Childhood, Pediatrics, 23:1091, 1959.

Salt, H. A., O. H. Wolff, June K. Lloyd, Audrey S. Fosbrooke, A. H. Cameron, and D. V. Hubble: On Having No Beta-Lipoprotein, a Syndrome Comprising a A-beta-lipoproteinemia, Acanthocytosis, and Steatorrhoea, Lancet, II:325, 1960.

Symposium on Amaurotic Family Idiocy (Tay-Sachs Disease), A.M.A. J. Diseases Children, 97:655, 1959.

Thannhauser, S. J.: "Lipidoses," New York, Grune & Stratton, Inc., 1958.

96 AMYLOIDOSIS
Kendall Emerson, Jr.

History. The widespread deposition of a homogeneous material throughout many organs of the body was first described in 1842 by Rokitansky. Virchow, in 1854, noted that, like starch, this material stained blue with iodine and sulfuric acid, and termed it *amyloid.* Actually it has no relation to starch but is a *protein* of variable composition, usually associated with a sulfate-bearing polysaccharide similar to, if not identical with, chondroitinsulfuric acid.

Incidence. Amyloidosis may be divided into primary and secondary types. Primary amyloidosis is of unknown etiology and of relatively rare occurrence. In some cases a familial incidence has been noted with the characteristics of a dominant trait. Rukavina has analyzed 154 cases in detail. Maximal age incidence of the disease is the fourth to the sixth decades. Secondary amyloidosis is associated with a chronic suppurative or inflammatory process such as tuberculosis, bronchiectasis, osteomyelitis, or rheumatoid arthritis. It was formerly much more frequent than the primary type, but with the decreasing incidence of chronic suppurative disease since the advent of antibiotics, the relative frequency of primary amyloidosis is increasing. The two types differ characteristically in the predominant localization of amyloid deposits in the various body tissues (Table 96-1). More recent observations, however, suggest a much higher incidence of primary amyloidosis of the kidney. A third type of amyloidosis is associated specifically with multiple myelomatosis. It resembles the primary type in its localization, but occurs more frequently in bones, joints, tendons, and muscles.

Etiology. The etiology of amyloidosis is uncertain. Experimentally, it may be induced by the repeated injection of sodium caseinate or by hyperimmunization with bacterial vaccine. It is generally considered that secondary amyloidosis results from

Table 96-1. LOCALIZATION OF AMYLOID DEPOSITS

Location	Per cent of cases	
	Primary amyloidosis*	Secondary amyloidosis†
Heart.................	85	1
Tongue.................	57	1
Gastrointestinal tract....	52	4
Skeletal muscle.........	41	
Kidney.................	26	72
Spleen.................	24	89
Adrenal gland..........	22	41
Liver..................	17	63
Bone and joint.........	11	

* Data from Eisen, Am. J. Med., 1:144, 1946 (46 cases).
† Data from Rosenblatt, Am. J. Med. Sci., 186:558, 1933 (110 cases).

the storage in the reticuloendothelial system of abnormal or incomplete protein breakdown products arising from areas of tissue damage or destruction. It is possible that these protein breakdown products may constitute antigen-antibody complexes.

Pathology. Amyloid is deposited initially around small blood vessels, and from this point it spreads gradually throughout the connective tissue stroma, encroaching upon and choking off the parenchymal cells in its path. The material is identified by its staining affinity for Congo red, iodine and sulfuric acid, or methyl violet. Secondary amyloid deposits nearly always stain characteristically with all three dyes, whereas primary amyloid and that associated with multiple myeloma may take only one or two of these dyes, and then much less intensely.

Clinical Picture. The signs and symptoms of amyloidosis depend principally upon the organs involved. The liver and spleen may be enlarged, with signs of hepatic insufficiency. Kidney involvement produces the picture of nephrosis with eventual renal failure and death, sometimes without hypertension. In the primary type, amyloid deposition in the heart and lungs may result in a picture of cardiac and pulmonary insufficiency indistinguishable, clinically, from the more common types of heart and pulmonary disease. Elsewhere, there may be only local, painless enlargement of an organ such as the tongue or thyroid, or visible infiltration of areas of the skin. Macroglossia is present in more than one-half and cutaneous lesions in approximately one-quarter of patients with primary amyloidosis, rarely in the secondary type. The skin of the face and periorbital regions is more frequently involved, the lesions appearing as yellowish papules or plaques resembling xanthelasma. There is no itching, but spontaneous ecchymoses may occur. Primary motor and sensory amyloid polyneuropa-

thies have been described. These usually present as sensory followed by motor disturbances of the legs, extending later to include the gastrointestinal tract and upper extremities. Enlargement of peripheral nerves may be noted on palpation. Usually there is evidence of amyloidosis elsewhere, but a familial form has been reported which affects the nervous system primarily. Vitreous opacities consisting of amyloid deposition extending out from around retinal blood vessels, with progressive decrease in visual acuity, have been described as diagnostic of familial primary amyloidosis.

Diagnosis. Secondary amyloidosis should always be looked for in the presence of any long-standing suppurative or inflammatory process, in chronic hemolytic anemias, and in the lymphomas, especially when there is an elevation of the serum globulin. Primary amyloidosis must be considered in any patient over the age of fifty exhibiting cardiac enlargement and congestive failure or pulmonary insufficiency, where the etiology is not evident. Chronic renal insufficiency in adults, especially if associated with the nephrotic syndrome, should raise the suspicion of primary renal amyloidosis. Elevation of the serum glucosamine and an abnormal peak in the α_2 fraction of the serum globulin may aid in the diagnosis. Congo red is taken up by amyloid, and if over 80 per cent of a standard dose of 10 ml of a 1 per cent solution of this dye disappears from the blood within 1 hr after intravenous injection, there is strong presumptive evidence for the presence of amyloidosis. In the presence of proteinuria the dye may appear in the urine and give a false positive test which is detected by acidifying the urine and noting the characteristic color change to blue of Congo red. A negative test does not rule out amyloidosis, since considerable quantities of amyloid must be present in order to retain a sufficient amount of dye to give a definitive test. Furthermore, certain types of amyloid appear not to have an affinity for Congo red. Under these circumstances a diagnosis may be established only by biopsy.

Cutaneous amyloidosis may be detected by the local injection of 1 ml subcutaneously or 0.1 ml intradermally of a 1.5 per cent solution of Congo red into the affected areas. After 24 to 48 hr the amyloid deposits will appear deep red, in contrast to the slight staining of the surrounding normal skin.

Treatment. The treatment of secondary amyloidosis should first be directed at the associated condition, cure of which may or may not be followed by disappearance of the amyloidosis. This treatment appears to be most beneficial in patients with relatively mild amyloidosis associated with rheumatoid arthritis or osseous tuberculosis. It is not effective in the severer forms of the disease. Remarkable benefit from the use of raw liver orally and crude liver preparations parenterally has been described recently; the amyloidosis may disappear in a matter of months even though the underlying disease process is unchanged. There is no known treatment of primary amyloidosis, beyond efforts to maintain the function of the organs involved.

REFERENCES

Hass, G. M., R. Huntington, and N. Krumdieck: Amyloid: Properties of Amyloid Deposits Occurring in Several Species under Diverse Conditions, Arch. Pathol., 35:226, 1943.

Jacobi, M., and H. Grayzel: Generalized Secondary Amyloidosis; Clinico-pathological Study of 84 Cases, J. Mt. Sinai Hosp., 12:339, 1945.

Kaufman, H. E., and L. B. Thomas: Vitreous Opacities Diagnostic of Familial Primary Amyloidosis, New Engl. J. Med., 261:1267, 1959.

Rukavina, J. G., W. D. Block, C. E. Jackson, H. F. Falls, J. H. Carey, and A. C. Curtis: Primary Systemic Amyloidosis: A Review and an Experimental, Genetic and Clinical Study of 29 Cases with Particular Emphasis on the Familial Form, Medicine, 35:239, 1956.

Symposium on Amyloidosis, U.S. Armed Forces Med. J.: 707, 1951.

97 HEMOCHROMATOSIS
George E. Cartwright

Definition. Idiopathic hemochromatosis (bronze diabetes, pigment cirrhosis) is characterized pathologically by excessive deposits of iron in the body and clinically by hepatomegaly with eventual liver insufficiency, pigmentation of the skin, diabetes mellitus, and frequently cardiac failure.

History. The first clinical description of the disease was given by Trousseau in 1865. In 1889 von Recklinghausen named the disease *hemochromatosis* and described the iron-containing pigment, hemosiderin. Sheldon, in a now classic monograph, reviewed the world's literature in 1935. Finch and Finch in 1955 reviewed the literature since 1935 and added 80 cases of their own.

Incidence. Hemochromatosis is a rare disease, recognized once in approximately 20,000 hospital admissions, and once in 7,000 hospital deaths. It is observed ten times as frequently in males as in females. Nearly 70 per cent of all patients with this disease develop their first symptoms between the ages of forty and sixty years. Hemochromatosis is rarely recognized below the age of twenty years.

Pathogenesis. One of the earliest measurable alterations in iron metabolism in hemochromatosis is the elevation of the plasma iron and saturation of the plasma iron-binding protein, transferrin. As the disease progresses, the amount of storage iron increases. In advanced disease, the tissues contain over 20 Gm iron, whereas total body iron in normal persons is in the range of 3 to 5 Gm. The increase in tissue iron can be accounted for in the two iron-storage compounds, ferritin and hemosiderin. Increased amounts of iron are found in almost all the body tissues, especially those in which there is organ dysfunction. Iron in the liver and pancreas is increased fifty to one hundred times, in the heart ten to fifteen times, in spleen, kidney, and skin about five times. It is generally accepted that the excessive deposition of iron is the cause of the tissue damage. Reasonable as this theory seems, it has yet to be proved. All attempts to produce hemochromatosis experimentally in animals by the administration of large amounts of iron have failed.

Since iron is not excreted from the body in appreciable amounts even in normal persons, the conclusion that iron absorption is increased in idiopathic hemochromatosis seems inescapable. The specific nature of the abnormality in absorption is unknown. The dietary intake of iron is normal in patients with idiopathic hemochromatosis. The chronicity of the disease, the absence of demonstrable gastrointestinal disease, and the familial incidence of the disorder suggest that the abnormality is an inborn error of metabolism.

Pathology. At autopsy the enlarged, nodular liver and pancreas present a striking ochre color. Histologically, hemosiderin is deposited in many organs, particularly the liver and pancreas. The liver shows considerable fibrosis. Testicular atrophy is frequently present, both grossly and histologically. There are hemosiderin deposits in the myocardium, and they may be associated with myocardial edema, fibrosis, and necrosis. The epidermis of the skin is thin, and melanin pigment is found in the cells of the basal layer. Hemosiderin is deposited almost entirely in the corium.

Clinical Manifestations. The symptoms and signs of hemochromatosis are related to the skin pigmentation, diabetes, liver impairment, and cardiac disease. Of these the cirrhosis of the liver is the most constant abnormality.

The initial symptoms most frequently encountered are related to the onset of diabetes. Weakness, lassitude, weight loss, change in skin color, abdominal pain, dyspnea, edema, ascites, loss of libido, and peripheral neuritis are also frequent initial symptoms. Hepatomegaly, pigmentation, spider angiomas, splenomegaly, ascites, evidences of congestive failure or cardiac arrhythmias, loss of body hair, testicular atrophy, jaundice, and hypertension are the most prominent physical signs, given in decreasing order of frequency.

The liver is the first tissue known to be damaged,

and hepatomegaly is present in about 93 per cent of symptomatic cases. Hepatic enlargement may exist in the absence of symptoms or in the presence of normal liver function test results. Indeed, over half the patients with symptomatic hemochromatosis have little or no laboratory evidence of functional impairment of the liver in spite of hepatomegaly and proved fibrosis. Loss of body hair, palmar erythema, testicular atrophy, gynecomastia, spider angioma, and, particularly, loss of libido are often seen and are related to the severity of the liver damage. Manifestations of portal hypertension and esophageal varices may occur but are less commonly observed than in Laennec's cirrhosis. A nontender, slightly enlarged spleen is present in approximately half the cases. Primary carcinoma of the liver develops in about 14 per cent. The incidence of this last complication increases greatly with age.

Excessive skin pigmentation is present in about 90 per cent of the patients at the time the diagnosis is established. Pigmentation may be due to deposition of melanin or iron or both. In general, melanin deposition gives rise to bronzing, iron deposition to a metallic gray hue. Pigmentation usually is diffuse and generalized, but frequently it is deeper on the face, neck, extensor aspects of the lower forearms, dorsae of the hands, lower legs, genital regions, and in scars. In only 10 to 15 per cent of cases is there demonstrable pigmentation of the oral mucosa.

About 82 per cent of all patients develop diabetes mellitus and symptoms therefrom. The diabetes may appear rapidly, and insulin requirements may increase rapidly. About 72 per cent of the patients require insulin for the control of the diabetes. In some instances severe insulin resistance develops, in others there may be sensitivity to insulin. In most instances, the diabetes is controlled with little difficulty. Since the diabetes is usually present for less than a decade, the late degenerative sequelae of this complication are not prominent.

Approximately one-third of patients with idiopathic hemochromatosis die of cardiac failure. The heart disease is extremely common in young adults, and symptoms may develop suddenly, with rapid progression to death. The most important manifestations of heart disease are congestive failure and cardiac arrhythmias, particularly ventricular extrasystoles and paroxysmal atrial tachycardia. Other arrhythmias may occur as well.

Diagnosis. The classical triad of skin pigmentation, diabetes mellitus, and hepatomegaly, especially in the presence of heart disease and evidence of hypogonadism, should always suggest the diagnosis. Confirmation of the presence of liver, pancreatic, heart, and gonadal disease should then be obtained by customary tests of the functions of these organs. It then remains to demonstrate that there is excessive storage iron.

The diagnosis is enhanced considerably if the plasma iron level is found to be elevated (above 150 μg per 100 ml) and the iron-binding protein of the plasma is 75 to 100 per cent saturated. However, the only definitive test is liver biopsy. Other procedures which indicate an excess of body iron stores are bone marrow aspiration for hemosiderin, examination of the urine sediment for hemosiderin, skin biopsy, and gastric mucosal biopsy.

Finch and Finch state that there are no unique features in idiopathic hemochromatosis by which it may be distinguished pathologically from the terminal stage of other iron-storage diseases, such as dietary or transfusion hemochromatosis. They define *hemosiderosis* as a focal increase in tissue iron or a general increase in iron stores without associated tissue damage, and *hemochromatosis* as a general increase in body iron stores with resultant tissue damage. From these definitions, the differentiation of hemosiderosis from hemochromatosis can be easily made by the presence or absence of organ dysfunction. Dietary and transfusion hemochromatosis can be differentiated from idiopathic hemochromatosis on the basis of a history of excessive iron intake by mouth, by injection, or intravenously in the form of blood. In evaluating dietary iron exposure, the dietary iron content, type of diet, type of cooking utensils, intake of medicinal iron, and iron content of the drinking water or other beverages must be considered.

At times it may be extremely difficult to differentiate hemochromatosis from alcoholic cirrhosis. Patients with alcoholic cirrhosis frequently develop skin pigmentation, splenomegaly, and even disturbances in glucose utilization, and in an occasional patient excess iron deposits may be present. In such cases differentiation can be made only by comparing the quantity of liver iron with that usually found in idiopathic hemochromatosis.

Prognosis. The life expectancy of patients after signs of clinical hemochromatosis have become manifest averages 4.4 years, but several instances have been recorded of patients living up to 20 or 30 years after manifestation of signs. The average duration of life after diabetes has developed is 3 years. The principal causes of death are cardiac failure (30 per cent), hepatic coma (15 per cent), hematemesis (14 per cent), hepatoma (14 per cent), and pneumonia (12 per cent). The most recent advance in the therapy of this disease, the introduction of methods for removal of iron, is expected to increase life expectancy further.

Treatment. The therapy of idiopathic hemochromatosis involves removal of the excess body iron by phlebotomy and supportive treatment of damaged organs. The management of the hepatic failure, cardiac failure, and diabetes differs little from the conventional management of these conditions. Loss of libido and change in secondary sex characteristics are relieved by testosterone therapy. Iron is best removed from the body by a weekly phlebotomy of 500 ml. Since the average amount of iron in a patient with hemochromatosis is approximately 25 Gm, about 2 years of weekly bleeding will be required to deplete the iron stores. Dietary restriction of iron is unnecessary and impractical, and chelating agents will not mobilize sufficient iron to be of any practical value.

REFERENCES

Finch, S. C., and C. A. Finch: Idiopathic Hemochromatosis, an Iron Storage Disease, Medicine, 34:381, 1955.

Sheldon, J. H.: "Hemochromatosis," London, Oxford University Press, 1935.

98 DISORDERS OF PIGMENT METABOLISM

Kendall Emerson, Jr.

CAROTENEMIA AND CAROTENODERMA

Definition. Carotenemia refers to the presence of an excessive amount of carotene in the blood which, when prolonged, leads to an excessive deposition of carotene in the skin, *carotenoderma.*

History. Carotenemia was first recognized during the First World War, when it became particularly prevalent in Europe. It was first publicized by Hess and Myers in 1919.

Etiology. High serum levels of carotene are seen in individuals who consume over long periods of time large quantities of leafy and yellow vegetables and fruits of high carotene content, such as carrots, spinach, squash, peaches, oranges, and apricots. The condition occurs most frequently in infants and children but is not uncommon in adults, particularly in obese individuals on reducing diets. It may also be found in patients with liver disease or myxedema, since carotene is converted to vitamin A in the liver and thyroid hormone is necessary for the conversion to proceed normally. In such cases the serum level of vitamin A will be decreased. The amount of both carotene and vitamin A in the serum tends to vary directly with the concentration of serum lipids, and in hyperlipemic states carotenemia is common. When the hyperlipemia is prolonged, as in uncontrolled diabetes mellitus, carotenoderma is likely to occur. In diabetes there is often the added factor of the ingestion of relatively large amounts of pigmented fruits and vegetables.

Clinical Picture. Carotene is a normal constituent of the skin and contributes, along with other pigments, to its natural yellow color. When the level of carotene in the blood exceeds the range of 0.21 to 0.8 mg per 100 ml, the excessive deposition of carotene in the skin known as carotenoderma becomes clinically manifest. Carotene is in part excreted by the sebaceous glands and reabsorbed by the stratum corneum. Thus the canary-yellow pigmentation is first noted in the nasolabial folds and over the forehead, where sebaceous glands are numerous, and in the palms and soles, where the stratum corneum is the thickest. In severe cases the pigmentation may be generalized, except that the scleras are never pigmented.

Diagnosis. The diagnosis of carotenemia and carotenoderma rests on the characteristic appearance and distribution of pigment, the history of excessive ingestion of yellow vegetables, and the demonstration of an elevated serum level of carotene. It is important to differentiate it from jaundice by the absence of pigmentation of the scleras, the localization of the pigmentation to the face, palms, and soles rather than the trunk, and normal icterus index following acetone precipitation or a normal serum bilirubin. The disorder should always be considered a possibility in patients exhibiting signs of hepatic insufficiency or hyperlipemia.

Treatment. This condition is harmless and produces no symptoms by itself. When due to excessive intake of carotene it will disappear within a few weeks upon correction of the dietary abnormality. It should lead the physician to direct his attention to the correction of its cause, whether this is a dietary idiosyncrasy, an underlying liver disease, hyperlipemia with or without diabetes mellitus, or a combination of these causes.

Lycopenemia. Lycopene is a real carotenoid distributed widely through fruits and vegetables. It is found in high concentration in ripened tomatoes, accounting for 90 per cent of the pigments. It does not form vitamin A. In the case of unusually high tomato juice intake over a period of months, high lycopene serum levels may occur, leading to an orange-yellow skin discoloration and lycopene vacuolization of the liver cells. Because of the close resemblance of this condition to carotenemia, a careful dietary history and direct isolation of the circulating pigments may be necessary for diagnosis. The serum is extracted with petroleum ether, and the carotenoids are separated on a calcium hydroxide column. Lycopene forms a distinct band on the column and may then be identified by spectrophotometry. It has an absorption maximum in carbon disulfide at 548 μ, while beta-carotene, the predominant pigment in carotenemia, has its peak at 520 μ. Lycopenemia has been associated with a mild derangement of liver function and bizarre vacuoles and crystals in liver cells; so the clinical picture may be accounted for in part by a failure of normal metabolism of the pigment.

MELANOSIS AND MELANURIA

Definition. The deposition of an abnormal quantity of the pigment melanin is termed *melanosis.* This occurs most commonly in the skin but may be seen in other organs such as the colon (melanosis coli), adrenal glands, retina, and leptomeninges. *Melanuria* signifies the excretion of melanin in the urine.

Metabolic Considerations. Melanin is formed by *melanocytes,* which are specialized cells probably arising from the neural crest and normally present in the basal layer of the epidermis at the junction of epidermis and dermis. The number and distribution of the melanin-producing cells of the body vary from one individual to another and are genetically determined.

The exact chemical composition of melanin is unknown, but it is generally considered to be a polymer of *tyrosine* formed by the action of a copper-containing enzyme, *tyrosinase.* Melanin producing cells contain an enzyme tyrosinase (identical with dopa oxidase) which acts upon tyrosine to form dihydroxyphenylalanine (dopa). This substance is then transformed by autooxidation to an indolequinone which ultimately polymerizes to form melanin. Electron microscopic studies have recently revealed that these reactions take place in organized structures, contained within the cytoplasm of the melanocyte, varying in size from 0.1 to 0.4 μ and resembling microsomes. These cell organelles in which tyrosinase is concentrated have been termed *melanosomes.* They gradually enlarge in the living cell, lose their tyrosinase activity, and are transformed into the typical granules of melanoprotein which impart to the melanocyte its characteristic dark color. This pigment is eventually lost from the body, largely through desquamation of the skin, and to a lesser extent through the intestinal tract, while none or only a very small amount is normally excreted through the kidneys. This is not remarkable, since it is a large molecule and very slightly water-soluble.

Melanoblastic activity is controlled by physicochemical, endocrine, and neurogenic factors. The enzymatic formation of melanin is dependent upon the availability of tyrosinase, its substrates tyrosine and dihydroxyphenylalanine, and molecular oxygen. The localized or generalized absence of tyrosinase in the skin gives rise to irregular, splotchy white areas of depigmentation known as *vitiligo,* or to a total lack of pigmentation of the skin, hair, and iris, a rare congenital condition termed *albinism.* Increased pigmentation will result from any condi-

tion causing prolonged hyperemia of the skin with increase in available oxygen for tyrosinase activity.

Inhibition of tyrosinase activity is brought about normally by the binding of its copper ion by sulfhydryl groups in the skin. Thus any process interfering with sulfhydryl metabolism will result in hyperpigmentation.

The *melanocyte-stimulating hormone* (MSH) of the pars intermedia of the pituitary increases pigmentation by causing dispersion of melanin granules throughout the cytoplasm of melanocytes, and probably also by increased melanin production. Recently Lerner has extracted and identified a chemical substance from pineal glands, N-acetyl-5-methoxytryptamine, which he has termed *melatonin* because of its chemical similarity to serotonin. This substance in minute quantities will cause clustering of melanin granules about the nucleus of the melanocyte in the frog's skin, which results in an apparent decrease in pigmentation. Thus far, it has not been shown to affect the dispersal of melanin granules in human skin. It has, however, been isolated from human sciatic nerve.

There appears to be some degree of control of melanin pigmentation by the gonadal hormones. The androgens tend to stimulate the melanoblasts generally, whereas the estrogens control the activity of certain specific melanoblastic cells, such as those in the areolas of the breasts and in the vulva and perianal region, but at the same time inhibit the stimulating action of the androgens on the melanophores generally.

Epinephrine and norepinephrine, inhibit the action of MSH in causing darkening of the frog's skin. Thus localized areas of hyperpigmentation (*café au lait* spots) may be the result of epinephrine lack associated with abnormalities of sympathetic innervation in the pigmented areas.

Etiology. Melanosis may be caused by either an increased activity of a normal number of melanocytes or an increased number of melanocytes. The vast majority of cases fall in the first category and may be classified, according to the factors controlling pigmentation described above, as genetic, physicochemical, hormonal, neurogenic, or neoplastic (Table 98-1).

Genetic factors are of primary importance in determining racial variations in pigmentation, the number, size, and location of freckles (ephelides), and the senile lentigines (liver spots) seen in older persons on areas exposed for many years to sunlight. In these instances the influences of heredity operate through the normal mechanisms stimulating melanoblastic activity. In the case of the pigmented nevus, an abnormal migration of melanocytes from the neural crest to the skin is genetically determined.

Any agent causing chronic hyperemia of the skin

Table 98-1. ETIOLOGY OF MELANIN PIGMENTATION
OF THE SKIN

Etiology	Number of melanocytes	
	Normal	Increased
Genetic.........	Racial factors	Pigmented
	Freckles	nevi
	Senile lentigines	
	Melanosis coli	
	Peutz-Jeghers syndrome	
Physicochemical .	Chronic irritation	
	Ionizing irradiation	
	Heavy metal intoxication	
	Vitamin deficiencies	
	Malnutrition	
	Scleroderma	
	Blood dyscrasias	
Endocrine.......	Addison's disease	
	Pregnancy	
	Acromegaly	
	Hyperthyroidism	
	Hepatic insufficiency	
Neurogenic......	Neurofibromatosis	
	Polyostotic fibrous	
	dysplasia	
	Café au lait spots	
Neoplastic......	Acanthosis nigricans	Melanoma

and thus making more oxygen available for tyrosinase activity will increase melanoblastic activity. Among these agents may be included thermal, mechanical, chemical, or infectious irritants and excess thyroid hormone.

Oxidation of sulfhydryl groups by ionizing irradiation such as ultraviolet light and x-ray may cause hyperpigmentation through failure of the normal sulfhydryl inhibition of tyrosinase activity. In a similar manner, increased melanin deposition may result from the binding of sulfhydryl groups by heavy metals, such as arsenic in chronic poisoning with this substance, or iron in hemochromatosis and after extensive subcutaneous extravasation of hemoglobin.

Vitamin deficiencies and localized nutritional disturbances such as scleroderma may produce melanosis by decreasing the supply of sulfhydryl groups available to inhibit tyrosinase activity. This may account for the increased melanin pigmentation seen in pellagra, in sprue, and less often, in vitamin A deficiency (Darier's disease) and scurvy. Diffuse melanosis occurs in about 10 per cent of patients with Hodgkin's disease but is less commonly seen in other blood dyscrasias. In these diseases it may be secondary to generalized pruritus with irritation from scratching, to malnutrition, or to x-ray or arsenic therapy.

Increased pigmentation of the skin is practically universal in pregnancy, because of increase in both circulating ovarian hormones and MSH. Usually most of this pigmentation disappears following termination of pregnancy, but some remains about the nipples, vulva, and anal regions. Marked pigmentation over the cheeks and forehead, known as *chloasma uterinum* may occur during pregnancy in individuals who are generously supplied with melanocytes in these regions. This pigmentation usually disappears following pregnancy but sometimes persists to a greater or lesser degree.

Increased melanin formation occurs in various forms of liver disease, in part because of failure of the liver to inactivate the gonadal hormones. The hyperpigmentation of acromegaly may be associated with increased pituitary MSH activity.

It is now known that MSH and adrenocorticotropic hormone (ACTH) are very similar in chemical composition. They both are long-chain polypeptides containing the same sequences of amino acids. ACTH has a longer chain but it is believed that it is capable, either directly or by being partially broken down to MSH, of exhibiting MSH activity. Thus, the pigmentation of Addison's disease can be explained by the increase in circulating ACTH which has been shown to occur in this condition. Suppression of ACTH by cortisone administration results in marked decrease of pigmentation in these patients. Adrenal insufficiency secondary to pituitary insufficiency, on the other hand, is usually associated with a decrease in skin pigmentation.

Among the neurogenic causes of skin hyperpigmentation, the best known are *von Recklinghausen's disease* (neurofibromatosis) and *Albright's disease* (polyostotic fibrous dysplasia). An area of pigmentation is frequently observed in the lumbar region over a spina bifida, and isolated areas of irregular pigmentation, *café au lait* spots, which are very commonly seen without associated disease, may be produced by congenital deficiency of sympathetic innervation in localized areas anywhere on the body.

Acanthosis nigricans constitutes a special form of melanosis in which increased melanin pigmentation is associated with hyperkeratosis and minute verrucous and papillomatous changes imparting a velvety feeling to the skin. The pigmentation usually begins and is most marked in the axillas but may become generalized and involve the mucous membranes of the mouth. About half the cases are associated with abdominal cancer, although in a few instances the condition has been reported accompanying cancer of the breast and lung. In the remaining cases, acanthosis nigricans is apparently a benign condition occurring primarily in children or at puberty and having an indefinite duration. Disturbances of hormonal function of the pituitary or gonads and vitamin deficiencies have been suggested as etiologic factors in this form of the disease. The microscopic picture of the skin is similar in both forms of the disease and is diagnostic.

Melanin deposits are occasionally seen in the colon, associated with intestinal obstruction or severe constipation in heavily pigmented individuals, particularly Negroes (*melanosis coli*). The *Peutz-Jeghers* syndrome is a rare familial condition characterized by spotty melanin pigmentation of the skin about the mouth and nose and on the buccal mucous membranes, hands, and fingers, in association with extensive small-intestinal polyposis.

The association of melanosis with an increased number of melanocytes is essentially confined to the pigmented nevi and melanotic carcinoma. This latter condition usually arises from a pigmented nevus but may occur in a nonpigmented mole, callus, normal skin, and especially in the pigmented cells of the retina. These malignancies may produce a diffuse melanin pigmentation of the skin in addition to the pigmentation of direct metastases.

Melanuria occurs chiefly in those cases of melanotic carcinoma with extensive primary or metastatic growths. It is seen very rarely in patients with Addison's disease and in heavily pigmented individuals with obstipation or chronic intestinal obstruction, and may be detected chemically following intense solar irradiation. At autopsy melanin may be detected in these conditions, by silver stain, as a granular deposit in the cells of the renal tubules, as well as in the reticuloendothelial cells of the liver, spleen, and lymph nodes. Its presence in the urine is indicated by a brown-black color. In some cases a colorless breakdown product of melanin, *pyrocatechol,* may be excreted which turns yellow on addition of ferric chloride. The dark urine occurring in porphyrinuria, alkaptonuria, and hemoglobinuria has occasionally been mistakenly reported as melanuria and should be carefully distinguished.

Symptomatology. The symptomatology of melanosis is that of the underlying disease which causes it. Its appearance varies widely, according to hereditary characteristics and etiologic factors. The pigmentary color may vary from light brownish yellow to blue-black, depending on the amount of pigment formed. It may be diffuse, covering the entire body, or localized to exposed or irritated surfaces, to skin folds, or to mucous membranes. It may occur in irregular splotches of any size or in sharply demarcated spots, such as in freckles and pigmented nevi.

Differential Diagnosis. Melanosis should be differentiated from pigmentation due to the absorption of metal, such as argyria, chrysiasis, and bismuthia, by the history, by the color and location of the pigment deposits, and by biopsy. Hemochroma-tosis, hemosiderosis, xanthomatosis, and carotenoderma may be distinguished by similar means.

Treatment. Melanosis in itself is a harmless condition and requires no treatment. It should be considered an important diagnostic sign of an underlying disease toward which treatment should be directed.

OCHRONOSIS

Ochronosis is an unusual metabolic pigmentary disorder, characterized by increased deposition of pigment in bone, cartilage, ligaments, and skin.

Incidence. It is a rare disease, less than 100 cases having been reported. Ochronosis is more frequent in men than in women.

Etiology. Increased pigment deposition characteristic of ochronosis may occur under three widely varying circumstances:

1. In association with an inborn error in the metabolism of tyrosine and phenylalanine, with resulting excretion of homogentisic acid. It is not unusual for several members of the same family to be affected (see Alkaptonuria, in Chap. 88).

2. Following prolonged external use of carbolic acid preparations.

3. In association with disturbed melanin metabolism.

Pathology. Excessive deposition of extracellular pigmentation in cartilage, bone, tendons, and other fibrous tissues throughout the body characterizes the condition of ochronosis. The cartilaginous structures may be so heavily pigmented as to be coal black in color. In its chronic form there is an increased tendency for degenerative changes such as arteriosclerosis and osteoarthropathies to take place, with resulting impairment in function. The pigment in the familial cases is a polymer of homogentisic acid closely related in structure to melanin. An excessive quantity of porphyrins has also been noted to contribute to the pigment deposits in bone.

Clinical Picture. Ochronosis may be asymptomatic. Early manifestations include bluish or bluish-black discoloration of the cartilages, particularly those of the ears and nose, and pigmentation of sclera, cornea, and skin of the face. Transillumination may reveal increased density of bones, particularly of the hands. One may observe greenish-brown axillary sebum and brownish-black cerumen. Characteristically, the urine turns from brown to black on standing or upon addition of alkali. The disease runs a chronic course, later being characterized by progressive development of degenerative changes, especially involving the larger joints, with premature systemic arteriosclerosis.

Diagnosis. The diagnosis is frequently first suggested by the observation of a brown discolorization of the linen stained by urine. In addition, the urine will turn from brown to black upon standing or upon addition of alkali. Later an observation of bluish-black discoloration of the cartilages makes the diagnosis quite evident.

Treatment. Obviously, carbolic acid preparations should be discontinued if they are being used. If homogentisic acid is demonstrated (alkaptonuria), vitamin C in large doses (500 mg daily) and a diet of restricted protein, high carbohydrate, and high fat may be used; the latter may be helpful if the ochronosis is associated with melanuria. In long-standing cases, therapy will be of little avail except for those measures directed toward correcting or relieving the degenerative changes.

REFERENCES

CAROTENEMIA AND CAROTENODERMA

Jeghers, H.: Medical Progress: Pigmentation of the Skin, New Engl. J. Med., 231:88, 1944.
Karrer, P., and E. Jucker: "Carotenoids," Amsterdam, Holland, Elsevier Publishing Company, 1950 (distributed by Elsevier Press, Inc., Houston, Tex.).
Reich, P., H. Shwachman, and J. M. Craig: Lycopenia, a Variant of Carotenemia, New Engl. J. Med., 262:263, 1960.

MELANOSIS AND MELANURIA

Becker, S. W., and M. E. Obermayer: "Modern Dermatology and Syphilology," pp. 3–7, Philadelphia, J. B. Lippincott Company, 1940.
Deutsch, S., and H. Mescon: Medical Progress: Melanin Pigmentation and Its Control, New Engl. J. Med., 257: Aug. 1 and Aug. 8, 1957.
Jacobsen, V. C., and G. H. Klinck: Melanin: I. Its Mobilization and Excretion in Normal and in Pathologic Conditions, Arch. Pathol., 17:141, 1934.
Jeghers, H.: Medical Progress: Pigmentation of the Skin, New Engl. J. Med., 231:88, 122, 181, 1944.
Lerner, A. B.: Melanin Pigmentation, Am. J. Med., 19:902, 1955.
——, and J. S. McGuire: Effect of Alpha- and Beta-Melanocyte Stimulating Hormone on the Skin Colour of Man, Nature, 189:176, 1961.

OCHRONOSIS

Oppenheimer, B. S., and B. S. Kline: Ochronosis: With Study of an Additional Case, Arch. Internal Med., 29:732, 1922.
Skinsnes, O. K.: Generalized Ochronosis: Report of Instance in Which It Was Misdiagnosed as Melanosarcoma with Resultant Enucleation of Eye, Arch. Pathol., 45:552, 1948.
Smith, J. W.: Ochronosis of Sclera and Cornea Complicating Alkaptonuria: Review of the Literature and Report of Four Cases, J.A.M.A., 120:1282, 1942.

PART FIVE

Disorders Due to Chemical and Physical Agents

Section 1: Chemical Agents

99 ALCOHOL

Maurice Victor and
Raymond D. Adams

Intemperance creates many problems in modern society, the importance of which can be judged by the repeated emphasis they receive in contemporary writings, both literary and scientific, as well as from health, social, and religious agencies. These problems may be divided into three categories—the psychologic, the medical, and the sociologic. The main psychologic problem is why a person drinks excessively, often with full knowledge that such action will result in physical injury to himself and irreparable harm to his family. The medical problem embraces all the diseases which relate to overindulgence in alcohol. The sociologic problem comprises the effects of sustained inebriety on the family and community.

The various problems raised by excessive drinking cannot be separated from one another, and the physician must therefore be conversant with all aspects of the subject. He may be asked to help the patient conquer his alcoholic tendency or to diagnose and treat the numerous diseases to which he is subject; often he must admit or commit the patient to a general or mental hospital, according to the nature of the clinical disorder that the patient presents; and lastly, he may be required to enlist the aid of available social agencies when their services are needed by either the patient or his family.

Alcoholism is the term applied to the state of addiction to alcohol as well as to the clinical abnormalities that result from the excessive consumption of alcohol. An *alcoholic* has been defined as one whose dependence upon alcohol has attained such a degree that it interferes with his health, his interpersonal relations, and his social and economic position. By this definition, there are in the United States about 5 million alcoholics. It requires little projection of the imagination to conceive the havoc wrought by alcohol in terms of decreased productivity, accidents, crime, mental and physical disease, and disruption of family life.

PHARMACOLOGY AND METABOLISM OF ALCOHOL

Ethyl alcohol, or ethanol, is the active ingredient in beer, wine, whisky, gin, brandy, and other less common alcoholic beverages. In addition, the stronger spirits contain enanthic ethers, which give the flavor but have no important pharmacologic properties, and impurities such as amyl alcohol (fusel oil) and acetaldehyde, which act like alcohol but are more toxic. Contrary to prevailing opinion, the content of B vitamins in American beer and other liquors is so low as to offer little or no protection against avitaminosis.

Alcohol is absorbed unaltered from the gastrointestinal tract, about 80 per cent from the intestine and the remainder from the stomach. Its presence may be detected in the blood within 5 min after ingestion, and the maximum concentration is reached in $\frac{1}{2}$ to 2 hr. The ingestion of milk and fatty foods impedes and water facilitates its absorption. In habituated persons the blood alcohol concentration actually rises somewhat faster and reaches a higher maximum than in abstainers.

Alcohol is carried chiefly in the plasma and enters the various organs of the body, as well as the spinal fluid, urine, and pulmonary alveolar air, in concentrations which bear a constant relationship to that in the blood. Elimination of alcohol is accomplished chiefly by oxidation, less than 2 per cent being lost through the lungs, skin, and kidneys. The energy liberated by the oxidation of alcohol (7 Cal per Gm) can be utilized as completely as that of the fats, sugars, and proteins, which it replaces isodynamically. It is important to emphasize that alcohol cannot be stored in the body or used in the replacement of destroyed tissue. Unless, therefore, the protein intake is adequate, a state of negative nitrogen balance will develop, a common finding in chronic alcoholics.

The oxidation of alcohol is accomplished mainly in the liver, where a series of catalytic enzymes metabolize alcohol, first to acetaldehyde, then to acetic acid, and finally to carbon dioxide and water. For practical purposes it may be accepted that once absorption is ended and an equilibrium established with the tissues, ethyl alcohol is oxidized at a constant rate, quite independent of its concentration in the blood. There are very few factors capable of affecting alcohol metabolism, although it would appear that animals with a high metabolism of carbohydrate are capable of oxidizing alcohol more rapidly than animals depleted of carbohydrate. On the other hand, the rate of oxidation of acetaldehyde does depend on its concentration in the tissues. The fact is of importance in connection with the drug disulfiram (Antabuse), which increases the tissue concentration necessary to metabolize a certain amount of acetaldehyde per unit of time. The patient taking both Antabuse and alcohol will accumulate an inordinate amount of acetaldehyde, resulting in nausea, vomiting, and hypotension sometimes pronounced and even fatal in degree. This pharmacologic principle underlies the treatment of alcoholism with Antabuse.

PSYCHOLOGIC AND PHYSIOLOGIC EFFECTS OF ALCOHOL

Alcoholic intoxication is such a universal phenomenon that there are few adults who do not know its effects from personal experience. A large body of data has accumulated regarding the psychomotor effects of alcohol, the nature of tolerance to alcohol, the relation of the blood alcohol level to intoxication, and the effect of alcohol on the various organs of the body. Only a few pertinent data will be presented here.

It is now generally accepted that alcohol is not a stimulant of the central nervous system, but a depressant. The early effects, seemingly of stimulation, are due to a depression of central inhibition, presumably a direct cerebral action; the later effects are attributed to a spread of the depression to other parts of the nervous system.

All manner of motor performance, whether simply the maintenance of a standing posture, the control of speech and eye movements, or the highly organized and complex motor skills such as typewriting, are adversely affected by alcohol. The movements involved in these motor acts are not only slowed but made more inaccurate and random in character and therefore less well adapted to the accomplishment of specific ends.

Similarly, alcohol impairs the efficiency of mental function, even after ingestion of a moderate quantity. Alcohol interferes with the learning process, which is slowed and rendered less effective. The faculty of forming associations, whether in the form of words or of figures, tends to be hampered, and the power of attention and concentration is reduced. The individual is not so versatile as usual in directing thought along new lines appropriate to the problems at hand. Finally, alcohol impairs the faculty of judgment and discrimination, and hence, all in all, the ability to think and reason clearly.

The immediate effect of alcohol on organs other than the central nervous system is relatively unimportant. With intoxicating doses the pulse rate rises, blood pressure falls, and there is cutaneous vasodilatation at the expense of splanchnic constriction. Increased sweating and vasodilatation cause a loss of body heat and a fall in temperature.

In low concentrations, by whatever route it is administered, alcohol is capable of stimulating the gastric glands to produce acid, apparently by causing the tissues to form or release histamine. With the ingestion of alcohol in concentrations of over 10 to 15 per cent the secretion of mucus is increased, the stomach mucosa becomes congested and hyperemic, and the secretion of acid then becomes depressed. This is a state of acute gastritis, from which recovery is relatively rapid. The increase in appetite following ingestion of alcohol is due to the stimulation of the end organs of taste and to a general sense of well-being. Similarly, the reviving effect of alcohol in fatigue states is a cerebral one, not due to a direct stimulating effect on muscle or other organs.

Alcohol also exerts a distinct effect on the renal excretion of water and electrolytes. The ingestion of 4 oz of 100-proof bourbon whisky, for example, results in a diuresis qualitatively indistinguishable from that which follows the drinking of large amounts of water. This diuresis is most likely due to the transient suppression of the release of antidiuretic hormone (ADH) from the neurohypophysis, since a relatively small amount of alcohol injected directly into a carotid artery evokes a prompt diuresis without a detectable rise in the concentration of alcohol in the systemic blood. The exact locus of action within the supraopticohypophyseal system is unknown. Alcohol does not alter the sensitivity of the kidney tubules to endogenous or exogenous ADH (Pitressin) and has no discernible effect on renal hemodynamic function in normal persons. The degree of diuresis seems to be more closely related to the duration of the rising blood alcohol level than to the rate of increase or the absolute level attained. In recumbent persons, the water diuresis following the ingestion of alcohol is associated with a diminished excretion of electrolytes (Na, K, Cl), presumably due to vasodilatation and the consequent redistribution of the circulating blood volume. There is also an increased urinary excretion of ammonium and titratable acidity following alcohol, owing to a mild degree of both metabolic and respiratory acidosis. The former is presumably due to an accumulation of acid metabolites and the latter to the direct action of alcohol on the respiratory center.

A scale relating the various degrees of clinical intoxication to the blood alcohol level in nonhabituated persons has been constructed by Miles. He found that at blood alcohol levels of 30 mg per 100 ml a mild euphoria was detectable, and at 50 mg per 100 ml, a mild incoordination. At 100 mg per 100 ml ataxia was obvious, at 300 mg per 100 ml the patient was stuporous, and a level of 400 mg per 100 ml was accompanied by deep anesthesia and could prove fatal. These figures are valid, provided that the alcohol content rises steadily over a 2-hr period. Such a scale has practically no value in the alcoholic patient, for it does not take into account the adjustment which the organism makes to alcohol, i.e., the phenomenon of tolerance. It is common knowledge that a habituated person can drink more and show fewer effects than the abstainer or moderate drinker. The organism is also capable of adapting itself to the presence of alcohol after a very short exposure. If the alcohol concentration in the blood is raised very slowly, no symptoms appear, even at quite high levels. Also, if the concentration is maintained at a constant level over a period of time, the symptoms of intoxication, originally present, disappear, despite a lack of change in the blood alcohol levels. It would appear that the important factor in this rapid adaptability is not so much the rate of increment or the height of the blood alcohol level, but the length of time the alcohol had been present in the body.

This type of tolerance accounts for the surprisingly large amounts of alcohol that can be consumed in a 24-hr period without significant signs of drunkenness. Three patients studied at the Addiction Research Center in Lexington, Ky., consumed 397 to 466 ml of 95 per cent alcohol per day without having any significant amounts of alcohol in the blood or clinical evidence of intoxication. In these patients, there was a very narrow margin between the doses associated with low blood alcohol levels and sobriety and the doses associated with high blood levels and drunkenness (between 430 and 479 ml daily). Observations such as these would tend to invalidate the use of a single estimation of alcohol concentration as a reliable index of drunkenness. It has also been shown that, if the dosage of alcohol which just causes blood levels to be high is held constant, the blood alcohol concentration falls and clinical evidence of intoxication disappears. The cause of this fall in alcohol concentration is not clear. This type of tolerance has been referred to as "metabolic" in contrast to "tissue tolerance," which refers to the adjustments made by the nervous system to long-continued exposure to alcohol. The latter seems to depend on an altered nervous tissue response, i.e., a biochemical adaptation of the habituated individual enabling him to function more effectively at a given alcohol concentration. The precise nature of the adaptation is still a matter of conjecture. Undoubtedly some inborn factor plays a part in determining relative susceptibility. It is also conceivable that there is a psychologic adjustment to high concentrations of alcohol in nervous tissues. The habituated individual may learn to compensate for his lack of coordination and the removal of his inhibitions in a manner that would be impossible for the abstainer.

CLINICAL MANIFESTATIONS OF ALCOHOLISM

The clinical effects of alcohol are mainly on the digestive organs and on the nervous system. Each of these will now be considered.

Effect of Alcohol on the Digestive Organs. The most common medical symptoms in alcoholics are gastrointestinal. Since these have been largely dealt with in other chapters, they will be only summarily treated here. Distinctive symptoms are *morning nausea and vomiting*, or the "dry heaves." These occur on first arising and may be spontaneous or provoked by food or cigarettes. They subside after one or several drinks, the patient then being able to consume large quantities of alcohol without recurrence of symptoms until the following morning. Since sufficient alcohol actually relieves the condition, the local effects of alcohol on the stomach are probably not responsible for this complaint. Gray, on the basis of a gastroscopic study of 100 alcoholics, concluded that this syndrome is not related to gastritis and postulated a central or "psychic" origin.

Many other gastrointestinal symptoms are common in the alcoholic patient. Particularly prominent are abdominal distention, epigastric distress, belching, and atypical or even typical ulcer symptoms and hematemesis. The pathologic basis for these symptoms is similarly diverse. Superficial gastritis is found in all alcoholics following a prolonged drinking bout; this lesion, which is usually reversible in a few days, may occasionally be the source of serious bleeding. The gastritis may be of all degrees of severity, however, and associated with erosions or with actual ulcerations. Lacerations at the cardioesophageal junction may cause profound or fatal hemorrhage (Mallory-Weiss syndrome). The lesion seems to be superimposed on the chronic gastritis of the alcoholic patient and follows severe retching. The incidence of peptic ulceration of the stomach and duodenum is exceptionally high in the alcoholic population.

The excessive ingestion of alcohol and the concomitant state of semistarvation bring about, within a few months, an enlargement of the liver, due to infiltration with fat. *Fatty hepatosis*, as this is called, is present in the majority of alcoholics who require admission to the hospital and is readily reversible. If the patient persists in his alcoholic and poor dietary habits, *alcoholic cirrhosis of the liver* may develop. This state, by virtue of its serious complications, such as anorexia, ascites, bleeding esophageal varices, and hepatic coma, is of prime medical importance. The relative importance of alcohol or deficient diet in the etiology of cirrhosis is still not settled; most likely these two factors act together.

Alcohol is also important in the production of *pancreatitis*. In its mildest form this condition is frequently attributed to acute gastritis, or it may go unnoticed, unless detected by a transient elevation of the serum amylase. Sometimes the patient presents symptoms of an acute abdominal condition, characterized by epigastric pain, vomiting, and rigidity of the upper abdominal muscles. These symptoms may so closely simulate those of perforated peptic ulcer that laparotomy is performed. Here the pancreas is tense and edematous, often with a serosanguineous exudation of fluid on its surface. In the absence of jaundice, surgical intervention is not indicated in alcoholic pancreatitis, and a needless operation might occasionally be avoided by the use of tests of pancreatic dysfunction. At times an acute hemorrhagic necrosis of the pancreas follows the ingestion of a large amount of alcohol. Curiously, such a catastrophe may afflict an individual who has had little or no previous indulgence in alcohol. A particularly troublesome clinical problem is a chronic recurrent type of pancreatitis. The etiology of pancreatic necrosis is discussed in Chap. 279). The fact that alcohol is a powerful stimulant of the gastric acidity is probably the important factor, since acid is the stimulus for the production of secretin, which in turn stimulates the pancreatic secretions.

Effect of Alcohol on the Nervous System. The neurologic disorders that complicate alcoholism can be classified as follows:

Table 99-1. CLASSIFICATION OF THE NEUROLOGIC DISORDERS THAT COMPLICATE ALCOHOLISM

I. Alcoholic intoxication
   A. Simple drunkenness
   B. Alcoholic coma
   C. Alcoholic excitement ("pathologic intoxication")
II. The abstinence or withdrawal syndrome
   A. Alcoholic tremulousness
   B. Alcoholic hallucinosis
   C. Acute and chronic auditory hallucinosis
   D. Alcoholic epilepsy
   E. Delirium tremens
III. Nutritional diseases of the nervous system
   A. The Wernicke-Korsakoff syndrome
   B. Polyneuropathy (neuritic beriberi)
   C. Alcohol (nutritional) amblyopia
   D. Pellagra
IV. Diseases in which the pathogenesis is uncertain
   A. Cerebellar degeneration
   B. Marchiafava-Bignami disease
   C. Central pontine myelinolysis

ALCOHOLIC INTOXICATION

Drunkenness is such a common phenomenon that its psychologic and physical effects require no elaboration. The signs of intoxication consist of varying degrees of exhilaration and excitement, loss of restraint, irregularities of behavior, loquacity, slurred speech, incoordination of movements and gait, irritability, combativeness, drowsiness, stupor, and coma. These signs are quite distinctive and as a rule present no problem in diagnosis or management. That alcohol may be an important cause of *coma* is not generally appreciated. This group of patients offers a serious problem in differential diagnosis. It should be stressed that the diagnosis of alcoholic coma is made not merely on the basis of a flushed face, stupor, and the odor of alcohol, but only after the careful exclusion of all other causes of coma. Furthermore, alcoholic coma is not always benign, as are the more common manifestations of intoxication. The ingestion of large amounts of alcohol over a short period of time may cause an irreversible depression of respiration. Such a state, heralded by the loss of corneal and pupillary reflexes, calls for the use of respiratory stimulants and the treatment of peripheral vascular collapse, if this should manifest itself.

In a small proportion of patients, acute intoxication results in greatly exaggerated rather than impairment of activity. In medical writings this abnormal reaction to alcohol is referred to as "pathologic intoxication" or "acute alcoholic paranoid state." This state is characterized by an outburst of irrational, combative, and at times destructive behavior and terminates when the patient falls into a deep stupor, after which he may have no memory for the entire episode. This unusual reaction may allegedly occur with the ingestion of small amounts of alcohol. It has been ascribed to constitutional differences in the susceptibility to alcohol, to previous craniocerebral trauma, and to an underlying epileptic predisposition, but there is little factual data to support any of these beliefs. An analogy may be drawn between this state of alcoholic excitement and a similar state which is provoked by barbiturates under some circumstances, as for example, when the latter drug is administered for the relief of pain.

The various manifestations of alcoholic intoxication are the result of a depressant action of the drug on nerve cells, acting in a manner akin to the general anesthetics. Unlike the general anesthetics, however, the margin between the dose of alcohol which produces surgical anesthesia and that which is dangerously depressant to respiration is a very narrow one. This fact accounts for the occasional fatality in cases of alcoholic narcosis.

THE ABSTINENCE
OR WITHDRAWAL SYNDROME

Of more serious consequence than the states of intoxication are the tremulous, hallucinatory, epileptic, and delirious states. Although prolonged inebriety is the underlying factor in these illnesses, the symptoms become manifest after a period of relative or absolute abstinence from alcohol. For this reason they may collectively be referred to as the abstinence or withdrawal syndrome. Each of these symptom complexes may occur distinct from the others and will be described as though it occurred in pure form. More frequently, however, they occur in various combinations; indeed, a single patient may show all the symptoms enumerated above. The prototype of the patients afflicted with these symptoms is the spree or periodic drinker, although the steady drinker is not immune if, for some reason, alcohol is withdrawn.

Alcoholic Tremulousness. By far the most common manifestation of the abstinence syndrome is a state of tremulousness, commonly referred to as "the shakes" or "the jitters," combined with a general irritability and gastrointestinal symptoms. The symptoms first show themselves after several days of drinking; they consist of tremulousness, nausea, and vomiting and occur in the morning, after the short period of abstinence that occurs during sleep. The patient needs to "quiet his nerves" by a few drinks; his symptoms are in fact relieved by alcohol, only to return the next morning with increasing persistence and severity. The usual spree lasts about 2 weeks, but this is variable. It is terminated not only because of recurrent tremor and vomiting, but for any one of many other reasons such as lack of funds, weakness, self-disgust, or collapse. The symptoms then become greatly augmented, reaching their peak intensity 24 to 36 hr after the complete cessation of drinking.

At this stage, the patient presents a distinctive clinical picture. He is alert and startles easily. His face is deeply flushed, the conjunctivas are injected, and there is usually a tachycardia. Anorexia, nausea, and retching are always in evidence. He may complain of insomnia and craves rest and sleep. He is preoccupied with his misery, inattentive and disinclined to answer questions; or he may respond in a rude or perfunctory manner. The patient may be mildly disoriented in time, but shows no significant confusion, being generally aware of his surroundings and of the nature of his illness.

Generalized tremor is an outstanding feature of this illness. It fluctuates widely, being hardly recognizable when the patient is calm, becoming gross and irregular upon attempted activity and during periods of emotional stress. The tremor may be so violent that the patient cannot stand without help, speak clearly, or feed himself. Sometimes there is little objective evidence of tremor, and the patient complains only of being "shaky inside."

Although the flushed facies, anorexia, tachycardia, and tremor subside largely within a few days, the patient does not regain his full composure for a much longer time. The overalertness, tendency to startle easily, and jerkiness of movement may persist for a week or longer; the curious feeling of uneasiness may not leave the patient completely for 10 or 14 days, and only at the end of this time is he able to sleep undisturbed, without sedation. An attempt should be made to keep the patient in hospital for this length of time; to discharge him after a few days increases the likelihood that he will turn to alcohol to suppress his still-present tenseness and sleeplessness.

Alcoholic Hallucinosis. Symptoms of disordered sense perception occur in about one-quarter of the tremulous patients. The patient may complain of what he calls "bad dreams." These are described as unnatural, nightmarish episodes associated with disturbed sleep, and only with difficulty can they be separated from real experience. Sounds and shadows may be misinterpreted, or familiar objects may be distorted and assume unreal forms. Although these are not hallucinations in the strict sense of the term, they represent the most common forms of disordered sense perception in the alcoholic. Of the actual hallucinations, the visual ones are the most common. There is little evidence to support the popular belief that certain visual hallucinations are specific to alcoholism. They are more commonly animate than inanimate and may comprise various forms of human, animal, or insect life. They may occur singly or in panoramas; they may appear shrunken or enlarged; they may be natural in appearance or take a distorted and hideous form.

Acute and Chronic Auditory Hallucinosis. This phenomenon in chronic alcoholics merits separate consideration. For many years, an alcoholic psychosis has been recognized in which vivid auditory hallucinations were the major abnormality. Kraepelin referred to this as the *hallucinatory insanity of drunkards* or *alcoholic mania,* and Wernicke, as the *acute hallucinosis of drunkards.* The central feature of the illness, in the beginning, is the occurrence of auditory hallucinations in an otherwise clear sensorium; that is, the patients are well oriented, not confused or obtunded, and have an intact memory. The hallucinations are almost always vocal in nature, although at times there are other auditory phenomena, such as the sound of running motors, buzzing, music, ringing of telephones, or dogs barking. When the voices can be identified, they are attributed to the patient's family, friends, or neighbors, rarely to God, radio, or radar. The voices may be directly addressed to the patient, or they may discuss him in the third person. In the majority of cases the voices are maligning, reproachful, or threatening in nature and are disturbing to the patient; a significant proportion, however, are not unpleasant and leave the patient undisturbed. The voices are intensely real and vivid, and they tend to be exteriorized; i.e., they come from behind the door, from the corridor, or through the wall. Another quality of these hallucinations, as of the visual ones, is the appropriateness of the patient's emotional response to the hallucinatory content. He may call on the police for protection or barricade and arm himself against invaders; even more dramatically, he may attempt suicide to avoid what the voices threaten. The hallucinations may be intermittent or continuous. Their duration varies greatly—they may be momentary, or they may last for days, and in exceptional instances for weeks or months.

Most patients, while actively hallucinating, have no appreciation of the unreality of their hallucinations. Insight is usually regained concomitantly with the cessation of the hallucinations. As the patient improves, he begins to doubt the reality of his hallucinations, is reluctant to talk of them, and may even question whether he had been sane during the episode. Full recovery is characterized by the realization that the voices were imaginary and by the ability to recall with remarkable clarity the abnormal thought content of the psychotic episode.

A unique feature of this psychosis is the evolution of a chronic auditory hallucinosis in a small proportion of the patients. At the outset, these patients show the characteristics of the more transient form of the illness, but after a variable period of time, the symptomatology is altered. In some patients the transition can be recognized after as short a period as 1 week. The patient becomes quiet and resigned, despite the fact that the hallucinations remain threatening and derogatory. Ideas of reference and influence and other poorly systematized paranoid delusions become prominent. At this stage these patients show many of the symptoms of schizophrenia—illogical thinking, vagueness, tangential associations, and a dissociation of affect and of thought content. There is some evidence that repeated attacks of acute auditory hallucinosis render the patient more vulnerable to this chronic form of the illness. Despite the similarities to schizophrenia, there are also points of difference. In the alcoholic illness the age of onset is considerably beyond that of "classic" schizophrenia; the past history reveals no evidence of schizophrenia or "schizoid" personality traits, and the symptoms develop in close temporal relationship to a drinking bout.

Alcoholic Epilepsy. The intimate connection between alcoholism and epilepsy has long been appreciated; the terms *alcoholic epilepsy* and "rum fits" are usually employed to designate the relationship. Unfortunately the former term lacks precision because of the variety of meanings that have been given to it. For example, the term is applied by some to patients with idiopathic epilepsy, in whom alcohol tends to increase the liability to seizures. Lennox found that, contrary to many previously expressed opinions, the incidence of heavy drinking is no greater in epileptic patients than in the general population; however, in approximately one-half of those who did use alcohol excessively there were more frequent seizures. This term is also used in instances of posttraumatic epilepsy, in which the number and severity of the seizures may be increased by even a short period of drinking.

There is, however, a clinical setting in which there exists a close relationship between alcoholism and epilepsy and to which the term "rum fits" most accurately applies. Patients in this category develop seizures for the first time after many years of excessive drinking. The seizures may occur singly, more often in bursts of two to six, and on rare occasions the patient may be found in status epilepticus. The seizures are grand mal in type, i.e., major generalized motor seizures with loss of consciousness.

The seizures, like tremulousness and hallucinations, do not occur when the patient is inebriated but are related to relative or absolute abstinence. The majority of seizures occur within the first 48 hr following the cessation of drinking. During this time there may be electroencephalographic abnormalities characteristic of seizure activity, particularly in response to hyperventilation and stroboscopic stimulation. In experimental subjects addicted to alcohol, this increased liability to seizures has been shown to occupy a discrete and brief period (17 to 33 hr) following the withdrawal of alcohol. After this period, and in the period between drinking bouts, the electroencephalographic patterns of patients with rum fits are normal. These observations would tend to discredit the widely held belief that alcohol causes seizures to become manifest only in those with "latent epilepsy" or with an "epileptic constitution."

The alcoholic complication most closely related to epilepsy is typical delirium tremens. In 101 consecutive patients whom the authors observed with delirium tremens, 30 also had seizures, always preceding the delirium. In the patients affected by both seizures and delirium the postictal confusional state may blend imperceptibly with the onset of delirium, or there may be a partial clearing of the postictal state before the delirium sets in; in a small group of patients the effects of the seizure may clear completely, the delirium showing itself within 12 hr to 5 days later.

"Rum fits" must be carefully distinguished from the various types of seizures which occur for the first time in adult life, viz., those due to cerebral trauma, infarction, abscess, infection, etc. If the alcoholic patient suffers focal seizures, one must invoke causes other than alcohol.

Delirium Tremens. This is the most dramatic and grave of all the alcoholic complications and is characterized by increased psychomotor and autonomic activity, disorientation, confusion, disordered sense perception, and at times a fatal outcome. The clinical features of delirium have been presented in detail in Chap. 38, The Acute Confusional States; only those features peculiar to the alcoholic variety (delirium tremens) are considered here. Delirium tremens develops in a variety of settings. The patient, an excessive and steady drinker of many years' duration, may have been admitted to the hospital for an unrelated illness, accident, operation, or infection, and 3 to 4 days later becomes delirious. Or following a prolonged spree, he may have already suffered through several days of tremulousness, hallucinosis, or seizures, and may even be recovering from these symptoms, when he suddenly develops delirium tremens.

In the majority of cases delirium tremens is benign and short-lived, ending as abruptly as it begins. Consumed by the relentless activity and wakefulness of several days' duration, the patient falls into a deep sleep; he awakens lucid, quiet, hungry, and exhausted, with virtually no memory for the events of the delirious period. Less commonly the delirious state subsides gradually; more rarely still there may be one or more relapses, several discrete episodes of delirium being separated by lucidity, the entire process lasting for as little as several days or as long as 4 or 5 weeks. The recurrent type presents the most confusing picture of all, for the delirious periods may be of varying severity and duration, and the lucid intervals of varying completeness. Where the delirium occurs as a single episode, the duration is 72 hr or less in over 80 per cent of the cases.

About 15 per cent of cases end fatally, and in the majority of these there is an associated infectious illness or injury. Other patients, even those without complicating illnesses, may develop hyperthermia or a state of peripheral circulatory collapse. In some, death comes so suddenly that the terminal events cannot be discerned.

Closely related to typical delirium tremens and about as common are the *atypical delirious-hallucinatory states*. These are bizarre variations in which one facet of the delirium tremens complex assumes prominence to the practical exclusion of the other symptoms. The patient may simply exhibit a transient state of quiet confusion, agitation, and peculiar behavior, or he may become violent and disturbed. Other patients present a vivid delusional state and abnormal behavior, consistent with their false beliefs. Such a patient may relate a loosely connected and fantastic tale of fighting pitched battles, participation in the Indian wars or bank robberies, or the like, although he may be superficially oriented and may later recall his delusions. Several of these symptoms may be combined, so that these states blend imperceptibly with fully developed delirium tremens. Unlike typical delirium tremens, these atypical states always present as a single circumscribed episode without recurrences, are only rarely preceded by epilepsy, and do not end fatally. This may be another way of saying that they are a partial or less severe form of the disease.

Pathologic examination is singularly unrevealing in the tremulous-hallucinatory-epileptic-delirious states. Edema and brain swelling have been absent in the authors' pathologic material except with shock, terminal hypoxia, or electrolyte imbalance, nor have there been any significant microscopic changes in the brain. Estimations of the blood sugar, nonprotein nitrogen, carbon dioxide, and the spinal fluid disclose no characteristic abnormalities. Low values of serum sodium, chloride, potassium, and magnesium occur unpredictably. The electroencephalographic findings have been discussed in relation to alcoholic epilepsy.

Etiology and the Role of Abstinence. Although chronic intoxication underlies all the illnesses included in this group, the mechanism by which alcohol produces its effects has been a matter of debate. That alcohol exerts a direct toxic effect would seem unlikely, since it nullifies symptoms such as nausea and vomiting, tremor, and hallucinosis. Furthermore, the signs of intoxication are in themselves distinctive and different from those under discussion. As has been indicated in the preceding descriptions, there exists a relation between the onset of the tremulous-hallucinatory-epileptic-delirious states and the relative or absolute withdrawal of alcohol. Aside from morning tremor and nausea, one can recognize three components of the abstinence syndrome: (1) tremulousness and hallucinations, (2) convulsive seizures, and (3) typical delirium tremens. The mildest degree of this syndrome, tremor and nausea, may arise after only a few days of drinking and after a relatively short period of abstinence. These symptoms may be controlled by reestablishing the blood alcohol level. The most severe form of this syndrome, delirium tremens, requires a background of months or years of inebriation and becomes manifest only after several days of abstinence. Any given patient may show one or all of the symptoms of abstinence, but in the latter instance they become manifest in a predictable sequence—first tremulousness, then seizures and hallucinosis, and finally delirium tremens.

This theory finds its strongest support in the experimental observations made at the Addiction Research Center, Lexington, Ky. In these studies, two groups of human volunteers were addicted over long periods of time to barbiturates and alcohol, respectively. On withdrawal of the drugs, these subjects quickly lost their symptoms of intoxication, and these symptoms were replaced by tremor, hallucinations, seizures, and delirium in this particular sequence.

A number of other theories have been suggested as causally important in this group of illnesses. A specific adrenal deficiency has been postulated. In the authors' experience adrenal cortical extract and ACTH have not altered the course of recovery in these patients in any way that could not be accounted for by the natural history of the disease. These observations would not allow the conclusion that there is an acute or constitutional deficiency in these substances; nor can other constitutional, traumatic, and infectious factors be regarded as more than predisposing causes. Nutritional deficiency has been invoked to explain these illnesses, since so many alcoholics eat poorly. Almost certainly, however, nutritional factors are not of primary importance here, for delirium tremens and its variants may develop in patients taking a normal diet. And as a corollary, these illnesses may subside uneventfully even though the patient receives no nutrients whatsoever. The low serum electrolyte values are probably associated abnormalities rather than causal.

NUTRITIONAL DISEASES OF THE NERVOUS SYSTEM

Nutritional diseases of the nervous system comprise a relatively small but serious group of illnesses in chronic alcoholics. In contrast to the abstinence syndrome, the role of alcohol is purely secondary, the nutritional disorders resulting from the displacement of food by alcohol. These illnesses and the role of alcohol in their production are discussed on pp. 1837 to 1838.

ALCOHOLIC DISEASES IN WHICH THE PATHOGENESIS IS UNCERTAIN

Included in this category are several rare and diverse disorders which are practically always encountered in alcoholic patients. The relationship of these disorders to the excessive use of alcohol is obscure, however, and probably not crucial, since all of them have been described in nonalcoholic patients. In all these disorders there is a suggestion that nutritional deficiency or some related factor is of etiologic significance, but as yet this etiology must be regarded as unproved.

Alcoholic Cerebellar Degeneration. This term is applied to a nonfamilial type of cerebellar ataxia which occurs in adult life against a background of prolonged ingestion of alcohol. The symptoms may progress slowly over a long period, but more frequently they evolve in a subacute fashion in several weeks or months, after which they remain stationary for many years. The signs are those of cerebellar dysfunction, affecting stance and gait predominantly. The legs are involved more frequently than the arms, and nystagmus and cerebellar speech disorders are rare. Once established, the cerebellar signs change very little, although some improvement of gait and recovery from complicating polyneuropathy may follow cessation of drinking. The essential pathologic change consists of a degeneration of varying severity of all the neurocellular elements of the cerebellar cortex, particularly the Purkinje cells, with a striking topographic restriction to the anterior and superior aspects of the vermis and hemispheres. The disorder of stance and gait seems to be related to the vermis lesion, and the ataxia of the limbs to the hemispheral involvement.

Marchiafava-Bignami Disease (Primary Degeneration of the Corpus Callosum). This is a rare complication of alcoholism occurring mainly, but not exclusively, in Italian men addicted to crude red wine. The symptomatology is a diverse one and includes psychic and emotional disorders, delirium and intellectual deterioration, convulsive seizures, varying degrees of tremor, rigidity, and paralysis, and ultimately coma. The duration is variable, from several months to years. The pathologic picture is more constant than the clinical one. It consists of symmetrically placed areas of demyelination in the corpus callosum, particularly the middle lamina, and less consistently of the anterior commissure and other parts of the white matter. Axis cylinders are better preserved than medullated fibers in these areas, and there are appropriate reactions in the macrophages and astrocytes.

Pontine Myelinolysis. This term refers to a rare pathologic change affecting the center of the basis pontis, in which the medullated fibers are destroyed in a single large symmetrical focus. In contrast, the axis cylinders, nerve cells, and blood vessels are well preserved. The disease may manifest itself by pseudobulbar palsy and quadriplegia, or the lesion may be so small as to cause no symptoms. The relationship of this condition to either alcoholism or malnutrition is obscure.

MANAGEMENT OF THE ALCOHOLIC PATIENT

The management of the various gastrointestinal complications of alcoholism is considered in the section dealing with these diseases. The management of the neurologic complications, coma, delirium tremens, and status epilepticus is considered in Chaps. 34 and 36. Here a few remarks will be made about alcoholic habituation. This presents quite a different and often a more difficult problem in management than the medical or neurologic illnesses associated with alcoholism. The patient may not have any disease that requires admission to a hospital but may nevertheless be seriously disabled in his marital, social, and economic life.

The only satisfactory solution to this problem is complete abstinence from all alcohol. This is extremely difficult to accomplish, and even the most experienced physicians and psychiatrists often fail to help the patient overcome his addiction. The following points seem to be of fundamental importance: The patient must accept the fact that he is incapable of drinking in moderation and that he cannot simply cut down on his alcoholic intake but must avoid liquor entirely. Also, the patient himself must have a genuine desire to overcome his drinking habit. If he is forced against his will to consult a physician and is not convinced that alcohol offers a problem, it is usually impossible to modify his alcoholic tendency. The only way to make such an individual discontinue drinking is to commit him to a psychiatric hospital for several weeks or months and to hope that as his health improves he will gain insight and will later accept psychiatric therapy.

If the patient realizes that his drinking habit is beyond his control and that he needs help, the chances of cure are reasonably good. Indeed, under these circumstances, many individuals stop drinking of their own volition. However, some of these patients despite the best of intentions will abandon the therapeutic program. Their will to overcome the alcoholic tendency may be bolstered by a number of methods such as the conditioned reflex technique, the use of Antabuse, psychotherapy, and the participation in social organizations for combating alcoholism.

The conditioned reflex technique consists of giving the patient a dose of emetine or apomorphine, followed by a dose of alcohol. The resultant nausea and vomiting become associated in the patient's mind with the imbibition of alcohol and supposedly create an aversion for the beverage. This form of treatment is usually carried out in special institutions and has therefore only limited value. The use of disulfiram (Antabuse) has been widely publicized in recent years. The principle upon which this treatment is based has been mentioned in the introductory part of this chapter. The patient is given a tablet containing 0.5 Gm daily and is warned of the severe and even fatal hypotension which may result if he drinks while he has the drug in his body. It should never be used in patients with cardiac or liver disease. Treatment with disulfiram has proved to be a useful adjunct in therapy.

There are many conflicting theories of causation of alcoholic addiction, and consequently there is no standard form of psychotherapy. An understandable formulation of the problem is that the alcoholic tendency is symptomatic of a personal weakness which is in the nature of a lack of satisfaction in family and social life, and to conquer it, satisfactory substitutive activities must be found. Supportive treatment should be directed toward improving general nutrition and health and the development of new spheres of activity and interest. Alcoholics Anonymous, an informal fellowship of former alcoholics, has been particularly successful in helping patients who are sincere in wishing to stop drinking. Perhaps the physician may best fulfill his duty by getting the patient to recognize the desirability of abstinence and by inducing him to accept outside help of the sort offered by Alcoholics Anonymous.

REFERENCES

Adams, R. D., Maurice Victor, and Elliott L. Mancall: Central Pontine Myelinolysis, A.M.A. Arch. Neurol. Psychiat., vol. 81, February, 1959.

Isbell, Harris, H. F. Fraser, Abraham Wikler, R. E. Belleville, and Anna J. Eisenman: An Experimental Study of the Etiology of "Rum Fits" and Delirium Tremens, Quart. J. Studies Alc., 16:1, 1955.

Miles, W. R.: "Alcohol and Man," chap. 10, Psychological Effects of Alcohol on Man, New York, The Macmillan Company, 1932.

Victor, M., and R. D. Adams: The Effect of Alcohol on the Nervous System, in "Metabolic and Toxic Diseases of the Nervous System," Research Publs. Assoc. Research Nervous Mental Disease, 32:526, 1953.

—— and J. Hope: The Phenomenon of Auditory Hallucinations in Chronic Alcoholism. J. Nervous Mental Disease, vol. 126, nos. 5 and 6, May-June, 1958.

——, R. D. Adams, and Elliott L. Mancall: A Restricted Form of Cerebellar Cortical Degeneration Occurring in Alcoholic Patients, A.M.A. Arch. Neurol., vol. 1, December, 1959.

100 OPIATES

Maurice Victor

The drugs included in this category are morphine, opium, heroin (diacetylmorphine), Dilaudid (dihydromorphinone), codeine (methylmorphine), Pantopon, dihydrocodeinone (Hycodan), dihydroxycodeinone (Eucodal), and 14-hydroxy-dihydromorphinone (Numorphan). The synthetic analgesics meperidine (Demerol), methadone (Dolophine or amidone), metopon (methyl-dihydromorphinone), racemorphan (Dromoran), alphaprodine (Nisentil), and phenazocine (Prinadol) will also be considered here, since they are similar to the opiates both in their pharmacologic effects and in the patterns of abuse, the differences being mainly quantitative. As with alcohol and the barbiturates, the opiates may be suitably considered from two points of view: (1) acute poisoning and (2) addiction.

OPIATE POISONING

Severe poisoning with morphine or related alkaloids is not a frequent accident, but moderate degrees are relatively common, the result of ingestion with suicidal intent, errors in the calculation of dosage, or unusual sensitivity. In children as well as in adults with myxedema, Addison's disease, chronic liver disease, or pneumonia, there may be an increased susceptibility to opiates, and relatively small doses may prove toxic. Acute poisoning may occur in addicts who are unaware that tolerance for opiates declines quickly after the withdrawal of the drug and who resume the habit at a formerly well-tolerated dose.

The clinical manifestations of acute poisoning are varying degrees of unresponsiveness, shallow respirations, miosis, bradycardia, and hypothermia. Mild intoxication is manifested by anorexia, nausea, vomiting, constipation, and loss of sexual interest. In the most severe degrees of intoxication, the pupils are dilated and cyanosis and circulatory collapse occur. The immediate cause of death is usually respiratory depression, with consequent asphyxia.

Treatment consists of gastric lavage if the drug was taken orally. This procedure may be efficacious many hours after ingestion, since severe pylorospasm may result in much of the drug being retained in the stomach. Other measures are directed toward the maintenance of an adequate airway and oxygenation, as described in the section dealing with barbiturate intoxication. If the patient does not respond rapidly to these measures, N-allylnormorphine (Nalline) should be administered. This is a specific antidote to the opiates and also to the synthetic analgesics. It is given in doses of 5 to 10 mg subcutaneously or intravenously. The improvement of circulation and respiration is usually dramatic; in fact, failure of Nalline to produce a striking improvement in respiration should cast doubt on the diagnosis of opiate intoxication. Nalline does little to restore consciousness, however, and the patient may remain drowsy for many hours. This is not harmful, provided that respiration is well maintained. Since the duration of action of Nalline is shorter than that of all the analgesics except Dilaudid and meperidine, respirations may again become depressed an hour or so after the administration of the antidote. It should then be given a second time, in smaller dosage.

Once the patient regains consciousness, usually in about 8 hr, other complaints such as severe pruritus, sneezing, persistent obstipation, and urinary retention may necessitate symptomatic treatment. Nausea and severe abdominal pain, due presumably to pancreatitis resulting from spasm of the sphincter of Oddi, are other troublesome symptoms.

OPIATE ADDICTION

Compared with the problems arising from the abuse of alcohol and barbiturates, narcotic addiction is not a great public health hazard. It is estimated that there are about 60,000 addicts in the United States, apart from patients who are addicted because of hopeless medical illnesses. Nevertheless, the problem of narcotic addiction is important for a number of reasons. To the patient and his family it is a tragedy which often brings about complete physical, social, and economic ruin. The physician must be constantly alert to the dangers of the long-term use of narcotic drugs and aware of the methods of legal control and treatment of addiction. Without the restraining influence of public health measures, addiction could conceivably assume epidemic proportions.

Etiologic Aspects. A number of factors, socioeconomic, psychologic, and pharmacologic, all contribute to the genesis of opiate addiction. In our culture, the most susceptible subjects are men or delinquent youths living in the economically depressed areas of large cities. Most of these individuals have psychoneurotic disorders, psychopathic personalities, or mental illnesses of other types. Many opiate addicts were formerly alcoholic and during their adolescence may have used marihuana before opiates. These so-called "social addicts" are introduced to drugs through their association with others already addicted. About 20 per cent of all addicts are patients who were introduced to drugs by their physicians in the course of an illness and who continued to use drugs following relief of their ailments. Judging from the studies at the Addiction Research Center, Lexington, Ky., only a few of these "medical" or "accidental" addicts can be regarded as normal, well-adjusted people. Instead the majority have psychologic abnormalities similar to those of the "social" addicts, the only difference being the original mode of contact with the drug.

According to Wikler, the problem of the abuse of opiate drugs progresses in three successive phases: (1) episodic intoxication or euphoria, (2) pharmacogenic dependence or addiction, and (3) the propensity to "relapse after cure" or habituation.

Some of the symptoms of opiate intoxication have already been considered. Of equal importance are the symptoms designated as "morphine euphoria," a term which refers to the pain- and anxiety-reducing abilities of this drug, as well as to the state of elation or sense of unusual well-being which it produces and which is especially prized by psychopathic thrill-seekers.

Individuals who take opiates for their euphoria-producing effects discover the need to increase the dose as time passes, in order to obtain an effect equivalent to that of the original dose. Expressed in another way, the effectiveness of a given dose of the drug decreases. This property, known as *tolerance*, is common to all the opiates and may be very marked in degree, so that enormous amounts, as high as 5,000 mg morphine daily, have been administered without the development of toxic symptoms. The mechanism of tolerance is not completely understood. There is some evidence that, during addiction, increasing amounts of morphine are destroyed or inactivated in the body.

With the continued administration of the drug, an organismal need for the drug develops, in so far as disagreeable symptoms develop when the drug is withheld. Ever-increasing doses of the drug are required for the suppression of these symptoms, and in this way also the use of opiates tends to become self-perpetuating. *Pharmacogenic dependence* or *addiction* refers to the state produced by the repeated administration of the drug, such that if administration of the drug is suddenly terminated, a drug-specific illness develops, termed the *abstinence syndrome*. The intensity of the abstinence syndrome depends mainly on the dose of the drug and duration of addiction, but also on individual factors. In respect to morphine it has been found that the majority of individuals receiving 240 mg daily for 30 days or more will show moderately severe abstinence symptoms following withdrawal, whereas mild grades of abstinence may be detected following as little as 80 mg daily for a similar period.

The abstinence syndrome which occurs in the morphine addict may be taken as the prototype of the opiate group. The first 8 to 16 hr of abstinence usually pass asymptomatically. At the end of this period yawning, rhinorrhea, sweating, and lacrimation become manifest. These symptoms are at first mild but increase in severity over a period of several hours and then remain constant for several days. The patient may be able to sleep during this early period but is restless, and thereafter insomnia remains a prominent feature. Dilatation of the pupils, recurring waves of gooseflesh, and twitchings of the muscles appear. The patient complains of severe aches in the back, abdomen, and legs, and of hot and cold "flashes," so that he covers himself with heavy blankets. By the end of about 36 hr the restlessness becomes more extreme, and nausea, vomiting, and diarrhea usually develop. The temperature, respiration, and blood pressure are slightly elevated. All these symptoms reach their peak intensity 48 to 72 hr after withdrawal, and then gradually decline. After 7 to 10 days, all objective signs of abstinence have disappeared, although the patient may complain of insomnia, nervousness, weakness, and muscle aches for several more weeks.

Wikler has divided the abstinence changes into two types—"nonpurposive" and "purposive." The former comprises the various autonomic and neuromuscular signs and is relatively transient in nature. That these symptoms represent an altered physiologic state and are not psychic in origin has been clearly demonstrated experimentally; physical dependence on morphine and methadone developed in the isolated segment of the spinal cord in chronic spinal and in chronic decorticated dogs. The "purposive changes" refer to the patient's craving for the drug and the manipulative activity directed to obtaining the drug. These symptoms may persist indefinitely and are important in relation to that characteristic of addiction referred to as *habituation, emotional dependence,* or *psychologic dependence.* These terms are used interchangeably and refer to the substitution of drug-seeking activities for all other aims and objects in life. Habituation is regarded by psychiatrists as the most important quality of addiction, since it is this feature which governs the initial use of the drug and relapse following apparent cure of addiction. An individual becomes addicted not because he needs the drug to prevent withdrawal symptoms but because of its euphoric-producing effect, i.e., the relief of pain and emotional discomfort. Similarly, relapse to the use of the drug may occur long after the nonpurposive abstinence changes have disappeared.

Opiates, barbiturates, and alcohol fulfill all three criteria of addiction. In the case of bromides, amphetamine, cocaine, and marihuana, only the factor of habituation is operative, and tolerance and pharmacogenic dependence do not develop.

The characteristics of addiction and of abstinence are qualitatively similar with all the drugs of the opiate group as well as the related synthetic analgesics. The differences are mainly quantitative and are related to the differences in potency and length of action. Heroin, Dilaudid, and metopon are more potent than morphine and have a shorter duration of action; hence the addict requires more doses per day, and the abstinence syndrome comes on and subsides more rapidly. The length of action of Dromoran is somewhat longer than that of morphine, so that withdrawal symptoms appear more slowly, are somewhat less intense, and subside more slowly. Abstinence symptoms from codeine, while very definite, are less intense than those from morphine, come on more slowly, and subside more slowly. Abstinence symptoms from methadone are even less intense and do not become evident until 3 or 4 days after withdrawal; furthermore, this drug is qualitatively different from morphine in so far as autonomic signs are lacking in the abstinence period. For these reasons methadone is used in the treatment of morphine addiction. Demerol addiction is of particular importance because of the high incidence among doctors and nurses and because there is still a widespread belief that this drug is nonaddicting. Tolerance to the toxic effects of Demerol is not complete, so that the addict may show tremors, twitching of the muscles, confusion, hallucinations, and at times convulsions. Signs of abstinence appear 3 to 4 hr after the last dose and reach maximum intensity in 8 to 12 hr, at which time they may be worse than those of morphine abstinence.

Diagnosis of Opiate Addiction. This is usually made by the patient's statement that he is addicted to and needs drugs. If the patient conceals his addiction, the diagnosis may be difficult. Miosis, needle marks, emaciation, or abscess scars are suggestive but not specific signs. Demerol addicts are likely to show dilated pupils and twitching of muscles. Test procedures for opiates in the urine are difficult and usually unavailable. Formerly it was necessary to isolate questionable cases and to observe the patient over a period of at least 2 days for signs of abstinence. By using the specific antagonist Nalline, a diagnosis of addiction to the opiates and related analgesic drugs can be made within an hour.

Nalline should be administered only in the presence of another physician or a nurse, with the full understanding and permission of the patient. Three milligrams of the antidote is given subcutaneously, and if no signs of abstinence have appeared in 20 min an additional 5 mg is given. If no signs have appeared in another 20 min, a final dose of 8 mg is given. Provided that the patient has taken more than occasional doses of the drug within a week of the test, the administration of Nalline will precipitate symptoms of abstinence. These become evident within 5 min of the first injection, reach their peak intensity in 20 min, begin to decline in 60 min, and disappear after 3 hr. Very severe symptoms of abstinence should be treated by small doses of morphine. Curiously, Nalline does not precipitate abstinence symptoms in Demerol addiction, unless the patient has been taking more than 1,600 mg daily.

The Management and Avoidance of Addiction. Once the diagnosis of narcotic addiction has been established, the patient should be persuaded to seek institutional treatment, preferably of the specialized type that is available in the Public Health Service hospitals at Lexington, Ky., and Fort Worth, Tex. Commitment to these institutions is purely voluntary, unless a Federal statute has been violated, and requests for admission should be made directly to the medical officers in charge. The ambulatory treatment of addiction never succeeds and should therefore not be undertaken. Addicts who are refused opiates may ask for methadone, Demerol, or Dromoran, on the grounds that these drugs are synthetic and nonaddicting. These drugs are addicting and have been legally defined as opiates. The physician should also be aware that he is breaking both the letter and the spirit of the regulations if he prescribes narcotics for an addict, merely for the purpose of preventing abstinence changes. Occasional exceptions may be made in cases of seriously ill addicts who are awaiting treatment, or in patients who are suffering from incurable painful disease.

Treatment of the hospitalized patient consists of the administration of morphine in doses just sufficient to prevent nonpurposive abstinence changes. Usually 30 mg four times daily suffices. After 3 days on this dosage, the drug is withdrawn by the so-called "rapid reduction" method in which successively smaller doses are administered over a 5- to 10-day period. A much longer time is required in the presence of serious medical disease. Flow baths, aspirin, intravenous fluids, and the cautious use of barbiturates help to control the abstinence symptoms.

An alternate method, once the patient has been stabilized on morphine, is to substitute methadone for morphine, in the ratio of 1 to 3 mg. After a period of a week, in which the patient receives 10 mg methadone four times daily, the drug is rapidly withdrawn. With this method the abstinence symptoms are relatively mild but long-lasting, so that some patients prefer the first method.

After withdrawal has been completed, the problem is one of preventing relapse. The period of institutional care should be prolonged to 4 to 6 months, if possible, and psychiatric help should be enlisted. Even under the most favorable conditions, continued abstinence is accomplished in only the minority of patients.

The physician must be constantly alert to the dangers of addiction, particularly in susceptible individuals, i.e., in those with psychoneurosis, psychopathic personality, or alcoholism. The use of opiates should be limited to cases where pain is the chief problem; they should not be used primarily as sedatives, or for the relief of asthma, or even in chronic pain until all other measures have been exhausted. It follows that it is most important to make a precise diagnosis of the cause or causes of pain, since in some cases measures other than opiates will suffice, while in others, such as hysteria and depression, narcotics are contraindicated.

If narcotics have to be used for the relief of chronic pain, then some consideration should be given to the choice of the appropriate drug and to the mode of administration. Morphine is still the drug of choice for most patients requiring relief of pain for periods of less than 14 days. Demerol is particularly useful in patients who cannot tolerate morphine and in pain associated with spasm of smooth muscle. Metopon is preferred in chronic painful diseases because of its effectiveness by the oral route and the slow development of tolerance. Methadone is utilized mainly in the treatment of the morphine abstinence syndrome. In general, the opiates should be administered orally whenever possible and the intravenous route should be avoided, since the latter method produces maximum euphoria and hence the greatest danger of addiction. One should prescribe the smallest dosage of drug effective in relieving the pain; doses should be spaced as far apart as possible and discontinued as soon as the need for pain relief has passed.

REFERENCES

Isbell, H., and W. M. White: Clinical Characteristics of Addictions, Am. J. Med., 14:558, 1953.

Vogel, V. H., H. Isbell, and K. W. Chapman: Present Status of Narcotic Addiction, J.A.M.A., 138:1019, 1948.

Wikler, A.: "Narcotics. The Effect of Pharmacologic Agents on the Nervous System," Research Publs.

Assoc. Research in Nervous Mental Disease, 37: 334, 1959.

101 BARBITURATES
Maurice Victor and Raymond D. Adams

The increasing incidence of addiction, suicides, and accidental deaths attributable to the improper use of the barbiturate drugs is a matter of growing concern to the medical profession. The production of barbiturates now appears to exceed greatly the amount needed for therapeutic purposes. It is estimated that in this country over 3 billion capsules of 0.1 Gm each (about 24 for each person) are used each year. Barbiturates account for 20 per cent of acute poisonings admitted to general hospitals; they are responsible for 6 per cent of suicides and 18 per cent of accidental deaths, figures exceeded by no other single poison. Despite a mortality rate of only 8 per cent of hospitalized cases, barbiturates cause about 1,500 deaths annually in the United States.

About 50 barbiturates have been marketed for clinical use, but only the following are encountered with any frequency: barbital (Veronal), phenobarbital (Luminal), diallylbarbituric acid (Dial), amobarbital (Amytal), aprobarbital (Alurate), pentobarbital (Nembutal), secobarbital (Seconal), and thiopental (Pentothal). These drugs are similar pharmacologically and differ only in their speed of onset and duration of action. The clinical problems posed by the barbiturates differ considerably, however, depending on whether the intoxication is acute or chronic, and these two types will be treated separately.

ACUTE BARBITURATE INTOXICATION

Acute barbiturate intoxication results from the ingestion of large amounts of the drug either accidentally or with suicidal intent, the incidence of the two types being about equal. An uncommon form of accidental poisoning occurs in individuals who are intoxicated with barbiturates or with alcohol and who, being confused, then ingest more of the drug. This type of poisoning has been termed *involuntary suicide* or *automatism*.

The ingestion of barbiturates with suicidal intent is most frequently the act of a depressed patient. An individual with hysteria or psychopathic personality may take an overdose as a suicidal gesture and sometimes become seriously intoxicated because of a miscalculation or ignorance of the toxic dosage. At times, no psychiatric disease is present, the drug being taken impulsively or while the patient is inebriated. The combination of alcohol and barbiturate intoxication is frequent and particularly dangerous, since these drugs have a potentiating effect.

The Site and Mode of Action of Barbiturates. Barbiturates decrease the excitability of nerve cells, although the mechanism is not fully understood. Attempts have been made to localize the action of barbiturates to certain anatomic regions, or even to specific nuclei within the nervous system, but it would appear that all parts are to some extent sensitive to the drug. Nevertheless, the reticular formation of the thalami and midbrain are particularly susceptible. There is little experimental evidence to support the clinical impression that with the administration of barbiturates the cerebral cortex is affected first and that lower centers are then successively affected. Reflex and other activity of the nervous system are probably depressed at all levels simultaneously and progressively, although, in the early stages of poisoning, spinal reflexes may be accentuated.

Symptoms and Signs. The symptoms and signs of acute barbiturate intoxication vary with the type and the amount of drug, as well as with the length of time that has elapsed since it was ingested. Pentobarbital and secobarbital produce their effects quickly, and recovery is relatively rapid. Phenobarbital induces coma slowly, and its effects tend to be prolonged. The duration of action of these drugs can be judged from the hypnotic effect of an average oral dose. In the case of the long-acting barbiturates, such as phenobarbital, barbital, and diallylbarbituric acid, it lasts 6 hr or more; with the intermediate-acting drugs, amobarbital and aprobarbital, 3 to 6 hr; with the short-acting drugs, secobarbital and pentobarbital, less than 3 hr.

In general, much larger doses of long-acting barbiturates are required to produce a depth of unconsciousness comparable to that produced by the short-acting ones. The ingestion by adults of more than 3 Gm secobarbital, pentobarbital, amobarbital, or diallylbarbituric acid at one time is usually fatal, whereas more than 6.0 to 9.0 Gm phenobarbital, 5.0 to 20.0 Gm barbital, and 15 Gm aprobarbital is required to produce a fatal outcome. Because of the many serious complications of prolonged coma, the fatalities are greater with the long-acting than with the short-acting drugs.

Clinically, it is useful to recognize three grades of severity of acute barbiturate intoxication, particularly in regard to prognosis and treatment. Mild intoxication follows the ingestion of approximately 0.6 Gm pentobarbital or its equivalent. The patient is drowsy or asleep, a state from which he is readily roused by calling his name loudly or by shaking.

The symptoms resemble those of alcoholic inebriation, except that the face is not flushed, the conjunctivas are not suffused, and there is no odor of alcohol. The patient thinks slowly, and there may be a mild disorientation, lability of mood, impairment of judgment, slurred speech, drunken gait, and nystagmus. Reflex activity and vital signs are not affected.

Moderate intoxication follows the ingestion of five to ten times the oral hypnotic dose. Here the state of consciousness is more severely depressed and is usually accompanied by depressed or absent deep reflexes and slow but not shallow respiration. Corneal reflexes are retained, with occasional exceptions. At times the patient can be roused by vigorous manual stimulation; when awakened, he is confused and dysarthric, and after a few moments he drifts back into coma. At other times the patient cannot be roused by this means. In the latter cases the depth of coma and seriousness of the respiratory depression may be roughly judged by the response of respiration to painful stimuli or to the inhalation of 10 per cent carbon dioxide. If these stimuli cause an increase in the depth and rate of respiration, the outlook for recovery is good and only symptomatic treatment is indicated. Similar information can be obtained by the injection of 5 ml of 10 per cent Metrazol; in moderate intoxication, the patient will respond with purposeful movements or a return of reflex activity.

Severe intoxication occurs with the ingestion of fifteen to twenty times the oral hypnotic dose. The patient cannot be roused by any of the means indicated. Respiration is slow and shallow or irregular, and pulmonary edema and cyanosis may be present. Deep reflexes are usually but not invariably absent, and in the most advanced cases the corneal and gag reflexes may also be abolished. Ordinarily the pupillary light reflex is retained in severe intoxication and is lost only if the patient is asphyxiated. The plantar responses are extensor. In the early hours of coma there may be rigidity of the limbs, hyperactive reflexes, ankle clonus, and decerebrate posturing; persistence of these signs indicates a severe degree of anoxia. The temperature may be subnormal, the pulse thready and rapid, and the blood pressure at shock levels.

Diagnosis. The diagnosis of barbiturate intoxication is made from the history and physical findings. If a reasonable suspicion of the diagnosis exists, then a careful search for drugs or their containers may be rewarding. One should also examine the mouth and gastric contents for any characteristically colored capsules. Acute barbiturate intoxication which presents as a state of coma must be distinguished from other forms of coma by the method outlined in Chap. 34, Coma and Related Disturbances of Consciousness. Actually there are few conditions other than barbiturate intoxication which cause a flaccid coma with reactive pupils, hypothermia, and hypotension. In the differential diagnosis, hysteria presents the main problem.

Reliable methods are now available for the *estimation of barbiturates in the blood*. The ultraviolet spectrophotometric method of Goldbaum is most widely used. The major virtue of this test is in identifying the etiology of coma, when this is in question. The blood level also helps to identify the drug as long- or short-acting, thus giving information as to whether the therapeutic problem will be short or prolonged. A blood barbiturate level of 2 mg per 100 ml in a *comatose* patient is usually due to poisoning with secobarbital or pentobarbital; although the immediate mortality is high in such instances, the therapeutic problem will be short. A level of 11.5 to 12.0 mg per 100 ml is usually due to poisoning with barbital or phenobarbital, and the comatose state will be prolonged. Because of the potentiating effects of alcohol and barbiturate, a patient who has ingested both may be comatose with relatively low blood barbiturate levels. For this reason, and also because of differences in individual tolerance, the correlation between blood barbiturate levels and depth of coma is not entirely dependable.

The *electroencephalogram* may also be useful in diagnosis, since characteristic patterns accompany barbiturate intoxication. In mild intoxication, the normal activity is replaced by fast activity, in the range of 20 to 30 cps, most prominent in the frontal regions. In more severe intoxication, the fast waves become less regular and interspersed with 3 to 4 per second slow activity. In the most advanced cases, there are short periods of suppression of all activity, separated by bursts of slow waves of variable frequency.

Management. The management of acute barbiturate intoxication depends on its severity. In mild or moderate intoxication, recovery is the rule and no vigorous treatment is required. The mildly intoxicated patient should be watched closely for signs of deepening coma, and analeptics such as coffee or parenteral caffeine sodium benzoate may be used. If the patient is unresponsive, special attention should be given to maintaining respiration and urinary excretion and to the prevention of infection. It is most important to place the patient in a prone position and to maintain a patent airway by the insertion of an endotracheal tube; suctioning should be used when necessary, and the patient should be turned frequently. Tracheotomy and bronchoscopic suctioning should be resorted to if atelectasis becomes manifest. The routine administration of oxygen is contraindicated in severe cases of respiratory depression, since the respiratory center loses its sensitivity to carbon dioxide, and respi-ration is maintained through the hypoxic stimuli from the aortic and carotid chemoreceptors; the administration of oxygen alone in such cases will remove the stimulus to respiration and cause the cessation of breathing.

Cases of severe respiratory depression, with cyanosis and pupillary dilatation, represent a serious medical emergency. A clear airway should be secured immediately and artificial respiration begun, preferably utilizing an automatic intermittent positive-pressure respirator. If the patient is in shock, the foot of the bed should be elevated, and norepinephrine and whole blood or plasma administered. Catheterization is required to determine the adequacy of urinary output, to obtain samples for laboratory examination, and to prevent distention of the bladder. Three to four liters of 5 per cent glucose in saline solution should be given daily to ensure an adequate output of urine; this is important because some barbiturates are excreted by the kidney and also because toxic amounts of barbiturate have an antidiuretic effect. Coma of any significant duration requires the administration of other electrolytes as well, the amounts being governed by their serum and urinary values. The occurrence of pulmonary and urinary infections should be treated by the appropriate antibiotic.

If ingestion has been recent, gastric lavage may be a therapeutic as well as a diagnostic measure. It must be performed within several hours of ingestion of the drug, since barbiturates are absorbed rapidly and completely. Laryngospasm may complicate this procedure but can be avoided by preliminary endotracheal intubation; the stomach must be entirely emptied to prevent aspiration.

The treatment of severe barbiturate intoxication with analeptic drugs has been a matter of contention and has not yet been settled to everyone's satisfaction. These drugs are antagonistic to barbiturates only in so far as they are powerful cortical stimulants as well as over-all nervous system excitants. Their effectiveness is most difficult to evaluate, since there is no precise way of quantitating the depth of central nervous system depression in any particular patient, and hence no way of predicting whether or not recovery would have occurred without analeptic therapy. Nor is the experimental evidence in agreement on this question. Because of this uncertainty, as well as the danger of convulsions with the use of these stimulants, some clinicians feel that the aim of therapy should be the maintenance of respiration, circulation, and excretion until the barbiturate has been excreted or metabolized.

The advocates of analeptic therapy, on the other hand, point out that a state of prolonged unresponsiveness, even if carefully managed, is frequently complicated by bronchopneumonia and atelectasis, and if the artificial kidney is not available, measures designed to shorten the coma are justified. Metrazol is the most widely used analeptic drug; it is given intravenously in doses of 500 mg every 15 to 20 min until consciousness or reflex activity returns. Picrotoxin is more difficult to use, because its action becomes evident only after a latent period of 10 to 15 min. A dose of 25 mg is given intravenously every 20 to 30 min, but this should be decreased if facial twitchings or convulsions occur. Other drugs such as Megimide (β,β-methyl-ethylglutarimide) and Doptazole (2-4-diamino-5-phenylthiozole) are about as effective as Metrazol and picrotoxin and seem to have a similar pharmacologic action. Dialysis of the blood by means of the artificial kidney has proved to be an effective form of therapy in some circumstances. This measure should be reserved for cases of profound intoxication due to long-acting barbiturates, in which a trial of symptomatic measures and analeptic drugs has failed. The use of nonconvulsive electrical stimulation has no particular advantage in the severely intoxicated patient. Recent reports have advocated the use of diuretic agents such as urea, along with alkalinization of the urine, as a means of increasing the rate of excretion of barbiturates. The effectiveness of this method of therapy has not yet been fully evaluated.

CHRONIC BARBITURATE INTOXICATION
(Barbiturate Addiction)

The problem of chronic barbiturate intoxication is quite different from acute intoxication, for it also embraces the phenomena of tolerance and addiction as well as the effects of ultimate withdrawal of the drugs. In these respects there is a remarkable similarity to the problem of chronic alcoholism. This concept of chronic barbiturate intoxication and the idea that it represents a true addiction have only become popular in recent years, mainly through the work of Isbell and his associates at the Addiction Research Center in Lexington, Ky. The following remarks are based largely on their studies.

Chronic barbiturate intoxication, like other addictions, usually develops on a background of some psychiatric disorder, most commonly psychoneurosis with symptoms of anxiety and insomnia, or a so-called character disorder. The patients with symptoms of anxiety and insomnia are originally given the drug by their physicians; and as the desired sleep-producing effect of the barbiturate is lost, the dose is slowly increased until the patient is taking an amount sufficient to produce symptoms when it is withdrawn. Individuals with character disorders are usually introduced to the drug by

associates; since the drug is taken for its intoxicating effect, the dose tends to be increased rapidly. Addiction to alcohol or to opiates may predispose to barbiturate addiction. Alcoholics find that barbiturates effectively relieve their nervousness and tremor and then may continue to take both alcohol and barbiturates, or the barbiturate may replace the alcohol. Morphine addicts may turn to barbiturates when they are unable to obtain opiates. As with other addicting drugs, the incidence of barbiturism is particularly high in individuals with ready access to drugs, such as physicians, pharmacists, and nurses.

The symptoms and signs of chronic barbiturate intoxication may be described in relation to (1) the toxic effects of the drug, (2) the development of tolerance, and (3) the effects of sudden withdrawal of the drug after a period of prolonged intoxication.

The toxic symptoms of chronic barbiturism are much the same as those of mild acute intoxication or of alcoholic inebriation. The barbiturate addict thinks slowly, shows an increased emotional lability, and becomes untidy in his dress and personal habits. The neurologic signs are quite characteristic and include dysarthria, nystagmus, and cerebellar incoordination. Both the mental and neurologic signs fluctuate greatly in the same individual, being more severe if the drug is taken in the fasting state and tending to increase during the day as more of the drug is ingested. If the dosage is elevated rapidly, the signs of moderate or severe intoxication become manifest.

A characteristic feature of chronic barbiturate intoxication is the development of tolerance, sometimes striking in degree. The average addict will ingest about 1.5 Gm daily of a potent barbiturate and will not develop signs of severe intoxication unless this amount is exceeded. Individual variations in the degree of tolerance make it difficult to state precisely the minimal amount of drug which must be ingested before the resulting condition is designated as chronic barbiturate intoxication. Most persons can ingest 0.2 Gm daily for years without obvious harm, although epileptic patients accustomed to this dosage may develop continuous seizures when the drug is withdrawn. With a dosage of 0.8 Gm daily, the efficiency at all tasks is greatly reduced, and after a period of 2 months on this dosage abrupt withdrawal will result in serious symptoms in the majority of patients. Even after 2 weeks of this dosage some patients will show mild withdrawal symptoms and paroxysmal electroencephalogram changes with photic stimulation. Individuals taking 0.3 to 0.7 Gm daily fall into an intermediate category; practically all show some mental dulling, and occasionally severe withdrawal symptoms may occur.

The Abstinence or Withdrawal Syndrome. Following the withdrawal of barbiturates from addicted individuals, characteristic symptoms occur. Immediately following withdrawal the patient seemingly improves, as he loses the symptoms of intoxication over 8 to 12 hr. After this short period a new group of symptoms appears, consisting of nervousness, tremor, and weakness. Generalized seizures, with loss of consciousness, may then occur, usually between the second and fourth day of abstinence, occasionally as long as 6 or 7 days after withdrawal. There may be a single seizure, or several, or rarely status epilepticus. A varying degree of improvement follows the convulsive phase, to be followed by a delusional-hallucinatory state or a full-blown delirium, indistinguishable from delirium tremens. Death has been reported under these circumstances. The abstinence syndrome may occur in all degrees of completeness, depending on the severity of addiction and the abruptness of withdrawal.

The *electroencephalogram* shows a number of changes in chronic barbiturate intoxication and following withdrawal. During chronic intoxication, the predominant pattern is that of fast activity of moderate voltage, interspersed with short bursts of high voltage, 6 to 8 per second rhythms, chiefly in the frontal and parietal regions. The electroencephalogram does not correlate closely with the degree of intoxication, nor does it reflect the development of tolerance. On withdrawal of barbiturates the fast activity diminishes. Also in the first few days of abstinence, paroxysmal bursts of mixed spike and slow waves or 4 per second spike and dome paroxysmal discharges occur, indicating the imminence of seizures. These changes disappear after 4 or 5 days, the record returning to a normal pattern. The most characteristic electroencephalogram findings in the abstinent period are paroxysmal changes evoked by photic stimulation. According to Wulff, these are far more common than the paroxysmal changes in the resting record.

The treatment of chronic barbiturate intoxication should always be carried out in the hospital. If the diagnosis of addiction is made before signs of abstinence have appeared, the first step in treatment should be the determination of the "stabilization dosage." This is the amount of a rapidly acting barbiturate required to produce mild symptoms of intoxication. Usually 0.2 to 0.3 Gm Seconal given orally every 6 hr is sufficient for this purpose. This method is preferable to a blind reduction of dosage, since patients frequently underestimate the amount of drug taken. Then a gradual withdrawal of the drug is undertaken, 0.1 Gm daily, the reduction being stopped for several days if abstinence symptoms appear. In this way a severely addicted person can be withdrawn in 14 to 21 days. Patients

undergoing withdrawal treatment require careful observation for symptoms of abstinence, and special precautions have to be taken to prevent the smuggling or concealment of drugs.

If the patient presents with severe symptoms of abstinence, such as seizures, he should be given 0.3 to 0.5 Gm sodium Luminal intramuscularly, and then enough to maintain mild intoxication. Withdrawal should then be carried out as indicated above. If the abstinence symptoms are not severe, it is not necessary to reintoxicate the patient, but treatment can proceed along the lines laid down for the delirious and confused patient (Chap. 38).

After recovery has taken place, whether from symptoms of chronic intoxication or of abstinence or from acute intoxication due to attempted suicide, the psychiatric problem requires evaluation and an appropriate plan of therapy. Many of the considerations in the management of alcoholism are equally applicable to barbiturate addiction (Chap. 99, Alcohol).

REFERENCES

Fazekas, J. F., and T. Koppanyi: Prevention and Treatment of Acute Barbiturate Intoxication, Gen. Practitioner, 6:79, 1952.

Goldbaum, L. R.: Determination of Barbiturates, Anal. Chem., 24:1604, 1952.

Isbell, H.: Acute and Chronic Barbiturate Intoxication, Veterans Admin. Tech. Bull., TB10-76, August, 1951.

Plum, F., and A. C. Swanson: Barbiturate Poisoning Treated by Physiological Methods, J.A.M.A., 163: 827, 1957.

Wulff, M. H.: "The Barbiturate Withdrawal Syndrome," Copenhagen, Ejnar Munksgaard, 1959, Suppl. No. 14. Electroencephalog. and Clin. Neurophysiol.

102 HEAVY METALS
Ivan L. Bennett, Jr., and Albert Heyman

Two highly effective chemicals, BAL and Versene, are available for the treatment of systemic poisoning with heavy metals by forming nontoxic, stable cyclic compounds with polyvalent metallic ions, thus permitting the offending material to be excreted safely in the urine.

The first to be developed was BAL (British anti-lewisite, 2,3-dimercaptopropanol, dimercaprol), which was originally intended as an antidote against the arsenical war gas, lewisite. Its tendency to combine with certain metallic ions such as arsenic, mercury, cobalt, nickel, antimony, and gold is so great that it can remove them from combination with the enzymes whose function they impair in the body. BAL is not useful in the treatment of lead poisoning. Because the effectiveness of BAL depends to some extent upon the speed with which its administration is begun, every attempt should be made to avoid delay in its use. For serious systemic intoxications, BAL should be given in doses of 4 mg per kg body weight intramuscularly as a solution in oil and 20 per cent benzyl benzoate. No single dose should exceed 300 mg. This dose should be repeated every 4 hr on the first day and every 6 hr on the second day. Thereafter, it should be given three times daily for several days; doses should then be tapered and discontinued about 10 days after acute poisoning. When the dose of poison has been relatively small, the schedule of BAL administration may be reduced by one-third. Because BAL is excreted in part by the kidneys, it can accumulate to toxic concentrations in anuric patients. Overdosage results in nervousness, hyperactivity, muscle twitching, and hyperreflexia. Large doses may produce convulsions. The presence of the material in tears sometimes causes blepharospasm. In patients with anuria or oliguria, therefore, BAL should be administered with caution and at a lower dosage than outlined above. If too much is given, sedatives should be administered; hemodialysis with an artificial kidney appears to remove some of the excess BAL and might be useful under these circumstances.

The second antidote to metal poisons is the chelating agent Versene (ethylenediaminetetraacetate, EDTA), which forms cyclic, stable, soluble, nontoxic compounds with most metals. Because Versene reacts with calcium in the same way as with other metals, it must be given as the calcium salt to avoid hypocalcemia. The material has been used with notable success in the treatment of lead poisoning.

Antimony. Symptoms of poisoning after the ingestion of antimony or acid food contaminated with antimony from cheap enamelware or "graniteware" are similar to those produced by arsenic except that antimony causes a more rapid onset of gastrointestinal symptoms. Treatment is the same as for arsenic, including BAL. Circulatory collapse occurs early and requires vigorous supportive treatment. The therapeutic injection of antimony (tartar emetic, etc.) can result in severe coughing, muscle and joint pains, or bradycardia. The last is an indication for stopping medication (see p. 1227).

Arsenic. Arsenic poisoning is usually the result of accidental or suicidal ingestion of insecticides or rodenticides containing paris green (copper acetoarsenate) or calcium or lead arsenate. Pesticides containing arsenic are a frequent source of poisoning in rural areas of the United States. Medications

such as Fowler's solution (potassium arsenite) and the organic arsenicals (arsphenamines and arsenoxides) were once common causes of intoxication.

The toxic dose of inorganic arsenic varies considerably and seems to depend upon individual susceptibility. Orchardists have been found to ingest as much as 6.8 mg of arsenic a day without any signs of intoxication. On the other hand, as little as 30 mg of arsenic trioxide has been fatal. Arsenic has a predilection for keratin, and the concentration of arsenic in the hair and nails is higher than that in other tissues. Arsenic reacts with the —SH groups in certain tissue proteins and thus interferes with a number of enzyme systems essential to cellular metabolism. Pathologic changes in fatal inorganic arsenical poisoning are fatty degeneration of the liver, hyperemia and hemorrhages of the gut, and renal tubular necrosis. The peripheral nerves often show fragmentation and resorption of myelin with disintegration of axis cylinders.

The symptoms of acute poisoning by the oral route are nausea, vomiting, diarrhea, severe burning of the mouth and throat, and agonizing abdominal pains. The vomitus often contains blood. Circulatory collapse is frequent, and death may ensue within a few hours. With chronic exposure, the first signs of poisoning are usually weakness, prostration, muscular aching, or nervous system involvement; gastrointestinal symptoms are minimal. In patients exposed to arsine gas (hydrogen arsenide), the outstanding features are hemolysis, chills, fever, and hemoglobinuria.

Patients who recover from acute poisoning and those with chronic intoxication usually develop skin and mucosal changes, peripheral neuropathy, and linear pigmentations in the fingernails. The *cutaneous manifestations* appear within 1 to 4 weeks and consist of a diffuse, dry, scaly desquamation, occasionally with hyperpigmentation, over the trunk and extremities. Hyperkeratoses of the palms and soles and edema of the face and extremities may also occur. The mucous membranes also show evidence of irritation, with conjunctivitis, photophobia, pharyngitis, or irritating cough. About 5 weeks after exposure to arsenic, a transverse white stria, 1 to 2 mm in width, appears above the lunula of each fingernail (*Mees lines*). Patients with more than one exposure to arsenic may show double lines several millimeters apart.

Symptoms of headache, drowsiness, confusion, and convulsions are seen in both acute and chronic intoxication. Evidence of peripheral neuropathy usually appears 1 to 3 weeks after exposure. There are numbness, tingling, and burning of the feet and hands followed by muscular weakness. The extremities show a decrease in touch, pain, and temperature sensations, in a symmetrical "stocking-glove" distribution, and distal weakness with inability to walk or stand, weakness of grip, and wrist drop. Tendon reflexes are absent or diminished, and atrophy of the affected muscles develops rapidly.

The laboratory findings usually consist of moderate anemia and a leukopenia of 2,000 to 5,000 white blood cells with mild eosinophilia. There is slight proteinuria, and liver function tests show mild abnormalities. The spinal fluid is normal.

None of the clinical or laboratory manifestations of arsenic poisoning is specific, and the diagnosis depends upon analysis of the hair and urine for arsenic. Normal individuals have an average concentration of 0.05 mg arsenic per 100 mg of hair, with a range of 0.025 to 0.088 mg. Concentrations of arsenic greater than 0.1 mg per 100 mg of hair are indicative of poisoning. As is the case with lead, the minimal level of arsenic in the urine indicating intoxication is difficult to establish. Normal persons have been found to excrete between 0.01 and 0.06 mg of arsenic per liter, and a few individuals as much a 0.2 mg per liter. Although there is considerable overlap, most patients with evidence of arsenic intoxication will be found to excrete more than 0.1 mg per liter; soon after acute exposure, many will show levels greater than 1 mg per liter.

The treatment for acute ingestion is gastric lavage (see p. 816). Replacement of lost fluids and elevation of blood pressure by vasopressor agents is often indicated. Immediate treatment with BAL should be instituted (p. 811). Patients with peripheral neuropathy rarely show significant improvement with BAL and continue to have sensory disturbances and weakness for many months. Dramatic responses, however, have been observed with the use of BAL in the treatment of exfoliative dermatitis, bone marrow depression, and encephalopathy caused by the arsphenamines and the organic arsenicals. BAL is of little value in the treatment of the hemolysis caused by inhalation of arsine.

Bismuth. Poisoning by bismuth is almost entirely a complication of antisyphilitic therapy. Toxic manifestations may appear in the mouth (gingivitis, followed by stomatitis), the kidneys (albuminuria and nephrotic syndrome), or the skin (exfoliative dermatitis), requiring immediate interruption of bismuth injections. The development of a bluish stippled line of pigmentation just at the margin of the gums is not dangerous but suggests that oral hygiene should be improved. Bismuth subnitrate occasionally gives rise to methemoglobinemia (p. 1310).

Cadmium. Poisoning is likely to occur after ingestion of an acid food prepared in a cadmium-lined vessel. The classic example is lemonade served from metal cans. Symptoms of nausea, vomiting, diarrhea, and prostration usually develop within 10 min after ingestion. Treatment is symptomatic, and symptoms ordinarily subside within 24 hr. The short incubation and the typical circumstances suggest the diagnosis. Inhalation of cadmium fumes in industry produces an acute, extremely severe pneumonitis (p. 1542). The use of BAL is not recommended for cadmium intoxication, as the BAL-cadmium complex dissociates in the kidneys and cadmium is nephrotoxic.

Copper. Acute poisoning due to ingestion of copper salts is rare. Copper sulfate (blue vitriol) is the chief offender, in which case the vomitus has a characteristic blue color. Manifestations are nausea, vomiting, bloody diarrhea, headache, severe thirst, and tachycardia. In fatal cases, death is preceded by convulsions. Treatment consists of gastric lavage with 1 per cent solution of potassium ferrocyanide, fluid replacement, and control of pain and diarrhea with opiates.

Gold. Because practically all cases of poisoning by gold are associated with its use in the treatment of arthritis, diagnosis is usually easy. Manifestations are skin rashes of various types, bone marrow depression, icterus, oliguria, nausea, vomiting, and gastrointestinal bleeding. Treatment consists of symptomatic relief of discomfort and the use of BAL, an effective antidote.

Lead. Poisoning results from ingestion of lead-containing materials such as paint or water which has stood in lead pipes or from inhalation of fumes from burning storage batteries, solder, etc. Lead-containing bullets or buckshot can cause poisoning years after becoming embedded in a serous cavity. Absorption is slow by any route, and prolonged exposure is required for the development of symptoms. Lead is a cumulative poison, excreted slowly. Acute poisoning is virtually nonexistent, although it was observed when lead was used for the treatment of malignant disease. Symptoms may develop suddenly after chronic exposure. Most of the absorbed lead is deposited in the bones; blood, urine, and feces contain only small amounts.

Manifestations of poisoning are colic, encephalopathy, peripheral neuritis, and anemia.

Lead colic, or painter's cramps, is characterized by agonizing, wandering, poorly localized abdominal pain, often with spasm and rigidity of the musculature of the abdominal wall. There is no fever or leukocytosis. Needless surgery has been carried out in these patients for supposed perforation of peptic ulcer or other catastrophe. Morphine has surprisingly little effect upon the pain; intravenous injection of calcium salts affords relief within a short time, although pain may recur. Attacks of colic seem to be brought on by intercurrent infection or alcoholic overindulgence.

Encephalopathy occurs chiefly in children and is manifested by convulsions, somnolence, mania, delirium, or coma. Mortality is high when convulsive seizures and coma occur. Mental enfeeblement is a common sequel.

Peripheral neuritis with paralysis, characteristically involving the muscles most used (e.g., wrist drop in painters, etc.), occurs in patients exposed to lead, often in the absence of other symptoms. It is rare in children.

Mild anemia, probably the result of increased brittleness of the erythrocytes as well as of a defect in cell maturation, is common. Pallor is out of proportion to anemia in patients with chronic plumbism and is attributed to spasm of small vessels in the skin. Anemia is almost never severe and is characterized by the presence of large numbers of erythrocytes with basophilic stippling. This is seen in other hematologic disorders, but a smear showing stippling should arouse suspicion of lead poisoning. In patients with poor oral hygiene a "lead line" of black lead sulfide may develop along the gingival margins. This is not seen in edentulous persons and is rare in children.

Patients with lead poisoning excrete increased amounts of coproporphyrin III in the urine (see p. 758). This is so consistent that examination of a urine specimen for porphyrin is the best screening test in suspected cases. A few milliliters of urine should be acidified with acetic acid and shaken with an equal volume of ether. Exposure of a specimen prepared in this manner under a Woods lamp will reveal reddish fluorescence of the ether layer if coproporphyrin is present. A positive test is strongly in favor of lead intoxication. Urinary lead determinations are of aid in confirming the diagnosis; a level of 0.2 mg per liter or more is usually regarded as significant, although interpretations vary.

Treatment consists of preventing further exposure and reduction of concentration of lead in the blood. In children, x-rays often show a "lead line" at the epiphyses, an aid in diagnosis. In the past, attempts to delead patients by giving a low calcium, acid-ash diet have resulted in symptomatic exacerbations without removal of enough lead to justify the risk. The development of chelating agents such as Versene permits deleading with safety. Versene should be administered immediately to patients with encephalopathy. A dosage of 500 mg given in 250 ml of 5 per cent glucose by intravenous infusion every 12 hr for 5 days is one "course." Several courses of therapy at intervals of 1 week should be given to patients with lead poisoning.

Acute symptoms usually subside within 48 to 72 hr after Versene is begun. Within 2 weeks, urinary excretion of coproporphyrin decreases and there may be dramatic improvement in neuritis, although this is not uniformly observed.

Occasional patients with severe encephalopathy and evidence of greatly increased intracranial pressure require surgical decompression of the skull as an emergency measure. The usefulness and safety of Versene on a long-term basis to prevent recurrence of acute symptoms in patients whose bones contain large amounts of lead have not yet been adequately evaluated.

Mercury. Poisoning occurs chiefly as a result of the acute ingestion of a soluble salt, usually mercuric chloride (bichloride of mercury). Toxic symptoms may occur with 0.1 Gm, and 0.5 Gm is almost always fatal unless immediate treatment is instituted. The mercuric ion is corrosive and produces severe local inflammation. Oral, pharyngeal, and laryngeal pain are severe; abdominal cramps with nausea and vomiting occur within 15 min. As mercury is absorbed, it is concentrated in the kidneys, where it poisons the tubular cells, producing a tendency to diuresis within the first 2 to 3 hr. The combination of vomiting, dehydration, shock, and progressive tubular damage, however, soon leads to anuria and uremia. The poison is also excreted into the colon and produces severe enteritis with bloody diarrhea and tenesmus. Death is usually from uremia. The chief objectives of treatment are to prevent the shock of dehydration and to remove mercury from the body. Early in treatment, copious quantities of fluid should be infused intravenously to prevent dehydration and to reduce the concentration of mercuric ion in the renal tubules. That the patient is anuric early is often simply the result of dehydration and shock. In such instances, forcing fluids is advisable. However, the gradual development of oliguria and anuria in a hydrated patient indicates renal damage by mercury, and at this stage a regimen for acute renal shutdown should be instituted (p. 1496).

Some poison can be removed from the body by gastric lavage, but more important in treatment is the binding of the mercuric ion in a harmless compound by BAL. The therapeutic usefulness of BAL depends on its immediate administration. Chronic poisoning from metallic mercury vapor occurs in individuals exposed to large amounts of the metal in laboratories or in industry and occasionally as a result of prolonged therapeutic use, as in vaginal douches. Manifestations may be those of subacute poisoning, with salivation, stomatitis, and diarrhea, or primarily neurologic, with parkinsonian tremors, vertigo, irritability, moodiness, and depression.

Silver. Most poisoning by silver involves silver nitrate, a caustic salt. There is intense nausea, vomiting, and diarrhea after swallowing nitrate (lunar caustic), and death from shock may occur within a few hours. The mouth is usually deeply stained by silver nitrate. Treatment is entirely supportive, with fluid replacement and control of pain.

Chronic exposure (usually to nose drops) produces a peculiar bluish skin discoloration (argyria).

Thallium. Thallium is a component of certain rodenticides and depilatories, and clinical poisoning is usually a result of accidental ingestion of these materials. The fatal dose is approximately 1.0 Gm. Manifestations are vomiting, diarrhea, and leg pains, followed by weakness and paralysis of the legs. There may be visual and mental disturbances. About 3 weeks after poisoning, the patient's hair falls out, providing a strong diagnostic clue if the etiology has not previously been determined. Treatment is symptomatic. The alopecia is temporary if the patient recovers.

REFERENCES

ARSENIC

Heyman, A., J. B. Pfeiffer, Jr., R. W. Willett, and H. M. Taylor: Peripheral Neuropathy Caused by Arsenical Intoxication: A Study of 41 Cases with Observations on the Effects of BAL (2,3-Dimercaptopropanol), New Engl. J. Med., 254:401, 1956.

Keusler, C. J., J. C. Abels, and C. P. Rhoads: Arsine Poisoning, Mode of Action and Treatment, J. Pharmacol. Exptl. Therap., 88:99, 1946.

Longcope, W. T., and J. A. Luetscher: The Use of BAL (British Antilewisite) in the Treatment of the Injurious Effects of Arsenic, Mercury and Other Metallic Poisons, Ann. Internal Med., 31:545, 1949.

BISMUTH

Heyman, A.: Systemic Manifestations of Bismuth Toxicity; Observations on 4 Patients with Pre-existent Kidney Disease, Am. J. Syphilis, Gonorrhea, Venereal Diseases, 28:721, 1944.

CADMIUM

Ross, P.: Cadmium Poisoning, Brit. Med. J., 1944, I:252.

GOLD

Margolis, H. M., and P. S. Caplan: BAL in Treatment of Toxicity from Gold, Ann. Internal Med., 27:353, 1947.

Strauss, J. F., Sr., R. M. Barrett, and E. F. Rosenberg: BAL Treatment of Toxic Reactions to Gold: A Review of the Literature and Report of Two Cases, Ann. Internal Med., 37:323, 1952.

LEAD

Aub, J. C., L. T. Fairhall, A. S. Minot, and P. Reznikoff: Lead Poisoning, Medicine, 4:1, 1925.

Byers, R. K., C. C. Maloof, A. DeSimone, and M. E. Morell: The Use of Calcium Disodium Versenate in the Treatment of Lead Poisoning in Children, Am. J. Diseases Children, 87:559, 1954.

Jones, R. R.: Symptoms in Early Stages of Industrial Plumbism, J.A.M.A., 104:195, 1935.

Kehoe, R. A., F. Thamann, and J. Cholek: Lead Absorption and Excretion in Relation to the Diagnosis

of Lead Poisoning, J. Indust. Hyg. & Toxicol., 15:320, 1933.

MERCURY

Doolan, P. D., W. C. Hess, and L. R. Kyle: Acute Renal Insufficiency Due to Dichloride of Mercury: Observations on Gastrointestinal Hemorrhage and BAL Therapy, New Engl. J. Med., 249:273, 1953.

Longcope, W. T., and J. A. Luetscher: Clinical Use of 2,3-Dimercaptopropanol (BAL): XI. The Treatment of Acute Mercury Poisoning by BAL, J. Clin. Invest., 25:557, 1946.

Peters, J. P., A. J. Eisenman, and D. M. Kydd: Mercury Poisoning, Am. J. Med. Sci., 185:149, 1933.

THALLIUM

Munch, J. C.: Human Thallotoxicosis, J.A.M.A., 102:1929, 1934.

103 OTHER CHEMICAL AGENTS

Richard J. Johns

The management of the poisoned patient challenges the skill and ingenuity of the physician. The diagnosis must be made swiftly, and proper therapy instituted as promptly as possible. Correct therapy requires a knowledge of the general principles of management as well as details of treatment for specific poisons. In addition to his immediate responsibilities to the patient, the physician has legal obligations in instances of attempted suicides or homicide, criminal abortion, and industrial exposure. Finally, the physician should not overlook his responsibilities in obtaining psychiatric care for the patient who has attempted suicide.

Emphasis here will be placed on clinical recognition, the general principles of management, and specific therapy of poisoning by common toxic substances.

GENERAL PRINCIPLES OF MANAGEMENT

In poisoning, as in all disease states, proper management must be based on correct diagnosis. Frequently, when the victim of poisoning first presents himself to the physician, the nature of his illness is not immediately apparent. The patient may be unaware of the exposure to poison, or he may be unable to communicate the fact because of stupor or coma. In attempted suicide or abortion, the patient may be reluctant to admit poisoning. Thus, the first step in the management of a poisoned patient is for the physician to *entertain the possibility of poisoning* as the cause of the clinical picture.

It is unusual for poisoning to be omitted from the diagnostic possibilities when the manifestations are those of coma, acute hepatic insufficiency, acute renal insufficiency, or aplastic anemia. Unfortunately, when the victim's major manifestation is abdominal pain, psychosis, tetany, acidosis, ataxia, or bronchiolitis, poisoning may not be considered. It is essential, then, that the physician not only know the treatment of specific poisonings but also recognize the varied symptomatology they produce.

The second step in management is to *identify the toxic agent*. Such identification is of obvious importance, since there are specific antidotes for some poisons. Furthermore, it is of medicolegal importance in the realms of homicide, suicide, criminal abortion, industrial exposure, and therapeutic misadventure that the poison be identified. The nature of the poison may be revealed by history of exposure or by a characteristic clinical picture. Toxicologic studies are usually not immediately available. Circumstantial evidence may be obtained by questioning relatives or acquaintances, by dispatching relatives or police to the scene of the poisoning in search of empty containers, by questioning the patient's private physician, a plant physician, or a pharmacist. Occasionally the offending agent is known only by its trade name. In such instances, manufacturers' agents, local or state toxicologic laboratories, poison control centers, or industrial hygiene commissions may be of aid in identifying the active ingredients. Included in the references at the end of this chapter are source books for determining the active ingredients in household products, pesticides, and toxic plants. Specimens of vomitus, gastric aspirant, urine, and feces should be labeled and saved for toxicologic examinations whenever diagnostic or medicolegal problems arise. Finally, treatment should not be withheld while confirming the suspected diagnosis of poisoning.

THERAPEUTIC CONSIDERATIONS

The essential features of treatment may be divided into (1) prevention of further absorption of the toxic substance, (2) symptomatic or supportive therapy, and (3) specific antidotal treatment. The first two types of procedure are applicable to virtually all types of poisoning, while the third can be employed only when the toxic agent is known and an antidote is available. The order in which these therapeutic measures are applied is governed by the clinical situation. Clearly, if the patient is in profound shock or manifests severe hypoxia, treatment must be first directed toward correcting these ill effects before attention is turned toward prevention of further absorption of the poison.

Prevention of Further Absorption of Ingested Poisons. Ingested poisons may be removed by emesis, gastric lavage, and purgation. The efficacy of these measures depends upon the site and rapidity of absorption of the poison and the interval between ingestion and attempted removal. Such variables as the delayed gastric emptying produced by shock or pylorospasm make it worthwhile to attempt removal in the absence of a contraindication. Since prompt removal is essential, it is more important to proceed with the means at hand than to wait for special equipment or solutions.

Emesis frequently follows the ingestion of gastric irritants. Vomiting may be induced by stimulating the pharynx, the administration of gastric irritants (hypertonic saline solution, mustard), or by the use of centrally acting emetic drugs such as apomorphine. These measures, however, are often ineffective, and the administration of large amounts of fluids may hasten passage of the poison through the pylorus before vomiting occurs. Whenever possible, it is better to rely upon gastric lavage than the vagaries of emesis.

Gastric lavage is associated with certain dangers. It should not be attempted after the ingestion of strong acids or alkalies, because of the danger of perforating the injured tissues. Clinical judgment must be used in deciding whether the advantages of lavage outweigh its dangers as a stimulus when the patient is convulsing. The danger of aspiration can be minimized by positioning the prone patient with head and shoulders lower than the hips and the head turned to one side. Careful removal of gastric contents in itself reduces the risk of aspiration in the unconscious patient. The orogastric tube should be of sufficient size (30 to 40 French) to permit aspiration of particulate matter. Passage into the esophagus is facilitated by flexing the patient's neck. After the initial aspiration, small amounts (in the range of 250 ml) of the lavage solution should be alternately instilled and aspirated. The use of larger volumes increases the risk of forcing gastric contents through the pylorus. Lukewarm water is a satisfactory irrigating liquid. *Universal antidote* (e.g., activated charcoal, 2 parts; tannic acid, 1 part; magnesium oxide, 1 part; water, 100 parts) may have some advantages. In some poisonings, lavage with a substance which destroys, precipitates, dissolves, or neutralizes the poison may be of help, but time should not be lost in the preparation of universal or specific antidotes if they are not immediately available. These agents will be mentioned in the discussion of specific poisons.

Cathartics may be used to hasten the passage of the remaining poison out of the lower gastrointestinal tract following removal of poison from the upper gastrointestinal tract. Saline cathartics such as magnesium sulfate in amounts of 15 to 30 Gm may be left in the stomach following lavage. Cathartics, in general, are contraindicated in strong acid and alkali poisoning.

Prevention of Absorption of Topically Applied Poisons. Removal of contaminated clothing should be followed by copious flooding of the involved area of skin or mucous membrane with water. While organic solvents, weak acids or bases may be more effective in certain instances (which will be noted), skin decontamination with water should proceed while they are being obtained. Wiping must be gentle to prevent inunction of poison remaining on the skin surface. If exposure is limited to an extremity, venous occlusion with a tourniquet may be helpful in delaying systemic absorption.

Prevention of Absorption of Injected Poison. Cruciate incision and suction will remove unabsorbed poison which has been injected, but this procedure is rarely feasible except in poisonous bites. Absorption from an extremity can be delayed by the application of cold and tourniquets and by immobilization of the limb.

Prevention of Absorption of Inhaled Poison. Further absorption of toxic gases, vapors, aerosols, and dusts can be prevented by removal of the victim to an uncontaminated atmosphere and by assuring adequate pulmonary ventilation. If the casualty cannot be moved, a protective mask should be applied.

Symptomatic and Supportive Therapy. For many poisons, no specific antidote is known. Therapy must then be directed toward control of manifestations as they appear. Even in instances where specific antidotes are available, such problems as hypotension and hypoxia must be attacked directly. Certain of these manifestations appear with sufficient frequency to justify their brief discussion here.

Coma, while an ominous sign, rarely requires specific therapy per se. The use of central nervous system stimulants in the management of drug induced coma continues to be debated. Concomitant depression of respiratory and vasopressor centers, however, frequently requires prompt and vigorous treatment if the patient is to survive. The comatose patient requires careful observation and meticulous nursing care (p. 318). The results of the Danish group indicate that attention to these factors are of greater importance than the administration of analeptics.

Hypotension may arise from any of a number of causes—anoxia, depression of the vasopressor centers, autonomic ganglionic blockade, loss of blood, water, or electrolytes, cardiac arrhythmia, or myocardial damage. Rational therapy is predicated upon correction of the underlying defect. Vasopressor amines, particularly norepinephrine, are helpful in combating the shock produced by central depression and ganglionic blockade. In the latter instance, the patient is unusually sensitive to vasopressor amines. For further discussion of the management of shock, see p. 103.

Hypoxia also may result from varied causes—poor pulmonary ventilation secondary to central respiratory depression, muscular paralysis, bronchospasm, retained secretions, or upper-airway obstruction, impairment of alveolar-capillary diffusion due to pulmonary edema, or deficient oxygen transport as in anemia, methemoglobinemia, carboxyhemoglobinemia, shock, and inhibition of cellular oxidation. When the hypoxia is produced by underventilation, the first step is to ensure a patent airway. Secretions should be removed by suctioning, and any obstruction relieved by the insertion of an oropharyngeal airway, endotracheal tube, or tracheotomy tube, depending upon the site of obstruction. If ventilation remains inadequate despite a clear airway and oxygen administration, or if there is respiratory arrest, the patient must be assisted manually or by mechanical means.

Pulmonary edema produced by injury to alveoli exposed to irritant gases is less responsive to treatment than the pulmonary edema associated with cardiac failure (p. 1383). Therapeutic measures include suppression of cough, frequent suctioning, high concentrations of oxygen under positive pressure, aerosols of surface-active agents, adrenal cortical steroids, bronchodilators, and if infection complicates the picture, antibiotics.

The management of methemoglobinemia, carboxyhemoglobinemia, and inhibition of cellular oxidation will be discussed under the specific poisons producing these changes.

Convulsions may be produced by a wide variety of poisons. The management of seizures is discussed, beginning on p. 340. In intoxications, respiratory depression may accompany or follow convulsions. Short-acting anticonvulsants are therefore preferable.

Electrolyte imbalance and *dehydration* are frequent sequelae to protracted vomiting and diarrhea. In addition, certain poisons produce more specific defects, for example, the acidosis of methanol poisoning and the hypocalcemia of fluoride and oxalate poisoning; these will be described under the appropriate poison.

Acute hepatic insufficiency is the primary manifestation of some poisonings (chlorinated hydrocarbons, cinchophen, phosphorus, and occasionally mushroom poisoning), and its management is described, beginning on p. 1689.

Acute renal insufficiency may appear as a result of such prerenal factors as shock, dehydration, and electrolyte imbalance or as the result of concentration and excretion of nephrotoxic substances by the kidney. When renal failure occurs, it should be managed as outlined on p. 1496.

Cardiac arrhythmias produced by poisons are managed in a manner similar to those otherwise produced (p. 1395).

SPECIFIC ANTIDOTAL TREATMENT

First, there are antidotes which *compete biochemically* with the toxic substance for its receptor site (e.g., vitamin K_1 in coumarin poisoning, or atropine in muscarine poisoning). Second are those antidotes whose pharmacologic action is *antagonistic* to that of the poison (e.g., Megimide in barbiturate poisoning). This latter type of antidotal treatment merges with symptomatic therapy in many instances. Third, there are those antidotes which exert their therapeutic effect by reducing the concentration of the toxic substance by promoting excretion (e.g., the administration of chloride or mercurial diuretics in bromism), by combining cyanide with methemoglobin, lead with ethylene diaminetetraacetate, or mercury with dimercaprol, or by precipitation in the gut (e.g., the use of sulfate to precipitate certain alkaloids).

Hemodialysis, peritoneal dialysis, and exchange transfusion have been used in increasing numbers of poisonings and should be considered to be another means of reducing the concentration of the poison. In theory, these methods should be effective in any instance in which the toxic manifestations are related to the concentration of the noxious substance and in which the toxic substance is distributed in the vascular compartment and diffusible (in the dialysis methods). These techniques are generally reserved for instances in which the course is unfavorable, or an unfavorable outcome is anticipated on the basis of the amount of substance ingested or its blood level. Peritoneal dialysis and exchange transfusion require the least equipment, but the latter is usually limited by availability of blood except in infants and children. Hemodialysis is perhaps the most effective; disposable and portable units have made its use more generally available.

CLINICAL MANIFESTATIONS OF SPECIFIC POISONINGS

In the discussions of specific toxic agents in this chapter, many details of drug action have been omitted except where pertinent to the problem of recognition or treatment of poisoning. Toxic manifestations due to drug hypersensitivity or allergy are discussed elsewhere (p. 1269). It has been necessary to eliminate from consideration a large number of toxic materials to which exposure occurs only in specialized industrial procedures. Instead, emphasis has been placed on toxic agents which may be encountered by the general population, including commonly used drugs, household products, solvents, pesticides, and poisonous plants. In the references at the end of the chapter will be found further details of toxicologic and historic interest.

Acetanilid, Acetophenetidin. Although symptoms resembling salicylate intoxication may follow overdosage of these agents, the most prominent finding is methemoglobinemia with dusky cyanosis, fatigue, and headache. Treatment is symptomatic. See p. 1310.

Acids. Since strong mineral acids are not commonly found in the home, ingestion is usually the result of suicidal attempt. Necrosis, sloughing, bleeding, and perforation of the gastrointestinal tract may be produced, and chemical burns are usually visible in the mouth and oropharynx. These lesions are more charred than the gelatinous burns produced by alkali and can often be differentiated from them by appearance alone. Because of the danger of perforation, lavage should not be attempted. Treatment consists of dilution of the acid, neutralization with weak alkali, relief of pain, and supportive measures if necessitated by shock or loss of blood and fluid. Alkalies such as sodium bicarbonate which evolve carbon dioxide should be avoided because of the possibility of rupture of an eroded stomach. Magnesium oxide or hydroxide and aluminum hydroxide are preferable. If weak alkali is not immediately available, the ingested acid should be diluted by administering water or milk. As with alkali burns, delayed perforation or stricture formation may occur, although the latter is said to be less common in acid burns.

Aconite (Wolfsbane, Monkshood, Larkspur). Aconite is the active principle of several members of the larkspur family; it is no longer used therapeutically because of its instability in solution. Poisoning is usually due to ingestion of one of these plants and is manifested by vagal and peripheral sensory nerve stimulation and medullary depression. Pathognomonic is intense tingling without erythema or evidence of inflammation. This is followed by nausea, vomiting, abdominal pain, diarrhea, bradycardia, hypotension, visual impairment, unconsciousness, and death due to respiratory depression. Treatment is purely supportive, with large doses of atropine (0.5 to 1.0 mg) to counter the vagal effects.

Alkali (Lye, Drano, Sodium Hydroxide, Caustic Potash, Potassium Hydroxide, Washing Soda, So-

dium Carbonate, Household Ammonia, Ammonium Hydroxide). The caustic action of lye and other strong alkalies results in deep, serious burns and subsequent scarring of the intestinal tract after ingestion. The immediate effects of oral ingestion are redness and soreness of mouth and pharynx, followed in several hours by sloughing of the mucosa and bleeding. The same process occurs in the esophagus and stomach. Treatment is directed toward cautious neutralization of the alkali with dilute acetic acid (10 per cent vinegar). Intubation during the acute stages should be avoided because of the likelihood of esophageal perforation. In severe cases, there is circulatory collapse as a result of pain and fluid loss. Occasionally, significant respiratory obstruction due to edema of the hypopharynx necessitates attention to the maintenance of airway. Pain should be relieved with meperidine (Demerol) or opiates. With subsidence of the acute phase of poisoning, esophageal dilatation and other measures such as corticosteroid administration for prevention of strictures should be carried out. Delayed perforation may occur.

Aminopyrine (Amidopyrine, Pyramidon). Overdosage of this drug may produce symptoms resembling those of salicylate intoxication; however, the drug is mainly of importance because of the frequency with which its use in therapeutic doses is followed by agranulocytosis, presumably because of a hypersensitivity reaction. See p. 1326.

Amphetamine (Benzedrine, Dexedrine). Amphetamine and its isomers are widely abused for their exhilarating effects. Besides its sympathomimetic action, amphetamine is a cerebral stimulant. Symptoms of overdosage are tremor, dry mouth, anorexia, nausea, diarrhea, irritability, hallucinations, and severe insomnia. Hypertension and angina occur, particularly in older patients. Although there has been a tendency to regard amphetamine as a relatively harmless stimulant which can be used safely in large amounts in comatose patients, such as those suffering from barbiturate poisoning, evidence indicates that in doses exceeding 300 mg daily there is danger of precipitation of fatal ventricular arrhythmias. Administration of any dosage level should cease with appearance of pulse irregularities. Treatment consists of barbiturates for sedation and appropriate agents such as quinidine or procaine amide for the purpose of controlling arrhythmias. See p. 1395.

Amygdalin (Cherry Laurel, Choke Cherry, Christmas Berry, Pin Cherry, Wild Black Cherry). While this glycoside is nontoxic per se, it is hydrolyzed to cyanide by the enzyme emulsin which occurs with it. Symptoms and management are as described under cyanide poisoning.

Aniline. This material is chiefly important as an industrial hazard, but its use in certain inks, dyes, crayons, and solvents such as paint removers causes occasional poisoning. It is absorbed as the vapor or through the skin, and poisoning has occurred in infants from exposure to inks used in marking hospital diapers. The main manifestation is methemoglobinemia. See p. 1310.

Antabuse (Disulfiram, Tetraethylthiuram Disulfide). See p. 803.

Antibiotics. See p. 871.

Anticoagulants (Heparin, Dicumarol, Warfarin). See p. 1455.

Antihistamines. The widespread and unsupervised use of antihistamines makes them readily available for accidental overdosage and suicidal attempts. There is wide individual variation in tolerance to these drugs. Death due to respiratory depression followed ingestion of only 200 mg of diphenhydramine (Benadryl) in one adult, whereas 2,000 mg produced only impaired mentation in another. In children, the usual toxic manifestations are excitement and convulsions, followed by central nervous system depression. In adults, depressive manifestations predominate, with lethargy, coma, and pupillary dilatation, although convulsions followed by further depression can occur. Initial treatment should be directed toward removal of unabsorbed drug and the maintenance of adequate respiration and blood pressure. Analeptics should be avoided if there is hyperreflexia. Should convulsions occur, they may be controlled with an ultra-short-acting barbiturate, such as thiopental, or with ether to avoid deepening postictal depression. Occasionally, patients intoxicated with antihistamine drugs which have prominent atropinelike properties may manifest toxic delirium, fever, mydriasis, dry mouth, and urinary retention (see Atropine).

Antihypertensive Drugs. Toxic effects of drugs used in the treatment of hypertension are described on p. 1358.

Antimalarial Drugs. See p. 1202.

Atropine (Hyoscine, Scopolamine, Hyoscyamine, Belladonna, Stramonium, Henbane, Jimson Weed Pods, Thorn Apple Pods). When these drugs have been used, poisoning is due to therapeutic overdosage in susceptible patients, the intranasal use of ophthalmic solutions, or ingestion of plants containing one of these alkaloids.

The manifestations of overdosage of atropine are those of parasympathetic blockade, central nervous system excitation followed by depression, dryness of mucous membranes, dysphagia, burning of eyes and throat with intense thirst, dilated and inactive pupils, tachycardia, marked flushing and dryness of the skin, hoarseness, strangury, restlessness, talkativeness, mental confusion, and hallucinations progressing to mania. Terminally, coma and circulatory collapse occur.

With scopolamine, the pulse is slow; there is no flushing of the skin, and central nervous system depression, with lethargy and somnolence, is seen rather than excitement of the type produced by atropine. The Babinski response is said to be present in scopolamine poisoning but absent after atropine.

Treatment consists of sips of water, instillation of "artificial tears" into eyes and nose to moisten mucous membranes, and the use of methacholine or pilocarpine to relieve peripheral symptoms. However, in the presence of a high degree of block these parasympathomimetic drugs have little or no effect. Indeed, the absence of effect following the subcutaneous injection of 5 or 10 mg methacholine will confirm suspected poisoning with belladonna alkaloids. Gastric lavage should be performed after oral ingestion. With atropine, cautious sedation may be necessary; with scopolamine, mild stimulation with caffeine or amphetamine combats depression. Catheterization is usually necessary. Hyperthermia may occur, particularly during hot weather because of inability to sweat. If the patient survives for 24 hr, death is unlikely, but manifestations may persist for several days, especially after an overdosage of atropine.

Barium. Poisoning occurs chiefly from ingestion of rodent poisons containing barium carbonate. Rarely, soluble barium salts have been given by mistake for x-ray purposes in place of the insoluble barium sulfate. Barium acts as a stimulant to contraction of all types of muscle, producing tremors and spasm in skeletal muscle and hypertension due to arteriolar spasm. Its action is particularly pronounced on the intestinal tract, where it is manifested by nausea, vomiting, and abdominal cramps. Death usually occurs from increased myocardial irritability with ventricular fibrillation. Muscle weakness persists for several days after recovery from acute poisoning. Treatment consists of gastric lavage and administration of Epsom salts (to precipitate the barium as insoluble sulfate), supportive measures, and the use of quinidine or procaine amide to reduce the danger of fatal cardiac arrhythmia.

Benzene. Exposure to this solvent occurs chiefly from its use in industry, but it may enter the home as a component of dry-cleaning solutions, paint remover, or rubber cement. In very large doses, it acts as an anesthetic, but its chief danger arises from bone marrow depression. Susceptibility to this poison appears to vary greatly, and exposures which are safe for most people may cause fatal disease in a few. Treatment is directed toward the hematologic defect (p. 1326) and *complete* protection from further exposure.

Beryllium. See p. 1547.

Bleaching Solutions (Sodium Hypochlorite, Clorox, Purex). The ingestion of sodium hypochlorite solution causes corrosion of the mucosa of the oropharynx and upper gastrointestinal tract. Local burning, nausea, and vomiting are produced. Laryngeal edema may occur. Lavage with sodium bicarbonate solution is indicated (weak acids should *not* be used). Perforation and stricture formation are rare.

Bromides. The bromide ion is a central nervous system depressant. Although seldom prescribed by physicians at the present time, it is still found in many proprietary headache remedies and "nerve tonics." Despite efforts in recent years to curtail the sale of bromides, chronic bromide intoxication, or bromism, is still relatively common. Acute poisoning is rare, because vomiting commonly follows ingestion of a single large dose. However, with continued administration, bromide accumulates in the body and symptoms of intoxication appear. These symptoms are caused by the bromide ion itself and are not a reflection of the decrease in chloride caused by displacement. Bromide is handled in the body like chloride, being excreted almost entirely via the kidneys, although tears, sweat, and gastric juice also contain the ion. Rapid tests for blood bromide are available. Although it is generally stated that a blood bromide level of 200 mg per 100 ml (25 mEq per liter) results in the appearance of symptoms, higher levels are sometimes well tolerated, and severe intoxication is often seen with lower quantities. In general, the finding of a level of 75 mg per 100 ml (9 mEq per liter) or more must be regarded as confirmatory of the diagnosis of bromism if the clinical picture suggests it.

Symptoms range from drowsiness, lethargy, and dysarthria to coma or mania with psychotic behavior. Many patients suffering from bromism were committed to mental institutions in the past. Often bromides were prescribed for control of symptoms of unrecognized bromide intoxication. A blood bromide determination is indicated in any patient with unusual mental symptoms or unexplained lethargy, particularly if a history of drug ingestion is elicited. Various types of skin eruptions ranging from acneform lesions to proliferative nodular lesions not unlike those of tertiary syphilis are also produced by bromides, but more than 75 per cent of patients with mental symptoms due to this drug have no dermatitis.

Treatment consists of sedation (paraldehyde being the drug of choice), careful nursing, and removal of the source of bromide. Chloride displaces the bromide ion and promotes its excretion; chloride administration may be pursued vigorously, but, in general, with cessation of bromide ingestion and mild chloride supplementation (2 to 4 Gm NaCl three times daily), symptoms subside readily and tremendous doses of sodium or ammonium chloride seem worthwhile only in extreme cases. The administration of mercurial diuretics hastens elimination of the drug by promoting a bromide as well as chloride diuresis. Hemodialysis with the artificial kidney hastens the excretion of the poison and is probably advisable in severe cases.

Caffeine. Although human fatalities due to caffeine are rare, overdosage leads to insomnia, mild delirium, tinnitus, tachycardia, and prominent diuresis. Because caffeine has a direct effect upon the myocardium, it may cause serious arrhythmias, and dosage should be limited to 6 Gm daily. A cup of coffee contains 100 to 150 mg of caffeine. The excitatory effects are easily controlled with barbiturates.

Camphor (Camphorated Oil). Formerly a popular stimulant, this drug is now rarely used therapeutically; however, occasional cases of poisoning are still seen as a result of ingestion of liniment or moth flakes. Manifestations are headache, sensation of warmth, confusion, clonic convulsions, and terminal respiratory depression. The characteristic odor of camphor facilitates the diagnosis. Treatment is supportive. Barbiturates should be used with caution in combating convulsions because of postictal respiratory depression. Camphor is closely related to thujone, formerly the active principle of absinthe, which was probably responsible for convulsions in absinthe addicts.

Cantharides (Spanish Flies, Blistering Beetles, Essence of Viper). Poisoning may follow accidental ingestion but is probably commonest after taking cantharides powder for abortion or as an aphrodisiac, often as a prank. It is a potent irritant and vesicant. Symptoms are severe burning pain in the mouth, esophagus, and abdomen, intense thirst, bloody diarrhea, and hematemesis. The vomitus contains shining particles if the powder has been taken. There is rapid onset of acute urethritis with painful micturition, priapism, oliguria, hematuria, anuria with uremia, hepatic failure, myocarditis, delirium, and death. Treatment consists of gastric lavage, avoidance of oils or fats (the active principle is fat-soluble), morphine for pain and tenesmus, and blood and fluid replacement. With anuria, which is due to glomerular and tubular damage, a regimen for acute renal failure (p. 1496) has been followed by recovery.

Carbon Monoxide. Carbon monoxide is a colorless, odorless gas formed by incomplete combustion of carbon-containing materials. It is a component of manufactured illuminating gas and automobile exhaust fumes. The effects of carbon monoxide arise from its ability to form a stable compound with hemoglobin (carboxyhemoglobin), reducing the oxygen-carrying capacity of the blood. Symptoms include decreased exercise tolerance, headache, irritability, reduced judgment and memory, confusion, collapse, and unconsciousness. The symptoms may all appear within a few minutes or may develop gradually if exposure is minimal but prolonged. Carboxyhemoglobin is bright red, and patients show a characteristic cherry-colored flush. Cyanosis is absent. Treatment is directed toward the breakdown of carboxyhemoglobin by adequate ventilation in the presence of high oxygen tension. The patient should therefore be removed from exposure immediately, and oxygen inhalation should be instituted. Recovery is usually rapid; but if tissue anoxia has been prolonged, irreversible nervous system damage may have occurred. A hemoglobin solution produced by diluting blood 1:20 with distilled water will turn brown upon the addition of an equal volume of 40 per cent sodium hydroxide, whereas a carboxyhemoglobin solution remains red.

Carbon Tetrachloride (and Other Halogenated Hydrocarbons). Halogenated hydrocarbons are widely used as industrial solvents. Inhaled in sufficient concentration, all are capable of inducing narcosis and in addition have varying amounts of hepatic and renal toxicity. Household exposure to carbon tetrachloride may occur through the use of "safe" (nonflammable) cleaning solvents or fire extinguishers. Absorption may occur following inhalation of fumes in a closed space, percutaneous absorption, or ingestion. Renal involvement is said to be more common after inhalation than after ingestion, which leads to absorption by the portal venous system. The toxic effects of this solvent are greatly enhanced in alcoholics. Manifestations are abdominal pain, nausea, vomiting, diarrhea, and headache within a few minutes, followed in hours or days by progressive damage to liver or kidneys or both. The renal lesion can progress to complete anuria; with proper fluid management and possibly the use of the artificial kidney, survival is possible despite this complication. Hepatic damage may be acutely progressive, with severe jaundice and rapid death. The hepatic lesion is a severe central necrosis. Death secondary to pulmonary edema, common in the past, was due to excessive fluid intake in anuric patients rather than any toxic action on the myocardium. Spraying carbon tetrachloride on an open flame results in the production of phosgene, an even more toxic substance which produces pulmonary edema. There is no specific therapy other than gastric lavage and stimulants. Management of the renal lesion (p. 1496) and a regimen designed to minimize the hepatic damage are indicated.

Castor Beans (Ricin). Poisoning by ricin, an extremely toxic protein, is usually a result of ingestion of castor beans by children. Castor bean plants are often raised as ornamental shrubs in this country. *Ricinism* is characterized by nausea, vomiting, and profuse diarrhea with severe dehydration beginning several hours after ingestion of the beans. Occasionally, convulsions and respiratory depression are a cause of death, but the usual picture is one of somnolence progressing to coma. Weakness is extreme. If the patient survives the acute symptoms, there may be anuria and uremia, with death after several days. There is evidence that this renal lesion is due to a direct action of the poison, but the early development of dehydration is undoubtedly an important factor also. Ricin has the property of agglutinating erythrocytes in vitro. It is uncertain whether this occurs in vivo, but isolated clinical reports of intravascular clotting make it seem likely that it can play a role in the development of symptoms.

Treatment consists of fluid replacement, sedation or stimulation as indicated, and management of anuria (p. 1496).

Chloral Hydrate. Poisoning due to this sedative is now rare. Differentiation from barbiturate poisoning is usually possible only by history, although miosis is said to be commoner with chloral poisoning. In addition to its action as a central nervous system depressant, chloral exerts a direct toxic effect upon heart, liver, and kidneys, particularly in the presence of preexisting disease. Patients who survive death due to respiratory depression during the first few hours may become icteric and die with acute yellow atrophy within a few days. Tolerance to chloral rarely develops; indeed, sudden increases in susceptibility to its effects may result in signs of poisoning in patients taking doses previously well tolerated. Chloral is a strong gastric irritant, and gastritis is prominent in habituated individuals, usually chronic alcoholics. There is probably no basis for stories of its potentiation by alcohol in "mickey finns."

Colchicine. Poisoning is due to accidental ingestion or therapeutic overdosage in the treatment of gout. Several hours after oral ingestion, nausea, vomiting, diarrhea (occasionally bloody), and abdominal pain appear. There are progressive weakness and lethargy, ascending paralysis with normal mental status, and terminal convulsions. Death is due to respiratory depression. Hematuria and anuria are common but usually transient. Treatment is symptomatic.

Coramine (Nikethamide). Poisoning due to Coramine is always the result of acute parenteral overdosage and is manifested by intense itching, sneezing, and, rarely, convulsions. Duration of action is so short that therapy is seldom indicated, although barbiturates may occasionally be helpful.

Croton Oil. This drastic cathartic has no therapeutic use, but poisoning by ignorant pranksters is occasionally seen. Croton oil is a strong irritant, producing vesiculation and pustulation if applied directly to the skin, and a severe hemorrhagic gastroenteritis within 1 to 3 hr after ingestion. Death is the result of dehydration, blood loss, and shock. A dose of 20 drops has been fatal for an adult. Treatment is supportive, with copious parenteral fluids, blood replacement, and morphine to quiet the bowel.

Cyanide. Hydrocyanic acid, a very volatile material, and its sodium or potassium salts are among the most rapidly acting poisons known. Hydrocyanic acid is sometimes used for fumigation. Cyanide salts are widely used in industry and may reach the home in photographic chemicals or as ingredients of certain types of silver polish. Cyanide has a typical bitter-almond odor (and has the property in extremely minute concentrations of giving tobacco smoke a peculiar taste; chemists working with cyanides often smoke during their exposure to facilitate recognition of minute leaks of the gas into the atmosphere). The fatal dose is small—as little as 300 mg salts or 100 mg hydrocyanic acid gas may cause death. Cyanides exert their physiologic effects by combining with iron-containing enzymes such as the cytochromes and catalase, with the result that hydrogen and electron transport are blocked (p. 482), the energy-releasing mechanisms of metabolism cease, and death occurs from tissue asphyxia. Since the metabolic block is in the tissues rather than the blood, the hemoglobin is saturated with oxygen, and cyanosis is not seen until respiratory depression supervenes. Symptoms depend on the mode of entry of the toxic material. When inhaled, absorption is so rapid that death may be almost instantaneous; hydrogen cyanide has been used for the execution of criminals. Oral doses act more slowly, requiring several minutes before the appearance of symptoms and as much as an hour for death. As the blood cyanide level increases, there is headache, ataxia, nausea, profound dyspnea, palpitation, convulsions, and unconsciousness. The diagnosis is suggested by the odor of bitter almonds and by the history of abrupt, catastrophic onset.

Treatment must be instituted immediately to be of value. The objective is to bind the cyanide in harmless form as the highly stable cyanmethemoglobin. This is accomplished by the production of methemoglobinemia by inhalation of amyl nitrite perles (one every 2 to 5 min unless blood pressure is below 80), followed by intravenous injection of 10 ml of 3 per cent sodium nitrite over a 2- to 4-min period. Since speed is essential, inhalation is preferable to injection in initiating treatment. The use of methylene blue has been advocated, but its action is too slow to be of great benefit, although it may be given if nitrates are not available. The production of methemoglobinemia should be followed by the slow intravenous injection of sodium thiosulfate (50 ml of a 25 per cent solution over a 10-min period) to convert cyanide liberated from the dissociation of cyanmethemoglobin to thiocyanate. Norepinephrine or epinephrine may be necessary to maintain blood pressure, particularly with the added hypotensive effect of nitrites. After nitrites have been given, supportive measures may be instituted, but unless a considerable degree of methemoglobinemia is produced promptly, the outlook is not improved by other forms of treatment.

Cyanide is rapidly destroyed in the body by oxidation to relatively harmless thiocyanate. If, therefore, the patient survives a few hours, recovery is likely. After the acute episode is over, there may be residual cerebral symptoms.

DDT (*p*-Dichlorodiphenyltrichlorethane, Chlorophenothane, and Similar Insecticides). This common ingredient of insecticide powders, sprays, and aerosols is poorly absorbed unless dissolved in a vehicle such as kerosene or carbon tetrachloride, but under these circumstances it readily enters the body through the skin, lungs, or gastrointestinal tract. Fatal poisoning has occurred from the absorption of 150 mg per kg body weight. The other related chlorinated diphenyl insecticides and the chlorinated indane insecticides (aldrin, Chlordane, dieldrin, heptachlor) produce toxic manifestations similar to those of DDT. Lindane (hexachlorbenzene) produces more striking liver damage. The symptoms of acute poisoning are central nervous system hyperexcitability, delirium, and convulsions, followed by progressive depression with paralysis, coma, and death. In chronically exposed patients, cerebellar symptoms and evidence of liver damage may develop. Treatment consists of gastric lavage, barbiturate sedation, support of respiration, and the alleviation of muscle contractions by intravenous injection of calcium salts. Epinephrine should probably be avoided, since animal studies indicate an increased susceptibility to epinephrine-induced ventricular fibrillation with DDT intoxication. Ingestion of fats should be avoided for several days. The potential toxicity of the vehicle in which DDT is dissolved should be remembered.

Digitalis. See p. 1388.

Ergot (Ergotamine, Ergonovine). Poisoning is usually due to illegal use as an abortifacient or to therapeutic overdosage. The latter is likely to occur in patients with severe infection, liver disease, or hyperthyroidism, which conditions are contraindications to the use of ergot derivatives. Symptoms are nausea and vomiting (relieved by atropine), diarrhea, burning abdominal pain (if orally ingested), weakness of legs, tingling of extremities, severe muscle pains (relieved by massage and calcium gluconate), psychotic behavior, and finally convulsions, coma, and ischemic peripheral gangrene. The vascular effects are due to a combination of prolonged vasoconstriction and obstructing intimal hyperplasia and thrombosis. Treatment is supportive, using nitrites, papaverine, and mechanical procedures designed to restore circulation, and morphine for pain which is often very severe.

Favism. Ingestion of fava beans or inhalation of its pollen by sensitive individuals results in an acute hemolytic anemia. Susceptibility to favism seems to run in families, although the disease sometimes appears with no family history of favism, often in patients who have eaten the beans for many years. Glucose 6-phosphate dehydrogenase deficiency in the erythrocytes has been demonstrated in some patients and families with this sensitivity. Treatment is purely supportive, with transfusions, etc. (p. 1294). The disease is rare in this country but has been common in Mediterranean countries, particularly Italy.

Fluoride. Fluoride salts are the chief toxic ingredient of many insect poisons. When kept in large quantities, expecially in institutional kitchens, they have been mistaken for baking powder or table salt and added to food, producing large epidemics of intoxication. Fatal poisoning occurs after the oral ingestion of about 2 Gm of the sodium salt. Fluoride acts in three ways: in the presence of an acid medium, e.g., the gastric contents, it forms hydrofluoric acid, an exceedingly corrosive material; it combines with plasma calcium, forming insoluble calcium fluoride, causing tetany; and it also blocks the glycolytic degradation of glucose, thus inhibiting carbohydrate metabolism in the initial steps (p. 476). Symptoms are nausea, vomiting of corrosive material, diarrhea, and abdominal pain. As the ionized plasma calcium falls, muscular hyperirritability progresses from increased reflex activity (positive Chvostek sign) to fasciculations and convulsive tonic spasms. There is circulatory collapse and death, usually several hours or, rarely, several days after ingesting the poison. Diagnosis is confirmed by the presence of tetany, by the fact that blood drawn from patients poisoned with fluoride clots poorly, and by the presence of a high blood glucose concentration. The hydrofluoric acid in vomitus may etch glass containers. The stomach should be washed at once with lime water, calcium chloride, or calcium gluconate. The skin of the face and perineum should be protected from the corrosive gastrointestinal contents. Tetany can be alleviated and some of the fluoride ion bound harmlessly by the constant slow intravenous injection of very large volumes of 10 per cent calcium gluconate or 1 per cent calcium chloride. The infusion rate should be adjusted so as barely to prevent a positive Chvostek sign. The hyperglycemia is not reduced by administration of insulin. Despite these measures, mortality is high in fluoride poisoning. The chronic ingestion of fluoride in moderate amounts (20 to 100 mg per day) produces mottling of dental enamel (fluorosis).

Formaldehyde. Poisoning due to this substance, which is a component of various germicides and fumigants, is usually diagnosed by the characteristic odor of formaldehyde in the vomitus. Manifestations are largely those of gastrointestinal irritation, with nausea,. vomiting, abdominal pain, tenesmus, difficult micturition, and central nervous system depression leading to coma. There is striking reduction in plasma carbon dioxide–combining power; presumably the acidosis is similar in etiology to that seen after methyl alcohol. Treatment is supportive, with gastric lavage using dilute ammonia and parenteral infusion of large amounts of sodium bicarbonate or lactate to combat acidosis. The fatal dose is about 30 ml.

Gases. Most fire fighters or victims who are "overcome" by smoke are in fact poisoned by carbon monoxide and respond rapidly to oxygen inhalation. In some instances, however, burning material releases irritant fumes, either by combustion or by the destruction of containers in which dangerous chemicals have been stored. Most of the irritant gases thus released cause immediate chemical burns of the upper respiratory tract and exposed skin. Ammonia, nitrogen oxides (which form nitric acid with water), hydrogen sulfide, and sulfur dioxide or trioxide (which form sulfurous and sulfuric acids, respectively, when hydrated) are chiefly dangerous for their local effects. Several hours after exposure has been terminated, and when the patient appears comfortable, severe pulmonary edema may develop. This is usually a result of inhalation of nitrogen dioxide or of phosgene, which is released when carbon tetrachloride fire extinguishers are played on hot surfaces. One should therefore watch carefully for complications in patients who have been exposed to smoke or burning fumes. Treatment includes administration of oxygen, control of cough, and use of steam inhalations.

Ferrous Sulfate. Taken in sufficient amount, ferrous sulfate produces gastrointestinal ulcerations, nausea, vomiting, abdominal pain, and diarrhea. The lethal dose is approximately 900 mg per kg body weight. There is systemic absorption of the iron through the damaged mucosa, and the serum iron rises rapidly. Systemic effects include acidosis, shock, drowsiness, coma, respiratory failure, and liver damage. In addition to supportive measures the stomach should be lavaged with a 10 per cent

sodium bicarbonate or disodium phosphate solution to precipitate the ferrous ion. Calcium disodium edathamil (Ca EDTA) has been used successfully in doses of 35 to 45 mg per kg per day orally, with the same dose intravenously. X-rays may be helpful in assessing the adequacy of removal of the radiopaque tablets.

Gasoline and Kerosene. Exposure to the fumes of gasoline in high concentration may lead to headache, vertigo, unconsciousness with typical muscle jactitations, convulsions, and death from respiratory depression. Treatment consists of administration of oxygen and control of seizures with barbiturates. Exposure to gasoline containing tetraethyl lead has the additional hazard of lead poisoning (p. 813).

Oral ingestion of gasoline or kerosene is almost invariably followed by bronchopneumonia, the management of which is the main therapeutic problem. The greatly increased mortality associated with aspiration of vomitus containing the hydrocarbon has been used as an argument for and against lavage.

Glycols. Propylene glycol is widely used as a vehicle for drugs and flavoring extracts and is relatively nontoxic. Ethylene and diethylene glycol are commonly used in permanent antifreeze compounds and are poisonous. Both are metabolized to oxalate in the body. Poisoning often results from intentional drinking of antifreeze for supposed alcoholic content. Ingestion of ethylene glycol is followed by nausea, vomiting, deep coma, bradycardia, clammy skin, hypothermia, and various neurologic findings such as nystagmus, anisocoria, absent reflexes, and convulsions. Death almost always occurs within 48 hr after massive ingestion from respiratory failure or pulmonary edema. Diethylene glycol produces severe hepatic and renal necrosis, with jaundice, anuria, and uremia. Because of the striking renal changes, mercury poisoning is often mistakenly suspected in these patients. There is no specific treatment, although calcium may be given intravenously in an attempt to reduce the oxalate level. Hemodialysis has proved successful in the management of ethylene and diethylene glycol poisoning.

Insecticides and Rodenticides. These toxic substances are commonly found in the home and are responsible for a significant number of fatal accidental and suicidal poisonings. The clinical manifestations produced depend upon the active ingredients and in some cases upon the toxicity of the solvent. Management is discussed under the active ingredients and solvents.

Insulin. See p. 661.

Iodine. Acute poisoning may follow ingestion of 1.0 ml tincture of iodine or of Lugol's solution, and five times this amount may be fatal. There is burning abdominal pain, nausea, vomiting, pallor, collapse, rapid pulse, albuminuria, and oliguria. Death may occur after an hour or may be delayed for a week. Salivation, conjunctivitis, and edema of the eyelids appear after a few hours. Vomitus is blue or black if the stomach contains starch. Treatment consists of gastric lavage with starch solution (the blue product is nontoxic), the injection of 10 ml of 10 per cent sodium thiosulfate intravenously every 4 hr to reduce free iodine to less toxic iodide, and supportive measures. Patients taking iodine for suicidal purposes rarely succeed.

Small doses of iodides produce salivation, lacrimation, coryza, fever, swelling of the eyelids, swelling and tenderness of the salivary glands (iodide mumps), and skin rash in susceptible individuals. Whether these manifestations of *iodism* are due to hypersensitivity or idiosyncrasy to the direct action of the drug itself is not definitely established.

Isopropyl Alcohol (Isopropanol, Rubbing Alcohol). The diagnosis of isopropyl alcohol intoxication is usually made by its characteristic odor or the finding of an empty bottle of this substance. It is approximately twice as toxic as ethyl alcohol and produces profound unconsciousness not unlike that produced by large amounts of its ethyl homologue. Coma rarely lasts longer than 8 to 14 hr, and treatment with mild stimulants and intravenous fluids is all that is indicated. The only threat to life is the irritating action in the stomach which makes vomiting with aspiration a great danger; gastric lavage is indicated in all patients. Transient acetonuria is common (isopropyl alcohol is oxidized to acetone in the body), but significant acidosis is not seen. If intravenous glucose has been given and glucosuria is present, the patient may be thought to have diabetes, although the confusion is soon corrected by observation of the patient's subsequent course. There are no sequelae; significant bleeding from gastritis has been reported to complicate convalescence.

Local Anesthetics (Procaine, Cocaine, Pontocaine, Nupercaine, etc.). The many drugs in this group vary greatly in toxicity, but manifestations of overdosage are so similar that a single description will suffice. Poisoning is almost always due to parenteral use of concentrated solution intended for topical use or to overdosage caused by confusion of names. Many persons are abnormally susceptible to local anesthetics and manifest symptoms with small doses of procaine, the least toxic of the group. In sufficient amounts these agents are toxic to the heart and respiratory center and stimulate the central nervous system. Mild reactions consist of dizziness, dyspnea, and pallor. In severe poisoning there are convulsions, circulatory collapse, mydriasis, and respiratory failure, which may supervene within

a period of a few minutes. Treatment consists of artificial respiration, injection of large doses (0.5 to 1.0 ml) of epinephrine, and intravenous injection of a short-acting barbiturate. Because barbiturates almost specifically counteract the toxic effects of local anesthetic, premedication with one of this group of sedatives is advisable before the use of these drugs.

Magnesium. The magnesium ion is a profound depressant of the central nervous system and of neuromuscular transmission. Poisoning is usually due to parenteral administration of magnesium sulfate for hypertension, or occasionally to oral or rectal use, particularly in patients with renal impairment. Manifestations of poisoning are disappearance of reflexes, fall in blood pressure, hypothermia, stupor, and respiratory failure. Magnesium is toxic for the myocardium, but significant cardiac depression is preceded in human beings by respiratory failure. The treatment is intravenous administration of a calcium salt, which immediately counteracts the untoward effects of magnesium. This antagonism between calcium and magnesium on neuromuscular and autonomic ganglionic transmission is due to their reciprocal effect on acetylcholine release.

Marihuana (*Cannabis sativa* or *indica*, Hashish, India Hemp, Reefers). This narcotic is smoked for its intoxicating and exhilarating effects. The sequence of events after exposure is not unlike that seen with alcohol, but there is more of a tendency to disorientation, hallucinations, paranoia, and particularly a loss of sensation of passage of time. The material does not produce tolerance, but smokers may become dependent on it for emotional support. Overdoses produce severe depression and coma, but death is unusual. There is no specific treatment. The effects are of short duration.

Mescaline (Peyote, Mescal Buttons). This drug is derived from a species of cactus and is used by Southwestern Indians for ceremonial purposes. Its ingestion produces symptoms very similar to those of acute schizophrenia. There are colorful, pleasurable hallucinations, loss of time sense, and mild anesthesia. Pupils are dilated, and there may be bloody diarrhea and unconsciousness after large doses. Death is due to respiratory failure. There is no treatment other than a supportive regimen.

Methyl Alcohol (Wood Alcohol, Methanol). Although industrial exposure by inhalation was formerly a hazard, methyl alcohol poisoning is now due almost entirely to its ingestion as a substitute for ethanol. The toxic dose is extremely variable; death has resulted from a dose as small as 20 ml, whereas 200 ml has been ingested with survival. Methanol is oxidized in the body slowly to formic acid via formaldehyde, and the manifestations of poisoning are believed to be due to accumulation of these toxic metabolites. This is borne out by the presence in most cases of a lag period of 12 to 24 hr between ingestion and onset of symptoms.

The prime manifestation of poisoning is severe acidosis, which is not fully explainable on the basis of accumulation of formic acid alone; at present, the best theory seems to be that formate exerts an inhibitory effect upon enzymes involved in the oxidation of carbohydrate, with the consequent accumulation of acid intermediates.

Symptoms of poisoning are visual disturbance, nausea, abdominal pain, muscle pain, dizziness, weakness, and various disturbances of consciousness ranging from deep coma to clonic seizures. Visual disturbance is almost universal and ranges from mild blurring to total loss of light perception. Often impairment of vision is transient, although as is well known, permanent blindness may follow survival of the acute symptoms. Abdominal pain is excruciating and is probably due to pancreatitis, which is commonly seen at necropsy. Serum amylase is elevated, and many cases have been erroneously thought to have surgical disease of the abdomen. Likewise, cerebrovascular accident is often suspected in sporadic instances of methanol coma. Kussmaul respiration may occur, but is absent in many severely acidotic patients. Abdominal tenderness and spasm are striking, and there may be rigidity of the neck. Eye findings are helpful; the pupils are dilated and nonreactive, and ophthalmoscopic examination usually shows typical hyperemia of the optic disk with retinal edema. There is no true papilledema, and vessel changes are not characteristic.

Death in severely acidotic patients is due to cessation of respiration in the phase of inspiration. Circulation is often well maintained for several minutes after breathing stops.

Treatment consists of intravenous infusion of alkali in large amounts. Five per cent sodium bicarbonate is convenient and effective. Plasma carbon dioxide–combining power is rapidly restored by this procedure, and symptoms of impaired vision, abdominal pain, etc., are dramatically relieved. Return of acidosis is frequent, and additional alkali may be needed; consequently continued observation of patients is advisable. Gastric lavage is useless, and administration of alkali by mouth is uncertain in nauseated patients. Despite considerable experimental evidence indicating that ethanol inhibits the oxidation of methanol to formic acid, limited clinical trials of ethanol in preventing acidosis have not seemed beneficial. Although administration of whisky or brandy is permissible, alkalinization is the mainstay of treatment and should be instituted immediately. Overtreatment alkalosis often occurs, but is not dan-

gerous and is preferable to undertreatment. Hemodialysis has been reported to be helpful, but amounts of methanol removed were not documented.

The use of barbiturates to control convulsions and various stimulants such as caffeine or amphetamine are helpful, but these procedures are only of transient benefit, and correction of acidosis is the primary aim of therapy.

Metrazol. Poisoning, manifested by convulsions, is due to therapeutic overdosage and is amenable to barbiturates. So violent are convulsions after Metrazol that fractures are a common sequel.

Milk Sickness (Snakeroot, Richweed, Rayless Goldenrod). The ingestion of these plants, which contain *trematol*, produces the disease in domestic animals known as "trembles." Human poisoning can result from eating the plant but is most frequent after consumption of the milk or meat of poisoned animals. Manifestations are weakness, stiffness of the legs, anorexia, nausea, and prostration. The tongue and mucosal surfaces are reddened, and the breath smells strongly of acetone. Circulatory collapse and unconsciousness occur terminally. Transient recovery with relapse is common. Biochemically, there is acidosis, acetonuria, hypoglycemia, and rise in nonprotein nitrogen, particularly of guanidine. The mechanism of action is not clear. Death rarely occurs in less than 48 hr, and symptoms can persist for several weeks. Gastric lavage is useless, because symptoms appear after a latent period of several hours. Treatment consists of administration of carbohydrate and supportive measures. Alcohol was long advocated as an almost specific antidote, but there is no basis for its use in therapy.

Moth Balls (Paradichlorobenzene, Naphthalene) (see also Camphor). These substances are relatively nontoxic except when prolonged massive exposure by inhalation has occurred. Under these circumstances, they produce central nervous system depression. Cataracts have been reported after severe chronic exposure, and paradichlorobenzene can produce liver damage, if sufficient quantities are absorbed. Both materials are relatively safe if swallowed, and no specific therapy other than gastric lavage is needed, although naphthalene in the form of moth balls or toilet bowl deodorant has been reported a number of times as causing hemolytic anemia after ingestion in patients with glucose 6-phosphate dehydrogenase deficient red cells.

Mushroom Poisoning (Mycetismus). There are many poisonous mushrooms, but in this country, most poisoning is due to *Amantia muscaria* or *Amanita phalloides*. After ingestion of *A. muscaria*, which contains muscarine, there is rapid onset of parasympathetic stimulation: nausea, vomiting, diarrhea, salivation, perspiration, lacrimation, bradycardia, dyspnea with increased bronchial secretion, wheezing expiration, dilated pupils, confusion, and excitability. Illness begins within 6 hr after eating the mushrooms. Recovery usually takes place within 24 hr.

Amanita phalloides contains a hepatotoxin and is far deadlier than the muscarine type. From 6 to 15 hr after eating there is explosive onset of violent abdominal pain, vomiting, and bloody diarrhea, with rapid dehydration and extreme thirst. The pupils are normal. Within 24 hr in the majority of cases, there is onset of jaundice and anuria, and death from acute yellow atrophy can occur within 4 days. Recovery is slow after this type of poisoning.

Treatment consists of fluid replacement, atropine in doses of 0.6 to 1.0 mg in the muscarine type, and barbiturates for persistent excitement. Morphine may be required for relief of pain.

Mussel Poison. During late spring and summer, the common Pacific Coast mussel sometimes contains a highly toxic material which produces illness and death within a few hours after ingestion of the shellfish. It has been determined that the toxin, which is not destroyed by cooking, is actually a component of certain dinoflagellates which form the diet of the mussel. Similar poisoning has been reported in other parts of the world. Manifestations, which come on within a few minutes, are paresthesias of the oral mucosa and extremities, progressing to complete anesthesia, weakness, incoordination, ataxia, dysarthria, and progressive central respiratory depression. Circulatory collapse is secondary to hypoxia. Survival for 12 hr indicates a good prognosis for life, but complete recovery may be prolonged for weeks. Treatment consists of gastric lavage, the use of artificial or mechanical respiration, and supportive measures.

Nicotine. This alkaloid is an ingredient of many insecticides. Poisoning may occur from 150 mg or less, equivalent to a few drops of nicotine sulfate (Black Leaf 40), by mouth or inhaled. The action of nicotine is a complex mixture of depression and stimulation of the autonomic system and depression of the central nervous system. Symptoms consist of gastrointestinal irritation combined with dizziness, headache, and tachycardia. Cortical irritability, culminating in convulsions, and myocardial irritability with arrhythmias precede death, which is usually the result of cardiac or respiratory arrest. Although atropine will counteract many of the peripheral autonomic disturbances (salivation, miosis, blurred vision) caused by nicotine, it is ineffective in preventing respiratory or cardiac failure. Supportive treatment directed toward maintenance of oxygenation and prevention of arrhythmias (p. 1395) is therefore of great importance.

Nitrites. These compounds are of importance chiefly because of their ability to produce methemoglobin (p. 1310). While these materials are usually administered therapeutically (the nitrites as amyl nitrite or nitroglycerin), accidental poisoning occasionally occurs from contamination of poorly capped wells with nitrate-producing soil bacteria or food adulteration.

Nitrogen Mustards. See p. 1341.

Organic Phosphate Insecticides. Numerous newly developed insecticides, including Parathion, TEPP, HETP, OMPA, EPN, Systox, Mipafox, and Malathion, are potent inhibitors of cholinesterase and have been responsible for fatal poisoning in man. These materials are usually prepared for use by dilution with inert powder, organic solvents, or water. They are rapidly absorbed by inhalation, through intact skin, or by ingestion. Since cholinesterase destroys the acetylcholine liberated by the central nervous system, autonomic ganglions, parasympathetic nerve endings, and motor nerve endings, symptoms are produced by the persistent action of acetylcholine at these sites. Clinical manifestations of poisoning are blurring of vision and miosis, rhinorrhea, salivation, sweating, nausea, vomiting, abdominal cramps, diarrhea, dyspnea, tightness of the chest, bronchospasm, bronchorrhea, cyanosis, muscular cramps and fasciculations followed by flaccid paralysis, convulsions, coma, and respiratory depression.

Management consists of removal of contaminated clothing and gentle cleansing of the skin with soapy water. Application of a tourniquet will delay systemic absorption from a contaminated extremity. Atropine will block parasympathetic and central neural effects. It should be given promptly and in large doses (1 to 2 mg intravenously). This dose may be repeated at 3- to 8-min intervals until parasympathetic manifestations are controlled (miosis often persists even with adequate atropinization). After control of symptoms, the interval between doses is judged by return of mild symptoms. Total doses of atropine as large as 20 mg per day are often necessary for severe poisoning. Since atropine has no effect on the muscular paralysis, artificial respiration may be necessary. Oximes are capable of reversing the effect of these poisons on skeletal muscle. 2-PAM (pyridine-2-aldoxime methiodide) 0.5 to 2 Gm may be administered intravenously over a 5-min period. Careful attention should be paid to the removal of bronchial secretions. Barbiturates may be required if convulsions persist despite full atropinization. Patients who survive for 24 hr usually recover without residua, although symptoms may persist for several days.

Oxalates. Poisoning from oxalates occurs chiefly from ingestion of ink eradicators or stain removers containing oxalic acid. They produce burning of the mouth, nausea, vomiting, and abdominal pain. Later, formation of insoluble calcium oxalate produces hypocalcemic tetany. Anuria from blockage of ureters by calcium oxalate has been reported. Treatment of acute poisoning consists of the oral administration of magnesium oxide or calcium salts and the intravenous administration of calcium gluconate or chloride, together with a supportive regimen.

Paraldehyde. The diagnosis of paraldehyde poisoning is made easy by its characteristic odor. An excellent sedative, this drug rarely produces respiratory depression even in tremendous dosage (up to 120 ml), although patients may remain unconscious for as long as 48 hr after overdosage. Treatment is supportive. Morphine and paraldehyde should be used together cautiously because of increased toxicity of this combination. Habituation to paraldehyde is occasionally observed among chronic alcoholics who hope to prevent delirium tremens by its use.

Phenol and Cresols (Lysol). Poisoning is usually due to ingestion with suicidal intent. Diagnosis is facilitated by the characteristic odor of phenol or Lysol. Manifestations of poisoning are the same, but Lysol requires larger doses for a fatal effect. Although poisoning with phenol can be fatal within 30 min, death may be delayed many hours. These substances produce severe erosion of the mucosa of the mouth, throat, esophagus, and gastrointestinal tract, the burned areas having a characteristic dead-white appearance. There is vomiting and later diarrhea, often with bleeding. An initial stage of excitement is followed by coma, circulatory collapse, and respiratory depression. Convulsions are commoner in children than in adults. If the patient survives long enough, small amounts of urine which darken on standing may be voided. Later, anuria due to tubular necrosis develops. There is often severe acidosis, with profound reduction in plasma carbon dioxide–combining power. The mechanism of this acidosis is unknown, but it may involve some defect in enzyme function such as is seen in methanol or formaldehyde poisoning.

Treatment is directed toward removal of the unabsorbed poison by gastric lavage and preventing obstruction of the glottis by edema due to the pharyngeal burns. Laryngoscopic inspection should be carried out early and intubation performed if necessary to maintain the airway. Rarely, tracheotomy may be needed. The stomach should be washed with olive oil. Because phenol is soluble in ethyl alcohol and alcohol is by far the best substance to use in removing phenol from the skin, it is often recommended as a lavage fluid. However, in contrast to olive oil, alcohol will speed the ab-

sorption of phenol and is definitely contraindicated for lavage. Other treatment consists of infusion of 5 per cent sodium bicarbonate intravenously to combat acidosis (this often produces dramatic improvement), replacement of blood, and the use of stimulants and measures to combat shock if blood pressure falls.

Chronic exposure to phenol results in pruritus, pigmentation of the skin, paresthesias, and gastrointestinal disturbances. Occasionally, discoloration of the cartilages similar to that in ochronosis is seen.

Phosphorus. Elemental phosphorus occurs in several allotropic forms. Of these, only one, yellow phosphorus, is appreciably toxic. It is an ingredient of certain rat poisons. The use of phosphorus in the manufacture of matches has been outlawed as a result of poisoning which occurred in workers in match factories and because of numerous instances of accidental poisoning in children. The exact fatal dose is not known.

There is burning of the mouth and throat after ingestion, and a garlic odor is noticeable on the breath. Abdominal pain and vomiting soon become intense. When sufficient quantities have been ingested, the vomitus glows in the dark. Often symptoms subside after a few hours, but after 24 to 48 hr, *subacute* effects on the liver become apparent, and jaundice develops rapidly. Death from acute yellow atrophy can occur in a few days.

Treatment consists of introducing 100 ml of 1 per cent copper sulfate solution into the stomach and performing gastric lavage. The removal of the copper by lavage is imperative. After subsidence of acute symptoms, a protective regimen for the liver should be instituted, and patients should be observed for several days.

Picric Acid. Poisoning by picrate can occur from systemic absorption after application to extensive burns, from accidental ingestion of solutions or ointments, or from exposure in industrial plants. Oral ingestion leads to severe gastroenteritis with yellow vomitus. There may be hemolysis, liver necrosis, or acute glomerular damage, with hematuria and oliguria, in severe cases. Picrate is also a central nervous system depressant in large doses. Treatment consists of gastric lavage and administration of egg white or cheese (to form insoluble protein picrates), fluid replacement, and symptomatic management of gastroenteritis. A regimen for acute renal shutdown (p. 1496) should be instituted if anuria occurs. High concentrations of picrate on the skin produce a severe itching eczema known as "picric itch."

Picrotoxin. Poisoning due to therapeutic overdosage of this drug produces convulsions which are controllable with barbiturates administered intravenously.

Pine Oil. This distillation product of pine resin is closely related to turpentine and is used in household cleansers and disinfectants. When taken internally it acts as an irritant producing nausea, vomiting, and diarrhea. Systemic symptoms include weakness, hypothermia, and central nervous system depression. In addition to supportive measures, exchange transfusion has been of benefit.

Pokeroot (Phytolacca). Poisoning is due to ingestion of the root or bark of this plant as a home remedy for arthritis; its leaves and berries are innocuous. Within 2 hr, nausea, vomiting, and diarrhea occur. They are followed by drowsiness, vertigo, and blurred vision. In fatal cases, death results from convulsions and respiratory paralysis. Treatment is purely supportive and should include gastric lavage if the patient is seen early.

Quinidine. See p. 1396.

Salicylates (Aspirin, Sodium Salicylate, Methyl Salicylate, Oil of Wintergreen). The derivatives of salicylic acid are used in larger amounts by the laity and by the medical profession than any other medication. Therapeutic poisoning usually results from the cumulative effect of prolonged high dosage for rheumatic fever, arthritis of other types, etc., but accidental poisoning or suicidal attempts account for an appreciable number of cases. There is considerable variation in susceptibility to the toxic effects of salicylates; idiosyncrasy is common, but instances of great resistance are also seen. Toxic symptoms may begin at dosages of 3 to 4 Gm per day or may not appear when as much as 10 Gm per day is given. The plasma salicylate level is almost always greater than 10 mg per 100 ml when symptoms appear, and the development of hyperventilation usually reflects a level of over 40 mg per 100 ml. The earliest manifestations are vertigo, tinnitus, and deafness. These signs may subside if treatment is interrupted briefly or even if administration is continued. If overdosage continues, nausea, vomiting, headache, and various types of mental aberration develop. Occasionally there may be great excitement, restlessness, and talkativeness, the so-called "salicylate jag." At this point the patient usually shows the typical salicyl dyspnea. Both vomiting and hyperventilation are due to an effect of the salicylate directly on the central nervous system. Early in the development of the syndrome, serum electrolytes and the carbon dioxide–combining power are usually normal, but as increased urinary loss of alkali compensates for the respiratory alkalosis, there is progressive diminution in both serum sodium and carbon dioxide–combining power. As this stage is reached, there is usually a mild ketosis, the result of dehydration and starvation. After ingestion of a single large dose of salicylates, the development of symptoms may be extremely rapid, so that the stage of dehydration, ketoacidosis, and hyponatremia is reached within a few hours. Urinalysis is helpful in that salicylates give a positive test with ferric chloride; the salicylate test is positive on boiled urine, serving to distinguish it from ketone bodies. While occasional instances of salicylate hypoprothrombinemia have resulted in bleeding, this is not a regular manifestation of intoxication.

Therapy is directed toward removal of unabsorbed salicylate by gastric lavage with sodium bicarbonate and promoting renal excretion by a water diuresis and alkalinization of the urine with oral sodium bicarbonate or intravenous sodium lactate. Exchange transfusion, peritoneal dialysis, and hemodialysis have all been highly effective in removing salicylate in seriously poisoned patients.

"Smog." This slang term is used to describe dense fog in which smoke and chemical fumes are also present. It is usually merely irritating, but under special circumstances, industrial waste gases such as hydrogen sulfide, sulfur dioxide, or the nitrogen oxides may introduce a definite risk of poisoning. Although morbidity is sometimes high, only among elderly patients with chronic cardiac or pulmonary disease is there danger of death. Treatment is removal from the smoky environment. If this is impractical, the use of an oxygen tent or mask may prevent serious difficulties in susceptible patients.

"Smoke." A large number of paint removers, lacquer thinners, antifreezes, and other solvent mixtures are ingested at one time or another for their supposed alcohol content. Because of their milky appearance when diluted with water, these mixtures are referred to as "smoke" in many localities, although other names are used. Some wholly unknown component of these materials occasionally causes a profound hypoglycemia, with coma, clammy skin, and bizarre neurologic signs. This disturbance should be considered in any alcoholic who remains stuporous after the usual treatments for alcoholic coma have been tried. The injection of 50 per cent glucose intravenously produces dramatic results in these patients and should not be delayed until the suspected diagnosis can be confirmed by laboratory test. Patients should be observed carefully for a few hours after treatment, because hypoglycemia may recur.

Solanine (Nightshades, European Bittersweet, Poisonberry, Irish Potato Sprouts). Ingestion of these solanaceous plants produces gastrointestinal irritation with nausea, vomiting, cramps, and diarrhea. Symptoms resembling atropine intoxication (p. 819) may also be seen, and it is not clear whether this is attributable to the glycoside solanine or to other toxic products.

Strychnine. Poisoning often results from ingestion of "A.S. and B." cathartic pills by children, eating poisoned grain, or suicidal attempts. The effect of strychnine is to increase the irritability of the entire nervous system and prolong the period of hyperexcitability after a normal stimulus. The patient remains conscious and acutely aware of his surroundings. After a period of heightened irritability and muscle twitching, tonic seizures occur in which there is opisthotonos, rigid extension of the legs, facial tetanus producing the risus sardonicus, and apnea due to spasm, both of the diaphragm and of muscles of the abdomen and thorax. Each convulsion lasts 1 to 2 min. Death from anoxia may follow two to five seizures.

Barbiturates should be given rapidly to control convulsions and hence prevent anoxia and death. Secondary measures, such as lavage, etc., must await sedation, for any stimulus may set off a seizure. Observation for 24 to 48 hr is necessary; any sign of increased irritability calls for more sedation. During this period supportive care is indicated as for any comatose patient. Morphine, which is a medullary depressant but a spinal cord stimulant, is contraindicated.

Sulfonamides. See p. 869.

Tranquilizers and Nonbarbiturate Sedatives. Drugs of this class are becoming increasingly important in suicidal attempts and accidental poisoning in children. In general, these drugs produce central nervous system depression with stupor, coma, respiratory depression, and death. Chronic intoxication and withdrawal symptoms also occur. Management of these problems is similar to the treatment of barbiturate intoxication (p. 809).

Two classes of compounds deserve particular mention. Large doses of *rauwolfia alkaloids* and *phenothiazine derivatives* have a potent hypotensive effect. The peripheral signs of shock, such as pallor and sweating, may be minimal or absent. Nevertheless, shock may be a major problem in management. Pressor amines are usually effective. These two types of drug may also produce a variety of dystonic movements. Some resemble parkinsonism with rigidity and tremor, while others closely simulate the writhing movements of choreoathetosis. Still other movements appear to be migratory painful spasms of muscle groups, especially the neck muscles. These dystonic manifestations are not clearly dose related and may not subside for months following cessation of the drug. Drugs useful in the management of parkinsonism (p. 1865) are often helpful in controlling these symptoms.

Turpentine. Turpentine is readily absorbed from the skin, intestine, or lungs and is excreted in the urine, which is said to have an odor of violets. Chronic exposure to turpentine leads to urethritis, a common symptom among painters. Ingestion of large amounts (usually for its supposed abortifacient effect) produces colic, nausea, vomiting, diar-

rhea, delirium, ataxia, and coma. If the acute stage of poisoning is survived, there may be painful micturition, albuminuria, hematuria, and, on occasion, anuria and acute renal shutdown due to tubular necrosis. Treatment is supportive; a regimen for anuria should be instituted (p. 1496), since the renal lesion is reversible.

Vitamins A and D. See pp. 550 and 553.

REFERENCES

GENERAL

Adams, W. C.: Emetics in Accidental Poisoning, Pediatric Clin. N.A., 8:351, 1961.

Clemmesen, C.: The Treatment of Poisoning during the Past Twenty-Five Years: A Retrospective Review, Danish Med. Bull., 6:209, 1959.

Conley, B. E.: Recommendations of Committee on Toxicology on First Aid Measures for Poisoning, J.A.M.A., 165:686, 1957.

Dack, G. M.: "Food Poisoning," 3d ed., Chicago, University of Chicago Press, 1956.

Dreisbach, R. H.: "Handbook of Poisons," Los Altos, Calif., Lang Medical Publications, 1955.

Editorial: Value of Gastric Lavage in Treatment of Acute Poisoning, J.A.M.A., 133:545, 1947.

Fairhall, L. T.: "Industrial Toxicology," Baltimore, The Williams & Wilkins Company, 1949.

Felts, J. H.: The Use of the Artificial Kidney in Poisonings, N. Carolina Med. J., 21:490, 1960.

Gold, H.: Household Poisonings, Am. J. Med., 6:238, 1949.

Goldman, L., and A. Gilman: "The Pharmacological Basis of Therapeutics," 2d ed., New York, The Macmillan Company, 1955.

Lucas, G. H. W.: "The Symptoms and Treatment of Acute Poisoning," Toronto, Clarke, Irwin & Company, Ltd., 1952.

Press, E.: "Accidental Poisoning in Childhood," Evanston, Ill., American Academy of Pediatrics (Committee on Accident Prevention), 1956.

Schreiner, G. E.: The Role of Hemodialysis (Artificial Kidney) in Acute Poisoning, A.M.A. Arch. Internal Med., 102:896, 1958.

Tatum, A. L., and M. H. Seevers: Theories of Drug Addiction, Physiol. Revs., 11:107, 1931.

Thienes, C. J., and T. J. Haley: "Clinical Toxicology," 2d ed., Philadelphia, Lea & Febiger, 1948.

Thomson, T. J., and S. Alstead: Treatment of Acute Poisoning, Brit. Med. J., 1960, II:726.

Von Oettingen, W. F.: "Poisoning, a Guide to Clinical Diagnosis and Treatment," 2d ed., Philadelphia, W. B. Saunders Company, 1958.

Yampolsky, J., and S. W. Perry: The Treatment of Poisoning in Children by Exchange Transfusion, Southern Med. J., 53:1169, 1960.

TOXIC PRODUCT IDENTIFICATION

"Clinical Memoranda on Economic Poisons," Savannah, Ga., Communicable Disease Center, Public Health

Service, U.S. Department Health Education and Welfare, 1956.

Frear, D. E. H.: "Pesticide Handbook," State College, Pa., College Science Publishers, 1960.

Gleason, M., R. Gosselin, and H. C. Hodge: "Clinical Toxicology of Commercial Products, Acute Poisoning (Home and Farm)," Baltimore, The Williams & Wilkins Company, 1957.

Langford, G. S.: "Entoma—Directory of Insect and Plant Pest Control," 9th ed., College Park, Md., American Assoc. Economic Entomologists, Department of Entomology, University of Maryland, 1951–1952.

Martin, H.: "Guide to the Chemicals Used in Crop Protection," 2d ed., London, Ontario, Canada, Department of Agriculture, 1955.

McCutcheon, J. W.: "Synthetic Detergent—Up to Date II," New York, MacNair-Dorland Company, 1952.

Muenscher, W. C.: "Poisonous Plants of the U.S.," 2d ed., New York, The Macmillan Company, 1951.

"Pesticide Official Publication and Condensed Data on Pesticide Chemicals," College Park, Md., Association of American Pesticide Control Officials, Inc., 1955.

Zimmerman, O. T., and I. Lavine: "Handbook of Material Trade Names," Dover, N.H., Industrial Research Service, 1953.

ACETANILID

Payne, S.: Acetanilid Poisoning: A Clinical and Experimental Study, J. Pharmacol. Exptl. Therap., 53: 401, 1935.

AMIDOPYRINE

Kracke, R. R.: Relation of Drug Therapy to Neutropenic States, J.A.M.A., 111:1255, 1938.

AMPHETAMINE

Bennett, I. L., Jr., and W. F. Walker: Cardiac Arrhythmias Following the Use of Large Doses of Central Nervous System Stimulants, Am. Heart J., 44:428, 1952.

Waud, S. P.: The Effects of Toxic Doses of Benzyl Methyl Carbinamine (Benzedrine) in Man, J.A.M.A., 110:206, 1938.

ATROPINE

Robertson, E. S.: Atropine Intoxication: Report of a Case with Recovery after Ingestion of One Half Grain (33 mg) Atropine Sulfate, Southern Med. J., 44:56, 1951.

BARIUM

Dean, G.: Seven Cases of Barium Carbonate Poisoning, Brit. Med. J., 1950, II:817.

BENZENE

Bowditch, M., and H. B. Elkins: Chronic Exposure to Benzene (Benzol): I. The Industrial Aspects, J. Ind. Hyg. Toxicol., 21:321, 1939.

Erf, L., and C. P. Rhoads: The Hematological Effects of Benzene (Benzol) Poisoning, J. Ind. Hyg. Toxicol., 21:421, 1939.

Hunter, F. T.: Chronic Exposure to Benzene (Benzol): II. The Clinical Effects, J. Ind. Hyg. Toxicol., 21: 331, 1939.

Mallory, T. B., E. A. Gall, and W. J. Brickley: Chronic Exposure to Benzene (Benzol): III. The Pathologic Results, J. Ind. Hyg. Toxicol., 21:355, 1939.

BROMIDES

Hanes, F. M., and A. Yates: Analysis of 400 Instances of Chronic Bromide Intoxication, Southern Med. J., 31:667, 1938.

Preu, P. W., J. Romano, and W. F. Brown: Symptomatic Psychoses with Bromide Intoxication, N. Engl. J. Med., 214:56, 1936.

Wagner, G. A., and D. E. Bunbury: Incidence of Bromide Intoxication among Psychotic Patients, J.A.M.A., 95:1725, 1930.

CANTHARIDES

Oaks, W. W., J. F. DiTunno, T. Magnani, H. A. Levy, and L. C. Mills: Cantharidin Poisoning, A.M.A. Arch. Internal Med., 105:574, 1960.

CARBON MONOXIDE

Drinker, C. K.: "Carbon Monoxide Asphyxia," New York, Oxford University Press, 1938.

Medical Research Council Report: Carbon Monoxide Poisoning, Use of Carbon Dioxide–Oxygen Mixture, Brit. Med. J., 1158, II:1408.

Pau, N., W. V. Consolazio, W. A. White, and A. R. Behnke: Formulation of the Principal Factors Affecting the Rate of Uptake of Carbon Monoxide by Man, Am. J. Physiol., 147:352, 1946.

CARBON TETRACHLORIDE

Dillenberg, S. M., and C. M. Thompson: Carbon Tetrachloride Poisoning: Report of 20 Cases with 1 Death, Military Surgeon, 97:39, 1945.

Friedberg, C. K.: Congestive Heart Failure of Renal Origin: Pathogenesis and Treatment in Four Cases of Carbon Tetrachloride Nephrosis, Am. J. Med., 9:164, 1950.

Myatt, A. V., and J. A. Salmons: Carbon Tetrachloride Poisoning, Arch. Ind. Hyg. Occupational Med., 6:74, 1952.

Norwood, W. D., P. A. Fuqua, and B. C. Scudder: Carbon Tetrachloride Poisoning, Arch. Ind. Hyg. Occupational Med., 1:90, 1950.

CYANIDE

Chen, K. K., and C. L. Rose: Nitrite and Thiosulfate Therapy in Cyanide Poisoning, J.A.M.A., 149:113, 1952.

——: Treatment of Acute Cyanide Poisoning, J.A.M.A., 162, 1154, 1956.

Ingegno, A. P., and S. Franco: Cyanide Poisoning: Successful Treatment of Two Cases with Intravenous

Sodium Nitrite and Sodium Thiosulfate, Ind. Med., 6:573, 1937.

DDT

Council on Pharmacy and Chemistry, A.M.A.: Pharmacology and Toxicologic Aspects of DDT (Chlorophenothane, U.S.P.), J.A.M.A., 145:728, 1951.

ERGOT

Gabbai, Lisbonne, and Purrquier: Ergot Poisoning at St. Esprit, Brit. Med. J., 1951, II:650.

von Storch, T. J. C.: Migraine Syndrome, Med. Clin. N. Am., 22:689, 1938.

Yater, W. M., and J. A. Cahill: Bilateral Gangrene of Feet Due to Ergotamine Tartrate Used for Pruritus of Jaundice: Report of Case Studied Arteriographically and Pathologically, J.A.M.A., 106:1625, 1936.

FERROUS SULFATE

Schafir, M.: The Management of Acute Poisoning by Ferrous Sulfate, Pediatrics, 27:83, 1961.

FLUORIDE

DeEds, F.: Chronic Fluorine Intoxication, Medicine, 12:1, 1933.

Peters, J. H.: Therapy of Acute Fluoride Poisoning, Am. J. Med. Sci., 216:278, 1948.

GASES

Cope, O.: Care of the Victims of the Cocoanut Grove Fire at the Massachusetts General Hospital, N. Engl. J. Med., 229:138, 1943.

Hardy, G. C., and A. L. Bachrach: Positive Pressure Respiration in the Treatment of Irritant Pulmonary Edema Due to Chlorine Gas Poisoning, J.A.M.A., 128:359, 1945.

GLYCOLS

Geiling, E. M. K., and P. R. Cannon: Pathologic Effects of Elixir of Sulfanilamide (Diethylene Glycol) Poisoning: A Clinical and Experimental Correlation: Final Report, J.A.M.A., 111:919, 1938.

Pons, C. A., and R. P. Custer: Acute Ethylene Glycol Poisoning: A Clinicopathologic Report of Eighteen Fatal Cases, Am. J. Med. Sci., 211:544, 1946.

Schreiner, G. E., J. F. Maher, J. March-Aurele, D. Knowlan, and M. Alva: Ethylene Glycol: Two Medications for Hemodialysis, Trans. Am. Soc. Art. Int. Organs, 5:81, 1959.

IODINE

Finkelstein, R., and M. Jacobi: Fatal Iodine Poisonings: Clinicopathologic and Experimental Study, Ann. Internal Med., 10:1238, 1937.

More, M.: Ingestion of Iodine as a Method of Attempted Suicide, N. Engl. J. Med., 219:383, 1938.

ISOPROPYL ALCOHOL

McCord, W. M., P. K. Switzer, and H. H. Brill: Isopropyl Alcohol Intoxication, Southern Med. J., 41:639, 1948.

KEROSENE

Olstad, R. B., and R. M. Lord: Kerosene Intoxication, Am. J. Diseases Children, 83:446, 1952.

Reed, E. S., S. Leiken, and H. D. Kerman: Kerosene Intoxication, Am. J. Diseases Children, 79:623, 1950.

MARIHUANA

Bromberg, W.: Marihuana Intoxication: Clinical Study of *Cannabis sativa* Intoxication, Am. J. Psychiat., 91:303, 1934.

MESCALINE

Stockings, G. T.: A Clinical Study of the Mescaline Psychosis, with Special Reference to the Mechanism of the Genesis of Schizophrenic and Other Psychotic States, J. Mental Sci., 86:29, 1940.

METHYL ALCOHOL

Bennett, I. L., Jr.: Poisoning Due to Substances Commonly Substituted for Ethyl Alcohol, Veterans Administration Tech. Bull., TB10-89, May 15, 1953.

——, F. H. Cary, G. L. Mitchell, Jr., and M. N. Cooper: Acute Methyl Alcohol Poisoning: A Review Based on Experiences in an Outbreak of 323 Cases, Medicine, 32:431, 1953.

Chew, W. B., E. H. Berger, O. A. Brines, and M. J. Capron: Alkali Treatment of Methyl Alcohol Poisoning, J.A.M.A., 130:61, 1946.

Stinebaugh, B. J.: The Use of Peritoneal Dialysis in Acute Methyl Alcohol Poisoning, A.M.A. Arch. Internal Med., 105:613, 1960.

MUSSEL POISON

Medcof, J. C.: Shellfish Poisoning—Another North American Ghost, Can. Med. Assoc. J., 82:87, 1960.

ORGANIC PHOSPHATE INSECTICIDES

Council on Pharmacy and Chemistry, A.M.A.: Symposium on Pharmacology and Toxicology of Certain Organic Phosphorus Insecticides, J.A.M.A., 144:104, 1950.

Grob, D.: The Manifestations and Treatment of Poisoning Due to Nerve Gas and Other Organic Phosphate Anticholinesterase Compounds, A.M.A. Arch. Internal Med., 98:221, 1956.

—— and R. J. Johns: Use of Oximes in the Treatment of Intoxication by Anticholinesterase Compounds in Normal Subjects, Am. J. Med., 24:497, 1958.

Harvey, A. M.: Potential Hazards of the Newer Insecticides, Am. J. Med., 8:1, 1950.

PHENOL

Bennett, I. L., Jr., D. F. James, and A. Golden: Severe Acidosis Due to Phenol Poisoning, Ann. Internal Med., 32:324, 1950.

PHOSPHORUS

Diaz-Rivera, R. S., P. J. Collazo, E. R. Pons, and M. V. Torregrosa: Acute Phosphorus Poisoning in Man; 56 Cases, Medicine, 29:269, 1950.

Rubitsky, H. J., and R. M. Myerson: Acute Phosphorus Poisoning, Arch. Internal Med., 83:164, 1949.

PINE OIL

Tauscher, J. W., and J. J. Polich: Treatment of Pine Oil Poisoning by Exchange Transfusion, J. Pediat., 55:511, 1959.

SALICYLATES

Crichton, J. U., and G. B. Elliott: Salicylate—a Dangerous Drug in Infancy and Childhood, Can. Med. Assoc. J., 83:1144, 1960.
Done, A., and L. Otterness: Exchange Transfusion in the Treatment of Oil of Wintergreen (Methyl Salicylate) Poisoning, Pediatrics, 18:80, 1956.
Graham, J. D. P., and W. A. Parker: Toxic Manifestations of Sodium Salicylate Therapy, Quart. J. Med., 17:153, 1948.
Greenberg, L. A.: Evaluation of Reported Poisonings by Acetylsalicylic Acid, N. Engl. J. Med., 243:124, 1950.
Schreiner, G. E., L. B. Berman, J. Griggin, and J.

Feys: Specific Therapy for Salicylism, N. Engl. J. Med., 253:213, 1955.
Singer, R. B.: The Acid-Base Disturbance in Salicylate Intoxication, Medicine, 33:1, 1954.
Tenny, S. M., and R. M. Miller: The Respiratory and Circulatory Actions of Salicylate, Am. J. Med., 19:498, 1955.

"SMOG"

McDonald, J. C., P. Drinker, and J. E. Gordon: The Epidemiology and Social Significance of Atmospheric Smoke Pollution, Am. J. Med. Sci., 221:325, 1951.

"SMOKE"

Brown, T. M., and A. M. Harvey: Spontaneous Hypoglycemia in "Smoke" Drinkers, J.A.M.A., 117:12, 1941.

STRYCHNINE

Aikman, J.: Strychnine Poisoning in Children, J.A.M.A., 95:1661, 1930.

Section 2: Physical Agents

104 DISORDERS DUE TO HIGH ENVIRONMENTAL TEMPERATURES

John H. Talbott

There are three clinical syndromes associated with high environmental temperatures: heat cramps, heat exhaustion, and heat pyrexia. Although the three entities may be identified clinically, there is considerable overlapping of the internal changes produced by a high environmental temperature. In each instance, they are the sequelae of excessive or prolonged physiologic response. The alterations are especially prevalent during the first few days of a heat wave before effective acclimatization. Prophylaxis, by means of augmented sodium chloride intake, prior to exposure to high environmental temperatures or restoration of the physiologic changes prior to the onset of overt morbidity, is helpful in preventing dire consequences. The child and the older person are more susceptible than the mature adult to heat stress. Strenuous physical activity or the presence of an acute or chronic disease may hasten the development of any one of the morbid states.

Acclimatization. Sweating is the most effective natural means of combating heat stress with little or no change in the core temperature of the body. So long as sweating continues, provided water and salt are replaced, man can withstand remarkably high temperatures. Two or three liters of sweat may be lost per day. Over short periods of time the loss per hour may approach this value. The most important constituents of sweat are water and sodium chloride. The concentration of sodium chloride may be low; at other times, it may approach that of interstitial body fluid. Since the sodium chloride concentration of sweat is less than body fluid, the excess salt must be retained in the body during the initial stages of sweating. Studies reveal the skin to be the repository. Dilatation of the peripheral blood vessels is a well-known phenomenon in high environmental temperatures. Histamine and histidine in the sweat may participate in the vasodilatation. Other alterations include a decrease in total circulating blood volume, a decrease in renal blood flow, and an increase of the antidiuretic substance in the urine (ADH). Aldosterone, the most potent mineralocorticoid, has also been detected in increased quantities in the urine following exposure. Vasodilatation, with an increased circulation in the blood vessels of the skin, permits dissipation of heat. The cardiac output is increased initially. As the stress persists there may be a decrease in cardiac output below normal, with forward failure. Subsequently, venous collapse may supervene. Failure of dissipation of heat with persistence of environmental temperatures greater than that of the body leads to retention of heat and hyperpyrexia.

Heat Cramps. Miner's cramps and stoker's cramps describe the syndrome associated with painful spasms of the voluntary musculature following strenuous exercise. Only subjects in good physical condition are candidates. External temperatures need not exceed the body temperature. Direct exposure to the sun is not necessary. Muscle cramps have been observed following excessive sweating, precipitated by strenuous exercise in cold environments in untrained persons heavily clothed. Muscles of the extremities that bear the brunt of physical activity show the highest incidence of involvement. Excruciating pain accompanies the spasms and subsides with cessation of cramps. Physical examination is essentially normal between the paroxysms. Examination of the blood reveals a concentration of the formed elements and a decreased concentration of total base, especially sodium and also of chloride. A diminished excretion of sodium chloride in the urine is characteristic. Cessation of cramps with replacement of sodium chloride and water is striking and supports the hypothesis that the etiology of heat cramps is associated with body depletion of these essential electrolytes.

Heat Exhaustion. Heat prostration or heat collapse is probably the most common heat syndrome. Weakness, vertigo, headache, nausea, anorexia, and faintness may precede collapse or participate as predisposing factors. The physically active as well as the sedentary person is susceptible. Onset may be sudden and the duration of collapse brief. During the acute stage, evidence of peripheral vascular collapse and poor venous return may be detected from the ashen gray appearance. The skin is cold and clammy. The pupils are dilated. The blood pressure may be decreased with a significant increase in the pulse pressure. Since prostration develops before exposure is prolonged, body temperature is subnormal or normal. The duration of exposure and the extent of sweat loss determine the degree of hemoconcentration. Treatment comprises supporting measures and removal to a cool area. Intravenous administration of saline solution or whole blood usually is not necessary. Although the pathogenesis of prostration is not primarily a depletion of water and salt, there are theoretical and practical reasons for maintaining an optimal concentration of these essential body constituents in persons exposed to high temperatures.

Heat Pyrexia. Heat hyperpyrexia, heat stroke, or sunstroke is most common in the person with a preexisting acute or chronic malady. Direct exposure to the sun is not a necessary prerequisite. A high relative humidity is an important predisposing factor. Heat pyrexia may develop during any period of hot weather, but the incidence in temperate climates appears to increase with the prolongation of a heat wave. A diminution or cessation of sweating before onset of acute symptoms may be observed and is indicative of a breakdown of the heat regulatory mechanism. The exact cause of the cessation of sweating in these patients is not known. Persons mildly afflicted may reveal no premonitory symptoms. Others may complain of headache, vertigo, faintness, or abdominal distress. Delirium may develop in the severely afflicted.

Pyrexia and prostration are the significant abnormal findings on physical examination. A rectal temperature greater than 106°F is a grave prognostic sign. Internal body temperatures as high as 110°F have been observed. The skin is hot and dry, and sweating is absent. The pulse rate is increased, and respirations are rapid and weak. There may be an elevation of systolic blood pressure. The tendon reflexes may be diminished. Circulatory collapse may be observed. If the patient survives 24 or 48 hr of pyrexia, recovery may be anticipated. One attack of heat pyrexia renders a person susceptible to future attacks. Extensive parenchymal damage to various organs either from hyperpyrexia per se or petechial hemorrhages may complicate recovery. The brain, heart, kidneys, and liver have been the site of petechial hemorrhages. Cerebral ataxia may persist.

Examination of the blood and urine may show few alterations from the normal. A leukocytosis is observed, but is not of diagnostic significance. There may be a temporary retention of nitrogenous products in the blood. Albumin and casts may be present in the urine. The electrocardiogram, in addition to tachycardia and sinus arrhythmia, may show flattening and subsequent inversion of the T wave and depression of the S-T segment. The roentgenogram may show detectable decrease in the size of the cardiac silhouette. Venous pressures more than double the control level have been observed in normal persons exposed to high temperatures. The extent to which such elevations are due to increased venous return to the heart, or to early failure of this organ, or to a combination of these mechanisms has not been clearly defined. It has been suggested that the elevation of venous pressure may be responsible for the diminished sweating, but proof for this concept is lacking.

The management of heat pyrexia requires heroic emergency measures. Time is most important. The patient should be placed in a cool place with adequate circulation of fresh air and with most of the clothing removed. Since the pathogenesis is a failure of the heat regulating mechanism with cessation of sweating, external means of heat dissipation must be substituted for those temporarily absent. An ice water bath is a drastic treatment for an acutely ill person, but there is no effective substitute. Emersion in ice water does not induce shock or stimulate cutaneous vasoconstriction. An ice tub bath should be given with a minimum of delay. The patient should be watched by a nurse or physician constantly, and the rectal temperature should be taken repeatedly. The bath may be discontinued when the core temperature falls below 103°F. The treatment should be resumed if there is a recrudescence. Ice water sponge baths, rubbing with ice, wet sheets, and electric fan are ineffective substitutes for an iced bath. Narcotics and stimulants such as adrenalin are contraindicated. Intravenous saline solution may be recommended if the patient is not in cardiac failure and if the prepyrexic clinical state does not contraindicate it. Following the bath the patient should be placed in a room that is cool and well ventilated. Massage of the skin, if effectively executed, aids in the acceleration of heat loss and stimulates return of the cool peripheral blood to the overheated brain and viscera. Several days of convalescence may be required after such an insult.

REFERENCES

Adolph, E. F.: "Physiology of Man in the Desert," New York, Interscience Publishers, Inc., 1947.

Daily, W., and T. R. Harrison: A Study of the Mechanism and Treatment of Experimental Heat Pyrexia, Am. J. Med. Sci., 215:42, 1948.

Essential Problems in Climatic Physiology, A Tribute to Professor Yaskuno, Edited by H. Yoshimura, K. Ogata, and S. Itoh, Kyoto, Nankodo, 1960.

Gold, Joseph: Heat Pyrexia, J.A.M.A., 173:1175, 1960.

Hoagland, R. J., and R. H. Bishop, Jr.: A Physiologic Treatment of Heat Stroke, Am. J. Med. Sci., 241: 415, 1961.

Schwartz, I. L., and S. Itoh: Fatigue of the Sweat Glands in Heat Stroke, J. Clin. Invest., 35:733, 1956.

Talbott, J. H.: Ill Effects of Heat, in "Modern Medical Therapy in General Practice," D. P. Barr (Ed.), Baltimore, The Williams & Wilkins Company, 1940.

105 HYPOTHERMIA AND COLD INJURY

Ralph W. Brauer and
Albert R. Behnke

HYPOTHERMIA

The development of methods for inducing and maintaining deep hypothermia in man with relative impunity call for the separate consideration of three aspects of the effect of cold on the mammalian organism: the destructive effects of severe lowering of temperature in relatively small portions of the body (this includes the problems of frostbite and of immersion foot), the effect of more widespread and generally more limited lowering of tissue temperatures (this is one aspect of the physiology of surgical hypothermia, and includes the important problem of the time dependence of the emergence of physiologic injury as well as the question of critical temperatures), and the effects of exposure to cold under conditions where temperature defense is still effective or at least where some temperature defense is still attempted by the body (this area might be thought of as including the discussion of cold acclimatization, as well as the analysis of the endocrine responses to local or to generalized cold exposure).

Lessons from Extreme Hypothermia Experiments. In its most extreme form the ability of the mammalian organism to survive deep hypothermia has been explored by two groups of investigators (Giaja, Andjus, and their associates in Yugoslavia, and A. Smith, Parks, and their associates in England). These workers have shown that in rodents a high percentage of animals can recover after their body temperature has been lowered to such an extent that a considerable fraction of the body water (as much as 30 per cent in the hamster) is converted to ice. From a practical point of view, particular interest attaches to two observations made in the course of this work: (1) the apparent importance of inducing hypothermia under conditions leading to marked hypercapnia—a conclusion supported by more recent work concerning surgical hypothermia—and (2) the observation that frostbite did not develop in the extremities of these animals unless they were subjected to manipulation or to mild trauma while in a state of cryorigidity. A third point, which may become of real importance in human medicine as technical improvements allow ever longer periods of sustained hypothermia for surgical and conceivably eventually for therapeutic purposes, is the observation of gastric lesions in test animals recovered after prolonged periods of maintenance at very low body temperatures. These lesions are attributed to changes in cell permeability which abolish the normal defense of cells lining the gastric mucosa against an extremely acid environment. Changes of this general type may well underlie the observation that, in general, survival rates decrease and morbidity of the survivors increase rather sharply as periods of deep hypothermia are extended.

Meryman has outlined the two avenues of approach to freezing biologic materials without injury, viz., (1) slow freezing with extracellular crystal formation and a resultant high concentration of electrolytes attending the extraction dehydration, and (2) rapid freezing, forming intracellular crystals sufficiently small so as to be benign. In slowly frozen blood, it appears to be dehydration and electrolyte concentration, and not ice crystal formation, which produce hemolysis (Lovelock). Minimizing these results by the addition of glycerol to the tissues prior to freezing has had wide application in the preservation of transplantable tissues in "organ banks."

Surgical Employment of Hypothermia. The employment of hypothermia in present-day surgery is based upon the observation that even rather extended periods of ischemia can be tolerated by such key organs as the brain or the liver provided the tissue temperature has been lowered sufficiently prior to interruption of the blood supply. This not only greatly enhances the margin of safety in operations such as certain procedures upon the heart and the great vessels where it might prove difficult to maintain an adequate general circulation, but also can be applied regionally to facilitate or even to permit procedures requiring temporary local ischemia. In the past, the overriding problem in the way of the application of this concept was posed by the dangers of ventricular fibrillation and of severe circulatory decompensation during the rather drastic measures necessary to cool and to rewarm the patient. Hypothermia can be induced with light anesthesia and surface cooling, by means of air, water, or blankets through which brine is circulated at freezing temperatures. French physiologists (Laborit, Huguenard), on the assumption that the above-outlined procedure is traumatic, attempted to provide pharmacologic means to induce hypothermia more smoothly through the administration of multicomponent solutions containing either chlorpromazine or certain hydrogenated ergot alkaloids. A review of 1,100 cases in which chlorpromazine was used as an adjunct to premedication is given by Lear, Chiron, and Pallin. Since then, however, the perfection of pump-oxygenators with suitable heat exchangers has reduced the danger of cardiac accidents to the point where one eminent authority refers to ventricular fibrillation in the course of extracorporeal induction of hypothermia as "a cosmetic defect of the electrocardiogram." At the same time, the availability of an extracorporeal source of cooled, oxygenated isologous blood at arterial pressures has encouraged the use of regional cooling in which general tissue temperatures elsewhere are reduced only moderately if at all. At the present stage of development, the principal medical problem attendant upon these procedures as a result of the induction of hypothermia alone consists in the danger of the distortion of the patient's acid-base balance, either deliberately to minimize the chance of ventricular fibrillation, or inadvertently as a result of altered blood gas equilibria. With further technical improvement in methodology the possibility should be envisioned of a medical use of more protracted periods of induced hypothermia in such conditions, for instance, as the treatment of severe burns. Whenever this becomes feasible, one must expect the appearance of a whole new family of medical complications of prolonged deep hypothermia, complications presaged at the moment merely by such observations as the gastric lesions in hamsters which have survived after extended periods of extreme hypothermia.

COLD INJURY AND COLD TOLERANCE

Physiologic Considerations and Tolerance Limits. *Vasoconstriction and Dilatation.* The effects of cold are inextricably bound up with vasoconstriction and vasodilatation. Unchecked or exaggerated, they are associated either with tissue anoxia or with fulminating vascular reactions destructive of tissue.

The immersion of fingers in ice water will demonstrate the relationship between vasoconstriction and pain and the periodic relief afforded by the local oscillatory vasodilatation and constriction, the "hunting" phenomenon of Sir Thomas Lewis. Blood flow in the extremities after reaching minimal values between 15 and 18°C (59 to 64.4°F) is greatly augmented apparently through arteriovenous shunts at temperatures between 0 and 8°C (32 to 46.4°F). In this temperature range arterialized blood can be withdrawn from the veins of the hand previously immersed in ice water. Blood flow in the chilled appendage can be greatly modified by warming or cooling the body as a whole (Spealman).

Blood and Metabolic Changes. Lung ventilation rate, arterial pressure, and pulse rate parallel oxygen consumption, with a rise during the "euphysiologic" state and a fall when compensation is broken, as in immersion hypothermia.

Blood volume changes, increased viscosity of blood, hemoconcentration, diuresis (apparently under posterior pituitary control), and increased hormonal activity are factors influencing the course of cold injury. Cold stimulation of the thyroid and adrenal glands may represent the acute response of unacclimatized animals or individuals, very similar to the stimulation induced in unacclimatized individuals subjected to altitude hypoxia (Chap. 106).

Limits of Tolerance to Cold. The opportunity to study participants during swimming trials (1955) in the English Channel by Pugh and Edholm and others focuses attention upon the remarkable ability of the trained athlete to maintain a normal deep body temperature for periods of 15 hr or more under conditions in which water and skin temperatures (about 15°C, 59°F) are some 38°F lower than deep body temperature. Such factual data lend support to the useful concept of a "body core" insulated by a "body shell." With vasoconstriction operative in cold water, a virtual cutoff of peripheral circulation serves to maintain deep body temperature by minimizing loss of heat and to effect what amounts to an autotransfusion. There is great individual variability in heat loss when the body is immersed in cold water. A relatively obese swimmer, for example, maintained a normal rectal temperature for 2 hr without shivering when he was immersed up to his neck in water with a temperature of 16°C. A lean man under the same conditions, despite violent shivering, experienced a fall in rectal temperature of several degrees and had to be assisted from the water tank because of partial incapacitation from rigor. In water colder than 10°C (50°F) man cannot produce sufficient heat to maintain thermal balance for long periods, and cooling proceeds rapidly toward temperature levels that cause serious functional impairment.

A skin temperature of the fingers of about 10°C (50°F) is the lower limit for the maintenance of a reasonable degree of manual dexterity in unacclimatized persons. However, Eskimos have been known to perform some remarkable manipulative feats with their bare hands at specific tasks in subzero weather.

In hypersensitive persons, exposure to ordinary degrees of cold may produce immediate or general reactions, such as asthma, hives, vascular spasm, vomiting, neuralgia, convulsions, and syncope, the latter apparently by a histamine-like effect on capillaries, with pooling of blood in the periphery.

The striking effects of actual exposure to cold air over a 4-day period were demonstrated by the response of three subjects at Lankenau Hospital, Philadelphia, exposed to a temperature of 46°F (8°C) and clad only in shorts with some protection of the feet by wool socks, tennis shoes, and a single blanket covering at night (Rodahl, et al.). The diet was restricted to 1500 Cal, with protein reduced to about 3 Gm. Under these conditions, shivering continued intermittently during the 24-hr period, metabolism was greatly elevated, and rapid physical deterioration took place. Resting pulse rate was elevated about 30 beats, and exercise pulse rate which was 110 to 120 normally was increased about 40 to 50 beats per minute. There were unusually high losses of urinary nitrogen which persisted in two individuals for several days after return to normal diet and environment. There was also increased excretion of catechol amines. By contrast, on the same restricted diet for 5 days at room temperature the subjects felt well and their physical performance was normal. The urinary nitrogen output in contrast with cold exposure showed a compensatory decrease of 50 per cent in response to the greatly reduced nitrogen intake.

The distressing sequel to the tests was an immersion-foot syndrome consisting of swelling of the feet, pain, and paresthesia. The development of this injury was insidious since there were no symptoms referable to the feet during the test period (cold anesthesia). Toe temperatures, however, were decreased to levels only a few degrees above ambient temperature, and the nail beds showed varying degrees of cyanosis. Termination of exposure to cold precipitated the severe foot discomfort, and the attendant swelling and tenderness of the metatarsal foot pads limited walking. The sensory disturbances which were disproportionately severe compared with physical signs of injury, gradually subsided over a period of 2 months. These tests demonstrate that cold exposure to air temperatures well above the freezing point can induce an insidious type of anoxic injury to the feet.

Rewarming. With respect to rewarming following hypothermia, Burton and Edholm conclude that the proper procedure is to restore normal body temperature either slowly or by rapid rewarming (water bath 45°C). There is no middle course. In acute immersion experiments there is no question about the beneficial effects of rapid rewarming in water 45°C (113°F) during the initial recovery period to circumvent the further drop in deep body temperature (DBT) caused by cold peripheral blood lowering the temperature of the body core. When the peripheral tissues are warm, however, the individual should be removed from the bath, even though deep body temperature is below normal, in order to forestall circulatory collapse from vasodilatation and excessive diversion of cardiac output to the periphery. Following long periods of immersion, the overall applicability of rapid rewarming is not conclusive, because of the probability of depletion of liver and cardiac muscle glycogen and of large fluid shifts resulting in a greatly decreased blood volume. In therapeutic hypothermia (Talbott), when low rectal temperatures of 25 to 27°C were maintained for as long as 48 hr, rewarming was carried out at room temperature.

Cold Acclimatization. The nice distinction has been made by Hart between acclimatization-changes in responses of an organism produced by continued alterations in the environment, acclimatization-alterations related to changes in a lifetime, and adaptation-changes occurring during several generations. Cold acclimatization represents a state of increased resistance to cold injury and is the result of exposure to a cold but tolerable environment. Thus broadly conceived, cold acclimatization may involve any or all of three types of adaptive responses: circulatory adjustments protecting the temperatures of exposed or of especially essential portions of the body; metabolic adaptation, resulting in greater heat production to compensate for increased heat losses; and behavioral and neural adaptations which either minimize the actual cold stress sustained in a given environment or minimize the discomfort resulting from physiologically still tolerable levels of local or of general hypothermia. There is a suggestion in the as yet rather incomplete data that a loose division of species can be made along the lines of the above three categories of cold adaptive mechanisms: in small mammals and possibly in some species of birds, metabolic responses predominate in the establishment of cold acclimatization; in larger mammalian species, possibly but not definitely including man, circulatory changes, including in particular changes resulting in the defense of body core temperatures and in the defense of dangerously undercooled tissues, are present and important in cold acclimatization; and finally in man, cold acclimatization appears to be based largely on neural and behavioral changes. Metabolic cold acclimatization of the rat was recently reviewed in detail, throwing into focus in particular the importance of nonshivering thermogenesis to successful cold adaptation in small rodents. Whether this phenomenon occurs to any extent in larger species is, however, questionable at the present time.

Although some primitive peoples live at zero or even subzero temperatures wearing little or no clothing, it has not been possible to provide conclusive data on human beings at these temperatures (though it has for lower animals) which clearly distinguish between the acclimatized, and even the adapted individual, compared with the unacclimatized person. The role of increased body insulation in cold acclimatization in man has been documented solely in connection with professional athletes preparing for long-distance swimming. Altered vascular responses to cold were at one time assumed on the basis of changes in skin temperature or in the response to hand or finger immersion into cold baths observed in men in the course of some sort of work or training regime entailing a certain amount of exposure to a cold environment. Subsequent work by and large has failed to support for man such assumption of specific cold adaptive changes of a vasomotor type. In part the results obtained are now interpreted as due to improvement of physical condition in the course of the "cold exposure" period. In part the changes observed are quite real but represent a change in the perceptual response to a given stress rather than a change in the conditions existing in the tissue. This is clearly evident for instance in the finger immersion test where local conditioning failed to produce any change whatever in the pattern of vascular response, but where pain perception was far less, and required far longer immersion in the case of the conditioned than in the case of the nonconditioned hand of the same subject.

In the same vein one should interpret perhaps the lessening of shivering and the concomitant lessening of extra oxygen consumption observed during test cold exposure in subjects after military training in the arctic, compared to their preconditioning responses. In this series of studies the interesting point was made that virtually the same changes could be observed without change in occupation by comparing the same subject during summer and toward the end of winter. Moreover, the winter comfort zone as defined by the American Association of Heating and Ventilating Engineers shows a decrease of some 5°F in winter temperatures compared with the summer level. Healthy individuals following infancy are remarkably tolerant to acute exposures in cold air or water in the benign range of temperature, and living in relatively cold rooms (60 to 65°F) has been consistent with good health and not attended by the respiratory difficulties associated with an indoor air environment of 80 to 85°F during the winter season. Finally, comparison of temperature patterns and shivering incidence during sleep has indicated two distinct patterns of cold adaptation: one, displayed by cold-acclimatized young Norwegian subjects, involves maintenance of relatively high skin temperatures at the expense of frequent and intense shivering throughout the night, coupled with the development of the ability to enjoy seemingly restful sleep even while shivering intensely. The second pattern, displayed in its extreme form by Australian aborigines, entails a marked temperature loss extending deeply into the body, with minimal shivering. For restoration, the subjects in this case apparently depend upon heat absorption from the environment in the morning. Thus the balance of evidence available at the present time would seem to lend support to the view of those who tend to discount the importance of specific cold adaptation in man, and to attribute such changes as are observed to an altered response to the perception of cold, or to general physical conditioning incidental to the cold exposure. In this respect, then, the response of man to a cold environment would appear to differ fundamentally from that to a warm environment: in the latter case heat acclimatization has been shown definitely to be associated with adaptive changes in the physiology of man.

Immersion Hypothermia. It is convenient to divide responses to cold water immersion into three stages: (1) stimulatory—deep body temperature, normal to 35°C (95°F); (2) depressant—deep body temperature, 35 to 30°C; (3) critical—deep body temperature, 30 to 25°C (86 to 77°F). Apparently, 30 to 25°C may be a critical zone rather than an absolute limit, since it is possible to cool small animals to 0°C (Andjus and Smith).

Cardiovascular Responses. With respect to cardiovascular responses of individuals immersed up to the neck in cold water (5 to 15°C), the initial vasoconstriction is followed by a slight rise of rectal temperature and a transient rise in blood pressure and heart rate. The heart rate then decreases in response to the action of low temperature on the pacemaker. In contrast with the bradycardia associated with the inhalation of oxygen at normal or at high pressures, bradycardia due to low temperature is not abolished by atropine or vagotomy. Bradycardia is a striking response to hypothermia.

At rectal temperatures of 30°C (86°F), arrhythmias may appear, and atrial fibrillation is common. When the deep body temperature reaches a level of about 25°C (77°F), there occurs in the dog a precipitous fall in blood pressure, and death supervenes at about 22°C from ventricular fibrillation. Of interest are experiments on dogs in which Lian and subsequently Riberi and Shumacker blocked the sinoatrial area with procaine and thereby lessened myocardial irritability and the occurrence of ventricular fibrillation. It is the depression of metabolism that renders hypothermia of value in surgery.

Blood flow and oxygen consumption may be reduced to about 25 per cent of the normal resting level (heart rate, 15 to 20 beats per minute) in the deep body temperature range of 25 to 30°C (77 to 86°F). In dogs, Rosomoff and Duncan found that cerebral blood flow decreased in proportion to the temperature fall; from 35 to 25°C (deep body temperature) there was a two-thirds reduction of blood flow to the brain.

Local Cold Injury. If the injurious responses to cold are divided into freezing (frostbite) and nonfreezing (immersion foot) types of injury, then Meryman's diagram (Fig. 105-1) outlines differences and similarities in both types of injury. The two types of injury may be observed in the same extremity or in different extremities in the same individual, e.g., trench foot, or freezing in the hands and nonfreezing in the feet of shipwreck survivors. Moreover, it is important to recognize the differences in clinical appearance, signs, and symptoms, underlying pathologic derangements, and sequelae of the two entities, which may require divergent courses of therapy. The diagnosis of freezing versus nonfreezing injury can be made generally on the basis of history and clinical signs and symptoms in the two conditions. For classical descriptions of the nonfreezing type of injury or immersion foot syndrome, reference is made to the excellent papers of White and of Ungley.

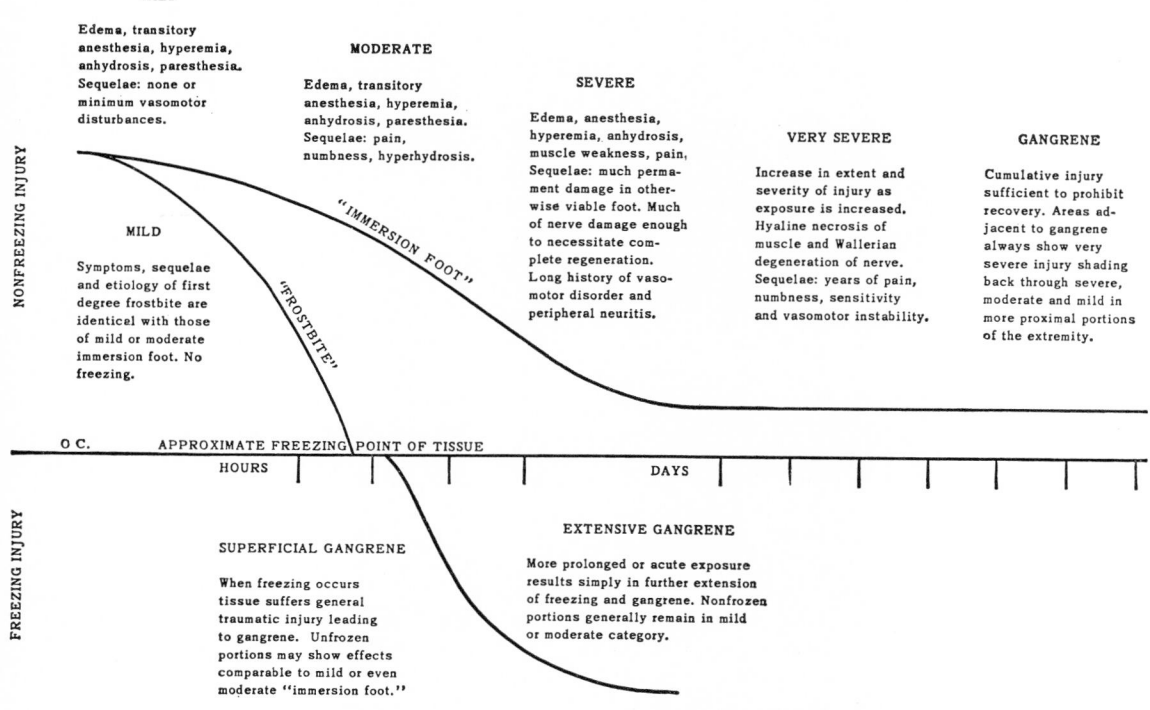

Fig. 105-1. Time-temperature relationship in clinical cold injury.

Immersion Foot. In this entity, observed in shipwreck survivors, or in soldiers (trench foot) whose feet have been wet but not freezing cold for prolonged periods, there is primarily injury to nerve and muscle tissue, with essentially no gross or irreparable pathologic changes in blood vessels and skin. The clinical picture is in harmony with the results to be anticipated from primary hypoxic trauma and lends itself to a description of three clearly recognizable states: (1) ischemia, denoted by a pale, pulseless extremity; (2) hyperemia, denoted by a bounding, pulsatile circulation, for example, in red, swollen, painful feet; and (3) a posthyperemic recovery period. The initial cold-induced vasoconstriction, increased blood viscosity, and impaired oxygen transport in the ischemic state are augmented by such factors as undernutrition, general hypothermia, dehydration, and trauma from relatively fixed, pendent extremities. The problem of rewarming pertains to these patients during the stage of ischemia, when overheating of tissue may lead to gangrene. In the stage of hyperemia, the red, swollen feet require judicious cooling, as indicated by White and by Ungley.

It may be helpful to consider this type of injury as a peripheral neuropathy following chilling, i.e., as giving rise to manifestations of the Raynaud syndrome, essentially free (to be sure, in the state of hyperemia) from the vascular restriction and occlusion seen in Buerger's disease. In its mildest form, it can be induced in the feet, for example, in whole-body immersion experiments of only 1-hr duration when the bath temperature is about 8°C (46.4°F). Under these conditions, intense vasoconstriction renders the toes exceedingly painful, and it is highly probable that the subsequent paresthesia of the feet, described as "burning sensation," which may persist for several years without functional impairment, is the result of the ischemia, induced during exposure by vasospasm.

Frostbite. In true frostbite in contrast with immersion foot, blood vessels may be severely or irreparably injured, the circulation of blood ceases, and the vascular beds of the frozen tissue are occluded by agglutinated cell aggregates and thrombi. The cutaneous injury consists in part of a separation of the epidermal-dermal interface. From his experiments, Kreyberg makes the distinction between direct injury to cells caused by cold, which may not be irreparable(if rapid rewarming serves to shorten the duration of the exposure to cold), and the subsequent fulminating vascular reaction and stasis which precede tissue necrosis. In the therapy of frostbite, medical and surgical measures to relieve vasospasm and restore circulation are of prime importance. Rapid rewarming may be the method of choice, with due concern for the initial elevation of deep body temperature. It would appear to serve no useful purpose to heat a cold extremity if the vascular bed cannot accommodate an adequate blood supply. In small animals whose extremities have been rapidly cooled to extremely low temperatures within a matter of minutes, rapid rewarming is the method of choice when ice crystals are present in tissues. It has not been proved convincingly to be so in soldiers whose feet have been exposed to wet cold over a period of days at freezing and nonfreezing temperatures.

With respect to therapy, Korean experience interdicted smoking, made bed rest mandatory, prescribed antibiotics, vitamins, and nicotinic acid (100 mg t.i.d.). An intravenous frostbite solution, consisting of 12 ml ethyl alcohol, 250 mg procaine hydrochloride, and 5 per cent glucose in water to make 250 ml, was given every 6 hr. To this solution, 100 mg heparin was added in the absence of bleeding injury. Of the vasodilator drugs, hexamethonium was the most effective.

One might conclude pessimistically that, except for terminating the cold exposure promptly and providing good supportive care and later medical and surgical treatment, little of value can be done in treating cold injury. Yet, it is necessary to recognize the type and underlying derangements of the cold injury one is confronted with; to be aware of the fact that cold injuries produce a galaxy of ever-changing physiologic and pathologic states which render routine therapy inadequate; and to be acquainted with the benefit and promise of spasmolytic agents and procedures and of judicious ambient temperature regulation. In addition, there emerge three important admonitions:

1. Avoid trauma to the cold extremity, including tight dressings, manipulation, and massage.

2. Leave blisters intact.

3. Observe absolute conservatism in any surgical procedure calling for amputation.

Sequelae of Frostbite Injury. Of the 5,600 cold injury casualties evacuated from Korea during the winter 1950–1951, it was possible for Blair, Schatzke, and Orr to report on a follow-up of 100 patients 4 years following injury. Although 90 per cent were gainfully employed, about 50 per cent were in some measure handicapped. Signs and symptoms associated with mild to fourth degree injury were cold feet (in winter), pain, numbness, excessive sweating, abnormal color, and impairment of joint mobility. The physical findings in patients who had a diagnosis initially of third and fourth degree injury were scars, tissue loss, and abnormal nails. With the exception of hyperhydrosis, the chronic injury may be similar to that produced by ionizing radiation (Chap. 108). Specific roentgenologic changes in bone were cystlike defects near the joint surfaces in the fingers and toes.

It should be emphasized that, although the

physical findings were negligible following first and second degree injury, the pain, sweating of extremities, and paresthesias were as intense as in the severely injured patients. The symptoms in these cases may be looked upon as real, not "psychocompensatory," but it would require refined functional tests to elicit abnormalities in these individuals.

Prevention of Cold Injury. The painstaking indoctrination and training of personnel and the excellent equipment now available should minimize future cold injury in American military units. Emphasis is to be placed, however, on the elimination of individuals susceptible to cold injury, and especially on the "hardening" and disciplined training possible only in cold environments. Although adaptation requires perhaps a period of several generations to confer on inhabitants of Patagonia the ability to exist with little protection in subzero weather, nevertheless, the degree of acclimatization possible over a period of months through proper training and graded exposure to cold should render resistant individuals who would otherwise become casualties. The nature of cold disability makes prevention mandatory. There is no specific treatment as yet for the mass disorganization and even disintegration of the biologic economy brought about by cold.

REFERENCES

Arctic Institute of North America: "Arctic Bibliography," Department of Defense, Washington, D.C., 1953.

Brauer, R. W.: The Liver in Hypothermia, Ann. N.Y. Acad. Sci., 80:395, 1959.

Burton, A. C., and O. G. Edholm: "Man in a Cold Environment," London, Edward Arnold & Co., 1955.

Dripps, R. D. (Ed.): "NRC Conference on the Physiology of Induced Hypothermia," October, 1955. (See papers by A. Riberi and H. B. Shumaker, H. L. Rosomoff, and D. A. Holaday, and by N. W. Shumway and F. J. Levis.)

Kreyberg, L.: Development of Acute Tissue Damage Due to Cold, Physiol. Revs., 29:156, 1949.

Laborit, H.: Resistance et soumission en physio-biologie, "L'Hibernation artificielle," Paris, Masson et Cie, 1954.

Lewis, F. J.: Repair of Atrial Septal Defects during Hypothermia, Post-graduate Med., 17:293, 1955.

"Macy Foundation Conferences on Cold Injury," Trans. I to V, Irene Ferrer (Ed.), and Trans. VI, S. Horvath (Ed.), New York, Josiah Macy, Jr., Foundation, 1951–1960.

Meryman, H. T.: The Freezing and Thawing of Whole Blood, Naval Med. Research Inst. Rept., 13:953, 1955.

——: The Mechanism of Local Cold Injury, 11:741, 1953.

Newburgh, L. (Ed.): "Physiology of Heat Regulation and the Science of Clothing," Philadelphia, W. B. Saunders Company, 1949.

Pugh, L. G. C., and O. G. Edholm: The Physiology of Channel Swimmers, Lancet, p. 761, Oct. 8, 1955.

Scholander, P. T., H. T. Hammel, J. S. Hart, and H. Le Mesurier: Cold Adaptation in Australian Aborigines, J. Appl. Physiol., 13:211, 1958; and 14:605, 1958.

Smith, A. U.: Viability of Supercooled and Frozen Mammals, Ann. N.Y. Acad. Sci., 80:29, 1959.

Smith, R. E., and D. J. Hoijer (Eds.): International Symposium on Cold Acclimation, Federation Proc., 19: Suppl. 5, 1960.

Ungley, C. C.: The Immersion Foot Syndrome, Advances in Surgery, 1:209, 1949.

Winslow, C. E. A., and L. P. Herrington: "Temperature and Human Life," Princeton, N.J., Princeton University Press, 1949.

Yaglou, C. P.: Abnormal Air Conditions in Industries: Their Effects on Workers and Methods of Control, J. Ind. Hyg. Toxicol., 19:12, 1937.

106 DISORDERS DUE TO ALTERATIONS IN BAROMETRIC PRESSURE

Albert R. Behnke

Several million individuals in the United States are continually subjected to unusual barometric pressures in sport diving, commercial and military diving, compressed air operations in tunnel construction, and aircraft. Severe and fatal injuries are not infrequent in sport diving if the participants are physically unfit, poorly trained, ill-equipped, and lack supervision and facilities for coping with accidents. Complicating the problem is the obsession to establish records pertaining to diving depth and to breath holding. Accidents arise chiefly from too rapid decompression and indirectly from high partial pressures of nitrogen, oxygen, and carbon dioxide and from anoxia. The skin and scuba (self-contained underwater breathing apparatus) diver is always in danger of drowning in case of mishap. Uncompensated pressure forces per se may cause traumatic air embolism, pneumothorax, emphysema, as well as painful but usually innocuous trauma to the eyes (face mask "squeeze"), middle ear, paranasal sinuses, gas containing viscera, and even diseased teeth. A few principles underlying the etiology, prevention, and management of disorders due to alterations in barometric pressure will be outlined and appropriate references given to definitive and detailed text.

PRIMARY PRESSURE PHENOMENA

Effect of Pressure Differences (Barotrauma). Normally some tissues of the body are subjected to compressive or distending pressure (the arteries, vertebras, and lower extremities) of the order of 100 to 200 mm Hg [1 to 2 lb per sq in. (psi)]. Pressure gradients may also exist in tissues when an individual is immersed in water up to his neck. By contrast, the pressure of the atmosphere at sea level (760 mm Hg, 14.7 psi, equivalent to 33 ft of sea water) can be increased to nearly 20 atm in diving operations or reduced to about 0.1 atm (53,500 ft) in the low pressure chamber without injury. In contrast to this uniform and innocuous application of great external pressure forces is the small difference in pressure of 50 mm Hg or less which serves to distend blood vessels and induce edema and hemorrhage in occluded sinal (aero-sinusitis) and aural (aero-otitis media) spaces. The mastoid air cells are involved in this type of aseptic trauma. The familiar "cupping" action, for example, is the result of a small difference in pressure due to absorption or utilization of oxygen from air trapped in an unaerated space. The most frequent cause of obstruction, which is usually partial, is acute and chronic infection in the nasopharynx. At any time in a group of apparently healthy men subjected to increased pressure, there will be an incidence of about 10 per cent of "ear block" and of sinal difficulty of 1.5 per cent. Even dental pain (aero-odontalgia) may be localized in teeth which are diseased or contain faulty fillings. The involvement of specific teeth, in the lower jaw, for example, in contrast to diffuse radiating pain emanating from maxillary sinusitis, suggests the presence of trapped gas which even in small quantities permits a "squeeze" of soft, sensitive pulp tissue during alteration of barometric pressure.

There is no specific therapy required for this type of barotrauma. Healing is spontaneous even following sinal hemorrhage and rupture of tympanic membranes. Hearing, temporarily impaired, returns to the preinjury level of acuity. There is absence or rarity of proved cases of deafness in contrast to permanent nerve deafness resulting from gunfire explosion.

Topical applications of astringent solutions and oral administration of ephedrine may aid professional personnel and others to accommodate rapidly to increased pressures in case of emergency.

Overdistention of the Lungs. If a diver breathing compressed air holds his breath during ascent to the surface, the intrapulmonic pressure becomes relatively higher than the hydrostatic pressure. A difference in pressure in excess of about 80 mm Hg may overdistend the lungs so that gas is forced or aspirated into the blood stream (traumatic air embolism). Gas emboli transported to the left ventricle are disseminated to the central nervous system to produce the most serious injury in diving. Fatal accidents have occurred during ascents from only 15 ft to the surface. On the other hand, free ascents (i.e., without breathing apparatus) have been made from a depth of 300 ft with due care taken to "vent" the lungs during ascent. Air embolism may also result from involuntary intrapulmonary trapping of air in the presence of a broncholith acting to produce a ball-valve mechanism (Liebow et al.).

Another type of pulmonary injury is the "squeeze" brought about when hydrostatic pressure exceeds intrapulmonic pressure during the descent of skin divers (i.e., without breathing apparatus) to depths greater than 100 ft (4 atm). The limiting factor is the reduction by the hydrostatic pressure of the thoracic volume to residual air volume.

Pneumothorax, mediastinal and subcutaneous emphysema are also sequelae of uncompensated pressure. Blebs and cysts on the lung surface predispose to this type of injury. Even straining incident to the Valsalva maneuver to clear ear block may provide sufficient force to rupture blebs or permit intrapulmonary gases to dissect pleural coverings along the large vessels and bronchi.

SECONDARY PRESSURE PHENOMENA ASSOCIATED WITH INCREASED GAS PRESSURES

Narcotic Action of Nitrogen. When the air pressure is raised to 4 atm or higher, the gaseous nitrogen induces a narcotic action manifest by a decreased ability to work and changes in mood, frequently a euphoria. A slowing up of mental activity and fixation of ideas are reported. Recollection requires greater effort, and concentration is difficult. Frequent errors may be made in arithmetical calculation and in recording of data. Motor performance is impaired. The responses are, in fact, similar to those associated with alcoholic intoxication. Although all individuals are to some extent narcotized at deep diving depths, stable persons react to the impairment by increased effort and carry out their tasks until consciousness is lost. The unstable individual, on the other hand, is rendered incapable of purposeful effort. The substitution of helium which has a lower oil-water solubility ratio than nitrogen diminishes the narcotic effect associated with high air pressures to about one-third. On helium-oxygen mixtures, diving depths of 600 ft have been attained, and the probable limit is perhaps about 1,000 ft. At this depth the narcotic action of the helium mixture should be equivalent to the inhalation of air at a depth of 300 ft.

A striking parallelism exists between the relative effects of nitrogen and helium in diving and the ability of these gases to protect mice against electroconvulsive seizures, as shown by Carpenter. The relative effect of these gases on bean roots exposed to ionizing radiation in the presence of oxygen (Ebert and Hornsey) is also of the same magnitude as their narcotic potency. The basic work of Carpenter and of Ebert and Hornsey is briefly outlined in "Medical Physics," vol. 3 (Behnke).

Oxygen Poisoning. The inhalation of oxygen at increased pressures following a latent period of variable duration may cause muscular twitching, nausea, narrowing of the fields of vision, impaired psychomotor performance, irritability, auditory hallucinations, and convulsive seizures similar to those observed in idiopathic epilepsy. Exercise and increased concentrations of carbon dioxide shorten the latent period and lower the oxygen tensions required to induce symptoms. In view of the fact that in scuba diving loss of consciousness may result in drowning, there is prevalent an ultraconservative attitude toward the use of oxygen in closed circuit breathing apparatus. Thus a U.S. Navy table incorporates the following exposure times for the inhalation of oxygen by scuba divers employing closed circuit apparatus: 45 min at a depth of 30 ft and 10 min at a depth of 40 ft. On the other hand, Lambertsen reported 5,000 man-hours of oxygen breathing in closed underwater circuits during the Second World War in which only five reactions indicative of oxygen poisoning occurred according to the following schedule: 120 min at 33 ft, 60 min at 60 ft, and 30 min at 66 ft. In experiments conducted by the author mainly in the dry chamber, healthy men in good physical condition have inhaled oxygen at simulated depths of 100 ft for 30 min and at 66 ft for several hours.

In the dry chamber, oxygen administered to moribund divers and caisson workers may be lifesaving. When toxic effects supervene, oxygen can be withdrawn. Recovery from initial toxic manifestations and even from convulsive seizures, if not induced too often, appears to be complete. Electroencephalographic recordings serve to monitor the advisability of administration of oxygen to susceptible individuals.

In the presence of elevated concentrations of carbon dioxide during the inhalation of oxygen at pressures of 1 atm and higher, consciousness may be suddenly lost (oxygen blackout). The response to the CO_2 enriched atmosphere is altered in the presence of oxygen. Dyspnea, for example, may not supervene as a warning of elevated CO_2.

Effect of Carbon Dioxide. Carbon dioxide enhances the toxicity of oxygen and the narcotic effect of nitrogen. In the diver's helmet the percentage of carbon dioxide must be reduced to a minimum.

During rapid descent in deep-sea diving, momentary vertigo and confusion are in part attributable to the accumulation of alveolar carbon dioxide as the air pressure rapidly rises in the lungs. The *effective* carbon dioxide percentage should not exceed 1.5 per cent, although percentages of carbon dioxide up to 5 are fairly well tolerated at normal barometric pressures for periods of at least 60 hr.

Uptake of Nitrogen at Increased Pressure. At atmospheric pressure (P_{N_2}, 570 mm Hg) about 9 ml of nitrogen is dissolved in 1 kg of body water and about 55 ml in 1 kg of body fat. In a lean, 70-kg man (7 kg of fat) about 400 ml of nitrogen is in body fluids, 100 ml in bone and spinal cord, and 400 ml in adipose tissue. About 5.2 liters of blood per minute perfuses the nonlipid cellular mass with its high water content, and only about 0.7 liter circulates through bone and adipose tissue. The half-time saturation of various nonlipid organs and tissues varies from 2 to 20 min (98.5 per cent saturation in 12 to 120 min), and for organs containing large amounts of lipid (long bones, spinal cord, adipose tissue) 60 to 120 min (98.5 per cent saturation in 6 to 12 hr). Duration of stay in diving and tunnel operations is such that nitrogen uptake is restricted mainly to nonlipid, rapidly saturating tissues, especially at higher pressures.

Decompression Procedures. After prolonged exposure (24 hr) at an equivalent diving depth of 33 ft (2 atm absolute), it is safe to decompress to 1 atm within a period of 2 min. Shorter exposures followed by rapid, continuous ascent are possible at deeper depths, e.g., 25 min (100 ft), 10 min (150 ft). This remarkable ability of the body to contain high pressures of nitrogen at least for short periods of time is probably responsible for the common error of decompressing divers and caisson workers too rapidly during the initial phase of decompression.

From 1 to 2 per cent or more of all decompressions are followed by symptoms of decompression sickness, and it is probable that all exposures in compressed air, following rapid decompression in the initial period, induce nascent bubble formation in the blood stream. Fortunately the pulmonary vascular bed can accommodate large quantities of gas transported in the veins, and there may be no symptoms initially from these "silent" bubbles.

The decompression procedure for divers follows a prolonged stage method that allows for increased time at each stop to the surface. By contrast, for caisson workers the decompression proceeds at a uniform rate following an initial rapid drop. This relatively shorter and uniform type of decompression may be conducive to the development of chronic bone lesions. The departures from current practice indicated are slower ascent in the early stage of decompression. For caisson workers it is proposed that they reside in the compressed air atmosphere for periods of 1 to 2 weeks followed by a slow decompression to the normal atmosphere over a period of 12 hr.

Factors Affecting Nitrogen Bubble Formation. After exposure to high pressure or high altitudes (in chambers and aircraft), the factors conducive to bubble formation fall into two groups. In the first are conditions which increase gas content of tissues, namely, the amount of fat, the degree and duration of exposure to pressure, the amount of work performed, and in rapid ascent to high altitudes, exercise which (among other effects) serves to introduce more carbon dioxide into the circulation. In the second group are variables affecting tissue perfusion and transport of gas from tissues. Thus age, time of day, temperature, fright, injury, and the postalcoholic state all affect "effective blood flow" through tissue.

Acclimatization. A sharp decline in disability during the initial weeks of tunnel operations is due in part to the elimination of susceptible individuals and to muscular training (Paton and Walder). A true acclimatization with a sharp decline in bends incidence has been reported for a specific group of workers exposed to a constant tunnel pressure for a period of weeks (Golding et al.). It is possible that embolic occlusion of blood vessels may stimulate the opening of new collateral channels. Acclimatization has not been observed in divers or during exposures in the altitude chamber.

SIGNS AND SYMPTOMS OF DECOMPRESSION SICKNESS

Acute injury may be designated as pain (bends), asphyxia (chokes), and paralysis. Minor effects are pruritus, rash, and fatigue. The parts of the body involved are the extremities (bends), cardiorespiratory system (chokes), and the spinal cord. Chronic lesions affect the spinal cord and the long bones.

Bends. The most common manifestation is a dull, throbbing type of pain, gradual in onset, progressive and shifting in character, and frequently felt in the joints, or deeply in muscles and bones. Pain of this nature constitutes a long-recognized clinical entity designated as "bends." The response to recompression therapy is rapid. There is no residual disability, although the chronic lesions of bone probably represent areas initially giving rise to bends.

Chokes and the Shock Syndrome. A serious manifestation of decompression sickness is a type of asphyxia designated by early caisson workers as "chokes." In comparison with bends, chokes occurs less frequently since it apparently requires the accumulation of rather large quantities of gas emanating from tissues and present in bubble form in the large veins, the right side of the heart, and

pulmonary vessels. Thus, several hours of complete well-being following decompression may elapse before the appearance of symptoms. The earliest symptom is a sensation of substernal distress elicited by deep inspiration and especially by the inhalation of tobacco smoke, which is frequently followed by paroxysmal coughing (Behnke).

Central Nervous System. Unless traumatic air embolism is present, there is a remarkable lack of cerebral involvement even under conditions of widespread embolism. Vertigo, deafness, aphasia, and transient visual disturbances have been reported. Convulsive seizures, loss of consciousness, and manifestations of focal cerebral involvement characterize traumatic air embolism associated with pulmonary overdistention. The most serious complication of decompression sickness is paralysis of spinal cord origin manifest as a spastic monoplegia or paraplegia usually confined to the lower extremities. Areas of hypersensitivity are present above the site of the lesion, and paresthesia or sensory paralysis is present below. There is incontinence of urine and feces in the transection type of lesion. Recovery may occur following prolonged decompression even following an interval of 2 hr between onset of symptoms and initiation of recompression treatment (Richter and Behnke). Prognosis as to ultimate recovery or partial recovery is difficult since improvement may occur over a period of 2 years following injury.

Bone Lesions. Bone infarction arising from disseminated emboli or bubbles forming *in situ* has become a major industrial compensation problem chiefly because roentgen visualization reveals islands of dense calcification in the shafts of long bones and frequently perichondral "snowcaps." In contrast to spinal cord involvement, the chronic osseous lesions, owing in part to their insidious and painless nature (unless there is joint involvement), are identified as sequelae of decompression sickness mainly on the basis of occupational history.

The roentgen manifestations of caisson disease in a full-blown case are almost pathognomonic due to their sites of predilection and sequence of occurrence in the lower femoral diaphysis, the upper tibial diaphysis, and the humeral head and neck; on the multiplicity of the lesions tending strongly to symmetrical bilaterality; and on the characteristic geographic maplike appearance of the diaphyseal lesions, so that one case is almost identical with a duplicate of the others. (Poppel and Robinson.)

The chronic lesions appear to be located in areas subjectively identified as the site of origin of bends pain. The bone changes, however, may be seen in individuals who have had no history of bends. Apparently, daily repeated exposures in compressed air are required in connection with aggravating factors such as alcoholism and generalized arteriosclerosis. Bone lesions have not been observed in divers. The problem poses the same difficulties as the etiologic relationship between cirrhosis of the liver, alcoholism, and other factors.

Treatment of Traumatic Air Embolism and Decompression Sickness. The prime objective in the treatment of decompression sickness is the rapid restoration of blood supply by immediate recompression which reduces the size of the gas emboli and increases oxygen supply (especially if oxygen is administered) to areas of infarction. Adequate recompression has been followed by complete recovery even when applied to the asphyxiated patient whose blood stream is occluded with multiple gas bubbles as well as to patients with incipient paralysis. Long periods of time measured in days are required for the absorption and elimination of gas bubbles. The absence of symptoms in a patient under recompression treatment does not signify freedom from "silent" bubbles. The most frequent errors in the treatment of decompression sickness are:

1. Inadequate recompression, especially of the serious cases

2. Failure to apply the test of recompression to "doubtful" cases and to delay treatment in the hope that spontaneous recovery will take place

3. Failure to keep the "treated" patient near the recompression chamber for a 24-hr period

4. Inadequate physical examination of the patient to detect pneumothorax and disabilities not directly caused by faulty decompression

SPECIFIC PROBLEMS

Skin and Scuba Diving. The problems are chiefly administrative, not medical, and involve proper training, adequate supervision, and provision for resuscitation, oxygen therapy, and recompression. In skin and scuba diving there is no place for the record breaker. A prime requisite is that individuals be good swimmers because without special equipment man is severally handicapped in an aqueous environment. The skin diver must rely under water on breath holding. As he descends to various depths, the hydrostatic pressure diminishes the volume of the thorax and increases the partial pressure chiefly of oxygen and nitrogen. During ascent the partial pressure of gases rapidly decreases as a result of the expanding thoracic volume. Should breath holding be prolonged at deep depths (100 ft), the partial pressure of oxygen during subsequent ascent to the surface may fall to asphyxial levels.

The scuba diver breathes unnaturally through a mouthpiece which increases salivation and air swallowing. A "demand" valve interposes inspiratory

resistance. Swimming underwater requires moderate to heavy exertion. In addition, cold and the narcotic action of nitrogen at deep depths may dissipate physical reserve to combat emergencies. The danger from drowning is always imminent. Facilities are usually not available for treatment of decompression sickness. Safety measures include the restriction of depth to 60 ft, except for men with special qualifications, and limitation of exposure underwater to periods of time that do not require decompression.

Caisson Work. The decompression of tunnel workers is much too rapid to prevent disability. Prolongation of the daily decompression does not appear to be feasible. However, the difficulty could be obviated as mentioned previously by prolonged residence in compressed air so that decompression is given at weekly or bimonthly intervals. In this way it should be possible to provide a 12- to 24-hr period of slow decrement in pressure. During the prolonged stay in compressed air, it should be possible to eliminate alcoholism and maintain the workers in prime physical condition.

Concluding Notes. In the physical examination of candidates for diving and caisson work, specific tests are required to ascertain vital capacity, maximal breathing capability, pulse response to short periods of exhaustive exercise, and examination of the lungs in the attempt to detect cysts and extensive calcification. In view of the possibility of bone lesions, it is essential to have x-ray visualization of the knee and humeral joint areas.

Following decompression, the deep inspiratory test (Behnke) should serve to indicate the presence of bubbles in the pulmonary vascular bed. Apart from frank signs of decompression sickness, the presence of rash, mottling of skin, pruritus, and an exhaustive, debilitating type of fatigue followed by prolonged sleep constitute signs and symptoms indicative of the presence of "silent" bubbles and the inadequacy of decompression.

Special care must be paid to the quality of air supplied to scuba divers; specifically carbon monoxide should not exceed 20 parts per million (about one-fifth of the allowable concentration for an 8-hr exposure in tunnels).

Lastly, facilities for recompression can be provided at reasonable cost if small chambers are employed. With strict enforcement of administrative procedures outlined, it should be possible to reduce drastically the accidents and injuries which attend sport diving and caisson operations.

DERANGEMENTS AT HIGH ALTITUDES

Physiologic Considerations. Pressure decrements expressed as a fraction of sea level barometric pressure (1 atm) may be enumerated for a number of altitudes under consideration in the following paragraphs: 5,000 ft (0.83), 10,000 ft (0.69), 15,000 ft (0.56), 18,000 ft (0.50), 25,000 ft (0.37), and 29,000 ft (0.31). These atmospheric fractions multiplied by 100 represent approximately the decrease in alveolar oxygen pressure in millimeters of mercury with altitude.

The mountain climber may acclimatize sufficiently to high altitudes during a period of 1 to 3 months so as to enable him to climb Mount Everest (29,002 ft) with supplemental oxygen and Nanga Parbat (26,660 ft) without added oxygen. These feats represent an ultimate in human acclimatization and endurance since rapid deterioration in a period of about 10 days takes place above 25,000 ft. Man cannot reside permanently above 18,000 ft. On the other hand, Andeans at 15,000 ft are well adapted for strenuous physical exertion in a hypoxic atmosphere.

Altitudes of 4,000 to 7,000 are noted for salubrious climate and undoubtedly provide the earth's most healthful atmosphere. The newcomer, however, forced to adapt to prolonged sojourn at altitudes of 10,000 ft or higher, initially experiences malaise, headache, insomnia, tachycardia, and dyspnea. These symptoms disappear as acclimatization takes place, and their disappearance is accelerated by exercise.

Hurtado and his coworkers at the Institute of Andean Biology have defined the morphologic and functional characteristics of the resident reared at high altitude, namely, (1) decreased body weight relative to stature, (2) increased vital capacity, thickening and enlargement of alveolar walls, and persistence of wall thickness in branches of the pulmonary artery, (3) increased pulmonary ventilation, (4) increased blood volume, hemoglobin, hematocrit, and myoglobin, (5) greatly increased tissue vascularization, and (6) increase in activity of tissue enzyme systems. The pulmonary-hematopoietic-circulatory adaptation apparently does not completely compensate for the decrement of 45 mm Hg in the sea level alveolar oxygen tension. There are data to support the observation that the Andean man, descended from generations of inhabitants living continuously at altitude, appears to have attained a degree of adaptation greater than the acclimatization achieved during the lifetime of the newcomer. The Andean is thus enabled to perform strenuous physical labor, e.g., cultivation of the slopes of the Andes, which is not excelled certainly at sea level. This is accomplished under conditions of normal oxygen metabolism and pH. With the exception of some degree of pulmonary hypertension, cardiovascular function is normal in terms of cardiac output, pulse rate, and peripheral blood pressure. Remarkable is the rarity in the Andean of peripheral hypertension, coronary thrombosis, and myocardial infarction. Arteriosclerosis of peripheral blood vessels is uncommon. Despite the normal condition of erythrocytosis, the type of erythremia associated with polycythemia vera is absent. The hypoxic stimulus at altitude affects strictly erythropoiesis. Generalized myeloid hyperplasia has not been reported.

Chronic Mountain Sickness (Seroche, Monge's Disease). The Andean, however, is affected by a clinical condition which represents a breakdown in compensation and adaptation to low oxygen tension. Loss of tolerance to the altitude environment as pointed out by Monge in 1928 may be observed in the striking accentuation of the erythrocytosis normally present. Hurtado has reported in detail derangements associated with this pathologic condition. In comparison with values (N) characteristic of the healthy native resident at altitude, there are increases of hemoglobin, 25 Gm per 100 ml (N 21 Gm per 100 ml), and in blood hematocrit, 80 per cent (N 60 per cent). The blood volume is increased 50 per cent, chiefly as a result of erythrocytosis. Plasma volume, however, is decreased. There are hyperplasia and hyperactivity of bone marrow erythroid cells, increased red cell destruction, but no derangements of the leukocyte series. The greatly impaired ability to work is associated with cyanosis, hypoventilation, lowered alveolar P_{O_2} and P_{CO_2}, increased cardiac output, a greater pulmonary hypertension and lower systolic blood pressure than are found in the healthy resident. Electrocardiographic findings are consistent with a diagnosis of cor pulmonale. With respect to etiology the mechanisms underlying the loss of sensitivity of the respiratory center and the accentuated hematopoietic response are obscure.

The signs and symptoms of Monge's disease have much in common with Ayerza's syndrome, or cardiaco negro (erythrocytosis, hyperplasia of bone marrow, cyanosis, dyspnea, and notably pulmonary arterial and arteriolar sclerosis). This entity appears to have a multiple etiology. Of interest is the fact that the same type of pulmonary injury with hypertension (pulmonary) is found in rats exposed for a month or longer in compressed air (4 atm).

Individuals who have a moderate degree of pulmonary hypertension associated with hypervolemia and hypoxia may gain relief when transported to sea level. Upon return to altitude, however, such patients may develop pulmonary edema.

Concluding Note. The studies of man and lower animals at altitude present many challenging problems. The remarkable physical performance of the Andean on a diet largely of vegetable protein and carbohydrate, the relative absence of peripheral cardiovascular disease despite work stress and the high viscosity and density of blood, and the dense vascularization of tissue have no precedent in a

European population at sea level. The cost of adaptation is measured in part by a high infant mortality. In horses and cattle introduced into the high altitude regions, it requires several generations of breeding to produce virile stock. Some of these problems are receiving intensive study which will serve to reveal the basic nature of the adaptations particularly in the biochemical reactions in tissue.

REFERENCES

HIGH PRESSURES

Reviews and Basic Investigations

Behnke, A. R.: Decompression Sickness, vol. 2, p. 257, in "Medical Physics," Otto Glasser (Ed.), Chicago, Year Book Publishers, 1950. (See also vol. 3, 1960, pp. 20 and 222).

Fulton, F. J. F.: "Decompression Sickness" (compilation of the National Research Council), Philadelphia, W. B. Saunders Company, 1951.

Hoff, E. C., and L. J. Greenbaum: "A Biographical Sourcebook of Compressed Air, Diving, and Submarine Medicine," vol. 11, Office of Naval Research and Bureau of Medicine and Surgery, November, 1954.

Jones, H. B.: Nitrogen Elimination, vol. 2, p. 855 in "Medical Physics," Otto Glasser (Ed.), Chicago, Year Book Publishers, 1950.

Central Nervous System

Haymaker, W., and A. D. Johnston: Pathology of Decompression Sickness: A Comparison of the Lesions in Airmen with Those in Caisson Workers and Divers, Military Med., 117:285, 1955.

Richter, R. W., and A. R. Behnke: Spinal Cord Injury Following a Scuba Dive to a Depth of 350 Feet, U.S. Armed Forces Med. J., 10:1227, 1959.

Bone Lesions

Meesters, J. N.: "Caissonziekte," Haarlem, Holland, De Erven F. Bohn N. V., 1958.

Poppel, M. H., and W. T. Robinson: The Roentgen Manifestations of Caisson Disease, Am. J. Roentgenol., 76:74, 1958.

Skin, Scuba, Deep Sea Diving

Current List of Diving Publications. Superintendent of Public Documents, Government Printing Office, Washington, D.C.

Duffner, G. J.: Medical Problems Involved in Underwater Compression and Decompression, Clinical Symposia (Ciba), 10:100 (July–August), 1958.

—— and E. H. Lanphier: "Science and Medicine of Exercise and Sports," p. 348, W. R. Johnson (Ed.), New York, Harper & Brothers, 1960.

Liebow, A. A., J. E. Stark, J. Vogel, and K. E. Schaefer: Intrapulmonary Air Trapping in Submarine Escape Training Casualties, U.S. Armed Forces Med. J., 10:265, 1959.

Skin and Scuba Diving Hazards and Medical Problems, Spectrum (Pfizer) 8:(July) 1960.

Caisson Operations

Golding, F. C., P. Griffiths, H. V. Hempleman, W. D. M. Paton, and D. N. Walder: Decompression Sickness during the Construction of the Dartford Tunnel, Brit. J. Indust. Med., 17:167, 1960.

Paton, W. D. M., and D. N. Walder: Compressed Air Illness, Med. Research Council Special Report Series No. 281, London, Her Majesty's Stationery Office, 1954.

DERANGEMENTS AT HIGH ALTITUDE

Carter, E. T.: Altitude: Pathologic Effects, vol. 3, p. 15 in "Medical Physics," Otto Glasser (Ed.), Chicago, Year Book Publishers, 1960.

Hurtado, A.: Pathological Aspects of Life at High Altitudes, Military Med., 117:273, 1955.

107 PROBLEMS OF AIR TRAVEL

Stuart Bondurant

The medical problems of aviation are caused by the unusual environmental conditions.

Altitude. An increase in altitude is equivalent to a decrease in barometric pressure, with a consequent reduction in the partial pressure of oxygen and an increase in the volume of gas trapped within the body (Table 107-1). The normal person, acclimatized to sea level, tolerates oxygen tension equivalent to altitudes of 10,000 to 12,000 ft with little change in arterial oxygen saturation. At altitudes above 12,000 ft, hypoxia becomes more marked and supplementary oxygen is usually used. While breathing 100 per cent oxygen, full oxygen saturation is maintained to altitudes of 30,000 to

Table 107-1. REPRESENTATIVE VALUES OF ARTERIAL OXYGEN AND RELATIVE VOLUME OF GAS AT VARIOUS ALTITUDES

Altitude, ft	Pressure, mm Hg	Arterial blood		Relative volume of gas
		Oxygen tension	Saturation	
0	760	94	98	1.0
5,000	632	66	92	1.2
8,000	564	60	89	1.25
10,000	523	53	86	1.5
14,000	446	44	79	1.7
18,000	379	36	71	2.0
37,500 up 100% O_2	159	74	94	4.8
44,000 up 100% O_2	116	36	72	6.5

35,000 ft. Many modern aircraft fly at altitudes of 20,000 to 40,000 ft, with cabins pressurized to maintain a maximum effective cabin altitude of 8,000 ft (jets) or 10,000 ft (reciprocating engines). An ascent of 5,000 ft or more may be followed by a period of lethargy, sleepiness, and headache. These symptoms subside within 24 hr.

A second consequence of decreased barometric pressure is expansion of gas trapped in body cavities. In the normal person, intestinal gas is passed as it expands and middle ear and sinus air escapes without difficulty during ascent. Gas which cannot escape (pneumothorax and pneumoperitoneum) may cause injury or death.

Acceleration. Acceleration is the instantaneous rate of change of velocity. The unit of acceleration, g, is the acceleration due to gravity of a body which is falling freely in vacuo. It represents a change in velocity of 32.2 ft per sec each second. Most of the physiologic consequences of acceleration are due to the force (inertia) which is equal in magnitude but opposite in direction to that causing the acceleration. Thus, headward acceleration causes footward displacement of soft tissues and blood. Duration, magnitude, direction, and rate of onset of acceleration determine the physiologic effects. In general, the longer and greater the acceleration, the less well it is tolerated. Prolonged forward or backward acceleration is tolerated better (approximately 14 to 20g, limited by apnea) than headward acceleration (4 to 7g, limited by blackout and cerebral ischemia), and footward acceleration (3 to 5g, limited by asystole, conjunctival and mucous membrane bleeding) is tolerated least well. Brief headward accelerations of 25g and backward accelerations of 40g are tolerated by normal subjects when well positioned and supported. In ordinary flight, linear accelerations greater than 1g are not encountered. Turbulent flight may cause brief linear accelerations of 10 to 12g which are great enough to cause fractures in persons who are not restrained. Angular accelerations of turns and the linear-angular accelerations of turbulent flight are of importance in causing motion sickness.

Miscellaneous. Some fuels and lubricants and their combustion products are toxic and may, with equipment failure, be concentrated in closed cabins. Reciprocating engines produce large quantities of carbon monoxide. Jet engines use fuels which are vesicants, with fumes that cause nausea, vomiting, and headache. Pyrolysis of lubricating oils produces fumes which cause conjunctival irritation.

Flight line personnel manifest hearing loss after prolonged exposure to jet noise unless protected by position or by mechanical devices. Noise levels inside aircraft are very low, and those in terminals and around airfields are apparently insufficient to cause hearing loss.

Little excess ionizing radiation is encountered in ordinary flight.

Aircrew Selection. Physical requirements for aircrews are described in appropriate governmental and airlines literature. Absence of circulatory, pulmonary, neurologic, visual, and auditory defects is of particular importance.

Air Transportation of Patients. Since it is now possible to fly without experiencing any physiologically significant departure from the usual environmental conditions, there are no absolute medical contraindications to moving patients by air. However, there are many instances in which patients should not be moved at all and others in which adequate aircraft with pressurized cabin and attending personnel may not be available. Commercial airlines will carry many patients subject to the discretion of the airline medical director. In addition to the condition of the patient, the comfort and convenience of other passengers must be a major factor in the decision of the commercial airlines. The following points apply to air transportation in general. Specific advice concerning commercial air transportation should be obtained from the appropriate airline medical director.

Circulatory Disease. The lower partial pressure of oxygen which may be encountered constitutes the major deterrent to flight for patients with circulatory diseases. There is no evidence that ordinary flying is associated with an increased incidence of angina, myocardial infarction, or cerebral vascular accidents. It is probably preferable to forego flying for 6 weeks after a myocardial infarction or a cerebral vascular accident. Coronary artery disease manifest by occasional angina or old myocardial infarction, minimal cerebral or peripheral vascular disease, hypertension, and compensated congenital or rheumatic heart disease appear to entail no added risk in flying. Patients with angina related to emotional stress may benefit from preflight sedation.

Patients with severe or frequent angina, severe hypertension, recent vascular accidents, or with cardiac decompensation at rest or with moderate exercise should fly only when a pressurized aircraft or supplementary oxygen is available to maintain ambient oxygen tension at levels of 150 mm Hg (sea level equivalent) or more.

Pulmonary Disease. It would seem wise to restrict flying during acute episodes in asthmatics who do not respond well to self-administered treatment. The likelihood of rupture of an emphysematous bleb does not appear to be increased by ordinary flight. Because of the increase in volume of bullae at altitude (Table 107-1), patients with marked bullous emphysema are not advised to fly above 6,000 ft. Generally, persons with pulmonary decompensation with only moderate (two flights of stairs) or severe exercise fly without difficulty to altitudes of 10,000 ft. Persons with pulmonary decompensation at rest or with mild exercise should fly only if ambient oxygen tension is maintained at levels of 150 mm Hg or more and facilities and personnel are available to treat acute decompensation. Pneumothorax constitutes a contraindication to flight in aircraft whose cabin pressure is not maintained at ground level equivalent. Expansion of the trapped gas causes, in effect, a tension pneumothorax. Several patients with therapeutic pneumothorax have died in flight.

Hematologic Disease. In the absence of cardiopulmonary disease, patients with hemoglobin of 7 to 9 Gm 100 ml usually tolerate flights at 4,000 to 6,000 ft without difficulty. If greater cabin altitudes are to be encountered, hemoglobin should be above 10 Gm per 100 ml.

Hypoxia causes increased sickling of erythrocytes containing hemoglobin S. There have been many well-documented reports of splenic infarction in patients with hemoglobin S during flights which usually exceeded 10,000 ft and lasted for several hours. Moreover, two patients with SC hemoglobin have had splenic infarctions during flights which did not exceed 6,000 ft. If ambient oxygen tension cannot be maintained at 150 mm Hg, flying is contraindicated for patients with SS (sickle-cell anemia) and SC hemoglobin and for those with SA (sickle-cell trait) who have large quantities of hemoglobin S. Others with hemoglobin S should be restricted to cabin altitudes below 10,000 ft. The occurrence of symptoms of splenic infarction (nausea, vomiting, left upper quadrant pain, shock) in flight is an indication for immediate return to ground level.

Pregnancy. A large experience has accumulated which suggests that ordinary flying has no adverse effects on the normal pregnant woman or fetus. Pregnant women should sit in rearward facing seats when possible and place the seat belt over the upper thighs and hips rather than around the abdomen. When pregnancy is complicated by preeclampsia, cardiopulmonary or hematologic disease, considerations similar to those discussed above for the nonpregnant patient apply.

Ear, Nose, and Throat Disease. Acute upper respiratory infections and chronic sinusitis may obstruct the eustachian tube or sinus ducts with barotitis or barosinusitis resulting when external pressure is increased during descent. If flight is necessary, use of a nasal spray (½ per cent Neo-synephrine) 6, 3, and ½ hr before flight and ½ hr before descent may help to maintain patency of the ducts.

A swallow or a Valsalva maneuver with the nose occluded will usually open the ducts. Children may be fed during descent to encourage swallowing. The treatment of barotrauma depends upon the severity and underlying cause. Intubation of the eustachian tubes is not advised. In most instances, conservative treatment with decongestants will suffice. Severe barotitis may be associated with hemorrhage into the middle ear requiring myringotomy and aspiration of blood to prevent ossicular ankylosis. Plastic repair of the ducts may be required to prevent recurrence.

Metabolic Disease. Control of the diabetic patient may be complicated by rapid movement from one time zone to another and by motion sickness. Careful planning of the flight in terms of elapsed rather than local time with consideration of the meals to be served and appropriate management of motion sickness should enable the well-controlled diabetic individual to fly without difficulty. Patients in diabetic acidosis may be transported after treatment is started if in-flight medical facilities are adequate.

Communicable Disease. Persons known to have a communicable disease may not enter a state or nation without the consent of the local health department.

Postoperative. Because of the expansion of abdominal gas with decrease in barometric pressure, it is generally considered preferable to forego flying for 10 days after abdominal or other major surgery. However, experience with air evacuation of military casualties suggests that, with proper facilities and personnel, practically all patients whose condition is stable can be moved by air if necessary. Most persons with fractures are flown without difficulty. Fracture of the mandible, particularly when immobilized, constitutes a special problem because of the possibility of vomiting and aspiration. A quick release wire support has been designed for in-flight use.

Epilepsy. Most patients with well-controlled epilepsy fly to altitudes of 10,000 ft without difficulty. Flight to greater altitude in unpressurized aircraft may precipitate seizures.

Motion Sickness. Modern aircraft have considerably reduced the incidence of motion sickness by minimizing turbulent flight and vibration. The problem remains because of occasional turbulent flights and persons who are extremely susceptible to motion sickness. Cyclizine (Marezine) 50 mg, meclizine (Bonine) 25 mg, and Dramamine 50 mg are effective prophylactic agents.

Aircraft Accidents. While there is evidence that rearward facing seats can minimize trauma and increase accident survival, it seems unlikely that such seating will be generally adopted by commercial airlines. Since aircraft occasionally encounter extreme turbulence without warning, passengers are well advised to fly with seat belt fastened.

REFERENCES

Armstrong, H. B.: "Aerospace Medicine," Baltimore, The Williams & Wilkins Company, 1960.

Gauer, O. H., and G. W. Zuidema: "Gravitational Stress in Aerospace Medicine," Boston, Little, Brown & Company, 1961.

McFarland, R. A.: "Human Factors in Air Transportation," New York, McGraw-Hill Book Company, Inc., New York, 1953.

Smith, E. W., and L. C. Conley: Sicklemia and Infarction of the Spleen during Aerial Flight, Bull. Johns Hopkins Hosp., 96:35, 1955.

108 RADIATION INJURY
Eugene P. Cronkite

TYPES OF RADIATION, INTERACTIONS WITH TISSUE, DOSE UNITS, DEFINITIONS

The types of radiation most likely to be concerned with injury are x-rays, gamma rays, alpha and beta rays, protons and neutrons. X-rays and gamma rays are identical, and a separate name was given to them only because of their difference in origin. The former are produced by x-ray machines and the latter by radioactive decay. In general, gamma rays are more energetic than x-rays. Beta rays are electrons. Ordinary electrons originate from the shells surrounding the atomic nucleus, and beta rays originate only from within the nucleus. Alpha rays are the stripped nuclei of the helium atom, with a mass of 4 and a charge of 2+. Protons are stripped nuclei of hydrogen atoms, with a mass of 1 and a charge of 1+. Protons are of interest since neutrons produce protons in tissue. Neutrons have a mass of 1 and a charge of 0. Biologic injury is produced primarily by ionization from secondary charged particles. Neutrons produce the secondary charged particles in diverse ways. Fast neutrons react principally with the hydrogen atoms, and as a result of the collision a portion of the energy is imparted to the hydrogen atom and a proton is ejected which does the damage. With thermal or slow neutrons the damage is done by actual capture of the neutrons and a secondary emission of ionizing radiation as the transmuted hydrogen, nitrogen, or other substance in tissue decays and emits radioactivity. These are the basic types of radiation with which a physician may be concerned.

Historically there are many theories about the mechanism of action of ionizing radiation on living tissues. All these concepts are discussed in the classic volume by Lea. In particular, the concepts of direct hits on the target molecules versus the indirect action mediated through products of reaction with the protoplasmic solvent water are analyzed lucidly. Today the most prevalent and acceptable view to account for a major part of the biologic effects of radiation may be divided into three interlinked steps. First, photons or particles penetrate the protoplasm, interacting to produce ion pairs. This reaction takes in the order of 10^{-13} sec. The second step is a primary radiochemical reaction of these ions primarily with water, producing "hot" radicals such as H and OH. These reactions take about 10^{-9} sec. These radicals produce a further chain of reactions with themselves and O_2 to produce H_2O_2. These products persist for microseconds or in part a few seconds. The last reaction is between these products and critical protoplasmic molecules. The nature of this last reaction is not known, but it sets into motion a series of observable histologic or chemical lesions that unfold with time. In addition to the effects observable within days, "bad invisible information" may be stored in the proliferative or nonproliferative cells presumably in deoxyribonucleic acid (DNA) that will not be manifested as a disease process for years.

In pharmacology, standardization of drugs has become scientific only when the structure is known and when one can measure the drug in an appropriate unit such as a milligram. With ionizing radiation, one is concerned not with the mass of the agent administered but with the *amount* of energy that has been absorbed by tissue at the *point of interest* (tumor, tissue essential for life, gonads, etc.).

Two dose units are essential for the understanding of the quantitative effects of radiation. The *roentgen* (r) is a measure of total dose in air and may be defined as the quantity of x-ray or gamma ray radiation such that the associated corpuscular emission per 0.001293 Gm of air at standard conditions produces in air ions carrying 1 electrostatic unit of either sign. For energy to be deposited there must be an interaction with matter. Hence, with x-rays passing through a vacuum no radiation dose would be delivered. We are interested in the energy imparted to tissue. This leads to the second unit, the *rad*, a unit of absorbed dose, which is equal to 100 ergs per Gm of tissue at the site of interest. The rad applies to all types of external or internal sources of radiation. For small pieces of tissue in an x-ray beam of 1 r per min, the absorbed dose will be very close to 1 rad per min. However, as irradiated objects become larger, one has to consider the diminution in intensity due to increasing distance (inverse square) and interaction of radiation with matter (build up and then exponential attenuation). This leads to a decreasing absorbed dose at successive levels after equilibrium is attained. Thus in addition to the exposure dose in roentgens and absorbed dose in rads, one must be concerned with the *distribution of the absorbed dose*. For example, if there is sufficient protection of bone marrow by shielding of one's own tissues to permit marrow regeneration and survival from what is considered an otherwise fatal *exposure dose*, one may ascribe incorrectly some great benefit to a procedure used therapeutically. Unfortunately, failure to consider the critical influence of the distribution of *absorbed dose* at the site of interest on the outcome of radiation injury has resulted in ascribing therapeutic benefit to various agents of no value at all.

The density of ionizations in tissue varies with the energy and type of radiation. The density of ionization is referred to as specific ionization (ions per unit track length) or as linear energy transfer (LET, kiloelectron volts deposited per unit track length). Amongst other things, the density of ionization influences the biologic effect for equivalent amounts of energy deposited, in general the effect being greater with more densely ionizing radiations. This leads to an important consideration, the relative biologic effectiveness (RBE), which may be defined as the ratio of a dose in rads of standard radiation, usually x-rays or gamma rays, to produce a given degree of biologic effect, to the dose in rads of an unknown radiation, to produce the same degree of biologic effect. For example, if the LD-50 dose of x-rays is 600 rads and for neutrons 300 rads, the RBE will be 2. The relative biologic effectiveness may vary with the biologic response. For example, when the same radiations are used, a different value may be obtained for mortality, cataract or tumor development, etc.

Also of importance is the dose rate. In a general sense the slower the dose rate, the less the effect for acute somatic effects. In a very crude sense, dose rates in excess of 5 r per min give essentially the same result. However, as the dose rate falls off below 5 r per min, there is a lesser effect per unit of radiation. In the past, genetic effects were believed independent of dose rate. This implies that all increments of radiation irrespective of when or how received by the gonads would add up directly as mutations to give a total effect ultimately to be measured as detectable effects in succeeding generations. However, it is now known that there is a dose rate dependence in respect to the production of mutations by irradiation of spermatogonia in mice and also for leukemogenesis in mice.

If the dose of radiation is sufficiently high, actual death of any living cell can be observed promptly in terms of classical pathologic criteria of cell necrosis. However, after lower doses of radiation (precise values vary with the tissue), disturbances in cell proliferation are seen. The rate at which cells divide is decreased. Deoxyribonucleic acid synthesis is impaired in two manners. First, the rate of synthesis is slower, and second, cells may continue DNA synthesis and become polyploid. It is reasonably certain that there are effects of radiation other than the outright killing of cells, the interference with mitosis, and DNA synthesis. However, other effects are not well defined. The Russians emphasize effects upon the nervous system and interference with various central functions. These are not yet generally accepted by western radiobiologists.

The diminution in the production of new cells in those tissues which are undergoing continual renewal (mucosa, blood, and gonads, etc.) results in a progressive hypoplasia to total atrophy, depending upon the dose. Some cells still capable of mitosis that were not killed outright may be so injured that they will go through one or two generative cycles, producing abnormal progeny such as giant metamyelocytes and hypersegmented neutrophils before dying. The atrophy of these "steady-state" cell renewal systems and direct injury of other tissues produce clearly defined clinical syndromes.

CLINICAL PHENOMENA AFTER EXPOSURE

Human experience is based on the effects of atomic bombs; accidental exposure to fallout from a hydrogen bomb; laboratory and reactor accidents in the United States, USSR, and Yugoslavia; and on "whole body" clinical radiotherapy. After any radiation accident, close cooperation of the physician and medical physicist is essential to obtain the best estimate of the radiation dose and to evaluate its probable effect in terms of the likely distribution of the *absorbed dose in rads*. However, clinical signs and symptoms remain paramount in the management of human disease and injury. Physical estimates of dose can never substitute for clinical judgment and experience.

For practical purposes, three acute radiation syndromes can be classified generally as *cerebral*, *gastrointestinal*, and *hematopoietic*.

The *cerebral syndrome* is produced by extremely high doses of radiation, i.e., in the vicinity of several thousand roentgens. It is always fatal, whether the radiation is delivered to the brain alone or to the whole body. Three processes have been described: a prodromal phase of nausea and vomiting; then listlessness and drowsiness ranging from apathy to prostration (probably traceable to nonbacterial inflammatory foci in the brain); and finally a more generalized component characterized by tremors, convulsions and ataxia, and death. This syndrome was observed in an industrial accident, death occurring 36 hr after exposure.

The *gastrointestinal syndrome* occurs when the dose of radiation is smaller. It is characterized by intractable nausea, vomiting, and diarrhea; these lead to severe dehydration, diminished plasma volume, vascular collapse, and death. The syndrome is initiated by a severe "intoxication" arising from necrosis of tissues diffusely throughout the body; it is extended by severe injury to the gastrointestinal tract. The latter development is caused by two factors: direct killing of a fraction of the crypt cells and inhibition of mitosis. The mature epithelial cells continue to migrate out in an orderly fashion, eventually being lost from the tip of the villi; this produces a progressive diminution in the number of cells covering the villi. Ultimately the intestinal villi are denuded, with massive loss of plasma into the intestine. If regeneration is possible after doses of radiation, massive plasma replacement during the first 4 to 6 days may keep animals alive so that sufficient time will be allowed for the gastrointestinal epithelium to regenerate. However, even if adequate plasma fluid and electrolyte replacement prolongs life over the critical period, respite is only temporary since hematopoietic failure will ensue, commencing within 2 to 3 weeks.

The *hematopoietic syndrome,* with anorexia, apathy, nausea, and vomiting, may be maximal for man within 6 to 12 hr after exposure to lower doses of radiation at the level of perhaps 600 to 800 r. These symptoms have been correlated with a period of rapid necrosis of radiosensitive tissues. Symptoms subside so that within 24 to 36 hr after exposure the subject is asymptomatic. The prodromes must be distinguished from the gastrointestinal syndrome described earlier and from that which occurs later on. After subsidence of the prodromes, a period of relative well-being arrives, during which atrophy of lymph nodes, spleen, and bone marrow progresses, leading to a pancytopenia. This atrophy is again the result of two clearly defined processes—direct killing of radiosensitive cells and inhibition of new cell production. In the peripheral blood lymphopenia commences immediately, becoming maximal within 24 to 36 hr. Thereafter the lymphocytes may remain essentially at the same level for months. Within a few hours after irradiation, a neutrophilic leukocytosis appears. Following this an oscillation in the neutrophil count occurs, the rate at which it falls to the minimum being a function of the dose of radiation. After sublethal and low lethal doses the minimal neutrophil values occur in 4 to 6 weeks, whereas after high lethal doses the granulocytes

diminish more rapidly and minimal values approaching zero appear within 7 to 10 days.

Thrombocytopenia and its relation to radiation bleeding have been studied extensively. After single doses of radiation a close correlation with the decrease in the platelet count and the tendency to bleed is evident. In animals and in human beings after various accidents, significant purpura was seen only when the platelet counts fell below 20,-000 per cu mm. The platelets remain steady or increase for 2 to 3 days after irradiation and thereafter diminish more or less linearly with time, the ultimate minimum and the rate it is attained being dose dependent. After about 200 rad whole body irradiation, it takes about 30 days for minimum platelet levels to develop. After 600 to 800 rad, minimal levels were observed within 10 to 12 days. Earlier observations in which bleeding in radiation injury was attributed primarily to hyperheparinemia have been refuted. There has been no evidence for hyperheparinemia and no indication for the use of antiheparin agents in the therapy of bleeding induced by radiation. Fresh viable platelet transfusions will stop bleeding, and maintenance of platelet levels by platelet transfusions will prevent development of bleeding in animals.

Decreases in the red blood cell count are prominent only after large doses of radiation which significantly interfere with new cell production and produce bleeding.

Studies of decreased resistance to infection have resulted in the following conclusions: There is (1) a dose-dependent decrease in circulating granulocytes and lymphocytes, (2) a dose-dependent impairment of antibody production, (3) impairment of granulocyte migration and phagocytosis, (4) decreased ability of the reticuloendothelial system to kill phagocytized bacteria, (5) diminished resistance to diffusion in subcutaneous tissues, and (6) hemorrhagic areas of the skin and bowel that present foci for entrance and growth of bacteria. Obviously an increased susceptibility to infection by both commensals and pathogens must be present.

The preceding syndromes may be produced when the whole body is uniformly exposed to radiation or if there is substantial inhomogeneous exposure of the whole body. An expression of the lethal dose range for man is desirable to assist in the management of casualties. In the case of inhomogeneous exposure one can see how misleading any single air or exposure dose may be. There is a hierarchy of effects that vary with time, dose, and organs involved. Ten thousand rad to the brain will be fatal, whereas 10,000 rad to a hand may only necessitate amputation. Since the bone marrow is somewhat more sensitive than other tissues, in large part ultimate survival is determined by the dose to this tissue. For uniform whole body exposure *without therapy* it has been estimated that the lethal dose curve will commence at about 200 rad and that survivals will be rare after doses in excess of 800 rad. Between these limits the per cent mortality dose curve is sigmoid. Even if the dose to an individual were known with precision, the individual prognosis must remain on a probability basis because one can never predict whether an individual belongs on the sensitive or resistant portion of the curve.

MANAGEMENT OF ACUTE RADIATION INJURY

Presumptive evidence of exposure to radiation and signs or symptoms described earlier must be recognized before there need be cause for concern. No therapy is available for the cerebral form. Whereas a small percentage of persons with the gastrointestinal syndrome may be kept alive until the affected tract regenerates, they must also face the hematopoietic syndrome; hence that is the real therapeutic problem. Therapy rests on the control of the sequelae of marrow aplasia and thus is similar to management of drug-induced and idiopathic marrow aplasia, suggesting that combined use of antibacterials and transfusions would be useful. The spontaneous course of radiation injury in man has clearly shown that the signs and symptoms develop at different times in different subjects after identical doses of radiation. Accordingly, the time of institution and type of therapy should be individualized. The following general therapeutic regimen is outlined.

1. Treat infection when it develops or recurs, using various antibiotics sequentially in doses two to three times the usual size. Use sulfonamides when antibiotics are exhausted. One is fighting for additional time to permit spontaneous regeneration.

2. Use fresh whole blood to control bleeding and to restore red cells. Fresh blood is defined as that which has been taken from the donor not more than 1 hr previously into plastic bags with Na_2EDTA. When the hematocrit is returned to normal range, use fresh platelet-rich plasma to control bleeding as clinically indicated and not on an inflexible schedule. Despite many claims concerning the value of lyophilized and frozen platelets, to date successful management of radiation bleeding has been obtained only by the use of fresh viable platelets that circulate in adequate numbers.

3. Watch the fluid and electrolyte balance closely and restore these as necessary with appropriate replacement solutions.

4. Maintain rigid asepsis. Bar visitors who show respiratory symptoms. In fact, it is best to use isolation technic. The preceding therapy has increased survival rate significantly in animals.

5. Unless infection or serious hemorrhage develops, therapy is not needed. Prophylactic therapy is contraindicated. Many human beings with epilation, severe pancytopenia, and purpura have recovered from doses of radiation ranging from 200 to 300 r without therapy.

Isogenic and *autologous* bone marrow transplantation will prevent death in almost all otherwise fatally irradiated animals. In fatally irradiated animals saved by homologous transplantation, the transplanted marrow will eventually produce a reaction presumably against the host, resulting in a severe late degenerative disease of the skin, kidneys, liver, and lymph nodes. A similar late fatal effect has been observed in children treated for leukemia with whole body irradiation in whom homologous marrow transplantation was successful. Although marrow transplantation has been widely acclaimed as a solution to fatal whole body radiation, the indications for attempting bone marrow transplantation are not clear. The author believes that it should be reserved for the cases where the dose is believed in excess of 600 r and in whom the signs and symptoms described before are persistent and the clinical condition continues to deteriorate during the first week. Rigid rules cannot be formulated in advance. Decisions can be made only at the bedside.

Prevention. Nothing can be substituted for prevention. Shielding from irradiation is the only really effective preventive measure in industry, medical practice, military or civil defense. A series of sulfhydryl drugs that will protect against radiation by an effective dose reduction up to 50 per cent is available. However, these must be administered within minutes preceding exposure. Accidents and warfare are not predictable. The severe toxic effects of these drugs prevent continuous administration under hazardous conditions.

Long-term Effects. Radiation alters the "information system" of proliferating somatic and germ cells. Thus the perpetuating cells of the blood, gastrointestinal tract, skin, lens, gonads, and other areas pass on either "bad or inadequate information" presumably in altered DNA to their progeny. With somatic cells this may be manifested ultimately as somatic disease, e.g., cancer, cataracts, degenerative disorders, or nonspecific shortening of life. Leukemia yield from radiation in human groups has been quantified. It is asserted but *not proved* that there is no threshold and that the yield of leukemia increases with dose. However, the greatest exposure of the American public comes from the medical uses of diverse types of radiation (predominantly diagnostic x-rays). If the assertion above is *correct,* then these medical uses of radiation are producing their small toll in an additional burden of leukemia and probably other diseases also. Therefore, it behooves the practitioner to be exceedingly cautious and to expose patients to radiation only when clearly indicated and needed diagnostically.

Radiation can produce mutations of genes, the information and transmission centers for heredity. Of this there is no doubt. Not all mutations are harmful, but the chances are overwhelming that a change will be detrimental to the species. All mutations do not produce visible immediately detectable effects. The concern is not only for an increase in the number of obvious freaks or cripples but with changes that would lead to such undesirable characteristics as lowered life expectancy, decreased fertility, a general increase in physical and mental disease, and an increase in fetal or neonatal death rates. It is the less obvious changes that are of the greatest importance. The more obvious changes usually lead to early death in the individual and reduced fertility in those who survive. Thus the harmful mutant is relatively quickly deleted from the population. The more subtle changes, however, are propagated longer and affect a very large number of persons. The mutation may be dominant or recessive. Most dominant mutations are also lethal, and many such mutations can be missed because the fertilized egg never develops far enough to be recognized as a new individual. If the mutation is completely recessive, it will be clear that for the manifestation to become apparent both parents of the individual must have the same mutation and must have transferred the affected gene to the individual concerned. It is extremely difficult to quantify these considerations. If the mutation rate were increased by a single exposure of the population to radiation, the effects would be spread through many generations. Half the total damage that would be manifested would not be observed until some 30 to 50 generations had been produced.

These are the practical considerations that make the problem particularly difficult to analyze. Damage that is inflicted now cannot be detected immediately and will become evident only many generations hence. These considerations also indicate why it is not possible to take negative evidence in populations that have been exposed to date as an indication that the degree of genetic damage is small. If there were, for instance, an obvious effect already in the children born of individuals irradiated in Japan by the atom bombs, it would be very obvious that the total genetic effect would have to be great indeed. These are sobering considerations for any thoughtful people. Although exposure to irradiation cannot be avoided in our modern industrial society or in the practice of medicine, it is mandatory that it be made minimal and rigidly controlled in order to protect future generations and the present generation due to the uncertainty about the quantitative effect in producing somatic or genetic effects.

EFFECTS OF SUN AND ULTRAVIOLET LIGHT

Injury from sunburn is probably the most widespread to which the human race is subject. Sunburn commonly does not go beyond erythema, sometimes accompanied by slight swelling of the affected skin, and is followed in the course of days or weeks by hyperpigmentation. Rarely is sunburn sufficiently severe to produce second-degree burns, although moderate first-degree burns are not infrequent. Systemic reactions are usually slight, although in more severe cases there may be fever and transient leukocytosis. Ultraviolet light may produce sunburn. The cornea is particularly sensitive to ultraviolet light, and even a brief exposure may lead to keratitis and conjunctivitis. Years of continuous exposure to insolation or ultraviolet light leads in other than very heavily pigmented skins to increased incidence of carcinoma, either epidermoid or basal cell in type.

RADIUM POISONING

It appears strange that radium water was used as a therapeutic agent not too long ago and resulted in poisoning. In addition radium watch-dial painters were poisoned during the First World War. The radium (often mesothorium) is deposited primarily on the surface of bones, and its distribution changes with the slow rebuilding of the osseous structure. Histologically one sees Haversian systems plugged with highly calcified material, gross regions of resorption, and osteocyte death as evidence by empty and highly calcified lacunas. Autoradiographs show both a "diffuse" distribution and "hot spots" of radioactivity. Pathologists consider the characteristic bony injury almost pathognomic of chronic radium poisoning. Many of the effects are due to direct radiation injury; some are secondary to vascular injury. Bone necrosis and interference with the normal processes of internal reconstruction of bone result in the formation of small and large cavities which give the characteristic radiolucency in radiographs of bone. Fibrosis of the bone is a constant feature usually limited to the endosteal surfaces of cortical and trabecular bone. The marrow may be spottily fibrotic. The disturbed structure of bone may so weaken it as to permit pathologic fractures. The long term irradiation is carcinogenic. Malignant bone tumors arise. The induction time is long—greater than 10 years, with an average of about 20 years. The types of tumors are not different from human bone tumors in general. In addition to bone tumors, carcinomas of the sinuses and nasopharynx have been seen in more greatly increased numbers than the expected rare incidence. Leukemias have been conspicuous by their almost total absence. Aplastic anemia has also been observed as a cause of death. There is no satisfactory treatment of late poisoning; prevention is the cure. Although mainly of historic interest, many elderly persons are still alive with significant body burdens of radium from therapy and from employment in the watch-dial industry.

REFERENCES

Bond, V. P., and J. S. Robertson: Vertebrate Radiobiology (Lethal Actions and Associate Effects), Ann. Rev. Nuclear Sci., 7:135, 1957.

Cronkite, E. P., and V. P. Bond: "Radiation Injury in Man," Springfield, Ill., Charles C Thomas, 1960.

——, ——, and C. L. Dunham: Some Effects of Ionizing Radiation on Human Beings: A Report of Fallout on the Marshallese, U.S. Government Printing Office, Washington, D. C.

Gerstner, H. B.: Acute Radiation Syndrome in Man, U.S. Armed Forces Med. J., 9:313, 1958.

Hine, G. J., and G. L. Brownell: "Radiation Dosimetry," New York, Academic Press, 1956.

Lea, D. E.: "Actions of Radiation on Living Cells," New York, The Macmillan Company, 1947.

Oughtersen, A. W., and S. Warren: "Medical Effects of the Atomic Bombs," New York, McGraw-Hill Book Company, Inc., 1956.

Report of the United Nations Scientific Committee on the Effects of Atomic Radiation, United Nations, N.Y., 1958.

The Effect of Radiation on Human Heredity, World Health Organization, Geneva, 1957.

Warren, S., and C. E. Dunlap: Effects of Radiation on Normal Tissues, Arch. Pathol., 34:562, 1942.

109   ELECTRICAL INJURY
Ivan L. Bennett, Jr.

The first human fatality from accidental electrocution occurred in 1879 and was produced by an alternating current of 250 v. Since that time, continuing increase in household and commercial uses of electrical power has made accidents almost inevitable. Injury and death from lightning have been occurring, of course, since time began.

Etiology and Pathogenesis. The end result of passage of an electrical current through the human body is unpredictable in the individual case. Certain generalizations are possible, however, and many of the factors that influence severity of injury by electricity are known. *Alternating currents* tend to produce tetanization of muscles and sweating (which lowers skin resistance), and *direct currents* produce electrolytic changes in the tissues. It has been estimated that alternating is about four or five times as dangerous as direct current; fatal electrocution can result from exposure to household circuits of 115 v at 60 cycles.

The electrical conductivity of tissues parallels their water content; consequently, the vascular system and musculature are good conductors, whereas bones, peripheral nerves, and skin offer high resistance. The resistance of normal skin is lowered by *moisture,* and this factor alone may convert what might ordinarily be a mild injury to fatal shock. The *grounding* of the body at the time of contact is important. It is well known that a person in water or on a wet surface is more susceptible to electrical injury. The *pathway of the current* through the body is crucial. Obviously, an accident involving passage of current between a point of contact on the leg and the ground is likely to be less injurious than one in which the poles of the circuit are the head and a foot. The *duration of contact* influences the outcome. Because, as mentioned, an electrical current can stimulate skeletal muscle to contract, a victim who has grasped an uninsulated wire may be unable to release it; this is far more likely with alternating than direct currents and accounts in part for the greater danger of alternating circuits. Sudden convulsive contraction of muscles can result in fractures of bone; sometimes, however, it throws the individual clear of contact. This can lead to additional mechanical trauma if the victim is thrown from a high place.

In traversing the skin, electrical energy of high-tension currents is converted to heat. When one considers that electric arcs with temperatures as high as 8000°C may be generated, it is not surprising that fourth or fifth degree burns often result. The term *electrical necrosis* is probably more appropriate than *burn* for this injury. It has been suggested that the immediate damage is aggravated by vasospasm in adjacent tissues.

The systemic effects of electricity are incompletely understood, but in general, low voltage produces ventricular fibrillation and death from circulatory failure, and high voltage produces respiratory arrest. High-tension currents produce cardiac standstill, but ventricular function resumes when the current stops, and death is presumably attributable to injury of medullary centers. Whether this neurologic damage is secondary to vasospasm or to increase in temperature of the brain, or whether it is the result of direct injury to neurones is not known.

A lightning flash is a rush of electrical energy (about 1 billion v and 20,000 amp) along a path more than a mile long and 18 to 20 ft in diameter. The duration of the current is about 0.001 sec. When the bolt reaches the earth, secondary flashes occur and objects within a radius of 100 ft may be struck. Direct contact usually results in immediate death. Persons nearby may be injured by the electrical current, by burning from heated air, or by the concussive force of compressed air.

If patients die immediately, autopsy findings are limited to burns and generalized petechial hemorrhage. If patients survive for a period of days or longer, postmortem examination reveals focal necroses of nerve, spinal cord, or brain, involving both neurones and white matter, with appropriate glial and vascular reactions.

Manifestations. Immediately after severe shock, patients are usually comatose and apneic, although the heart may continue to beat until anoxia leads to circulatory failure. Surviving this stage, patients are often disoriented and combative; convulsions are frequent. Blackened, charred areas at the points of entrance and exit of the current may appear to be relatively small and well localized. After a few days, however, huge sloughs, often involving major blood vessels, reveal the true extent of the destruction. A frequent finding in victims of lightning is a characteristic, lacy network of superficial "arborescent burns," or "lightning prints," on the skin. These fade within 24 to 48 hr. Late effects include various neurologic disabilities, visual disturbances, and, of course, the residual damage left by burns. A curious finding in many victims of lightning is temporary flaccid paralysis of the lower extremities with loss of sensation, so-called "keraunoparalysis," which passes off in 12 to 24 hr. This condition is often accompanied by blanching and coldness of the legs and is believed to be a result of severe vasoconstriction. Hysterical symptoms are common after exposure to lightning. Injuries to peripheral nerve, spinal cord, and brain often leave symptoms which may be confused with peripheral neuritis and multiple sclerosis. The development of cataracts is another late complication.

The wide use of electric shock in the treatment of psychiatric diseases (p. 370) has led to occasional accidents. These have been of two types. Sudden death, attributed to ventricular fibrillation, has been observed in elderly patients with heart disease. Fracture of vertebral bodies during the convulsive seizure has occurred; this is preventable by the use of relaxant drugs.

Laboratory Findings. Leukocytosis with many large, immature granulocytes in the peripheral blood is common after severe electrical shock. Albuminuria is the rule; hemoglobinuria has been reported in many cases, probably secondary to severe burns. Although elevation of cerebrospinal fluid pressure is often mentioned in electrical shock, it is an inconstant finding; bloody spinal fluid occurs in some cases as a result of widespread vascular injury.

Management. Immediate *removal of the victim from contact* with the current is obviously important; this should always be preceded by cutting off the source of the current, when possible. Rescuers should be insulated by rubber gloves or a thick layer of dry cloth or newspapers. Many needless deaths have followed ill-planned attempts to rescue the body of an individual already dead from electrical shock.

Artificial respiration should be instituted immediately if the victim is not breathing. The importance of this maneuver cannot be overemphasized. In one series of 700 cases of electrical injury (Maclachlan), there were 479 with respiratory arrest, of which 323 responded to artificial respiration. The majority of patients who respond do so within 20 min, but recovery after longer periods of time is frequent enough that manual or mechanical respiration should be continued for a minimum of 4 hr before giving up. It has been estimated that a delay of 6 min in the institution of resuscitative measures increases the death rate in electrical shock by 80 per cent.

Other treatment is supportive. Stimulants should be used with caution during the first few hours because of the tendency of many patients to convulse. There is no evidence that the frequently advocated procedure of cerebrospinal fluid drainage is beneficial. Survivors of the acute episode often require extensive treatment for electrical burns, secondary infection, and massive hemorrhage as the devitalized tissues slough.

Prevention. An awareness of the danger of electricity is the most important factor in preventing accidents. Proper insulation of appliances in the home and the use of rubber gloves and dry shoes when working with circuits will avoid disability and death. Proper grounding of telephone and radio aerials against lightning should be routine. In a thunderstorm, the safest shelter is a house with windows and doors closed. A closed automobile, cave, ditch, or depression is relatively secure. Hilltops, riverbanks, hedges, and wire fences should be avoided. Although a tree standing alone is dangerous, the center of a wooded area is fairly safe.

REFERENCES

Glaister, John: "Medical Jurisprudence and Toxicology," 9th ed., chap. 7, Baltimore, The Williams & Wilkins Company, 1950.

Jex-Blake, A. J.: The Goulstonian Lectures on Death by Electric Currents, Brit. Med. J., I:425, 1913.

Langworthy, O. R., and W. B. Kouwenhoven: An Experimental Study of Abnormalities Produced in the Organism by Electricity, J. Ind. Hyg., 12:31, 1930.

Lightning Injuries, Lancet, I:351, 1946.

Maclachlan, W.: Electrical Injuries, J. Ind. Hyg., 16:1, 1934.

Section 1: Basic Considerations

110 AN APPROACH TO INFECTIOUS DISEASES

Ivan L. Bennett, Jr., and
David E. Rogers

The vast majority of human and animal diseases of known etiology are produced by biologic agents, viruses, rickettsias, bacteria, fungi, protozoa, or nematodes. No small part of the past and present importance of infectious diseases in medical practice is attributable to their enormous frequency and the public health implications of the contagiousness of many of them. It is also of note, however, that development in sanitary engineering, vector control, techniques of immunization, and specific chemotherapy have modified the situation favorably. While important exceptions remain, infectious diseases as a class are more easily prevented and more easily cured than any other major group of disorders. Despite the virtual elimination of certain infectious diseases and profound reduction in the morbidity and mortality produced by other biologic agents, human beings have not been rendered free of infection. It is important to point out that the *total human load of disease produced by microbial parasites has been only moderately, if at all, decreased.* As certain specific microbial infections have been controlled, others have emerged as troublesome therapeutic and epidemiologic problems. As Dubos has pointed out, microbial infections appear to form an inherent part of human life.

Because better environmental sanitation and other measures now prevent contact with many microbial agents and the development of acquired immunity early in childhood, certain infections have been seen more frequently in adults in our Western culture. For example, as contact with poliomyelitis virus in childhood has declined, paralytic poliomyelitis has become more common in young adults. Similarly, decreasing infection with the tubercle bacillus has raised important questions regarding the status of adult antituberculous immunity. Childhood infection with the tubercle bacillus was commonplace 20 years ago, and over 70 per cent of young adults had positive tuberculin tests. Today less than 5 per cent of young adults manifest tuberculin hypersensitivity.

As antimicrobial agents have sharply reduced the mortality associated with certain common infections, other microbes have emerged as important causations of human disease. It is now unusual for patients to die of pneumococcal pneumonia—a disease readily handled with agents currently available. However, it is now common to see sick patients develop serious disease produced by microorganisms which form part of man's normal microbial flora. These include infections produced by staphylococci, enteric bacilli, and fungi.

THE PARASITE AND THE HOST

The complex interaction between microorganism and man that results in infection and disease has been subjected to extensive study. Much has been learned about the initiation of the process, the ways in which microbes produce tissue injury, the influence of specific immunity and "nonspecific" resistance of the host, and mechanisms of recovery. Unfortunately, it is not yet possible to transfer in any specific way much of the information thus far acquired to the individual human patient with an infectious disease. In a textbook of medicine, therefore, it seems appropriate to emphasize those general aspects of the host-parasite relationship that form a basis for diagnostic procedures, that are of importance in deriving therapeutic principles, or that help explain the epidemiology of infection and infectious disease. This necessitates omitting from these pages discussion of many highly significant and interesting experimental studies, controversial issues, and theoretic or incompletely established concepts. The bibliography at the end of the chapter contains excellent reviews of these important subjects.

Infection and Clinical Disease. It is well known that microorganisms of different species or different strains of the same species vary widely in their capacity to produce disease and that human beings are not equally susceptible to the disease caused by a given bacterium or virus. Furthermore, while a specific infectious disease will not occur in the absence of the causative organism, the mere presence of the organism in the human body does not lead invariably to clinical illness. Indeed, it is now obvious that the production of symptoms in man by many parasites is an exceptional event rather than the rule, a "subclinical infection" or "carrier state" being the usual host-parasite relationship. *Disease* in a clinical sense is not synonymous with the presence of the organism or *infection* in a microbiologic sense. The ratio of subclinical infection to overt clinical disease varies widely in different microbial species. For example, subclinical infections with the virus of poliomyelitis are the rule. Less than one in a thousand infected individuals develop overt poliomyelitis—the clinical disease. By contrast, active human infection with the rabies virus probably almost always produces progressive fatal disease. Subclinical infections with rabies have not been observed.

Mechanisms of Injury. It is customary to refer to bacteria or other microorganisms that are capable of producing disease as *pathogenic. Virulence,* the ability to produce harmful effects in the host, is distinguished carefully from *invasiveness,* the ability to spread and disseminate in the body. For example, *Clostridium tetani* is pathogenic and, by virtue of its exotoxin, highly virulent, but it is almost completely lacking in invasiveness. These distinctions are valuable in microbiology and experimental pathology, but they often mean relatively little at a clinical level in an individual patient. Under certain circumstances and in certain anatomic locations, mildly "pathogenic" organisms can produce fatal disease, or highly "pathogenic" species can dwell and multiply without producing any harmful effect.

A few parasites produce *toxins* that account for the tissue damage and physiologic alterations of infection. *Hypersensitivity* to components of the parasite is demonstrable in several infections, but in relatively few has sensitization been shown to account for the manifestations of disease. For a large proportion of pathogenic agents, an explanation of their damaging effects upon the host is incomplete or wholly lacking. Generally, therefore, the aim of therapy is to stop multiplication or to kill the parasites with appropriate drugs; in diseases caused by toxin-producing organisms, the use of antiserum (as in tetanus or diphtheria) is the definitive procedure, chemotherapy being secondary.

The *tropism* of certain pathogenic organisms, their tendency to *localize in certain cells or organs* and to produce damage is unexplained in most instances. Clinically, however, the presence of disease in a specific anatomic site or a combination of symptoms referable to certain organs often suggests the identity of the causative organism. Similarly, in the presence of disease known to be caused by a given agent, complicating involvement of other tissues can be anticipated or predicted.

Frequently, the proper management of infectious disease involves the use of techniques completely unrelated to microbiology or chemotherapy, in an effort to support the function of damaged organs. Survival in poliomyelitis may depend upon treatment of respiratory failure, the management of heart failure in endocarditis is sometimes a greater problem than the eradication of the causative organism, and in epidemic hemorrhagic fever, or Weil's disease, maintenance of fluid and electrolyte balance during the stage of acute renal failure is the important therapeutic objective.

Resistance and Susceptibility. Many so-called "host factors" are known to influence the likelihood that disease will occur if organisms enter the tissues or, if infection becomes established, to play a determining role in the final outcome—recovery or death.

In experimental animals, *sex, strain, age, route of infection,* the presence of *specific antibody, other diseases, nutritional state,* and the use of such procedures as exposure to ionizing radiation or high environmental temperature or administration of mucin, nitrogen mustard, adrenal steroids, epinephrine, xerosin, and metabolic analogues can be shown to exert a profound effect upon infection by bacteria, viruses, and other agents.

In man, these factors are no less impressive, although controlled studies are lacking for many. Alcoholism, diabetes, agammaglobulinemia, the nephrotic syndrome, malnutrition, chronic administration of adrenal hormones, chronic lymphedema, ischemia, the presence of foreign bodies such as bullets, calculi, or bone fragments, obstruction of a bronchus, the urethra, or any hollow tube, agranulocytosis, various blood dyscrasias, and many other circumstances influence susceptibility to systemic or local infection. Furthermore, in those instances where the extenuating condition is remediable, the probability of recovery is enhanced.

Racial differences in susceptibility, such as the poor resistance of the Negro to tuberculosis or the peculiar resistance of Negroes to malaria caused by *Plasmodium vivax,* are well established in several infections. The increased frequency and severity of some infections in children, others in pregnant women, still others in the aged are familiar clinical facts.

Prior contact with an organism, whether by active infection or by artificial immunization, increases resistance to some infections, such as measles and poliomyelitis, but seems to have little influence on resistance to others, such as gonorrhea and acute coryza.

In the chapters that follow, the variations in human resistance to specific infectious agents are discussed in detail.

Finally, it must be emphasized that present knowledge of the factors involved in human resistance and susceptibility extends little beyond an *empirical tabulation of clinically observed relationships.* The attractive explanations that have been suggested, including changes in physical or chemical activity of phagocytes, antibacterial substances such as lysozyme, properdin, and phagocytin, qualitative or quantitative alterations in serum proteins, disordered metabolism at the cellular level, "products of tissue injury" that influence vascular permeability, and several others, remain for the most part in the realm of hypothesis.

The profound influence of "host factors" upon the infectious process makes it clear, however, that if our understanding of them ever reaches a point that enables us to control them in a predictable fashion, we will enter a new era in the management and control of infectious disease. There is no more important and fertile field for investigation in medicine.

PATHOGENESIS OF INFECTION

With relatively minor variations, the development of an infectious disease follows a consistent pattern. The parasites enter the body through the skin, nasopharynx, lung, intestine, urethra, or other portal, and a regular sequence ensues. Once established in the host, the organisms can multiply and, in so doing, establish a *local* or *primary lesion*. From this site, there may be *local spread* along fascial planes or tubular structures, such as a bronchus or ureter. The next step is *systemic spread* of the microorganisms by the circulating blood, which they reach by direct invasion of vessels (a relatively unusual occurrence) or by the common method of being borne in lymph to the thoracic duct and entering the venous system. In the blood stream, they spread to other tissues and can produce *distant*, or *secondary*, *lesions*. In infections such as tetanus and diphtheria, distant lesions are produced by toxins elaborated at the primary lesion without systemic spread of the parasites. The infectious process may terminate in recovery or death at any stage, the local lesion, systemic spread, or distant lesion.

The apparent inconsistency of this pattern in clinical medicine is attributable to the fact that the infection has been recognized as a *clinical entity* only at the stage when symptoms are most likely to appear. For example, pneumococcal pneumonia is a local lesion, and the distant lesion, pneumococcal meningitis, is referred to clinically as a *complication*. In meningococcal infections, the local lesion, a nasopharyngitis, is rarely symptomatic and has no status as a clinical entity, but the stage of spread, meningococcemia, and the commonest distant lesion, meningitis, are clinical entities. A rarer distant lesion, arthritis, is called a complication. In subacute bacterial endocarditis both the local lesion in the gums and the stage of spread are insignificant; the distant lesion is the clinical disease. In a patient who has osteomyelitis, a clinical entity, a recent furuncle may be referred to as a *predisposing factor*. In another patient with extensive furunculosis who develops osteomyelitis, the infection in bone may be regarded by the clinician as a complication of the superficial infec-

tion. The stages mentioned are in no way limited to bacterial diseases; the primary lesion of poliomyelitis is intestinal, viremia may occur without neurologic involvement, or a distant lesion, the classic "infantile paralysis," may be established.

Because of established clinical usage and terminology based upon the symptomatic illness that leads patients to seek medical aid, the consistency of this general sequence in the pathogenesis of infection is often not recognized. However, the concept is useful to the clinician and offers some basis for systematizing what may otherwise seem to be a miscellaneous collection of unrelated clinical signs and symptoms.

CLINICAL MANIFESTATIONS OF INFECTIONS

So varied are the disorders attributable to infection or infestation of man by lower organisms that generalization about them is difficult. The clinical manifestations of infection can duplicate those of diseases of any other etiology. On p. 65, there is a discussion of certain clinical features highly suggestive of infection, including abrupt onset, fever, chills, myalgia, photophobia, pharyngitis, acute lymphadenopathy or splenomegaly, gastroenteritis, and leukocytosis or leukopenia. It is obvious that the presence of one, several, or all of these features does not constitute proof of the microbial origin of illness in a given patient. Conversely, serious, even fatal, infectious disease can exist in the absence of fever or the other signs and symptoms mentioned.

While there is no infallible clinical criterion of infection, it is still possible to recognize accurately many specific infectious diseases from information obtained by *history, physical examination, blood count,* and *urinalysis*. The importance of interrogation about past illness, predisposing factors such as alcoholism, familial disease, exposure to ill persons, contact with animals or insects, ingestion of contaminated food, type and order of onset of symptoms, and recent or remote residence in endemic areas is discussed in subsequent chapters for specific diseases and etiologic agents. Cardinal physical signs are also described for each entity.

It is fitting to acknowledge our ignorance of the mechanisms that produce most of the signs and symptoms of human infection. As discussed on p. 61 the pathogenesis of fever is poorly understood. The physiologic alterations underlying "malaise," "postinfectious asthenia," "toxicity," and other common complaints are completely mysterious. We have little or no idea about the factors responsible for the leukocytoses or leukopenias that characterize certain infections. Why the rash of typhus begins on the trunk while that of another rickettsiosis, Rocky Mountain spotted fever, begins on the extremities is unanswered. It cannot be said that failure to understand the production of these manifestations impairs their clinical usefulness in differential diagnosis, but it is probable that understanding would bring with it clues to more accurate diagnosis and better management.

DIAGNOSTIC PROCEDURES

When dealing with diseases produced by living agents, it is soon evident that confirmation of a presumptive diagnosis, or sometimes the first suggestion as to the etiology of illness, often depends upon laboratory procedures. The availability of a multitude of laboratory tests in the modern hospital has not made it possible to substitute a "routine lab work-up" for history, physical examination, and observation of a patient's course. Indeed, the information derived from these procedures is the only reasonable basis for selecting the tests to be performed by the laboratory.

The importance of roentgenographic changes, alterations in chemical constituents of the blood, and tests of the functional capacity of organs such as the liver and kidney is as great in infectious disease as in illnesses of other etiologies and needs no discussion here.

The specific procedures for the diagnosis of infectious disease involve *direct demonstration of the causative organism* or *proof of its presence by indirect means.*

Demonstration of the Organism. In bacterial diseases, it is often possible to find the causative organism by *microscopic examination of properly stained preparations of sputum, spinal fluid, and other body fluids.* This simple procedure is often neglected as an unnecessary bother when material is being sent for bacteriologic culture, but it is a most valuable source of immediate information. In many diseases, the etiologic agent cannot be cultured (bartonellosis), and in others, isolation is time-consuming (tuberculosis, blastomycosis). The diagnosis of meningococcal infection (p. 926) by finding the organism in fluid from skin lesions or in the buffy coat or the finding of *Hemophilus influenzae* in stained smears of cerebrospinal fluid enables the clinician to initiate specific chemotherapy immediately with assurance that the regimen is the proper one.

Direct examination of bone marrow is a useful method for demonstrating organisms in some diseases, kala-azar, histoplasmosis, and tuberculosis being examples. In protozoan (amebiasis, malaria) and parasitic diseases (schistosomiasis, filariasis), *direct examination of blood, feces, or urine* is the only specific method for establishing a diagnosis.

There are also infections in which the *detection of characteristic cytologic changes or the causative organism itself in smears or histologic sections of biopsy material* can be the quickest method for diagnosis. Tubercles and tubercle bacilli in lymph nodes or liver biopsy material, leprosy bacilli in skin or nasal scrapings, inclusion bodies in the skin lesions of varicella or variola, and exudate of inclusion blenorrhea, "Warthin" cells from the nasal mucosa in measles, schistosome ova in pinch biopsies of rectal mucosa, and the Councilman bodies of yellow fever in liver are examples. In addition, characteristic histologic changes make it feasible to identify the lesions of chancroid, syphilis, lymphogranuloma venereum, cat-scratch disease, or viral hepatitis in biopsy specimens. Indeed, even in diseases where other reliable tests are available, diagnosis by histologic examination is sometimes the most rapid method, an example being the characteristic muscle lesion of Weil's disease (p. 1084).

Special Microscopic Techniques. *Dark-field examination* of material from genital lesions for the spirochete of syphilis is a well-known procedure. In several other spirochetal diseases, including leptospirosis, the dark-field technique can be useful, but experience in recognition of the organisms is necessary for correct interpretation of findings.

Fluorescence microscopy, in which the causative organisms can be recognized and identified rapidly by the use of fluorescent-antibody preparations (the Coons technique) has not been applied to general clinical work. With further refinement and simplification, it may eventually prove to be extremely useful in diagnosis.

Culture and Animal Inoculation. Specimens for bacteriologic culture should be collected *before the initiation of chemotherapy.* The material to be cultured—sputum, pus, blood, or bone marrow—should be selected on the basis of the suspected infections, and the precise cultural techniques employed—media, CO_2 incubation, anaerobic incubation, etc.—must be decided upon in a similar fashion.

In several infections, including Weil's disease, rat-bite fever, certain mycoses, tuberculosis, and the rickettsioses, isolation of the etiologic organism can be made by *inoculation of appropriate material into mice or guinea pigs.* This is a cumbersome procedure for routine use, but in selected instances it should be employed. As mentioned in subsequent chapters, many viruses can be isolated by inoculation of appropriate animals. This is rarely feasible for ordinary clinical diagnosis and, for several agents, is hazardous.

Facilities for isolating viruses by *inoculation of tissue cultures* are available in a few centers, but this method is likely to remain an investigative tool until it can be simplified and adapted to general use at a clinical level.

Blood Cultures and Bacteremia. Because of the peculiar clinical importance of demonstrating bacteria in the blood stream and because there are varying opinions about optimal timing and sites of sampling for blood cultures, it is of practical importance to the clinician to understand something about the mechanisms of bacteremia.

Excepting intravascular infections (bacterial endocarditis or endarteritis, mycotic aneurysm, suppurative thrombophlebitis), the entry of bacteria into the circulation occurs almost invariably through the lymphatic system. Consequently, when bacteria multiply at a site of local infection in the tissues, the likelihood of bacteremia parallels the occurrence of local conditions that favor drainage of lymph from the area to the thoracic duct and eventually, the venous blood. These factors include the number and anatomic arrangement of local lymph vessels, accumulation of fluid and increase in tissue pressure (a prominent feature of the inflammatory response), and exercise or massage of the part.

Once bacteria enter the blood, they are removed rapidly by the fixed phagocytes of the reticuloendothelial system in the liver and spleen and by engulfment in polymorphonuclear leukocytes in capillaries, especially those of the lung.

Clinically, bacteremia can be transient, intermittent, or continuous. Many transient bacteremias result from manipulation of infected or contaminated tissues, common examples being instrumentation of the genitourinary tract, tonsillectomy, dental procedures, and massage or surgical incision of furuncles or abscesses. In the vast majority of instances, the sudden discharge of bacteria into the blood produces no symptoms or, at most, a rigor and brief fever, and the organisms are promptly dealt with by the removal mechanisms already mentioned. The great importance of these "man-made" bacteremias is their role in producing bacterial endocarditis (p. 1039) in patients with endocardial damage.

Transient bacteremia accompanies the early phase of many infections. In pneumococcal pneumonia, the typical rigor at onset is a result of transient bacteremia. In most cases, with localization of the pulmonary lesion, blood cultures rapidly revert to negative. The poor prognosis assigned to patients with pneumonia who continue to have positive blood cultures is not based upon any danger from the mere presence of organisms in the blood as much as it is upon bacteremia as a reflection of spreading infection in the lung itself.

A sudden single influx of microorganisms into the blood stream may be followed by a shaking chill and fever. However, there is a "lag period" of 30 to 90 min before the febrile response (similar to the lag in pyrogen fever, p. 62). During this delay, the bacteria are usually promptly removed from the circulation by phagocytosis and, consequently, a blood culture taken at the time of the rigor may be negative. Failure to recognize this sequence led for many years to the idea that chilling after instrumentation of the urethra was the result of some peculiar property of the bladder, and even today, the term "catheter fever" is sometimes employed. *Failure to obtain growth in a blood culture taken during a chill does not rule out bacteremia as a cause of the fever.* Another frequent effect of transient bacteremia is the production of transient severe leukopenia followed by a polymorphonuclear leukocytosis for a few hours. *Peripheral leukocyte counts made during the few hours after a chill may give information that is erroneously interpreted in diagnosis.*

Continuous bacteremia is a feature of the first several days of typhoid fever, of brucellosis, and of intravascular infections such as endocarditis.

Blood cultures should be taken at frequent intervals in patients with febrile disease of unknown etiology; in general, an attempt should be made to obtain blood *before* an expected rise in fever or chill. When a patient is suspected of bacterial endocarditis or another of the diseases in which bacteremia is constant, two to four cultures daily for 2 to 3 days are more than sufficient to establish diagnosis, and treatment in such cases should not be withheld for a longer period.

There is no evidence that arterial blood possesses any advantage over blood from the antecubital veins for culture. Suspected bacteremia is sometimes mentioned as a contraindication to diagnostic lumbar puncture because of the possible development of meningitis, but clinical evidence does not support this idea. Culture of bone marrow is occasionally superior to peripheral blood for recovery of organisms in typhoid, brucellosis, and rare cases of subacute bacterial endocarditis. While it is common practice to make pour plates of blood and to quantify bacteremia in terms of a certain number of colonies per milliliter of blood, the results of this rather cumbersome procedure have no diagnostic or prognostic significance, and it has no advantage for routine use. In typhoid, for example, the number of bacilli in the blood rarely exceeds 25 to 30 per ml and bears no relationship to the severity of illness. When blood cultures are taken for diagnostic purposes, some should be incubated in carbon dioxide, and a sample of blood should also be cultured in thioglycollate broth or some other anaerobic medium. Anaerobic cultures are especially important in women with puerperal or postabortal infections.

Immunologic Methods. These diagnostic methods are intended to supply evidence of past or present infection by demonstrating antibodies in serum or other body fluids, by showing changed reactivity of the host (hypersensitivity, allergy) to products of the organism, or rarely, to detect components of the causative organism in the body. The reader is referred to standard texts of immunology for detailed discussion of the nature of antigens and antibodies, the cellular origin of antibody, and the complex interactions of antigen-antibody systems. Emphasis here is directed toward the interpretation of immunologic tests commonly used for clinical diagnosis.

Serologic Tests. The finding on a single occasion that a patient's serum contains antibody that reacts with a certain antigen merely indicates that the patient has had previous contact with the antigen or a closely related substance. For this reason, with rare exceptions, the clinical interpretation of serologic tests depends upon serial determinations. If the antibody titer is found to *rise or fall significantly,* one can then be reasonably sure that the response is a result of recent or current contact with the antigen. In subsequent chapters, the need for serologic testing of acute phase and convalescent serum is emphasized repeatedly. *In any patient with a puzzling illness, a sterile specimen of serum should be preserved in a frozen state so that it can, if necessary, be studied and compared with serum collected at a later date.*

Prior contact with an antigen can be the result of past artificial immunization with vaccines; interpretation of serum agglutinin titers for typhoid bacilli is often made difficult or impossible by prior immunization. The occurrence of the so-called "anamnestic reaction," a supposed nonspecific stimulation of antibody formation by an acute illness (e.g., a rise in brucella agglutinins in a patient with acute tularemia), is now known to result only when the two organisms are antigenically related and rarely presents a serious problem. The vibrio of cholera contains an antigen similar to that of brucella, and surprisingly high levels of brucella agglutinins have been seen in servicemen immunized with cholera vaccine.

The exact methods employed for detecting antibody rises in various infections have been selected empirically on the basis of the ease of performing the test, as well as on careful study to correlate the results of the test with other diagnostic criteria in patients. Therefore, the fact that one agent is detected by a precipitin technique, another by agglutination of whole organisms or the production of capsular swelling, and still another by complement fixation is a practical matter of convenience and bears no necessary relationship to the agent, the type of infection produced, or basic pathogenesis.

By coating some particulate material, such as erythrocytes or collodion particles, with antigen derived from a certain organism, antibody can sometimes be demonstrated by an agglutination test rather than by some more complex method.

Particular properties of the causative organism can sometimes be utilized to devise a simplified clinical test for antibody. Two striking instances of this are widely used. The ability of influenza and related viruses to clump erythrocytes (see p. 1123) makes possible the demonstration of antibody to virus by merely testing the capacity of a patient's serum to prevent the agglutination of red cells by suspensions of virus, the so-called "hemagglutination-inhibition" reaction. Similarly, because many microorganisms possess hemolytic components or toxins, the assay of a patient's serum for capacity to prevent lysis of red cells is a convenient and simple clinical test for antibody. The antistreptolysin O test in group A beta-hemolytic streptococcal infections (p. 902) is an example of this.

In a few infections, predominantly those caused by viruses, the only reliable serologic test is a *neutralization* or *protection* test, an assay of the protection afforded by the patient's serum against active infection in experimental animals or in tissue culture. This technique is time-consuming and is usually performed only in special diagnostic centers.

Some mention of "nonspecific" serologic changes may serve to emphasize again that clinical laboratory tests have come into use *only because they have been found to correlate reasonably well with clinical findings.* In several diseases, it has been found, often accidentally, that there develops serum antibody that will react with antigens derived from sources other than the etiologic agent (which may actually be unknown). Common examples are heterophil agglutinins in infectious mononucleosis (p. 1250), cold agglutinins in some forms of nonbacterial pneumonia (p. 1120), and the agglutination of certain strains of proteus bacilli by serum of patients with rickettsial diseases (p. 1094). The outstanding example of a clinically useful nonspecific serologic test is the Wassermann reaction for syphilis. This test and its modifications are performed with antigens derived from sources completely unrelated to the spirochete that causes the disease. Because of their simplicity, they are still used in preference to more complicated and admittedly more accurate techniques that utilize the *Treponema pallidum* itself (p. 1077).

In summary, the results of serologic tests must be interpreted in the light of other information about the patient, including such factors as previous immunizations and illnesses, the possibility of exposure to chemically but etiologically unrelated antigens, and the importance of a changing titer in serial tests as opposed to a single isolated observation.

Skin Tests. Exposure to antigens of certain types, by various routes, and under circumstances not completely understood often results in the development of *immediate* (*anaphylactic, atopic*) *hypersensitivity* or *delayed* (*bacterial, tuberculin*) *hypersensitivity* (see p. 1257 for further details).

Active infection with some, but not all, bacteria and viruses results in delayed hypersensitivity to the infecting agent in some, but not all, individuals. Clinically, the detection of this allergic state is accomplished by intradermal injection of the organisms or some component of them; in a sensitive person, there will appear induration and erythema at the local site within 24 to 48 hr. If an individual is highly sensitive or if the amount of antigen injected is excessive, there may be extensive local inflammation with necrosis, vesicle formation, edema, regional lymphadenopathy, and even systemic manifestations of malaise and fever. Antigens prepared in concentrations unlikely to provoke severe reactions are generally available for intradermal testing for tuberculosis, leprosy, mumps, lymphogranuloma venereum, cat-scratch disease, chancroid, brucellosis, tularemia, glanders, toxoplasmosis, blastomycosis, histoplasmosis, coccidioidomycosis, and many other infections. The "immune reaction" to vaccination (p. 1165) is also an example of delayed dermal hypersensitivity.

The reliability, specificity, and usefulness of the individual tests differ and are discussed in the chapters on specific infections. However, certain general principles apply to their use and interpretation:

1. They are highly useful in epidemiologic surveys as indicators of the incidence of infection in a population.

2. In most individuals, dermal reactivity persists for many years or for life. A single positive test means only that at some past time the individual was exposed to the organism (or a closely related one). Unless supplementary information in the form of clinical findings, cultural studies, or more specific serologic data bear out the presence of active infection, a diagnosis of the disease is not justified.

3. The appearance of a positive dermal reaction in an individual known to have been nonreactive a short time before is good evidence of recent infection; this is becoming a useful method for detecting early tuberculosis.

4. A *negative intradermal test does not rule out past or present infection.* For unknown reasons, patients with measles, Hodgkin's disease, or sarcoidosis often develop a state of "anergy," or inability to react to intradermally injected antigens. In several diseases, dermal sensitivity develops after weeks or months of infection; an important example of this is acute histoplasmosis (p. 1059), in which

patients can be acutely ill for many weeks without showing a positive skin test. The skin test to coccidioidin is always negative in disseminated coccidioidomycosis (p. 1056), and in far-advanced or miliary tuberculosis in elderly patients, failure to react to intradermal tuberculin in the usual amounts employed for testing occurs in as many as 10 to 15 per cent of the cases.

Intradermal injection of antigens derived from sources other than microorganisms usually produces an immediate "wheal and erythema" reaction which subsides promptly. The greatest clinical usefulness of this type of reaction is in the detection of allergy to foreign serums, pollens, and animal dander (see p. 1261). The skin tests developed for demonstrating infestation with helminths (trichinosis, filariasis) produce reactions of the immediate type in allergic individuals, but the antigens employed are so nonspecific that they are of little use in diagnosis.

THE IMPORTANCE OF SPECIFIC DIAGNOSIS IN INFECTIOUS DISEASES

Medicine and Microbiology. The diagnostic procedures employed for infectious diseases are no more absolute than those in other diseases; they cannot be blindly equated with the science of microbiology. The responsibility for interpreting the facts supplied by the bacteriologist, immunologist, and virologist in the total context of a patient's illness remains that of the physician. A positive tuberculin skin test certainly does not indicate that a patient has active tuberculosis. The finding of *Candida albicans* (monilia) in a stool culture does not necessarily mean that a patient's diarrhea is caused by intestinal moniliasis. The presence of staphylococci in nasal cultures from a patient with headaches does not establish a diagnosis of staphylococcal sinusitis. A throat culture containing beta-hemolytic streptococci does not rule out diphtheria; nor does such a culture establish that a febrile illness in a patient with mitral stenosis is a recurrence of acute rheumatic fever and not bacterial endocarditis. A positive serologic test for syphilis may be the first sign of incipient lupus erythematosus. The decisions in such matters must be made by the patient's physician.

Chemotherapy. The next chapter discusses the antimicrobial drugs in detail. The impact of chemotherapy upon mortality and morbidity from infection and upon epidemic disease is now a matter of historical record. These therapeutic agents, however, have in no way lessened the importance of specific diagnosis; indeed their availability has increased the need for obtaining exact etiologic information. It requires but a moment's reflection to realize that the substitution of a prescription for a "broad-spectrum" antibiotic or a quick injection of penicillin for the systematic collection of facts and thoughtful consideration of diagnostic possibilities is fallacious, unwise, and dangerous. Numerous antibiotics with overlapping spectrums are now available, dosages for different infections vary widely, certain diseases are best treated with combinations of drugs, and the drugs themselves are potentially dangerous. They should never be prescribed as placebos, antipyretics, or substitutes for diagnosis. In the vast majority of instances where this is done, patients recover just as they would if no "therapy" had been given and the drugs are wasted. More important, inadequate dosage or the wrong agent given blind may suppress symptoms temporarily without curing, make isolation of the etiologic agent difficult, and delay the recognition of the true nature of an illness and the institution of curative treatment. Finally, to expose a patient to the risk of drug reaction without proper indication is inexcusable on the part of the physician, whether the drug is an antibiotic, a sedative, a laxative, or a narcotic.

Epidemiologic and Other Considerations. Just as the decision to administer antibiotics to a patient with a febrile illness of presumed infectious etiology must be made on an individual basis, the selection of cases in which extensive cultural and serologic testing is required is a matter of judgment. The majority of common "grippelike" illnesses subside spontaneously, and symptomatic treatment is sufficient. However, because of this tendency toward spontaneous recovery and also because the results of serologic tests, even if diagnostic, may not be available until a patient is convalescent, there are many who regard continued effort to determine the specific etiology of illness as an impractical, "academic" procedure. Such an attitude fails to recognize that the responsibility of the physician extends beyond the individual patient to include the community. Furthermore, the physician has a responsibility to himself. For example, a patient recently recovered from "viral pneumonitis" may feel that his physician has cared for him competently and well. The doctor himself may feel that he has discharged his professional duties properly and that his having refrained from giving the patient antibiotics for what was clinically a virus disease and therefore unlikely to benefit from chemotherapy was a laudable act of forbearance. However, if a serologic test is reported a few days later as showing that the patient's serum has shown a rise in complement-fixing antibody against psittacosis virus, the situation might change. The patient himself would continue to be well, but a search for the source of the disease, such as the patient's pet parakeet, would certainly be indicated, and future illnesses in others might be prevented. Furthermore, the physician would benefit from being reminded that antibiotics are effective in a few of the viral diseases and that "pneumonitis" is one of the clinical situations in which this possibility should be considered.

Other examples of the practicality of "academic" procedures could be cited. There are extremes in everything, and, in the final analysis, the decision about the individual case must be made by the attending physician using his best judgment, based on some of the factors that have been mentioned.

REFERENCES

Bennett, I. L., Jr., and P. B. Beeson: Bacteremia: A Consideration of Some Experimental and Clinical Aspects, Yale J. Biol. and Med., 26:241, 1954.

Burnet, M.: "Natural History of Infectious Disease," New York, Cambridge University Press, 1953.

Dubos, R. J.: "The Bacterial Cell," Cambridge, Mass., Harvard University Press, 1947.

——: "Biochemical Determinants of Microbial Diseases," Cambridge, Mass., Harvard University Press, 1954.

MacLeod, C. M., and L. E. Cluff (Eds.): Symposium on Non-specific Resistance to Infection, Bacteriol. Rev., 24:1, 1960.

Rich, A. R.: "The Pathogenesis of Tuberculosis," 2d ed., Springfield, Ill., Charles C Thomas, Publisher, 1951.

Rogers, D. E.: The Changing Pattern of Life-threatening Microbial Disease, N. Engl. J. Med., 261:677, 1959.

Wood, W. B., Jr.: Studies on the Cellular Immunology of Acute Bacterial Infections, Harvey Lectures, 47:72, 1951–1952.

111 CHEMOTHERAPY OF INFECTION

Louis Weinstein

The chemotherapy of infection as discussed in this chapter may be best defined as the use of drugs to suppress the growth of or kill pathogenic microorganisms in the animal body. The chemotherapeutic agents at present available for the treatment of infectious diseases can be divided into two main groups, on the basis of their origin: (1) those which are totally synthetic substances, such as sulfonamides, sulfones, quinacrine, arsenic compounds, and isonicotinic acid hydrazide; and (2) those which are elaborated by various types of microorganisms (some have been synthesized subsequent to their initial isolation), such as penicillin, streptomycin, chlortetracycline (Aureomycin), and chloramphenicol (Chloromycetin). The latter are called antibiotics.

THE CHEMOTHERAPEUTIC AGENTS

To be of practical value in the treatment of infection, a drug must exert its effect upon the invading microorganism without seriously damaging the cells of the host. It is remarkable that so many agents with this selective activity have been developed. As far as is known, all chemotherapeutic agents exert their effects by acting directly upon the parasite, and not by enhancing the natural defense mechanisms of the host. The principal action is a retarding of the rate of growth of bacteria which enables the normal defense mechanisms of phagocytosis, antibody, etc., to deal with them. When present in sufficient concentration, some drugs can kill bacteria in vivo and in vitro. When chemotherapeutic substances are given in large doses early in some diseases, depression, delay, or elimination of the immune response to the invading microorganism may follow.

Quinine, emetine, heavy metals, organic iodides, and other synthetic agents are used extensively in the treatment of protozoal and helminthic infections; information concerning these agents is presented in the chapters dealing with these specific diseases. The discussion to follow will be limited to two classes of chemotherapeutic substances: the sulfonamides (effective for the most part only against bacteria) and the antibiotics (active against bacteria, rickettsias, amebas, and some of the larger viruses). Tuberculostatic drugs, some of which are neither sulfonamide compounds nor antibiotics, are also discussed.

THE SULFONAMIDES

The sulfonamide compounds have been used in clinical medicine since 1937. The important sulfonamides are Sulfadiazine, Sulfamerazine, sulfisoxazole (Gantrisin), sulfamethoxypyridazine (Kynex, Midicel), sulfamethoxypyrimidine (Madribon), succinylsulfathiazole (Sulfasuxidine), and phthalylsulfathiazole (Sulfathalidine).

The sulfonamides, despite the availability of more effective antibacterial agents, are very valuable in the management of certain infections. They are the drugs of choice in meningococcal meningitis and bacillary dysentery. They are often applied, with varying success, in urinary tract infections which have not responded to various antibiotics. Sulfonamides can be employed in the prophylaxis of recurrent rheumatic fever. Although there is a

strong clinical impression that an additive chemotherapeutic effect may be produced by a combination of sulfonamide and antibiotics, data from controlled studies are meager.

The sulfonamide compounds at present employed for the treatment of systemic infections are readily absorbed from the gastrointestinal tract and are probably best administered by this route to the conscious patient. Sodium salts for either intramuscular or intravenous use are also available. Liquid preparations made palatable by the addition of flavoring materials are useful in treating young children. For most of the infectious diseases in which the sulfonamides are of value, the duration of therapy should be no less than 1 week.

An adequate concentration of the sulfonamides must be maintained in the blood and tissues to produce effective bacteriostasis. A blood level of 10 to 12 mg per 100 ml is sufficient for the management of most of the susceptible infections. The interval between separate doses is usually short, 4 to 6 hr, except for sulfamethoxypyridazine and sulfamethoxypyrimidine which need to be given only once daily usually. If the drugs are given by the parenteral route, the size of each dose should be reduced and the interval between doses should be increased. The concentration of drug in the blood must be estimated at frequent intervals; this is relatively simple and can be accurately determined by colorimetric methods.

Most of the sulfonamide compounds are *widely distributed* in the body. After absorption, the major metabolic alteration is acetylation of the primary amino group. Sulfonamides are excreted by the kidney, chiefly by glomerular filtration. Derivatives which are not firmly bound to plasma or tissue proteins tend to be distributed evenly in total body water and thus reach high concentrations in tissue cells, whereas those with a tendency to bind are concentrated in the plasma.

The *bacteriostatic* activity of the sulfonamides is presumed to be related to their antimetabolic properties. Para-aminobenzoic acid (PABA), which inhibits the antibacterial effect of most of these agents, is an essential metabolite of many microorganisms. PABA is part of the molecule of folic (pteroylglutamic) acid. It has been suggested that the sulfonamides prevent the incorporation of PABA into the pteroylglutamic acid molecule, but it is likely that they do not always act on a single state in the chain of enzymatic reactions involved in cell metabolism but may inhibit several steps.

The principal *toxic effects* of the sulfonamides are hypersensitivity reactions and injury to the kidneys. Hypersensitivity may be manifested by fever, rash, granulopenia, or depression of other components of the bone marrow. These reactions may develop any time after the first week of therapy, or even earlier in patients who have received the drugs previously. Sensitivity to one type of compound frequently confers sensitivity to others. Crystallization of the drug in the renal tubules is not likely to occur when an inadequate quantity of fluid has been ingested or when the reaction of the urine is acid, since the solubility of both acetylated and free forms is considerably greater in a neutral or alkaline medium. One obvious method of avoiding renal injury is to maintain a copious urine output—at least 1,200 ml per day. Another procedure is to produce an alkaline urine by the oral administration of 12 to 15 Gm sodium bicarbonate per day. With the increase in solubility of the sulfonamide in the urine, the excretion of the drug is simultaneously more rapid. The concentration is thus lowered in the blood, and this makes necessary the administration of larger quantities in order to raise the blood level to the point of maximal effectiveness. In many clinics, therefore, alkalinization of the urine is not carried out. Another method of preventing precipitation in the urinary tract is to administer two or three sulfonamides concomitantly, since the solubility of each is independent of the presence of the others. *Acute tabular necrosis*, a rare complication of sulfonamide therapy, usually occurs in patients who have taken one of these drugs in the past; it may follow the ingestion of as little as 1 Gm of the agent. It is a totally unpredictable and unavoidable accident for which there is no specific therapy. Another rare but serious manifestation of sulfonamide toxicity is *acute hemolytic anemia*. This may develop within 48 hr of therapy and is manifested by a rapid fall in the number of erythrocytes, icterus, fever, and hemoglobinuria. Drug administration should be discontinued at once and blood transfusions given.

Sulfadiazine (2-sulfanilamidopyrimidine) is absorbed from the gastrointestinal tract slowly and incompletely, and renal excretion is relatively slow. The tissue concentration is 60 to 75 per cent of that in the plasma. Sulfadiazine appears in the urine in both the free and acetylated forms; neither is very soluble, and crystalluria is common. For most systemic infections in adults, Sulfadiazine is administered in a dose of 4 to 6 Gm per day following an initial dose of 4 Gm. In young children 0.065 to 0.1 Gm per lb body weight per 24 hr usually produces an adequate effect; the initial dose should be about one-half of this quantity.

Sulfamerazine (4-methyl-2-sulfanilamidopyrimidine) is absorbed more rapidly and completely from the gastrointestinal tract than Sulfadiazine. For these reasons the "loading" dose need be only 2 Gm in most cases, and effective blood levels may be maintained by the administration of 1 Gm only every 6 to 8 hr. The concentration in the tissues is 50 to 75 per cent of that in the plasma. Very little acetylation of Sulfamerazine occurs, and the tendency to renal tubular damage is less than with Sulfadiazine.

Succinylsulfathiazole (Sulfasuxidine: 2-N⁴-succinylsulfanilamidothiazole) and phthalylsulfathiazole (Sulfathalidine: 2-N⁴-phthalylsulfanilamidothiazole) are poorly absorbable from the intestinal tract and are used primarily, therefore, for the suppression of bacterial growth in the intestine.

Gantrisin (3, 4-dimethyl-5-sulfanilamidoisoxazole) is more soluble than any of the sulfonamide compounds described above. It is absorbed rapidly from the gastrointestinal tract and is distributed only in the extracellular water of the body. Therefore, the administration of the same quantity of drug will yield a plasma concentration of Gantrisin three times that for sulfanilamide and about twice that for Sulfadiazine and Sulfamerazine. The dosage and clinical effectiveness of Gantrisin are of the same order as those of Sulfadiazine.

Sulfamethoxypyridazine (3-sulfanilamido-6-methoxypyridazine, Kynex) is well absorbed from the gastrointestinal tract and is excreted slowly in the urine. It penetrates the cerebrospinal fluid well and has antibacterial activity about equal to that of Sulfadiazine. A dose of 1 Gm every 48 hr produces blood levels of 5 to 12.5 mg per 100 ml. Sulfamethoxypyridazine is most useful for prolonged therapy or prophylaxis. The dose recommended for therapy is 1 Gm initially and 0.5 Gm every 24 hr. When higher blood levels are required, the dosage can be raised to 2 Gm followed by 1 Gm daily. A weekly dose of 30 mg per kg body weight has been suggested for prophylaxis against streptococcal infections in rheumatic patients. Blood levels should be determined if therapy is continued for more than 1 week. This is mandatory in patients with impaired renal function. The risk of severe reactions from sulfamethoxypyridazine is probably related to dosage, and caution should be exercised against giving excessive quantities.

Sulfamethoxypyrimidine (sulfadimethoxine, Madribon) is also a rapidly absorbed sulfonamide which is excreted relatively slowly. The activity of the drug is not reversed by PABA in vivo. The anti-infective effectiveness of Madribon is comparable to that of methoxypyridazine. It diffuses poorly into the cerebrospinal fluid.

The dose of Madribon for individuals weighing over 80 lb is 2 Gm initially followed by 1 Gm once daily; for those about 40 lb in weight, the primary quantity is 1 Gm followed by 0.5 Gm every 24 hr; for children who weigh about 20 lb, 0.5 Gm is given first and then 0.25 Gm is administered once a day. Untoward reactions similar to those with other sulfonamides have followed the use of sulfamethoxypyrimidine.

Although both Kynex and Madribon have been recommended for the therapy of acute infections due to sulfonamide-susceptible organisms, these "long-acting" drugs have no advantages over the rapidly absorbed and excreted ones except for the convenience associated with the fact that they need to be taken only once daily. This does not appear to be sufficient grounds on which to recommend them for the treatment of acute infections in place of such well-tested agents as Sulfadiazine or Gantrisin. The greatest area of usefulness of the slowly excreted agents appears to be in situations in which a sulfonamide needs to be given for a long period of time, as in the control of chronic urinary tract infections or the prophylaxis of rheumatic fever recurrence. These drugs probably also have a place in the prevention of bacillary dysentery and meningococcal meningitis.

ANTIBIOTICS

The development of antibiotics for the treatment of infections constitutes one of the most important advances in modern medicine. Among those which are presently available are penicillin, streptomycin, tetracycline, chlortetracycline, oxytetracycline, demethychlortetracycline, chloramphenicol, erythromycin, bacitracin, neomycin, polymyxin, amphotericin, kanamycin, vancomycin, ristocetin, and paromomycin.

Testing Organisms for Sensitivity to Various Antibiotics

The sensitivities of bacteria to various chemotherapeutic agents are usually determined by bacteriologic techniques. The most accurate method for use in the routine bacteriology laboratory involves inoculation of the organism into culture medium in test tubes containing serial dilutions of the drug. After a suitable period of incubation, the lowest concentration of antibiotic which inhibits growth of the bacteria is expressed as the "sensitivity." A more rapid method uses filter paper disks which have been infiltrated with a known quantity of drug. These are placed on the surface of agar plates on which the organism has been streaked. The smallest quantity of antibiotic around which inhibition of growth is present is the level of sensitivity of the bacteria. This procedure is relatively crude, and although useful in clinical practice for the rapid determination of relative sensitivities of organisms, it does not take the place of the test tube serial dilution technique. Clinical laboratories should always be able to carry out these tests

reliably. They are not necessary in all cases; furthermore, there is only a rough correlation between clinical response to drug and the test result. Nevertheless, the procedure may be invaluable in indicating which therapeutic agent to employ and the general level of dosage required.

Resistance of Bacteria to Antibiotics

Each chemotherapeutic agent has a certain range of effectiveness. Presumably, a principal determining factor in this is whether the microbial enzyme system affected by the drug is an essential one. Another factor is the elaboration by the parasites of substances which inactivate the chemotherapeutic agent. For example, the pseudomonas group of bacteria, which are naturally resistant to penicillin, produce a penicillinase which, when added to a culture medium, will inhibit the bacteriostatic action of that drug for organisms normally susceptible to it. Some naturally resistant strains of staphylococcus also have been found to elaborate penicillinase.

Acquired Resistance. Bacteria growing in the presence of chemotherapeutic agents may develop the ability to grow in concentrations of drug which originally would have suppressed them completely. This kind of change can occur within the animal body as well as in the test tube. The rapidity with which it develops varies with different strains and drugs.

The development of drug resistance may be the result of selective survival of naturally occurring variants or possibly the production of mutants in the culture. The presence of the chemotherapeutic agent does not increase the rate of appearance of these insensitive forms, which are at first in such a minority that they escape detection. However, as the growth of susceptible bacteria is inhibited, the resistant variants multiply and eventually outnumber the susceptible ones.

The acquisition of drug resistance is observed more and more frequently in vivo. A most important problem is the increasing number of staphylocci which are insensitive to penicillin and other antibiotics.

Streptomycin treatment very commonly induces resistance in organisms. Some of the bacteria involved in urinary tract infections and *Hemophilus influenzae,* for example, may become totally insensitive to streptomycin within 3 or 4 days after the initiation of therapy. An increasing number of bacteria, both gram-negative and gram-positive, have been shown to develop varying degrees of lack of susceptibility to Aureomycin, Chloromycetin, Terramycin, and erythromycin.

Organisms which become insensitive to one antibiotic may simultaneously develop resistance to another. Thus, not infrequently, bacteria which lose their susceptibility to Aureomycin simultaneously exhibit insensitivity to Terramycin, Chloromycetin, and Achromycin. The development of neomycin resistance is quite readily associated with a significant loss of sensitivity to streptomycin. The reverse does not occur so regularly.

Combination of antibiotics may result in a diminution in the speed of emergence of bacterial resistance to any of the drugs in the mixture. For example, clinical experience indicates that the emergence of resistance in the tubercle bacillus to streptomycin is considerably delayed by the simultaneous administration of para-aminosalicylic acid or isonicotinic acid hydrazide (p. 1010).

DETERMINATION OF DRUG CONCENTRATIONS IN BODY FLUIDS

Knowledge of the absorption, distribution, and excretion of chemotherapeutic agents is of the greater importance in determining methods of clinical use. Sulfonamide and Chloromycetin concentrations in various body fluids can be determined chemically, using colorimetric techniques. For most of the antibiotics, however, there is no means of chemical analysis, and tedious bioassay is required.

PENICILLIN

Penicillin is an antibacterial substance produced by various strains of *Penicillium*. Although this mold elaborates several penicillins which are closely related chemically and in biologic activity, the one used most extensively in clinical medicine at the present time is penicillin G, or benzyl penicillin. Several modifications of the drug have been produced primarily for the purpose of prolonging the duration of antibacterial activity or increasing resistance of the drug to gastric acidity; these include the procaine ester, dibenzylethylenediamine dipenicillin (Bicillin), and phenoxymethyl penicillin (penicillin V). Two new penicillins are semisynthetic derivatives of 6-amino-penicillanic acid; these are 6-(alpha-phenoxypropionamido) penicillanate or phenoxyethyl penicillin (phenethicillin, Syncillin, Broxil) and 6-(2,6-dimethoxybenzamido) penicillanate monohydrate (Staphcillin).

Penicillin in low concentrations is bacteriostatic; large quantities are bactericidal. Organisms are killed only if they are exposed to the drug while they are in an active phase of multiplication. The mode of action of penicillin is interference with the formation of bacterial cell walls by inhibiting the incorporation of a compound containing a uridine nucleotide, an acetyl amino sugar, and a peptide of three amino acids (DL-alanine, D-gluta-

mate, and lysine) which is an intermediate in cell wall production.

Penicillin may be administered by several routes: orally, intramuscularly, subcutaneously, intravenously, or by inhalation. It has also been applied topically. Application to the skin, especially if preparations dissolved in oily bases are employed, is to be avoided wherever possible, because the degree of sensitization to the drug produced by this type of therapy is very high. The procaine salt of the antibiotic is probably the most extensively used preparation because absorption is slowed, and detectable blood levels may be present for as long as 24 hr. The addition of aluminum monostearate to procaine penicillin may allow detectable blood levels to be maintained for as long as 48 to 72 hr. Solutions of crystalline penicillin G in physiologic saline may be inhaled for the treatment of various acute or chronic pulmonary infections.

Bicillin may be administered either by mouth or parenterally. When given orally, however, the absorption of this agent is more erratic than that of buffered penicillin G, which yields three to six times the penicillin activity of Bicillin. The intramuscular injection of Bicillin has the advantage over penicillin G of prolonging the duration of blood levels; the administration of 200,000 to 500,000 units may produce a detectable concentration of antibiotic in the blood for as long as 2 weeks. Penicillin V differs from G in a single oxygen molecule. The free acid and potassium salt are more stable and much less soluble at the pH of gastric juice than is penicillin G. Penicillin V is, however, rapidly dissolved in alkaline solution and is readily absorbed from the upper portion of the small intestine. Taken by mouth, penicillin V produces higher and more prolonged blood levels than the same quantity of penicillin G. The intramuscular injection of penicillin V produces lower blood levels than penicillin G given by the same route.

Only about 20 per cent of an orally administered dose of penicillin G is absorbed into the blood stream, the remainder being destroyed by gastric acidity and by penicillinase in the lumen of the intestines. As a consequence, much larger doses are needed for oral than for parenteral therapy. Penicillin should not be given by mouth later than 1/2 hr before or earlier than 2 1/2 hr after a meal. When penicillin is injected subcutaneously or intramuscularly it causes little or no local irritation and is absorbed very rapidly into the blood stream, from where it is either excreted by the kidneys or distributed evenly in the plasma and extracellular fluid. Normally, only minute amounts penetrate into the cerebrospinal fluid, but in the presence of meningeal inflammation, appreciable levels of the drug may be obtained.

Penicillin is excreted by the kidneys with great rapidity, mainly by a tubular mechanism, about 10 per cent being cleared in the glomerular filtrate. The renal clearance approximates the total renal blood flow. Attempts have been made to delay renal excretion by concurrent administration of substances which compete for available tubular excretory structures. Diodrast, para-aminohippuric acid, and Benemid (*p*-di-*n*-propylsulfamyl-benzoic acid) retard penicillin excretion to a variable degree. Benemid appears to be the most effective in reducing the rapidity of excretion of penicillin; the dose is 0.5 Gm four times a day.

Phenethicillin [6-(alpha-phenoxypropionamido) penicillanate, phenoxyethyl penicillin, Syncillin] is absorbed when taken by mouth and is resistant to gastric acidity. However, it is absorbed less well than penicillin V if it is taken with or shortly after a meal. Blood levels of phenethicillin are higher than those produced by penicillin V, but these do not lead to a greater degree of antibacterial activity. In fact, the blood levels obtained by administration of the semisynthetic compound may actually be lower than those present after giving penicillin V in terms of activity against bacteria when the two agents are compared with the same standard penicillin and the results are expressed in terms of penicillin G activity. Intramuscularly injected penicillin G is superior to phenethicillin; the former produces higher and more sustained blood levels. Although in vitro studies have suggested that phenethicillin is active against penicillin-resistant staphylococci, this probably has no significance in the treatment of infections due to this type of organism. The "synthetic" compound may produce allergic reactions in individuals previously sensitized to other penicillins.

Dimethoxyphenyl penicillin (Staphcillin) appears to be effective both in vitro and in vivo against all strains of penicillinase-producing *Staphylococcus aureus* thus far studied. The drug is, however, only $\frac{1}{20}$ to $\frac{1}{40}$ as active against group A beta-hemolytic streptococci and neisseria, about $\frac{1}{10}$ as active against *Diplococcus pneumoniae* and *Streptococcus viridans*, inactive against gram-negative bacilli, even those which are moderately sensitive to penicillin G, and only slightly inhibitory for *Hemophilus influenzae*. It is 50 times more active than benzyl penicillin for penicillinase-elaborating staphylococci, but probably only $\frac{1}{50}$ as effective for strains which do not produce this enzyme. Dimethoxyphenyl penicillin is little if at all inactivated by staphylococcal penicillinase, but it is inhibited by the penicillinases of *Bacillus licheniformis* and *B. cereus* (Neutrapen), although more slowly than penicillin G. Exposure of staphylococci to this antibiotic in vitro or in vivo does not lead to the development of resistance.

A number of serious systemic staphylococcal infections have been treated successfully with dimethoxyphenyl penicillin. The recommended dose for adults is 1 Gm every 4 hr, and for children 100 mg per kg body weight per day in equally divided quantities. The agent must be given parenterally; either intramuscular or intravenous injection leads to rapid excretion, useful levels being demonstrable for 4 hr when the former route is used and for 3 hr when the latter is employed. Benemid does not retard the excretion of this type of penicillin. Large quantities must be administered before the antibiotic will diffuse into the cerebrospinal fluid. Among the untoward effects which have been observed following the use of dimethoxyphenyl penicillin are pain and tenderness at the site of injection, local reactions, hypersensitivity phenomena (in patients allergic to other forms of penicillin) and superinfections.

The development of dimethoxyphenyl penicillin unquestionably represents a major advance in the treatment of infections due to penicillinase-producing staphylococci. This agent is yet too new to have undergone complete evaluation, however, and the conclusions drawn presently may be modified by longer experience.

Penicillin is almost devoid of toxicity in the human being. It does produce, however, a number of untoward effects, many of which are due to the development of hypersensitivity. These are discussed below.

The clinical use of penicillin in treating specific infections is discussed in detail in other chapters of this book.

STREPTOMYCIN

Streptomycin, an antibiotic produced by *Staphylococcus griseus*, is active against the tubercle bacillus and both gram-positive and gram-negative bacteria. Dihydrostreptomycin, a hydrogenated derivative of streptomycin, is no longer used in clinical practice because of its propensity to produce irreparable nerve deafness. The exact mode of action of the drug is not known. For antibacterial activity to be present, the exposed organisms must be metabolically active but do not need to be growing. The drug interferes with normal cell division without disturbing cell growth. It has been suggested that streptomycin interferes with the formation of adaptive enzymes in inhibiting respiration.

Streptomycin salts are readily soluble in water. The drug is poorly absorbed from the gastrointestinal tract but when given parenterally is well absorbed and distributed evenly in extracellular fluids. It penetrates the blood–spinal fluid barrier poorly unless meningeal inflammation is present. Renal excretion is largely by filtration, 80 per cent of the antibiotic appearing in the urine over a period of 24 hr.

The main route of administration of streptomycin is intramuscular. When a local effect in the intestinal tract is desired, the drug is given orally: it is not absorbed in appreciable quantities when given in this manner. The infections in which streptomycin may be of value are those produced by *Hemophilus influenzae,* some strains of *Escherichia coli, Aerobacter aerogenes,* and uncommonly proteus, the tubercle bacillus, and some strains of *Staphylococcus aureus* and *Streptococcus viridans.* The usual dose for adults is 1 to 2 Gm per day in equally spaced and divided quantities; in tuberculosis, the entire daily dose may be given as a single injection. For oral administration, the recommended dose is 0.25 to 0.5 Gm every 6 hr. Intrathecal administration may be important in the management of meningitis due to organisms susceptible to streptomycin. The most important untoward reactions are fever, rashes, urinary tract infection, vestibular dysfunction, and deafness.

Specific indications for the use of streptomycin in various diseases are discussed in other chapters of this book.

CHLORTETRACYCLINE (Aureomycin)

This antibiotic, a product of *Streptomyces aureofaciens,* has a wide range of activity, encompassing not only many gram-positive and gram-negative bacteria, but also the *rickettsias* and some of the larger "viruses." Many strains of *Staphylococcus aureus* and some of the gram-negative bacteria such as *Proteus vulgaris* and pseudomonas may become rapidly insensitive to the drug. Absorption from the gastrointestinal tract is rapid but inefficient, as a result of destruction of the antibiotic by intestinal contents. After a single oral dose, it can be demonstrated in the urine for as long as 24 hr. Concentration in the plasma falls rapidly below detectable level. Only a small proportion of the quantity injected parenterally can be demonstrated in the urine. Aureomycin diffuses into the spinal fluid but in smaller amounts than into the plasma. Subcutaneous and intramuscular injections are not practical because of local irritation. When the drug is given by mouth, nausea and vomiting occur occasionally. Attempts to overcome this gastric irritation by the administration of aluminum hydroxide lead to a reduction of the serum concentration of Aureomycin by 80 per cent or more; these two agents should not be used together. The ingestion of milk or food reduces gastric irritation without altering plasma levels of the drug. Mild diarrhea, associated with loose, bulky stools, may be caused by the local irritation or alteration in the bacterial flora of the intestinal tract due to the antibiotic.

The dose of the antibiotic is 1 to 2 Gm per day, given in divided doses at 6-hr intervals. The dose for intravenous administration (buffered solutions) in adults should not exceed 2 Gm per day because of the risk of "toxic" hepatitis.

OXYTETRACYCLINE (Terramycin)

Terramycin, an antibiotic produced by *Streptomyces rimosus,* is very closely related chemically to Aureomycin. It may be administered orally or intravenously. The most commonly used form of Terramycin is the capsule of the crystalline hydrochloride salt for oral use. Intravenous injection of this antibiotic should be reserved for instances of severe illness or for cases in which it cannot be taken by mouth. Solutions of Terramycin must be properly buffered.

Terramycin is absorbed rapidly from the gastrointestinal tract. No significant difference is present in the plasma concentration when the agent is given in the fasting or nonfasting state. A single oral dose may produce detectable concentrations in the blood for as long as 24 hr. When 250 mg of the drug is given at 6-hr intervals, blood levels are usually in the order of 5 to 10 μg per ml throughout the 24-hr period. Intravenous injection produces serum levels ranging between 5 and 10 μg per ml at the end of 1 hr and from 1 to 5 μg per ml after 12 hr.

The clinical applications of Terramycin are practically the same as those of Aureomycin.

TETRACYCLINE (Achromycin)

Achromycin is closely related chemically to both Aureomycin and Terramycin. It is essentially the skeleton structure of these two antibiotics and is prepared synthetically. The biologic activity of Achromycin is equal to that of Aureomycin and Terramycin. Achromycin is useful in the same infections as are known to respond favorably to either Aureomycin or Terramycin. The incidence of side reactions, such as nausea, vomiting, and diarrhea, is said to be lower following the use of Achromycin than has been observed with the other related drugs. The development of bacterial resistance to Achromycin is accompanied by simultaneous loss of sensitivity to other agents.

Achromycin is stable in solution. The drug is available in the form of the crystalline hydrochloride in capsules and as a dispersible powder, for intravenous use. Intravenous therapy should be employed only in patients who are unable to take medication by mouth. The average adult dose is 500 mg intravenously at 12-hr intervals. This dosage may be increased to a maximum of 500 mg every 6 hr. For oral treatment a dose of 1 to 2

Gm divided into four doses per day is usually adequate.

DEMETHYLCHLORTETRACYCLINE (Declomycin)

Demethylchlortetracycline is a fermentation product of a mutant strain of *Streptomyces aureofaciens*. It differs from chlortetracycline in the absence of a methyl group. Declomycin is highly stable and is about twice as active as Achromycin against most organisms. The rate of renal excretion is less than half of Achromycin. Smaller doses of Declomycin are required than of Achromycin to obtain the same clinical result. The demethylated compound needs to be given less frequently; two doses per day are said to suffice. Large quantities may produce diarrhea. Photosensitivity may develop during ingestion of Declomycin.

CHLORAMPHENICOL (Chloromycetin)

The initial preparations of Chloromycetin, a fermentation product of *Streptomyces venezuelae*, have been isolated in pure crystalline form and synthesized. There is no difference in the antibacterial activity of the synthetic and the natural products. Chloromycetin affects the amino acid metabolism and drastically inhibits protein synthesis in sensitive organisms.

Chloromycetin is stable in the dry state. It is highly soluble in water. Some of its salts are soluble.

Most treatment with Chloromycetin is carried out by the oral route, although preparations are available for intramuscular or intravenous injection. The demonstration that this agent may on occasion depress the bone marrow suggests caution in its administration. The drug is rapidly absorbed from the gastrointestinal tract, appearing in the blood within a few minutes. The maximal concentration occurs at the end of 2 hr, but some may still be found after 16 or 24 hr. About 80 per cent of the quantity administered orally can be demonstrated in the urine; however, only about 15 per cent is biologically active. Inactivation appears to be due to conjugation with glucuronic acid.

A large number of organisms are susceptible to Chloromycetin. Although it is active against some types of gram-positive bacteria, it is most effective against the rickettsias and gram-negative organisms. *Staphylococcus aureus*, coliform bacilli, and other enteric organisms are known to become resistant to this antibiotic.

Aside from the mild gastrointestinal irritation produced by Chloromycetin, the most serious untoward effect which results is depression of the bone marrow. Granulopenia develops first and may be followed by aplastic anemia if administra-

tion of the drug is continued; this is rare. The other complications of Chloromycetin therapy are discussed below.

ERYTHROMYCIN (Ilotycin)

Erythromycin, an antibiotic elaborated by *Streptomyces erythreus*, has been produced in crystalline form. It is soluble only to the extent of 2 mg per ml in water, but it is highly soluble in alcohols and in a number of other organic solvents.

The usual route of administration of erythromycin is by mouth; the drug is absorbed from the intestinal tract. There is a rough correlation between maximal blood level and the dose of antibiotic ingested. Peak serum concentrations appear 1 to 2 hr after ingestion of a dose and decline rapidly so that the agent is no longer demonstrable after 4 to 6 hr. Only small amounts are recovered from the urine.

Gram-positive organisms, including *Staphylococcus aureus*, are highly sensitive to erythromycin, being inhibited, on the average, by concentrations of less than 1 μg per ml.

In clinical practice, the use of erythromycin should be restricted to the treatment of infections due to staphylococci or other penicillin-resistant gram-positive organisms. It is also of value in the therapy of beta-hemolytic streptococcal and pneumococcal infections in individuals sensitized to penicillin.

Bacteria exposed to erythromycin either in vitro or in vivo become resistant to the drug quite rapidly.

BACITRACIN

Bacitracin, a polypeptide antibiotic produced by a strain of *Bacillus subtilis*, has an antibacterial spectrum resembling that of penicillin. The drug is soluble in water or physiologic saline solution. For systemic administration it is usually dissolved in 2 per cent procaine solution in physiologic saline solution.

Very little bacitracin is absorbed from the gastrointestinal tract, although it inhibits the growth of many bacteria in the bowel, including clostridia and gram-positive cocci. The antibiotic appears in the blood and tissues, but very little diffuses into the cerebrospinal fluid after intramuscular injection. The renal clearance of the drug is low and approximates the glomerular filtration rate. Bacitracin is excreted slowly; plasma concentrations may remain elevated for several hours.

Bacitracin has its greatest clinical application in the therapy of infections due to *Staphylococcus aureus* and other gram-positive bacteria, particularly those resistant to other antibiotics. The intramuscular dose is 15,000 to 20,000 units given four times a day. Larger quantities increase the risk of serious renal damage. Careful attention must be given to the development of nephrotoxic manifestations; if kidney dysfunction becomes appreciable, the drug should be discontinued.

POLYMYXIN (Aerosporin)

Polymyxin is a polypeptide antibiotic obtained from *Bacillus polymyxa*. The principal effect is upon gram-negative bacilli, for which it is one of the most potent chemotherapeutic agents available; strains of *Proteus* are, however, resistant. The drug can be administered intramuscularly at intervals of 8 or 12 hr, the total daily dose being 0.2 to 0.5 Gm. It is not absorbed from the bowel, but it eliminates sensitive organisms from the intestinal flora. Following parenteral use it disappears from the blood quickly. It does not pass into the cerebrospinal fluid and cannot be detected in the bile or in the urine in biologically active form. Considerable limitation of usefulness arises from its toxicity for the kidney, and because of the danger of renal damage, this chemotherapeutic agent should be employed only when others are ineffective and when the patient's life is in jeopardy. Impressive clinical results have been produced in some cases of *Pseudomonas aeruginosa* bacteremia or meningitis.

NEOMYCIN

Neomycin, an antibiotic derived from a strain of *Streptomyces* closely related to *Streptomyces fradiae*, is a basic compound, heat stable, and resistant to the action of acid (pH 2). It is bactericidal in vitro against a wide variety of gram-negative and gram-positive organisms. There is some indication that it is highly effective in the treatment of infections due to *Proteus vulgaris*. The drug has been administered by oral and parenteral routes. Absorption from the intestinal tract is relatively poor. The usual oral dose of neomycin is 2 Gm in divided doses per day. The antibiotic may also be administered intramuscularly; the daily dose is 1 to 2 Gm.

Although the in vitro antibacterial effectiveness of neomycin is impressive, its clinical usefulness is sharply limited by high toxicity when it is given parenterally. Kidney and eighth nerve damage occur in a significant number of patients. In view of these untoward effects, neomycin should *never* be the first drug employed in the treatment of any infection. It should be reserved for those diseases in which no other antibiotic is effective and in which the infection threatens life.

NOVOBIOCIN

Novobiocin (Cathomycin, Streptonivicin, Albamycin, Cardelmycin) is elaborated by both *Streptomyces niveus* and *Streptomyces spheroides*. It is a dibasic substance. Salts formed with metal ions dissolve readily in aqueous solution. In vitro, the drug inhibits the growth of strains of *Staphylococcus aureus* resistant to other antibiotics as well as hemolytic streptococci, brucellas, the pneumococcus, the meningococcus, *Hemophilus pertussis*, pasteurella, and proteus organisms. There is a marked decrease in antibacterial activity in the presence of serum; more than 90 per cent of novobiocin appears to be bound to serum protein. The drug is rapidly absorbed from the intestinal tract; it may also be given parenterally. It is excreted slowly in the urine; appreciable amounts are detectable in the serum for 24 hr.

The use of novobiocin should be restricted to the treatment of staphylococcal infections due to strains which are insusceptible to other antibiotic agents, because it has no advantages over other drugs when employed for the eradication of other sensitive organisms. However, proteus is sometimes sensitive to novobiocin, and its use has proved effective in infections produced by strains of this organism insensitive to other antibiotics. Staphylococci become resistant to novobiocin rapidly. For this reason, it should not be administered alone but should be given concurrently with another antibiotic to which the infecting strain is sensitive. The usual dose of novobiocin is 0.5 Gm at 6-hr intervals orally, or 1 to 2 Gm, in equally divided doses, intramuscularly. Nausea, vomiting, dermatitis, and fever have been noted following its administration.

KANAMYCIN (Kantrex)

Kanamycin is a water-soluble basic antibiotic obtained as a fermentation product of *Streptomyces kanamyceticus*. It is distinct from but related closely to neomycin and has a lesser but definite relationship to streptomycin. It is active against gram-negative bacteria such as *Escherichia coli*, *Aerobacter aerogenes*, salmonella; gram-positive organisms, such as *Staphylococcus pyogenes* var. *aureus*, and the tubercle bacillus. It is ineffective against streptococci, *Diplococcus pneumonia*, and clostridia. In high concentrations the drug is bactericidal, in lower ones bacteriostatic.

Kanamycin has been shown to be of use in a limited number of cases of urinary tract infection, shigellosis, typhoid fever, bacteremia due to gram-negative bacteria, peritonitis, systemic staphylococcal infections, and some types of tuberculosis. It must be stressed that, although kanamycin is a so-called "broad-spectrum" antibiotic, it is not a substitute for all other antimicrobial agents. This drug should be reserved for the management of infections due to organisms not susceptible to those antibiotics with which there has been a much broader and extensive experience. Kanamycin has been suggested for the reduction of intestinal bacteria; for this purpose it is given orally, since, by this route, it is very poorly absorbed and the risks of toxicity are minimal.

For the treatment of systemic infection in adults, the recommended dose of kanamycin is 0.25 to 0.5 Gm every 4 hr intramuscularly. When this antibiotic is given orally, the suggested dose is 4 to 12 Gm per day. Intramuscular injection of the drug yields peak blood levels at 1 to 2 hr, the concentration varying with the quantity administered. Kanamycin is secreted into the cerebrospinal fluid, bone, and heart very poorly. The concentrations in the kidneys and muscle approximate those in the blood.

Among the untoward effects of the parenteral administration of kanamycin are pain at the site of injection, skin eruptions, damage to the eighth nerve, and nephrotoxicity. The latter two are the most important; their incidence is related to the total dose of the drug given. The risk is less with 25 mg per kg than with 50 mg per kg. Most patients who receive kanamycin develop cylindruria, and many develop albuminuria.

VANCOMYCIN (Vancocin)

Vancomycin, a water-soluble antibiotic elaborated by *Streptococcus orientalis,* is active mainly against the beta-hemolytic streptococcus, *Streptococcus faecalis, Diplococcus pneumoniae, Neisseria gonorrhoeae, Corynebacterium diphtheriae, Clostridium tetani,* and staphylococcus and ineffective against all gram-negative rods, such as *Escherichia coli, Aerobacter aerogenes,* pseudomonas, and proteus, and the tubercle bacillus, yeasts, and fungi. The majority of strains of staphylococcus are inhibited by a concentration of 2 μg per ml. Resistance to vancomycin develops in staphylococci only to a very small degree, if at all.

Vancomycin is not absorbed from the gastrointestinal tract and must be administered intravenously to produce the desired clinical effect. The usual parenteral dose for adults is 1 to 2 Gm, divided into four equal parts per day. The administration of 500 mg intravenously every 6 hr is recommended for the treatment of staphylococcal bacteremia. This is increased to 1 Gm every 6 hr in cases of endocarditis or meningitis due to *Staphylococcus pyogenes* var. *aureus.* The usual period of therapy is 2 to 4 weeks. The drug is best dissolved in distilled water, 20 ml for 1 Gm for intravenous administration.

Pain at the site of intravenous injection of vancomycin is relatively frequent. Thrombophlebitis is common, especially in children and adults with small veins. Skin eruptions, usually morbilliform in character, may result from sensitization to the drug. Most patients receiving vancomycin have a large number of hyaline and granular casts and albumin in the urine, and nitrogen retention can appear. Nerve deafness may also occur.

RISTOCETIN (Spontin)

Ristocetin, an antibiotic elaborated by *Nocardia lurida,* contains two components, ristocetin A and ristocetin B, the latter being about three times more active than the former. The drug is bactericidal at the same level as it is bacteriostatic and is active against gram-positive organisms including staphylococci, enterococci, beta-hemolytic streptococcus, clostridia, *Diplococcus pneumoniae, Actinomyces bovis,* listerias, and mycobacteria including the tubercle bacillus. It is said to be especially effective against staphylococci resistant to a variety of other antibiotics. There is no cross resistance with erythromycin or penicillin.

The main application of ristocetin at present is the treatment of staphylococcal infections produced by strains of organisms insensitive to the more commonly used antibiotics. It is not the drug of choice in the management of disease due to pneumococci or beta-hemolytic streptococci. Infections produced by enterococci resistant to other antibiotics may respond to the administration of ristocetin, and the use of this agent should be considered in instances of endocarditis due to strains of this organism insensitive to penicillin. The drug is of no value in the management of disease due to gram-negative bacilli, such as *Escherichia coli, Aerobacter aerogenes,* proteus, and pseudomonas.

Ristocetin is not absorbed from the gastrointestinal tract and requires intravenous or intramuscular injection when used to treat systemic infections. The dose for serious infections is 50 mg per kg body weight divided in two equal parts given at 12-hr intervals; for less serious disease, the dose is reduced to 25 to 37 mg per kg. The intravenous route yields the highest blood levels, but intramuscular administration of large doses produces satisfactory serum concentrations.

Ristocetin is excreted largely in the urine. It does not penetrate the normal meninges, and cerebrospinal fluid levels are not produced or are very low. The action of ristocetin is enhanced in the presence of globulin.

Thrombophlebitis occurs at the site of intravenous injection of ristocetin. Skin eruptions and fever have followed use of the drug. Rarely, depression of the white blood count with the development of neutropenia may occur. Thrombopenia, with and without bleeding into the skin and mucous membranes, has also been observed. Patients receiving ristocetin should have white blood counts carried out every other day. Smears of the blood should be studied carefully for the presence of an adequate number of neutrophils and thrombocytes; in questionable cases, it is important to determine the total number of platelets.

PAROMOMYCIN (Humatin)

Paromomycin, an antibiotic produced by a strain of *Streptomyces,* is presently employed for reduction of the number of bacteria in the intestinal tract and for the treatment of intestinal infections due to salmonellas, shigellas, and *Endamoeba histolytica.* This drug is effective in vitro against gram-positive organisms including *Corynebacterium diphtheriae, Staphylococcus aureus,* and *Streptococcus fecalis* and gram-negative bacilli such as *Escherichia coli, Aerobacter aerogenes,* paracolon bacillus, *Klebsiella pneumoniae, Pasteurella multocida,* brucellas, and some species of *Proteus.* It is also active both in vitro and in vivo against the tubercle bacillus. *Pseudomonas aeruginosa* is not affected.

Data concerning the effects of parenteral administration of Humatin are too meager to allow any conclusions concerning its range of therapeutic activity and untoward effects at the moment. Most of the available information concerns the oral administration of this agent which, given by this route, has a low degree of toxicity and is absorbed from the gastrointestinal tract to only a very limited degree.

Paromomycin is effective in the management of enteritis due to strains of *Salmonella* or *Shigella.* It has also been shown to eradicate the chronic carrier state with these organisms: failures after one course of therapy for 2 weeks frequently clear following a second exposure to the drug; the dose usually employed is 2 Gm per day orally. Humatin is a direct amebicidal agent: infections of the colon due to *Endamoeba histolytica* respond rapidly and with a high degree of success to the daily ingestion of 15 to 25 mg per kg body weight of the drug for 7 to 10 days. Both trophozoites and cyst forms are eliminated. This drug is presently thought to be the most effective of the antibiotics, with the exception of fumagillin, for the management of amebiasis.

NYSTATIN (Mycostatin)

Nystatin, elaborated by *Streptomyces noursei,* is insoluble in fat solvents, highly soluble in methanol, and soluble to the extent of 10 to 20 units per ml in water. It is poorly absorbed from the gastrointestinal tract. High blood levels follow intravenous injection. This antimycotic agent is employed for local application in the form of ointments, solutions, powders, suppositories, and gels. Topical use in the treatment of candida infections of the skin and vagina has been reported to be successful.

The usual oral dose of nystatin is 150 mg (500,-000 units) three times a day. Although an occasional case of disseminated mycotic infection has been treated parenterally with nystatin with reported good results, the place of this agent in the therapy of deep-seated mycoses still remains to be determined.

AMPHOTERICIN (Fungizone)

Amphotericin B is the only agent presently available for the treatment of deep-seated mycotic infections. This agent produces cure in most cases of cryptococcosis, histoplasmosis, blastomycosis, disseminated candidiasis, and coccidiomycosis. It may be administered either intravenously or intramuscularly, and must not be dissolved in saline because it precipitates in this medium. For intravenous administration, the drug is dissolved in 5 per cent glucose to a concentration of 1 mg per 10 ml and infused over a period of 6 hr. Solutions maintained at room temperature over 24 hr must be discarded. The initial intravenous dose is 0.25 mg per kg body weight; this is increased by an increment of 0.25 mg per kg per day until a dose of 1 mg per kg is reached, when therapy is continued at this level for 30 to 60 days. In infections which do not respond favorably the dose may be increased to 1.5 mg per kg per day. If therapy is stopped and later reinstituted, it is best to begin again with 0.25 mg per kg. The intramuscular dose is 20 mg dissolved in 2 ml of 5 per cent glucose to which a local anesthetic is added; this quantity is given daily. In mycotic meningitis the intrathecal injection of 0.5 to 1 mg of the drug dissolved in 5 ml of water every 48 hr has been recommended. The initial intravenous administration of amphotericin is frequently associated with a febrile response often accompanied by chills. These reactions tend to diminish with each succeeding infusion, and their frequency and intensity may be reduced by giving an antipyretic or antihistaminic agent prior to treatment. The drug should be omitted during a febrile reaction. Among the other untoward effects of amphotericin are headache, nausea, vomiting, phlebitis, hepatitis, and azotemia. Increase in nonprotein nitrogen should not be allowed to exceed 40 mg per 100 ml. If the nonprotein nitrogen rises, the antibiotic should be withheld temporarily or given on alternate days.

GRISEOFULVIN

Griseofulvin is an antifungal agent produced by several species of *Penicillium*. Exposure of certain fungi to this agent leads to shriveling of the hyphae which become stunted, the so-called "curling" phenomenon. The drug probably acts by interfering with nucleic acid synthesis. It is absorbed from the gastrointestinal tract and incorporated in newly growing cells: it is found in the hair of persons under treatment.

Griseofulvin is effective in the treatment of infection due to dermatophytes. Thus, tinea capitis, corporis, and cruris, onychomycosis, and dermatophytosis respond well to the administration of this agent. The drug is fungistatic but not fungicidal for *Trichophyton gypseum, rubrum, schoenlenii, sulfureum, tonsurans,* and *verrucosum; Epidermophyton floccosum;* and *Microsporum audounii, canis,* and *gypseum*. Infections due to these organisms respond to the use of griseofulvin. Candidiasis, blastomycosis, actinomycosis, torulosis, pityriasis versicolor, and mucormycosis are unaffected by the drug.

The dose of griseofulvin is 250 mg given orally three to four times a day in adults; in children, one-half the adult quantity is administered. Therapy must be continued for an adequate period. The average duration of treatment for tinea capitis, cruris, and corporis is 2 to 8 weeks; infections of the palms and soles require a longer period of exposure to the drug. Griseofulvin must be given for 4 to 6 months to eradicate onychomycosis; involvement of the toenails requires longer treatment than that of the fingernails. Attempts to reduce the duration of therapy have been made using topical application of the antibiotic (1.5 per cent in suspension with surfactants, stabilizer, and urea in glyceride oil) or by a short oral administration followed by surgical removal of the affected nail. Relapses are not infrequent but usually respond to re-treatment.

Although griseofulvin has been used for only a short period of time, the untoward reactions which have been observed include nausea, vomiting, epigastric discomfort, dizziness, insomnia, anorexia, fatigue, diarrhea, stomatitis, albuminuria without decrease in renal function, transient leukopenia, and urticarial, vesicular, and maculopapular rashes. Although suppression of spermatogenesis occurs in animals, this has not been observed in man. Superinfection with candida may develop.

NITROFURANTOIN (Furadantin)

Nitrofurantoin [N-(5-nitro-2-furfurylidene)-1-aminohydantoin] is an antibacterial agent of value primarily in the treatment of some types of urinary tract infection. It is poorly soluble in water. The drug is bacteriostatic and, in high concentrations, is bactericidal. It is most active against *Escherichia coli* (bactericidal), of intermediate effectiveness against *Aerobacter aerogenes,* and completely without effect against *Pseudomonas aeruginosa* (*P. pyocyanea*). The activity of the drug against *Proteus* is variable, although many strains are quite sensitive. *Staphylococcus aureus* and enterococci are inhibited by low concentrations.

Nitrofurantoin is administered orally, usually in a dose of 7 to 10 mg per kg body weight (100 to 200 mg four times a day). Useful blood levels cannot be produced. The drug is excreted in the urine. Within 4 to 6 hr after a maximal clinical dose, the concentration in the urine is 25 to 50 mg per 100 ml; 8 hr after a dose, the levels are low. With highly alkaline urine, as is the case in proteus infection, the inhibitory effect of nitrofurantoin appears to be depressed; for this reason, the simultaneous administration of an acidifying agent has been suggested. The development of bacterial resistance to the drug has not been noted.

The infections of the urinary tract which respond most favorably to therapy with nitrofurantoin are the acute and uncomplicated ones. Infections produced by *E. coli* are the most easily eradicated by this agent. Those due to *P. aeruginosa* are totally unaffected, and infections caused by *Aerobacter aerogenes* occupy an intermediate position. *Pseudomonas aeruginosa* may appear in the urine for the first time during a course of treatment with nitrofurantoin. Although the drug has been said to be most active against proteus infection, the results are quite variable. Not infrequently, this organism is only temporarily suppressed and reappears after cessation of therapy.

Nitrofurantoin is relatively nontoxic. Nausea, with or without vomiting, is the commonest untoward reaction. Various types of rashes have been described. Leukopenia occurs rarely.

TUBERCULOSTATIC DRUGS

Although streptomycin is effective in the treatment of all types of tuberculosis, the use of this agent alone leaves much to be desired in the way of maximal antibacterial effect as well as in preventing the emergence of drug-resistant strains of *Mycobacterium tuberculosis*. For these reasons, attempts have been made to develop other compounds possessing tuberculostatic activity which might be given concurrently with streptomycin. Two such agents are para-aminosalicylic acid and isonicotinic acid hydrazide.

Para-aminosalicylic Acid (PAS). Para-aminosalicylic acid, a white crystalline powder, is sparingly soluble in water but easily dissolved in the form of its sodium salt. This agent has a bacteriostatic effect in vitro against many strains of *Mycobacterium tuberculosis,* even those which have become streptomycin-resistant. The antibacterial activity is not inhibited by serum or sodium salicylate but is partially decreased by para-aminobenzoic acid (PABA).

Para-aminosalicyclic acid and its sodium salt when given orally are rapidly absorbed and quickly excreted. It is necessary to give the drug frequently in order to reach and maintain adequate blood levels. A single dose produces maximal serum concentration within 30 to 60 min of administration; thereafter there is a gradual fall so that the agent disappears from the blood in 2 to 3 hr.

Para-aminosalicyclic acid is usually given orally. Since considerable gastric irritation may result from the large quantities necessary, the concurrent administration of various types of alkali or milk is advisable. Various mixtures containing flavoring and alkaline compounds have been employed. Preparations for intravenous use are also available; these should be reserved for patients in whom severe gastric distress prohibits oral use or for those in coma. The usual quantity given by mouth is 8 to 12 Gm per day in divided doses. Although it has been reported that PAS alone may be effective in the treatment of mild tuberculous infections, it is best to give this agent together with streptomycin. The details of this type of treatment are described on p. 1010. Tubercle bacilli may become resistant to PAS if this drug is used alone.

The most common toxic effects produced by PAS are nausea, vomiting, and burning epigastric distress. Diarrhea occurs occasionally. Toxic damage to the liver and potassium deficiency have been recorded. Occasionally tinnitus and reduction in the acuity of hearing may develop; they usually disappear rapidly after cessation of treatment.

Isonicotinic Acid Hydrazide. Of all the tuberculostatic agents, isonicotinic acid hydrazide has the highest activity in vitro. It is not effective against organisms other than *Mycobacteria.*

Isonicotinic acid hydrazide is administered orally, as a rule, and is almost completely absorbed from the digestive tract. One-half to three-quarters of the amount ingested is recovered from the urine in 24 hr, and not more than 5 to 10 per cent appears in the feces. The peak serum concentration may occur 1 to 3 hr after administration, and minimal detectable concentrations persist for 6 to 24 hr. The drug is well distributed in the various body fluids and is not inactivated by them; it is present in sputum, urine, pleural exudate, plasma, and cerebrospinal fluid in active form. It passes the blood-brain barrier readily, and in cases of meningeal inflammation the quantities in the spinal fluid may be larger than those in the plasma, making it extremely valuable in tuberculous meningitis.

Cultures of tubercle bacilli acquire resistance to isonicotinic acid hydrazide readily. Insensitive strains are recovered from the majority of tuberculous patients who receive this drug alone for 1 to 2 months. There is no cross resistance between isonicotinic acid hydrazide and streptomycin or PAS. Isonicotinic acid hydrazide should be given in combination with streptomycin or PAS.

There is a great deal of variation in the metabolism of isonicotinic acid hydrazide in man. Some individuals inactivate the drug slowly, while others inactivate it rapidly. The slow inactivator is an autosomal homozygous recessive, while rapid inactivators are of two types, heterozygotes and homozygous dominants. The process of inactivation is probably enzyme mediated and may consist in a facilitation or speeding of acetylation of the drug. The development of polyneuritis and reversal of infectiousness are more frequent and earlier in slow than in rapid inactivators. There appears to be no association between the isonicotinic acid hydrazide inactivator type and the appearance of drug resistance in tubercle bacilli.

The dosage of this drug is discussed on p. 1010.

Although isonicotinic acid hydrazide is relatively nontoxic, a number of untoward effects may develop. These include drowsiness, hyperreflexia, tremor of the limbs, twitching of the legs, weakness, difficulty of micturition, nausea, abdominal discomfort, transient flushing of the face, pruritic skin eruptions, peripheral neuropathy, acute pellagra, toxic hepatitis with jaundice, temporary arterial vasospasm, epileptiform seizures, and psychotic reactions. The administration of 100 mg per day of pyridoxine virtually eliminates the appearance of reactions related to dysfunction of the nervous system and does not alter the serum concentrations of antimicrobially active isonicotinic acid hydrazide.

Pyrazinamide and Cycloserine. Two of the more recently developed antituberculous agents are cycloserine, a fermentation product of *Streptomyces orchidaceus,* and pyrazinamide (Aldinamide), a synthetic compound. Both have been used in the treatment of human tuberculosis, especially that due to organisms resistant to streptomycin or isonicotinic acid, or both, with promising results; they should not constitute primary therapy. Their effectiveness when given in combination with other tuberculostatic agents is under investigation. The usual dose of cycloserine is 0.75 Gm given four times daily, while that of pyrazinamide is 0.05 Gm per kg body weight per day. Although of low toxicity, cycloserine has been thought to cause epileptiform seizures (10 per cent), changes in personality, or definite depression in some patients. The administration of 100 mg of pyridoxine per day may eliminate all these manifestations. The most serious untoward reaction to pyrazinamide is acute hepatitis; joint pains, nervousness, palpitation, feeling of tightness in the chest, febrile reactions, and eosinophilia have also been noted.

SELECTION OF A CHEMOTHERAPEUTIC AGENT

In the therapy of infections the physician has to choose among an ever-increasing number of antibacterial drugs. In order to obtain the best results, it is essential that he have a working knowledge of the common pathogenic microorganisms. While cultural studies are perhaps theoretically desirable in every case, they are not always practicable. In many instances the etiology can be inferred from the onset and the clinical features of the disease. Nevertheless, it must be stressed that there are situations in which careful bacteriologic studies are essential to proper treatment, and the conscientious physician must take whatever steps are required to obtain experienced bacteriologic help.

Even when the etiology of an infectious process is determined, selection of an appropriate drug does not follow automatically, because there may be wide variations in susceptibility among organisms of the same or related species. For example, in treating a series of proteus infections, it will be found that some strains respond only to streptomycin, others to sulfonamides, Aureomycin, Chloromycetin, or even neomycin. The cost of the different drugs has to be considered at times, since there are very wide differences. The nature of the illness may also affect the choice of agent; for example, an orally administered drug may be unsatisfactory in a patient who is vomiting. In critically ill patients it is sometimes wisest to give a combination of drugs until cultural and sensitivity studies reveal which is specifically indicated. In such cases, cultures should always be taken *before initiation of therapy*. If an individual has previously shown hypersensitivity or any other serious reaction to a drug, or if he develops such untoward effects during therapy, a different agent should be used, if possible. The approximate order of preference of various antibacterial drugs will not be tabulated, as is the usual custom, in this chapter. Instead, the reader is referred to the discussions of the therapy of specific infections in other parts of this book, where the agents of primary and secondary value in treatment are indicated.

COMBINATIONS OF ANTIBACTERIAL AGENTS

Treatment of Mixed Bacterial Infections. In bronchiectasis, peritonitis, and some cases of acute or chronic otitis media and urinary tract infection, two or more organisms are often involved. In some instances, the responsible bacteria, although of different species, are sensitive to a single antimicrobial agent, while in others they have distinctly different drug susceptibilities. This emphasizes the need for determination of the drug sensitivity of each of the components of a mixed flora individually before therapy is initiated. The antibiotics to be given are selected on the basis of these studies and administered in *full doses*. In some cases it may be unnecessary and even dangerous to delay initiation of treatment until definitive bacteriologic data are available. Peritonitis is an outstanding example. Because both gram-positive and gram-negative organisms may be acting synergistically to produce this disease and because delay in therapy may result in a rapidly fatal outcome, treatment should be started immediately with maximal quantities of the antibiotics known to be most effective against these types of bacteria. Many clinicians prefer to give penicillin (5 to 10 million units per day) together with streptomycin (1 to 2 Gm per day). In bronchiectasis and in chronic otitis media and urinary tract infections, except when acute exacerbations occur, therapy need not be initiated before diagnostic bacteriologic information becomes available because these infections have usually been present for such a long time that a delay of 2 or 3 days makes little or no difference in their outcome.

Reduction of Dose of Drug and Duration of Therapy. The simultaneous administration of penicillin and streptomycin in subacute bacterial endocarditis due to an organism sensitive to both of these agents is said to permit the use of smaller doses of penicillin and allows reduction of the period of therapy from the usual 4 weeks to 2 weeks. This type of therapy requires more confirmation, however, before it can be recommended for general adoption in the management of this disease. The administration of antibiotic combinations to reduce the total dose of drug and the duration of therapy has also been recommended in brucellosis. Whether this principle is applicable in other infections is not known. Therapy for these purposes should be used with caution, however, since the level of antimicrobial activity of a mixture of antibiotics is often unpredictable and may, in fact, be lower than that which obtains when a single drug is given in full therapeutic dose.

Removal of Superficially Located Bacteria. The use of antibiotic combinations has been recommended for treatment of superficial infections, as of the skin, for example, especially when these are due to more than one species of bacteria. On this basis, mixtures of neomycin, polymyxin, and bacitracin have been applied topically because these agents possess a low level of sensitizing capacity.

Some dermatologists have pointed out the lack of evidence in support of such therapy, however. The area of superficial "infection" in which combined therapy appears to be superior to single agents is the intestinal tract. The degree of reduction in the number of organisms in the bowel flora is greater with a combination of neomycin and polymyxin administered orally than when either is given alone. The same is true for polymyxin and streptomycin.

Delay in Rate of Emergence of Bacterial Resistance. Clinical investigations have indicated that delay of emergence of antibiotic resistance is produced by combinations of antimicrobial drugs in some types of infection but not in all. Thus, the concomitant administration of two or more drugs suppresses strikingly the development of resistance in the tubercle bacillus. Tuberculosis is best treated, therefore, with at least two and in some instances (miliary tuberculosis and tuberculous meningitis) with three tuberculostatic agents simultaneously. The same appears to be true in *Hemophilus influenzae* meningitis in which it has been shown that the injection of streptomycin together with the exhibition of sulfonamide eliminates the appearance of streptomycin resistance in the organism.

It is common practice to treat all systemic staphylococcal infections with more than one antibiotic. The need for this type of therapy has recently been questioned, however, because evidence that *Staphylococcus pyogenes* var. *aureus* becomes drug resistant in vivo is difficult to substantiate. In "closed" infections, endocarditis, for example, the administration of a single potent antibiotic rarely leads to the appearance of insensitive staphylococci. In "open" infection, such as wounds or pneumonia, on the other hand, resistance appears to develop. It has been postulated that this is not due to a change in the organism responsible for the infection initially but results from the introduction of a new drug-insensitive strain from the patient's environment. In accordance with this concept, some physicians are now treating staphylococcal infections with a single effective drug. It must be pointed out, however, that until it has been definitely proved that combined chemotherapy is not necessary for certain types of staphylococcal infection, it is best to use more than one antibiotic in the treatment of all forms of this disease. Clinical experience suggests that, when this is done, the appearance of resistant strains is a relatively uncommon problem. Combinations of drugs may be effective in preventing the implantation of new strains or eradicating them if they have managed to gain a foothold. When more than one drug is administered, the infecting organism must be sensitive to both agents.

"Fixed Dose" Combinations. A valid experimental approach to the study of the in vivo activity of antibiotic combinations versus single agents is the determination of the antibacterial capacity of the blood of patients receiving the drugs. On the basis of a series of studies using this technique, the following conclusions have been drawn:

Combinations encourage the use of inadequate treatment, since there is an inevitable tendency to use the same total dose of the combination as of the single agent, and this does not provide the expected effective dose of either, particularly of the inferior drug. They provide a false sense of security as offering a wider coverage or broad spectrum of activity when in fact they provide a narrower effective coverage by substituting less active agents and smaller amounts of individual agents than if antibiotics were chosen individually each for its own purpose and given in the proper dose for that purpose. They reduce the therapeutic effectiveness that might be expected from proper dosage of individual agents or from the proper selection of combinations of agents according to specific requirements, particularly when care is taken to choose only agents that may be expected to be the most active against the causative organism.

Therapy of Severe Infections in Which Specific Etiology Is Unknown. The commonest use of antibiotic combinations is for the treatment of infections the etiology of which is not immediately apparent. The physician with a patient whom he suspects of having bacterial infection often decides that chemotherapy is necessary. Because the exact cause cannot be immediately determined, more than one agent is given in the hope that this will "cover" the situation: "fixed dose" mixtures are very often used for this purpose. In not a small number of cases, the infectious process is due to some virus and the application of any antimicrobial agent is not indicated.

When "full dose" combinations are to be given in the absence of a specific bacteriologic diagnosis, the physician must decide, on the basis of the clinical features of the disease, a detailed history, and laboratory investigations, including examination of stained preparations, if possible, not only that a patient has a bacterial infection but also the type of organism which is most likely to be involved. *Under no circumstances must chemotherapy be initiated until all the necessary bacteriologic investigations have been started.*

THE PROPHYLAXIS OF INFECTION

The chemotherapeutic agents now available offer an excellent means of prophylaxis in some but not all infectious diseases. Chemoprophylaxis has been used primarily for four purposes: (1) to protect healthy individuals, either singly or in groups of varying size, against invasion by specific micro-organisms; (2) to prevent bacterial infection in individuals acutely ill with diseases, often of viral origin, for which antimicrobial agents are not effective; (3) to reduce the risk of infection in patients with various types of chronic illness; and (4) to inhibit the spread of disease from areas of localized infection, or to prevent infection in general, in persons who have been subjected to accidental or surgical trauma. Experience over the years has indicated the areas in which chemoprophylaxis is of proved value and those in which it is totally ineffective and may, in fact, be associated with an increased risk of infection. There still remain, however, instances in which opinion concerning the efficacy of antimicrobial agents in preventing bacterial invasion is unsettled. In general, it may be said that, when the purpose of chemoprophylaxis is the prevention of implantation or early eradication of a single specific organism by the use of a single potent drug, it has a high degree of success. If, on the other hand, the purpose is to prevent implantation of any or all bacteria that happen to be in the patient's internal or external environment, failure is the usual results.

Table 111-1 lists the diseases or situations in which chemoprophylaxis is of proved or unsettled degree of value and those in which experience has indicated lack of success. The antibiotics used are indicated; the doses and methods of administration are discussed in the sections dealing with the specific disease entities discussed elsewhere in this book.

Table 111-1. VALUE OF CHEMOPROPHYLAXIS

I. *Chemoprophylaxis of proved value*
  1. Streptococcal (group A) infections and rheumatic fever recurrences: sulfonamides, various forms of penicillin, erythromycin
  2. Bacillary dysentery: sulfonamides, chloramphenicol
  3. Diarrhea due to enteropathogenic *Escherichia coli:* neomycin orally
  4. Gonorrhea—acute urethritis and ophthalmia: penicillin
  5. Congenital syphilis (treatment of mother): penicillin
  6. Meningococcal infections: sulfonamides
  7. Dental extraction in presence of heart disease: penicillin
  8. Mucoviscidosis: tetracycline compounds
  9. Hepatic coma: neomycin or paromomycin orally
  10. Contaminated or infected wound surgery: penicillin plus streptomycin
  11. Labor when membranes ruptured over 24 to 48 hr: penicillin plus streptomycin
  12. Steroid therapy in patients with high risk of tuberculosis

Table 111-1. VALUE OF CHEMOPROPHYLAXIS (*Continued*)

II. *Chemoprophylaxis of no value*
  1. Viral infections of upper respiratory tract including common cold, influenza, and CA, CCA, JH, ECHO, Coxsackie, and adenovirus infections
  2. "Atypical viral pneumonia"
  3. Psittacosis
  4. "Childhood" viral diseases—mumps, measles, rubella, chickenpox, vaccinia
  5. Poliomyelitis
  6. Infectious mononucleosis
  7. Smallpox
  8. "Clean" surgical and obstetric procedures
  9. Pertussis
  10. Burns
  11. Shock
  12. Coma
  13. Cardiac failure
  14. Catheterization or other instrumentation of urinary tract
  15. Premature infants
  16. X-ray irradiation
  17. Administration of steroids, except in instances with high risk of tuberculosis

III. *Chemoprophylaxis of unsettled value*
  1. Surgical procedures on heart or urinary tract in presence of chronic cardiac disease
  2. Acute diffuse glomerulonephritis
  3. Syphilis—venereal contact
  4. Chronic nontuberculous pulmonary disease
  5. Tuberculin-negative contacts of active case of tuberculosis
  6. Staphylococcus carrier state
  7. Transmission of *Staphylococcus aureus* in nurseries and other hospital areas
  8. Reduction of number of intestinal bacteria prior to bowel resection
  9. Cardiac catheterization
  10. Exchange transfusion

Dangers of Chemoprophylaxis. It is important to point out that the same untoward effects which occur when antibiotic agents are used for therapeutic purposes are observed when patients who have no active infection are given these drugs. The risk of development of reactions and the difficulties which they involve must always be taken into consideration in planning a program of chemoprophylaxis. When there is no evidence that chemoprophylaxis will be effective, it should not be used.

COMPLICATIONS OF CHEMOTHERAPY

Complications resulting from the widespread use of various chemotherapeutic agents are steadily increasing in frequency. All the available drugs produce one or another type of untoward effect. Some of these effects are directly toxic, some are allergic, and others are related to the biologic activities of the chemotherapeutic substances.

The list of the undesirable effects actually observed and attributed to therapy with the widely used antimicrobial agents is long and varied and involves most of the organ systems. Not all the complications have been observed with each of the chemotherapeutic substances, and some have been noted with only one of them. For purposes of convenience these reactions are discussed here in relation to organ systems. In order to conserve space they are presented in tabular form (Table 111-2).

Table 111-2. COMPLICATIONS OF CHEMOTHERAPY

I. Cutaneous manifestations
   Mostly due to hypersensitivity. Occur with all antibacterial drugs
   1. Morbilliform rashes—commonest
   2. Scarlatiniform, urticarial, vesicular, or bullous eruptions
   3. Purpura, with or without thrombopenia
   4. Erythema multiforme
   5. Stevens-Johnson syndrome (mainly sulfonamides and penicillin)
   6. Erythema nodosum
   7. Exfoliative dermatitis
   8. Inflammatory reactions at site of infection

II. Oral lesions
   Thirty-three different ones described. Noted with many antibiotics. Commonest with broad-spectrum drugs
   1. Dryness, burning, soreness, and itching of mouth and tongue
   2. Vesicular stomatitis
   3. Acute glossitis
   4. Angular stomatitis (cheilosis)
   5. Black or brown "furred" tongue

III. Other manifestations of hypersensitivity
   1. Fever
   2. Contact dermatitis—handling of drugs
   3. Angioedema
   4. Serum sickness (penicillin)
   5. Arthus reaction
   6. Acute anaphylactic shock (rare but commonest with penicillin)
   7. "Allergic" vasculitis
   8. ?Polyarteritis nodosa
   9. ?Systemic lupus erythematosus
   10. Pruritis ani or vulvae

IV. Gastrointestinal and hepatic complications
   Commonest with broad-spectrum antibiotics
   1. Nausea
   2. Vomiting
   3. Heartburn
   4. Diarrhea due to irritation or transformation of bowel flora
   5. *Staphylococcus aureus* enteritis
   6. Pseudomembranous colitis
   7. Stomatitis and pharyngitis due to candida
   8. Jaundice and hepatitis (sulfanilamide)

Table 111-2. COMPLICATIONS OF CHEMOTHERAPY *(Continued)*

   9. Liver damage (tetracyclines intravenously in doses larger than 2 Gm per day, isonicotinic acid hydrazide, pyrazinamide)
   10. Proctitis
   11. Steatorrhea (neomycin)
   12. Malabsorption syndrome (neomycin)

V. Urinary tract complications
   1. Hematuria and crystalluria (sulfonamides)
   2. Acute tubular necrosis (sulfonamides, kanamycin)
   3. Obstruction to urine flow (sulfonamides)
   4. Albuminuria and cylindruria (streptomycin in acid urine, bacitracin, polymyxin, neomycin, vancomycin, kanamycin)
   5. Nephrotoxicity with renal failure (bacitracin, polymyxin, neomycin, kanamycin, vancomycin, amphotericin)

VI. Nervous system complications
   1. Injury to peripheral nerves by direct injection of antibiotic solution
   2. Arachnoiditis (intrathecal injection of antibiotics)
   3. Peripheral neuritis (broad-spectrum antibiotics, isonicotinic acid hydrazide)
   4. Paresthesias (streptomycin, polymyxin)
   5. Damage to eighth cranial nerve (streptomycin, kanamycin, neomycin, vancomycin)
   6. Encephalitis (some sulfonamides)
   7. Encephalopathy (due to *excessive* intrathecal doses of penicillin or streptomycin)
   8. Convulsions (isonicotinic acid hydrazide, cycloserine)
   9. Psychoses (isonicotinic acid hydrazide, cycloserine)
   10. Hyperreflexia, tremors, twitching, difficulty in micturition (isonicotinic acid hydrazide)

VII. Complications in blood and blood-forming organs
   1. Acute hemolytic anemia (sulfonamides)
   2. Eosinophilia (sensitization to any of the drugs)
   3. Thrombopenia (streptomycin, chloramphenicol)
   4. Anemia with absence of reticulocytosis (chloramphenicol)
   5. Granulopenia or aplastic anemia (chloramphenicol, streptomycin, nitrofurantoin, ristocetin)
   6. LE phenomenon (sensitization to penicillin)

VIII. Miscellaneous complications
   1. Negative nitrogen balance (tetracyclines)
   2. Increased riboflavin excretion (tetracyclines)
   3. Hypoprothrombinemia (broad-spectrum drugs given orally)
   4. Decreased or absent formation of urobilinogen (broad-spectrum drugs)
   5. Electrolyte disturbances (streptomycin)
   6. Herxheimer reaction (penicillin in syphilis)
   7. Kernicterus (sulfisoxazole in premature babies)
   8. "Gray" sickness (doses of more than 50 mg per kg body weight of chloramphenicol in

Table 111-2. COMPLICATIONS OF CHEMOTHERAPY
(*Continued*)

    neonates—due to failure of liver to conjugate drug with glucuronic acid—may lead to death)

  9. Photosensitivity (demethylchlortetracycline)

10. "Hypersensitivity" myocarditis (sulfamethoxypyridazine)

11. Acute pellagra (isonicotinic acid hydrazide)

12. Sterile abscesses (intramuscular injection of most antibiotics)

13. Pulmonary embolism (accidental intravenous injections of solutions in oil or insoluble salts of antibiotics)

14. Thrombophlebitis (intravenous injection of tetracycline, erythromycin, vancomycin, ristocetin, amphotericin)

15. Suppression of immune response (antibiotics given in large doses early in course of infection)

16. Changes in bacterial flora of body

17. Transient arterial vasospasm (isonicotinic acid hydrazide)

IX. Superinfections

    These occur with all chemotherapeutic agents. They are due to invasion by normally present organisms or by those acquired by contact with other patients or attendants, or they may result from the accidental introduction of bacteria during injection of the drug; in all instances, the new infections are produced by strains of organisms insensitive to the antibiotic being administered at the time they first appear. Infections due to organisms of the genus *Candida* (*Monilia*) may also occur during chemotherapy; they may involve the mouth, pharynx, or lung, or they may become generalized, when they may be fatal. This type of superinfection is being reported more frequently and is particularly important because no specific agent for treatment of systemic involvement is presently available.

    Superinfections occur in about 2 per cent of patients who receive a chemotherapeutic agent. The organs involved in the secondary infection are most frequently the same as those affected in the primary disease. The organisms responsible for superinfections are often difficult to treat with the presently available antibacterial drugs. The factors which predispose to the development of superinfection are (1) age of three years or less, (2) primary disease of the lower respiratory tract, (3) infection of the middle ear, and (4) the use of a drug or combination of antibiotic agents which tend to have a "broad" antibacterial effect; the "wider" the antimicrobial "spectrum," the greater is the danger of secondary bacterial invasion. Superinfections appear most frequently on the fourth or fifth day after initiation of chemotherapy and may convert a benign, self-limited disease into a serious, prolonged or even fatal one. It is essential to carry out frequent bacteriologic studies, whenever possible, to determine changes in bacterial flora that may subsequently be responsible for a

Table 111-2. COMPLICATIONS OF CHEMOTHERAPY
(*Continued*)

secondary infection. The administration of an antibiotic active against the predominating organism and its elimination before it is responsible for infection may prevent the appearance of a complicating disease.

X. Development of a resistance by some bacteria to any of the chemotherapeutic drugs

    None of the available antibacterial substances is free of the potentialities of producing trouble. With some, like the sulfonamides, the risk of development of serious reactions is great; with others, like penicillin, it is relatively small in comparison to the beneficial effects of the agent. Two types of reaction are common to all the chemotherapeutic agents: (1) the development of hypersensitivity and (2) the production of superinfections by resistant organisms.

    The fact that harmful effects may follow the use of these drugs should not discourage the physician from applying them in situations where they are definitely indicated. It should, however, make him hesitant to employ them in cases where indications for their use are entirely absent or at most only slightly suggestive. Moreover, the appearance of reactions during the course of treatment does not always make the cessation of therapy mandatory, especially if the drug used happens to be the only effective one available for the purpose required. The severity and type of the reactions, their expected course, and the possibility of influencing them by proper management must all be weighed against the importance of the infection under treatment.

MISUSES OF CHEMOTHERAPY

    There is little doubt that the antimicrobial agents are used in many situations where they are not required and that, even when they are indicated, failure to utilize them properly may lead to a poor clinical result. Listed below are the most common misuses of the chemotherapeutic compounds.

  1. Treatment of fever of obscure origin

  2. Choice of ineffective antibiotic

  3. Inadequate or excessive doses

  4. Improper route of administration

  5. Continuation of therapy with drug to which bacterial resistance develops

  6. Failure to stop treatment in presence of serious toxic or allergic reaction

  7. Failure to alter therapy when superinfection occurs

  8. Prophylaxis of unpreventable secondary bacterial infection (see above)

  9. Therapy of insusceptible infections—infections produced by true viruses

10. Use of combinations of drugs when not specifically indicated

11. Reliance on chemotherapy or prophylaxis to the exclusion of necessary surgical intervention, e.g., drainage of localized areas of infection

Probably the most frequent misuse of antimicrobial drugs is in the therapy of fever of unknown origin. The mere presence of fever, in the absence of localizing signs, does not necessarily indicate that it is due to an infectious process (see p. 65). In the absence of strong clinical evidence that a febrile episode is infectious in origin, particularly when there is no detectable focus, chemotherapy should be delayed until adequate clinical and laboratory studies have been performed.

REFERENCES

British Medical Research Council: The Treatment of Pulmonary Tuberculosis with Isoniazid, Brit. Med. J., II:735, 1952.

Coffey, G. L., L. E. Anderson, M. W. Fisher, et al.: Biologic Studies of Paromomycin, Antibiotics & Chemotherapy, 9:730, 1959.

Coles, H. M. T., B. McNamara, L. Mutch, R. J. Holt, and G. T. Stewart: Paromomycin in the Treatment of Shigella and Salmonella Infections in Children, Lancet, II:944, 1960.

Dooner, H. P.: The Treatment of Amebiasis with Paromomycin (Humatin), Antibiotics & Chemotherapy, 7:486, 1960.

Dowling, H. F.: "Tetracycline," New York, Medical Encylopedia, Inc., 1955.

Epstein, I. G., K. G. S. Nair, and L. J. Boyd: Cycloserine, a New Antibiotic in the Treatment of Pulmonary Tuberculosis, Antibiotic Med., 1:80, 1955.

Evans, D. A. P., K. A. Manley, and V. A. McKusick: Genetic Control of Isoniazid Metabolism in Man, Brit. Med. J., II:485, 1960.

Finland, M.: Chemoprophylaxis of Infectious Disease, Disease-a-Month, Chicago, Year Book Publishers, Inc., December, 1959, July, 1960, September, 1960.

——— and L. P. Garrod: Demethylchlortetracycline, Lancet, II:959, 1960.

——— and T. J. Haight: Antibiotic Resistance of Pathogenic Staphylococci, A.M.A. Arch. Internal Med., 91:143, 1953.

——— and L. Weinstein: Complications Induced by Antimicrobial Agents, New Engl. J. Med., 248:220, 1953.

Fisher, M. W., M. C. Manning, L. A. Gagliardi, M. R. Gaetz, and A. L. Erlandson: Paromomycin: Experimental Antibacterial Activity, p. 293, Antibiotics Annual, Antibiotica Inc., New York, 1959–1960.

Gocke, T. M., and M. Finland: Cross Resistance to Antibiotics, J. Lab. Clin. Med., 38:719, 1951.

Goldman, L., J. Schwarz, R. H. Preston, A. Beyer, and J. Loutzenhiser: Current Status of Griseofulvin, J.A.M.A., 172:532, 1960.

Herrell, W. E.: "Erythromycin," New York, Medical Encyclopedia, Inc., 1955.

Hirsh, L. H., and L. E. Putnam: "Penicillin," New York, Medical Encyclopedia, Inc., 1958.

International Symposium on Griseofulvin and Dermatomycoses, A.M.A. Arch. Dermatol., 81:649, 1960.

Jawetz, E.: "Polymyxin, Neomycin, Bacitracin," New York, Medical Encyclopedia, Inc., 1956.

Jones, W. F., Jr., and M. Finland: Blood Levels from Orally Administered Penicillins G and V, New Engl. J. Med., 253:754, 1953.

Kirby, W. M. M., D. G. Hudson, and W. D. Noyes: Clinical and Laboratory Studies of Novobiocin, a New Antibiotic, A.M.A. Arch. Internal Med., 98:1, 1956.

Lavener, H., and G. Favez: The Inhibition of Isoniazid Inactivation by Means of PAS and Benzoyl-PAS in Man, Am. Rev. Respirat. Diseases, 80:26, 1959.

Lepper, M. H.: "Aureomycin (Chlortetracycline)," New York, Medical Encyclopedia, Inc., 1956.

Madigan, D. G., L. L. Griffiths, M. J. G. Lynch, R. A. Bruce, S. Kay, and G. Brownless: Para-aminosalicylic Acid in Tuberculosis, Lancet, I:239, 1950.

Mandel, W., A. D. Heaton, W. F. Russel, Jr., and G. Middlebrook: Combined Treatment of Tuberculosis: II. Studies of Antimicrobially-active Isoniazid and Streptomycin in Adult Tuberculosis, J. Clin. Invest., 38:1356, 1959.

McCarthy, C. G., and M. Finland: Absorption and Excretion of Four Penicillins, Penicillin G, Penicillin V, Phenethicillin and Phenylmercaptomethylpenicillin, New Engl. J. Med., 263:315, 1960.

Musselman, M. M.: "Terramycin (Oxytetracycline)," New York, Medical Encyclopedia, Inc., 1956.

Nichols, R. L., and M. Finland: Novobiocin: A Limited Bacteriologic and Clinical Study of Its Use in Forty-Five Patients, Antibiotic Med., 2:241, 1956.

Peters, J. H.: Studies on the Metabolism of Isoniazid: II. The Influence of Para-aminosalicylic Acid on the Metabolism of Isoniazid by Man, Am. Rev. Respirat. Diseases, 82:153, 1960.

Richards, W. A., E. Riss, E. H. Kass, and M. Finland: Nitrofurantoin: Clinical and Laboratory Studies in Urinary Tract Infection, A.M.A. Arch. Internal Med., 96:437, 1955.

Rutenberg, A. M., H. L. Greenberg, and F. B. Schweinburg: Clinical Experience with 2,6-dimethoxyphenyl Penicillin Monohydrate in Staphylococcal Infections, New Engl. J. Med., 263:1174, 1960.

Stewart, G. T.: Microbiological Studies on Sodium 6-(2,6-dimethoxy-benzamido) Penicillanate Monohydrate (BRL 1241) in Vitro and in Patients, Brit. Med. J., II:694, 1960.

———, H. H. Nixon, H. M. T. Coles, with 7 collaborators: Report on Clinical Use of BRL 1241 in Children with Staphylococcal and Streptococcal Infections, Brit. Med. J., II:703, 1960.

Waisbren, B. A., and W. Crowley: Nitrofurantoin: Clinical and Laboratory Evaluation, A.M.A. Arch. Internal Med., 95:653, 1955.

—— and W. W. Spink: A Clinical Appraisal of Neomycin, Ann. Internal Med., 33:1099, 1950.

Weinstein, L.: The Complications of Antibiotic Therapy, Bull. N.Y. Acad. Med., 31:500, 1955.

——: The Chemoprophylaxis of Infection, Ann. Internal Med., 43:287, 1955.

——: A Clinical Evaluation of the Therapeutic Application of Antibiotic Combinations, Conn. State Med. J., 24:87, 1960.

——: Recent Advances in the Chemotherapy of Infection, A.M.A. Arch. Environmental Health, 121:487, 1960.

—— and N. J. Ehrenkranz: "Streptomycin and Dihydrostreptomycin," New York, Medical Encyclopedia, Inc., 1958.

——, M. Goldfield, and T. W. Chang: Infections Occurring during Chemotherapy: A Study of Their Frequency, Type and Predisposing Factors, New Engl. J. Med., 251:247, 1954.

——, M. A. Madoff, and C. M. Samet: The Sulfonamides, New Engl. J. Med., 263:793, 842, 900, 952, 1960.

Welch, H.: The Newest Addition to the Repository Penicillins (Dibenzylethylenediamine Dipenicillin), Antibiotics & Chemotherapy, 3:357, 1953.

—— and M. Finland: "Antibiotic Therapy for Staphylococcal Disease," New York, Medical Encyclopedia, Inc., 1959.

Woodward, T. E., and C. L. Wisseman, Jr.: "Chloromycetin (Chloramphenicol)," New York, Medical Encyclopedia, Inc., 1958.

Yeager, R. L., W. G. C. Monroe, and F. I. Dessau: Pyrazinamide in the Treatment of Pulmonary Tuberculosis, Am. Rev. Tuberc., 65:523, 1952.

Section 2: Diseases Produced by Gram-positive Cocci

112 PNEUMOCOCCAL INFECTIONS

Ivan L. Bennett, Jr.

Etiology. The pneumococcus is a gram-positive, encapsulated coccus that usually grows in pairs or short chains. In the diplococcal form, the adjacent margins are rounded and the opposite ends slightly pointed, giving the organisms a "lancet" shape. In stained preparations of exudate, gram-negative forms are often present. Because pneumococci produce greenish discoloration of blood agar, they are sometimes confused with alpha-hemolytic streptococci. The two organisms can be distinguished by the bile solubility and mouse virulence of the pneumococcus or by serologic typing. A simpler method, utilizing inhibition of pneumococci by Optochin-impregnated paper disks, is accurate and less cumbersome for routine use.

The capsular substances are complex polysaccharides and are the basis for dividing pneumococci into serotypes. Organisms exposed to type-specific antiserum show capsular swelling, the *Neufeld quellung reaction;* by this means, about 75 serotypes have been identified. All are pathogenic for man, but types 1, 2, 3, 5, 7, and 8 are encountered most frequently in clinical practice. Type 14 causes pneumonia in children but is rare in adults.

Specific typing of pneumococci was of great clinical importance when therapeutic antiserum was used but has been largely abandoned because sulfonamides and antibiotics are effective against pneumococci of all types.

Epidemiology. Pneumococci are normal inhabitants of the upper respiratory tract in 5 to 60 per cent of the population, depending upon the season. Pneumococcal infection occurs predominantly during the winter months; the ratio of infection in males and females is 3:2, and morbidity and mortality are higher for Negroes than whites. Person-to-person transmission by droplets is undoubtedly common, but true epidemics of pneumococcal pneumonia are rare, even in closed populations. Patients with pneumococcal infection can be managed without isolation precautions.

Pathogenesis. The mechanism by which pneumococci damage tissue is obscure. It is conceivable that toxic substances may be elaborated when they multiply in the body, but no such toxin has been demonstrated. It has been suggested that rapid growth of pneumococci interferes with essential metabolic processes in the host, but this is supported by no firm evidence. The capsular substance is known to be a necessary factor in virulence, and it also protects the organism to a certain extent from engulfment by phagocytes.

Invasion of the tissues of the nasopharynx rarely, if ever, occurs, and "pneumococcal pharyngitis" is always a questionable diagnosis. The organisms multiply readily and produce acute inflammation in the lung, serous cavities, and the endocardium. The factors that ordinarily protect the lung from pneumococci include the mucus of the respiratory epithelium, the direction and velocity of air currents, and ciliary action. Under circumstances which impair the effectiveness of these barriers, pneumococci are carried to the alveoli in droplets of saliva or mucus and infection occurs; pneumonia usually begins in the right lower, right middle, or left lower lobe. Susceptibility to pneumococcal pneumonia seems to be related to common respiratory disease, fatigue, chilling, and depression of the cough reflex. Intoxication with alcohol is a well-known predisposing factor, and the infection is likely to be severe in alcoholics. Patients with multiple myeloma are peculiarly susceptible to pneumococcal infection, especially pneumonia, and pneumococcal peritonitis is a frequent complication of the nephrotic syndrome in children. In some parts of the world, the pneumococcus is said to be a common cause of secondary infection in patients with brucellosis or trypanosomiasis. Experimentally, the production of pulmonary edema increases the susceptibility of animals to pneumococcal pneumonia, and the frequency and severity of pneumonia in patients with chronic heart disease suggests that a similar situation also holds for man.

In the pulmonary alveoli, the organisms cause an outpouring of polymorphonuclear leukocytes and edema fluid. The studies of Wood have shown that this fluid, which contains myriads of pneumococci, spreads rapidly through bronchioles, bronchi, and the alveolar pores of Cohn. As the infection develops, neutrophils and macrophages begin to ingest pneumococci, and the alveoli are filled with a fibrinous exudate containing many white cells but fewer and fewer organisms. The peripheral zone of spreading edema can advance to involve additional lung tissue at a time when the older part of the lesion is actually undergoing resolution. The outcome of the infection depends upon the rate at which bacteria in the edema fluid can multiply and spread into new areas as compared with the host's ability to immobilize and destroy them by phagocytosis.

Bacteremia, the result of entry into the blood by way of lymphatic vessels, is common during the stage of spreading pulmonary infection; indeed transient bacteremia probably occurs at the onset of nearly every pneumococcal infection in the lung. Continued bacteremia is a poor prognostic sign, not only because of the danger of metastatic infection, but because it indicates poor localization of the pneumonic process.

The resistance of the host to pneumococcal infection is greatly enhanced by specific antibody, which not only increases phagocytosis by "opsonizing" the organisms but, as Rich has shown, also retards the spread of bacteria in the tissues. Recovery is not entirely dependent upon the immune response, since antibody is not invariably demonstrable in patients who recover with or without chemotherapy. However, the dramatic recovery by crisis that used to occur before specific treatment became available usually coincided with the appearance of antibody in the blood. With arrest of the infection, the alveolar exudate undergoes liquefaction and the process resolves, apparently by lymphatic removal of the inflammatory debris. Pneumococcal pneumonia rarely produces necrosis of alveolar walls or bronchi, and the lung is often restored to normal within a few days.

In addition to producing pneumonia, the pneumococcus can extend from the nasopharynx to produce otitis or mastoiditis, paranasal sinusitis, or meningitis; from the lung it can extend to infect pleura, pericardium, or mediastinum, and bacteremia may give rise to meningitis, peritonitis, arthritis, endocarditis, or other metastatic infections.

PNEUMOCOCCAL PNEUMONIA

Pneumococcal pneumonia is a disease remarkable for its uniformity, in contrast to other infections such as typhoid fever and tuberculosis. The diseases produced by different pneumococcal serotypes show little variation in severity or in clinical manifestations. The prognosis in type 3 pneumococcal pneumonia is usually regarded as poor; this is in large measure attributable to the frequency with which type 3 infections occur in patients with other debilitating diseases such as diabetes or congestive heart failure. However, the type 3 pneumococcus possesses an unusually thick capsule, is especially difficult for neutrophils to engulf, and is the pneumococcus most likely to produce abscess formation in the lungs of man and experimental animals; these facts suggest that its virulence is partly intrinsic and not wholly the result of its attacking susceptible hosts. It is still customary to classify pneumococcal pneumonias as *lobar*, a process involving one or more large segments or lobes of the lung, or *bronchopneumonia*, in which there is patchy involvement, usually of both lungs. This distinction now has little clinical importance; treatment is the same for both anatomic types when the etiologic organism is the same, and prognosis depends upon other factors. The usual lesion in adults is lobar in distribution, but in children and the aged, bronchopneumonias are frequent.

Manifestations. Pneumonia is frequently preceded for a few days by coryza or some other form of common respiratory disease. The onset is usually so abrupt that patients can often state the exact hour that illness began. There is a sudden *shaking chill* in more than 80 per cent of the cases, rapid rise in temperature, and corresponding tachycardia. It is unusual for patients with pneumococcal pneumonia to experience more than a single rigor unless antipyretic drugs are administered, and repeated chills should suggest another etiologic agent.

About 75 per cent of patients develop severe *pleuritic pain* and *cough,* productive of pinkish or "rusty" mucoid sputum within a few hours. The chest pain is agonizing, and respirations become rapid, shallow, and grunting as the patient tries to splint the affected side. Many patients are mildly cyanotic and show dilatation of the alae nasae when first seen. Patients appear acutely ill, but nausea, headache, malaise, and other complaints are unusual, and most individuals are alert. The pleuritic pain is the dominant complaint.

Physical examination reveals restricted motion of the affected hemithorax, impaired or flat percussion note with increased fremitus over the involved area and, usually, decreased breath sounds. Later, bronchial breathing, pectoriloquy, and fine moist rales are evident.

In the untreated disease, there are sustained fever with a temperature of 102.5 to 105°F, continued pleuritic pain, cough, and sputum, and gaseous distention is frequent. Herpes labialis is a common complication. After 7 to 10 days, there are diaphoresis, abrupt defervescence, and dramatic improvement in manifestations, the "crisis."

In cases which terminate fatally, there is usually extensive pulmonary involvement, and dyspnea, cyanosis, and tachycardia are prominent. Circulatory collapse or a picture resembling "forward" heart failure is common. Death in a few patients is associated with empyema or some other suppurative complication.

Effect of Specific Chemotherapy. Pneumococcal pneumonia usually terminates promptly when an appropriate antimicrobial drug is given. Within 12 to 36 hr after initiation of treatment with penicillin, temperature, pulse, and respiration fall to normal, pleuritic pain subsides, and the spread of the inflammatory process is halted.

Complications. The typical course of pneumococcal pneumonia just described can be modified by the development of one or more local or distant complications:

In the Lung. Atelectasis of all or part of a lobe may occur during the active stage of pneumonia or after treatment has been instituted. The patient may complain of sudden recurrence of pleuritic pain and show rapid respirations. Small areas of atelectasis are sometimes detected by x-ray in the absence of symptoms. These areas usually clear with coughing and deep breathing, but bronchoscopic aspiration is occasionally necessary. If atelectasis is allowed to persist, the affected area becomes fibrotic and functionless. *Delayed resolution:* The removal of exudate from the lung following pneumococcal infection is usually complete within a few days, but occasionally, especially in elderly individuals, consolidation persists for longer periods. Sometimes the involved area never becomes reaerated, and fibrosis results. *Lung abscess* is a rare sequel to pneumococcal infection. It is manifested clinically by continued fever and profuse expectoration of purulent sputum. X-ray shows one or more cavities. This complication is exceedingly rare in patients who receive penicillin therapy and is more likely to result from type 3 infections.

In Adjacent Structures. Pleural effusion is noted in about 5 per cent of patients with pneumococcal pneumonia, even with specific therapy. The amount of fluid is usually not sufficient to cause obvious displacement of mediastinal structures. If it does not become infected, it is spontaneously reabsorbed within a week or two.

Prior to the introduction of effective chemotherapy, pneumococcal infection of the pleura with *empyema* occurred in 5 to 8 per cent of patients with pneumococcal pneumonia; it is now observed in far less than 1 per cent of treated cases. It is manifested by persistent fever or pleuritic pain, together with signs of pleural effusion. In the early stages, the gross appearance of infected fluid may not differ from that of a sterile pleural effusion; later, however, there is profuse outpouring of polymorphonuclear leukocytes and fibrin, resulting in an exudate of thick, greenish pus containing large plaques of fibrin. The quantity of exudate may become large enough to compress the lung and displace mediastinal structures. In neglected cases this leads to extensive pleural scarring, with limitation of chest movement. Rupture and drainage through the chest wall (*empyema necessitatis*) can occur. Metastatic *brain abscess* is an occasional complication of chronic pleural empyema; the origin of this appears to be the passage of septic thrombi through the intercostal and vertebral veins.

Pericarditis. A particularly serious complication is spread of infection to the pericardial sac. This may be manifested by pain in the precordial region, and a friction rub synchronous with the heartbeat, although neither of these is always present. The possibility of coexisting purulent pericarditis should be considered whenever there is pleural empyema, especially when the patient appears gravely ill.

Metastatic Infections. Arthritis occurs more often in infants than in adults. The affected joint is swollen, red, and painful, with a purulent effusion. It subsides promptly with systemic administration of penicillin.

Acute bacterial endocarditis complicates pneumococcal pneumonia in less than 0.5 per cent of cases. Its manifestations and treatment will be discussed later in this section.

Meningitis, another complication of pneumococcal pneumonia, will also be discussed subsequently.

Paralytic Ileus. As already noted, gaseous abdominal distention is commonly present. In severely ill patients this may assume serious proportions, such that the term *paralytic ileus* is justified. This complication further impairs respiratory movement and constitutes a difficult problem in management.

Impaired Liver Function. Alterations in liver function are very common during the course of pneumococcal pneumonia, and jaundice is not at all rare. The mechanism of the jaundice cannot be precisely defined.

Laboratory Findings. *X-ray* of the chest reveals a homogeneous density in the affected area of lung. In well-established cases, the density may occupy one or more entire lobes, whereas in early cases only a portion of one lung may be involved. The white blood count usually shows a polymorphonuclear *leukocytosis* ranging from 12,000 to 25,000 cells per cu mm. Normal leukocyte count or leukopenia is sometimes observed in old people or in those with overwhelming infection and bacteremia. The *blood culture* is positive for pneumococci during the first 3 or 4 days of illness in 20 to 25 per cent of cases. The *sputum,* when stained by Gram's method, shows polymorphonuclear leukocytes and moderate numbers of gram-positive cocci, singly and in pairs. These can be typed directly, by the Neufeld capsular swelling technique, but this procedure is not essential for present methods of therapy.

DIFFERENTIAL DIAGNOSIS OF PNEUMONIA

Fever, cough, and pulmonary consolidation on physical or x-ray examination form a symptom complex that can be produced by many diseases of infectious, toxic, or other etiology.

Staphylococcal pneumonia (p. 897) is likely to be encountered in children, in adults during or after an epidemic of influenza, and in debilitated, elderly individuals as a nosocomial infection. The clinical picture is less uniform than that of pneumococcal pneumonia, varying from bronchitis with few systemic symptoms to a fulminating infection. Multiple chills, hectic fever, early formation of lung abscesses, empyema, and, in infants, pneumatoceles or pyopneumothorax, suggest the diagnosis. The sputum is often grossly bloody or purulent; culture of sputum and blood establishes the diagnosis. Positive blood cultures should alert the clinician to the possibility that pulmonary involvement is secondary to a focus of staphylococcal infection elsewhere in the body.

Hemolytic streptococcal pneumonia (p. 908) can also occur in association with influenza. The clinical picture closely resembles that of pneumococcal pneumonia, but multiple chills, hectic fever, early prostration, and rapid pleural involvement with accumulation of fluid, or associated streptococcal pharyngitis, are often helpful signs. Diagnosis can be made by blood and sputum culture or by finding a rise in antistreptolysin O titer in convalescent serum.

Friedländer bacillus pneumonia (p. 938) is commonest in men past middle age, especially in alcoholics. The patient is usually severely ill, the sputum tends to be thick and tenacious, physical findings in the chest are often surprisingly scanty despite massive consolidation by x-ray; nausea, diarrhea, jaundice, and delirium are more frequent than in pneumococcal infections, and large numbers of gram-negative bacilli are usually present in stained smears of sputum.

Tularemia (p. 964) of the ulceroglandular or typhoidal type is often accompanied by pulmonary lesions. There may be no respiratory symptoms and a paucity of physical signs, or pleurisy, hemoptysis, and consolidation may dominate the clinical picture. Patients are usually very ill, with temperatures of 104 to 106°F, and the disease does not respond to penicillin. Agglutinins for the organism may not appear until the third week. A history of contact with wild rabbits or the finding of a cutaneous ulcer and regional lymphadenitis is helpful in diagnosis.

Infection by other bacteria can produce pneumonia. Pulmonary involvement is frequent in patients with salmonella bacteremia, especially in *Salmonella suipestifer* infections (p. 948). *Hemophilus influenzae* is a common cause of lung disease in children; in adults it occasionally produces a necrotizing bronchiolitis, and in elderly patients with chronic lung disease, it may produce bronchopneumonia (p. 954). The diagnosis is usually made only by culture of sputum. Pulmonary lesions with cough and hemoptysis can be prominent in Weil's disease (p. 1085), and, of course, the plague bacillus can cause an overwhelming and rapidly fatal pneumonia, especially when plague becomes epidemic (p. 968); sporadic infection by *Pasteurella pestis* is more likely to be the "bubonic" form.

Primary atypical pneumonia (p. 1120) is usually more insidious in onset than bacterial pneumonias, chills are infrequent, fever is usually lower, pleuritic pain and effusions are unusual, headache and malaise are prominent, the cough is hacking, irritating, and productive of small amounts of mucoid sputum, rarely blood-tinged, and physical signs are scanty in comparison with x-ray changes. Herpes labialis is unusual. The leukocyte count is usually normal, although it may be increased during the second week of illness, and in 30 to 50 per cent of cases, cold agglutinins are demonstrable during the second week.

Psittacosis (p. 1126) is often described as a "severe form of atypical pneumonia." Actually, most patients with this disease are febrile and have systemic symptoms of headache, lethargy, and malaise for several days before pulmonary lesions develop. The pulse is usually slow in proportion to fever, and patients are sometimes suspected of having typhoid. A history of contact with parrots, poultry, or other birds may be helpful. The leukocyte count is normal, and diagnosis is established by finding complement-fixing antibodies in rising titer. Splenomegaly is present in a variable proportion of patients with psittacosis and is sometimes a clue to diagnosis.

Q fever (p. 1107) is characterized by severe headache, sustained fever, and, usually, minimal symptoms of respiratory disease, although a large proportion of patients show roentgenographic evidence of patchy pulmonary involvement. A history of contact with cattle suggests the possibility of Q fever, which is widely distributed in this country.

Acute tuberculous pneumonia (p. 1005) may be difficult to recognize because, in the early stages, tubercle bacilli may not be demonstrable in the sputum; the early consolidation is often the result of an inflammatory response to discharge of tuberculin-containing material into the lung. Fever is usually remittent or intermittent, and the temperature may not exceed 102°F. Many patients with tuberculous pneumonia feel surprisingly well, despite consolidation of an entire lobe. *Pleurisy with effusion* is seldom abrupt in onset, its course is prolonged, and physical and x-ray findings are those of accumulating pleural fluid rather than parenchymal consolidation. The leukocyte count is usually normal. Herpes labialis is rare in tuberculosis.

Blastomycosis (p. 1055) can produce acute lobar or bronchopneumonia, with high fever, pleuritic pain, dyspnea, and pleural fluid. The organisms are usually easily found in the sputum, and cavitation develops early in the illness. The usual course of pulmonary blastomycosis is less acute, with low-grade fever and slow evolution of the pulmonary findings. Typical skin lesions of blastomycosis or concomitant involvement of bone are aids in diagnosis.

Actinomycosis of the lung (p. 1052) is usually a more chronic disease than bacterial pneumonia and is more likely to be confused with tuberculosis or lung tumors. The diagnosis is made by finding sulfur granules in sputum or by culturing the organism. Other mycotic infections of the lung include *primary histoplasmosis* (p. 1060), which can produce an acute illness with fever, cough, and multiple nodular pulmonary densities that lasts for several weeks; and *primary coccidioidomycosis* (p. 1056), distinguishable in endemic areas by pulmonary infiltration, fever, eosinophilia, and, often, erythema nodosum.

Lung abscess may have an abrupt onset, with chill, fever, and pleuritic pain and can be confused with acute pneumonias. The development of cavitation in a well-circumscribed pulmonary density and profuse, purulent sputum makes the diagnosis clear. In individuals with chronic abscess, weight loss is prominent and cavitation readily apparent. There is usually intermittent or remittent fever. A history of epilepsy, alcoholic intoxication, anesthesia, dental extraction, tonsillectomy, or aspiration of a foreign body may be elicited. Abscess may be the first sign of bronchogenic carcinoma.

Atelectasis may occur in patients confined to bed, especially if respiratory motion is limited (as after an abdominal operation) or when the cough reflex is depressed by drugs or central nervous system disease. Infection of the collapsed pulmonary segment leads to fever, pleuritic pain, and purulent sputum. There is often a shift of the mediastinum toward the affected side. Tumor, enlarged hilar nodes, and foreign body are important causes of persistent collapse, although plugging of bronchi by inspissated mucus is by far the most frequent cause.

Pulmonary adenomatosis (p. 1561), a diffuse neoplastic disease, can be accompanied by fever, profuse, glairy sputum, and hemoptysis, with various x-ray findings, and is sometimes mistaken at first for acute bacterial pneumonia or tuberculosis.

Pulmonary infarction is especially frequent in patients with congestive heart failure and after surgical procedures. Prostatic surgery and parturition are particularly likely to lead to embolization from the pelvic veins. Pulmonary embolization may be asymptomatic, but in many patients, there are sudden pleuritic pain, dyspnea, anxiety, transient hypotension, and hemoptysis. Fever is common, but true chills are rare. Icterus may accompany pulmonary infarcts in individuals with congestive heart failure. Signs of consolidation and pleural fluid are common, and often evidence of phlebothrombosis can be detected in the legs.

Septic pulmonary infarcts with abscess formation and cavitation should always suggest puerperal sepsis or infected abortions with pelvic thrombophlebitis in a woman. For reasons that are obscure, phlebothrombosis and pulmonary infarction are relatively frequent complications of convalescence from psittacosis.

The lungs of patients with *uremia* sometimes show x-ray changes consisting of infiltrations that flare toward the periphery from both hilar areas.

Roentgenographically, the changes in the lungs of patients with *acute pulmonary edema* and *heart failure* are sometimes surprisingly well localized to a segment or lobe of one lung.

The inhalation of *noxious materials or irritants* (p. 1542), including smoke, chlorine, phosgene, cadmium fumes, bagasse fibers, and other organic dusts, can lead to bronchitis, bronchiolitis, and patchy or even lobar infiltration in the lung, dyspnea, and low-grade fever. The diagnosis is usually made by eliciting a history of exposure. The ingestion of gasoline or kerosene (p. 824) is almost invariably complicated by severe chemical bronchopneumonia.

Pneumonitis is detectable by physical examination or x-ray in some patients with erythema multiforme (p. 1924), lupus erythematosus (p. 1893), rheumatic fever (p. 916), or intestinal helminthiasis (pp. 1217 and 1218). Infectious mononucleosis (p. 1248) and lymphocytic choriomeningitis (p. 1137) are sometimes accompanied by pulmonary infiltrations and, occasionally, by signs of respiratory irritation with cough and sputum. Pulmonary lesions, usually in the form of scattered nodular densities, with accompanying cough, dyspnea, and cyanosis, occur in a small proportion of patients with smallpox (p. 1164), chickenpox (p. 1167), or measles (p. 1158); the involvement in these diseases is believed to be caused by the virus rather than by secondary bacterial invaders. Rupture of amebic abscess into the pleural cavity can be mistaken for acute pneumonia (p. 1198), and in a few patients with estivo-autumnal malaria, blockage of pulmonary capillaries by parasites can lead to confusion with respiratory infections of various types (p. 1200).

PNEUMOCOCCAL MENINGITIS

The pneumococcus is second only to the meningococcus as a cause of purulent meningitis in adults; in children, influenzal meningitis is also more frequent than pneumococcal infection.

Pneumococcal meningitis can develop as a "primary" disease without preceding signs of infection elsewhere, as a complication of pneumococcal pneumonia, by extension from otitis, mastoiditis, or sinusitis, or following a skull fracture which creates an opening into the nasal cavity or paranasal sinuses. Patients with pneumococcal endocarditis frequently develop meningeal infection. Patients with multiple myeloma seem to be prone to pneumococcal infection of the meninges, just as they are to pneumonia.

The *manifestations* are those of any acute pyogenic meningitis and include chills, fever, headache, nuchal rigidity, Kernig and Brudzinski signs, delirium, and cranial nerve palsies. Evidence of otitis,

sinusitis, or pneumonia should be carefully sought by physical and roentgenographic examination in all patients.

The *spinal fluid* is under increased pressure, appears cloudy, often with a greenish tint, and shows a high protein and low glucose content. Stained smears usually reveal myriads of gram-positive diplococci and polymorphonuclear leukocytes; in some patients, the number of cells in the spinal fluid is surprisingly small, much of the cloudiness being produced by the bacterial content.

With appropriate chemotherapy, recovery can be expected in 70 to 85 per cent of cases. Before penicillin was available, the mortality rate exceeded 95 per cent, and sulfonamides did little to reduce this. Relapse can occur but is unusual if adequate treatment is carried out. Subarachnoid block, the result of accumulation of large amounts of thick exudate in the meningeal space and at the base of the brain, is now an unusual complication.

PNEUMOCOCCAL ENDOCARDITIS

Endocarditis is almost always a complication of pneumonia. The clinical picture is that of acute bacterial endocarditis (p. 1039), with remittent fever, petechial hemorrhages, splenomegaly, and metastatic infection of the lungs, meninges, joints, eye, and other tissues. The infection can attack normal valves and is particularly likely to occur on the aortic valve. The valvular infection is destructive, and loud murmurs and heart failure develop rapidly. Rupture or perforation of cusps or even rupture of the aorta can occur. The blood culture is consistently positive for the pneumococcus; yet at the same time antibodies for the infecting organism can usually be demonstrated in the blood, a combination of findings seldom observed except in endocarditis or brucellosis. The rapid destruction of the valvular structures combined with a striking tendency to the development of myocardial abscess in the region of the valve ring makes pneumococcal endocarditis a difficult disease to cure, despite the sensitivity of the organism to penicillin.

PNEUMOCOCCAL PERITONITIS

Pneumococcal peritonitis occasionally occurs in young girls; presumably the vagina and fallopian tubes are the portal of entry. Symptoms are fever, pain, abdominal distention, vomiting, and accumulation of peritoneal fluid. The diagnosis is made by examination of the purulent ascitic fluid; blood cultures are often positive, and a polymorphonuclear leukocytosis is the rule.

Peritonitis is also a frequent complication of the nephrotic syndrome, particularly in children, in whom there may be repeated episodes of this infection.

TREATMENT

Specific Chemotherapy. Penicillin is the drug of choice in all pneumococcal infections. The minimum curative dosage for *pneumonia* is less than 60,000 units daily, and a total daily dose of 600,000 units, as one injection of a depot preparation or multiple injections of aqueous crystalline penicillin, provides a good margin of safety. Treatment should be continued until the patient has been afebrile for 48 to 72 hr. The response is usually dramatic, and relapse is virtually unheard of. Pneumococcal pneumonia can be treated adequately with oral penicillin in a dosage of 1.2 to 2.4 million units daily.

Peritonitis usually responds within 36 to 48 hr to 600,000 units of penicillin daily.

Pneumococcal *meningitis* is best treated with massive amounts of penicillin intramuscularly; a minimum dosage is 12 million units of aqueous penicillin daily, and, in many clinics, larger amounts are used and Benemid is also given to impede renal excretion of the antibiotic. There is convincing evidence that the addition of sulfadiazine to this regimen affords no advantage and that the supplementary administration of chlortetracycline (and presumably, other broad-spectrum drugs) actually exerts a deleterious effect, producing antibiotic "antagonism" (see p. 881). In the presence of sinusitis or otitis, surgical drainage should be carried out as soon as feasible. The response of meningitis is usually less dramatic than that of pneumonia; patients often remain febrile and disoriented, and signs of meningeal irritation may persist for several days, improvement becoming gradually evident with continued treatment.

In *pneumococcal endocarditis* also, large doses are required—6 to 12 million units daily by intramuscular injection. Rapidly developing heart failure in these patients and the tendency to myocardial abscess formation, however, often lead to a fatal outcome despite large doses of antibiotics.

Sulfonamides are effective in pneumococcal pneumonia, but their action is not so prompt or dramatic as that of penicillin; they are virtually useless in meningitis and endocarditis.

The *tetracycline* drugs and *chloramphenicol* are effective in the treatment of pneumonia in doses of 1.0 to 2.0 Gm daily. They are recommended only for patients who have exhibited an untoward reaction to penicillin.

Arthritis responds to systemic penicillin; aspiration and intraarticular instillation of the drug are rarely necessary. *Empyema* should be watched for and treated as early as possible. When an effusion is detected, the fluid should be examined for organisms, and if they are found, 50,000 to 200,000 units of penicillin should be injected intrapleurally. Daily aspiration of fluid and instillation of penicillin should be carried out until cultures are persistently negative. Fluoroscopic guidance may be needed for aspiration of small empyema pockets. If the exudate becomes especially thick and viscid, streptokinase-streptodornase (Varidase) may facilitate its withdrawal. Aspiration of exudate and instillation of penicillin is the treatment of choice in *pericarditis* also. In empyema or pericarditis, the development of loculation and thick exudate with difficulty in aspiration should lead to consideration of surgical drainage. While there has been good success in the medical management of these infections of serous cavities, thoracotomy will sometimes shorten a patient's hospital course and should not be neglected when difficulties develop in medical treatment.

Other Measures. *Oxygen* may be used for intense cyanosis in pneumonia but is likely to aggravate abdominal distention. Codeine, 30 to 60 mg every few hours, will usually control mild *pleuritic pain*. A chest binder or adhesive strapping of the affected side may diminish pain but increases the likelihood of atelectasis and interferes with subsequent examinations. When pain is severe, intercostal nerve block by injection of 2.0 ml of 1 per cent procaine beneath the rib margins proximal to the site of pain is usually effective. The procedure is not technically difficult or dangerous. Other methods of relieving pleuritic pain are usually transient in their effect but are sometimes worth trying; they include ethyl chloride spray over the painful area, intravenous injection of calcium gluconate, and intravenous injection of tetraethylammonium chloride.

PROGNOSIS

With proper chemotherapy, the mortality from pneumococcal pneumonia has fallen to less than 5 per cent, and in many clinics to less than 1 per cent. The recovery rate in meningitis is 70 to 85 per cent. Pneumococcal endocarditis is still fatal in at least half the cases.

Signs of poor prognosis in pneumonia include leukopenia, circulatory collapse, multilobar involvement, and persistent bacteremia. Jaundice is often prominent in fatal cases, but icterus alone is not a poor prognostic finding.

REFERENCES

Austian, R.: Pneumococcal Endocarditis, Meningitis, and Rupture of Aortic Valve, A.M.A. Arch. Internal Med., 99:539, 1957.

—— and A. L. Winston: Efficacy of Penicillin V (Phenoxymethylpenicillin) in Mild and Moderately Severe Pneumococcal Pneumonia, Am. J. Med. Sci., 232:624, 1956.

Dowling, H. F., and M. H. Lepper: The Effect of Antibiotics (Penicillin, Aureomycin, and Terramycin) on the Fatality Rate and Incidence of Complications in Pneumococcic Pneumonia, Am. J. Med. Sci., 222:396, 1951.

Finland, M.: Pneumonia: Present Status of Diagnosis and Treatment, Veterans Admin. Tech. Bull., TB-1084, Nov. 30, 1952.

—— and H. I. L. Lovernd: Massive Atelectatic Collapse of the Lung Complicating Pneumococcus Pneumonia, Ann. Internal Med., 10:1828, 1937.

Lepper, M. H., and H. F. Dowling: Treatment of Pneumococcic Meningitis with Penicillin Compared with Penicillin Plus Aureomycin, A.M.A. Arch. Internal Med., 88:489, 1951.

Rich, A. R.: The Mechanism Responsible for the Prevention of Spread of Bacteria in the Immune Body, Bull. Johns Hopkins Hosp., 52:203, 1933. (Describes retarding of spread of pneumococci by specific antibodies.)

Wood, W. Barry, Jr.: Studies on the Mechanism of Recovery in Pneumococcal Pneumonia: I. The Action of Type Specific Antibody upon the Pulmonary Lesion of Experimental Pneumonia, J. Exptl. Med., 73:201, 1941.

Zimmerman, H. J., and L. J. Thomas: The Liver in Pneumococcal Pneumonia: Observations in 94 Cases on Liver Function and Jaundice in Pneumonia, J. Lab. Clin. Med., 35:556, 1950.

Zinneman, H. H., and W. H. Hall: Recurrent Pneumonia in Multiple Myeloma, Ann. Internal Med., 41:1152, 1954.

113 STAExPHYLOCOCCAL INFECTIONS

David E. Rogers

Staphylococci cause most superficial suppurative infections in man. They also produce certain serious infections of the lungs, pleural space, long bones, kidneys, and surgical wounds.

Staphylococcal infections have assumed increasing clinical importance since the development of antibiotics. Between 50 and 80 per cent of serious staphylococcal infections now arise in hospitalized patients. Certain characteristics of staphylococci appear to have led to this situation. These are: (1) the frequency of potentially pathogenic strains as part of man's normal flora, (2) the capacity of staphylococci to develop resistance to each new antimicrobial in wide use, and the sluggish response of established staphylococcal disease to antibacterial therapy, (3) the tendency of staphylococci to produce disease in debilitated patients, and (4) the rapid tissue destruction and abscess formation which characterize staphylococcal infections.

Bacteriology. Staphylococci are spherical gram-positive cells which grow abundantly in the usual meat extract or infusion media. On solid agar media, staphylococcus colonies develop characteristic pigmentation by which three species can be differentiated: *Micrococcus pyogenes* var. *aureus* (*Staphylococcus aureus*), golden yellow, *Micrococcus pyogenes* var. *albus* (*Staphylococcus albus*), ivory white, and *Micrococcus citreus,* lemon yellow. Most human infections are caused by S. *aureus.* The name staphylococcus derives from the characteristic grapelike clusters of organisms seen in stained smears prepared from colonies on solid media (Greek *staphule,* grape). In stained smears obtained from pus, smaller clusters, diploids, and short chains are seen. In such preparations, staphylococci characteristically retain their uniform round shape, in contrast to the boatlike forms assumed by pneumococci. Staphylococci may be seen within the cytoplasm of polymorphonuclear cells in pus, a finding not common in other gram-positive coccal infections.

In general, pathogenic strains possess a broader complement of biochemical activities, and several laboratory methods are commonly used to recognize these pathogenic strains. Most staphylococci isolated from active infections produce yellow pigment and hemolyze rabbit or sheep red blood cells in blood agar plates. The ability to produce *coagulase,* a substance which clots the plasma of certain animals and man, the elaboration of *alpha toxin,* the fermentation of *mannite,* and the hydrolysis of *phenolphthalein phosphate* are characteristics of infection-producing strains. The ability of a given strain to produce coagulase is generally considered the best simple evidence of probable pathogenicity.

Different strains of pathogenic staphylococci can be recognized by the patterns of lysis produced by staphylococcal bacteriophages. Although techniques are cumbersome, phage typing of staphylococci now allows more precise strain characterization and is commonly used in studies of intrahospital disease and epidemics of staphylococcal infection.

Pathogenesis. Little is known of the events which allow staphylococci to become invasive and produce active disease. Enormous numbers of staphylococci must be used to establish experimental infections in animals or man. Strains of staphylococci capable of producing infection are common skin and mucous membrane inhabitants, and over 50 per cent of serious staphylococcal infections of deep tissues arise from skin foci of infection. A lesser number of staphylococcal infections originate in the respiratory or genitourinary tract.

Certain situations are known to predispose to staphylococcal disease. *Diabetics* have a high incidence of staphylococcal infections. Under circumstances of severe *debilitation* and/or *malnutri-*

tion, staphylococcal infections are common. Staphylococcal infections commonly arise when skin continuity is broken. *Abrasions, wounds, burns,* and skin areas denuded by *exfoliative dermatitis* are commonly infected with staphylococci. Individuals who work with greasy skin irritants have a greater incidence of superficial staphylococcal infections. *Influenza* and *measles* appear to predispose to staphylococcal invasion of the lower respiratory tract. *Broad-spectrum antimicrobial therapy* may allow the implantation or overgrowth of antimicrobial resistant strains of staphylococci in the gastrointestinal tract and the production of active staphylococcal disease.

Staphylococci appear to invade the human integument via hair follicles and sebaceous glands. When the skin continuity has been breached, active local microbial multiplication is accompanied by inflammation and tissue necrosis at local sites of infection. Polymorphonuclear leukocytes rapidly enter the area and ingest large numbers of staphylococci. Thrombosis of surrounding capillaries occurs, fibrin is deposited about the periphery, and later, fibroblasts create a relatively avascular wall about the area. The fully developed staphylococcal lesion consists of a central core of dead and dying leukocytes and bacteria which gradually liquefies to form characteristic thick, creamy staphylococcal pus, surrounded by a fibroblastic wall, the "pyogenic membrane."

When host mechanisms fail to contain the cutaneous or subcutaneous infection, staphylococci may enter the blood stream. Common sites of metastatic seeding are the diaphyseal ends of long bones in children, the lungs, kidneys, endocardium, liver, spleen, and brain.

Certain biologic properties of staphylococci appear to contribute to pathogenicity. Many pathogenic strains elaborate an *exotoxin* (alpha toxin) capable of causing dermal necrosis in animals. Fever, tachycardia, cyanosis, shock, and death ensue when exotoxin is administered to experimental animals intravenously. A similar picture has been observed in certain fulminating cases of staphylococcal bacteremia in man.

The high correlation between *coagulase* production and virulence suggests that this substance is important in the pathogenesis of staphylococcal infections. Although coagulase has been said to protect staphylococci from leukocytes, active phagocytosis of staphylococci is readily demonstrated in systems containing human plasma or serum. Abscess formation is said to be less common in animal species who lack a coagulable plasma and in infants who show low titers of serum coagulase reacting factor. The thesis that coagulase may play a role in focal abscess formation is weakened by the demonstra-

tion that mice, who lack a coagulable plasma, develop typical abscesses during staphylococcal infections. Certain studies indicate that coagulase may protect staphylococci from bacteriostatic substances present in normal serum. Thus while coagulase may be important in the initiation of staphylococcal infections, its precise role has not been established.

Certain pathogenic staphylococci produce a *leukocidin* which destroys human and rabbit leukocytes in vitro. Some strains elaborate *hyaluronidase.* Many staphylococci produce an *enterotoxin* which produces nausea, vomiting, and diarrhea in certain experimental animals and man.

In vitro studies have demonstrated that pathogenic staphylococci can survive within human leukocytes while nonpathogenic strains do not. Such intracellular survival may be a means of transporting staphylococci and spreading to distant tissues.

Immunity. Clinical observation suggests that some degree of resistance to staphylococcal infections develops with age and experience with staphylococci. Primary staphylococcal pneumonia is common in infants, but rare in adults. Acute staphylococcal osteomyelitis is almost exclusively a disease of children. Abscess formation appears to be less usual and bacteremia more frequent in infants than in adults.

Pathogenic strains may possess a capsular structure or surface component which impedes phagocytosis. Several studies suggest that specific opsonizing antibody is required for the phagocytosis of pathogenic staphylococci. Antistaphylococcal antibody has been shown to pass from mother to fetus, and the incidence of demonstrable hemagglutinating antibody rapidly rises with age. Virtually 100 per cent of adults possess antistaphylococcal antibodies in their serum. Nevertheless the role of humoral immunity in modifying or protecting against staphylococcal infection is uncertain. Serologic techniques have thus far failed to demonstrate a significant increase in antistaphylococcal antibody following prolonged staphylococcal infections. Immunization of animals with exotoxin, coagulase, or whole staphylococci may prolong experimental staphylococcal infection, but does not protect against eventual death. At present there is no satisfactory evidence to suggest that human staphylococcal infections can be significantly modified by vaccination or "desensitization."

Epidemiology. Pathogenic strains of staphylococci reside in the anterior nares and upon the skin of 30 to 60 per cent of human beings. Hospital patients and personnel have significantly higher staphylococcal carrier rates than the general population. Over 90 per cent of newborn infants acquire staphylococci within the anterior nares within

2 weeks. Such infants are colonized by the same staphylococcal phage types found in nursery personnel.

Staphylococci remain viable for long periods in dust, blankets, or clothing. Whether nasal discharges and contaminated airborne dust particles or direct contact represent the more important means of transmission of staphylococci from person to person remains a subject of controversy. Active staphylococcal infections are probably a more serious source of cross infection than the simple carrier state.

Certain phage types of staphylococci are responsible for the majority of intrahospital infections. The so-called "epidemic strain" 80/81 causes 30 to 70 per cent of serious intrahospital infections. Epidemics of staphylococcal disease in newborn units or surgical services are almost always produced by antimicrobial resistant 80/81 strains, more occasionally by other antimicrobial resistant phage group III strains. The high incidence of active staphylococcal disease in carriers of 80/81 strains suggests that this strain may possess higher virulence for human beings than do most strains of staphylococci.

Antimicrobial Resistance. The introduction of each new drug active against staphylococci has been followed by the appearance of staphylococci specifically resistant to that agent. When penicillin was first introduced, less than 10 per cent of staphylococcal strains isolated from patients or carriers were resistant to penicillin in vitro. By 1961, 60 to 90 per cent of staphylococci isolated from hospitalized patients throughout the world were insusceptible to penicillin. This pattern of the emergence of resistant strains has followed the use of streptomycin, the tetracyclines, chloramphenicol, erythromycin, oleandomycin, and novobiocin. The incidence of resistance to a specific antimicrobial has correlated closely with the frequency of its administration. Resistance to bacitracin, neomycin, kanamycin, ristocetin, and vancomycin has been rare.

Most of the observations on the incidence of antimicrobial resistant strains have been made within hospitals where antimicrobial use is heaviest. It has been shown that drug susceptible strains carried by patients may be replaced by drug resistant group III or type 80/81 staphylococci present in the hospital environment during antimicrobial treatment. These strains are in turn acquired by hospital personnel who serve as a reservoir of potentially pathogenic, antimicrobial resistant strains. Staphylococci isolated from population groups outside the hospital have not shown such a striking increase in the incidence of antimicrobial resistant strains. This fact is of great importance in preliminary decisions regarding the therapy of staphylococcal infections.

SUPERFICIAL INFECTIONS

Simple infection of hair follicles manifested by a minute erythematous nodule without involvement of the surrounding skin or deeper tissues is termed *folliculitis*. Chronic recurrent folliculitis of the beard area is termed *sycosis barbae*.

A more extensive and invasive follicular or sebaceous gland infection with some involvement of subcutaneous tissues is termed a *furuncle* or *boil*. Itching and mild pain are followed by progressive local swelling and erythema. The overlying skin becomes thinned, tense, shiny, and exquisitely painful on pressure or motion. Relief of pain occurs promptly after spontaneous or surgical drainage.

Furuncles are most frequent on the face, neck, axillas, forearms, buttocks, thighs, breasts, upper back, and labia. The acne of adolescence is frequently complicated by secondary furunculosis. Staphylococcal infection can involve the sweat glands in the axillas (*hidradenitis suppurativa*). These infections may be deep seated, slow to localize and drain, and are prone to recurrence and scarring.

Staphylococcal infections within the thick, fibrous, inelastic skin of the back of the neck and upper back lead to formation of a *carbuncle*. The relative thickness and impermeability of the overlying skin lead to lateral extension and loculation, and a large indurated, painful lesion with multiple ineffective drainage sites results. Carbuncles produce fever, leukocytosis, extreme pain, and prostration. Bacteremia is common.

OSTEOMYELITIS

Staphylococci are responsible for the majority of cases of *acute osteomyelitis*. This infection occurs almost exclusively in children under the age of twelve and has dropped sharply in incidence since the introduction of antibiotics. Males are affected more commonly than females. Approximately 50 per cent of patients give a history of a furuncle or superficial staphylococcal infection preceding osteomyelitis. Bone involvement follows hematogenous dissemination of bacteria. The frequent localization in the diaphyseal end of long bones is thought to be due to the endarterial circulation of the diaphysis. Many patients give a history of preceding trauma to the involved area.

Once established, infection spreads through the newly formed juxta-epiphyseal bone to the periosteum or along the marrow cavity. If the infection reaches the subperiosteal space, the periosteum is lifted, a subperiosteal abscess forms, and rupture with infection of the subcutaneous tissues may occur. Rarely, the joint capsule is penetrated, producing a pyogenic arthritis. There is death of bone producing *sequestrum* followed by new bone formation (the *involucrum*).

Occasionally indolent staphylococcal infections of bone remain localized within dense granulation tissue about a central necrotic cavity. Such a local infection may persist for years as a so-called *Brodie's abscess*.

Osteomyelitis in children usually begins abruptly with chills, high fever, nausea, vomiting, and progressive pain at the site of bony involvement. Muscle spasm about the affected bone is a common early sign of osteomyelitis, and the child may refuse to move the affected limb. Leukocytosis is the rule. Blood cultures are positive for staphylococci in 50 to 60 per cent of cases early in the disease. The tissues overlying the involved bone become edematous and warm, the skin becomes erythematous and shiny. Anemia develops during the course of untreated disease. Roentgenograms are usually normal during the first week. Bony rarefaction, local periosteal elevation, and new bone formation can frequently be seen during the second week.

Diagnosis. Osteomyelitis should be suspected in any child with fever, limb pain, and leukocytosis. History of a preceding cutaneous infection, local tenderness over the end of a long bone, and the finding of *Staphylococcus aureus* in blood cultures are confirmatory. In early stages, osteomyelitis must be differentiated from acute rheumatic fever, poliomyelitis, pyogenic arthritis, scurvy, and syphilitic periostitis.

Prognosis. Prior to the advent of antimicrobials, the over-all mortality was approximately 25 per cent. Death was more common in individuals with demonstrable bacteremia. Chronic osteomyelitis with recurrent activation and metastatic foci in other bones was common. Today acute staphylococcal osteomyelitis is declining in incidence, death is rare, and chronic osteomyelitis is disappearing.

STAPHYLOCOCCAL PNEUMONIA

Staphylococci are the cause of 1 to 5 per cent of bacterial pneumonias. This disease occurs sporadically except during epidemics of influenza when staphylococcal pneumonia is more common.

Primary staphylococcal pneumonia in infants and young children is a frequent cause of pyopneumothorax. This complication occurs early and should suggest *Staphylococcus aureus* infection. In older children and adults, primary staphylococcal pneumonia is usually secondary to influenza or measles. More recently, staphylococcal pneumonia has been seen with increasing frequency in hospitalized patients with leukemia, mucoviscidosis, diffuse collagen disease, or other chronic debilitating disease.

In adults, pneumonia is generally preceded by an influenza-like respiratory infection. Onset of staphylococcal involvement is abrupt with chills, high fever, progressive dyspnea, cyanosis, cough, and pleural pain. Early peripheral vascular collapse is common, and examination frequently reveals a patient who seems sicker than his physical findings would suggest. Sputum in the early phases is not characteristic but may become frankly purulent. Admixture with blood may produce a thick, creamy, pink sputum.

Staphylococcal pneumonia arising in hospitalized patients may begin more insidiously. Increasing fever, tachycardia, and an elevated respiratory rate may be the only indications of infection. Typical pneumonic symptoms may also be absent when pulmonary involvement occurs during the course of staphylococcal bacteremia.

Staphylococci generally produce patchy, centrally located areas of pneumonia. Pleural involvement and empyema are common.

Because of the central pulmonary involvement, chest findings are variable. Signs of frank consolidation are rare. Scattered fine to coarse rales and rhonchi may be heard over the involved areas. Empyema produces typical signs of pleural fluid. Signs of abscess may appear late in the course of the disease. Bacteremia is unusual (less than 20 per cent of patients), and its presence should suggest that the pneumonic involvement is metastatic and secondary to foci of infection elsewhere. Chest x-rays commonly reveal a patchy pneumonic process about the hilar area and may show early evidence of pleural fluid accumulation.

The course of staphylococcal pneumonia may be stormy despite adequate antimicrobial therapy. Gradual defervescence starting 48 to 72 hr after the initiation of therapy is the rule. Pulmonary abscesses or empyema cavities frequently require local surgical treatment.

Diagnosis. Staphylococcal pneumonia must be differentiated from other pneumonias. The preceding influenza-like illness, rapid onset of pleural pain, cyanosis, and prostration out of proportion to physical findings should suggest primary staphylococcal pneumonia. The finding of masses of polymorphonuclear leukocytes and gram-positive intraleukocytic cocci strongly suggests the diagnosis. The blood leukocyte count is generally above 15,-000. The sudden or insidious development of pneumonia with high fever, tachycardia, and leukocytosis in debilitated, hospitalized patients receiving antimicrobials should be considered staphylococcal in origin.

Prognosis. Prior to 1942, mortality ranged from 50 to 95 per cent. The presence of bacteremia was almost invariably associated with a fatal outcome. The prognosis has improved with the use of antimicrobials but continues to range from 15 to 20 per cent in primary staphylococcal pneumonia. Higher mortality is seen in debilitated individuals acquiring staphylococcal pneumonia in the hospital. Abscess formation and pleural involvement often prolong convalescence.

STAPHYLOCOCCAL BACTEREMIA

Staphylococcal bacteremia may arise from any local staphylococcal infection. Infections of the skin, respiratory tract, long bones, or genitourinary tract precede bacteremia in descending order of frequency. Trauma to local lesions, such as pinching, or surgical drainage before adequate localization may precipitate bacteremia.

Rarely, patients with bacteremia die in 12 to 24 hr with high fever, tachycardia, cyanosis, gastrointestinal symptoms, and vascular collapse. More commonly, the course of the disease is slower, with hectic fever and metastatic abscess formation in the skin, bones, kidneys, brain, myocardium, spleen, or other tissues. *Meningitis* is an occasional complication.

Endocarditis of the malignant or ulcerative type occurs in 20 to 60 per cent of patients with protracted bacteremia. Normal heart valves are frequently involved. Typically, staphylococcal endocarditis runs an acute course with high fever, progressive anemia, and metastatic abscesses in the skin and deeper structures. Rupture of the valve leaflets and valve ring abscesses are common. Specific diagnosis of endocardial involvement is difficult. Its presence should be assumed in patients with staphylococcal bacteremia with demonstrable cutaneous lesions (petechiae or cutaneous pustules) and a significant heart murmur.

Both coagulase positive and coagulase negative staphylococci can occasionally produce a subacute endocarditis indistinguishable from that produced by *Streptococcus viridans*. Coagulase negative staphylococcal endocarditis has been seen with increasing frequency in patients undergoing cardiac surgical procedures. This fact should be remembered when blood cultures are reported as "contaminated" with *Staphylococcus albus* strains.

Staphylococcal bacteremia is generally accompanied by a polymorphonuclear leukocytosis of 12,000 to 20,000, but a normal leukocyte count or leukopenia is occasionally seen. Anemia develops rapidly during the course of the illness.

Prognosis. Staphylococcal bacteremia is an extremely serious disease. Prior to the development of antimicrobials, over 80 per cent of individuals succumbed, the majority within 10 days of the onset of illness. The development of endocarditis or meningitis during bacteremia was almost invariably fatal. The sulfonamides produced little alteration in this mortality. From 50 to 60 per cent of patients now survive with the administration of effective antibiotics and appropriate surgical treatment of local sites of infection.

STAPHYLOCOCCAL FOOD POISONING

Certain strains of staphylococci produce an enterotoxin which is responsible for the majority of outbreaks of acute gastroenteritis. Foods are commonly contaminated from superficial infections in food handlers or by nasal droplets containing pathogenic staphylococci. Cream-filled pastries, custards, cottage cheese, milk products, or meats subjected to improper refrigeration allowing staphylococcal multiplication are the common offenders.

Symptoms typically appear 1 to 6 hr after ingestion of enterotoxin. The onset is usually abrupt, with severe nausea, vomiting, cramping abdominal pain, diarrhea, and prostration. The disease is brief and requires only rest and sedation. Rare fatalities have occurred in the aged. Diagnosis can be surmised from the short incubation period, the epidemic nature of the disease, the short duration of symptoms, and the lack of fever. Etiology can be proved only if specimens of ingested food can be shown to contain large numbers of enterotoxin-producing staphylococci.

STAPHYLOCOCCAL ENTERITIS

Staphylococcal enteritis, a true infection of the gut that sometimes complicates antimicrobial therapy, is described on p. 1657.

MISCELLANEOUS INFECTIONS

Staphylococci may cause otitis, sinusitis, or mastoid infections. Certain strains elaborate an erythrogenic toxin that results in a rash indistinguishable from streptococcal scarlet fever. Pyelonephritis or lower urinary tract infections may be staphylococcal in origin. Epidemics of staphylococcal pyoderma in newborn infants and maternal breast abscesses are a recurring problem in many maternity units.

THE CHANGING PATTERN OF STAPHYLOCOCCAL INFECTIONS

Changes have occurred in the relative incidence of some staphylococcal syndromes. There is evidence to indicate that circumstances existing within modern hospitals may contribute to the incidence of staphylococcal disease.

In prolonging the life span of many patients with serious illnesses, a group of individuals with increased susceptibility to many infections has emerged. The adrenal steroids, corticotropins, nitrogen mustards, or the folic acid antagonists appear to alter host defense mechanisms. Many surgical procedures create portals of entry for microorganisms.

In this setting, staphylococcal infections (along with gram-negative bacillary infections and certain fungous infections) have become an increasing problem. Thus, staphylococcal infections now fall into two relatively distinct groups.

Individuals who develop infections outside the hospital commonly present with the typical acute staphylococcal syndromes already discussed. The staphylococcal strains isolated from such infections have generally been susceptible to antimicrobial drugs.

Individuals who acquire staphylococcal infections within hospitals often develop atypical disease caused by antimicrobial resistant strains of staphylococci. Staphylococcal pneumonia, formerly rare, now occurs as a terminal complication of many disease states. Postoperative wound infections due to staphylococci have increased in frequency. Staphylococcal bacteremia arising in the hospital is a common problem, and staphylococcal enteritis is almost exclusively a hospital disease.

There is little to suggest that staphylococcal strains resistant to antimicrobials are any more invasive than those which have always been prevalent. Nevertheless, the disease states in which staphylococcal infections now commonly arise as complications are often of themselves critical. Staphylococcal infections in these situations continue to carry a high mortality.

TREATMENT

Features of Staphylococcal Infection Which Influence Therapy. Certain characteristics of staphylococcal disease should be borne in mind in planning therapy.

1. The setting in which infection arises is of considerable therapeutic importance. Acute staphylococcal infections arising outside the hospital are often caused by penicillin susceptible strains, although the incidence of antimicrobial resistant strains in urban communities is increasing. Most intrahospital infections are produced by strains which are insusceptible to penicillin.

2. Staphylococci produce rapid necrosis of tissues. Delays in effective therapy may allow a reversible infection to become a chronic suppurative process that responds slowly, if at all, to antimicrobials.

3. Frank abscess formation is common. While most antimicrobials probably reach abscess cavities in adequate concentrations, the physiologic insusceptibility of microorganisms residing in areas of extensive necrosis or suppuration render these agents almost completely ineffective in this situation. Surgical drainage of local lesions is often of primary importance.

4. Staphylococci are killed slowly by antimicrobials. Infections tend to become chronic, and relapses are frequent. Thus antimicrobial therapy should be continued longer than in many bacterial infections.

5. While treatment must be initiated on the basis of past experience, rational therapy requires that the antibiotic susceptibility of the infection strain be known in planning changes in treatment.

6. No single antimicrobial regimen has been found universally effective, and treatment is continuously changing.

It is now a common practice to administer more than one antimicrobial drug to patients with staphylococcal infections. Such multidrug therapy has emerged because of two considerations: (1) The large number of therapeutic failures on any single antimicrobial program has led to an unwillingness to withhold any agent of possible benefit to the patient. (2) There is in vitro evidence that the emergence of resistant microorganisms can be delayed by the simultaneous use of two or more antibiotics. It should be noted, however, that at present there is no convincing proof that combined antibiotic therapy is superior in the treatment of staphylococcal infection and that increasing resistance of strains in deep-seated lesions under treatment is actually rare. It is the impression of many that the so-called "bactericidal" antimicrobials (penicillin, streptomycin, bacitracin, vancomycin) are more effective than the "bacteriostatic" agents in treating serious staphylococcal disease.

Infections Arising outside the Hospital. When serious staphylococcal infection is suspected, appropriate cultures should be obtained and treatment started immediately with aqueous penicillin, 6 million to 20 million units daily. Smaller doses may be administered intramuscularly every 2 hr. When daily doses over 10 million units are administered, a continuous intravenous drip using a small scalp vein needle is generally required. Surgical drainage of local foci should be carried out. The addition of a companion antimicrobial such as erythromycin, novobiocin, or chloramphenicol may be advisable in view of the increasing number of extrahospital infections insusceptible to penicillin.

Infections Arising within the Hospital. When staphylococcal infection has arisen within the hospital or in other situations where antimicrobial resistant strains are common, therapy should be initiated with drugs other than penicillin. Agents which have been employed in such infections include vancomycin, chloramphenicol, erythromycin, novobiocin, kanamycin, ristocetin, streptomycin, the tetracyclines, bacitracin, and neomycin.

It is now clear that *dimethoxyphenyl penicillin* or Staphcillin (p. 873) is the drug of choice in the initial treatment of severe staphylococcal disease. It is given intravenously or intramuscularly in a dosage of 1 Gm every 4 to 6 hr for adults and 100 mg per kg of body weight per day for children. Vancomycin is the one other antibiotic that can be used in initial therapy in serious intrahospital infections. From 1 to 4.0 Gm should be administered daily by vein in divided doses in rapid 100 to 200 ml intravenous infusions, or by continuous intravenous drip.

Numerous other therapeutic programs have been employed, depending on the characteristic antimicrobial sensitivity patterns of the strains prevalent in the area and the familiarity of the physician with the antimicrobial agent. These include the following: (1) Both chloramphenicol and novobiocin or erythromycin, 2 to 4 Gm daily, in divided doses by the oral route. (2) Kanamycin 2.0 Gm daily administered in 0.5 Gm doses intramuscularly every 6 hr. In some clinics a companion antimicrobial, active against staphylococci, is administered simultaneously.

Changes in Therapy. Established staphylococcal infections respond slowly to the most effective antimicrobial regimens, making it difficult to know when therapy should be considered inadequate. Characteristically, 24 to 48 hr elapses before a decline in fever is noted, and recovery is accompanied by slow return of the temperature to normal in 7 to 10 days. If the disease process shows evidence of rapid progression during the first 24 to 48 hr of treatment, or fever remains high for over 96 hr in the absence of detectable abscess formation, antimicrobial therapy should be revised.

While in vitro sensitivity studies are of great value, the clinical response of the patient is the most important index on which to base changes in therapy. If the response to initial therapy is satisfactory, it should be continued regardless of in vitro evidence of resistance of the staphylococcus isolated. If changes in therapy are indicated by the clinical course, other antimicrobials should be selected on the basis of the in vitro activity against the strain under treatment. Most strains of staphylococci now isolated (1961) are sensitive to vancomycin, kanamycin, ristocetin, and bacitracin. The incidence of susceptibility to novobiocin

and chloramphenicol remains above 60 per cent in most hospitals. Strains susceptible to erythromycin, the tetracyclines, streptomycin, and penicillin are less commonly isolated in hospital centers.

The therapeutic regimens outlined above apply to the management of staphylococcal pneumonia or bacteremia. Treatment should be continued for a minimum of 4 to 6 weeks. Any suggestion of inadequate response or the presence of staphylococcal endocarditis should prolong treatment to 8 weeks to 4 months.

Superficial Infections. Superficial infections frequently do not require the use of antibiotics. There is currently no adequate therapy for recurrent furunculosis, but if the disease is severe, antimicrobial treatment may be attempted. Antibiotics to which the strain is susceptible should be administered for a minimum of 10 to 14 days. Local moist heat, immobilization of the infected part, and incision and drainage should be utilized. The surrounding skin should be protected with a coating of zinc oxide to prevent maceration. Treatment of the nasal carrier state by the local application of topical antibiotics of low sensitizing potential in a water soluble base (i.e., bacitracin, polymyxin, neomycin) may be advisable. Careful daily baths with germicidal soaps, attention to personal hygiene, and the passage of time appear to be measures most likely to interrupt the process. Attempts to prevent recurrence by autogenous or other vaccines have not proved generally effective.

Empyema. Empyema should be treated by aspiration. In penicillin sensitive infections the instillation of 200,000 to 500,000 units of penicillin may be worthwhile. Streptomycin, 200 to 1,000 mg, may be utilized. If loculation and thick exudate prevent adequate needle drainage, the local instillation of proteolytic enzymes may aid in liquefying the exudate. The removal of exudate is the most important aspect of treatment. Surgical drainage is frequently necessary and should be undertaken promptly if needle drainage is inadequate.

Osteomyelitis. Acute osteomyelitis is generally produced by penicillin susceptible strains. Aqueous penicillin, 300,000 to 1,000,000 units, should be given every 4 hr and continued for 14 to 28 days. If the illness is rapidly progressing or an antimicrobial resistant strain is suspected, vancomycin, chloramphenicol, novobiocin, erythromycin, or streptomycin should be administered along with penicillin. Bacitracin may be of value in certain cases. Local drainage of abscess cavities in soft tissues or bones should be considered in all patients where response to antimicrobials is inadequate or delayed, but the need for surgical intervention is rare. If sequestration occurs, devitalized bone should be removed.

REFERENCES

Blair, J. E.: The Staphylococci, chap. 12, in "Bacterial and Mycotic Infections of Man," 3d ed., R. Dubos (Ed.), Philadelphia, J. B. Lippincott Company, 1958.

Chickering, H. T., and J. H. Parks: *Staphylococcus aureus* Pneumonia, J.A.M.A., 72:617, 1919.

Dack, G. M.: Staphylococcus Food Poisoning, chap. 5 in "Food Poisoning," Chicago, The University of Chicago Press, 1949.

Dearing, W. H., and F. R. Helman: Micrococci (Staphylococcic) Enteritis as a Complication of Antibiotic Therapy: Its Response to Erythromycin, Proc. Staff Meetings Mayo Clinic, 28:121, 1953.

Elek, S. D.: "Staphylococcus Pyogenes," Edinburgh, E. & S. Livingstone, Ltd., 1959.

Fisher, A. M., H. N. Wagner, and R. S. Ross: Staphylococcal Endocarditis: Some Clinical and Therapeutic Observations on 38 Cases, A.M.A. Arch. Internal Med., 95:427, 1955.

Howe, C. W.: Post-operative Wound Infections Due to *Staphylococcus aureus*, New Engl. J. Med., 251: 441, 1954.

Rogers, D. E.: "Staphylococcal Infections," pp. 1–48, Disease-a-Month Series, Year Book Publishers, Inc., Chicago, April, 1958.

—— and Louria, D. B.: Current Concepts in Therapy. Treatment of Staphylococcal Infections, New Engl. J. Med., 261:88, 1959.

Schreck, K. M.: Observation on the Epidemiology of Staphylococcal Infections, Am. J. Med. Sci., 240: 171, 1960.

Skinner, D., and C. S. Keefer: Significance of Bacteremia Caused by *Staphylococcus aureus*: A Study of One Hundred and Twenty-two Cases and a Review of the Literature Concerned with Experimental Infections in Animals, Arch. Internal Med., 68: 870, 1941.

Spink, W. W.: Staphylococcal Infections and the Problem of Antibiotic Resistant Staphylococci, A.M.A. Arch. Internal Med., 94:167, 1954.

114   HEMOLYTIC STREPTOCOCCAL INFECTIONS (Including Rheumatic Fever and Glomerulonephritis)

Charles H. Rammelkamp, Jr.

Aerobic streptococci, as a group, are probably among the most important bacterial pathogens for man. These bacteria may invade any tissue or organ and, depending on the site of invasion and the parasite-host relationship, produce different clinical syndromes. Streptococcal infections may be divided conveniently into two large groups. The acute and often dramatic illnesses, such as sore throat, scarlet fever, erysipelas, puerperal fever, and lymphangitis, are included in the first group. These infections occur frequently and are characterized by certain toxic, septic, or suppurative features. The second group of diseases have been called the late, nonsuppurative complications of streptococcal infections. These illnesses, which include acute rheumatic fever and acute glomerulonephritis, commonly become manifest 2 to 3 weeks after an acute streptococcal infection. These diseases assume major importance because they may be followed by chronic valvular heart disease or possibly by chronic nephritis.

History. Although scarlet fever was recognized in 1676 by Sydenham, rheumatic fever and acute nephritis were not well described until 1805 and 1836, respectively. The role of the streptococcus as the inciting agent of scarlet fever was established in 1924. With the realization that rheumatic fever and nephritis were related to streptococcal infections, methods for the control and management of these nonsuppurative complications developed rapidly.

Bacteriology. Streptococci are gram-positive and tend to form chains. When streptococci are grown on a sheep blood agar plate, it is possible to divide them into three groups. *Alpha* colonies show a zone of incomplete or green hemolysis; *beta* streptococci exhibit a clear zone of complete hemolysis; and finally, *gamma* streptococci produce no visible change in the blood agar. Such a simple procedure as streaking a culture on a blood agar plate is sufficient to indicate the important pathogenic streptococci, because those exhibiting *beta*-hemolysis are responsible for the majority of infections in man.

On the basis of a specific carbohydrate, 12 groups of streptococci have been identified and designated Lancefield groups A, B, C, D, E, F, G, H, K, L, M, and N. Respiratory infections are caused by group A and only rarely by groups C and G streptococci. Group D streptococcus, previously referred to as *Streptococcus faecalis* or enterococci, inhabits the gastrointestinal tract and is responsible for infections of the abdominal cavity and the urinary tract.

Not only may streptococci be classified by grouping, but also most groups contain several different types. Group A, of primary interest to the clinician, comprises at least 40 specific types. Typing is based either on an agglutinin reaction or on the precipitin test. The type-specific antigen is the T-substance in the former method, the M-substance in the latter.

By grouping and typing streptococci, considerable information has been accumulated concerning streptococcal infections from both a theoretic and a practical standpoint. The carbohydrate responsible for the group characteristics is nontoxic and unassociated with virulence or immunity. In contrast, the M-protein, which tags the organism as the polysaccharide tags the pneumococcus, is identified by typing, is antigenic, and is probably responsible in part for the virulence of the organism as well as for type-specific immunity. Glossy forms of group A streptococci which contain no M-substance are avirulent, whereas virulent organisms always contain this specific protein. The T-substance is not related to virulence.

Several substances produced during the growth of beta streptococci serve to differentiate these organisms from other streptococci, as well as to explain, in part, their pathogenic effects. The type of hemolysis has been used, as described above, for classification of these bacteria. Of the various hemolysins produced by streptococci, at least two types have been recognized and termed *streptolysin O* and *streptolysin S*. They are produced by streptococci of Lancefield groups A, C, and G, the three organisms which cause the majority of human infections. The role of these hemolysins in infections in man is not definitely known, but they may be responsible for the anemia observed during the course of certain streptococcal diseases. In man, infections due to streptococci of groups A, C, and G result in the production of antistreptolysin O. Approximately 85 per cent of patients develop antistreptolysin O during the second to third week of convalescence. It is apparent, then, that the determination of the antistreptolysin titers of acute and convalescent serums may establish the diagnosis, since an increase in titer occurs following a streptococcal infection.

Another filtrable toxin produced by group A streptococci is the erythrogenic or *scarlatinal toxin*. It is so named because it causes a scarlatiniform rash when injected into man, and if sufficient quantities are given, there may be fever and nausea. That this toxin is responsible for the rash and toxic features of scarlet fever is well established. Trask and Blake were able to demonstrate a toxin in the circulating blood of patients with scarlet fever and showed that it was neutralized by specific antitoxin. Using the erythrogenic toxin as an antigen, a skin test for susceptibility to scarlet fever was developed by the Dicks. When one skin test dose is injected intradermally, persons susceptible to the erythrogenic toxin respond with an area of erythema which reaches its maximum within 24 hr. Persons exhibiting this skin reaction are susceptible to scarlatiniform rashes when infected by streptococci which produce erythrogenic toxin. It should be emphasized that individuals exhibiting a negative Dick skin test, although generally immune to scarlet fever, are not immune to infection by group A streptococci. The occasional occurrence of second attacks of scarlet fever may be explained by the fact that there are at least two types of immunologically distinct erythrogenic toxins.

In 1933, it was observed that hemolytic streptococci rapidly liquefied human fibrin. The extracellular substance responsible for this action is termed *streptokinase*. Streptokinase does not lyse the fibrin directly but activates a serum enzyme, plasminogen, which in turn lyses the clot. Streptokinase is produced by strains of Lancefield groups A, C, and G, and only occasionally in small amounts by groups B and F.

The exact role of streptokinase in the infectious process is not known. The spreading nature of streptococcal infections has been thought to be due to streptokinase which breaks down the fibrin barrier.

Following infection in man by a strain of group A streptococcus which produces large amounts of streptokinase, antibody usually develops which specifically prevents the lysis of fibrin. Thus, the measurement of antistreptokinase may aid in diagnosis. This serologic test is not so useful a diagnostic tool as the antistreptolysin test because not all group A streptococci produce sufficient streptokinase to stimulate antibody formation.

Streptodornase (deoxyribonuclease) is an enzyme produced by several groups of streptococci. Group A organisms produce three (A, B, and C) immunologically distinct deoxyribonucleases which depolymerize deoxyribonucleoprotein and deoxyribonucleic acid, the two substances which account for the high viscosity of exudates. A preparation of streptokinase-streptodornase (SK-SD) is now available for injection into body cavities containing pus or blood. Such therapy results in the liquefaction of the fibrin and cellular debris.

Other substances produced by streptococci are leukocidin, hyaluronidase, and streptococcal proteinase. Leukocidin, which is probably identical with streptolysin O, is able to inhibit phagocytosis in vitro. The enzyme hyaluronidase, or spreading factor, undoubtedly facilitates the spread of bacteria by increasing tissue permeability. It is produced in large quantities by types 4 and 22 of group A streptococci.

ACUTE STREPTOCOCCAL INFECTIONS

Epidemiology

Aerobic streptococcal infections are observed in all races, in both sexes, and at all ages. Furthermore, they occur during any season of the year throughout the world. The *incidence* and the *clinical manifestations* are altered by certain of the above factors. Thus streptococcal respiratory infections, including scarlet fever, are encountered especially during the colder months of the year. Scarlet fever is rare in the tropics. Under the age of three months, streptococcal infections are rare and, when they occur, are associated with a high mortality. Between the ages of six months and ten years, scarlet fever occurs frequently. Tonsillitis and pharyngitis are especially prevalent throughout childhood and early adult life. In women during the child-bearing period, puerperal infections caused by streptococci are occasionally observed. Finally, erysipelas, which may occur at any age, appears to be more prevalent in infants and the older age groups.

Soon after birth, alpha streptococci appear in the upper respiratory tract and may be isolated therefrom throughout life. Streptococci of Lancefield groups C and G and, more rarely, organisms of groups other than A may be isolated from the oropharynx of 5 per cent or more of the normal population. Occasionally group C and G streptococci cause tonsillitis.

The group A flora of the oropharynx of any population group is made up of many different specific types, but usually several types predominate. In general, at least 5 per cent of the people of any community harbor group A streptococci. The prevalence varies and depends upon the cultural methods used as well as upon environmental, host, and bacterial factors. Persons under twenty years of age, especially if the tonsils are present, are most likely to harbor group A streptococci.

Studies of carriers of group A streptococci suggest that many are convalescent carriers; that is, they recently suffered either an apparent or an unapparent infection. This appears to be especially likely if large numbers of streptococci are isolated from the oropharynx. Such individuals frequently give a history of a recent illness, and the antistreptolysin titer of their serum is high. These data suggest that streptococci of group A rarely occur in the throat in large numbers except immediately before, during, or after an infection. Once an individual has been infected, he may remain a carrier for many months. As the carrier state progresses, the streptococci lose their ability to produce M-protein.

Ability to spread disease appears to be an attribute of individuals who have recently been infected. Whether this is because such persons harbor numerous streptococci in the nose and throat or because the organisms are especially capable of parasitizing another person cannot be determined from the available evidence. It is established that nasal carriers of group A streptococci are especially likely to spread disease.

Respiratory pathogens are believed to be spread by two mechanisms: (1) *directly* between two persons by physical contact or by droplets passing through the air for short distances, (2) *indirectly* by droplet nuclei, dust, and fomites. Recent studies have shown, however, that group A streptococci

naturally deposited in dust and on blankets will not produce respiratory infections in man. The evidence implicates the direct mode of transfer as primarily responsible for dissemination of such infections.

The spread of streptococci in any population group must also be related to the degree of exposure. Thus, during the winter months when people are confined to enclosed areas and under crowded conditions, dissemination of bacteria is especially likely to occur.

Outbreaks of streptococcal infection occasionally occur following the contamination of food. Such outbreaks are dramatic in that a large number of persons are affected almost simultaneously. Formerly this type of infection was termed *septic sore throat;* aside from the fact that the infection is caused by a single type of streptococcus, it varies clinically in no way from other streptococcal epidemics.

Clinical studies have demonstrated that reinfection may occur by a second type of group A streptococcus in a patient recovering from streptococcal pharyngitis and tonsillitis.

Primary infection of the upper respiratory tract is undoubtedly the most common form of streptococcal infection in man. It is doubtful whether anyone in the United States escapes one or more of these infections. The disease occurs especially in individuals between the ages of one and twenty years, but it may develop at any age. It is especially prevalent in the Temperate Zones during the winter and early spring seasons. In most areas the disease is endemic. Epidemics are usually due to one or, at the most, several types of group A streptococci, whereas many different types are responsible for cases of pharyngitis and tonsillitis occurring sporadically.

Tonsillitis and *pharyngitis* due to the beta streptococcus are characterized by an acute sore throat which may or may not be accompanied by a cutaneous rash. If a rash is observed, a diagnosis of *scarlet fever* is made. The occurrence of a rash is related to antitoxic immunity, which may be measured by the Dick test.

Studies of the Dick reaction in various population groups have shown that at birth and up to three months of age the test is usually negative. By the age of one to two years, 85 per cent of the reactions are positive. There is a rapid decline in the positive reactors to a level of approximately 15 per cent at the age of ten. During the rest of life the decline is gradual. These results would indicate that children under the age of ten are most susceptible to scarlet fever, and this is the age period when most scarlet fever occurs. Following an attack of scarlet fever, the Dick reaction usually becomes negative.

The incidence of scarlet fever has not changed significantly in the past 30 years, but there has been a spectacular decline in mortality. Top reports a fatality rate in Detroit of 2.7 in 1920, 1.3 in 1930, and 0.3 in 1940. The reason for the apparent decreasing severity of scarlet fever is not entirely clear.

Infections of the *paranasal sinuses* and middle ear often develop following infection of the tonsils or pharynx. Not only may they occur as a complication of streptococcal sore throat, but they are also commonly seen following measles, influenza, pertussis, and other respiratory infections.

Bacterial pneumonia caused by aerobic streptococci accounts for less than 5 per cent of all cases of pneumonia. The disease is almost invariably caused by group A streptococci and may arise secondarily to an infection of the upper respiratory tract. Epidemics have been observed following influenza and measles. It also is likely to occur in those individuals with chronic lung disease, including asthma and bronchiectasis. Streptococcal empyema, a complication of pneumonia in most instances, is observed most frequently in patients under thirty years of age.

Formerly it was thought that *erysipelas* was caused by a specific strain of beta-hemolytic streptococcus, but it is now known that group A, C, or G streptococci may be isolated from the skin lesions. Group A organisms are responsible for the majority of infections, and the organisms may belong to any of the various types in this group. Although there are examples of several people having contracted erysipelas following contact with a case, in most instances it has been impossible to trace the infection to such contact. Erysipelas tends to occur in the older age groups, especially in those individuals with chronic disabling diseases. Immunity does not develop; in fact, individuals who have suffered from one attack are more susceptible than the normal population. In some of the recurrences, however, the organisms cannot be isolated from the skin lesions but may be found in the oropharynx. It is suggested that in such instances the disease is due to absorption of some toxic product of the streptococcus which, in turn, causes the local inflammatory lesion in the skin that is altered in its reactivity.

Wounds may be infected by contamination at the time of dressing by droplets from either the patient or the attending physician. Another possible source of infection is dust. *Lymphangitis* may arise from a minute abrasion.

Numerous studies have indicated that either aerobic or anaerobic streptococci cause *puerperal sepsis*. Approximately 70 per cent of fatal cases are due to beta-hemolytic streptococci. Most of the infections are caused by group A, although an occasional case is due to streptococci belonging to group B, C, D, or G. Since the group A streptococcus is rarely isolated from the genital tract either before or after labor, it is assumed that infection is extrinsic. Careful study of the patient and all persons coming in contact with her has shown that similar types of group A streptococci can be isolated from 75 per cent of cultures obtained from the oropharynx of such a patient or those attending her. It appears from these studies that infection is usually contracted from an outside source and occasionally from the respiratory tract of the patient herself.

Pathogenesis

Streptococci gain entrance to the body primarily through the upper respiratory tract. The organisms, lodging on the mucous membranes or on other tissues, probably remain viable for relatively short periods unless they actually invade the tissues. In the nose and throat there is ample opportunity for invasion. The organisms usually gain entrance through the lymphoid tissues of the throat, especially the tonsils, whose crypts apparently offer an ideal locus. Occasionally the primary infection may be in the paranasal sinuses.

The factors which determine whether an infection follows exposure to the organism are multiple. The *dosage* or number of streptococci is apparently a decisive factor. Infection usually results when there is exposure to large numbers of group A streptococci, as occurs in food-borne outbreaks. Under natural conditions of spread, the number of organisms acquired is dependent in part on the duration and intimacy of exposure to the organism.

The second factor in relation to the organism is *virulence*. In general, little is known concerning this important feature. Streptococci of groups other than A may be considered relatively avirulent when implanted in the lymphoid tissues of the throat. The virulence of the group A organism may be related to their M antigenic component. Whether there is variation in the virulence of the group A streptococci according to the specific type is not definitely known, nor is there much evidence that rapid passage of a given type from man to man increases the virulence of the organisms, although this is a common belief.

Perhaps as important as the organism itself is the susceptibility of the host. It is stated that a recent or simultaneous infection with one of the common respiratory viruses renders the host more susceptible to bacterial invasion. Experience during the First World War would seem to indicate that influenza does indeed make one more susceptible to bacterial infections. Whether the common cold or acute respiratory disease acts in a similar fashion is not known.

Whether the group A streptococcus gains a foothold in the tissues is also governed by the immune status of the host. The presence of type-specific antibodies undoubtedly protects the individual against infection.

When the bacteria begin to multiply in the infected tissues, they produce certain toxic substances which account for the clinical manifestations of disease. For example, some of the constitutional symptoms observed in patients with scarlet fever are believed to be due to the erythrogenic toxin. Usually the mucous membrane is denuded and covered by a thin yellow, white, or gray exudate. Edema and hyperemia of the lymphoid tissues are present. The lymphatics are dilated. The regional cervical lymph nodes are enlarged.

The organisms may invade the blood stream if the local defense mechanism is not functioning adequately and cause either metastatic infections, such as meningitis, brain abscess, and endocarditis, or a generalized infection, which without treatment almost invariably results in death. Mallory and Keefer have studied the cellular changes in such patients as well as the disease process in patients dying during the acute phase of streptococcal infections without bacteremia. In fulminating streptococcal infections the streptococci may be seen in blood vessels throughout the body, as well as in the endothelial cells of the endocardium and in the perivascular areas. There is little cellular reaction around the organisms, but their distribution is similar to the distribution of those lesions observed in patients dying several days after onset of the infection. In the latter cases, foci of lymphocytes, plasma cells, and histiocytes are commonly found in the heart, especially just under the surface endothelium and endocardium. Such collections occur also in the perivascular connective tissues, myocardium, and pericardium. Occasionally some of the foci show polymorphonuclear leukocytes. In the kidneys, interstitial nephritis is observed, with focal areas of round-cell infiltration in the tissue surrounding the tubules, glomeruli, and blood vessels. Similar lesions may be observed in other organs, including the lung, portal areas of the liver, and pancreas.

Most streptococcal infections are of short duration, the acute phase ending within 5 to 7 days. The exact mechanism for recovery at this time has not been defined, but, as in other bacterial infections, it is assumed that antibodies develop which aid in the destruction of the organism. Perhaps the most important of these are the antibacterial substances. Techniques for measuring these antibodies are difficult, but it is apparent that following infection there is an increase in the bactericidal power of whole blood. Such bactericidal action is type-specific; the patient is protected only against the infecting type of group A streptococci and not against other types of this group of organisms. Such antibacterial immunity may persist for years.

Acute Tonsillitis, Pharyngitis, and Scarlet Fever

The terminology used to classify streptococcal infections of the upper respiratory tract has been in use for many years and was introduced prior to the time that it was realized that *scarlet fever, septic sore throat, acute tonsillitis,* and *pharyngitis* with or without exudate were all caused by any of the numerous types of group A streptococci. In these diseases the organism establishes itself in the lymphoid tissue; *streptococcal lymphoiditis* might well be substituted for the above names. As far as is known, the course of the illness, complications, and sequelae are similar in scarlet fever, septic sore throat, and streptococcal tonsillitis.

Symptoms. The incubation period varies from 1 to 10 days but is usually 3 to 5 days. The illness begins abruptly in most cases with symptoms of feverishness, chilliness, headache, and sore throat. Nausea and vomiting are especially common in children. A few patients complain of diarrhea. Within a period of 24 to 48 hr the disease reaches its maximum intensity. Chilliness is a constant symptom, but true rigors are rarely observed. Approximately 75 per cent or more of the patients complain of such constitutional symptoms as headache, malaise, and loss of appetite.

The symptom which is very annoying and almost constantly present within 24 hr of onset is sore throat. The soreness is aggravated by swallowing and may be referred to the neck, so that even turning of the head is accompanied by pain. Nasal obstruction and discharge are minor complaints but occur in 60 per cent of patients. About half the patients develop very mild symptoms referable to the lower respiratory tract, including cough and hoarseness. The cough is not productive and is rarely associated with chest pain. Loss of voice due to laryngitis does not occur. Earache is common and may last a few hours to several days. Occasionally, epistaxis is observed.

During the period of maximum temperature there may be a diffuse blush of the skin. In some cases it becomes more pronounced, and a diagnosis of *scarlet fever* is made. The rash may appear 1 to 5 days after onset of illness and is first noticed over the neck and upper chest. It spreads rapidly to include the skin over the abdomen and upper and lower extremities. The face appears flushed, and a circumoral pallor is prominent in many cases. Itching occasionally occurs but is rarely severe.

Physical Signs. The degree of prostration varies, but the majority of patients appear mildly or moderately ill. The temperature is usually elevated to 102 to 104°F; occasionally it may be as high as

106°F. A few patients have no fever. In children the pulse rate is between 140 and 160, in adults between 120 and 140 per minute. Usually the respirations are not greatly increased.

Various degrees of diffuse redness of the mucous membranes of the posterior pharynx, faucial tonsils, and soft palate are invariably present. The uvula is frequently edematous, as are the tonsils and pharynx but to a lesser degree. Lymphoid hyperplasia and edema, which gives the posterior pharynx a cobblestone appearance, are present. Characteristically there is discrete to confluent exudate on the tonsils, and variable numbers of pinhead-size areas of exudate appear on the pharynx. In severely ill patients the latter are seldom seen, because nasal secretions cover the posterior wall. The exudate is often yellow, sometimes gray or white, and is relatively easily removed by swabbing. In about 20 per cent of adults, and more frequently in infants, exudative lesions on the mucous membranes do not develop. Occasionally, and especially if sinusitis and rhinitis are coexistent, there is a thick mucopurulent nasal discharge which may be tinged with blood. In children the nares may be excoriated. The cervical lymph nodes are swollen and frequently tender. The lymph nodes just below the angle of the jaw are the first to enlarge; rarely they attain such size that the head is thrown back. Marked adenopathy is frequently followed by suppuration.

In those patients with *scarlet fever* the signs include both an enanthem and an exanthem. The appearance of the throat is similar to that seen in tonsillitis and pharyngitis without rash, except that diffuse redness is more intense and has been described as "boiled-lobster" red. There may be punctate redness of the soft and hard palate. The buccal mucous membranes appear red and swollen, as do the lips. About the second to fifth day, small, milk-white patches may be seen on the buccal mucous membranes. They represent desquamation of the epithelium and are easily peeled off.

Early in the course of the infection the tongue is heavily coated and grayish. Soon the tip and edges become an angry red. Fungiform papillae become swollen and emerge through the gray surface of the tongue. By the fourth to fifth day there is complete lingual desquamation which leaves multiple papillary elevations, the so-called "strawberry tongue."

The color of the exanthem varies and has been described as scarlet, bright red, rose-colored, or dull, dusky red. At a distance there appears to be a uniform blush, but upon close inspection innumerable small reddish points are seen. Because of pin-point elevations at the site of the hair follicles, the skin may feel like sandpaper. This sign is of special importance in races where the skin is heavily pigmented. When the eruption is intense, there may be many small miliary vesicles over the chest and abdomen. The face may be free of rash, but ordinarily the temples and cheeks are deep red, leaving an area of pallor around the mouth and nose. The rash is due to hyperemia, and pressure causes it to fade. In some areas there may be punctate hemorrhages which do not fade; these are commonly seen in the creases at the elbow flexure (Pastia's sign), groin, and axillary folds.

Course of Illness (Fig 114-1). The majority of upper respiratory illnesses caused by group A streptococci are self-limited. In adults the temperature usually returns to normal by the third to fourth day, whereas in children fever may persist for 5 to 9 days. The temperature curve is not characteristic, although there is usually a slight morning remission. In patients with scarlet fever the temperature remains elevated until the rash has reached its maximum intensity. Fever may last for several weeks, but in such instances it is well to search for some suppurative complications. The constitutional symptoms, as well as the localizing symptom of sore throat, usually disappear shortly after the fever subsides.

The edema, redness, and exudate disappear rap-

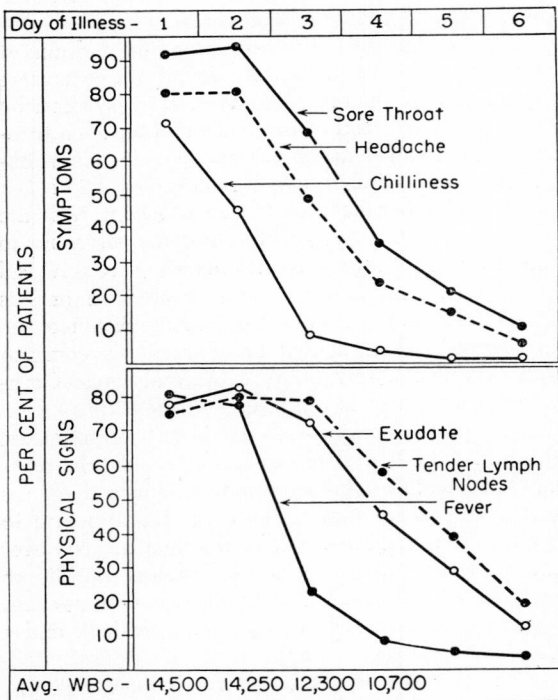

FIG. 114-1. The natural course of group A streptococcal tonsillitis.

idly, and except for a few small isolated spots of exudate and a slight degree of redness, the throat appears essentially normal shortly after the fever subsides. The lymphoid tissues of the posterior pharynx as well as the tonsils decrease in size and by the third to sixth week appear to be normal. The lymph nodes may not return to normal size for 6 weeks.

When rash does occur, it usually makes its appearance on the second day, reaches its maximum intensity shortly thereafter, and then begins to fade. The exfoliation of the epithelium begins during the decline of the eruption and is seen first in those areas where the rash originally appeared. By the sixth to seventh day it is more or less generalized. On the hands and feet the skin sheds in flakes, or, more rarely, an entire cast of the hand or foot may be observed. The skin in these areas becomes dry, hard, and wrinkled. The most typical form of desquamation is seen beneath the free edge of the fingernails. A fissure appears under the edge of the nail and then widens, revealing the soft, pinkish underlying skin.

Before the introduction of specific chemotherapeutic agents, the mortality rate was in the neighborhood of 3 per cent; it is now less than 0.5 per cent. This may be because of treatment or because few severe forms of scarlet fever are seen today. Streptococcal infections are likely to be fatal in the extremes of life and in those individuals with severe suppurative complications.

Laboratory Findings. In 80 per cent of patients the total leukocyte count is increased. During the first 2 days of disease the average count is 14,000, and as the illness progresses, it returns to normal values. If the number of leukocytes remains elevated after 1 week, evidence of a complication may be found. During the first 2 days of illness eosinophils are rarely seen, but convalescence is characterized by an increase of these cells. Patients with scarlet fever are especially likely to exhibit an elevation of eosinophils. Not infrequently a trace of albumin may be found in the urine during the acute phase of the illness. Rarely, such specimens show a few red cells or casts. Proteinuria occurring during the first 5 days of illness is transient and is not attended by serious sequelae.

Cultures made on blood agar plates from a swab rubbed over the tonsils and oropharynx usually show a predominant growth of beta-hemolytic streptococci. Occasionally only a few colonies are observed. Rarely, no streptococci are isolated. In the latter instance, repeated cultures should be obtained. The convalescent carrier state may continue for several months.

Diagnosis. Important features in the diagnosis of streptococcal pharyngitis and tonsillitis are the his-

tory of an acute onset of soreness on swallowing, associated with feverishness and other constitutional symptoms. The physical signs of diffuse redness and edema of the mucous membranes of the oropharynx, tonsils, and soft palate, the presence of discrete to confluent exudate, and enlargement and tenderness of the lymph nodes at the angle of the jaw are especially helpful. These findings, together with a leukocyte count of at least 12,000, suggest a streptococcal infection. If the culture of the local lesion shows a predominant growth of beta streptococci, the diagnosis is almost certainly established. When only a few colonies grow on the blood agar plate, it is impossible to be sure whether the patient is a carrier or actually has an infection due to the streptococcus. In such cases it is of considerable help to obtain acute and convalescent blood specimens for determination of the antistreptolysin titer.

When a rash is associated with the above clinical and laboratory findings, the diagnosis is scarlet fever. Confirmation is obtained if later the skin desquamates. Occasionally, however, the diagnosis is doubtful, and in such cases the Schultz-Charlton test may be of considerable aid. In this test 0.1 ml scarlet fever antitoxin or 0.2 to 0.5 ml scarlet fever convalescent serum is injected subcutaneously into the area of the skin where the heaviest rash appears. If the rash is due to the erythrogenic toxin, blanching is observed within 2 to 8 hr. The test should be employed soon after the eruption appears, because blanching may not occur after the second day of rash. The Dick test may also be of some use in establishing the diagnosis; early in the disease it is positive, whereas during convalescence it usually becomes negative.

Differential Diagnosis of Sore Throat. *Nonbacterial exudative tonsillitis and pharyngitis* must be differentiated from streptococcal infections of the oropharynx (see p. 1118). The agents responsible for these infections have not been completely defined, but it is known that some of the adenoviruses will produce respiratory infections associated with exudative lesions, and in some outbreaks there is involvement of the conjunctiva. In general the onset of illness is not rapid, soreness of the throat is seldom marked, and constitutional symptoms are mild. Hoarseness and cough are likely to occur several days after the onset. The exudate is rarely confluent. Diffuse redness and edema of all the mucous membranes are rare. The lymph nodes may be slightly enlarged, but they are not remarkably tender.

The leukocyte count is usually normal, although in a few cases it may be slightly elevated. Cultures of the throat fail to show beta-hemolytic streptococci. Occasionally a few streptococci are recovered, but these organisms usually belong to groups other than A and occur only in small numbers.

Infectious mononucleosis is most frequently observed in young adults and, because of the local reaction in the throat, is likely to be confused with streptococcal pharyngitis (see p. 1248). The onset may be insidious, and malaise is prominent. Sore throat with exudative lesions of the tonsils is observed in over half the cases. The exudate is usually white and pasty and persists for 1 to 3 weeks. The temperature tends to be very irregular, and fever continues for a longer period than is usual in streptococcal infections. Lymph node enlargement is more generalized, but suppuration is not observed. The spleen may be palpable. In 10 to 15 per cent of cases a fleeting skin rash occurs which may be identical with that seen in scarlet fever. In such cases a negative Schultz-Charlton test may be helpful. The blood changes are characteristic, and a positive heterophil antibody test is usually obtained.

Vincent's angina is not easily confused with streptococcal infections. The disease is characterized by insidious onset without constitutional symptoms. Fever is rare. The area surrounding the exudate shows little inflammatory reaction, and only one tonsil is involved. Cervical adenopathy is usually unilateral.

In contrast to streptococcal pharyngitis, the onset of *diphtheria* is rarely sudden and the symptoms are not severe (see p. 982). Sore throat is not a constant feature of the disease. The exudate is smooth and cream-colored and appears to be incorporated in the mucous membranes. The membrane is removed with difficulty, leaving a bleeding bed. Cutaneous rashes are absent. Cultures show *Corynebacterium diphtheriae*.

In patients with a rash, the disease must be differentiated from *German measles* and *measles*. In German measles the posterior cervical lymph node enlargement is helpful, as well as the fact that the rash tends to be macular and discrete. The tongue never peels, and a leukopenia is characteristic. In measles there are prodromal respiratory symptoms, and the maculopapular rash occurs chiefly on the face and neck. There is no blanching of the skin following a Schultz-Charlton test. The presence of Koplik's spots aids in establishing the diagnosis.

Streptococcal infections without exudate or a cutaneous rash must be differentiated from *influenza virus infections* and *common respiratory diseases*. In general, such differentiations cannot be made on clinical evidence alone, so that the leukocyte count, culture studies, and serologic tests must be employed.

Primary *herpes simplex pharyngitis* (see p. 1171) and *herpangina* (see p. 1173) are characterized by vesicles which rupture and produce small ulcers covered with exudate. Herpetic lesions are scattered over all mucous membranes of the mouth, and the kissing ulcer under the tip of the tongue is typical. The ulcers of herpangina, caused by Coxsackie A viruses, are observed on the anterior pillars and the soft palate. In both diseases the leukocyte count is usually normal.

Sinusitis, Otitis Media, Mastoiditis, and Peritonsillar Abscess

Infection of the paranasal sinuses probably occurs to a minor degree in all patients with streptococcal respiratory infections. Sinusitis and otitis media presenting overt clinical signs develop in approximately 3 per cent of patients whose tonsils and adenoids are intact. Mastoiditis is observed in less than 1 per cent of patients. Peritonsillar cellulitis is observed in 2.5 per cent of patients with tonsils, but it rarely occurs in those whose tonsils have been removed or in those patients who receive proper therapy with antibiotics. The diagnosis and management of these suppurative complications are described on p. 1031.

Pneumonia and Empyema

The natural course of pneumonia caused by Lancefield group A streptococci is extremely variable, probably because in many instances it is secondary to such infections as influenza, tonsillitis, measles, and erysipelas. It may be associated with pneumococcal infection of the lung or may arise as a metastatic complication of streptococcal bacteremia. Although it is not a common complication of streptococcal sore throat, about 25 per cent of pneumonia cases follow this infection. Characteristically, this organism produces an interstitial or confluent pneumonia. The reported mortality rate varies from 15 to 60 per cent.

The onset of pneumonia may be abrupt, with such constitutional symptoms as chills, feverishness, anorexia, and vomiting. Symptoms include cough, expectoration of purulent sputum, and chest pain. The pulse and respiratory rates are increased, and cyanosis may be prominent. The temperature tends to be high (104°F) and septic in type. Examination reveals local signs of pneumonia, with scattered fine rales and occasional areas of dullness. Frank signs of lobar consolidation are rare.

The leukocyte count is almost invariably elevated to 20,000 to 30,000, and the sputum is found to contain large numbers of group A organisms. Usually the blood cultures are sterile; when bacteremia occurs, the prognosis is poor.

The untreated disease runs a variable course. In most instances recovery is delayed for several weeks, and lung abscess and bronchiectasis are not uncommon complications. In fatal cases mediastinitis and pericarditis may occur. The most frequent complication is empyema, which occurs in 20 per cent of the cases.

Streptococcal *empyema* is usually secondary to pneumonia caused by the same organism, but occasionally it arises following other infections of the lung, infarcts, or lung tumors. It is most likely to occur under the age of thirty years, and the mortality rate in untreated cases is high. Early in the disease the pleural fluid may be hemorrhagic. It becomes thick and purulent slowly, in contrast to the exudate seen in pneumococcal empyema.

Pericarditis, Arthritis, Peritonitis, and Meningitis

Streptococcal infections of the various body cavities result from bacteremia or from extension from a local lesion. *Pericarditis,* a rare complication, is especially likely to occur during the course of pneumonia or empyema. The diagnosis is difficult, since the symptoms arising from pericarditis are overshadowed by the primary disease. The first sign may be a sudden increase in pulse rate and the development of an audible pericardial friction rub. Roentgenograms are of great aid in establishing the diagnosis. Once the diagnosis is suspected, aspiration and culture of the fluid are indicated.

Suppurative arthritis is secondary to bacteremia or to extension of a local cellulitis. It is a rare complication of streptococcal sore throat. Pain is the most common symptom, and usually only one joint is involved. The pain is first noticed on motion, but within a short period redness, swelling, and tenderness develop and the pain becomes intense. Aspiration reveals a fluid containing polymorphonuclear leukocytes and streptococci. Nonsuppurative arthritis is seen in patients with scarlet fever during the first week of illness.

Infection of the peritoneum with the hemolytic streptococcus is rare but is especially apt to be associated with such local infections as erysipelas and scarlet fever. In these cases the organism belongs to Lancefield group A. Symptoms develop rapidly, and in addition to fever and other constitutional symptoms, prostration, abdominal pain, and vomiting are prominent. The pulse is rapid and weak. The abdomen is distended, tender, and rigid to palpation.

Streptococcal *meningitis* is usually caused by group A organisms, but occasionally members of other groups may be isolated from the spinal fluid. In most instances the meningitis arises by extension and invasion of the blood stream from an otitis media, mastoiditis, or petrositis, which are especially likely to develop following infection of the respiratory tract and are most frequently seen in the young age groups. Prior to the introduction of specific therapy these infections were always fatal. The symptoms of streptococcal meningitis are not distinguishable from other types of bacterial meningitis. It should be emphasized that all patients, especially infants, with infections of the middle ear should be watched for signs of meningeal irritation. Once such signs develop, lumbar puncture and culture of the spinal fluid establish the diagnosis.

Wound and Skin Infections, Lymphangitis, Puerperal Fever, and Erysipelas

As indicated earlier, *wound and skin infections* are usually the result of contamination. Children with chickenpox, impetigo, and other skin lesions may become infected with group A and C streptococci.

Hemolytic streptococci are responsible for the majority of cases of the familiar form of *lymphangitis.* The disease is characterized by the rapid development of one or more fine red streaks extending upward from the hand or foot. Usually the process continues up to the axilla or groin, and the lymph nodes in these areas become enlarged and tender. Associated with the spread of the infection in the lymphatics, such symptoms as rigor, fever, malaise, headache, and vomiting occur. Occasionally the blood stream is invaded. The original site of infection in these cases of lymphangitis may be unapparent. Although these infections may be serious, the course of the illness is usually short, and suppuration seldom occurs along the course of the lymphatics or in the regional lymph nodes.

Puerperal infections caused by hemolytic streptococci are always serious. Following abortion or delivery, the streptococci invade the endometrium and lymphatics. The infection may spread to the surrounding structures, producing cellulitis, phlebitis, abscess, peritonitis, or bacteremia. The patient develops a high, irregular fever associated with rigors. The pulse is rapid. The diagnosis is based on local signs of infection as well as on such laboratory findings as leukocytosis and isolation of streptococci from the blood stream or from the cervical discharge.

Erysipelas is an acute streptococcal infection of the skin and, to a lesser extent, of the mucous membranes. The onset is usually abrupt, beginning after an incubation period of approximately 1 to 4 days. In some patients a history of preceding respiratory infection is obtained. The initial symptoms include chilliness, feverishness, headache, malaise, anorexia, and vomiting. The first symptom may be a true rigor. At the onset the local cutaneous lesion may not be apparent, although there may be slight redness in those instances where it arises in conjunction with an abrasion of the skin. The skin may itch and feel sore around the point of entry of the organisms. Within a few hours, and usually by 24 hr, the cutaneous lesion becomes obvious.

The skin of the face is most commonly involved,

but any area of the body may be infected. The point of entry around the face may be just anterior to the ear, at the inner canthus of the eye, around the lips and nose, or over the cheeks. From these points the lesion spreads rapidly, reaching its maximum extent within 3 to 6 days. On the face, erysipelas frequently involves the butterfly area, i.e., the cheeks and nose. The lesion consists of an advancing border which is raised from the surrounding normal skin and may be purple. Within this border the skin is tense and usually a dark, dull red. If the infection occurs in areas where the skin is lax, such as around the eyes, edema is pronounced. The eyelids frequently become so swollen that they cannot be opened. Blebs or even necrotic areas may appear as the disease progresses.

At the height of the infection the temperature is usually high (104 to 105°F), although occasionally the febrile response is slight. The blood stream is not uncommonly invaded during this period. The disease lasts for a variable length of time, but in most instances recovery is apparent by the sixth to seventh day. The local lesion begins to fade in the center and is usually accompanied by some desquamation and pigmentation. No scarring results unless abscesses develop.

Before the introduction of chemotherapy, the fatality rate was about 15 per cent. During the first 6 months of life approximately 65 per cent succumb, whereas in children and young adults the death rate is low. In patients with fatal infections the lesion is likely to involve the trunk, and, in addition, the blood stream is invaded.

Bacteremia

Strepococci are a common cause of bacteremia, but in uncomplicated tonsillitis and pharyngitis the organisms rarely invade the blood stream. Bacteremia occurring under the age of twenty usually is secondary to otitis media, mastoiditis, or thrombosis of the lateral or cavernous sinuses. In the adult, invasion of the blood stream is especially likely to occur in women with puerperal infections, whereas after the age of forty bacteremia is usually secondary to cellulitis and erysipelas. Metastatic abscesses develop infrequently during the course of bacteremia.

The diagnosis of bacteremia is difficult and can be made only by culturing the organisms from the blood. The sudden development of chills and high fever, either irregular or continuous, suggests invasion of the blood stream. Severe headache, nausea, vomiting, and delirium are common symptoms. In streptococcal bacteremia there may be arthritis, signs of pneumonia, petechiae, or skin eruptions. In fulminating cases anemia develops rapidly and jaundice may occur. Without specific therapy the mortality rate is 70 per cent.

Pyelonephritis

Infections of the kidney and urinary passages will be discussed in more detail in Chap. 258. Here it should be emphasized that streptococci usually belonging to group D may be isolated from the urine of patients with infection of the urinary tract. When the organisms are present in large numbers, there is usually dysuria, frequency, flank pain, fever, and pyuria.

Treatment

There are now several agents which may be employed in the therapy of aerobic streptococcal infections. The sulfonamides have been widely employed. These compounds exert a bacteriostatic effect against all Lancefield groups except D. However, there are strains of group A streptococci that have acquired resistance. Most antibiotic compounds exhibit a more marked effect than the sulfonamides, but penicillin displays the maximal antistreptococcal activity. Penicillin actually kills group A organisms, and if it is administered for at least 10 days, all streptococci are eliminated in most instances. Therapeutic measures which do not result in the eradication of the infecting organism do not alter the attack rate of rheumatic fever.

The administration of penicillin or other antibiotics within 24 hr of the onset of streptococcal respiratory infections results in a definite favorable effect on the symptoms and signs associated with the acute illness. When therapy is instituted after 48 hr a favorable effect is difficult to demonstrate, but suppurative complications, including sinusitis, otitis media, and peritonsillar cellulitis are still prevented. The time that treatment is started is not decisive in the reduction of rheumatic fever; however, early therapy may be important in the prevention of nephritis.

In the average case of streptococcal infection, whether scarlet fever, tonsillitis, or erysipelas, sufficient concentration of antibiotic can be maintained most readily by a single injection of 600,000 to 900,000 units of benzathine penicillin. In patients who exhibit rheumatic heart disease and who develop a streptococcal infection, it may be advisable to administer 600,000 units of procaine penicillin twice daily for 2 weeks.

Oral therapy may by prescribed, but it should be emphasized that many patients discontinue the medication when the acute phase symptoms subside. Under these circumstances the organism frequently invades the tissues again, and a clinical relapse occurs. More important, the attack rate of the nonsuppurative complications is not altered. All forms of oral medication must be taken in full doses for at least 10 days and preferably for 2 weeks. Oral preparations of penicillin are given in doses of 250,000 units four times daily. If the patient is sensitive to penicillin, then erythromycin in doses of 0.2 Gm is administered every 6 hr. Tetracycline is given every 4 hr in a dose of 0.25 Gm.

The *sulfonamides* should never be employed in the treatment of streptococcal infections since they fail to eliminate the infecting organism and do not alter the subsequent attack rate of rheumatic fever. Application of penicillin or other drugs by means of troches or sprays has little effect on the local inflammatory lesion or on the infecting organism.

Penicillin appears to exert a definite effect on the incidence of suppurative complications of tonsillitis and pharyngitis. Complications such as mastoiditis are rare during this form of therapy. Infections of the mastoid and paranasal sinuses should likewise be treated by the parenteral administration of penicillin. Streptococcal pneumonia should be treated with somewhat larger amounts of penicillin; a dose of 100,000 units every 3 hr is suggested. Similar amounts administered every 2 hr should be given to patients with puerperal sepsis and bacteremia. Empyema, purulent pericarditis, and arthritis are best treated by local instillation of 10,000 to 50,000 units of penicillin every 48 to 72 hr until cultures are sterile. In addition, full doses of parenteral penicillin should be administered. In these infections early treatment is required if surgical drainage is to be avoided.

General measures for the supportive and symptomatic therapy of infections should be employed. The use of saline gargles and irrigations of the throat may be effective in the relief of the angina associated with tonsillitis. The use of cold applications to erysipelas or to tender and enlarged cervical lymph nodes frequently affords symptomatic relief.

Prevention

It may be stated that there is no completely adequate method for the prevention of streptococcal infections. A number of procedures will limit the spread of the organism to some extent. The problem is exceedingly complicated because group A streptococci occur in the upper respiratory tract of many individuals.

In the past it has been customary to isolate all patients with scarlet fever, but today such procedures seem unwarranted, for no precautions are taken for sore throat without a rash caused by the same bacterium. Any patient with a streptococcal infection of the upper respiratory tract may be a source of infection. During the acute stage of all such illnesses the patient should be advised against intimate contact with others.

Approximately 90 per cent of patients with streptococcal infections continue to carry the organism in the pharynx 3 months after the acute infection. Usually the number of organisms is small. Individuals with suppurative complications of the sinuses are likely to harbor large numbers of streptococci and would appear to be a dangerous source of infection. Proper therapy of acute infections with penicillin prevents the development of the carrier state and promptly eliminates the organism.

There is no specific immunizing procedure which will protect against streptococcal infections. This is not surprising, since the evidence today is that immunity is largely type-specific.

Individuals or groups of individuals may be protected from streptococcal infections by the prophylactic use of sulfonamide drugs. For this purpose 1 Gm sulfadiazine is administered daily. Such prophylaxis, when given to populations already experiencing an epidemic, will control the outbreak as long as the drug is administered. When therapy is stopped, streptococcal infections again occur because of the failure of sulfonamides to eliminate the infecting organism. For this reason oral penicillin in doses of 250,000 units two or three times daily for 10 days or the injection of 1,200,000 units of benzathine penicillin is a preferred form of prophylaxis in large population groups. Benzathine penicillin in doses of 600,000 and 1,200,000 units will protect the individual from new infections for from 3 and 4 to 6 weeks, respectively.

Tonsillectomy has been employed widely as a prophylactic measure for streptococcal infections. It is obvious that tonsillitis cannot occur if the organ is removed, but there is no protection afforded against streptococcal pharyngitis. Indeed, the only measurable effect is that tonsillectomy makes subsequent recognition of the cause of the respiratory illness difficult.

Many attempts have been made to control respiratory disease by altering certain environmental factors, by using, for example, ultraviolet light, aerosols, and various dust-holding procedures and by treating bed clothing with oils. It has been demonstrated that such methods decrease the contamination of the air, but the degree of their effectiveness in preventing infection is slight.

LATE NONSUPPURATIVE COMPLICATIONS OF GROUP A STREPTOCOCCAL INFECTIONS

As indicated previously, beta-streptococcal infections assume importance not only because of the high morbidity and the immediate suppurative complications, but also because of the late sequelae.

There is considerable evidence that rheumatic fever, acute glomerulonephritis, and scleredema adultorum (see p. 1901) are precipitated by, if not directly related to, infection with the beta streptococcus. Rheumatic fever may be followed by valvular disease, and therefore this sequela of streptococcal infection assumes importance as a cause of chronic illness.

Etiology and Pathogenesis

Although group A streptococci are considered to be the inciting agent of both rheumatic fever and glomerulonephritis, these two diseases have never been reproduced in animals, nor have the mechanisms involved been defined. Therefore, it is not surprising that numerous theories have been proposed to explain the nature of the cardiac and renal complications.

Streptococcal infections are characterized by an acute toxic or septic phase which last 3 to 7 days. Following the acute illness, the patient seemingly recovers completely, except for those few individuals who have developed a suppurative complication. After a latent period, the patient may again present symptoms and signs of illness, but this time the manifestations are related to involvement of new areas of the body, and the illnesses developing after the latent period present a varied clinical picture. These illnesses have been collectively termed the late nonsuppurative complications of hemolytic streptococcal infections (Fig. 114-2). The latent period and the resemblance of certain manifestations to serum sickness suggest some altered or unusual tissue reaction, but to ascribe hypersensitivity as the responsible mechanism on the basis of this evidence alone is not warranted.

The spectrum of the nonsuppurative illnesses is broad. Certain patients develop fever with no localizing signs. Others exhibit lymphadenitis with fever. Such illnesses have been called streptococcal fever, but it seems probable that they represent

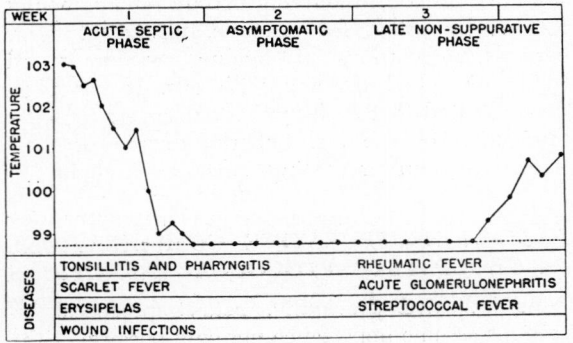

FIG. 114-2. The various phases of hemolytic streptococcal infections.

mild rheumatic attacks. Approximately 3 per cent develop signs of involvement of the joints or heart, and a diagnosis of rheumatic fever is evident. In a few, depending on the serologic type of infecting streptococcus, acute glomerulonephritis becomes manifest. Skin eruptions, such as erythema marginatum, erythema nodosum, and scleredema adultorum, occasionally appear.

This sequence of (1) an acute streptococcal respiratory illness, (2) a latent period of 1 to 5 weeks, and (3) the development of nonsuppurative illness occurs with sufficient frequency to suggest a causal relationship to the group A streptococcus. In the family unit experiencing streptococcal infections, in patients with scarlet fever, and in food- and milk-borne outbreaks, it is not uncommon to observe rheumatic fever and nephritis. Other nonbacterial respiratory infections are not followed by these complications.

Further evidence that rheumatic fever and nephritis are related to group A streptococcal infections is obtained from study of patients with these diseases. Usually a history of a recent infection of the throat is obtained, and cultures frequently exhibit hemolytic colonies. Antistreptolysin titers of the serum are elevated. Measures known to protect the individual from streptococcal infections reduce the incidence of rheumatic fever and nephritis.

The exact mechanism whereby rheumatic fever and acute glomerulonephritis are produced is not known. The majority of students favor some form of hypersensitivity mechanism, but it is now apparent that the substances responsible for the tissue reactions are not identical in nephritis and rheumatic fever. Furthermore, the host response to infection with the streptococcus in patients with nephritis is different from that in patients with rheumatic fever; in the first instance a recurrence is rare, in the second it is common. In nephritis the observation that hematuria is observed during the acute streptococcal illness suggests the direct action of some nephritotoxic substance; however, the hematuria clears and subsequently becomes apparent again. In rheumatic fever and to a less extent in nephritis, the patient responds to the initiating infection by the production of large amounts of antibody to various streptococcal antigens. Why such a response is more likely to be associated with a nonsuppurative complication is unknown, but this observation contributes to the interest in the antigen-antibody reaction in relation to the mechanisms involved in tissue damage.

In experimental models, tissue reactions in the kidneys and to a less extent in the heart have been produced by a variety of procedures. These observations have contributed to the emphasis on altered reactivity of the tissues, but it is difficult to translate these studies to the diseases nephritis and rheumatic fever as they occur in man. Indeed, in cases of rheumatic valvular heart disease there is some evidence indicating that the streptococcus produces its damage directly. Green and others have recovered hemolytic streptococci from the valves of patients dying with acute rheumatic fever.

Epidemiology of Rheumatic Fever and Nephritis

There are no reliable figures of the incidence of rheumatic fever and glomerulonephritis because the diseases are not reportable, and, in many instances, their manifestations are so mild that the illnesses are not recognized. That rheumatic fever occurs frequently is indicated from reports which show that approximately 2 to 3 per cent of patients with streptococcal infections subsequently develop rheumatic fever. Since most people experience one to several streptococcal infections in a lifetime, it can be assumed that rheumatic fever is common but frequently goes unrecognized. More accurate information is available from studies of heart disease; 1 to 6 per cent of the population exhibits specific valvular defects. Since many patients with rheumatic fever recover completely, such high rates of valvular defects must represent many cases of rheumatic fever in the population. In contrast to rheumatic fever, attack rates for nephritis following streptococcal infections vary from 0 to 90 per cent. Determination of the number of cases of chronic nephritis gives no indication of the past experience of the population with the acute disease or with streptococcal infections, since the relationship of the chronic disease to the streptococcal infection is not clear.

Rheumatic fever occurs with equal frequency in the two sexes, whereas clinical manifestations of nephritis are observed more frequently in the male. Both complications occur primarily between the ages of two and thirty, with a peak of incidence at seven. Nephritis is somewhat more frequently observed in the young infant than rheumatic fever. Acute rheumatic fever in the adult is likely to be a recurrence rather than an initial attack. Age does not alter susceptibility to rheumatic fever, but streptococcal infections are less likely to be acquired in adult life.

Individuals who have experienced one attack of rheumatic fever are especially susceptible to subsequent attacks. It has been estimated that as many as 40 per cent of patients will experience a recurrence within 1 year after the initial attack. However, as time progresses, the risk of recurrence decreases.

Wilson has stated that the attack rate of rheumatic fever in siblings of rheumatic parents is higher than in siblings of parents free of the disease, but recent data show that following a streptococcal infection the attack rate is 3 per cent, irrespective of the presence or absence of the rheumatic state in the parents. These results would indicate that there is no increased susceptibility to rheumatic fever in such families.

The other epidemiologic features of acute rheumatic fever and acute nephritis are those of streptococcal infections in general. In addition, the epidemiology of nephritis is governed by the fact that not all strains of group A streptococci are capable of producing renal disease. The evidence at present indicates that strains belonging to type 12 account for the majority of cases throughout the world. In addition, strains of type 1, 4, 6, 25, and a newly recognized type termed *Red Lake* may produce nephritis. The attack rate of nephritis following infection with these nephritogenic strains is not constant, suggesting that either the strains vary in their nephritogenic capacity or some other factor is operative. Since the attack rate may approach 90 per cent following infection, multiple cases within the family unit are common.

Pathology

The tissue changes occurring during the course of *rheumatic fever* are found throughout the body. Because alterations in certain organs result in abnormal function, the clinician and pathologist have focused their interest on the heart, joints, and brain. The characteristic change evoked by acute rheumatic fever is the development of minute nodules, called *Aschoff bodies*. These lesions are considered specific for rheumatic fever. It has been universally accepted that the Aschoff nodule develops as a result of swelling and fusion of the collagenous ground substances of the connective tissues. More recently, Murphy has presented considerable evidence indicating that these Aschoff nodules result from rheumatic injury to the heart muscle cell. The sarcoplasmic fragments of myofibers lose their striations and therefore have been confused with collagen. A multinucleated mass is associated with the disintegrating sarcoplasm. As the lesion ages, fibrosis occurs, leaving a minute scar. Damage to the media of the arteries in the heart is manifested by edema, necrosis, fibrosis, and multinucleated cells.

In patients dying with acute rheumatic myocarditis, the heart shows few gross abnormalities. The left ventricle is enlarged, and there is widening of the atrioventricular valves. The leaflets of the mitral valve may be slightly swollen and thickened, and along the point of contact of the cusps a row of small, beadlike vegetations is observed. In patients with pericarditis, there may be fluid in the pericardial sac, and the heart may be covered with a fibrinous exudate. Microscopic examination shows focal or diffuse infiltration of the myocardium with inflammatory cells and variable degrees of necrosis of muscle cells.

The joints become red, swollen, and tender. The periarticular tissues and synovia are edematous and show collections of mononuclear cells. The synovial fluid becomes increased. Involvement of the tendons, especially the hamstring and Achilles tendons, gives rise to the so-called "growing pains" of childhood. Subcutaneous nodules, loosely connected to the tendon sheaths, are likely to be found during the acute phase of the disease in children.

In the brain, true Aschoff bodies are seldom observed; instead, there is a perivascular collection of round cells. There may be proliferation of the intima and thrombosis of vessels.

Inflammatory reactions have been described in the tissues of other organs of the body. In the lung there may be an interstitial pneumonia and hemorrhage.

In *acute glomerulonephritis,* the kidneys are normal or slightly enlarged and appear pale. Over the surface small punctate hemorrhages are observed. Histologically, the earliest lesion is an increased cellularity of the glomerulus, with infiltration with polymorphonuclear cells. Red cells and leukocytes appear in Bowman's space and in the tubules. The basement membrane is thickened. The tubular cells may show some swelling. Acute fibrinoid necrosis of the arterioles and glomerular tufts is seen. Lesions observed at autopsy after several weeks or months of illness show epithelial crescents, fibrinoid necrosis, tubular degeneration, and inflammatory infiltration around the glomerulus. Fibrosis is a late manifestation. The relation of these latter changes to nephritis following group A infections has not been well defined.

Acute Rheumatic Fever

Clinical Manifestations. One of the outstanding characteristics of the late nonsuppurative complications of streptococcal infections is the variation of the clinical features. Frequently, a definite diagnosis of rheumatic fever is easily made, but there are also many instances where such a diagnosis is difficult, if not impossible. The correct diagnosis may become apparent only after a long period of observation.

Streptococcal fever is a term applied when there is fever, usually of mild degree, without other signs of rheumatic activity or of a suppurative process. A history of a preceding pharyngitis is usually obtained. There may be some cervical lymphadenitis, but in many instances the glands are not prominent or tender. In some patients the temperature may be normal except during the late afternoon. An increase in the total leukocyte count or in the sedimentation rate may accompany the fever.

Rheumatic fever may be insidious in onset, or it may develop rapidly. Although it is common for patients to give a history of a preceding streptococcal respiratory infection followed by a latent period of several days to 6 weeks, occasionally symptoms of rheumatic fever develop without a latent, symptom-free period. Usually the patient complains of malaise which is soon followed by feverishness, perspiration, prostration, and polyarthritis.

In the absence of a specific diagnostic test, the recognition of rheumatic fever depends upon the presence of a combination of symptoms and signs, of which the most important are polyarthritis, carditis, chorea, subcutaneous nodules, erythema marginatum, fever, and dramatic improvement of pain and fever following the administration of salicylates. It is important to stress that many of these manifestations may be absent in a given instance.

Although *migratory polyarthritis* is considered one of the typical symptoms of rheumatic fever, it is also a confusing symptom, since arthralgia may be caused by other diseases. In rheumatic fever, painful joints develop rapidly, and the ankles, knees, hips, shoulders, elbows, and wrists are likely to be involved. Occasionally the small joints become inflamed. Several joints may become involved simultaneously, or they may be affected in rapid succession. As one joint becomes involved, the pain and swelling in another may be receding. Arthralgia in any one joint may last a few hours to several days or, rarely, weeks. Commonly there are all the signs of acute inflammation with redness, swelling, heat, pain, and tenderness.

In children arthritis may be atypical, the manifestations being pain and tenderness without swelling of the joint. The arthritis of rheumatic fever does not suppurate, and normal function is restored following subsidence of symptoms and signs of inflammation.

Acute carditis is responsible for death in active rheumatic fever. The severity of the initial injury may vary from the mildest forms which give rise to no clinical manifestations to the types in which extensive pathologic changes in the heart are unmistakably displayed by abnormal clinical signs. Usually, the term active carditis is limited to those instances where the clinical signs of impairment of the heart are definite.

The recognition of acute carditis is often not a simple matter. Unquestionable injury to the heart is evidenced by the appearance of congestive failure, enlargement of the heart, pericarditis, or "significant" murmurs. The problem is simplified if it is borne in mind that the development of significant murmurs is the unfailing sign of acute carditis.

Acute pericarditis, congestive failure, definite cardiac enlargement are all indicative of serious cardiac damage, but since each one of these signs is usually associated with the appearance of murmurs, it is primarily with the discovery of significant murmurs that one is most concerned.

What are the significant murmurs? A diastolic murmur, not previously present, constitutes unequivocal evidence of cardiac damage. This may be either the faint blow of aortic insufficiency heard best at the second right parasternal border or along the left parasternal border; or it may be the mid- or late-diastolic rumble heard best at the apex. There are some who consider the diastolic murmur the only one of indubitable significance. A *loud* systolic murmur at the mitral area which is transmitted well into the axilla has practically the same significance. It is important to bear in mind that these murmurs do not invariably imply permanent valvular damage. Even the diastolic murmur may vanish, and we must assume that dilatation of the cardiac chambers or of the valve rings or a transitory distortion of the cusps has disappeared. The greatest difficulty comes from estimating the importance of a less intense mitral systolic murmur, which may be due to alteration either of the valve leaflets or of the myocardium sufficient to cause enlargement of the mitral ring; or it may be caused simply by the fever and tachycardia without necessarily implying serious endocardial damage.

Cardiac enlargement is frequently encountered in children but seldom observed in the adult. The diagnosis of involvement of the myocardium is usually based on the recognition of disturbances of rhythm and electrocardiographic abnormalities. Most patients with rheumatic fever, if examined frequently, will show evidence of myocardial involvement. Tachycardia is frequent. Gallop rhythm, usually heard during the acute phases of the illness, is especially apt to occur. The heart sounds may be muffled, or the first sound may vary in intensity. The finding of dropped beats suggests a partial heart block (Wenckebach phenomenon). Atrial fibrillation, uncommon in children, may be associated with recurrent attacks of rheumatic fever in the adult.

The electrocardiographic change most frequently encountered during the course of acute rheumatic fever is prolongation in the P-R interval. This interval usually becomes normal as signs of infection disappear, but prolongation may persist. Other abnormalities include partial atrioventricular heart block, atrioventricular dissociation, inversion of T waves, and bundle branch block.

Discomfort over the precordial area does not always indicate acute pericarditis, but the detection of a harsh to-and-fro friction rub is pathognomonic.

Frequently the precordial pain is severe in patients exhibiting a friction rub. Rheumatic pericarditis in children is often associated with little pain. Effusion into the pericardial sac may develop and must be differentiated from cardiac dilatation.

One of the major manifestations of rheumatic fever is *chorea,* or St. Vitus' dance. In children it is observed in approximately one-half the patients, whereas in adults it is rare. Commonly, chorea appears late in the illness, so that it may be the only manifestation of the rheumatic state. Chorea usually develops slowly, so that a week or two is required before the parents realize the child is ill. Typically, the patient is restless, nervous, and emotionally unstable, and performs many purposeless movements. The manifestations of chorea are usually mild, and careful observation is required to detect the incoordination. Hyperextension of the fingers, grimacing, and purposeless movements of the tongue, extremities, and fingers are characteristic (see p. 254).

One of the most characteristic features of rheumatic fever is the development of *subcutaneous nodules*. These nodules, which vary in size from 1 mm to 2 cm, are especially likely to develop over the extensor tendons of the hands and feet, over the extensor aspects of the knee and elbow, and over the spine, scapulas, and skull. Usually they are distributed symmetrically and may occur in crops. They lie deep in the tissue, and the skin is movable over their surfaces. They are not painful. Detection of these nodules is best accomplished by inspection of the skin when drawn taut by flexion of the joints. The nodules persist for a few days to several weeks but always disappear. Since subcutaneous nodules are especially likely to develop in patients with severe carditis, they are seldom helpful from the standpoint of diagnosis.

The tendency toward *recurrent attacks* is a striking feature of rheumatic fever. Approximately three-fourths of all patients with recognizable rheumatic fever will develop a recurrence of the disease, so that a previous history of an attack aids in the establishment of the proper diagnosis.

Numerous symptoms, physical signs, and abnormalities in laboratory examinations aid in the establishment of proper diagnosis. *Fever* is usually associated with acute rheumatic fever, although it may be absent in patients with chorea. Fever may be the only clinical manifestation of the disease, other studies, such as serial electrocardiograms and detection of endocardial murmurs, being required to establish the diagnosis. A diagnosis of rheumatic fever made solely on the basis of low-grade fever is not warranted, but it should be emphasized that fever may be the only sign of rheumatic activity.

Little experience is required to appreciate the protean character of rheumatic fever. Studies of

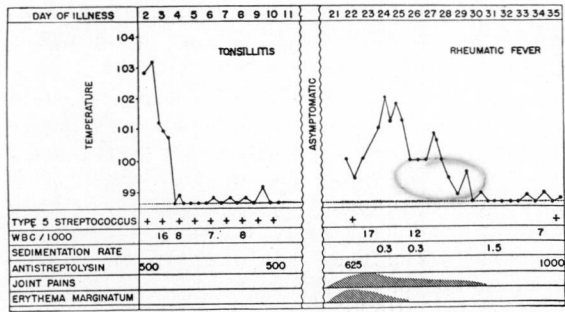

FIG. 114-3. The time sequence of streptococcal tonsillitis and rheumatic fever.

outbreaks of streptococcal infection emphasize that nonsuppurative sequelae include typical rheumatic fever and a low-grade, often continuous, fever without signs of rheumatic activity. It is natural to assume that such cases of so-called streptococcal fever are produced by the same mechanism responsible for the clinically recognizable form of rheumatic fever. A history of a preceding streptococcal infection is of help in diagnosis (Fig. 114-3).

During the acute phase of rheumatic fever various *rashes* may appear. Most typical is *erythema marginatum*. This rash is said to occur in 15 per cent of patients with acute rheumatic fever and probably should be considered indicative of active rheumatic infection. It is characterized by a depressed center and an erythematous margin, which may form rings. When the lesions fuse, various gyrate patterns are observed. The rash is evanescent and may become apparent only by warming the body. Other rashes include erythema nodosum, urticaria, and various purpuric lesions.

Abdominal pain occurs frequently and may be incorrectly diagnosed as resulting from acute appendicitis. Since a leukocytosis occurs in both rheumatic fever and appendicitis, operation is frequently performed. Careful search for other signs of rheumatic activity should be made in all children and young adults complaining of abdominal pain and fever.

Not only does abdominal pain occur as a manifestation of acute rheumatic fever, but also pleuritic pain is observed. *Pleurisy* is usually associated with severe rheumatic fever and gives rise to pain on respiration. Rarely, it is the initial manifestation of the illness. Usually the pleurisy does not persist for more than a few days, and symptoms may be relieved as fluid accumulates in the intrapleural space. In some patients, and again especially in those with a severe illness, symptoms and signs of *pneumonia* may develop. The sputum may become blood-streaked. Physical signs are frequently difficult to interpret, for there is usually concomitant

myocarditis and cardiac failure. Roentgenographic examination of the lungs is a most valuable procedure in patients suspected of having pneumonia.

Epistaxis is commonly observed in patients with acute rheumatic fever. The exact cause of these recurrent attacks of bleeding is not known. Hypoprothrombinemia may be due to salicylate administration.

Laboratory Findings. The urine is usually normal. Traces of albumin may occur during the febrile period, and microscopic hematuria is observed on occasion. In patients with severe or prolonged infections various degrees of anemia are common. A leukocyte count of 15,000 to 30,000 is the rule during the acute phases of infection, but in some patients the count may be normal.

The sedimentation rate is an excellent index of rheumatic activity and is generally considered more reliable than the leukocyte count. The rate of sedimentation of the cells almost invariably increases during the acute phases of the infection; with clinical improvement the rate decreases and returns to normal. In patients with carditis and cardiac failure, normal values may be obtained, but as failure disappears the sedimentation of the cells increases.

The determination of C-reactive protein content of the blood is a useful procedure in judging rheumatic activity. Since this protein also appears in the blood during the course of acute bacterial infections, the reaction must not be considered specific. Culture of the tonsils and oropharynx may show beta streptococci of Lancefield group A, but failure to isolate these organisms even early in the course of the disease is not unusual. Of significance is the finding of a high antistreptolysin titer which falls during the convalescent period. Antistreptolysin titers of 200 or more indicate a recent infection by group A streptococci; they are not diagnostic of rheumatic fever. Early in the course of rheumatic fever titers of less than 100 are rare.

Diagnosis. There is no laboratory test available that establishes the diagnosis of acute rheumatic fever. *Polyarthritis, carditis, chorea, subcutaneous nodules, erythema marginatum,* and *recurrent attacks* characterize the disease. According to Jones, the diagnosis of rheumatic fever becomes established when two or more of the above manifestations coexist. It should be emphasized that rheumatic fever undoubtedly occurs in the absence of these conditions, but only by long observation is it usually possible to make certain of the diagnosis.

Rheumatic fever must be differentiated from other forms of acute arthritis. Under the age of twenty, *gonococcal arthritis* may be confused with rheumatic fever (see p. 929).

Rheumatoid arthritis, although relatively rare in children, is generally polyarticular in its manifestations, so that it is commonly confused with acute rheumatic fever (see p. 1914). Temporomandibular joint involvement is rare in rheumatic fever and common in rheumatoid arthritis. The development of deformities or ankylosis clearly indicates rheumatoid arthritis.

Septic or *purulent arthritis* is recognized readily in most instances, and cultures of the blood and joint fluid establish the correct diagnosis. *Tuberculous arthritis* is usually monoarticular in distribution and subacute in its course. Some cases of acute *disseminated lupus erythematosus* may be difficult to distinguish from acute rheumatic fever. The former disease almost invariably occurs in females and is associated with leukopenia, hematuria, and, in most instances, a rash over the face (see p. 1893).

In the adult, and especially in men, *gout* must be considered. The occurrence of tophi, podagra, and an increased uric acid content of the blood, as well as the appearance of erosions of the bone in the roentgenograms serve to differentiate gout from rheumatic fever.

The administration of salicylic acid compounds is often helpful in differential diagnosis. In rheumatic fever these drugs produce rather marked symptomatic relief, the temperature decreases, and the pulse slows.

In patients with fever and valvular heart disease *subacute bacterial endocarditis* may mimic rheumatic fever. Here the presence of petechiae, enlarged spleen, hematuria, or a positive culture of the blood assist in establishing the diagnosis.

Course and Prognosis. Approximately 4 per cent of hospitalized patients die during their initial attack of rheumatic fever, and in every instance death is due to active carditis. The course of the acute illness is extremely variable, and prognosis should be guarded. In a few patients a normal status is apparent within 1 week, but the majority require 4 to 6 weeks before the clinical and laboratory signs of activity disappear. In the past there was an appreciable number of patients who continued to exhibit signs of rheumatic fever, either progressive or cyclic in nature. Today, such a course is rarely observed, presumably because of better therapy rather than because of a fundamental change in the character of the rheumatic process.

The most important feature of rheumatic fever is carditis. If the patient is going to manifest disease of the heart, signs are readily detected early in the acute illness. Patients who subsequently develop chronic valvular heart disease usually exhibit murmurs during the acute illness. Although there is some correlation between the severity of acute carditis and chronic valvular deformities, it is difficult to make a prognosis until the patient has been observed for many months. The occurrence of re-

peated attacks of rheumatic fever alters the prognosis considerably. Repeated attacks usually result in serious cardiac injury.

Although death in the child is usually due to active carditis, in the adult mechanical failure of the heart results from marked valvular deformities. The adult patient succumbs to heart failure with atrial fibrillation, embolic episodes, or bacterial endocarditis. The latter complication develops most frequently in patients who do not exhibit signs of failure during the acute illness. In all patients showing signs of cardiac failure, active rheumatic fever should be suspected.

Treatment. During an attack of acute rheumatic fever attention is directed toward providing nursing care, a good diet, adequate fluid intake, and rest in bed. Most physicians believe that *bed rest* is an important feature of treatment, and it undoubtedly is in patients with severe carditis. Absolute bed rest is difficult to maintain during therapy because the drugs employed relieve all symptoms in the majority of instances. It is common practice to require bed rest until clinical signs of activity have disappeared. The pulse rate, leukocyte count, sedimentation rate, and C-reactive protein are employed as an index of activity of the disease. Some restriction of physical exertion is advised until these indices return to normal values.

Patients with severe arthritis or substernal pain may require codeine or morphine for immediate relief. The development of cardiac failure is an indication for digitalis therapy, although occasionally such treatment is not followed by rapid improvement.

Chorea requires special attention. The patient should be placed in bed in a quiet room. Precautions must be instituted so that the patient does not injure himself. Feeding, if difficult, requires an understanding nurse. Sedation, usually phenobarbital, should be administered in sufficient quantities to supply required rest.

Once the diagnosis of rheumatic fever is established, all patients should receive a course of penicillin therapy in amounts necessary to eliminate the group A streptococcus. Penicillin is not withheld in patients whose oropharyngeal cultures are negative, since studies have shown that the streptococci may be in inaccessible areas. At present 500,000 units of penicillin is administered intramuscularly every 4 hr for 2 weeks. This is followed by a single injection of 1,200,000 units of benzathine penicillin. An alternative method is the injection of 600,000 units of procaine penicillin twice daily for 2 weeks to be followed by an injection of benzathine penicillin. It is possible that elimination of the streptococcus by such therapy will alter the further development of valvular heart disease.

Symptomatic therapy of acute rheumatic fever is accomplished by the use of salicylates or one of the steroid hormones. All these agents exert a favorable effect on the arthritis and constitutional symptoms. Hormone therapy, in addition, may alter the evolution of valvular heart disease if instituted within a week of onset. If the illness is of over 2 weeks' duration, steroid therapy is of doubtful value. There is some evidence suggesting that steroids are effective in the patient with acute carditis.

Sodium salicylate or acetylsalicylic acid rapidly relieves such symptoms as joint pain, tachycardia, and anorexia. Unfortunately, symptoms of salicylism appear early, so that careful adjustments are necessary to obtain maximum relief of symptoms. Small doses of these compounds given at frequent intervals are preferable to large doses. In the adult 8 to 10 Gm during a 24-hr period may be required for maximal effect. Enteric-coated pills may be employed when there is intolerance.

Hormone therapy is advised for all patients whose illness is of less than 1 week duration. Hydrocortisone is given in divided doses of 300 to 600 mg daily. Prednisone 60 to 160 mg or triamcinolone 50 to 100 mg daily in divided doses may be substituted for hydrocortisone. With any of these steroids the dose is gradually reduced over a 3- to 6-week period. In general, therapy is continued until there is no further improvement of cardiac murmur. After the drug is discontinued, signs of activity may recur, the so-called "rebound phenomenon." If the rebound is not accompanied by severe symptoms, it is not necessary to resume therapy. Prednisone may be substituted for cortisone and has the advantage that it entails less risk of fluid retention.

In all patients with active rheumatic fever and especially those receiving hormone therapy, continuous prophylactic administration of sulfadiazine or penicillin should be instituted immediately after the first 2 weeks of therapy. The physician should be careful in the management of each patient to make certain that a psychologically crippled individual is not produced. Likewise, the importance of continuous observation and prevention of recurrences should be stressed.

Acute Glomerulonephritis

Most of the knowledge of acute glomerulonephritis has accumulated from study of hospitalized patients and, of necessity, has been derived only from individuals with symptoms. Observation of patients infected with nephritogenic streptococci reveals that the spectrum of nephritis is broad; many individuals exhibit signs of the disease without associated symptoms. Since relatively few patients have been observed throughout life after the streptococcal infection, knowledge concerning the evolution of the renal lesion is limited. With the introduction of needle biopsy of the kidney, the relationship of chronic nephritis to acute nephritis can be expected to be clarified in the future.

Symptoms and signs of acute nephritis can be produced by a number of stimuli in addition to infection by nephritogenic streptococci. Pneumococcal and other bacterial infections may be associated with hematuria and albuminuria, with or without edema and hypertension. Some of these illnesses are undoubtedly acute exacerbations of chronic nephritis, whereas others may have resulted from infection with group A streptococci, but the techniques for isolating the organism were not adequate. In addition, signs of nephritis may be produced by bee stings, chemical poisons, and bacteremia. However, most acute glomerulonephritis is caused by a few serologic types of group A streptococci.

Clinical Manifestations. An acute respiratory illness is an integral feature of acute glomerulonephritis. Approximately 80 per cent of patients infected with group A streptococci experience clinical manifestations. Since such infections are not always associated with a recognizable illness, it is not surprising that a few patients exhibit no symptoms. In addition, in children the symptoms referable to the respiratory system may be overshadowed by infection of the skin. Eczema or small abrasions may become infected by nephritogenic streptococci and may dominate the initial clinical picture presented by the patient. In such instances, bacteriologic studies of the oropharynx usually reveal group A streptococci.

Symptoms of nephritis may develop during the acute respiratory illness, but commonly they develop 10 days later. Thus, the symptoms of the acute respiratory illness subside or disappear completely prior to the onset of the nonsuppurative complication. Occasionally, the latent period may be as long as 4 weeks.

As already stated, most knowledge of acute glomerulonephritis is derived from the study of hospitalized patients. In this population the manifestations are of such a nature that they are considered to be serious by the patient as well as by the physician. Actually, nephritis frequently produces few or no symptoms, the only sign being an increased excretion of red blood cells. Symptoms, if present, include vague lumbar soreness, transient pain in the groins or abdomen, anorexia, and general malaise.

In patients seeking medical care because of the development of nonsuppurative disease of the kidney, the symptoms include puffiness of the eyes, gross hematuria, and headache. Less commonly the initial symptom may be pain in the lumbar area, severe pain in the groin or deep in the abdomen, convulsions, pulmonary edema, and coma. Any combination of the above symptoms may be associated with anorexia, vomiting, oliguria or anuria, and nitrogen retention.

Edema is one of the most common manifestations of acute nephritis. Characteristically, the parents observe that the face is swollen, especially around the eyes. The edema is most apparent upon arising in the morning. Edema fluid frequently becomes manifest in the lower extremities, over the sacrum, or in the body cavities. The exact mechanism involved in production of edema in acute nephritis is unknown, but presumably it is due to sodium retention. Other factors which may play a role are capillary damage and congestive heart failure. Since the edema fluid exhibits a low protein content, it is difficult to explain the accumulation of fluid by capillary damage.

Some degree of *hematuria* is observed in all patients, and the diagnosis of nephritis should not be made in its absence. Individuals infected with group A streptococci exhibit an increased number of red cells in the urine during the febrile period. If the organism is nephritogenic, the "febrile hematuria" is even more marked; 20 per cent may show over 20 cells per cu mm in the uncentrifuged specimen. This initial hematuria disappears, only to recur in a few days in those patients who develop acute glomerulonephritis. There is some evidence that "febrile hematuria" is especially likely to occur in patients who subsequently develop nephritis.

Gross hematuria, especially when it occurs in the male, may be the presenting symptom. Somewhat less than half the patients observe brown urine which lasts only a few days. Since the blood must travel a long distance through the nephrons, the color of the urine differs from that observed in hemorrhage from the bladder. The red cells have been exposed to an acid environment, which produces the brown or coffee grounds appearance. Microscopic hematuria may persist for weeks and occasionally for months. There is poor correlation between the severity of nephritis and the degree of hematuria.

One of the characteristic signs of acute nephritis is *hypertension.* The blood pressure tends to be extremely labile, especially during the initial phase of the disease. Patients with a normal pressure have been observed to develop marked hypertension, edema, cardiac dilatation, and signs of failure immediately following stimuli such as an alcohol sponge bath administered as treatment for fever. Observations such as this suggest that arteriolar spasm is responsible for elevated pressures. Hypertension, if it develops, is likely to become manifest within a week or so of onset.

Convulsions, visual disturbances, and coma appear to be related to the general vascular instabil-

ity. Sudden elevation of pressure is associated with severe headache, nausea, vomiting, and rarely results in actual rupture of a cerebral vessel. Generalized convulsions, which occur mainly in young children, may be the first or major symptom. Blurring of vision or even amaurosis may be experienced. Examination shows papilledema, rarely hemorrhages into the retina, and constriction of the arteries.

The patient who develops hypertension is especially susceptible to vascular congestion. The symptoms of congestive failure may develop rapidly, reaching a critical stage within a few hours. Death in the early phase of the disease is commonly due to congestive failure. The symptoms vary considerably, from moderate dyspnea to frank signs of pulmonary edema and acute congestion with enlargement of the liver, rapidly accumulating edema, and elevated venous pressure.

Laboratory Findings. The function of the kidney is altered in many patients, but specific data are meager concerning function in the patient without edema or hypertension and in the very early stages of poststreptococcal nephritis. The ability to excrete water may be normal or impaired. In the initial phases the ability to concentrate is usually maintained. During convalescence the specific gravity may remain relatively fixed near 1.010 for several weeks or months. The urea clearance may be depressed and the excretion of phenolsulfonphthalein decreased. The discrete measurements show that the glomerular filtration rate is reduced in most cases; renal plasma flow is normal or slightly depressed; and there is a low filtration fraction. There is evidence of some dysfunction of the tubular cells. In patients with small urinary volumes and edema, there may be azotemia.

As stated under Clinical Manifestations, *hematuria* of varying degrees is a constant finding in acute glomerulonephritis. Microscopic examination shows red cells of normal size, but in addition, there are many small, distorted erythrocytes and red cell stroma. Identification of the distorted cells and stroma can best be accomplished in a fresh, uncentrifuged specimen. Bleeding from other areas of the urinary tract is not associated with abnormal cells or stroma. For the proper interpretation of hematuria, as well as for the long-term management of the patient, quantitative measurements of red cell excretion are required. In the past these values have been expressed on the basis of 24-hr excretions by the method of Addis. A much simpler technique is the enumeration of cells in the hemocytometer employing a fresh morning specimen which has not been stored in the icebox. The cells are not sedimented prior to counting, since this procedure ruptures many abnormal cells and makes the cell membranes stick together in a homogeneous mass.

Normal individuals excrete less than 10 red cells per cubic millimeter. Patients with acute nephritis usually excrete over 100 cells, although in very mild attacks or during the convalescent stages the number of cells may vary between 10 and 100. Normal individuals, especially females, will occasionally exhibit counts between 10 and 100, but subsequent examinations will show normal counts. Some increase in cells occurs in urine containing sperm, and such urine should not be considered abnormal. Likewise, during acute infections, heart failure, and infections of the urinary tract an increased number of cells is observed. The presence of bacteria, leukocytes, and epithelial cells should be recorded. The number of leukocytes is usually increased in acute nephritis. If abnormal numbers of erythrocytes are observed, an aliquot of urine is centrifuged and the sediment examined for casts. The presence of red cell casts indicates bleeding from the glomerulus.

Proteinuria is common and is always present in patients exhibiting edema or hypertension. In contrast to common belief, protein may be absent or present in very small quantities in patients without hypertension or edema. In patients exhibiting marked degrees of proteinuria without hypertension or signs of edema, the illness most likely represents an acute exacerbation of chronic nephritis or some other form of renal disease.

In each patient a careful search for evidence of a streptococcal infection should be made. Several cultures of the throat should be obtained before institution of chemotherapy. The culture is inoculated on the surface and subsurface of sheep blood agar, since nephritogenic organisms frequently fail to produce typical hemolytic zones by other techniques. Specimens from all members of the immediate family and other household contacts should be cultured to obtain evidence of infection in this group. Those with positive cultures should be followed for urinary abnormalities. Blood for antistreptolysin determinations should be taken especially in those who exhibit a negative throat culture. A very high titer or a rising titer indicates a recent streptococcal infection.

In acute nephritis during the active phase of the disease the sedimentation rate is increased and there may be anemia.

Diagnosis. The problems of diagnosis of various forms of nephritis are discussed in detail elsewhere (see p. 1479). Here, it should be emphasized that exacerbations of chronic nephritis present the most difficult problem. It is important for the physician to differentiate between initial attacks of acute glomerulonephritis and exacerbations of chronic nephritis because the prognosis is excellent in the former and poor in the latter group. Chronic renal disease is suspected whenever there is marked proteinuria in the absence of edema or hypertension. Any infection may precipitate an exacerbation, but only infection with nephritogenic streptococcal types produces classical acute glomerulonephritis. Thus, the isolation of a type of streptococcus which is not nephritogenic suggests that the illness represents an exacerbation of chronic nephritis.

Increased excretion of red cells is observed in many patients with acute infections. In the majority of these, the hematuria, along with slight albuminuria, disappears soon after the temperature returns to normal. In contrast, following infection with nephritogenic streptococci, the hematuria returns and persists for several days or weeks. During this second episode of hematuria, proteinuria is not a characteristic feature. It seems likely that such cases represent a mild form of acute nephritis.

Course and Prognosis. The course of acute nephritis is extremely variable. In hospitalized cases 3 to 5 per cent die. In most instances death occurs in patients presenting a syndrome resembling heart failure. Since these patients exhibit retention of water, oliguria, and hypertension, it is difficult to determine the pathogenesis of the apparent heart failure. Occasionally death is due to uremia, convulsive seizures, infection, or rupture of a cerebral vessel.

Two different courses of illness are observed in patients who do not die during the acute phase. In one complete recovery is the rule, whereas in the other group the majority develops chronic, progressive renal disease. There is reason to believe that acute nephritis caused by nephritogenic streptococci does not lead to chronic nephritis. Patients who give a classical history of a preceding respiratory infection or develop nephritis following scarlet fever rarely develop chronic nephritis (Ellis type I). These patients usually seek medical attention within a few days after the onset of symptoms of nephritis. In contrast, the patient who exhibits an insidious onset of nephritic symptoms, gives no evidence of a recent streptococcal infection, shows large amounts of protein in the urine, or develops hematuria without a latent period is especially likely to exhibit chronic progressive renal disease. The illnesses in this group of patients (Ellis type II) may represent exacerbations of chronic nephritis. Recent studies show that the serum from these patients contains no antibody against nephritogenic organisms, whereas such antibodies can be demonstrated in many patients who have recovered following an attack of type I nephritis.

The clinical signs of nephritis observed following infection with nephritogenic streptococci last only a few weeks. Edema, hypertension, and gross hematuria disappear within a few days or weeks. Persistence of these signs for more than 2 months is a bad prognostic sign and may indicate chronic renal disease. Abnormal numbers of red cells and moderate proteinuria may persist for months in a few patients. Individuals who recover from acute nephritis rarely experience another attack.

Treatment. *Bed rest* is necessary in the early phases of an attack of acute nephritis. During the first week or two, physical exertion or sudden stimuli, such as an alcohol rub or news of death in the family, may precipitate severe hypertension, pulmonary edema, convulsions, cerebral hemorrhage, or coma. If possible, the patient should be placed in a single room, mild sedation should be administered, few or no visitors should be permitted, and the number of examinations and procedures should be kept to a minimum. Bed rest should be enforced until the blood pressure has become stabilized and signs of edema have disappeared. Restricted activity is advisable until the sedimentation rate is normal and the number of red cells excreted is not altered significantly by exercise. There is no evidence indicating that activity is harmful to the patient who continues to excrete red cells in moderate numbers during the convalescent period.

Patients infected with nephritogenic streptococci who subsequently develop nephritis are especially likely to exhibit abnormal degrees of hematuria during the acute respiratory infection. Since this may indicate that some product of these organisms damages the glomerulus directly, the organism should be eliminated. This is best accomplished by the administration of procaine penicillin in doses of 600,000 units twice daily for 2 weeks.

During the first 2 weeks of illness, and especially in patients exhibiting edema, hypertension, or oliguria, the nutrition, fluid, and electrolyte intake should be carefully controlled. The value of a low protein diet has not been established in man, but in experimental nephritis in rats a high protein diet produces an adverse effect. Another reason to limit the protein is the high potassium content. Fluid should never be forced and should be limited in patients showing edema or hypertension. Potassium intake should also be limited.

In the treatment of *circulatory congestion* digitalis is of little value. Diuretics are seldom employed, but phlebotomy of 400 ml may prove beneficial.

Hypertension and convulsions are difficult to control. As mentioned above, bed rest and limitation of sodium intake are important preventive measures. In severe hypertension, 1 to 3 mg reserpine is administered intramuscularly and may be repeated as necessary. If convulsions are frequent, 250 ml of a 2 per cent solution of magnesium sulfate is administered intravenously.

Prevention of Rheumatic Fever and Nephritis

Both initial and recurrent attacks of rheumatic fever and nephritis can be prevented. Prompt and adequate treatment of group A streptococcal infections will prevent both complications, and continuous prophylaxis will greatly reduce the number of recurrences in patients who have already had an attack of rheumatic fever.

It is now well established that therapy of streptococcal infections which eliminates the infecting organism will prevent initial attacks of rheumatic fever and nephritis. If the organism is not eliminated, the attack rate of rheumatic fever is not altered. The preferred method of therapy is either a single injection of 900,000 units of benzathine penicillin or 200,000 to 250,000 units of penicillin V four times daily for at least 10 to 14 days. If the patient is sensitive to penicillin, erythromycin or the tetracyclines are given in full doses for 10 to 14 days. Treatment should be instituted promptly, especially if acute nephritis is to be prevented. Therapy instituted after symptoms of the acute respiratory illness have subsided will still prevent the onset of rheumatic symptoms. Since the sulfonamide drugs are bacteriostatic, they should never be employed for the treatment of streptococcal infections.

Once rheumatic fever develops, penicillin should be administered in full therapeutic doses in order to eliminate the streptococcus. This therapy is advised under the assumption that the organism may be contributing to the rheumatic process. Eradication of the streptococcus should alter the disease in a favorable fashion, but evidence establishing the efficacy of such therapy is not available.

From 20 to 80 per cent of streptococcal infections which occur in individuals who have had an initial attack of rheumatic fever are followed by recurrences. Since many streptococcal infections produce no symptoms, it is not possible to rely on treatment of the infection for the prevention of recurrences. For this reason patients with rheumatic fever or established rheumatic heart disease should be protected continuously against streptococcal disease. This is best accomplished by the intramuscular administration of 1,200,000 units of benzathine penicillin once each month. Oral prophylaxis, which depends upon full cooperation of the patient, is obtained by the daily administration of 0.5 to 1.0 Gm sulfadiazine. Penicillin may be employed, but medication must be given twice daily in doses of 250,000 units. Prophylaxis is maintained throughout the year. Except in individuals who show no evidence of valvular heart disease or in a few patients in whom the risk of contracting a streptococcal infection is considered negligible, prophylaxis is continued indefinitely.

Patients with rheumatic valvular heart disease subjected to surgical procedures, especially tooth extractions, should receive penicillin as a prophylactic measure before and several days after the operation. It is believed that such treatment will prevent the development of subacute bacterial endocarditis.

The problem presented by the patient with acute nephritis differs from that posed by the patient with rheumatic fever. The appearance of a case of acute nephritis in the hospital or physician's office indicates that a nephritogenic type of streptococcus is circulating in the population. Since the attack rate of nephritis may be very high following infection with these organisms, the physician has a duty to the public to eliminate the streptococcus from both the patient and all contacts. Spread of streptococci is especially likely to occur in the home and school. Therefore, cultures of the throat should be obtained from contacts in these two areas. Individuals with positive cultures should receive therapy in a form sufficient to eliminate the organism. In addition, the urine should be examined microscopically, for unapparent cases of nephritis will be found in persons found to have a positive culture.

Once the patient has *recovered* from the acute phase of nephritis, it is not necessary to institute prophylaxis against streptococcal infection. Recurrences are rare, if they occur at all. The most likely explanation for this fact is that the patient acquires lasting immunity against the infecting type of streptococcus and, statistically, has little chance to be infected with another type possessing nephritogenic qualities. It is also possible that the substance responsible for nephritis is antigenic, thus antibody against the hypothetical nephritogenic toxin might afford a protective mechanism.

Individuals who present signs of chronic glomerulonephritis may suffer exacerbations following bacterial infections, including those caused by any type of group A streptococcus. In these patients the monthly injection of 1,200,000 units of benzathine penicillin may be advisable.

Tonsillectomy has been considered effective in preventing rheumatic fever and nephritis. There is no evidence to substantiate this suggestion. On the contrary, the risk of developing rheumatic fever or nephritis is increased because after tonsillectomy the physician is less likely to make the correct diagnosis and, therefore, less likely to prescribe adequate treatment.

REFERENCES

Denny, F. W., L. W. Wannamaker, and E. O. Hahn: Comparative Effects of Penicillin, Aureomycin and Terramycin on Streptococcal Tonsillitis and Pharyngitis, Pediatrics, 2:7, 1953.

Earle, D. P., and D. Seegal: Natural History of Glomerulonephritis, J. Chronic Diseases, 5:3, 1957.

Ellis, A.: Natural History of Bright's Disease, Lancet, I:1, 34, 72, 1942.

Jones, T. D.: The Diagnosis of Rheumatic Fever, J.A.M.A., 126:481, 1944.

Lancefield, R. C.: Specific Relationship of Cell Composition to Biological Activity of Hemolytic Streptococci, Harvey Lectures, 36:251, 1940–1941.

McCarty, M.: Nature of Rheumatic Fever, Circulation, 14:1138, 1956.

Mortimer, E. A., and C. H. Rammelkamp, Jr.: Prophylaxis of Rheumatic Fever, Circulation, 14:1144, 1956.

Murphy, G. E.: Nature of Rheumatic Heart Disease with Special Reference to Myocardial Disease and Heart Failure, Medicine, 39:289, 1960.

Rammelkamp, C. H., Jr.: Epidemiology of Streptococcal Infections, Harvey Lectures, 51:113, 1957.

Rantz, L. A., and W. M. M. Kirby: Enterococcic Infections: An Evaluation of the Importance of Fecal Streptococci and Related Organisms in the Causation of Human Disease, Arch. Internal Med., 71:516, 1943.

115 OTHER STREPTOCOCCAL INFECTIONS

Ivan L. Bennett, Jr.

Definition and Etiology. Beta-hemolytic streptococci of Lancefield group A, discussed in the preceding chapter, are responsible for the vast majority of human streptococcal disease, but four other general types of streptococcus can infect man. Organisms of *Lancefield group C*, primarily pathogens of domestic animals, sometimes produce otitis, pharyngitis, sinusitis, or bacteremia and, indeed, any of the other groups can elicit human disease on occasion. More important, however, are *Lancefield group D (enterococci), the viridans group,* and *anaerobic streptococci.* All three occur as part of the normal bacterial flora of the mouth, intestine, or genital mucosa, and their ability to produce disease is evident only when injury to tissue or other circumstances have impaired the resistance of the host. Because these streptococci are normal inhabitants of body surfaces, their presence in cultures, especially cultures containing other bacteria, is not necessarily of etiologic significance and must be interpreted in the light of clinical manifestations.

Viridans or Green Streptococci. These normal inhabitants of the mouth, intestine, and vagina possess no C carbohydrate and cannot be classified by the Lancefield method. *Alpha* strains produce green discoloration on blood agar, very similar to that surrounding colonies of pneumococci, and differentiation from pneumococci is often a problem (see p. 887). *Gamma* strains are nonhemolytic. Strains isolated in the clinical laboratory are usually simply designated S. *viridans,* although S. *salivarius* (S. *hominis*) and S. *mitis* are sometimes differentiated. Chewing, etc. (see p. 865), leads to repeated entry of these bacteria into the blood of most individuals without harmful effect. However, in the presence of damage to heart valves or of arteriovenous shunts, these organisms can cause bacterial endocarditis or endarteritis, and it is as the etiologic agents of this type of disease that they have achieved medical importance. (See p. 1039 for discussion of bacterial endocarditis.) They are uniformly susceptible to penicillin.

Enterococci (Lancefield Group D). These normal inhabitants of the intestine differ from the viridans streptococci by possessing a group specific antigen, by their ability to grow in 6.5 per cent NaCl and to reduce methylene blue, and by their greater pathogenicity or tendency to produce disease. Most strains are alpha-hemolytic, although beta and gamma organisms are frequent. Organisms isolated by clinical laboratories are usually designated as "enterococci," S. *faecalis,* or if they liquefy gelatin, S. *liquefaciens.*

Enterococci cause 5 to 10 per cent of bacterial endocarditis, sometimes attacking normal heart valves. The course of this disease and its therapy with a synergistic mixture of penicillin and streptomycin are discussed on p. 1043. Enterococci can produce local infections of the meninges, mastoids, the post-partum uterus, and (usually with other bacteria) the peritoneum. These organisms are frequent in urine cultures and are sometimes the sole cause of cystitis or pyelonephritis. Entry of enterococci into the blood is frequent in elderly men with prostatic enlargement, and a large proportion of endocarditis occurs in this age group.

The greater pathogenic potential of S. *faecalis* than that of S. *viridans* is illustrated by the former's ability to incite disease in tissues other than the vascular system as well as the fact that embolic lesions in S. *faecalis* endocarditis often suppurate while those produced by S. *viridans* do not.

Most strains are sensitive to the tetracyclines and chloramphenicol, and these drugs, as well as combined penicillin and streptomycin, can be used to treat infections other than endocarditis.

Anaerobic Streptococci. Among the body's normal inhabitants are many streptococci that cannot be cultured at atmospheric concentrations of oxygen, although most are not obligate anaerobes and are properly termed *microaerophilic.* They are often found in exudates with other organisms, especially *Bacteroides,* coliform bacilli, and clostridial species.

They infect soft tissue wounds and compound fractures, sometimes producing a crepitant myositis that resembles clostridial gas gangrene. Postabortal and puerperal sepsis with pelvic thrombophlebitis and septic lung infarcts, peritonitis, thoracic empyema, abscesses of the lung and liver, perirectal abscesses, mastoiditis, dental infections, and wounds produced by human bites are the most frequent lesions from which anaerobic streptococci in pure or mixed cultures are isolated.

Certain characteristics of anaerobic streptococcal infections are distinct enough to arouse strong suspicion clinically. They cause the production of copious amounts of dirty brown, thin pus. Indeed, the gas-producing infections in wounds that may mimic clostridial gangrene are often distinguished by this intense exudation. This pus, the lochia in uterine infection, and the breath of patients with lung abscess possesses a penetrating, overwhelmingly foul odor that can only be described as hideous. The fetor often ascribed to colon bacillus exudates is a result of the concomitant presence of anaerobic streptococci or *Bacteroides* bacilli. While classification is still imperfect, some of the species names that have been suggested emphasize the feculent characteristics of anaerobic streptococcal exudates including S. *foetidis* (stinking) and S. *putridus* (rotten). *Streptococcus foetidus* is sometimes recognizable in stained smears by its tendency to grow in curious parallel chains, and another species, S. *parvulus,* produces black pigment on agar plates.

Patients with pleural empyema caused by anaerobic streptococci often develop painful areas of cellulitis around the site of thoracentesis needle punctures, a rare event in other empyemas.

Two more or less distinct clinical entities have been attributed to anaerobic streptococci: *burrowing ulcer* and *progressive bacterial synergistic gangrene.* Both are unusual but sufficiently characteristic to be recognized by inspection. Burrowing ulcer occurs on the trunk or extremities and consists of a ragged ulceration from which necrotic sinuses extend subcutaneously with occasional breaking through to the surface. The process is chronic, accompanied by pain, fever, and emaciation, and death from necrosis of a major blood vessel has occurred. It does not attack muscle, stopping at the fascial layer. Anaerobic streptococci in pure culture are usually obtained from the exudate. Progressive bacterial synergistic gangrene usually complicates surgical operations upon the abdomen and consists of progressive, spreading ulceration, often around a stay suture. It is caused by mixture of hemolytic staphylococci and anaerobic streptococci. The lesion is distinguished by a bright red peripheral zone enclosing a ring of purplish discoloration and a gangrenous, granulating center.

Surgical drainage and debridement are important in the management of anaerobic streptococcal infections. Penicillin in large doses is the drug of choice; tetracyclines and bacitracin may be efficacious in certain cases.

REFERENCES

Evan, A. C., and A. L. Chinn: The Enterococci: With Special Reference to Their Association with Human Disease, J. Bacteriol., 54:495, 1947.

Fisher, A. M., and T. J. Abernathy: Putrid Empyema with Special Reference to Anaerobic Streptococci, Arch. Internal Med., 54:552, 1934.

Kerr, A., Jr.: "Subacute Bacterial Endocarditis," Springfield, Ill., Charles C Thomas, Publisher, 1955.

Rantz, L. A., and W. M. M. Kirby: Enterococcic Infections, Arch. Internal Med., 71:516, 1943.

Rosebury, T., and A. C. Sonnenwirth: Bacteria Indigenous to Man, p. 626 in "Bacterial and Mycotic Infections of Man," R. J. Dubos (Ed.), Philadelphia, J. B. Lippincott Company, 1958.

Smith, L. D. S.: "Introduction to the Pathogenic Anaerobes," Chicago, University of Chicago Press, 1955.

Section 3: Diseases Produced by Gram-negative Cocci

116 MENINGOCOCCAL INFECTIONS

Ivan L. Bennett, Jr.

Definition. The commonest infection produced by the meningococcus is a subclinical nasopharyngitis or upper respiratory carrier state. In a relatively few individuals, this is followed by invasion of the blood stream, with involvement of the meninges and other sites, or fulminating sepsis with rapid circulatory collapse and death.

Etiology. *Neisseria meningitidis* or *intracellularis*, a gram-negative coccus, was shown to be the cause of cerebrospinal or "spotted fever" by Weichselbaum in 1887. In stained smears of exudates, the organisms appear as biscuit-shaped single cocci or diplococci, often within polymorphonuclear cells. The meningococcus grows best when fresh inoculums are incubated in carbon dioxide (candle jar) on media containing blood, serum, or ascitic fluid; chocolate agar is frequently used. Like other *Neisseria*, the organism gives a positive "oxidase" test, its colonies on solid medium turning purple when exposed to 1 per cent *p*-aminodimethylanilidemonochloride. The meningococcus is identified by its ability to ferment glucose and maltose. The gonococcus ferments glucose only, and nonpathogenic neisserias (*N. flava, N. sicca, N. catarrhalis*) ferment glucose, maltose, and sucrose, or none of these sugars. Meningococci have been classified into serologic types, but these types are presently of interest only on epidemiologic grounds. The clinical diseases produced by all serotypes are identical, and all are susceptible to sulfonamides, penicillin, and several other antibiotics.

Epidemiology. Under ordinary circumstances, 2 to 5 per cent of normal individuals harbor meningococci as part of the flora of the nasopharynx. Studies such as that of Phair and Schoenbach in 1944 have shown that crowding during the winter months can be associated with a rise in the carrier rate to as high as 40 to 90 per cent. As the rate rises, cases of systemic meningococcal infection appear, but it is clear that fewer than 1 per cent of parasitized individuals develop serious illness. The circumstances leading to spread of infection beyond the nasopharynx are unknown, although several factors have been suggested: (1) failure of nasopharyngeal infection to confer immunity—this is unlikely to play a role in that relatively few carriers are found to possess serum antibodies; (2) in vivo development of invasive mutants; (3) sudden introduction of a virulent strain into a population group; (4) concomitant viral infection of the nose and throat—in army outbreaks, recruits have been more susceptible to meningococcal infections during the "seasoning period," when upper respiratory infections are numerous. Malnutrition, trauma, and debilitating disease seem to play little or no role. Disseminated meningococcal infection is commoner in males and below the age of five years. Mortality is greatest at the extremes of life. Case-to-case transmission is rarely demonstrated, and the frequency of asymptomatic carriers makes it obvious that strict isolation of clinical cases is unjustified. Administration of sulfonamides or penicillin to a patient results in rapid disappearance of

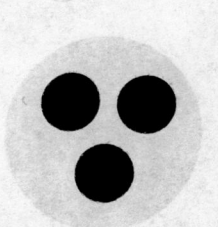

253-9068

Michele Withrow

333 Dodd Unit

a.s.a.—

Sed Rate

9 mm

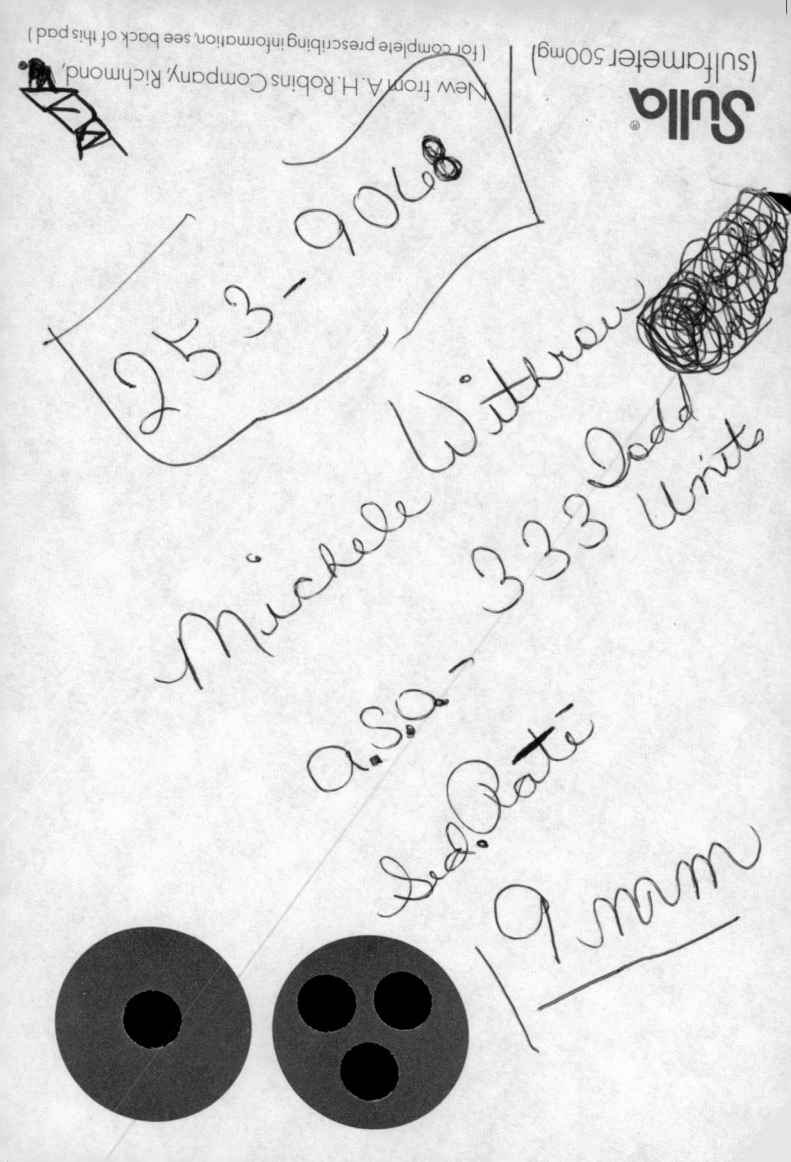

meningococci. The prophylactic use of oral sulfadiazine in a dose of 1 to 2 Gm to a population reduces the carrier rate abruptly and can abort an epidemic in a school, army post, or other limited group.

Pathogenesis. Spread of organisms occurs by droplet infection; the upper respiratory tract is the usual portal, although there are rare instances of isolated meningococcal conjunctivitis, in which the eye was apparently a primary point of entry. About 75 per cent of systemic infections are preceded by upper respiratory symptoms, but the role of the meningococcus in these is difficult to assess. Spread of infection beyond the nasopharynx is now known to occur almost exclusively via the blood stream. Purulent meningitis, the commonest metastatic complication, is preceded by a bacteremia, as are arthritis and rarer localizations such as ophthalmitis, pneumonia, pericarditis, endocarditis, empyema, orchitis, salpingitis, and epididymitis. Bursitis and tenosynovitis may accompany articular involvement, which, next to meningitis, is the most frequent complication of meningococcemia, occurring in about 3 per cent of cases.

The meningococcus possesses an endotoxin similar to those of gram-negative bacilli; injection of this material into experimental animals results in fever, vascular damage, shock, and other toxic changes. There is much to indicate that endotoxin may be responsible for the rapidly fatal course of fulminating meningococcemia with hemorrhagic skin lesions and circulatory collapse.

Autopsy findings include widespread dermal and visceral hemorrhage, purulent basilar meningitis, and, in older cases, extensive meningeal scarring and hydrocephalus. Meningitis is often absent or minimal in cases of fatal meningococcemia, the main findings consisting of large hemorrhages in the various organs and tissues. Histologic examination reveals widespread thrombosis of small vessels and numerous areas of necrosis containing large numbers of meningococci. The adrenal cortex may be grossly hemorrhagic and almost invariably contains microscopic lesions of severe and extensive degeneration.

Clinical Manifestations. The course of disseminated meningococcal infection is highly variable. Clinically, there are three main types: *meningococcemia, meningitis,* and *fulminating sepsis.*

Meningococcemia. Invasion of the blood by meningococci may be followed almost immediately by meningitis, or patients may be seen during the bacteremic stage. Prodromal symptoms of upper respiratory irritation are followed by abrupt onset of fever, often with a rigor, myalgia, headache, nausea, and particularly in children, diarrhea. Extreme tenderness of the soles of the feet, without signs of local inflammation, is highly suggestive of the disease; many patients are thought in the beginning to have influenza or some other grippelike illness. The diagnosis is facilitated by the development of *skin lesions* in about three-fourths of the cases. The rash, from which the disease derived the name "spotted fever," consists of petechiae of the skin and mucous membranes and typical bright pink, nonpruritic, tender macules or papules 2 to 10 mm in diameter over the extremities and trunk. These lesions sometimes have hemorrhagic centers. Hemorrhagic vesicles and larger cutaneous ecchymoses ("suggillations") sometimes occur. Lesions may be few, and careful search is essential; in some cases, the eruption is so profuse and rapid in onset that new lesions can be seen to appear within minutes.

Splenomegaly is inconstant in the early stage; conjunctivitis, hemorrhages in the fundus oculi, and arthritis are sometimes present, but joint involvement is more frequent in the chronic form of the disease.

Chronic meningococcemia is characterized by periodic bouts of fever, arthralgia or arthritis, and recurrent cutaneous lesions. The disease may continue for many months. Splenomegaly is usually present, and each recurrence is accompanied by polymorphonuclear leukocytosis. Patients with this peculiar infection are usually asymptomatic between attacks. The disorder is sometimes mistaken for malaria or allergic purpura. The skin lesions can take any of the forms described above. The majority of patients become asymptomatic after several weeks or months even without treatment; a few finally develop endocarditis or meningitis.

Meningitis. In most patients, the bacteremic stage is followed within a few hours or days by the onset of acute purulent meningitis with severe headache, nuchal rigidity, nausea, vomiting, disorientation, and stupor. Impairment of hearing occurs early, and what appears to be lack of cooperation or inability to answer questions is sometimes attributable to this. There is high fever, respirations may be periodic, and skin lesions are frequent. Signs of meningeal irritation are prominent, but papilledema is unusual.

Fulminating Infections. Meningococcemia can produce death within a few hours with the Waterhouse-Friderichsen syndrome of bacteremia, massive skin hemorrhage, and shock. This triad can result from pneumococcal, streptococcal, or other infections, but the meningococcus is the usual etiologic agent. The complex is commoner in children below the age of five years.

The onset is abrupt, with fever and nonspecific discomfort until dermal petechiae appear and rapidly enlarge into areas of confluent purpura.

The blood pressure falls rapidly, although the skin may remain warm to the touch. Patients usually remain alert. Ordinarily, the infection leads to death within several hours. Because bilateral adrenal hemorrhage is frequently present at autopsy, and microscopic adrenal necrosis is almost invariable, the role of acute adrenal insufficiency in this infection has been much argued. The use of adrenal steroids is justified, but therapeutic regimens have not been evaluated systematically. In patients who recover, oliguria may persist for 18 to 24 hr after blood pressure stabilizes, and extensive sloughing of the skin lesions or loss of extremities from gangrene often prolongs convalescence. Meningitis is not a usual feature.

Rarely, meningococcal infection may take an *encephalitic* course, in which signs of meningeal infection are scanty but extensive cerebral involvement leads to stupor, coma, and death within a few days. Circulatory collapse is not a prominent part of the picture, except terminally. Progressive signs of neurologic disturbance and papilledema are the outstanding manifestations.

Laboratory Findings. Polymorphonuclear leukocytosis of 12,000 to 40,000 cells per cu mm is the rule. In meningitis, there is elevation of spinal fluid pressure, and the fluid is cloudy (it may be clear early in the disease), containing from a few hundred to 40,000 polymorphonuclear cells per cu mm. Protein is elevated, and the glucose content is low. Albuminuria and microscopic hematuria are not infrequent, and transient glucosuria is sometimes present.

Specific diagnosis depends upon demonstration of the meningococcus in smears or cultures of spinal fluid or material aspirated from skin lesions or joints. Smears of body fluids stained with methylene blue are useful for detection of the organism, which is frequently contained in polymorphonuclear leukocytes; its gram-staining reaction should be confirmed. Confusion sometimes arises with *Hemophilus influenza* (p. 954), or Mimae (p. 972), which are gram-negative and pleomorphic. It is sometimes impossible to find meningococci in stained sediment of spinal fluid; this absence of organisms is more likely to occur in this disease than in any other pyogenic infection of the meninges.

So numerous are meningococci in the blood that it is not unusual to find them in smears of buffy coat material. The skin lesions often contain many organisms also; the skin around the lesion should be pinched up, the lesion punctured, and a drop of tissue fluid (not blood) smeared and stained.

Material taken for culture should be inoculated immediately (preferably at the bedside) onto chocolate agar and incubated in a candle jar. Meningococci can usually be cultured from the nasopharynx.

Complications. *Herpes labialis* is common in meningococcal infections, particularly in meningitis. Urinary retention is often a problem, and patients must, of course, be guarded against the usual complications of coma, including aspiration.

Chronic hydrocephalus was formerly seen with considerable frequency; it is now rare. Transient *palsies of cranial nerves* occur and usually clear completely within 6 weeks. *Blindness, hemiplegia, myocarditis* with heart failure, and *localized meningococcal infections* in other sites are all very rare. *Deafness* of a degree detectable by audiometry is present in about 5 per cent of patients who recover from meningitis; it is usually unilateral, and severe impairment of hearing is now unusual.

It is not unusual for patients to complain of fatigability, headache, dizziness, and insomnia for many months after recovery. It is believed that many of these symptoms result from injudicious psychologic management of patients during convalescence.

Among patients who recover from the Waterhouse-Friderichsen syndrome, it is exceedingly rare to observe any evidence of adrenal insufficiency.

Diagnosis. The clinical diagnosis of meningococcal infection is easily made in patients with fever, skin lesions, and meningitis. Diseases with which confusion can arise include other forms of meningitis, bacterial and nonbacterial, endocarditis, the common exanthems, subarachnoid hemorrhage, rickettsioses, thrombocytopenic and other purpuras, and drug eruptions. Once the meningococcus is suspected as the etiologic agent, the diagnosis can usually be established by demonstration of the organisms.

Treatment. When the clinical diagnosis of meningococcal infection has been made and specimens have been obtained for culture, *specific antimicrobial* therapy should be instituted immediately. Sulfonamides and penicillin are equally effective. Sulfadiazine, sulfamerazine, and sulfisoxazole (Gantrisin) are excellent agents. In patients with hypotension and oliguria, dosage should be reduced until urine flow is reestablished. Penicillin in a dosage of 1.2 to 2.4 million units per day, in divided doses, has the advantage of immediate bactericidal action, in contrast to the 4- to 6-hr delay before sulfonamides begin to act; for this reason, penicillin is preferable in fulminating infections where a slight delay may be crucial. The initial dose of penicillin should be given intravenously to patients with circulatory collapse. Chloromycetin, the tetracyclines, and other antibiotics are effective in meningococcal infections but have not replaced sulfonamides and penicillin as the drugs of choice. There is no advantage to combining sulfonamides and penicillin, although this is frequently done.

Supportive therapy includes the usual precautions in patients who are delirious or stuporous, sedation, and relief of headache with Demerol, which is less likely to aggravate urinary retention than are opiates. Maintenance of fluid balance is particularly important if sulfonamides are given; the majority of patients are dehydrated when first seen because of vomiting and lack of intake. There is nothing to be gained by overloading hypotensive patients with fluid during the oliguric phase of fulminating meningococcal infection. It is extremely important to keep a careful *record of blood pressure and fluid balance* in all patients with meningococcal disease until a definite therapeutic response is evident.

In patients with overwhelming meningococcemia and circulatory collapse, prompt and vigorous antimicrobial therapy is the most important step. Pressor amines may be given by intravenous infusion, as may adrenal steroids; the evidence for the effectiveness of these hormones is incomplete, and recovery has been reported without their use, but the usual practice at present is to give them. It is worth remembering that individuals with the Waterhouse-Friderichsen syndrome are extremely susceptible to the local necrotizing action of pressor amines, and extravasation into the tissues should be carefully avoided. Large amounts of blood and plasma will not influence the hypotension and should not be given.

The response of meningococcemia to treatment is dramatic; defervescence usually occurs within 24 hr. Patients with meningitis may continue to have some fever, disorientation, and meningeal signs for 2 to 5 days; this should not lead to a change in chemotherapy. Relapse is almost never seen, and although documented second attacks of meningococcal meningitis have been reported, they are extremely rare.

Prevention. The frequency of carriers and the effectiveness of chemotherapy in rendering patients noninfectious makes the use of strict isolation technique for meningococcal infections both ineffectual and fallacious. As has been mentioned, the wholesale administration of 1 to 2 Gm sulfadiazine will reduce the carrier rate and abort an epidemic in a closed population. When continued contacts with the general public are maintained, however, the effectiveness of this procedure is likely to be transient.

REFERENCES

Applebaum, E.: Chronic Meningococcic Septicemia, Am. J. Med. Sci., 193:96, 1937.

Banks, H. S.: Meningococcal Fever, in "Modern Practice in Infectious Fevers," vol. I, New York, Paul B. Hoeber, Inc., Medical Department of Harper & Brothers, 1951.

Buzzard, E. M., et al.: Management of Adrenal Cortical Failure in Meningococcal Septicemia, Lancet, II:907, 1953.

Lepper, M. H., et al.: Meningococcic Meningitis: Treatment with Large Doses of Penicillin Compared to Treatment with Gantrisin, J. Lab. Clin. Med., 40: 891, 1952.

Phair, J. J., and E. B. Schoenbach: The Dynamics of Meningococcal Infections and the Effect of Chemotherapy, Am. J. Hyg., 40:318, 1944.

Weiner, H. A.: Gangrene of the Extremities: A Recently Recognized Complication of Severe Meningococcic Infection, A.M.A. Arch. Internal Med., 86:877, 1950.

117 GONOCOCCAL INFECTIONS

Ivan L. Bennett, Jr.

Definition. Gonorrhea, perhaps the commonest bacterial disease of man, is a purulent inflammation of the mucosa of the genital tract caused by *Neisseria gonorrhoeae*, the gonococcus. Transmission occurs almost exclusively by direct sexual contact. Other gonococcal infections, all now rare, include ophthalmia neonatorum, and several which complicate venereal infection including perihepatitis, arthritis, tenosynovitis, periostitis, endocarditis, pericarditis, meningitis, suppurative myositis and abscesses of the brain, liver, pleura and other tissues.

Etiology. *Neisseria gonorrhoeae* is a gram-negative coccus which closely resembles the meningococcus in its nutritional requirements and in giving a positive "oxidase" test. It is distinguishable from all other *Neisseria* species by its ability to ferment only glucose. In preparations of infected tissue or exudate, gonococci appear as reniform single cocci or diplococci, frequently within granulocytes. Most strains are now resistant to sulfonamides but are susceptible to penicillin, the tetracyclines, and several other antibiotics.

Epidemiology and Control. Man is the only reservoir of *N. gonorrhoeae* and, excepting ophthalmia neonatorum which is acquired from the mother at parturition, venereal transmission is so universal that the presence of infection is *prima facie* evidence of sexual contact. Gonococci die rapidly outside the body, and save in extraordinarily rare instances, the disease is not acquired from toilet articles, instruments, or fomites.

Acute gonorrhea in either sex may become virtually asymptomatic for months or years without disappearance of the bacteria, a fact of much epidemiologic importance. Immunity to reinfection is negligible; chronic carriers can be reinfected experimentally with acute gonorrhea, and particularly among males, repeated attacks are common. For statistical purposes, public health authorities usually differentiate *relapse* and *reinfection* on the arbitrary basis of recurrence of acute symptoms less (relapse) or more (reinfection) than 1 year after the initial disease.

All males exposed to an infected female are not necessarily infected; prolonged coitus and acute alcoholism are believed to enhance contagion. The intraurethral inoculation of gonococci in nearly 250 male volunteers was followed by clinical gonorrhea with laboratory confirmation of infection in only about one-third of the subjects. The incidence of gonorrhea among prostitutes is about 20 per cent.

There are probably between 1 million and 2 million new gonococcal infections in the United States annually. Acute gonorrhea can be cured with relatively small doses of penicillin, but while its reported incidence in the years since chemotherapy came into use is lower, the decrease is in no way as dramatic as that of syphilis. The major reason for this is incomplete reporting of the disease. This, in turn, is attributable to the ready availability of curative drugs from nonmedical sources, to the widespread belief that gonorrhea is a trivial affliction, to the difficulty of diagnosing all cases in females, and to the efforts of some physicians to "protect a patient's good name" by not reporting the disease. Even the use of intensive, specialized techniques such as so-called "speed zone" epidemiology which is successful in locating and treating 85 per cent of contacts of known cases within 72 hr has not overcome this difficulty.

The peculiarities of gonorrhea as a public health problem have been well summarized by Garson and Thayer who point out the four principles in controlling contagion: quarantine, immunization, eradication of animal reservoirs or vectors, and specific therapy. *Quarantine* is out of the question politically, let alone impossible in view of incomplete case finding. Artificial *immunization* is lacking, and more important, an attack of gonorrhea confers no natural resistance to reinfection. Man is the only *reservoir*. The end result of *specific treatment* of gonorrhea, then, is a return to the population of nonimmune susceptibles within a few days and a sharp increase in reinfections in any given year. These reinfections increase incidence and morbidity figures, and the disease maintains itself in the population. There is probably no more striking illustration than gonorrhea of the failure of specific treatment alone to eradicate a communicable disease.

Pathogenesis and Anatomic Changes. Gonococci multiply on columnar epithelium, accounting for "skip areas" such as the vagina in genital infections. In tortuous passages, where drainage is poor, copious amounts of purulent exudate will accumulate; there is no pathognomonic histologic change. Urethritis in the male becomes established as the urethral glands are involved; spread to the prostate, seminal vesicles, Cowper's glands, epididymis, and, rarely, the testicle can occur. Female urethritis is usually transient, presumably a result of the absence of urethral glands. The vagina in adults is spared (although in children, vaginitis is frequent). Gonorrhea persists as a cervicitis. Abscesses of Skene's or Bartholin's glands occur, but gonorrhea is *not* the commonest cause of this type of infection. The endometrium is spared, but salpingitis, oophoritis, pelvic or general peritonitis, and perihepatitis can occur. Proctitis is commoner in females; cystitis, pylonephritis, and perinephric abscess have always been very rare.

Gonococcal inflammations tend to heal by dense scarring, and residuals such as urethral stricture, nonpatency of fallopian tubes, sterility after epididymitis, and "violin-string" peritoneal adhesions may result.

It is probable that transient, asymptomatic gonococcemia accompanies many genital infections. Occasionally, a syndrome resembling meningococcemia occurs. All metastatic gonococcal infections are becoming very rare including arthritis, tenosynovitis, bursitis, suppurative myositis, periostitis, meningitis, brain and liver abscess, endocarditis, pericarditis, suppurative myocarditis, pneumonia, empyema, and keratodermia blennorrhagica, a peculiar necrotizing hyperkeratosis of hands and feet.

Manifestations. Genital and joint disease are the only gonococcal infections often encountered, at present, and even arthritis is diminishing rapidly in frequency. Gonococcemia, endocarditis, perihepatitis in females, and ophthalmitis are clinical curiosities, but because of the importance of recognizing these rare syndromes, they are described below.

Gonorrhea in the Male ("Clap" or "Strain"). The incubation period is 3 to 7 days. Severe burning on urination and copious purulent urethral discharge are followed by retention, stranguria, perineal pain, hematuria, chordee, and local spread. Acute prostatitis is unusual as is seminal vesiculitis, but unilateral epididymitis complicates 5 to 10 per cent of untreated cases. Ordinarily, the untreated disease subsides gradually within 6 weeks with disappearance of gonococci or development of a chronic carrier state, organisms usually persisting in the prostate.

Urethral stricture is a common sequel, especially if there are repeated attacks. Gonorrhea is an afebrile disease but high fever, even chills, accompany epididymitis. A slight urethral discharge, evident in the morning, may persist for many months (the so-called gleet).

Gonorrhea in the Female (Pelvic Inflammatory Disease, P.I.D.). Gonococcal infection in the female often involves transient urethritis, but medical advice is sought usually for *cervicitis,* manifested by copious, irritating leukorrhea, *acute salpingitis* with or without tubal abscess ("pus tube"), *pelvic peritonitis* with abdominal pain and fever, or more rarely, *proctitis,* manifested by tenesmus and bloody, mucoid stools. The end result of the infection in females is very likely to be sterility.

Arthritis. Gonococcal arthritis, although classically characterized as monoarticular, is polyarticular in 80 per cent of the cases. It may begin with insidious, fleeting arthralgias or the sudden onset of fever and red, hot, swollen, exquisitely painful arthritis. The joints involved in order of frequency are knees, ankles, wrists, hips, shoulders, spine (especially cervical), sternoclavicular, and temporomandibular. Tenosynovitis accompanies 50 per cent of cases, and its presence should immediately alert the clinician to the possibility of gonococcal etiology.

Careful bacteriologic study reveals gonococci in, at best, about one-half of joint fluids, and the synovial exudate ranges from frankly purulent to straw-colored, containing only a few granulocytes. The severity of genital disease seems to play no part in arthritis. A history of recent gonorrhea is occasionally obtained, but arthritis may precede venereal manifestations or may follow them by several months. Perhaps because of tenosynovitis as well as the agonizing pain that accompanies the slightest movement, flexion contractures and muscle atrophy develop with great rapidity in gonococcal arthritis, an important factor in rehabilitation. Response of symptoms to penicillin may be dramatic or very gradual.

There is still some support for the occurrence of two forms of arthritis in gonorrhea, one a local infection, the other a "hypersensitivity" response. The facts are unknown. Occasionally, confirmed gonococcal arthritis appears to undergo a direct transition into clinically typical rheumatoid arthritis, especially in young women. Rather than interpreting this as evidence for gonococcal etiology of some cases of rheumatoid disease, it is best to regard this event as coincidence.

Ophthalmitis. From 15 to 20 per cent of patients with gonococcal arthritis have a nonpurulent conjunctivitis from which bacteria cannot be cultured. Purulent gonococcal ophthalmia in adults is extremely rare and responds well to treatment.

Ophthalmia neonatorum was formerly responsible for about 12 per cent of blindness throughout the world. Characterized by onset within 72 hr after birth of periorbital edema, purulent conjunctivitis, and a tendency to rapid corneal ulceration, the disease has been virtually eliminated by Credé prophylaxis, the instillation of 1 per cent silver nitrate or, presently, penicillin into the eyes of all newborn infants. Inclusion blennorrhea (p. 1175), a viral disease, rarely appears less than 5 days after birth and should never cause diagnostic confusion.

Perihepatitis (Fitzhugh-Curtis Syndrome). This is an unusual complication resulting from spread of the gonococcus to the upper abdomen in females. From 1 to 2 months after venereal infection, there is abrupt onset of fever, leukocytosis, and right upper quadrant manifestations of pain, tenderness, and muscle spasm. Right shoulder pain is frequent, and a friction rub is often audible over the liver. Cholecystograms usually show no filling of the gallbladder, leading to confusion with cholecystitis in many patients. There is no jaundice.

Symptoms subside promptly with specific treatment or gradually within 2 weeks without treatment. This complication is the cause of violin-string perihepatic adhesions.

Bacteremia and Endocarditis. Very rarely, *gonococcemia* results in a febrile illness, occasionally relapsing, that is so closely similar to meningococcemia that differentiation on clinical grounds is not possible. Chills, fever, transient arthritis, leukocytosis, and a papular, purpuric, petechial rash (from which lesions gonococci can be smeared or cultured) complete the picture.

Gonococcal *endocarditis* was five times as common in males as in females, accounted for 10 to 20 per cent of cases of acute bacterial endocarditis, and has virtually disappeared with the availability of specific treatment for gonorrhea. The course is sometimes subacute, but gonococci usually attack valves that are previously normal. The infection is commonest on the aortic valve, and the gonococcus is the organism most likely to affect the tricuspid or pulmonary valve. In addition to petechiae, glomerulonephritis, embolic phenomena, anemia, and splenomegaly, two clinical features of gonococcal endocarditis may suggest the diagnosis. *Jaundice* is very common (presumably a "toxic" hepatitis), and more than one-half of patients show a characteristic febrile pattern consisting of two distinct spikes of fever during each 24-hr period (the church-steeple or double quotidian pattern; the double daily hump). This pattern is not seen in gonococcemia without endocarditis; it occurs in kala-azar (p. 1202) and in occasional patients with miliary tuberculosis.

Laboratory Findings and Diagnosis. The diagnosis of gonococcal infections is established by demonstration of *N. gonorrhoeae* in smears or cultures of exudate from urethra, cervix, eye, serous cavity, or blood. Cultures should be planted quickly on Pizer's agar, chocolate agar, or one of several available commercial media for neisserias and incubated in a candle jar at 37°C. Large inoculums will facilitate isolation. The *gonore-action* (gonococcal complement fixation test) is sometimes helpful in differentiating gonococcal from other types of arthritis, but it has never been standardized.

Reiter's disease consisting of urethritis, arthritis, and conjunctivitis is discussed on p. 1907. Pelvic tuberculosis can cause a picture not unlike that of "P.I.D." but, along with acute appendicitis, another disorder that may cause confusion, it can usually be distinguished from gonorrhea.

The diagnosis of gonococcal arthritis often comes from a therapeutic trial of penicillin, although culture of the gonococcus, presence of tenosynovitis, positive gonoreaction, failure to demonstrate rheumatoid factor (p. 1911), lack of diagnostically significant response to salicylates or colchicine, and absence of carditis are all helpful in recognition.

Treatment. Penicillin is the drug of choice in all gonococcal infections.

For *gonorrhea* in males, a single injection of 600,000 to 1.2 million units of depot penicillin and for females, two weekly injections of 1.2 million units are sufficient. A repetition of therapy will cure nearly all relapses. A similar regimen suffices for ophthalmia.

Gonococcal arthritis should be treated with 1.8 to 2.4 million units of aqueous penicillin parenterally for 7 to 14 days. Response may be gradual, and therapy should not be stopped because symptoms are slow to subside. Intrasynovial penicillin is not required.

The optimum dosage in gonococeal endocarditis is not known, but 4 million to 10 million units daily for 4 to 6 weeks is recommended.

Appropriate surgical procedures for localized suppurations, urethral strictures, and scarring of the female internal genitalia and attention to restoration of muscle strength and joint mobility in arthritis (see p. 1914) are, of course, important.

One of the tetracyclines can be substituted in patients with hypersensitivity to penicillin.

Artificial fever is no longer needed in the management of gonococcal disease.

When *both syphilis and gonorrhea* are contracted by the same exposure, as has occurred in the past in as many as 3 per cent of cases, gonorrhea be- comes clinically evident during the incubation period of syphilis. Incipient syphilis is usually aborted by the dosage of penicillin given, but masking without cure can occur, and serologic tests for syphilis should be performed on *all* patients treated for gonorrhea before therapy and at regular intervals for 6 months. The onset of chills and fever in a patient given penicillin for gonorrhea is highly suggestive of a syphilitic Herxheimer reaction (p. 1079).

Prevention. The problems of control have been discussed under Epidemiology. The administration of 250,000 units of oral penicillin to all individuals given furlough or to all individuals reporting sexual exposure has been employed in the Armed Forces, not, however, without strenuous objections on moral grounds by civilian groups. Presently, it is common practice in clinics to administer penicillin to every sexual contact of a diagnosed case of gonorrhea without awaiting laboratory confirmation of the diagnosis in these contacts. Considering the numbers of individuals involved, this seems entirely permissible and, in practice, allergic reactions to the drug have not proved to be a significant drawback.

REFERENCES

Fitzhugh, T., Jr.: Acute Gonococcic Peritonitis of the Right Upper Quadrant in Women, J.A.M.A., 102: 2094, 1934.

Fromer, S., J. C. Cutler, and S. Levitan: Masking of Early Syphilis by Penicillin Therapy in Gonorrhea, J. Venereal Disease Inform., 27:174, 1946.

Futcher, P. H.: The Double Quotidian Temperature Curve of Gonococcal Endocarditis: A Diagnostic Aid, Am. J. Med. Sci., 199:23, 1940.

Garson, W., and J. D. Thayer: The Gonococcus, p. 505 in "Bacterial and Mycotic Diseases of Man," 3d ed., Philadelphia, J. B. Lippincott Company, 1958.

Keefer, C. S.: Gonococcic Infections, in "Oxford Medicine," vol. 5, pt. 1, p. 39, New York, Oxford University Press, 1949.

—— and W. W. Spink: Gonococcic Arthritis; Pathogenesis, Mechanism of Recovery Treatment, J.A.M.A., 109:1448, 1937.

Keil, H.: A Type of Gonococcal Bacteremia with Characteristic Hemorrhagic, Vesiculo-pustular and Bullous Skin Lesions, Quart. J. Med., 31:1, 1938.

Mahoney, J. F., C. J. Van Slyke, J. C. Cutler, and H. L. Blum: Experimental Gonococcic Urethritis in Human Volunteers, Am. J. Syphilis, Gonorrhea, and Venereal Diseases, 30:1, 1946.

Section 4: Diseases Produced by Enteric Gram-negative Bacilli

118 COLIFORM BACTERIAL INFECTIONS

Ivan L. Bennett, Jr.

Etiology. The coliform bacteria are gram-negative bacilli which normally inhabit the human intestinal tract; similar organisms that occur in soil or vegetation are often included in the group. The best-known coliform bacilli are *Escherichia coli* (the colon bacillus) and *Aerobacter (Klebsiella) aerogenes* (p. 938). These two species ferment lactose, and although they are harmless saprophytes in the intestinal tract, both are capable of producing severe infections if introduced into other tissues. The ability to ferment lactose was formerly regarded as an important differentiating characteristic between the saprophytic coliforms and the non-lactose-fermenting enteric pathogens of the salmonella and shigella groups. It is still a useful property in the laboratory, but it is now recognized that there is no sharp biochemical and antigenic dividing line between pathogenic and nonpathogenic species, but rather there is a gradual transition through an intermediate group of organisms, the "paracolon" bacilli. These organisms ferment lactose slowly or not at all; the so-called Arizona, Ballerup, Bethesda, and Providence bacteria are paracolon bacilli. Biochemically or even serologically, many of them are extremely difficult to distinguish from *Salmonella* species. The paracolon bacilli can produce pyogenic infections in extraintestinal sites, and evidence indicates that some are capable of producing gastroenteritis in man.

The tests commonly employed in differentiating the members of the coliform group are sugar fermentation, the Voges-Proskauer reaction, methyl red test, citrate utilization, and serologic identification. *Alcaligenes faecalis* is another normal coliform inhabitant of the bowel which does not ferment lactose and is sometimes confused with enteric pathogens on SS or desoxycholate agar plates.

Because the types of infections produced, susceptibilities to chemotherapeutic agents, and general clinical import are closely similar for *E. coli* and *A. aerogenes,* it is customary in many laboratories to report a culture as containing "coliaerogenes" bacilli without differentiating between them.

The presence of coliforms in water or milk is presumptive evidence of fecal contamination in public health and sanitary bacteriologic testing.

Pathogenesis. These organisms can be transported from the intestinal tract to other parts of the body by way of the lymphatic vessels or blood stream, or they may be spread by fecal contamination. Histologically, the lesions produced in various body tissues show typical acute inflammation with pus and abscess formation. There is a common misconception that coliform bacterial infections are characterized by a foul-smelling, feculent exudate. Such an odor is caused by anaerobic streptococci or *Bacteroides* species which are often associated with coliform bacteria in mixed infections.

Manifestations. *Urinary Tract Infections.* Coliform bacilli are the commonest infecting agents in pyelonephritis and cystitis. The route by which these organisms reach the urinary tract from the bowel is usually by introduction into the urethra, often by catheters or other instruments. The frequency of pyelonephritis in young girls is believed to be accounted for by the combination of a short urethra and fecal soiling. The pathogenesis, clinical manifestations, complications, and treatment of pyelonephritis are discussed in detail on p. 1035.

Appendicitis and Peritonitis. Coliform organisms can nearly always be cultured from the exudate of an appendiceal infection, from diverticulitis, and from the peritoneum after perforation of a viscus. Often, they are found in mixed culture with anaerobic streptococci and clostridia. It is difficult to assess the role of various bacteria in mixed infections of this type, but there is no doubt about the ability of coliforms to infect serous cavities.

Biliary Tract Infections. Coliform bacilli are the common etiologic agents in obstructive cholangitis. So-called "Charcot's intermittent fever" may be seen in this condition, and liver abscess is one of its complications (see p. 1698).

Omphalitis. Infection of the umbilical stump in newborn infants by colon bacilli can lead to fatal bacteremia (Winckel's disease).

Bacteremia. While organisms can invade the blood in almost any type of coliform infection, bacteremia is especially common in pyelonephritis. It often begins with a rigor and high fever. Most patients are prostrated, slight icterus is not uncommon, and even after a single transient episode, hypotension of several hours duration is often observed.

Profound circulatory collapse is far more likely to complicate bacteremias due to gram-negative organisms, including coliform bacilli, pseudomonas, proteus, salmonellas, and others (see Meningococcemia, p. 925), than it is with gram-positive species. Shock is more frequent in older individuals and carries a poor prognosis. This type of infection is especially likely to occur in elderly men following operative procedures on the genitourinary tract. There is no specific treatment; pressor amines and adrenal steroids should be given and moderate amounts of whole blood or plasma are permissible. These measures should not lead to neglect of the important step of initiating vigorous antibacterial therapy.

Circulatory collapse, especially that attended by severe dyspnea with or without pulmonary edema, is often the first manifestation of gram-negative bacteremia. In elderly patients, fever may be absent or low, and there may be no peripheral leukocytosis, leading to delay in recognition of the infectious etiology of the circulatory disturbance which is often first attributed to pulmonary embolism, coronary occlusion, cerebrovascular accident, or internal bleeding.

The sudden onset of *shock, dyspnea,* or *pulmonary edema* in a patient with *diabetes, urinary tract infection,* disease of the *biliary tract, leukemia* or other blood dyscrasia, or history of recent *abortion* or *abdominal suppuration* should immediately call to mind the possibility of infection.

Escherichia coli bacteremia is occasionally seen in patients with hepatic cirrhosis in the absence of any obvious primary focus of infection. The mechanism of entry of the bacilli into the blood in these patients is unknown.

Pyogenic Infections. Coliform organisms are capable of producing abscesses in various parts of the body (see p. 1029). Diabetic patients are particularly prone to infection by these organisms, and small abscesses at the sites of insulin injections are sometimes seen. Coliform infection frequently complicates and greatly worsens ischemic gangrene of the extremities. An interesting and important feature of coliform infections and abscesses in diabetes (and occasionally in nondiabetic patients) is the production of large amounts of gas in the tissues; crepitation is often detectable, and the gas may be visualized by x-ray. It has been suggested that the gas production is related to high glucose content of diabetic tissues. An erroneous diagnosis of clostridial infection is often made in these circumstances.

Gastrointestinal Disease. There are several good epidemiologic studies incriminating certain strains of *E. coli* in the etiology of epidemics of neonatal diarrhea. In several outbreaks of adult gastroenteritis, there has been highly suggestive evidence that a paracolon bacillus produced the illness. In view of the close resemblance of some paracolon bacilli to the salmonella group, it is not surprising that occasional strains might produce gastroenteritis in man.

Treatment. The management of bacteremic shock has been discussed. The incision and drainage of localized suppurations are important in coliform infections. The general measures for pyelonephritis are discussed on p. 1038.

A variety of chemotherapeutic agents is available, but none is regularly effective against all coliform bacilli, and in any serious infection, the drugs should be chosen with the guidance of sensitivity tests of the infecting strain. Chloramphenicol or one of the tetracycline derivatives in an oral dosage of 2 Gm daily, alone or in combination with 1 to 2 Gm streptomycin intramuscularly, is likely to be effective. Nitrofurantoin and the sulfonamides are sometimes effective for urinary tract infections. Neomycin and kanamycin are toxic but are usually highly effective against organisms of this group and are worth using in any serious, uncontrolled infection.

REFERENCES

Felty, A. R., and C. S. Keefer: *Bacillus coli* Sepsis, J.A.M.A., 82:1430, 1924.

Hall, W. H., and D. Gold: Shock Associated with Bacteremia, A.M.A. Arch. Internal Med., 96:403, 1955.

Martin, W. J., et al.: Severe Liver Disease Complicated by Bacteremia Due to Gram-negative Bacilli, A.M.A. Arch. Internal Med., 98:8, 1956.

Morse, K. T., and F. N. Furness (Eds.): Epidemic and Endemic Diarrheal Diseases of the Infant, Ann. N.Y. Acad. Sci., 66 (1):3, 1956.

Simmons, D. H., J. Nicoloff, and L. B. Guze: Hyperventilation and Respiratory Alkalosis as Signs of Gram-negative Bacteremia, J.A.M.A., 174:2196, 1960.

Spittel, J. A., Jr., W. J. Martin, and D. R. Nichols: Bacteremia Owing to Gram-negative Bacilli, Ann. Internal Med., 44:302, 1956.

Spring, M., and S. Kahn: Nonclostridial Gas Infection in the Diabetic, A.M.A. Arch. Internal Med., 88:373, 1951.

Studdiford, W. E., and G. W. Douglas: Placental Bacteremia: A Significant Finding in Septic Abortion Accompanied by Vascular Collapse, Am. J. Obstet. Gynecol., 71:842, 1956.

Waisbren, B. A.: Bacteremia Due to Gram-negative Bacilli Other than the *Salmonella,* A.M.A. Arch. Internal Med., 88:467, 1961.

Whipple, R. L. Jr., and J. F. Harris: *Bacillus coli* Septicemia in Laennec's Cirrhosis of Liver, Ann. Internal Med., 33:462, 1950.

119 PROTEUS INFECTIONS

Robert G. Petersdorf and
Ivan L. Bennett, Jr.

Etiology. The genus *Proteus* consists of pleomorphic gram-negative bacilli which do not ferment lactose and are characterized by their active motility and spreading growth upon solid media. There are four pathogenic species: *P. mirabilis, P. vulgaris, P. morganii,* and *P. rettgeri. Proteus mirabilis* is the most frequent cause of infections in man and is distinguishable from the other three species by its inability to form indole. All species split urea, with production of ammonia. Some strains of *P. vulgaris* share a common antigen with certain rickettsias, accounting for the appearance of antibodies against proteus organisms (Weil-Felix reaction) in typhus, scrub typhus, and Rocky Mountain spotted fever.

Epidemiology and Pathogenesis. Members of the genus *Proteus* are normally found in soil, water, and sewage and are part of the normal fecal flora. Occasionally, proteus organisms have been implicated as a cause of epidemic diarrhea in infants, but the evidence for this is inconclusive. The organism is frequently cultured from superficial wounds, draining ears, and sputum. It tends to form colonies in patients who have received antibiotics and replaces the more susceptible flora eradicated by these drugs. Proteus often localizes in already damaged tissues where it produces a typical exudative inflammatory reaction.

Manifestations. Proteus is rarely a primary invader but produces disease in locations previously infected by other organisms. These include the skin, ears and mastoid sinuses, eyes, peritoneal cavity, urinary tract, meninges, and blood stream.

Cutaneous Infections. Proteus organisms are frequently isolated from surgical wounds, particularly following antimicrobial therapy. They do not interfere with normal wound-healing provided that the tissues are viable and foreign bodies are not present. Burns, varicose ulcers, and decubiti may become contaminated with proteus often in company with other gram-negative organisms or staphylococci.

Infections of the Ears and Mastoid Sinuses. Otitis media and mastoiditis in which proteus is present may result in extensive destruction of the middle ear and mastoid sinuses. Fetid otorrhea, cholesteatoma formation, and development of granulation tissue contribute to a chronic focus of infection in the middle and inner ears and mastoid and may culminate in deafness. Paralysis of the facial nerve is an occasional complication. The great danger of these infections lies in intracranial extension, leading to thrombosis of the lateral sinus, meningitis, brain abscess, and septicemia.

Ocular Infections. Proteus may cause corneal ulcers, usually following trauma to the eye. If extensive, these ulcers may terminate in panophthalmitis and destruction of the eyeball.

Peritonitis. Proteus organisms may be isolated from the peritoneal cavity following perforation of the appendix and bowel or mesenteric infarction. Presumably this represents soilage of the peritoneum by intestinal flora.

Urinary Tract Infections. Proteus organisms are common pathogens in the urinary tract and account for 15 to 25 per cent of all urinary tract infections. In general, these organisms are isolated from patients with recurrent pyelonephritis—most commonly those with obstructive uropathy, a history of instrumentation of the bladder, and repeated courses of chemotherapy. At times, proteus is found in patients with ostensibly normal excretory systems. Many of these patients have diabetes mellitus, suggesting a predisposition to proteus urinary tract infections in patients with this metabolic disorder. Proteus is also often cultured in patients with renal or bladder calculi. This may be due to the ammoniagenic property which renders the urine alkaline and provides a fertile medium for formation of the ammonium-magnesium-phosphate stones.

Bacteremia. Blood stream invasion by proteus is the most serious manifestation of infection with this organism. In 75 per cent of cases, the urinary tract serves as the portal of entry; in the remainder the biliary tree, gastrointestinal tract, ears and sinuses, and skin are the primary foci. Proteus bacteremia is frequently preceded by cystoscopy, urethral catheterization, transurethral prostatic resection, or other operative procedures. Clinically, the signs, symptoms, and laboratory findings of proteus sepsis —high fever, chills, shock, metastatic abscesses in remote locations, leukocytosis, and occasionally thrombocytopenia—are indistinguishable from blood stream infections with other gram-negative bacteria.

Diagnosis. The diagnosis of proteus infection depends on culture of the organism from blood, urine, or exudate and its identification by appropriate biochemical tests. It is especially important to separate *P. mirabilis,* the indole-negative species, from *P. morganii, rettgeri,* and *vulgaris,* which are indole-positive, since only *P. mirabilis* is susceptible to the action of penicillin. Proteus is often present in mixed infections with other pathogens. Particular care should be exercised in the isolation of other organisms growing in the same medium with proteus lest they be masked by its spreading growth.

Treatment. The majority of strains of *P. mirabilis* is sensitive to 10 units of penicillin per milliliter, a level which can be easily attained in blood and tissues by the use of large intravenous doses coupled with probenecid. Most strains of this species are also inhibited by chloramphenicol and a few by streptomycin. There is some evidence that penicillin and chloramphenicol exert a synergistic antibacterial effect against some strains. On the basis of these data, mild *P. mirabilis* infection should be treated with chloramphenicol, 0.5 Gm every 6 hr by mouth. Streptomycin can be added to this regimen if the organism is sensitive to this agent. In life-threatening or refractory *P. mirabilis* infections, 20 million units of penicillin a day should be given intravenously and 2.0 Gm probenecid administered. It should be pointed out that most antibiotic-sensitivity disks contain less than 10 units penicillin per milliliter, and tube dilution tests should be used to determine the sensitivity of proteus to penicillin. Most strains of proteus other than *P. mirabilis* are highly resistant to all antibiotics including penicillin and are susceptible only to kanamycin. This agent should be given intramuscularly in dosage of 0.5 Gm every 6 hr to all patients with serious penicillin-resistant proteus infections. Its toxicity to the eighth nerve and kidneys places a limitation on the duration of therapy. As with all patients with severe infection, close attention must be given to fluid and electrolyte status, adequate protein intake, and drainage of pus. In some urinary tract infections, the organism is sensitive only to nitrofurantoin, which may be given in dosage of 100 mg four times a day.

REFERENCES

Hook, E. W., and R. G. Petersdorf: In Vitro and in Vivo Susceptibility of Proteus Species to the Action of Certain Antimicrobial Drugs, Bull. Johns Hopkins Hosp., 107:337, 1960.

McGovern, F. H., and A. A. Khuri: Chronic Otitis Media and Mastoiditis Due to *Proteus vulgaris* (*Bacillus proteus*), A.M.A. Arch. Otolaryngol., 67:403, 1958.

Spittel, J. A., W. J. Martin, Jr., and D. R. Nichols: Bacteremia Owing to Gram-negative Bacilli: Experience in the Treatment of 137 Patients in a 15-year Period, Ann. Internal Med., 44:302, 1956.

Stein, M. N., and E. Gechman: Blood Stream Infection Due to *Proteus vulgaris* and Causing Thrombocytopenic Purpura, New Engl. J. Med., 252:906, 1955.

Waisbren, B. A.: Treatment with Large Doses of Penicillin in a Case of Severe Bacteremia Due to Proteus, A.M.A. Arch. Internal Med., 91:138, 1953.

—— and C. Carr: Penicillin and Chloramphenicol in

the Treatment of Infections Due to Proteus Organisms, Am. J. Med. Sci., 223:418, 1952.

120 PSEUDOMONAS INFECTIONS

Robert G. Petersdorf and Ivan L. Bennett, Jr.

Etiology. *Pseudomonas aeruginosa* is a gram-negative motile rod which is not encapsulated and forms no spores. It grows readily in all ordinary culture media and on agar it forms round, smooth, glistening colonies which have a fluorescent yellow-green color because of diffusion into the medium of a bluish-green pigment composed of two substances: pyocyanin and fluorescin. Pseudomonas produces acid but no gas in glucose; it liquefies gelatin, produces ammonia, and grows in citrate medium. It is indole, methyl red, and Voges-Proskauer negative. Of more than 30 species, *P. aeruginosa* is the only one pathogenic for man.

Epidemiology. Pseudomonas organisms are present on the skin of some normal individuals, particularly in the axillas and anogenital regions. They are uncommon in the stools of adults unless they are receiving antibiotics. In the majority of instances, pseudomonas is cultured as a relatively avirulent secondary contaminant in superficial wounds. It is also not uncommon to find this organism in the respiratory tract of patients treated with antibiotics. Ordinarily this is of no consequence, since the organisms merely fill the bacteriologic vacuum left by the elimination of more sensitive bacteria. Occasionally, however, superinfections (p. 885) with pseudomonas occur in the ear, lung, or skin of patients after the primary pathogen has been eradicated by antibiotics. Serious infections with pseudomonas are almost invariably associated with damage to local tissue or diminished resistance in the host. Premature infants, children with congenital anomalies, patients with leukemia—usually receiving antibiotics, adrenal steroids, or antimetabolites—and geriatric patients with debilitating diseases—are prone to develop infection with this organism. Most pseudomonas infections occur in the hospital environment, and the organisms have been cultured from a variety of sources in hospitals, including water from laboratory sinks and wash basins, antiseptic solutions, particularly alkyl-dimethyl-benzyl ammonium chloride (Zephiran), fluorescein, saline, penicillin, and a variety of other medications. It is particularly prevalent in urine receptacles, catheters, and on the hands of orderlies, nurses, and surgeons on urologic wards, and several outbreaks of pseudomonas urinary tract infections have been reported in this locale—presumably transmitted from patient to patient by human carriers. Similar epidemics have been reported in premature nurseries. By means of bacteriophage and serotyping techniques, these epidemics have been traced to a few specific strains and resemble the spread of nosocomial strains of staphylococci in hospitals.

Pathogenesis. The portal of entry of pseudomonas varies with the patient's age and underlying disease. In infancy and childhood, the skin, umbilical cord, and gastrointestinal tract predominate, while the urinary tract is most often the primary focus in old age. Many superficial pseudomonas infections remain localized to the skin or subcutaneous tissues. Hematogenous dissemination is characterized by a typical histologic picture consisting of infiltration of the arterioles with bacteria, thrombosis of the vessels, and infarction and necrosis of tissue accompanied by sparse cellular exudation.

Manifestations. Pseudomonas infections occur in many locations, including the skin, subcutaneous tissue, bone and joints, eye, ears, mastoid and paranasal sinuses, meninges, and heart valves. Sepsis without a predominating primary focus may also occur.

Infections of the Skin and Subcutaneous Tissues. Pseudomonas is frequently cultured from surgical wounds, varicose and decubitus ulcers, and burns. Draining tuberculous or osteomyelitic sinuses also tend to become secondarily infected with this organism. The mere presence of pseudomonas in these sites is of little significance provided that bacteremia does not ensue. Cutaneous infections usually heal following removal or slough of devitalized tissue.

Infections of the Ear, Mastoid and Paranasal Sinuses. Otitis externa is the most common form of pseudomonas infection involving the ear. It is particularly troublesome in tropical climates and is characterized by chronic serosanguineous and purulent drainage from the external auditory canal. Hearing may be impaired. Otitis media or mastoiditis is usually a superinfection following eradication of pneumococci, streptococci, or staphylococci by antimicrobial agents. Frequently pseudomonas is present in association with other gramnegative organisms.

Infection of the Eye. Corneal ulceration is the most severe form of ocular pseudomonas infection. It usually follows a traumatic abrasion and may terminate in panophthalmitis and destruction of the globe. Purulent conjunctivitis may occur as a manifestation of pseudomonas infection in premature infants.

Urinary Tract Infections. Pseudomonas is a common pathogen in the urinary tract and is usually found in complicated infections, i.e., in patients with obstructive uropathy or other structural abnormality who have been subjected to repeated urethral manipulations or surgery and who have received multiple courses of antibiotics. In this situation, pseudomonas is often present in association with other urinary pathogens such as *Escherichia coli* or organisms of the genus *Klebsiella* or *Proteus.* A detailed description of pyelonephritis is given on p. 1035.

Gastrointestinal Tract. Pseudomonas has been implicated as the cause of epidemic diarrhea of infancy. In addition, a number of infants dying from unexplained causes have the classical necrotic, avascular ulcers of pseudomonas infection in the bowel at autopsy. Antibiotic therapy may predispose to development of pseudomonas enteritis. A "typhoidal" form of pseudomonas infection characterized by fever, myalgia, and diarrhea occurs predominantly in the tropics. This illness, also called "thirteen-day fever" or "Shanghai fever" is self-limited, and the prognosis is good.

Respiratory Tract. Primary pseudomonas pneumonia probably does not occur, and culture of this pathogen from the sputum usually represents secondary invasion. The organism is generally isolated from patients with bronchiectasis, chronic bronchitis, and cystic fibrosis who have lingering infections punctuated by multiple courses of chemotherapy. Pseudomonas bronchitis and bronchiolitis followed by hematogenous spread is a frequent mode of death in cystic fibrosis.

Meningitis. Spontaneous pseudomonas meningitis is most unusual, but the bacilli may be introduced into the subarachnoid space by lumbar puncture, spinal anesthesia, or head trauma. Ventriculomastoid shunts performed for hydrocephalus may be contaminated with pseudomonas. Meningitis is often a terminal phenomenon in pseudomonas sepsis.

Bacteremia. Blood stream invasion by pseudomonas tends to occur in debilitated patients—premature infants, children with congenital defects, patients with lymphomas and leukemias, and elderly patients who have undergone surgery of the biliary or urinary tracts. Pseudomonas bacteremia is an important cause of death in patients with severe burns. In adults, pseudomonas bacteremia is indistinguishable from blood stream infection with other bacterial species. Hectic fever, true rigors, shock, and leukocytosis are present in most cases. Metastatic abscesses in the kidneys, lungs, adrenals, and intestine are common. Dissemination of the organism to the skin may result in the classical lesions of *ecthyma gangrenosum.* These are round, indurated, ulcerated areas with black necrotic centers surrounded by a zone of erythema. They are most commonly located in the anogenital region. Organisms can be cultured from these lesions which are thought to represent a Shwartzman phenomenon (p. 1269). Other eruptions described in pseudomonas bacteremia include vesicles filled with cloudy fluid containing the organisms, large areas of hemorrhagic cellulitis, and macular lesions on the trunk similar to "rose spots."

Miscellaneous. Pseudomonas endocarditis has been observed in a patient with acquired arteriovenous fistula, one who underwent open-heart surgery, and a number with normal hearts. Septic arthritis and osteomyelitis are rare complications. Several cases of fetal intrauterine death in women with pseudomonas sepsis during pregnancy are on record.

Treatment. Localized pseudomonas infections are best treated by irrigation with 1 per cent acetic acid or topical therapy with nitrofurazone, polymyxin B, or neomycin. Removal of devitalized tissue is essential. The outcome of systemic pseudomonas infection is intimately associated with the course of the underlying disease. For example, pseudomonas sepsis in patients with leukemia can be controlled only if remission of the leukemic process occurs concomitantly. Drainage of pus, removal of obstructive foci, and improvement of the patient's over-all condition are important in controlling pseudomonas sepsis. Specific chemotherapy is dependent upon sensitivity studies. Approximately one-third of strains are susceptible to streptomycin, and this agent should be used whenever possible. The tetracyclines are effective against 25 per cent of strains; the antibacterial activity of chloramphenicol, kanamycin, and neomycin is unpredictable. The majority of strains are inhibited by polymyxin B and an analogue of this drug, colistin. The antimicrobial activity of these two is quite similar, but the neurotoxic and nephrotoxic effects of polymyxin B are considerably greater than those of colistin. With both of these agents in vitro blood levels exceed minimal inhibitory concentrations only twofold, which may explain their inconsistent effectiveness in bacteremia. Colistin is excreted largely in the urine and is the drug of choice for pseudomonas infection of the urinary tract.

If sensitivity studies warrant, patients with pseudomonas bacteremia should receive streptomycin 2.0 Gm daily and tetracycline in the same dosage simultaneously. In more resistant cases, colistin or polymyxin B should be used. Both these drugs must be given intramuscularly. The dosage is 30 to 75 mg intramuscularly every 6 hr for colistin and 50 to 100 mg intramuscularly every 6 hr for polymyxin B. Occasionally the organism is sensitive only to kanamycin, which should be administered in dosage of 0.5 Gm intramuscularly every 6 hr.

There is some experimental evidence that γ-globulin enhances resistance to pseudomonas infection in mice. This has not been observed in man.

Prognosis. The mortality rate in pseudomonas bacteremia is over 75 per cent. The prognosis is dependent more on the nature of the associated disease than the infection or the antibiotics employed. In general, the outcome is more favorable in patients with pseudomonas bacteremia following surgery of the urinary tract than in premature infants, children with cystic fibrosis, or leukemia. Localized pseudomonas infections do not present a threat to life unless hematogenous dissemination occurs.

REFERENCES

Curtin, J. A., R. G. Petersdorf, and I. L. Bennett, Jr.: Pseudomonas Bacteremia: Review of 91 Cases, Ann. Internal Med., 54:1077, 1961.

Forkner, C. E., Jr., E. Frei, III, J. H. Edgcomb, and J. P. Utz: Pseudomonas Septicemia, Am. J. Med., 25:877, 1958.

Gould, J. C., and M. W. McLeod: A Study of the Use of Agglutinating Sera and Phage Lysis in the Classification of Strains of *Pseudomonas aeruginosa*, J. Pathol. Bacteriol., 79:295, 1960.

Jawetz, E.: Infections with *Pseudomonas aeruginosa* Treated with Polymyxin B, Arch. Internal Med., 89:90, 1952.

Markely, K., G. Gurmendi, P. M. Charez, and A. Bazan: Fatal Pseudomonas Septicemias in Burned Patients, Ann. Surg., 145:175, 1957.

McLeod, J. W.: The Hospital Urine Bottle and Bed Pan as Reservoirs of Infection by *Pseudomonas pyocyanea*, Lancet, 1:1017, 1958.

Petersdorf, R. G., and E. W. Hook: The Use of Colistin in Infection of the Urinary Tract, Bull. Johns Hopkins Hosp., 107:133, 1960.

Plotkin, S. A., and R. Austrian: Bacteremia Caused by Pseudomonas Species Following the Use of Materials Stored in Solutions of a Cationic Surface-active Agent, Am. J. Med. Sci., 235:621, 1958.

Stanley, M. M.: *Bacillus pyocyaneus* Infections, Am. J. Med., 2:253 and 347, 1947.

121 BACTEROIDES INFECTIONS (Necrobacillosis)

Edward W. Hook and
Ivan L. Bennett, Jr.

Etiology. The genus *Bacteroides* includes a group of gram-negative, non-spore-forming, strictly anaerobic bacilli that are normal inhabitants of the mouth, intestinal tract, and vagina. These organisms are found in large numbers in feces, sometimes outnumbering *Escherichia coli* by 100-fold or more.

Bacteroides funduliformis (*B. necrophorus*), *B. fragilis,* and *B. nigrescens* (*B. melaninogenicus*) are the species usually responsible for local or systemic infection of man.

Pathogenesis. Bacteroides are not highly invasive microorganisms, and infection is usually secondary to an underlying process that impairs the normal defenses of the host. The initial reaction to infection results in a localized suppurative lesion characterized by the formation of fetid pus. Infection usually remains localized, but blood stream invasion may occur. In instances of bacteremia, suppurative thrombophlebitis adjacent to the site of initial infection is a frequent occurrence, and emboli harboring viable bacilli may be dislodged, resulting in septic pulmonary infarction. Organisms of the genus *Bacteroides* elaborate a heparinase, but the role of this enzyme in the formation of thrombi is unknown. Localization of blood-borne organisms at distant sites is not unusual and may result in abscess formation in the lungs, liver, joints, kidneys, brain, or other organs.

Although bacteroides may be isolated in pure culture from infected tissue or pus, another organism is present in the majority of cases, usually anaerobic or aerobic streptococci, coliform species, or staphylococci. It is not known whether a symbiotic relationship exists between bacteroides and other bacterial species in infections of man. However, bacteroides and anaerobic streptococci have been shown to act synergistically in the induction of abscesses in mice.

Manifestations. *Local Infections.* Bacteroides may be isolated from local suppurative lesions of any tissue liable to contamination with the flora of the intestinal tract or vagina. For example, members of this genus have been isolated from peritonsillar, appendiceal, ischiorectal, or pelvic abscesses and from infected Skene's or Bartholin's glands. These organisms can also be cultured from the surfaces of acutely inflamed appendixes, from exudate in localized or generalized peritonitis, and from purulent discharges in patients with endometritis. Surgery of the gastrointestinal or genitourinary tract may be complicated by bacteroides wound infection.

Local infection is usually manifested by pain and tenderness, and the course and outcome depend on the site of involvement and extent of infection. Necrosis of blood vessels in an abscess cavity occasionally results in severe hemorrhage.

Systemic Infection. Invasion of the blood stream by bacteroides is usually secondary to local infection of the tonsils, female genital tract, or peritoneum. The initial manifestations are determined by the portal of entry and may be those of peri-

tonsillar abscess, endometritis, or appendicitis. When blood stream invasion occurs, the patient becomes extremely ill. Severe chills, hectic type of fever ranging from 101 to 106°F, and severe diaphoresis are common. In septicemia complicating tonsillar infection, the internal jugular vein may be the site of suppurative thrombophlebitis, and in pelvic infections the iliac and femoral veins may be involved. Palpation along the course of an involved vein, such as the internal jugular, may disclose a firm, tender cord, indicating the presence of a thrombus. Emboli may be dislodged, resulting in multiple septic pulmonary infarcts manifested by rales, dyspnea, cough, hemoptysis, pleurisy, and roentgenographic evidence of consolidation. Lung abscess and empyema may complicate pulmonary infection. Metastatic infection at other sites is not unusual and may be manifested as brain abscess, liver abscess, or septic arthritis. A diffuse hepatitis may develop, leading to enlargement and tenderness of the liver and jaundice. The prognosis in systemic bacteroides infection is grave, and death may occur in a few days.

Bacteroides have also been implicated in certain other serious systemic infections. Meningitis secondary to otitis media or mastoiditis and subacute bacterial endocarditis have been described, and aspiration of secretions harboring bacteroides may lead to pneumonia, abscess formation, or empyema. Bacteroides are a rare cause of urinary tract infection.

Laboratory Findings. Leukocytosis of 12,000 to 25,000 cells per cu mm may occur in localized bacteroides infection and is almost always present in systemic infection. Patients with liver abscesses or hepatitis have elevated serum bilirubin values and other aberrations of hepatic function.

Bacteroides infection should be considered whenever pus with an extremely foul odor is encountered. A smear of the pus reveals slightly elongated gram-negative bacilli, and often another organism, usually a gram-positive coccus. Definitive diagnosis depends on isolation of an anaerobic, non-spore-bearing, gram-negative bacillus. These organisms grow slowly and may be difficult to detect, especially when associated with another organism. Agglutinins against the strain responsible for an infection develop during the second or third week of infection, but because of the variable antigenic composition of bacteroides serologic methods are rarely of diagnostic aid.

Treatment. Surgical drainage of abscess cavities is of prime importance and should be carried out as soon as fluctuation and localization occur. Antimicrobial therapy is indicated when infection is not localized. Tetracycline in a concentration of 3 μg per ml or less inhibits almost all strains of *Bacteroides* and is the antibiotic of choice. Chloramphenicol is also active against the majority of isolates from human infections. Practically all strains of the genus *Bacteroides* are resistant to the action of streptomycin or neomycin.

Venous ligation and anticoagulant therapy should be considered in patients with thrombophlebitis and multiple septic pulmonary infarctions.

REFERENCES

Alston, J. M.: Necrobacillosis in Great Britain, Brit. Med. J., II:1524, 1955.

Beigelman, P. M., and L. A. Rantz: Clinical Significance of Bacteroides, Arch. Internal Med., 84:605, 1949.

Carter, B., C. P. Jones, R. L. Alter, R. N. Creadick, and W. L. Thomas: Bacteroides Infections in Obstetrics and Gynecology, Obstet. and Gynecol., 1:491, 1953.

Fisher, A. M., and V. A. McKusick: Bacteroides Infections: Clinical, Bacteriological and Therapeutic Features of Fourteen Cases, Am. J. Med. Sci., 225: 253, 1953.

Gillespie, W. A., and J. Guy: Bacteroides in Intraabdominal Sepsis, Lancet, I:1039, 1956.

McVay, L. V., Jr., and D. H. Sprunt: Bacteroides Infections, Ann. Internal Med., 36:56, 1952.

122 FRIEDLÄNDER BACILLUS (Klebsiella) INFECTIONS

Ivan L. Bennett, Jr.

Etiology. The Friedländer bacilli (*Klebsiella pneumoniae* or *friedlanderi*) are encapsulated gram-negative bacilli, found among the normal flora of the mouth and respiratory and intestinal tracts. They are closely related to *Aerobacter aerogenes* (see p. 931) and cannot be differentiated by biochemical reactions. Indeed, there is general agreement that separation of the *Aerobacter* genus from *Klebsiella* is not justified, although clinical usage will continue to refer to the strains from the respiratory tract as Friedländer bacilli and those from other regions as *Aerobacter*. The klebsiellas isolated from respiratory infections usually form large mucoid colonies on solid media and are virulent for mice. These characteristics, however, are not invariable enough to differentiate them from intestinal strains. The capsular polysaccharides of Friedländer bacilli are similar to those of pneumococci; in fact, serologic cross reactions occur between certain Friedländer strains and pneumococci. Friedländer bacilli have been divided serologically into groups. Most infections in human beings are due to members of group A.

Pathogenesis. Infections of the urinary and biliary tracts, the peritoneal cavity, and other serous membranes comprise the bulk of diseases caused by the Friedländer bacilli. These are similar in manifestations and pathogenesis to those produced by the coliform organisms, discussed on p. 931. In the lungs, however, Friedländer infections take the form of an acute, rapidly progressive, and often fatal pneumonia, or of a chronic lung disease, with bronchitis, bronchiectasis, and cavity formation.

Manifestations. As already mentioned, the majority of infections caused by the Friedländer bacilli are similar to those due to the coliform bacteria. Thus Friedländer bacilli may be among the infecting organisms in general peritonitis, or they may be the etiologic agents in pyelonephritis or cholangitis. Occasionally, they cause infections of the middle ear, mastoids, or paranasal sinuses, or meningitis secondary to one of these. A significant proportion of all reported cases of Friedländer bacillus meningitis has involved persons with diabetes mellitus. Another kind of Friedländer bacillus meningitis is that which complicates traumatic perforation of the skull or spinal canal, especially as encountered in war wounds.

Acute Pneumonia. About 1 per cent of all cases of bacterial pneumonia are caused by Friedländer bacilli. The disease is most common in men over forty years of age and is frequent in alcoholic addicts. The manifestations are similar to those of pneumococcal pneumonia, with sudden onset of chills, fever, and severe pleuritic pain. Patients are more likely to be delirious and prostrated, and fever is more often remittent than in pneumococcal pneumonia. In about half the cases the sputum is dark brown or red and is so sticky that the patient has difficulty in expelling it from his mouth and lips. The pulmonary lesion usually progresses rapidly, spreading from lobe to lobe and from one lung to the other within a few days. Cyanosis and dyspnea develop rapidly, and jaundice, vomiting, and diarrhea are often present. Although x-rays may show extensive consolidation in the lungs, physical signs may be deceptively few. The blood leukocyte count may be elevated but is often low or in the normal range. Lung abscess and empyema are frequent complications. Previous to the introduction of sulfonamides and streptomycin, the fatality rate reported in different clinics varied from 50 to 80 per cent; death within 48 hr was not infrequent.

Chronic Infection of the Lung. This disease is now rare. It may follow acute Friedländer pneumonia but is also seen in patients who give no history of acute onset. The principal manifestations are productive cough, weakness, and anemia. Hemoptysis is not common. Chronic empyema or sterile serous effusion is observed in about one-fourth the cases. Cavity formation frequently occurs and is usually located in the upper lung fields. There is very little inflammatory reaction around the cavities, so that in roentgenograms they appear to have thin walls. A number of patients with chronic Friedländer infection of the lung have had an erroneous diagnosis of pulmonary tuberculosis and have been give sanatorium treatment. The course of this disease is quite variable. Some cases have been observed for 10 or 20 years with very little change in symptoms and signs, whereas others have shown gradual improvement after several months.

Diagnosis. Diagnosis can be made only by the isolation of Friedländer bacilli. A presumptive diagnosis of Friedländer pneumonia can be made on the basis of Gram stain of the sputum; this shows numerous short, plump, gram-negative bacilli, each surrounded by a clear space because of the capsule. Indeed, one of the most important reasons for examination of stained sputum smears is the detection of a predominance of gram-negative bacilli rather than, as many seem to think, to differentiate among gram-positive cocci. In any patient with acute pneumonia whose sputum is found to contain a predominance of gram-negative bacilli, a presumptive diagnosis of Friedländer infection should be made and appropriate therapy instituted. Culture of the sputum on a solid medium shows almost pure growth of Friedländer colonies. Certain proof is afforded by isolation of the organisms from the blood, pleural exudate, or fluid aspirated from the lung.

Treatment. In view of the age group involved and the frequent association with alcoholism and malnutrition, the fatality rate in acute Friedländer pneumonia will doubtless remain fairly high, i.e., 25 to 50 per cent. Specific antiserums have been employed in the treatment of acute Friedländer pneumonia, but the results have not been encouraging. In vitro, Friedländer bacilli are usually susceptible to sulfonamides, streptomycin, chlortetracycline, and chloramphenicol, and results of therapy of experimental Friedländer infections with all these agents have been quite satisfactory. The best regimen employs streptomycin in large doses (3 to 4 Gm daily) with chloramphenicol or a tetracycline. Resistance to streptomycin develops rapidly, and if the response is satisfactory, the dose can be reduced or it can be discontinued after 3 to 5 days. Chloramphenicol or tetracycline should be continued for a minimum of 10 to 14 days.

REFERENCES

Barber, J. M., and A. P. Grant: Friedländer's Pneumonia, Brit. Med. J., II:752, 1952.

Hyde, L., and B. Hyde: Primary Friedländer Pneumonia, Am. J. Med. Sci., 205:660, 1943.

Kirby, W. M. M., and D. H. Coleman: Antibiotic Therapy of Friedländer Pneumonia, Am. J. Med., 11: 179, 1951.

Ritvo, M., and F. Martin: The Clinical and Roentgen Manifestations of Pneumonia Due to *Bacillus mucosus capsulatus* (Primary Friedländer Pneumonia), Am. J. Roentgenol., 62:211, 1949.

Solomon, S.: Chronic Friedländer Infections of the Lungs, J.A.M.A., 115:1527, 1940.

Thompson, A. J., E. B. Williams, Jr., E. D. Williams, and J. M. Anderson: *Klebsiella pneumoniae* Meningitis: Review of the Literature and Report of a Case with Bacteremia and Pneumonia, with Recovery, A.M.A. Arch. Internal Med., 89:405, 1952.

123 TYPHOID FEVER

*T. E. Woodward and
Richard B. Hornick*

Definition. Typhoid fever is a systemic infection caused by *Salmonella typhosa*. Anatomically there are hyperplasia and ulceration of the intestinal lymph follicles and Peyer's patches, mesenteric lymphadenopathy, splenomegaly, and parenchymatous changes in various organs, including the liver. The illness is characterized by fever of several weeks' duration, headache, cough, toxemia, abdominal pain, a characteristic skin eruption (rose spots), leukopenia, bacteremia, and the appearance in the patient's blood of agglutinins to the somatic (O) and flagellar (H) antigens of the bacillus.

Epidemiology. *Salmonella typhosa* resides solely in man and is perpetuated in nature by its transmission to healthy persons from patients or carriers. Water, milk, and food are contaminated from infected feces. The principal source of the sporadic case is the typhoid carrier who may shed virulent organisms indefinitely in spite of apparent good health. Infected persons who handle food are a potential serious threat to families or larger groups. Typhoid carriers, once identified, should be prevented from handling food until they have been rendered free of harboring *S. typhosa*.

Flies are active agents of dissemination; they mechanically transmit the typhoid bacillus to food, water, or milk. Formerly, typhoid fever was especially prevalent during the summer months. In many countries, sizable outbreaks no longer occur and there is no definite seasonal variation since carriers are the principal source of infection. The disease has not been controlled in some countries primarily because of crowded living conditions and poor sanitation.

Typhoid fever has figured prominently as a major cause of disability and death during times of war or privation, with a heavy toll of suffering among civilian and military populations. The disease prevailed in the United States during all the wars prior to the First World War. The decades since 1900 have witnessed a steadily declining incidence which can be attributed largely to sanitary advances.

History. In 1829, Louis described the findings in 158 cases, including intestinal lesions, enlarged mesenteric lymph glands, splenomegaly, rose spots, and intestinal hemorrhage and perforation. This great clinician first employed the term "typhoide." The British, however, continued to view the intestinal lesion as an incidental complication of typhus. William Gerhard of Philadelphia, a former student of Louis, presented the first clearly defined differences between typhus and typhoid based on precise clinical and anatomic findings in 1836.

Budd, an English practitioner, in a series of publications extending from 1856 to 1870, suggested the contagiousness of typhoid and stressed the importance of spread by the bowel discharges of infected persons. His prophecy was not fulfilled until 1885, when Pfieffer reported the first stool isolate. Eberth is credited with discovering the organism in 1880, reporting the presence of bacteria in smears of mesenteric lymph nodes and spleen.

Widal described the test for agglutinins in the serum of patients in 1896.

Pathogenesis and Pathologic Changes. The organism gains entrance by ingestion of food or liquids previously contaminated by feces or urine. Typhoid bacilli are not destroyed by gastric secretions, invade the mucosa of the small intestine, and soon traverse the intestinal lymphatics and mesenteric nodes to reach the blood. Bacteremia has been demonstrated in man prior to the onset of significant clinical signs, i.e., 3 to 4 days after ingestion of viable bacteria. *Salmonella typhosa* is present in the feces at this time and can be detected for several days. Secondary areas of inflammation are established in the liver, spleen, bone marrow, gallbladder, and other lymph nodes, presumably as a sequel to the circulatory spread.

Bacteremia continues until late in the second week. Antibodies appear at this time, overlapping the bacteremia by several days. Subsequently, the infection is firmly established in the liver, gallbladder, and Peyer's patches. Typhoid bacilli are shed into the upper small intestine from the biliary tract, rendering the stools bacteriologically positive from the second week upward to several months. In about 3 per cent of patients, a permanent carrier state persists.

The Peyer's patches are swollen and ultimately undergo necrosis, forming oval-shaped ulcers which are most numerous in the terminal 24 in. of the ileum. Ulceration can occur in the jejunum and

lymphoid follicles of the cecum and colon. The two most common complications of typhoid fever are hemorrhage and perforation which result from necrosis in such lesions, usually during the third week of illness. The intestinal ulcer eventually heals completely without scar formation.

In the intestinal lesion the histologic changes are proliferation of large mononuclear cells and edema. Typhoid bacilli are seen within macrophages or plasma cells; the intracellular residence of *S. typhosa* may protect them from the antibacterial action of antibiotics or antibodies and helps explain their continued presence in the host after improvement or full recovery. The marked monocytic hyperplasia involves the mesentery nodes, spleen, bone marrow, and liver. Lymph nodes often exhibit necrosis showing marked proliferation of the sinusoidal cells, and the sinusoids are filled with macrophages.

Focal metastatic infection may be responsible for cholecystitis, osteomyelitis, chondritis, meningitis, endocarditis, or nephritis. The gallbladder is frequently infected, although acute cholecystitis is less common. Bronchitis frequently accompanies the disease, and pneumonia due to *S. typhosa, Diplococcus pneumoniae,* or pyogenic bacteria occasionally occurs.

Considerable evidence supports the thesis that *S. typhosa* endotoxin, a lipid-polysaccharide-protein complex of the somatic fraction, is responsible for the morphologic alterations as well as the clinical manifestations. The intravenous infusion of endotoxin in rabbits results in congestion and hemorrhagic necrosis of the intestinal mucosa, liver, spleen, and bone marrow, with damage to the vascular endothelium similar to that in fatal typhoid cases.

Studies in man confirm the fact that significant tolerance to the endotoxic effects of *S. typhosa* and *Escherichia coli* develops early in convalescence, i.e., 2 to 3 days after defervescence following chloramphenicol therapy. Moreover, during the active stages of typhoid fever, when the endotoxic reaction is augmented, there is increased sensitivity of the capillary vessels to minute doses of norepinephrine. Each of these parameters, (1) the development of tolerance to pyrogenic activity and (2) vascular hyperreactivity to catechol amines, is an indicator of endotoxin effects.

The intestinal lesions subside ultimately, whereas the infection of the liver and biliary tract may continue indefinitely without any apparent ill effect on the host. Typhoid carriers have been observed to shed 50 million *S. typhosa* per milliliter of bile. The specific mechanisms responsible for the manifestations of typhoid fever will remain a mystery until (1) the factors leading to microbial persistence of *S. typhosa* in the host are known, (2) the biochemical and dynamic actions of endotoxin are fully characterized, and (3) the cellular response of the host and the mechanisms leading to endotoxin tolerance are defined.

Manifestations. The *incubation period* averages about 10 days, with a range of 3 to 25 days. This information is derived from analysis of typhoid epidemics as well as from observations made during volunteer studies. Mild prodromata include headache, weakness, and anorexia, which are not incapacitating.

In most instances recognized clinically as typhoid fever and given no therapy, the course of pyrexia is 3 weeks or more, with an extended period of convalescence. However, typhoid can masquerade in many forms, one so mild as to elude diagnosis and another so severe as to outdistance ordinary treatment. In mild cases, the fever and other manifestations may abate within 2 weeks.

The *onset* is usually gradual, with initial features of headache, anorexia, weakness, abdominal pain, diarrhea or constipation, epistaxis, and fever. The temperature increases steadily, rising each day to an afternoon level of 103 to 105°F. For 10 days to 2 weeks, the febrile pattern is either continuous or remittent, fluctuating between 103 to 105°F.

During the third and fourth weeks there are wider fluctuations of temperature, with morning levels often reaching normal and gradual defervescence by slow lysis.

Headache is a dominant complaint and, with fever, usually ushers in the disease. It is severe, generalized, and unrelenting. With high fever there may be nocturnal mental confusion. *Chills,* including shaking rigor, occasionally occur early in the disease but are not usual.

Cough and *bronchitic symptoms* are common at the onset and may be mistaken for a "nonspecific" viral type of pneumonitis. Anorexia without vomiting is characteristic. In the first week the patient suffers from diffuse abdominal pain which is occasionally colicky. The bowel may be constipated, or there may be loose, mushy movements. Later, at the height of illness, diarrhea may ensue, with watery or typical "pea soup" stools.

In the *second week,* all symptoms are aggravated. The temperature remains high, with slight morning remissions. Apathy, mental dullness, and delirium are now apparent. The face is frequently expressionless, the eyes are glassy, and the skin, tongue, and mucous membranes are dry. There is usually abdominal distention, with diffuse tenderness frequently accentuated on the right side. Cough and rales may persist. The pulse is usually rapid but may be slow and dicrotic.

During the *third week* there is accentuation of all manifestations, with an intermittent febrile pattern showing a gradual decline with morning remissions. The pulse ranges from 110 to 130 and is of poor quality. Weakness and weight loss are noticeable. Diarrhea, abdominal pain and distention may be troublesome, and other unfavorable features such as pulmonary complications and feeble heart sounds mark the seriously ill patient. Hemorrhage or perforation of the intestinal lesion is more prone to occur at this stage. Typhoidal psychoses with delirium or mania may become manifest early in the illness or at the height of the febrile-toxic period.

Several characteristic features merit special attention. The *eruption,* or "rose spots," are found often on the trunk over the upper abdomen or lower chest or anterior axilla. They are seldom numerous and appear as rose-pink hyperemic papules 2 to 4 mm in diameter, the central peak being felt on light palpation. They make their first appearance during the second febrile weeks, or at the time of relapse, and come out in successive crops lasting for 2 or 3 days, usually leaving a faint brownish discoloration. They are found rarely on the back, arms, and hands.

The *spleen* is frequently enlarged late in the first week of illness, but unless the examiner employs light palpation, it may not be felt. The organ is often tender, and occasionally a friction rub may indicate the presence of perisplenitis. Splenomegaly abates with defervescence.

Convalescence in typhoid patients is gradual, with a slow return of appetite and vigor. Weakness usually persists for weeks. Prior to the advent of antibiotics, such complications as thrombophlebitis, peripheral neuritis, and various pyogenic infections developed as sequelae of the protracted illness, malnutrition, and vitamin depletion.

Gastrointestinal Hemorrhage. Gross hemorrhage of the typhoidal ulcer occurs in approximately 10 per cent of cases; occult bleeding is present in about 20 per cent. Characteristically it occurs late in the second or during the third week of disease. There may be a sudden large hemorrhage or continuous slow oozing. Clinical signs indicative of blood loss are apprehension, sweating, pallor, depression of cutaneous temperature, rapid weak pulse, hypotension, and narrow pulse pressure. This complication occurs in spite of the favorable effect of chloramphenicol.

Intestinal Perforation. Intestinal perforation occurs in about 3 per cent of untreated cases and was formerly an important cause of death. Rupture of the intestinal ulcer with resultant peritonitis still occurs, although antibiotics have reduced the number of fatalities sharply. The part of the gut to perforate is the lower ileum in most instances. It may occur in the first week, but usually occurs at the height of disease in the third week, particularly in those patients with tympanites, diarrhea, and hemorrhage. It may strike with lightning suddenness in patients presumably progressing favorably. A sudden, sharp pain in the right lower quadrant is typical. Abdominal distention may increase rapidly, with signs of muscle rigidity, rebound tenderness, and diminished peristalsis. Obliteration of liver flatness with excessive tympanites is a valuable sign of free abdominal air. Pallor, clammy perspiration, tachycardia, and lowered blood pressure all herald impending shock. At this stage, the temperature is low and the blood leukocyte count ranges from 9,000 to 13,000 cells per cu mm. Perforation may be mistaken for appendicitis, acute cholecystitis, phlebitis of the iliac vein, or merely an accentuation of the abdominal pain in the debilitated typhoid patient. Under these circumstances frequent examinations and serial leukocyte counts can be very helpful in reaching a decision. Rarely, typhoidal peritonitis can result from rupture of a softened mesenteric gland.

Other Complications. Bacterial or lobar pneumonia developing at the height of the disease was formerly a serious complication of typhoid fever. Pneumococci or pure cultures of typhoid bacilli have been isolated from the sputum or consolidated lungs. The diagnosis should be verified by appropriate physical signs, bacteriologic findings, and roentgen examination. Other pyogenic complications include parotitis, sinusitis, and furunculosis. Typhoidal meningitis is rare but serious. *Chondritis* or *periostitis* are indolent focal infections from which typhoid bacilli may be isolated. Monoarticular and polyarticular arthritis are rare sequelae. Cholecystitis manifested by abdominal tenderness, muscle spasm, rigidity, and mild leukocytosis may occur during the acute illness. Months or years later, there may be chronic cholecystitis or gallstones from which viable *S. typhosa* may be isolated. Acute nephritis or pyelonephritis is seen occasionally at the height of illness or during convalescence. Deafness is common but seldom permanent. For some strange reason, herpes labialis is rare in typhoid patients.

Recrudescence (Relapse). In typhoid fever, the incidence of relapse varies in untreated patients from 5 to 15 per cent. Several important clinical features, such as stepwise temperature at onset, headache, intestinal symptoms, rose spots, and splenomegaly highlight the relapse. Bacteremia is usually demonstrable, and as a rule the manifestations are milder than those of the initial illness. In spite of the therapeutic efficacy of chloramphenicol, relapse has occurred in as many as 20 per cent of patients in some series. On an average, the relapse occurs approximately 15 days after cessation of chloramphenicol therapy, regardless of the duration of treatment or the stage at which the antibiotic is first given. The development of chloram-

phenicol-resistant strains of *S. typhosa* as a result of treatment is rare. There appears to be no correlation between the susceptibility of patients to relapse and the presence or absence of somatic (O) or flagellar (H) antibodies; immunity is not gauged by the serologic response of the patient to these antigens of *S. typhosa.*

The Typhoid Carrier. Typhoid bacilli may persist in the bile passages indefinitely and in the intestines in about 3 per cent of patients who recover from the disease. Many carriers have no history of prior infection, and all are in apparent good health. The carrier state is due to the persistence of infection in the biliary tract, and neither cholecystectomy or chemotherapy are invariably successful in rendering the carrier free of the organism. Urinary carriers are infrequent and represent a minor health hazard. Four therapeutic methods: (1) cholecystectomy; (2) penicillin treatment in the dosage of 12 million units daily, supplemented with Benemid for 12 to 14 days; (3) combined treatment with chloramphenicol (1.0 Gm every 8 hr) and streptomycin (1.0 Gm twice daily) for 3 weeks; and (4) chloramphenicol therapy with simultaneous vaccine administration have been successful in eradicating the carrier state in some subjects. Cholecystectomy should not be performed until chemotherapy has been attempted.

Laboratory Diagnosis. One of the distinctive hematologic features of typhoid fever is leukopenia, with white blood cell counts ranging from 4,000 to 6,000 cells per cu mm during the first two weeks and 3,000 to 5,000 cells per cu mm during the third and fourth weeks. In the presence of intestinal perforation or pyogenic complications, the leukocyte count rises moderately to 10,000 to 14,000 cells per cu mm. Normocytic anemia is present in many patients; with blood loss, it is hypochromic and microcytic. Except for transient albuminuria during the febrile stage, the urine is normal. Occult blood is present in the feces, beginning in the second week.

Isolation of *S. typhosa* from the blood and feces is the most dependable diagnostic test. Blood cultures are positive in most cases during the first and part of the second febrile week. Bacteremia is also demonstrable during relapse. *Salmonella typhosa* can be grown from the feces usually after the tenth day, and the incidence of isolations increases up to the fourth or fifth weeks.

The Widal test is a readily available and adequate serologic test for the diagnosis of typhoid fever. Specific agglutinins appear in the serum after 7 to 10 days of illness. The titer rises steadily to a peak from the third to fifth weeks and falls gradually over several weeks. It does not rise appreciably during a relapse. The titer of the flagellar

(H) agglutinin is usually higher than the somatic (O) antibody. As in most serologic diagnostic procedures, the demonstration of a rise in titer is of prime importance in establishing the laboratory confirmation.

Differential Diagnosis. No single symptom or clinical feature is pathognomonic at the time of onset. Manifestations such as headache, fever, malaise, weakness, anorexia, cough, and abdominal pain are common to many diseases. These include the major rickettsioses, brucellosis, tularemia, leptospirosis, infectious hepatitis, infectious mononucleosis, primary atypical pneumonia, miliary tuberculosis, malaria, lymphoma including Hodgkin's disease, and rheumatic fever. The *rose spot* is the most valuable single sign, and when coupled with the presence of fever, splenomegaly, and leukopenia usually clinches the diagnosis. Differentiation of typhoid fever from those diseases which it resembles depends upon laboratory confirmation by (1) culture of the blood, feces, and urine and (2) the demonstration of a positive Widal test. Repeated negative cultures of the blood and feces and negative agglutination tests should suggest other illnesses. Rarely are the bacteriologic and serologic tests repeatedly negative.

Management. The mortality and prolonged morbidity of typhoid fever has been reduced effectively by the combined application of antibiotics and supportive measures. In spite of specific therapeutic advances, such complications as intestinal hemorrhage, perforation, and relapse occur in a small percentage of patients. The point is unsettled whether treatment with chloramphenicol, initiated very early in the illness (during the first week), leads to a higher incidence of relapse. Regardless of this consideration, it is advisable to begin specific therapy as early as possible to prevent the development of more serious complications.

Specific Treatment. Chloramphenicol is highly effective and administration should be continued for 2 weeks. After an initial oral dose of 50 mg per kg body weight, the subsequent daily requirement is calculated on the same basis, divided in equal doses, and given at 8-hr intervals. After an apparent clinical response, with defervescence, the daily dose may be reduced to 2.0 Gm. In some patients, the sodium succinate ester of chloramphenicol may be given intravenously or intramuscularly, based on a daily dose of 25 mg per kg. Daily intravenous doses exceeding 3.0 Gm are not advised, and the oral route is preferred.

Shown in Fig. 123-1 is the pattern of response in a patient given chloramphenicol on the ninth day of illness. The patient was subjectively improved, with lessened headache and toxemia within 48 hr after beginning therapy, and the temperature reached normal in less than 4 days. This is the usual pattern. At this stage the patient is more vigorous, the appetite has returned, and abdominal

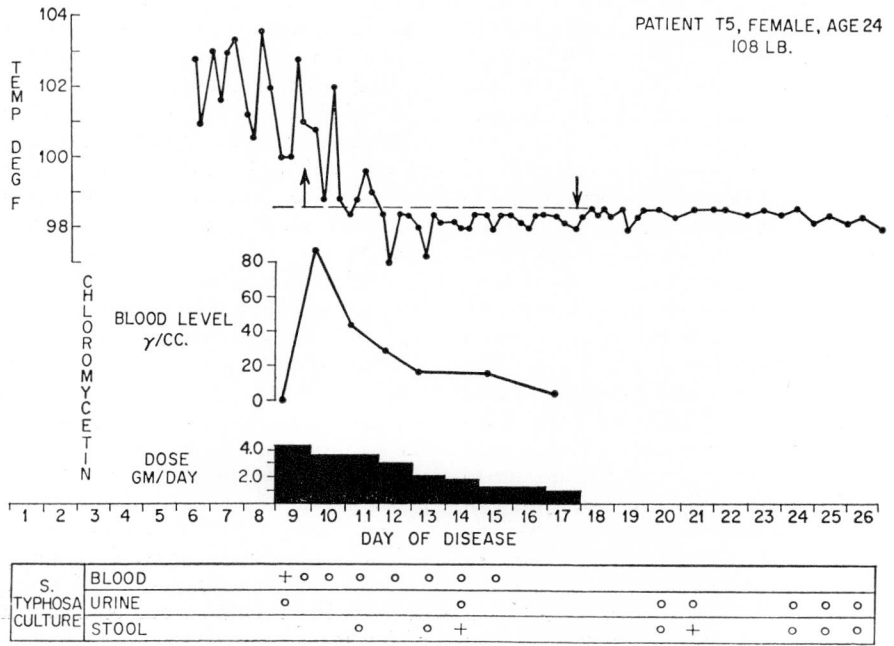

FIG. 123-1. Typical febrile response following chloramphenicol therapy in typhoid fever. (*Ann. Internal Med.,* 29:133, 1948.)

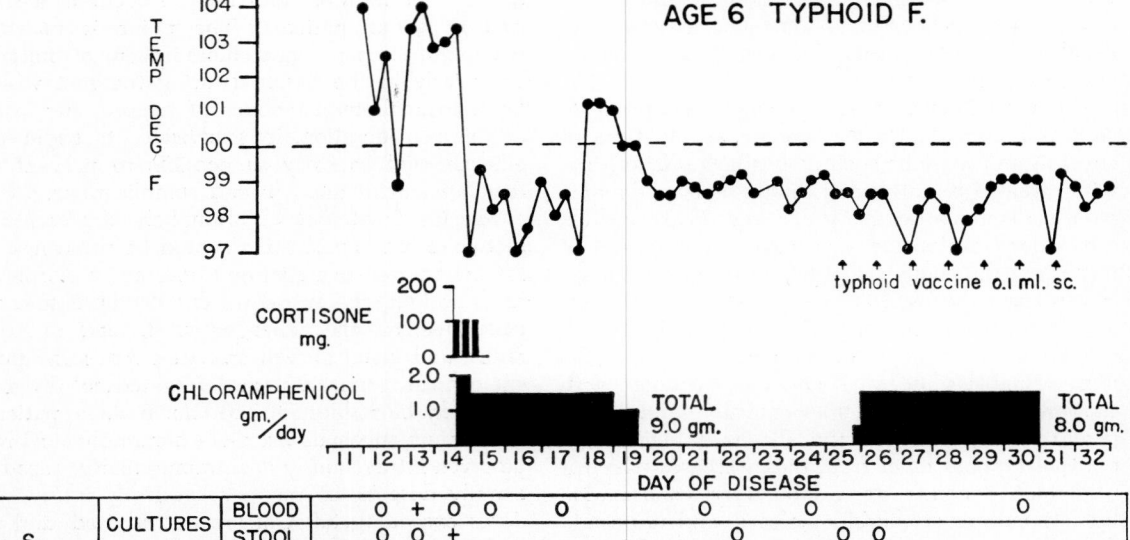

FIG. 123-2. Dramatic demonstration of the effect of steroids in producing lysis of fever in typhoid. Note the "rebound," a common finding following steroid therapy. (*Med. Clinics N. Am., March*, 1954, *vol. 38, no. 2.*)

pain has abated. Bacteremia is no longer demonstrable several hours after beginning treatment, although stool cultures may be intermittently positive throughout the course.

Failure of typhoid patients to respond to chloramphenicol treatment is unusual. Under these circumstances penicillin in doses not less than 12 million units daily has been reported to be effective in small numbers of patients. The effect of the tetracyclines is unpredictable.

Antitoxemic Effects of Steroids. In severely ill patients, there is a period of 3 to 4 days after institution of chloramphenicol therapy before toxemia and pyrexia disappear. This interval can be shortened appreciably if chloramphenicol is supplemented with steroids. Note in Fig. 123-2 the dramatic febrile response of a six-year-old patient who received combined treatment beginning on the fourteenth day of disease. The temperature reached normal levels within 12 hr, and the headache and toxic signs abated simultaneously.

Cortisone, 200 to 300 mg, or prednisone, 40 to 60 mg, is given daily. Three days of treatment with steroids is sufficient. European investigators have reported a "typhoid-shock" syndrome following chloramphenicol treatment presumably as a result of excessive endotoxin release. Under these conditions steroid treatment would exert a protective effect. Steroids should be reserved for those clinical situations associated with severe typhoidal toxemia.

Supportive Therapy. General supportive care is vital to supplement antibiotic therapy. Bed rest extending into early convalescence is essential. Ambulation should be gradual to avoid undue fatigue or exertion. Laxatives and promiscuous use of enemas are ill advised because of the danger of perforation or hemorrhage. Analgesics aid in ameliorating headache, although *salicylates should be avoided* because of the propensity of typhoid patients to show exaggerated reactions to the antipyretic action of these drugs. Tepid sponge baths are effective in lowering body temperature and should be employed when excesses of 104°F appear.

Good nursing care is essential and includes special attention to oral hygiene and adequate bathing. The observations of pulse rate, onset of severe abdominal pain, the presence of tarry or bloody stools, or the occurrence of vomiting are of utmost importance in the early recognition of complications.

A bland or liquid diet consisting of 3000 Cal is prescribed until the appetite improves. Attention to fluid and electrolyte balance is essential. The judicious transfusion of whole blood given slowly, and in small amounts, may be lifesaving in severely ill, anemic patients encountered late in the course of illness.

Intestinal Hemorrhage. An awareness of this complication and its early detection are essential for proper management. The prevention of shock or its early treatment by blood transfusions is of prime importance. The extent and duration of bleeding should be assessed by frequent determinations of the hematocrit and tests for the presence of occult blood. Adequate reserves of blood should be readily available. Strict bed rest should be enforced and oral alimentation restricted. Under these conditions the antibiotics may be given parenterally.

Intestinal Perforation. A severely damaged intestine requires time for healing. Hence, the threat of intestinal perforation exists for several days after specific therapy is instituted. The debilitated toxic condition of the patient, the weakened circulation, the friability of the intestinal lesion, the stress of anesthesia and operative procedure make the typhoid patient a poor surgical risk. It is justified to place greater emphasis upon medical management, i.e., combat shock by routine measures, institute means effectively to decompress the bowel, and continue antibiotic treatment adding penicillin and streptomycin. Should it become obvious to

the physician and surgeon in attendance that the process is failing to localize as evidenced by the findings on examination, persistence of shock, continued leukocytosis, and other signs, it may be surmised that the ulcer is not healing and that surgical intervention is indicated.

Relapses. The greatest incidence of relapse occurs about 2 weeks after the cessation of chloramphenicol therapy. Patients should be followed for 3 weeks after becoming afebrile. Figure 123-3 illustrates the course of illness in a patient with relapse which was moderately severe and self-limiting. Chloramphenicol would have provoked rapid defervescence and clearing of bacteremia. Specific treatment should be instituted and continued for a week when symptoms and fever persist beyond 24 hr. There are no reliable data which indicate that the administration of chloramphenicol utilizing intermittent regimens, with antibiotic rest periods, prevents relapses.

Control and Immunization. All typhoid patients should be reported to appropriate health authorities in order that the source of illness and infection

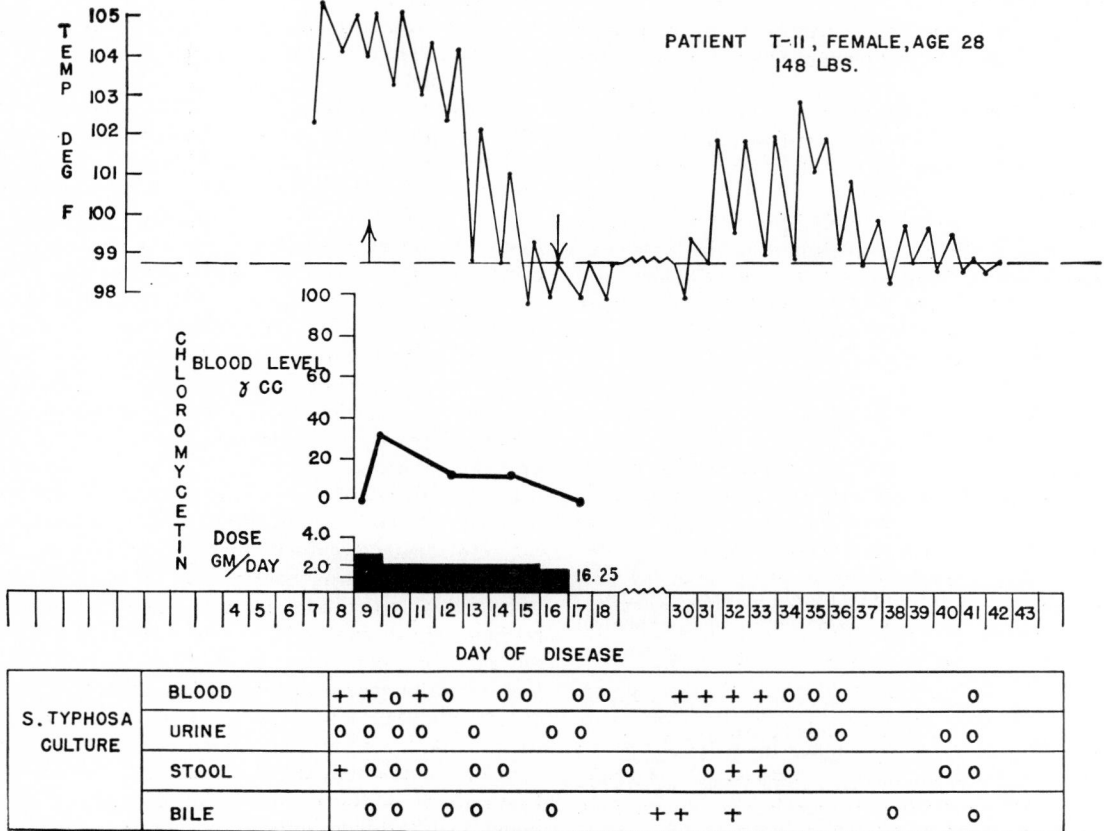

FIG. 123-3. Relapse of typhoid fever occurring 2 weeks after chloramphenicol therapy. Note that the relapse was less severe than the initial illness and responded without specific therapy. In 1948, when the patient was treated, the supply of chloramphenicol was exhausted at the time of relapse.

among contacts may be investigated. Patients should be hospitalized until at least three consecutive stool cultures are negative for S. typhosa. Hospital attendants should protect their clothes with clean gowns. Stools should be discarded in flush toilets; otherwise disinfection should be accomplished with phenol or formalin. Urinals, bedpans, linens, and eating utensils should be sterilized by boiling in water or by autoclaving.

Typhoid vaccine is effective, but it is not an absolute prophylactic agent. The standard phenolized vaccine is the most effective biologic for reducing the morbidity of typhoid. Persons at risk because of travel or occupation should receive TAB vaccine (typhoid, paratyphoid A and B). Weekly doses of 0.5, 1.0, and 1.0 ml given subcutaneously are recommended. A booster injection of 0.5 ml subcutaneously or 0.1 ml intradermally each year is indicated under conditions of high risk. Attention to proper hygienic measures is the best effective preventive measure.

All carriers should be followed periodically and their occupations carefully regulated.

Prognosis. The mortality rate in typhoid fever in the United States prior to the introduction of antibiotic therapy was about 12 per cent. Most deaths occurred from intestinal perforation, hemorrhage, or both. Toxemia, with resultant inanition, was responsible for some fatalities. Despite the efficacy of chloramphenicol in therapy, a certain number of deaths from typhoid fever still occur. This may be expected to be reduced to a minimum if early diagnosis is made and adequate prompt specific and supportive treatment is instituted before extensive lesions develop. The highest incidence of death is in the aged, in young infants, and in those patients previously malnourished and anemic.

REFERENCES

Edsall, G., S. Gaines, M. Landy, W. D. Tigertt, H. Sprinz, R. J. Trapani, A. D. Mandel, and A. S. Benenson: Studies on Infection and Immunity in Experimental Typhoid Fever: I. Typhoid Fever in Chimpanzees Orally Infected with Salmonella typhosa, J. Exptl. Med., 112:143, 1960.

Friedman, A.: An Evaluation of Chloramphenicol Therapy in Typhoid Fever in Children, Pediatrics, 14:28, 1954.

Goodpasture, E. W.: Concerning the Pathogenesis of Typhoid Fever, Am. J. Pathol., 13:175, 1937.

Greisman, S. E., T. E. Woodward, R. B. Hornick, and M. J. Snyder: Studies on Pathogenesis of Typhoid Fever: Endotoxin and Vascular Reactivity, Bull. N.Y. Acad. Med., 37:493, 1961.

McCrae, T.: The Symptoms of Typhoid Fever, chap. 4 in "Modern Medicine," vol. 2, Infectious Diseases, p. 104, W. Osler, and T. McCrae (Eds.), Philadelphia, Lea Brothers and Company, 1907.

Stuart, B. M., and R. L. Pullen: Typhoid: Clinical Analysis of 360 Cases, Arch. Internal Med., 78: 629, 1946.

Woodward, T. E., J. E. Smadel, R. T. Parker, and C. L. Wisseman, Jr.: Treatment of Typhoid Fever with Antibiotics, Ann. N.Y. Acad. Sci., 55:1043, 1952.

124 OTHER SALMONELLA INFECTIONS

*Edward W. Hook and
Ivan L. Bennett, Jr.*

Since the first description of *Salmonella* was published in 1886 by Salmon and Smith, over 400 members of the genus have been identified. Although there is striking variation in the pathogenicity of the various serotypes, almost all are capable of producing human disease. The infections in man are *acute gastroenteritis* or *food poisoning*, *enteric* or *paratyphoid fever*, *bacteremia*, and a multitude of *localized infections* ranging from osteomyelitis to endocarditis.

Etiology and Epidemiology. The salmonellas are motile gram-negative bacilli that ferment dextrose, maltose, and mannite with production of gas and do not utilize lactose or sucrose. These organisms are classified by serologic methods on the basis of their somatic (O) and flagellar (H) antigens. Accurate identification is technically complex and can be carried out only in a few typing centers but is very important for epidemiologic studies.

Salmonellas inhabit the intestinal tracts of man and many lower animals. The incidence of asymptomatic human carriers in the general population is about 0.2 per cent, and a much larger reservoir of infection is present in lower animals. An incomplete list of the lower species from which these organisms have been isolated includes the mouse, rat, cat, dog, pig, cow, chicken, duck, turkey, parakeet, snake, tick, flea, and cockroach.

Infection is acquired by the oral route, usually by ingestion of contaminated food or drink. Almost any food product, especially those of animal origin, is a potential source of human infection. The meat of infected animals, eggs or egg products, and food, milk, or water contaminated by excreta of man or animals may serve as vehicles of infection. By-products of the meat-packing industry such as bone meal, fertilizer, and domestic animal feed also constitute an important medium for spread of salmonellas.

The incidence of salmonella infections has increased strikingly in the last 10 years. Although the observed increase may represent only better detection and more efficient recording, it emphasizes the fact that salmonellosis is a health problem of considerable magnitude. Large epidemics of gastroenteritis are common but are greatly outnumbered by sporadic cases and family outbreaks, many of which have been unrecognized.

There is a close correlation between the species of *Salmonella* predominating in animals and those isolated from man in a specific geographic area. In the United States the most frequent causes of human infections are *S. typhimurium, S. newport, S. montevideo, S. oranienburg, S. choleraesuis, S. schottmuelleri,* and *S. anatum.*

The incidence of infection due to *Salmonella* is greatest during the summer months. *Salmonella choleraesuis* infections do not follow this seasonal distribution and occur at a fairly constant rate throughout the year.

Pathogenesis. The course of events after salmonella organisms have gained access to the gastrointestinal tract is determined by the dose, species, and invasive potential of the organism and the resistance of the host. Multiplication of ingested organisms in the intestinal tract may be followed by symptoms of food poisoning which, in the majority of instances, subside after a few days. The intestinal irritation and inflammation are probably produced by true infection of the mucosa, and penetration of the intestinal wall with resulting transient bacteremia or more serious systemic illness occurs in a few patients. With the development of systemic infection, there may be histologic changes similar to those of typhoid fever or multiple foci of suppuration in bone, joints, endocardium, pleura, meninges, etc.

Studies in healthy human volunteers suggest that large numbers of organisms must be ingested to produce disease, although the minimum infectious dose varies strikingly among different serotypes. The coliform bacteria of the intestinal microflora apparently exert a protective action by suppressing the multiplication of salmonellas if the number ingested is small. This suggestion is based upon the demonstration that elimination of intestinal saprophytes by giving antibiotics increases the susceptibility of mice to infection with *S. typhimurium* 100,000-fold. Salmonella enteritis has been reported as a rare complication of the administration of broad-spectrum antibiotics to man. Alteration in intestinal microflora has also been suggested as a mechanism of the increased susceptibility of patients convalescent from gastrointestinal surgery, especially gastrectomy and gastroenterostomy, to intestinal infection with salmonellas.

In previously healthy individuals, blood stream invasion is unusual in infections produced by most species of *Salmonella.* However, the marked invasiveness of *S. choleraesuis* sets it apart from other species. About 50 per cent of *S. choleraesuis* infections are accompanied by bacteremia, and the mortality rate is about 20 per cent. The infrequent occurrence of gastroenteritis and a carrier state due to *S. choleraesuis* also reflects the invasiveness of this organism.

Severe salmonella infection has been described as a complication of many acute and chronic diseases, such as streptococcal pharyngitis, meningococcal meningitis, beriberi, hepatic cirrhosis, various lymphomas, and lupus erythematosus. Such occurrences are sometimes coincidence but more often reflect a generally decreased resistance to bacterial infection. In a few diseases there is strong evidence to indicate a specific predisposition to infection by salmonellas that far exceeds any general susceptibility to other bacterial species. Patients with sickle-cell anemia, and other hemoglobinopathies, are unusually susceptible to salmonella infection, and there is a strong tendency for localization in bone, with the production of osteomyelitis. The high mortality in acute bartonellosis is almost entirely accounted for by secondary salmonellosis (see p. 976), and the effectiveness of chloramphenicol in bartonellosis is attributable to its action against the secondary infection rather than the bartonella organisms. Salmonellosis is also an unusually frequent complication of malaria and relapsing fever.

Clinical Manifestations. *Salmonella Food Poisoning.* Gastroenteritis often occurs in epidemics among individuals who have partaken of the same contaminated food, although sporadic cases are not infrequent. After an incubation period of 8 to 48 hr, there is sudden onset of colicky abdominal pain and loose, watery diarrhea, occasionally with mucus or blood. Nausea and vomiting are frequent but are rarely severe or protracted. Temperature of 101 to 102°F is common, and there may be an initial chill. Symptoms usually subside promptly within 2 to 5 days, and recovery is uneventful. Fatalities rarely exceed 1 or 2 per cent of the affected population and are limited almost entirely to infants, the aged, and the debilitated.

The causative organism can often be isolated from the suspected food and from feces during the acute illness. Stool cultures usually become negative for salmonellas within a few days, but it is not unusual for patients to continue to excrete organisms for weeks or months. The leukocyte count is usually normal.

Enteric or Paratyphoid Fever. Certain species of *Salmonella* can produce an illness which is clinically indistinguishable from typhoid fever, i.e., a prolonged febrile illness with rose spots, spleno-megaly, leukopenia, gastrointestinal symptoms, and positive blood and stool cultures (see p. 939). The organisms most likely to produce this picture are *S. paratyphi* (*S. paratyphi A*), *S. paratyphi B* (*S. schottmuelleri*), and *S. choleraesuis* (*S. suipestifer*). Occasionally a typical attack of food poisoning is followed in a few days by paratyphoid fever. Generally, paratyphoid fevers tend to be milder than *S. typhosa* infections, but differentiation on clinical grounds alone is not possible in the individual case. Recovery may be followed by continued excretion of the causative organism in the stools for several months, although the carrier state is less frequent and less prolonged than in typhoid.

Bacteremia. *Salmonella choleraesuis* is the species most likely to produce bacteremia, but prolonged illness with positive blood cultures has also resulted from infection with many other types, particularly in patients with another debilitating illness. Although symptoms of gastroenteritis can precede bacteremia, they are usually lacking, and most cases arise sporadically. In many instances, the only manifestations are prolonged fever, sometimes low-grade, but often spiking and accompanied by repeated rigors, sweats, aching, anorexia, and weight loss. The characteristic features of typhoid and paratyphoid fever, such as rose spots, persistent leukopenia, and sustained fever, are absent. Stool cultures are usually negative. Discharge of organisms into the blood stream is intermittent (in contrast to the constant bacteremia of typhoid-paratyphoid), and repeated blood cultures are often required to demonstrate the causative organism. At some time in the course of the illness, localizing signs of infection appear in one-fourth of the cases. Pulmonary infection in the form of bronchopneumonia or abscess, pleurisy, empyema, pericarditis, endocarditis, pyelonephritis, meningitis, osteomyelitis, and arthritis are relatively common. The blood leukocyte count is usually normal, but with the development of focal lesions, polymorphonuclear leukocytosis as high as 20,000 to 25,000 cells per cu mm occurs. Salmonella bacteremia can be a very puzzling disorder, especially before localization takes place, and should be considered in cases of fever of unknown origin.

Local Pyogenic Infections. In addition to the suppurative lesions already mentioned, salmonella organisms can produce abscesses in almost any anatomic site. These can occur independently of previous symptoms of gastroenteritis or other illness or as complications of bacteremias. There is nothing characteristic about the suppurative lesions, and the correct etiologic diagnosis is rarely made on the basis of clinical findings alone. There is a strong tendency for salmonellas to localize in tissues that are the site of preexisting disease. For example, in patients with systemic salmonellosis, localization has been described in aneurysms, bone adjacent to aortic aneurysms, hematomas, and many different tumors including hypernephroma, ovarian cyst, and pheochromocytoma. Meningeal localization of salmonella infection is common in newborns and infants, and occasional small outbreaks of salmonella infection in nurseries have consisted almost entirely of cases of meningitis.

Diagnosis. Febrile gastroenteritis produced by presumed viral agents (see p. 1134), and shigellosis can be distinguished from salmonella food poisoning only by appropriate stool cultures in most instances, especially in sporadic cases. The bacteriologic methods are described on p. 950. Staphylococcal food poisoning is usually an afebrile disease, and vomiting is a more prominent feature than in most salmonella infections. Systemic manifestations are usually absent in patients with gastroenteritis caused by *Clostridium welchii* (*C. perfringens*). Many toxic agents and drugs can produce diarrhea, nausea, and abdominal pain, but fever is rarely a feature of these disorders, and the diagnosis depends upon a history of exposure or ingestion.

The diagnosis of paratyphoid fever or salmonella bacteremia depends upon isolation of the causative organism. Agglutination tests with acute and convalescent serums as performed in the usual clinical laboratory are usually not very helpful.

Treatment. The treatment of salmonella food poisoning is supportive. Dehydration should be corrected by parenteral administration of fluids and electrolytes. The abdominal cramps and diarrhea can be alleviated by small doses of morphine or paregoric and are frequently much improved if the patient takes nothing by mouth for 8 to 12 hr. There is no evidence that antimicrobial drugs modify the course of the disease.

Chloramphenicol is the antibiotic of choice in systemic infections, the dosage being 3 to 4 Gm daily. Its effectiveness is variable and unpredictable. The tetracycline derivatives have sometimes appeared to exert a beneficial effect, but streptomycin, polymyxin, neomycin, and the sulfonamides are generally ineffective. Occasional dramatic results have been obtained with massive doses of penicillin (40 to 100 million units daily), and this should be tried in any patient who is seriously ill with a refractory infection such as endocarditis or meningitis.

Antibiotic therapy is usually ineffective in terminating the carrier state in persons continuing to excrete salmonellas after an acute illness. Cholecystectomy is often effective in eradicating the chronic carrier state in patients with gallbladder disease.

Surgically accessible suppurative lesions should be drained.

REFERENCES

Bengston, E., et al.: Epidemic Due to *Salmonella typhimurium* (Breslau) Occurring in Sweden in 1953: With Special Reference to Clinical Complications, Bacteriology, Serology, Antibiotic Treatment and Morbid Anatomy, Acta. Med. Scand., 153:1, 1955.

Bennett, I. L., Jr., and E. W. Hook: Some Aspects of Salmonellosis, Ann. Rev. Med., 10:1, 1959.

Black, P. H., L. J. Kunz, and M. N. Swartz: Salmonellosis—A Review of Some Unusual Aspects, New Engl. J. Med., 262:811, 864; 921, 1960.

Harvey, A. M.: *Salmonella suipestifer* Infection in Human Beings, Arch. Internal Med., 59:118, 1937.

Gezon, H. M.: "Salmonellosis," Disease-a-Month Series, Chicago, Year Book Publishers, July, 1959.

Saphra, I., and M. Wasserman: *Salmonella choleraesuis:* A Clinical and Epidemiological Evaluation of 329 Infections Identified between 1940 and 1954 in the New York Salmonella Center, Am. J. Med. Sci., 228:525, 1954.

Seligman, E., I. Saphra, and M. Wasserman: Salmonella Infections in the U.S.A., J. Immunol., 54:69, 1946.

125   BACILLARY DYSENTERY (Shigella Infections)

Ivan L. Bennett, Jr.

Definition. With rare exceptions, human infection by bacteria of the genus *Shigella* (often called the "dysentery bacilli") is limited to the intestinal tract and is characterized by fever, abdominal pain, and diarrhea. In clinical practice this disease is usually called "bacillary dysentery"; a preferable term is "shigellosis," but this has not achieved wide usage.

Etiology. The shigellas are short, nonmotile, gram-negative bacilli which either fail to ferment lactose or do so only slowly. Their biochemical characteristics are sufficiently constant to serve as a reliable guide in identification, although definitive typing into species is dependent upon complex antigenic analysis. There is considerable confusion about the nomenclature of this genus. The official classification (Kauffmann) consists of group A, the shigella unable to ferment mannite, and groups B, C, and D, the mannite fermenters. There are several numerically designated types in each group. The organisms are still widely referred to by earlier terminology. The most important species from a clinical viewpoint are *Shigella shigae* (*S. dysenteriae;* the Shiga-Kruse bacillus), *S. flexneri* (*S. paradysenteriae*), *S. boydii*, and *S. sonnei*. Two

species, *S. alkalescens* and *S. dispar,* are almost never associated with outbreaks of diarrheal disease and are thought by many to be better classified as saprophytic coliforms than as enteric pathogens. Isolation of either from the stool of a patient with diarrhea does not establish a diagnosis of bacillary dysentery.

Shigella shigae contains a substance that is neurotoxic for animals and resembles a true exotoxin. Evidence for a significant role of this toxin in human disease is lacking. All shigellas possess endotoxins, similar to those of other gram-negative bacilli, but the manifestations of bacillary dysentery cannot be attributed to these substances, either.

Epidemiology. In contrast to the salmonella group, which is widespread throughout the animal kingdom, shigellas live primarily in the gut of man, although monkeys and, rarely, dogs may excrete the organisms. The convalescent or asymptomatic carrier is the principal reservoir of the disease. The only important route of spread is fecal-oral; transmission is indirect by means of food, utensils, towels, etc. Watt and Hardy have conducted cultural surveys in this country and have found carrier rates ranging from 10 per cent of the population in certain parts of New Mexico to 0.1 per cent in New York City. Studies such as that of Philbrook have shown that excretion of shigellas by carriers is so intermittent that, practically speaking, their detection and treatment on any large scale is impossible.

In regions of the world where sanitation is poor and under conditions such as mobilization of troops in the field, epidemics of dysentery are common. Outbreaks are rarely explosive but develop over a period of several weeks. The ability of some shigella strains to survive in sea water for 3 days was shown by Cheever to be responsible for ship-to-ship spread of dysentery among naval personnel. Flies can transmit the infection by mechanical contamination, and in warm climates where sewerage is primitive, the number of cases of dysentery parallels the fly count, and fly control is important in prevention.

In the civilized countries of the world, large outbreaks of shigella dysentery are now rare, with the exception of so-called "asylum" dysentery, occurring in mental institutions and orphanages where there are close contact and unusual opportunity for fecal soiling among the feebleminded or youthful inmates.

Pathogenesis. The monkey is the only laboratory animal in which shigella dysentery can be produced with regularity. In volunteer studies, it has required the ingestion of surprisingly large numbers of bacilli to establish infection in man.

Multiplication of ingested bacilli in the intestinal tract is followed by a diffuse enteritis. The rectum and sigmoid are almost always involved, and in severe cases, the entire colon and terminal ileum may be diseased. The infection remains localized in the intestinal wall, there being no tendency to invasion of the blood stream or biliary tract as in typhoid fever or other salmonella infections. The lumen of the affected segments is covered by a fibrinous exudate containing large numbers of neutrophils, and as necrosis of mucosal cells develops, superficial ulcerations that bleed easily appear. In severe cases, the ulcers enlarge and coalesce until only a few scattered patches of intact mucosa remain on the raw and inflamed surface. While the inflammatory process sometimes involves the submucosa and muscularis, with resulting edema and thickening of the intestinal wall, perforation is very rare. The systemic effects of the disease result almost entirely from losses of fluid and electrolytes with the diarrhea.

Even in untreated cases, spontaneous recovery usually occurs within a few days, with rapid restoration of the intestinal mucosa to normal. The mechanism of this is not known. It is clearly unrelated to serum antibody formation, and the suggestion that bacteriophage may be involved is unsupported.

Relapses are sometimes seen, and second attacks are not infrequent. These are, again, unrelated to serum antibody levels. Residency in endemic areas in the tropics is well known to lead to resistance to clinically apparent attacks of bacillary dysentery. The basis for this "seasoning" is also unknown.

Manifestations. The incubation period is usually 24 to 48 hr. Colicky abdominal pain is followed within an hour by profuse diarrhea. Fever up to 104°F, occasionally with chills, occurs, and nausea, vomiting, headache, and malaise develop rapidly. Stools are watery, greenish, and irritating and contain shreds of mucus and, often, flecks of blood. In a few patients, there may be profuse bleeding. Tenesmus and straining are prominent accompaniments of the diarrhea. Depending upon fluid losses, the patient may become profoundly dehydrated, and circulatory collapse can occur, especially in elderly or debilitated patients. There is generalized abdominal tenderness without rigidity or localizing signs. Rarely, the spleen is palpable. Sigmoidoscopic examination reveals diffuse mucosal inflammation, often with multiple ulcerations. The ulcers are not so large and sharply demarcated as those of amebic colitis, and in amebiasis the intervening mucosa is usually uninflamed.

Spontaneous recovery within 2 to 7 days is usual, with relapses in about 10 per cent of the cases unless chemotherapy is given. Children under two years of age and elderly individuals are usually more severely ill, and the mortality rate is highest in these groups.

Shigella shigae produces the severest infections; mortality rates of 25 to 50 per cent have been recorded in epidemics produced by this species, which is, fortunately, very uncommon in the United States.

Chronic bacillary dysentery is virtually unheard of in this country, but it is said to occur in the tropics, especially after Shiga infections. The role of reinfection in such cases has not been evaluated, and many of these cases probably represent amebic infections. Patients may continue to shed shigellas after convalescence; the true incidence of the carrier state is probably higher than has been realized, in view of the intermittency with which positive cultures have been obtained in carefully controlled follow-up studies.

Complications include acute *arthritis*, usually involving a single, large, weight-bearing joint during convalescence. Joint fluid is sterile. This complication is unusual in patients given chemotherapy and is most likely to follow infections with S. *shigae* which have a protracted course. *Reiter's syndrome*, the triad of arthritis, conjunctivitis, and urethritis, is thought by some to be a sequel of shigella infections. This is discussed on p. 1907.

There is no convincing evidence to support the assertion that bacillary dysentery and chronic ulcerative colitis are etiologically related.

A few instances of perforation of the colon have been reported. Shigella organisms have been isolated from abscesses, but this is very uncommon. *Shigella alkalescens* has been reported as the causative agent in acute pyelonephritis and has been isolated from the blood in rare instances; many of these infections have been in children.

Laboratory Findings. The blood leukocyte count in bacillary dysentery is normal. Changes in erythrocytes and urine are secondary to dehydration. Microscopic examination of the stool reveals shreds of mucus, erythrocytes, and polymorphonuclear leukocytes. Pus cells are not characteristic of the stools in amebiasis, although they occur in salmonella enteritis.

The causative organism can be isolated in most cases from stool cultures, using feces emulsified in saline solution. A better technique for obtaining cultures is to swab the rectal mucosa. Preliminary incubation in a medium such as selenite F is helpful, but cultures can be streaked directly onto SS or desoxycholate citrate agar plates. A positive diagnosis should be obtained in at least 80 per cent of cases of bacillary dysentery.

Serologic changes are not diagnostic because of the many cross reactions within the shigella group and with other enteric bacilli.

Diagnosis. Shigella infection should be suspected in every febrile diarrheal illness, especially if it occurs in epidemic form. Outbreaks of staphylococcal food poisoning or salmonella gastroenteritis are usually more explosive than those of bacillary dysentery. Staphylococcal food poisoning is ordinarily an afebrile disease in which nausea and vomiting are very severe; salmonella infection can be differentiated with certainty only by bacteriologic studies. Amebic colitis is rarely epidemic; its onset is not usually abrupt and prostrating, and motile amebas are found in the stools. Diarrheas of viral origin are usually unaccompanied by mucus and blood in the stools, but this is not invariable (see p. 1134).

In children, the onset of otitis, tonsillitis, pneumonia, poliomyelitis, or osteomyelitis is often accompanied by diarrhea, but careful clinical examination usually clarifies the situation.

Treatment. The sulfonamides are highly effective in shigella infections. Sulfadiazine, 4 Gm initially, followed by 1 Gm every 4 to 6 hr, is adequate. Fluid intake is very important in patients with diarrhea given sulfonamides. Poorly absorbed drugs such as Sulfasuxidine (3 to 4 Gm every 6 hr) are effective but offer no advantage. Treatment should be continued for 7 to 10 days. Many strains of *Shigella* are resistant to sulfonamides. Oral chloramphenicol and tetracyclines are effective in a dosage of 1 to 2 Gm daily. Streptomycin and polymyxin B have been used in a dosage of 0.5 to 1.0 Gm daily by the oral route with good success.

Fluid replacement sufficient to maintain urine output of 1,000 ml per day is important; intravenous infusion is sometimes needed, and rarely, blood transfusion is required because of excessive blood loss.

The diet is unimportant. In many patients, symptoms are aggravated by ingestion of food or fluid, and it is advisable to rely on the parenteral route during the acute phase of the disease. Paregoric, codeine, or morphine often alleviates abdominal cramping, diarrhea, and tenesmus.

Chloromycetin is more effective in eliminating shigellas from the stools of chronic carriers than are the sulfonamides.

Prevention. The most important prophylactic measures are the maintenance of proper sanitation and adequate sewage disposal. The detection and elimination of carriers is difficult and rarely practicable. Various vaccines, oral and parenteral, have been used, but extensive experience offers no indication that parenteral vaccine exerts a significant protective effect. The wide range of potentially pathogenic species, necessitating a polyvalent vaccine, is another discouraging aspect of this approach to prophylaxis.

REFERENCES

Cheever, F. S.: Bacillary Dysentery and the Shigella, in "Bacterial and Mycotic Infections of Man," 3d ed., R. J. Dubos (Ed.), Philadelphia, J. B. Lippincott Company, 1958.

Garfinkel, B. T., et al.: Antibiotics in Acute Bacillary Dysentery: Observations in 1,408 Cases with Positive Cultures, J.A.M.A., 51:1157, 1943.

Hardy, A. V., T. DeCapito, and S. P. Halbert: Studies of the Acute Diarrheal Diseases XIX: Immunization in Shigellosis, Pub. Health Repts. (U.S.), 63: 685, 1948.

Lieberman, D., and E. Jawetz: Treatment of Chronic *Shigella* Infections in Children with Oral Polymyxins, Pediatrics, 8:249, 1951.

Philbrook, F. R., et al.: Prolonged Laboratory Observations on Clinical Cases and Carriers of *Shigella flexneri III* Following an Epidemic, U.S. Naval Med. Bull., 48:405, 1948.

Shaugnessy, H. J., et al.: Experimental Human Bacillary Dysentery, J.A.M.A., 132:362, 1946.

126 CHOLERA
Ivan L. Bennett, Jr.

Definition. Cholera is an acute infection of the gastrointestinal tract caused by *Vibrio comma*. The disease is characterized by its epidemic occurrence and the production of vomiting, massive diarrhea, and rapid, severe dehydration.

Etiology and Epidemiology. *Vibrio comma* is a curved, aerobic gram-negative bacillus with a polar flagellum. It is motile and possesses both O and H antigens. Serologic identification of several strains of cholera vibrios is based upon secondary antigenic differences.

Cholera is endemic and often epidemic in South and Southeast Asia, particularly in India and Pakistan. The disease has not been epidemic in the United States since 1873, but its potential distribution is world-wide. The last significant European outbreaks occurred during the First World War.

The organisms are transmitted in food or beverage contaminated by infected feces. Flies are important in spreading the disease, and many epidemics have been waterborne. Spread of the disease is highly unlikely where adequate sanitation exists, and although poor diet and prior enteric disease probably predispose to cholera, crowding and poor sanitation are primarily responsible for its continuing presence in Asia.

The reservoir of infection between epidemics is a mystery. It has been postulated that the organism survives in nature in a lower animal host or in a "masked form," but this has not been established. Chronic carriers of the organism have not been found and, presently, the spread of the disease from person to person by patients in the incubation or convalescent stages of illness or by patients with "subclinical" infection is the most acceptable explanation of the persistence of infection. The frequency of subclinical infection is not actually known, but there is enough variation in the severity of the disease in its recognizable form to suggest strongly that asymptomatic infections occur.

Pathogenesis. The mechanism of the injurious action of the cholera vibrio upon the intestine is unknown. Fractionation of the bacillus has yielded preparations that are toxic or lethal when injected into animals, but none of these elicits any effect that seems related to the disease in man. The vibrio possesses a highly active mucolytic enzyme, and it has been postulated that this substance produces extensive desquamation of intestinal epithelium with resultant massive exudation of fluid into the lumen through the denuded surface. Autopsy descriptions of extensive mucosal loss in cholera have been frequent. However, study of serial intestinal biopsies obtained during the course of cholera has made it clear that there is no mucosal defect (autopsy findings presumably having been postmortem autolytic phenomena), although goblet cell activity is increased and the submucosa is nonspecifically inflamed. The stools of patients with cholera are profuse, nonbloody, and watery, containing numerous flecks of mucus (*not* mucosal cells) which impart a characteristic "rice water" appearance. The stool is a transudate, containing very little protein; the concentrations of sodium and chloride are less than those of plasma whereas both bicarbonate and potassium are lost in concentrations well above those of plasma, indicative of the fact that something more than simple filtration of plasma is involved. Although understanding of the defect in intestinal function is incomplete, these findings have important bearing upon therapy of the disease.

Manifestations. After an incubation period of 1 to 3 days, during which time there may be some malaise or mild diarrhea, there is the explosive onset of massive diarrhea and vomiting. Tenesmus and nausea are usually absent. Several liters of fluid may be lost within hours, and because patients can retain nothing ingested, dehydration is rapid and muscle cramps are frequent and severe. Urine output ceases, patients become lethargic and weak with cold skin, tachycardia, and hypotension. Cholera is not a febrile disease, and patients are usually oriented and responsive.

In any epidemic, there are many milder cases in which diarrhea and vomiting are not severe enough to lead to hospitalization; the importance of these in spread of the disease is obvious.

The disease runs its course in 72 to 96 hr, and with adequate fluid replacement patients often return to normal with surprising speed. The important complications are uremia, a result of tubular necrosis, in patients whose dehydration and hypo-tension go too long uncorrected, and secondary infection. Cholera tends to affect populations where health and nutrition are generally poor, and, occasionally, convalescence is marked by the sudden appearance of clinical signs of vitamin deficiency.

Laboratory Diagnosis. In epidemics or in endemic areas, the clinical picture should arouse strong suspicion immediately. Sporadic confusion of cholera, especially a milder attack, with other diarrheal diseases is not infrequent. Stool specimens stained with carbolfuchsin will show a typical swarm of vibrios, the so-called "fish-in-stream" appearance. Culture of stool in alkaline (pH 8.4) peptone water at 37°C results in typical surface growth within 8 hr. Further confirmation requires subculture and agglutination with specific serum.

Therapy. Fluid replacement should be generous and prompt. It was long the custom to give limited amounts of fluid because it was held that the diarrhea would be aggravated by attempts at complete restoration. Generous amounts of physiologic saline should be infused. The addition of glucose or thiamine is permissible but not mandatory. Acidosis is rather frequent after a day or two and is best corrected by sodium bicarbonate or lactate. Occasionally, hypertonic solutions may be needed later in the course to correct a deficit resulting from continued electrolyte loss or overdilution. Some patients may require as much as 25 liters of fluid within 72 hr; in one series, the average amount infused was 16 liters. While the hematocrit has been used as a rough guide in fluid therapy, the fact that so many patients with cholera are already anemic makes it unreliable. By far the best indicator is the blood specific gravity, easily determined by the copper sulfate method. The goal should be to reduce this value to normal (1.056); it is often as high as 1.070 when patients are first seen.

While sulfonamides, tetracyclines, and chloramphenicol are effective in vitro against V. *comma*, they do not shorten the course of cholera in man and do not influence mortality. Stools become negative for cholera vibrios sooner in patients given these drugs, however, an important point in terms of reducing infectiveness. Presently, it can be said that use of these antibacterial drugs is justified, but they are no substitute for and do not modify the need for vigorous replacement of fluids and electrolytes.

Prognosis. Under ideal conditions, prompt therapy will reduce mortality to 5 per cent or less. However, because of the remoteness of areas in which epidemics occur, because emergency facilities almost always involve compromises, and because of difficulties in initiating treatment promptly when large numbers of cases are occurring in poverty-stricken populations, death rates as high as 50 per cent are still to be expected, especially in initial phases of an outbreak.

Prevention. Vaccination is effective in preventing infection. After an initial course of two or three injections, a booster should be given at 6-month intervals as long as an individual resides in an endemic zone. The final control of the disease will come only with proper sanitary facilities and practices.

REFERENCES

Benyajati, C., M. Keoplug, W. R. Beisel, E. J. Gangarosa, H. Sprinz, and Sitprija: Acute Renal Failure in Asiatic Cholera: Clinicopathologic Correlations with Acute Tubular Necrosis and Hypokale-

mic Nephropathy, Ann. Internal Med., 52:960, 1960.

Bloomfield, A. L.: A Bibliography of Internal Medicine: Cholera, A.M.A. Arch. Internal Med., 96:734, 1955.

Fuhrman, G. J., and F. A. Fuhrman: Inhibition of Active Sodium Transport by Cholera Toxin, Nature (London), 188:71, 1960.

Gangarosa, E. F., W. R. Beisel, C. Benyajati, H. Sprinz, and P. Piyaratn: The Nature of the Gastrointestinal Lesion in Asiatic Cholera and Its Relation to Pathogenesis: A Biopsy Study, Am. J. Trop. Med., 9:125, 1960.

Watten, R. H., F. M. Morgan, Yachai-Na-Songkhla, B. Vanikiati, and R. A. Phillips: Water and Electrolyte Studies in Cholera, J. Clin. Invest., 38:1897, 1959.

Section 5: Diseases Produced by Other Gram-negative Bacilli

127 HEMOPHILUS INFECTIONS

Louis Weinstein

The genus *Hemophilus* consists of nonmotile, gram-negative rods or coccobacilli which require specific growth factors (X and V) for multiplication. The organisms of importance in human disease are *H. influenzae*, *H. pertussis*, *H. ducreyi*, the Koch-Weeks bacillus, and *Moraxella lacunata*. Two other species are found in the pharynx of normal individuals and, rarely, may produce pharyngitis (*H. hemolyticus*) or endocarditis (*H. parainfluenzae*). The site invaded most frequently is the respiratory tract, and the organisms responsible for the bulk of infections are *H. influenzae* and *H. pertussis*.

HEMOPHILUS INFLUENZAE INFECTIONS

Hemophilus influenzae produces a wide variety of diseases in many organ systems. The organism was first isolated by Pfeiffer during a pandemic of influenza in 1890, and was thought to be the causative agent of this disease. During the 1918 influenza pandemic, extensive bacteriologic investigations revealed a high incidence of *H. influenzae* in the nasopharynx and lungs of patients in many parts of the world.

Etiology. *Hemophilus influenzae* is a gram-negative, nonsporulating, pleomorphic rod. In exudates, the organisms are usually predominantly coccobacillary and can be mistaken for pneumococci or meningococci. Some strains demonstrate bipolar staining, and bacillary forms that vary from short rods to long filamentous ones occur. The pleomorphism of the organism is its most striking feature.

Hemophilus influenzae grows well on chocolate agar and Levinthal's medium, which has the advantage of being transparent. On Levinthal's agar, typical colonies are iridescent when viewed by obliquely transmitted light when they are about 4 to 6 hr old; this property disappears after 24 hr.

Virulent strains of the influenza bacillus are encapsulated. Although it had been thought that strains without capsules were nonpathogenic, recent observations have implicated such strains in infections of the respiratory tract. On the basis of specific capsular polysaccharides, *H. influenzae* may be classified into six types. Type B produces about 95 per cent of human infections. Three of the types are immunologically related to certain pneumococci. Influenza bacilli lack certain enzyme systems common to most bacterial species, and very little fermentation of carbohydrates takes place. Like pneumococci, this organism is soluble in bile.

Epidemiology. *Hemophilus influenzae* infects only man naturally. It is not ordinarily invasive for any of the smaller animals, although monkeys can be infected experimentally. Although the pathogenicity of the influenza bacillus is closely related to the presence of the capsule, nonencapsulated strains can also produce disease.

The incidence of *H. influenzae* infections is greatest in the winter and early spring. Nose and throat cultures during these seasons reveal encapsulated or nonencapsulated strains in many asymptomatic individuals. Penicillin therapy increases the incidence of positive throat cultures in a population.

Children in the first 2 months of life have a high level of bactericidal antibody for *H. influenzae*, passively transferred from the mother. Between the ages of two months and three years, most children show little serum bactericidal capacity, but with aging, the number of individuals whose blood exerts a lethal action against the organism increases.

The influenza bacillus is transmitted by way of the respiratory tract from carriers or active cases of infection.

Pathology. The characteristic tissue response produced by *H. influenzae* is acute suppurative inflammation. Infections of the larynx, trachea, and bronchial tree are characterized by inflammation and edema of the mucosa and the presence of thick exudate, and invasion of the lungs results in a bronchopneumonia similar to that produced by other bacteria. Swelling of the small radicles of the bronchial tree is common, and particularly in young children, a severe, diffuse bronchiolitis can occur. In influenzal meningitis, the vertex of the brain is covered with thick, greenish-yellow exudate.

Microscopic examination of the lesions produced by *H. influenzae* reveals an exudate consisting primarily of polymorphonuclear leukocytes and large numbers of organisms enmeshed in fibrin.

Clinical Manifestations. Infections due to *H. influenzae* are usually accompanied by a constitutional reaction. In severe disease, there is high fever, usually without rigors, and generalized malaise. In milder infections, systemic manifestations are slight and fever is inconstant.

The most important manifestations of influenzal infection result from disturbances at the primary sites of bacterial multiplication. The commonest diseases produced by *H. influenzae* are pharyngitis, epiglottitis, laryngotracheitis, pneumonia, bronchitis and bronchiolitis, otitis media, and meningitis. The symptoms and signs of influenzal invasion of the respiratory tract or meninges are similar to those of infection of these areas by other organisms, and differential etiologic diagnosis depends upon epidemiologic background, the age of the patient, and demonstration of the causative agent.

Pharyngitis. Hemophilus influenzae is a relatively common cause of pharyngitis in children, and acute influenzal pharyngitis is being observed with in-

creasing frequency in adults, where it often occurs as a complication of the chemotherapy of other infections. Examination of the throat usually reveals only marked redness and injection. Very rarely, patches of soft yellow exudate may be present. The pharyngitis tends to persist for many days unless properly treated. Discomfort in the pharynx is often out of proportion to the physical findings.

Epiglottitis. Disease of the upper respiratory tract produced by *H. influenzae* is sometimes limited to the epiglottis, which becomes reddened, swollen, and stiff. Discomfort in the hypopharynx and "croupy" breathing may progress to a point at which tracheotomy becomes necessary. This disease is rare in adults.

Laryngotracheobronchitis. The entire laryngotracheobronchial tree may be the site of infection, with resulting rapidly progressive obstruction of the airway. "Croupy" cough is accompanied by increasing signs of respiratory embarrassment, and tracheotomy is sometimes necessary. Influenzal laryngotracheitis is very rare in adults. The disease can lead to death within 18 to 24 hr.

Pneumonia. Primary pneumonia due to *H. influenzae*, with rare exceptions, is a disease of children. In the adult, it is usually secondary to viral influenza, measles, or bacterial pneumonitis. It may complicate rubeola or pertussis in the young. Bacteremia occurs in approximately one-third of the cases.

Bronchitis and Bronchiolitis. Severe, diffuse bronchiolitis characterized by persistent nonproductive cough, wheezing, and dyspnea occurs in children. Physical examination usually reveals lowering and fixation of the diaphragms, prolonged expirations, and typically asthmatic breathing. Roentgenographic examination of the chest reveals increased radiolucence, and flattening of the diaphragms consistent with emphysema. This is an extremely serious illness and unless promptly recognized and treated may be rapidly fatal.

The factor of infection contributes significantly to the clinical manifestations and progressive deterioration in established chronic bronchitis or "senile emphysema" in adults. Among the bacteria involved, the pneumococcus and *H. influenzae* are the commonest; the latter has been isolated from the respiratory tracts of 80 to 90 per cent of patients in some groups.

Otitis Media. Hemophilus influenzae is a common cause of suppurative otitis media in children; the infection is uncommon in adults. Influenzal middle ear disease is indistinguishable on clinical grounds from infection due to other bacteria.

Meningitis. The influenza bacillus is the commonest cause of meningitis between the ages of six months and two years and is frequent in later childhood. In adults, it may follow operation on or injury to the head. The author has studied one adult in whom spinal anesthesia, in the presence of a severe sore throat, was followed within 24 hr by meningitis due to type B *H. influenzae.* Ninety-five per cent of cases are produced by type B organisms, a few by type A, and a rare one by nonencapsulated strains. About two-thirds of the patients have a preceding infection of the upper respiratory tract, and about one-third have broncho-pneumonia. Signs of meningeal irritation, stiff neck and back, and positive Kernig and Brudzinski signs are usually prominent, except in very young babies in whom bulging of the fontanels may be the only sign. The diagnosis should be suspected because of the age of the patient and the frequent prodrome of respiratory infection; it is confirmed by identification of the organisms from the spinal fluid or blood.

Other Diseases. Subacute and acute bacterial endocarditis may be produced by *H. influenzae,* although more infections of the heart valves have been due to *H. parainfluenzae.* The influenza bacillus is a rare cause of suppurative *pericarditis.* In the winter, *acute conjunctivitis* may be due to *H. influenzae.* While there are no clinical features which distinguish this from "pink eye" produced by the Koch-Weeks bacillus, epidemics of conjunctivitis due to the latter are most common in the summer. Although it has been suggested that *H. influenzae* and the Koch-Weeks bacillus are identical, more recent observation has indicated that, although they are antigenically related, they are distinct species. *Moraxella lacunata* is also an occasional cause of acute purulent conjunctivitis. Acute pyogenic *arthritis* due to *H. influenzae* has been reported. One of the very important lesions in which this organism plays a role in the adult is *bronchiectasis.* Together with other pyogenic bacteria, it can be responsible for the perpetuation of this disease.

Laboratory Findings. As a rule, infections due to *H. influenzae* are accompanied by polymorphonuclear leukocytosis ranging from 15,000 to 30,000 per cu mm. In young children with severe disease, leukopenia (2,000 to 3,000 leukocytes per cu mm) with a deficiency of polymorphonuclear leukocytes can occur. Bacteremia is of irregular occurrence in influenzal infections of the respiratory tract but is demonstrable in about 50 per cent of cases of meningitis.

Course and Complications. The course of *H. influenzae* infections is influenced completely by the location of the disease. Epiglottitis, laryngo-tracheobronchitis, bronchiolitis, or pneumonia may be fulminating, particularly in young children. Some of these patients succumb to the uncontrolled infection, but in many, the cause of death is obstruction of the airway. This cannot always be relieved by surgical methods, because impediment to flow of air is most marked in the smaller radicles of the bronchial tree. Virtually 100 per cent of untreated cases of influenzal meningitis terminate fatally. Internal and external hydrocephalus, brain abscess, subdural empyema, diffuse cortical necrosis, and shock (the Waterhouse-Friderichsen syndrome) are possible complications. With specific therapy the incidence of complications is generally sharply reduced. However, if subdural aspiration is carried out routinely in children with influenzal meningitis which is responding to antibiotics, sterile fluid is demonstrable in about half the cases. Neurologic disturbances from subdural effusions are uncommon. Epileptiform seizures can occur while the disease is responding favorably to chemotherapy.

Treatment. Specific serotherapy is presently used only in unusual situations. The sulfonamides, streptomycin, the tetracyclines, and chloramphenicol inhibit *H. influenzae.* Streptomycin is very effective but has the disadvantage of leading to the rapid development of bacterial resistance. Sulfadiazine or sulfisoxazole (Gantrisin) is effective in influenzal pharyngitis, but the tetracycline compounds are more active than the sulfonamides and are preferred for the therapy of lesions involving the respiratory tract. There is controversy concerning the treatment of influenzal bacterial meningitis, but several facts are clear. The sulfonamides should never be used alone. Streptomycin, given both intramuscularly and intraspinally, reduces the mortality rate, but about 10 per cent of patients develop drug-resistant organisms 48 to 72 hr after initiation of treatment. The tetracyclines alone do not eradicate the meningeal infection. Chloramphenicol (50 to 75 mg per kg body weight per day) and sulfadiazine (0.1 Gm per lb body weight per day, the initial dose being one-half the quantity required daily) constitute the preferred regimen in many clinics. Death or complications still occur, and clearing of the organisms from the spinal fluid may be delayed. In the author's experience, the most effective therapy is as follows. Streptomycin (no more than 25 mg in children under age three and 50 mg in older ones) diluted in 10 ml saline is injected intraspinally at the time the diagnosis is established and once again 12 hr later; the drug is *not* administered intraspinally after the second dose. Streptomycin (0.5 to 1.0 Gm daily in divided doses, depending on the age and size of the patient) is given intramuscularly, and sulfadiazine or Gantrisin is administered in quantities sufficient to produce a blood level of 12 to 15 mg per 100 ml. Treatment is continued for 2 weeks. In about 100 consecutive cases of influenzal meningitis so treated there have been no deaths and no detectable complications.

PERTUSSIS

Whooping cough is a common disease which affects about 85 per cent of all unimmunized children. It is characterized by an inflammatory reaction involving the entire respiratory tract which produces paroxysmal cough and the typical inspiratory stridor, or "whoop."

Etiology. The causative agent is *Hemophilus pertussis* (also called *Bordatella pertussis*), a short or ovoid gram-negative, nonmotile, nonsporulating, facultatively anaerobic bacillus. It shows very little tendency toward pleomorphism. Bipolar staining is frequent, and encapsulation can be demonstrated by special stains.

The pertussis bacillus requires both the X and V factors for growth, especially for initial isolation, and multiplies best on Bordet-Gengou medium.

Hemophilus pertussis is a uniform antigenic species, without fixed variation or types.

The pertussis bacillus produces no demonstrable endotoxin, although it has been postulated that some of the clinical features of whooping cough may be due to such material; definite evidence for this is lacking.

Epidemiology. Pertussis is world-wide and may be endemic or epidemic. If the disease has not been present for several years, it tends to assume epidemic proportions when it reappears. In some geographic locations the disease is most common during the winter, and in others it is seen with greatest frequency in the late summer and fall. The index of contagion is 80 to 100 per cent; about 200,000 cases occur in the United States each year.

Approximately 40 per cent of cases of pertussis occur in the first two years of life; the same number is observed between two and five years. At least 50 per cent of all children have had whooping cough before they reach the age of five and 75 per cent by the age of seventeen.

Pertussis is spread by droplets from the respiratory tract. It has been suggested that, rarely, the organisms may be transmitted by fomites. The infectivity of the disease during the incubation period is questionable; it is most contagious during the catarrhal stage. Healthy carriers play no role in dissemination; mild or missed cases are of great importance. The duration of contagiousness is about 4 to 6 weeks.

Pathology. The initial lesion in whooping cough is hyperplasia of the peribronchial lymphoid tissue and tracheobronchial lymph nodes. Subsequently or perhaps coincidentally, the bronchi, trachea, larynx, and nasopharynx are involved in a necrotizing inflammatory reaction. The organisms are present in large numbers between the cilia of the epithelial cells lining the trachea and bronchi. It has been thought that the pulmonary alveoli are not involved in pertussis, but there is often a diffuse bronchopneumonia with marked desquamation of the alveolar epithelium, and lymphocytic infiltration of the peribronchial tissues and alveolar walls.

Clinical Manifestations. The incubation period of whooping cough averages 12 to 15 days, although it can be as long as 20 days. The first clinical manifestations are nonspecific, consisting of slight nasal discharge, conjunctivitis, and mild cough without fever. This *catarrhal stage* lasts for 7 to 14 days.

The *paroxysmal phase* of pertussis follows the *catarrhal stage* and is characterized by paroxysms of coughing ending in a loud, crowing inspiratory noise (the whoop), the expulsion of varying quantities of thick, mucoid sputum from the respiratory tract, and vomiting. Episodes of cough may be as few as 1 or 2 or as many as 40 to 50 per day. Children under the age of six months frequently do not whoop. The mere presence of a whoop is in itself not diagnostic of pertussis. Rarely, the paroxysms of coughing and whooping are replaced completely by sneezing.

Fever of appreciable degree does not occur in the paroxysmal phase of pertussis unless complications are present. Vomiting frequently follows spells of coughing but is not a specific manifestation of the disease. Soreness over the trachea and main bronchi are common. Spasm, ulcer, and, more rarely, edema of the glottis sometimes occur. In cases with severe vomiting and inability to retain food, serious inanition, wasting, and tetany may appear.

There is a bleeding tendency in pertussis. This has been attributed to the effect of an angiotoxin (not proved) elaborated by the organism which increases the ease of rupture of blood vessel walls. Hemoptysis, epistaxis, purpura, and subconjunctival or intestinal hemorrhages may occur but are usually of little clinical significance.

Physical examination in pertussis is often entirely normal. There may be redness and injection of the blood vessels of the nose and pharynx. Although there are usually no abnormal findings in the lungs, fine, crackling, "sticky" rales are sometimes present. There are ulcers of the frenum of the tongue in about 20 per cent of cases; these occur only when the lower central incisor teeth are present.

The paroxysmal stage of pertussis usually lasts from 1 to 6 weeks. When coughing persists beyond 6 weeks, it is usually due to the development of a so-called "habit whoop" and not to continuation of the disease.

Laboratory Findings. The peripheral white blood count is, as a rule, elevated in pertussis. The total count may be over 100,000 cells per cu mm, and lymphocytes may constitute 90 per cent of the cells. All the lymphocytes are mature. This helps to distinguish the blood picture from that of acute leukemia but not from acute lymphocytosis. Blood cultures are sterile. Cultures of the upper part of the nasopharynx reveal *H. pertussis*, the incidence of positive isolations varying with the stage of the disease. X-ray study of the lungs in the uncomplicated case usually reveals only hilar lymphadenopathy and increase in the density of the bronchovascular markings.

Complications. Bronchopneumonia occurs in from 1 to 10 per cent of cases; the organisms most frequently involved are the beta-hemolytic streptococcus, *Diplococcus pneumoniae, Staphylococcus aureus, H. influenzae,* and *H. pertussis.* When pneumonitis appears during the course of chemotherapy, the bacteria most often responsible are *Escherichia coli, Proteus* strains, *Aerobacter aerogenes,* or *Pseudomonas aeruginosa.* Another important complication is atelectasis; small areas of collapse are an almost constant finding in this infection, but major portions or even a whole lung may be involved. Pneumothorax is rare.

The severe coughing of pertussis may lead to several complications. Hemorrhage may appear in the anterior chamber of the eye or in the retina. Detachment of the retina and blindness develop in rare cases. Prolapse of the rectum and inguinal or umbilical hernias have been noted. Otitis media is observed in about 10 per cent of cases; the organisms most frequently involved are the beta-hemolytic streptococcus and *Staphylococcus aureus,* although *H. pertussis* is sometimes responsible.

Nervous system manifestations are not rare in pertussis. The commonest is convulsions; they often come with the sudden fever of secondary bacterial infection. Other causes of seizures are encephalopathy (1 to 14 per cent of cases), multiple petechial or gross hemorrhages of the brain, and cerebral hypoxia due to the combined effect of anoxic anoxia and venous stasis in the brain. The encephalopathy is characterized by an increase in the protein and cell content of the spinal fluid. Its etiology is unknown. Hyperreflexia, nuchal rigidity, cranial nerve palsies, areflexia, extensor plantar responses, flaccid hemiplegia, spasticity of the extremities, opisthotonos, difficulty in speaking, twitching, papilledema, nystagmus, blindness, strabismus, and difficulty in swallowing can all occur. Some of the more important residua are mental retardation, recurrent convulsions, behavior and personality disorders, amnesia, aphasia, diffuse cerebral atrophy, chorea, athetosis, hydrocephalus, epilepsy, and idiocy.

Diagnosis. The diagnosis of pertussis can frequently be made on clinical grounds alone. A known contact is helpful, but the appearance of paroxysms of typical coughing and whooping, after a short period of an undefined upper respiratory tract infection, is strongly suggestive. It must be stressed, however, that in babies under the age of six months there is usually only paroxysmal coughing, without the characteristic whoop.

An increased white blood count with a large increase in lymphocytes is characteristic; the lymphocyte count must, however, be evaluated in relation to the age of the patient.

Isolation of *H. pertussis* from the respiratory tract establishes the diagnosis; unfortunately this is not possible in many cases. Using cough plates and nasopharyngeal swabs, positive cultures can be obtained in 90 per cent of patients in the catarrhal stage of the disease; pertussis, however, is rarely seen by the physician in this phase. The incidence of positive cultures is lower after paroxysmal coughing appears, and decreases with the duration of symptoms.

Serologic studies are of little or no help in establishing the presence of pertussis.

Prevention. Active immunization is effective in preventing pertussis in the majority of individuals who are given vaccine. Immunization may be started at the age of three months; both antibody production and protection against invasion by *H. pertussis* result. If the procedure is carried out at this early age, a "booster" injection should be administered at the end of the first year of life, and again just before the child starts to school. Although it is not commonly practiced, passive immunity can be conferred on the newborn child by active immunization of the mother beginning in the sixth or seventh month of pregnancy. Vaccine should not be given in the presence of the active disease; not only is it useless, but it may provoke serious neurologic reactions. There is evidence that the administration of "quadruple" vaccine—poliomyelitis virus, tetanus and diphtheria toxoid, and *H. pertussis*—leads to some degree of suppression of the response to the pertussis bacillus. For this reason, it is suggested that poliomyelitis vaccine (formalinized) be given separately from the commonly used "triple" vaccine.

In children who have been exposed to a case of pertussis but have not been actively immunized, passive protection may be given by the injection of 20 to 30 ml human hyperimmune pertussis antiserum, or 2 ml immune γ-globulin as soon as possible after exposure, and again 1 week later. Such prophylaxis is 75 to 85 per cent effective.

Treatment. Although most of the antimicrobial drugs have been employed in the treatment of pertussis, there is no incontrovertible evidence that they are strikingly beneficial. Chlortetracycline, chloramphenicol, oxytetracycline, and erythromycin have been used, but the results obtained in controlled studies are not remarkable.

There are few controlled studies of serum therapy

in whooping cough, but in many clinics it is the practice to administer human hyperimmune serum (20 ml every 48 hr for three doses), or immune γ-globulin (2 ml every 48 hr for three doses) to all children with pertussis under the age of two years.

Most important in the program of therapy is repair of the water and salt loss which follows severe and frequent vomiting. If failure to retain food is combated by prompt refeeding, whooping cough patients can be made to maintain or gain weight.

Early detection and treatment of complications is one of the most important factors in the reduction of mortality in pertussis. The prompt recognition of secondary bacterial infections of the lungs or middle ear and therapy with a properly selected antibiotic agent lead to cure in practically all cases. When gross atelectasis occurs, correction by tracheal catheter suction or bronchoscopy may be lifesaving. Little can be done to influence the course or outcome of such complications as gross cerebral hemorrhage or encephalopathy.

Proper management of whooping cough has made the outlook for complete recovery excellent. There have been only two fatalities in 500 patients with this infection in the last 8 years in the author's clinic; neither was due to a preventable or treatable complication.

REFERENCES

Alexander, H. E.: Experimental Basis for Treatment of *Haemophilus influenzae* Infections, Am. J. Diseases Children, 66:160, 1943.

Baty, J., and M. Kreidberg: Acute Laryngotracheobronchitis, Med. Clin. N. Am., 36:1279, 1952.

Bell, J. A.: Pertussis Immunization, J.A.M.A., 137:1276, 1948.

Crowell, J., and S. D. Loube: Primary *Hemophilus influenzae* Pneumonia, A.M.A. Arch. Internal Med., 93:921, 1954.

Felton, H. E.: The Status of Passive Immunization and Treatment in Pertussis, J.A.M.A., 128:26, 1945.

Lapin, J.: "Whooping Cough," Springfield, Ill., Charles C Thomas, Publisher, 1943.

Litvack, A. M., H. Gibel, S. E. Rosenthal, and P. Rosenblatt: Cerebral Complications in Pertussis, J. Pediat., 32:357, 1948.

Lucchesi, P. F., and A. C. LaBoccetta: Whooping Cough Treated with Pertussis Immune Serum (Human): Report of a Controlled Series of 52 Patients under One Year of Age, Am. J. Diseases Children, 77:15, 1949.

Mulder, J., W. R. O. Goslings, M. C. van der Plas, and P. L. Cardozo: Studies on the Treatment with Antibacterial Drugs of Acute and Chronic Mucopurulent Bronchitis Caused by *Hemophilus influenzae*, Acta Med. Scand., 143:32, 1952.

Rose, H. M.: *Hemophilus influenzae* Type A Endocarditis, Am. J. Med. Sci., 202:187, 1941.

Sako, W., W. L. Treuting, D. B. Witt, and S. J. Nichamin: Early Immunization against Pertussis with Alum Precipitated Vaccine, J.A.M.A., 127:379, 1945.

Schoenbach, E. B., H. C. Spencer, and J. Monnier: Treatment of *H. influenzae* Meningitis with Aureomycin and Chloramphenicol, Am. J. Med., 12:263, 1952.

Weinstein, L., R. Seltser, and C. T. Marrow: The Treatment of Pertussis with Aureomycin, Chloramphenicol and Terramycin, J. Pediat., 39:549, 1951.

—— M. Goldfield, and D. Adamis: A Study of the Intrathecal Chemotherapy in Bacterial Meningitis, Med. Clin. N. Am., September:1363, 1953.

128 CHANCROID
Albert Heyman

Definition. Chancroid is an acute, localized, venereal disease caused by the Ducrey bacillus (*Hemophilus ducreyi*). It is characterized by ulceration at the site of inoculation and by enlargement and suppuration of the regional lymph nodes.

Etiology. The etiologic agent of chancroid, the Ducrey bacillus, is a short, plump, gram-negative organism with rounded ends. When stained by special methods, the bacillus exhibits bipolar staining. In the stained smears of genital lesions the organisms usually appear singly or in small clusters, but they may be arranged in long parallel columns between cells or shreds of mucus. Occasionally, the bacilli are situated intracellularly. The organism can be cultivated in whole defibrinated blood or nutrient broth containing blood. When grown in pure culture in a liquid medium, the Ducrey bacillus appears in long, tangled chains composed of both coccal and bacillary forms.

Incidence. The number of cases of chancroid occurring every year cannot be determined satisfactorily, since accurate diagnosis of this condition is not generally attempted. A diagnosis of chancroid is frequently applied to genital lesions improving with sulfonamide therapy in which the *Treponema pallidum* cannot be demonstrated. The disease is encountered in the West Indies, North Africa, and the Orient, particularly in the lower economic groups of the population. It is also prevalent in the Southeastern part of the United States and is more frequent in Negroes than in whites. Approximately 1,600 cases were reported in the United States in 1959; the true incidence is probably considerably higher.

Pathogenesis. Chancroid is usually contracted by sexual intercourse, and the lesions are almost always located about the genitalia. The disease can apparently be acquired from sexual partners who show no evidence of an active chancroidal infection. The organism has been cultivated from the smegma and vaginal secretions in patients without clinical manifestations of the disease. Such individuals may be carriers of the Ducrey bacillus. The organism readily produces an infection when inoculated into open or slightly abraded areas of the skin or mucous membranes. Chancroidal ulcerations frequently occur in areas of the genitalia, where minor abrasions may be present (fourchette of the vulva, edge of phimotic prepuce, and frenum). After an incubation period of 2 to 5 days, a localized ulceration appears at the site of inoculation. This may be followed later by inflammation and suppuration of the regional lymph nodes.

Chancroidal infection produces a distinct histologic appearance. The base of the ulcer is a shallow zone made up of polymorphonuclear leukocytes, fibrin, red blood cells, and necrotic tissue. Below this is a fairly wide layer, consisting chiefly of proliferating endothelial cells and newly formed blood vessels, some of which show degeneration of their walls. Finally, there is a deep zone in which a dense infiltration of plasma cells and lymphocytes occurs. This histologic pattern is sufficiently characteristic to permit differentiation from other genital lesions. Biopsy is a valuable diagnostic procedure.

Clinical Manifestations. The typical chancroidal lesion is a painful, shallow, irregular ulcer with ragged undermined edges, a granular, friable base, and a dirty-yellow exudate. The lesion is characteristically nonindurated and for this reason has been called *soft chancre*. The size of the ulceration varies but seldom exceeds 2 cm in diameter. Multiple lesions resemble a folliculitis or pyogenic infection. Almost any portion of the genitalia may be involved, but extragenital lesions are rare. In about 50 per cent of the patients inflammation and suppuration of the inguinal lymph nodes will occur. The term *bubo* is given to this type of lymphadenitis. The chancroidal bubo develops rapidly and becomes a very painful, inflammatory inguinal mass. When suppuration occurs, the mass may become tensely fluctuant and may rupture spontaneously, leaving a large, single, craterlike abscess. Mild constitutional symptoms may accompany the involvement of the inguinal lymph nodes, and the patient may complain of headache, malaise, fever, or anorexia.

Diagnosis. Although the clinical appearance of chancroid is often sufficiently characteristic to suggest the correct diagnosis, laboratory confirmation is desirable. Stained smears or culture of the exudate taken from the undermined edge of the lesion will reveal the Ducrey bacillus in the majority of the early cases. The organism is not easily demonstrated, however, in larger lesions when secondary bacterial contamination has occurred. Biopsy is feasible in such cases and is an efficient method of diagnosis. Attempts to demonstrate the organism in the buboes by either culture or smear usually are not successful. The majority of patients with chancroidal infection will exhibit a positive skin reaction to an intradermal injection of killed Ducrey bacilli. The value of this skin test is limited by the fact that a positive reaction persists for years after exposure to the infection. One cannot be certain, therefore, whether a positive skin test in an individual patient represents the existing chancroidal infection or a previous one. Early syphilis may be present concurrently with chancroid in these patients. Serologic tests and dark-field examination of the lesions and regional lymph nodes should be done to rule out this possibility.

Treatment. Sulfadiazine or Gantrisin is the drug of choice in the treatment of chancroid; doses of 4 Gm a day for 7 to 12 days are usually curative. Local medication is not necessary, but saline soaks and cleanliness are advised. Although the buboes usually subside with sulfonamide therapy, fluctuation may persist, and the node should be aspirated in order to prevent spontaneous rupture. Streptomycin, chloramphenicol, and the tetracyclines in doses of 2 Gm a day for 7 to 10 days will each produce satisfactory healing of the lesions of chancroid. The use of these agents is rarely necessary since sulfadiazine is equally effective. The antibiotics with treponemicidal properties should not be used in the treatment of chancroid until repeated dark-field examinations and serologic tests have ruled out the possibility of early syphilis.

REFERENCES

Heyman, A., P. B. Beeson, and W. H. Sheldon: Diagnosis of Chancroid, J.A.M.A., 129:935, 1945.

Sullivan, M.: Chancroid, Am. J. Syphilis, Gonorrhea, Venereal Diseases, 24:482, 1940.

129 BRUCELLOSIS (Undulant Fever)

Wesley W. Spink

Definition. Brucellosis is an infectious disease due to microorganisms belonging to the genus *Brucella*, and is transmitted to man from lower animals. The acute form of the illness is frequently characterized by a febrile illness without localizing findings, while the chronic form is featured by fever, weakness, and vague complaints, which may persist for months and years.

History. Accurate clinical descriptions of brucellosis have been ascribed to Hippocrates, but the first clear-cut picture of the disease was presented in 1863 by Marston, who, as a British Army surgeon in Malta, detailed his own case and those of others. The etiologic agent was discovered by Bruce in 1886. The outstanding clinical description of the disease is contained in the monograph by Hughes published in 1897. Wright and Semple in 1897 demonstrated agglutinins for brucella in human blood. In the same year, Bang reported that *Bacillus abortus* was the cause of contagious abortion in cattle in Denmark. The Mediterranean Fever Commission Reports of 1905 to 1907 detail the classic studies on epidemiology. The first recognized human case of brucellosis in the United States occurred in a nurse in Washington, D.C., and was described by Craig in 1906. In 1911 brucellosis was found to be endemic in the goats of Texas, and Gentry and Ferenbaugh traced human cases to this source. Traum first identified brucella organisms from aborting sows in 1914, and Evans in 1918 distinguished the difference between *Brucella melitensis* and *Brucella abortus*, and suggested that raw milk from infected cows could be the source of human cases. In 1924 Keefer described the first human case of brucellosis in this country due to organisms other than *B. melitensis*.

Etiology. Human brucellosis is due to one of three species of *Brucella*—viz., *B. melitensis* (goats), *B. suis* (hogs), and *B. abortus* (cattle). Brucellas are small, nonmotile, non-spore-forming rods staining gram-negative. Growth is best supported at 37°C in trypticase soy broth or tryptose phosphate broth having a pH of 6.6 to 6.8. The primary isolation of *B. abortus* requires displacement of 10 per cent of the air by carbon dioxide. The differentiation of the three species is dependent upon biochemical and serologic reaction. In general, *B. melitensis* is the most invasive of the three species, which fact is reflected in the severity of human infections, while *B. abortus* is the least virulent.

Epidemiology. The natural reservoir of brucellosis is in domestic animals, particularly cattle, swine, goats, and sheep. The disease is very rarely transmitted from human to human. By and large, man acquires brucellosis through the ingestion of milk or milk products containing viable brucellas, or through contact of the skin with infected tissues, excretions, and secretions. Recent epidemiologic studies in the United States indicate that the majority of cases are acquired through contact, and fewer and fewer cases are caused by the ingestion of milk. This trend is due to the enactment of local and state ordinances requiring all milk sold for human consumption to be pasteurized. There is some evidence that brucellosis may be air-borne, with the disease resulting from the inhalation of brucella. Infections caused by *B. abortus* are spread through cow's milk or through dermal contact with brucella. Epidemics of brucellosis traced to raw cow's milk have been caused by *B. abortus*. Contact with infected porcine tissue is a common cause of infections due to *B. suis*. While infections due to *B. melitensis* result from eating goat's cheese or drinking unpasteurized goat's milk, studies in Minnesota and Iowa have shown that contact with infected hogs has been the source of *melitensis* infections. It is readily appreciated why brucellosis is primarily a disease of rural areas and why it is considered an occupational disease involving meat-packing plant employees, farmers, veterinarians, and livestock producers.

Pathogenesis. Following invasion of the body by brucellas through the oropharynx or through the skin, the organisms tend to localize in tissues of the reticuloendothelial system, such as the bone marrow, lymph nodes, liver, spleen, and also the kidneys. A characteristic but nonspecific reaction of these tissues to the brucella is the appearance of epithelioid cells, giant cells of the foreign body and Langhans' types, and lymphocytes and plasma cells. Necrosis and caseation rarely occur in these granulomatous areas. When caseation is encountered, it is usually caused by *B. suis*. The granulomas are similar to those of sarcoidosis and tuberculosis. Other less frequent sites of localization of brucella organisms are the bones, especially the spine, the endocardium, and the testes. While the central nervous system and peripheral nerves are commonly affected deleteriously by brucellas, the mechanism whereby this takes place is not known. Like other blood-borne infections, brucellas may on occasion localize in any tissue or organ in the body. Though brucellosis is a common cause of abortions in cattle, swine, and goats, authentic cases of human abortions occur no more frequently with this disease than with other bacteremias. Orchitis in the male is rarely the cause of subsequent sterility.

Manifestations. The incubation period varies between 5 and 21 days, though many months may elapse between the time of infection and the first appearance of symptoms. The onset in many instances may be insidious, the patients exhibiting a low-grade fever with no localizing findings, and complaining of headache, weakness, insomnia, sweats, anorexia, constipation, pain over the spine, and generalized aches and pains. Less frequently, the disease may be ushered in by chills, high fever, and prostration, but, again, localizing abnormal physical findings may be absent. In general, about 50 per cent of the patients exhibit enlarged lymph nodes, especially of the cervical region, and splenomegaly is detected in about one-third of the cases. An enlarged and tender spleen is usually associated with the more severe cases. Pain on pressure over the vertebras occurs occasionally. Pain distributed over the course of the peripheral nerves, particularly the sciatic nerve, is encountered. Orchitis appears after several days of illness and, like the orchitis of mumps, is ushered in with a chill or chilliness, high fever, and tender and enlarged testes. Painful and swollen joints are seen occasionally, but persistent and deforming arthritis is not specific for the disease. Signs and symptoms referable to the lungs and pleurae are uncommon. A rare but serious complication is subacute bacterial endocarditis. Ocular disorders are associated with the more chronic forms of the disease.

The initial febrile stage of the illness may endure for only a few days or up to several weeks. The persistence of fever and symptoms is definitely related to physical activity. Rest in bed during the acute illness is frequently associated with prompt improvement. The natural course of the disease in the majority of patients is marked by a permanent remission of fever and symptoms within 3 to 6 months. A small number of bacteriologically proved cases may have an illness that persists longer than 1 year.

The present status of chronic brucellosis is extremely difficult to assess. There is no doubt that the infection may persist in some individuals for months and years. Such patients exhibit a state of ill health manifested by weakness, fatigue, mental depression, vague aches and pains, and no abnormal physical findings. Intermittent fever may occur. The precise incidence of chronic brucellosis awaits further investigation. Much of the data now available are based upon uncritical clinical and laboratory studies.

Laboratory Procedures. A precise diagnosis of brucellosis is dependent upon the results of laboratory procedures.

Blood. The total leukocyte count is usually normal or slightly reduced but is rarely over 10,000 cells per cu mm. The differential count reveals a relative lymphocytosis. The erythrocyte sedimentation rate is of no specific diagnostic aid, the rates being normal or accelerated.

The most practical method for screening suspected cases of brucellosis is the *agglutination* reaction. Agglutinins usually appear during the second or third week of illness. If proper techniques and antigen are employed, agglutinins are demonstrated in the vast majority of bacteriologically proved cases. Active brucellosis is usually associated with titers of 1:100 or above. Agglutinins for brucellosis are not always specific, since cross reactions occur with the cholera vibrio and with *Pasteurella tularensis*. Agglutinins may persist in the blood long after the patient has recovered.

At least one *culture* of blood, and preferably more, should be carried out in every suspected case of brucellosis. Cultures of *Brucella* have been isolated from aspirated sternal bone marrow, when simultaneous blood cultures remained sterile. It is too impractical for routine purposes to attempt to isolate brucellas from the urine, bile, or feces.

The *opsonocytophagic test,* which is a measure of the phagocytosis of brucellas by polymorphonuclear neutrophil leukocytes, is of extremely doubtful diagnostic aid. The *complement fixation test* does not contribute enough additional information to warrant its use.

Intradermal Tests. Various antigenic preparations, including killed organisms, are used widely for diagnostic purposes. A positive reaction has no more significance than that obtained with tuberculin in suspected cases of tuberculosis. A positive reaction indicates previous invasion of the body by brucellas and does not mean that active disease is present. Unfortunately, many instances of chronic brucellosis are being diagnosed on the basis of a vague illness and positive intradermal tests. When agglutinins are absent and cultures remain sterile, considerable caution must be exercised before making a diagnosis of brucellosis, even though the skin test is positive. Negative skin tests are encountered in severe cases of brucellosis where a high titer of agglutinins is present and a bacteremia is demonstrated.

In summary, the diagnosis of brucellosis depends upon a correlation of epidemiologic data, the nature of the illness, and laboratory information, such as the presence of agglutinins and isolation of brucellas from the tissues or blood.

Differential Diagnosis. Brucellosis must be differentiated from other acute febrile illnesses such as *influenza* and other *upper respiratory diseases* of doubtful etiology. Brucellosis is not commonly associated with coryza or pharyngitis. Other diseases from which it must be differentiated include *malaria* and *typhoid fever*. Brucellosis may be confused with *infectious mononucleosis*, but the characteristic blood picture and the elevated titer of heterophil antibodies in the latter disease are helpful differential aids.

Chronic brucellosis simulates *psychoneurosis, anxiety states,* and *chronic nervous exhaustion.* Indeed, a patient with brucellosis may suffer from the foregoing nervous disorders. Some confusion may arise in differentiating it from other diseases, including tuberculosis and lymphoblastoma, especially Hodgkin's disease.

Treatment. Unfortunately, much information of a popular nature on brucellosis has been disseminated widely. The general public has heard or read that brucellosis is a chronic disease which may last for years and that no satisfactory treatment is available. Therefore, any physician who believes that he is dealing with a case of brucellosis should reassure the patient that the disease is self-limiting, and that complete recovery will ensue. Psychotherapy is extremely important in the management of these mentally depressed and tired patients. The acutely ill and febrile patient should be kept in bed. Many patients will recover completely following a period of rest.

Over the years the lack of specific treatment for brucellosis has been emphasized by the number of agents and procedures that have been recommended and then discarded, one by one. Although sulfanilamide and its various derivatives can suppress the growth of brucellas, these agents are unsatisfactory for the treatment of human brucellosis. Penicillin is an ineffective drug for brucellosis. Streptomycin and dihydrostreptomycin are unusual drugs in that they not only inhibit growth of brucellas, but they can kill large numbers of the organisms within a relatively short period of time. However, streptomycin is a poor therapeutic agent in brucellosis, because, while the antibiotic is quite lethal for extracellular brucellas, intracellular brucellas are protected against the drug. But there is no question that simultaneous treatment with streptomycin or dihydrostreptomycin and sulfadiazine is much more effective in human brucellosis than the administration of either the antibiotic or sulfonamide alone. Streptomycin or dihydrostreptomycin can be given intramuscularly in a dose of 0.5 Gm every 12 hr for 2 weeks. At the same time 1 Gm sulfadiazine is administered orally four times daily and continued for 3 weeks.

Although the combination of streptomycin and sulfadiazine proved to be a definite advance in the therapy of brucellosis, superior results have been obtained with the use of any one of the tetracyclines in an oral dose of 0.5 Gm four times daily for at least 3 weeks. Relapses can be successfully treated in the same manner. Chloramphenicol does not appear to be so satisfactory an antibiotic for brucellosis as the tetracyclines, and its use is not recommended.

There is evidence that *a combination of streptomycin or dihydrostreptomycin with one of the tetracycline drugs* provides a more efficient form of therapy than the tetracyclines alone. The policy at the University of Minnesota clinics is to use one of the tetracycline antibiotics alone for the average case of brucellosis due to *B. abortus* in doses as recommended above. However, for more severe cases, and for all those due to *B. melitensis* or *B. suis*, streptomycin or dihydrostreptomycin is given intramuscularly in a dose of 0.5 Gm every 12 hr for 2 weeks, along with an oral dose of 0.5 Gm tetracycline administered four times daily. Treatment with the latter drug is usually kept up for 3 weeks.

Patients with acute brucellosis often exhibit a severe toxic state which simulates typhoid fever and which gradually subsides after several days of therapy with antibiotics. However, rapid and dramatic improvement, occurring within 8 to 12 hr, can be obtained with the use of one of the adrenocorticoid steroid preparations. An initial dose of 100 mg hydrocortisone can be given intravenously, followed by an oral dose of 25 mg four times daily. Other steroid preparations, such as cortisone and prednisone, can be given orally in equivalent doses. Any steroid therapy should be discontinued after 72 to 96 hr, and appropriate antibiotics should always be administered simultaneously.

A common therapeutic practice in the more chronic cases is to attempt desensitization of the tissues to brucella organisms by treating patients with one of the several antigenic preparations, such as heat-killed brucella cells or filtrates of brucella cultures. While hypersensitivity to brucellas is a factor in the symptomatology, and the use of ascending doses of antigenic material may be sound therapy, the results are difficult to evaluate, and treatment must often be continued for several months. Violent local and systemic reactions often occur, even following the injection of minute amounts of antigen.

For the relief of headache and the generalized aches and pains, salicylates may be prescribed; the occasional use of barbiturates is desirable for the insomnia which is so commonly a part of the disease.

Prognosis. While brucellosis may be a chronic and disabling disease, the over-all mortality rate is not more than 2 to 3 per cent and is negligible when appropriate antibiotic therapy is promptly employed. The physician today may learn a great deal about the prognosis of this disease by turning back and looking over the rich experience of the Mediterranean Fever Commission, which was recorded in 1905 to 1907. In a day when specific treatment was lacking, careful clinical observations were made. In an analysis of hundreds of *B. melitensis* cases, Eyre stated the following, in 1908:

One may safely say that not more than 10 per cent are convalescent in a shorter period than one month from the onset of symptoms. In 50 per cent, the disease extends over two months, in 25 per cent to three months, and in fully 15 per cent, a duration of three months is exceeded.

Over the succeeding years, it has been observed that a relatively small, but important, number of cases will have a protracted illness. Cases of bacteriologically proved brucellosis in which the disease has continued for over a year have been studied at the University of Minnesota Hospitals. But such cases are not commonly encountered. One cannot escape the conviction that so-called chronic brucellosis is being mislabeled too often on the basis of procedures of doubtful value, especially the intradermal test with brucella antigen.

Relapses do occur in the more chronic cases of brucellosis. These recurrences are manifested by fever and by mental and physical disability, with generalized aches and pains. But too little attention has been given to the problem of reinfections. Clinical observations in meat-packing plant employees have confirmed studies made with experimentally infected animals, in that the immunity induced by one attack of brucellosis is only relative. Second and third infections do take place. Thus, in individuals who continue to be exposed to the disease, it may be quite difficult to differentiate between relapses and reinfections.

Prevention. As long as the reservoir of brucellosis persists in domestic animals, human brucellosis will occur. The only practical means of eliminating the disease in human beings is to eradicate the disease from cattle, hogs, sheep, and goats. Control measures in animals are being worked out in several areas in the United States. Since human brucellosis is contracted through the ingestion of contaminated milk and milk products, it is essential that only properly pasteurized milk be utilized for human consumption. Brucellosis is an occupational disease involving farmers, livestock workers, veterinarians, and those working in meat-packing plants. There are no dependable and safe means available for immunizing these groups against the disease.

REFERENCES

Eyre, J. W. H.: Melitensis Septicemia, Lancet, I:1677, 1747, 1826, 1908.

Hardy, A. V., C. J. Jordan, I. H. Borts, and G. C. Hardy: Undulant Fever with Special Reference to a Study of Brucella Infection in Iowa, Natl. Insts. Health Bull., 1:58, 1931.

Hughes, M. L.: "Mediterranean, Malta or Undulant Fever," London, The Macmillan Company, Ltd., 1897.

"Reports of the Commission for the Investigation of Mediterranean Fever," pts. 1 to 7, London, Harrison & Sons, Ltd., 1905–1907.

Spink, W. W.: "The Nature of Brucellosis," Minneapolis, University of Minnesota Press, 1956.

130 TULAREMIA
Leighton E. Cluff

Definition. Tularemia (rabbit fever, deer-fly fever, Ohara's disease) is an infectious disease of animals transmitted to man by direct contact or by insect vectors. A cutaneous or mucous membrane lesion at the site of inoculation and regional lymph node enlargement are the characteristic manifestations of the disease in the human being.

History. The microorganism responsible for tularemia was identified by McCoy and Chapin in 1912 among infected ground squirrels in Tulare County, California. The first description of tularemia in man was that by Wherry and Lamb in 1914.

Etiology. *Pasteurella tularensis* is a pleomorphic, nonsporulating, gram-negative bacillus. It can be cultured only on media containing glucose, cystine, and serum. Thorough cooking renders meat from infected animals safe for consumption, but tularemia can develop in persons handling carcasses that have been frozen for many days. *Pasteurella tularensis* is related antigenically to the causative organisms of brucellosis and plague and possesses an endotoxin similar to those of many other gram-negative bacteria.

Epidemiology and Pathogenesis. Contact with infected animals is the commonest source of tularemia in man, but the disease also may be acquired from insects or by exposure to the organism in the laboratory. A variety of rodents, carnivores, ungulates, birds, and arthropods are naturally infected by *P. tularensis,* including rabbits, squirrels, woodchucks, muskrats, skunks, coyotes, foxes, opossums, mice, rats, quail, chickens, pheasants, snakes, ticks, and flies. The Rocky Mountain tick, western wood tick, eastern dog tick, and the Lone Star tick (*Dermacentor andersoni, D. variabilis, D. occidentalis,* and *Amblyomma americanum*) may act as reservoirs of infection. One species of deer fly (*Chrysops discalis*) and a mosquito (*Aedes cinereus* in Sweden) can transmit tularemia to man. Ticks are an important reservoir of the disease because the microorganism is transferred transovarially from the female to her progeny. Sporadic and epidemic tularemia have occurred following contact with water and fish contaminated by infected animal carcasses. However, human-to-human transmission of infection probably does not occur. Wild cottontail rabbits are the principal source of tularemia in the United States.

Man is highly susceptible to tularemia; the organism usually invades through the skin, mucous membrane, or gastrointestinal tract. Hunters, butchers, and housewives are most often affected, through exposure to infected animals.

Pathology. Microscopically, the primary cutaneous lesion shows neutrophilic infiltration, granulomatous reaction, and necrosis. The regional lymph nodes develop similar changes and often suppurate. The granulomatous reaction in tularemia consists of giant and epithelioid cells, and lesions resembling tubercles may occur in liver, spleen, lung, and kidney. *Pasteurella tularensis* has been recovered from lymph nodes many days after apparent subsidence of the disease.

Manifestations. The incubation period is 3 to 7 days. A typical lesion of skin or mucous membranes is not invariably present, and, therefore, tularemia has classically been separated into several clinical types.

More than 80 per cent of infections by *P. tularensis* are associated with a lesion of the skin or mucous membranes which has no distinguishing characteristics. It begins as a reddened papule that may be pruritic and soon ulcerates. The primary lesion in this *ulceroglandular* form of the disease is rarely very painful, is usually present before onset of systemic symptoms, and may not heal until convalescence is well under way. Frequently it is overlooked, or its relationship to severe systemic symptoms is not recognized. Regional lymph node enlargement is a constant feature and is usually more prominent than that accompanying infections of similar severity produced by other microorganisms. The involved nodes are often exquisitely tender and fluctuant. The overlying skin may be hot and reddened. Fistula formation and drainage can occur spontaneously. Generalized lymphadenopathy is present in some cases, but the regional nodes are most prominently involved. There is considerable variation in the intensity of the systemic symptoms of ulceroglandular tularemia; the patient may be almost asymptomatic or severely prostrated. Clinical and roentgenographic evidence of pneumonitis can accompany this form of the disease, illustrating its disseminated character, but bacteremia is rarely demonstrable.

Localized lymph node enlargement without detectable skin lesion is referred to as *glandular* tularemia. The pathogenesis of this form of the disease is probably identical with that of ulceroglandular tularemia, and the features of the illness are also the same.

Rarely, the portal of entry of the organism is the conjunctiva, where there develops an ulcer, with edema, congestion, lacrimation, photophobia, and pain. In this *oculoglandular* type of tularemia the preauricular, submaxillary, and anterior cervical lymph nodes enlarge in some patients. Corneal ulceration and scarring or perforation of the globe can occur.

Ingestion of contaminated meat or water can result in primary lesions of tularemia in the *gastrointestinal* tract. This rare form of the disease is characterized by pronounced diarrhea, abdominal pain, nausea, vomiting, melena, and hematemesis, but otherwise differs little from tularemia introduced through other portals. Ulcerative lesions are often found in the buccal mucosa, pharynx, or intestine, and the mesenteric or cervical lymph nodes are involved early in the disease.

Tularemia without obvious primary ulcer or localized lymphadenitis is referred to as the *typhoidal* type. Constitutional symptoms in typhoidal tularemia differ in no way from those in other types of the disease, although patients are, as a rule, more prostrated. In the absence of localized manifestations the clinical recognition of tularemia is, of course, more difficult and diagnosis is likely to depend principally upon serologic tests or isolation of the organism.

Pneumonia can accompany any of the various clinical types of tularemia. Involvement of the lung is secondary to hematogenous dissemination. Even in situations where infection is probably acquired by inhalation of the organism (as in bacteriology laboratories), there is no convincing evidence that primary tularemic pneumonia occurs. Pneumonitis in tularemia can lead to prominent signs of cough, mucoid sputum, hemoptysis, pleuritic pain, dyspnea, and cyanosis, but extensive x-ray evidence of pneumonitis is sometimes present in the absence of any symptoms of pulmonary disease. Physical findings often correlate poorly with the roentgenologic changes, which consist of diffuse patchy or lobar infiltrations and inconstant hilar adenopathy. Pleural effusion can occur in tularemic pneumonia, but lung abscess is rare.

Among the unusual infections produced by *P. tularensis* are endocarditis, pericarditis, peritonitis, appendicitis, osteomyelitis, and meningitis.

Fever in tularemia develops abruptly, often with rigors, and in the untreated patient may persist with temperatures at levels of 104 to 106°F for as long as 4 weeks. The fever is sustained or mildly remittent, and defervescence is by lysis. Headache, myalgia, anorexia, and nausea are common.

Splenomegaly of moderate degree is detectable in many patients. An evanescent macular or papular *rash* is sometimes present on the trunk and extremities early in the disease.

Convalescence in untreated tularemia is prolonged, and fever, lassitude, fatigability, myalgia, irritability, or anorexia may persist or recur for many months. Recovery is usually prompt if acute tularemia is treated with antibiotics before the third week of disease. When therapy is delayed beyond this period, patients are more likely to be left with mild debilitation that is unresponsive to further administration of antimicrobial drugs.

Recovery from tularemia is usually followed by immunity in the sense that recurrence of severe disease is unlikely. However, immunity to reinfection is not complete, and several instances of second, even third attacks of tularemia have been recorded. Almost invariably, they have consisted of the development of a local lesion and mild regional adenopathy without systemic symptoms and with little or no fever.

Laboratory Findings. Agglutinins for *P. tularensis* are present in serum after the second week of illness. Although it has been said that cross agglutination may occur with antigens of *Brucella*, this is by no means a constant finding.

Pasteurella tularensis can be recovered from the infected patient by appropriate cultures or animal inoculation. It is rarely found in blood cultures, but it can be isolated from the mucocutaneous ulcer or regional lymph nodes with regularity. The organism has been cultured from the sputum and gastric washings in several patients, some of whom have shown no roentgenographic evidence of pneumonitis; this can be a useful diagnostic procedure. Although *P. tularensis* is highly infectious, the hazards of isolating it have been overemphasized, and with reasonable care, accidental infection of personnel in diagnostic laboratories is unlikely.

Skin test with a diluted suspension of killed *P. tularensis*, or purified antigen, becomes positive during the first week of disease. The cutaneous hypersensitivity response is "delayed" and resembles the tuberculin reaction.

The total blood leukocyte count is usually normal. The erythrocyte sedimentation rate is normal in ulceroglandular or mild disease but is frequently elevated in severe typhoidal tularemia.

Differential Diagnosis. Brucellosis, typhoid fever, disseminated tuberculosis, the early stage of several rickettsial diseases, and infectious mononucleosis can closely resemble typhoidal tularemia. History of possible contacts is important, and appropriate serologic and cultural studies are usually successful in differentiating these infections. Pneumonic tularemia must be distinguished from viral, mycotic, and other bacterial infections of the lung. The differential diagnosis of pneumonia is discussed on p. 890. Oculoglandular syndromes likely to be confused with tularemia are described on p. 890.

The common ulceroglandular type of tularemia must be distinguished from a variety of infections in which a *local cutaneous ulcer with regional lymphadenopathy* can occur. Besides ordinary pyoderma caused by streptococci or staphylococci, these include lymphogranuloma venereum, cat-scratch fever, rat-bite fever, bubonic plague, anthrax, glanders, several rickettsioses of which the important one in this country is rickettsialpox, several viral infections of the skin such as orf, cowpox, etc., and inoculation syphilis or tuberculosis. In all these, with the exception of lymphogranuloma venereum and cat-scratch fever, the regional lymph node involvement is usually proportional to the size of the cutaneous ulcer. Extragenital lymphogranuloma is rare; fever and systemic symptoms in cat-scratch fever are rarely severe for more than a few days.

Treatment. Streptomycin is the antibiotic of choice for tularemia. The dosage is 0.5 to 1.0 Gm every 12 hr for 10 days. Response to treatment is almost invariably prompt, with the temperature usually returning to normal in 3 days. *Pasteurella tularensis* cannot be recovered from lymph nodes or skin lesions after 24 to 48 hr of therapy. However, the regional lymph nodes may continue to enlarge and suppurate for several days. Pulmonary lesions usually subside rapidly, although the evolution of the cutaneous lesion is not interrupted. The tetracycline antibiotics, chloramphenicol, and novobiocin also are effective, although fever and other manifestations may recur 7 to 14 days after cessation of therapy. Recrudescent illness, however, responds rapidly to readministration of the antibiotic. Aspiration of pus from suppurating nodes rarely is necessary; but if fistulas persist, total surgical removal of the involved tissue can be carried out. Surgery may be followed by transient recurrence of fever despite failure to demonstrate the organism in excised tissues.

Prophylaxis. A killed bacterial vaccine developed by Foshay has been shown to stimulate serum agglutinins and induces positive skin reactions to the bacterial antigens, but produces little immunity to infection with *P. tularensis*. An attenuated live bacterial strain prepared in Russia has been developed, however, and shown to be effective in inducing protection against infection. The live attenuated vaccine undoubtedly will replace the killed vaccine for prevention of tularemia in hunters, butchers, and laboratory workers exposed to the organism.

Antibiotic prophylaxis with streptomycin following exposure to tularemia will protect against infection. Chloramphenicol and tetracycline, however, only prolong the incubation period of the disease and do not prevent its occurrence.

Avoidance of contact with possible sources of infection is important in prevention, and the incidence of tularemia in several localities has fallen sharply with the introduction of laws prohibiting the sale of wild rabbits by butchers.

Prognosis. The mortality rate in untreated tularemia is 6 to 7 per cent. However, with specific antimicrobial therapy, death is rare. A fatal outcome is more likely in typhoidal tularemia than in other types, possibly because the disease may be unrecognized.

REFERENCES

Eigelsbach, H. T., C. M. Downs, and R. O. Herring: Comparative Immunogenicity of Live and Killed

Tularemia Vaccines for the Mouse and Guinea Pig, Bacteriol. Proc., 74:1958.

Foshay, L.: Treatment of Tularemia with Streptomycin, Am. J. Med., 2:467, 1947.

Francis, E.: Tularemia, in "Oxford Medicine," New York, Oxford University Press, 1948.

McCrumb, F. R., Jr., M. I. Snyder, and T. E. Woodward: Studies on Human Infection with *Pasteurella tularensis:* Comparison of Streptomycin and Chloramphenicol in the Prophylaxis of Clinical Disease, Trans. Assoc. Am. Phys., 70:74, 1957.

Stuart, B. M., and R. L. Pullen: Tularemic Pneumonia: Review of American Literature and Report of Fifteen Additional Cases, Am. J. Med. Sci., 210:233, 1945.

Woodward, T. E., W. T. Raby, W. Eppes, W. A. Holbrook, and J. A. Hightower: Aureomycin in Treatment of Experimental and Human Tularemia, J.A.M.A., 139:830, 1949.

131 PLAGUE
Edward S. Miller

Definition. Human plague is an acute, severe, frequently fatal infection characterized by fever, prostration, and suppurative lesions of the lymphatic system. Sometimes there is an associated pneumonia. *Pasteurella pestis* is the etiologic agent, rodents are the primary hosts, and the usual vectors are fleas.

History. Plague is one of the ancient pestilences of man. Descriptions of a plaguelike disease are found in the Old Testament. Early Greek and Roman manuscripts testify to its existence in the Mediterranean region long before the Christian era. For many centuries the disease was endemic in Asia and in Europe, where from time to time great pandemics destroyed large segments of the human population. The last major outbreak originated in China in the late nineteenth century, spread to all the continents, and was first recognized in the United States in 1900. Some authorities believe that it was initially introduced into this country at that time through the Port of San Francisco. However, other evidence suggests that rodent plague actually was present long before. In any event, it has certainly now become well established.

Etiologic Agent. *Pasteurella pestis* is an encapsulated, nonmotile, gram-negative bacterium which produces no spores and will grow under either aerobic or anaerobic conditions. Though it is predominantly bacillary in shape, coccal, ovoid, and other pleomorphic forms are often seen. When stained with carbolfuchsin or carbolthionin, the organisms display a characteristic bipolar appear-

ance. Growth occurs on ordinary media. On agar the colonies are small, round, transparent, colorless, and viscous. There are no important antigenic differences among strains collected from different animal species in various parts of the world.

Epidemiology. As with other infectious organisms spread through the agency of vectors, *P. pestis* is enabled to survive and be transmitted by means of a series of intricate ecologic adaptations. Plague is fundamentally an affection of rodents; from them it is sometimes, and quite incidentally, transmitted to man. In so far as human plague is concerned, domestic rats (*Rattus rattus* and *R. norvegicus*) are the most important animal hosts. They are found all over the world, travel widely, and live in close association with man. In rural or wooded regions in many areas of the world, plague is enzootic in numerous other species of vertebrate hosts, chiefly rodents. Such infection is referred to as *sylvatic plague*, in contrast to *rat* or *murine plague*. In the United States the endemic reservoir encompasses at least 38 species, including rats, mice, marmots, owls, gophers, badgers, rabbits, prairie dogs, squirrels, and chipmunks. Worldwide, the list has been expanded to 344 species of mammals and 2 species of birds, which have been naturally infected, experimentally infected, or have been found to harbor infected fleas.

Murine plague and sylvatic plague follow different but sometimes overlapping patterns. The chief permanent reservoirs of disease are in the rural rodents and their ectoparasites. Certain species are relatively resistant and thus maintain a smoldering nidus of infection through interepidemic periods. An epizootic of sylvatic plague in an area may involve a number of different animal species and a complex exchange of ectoparasites. Such outbreaks may be devastating to the rodent populations, yet may give rise only to sporadic human cases simply because man rarely comes into close contact with these animals. Since 1900 approximately 500 cases of human plague have been reported in the United States, of which less than 100 have resulted from contact with rural rodents; the remainder developed in association with domestic rats. Plague is widely and permanently entrenched in the rodent population of the United States, chiefly in the West, as well as in western Mexico and Canada. Infected animals have been found in California, Oregon, Washington, Utah, Idaho, Nevada, New Mexico, Texas, Louisiana, Florida, Michigan, Arizona, Colorado, Montana, Wyoming, Kansas, and North Dakota. Human cases have occurred in the first eleven of these states.

As indicated above, most cases of human plague arise in urban areas and in the wake of rat epizootics. Under circumstances of poor sanitation, a concentration of people and of rats provides an opportunity for the transmigration of fleas from rats to man. It is becoming increasingly apparent that domestic rat populations in the United States tended to acquire their infections by commingling with rural rodent reservoirs. Sylvatic plague is impossible to eradicate and offers a constant threat of extension into urban rat communities, and thence to man.

The flea is the usual transmitting agent. In murine and human infections the most important species is the Oriental rat flea, *Xenopsylla cheopis*. Other arthropods occasionally function as vectors, including lice, ticks, and possibly bedbugs. The flea becomes infected by ingesting the blood of a bacteremic animal. The organisms multiply in the alimentary tract of the insect and eventually plug the stomach so that no more blood can enter. When the flea feeds on a new host, the bite wound is inoculated by the regurgitation of organisms or as a result of mechanical contamination by the mouth parts. Plague bacilli are also present in flea feces, and infection may follow the scratching of this material into the skin. Oriental rat fleas will accept other hosts, including man, particularly if rats are not immediately available. When an epizootic decimates the rat population, fleas are encouraged to transfer from the dead hosts to humans.

Human bubonic plague results chiefly from the bite of the rat flea, but infection can also be acquired by direct contact with the tissues of an infected animal or by its bite. The organisms can penetrate through skin abrasions and through intact mucous membranes. Not a few accidental infections have occurred in laboratory workers as a result of handling cultures and infected animals. Direct transmission of the bubonic form from man to man is unusual, in contradistinction to the mode of spread of primary pneumonic plague. The latter type of epidemic is initiated by a patient with bubonic disease who develops a secondary plague pneumonia and thereafter excretes large quantities of organisms in his sputum. The infection may then be air-borne in droplet nuclei directly to a human contact. This type of plague is highly contagious, secondary cases are common among those attending a patient, and under suitable circumstances, tremendous outbreaks may occur.

A close relationship exists between the distribution of murine plague and that of the Oriental rat flea. This flea flourishes under certain optimal climatic conditions, which are found in the United States along the Pacific Coast and the Gulf, in the southern Atlantic Coast states, and in certain valleys radiating from these regions. Sylvatic plague involves other arthropod vectors and other animal hosts and, therefore, has a somewhat different and wider distribution. Since susceptible hosts exist in all parts of the country, the appearance of this disease elsewhere is a possibility, especially under circumstances of a national disaster.

Pathogenesis. Following the bite of an infected flea, organisms are carried by the lymphatics to the thoracic duct and thence to the blood stream. There is a brief initial bacteremia, during which organisms are disseminated to all the organs. The chief defense of the body is the mechanism of phagocytosis, aided by the development of circulating antibodies, which react with the capsular substance of the organisms and thus facilitate phagocytosis. Plague infection is accompanied by the production of an endotoxin which has seriously damaging effects on the tissues of the host. Modern chemotherapeutic agents may result in control of the infection bacteriologically, yet the patient may die from the toxemia.

The most prominent lesions are ordinarily in the lymphatic system. In bubonic plague a hemorrhagic zone of edema surrounds an inflamed and suppurating group of regional lymph glands. The latter are hyperplastic and show areas of focal necrosis containing many organisms. Similar metastatic lesions may develop in distant groups of glands or in other viscera. In pulmonic infections there is a lobular pneumonia with hemorrhagic exudate in the alveolar spaces, with accompanying pleuritis and bronchitis. Hemorrhages may be found in any organ or beneath epithelial surfaces.

Manifestations. Symptoms appear after an incubation period of 1 to 12 days. The disease can assume several different clinical forms, of which the *bubonic* variety is the most common. Illness begins abruptly, with chills, a rise in temperature to 102 to 105°F, tachycardia, headache, vomiting, uncertain gait, marked prostration, and delirium. The spleen is sometimes palpable. The fleabite which represents the portal of entry rarely can be seen; if present it is marked by a papule or vesicle which ultimately becomes pustular. Pain and tenderness point to the regional glandular lesions, which give the disease its name. They are in the inguinal or femoral regions in the majority of cases, less often in the axilla or neck, and are uncommon elsewhere. The infection may extend secondarily to other superficial or deeply situated groups of glands. The bubo consists of a firm, matted group of glands, measuring 2 to 5 cm in diameter, and surrounded by a boggy and frequently hemorrhagic zone of edema. It usually suppurates and drains spontaneously after 1 or 2 weeks, though in some instances there is complete resorption.

There is a marked hemorrhagic tendency, presumably due to an endotoxic effect on blood vessels. Petechiae or ecchymoses are often seen beneath cutaneous or mucous surfaces. Bleeding may occur into a viscus or a serous cavity, or from the nose, alimentary, respiratory, or urinary tracts.

The course of bubonic plague is marked by an irregular or remittent fever. It often drops at the time of appearance of the bubo, only to rise again. In favorable cases the temperature falls gradually during the second week, concomitant with improvement in the general clinical condition. A rise to hyperpyrexic levels, or a precipitous fall to normal or to subnormal, frequently heralds approaching death. Most fatalities occur during the first week of illness. Though bubonic plague is usually a severe illness, mild cases are sometimes seen during epidemics; to these is applied the name *pestis minor*.

The second clinical form of plague is the so-called "primary septicemic" form, which is actually a variant of bubonic plague. The patient experiences a sudden and overwhelming systemic illness. There is a marked constitutional reaction, with chills, fever, rapid pulse, severe headache, nausea, vomiting, and delirium. Death terminates the course within a few days, before localizing lesions become clinically apparent. Nevertheless, autopsy usually reveals inflammation in some part of the lymphatic system.

The third form which plague may take is that of *pneumonia*. The initial cases appear in patients with bubonic plague, of whom as many as 5 per cent develop secondary lesions in the lungs. These individuals may provide the starting point for a man-to-man epidemiologic cycle of air-borne primary pneumonic plague. It is a fulminating infection accompanied by great prostration, cough, dyspnea, and, in the later stages, cyanosis. The sputum is abundant, bloodstained, and teeming with *P. pestis*. Often there are no clear-cut pulmonary signs, though scattered rales or areas of dullness may be found. In the absence of specific therapy, plague pneumonia invariably ends in death within 1 to 5 days.

The infectious process may localize in other regions of the body. Subcutaneous abscesses and cutaneous ulcerations sometimes occur, and the meninges are occasionally invaded.

Laboratory Findings. Since plague is an uncommon disease in the United States, the diagnosis often has been overlooked until the patient has succumbed, or until multiple cases have developed. Nevertheless, the epidemiology and the clinical features provide highly characteristic leads to the clinician. Once a suspicion of plague is entertained, it can readily be verified by smear, culture, and animal inoculation of appropriate specimens. The technique of staining a suspected specimen with fluorescent specific antiserum provides an elegant method for rapid identification of *P. pestis*. If a bubo is present, a small quantity of interstitial fluid should be aspirated from its center. Large numbers of morphologically characteristic bacilli are usually seen in a stained smear. Infected sputum likewise contains many organisms. Bacteremia of varying degrees occurs at some time during the course of the disease in nearly all cases. Pus and sputum should be cultured on blood agar plates, while blood is inoculated into hormone-cystine or other nutrient broth. Organisms are identified by their morphologic and colonial characteristics and by agglutination with specific antiserum. Guinea pig inoculation is the final step in identification. In this animal the gross and microscopic lesions are highly characteristic. It is to be emphasized that the handling of infected materials or animals involves great danger of infection of the laboratory workers. Hemagglutinating antibody appears in the serum of patients and provides another diagnostic method.

The white blood cell count is elevated to levels of 20,000 to 40,000 cells per cu mm, with a predominance of polymorphonuclear leukocytes. There is little or no change in the red blood corpuscles.

Differential Diagnosis. Before the appearance of localizing signs, plague may be confused with severe systemic illnesses such as typhoid or typhus. The bubonic form bears certain resemblances to other varieties of infectious lymphadenitis, including tularemia, syphilis, and lymphogranuloma venereum, and to those of staphylococcal or streptococcal origin. Pneumonic plague must be distinguished from tularemic, pneumococcal, and other bacterial pneumonias, as well as from psittacosis and primary atypical pneumonia. A consideration of epidemiologic factors, plus bacteriologic studies, will aid in the differentiation.

Treatment. The therapy and the prognosis of plague have been vastly improved by the introduction of streptomycin and other chemotherapeutic agents. Even pneumonic and septicemic cases can be salvaged if treatment is initiated early (within the first 20 hr after onset). Streptomycin is the drug of choice; it is given in divided doses of 2 to 4 Gm daily until the patient has been afebrile at least 3 days. Sulfadiazine is almost as effective in uncomplicated bubonic plague, but definitely less so in septicemic and pneumonic cases. Chloramphenicol, oxytetracycline, chlortetracycline, neomycin, and polymyxin are all potent antiplague substances; the first two have been used successfully in treating pneumonic plague. Antiplague serum also has value as an antitoxic agent. Various combinations of these medicines can be used to advantage, depending on their availability, the severity of illness, and the duration of illness before treatment is begun.

Buboes are treated with hot, moist applications.

Incision and drainage should be postponed until the lesion becomes well localized.

Prophylaxis and Control. The control of plague in endemic urban areas demands unceasing vigilance in detecting rodent epizootics and vigorous measures in combating such outbreaks. These include the extermination of rats, the eradication of ectoparasite vectors, and sometimes the immunization of the human population. Rats are attacked by poisoning and trapping, by elimination of harborage areas, and by separating them from their food supplies. DDT has been used with brilliant success in diminishing the flea population infesting both rodents and humans. Other insecticides such as Aldrin, Dieldrin, and Chlordane are also useful. The complete elimination of sylvatic plague is an impossibility. The object of a control program is limited to the eradication of foci of wild rodent infection around areas of human habitation. In these peripheral zones the wild and the domestic rodents live commensally, exchange fleas, and thus threaten the human community.

Patients must be disinfested and carefully isolated, while other intimately exposed persons should be quarantined. Excellent prophylaxis is provided to contacts by administering sulfadiazine in a dose of 3 Gm per day or streptomycin in a dose of 1 Gm per day. This often protects even against exposure to pneumonic patients. Three types of vaccines are used, one composed of dead organisms, one containing an avirulent live strain of organism, and the third consisting of a chemical extract. They each provide limited and transitory immunity. General vaccination of a population is a worthwhile procedure in an area under serious threat of an epidemic.

Prognosis. Formerly the fatality rate of bubonic plague varied from 50 to 90 per cent, while the pneumonic, septicemic, and meningitic forms were almost invariably fatal. However, even the gravest varieties of infection respond to chemotherapy if treated early enough. The over-all fatality rate has been reduced to 5 to 10 per cent.

REFERENCES

Girard, G.: Plague, Ann. Rev. Microbiol., 69:253, 1955.

Hirst, L. F.: "The Conquest of Plague: A Study of the Evolution of Epidemiology," New York, Oxford University Press, 1953.

Kartman, L., F. M. Prince, S. F. Quan, and H. E. Stark: New Knowledge on the Ecology of Sylvatic Plague, Ann. N.Y. Acad. Sci., 70:668, 1958.

Meyer, K. F., S. F. Quan, F. R. McCrumb, and A. Larson: Effective Treatment of Plague, Ann. N.Y. Acad. Sci., 55:1228, 1952.

Pollitzer, R.: "Plague," World Health Organization Monograph Series, No. 22, Geneva, 1954.

132   GLANDERS
Edward S. Miller

Definition and Etiology. Glanders is a grave infectious disorder characterized by the development of numerous granulomatous abscesses throughout the body. The causative agent is *Malleomyces mallei* (*Actinobacillus mallei*), a small aerobic, nonmotile, nonsporulating, gram-negative bacillus.

Epidemiology and Pathogenesis. This is another of the group of infectious diseases of animals which are sometimes transmitted to man. In this instance, the principal natural hosts are horses, mules, and asses. Glanders once was a common equine disease in America, but stringent control measures have virtually eradicated it. However, it is still prevalent in certain sections of Central Europe, North Africa, and Asia. The infection may be acquired by handling diseased animals. Organisms gain entry through cutaneous abrasions, by implantation on the conjunctiva, by ingestion, or by inhalation. Human beings are highly susceptible, as evidenced by the large number of laboratory workers who have contracted the disease. With the elimination of animal glanders in the United States, the infection has become rare in man also.

Manifestations. Human glanders usually runs an acute and stormy course. After an incubation period of several days to several weeks, illness begins abruptly, with chills, high fever, and marked prostration. At the portal of entry, commonly on the skin, a nodule forms and breaks down to become a painful ulcer. Such ulcers show irregular, sharply demarcated borders, with little tendency to heal. The regional lymph nodes are involved, and lymphatic and vascular dissemination soon results in a generalized spread. Miliary lesions develop along the course of lymphatics, in subcutaneous and submucous tissues, in muscle, in the lungs, and in other viscera. The lesions gradually enlarge, coalesce, and undergo central caseous necrosis. The superficial nodules ulcerate, while more deeply situated abscesses often form fistulous tracts which exude discharges onto the surface. Areas of consolidation appear in the lungs, and the liver and the spleen become inflamed and enlarged. Many patients exhibit ulcerations of the upper respiratory tract with erosion of adjacent cartilaginous and bony structures. An eruption sometimes becomes evident, either localized to one area or generally distributed. At first it is a macular rash, then it becomes papular and pustular, and the lesions may ulcerate. Among other septic manifestations are meningitis, osteomyelitis, and purulent polyarthritis. Infection may extend to the sinuses, ears, conjunctiva, mouth, pharynx, and trachea.

Acute glanders progresses with great rapidity, ending fatally in 1 to 3 weeks in the majority of cases. A milder syndrome has been described in a group of laboratory workers who were accidentally infected via the respiratory tract. In these cases, the clinical picture was not unlike that of viral pneumonia of average severity, and all patients recovered.

A chronic form of glanders sometimes is seen. The onset is generally insidious, with low-grade fever and mild initial symptoms. The course is characterized by exacerbations and remissions and punctuated by the irregular appearance of painful ulcers and draining abscesses. Chronic glanders may at any time assume the fulminating qualities of the acute form. More than half the patients die after months or years of exhausting illness.

Diagnosis. Specific diagnosis can be established by culture, by animal inoculation, by serologic testing, by the demonstration of dermal sensitivity, and by biopsy. *Malleomyces mallei* can be recovered from exudates, sputum, scrapings from a local lesion, and terminally from the blood. Straus's reaction is elicited by injecting infected material into the peritoneal cavity of a male hamster or a male guinea pig. Scrotal swelling becomes apparent in 2 to 4 days, and organisms then can be recovered from the tunica vaginalis. Both agglutinating and complement-fixing antibodies appear in the blood during the second to fourth weeks of illness; they are specific when present in high titer (agglutination titer of 1:640 or higher; complement-fixing titer of 1:20 or higher), except for some cross reaction with the antigens of *Pseudomonas pseudomallei*. The latter organism causes melioidosis, a disease closely related to glanders (see Chap. 133). Patients who survive the initial onslaught of illness develop a persistent skin sensitivity to mallein, which is an antigen prepared from cultures of *M. mallei*. The test is performed by intradermal injection of 0.1 ml of a 1:10,000 dilution of commercial mallein; it is considered positive if an erythema is present 48 hr later. Skin and mucous membrane lesions show characteristic histologic features and are readily accessible to biopsy.

Treatment. Sulfadiazine has proved to be a potent chemotherapeutic agent in experimental animal infections and has been used successfully in several human cases. The drug should be administered for a minimum of 20 days, in doses sufficient to maintain blood levels of 10 to 15 mg per 100 ml. Penicillin is ineffectual. Streptomycin was of only slight benefit in an experimental study but appeared to be useful in the treatment of one reported human case. Little or no information is available on the therapeutic activity of the newer antibiotics. It is evident that strains isolated from patients should be subjected to careful studies of in vitro sensitivities, and treatment should be guided thereby. Other antibiotics, singly or in combination, may prove even more effective than sulfadiazine. It is probable that prolonged administration of antimicrobial agents will be necessary to eradicate infection and to prevent relapses.

REFERENCES

Howe, C., and W. R. Miller: Human Glanders: Report of Six Cases, Ann. Internal Med., 26:93, 1947.

McGilvray, C. D.: Glanders, p. 119–133 in "Diseases Transmitted from Animals to Man," 3d ed., T. G. Hull (Ed.), Springfield, Ill., Charles C Thomas, Publisher, 1947.

Miller, W. R., L. Pannell, L. Cravitz, W. A. Tanner, and M. S. Ingalls: Studies on Certain Biological Characteristics of *Malleomyces mallei* and *Malleomyces pseudomallei*: I. Morphology, Cultivation, Viability, and Isolation from Contaminated Specimens, J. Bacteriol., 55:115, 1948.

——, —— and M. S. Ingalls: Experimental Chemotherapy in Glanders and Melioidosis, Am. J. Hyg., 47:205, 1948.

133 MELIOIDOSIS
Edward S. Miller

Definition. Melioidosis is a fulminating, usually fatal, infectious disease in which granulomatous lesions develop throughout the body. Etiologically, pathologically, and clinically it bears a striking resemblance to glanders.

Etiology. The causative organism is *Pseudomonas pseudomallei* (until recently designated as *Malleomyces pseudomallei*), a motile, aerobic, gram-negative bacillus. This bacterium is closely related to *Malleomyces mallei* (*Actinobacillus mallei*), the causative agent of glanders, but the two can be differentiated by bacteriologic and serologic methods. They are also epidemiologically dissimilar, for glanders is principally a disease of horses, whereas melioidosis is found in other species (see below). The organism also resembles *Pseudomonas aeruginosa*. In tissues the pathologic lesion produced is a tiny pus-filled abscess with a granulomatous margin.

Epidemiology. The disease was first identified in Rangoon in 1911, and over 300 human cases have since been reported, chiefly from Indo-China, the Malay States, Thailand, Ceylon, and contiguous regions. There are indications that the geographic distribution is actually much broader, for a few human cases have been reported as originating in the United States, Panama, Guam, and the Philippine Islands. Infected animals have been found in

Australia, Madagascar, and the Netherland Antilles (near South America). The principal reservoir of melioidosis is said to be in rats, but this has not been proved. Natural infections have been found in a number of animal species, including rats, rabbits, sheep, goats, horses, swine, cats, and dogs. It has been suggested that disease is transmitted via food and water contaminated by excreta and fomites of rodents, the usual portal of entry being the alimentary tract. Organisms have been recovered from surface waters. Man to man transmission has not been known to occur.

Manifestations. The clinical course of melioidosis is much like glanders, except that it is even more virulent and lethal. Nearly all cases not treated with antimicrobial agents have ended fatally. In the most acute form (90 per cent of reported cases), illness is sudden in onset, with shaking chills, high fever, and marked prostration, often associated with vomiting and severe diarrhea. Bacteremia occurs early and results in the development of widely disseminated granulomatous abscesses. The patient passes into a state of stupor and dies within 3 to 4 days. In subacute cases, the course of disease is similar except that the patient survives sufficiently long (3 to 4 weeks) for some of the disseminated lesions to become clinically evident. These are likely to develop in the lungs, bones, liver, spleen, skin, and subcutaneous tissues. Pyelonephritis, orchitis, epididymitis, and prostatitis sometimes are seen. A pustular rash has been observed. In rare cases melioidosis becomes chronic, with deep-seated lesions and draining sinuses which persist for years. A few cases have been apparently cured.

Diagnosis. Cultural methods afford the best means of prompt diagnosis. *Pseudomonas pseudomallei* can be recovered from blood, sputum, exudates, and urine. As in glanders, Straus's reaction can be elicited by intraperitoneal injection of infected material into male hamsters or guinea pigs. The agglutination and complement fixation tests become positive in 2 to 4 weeks. The white blood cell count ranges from normal up to 20,000 cells per cu mm. Biopsy specimens reveal characteristic changes indistinguishable from those seen in glanders.

Treatment. The reported fatality rate of 95 per cent attests to the inefficacy of older methods of treatment. Localized lesions should be incised and drained. Experimental studies and a few clinical reports indicate that chloramphenicol, sulfonamides, tetracyclines, novobiocin, penicillin, and streptomycin exhibit some antimicrobial activity, but there is great variation in strain susceptibility and in clinical response. It is imperative that treatment be guided by prompt identification of the organism and by in vitro sensitivity tests. In a disease as dangerous as this it is justifiable to use multiple antibiotics and to administer them for long periods of time.

REFERENCES

Couture, E. L.: La melioidose: état actuel de la question, Rev. hyg. et méd. prévent., 57:190, 1935.

Garry, M. W., and M. L. Koch: Chronic Melioidosis: Bacteriologic and Clinical Correlation and Diagnosis, J. Lab. Clin. Med., 38:374, 1951.

Miller, W. R., L. Pannell, L. Cravitz, W. A. Tanner, and M. S. Ingalls: Studies on Certain Biological Characteristics of *Malleomyces mallei* and *Malleomyces pseudomallei:* I. Morphology, Cultivation, Viability, and Isolation from Contaminated Specimens, J. Bacteriol., 55:115, 1948.

Prevatt, A. L., and J. S. Hunt: Chronic Systemic Melioidosis, Am. J. Med., 23:810, 1959.

134　VIBRIO FETUS INFECTION

Robert G. Petersdorf and Ivan L. Bennett, Jr.

Vibrio fetus is an important cause of infectious abortion in sheep and cattle, which occasionally produces disease in man.

Etiology. The etiologic agent, *V. fetus*, is a motile, comma-shaped or spirillar, gram-negative rod with a single unipolar flagellum. Identification is best made on smears from cultured material. The organism grows well in trypticase soy broth under increased carbon dioxide tension. Several serotypes have been isolated by agglutination with antiserums from both human and bovine strains. Cross agglutination reactions occur with other bacterial species, particularly *Brucella abortus*.

Epidemiology. Vibriosis is a venereal infection of cattle, sheep, and goats and is transmitted to gravid heifers or ewes, resulting in abortion. Although the male does not become symptomatic, he acts as a carrier of *V. fetus* which has been isolated from the genitalia and semen of bulls. Vibriosis in man is probably rare, 17 cases having been reported prior to 1960. Farmers and meat handlers have been infected occasionally, but the majority of patients have not been in direct contact with animals. There is no evidence that *V. fetus* is transmitted to man through milk. Because some patients have developed endocarditis with *V. fetus* following dental extraction, the mouth has been postulated as the portal of entry of the organism. In the majority of instances, however, the mode of infection in man is obscure.

Manifestations. Vibriosis in man can present a variety of clinical syndromes. Fever is uniformly present, but the remainder of the clinical picture varies widely. Three women were pregnant, and two of the three aborted or delivered prematurely. Three patients had classical signs and symptoms of subacute bacterial endocarditis, and in two the illness followed dental extractions. In two others vibrio infections were indistinguishable from brucellosis. Thrombophlebitis associated with fever was a prominent finding in four cases; both upper and lower extremities were involved.

Diagnosis. Identification of the organism in smears from cultures is the only definitive method of making the diagnosis. Failure to incubate blood cultures under increased CO_2 tension may delay correct identification of the organism. Agglutination by specific antiserums strongly supports the diagnosis of *V. fetus* infection. On clinical grounds, vibriosis should be suspected in pregnant women with chills and fever, particularly in association with abortion or premature delivery, farmers and slaughterhouse workers with obscure febrile illnesses, and patients with fever and thrombophlebitis. Despite a high index of suspicion, the diagnosis will come as a surprise to the clinician most of the time.

Treatment. *Vibrio fetus* has been found to be sensitive to tetracycline, chloramphenicol, streptomycin, kanamycin, erythromycin, and sulfadiazine. Penicillin, novobiocin, vancomycin, and polymyxin B are ineffective. A 10-day course of tetracycline in dosage of 2.0 Gm per day coupled with streptomycin 1.0 Gm per day will probably eradicate the organisms in most instances. In cases of endocarditis this regimen should be continued for 6 weeks.

REFERENCES

Kahler, R. L., and H. Sheldon: *Vibrio fetus* Infection in Man, N. Engl. J. Med., 262:1218, 1960.

Spink, W. W.: Human Vibriosis Caused by *Vibrio fetus*, J.A.M.A., 163:18, 1957.

135 *MIMA POLYMORPHA* INFECTIONS

Robert G. Petersdorf and Ivan L. Bennett, Jr.

Mima polymorpha is a gram-negative pleomorphic organism, which is easily confused with members of the genus *Neisseria*. It has been isolated from patients with meningitis, subacute bacterial endocarditis, and fulminating septicemia.

Etiology. *Mima polymorpha*, described by De Bord in 1939, is one of three species within the tribe Mimae, the others being *Herellea vaginicola* and *Colloides anoxydana*. More recently *Bacterium anitratum* and a fifth species B5W, both closely related to the tribe Mimae, have been classified with this group and the five species assigned to the family Parvobacteriaceae. These organisms are pleomorphic, gram-negative, encapsulated, and of variable motility. They grow well on ordinary media, forming white, convex, smooth colonies. Diplococcal forms predominate in colonies grown on solid media, while rods and filamentous forms are more common in liquid media. The species can be differentiated from one another by their capacity to attack different carbohydrates and give a negative oxidase reaction, separating them from the neisseria, from which they can also be distinguished by means of specific typing serums.

Epidemiology and Pathogenesis. Mimas have been recovered from a variety of human sources including vaginal, urethral, and conjunctival secretions; war wounds, chancroid lesions, and urine; sputum, blood, brain, meninges, cerebrospinal fluid, petechiae and bone marrow, and synovial fluid. Although they have been incriminated as causes of conjunctivitis, vaginitis, and nongonococcal urethritis, they have also been found in the conjunctiva, vagina, and urethra of many normal persons, casting doubt upon their significance as a cause of infection in these sites. In contrast, mimas have been cultured from well-documented cases of meningitis, endocarditis, and septicemia, *Mima polymorpha* being the causative pathogen in most instances. The upper respiratory tract was the presumed portal of entry in most of these cases. In one patient with subacute bacterial endocarditis the infection emanated from the prostate.

Manifestations. Meningitis caused by *M. polymorpha* closely resembles meningitis caused by the more common pathogens, such as meningococcus (p. 924) and pneumococcus (p. 887) and cannot be differentiated from them on clinical grounds. Subacute bacterial endocarditis has usually been reported in patients with congenital or rheumatic heart disease and tends to pursue an indolent course; one patient had symptoms for 18 months. Occasionally *M. polymorpha* may be the cause of fulminating septicemia characterized by high fever, marked toxicity, vascular collapse, petechiae, and ecchymoses, indistinguishable from the Waterhouse-Friderichsen syndrome. One such patient showed adrenal hemorrhages at autopsy. *Bacterium anitratum* has also been implicated as a cause of bacteremia in patients with Laennec's cirrhosis and of urinary tract infections. It does not seem likely that either mimas or *B. anitratum* are important causes of vaginitis, urethritis, and purulent conjunctivitis.

Diagnosis. The diagnosis depends upon isolation of the organism from blood, cerebrospinal fluid, or urine. Mimas have been reported only rarely in cultures from patients with meningitis or subacute bacterial endocarditis, probably because most strains are identified as *Neisseria meningitidis.* In fact, the name Mimae was chosen because of the organisms' tendency to mimic other more common gram-negative species. The separation of mimas from neisserias is of more than academic importance since the antibiotic sensitivities of the two groups differ considerably. *Mima polymorpha* can be differentiated from other species of the tribe as well as neisserias by its inability to ferment carbohydrates. In general, mimas give a negative oxidase reaction. The development of type-specific antiserums affords the simplest and most accurate method for differentiating mimas from neisserias.

Treatment. Most strains of Mimae have been sensitive to oxytetracycline and chlortetracycline and resistant to penicillin and streptomycin. Sensitivity to chloramphenicol and the sulfonamides has been variable. Oxytetracycline in dosage of 2.0 Gm per day orally or 100 mg every 6 hr intramuscularly would seem to be the drug of choice in *M. polymorpha* meningitis or endocarditis. Sensitivity to the newer antibiotics, kanamycin and colistin, has not been determined.

REFERENCES

De Bord, G. G.: Descriptions of Mimae Tribe with Three Genera and Three Species and Two New Species of Neisseria from Conjunctivitis and Vaginitis, Iowa State Coll. J. Sci., 16:471, 1942.

Minzter, A.: Human Infection Caused by the Mimae Organisms: Report of Case of a Presumably Healed Bacterial Endocarditis Due to *Herellea vaginicola*, A.M.A. Arch. Internal Med., 98:352, 1956.

Olaffson, M., C. Y. Lee, and G. J. Abernethy: *Mima polymorpha* Meningitis, N. Engl. J. Med., 258:456, 1958.

Section 6: Miscellaneous Bacterial Diseases

136 ANTHRAX
Leighton E. Cluff

Definition. Anthrax (malignant pustule, charbon, splenic fever, milzbrand, woolsorter's disease) is a disease of wild and domesticated animals that is transmitted to man by contact with infected animals or their products and, rarely, by insect vectors which act as mechanical carriers of the etiologic organism. The characteristic lesion of human anthrax is a necrotic cutaneous ulcer, the "malignant pustule."

Etiology. *Bacillus anthracis* is a large, encapsulated, gram-positive, aerobic, spore-forming microorganism that grows well in most nutrient media. Its pathogenicity for laboratory animals differentiates it from *Bacillus subtilis*, which it closely resembles. The spores are killed by boiling for 10 min but can survive for many years in soil and in animal products, an important factor in persistence and spread of the disease. The anthrax bacillus possesses a capsule of glutamyl polypeptide which interferes with phagocytosis of the microorganism. In addition, it contains an anticomplementary substance and elaborates a "protective" antigen and toxin of importance probably in determining virulence.

The anthrax bacillus was identified by Royer and Davaine in sheep in 1849 and was, therefore, the first causative agent of an infectious disease ever demonstrated. The classic studies of Robert Koch in 1877, showing that *B. anthracis* was indeed the cause of anthrax, serve as the prototype for the establishment of etiology of infectious diseases.

Epidemiology. Anthrax is world-wide; repeated outbreaks have occurred in Southern Europe, Africa, Australia, Asia, and on both American continents.

Cattle, horses, sheep, goats, and swine are most commonly infected. Between 1945 and 1955, there were 3,447 recognized outbreaks of anthrax among animals in the United States, centering mostly in South Dakota, Nebraska, Arkansas, Mississippi, Louisiana, Texas, and California. The tendency of the disease to occur in animals in late summer and early fall is related to grazing conditions and the abundance of flies.

The disease in man is acquired by butchering, skinning, or dissecting infected carcasses or by handling contaminated hides, wool, hair, or other materials. It is seen principally in agricultural and industrial employees. Of the 483 reported cases of human anthrax in this country between 1945 and 1955 the majority involved workers handling imported and unprocessed wool, hair, or hides. The usual form of human disease follows inoculation of bacilli or spores into the skin, often, if not always, through a wound or abrasion. However, intestinal infection has followed ingestion of contaminated meat, and anthrax may develop after inhalation of spores.

Pathogenesis. The "malignant pustule" which follows cutaneous inoculation of anthrax organisms is characterized microscopically by vesiculation, neutrophilic infiltration, and gelatinous edema in surrounding structures. Suppuration is rare in the absence of secondary pyogenic infection. Spread of the bacilli to the regional lymph nodes may be followed by systemic dissemination. Examination of tissues from fatal human cases reveals masses of the bacteria in blood vessels, lymph nodes, parenchyma of various organs, and in connective tissues. There is scanty or absent cellular exudation at these foci, the predominant changes being widespread hemorrhage and edema. So-called "anthrax pneumonia" and "anthrax meningitis" are, in all probability, an expression of this generalized hemorrhage and edema in an easily detectable clinical site, rather than selective localization of bacterial multiplication in these tissues.

Although it was at one time thought that in anthrax death might be the result of occlusion of vessels by masses of bacilli, studies have now shown that the blood of fatally infected experimental animals contains a lethal toxin which can be neutralized by appropriately prepared antiserums. This toxin has been isolated in vitro, but its exact role in the pathogenesis of the disease requires further study.

Manifestations. The "malignant pustule" of human anthrax begins, usually on an exposed body surface, as a painless, pruritic erythematous papule, which soon vesiculates and ulcerates to form a black eschar. Tiny satellite vesicles are frequent. The ulcer may be surrounded by extensive edematous swelling, which is nontender, nonpitting, and so characteristic of anthrax that it is a valuable diagnostic sign. After about 5 days the ulcer begins to subside, but edema may persist for many days or even weeks. Mild tenderness and enlargement of regional lymph nodes is frequently present, but the involvement is not so striking as in tularemia or cat-scratch disease. Constitutional symptoms are often absent despite extensive local changes, but there may be mild fever, headache, and malaise. In the infrequent fulminant case of disseminated anthrax, high fever, prostration, and a rapidly fatal course are seen. So-called "woolsorter's disease," a highly fatal disseminated infection, is

characterized by cyanosis, dyspnea, mediastinitis, and hemoptysis, and this type of infection probably is dependent upon the pulmonary route of inoculation. As has been mentioned, human infection can occur from ingestion of the uncooked meat of infected animals. However, enormous numbers of organisms are probably necessary to produce the disease by this route in man, and it does not occur in the United States.

Laboratory Findings. The serosanguineous fluid from the cutaneous lesion frequently contains many bacilli, demonstrable by Gram's stain and culture. Bacilli may be found on direct examination or culture of the blood of patients with bacteremia. The blood leukocyte count is normal in mild cases, but there is polymorphonuclear leukocytosis in severe disease. Similarly, the erythrocyte sedimentation rate may be increased, but changes are irregular. There are no characteristic abnormalities of the urine. Patients with meningeal involvement usually show bloody spinal fluid in which the organisms are easily found by direct examination or culture.

Diagnosis. A serologic agar-gel precipitin inhibition test has been devised which has proved useful in epidemiologic studies of anthrax, showing that subclinical anthrax infection may occur in persons exposed to the microorganism in industry and demonstrating increasing serum antibody titers following immunization. A positive diagnosis of anthrax can be made by isolation of the organism in culture. However, a history of occupational exposure and characteristic eschar and edema should suggest the proper diagnosis. Pyogenic infections of the skin are usually painful, whereas the "malignant pustule" is not. In addition, cutaneous anthrax is rarely purulent. The differential diagnosis of other diseases characterized by local ulceration at the portal of entry is discussed on p. 965.

Treatment and Prophylaxis. Many antibiotics are effective in the treatment of human anthrax, including penicillin, chloramphenicol, tetracycline derivatives, erythromycin, and streptomycin. A dosage of 600,000 units of aqueous crystalline or repository penicillin should be given once or twice daily until the local edema subsides. The eschar goes through its natural evolution in spite of treatment, and lymph node enlargement may persist for several days. *Bacillus anthracis* cannot be recovered from the skin lesion after 24 to 48 hr of penicillin therapy, but it may persist for a longer period when chloramphenicol or tetracycline is used.

Exposure of personnel in industrial plants where contaminated animal products are handled still occurs in spite of measures to control it. An outbreak of inhalation anthrax with a high mortality rate was reported in a goat hair processing mill. Sterilization of all raw wool, mohair, etc., would probably remove this hazard but has had only limited application in the United States. A vaccine prepared from the "protective" antigen of *B. anthracis* is available, and it has been shown to be effective in reducing the incidence of infection in an exposed population. Spore vaccines of various types are used with good effect in domestic animals in endemic areas, but are not suitable for use in human beings.

Transmission of anthrax from one human being to another has never been recognized. Whereas the cutaneous disease was fatal in 20 to 30 per cent of cases before antimicrobial drugs were available, the mortality now is less than 1 per cent in the United States.

REFERENCES

Brachman, P. S., S. A. Plotkin, F. H. Bumford, and M. A. Atchison: An Epidemic of Inhalation Anthrax: II. Epidemiologic Investigation, M. J. Hyg., 72:6, 1960.

Gold, H.: Anthrax: Report of 117 Cases, A.M.A. Arch. Internal Med., 96:387, 1955.

Howe, C.: Anthrax, in "Oxford Medicine," New York, Oxford University Press, 1950.

Norman, P. S., J. G. Ray, P. S. Brachman, S. A. Plotkin, and J. S. Pagano: Serologic Testing for Anthrax Antibodies in Workers in a Goat Hair Processing Mill, Am. J. Hyg., 72:32, 1960.

Smith, H., and J. Keffie: Observations on Experimental Anthrax: Demonstrations of a Specific Lethal Factor Produced *in vivo* by *Bacillus anthracis*, Nature, 173:869, 1954.

137 STREPTOBACILLUS MONILIFORMIS INFECTION

Edward W. Hook and Ivan L. Bennett, Jr.

Streptobacillus moniliformis causes an acute febrile disease characterized by skin rash and arthritis. Infection is usually transmitted to man through the bite of a rat, and the disease acquired in this manner is sometimes termed "rat-bite fever." In rare instances infection is acquired by the oral route by ingestion of contaminated food or drink.

History. *Streptothrix muris ratti* was isolated from the blood of a patient with rat-bite fever by Schottmüller in 1914, and this organism, subsequently termed *Streptobacillus moniliformis*, was first isolated in the United States by Blake in 1916. Further studies showed that *Spirillum minus* was also responsible for certain cases of rat-bite fever and that the clinical manifestations of *Streptobacillus moniliformis* and *Spirillum minus* infections are sometimes indistinguishable.

Etiology. *Streptobacillus moniliformis* is a microaerophilic gram-negative bacterium that grows in artificial media as chains of bacilli of variable length interspersed with beeded or fusiform swellings. Long filamentous forms 0.4 to 0.6 μ wide growing in interwoven masses may be observed. Primary isolation is best achieved in a fluid medium such as tryptose phosphate broth enriched with 10 to 20 per cent blood or ascitic fluid. In blood cultures growth may not be apparent for 48 hr or more when it appears as minute "fluff balls" on the surface of sedimented red blood cells.

A pleuropneumonia-like L_1 (L = Lister Institute) variant can be isolated from the bacterial phase of most strains of *Streptobacillus moniliformis*. The L_1 component can be maintained in pure culture and transformed back to the bacterial phase. The L_1 variant has been isolated from the blood of man as long as 10 weeks after onset of *Streptobacillus moniliformis* infection.

Streptobacillus moniliformis is highly pathogenic for mice and chicken embryos, and in these hosts shows a striking affinity for joints and periarticular tissues where it produces arthritis and osteomyelitis.

Epidemiology. *Streptobacillus moniliformis* is a normal inhabitant of the nasopharynx of wild or laboratory rats; the carrier rate sometimes exceeds 50 per cent. Although the majority of sporadic cases of streptobacillus infection follows the bite of a wild rat, infection may be transmitted by the bite of a laboratory rat, squirrel, or weasel. Occasionally there is no history of rodent bite or animal contact. Infection with this organism occurs primarily in infants, children, and men and women whose occupations involve exposure to rats or rat-infested areas.

Streptobacillus moniliformis infection also occurs in an epidemic form related to ingestion of contaminated food or milk. The outbreak in Haverhill, Mass., in 1926 involved 86 persons and was apparently caused by streptobacillus in raw unpasteurized milk or ice cream from a single source. The clinical manifestations of food-borne infection are similar to those of sporadic cases after rat bite except for the absence of a local lesion. The names *Haverhill fever* and *erythema arthriticum epidemicum* have been applied to cases in which there was no history of rodent bite.

Streptobacillus infection is not transmitted from person to person, and isolation is not required.

Manifestations. The incubation period is short, usually 1 to 3 days, although extremes of a few hours to 22 days have been described. The onset of the disease is sudden with fever, headache, myalgia, and malaise. Chills occur in about 60 per cent of the patients. A lesion may be observed at the site of the rat bite, which is usually on an extremity, the face, or tongue. Regional lymphadenopathy may be present but is usually not a prominent feature. A discrete macular rash which fades on pressure develops 1 to 3 days after onset of symptoms in about 90 per cent of the patients. The rash is most marked on the extremities, sometimes involves the palms or soles, and may be generalized. The cutaneous lesions may occasionally become confluent, papular, pustular, or petechial. Arthritis of multiple joints appears in the majority of patients during the first week of disease. Large joints are usually involved, but small joints such as those of the fingers and toes may also be affected. The joints are swollen, hot, and tender, and effusion may occur, especially in the knees.

Manifestations of disease usually subside after about 1 week, although in the absence of antimicrobial therapy convalescence may be prolonged for several weeks because of arthritis and recurrent fever.

Bacterial endocarditis and abscess formation in brain, myocardium, or other tissues are rare but serious complications.

Laboratory Findings. The blood leukocyte count ranges from 6,000 to 30,000 cells per cu mm, but the average count is about 12,000. Differential leukocyte count may reveal an increase in the proportion of neutrophils. The platelet count is normal, although the tourniquet test may be positive. *Streptobacillus moniliformis* can usually be isolated from blood, joint fluid, or pus during the acute febrile phase of the disease and occasionally for 1 to 2 weeks after subsidence of fever. Agglutinins against *Streptobacillus moniliformis* develop during the second to third week of illness and are of diagnostic importance if an increasing titer is demonstrated. A false-positive serologic test for syphilis occurs in about 15 per cent of the cases.

Differential Diagnosis. *Streptobacillus moniliformis* and *Spirillum minus* infections both occur after rat bite and present remarkably similar manifestations. Differentiation on the basis of clinical data is difficult, sometimes impossible. However, *Streptobacillus moniliformis* infection is characterized by an incubation period that is usually less than 10 days, prompt healing of the primary lesions without flare-up at the onset of systemic symptoms, a high incidence (70 per cent) of arthritis, and a low incidence (16 per cent) of false positive serologic tests for syphilis. In contrast, *Spirillum minus* infection is distinguished by an incubation period of 1 to 4 weeks, recurrence of pain and induration at the site of the bite during the acute phase of illness, a low incidence of arthritis, and a high

incidence (51 per cent) of false positive tests for syphilis.

Streptobacillus moniliformis infection must also be differentiated from other forms of acute infectious arthritis, rheumatic fever, meningococcemia, and many other processes characterized by macular eruption and fever.

Treatment. *Streptobacillus moniliformis* infections usually respond promptly to therapy with penicillin in moderate doses. A suitable schedule for an adult is procaine penicillin, 600,000 units intramuscularly twice daily for 7 to 10 days. The organism is also sensitive to most of the other commonly used antimicrobials, and streptomycin or erythromycin can be substituted in therapy if penicillin is contraindicated. Patients with endocarditis should receive penicillin in a dose of 12 to 15 million units per day for 3 to 4 weeks.

Prognosis. The mortality rate in sporadic cases prior to the advent of effective antimicrobial therapy was about 10 per cent. Death was usually related to the presence of bacterial endocarditis and occasionally to myocarditis, myocardial abscesses, or bronchopneumonia. In patients treated with penicillin or other effective antibiotics, the mortality rate is quite low.

REFERENCES

Brown, T. McP., and J. C. Nunemaker: Rat-bite Fever: A Review of the American Cases with Re-evaluation of Etiology, Bull. Johns Hopkins Hosp., 70: 201, 1942.

Dolman, C. E., D. E. Kerr, H. Chang, and A. R. Shearer: Two Cases of Rat-bite Fever Due to *Streptobacillus moniliformis*, Can. J. Pub. Health, 42:228, 1951.

Hamburger, M., and H. C. Knowles: *Streptobacillus moniliformis* Infection Complicated by Acute Bacterial Endocarditis, A.M.A. Arch. Internal Med., 92:216, 1953.

Levine, B., and W. H. Civin: *Streptobacillus moniliformis* Bacteremia with Minor Clinical Manifestations, Arch. Internal Med., 80:53, 1947.

Watkins, C. F.: Rat-bite Fever, J. Pediat., 28:429, 1946.

138 BARTONELLOSIS
Ivan L. Bennett, Jr.

Definition. Bartonellosis (Carrion's disease) is an infection with *Bartonella bacilliformis*. Two well-defined clinical types may develop—an acute febrile anemia of rapid onset and high mortality, designated *Oroya fever;* and a benign eruptive form with chronic cutaneous lesions called *verruga* *peruana.* Either of these types may be mild, and asymptomatic cases constitute the greatest epidemiologic hazard.

Etiology. *Bartonella bacilliformis* is a small, motile, pleomorphic, gram-negative bacillus which stains reddish violet with Giemsa's stain. It can be cultured on enriched media and chick embryos.

Epidemiology. The disease is limited to certain valleys in the Andes Mountains comprising parts of Peru, Ecuador, and Colombia. It occurs in regions between the altitudes of 2,400 and 8,000 ft where the sandfly vector, *Phlebotomus,* propagates. The reservoir of infection in nature is not known, but certain plants and lower animals have been suspected, since the disease is often contracted in regions which are practically uninhabited. Epidemics occur more frequently during the rainy season and often coincide with immigration of workers from uninfected areas.

Manifestations. The incubation period is approximately 3 weeks but may be longer. The initial symptoms are fever and pains in the bones, joints, and muscles. In the early stages the disease often resembles influenza or malaria, but blood cultures for bartonella organisms are positive even in the absence of anemia. Following this initial stage the patient develops one of the two classic types of the infection.

Oroya Fever

This type is characterized by sudden onset of high fever, extreme pallor, weakness, and a precipitous drop in the red blood cells. The count may fall from normal to 1 million per cu mm within 4 or 5 days. Muscle and joint pain and headache are severe, and insomnia, delirium, and coma are the terminal manifestations. Death can occur within 10 days to 4 weeks. Organisms are numerous in the blood, and stained smears may show 90 per cent of the erythrocytes heavily invaded. They are also present in the circulating monocytes and fixed phagocytes of the reticuloendothelial system. Secondary infection with salmonellas is an important factor in fatal cases. Neither hemolysins nor agglutinins for bartonellas are found in the serum of patients. Recovery results if the organisms decrease and fever abates. The red cell count stabilizes, then approaches normal values in about 6 weeks, when convalescence begins.

Verruga Peruana

This form of the disease, characterized by a profuse skin eruption, may follow the anemic form or may occur in patients without previous symptoms. The verrugas vary in color from red to purple and vary in size and location. They may be miliary, nodular, or eroding, and they range in size from 2 to 10 mm up to 3 or 4 cm in diameter. The three types of verrugas may occur together, since eruption takes place in successive crops; verrugas of all types and in all stages of development may be found on the same patient. The chief sites involved are the limbs and face, and less frequently the genitalia, scalp, and mucosa of the mouth and pharynx. They may persist for 1 month to 2 years. The eruption is accompanied by pain, fever, and moderate anemia. Bartonellas may be demonstrated in the lesions and cultured from the blood.

Treatment. Chloramphenicol, orally or intravenously, is highly effective, particularly when salmonella infections are also present.

REFERENCES

Cuadra, M. C.: Salmonellosis Complication in Human Bartonellosis, Texas Repts. Biol. and Med., 14:97, 1956.

Ricketts, W. E.: Clinical Manifestations of Carrion's Disease, Arch. Internal Med., 84:751, 1949.

Urteaga, O. B., and E. H. Payne: Treatment of the Acute Febrile Phase of Carrion's Disease with Chloramphenicol, Am. J. Trop. Med. Hyg., 4:507, 1955.

139 GRANULOMA INGUINALE

Albert Heyman

Definition. Granuloma inguinale is a chronic, ulcerative granulomatous disease, usually confined to the skin and mucous membranes of the genitoinguinal area but occasionally appearing in other portions of the body.

Etiology. The etiologic agent of this disease is the Donovan body (*Donovania granulomatis*), a nonmotile, gram-negative bacillus. In stained smears of the lesions the organisms appear as encapsulated, bipolar bodies situated within large mononuclear cells. In chick embryo cultures, the morphology of the organism is variable and may consist of bipolar forms, curved rods, chains, or unencapsulated bodies. The organism is not pathogenic for laboratory animals and can be cultivated only in artificial media containing yolk material.

Incidence. Granuloma inguinale was once regarded as occurring only in tropical or subtropical areas, but it has been shown to exist in almost every country and climate. The majority of the cases in the United States are found in the Southeastern section, usually among Negroes. The incidence of the disease has decreased significantly in this country during recent years. Approximately 280 cases were reported in 1959.

Pathogenesis. Granuloma inguinale is generally believed to be acquired by sexual intercourse. The disease is apparently not highly infectious, however, since it is frequently not transmitted to sexual partners. The factors predisposing to invasion of the organism are not definitely known, but the disease is found most frequently among sexually promiscuous individuals and in association with other venereal diseases. The incubation period varies from 3 to 40 days. Although the majority of infections appear on or near the external genitalia, lesions about the face, hands, and neck are not uncommon. Systemic complications of granuloma inguinale (such as invasion of the bones, joints, and viscera) have also been noted, suggesting that the infecting agent can spread throughout the body by way of the blood stream.

Clinical Manifestations. The lesion of granuloma inguinale usually is a painless, sharply demarcated ulcer having an exuberant, red, granulating base which bleeds easily on trauma. The disease is extremely chronic, and the ulcers slowly enlarge and coalesce. Secondary infection frequently is present and produces a foul-smelling, seropurulent discharge. Interference with lymphatic drainage may occur, leading to swelling and elephantiasis of the genitalia, similar to that caused by lymphogranuloma venereum. When healing occurs, further scarring and deformity may appear. Lesions of the cervix of the uterus are frequent and sometimes are mistaken for carcinoma. Lesions about the perianal area closely resemble condylomata lata of secondary syphilis, and dark-field examinations and serologic tests for syphilis are often necessary to differentiate the two conditions.

The disease occasionally produces widespread manifestations such as arthritis and osteomyelitis. In such instances there may be general debility, anemia, and malnutrition; occasionally, these have resulted in death.

Diagnosis. The diagnosis of granuloma inguinale is based upon demonstration of the presence of Donovan bodies. Impression smears of early lesions stained by Wright's method usually will show Donovan bodies lying within the cytoplasm of large mononuclear cells. The smear is of less value in chronic cases. The diagnosis can also be made by histologic examination of fixed tissues. The microscopic appearance of granuloma inguinale is essentially that of a richly vascularized granulation tissue with marked inflammatory cell infiltration. Polymorphonuclear leukocytes are scattered throughout the tissue and form small microabscesses. Numerous large mononuclear cells are also present and show finely reticulated or vacuolated cytoplasm. Phagocytosis of polymorphonuclear leukocytes and other cellular debris by these cells is common. Intracellular or extracellular Donovan bodies are readily seen in tissue sections, particularly in acute cases. In chronic cases they may be found only after considerable search, but the histologic pattern is sufficiently characteristic to permit a tentative diagnosis, even when organisms are not found. Specific serologic tests (complement fixation) and skin tests have been developed, but their diagnostic value is yet to be determined.

Treatment. Healing of granuloma inguinale will usually occur promptly following treatment with streptomycin, chloramphenicol, or the tetracyclines. Streptomycin has the disadvantage of requiring parenteral administration. The other antibiotics seem to be more effective and are given orally in doses of 2 Gm a day for approximately fifteen days. These antibiotics have treponemicidal properties and should not be given until repeated dark-field examinations and serologic tests have excluded the diagnosis of early syphilis.

REFERENCES

Anderson, K., W. A. DeMonbreun, and E. W. Goodpasture: An Experimental Investigation of the Etiology and Immunology of Granuloma Inguinale, Am. J. Syphilis, Gonorrhea, Venereal Diseases, 29: 165, 1945.

Pariser, H., and H. Beerman: Granuloma Inguinale, Am. J. Med. Sci., 208:547, 1944.

Rajam, R. V., and P. N. Rangiah: Donovaniosis (Granuloma Inguinale and Granuloma Venereum), World Health Organization Monograph Series, No. 24, 1954.

Sheldon, W. H., B. R. Thebaut, A. Heyman, and M. J. Wall: Osteomyelitis Caused by Granuloma Inguinale, Am. J. Med. Sci., 210:237, 1945.

140 LISTERIA INFECTIONS
Paul D. Hoeprich

Listeria monocytogenes infections have been demonstrated in at least 30 animal species, including man. Occasional or even chronic involvement of the genital tract of the fertile female with consequent perinatal fetal infection is emerging as the most nearly singular of the many clinical syndromes known collectively as listerosis.

Etiology. When isolated from disease, listerias are gram-positive, non-acid-fast, nonsporulating, microaerophilic, motile bacilli (0.3 to 0.6 by 0.8 to 2.5 μ). Listerias are readily and frequently confused with nontoxigenic corynebacteria, erysipelothrix, and occasionally streptococci. Antigenic distinction is clearly drawn, even to the point of distinguishing four types of listerias; unfortunately typing serums are not commonly available. Motility and ability to reduce 2,3,5-triphenyltetrazolium chloride set off listeria from erysipelothrix; yet, demonstration of characteristic animal pathogenicity must support morphologic and cultural data. Swabbing the conjunctiva of the rabbit with listerias regularly leads to a keratoconjunctivitis in 3 to 5 days. The process usually remains localized to the eye and is caused by no other bacteria save rare strains of *Erysipelothrix*. Generalized listeria infection in the rabbit provokes a monocytosis maximal 3 to 7 days after inoculation. Intraperitoneal injection of 10^4 listerias is lethal to mice in 1 to 3 days; myriads of tiny hepatic abscesses are characteristic, and these commonly border on central lobular veins.

Epidemiology and Pathogenesis. World-wide in distribution, organisms of the genus *Listeria* appear to be primarily parasites of a variety of birds and mammals, both wild and domestic. With the exception of type 2, all serotypes infect both human and infrahuman hosts in several countries. In the United States, 75 per cent of listerias fall into type 4 (71 per cent 4b), while in Germany type 1 isolates are most common.

While wildlife may be the reservoir of listerias, mechanisms making for sporadic listerosis in domestic animals and in man are obscure. Transplacental infection occurs in many species, including man, and represents the only as yet proved example of human transmission of listerias. Inhalation of infected dust, ingestion of contaminated milk, and contact with the fluids of infected animals have all been implicated as means for human infection on the basis of a few proved cases of listerosis.

Whatever the route of infection with listerias, in the gravid mammal, fetal infection proceeds via the placenta. Dissemination of listerias by fetal bacteremia originating in the infected placenta results in widespread disease.

Manifestations. Fetal listerosis (also known as septic or miliary granulomatosis, granulomatosis infantiseptica, argentophile-rod infection, pseudotuberculosis) is the most frequent of human infections known to be due to listerias. Described as a pathologic entity by Henle in 1893, this disease was found in aborted, premature, stillborn, and neonatal children. Clinical attributes were described by several German workers in the 1950s. The disease may be asymptomatic in the mother, or a week to a month prepartum there may have been malaise, a shaking chill, perhaps with diarrhea, pain in the back or flanks, and itching of the skin. When symptomatic, the disease is benign and self-

limited in the mother; however, as symptoms subside, fetal movement may be noted to have decreased or stopped. Infection of the fetus may occur as early as the fifth month of gestation. Delivery is normal, although before term. Fetal infection is usually lethal ante partum. Of those children born alive, most succumb within minutes post partum, while the remainder usually do not survive beyond 2 weeks. Infants in the latter group are critically ill with cardiorespiratory distress, vomiting, and diarrhea. There is hypothermia and hepatosplenomegaly, and mutiple granulomas may be seen on the posterior pharyngeal wall. Often, dark-red skin papules appear—particularly on the lower extremities. When infection becomes symptomatic more than 2 weeks after delivery, the onset is usually that of respiratory tract affliction with pneumonitis. Purulent meningitis may also occur.

At postmortem examination the findings are characteristic and mimic those seen in rodent listerosis —widely disseminated abscess formation with lesions varying in size from grossly visible to microscopic, involving (in decreasing frequency) liver, spleen, adrenal glands, lungs, pharynx, gastrointestinal tract, central nervous system, and skin. Typically, the lesions are abscesses, but classic granuloma formation may be seen, depending principally on the duration of infection before death. Gastrointestinal involvement in fetal listerosis offers the possibility of rapid diagnosis, the essential to early institution of vigorous therapy which may salvage some of the infants born alive but infected. Microscopic examination of a gram-stained smear of meconium from the newborn normally does not disclose bacteria; enteric fetal listerosis results in meconium laden with gram-positive bacilli. Alex in East Germany recommends smear-gram-stain examination of meconium of all newborns whose mothers had fever before or at onset of labor or who were born prematurely.

Intrauterine fetal infection results in abortion or premature delivery. Accordingly, the possibility of repeated or habitual abortion in women having its basis in chronic, asymptomatic genital tract listerosis (as is known to occur in animals—rabbit) must be considered. The serologic studies of Rost and coworkers in Germany and the cultural data of Rappaport et al. (Austria and Israel) both indicate that genital tract listerosis occurs not infrequently in women who have had repeated abortions. The significance of these findings to the over-all problem of spontaneous abortion remains to be defined. A report of listeric urethritis in men raises the possibility of venereal spread of listerosis—another aspect requiring further study.

Leptomeningitis, if not the most common, is the best known form of listerosis encountered in the adult human. Clinically, meningitis due to *Listeria monocytogenes* cannot be distinguished from meningitis due to other kinds of bacteria.

Oculoglandular listerosis is the uncommonly met with human analogue of the illness initiated in the rabbit by conjunctival inoculation of listeria. There is a purulent conjunctivitis which may lead to corneal ulceration. Regional node involvement usually spells the limit of spread from the eye; however, listeric meningitis has been reported as a complication to oculoglandular listerosis.

Other syndromes caused by listeria, but rare in occurrence, include generalized illness with bacteremia and high fever, endocarditis, polyserositis, and cutaneous infection.

Listeria monocytogenes does not cause infectious mononucleosis as the disease is defined in this country.

Laboratory Findings. The major difficulty in the laboratory diagnosis of listeria lies in distinguishing it from diphtheroids. Listerias grow well on the usual laboratory media; however, specimens from sites where normally many other kinds of bacteria are present are best cultured on selective media, after enrichment. If the numbers of listerias in a specimen are likely to be few, greater success in isolation results when the specimen is kept in glucose broth at 4°C and subcultured weekly.

Monocytosis is not commonly found in human listerosis. Leukocytosis with neutrophilia, as in any acute bacterial infection, is seen in listeric meningitis, oculoglandular infection, bacteremia, and endocarditis. Other laboratory findings, e.g., cerebrospinal fluid in meningitis, are in keeping with the clinical syndromes engendered.

Differential Diagnosis. Fetal listerosis and possibly habitual abortion are clinical syndromes which should call to mind infection due to *Listeria monocytogenes*. Abortion, premature delivery, stillbirth, and neonatal death may be due to causes other than listerosis—Rh incompatibility, syphilis, toxoplasmosis.

In patients with leptomeningitis, conjunctivitis, endocarditis, bacteremia, or polyserositis, reports of isolation of "diphtheroids" or "nonpathogens" must always be challenged with the possibility that these may be listerias.

Treatment. *Listeria monocytogenes* are susceptible by in vitro testing to sulfonamides, penicillin, streptomycin, chloramphenicol, the tetracyclines, erythromycin, and novobiocin in concentrations attainable in the blood of patients. Sulfonamides, penicillin, streptomycin, the tetracyclines, and erythromycin have had most frequent clinical trial. On the basis of potency, bactericidal potential, safety, and cost, a combination of penicillin and erythromycin is optimal. Dosage and duration of therapy should vary according to the kind of infection. Thus, in fetal listerosis, where therapy must be rapidly effective to be of value, a successful regimen is yet to be devised. For listeric meningitis in the adult, 20 to 30 megaunits potassium benzylpenicillin by continuous intravenous infusion per day plus 3 to 4 Gm erythromycin propionate by mouth (or one-half as much erythromycin by intramuscular injection) per day—both are given for 5 to 7 days beyond defervescence. Oculoglandular listerosis warrants less massive therapy: 600,000 units procaine benzylpenicillin by intramuscular injection twice daily plus 2 to 3 Gm erythromycin propionate by mouth per day. Endocarditis and bacteremia from an unknown site have been infrequently treated but would be justification for vigorous therapy: 5 to 10 megaunits potassium benzylpenicillin by intramuscular or intravenous injection per day plus 2 to 3 Gm erythromycin propionate by mouth per day. There is little reported experience in the treatment of chronic female genital tract listerosis. Administration of single agents and combinations of penicillin (600,000 units procaine benzylpenicillin, twice daily, intramuscularly, for 14 days), sulfamethoxypyridazine (1 Gm per day for 14 days), tetracycline (1 to 2 Gm per day for 14 days) has rendered vaginal and cervical cultures free of listeria.

Prognosis. Prompt antibiotic therapy of the acute forms of listerosis, excepting fetal listerosis, is highly effective. On the basis of agglutinin titers, circulating antibody disappears during the months following cure of listeria infections.

The results of antibacterial chemotherapy in chronic genital tract listerosis, while initially optimistic, have yet to be evaluated.

REFERENCES

Hoeprich, P. D.: Infection Due to *Listeria monocytogenes,* Medicine, 37:142, 1958.

Rappaport, F., M. Rabinovitz, R. Toaff, and N. Krochik: Genital Listerosis as a Cause of Repeated Abortion, Lancet, I:1273, 1960.

Seeliger, H. P. R.: "Listeroise," Leipzig, J. A. Barth, 1955.

141 ERYSIPELOTHRIX INFECTIONS

Paul D. Hoeprich

The parasitic incursions of *Erysipelothrix rhusiopathiae* (*E. insidiosa*) are more frequently expressed in some 20 species of animals than in man.

Clinically, unique cutaneous infection is the most common form of human illness; while endocarditis and arthritis have been described, these are but rarely encountered.

History. Although isolated from mice by Koch in 1880 and from pigs (swine erysipelas) by Loeffler in 1882, erysipelothrix was first related to human disease in 1884 when Rosenbach cultured erysipelothrix from a skin lesion in a patient. This cutaneous disease which Rosenbach labeled erysipeloid was proved to be caused by erysipelothrix by his reproduction of it by self-inoculation.

Etiology. As isolated from human disease, erysipelothrix are gram-positive, non-acid-fast, non-sporulating, microaerophilic, nonmotile bacilli (0.2 to 0.4 by 0.5 to 2.5 μ). Confusion with non-toxigenic organisms of the genus *Corynebacterium* or *Listeria* is not certainly resolved on morphologic grounds alone. Serologic differentiation is reliable when available. Generally, animal inoculation is required, conjunctival inoculation in the rabbit only rarely leads to a conjunctivitis; generalized infection in the rabbit may cause some monocytosis, a much less marked reaction than caused by listeria; intraperitoneal injection in mice leads to death in 2 to 4 days, there is little gross hepatic abscess formation whereas purulent conjunctivities is common.

Epidemiology and Pathogenesis. Widespread in nature, erysipelothrix organisms gain foothold through injuries to the skin. Erysipeloid is the usual result and is virtually restricted to persons who in their occupations handle animals, fish, shellfish, or materials derived from animals. The incidence of erysipeloid parallels the incidence of swine erysipelas, being highest in summer and early fall. Yet, the individuals who tend pigs, even pigs ill with porcine erysipelas, do not commonly develop erysipeloid. If dermal containment of erysipelothrix is not accomplished, the seeding of damaged cardiac valves may eventuate in endocarditis.

Manifestations. From 2 to 7 days after injury (healing has usually occurred), a maculopapular, nonvesiculated, sharply defined, raised, purplish-red zone surrounds the site of entry. An itching, burning, painful irritation may precede and always accompanies this typical skin lesion. There is local swelling, and nearby joints may become stiff and painful. Centrifugal spread from the site of inoculation is apparent in a day or so. Movement is slow, ½ in. per 24 hr maximally, and more rapid proximally than distally; involvement of the terminal phalanx is rare, while spread to other fingers and the hand (but not above the wrist) is common. With extension, the original center fades without desquamation or suppuration, but with subsidence of local symptoms. There are usually no systemic signs or symptoms; regional lymphangitis and lymphadenitis are rarely seen. Untreated, the disease subsides within 3 weeks in most patients, although relapse has been observed.

The manifestations of erysipelothrix endocarditis may be either acute or subacute, depending on the virulence of the infecting strain of bacilli and on the state of resistance of the host. Usually there are no classic erysipeloid skin lesions to suggest the etiology at the time endocarditis is clinically evident. However, a history of recent erysipeloid, when obtained, may be helpful.

Erysipelothrix arthritis is not clinically characteristic but usually can be related to erysipeloid or erysipelothrix bacteremia. Isolation of erysipelothrix organisms from synovial fluid has not been reported.

Laboratory Findings. Isolation of erysipelothrix depends primarily upon awareness of the possibility of the presence of these bacteria. The usual laboratory culture media are adequate for growth of erysipelothrix, but recognition of their significance on culture requires distinction from diphtheroids. In erysipeloid, erysipelothrix are best recovered in glucose containing broth cultures of a full thickness of skin removed from the advancing edge of a lesion. Culture of aspirate obtained without removing the needle after injection of saline into the periphery of a lesion may also yield erysipelothrix.

With endocarditis and arthritis, findings (other than culture of erysipelothrix) are in keeping with these clinical syndromes and are not characteristic of a specific etiology.

Differential Diagnosis. The appearance and location of erysipeloid, its slow and limited spread, the lack of constitutional reaction, the history of occupation and injury all serve to identify this disease. Thus, the afflicted skin in erysipelas is quite erythematous and is usually on the face and scalp; there is regional lymphangitis and lymphadenitis, leukocytosis, fever, and malaise. Eczematous lesions may itch, but display vesicles and little abnormal color. The various erythemas have a different location and while red do not itch or burn and are more apt to be chronic and not even slowly migratory.

Treatment. Erysipelothrix are inhibited by penicillin, the tetracyclines, chloramphenicol, erythromycin, and novobiocin. The agent of choice is penicillin. Erysipeloid is adequately treated by injection of 1,200,000 units benzathine penicillin G. Cure of erysipelothrix endocarditis has followed benzylpenicillin therapy in dosages of 2 to 20 megaunits per day for 4 to 6 weeks. General supportive measures must not be neglected.

Prognosis. Prompt antibiotic therapy is highly effective in eradicating erysipelothrix. Second attacks of erysipeloid have been reported—apparently a solid immunity does not result from clinical infection. As with bacterial endocarditis from any cause, prognosis rests primarily on the extent of valvular dysfunction as it may be aggravated by bacterial growth on valves that are already damaged.

REFERENCES

Nelson, E.: Five Hundred Cases of Erysipeloid, Rocky Mt. Med. J., 52:40, 1955.

Wilson, G. S., and A. A. Miles: "Topley and Wilson's Principles of Bacteriology and Immunity," 4th ed., pp. 479–488, Baltimore, The Williams & Wilkins Company, 1957.

Section 7: Diseases Caused by Toxin-producing Bacteria

142 DIPHTHERIA
Louis Weinstein

Definition. Diphtheria is an acute infectious disease produced by *Corynebacterium diphtheriae* and characterized by a local inflammatory lesion, usually in the upper respiratory tract, and by remote effects resulting from the absorption of toxin which may affect particularly the heart and peripheral nerves.

History. The earliest precise description of diphtheria is attributed to Bretonneau who, in 1821, separated diphtheria from other clinical entities with which it had been grouped together as "the croup." Klebs reported the morphologic appearance of *C. diphtheriae* in 1883, and the next year Loeffler isolated the organism in pure culture. The *toxin* of diphtheria was defined in 1888 by Roux and Yersin who demonstrated that some of the manifestations of the disease could be produced in guinea pigs by the injection of sterile culture filtrates. Diphtheria antitoxin was produced by von Behring in 1890; this was soon followed by application of serotherapy in the human disease. The skin test for susceptibility to diphtheria was developed by Schick in 1913. In 1923 Ramon showed that the toxin could be altered in such a way that it lost its poisonous effects but retained its ability to provoke the development of antitoxin; this was the first diphtheria *toxoid* and served as the basis for the present methods of immunization against the disease.

Etiology. *Corynebacterium diphtheriae* is a grampositive, nonsporulating, nonmotile, unencapsulated rod. It is pleomorphic, slender, and slightly curved. Pseudobranching and "palisade" formations are often seen in stained smears. Characteristically, there is a swelling at one end of the bacillus which gives it a "club" shape. Diphtheria bacilli have been classified into three groups on the basis of their colonial appearance on tellurite medium, their fermentation reactions, and their ability to produce hemolysis. The *mitis* type grows as a black, shiny, round, regular colony; the organisms are long, contain metachromatic granules, are hemolytic, and do not ferment glycogen or starch. The *gravis* strain produces large, gray colonies which resemble a daisy head and which are composed of short, uniformly staining rods which are nonhemolytic and ferment starch and glycogen. The *intermedius* type is a long, clubbed bacillus which produces a moderate-sized, dull black colony, is nonhemolytic, and does not attack either starch or glycogen. European workers, particularly those in the British Isles, believe that there is a significant difference in the clinical manifestations and severity of the disease related to the strain; *gravis* and *intermedius* infections are thought to be accompanied by more severe toxic manifestations and a higher death rate than those due to *mitis* strains; the latter have been featured mainly by the development of laryngeal obstruction. In the United States, the *gravis* strain is comparatively uncommon, and less significance is attached to the relationship of the type of organism to the clinical form of the disease.

Corynebacterium diphtheriae produces a potent toxin which is responsible for many of the clinical manifestations. This material has been purified and is a protein; as little as 0.0001 mg is a lethal dose for guinea pigs. Strains of diphtheria bacilli which elaborate exotoxin are lysogenic, that is, they carry bacteriophage ("prophage"). Absence of lysogeny is associated with lack of toxin formation and virulence. The lysogenic state results in altered metabolism of the avirulent cell, an alteration manifested as toxin production.

Epidemiology. Diphtheria occurs primarily in the Temperate Zone and has been very common in Europe for many years. In general, the number of cases of diphtheria in the United States and the British Isles has been decreasing steadily during the past 20 years.

Prior to 1927, the disease occurred primarily in the preschool child. Since 1927, the highest frequency has been in children over six years of age and adults have been involved more commonly. Another striking change has been a decrease in the incidence of laryngeal involvement.

Diphtheria is acquired by droplet transmission from active cases or asymptomatic carriers. Fomites play little or no role in spread of the infection, but *C. diphtheriae* may remain alive and virulent in the dust of a darkened room for several weeks; this may act as a source for dissemination of the organisms.

Pathogenesis and Pathology. The commonest portal of entry for the diphtheria bacillus is the upper respiratory tract. The skin, genitalia, eye, or middle ear may also be primary sites of invasion. Growth of the organism is limited to a superficial area in most cases, there being little tendency to invade deeper tissues or to enter the lymphatics or blood stream except in the terminal stages of the disease. The exotoxin elaborated by the bacilli in the local lesion is carried by the blood to all parts of the body. Dissemination of toxin with damage to remote areas appears to be greater when the primary lesion is in the nasopharynx, less when it is limited to the larynx, and least when it is confined to the nasal mucous membrane; the most intense intoxication is observed when lesions are present in the pharynx, larynx, trachea, and bronchial tree simultaneously.

The *primary lesion* of diphtheria is the membrane. It is thick, homogenous, leathery, and blue-white and is composed of bacteria, necrotic epithelium, phagocytes, and fibrin. The membrane is surrounded by a narrow zone of inflammation and is firmly adherent to the underlying tissues; when it is removed forcibly, bleeding follows. Ulceration is not a feature; if it occurs, it is very superficial. Regional lymphadenitis is frequent, especially with *gravis* infections.

The systemic lesions of diphtheria result from the activity of the exotoxin and are detectable primarily in the heart, kidneys, and peripheral nerves. The brain may rarely be affected. Cardiac enlargement is frequent; this appears to be related to the presence and degree of myocarditis and not to myocardial hypertrophy. The kidneys reveal acute degeneration of the epithelium, cloudy swelling, and interstitial changes; they may be quite enlarged. In some cases, particularly those with laryngeal involvement, there is a bronchopneumonia which may be due to *C. diphtheriae* or to secondary invading organisms. When the pneumonitis is caused by the diphtheria bacillus, membrane is present throughout the bronchial tree. The peripheral nerves may reveal fatty degeneration, breaking up of the medullary sheaths, and involvement of the axis cylinder. Both motor and sensory fibers may be affected, but the main impact is on motor innervation. The anterior horn cells and the posterior columns of the spinal cord may be damaged. Other central nervous system involvement includes cerebral hemorrhage, meningitis, degeneration of ganglion cells and nerve tracts, and encephalitis. Petechial hemorrhages and purpuric lesions are occasionally present in the kidneys, skin, and adrenals. Bacterial endocarditis due to the diphtheria bacillus is a rare finding.

Death in diphtheria may result from respiratory tract obstruction by membrane or edema or from the action of toxin on the heart, nervous system, or other organs.

Immunity. Susceptibility to diphtheria is determined by the presence or absence of circulating antibody to exotoxin. The *Schick test* yields a rough estimate of the quantity of antitoxin in the circulation. The present method of carrying out this test is as follows: 0.1 ml of purified diphtheria *toxin* ($\frac{1}{50}$ MLD) dissolved in buffered human serum albumin is injected intradermally in the volar surface of the forearm; 0.1 ml of purified diphtheria *toxoid* (0.01 Lf) is injected into the other arm as a control. These areas are examined at 24 and 48 hr and between the fourth and seventh days:

1. When the reaction is *positive*, the site of toxin injection begins to redden in 24 hr; this increases and reaches a maximum in about a week, at which time the lesion may be as large as 3 cm in diameter and moderately swollen and tender. There is usually a small (1 to 1.5 cm) dark red central zone which gradually turns brown, desquamates, and leaves a pigmented area. The area of *toxoid* injection shows *no reaction*. A *positive* test indicates little or no circulating antitoxin or immunity.

2. In a *negative* test, there is *no reaction* at the site of either *toxoid* or *toxin* instillation. This is consistent with a blood antitoxin level of $\frac{1}{30}$ to $\frac{1}{100}$ units and immunity to ordinary exposure.

3. Inflammation at both sites of injection within 12 to 14 hr, which reaches a maximum in 48 to 72 hr, and then fades constitutes a *pseudoreaction*. This practically always indicates immunity plus hypersensitivity to the toxin or other materials in the solution.

4. The *combined reaction* begins like the *pseudoreaction*, but the inflammatory response at the toxin site persists for some time after that in the area of toxoid injection has faded. This type of reaction is uncommon with the use of purified Schick testing materials and indicates delayed sen-

sitivity to toxin or other proteins. Circulating anti-toxin is either absent or low in these cases. *Combined reactions* are uncommon in children and probably result from previous unapparent diphtheritic infection; their frequency increases with age and is highest in unimmunized groups living in areas where diphtheria is prevalent.

Individuals with negative Schick tests occasionally contract diphtheria, and some persons with positive Schick reactions do not develop the disease after exposure. Less than 50 per cent of *adults* in some parts of the United States have "protective" levels of circulating antitoxin.

Second attacks of diphtheria are very rare despite the fact that only about 90 per cent of patients who have had the disease become Schick-negative. This suggests that factors other than antitoxin may play a role in protection against infection.

The risk of death is sharply reduced although the disease may be quite severe and complications develop in Schick-negative persons. In general, immunized patients have a milder illness than unimmunized ones when the initial clinical picture and level of circulating antitoxin are the same. Early therapy of cases of diphtheria with antibiotics may lead to recurrence of the disease if exposure to fresh infections occurs shortly after discontinuation of treatment. Although proof is lacking, this suggests the possibility that the development of antitoxic immunity is suppressed in these instances.

Clinical Manifestations. The *incubation period* is 1 to 7 days. The local symptoms vary with the site of the primary lesion. Systemic reactions, in the uncomplicated disease, are usually of only minor to moderate severity. Although fever may be present, it is usually low (100 to 101°F) unless infection with another organism (often the beta-hemolytic streptococcus) supervenes; when this happens the temperature may rise to high levels. When toxic manifestations are absent, patients feel well except for a varying degree of discomfort at the site of the local lesion. Pallor, listlessness, tachycardia, and weakness are common and striking in more severe cases. Peripheral vascular collapse often develops in the terminal stages of the disease.

Nasal Diphtheria. Diphtheria is occasionally restricted to the nasal mucous membrane. The infection is usually localized to one side, and a unilateral serosanguineous discharge which lasts for weeks is characteristic. Membrane is present on the septum or turbinates in the anterior portion of the nose and may persist for a long time without the development of toxic manifestations. When the disease is located in the posterior nasal areas, extension to the pharynx is frequent and is followed by absorption of toxin. The presence of a foreign body must be ruled out in all cases of suspected nasal diphtheria.

Pharyngeal Diphtheria. The very early diphtheritic membrane in the pharynx consists of small areas of soft exudate which wipe off easily and leave no bleeding points. As the disease progresses, these coalesce to form an easily removable thin sheet which spreads to cover both tonsils or the pharynx, or both. Later, it becomes more dense, bluish-white, gray, or black, depending on the degree of hemorrhage, and is firmly attached to the underlying mucous membrane so that when it is taken off bleeding occurs. There is usually a small zone of inflammatory reaction about the periphery of the membrane. If infection with organisms such as the beta-hemolytic streptococcus is superimposed, the pharynx is diffusely red and edematous. There is very little soreness of the throat in the average case of diphtheria; discomfort is often severe, however, when pharyngeal inflammation is marked. There is usually only a moderate degree of leukocytosis, 15,000 or less white blood cells per cu mm.

Marked local spread of the pharyngeal membrane may take place, and the throat, tonsils, and soft and hard palates may be completely covered. Patients with severe disease may show the picture of so-called "malignant" diphtheria. In this, there is great swelling of the submandibular areas and the anterior neck, giving the characteristic "bull-neck" appearance. The breathing is noisy and carried on through the open mouth, the tongue protrudes, the breath is foul, and the speech thick. The pharyngeal tissues are red and edematous, and the cervical lymph nodes are enlarged. The skin is pale and cool. There is great weakness. Occasionally, purpuric eruptions of the skin may appear, particularly on the neck and anterior chest wall. Drowsiness and delirium are common.

Laryngeal Diphtheria. Involvement of the larynx in the course of diphtheria usually results from extension of membrane from the pharynx. Rarely, however, the infection may begin in and be limited to the larynx or trachea. This possibility should be considered in the differential diagnosis of all cases of "croup"; it can be ruled out only by direct examination of the airway. The clinical features of this type of disease are described below.

Skin Diphtheria. Although skin diphtheria is a problem primarily in tropical areas where it is responsible for some cases of "jungle sore" and may become epidemic, it occurs occasionally in the Temperate Zone. *Corynebacterium diphtheriae* is unable to penetrate unbroken skin and invades, as a rule, only when epithelial integrity has been destroyed as in wounds, burns, etc. Although the lesions develop most often on the lower extremities, they may appear at any site, including the perianal region.

The typical lesion of skin diphtheria is a round,

deep, "punched out" ulcer varying from 0.5 cm to several centimeters in diameter. In the early stages, the lesions are covered by a gray, yellow, or gray-brown membrane which strips off easily to reveal a clean hemorrhagic base which dries quickly and becomes covered by thin, leathery, dark-brown or black, adherent membrane. This separates spontaneously 1 to 3 weeks after infection. The margin of the fully developed ulcer is usually slightly undermined, purple, rolled, and sharply defined. Breakdown, either after minor trauma or spontaneously, is frequent, and the development of anesthesia, after a few weeks, is characterstic. Healing of the lesions is usually slow. Scarring is the rule. Myocarditis occurs in about 5 per cent and peripheral neuritis in about 20 per cent of cases of skin diphtheria; the Guillain-Barré syndrome may develop.

Diphtheria Lesions in Other Areas. Diphtheria may involve the uterine cervix, vagina, vulva, and penis (after circumcision). Diphtheritic cystitis and urethritis have been observed following prostatectomy. These lesions are often secondary to respiratory tract involvement but may be primary. Toxic manifestations are common. The tongue, buccal mucous membrane, gums, and esophagus may also be affected. Infection of the conjunctiva occurs rarely. Otitis media may occur as an isolated syndrome or secondary to diphtheria in the upper respiratory tract; aural discharge from which virulent organisms can be isolated may persist for many months.

Complications of Diphtheria. The complications of diphtheria are of two types: those which result from spread of the membrane in the respiratory tract and those which are due to the activity of the toxin absorbed from the local lesion.

Extension and Spread of Membrane. The membrane of diphtheria may spread from the fauces over the posterior pharyngeal wall into the nasopharynx and anterior portion of the nose. This usually produces severe illness and is accompanied by a high risk of toxic manifestations. With extension of membrane into the larynx or trachea, or both, there is gradual occlusion of the airway. This is first manifested by tachypnea and, as obstruction increases, restlessness, use of accessory muscles of respiration, and finally cyanosis and, if relief is not produced, death. This progression of events occurs most frequently in children. In some cases, the diphtheritic membrane extends from the trachea diffusely into the bronchial tree and produces clinical manifestations of pneumonia. Bronchopulmonary diphtheria is very serious not only because of respiratory tract obstruction but also because of the large area of surface from which toxin can be absorbed; the death rate is very high. When the pulmonary lesion regresses, pieces of membrane

may break off and produce sudden occlusion of the airway; a complete cast of the bronchial tree may be coughed up. On occasion, pharyngeal membrane has extended into the esophagus and cardia of the stomach.

Toxic Complications of Diphtheria. Myocarditis develops in about two-thirds of patients with diphtheria but is clinically evident in about 10 per cent. In these, alterations in the intensity of the heart sounds (softening of the mitral valve sounds), systolic murmurs, bundle branch block, incomplete or complete heart block (rate as low as 30), atrial fibrillation, ventricular premature beats or tachycardia, or both, are detectable. Ventricular fibrillation is a constant threat and is frequently the mechanism responsible for sudden death. Ninety per cent of the cases with atrial fibrillation, ventricular tachycardia, or complete heart block die. Frank congestive failure due to diphtheritic myocarditis occurs infrequently. Evidence of failure of the right heart usually develops first, and the commonest symptoms is pain in the right upper quadrant of the abdomen due to rapid engorgement of the liver. Decompensation of the left heart with dyspnea and rales may appear later. Diphtheritic heart disease is not "benign" in some individuals who survive the acute stage. Permanent cardiac damage may sometimes occur. Fibrosis of the myocardium has been observed in young adults and in children who have expired several weeks after mild myocarditis was detected by electrocardiographic study; the degree and extent of fibrotic change are frequently greater than would be predicted from the type of abnormality in the tracing.

Peripheral neuritis occurs at three different times in the course of diphtheria. Paralysis of the soft palate and posterior pharyngeal wall occasionally appears very early in the disease (2 to 3 days) when there is extensive membrane in the pharynx. This is probably due to direct action of toxin on the motor nerve endings in the thorax. Neuritis develops during the second to sixth week most frequently (10 per cent). At this time, cranial nerve dysfunction is commonest, the third, sixth, seventh, ninth, and tenth nerves being involved most often. Loss of accommodation, nasal voice, and difficulty in swallowing are the most frequent manifestations. However, any of the peripheral nerves may be affected, with resulting paralysis of the extremities, diaphragm, or intercostal muscles; death may occur from failure of respiration. The peripheral neuritides which appear in the second to the sixth week of the disease are featured almost completely by motor loss; sensory changes are uncommon and, when present, are minor in degree. Peripheral neuritis may not appear until 2 to 3 months after the onset of diphtheria. In these cases, the clinical picture and course resemble infectious polyneuritis. The outstanding findings are symmetrical loss of sensation in a "glove and stocking" distribution and albuminocytologic dissociation in the cerebrospinal fluid identical with that observed in the Guillain-Barré syndrome. Motor weakness and areflexia may develop with progression of involvement but need not be present. Very rarely, a fatal ascending paralysis of the Landry type may develop. Complete recovery is the rule; this may require as long as a year.

Encephalitis is a rare toxic complication of diphtheria; clinical manifestations are usually absent. *Shock*, which develops suddenly and without warning, is an occasional cause of rapid death in this disease. In some instances, this may be a consequence of myocarditis; in others, no cause can be discovered.

Other Complications. Cerebral infarction with hemiplegia occurs rarely in diphtheria; it is probably due to embolization from atrial thrombi in patients with myocarditis and cardiac dilatation. Bronchopneumonia due to pyogenic organisms sometimes supervenes, especially in cases in which laryngotracheal or bronchial diphtheria is present. Superinfection of the lungs is a risk in all patients with diphtheria who are given antimicrobial agents. Purpuric skin eruptions may be seen in severe cases, especially those with the malignant or "bull-neck" form of the disease. Thrombopenia is a rare finding. A mild morbilliform rash may be present during the early stage of development of the diphtheritic membrane. Beta-hemolytic streptococcal pharyngitis may occur; it is presently uncommon because antibiotics are usually administered from the beginning of the disease to eradicate the carrier state. Serum sickness occasionally follows the use of antitoxin. Relapses of diphtheria may occur when patients given antimicrobial agents are exposed to fresh cases soon after the drug has been stopped. Bacteremia, endocarditis, and meningitis are rare complications.

Course and Prognosis. The membrane may be present for only 3 to 4 days in mild faucial diphtheria, even when no antitoxin is given; it usually lasts for about a week in cases of moderate severity. It is quite common for the pharyngeal lesion to increase in extent and thickness during the first 24 hr after the administration of antitoxin. As the disease begins to recede, the exudate softens, wipes off easily leaving no bleeding areas, becomes patchy so that it resembles the picture of "follicular" tonsillitis, and finally disappears, leaving normal underlying mucous membrane. Local lesions in areas other than the pharynx behave in the same fashion.

The fatality rate in diphtheria prior to the use of specific antitoxin was about 35 per cent in average cases and 90 per cent in those with laryngeal involvement. Since specific serotherapy has been employed, this has been reduced to a range of 3.5 to 22 per cent, but it is still highest when the larynx is affected. The over-all death rate in the United States is about 10 per cent. In the author's experience the severity of cardiac involvement and the incidence of death appear to be related to the strain of *C. diphtheriae*. The author has observed that, while there is no difference in the distribution of *gravis* and *mitis* strains in the mild forms of myocarditis, the incidence of the *gravis* type is three times higher than that of *mitis* in cases in which physical evidence of heart disease and a very high death rate (90 per cent) are present. Age influences the outcome of diphtheria, death being most frequent in the very young and old, and lowest in those ten to thirty years old. Immunization is a factor of great importance in determining prognosis. The fatality rate in immunized individuals is one-tenth that in the unimmunized population. Paralysis is five times and "bull-neck" fifteen times less common in immunized patients. As a rule, the longer the delay in the use of serotherapy, the greater the incidence of complications and death.

Diagnosis. The features of the fully developed diphtheritic membrane, especially in the pharynx, are sufficiently characteristic to suggest the possibility of the disease in most instances. It must be emphasized, however, that because many clinicians have had little experience with this infection too much reliance must not be placed on the appearance of the pharyngeal exudate alone in establishing the diagnosis. There are a number of other infections in which pseudomembranes which may be confused with those of diphtheria are present; among these are infectious mononucleosis, streptococcal pharyngitis, viral exudative pharyngitis, fusospirochetal angina, acute moniliasis, and staphylococcal infections of the thorax secondary to chemotherapy.

The only positive method of establishing the presence of diphtheria is by demonstrating the typical organisms in stained smears and cultures. With some experience, it is possible to make a positive diagnosis from methylene blue stained preparations in 75 to 85 per cent of cases. These observations require confirmation by isolation of the organisms. Diphtheria bacilli can be recovered from patients who have not been given antibiotic agents in 8 to 12 hr on Loeffler's medium incubated at 37°C; *C. diphtheriae* also multiplies, but more slowly, on ordinary blood agar. If drugs, especially penicillin or erythromycin, have been administered prior to obtaining material for culture, the organisms may not grow out for as long as 5 days or may fail to grow at all. All strains of the diphtheria bacillus recovered from patients should be examined for toxin production. This can be accomplished using antitoxin-protected and unprotected guinea pigs or by means of an in vitro technic.

Treatment. Patients with diphtheria should be isolated and kept at strict bed rest, with reduction of physical effort during the acute and early convalescent stages. Local therapy of the diphtheritic lesion is usually not required because pharyngeal discomfort is mild. A liquid or soft diet is preferable. There is no evidence that a high intake of carbohydrate and vitamin C, as has been recommended, is necessary. There is no indication for parenteral feeding if the patient is able to take adequate calories and fluid by mouth.

The only specific treatment for diphtheria is *antitoxin.* Although the dosage schedules are somewhat empiric, experience has suggested the use of certain quantities in the therapy of lesions of varying severity, extent, and location. Antiserum must *never* be given until the absence or presence of sensitivity to horse serum, using the eye and skin tests, has been determined. Despite a failure to find hypersensitivity, it is probably best to administer the antiserum in divided doses to adults. The following dosage schedule is widely used: When exudate is present on only one tonsil, 5,000 units of antitoxin are given; for lesions covering both tonsils, 10,000 units are administered. When the entire pharyngeal wall and the tonsils are involved, the quantity is increased to 20,000 to 50,000 units. Laryngeal diphtheria is treated with 50,000 to 100,000 units of antitoxin. Because of the length of time required for antibody to reach maximal levels in the blood after intramuscular injection, one-half of the calculated dose is given by this route. If no reaction occurs, the rest of the antitoxin is infused slowly by vein. Desensitization should be attempted if the initial skin or eye tests are positive. A rare patient may be sensitive to such a high degree that the antiserum cannot be administered without the risk of death. Nothing is gained by repeated injections of antitoxin.

Antitoxin should be given as early in the course of diphtheria as possible. It has been suggested that larger quantities of antiserum than those recommended above should be used when therapy is given late; since toxin is fixed instantaneously to tissues and then cannot be neutralized by antitoxin, no matter how large the dose, the effectiveness of this practice is questionable. Antimicrobial agents do not alter the course, incidence of complications, or outcome of diphtheria.

Patients with *laryngeal obstruction* should be watched very carefully. In mild cases, inhalation of warm or cool vapor may be of some benefit. If advancing signs of airway obstruction develop, intubation or tracheostomy should be performed. These procedures must *never* be delayed until

cyanosis appears because, at this point, stimulation of the pharynx or trachea may result in sudden cardiac standstill and death. Sedative or hypnotic agents should *never* be given because their effects may obscure increasing respiratory difficulty. Intubation is the preferred method of relieving diphtheritic laryngeal obstruction. This requires experienced medical and nursing staff. When such personnel are not available, tracheostomy is probably the safer measure. Since patients with tracheal tubes in place cannot call for help, special nurses should be on duty at all times to ensure prompt and proper care. Tracheostomy or intubation has to be maintained for at least 3 or 4 days.

The pulse and blood pressure should be determined frequently. Little can be done to alter the course of the myocarditis once it develops. Quinidine has been used to prevent some of the arrhythmias, but little has been accomplished. This drug has also been given when potentially lethal abnormal cardiac rhythms have appeared; the results have not been striking, and deleterious effects have been suspected in some instances. The use of procaine amide when ventricular premature beats or tachycardia supervene suggests itself, but no documented observations of its effect have been recorded. The administration of digitalis when cardiac failure occurs in diphtheria is controversial. Some observers consider this drug completely contraindicated and employ fluid and salt restriction and diuretics. Others feel, however, that, used carefully, digitalis may be given safely and with beneficial effects. Shock is best treated with vasoconstricting agents such as ephedrine, norepinephrine, mephentermine sulfate, or metaraminol bitartrate; in many cases, however, such therapy is of no avail and death occurs. There is no evidence that corticosteroids or corticotropin are of any value in the treatment of diphtheria or any of its complications.

Treatment of the Carrier. *Corynebacterium diphtheriae* usually disappears from the upper respiratory tract between the second and fourth weeks in patients who do not receive antimicrobial drugs; in a small number of such individuals the organism may persist for a long time or be present permanently. The most effective treatment of the acute and chronic carrier state is penicillin or erythromycin. The administration of 300,000 to 400,000 units of penicillin G in divided doses per day for 10 to 12 days eliminates the diphtheria bacilli in practically 100 per cent of cases. A single injection of 600,000 units of procaine penicillin per day produces about the same results. Erythromycin, 25 to 50 mg per kg body weight per day orally, is also highly effective and is the drug of choice in persons known to be sensitive to penicillin. Re-treatment is indicated for carriers who do not clear on the first trial. This is preferable to tonsillectomy, which may be considered as a last resort should the carrier state persist despite repeated exposure to antibiotics.

Prevention of Diphtheria. Diphtheria is, for the most part, a preventable disease. Immunization at the age of three months should be routine. Diphtheria toxoid is best given together with tetanus toxoid and pertussis vaccine (DPT) because antibody titers are higher with combined immunization than with either agent alone. "Booster" doses should be administered at the age of one year and again just before a child goes to school. Although it has been suggested that Schick testing is not necessary in those who have been immunized, many physicians still carry this out to determine the status of antitoxic immunity. A Schick test acts as a "booster." It must be reemphasized that a negative reaction does not indicate absolute protection against diphtheria. The old objection to the immunization of adults because of the frequency of severe reaction to the toxoid is no longer valid. The development of highly purified toxoid has made it possible to protect these individuals with little or no risk of untoward sequelae. The usual procedure is to inject 0.1 ml of purified toxin subcutaneously. If there is no reaction in 24 to 48 hr, the regular immunization procedure is carried out.

Unimmunized persons exposed to an active case of diphtheria should be given 2,000 units of antitoxin intramuscularly, after appropriate skin and eye tests. In those who have been previously immunized, a "booster" dose of "fluid" toxoid is usually sufficient. Patients with diphtheria should be quarantined until three successive cultures of the nose, throat, or other infected areas, taken at 24-hr intervals, are negative. When antibiotics have been administered, cultural studies should not be initiated until at least 24 hr after cessation of therapy.

REFERENCES

Beach, M. W., W. B. Gamble, Jr., C. H. Zemp, Jr., and M. Q. Jenkins: Erythromycin in the Treatment of Diphtheria and Diphtheria Carrier State, Pediatrics, 16:335, 1955.

Boyer, N. H., and L. Weinstein: Diphtheritic Myocarditis, New Engl. J. Med., 239:913, 1948.

Dolgopol, V. B., and S. H. Katz: Encephalitis in Diphtheria, Am. J. Diseases Children, 79:640, 1950.

Gore, I.: Myocardial Changes in Fatal Diphtheria: A Summary of Observations in 221 Cases, Am. J. Med. Sci., 219:257, 1948.

Hollander, M. H.: Diphtheria of the Skin, U.S. Air Force Med. J., 2:229, 1951.

Ipsen, J.: Circulating Antitoxin at the Onset of Diphtheria in 425 Patients, Medicine, 251:459, 1954.

——: Immunization of Adults against Diphtheria and Tetanus, New Engl. J. Med., 251:459, 1954.

King, E. O., M. Frobisher, Jr., and E. I. Parsons: The in Vitro Test for Virulence of *Corynebacterium diphtheriae*, Am. J. Pub. Health, 39:1314, 1949.

McLeod, J. W.: The Types *Mitis, Intermedium,* and *Gravis* of Corynebacterium Diphtheriae: A Review of Observations during the Past Ten Years, Bacteriol. Rev., 7:1, 1943.

——: A Survey of the Epidemiology of Diphtheria in North-West Europe and North America in the Period 1920–1946, J. Pathol. Bacteriol., 74:130, 1950.

Naiditch, M. J., and A. G. Bower: Diphtheria: A Study of 1,433 Cases Observed During a Ten-year Period at the Los Angeles County Hospital, Am. J. Med., 17:229, 1954.

Pappenheimer, A. M., Jr.: "Bacterial and Mycotic Infections of Man," 3d ed., chap. 8, The Diphtheria Bacillus and the Diphtheroids, Philadelphia, J. B. Lippincott Company, 1958.

——, G. Edsall, H. S. Lawrence, and J. J. Banton: A Study of Reactions following Administration of Crude and Purified Diphtheria Toxoid in an Adult Population, Am. J. Hyg., 52:323, 1950.

Parsons, E. I.: Induction of Toxigenicity in Non-Toxigenic Strains of *C. Diphtheriae* with Bacteriophages Derived from Non-toxigenic Strains, Proc. Soc. Exptl. Biol. Med., 90:91, 1955.

——, M. Frobisher, M. Moore, and M. A. Aiden: Rapid Virulence Test in Diagnosis of Diphtheria, Proc. Soc. Exptl. Biol. Med., 88:368, 1955.

Scheid, W.: Diphtherial Paralysis: An Analysis of 2292 Cases of Diphtheria in Adults Which Included 174 Cases of Polyneuritis, J. Nervous Mental Disease, 116:1095, 1952.

Weinstein, L.: The Treatment of Acute Diphtheria and the Chronic Carrier State with Penicillin, Am. J. Med. Sci., 213: 308, 1947.

143 TETANUS
Edward S. Miller

Definition. Tetanus is a severe intoxication characterized by generalized hypertonicity of skeletal muscles and convulsive seizures. The manifestations result from the action of an exotoxin produced by *Clostridium tetani*.

History. Tetanus was described by Hippocrates and has been known since ancient times as a scourge of parturient women, newborn babies, and wounded soldiers. As recently as the eighteenth century one out of every six infants born in the Rotunda Hospital in Dublin died of tetanus neonatorum. The record was no more enviable in other parts of the world. Studies beginning in 1884 demonstrated that the disease is caused by a toxin-producing *Clostridium*. In succeeding years immunologic methods were developed for the prevention of the disease.

Etiologic Agent. *Clostridium tetani* is a large, motile, spore-forming, gram-positive bacillus without a capsule. It is an obligate anaerobe and can be cultivated on artificial media in the absence of atmospheric oxygen. Characteristic spherical terminal spores are produced, which are highly resistant; if protected from direct sunlight, they can survive for many years. Tetanus spores are often present in the intestinal contents of man and animals and have been found in soil and street dust in many parts of the world. Under suitable conditions of growth *C. tetani* elaborates a powerful exotoxin. At least 10 antigenic types of the organism have been distinguished, but differentiation is of no practical importance, since the exotoxins of all have the same immunologic properties.

The vegetative forms of *C. tetani* and the exotoxin are destroyed by heating to 65°C for 10 min. Spores can be killed by autoclaving at a temperature of 115°C for 20 min.

Pathogenesis and Epidemiology. The etiologic agent is carried into human tissues by contamination of a wound. A variety of lesions, both large and small, may offer a suitable haven for growth: lacerations, compound fractures, gunshot wounds, burns, frostbites, bedsores, and penetrating lesions produced by nails, human and animal bites, and slivers. Cases have resulted from the use of unsterile surgical supplies and biologic materials. Infections of the post-partum uterus and the umbilical stump (tetanus neonatorum) were once extremely common but became rare after the introduction of aseptic obstetric techniques. *Clostridium tetani* is so ubiquitous in the human environment that almost any contaminated wound may contain the organisms.

The mere fact that *C. tetani* is present does not necessarily mean that tetanus will develop; local conditions in the wound must be suitable. The organisms will proliferate only in the presence of an oxidation-reduction potential far lower than that existing in normal living tissue. Such a fall in potential may occur as a result of the presence in the wound of necrotic tissue, soil, cloth, metal, wood, or of tetanus toxin. Once the organism begins to grow, it produces toxin and thereafter can itself maintain the conditions necessary for continued multiplication. If the conditions for growth are not optimal, tetanus spores may persist in the tissues for many months in a dormant but viable state. Some may be carried by phagocytes to distant parts of the body. If such tissues are later traumatized (as by surgical procedure), tetanus may then develop.

Tetanus bacilli grow locally in a wound, show little capacity to invade, and are in themselves harmless. They cause disease by virtue of a soluble exotoxin elaborated in the course of growth. Actu-

ally, two toxins are produced, tetanolysin and tetanospasmin. Tetanolysin has a lytic effect on red corpuscles in vitro and may also be damaging to leukocytes. Its exact clinical effect is unknown, but it may contribute to tetanus infection by causing local tissue necrosis and by antiphagocytic action. Tetanospasmin is a protein substance with potent neurotoxic properties. It is estimated that a dose of 0.13 mg is lethal for man. The toxin acts at two points in the body: on the neuromuscular end organs, causing sustained muscle spasm, and on the motor nerve cells of the spinal cord, medulla, and pons, causing convulsive seizures. Tetanospasmin has a strong affinity for nerve tissue of susceptible animals, and when once combined with it in vivo cannot be neutralized by any amount of antitoxin. The means by which toxin travels from the local lesion to the nervous system is still a matter of controversy. According to one theory, the toxin enters the neuromuscular end organs, passes centripetally up the axones of motor nerves to the cord, then spreads throughout the nervous system. However, other evidence supports the theory that the toxin is carried to the nervous system via the circulating blood.

Manifestations. The incubation period varies from 2 days to several months, but in two-thirds of cases it falls within the range of 6 to 15 days. Some patients have prodromal symptoms of restlessness and headache. In others the first symptoms are those stemming from the developing muscular rigidity, with vague discomfort in the jaws, neck, or lumbar region. Among the first muscles to show involvement are those innervated by the cranial nerves, particularly the fifth, seventh, ninth, tenth, eleventh, and twelfth. Spasm of the muscles of mastication causes trismus and difficulty with chewing. This highly characteristic phenomenon gives to the disease its common name of *lockjaw*. Sustained contraction of the facial muscles produces a distorted grin, called *risus sardonicus*. Spasm of the pharyngeal muscles makes swallowing difficult. Stiff neck and opisthotonos are also among the early signs. Progressively, other muscle groups become involved, with tightness of the chest and rigidity of the abdominal wall, the back, and the limbs.

The patient is conscious and mentally clear, suffering great pain from muscular spasms. There is profuse perspiration. Fever may or may not be present. The wound through which *C. tetani* was introduced is usually evident, although in 10 to 20 per cent of patients it cannot be found. Neurologic examination discloses hyperactive tendon reflexes, often with sustained clonus. There are no sensory changes.

The symptoms and signs increase in severity for several days. Generalized tonic convulsions appear in all but the milder cases and are accompanied by spasm of the larynx and the respiratory muscles. The resulting acute asphyxia may end fatally. Convulsions are precipitated by various noxious stimuli such as a sudden noise, a hypodermic injection, or jostling of the bed. If the patient survives, the intensity of muscle spasm begins to diminish slowly during the second week. Complete recovery may take several months.

Occasionally *mild cases* occur in which there is only moderate muscle rigidity without tetanic seizures. Sometimes the administration of tetanus antitoxin forestalls the development of generalized tetanus but not of *local tetanus* involving the muscles around the site of injury.

Complications are frequent in tetanus. Pulmonary atelectasis is common and may be followed by pneumonia, which is especially to be dreaded, for it seriously lessens the chances of recovery. Constipation, fecal impaction, and urinary retention are often encountered. Cystitis and pyelonephritis may develop in patients requiring catheterization. Traumatic glossitis is seen frequently. Compression fractures of vertebras may result from the convulsive seizures. Decubitus ulcers are likely to occur in patients under heavy sedation. Serum sickness may appear 1 to 3 weeks after administration of antitoxin. Foot drop and muscle contractures may follow prolonged unconsciousness with the limbs in poor position. Asphyxia from respiratory muscle or laryngeal spasm, or from aspiration of secretions, vomitus, or food may be the immediate cause of death.

Laboratory Findings. The diagnosis of tetanus must be based on the clinical picture, for laboratory examinations are of little assistance. It is difficult to isolate the organism from the local lesion, and it is a laborious task to identify it precisely. Furthermore, the presence of *C. tetani* in a wound does not necessarily indicate that the patient has tetanus. The intoxication itself produces no change in the leukocyte count, but leukocytosis may accompany secondary infection. The cerebrospinal fluid is often under increased pressure but is otherwise not remarkable. The urine is normal unless secondary urinary tract infection is present.

Differential Diagnosis. The incipient stages may resemble certain other conditions, but fully developed tetanus is likely to be confused with few other diseases. A frequent diagnostic problem is differentiation of *serum sickness* from early tetanus. Many patients with injuries are given tetanus antitoxin, and some subsequently develop serum sickness with temporomandibular arthralgia and trismus. Usually arthralgia of other joints is also present, together with urticaria and generalized adenitis. Other conditions in which trismus occurs include *peritonsillar* abscess and local infections of the mouth and cervical region. The finding of a normal spinal fluid in tetanus eliminates confusion with *meningitis*. The clinical picture of *strychnine poisoning*, with hyperexcitability of the muscles, opisthotonos, "risus sardonicus," and tonic convulsions, may closely mimic tetanus, except that the muscles are relaxed between seizures in strychnine intoxication, while spasm tends to persist in tetanus. In *rabies* inability to swallow is often an early symptom, with drooling of saliva and spasms of the muscles of deglutition, followed by fever, anxiety, excitement, delirium, hyperesthesia, and convulsions. A history of animal bite usually is obtainable.

Treatment. This is a grave disease for which, unfortunately, there is no specific treatment. Nevertheless, careful and constant attention to certain supportive measures often will change the outcome from death to recovery.

Sedatives and Muscle Relaxants. A most important feature in therapy involves the utilization of techniques to induce relaxation of muscle spasm and to prevent the dangerous acute tetanic seizure. Traditionally this has been accomplished by the use of sedatives, and often it has been necessary to use doses so large as to render the patient unconscious for long periods of time. This complicates management, as it introduces the dangers of respiratory depression and the problems inherent in the care of an unconscious individual. Various drugs have been used, including barbiturates, paraldehyde, chloral hydrate, magnesium sulfate, and tribromoethanol. Some of the newer muscle relaxants and tranquilizers have proved to be extremely useful in controlling spasms and seizures, and at the same time they permit a reduction in the amount of ancillary sedative medication required. The patient need no longer be narcotized. Meprobamate (400 mg every 4 hr) appears to be the preferred medication for basic use. If satisfactory control is not obtained with it, then chlorpromazine (25 to 50 mg every 4 hr) is added to the regimen. However it may cause excessive hypotension and somnolence. A barbiturate such as sodium pentobarbital is also given periodically (100 mg every 4 to 8 hr) to induce suitable sedation. These preparations are given parenterally during the acute phase of illness. Precise dosage schedules must of course be determined empirically. Neuromuscular blocking agents such as curare are considered by many clinicians to be too dangerous, because of the possibility of precipitating respiratory paralysis.

Antiserum. As soon as the patient has received adequate sedation, he is given 50,000 units of tetanus antitoxin intramuscularly and 50,000 units intravenously, the latter being added to 250 cc of normal saline, which also contains 1 cc of 1:1,000 solution of aqueous epinephrine. It has been shown that the plasma titer of antibody rises slowly over a 2-day period after intramuscular injection; so it is prudent to give some of the antiserum intravenously. Ten thousand units of antitoxin is infiltrated around the local lesion, because a considerable reservoir of toxin is present in this region. Serum never should be given intraspinally. The usual tests for serum sensitivity must be performed beforehand. Bovine antiserum is available if the patient is allergic to horse serum. This dose is sufficiently large to provide a safe excess of circulating antitoxin for 7 weeks or longer. Repeated doses are not necessary except in unusual cases involving extensive, slow-healing wounds, where readministration may have to be considered. Antitoxin has no curative action in tetanus, for it has no effect on the toxin which is already combined with nerve tissue. Its only action is to neutralize newly formed toxin as it is produced in the lesion and before it has reached susceptible nerve cells.

Treatment of Local Lesion. The patient should receive sedatives and antiserum before the site of infection is manipulated. The lesion is then treated according to the same surgical principles that would be applicable if tetanus were not present. Specifically, a limb should not be amputated simply because the patient has tetanus.

Nursing Care. There is no disease in which meticulous, gentle nursing care is of greater importance. Constant attendance by special nurses is essential. The patient should be in a quiet, darkened room, where all external stimuli, such as noise, drafts, and jarring, are kept to a minimum. Secretions which accumulate in the pharynx must be removed by suction and postural drainage. It has been shown that a 25° elevation of the foot of the bed is necessary to achieve successful postural drainage. A padded tongue depressor should be placed between the teeth to prevent biting of the tongue during convulsions. Bedsores can be avoided by use of a foam rubber mattress, by changing the patient's position frequently, and by special attention to care of the skin. Catheterization may be necessary, but an indwelling catheter is best avoided, as it precipitates convulsive seizures. Enemas are given as needed. Foot drop and wrist drop can be prevented by suitable positioning with pillows, sandbags, or splints.

Feeding. Oral feeding is impossible because of trismus. Intravenous feeding must be used during the first few days of illness, and particularly in heavily sedated or unconscious patients. It is best not to give fluids subcutaneously because the attendant pain stimulates the patient unduly. After his condition has stabilized, and if he is conscious, he may be fed by nasogastric tube.

Management of Respiratory Tract. It is essential that respiratory tract obstruction be prevented or corrected. This complication can result from the presence of excessive secretions, from spasm of the larynx or the muscles of respiration, or from failure of the respiratory center. It leads to anoxia, pulmonary edema, atelectasis, and pneumonia. Tracheotomy has proved to be a safe and an extremely valuable therapeutic adjunct, and it may be used to advantage in most moderately to severely ill patients. The orifice should be bathed, cleansed, and suctioned frequently. Alevaire and oxygen are administered as needed, and bronchoscopy is readily performed when indicated. Following tracheotomy it is often found that convulsive seizures are fewer, while at the same time smaller doses of sedatives are required.

Chemotherapy. The tetanal infection itself requires the use of an antibiotic, since antitoxin does not have antimicrobial properties. Conversely, antibiotics do not possess antitoxic properties. Experimental studies indicate that oxytetracycline is the drug of choice, though other tetracyclines or penicillin are also effective. One of these should be given during the first week.

Prophylaxis. In the prevention of tetanus it is important that all contaminated wounds receive thorough and prompt cleansing and debridement. Certain types of wounds are prone to develop tetanus infections, including those contaminated by soil, those over 3 hr old, those already infected, deep and puncture wounds, and those containing devitalized tissue. The physician must exercise his clinical judgment in determining which will be given tetanus prophylaxis.

As noted above, oxytetracycline or penicillin is given to prevent or to cure an incipient tetanal infection. In addition, either passive or active immunization is used to raise the resistance of the patient. If he has not had the benefit of previous active immunization, he must be given immediate passive protection with horse serum antitoxin. This is administered subcutaneously in a dose of 1,500 to 10,000 units. The traditional dose is 1,500 units, and only rarely does tetanus follow this treatment. Nevertheless, many authorities now believe that the minimum dose should be 3,000 units, and that the amount should be increased if there is delay in treatment or in the presence of a serious injury such as a compound fracture, a gunshot wound, or a heavily contaminated wound.

However, there are serious disadvantages to the use of antitoxin. It provides protection for only a few weeks. A significant proportion of patients exhibit allergic reactions, including local hypersensitivity, serum sickness, and rare but catastrophic anaphylactic shock. Hypersensitivity reactions are reported in 2.5 to 9 per cent of patients who have not had previous serum injections, and in up to 24 per cent of those who had them. Furthermore, patients who have had previous experience with horse serum often exhibit great acceleration in the rate of removal of antibody from the blood, so that passive protection in them is short-lived. Another limitation to the use of antitoxin is the fact that not all who need it receive it. In one-third to one-half of cases of tetanus, illness follows a wound so trivial that it is disregarded by the patient or is considered by the physician to be too insignificant to warrant antitoxin prophylaxis.

Active immunization provides the most satisfactory and safest type of prophylaxis. A toxoid is used, and primary immunization is achieved by giving two doses of an alum-precipitated toxoid or three doses of fluid toxoid at monthly intervals. A reinforcing dose is given after 6 to 12 months, thus achieving basic immunization. Thereafter immunity is maintained with a booster dose every 3 to 5 years. The antibody response to primary immunization is slow, so that if active immunization is initiated at the time of injury the patient will not get the immediate protection he needs. However, if he has previously had basic active immunization, a satisfactory rise in serum antibody titer will occur within 4 to 7 days after a booster dose. Ordinarily a booster dose may be relied on as late as 10 years after the last previous toxoid injection, provided one is certain the patient has had basic immunization, and provided it is given within 24 hr after the injury. However, there are occasional situations involving actively immunized individuals in which conservative judgment indicates the simultaneous administration of both toxoid and antitoxin (utilizing opposite arms). This should be done in massively contaminated, large or multiple wounds, particularly if they involve the head or neck. It should also be done if there is doubt regarding previous active immunization, or if there is delay beyond 24 hr in administering the booster in the presence of a serious wound.

It is of interest to note that, in an individual who has had previous active immunization, the simultaneous administration of a booster dose of toxoid and of up to 1,500 units of antitoxin (in different arms) will not interfere with the antibody response to toxoid. In the previously unimmunized individual it may. Therefore, the first dose of toxoid should be given several weeks after the antitoxin, or if given simultaneously an extra dose of toxoid should be given in the basic series.

The foregoing discussion supports the proposition that all persons should receive the benefit of routine active immunization. Not only will this provide protection against tetanus, but of even greater practical importance is the fact that it will obviate the frequent necessity of administering antitoxin, with all the attendant hazards of sensitization. A large pool of actively immunized individuals already exists in the United States, including those who served in the Armed Forces, and the many children who have benefited from pediatric immunization programs during the past 25 years. Their immunity should not be permitted to wane. It is particularly urgent that toxoid be administered to all patients who have allergies, to all who have received injections of horse serum, and to those who are occupationally prone to injuries.

Prognosis. Case fatality rates average 30 to 40 per cent, but vary markedly with the character of the cases. The rate is much higher in young children, in the aged, in drug addicts, and in those who develop pneumonia or other secondary infections. It is much higher if the incubation period is less than 7 days or if tetanal spasms supervene within 2 days after onset. Most deaths occur within the first 10 days of illness. Survivors make a complete recovery. Interestingly, they are not immune to reinfection.

REFERENCES

Drew, A. L.: Tetanus: Historical Review of Treatment, Neurology, 4:449, 1954.

Edsall, G.: Specific Prophylaxis of Tetanus, J.A.M.A., 171:417, 1959.

Perlstein, M. A., M. D. Stein, and H. Elam: Routine Treatment of Tetanus, J.A.M.A., 173:1536, 1960.

Smith, L. DeS.: *Clostridium tetani* in "Introduction to the Pathogenic Anaerobes," pp. 88–107, Chicago, University of Chicago Press, 1955.

Wright, G. P.: The Neurotoxins of *Clostridium botulinum* and *Clostridium tetani*, Pharmacol. Rev., 7: 413, 1955.

144 BOTULISM
Edward S. Miller

Definition. Botulism is an intoxication resulting from absorption of a poisonous substance produced by *Clostridium botulinum*. The illness is characterized by generalized muscular weakness and frequently ends in death.

History. This disease was first described in Europe over 200 years ago. It was sometimes seen in individuals who had eaten contaminated sausages. For this reason the name of the illness is derived from the Latin word for sausage. Outbreaks of botulism have been observed in the United States for many years, chiefly in association with the consumption of inadequately processed canned foods.

Etiology. *Clostridium botulinum* is a motile, gram-positive bacillus which produces subterminal spores. It grows readily on artificial media but only under anaerobic conditions. The organisms are natural inhabitants of the soil and are found in abundance in many parts of the world. In the United States the soils of the Rocky Mountain and the Pacific Coast regions are most heavily infested. Organisms are frequently present on fruits and vegetables and thus are carried into the gastrointestinal tracts of animals and of man. However this species is unable to establish itself and grow in the human intestine, in contrast to other kinds of clostridia.

Clostridium botulinum produces a remarkably potent exotoxin (called *botulin*), under suitable conditions of anaerobic growth, in a variety of foodstuffs of animal and plant origin. There are five different immunologic varieties of this organism, designated as types A, B, C, D, and E. They differ in that each produces a specific exotoxin which is antigenically distinct from the others. These toxins are by far the most potent poisons known, the lethal dose for man being estimated in terms of a fraction of a gamma. Only tetanus and shigella toxins are of the same order of toxicity. Type A and type B toxins have each been obtained in presumably pure states and identified as globulins of large molecular weight. Botulin has the capacity to hemagglutinate red blood cells. There are no qualitative differences in the effects of the different types of toxins, but there are marked species differences in host susceptibility. Human cases are usually due to type A or type B, and rarely to type E; only two outbreaks of type C have been reported, and only one of type D.

Some spores can withstand boiling at 100°C for as long as 22 hr, but are killed by moist heat at 120°C in 4 to 20 min. The exotoxin is more labile and is inactivated by boiling at 100°C for 10 min.

Pathogenesis. Botulism occurs as a result of the ingestion of toxin which has previously been formed in food. The botulinus bacillus does not produce toxin in the alimentary tract and therefore is harmless when ingested. This organism frequently contaminates foodstuffs, but no human disease has resulted from the consumption of fresh food. However, the spores will survive and produce toxin if improper methods of food preservation are employed. The products implicated are canned fruits and vegetables and canned or preserved fish and meats, as well as cheeses. Commercial packers in this country now use sterilizing techniques which are adequate to destroy all spores. The chief danger lies in home-canned products, particularly when high-pressure steam methods are not utilized. Because of this, most outbreaks in the United States have occurred in individual families or other small groups. About 15 such outbreaks are reported annually in this country, the majority of them in California, Washington, and Colorado.

Spoilage of food may be suspected because of abnormal taste, odor, gas, turbidity, or softening, but there may be no observable alterations. Therefore, when possible, home-preserved products should be boiled for 10 min before use. Needless to say, any item which appears to be spoiled must be destroyed without being tasted. Care must be taken to prevent contact of contaminated food with cuts on the hands, for a dangerous quantity of botulin might conceivably be absorbed.

The natural and usual portal of entry of botulin is via the gastrointestinal tract. The toxin is a protein; yet somehow it is able to preserve its identity in the gastrointestinal tract, traverse the intestinal wall, and enter the circulation. The mechanism of this remarkable accomplishment is not understood. A possible explanation is as follows: only a minute fraction of the ingested toxin escapes digestion and is absorbed, but botulin is so potent that this tiny amount is sufficient to produce disease. The major site of absorption is thought to be in the small intestine. Until recently it was believed that this represented the only natural means by which human beings acquire botulism, though it has long been known experimentally that animals are far more susceptible when challenged parenterally or via the respiratory tract. It is of interest to note several case reports which indicate that *C. botulinum* can sometimes proliferate in contaminated wounds, produce toxin, and thus cause clinical botulism in man. This is an entirely new concept of pathogenesis, and it demands a careful evaluation of the course of illness in patients with wound infections, particularly in the presence of gas gangrene.

Botulinus toxin has a highly specialized biochemical effect. It acts only on the cholinergic system, that is, only at the myoneural junctions of somatic motor nerves and at the synapses of efferent parasympathetic nerves, thus blocking the transmission of nerve impulses along these pathways. It interferes either with the production or with the release of acetylcholine from the terminal fibers. It has no effect on the central nervous system; it does not abolish conduction in the nerve itself, it does not affect the reactivity of the end plate, nor does it affect the muscle fibers.

Botulism is not limited to man. The natural disease occurs in a varied assortment of wild and domesticated animals and birds, while still others are susceptible to experimental inoculation. The disease is sometimes seen in chickens or cats in relation to human outbreaks, when these animals are fed scraps from the table.

Manifestations. Following ingestion of botulin, there is a latent period, usually in the range of

12 to 36 hr, though it may be as short as 2 hr or as long as 14 days. The incubation period is shortened and the severity of illness increased as the size of the dose is increased.

Illness begins insidiously, with fatigue, weakness, headache, and dizziness. Digestive complaints are observed in only one-third of cases and probably are due to local irritation from other substances in the spoiled food, rather than to the toxin. They consist of nausea, vomiting, upper abdominal discomfort, and diarrhea. Such symptoms subside after a few hours, and thereafter there is obstipation, with abdominal distention but without tenderness or pain. Botulism is essentially a generalized paralytic disease, and these manifestations soon dominate the clinical picture. Weakness is noted during the first 24 hr in the muscles innervated by the cranial nerves. Soon it spreads to the rest of the skeletal system. Except for headache, botulism does not give rise to pain.

The patient is clear mentally and remains so throughout the course of his illness. There is no fever unless secondary infection occurs. Initially, there may be hypersecretion of the lacrimal, salivary, and sweat glands, but this is soon followed by diminished function. Early in the illness excessive vagal tone sometimes causes the pulse rate to drop below 50 per minute. Subsequently, there are vagal depression and tachycardia. Hypotension may occur as a result of peripheral vascular dilatation.

The most significant physical alterations are seen in the nervous system. Nearly all patients exhibit cranial nerve palsies involving any except the olfactory and optic nerves. Weakness of the intrinsic and extrinsic eye muscles results in loss of the light and accommodation reflexes, mydriasis, ptosis, strabismus, diplopia, or nystagmus. The face becomes expressionless because of the seventh nerve paralysis. Chewing, swallowing, and phonation are interfered with, and the tongue cannot be controlled. The neck muscles are unable to support the head. The limbs become progressively weaker, and movements may be incoordinated. Complete paralysis of a limb is rarely encountered, since death supervenes before this occurs. Pulmonary ventilation is diminished as a result of weakness of the intercostal muscles and the diaphragm, and cyanosis appears. The superficial and deep reflexes are diminished but rarely absent. The sensory system is intact.

The paralysis may progress to a fatal termination after 2 to 10 days of illness. Death results from paralysis of the respiratory muscles, from obstruction of the airway, or from attendant pulmonary infection. In nonfatal cases the muscular weakness increases over a period of 10 days; then, almost imperceptibly, function begins to return. The muscles involved in respiration, deglutition, and speech are the first to show improvement. Visual abnormalities persist for weeks or months. From 2 to 6 months elapse before all symptoms disappear.

Laboratory Findings. The clinical diagnosis can be substantiated by identifying botulinus toxin either in the food or in the body of the patient. A suspected specimen is suspended in saline solution and inoculated into mice. If toxin is present, the animals become paralyzed, whereas control mice, passively immunized with specific antiserum, are protected. The toxin can occasionally be demonstrated in the stomach or intestinal contents, in the peripheral blood during life, or in organ extracts after death. Additional evidence may be gained by culturing *C. botulinum* from the food, although it must not be forgotten that the organism may be a harmless contaminant.

The disease produces no characteristic changes in the leukocyte or erythrocyte counts, in the urine, or in the spinal fluid. The electrocardiogram may show flattening of T waves and depression of S-T segments.

Differential Diagnosis. Botulism may be confused with other diseases of toxic or infectious origin. One should seek a history of recent consumption of home-preserved foods, and of coincident illness among other human beings or animals that shared the food. Cranial nerve palsies and other paralytic phenomena are seen at times in poliomyelitis, in viral encephalitis, and in acute infectious polyneuritis. These diseases are often accompanied by fever and by spinal fluid abnormalities. In postdiphtheritic paralysis a history of preceding sore throat usually can be obtained. The paralysis of shellfish poisoning appears a few minutes after ingestion of the sea food and is accompanied by paresthesia, giddiness, and somnolence. In mushroom poisoning there are severe pains with marked vomiting and diarrhea. Intoxication with the belladonna group of alkaloids leads to fever, tachycardia, and delirium. An overdose of curare results in the rapid onset of widespread paralysis, with death or recovery in the course of minutes or a few hours. Myasthenia gravis is usually easily differentiated.

Treatment and Prophylaxis. Botulism is most satisfactorily controlled by prevention, for methods of treatment are inadequate. Practically all human cases are due to either type A or type B toxin, and a bivalent antitoxin is available for prophylaxis and for therapy. When the diagnosis is suspected on clinical grounds, the antitoxin should be administered immediately by the intravenous route in a total dose of 100,000 units. The antiserum will not reverse the effects of toxin which has already become bound to receptor cells, but it will neutralize that which has not yet been fixed. Early administration, therefore, is important. The same dose should be given prophylactically to other individuals who have eaten the contaminated food but have not yet developed symptoms.

The patient should be kept at strict bed rest. There may be residual toxin in the gastrointestinal tract; therefore it should be emptied by gastric lavage, by enema, and by catharsis. Hypotension and shock can be counteracted by appropriate measures. Careful and continuous nursing care is essential.

Respiratory failure and airway obstruction are fundamental features which lead to death, and every effort must be made to overcome these dangers. The problems are similar to those encountered in poliomyelitis with respiratory paralysis. Many of the newer therapeutic techniques which have proved successful in that disease are applicable to the treatment of botulism (see p. 1145). When the swallowing reflex is lost, oral feeding becomes dangerous and must be replaced by nasogastric tube or intravenous feeding. Pharyngeal secretions are removed by suction and by postural drainage. The patient should be placed in a mechanical respirator with the first signs of weakness of the respiratory muscles. Tracheotomy is an essential part of the program, providing an unobstructed airway and a means of removing tracheal secretions.

Narcotics, sedatives, and other respiratory depressants are strictly contraindicated, even though patients are often apprehensive and restless.

Effective toxoids have been developed for protection against all five types of toxin. They are useful chiefly in protecting laboratory workers.

Prognosis. The fatality rate in type A cases is 70 per cent, while in type B cases it is 20 per cent or less. If a patient survives the first 10 days of illness, his chances of recovery are good. Convalescence may take as long as 6 months, but it leads eventually to complete restoration of function.

REFERENCES

Dack, G. M.: "Food Poisoning," 3d ed., pp. 59–108, Chicago, University of Chicago Press, 1956.

Lamanna, C.: The Most Poisonous Poison, Science, 130:763, 1959.

Smith, L. DeS.: "Introduction to the Pathogenic Anaerobes," pp. 108–133, Chicago, University of Chicago Press, 1955.

145 OTHER CLOSTRIDIAL INFECTIONS

Edward W. Hook

Bacteria of the genus *Clostridium* are normal inhabitants of soil and the gastrointestinal tracts of man and animals. Most of the 50 species that have been recognized are saprophytic, but others are infectious for man and animals, usually under conditions of lowered host and tissue resistance. Infections with these organisms are often associated with profound systemic manifestations, and all pathogenic clostridia, except *Clostridium tetani* (p. 988) and *C. botulinum* (p. 992), are capable of causing extensive tissue destruction at the site of invasion. Diseases caused by these other clostridia include gas gangrene, cellulitis, postabortal and puerperal sepsis, and rarely, pneumonia, pleurisy, peritonitis, meningitis, endocarditis, cystitis, or bursitis. In addition, ingestion of food contaminated with certain clostridia may cause enterocolitis without the neurologic manifestations of botulism.

Hippocrates and Celsus were aware of the relationship between penetrating wounds and gas gangrene, but the nature of this disorder was not appreciated until the discovery of pathogenic clostridia by Pasteur, Novy, and Welch. The incidence of gas gangrene diminished markedly with the advent of antiseptic surgery in the latter half of the nineteenth century, only to rise again to epidemic proportions during the trench warfare of the First World War. The rarity of serious clostridial infections in United Nations troops in Korea attests to the advances in surgical management of war wounds. Gas gangrene and clostridial cellulitis are still encountered in neglected civilian injuries, and clostridial infections of the uterus account for a large proportion of deaths from criminal abortions.

Etiology. Wounds complicated by gas gangrene usually contain a mixture of pathogenic and saprophytic clostridia, often including *C. tetani,* as well as a variety of other organisms. *Clostridium welchii* (*C. perfringens*), *C. oedematiens* (*C. novyi*), or *C. septicum* (*Vibrion septique*) can be cultured from most cases of gas gangrene and clostridial cellulitis, and *C. welchii* causes virtually all clostridial infections of the uterus. *Clostridium bifermentans, C. sporogenes, C. histolyticum, C. tertium,* and *C. fallax* are less virulent organisms that occasionally cause gas gangrene but are more commonly associated with localized cellulitis. *Clostridium botulinum* has been isolated from wound infections of several patients with clinical manifestations of botulism (see p. 993).

The clostridia of gas gangrene and related infections are anaerobic or microaerophilic gram-positive bacilli that produce abundant gas in artificial media and form subterminal endospores. *Clostridium welchii* is encapsulated and nonmotile, rarely sporulates in artificial media, and its spores can usually be destroyed by boiling.

Epidemiology and Pathogenesis. Clostridia do not penetrate intact skin or mucous membranes, but gain entrance to the tissues through wounds or perforated abdominal viscera. Gas gangrene develops only in devitalized tissues in which the arterial circulation has been compromised by trauma, by constricting tourniquets or casts, or by obliterative arterial disease. Infection is most frequent after severe muscle injuries, particularly of the thigh, and is more common in wounds complicated by compound fractures or lodgment of foreign bodies. The importance of host factors in the pathogenesis of clostridial infections is emphasized by the observation that pathogenic clostridia can be cultured from one-third to two-thirds of severe traumatic wounds whereas gas gangrene develops in only an occasional case.

Gas gangrene and related infections are characterized by extensive necrotizing myositis, edema, thrombosis of small vessels, interstitial gas bubbles, and minimal infiltration of leukocytes. Although bacteremia may occur, infection at distant sites is rare. Clostridia produce potent toxins during the course of infection; spores or vegetative forms washed free of toxin are completely innocuous when injected into undamaged tissues of experimental animals. The nature and the amounts of toxin produced vary considerably for different species and strains. Clostridium welchii elaborates alpha toxin, a lecithinase which is the principal tissue-destroying, hemolytic, and "lethal" toxin. Other C. welchii toxins include collagenase, hyaluronidase, hemolytic theta toxin, a substance that damages vascular endothelium, and a factor that inhibits leukocyte migration and phagocytosis. None of these organisms produces a neurotoxin; muscle spasm or paralysis in a patient with gas gangrene suggests concurrent tetanus or botulism.

Clostridial Myonecrosis (Gas Gangrene, Clostridial Myositis)

Gas gangrene occurs as a complication of extensive injury and ischemia of skeletal muscle. The incubation period is usually 1 to 4 days but may vary from 6 hr to 6 weeks or longer. The earliest symptom is sudden, severe pain in the injured part. The distal portion of an involved limb becomes cold and edematous within a few hours, and eventually pulseless and gangrenous. The wound drains a watery, brown material with a peculiar sweet, foul odor. The appearance of the wound is usually not that of a pyogenic inflammatory lesion. Depending on the duration of the process, the surrounding skin may be normal, white and tense, or dusky brown and reddish. Vesicles or hemorrhagic bullae may develop, particularly in C. septicum infections. Gas is usually not detectable in the tissues by palpation except in advanced lesions. Occasionally tiny bubbles may be seen in the discharge from the wound, and rarely crepitation can

be detected at an early stage by auscultation with the stethoscope. The involved muscle appears dark red or black, herniates through the wound, and sloughs at the surface.

Systemic manifestations developing shortly after onset of severe pain and swelling of an injured extremity strongly suggest gas gangrene. The patient is prostrated, pale, and motionless but is usually well oriented, alert, and extremely apprehensive. The temperature usually does not exceed 101°F and may be normal. As the illness progresses, there may be anorexia, vomiting, profuse watery or bloody diarrhea, and eventually, circulatory collapse with clammy skin, tachycardia, hypotension, and sometimes wide pulse pressure and dicrotic pulse. The pulse rate is elevated out of proportion to the temperature. Massive intravascular hemolysis is rare with C. welchii myositis. Pericardial effusion is sometimes noted. Delirium and coma may precede death, but more commonly the patient dies suddenly several days after the onset of illness, often during surgery or anesthesia or while only being moved. Acute renal failure is occasionally a late complication.

Gas gangrene must be differentiated from nonclostridial infections of gangrenous limbs caused by anaerobic streptococci (p. 923) or aerobic gas-forming coliform bacilli (p. 932).

Clostridial Cellulitis

This is a relatively benign infection of skin and subcutaneous tissues that occurs in approximately 5 per cent of wounds contaminated with pathogenic clostridia. The disease is characterized by spreading necrosis of superficial tissues and a profuse, foul-smelling, brown, seropurulent exudate. Gas, which crepitates on palpation, invariably forms in the subcutaneous tissues and may involve an entire limb or form a localized gas abscess. In clostridial cellulitis, the underlying skeletal muscle is not involved, pain is not severe, and the only systemic manifestations are slight fever and moderate tachycardia. It can usually be differentiated from streptococcal cellulitis by the presence of subcutaneous gas and the absence of erythema.

Postabortal and Puerperal Sepsis

Uterine infections with C. welchii usually occur after incomplete abortions induced under unsterile conditions and, occasionally, after spontaneous abortions, prolonged labor at term, ruptured membranes, or operative interference with pregnancy. The organisms presumably invade the damaged endometrium through the retained products of conception. The earliest symptoms may be caused by instrumentation and consist of metrorrhagia, suprapubic and back pain, chills, and fever. Fever with a temperature of 100 to 103°F, often with chills, usually recurs several days after abortion, but the incubation period can be as short as 6 hr. Vaginal bleeding is almost invariably present, and there is often a brown, foul-smelling vaginal discharge containing necrotic tissue. The cervix is soft and patulous, and the uterus and adnexas are usually very tender. The lower abdominal wall is often tense, or signs of generalized peritonitis may be present, secondary to perforation of the uterus or parametrial extension of infection. Nausea, vomiting, and profuse diarrhea are often prominent.

Systemic manifestations usually appear with dramatic suddenness. Massive intravascular hemolysis, accompanied by hemoglobinemia, hemoglobinuria, and jaundice, is often the most striking feature of the disease. Icterus may appear within hours after the onset of illness. As in gas gangrene, the clinical picture may be dominated by circulatory collapse with hypotension, extreme tachycardia, cyanosis, hyperpnea, and pulmonary edema. Despite severe prostration, the patient is well oriented, alert, and apprehensive almost to the end. The mortality rate in postabortal or puerperal sepsis caused by *C. welchii* is 40 to 70 per cent. Death may occur a few hours after onset or be delayed for several days. Patients who recover from the acute episode of shock, dehydration, and hemolysis frequently develop acute renal failure.

Unusual local complications of the uterine infection are gas gangrene of the vagina and rectum with formation of a cloaca and clostridial cellulitis of the anterior abdominal wall following caesarean section or hysterectomy. At times, the infectious process is confined to the endometrium and myometrium, with intrauterine gas formation (physometra).

Diseases to be considered in the *differential diagnosis* include perforated uterus, ruptured ectopic pregnancy, ingestion of toxic abortifacients, streptococcal or staphylococcal puerperal sepsis, pelvic thrombophlebitis with septic pulmonary emboli, acute hepatic necrosis of pregnancy, sickle-cell crisis, and Weil's disease.

Clostridium welchii *Food Poisoning*

temperature for several hours after cooking. Nausea is common, but vomiting is rare. Systemic manifestations are usually absent, and recovery is uneventful after 12 to 24 hr. A severe form of the disease in Germany, known as "enteritis necrotans," has been associated with a high incidence of intestinal obstruction, severe dehydration, shock, and death.

Clostridium welchii food poisoning can be reproduced experimentally in man by feeding the organism actively growing in meat or soup. However, gastroenteritis does not occur after ingestion of bacteria-free filtrates of cultures of food-poisoning strains.

Miscellaneous Clostridial Infections

Pathogenic clostridia are occasionally introduced into the abdomen, thoracic cavity, or cranium through penetrating wounds or surgical incisions. Actual visceral infections with these organisms are exceedingly rare and almost invariably associated with a mixed bacterial flora. Primary pneumonia in the absence of a penetrating wound or distant focus has been described. Clostridial pleurisy may involve the underlying lung but is usually an indolent localized infection with minimal systemic manifestations. Meningitis is usually secondary to a puncture wound of the skull and is often associated with a necrotizing cerebritis. Clostridial peritonitis may follow perforation of the gallbladder, appendix, or other viscus and is usually rapidly fatal. Clostridial septicemia occurs occasionally in patients with leukemia or other neoplastic processes who are treated with antimetabolites and anti-inflammatory glucocorticoids. The primary infection is in the gastrointestinal tract, which is usually the site of extensive neoplastic disease. Cystitis with pneumaturia, endocarditis, and bursitis after needle aspiration are other examples of rare clostridial infections.

Laboratory Findings. The diagnosis of gas gangrene, clostridial cellulitis, postabortal sepsis or other clostridial infections quently in gas gangrene and invariably in post-abortal sepsis; total blood leukocyte counts range from 15,000 to 40,000 cells per cu mm, and occasionally exceed 60,000 cells per cu mm. Marked thrombocytopenia develops in about 50 per cent of patients with clostridial sepsis. The urine frequently contains protein and casts. Renal insufficiency may lead to severe and irreversible azotemia, hyperpotassemia, hyperphosphatemia, and acidosis.

X-ray examination sometimes provides the first clue leading to the correct diagnosis by revealing the presence of gas in muscle, subcutaneous tissue, or uterus; however, demonstration of gas in tissues is not diagnostic of clostridial infection. Other bacteria, especially of the genus *Aerobacter* or *Escherichia,* may be responsible for gas production, and occasionally air is sucked into a wound at the time of penetrating injury.

Profound alterations of circulating erythrocytes are common in postabortal sepsis but are much less frequent in other clostridial infections. Anemia may develop with almost unbelievable rapidity; the red blood cell count occasionally decreases by 2 million cells per cu mm in less than 24 hr. Hemolysis results in severe anemia, hemoglobinemia, hemoglobinuria, and elevated levels of indirect serum bilirubin. Spherocytosis, increased osmotic and mechanical fragility of the red blood cells, erythrophagocytosis, and methemoglobinemia have also been described.

Treatment. Serious clostridial infections require prompt surgical intervention. If clostridial myonecrosis is strongly suspected, early surgery aids diagnosis, permits decompression of fascial compartments and excision of devitalized muscle, and may circumvent amputation. In addition, early debridement of an involved extremity may afford dramatic relief of the systemic manifestations of gas gangrene. Curettage of the uterus should be performed for diagnosis and treatment of postabortal clostridial infections. Hysterectomy should be considered if myometritis is present. Simple excision and adequate drainage usually suffice for treating clostridial cellulitis.

Penicillin is the antibiotic of choice for all clostridial infections and should be administered in doses of at least 20 million units a day. Tetracycline is also active against most strains of *Clostridium* and has been recommended as an adjunct to penicillin therapy. Despite the fact that clostridial toxins are rapidly fixed in the tissues and cannot be demonstrated in the blood, early treatment with antitoxin appears to reduce the mortality from gas gangrene complicating war wounds. It is recommended that 100,000 units of polyvalent gas gangrene antitoxin be given intravenously as an initial dose, followed by 50,000 units every 4 to 6 hr to all patients with suspected gas gangrene or clostridial postabortal sepsis.

The use of clostridial toxoids for prophylactic immunization of individuals in hazardous occupations awaits evaluation. Antitoxin is apparently ineffective as a prophylactic agent and is not recommended. The most reliable protection against gas gangrene is achieved by early and adequate wound debridement.

Intravenous infusions of blood, plasma-volume expanders, fluids, and electrolytes are often required to combat shock, anemia, and dehydration. Renal insufficiency should be treated in the same manner as acute tubular necrosis from other causes (see p. 1496).

REFERENCES

Altemeier, W. A., and W. L. Furste: Gas Gangrene, Intern. Abstr. Surg., 84:507, 1947.

Boggs, D. R., E. Frei, and L. B. Thomas: Clostridial Gas Gangrene and Septicemia in Four Patients with Leukemia, New Engl. J. Med., 259:1255, 1958.

Editorial: *Clostridium welchii* Food-Poisoning, Brit. Med. J., I:711, 1960.

Hill, A. M.: Post-abortal and Puerperal Gas Gangrene: Report of 30 Cases, J. Obstet. Gynaecol. Brit. Empire, 43:201, 1936.

MacLennan, J. D.: Anaerobic Infections of War Wounds in the Middle East, Lancet, II.63, 94, 123, 1943.

Mahn, E., and L. M. Dantuono: Postabortal Septicotoxemia Due to *Clostridium welchii:* Seventy-five Cases from the Maternity Hospital, Santiago, Chile, 1948–1952, Am. J. Obstet. Gynecol., 70:604, 1955.

Smith, L. DeS.: Clostridia in Gas Gangrene, Bacteriol, Revs., 13:233, 1949.

Section 8: Mycobacterial Diseases

146   TUBERCULOSIS
William M. M. Kirby

Definition. Tuberculosis is an infectious disease of protean manifestations which is widespread among man and animals. The initial lesion is usually located in the lung, and from it tubercle bacilli may spread by intrabronchial dissemination, or by direct extension; or they may be carried in the blood stream to many organs throughout the body, causing destructive lesions at the time of dissemination or after long periods of latency. In the majority of individuals the primary infection becomes arrested, but it causes alterations in the immunologic state of the host which modify the response of the tissues to subsequent reinfection or to exacerbation of the primary infection. Pathologically, varying degrees of exudation, production, tubercle formation, necrosis, and fibrosis are observed, depending on the organ involved, the number of infecting bacilli, the virulence of the organisms, and the immunologic state of the patient.

History. The discovery of lesions involving the bones of a Neolithic man and of Egyptian mummies indicates that man has been afflicted with tuberculosis during much of his evolutionary development. The contagiousness of tuberculosis was recognized by Aristotle, and the name *phthisis* was conferred by Hippocrates because of the marked bodily wasting produced by the disease. An important advance occurred in 1819 when Laennec asserted in his treatise on the use of the stethoscope that tubercles, wherever present, were manifestations of a single disease process. This disputed doctrine was supported by the inoculation experiments of Villemin in 1865 and was finally proved by the discovery of the tubercle bacillus by Koch in 1882. Subdivision of the tubercle bacilli pathogenic for man into three types followed, the avian bacillus being isolated by Magucci in 1890 and human and bovine types being differentiated by Theobald Smith in 1898.

A most important development in the history of tuberculosis was the discovery of streptomycin by Waksman and his associates in 1944. The early studies of Hinshaw and Feldman indicated that streptomycin possessed therapeutic potentialities unapproached by earlier chemotherapeutic agents. Lehmann, working with derivatives of benzoic acid, was responsible in 1943 for experiments leading to the synthesis and eventual clinical utilization of para-aminosalicylic acid. Isoniazid was discovered independently in 1951 by three groups of chemists who were studying the tuberculostatic action of derivatives of nicotinic acid.

Prevalence and Incidence. Tuberculin surveys and autopsy studies 50 years ago indicated that virtually 100 per cent of the population was infected prior to the age of twenty. The situation has changed greatly since that time; in the United States, for example, tuberculin surveys now reveal less than 20 per cent of positive reactors in young adults, and it is estimated that less than 50 per cent of the total population is infected. Skin hypersensitivity is known to disappear in a certain percentage of individuals, and consequently, autopsy studies yield higher figures than tuberculin surveys. Autopsies performed by Medlar in New York City from 1944 to 1946 showed that the incidence of infection in individuals over fifty years of age was above 80 per cent. These studies indicate that the decline in the incidence of infection has occurred chiefly among the younger age groups.

The *morbidity*—i.e., the frequency of actual tuberculous disease—is difficult to estimate accurately, but most authorities agreed that there were approximately 350,000 active cases in the United States in 1957. Thus, although almost half the total population was infected by the tubercle bacillus, clinically significant disease develops in only a relatively small number of individuals.

There has been a striking decline in the *mortality rate* from tuberculosis during the past 50 years. From first place in 1900 with over 200 deaths per 100,000 population, tuberculosis by 1940 had fallen to seventh place as a leading cause of death, with a mortality rate of 45.9 per 100,000. By 1950, the figure had fallen to only 22, and in 1958 it was 7.1. The most important factors in this decline have been the improvement in living standards, with better nutrition and housing, shorter working hours, and earlier diagnosis and treatment. Tuberculosis remains one of the major causes of death in young adults, ranking fourth in the age group fifteen to thirty-four.

Since 1945, the mortality rate has declined more precipitously than during the preceding two decades, because of the advent of chemotherapy. From 1938 through 1945 the death rate declined about 3 per cent each year. From 1946 through 1951 the average annual decline increased to 11 per cent, and in 1952 (when isoniazid was introduced) through 1954 it was 20 per cent. The figure for 1958 was 9 per cent.

Unfortunately, there has not been a proportionate decrease in the number of newly discovered active infections. Since 1930, for example, the death rate has fallen from 70 to 10 per 100,000 persons, while the new-case rate has declined only from 100 to 60. Thus the situation has reached the point where the mortality rate is no longer an accurate index of the prevalence of tuberculous infection. The large number of new cases discovered each year (over 60,000) indicates that many individuals with undiagnosed active tuberculosis are still at large in the community. Of the estimated 350,000 cases of active tuberculosis in the United States today, 125,000 remain unrecognized.

The tendency for active tuberculosis to occur among older age groups deserves special mention. In only 20 years the percentage of newly discovered cases in individuals under the age of thirty has dropped from more than 50 per cent to 20 per cent. During the same period the percentage of patients in tuberculosis hospitals who are over sixty years of age has increased from 6 to almost 25. The rate of newly reported active cases of tuberculosis among men is nearly twice that among women; in patients over fifty years of age the ratio is 4:1. Homeless, alcoholic men make up a large proportion of the new cases.

ETIOLOGY

Three types of tubercle bacilli—human, bovine, and avian—are known to infect man. The last is of least importance; only a small number of proved cases of avian infection have been reported in humans. Morphologic and cultural differences between the three types are somewhat variable, and animal inoculation is resorted to for positive identification. The human type causes disease in the guinea pig but not in the rabbit, the bovine type in both the guinea pig and the rabbit, and the avian type in birds and rabbits, but not in the guinea pig.

The tubercle bacillus is about 1.0 to 4.0 μ in length and 0.3 μ in thickness. Beaded and granular forms have been observed with both modified Gram and acid-fast stains, but evidence indicates that many of these are artefacts of the staining process. True granular forms do occur, particularly in older cultures, and are identified by their red rather than purple color, lack of distention of the cell wall, and failure to disappear with the addition of alcohol. Evidence for a filtrable virus or zoogleic stage in the life cycle of the tubercle bacillus is not entirely convincing; for the present it must be assumed that reproduction occurs by fission. The distinguishing tinctorial property of the tubercle bacillus—namely, its ability to resist decolorization by acid alcohol when stained with basic fuchsin—is known to be related to the waxy component, and probably specifically to mycolic acid. Curiously, the structural integrity of the cell is also involved, for grinding the bacilli between glass slides destroys acid-fastness, whereas prolonged extraction with fat solvents does not alter this property.

Avirulent dissociates of virulent strains of tubercle bacilli may be produced by appropriate cultural techniques, and occasionally tubercle bacilli of unusually low virulence for laboratory animals have been isolated from man. It has not been definitely established, however, that true dissociation can occur in the human body. A simple morphologic differentiation between virulent and avirulent dissociates has been described by Middlebrook and Dubos—namely, that virulent cultures grow in long, tightly formed cords, with individual bacilli parallel to each other, whereas avirulent organisms are haphazardly arranged. The correlation between cording and virulence is not absolute, however.

Chemically, the tubercle bacillus is unique in its high lipid content, which makes up one-fourth to one-third of its dry weight. The lipids are composed of phosphatides, acetone-soluble fats, and waxes. These substances probably account for the unusual resistance of the tubercle bacillus to bactericidal agents, to drying, and to wide temperature variations. They are not, however, as was once thought, situated on the surface of the cell as a thick capsule but are distributed throughout the body of the bacillus.

Tubercle bacilli are strict aerobes and are usually isolated on solid media containing potato, egg yolk, and glycerin. Growth is slow, 4 to 6 weeks being required for colonies to develop. Because of their high lipid content, tubercle bacilli are hydrophobic and grow in clumps on the surface of ordinary liquid media. Dubos has developed a liquid medium containing a complex ester of oleic acid, Tween 80, which coats the bacilli, making them hydrophilic, and provides rapid, diffuse, submerged growth. This medium has become a standard tool for quantitative laboratory studies.

TRANSMISSION

Inhalation of air containing tubercle bacilli is the most important means of acquiring tuberculous infection in man. The bacilli may be transmitted in droplets of saliva or sputum. Transmission may occur also from inhalation of particles of dust laden with viable organisms, a method which is possible because of the peculiar resistance of the tubercle bacillus to desiccation and exposure. Tubercle bacilli are killed within a few hours in direct sunlight, but survive up to 5 days in a well-lighted room, up to 5 months in the dark, and as long as a year and a half in the refrigerator.

In addition to inhalation, tubercle bacilli may enter the mouth and pharynx by direct or indirect contact with infected material. Tuberculous food handlers, for example, may deposit organisms on food or eating utensils, which are then placed in the mouths of uninfected subjects. Similarly, tuberculous sinuses, and urine and feces, may occasionally be sources of infection. Kissing is an example of transmission by direct contact and is probably an important source of infection in infants. Dogs are susceptible to both the human and the bovine bacillus and may occasionally transmit tuberculosis. Cats are said to be highly resistant to the human type of bacillus but susceptible to the bovine form. Placental transmission of tuberculosis in the human occurs but is rare.

The various sources of infection described above apply chiefly to the human bacillus, which is responsible for over 95 per cent of tuberculous infections in this country. The intensive campaign to destroy tuberculous cattle and to encourage pasteurization of milk has practically eliminated the milk-borne bovine type of tuberculosis in the United States. In some countries, ingestion of contaminated milk is still responsible for a large number of cases of cervical adenitis and abdominal tuberculosis in infants and children. Infection of the lungs by the bovine bacillus is uncommon, even in areas in which it is responsible for a high incidence of intestinal tuberculosis. The tubercle bacillus is destroyed by boiling in water for 2 min, or by pasteurization at 60°C for 20 min.

PATHOLOGIC ANATOMY

This subject is considered exhaustively in textbooks of pathology; a brief summary will provide adequate reorientation for the purposes of this discussion. In general, two types of tissue response predominate in tuberculosis—exudative and productive. According to Pinner, exudative reactions tend to occur in association with loose tissue structure, large doses of highly virulent organisms, and bronchogenic spread to parenchymal tissues. Productive reactions are commonly observed with small doses, low virulence, and firm tissue structure, and in lesions in interstitial tissues resulting from hematogenous dissemination.

In the exudative lesion in the lung, polymorphonuclear leukocytes, large mononuclear cells, and fibrin infiltrate the alveolar spaces. After a variable period of time this pneumonic type of lesion may undergo partial or complete resorption, or it may caseate. If caseation occurs, areas of caseous pneumonia become liquefied, a process which leads to cavitation, with leukocytes and exudative material being expelled as sputum. Caseous areas may also be replaced gradually by fibrosis and calcification. It should be emphasized that the exudative reaction may be misdiagnosed easily, even by histologic examination, since epithelioid cells, Langhans giant cells, and caseation may be absent.

The productive lesion, or *tubercle,* involves growth of new granulation tissue, supported by a definite reticulum which pushes the normal tissue aside. The tubercle consists of Langhans giant cells, epithelioid cells, and a surrounding layer of lymphocytes. Later, the granulation tissue making up the tubercle forms a fibrous capsule around the periphery, differing in this respect from the exudative lesion, in which the surrounding fibrosis is produced by collagenous tissue normally present in the peribronchial, perivascular, and septal spaces. Productive lesions rarely undergo resolution to the extent observed with exudative lesions.

Rarely, primary tissue necrosis may occur in tuberculous infection. This is observed in the so-called "acute caseating miliary tuberculosis" and presumably results from the sudden hematogenous dissemination of large numbers of tubercle bacilli in extremely hypersensitive individuals.

IMMUNITY

Native Resistance. Man possesses a relatively high degree of native resistance to tuberculosis, as manifested by his ability to arrest the infection in the great majority of instances. Susceptible animals, such as the guinea pig, have little resistance and almost invariably succumb to the disease. There are probably no differences in actual native resistance among white races; the higher mortality rate of city-dwelling Irish, as compared with Jews, is probably due to natural selection of resistant individuals among the latter. Negroes and Indians possess distinctly lower native resistance than whites. Resistance is influenced by age and sex; examples are the high mortality rate in infants, and in females during the child-bearing period. The effect of environmental influences such as poor nutrition and overcrowding is clearly demonstrated by the close correlation of tuberculous mortality with economic and hygienic alterations during wartime.

Acquired Resistance. Koch observed that cutaneously inoculated guinea pigs developed an indolent ulcer at the local site, with rapid spread to, and marked enlargement of, the regional lymph nodes and eventual death from generalized tuberculosis. In contrast, animals previously infected developed an intense local skin reaction within a day or two, followed by ulceration and healing. Spread from the local site was greatly inhibited, and there was little involvement and enlargement of the tributary lymph nodes. Subsequent studies have confirmed and elucidated the chief characteristics of the lesion of reinfection in animals and man, namely, (1) an intense local inflammatory reaction, which develops much more rapidly than with the primary infection; (2) suppression of multiplication of the organism; and (3) inhibition of spread of the bacilli, with little or no involvement of the regional lymph nodes, and a greatly decreased tendency toward hematogenous dissemination.

Tuberculin hypersensitivity appears at approximately the same time as acquired resistance, from 2 to 6 weeks following the initial infection. The two are closely associated, although the degree of hypersensitivity is not a measure of immunity. In man, a definite but limited degree of acquired resistance occurs as a result of a primary infection.

Mechanisms of Resistance. The basic mechanisms underlying native and acquired resistance to the tubercle bacillus are unknown. Native resistance seems to be determined by conditions existing within the mononuclear phagocytes, in which large numbers of tubercle bacilli become segregated soon after entering the body. In the susceptible body, bacilli multiply freely in the monocytes, while in the natively resistant body the environment is, for some unknown reason, unfavorable, causing the organisms to be inhibited and gradually to die.

In acquired resistance, humoral immunity has not been found to play the important role it does in most other infections. Humoral antibodies have been demonstrated repeatedly in animals and patients infected with the tubercle bacillus, but they appear irregularly, do not increase the resistance of normal animals to tuberculosis, and have not been found in vitro to render tubercle bacilli more easily phagocytable by opsonization.

Lurie has observed an increased metabolic activity of phagocytes in natively resistant or immunized rabbits, and studies indicate that hormones may play an important role in immunity. Genetically susceptible rabbits have been found to secrete about twice as much hydrocortisone as animals which are genetically resistant. These observations may lead to a better understanding of immunity in tuberculosis.

PATHOGENESIS

Primary Tuberculosis. Most tissues exposed to direct contact with bacilli are protected by local mechanical defenses under ordinary circumstances but may become infected when these defenses are broken. Thus, the primary focus is observed occasionally on the fingers, on ear lobes that have been pierced, on the tonsils, and on the conjunctiva.

In the lung, the primary focus is usually near the pleura and occurs most frequently in the upper part of the lower lobe or the lower part of the upper lobe. Initially exudative in character, the primary focus rapidly undergoes caseation. Tubercle bacilli escape freely and are carried to the bronchopulmonary and tracheobronchial lymph nodes, which become greatly enlarged and undergo exudation and caseation. The combination of the primary focus and the enlarged regional lymph nodes is commonly referred to as the *primary complex.*

It has become increasingly common for individuals to attain adult life without contracting a primary tuberculous infection. It is a curious fact, however, that, in white adults, it is unusual to observe the x-ray enlargement of the tracheobronchial lymph nodes so characteristic of primary infections in childhood. From the standpoint of both x-ray appearance and clinical course, lesions in recently tuberculin negative adults are indistinguishable from those clearly due to reinfection tuberculosis. Exceptions have been observed but are uncommon. In Negroes, typical primary complexes are observed in adults as well as in children. This racial difference suggests that an age-determined native resistance may modify the characteristics of primary infections in white adults, while in Negroes, who have a lower degree of native resistance, the age-determined difference is lacking.

Deviations from the classic primary complex have been described by Terplan. The parenchymal focus and the lymph node component have been observed to occur separately, and new typical primary complexes have been noted in lungs in which the true initial complexes are in a relatively advanced state of healing.

In the great majority of instances the primary complex undergoes gradual healing, with encapsulation of the parenchymal and lymph node components, and eventual calcification. By x-ray the lesions gradually recede from the periphery, and eventually leave small areas of calcific density, usually less than 1 cm in diameter. Bacteriologically, in over 80 per cent of adults who have arrested a primary infection in childhood, the calcified primary complex is sterile. In these instances the possibilities of endogenous exacerbation are not completely excluded, however, for tubercle bacilli may remain viable in lesions of the paratracheal or upper mediastinal nodes.

In a small percentage of cases there is progression of the primary complex; this accounts for most of the fatalities in infants and children. Progression occurs in the following ways: (1) direct extension or intrabronchial spread; (2) massive lymph node caseation with rupture into a bronchus, resulting in tuberculous pneumonia; and (3) hematogenous dissemination. Hematogenous dissemination occurs frequently during the course of primary tuberculosis, and may result in the full-blown picture of miliary tuberculosis, with death in a few weeks, or may merely give rise to seeding in various organs. Seeding is common in the upper parts of the lungs, producing lesions which appear in x-rays as small, indistinct areas of increased density. These foci tend to heal with fibrosis and calcification. Focal hematogenous lesions in other organs may regress and heal, or they may lie dormant for many years, and eventually cause progressive destructive lesions.

Reinfection Tuberculosis. Tuberculosis in the adult is regarded as usually being reinfectious in character, i.e., infection in individuals whose immunologic state and tissue response have been altered by previous contact with the tubercle bacillus. The basic manifestations of this altered response are, as indicated in the section on Immunity, an intense local inflammatory reaction, suppression of proliferation of the bacilli, and inhibition of their spread. These features are observed in cases of reinfection tuberculosis in human beings just as they are in experimental animals in the Koch phenomenon; in fact, adult reinfection pulmonary tuberculosis (phthisis) is in essence, as pointed out by Pinner, a Koch phenomenon in the lung. There is an intense local reaction of the tissues with a tendency to chronicity, marked fibrosis, excavation, and restriction in the involvement of lymph nodes.

Reinfection tuberculosis in the adult usually begins as a small caseopneumonic focus in the posterior portion of the upper lobe; less commonly, it may be present in the apical portion of a lower lobe. While the patient is still asymptomatic, this lesion can often be seen as a small area of density with indistinct borders in the infraclavicular region between the first and third anterior ribs. This focus is commonly referred to as an *early infiltrate.*

One of the unsolved problems of tuberculosis is the source of the tubercle bacilli which are responsible for the early infiltrate. There are two possibilities: One is inhalation of bacilli from without, giving rise to an entirely new infection in the upper portion of the lung—i.e., the establishment of a true exogenous reinfection. The other possibility is local exacerbation, or transmission to the local site of bacilli which have lain dormant somewhere in the body following subsidence of the primary infection; this is known as endogenous exacerbation. The relative frequency with which exogenous reinfection and endogenous exacerbation are responsible for the early infiltrate is not known; both undoubtedly occur.

Adult tuberculosis as discussed in the preceding paragraphs is assumed to be largely reinfectious in nature. It should be stated again, however, that an increasing number of cases of adult tuberculosis are instances of primary infection, and unequivocally exogenous in origin.

Pulmonary tuberculosis in the adult usually, but not invariably, begins as an early infiltrate. In an occasional instance tuberculous pneumonia may follow the rupture of a caseous hilar lymph node; this is seen with increasing frequency in older individuals. Clinically suggestive evidence also indicates that pneumonic lesions may develop when a large inoculum of bacilli is carried suddenly to a portion of the lung from some endogenous focus. Contiguous spread from nodular foci at the extreme pulmonary apex, a mode of development thought at one time to account for virtually all phthisis, unquestionably occurs in some cases. Finally, hematogenous seeding may give rise to bilateral foci, usually in the upper parts of the lungs, which remain interstitial and cause relatively few symptoms, or ulcerate through the bronchi and gradually produce bronchogenic phthisis.

Once formed, the early infiltrate may regress and heal completely. This may occur in ambulatory, asymptomatic individuals, but the value of bed rest in aiding this process is well established. All too often, the early infiltrate progresses to the characteristic chronic, destructive form of pulmonary tuberculosis. Caseation is followed by liquefaction and cavitation. Intrabronchial aspiration gives rise to new parenchymal foci where the process is repeated. The presence of bacilliferous sputum also leads in a large percentage of cases to lesions of the bronchial and tracheal mucosa. Reparative processes supervene, with resorption and fibrosis, but the nature of the lesions, especially the cavities which continually discharge infective material into the bronchial passages, tends to foster chronicity and gradual extension of the disease.

As pulmonary tuberculosis progresses, increasingly large numbers of tubercle bacilli are expelled in the bronchopulmonary secretions and are responsible for lesions in the larynx, the mouth, and the intestinal tract. The pathogenesis of other forms of extrapulmonary tuberculosis may be stated briefly. Tuberculosis of the kidneys, epididymis, prostate, fallopian tubes, adrenals, bones, brain, eyes, lymph nodes, and other organs not in direct contact with the external environment is lymphohematogenous in origin. Seeding of these organs may occur during the active primary stage of infection, causing progressive, destructive lesions at that time, or after many years of latency. Hematogenous dissemination may also occur during reinfection tuberculosis in adults. The internal organs vary considerably in their susceptibility to tuberculous infection. Some, such as those listed above, are relatively frequently involved, while others, including the pancreas, thyroid, ovary, spleen, heart, liver, and skeletal muscles, are rarely the site of progressive lesions.

PULMONARY TUBERCULOSIS

Manifestations

The onset of symptoms of pulmonary tuberculosis is in many instances *insidious*. In the early stages, and at times when moderate progression has occurred, the patient is usually *entirely asymptomatic* and may remain so for a considerable period. This cannot be emphasized too strongly; more and more early asymptomatic cases are being discovered as a result of routine films and x-ray surveys.

The earliest symptoms are constitutional and probably result chiefly from the absorption of tuberculoprotein into the circulation of the hypersensitive body. *Fever* is one of the commonest manifestations of tuberculosis and usually begins as a slight elevation of the temperature in the late afternoon or evening. This elevation may occur daily, gradually attaining higher levels over a period of weeks or months, or it may subside altogether and reappear intermittently as the patient passes through a series of grippelike episodes. It is characteristic for fever to be relatively well tolerated in patients with tuberculosis, even with a temperature elevation to 102 or 103°F. Except for sensations of warmth and flushing, the patient is often quite comfortable and in some instances is even euphoric.

Fatigue and malaise are among the earliest symptoms noticed by the patient. They usually first manifest themselves as excessive tiredness at the end of the day and may lead the patient to restrict his activities in the evening in order to get more rest. In other instances, particularly when the subject refuses to modify his routine, he may become irritable and morose. Eventually, in far-advanced disease, profound asthenia is often present.

Weight loss is usually noted somewhat later than the above symptoms and may not be present for many months unless the disease runs a malignant course. Anorexia and indigestion are associated symptoms and seem to vary with the severity of the other manifestations. Anorexia may provide a clue from the standpoint of differential diagnosis; tuberculosis at this stage can be confused with diabetes and thyrotoxicosis, and in both these conditions loss of weight is characteristically associated with an increase in appetite.

Chilly sensations may be noted as the toxemia progresses, particularly when the temperature rises abruptly in the evening. *Night sweats* are considered classic manifestations of tuberculosis but actually do not occur in most instances until the disease is fairly far advanced. *Tachycardia* occurs along with the fever. *Headache* is noted in some individuals in the evening when the temperature is elevated but the symptom usually subsides by morning and is absent during the daytime.

Menstruation is said to be disturbed in tuberculosis, but this statement is based upon the situation occurring in far-advanced disease. In the early stages the menses are usually normal and become irregular and scanty only as the disease progresses. Amenorrhea may occur in the later stages, particularly when the condition becomes terminal. For reasons not entirely clear, hemoptysis seems to occur more frequently during the menstrual period.

Since examination of the lungs in the early stages is negative in most instances and the blood count and sedimentation rate may be entirely normal, the importance of the chest x-ray in diagnosis cannot be overemphasized.

In many patients with pulmonary tuberculosis, the onset of symptoms is *relatively sudden*. A characteristic story is that of a "bad cold," or "influenza," without awareness of any prior disability. The "cold"—especially the cough—persists, while the constitutional manifestations may subside temporarily, giving the patient the feeling that he is recovering. Some individuals may recall a slight morning cough of some months' duration, attributed usually to irritation from smoking. Cough is characteristically first noted in the morning, because secretions formed in the lungs during the night flow into the bronchi and trachea and stimulate the cough reflex on arising. Once these passages are cleared, the patient coughs infrequently or not at all until the next morning, when another mild paroxysm occurs. As the disease progresses, the secretions are formed in larger amounts, and the cough becomes more troublesome, occurring throughout the day and night.

Along with cough, there is expectoration of *sputum*. In early cases a few flecks of pus may be seen in the mucus, and later the sputum becomes predominantly purulent in character. As cavitation progresses, liquefied caseous material is formed in increasing amounts, until 2 or 3 oz of sputum is produced daily. In caseous pneumonic lesions with cavitation and liquefaction, the purulent matter is usually green or greenish yellow. Later, as the clinical condition improves, the sputum is yellowish and more mucoid. Tuberculous sputum is not foul except in rare instances in which the pulmonary lesions become secondarily infected with anaerobes. Layering does not usually occur, a feature which is at times helpful in differentiating tuberculosis from lung abscesses. Late in the course of the disease, secondary infection of tuberculous cavities does occasionally occur, and the patient may become exhausted by his efforts to bring up 300 or 400 ml of sputum daily.

Hemoptysis is commonly associated with cough and expectoration, and ordinarily consists of streaking of the sputum with small amounts of blood. Occasionally, a gross hemoptysis may usher in the disease, the patient being unaware of any previous symptoms. Bleeding results usually from the ulceration of vessels in tuberculous cavities, and the natural tendency of the infectious process to cause vascular thrombosis is an important factor in preventing massive hemorrhages in the majority of patients with cavitary disease. Large hemoptyses usually occur without warning and frequently begin when the patient is asleep. Ordinarily, not more than 300 ml of blood is produced. Dark clots of blood are usually brought up for several days; if the cough mechanism is inadequate, there may be blockage of a main bronchus with collapse of one or more lobes. Bleeding may recur at frequent intervals, and transfusions may be needed. In an occasional instance the hemorrhage is massive and fatal; this usually occurs with old fibrotic disease, and the patient drowns within a few minutes. One of the greatest hazards of hemoptysis is the danger of spreading the infection throughout the lungs. Depending on the number of tubercle bacilli present in the bloody fluid, posthemoptysic spreads vary in extent from scattered, finely mottled infiltrations to massive tuberculous pneumonia.

As pulmonary tuberculosis progresses, and especially with cavitary disease, ulcerations or granulomatous infiltrations frequently appear in portions of the tracheobronchial tree draining affected lung tissue, with *wheezing* as a common symptom. Endobronchial disease may alter the treatment, and therefore this symptom should be carefully sought for. Wheezing may also occur in the absence of demonstrable ulcerations or granulations and is then presumably caused by mucosal swelling or retained secretions. It should be noted that tuberculous tracheobronchitis occasionally occurs in the absence of demonstrable parenchymal disease.

Tuberculous Pneumonia. The clinical onset of tuberculosis occasionally may be an acute pneumonic episode, especially in Negroes, in children, and in elderly individuals both white and colored. The sudden aspiration of a dose of bacilli sufficiently large to cause a pneumonic lesion results usually from the abrupt emptying of a cavity, from a hemoptysis, or from the rupture of a caseous node into a bronchus. Fever, chilly sensations, cough, and chest pain are noted, and the condition can easily be confused with primary atypical pneumonia. The temperature is usually not above 102°F, though it may rise to 104 or 105°F, and the white blood count is in most instances not elevated above 15,000. Untreated, tuberculous pneu-

monia may run a malignant course, with death in 1 to 3 months, or the process may gradually subside and become chronic.

Pleurisy with Effusion. This condition is common among young adults, and its pathogenesis and significance need emphasis. The pleura usually becomes involved as a result of direct or lymphatic extension from an underlying parenchymal process, and the lesion in the lung often is not of sufficient size to be visible on the x-ray. Whether the pleura can also be infected directly by way of the blood stream is a matter of dispute. Animal experiments indicate that parenteral injections of tubercle bacilli rarely result in direct infection of serous cavities. The not infrequent occurrence of bilateral effusions, on the other hand, is often cited as evidence that infection of the pleural surfaces may result from direct hematogenous seeding. Chest pain and fever are the initial symptoms; the pain may be sharp and pleuritic in character, or it may begin as a dull ache or uncomfortable sensation in the lower chest. In the more acute cases there is marked prostration with a high fever and a stormy course for 2 or 3 weeks. More commonly the temperature is only moderately elevated, and the patient does not feel particularly ill except for the pain in the chest. Clear yellow fluid is obtained by aspiration, and tubercle bacilli are recovered by culture or guinea pig inoculation in approximately 50 per cent of the cases. Whether the organism is recovered or not, experience has shown that, without treatment, 30 to 50 per cent of the patients develop clinical and x-ray signs of active pulmonary tuberculosis within 5 years. These figures are sufficiently high to warrant the assumption that all cases of "nonspecific" pleurisy with effusion are caused by tuberculosis, and they should be treated accordingly. Details of management will be outlined in a subsequent section.

Physical and X-ray Examination

The widespread use of the x-ray during the past 25 years has demonstrated the marked limitations of physical examination in detecting and appraising the lesions of pulmonary tuberculosis. As a result, the tendency at present in many quarters is virtually to ignore the physical examination altogether; this is lamentable, for the physical signs contribute information which, when correlated with the x-ray findings, gives a more complete understanding of the nature and activity of the parenchymal disease.

Early asymptomatic infiltrations are usually missed on routine physical examination, and indeed it is often surprising how extensive the x-ray infiltrations may become before definite physical abnormalities are detected. Crepitant posttussic rales may be noted over a small area in minimal lesions, although rales are not of themselves conclusive evidence of activity. With larger lesions, especially after cavitation develops, dullness and moderately coarse rales are usually elicited. With pneumonic lesions the classic signs of consolidation are noted, and as cavitation develops, coarse bubbling rales appear, especially at the base of the cavities where liquefied pus tends to accumulate. Even with large cavities demonstrable on the x-ray, however, the classic signs of tympany and amphoric breathing are often absent because the soft, shaggy cavity walls and surrounding structures do not act as good resonators. In old fibrocaseous lesions the walls are relatively thick and rigid, and the classic signs of cavitation may be present. Tension cavities, associated with bronchial disease preventing normal egress of air during expiration, also produce atypical signs. With long-standing disease, extensive fibrosis causes contraction and distortion of the pulmonary tissue. In such instances, a wide variety of physical signs, such as bronchial breath sounds, coarse rales, deviation of the trachea, spasm and atrophy of various chest and neck muscles, and diminished movements of one hemithorax, are noted.

From an x-ray standpoint, the early infiltrate is usually observed in the infraclavicular region, although it may be located entirely above the clavicle, or in the midlung field. As the infiltrations progress and enlarge, the x-ray appearance of pulmonary tuberculosis may be indistinguishable from various nontuberculous conditions. Tuberculous cavities, especially when located in the lower lung fields, closely simulate nontuberculous lung abscesses. Similarly, the tuberculous nature of bronchopneumonic or lobar consolidations cannot be determined on the basis of the x-ray alone. The limitations of a single film in determining whether an infiltration is tuberculous, and of assessing its activity, leads to serious diagnostic and therapeutic errors.

Aside from its diagnostic limitations, the x-ray film may at times give misleading impressions concerning the functional status of the lungs. For example, in patients who have had pleural effusions, or extensive nodular bronchogenic disseminations following hemoptysis, the lung fields may eventually become almost entirely clear by x-ray, although pulmonary function remains markedly impaired. Careful physical examination will reveal the presence of impaired function in such cases and will lead to more precise pulmonary function studies if surgery is contemplated.

Tuberculin Test

Tissue hypersensitivity to tuberculoprotein results from the production of tuberculous tissue in the body by intact whole tubercle bacilli, living,

attenuated, or dead. A positive tuberculin test indicates, therefore, that an individual has, or has had, such a focus of tuberculous tissue in his body. It does not indicate that he harbors a clinically significant lesion, or that any of his present signs or symptoms are necessarily due to tuberculosis, active or inactive. The chief value of the test lies in exclusion. If negative, it can be fairly reliably concluded that the patient does not have active tuberculosis; virtually all individuals with active tuberculosis have a positive tuberculin reaction. Exceptions are sometimes noted during the course of intercurrent infections, especially measles and influenza, late in the course of pregnancy, and in some terminal cases of tuberculosis. The tuberculin skin reaction may turn negative after a period of years in individuals who have arrested and healed a primary tuberculous infection; the frequency with which this occurs is not known, but many well-documented instances are on record. The increasing incidence of negative tuberculin reactions in young adults has enhanced the diagnostic value of the test in recent years. Only 20 to 30 per cent of young men in the Armed Forces during the Second World War were tuberculin positive; in this age group, the skin reaction is particularly helpful in ruling out tuberculosis in the presence of obscure fevers and undiagnosed pulmonary conditions.

The most reliable and accurate method of performing the tuberculin test is the intracutaneous, or Mantoux, test, in which 0.1 ml of suitably diluted tuberculin is injected intradermally into the skin of the forearm. If positive, induration (5 mm or more) appears at the local site in 24 to 72 hr and is surrounded by an area of inflammation varying from one to several centimeters. Intense local reactions occur if the dose of tuberculoprotein is too large, causing tissue necrosis and lymphangitis extending to the regional nodes. Absorption of tuberculoprotein into the circulation of the highly hypersensitive body causes constitutional symptoms, chiefly malaise and fever, and may produce focal reactions around tuberculous lesions throughout the body. To avoid these untoward reactions, small doses of tuberculin should be used for the initial test, with gradually increasing amounts thereafter at intervals of 3 or 4 days until the test becomes positive. If old tuberculin (OT) is used, the initial dose is usually 0.01 mg (0.1 ml of a 1:10,000 dilution); in individuals suspected of being unusually hypersensitive, the initial dose may be reduced to 0.001 mg. If the reaction is negative, tenfold increments in the amount of OT are employed for subsequent tests. An individual is ordinarily considered tuberculin negative if he fails to react to 1.0 mg, although some observers prefer to increase the amount to 10 mg. In recent years the purified protein derivative (P.P.D.) of Seibert has partially replaced OT because it gives more uniform results and minimizes false positive reactions. It is available commercially in two strengths, the first (0.00002 mg) being roughly equivalent to 0.01 mg OT, and the second (0.005 mg) corresponding to 1.0 mg OT. Recent evidence indicates that the second strength sometimes gives false positive reactions, and the present trend is towards using a single, intermediate strength concentration of P.P.D., namely, 0.001 mg.

The tuberculin patch test is often used in children to avoid the use of needles. It is less reliable, however, and, if negative, should be followed by the intracutaneous test if an accurate appraisal of the skin reactivity is desired.

Laboratory Findings

Recovery of Tubercle Bacillus. Aside from the x-ray, the most important laboratory procedures used in the diagnosis and management of patients with tuberculosis are those concerned with the isolation of tubercle bacilli from sputum, gastric washings, urine, feces, spinal fluid, serous and purulent effusions, abscesses, and draining sinuses.

Sputum may be absent, or present in only small amounts early in the morning in patients with minimal tuberculosis, and a few flecks of mucopurulent material obtained at this time may be adequate to make the diagnosis. The material is usually examined first by the direct smear. The Ziehl-Neelsen method of staining is the most widely used, although a fluorescent dye, carbolauramine, has become popular in recent years. Fairly large numbers of tubercle bacilli must be present to be seen on the direct smear. Therefore, if this is negative, 20 ml or more of sputum is collected, digested with acid or alkali, concentrated by centrifugation, neutralized, and the sediment smeared, stained, and examined. With this technique a significantly higher percentage of specimens is positive than on direct smear. If negative on smear, the concentrated sediment is cultured or inoculated into guinea pigs, or both. Twenty to thirty per cent more positives are obtained by culture or guinea pig inoculation than by smear of the concentrated sediment. The relative merits of cultures and guinea pig inoculations are debated, but the results with cultures are so favorable that in many laboratories the more laborious and expensive guinea pig method has been abandoned.

If no sputum is produced, the *gastric contents* should be aspirated shortly after the patient awakens in the morning. Smears of the gastric contents may give false positive results; therefore, the material is digested, concentrated, and cultured or inoculated into guinea pigs. In minimal cases of pulmonary tuberculosis, prior to the development of cavitation, discharges carried into the bronchial tree and swallowed by the patient are small in amount, and many cultures of the gastric contents may be necessary to recover tubercle bacilli. For example, in one study it was found that 68 per cent of minimal cases had at least 3 negative specimens before a positive was obtained, and in another series of 61 patients, 5 to 14 negatives were reported prior to the first positive culture. Once cavitation develops, the discharges increase in amount, and bacilli can be recovered by cultures of the sputum or gastric contents with comparative ease. A series of negative sputum or gastric cultures in the presence of cavitation provides strong presumptive evidence against the diagnosis of active pulmonary tuberculosis.

The basic principles outlined for sputum and gastric contents apply to the recovery of tubercle bacilli from other sources. Minor modifications are necessary, especially in preparing and concentrating urine and stool specimens. With spinal fluid, tubercle bacilli are often detected by smear or culture of the pellicle which forms if the specimen is left in the icebox overnight.

Sedimentation Rate. The sedimentation rate is normal in the majority of individuals with minimal tuberculosis. In more advanced febrile cases, the sedimentation rate usually is elevated and often is used as an index of the progression or regression of the disease. This use has definite limitations, however, since the rate may be normal in patients on absolute bed rest in spite of progressive intrabronchial disseminations, and, conversely, a sudden increase in the rate may accompany the onset of a relatively insignificant complication such as mild pleurisy.

Blood. Hematologic changes in tuberculosis are relatively slight. In minimal cases the blood count is usually normal, but as the disease progresses, there may develop a mild normochromic normocytic anemia. Even in far-advanced cases the anemia usually is not marked except in the presence of extrapulmonary complications such as intestinal tuberculosis or amyloidosis. A mild leukocytosis may be present in progressive, febrile stages, with a count of 10,000 to 15,000, but even in acute tuberculous pneumonia the total white count is rarely above 15,000. An increase in monocytes with a decrease in lymphocytes is regarded by some observers as indicative of progression of the disease, and in experimental animals this appears to be well substantiated. In man, however, the lymphocyte-monocyte ratio and other prognostic guides, such as the Medlar index, are of limited value. Exceptions to some of the above statements should be noted; in widespread acute tuberculous pneumonia, for example, the total white count may occasionally be well above 20,000, with a polymorphonuclear count of over 95 per cent. Similarly, in acute miliary tuberculosis, there may occur a high-grade leukocytosis and at times even a leukemoid blood picture, or there may be a marked leukopenia.

Urine. Changes in the urine in pulmonary tuberculosis, as in other chronic febrile diseases, consist chiefly of intermittent traces of albumin without other significant abnormalities. Renal tuberculosis is not uncommon, and frequent urine examinations should be made, noting especially persistent proteinuria and an abnormal number of erythrocytes and leukocytes. If these are present, pyelograms are indicated, and concentrated urine specimens should be cultured and inoculated into guinea pigs. Except in rare cases, an active renal lesion is present if tubercle bacilli are recovered repeatedly from the urine, and drug therapy is indicated.

Other Tests. A number of serologic tests have been employed in tuberculosis, but none has been found to be of practical diagnostic or prognostic value. The complement fixation reaction, for example, is positive in less than 50 per cent of patients with minimal lesions, and false positive reactions are obtained in over 10 per cent of individuals with no evidence of active tuberculosis.

Differential Diagnosis

The onset and course of pulmonary tuberculosis vary widely and may simulate a great number of other diseases. The outstanding conditions which may be confused with tuberculosis, and the main differential features, will be considered briefly.

Psychoneurosis. Patients with purely functional disorders frequently present complaints similar to those of early pulmonary tuberculosis. Malaise, easy fatigability, and inability to concentrate are common symptoms, and there may be anorexia with slight weight loss. A chronic hacking cough may be present, due to irritation of the respiratory passages from smoking. A careful evaluation of these complaints will usually give a clue to the correct diagnosis. A chest x-ray is an essential part of the examination of patients with the symptoms described above.

Endocrine Disorders. Two endocrine disorders, *hyperthyroidism* and *diabetes*, are commonly manifested by weight loss and easy fatigability. In contrast to tuberculosis, however, the weight loss is associated with an increased appetite rather than with anorexia. Negative chest x-rays, in addition to glycosuria and an abnormal glucose tolerance test in diabetes, and an elevation of the basal metabolic rate in hyperthyroidism, lead to the correct diagnosis.

Obscure Fevers. Tuberculosis is always to be considered in the differential diagnosis of fevers of unknown origin. With a negative chest x-ray, the fever may be caused by early miliary tuberculosis, or by an extrapulmonary tuberculous focus, and localizing signs should be sought for (see p. 66).

Pulmonary Fibrosis and Emphysema. Pulmonary fibrosis and emphysema with cough, weakness, dyspnea, and at times streaking of the sputum, are relatively common in older individuals. Tuberculosis is in some cases the cause, or is an associated condition, and therefore the sputum should be examined carefully for tubercle bacilli. Pneumoconioses, especially silicosis, should be kept in mind, and the patient questioned concerning possible industrial exposure. Nodulation, more dense near the hilar regions and extending peripherally through both lung fields, is the characteristic x-ray appearance of silicosis. With the development of a superimposed tuberculous infection, larger confluent shadows appear, and the constitutional manifestations of tuberculosis are usually present, although it may be very difficult to recover tubercle bacilli from the sputum.

Nontuberculous Lung Abscess. This affection, which may be roentgenologically indistinguishable from tuberculosis, usually has an acute onset with chills, fever, and leukocytosis. The sputum may or may not be foul, depending on the organisms involved. The differential diagnosis is usually relatively simple, since acid-fast bacilli are almost always readily demonstrable in patients with tuberculous cavities. Clubbing of the fingers may develop in 4 to 8 weeks in the presence of a nontuberculous abscess. Nontuberculous abscesses may become chronic and, when seen at this stage, especially in conjunction with hemoptysis, may be very suggestive of tuberculosis. Sputum studies, plus a careful review of the original signs and symptoms, usually will clarify the situation (see p. 1554).

Bronchiectasis. Bronchiectasis is usually associated with a chronic productive cough and is one of the commonest causes of hemoptysis. Clubbing of the fingers is common, while in tuberculosis it is rare. Bronchiectasis usually involves the lower portions of one or both lungs but is sometimes situated at the apex. The x-ray may be completely negative, or there may be increased linear densities extending outward and downward from the hilar regions. Moderately coarse rales usually are noted over the involved areas. The failure to find acid-fast bacilli in the sputum and the demonstration of radiographic abnormality by bronchogram confirm the diagnosis. Not infrequently, tuberculosis and bronchiectasis are found to coexist.

Primary Atypical Pneumonia. This presents a clinical and x-ray picture which may be indistinguishable from pulmonary tuberculosis. The absence of cavitation, the failure to find tubercle bacilli in repeated examinations of the sputum, and the eventual complete clearing of the parenchymal lesions are the important differential features.

Mycotic Diseases. *Coccidioidomycosis* presents a clinical and x-ray picture similar to pulmonary tuberculosis. This condition is of national importance because of the large number of individuals who were in the endemic areas of the Southwest during the Second World War. A history of possible exposure, the coccidioidin skin test, smears and cultures of the sputum for *Coccidioides immitis,* and precipitin and complement fixation tests of the patient's serum are the procedures used in confirming or excluding the diagnosis. *Histoplasmosis* recently has been suspected of causing pulmonary calcifications similar to those occurring in tuberculosis, because of the observation that many individuals in the South Central states with pulmonary calcifications have positive histoplasmin skin tests and negative tuberculin reactions. Other mycotic infections, such as *actinomycosis* and *blastomycosis,* may at times simulate tuberculosis, but the fungi involved usually can be readily recovered from the sputum.

Sarcoidosis. Typically, the patient with sarcoidosis is afebrile and has a negative tuberculin test, and biopsy of lymph nodes reveals tubercles without caseation. Fever may be present, however, and in about 20 per cent of cases the tuberculin test is positive. Pulmonary infiltrations vary from hilar adenopathy to extensive parenchymal involvement which can resemble tuberculosis very closely. In some cases differentiation is extremely difficult, and the situation is further complicated by the fact that some patients with a diagnosis of sarcoidosis eventually die of tuberculosis.

Carcinoma of Lung. Carcinoma of the lung, with chronic cough, blood-streaked sputum, fever, and weight loss, may present a clinical picture very similar to tuberculosis in older individuals. Carcinomas located peripherally produce fewer symptoms but may present an x-ray appearance indistinguishable from that of tuberculosis. Patients with lesions suspected of being carcinomatous, from whom tubercle bacilli cannot be recovered, should be subjected to early thoracotomy. It should be noted that both tuberculosis and carcinoma are occasionally present in the same patient.

Cardiovascular Disorders. These may produce symptoms suggestive of tuberculosis. Hemoptysis occurs frequently with mitral stenosis and is occasionally observed with hypertension. Long-standing pulmonary congestion, such as occurs in patients with mitral stenosis, causes pulmonary fibrosis; infected pulmonary infarcts may develop into abscesses suggestive of tuberculous cavitation.

Other Conditions. Mediastinal cysts, bacterial pneumonia, lipoid granuloma, lymphomas, amebiasis, aortic aneurysms, and metastatic neoplasms may be confused with tuberculosis. Careful evaluation and study, including the exclusion of tuberculosis by the failure to find tubercle bacilli, usually will lead to the correct diagnosis.

Evaluation of Need for Treatment

In patients with progressive symptomatic pulmonary tuberculosis the clinical and x-ray findings are usually characteristic, and the diagnosis and need for treatment are established readily. In some situations, however, the diagnosis and degree of activity and, therefore, the need for treatment are more difficult to ascertain. At the outset it may be stated that old calcified primary complexes, nodular fibrotic areas at the extreme apices, and adhesions and scarring due to old pleurisy are not indications for treatment. Individuals with these lesions should have yearly x-ray examinations, since dormant foci can give rise to active disease during periods of lowered resistance.

Minimal infraclavicular infiltrations, often detected as a result of x-ray surveys, require careful evaluation, which in most instances should be carried out with the patient at bed rest. This is particularly true of individuals under twenty-five years of age. Hazy, poorly circumscribed shadows indicate exudative, unstable lesions, while dense, sharply circumscribed infiltrations usually represent old arrested disease which is unlikely to progress. Serial x-rays are the best means of following a lesion and determining its activity. These should be made at least once a month, and sometimes more frequently in young adults with exudative lesions. Gastric washings should be cultured repeatedly. Careful clinical observations and serial roentgenograms over a period of at least 6 months are usually adequate to determine the activity of the lesion. Chemotherapy may be instituted at the outset if clinical and x-ray findings indicate that the lesion is almost certainly active.

Treatment

The advent of effective chemotherapeutic agents has brought about great changes in the treatment of tuberculosis during the past two decades. It is now generally agreed that all patients with active tuberculosis should receive prolonged chemotherapy and that bed rest is necessary for only the first part of the treatment period. Collapse therapy is used infrequently, so that initial treatment for most patients consists of rest and the administration of antimicrobial drugs. If, after several months, the sputum remains positive or if there are open cavities or large residual necrotic foci, surgical excision of the involved areas may be performed. The basic principles of therapy can thus be stated very simply, but much is still being learned about optimal indications for, and details of, bed rest, chemotherapy, and surgical management of the disease.

Bed rest was once considered the most important single measure in the therapy of tuberculosis. The course of the disease is so changed by chemotherapy, however, that the formerly strict regimens have been greatly modified. Fever and toxicity are still definite indications for bed rest. When the temperature has returned to normal, sufficient rest to avoid fatigue is all that is necessary. It has even been shown that, with adequate drug therapy, moderate physical exertion is not harmful. Some authorities still maintain a much more conservative attitude, insisting on complete bed rest except for bathroom privileges as long as the sputum is positive and chest x-rays show continuing changes. A middle ground is now the usual practice.

Under ideal circumstances treatment at home is feasible, but therapy should usually be instituted in a sanatorium or in an isolation unit of a general hospital, and the patient should remain there for at least a few months. The chief advantages of hospitalization are that a careful program of daily activities can be carried out in a neutral environment under expert supervision and the patient's progress can be followed closely with both clinical and laboratory observations. Other advantages are that the patient is removed from the community during the infectious period and opportunities for education, orientation, and rehabilitation are provided.

Climate was at one time considered an important part of the treatment of pulmonary tuberculosis, but it is now thought to exert an insignificant influence on the course of the disease. Aside from the elements comprising a good, well-balanced diet, no vitamins or other substances are known which specifically promote healing. The total caloric intake should be designed to enable the patient to regain and maintain his ideal weight.

Chemotherapeutic Agents. Factors affecting resistance, which have been described above, are often inadequate by themselves to control tuberculous infection. The remarkable effectiveness of drugs in decreasing the number of tubercle bacilli so tips the balance in favor of the host, however, that many patients are now salvaged who would previously have succumbed to the disease.

Three drugs are now in widespread use in the treatment of tuberculosis: streptomycin, para-aminosalicylic acid (PAS), and isoniazid. Other agents which may be used when these drugs are poorly tolerated, or when bacterial resistance has developed, are viomycin, oxytetracycline, cycloserine, and pyrazinamide. Viomycin is somewhat less effective than streptomycin and is quite toxic. It has proved to be a valuable agent, however, when isoniazid and streptomycin are poorly tolerated or ineffective. Oxytetracycline exerts a weak action but can be used in doses of 2 to 4 Gm daily if necessary as an alternative to PAS. Pyrazinamide

and cycloserine are quite effective but are also toxic, cycloserine to the central nervous system and pyrazinamide to the liver. The principal drugs will be considered separately, and then the combinations used in therapy will be described.

Either streptomycin or its hydrogenated derivative dihydrostreptomycin may be employed; the latter is seldom used now because of its greater tendency to cause deafness. Streptomycin was at first given alone and was effective for only 2 or 3 months because of the appearance of drug-resistant tubercle bacilli. It was then learned that the emergence of resistant organisms could be markedly delayed by the concomitant administration of PAS. As a result, the duration of effective drug therapy has been greatly lengthened. For most patients with pulmonary tuberculosis, when streptomycin is combined with PAS, 1 Gm twice weekly has been found to be as effective as the daily administration of the same dose. For more serious forms of the disease, such as miliary tuberculosis and tuberculous meningitis, streptomycin is given every day at least for the first 2 or 3 months.

Para-aminosalicylic acid, commonly referred to as PAS, is a relatively weak tuberculostatic agent when used alone but is very effective in delaying the emergence of streptomycin-resistant and isoniazid-resistant tubercle bacilli. The optimal regimen is unknown, but the usual procedure is to administer 12 Gm daily by mouth in three or four doses. Gastrointestinal irritation is common, causing anorexia, nausea, vomiting, and abdominal pain. The sodium salt causes fewer reactions than the free acid and is the form of the drug most commonly used. To administer 12 Gm of the free acid, 16.5 Gm of the sodium salt must be prescribed. A lyophilized preparation of the sodium salt is available for parenteral administration, and as much as 30 Gm a day can be given intravenously without causing anorexia and nausea. Serious toxic reactions are rare. Dermatitis and drug fever are encountered occasionally and can usually be controlled by desensitizing the patient with increasing doses of the drug. Para-aminosalicylic acid is sometimes goitrogenic, but thyroid enlargement from this cause can usually be prevented or ameliorated by the administration of desiccated thyroid. This is rarely necessary. The emergence of drug-resistant organisms has been observed when PAS is given alone but is less common when it is administered with streptomycin.

Isoniazid, a derivative of nicotinic acid, is more effective than either streptomycin or PAS and is the mainstay of drug therapy. In contrast to streptomycin, it penetrates mononuclear phagocytes and is active against intracellular as well as extracellular tubercle bacilli. Like streptomycin, isoniazid is bactericidal only against actively multiplying tubercle bacilli. Under these conditions, Koch-Weser has shown that isoniazid is irreversibly bound to the organisms, which after several days become non-acid-fast and lose their ability to produce tuberculin hypersensitivity. With metabolically inactive organisms such as occur in poorly oxygenated lesions or after previous therapy, isoniazid is taken up reversibly and does not interfere with acid-fastness or sensitizing ability. These observations undoubtedly explain in part why tubercle bacilli are not often eradicated from tuberculous lesions in patients. During therapy, drug-resistant organisms emerge quite rapidly, and it is customary therefore to administer another antimicrobial agent simultaneously. With isoniazid, however, the appearance of resistant mutants is not so clearly related to a failure to show continued improvement as it is with streptomycin. This may be related to Middlebrook's observation that some isoniazid-resistant tubercle bacilli do not form catalase and have little or no virulence when injected into guinea pigs. Failure of these organisms to grow in tissues may be due to susceptibility to the toxic effects of hydrogen peroxide. Catalase-positive, isoniazid-resistant mutants which are fully virulent also occur and probably account for progression of the disease which is observed after isoniazid resistance has developed.

Isoniazid is usually given orally in a total daily dose of 3 to 10 mg per kg body weight. For adults, the arbitrary selection of a daily dose of 300 to 400 mg, given in divided doses at 8- or 12-hr intervals, is satisfactory. Some patients (about 40 per cent) acetylate the drug at an unusually rapid rate, but controlled studies have failed to demonstrate that high doses of isoniazid (800 to 1,200 mg daily) produce significantly better therapeutic results in these "rapid inactivators." Higher doses are, however, used routinely in some clinics. When high doses are employed, 50 to 100 mg pyridoxine should also be given daily to prevent peripheral neuritis (see p. 1873).

Drug Regimens. With few exceptions, two and sometimes three drugs should be administered simultaneously in the treatment of all forms of tuberculosis. The exceptions apply to isoniazid, which is adequate when used alone for the treatment of tuberculin converters, minimal pulmonary tuberculosis, and tuberculous pleurisy with effusion. Isoniazid is also used alone in many patients for a year or two, or indefinitely, following an initial period of multiple-drug therapy.

Of the regimens available, it has been definitely shown that those containing isoniazid produce superior results. Thus, the combination of streptomycin and PAS, which was so widely used for a few years, is now employed for initial therapy only under unusual circumstances. Isoniazid-PAS is most widely used for the initial treatment of pulmonary tuberculosis at the present time. The results are comparable, or nearly so, to those obtained with any other combination, and both drugs are taken by mouth. Another important advantage is that streptomycin is held in reserve for use later in conjunction with surgery if it is needed. In some patients, serum concentrations of isoniazid are slightly elevated by the concomitant administration of PAS. This is probably not due to competition for the same acetylation mechanisms, as was at first thought.

Results with isoniazid-streptomycin are perhaps slightly superior in far-advanced cases to those obtained with isoniazid-PAS, particularly when streptomycin is injected daily rather than twice a week. The chief disadvantage, namely, that the two most potent drugs are likely to become ineffective because of the development of resistant organisms, is not of great importance since the relapse rate is only about 5 per cent. Furthermore, the combination of viomycin-PAS is available if needed for surgical coverage. In older individuals, who are more susceptible to the toxic effects of streptomycin, some experts prefer to avoid this drug and to select isoniazid-PAS instead. It is apparent from what has been said that both isoniazid-PAS and isoniazid-streptomycin have their advantages, and it is desirable to select the combination most suitable for each individual patient. The use of three drugs simultaneously (isoniazid, streptomycin, and PAS) has not been found superior for the treatment of pulmonary tuberculosis. For certain extrapulmonary forms of the disease to be considered later, triple-drug regimens are commonly used.

Steroid Therapy. Because of their tendency to reactivate the disease, adrenal corticosteroids were at first thought to be contraindicated in patients with tuberculosis. It was then learned that, with effective chemotherapy, steroids were not harmful and indeed might have a beneficial effect. Controlled studies have shown that, in pulmonary tuberculosis, steroids cause more rapid x-ray clearing and decrease in fever and toxicity but that there is little or no superiority when comparisons are made after 8 to 12 months. In patients with miliary tuberculosis and tuberculous meningitis, however, steroids often cause a marked defervescence of fever and toxicity and should be administered for 2 to 4 weeks in patients seriously ill with these forms of the disease.

Duration of Chemotherapy. The optimal duration of therapy cannot be stated with finality. The most important trend to be noted is a gradual lengthening from 2 to 3 months in the years prior to 1949 to regimens which call for at least 1 to 2 years of drug therapy. Combined therapy, which is associated with a marked delay in development of bacterial resistance, has been chiefly responsible for the change. It is probaby safe to follow the policy of continuing drug therapy for a least 6 months after clinical and laboratory observations indicate that the disease has become inactive. The minimal period should not be less than 12 months, and 2 years seems a reasonable maximum. There are many patients, however, with extensive disease not amenable to surgical therapy, to whom it may be wise to administer antimicrobial therapy indefinitely.

Collapse Therapy. This is another area in which older concepts have undergone radical changes. At one time statistical studies of pulmonary tuberculosis invariably showed a worse prognosis in patients with open cavities than in those without cavitary disease. Large cavities closed occasionally on bed rest alone, but usually they did not, and it was primarily in this type of case that artificial collapse therapy had its greatest usefulness. Now, however, collapse therapy is indicated in only a small percentage of patients with pulmonary tuberculosis, even when cavities are present. The various forms of collapse therapy will be reviewed briefly and the indications for each will be presented.

Pneumoperitoneum. Although used widely until very recently, even this form of collapse therapy has been virtually abandoned in most clinics. Administration of air into the peritoneal cavity is simple from a technical standpoint, and complications are rare. Pneumoperitoneum can be maintained for a long period of time and yet can be abandoned at any time. The chief indication is extensive exudative disease with bilateral cavitation. In such cases pneumoperitoneum may aid in improving the patient's condition to the point where resection of residual cavities and necrotic foci is feasible. In patients unable to withstand surgery, refills may be continued indefinitely.

Artificial Pneumothorax. Designed originally for predominantly unilateral disease with cavitation, this form of therapy produced brilliant results in carefully selected cases. Because of the high incidence of pleural complications, however, it is rarely used today.

Phrenemphraxis. Temporary paralysis of the diaphragm is effected by crushing the phrenic nerve. The diaphragm remains elevated and immobile for 6 or 8 months and then gradually resumes its normal function. The main disadvantages of phrenemphraxis are gastrointestinal disturbances, especially when it is performed on the left side, failure of the nerve to regenerate in about 10 per cent of cases, and reduction in respiratory reserve. This procedure is rarely used at present.

Thoracoplasty. Until recently, the classic indication for thoracoplasty was chronic fibroid disease at or near the apex of one lung, with a cavity which could not be closed effectively or safely by other means. Now, however, surgical excision is performed in the great majority of patients who formerly would have undergone thoracoplasty. Primary thoracoplasty is now reserved chiefly for patients with an apical cavity in whom resection is not possible and in whom other measures have failed.

Resection. Surgical resection has become an important part of the management of selected cases of pulmonary tuberculosis. The principal indications for resection have been the persistence of open cavities and large residual necrotic foci, with or without positive sputum, following several months of rest and chemotherapy. These indications are gradually being modified. For example, many patients with large cavities and negative cultures do as well with prolonged chemotherapy as when cavities are removed, and the avoidance of surgery is obviously of advantage when the risks of resection are great because of poor pulmonary function. In addition to open cavities, solid areas with a diameter greater than 4 cm are often resected. This problem will be considered in greater detail below in relation to viability of the tubercle bacilli.

Following prolonged chemotherapy, it is relatively simple to remove small wedges of lung tissue, and often several can be resected at one time. Little functioning pulmonary tissue is sacrificed, and these subsegmental resections can be performed on both lungs. With more extensive involvement, segmental resection, lobectomy, or pneumonectomy are indicated. Except when lobectomy or pneumonectomy is necessary, the mortality rate from surgery should be well under 1 per cent.

Bronchopleural fistula and empyema are the most serious problems following resection. These can be minimized by deferring surgery until endobronchial disease is well controlled. Postoperative spread of the disease, formerly a major hazard, now occurs in less than 2 per cent of resections. If a large amount of lung tissue, such as a whole lobe, is removed, overdistention of the remaining lung tissue may be prevented by performing a thoracoplasty. The need for thoracoplasty following lobectomy, or even pneumonectomy, is open to serious question, however, and it is now customary to perform the procedure only if signs of overdistention appear during the first month or two after the resection.

Viability of Tubercle Bacilli in Resected Lesions. When residual necrotic foci are removed following prolonged chemotherapy, they often contain large numbers of tubercle bacilli which appear normal on smear but do not grow on culture media and do not cause disease in guinea pigs. This phenomenon was also observed prior to the introduction of chemotherapy and is invariably associated with closed lesions. Since the organisms appear normal and healthy, the possibility has been raised that they are actually viable but have been so altered by the chemical composition of the closed necrotic lesion that they are incapable of multiplying when subjected to the usual tests. Hobby has shown that growth can often be obtained after many months of incubation in special culture media. The need for resecting necrotic foci remains unsettled, however, since the danger from these metabolically inactive organisms probably decreases with the passage of time. Controlled studies have not shown a higher incidence of relapse in patients with closed lesions who receive prolonged chemotherapy without surgery. Some authorities continue to advocate the resection of the larger residual necrotic foci (over 3 or 4 cm in diameter); others do not.

Correlation of Rest, Chemotherapy, and Resection. The manner in which various forms of therapy are correlated, especially from the standpoint of time relationships, can be considered briefly. The statements which are made are somewhat tentative, but will serve to illustrate the principles employed and will emphasize the shorter period of hospitalization which is necessary.

Following 3 to 6 months of rest and chemotherapy, the average patient with moderately advanced pulmonary tuberculosis will have attained maximal improvement from an x-ray standpoint, and cultures of sputum and gastric washings will be negative for tubercle bacilli. At this point tomograms are made, and if the residual lesions are insignificant in size and extent, ambulation is increased. This is a gradual process, requiring at least 3 months before the patient is up for the whole day. Another 3 months is allowed before he returns to work. Most patients of this type are discharged from the hospital 6 to 8 months after admission, and continue drug therapy on an outpatient basis for at least another 6 to 12 months.

If tomograms reveal the presence of cavities or other significant lesions, the diseased lung tissue may be resected. In the type of case under consideration, surgery is ordinarily performed between 4 to 8 months after admission to the hospital. If the postoperative course is uneventful, ambulation is begun 2 to 4 weeks later, and the subsequent course is as outlined above.

This example illustrates the usual procedure in the average, uncomplicated case. Patients with minimal lesions probably require less therapy, and in patients with far advanced bilateral disease the situation is often much more complex and time-consuming. In such cases the sputum often remains positive, and new drugs are added before surgery is performed. On the average, however, the period of hospitalization is much shorter than it formerly was. For example, in many tuberculosis hospitals the average hospital stay is only 8 months, as opposed to 20 months formerly. Providing facilities for administering chemotherapy on an outpatient basis is an important feature of the program.

Treatment of Special Conditions. The general principles underlying the treatment of pulmonary tuberculosis have been described above, but the management of certain features deserves special consideration.

Hemoptysis. Pulmonary hemorrhages are not infrequent in patients with pulmonary tuberculosis, and represent a dangerous and alarming complication. Fortunately, closure of the ulcerated blood vessel occurs promptly in most instances. Allaying fears of the patient concerning a possible fatal termination of the episode is an important part of the management of hemoptysis. The patient is instructed to lie on the affected side, to prevent material laden with bacilli from flowing into other parts of the lungs and spreading the disease. If the side from which the blood is coming is not known to the physician from previous examination and x-rays, the patient often can sense it from a peculiar feeling in one side of the chest. Although he lies mostly on the affected side, for a few minutes every hour, the patient should roll onto the other side, so that bloody discharges may drain into the trachea and be removed by gentle coughing. The time-honored warning against injudicious use of opiates is sound, but small doses of codeine may be a valuable aid in preventing spread of the disease by converting a severe intractable cough into one that is mild but effective. The patient usually brings up dark clots of blood over a period of several days as the episode subsides. In some instances the bleeding continues or recurs, and in such cases it may be necessary to institute artificial pneumothorax, which allows the bleeding vessel to contract and usually terminates the hemorrhage. If possible, pneumothorax should be avoided, since collapsing the lung during the acute episode impairs drainage of the retained secretions and the danger of pleural complications is great. If artificial pneumothorax is unsuccessful, phrenemphraxis or pneumoperitoneum is occasionally instituted in an attempt to stop the bleeding. If bleeding persists, transfusions should be given. Many drugs, such as calcium gluconate, atropine, ascorbic acid, vitamin K, and nitroglycerin, have been thought to be effective in isolated cases of hemoptysis, but their general use cannot be recommended. Fresh exudative lesions which follow hemoptysis respond extremely well to chemotherapy. In many instances, of course, the exudative "spread" is mostly blood, which would disappear on rest alone within a few weeks.

Spontaneous Pneumothorax and Bronchopleural Fistula. Spontaneous pneumothorax is a relatively common occurrence in young adults. It usually begins suddenly with a sharp pain in the anterior chest and in the majority of instances is due to the rupture of a subpleural bulla. The bulla may be secondary to fibrosis caused by tuberculosis or other infections, or it may be congenital. The available evidence indicates that only a small percentage of spontaneous pneumothoraxes are tuberculous in origin, and therefore bed rest is not prescribed unless a parenchymal focus is demonstrated or tubercle bacilli are recovered (see p. 1565).

When tuberculous in origin, spontaneous pneumothorax results from the ulceration of a subpleural caseous focus, or the rupture of a tuberculous cavity directly into the pleural space. If possible, the lung should be reexpanded at once, using catheter drainage with controlled suction, for this is a much more serious situation than is the rupture of a bulla. In this instance the fistula carries large numbers of tubercle bacilli into the pleural cavity, causing infection, fluid formation, and the development of empyema. This may be a simple tuberculous empyema, or other organisms, such as streptococci and staphylococci, may pass through the fistulous opening to form a mixed infection empyema. An open bronchopleural fistula with empyema is a dangerous situation; the empyema fluid may drain slowly through the fistula into the bronchi and lungs, causing widespread dissemination of the disease, or if the fistula suddenly enlarges, several hundred milliliters of pus may flood into the bronchial tree, causing the patient to drown in his own secretions. A patent bronchopleural fistula should be suspected when the patient coughs up material similar to pus aspirated from the chest and may be proved by injecting methylene blue into the empyema cavity and subsequently observing the dye in the sputum. Once diagnosed, a bronchopleural fistula is an indication for surgical drainage because of the dangers mentioned above and because of the failure of mixed-infection empyemas to respond to aspiration and irrigations.

Tuberculous Empyema. This condition is considered separately, for its management differs somewhat from that of bronchopleural fistula with mixed-infection empyema. Pure tuberculous empyema may appear spontaneously, or as a complication of artificial pneumothorax or surgical resection. There is a tendency to regard all effusions as empyemas if tubercle bacilli can be recovered. This is mis-

leading, for with clear effusions the prognosis is much more favorable than in true empyemas, in which the fluid is thick, purulent, and swarming with bacilli. With chemotherapy, aspiration and irrigation, and instillation of streptokinase and streptodornase, considerable improvement may occur, but the empyema is usually not obliterated. The procedure of choice at the present time is to excise the entire empyema cavity, proceeding extrapleurally as much as possible. Diseased lung tissue is resected at the same time. To obliterate the space and prevent a recurrence of the empyema, a thoracoplasty is usually performed. An unroofing procedure of the Schede type, which is dangerous and deforming, is rarely necessary.

Fibrinous and Serofibrinous Pleurisy. Pleural involvement occurs in most cases of pulmonary tuberculosis. One indication of this is the high incidence of pleural adhesions in patients receiving artificial pneumothorax. The adhesions result from localized areas of fibrinous pleurisy overlying peripherally located parenchymal foci, and the apposition of the two pleural surfaces aids in localization of the process. With fibrinous pleurisy, symptoms may be absent, or there may be sharp, pleuritic pain, and a friction rub may be detectable. The course of fibrinous pleurisy is usually mild, and, except for local palliative measures, attention should be directed at the underlying parenchymal disease.

Five to ten per cent of patients with pulmonary tuberculosis develop serofibrinous pleurisy, which is discussed on p. 1005. Care must be taken to exclude other causes of serous effusions, such as pneumonia; a careful analysis of clinical signs and symptoms prior to the onset of the effusion is usually adequate to make this differential.

Fluid is aspirated initially for diagnosis. After removal of most of the effusion, 100 ml of air may be injected into the pleural space, allowing the remainder of the fluid to fall to the base so that the pulmonary parenchyma can be visualized clearly on the x-ray. Opinion is divided as to whether repeated aspirations should be performed if the fluid persists and increases in amount after the first tap. The author feels that fluid should be removed repeatedly to prevent incarceration of the lung. The fluid usually does not reappear after several thoracenteses have been performed, and there is a minimal degree of mediastinal shift and pleural thickening. It is generally agreed that artificial pneumothorax is contraindicated, because the presence of air impedes healing and the lung often does not reexpand after being collapsed for a prolonged period in the presence of fluid.

In addition to aspirations, the treatment is that prescribed for an active case of minimal tuberculosis, namely, rest and chemotherapy. Isoniazid alone is probably adequate in such cases, but most authorities prefer to administer PAS in addition.

EXTRAPULMONARY TUBERCULOSIS

Laryngeal and Tracheobronchial Tuberculosis. Tuberculous laryngitis usually occurs in patients with advanced pulmonary tuberculosis, the infection resulting from the continual passage of bacilliferous sputum over the vocal cords and accessory structures, which are irritated by the chronic cough. Rarely, laryngeal lesions are seen in patients with little or no active pulmonary tuberculosis, and the infection then is presumably hematogenous or lymphogenous in origin. Hoarseness and a dry sensation in the throat are the common symptoms; the diagnosis can be confirmed by direct or indirect laryngoscopy, and a biopsy. The posterior part of the larynx and vocal cords are first involved, and later there are deep, extensive ulcerations of the laryngeal cartilages, including the epiglottis. With the latter there is severe pain on swallowing, which interferes with eating. Heretofore, treatment consisted of complete voice rest, cauterization of granulations or deep ulcerations, anesthetic sprays to relieve pain, and antibiotics to reduce secondary infection. With chemotherapy, however, the condition usually responds so well that most of the palliative measures mentioned above are unnecessary. Pain subsides within a few days, and the ulcers heal within a few weeks.

Chemotherapy exerts a similarly favorable influence in tuberculous tracheobronchitis. Tracheobronchial lesions consist of ulcerations or of granulomatous infiltrations which tend to occlude the bronchial lumen as they undergo fibrosis and healing. Stenosing bronchial lesions are to be suspected in the presence of wheezing, especially when this is localized over one lung or over a single lobe. Episodes of pneumonitis occur distal to the stenosis owing to impairment of the normal drainage of secretions, and bronchiectasis may appear in the affected lobe. Bronchoscopy aids in determining the nature and extent of the tracheobronchial disease, and in assessing the efficacy of antimicrobial therapy. Old fibrotic cicatricial stenoses are not benefited by chemotherapy, and resection is usually necessary.

Generalized Miliary Tuberculosis. Resulting from the sudden entry of large numbers of tubercle bacilli into the blood stream, miliary tuberculosis is characterized by seeding throughout the tissues of small foci of roughly the same age and size. The source of the bacilli is probably, in most instances, a caseous hilar or mediastinal lymph node which erodes into a blood or lymph vessel. Caseous foci in other organs, such as the kidneys, bones, ad-renals, and prostate, may also give rise to massive blood stream invasion. Tubercle bacilli are carried to every part of the body, but some organs, such as the pancreas, thyroid, skeletal muscles, brain, and stomach, show little or no involvement.

Miliary tuberculosis occurs most frequently during the period when the primary complex is active; the peak is during early childhood. The condition is not rare, however, in adults. The onset may be sudden, with high fever, aching, chilliness, and prostration, or it may be gradual, with an initial period of general malaise and weakness. Cough is not a striking feature and, if present, is usually mild and nonproductive. The diagnosis often remains obscure until characteristic miliary lesions appear on the roentgenogram, which may not be until several weeks following the onset of symptoms. In general, when there is an acute onset with high fever and marked prostration, the lesions are exudative, while in patients with a more insidious onset and low fever, a productive reaction is predominant. The white blood count may vary from agranulocytosis to marked leukocytosis, or there may even be a leukemoid reaction. Other conditions which may present a clinical and x-ray picture similar to that of miliary tuberculosis are presented elsewhere (see p. 1509). Because the lesions are interstitial, the recovery of tubercle bacilli is often delayed for many weeks. Tubercle bacilli can often be cultured from the bone marrow and, sometimes, the blood.

Heretofore, miliary tuberculosis has been a highly fatal condition, with death characteristically occurring 6 to 10 weeks following the onset. This situation has been altered dramatically by chemotherapy. Fever and toxemia usually subside within a few days, and within a few weeks the pulmonary lesions begin to show regression. In the early days of streptomycin therapy, when treatment was continued for only 2 or 3 months, over half the cases relapsed and died. With prolonged, combined chemotherapy, recovery occurs in more than 85 per cent of cases, and relapses are rare. This is one of the forms of tuberculosis in which all three of the antimicrobial agents—isoniazid, streptomycin, and PAS—are administered simultaneously. One gram of streptomycin is injected every day for the first 4 months, then twice weekly. The daily dosages of isoniazid and PAS are 0.3 to 0.6 Gm and 12.0 Gm, respectively. Treatment is continued for 2 years.

Tuberculous meningitis often occurs during the course of miliary tuberculosis, even when the patient is receiving streptomycin therapy. Since the addition of isoniazid to the chemotherapeutic regimen, however, this complication has rarely been observed. It is, therefore, less important to perform frequent lumbar punctures in patients with miliary tuberculosis than it was a few years ago.

Subacute and Chronic Hematogenous Tuberculosis. Instead of a single, massive invasion of the blood stream, smaller numbers of tubercle bacilli may escape intermittently into the circulation, and give rise to a variety of clinical manifestations. Among the more common manifestations are low-grade fever, local or generalized lymphadenopathy, effusions into the pleural and peritoneal cavities, splenomegaly, and destructive lesions of the bones, kidneys, skin, and eyes.

The protean manifestations and bizarre clinical picture caused by subacute and chronic forms of hematogenous tuberculosis provide diagnostic puzzles which often can be solved only by cultures of secretions or discharges, or by biopsy of the affected tissues. It should be borne in mind that hematogenous foci may remain latent in various organs for many years.

Tuberculous Meningitis. As in miliary tuberculosis, tuberculous meningitis is more common during early childhood than at any other age period. The percentage of adults infected with the tubercle bacillus who die of tuberculous meningitis is relatively small. The evidence of Rich indicates that the meninges are infected by direct extension from an adjacent focus. In miliary tuberculosis, Rich showed that meningitis results not from the direct escape of large numbers of bacilli into the meninges from the blood stream but from miliary meningeal tubercles which gradually enlarge to produce direct extension, or that it arises from older, dormant foci which became reactivated and extend into the meningeal spaces. Pathologically, the reaction consists of tubercles, edema and congestion, and a fibrinous exudate, most marked over the base of the brain. Various cranial nerves are commonly affected.

Tuberculous meningitis may appear in individuals who previously were apparently entirely well. The symptoms of miliary tuberculosis usually precede those of tuberculous meningitis by several weeks, when the two occur together. The early symptoms of tuberculous meningitis are headache, restlessness, and irritability, and, on examination, typical signs of meningeal irritation are usually elicited. The spinal fluid pressure is elevated, and there is an increase in protein and cells, most of which are mononuclear. The chlorides and sugar are depressed, moderately in some cases, markedly in others. On standing, a pellicle usually forms. Smears of the centrifuged sediment, or pellicle, may reveal tubercle bacilli, but in the majority of cases they do not. Repeated cultures and guinea pig inoculations usually are necessary to recover the causative organism.

Until streptomycin became available, there was no urgency about establishing the diagnosis of tuberculous meningitis; treatment was purely supportive and the outcome almost always fatal. Now, however, treatment must be started in many cases before the organisms are recovered. Early differentiation between tuberculous meningitis and meningitis due to other agents, chiefly fungi and viruses, is at times impossible; in such cases chemotherapy should be administered if tuberculosis seems the probable cause on the basis of a positive tuberculin test, marked depression of the spinal fluid sugar and chloride, and the general clinical picture.

The treatment of tuberculous meningitis is identical with that outlined above for miliary tuberculosis, except that streptomycin should probably be given in daily doses of 2 Gm, rather than 1 Gm, for the first 4 months. Intrathecal administration of streptomycin has been largely abandoned, greatly simplifying therapy. Intrathecal administration of tuberculin has given dramatic results in some cases but cannot be recommended until the benefits and dangers are more clearly defined. Corticosteroids produce a dramatic decrease in fever and toxicity, and may diminish the formation of exudate about the base of the brain. Their use is probably indicated in most if not all cases; these hormones can usually be discontinued by the end of the first month.

With the availability of isoniazid, the cure rate is in the neighborhood of 80 to 90 per cent in many clinics, and poor results occur mostly in patients who are treated late in the course of the disease. Many patients make a complete clinical recovery, without mental impairment or neurologic defects.

Tuberculosis of Lymph Nodes. Tuberculosis of hilar and mediastinal nodes, which is the commonest form of tuberculous lymphadenitis, has its inception during the primary infection, when tubercle bacilli escape freely from the initial pulmonary lesion. Children with a primary infection may have massive lymph node involvement with few constitutional manifestations. The symptoms in such cases are due chiefly to pressure on surrounding structures and consist of wheezing, dyspnea, and hacking cough. In addition, compression of a bronchus may cause collapse of one or more lobes, with pneumonitis caused by other bacteria distal to the site of narrowing. Except when there is perforation into a bronchus or when death results from progressive tuberculosis, the involved nodes show a marked tendency to heal and become calcified. Even with apparent healing, however, viable tubercle bacilli may remain in the nodes for long periods. Aside from rest and chemotherapy, x-ray and tuberculin therapy are sometimes recommended but are of questionable value and are potentially dangerous because excessive doses may aggravate tissue necrosis. Chemotherapy was at first unimpressive, probably because of poor penetration of streptomycin into the large caseous nodes. Isoniazid is effective, however, not only in promoting healing of the mediastinal nodes but in preventing spread to other organs. Isoniazid is often used alone in milder cases in children, but with extensive involvement streptomycin or PAS should be added. Calcified nodes occasionally perforate into a bronchus many years after the primary complex apparently has become arrested. This condition, known as *broncholithiasis*, is characterized by pneumonitis, hemoptysis, and expectoration of small bits of calcified material.

Cervical adenitis, or scrofula, has become relatively uncommon in the United States in the past 50 years as a result of the elimination of tuberculous cattle and the widespread pasteurization of milk. Direct infection by tubercle bacilli through the tissues of the pharynx or tonsils has been virtually eliminated, but cervical adenitis of lymphohematogenous origin is still observed in both adults and children. The swelling usually begins insidiously and may involve one or many nodes. The lymph nodes tend to be matted, but this is not a reliable diagnostic feature. The skin often perforates at one or more sites, permitting the drainage of thick, greenish yellow pus. The treatment of tuberculous cervical adenitis consists of rest and chemotherapy, with surgical removal of the residual nodes after several months if they are still enlarged. Results with isoniazid and PAS, or with isoniazid alone, have been so good that surgery usually is unnecessary.

Gastrointestinal Tuberculosis. Tuberculous ulcers occur occasionally on the tongue, lip, pharynx, and tonsils. The diagnosis is made by curetting or excising a small portion of the involved tissue and preparing microscopic sections. These lesions respond very well to chemotherapy.

Tuberculosis of the esophagus and stomach is rare. The *intestine,* however, especially the lower ileum and cecum, is frequently involved in patients with advanced pulmonary tuberculosis as a result of swallowing bacilli. The symptoms of ileocecal tuberculosis are variable, consisting chiefly of intermittent indigestion, colicky pain, constipation, and diarrhea. The appearance of any unusual gastrointestinal complaints should arouse suspicion, especially in patients with far advanced pulmonary involvement. A moderate anemia is common, and should direct attention to the intestinal tract whenever present in patients with pulmonary tuberculosis. X-ray studies of the ileocecal region provide

valuable confirmatory evidence of spasticity and hypermotility. The treatment is directed at both the pulmonary lesions and the ulcers in the bowel. For the latter a low-residue, bland diet diminishes irritation of the bowel wall, and opium derivatives or bismuth compounds are given to relieve the pain and diarrhea. Chemotherapy which is prescribed for the pulmonary disease usually brings about healing of the intestinal lesions. In some cases an excessive amount of irritation is caused by PAS, and it is wise in most instances, therefore, to administer streptomycin and isoniazid.

Tuberculous Peritonitis. This condition results from extension of local lesions in the intestine, lymph nodes, or genital tract, or it may be caused by hematogenous spread from other parts of the body. Serofibrinous peritonitis usually has an insidious onset, with mild constitutional symptoms and vague intestinal complaints. As with serofibrinous pleurisy, however, the onset may in some cases be acute, with high fever, severe abdominal pain, and marked prostration. Fluid often appears, especially in the more toxic cases, and may require repeated aspirations to relieve distention and discomfort. Treatment consists of rest and chemotherapy, using the same regimen as for pulmonary tuberculosis. As healing occurs, thick adhesions may form, matting the intestines and omentum together, interfering with normal peristalsis, and causing stenosis of various portions of the bowel. Unless the adhesive process is localized and surgically resectable, as it sometimes is in the region of the cecum, the treatment is symptomatic and palliative. Fortunately this complication is uncommon.

Tuberculosis of the Kidney. In most instances this occurs by hematogenous dissemination from foci in the lungs or lymph nodes; occasionally infection may come from the genital tract. Small foci may remain latent in the kidneys for long periods before causing destructive lesions; many patients with renal tuberculosis show no evidence of active pulmonary disease. As the ulcerative lesions in the kidney enlarge, tubercle bacilli escape into the urinary tract and often infect the ureters and bladder. Dysuria and hematuria are the main symptoms, but cases of renal tuberculosis are not infrequently diagnosed before symptoms appear. Blood and pus are found in the urine, and tubercle bacilli are recovered from the centrifuged sediment by culture or guinea pig inoculation. Intravenous and retrograde pyelograms often show characteristic renal ulcerations; retrograde studies are particularly helpful in determining whether the involvement is bilateral. Lattimer has shown that chemotherapy of renal tuberculosis is so effective that surgery is now rarely necessary. Triple-drug therapy (isoniazid, streptomycin, and PAS) was used in his studies and was continued for 1 to 2 years. It is now felt that damaged kidney tissue should be removed only if there is a relapse after prolonged drug therapy.

Genital Tuberculosis. Genital tuberculosis is almost invariably hematogenous in origin, and in the male involves the prostate, seminal vesicles, epididymides, and occasionally the testes. Infection of the genital tract may, in occasional instances, be secondary to renal tuberculosis. Clinically, involvement of the epididymis is diagnosed most frequently, although pathologic examinations reveal a higher incidence of tuberculosis of the prostate and seminal vesicles. Tuberculous epididymitis often begins insidiously, with a gradual development of nodular infiltrations which are moderately tender. The onset is sometimes acute, with sudden swelling, redness, and marked tenderness of the epididymis and surrounding structures. Rest and chemotherapy are indicated, and the epididymis and seminal vesicles are removed only if there are large residual masses of inflammatory tissue.

Genital tuberculosis in the female involves the fallopian tubes more frequently than the other organs, and the lesions are more often unilateral than bilateral. Less commonly, the ovaries and uterus may be the site of destructive lesions; the cervix, vagina, and labia are rarely affected. Vague, irregular lower abdominal pain may be the only symptom of tuberculous salpingitis, and an adnexal mass may be found on pelvic examination. If the uterus is involved, tubercle bacilli may be present in the vaginal discharge, or tuberculous tissue may be removed by curettage. The menses may be normal, but in advanced cases are usually scanty or absent. Tuberculous salpingitis is potentially dangerous, because it may cause diffuse peritonitis. Again, the trend is toward prolonged chemotherapy, with surgery only if there are large residual masses.

Pericarditis. The pericardium can become infected in tuberculosis by discharge of the contents of a caseous mediastinal lymph node into this space, by hematogenous dissemination (involvement of serous surfaces by this means is relatively rare), or by direct extension from nearby pleuropulmonary lesions. The inflammatory process in the pericardium varies from a serofibrinous reaction containing relatively few bacilli (presumably a response to sudden discharge of tuberculoprotein onto a sensitized serous surface similar to that in pleurisy with effusion) to extensive fibrocaseous lesions containing myriads of acid-fast organisms.

The clinical picture produced by tuberculous infection of the pericardium is extremely variable. The sudden onset of substernal pain and fever with accompanying signs such as a to-and-fro friction rub. Ewart's sign, etc. (see p. 1467), in a patient known to have had tuberculosis makes the diagnosis relatively easy. However, the disease may be entirely asymptomatic, attention being drawn to it by the finding of enlargement of the cardiac shadow in a routine x-ray of the chest. Again, because of epicardial and myocardial involvement, or tamponade, patients may be thought to have congestive heart failure of many etiologies. Low-grade fever, vague complaints of discomfort in the chest, and mild weight loss may be the only complaints. The finding of pericardial adhesions in many tuberculous patients at autopsy suggests that many instances of minimal pericardial tuberculosis may spontaneously subside and become inactive. While occasional patients may accumulate large amounts of fluid in the pericardium, sometimes bloody, and require repeated aspirations to avoid serious circulatory difficulties, this is not usual. In such cases, there is often simultaneous involvement of one or both pleural spaces, leading to confusion with such diseases as systemic lupus erythematosus, pyogenic infections, and "benign idiopathic" pericarditis. Occasional patients with tuberculosis of the pericardium run an intermittent course, experiencing several bouts of pain and fever, with friction rubs, reaccumulation of fluid, etc.

Tuberculosis of the pericardium is the commonest cause of constrictive pericarditis. The fibrosis and calcification that accompany the healing process in this infection can lead to encasement of the heart in an unyielding tunic of dense scar with serious effects upon the circulation (see p. 1471).

Diagnosis by demonstration of tubercle bacilli in smears or cultures of aspirated fluid is often difficult, and in cases of doubtful etiology pericardial biopsy is becoming an increasingly feasible and useful procedure. The institution of chemotherapy of the type recommended for pulmonary tuberculosis before operation makes spread of infection unlikely. It is not uncommon to find a surprising amount of pericardial scar when operation for biopsy is carried out, and in such instances many feel that pericardiectomy can and should be done. The final place of early surgical treatment in tuberculous pericarditis remains to be determined. It is clear, however, that in some cases where infection is arrested or eradicated by chemotherapy, sufficient mechanical difficulty can remain to warrant excision of the thickened membrane. The duration of drug treatment should be at least a year, and indications for rest, proper diet, etc., differ in no way from those in other forms of tuberculosis.

Skeletal Tuberculosis. Bone and joint tuberculosis is usually hematogenous in origin and is most likely to occur in young children. In adults the incidence is higher in males, and it is more frequent in Negroes than in whites. With joint involvement, diagnosis depends on study of aspirated fluid or pus and on surgical biopsy. Destructive bone changes visible on roentgenograms often occur late.

In over half the cases there is active pulmonary tuberculosis, and a presumptive diagnosis can often be made on this basis.

Chemotherapy, if started early, often results in a complete return of function of the involved joints. With marked bone destruction, surgical immobilization (arthrodesis) is usually necessary, but this is carried out only after a period of drug therapy. Triple-drug regimens similar to those used for genitourinary tuberculosis should be employed. Details of orthopedic procedures are beyond the scope of this presentation. Close cooperation between the internist and orthopedist is obviously desirable.

PROGNOSIS

The outlook for the great majority of patients with tuberculosis has been vastly improved by the availability of effective chemotherapeutic agents and advances in surgical management. The case fatality rate is falling rapidly, and there has been a marked decrease in the number of domiciliary cases. Further advances in therapy can be expected, and it is probable that it will eventually be possible to arrest the disease permanently in most patients.

One deterrent to this optimistic outlook is the fact that socioeconomic factors are becoming increasingly important. Most patients with tuberculosis are among the lower-income groups and are individuals who have adjusted themselves poorly to the stresses and strains of modern society. The aid of social service workers, occupational therapists, and psychiatrists is therefore of the greatest importance in the over-all plan of rehabilitation.

PREVENTION AND ERADICATION OF TUBERCULOSIS

The remarkable decline in the mortality rate from tuberculosis during the first two decades of the twentieth century led a number of careful students of the problem to predict the virtual eradication of the disease by 1950 or earlier. The fallacy in the prediction lay in the assumption that the number of individuals harboring active lesions would fall to the point that the disease would cease to propagate itself. This has not occurred; as pointed out in the section on Prevalence and Incidence, the decline in the mortality rate is probably due chiefly to improved living conditions and other factors which tend to increase resistance, but the incidence of infection of the population as a whole remains relatively high. This means that a large number of individuals with active disease are not hospitalized and remain at large to infect the general populace. Evidence indicating the occurrence of such "carriers" is provided by the fact that no apparent source of contact can be found for most adults with pulmonary tuberculosis. Autopsy studies further indicate that undiagnosed cases of active tuberculosis are common in older persons, especially men.

Preventive measures in addition to the improvement in living conditions which have contributed greatly to the advances accompanying the antituberculosis campaign are earlier diagnosis and treatment, isolation of active cases, better hospital facilities, programs for the rehabilitation of patients with arrested disease to prevent relapse, examination of close contacts of tuberculous patients, large-scale x-ray surveys, elimination of tuberculous cattle, and pasteurization of milk. Much has been accomplished, but in almost every one of the above categories present efforts and results fall far short of what is desired.

In 1960 the Report of the Arden House Conference on Tuberculosis was published. A group of national leaders in public health and tuberculosis control concluded that the time was ripe to push for the elimination of tuberculosis in the United States. It was agreed that the principal weapon is modern drug treatment, and 11 recommendations were made concerning the establishment of intermediate goals and performance standards that will lead to eventual eradication. The impetus resulting from this conference has unquestionably accelerated the pace and efficiency of tuberculosis control programs.

BCG (bacillus Calmette-Guérin), an attenuated bovine tubercle bacillus, has been used widely abroad for vaccination against tuberculosis. Controlled studies of its efficacy are difficult to conduct, but the experiments which have been made seem to provide some evidence of its value. Protection is by no means complete, but a sufficient degree of acquired resistance is conferred to warrant consideration of its use among tuberculin negative groups in which exposure to tuberculosis is especially likely to occur. Examples are tuberculin negative nurses, medical students, and individuals living under poor economic conditions in overcrowded urban areas. In many medical and nursing schools, the incidence of tuberculosis is so low that the use of BCG has been abandoned. In the opinion of the author, the use of BCG is rarely if ever indicated in the United States at present.

REFERENCES

Dubos, R. J.: Unsolved Problems in the Control of Tuberculosis, Am. Rev. Tuberc., 70:391, 1954.

Harris, H. W.: High-dose Isoniazid Compared with Standard-dose Isoniazid, with PAS, in Cavitary Pulmonary Tuberculosis, Trans. 20th Conf. on Chemotherapy of Tuberculosis, V.A. Central Office, Washington, D.C., 1961.

Hobby, G. L., O. Auerbach, T. F. Lenert, M. J. Small, and J. V. Comer: The Late Emergence of *M. tuberculosis* in Liquid Cultures of Pulmonary Lesions Resected from Humans, Am. Rev. Tuberc., 70:191, 1954.

Koch, R.: Die Aetiolgie der Tuberculose, Klin. Wochschr., 19:221, 1882 (translation published by the National Tuberculosis Association, New York, 1932).

Laennec, T. R. H.: "Traité de l'ausculation médiate et des maladies des poumons et du coeur," Paris, J. S. Chaude, 1826.

Lurie, M. B.: Studies on the Mechanism of Immunity in Tuberculosis, J. Exptl. Med., 75:247, 1942.

—— and G. S. Ninos: The Effect of Triiodothyronine and Propyl Thiouracil on Native Resistance to Tuberculosis, Am. Rev. Tuberc., 73:434, 1956.

McDermott, W., L. Ormond, C. Muschenheim, K. Deuschle, R. M. McCune, Jr., and R. Tompsett: Pyrazinamide-isoniazid in Tuberculosis, Am. Rev. Tuberc., 69:319, 1954.

Medlar, E. M.: Primary and Reinfection Tuberculosis as the Cause of Death in Adults, Am. Rev. Tuberc., 55:517, 1947.

——: The Pathogenesis of Minimal Pulmonary Tuberculosis, Am. Rev. Tuberc., 58:583, 1948.

Middlebrook, G., R. J. Dubos, and C. Pierce: Virulence and Morphologic Characteristics of Mammalian Tubercle Bacilli, J. Exptl. Med., 86:175, 1947.

Pinner, M.: "Pulmonary Tuberculosis in the Adult," Springfield, Ill., Charles C Thomas, Publisher, 1951.

Rich, A. R.: "The Pathogenesis of Tuberculosis," 2d ed., Springfield, Ill., Charles C Thomas, Publisher, 1951.

Rothstein, E.: The Chemotherapy of Tuberculosis, New Engl. J. Med., 263:588, 1960.

Terplan, K.: Anatomical Studies on Human Tuberculosis, Am. Rev. Tuberc., 42:Suppl., August, 1940.

Tucker, W. B., and D. G. Livings: Isoniazid, Streptomycin, and Para-aminosalicylic Acid Compared as Two-drug Regimens in the Treatment of Pulmonary Tuberculosis among Previously Untreated Patients: III. An Account of the Cooperative Investigation of the Veterans Administration, Army, and Navy, August, 1952, to September, 1954, Am. Rev. Tuberc., 72:756, 1955.

Waksman, S. A., and A. Schatz: Streptomycin: Origin, Nature and Properties, J. Am. Pharm. Assoc. (Sci. Ed.), 34:273, 1945.

147 LEPROSY
(Hansen's Disease)

Gustave J. Dammin

Definition. Leprosy is a specific infectious disease of man caused by the *Mycobacterium leprae*. It is usually characterized by a long incubation period, a long course with exacerbations and remissions, and involvement primarily of the skin and mucous membranes and/or the peripheral nervous system. The major forms of the disease are the polar forms, the lepromatous and the tuberculoid; in addition, there are dimorphous and indeterminate forms.

History. Whether leprosy as it is understood today was described in the ancient records has been questioned (Lendrum). In Europe, leprosy appeared first in Greece in the fourth century B.C., probably having been introduced from the East. It spread northward and westward and had affected most of Europe by the end of the tenth century A.D. Leprosy was prevalent in Europe until the fourteenth century and then began slowly to decline.

As leprosy was declining in Europe, it was being spread to the Western Hemisphere by the slave traders and the discoverers from Portugal and Spain. In the United States, leprosy appeared first in Louisiana in 1758, presumably spread from the West Indies. Additional foci were established from other sources: in Minnesota from Norway, in California and Hawaii from China and India.

There are about 2 million cases of leprosy registered throughout the world, but many authorities place the actual number of affected individuals at 10 or 12 million.

Etiology. *Mycobacterium leprae*, described by Hansen in 1874, is accepted as the causal agent of human leprosy even though the organism has not been cultivated on artificial media or in tissue culture and the disease has not been transmitted artificially to man or to lower animals. Despite encouraging preliminary results obtained by inoculation of the ears and testes of hamsters (Binford) and the footpad of the white mouse (Shepard), repeated passage has not been achieved. Obviously, the evaluation of chemotherapeutic agents for the disease would be greatly facilitated by the development of a model disease in animals.

Mycobacterium leprae is a pleomorphic, acidfast, non-spore-forming, gram-positive bacillus. Lepra bacilli differ from tubercle bacilli in that they (1) are found in tremendous numbers in lesions (lepromatous) in the form of packets, palisades, and globular masses (globi) both intra- and extracellularly; (2) decolorize more readily; (3) may be stained with the stronger bacterial stains; (4) cannot be cultivated and do not produce disease in animals following inoculation.

Epidemiology and Pathogenesis. The exact mode of transmission is not known. A history of prolonged direct contact usually beginning in childhood is common. Leprosy may not manifest itself clinically until 1 to 5 years after the period of exposure, and appears most often during the third decade of life. Resistance to leprosy appears to increase with age.

Leprosy is not transmitted to the offspring, and it is well known that infants born of leprous parents, if removed and reared in an environment permitting no contact, do not develop the disease. Those not separated are likely to develop leprosy in early life; even when separated at six months of age, 50 per cent of the children had clinical manifestations by the age of five years.

Of interest are cases recognized as accidental-inoculation leprosy. One report concerns two marines who "were tattooed successively by the same man in Melbourne, Australia, on the same day in June, 1943. Both developed maculoanesthetic leprosy in the tattoos about 2½ years later" (Porritt and Olsen).

Lepra bacilli leave the body by many routes. In lepromatous leprosy they may escape in the secretions and excretions and through any interruption in the involved skin and mucous membranes. The route by which they enter a new host is not known, but it is believed that infection occurs by way of the skin and mucous membranes following direct contact.

Once in the body, the bacilli are probably spread by way of the lymphatics and blood stream and by autoinoculation. Localization occurs primarily in the skin and/or nerves, and in advanced cases of lepromatous leprosy, bacilli are found in many of the viscera. Bacillemia occurs more commonly in the lepromatous type.

Pathology. The lesions of leprosy have been classified according to their microscopic appearance into four principal types: (1) lepromatous, (2) tuberculoid, (3) dimorphous, and (4) indeterminate.

In the *lepromatous type*, bacilli are numerous, there is relatively little cellular response and cutaneous nodules, papules, macules, and diffuse infiltrations are distributed symmetrically in large numbers. A distinctive feature is the "lepra cell," a large macrophage containing many bacilli and fat droplets. In large accumulations the bacilli form globi and rosettes.

The *tuberculoid* lesions are observed in cutaneous leprids and the affected nerves. The leprids are often macules and are usually asymmetric in distribution. Bacilli are few or absent, and epithelioid cells, giant cells, lymphocytes, and plasma cells are present, often in the form of tubercles.

The *dimorphous* lesion, which is uncommon and presumably represents a transient state, has microscopic features of both the lepromatous and tuberculoid forms.

The *indeterminate type* of lesion contains few bacilli and shows a slight cellular reaction which is limited to the perivascular and perineural areas.

The gross lesions in the skin and nerves are not characteristic or advanced enough to permit classification with the two principal clinical types.

Clinical Classification. A combined clinicopathologic classification is recommended, since it makes more direct clinical, immunologic, bacteriologic, and epidemiologic correlations possible. That is, regardless of the sites involved, the lepromatous type is characterized by a relatively rapid course, a negative lepromin reaction, and lesions containing many bacilli, and because of this, is an "open" or dangerous type for the community. The tuberculoid type has a more chronic course, shows more resistance to the disease, has a positive lepromin reaction, has few bacilli in the lesions, and is therefore a "closed" type and less of a community hazard. The indeterminate type is viewed as a transitional form. The lepromin reaction in this type has prognostic significance, since many cases with negative reactions develop into the lepromatous type and those with positive reactions into the tuberculoid type. The dimorphous type is a macular lesion not representative of a particular clinical group.

The distribution of types varies in different geographic areas. The tuberculoid type is often preponderant in areas known to have had leprosy for long periods and where control has shown some degree of effectiveness; the lepromatous type may predominate in newly involved areas and those in which control has been less effective.

Clinical Course. The onset is often unheralded and difficult to date. The incubation period averages about 3 to 5 years. Claims of very long incubation periods must be scrutinized, since minor lesions are likely to remain unrecognized for long periods.

Initial skin lesions of the lepromatous type usually are found on the extensor surfaces, the forehead, cheeks, and ears. Their development may be so gradual that the changes may be noted by others before the patient himself is aware of them.

Early signs of mucosal involvement in the upper respiratory and intestinal tracts may be evidenced by nasal discharge and dysphagia. Hoarseness and dyspnea may be due to laryngitis.

The patient with the tuberculoid type is more likely to be aware of the disease early. The initial lesions usually take the form of hypopigmented or erythematous anesthetic macules. Subjective manifestations due to neural involvement consist of numbness, tingling, and formication, and the skin may show burns or other lesions which the patient states are painless.

The progressing cutaneous leprids of tuberculoid leprosy enlarge and clear centrally. The central area is anhidrotic and anesthetic to light touch, pain, and thermal stimuli. The nerves later are thickened and tender if the disease progresses. Before nerve destruction and atrophy occur, pain of a neuritic type may be prominent. Late stages are characterized by resorption of the small distal bones of the hands and feet and painless ulcers of the extremities.

This distal resorption of bone is not appreciably influenced by chemotherapy, and its crippling effects constitute a great problem in rehabilitation of arrested cases.

Although more marked in lepromatous leprosy, generalized lymph node enlargement is common in all types of leprosy.

The lepromin skin test is primarily of prognostic value. The test material is prepared from lepromatous nodules. Those with tuberculoid leprosy generally show positive reactions; and lepromatous cases, negative reactions. A satisfactory therapeutic response is shown by the transformation of a negative to a positive reaction in the lepromatous type. Those patients with the indeterminate type of lesion who have positive lepromin tests are likely to develop tuberculoid lesions if the disease progresses, and those who have negative lepromin reactions, lepromatous lesions.

Recent studies have defined better the relationship between tuberculosis and leprosy. The guinea pig, normally lepromin-negative, becomes lepromin-positive after BCG (bacillus Calmette-Guérin) administration. Patients who have remained lepromin-negative after sulfone treatment may become lepromin-positive following BCG administration. In some instances clinical improvement has accompanied this change. The place of BCG in the treatment of leprosy is yet to be defined, but its contribution to control has been accepted in many countries and particularly where tuberculosis is common. BCG vaccination in children results in most instances in positive early, or Fernandez, reactions, and late, or Mitsuda, reactions.

The histamine test may be of assistance when the skin lesions are atypical or the neurologic examination cannot be satisfactorily performed. The normal cutaneous response to a needle prick through a drop of 1:1,000 histamine consists of a wheal with surrounding erythema. When there is impairment of neural function in leprosy, only the wheal and no erythematous halo appears.

The pilocarpine test, showing impairment of the sweating response to intradermally injected pilocarpine, is helpful in identification of the leprid.

Laboratory Diagnosis. Although clinical findings may be sufficient for diagnosis, demonstration of the bacilli or the histologic lesion is desirable for confirmation or to observe response to therapy. In searching for bacilli in a suspected lepromatous case in which the skin lesions are not distinctive, the ear lobule should be examined. The lobule is held firmly enough to cause blanching. A small incision is made with a sharp scalpel and the material which can be scraped from the edges is spread on a slide. Stained by the Ziehl-Neelsen or fuchsin method, a positive lesion will show numerous acid-fast bacilli. In suspected tuberculoid leprosy, a biopsy is usually necessary.

The erythrocyte sedimentation rate is elevated in all types of leprosy but is most increased in the lepromatous type. Serologic tests for syphilis performed with the beef heart antigens may be positive in 10 to 40 per cent of cases of leprosy, whereas with cardiolipin antigens, only 1 to 2 per cent may be positive. TPI (*Treponema pallidum immobilization*) tests have been negative in most cases of leprosy unless syphilis also was suspected. The β-globulin, C-reactive protein, is present in most cases of active leprosy and absent in most cases of arrested leprosy (Rabson).

Differential Diagnosis. In nonendemic areas, leprosy is seldom diagnosed early. Once leprosy is suspected, clinical and laboratory procedures are usually successful in establishing the presence or absence of the disease. It must be differentiated from syphilis, superficial fungous infections, lupus vulgaris, lupus erythematosus, vitiligo, dermal leishmaniasis, yaws, seborrheic dermatitis, psoriasis, Boeck's sarcoid, rheumatoid arthritis, nonspecific neuritis, syringomyelia, and neurofibromatosis. Differentiation from syphilis may be difficult because of clinical similarity and the frequent appearance of positive serologic tests for syphilis in leprosy. Important procedures in differential diagnosis are (1) the examination of cutaneous and mucosal lesions for *Mycobacterium leprae*, (2) study of skin sensation and reaction to histamine and pilocarpine, and (3) examination of the peripheral nerves for thickening and tenderness.

Treatment. Several considerations must be heeded in evaluating the efficacy of therapy. (1) Leprosy is an intermittently progressive chronic disease during which temporary and even permanent spontaneous arrest can occur. (2) The patient seeks treatment during and toward the end of an exacerbation which may naturally be followed by a remission of variable duration. (3) The initial appearance of an exacerbation may be precipitated by a more or less self-limited disease—e.g., malaria or dysentery—or by an unfavorable nutritional and hygienic state, which, when corrected, may be followed by a remission. Clinical and laboratory observation over a period of years is, therefore, necessary for proper evaluation of therapy.

The general therapeutic regimen should resemble that for tuberculosis, since much can be accomplished by good diet and regulated rest and exercise. Chaulmoogra (hydnocarpus) oil was long used in Asia in the treatment of leprosy, but only during the latter part of the nineteenth century was it introduced into Western medicine. The Cairo Congress in 1938 regarded chaulmoogra oil and its esters as the most efficacious drugs for the treatment of leprosy. Although many cases appeared to be benefited, this opinion was not concurred in generally.

The history of effective chemotherapy began in 1908 with the discovery of sulfone, but the value of this drug in the treatment of bacterial infections was not demonstrated until 1937. The efficacy of the sulfone derivative, Promin, in the treatment of leprosy was first reported in 1943. It was found later that the parent sulfone, dapsone or DDS (4,4'-diaminodiphenylsulfone), also was effective, was well tolerated, and was the least expensive of this group of drugs. It is rapidly absorbed after oral administration and slowly excreted, cumulative effects therefore occurring when large doses are given. Initially 100 mg is given orally twice a week and the dose increased by the same amount each week until the dose of 400 mg twice a week is reached. This amount is continued, and the patient is observed for toxic effects such as hemolytic anemia, hepatitis, drug fever, dermatitis, and psychosis. Muir has reported that vitamin B_{12} increases the tolerance for DDS.

Promising results have been reported with Etisul (diethyl dithioisophthalate), administered by inunction.

The response to therapy is estimated by periodic bacteriologic examinations and objective clinical studies. Early cases and those with low bacteriologic indices can be expected to show improvement after about 1 year of treatment; others may require 3 to 4 years; and some, approximately 20 per cent of all clinical cases, will show no recognizable improvement.

The thiosemicarbazones are not so effective as DDS but are occasionally useful as alternative agents. The response to isoniazid has been poor in most cases. ACTH and cortisone have been found to produce desirable temporary effects but unfortunately have been followed by aggravation of neural and cutaneous lesions. Their use is justified in treatment of the drug fever induced by sulfones. In leprous ophthalmitis cortisone applied locally is advised (Lowe).

Hanks has reviewed the problem of immunity in leprosy and the approaches to stimulation and/or enhancement of the specific immune response. The present status of therapy would make it highly desirable to use adjuvants with antigens in the hope that the efficacy of chemotherapy might be increased.

Prognosis. This is dependent upon the type of leprosy, the stage in which treatment is begun, and the general health of the patient. The occurrence of temporary and occasionally permanent spontaneous disease arrest must be kept in mind.

The tuberculoid type has a relatively better expectancy, although disability is common, and the prognosis is relatively better in so far as disease arrest is concerned. The lepromatous type has the poorer outlook. With the hope which the sulfone derivatives hold, it should become easier to induce patients to seek treatment earlier. Generally, pneumonia and tuberculosis are common causes of death. In the United States, over one-third of the cases die with renal insufficiency due to amyloidosis. The average duration of life after diagnosis is 20 years, and the average age at death is fifty-nine years.

Control. Segregation and early treatment of patients, particularly those with the lepromatous type, are essential. A program of control should be directed toward encouraging voluntary admission to a leprosarium. The harm the patient may do to himself and his immediate contacts by delaying treatment, and the hopefulness with which treatment can now be regarded, should be emphasized. Mention has been made of the enlarging role which mass BCG vaccination has been given in control. Efforts to identify and define the carrier state should be intensified, and the efficacy of the sulfones in controlling the carrier determined. Cultivation of a more objective and less emotional public attitude toward the disease is fundamental to any control program.

REFERENCES

Binford, C. H.: Histiocytic Granulomatous Mycobacterial Lesions Produced in the Golden Hamster (*Cricetus auratus*) Inoculated with Human Leprosy, Lab. Invest., 8:901, 1959.

Doull, James A.: Leprosy, Veterans Administration Tech. Bull., TB10-98, Mar. 15, 1954.

Gay Prieto, J.: International Work in Leprosy, WHO Chronicle, 14:3, 1960.

——: Excitation of Specific Immune Response in Leprosy Patients, Intern. J. Leprosy, 26:9, 1958.

Hanks, J. H., and C. T. Gray: The Metabolic Properties of Mycobacteria and the Pathogenesis of Mycobacterial Disease, Advances in Tuberculosis Research, 7:1, 1956.

Hansen, G. A.: Spedalskhedens Arsager (Causes of Leprosy), Intern. J. Leprosy, 23:307, 1955. (English translation of report published in 1874.)

Lendrum, F. C.: The Name "Leprosy," Am. J. Trop. Med. Hyg., 1:999, 1952.

Lowe, J.: ACTH and Cortisone in the Treatment of Complications of Leprosy, Brit. Med. J., p. 746, Oct. 4, 1952.

Muir, E.: Treatment of Leprosy with DDS, Trans. Roy. Soc. Trop. Med. Hyg., 46:113, 1952.

Powell, C. S., and L. L. Swan: Leprosy: Pathologic Changes Observed in Fifty Consecutive Autopsies, Am. J. Pathol., 31:1131, 1955.

Shepard, C. C.: Acid-fast Bacilli in Nasal Excretions in Leprosy, and Results of Inoculation of Mice, Am. J. Hyg., 71:147, 1960.

148 OTHER MYCOBACTERIAL INFECTIONS

Ivan L. Bennett, Jr.

Acid-fast bacteria morphologically similar to tubercle bacilli are widely distributed in nature as saprophytes or as pathogens of lower animals. Many examples are known of parasitism of amphibians and fishes by mycobacteria that cannot multiply at mammalian body temperatures. Among animal diseases that have been studied extensively are *Johne's disease,* an enteritis in cattle caused by *Mycobacterium paratuberculosis* (*M. johnei*), a leprosy-like illness in water buffalo and oxen called *lepra bubalorum* or *lepra bovinum,* and murine leprosy. The long-standing view that all other acid-fast bacilli were of importance in clinical medicine only because they might be confused with *M. tuberculosis* or *M. leprae* in smears or cultures of human material has gradually given way to the realization that many are pathogenic for man, producing *chronic cutaneous ulceration* or *pulmonary disease.* Despite the unsatisfactory status of terminology and bacteriologic criteria for identifying mycobacteria, the clinical manifestations of the two groups of disorders are sufficiently well defined to permit their recognition and treatment.

Mycobacterium balnei ("Swimming-pool Bacillus"). This acid-fast organism inhabits fresh-water swimming pools, where it gains entry to the human body through cutaneous abrasions from rough concrete and causes a type of superficial ulceration known as "swimming-pool disease" or "sore elbow." The ulcers occur on elbows, ankles, toes, and hands; they are not extensive or destructive, tend to bleed easily, are moderately painful, and heal slowly, partly because of their tendency to localize in areas that are subject to repeated trauma. The organism was discovered during investigations of epidemics of what was initially thought to be tuberculosis of the skin in Scandinavia; sporadic cases as well as epidemics have occurred in many countries, including the United States. *Mycobacterium balnei* grows optimally at 31°C and multiplies poorly or not at all in cultures kept at 37°C. This temperature range probably accounts for the lack of systemic spread; indeed regional lymph nodes remain uninvolved unless secondary pyogenic infection occurs.

The diagnosis is made by culturing the organisms, usually from biopsy material. Histologically, the lesion is a nonspecific granuloma containing acid-fast bacilli. Most patients do not react to tuberculin although positive reactions to skin tests can be elicited using a tuberculin-like extract of *M. balnei.* The circumstances of infection and the absence of evidence of tuberculosis in a patient with cutaneous ulceration containing acid-fast bacilli usually suffice to establish the diagnosis.

Treatment with antituberculous drugs does not appear to speed healing, which finally occurs spontaneously (although the organisms are sensitive to streptomycin).

Prevention consists of disinfecting pools where cases have occurred and rigid exclusion of individuals with skin lesions.

Mycobacterium ulcerans. This acid-fast bacillus, which grows optimally at 30 to 33°C and poorly or not at all at 37°C, was first isolated from extensive ulcers of the extremities in the town of Bairnsdale, Australia, and the skin lesions are often called "Bairnsdale disease." *Mycobacterium ulcerans* produces spreading granulomatous ulceration which is far more extensive than that produced by *M. balnei* and often destroys the subcutaneous tissue down to fascia and muscle. The reservoir in nature and the source of infection are unknown. Sporadic cases have been reported in Europe, Great Britain, and the United States. Systemic dissemination does not occur, again, it is thought, because of the temperature requirements of the organism. Antituberculous drugs, with the possible exception of streptomycin, do not inhibit appreciably the progressive extension of necrosis; prompt surgical excision of all involved tissue, followed by grafting of the defect, has been uniformly curative.

Mycobacterial Ulcers in Africa. Acid-fast bacilli have been isolated from a distinctive cutaneous ulceration that appears to be widespread among eastern Congolese natives and has been observed also in Europeans living in central Africa. Two bacterial strains, tentatively designated *M. kakerifu* and *M. kasongo* (for geographic areas) have been studied and shown to differ from *M. ulcerans.* The lesions begin on the extremities, thorax, or face as acutely inflamed blebs or more indolent ulcers which extend progressively, burrowing through the subcutaneous tissues, destroying muscle, and occasionally producing osteitis with slow lysis of underlying bone. Lymphatic and systemic spread do not occur (the organisms will not grow at 37°C). While the process sometimes subsides spontaneously, its inexorable course often necessitates block excision to save an eye or prevent amputation of an extremity. The bacilli are more likely to be sensitive to isoniazid than to streptomycin, but drug therapy is only an adjuvant to surgery. Two peculiar features are the early occurrence of extensive, completely reversible calcification in diseased tissues and the finding of small, nonulcerating, subcutaneous granulomas at distant sites. These nodules are almost invariably marked by a patch of extensive hirsutism in the overlying skin.

PULMONARY DISEASE PRODUCED BY "ATYPICAL" OR "ANONYMOUS" MYCOBACTERIA

Definition. Many mycobacterial species that were long believed to be nonpathogenic or, at best, very rarely pathogenic for man are now known to be capable of causing chronic progressive pulmonary disease with fibrosis or cavitation closely resembling that of tuberculosis.

Etiology. The generally preferred term for the acid-fast bacilli which cause nontuberculous pulmonary disease is "anonymous" rather than "atypical" mycobacteria. Until methods for identification of species are greatly improved, this heterogeneous collection of microorganisms allows few general statements; the best classification at present is that devised by Runyon in cooperation with the Veteran's Administration and the National Tuberculosis Association.

Anonymous mycobacteria differ from tubercle bacilli by failure to elicit progressive disease in guinea pigs, by the development of pigment in cultures, by relative insusceptibility to isoniazid and para-aminosalicylic acid (less often to streptomycin), by failure to produce nicotinic acid in culture (determined by the simplified Konno test), and by certain less-regular morphologic variations.

The Runyon schema classifies these organisms into four groups. Group I, the *Photochromogens,* produce no pigment when cultured in the dark but assume a yellow-to-orange hue on short exposure to light. Two species, *M. luciflavum* and *M. kansasii,* are believed to predominate in this relatively homogeneous group. Group II, the *Scotochromogens,* produce pigment whether grown in light or dark. Group III, the *Nonphotochromogens,* produce little or no pigment. The "Battey" bacilli (so called after a tuberculosis hospital in Georgia) belong in this group. Group IV, the *Rapid Growers,* include organisms which grow out within 48 hr. *Mycobacterium fortuitum* is at least one of the species in this group, and it is believed that several strains of *Nocardia* (see p. 1063) have accidentally been included within it.

Group I and group III are responsible for the vast majority of human disease, although a few verified instances of infection by groups II and IV organisms are on record and studies throughout the world are so incomplete that no conclusions can be drawn about incidence.

Epidemiology. The mode of transmission and the question of animal reservoirs of infection are unsettled. Skin tests utilizing tuberculin and similar preparations from anonymous mycobacteria have shown that a large proportion of cross reactions occur but that patients usually react more strongly to the preparation derived from the organism responsible for their disease. Surveys of populations in limited areas have likewise revealed that tuberculin skin sensitivity is not always derived from contact with *M. tuberculosis,* that asymptomatic infection with anonymous bacilli is common between the ages of seven and fifteen years, and the ratio between subclinical infection and clinical disease is much higher for anonymous bacilli than for tubercle bacilli, indicating a lesser order of pathogenicity for man than exists in tuberculosis.

A striking predominance of infections in certain areas is produced by organisms of one group. In Texas, group I disease predominates; in Georgia, Alabama, and Florida, group III infections form the majority.

In all areas, most cases of symptomatic pulmonary disease are in white males thirty to sixty years of age and illness is unusual in Negroes. Two limited culture surveys are worthy of note. In Georgia, unclassified acid-fast bacilli were isolated from saliva or sputum in 14 per cent of the normal individuals studied. In Texas, group I bacilli have been grown from the pharynx of many normal children and have also been recovered from the exudate of draining cervical lymph nodes in tuberculin-positive children. The relationship of this type of infection in children to cat-scratch disease (p. 1178) is uncertain.

Pathology. Limited studies of pulmonary tissue from cases of group I (Photochromogen) infection have shown a general resemblance to tuberculosis, with several differences: (1) there is more tendency to acute inflammation admixed with caseation; (2) cavities tend to be irregular and thin-walled; (3) fibrosis elsewhere is more intense; (4) endobronchial disease, often acute, is very common but endobronchial spread of infection is unusual; (5) large amounts of free and phagocytosed fat are present; and (6) asteroid, or Schaumann, bodies occur in 30 to 40 per cent of the cases.

Manifestations and Diagnosis. The symptoms and signs are those of pulmonary tuberculosis (see p. 1004). There is a tendency for manifestations to be milder than those of tuberculosis in the presence of extensive x-ray changes, cavitation is more likely to occur and the cavities are thin-walled, and calcification of lesions is more frequent.

These findings in a middle-aged white male should arouse suspicion. The diagnosis is established by isolating anonymous mycobacteria from sputum.

Skin tests are not specific enough to allow differentiation from tuberculosis in the individual patient.

Treatment. Antituberculous drugs are usually less effective in anonymous bacterial infections than in tuberculosis. However, many patients heal slowly on isoniazid and streptomycin. Para-aminosalicylic acid is rarely useful. In general, a vigorous medical regimen and early surgery for cavitary disease have given the best results.

REFERENCES

Chapman, J. S., and R. L. Guy: Scrofula Caused by Atypical Mycobacteria, Pediatrics, 23:323, 1959.

Feldman, W. H., and A. G. Karlson: *Mycobacterium ulcerans* Infection: Response to Chemotherapy in Mice, Am. Rev. Tuberc. and Pulm. Dis., 72:266, 1957.

Jenkins, D. E., D. Bahar, and I. Chofnas: Pulmonary Disease Due to Atypical Mycobacteria: Current Concepts, Trans. 19th Veterans Administration–Armed Forces Conference on the Chemotherapy of Tuberculosis, p. 224, 1960.

Linell, F., and A. Norden: *Mycobacterium balnei*: A New Acid-fast Bacillus Occurring in Swimming Pools and Capable of Producing Skin Lesions in Humans, Acta Tuberc. Scandinav., Suppl. No. 33, 1954.

MacCallum, P., J. C. Tolhurst, G. Buckle, and H. A. Sissons: A New Mycobacterial Infection in Man, J. Pathol. and Bacteriol., 60:93, 1948.

Runyon, E. H.: "The Anonymous Mycobacteria in Human Disease," Springfield, Ill., Charles C Thomas, Publisher, 1960.

Section 9: Infections of Specific Tissues and Anatomic Sites

INTRODUCTION

Ivan L. Bennett, Jr.

It is traditional and convenient to classify bacterial diseases in terms of etiologic agents. This is adequate for those that follow more or less consistent patterns as do typhoid, anthrax, brucellosis, tularemia, or tetanus, but there are other important disorders that lend themselves poorly to categorization on the basis of causative organisms. Because many microbial agents are able to invade and to localize in almost any tissue, they are not regularly associated with a single symptom complex. Furthermore, infection of an anatomic site such as the urinary tract or the meninges by any one of a wide variety of unrelated bacterial species produces essentially the same symptoms and clinical signs. Recognition of the basic pathologic process by the clinician is, in most instances, independent of microbiological techniques. This statement is not intended to direct emphasis away from the important procedure of specific identification of infecting bacteria as a basis for choosing the appropriate antimicrobial drugs.

In this section, many clinical entities are described. Several are more likely to be caused by certain microorganisms than others, but all can be produced by many species. Most can be recognized in their typical forms by history, physical examination, and clinical tests of blood and urine. Final identification of the infecting agent may depend upon time-consuming bacteriologic tests, but a knowledge of the likely pathogens often enables the physician to initiate appropriate therapy before this information is available. Surgical drainage is an essential part of proper management for several of the disorders to be described; indeed, surgery may be an emergency procedure for many of them, necessitated not by the species of the infecting organisms but by the anatomic location of the infection.

For these reasons, it seems logical to describe these afflictions in terms of their manifestations in the patient. Cross references to other sections of the book for details of bacteriology have been given where specific causative agents are mentioned for the diseases.

149 LOCALIZED INFECTIONS AND ABSCESSES

Ivan L. Bennett, Jr.

Localized pyogenic infection can develop in any region or organ of the body. This may be initiated by *trauma* and secondary bacterial contamination, by some *alteration in local conditions* that renders a tissue susceptible to organisms already present as part of the "normal flora" to which it is ordinarily immune, by *contiguous spread* from a nearby lesion, or by *metastatic implantation* of microorganisms carried in blood or lymph.

Infection is more likely to occur in some anatomic sites than in others because of structural differences favoring localization or because of greater exposure to the risk of trauma (for example, the hand).

The symptoms and signs of infection in several areas are characteristic enough to allow their clinical recognition and also to enable one to predict the pathways likely to be traversed as adjacent or distant structures become involved. The definitive treatment of many circumscribed infections, particularly if abscess formation occurs, is primarily surgical. Several, however, are complications of diseases that are ordinarily cared for by the internist and the treatment of any of the serious types may call for careful integration of medical and surgical measures. It is important, therefore, that the physician be able to recognize the major types of localized suppurative disease and know something of the principles of their management.

Etiology. Under appropriate conditions of lowered tissue resistance, almost any of the common bacteria can initiate the infectious process. Cultures from open lesions such as those of the skin or from intraabdominal foci arising from perforations of the gastrointestinal tract frequently contain several bacterial species; as might be expected, the organisms found most frequently are the "normal flora" of these regions.

Infection in some areas is more likely to be caused by certain organisms (examples being staphylococci in the skin and coliform bacteria in the urinary tract) and special features of the tissue reaction produced by some bacterial species make it possible to recognize infection by them with considerable accuracy. The *staphylococci* produce rapid necrosis and early suppuration with large amounts of creamy yellow pus (see p. 894). Group A beta-hemolytic streptococcal infections (p. 901) tend to spread rapidly through tissues, causing intense inflammatory edema and striking erythema but relatively little necrosis and thin, serumlike exudates; anaerobic streptococci (p. 922) and members of the *Bacteroides* group (p. 936) produce necrosis and profuse, brownish, foul-smelling pus. *Pseudomonas* infections (p. 934) are often rather indolent, and their thick, bluish green exudate is familiar to most clinicians; the *pneumococcus* (p. 887) stimulates the production of viscid greenish pus containing large plaques of fibrin and denatured protein.

The causative agents of many other diseases are capable of producing localized infection in tissues that are not usually involved in the specific "clinical entities" ascribed to them. Examples include the typhoid bacillus, *Corynebacterium diphtheriae* (cutaneous ulcers), the *brucellas, Pasteurella tularensis,* and many others.

The identification of the infecting organism or organisms is an important procedure in the choice of local or systemic chemotherapy and should not be neglected. However, when one is dealing with infection in an area where exposure to the microflora of the body is constant (sputum, paranasal sinusitis, cutaneous ulcers), it is unlikely that cultures will ever become *sterile,* and the interpretation of the findings in serial cultures during therapy must be tempered by this realization.

Pathogenesis. Factors predisposing to the initiation and persistence of infection in a tissue include trauma, obstruction of normal drainage (sweat glands, biliary tract, bronchial tree, urinary tract), ischemia (infarction, gangrene), chemical irritants (gastric contents, bile, intramuscularly injected drugs), hematoma formation, accumulation of fluid (lymphatic obstruction, cardiac edema), foreign bodies (bullets, splinters, sutures), and others such as the occurrence of turbulence in the vascular system (see Bacterial Endocarditis, p. 1039).

Infection in soft tissue usually begins as a *cellulitis,* a diffuse acute inflammation with hyperemia, edema, and leukocytic infiltration but little or no necrosis and suppuration. With some organisms, this is followed by necrosis, liquefaction, accumulation of leukocytes and debris, suppuration, loculation and walling off of the pus, and formation of one or more *abscesses.* Abscess formation is particularly prone to follow infection in a preexisting circumscribed space or cavity, examples being the fallopian tubes, lung cysts, and pilonidal sinuses. Ureteral obstruction in the presence of pyelonephritis is sometimes followed by accumulation of large quantities of thick pus in the renal pelvis, a *pyonephrosis.*

The local spread of infection generally follows the path of least resistance along fascial planes; proper surgical treatment is based upon a knowledge of these routes, which will be described for specific infections later in this chapter. Lymphatic spread can lead to lymphangitis, lymphadenitis, or, if the regional nodes suppurate, to the formation of a *bubo.* Involvement of local venules or large veins can lead to infective thrombophlebitis with resulting bacteremia, septic embolization, and systemic dissemination of infection. Staphylococci, streptococci, and bacteroides are notorious for the frequency with which they produce vascular lesions of this type.

Depending upon the infecting organism and the anatomy of the affected region, a small abscess may subside completely, there may be gradual encapsulation of the accumulated pus and persistence of the focus in a chronic or quiescent state, or the lesion may "point" and rupture into adjacent tissues or to the outside surface of the body, as usually happens with furuncles and, occasionally, with pleural abscess (*empyema necessitatis*). Spontaneous drainage of the pus to the outside ordinarily leads to subsidence and healing of a superficially situated suppurative focus. However, if the abscess is deeply situated and well encapsulated, there is often persistence of a fistulous tract and the formation of a chronic, draining sinus. *The development of persistent sinuses over an area of suppuration produced by ordinary pyogenic bacteria should always suggest involvement of underlying bone or the presence of a foreign body.* Fistulas that open onto the skin are, of course, soon colonized by microorganisms from the external environment. Ordinary bacterial cultures of drainage fluid almost invariably show a mixed flora and should never be relied upon for the etiologic diagnosis of the underlying disease. This is particularly important when one considers those disorders that characteristically lead to persistent sinus formation: tuberculosis, mycotic infection (actinomycosis, blastomycosis), melioidosis, glanders, tularemia, and, rarely, amebic abscess of the liver or cecum.

Therapeutic Considerations. Recognition of the subsidence of inflammation and striking symptomatic improvement that follow spontaneous evacuation of a suppurative focus led long ago to the adoption of *surgical incision* for the treatment of abscesses. The exact reasons for the amelioration of local and constitutional manifestations that results from drainage of pus are still unknown, but, clinically, the benefits of adequate incision and drainage are unequivocal.

It has been learned by experience that incision of infected tissue before the stage of liquefaction and accumulation of pus is well established is often deleterious, failing to relieve discomfort and facilitating spread of infection. For this reason, it is sometimes necessary to wait until an abscess "ripens," that is, localizes and "comes to a head." It has long been known that the *application of heat* to an area of inflammation will relieve pain and often speed the subsidence of cellulitis without suppuration. If necrosis of tissue is already under way, hot applications appear to facilitate localization of the process and accumulation of pus, making incision and drainage feasible at an earlier time. Another procedure that aids in reduction of swelling and relief of pain is *elevation of the affected part*.

The availability of specific chemotherapeutic drugs has modified the need for heat, elevation, and incision surprisingly little. The early administration of sulfonamides or antibiotics has reduced the incidence of suppurative complications in many disorders, but once suppuration has appeared, antimicrobial drugs become remarkably incapable of eradicating the infecting organisms. It is known that pus contains substances which effectively inactivate the sulfonamides, and this fact alone accounts adequately for the failure of these drugs to influence localized suppurations.

Antibiotics, however, can be demonstrated in vitro to retain their antibacterial activity in the presence of pus and necrotic tissue, and the explanation of the deleterious effect of suppuration upon their therapeutic effectiveness is not simple. Several factors undoubtedly contribute to the final result. It is probable that failure of the drug to penetrate into an area of suppuration is rarely the reason for therapeutic failure. Although this possibility exists in such infections as osteomyelitis, it is usually overcome by increasing dosage. Because direct instillation of the antibiotic into an infected area is not, by itself, a curative procedure, other factors are probably more important than faulty diffusion of the agent into the focus. The experiments of Eagle and of Wood have shown clearly that an established inflammatory exudate is a relatively poor environment for bacterial multiplication. Because penicillin's bactericidal action is exerted only against rapidly multiplying organisms, it is now believed that failure of this antibiotic to eradicate bacteria in an abscess is related to their relatively inactive metabolic state. Because a bacteriostatic agent such as tetracycline or chloramphenicol is capable only of inhibiting multiplication of bacteria and usually exerts no direct lethal action, the final death of organisms in any infection treated with agents of this type is dependent upon other mechanisms. For most pyogenic bacteria, phagocytosis is one of the most important of these mechanisms (although there must be others that have not been as carefully studied), and it is now known that, in the absence of phagocytes or in circumstances which inhibit their activity, bacteriostatic drugs are relatively ineffective. In fluid-filled cavities, and particularly in the metabolically unfavorable milieu of an abscess, phagocytosis is greatly reduced, and, consequently, despite inhibition of multiplication, bacteria can remain dormant and survive for long periods of time. It is probably a combination of these two circumstances, decreased multiplication of bacteria and decreased phagocytosis, that makes infection on the heart valves, in the kidney, or in the meninges as well as soft tissue abscesses so resistant to antibiotic therapy. Administration of large doses of bactericidal drugs for long periods often becomes necessary to achieve cure.

From a practical viewpoint, antimicrobial drugs can be expected to prevent suppuration if given early enough or to prevent spread of an already existent abscess, but they cannot be substituted for surgical drainage. Indeed, their use in the face of a lesion requiring evacuation of pus is one of the most common serious errors in treating infections.

In thoracic empyema, suppurative pericarditis, or pyarthrosis, excellent therapeutic results are sometimes achieved by aspiration of pus through a needle and instillation of antibiotics into the infected area. The success of this procedure, however, is fully as dependent upon the adequacy of the drainage that it achieves as it is upon the local application of the antibiotic, and if there is loculation or the exudate becomes too viscid to allow removal, surgical incision becomes mandatory.

In the presence of infective thrombophlebitis, surgical interruption of the veins by ligation or, in certain instances, by total excision of an infected segment is often indicated to prevent seeding of other organs by infected emboli.

Manifestations. Secondary infection of wounds and cutaneous ulcers is usually recognizable by inspection. Infections of the skin and subcutaneous tissues almost invariably produce the classic manifestations, *redness, tenderness, heat,* and *swelling.* Reddish streaks extending proximally and associated with tender enlargement of regional lymph nodes indicate lymphangitis. Systemic symptoms can be absent or mild, or there can be fever, malaise, prostration, and leukocytosis.

Infection and suppuration in deeper tissues or in body cavities is often manifested by local pain and tenderness, but the task of locating and determining the exact nature of the lesion can be difficult. The palpation of a tender mass is helpful, but muscle spasm and intervening structures often interfere. Abdominal or pelvic examination under anesthesia is sometimes useful in these circumstances.

Auscultation may reveal a friction rub over an abdominal viscus, the pleura, or the pericardium. The rapid development of an effusion in the pericardium, pleura, abdomen, or a joint should suggest infection. Similarly, fluid detected by transillumination of paranasal sinuses or inspection of the tympanic membrane can be the first sign of infection.

Depending upon the location of an abscess, symptoms and signs referable to encroachment upon adjacent structures may dominate the picture. Respiratory obstruction may be the first sign of mediastinal abscess; dysphagia often first calls attention to peritonsillar or retropharyngeal abscesses; and acute tamponade is sometimes the initial clue to pericardial infection. Localizing signs of dysfunction are especially striking and important with suppurations of the brain and spinal cord (see p. 1044).

Local pain and tenderness or signs of dysfunction are relatively mild or equivocal in some patients, *constitutional manifestations of fever, prostration, and weight loss* dominating the picture. The fever can be low-grade but is often hectic with repeated rigors and drenching night sweats. Fatigue and anemia are frequent, and weight loss may be so rapid as to result in emaciation within a few weeks. A patient with these symptoms and signs may have chronic subphrenic, perinephric, or other abscess in the complete absence of any detectable physical sign pointing to the location of a huge accumulation of pus.

Fluctuation of a mass on palpation is a reliable sign that it contains fluid, perhaps pus, but failure to detect this sign when deeper structures are examined is no guarantee that suppuration is absent and should not be taken by itself to indicate that the mass is noninfectious in origin or that drainage is not required.

Laboratory Findings. Peripheral polymorphonuclear leukocytosis is frequent with abscesses, and unexplained elevation of the white count in any patient should lead to a search for localized suppuration. Depending upon the severity and duration of infection, there may be a chronic normocytic, normochromic anemia. Mild albuminuria is occasionally noted in febrile patients and has no diagnostic import.

Pus or fluid obtained by needle aspiration or incision of a suspected lesion should *always* be stained and examined directly in addition to being cultured aerobically and anaerobically. As has been mentioned, pus is a poor metabolic substrate, for many bacteria and organisms may fail to grow in cultures, particularly from an abscess of long standing. In such instances, the findings on microscopic examination may be the only guide in choosing proper chemotherapy for the disease.

Blood cultures are often positive in intravascular infections such as endocarditis (p. 1039), in pyelonephritis (p. 1035), and in pyogenic infections in which localized abscesses are metastatic, as in staphylococcal (p. 894), streptococcal (p. 901), and salmonella (p. 946) bacteremias. It should be remembered that manipulation, including surgical incision, of any localized infection can be followed by transient bacteremia.

CLINICAL FEATURES OF INFECTIONS IN VARIOUS REGIONS

The pathogenesis, diagnosis, and treatment of several important infections in specific anatomic sites and organs are discussed in detail in other parts of this book. These include lung abscess (p. 1554), mediastinitis (p. 1567), bacterial endocarditis (p. 1039), pericarditis (p. 1467), infections of the brain and spinal cord (p. 1044), osteomyelitis (p. 896), pyelonephritis (p. 1035), appendicitis and appendiceal abscess (p. 1636), pylephlebitis and hepatic abscess (p. 1698), pancreatic abscess (p. 1663), and diverticulitis (p. 1645).

The remainder of this chapter is devoted to some features of dermal infection, chronic ulcerations, and a consideration of a number of other important regional infections including those of the neck, spleen, subphrenic space, kidney, perirenal space, retroperitoneal space, and rectum.

Skin and Subcutaneous Tissues

Impetigo is a superficial infection caused by hemolytic staphylococci and Group A hemolytic streptococci. It is primarily a disease of children, common in warm weather, characterized by multiple erythematous lesions which vesiculate and are intensely pruritic. Local spread occurs through scratching and release of infected vesicle fluid. Serious complications are metastatic abscesses and hemorrhagic nephritis (p. 918). Treatment consists of local and general cleansing of the skin, application of bacitracin-neomycin ointment, covering with a loose dressing to prevent further contamination, and appropriate systemic antibiotics.

Deeper infections of the skin are almost invariably staphylococcal in origin and are described in the chapter beginning on p. 894. Erysipelas, a characteristic dermal lesion produced by Group A streptococcus, is described on p. 909, and erysipeloid is described on p. 980.

Lymphadenitis with or without suppuration can complicate any pyogenic skin lesion and is often striking with superficial streptococcal infections. Specific diseases characterized by suppurative regional lymphadenitis include lymphogranuloma venereum (p. 1177), cat-scratch disease (p. 1178), tularemia (p. 963), and bubonic plague (p. 966).

Infections of the Hand

These are almost invariably secondary to trauma and are very common. Because of the rapidity with which infection can spread through the complex fascial spaces of the hand, wrist, and forearm with the production of irreparable functional damage, *any deep infection in this area should receive expert surgical attention immediately*. The importance of this has in no way been lessened by the availability of antibiotics.

The ordinary *paronychia,* or "run-around," is a superficial infection of the epithelium lateral to a nail, usually a result of tearing a "hangnail" and most frequently caused by the staphylococcus. Hot applications will lead to subsidence of paronychial cellulitis, but often a superficial blister of pus appears or the infection burrows beneath the nail to form a painful *subungual abscess*. Incision and

drainage with partial or complete removal of the nail are then necessary. Recurrence is common, especially in nail biters, and this seemingly trivial infection can cause painful disability. Chronic paronychial inflammation produced by various fungi occurs in diabetics, and a similar lesion is seen in psoriasis and some types of pemphigus.

What appears to be a small furuncle of the webs of the fingers sometimes produces a *collar-button abscess,* consisting of a superficial and a deep compartment connected by a narrow tract; evacuation of the shallow pocket without emptying the deeper abscess can lead to puzzling persistence of infection.

Infection of the distal phalanx of a finger, usually acquired by pinprick, thorn prick, etc., can lead to the formation of a *felon* or *whitlow*. This is a suppurative infection in the tightly enclosed fibrous compartments of the finger pulp (the "anterior closed space") which can soon compromise the distal blood supply by compression of the digital arteries with consequent necrosis of bone and the development of osteomyelitis. The manifestations are swelling, extreme pain, and tenderness of the palmar surface of the finger tip. The treatment is immediate incision, using a lateral approach and cutting all the fibrous septa that radiate from the periosteum to the subcutaneous fascia.

Suppurative tenosynovitis, usually a complication of a puncture wound, is an even more serious infection of the hand from the point of view of functional damage; early diagnosis and treatment are mandatory to prevent permanent disability from destruction of the tendon or its sheath. The three cardinal manifestations of tenosynovitis listed by Kanavel, the father of modern surgery of the hand, are (1) exquisite tenderness limited to the course of the sheath; (2) the fingers held in flexion; (3) extension of the involved finger producing excruciating pain, most marked at the base of the digit. *Immediate incision* of the sheath is indicated not only to prevent damage to the tendon itself but to avoid proximal extension of the process into the major fascial spaces of the hand or forearm. Vigorous antibiotic treatment should accompany the surgery.

The definitive treatment of any serious infection of the hand is a matter for a skilled surgeon, but the early recognition of the need for surgery often falls to the physician. One last infection of the hand that is very important is that complicating *human bites*. Neglected injuries of this type almost invariably produce a highly destructive, necrotizing lesion, the result of infection by a mixture of aerobic and anaerobic organisms. A deliberately inflicted bite on the hand or elsewhere is usually recognized as dangerously contaminated, but wounds on the knuckles produced by striking an opponent's teeth with the fists may not be recognized as potentially dangerous. In general, bite wounds should be cleaned thoroughly and *not* sutured; patients should be given prophylaxis for tetanus and antibiotics, preferably penicillin and streptomycin, and observed carefully.

Chronic Cutaneous Ulcers

A partial list of the causes of chronic ulcers of the skin includes circulatory disturbances such as varicose veins and obliterative arterial disease, extensive injury from frost bite or burns, trophic changes accompanying many neurologic disorders, bedsores, or decubiti, systemic diseases such as sicklemia and myxedema, neoplasms, and several infections of mycotic and spirochetal origin. No matter what the underlying disease responsible for the lesion, secondary infection is very likely to occur and to interfere with healing, complicate grafting or other restorative procedures, or produce extension of the process.

The management of secondary bacterial infection in skin ulcers associated with obliterative arterial disease, a common problem in diabetics, is especially important, because infection is frequently the factor that precipitates spreading gangrene and makes amputation necessary.

Studies of the microflora of chronic cutaneous ulcers have almost invariably shown bacteria of many species including staphylococci, aerobic and anaerobic streptococci, coliform bacilli, and members of the proteus and pseudomonas groups. Depending upon the patient's environment and upon systemically or locally administered antimicrobial drugs, the predominating bacterial species show great variation when lesions are cultured serially. Particularly noteworthy is the replacement of sensitive organisms by resistant strains or species in the course of chemotherapy.

Treatment of chronic dermal ulcers should be directed toward the underlying disorder but should also include *local debridement* and *chemotherapy*. Debridement by surgical excision is often needed, but the local application of proteolytic enzymes such as Varidase, a mixture of streptokinase and streptodornase, or trypsin, so-called "chemical or medical debridement," is sometimes sufficient. Intensive systemic administration of antibiotics should be carried out only in conjunction with definitive surgical procedures or when infection can be controlled in no other way, but the prevention of infection by "prophylactic" administration of antimicrobial drugs is a hopeless task. The result will be the development of a flora resistant to the drugs being used. The *local application of antibiotics* is sometimes highly effective, and it is in the management of chronic mixed infections of this type that several potent but toxic antibiotics

have great value. The topical use of an ointment or solution containing neomycin, bacitracin, and polymyxin results in a bactericidal effect against a wide variety of organisms and will sometimes temporarily sterilize a chronic lesion. Other useful topical medications are Furacin and 3 per cent acetic acid, the latter being especially helpful in pseudomonas infections.

Diphtheritic ulcer of the skin is discussed on p. 984.

Infections of the Head and Neck

Mention may first be made of the peculiar danger of pustules of the nose and upper lip because of the likelihood of extension of infection intracranially through the angular vein to the cavernous sinus (see p. 1046). Such lesions should be treated conservatively, manipulation or incision being avoided if possible, and systemic antibiotics being given if local swelling or redness appears.

Suppurative parotitis is usually a complication of chronic debilitating disease or blockage of Stensen's duct by a calculus and is largely avoidable by maintenance of hydration and oral hygiene. Its onset is heralded by local pain and swelling; fever and chills are frequent. Frank pus can sometimes be expressed from the duct, and the gland itself is firm and tender, often with pitting edema of the overlying skin. In severe cases there may be facial palsy on the involved side. Removal of any obstruction in the duct, application of heat, and administration of antibiotics sometimes leads to prompt subsidence of local and systemic signs. However, incision is still required in many cases, and *failure of a patient to respond promptly to these more conservative measures is an indication for surgical drainage.* Abscess formation may be far advanced without there being detectable fluctuation because of the dense fibrous capsule of the gland. Before chemotherapy was available, the mortality rate in pyogenic parotitis was 30 to 50 per cent.

The use of penicillin and other antibiotics has reduced the incidence of many formerly common suppurative complications of streptococcal pharyngitis (see p. 908). However, as a result of streptococcal sore throat, bacteroides infections of the pharynx (see p. 937), or introduction of infection by trauma to the floor of the mouth or the pharyngeal wall, abscesses of the deep cervical structures still occur. *Suppurative cervical adenitis,* once an all-too-common sequel to streptococcal pharyngitis in children, is now rare. *Peritonsillar abscess,* or *quinsy,* is manifested by fever, sore throat, unilateral pain radiating to the ear on swallowing, and enlargement of the tonsil with redness and swelling of the adjacent soft palate. Treatment with penicillin and irrigations of warm saline sometimes leads to subsidence of the process, but if digital palpation reveals fluctuation, surgical drainage with or without tonsillectomy is indicated.

The course of *deep cervical infections* is fully as dependent upon the anatomic arrangement of fascial planes as is that of infections of the hand. There are five important potential compartments in the anterior neck; these are described in detail in the article by Barnhill listed at the end of the chapter. Infection in any of these areas is serious and attended by fever, prostration, and leukocytosis. A tender mass may be palpated, but it is to be emphasized that *surgical evacuation of such an infection should not be delayed because of failure to detect fluctuation,* which is usually absent because of the dense fascial layers.

Infection of the *sublingual space,* so-called "Ludwig's angina," is characterized by brawny induration of the submaxillary region, edema of the floor of the mouth, and elevation of the tongue. There is severe pain, dysphagia, and, within hours, dyspnea from respiratory obstruction. The usual causative organism is the streptococcus. Mortality was formerly about 50 per cent. *Treatment* consists of large doses of penicillin and careful observation. If there is significant progression of obstruction during the 4 to 6 hr after treatment is instituted, wide incision is indicated for relief of pressure; rarely is there extensive suppuration.

The retropharyngeal space lies between the muscles anterior to the cervical vertebrae and the pharyngeal mucosa. *Retropharyngeal abscess,* formerly common in children, is manifested by dysphagia, progressive stridor, pain, and fever. The bulging mass is easily seen and can completely occlude the airway within hours. Incision and drainage are mandatory; spontaneous rupture can lead to death by aspiration. Tuberculous abscess, secondary to spinal disease, occasionally presents in the retropharyngeal space; it is painless, and relief of obstruction follows surgical incision. The pharyngomaxillary and submastoid spaces lie high and lateral in the neck, the latter slightly posteriorly. Suppuration in the submastoid space, a *Bezold abscess,* is usually secondary to otitis and produces nuchal rigidity, which may lead to a mistaken diagnosis of otogenous meningitis. Infection can extend down the carotid sheath to the mediastinum. A suppurative thrombophlebitis of the jugular vein usually accompanies this type of spread, and the vessel is easily felt as a tender cord. Bacteremia and systemic spread of infection makes this a dangerous complication; there are many who advocate excision of the involved venous segment. Spontaneous rupture of the carotid artery and rapid death from exsanguination is a rare complication of infections of this type.

Splenic Abscess

The majority of splenic abscesses are produced by hematogenous dissemination of infection from a focus in the skin, endocardium, or elsewhere. Trauma to the spleen with formation of a subcapsular hematoma or bland infarction of the organ can lead to infection in the course of transient bacteremia. Occasionally, extension of a nearby infection (usually left subphrenic abscess), or perforation of the colon or stomach into the spleen is the source. Onset is sudden, with chills, fever, and left upper quadrant pain. There is tenderness and muscle spasm, and the skin and subcutaneous tissues overlying the spleen may be edematous. Involvement of the upper pole commonly leads to left pleuritic pain, radiating to the shoulder, with elevation of the diaphragm or left pleural effusion. Lower pole abscess gives signs of peritoneal inflammation. The spleen is usually palpable and tender; a friction rub is often audible. Disorders to be considered in differential diagnosis are subphrenic abscess, infection of the left lung, bland infarction of the spleen, pancreatic pseudocyst, and abscess secondary to perforation of the transverse colon. *Treatment* consists of antibiotics, and splenotomy or, if the organ is easily mobilized, splenectomy. If the abscess is a complication of generalized pyogenic infection, immediate surgery may be contraindicated. Splenic infarction in subacute bacterial endocarditis caused by *Streptococcus viridans* almost never suppurates, but in endocarditis, infected splenic infarcts are a rare cause of continued bacteremia in the face of massive chemotherapy, and splenectomy may then be the treatment necessary to achieve the final eradication of the organism.

Subphrenic Abscess

Peritoneal infections show a striking tendency to localize in the upper part of the abdomen between the transverse colon and the diaphragm. In a few instances, suppuration in this area seems to be hematogenous in origin, but the vast majority of subphrenic abscesses are the result of extension from perforations of the gastrointestinal tract or from biliary tract infections. The most frequent sources of infection are appendicitis, perforations of the stomach and duodenum, and ascending cholangitis. *Any patient with persistent fever and a history of recent intraabdominal sepsis should be suspected of having a subphrenic abscess.* In considerably more than half of the cases, the patient has undergone recent laparotomy. The avenues by which infection reaches the subphrenic region are the same as those described for hepatic abscess (p. 1698) and appendiceal abscess (p. 1636). Subphrenic abscess is at least five times more frequent on the right side.

The *manifestations* include fever, upper quadrant pain, and tenderness. The localizing signs are by no means striking in all cases, however. It is becoming evident that the widespread practice of "covering" postoperative patients with antibiotics prophylactically can attenuate subphrenic infection without eradicating it and that the result may be an insidiously progressive illness with weight loss and low-grade fever beginning weeks or months after a laparotomy. Faxon has emphasized the following findings in the diagnosis of subphrenic infection: point tenderness over the lower ribs; tenderness of the area when the lower rib cage is compressed or percussed; elevation and fixation of the diaphragm, confirmed by x-ray; other signs of diaphragmatic pleurisy such as pain referred to the shoulder, hiccups, or pleural effusion. X-rays will show an air-fluid level beneath the diaphragm eventually in about one-fourth of the cases, but this finding is less frequent in early abscess. The gas is usually from a perforated viscus or enters through an external sinus and is only rarely the result of bacterial multiplication.

In the presence of frank suppuration, the treatment is surgical drainage. Actually, there are several subphrenic "spaces," anterior and posterior, and the exact incision employed is dependent upon the compartment involved. Often, subphrenic infection becomes evident before suppuration ensues, and such cases of *subphrenic cellulitis* often subside without drainage, antibiotics alone being sufficient to control the process. It is important to avoid incision of an area of subdiaphragmatic cellulitis, and many surgeons prefer to explore the area by needle aspiration before operation.

Retroperitoneal Infections

Strictly speaking, all perinephric and many subphrenic abscesses are located outside the peritoneum, but the term *retroperitoneal abscess* usually refers to infection in the lumbar and iliac regions. Suppuration in these areas is relatively rare, but the importance of recognizing its existence in patients with fever and low back pain in terms of instituting surgical drainage is great. In the review of retroperitoneal infections published by Neuhof and Arnheim, listed in the references at the end of this chapter, the average duration of illness in 65 patients before diagnosis was approximately 1 month.

Infection in the retroperitoneal spaces appears to arise rather frequently as a complication of bacteremia, particularly in staphylococcal disease. Other sources are extension from posterior perforations of the appendix or colon, renal or spinal infections, and suppurative lymphadenitis in the iliac area, usually secondary to streptococcal infections of the lower extremity in children.

In *lumbar abscess,* there is tenderness and spasm of the back muscles on the affected side, and a mass is usually palpable in the lumbar region or in the abdomen. There may be a prominent, tender abdominal mass without lumbar pain or spasm. Flexion of the hip (psoas sign) occurs in a few cases but is more often present with infections lower in the retroperitoneal area. *Fever, leukocytosis,* and *lumbar spasm* should suggest the diagnosis. The absence of a palpable mass can lead to protracted observation, and it is in these instances that palpation under anesthesia is often helpful.

In *iliac abscess,* there is abdominal pain in the iliac or inguinal region and, particularly when the psoas muscle is involved, there may be severe pain referred to the hip, thigh, or knee. Careful palpation of the lower abdomen usually reveals a mass, and fullness and tenderness on rectal examination are common. Hip spasm (psoas sign) is often present.

X-ray may delineate the inflammatory mass; pyelography shows displacement of the kidney in some cases of lumbar infection; scoliosis with concavity on the side of the infection and blurring of the psoas shadow are also useful findings.

Treatment consists of surgical drainage and appropriate antibiotic therapy.

Renal Abscess

Single or multiple abscesses of the renal cortex are almost invariably the result of metastatic implantation of staphylococci from another focus. It is believed by many that the infection is initiated in glomeruli. There is no relationship to previous renal disease; the infection occurs in younger individuals, is usually unilateral, and occurs on the right side oftener than the left. Many patients give a history of recent superficial infection such as furuncle. The onset is abrupt, with chill and fever, followed by costovertebral pain and tenderness of moderate severity. The urine contains *no white cells,* usually a few red cells, and a trace of albumin. Stained urinary sediment will show myriads of gram-positive cocci, and this finding is diagnostic. Transient gross hematuria can occur at the onset. The white blood count is usually elevated and may exceed 30,000 cells per cu mm. Physical signs are usually localized to the region of the kidney, but abdominal spasm can lead to confusion with appendicitis or cholecystitis. Early in the disease, ureteral calculus or acute hydronephrosis may be considered as possible diagnoses. Sudden onset of *fever, leukocytosis,* and *renal pain in the absence of pyuria* suggest the diagnosis, especially in a patient with infection elsewhere. *Treatment* consists of appropriate antibiotics, adequate fluids, and relief of pain. An abscess may suddenly discharge into the renal pelvis with relief of pain and the passage of cloudy urine containing enormous numbers of leukocytes and bacteria. *Complications* include formation of a thick-walled chronic renal "carbuncle," requiring surgical removal, rupture into the perirenal space, and secondary pyelonephritis, usually produced by coliform bacilli. Recovery is ordinarily prompt and chronic sequelae are rare.

Perinephric abscess is virtually always secondary to infection elsewhere in the body, usually superficial staphylococcal or streptococcal infection. The perirenal tissue may be seeded directly in the course of bacteremia, by rupture of a renal cortical abscess into the perinephric space, or by chronic pyelonephritis, particularly when renal calculus or pyonephrosis is present. Flank pain with radiation to the upper abdomen or even the shoulder, nausea, vomiting, fever, leukocytosis, tenderness with spasm of flank and upper abdominal muscles, and a palpable mass which moves with respiration are the main manifestations. Except where there is pre-existing pyelonephritis, perinephric abscess is *not* accompanied by urinary symptoms. In a few patients, elevation of the diaphragm on the diseased side occurs and leads to confusion with subphrenic infection. The psoas muscle is involved by the inflammatory process, and patients are frequently more comfortable with the thigh held in flexion. X-ray occasionally will reveal a mass; there is usually blurring of the kidney silhouette; and the psoas shadow is indistinct on the involved side. *Treatment* by surgical drainage and systemic administration of antibiotics (*not* urinary antiseptics) is usually followed by dramatic subsidence of pain and fever, and unless intrinsic renal disease is present, recovery is complete.

Rectal Abscess

Suppurations of the anorectal region have been classified anatomically in several ways, most of the classifications being based upon the surgical approaches required for drainage. Infection in the apocrine glands (hidradenitis) or folliculitis in the perianal region, extension of cryptitis or obstructions in the "anal glands" which open into the crypts of Morgagni, and contamination of submucosal hematomas, sclerosed hemorrhoids, or anal fissures can lead to abscess formation. These are usually painful, easily palpable, often visible on inspection, and yield readily to hot applications and drainage.

Difficulties in diagnosis are more likely to arise with infections higher in the rectum, especially those above the pelvic diaphragm, the types that Gaston and Warren have called *supralevator abscess*. Patients with this type of infection often have fever, malaise, and leukocytosis for several days or even weeks before any symptoms referable to the rectum develop. There is vague pelvic discomfort, relieved by defecation, and constipation punctuated by short episodes of diarrhea is common. In males, the inflammation often involves the base of the bladder, and urinary urgency and, finally, retention is not infrequent. This, of course, centers attention upon the urinary tract as a source of fever and malaise. Eventually, the abscess becomes known by severe pain, chills, and fever; palpation and instrumentation will reveal the swelling in the rectal ampulla. Such an abscess can surround the rectum and produce narrowing that is differentiated from that caused by neoplasm by the fact that the mucosa remains intact. A useful sign of deep rectal abscess is the eliciting of severe pain by pressure in the region between the anus and the coccyx. The supralevator space is continuous with the ischiorectal space, with both the gluteal and obturator regions, and with the retroperitoneal space. In neglected cases, the abscess may drain through the skin of the perineum, the groin, or the buttock or may extend as high as the perirenal areas. Rectal abscesses are not uncommon in patients with diabetes, and infections in this area are also peculiarly frequent in patients with monocytic leukemia. Because the clinical picture may be that of "fever of unknown origin" for a long period, it is important that thorough digital and endoscopic examination of the rectum be carried out in febrile patients. A rectal examination should be made in all patients with diabetes, especially if ketosis is present; failure to observe this rule has more than once led to delay in detecting the infection responsible for diabetic ketosis or coma.

Treatment consists of incision and drainage, hot sitz baths, analgesics, and penicillin and streptomycin or other antibiotics as indicated by culture of the exudate.

REFERENCES

GENERAL

Bunnell, S.: "Surgery of the Hand," 3d ed., Philadelphia, J. B. Lippincott Company, 1956.

Eagle, H.: Experimental Approach to the Problem of Treatment Failure with Penicillin: I. Group A Streptococcal Infection in Mice, Am. J. Med., 13: 389, 1952.

Moseley, H. F. (Ed.): "Textbook of Surgery," St. Louis, The C. V. Mosby Company, 1952.

Richards, J. H.: Bacteremia Following Irritation of Foci of Infection, J.A.M.A., 99:1496, 1932.

Smith, M. R., and W. B. Wood, Jr.: An Experimental Analysis of the Curative Action of Penicillin in Acute Bacterial Infections: III. The Effect of Suppuration upon the Antibacterial Action of the Drug, J. Exptl. Med., 103:509, 1956.

Wood, W. B., Jr.: Studies on the Cellular Immunology of Acute Bacterial Infections, Harvey Lectures, 47:72, 1951.

SPECIFIC INFECTIONS

Barnhill, J. F.: Deep Abscess of the Neck: Surgical Treatment, Am. J. Surg., 42:207, 1938.

Beck, A. L.: A Study of Twenty-four Cases of Neck Infection, Trans. Am. Acad. Ophthalmol. Otolaryngol., 37:342, 1932.

Blades, B.: Subphrenic Abscess, editorial, Surg. Gynecol. Obstet., 103:765, 1956.

Eisenhammer, S.: The Internal Anal Sphincter and the Anorectal Abscess, Surg. Gynecol. Obstet., 103:501, 1956.

Faxon, H. H.: Subphrenic Abscess: A Report of 111 Consecutive Operative Cases, New Engl. J. Med., 222:289, 1940.

Gaston, E. A., and L. O. Warren: Supralevator Abscess, New Engl. J. Med., 229:613, 1943.

Lingeman, C. J., et al.: Subacute Bacterial Endocarditis: Splenectomy in Cases Refractory to Antibiotic Therapy, A.M.A. Arch. Internal Med., 97:309, 1956.

Nesbit, R. M.: Acute Staphylococcal Infections of the Kidney: Their Clinical Aspects and Treatment, J.A.M.A., 98:708, 1932.

Neuhof, H., and E. E. Arnheim: Acute Retroperitoneal Abscess and Phlegmon: A Study of Sixty-five Cases, Ann. Surg., 119:741, 1944.

—— and E. E. Jemerin: "Acute Infections of the Mediastinum," Baltimore, The Williams & Wilkins Company, 1943.

Pearse, H. E., Jr.: Mediastinitis Following Cervical Suppurations, Ann. Surg., 108:588, 1938.

Richards, L.: Retropharyngeal Abscess, New Engl. J. Med., 215:1120, 1936.

Simeone, F. A.: Perinephric Abscess, Arch. Surg., 45:424, 1942.

Taffel, M., and S. C. Harvey: Ludwig's Angina: Analysis of 45 Cases, Surgery, 11:841, 1942.

Vicher, E. E., J. W. Soska, and G. G. Jackson: Microbiologic Flora of Chronic Cutaneous Ulcers: *In Vitro* Sensitivity of Microbiologic Flora to Three Antibiotics—Penicillin, Streptomycin, and Bacitracin, A.M.A. Arch. Surg., 66:283, 1953.

Waldapfel, R.: Post-tonsillitis Pyaemia, Trans. Am. Acad. Ophthalmol. Otolaryngol., 33:291, 1928.

Wolfson, I. N.: Abscess of the Spleen, New Engl. J. Med., 230:135, 1944.

150 PYELONEPHRITIS AND OTHER INFECTIONS OF THE URINARY TRACT

Paul B. Beeson and
Lawrence R. Freedman

Bacterial infections of the urinary tract constitute one of the major medical problems, encompassing all fields of practice. They may present themselves as primary acute infectious diseases, as complications of other disorders, or as chronic symptomless processes chiefly dangerous because of the threat of destruction of the kidney. They are notoriously resistant to treatment and prone to relapse and recurrence.

Etiology. Many different microorganisms can infect the tissues and fluids of the urinary organs, but by far the commonest are the coli-aerogenes group of gram-negative bacilli. Other microorganisms which may be found include enterococcus, proteus, pseudomonas, chromobacteria, staphylococcus, and certain yeasts. Infection by other than the coli-aerogenes organisms is generally related to previous instrumentation of the urinary tract, with or without the use of chemotherapeutic agents. Proteus and pseudomonas urinary infections, for example, are virtually never seen except in patients who have had catheters or other instruments passed through the urethra. The relative importance of staphylococcal infections has probably been exaggerated in the past, because of the prevalent custom of culturing urine only in a liquid medium, a procedure which negates any possibility of estimating the numbers of bacteria present in a given quantity of urine. Since staphylococci are commonly present in the urethra, they may therefore be recovered in such cultures. The employment of quantitative bacteriologic techniques reveals that staphylococci play a minor role in the total problem of urinary tract infection.

Pathogenesis. *Sources of Infection.* The entire urinary tract should be looked upon as an anatomic unit in which infection of one part can easily spread to another. While it is probable that the source of infecting bacteria is the intestinal tract, there is considerable disagreement regarding the routes by which microorganisms usually get from there to the urinary tract. One view holds it to be by way of the circulating blood; another favors the concept that bacteria gain entry by way of the urethra and pass upward to the kidneys through the bladder and ureters. The latter seems especially plausible as an explanation of the far greater frequency of spontaneously occurring infections in females, since the short urethra and its nearness to the anus should provide more opportunity for fecal bacteria to reach the bladder cavity. A third hypothesis, that lymphatic connections between the bowel and the urinary tract or between the lower and upper urinary tracts are important avenues for spread of infection, has little to support it. On the basis of clinical correlations there is much evidence favoring the view that the ascending route, i.e., lower to upper urinary tract via the urinary passages, is the most important one. The possibility remains, however, that bacteria occasionally are carried to the kidney by way of the blood stream, thus inciting an infection which later spreads downward along the course of urinary flow.

Associated Conditions. AGE AND SEX. Precise estimates cannot be given, but it can be said with assurance that urinary tract infections are far more frequent in females than in males except in older age groups, where prostatic obstruction accounts for a high incidence in men. There is also a high incidence in children between the age of six months and two years, especially girls; this is thought to be related to fecal soiling of the urethral meatus during the diaper period.

PREGNANCY. Acute pyelonephritis occurs in about 2 per cent of pregnant women, usually after the fourth month, at a time when some dilatation of the ureters and kidney pelves occurs physiologically. Urinary tract infection can be demonstrated in about 20 per cent of patients with toxemia of pregnancy.

DIABETES MELLITUS. Urinary tract infection is three or four times as common in diabetics as in other persons of comparable age. Factors which may contribute to this include the supposed increased susceptibility to infection in diabetics, liability to catheterization, and poor bladder emptying due to autonomic neuropathy. About half of all reported cases of the fulminating form of pyelonephritis called *necrotizing papillitis* have been in patients with diabetes.

OBSTRUCTIVE UROPATHY. Any impediment to the free flow of urine—tumor, stricture, or stone—results in hydronephrosis and a greatly increased frequency of urinary tract infection. Autopsy statistics indicate that pyelonephritis occurs about a dozen times more often when there is hydronephrosis than when the kidneys show no sign of increased hydrostatic pressure.

INSTRUMENTATION. Infection of the lower urinary passages is sometimes initiated by bacteria carried on catheters or other instruments being passed through the urethra into the bladder.

METABOLIC DISORDERS. There appears to be an unusually high incidence of pyelonephritis in patients with nephrocalcinosis and in those with chronic hypopotassemia. The relation of the latter is obscure; in nephrocalcinosis the important factor may be production of tubular obstruction by the deposits.

NEUROGENIC BLADDER DYSFUNCTION. Interference with the nerve supply to the bladder, as in spinal cord injury, tabes dorsalis, multiple sclerosis, etc., is likely to be associated with urinary tract infection. The infection may be initiated by the use of catheters for bladder drainage and favored by the prolonged standing of urine in the bladder. Additional factors which often operate in these patients are bone demineralization due to immobilization, causing hypercalcuria, calculus formation, and obstructive uropathy.

EXPERIMENTAL EVIDENCE. Urinary tract infections can be produced in experimental animals by several methods, including inoculation of bacteria into the pelvis or substance of the kidney, or into the bladder urine. Certain organisms such as staphylococci and monilias are capable of causing infection in the normal kidney when they are injected by the intravenous route. Coliform organisms will not do this unless the kidney has previously been injured, as by mechanical bruising or acute obstruction of the ureter. It has also been shown that the renal scarring resulting from a staphylococcal infection can render the kidney susceptible to infection by colon bacilli injected intravenously.

The frequent association of urinary tract infection with an obstructive lesion has led to the widespread view that stasis of urinary flow is a prime factor in the development of infection. In support of this is the fact that urine is a good medium for growth of bacteria; hence, prolonged opportunity for multiplication during slow passage along the tract would provide a heavier inoculum to which the kidneys and other tissues of the tract are exposed. This concept is the basis for the custom of "forcing fluids" in treating urinary infections. There may be an additional factor to explain the association between obstruction and urinary infection: the effect of increased hydrostatic pressure. One can cite several examples where clinical experience demonstrates that blockage to an excretory duct seems to render an organ more susceptible to the development of pyogenic infection. For instance, bacterial cholangitis is seldom encountered except when there is obstruction to the biliary passages. It seems unlikely that the mere flushing out of bacteria in the excretory fluid could be the sole factor of protection against these infections. To assess the relative importance of stasis and increased pressure is difficult, since slowing of flow of the fluid is an inevitable accompaniment of obstruction and dilatation of the passages above the level of obstruction. It can be said with assurance that, even when a profuse diuresis is obtained in a patient with partially obstructed urinary tract, this seldom achieves cure of an infection, whereas relief of the obstruction, with or without diuresis, frequently is followed by subsidence of infection.

In urinary tract infection, two different areas are interacting: the tissues and the urine itself. On the basis of animal experiments and clinical observations it seems clear that infection beginning in one can spread to the other. The complexity and extent of the urinary system may be responsible, then, for the tenacity of infection in it. One conceives of chronic pyelonephritis as an indolent process consisting of many isolated microabscesses, some of them within single tubules. Here bacterial growth may be slow, phagocytosis inefficient, and antibacterial drugs may not be capable of exerting optimal effect. Yet such areas may, from time to time, discharge their contents into the urinary passages, affording opportunity for rapid bacterial multiplication and spread to other parts of the system. In the urine phagocytosis is probably even less effective than it is in tissues, and elimination of bacteria may call for more than simple bacteriostasis. This line of reasoning leads to the conclusion that optimal results in drug treatment require the use of an agent or a combination of agents capable of killing the infecting bacteria both in the tissues and in the urine.

Manifestations. *Cystitis* is accompanied by pathognomonic local symptoms: frequency and urgency of micturition, and burning pain felt in the urethra during and immediately following the act. Cystitis alone almost never gives rise to prominent systemic manifestations of infection such as fever above 101°F, muscular pain, nausea, vomiting, and prostration, and when present these should cause the physician to suspect concomitant infection in the kidney, prostate, or some other part of the body.

The symptoms of *acute pyelonephritis* generally develop rapidly, over a period of a few hours or a day or two. The characteristics are aching pain in one or both lumbar regions, and fever which may be high (103 to 105°F), often with one or more shaking chills. There may be nausea, vomiting, and diarrhea or, occasionally, constipation. Symptoms of cystitis are usually associated, and either one may precede the other.

On physical examination, in addition to fever and some generalized tenderness of the muscles, the key finding is tenderness on deep pressure in one or both costovertebral areas or on bimanual palpation of the kidney region. Occasionally, even this sign is absent in acute pyelonephritis.

Except in individuals with ureteral obstruction, as by stone, the manifestations of acute pyelonephritis usually subside within a few days, even without specific antibacterial therapy, the patient becoming symptom-free, although laboratory tests may show that bacteriuria with or without pyuria is still present. It would seem, therefore, that after the first acute inflammation in the renal parenchyma, with swelling and perhaps intermittent plugging of the ureter by inspissated pus to account for the pain, there ensues a change in character of the disease, with the parenchymal infection going over to a more indolent process involving many small foci in the kidney substance, but with continuing growth of bacteria in the kidney pelvis and the descending urinary passages.

Undoubtedly some individuals recover completely and permanently after an attack of acute pyelonephritis, but in a considerable proportion of cases there are repeated attacks, at irregular intervals, sometimes over a period of many years; between these the patient is symptom-free. It is possible, however, that bacilluria and pyuria could be demonstrated during these free intervals, if looked for repeatedly. The important point to be stressed is that infection in any part of the urinary tract is capable of subclinical continuation, which may persist for months or years and which, in the kidney, eventually may cause serious destruction of essential tissue. Such a patient may exhibit no symptoms and may live an apparently normal life for long periods, even though urine examination gives continuing evidence of active infection. This is the feature which makes it so treacherous and such an important cause of serious renal disease.

In the *chronic, progressive form of pyelonephritis* there are no distinctive manifestations until one of the serious complications makes its appearance, i.e., renal failure or hypertension. Before this time, there may be some lassitude, lack of energy and mild normochromic anemia. Occasionally, patients with long-standing pyelonephritis are found to have large spleens, the pathogenesis of which is obscure.

Laboratory Findings. In acute pyelonephritis there is a polymorphonuclear leukocytosis; in cystitis and in chronic urinary tract infection the white blood cell picture is normal. The urine sediment in acute pyelonephritis or cystitis usually reveals numerous leukocytes occurring singly, in clumps, and in casts, and occasionally some red blood cells. Sometimes there is gross hematuria. Bacteria can easily be demonstrated by suitable stains. In chronic infections of low-grade activity, diagnosis may be very difficult on the basis of urine sediment. There may be a few pus cells, or they may be found only intermittently during repeated urinalyses. Special stains for the so-called "glitter cell" are thought by some to be of value in pointing to the presence of chronic pyelonephritis, although the demonstration of this cell cannot be regarded as diagnostic.

Culture of the urine is the most important diagnostic procedure. In acute pyelonephritis bacteria are nearly always demonstrable in large numbers, sometimes hundreds of millions of them per milliliter. In subacute and chronic infections bacteria may appear in the urine intermittently. Inasmuch as urine cultures may be contaminated by small numbers of bacteria lying in the urethral canal even in a specimen obtained by catheter, it is important that the laboratory employ some quantitative method for determining the number of organisms present in the urine, and that the urine be cultured on a solid medium, in order to estimate the relative preponderance when mixed growth is obtained. A rough quantitative estimate of the situation can be made by means of a Gram stain on uncentrifuged freshly voided urine. If bacteria can be found by this method, it can be assumed that the number present is greater than would be expected to occur as a result of urethral contamination. If quantitative cultures reveal more than 10,000 bacteria per milliliter of freshly passed urine, it can be assumed that active infection is present. If less than 1,000, they are likely to be of no significance. Between these two figures one cannot draw a positive conclusion. *Intravenous pyelogram* may be of value in the diagnosis of pyelonephritis, evidenced by an asymmetry between the kidneys as judged by their size and the density of the renal shadows. This, of course, is a reflection of the patchy distribution of the pyelonephritis lesion. It is said also that careful radiographic studies will show hypotony of the calyxes, pelvis, and ureters in a high proportion of these cases. *Biopsy of the kidney* by needle may be the only means of demonstrating low-grade pyelonephritis, but its value is also limited by the spotty distribution of the lesions.

Treatment. The soundest approach to treatment is based upon a conception of the urinary tract as a complex system wherein infection introduced into, or persisting in, any one part may spread to all the others. For example, certain drugs which have been recommended for treatment of urinary tract infection appear to be capable of acting only in urine. These, which include mandelic acid, Urotropin, and nitrofurantoin (Furadantin), often suppress but do not eradicate infection. The antibiotics are generally also effective in tissues, although some are more likely to exert a bactericidal action than others. Sulfonamides are principally bacteriostatic. Another essential principle in management is to consider what factors in the patient may be contributing to the infection, such as obstruction, faulty bladder innervation, diabetes, etc.; these were mentioned in a preceding section. Relief of obstruction or correct management of diabetes may be the essential factor in eradicating the infection. Although no further space will be devoted to this aspect of treatment, its importance cannot be overemphasized.

In antibacterial therapy, best results are obtained when there is individualization of the treatment. Advertisements and medical articles which describe the effectiveness of any one agent in the treatment of urinary infections are misleading. There is a wide choice of agents which may be used, and the best results are obtained by employing the therapy suited to the microbes operating in the individual patient.

In view of the varying conditions under which bacteria grow in urine and in urinary tract tissues, it seems probable that the ideal chemotherapeutic attack is to employ a form of treatment which is capable of bactericidal, not simply bacteriostatic, action. Determination of possible synergistic or antagonistic effects of combinations of agents on the bacteria to be attacked is sometimes necessary. Streptomycin is perhaps the most valuable of all agents available, its main defect being the rapidity with which bacteria develop resistance to it; this defect can be lessened, however, by giving streptomycin in combination with another antibiotic such as tetracycline. Enterococcus infections may yield to a combination of penicillin and streptomycin. For proteus infections, the antibiotics most likely to be beneficial are penicillin in massive doses or neomycin. For pseudomonas infection, polymyxin may be required. Since the use, contraindications, dosages, etc., of these agents are covered in detail in another chapter (p. 868), they will not be repeated here.

In view of the nature of urinary tract infection, it seems possible that prolonged treatment, for from 2 weeks to several months, might be ideal. This, however, is impractical in many situations. Nevertheless, every effort should be made to administer the appropriate drug or drugs for 7 to 10 days, no matter how prompt the symptomatic response may be. It is essential to obtain follow-up urine cultures several months after discontinuing of treatment, to avoid overlooking smoldering asymptomatic infection with its potentialities for eventual development of serious disease. It is unwise to employ catheter specimens for these follow-up examinations, since they may actually cause reinfection of the urinary tract and are not wholly reliable as methods of obtaining uncontaminated urine from the bladder. With proper care it is possible to obtain suitable "clean-voided" specimens of urine from females as well as males.

Prognosis. It is usually possible to obtain a dramatic cessation of symptoms in the treatment of acute urinary tract infection not complicated by other diseases. The dangerous feature is persistence of chronic asymptomatic infection which will gradually destroy the kidney or lead to development of hypertension (p. 1346). It is not possible to state what the risk is that a simple cystitis may spread to one or both kidneys and it is often extremely difficult to decide whether infection is limited to the lower urinary tract. Nevertheless, the fact that a significant proportion of patients coming to autopsy show evidence of pyelonephritis and some degree of renal damage indicates the great importance of this problem. In patients with some of the complicating diseases mentioned above, particularly neurogenic bladder, irremediable obstruction, or multiple stones, eradication of urinary tract infection is exceedingly difficult, if not impossible. Even here, however, the extent of the process can be minimized by comprehensive care, including surgical measures, prevention of stone formation, and appropriate chemotherapy guided by reliable laboratory procedures.

REFERENCES

Beeson, P. B.: Factors in Pathogenesis of Pyelonephritis, Yale J. Biol. and Med., 28:81, 1955.

Kleeman, C. R., W. L. Hewitt, and L. B. Guze: Pyelonephritis, Medicine, 39:3–116, 1960.

A Symposium on "The Biology of Pyelonephritis," Boston, Little, Brown and Company, 1960.

151 BACTERIAL ENDOCARDITIS

Paul B. Beeson

Bacterial endocarditis includes a variety of clinical syndromes, some of which pursue a rapid and acute course whereas others evolve slowly over a period of many months. By far the commonest type of bacterial endocarditis is the subacute variety caused by streptococci of the *viridans* group.

SUBACUTE BACTERIAL ENDOCARDITIS DUE TO *VIRIDANS* STREPTOCOCCI

Definition. This is a prolonged, febrile, often fatal disease, resulting from streptococcal infection of a heart valve, characterized by fever, heart murmur, splenomegaly, embolic phenomena, and bacteremia.

Etiology. The *viridans* group of streptococci includes several different varieties (p. 922). Those which are important causes of subacute bacterial endocarditis are *Streptococcus salivarius, S. mitis,* and *S. bovis,* normally present in the mouth; the enterococcus *S. fecalis* normally present in the intestinal tract; and *S. sanguis,* which has been encountered mainly in cases of bacterial endocarditis.

Pathogenesis. In the great majority of cases, bacterial infection is established on a valve which has been previously damaged by rheumatic fever. Changes caused by arteriosclerosis or syphilis may also provide the foundation for this infection. The mitral valve is the one most often involved; the

aortic is second in frequency. The valves on the right side are affected far less often, i.e., in only about 15 per cent of cases, including those in which the mitral and aortic are also involved. This corresponds with the frequency of involvement of the four valves in rheumatic heart disease. Valves only slightly damaged appear to be more frequently affected than those which are extensively scarred. This is partly attributable to the fact that people live longer with slightly damaged than with severely damaged valves, and hence have more opportunity to contract the infection; but other factors which may play a part include turbulence of blood flow over the valve, the circulation within the valve, and the amount of scar tissue present. It is generally agreed that bacterial endocarditis rarely occurs in persons with chronic atrial fibrillation.

Bacterial endocarditis is a frequent complication of some forms of congenital heart disease, notably patent ductus arteriosus and ventricular septal defect. It rarely develops on an atrial septal defect.

Arteriovenous fistula may be the seat of a similar process: this is called subacute bacterial endarteritis.

Bacteria must reach the heart valves by way of the blood stream. There is abundant evidence to show that entry of bacteria into the circulation is not infrequent. For example, it is a common occurrence in minor surgical procedures such as tooth extraction and tonsillectomy. Bacteremia can occur in persons with periapical dental infection simply as a result of grinding the teeth together. Ordinarily, such brief episodes of bacteremia are not serious, because the organisms are quickly phagocytized by the reticuloendothelial system. If, however, living bacteria happen to lodge in or on a damaged heart valve, the stage has been set for the establishment of a grave infection. The manner in which a colony of bacteria becomes established in such a location is not known with certainty. The fact that preexisting deformity of the valve is usually a requirement brings up the possibility that roughening of the endocardial surface or some change in blood supply to a valve may predispose to implantation of the infection. Possibly the bacteria become lodged beneath small platelet thrombi on the surface of a valve. Possibly they are carried into a valve through its blood supply and deposited beneath the endocardium. In any event, the primary site of bacterial growth is usually near the free edge of the valve at the line of closure, and on the outflow surface. This growth stimulates the deposition of platelets and fibrin and leads to the formation of a *vegetation.* This structure increases in size and may extend onto the adjacent mural endocardium. Meanwhile, the valve leaflet is undergoing gradual necrosis. Granulation tissue grows into the vegetation from the valve, but capillaries seldom reach the periphery of the infected necrotic area. Nests

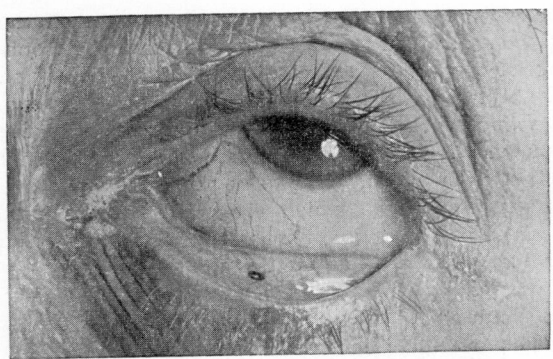

FIG. 151-1. White-centered conjunctival petechia in a patient with subacute bacterial endocarditis. (*Courtesy, Dr. John Wedgwood, Cambridge, England.*)

of growing bacteria are scattered through the vegetation; those which are in the avascular outer portion of the vegetation are protected from phagocytosis, since leukocytes do not seem able to penetrate the area. This protection from phagocytosis may be the principal factor which permits survival of bacteria and persistence of the infection and which accounts for the unsatisfactory therapeutic results obtained with drugs which are only bacteriostatic.

Organisms are constantly shed into the blood from the vegetation, but their stay in the circulation is very short, since studies have shown that one-half to one-third the organisms entering the arterial blood are removed during each circuit of the body. The principal sites of removal are organs rich in reticuloendothelial elements—i.e., liver, spleen, and bone marrow.

Vegetations of bacterial endocarditis are friable, and fragments are occasionally broken off by motion and the current of blood passing over them. These particles are carried in the blood to all parts of the body, where they eventually lodge as emboli. The damage produced by an embolus depends principally on its size and the vessel which happens to receive it. Emboli which lodge in the brain, in the mesentery, or in arteries of the extremities are most likely to have serious effects. Those carried into the walls of large arteries by vasa vasorum can cause mycotic aneurysms which may rupture at a later time.

It should be noted that the infected emboli and the free bacteria which are constantly disseminated throughout the body very seldom create metastatic abscesses. The infecting organisms are usually of low pathogenicity, and when separated from the protection of the vegetation, they are readily destroyed. An exception should be made for cases in which enterococcus is the infecting organism, since they may develop suppuration at sites of embolization, especially in the spleen.

The *myocardium* may be the site of a low-grade inflammatory process which is probably an embolic myocarditis. The *spleen* is nearly always enlarged, and in most instances shows areas of infarction. The *kidneys,* which, because of their rich blood supply, constantly receive small emboli, show changes of focal embolic nephritis. In addition, a diffuse glomerulitis is commonly encountered. These processes may result in renal insufficiency, which can be fatal.

Manifestations. In about one-third of cases, symptoms begin 1 to 3 weeks after some other illness such as acute respiratory infection or septic abortion, or some operative procedure such as dental extraction, tonsillectomy, or urethral instrumentation.

The symptoms and course of subacute bacterial endocarditis do not conform to any single typical picture, since they depend upon many factors, including the extent of the preexisting valve damage and the chance distribution of emboli. The symptoms of congestive failure may be superimposed at any time during the course of the disease.

In only about 25 per cent of cases is the onset of symptoms sufficiently dramatic that it can be recalled with certainty by the patient. More often, the illness begins very insidiously, and the patient cannot name the exact time of onset. The principal *symptoms* are weakness, malaise, feverishness, chills (occasionally), sweating, weight loss, anorexia, nausea, joint pains, paresthesias, and paralysis.

The patient usually appears chronically ill. The skin is pale and sometimes has a tan color, the so-called *café au lait* appearance. The skin may be flushed and hot, or it may be wet with perspiration. Tiny *petechial hemorrhages* may be visible in any part of the body; they are particularly evident on mucosal surfaces: the conjunctiva, the palate, or the buccal mucosa. Some of the petechiae in the conjunctiva have white or gray centers (see Fig. 151-1); these are considered by many to be of diagnostic significance but are occasionally seen in other conditions. A distinctive lesion can sometimes be seen in the ocular fundus—the "Roth spot." This consists of a circular, or oval, pale area surrounded by a ring of hemorrhage, usually near the disk. (Similar lesions occur in acute myelogenous leukemia and in septicemia.) Petechiae may be found on any area of the skin; they have to be distinguished from other lesions, such as small angiomas. The latter usually blanch when pressed with a glass slide. It is sometimes helpful to circle all suspicious lesions with ink and reexamine them later. Old petechiae fade in a day or two, and new ones appear in other areas, whereas angiomas do not change. Petechial hemorrhages in the nail beds usually are located near the distal margin and have a linear shape resembling embedded splinters; hence the name *splinter hemorrhages*. Small, painful, reddish or purplish areas in the pulps of the fingers (*Osler's nodes*) may develop during the course of the disease; they usually disappear within a day or two. Larger painful erythematous areas may appear from time to time on the palms of the hands or soles of the feet. Embolization of small arteries in the digits or in the nose occasionally produces a local area of gangrene. In cases of long duration, *clubbing of the fingers* is likely to be present. Examination of the heart reveals the signs of the preexisting valvular defect. Changing murmurs have often been mentioned as helpful in diagnosis, but too much stress should not be given this sign. The changes which do occur are most often due to the circulatory effect of anemia and fever. Occasionally, however, there are rather striking fluctuations; these are especially likely to occur in patent ductus endarteritis. The *spleen* is palpable in more than one-half of all cases; following an infarction there may be severe pain and tenderness in the left upper quadrant, and a friction rub may be audible over the left lower costal margin. Inflammation of *joints* occurs in about one-fourth of all cases and may simulate acute rheumatic fever. The pathogenesis of these arthritides is not clear.

Symptoms and signs of congestive heart failure may be present from the onset or may appear at any time during the course of subacute bacterial endocarditis. There may be orthopnea, distention of the neck veins, peripheral edema, rales in the lungs, pleural effusion, and a large, tender, swollen liver. When present, these manifestations may dominate the clinical picture and may in fact obscure the diagnosis.

The *manifestations of embolic phenomena* depend upon the tissues involved. There may be hemiplegia; meningeal inflammation; infarction of lung, myocardium, mesentery, spleen, or kidney; or occlusion of peripheral arteries. In right-sided endocarditis or patent ductus endarteritis, emboli are carried to the lungs; these may be responsible for an erroneous diagnosis of pneumonia.

The *course* of subacute bacterial endocarditis is variable and may last 1 month to 2 years. Before effective methods of treatment were available, the majority of patients died within 9 months of the onset.

Intercurrent infections are not very common, although bronchopneumonia occurs occasionally. In rheumatic subjects, the development of arthritis produces a clinical picture which may be indistinguishable from acute rheumatic fever.

Since the introduction of penicillin therapy, which controls the infection in most instances, the principal *cause of death* in subacute bacterial endocarditis is progressive, intractable cardiac decom-

pensation. This is probably the result of valvular damage which renders the heart mechanically less efficient, together with myocarditis and increased demand for cardiac work occasioned by fever and anemia. Some patients die following cerebral, myocardial, or mesenteric embolism, while others succumb to a progressive "toxemia" of infection without localizing manifestations. Rarely, death is due to uremia caused by a progression of the nephritis; this is more likely to occur in the relatively inactive cases. Sometimes, coma and death are the result of multiple small cerebral emboli which do not give localizing signs.

Laboratory Findings. The *leukocyte count* in the peripheral blood is usually moderately elevated but may be within the normal range. *Circulating macrophages* may be found in smears of the peripheral blood, particularly when the specimen is obtained by puncture of an ear lobe instead of the finger tip. This finding may be of some diagnostic value. In cases of long standing, a moderately severe normochromic *anemia* may be present. There may be an *increase in serum globulin,* and *cold-precipitable globulins* are found in some cases. The erythrocyte *sedimentation rate* is elevated. Microscopic hematuria is very common and is helpful in diagnosis. Albumin may also be found in the urine. The *blood culture* is positive for *Streptococcus viridans* in about 85 per cent of cases. In these cases the number of colonies of bacteria per milliliter of blood is usually approximately the same from day to day. In a minority of instances the blood culture is consistently negative, for reasons which are not clear. It may be that in these cases the bacteria grow more deeply in the vegetations and hence do not have free access to the circulating blood. It is often said that bacterial endocarditis located on the right side of the heart is more likely to be associated with negative blood cultures, but there is little foundation for this assertion. Actually it is not at all uncommon for bacteremia to be present in cases of right-sided bacterial endocarditis.

Differential Diagnosis. The diagnosis of subacute bacterial endocarditis may be very easy or may be extremely difficult, depending on the prominence of the various manifestations. In a patient with the cardinal manifestations of fever, heart murmur, splenomegaly, petechiae, and clubbing of the fingers, the diagnosis is obvious. On the other hand, subacute bacterial endocarditis can be a most difficult diagnostic problem, since it can simulate a variety of diseases. *The possibility of subacute bacterial endocarditis should be considered in every patient with fever and heart murmur.* The diagnosis is missed most often in elderly patients, especially those whose presenting complaint is the result of a cerebral embolic accident; in such individuals a diagnosis of cerebral thrombosis or hemorrhage is likely to be made and little consideration given to the presence of a systolic murmur or low-grade fever. Heart murmur is present in the great majority of patients, and its absence is a strong point against this diagnosis. Occasionally, in middle-aged men without previous heart disease, endocarditis develops on the aortic valve, and the murmur of aortic insufficiency is not detected until infection has been present for some days. Also, in bacterial endocarditis limited to the tricuspid or pulmonic valves, heart murmurs may not be easily detected.

This disease is one of the classic causes of "fever of undetermined origin," the important differential diagnostic points of which are covered elsewhere (p. 65). Chief among the disorders which can be confused with it are systemic lupus erythematosus, Hodgkin's disease, miliary tuberculosis, brucellosis, periarteritis nodosa, and acute rheumatic fever.

Prognosis. The natural course of the disease almost invariably leads to death, the incidence of spontaneous recovery being less than 1 per cent. In the past, many forms of therapy were tried but found ineffective; these included transfusions from immunized donors, autogenous vaccines, antiseptic drugs, irradiation of the heart valves, and so on. With sulfonamide therapy a small proportion of patients, probably not more than 4 per cent of those treated, recovered. The advent of antibiotic treatment brought about a great change in outlook, and at present about 70 per cent of these infections can be brought under control. Factors which point to a favorable outcome, in order of importance, are penicillin-sensitive organism, freedom from signs of heart failure, positive blood culture, and short duration of illness. The outlook is better when the mitral valve is affected than in aortic valvulitis, because early and intractable heart failure is more likely to result from damage to the aortic cusps.

Treatment. The following general statements deserve emphasis:

1. Eradication of the infection requires employment of chemotherapeutic agents which exert a bactericidal action, presumably because, in their protected location, the organisms must be killed without the aid of phagocytosis.

2. Penicillin is the antibiotic of prime importance. The special properties which make it so valuable in this situation are that huge doses can be tolerated by man, that it diffuses into the vegetation in high concentration, that organisms do not rapidly develop resistance to it, and, most important of all, that it can be bactericidal and can eradicate the causative organisms without aid of phagocytes. With most other antibiotics the situation is less favorable. Even though capable of inhibiting bacterial growth in vitro, the bacteriostatic antibiotics such as the tetracyclines and chloramphenicol rarely achieve a cure in this infection. Therefore, even when sensitivity tests indicate that the organism is as sensitive, or even more sensitive, to some other antibiotic, penicillin may be the only agent capable of eliminating the infection.

3. Streptomycin, almost worthless when used alone, has a place in treatment, as an adjunct to penicillin. This pertains especially to infections due to enterococcus, which is relatively resistant to penicillin alone. In the case of other varieties of S. viridans the value of the combination therapy is less certainly established, but since it may be beneficial and almost certainly does not detract from the efficacy of penicillin, current practice in most places is to use both drugs in all cases of S. viridans endocarditis.

4. In an occasional case, either because the organism is totally unaffected by penicillin (and streptomycin) or because the patient is so allergic to penicillin that this therapy in itself would threaten his life, some other antibiotic regimen has to be employed. Sensitivity tests with various combinations of antibiotics, with special attention to bactericidal effect, must be employed. Bacitracin, vancomycin, and neomycin, despite their greater toxicity, are usually preferable to chloramphenicol or the tetracycline compounds. Erythromycin and novobiocin may be effective, especially when combined with other drugs.

5. Antibiotic treatment must be continued for a considerable period of time. In early experience with penicillin, the impression was formed that treatment had to be maintained for 6 to 8 weeks, and some authorities still regard this as the safest practice in all cases. However, later experience, based upon use of much larger daily doses of penicillin in combination with streptomycin, indicates that courses of treatment of 2 to 4 weeks are sufficient in most instances. These shorter courses are justified in cases where the duration of illness is less than 3 months, the organism is sensitive to penicillin, and where there is prompt clinical improvement following the beginning of treatment. Without these favorable indications it is safest to continue treatment for up to 8 weeks.

Since the diagnosis can often be made with reasonable certainty on clinical grounds before bacteremia can be demonstrated, and since in perhaps 15 per cent of cases blood cultures remain negative, the question which often arises is how soon to begin chemotherapy. An accurate bacteriologic diagnosis, including antibiotic sensitivities, is of great value and should be achieved if possible, but undue delay of treatment must be avoided because of the possibility of embolic accident and progressive destruction of a cardiac valve. A reasonable practice is to collect four to six blood cultures during a 48-hr period, then begin treatment with penicillin and streptomycin, observing the clinical response and modifying the chemotherapeutic regimen later as dictated by bacteriologic findings.

When the infecting organism is penicillin-sensitive, a suitable dosage schedule is 2,400,000 units penicillin and 1 Gm streptomycin per day. If the clinical response is not satisfactory or if the organism is only slightly sensitive to penicillin, very much larger doses of penicillin, up to 100,000,000 units per day, may have to be given. The dosage of streptomycin probably should seldom exceed 2 Gm per day. The administration of very large amounts of penicillin is technically difficult, since the pain of intramuscular injections is often severe and their intravenous administration may cause chemical phlebitis. In order to maintain such a program of treatment for several weeks it is usually necessary to employ a variety of methods, including continuous and intermittent intravenous and intramuscular injections. Adjuvants such as Benemid may be used to reduce the rate of excretion of penicillin by the kidneys. Ingenuity, technical skill, and stubborn persistence on the part of the doctor may be life-saving.

Embolic accidents, resulting in hemiplegia, mesenteric infarction, or occlusion of a peripheral artery, may take place many days after the beginning of effective antimicrobial therapy.

The course of the fever after beginning chemotherapy is somewhat variable. In most instances there is a defervescence within the first day or two, but sometimes, even when the end result is satisfactory, a low-grade fever continues for as long as 2 or 3 weeks.

The treatment of congestive heart failure in bacterial endocarditis does not differ from that of other kinds of congestive heart failure (see p. 1385).

In infections located on a patent ductus arteriosus or an arteriovenous fistula, cure can sometimes be achieved by surgical excision or obliteration of the fistulous tract. Such operative treatment can be carried out during, or at the conclusion of, an appropriate course of chemotherapy.

Relapse may occur after the cessation of penicillin therapy, especially when the period of treatment has been short. The great majority of relapses occur within the first 4 weeks after cessation of treatment. It is usually safe to consider a patient's infection eradicated if he is free of symptoms and signs of the disease and if his blood cultures show no growth 6 weeks after the conclusion of therapy. A recrudescence after that time may be due to a new infection rather than to persistence of the initial one.

In the event of relapse, additional chemotherapy is indicated. It is particularly important to check the sensitivity of the infecting organism and to adjust the dose of penicillin or other antibiotic accordingly.

Persons who have recovered from subacute bacterial endocarditis should be given prophylactic penicillin therapy before any operative procedure in an infected area, such as tonsillectomy or tooth extraction. It is advisable to administer penicillin orally in a dosage of 1 million units daily for 2 days prior to the procedure and for 1 day afterward.

OTHER ETIOLOGIC AGENTS IN BACTERIAL ENDOCARDITIS

Although streptococci of the *viridans* type are by far the commonest cause of bacterial endocarditis, a wide variety of other microorganisms may be the cause of subacute or acute bacterial endocarditis. These include nonpathogenic bacteria, such as *Staphylococcus albus, Hemophilus parainfluenzae,* which give rise to the subacute pattern of disease just described, and many genuinely pathogenic organisms, such as S. *aureus,* hemolytic streptococcus, brucella, the gonococcus, meningococcus, and pneumococcus, which are likely to give a more fulminating disease picture. In addition to bacteria, certain of the fungi, such as *Histoplasma capsulatum,* have been shown to cause bacterial endocarditis.

Narcotic addicts, who inject themselves intravenously, usually without aseptic technique, are liable to develop acute bacterial infections on previously normal heart valves.

Bacterial endocarditis due to S. *aureus* or S. *albus* is now a well-recognized hazard of surgical treatment of rheumatic or congenital heart disease, the incidence being perhaps 1 to 3 per cent. Diagnosis in these cases may be delayed because of antimicrobial drug therapy for other indications and difficulty in differentiating the manifestations from those of postcardiotomy syndromes.

The term *acute bacterial endocarditis* is usually given to those cases in which the etiologic organism is a true pathogen, such as S. *aureus* or the pneumococcus, and in which the course is relatively rapid—i.e., a few weeks. This type of infection may involve previously normal valves; hence a heart murmur may not always be present at the onset of illness. The clinical picture is characterized not only by a short course but also by high fever, multiple petechial hemorrhages and other embolic manifestations, development of metastatic abscesses in other parts of the body, and rapid destruction of the heart valve.

Acute pneumococcal endocarditis should be watched for during convalescence from pneumococcal meningitis. Rupture of an aortic valve cusp, with rapidly progressive heart failure, is a well-known sequel to pneumococcal meningitis.

The results of chemotherapy in these fulminating infections are still unsatisfactory. Probably not more than 20 per cent of patients with acute staphylococcal or pneumococcal endocarditis recover, even though the organism may appear to be sensitive to penicillin in the test tube. Autopsies often reveal healing of the ulcerative endocarditis but the presence and persistence of one or more abscesses elsewhere. Especially noteworthy are myocardial abscesses, located in the region of the valve ring. Apparently, the sterilization of infection in such an abscess is very difficult to achieve with chemotherapy, and this seems to be one of the reasons for the poor results obtained in this disease.

REFERENCES

Austrian, R.: Pneumococcal Endocarditis, Meningitis, and Rupture of the Aortic Valve, A.M.A. Arch. Internal Med., 99:539, 1957.

Kerr, A. J., Jr.: "Subacute Bacterial Endocarditis," Springfield, Ill., Charles C Thomas, Publisher, 1955.

Sheldon, W. H., and A. Golden: Abscesses of the Valve Rings of the Heart, A Frequent but Not Well Recognized Complication of Acute Bacterial Endocarditis, Circulation, 4:1, 1951.

Tumulty, P. A.: The Management of Bacterial Endocarditis, A.M.A. Arch. Internal Med., 105:126, 1960.

152 PYOGENIC INFECTIONS OF THE NERVOUS SYSTEM

John N. Walton

Since many of the infective disorders of the central nervous system have already been dealt with elsewhere, this chapter will be limited to a discussion of specific neurologic syndromes which arise when pyogenic bacteria or their products encroach upon nervous tissue. The neurologic effects of suppuration within the cranial cavity or vertebral canal and certain neurologic aspects and complications of meningitis will be considered.

Pyogenic organisms may gain access to the cranial cavity or spinal canal in a number of ways. So far as the cranium is concerned, direct spread of an infective process beginning in the middle ear or in a paranasal sinus may cause an osteomyelitis of cranial bones. This in turn will often affect the extradural space, whence further spread is possible through the meninges to the brain itself. Septic thrombosis of diploic and emissary veins may play

an important part in this process. In the vertebral column, osteomyelitis of a vertebra plays a similar role. The next most frequent source of suppuration around or within the neuraxis is metastatic infection with blood-borne organisms arising from a remote septic focus, often in the skin or lung. Lymphatic spread from a nearby locus of infection may account for certain cases of intraspinal suppuration but is virtually unknown as a cause of intracranial abscess formation. In other cases, organisms may be introduced by foreign bodies such as projectiles, while rarely faulty aseptic technique in such procedures as lumbar puncture or cranial exploration may be responsible. Of all the mechanisms described, direct spread from the enveloping bony cage and metastatic infection are by far the most common in civilian medical practice.

NEUROLOGIC ASPECTS OF BACTERIAL MENINGITIS

Bacterial meningitis, as typified by that due to the meningococcus, is regarded by many as a disease in which the pathologic changes are limited to the subarachnoid space and do not encroach upon nervous tissue. It is also generally believed that these changes are entirely reversible with adequate treatment. While both these views have considerable substance, it is also true that sometimes lasting disability or a fatal outcome is due not to the meningitis but to certain distinctive pathologic changes which the disease produces in the nervous parenchyma. Indeed, it is probable that such changes may be far more frequent than is generally realized. Similarly, certain other neurologic manifestations are now known to depend upon vascular changes which are a part of the inflammatory process, while others, as well as some common sequelae, may be attributed to incomplete resolution of the meningeal inflammation.

Having accepted these generalizations, it is possible to say that modern antibiotic and chemotherapeutic methods of treatment have greatly reduced the incidence of complications, particularly in meningococcal meningitis. However, they are still of considerable importance in the other forms which show a less uniformly favorable response to treatment. In tuberculous meningitis, complications are an outstanding feature.

It is perhaps justifiable to consider the pathologic findings in fatal cases of influenzal meningitis as typifying the changes observed. There are wide variations in the pathologic picture, which can probably be related in most cases to the duration of the illness but in others are dependent on numerous factors, particularly the resistance of the patient and the efficacy of treatment.

The outstanding changes may be classified as follows:

1. Subdural effusions, serous or purulent
2. Severe brain swelling with tentorial or cerebellar herniation
3. Acute hydrocephalus without blockage of cerebrospinal fluid pathways
4. Ischemic necrosis of cerebral cortex or, in more chronic cases, nerve cell degeneration with marked glial reaction
5. Subependymal perivascular cellular infiltration with astrocytic and microglial proliferation
6. Subpial degeneration of spinal cord; superficial as well as irregular parenchymatous degeneration of cranial and spinal nerves
7. Vascular changes:
    a. Cortical thrombophlebitis
    b. Endothelial swelling and cellular infiltration in meningeal arteries; in some cases there is a severe arteritis leading to thrombosis
8. Organization of exudate with meningeal fibrosis

Subdural empyema is a relatively uncommon complication of bacterial meningitis and will be considered in detail shortly. *Serous subdural effusions* have been recognized recently as an important complication of meningitis in infancy. McKay, Ingraham, and Matson found such collections in 60 per cent of all patients under one year of age who were suffering from meningococcal, influenzal, or pneumococcal meningitis. They suspect that such collections may be present if any of the following features are noted: (1) persistent high temperature after 72 hr of adequate treatment, (2) positive cerebrospinal fluid culture after 48 hr of treatment, (3) convulsions during convalescence, (4) focal convulsions at any time, (5) vomiting during the convalescent period, (6) gross neurologic abnormality, (7) clinical impression that the course is unsatisfactory. Any one of these findings is, they believe, an indication for aspiration of the subdural space, carried out by needling in the lateral angle of the anterior fontanel. If a subdural effusion is present, fluid will readily be withdrawn. It is always xanthochromic and may even be frankly bloody; it usually contains up to 2 or 3 Gm per 100 ml of protein and several hundred white cells per cubic millimeter. It is sterile on culture in most cases. Many workers believe that this complication is best treated by daily aspiration while antimicrobial therapy is continued. Others, however, suggest that in these patients a subdural membrane, similar to that of chronic subdural hematoma, is present and should be removed surgically; McKay, Ingraham, and Matson believe that, if such a membrane is left, it will interfere with the growth of the brain. In the absence of

any conclusive evidence that this does in fact occur, it seems that repeated aspiration is the treatment of choice and that surgery should be reserved for those cases which fail to respond to this regimen.

In a proportion of the cases of acute meningitis which die within 24 to 48 hr of the onset, an *acute brain swelling* or, alternatively, *hydrocephalus* may be seen, producing fatal tentorial or cerebellar herniation. The exact cause of these changes is unknown, though they seem to be related in some way to the acuteness of the disease process.

The etiology of the cortical and subependymal changes is also obscure. The diffuse nerve cell degeneration and subpial glial reaction are probably evidence of a *noninfectious encephalomyelopathy* due to a number of circulatory and toxic factors, but the subependymal changes may be the result of direct bacterial invasion. This encephalopathy is probably responsible for the stupor, coma, and the generalized convulsions of the disease. The areas of *cortical necrosis* probably explain many of the focal neurologic symptoms and signs, such as focal seizures or hemiplegia. Pain in the limbs, blindness, and deafness or other cranial nerve palsies can be attributed to *degenerative changes in the nerves or roots*. Chronic meningeal fibrosis, so-called *adhesive arachnoiditis*, may sometimes produce similar effects as a late sequel, through constriction of nerve trunks.

The *arterial infiltration* already described does not appear to be responsible for important nervous lesions in pyogenic meningitis. *Thrombophlebitis* may give rise to focal convulsions, neurologic signs, or subarachnoid bleeding through cortical infarction. The thrombophlebitis is generally aseptic and occasionally involves the sagittal sinus, giving a syndrome which will be discussed later in this chapter.

Meningeal fibrosis and organization of exudate can block the aqueduct, the foramina in the roof of the fourth ventricle, or the tentorial hiatus. Obstructive or communicating hydrocephalus results. Similar dense meningeal thickening around the brain stem may sometimes be responsible for the tonic spasms which occasionally accompany and follow meningitis, and it is conceivable that they may even be the basis for the terminal decerebrate state of some such patients.

Although these changes have been most carefully studied in influenzal and pneumonococcal meningitis, it is probable that the complications and sequelae of most forms, including tuberculous meningitis, are similarly determined. Tuberculosis may be complicated by infarction due to arterial occlusion, since the basal arteritis, which has been well described by Doniach, is more striking in this than in other types of meningitis.

INTRACRANIAL SUPPURATIVE DISORDERS

If bacterial meningitis is excluded, it can be said that suppurative disease within the cranial cavity occurs in one of five situations. The process may occur external to the dura, in which case an *extradural abscess* results, or it may penetrate the dura to give a *subdural abscess* or *empyema;* very rarely, a localized *subarachnoid abscess* may occur within the subarachnoid space. In other instances the inflammation may affect principally an intracranial venous sinus or its radicals, giving *suppurative thrombophlebitis.* Most commonly of all, the inflammatory process involves brain tissue, beginning as a diffuse process of *suppurative encephalitis.* This inflammatory process may continue to spread until the patient dies, but more often, the infected area or areas become surrounded by reactive tissue to give one or more *brain abscesses.*

Practically all extradural and subdural abscesses and more than 50 per cent of brain abscesses are produced by centripetal spread of suppuration from the cranial bones.

Extradural Abscess

The cranial osteomyelitis responsible for producing an extradural abscess is generally due to otitis media, sinusitis, or trauma. Pus accumulates on the inner side of the cranium and strips off the dura, which becomes lined on its external surface by a layer of granulation tissue. An abscess in this situation is difficult to diagnose, since it is rarely large enough to produce a severe increase in intracranial pressure or focal neurologic signs. It may, however, be suspected in the presence of irregular pyrexia and headache which radiates from either the mastoid (in otitis media) or frontal region (in frontal sinusitis); there is often marked tenderness of the skull in the affected region. The cerebrospinal fluid may be normal but usually shows a slight polymorphonuclear or mononuclear pleocytosis. This condition can be treated effectively by antibiotic therapy and surgical drainage.

Subdural Abscess or Empyema

This syndrome is usually a complication of frontal sinusitis; it sometimes occurs in otitis but is rarely metastatic.

In most cases, infection of the subdural space is effected by direct extension through the dura, but in others it is the result of septic thrombophlebitis of venous sinuses, particularly the superior longitudinal. The subdural pus usually covers the greater part of the lateral surface of the affected hemisphere and tends to accumulate over the lateral aspect of the frontal lobe. In fatal cases, ischemic necrosis of subjacent cortical gray matter is found, and thrombosis of subarachnoid and cortical veins is frequent.

The symptomatology of this disease follows a relatively stereotyped pattern. When it complicates sinusitis, there is usually exacerbation of frontal pain and nasal discharge followed by orbital swelling; headache is at first localized to the frontal region but later becomes generalized and increases in severity. Concurrently, high fever, neck stiffness, and drowsiness or stupor develop and are followed by focal neurologic signs. Jacksonian seizures are common, aphasia is seen in left-sided lesions, paralysis of contralateral ocular deviation is frequent, and all patients have a *hemiparesis* or *hemiplegia.* Clinical manifestations in cases not caused by sinusitis are identical save for the absence of signs of sinus infection and orbital swelling.

Most cases show a marked increase in cerebrospinal fluid pressure, and the total protein content is raised, often to about 100 mg per 100 ml, though the sugar remains normal and the fluid is sterile on culture. A cell count of several hundred per cubic millimeter is usual, and the majority of the cells are polymorphonuclear leukocytes.

If not treated, the condition is fatal within about 10 to 14 days after the onset of headache or 3 to 4 days after the accession of focal neurologic signs. Elective treatment consists in administration of the appropriate antibiotic, combined with drainage of the abscess through one or more burr holes. Attempts to drain the abscess through the frontal sinuses or ear almost invariably fail.

It is sometimes difficult to distinguish this condition from intracranial thrombophlebitis or from necrotizing encephalopathy with predominant involvement of one hemisphere.

Intracranial Thrombophlebitis

This most often affects the lateral, cavernous, or superior longitudinal sinuses, owing to centripetal spread of infection from the middle ear, the skin of the face, or the frontal sinus, respectively. In all three conditions the patients are acutely ill with high remittent fever.

In *lateral sinus thrombosis* there is usually headache in the temporal region. Papilledema may sometimes occur, but focal neurologic signs are generally absent, and the clinical picture is dominated by the manifestations of pyemia. Compression of the homolateral internal jugular vein may produce no rise in pressure during spinal manometry, whereas a normal rise occurs during compression on the opposite side (Tobey-Ayer test).

Cavernous sinus thrombosis gives homolateral frontal headache and facial pain followed by proptosis, edema of the eyelids, chemosis, and paresis of oculomotor nerves. Often the infection spreads through the circular sinus to the other cavernous sinus. This may sometimes be prevented by early treatment.

Suppuration within the *superior longitudinal sinus* usually produces headache and marked papilledema with edema and engorgement of the scalp over the vertex. A monoplegia of one leg or a paraplegia may result from infarction of the leg area or areas of the motor cortex, but this is uncommon. More often a subdural empyema results.

Septic thrombosis in any of the three situations requires vigorous chemotherapy, and this is the only method of treatment in cavernous sinus disease. Surgical exposure and drainage of the lateral sinus or ligation of the internal jugular vein may sometimes be required.

Aseptic thrombosis of intracranial venous sinuses, particularly the lateral and superior longitudinal, is an occasional complication of otitis media, and in many such cases there is no evidence of intracranial spread of microorganisms. The resulting syndrome is characterized by severe papilledema and increase in the intracranial pressure with comparatively little headache; it has been called *otitic hydrocephalus* by Symonds. In severe cases (when the process extends to cortical veins) seizures, focal neurologic signs, and even profuse subarachnoid hemorrhage may result from cortical infarction. An identical syndrome not uncommonly occurs in marasmic infants, in cachectic patients, during pregnancy, following closed head injury, or in individuals with heart disease or blood dyscrasias.

Brain Abscess

Incidence. Brain abscess may occur at any age and is equally common in the two sexes. It is probably that fewer cases of otitis and intrathoracic suppuration have been complicated in this way since the advent of antibiotic therapy, but certain patients who would previously have died from the primary infection now survive to develop a brain abscess.

Etiology and Location. About 40 per cent of brain abscesses are secondary to middle ear disease, and of these about a third arise in the anterior part of the lateral cerebellar lobe, the remainder lying in the middle part of the temporal lobe above the tegmen tympani. Frontal sinusitis accounts for roughly 10 per cent of cases, and the abscess is almost invariably situated in the anterior part of the frontal lobe. Of the remaining 50 per cent of cases, a small proportion are due to penetrating wounds, and the remainder are metastatic; in about half of these the primary septic focus is in the lung (bronchiectasis, empyema, lung abscess), and in the others it may be in the skin or other diverse locations such as bone or the heart. Brain abscesses are particularly frequent in patients with congestive heart failure or cyanotic congenital heart disease, even without evidence of bacterial endocarditis. In traumatic cases the site of the abscess will clearly depend upon the area which has been traumatized, but a metastatic abscess may be situated anywhere within the cranium, though it is usually above the tentorium. Most abscesses lie within the distribution of the middle cerebral artery, beginning at the junction of the gray and white matter; they are not infrequently multiple or multilocated, a finding which is less frequent in the case of otitic abscesses.

Almost any of the common organisms may cause a cerebral abscess, the most frequent being streptococci, pneumococci, and staphylococci, while fusiform bacilli and oral spirochetes are sometimes found. Less commonly such organisms as *Escherichia coli*, actinomyces, or even *Endamoeba histolytica* may be responsible.

Pathology. Invasion of nervous tissue by the causal organism leads initially to focal necrosis and liquefaction accompanied by edema of the surrounding brain; this stage is called *suppurative encephalitis*. If the patient survives, pus accumulates, and a capsule begins to form from fibroblasts derived from proliferating capillaries. In due course, a firm, thick fibrous capsule forms and may be several millimeters in diameter; it is lined by a layer of granulation tissue containing polymorphonuclear leukocytes, histiocytes, lymphocytes, and proliferating capillaries. In brain tissue surrounding the fibrous wall are found reacting microglia, fibroblasts, and astrocytes in profusion.

Clinical Manifestations. The physician should be aware of the many ways in which a brain abscess may develop, for early diagnosis is the key to effective treatment. Early in the illness the patient's symptoms are all-important, since physical signs may not develop until a relatively late stage. When a known sufferer from otitis media experiences a suppression of aural discharge following a period of exacerbation and this is succeeded by headache, vomiting, and confusion, it is reasonable to suspect that inflammation has spread intracranially. In many cases, however, the symptoms are not striking, and the patient may seem to recover from a flare-up of his otitis but remains unwell, experiencing attacks of depression and irritability, vague intermittent headache and nausea, anorexia, weight loss, and mild fever. Symptoms and signs of meningeal irritation are usually minimal. A history of this type in a patient with paranasal sinusitis should also make one suspicious of intracranial suppuration; the cerebrospinal fluid should be examined immediately.

In hematogenous abscess, the onset is sometimes dramatic with sudden focal seizures and neurologic signs, followed, after an interval of days or weeks, by increasing pyrexia and evidence of mounting intracranial pressure. This may be seen when an infected embolus becomes impacted in a large vessel. Far more often, however, the onset is insidious, with minimal headache, slight, intermittent pyrexia, and gradual personality change. When there is an evident septic focus in the skin or lung, the possibility of abscess may come to mind, but in many other instances the patient may be felt to be suffering from an intracranial tumor. This is particularly common when antibiotic therapy effectively masks the patient's symptoms throughout the stage of suppurative encephalitis.

When the clinical manifestations of brain abscess are more fully developed, they fall into three groups: (1) general symptoms of infection, (2) symptoms and signs of increased intracranial pressure, and (3) focal symptoms and signs.

The severity of the *general symptoms of infection* is related to the acuteness of the disease process. In cases of acute suppurative encephalitis, they may be severe; in patients in whom the onset is more insidious, a low intermittent pyrexia is the rule, while in more chronic cases the temperature may be normal throughout.

Some evidence of *increased intracranial pressure* is usually found, although in a few patients with large chronic abscesses it may be lacking. In general, the patients have headache, which may occasionally be localized over the suppuration. More often it is of the type usually seen in increased intracranial pressure, being paroxysmal, worse in the mornings, and increased by movement. Nausea is frequent and is followed by vomiting in the later stages. The pulse is more likely to be slow in patients with abscess than in any other form of intracranial disease. Papilledema is usually a late sign, but mental changes consisting of mild confusion and irritability or other change in temperament, progressing to severe confusion, drowsiness, stupor, and coma, are commonly present.

Temporal Lobe Abscess. If the abscess affects the dominant hemisphere, dysphasia, which is often of "normal" or "amnesic" type, is frequent; the patient finds difficulty in naming familiar objects. A homonymous upper quadrantic field defect is often seen because of involvement of the optic radiation. Evidence of pyramidal tract involvement is usually minimal and may be a little more than slight contralateral facial or finger weakness, though extensive lesions may give a hemiparesis. Herniation of the temporal lobe through the tentorial hiatus may lead to a homolateral third nerve palsy, to coma, and to signs of bilateral disease of the pyramidal tracts.

Cerebellar Abscess. Headache in the suboccipital region is common, and the neck may be stiff or held to one side. Evidence of increased intracranial pressure is often more striking in these patients than in those with abscesses situated elsewhere. Signs of cerebellar deficiency such as hypotonia, incoordination, past pointing, and slow performance of rapid alternating movements may be seen in the limbs on the affected side. The patient may tend to fall or stagger to this side on walking. Nystagmus is usually present, being most marked on lateral gaze to the side of the lesion; there may also be compression of the brain stem, leading to cranial nerve pareses and contralateral pyramidal signs, but these manifestations are most variable. Homolateral pyramidal signs may occur, probably because of compression of the contralateral cerebral peduncle against the free edge of the tentorium.

Frontal Lobe Abscess. Patients with frontal lobe abscess often show no focal neurologic signs. Headache, drowsiness, and impairment of memory, attention, and intellectual function are prominent. In some cases there is a grasp reflex and contralateral deviation of the head and eyes. If the abscess is large, a hemiparesis and dysphasia (in dominant hemisphere lesions) may result.

Diagnostic Procedures. Examination of the *cerebrospinal fluid* may be of great diagnostic value, but this procedure should be carried out with care, particularly in those cases in which a temporal or cerebellar abscess is suspected. In such a case, removal of even a moderate quantity of fluid can lead to herniation of the temporal lobe through the tentorial hiatus or of the cerebellum through the foramen magnum, with fatal results. Whenever there is evidence of increased intracranial pressure, only a small amount of fluid should be removed, and in the presence of marked papilledema, the procedure is contraindicated. The fluid usually shows an increased pressure, and its protein content is often higher than 100 mg per 100 ml; it rarely contains more than 100 white cells per cubic millimeter and the majority are mononuclear, though a number of neutrophils may be present in the early stages. The sugar content of the fluid is normal, and no bacteria are seen in smears or isolated by culture. *Electroencephalography* may be of considerable value in diagnosis and localization, since an abscess in one cerebral hemisphere usually gives a focus of extremely slow and irregular delta activity of high amplitude. *Radiography* of the skull may show displacement of the pineal body. *Angiography* may localize it accurately, but many surgeons prefer *ventriculography. Air encephalography* by the lumbar route is dangerous when the intracranial pressure is raised. After treatment of the abscess, instillation of Thorotrast into the cavity may demonstrate its progressive decrease in size.

Diagnosis. In the chronic abscess with no clear primary focus of infection, differentiation from intracranial tumor may be impossible except by cerebrospinal fluid examination or exploration. In the more acute cases, the condition is distinguished from meningitis by the absence of meningeal irritation and by the cerebrospinal fluid changes. In patients with otitis media there may be confusion between temporal abscess and lateral sinus thrombosis, or between cerebellar abscess and labyrinthitis. However, septic thrombosis of the lateral sinus is usually a more dramatic febrile illness than temporal abscess and rarely produces focal neurologic signs; in a proportion of cases the Tobey-Ayer manometric test will be positive. Labyrinthitis can usually be recognized, since it tends to give more vertigo and less headache than does cerebellar abscess and does not produce papilledema or changes in the cerebrospinal fluid.

Prognosis. Without treatment, brain abscess is an almost uniformly fatal disease save for the very rare cases in which the lesion becomes quiescent and thickly encapsulated and a few in which spontaneous drainage occurs via the middle ear or frontal sinus. Death usually results from diffuse suppurative encephalitis, increased intracranial pressure, brain herniation, or rupture of the abscess into the ventricular system or subarachnoid space. Before the days of antibiotics, about 50 per cent of patients died despite surgical treatment; after penicillin became freely available, the mortality rate dropped to under 30 per cent.

Late Prognosis. Not all the 70 per cent of patients who survive after treatment of a brain abscess recover completely. Some are left with signs of neurologic deficit, varying from a mild field defect to hemiplegia. Recurrent headaches, intellectual impairment, and anxiety states are common, and about 50 per cent of surviving patients develop seizures as a sequel.

Treatment. During the stage of acute suppurative encephalitis, to carry out an intracranial operation is to court disaster through wider dissemination of the inflammatory process. At this stage every attempt should be made to isolate the responsible organism from either the cerebrospinal fluid or the primary septic focus. Vigorous antibiotic therapy with the appropriate agent, given systemically and, if safe, intrathecally, is indicated. Sometimes a patient who appears to have all the typical symptoms and signs of a brain abscess recovers on medical therapy alone. The great majority, however, require surgical intervention. Occasionally, in the presence of deepening coma and progressive neurologic signs, operation may be necessary even in the acute stage. More often it is possible to wait until the inflammatory process has become localized. All abscesses presenting in the chronic stage should be operated upon promptly. Details of surgical treatment are beyond the scope of this volume, but it can be said that some surgeons prefer to aspirate the abscess and instill antibiotics, while others believe in its total extirpation. In the former

method, it is easy to overlook multiple abscesses or separate loculi, and recurrences are possible, but extirpation may give more severe sequelae than would have occurred after aspiration. Both methods have proved successful in the hands of their proponents.

INTRASPINAL SUPPURATIVE DISORDERS

Of the suppurative conditions within the spinal canal, epidural abscess is the commonest by far. Very rarely an abscess may form within the subdural space, following a penetrating wound or localization of a purulent meningitis; however, its clinical manifestations do not differ significantly from those of epidural abscess, and in both conditions surgical exploration is required. *Intramedullary spinal abscess* is also extremely rare; it is almost invariably metastatic in origin, tends to run a more rapid course than most cases of epidural suppuration, and is attended by less pain than is the latter. It often presents with paresthesias in the lower limbs, followed by progressive flaccid paralysis. Many cases of this type cannot be distinguished from other forms of acutely progressive myelopathy, and few are diagnosed during life. Foley has pointed out that the diagnosis may be suspected when clinical, manometric, and radiologic findings suggest an intramedullary tumor and there is also a clear focus of infection elsewhere in the body. In such cases, improvement and certainly survival may follow aspiration or incision and drainage of the abscess, together with antibiotic therapy. In view of the rarity of subdural and intramedullary suppuration in the spinal canal they will not be considered further. Nor will tuberculous epidural abscess be given separate consideration, since its presentation and management are best considered along with tuberculous spinal disease.

Spinal Epidural Abscess

The recognition of this condition is a matter of paramount importance since surgical intervention in the early stages is usually rewarded by total recovery, whereas even brief delay may lead to paraplegia or death. There are few disorders in which early diagnosis is so imperative, and for this reason alone it merits detailed description.

Etiology. Vertebral osteomyelitis is the cause of this syndrome in about a third of cases. Hematogenous spread from an infective focus, often cutaneous sepsis, and sometimes pyelonephritis are presumably responsible for most of the remaining cases. Much more rarely the abscess may arise through lymphatic spread from a paraspinous lesion such as a mediastinal or retropharyngeal abscess, and it is also possible for it to be caused by direct inoculation (lumbar puncture needle) or by a penetrating wound. Almost invariably *Staphylococcus aureus* is the responsible organism.

Pathology. Granulomatous tissue, with a variable amount of pus, tends to accumulate in the epidural fat over the dorsal aspect of the dura and to spread longitudinally. In osteomyelitic cases aggregations of purulent material are often found in the lateral epidural regions in relation to the bony lesion, but an anterior accumulation is rare owing to the intimate relationship of the dura and the intervertebral ligaments. Large collections of pus are uncommon; more often it is found as multiple small pockets in exuberant granulation tissue. The inflammatory process may extend axially so as to overlie as many as seven bony segments but is usually limited to three or four; extension is less marked in the osteomyelitic cases. The inflammatory process may also spread laterally and dorsally to involve paravertebral structures, spinal muscles, and even the subcutaneous tissue, but anterior extension is virtually unknown. Nor does the process often traverse the dura; its effect upon the spinal cord seems to depend upon a combination of a simple compression and interference with the circulation in epidural veins, leading to derangement of its blood supply.

Clinical Manifestations. Heusner has pointed out that, although spinal epidural sepsis produces clinical syndromes which differ in tempo, there is a basic clinical pattern common to all variants. It consists of the following march of events:

Phase I: Spinal ache
Phase II: Fever, root pain, spinal tenderness
Phase III: Weakness of voluntary muscles, sphincters, sensibilities
Phase IV: Paralysis

Sometimes the symptoms and signs of severe infection may partially mask the above features, but they are always present if looked for with care. The initial aching pain is usually accompanied by fever, and the spine is tender in the affected region. Within 2 or 3 days, root pains are added, which radiate from the affected segment, and the spine is then exquisitely tender. If the condition remains untreated, the general signs of infection increase, the spinal ache becomes excruciating, neck stiffness develops, and soon afterward weakness, ascending numbness of the limbs, and impairment of sphincter control appear. Between this stage and that of irreversible flaccid paralysis there may be an interval of only a few hours.

Many authors distinguish the acute metastatic from the acute osteomyelitic syndrome on clinical grounds; the interval between phase I and phase II is very much longer in the osteomyelitic cases, lasting days or even weeks, but thereafter the disease progresses with extreme rapidity. It is also true that there occur occasional chronic cases in which the march of events and the clinical picture are both attenuated, and the illness lasts weeks or months, with much less pain and few or no general signs of infection. Despite these variations the condition is a well-defined clinical syndrome; the diagnosis must be made in phase II or early in phase III if the patient is to survive without residual paralysis.

Diagnostic Procedures. While radiography of the spine may be of great value in diagnosis, particularly of the osteomyelitic cases, there will be many instances in which an epidural abscess is present before the characteristic radiologic changes of osteomyelitis have had time to develop. The most important investigation is spinal puncture. It must be stressed, however, that when this condition is suspected, spinal puncture should be performed by a skilled physician who is fully acquainted with the pathology of the probable lesion. Lack of adequate care may mean that the needle will carry organisms from the extradural to the subarachnoid space. If the puncture is performed at the level of the lesion, pus will be found in the epidural space; if not there will be a complete manometric spinal block, and the spinal fluid will be xanthochromic, containing a large amount of protein and only a few white cells. With a characteristic clinical picture, either of these findings is a sufficient indication for surgical exploration. Myelography, however, is often necessary for accurate localization, and the operator should be prepared to inject contrast medium when the spinal puncture is performed; for an attempt to inject this material into the subarachnoid space some hours or days after cerebrospinal fluid has been removed from below a spinal block may be unsuccessful.

Diagnosis. In phase I, cases of this type are often dismissed as examples of arthritis, lumbago, or spinal strain. In phases II and III, however, the characteristic combination of fever, root pain, and exquisite spinal tenderness is sufficient to exclude such conditions as prolapsed intervertebral disk, meningitis, poliomyelitis, transverse myelitis, and acute postinfective polyradiculopathy (the Guillain-Barré syndrome). In the uncommon chronic cases, differentiation from intrathecal neoplasm may be difficult on clinical grounds, but the changes found on spinal puncture will indicate the need for surgical exploration.

Treatment. Once the diagnosis is established, the great majority of patients require immediate laminectomy for drainage of the epidural space, and vigorous antibiotic therapy should be continued. Very occasionally, if the abscess is situated below the termination of the spinal cord, there may be recovery with antibiotics alone. Scrupulous observation is necessary, and neurologic signs are an indication for immediate surgery.

REFERENCES

Adams, R. D., and C. S. Kubik: The Effects of Influenzal Meningitis on the Nervous System, N.Y. State J. Med., 47:2676, 1947.

Doniach, I.: Changes in the Meningeal Vessels in Acute and Chronic (Streptomycin-treated) Tuberculous Meningitis, J. Pathol. Bacteriol., 61:253, 1949.

Elsberg, C. A.: "Surgical Diseases of the Spinal Cord, Membranes and Nerve Roots," New York, Paul B. Hoeber, Inc., Medical Department of Harper & Brothers, 1941.

Foley, J.: Intramedullary Abscess of the Spinal Cord, Lancet, II:193, 1949.

Heusner, A. P.: Nontuberculous Spinal Epidural Infections, New Engl. J. Med., 239:845, 1948.

Jooma, O. V., J. B. Pennybacker, and G. K. Tutton: Brain Abscess: Aspiration Drainage or Excision? J. Neurol., Neurosurg., Psychiat., 14:308, 1951.

Kubik, C. S., and R. D. Adams: Subdural Empyema, Brain, 66:18, 1943.

McKay, R. J., F. D. Ingraham, and D. D. Matson: Subdural Fluid, Complicating Bacterial Meningitis, J.A.M.A., 152:387, 1953.

Pennybacker, J.: Abscess of the Brain, pp. 257–290 in "Modern Trends in Neurology," A. Feiling (Ed.), London, Butterworth & Co. (Publishers) Ltd., 1951.

Symonds, C. P.: Otitic Hydrocephalus, Neurology, 6:681, 1956.

Section 10: Diseases Produced by Fungi

INTRODUCTION

Abraham I. Braude

Except for their etiology, fungous infections differ little from bacterial infections. The close relationship between bacteria and fungi is apparent from transitional forms connecting the two classes, and from the similarity of the pathologic changes and clinical manifestations induced by them.

The intermediate, or transitional, forms are represented by the *Actinomyces*. These possess the characteristic branched mycelium of fungi but divide by segmentation into gram-positive bacillary or coccoid forms. The acid-fast property of one species, *Nocardia asteroides*, indicates a relationship to the tubercle bacillus. Although actinomycosis and nocardiosis are placed among the fungous diseases in this book, the causative agents remain in an uncertain position between fungi and bacteria.

An important characteristic of pathogenic fungi is dimorphism, growth in two distinct forms under different environmental conditions. The fungi responsible for blastomycosis, sporotrichosis, and histoplasmosis assume unicellular "yeast" forms in infected tissues but grow as mycelia and produce asexual spores on Sabouraud agar. The reverse is true for the fungus causing moniliasis. Another type of dimorphism is found in coccidioidomycosis. The organism responsible for this infection is multicellular in vivo and in vitro, but its form differs under the two conditions. In the tissues it is a sac filled with spores, but the growth on agar is a seg-

mented mycelium. *Cryptococcus neoformans* is the only pathogenic fungus that fails to change form when environmental conditions vary.

Mycotic diseases are not transmitted from one person to another. Many fungous infections are acquired by inhalation of spores growing freely in nature. These spores may be rectangular unicellular mycelial fragments known as *chlamydospores,* or spherical bodies borne on thin mycelial stalks and called *conidia.* Other infections, such as sporotrichosis, result from inoculation of spores directly into the skin.

A few fungous diseases are endogenous in origin. *Actinomyces bovis* and *Candida albicans* are normal residents of the bowel and mouth. When resistance is lowered, endogenous infection by either agent can develop. Actinomycosis is often preceded by tooth extraction, and overgrowth of normal saprophytic bacteria by *C. albicans* in the course of antibiotic therapy can lead to moniliasis.

The mechanisms whereby fungi produce disease are obscure. *Cryptococcus neoformans* possess a polysaccharide capsule similar to that of the pneumococcus which seems to protect the yeast from phagocytosis. This capsular material also produces mechanical injury in the nervous system. It is possible that the thick walls of other fungi such as *Blastomyces dermatiditis* and *Coccidioides immitis* function similarly as a protection against leukocytes. Some fungi are ingested by phagocytes but seem to flourish within these cells. In histoplasmosis, for example, the parasites are found in enormous numbers within reticuloendothelial cells. The endothelium of small vessels can become so packed with histoplasma organisms that blood flow is compromised.

Another possible factor in the pathogenesis of these infections is hypersensitivity. In most fungous diseases the patient exhibits marked local or even systemic reactivity to intradermal injection of the causative organism. In coccidioidomycosis this type of reaction is closely associated with the development of erythema nodosum and pleural effusions. The occurrence of necrosis at the site of injection of fungous antigens suggests that hypersensitivity may be responsible for necrosis of infected tissues. In other patients, however, widespread destruction of tissue can occur despite absence of dermal sensitivity.

Despite the differences in morphology and life cycle of fungi and bacteria, both elicit similar pathologic changes and clinical manifestations. For this reason, specific diagnosis can seldom be made with certainty without demonstration of the causative organism. Fortunately, most pathogenic fungi are easily seen in infected tissues or exudates. In a few circumstances, however, it is necessary to rely upon epidemiologic and immunologic methods for diagnosis.

The following chapters deal only with those infections in which fungi penetrate beneath the skin and mucous membranes to involve the underlying tissues and viscera.

153 ACTINOMYCOSIS
Abraham I. Braude

Definition. Actinomycosis is a noncontagious suppurative infection produced by an anaerobic organism normally resident in the mouth. The disease is characterized by chronic inflammatory induration and sinus formation.

Etiology. The causative agent is a branching gram-positive filamentous organism. Attempts have been made to recognize two separate anaerobic species of the genus *Actinomyces* on the basis of pathogenicity for man or cattle. Those who would make this differentiation have designated *Actinomyces bovis*, the culturally smooth form, as the agent responsible for actinomycosis in cattle and *A. israeli*, the rough form, as the etiologic agent of human actinomycosis. Because these smooth and rough forms are probably variants of the same species, the term *Actinomyces bovis* will be used here for all pathogenic anaerobic actinomyces.

Actinomyces bovis differs from other actinomyces in its intolerance of free oxygen and its failure to grow on Sabouraud's medium. It also has a much

greater tendency to fragment into short gram-positive rods (arthrospores). On blood agar, colonies require 4 to 6 days of anaerobic incubation at 37°C to reach a size of 1 to 2 mm. Although most strains require anaerobic conditions for isolation, some can be subcultured aerobically in 10 to 20 per cent carbon dioxide. *Actinomyces bovis* has never been found outside the human or animal body, and case-to-case transmission is unknown.

Pathogenesis. The oxidation-reduction potential of normal tissues is probably too high for multiplication of *A. bovis*, but devitalized tissues allow it to reproduce and gain a foothold from which it can spread. The frequency of actinomycotic lesions of the face and neck may be explained by the greater population of *A. bovis* on surfaces of teeth, in carious teeth and tonsillar crypts and by the frequent trauma to which these tissues are subjected by eating, by dental procedures, or by infection with oral bacteria. Anaerobic conditions also prevail in atelectatic areas of the lung after aspiration of *A. bovis* so that pulmonary actinomycosis can develop. It is also possible that pulmonary actinomycosis may arise hematogenously from an infected focus in the mouth. The exact mode of development of abdominal actinomycosis is unknown, but the frequency with which the cecal region is involved suggests that the conditions here favor devitalizing injury. Occasionally, perforation by a foreign body precedes infection.

From foci in the jaw, lung, or bowel, actinomycosis may spread by contiguity or through the blood to the liver, spine, brain, kidneys, internal genitalia, spleen, and subcutaneous tissues. Lymphatic spread is rare.

The inflammatory reaction to *A. bovis* is characterized by three features: (1) chronic suppuration, (2) extensive necrosis, and (3) intense fibrosis. The so-called "sulfur granules" which occupy a prominent place in the inflammatory lesion of actinomycosis are composed of intertwined mycelial filaments.

Clinical Manifestations. The essential feature of actinomycosis is a painful, indurated swelling. This lesion may appear over the jaw a week or more after such trauma as tooth extraction or compound fracture of the mandible. As it increases in size, points of suppuration, the openings of fistulas, appear on the bluish red surface of the edematous skin. Cervical lymphadenopathy is rare.

The lower lobes of the lung are frequently affected, and the disease can suddenly become evident only when the pleura and chest wall are involved by direct extension from the lung. Until then the patient may notice only fever, cough, and expectoration. Physical examination at this time reveals a diffuse, tender, indurated thoracic swelling with evidence of pulmonary consolidation and empyema. Actinomycosis of the lower chest can extend through the diaphragm to produce subphrenic or hepatic abscess.

Abdominal actinomycosis is often mistaken for appendicitis, carcinoma of the cecum, tuberculosis, or amebiasis. Patients with abdominal actinomycosis have been subjected to surgery for drainage of a supposed appendiceal abscess, the true nature of the disease being recognized only when an indurated draining sinus remains and stubbornly refuses to heal. Actinomycosis may also be mistaken for tumor of the reproductive organs in women or for tuberculous psoas abscess. Peritonitis is rare.

In the rare case of disseminated actinomycosis, lesions appear in all parts of the body as a result of hematogenous spread. Painful indurated nodules under the skin of the legs, arms, back, and scalp are prominent.

Diagnosis. The disease is easily recognized by detecting *A. bovis* in pus obtained from sinuses, empyema fluid, or abscess cavities. Interpretation of the finding of actinomyces in sputum is difficult, of course, because the organisms are normal inhabitants of the mouth. Sulfur granules vary in size from several microns to 3 mm in diameter. Large granules are nearly always found if a thorough search is made by diluting the pus with saline and filtering through gauze. They are white, yellow, or brown and stand out sharply against the background of blood-tinged pus. The conclusive finding, of course, is the demonstration of gram-positive filaments or bacilli which fail to grow aerobically on conventional laboratory media. Granules of other organisms (staphylococci, nocardias, monosporia), fragments of caseous material, and clumps of pus cells or fibrin may be confused with actinomycotic granules. The technique for recovery of *A. bovis* from the infected material differs from that of most other pathogenic fungi in two important respects: (1) Animal inoculation is of no value, and (2) Sabouraud medium will not support its growth. Cultural isolation of *A. bovis* is not difficult if any of several anaerobic methods is used. Inoculation of Brewer's thioglycollate medium or glucose-agar shake cultures is simple and satisfactory.

Biopsy examination may establish the diagnosis if the actinomycotic colony ("ray fungus") is observed microscopically. Demonstration of the organism can be exceedingly difficult, requiring careful search of many sections.

Intradermal or serologic tests with *A. bovis* or its fractions are of no diagnostic aid. Radiologic examination is rarely of specific value, because the intrathoracic lesions resemble tuberculosis or tumor and those in bone cannot be distinguished from bacterial osteomyelitis.

Treatment. Penicillin and the tetracycline antibiotics are effective. When either is administered in large doses over long periods of time, remarkable improvement may be expected even when the purulent processes are inaccessible to surgical drainage. Many reports indicate that the tetracycline drugs (chlortetracycline, oxytetracycline, tetracycline) are superior to penicillin. When the tetracyclines are given in doses of 500 mg every 6 hr, there is a reduction in pain and swelling within a few days as well as gain in strength, increase in weight, and prompt defervescence. Treatment should be continued for several weeks after the patient appears cured. Because penicillin is no more effective than the tetracyclines and because it requires repeated intramuscular or intravenous injection of large doses for long periods of time, it should be reserved for patients who cannot tolerate tetracycline drugs. The optimum dose of penicillin is not known. At least 1 million units daily should be given intramuscularly.

Surgical drainage or excision of accessible actinomycotic lesions is a valuable adjunct to chemotherapy, although surgery alone is of little value. Older treatments such as iodides, irradiation, or the sulfonamides have no place in the current therapeutic regimen for actinomycosis.

REFERENCES

Cope, V. Z.: "Actinomycosis," London, Oxford University Press, 1938.

Drake, C. H., M. T. Sudler, and R. I. Canuteson: A Case of Staphylococcic Actinophytosis (Botryomycosis) in Man, J.A.M.A., 123:339, 1943.

Garrod, L. P.: Actinomycosis of the Lung: Etiology, Diagnosis, and Chemotherapy, Tubercle, 33:258, 1952.

Lane, S. L., A. Kutscher, and R. Chaves: Oxytetracycline in the Treatment of Orocervical-Facial Actinomycosis: Report of Seven Cases, J.A.M.A., 151:986, 1953.

McVay, L. V., Jr., and D. H. Sprunt: A Long-term Evaluation of Aureomycin in the Treatment of Actinomycosis, Ann. Internal Med., 38:995, 1953.

Nichols, D. R., and W. E. Herrell: Penicillin in the Treatment of Actinomycosis, J. Lab. Clin. Med., 33:521, 1948.

Rosebury, T.: The Parasitic Actinomycetes and Other Filamentous Microorganisms of the Mouth: A Review of Their Characteristics and Relationships of the Bacteriology of Actinomycosis and of Salivary Calculus in Man, Bacteriol. Revs., 8:189, 1944.

154 CRYPTOCOCCOSIS
Abraham I. Braude

Definition. Cryptococcosis is a highly fatal infection caused by *Cryptococcus neoformans*, an encapsulated yeast with a special predilection for the central nervous system. Cryptococcosis can also involve the lungs, bones, and skin and occurs with increased frequency in patients with leukemias or lymphomas.

Etiology. Members of the genus *Cryptococcus*, to which *C. neoformans* belongs, form neither mycelia or spores and reproduce entirely by budding. The cells of *C. neoformans* are spherical, measure 5 to 15 μ in diameter, retain the Gram stain, and are surrounded by a capsule which may become so large that its total diameter is three times that of the cell proper. The capsular material contains a polysaccharide which is responsible for the slimy appearance of the yeast in culture and for the myxomatous character of cryptococcal lesions.

The organisms grow readily on various media at room temperature and at 37°C. On Sabouraud glucose agar, visible growth appears within a few days at 37°C and gradually assumes a characteristic brownish, slimy appearance. Unlike other pathogenic yeastlike fungi, cryptococci never form mycelia regardless of temperature of incubation or culture medium. Most cells of *C. neoformans* are killed in 24 hr at temperatures of 40.6°C or higher.

Pathogenesis and Pathology. Cryptococci resembling *C. neoformans* have been isolated from soil, pigeon droppings, the surface of fruit, and from the skin and intestinal tract of normal man. Hence is it possible for infections to be either of endogenous or exogenous origin. Whatever the mode of entry may be, the organism ultimately finds its way to the nervous system in most cases of cryptococcosis. Although the neurologic disturbances overshadow those produced elsewhere, there is good evidence that foci of infection are usually established in the lung and other viscera before dissemination to the brain and the meninges occurs. Often the pulmonary foci give rise to no clinical findings, although they can be detected if a careful search is made at postmortem examination.

Penetration of tissues by the cryptococcus does not evoke the active inflammatory response observed with other fungi or bacteria. The cellular reaction is very slow to develop and is seldom intense. The cryptococcus seems to meet little resistance and frequently proliferates so freely that macroscopic masses of gelatinous yeasts fill the lesions. Older lesions occasionally show granulomatous reactions. The small number of cryptococci observed within granulomas suggests that they can destroy the organism. This may account in part for the fact that lymphomatous diseases involving the mononuclear cells lower resistance to cryptococcal infection. At other times, however, many cryptococci are present within mononuclear and giant cells. It is unusual to see necrosis of the host tissue in cryptococcosis.

Granulomas or gelatinous cryptococcal masses can appear in the nervous system, lungs, bones, or skin. In the nervous system, lesions usually develop in the meninges at the base of the brain with resulting involvement of the brain stem, cranial nerves, and cerebellum. Large masses of yeast may accumulate in the subarachnoid space and extend diffusely along perivascular spaces into the brain substance to produce cystic nodules. Because the fungal masses shrink after fixation of the brain in formalin, cystlike spaces remain. These spaces were thought to result from a histolytic action of the fungus by early observers who named the yeast *Torula histolytica*. In the lung, either scattered miliary nodules, diffuse pneumonic infiltrations, or solitary masses easily mistaken for pulmonary neoplasms may occur. Pulmonary cavitation, calcification or hilar lymphadenopathy is extremely rare. These characteristics of the cryptococcal pulmonary lesions are helpful in distinguishing the disease from tuberculosis, sarcoidosis, and other mycoses.

Clinical Manifestations. Most patients with cryptococcal infection come under the care of a physician after the onset of neurologic manifestations. Complaints of severe headache, diplopia, dizziness, ataxia, vomiting, tinnitus, memory disturbances, or Jacksonian convulsions are common. Fever is usually low and can be absent. Many patients die within a few months, but some have lived for many years as the disease undergoes remissions and relapses.

When pulmonary infection is present in the absence of meningoencephalitis, the patient is generally free of constitutional symptoms. The disease is detected when roentgenographic examination of the chest shows a dense, usually solitary infiltration of the lower portions of the lung. Cough may be a prominent feature of diffuse cryptococcal pneumonia.

Involvement of bones in the absence of disseminated disease is rare, and cryptococcosis of joints is almost always secondary to adjacent osseous lesions.

Disseminated infection may also produce multiple nodules or papules in the skin. These range from a few millimeters in diameter to masses resembling strawberries in size and color.

The possibility of underlying Hodgkin's disease, lymphosarcoma, or leukemia should be considered in every patient with cryptococcosis.

Diagnosis. Cryptococcal meningitis must be distinguished from other diseases which present the syndrome of aseptic meningitis (p. 1136) such as brain abscess, tuberculous meningitis, and coccidioidal meningitis. In each of these, the spinal fluid is sterile by ordinary cultural methods and may contain from a few to several hundred mononuclear cells, an increased amount of protein, and a reduced concentration of glucose. Because *C. neoformans* is recovered with much greater ease than the etiologic agents of the other diseases, culture of the spinal fluid is the decisive procedure in differential diagnosis. The cryptococcus is isolated on Sabouraud's agar at room temperature and can usually be recognized after 1 to 2 weeks. In tuberculous and coccidioidal meningitis positive cultures are much fewer, and in uncomplicated brain abscess the spinal fluid is sterile. Cryptococcal cells may also be found by direct microscopic examination of sediment from centrifuged spinal fluid. Mixing a drop of sediment with India ink on a glass slide facilitates the recognition of the mucinous capsule. The organism can also be seen in tissue removed by biopsy. Intracellular forms with small capsules can resemble *Histoplasma capsulatun* but may be differentiated by mucicarmine, which stains the capsular mucopolysaccharide peculiar to *C. neoformans*. Biopsied material should also be inoculated intraperitoneally in white mice. *Cryptococcus neoformans* is highly pathogenic for these animals and readily demonstrated microscopically in sections or smears of their brains. Serologic or skin tests are of no value in diagnosis.

Treatment. All forms of cryptococcosis usually improve after intravenous infusions of 75 to 125 mg amphotericin B daily. Patients without meningoencephalitis can be cured with total doses of less than 1.5 Gm, but 3.0 Gm is probably required for infections of the nervous system. If meningeal relapse occurs after intravenous treatment, amphotericin B may be dissolved in the spinal fluid and 0.5 mg injected intrathecally on alternate days in conjunction with intravenous administration. Strict precautions must be taken during intrathecal injection to avoid bacterial contamination and drug overdosage. One milligram amphotericin B intrathecally may cause fever, temporary paralysis of the bladder and legs, and arachnoiditis.

Because of the susceptibility of cryptococci to heat, hyperthermia has been suggested as a form of treatment but has received little trial.

REFERENCES

Beeson, P. B.: Cryptococcic Meningitis of Nearly Sixteen Years' Duration, A.M.A. Arch. Internal Med., 89:797, 1952.

Kuhn, L. R.: Growth and Viability of *Cryptococcus hominis* at Mouse and Rabbit Body Temperatures, Proc. Soc. Exptl. Biol. Med., 41:573, 1939.

Littman, M. L., and L. E. Zimmerman: "Cryptococcosis," New York, Grune & Stratton, Inc., 1956.

155 NORTH AMERICAN BLASTOMYCOSIS

Abraham I. Braude

Definition. North American blastomycosis is a fungous infection of the skin and viscera caused by *Blastomyces dermatiditis*.

Etiology. In infected tissues, *B. dermatiditis* has the appearance of a yeast, forming single buds from 3 to 24 μ in diameter. Two features aid in recognition: (1) its thick wall, spoken of as "double-contoured," because the inner and outer margins can be seen, and (2) the wide opening between parent cell and bud at the base of attachment.

In culture, the fungus is dimorphic and appears as the wrinkled, waxy yeast form on blood agar incubated at 37°C, or as a mold with branching hyphae on Sabouraud's agar at room temperature. On microscopic examination the cultured yeast may be identical with that in the infected lesions or may have abortive mycelia. The mycelia give rise to oval or pear-shaped exogenous spores.

Pathogenesis and Pathology. The skin has been proposed as a portal of entry because cutaneous lesions are prominent and because infections have followed injury to the skin. The lung is also a likely portal but the fungus has never been cultured from the soil. During the epidemic in Grifton, N.C., in 1954 (Smith, Harris, Conant, and Smith), all patients had pulmonary disease, and only one had a blastomycotic lesion of the skin; yet a respiratory mode of transmission could not be proved.

The characteristic pathologic features are found in the lung and skin. Pulmonary lesions consist of focal granulomas or diffuse purulent pneumonia and vary in size from miliary nodules to confluent areas involving an entire lobe. The granulomas can undergo caseation and fibrosis. *Blastomyces dermatiditis* is often found within giant cells or other phagocytes, facilitating differentiation from tuberculosis.

The characteristic cutaneous lesion consists of microabscesses just beneath the epidermis, surrounded by a granulomatous reaction. The epidermis itself often becomes so hyperplastic that it resembles an epithelioma.

The infection can spread to the brain, bones, urogenital tract, liver, spleen, and lymph nodes.

Clinical Manifestations. In the typical case of systemic blastomycosis the onset is insidious. The patient may seek medical attention because of a persistent "chest cold," low-grade fever, weight loss, or progressive disability. Physical examination and roentgenogram of the chest disclose evidence of pneumonia, which can involve any segment or lobe of the lung. Cavitation is frequent, and mediastinal lymph nodes may be prominently enlarged. Hemoptysis, purulent sputum, chest pain, and dyspnea appear as the disease progresses. Although the pulmonary infection can subside spontaneously, extrapulmonary lesions of the skin, bones, joints, and viscera eventually call attention to dissemination in many patients. These metastatic suppurative lesions are accompanied by an increase in fever, sweats, chills, and weakness. Death in the untreated infection sometimes occurs in less than 6 months, but most patients live for a year or two. The over-all mortality rate in systemic blastomycosis is said to be 92 per cent in patients who have been followed for 2 years or longer without specific therapy.

Primary infection of the skin (Gilchrist's disease) first appears on an unclothed area such as the hands, face, or forearm but not the scalp, palms, or soles. The infection begins as a firm nodule surrounded soon by similar lesions which tend to coalesce. Suppuration in the center of the nodule is followed by partial healing, and fibrosis as extension occurs peripherally. The hyperplasia of the epithelium gives these lesions a hard, raised, wartlike margin. When fully developed, blastomycosis of the skin presents the appearance of one or more ragged ulcers with partially healed centers and thick raised margins. The primary cutaneous infection may be confined to the skin for months or years before it spreads to the viscera.

Diagnosis. Pulmonary blastomycosis closely resembles tuberculosis, carcinoma of the lung, aspiration pneumonitis, and other fungous infections including coccidioidomycosis, actinomycosis, nocardiosis, and histoplasmosis. Differentiation must be based on the recovery of the etiologic agent, because neither clinical nor epidemiologic features are specific. Most cases of North American blastomycosis are found in the Southeastern United States and in the Mississippi River Valley, but the disease occurs throughout the United States and Canada. Occupational history, sex, race, and age are of no diagnostic aid.

It is usually possible to find *B. dermatiditis* by microscopic examination of biopsied material, sputum, or pus. The thick-walled, yeastlike form can be readily observed if a drop of purulent material is first mixed on a slide with a drop of 20 per cent potassium hydroxide and kept at room temperature for 30 min. *Blastomyces dermatiditis* is readily isolated by culturing pus on Sabouraud's agar at room temperature and on blood agar at 37°C. Inoculation of mice or other animals is usually not a successful method for recovering the fungus because of low pathogenicity for laboratory animals.

The value of the skin test for blastomycosis, using killed cells or blastomycin, is limited because of negative reactions in patients with disseminated infection and cross reactions in persons with hyper-sensitivity to coccidioidin or histoplasmin. The complement fixation test is positive in high titer with sera of patients who have systemic infections. The results of intradermal and serologic tests may be of prognostic value. Patients with marked dermal hypersensitivity and low serum titers of complement-fixing antibody are said to have a better prognosis than those with negative skin tests and high complement fixation titers. Neutrophilic leukocytosis and hypochromic anemia are usually present in systemic blastomycosis.

Treatment. Amphotericin B is probably superior to 2-hydroxystilbamidine. Either drug is given daily or every other day by slow intravenous drip in increasing doses. The maximum daily dose of amphotericin B is 75 to 100 mg and that of 2-hydroxystilbamidine is 250 mg. Complete arrest has been observed after a total of 1.0 Gm amphotericin B, while 4 to 10 Gm of 2-hydroxystilbamidine may be required. Nausea, vomiting, azotemia, and hepatic dysfunction often develop from injections of amphotericin B but disappear when treatment is stopped. Anesthesia over the distribution of the trigeminal nerve is the main untoward reaction from 2-hydroxystilbamidine and persists after treatment. Surgical excision of pulmonary cavities or destroyed tissues is sometimes necessary in addition to chemotherapy.

REFERENCES

Harrell, E. R., and A. C. Curtis: North American Blastomycosis, Am. J. Med., 27:750, 1959.

Martin, D. S., and D. T. Smith: Blastomycosis (American Blastomycosis, Gilchrist's Disease): Review of the Literature, Am. Rev. Tuberc., 39:257, 1939.

Smith, J. G., J. S. Harris, N. F. Conant, and D. T. Smith: An Epidemic of North American Blastomycosis, J.A.M.A., 158:641, 1955.

156 COCCIDIOIDOMYCOSIS
Abraham I. Braude

Definition. Coccidioidomycosis is an infection acquired by inhalation of *Coccidioides immitis*, a fungus existing only in the mycelial phase in nature and converted to a spherule in tissues. Although most infections are mild or unapparent, *C. immitis* may produce a fatal disseminated disease with destructive lesions in the lungs, lymph nodes, spleen, liver, bones, kidneys, and brain.

Etiology. Unlike other dimorphic pathogenic fungi, *C. immitis* can be cultured only in the mycelial phase. It grows readily at room temperature or at 35°C and produces white, cottony mycelia. As a culture ages, the segmented mycelium breaks up into thick-coated rectangular *arthrospores,* 2 by 4 μ in size. These arthrospores can survive in stored cultures and are highly infectious for laboratory personnel. The mycelium and its spores are pathogenic for various laboratory animals. The mycelial form is converted to a thick-walled spherule filled with endospores in animal tissues.

Pathogenesis and Pathology. Coccidioidomycosis is acquired by inhalation of *chlamydospores* in endemic areas in the semiarid regions of the Southwestern United States and the Chaco district of Argentina. The majority of infections occur during the dry seasons, particularly after exposure to dust storms. The fungus is thought to grow in the soil in rainy weather and become disseminated in dust during dry weather. This concept is supported by isolations of *C. immitis* from soil and from desert rodents. These animals are thought to be a reservoir for contamination of soil.

The inhaled spores are carried to the terminal bronchioles and alveoli, where the first reaction is an outpouring of polymorphonuclear leukocytes, fluid, and a few mononuclear cells. In most cases, the organism is probably killed, or at least arrested at a stage when the lesion is too small to be detected by clinical means. In others, the organisms proliferate and elicit a varying inflammatory response which appears to depend on the rate of multiplication of the fungus. The phase of rapid multiplication, as manifested by frequent discharge of endospores from the ripened spherules, elicits suppuration and an exudate rich in polymorphonuclear leukocytes. The phase of slow multiplication, with infrequent rupture of spherules, produces a granulomatous reaction in which epithelioid cells and giant cells predominate. Although polymorphonuclear leukocytes congregate about the point of rupture of a spherule and actually invade the broken capsule, attempts at phagocytosis by these cells are unsuccessful. As the released endospores develop into spherules, the neutrophilic reaction gives way to proliferating mononuclear cells which often are able to ingest the fungus.

Either phase of this inflammatory cycle may predominate, or a mixture of the two may be found. Rapidly progressive infections produce large areas of confluent suppurative pneumonia and necrosis of adjacent bronchi. In contrast, granulomatous lesions contain exudates composed almost exclusively of mononuclear cells and giant cells which fill the alveoli but leave their walls intact. Both reactions are accompanied by involvement of the overlying pleura and of the hilar and mediastinal lymph nodes. Ultimately the bronchopneumonia in most patients resolves or heals by fibrosis; in others, the lesions are permanently arrested but persist as cavities or solid nodules.

Recovery is accompanied by the development of hypersensitivity to the fungus. This hypersensitivity is apparently responsible for at least two special pathologic manifestations: (1) *erythema nodosum;* this is a sterile focal nodular granulomatous reaction usually limited to the skin of the lower extremities and characterized by extravasation of red cells into the lesion (p. 1924); (2) *pleural effusion.* It is believed that rupture of a pleural granuloma discharges antigenic material onto the sensitized pleural membranes.

In patients who do not tend to develop dermal hypersensitivity, the infection spreads systemically to involve lymph nodes, spleen, bones, liver, kidney, meninges, skin, adrenals, and pericardium. In the meninges, the two inflammatory reactions can take special forms: (1) the granulomatous reaction is commoner and produces a firm plastic lesion which encloses the brain stem and other structures in a rigid mass of tissue; (2) the suppurative reaction results in outpouring of polymorphonuclear leukocytes with little granulomatous change. In either type, but especially in the granulomatous, the involvement of the brain stem can lead to severe hydrocephalus.

Clinical Manifestations. The infection may be either benign or disseminated. The benign infection, so-called "desert fever," is self-limited. As many as 50 per cent of benign infections are asymptomatic. The remainder are accompanied by symptoms like those of influenza or pneumonia. After an incubation period of 1 to 3 weeks, the patient experiences fever, chills, fatigue, headache, severe arthralgia, and symptoms of respiratory infection. The most frequent complaint is poorly localized chest pain, aggravated by breathing or coughing. Some patients also experience substernal pain on swallowing of sufficient severity to prevent eating solid food. A nonproductive cough is common but hemoptysis is infrequent. Physical findings are scant except in those patients (3 to 20 per cent) who develop erythema nodosum or pleural effusion. Although hydrothorax may be massive and require repeated thoracenteses, it eventually resorbs without further difficulty.

Despite the paucity of signs in the chest, prominent abnormalities are found in roentgenograms. These include focal areas of pneumonic infiltration, hilar and mediastinal lymphadenopathy, pulmonary nodules or cavities, and pleural effusion. The commonest are single or multiple infiltrations which may appear in any segment and can simulate secondary tuberculosis if the upper lobe is involved. They usually resolve after several weeks.

In about 2 per cent of benign infections a solid or cavitary pulmonary lesion remains after the active stage is over. The typical cavity of coccidioidomycosis is peripheral, has a thin wall, and gives a cystlike appearance in roentgenograms. Bronchoscopic examination may disclose stenosis and ulceration of the bronchus leading to the corresponding lobe. This deep bronchial disease is responsible for the distention of the cavities. Residual solid lesions can be as large as 3 cm in diameter. Both solid and cavitary lesions are commoner in the upper lobes. Calcification is rare.

In a relatively few individuals (0.05 to 0.2 per cent), the primary infection progresses to the disseminated form of the disease. Dissemination usually occurs within a few months of infection. Dark-skinned persons are more vulnerable to this type of spread and experience a higher death rate. Among Negroes and Filipinos, 85 to 90 per cent with dissemination succumb, as compared to 50 per cent of whites. Patients who develop progressive coccidioidomycosis do not give a history of erythema nodosum.

The course of disseminated infection is marked by the appearance of fungating or ulcerating skin lesions, multiple pulmonary nodules or cavities, widespread destructive lymphadenopathy, osteomyelitis, and meningitis. Weight loss, fever, and weakness are the outstanding systemic manifestations, and the course is often rapid with death occurring in less than a year. If vital organs are spared, however, patients with disseminated coccidioidomycosis may feel surprisingly well, continue to work, and even gain weight despite the presence of large numbers of *C. immitis* in the sputum or subcutaneous abscesses. The meningeal form is invariably fatal, but even this is compatible with survival for several years. In the presence of meningitis with progressive hydrocephalus, patients experience severe headaches, cranial nerve palsies, memory disturbances, and disorientation. The spinal fluid shows 100 to 200 cells, mostly mononuclear, elevated protein, and frequently a reduction in glucose concentration.

Diagnosis. With the exception of meningitis, *C. immitis* is easily recovered from the lesions of disseminated coccidioidomycosis by direct examination and cultures of exudates or biopsied tissues. The characteristic spherule with endospores is best seen in purulent material treated with 20 per cent potassium hydroxide. Occasionally, in biopsied tissue, spherules may all be immature and contain no endospores, making them indistinguishable from *Blastomyces dermatiditis*. Cultural identification becomes essential for diagnosis. On Sabouraud agar, mycelial growth appears in 4 to 8 days, and inoculation of mice produces multiple necrotic lesions containing spherules. In meningitis, only a few spherules appear in the spinal fluid, despite the presence of large numbers in the granulomatous exudate around the brain stem. Occasionally, the culture of 20 to 30 ml of spinal fluid yields positive results, but

sometimes the diagnosis can only be based on serologic tests.

Serologic tests are performed with coccidioidin, a filtrate from cultures of *C. immitis*. By the third week of primary infection, precipitins are found in the serum of 91 per cent of patients with symptomatic infection but in only 7 per cent of asymptomatic individuals. Complement-fixing antibodies appear later and persist longer than precipitins in nondisseminated coccidioidomycosis; they are almost always present in the disseminated disease. Intradermal tests with coccidioidin are of value in the recognition of primary benign infections because they become positive before the precipitins appear, but in disseminated infection the skin test is frequently negative.

The roentgenographic appearance of pulmonary lesions is suggestive of primary coccidioidomycosis if hilar lymphadenopathy progresses while the parenchymal infiltrate is subsiding or if the adenopathy is associated with multiple areas of pneumonitis. A residual smooth, thin-walled cavity without surrounding parenchymal infiltration is also characteristic of the primary form of the disease. Other residual lesions include calcified or noncalcified nodular foci and localized bronchiectasis. In disseminated pulmonary infection the commonest picture is that of multiple infiltrations accompanied by pleural involvement and prominent hilar or mediastinal lymphadenopathy.

The only remarkable hematologic finding is eosinophilia, which may reach 35 per cent of the total leukocyte count in the primary disease.

Treatment. Intensive intravenous treatment with amphotericin B in daily doses of 1.0 mg per kg body weight appears to be highly effective in extrameningeal coccidioidomycosis. Coccidioidal meningitis requires repeated intrathecal injections of 0.5 mg amphotericin B. The total dose necessary for successful treatment varies from less than 1.0 Gm to more than 10.0 Gm intravenously and as much as 45 mg intrathecally. Severe nausea, venous thrombosis, and reversible impairment of renal and hepatic function often interrupt the treatment schedule, but persistent administration of amphotericin B in the face of troublesome side effects is required for favorable clinical results. A fall in titer of complement-fixing antibodies and a return of coccidioidin skin sensitivity are signs of effective treatment. Drug therapy should be supplemented if possible by surgical removal of peripheral granulomas.

Primary surgical excision of residual pulmonary foci is indicated if these lesions become troublesome because of secondary infection or hemoptysis. Dissemination of the disease from these foci almost never occurs.

REFERENCES

Baker, O. B., and A. I. Braude: A Study of Stimuli Leading to the Production of Spherules of Coccidioidomycosis, J. Lab. Clin. Med., 47:169, 1956.

Emmons, C. S.: Isolation of *Coccidioides* from Soil and Rodents, U.S. Public Health Repts., 57:109, 1942.

Fiese, M. J.: "Coccidioidomycosis," Springfield, Ill., Charles C Thomas, Publisher, 1958.

Forbus, W. D., and A. M. Bestebreurtje: Coccidioidomycosis: A Study of 95 Cases of the Disseminated Type with Special Reference to the Pathogenesis of the Disease, Military Surgeon, 99:654, 1946.

Forsee, J. H., and R. B. Perkins: Focalized Pulmonary Coccidioidomycosis: A Surgical Disease, J.A.M.A., 155:1223, 1956.

Peck, W. A., and S. S. Romendick: Coccidioidomycosis: A Roentgen Study, Texas State J. Med., 52:86, 1956.

Smith, C. E., M. T. Saito, and S. A. Simons: Pattern of 39,500 Serologic Tests in Coccidioidomycosis, J.A.M.A., 160:546, 1956.

Taylor, A. B., and A. K. Briney: Observations on Primary Coccidioidomycosis, Ann. Internal Med., 30:1224, 1949.

157 HISTOPLASMOSIS
Abraham I. Braude

Definition. Histoplasmosis is a protean infection caused by the dimorphic fungus *Histoplasma capsulatum,* an organism found as a tiny body within reticuloendothelial cells. The disease varies from mild or unnoticed respiratory infection to widely disseminated lethal disease characterized by fever, anemia, hepatomegaly, splenomegaly, leukopenia, pulmonary lesions, ulcerations of the gastrointestinal tract, and adrenal necrosis.

Etiology. Although *H. capsulatum* grows on Sabouraud's agar at room temperature as a spore-bearing mold, it is transformed upon animal inoculation into nonencapsulated oval yeastlike cells measuring 2 by 4 μ. In histologic section the protoplasm is shrunken so that the unstained space beneath the cell wall has the appearance of a capsule. The name *capsulatum* is based on a misinterpretation of the nature of this unstained space. The fungus also grows in the yeastlike phase if incubated at 37°C in sealed tubes of blood agar. The most distinctive cultural feature, however, is the tuberculate *chlamydospore* found only on mycelia; it is round, 10 by 20 μ in diameter, and covered with warty projections. Another smaller spore, not distinguishable from that of *Blastomyces dermatiditis,* is also present on the mycelium.

Pathology and Pathogenesis. The source of human infection is probably soil containing spores of *Histoplasma.* Several studies have emphasized the isolation of the fungus from soil in areas inhabited by chickens. In most cases the portal of entry is probably the lung, where a primary complex may be formed by extension of infection from the pulmonary focus to the regional lymph nodes. Infection through the gastrointestinal tract must also be considered in patients whose initial lesions are in the mouth and pharynx.

The basic pathologic process is the multiplication of *H. capsulatum* in cells of the reticuloendothelial system. The yeast form multiplies extensively and greatly distends the cells. As proliferating histiocytes encroach on parenchymal cells, the infected organ becomes enlarged. The liver, lymph nodes, lung, spleen, adrenal, bowel, and marrow may be affected by this diffuse reticuloendothelial disturbance in disseminated histoplasmosis.

In addition to the diffuse lesions of the reticuloendothelial system, the tissues contain nodular accumulations of epithelioid cells and giant cells of the Langhans type. The noncaseous granuloma probably represents an effective defensive action, and histoplasma organisms are difficult to demonstrate in the epithelioid cells of such a lesion. Caseous necrosis may accompany both types of lesion. The adrenals, which are involved in nearly all disseminated infections, are often massively enlarged. Caseous necrosis is usually present in the center of the pulmonary granulomas, which resemble those of cavitary pulmonary tuberculosis. Necrotizing histoplasmosis may also take the form of renal papillitis. Extracellular forms of histoplasma are readily found in the necrotic areas of all organs by special stains (periodic acid–Schiff, Gridley). These extracellular organisms may be much larger than the intracellular ones, appear distorted, and occasionally assume the mycelial form.

Clinical Manifestations. The signs and symptoms of histoplasmosis range from those of a slight self-limited infection to the overwhelming disturbances of fatal disseminated disease. The high incidence of positive intradermal reactions to histoplasmosis in healthy persons in many parts of the world indicates that most infections by *H. capsulatum* are inapparent or very mild. This variability in severity is observed among different persons involved in the same outbreak. Severe infections are characterized by prolonged fever, dyspnea, chest pain, weight loss, prostration, widespread pulmonary infiltrates, hepatomegaly, and splenomegaly. Other infected persons may exhibit only a benign acute pneumonitis lasting a week or less, while still others are entirely free of symptoms. Widespread ill-defined noncalcified pulmonary infiltrates of miliary size or larger are found in symptomatic infections and may also be present, although less extensively, in the asymptomatic ones. Eventually, pulmonary lesions either disappear or calcify. In the east central part of the United States there is a high incidence of pulmonary calcification in persons who have negative tuberculin and positive histoplasmin skin tests.

Least resistance to histoplasmosis is encountered in young infants and adults after the fifth decade. Most cases of disseminated infection have occurred at these extremes of life, but with somewhat different clinical manifestations in the two groups. In the infant there are fever, emaciation, anemia, and leukopenia, and evidence of widespread involvement of many viscera including the liver, spleen, lung, bowel, lymph nodes, adrenals, skin, kidney, brain, eye, or endocardium. While the same degree of dissemination may occasionally occur in the adult, usually the visceral involvement is less widespread. Unlike the disease in infancy, adult histoplasmosis shows a marked predilection for men. Histoplasmosis of the lips, mouth, nose, and larynx occurs almost exclusively in adults and is the initial manifestation in about one-third of the fatal cases. Among the various syndromes encountered are subacute vegetative endocarditis, massive lymphadenopathy resembling tuberculosis or lymphoma, various forms of pneumonia including an interstitial type with capillary-alveolar block, and meningitis. The last is characterized by signs of basilar localization with spinal fluid findings and a clinical course identical with those of tuberculous meningitis.

In addition to the acute benign and disseminated infections, chronic localized histoplasmosis occurs in adults. Although frequently accompanied by necrosis or ulceration, this form is basically a granuloma, and its tendency to remain localized is probably related to the effective defensive activity of the granulomatous reaction.

Two main clinical types of chronic localized histoplasmosis are encountered: (1) *Pulmonary.* This may resemble pulmonary tuberculosis in all respects. The patient can be asymptomatic or complain of a chronic and occasionally productive cough. Roentgenograms will show lesions identical with those of reinfection tuberculosis, sometimes with cavitation, and accompanied by consistently positive cultures of sputum for *H. capsulatum.* (2) *Mucocutaneous.* Ulcers of the mouth, tongue, pharynx, gums, larynx, penis, or bladder are rare lesions found only in adults. Regional lymphadenopathy is common in these types.

Diagnosis. Isolation of *H. capsulatum* is not difficult in disseminated or chronic localized infections if cultures are made of bone marrow, blood, biopsied lesions, sputum, or exudate from an ulcer. After incubation of infected material on Sabouraud agar at room temperature there appears a white cottony colony which later turns brown and produces the diagnostic tuberculate chlamydospores. Material may also be cultured at 37°C on Francis' medium or blood agar, but the growth is yeastlike, and the diagnostic spores are not found. Isolation from sputum is best accomplished in mice, because contaminants are suppressed and the mouse is extremely susceptible to infection by histoplasmas. The animal does not die, but subculture of the spleen one month later on Sabouraud agar yields the organism. Histoplasmas may also be seen in bone marrow, material from open or biopsied lesions, and occasionally in blood smears of terminally ill patients. Special fungus stains (periodic acid–Schiff, Gridley) should be used. Certain intracellular forms of *Cryptococcus neoformans* may be indistinguishable from histoplasma in histologic sections, unless strains for the cryptococcal mucinous capsule are employed.

In those cases from which *H. capsulatum* cannot be isolated, indirect clues to identification are: (1) history of exposure to soil or dust in an endemic area, (2) positive complement fixation tests, (3) positive histoplasmin skin tests, and (4) development of miliary calcifications in the lung. Although these criteria are not dependable individually, they appear to be reliable when used together. The serologic and skin tests are frequently negative in culturally proved cases of histoplasmosis, and their specificity is not fully established.

Histoplasmosis must be differentiated from tuberculosis, sarcoid, leukemia, infectious mononucleosis, Hodgkin's disease, brucellosis, and kala-azar. Because cortisone is frequently of value in sarcoid, but can cause dissemination in histoplasmosis, differential diagnosis between these two diseases is critical. Biopsied tissue in both diseases contains morphologically identical granulomas. For this reason the diagnosis of sarcoid should be withheld until tissues have been examined with special fungus stains. In kala-azar the intracellular Leishman-Donovan body bears a close resemblance to *H. capsulatum,* and cultural isolation of the fungus may be important in distinguishing between the two.

Treatment. Amphotericin B, in intravenous doses of 50 to 100 mg daily, is effective in all forms of histoplasmosis. Treatment given daily, or on alternate days, must be continued for periods varying from one month to many months. Sulfadiazine or triple sulfonamides have also been effective in adults in oral doses of 6 Gm daily and may be given in conjunction with intravenous amphotericin B.

REFERENCES

Binford, C. H.: Histoplasmosis: Tissue Reaction, and Morphologic Variations in the Fungus, Am. J. Clin. Pathol., 25:25, 1955.

Emmons, C. W.: Histoplasmosis, Bull. N.Y. Acad. Med., 31:627, 1955.

Loosli, C., G. T. Grayston, E. R. Alexander, and F. Tanzi: Epidemiological Studies of Pulmonary Histoplasmosis in a Farm Family, Am. J. Hyg., 55: 392, 1952.

Parsons, R. J., and C. J. D. Zarafonetis: Histoplasmosis in Man: Report of Seven Cases and Review of Seventy-one Cases, Arch. Internal Med., 75:1, 1945.

Shapiro, J. L., J. J. Lux, and B. E. Sprofkin: Histoplasmosis of the Central Nervous System, Am. J. Pathol., 31:319, 1955.

Sweany, Henry C.: "Histoplasmosis," Springfield, Ill., Charles C Thomas, Publisher, 1960.

158 SPOROTRICHOSIS
Abraham I. Braude

Definition. Sporotrichosis is a chronic infection due to *Sporotrichum schencki*. It is characterized by the formation of suppurating nodules along the lymphatics of the skin and subcutaneous tissues. Hematogenous dissemination is rare.

Etiology. The fungus *S. schencki* is dimorphic. On Sabouraud's agar at room temperature its growth is mycelial, but in the tissue it takes the form of tiny, cigar-shaped yeast cells. The yeast phase also develops in vitro by incubation at 37°C on blood agar containing cystine.

Pathogenesis and Pathology. The fungus lives as a saprophyte on vegetation and penetrates the hands when the skin is broken. Many cases have followed injury by thorns, and an outbreak of sporotrichosis occurred among South African natives exposed to *S. schencki* growing on timbers supporting a gold mine.

After penetrating the skin, the fungus spreads up the extremities and evokes nodular lesions along the thickened lymphatics. Microscopically the nodules are granulomas with central necrosis. In exceedingly rare infections the organism may become disseminated throughout the subcutaneous tissues, the liver, testicles, bone, and kidney. Disseminated disease is not usually accompanied by primary infections of the extremities, and its portal of entry, therefore, is believed to be in the gastrointestinal tract.

Clinical Manifestations. There is a marked disproportion between symptoms and findings. A chain of hard, reddened discrete lumps extends up the arm or leg to the axilla or groin, and the intervening lymphatics are red and thickened, but there is no pain, fever, or other constitutional symptoms. Older nodules often rupture to produce fistulas or ulcers. In the rare patient with disseminated sporotrichosis, constitutional symptoms may be marked and the disease rapidly fatal. Unlike other disseminated mycoses, sporotrichosis almost never involves the lungs or central nervous system.

Without treatment, sporotrichosis does not heal, and the lesions often become secondarily infected with bacteria.

Diagnosis. The fungus cannot be seen upon microscopic examination of biopsied material or pus in most cases. Cultural isolation is invariably successful, however, if pus is aspirated from an unbroken nodule and inoculated onto Sabouraud agar. The growth at first has the soft creamy character of bacterial colonies and later develops a wrinkled dark brown appearance without the cottonlike filament of most molds. Microscopically, typical clusters of pear-shaped spores are found at the tips of conidiophores arising from the tangled mass of delicate branched mycelia. If the mold, or the pus is inoculated intraperitoneally into mice or rats, numerous yeast forms will be seen in lesions of the peritoneal cavity or testicle, where they take the form of gram-positive cigar-shaped rods within polymorphonuclear leukocytes.

Recovery of the organism by these techniques permits ready differentiation of sporotrichosis from other chronic infections of the subcutaneous tissues such as syphilis, tularemia, blastomycosis, coccidioidomycosis, and tuberculosis (see p. 999). The hard sporotrichotic lesions are sometimes mistaken for syphilitic gummas, and their response to iodides can be interpreted as therapeutic proof of the diagnosis.

Treatment. Sporotrichosis is almost invariably dramatically cured by saturated potassium iodide. This should be given orally in starting doses of 10 drops t.i.d. after meals and gradually increased to the point of maximum tolerance. Treatment should be continued for a month after lesions disappear. Additional local therapy may be required for cutaneous ulcers, which should be painted with tincture of iodine. It may also be necessary to excise the epidermal lesions, as these do not usually subside with oral iodides.

REFERENCES

Cawley, E. P.: Sporotrichosis, a Protean Disease: With Report of a Disseminated Gummatous Case of the Disease, Ann. Internal Med., 30:1287, 1949.

Forester, R. H.: Sporotrichosis: An Occupational Dermatosis, J.A.M.A., 87:1605, 1926.

Ruediger, G. F.: Sporotrichosis in the United States. J. Infectious Diseases, 11:193, 1917.

159 MONILIASIS (Candidiasis)
Abraham I. Braude

Definition. Moniliasis is a common mild mucocutaneous infection due to *Candida albicans*. This fungus is also an unusual cause of widespread visceral infection.

Etiology. Among the many species of *Candida*, only *C. albicans* is pathogenic for man. On the usual nutrient laboratory media *C. albicans* grows as a budding yeast in creamy white colonies, but produces both mycelia and yeastlike cells in infected tissues.

Pathogenesis. *Candida albicans* resides normally on the mucous membranes and is frequently cultured from the mouth and feces of persons in good health. The rate of cultural isolation from feces in numerous surveys has ranged from 14 to 19 per cent. In debilitated infants, and sometimes in adults, the fungus may produce white patches on the buccal mucosa and initiate mild inflammatory reaction in the underlying tissues. In pregnancy and diabetes, *C. albicans* frequently establishes a mild superficial infection of the vagina. Presumably, the high glycogen content of the vaginal mucosa in pregnancy and the glycosuria of diabetes favor its growth. Candida multiplies excessively in the bowel or mouth if the normal bacterial flora are suppressed by chemotherapy. Although true infection seldom accompanies this overgrowth of candida, the large inoculum provides a threat in debilitated persons who may develop aspiration pneumonia or even candida septicemia. The kidney and brain bear the brunt of hematogenous infection, but lesions also occur in the thyroid, myocardium, endocardium, pancreas, adrenals, and liver. The visceral lesions are granulomatous nodules or abscesses containing both mycelia and yeastlike cells.

Clinical Manifestations. No systemic disturbances accompany the local signs of mucocutaneous infection. Infection of the mucous membranes, known as *thrush*, gives rise only to soft white patches on the tonsils, cheeks, gums, and tongue. These patches are easily removed and leave a reddened surface. Although usually self-limited, the disease may become chronic and spread to other mucosal surfaces or intertriginous areas in the groins, the antecubital fossae, the interdigital folds, the inframammary areas, the umbilicus, and the axillas. Eczematoid lesions and vesicles are also found in vulvovaginal moniliasis of pregnancy or diabetes.

Aspiration pneumonia is probably the chief form of visceral moniliasis. It is seen in debilitated persons, often in the course of intensive therapy with tetracycline or other antibiotics, and may be accompanied by mixed infection with bacteria. Cough, chest pain, and high fever are prominent. Less extensive involvements of the lung are said to heal completely or progress to chronic infections, but the disease is sometimes fatal.

Septicemic infections are seen in the late stages of severe debilitating disease and seem to occur most commonly in children receiving intensive antibiotic therapy. Acute disseminated moniliasis may be suspected in debilitated adults who suddenly develop fever, shock, azotemia, depressed sensorium, and gastrointestinal bleeding after receiving continuous antibiotic treatment. Septicemic moniliasis also accompanies vegetative endocarditis, a disease that has been described mainly in narcotic addicts. Meningitis is another rare form of moniliasis; it produces a clinical syndrome similar to tuberculous meningitis.

Diagnosis. In thrush, the organisms are seen upon microscopic examination of the white patches as a tangled mass of mycelia and yeastlike cells. They grow readily on Sabouraud agar. In septicemias the fungus can be isolated repeatedly from the blood. Pulmonary moniliasis may be difficult to recognize, because *C. albicans* is a normal resident of the oropharynx and may appear in the sputum in the absence of respiratory infection. For this reason, it is often impossible to be certain of the diagnosis of pulmonary moniliasis unless the organism is demonstrated in pulmonary lesions at autopsy or surgery.

Treatment. Thrush and vaginal moniliasis are best treated by nystatin administered orally in doses of 500,000 units t.i.d. Topical therapy with nystatin ointments or with alcoholic solutions of gentian violet is effective in cutaneous moniliasis. Nystatin may also be of some benefit in preventing candidal pneumonia or septicemia in debilitated persons whose mouth and intestines have become overgrown with candida during treatment with antibiotics. Intravenous amphotericin B in doses of 1.0 mg per kg body weight daily is said to be effective in treating systemic moniliasis.

REFERENCES

Benham, R. W., and A. M. Hopkins: Yeast-like Fungi Found on the Skin and in the Intestines of Normal Subjects, Arch. Dermatol. Syphilol., 28:532, 1933.

Braude, A. I., and J. Rock: The Syndrome of Acute Disseminated Moniliasis in Adults, A.M.A. Arch. Internal Med., 104:91, 1959.

Klegler, A. M.: Are Fungus Infections Increasing as a Result of Antibiotic Therapy?, J.A.M.A., 149:979, 1952.

Merchant, R. K., D. B. Luria, P. H. Geisler, J. H. Edgcomb, and J. P. Utz: Fungal Endocarditis: Review of the Literature and Report of Three Cases, Ann. Internal Med., 48:242, 1958.

160 MUCORMYCOSIS
Abraham I. Braude

Definition. Mucormycosis is a rare but malignant infection of cranial, pulmonary, and abdominal blood vessels in diabetic and other acidotic patients. It is due to a fungus assumed to be a member of the order Mucorales on the basis of its morphology in fixed tissues and the rare isolation of *Rhizopus oryzae*. The most frequent manifestations are ophthalmoplegia and meningoencephalitis.

Etiology. The etiologic agent has never been cultured from the brain or spinal fluid even when expert mycologic techniques were used with fresh cerebral tissues known to harbor the characteristic mycelium. The mycelium is broad, branching, and aseptate, with a diameter of 6 to 15 μ. The fungus *Rhizopus oryzae*, a species of the order Mucorales, has been recovered from paranasal sinuses of fatal cases, and the mycelia in culture were identical in appearance with those in the brain. Because known members of the order Mucorales grow readily on ordinary media, the failure of cultural isolation from the brain remains a puzzle.

Pathogenesis. These fungi abound in soil, manure, and starchy foodstuffs, but only become pathogenic for man in rare cases of diabetic acidosis and even less commonly in patients debilitated by uremic acidosis, leukemia, or massive corticosteroid therapy. The usual portal of entry appears to be the paranasal sinuses; from there the organism is thought to extend along the invaded vessels to the retroorbital tissues and cerebrum. Thrombosis of arteries and veins leads to multiple infarcts throughout the brain but only minimal inflammatory response to the mycelia. Cerebral mucormycosis may be associated with hematogenous spread to pulmonary and intestinal vessels. Pulmonary and intestinal infarction may also develop as a primary infection apparently after inhalation or ingestion of the fungus. Organisms probably penetrate the walls of bronchi or intestine and infect the adjacent hilar or mesenteric vessels. Intestinal mucormycosis takes the form of hemorrhagic segmental infarction of the ileum or colon.

Clinical Manifestations. Cerebral mucormycosis is characterized by three features: (1) uncontrolled diabetes with acidosis, (2) ophthalmoplegia, and (3) signs of acute diffuse cerebrovascular disease. When the patient is first seen, drowsiness and semi-stupor are usually attributed to the metabolic disturbance, but the cerebral manifestations persist and progress after the acidosis is corrected. Headache and fever are prominent.

In addition to complete internal and external ophthalmoplegia, there may be edema of the eyelids and retina and signs of retinal vascular occlu-sion. Nuchal rigidity and mild mononuclear pleocytosis in the spinal fluid have also been described. Pulmonary mucormycosis may start gradually or suddenly with chest pain, fever, hemoptysis, and a friction rub. A few cases have been described in which the orbit or sinuses were infected without extension to the brain.

Diagnosis. The syndrome of cerebral mucormycosis is so characteristic that it can be recognized by its clinical features alone.

Prognosis. Mucormycosis is almost invariably fatal. Rare cases of recovery have followed control of diabetic acidosis.

Treatment. There is no specific chemotherapy. Treatment should be directed toward rapid correction of the hyperglycemia and acidosis with the hope that remission will occur in patients who have not suffered irreparable neurologic damage. Surgical removal of infected lung has been successful.

REFERENCES

Baker, R. D.: Mucormycosis—a New Disease? J.A.M.A., 163:805, 1957.

Bauer, H., L. Ajello, E. Adams, and D. Hernandez: Cerebral Mucormycosis: Pathogenesis of the Disease: Description of the Fungus *Rhizopus oryzae* Isolated from a Fatal Case, Am. J. Med., 18:822, 1955.

Gregory, J. E., A. Golden, and W. Haymaker: Mucormycosis of the Central Nervous System, Bull. Johns Hopkins Hosp., 73:405, 1943.

161 NOCARDIOSIS
Abraham I. Braude

Definition. Nocardiosis, an infection caused by an aerobic actinomycete, may produce lung abscesses and spread to the brain and elsewhere; or it may appear as a chronic deforming granulomatous infection limited to the foot (maduromycosis).

Etiology. Pulmonary and disseminated nocardiosis usually result from infection with *Nocardia asteroides*. This organism is relatively acid-fast, and its bacillary form resembles the tubercle bacillus. The following properties of *N. asteroides* permit easy differentiation from the tubercle bacillus: (1) rapid growth on Sabouraud's medium or on 10 per cent blood agar with colonies appearing in 3 to 14 days at room temperature; (2) the presence in exudates of long-branched mycelial forms in addition to the bacillary forms; (3) rapid killing of guinea pigs and rabbits inoculated intraperitoneally and the recovery of *N. asteroides* from miliary nodules in the abdominal viscera; death of guinea pigs occurs in less than a week from pathogenic strains; (4) gram-positive staining reaction.

Pathogenesis. *Nocardia asteroides* can be recovered readily from soil. Nocardiosis appears, therefore, to be an exogenous infection usually having its portal of entry in the lungs. In almost every patient with nocardiosis (other than maduromycosis) the earliest and most extensive lesions are pulmonary. These lesions are accompanied by neither the intense fibrosis nor the granulomatous reaction of pulmonary actinomycosis; they are acute suppurative foci containing acid-fast, branching, nocardial filaments. A well-defined wall is absent, a fact which probably accounts for the marked tendency of nocardial abscesses to spread to the brain and to a lesser extent to the spleen, skin, peritoneum, and kidney.

Clinical Manifestations. The chief symptom is cough, usually productive of a thick, sometimes bloody, sputum. Chest pain and dyspnea are common. These symptoms are usually accompanied by fever, sweats, chills, leukocytosis, weakness anorexia, and weight loss. The illness may be prolonged and present the picture of a chronic pulmonary infection resembling tuberculosis, lung abscess, or unresolved suppurative pneumonia. In nearly one-third of the patients this syndrome is interrupted suddenly by the acute neurologic changes of metastatic brain abscess. At this time the patient may experience severe headache and focal sensory or motor disturbances. The protein, cells, and pressure of the spinal fluid are increased, but the concentration of glucose is not reduced unless the meninges are also infected. Infection of the skin is frequent and produces numerous scattered abscesses or single draining sinuses of the hand, chest wall, or buttocks.

The disease is usually fatal, but the duration varies from months to years.

Diagnosis. Because patients with nocardiosis are usually suspected of having tuberculosis, their sputums are likely to be examined for tubercle bacilli. The usual methods for concentrating tubercle bacilli often inactivate *N. asteroides,* however, and the fungus may not be recovered after such treatment despite the readiness with which it otherwise grows on a variety of media. *Nocardia asteroides* may also be overlooked in smears stained by the Ziehl-Neelsen method, because it is less resistant than the tubercle bacillus to the decolorizing action of acid alcohol. If nocardiosis is suspected on clinical grounds, precautions must be taken, therefore, against killing the organism by sputum concentration methods and against overdecolorizing it. The first can be avoided by concentrating with trisodium phosphate; the second by using a weak solution of acid alcohol.

Although sulfur granules are not found in pulmonary or disseminated nocardiosis, the gram-positive filamentous organisms in nocardial exudates often resemble those found in infections due to *Actinomyces bovis.* The two pathogens can be distinguished, however, by the ease with which *N. asteroides* is cultivated on Sabouraud or blood agar aerobically, by its acid-fast staining characteristics, and by its pathogenicity for guinea pigs and rabbits. If biopsy material is available, the nongranulomatous and minimally fibrotic character of the nocardial suppurative reaction also helps to distinguish it from that seen in infections due to *A. bovis.* The absence of tubercles, of course, is valuable in differential diagnosis from tuberculosis.

The isolation of a few colonies of nocardia from sputum or gastric juice is by no means diagnostic of nocardial infection. This organism is widely distributed as a saprophyte and only rarely achieves pathologic significance.

Treatment. Sulfadiazine is sometimes successful in the treatment of nocardiosis. Penicillin and the tetracycline derivatives appear ineffective, although the number of cases treated have been too few for definite evaluation of these agents. The resistance of a patient with nocardiosis to the tetracyclines and penicillin may be used in distinguishing it from actinomycosis due to *A. bovis* and other pulmonary infections which respond to these antibiotics. Patients with nocardiosis should receive 8 to 12 Gm sulfadiazine daily. Despite the poor clinical results with penicillin and oxytetracycline, in vitro tests are warranted to determine the sensitivity of each new strain of *N. asteroides* to various antibiotics. An antibiotic selected on this basis can be used to supplement the sulfonamides.

REFERENCES

Bobbitt, O. B., I. H. Friedmen, and C. Lupton: Nocardiosis, New Engl. J. Med., 252:893, 1955.

Henrici, A. T., and E. L. Gardner: The Acid-fast Actinomycetes: With a Report of a Case from Which a New Species Was Isolated, J. Infectious Diseases, 28:232, 1921.

Weed, L. A., H. A. Andersen, C. A. Good, and A. H. Baggenstos: Nocardiosis: Clinical, Bacteriologic and Pathologic Aspects, New Engl. J. Med., 253:1138, 1955.

162 OTHER DEEP MYCOSES
Abraham I. Braude

ASPERGILLOSIS

Definition. Aspergillosis is an uncommon infection produced by *Aspergillus fumigatus* and other species of *Aspergillus,* a group of fungi of low pathogenicity for man unless resistance is overcome by an overwhelming inoculum or debilitating illness. The disease may become disseminated or remain localized to the lung, ear, orbit, or paranasal sinuses.

Etiology. Aspergilli assume the mycelial form both in culture and infected tissues. They are hardy, widely prevalent organisms and grow rapidly on all culture media at room temperature or 35°C as colored woolly colonies peppered with black dots. They are composed of segmented mycelia that bear masses of small round spores on a knoblike swelling at the end of specialized mycelial stalks known as conidiophores.

Pathogenesis and Pathology. Primary infection of the lung usually develops after inhalation of massive numbers of spores from mycelia growing on grain. Pulmonary aspergillosis was an occupational disease in persons who fattened squabs by forcing masticated grain from their mouths into the esophagus of the birds. Secondary pulmonary infection may be superimposed on tuberculous cavities, bronchiectasis, and bronchogenic carcinoma or may become established after resistance is lowered by leukopenia, Hodgkin's disease, irradiation, and other debilitating processes. Excessive use of adrenal steroids or antibiotics is also thought to favor secondary invasion by aspergilli. The most distinctive pulmonary lesion is the aspergilloma, a mycelial mass in a fibrous cavity lined with bronchial epithelium. Chronic granulomatous lung lesions resembling tuberculosis have also been described. More destructive infections take the form of bronchopneumonia and lung abscesses. Thrombosis of pulmonary vessels by invading mycelia leads to local necrosis with hemorrhage and to hematogenous abscesses in the brain, lung, kidney, spleen, heart, and thyroid. Primary infections of the ear, orbit, and nasal sinuses may also be invasive and extend locally into the middle ear and brain. In all lesions, mycelia are prominently observed in tissues stained with Schiff's periodic acid or Gram's stain.

Clinical Manifestations. In pulmonary aspergillomas the chief symptom is hemoptysis. Aspergillus lung abscesses and granulomas are associated with cough and fever. In fulminating disseminated infections, pulmonary manifestations are often overshadowed by coma and other signs of cerebral infection. Fever, joint pains, and skin eruptions lasting for a few weeks or months may also accompany disseminated aspergillosis.

Diagnosis. Cultures of aspergilli has no diagnostic value unless they are obtained directly from infected tissues. They are frequently present in the mouth and in sputum cultures in the absence of aspergillus infection. They are also present in the air and may contaminate uninfected biopsy specimens unless strict sterile precautions are observed. Cultural findings should be confirmed by demonstration of the characteristic septate mycelia in biopsy material. Diagnosis should not be based alone on the morphology of the fungus in tissue section without simultaneous culture because its mycelia may be confused with those found in the tissues in candidiasis and mucormycosis.

Aspergillomas of the lung can usually be recognized by the unique appearance in roentgenograms of a crescentic radiolucency surrounding a circular mass. In other forms of pulmonary aspergillosis the roentgenogram is not diagnostic and may resemble bronchogenic carcinoma, bacterial lung abscess, and tuberculosis.

Treatment. Localized lesions have been successfully excised from both the lung and the brain. The value of chemotherapy remains to be established.

GEOTRICHOSIS

Definition. Geotrichosis is the name given to certain disorders of the mouth, bronchi, and intestinal tract from which *Geotrichium candidum* has been isolated. This fungus has not been established as a human pathogen, and the validity of geotrichosis as a disease entity remains questionable.

Etiology. The fungus *Geotrichium candidum* may resemble *Coccidioides immitis* in culture because its septate mycelium fragments into large square-ended arthrospores. *Geotrichium candidum* does not form sporangia in vivo, however, and its soft creamy colonies on solid medium are easily distinguished from those of *C. immitis.*

Pathogenesis. Geotrichium is a normal inhabitant of the pharynx and bowel and may proliferate locally to produce visible white colonies on the mucous membranes. It may also appear in devitalized tissues and secretions of the nasopharynx, bronchopulmonary tree, and colon but probably not as a primary pathogen.

Clinical Manifestations. Geotrichosis is reported to cause pulmonary cavities and colitis. In bronchopulmonary geotrichosis, the patient is said to cough up gelatinous sputum tinged with blood, and in rare cases thin-walled cavities like those of coccidiomycosis have been described.

Diagnosis. In secretions and exudates, *G. candidum* has the appearance of oval or barrel-shaped spores measuring up to 8 to 10 mm in diameter. They are easily recovered on Sabouraud's agar at room temperature.

Treatment. Lesions resembling thrush respond to local application of 1:10,000 solution of gentian violet. Bronchopulmonary geotrichosis is said to respond to oral treatment with potassium iodide, and intestinal geotrichosis is treated by oral administration three times daily of capsules containing 0.32 mg gentian violet.

MADUROMYCOSIS (Madura Foot)

Definition. Maduromycosis is a chronic destructive infection of the foot, characterized by the presence of multiple fistulas which extrude mycotic granules. The term *maduromycosis* is used here synonymously with *mycetoma* and includes not only infections caused by *Nocardia* but also those caused by higher fungi with larger hyphae.

Etiology. The most frequent cause of maduromycosis in the United States is a higher fungus known as *Monosporium apiospermum*, the "imperfect" form of the ascomycete *Allescheria boydii*. It grows rapidly on Sabouraud's agar as a cottony mycelium bearing asexual spores borne singly or in small groups at the tips or sides of conidiophores. Other higher fungi isolated in maduromycosis include members of such diverse genera as *Aspergillus*, *Penicillium*, *Madurella*, *Cephalosporium*, and *Phialophora*.

Members of the genus *Nocardia* are important causes of Madura foot outside the United States. *Nocardia madurae* is found in southeastern Asia and *N. brasilinesis* in South America.

Pathogenesis and Pathology. The fungi found in mycetoma are inhabitants of the soil and enter the tissues of the bare foot presumably after trauma. In rare instances the hand may also be infected.

The infection begins in the outer tissues and burrows throughout the foot to destroy bone, muscle, and connective tissue indiscriminately. The areas of destruction show chronic suppuration with fibrosis and are connected by multiple fistulas which rupture to the outside. Mycotic granules are seen in the suppurative foci. The prolonged proliferation of granulation and scar tissue leads to enlargement of the affected part.

Clinical Manifestations. The earliest sign is usually a small swelling on the sole or dorsum of the foot. This undergoes a recurring cycle of swelling, suppuration, and healing. Later, similar lesions appear on other parts of the foot, and over a period of months the destruction of deeper tissues is manifested by slight or moderate pain, generalized swelling, and redness. The course is intermittently progressive, and there may be periods of remission. Ultimately the foot becomes a swollen, deformed mass of destroyed tissue with many fistulous openings through which mycotic granules are discharged. The infection does not spread hematogenously to other parts, but in rare instances there is direct extension along lymphatics. Death can occur from secondary bacterial infection.

Diagnosis. The characteristic granules are 0.5 to 2 mm in diameter and may be white, yellow, black, or red. Nocardial granules are easily distinguished from those of *Aspergillus boydii* and other higher fungi by direct microscopic examination. They are masses of radiating gram-positive filaments; those of higher fungi contain large segmented hyphae and numerous chlamydospores. Either type of granule grows rapidly on Sabouraud agar.

Roentgenograms of the foot disclose destruction of bone which is more extensive than the external appearance and pain might indicate.

Treatment. Wide excision of infected tissues may slow the progress of the disease, and antibacterial chemotherapy is valuable in arresting secondary infection. There is no known cure, however, and most cases eventually require amputation of the foot.

CHROMOBLASTOMYCOSIS

Definition. Chromoblastomycosis is an infection of the skin produced by several species of the genus *Phialophora* and characterized by slowly progressive cauliflowerlike lesions of the legs of agricultural workers in tropical or subtropical regions.

Etiology. The three species *P. pedrosi*, *P. compactum*, and *P. verrucosa* cannot be distinguished upon microscopic examination of infected tissue, in which all appear as small clusters of spores with thick, dark brown walls. On culture, however, the three differ in their methods of sporulation. The species most commonly found, *P. pedrosi*, exhibits three types of spore formation: (1) branching chains of spores borne at the tips of long conidiophores, (2) clusters of spores forming sleeves about the hyphae, and (3) balls of spores arising in the cuplike ends of very short flask-shaped conidiophores. *Phialophora verrucosa* forms only the third type of spore, and *P. compactum* is recognized by chains of spores arranged in compact masses. On Sabouraud's agar all three grow very slowly and will produce deeply pigmented olive or black colonies.

Pathogenesis and Pathology. The fungi undoubtedly live in the soil or vegetation and enter the skin of agricultural workers.

Three pathologic processes are found: (1) microabscesses in the dermis containing numerous fungi, (2) extensive fibrosis, and (3) epidermal hyperplasia and hyperkeratosis. The lesions progress along the lymphatics but not beyond them; dissemination through the blood or deep penetration into bone does not occur.

Clinical Manifestations. The earliest lesion is a papule, which develops into a well-circumscribed bluish lesion with a warty, raised margin. Although it resembles the cutaneous form of North American blastomycosis at this early stage, it does not spread peripherally. Instead, adjacent new lesions appear over a period of years and, as the epithelial hyperplasia and hyperkeratosis increase, the entire area assumes a cauliflowerlike appearance. Eventually the whole extremity is covered. Pain and constitutional symptoms are absent unless secondary bacterial infection occurs or elephantiasis develops as a result of lymphatic scarring.

Diagnosis. The typical dark brown septate bodies are seen in large numbers in biopsied tissue or pus, and brown hyphae can be found in crusts treated with 10 per cent potassium hydroxide. For specific identification, however, it is necessary to culture the slowly growing fungus on Sabouraud's agar.

Treatment. Early in the disease, the lesions may be destroyed by electrocoagulation or removed by surgical excision. Later in the course, excision of the larger nodules leaves indolent ulcers which heal very slowly.

Except for treatment of secondary infection, there is no specific medical therapy. The disease is never fatal, however, and the usefulness of the limb is retained despite its unsightly appearance.

SOUTH AMERICAN BLASTOMYCOSIS

Definition. South American blastomycosis is a highly destructive but curable infection that results from invasion of the nasopharynx by *Blastomyces brasiliensis.* It occurs only in South America. From the pharynx the disease can extend locally to regional nodes or spread to the lungs and abdominal viscera.

Etiology. Multiple buds on the yeastlike cell of *B. brasiliensis* distinguish it morphologically from its North American counterpart, *B. dermatiditis.* The tiny multiple buds have the appearance of a crown of small beads attached to the cell wall. The fungus reproduces by budding both in tissues and when cultured at 37°C. At room temperature it produces mycelia which bear spores resembling those of *B. dermatiditis.*

Pathogenesis. In most cases the portal of entry of this exogenous fungus is the nasopharynx. Here it produces a destructive lesion with gross swelling and ulceration and eventual extension to the cervical lymph nodes. Occasionally, the primary lesion is inconspicuous, and massive enlargement and suppurative necrosis of the regional lymph nodes are the predominant pathologic changes. Hematogenous spread to other lymph nodes, liver, spleen, and bone eventually leads to suppurative or granulomatous nodules in those organs. In addition to the nasopharynx, primary lesions can occur in the lymphoid tissue of the cecal and appendiceal regions.

Clinical Manifestations. The first symptoms usually result from painful ulcers of the mouth or nose, although loss of appetite, abdominal pain, vomiting and diarrhea may be the first complaints when ulceration begins in the gut. In other cases, massive lymphadenopathy precedes other manifestations. In the usual infection, however, there is a progressive extension of lesions from the mouth and neighboring skin. The lymph nodes undergo suppurative necrosis, and sinuses rupture through the overlying skin. The patient suffers from severe pain, fever, inability to eat, and cachexia. Depending on the rapidity of spread to the viscera, bones, and central nervous system, the disease is fatal after periods ranging from a few months to 3 years or more if untreated.

Diagnosis. Microscopic examination of pus or tissue treated with 10 per cent potassium hydroxide will reveal the characteristic multiple budding cells of *B. brasiliensis,* in addition to cells with single buds. The multiple budding cells are also found in cultures on blood agar incubated at 37°C, but growth is very slow and more than a month may elapse before colonies appear.

Treatment. The infection responds dramatically to sulfonamide drugs. Sulfadiazine or sulfamerazine in doses of 4 to 6 Gm daily has been used successfully in arresting or curing the disease.

RHINOSPORIDIOSIS

Definition. Rhinosporidiosis produces small tumorlike masses usually confined to the nose and nasopharynx. An endosporulating fungus seen in the tissues cannot be cultured on laboratory media.

Etiology. The fungus *Rhinosporidium seeberi* is placed in the class Phycomycetes and family Coccidioidaceae because characteristic giant sporangia develop in the tissues. These thick-walled endospore-filled sporangia may reach 500 μ in diameter but otherwise resemble the smaller spherules of *Coccidioides immitis.*

Pathogenesis and Pathology. The disease is probably acquired by bathing or diving into infected water. In India, where rhinosporidiosis reaches endemic proportions, its rarity in women is attributed to social taboos that prohibit their bathing in open places. The characteristic lesion is a vascularized papillomatous proliferation of the nasal or pharyngeal mucous membrane containing sporangia in various stages of maturity. Red cells, inflammatory cells, and extruded endospores fill the interstitial tissue. As sporangia enlarge they compress the columnar epithelium of the nose or the squamous epithelium of the pharynx and allow endospores to escape and reinoculate the adjacent tissue.

Clinical Manifestations. Single or multiple pedunculated fleshy red masses appear in the nares or pharynx and produce symptoms of rhinitis, epistaxis, and nasal obstruction. In exceptional cases hoarseness may develop from laryngeal infection.

The conjunctivas and lacrimal sac may also be involved.

Diagnosis. The characteristic sporangia are easily identified in biopsied tissue section. Because the only endemic foci are in India, most patients are Asiatic.

Treatment. The lesions can be completely removed surgically or by electrocautery. Electrocautery is preferred because surgery leaves open incisions in which spores can be implanted.

REFERENCES

ASPERGILLOSIS

Finegold, S. M., D. Well, and J. F. Murray: Aspergillosis: A Review and Report of Twelve Cases, Am. J. Med., 27:463, 1959.

Grcevic, N., and W. F. Mathews: Pathologic Changes in Acute Disseminated Aspergillosis, Am. J. Clin. Pathol., 32:536, 1959.

Naji, A. F.: Bronchopulmonary Aspergillosis, A.M.A. Arch. Pathol., 68:282, 1959.

CHROMOBLASTOMYCOSIS

Barwasser, N. C.: Chromoblastomycosis: Thirteenth Reported Case in the United States, J.A.M.A., 153:556, 1953.

Binford, C. H., G. Hess, and C. W. Emmons: Chromoblastomycosis, Arch. Dermatol. Syphilol., 49:398, 1944.

Conway, H., and W. Berkeley: Chromoblastomycosis (Mycetoma Form) Treated by Surgical Excision, A.M.A. Arch. Dermatol. Syphilol., 66:695, 1952.

GEOTRICHOSIS

Smith, D. T.: Geotrichosis, J. Chronic Diseases, 5:532, 1957.

Kunstadter, R. H., A. Milzer, and F. Whitcomb: Bronchopulmonary Geotrichosis in Children, Am. J. Diseases Children, 79:82, 1950.

MADUROMYCOSIS

Ajello, L.: Soil as Natural Reservoir for Human Pathogenic Fungi, Science, 123:876, 1956.

RHINOSPORIDIOSIS

Purandare, N. M., and S. M. Deoras: Rhinosporidiosis in Bombay, Indian J. Med. Sci., 7:603, 1953.

SOUTH AMERICAN BLASTOMYCOSIS

Moore, M.: Blastomycosis: Coccidioidal Granuloma and Paracoccidioidal Granuloma, Arch. Dermatol. Syphilol., 38:163, 1938.

Section 11: Spirochetal Diseases

163 SYPHILIS
Albert Heyman

Definition. Syphilis is a chronic, systemic, infectious disease caused by the *Treponema pallidum* and usually transmitted by sexual contact. It is capable of producing tissue destruction and chronic inflammation in almost any organ in the body and can express itself in a great diversity of clinical manifestations.

History. Considerable knowledge of the pathology and clinical aspects of syphilis was accumulated in the sixteenth to nineteenth centuries, but it was not until early in the present century that most of the fundamental information about the disease was uncovered. The etiologic agent, the *T. pallidum*, was discovered by Schaudinn and Hoffmann in 1905. Soon afterward, Wassermann and his associates introduced serologic methods of diagnosis. In 1949, Nelson and Mayer introduced the *T. pallidum* immobilization test, following which other tests for demonstrating humoral antibodies were subsequently developed.

In 1910 Ehrlich announced the discovery of arsphenamine, and in 1917 Wagner von Jauregg demonstrated the value of malarial fever therapy for paresis. These were the two most important advances in the treatment of syphilis until 1943, when penicillin was found by Mahoney and his associates to be effective in the early stages of the disease. This drug has replaced the other forms of chemotherapy in syphilis.

Etiology. The *T. pallidum* is a slender spirochete with regular, evenly spaced spirals. It varies in length from 5 to 20 μ. When viewed under the dark-field microscope, *T. pallidum* shows characteristic motility, rotating on its long axis and moving slowly backward and forward. The spirals usually keep their uniform shape and size, although the body of the organism may bend at the middle. It does not have the quick, whipping movements of other spirochetes which are often found in ulcerative lesions. The organism does not stain well with ordinary dyes but can be demonstrated by silver impregnation methods in fixed tissues. For clinical purposes it can be demonstrated by dark-field microscopy of material from primary or secondary syphilitic lesions.

Treponema pallidum is readily killed by soap, ordinary antiseptics, drying, and heat. It may resist cold temperatures, however, and can be frozen and stored for long periods without its virulence being affected. The organism does not remain viable, however, in whole blood or plasma which has been stored at refrigerator temperature for more than 96 hr.

Pathogenic forms of *T. pallidum* have not been cultivated and passed serially on artificial media. Strains of the organism which have been cultured are not virulent in animals and differ morphologically from pathogenic *T. pallidum*. Rabbits and monkeys can be experimentally infected with syphilis.

Frequency. Exact information is not available as to the number of persons infected with syphilis in the United States (i.e., *prevalence*) or the number of new infections occurring each year (i.e., *incidence*). Both the incidence and prevalence of the disease have decreased considerably since the Second World War. In 1947, approximately 108,000 cases of primary and secondary syphilis were reported in this country to the Public Health Service, whereas in 1957 only 6,250 cases were reported. In the following 3 years, however, a disturbing rise in the incidence of new cases of syphilis appeared. It was predicted that in 1961 more than 10,000 cases of primary and secondary syphilis would be reported. The dramatic postwar decline in the incidence of syphilis was largely the result of the development of rapid-treatment methods, mass blood testing, and large-scale epidemiologic measures. Another factor responsible for the decline was the widespread use of penicillin for other diseases. As a result of this decrease in syphilis case rates, many of the states abandoned their public health control measures. The rise in the incidence of new cases leaves no doubt as to the need for continuing intensive control programs. It is of interest that the incidence of new cases of syphilis has risen in the teen-age population, particularly in certain racial groups and in the lower socioeconomic classes.

Pathogenesis. Syphilis is usually transmitted by direct and intimate contact with moist infectious lesions of the skin and mucous membranes. Sexual contact is by far the commonest means of infection, but transfer of the disease by kissing or biting occasionally occurs. Indirect transmission—i.e., by contaminated objects—is exceptional, since the organisms quickly die if allowed to dry. The disease can be spread by inoculation with infected blood, as in transfusion syphilis. Infection is transmitted to the fetus through the placenta. *Treponema pallidum* is apparently capable of penetrating the intact mucous membrane, but a small abrasion is probably required for inoculation to occur through the skin. Once the spirochete has penetrated the epithelium, it enters the lymphatics and can be demonstrated in the regional lymph nodes a few hours after experimental inoculation. From the lymph nodes the organism spreads rapidly throughout the body by way of the blood stream. This spirochetemia may occur several weeks before appearance of the primary lesion at the site of inoculation. The early seeding of *T. pallidum* in various tissues is the basis for many of the later manifestations of the disease.

About 3 to 6 weeks after the organism has entered the body, a primary lesion, the *chancre*, develops at the site of inoculation. The chancre is usually a single ulceration of the skin or mucous membrane; it heals spontaneously. About 6 weeks after its appearance a generalized skin eruption, known as *secondary syphilis*, develops. In this stage, systemic manifestations are common. The signs of secondary syphilis also disappear spontaneously.

This sequence of events in early syphilis is variable. Infection without noticeable lesions probably occurs in a high percentage of cases, and many individuals with late syphilis are unable to recall either primary or secondary manifestations.

Following healing of the primary and secondary manifestations, the patient may show no outward signs of the infection (*latent syphilis*). Nevertheless, chronic, progressive, inflammatory changes may be taking place in the visceral organs or in the cardiovascular or central nervous system. Clinical evidence of cardiovascular syphilis or neurosyphilis may not develop for 10 to 20 years or more after the onset of the disease. Occasionally, the tissues of the host seem to become sensitized to the spirochetes, and large destructive lesions, called *gummas*, result. These lesions, which contain very few spirochetes, can occur in almost every organ of the body but are most frequent in the skin or bones.

Many patients with latent syphilis do not develop late manifestations and show no evidence of syphilis at autopsy. A study of patients with untreated early syphilis followed for a number of years showed that approximately one-third of them achieved spontaneous cures with the development of negative serologic tests. An equal number died of causes other than syphilis or developed latent syphilis with no clinical evidence of the disease other than a positive serologic test. The remaining third developed serious lesions of the cardiovascular or central nervous system or benign gummatous lesions of the skin or bones.

Histopathology. The early lesions of syphilis are characterized by infiltration of the blood vessel walls and perivascular spaces with plasma cells, large mononuclear cells, and lymphocytes. Spirochetes can be demonstrated by silver impregnation stains. In the late lesions of syphilis there may be necrosis with granuloma or gumma formation. The necrosis is thought to be the result of an exaggerated or hypersensitive response to a small number of organisms. Spirochetes are rarely found. These lesions heal slowly and often produce large scars.

Immunity and Resistance. The development of immunity in a syphilitic patient can be considered from two standpoints: the resistance the patient develops to his own infection and the immunity he develops to reinfection.

Practically every patient with syphilis develops some resistance to his own infection. The degree of immunity determines whether the patient will achieve a spontaneous cure, the disease will remain latent, or late complications will develop. The factors responsible for the development of this type of immunity and the destruction of spirochetes are largely unknown. The serum of experimentally infected animals and patients with syphilis contains antibodies which immobilize and render noninfectious virulent strains of *T. pallidum*. These antibodies can be demonstrated in vitro by means of the *T. pallidum* immobilization (TPI) test developed by Nelson. In human beings this immobilizing antibody appears during the early stages of syphilis and will usually persist indefinitely unless early adequate treatment for syphilis is instituted. The antibody is not present in the serum of normal persons nor in those with nonspirochetal diseases, but it occurs in the serum of patients with various treponematoses, such as bejel, yaws, and pinta. The exact relationship between this antibody and the development of immunity has not yet been determined.

Humoral antibodies in syphilis have also been demonstrated by newer techniques such as the *T. pallidum* complement fixation test, the fluorescent antibody test, and the Reiter protein complement fixation test. These procedures for detecting syphilitic antibodies are still in the experimental stage, but some of them are being used as diagnostic tests, particularly in cases in which there is doubt as to the validity of the routine serologic methods.

Apparently the outcome of the syphilitic infection is influenced to some extent by the sex and race of the individual. Neurosyphilis, for example, occurs more frequently in men than in women, and in a higher proportion of white individuals than Negroes. Bone and cardiovascular syphilis are more common in Negroes.

Immunity to reinfection develops soon after the onset of the disease. In animals, immunity has been found to appear within 3 weeks after the initial infection and to increase progressively during a period of 6 months. In human beings, reinoculation usually results in a chancre if carried out within 15 days after the appearance of the primary lesion of the initial infection. Later than this a chancre seldom develops, but this resistance is relative.

Adequate treatment of patients with early syphilis may abort the development of immunity, and reinfections can occur. If treatment is delayed until after this period, immunity to reinfection becomes established and may remain throughout the lifetime of the individual.

If inadequate treatment is given during early syphilis and complete destruction of the patient's spirochetes is not obtained, redissemination of the organisms may occur and produce infectious skin and mucosal lesions. This is the basis for the statement that poor treatment is worse than none at all. Once the patient has developed immunity to his own infection (usually within 4 years after the onset of the disease), inadequate treatment does not result in redissemination of organisms.

CLINICAL MANIFESTATIONS OF EARLY ACQUIRED SYPHILIS

Primary Stage. The period of incubation may vary from 10 to 90 days. The typical chancre is a solitary, indurated, nonpainful ulceration, which heals slowly with scar formation. It is often accompanied by painless enlargement of the regional lymph nodes, the *satellite bubo*. It must be emphasized that primary syphilis is often atypical and may be manifested by small, multiple, or painful lesions which resemble many other conditions. Because of the frequent atypical appearance of the chancre, the clinical diagnosis or exclusion of primary syphilis can never be relied upon, and every genital lesion should have a dark-field examination.

Approximately 95 per cent of primary lesions are found on or near the genitalia. In the male, the chancre frequently appears on the coronal sulcus or on the prepuce. Any part of the genitalia may be involved, however. Chancres of the external genitalia must be differentiated from chancroid, granuloma inguinale, lymphogranuloma venereum, carcinoma, and many other lesions which appear in this area. In the female, the primary lesion often appears on the labia and in the fourchette, but the perineum, pubis, clitoris, or urethra may be involved. Chancres of the cervix are frequent and are often mistaken for nonspecific erosions. About 5 per cent of primary lesions occur on the lips, female breasts, or in the mouth.

In the diagnosis of primary syphilis, serologic tests cannot be relied upon entirely, since they are often negative in this stage of the disease. Moreover, a positive serologic reaction in a patient with a genital lesion may represent either latent infection associated with nonsyphilitic lesion or else a biologic false positive reaction caused by another disease (i.e., lymphogranuloma venereum or chancroid). For this reason, a dark-field examination is of greatest importance in the diagnosis of this stage of the disease and should be done on the first visit of every patient suspected of having primary syphilis. If the initial dark-field examination is negative, material from the regional lymph nodes should be aspirated and examined. All local medication as well as antibiotics with treponemicidal activity should be withheld, but oral sulfonamides may be administered during this period of time. If the dark-field examinations and serologic tests for syphilis are negative, the serologic test should be repeated several times during the first 2 or 3 weeks and every few weeks thereafter for 3 months after the appearance of the lesion. If the patient develops a positive serologic reaction in a high or rising titer (with or without evidence of secondary manifestations), then antisyphilitic therapy should be begun. A single serologic test of low titer is not sufficient evidence for beginning antisyphilitic treatment if dark-field examinations are negative. Such tests should be confirmed several times for at least 2 weeks before treatment for syphilis is justified.

Penicillin or other spirocheticidal drugs should not be given as a therapeutic test to patients suspected of having primary syphilis. Healing of the genital lesion following such tests does not necessarily indicate the presence of syphilis, since nonsyphilitic lesions sometimes heal spontaneously. Biopsy of the genital lesions is often of value in the diagnosis of these patients.

Secondary Stage. The secondary stage of syphilis usually develops about 6 weeks after appearance of the chancre and is manifested by a generalized skin eruption and systemic symptoms. Some patients exhibit secondary lesions without ever being aware of a primary; others never develop secondary manifestations and enter the latent stage directly following the healing of the chancre.

The appearance of the *cutaneous lesions* of secondary syphilis varies considerably and may be confused with many other skin eruptions. The lesions most often found are papules, maculopapules, or follicular papules. Occasionally, annular, pustular or rupial lesions occur. Indeed, almost any type of skin eruption may appear except a vesicular one. The rash is usually widespread and frequently involves the palms, soles, and face, in addition to the trunk and extremities. The lesions are sometimes pruritic.

The *mucous membranes* of the mouth and genitalia are often involved in secondary syphilis. Syphilitic lesions of the mouth appear as painless, superficial erosions on the buccal surfaces, on the tongue, or inside the lip. When these lesions are covered with a thin, grayish exudate, they are *mucous patches*. They contain a large number spirochetes but may be very inconspicuous, and patient may not be aware of them. Lesions of the palate and tonsillar area can cause a persistent *sore throat*. So-called *split papules* are occasionally seen in secondary syphilis and may be mistaken for herpes, benign fissures, or the lesions of riboflavin deficiency.

Syphilitic mucosal lesions of the genitalia or perianal regions often become hypertrophic and are called *condylomata lata*. These lesions are broad, flat, wartlike excrescences which are found on the labia majora, perineum, and anal region. They are highly infectious and should be differentiated from condylomata acuminata, which are nonvenereal, pedunculated lesions.

Although the clinical findings of secondary syphilis are often confined to the skin and mucous membranes, many patients will present evidence of *constitutional symptoms* and widespread spirochetal dissemination. Malaise, lassitude, headaches, fever, and myalgia are often noted. There may be a *generalized lymphadenopathy*. Localized areas of *alopecia* also occur, causing a "moth-eaten" appearance of the scalp.

Approximately 4 per cent of patients with secondary syphilis have involvement of the eye, usually *iritis* or *neuroretinitis*.

Skeletal lesions occasionally occur in secondary syphilis and are manifested by localized areas of swelling and tenderness. *Arthralgia* and *hydrarthrosis* also occur, but changes in the joints cannot be detected by x-ray examination. An acute *nephrosis* with marked proteinuria, edema, and hypercholesteremia is sometimes seen in secondary syphilis. Evidence of *central nervous system involvement*, such as paralysis of the cranial nerves or meningitis, may also appear in this stage of the disease.

It is apparent from the above description that secondary syphilis may be manifested by a great variety of apparently unrelated clinical symptoms. Although isolated lesions, such as iritis or periostitis, may not in themselves suggest the diagnosis, the recognition of other symptoms, such as sore throat, lymphadenopathy, or skin lesions will often make the diagnosis of secondary syphilis obvious. Whenever secondary syphilis is suspected, blood should be taken for a serologic test. This will be positive in practically 100 per cent of the cases. Conversely, if the serologic test is negative (and technical errors excluded), secondary syphilis can be ruled out.

INFECTIOUSNESS AND EPIDEMIOLOGY

Syphilis is most infectious during the primary and secondary stages, when there are moist skin or mucosal lesions. The genital condylomas and the

osal lesions contain large numbers of spiro-
and are more infectious than the dry skin
ons. The transmission of the disease by individ-
als or marital partners who deny having had open
lesions is probably by way of small mucosal lesions
which appear during the recurrent episodes of spirochetemia. Some secretions, such as saliva and
semen, are frequently in contact with infectious
mucosal lesions and may thus contain *T. pallidum*.
The blood of patients with early syphilis has been
shown to contain spirochetes and should not be
used for transfusion. The serologic test is not always
an indication of the infectiousness of the blood,
since transfusion syphilis can be transmitted from
patients in the incubation period or in the sero-
negative primary stage of the disease. The danger
of transmitting syphilis either by transfusion or by
direct contact is greatest in the first 4 years of the
disease and is negligible after this period of time.
In pregnancy, however, the disease can apparently
be transmitted to the fetus for as long as 10 years
or more after the onset of the disease, although the
vast majority of congenital infections are acquired
during the first 4 years of maternal infection.

It is important that the physician make an effort
to determine the source of infection of his patients
with syphilis, particularly those with primary and
secondary manifestations. It is equally important
that the individuals to whom the patient may have
transmitted the infection be located.

LATENT SYPHILIS

Latent syphilis is that stage of the disease in
which there are no clinical signs or symptoms of
the infection. Patients without signs or symptoms
but with abnormal spinal fluid findings have a much
more serious prognosis and are not regarded as having latent syphilis but are classified instead as having asymptomatic neurosyphilis.

Latent syphilis is by far the most frequent type
of syphilis. Routine serologic testing is the only way
in which the majority of patients with latent syphilis can be recognized.

Although the syphilitic infection is not clinically
evident during the latent period, it may be producing serious changes in the viscera. Often the spirochete exists within the body throughout the entire
lifetime of the host without producing any apparent effects upon health and longevity. Most of the
patients with late latent syphilis develop sufficient
resistance to their infection to prevent late clinical
manifestations.

The diagnosis of latent syphilis is one of exclusion, and a careful history and physical examination should be made for clinical evidence of this
disease. Since the diagnosis of latent syphilis is dependent upon the serologic test, false positive re-

actions must be ruled out. *Treponema pallidum* immobilization (TPI) tests or the newer treponemal
antigen tests should probably be carried out routinely in patients with positive serologic tests in
whom there is no history or clinical evidence of
syphilis and in whom the diagnosis seems unlikely.

CLINICAL MANIFESTATIONS OF
LATE ACQUIRED SYPHILIS

Skin and Mucous Membranes. Late syphilis of
the skin may appear either as small nodules or
ulcerating gummas. The gumma begins as a painless, subcutaneous tumor which gradually softens
and ruptures, exuding a viscous, gummy material.
Spirochetes are seldom found in these lesions. The
nodular form of late syphilis consists of slightly
raised, reddish brown lesions on the skin, which
often coalesce to form arciform or serpiginous configurations.

Gummas also occur in the mucous membranes of
the nose and throat, and may produce painful destructive lesions in the palate and nasal septum.

Skeletal System. Late osseous syphilis often presents a difficult diagnostic problem. The chief symptoms are pain, tenderness, and local warmth. The
bones usually involved are the skull and tibia, although the clavicle, humerus, ribs, and nasopalatine
structures are sometimes affected.

Syphilis of the skeletal system is often confused
with other types of subacute or chronic osteomyelitis, primary or secondary neoplasms, or Paget's
disease. The diagnosis can usually be made by close
correlation of the serologic, clinical, and roentgenographic findings. In some instances, biopsy may be
necessary.

The most common joint manifestation occurring
in late syphilis is the *Charcot joint*. This condition
is not caused directly by *T. pallidum* but develops
as a consequence of destruction of the proprioceptive nerves in tabes dorsalis. It also occurs in other
neurologic disorders, such as syringomyelia. The
Charcot joint is usually confined to a single weight-
bearing joint, such as the knee, ankle, or hip, and
occasionally the spine. It begins as a painless swelling of the joint and is later manifested by hypermo-
bility and loss of contour. The joint surface disintegrates, so that fragments of bone and cartilage
can be felt within the joint capsule. Charcot joints
often appear in arrested or "burnt-out" cases of tabes
dorsalis—i.e., patients with normal blood and spinal
fluid findings. Antisyphilitic drugs are of little value
in treatment, and orthopedic measures are usually
necessary.

Liver. In patients with late syphilis the liver may
contain multiple, minute, gummatous lesions or several very large ones. On healing, these lesions produce scarring and contraction of the surface, giving

the liver the appearance of having several additional lobes—hence the name *hepar lobatum*. The most common finding on physical examination is a large, coarsely nodular, irregular liver. Ascites, jaundice, and splenomegaly are occasionally present. The serologic test for syphilis is almost always positive. Response to treatment is often dramatic, with rapid reduction in liver size and relief of symptoms.

Stomach. Late syphilis of the stomach consists of a diffuse granulomatous infiltration of the stomach wall or a localized annular constriction about the pyloric area. Secondary ulceration and obstruction may occur, so that differentiation from carcinoma by roentgenographic examination is often impossible. Syphilis of the stomach may be suspected in young individuals on the basis of the roentgenographic appearance of the lesion and a positive serologic test, but exploratory laparotomy is usually indicated to confirm the diagnosis.

Larynx. Syphilis of the larynx produces hoarseness without pain. Laryngoscopic examination may reveal gummatous infiltration of the vocal cords with secondary ulceration. The lesions may simulate carcinoma or tuberculosis, and biopsy is necessary for differential diagnosis. Treatment of this condition should be cautious, since intensive therapy has been known to produce edema, stridor, and suffocation. Patients with late syphilis may also develop hoarseness without pain as a result of recurrent nerve paralysis caused by aneurysm of the aorta.

Kidney and Genitourinary Tract. An acute nephrotic syndrome occasionally appears in early syphilis. In late syphilis, a specific type of interstitial nephritis may be present on postmortem examination without having produced a characteristic clinical picture. Gumma of the kidney is rare, but late syphilis of the bladder, testes, and penis is occasionally reported. Paroxysmal hemoglobinuria is sometimes caused by syphilis. It is discussed in another section (see p. 1295).

In the female, late syphilis rarely involves the internal genital organs, but gummatous lesions sometimes appear in the breast.

Involvement of the endocrine glands, such as the adrenals, thyroid, and pituitary gland, is also infrequent.

Cardiovascular Syphilis. Since cardiovascular syphilis is discussed fully elsewhere (p. 1435) it will be mentioned only briefly at this point. Cardiovascular syphilis is one of the most important of the late lesions of syphilis and probably accounts for the majority of deaths resulting from this disease. It is much more common in men than in women and seems to be more frequent in Negroes than in whites. It usually appears in the second to third decade after infection and may be associated with neurosyphilis and other late manifestations.

The fundamental lesion of cardiovascular syphilis

is *aortitis. Treponema pallidum* causes destruction of the media, fragmentation of the elastic material, and eventual dilatation of the vessel. The base of the aorta is often involved, with dilatation of the valve ring and *aortic insufficiency*. If the weakening is localized, a saccular *aneurysm* may develop. The intima of the aorta becomes thickened, and occlusion of the orifices of the coronary arteries may occur. A few cases of multiple gummas of the myocardium have been reported, but the existence of a diffuse syphilitic myocarditis is a matter of controversy.

Central Nervous System. Neurosyphilis, together with cardiovascular syphilis, accounts for about 90 per cent of deaths caused by syphilis. Although all the tissues of the central nervous system are invaded by the spirochetes, the clinical symptoms may be arbitrarily divided into meningeal, vascular, and parenchymatous. Meningeal and vascular symptoms usually develop early in the course of the disease, whereas parenchymatous involvement, as manifested by tabes dorsalis and paresis, usually does not appear until 10 to 20 years after the primary infection. Meningeal lesions are inflammatory and often reversible. Parenchymatous lesions, however, are likely to be degenerative with irreversible damage. The type of lesion which predominates, the structures involved, and the exact location of the lesion within the central nervous system are the three important factors which influence prognosis and response to treatment.

Gummas of the brain and spinal cord are occasionally observed. They produce symptoms similar to tumors of the central nervous system, and differentiation is difficult.

Asymptomatic Neurosyphilis. Asymptomatic neurosyphilis is that stage of the disease in which an abnormal spinal fluid exists without clinical signs or symptoms to indicate that the function of the central nervous system has been affected.

The outcome of asymptomatic neurosyphilis and the extent of the spinal fluid abnormalities appear to be definitely related, since patients exhibiting marked changes are more likely to develop signs and symptoms. The activity of the neurosyphilitic process is often related to the spinal fluid cell count and protein level. The presence of a positive spinal fluid Wassermann reaction indicates that infection of the central nervous system has occurred; the cells and protein indicate the activity of the condition. This concept maintains that if the spinal fluid is inactive—i.e., if the cell count and protein are normal—the syphilitic infection in the central nervous system has been arrested, and no further therapy is needed. Although this concept is not completely accepted, it seems to hold true in the majority of patients.

The serologic reaction of the blood does not always parallel the spinal fluid findings. Patients with previous treatment may have a negative blood test and a strongly positive spinal fluid. This combination seldom occurs in untreated cases.

If the spinal fluid is completely negative 5 years after the onset of the disease, it rarely if ever becomes positive again.

Meningitis. In a small number of patients, involvement of the central nervous system may be manifested by an acute meningitis. This condition usually appears within the first 2 years after the onset of syphilis. It nearly always occurs in patients who have previously had inadequate therapy and may be associated with an infectious or mucocutaneous relapse.

The symptoms usually consist of headache, cranial nerve lesions, delirium, convulsions or signs of increased intracranial pressure. *Papilledema* is frequently found in patients with syphilitic meningitis, and these cases are often diagnosed erroneously as having brain tumors.

The serologic test for syphilis and the spinal fluid Wassermann are usually strongly positive. The spinal fluid may show a marked lymphocytosis, counts as high as 2,000 cells per cu mm having been observed. This condition is often confused with other forms of lymphocytic meningitis, such as tuberculous or virus meningitis. The immediate prognosis is good, but the ultimate prognosis is much more serious. If the patient does not receive adequate treatment, late manifestations of neurosyphilis or paresis are likely to develop.

Meningovascular Syphilis. Meningovascular syphilis is usually manifested by signs of thrombosis of one or more of the branches of the cerebral or spinal arteries. Since there is almost always some evidence of leptomeningitis, the term meningovascular syphilis is used to describe these cases.

The symptoms of this condition depend upon the location and size of the vessels involved. Monoplegia or hemiplegia, hemianesthesia, aphasia, or hemianopsia may occur. Cranial nerve palsies are frequent and convulsions are often observed. Syphilitic endarteritis may also involve the cerebellar vessels. Patients with meningovascular syphilis sometimes develop psychotic behavior, and differentiation from paresis is often difficult.

In older patients it is often impossible to differentiate clinically between syphilitic vascular disease and a cerebral thrombosis of other etiology. In such cases the blood and spinal fluid findings provide the only means of differentiation. The blood serologic test is positive in the majority of patients with vascular neurosyphilis, and the spinal fluid usually shows a moderate increase of cells and protein with a positive serologic reaction. A diagnosis of meningovascular syphilis should not be made if the spinal fluid is normal.

The vessels and meninges of the spinal cord undergo changes identical with those in the brain. With thrombosis of the anterior spinal artery, the patient may suddenly develop signs of an acute *transverse myelitis* with paraplegia, loss of sensation, and fecal or urinary incontinence. Usually, however, meningovascular lesions of the spinal cord are insidious and produce chronic progressive paralyses and sensory disturbances. A number of neurologic syndromes result from more or less localized spinal cord lesions: syphilitic involvement of the pyramidal tract produces the so-called *Erb's spastic spinal paraplegia;* anterior horn cell degeneration causes a picture similar to *progressive muscular atrophy;* while a single localized *gumma* may simulate cord tumor.

The term *meningovascular syphilis* is also employed for a large group of patients with diverse signs and symptoms, such as *epilepsy, eighth nerve deafness,* other cranial nerve lesions, or chronic headaches. Pupillary abnormalities are frequently present and may consist of a variety of changes, such as miosis, dilatation, anisocoria, fixed pupils, or typical Argyll Robertson phenomena.

Tabes Dorsalis (Locomotor Ataxia). Tabes dorsalis is a form of neurosyphilis in which there is selective degeneration in the posterior roots of the spinal nerves and the posterior columns of the spinal cord. Microscopically the dorsal roots may appear completely demyelinated, and there is marked loss of nerve fibers. The posterior columns of the spinal cord also show a loss of myelin and degeneration of the axons. Spirochetes are rarely found in these lesions. In the majority of cases tabes appears 20 to 30 years after the initial infection. It is found more commonly in men than in women.

Patients with tabes frequently develop severe, agonizing *shooting* or *"lightning"* pains in the legs. Girdle pains also occur in tabetics, along with paresthesias, numbness, and tingling of the trunk, hands, or feet. Another type of severe pain occurs in attacks of *gastric crisis.* About 10 per cent of tabetic patients develop severe episodes of abdominal pain associated with nausea and vomiting. These attacks may last for days, resulting in dehydration and exhaustion. Patients with gastric crises are sometimes diagnosed as having acute surgical conditions, and unnecessary operations have been performed on these individuals.

Ataxia is a major symptom in tabes and may be so severe that the patient is unable to walk or stand. Some patients develop a typical tabetic gait, which consists of slapping of the feet and walking on a broad base. The ataxia is worse in the dark, and the patient may sway or fall when standing with his eyes closed (Romberg's sign). The damage to the nerve fibers in the posterior columns not only results in ataxia but also produces loss of position sense, and the patient does not know without visual assistance the exact position of his toes or feet. Vibratory sensation in the legs is diminished or absent. There may be diminution of deep pain sensation to pressure on the testes or Achilles tendon, and areas of hypesthesia may be present on the trunk or in the hands and feet. The patella and Achilles tendon reflexes are sluggish or absent. Patients with tabes often show evidence of hypotonia and hyperextensibility of the joints. Degenerative lesions, such as chronic, nonhealing lesions of the skin and *Charcot joints,* are also found.

Involvement of the autonomic nervous system may occur in patients with tabes, and *postural hypotension* is occasionally present. Severe *paroxysmal hypertension,* associated with gastric crises, has also been observed and may simulate paroxysmal hypertension caused by pheochromocytoma.

Urinary difficulties occur in approximately 50 to 60 per cent of patients with tabes. These often appear early in the disease and consist of hesitancy or difficulty in starting micturition. Later the patient develops complete loss of bladder sensation. Patients with tabetic bladder often give no history of urinary symptoms, and catheterization for residual urine should be done in all who have evidence of tabes. *Impotence* and loss of sexual desire are frequently noted.

Paralysis of the oculomotor nerves is common in tabes, resulting in diplopia, ptosis of the lids, or ophthalmoplegia. Pupillary abnormalities are also extremely common and may be manifested by the classic *Argyll Robertson phenomena,* that is, miosis, reaction to accommodation but no reaction to light, poor response to atropine, and absence of ciliospinal reflex. This condition must be differentiated from *Adie's pupil,* which is usually unilateral, is larger than the normal pupil, and reacts slowly to both light and accommodation. Patients with Adie's pupils may also have absent or diminished tendon reflexes.

Atrophy of the optic nerve occurs in about 10 to 15 per cent of patients with tabes. About 70 per cent of patients with untreated optic atrophy become blind in 3 years and 90 per cent in 5 years. On ophthalmoscopic examination the optic disk appears white and sharply defined. The physiologic cup is prominent and the lamina cribrosa is abnormally conspicuous. Visual field defects and diminution of vision may be present with only slight changes in the color of the disks. To detect such cases of optic atrophy early, careful perimetry and visual acuity examinations should be made in all cases of neurosyphilis. Although improvement in vision is not to be expected in patients with optic atrophy, arrest of the atrophic process can usually be obtained by penicillin therapy in patients with early involvement.

In early cases of tabes the serologic test for syphilis is often strongly positive, and the spinal fluid may show definite abnormalities, such as increased cells and protein and a positive Wassermann. In patients with long-standing tabes, however, the blood and spinal fluid findings may be misleading. Approximately one-fourth of such patients have negative blood serologic tests, while as many as 20 per cent have normal spinal fluids. Tabes dorsalis must be differentiated from numerous other diseases of the spinal column, such as cord tumor, combined system disease, and syringomyelia, as well as various types of peripheral neuritis (particularly diabetic neuropathy). The response of tabes to treatment is often poor, and symptoms may progress despite all forms of therapy.

Paretic Neurosyphilis (Dementia Paralytica, Paresis, General Paralysis of the Insane). General paresis is a psychosis caused by extensive spirochetal invasion of the brain. On histologic examination the most prominent feature is degeneration of the nerve cells. Perivascular infiltration and endothelial proliferation of the small vessels is seen. *Treponema pallidum* can be demonstrated in the cerebral cortex and other portions of the brain.

Paretic neurosyphilis is more common in men than in women and usually develops between the ages of thirty-five and fifty years. The onset is most often insidious; prodromal symptoms consist of headache, insomnia, difficulty in concentration and easy fatigability. As the disease progresses, a gradual change in personality takes place, with increased irritability, memory loss, poor judgment, lack of personal care, and deviations in character. These alterations may occur over a period of several months. Many of them are noted by the patient's family only in retrospect and elicited only by close questioning. The onset of paresis is sometimes sudden and may be ushered in by convulsions, syncope, or a cerebral vascular accident.

The simple, demented type of psychosis is the most common. These patients show confusion, apathy, impaired memory, and defects in judgment. Memory is particularly poor for recent events. They are often unable to concentrate on simple calculations and show little insight or concern about their illness. The grandiose form of paresis is manifested by euphoria, overactivity, ideas of grandeur, and megalomania. Auditory and visual hallucinations are not common in these patients, but delusions of wealth and prowess are frequent. The type of psychosis that prevails in a given case depends to a great extent upon the preparetic personality of the individual. As the disease progresses, however, the symptoms of euphoria, paranoia, or mania recede, and simple deterioration and dementia become the outstanding features.

Eventually the patients become completely bedridden and are unable to move and feed themselves.

On neurologic examination these patients may present various motor disturbances, such as *tremors* of the facial muscles, tongue, and outstretched hands. The patient's handwriting is altered because of the tremors and incoordination. The speech becomes slurred, and test phrases are mispronounced. Pupillary abnormalities are common, and deep reflexes are usually exaggerated. Some patients with paresis also have signs and symptoms of tabes—i.e., *taboparesis.*

The demented form of paresis must be differentiated from senile dementia and Alzheimer's disease. The manic and paranoic types must be distinguished from manic depressive psychoses and schizophrenia. In the early stages of paresis, differentiation from neurasthenia is sometimes difficult, and spinal fluid examination may be the only means of diagnosis.

The spinal fluid in general paresis shows marked changes, with increased cells and protein, positive serologic test, and first-zone colloidal reaction. The diagnosis of paresis should never be made in the presence of a normal spinal fluid; a positive spinal fluid is present in 100 per cent of untreated cases.

The course of untreated paresis is progressive, and death usually occurs within a few years after the onset of symptoms. The prognosis improves considerably with therapy, but the chances for complete recovery are at best about 50 to 60 per cent.

SYPHILIS IN PREGNANCY

Syphilis in pregnancy is a special problem, because the fetus becomes infected after the fifth month of pregnancy by passage of *T. pallidum* through the placenta. This usually occurs in women with early untreated syphilis, but is sometimes observed in late syphilis. Pregnancy complicated by syphilis may terminate in a spontaneous abortion, a stillborn infant, or a premature or full-term infected child. The maternal infection, however, becomes attenuated as the duration of the disease increases, and the chances of the fetus being infected are less with each succeeding pregnancy.

Pregnancy is believed to have a beneficial influence upon the course of the syphilitic infection, and late manifestations of the disease seem to occur less frequently in multiparous women than in others. A serologic test for syphilis should be taken routinely at the first prenatal visit of every pregnant woman. The early recognition of syphilis in pregnancy followed by adequate treatment will prevent congenital syphilis in almost every instance.

CONGENITAL SYPHILIS

Infantile congenital syphilis is often an overwhelming infection; such infants are severely ill,

malnourished, and dehydrated. The most common manifestations of the disease in infants are skin lesions, fissures, condylomas, persistent rhinitis, tenderness over the long bones, and pseudoparalysis.

The diagnosis of syphilis in the infant is best established by dark-field demonstration of *T. pallidum* from the cutaneous or mucosal lesions. A positive serologic test in the first two months of life does not always indicate syphilis in the infant, since reacting substances may have been transferred from the maternal circulation. A very high titer of the serologic reaction or a steady rise in titer, however, is indicative of congenital syphilis. Roentgenographic examination of the long bones may show characteristic areas of bone destruction and *osteochondritis.*

Late congenital syphilis frequently manifests itself in the second decade with signs of central nervous system involvement, such as eighth nerve deafness, optic atrophy, and *juvenile paresis.* The prognosis of congenital neurosyphilis is serious; these patients commonly show little response to treatment. Cardiovascular syphilis is rare in the congenital infection.

Patients with late congenital syphilis often exhibit typical stigmas, such as hypoplasia, wide spacing and notching of the central incisors (*Hutchinson teeth*), frontal bossing, a highly arched palate, and *saber shins.* The first permanent molar is also frequently affected in congenital syphilis and shows a characteristic appearance, with several small atrophic cusps on the occlusal surface. This is known as a "mulberry molar." *Interstitial keratitis,* a frequent complication, usually appears in the second decade. It is characterized by pain, lacrimation, circumcorneal injection, and corneal opacity. The response to therapy is poor, and serious impairment of vision often results. Occasionally, hydrarthrosis of the knee joint (*Clutton's synovitis*) is associated with interstitial keratitis.

LABORATORY DIAGNOSIS

Dark-field demonstration of *T. pallidum* is most useful in the early stages of syphilis. It should be employed routinely on every genital lesion and on all cutaneous and mucosal lesions suspected of being syphilitic. In the hands of a competent microscopist, dark-field examination is reliable and establishes without doubt the diagnosis and stage of the infection.

Serologic Tests. Serologic tests for syphilis (STS) are the most commonly used diagnostic procedures. In latent syphilis they are the only means by which the diagnosis can be made. The serologic tests are based upon the presence of an antibodylike substance (sometimes called *reagin*), which appears in the patient's serum soon after the onset of the disease. Syphilitic serum reacts with a lipoidal antigen made from an alcoholic extract of beef heart. Various modifications of flocculation tests for syphilis have been named after their originators (Kahn, Kline, and Hinton). The complement fixation technique or Wassermann test employs the same type of antigen, the Kolmer modification being the most commonly used in this country. The VDRL (Venereal Disease Research Laboratory) test is a rapid slide technique employing cardiolipin antigen. It has a high degree of sensitivity and specificity and has become the flocculation test of choice in most state laboratories and hospitals.

In addition to these serologic tests for syphilis (STS) using lipoidal or cardiolipin antigens, a number of other techniques have been developed since 1949 which employ antigens made from whole body virulent *T. pallidum* or from chemical fractions of this organism. These include the *T. pallidum* immobilization (TPI), agglutination (TPA), complement fixation (TPCF), and the fluorescent treponemal antibody (FTA) reactions. In addition, a standardized antigen of the Reiter strain of the cultivated spirochete is now commercially available and is being used in the Reiter protein complement fixation test (RPCF). Although many new serologic procedures are now available, it is recommended that the standard reagin tests continue to be used for the routine serologic diagnosis of syphilis since they are highly standardized, easily reproducible, and inexpensive. Moreover they are widely used, and the results are readily understood and interpreted by the physician. The current treponemal tests do not offer sufficient advantages over the standard reagin tests to supplant them as routine diagnostic procedures, but they are very helpful as confirmatory tests and in the diagnosis of biologic false positive reactions. The Reiter protein complement fixation test has been suggested as a feasible method of confirming a positive standard serologic test in individuals who previously had not been suspected of having the disease. When there is a discrepancy between the results of the standard serologic test and the Reiter protein complement fixation test, a biologic false positive reaction should be considered and the patient's serum tested with one of the treponemal procedures which employ virulent organisms as an antigen.

The rapid plasma reagin (RPR) test has the advantage of being a very rapid serologic procedure since it uses unheated plasma or serum. It is more sensitive than the standard serologic tests and has been recommended as a routine screening technique for laboratories performing large numbers of tests or for surveys requiring on-the-spot results.

It has been recommended that the results of serologic tests be reported as "reactive," "weakly reactive," and "nonreactive" in substitution or in place of the previous terms "positive," "doubtful," or "negative." The presence of a nonreactive or negative standard reagin test does not always exclude syphilis nor is a reactive or positive test always proof of the existence of the disease. Serologic tests are nonreactive in the incubation period of syphilis during the early weeks of the primary stage and in many of the late manifestations such as cardiovascular and neurosyphilis (tabes dorsalis in particular).

The height of the titer in serial serologic tests is of value in the diagnosis and management of the various stages of the disease. A sharply rising titer is usually found in recently acquired syphilis, while a stationary titer indicates an infection of some duration. A rapidly falling titer in the absence of therapy is evidence against the diagnosis of syphilis and may indicate a false positive reaction. The height of the titer has no bearing on the prognosis or outcome of the disease. Carefully titered tests are also important in determining the results of therapy; a continuing falling titer indicates a satisfactory response.

Biologic False Positive Serologic Tests for Syphilis. Positive reactions appear in a great variety of illnesses and are due presumably to the appearance in the patient's serum of substances which act like reagin and give positive flocculation and complement fixation reactions for syphilis. These reactions are usually transient, but in some instances may be positive for months or years.

Biologic false positive reactions are frequently observed in patients with vaccinia, infectious mononucleosis, malaria, leprosy, and upper respiratory diseases, as well as in spirochetal infections, such as yaws, pinta, and relapsing fever. Other infections which are occasionally associated with false positive reactions are lymphogranuloma venereum, chancroid, measles, chickenpox, atypical pneumonia, infectious hepatitis, rat-bite fever, and disseminated lupus erythematosus. In fact, any febrile disease or immunization is a potential cause of false positive tests. There is evidence that individuals with biologic false positive reactions of long duration may have serious illnesses such as collagen disorders, sarcoid, or lymphomas.

The *Treponema pallidum*–immobilizing (TPI) test of Nelson and other treponemal tests are often of considerable aid in the diagnosis of false positive reactions. These tests are almost always positive in late syphilis. A negative treponemal test is, therefore, of value in excluding the diagnosis of syphilis. A positive test on the other hand indicates the existence of a syphilitic infection even if the standard serologic tests are negative. In most cases, the false positive reaction will become negative within 6 months. If the patient continues to show a positive serologic test and if the adjunct procedures do not indicate a false positive reaction, antisyphilitic therapy should be instituted. If the patient becomes pregnant or is to be married, immediate treatment is indicated.

Seroresistance. In many patients with syphilis the serologic test remains positive despite prolonged, intensive therapy. These patients are called sero-resistant, or Wassermann-fast. One of the aims of therapy in early syphilis (particularly during the first 2 years of the disease) is to procure and maintain a negative serologic reaction. In late syphilis, however, seroresistance is of little clinical importance and has no relationship to the outcome of the disease.

In most patients with early syphilis the serologic test becomes negative within 6 months after beginning therapy. Occasionally the titer of the serologic reaction falls very slowly and the tests remain positive in low titer (i.e., less than 1:4 dilution) for as long as 1 to 2 years. In some patients with early syphilis there is very little serologic response to treatment, and the titer remains high for 6 to 9 months or more. This type of seroresistance is usually followed by clinical relapse, and these patients should be re-treated.

Neurosyphilis is frequently associated with sero-resistance in both early and late cases, and the spinal fluid should be examined in every patient with a persistently positive serologic reaction.

The seroresistant patient is often discouraged over the failure to reverse the serologic test and becomes deeply concerned for fear that the infection is not arrested. In addition, he may be embarrassed in applying for a marriage license or employment when blood tests are a part of the premarital or preemployment examination. The physician should make every effort to reassure such patients that the outcome of the disease is not related to the persistence of a positive serologic test. Seroresistance should not be an obstacle to marriage.

Spinal Fluid Tests. The spinal fluid must be examined in every patient with syphilis. This is the only method of detecting involvement of the central nervous system in the asymptomatic stage, of determining the efficacy of treatment, and of confirming the diagnosis of symptomatic neurosyphilis.

The spinal fluid cell count should be done within an hour after the fluid is withdrawn. A count of more than 8 lymphocytes per cubic millimeter is usually considered abnormal. Even a small amount of blood in the spinal fluid will affect the accuracy of the various examinations. A quantitative determination of the spinal fluid protein should be done in every case.

Complement fixation tests for syphilis are generally regarded as being more sensitive than floc-culation tests for examination of spinal fluid. The spinal fluid of patients with neurosyphilis has been found to contain immobilizing antibodies for *T. pallidum.*

The spinal fluid may also show biologic false positive complement fixation or flocculation reactions. This may be caused by a bloody tap or any condition which produces an increased protein in the spinal fluid. Brain tumor, bacterial or virus meningitis, encephalitis, or subarachnoid hemorrhage can produce a false positive test for syphilis in either syphilitic or nonsyphilitic patients.

The value of colloidal precipitation tests (gold and mastic reactions) has been overemphasized in the diagnosis of neurosyphilis. The zone of precipitation or the shape of the colloidal curve has little diagnostic significance.

Biopsy. Biopsy is a valuable diagnostic procedure, especially for cutaneous lesions. In late syphilis involving the lymph nodes, testes, or larynx, it is indispensable.

TREATMENT

In patients with early syphilis adequate treatment can produce an absolute, or biologic, cure, with complete healing of lesions and reversal of serologic tests and spinal fluid findings. These patients become entirely well, are not infectious, and do not develop any of the late manifestations of the disease.

Treatment of late syphilis may not achieve these goals. Despite long and vigorous therapy the serologic tests in late syphilis often remain positive. Late syphilitic lesions are often associated with permanent damage, and treatment may produce little or no return of function.

Early Syphilis. In 1943 penicillin was found to be effective in the treatment of syphilis. The use of arsenicals, bismuth, or mercurials is rarely, if ever, indicated. Other antibiotics, such as chloramphenicol and the various tetracyclines have trep-onemicidal activity and produce healing of both early and late syphilitic lesions. The ultimate place of these drugs in the treatment of syphilis has not yet been established. They are probably not so effective as penicillin, but doses of 3 to 4 Gm daily for 10 to 12 days are recommended. Erythromycin and carbomycin have also been shown to have some treponemicidal action.

Procaine penicillin and benzathine penicillin G have generally replaced crystalline penicillin in aqueous solution, except perhaps in the very serious or far-advanced stages of syphilitic infection. The minimal effective total dosage of penicillin has been found to be approximately 2.4 million units. Increasing the total amount of penicillin from 2.4 to

9.6 million units does not decrease the failure rate in early syphilis.

The total dosage of depot penicillin usually prescribed is approximately 4 to 6 million units given over a period of 8 to 12 days. This schedule will produce satisfactory results in about 90 per cent of patients. The remaining 10 per cent will show clinical or laboratory changes of either a relapse or reinfection. Benzathine penicillin G has also been found to be effective in early syphilis when given as a single injection of 2.4 million units or in two or three weekly doses. It has the advantage from the public health standpoint of completing treatment in a minimum period of time but is not recommended as a routine method of treatment. Oral penicillin products are not recommended for the treatment of syphilis. The other antibiotics with treponemicidal activity should be used only in patients in whom penicillin is contraindicated.

Jarisch-Herxheimer Reaction. Within a few hours after the first injection of either an arsenical or penicillin, about 50 per cent of patients with early syphilis experience fever, malaise, headache, myalgia, and a flare-up of cutaneous lesions. This is presumed to be caused by release of breakdown products of spirochetes following the injection of treponemicidal agents. In early syphilis these symptoms disappear within several hours and leave no permanent tissue damage. In late syphilis such reactions can be disastrous if the lesions are located in such areas as the ostiums of the coronary arteries, the wall of an aneurysm, or the central nervous system.

Posttreatment Observation. After completing treatment, patients should return every month during the first year for quantitative serologic tests and examination for relapsing lesions. If the patient develops a recurrence of syphilitic lesions or evidence of neurosyphilis, or if there is a birth of a syphilitic child, re-treatment is necessary. If the serologic test in patients with early syphilis shows no appreciable decrease within 6 months or if the titer is elevated (arbitrarily a dilution of 1:4 or higher) 1 year after completion of therapy, further treatment is indicated. A positive reaction in any dilution 18 months or more after completion of treatment of primary or secondary syphilis should be considered as evidence of treatment failure, and another course of therapy with penicillin is indicated.

Serologic tests should be taken at 3-month intervals during the second year after treatment and at 6-month intervals during the third, fourth, and fifth years. If at the end of 5 years the patient has no clinical evidence of syphilis and has a normal blood and spinal fluid, he may be considered completely cured.

A *spinal fluid examination should be performed 6 months after the completion of treatment for early syphilis.* If it is normal at this time and if the patient continues to show no evidence of clinical or serologic relapse, it need not be repeated until approximately two years following treatment. Patients having positive spinal fluid tests for syphilis 6 months or more after treatment for early syphilis should be re-treated.

Relapse and Reinfection. Evidence of relapse in early syphilis may occur as early as 4 weeks or as late as 2 years after treatment.

The prognosis of relapsing syphilis is more serious than the initial infection, and such patients should be re-treated with twice the original dose of penicillin, given over a longer period of time. Many patients with recurrent syphilis actually have a new infection rather than a relapse of their original infection. Although various criteria have been set up to distinguish relapse from reinfection, differentiation is often impossible.

Syphilis in Pregnancy. Congenital syphilis can be prevented by proper treatment of syphilis in pregnancy. Although women with syphilis of many years' duration are not likely to bear syphilitic children, further treatment of such patients during pregnancy is recommended. Although treatment with penicillin is of considerable value when given during the last months of pregnancy, it is best given before the fetus becomes grossly infected, i.e., before the last trimester.

All patients treated for syphilis in pregnancy should be observed very closely, and quantitative serologic tests for syphilis taken at least every month. Re-treatment during pregnancy is indicated if there is a rise in serologic titer following therapy, if a definite decrease in titer fails to occur in patients with early syphilis, or if the patient develops recurrent syphilitic lesions. A positive serologic test at the time of delivery does not necessarily indicate that treatment has been inadequate. The child born of a mother treated for syphilis should have a serologic test every 2 to 4 weeks until it is at least six months of age. Once the woman has received adequate amounts of penicillin for syphilis, it is not necessary to re-treat her during succeeding pregnancies if the titer of the serologic test is negative or remains low (less than 1:4).

Congenital Syphilis. Infants with congenital syphilis should receive careful supportive care and adequate nutrition, in addition to antisyphilitic treatment. Penicillin is very effective; a total dosage of 200,000 units per kg body weight given in equally divided amounts every 3 hr for 7 to 10 days is adequate. Although the use of procaine penicillin in a large series of these cases has not been reported, this type of penicillin should also give satisfactory results. Doses of 150,000 units of procaine penicillin in aqueous solution given every day for eight injections are recommended. Follow-up blood tests and the indications for retreatment in early congenital syphilis are the same as in early acquired syphilis.

Treatment of interstitial keratitis is not altogether satisfactory. Penicillin therapy is recommended, but it does not always result in reduction of the inflammation or clearing of the corneal opacities. Occasionally, interstitial keratitis appears for the first time during, or immediately after, what appear to be adequate dosages of penicillin. It seems probable that this ocular manifestation represents a type of hypersensitivity phenomenon. Cortisone in aqueous suspension (5 mg per ml) or in ointment form should be applied to the involved eye every few hours day and night for several weeks. The inflammatory reaction often recurs, however, after the drug is discontinued, and repeated courses may be necessary until spontaneous regression of the condition appears. Hydrarthrosis (Clutton's synovitis) responds slowly to penicillin therapy.

Late Syphilis. *Latent Stage.* The chief purpose in treating late latent syphilis is to prevent the development of gummatous lesions and cardiovascular syphilis. Patients with late latent syphilis have negative spinal fluids and rarely, if ever, develop neurosyphilis.

Penicillin has not been fully evaluated in late latent syphilis. Since the prognosis of this stage of the disease is so good and since the drug is known to be effective in both early and late symptomatic syphilis, it is presumed to be of value in patients with latent infection. The treatment schedules suggested for early syphilis, employing 4 to 6 million units of penicillin, are recommended. Failure of the serologic test to revert to negative after adequate treatment—i.e., *seroresistance*—is not necessarily a forerunner of late complications. Once the patient with late syphilis has had adequate treatment, additional penicillin therapy will not contribute significantly toward reversal of the blood test.

Skin, Bones, and Viscera. Gummatous lesions of the skin, mucous membranes, bones, and viscera usually respond promptly to penicillin therapy. The recommended total dosage of penicillin is greater than that employed in early syphilis and should be approximately 10 million units. This can be administered as 900,000 units of procaine penicillin given every 48 hr for 12 injections. The posttreatment observations and indications for re-treatment of these patients are the same as those recommended above. A high percentage of patients with late syphilitic lesions have abnormal spinal fluid findings, and a lumbar puncture is indicated in every patient before treatment is instituted.

Cardiovascular Syphilis. The value of antisyphilitic therapy in late cardiovascular syphilis is difficult to determine. Many syphilologists believe that treatment does not delay the ultimate development

of myocardial failure or aneurysmal rupture. Treatment appears to be of some value, however, in early aortic insufficiency, uncomplicated aortitis, or small asymptomatic aneurysms. The risk of a serious Herxheimer reaction following initiation of penicillin treatment of these cases has been found to be minimal. Preparatory bismuth therapy is probably of little value in preventing this type of reaction, and most workers begin treatment with penicillin. The total dosage is 10 to 15 million units of penicillin, given in schedules similar to those recommended for gummatous lesions. As in other types of late syphilis, the serologic test often remains positive after therapy. Proper management of congestive failure and restriction of physical activity of these patients is of paramount importance.

Neurosyphilis. The results of treatment of neurosyphilis depend largely upon the type and duration of the neuropathologic process. If the predominant lesion of the central nervous system is degenerative, as in tabes and optic atrophy, little response to any form of treatment can be expected. If the tissue reaction is chiefly inflammatory, as in syphilitic meningitis, rapid and almost complete return of function will occur.

Penicillin treatment of neurosyphilis is often followed by dramatic clinical response with prompt and favorable changes in the spinal fluid. Shortly after penicillin therapy, there is a rapid reduction in the spinal fluid cell count and protein. The spinal fluid serologic reaction, however, may not become negative for 5 years or more. Penicillin produced normal spinal fluid cell counts in 85 to 90 per cent of patients treated for various types of neurosyphilis. The remaining 10 to 15 per cent showed abnormal spinal fluid cell counts 6 to 12 months following treatment and were considered treatment failures.

It is generally agreed that the improvement in the clinical manifestations of neurosyphilis as well as the spinal fluid abnormalities following penicillin is as good as that obtained with fever therapy. Penicillin alone is the treatment of choice in patients with asymptomatic neurosyphilis, syphilitic meningitis, meningovascular syphilis, and tabes. The optimum dosage schedule has not been definitely established, but doses of 10 to 15 million units are usually recommended either as the aqueous solution, 100,000 units every 3 hr, or as repository penicillin 900,000 units a day.

Treatment of the tabetic bladder may be very discouraging. Drugs, such as Mecholyl chloride and ergotamine, have been employed to increase bladder tone and contraction, but the results are variable. In early cases the patient can be trained to micturate at regular intervals and empty the bladder by pressure on the lower abdomen. In late cases, surgical procedures (transurethral resection of the vesical neck, suprapubic cystotomy) may be necessary. Urinary tract infection should be prevented and instrumentation avoided as much as possible. Charcot joints are rarely improved by antisyphilitic therapy, and special orthopedic treatment is necessary. The management of patients with gastric crisis is sometimes very difficult. In the acute attack the patient should be heavily sedated. Morphine should be avoided. Large doses of atropine are said to be of value in relieving the symptoms of gastric crisis.

In most cases of advanced optic atrophy the use of penicillin or fever, alone or in combination, does not prevent the development of blindness. Patients with optic atrophy should be admitted to the hospital and given penicillin in aqueous solution, 200,000 units every 4 hr for 13 to 17 days, for a total dosage of 15 to 20 million units.

In paresis, penicillin alone often results in marked improvement in tremor, mental state, and speech and writing defects. It has been reported to produce entirely satisfactory results in about 20 per cent and significant improvement in an additional 35 per cent of a large series of patients with paresis treated in general hospitals. Early penicillin treatment of incipient paresis has resulted in clinical remission and ability to return to work in more than 80 per cent of patients. Large amounts of penicillin —15 to 20 million units—are generally recommended, but doses as low as 6 million units have been found to be of value. Although the repository type of penicillin is said to be as effective as aqueous penicillin in paresis or optic atrophy, the aqueous preparation is preferred in the moderately or severely affected cases. It should be given in schedules similar to those recommended for optic atrophy.

Fever therapy is rarely used at present in either optic atrophy or paresis since recent evidence indicates that its possible additive effects are not sufficient to justify the hazards associated with it. In selected patients with these disorders, however, in whom the neurosyphilitic process progresses despite adequate initial penicillin therapy, re-treatment with fever therapy and penicillin should be considered. Re-treatment with penicillin alone, however, is indicated in progressive paresis if the initial course of treatment consisted of less than 6 million units. Penicillin alone should also be used to re-treat patients who show elevated spinal fluid cell counts a year or more after the initial therapy or in whom there was temporary clinical improvement after treatment but subsequent progression.

Careful neuropsychiatric and spinal fluid observations should be made following treatment of all patients with neurosyphilis. These should be done every 4 months during the first year, twice during the second year, and once a year thereafter, or until the spinal fluid is completely negative and permanent regression of symptoms seems apparent. In late neurosyphilis the spinal fluid serologic reaction often remains positive for many years, despite repeated courses of chemotherapy or fever; this does not in itself indicate progression or relapse of the neurosyphilitic process.

Herxheimer Reactions in Late Syphilis. Exacerbations of late syphilitic lesions are not infrequently observed following the initial administration of arsenicals or penicillin. Approximately one-half the patients treated for paresis become temporarily worse and show increased agitation and mental confusion during the first 24 hr of penicillin treatment. Other manifestations of Herxheimer reaction, such as myelitis, convulsions, and exacerbation of lightning pains, have been reported.

There have been very few cases in which penicillin therapy has appeared to produce an acute exacerbation of clinical manifestations of cardiovascular syphilis. Neither the use of small initial doses of penicillin nor preparatory treatment with bismuth seems indicated in an attempt to prevent Herxheimer effects.

Effect of Penicillin and Other Antibiotics When Used for Other Diseases. The widespread use of penicillin and antibiotics with treponemicidal properties in the treatment of various other infections has created confusion in the diagnosis and management of syphilis. This is particularly true when gonorrhea is treated. Patients with gonorrhea may have acquired syphilis simultaneously. Although there is reason to believe that the use of penicillin and perhaps the other antibiotics frequently abort the syphilitic infection completely, they may at times only delay the appearance of the lesions or prevent their development. For these reasons it is recommended that all persons with gonorrhea treated with penicillin or the other spirocheticidal antibiotics should have serologic tests for syphilis at monthly intervals for at least 4 months. The appearance of fever several hours after the administration of penicillin for gonorrhea is suggestive of a Herxheimer reaction and the presence of syphilis.

The management of patients with positive serologic tests who have had previous penicillin therapy for other nonrelated infections is sometimes difficult. If syphilitic infection is thought to be present, the decision as to further therapy should be based upon the amount of penicillin already administered, the type and duration of syphilitic infection, the result of the spinal fluid examination, and the titer of the serologic test.

PROPHYLAXIS

Syphilis and the other venereal diseases can be prevented in most instances by the proper prophylactic measures during and following sexual intercourse. Protection from contact with infectious genital lesions can be obtained to some degree by the use of a condom. The danger of infection can also be reduced if the genitalia are washed thoroughly with soap and water immediately after exposure. Although ointments containing various treponemicidal substances have been employed for many years as local prophylactic agents, the use of such compounds is no longer recommended. In small series of cases, penicillin has been shown to prevent infection in individuals who are known to have been sexually exposed to patients with primary or secondary syphilis. The use of penicillin in these cases is justified not only as an attempt to abort the infection in the exposed individual, but also to prevent reinfection of the original patient who often maintains sexual relations with the contact despite instructions to the contrary.

Procaine penicillin or benzathine penicillin G in doses of 1.2 million units should be given soon after exposure to persons who have had sexual contact with known or suspected cases of infectious syphilis. The administration of penicillin as a routine prophylactic measure following every extramarital sexual exposure is neither practical nor advisable. Persons receiving prophylactic treatment should be kept under observation, if possible, and should have repeated serologic tests for at least 6 months.

The prophylactic treatment of nurses, physicians, or laboratory workers accidentally exposed to, or inoculated with, infectious material will depend largely upon the risk of infection in the individual case. Another indication for prophylactic treatment is in pregnant women who are sexually exposed to infectious patients. A full course of penicillin treatment in these cases is indicated in an effort to prevent fetal infection.

PSYCHOTHERAPY

There is still considerable stigma and psychologic trauma attached to the diagnosis of syphilis, and proper treatment requires more than the mere administration of chemotherapeutic agents. The physician must be aware of the sociologic and psychologic aspects of this disease. Patients often have a sense of shame and guilt, and some of them postpone or discontinue medical care. Others develop serious anxiety states and return to the physician repeatedly for reassurance that the disease has been arrested. Some individuals develop syphilophobia as a result of having heard or read of the serious effects of the disease. The physician should make every effort to relieve these patients of their anxiety by correcting mistaken ideas regarding the infection and by emphasizing the good prognosis whenever possible. His attitude toward the patient should be free of censure.

Upon learning the diagnosis, many patients either condemn their marital partners and threaten divorce or separation or else refuse to impart the information to their spouse. The physician should not enter into the moral aspects of the disease but should make certain that the marital partners of patients with infectious syphilis are examined at regular intervals for evidence of the disease.

REFERENCES

Clark, E. G., and N. Danbolt: The Oslo Study of the Natural History of Untreated Syphilis: An Epidemiologic Investigation Based on a Restudy of the Boeck-Bruusgaard Material: A Review and Appraisal, J. Chronic Diseases, 2:311, 1955.

Garson, W.: Recent Developments in the Laboratory Diagnosis of Syphilis, Ann. Internal Med., 51:748, 1959.

Hahn, R. D.: Tabes Dorsalis, with Special Reference to Primary Optic Atrophy, Brit. J. Venereal Diseases, 33:139, 1957.

—— et al.: Penicillin Treatment of General Paresis (Dementia Paralytica), A.M.A. Arch. Neurol. and Psychiat., 81:557, 1959.

Heyman, A., W. H. Sheldon, and L. D. Evans: The Pathogenesis of the Jarisch-Herxheimer Reaction, Brit. J. Venereal Diseases, 28:50, 1953.

Magnuson, H. J.: Current Concepts of Immunity in Syphilis, Am. J. Med., 5:641, 1948.

Merritt, H. H., R. D. Adams, and H. C. Solomon: "Neurosyphilis," New York, Oxford University Press, 1946.

Montgomery, C. H., and J. M. Knox: Antibiotics Other than Penicillin in the Treatment of Syphilis, New Engl. J. Med., 261:277, 1959.

Moore, J. E., and C. F. Mohr: Biologically False Positive Serologic Tests for Syphilis: Type, Incidence, and Cause, J.A.M.A., 150:457, 1952.

—— and W. B. Lutz: The Natural History of Systemic Lupus Erythematosus: An Approach to Its Study through Chronic Biologic False Positive Reactors, J. Chronic Diseases, 1:297, 1955.

Nelson, R. A.: Changing Concepts in the Serodiagnosis of Syphilis: Specific Treponemal Antibody versus Wassermann Reagin, Brit. J. Venereal Diseases, 28:160, 1952.

Nielson, H. A., and A. Reyn: The *Treponema pallidum* Immobilization Test, Bull. World Health Organization, 14:262, 1956. (This issue of the Bulletin contains other pertinent articles on serologic diagnosis.)

164 YAWS
Albert Heyman

Definition. Yaws is an infectious tropical disease caused by the *Treponema pertenue*. It is characterized by a primary cutaneous lesion, which is followed by a granulomatous skin eruption and, in some instances, by late destructive lesions of the skin and bones. The disease is also known as *frambesia, pian, bouba,* and *parangi.*

Etiology. The etiologic agent of yaws, the *T. pertenue,* is morphologically indistinguishable from *Treponema pallidum;* it further resembles the spirochete of syphilis, as it produces a positive reaction with the Wassermann and flocculation tests for syphilis, and is also susceptible to arsenicals, bismuth, and penicillin. Cross immunity between the two diseases has been observed in both man and experimental animals. There has been considerable controversy as to whether the two diseases were at one time identical and have been modified over the years by climate, race, and other factors.

Epidemiology. Yaws is confined entirely to the tropics and is prevalent in the West Indies, South Pacific islands, equatorial Africa, and South America. The disease is usually acquired before puberty and is spread by direct contact with open lesions containing the spirochete. Transmission of the disease occurs rarely by sexual contact. Certain species of flies are also thought to be vectors of this infection. The disease is more common in natives with poor personal hygiene.

Manifestations. Following an average incubation period of 3 to 4 weeks, a primary lesion, the *mother yaw,* appears at the site of inoculation. This is almost invariably extragenital and usually occurs on the legs. This lesion is a granuloma, which later ulcerates and heals with scar formation. About 6 to 12 weeks after the appearance of the lesion, a generalized eruption develops, consisting of large papules or granulomas on the face, neck, extremities, and buttocks. These lesions often occur about the mucocutaneous junctions, such as the mouth, nose, and rectum, and resemble condylomas of secondary syphilis. They heal slowly, but relapses may occur months or years after the onset of the initial yaw. The lesions of yaws often appear on the soles of the feet and produce painful ulcerations, so-called "crab yaws."

After several years, late destructive lesions may appear in the skin and bones. Periostitis and osteitis are found in the bones of the hands, arms, and legs, producing characteristic dactylitis and "saber shins." Destructive lesions appear about the nose and result in severe ulcerative areas (*gangosa*). Proliferative exostoses develop in the nasal portion of the maxillary bones; this is known as *goundou.* Juxtaarticular nodules are also seen in the late stage of the disease. Involvement of the aorta and the central nervous system has been reported, but these complications are rare.

Diagnosis. The diagnosis of yaws can often be made on the appearance of the generalized skin eruption alone, but *T. pertenue* is easily demonstrated in the lesions. The Wassermann and flocculation tests for syphilis are usually positive. The lesions of yaws may be confused with those of leishmaniasis, leprosy, and tuberculosis. It is often impossible to differentiate between late lesions of yaws and late gummatous syphilis.

Treatment. Penicillin is the drug of choice in the treatment of yaws and produces prompt disappearance of the treponemes on dark-field examination and rapid healing of the lesions. The recommended dosage is a single injection of 1.2 million units of procaine penicillin in adults with early active lesions and proportionally less in children and latent cases. The tetracyclines are thought to be less effective in the management of this condition. The World Health Organization has conducted large-scale campaigns to eradicate the disease in endemic areas, and some 40 million persons have been treated under their auspices. In high-prevalence areas, treatment has been given to the total population, with dramatic reduction in the incidence of new cases. As a result of these control measures and improvement in living standards of the native populations, yaws is rapidly receding in the equatorial portions of the world.

REFERENCES

Hackett, C. J.: An International Nomenclature of Yaws Lesions, World Health Organization Monograph Series, No. 36, 1957. (An atlas containing numerous photographs illustrating recommended terminology.)

Hackett, C. J., and T. Guthe: Some Important Aspects of Yaws Eradication, Bull. World Health Organization, 15:869, 1956. (This reference is part of a symposium on treponematoses as a world-wide problem.)

Manson-Bahr, P. M.: "Manson's Tropical Disease," London, Cassell and Company, Ltd., 1954.

Turner, T. B., and D. H. Hollander: Biology of the Treponematoses, World Health Organization Monograph Series, No. 35, 1957.

165 PINTA
Albert Heyman

Definition. Pinta is an infectious disease of the skin caused by *Treponema carateum.* It is characterized by an initial papular lesion of the skin, followed by depigmented areas on the extremities and hyperkeratosis on the soles and palms. The disease is also known as *mal del pinto, azul,* and *carate.* Pinta is found almost entirely in the Western Hemisphere and is especially prevalent in Mexico and Colombia.

Etiology. *Treponema carateum,* the etiologic agent of pinta, is morphologically indistinguishable from *Treponema pallidum.* The exact relationship of this disease to other treponematoses (syphilis, yaws, and bejel) has not been definitely determined, and there are many similarities in the clinical manifestations of these infections. Pinta is usually transmitted from person to person by direct contact. It may also be spread by an insect vector.

Manifestations. The primary lesion of pinta appears after an incubation period of 7 to 20 days as a nonulcerative papule at the site of infection. This is followed 5 to 18 months later by a secondary eruption characterized by flat erythematous and hyperpigmented lesions, called *pintids.* Late lesions develop after several years and appear as vitiligoid, slate blue, or variously colored patches of the skin. The hands, wrists, knees, and ankles are commonly involved, and hyperkeratoses of the palms and soles are also seen. Aortitis and spinal fluid abnormalities similar to those found in neurosyphilis have been observed in some pinta patients. The Wassermann reaction of the blood and flocculation tests for syphilis are usually positive in the late stages of the disease.

Treatment. A single injection of 1.2 million units of procaine penicillin or benzathine penicillin G produces rapid disappearance of the *T. carateum* from the lesions of pinta and a decline in serologic titer. It is the treatment of choice in this disease and is more effective than chloramphenicol or the tetracyclines.

REFERENCES

Beerman, H.: Pinta: A Review of Recent Etiologic and Clinical Studies, Am. J. Med. Sci., 205:611, 1943.

Marquez, F., C. R. Rein, and O. Arias: Mal Del Pinto in Mexico, Bull. World Health Organization, 13: 299, 1955.

166 BEJEL
Albert Heyman

Definition and Etiology. Bejel is a chronic infectious disease caused by a spirochete indistinguishable from *Treponema pallidum.* It is found chiefly among the children of Arab tribes in the Eastern Mediterranean area, being particularly prevalent in some sections of Iraq, Syria, and Jordan. The illness is first manifested by ulcerations of the mucous membranes in the mouth and is thought to be spread by the use of common drinking utensils. It is rarely transmitted by sexual contact and is usually acquired by adults through close contact with an infected child as by kissing and fondling.

Treponemes are readily found on dark-field examination of the lesions of the skin and mucous membranes. The disease is thought by Hudson to be an example of nonvenereal syphilis, the causative organism and the clinical manifestations having been modified for many generations by special epidemiologic and climatic factors. Bejel resembles in many respects the cases of endemic syphilis which appeared for many years in certain areas of South Africa and Yugoslavia.

Manifestations. The illness begins with ulcerations in the mouth and lips, but there may also be a diffuse papular eruption with moist lesions on the mucocutaneous surfaces and skin folds. The late lesions resemble gummatous syphilis and are manifested as ulcerations in the skin and mucous membranes. Osteitis and periostitis of the long bones and skull may develop. The nasal bones, palate and pharynx, particularly, may be involved in a destructive process. The heart and nervous system are rarely, if ever, affected. The illness also differs from venereal syphilis in that it is apparently not spread to the child in utero from an infected mother. The diagnosis can be made by dark-field examination of the lesions or by the usual serologic tests for syphilis (see p. 1076).

Treatment. A single injection of 1.2 million units of procaine penicillin seems to be effective. In patients with late osseous or ulcerative lesions, additional penicillin may be required.

REFERENCES

Guthe, T., and R. R. Willcox: Treponematoses—A World Problem, Chronicle of the World Health Organization, 8:39, 1954.

Hudson, E. H.: "Non-venereal Syphilis," Edinburgh, E. S. Livingston, Ltd., 1958.

Simons, R. D. G. Ph.: "Handbook of Tropical Dermatology and Medical Mycology," New York, Elsevier Publishing Company, 1952.

167 LEPTOSPIROSIS
Fred R. McCrumb, Jr., and
T. E. Woodward

Etiology. Leptospiral infections are caused by a large group of antigenically distinct microorganisms comprising the genus *Leptospira.* The organisms exhibit a fine spiral configuration about an axial filament and vary in length from 4 to 20 μ. Leptospiras pathogenic for man are indistinguishable morphologically and are separable only by antigenic structure. They are actively motile and may exhibit hooklike bending of one or both ends. The genus *Leptospira* is made up of at least 20 serogroups, each comprised of several specific serotypes. Of the 12 serotypes presently known to occur in the United States, 8 have been associated with leptospiral infection of man.

Epidemiology. Leptospirosis is primarily a disease of lower animals. Natural infection of rats, mice, voles, opossums, cattle, swine, and dogs leads to the development of a renal carrier state and shedding of leptospiras in the urine of these hosts. Man may become infected whenever his occupational or pastime activities bring him into an area inhabited by animal carriers. Infected rats and mice usually exhibit no evidence of disease, and adult pigs may experience only an increased incidence of abortion. On the other hand, well-defined clinical illness, sometimes fatal, occurs in dogs and cattle. Predilection of specific leptospiras for certain lower animals limits the number of serotypes encountered in some regions. Transmission of leptospiras to man usually is accomplished through the medium of water contaminated by the urine of these animals, although direct contact with infected tissues is important in veterinarians and slaughterhouse workers. The disease is most frequently observed in veterinarians, farmers, swineherds, cane cutters, rice-field workers, abattoir workers, miners, sewer workers, and military personnel. Age and sex distribution of leptospiral infection is determined by the age and sex of persons engaged in these activities. Thus, the preponderance of men in groups affected with leptospirosis merely reflects the predominance of men among those at risk.

By 1956, less than 500 cases of leptospiral infection of man had been reported in the United States. Of the 12 serotypes associated with infections in lower animals, *L. icterohemorrhagiae, L. canicola, L. pomona, L. autumnalis, L. grippotyphosa, L. bataviae, L. australis A,* and *L. ballum* have been recognized as causes of human disease in this country. The first three of these serotypes are most frequently associated with infection of man.

Pathogenesis. Leptospiras gain access to the human body by way of the skin and mucous membranes. Cutaneous transmission of leptospiras must occur more commonly since skin is exposed frequently to the media through which this disease is acquired. The role of cutaneous breaks in transmission is clear from the increased incidence of leptospirosis in workers whose occupation results in trauma to skin of the hands and lower extremities. Accidental contamination of the buccal mucous membranes or conjunctivas has been followed by leptospiral infections in laboratory workers, and outbreaks of this disease have been related to the consumption of contaminated food or water. Transmission from man to man is rare; this may be explained by the failure of leptospiras to survive in acid urine.

Infection in man is regularly associated with entry of leptospiras into the blood and dissemination to various organ systems. Adequate histopathologic studies have been limited to fatal cases wherein tissue changes were of an extreme nature. Renal changes consist of cloudy swelling of tubular epithelium and focal areas of interstitial nephritis composed principally of lymphocytes and plasma cells. Dissociation of hepatic cords and cloudy swelling of parenchymal and Kupffer cells are frequent in patients dying of leptospirosis. Obstruction of bile capillaries may be observed but is not a consistent finding. Hepatic dysfunction can be much more severe than histopathologic abnormalities would suggest. The mechanism of hemorrhagic manifestations of leptospirosis is not clearly understood. Inflammatory lesions are observed in skeletal muscle as well as myocardium. Perivascular inflammation is present in the brain and meninges of patients exhibiting signs of central nervous system involvement during life. Leptospiras are demonstrated irregularly in renal and hepatic tissues by silver impregnation staining, but this procedure is not a suitable substitute for cultural methods.

Clinical Manifestations. Leptospirosis was first recognized and described as a distinct clinical entity in 1883 by Landouzy. Three years later, Weil observed several patients with fever, jaundice, and hemorrhages associated with hepatic and renal failure. This form of leptospirosis, since known as *Weil's disease,* is characterized by unusual severity and mortality. One of the causative organisms of this disease was discovered by Inada in 1915, and 2 years later, Noguchi proposed the generic name *Leptospira.* Most leptospiral serotypes produce self-limiting disease of varying severity rarely lasting more than 7 days. The vast majority of infections are benign and do not conform to Weil's description of severe leptospirosis.

Leptospiral infections in man are characterized by the abrupt onset of high fever, prostration, headache, nausea and vomiting, conjunctival injection, and myalgia after an incubation period of 3 to 19 days, usually 7 to 13 days. The febrile phase of the illness usually ends after 1 week, and in milder infections, other evidence of disease subsides with defervescence. Mild relapses lasting 2 to 3 days are not uncommon. Although the term Weil's disease is used to describe severe leptospiral illnesses caused by *L. icterohemorrhagiae,* it should be noted that milder infections with this organism are not rare and that other leptospiral serotypes can produce severe and even fatal forms of the disease. The frequency with which *icterus* and *renal decompensation* occur varies with the geographic area, as certain serotypes commonly associated with severe infections are more prevalent in some countries than in others.

Headache is present in nearly all patients with leptospirosis, and about 50 per cent complain of severe retrobulbar pain. *Conjunctival injection* is noted in 85 per cent of patients, and it is marked in the severely ill. *Rash* appears between the fourth and eighth day of disease in about 25 per cent of patients, and there is a tendency for it to become hemorrhagic in those with a serious infection. The eruption usually consists of small macules or maculopapules distributed over the trunk and extremities. Gastrointestinal disturbances consisting of *anorexia, nausea, vomiting,* and *abdominal pain* occur in nearly all patients with leptospirosis, and protracted vomiting and headache frequently constitute the most distressing features of the illness. *Cough* is a common complaint and is productive of blood-streaked sputum in about 25 per cent of those with this symptom. Roentgen examination of the chest may reveal *pneumonitis,* a feature of the disease which has not received much attention.

Severe *hemorrhagic manifestations* of leptospirosis are uncommon except in profoundly ill patients; however, some evidence of bleeding is observed in 30 to 50 per cent of all patients. Hematemesis and hemoptysis are the most common hemorrhagic manifestations, followed in frequency by conjunctival hemorrhage, epistaxis, petechiae, and melena. There may be moderate lymphadenopathy, but splenomegaly is rare.

Nuchal rigidity occurs in 30 to 40 per cent of patients. In some instances, the clinical picture is that of *aseptic meningitis* and may be indistinguishable from the same syndrome caused by mumps, lymphocytic choriomeningitis, and certain enterovirus infections (see p. 1136). When other evidence of leptospirosis is inconspicuous or absent in patients with aseptic meningitis, some time may elapse before the true etiology is suspected. *Iridocyclitis* manifested by photophobia and circumcorneal injection occurs in less than 5 per cent of patients with leptospirosis.

The incidence of clinically overt *jaundice* varies considerably, depending upon the infecting serotypes encountered. Icterus is found in 75 per cent of patients infected with *L. icterohemorrhagiae* but only in 5 to 10 per cent of persons infected with serotypes such as *L. grippotyphosa, L. canicola,* and *L. pomona.* Jaundice usually appears toward the end of the first week of illness as the fever is subsiding. Those with marked liver involvement show evidence of progressive hepatic dysfunction, and recovery may not be evident for 2 or 3 weeks. Hepatomegaly and liver tenderness are common findings in patients with jaundice.

Severe leptospiral infections are also characterized by renal decompensation manifested by oliguria, proteinuria, and azotemia. Fatal leptospirosis is almost always ascribable to renal failure, although hepatic insufficiency complicates the illness and massive hemorrhage may cause death. Mortality ranges from less than 1 per cent to as high as 10 per cent in different regions, depending upon the incidence of severe forms of the disease.

Laboratory Findings. Although normal peripheral blood leukocyte counts are the rule in uncomplicated leptospirosis, neutrophilic leukocytosis of 12,000 to 15,000 cells per cu mm may be observed in severely ill patients and counts of 25,000 to 40,000 cells per cu mm occur in Weil's disease. Urinary abnormalities are noted in about 80 per cent of patients with leptospirosis; proteinuria, cylindruria, pyuria, and hematuria are frequent and constitute important diagnostic clues. Return to normal renal function usually is rapid, and there is no evidence that permanent renal damage results from leptospiral infections.

Hyperbilirubinemia, abnormal flocculation tests, reversal of albumin/globulin ratio, and increase in alkaline phosphatase can be demonstrated in over 50 per cent of patients without clinical evidence of liver disease. Recovery of normal liver function is rapid as the clinical manifestations of the illness subside.

Leptospirosis has been shown to be the cause of approximately 4 per cent of all cases of aseptic meningitis in several well-studied series. However, the frequency with which the central nervous system is involved in leptospirosis is not known. Pleocytosis of a mild variety (40 to 500 cells) composed chiefly of mononuclear cells characterizes leptospiral aseptic meningitis. Modest elevation of cerebrospinal fluid protein is usual, but glucose and chloride concentrations remain normal. The cerebrospinal fluid quickly reverts to normal during early convalescence.

Leptospiras can be isolated from the blood of most patients during the acute phase of illness. Many leptospiral serotypes do not produce overt disease in guinea pigs and hamsters, and isolation of these organisms ultimately requires the use of cultural techniques. For this reason, the use of laboratory animals to diagnose leptospirosis should be limited to situations where the only material available for isolation of the causative organism is contaminated. The simplest of artificial media for the culturing of leptospiras is prepared by mixing a small amount of peptone with distilled water and adding sterile inactivated rabbit serum in a final concentration of 7 to 10 per cent. This medium is dispensed in 10-ml amounts into screw-capped tubes or rubber-stoppered bottles and may be stored in a refrigerator for several months. It is imperative to use small inoculums when attempting to recover leptospiras to avoid inhibition of these organisms by excessive quantities of blood. When single drops of whole venous blood are inoculated into each of five tubes at the bedside, positive results may be expected in 75 to 90 per cent of cultural attempts made during the first 3 days of illness. As the disease progresses, the intensity and regularity of leptospiremia decrease. Because of the intermittent nature of leptospiruria and the adverse effect of low pH and bacterial contamination, culture of urine is not recommended. Leptospiras have been recovered from cerebrospinal fluid.

Incubation of cultures is carried out at 32°C, and in order to avoid the risk of contamination of the medium, dark-field examination of the cultures is performed at weekly intervals, beginning 10 days after inoculation.

Several serologic tests are employed in the diagnosis of this disease. The classical *agglutination-lysis* test is cumbersome because of its type specificity and the need to employ numerous antigens and should be confined to reference centers and research laboratories. Tests employing broadly reactive antigens with generic specificity permitting the recognition of antibody against any leptospiral serotype should be employed by diagnostic laboratories. Two such antigens are available currently. A trivalent antigen prepared by sonic vibration of *L. icterohemorrhagiae, L. grippotyphosa,* and *L. hyos* has been found adequate in *complement fixation* tests. The best test employs antigen prepared from *L. biflexa* and adsorbed onto sheep erythrocytes. *Hemolysis* is observed in the presence of leptospiral antibody and complement. Antibody titers of 1:1,000 to 1:40,000 are frequently observed in the serum of patients convalescing from leptospirosis caused by any serotype. At the present time, the hemolysis test is the routine serodiagnostic procedure of choice.

Diagnosis. Leptospirosis should be considered a possible cause of any febrile disease characterized by headache, gastrointestinal disorder, conjunctival injection, and myalgia. The presence of urinary abnormalities and a history of contact with natural bodies of water frequented by rodents or domestic animals should arouse further suspicion. The diagnosis should not be reserved for patients with jaundice, as a majority of leptospiral infections are not associated with clinically overt icterus. Leptospirosis should be considered in the differential diagnosis of all cases of aseptic meningitis (p. 1136). Other acute febrile illnesses with which leptospirosis may be confused include influenza (p.

1123), rickettsioses (p. 1090), enteric fevers (p. 123), brucellosis (p. 959), and dengue (p. 1188). Late manifestations of Weil's disease may resemble infectious hepatitis, hemolytic and obstructive jaundice, and acute glomerulonephritis.

Treatment. Evaluation of antibiotics in human leptospirosis is complicated by the relatively short course of the acute infection and the lack of suitably controlled studies to date. Penicillin, streptomycin, and the tetracyclines inhibit the growth of leptospiras in vitro and will control experimental infections in hamsters and guinea pigs. Streptomycin and tetracyclines eliminate leptospiras from the kidneys of canine carriers of *L. canicola.*

There are differences of opinion regarding the usefulness of penicillin and tetracyclines in the treatment of human leptospirosis. All observers agree that chloramphenicol does not favorably alter the course of this disease. The use of tetracyclines, penicillin, streptomycin, and chloramphenicol in one controlled study failed to reveal a shortening of the febrile course or a reduction in the incidence of complications as a result of antibiotic therapy. Other evidence supports the concept that penicillin affects a reduction in the duration of fever and complications. At the present time, the use of 4 to 6 million units of penicillin daily during the febrile phase of the illness is probably indicated.

Most leptospiral infections are not severe and subside without complications even in the untreated patient. As the renal dysfunction of leptospirosis is reversible, management of the acute phase of renal decompensation should make use of all available therapeutic aids (see p. 1496). Rarely, hemorrhage may result in enough blood loss that replacement is necessary.

REFERENCES

Alston, J. M., and J. C. Broom: "Leptospirosis in Man and Animals," London, E. Livingstone, 1958.

Cox, C. D., A. D. Alexander, and L. C. Murphy: Evaluation of the Hemolytic Test in the Serodiagnosis of Human Leptospirosis, J. Infections Diseases, 101:210, 1957.

Doherty, R. L.: A Clinical Study of Leptospirosis in North Queensland, Australasian Ann. Med., 4:53, 1955.

Fairburn, A. C., and S. J. G. Semple: Chloramphenicol and Penicillin in the Treatment of Leptospirosis among British Troops in Malaya, Lancet, 1:13, 1956.

Hall, H. E., J. A. Hightower, R. Diaz Rivera, R. J. Byrne, J. E. Smadel, T. E. Woodward: Evaluation of Antibiotic Therapy in Human Leptospirosis, Ann. Internal Med., 35:981, 1951.

McCrumb, F. R., Jr., J. L. Stockard, C. R. Robinson, L. H. Turner, D. G. Levis, C. W. Maisey, M. F. Kelleher, C. A. Gleiser, and J. E. Smadel: Leptospirosis in Malaya: I. Sporadic Cases among Military and Civilian Personnel, Am. J. Trop. Med. Hyg., 6:238, 1957.

Wolff, J. W.: "The Laboratory Diagnosis of Leptospirosis," Springfield, Ill., Charles C Thomas, Publisher, 1954.

168 RELAPSING FEVER
Ivan L. Bennett, Jr.

Definition. Relapsing fever is an acute infectious disease caused by spirochetes belonging to the genus *Borrelia*. The outstanding clinical characteristic is a relapsing type of fever.

Etiology. Members of the genus *Borrelia* are slender, flexible spirochetes, 10 to 20 μ in length which move with a corkscrewlike action. *Borrelia* species are pathogenic for many rodents, including rats, mice, and squirrels. They can be cultured in media enriched with serum or blood. The strain encountered most commonly in North America is *Borrelia recurrentis*. In other areas *B. novyi* and *B. duttonii* are of clinical importance.

Epidemiology and Pathogenesis. Relapsing fever occurs in many parts of the world, including Asia, Africa, Europe, and South and North America. Wild rodents appear to be the natural reservoirs of the infection. The disease is transmitted to man by insect vectors. In some parts of the world human beings are infected by the bite of ticks (*Ornithodori*), while in other localities, as in Asia, the principal vector is the body louse. Disease in man can follow the crushing of a louse on the skin, especially when the area is scratched. Fleas and bedbugs have been suspected of transmitting relapsing fever. It is likely that an animal reservoir is not always necessary for perpetuation and that infection is transmitted from man to vector to man. In the United States, relapsing fever has been recognized predominantly in the West and in Texas; in these areas, ticks are the vectors and wild rodents are reservoirs.

After inoculation into man by contact with the excreta or by the bite of an arthropod, borrelias are apparently disseminated by way of the blood stream and lymphatics. The large number of spirochetes present in the blood of an infected person suggests that these organisms are capable of growing in the blood itself. They have been demonstrated in the cerebrospinal fluid during the acute stage of relapsing fever, and autopsy discloses them in the brain, spleen, kidneys, and liver.

Manifestations. It is usually difficult to determine an *incubation period* in individual cases, but epidemiologic evidence suggests that 5 to 11 days is the usual time. *Symptoms* develop abruptly, with chilliness, fever, headache, muscle aching, and nonproductive cough. Nausea and vomiting are frequent. Some patients complain of paresthesias of the face and tongue. The patient appears acutely ill, with flushed face and injected conjunctival and pharyngeal mucous membranes. At the height of the fever there may be dizziness, mental cloudiness, or delirium. Signs of extracellular fluid deficit—dry, inelastic skin and wrinkled tongue—are often present. *Tenderness of the calf muscles* is a characteristic physical finding. *Jaundice* occurs in a small proportion of cases, usually after several days of fever. A transitory erythematous *rash* may be observed, especially about the neck and shoulders. In severe cases there may be *petechiae. Enlargement of the spleen* is observed in about half of all cases. The pattern of the temperature curve is somewhat variable. Usually there is an elevation to 103 to 105°F. The fever may be sustained or remittent.

Course of Disease. The initial fever persists for 4 to 15 days and subsides spontaneously. At the termination of fever there is usually profuse sweating, and the temperature may fall to 96 or 97°F, gradually returning to normal during the succeeding day or two. A relapse is to be expected several days later, with a repetition of the same series of events. It is usual for untreated patients to have three to five attacks of fever, after which the disease ceases spontaneously. Additional relapses may occur, but the usual end result is complete cure of the infection. Death from relapsing fever is usually a result of hyperpyrexia, massive bleeding, circulatory failure, splenic rupture, or some secondary infection. Nose bleed and gastrointestinal bleeding occur in severe cases. Pneumonia may be observed at the time of death. Orchitis and iridocyclitis are rare complications. In the Orient, salmonella bacteremia occurs with great frequency in patients with relapsing fever.

Laboratory Findings. The leukocyte count is usually between 10,000 and 15,000 cells per cu mm. The spinal fluid may show increased protein and a mononuclear pleocytosis.

A *specific diagnosis* nearly always can be made during febrile periods, and occasionally during remissions, by the finding of borrelias in smears of the peripheral blood stained with Giemsa or Wright's stain. If the organisms cannot be found by this method, mice should be inoculated intraperitoneally with the patient's blood. Borrelias will be present in the blood of these animals from 16 hr to 3 days later, if the patient is suffering from relapsing fever.

Because of the ease with which a specific diagnosis can be made from the blood smear, serologic diagnostic tests are not needed. It is worth noting, however, that false positive serologic tests for syphilis are obtained in about 10 per cent of patients with relapsing fever and that nearly all patients develop agglutinins for *Proteus OX-K.*

Differential Diagnosis. Relapsing fever must be differentiated from other acute infectious diseases, particularly those which may be associated with a relapsing type of fever, such as malaria, meningococcemia, and rat-bite fever. At the onset of the disease the picture simulates that of Weil's disease. Under conditions of poverty and famine, the problem of diagnosis may be increased by concurrent epidemics of typhus, malaria, and tuberculosis.

Treatment. Excellent results have been reported in small series of cases treated with 800,000 units or more of penicillin daily. Tetracyclines are perhaps even more effective and appear now to be the agents of choice. Dosage recommended is 2 Gm daily for 7 to 10 days.

Therapy with arsenical preparations such as Mapharsen (arsenoxide) is regarded as highly effective in relapsing fever observed in some parts of the world. It is recommended that two injections of this drug be given intravenously, 3 to 5 days apart, the dose being 0.04 Gm for adults. Arsenical therapy is likely to cause a Herxheimer-like reaction 4 to 12 hr after the injection, evidenced by rise in temperature, malaise, and intensification of symptoms. This reaction can cause death of the patient when superimposed at the height of a severe febrile attack. Consequently, it is usually recommended that specific therapy be withheld in severely ill patients until a natural crisis occurs. The patient should be given supportive therapy meanwhile, in the form of parenteral fluids and electrolytes. Mapharsen is then administered at the onset of the next febrile period, or a day or two before it is expected. Further treatment is indicated in the event of a relapse.

Prognosis. Relapsing fever is not in itself a highly fatal infectious disease. However, because it occurs frequently under conditions of famine and extreme poverty and therefore may be associated with other infections and malnutrition, a significant fatality rate is usually ascribed to it. Reported fatality rates have varied from 2 to 50 per cent; they would probably be less than 2 per cent among otherwise healthy persons given proper treatment.

REFERENCES

Anderson, T. R., and L. E. Zimmerman: Relapsing Fever in Korea: A Clinicopathologic Study of Eleven Fatal Cases with Special Attention to Association with Salmonella Infection, Am. J. Pathol., 31:1083, 1955.

Chung, Hui-Lan, and F. C. Chang: Relapsing Fever: Clinical and Statistical Study of 337 Cases, Chinese Med. J., 55:6, 1939.

Schuhardt, V. T.: Treatment of Relapsing Fever with Antibiotics, Ann. N.Y. Acad. Sci., 55:1209, 1952.

Wolff, B. P.: Asiatic Relapsing Fever: Report of 134 Cases Treated with Mapharsen, Ann. Internal Med., 24:203, 1946.

169 RAT-BITE FEVER (*Spirillum minus* Infection)

Ivan L. Bennett, Jr.

Definition. Rat-bite fever (sodoku) is an acute infectious disease caused by *Spirillum minus* and characterized by relapsing fever, arthritis, and a skin eruption.

Etiology. The causative organism is a spirillum 2 to 5 μ in length; it has two to five broad spirals, and is propelled by flagella. The organism is easily identified in dark-field preparations by its quick, darting motility. It is found occasionally in the blood of apparently healthy rats, mice, and guinea pigs.

Epidemiology. In man, infection by S. *minus* is almost always acquired through the bite of a rat. It is commonest in infants and young children but may also occur in adults. Rats may attack sleeping persons and will bite anyone attempting to catch or handle them. Documented examples of infection from the bite of a mouse are known.

Manifestations. The incubation period varies from 1 to 6 weeks. With the onset of symptoms, the site of the original bite usually becomes swollen, tender, and purplish and regional lymphadenitis appears. A chill may occur at the onset of a febrile period. Bouts of fever last 2 to 4 days and are separated by afebrile periods, also lasting 2 to 4 days. During febrile episodes there are malaise, headache, sweating, photophobia, nausea, and vomiting. In about 50 per cent of cases there is *arthritis*, with redness and swelling of one or more large joints. In a similar proportion of cases a *skin eruption* occurs, usually on the extremities. The rash is frequently asymmetric in its distribution and most commonly consists of reddish or purplish plaques, which may become large and confluent. The disease tends to run a prolonged course, usually 4 to 8 weeks, but cases have been reported in which clinical manifestations continued for more than a year. Subacute bacterial endocarditis due to this organism has been observed.

Laboratory Findings. The total leukocyte count may be normal, or there may be a moderate leukocytosis. In prolonged cases there is a normochromic anemia. Biologic false positive serologic tests for syphilis are frequent. The *S. minus* seldom can be found in the blood or tissues of patients by direct examination. Mice or guinea pigs should be inoculated intraperitoneally with the patient's blood. *Spirillum minus* can usually be found in the blood of the animal by dark-field examination 1 to 3 weeks later. Laboratory animals may be naturally infected with *S. minus,* and precautions must be taken to ensure that the animals are free of infection before inoculation.

There are reports of isolation of this spirillum from the blood by culture, using routine bacteriologic blood culture technique.

Differential Diagnosis. It is important to inquire about rat bite in all patients with a relapsing type of fever. In patients with a history of rat bite, the principal problem is in differentiating between *S. minus* infection and *Streptobacillus moniliformis.* This cannot be done with certainty on clinical grounds, but a prolonged incubation period and few or no manifestations of arthritis suggest a diagnosis of *S. minus* infection. Laboratory tests should be made for both organisms. The significance of a previous rat bite may not be appreciated in cases with a long incubation period, and the disease may be confused with other infections characterized by relapsing fever, such as malaria, meningococcemia, and *Borrelia recurrentis* infection.

Treatment. This infection usually responds promptly to treatment with arsenical preparations such as arsenoxide (Mapharsen) or neoarsphenamine. Doses appropriate to the patient's age and size and equivalent to those used in the treatment of syphilis are satisfactory. The usual practice is to give two or three injections at 3- or 4-day intervals. Penicillin, streptomycin, and the tetracyclines have been effective in the few cases in which there has been opportunity to use them.

Prognosis. In the absence of serious complicating illnesses, rat-bite fever caused by *S. minus* is never fatal.

REFERENCES

Brown, T. McP., and J. C. Nunemaker: Rat-bite Fever: A Review of the American Cases with Re-evaluation of Etiology; Report of Cases, Bull. Johns Hopkins Hosp., 70:201, 1942.

Farquahar, J. W., P. N. Edmunds, and J. B. Tilley: Sodoku in a Child: Result of Mouse Bite, Lancet, 2:1211, 1958.

Sen, S., B. C. Basu, and D. Banerju: Streptomycin and Terramycin in the Treatment of Rat-bite Fever Due to *Spirillum minus,* Indian Med. Gaz., 89:3, 1954.

Shwartzman, G., A. L. Florman, M. H. Bass, S. Karelitz, and D. Richtberg: Repeated Recovery of a Spirillum by Blood Culture from Two Children with Prolonged and Recurrent Fevers, Pediatrics, 8:227, 1951.

Section 12: The Rickettsioses

170 GENERAL CONSIDERATIONS AND PATHOLOGY

*Theodore E. Woodward and
J. E. Smadel*

The rickettsial diseases of man consist of a variety of clinical entities caused by microorganisms of the family Rickettsiaceae. The rickettsias are obligate intracellular parasites about the size of bacteria and are usually seen microscopically as pleomorphic coccobacillary organisms. Each of the rickettsias pathogenic for man is capable of multiplying in one or more species of arthropod as well as in animals and man. Indeed, the majority of the rickettsias are maintained in nature by a cycle which involves an insect vector and an animal reservoir, and infection of man is unimportant in the cycle. Q fever is a partial exception to this generalization, since man usually contracts the infection via the respiratory route by inhaling rickettsias as an aerosol derived from infected animal or tick excretions; however, this rickettsiosis is also maintained in nature in ticks and their animal hosts. Epidemic typhus presents a number of points of dissimilarity to most of the other rickettsioses, since the natural cycle of infection involves only man and the louse. Moreover, the agent of epidemic typhus, unlike the other rickettsias, has not established a well-organized parasitic relationship which ensures its perpetuation either in its mammalian host and reservoir (man) or in its arthropod host (louse). Man frequently dies from epidemic typhus, and only rarely do recovered patients serve as a suitable reservoir (i.e., suffer a recurrence in later years, resulting in what is known as Brill's disease) and infect their body lice. Furthermore, the louse is relatively poorly adapted to perpetuation of the rickettsias which induce a fatal

Table 170-1. RICKETTSIAL DISEASES

Disease				Natural cycle		Transmission to man	Serologic diagnosis	
Group	Type	Agent	Geographic distribution	Arthropod	Mammal		Weil-Felix reaction	Complement fixation
Spotted fever	Rocky Mountain spotted fever	*R. rickettsii*	Western Hemisphere	Ticks	Small wild rodents; dogs	Tick bite	Positive OX-19 OX-2	Positive group- and type-specific
	African tick fever	*R. conorii*	Mediterranean and Africa					
	Rickettsialpox	*R. akari*	North America Europe Africa	Blood-sucking mite	House mouse	Mite bite	Negative	
Typhus	Endemic	*R. mooseri*	World-wide	Flea	Small rodents	Infected flea feces into broken skin	Positive OX-19	Positive group- and type-specific
	Epidemic	*R. prowazeki*	World-wide	Body louse	Man	Infected louse feces into broken skin	Positive OX-19	
	Brill's disease		World-wide	Recurrence years after original attack of epidemic typhus			Usually negative	
	Scrub	*R. tsutsugamushi*	Asia Australia Pacific islands	Trombiculid mites	Small rodents	Mite bite	Positive OX-K	Positive in 50% of cases
Q fever		*R. burneti*	World-wide	Ticks	Small mammals, cattle, sheep, goats	Inhalation of dried infected material	Negative	Positive
Trench fever		*R. quintana*	North America Europe Africa	Body louse	Man	Infected louse feces into broken skin	Negative	None available

disease in this arthropod. In contrast, most rickettsias cause only a mild disease in their mammalian hosts and do not affect their arthropod host adversely; indeed, a number are transmitted transovarially in insects from one generation to another.

The rickettsial infections of man encountered in the United States are, in order of their frequency, Rocky Mountain spotted fever, murine typhus, rickettsialpox, Q fever, and Brill's disease (recurrent epidemic typhus). These diseases will receive particular emphasis; however, students and practitioners of medicine in this generation must be familiar with infections which they may encounter in other parts of the world or which might reappear in the United States; therefore, some space will be devoted to epidemic typhus, scrub typhus, and certain of the foreign diseases of the spotted fever group.

A compendium of information on the rickettsial diseases is presented in Table 170-1. Since each of the rickettsioses encountered in America responds therapeutically to the broad-spectrum antibiotics, the table contains no mention of therapy. Procedures for diagnostic isolation of the rickettsias are

omitted from the table because they generally are less useful than serologic methods, and the techniques which they require are highly specialized and hazardous for laboratory personnel. Information on isolation procedures may be found in textbooks devoted to viral and rickettsial diseases.

History of the Rickettsial Diseases. Of all the afflictions of mankind the rickettsial diseases, particularly epidemic typhus, rank among the foremost as a cause of human suffering and death. Classical typhus fever undoubtedly existed during ancient times, although Zinsser cites an outbreak of illness in 1083 in a monastery near Salerno, Italy, as the first probable recorded incidence of this disease. Typhus fever, through its able transmitter the body louse, has always identified itself intimately with wars, famines, and human catastrophes of all kinds. Alone it has cast a decisive vote in the outcome of many military campaigns.

The record of deaths from epidemic typhus in this century in the Balkan countries and in Poland and Russia reaches astounding figures. Serbia in 1915 suffered an epidemic of major proportions with 150,000 dead, and a mortality rate ranging from 20 to 60 per cent. Typhus ravaged Russia and eastern Poland from 1915 to 1922, infecting 30 million of the inhabitants and causing deaths estimated at 3 million.

The past two decades have seen the development of amazingly satisfactory methods for the prevention and treatment of the rickettsioses of man. In fact, these measures have been so successful that the rickettsioses have become of minor importance in the United States and in a number of other countries. Although conquered, the rickettsioses have not been eliminated, and they could again become rampant if the will to control them, the present high standards of sanitation, and the necessary industrial capacities for production of effective insecticides and therapeutic agents should be decreased through war or disaster. It is worthwhile to review the classical milestones representing the clinical and scientific contributions which have resulted in the understanding and conquest of the rickettsial infections.

Gerhard in 1836 differentiated typhoid fever from louse-borne typhus fever. In 1899 Maxcy described the clinical manifestations of Rocky Mountain spotted fever. In a series of studies from 1906 to 1909 Ricketts, for whom the rickettsia microorganisms are named, successfully transmitted the disease to guinea pigs, incriminated the wood tick as a vector, and observed rickettsias in smears prepared from tick tissues.

Nicolle in 1909 reproduced typhus fever in monkeys and demonstrated transmission by the body louse. Von Prowazek in 1914 and Da Rocha-Lima in 1916 demonstrated small microorganisms in the tissues of lice taken from typhus patients.

Brill in 1910 recognized a febrile disease in patients in New York City as an example of mild epidemic typhus unassociated with lousiness. Zinsser in later years (1934) postulated that Brill's disease was a recurrent form of typhus occurring in patients during periods of stress or waning immunity. Subsequent studies have essentially confirmed Zinsser's hypothesis.

Weil and Felix working with typhus patients in Poland in 1915 recognized that agglutinins for certain proteus organisms appeared in the serum of convalescent patients. The Weil-Felix reaction, although nonspecific in character, affords a simple and valuable screening method for the diagnosis of certain rickettsioses.

In 1926 Maxcy, on purely epidemiological evidence, surmised that typhus in this country had its reservoir in rodents and was transmitted to man by ticks or fleas. Confirmation of Maxcy's hypothesis was obtained in Baltimore in 1930 by Dyer and others when they isolated rickettsias from the brains of rats and shortly thereafter incriminated the flea as a vector. This disease, caused by *Rickettsia*

mooseri and now designated endemic, or murine, typhus, is distinct from epidemic typhus and Brill's disease.

The development of suitable vaccines and specific diagnostic antigens was impeded until it was possible to prepare appreciable quantities of highly infectious rickettsial material in the laboratory. The most important steps were (1) the Weigl vaccine (1930), which was a phenolized suspension of gut tissue obtained from body lice which had been injected intrarectally with the rickettsiae of epidemic typhus; (2) the killed murine typhus vaccine prepared by Castaneda (1939) from lung tissues of rats injected intranasally; and (3) the inactivated Rocky Mountain spotted fever vaccine obtained by Cox (1941) from infected yolk sacs of embryonated hen's eggs. Each of the developments was applied in principle to other rickettsial agents, but the low cost and relative simplicity of the egg techniques have led to their general use for preparation of vaccines and diagnostic antigens. The specific diagnostic complement fixation tests for the rickettsial diseases now used in the United States stem directly from the pioneering work of Bengtson in Q fever and of Plotz on the spotted and typhus fevers during the early 1940s.

The years of the Second World War saw many strides in the conquest of the rickettsioses; perhaps greatest among these were the highly successful attacks on the insect vectors of disease. The lousicide DDT proved to be ideal for control by dusting on the clothes of infested persons. The epidemic at Naples during the winter of 1943 to 1944 established a milestone, since it was the first to be suppressed within several weeks mainly by the use of insecticides. On the other side of the world, scrub typhus (mite-borne typhus) was creating a major problem in military medicine in the Pacific area. Here too, the major contributions to successful control were concerned with application of miticidal chemicals to the person and his clothes.

Specific therapy of rickettsial infections is a rather recent development. Although hyperimmune rabbit serum (Topping, 1939) ameliorated the course of Rocky Mountain spotted fever if given during the early stages and para-aminobenzoic acid (Yeomans, 1944) was found to be effective in typhus fever, the advent of broad-spectrum antibiotics, first chloramphenicol, then chlortetracycline in 1948, and later oxytetracycline provided the dramatic therapeutic results in each of the rickettsioses.

Table 170-1 lists several rickettsial diseases which have not been mentioned in this historical review. While important in themselves, except for Q fever, these have not been the subject of work which contributed broad principles applicable to the group.

Pathogenesis. Rickettsial diseases of man develop following infection by one of two routes, i.e., the skin or the respiratory tract. Agents of the typhus and spotted fever group of rickettsias are introduced into the skin through the bite of the infected arthropod vector. Ticks and mites which transmit the spotted fevers and scrub typhus inoculate the rickettsias directly into the dermis during feeding. The louse and flea, which transmit epidemic and murine typhus, respectively, deposit infected feces on the skin; infection occurs when organisms are rubbed into the puncture wound made by the arthropod, a process facilitated by scratching the itching bitten area. The rickettsia of Q fever gains entry through the respiratory tract by inhalation of infected dust; moreover, the respiratory route may occasionally be indicted in epidemic typhus when infection results from inhalation of dried infected louse feces.

While multiplication of organisms probably takes place at the original site of entry in all instances, local lesions appear with considerable regularity only in certain diseases, viz., the initial cutaneous lesions of scrub typhus, rickettsialpox, and African tick typhus, and the pneumonitis which develops in about half the persons infected with Q fever. Investigations have demonstrated that volunteers infected with either scrub typhus or Q fever develop rickettsemia late in the incubation period, often some hours before the onset of fever. Similar events probably occur in all the rickettsial diseases; certainly circulating rickettsias can be detected during the early febrile period in practically all patients. Little is known about the pathogenesis of infection during the midportion of the incubation period. However, it is reasonable to assume that, during this time in patients with typhus or spotted fever, a transient, low-grade rickettsemia results from release of organisms multiplying at the initial site of infection and that this seeds infection in the endothelial cells of the vascular tree. Vascular lesions developing at such sites could account for the pathologic changes including the rash (see following discussion of Pathology).

The underlying cause of the toxic-febrile state which characterizes the rickettsial diseases, as well as most infectious diseases, remains unknown. If the products of destruction of infected cells contribute to the state, then fairly extensive damage is required, i.e., more than that occurring late in the incubation period of scrub typhus, when enough infected cells are destroyed to liberate appreciable numbers of rickettsias into the circulation yet the patient remains afebrile and feels well. Several rickettsial species contain type-specific toxins which are lethal for mice; what role these play in the toxic-febrile state of patients remains unknown. Cortisone suppresses the febrile response in patients but does not prevent death of mice injected with rickettsial toxins.

Pathology. The basic pathologic lesions in the spotted and typhus fever groups of diseases are in the small vessels. The most diverse and extensive of these are found in Rocky Mountain spotted fever. Here swelling, proliferation, and degeneration of the endothelial cells occur, frequently with thrombus formation which partially or completely obliterates the lumen. The muscle cells of the arteriole undergo degeneration represented by swelling and fibrinoid changes. The adventitial tissues are infiltrated with mononuclear leukocytes, lymphocytes, and plasma cells. Such vascular damage is scattered in localized regions along the arteries, veins, and capillaries with normal architecture prevailing throughout most of the vascular bed. The changes in murine, epidemic, and scrub typhus fevers resemble those in Rocky Mountain spotted fever as regards the endothelial swelling and the adventitial inflammatory infiltrations; however, thrombosis is uncommon, and involvement of the musculature is rare.

The vascular changes with resultant lesions in adjacent parenchymatous tissues occur throughout the vital organs but are most conspicuous in the heart, lung, and brain. Interstitial myocarditis occurs in each member of this group of diseases but is usually most extensive in Rocky Mountain spotted fever and in scrub typhus. In the brain, the glial nodule is found in all members of the group; but microinfarcts in the brain tissue or in the myocardium are most often observed in spotted fever. The glial nodule represents a cellular response in an area adjacent to a small vascular lesion. The microinfarct, on the other hand, constitutes anemic necrosis in an area whose supplying vessel has been occluded by the intimal reaction or thrombosis. Visceral lesions in most of the other organs are similarly dependent upon the primary vascular abnormalities, or are those nonspecific changes associated with severe febrile illnesses.

A rickettsial pneumonitis occurs at least to some extent in many patients with spotted or typhus fever and is the characteristic pathologic change in patients with Q fever. This is an interstitial pneumonitis which closely resembles that encountered in primary atypical pneumonia and viral influenzal pneumonia. The process is patchy and consists macroscopically of areas of congestion and edema with gray granular consolidation. Microscopically, in the consolidated areas the alveoli are filled with compact fibrinocellular exudate containing lymphocytes, plasma cells, large mononuclear cells, and erythrocytes, but few if any polymorphonuclear leukocytes. The alveolar epithelium is hyperplastic, and the intraalveolar septums, as well as the peribronchial and perivascular tissues, are thickened by accumulations of leukocytes such as are found within the alveolar lumena.

Table 170-2. SEROLOGIC DIAGNOSIS OF RICKETTSIAL DISEASES IN THE UNITED STATES

Group	Disease	Weil-Felix reaction				Complement fixation tests with type-specific antigen				
		Proteus	Illustrative titer		Cases with diagnostic titer	Rickettsial antigen	Illustrative titer			Cases with diagnostic titer
			10th day	20th day			10th day	20th day	30th day	
Spotted fever group	Rocky Mountain spotted fever	OX-19 OX-2	40 20	320 160	Most	*R. rickettsii*	20	160	80	Most
	Rickettsialpox	OX-19 OX-2	0 0	0 0	None	*R. akari*	0	64	128	Most
Typhus group	Murine typhus	OX-19 OX-2	160 10	640 40	Most	*R. mooseri*	0	160	160	Most
	Brill's disease	OX-19 OX-2	20 0	320 0	Infrequent	*R. prowazeki*	640	1280	320	Most
	Q fever	OX-19 OX-2	0 0	0 0	None	*R. burneti*	10	80	160	Most

Rickettsias can occasionally be observed microscopically in sections of tissue from persons dying from rickettsial diseases. However, special fixation of tissues, special staining techniques, infinite patience for work with the oil immersion objective, and luck are required for success. The failure to demonstrate rickettsias in histologic section is of no diagnostic significance.

Laboratory Diagnosis. Diagnostic procedures which depend on isolation of the etiologic agent from blood or other clinical material are expensive, time-consuming, and hazardous to laboratory personnel. Except in unusual circumstances the currently available serologic tests are adequate for laboratory confirmation of the clinical diagnosis in each of the rickettsial diseases.

As in most serologic diagnostic procedures the demonstration of a rise in titer of specific antibody during convalescence is of prime importance in establishing the laboratory confirmation. Table 170-2 summarizes the serologic results usually encountered in persons who suffer from rickettsial diseases in the United States. The Weil-Felix test employing *Proteus* strains OX-19 and OX-2 gives positive results in patients with spotted fever and murine typhus and negative results in those with rickettsialpox and Q fever. It is useful as a screening procedure but cannot be relied upon to differentiate spotted fever from murine typhus.

Complement fixation tests employing group-specific rickettsial antigens provide data which clearly differentiate the most common infections, i.e., murine typhus, Rocky Mountain spotted fever, and Q fever. Moreover, if type specific rickettsial antigens are employed, it is generally possible to distinguish rickettsialpox from spotted fever and Brill's disease from murine typhus.

Specific antibiotic therapy has little effect on the time of appearance of antibodies or on their ultimate titer, provided treatment is begun some days after onset of the rickettsial disease. However, if the illness is cut short by early and vigorous treatment, then antibody production may be delayed for a week or so, and also the maximal titers attained may be below those illustrated in Table 170-2. Under these circumstances a sample of blood taken 4 to 6 weeks after onset of illness should be examined.

Except for normochromic anemia, which occurs in patients severely ill with rickettsial diseases, there are no other distinctive alterations of the hematologic picture. The white blood cell count in Rocky Mountain spotted fever, rickettsialpox, murine and epidemic typhus, Brill's disease, Q fever, and others is usually within the normal range: 6,000 to 10,000 cells per cu mm. Leukopenia is occasionally observed, and in the presence of complications, such as superimposed infections and extensive vascular lesions, moderate leukocytosis occurs. The differential blood count is usually normal.

REFERENCES

Allen, A. C., and S. Spitz: A Comparative Study of the Pathology of Scrub Typhus (Tsutsugamushi Disease) and Other Rickettsial Diseases, Am. J. Pathol., 21:603, 1945.

Bayne-Jones, S.: Epidemic Typhus in the Mediterranean Area during World War II, with Special Reference to the Control of the Epidemic in Naples in the Winter of 1943–44, pp. 1–15 in "The Rickettsial Diseases of Man," Washington, American Association for the Advancement of Science, 1948.

Bengtson, I. A.: Complement Fixation in "Q" Fever, Proc. Soc. Exptl. Biol. Med., 46:665, 1941.

Cox, H. R.: The Spotted-fever Group, pp. 828–868 in "Viral and Rickettsial Infections of Man," 3d ed., T. M. Rivers and F. L. Horsfall, Jr. (Eds.), Philadelphia, J. B. Lippincott Company, 1959.

Harrell, G. T.: Rickettsial Involvement of the Nervous System, Med. Clin. N. Am., 37:395, 1953.

Lillie, R. D., T. L. Perrin, and C. Armstrong: An Institutional Outbreak of Pneumonitis: III, Histopathology in Man and Rhesus Monkeys in the Pneumonitis Due to the Virus of "Q" Fever, U.S. Pub. Health Repts., 56:149, 1941.

Plotz, H.: Complement Fixation in Rickettsial Diseases, Science, 97:20, 1943.

—— B. L. Bennett, K. Wertman, M. J. Snyder, and R. Gauld: Serological Pattern in Typhus Fever: I. Epidemic, Am. J. Hyg., 47:150, 1948.

Smadel, J. E.: Influence of Antibiotics on Immunologic Responses in Scrub Typhus, Am. J. Med., 17:246, 1954.

——: Rickettsial Diseases, pp. 513–552 in "Diagnostic Procedures for Virus and Rickettsial Diseases," New York, American Public Health Association, 1956.

——: Status of the Rickettsioses in the United States, Ann. Internal Med., 51:421, 1959.

Snyder, J. C.: The Typhus Fevers, pp. 799–827 in "Viral and Rickettsial Infections of Man," 3d ed., T. M. Rivers and F. L. Horsfall, Jr. (Eds.), Philadelphia, J. B. Lippincott Company, 1959.

Tigertt, W. D., and A. S. Benenson: Studies on Q Fever in Man, Trans. Assoc. Am. Physicians, 69:98, 1956.

Wolbach, S. B.: Studies on Rocky Mountain Spotted Fever, J. Med. Research, 41:1, 1919.

——: The Rickettsial Diseases: A General Survey, pp. 789–816 in "Virus and Rickettsial Diseases," Cambridge, Mass., Harvard University Press, 1940.

Zinsser, H.: "Rats, Lice and History," Boston, Little, Brown & Company, 1935.

171 ROCKY MOUNTAIN SPOTTED FEVER

*T. E. Woodward and
J. E. Smadel*

Definition. Rocky Mountain spotted fever, an acute febrile illness caused by *Rickettsia rickettsii*, is transmitted to man by ticks. The disease is characterized by sudden onset with headache and chills and by fever which persists for 2 to 3 weeks. A characteristic exanthem appears on the extremities and trunk about the fourth day of disease; this rash, like other anatomical manifestations of the disease, stems from focal areas of endangiitis scattered throughout the body. Delirium, shock, and renal failure occur in the severely ill. Agglutinins for the proteus organisms and specific complement-fixing antibodies appear in the patient's serum during the second or third week of disease. The broad-spectrum antibiotics are highly specific therapeutically. A review of the pertinent historical features is given in Chap. 170.

Etiology and Epidemiology. The causative microbe, *Rickettsia rickettsii*, represents the prototype for the rickettsial group of agents. The minute organisms, about 1 μ in length and 0.2 to 0.3 μ in width, are purple when stained by Giemsa's method or red by Macchiavello's technique and often occur in pairs surrounded by a halo as if encapsulated. The rickettsias grow in the nucleus as well as in the cytoplasm of infected cells of ticks, mammals, and embryonated eggs; the intranuclear situation of the organisms is shared by the other members of the spotted fever group, but not by rickettsias of the typhus group. *Rickettsia rickettsii* are readily distinguishable from the agents of the typhus fevers by cross immunity tests in guinea pigs and by complement fixation tests employing antigens prepared from infected yolk sac tissues. The differentiation of *R. rickettsii* from closely related members of the spotted fever group frequently requires elaborate procedures. Strains of the agent of Rocky Mountain spotted fever vary considerably in their virulence for man and animals.

The first reports of spotted fever in Idaho and Montana during the final decade of the last century led to the name Rocky Mountain spotted fever. However, the disease has been reported in all states except Maine and Vermont, as well as in Canada, Mexico, Colombia, and Brazil. Although related diseases are found on other continents, this particular infection is limited to the Western Hemisphere. Formerly about 500 but currently about 300 cases of spotted fever occur annually in the United States; the mortality which in the days before specific therapy was about 20 per cent decreased to 3 per cent in 1955 but has since risen to about 7 per cent. The attack rate per unit of population is highest in Wyoming, but the rates in Delaware, Maryland, Virginia, and North Carolina are about the same as those in Montana, Idaho, Nevada, and Utah. Moreover, approximately two-fifths of all cases in the United States occur each year in the Middle Atlantic states just mentioned.

A number of species of ticks are found infected with *R. rickettsii* in nature, but only two species are important in transmitting spotted fever to man. These are *Dermacentor andersoni,* the wood tick which is the principal vector in the West, and *D. variabilis,* the dog tick which assumes this role in the East. Ricketts almost half a century ago demonstrated that infected adult female ticks transmit the agent transovarially to at least some of their offspring. Ticks which become infected, either through the egg or at one of the stages during their developmental cycle by feeding on an infected mammal, harbor the rickettsias throughout their lifetime, which may be as long as several years. Thus the tick probably serves as a reservoir in addition to being a vector. Small wild mammals are suspected of playing an important role in spreading the rickettsias in nature by infecting those new ticks which feed on them during that period of the disease when rickettsemia is occurring.

Disease in man is generally acquired from the bite of an infected tick. However, transmission is unlikely unless the tick remains attached for a number of hours. Infection may also be acquired through abrasions in the skin which become contaminated with infected tick feces or tissue juices; hence the hazard associated with crushing ticks between the fingers when removing them from persons or animals.

There are seasonal variations in the incidence of cases of spotted fever, as well as differences in age and sex distribution of cases. In each instance these differences are related to exposure to ticks. Thus most patients are seen during the period of maximal tick activity, i.e., late spring and early summer. Topping found that about half the cases in the Western states occurred in men over forty, whereas half those in the Eastern states were in children under fifteen. This age distribution is undoubtedly influenced by propinquity to the wood and dog ticks, respectively. Mortality increases with age of the patient; hence the crude fatality rates in the West are generally higher than those in the East. However, when corrected for age, the rates in comparable groups are similar.

Clinical Manifestations. *Incubation Period and Prodromata.* A history of tick bite is elicited in approximately 80 per cent of patients. The incubation period varies between 3 and 12 days with a mean of 7. A short incubation period usually indicates a more serious infection.

Onset and Symptoms. In nonvaccinated persons, the onset is usually abrupt, with severe headache, a sudden shaking rigor, prostration, generalized myalgic pains especially localized in the back and leg muscles, nausea with occasional vomiting, and fever which reaches 103 to 104°F within the first 2 days. Pain in the abdominal muscles may be severe, and arthralgia is not uncommon. Deep muscle palpation often elicits tenderness. Occasionally the debut of illness in children and adults is mild, accompanied by lethargy, anorexia, cephalgia, and low-grade fever. These symptoms are similar to those of many acute infectious diseases, making specific diagnosis difficult during the first few days.

Pyrexia. Fever continues for approximately 15 to 20 days in untreated cases. The febrile course in children may be shorter. The pyrexia is high, with morning remissions that do not reach normal levels. Hyperthermia of 105°F or greater is of unfavorable prognostic significance, although fatalities may occur when the patient is hypothermic, with concurrent vasomotor collapse. Fever generally terminates by lysis over a period of several days, but rarely it does so by crisis. Recurrent fever is quite uncommon except in the presence of secondary pyogenic complications.

The headache is generalized and excruciating, and frequently more intense over the frontal area. It persists throughout the first and second week of illness in untreated cases. Malaise continues for the first week; irritability is notable, and the patient shuns distractions such as questioning and examination.

Cutaneous Manifestations. The rash which is present in practically all cases is the most characteristic and helpful diagnostic sign. It usually appears on the *fourth* febrile day: range, 2 to 6 days. The initial lesions are on the wrist, ankles, palms, soles, and forearms. The first lesions are macular, nonfixed, pink, irregularly defined, and 2 to 6 mm in width. A warm compress applied to the extremity accentuates the rash in the early stages. The exanthem is most prominent when the temperature is elevated. After 6 to 12 hr, the rash extends centripetally to the axilla, buttocks, trunk, neck, and face. (This is in contrast to the eruption of typhus fever, which begins on the trunk and spreads centrifugally, rarely involving the face, palms, or soles.) The rash becomes maculopapular after 2 to 3 days (it may be felt by light palpation) and assumes a deeper red hue. By about the fourth day it is petechial and fails to fade on pressure. Not uncommonly the hemorrhagic lesions coalesce to form large ecchymotic blemishes; these lesions tend to form over bony prominences and may ultimately slough to form indolent slow-healing ulcers. Patients who have had the typical rash show brownish pigmented discolorations at the site of the previous lesions for several weeks during convalescence. In milder cases the rash does not become purpuric and may disappear within several days. Modern antibiotic therapy may abort the early exanthem, whereas the later fixed lesion fades less rapidly under specific therapy.

The application of tourniquets for several minutes, or the occasional taking of the blood pressure, may provoke additional petechiae (Rumpel-Leede phenomenon), which is further evidence of capillary abnormalities.

Cardiovascular and Respiratory Features. During the early stages, the pulse is full and regular but accelerated in proportion to the height of the temperature, and the blood pressure is well sustained. During the peak of illness in seriously ill children and adults, the pulse is rapid and feeble, and hypotension of 90 mm Hg is common. If circulatory failure is long sustained, the resultant hypoxia and shock lead to agitation and delirium and contribute to the formation of ecchymoses and gangrene of fingers, toes, genitalia, buttocks, ear lobes, and nose. Cyanosis of the peripheral parts of the body is common. Venous pressure determinations do not reveal elevations indicative of congestive heart failure per se, nor is the venous pressure elevated following the careful administration of intravenous fluids. A reduction of the total blood volume is occasionally found, as are evidences of myocardial impairment as shown by electrocardiography, i.e, low voltage of ventricular complexes, minor S-T segment deflections, and occasionally delay in atrioventricular conduction time (Harrell). These changes are transient and similar to those encountered in patients with pneumonia, typhoid fever, or uremia. Severely ill patients present a puffy appearance of the face, hands, ankles, feet, and lower sacrum.

Respirations are either normal or slightly accelerated. Cough may be harassing and nonproductive, and localized pneumonitis may occur, whereas pulmonary consolidation is extremely uncommon. Pulmonary edema may develop particularly after the injudicious use of intravenous fluids.

Hepatic and Renal Manifestations. In the majority of moderately ill patients, there is little alteration in the renal or hepatic function. The liver may be enlarged, but jaundice is unusual. Oliguria commonly occurs in the seriously ill, and anuria may mark the critical case. Azotemia is common but when marked is a very unfavorable sign. Abnormalities in liver function are probably responsible for the hypoproteinemia, with reduction in the albumin fraction.

Neurologic Manifestations. The principal neurologic manifestations are headache, restlessness, and varying degrees of insomnia. Stiffness of the back is common. The cerebrospinal fluid is clear, with normal dynamics and normal chemical constituents. Coma and muscular rigidity may occur. Athetoid movements, convulsive seizures, and hemiplegia are grave manifestations. Deafness during the active stages of the disease is not uncommon. As a rule, all neurologic signs abate without residual. Findings based upon follow-up examinations and electroencephalograms may be interpreted as indicative of minor residual brain damage for a year or more following recovery of certain patients from Rocky Mountain spotted fever.

Other Physical Manifestations. Patients become dehydrated, with extreme dryness of lips, gums, tongue, and pharynx. The skin is hot and dry, the conjunctivae are frequently injected, and the eyes suffused. Photophobia is common in the early stages of illness. Petechial hemorrhages may be noted in the conjunctivas or in the retina. The spleen is enlarged in approximately one-half the cases and is firm and nontender. Abdominal distention is frequent, and occasionally some degree of intestinal ileus is observed. Constipation is usual.

Course of Disease. In mild and moderately severe cases given no specific antibiotic therapy, the disease abates within 2 weeks, and convalescence is rapid. In fatal cases death usually occurs during the latter part of the second week as a result of toxemia, vasomotor weakness, and shock or renal failure with azotemia.

In vaccinated individuals who contract the disease, the illness is mild, with a short febrile course and an atypical rash.

Complications and Prognosis. If the serious manifestations of spotted fever mentioned above are regarded as intrinsic parts of the disease, then complications are uncommon and consist mainly of secondary bacterial infections, viz., bronchopneumonia, otitis media, and parotitis. Thrombosis of major blood vessels may result in gangrene of a portion of an extremity. Hemiplegia and peripheral neuritis are important but rare sequelae.

The over-all mortality rate for spotted fever was formerly about 20 per cent. Fatal outcome occurred in more than half of persons over forty years of age but was appreciably lower in children and young adults. Since the introduction of the broad-spectrum antibiotics and the development of more precise knowledge regarding correction of the physiologic abnormalities which develop during the disease, deaths rarely occur from this infection even among the patients who first come under medical care rather late in the disease.

Differential Diagnosis. During the early stages of infection before the rash has appeared, differentiation from other acute infections is difficult. History of tick bite while living or traveling in a highly endemic area is helpful. The rash of meningococcemia resembles Rocky Mountain spotted fever in certain aspects, since it is macular, or maculopapular, or petechial in the chronic form, and petechial, confluent, or ecchymotic in the fulminant type. The meningococcic skin lesion is tender and develops with extreme rapidity in the fulminant form, whereas the rickettsial rash occurs on about the fourth day of disease and gradually becomes petechial. The exanthem of rubella rapidly becomes confluent, while that of rubeola almost never becomes petechial. The exanthem of varicella or variola is first erythematous and later becomes vesicular. The rose spots of typhoid fever are usually on the lower chest or abdomen and remain delicate, without hemorrhagic character. Rocky Mountain spotted fever skin lesions, in contrast to those of typhoid, begin on the periphery of the body and later become petechial. The rash of infectious mononucleosis is usually morbilliform on the trunk and rarely becomes petechial. Moreover, in this disease, angina, lymphadenopathy, and atypical lymphocytes in the blood are differentiating features.

Murine typhus is a milder disease than Rocky Mountain spotted fever; the rash is less extensive, nonpurpuric, nonconfluent; and renal and vascular complications are uncommon. Not infrequently differentiation of these two rickettsial infections must await the results of specific serological tests. Epidemic typhus fever is capable of causing all the pronounced clinical, physiologic, and anatomic alterations seen in patients with Rocky Mountain spotted fever, i.e., hypotension, peripheral vascular failure, cyanosis, skin necrosis and gangrene of digits, renal failure with azotemia, and neurological manifestations. However, the rash of classical typhus is noted initially in the axillary folds and on the trunk and later extends peripherally, rarely involving the palms, soles, or face. The serologic patterns in these two diseases are distinctive when specific rickettsial antigens are employed in tests. Moreover, louse-borne typhus is not recognized in the United States except in the form of Brill's disease (recurrent typhus fever). Rickettsialpox, although caused by a member of the spotted fever group of organisms, is usually readily differentiated from Rocky Mountain spotted fever by the initial lesion, the relative mildness of the illness, and the early vesiculation of the maculopapular rash. The Weil-Felix reaction is positive in Rocky Mountain spotted fever and in murine and epidemic typhus, but is negative in rickettsialpox. Agglutinins against *Proteus* OX-19 and OX-2 appear in the serum of patients with spotted fever but only those against OX-19 are generally found in murine and epidemic typhus.

Therapy

General. Certain physiochemical changes occurring in the patient seriously ill with one of the diseases of the typhus spotted fever group should be understood before outlining a therapeutic regime. These changes are circulatory collapse, coma, oliguria and anuria, azotemia, anemia, hypoproteinemia, hypochloremia, and edema of the underlying tissues. These alterations are often absent in the mildly ill, and in them management is much less complicated. The therapeutic principles necessary for the treatment of all rickettsioses are (1) specific chemotherapy and (2) supportive care. Attention to both is mandatory for the seriously ill patient first recognized late in the disease. Contrariwise, during the first week and in the moderately ill patient, supportive therapy may be less energetic, since specific chemotherapy usually suffices. The early mild case may be successfully treated at home, whereas the later case should receive hospital care.

Therapeutic measures advisable for the management of Rocky Mountain spotted fever will be described in detail. Variations of this regimen which apply to the other rickettsioses are described in subsections relegated to other diseases of the typhus–spotted fever group and Q fever.

Specific Therapy. Specific therapy is most effective when initiated during the early stages of disease coincident with the appearance of the rash. When therapy is delayed until the rash has become hemorrhagic and widespread, the response is less dramatic. The antibiotics of choice are chloramphenicol, chlortetracycline, and oxytetracycline, which are effective because of their rickettsiostatic properties. They are not rickettsiocidal. Each of the antibiotics is supplied for oral and intravenous use.

Chloramphenicol. The initial oral dose is calculated on the basis of 50 mg per kg body weight, and subsequent doses of 1.0 Gm are given every 8 hr or 0.5 Gm every 4 hr for adults. Daily requirement for children is calculated on the basis of 75 mg per kg body weight per day. The succinate ester of chloramphenicol available in 1.0-Gm ampules may be given intravenously, incorporating the solution in either 5 per cent glucose or in physiological saline in volumes not exceeding 200 ml. Daily doses exceeding 3.0 Gm are not advised, and the oral route should be utilized when feasible. Chloramphenicol powder obtained from the gelatin-sealed capsules may be suspended in saline or distilled water for administration via stomach tube. Chloromycetin palmitate, a palatable liquid preparation suitable for children, may be given for maintenance therapy calculated on the basis of 100

Table 171-1. EFFECT OF SPECIFIC ANTIBIOTICS ON THE COURSE OF THE MAJOR RICKETTSIOSES

Disease	Untreated		Treated	
	Average duration of fever, days	Mortality, per cent	Average duration of fever after Rx, days	Mortality, per cent
Rocky Mountain spotted fever....	16	21	3	0
Epidemic typhus...	14	30	2	0
Murine typhus....	12	2	2	0
Scrub typhus......	14	15	1	0

mg per kg body weight per day divided in equal doses at 6- to 8-hr intervals.

Tetracyclines. The earlier studies showed that chlortetracycline and oxytetracycline were effective. All the tetracycline group of antibiotics are now used with equal effectiveness. The initial oral dose is calculated on the basis of 25 mg per kg body weight. Subsequent daily doses of 25 mg per kg body weight are divided equally and given at 4 to 6-hr intervals. Parenteral forms of these antibiotics are available for use in the daily doses indicated above. Under no circumstances should more than 2.0 Gm be given intravenously per day, and the oral route is preferred.

Table 171-1 summarizes information on the duration of disease and the mortality in the major rickettsioses prior to and since the introduction of specific antibiotic therapy.

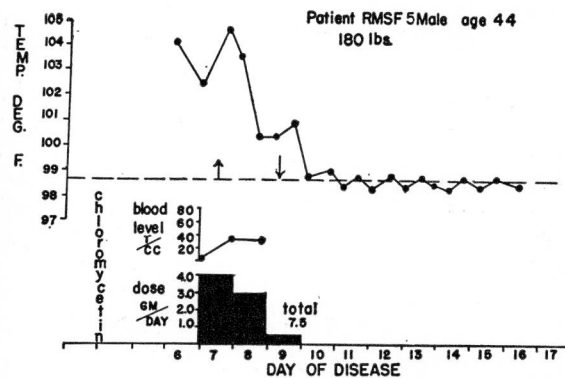

FIG. 171-1. Rocky Mountain spotted fever. Course of illness in a moderately ill adult patient treated with chloramphenicol. Patient became afebrile in 2.5 days.

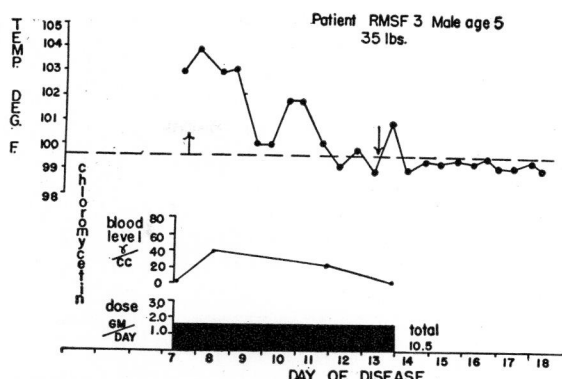

FIG. 171-2. Rocky Mountain spotted fever. Clinical course in a severely ill, semicomatose boy who received energetic supportive therapy as well as chloramphenicol. The temperature reached normal levels 6 days after treatment was instituted. Convalescence was uncomplicated.

Duration of Therapy and Therapeutic Response. Therapy with antibiotics is continued until the toxemia has abated, the general condition has markedly improved, and the temperature has remained at normal levels for 24 hr. In uncomplicated cases of spotted fever, there is symptomatic improvement within 24 hr and normal temperature in 60 to 72 hr.

Figure 171-1 illustrates the typical response in a moderately ill adult in whom specific therapy was augmented by a moderate supportive regimen. Figure 171-2 summarizes the findings in a severely ill child who required a longer course of antibiotic treatment as well as vigorous supportive care.

Supportive Care. *Nursing Care.* Frequent turning of the patient relieves pressure from prominent bony parts such as the lower spine, hip, elbows, and heels, thereby lessening superficial skin lesions. In comatose patients frequent turning also militates against the development of hypostatic pneumonia. Proper mouth hygiene with frequent swabbing of the oral cavity may avert the development of parotitis and gingivitis. Sucking of the juice of a lemon or the oral use of glycerin or mineral oil is helpful.

Protein Balance. A generous intake of protein should be provided by frequent feedings as soon as the disease is suspected, in order to avoid subsequent protein deficiency. Usually food is well tolerated by patients with rickettsial disease, and the daily diet should provide 3 to 5 Gm protein per kg normal body weight, with adequate carbohydrate and fat to make it palatable. When the patient is uncooperative, the diet may be supplemented by hourly liquid protein feedings via stomach tube, provided that there is no abdominal distention.

At the critical stage, when hypoproteinemia is present and changes in capillary permeability lead to edema and vascular embarrassment, careful attention is given to the parenteral administration of protein supplements. When indicated by hematologic studies, whole-blood transfusions given slowly are helpful, or if the total red cell mass is adequate, one of the preformed protein supplements is beneficial. Intravenous albumin may be particularly useful, since it also aids in the reduction of tissue edema. The judicious administration of one of the plasma expanders at this stage may have a definite favorable effect upon the impending circulatory collapse. If the patient is anuric and azotemia is pronounced, overloading the circulation with protein supplements and fluids is to be avoided. The type and amount of parenteral therapy should be governed entirely by clinical judgment and very careful laboratory studies. Frequent determinations of hemoglobin, hematocrit, electrolytes, and protein, sometimes at intervals of a few hours during crucial periods, are necessary in order to ascertain abnormalities and to permit institution of corrective measures.

Fluid Balance. Special attention should be given to the total daily fluid requirement. In the presence of coma, 3 to 5 liters of parenteral fluids may be required, particularly in severely dehydrated patients. Using the laboratory results as a guide, intravenous physiologic saline may be used to correct the hypochloremia. As a rule the proper administration of intravenous saline and glucose infusions will correct the electrolytic imbalance. Efforts should be directed toward ensuring a daily urinary output of approximately 1,500 ml. Too rapid administration of intravenous fluids may provoke additional tissue edema and greatly increase the load upon a weakened myocardium.

Complications

Pyogenic complications, including otitis media and parotitis, are encountered in patients severely ill with Rocky Mountain spotted fever and other rickettsioses. These localized infections respond to therapy with the broad-spectrum antibiotics when combined with ordinary supplemental surgical measures. The sulfonamides are unnecessary for treatment of pyogenic complications and actually exert a detrimental effect on patients with rickettsial infections.

Pneumonitis usually develops as a result of specific rickettsial action. The sputum is scant but should be examined to determine whether superimposed infection is present. Specific therapy is guided by the results of these laboratory studies.

The pneumonitis generally responds to the antibiotic therapy already outlined, and penicillin or supplemental antibiotics are rarely required for secondary bacterial pneumonia.

Circulatory failure of peripheral or central origin is combated by careful administration of electrolytic and protein supplements as described. Myocardial failure may develop rarely from the disease or as a result of overzealous intravenous alimentation and is recognized by the common signs of rapid pulse, gallop rhythm, increase in venous pressure, and muffled cardiac sounds. This complication under present regimens is unusual. When the clinical signs reveal unmistakable evidence of cardiac failure, digitalis may be employed in the usual manner. Oxygen therapy by nasal tube, mask, or tent improves the cardiac and circulatory status and is helpful in hypoxic patients with involvement of the central nervous system.

Prevention

Prevention is attained primarily by avoidance of tick-infested areas. When this is impractical, prophylactic measures include (1) spraying the ground with dieldrin for area control of ticks, (2) application of repellents such as diethyltoluamide or dimethylphthalate to clothing and exposed parts of the body, or in very heavily infested areas the wearing of clothing which interferes with attachment of ticks, i.e., boots and a one-piece outer garment, preferably impregnated with repellent, and (3) daily inspection of the entire body, including the hairy parts to detect and remove attached ticks. In removing attached ticks great care should be taken to avoid crushing the arthropod, with resultant contamination of the bite wound; touching the tick with gasoline or whisky encourages detachment but gentle traction with tweezers applied close to the mouth parts may be necessary; the skin area should be disinfected with soap and water or other antiseptics. Similarly, precautions should be employed in removing engorged ticks from dogs and other animals, since infection through minor abrasions on the hands is possible. Vaccines containing *R. rickettsii* are available commercially and should be used for those exposed to great risk, viz., persons frequenting highly endemic areas and laboratory workers exposed to the agent. Since the broad-spectrum antibiotics were shown to be such excellent therapeutic agents in spotted fever, there has been less impetus for vaccination of persons who run only a minor risk of infection.

REFERENCES

Cox, H. R.: The Spotted-Fever Group, pp. 828–868 in "Viral and Rickettsial Infections of Man," 3d ed., T. M. Rivers and F. L. Horsfall, Jr. (Eds.), Philadelphia, J. B. Lippincott Company, 1959.

Harrell, G. T.: Rocky Mountain Spotted Fever, Medicine, 28:333, 1949.

Ley, H. L., Jr., and J. E. Smadel: Antibiotic Therapy of Rickettsial Diseases, Antibiotics & Chemotherapy, 4:792, 1954.

Parker, R. R.: Rocky Mountain Spotted Fever, J.A.M.A., 110:1185, 1938.

Pincoffs, M. C., E. G. Guy, L. M. Lister, T. E. Woodward, and J. E. Smadel: The Treatment of Rocky Mountain Spotted Fever with Chloromycetin, Ann. Internal Med., 29:656, 1948.

Powell, A. M., M. J. Snyder, J. V. Minor, Jr., J. F. Benson, and T. E. Woodward: The Use of Terramycin in Rocky Mountain Spotted Fever, Bull. Johns Hopkins Hosp., 89:30, 1951.

Ricketts, H. T.: "Contributions to Medical Science by Howard Taylor Ricketts 1870–1910," Chicago, University of Chicago Press, 1911.

Ross, S., E. B. Schoenbach, F. G. Burke, M. S. Bryer, E. C. Rice, and J. A. Washington: Aureomycin Therapy of Rocky Mountain Spotted Fever, J.A.M.A., 138:1213, 1948.

Wolbach, S. B.: Studies on Rocky Mountain Spotted Fever, J. Med. Research, 41:1, 1919.

172 RICKETTSIALPOX
T. E. Woodward and J. E. Smadel

Definition. Rickettsialpox is a mild, nonfatal, self-limited, acute febrile illness caused by *Rickettsia akari,* which is transmitted from mouse to man by mites. It is characterized by an initial skin lesion at the site of the mite bite, a week's febrile course, and a papulovesicular rash.

Etiology and Epidemiology. Rickettsialpox was first recognized in New York City in 1946 and later in several areas in New England. It has an annual incidence of approximately 200 cases. The vector is a small, colorless mite, *Allodermanyssus sanguineus* (Hirst), which infests small mice and rodents. House mice serve as the reservoir of infection.

Rickettsia akari is morphologically and biologically similar to other rickettsias and is antigenically related to, but distinct from, *R. rickettsii,* the cause of Rocky Mountain spotted fever. Mice, guinea pigs, and fertile hen's eggs are susceptible to experimental infection, and diagnostic antigens prepared from infected yolk sacs are used in complement fixation tests.

Clinical Manifestations. The initial skin lesion appears about 7 to 10 days after the mite bite as a firm red papule 1 to 1.5 cm in diameter. In a few days the center vesiculates, and the papule is surrounded by an area of erythema. The regional lymph glands are moderately enlarged. The primary lesion, which is never painful, becomes covered with a black scab; it heals slowly, and a small scar is visible on separation of the crust.

The febrile phase begins 3 to 7 days following the initial lesion, and a body exanthem may accompany the fever or begin several days later. The onset of fever is sudden, with chilly sensations or frank chills, headache, sweats, myalgia, anorexia, and photophobia. The pyrexia ranges from 103 to 104°F and continues for about a week, occasionally with morning remissions.

The exanthem is maculopapular-vesicular, generalized in distribution, and may be abundant or scant. The lesions may involve the oral cavity but not the palms or soles. In a week, the vesicles dry and form scabs which eventually scale but leave no scar.

The constitutional symptoms are generally mild, and the course of illness uncomplicated. No fatal cases have been reported.

The disease may be confused with varicella (chickenpox), which is different in that it occurs usually in childhood and has no initial lesion, and the papular cutaneous lesion is entirely transformed into a vesicle. Variola (smallpox) is accompanied by a more severe constitutional reaction, and the vesicles become pustules. The skin lesions of the other rickettsioses differ in their lack of vesiculation. The Weil-Felix reaction remains negative in this rickettsial disease, but the specific complement fixation test is a useful laboratory diagnostic aid even though there is considerable crossing with materials from Rocky Mountain spotted fever.

Treatment and Prevention. Chloramphenicol and the tetracycline antibiotics are all effective for treating patients with rickettsialpox. The temperature reaches normal levels in about 2 days, and recovery is rapid. The therapeutic procedures are comparable to those used in spotted fever, which are described in detail on p. 1098.

Control measures should be directed toward elimination of house mice and the vector mites responsible for transmitting the disease.

REFERENCES

Greenberg, M.: Rickettsialpox in New York City, Am. J. Med., 4:866, 1948.

Huebner, R. J., W. L. Jellison, and C. Pomerantz: Rickettsialpox, a Newly Recognized Rickettsial Disease: IV. Isolation of a Rickettsia Apparently Identical with the Causative Agent of Rickettsialpox from *Allodermanyssus sanguineus,* a Rodent Mite, U.S. Pub. Health Repts., 61:1677, 1946.

Rose, H. M.: The Clinical Manifestations and Laboratory Diagnosis of Rickettsialpox, Ann. Internal Med., 31:871, 1949.

——: The Treatment of Rickettsialpox with Antibiotics, Ann. N.Y. Acad. Sci., 55:1019, 1952.

Zdrodovskii, P. F., and E. M. Golinevich: Vesicular and Varicelliform Rickettsiosis, pp. 276–286 in "Uchenie and Rikketsiakh i Rikkesiozakh" (The Study of Rickettsiae and Rickettsioses), Moscow, Medgiz, 1956.

173 AFRICAN TICK-BORNE FEVER

T. E. Woodward and
J. E. Smadel

Definition. African tick-borne fever, also called *boutonneuse fever, South African tick-bite fever,* is a mild to moderately severe, nonfatal illness characterized by an initial lesion (called the *tache noir* in boutonneuse fever), fever of several days to 2 weeks, and a generalized maculopapular erythematous rash which appears on about the fifth day and usually involves the palms and soles. Specific complement fixing antibodies appear in the patient's serum during convalescence, but agglutinins to *Proteus* OX-19 (Weil-Felix reaction) are frequently found only in low titer.

Etiology and Epidemiology. The causative agent, *Rickettsia conorii,* is a member of the spotted fever group of rickettsias and is transmitted to man by infected ticks. In the Mediterranean area, the bite of infected *Rhipicephalus sanguineus,* the brown dog tick, is responsible, whereas in South Africa a number of ticks are assumed to be vectors, viz., *Haemaphysalis leachi, Amblyomma hebraeum, Rhipicephalus appendiculatus, Boophilus decoloratus,* and *Hyalomma aegyptium.*

The disease occurs in the Mediterranean and Black Sea area and in Africa, but not in the Western Hemisphere. It is more prevalent during summer months in temperate zones, whereas it occurs throughout the year in the tropics.

Clinical Manifestations. The clinical course is usually milder than in spotted fever, with a shorter febrile period and fewer severe complications; fatalities are few and generally limited to the aged or debilitated. The initial lesion heals slowly, and the regional lymph nodes are enlarged. The rash usually remains papular and rarely becomes hemorrhagic as it does in spotted fever.

Treatment and Prevention. Chloramphenicol, chlortetracycline, and oxytetracycline are equally effective therapeutic agents for African tick-borne fever. Patients generally become afebrile after 2 days of treatment, and recovery is rapid. The therapeutic procedures are comparable to those used in spotted fever, which are described in detail on p. 1098.

The major effective methods of control are concerned with avoidance of tick bites; these include application of newer repellents and prompt removal of attached ticks. Effective vaccines are not available commercially.

REFERENCES

Conor, A., and A. Bruch: Une fièvre éruptive observée en Tunisie, Bull. soc. pathol. exotique, 3:492, 1910.

Gear, J. H. S., and C. Bevan: An Outbreak of Tick-bite Fever, S. African Med. J., 10:485, 1936.

—— and A. L. Harington: Tick-bite Fever: Two Cases Treated with Aureomycin (Lederle), a New Antibiotic, S. African Med. J., 23:507, 1948.

Joint OIHP/WHO: Study Group on African Rickettsioses: Report on the First Session, World Health Organization, Tech. Rept. Ser. No. 23, Geneva, World Health Organization, December, 1950.

LeGac, P., and M. Rouby: Aureomycine dans le traitement de la fièvre boutonneuse en Afrique equatoriale, Bull. soc. pathol. exotique, 43:678, 1950.

174 MURINE (Endemic) TYPHUS FEVER

T. E. Woodward and
J. E. Smadel

Definition. Murine typhus fever is an acute specific febrile disease caused by *Rickettsia mooseri* (*R. typhi*) and transmitted to man by fleas. The clinical illness is characterized by fever of 9 to 14 days, headache, a maculopapular rash appearing on the third to fifth day, myalgia, moderate neurologic manifestations, and the appearance during convalescence of agglutinins for certain strains of *Proteus* bacteria (Weil-Felix reaction) and of specific complement fixing antibodies which react with the causal rickettsiae. Treatment with the broad-spectrum antibiotics is highly efficacious.

Etiology and Epidemiology. *Rickettsia mooseri* resembles other rickettsias as regards morphologic properties, staining characteristics, and intracellular parasitism. Under the electron microscope *R. mooseri* contains dense masses of nuclear material in a less dense homogeneous protoplasmic substance, the whole of which is surrounded by a limiting membrane. It differs from *R. rickettsii* in that it always multiplies within the cytoplasm of cells, in contrast to the intranuclear and cytoplasmic positions of spotted fever rickettsias.

Invasion of the body by *R. mooseri* provokes specific and nonspecific immunologic responses. Utilizing highly purified antigens, specific antibodies may be demonstrated readily by complement fixation and agglutination reactions. The positive Weil-Felix reaction which occurs in this disease is essentially nonspecific, since it is attributable to the presence of a common carbohydrate antigen in *Proteus* OX-19 and *R. mooseri* and since the reaction is also positive in epidemic typhus and spotted fever. A number of investigators have demonstrated group specific rickettsial antigens common to both *R. mooseri* and *R. prowazeki*, viz., a heat-stable complement-fixing substance. Furthermore, both murine and epidemic rickettsias possess a toxic factor which is lethal to mice and rats and may be neutralized by convalescent serum from man or lower animals.

The common vector of *R. mooseri* for rats and man is the rat flea (*Xenopsylla cheopis*). Blanc is of the opinion that infection may be spread from man to man by the pest flea (*Pulex irritans*). In nature the rat louse (*Polypax spinulosis*) may transmit the agent among rodents. Customarily rat fleas become infected on ingestion of blood from diseased rats; the rickettsias multiply within the intestinal cells of the arthropod and are excreted in the feces. Infection in man occurs following the flea bite and contamination of the broken skin by rickettsia-laden feces. Dried flea feces may infect via the conjunctivas or upper respiratory tract.

Rats and mice are naturally infected with murine typhus, and although the rodent disease is nonfatal, viable rickettsias persist in the brain for variable periods.

Murine typhus is one of the most benign and widespread of the rickettsioses in the United States. Prevalent in the Southeastern and Gulf Coast states, it has been identified in most of the other states and in harbor centers throughout the world wherever rats and fleas abound. Through control of rats and their fleas a sharp decline in incidence has occurred since 1951, particularly in the Southern United States. In urban areas the disease is more prevalent during the summer and fall months and occurs predominantly among persons working in proximity to granaries or food depots. Recently there has been an extension to certain rural areas because changing agricultural practices have provided rats with ready access to adequate food supplies.

Clinical Manifestations. *Incubation Period and Prodromata.* Based upon experimental observations the incubation period ranges from 8 to 16 days, with a mean of 10. Common prodromata are headache, backache, arthralgia, and chilly sensations. Nausea, malaise, and insufficient temperature rises may actually precede the true onset of disease.

Onset and General Symptoms. A frank shaking chill and often repeated rigors are present at onset, associated with a severe frontal headache and fever. This triad of headache, chill, and pyrexia is usually followed within a few hours by nausea and vomiting. Prostration, malaise, and weakness are sufficient to enforce cessation of activity in adults in contrast to children, whose illness is less severe. Occasionally, mild symptoms make it difficult to define the actual onset.

Pyrexia. The usual febrile course in murine typhus lasts for about 12 days in adults, and the temperature ranges from 102 to 104°F but may reach 105 to 106°F in children. The temperature may reach high levels abruptly after onset or ascend in a stepwise manner during the first few days. With the appearance of the rash, fever is usually sustained, with partial daily remissions which occasionally reach normal levels in the morning. Defervescence is generally by lysis over several days but sometimes occurs by abrupt crisis. Transient mild fever of 100°F is not uncommon during early convalescence. A few patients experience only low-grade fever throughout, but this does not necessarily connote a mild illness.

Cutaneous Manifestations. The early lesions, which are sparse and discrete, are hidden in the axillae and inner surface of the arm. Most patients then develop with surprising suddenness a generalized, dull red macular rash of the upper abdomen, shoulders, chest, arms, and thighs. The individual lesions are discrete and pea-size, with an ill-defined border, and fade on pressure during the first 24 hr. They later become maculopapular in contrast to the exanthem of epidemic typhus, which is persistently macular. The distribution over the trunk with sparse involvement of the extremities, palms, soles, and face differs from the peripheral distribution and facial involvement of Rocky Mountain spotted fever. The murine rash generally appears initially on the fifth febrile day, but rarely is it seen concurrently with the onset or developing as late as the seventh day.

Eighty per cent of patients develop a rash which usually persists for 4 to 8 days and fades before defervescence. The cutaneous manifestations vary greatly in intensity and duration and may be fleeting. They are readily overlooked in dark-skinned patients, in whom they should be searched for by light palpation and indirect lighting.

Cardiovascular and Respiratory Features. An irritating nonproductive cough is frequent and is occasionally associated with moderate hemoptysis. Early in the second week rales may be detected in the basilar lung areas. These changes are generally rickettsial rather than bacterial in origin and respond to the broad-spectrum antibiotics but not to penicillin or sulfonamide therapy. Pulmonary congestion occurs in extremely ill and elderly patients.

Accelerated pulse, hypotension, and general circulatory weakness occur in this disease, although less frequently than in patients with the more severe epidemic typhus or Rocky Mountain spotted fever. The reader is referred to the chapter on Rocky Mountain spotted fever (Chap. 171) relative to the details of the cardiovascular features.

Neurologic Manifestations. Headache is the most common neurologic manifestation of murine typhus and may dominate the clinical picture. It is frontally localized and continues into the second week of illness. In the early stages the facial expression is strained, and the patient resents distraction. Stupor and prostration may occur in the second week, and in severe cases there may be muttering delirium and extreme agitation, and coma similar to the more severe louse-borne typhus. Coma in elderly patients after 2 weeks of illness presages death. Nuchal rigidity and general spasticity often suggest meningitis, although the spinal fluid is essentially normal except for slight increases in pressure and lymphocytes (5 to 30 per cu mm). Transient partial deafness occurs occasionally in murine typhus patients, but rarely is there localized neuritis or hemiplegia. Neurologic sequelae are unusual. Children experience minimal neurologic changes.

Other Physical Manifestations. During the first 2 days of illness the patient may be nauseated and vomit, but vomiting later in the illness should arouse suspicion of an intercurrent complication. Abdominal pain, particularly in dehydrated patients, is bothersome, and when associated with diarrhea responds to intravenous alimentation. A sluggish, constipated bowel is occasionally observed. Hepatomegaly and jaundice are unusual. There is splenomegaly in approximately 25 per cent of patients.

Photophobia, retroocular pain, suffusion of the eyes, and congestion of the conjunctivas are common manifestations but are less severe than in the other typhus and spotted fevers. Dehydrated patients often have a furred, brown tongue and crusting of the gums and mucous membranes.

Renal function is usually unaltered except in elderly patients with prolonged hypotension and vascular weakness. Under these circumstances in seriously ill patients, azotemia may develop to the degree observed in epidemic typhus. The blood chlorides are low in severe murine typhus as in the epidemic type; hypochloremia of 80 mEq per liter may be observed. Hypoproteinemia, resulting from lowered serum albumin, is encountered.

Course of Disease and Complications. After defervescence murine typhus patients recover rapidly. Fatalities occur between the ninth and twelfth days in elderly or debilitated patients, usually as a result of circulatory and renal failure, thrombosed blood vessels, or intercurrent infection.

Complications are usually pyogenic, such as otitis media and parotitis, and a superimposed pneumonitis may be difficult to differentiate from pulmonary congestion. Fortunately the average course of murine typhus fever is quite uncomplicated.

Prognosis. The mortality in murine typhus was low even before the introduction of modern specific therapy. Only one death occurred in the 114 cases studied by Maxcy and none in the 180 reported by Stuart and Pullen.

Differential Diagnosis. See the discussion in the chapter on Rocky Mountain spotted fever (p. 1098). The geographic and seasonal occurrence of murine typhus and spotted fever differ and may help in diagnosis.

Treatment and Prevention. The therapeutic procedures are comparable to those used in spotted fever, which are described in detail on p. 1098. Chloramphenicol and the tetracycline antibiotics have each controlled the disease.

Prevention of murine typhus in man is attained by reducing the natural reservoir and vector by applying measures for eliminating rodents and employing DDT in rat-infested areas to control fleas.

REFERENCES

Bradley, G. H., and J. S. Wiley: The Control of Murine Typhus in the United States, pp. 229–240 in "The Rickettsial Diseases of Man," Washington, American Association for the Advancement of Science, 1948.

Ley, H. L., Jr., and J. E. Smadel: Antibiotic Therapy of Rickettsial Diseases, Antibiotics & Chemotherapy, 4:792, 1954.

—— T. E. Woodward, and J. E. Smadel: Chloramphenicol (Chloromycetin) in the Treatment of Murine Typhus, J.A.M.A., 143:217, 1950.

Maxcy, K. F.: Typhus Fever in the United States, U.S. Public Health Repts., 44:1735, 1929.

Stuart, B. M., and R. L. Pullen: Endemic (Murine) Typhus Fever: Clinical Observations of One Hundred and Eighty Cases, Ann. Internal Med., 23: 520, 1945.

Woodward, T. E.: Endemic (Murine) Typhus Fever: Symptomatology, pp. 134–138 in "The Rickettsial Diseases of Man," Washington, American Association for the Advancement of Science, 1948.

175 EPIDEMIC (Louse-borne) TYPHUS FEVER

T. E. Woodward and
J. E. Smadel

Definition. The classical epidemic form of typhus is a severe acute febrile disease caused by *Rickettsia prowazeki* and transmitted to man by the body louse. Intense headache, continuous pyrexia of about 2 weeks, a macular skin eruption appearing on about the fifth febrile day, malaise, and vascular and neurologic disturbances represent the principal clinical features. Confirmation of the diagnosis is made by demonstration of *Proteus* OX-19 agglutinins and of specific complement fixing antibodies in convalescence. The broad-spectrum antibiotics are specific therapeutic agents.

Etiology and Epidemiology. The causative microbe, *R. prowazeki,* is closely related to *R. mooseri* (*R. typhi*) which causes murine typhus; indeed, the two have a number of common antigens. *Rickettsia prowazeki* was the first of the rickettsias shown to have its own enzyme system, which permits it to respire independently of the host cell (Bovarnick and Snyder, 1949).

Man generally is infected when rickettsia-laden louse feces are rubbed into the broken skin; scratching the louse bite facilitates this process. *Pediculus humanus corporis,* which is peculiarly adapted to man, is the only important vector of epidemic typhus. It dies of its infection and fails to transmit rickettsias to its offspring. There is no known animal habitat of *R. prowazeki;* it is maintained by a cycle involving man-louse-man. New epidemics apparently originate from patients with Brill's disease (recurrent epidemic typhus). Inhalation of dust containing dried louse feces may rarely cause infection.

Epidemic typhus, if uncontrolled, behaves as a cyclic disease in a susceptible population, extending over a 3-year period. During the first year there is a gradual seeding of cases throughout the group; during the second there is epidemic spread; and during the third the epidemic tapers off, because the majority of persons have already become immune. Outbreaks of epidemic typhus last occurred in the United States in the nineteenth century, and its presence is now recognized only in the form of Brill's disease (see p. 1106).

Clinical Manifestations. A classic clinical description of Old World typhus is provided in Wolbach, Todd, and Palfrey's monograph of 1922. Epidemic typhus resembles murine typhus, but is more severe. After an incubation period of about 7 days an abrupt onset of headache, chill, and rapidly mounting fever ushers in the illness. Cephalgia, malaise,

and prostration continue unabated until the rash appears on the fifth febrile day. It is initially macular in the axillary folds but ultimately invades the trunk and extremities as a pink, irregular macular lesion which becomes fixed, petechial, and confluent in the later stages.

Neurologic features range from headache and general spasticity to extreme agitation, stupor, and coma. Circulatory disturbances consisting of tachycardia, hypotension, and cyanosis are more profound than those observed in murine typhus and are almost as severe as in Rocky Mountain spotted fever. Ultimately in untreated cases azotemia often reaches high levels as a result of vascular and renal failure, and death occurs late in the second week of illness. Furthermore, thrombosis of major blood vessels and cutaneous gangrene develop in a manner similar to that seen in the virulent form of Rocky Mountain spotted fever.

The complications and sequelae in epidemic typhus are more severe than those in murine typhus, but not so severe as those in Rocky Mountain spotted fever. However, during certain outbreaks epidemic typhus was fatal to 60 per cent of those infected, and convalescence in survivors was prolonged. Broad-spectrum antibiotics have essentially eradicated mortality in this dread disease, provided therapy is instituted before irreversible changes have been established in the tissues.

Differential Diagnosis. Differentiation of epidemic typhus from the various rickettsioses and other diseases with which it may be confused is described in Chap. 171, Rocky Mountain Spotted Fever. The disease in epidemic form never occurs in the absence of lousiness in the general population. Under the conditions in which typhus epidemics are likely to occur other diseases which may cause confusion include malaria, relapsing fever, pneumonia, and tuberculosis. Classic typhus contracted by a previously vaccinated person is usually mild and may be clinically indistinguishable from murine typhus except by serologic methods.

Treatment and Prevention. Chloramphenicol and the tetracycline antibiotics have each been found to be highly efficient therapeutic agents in epidemic typhus. Usually the patient becomes afebrile after 2 days of treatment. The therapeutic procedures are comparable to those used in spotted fever, which are described in detail on p. 1098.

The most effective measures for controlling epidemic typhus are those which eliminate lousiness. DDT or lindane powder when dusted into clothing is suitable for this purpose. If resistant lice are found, malathione may prove effective.

A commercially available vaccine prepared from

formalin-treated infected yolk sac tissue is an effective immunizing agent.

REFERENCES

Nicolle, C.: Reproduction expérimentale du typhus exanthématique chez le singe, Compt. rend., 149: 157, 1909.

Payne, E. H., E. A. Sharp, and J. A. Knaudt: Treatment of Epidemic Typhus with Chloromycetin, Trans. Roy. Soc. Trop. Med. Hyg., 42:163, 1948.

Snyder, J. C.: The Typhus Fevers, pp. 799–827 in "Viral and Rickettsial Infections of Man," 3d ed., T. M. Rivers and F. L. Horsfall, Jr. (Eds.), Philadelphia, J. B. Lippincott Company, 1959.

Wolbach, S. B., J. L. Todd, and F. W. Palfrey: "The Etiology and Pathology of Typhus," Cambridge, Mass., Harvard University Press, 1922.

Woodward, T. E., and E. F. Bland: Clinical Observations in Typhus Fever with Special Reference to the Cardiovascular System, J.A.M.A., 126:287, 1944.

Yeomans, A.: The Symptomatology, Clinical Course and Management of Louse-borne Typhus Fever, pp. 126–133 in "The Rickettsial Diseases of Man," Washington, American Association for the Advancement of Science, 1948.

176 BRILL'S DISEASE (Recrudescent Typhus)

T. E. Woodward and J. E. Smadel

Definition. Brill's disease is a recrudescent episode of epidemic typhus fever which occurs years after the initial attack. Nathan Brill in 1898 observed a sporadic disease which resembled typhus fever among nonlousy inhabitants of New York City. Zinsser, in 1934, suggested on the basis of epidemiologic and immunologic considerations that this malady was a recurrent form of typhus encountered in persons who had recovered from the epidemic disease while residing in countries where it was prevalent. Additional information has gradually accumulated in support of this hypothesis.

Murray and Snyder (1951) were successful in regularly isolating rickettsias indistinguishable from *Rickettsia prowazeki* in lice fed on patients during the active stages of illness.

Clinical Manifestations. The clinical entity, not always mild, resembles epidemic typhus fever as pertains to character of the rash, circulatory disturbances, hepatic, renal, and nervous system changes. Recovery is the rule. The Weil-Felix reaction with the various *Proteus* antigens is usually

negative, or positive in very low titer, in Brill's disease. The specific complement fixation reaction is valuable in establishing the diagnosis. The therapeutic procedures are comparable to those used in spotted fever, which are described in detail on p. 1098.

REFERENCES

Brill, N. E.: An Acute Infectious Disease of Unknown Origin: A Clinical Study Based on Two Hundred and Twenty-one Cases, Am. J. Med. Sci., 39:484, 1910.

Murray, E. S., G. Baehr, G. Shwartzman, R. A. Mandelbaum, N. Rosenthal, J. C. Doane, L. B. Weiss, S. Cohen, and J. C. Snyder: Brill's Disease: I. Clinical and Laboratory Diagnosis, J.A.M.A., 142: —— and J. C. Snyder: Brill's Disease: II. Etiology, Am. J. Hyg., 53:22, 1951. 1059, 1950.

177 SCRUB TYPHUS

T. E. Woodward and J. E. Smadel

Definition. Scrub typhus is limited to eastern and southeastern Asia, India, northern Australia, and the adjacent islands. It is caused by *Rickettsia tsutsugamushi* and characterized by a primary lesion at the site of the bite of an infected mite, a fever of about 2 weeks' duration, a cutaneous rash which develops about the fifth day, and the appearance late in the second week of agglutinins against the OX-K strain of *Proteus* bacillus. The broad-spectrum antibiotics are specific therapeutic agents.

Etiology. The agent of scrub typhus resembles other rickettsias in its physical properties but differs from them in antigenic structure, vector, and reservoir. The disease is transmitted by larvae of several species of mites, especially *Trombicula akamushi* and *T. deliensis*. These tiny chiggers attach themselves to the skin and during the process of obtaining a meal of tissue juice may acquire infection from the host or transmit rickettsias to the vertebrate. The infection is maintained in nature by a cycle involving mites and small rodents and by transovarial transmission in mites; human infection represents an accident attributable to propinquity.

Clinical Manifestations. About 10 to 12 days after infection, illness begins abruptly with chilliness, severe headache, fever, conjunctival injection, and moderate generalized lymphadenopathy which is most prominent in the nodes draining the area of the primary lesion. The initial lesion at the beginning of fever is evidenced by an erythematous indurated area 1 cm in diameter, surmounted by a multiloculated vesicle; within a few days the vesicle ulcerates and becomes covered with a black crust.

Fever increases progressively during the first week, generally reaching 104 to 105°F, but the pulse remains relatively slow, i.e., 70 to 100 per minute. The red macular rash, which begins on the trunk about the fifth day and spreads to the extremities, sometimes becomes maculopapular but usually fades in a few days. The course of the disease and the complications resemble those of endemic and epidemic typhus; however, interstitial myocarditis is more prominent than in the other typhus fevers.

Prognosis. Prior to the introduction of the broad-spectrum antibiotics the mortality varied from 1 to 60 per cent, depending on the geographic area and the virulence of the local strains of *R. tsutsugamushi,* and convalescence was prolonged. With modern therapeutic methods deaths are extremely rare and convalescence is short.

Differential Diagnosis. Scrub typhus is to be differentiated from the other members of the typhus and the spotted fever group of diseases as well as from measles, typhoid fever, and meningococcal infections (see Chap. 171, Rocky Mountain Spotted Fever). The geographic localization of scrub typhus, the primary lesion, and the occurrence of OX-K agglutinins are especially useful in establishing the diagnosis.

Treatment and Prevention. Chloramphenicol and the tetracycline antibiotics are valuable specific therapeutic agents in scrub typhus. The therapeutic procedures are comparable to those used in spotted fever, which are described in detail on p. 1098. In fact, scrub typhus is more amenable to drugs than are the other rickettsial infections, since patients with this disease regularly become afebrile and are decidedly improved within 24 to 36 hr after beginning treatment, irrespective of the stage of disease.

Prevention of disease in the individual is accomplished by the application of miticidal chemicals (dibutyl phthalate, benzyl benzoate, and others) to clothing and the skin. There is no satisfactory vaccine.

REFERENCES

Audy, J. R., and J. L. Harrison: A Review of Investigations on Mite Typhus in Burma and Malaya, 1945–1950, Trans. Roy. Soc. Trop. Med. Hyg., 44:371, 1951.

Blake, F. G., K. F. Maxcy, J. F. Sadusk, Jr., G. M. Kohls, and E. J. Bell: Studies on Tsutsugamushi Disease (Scrub Typhus, Mite-borne Typhus) in New Guinea and Adjacent Islands: Epidemiology, Clinical Observations, and Etiology in the Dobadura Area, Am. J. Hyg., 41:243, 1945.

Fletcher, W., J. E. Lesslar, and R. Lewthwaite: The Aetiology of the Tsutsugamushi Disease and Tropical Typhus in the Federated Malay States, Part II, Trans. Roy. Soc. Trop. Med. Hyg., 23:57, 1929.

Kawamura, R.: Studies on Tsutsugamushi Disease (Japanese Flood Fever), The Medical Bulletin, College of Medicine, University of Cincinnati, 4: Spec. Nos. 1 and 2, 1, 1926.

Smadel, J. E.: Influence of Antibiotics on Immunological Response in Scrub Typhus, Am. J. Med., 17: 246, 1954.

———: Scrub Typhus, pp. 869–879 in "Viral and Rickettsial Infections of Man," 3d ed., T. M. Rivers and F. L. Horsfall, Jr. (Eds.), Philadelphia, J. B. Lippincott Company, 1959.

——— and E. B. Jackson: Chloromycetin: An Antibiotic with Chemotherapeutic Activity in Experimental Rickettsial and Viral Infections, Science, 106:418, 1947.

——— T. E. Woodward, H. L. Ley, Jr., and R. Lewthwaite: Chloramphenicol (Chloromycetin) in the Treatment of Tsutsugamushi Disease (Scrub Typhus), J. Clin. Invest., 28:1196, 1949.

178 Q FEVER
T. E. Woodward and J. E. Smadel

Definition. Q fever is an acute infectious disease caused by *Rickettsia burneti* characterized by a sudden onset of fever, malaise, headache, weakness, anorexia, and usually an interstitial pneumonitis. Rickettsemia occurs during the febrile period, and specific complement fixing antibodies are present during convalescence. In contrast to the other rickettsioses, the disease is not associated with a cutaneous exanthem or agglutinins for the proteus bacteria (Weil-Felix reaction).

Etiology and Epidemiology. *Rickettsia burneti* (Derrick, 1939) possesses the general properties of other rickettsias but is somewhat more resistant to inactivation in unfavorable environments and more pleomorphic than the others. Its infectivity after drying under natural conditions is of importance in the spread of infection to man. Its pleomorphism, which ranges from diplobacillary structures measuring 1.5 μ in length to tiny spheres about 0.2 μ in diameter, contributes to its filterability through Berkefeld N candles. This filterability led Cox (1939) to suggest the name *R. diaporica* for the first American isolate, but the name was subsequently abandoned when this agent was found to be identical with that causing Q fever in Australia. *Rickettsia burneti* has a wide host range in nature, but guinea pigs and embryonated eggs are the common laboratory hosts employed for its propagation.

Human cases of Q fever are contracted by inhalation of infected dusts, by handling infected materials, and by drinking milk contaminated with *R. burneti.* The disease in Australia is enzootic in animals, especially bandicoots, and is transmitted in nature by ticks. Rickettsia laden tick feces may contaminate cattle hides, and inhalation of such material has caused infection in man. In the United States, a number of species of ticks are naturally infected, among them *Dermacentor andersoni* and *Amblyomma americanum,* and in North Africa transovarial transmission of the agent in indigenous ticks has been demonstrated by Blanc. Sheep, goats, and cows have been found naturally infected in *North America* and in *Europe. Rickettsia burneti* has been recovered from the milk of such animals (Huebner et al., 1948; Caminopetros, 1948; Marmion and Stoker, 1950). Such milk, as well as infected excretions from livestock, probably acounts for certain outbreaks of human disease which appear attributable to inhalation of infected dust from barns and pens (Lennette and Welsh, 1951). The method of spread of outbreaks of Q fever was not clearly established among stockyard workers in Texas and Illinois, wool processors in Pennsylvania, employees in a rendering plant in New York, and laundry workers in Montana who hauled dirty linen from a laboratory engaged in studies in Q fever; however, the air-borne route for dried contaminated material seems the most likely. A number of epidemics have occurred among laboratory workers engaged in studies on *R. burneti* in various institutions throughout the world. The disease is not transmitted from man to man.

Clinical Manifestations. After incubation of approximately 19 days (the range is 14 to 26) the disease begins with headache, chilly sensations, fever, malaise, myalgia, and anorexia. For several days, the temperature ranges from 101 to 104°F; the entire course may not exceed 2 weeks and usually ranges from 3 to 6 days. There may be wide fluctuations of the fever. Respiratory and gastrointestinal symptoms are not conspicuous in the early stages. Headache and fever predominate. A dry cough and chest pain occur after about 5 days, when rales are usually audible. Roentgenographic findings indistinguishable from those of primary atypical pneumonia are present usually by the third to fourth day of disease, first as patchy areas of consolidation involving a portion of one lobe, giving a homogeneous ground-glass appearance. These manifestations persist beyond the febrile period and may appear in patients who are unaware of pulmonary involvement. Complications are rare, and coincident with defervescence the appetite begins to return, and convalescence progresses slowly for several weeks, during which time the principal disability is weakness. It is not uncommon for patients to lose 15 to 20 lb during the active stages of disease. Several investigators have emphasized that the disease may be protracted in approximately 20 per cent of cases, with fever persisting for longer than 4 weeks, particularly in elderly patients. Occasionally relapse occurs, particularly in patients treated with antibiotics during the first several days of disease. Moreover, hepatitis with the development of clinically detectable icterus occurs in approximately one-third of patients with the protracted form.

Prognosis. The prognosis from the point of view of mortality is excellent, and few fatalities have been recorded in the modern literature. Except for the patient with the protracted type of illness and hepatic involvement, the course of disease is generally uncomplicated and benign.

Treatment and Control. The tetracycline antibiotics and chloramphenicol are effective in the treatment of patients with Q fever. Most patients, when treated early in the course of disease, respond promptly and recover without relapses. The therapeutic procedures are comparable to those used in spotted fever, which are discussed in detail on p. 1098. It should be emphasized that patients with hepatic involvement should receive careful attention to their dietary requirement, particularly with relation to protein and carbohydrate intake. Oxygen is beneficial in patients with severe interstitial pneumonitis.

REFERENCES

Bell, J. A., M. D. Beck, and R. J. Huebner: Epidemiological Studies of Q Fever in Southern California, J.A.M.A., 142:868, 1950.

Clark, W. H., and E. H. Lennette: Treatment of Q Fever with Antibiotics, Ann. N.Y. Acad. Sci., 55:1004, 1952.

Derrick, E. H.: "Q" Fever, a New Fever Entity: Clinical Features, Diagnosis, and Laboratory Investigation, Med. J. Australia, 2:281, 1937.

Hornibrook, J. W., and K. R. Nelson: An Institutional Outbreak of Pneumonitis: I. Epidemiological and Clinical Studies, U.S. Public Health Rept., 55:1936, 1940.

Lennette, E. H.: Q Fever, pp. 880–895 in "Viral and Rickettsial Infections of Man," 3d ed., T. M. Rivers and F. L. Horsfall, Jr. (Eds.), Philadelphia, J. B. Lippincott Company, 1959.

—— and W. H. Clark: Observations on the Epidemiology of Q Fever in Northern California, J.A.M.A., 145:306, 1951.

Tigertt, W. D., and A. S. Benenson: Studies on Q Fever in Man, Trans. Assoc. Am. Physicians, 69:98, 1956.

Section 13: Introduction to Viral Diseases

179 GENERAL PRINCIPLES AND CLASSIFICATION

Robert R. Wagner

Biologic Properties. Viruses are distinct biologic entities, but they are not organisms; this fact is basic to an understanding of viral diseases. Unlike bacteria and fungi, viruses are completely dependent for their existence on the cells that they infect. Immediately upon entering a cell, a virus loses its identity and becomes an integral part of the genetic apparatus of that cell. In its extracellular form each virus has a recognizable shape, size, mass, and other distinguishing features that differ in many respects from normal cell constituents such as genes or enzymes. The small viruses are comparatively simple macromolecules composed entirely of nucleic acid and protein. The larger, more complex viruses may also contain carbohydrates, lipids, enzymes, and coenzymes. All viruses are surrounded by a protein coat and many, if not all, contain a distinct internal nucleoprotein. Together, these proteins impart antigenic identity to each virus.

All animal viruses contain either deoxyribonucleic or ribonucleic acid; none of the true viruses is known to contain both. In common with organisms, virus progeny resemble their parents except for mutations that occur spontaneously or under the influence of mutagenic agents. Two related viruses that infect a single cell may also mate within that cell and give rise to progeny that are identical to neither parent. This process is known as *virus recombination*. New genetic forms, that arise by mutation or recombination, may have new antigens in their protein coats or may be capable of infecting different hosts or tissues.

Infection at the Cellular Level. The major contributions to our knowledge of the nature of virus-cell interactions have come from the study of bacteriophages, viruses that infect bacteria. Similar techniques are being devised for the study of animal viruses. It is now known that viral infection occurs only after random collision between a virus particle and a susceptible cell. The concept of virus tropism, implying attraction of virus to a particular cell, is no longer tenable and should be discarded. Once attached to the cell surface, a bacterial virus injects its nucleic acid into the cell, whereas the entire animal virus particle enters the

cell by a process known as *viropexis*. Thereafter, the protein coat of the infecting virus plays no role in the infectious process.

After penetration into a susceptible cell, virus nucleic acid imparts new genetic information to that cell. In general terms, the virus nucleic acid diverts the normal biosynthetic pathways of the cell to the production of virus nucleic acid and virus protein. These new genetic and metabolic processes occur at the expense of, but not necessarily to the exclusion of, synthesis of cellular nucleic acid and protein. Virus nucleic acid and protein are formed separately inside the cell during the stage of infection known as *virus eclipse*. At this stage, infectious virus cannot be extracted from the cell, nor can virus particles be seen by electron microscopy. Only later in the course of infection are the independent nucleic acid and protein moieties assembled within the cell to make mature virus particles which the cell may release and which are capable of infecting other cells. Under certain conditions (such as infection of mouse brain with most strains of influenza virus) nucleic acid is not readily incorporated into the protein coat, resulting in the formation of "incomplete" or noninfectious virus.

Different viruses mature in different parts of the cells that they infect. Herpes simplex virus and adenoviruses, for example, form within the nucleus as a crystalline array in which the individual virus particles assume a regular pattern when viewed by electron microscopy. These crystals are the intranuclear inclusion bodies seen in stained cells. In contrast, influenza and other myxoviruses develop at the periphery of the cell just under the cytoplasmic membrane. As they mature, myxovirus particles extend from the cell surface as fingerlike projections, which then detach to become extracellular virus.

Certain other cytopathologic changes appear to be common to many viral infections. Dissolution of nucleoli and clumping and margination of chromatin are frequently seen within the nucleus. Ribonucleic acid granules often appear in the cytoplasm and are extruded into the surrounding medium. Eventually, the cytoplasm may disappear, leaving a densely staining pyknotic nucleus. However, not all viral infections result in cell death. Measles virus can also spread to contiguous cells by inducing fusion and dissolution of cytoplasmic membranes. This process leads to the formation of multinucleated syncytia, or giant cells, which are characteristic of infection with measles and certain other viruses.

Pathogenesis. The events that occur during the course of viral infection in a single cell do not differ in any important respect from the sequence of events that leads to infection of a multicellular organism, including man. To initiate an infection, a virus must make contact with a susceptible cell in the respiratory tract, intestine, skin, eye, or mucous membranes. Newly formed virus is then released and transmitted to adjacent cells at the primary focus. Certain viruses remain localized to the original site of infection and draining lymph nodes. Others invade the blood stream, usually by way of lymphatics, and are disseminated to distant organs. Viremia is often accompanied by prodromal manifestations. A secondary cycle of infection may then be established at single or multiple tissue sites. Whether infection remains localized or becomes generalized or whether localized or systemic infection results in disease is determined largely by the genetic constitution of the virus and of the host. Immunologic responsiveness, other host factors, the infecting dose, and environmental conditions may also determine the outcome of infection.

Most viral infections of man do not cause recognizable disease. The term *virulence* is an expression of the disease-producing capacity of a particular virus that infects a particular host. Virulence usually reflects the degree of tissue damage caused by the infection, which in turn is a function of the degree to which the virus multiplies. A strain of poliovirus, for example, is said to be virulent for man if infection of the intestine leads sequentially to viremia, dissemination to the central nervous system, multiplication of virus in anterior horn cells, cell death, and paralysis in a high proportion of cases.

Tissue reactions to viral infections vary from rapid cell destruction to indetectable histologic changes. Inflammatory responses are usually characterized by the presence of macrophages, but polymorphonuclear leukocytes may predominate after infection with viruses that cause extensive tissue necrosis or hemorrhage. Hemorrhagic lesions often signify involvement of endothelial cells. Although the extent of tissue damage, and hence the severity of the disease, varies considerably, the types of responses to different viruses are often quite similar. For example, many viruses can infect the meninges and produce virtually indistinguishable clinical syndromes of aseptic meningitis (see p. 1137). Conversely, a single virus such as Coxsackie B may cause a variety of illnesses ranging from fatal myocarditis, pleurodynia, meningitis, and encephalitis to nonspecific fevers.

Rather than causing tissue necrosis, certain viruses can stimulate cellular proliferation. Vaccinia virus may sometimes induce hyperplasia, and influenza virus regularly causes squamous metaplasia of bronchial epithelium. Hundreds of viruses have now been found to be capable of causing neoplasms in animals. The Stewart-Eddy polyoma virus has been particularly well studied and has been found to be responsible for widespread epizootics of malignant tumors in mice. Polyoma virus is also infectious for other rodents, including newborn hamsters which may develop sarcomatous lesions of virtually any organ weeks or months after subcutaneous inoculation. Neoplastic viruses with widely varying biologic properties have been isolated from vertebrate species ranging from fish to primates. Thus far, only warts have been proved to be virus-induced tumors of man. It will be surprising if more human neoplasms are not found to be caused by viruses.

Classification. Virologists have been slow to accept taxonomic systems, but a movement to classify viruses by genera and species has been gaining ground. Group classification is based largely on physical, chemical, and biologic properties, whereas subdivision within major groups is most logically based on antigenic composition. Although names of viruses are often derived from the diseases that they cause, classification based on disease alone is unrealistic. However, it is feasible and convenient to categorize viruses that infect man by their portal of entry and initial site of multiplication. Such a system has the advantage for the clinician of characterizing viruses by their usual mode of transmission and epidemiology. Table 179-1 lists the most common viruses infectious for man under the generic names that are most widely accepted and summarizes some of their salient epidemiologic, cultural, and clinical features. In general, the large and complex viruses are listed first, followed in descending order by the smaller and simpler viruses. The agents that fall into the psittacosis group are classified as viruses only by custom; they belong more properly with the rickettsias. It should be emphasized that the classification offered here is tentative and meant only to be a guide that will be modified by future studies. This system is frankly anthropocentric and fails to account satisfactorily for all physical and chemical differences among viruses. The reader is referred to the classification of animal viruses proposed by Cooper (1961), which is based wholly on nucleic acid type (DNA or RNA), sensitivity to ether (lipid content), size, and antigenic relationships.

Immunity to Viral Diseases. Acquired resistance to viral infections may take several forms. Probably the most important is specific immunity induced by natural exposure to a virus or by vaccination. The presence of antibody in the circulation and extra-cellular fluids serves as a barrier to cross infection of cells and, therefore, limits virus multiplication. If reinfection with the same or an antigenically related virus occurs even after a long interval, a prompt anamnestic response often prevents spread of infection from the primary focus and the host's reaction to infection is mild or asymptomatic. Similarly, viruses that persist in the tissues for many years after a primary infection are prevented from causing widespread disease by continual formation of antibody. Secondary herpes simplex, for example, usually remains localized to the lips rather than becoming disseminated as may occur in primary infection.

Factors other than antibody production also influence the outcome of infection on first exposure to a virus. It is a common experience to find that the acute manifestations of a viral disease have abated before neutralizing antibody can be detected in the circulation. Moreover, children with agammaglobulinemia have been noted to recover from measles, mumps, chickenpox, poliomyelitis, and viral respiratory infections in the same manner as do normal individuals. Furthermore, these children rarely show evidence of reinfection with a virus, in contrast to their tendency to undergo repeated infections by the same bacteria. However, vaccinia gangrenosa and severe viral hepatitis appear to be unusually frequent in children with agammaglobulinemia.

A form of immunologic tolerance may play a significant role in resistance to congenital viral infections. Mice infected in utero, or a few hours after birth, with lymphocytic choriomeningitis virus resist reinfection with the same virus for many months. These resistant animals form no antibody to the virus even though viremia persists throughout their lives. An analogous situation may obtain in congenital infections of man with salivary gland virus. This virus often lies dormant in the tissues for many years without causing cytomegalic inclusion disease or other manifestations of infection. Only when virus appears in the urine or saliva, suggesting loss of resistance, can antibody be regularly detected in the circulation.

Infection with one virus may also confer resistance to infection with an antigenically unrelated virus, a phenomenon known as *viral interference*. This observation is of practical significance in scheduling the sequence of oral vaccination with the Sabin strains of attenuated polioviruses. If all three poliovirus types are administered together, type 2 may inhibit enteric multiplication of the other two types, with consequent depression of antibody response to them. Latent enteric infection with ECHO or other enteroviruses has also been noted to prevent infection with virulent polioviruses. Experimental studies indicate that viral interference is caused by a nonviral protein, called *interferon*, which is produced by infected cells. The suggestion has been made that recovery from certain viral infections may be attributable to endogenous production of interferon.

Vaccination. Purified concentrated virus inactivated by formalin or attenuated infectious virus can be used as vaccines. Their success depends, in large measure, on the antigenic mass originally injected or on the multiplication of attenuated virus to equivalent titers. Repeated administration is often required, and even then, immunity is likely to be less pronounced and of shorter duration than that following recovery from natural infection.

The efficacy of a vaccine is judged from several standpoints. The first consideration is its safety for those receiving it and for their contacts. Secondly, a vaccine must induce a significant antibody response and, in so doing, reduce morbidity and mortality after natural exposure to the virus. Rarely is prevention of infection per se considered to be an important goal of vaccination. In fact, asymptomatic infection after vaccination can serve to enhance and prolong the immune response.

Administration of attenuated poliomyelitis and influenza virus has also been advocated to halt epidemics in progress. The rationale of this procedure is to replace the virulent viruses with attenuated strains by the mechanism of viral interference. However, additional supporting data are required to prove that vaccination is efficacious in terminating viral epidemics.

Persistence and Latency. Many viruses persist in host tissues for months or years without causing overt disease. A flare-up of these latent infections may be induced by trauma, intercurrent disease, decline in antibody titers, or unknown stimuli. Experiments with tissue cultures and laboratory animals reveal that persistence of virus in tissues results from an interplay of various factors peculiar to each virus and its host. Latency is promoted by the presence of antibody or other viral inhibitors that prevent extensive cell-to-cell spread of virus. If antibody is withdrawn, virus multiplication often resumes, with concomitant cellular necrosis. Other extracellular factors, such as temperature and electrolyte concentration, may also promote virus persistence. Congenital viral infections tend to be latent for long periods of time, possibly through the mechanism of immunologic tolerance. One of the most important causes of virus persistence is thought to result from endogenous production of interferon by chronically infected cells. Apparently, an equilibrium can be established in tissue culture

Table 179-1. A CLASSIFICATION OF VIRUSES THAT INFECT MAN

"Group" or *generic* name	Prototype viruses (common name)	Known major antigenic types	Best available methods of virus isolation	Principal routes of transmission	Usual clinical manifestations
"Psittacosis"*	Psittacosis Lymphogranuloma Trachoma Inclusion blenorrhea	1 ?	Mice, chick embryos Yolk sac of chick embryos	Respiratory Venereal Eye Venereal, eye	Pneumonia Bubo, proctitis Conjunctivitis Conjunctivitis
"Primary atypical pneumonia"*	Eaton agent	1 or more	Chick embryos + fluorescent antibody	Respiratory	Pneumonia
Poxvirus	Smallpox Vaccinia Cowpox Molluscum contagiosum	1 1 1 ?	Mice, chick embryos, rabbits Human volunteers	Respiratory Skin Skin Skin	Pustular exanthem Local papule and pustule Papules
Herpesvirus	Herpes simplex Monkey "B"	1 1	Tissue culture Tissue culture	Mucous membranes Skin (monkey bite)	"Cold sores," stomatitis Encephalitis
Myxovirus	Influenza A, B, C Parainfluenza Mumps Newcastle disease	3 4 1 1	Chick embryos, tissue culture	Respiratory Respiratory Respiratory Eye (man)	Influenza, pneumonia URI, pneumonia (newborns), croup Parotitis, orchitis, meningitis Conjunctivitis
"Common respiratory viruses"	Many, including common cold Respiratory syncytial (RS)	Unknown 1	Human volunteers, tissue culture Tissue culture	Respiratory Respiratory	URI Bronchiolitis, croup, pneumonia
"Respiratory exanthematous viruses"	Measles Chickenpox— herpes zoster German measles	1 1 1	Tissue culture Tissue culture Human volunteers	Respiratory Respiratory Respiratory (Transplacental)	Macular rash, pneumonia Multiform rash, pneumonia Radiculitis, vesicles Macular rash (congenital malformations)
"Salivary gland viruses"	Human salivary gland virus	1	Tissue culture	Congenital (Transplacental?)	Cytomegalic inclusion disease
Adenovirus	Adenoviruses (APC)	26–31 or more	Tissue culture	Respiratory, eye, ? enteric	Pharyngitis, pneumonia, conjunctivitis
Reovirus	Reoviruses	3 or more	Tissue culture	Respiratory, enteric	URI, fever, enteritis
Enterovirus	Poliovirus Coxsackie A Coxsackie B ECHO	3 23 or more 6 28 or more	Tissue culture Infant mice Tissue culture, mice Tissue culture	Enteric Enteric Enteric Enteric	Paralysis, meningoencephalitis Herpangina, fever Pleurodynia, myocarditis, meningitis Meningitis, macular rash
"Miscellaneous human viruses"	Infectious hepatitis Serum hepatitis Nonbacterial gastroenteritis Exanthem subitum Erythema infectiosum "Warts" (verrucae)	1 1 2 or more 1 (?) 1 (?) ?	Human volunteers Human volunteers Human volunteers Human volunteers Human volunteers Human volunteers	Enteric Injection, congenital? Enteric Probably enteric Probably enteric Skin	Hepatitis Hepatitis Gastroenteritis Macular rash, fever Macular rash Warts
"Arbor, group A"..... "Arbor, group B"..... "Arbor, group C"..... "Arbor, ungrouped"...	Equine encephalitis and others Japanese B West Nile Russian tick-borne Yellow fever Dengue Clinically unimportant Rift Valley Colorado tick fever Sandfly fever	Many related Many related Several Many unrelated	Cerebral injection of mice, some in tissue culture	Skin (mosquito) Skin (mosquito) Skin (tick) Skin (mosquito) Skin (mosquito) Skin (mosquito, tick, sandfly)	Encephalitis, denguelike fever, mild fever, hemorrhagic fever, hepatitis, or no disease
"Miscellaneous animal viruses" (vary widely in size and biological properties)	Lymphocytic choriomeningitis Rabies Encephalomyocarditis Foot-and-mouth disease Vesicular stomatitis	1 1 1 1 1	Mice Mice Mice Guinea pigs Tissue culture	Respiratory Skin (bite) Unknown Skin and mucous membranes	Meningitis Encephalitis Fever, encephalitis Vesicles Vesicles

* Not true viruses. The Eaton agent is now known to be a pleuropneumonia-like organism (PPLO).

when a small proportion of the cells in a population produces infectious virus and the same or different cells produce interferon.

Diagnosis. Although similar in principle to diagnostic bacteriology, laboratory diagnosis of viral diseases often entails procedures that are far more time-consuming and costly. Therefore, the decision to undertake virus diagnostic studies must be based on sound clinical judgment and a carefully reasoned evaluation of the public health implications of the disease in question. Specimens sent to the virus laboratory as part of a "complete" diagnostic work-up are usually valueless. The laboratory procedures to be followed vary considerably for different viral diseases and frequently depend on the duration of illness and whether the infection has occurred sporadically or during an epidemic. The virologist often relies heavily on knowledge of diseases endemic in a community, their seasonal incidence, the geographic distribution of certain viruses, and the potential animal reservoirs and insect vectors of an area. The presence of characteristic histopathologic lesions may contribute more to a retrospective diagnosis of diseases such as rabies, yellow fever, measles, cytomegalic inclusion disease, and poliomyelitis than will be gained by virus isolation and serologic studies. The diagnosis of infectious hepatitis, German measles, and several other viral diseases is based entirely on clinical or pathologic findings.

The advent of tissue culture and cell culture methods has greatly facilitated isolation of certain viruses (see Table 179-1). Standard cell strains originating from human carcinomas and monolayer cultures of monkey kidney epithelial cells have been particularly useful for cultivation of enteroviruses, adenoviruses, herpesviruses, myxoviruses, and some of the common exanthematous viruses. However, because of variation in cellular susceptibility to viral infection, it is often essential to choose the type of tissue culture on the basis of the virus anticipated to be present. Despite continuing advances in technique, viruses are generally difficult to isolate and even more difficult to identify. Some cause characteristic cytopathology in culture, but cellular reactions to others often lack specificity. The histochemical technique of immunofluorescence is another reliable means for rapid identification of virus antigen within cells.

A serious problem in diagnostic virology is the frequency with which uninoculated tissue cultures are contaminated with latent viruses that may induce cytopathic effects indistinguishable from those caused by the virus one is attempting to isolate. For example, cultures of renal epithelium from presumably healthy monkeys often contain measles or other viruses. Another major difficulty stems from the observation that feces and nasopharyngeal secretions may contain viruses other than, or in addition to, those originally suspected of causing a patient's illness. To cite but two examples, the ECHO viruses were discovered during investigative studies of poliomyelitis, and some of the parainfluenza viruses were originally isolated during an influenza epidemic. In several instances, identification of new viruses has led to recognition of new disease entities, the existence of which had not been suspected on clinical grounds alone.

Final identification of viruses and the diagnosis of viral diseases almost invariably depend on immunologic tests. Each diagnostic laboratory maintains a supply of viral antigens and standard reference antiserums. When a virus is isolated, it is identified in terms of its immunologic reactivity compared with known viruses. The most useful serologic procedures in virology are complement fixation and neutralization of infectivity. Virus neutralization is the most sensitive immunologic test yet devised, because a single molecule of antibody can theoretically be detected by this method. Precipitin reactions in fluid medium or by agar gel diffusion can be performed only with highly concentrated preparations of virus and specific antibody. For those viruses which readily agglutinate erythrocytes, such as the myxoviruses, antibody can be assayed by hemagglutination inhibition or by hemadsorption inhibition. It is important to keep in mind that different serologic tests may measure different antigenic components of the same virus. All 30 members of the adenovirus group, for example, share a common complement-fixing antigen, but each can be typed by specific neutralizing antibody.

In the final analysis, only an antibody response in the host constitutes definitive evidence of infection with a specific virus. Therefore, it is essential to obtain serum specimens at properly spaced intervals. The result of a single serologic test is often misleading because it may be impossible to determine whether the antibody is a response to infection in the recent or distant past.

REFERENCES

Bang, F. B.: Virus Disease: Some Aspects of Host and Tissue Specificity, Ann. Rev. Med., 11:1, 1960.

Beard, J. W. (Ed.): "Symposium: Phenomena of the Tumor Viruses," National Cancer Institute Monograph No. 4, U.S. Department of Health, Education and Welfare, Public Health Service, 1960.

Cooper, P. D.: A Chemical Basis for the Classification of Animal Viruses, Nature, 190:302, 1961.

Dudgeon, J. A.: Modern Aids to Diagnosis of Virus Diseases, Brit. Med. J., 1, 1269, 1961.

Luria, S. E.: The Reproduction of Viruses: A Comparative Survey, in vol. 1, p. 549, "The Viruses: Biochemical, Biological, and Biophysical Properties," F. M. Burnet and W. M. Stanley (Eds.), New York, Academic Press, Inc., 1959.

Lwoff, A.: Bacteriophage as a Model of Host-Virus Relationship, in vol. 2, p. 187, "The Viruses: Biochemical, Biological, and Biophysical Properties," F. M. Burnet and W. M. Stanley (Eds.), New York, Academic Press, Inc., 1959.

Najjar, V. A. (Ed.): "Immunity and Virus Infection," New York, John Wiley & Sons, Inc., 1959.

Swartz, M. N., and J. W. Littlefield: Biochemistry of Viral Infection, New Engl. J. Med., 262:287 and 342, 1960.

Wagner, R. R.: Viral Interference: Some Considerations of Basic Mechanisms and Their Potential Relationship to Host Resistance, Bacteriol. Rev., 24:151, 1960.

Weidel, W.: "Virus," Ann Arbor, Mich., The University of Michigan Press, 1959.

Section 14: Viral Diseases of the Respiratory Tract

180 COMMON RESPIRATORY DISEASE (Including Viral Pneumonia)

Alto E. Feller

The acute respiratory infections may be considered as a spectrum of clinical conditions with gradations from mild or minimal involvements of the respiratory passages to prostrating illnesses with or without pulmonary infiltration. The spectrum encompasses certain well-known specific infections, i.e., influenza, beta-hemolytic streptococcal infections, and the bacterial pneumonias. But the greater part of the spectrum, in terms of frequency of occurrence of cases, is comprised of the large group of illnesses variously called the common cold, coryza, head cold, nasopharyngitis, laryngitis, catarrhal fever, flu, grippe, tracheitis, bronchitis, primary atypical pneumonia, virus pneumonia, etc. The term *common respiratory disease* is employed in this chapter to refer collectively to this large and heterogeneous segment of the acute respiratory infections.

Despite extensive investigation of these infections, relatively little is yet known about their relationships and causation. The problem of the common respiratory diseases might be presented from the clinical, etiologic, or epidemiologic point of view. None of these approaches is satisfactory at present because of insufficient data. But data are accumulating rapidly; some 70 viruses, either directly or indirectly related to respiratory illness, have been isolated. Studies show that most of the so-called clinical entities may be caused by any one of several viruses and that infection with one of these viruses may produce a clinical picture varying from inapparent to severe.

The ultimate aim is to consider the various respiratory illnesses in terms of the agents that cause them. However, it is unusual to be able to make an etiologic diagnosis from the clinical picture, and laboratory tests for many of the known agents are not available except in a relatively few laboratories.

Occurrence

The common respiratory diseases are world-wide in distribution, and no geographic area is known to be consistently free of them. Certain isolated communities have been without respiratory illness for variable lengths of time, but resumption of intercourse with the outside world usually is followed by its reappearance. It is commonly believed that respiratory diseases are less prevalent in the warmer areas of the earth, but there are insufficient data to determine whether the presumed difference is due to an actual decrease in attack rate, to the occurrence of less severe illnesses, to less crowding in the tropics, or to other factors.

Viral respiratory disease is seasonal. In the temperate zone, waves of increased prevalence occur in the fall, winter, and spring.

The respiratory diseases are highly prevalent in the United States. Data from industry show that they are among the leading causes of absenteeism from work. Most persons have two or three acute respiratory infections each year.

Epidemiology

Since recognition of the common respiratory diseases is dependent mainly upon clinical features, epidemiologic concepts are applicable only to the problem as a whole. Nevertheless, certain concepts have become established and may be summarized as follows:

1. The air-borne route of transmission appears to

Table 180-1. NEWLY ISOLATED VIRUSES WHICH CAUSE RESPIRATORY DISEASE

Name	Synonyms	Associated disease
Parainfluenza 1	HA 2, Sendai, HV J, influenza D	Pneumonia, croup, upper respiratory illness of varying severity
Parainfluenza 2	CA	Laryngotracheobronchitis, croup
Parainfluenza 3	HA 1	Croup, pneumonia, upper respiratory illness of varying severity
Respiratory syncytial	CCA, RS	Bronchopneumonia, laryngotracheobronchitis, bronchiolitis, acute respiratory illness
2060, JH......	?ECHO 28	Coryza, mild, with or without fever

be an important, but not necessarily the only, mode of transfer.

2. "Carriers" or individuals with very mild illness are capable of transmitting respiratory infections.

3. Highest attack rates occur in children under the age of five years. Infants under the age of one year have relatively low rates. The lowest attack rates occur in the second decade of life. The curve rises slowly to a small peak in the ages from twenty-five to thirty-five years and then gradually declines.

4. In segregated populations, such as military recruits or boarding school children, a wave of respiratory infections may sweep through the population shortly after the individuals are brought together. These outbreaks are followed by mass insusceptibility, which can last for months or even years. The explanation for this "seasoning" is not entirely clear, but aging and immunologic phenomena are probably important factors.

5. Rigorous life or exposure to inclement weather per se is not an important factor in provoking the occurrence of the common respiratory diseases.

6. An increased prevalence of the common respiratory diseases is often associated with an increased occurrence of the bacterial pneumonias.

CLASSIFICATION

Clinical classification of the common respiratory diseases presents a difficult problem because (1) the clinical picture in individual cases often is not distinctive and may not differ from that of several specific diseases (for example, influenza A) and (2) when studied in the mass, the illnesses present smooth gradations in severity, rather than sharp differences, and there are many combinations of symptoms and physical signs.

The most useful clinical classification employs as criteria the site of localization of the prominent symptoms or physical signs, the severity of illness, the presence of exudate in the thorax, and the presence of pneumonia:

CLASSIFICATION OF COMMON RESPIRATORY DISEASE

1. Common cold
2. Acute undifferentiated respiratory disease (ARD)
3. Nonbacterial pharyngitis or tonsillitis
4. Primary atypical pneumonia

It should be emphasized that this classification is artificial and is employed mainly for convenience in describing the disease picture. Many patients with common respiratory disease present manifestations which cannot be assigned clearly to any single group.

Etiology

Many viruses have now been isolated from the respiratory tract secretions of patients with respiratory infection. Table 180-1 lists the viruses for which sufficient data are available to indicate that they cause respiratory disease. The *parainfluenza viruses* have been studied mostly in infants and children and have been found associated with severe respiratory illnesses but also have been found in milder and even inapparent infections in children and adults. Parainfluenza 1 has caused an epidemic of influenza-like illnesses in Russia. *Respiratory syncytial* virus also has been related to relatively severe pneumonic illnesses in children, as well as to illnesses apparently confined to the upper respiratory tract. The 2060 and JH viruses are either identical or closely related and have been

Table 180-2. NEWLY ISOLATED VIRUSES WHICH MAY BE ASSOCIATED WITH COMMON RESPIRATORY DISEASE

Name	Synonym	Associated disease
ECHO 11	Philipson's U virus	Nondiphtheritic croup, ? common cold
Coe..........	....	Pharyngitis, common cold, illnesses quite mild
Reoviruses, types 1, 2, and 3	ECHO 10	Uncertain
Salisbury common cold viruses	H.G.P., P.K., F.E.B.	Common cold
Parainfluenza 4	M 25	Mild upper respiratory illness
JV 1.........	ECHO 20	Children with respiratory and/or gastrointestinal illness

associated mainly with the common cold although they account for only a small proportion of the total number of colds in the population. Table 180-2 lists the viruses which may be associated with common respiratory disease, but data are too limited to be certain of their role. The Salisbury common cold viruses have been induced to grow in tissue cultures and will undoubtedly be studied intensively.

ADENOVIRUSES

These agents have been variously called the AD, APC, or RI viruses but are now widely known as the adenoviruses. They have been isolated from a variety of diseases. They are associated with certain clinical entities with regularity, but it should be remembered (1) that the clinical syndromes to be noted are not always due to adenoviruses and (2) that a particular type of adenovirus may cause a certain illness in one person and an entirely different clinical picture, or no illness, in another. Uniformity of illnesses is more often observed in epidemics than in sporadic adenovirus infections.

Eighteen or more types have been isolated from human sources and can be distinguished by specific antibody neutralization. All strains share a common complement-fixing antigen. Thus, human infection by these viruses can be recognized serologically, employing acute-phase and convalescent-phase serums. Isolation of the agents from respiratory secretions employing tissue cultures can be carried out but is less reliable for diagnosis than serologic methods.

The clinical entities and the types of adenoviruses found in association with them are presented in Table 180-3. Adenoviruses, principally types 1, 2, and 5, have also been isolated from 50 per cent or more of tonsils and adenoids which have been surgically removed. The significance of this finding remains to be determined. In addition, serologic surveys of civilian populations have shown that by middle age more than 50 per cent of persons have

Table 180-3. ADENOVIRUSES AND DISEASE

Types*	Associated disease
3, **4**, **7**, 14	Acute respiratory disease of military recruits (ARD)
1, **3**, 7A	Pneumonia in infants
3, **4**, **7**, 14	Pneumonia in adults with acute respiratory disease
1, 2, **3**, **4**, 5, 6, 7A, 14	Pharyngitis and pharyngoconjunctival fever
2, **3**, 4, 6, 7A, 9, 10, 15	Follicular conjunctivitis
3, **8**, 7A	Epidemic keratoconjunctivitis (EKC)

* The types in boldface are most commonly found in the indicated disease.

antibodies to four or more types and 80 per cent of children may have antibody to at least one type by the age of five years. However, less than 3 per cent of all respiratory illnesses in civilian populations are caused by adenoviruses when the individual illnesses are studied by laboratory methods. In military recruits, the adenoviruses, especially types 4 and 7, are the most important cause of acute respiratory disease (ARD). As many as 80 per cent of recruits may be infected in winter months and 20 to 40 per cent may require hospitalization. Why such epidemics do not occur in civilian populations remains a mystery. Adenovirus pharyngitis, pharyngoconjunctival fever, and follicular conjunctivitis may occur in epidemics, especially in summer camps for children. Adenovirus pneumonia is most often associated with acute respiratory disease of recruits but has been described in children. A few cases have been fatal in children. Type 8 has been found so regularly in epidemic keratoconjunctivitis that it may now be accepted as an etiologic entity.

COMMON COLD

Definition. The common cold is an acute infection of the upper respiratory tract in which coryza is the prominent feature. Constitutional symptoms are characteristically mild, and there is little or no fever. The acute symptoms usually last for only a few days.

Etiology. Data now indicate that there are multiple agents, presumably viruses, which can cause the common cold. Extensive studies have shown that the common cold can be transmitted to volunteers by using bacteria-free filtrates of respiratory tract secretions. Curiously, the attack rate in these experiments rarely has exceeded about 50 per cent. Attempts to isolate viruses from such filtrates have generally been unsuccessful, but certain of the Salisbury common cold viruses have now apparently been propagated in tissue cultures. Several of the viruses listed in Tables 180-1 and 180-2, particularly the JH and 2060 viruses, have been associated with the common cold by means of virus isolations, antibody studies, and inoculation of volunteers.

Manifestations. The onset is gradual, with a sensation variously described as irritation, dryness, rawness, or tickling in the nasopharynx or the nose. Frequently, chilliness or malaise accompanies the local discomfort. During the next 24 to 48 hr, symptoms progress to those of the "full-blown" cold (Fig. 180-1). There are coryza, sneezing, nasal obstruction, thin nasal discharge, and watery eyes. Malaise, lassitude, chilliness, headache, and the subjective feeling of feverishness with little or no change in body temperature add to general discomfort and irritability. Patients may be described

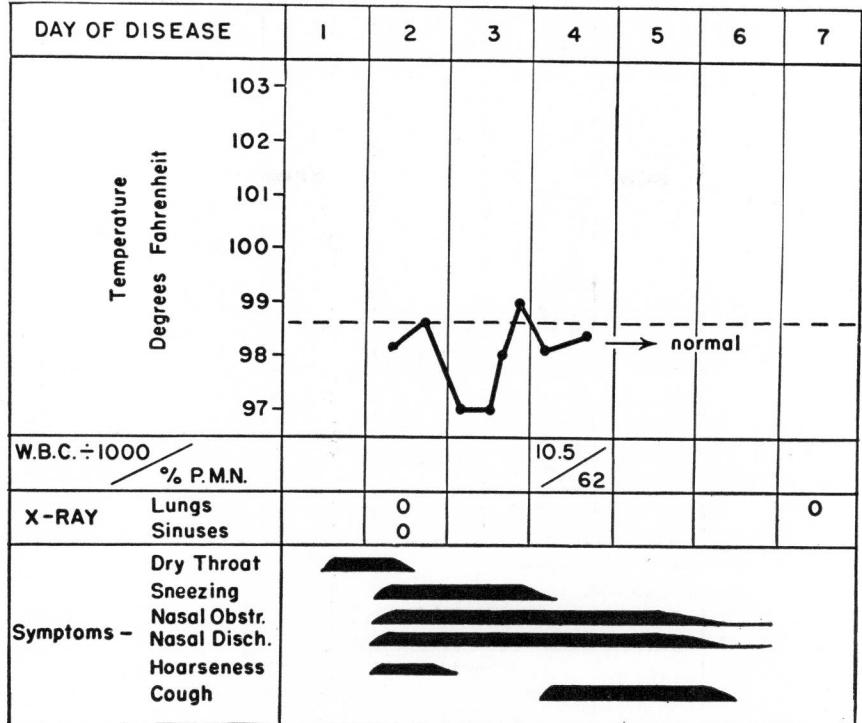

FIG. 180-1. Clinical chart of a patient with a common cold. (*Commission on Acute Respiratory Diseases, Fort Bragg, N.C., J. Clin. Invest.*, 26:959, 1947.)

as not feeling well enough to work efficiently but not sufficiently ill to submit to bed rest. During the next 2 or 3 days, systemic symptoms gradually subside, the nasal discharge becomes mucoid or purulent, the coryza and nasal irritation become less troublesome. Some discharge may persist for several days, or even for weeks; the frequency with which complicating paranasal sinusitis contributes to this picture is not certain.

On physical examination, the nasal mucosa is reddened and edematous and nasal discharge is usually obvious. The nares may be reddened or excoriated, and slight tenderness over the maxillary and frontal sinuses is frequent.

Laboratory Findings. The leukocyte count and erythrocyte sedimentation rate are normal. Cultures of the nasal secretion, nasopharynx, or oropharynx usually reveal the bacteria which are common inhabitants of these areas. The urine is normal.

Differential Diagnosis. During the first 24 or 48 hr of illness, it may be difficult to distinguish the common cold from the prodromal symptoms of the acute exanthems, particularly measles. Coryzal symptoms or signs in a young person should always lead to a search for Koplik spots and to inquiry about possible exposure.

The sudden onset of sneezing, itching in the nose, and lacrimation, characteristic pale, boggy appear-

ance of the turbinates, and a history of similar episodes are features which suggest allergic rhinitis rather than the common cold.

ACUTE UNDIFFERENTIATED RESPIRATORY DISEASE (ARD)

Definition. Acute undifferentiated respiratory disease is an infection of the respiratory tract in which constitutional symptoms and fever are prominent. Respiratory symptoms are likely to be localized to the throat, trachea, or bronchi and tend to be rather mild. The illnesses in this group differ from the common cold in that they are more severe, and systemic manifestations predominate. As employed here, the term acute undifferentiated respiratory disease includes the illnesses commonly called "grippe" or "flu" but does not include influenza A or influenza B.

Etiology. In military recruit populations where the disease is particularly common and often occurs in epidemics, the adenoviruses, types 4 and 7, and to a lesser degree, type 3, are the cause of most but not all such illnesses. In some outbreaks, only a small proportion of cases of clinically similar disease can be shown to be caused by these viruses. In civilian populations several studies have revealed that adenovirus infections constitute a very small

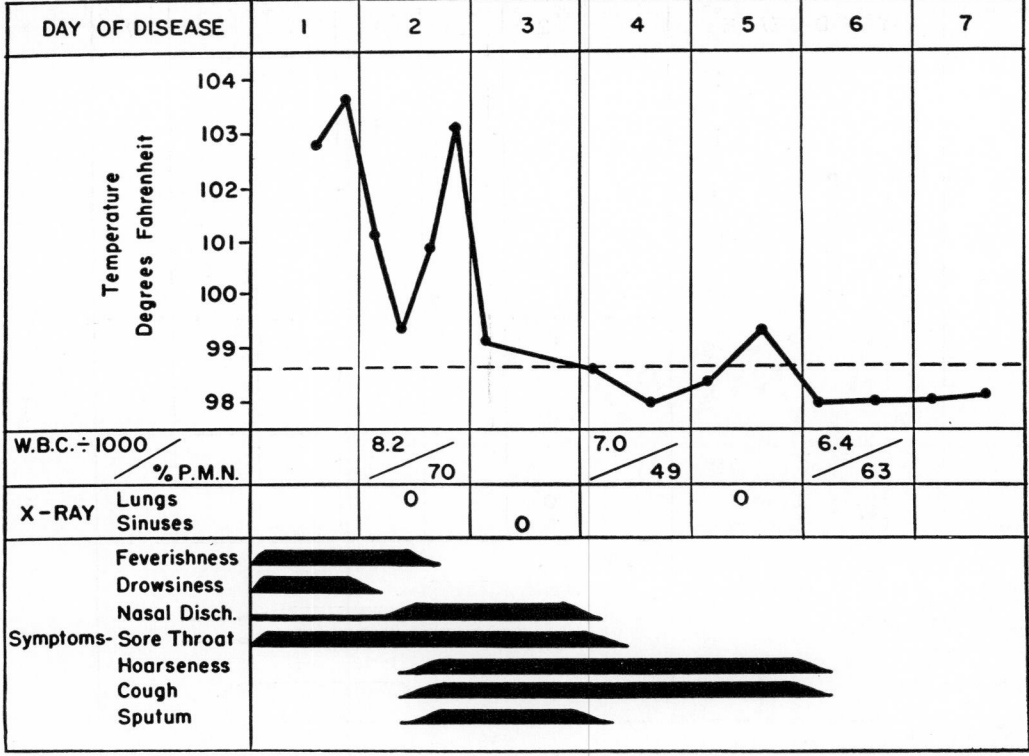

Fig. 180-2. Clinical chart of a patient with acute undifferentiated respiratory disease. (*Commission on Acute Respiratory Diseases, Fort Bragg, N.C., J. Clin. Invest.*, 26:959, 1947.)

proportion of acute undifferentiated disease. The etiologic role of the viruses listed in Tables 180-1 and 180-2 is as yet unknown. Some illnesses, both naturally occurring and induced in volunteers, associated with the parainfluenza viruses, have had symptoms and signs compatible with the clinical picture of acute undifferentiated respiratory disease.

Manifestations. The onset is gradual. The prominent constitutional symptoms are feverishness, chilliness, and headache; in addition, malaise and anorexia are present in approximately 50 per cent of the patients. The amount of fever varies, but the temperature averages 101°F. Sore throat, with discomfort rather than actual pain on swallowing, is the earliest and most salient respiratory symptom. Hoarseness, cough, and discomfort in the chest are frequent. Nasal discharge and sneezing are usually minor. Fever and malaise generally subside by the third day, but sore throat and hoarseness often persist for a few days, and it is not uncommon for cough to persist for one or more weeks.

Physical signs are not characteristic. The pharynx and fauces may be moderately reddened, with prominent lymphoid follicles. There is usually no pharyngeal exudate. There is often mild cervical lymphadenitis. The lungs are usually clear, but there may be tenderness or soreness to pressure over the sternum. Pneumonitis occurs in a small proportion of cases.

Acute undifferentiated respiratory disease is a more severe illness than the common cold (Fig. 180-2). Patients are usually only moderately ill but occasionally may be prostrated. Complete restoration of well-being usually requires several days.

Laboratory Findings. The leukocyte count is normal, although occasionally a count of 10,000 to 12,000 cells per cu mm may be found. The erythrocyte sedimentation rate is normal or only moderately increased. Bacteriologic studies usually reveal only the organisms which are common residents of the respiratory tract.

Differential Diagnosis. The differential diagnosis includes the common cold, viral influenza (p. 1123), infectious mononucleosis (p. 1248), primary atypical pneumonia, bacterial pneumonia, and the acute exanthemas (p. 1157).

NONBACTERIAL PHARYNGITIS OR TONSILLITIS

Definition. Nonbacterial pharyngitis or tonsillitis is an acute respiratory disease of unknown etiology in which exudate on the tonsils or pharynx is a

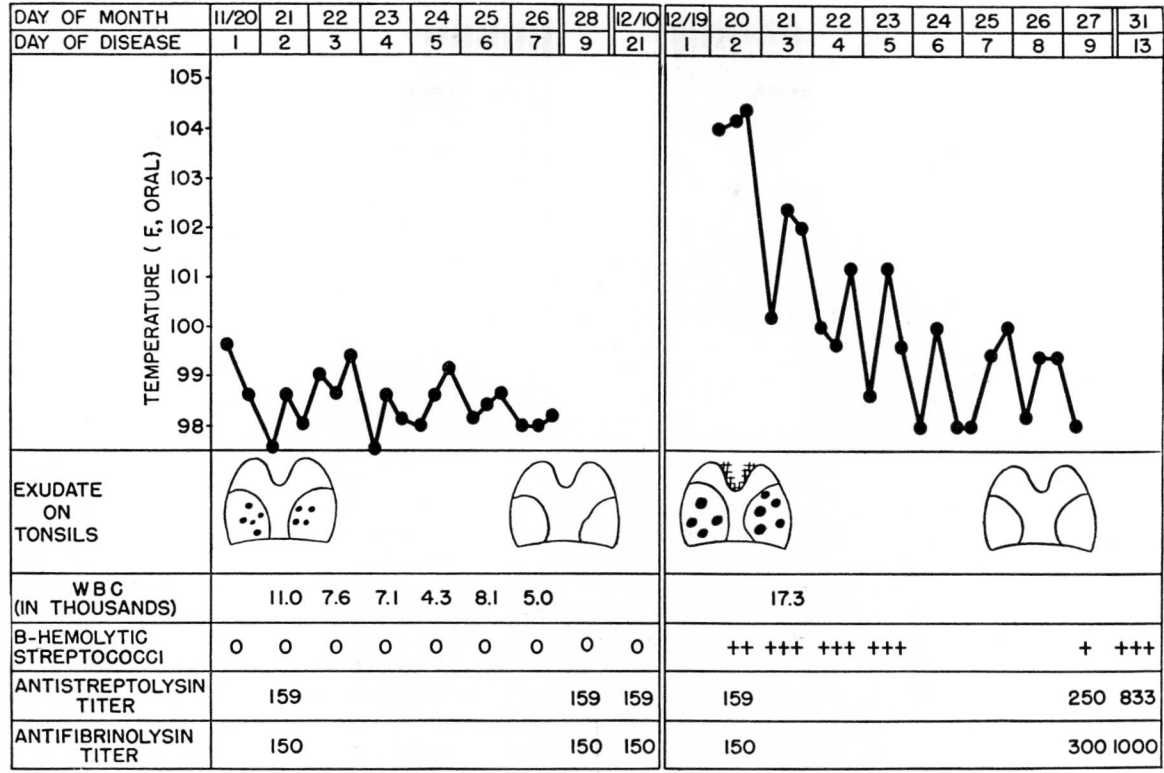

DAY OF MONTH	11/20	21	22	23	24	25	26	28	12/10	12/19	20	21	22	23	24	25	26	27	31
DAY OF DISEASE	1	2	3	4	5	6	7	9	21	1	2	3	4	5	6	7	8	9	13

WBC (IN THOUSANDS)		11.0	7.6	7.1	4.3	8.1	5.0				17.3								
B-HEMOLYTIC STREPTOCOCCI	0	0	0	0	0	0	0	0	0		++	+++	+++	+++				+	+++
ANTISTREPTOLYSIN TITER		159						159	159		159							250	833
ANTIFIBRINOLYSIN TITER		150						150	150		150							300	1000

FIG. 180-3. Clinical and laboratory data from a patient with nonstreptococcal exudative pharyngitis and tonsillitis of average severity (*left*), and from a patient with beta-hemolytic streptococcal tonsillitis and pharyngitis (*right*). Note the absence of beta-hemolytic streptococci in repeated throat cultures in the former and their presence in large numbers in the latter; the rise in titer of antistreptolysin and antifibrinolysin (expressed in units) in convalescent phase serums in the latter; the definite leukocytosis in the latter; the differences in the amount of exudate on the tonsils; and the presence of edema of the uvula and soft palate in the latter. (*Commission on Acute Respiratory Diseases, Fort Bragg, N.C., J.A.M.A., 133:588, 1947.*)

distinctive feature. In other respects it resembles acute undifferentiated respiratory disease rather closely, but occasionally it presents symptoms and signs suggestive of beta-hemolytic streptococcal pharyngitis.

Etiology. The beta-hemolytic streptococcus is excluded by definition. Bacteriologic and limited serologic studies have indicated that other bacteria are not causative. Adenovirus type 3 and occasionally other types (see Table 180-3) have been found in several outbreaks of nonbacterial pharyngitis occurring principally in children in the summertime. Some of these patients have had an associated conjunctivitis, and Huebner and associates have employed the term pharyngoconjunctival fever for the condition. Only a minority of cases of nonbacterial pharyngitis in adults is caused by adenoviruses. The parainfluenza viruses have been found associated with illnesses diagnosed as pharyngitis or tonsillitis in a few instances. The etiologic role of the other viruses (Tables 180-1 and 180-2) is unknown.

Manifestations. Nonbacterial tonsillitis or pharyngitis is a mild disease of short duration (Fig. 180-3). The onset is gradual, as a rule. The early symptoms in most cases are referable to the throat, but fever or malaise is sometimes the presenting complaint. The great majority of patients have malaise, headache, and anorexia. The average maximum temperature is 101 to 102°F, and fever lasts 2 or 3 days but may be longer.

Sore throat is the most prominent respiratory symptom and is described as discomfort, rawness, or soreness, rather than as actual pain or dysphagia. Hoarseness, cough, and substernal discomfort are common.

The chief signs are in the throat. Hyperemia is usually "streaky," and only rarely diffuse or intense. The lymphoid follicles of the pharyngeal wall are usually enlarged and reddened and frequently surmounted by small patches of exudate. Edema of the soft palate or fauces is rarely prominent. The lymph nodes in the anterior triangles of the neck are sometimes enlarged and tender.

Laboratory Findings. The total leukocyte count is usually normal but exceeds 10,000 cells per cu mm in approximately one-third of the cases. Throat cultures reveal normal flora.

Differential Diagnosis. (See p. 907.)

PRIMARY ATYPICAL PNEUMONIA

Definition. Primary atypical pneumonia is an acute respiratory infection characterized by pulmonary lesions, a paucity of physical findings in the chest, constitutional symptoms, cough, sputum, and prolonged convalescence.

Etiology. The etiology of primary atypical pneumonia has been a difficult problem for many years. Several different viruses have been recovered from patients, but only two, the adenoviruses and the Eaton agent, have been generally accepted as causative agents of the human disease. Cases of primary atypical pneumonia can now be divided into at least three groups: (1) Adenovirus infections, many of which have pulmonary infiltrates and therefore are recognized as primary atypical pneumonias. These infections have occurred principally in military recruits. Patients with these infections have developed neither cold hemagglutinins or agglutinins for streptococcus MG in their serums. (2) Primary atypical pneumonia with cold hemagglutinins or streptococcus MG agglutinins, or both. This disease has been transmitted to volunteers with bacteria-free filtrates of sputum and throat washings and was presumed to be caused by a virus. Many such patients, but not all, have developed antibodies to the Eaton agent in their convalescent-phase serums demonstrable by fluorescent antibody techniques. Also, the Eaton agent, first isolated in 1944, has again been isolated from the respiratory tract secretions of some patients with this illness. The Eaton agent is now known to be a pleuropneumonia-like organism (PPLO) rather than a true virus. (3) Cases falling into neither of the above groups. The etiologic role of the new respiratory tract viruses (Tables 180-1 and 180-2) in primary atypical pneumonia is unknown.

Manifestations. The onset is insidious; most patients have minor respiratory or constitutional symptoms for several days before consulting a physician. Sudden onset is unusual.

Early in the illness, feverishness, chilliness, headache, and malaise are the outstanding complaints. Anorexia is common. Shaking chills are very unusual. The headache is aggravated by cough, which is paroxysmal and harassing, interfering with sleep. It is nonproductive at first, but mucoid or mucopurulent sputum is raised after a few days. Streaks of bright red blood can appear in the sputum, but grossly bloody, rusty, or "prune juice" sputum is rare. Substernal discomfort is common, but pleural pain is very unusual.

Physical signs are not prominent, especially early in the illness. The patient appears mildly or moderately ill. The temperature rarely exceeds 104°F. Examination of the chest may reveal few signs in spite of the extensive pulmonary lesions by x-ray. Early in the disease, rales are audible only at the height of inspiration; later, rales and rhonchi are often widespread. Other signs of consolidation are rarely prominent.

Roentgenographic examination of the chest is the most reliable method of detecting the pulmonary lesions. The pulmonary infiltrates are typically soft, diffuse, patchy, or nodular and poorly outlined. The earliest lesions often begin as a hilar enlargement, which then "fans out." The lower lobes are most frequently involved, but multilobar disease is common. The lesions vary from slight, stringy peribronchial shadows to extensive infiltration that is indistinguishable from that of pneumococcal pneumonia. One to three weeks is usually required for resolution.

In the usual case (Fig. 180-4), fever and acute illness last 5 to 8 days. Convalescence is typically prolonged. There is continued cough, and return of strength and well-being is slow. Complete recovery without residual disability is the rule, although occasional patients succumb with dyspnea, cyanosis, and prostration.

Laboratory Findings. The laboratory findings in the average case of primary atypical pneumonia are usually within normal limits. A leukocyte count of 20,000 per cu mm, or higher, can occur after the first week, but early leukocytosis should suggest some other disease. The erythrocyte sedimentation rate may be increased, but this is not consistent.

The appearance of cold hemagglutinins for human group O erythrocytes or of agglutinins for streptococcus MG in the blood are of value in the retrospective diagnosis of primary atypical pneumonia. These agglutinins do not increase in titer until the second or third week after onset and are, therefore, not useful at the time therapeutic considerations are paramount. Cold hemagglutinins are

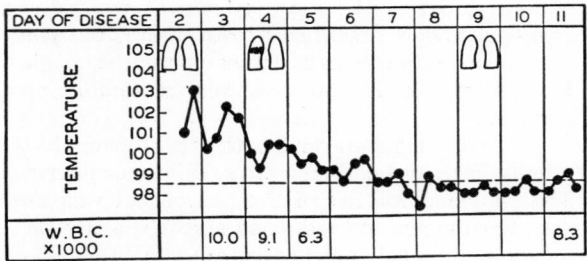

FIG. 180-4. Clinical chart of a patient with primary atypical pneumonia of moderate severity. (*Dingle et al.: War Medicine*, 3:223, 1943.)

demonstrable in approximately 50 per cent of cases. The incidence of cold hemagglutinins is increased in the more severe illnesses, as judged by the height and duration of fever and the number of lobes of the lung which are involved. Agglutinins for streptococcus MG are present in approximately 25 per cent of cases, but the incidence increases with the severity of illness.

False positive Wassermann reactions occur in a few patients with primary atypical pneumonia. The occurrence of several other serologic reactions in convalescent-phase serums indicates that serologic tests in general should be interpreted with caution in this disease.

Differential Diagnosis. (See p. 890.)

COMPLICATIONS OF COMMON RESPIRATORY DISEASE

Purulent paranasal sinusitis, otitis media, mastoiditis, and bacterial pneumonia are frequent and often serious complications of the common respiratory diseases. Pneumococci, staphylococci, and streptococci are the chief offenders. Secondary bacterial infection should be suspected if fever persists and leukocytosis occurs.

Copious, thick nasal exudate, postnasal discharge, laryngitis, hoarseness, and chronic cough occur so frequently that they may well be an integral part of the clinical picture. Painful involvement of the paranasal sinuses during the acute illness seems in many instances properly to be regarded as an extension of the original inflammatory process. There is much uncertainty about the role of bacteria as "secondary invaders" in these conditions.

Herpes simplex of the lips or face is particularly frequent in the common cold group. However, in primary atypical pneumonia, herpes is so unusual that its presence strongly suggests a bacterial etiology of pneumonia.

Complications of primary atypical pneumonia are unusual. Pleural effusion is rare and when it occurs is almost invariably small, bacteriologically sterile, and readily absorbed. Encephalitis, meningoencephalitis, or myocarditis has occurred in the rare severe cases with a fatal outcome. Hemolytic anemia has been observed during the acute illness.

There is uncertainty concerning the role of bacteria in the pathogenesis of the common respiratory diseases, but the weight of evidence indicates that bacteria are not primary incitants. The chief points in favor of the hypothesis that bacteria commonly act as "secondary invaders" are (1) there are reports that the total bacterial population increases as the inflammatory process proceeds, especially when the secretions become thick, and (2) certain specific organisms are present in large numbers in the secretions.

Evidence that "allergy" or "bacterial allergy" is an important factor in the pathogenesis of common respiratory disease is neither substantial nor convincing.

IMMUNITY

Repeated or successive respiratory infections in an individual do not necessarily imply lack of immunity unless it can be established that a single agent is responsible. Such information is available in very few instances.

Experiments with volunteers employing common cold filtrates for challenge have yielded conflicting results. In one study, rechallenge in the early postconvalescent period induced some second illnesses. Similar studies by others employing several different common cold filtrates have demonstrated definite resistance on reinoculation with the same filtrate.

Studies in volunteers with the JH and 2060 viruses have shown definite but incomplete resistance to challenge reinoculation. The data also showed that the two viruses gave good cross immunity.

Many studies have shown that adenovirus infections of military recruits due to the types 3, 4, and 7 viruses provide good immunity, though the duration of the immunity is unknown.

There is not enough information to allow reliable conclusions concerning immunity to the viruses listed in Tables 180-1 and 180-2. It appears, however, that illnesses from some of these agents may occur in individuals who already possess specific serum antibody.

Numerous reports indicate that second attacks of primary atypical pneumonia may occur even though only a few weeks or months have elapsed since the first attack. Evaluation of these data is not possible because information concerning the number of agents which may cause primary atypical pneumonia is lacking.

The existence of "local immunity" in the respiratory tract has been suggested but not proved.

PREVENTION

Adenovirus vaccines containing types 3, 4, and 7 virus have been successful in preventing acute undifferentiated respiratory disease in military recruits. The protective effect has approximated 80 to 90 per cent, and the vaccine has now been adopted for routine use in the armed services. It is effective only for adenovirus infections and not for other respiratory illnesses. Adenovirus infections constitute a very small proportion of total respiratory illnesses in civilians, and the vaccine is not recommended for general use.

Except for the adenovirus vaccines just noted,

there are no established methods or immunizing agents effective for preventing common respiratory disease. Various "cold vaccines" or "cold shots" are widely employed, but none has yet been shown to be of value when tested under controlled conditions. The viruses listed in Tables 180-1 and 180-2 raise the possibility that effective vaccines containing certain of these agents may be developed in the future.

Adequate rest, a nutritious diet, sensible avoidance of undue exposure to cold or wet, and avoidance of exposure to those with respiratory infections seem reasonable and advisable but cannot be relied upon to prevent the common respiratory diseases.

PROGNOSIS

In the absence of complications, the prognosis for life is uniformly good, although primary atypical pneumonia in the debilitated or in patients with chronic illness, e.g., cardiac disease, asthma, etc., may be serious or fatal. Fatalities in young adults occur in approximately one in a thousand cases of primary atypical pneumonia; the fatality rate in children and the aged is not established but is probably higher.

TREATMENT

There is no specific treatment for common respiratory disease; the sulfonamides and antibiotics are not of value for the treatment of the primary illness.

Symptomatic therapy is often overdone. Aspirin is as good as any of the various compounds employed for the relief of feverishness, headache, and malaise. The "antihistaminic" drugs are of little value for the treatment of the common cold or other common respiratory diseases.

Routine use of the sulfonamides or antibiotics for the prophylaxis of the bacterial "secondary invaders" is to be condemned. Their use in therapeutic doses is justified if bacterial complications are present.

Patients with severe primary atypical pneumonia may be dyspneic or cyanotic; the use of oxygen is very helpful, and occasionally it appears to be life-saving. In general, bed rest for a few days after the temperature is normal is advisable, but resolution of the pulmonary process does not appear to be necessary before ambulation.

Several reports suggest that the tetracycline drugs are of value in the treatment of primary atypical pneumonia, although there is general agreement that the sulfonamides and penicillin are ineffective. The tetracyclines have been of benefit in cases caused by the Eaton agent, but in others no effect has been obtained. Thus, while no definitive recommendation for the use of the broad-spectrum antibiotics can be made at present, their use in primary atypical pneumonia is justified, particularly in the more severe illnesses.

REFERENCES

Adams, J. M.: "Newer Virus Diseases: Clinical Differentiation of Acute Respiratory Infections," New York, The Macmillan Company, 1960.

Badger, G. F., J. H. Dingle, A. E. Feller, R. G. Hodges, W. S. Jordan, and C. H. Rammelkamp: A Study of Illness in a Group of Cleveland Families: II. Incidence of the Common Respiratory Diseases, Am. J. Hyg., 58:31, 1953.

Chanock, R. M., A. Vargosko, A. Luckey, M. K. Cook, A. Z. Kapikian, T. Reichelderfer, and R. H. Parrott: Association of Hemadsorption Viruses with Respiratory Illness in Childhood, J.A.M.A., 169:548, 1959.

Commission on Acute Respiratory Disease: The Transmission of Primary Atypical Pneumonia to Human Volunteers, Bull. Johns Hopkins Hosp., 79:97, 1946.

——: Experimental Transmission of Minor Respiratory Illness to Human Volunteers by Filter-passing Agents, J. Clin. Invest., 26:957, 1947.

Denny, F. W., Jr.: Viruses Newly Isolated from the Upper Respiratory Tract, Pediat. Clin. N. Am., 7:295, 1960.

Dingle, J. H., and A. E. Feller: Noninfluenzal Viral Infections of the Respiratory Tract, New Engl. J. Med., 254:465, 1956.

Feller, A. E., and M. R. Hilleman: Primary Atypical Pneumonia, in "Diagnostic Procedures for Virus and Rickettsial Diseases," 2d ed., New York, American Public Health Association, 1956.

Hilleman, M. R.: Adenovirus Vaccine: Development, Field Evaluation, and Appraisal of the Need for Vaccination in Military and Civilian Populations, Arch. Internal Med., 101:47, 1958.

Huebner, R. J., W. P. Rowe, T. F. Ward, R. H. Parrott, and J. A. Bell: Adenoidal-pharyngeal-conjunctival Agents: A Newly Recognized Group of Common Viruses of the Respiratory System, New Engl. J. Med., 251:1077, 1954.

Jackson, G. G., and H. F. Dowling: Transmission of the Common Cold to Volunteers under Controlled Conditions: IV. Specific Immunity to the Common Cold, J. Clin. Invest., 38:762, 1959.

Jordan, W. S.: "Newer Viruses," Disease-a-Month Series, Chicago, Year Book Publishers, Inc., February, 1959.

Tyrrell, D. A. J., M. L. Bynoe, G. Hitchcock, M. G. Pereira, and C. H. Andrewes: Some Virus Isolations from Common Colds: I. Experiments Employing Human Volunteers, Lancet, 1:235, 1960.

—— and R. Parsons: Some Virus Isolations from Common Colds: III. Cytopathic Effects in Tissue Cultures, Lancet, 1:239, 1960.

Von Volkenburgh, V. A., and W. H. Frost: Acute Minor Respiratory Diseases Prevailing in a Group of Families Residing in Baltimore, Maryland, 1928–1930: Prevalence, Distribution and Clinical Description of Observed Cases, Am. J. Hyg., 17: 122, 1933.

181 INFLUENZA
Robert R. Wagner

Definition. Influenza is an acute respiratory infection of specific viral etiology characterized by sudden onset of headache, myalgia, fever, and prostration. The terms *influenza* and "flu" should not be loosely applied to all common respiratory diseases with systemic manifestations but should be restricted to those cases with clear-cut epidemiologic or laboratory evidence of infection with influenza viruses.

History. Influenza is an Italian word meaning "influence" (originally referring to the influence of the stars or the cold), which first came into common English usage during the European epidemic of 1743. In most non-English-speaking countries, the disease is usually referred to by the French word "grippe," or its equivalent. According to the best available records, influenza was uncommon in Europe during the nineteenth century until the pandemic of 1889. Subsequently, the frequency and severity of epidemics increased, culminating in the disastrous pandemic of 1918, which caused an estimated 20 to 40 million deaths. The isolation of the causative virus in 1933 by Smith, Andrewes, and Laidlaw led to the development of simple diagnostic tests, which have greatly advanced knowledge of the clinical variations, epidemiology, and pathogenesis of the disease. The next pandemic occurred in 1957 and was, perhaps, the most thoroughly studied and documented major epidemic in the annals of medicine.

Etiology. There are, at present, three distinct antigenic types of influenza virus, designated A, B, and C, in the order in which they were discovered. The Sendai virus, formerly designated as influenza D, is now classified with the parainfluenza group (see p. 1115). Infection with one type confers no immunity to infection with the other two. They are all approximately 100 mμ in diameter, visible as spheres or filaments by electron microscopy, and are biologically related by their infectivity for chick embryos, capacity to agglutinate erythrocytes, and affinity for the respiratory epithelium of various mammals. Influenza viruses are the prototypes of the myxovirus group, which also includes mumps, Newcastle disease, fowl plague, and the four types of parainfluenza viruses.

Epidemiology. Influenza B and C usually occur sporadically or in localized outbreaks, particularly in schools and military camps. Influenza A viruses are the cause of major epidemics which tend to recur at intervals of 2 to 4 years, usually in the winter months. The factors responsible for this periodicity are the decline in effective immunity of a population in interepidemic periods and the emergence every few years of new strains of virus slightly different antigenically from the former strains. A marked change in the antigenicity of type A viruses occurred in 1946–1947, when viruses extant between 1933 and 1945 completely disappeared and were replaced by strains designated as influenza A' or A$_1$.

A further, more pronounced, alteration in the serotype of influenza A viruses was detected in China early in 1957. These A$_2$ or "Asian" influenza viruses were widely disseminated in the Orient in the following spring, giving rise to the Asian influenza pandemic of 1957. On the basis of laboratory studies and international epidemic intelligence, accurate predictions were made within a month of the first outbreaks in East Asia that influenza would spread throughout the world. A second pandemic wave occurred early in 1958, and major epidemics of the same type recurred in the winter of 1959–1960. These A$_2$ variants of influenza A virus almost undoubtedly will be the prevalent epidemic strains until 1970.

Influenza A epidemics start abruptly, reach a peak in 2 to 3 months, and subside almost as rapidly. The attack rate is variable but was noted in 1957 to exceed 50 per cent of urban populations. An additional 25 per cent of individuals may show serologic evidence of infection without clinical manifestations. The prevalence of influenza in winter months and the simultaneous appearance of epidemics in widely separated areas were formerly attributed to external factors, such as cold and inclement weather. Experiences in 1957 proved conclusively that crowding, even in summer months or in tropical countries, is the major factor predisposing to epidemics. School children, in particular, are the primary focus and disseminators of infection in the United States. The end of summer recess in September brings a highly susceptible population into close proximity, which facilitates rapid spread of infection in the classroom and beyond. If the general immunity of a population is at low levels, as was true in 1957, community-wide epidemics may occur within a few weeks of the opening of schools. If, on the other hand, immune individuals predominate, the case rate will rise slowly and may not reach epidemic proportions, or may do so later in the winter.

Pathogenesis. Influenza is primarily an infection of the respiratory epithelium that is transmitted from man to man by inhalation of infective droplet nuclei. Influenza A viruses have been recovered in nature from swine and horses, but these animals probably do not transmit the infection to man. Detailed experimental studies of the pathogenesis of the disease have been made in ferrets and mice. After intranasal inoculation, the virus multiplies to maximum titers in 24 to 48 hr and rapidly involves the entire tracheobronchial tree. At first, the mucosa becomes boggy and hyperemic and loses its normal ciliary activity. This may shortly be followed by necrosis of respiratory epithelium, invasion by leukocytes, pulmonary consolidation, and abnormal regeneration of metaplastic squamous epithelium in the bronchi and bronchioles. The infection is largely confined to the respiratory tract and hilar lymph nodes of adult animals; viremia is a transient and inconstant feature. However, virus has been isolated from heart, kidney, and other extrapulmonary tissues in fatal human infections, a finding which suggests that virus products can enter the circulation and may account for systemic manifestations of the disease.

The most characteristic findings at autopsy are pulmonary hemorrhages, necrosis of bronchial epithelium, bronchiolitis, squamous metaplasia of respiratory epithelium, and marked edema of alveolar septa and spaces. Fatal human infections can be caused by the influenza virus itself or by combined viral and bacterial infections.

Manifestations. The disease assumes its most typical form during major epidemics of influenza A, but clinical differentiation between influenza A and B is not possible in localized outbreaks. Sporadic infections with either influenza A or B are likely to result in relatively minor illnesses, with predominantly respiratory symptoms, similar to those of common respiratory disease (see p. 1114). Influenza C is particularly difficult to recognize because of its mildness. Although the manifestations and severity of influenza A vary from year to year, cases in a single epidemic often follow a remarkably similar pattern. The clinical description that follows is a composite picture of epidemic influenza A of the past decade.

The *incubation period* is usually 18 to 36 hr but may be as long as 3 days. Mild prodromal symptoms of cough, malaise, and chilliness are sometimes present, but extremely sudden onset is often such a characteristic feature that many patients can recall its exact time. The most common initial symptom is severe generalized or frontal *headache*, frequently accompanied by stabbing retroorbital pain that is accentuated by lateral or upward gaze. Dif-

fuse *myalgia*, particularly marked in the legs and over the lumbosacral area, occurs in more than half the cases; this is often so severe that the patient is reluctant to move. Pain and spasm localized to the abdominal muscles may simulate acute peritonitis, and incapacitating periarticular pains are sometimes confused with acute arthritis. Some observers have commented on the frequency of faintness and dizziness as early symptoms. *Feverishness* and *chilliness*, or occasionally true rigors, may be the first manifestations, but more often they are preceded by headache and myalgia. The temperature rises abruptly to a maximum of 100 to 103°F several hours after onset; rarely it may reach 106°F. Thereafter, the fever and pain usually subside over a 2- to 3-day period but can persist for as long as a week. A common variant in the temperature course is rapid defervescence after the initial peak, with a secondary rise to the original level on the following day. In general, severity of illness parallels the height and duration of the fever. The pulse rate is usually slow in relation to the fever, but marked tachycardia can occur in severely ill patients.

Prostration of some degree is almost invariable and is often the most prominent and alarming manifestation. The face is usually flushed, and the skin is hot and dry; however, profuse sweating and cold, mottled extremities are sometimes noted. A peculiar type of "heliotrope" facial cyanosis occurred during the 1918 pandemic, but it is rarely seen at present. Anorexia, nausea, and constipation are frequent secondary symptoms, but vomiting and diarrhea are rare. There is no evidence that influenza viruses infect the gastrointestinal tract, and the term *intestinal flu* is a misnomer. Meningoencephalitis, polyneuritis, cranial nerve palsies, transient nerve deafness, aphasia, hemiplegia, psychoses, and other neurologic disorders have been described in association with influenza but are very unusual. Hypotension, heart block, peripheral vasoconstriction, and fatal myocarditis have also been reported in a few cases. The exact relationship of these neurologic and cardiovascular disorders to influenza viral infection has not been determined. The incidence of abortion appears to be increased when influenza occurs during the first trimester of pregnancy.

Respiratory symptoms may be present at the onset but become most prominent when the systemic manifestations and fever begin to subside. They are frequently less pronounced than in common respiratory disease and can be entirely absent. Sneezing, watery nasal discharge, or stuffy nose occurs in most cases; hoarseness and epistaxis are less frequent. Conjunctival suffusion and burning, and itching, watery eyes are often noted. Sore throat is not a usual complaint, although the throat may feel dry and the pharynx often appears slightly injected. *Cough* develops during the course of the illness in more than three-fourths of the cases, and in about a third of these it is productive of small amounts of tenacious, mucoid sputum. *Chest pain,* usually substernal in location and accentuated by coughing but not by breathing, is present in almost half the patients. Pleurisy and pleural effusion are uncommon. Slight hyperpnea is often noted, but the most ominous, although infrequent, signs are dyspnea and cyanosis, which signal bronchiolar or pneumonic involvement. Physical examination of the lungs is often negative in uncomplicated influenza, but scattered rhonchi, wheezes, and showers of moist rales have been reported in 5 to 40 per cent of cases in different epidemics. Influenzal bronchiolitis should be suspected if rales persist in the absence of x-ray evidence of pneumonitis and if the patient raises mucopurulent or blood-tinged sputum.

The chief *complications* of influenza are secondary bacterial infections of the paranasal sinuses, middle ear, bronchi, and lungs. The incidence of bacterial pneumonia is greatly increased during influenza epidemics; even mild or asymptomatic infections with influenza viruses predispose to pneumococcal and other types of pneumonia. The most serious complication is staphylococcal pneumonia, which tends to run a fulminant, often fatal, course. Superinfection with *Hemophilus influenzae,* so common in the pandemic of 1918, is rarely encountered now.

Recovery from uncomplicated influenza is often complete in 2 to 3 days or, occasionally, in a week, but convalescence may be prolonged by "postinfectious asthenia" and depression, particularly in elderly persons. Minor relapses with fever can occur but are uncommon.

The *mortality* rate from all causes always increases markedly during epidemics of influenza. In the fall and winter of 1957–1958 it was estimated that 80 million persons in the United States became ill with influenza, and the total number of influenza-associated deaths was reported to be in excess of 8,000. In addition, approximately 60,000 more deaths from various causes occurred during this period than would be expected under normal conditions. The greatest incidence of excess mortality occurred among infants under one year of age and adults over sixty years of age. The high mortality in young adults that characterized the pandemic of 1918 fortunately did not recur. However, data from small series of cases clearly indicate that influenza is all too frequently a fatal infection in individuals with preexisting pulmonary or cardiac disease, regardless of age. Chronic rheumatic heart disease with mitral stenosis, in particular, appears to predispose to fatal influenzal pneumonia.

Laboratory Findings. Virus is isolated most readily during the acute phase of the disease by inoculation of broth garglings into the amniotic cavity of chick embryos or into tissue cultures of monkey kidney or human cells. Serologic diagnosis can be made most reliably by hemagglutination-inhibition or complement fixation tests, using paired serum samples obtained in both the acute and convalescent phases. However, type-specific antibody against soluble complement fixing antigens of influenza A virus often appears in the circulation of patients during the acute illness.

X-ray of the lungs in uncomplicated influenza is usually normal but occasionally reveals increased vascular markings, basilar streaking, small areas of patchy infiltration, atelectasis, nodular densities, or pleural effusion. The blood leukocyte count may be low 2 to 4 days after onset of illness, but is often normal or slightly elevated. Leukocytosis with counts above 15,000 cells per cu mm indicates secondary bacterial infection, but it is well to remember that leukopenia can occur in severe staphylococcal pneumonia. Slight proteinuria is common during the height of the febrile illness.

Differential Diagnosis. Many bacterial and viral infections simulate influenza at their onset, but few febrile diseases have such a self-limited course. The pattern of clinical manifestations becomes readily apparent during an epidemic, but many influenza outbreaks are associated with an increased incidence of other respiratory infection or viral and bacterial etiology. Noninfluenzal respiratory diseases (see p. 1114) are generally characterized by more gradual onset, milder systemic manifestations, and predominant symptoms of coryza, rhinorrhea, pharyngitis, and conjunctivitis.

Treatment. Antibiotics do not affect the course of uncomplicated influenza, nor is there any evidence that they prevent complications. Specific chemotherapy should be reserved for secondary bacterial infections. Codeine affords relief from incapacitating cough and is more effective than salicylates for symptomatic treatment of headache and myalgia; salicylates often increase discomfort by causing drenching sweats and chills. Bed rest and gradual return to full activity are advisable to prevent prolonged postinfectious asthenia.

Prophylaxis. Formalinized egg vaccines containing a mixture of influenza A, A_1, A_2, and B viruses are the standard preparations available commercially in the United States. The British favor the use of a monovalent vaccine presently prepared from a more concentrated suspension of influenza A_2 virus. Infectious attenuated virus administered intranasally has been widely used for influenza immunization in the Soviet Union, but its safety and efficacy have not been thoroughly proved. The most promising results have been obtained in the American Armed Forces by preliminary trials of adjuvant influenza vaccines emulsified with mineral oil and

Arlacel A. Although they stimulate the production of serum antibodies, the prophylactic value of influenza vaccines is limited by the following factors: (1) infection can occur in spite of high levels of serum antibody; (2) antibody concentration is low at the site of infection in the respiratory tract; (3) vaccines sometimes do not contain antigens prepared from the most recent strains of virus; and (4) even under optimal conditions, their protective effect often lasts for only a few months.

Nevertheless, there is ample evidence that vaccines currently available reduce the incidence and severity of influenza, particularly during epidemics in closed populations (such as boarding schools and military camps). The U.S. Public Health Service strongly recommends routine yearly immunization with polyvalent influenza vaccine for high-risk groups, including: persons of all ages who suffer from chronic rheumatic heart disease, other cardiovascular diseases, chronic bronchopulmonary diseases, diabetes mellitus, or Addison's disease; also pregnant women and persons sixty-five years of age, or older, regardless of their previous state of health. For initial immunization it is advisable to administer the vaccine subcutaneously in two divided doses of 1 ml each, the first injection in September and the second several weeks or months later. A single subcutaneous dose of 1 ml given each autumn is satisfactory as a yearly booster. Intradermal injection of vaccine is far less satisfactory because a sufficient antigenic mass cannot be administered by this route.

Influenza vaccination is generally safe but not completely innocuous. Fatal anaphylactic reactions and purpura have been reported in individuals sensitive to egg proteins, and inactivated virus itself is pyrogenic and can sometimes produce an illness similar to active influenza. Influenza vaccine should be administered only advisedly and in much smaller doses to infants and young children, in whom severe febrile reactions may result in convulsions and death.

REFERENCES

Jensen, K. E., F. L. Dunn, and R. Q. Robinson: Influenza, 1957: A Variant and the Pandemic, pp. 165–209 in "Progress in Medical Virology, I," E. Berger and J. L. Melnick (Eds.), New York, Hafner Publishing Company, 1958.

Loosli, C. G. (Ed.): Proceedings of the International Conference on Asian Influenza, Bethesda, Maryland, February, 1960, Am. Rev. Respirat. Diseases, 83: part 2, February, 1961.

Louria, D. B., H. L. Bumenfeld, J. T. Ellis, E. D. Kilbourne, and D. E. Rogers: Studies on Influenza in the Pandemic of 1957–1958: II. Pulmonary Complications of Influenza, J. Clin. Invest., 38: 213, 1959.

Trotter, Y., Jr., F. L. Dunn, R. H. Drachman, D. A. Henderson, M. Pizzi, and A. D. Alexander: Asian Influenza in the United States, Am. J. Hyg., 70:34, 1959.

Zhdanov, V. M., V. D. Solov'ev, and F. G. Epshtein: "The Study of Influenza: A Translation from the Russian *Ucheniye o Grippe*," Public Health Service Publication No. 792, U.S. Department of Health, Education, and Welfare, Bethesda, Md., 1960.

182 PSITTACOSIS
Robert R. Wagner and Ivan L. Bennett, Jr.

Definition. Psittacosis is an infectious disease of birds caused by a large virus. Transmission of the virus from birds to man results in a febrile illness characterized by pneumonitis and systemic manifestations. The name *ornithosis* is sometimes applied to infections contracted from birds other than parrots or parakeets, but *psittacosis* is the more common and preferred term for all forms of the disease.

History. In 1880 a Swiss physician, Ritter, reported a fatal pneumonic illness in patients who had been in contact with sick birds. Psittacosis was considered to be a rare and exotic disease until 1929–1930, when almost 800 cases occurred in Europe, Asia, and America. This "pandemic" was traced to a shipment of South American parrots (Meyer, 1942). During the past 30 years psittacosis has been reported with increasing frequency. At least 1,000 cases occur each year in the United States, and many more probably go unrecognized.

Etiology. The causative organism is an obligate intracellular parasite which is usually referred to as a virus, although it more nearly resembles a rickettsia in size, staining properties, susceptibility to antibiotics, and its capacity to multiply by binary fission. It is closely related to the virus of lymphogranuloma venereum and to a wide variety of mammalian viruses which have not been shown conclusively to produce human disease, except for rare laboratory-acquired infections.

Epidemiology. Psittacosis is widely distributed throughout the world, and almost any avian species can harbor the virus. Psittacine birds are most commonly infected, but human cases have been traced to contact with pigeons, ducks, turkeys, chickens, and many other birds. Psittacosis can be considered an occupational disease of pet-shop owners, poultry raisers, pigeon fanciers, taxidermists, and zoo attendants. The incidence of human infection has steadily risen during the past decade owing in large part to the increasing popularity of parakeets and related birds as pets and the easing of regulations banning their importation and interstate shipment.

The virus is present in nasal secretions, excreta, tissues, and feathers of infected birds. Although the disease can be fatal, infected birds frequently show only minor evidences of illness such as ruffled feathers, lethargy, and anorexia. Asymptomatic avian carriers are common, and complete recovery can be followed by continued shedding of virus for many months. Prolonged oral administration of feed impregnated with chlortetracycline may eradicate the infection in many birds, but not all. Campaigns to educate breeders to treat all young parakeets with adequate doses of antibiotics have met with indifferent success.

Psittacosis is almost always transmitted to man by the respiratory route. On rare occasions the disease may have been acquired from the bite of a pet bird. Intimate and prolonged contact is not essential for transmission of the disease; a few minutes spent in an environment previously occupied by an infected bird has resulted in human infection. The severity of the disease in man bears no apparent relationship to closeness or duration of contact. Human-to-human transmission of psittacosis has occurred particularly among hospital personnel, and the resulting infections are usually severe, often fatal. There is evidence that these "human" strains are more virulent than native avian viruses. There is no record of infection acquired by eating poultry products.

Pathogenesis. Psittacosis virus gains entrance to the body through the upper respiratory tract and eventually localizes in the pulmonary alveoli and the reticuloendothelial cells of the spleen and liver. Invasion of the lung parenchyma probably takes place by way of the blood stream rather than by direct extension from the upper air passages. A lymphocytic inflammatory response occurs on both the interstitial and respiratory surfaces of the alveoli as well as in the perivascular spaces. The alveolar walls and interstitial tissues of the lung are thickened, edematous, necrotic, and occasionally hemorrhagic. Histologically, the affected areas show alveolar spaces filled with fluid, erythrocytes, and lymphocytes. The picture is not pathognomonic of psittacosis unless macrophages containing characteristic cytoplasmic inclusion bodies (LCL bodies) can be identified. The respiratory epithelium of the bronchi and bronchioles usually remains intact.

Manifestations. The clinical manifestations and course of psittacosis are extremely variable. After an *incubation period* of 7 to 14 days, or longer, the disease may start abruptly with shaking chills and high fever, but the onset is often gradual with increasing fever and malaise over a 3- to 4-day period. Headache is almost always a prominent symptom; it is usually diffuse and excruciating and often the patient's chief complaint. Generalized myalgia is also common. Spasm and stiffness of the muscles of the back and neck can lead to an erroneous diagnosis of meningitis. A faint, macular rash (Horder's spots) simulating the rose spots of typhoid fever has been described. Lethargy, mental depression, agitation, insomnia, and disorientation have been prominent features of the illness in some epidemics, but not in others; delirium and stupor occur near the end of the first week in severe cases. Occasional patients are comatose when first seen by a physician, and the diagnosis of psittacosis may be missed in this circumstance. Gastrointestinal complaints such as abdominal pain, nausea, vomiting, or diarrhea are present in some cases; constipation and abdominal distention sometimes occur as late complications. Icterus, the result of severe hepatic involvement, is a rare and ominous finding. Symptoms of upper respiratory infection are not prominent, although mild sore throat, pharyngeal injection, and cervical adenopathy are often present. Epistaxis is encountered early in the course of nearly one-fourth of the cases. Photophobia is also a common complaint.

The dry, hacking cough of atypical pneumonia is characteristic of psittacosis; it is usually nonproductive, but small amounts of mucoid or bloody sputum may be raised as the disease progresses. Cough may appear early in the course of the disease or as late as 5 days after the onset of fever. Chest pain, pleurisy with effusion, or a friction rub can all occur but are not usual. Pericarditis and myocarditis have been reported. Most patients have a normal or slightly increased respiratory rate; marked dyspnea with cyanosis occurs only in severe psittacosis with extensive pulmonary involvement. In psittacosis, as in most nonbacterial pneumonias, the physical signs of pneumonitis tend to be less prominent than symptoms and x-ray findings would suggest. The initial examination may reveal fine, sibilant rales, or clinical evidence of pneumonia may be completely lacking. Rales usually become audible and more numerous as the illness progresses. Signs of frank pulmonary consolidation are usually absent.

Patients without cough or other clinical evidence of respiratory involvement present the problem of a fever of unknown origin. The pulse rate in psittacosis is slow in relation to the fever. Splenomegaly, when present in a patient with acute pneumonitis, strongly suggests psittacosis. Inability to feel the spleen is of no diagnostic significance, however; the reported incidence of splenomegaly has ranged from 10 to 70 per cent in different series of proved cases. It should be remembered that the spleen is only slightly enlarged and is more frequently palpable late in the course of the disease. Nontender hepatic enlargement also occurs, but jaundice is rare. Thrombophlebitis is not unusual during convalescence; indeed, pulmonary infarction is sometimes a late complication and may be fatal.

In untreated cases of psittacosis, sustained or mildly remittent fever persists for 10 days to 3 weeks, or occasionally as long as 3 months. Defervescence is by lysis, rarely by crisis, and is accompanied by abatement of respiratory manifestations. Psittacosis contracted from parrots or parakeets is more likely to be a severe, prolonged illness than infections acquired from pigeons or barnyard fowl. Relapses occur but are rare. Secondary bacterial infections are uncommon. Immunity to reinfection is probably permanent.

Laboratory Findings. The x-ray of the lungs in psittacosis mimics a great variety of pulmonary diseases. The pneumonic lesions are usually patchy in appearance but can be hazy, diffuse, homogeneous, lobar, atelectatic, wedge-shaped, nodular, or miliary. The white blood cell count is normal or moderately decreased in the acute phase of the disease but may rise in convalescence. The erythrocyte sedimentation rate is frequently not elevated. Transient proteinuria is common. The cerebrospinal fluid sometimes contains a few mononuclear cells but is otherwise normal. Cold agglutinins are rarely present in the serum of patients with psittacosis.

The diagnosis of psittacosis can be confirmed only by virus isolation or serologic studies. The virus is present in the blood during the acute phase of the disease and in the bronchial secretions for weeks or sometimes years after infection, but it is often difficult to isolate. Psittacosis is most readily diagnosed by the demonstration of a rising titer of complement fixing antibody in the patient's blood. An acute and convalescent specimen should always be tested. Even a low titer of antibody during the acute febrile phase constitutes presumptive evidence of psittacosis. The prompt initiation of treatment with tetracycline has been shown to delay antibody rise in convalescence for several weeks or months. Interpretation of a single complement fixa-tion test can sometimes be difficult because of the antigenic cross reaction between the viruses of psittacosis and lymphogranuloma venereum.

Differential Diagnosis. A history of exposure to birds may be the only clinical basis for differentiating psittacosis from a great variety of infectious and noninfectious febrile disorders. A partial list of pneumonic diseases that can be confused with psittacosis includes primary atypical pneumonia, Q fever, coccidioidomycosis, tuberculosis, carcinoma of the lung with bronchial obstruction, and bacterial pneumonias. In the early stages, before pneumonitis appears, psittacosis can be mistaken for influenza, typhoid fever, miliary tuberculosis, infectious mononucleosis and, less commonly, rheumatic fever or bacterial endocarditis.

Treatment. The tetracyclines are consistently effective in the treatment of psittacosis. Defervescence and alleviation of symptoms usually occur in 24 to 48 hr after instituting therapy with 2 to 3 Gm daily. To avoid relapse, treatment should probably be continued for at least 7 days after defervescence. The disease will usually respond to penicillin if a daily dose of at least 2 million units is used. In severe cases, oxygen and other supportive measures are indicated.

REFERENCES

Beaudette, F. R. (Ed.): "Progress in Psittacosis Research and Control," New Brunswick, N.J., Rutgers University Press, 1958.

Meyer, K. F.: The Ecology of Psittacosis and Ornithosis, Medicine, 21:175, 1942.

——: Psittacosis-Lymphogranuloma Group, pp. 701–728, in "Viral and Rickettsial Infections of Man," 3d ed., T. M. Rivers and F. L. Horsfall, Jr. (Eds.), Philadelphia, J. B. Lippincott Company, 1959.

Seibert, R. H., W. S. Jordan, Jr., and J. H. Dingle: Clinical Variations in the Diagnosis of Psittacosis, New Engl. J. Med., 254:925, 1956.

—— et al.: Epidemiological Studies of Psittacosis in Cleveland, Am. J. Hyg., 63:28, 1956.

Section 15: Enteric Viruses

INTRODUCTION

Robert R. Wagner

The term *enterovirus* has a very specific meaning to the virologist. Under this designation are classified the related viruses of poliomyelitis, Coxsackie A, Coxsackie B, and the ECHO group (see Table 179-1). The more inclusive term "enteric viruses," which has no official status in virus nomenclature, is often used by the clinician to lump together the enteroviruses and other unclassified viruses that infect the intestinal tract of man. Among the latter are certain unidentified causative agents of gastroenteritis and the virus of infectious hepatitis.

The history of the *enteroviruses* is intimately associated with research in *poliomyelitis*. The existence of *Coxsackie viruses* was first recognized in 1948 during attempts to isolate viruses from patients with poliomyelitis by injecting stool suspension into suckling mice. The Coxsackie viruses were then divided into groups A and B largely on the basis of differences in pathologic lesions in infected mice. The *ECHO viruses* were discovered when tissue culture methods became readily available for studying polioviruses. During the decade 1950–1960, dozens of hitherto unsuspected viruses were recognized, most of which could not be associated with any specific disease. The resulting chaos prompted the formation of a clearing house (Committee on the Enteroviruses) for classification of these "orphan" viruses. The term *enterovirus* was officially coined in 1957 when it became apparent that these agents shared certain physicochemical and biologic properties. All viruses of the polio, Coxsackie, and ECHO groups are strikingly resistant to inactivation by heat, drying, and certain chemical agents. In addition, those which have been carefully studied are relatively small spherical viruses, 25 to 35 mμ in diameter, and are composed entirely of ribonucleic acid and protein in a ratio of about 1:3.

The major problems have been to subdivide the enteroviruses into meaningful categories and to relate them to human disease. Originally, the general policy was to classify newly discovered intestinal viruses as Coxsackie A if they infected only suckling mice, Coxsackie B if they infected both suckling mice and tissue culture, or ECHO if they infected only tissue culture and were not antigenically related to the three poliovirus types. Unfortunately, these criteria were too crude, and the system of classification soon began to break down. For example, Coxsackie A type 9 and other types were found to infect tissue culture, some Coxsackie B viruses are not pathogenic for suckling mice when first isolated but readily infect monkey kidney and certain human cell lines, and a few ECHO viruses cause disease in suckling mice. ECHO virus type 10 turned out not to be an enterovirus at all and has been reclassified, along with other similar agents, in the *reovirus* group (respiratory-enteric viruses). Recovery of adenoviruses from feces and enteroviruses from the respiratory tract even raises the question of the adequacy of the site of infection as a basis for classification.

Perhaps the major problem in arriving at a meaningful nomenclature, particularly for the clinician, is increasing awareness that enteroviruses do not fall into neat etiologic categories of disease. It was soon recognized that designation of aseptic meningitis as "nonparalytic poliomyelitis" was often a misnomer. Then came the realization that Cox-

sackie and ECHO viruses may occasionally cause diseases clinically indistinguishable from paralytic or bulbar poliomyelitis. It now seems apparent that all members of the enterovirus family can sometimes be causative agents of illnesses that were formerly considered to be specific reactions to infection with Coxsackie, ECHO, or polioviruses. An indication of this etiologic diversity is presented in the following table.

SPECTRUM OF MAJOR CLINICAL DISORDERS
ATTRIBUTED TO ENTEROVIRUSES

Clinical syndrome	Associated enteroviruses		
	Poliovirus	Coxsackie	ECHO
Aseptic meningitis...	+	+	+
Carditis (pericarditis or myocarditis)....	+	++	+
Encephalitis........	+	+	+
Febrile exanthem....	(?)+	+	++
"Flu" syndrome.....	+	+	+
Gastroenteritis......	+	+	++
Herpangina.........	0	+	(?)+
Pleurodynia........	(?)0	++	+
Poliomyelitis........	++	+	+

SOURCE: Adapted from J. P. Sanford and S. E. Sulkin, New Engl. J. Med., 261:1113, 1959.

Inability to establish absolute biologic and clinical criteria for classifying enteroviruses has prompted the suggestion that the terms Coxsackie A, Coxsackie B, ECHO, and poliovirus be abandoned. The proposal to substitute a numerical system for designating the enteroviruses based largely on antigenic constitution, however, seems both premature and unmanageable. Despite overlap in biologic and clinical properties, the present nomenclature is useful for both the clinician and the virologist. Coxsackie B viruses, for example, can still be considered the most common, although not the only, cause of pleurodynia.

In considering the *epidemiology* of the enteroviruses, it was formerly presumed that they were normal inhabitants of the intestinal tract in much the same manner as are the Enterobacteriaceae. This does not appear to be correct. Enteroviruses may be excreted in the feces for weeks or months after infection, but they do not persist indefinitely. Infections are far more prevalent during summer and autumn; as anticipated, these are the seasons of highest incidence of poliomyelitis, pleurodynia, and aseptic meningitis. In addition, enteroviruses are more widespread in populations with inadequate sanitary facilities. Under these conditions, mixed infections with two or more enteroviruses are not unusual. There are undoubtedly multiple modes of transmission, including sewage, water, food, and flies. However, the most important factor predisposing to communicability of enteroviruses is intimate and prolonged personal contact, particularly within family groups or in institutions.

The *pathogenesis* of infection with the known enteric viruses is characterized by multiplication of virus in the intestinal tract. This is sometimes accompanied by mild gastroenteritis, but most intestinal infections with Coxsackie, ECHO, hepatitis, and polioviruses are asymptomatic. Infections with enteric viruses generally come to the attention of the physician only on those relatively rare occasions when viremia and systemic dissemination result in a characteristic disease picture. Therefore, descriptions of the clinical manifestations of infection with these viruses more properly belong in other sections of a textbook of medicine and will be found on the following pages: infectious hepatitis, p. 1670; poliomyelitis, p. 1139; aseptic meningitis, p. 1135; herpangina, p. 1173, and enteroviral exanthems, p. 1162.

REFERENCES

Committee on the Enteroviruses, National Foundation for Infantile Paralysis: The Enteroviruses, Am. J. Pub. Health, 47:1556, 1957.

Dalldorf, G.: The Enteroviruses and Paralytic Disease, p. 128 in "Viral Infections of Infancy and Childhood," H. M. Rose (Ed.), New York, Paul B. Hoeber, Inc., Medical Department of Harper & Brothers, 1960.

Davis, E. V.: Isolation of Viruses from Children with Infectious Hepatitis, Science, 133:2059, 1961.

Kibrick, S.: The Role of Coxsackie and ECHO Viruses in Human Disease, Med. Clin. N. Am., 43:1291, 1959.

Macrae, A. D.: Enteroviruses, Brit. Med. Bull., 15:210, 1959.

183 COXSACKIE A VIRUSES
Robert R. Wagner

The enteroviruses relegated to the classification of Coxsackie A are divided into 23 or more distinct antigenic types. The salient biologic property of Coxsackie A viruses is their infectivity for suckling mice which develop flaccid paralysis and die with characteristic necrotizing, inflammatory lesions specifically confined to striated muscle. Unlike other enteroviruses, most members of the Coxsackie A group have only limited capacity to induce cytopathic changes in tissue culture. Type 9 and some strains of type 16 infect cultures of monkey kidney or human amnion cells but not HeLa carcinoma cells of human origin. Of considerable interest is the fact that some Coxsackie A viruses can produce paralysis and neuropathologic lesions in monkeys that are difficult to distinguish from the effects of poliovirus. It is not surprising, therefore, that a virus isolated from patients with paralytic poliomyelitis and originally thought by Russian investigators to be a new type of poliovirus turned out to be Coxsackie A type 7.

Coxsackie A viruses are widespread in human populations and have been implicated as causative agents of a variety of childhood diseases (see Table 179-1). The first recognized etiologic relationship was with herpangina; this disease is probably still the most readily identified syndrome caused by at least six immunologic types of Coxsackie A virus (see p. 1173). Perhaps the most frequent, but least dramatic, manifestations of infection with Coxsackie A viruses are obscure epidemic febrile disorders occurring among children during the summer that go under such names as "3-day fever," "summer complaint," and "summer grippe and sore throat." An increasing number of isolated reports indicates that Coxsackie A viruses may also occasionally cause the following disorders: aseptic meningitis (p. 1135), fatal myocarditis (p. 1132), pericarditis (p. 1132), encephalitis (p. 1152), febrile exanthem (p. 1162), pleurodynia (p. 1131), and gastroenteritis (p. 1134). Undoubtedly, all these diseases are uncommon when compared with the overwhelming incidence of asymptomatic infection.

None of the 23 types of Coxsackie A viruses is known to be the sole cause of any specific disease. However, it is worth noting that type 9 virus is one member of the group that is not infrequently associated with severe illness. Children studied during a Coxsackie A type 9 epidemic exhibited a recognizable disease pattern characterized by fever, vesicular or petechial rash, pharyngitis, and pneumonia. A causative agent of respiratory infections known as Coe virus has recently been reclassified as Coxsackie A type 21. Another investigation suggests that Coxsackie A virus type 4 may be responsible for some cases of "sudden, unexplained death" of infants. This enigma has plagued pathologists because respiratory and cerebral lesions discernible at autopsy are relatively inconsequential.

REFERENCES

Gold, E., et al.: Viral Infection: A Possible Cause of Sudden, Unexpected Death in Infants, New Engl. J. Med., 264:53, 1961.

Lerner, A. M., et al.: Infections Due to Coxsackie Virus Group A, Type 9, in Boston, 1959, with Special Reference to Exanthems and Pneumonia, New Engl. J. Med., 263:1265, 1960.

Wenner, H. A., et al.: Experimental Infections with Coxsackie Viruses, I and II, Arch. ges. Virusforsch., 10:426 and 451, 1961.

184 COXSACKIE B VIRUSES
Robert R. Wagner

Coxsackie B viruses were originally differentiated from the Coxsackie A group on the basis of distinctive pathogenicity for suckling mice. Infection of these animals with most strains of Coxsackie B virus results in encephalitis, necrotizing steatitis with degeneration of brown fat, hepatitis, and carditis. Pancreatitis often occurs in both adult and suckling mice. Inflammation and necrosis of skeletal muscle are less common and less prominent than they are after infection of suckling mice with Coxsackie A viruses. All Coxsackie B viruses produce cytopathic changes in monkey kidney tissue cultures; this is usually the most sensitive method for detecting virus in feces or throat washings. Final identification is based on serologic studies, primarily by tissue culture neutralization or by complement fixation, procedures which are less formidable than those for identification of Coxsackie A or ECHO viruses because only six types of Coxsackie B virus have been recognized.

It must be borne in mind that Coxsackie B viruses are not the sole etiologic agents of pleurodynia, pericarditis, and myocarditis of the newborn, as was once thought. Clinically indistinguishable syndromes are occasionally associated with infections by Coxsackie A, ECHO, and probably other viruses. Nevertheless, descriptions of these diseases are presented in this chapter because Coxsackie B viruses are by far their most common cause. The role of Coxsackie B viruses in aseptic meningitis (p. 1135) and enteroviral exanthems (p. 1162) is discussed elsewhere.

PLEURODYNIA

Definition. This is an acute infectious disease characterized by sudden onset of paroxysmal lower thoracic and abdominal pain and fever. Common synonyms are Bornholm disease, epidemic myalgia, and devil's grip.

Epidemiology. Pleurodynia is a disease of the summer and autumn that occurs in epidemic form throughout the world. All age groups are affected, but the highest incidence is in children and young adults. Explosive outbreaks with high attack rates have been reported, particularly in institutions, but it is more usual for epidemics to start insidiously, reach a peak in several weeks, and subside over a period of months. Multiple cases in a single household are infrequent, indicating a predominance of asymptomatic infections and carriers. Infection is spread by close personal contact, probably by the fecal-oral route through fomites, food, and water. Other modes of transmission are suggested by isolation of Coxsackie viruses from respiratory secretions, sewage, and flies.

Manifestations. The incubation period is usually 2 to 5 days but may be as long as 2 weeks. Mild prodromal symptoms, such as malaise, sore throat, coryza, anorexia, or myalgia, may be present for several days. However, the most characteristic feature of the disease is the sudden onset of severe, sharp, paroxysmal pain over the lower ribs or in the substernal area. It is accentuated by moving, breathing, coughing, sneezing, or hiccuping and may be referred to the shoulders, neck, or scapulas. Pain and spasm of the anterior abdominal muscles occur in about half the cases, often in combination with chest pain but sometimes limited entirely to the lower abdomen. Muscle tenderness is usually not prominent, but some patients complain of intense cutaneous hyperesthesia and paresthesias over the affected area. Headache is frequent and is sometimes of excruciating severity. The disease may be accompanied by delirium, dizziness, and true vertigo. Fever with temperatures of 100 to 105°F develops shortly after the onset of pain and is often preceded by chilliness or shaking chills. The temperature may be elevated in the early morning, fall to normal at midday, and rise again in the evening. Respiratory manifestations are not prominent, but there may be mild pharyngeal injection and nonproductive cough. Conjunctivitis and photophobia are rare. A pleural friction rub is detectable in 10 to 25 per cent of patients and can persist after the pain subsides. Transitory erythematous rashes have occasionally been noted. Anorexia and nausea are frequent, and vomiting and diarrhea often occur in children.

The complications of pleurodynia are largely the result of disseminated infection with the causative virus. *Meningitis* can occur several days after the onset of pain and fever, or it may be the sole manifestation of infection, indistinguishable from other forms of benign aseptic meningitis (see p. 1135). *Orchitis* developing in the second week of the disease has been a frequent complication in certain outbreaks but is rare in others. *Arthritis* and *jaundice* have also been reported.

The average duration of illness is 4 days but varies from 1 day to several weeks. Relapses occur in 25 to 50 per cent of cases, usually 2 to 3 days after subsidence of the initial episode but sometimes after an interval of several weeks. Some patients experience multiple attacks of equal severity. Complete recovery may be delayed for weeks by generalized weakness, but convalescence is otherwise uneventful, and there are no known sequelae. Immunity is type specific, and reinfection can occur with other types of Coxsackie virus.

Laboratory Findings. Coxsackie B viruses can be isolated from blood, urine, skeletal muscle, cerebrospinal fluid, spinal cord, and myocardium. However, isolation of Coxsackie B virus from the feces or throat washings does not constitute valid proof of infection unless supported by strong epidemiologic evidence. Definitive diagnosis can be made by demonstrating a rising titer of neutralizing or complement-fixing antibodies in the serum. X-ray of the chest is normal except for rare instances of pneumonitis or pleural effusion. The blood leukocyte count is usually normal but can be low or moderately elevated. Slight eosinophilia sometimes occurs several days after onset or in convalescence. The cerebrospinal fluid may be normal or may contain as many as 300 cells, most of them mononuclear.

Differential Diagnosis. Pleurodynia is often confused with early bacterial pneumonia when pain is localized to the chest, and with intraabdominal disease, particularly acute appendicitis, when abdominal pain predominates.

Treatment. Coxsackie viruses are not affected by antibiotics. Aspirin, codeine, or morphine is often required for symptomatic relief of pain. The usual measures for relief of pleurisy (p. 1564) may be helpful.

COXSACKIE PERICARDITIS

Coxsackie viruses, particularly group B, appear to be a major cause of acute benign pericarditis. This disease has been reported predominantly in young adult males but may occur in either sex at any age. Pericarditis is sometimes the sole manifestation of infection with Coxsackie viruses, or it may be seen in association with pleurodynia and its complications. The principal manifestations are slight or moderate fever for several days, substernal soreness or oppressive anterior chest pain radiating to the left arm, splinting of the chest, mild dyspnea, and apprehension. The diagnosis is usually suggested by the presence of a pericardial or pleuropericardial friction rub. Chest x-ray often reveals an enlarged cardiac silhouette and signs of pleural effusion. Pericardial paracentesis may yield moderate amounts of serous or serosanguineous fluid which frequently is free of virus. Electrocardiography usually confirms the diagnosis of pericardial disease. The presence of cardiac decompensation and conduction defects have been cited as evidence of myocardial as well as pericardial involvement. However, myocarditis is rarely severe in adults and does not appear to be a major component of Cox-

sackie pericarditis. No fatalities have been reported, but relapses occur and several weeks may be required for complete recovery. Insufficient data are available to determine the incidence of sequelae, if any. Establishment of an etiologic diagnosis depends on virus isolation from the feces or pharyngeal secretions, or rarely from other sites, and demonstration of a rising antibody titer to the virus isolated.

MYOCARDITIS OF THE NEWBORN

Coxsackie B viruses also cause a severe, often fatal, myocarditis of newborn infants which becomes manifest in the first few days or weeks of life. In several reported cases the infection appears to have been acquired in utero subsequent to a Coxsackie infection of the mother near or at term. The disease may start abruptly and terminate in death within a few hours. Not infrequently, however, the illness is biphasic with insidious onset of low-grade fever, diarrhea, apathy, and refusal to feed. There may then be a period of apparent recovery for 1 to 7 days followed by high fever, cardiac decompensation, cyanosis, shock, extreme tachycardia, and arrhythmias. The electrocardiogram may show conduction defects. Deterioration is rapid, and the outcome is usually fatal. Many of these infants also exhibit clinical signs of generalized infection, particularly of the brain and liver, a syndrome designated as *encephalohepatomyocarditis neonatorum*.

Autopsy often reveals extensive necrosis and inflammation of myocardium, liver, brain, and spinal cord and interstitial pneumonitis. Coxsackie B viruses, types 2, 3, 4, or 5, can usually be recovered from these tissues in large amounts.

REFERENCES

Dalldorf, G., J. L. Melnick, and E. C. Curnen: The Coxsackie Virus Group, p. 519 in "Viral and Rickettsial Infections of Man," 3d ed., T. M. Rivers and F. L. Horsfall, Jr. (Eds.), Philadelphia, J. B. Lippincott Company, 1959.

Finn, J. J., Jr., T. H. Weller, and H. R. Morgan: Epidemic Pleurodynia: Clinical and Etiological Studies Based on One Hundred and Fourteen Cases, Arch. Internal Med., 83:305, 1949.

Gear, J. H. S.: Coxsackie Virus Infections of the Newborn, Progr. Med. Virology, 1:106, 1958.

Gordon, R. B., E. H. Lennette, and R. S. Sandrock: The Varied Clinical Manifestations of Coxsackie Virus Infections, A.M.A. Arch. Internal Med., 103: 63, 1959.

Kibrick, S., and K. Benirschke: Generalized Disease (Encephalohepatomyocarditis) Occurring in the Newborn Period and Due to Infection with Coxsackie Virus, Group B, Pediatrics, 22:857, 1958.

Sylvest, E.: "Epidemic Myalgia: Bornholm Disease," London, Oxford University Press, 1934.

van Crevald, A.: Virus Myocarditis in Infancy—Acute Phase and Possible Late Sequels, p. 33 in "Viral Infections in Infancy and Childhood," H. M. Rose (Ed.), New York, Paul B. Hoeber, Inc., Medical Department of Harper & Brothers, 1960.

185 ECHO VIRUSES
Robert R. Wagner

The term ECHO viruses is derived from an early description of these agents as *enteric cytopatho-genic human orphan* viruses. The name is still apt but must be qualified in the light of later studies. In common with other enteroviruses, the ECHO viruses primarily infect the intestine of man and are transmitted by the fecal-oral route, but they also multiply in the upper respiratory tract and can be disseminated to virtually any organ. Another characteristic is their ability to induce cytopathic changes in tissue cultures of monkey kidney and human amnion cells but not in HeLa carcinoma cells. ECHO viruses isolated directly from man are less pathogenic for suckling mice and monkeys than are Coxsackie and polioviruses; these criteria form the essential basis for classification of enteroviruses. When newly isolated strains of ECHO virus type 9 were found to be virulent for suckling mice, they were reclassified as Coxsackie A type 23. Some types agglutinate human erythrocytes.

Despite similarities in their biologic and epidemiologic properties, the ECHO viruses do not share a common complement-fixing antigen, as do the adenoviruses, and can be separated into at least 28 immunologic types on the basis of complement fixation and neutralization tests. Type specificity is not absolute in that serologic cross reactions have been demonstrated between several types and to a slight extent with polioviruses. ECHO virus type 9 also exhibits an interesting antigenic relationship to herpes simplex virus. Enteroviruses similar to the ECHO group in man have been isolated from animals and have been given names such as ECBO (bovine) or ECMO (monkey) viruses. None of these animal viruses has been implicated as an agent of human infection.

The original concept of ECHO viruses as "orphans," or "viruses in search of disease," has also undergone modification. In fact, we are now confronted with the converse problem of sorting out the diverse clinical manifestations caused by these agents that were formerly considered to be largely saprophytic. Although some ECHO types are still of doubtful etiologic significance and can be isolated from apparently healthy individuals, others have been shown to induce a wide variety of pathologic effects. Many of these disorders can also be caused by unrelated viruses (see p. 1112) and are discussed in other chapters of this book. Among the disease entities in which ECHO viruses have been found to play an etiologic role are enteroviral exanthems (p. 1162), aseptic meningitis (p. 1135), viral enteritis (p. 1134), and rarely, various forms of encephalomyelitis, some of which can simulate poliomyelitis (p. 1139). Some epidemics have been characterized by the occurrence of combinations of these symptom complexes in the same infected individuals. Although it is not possible to associate each type of ECHO virus with a specific illness, circumscribed outbreaks usually exhibit a preponderance of one clinical syndrome. For example, infections with ECHO virus type 16 often result in febrile exanthem and enanthem (Boston exanthem), whereas type 6 virus has caused epidemic meningitis without rash. ECHO virus type 9 has been associated with both meningitis and febrile exanthems in the same epidemic, or either clinical entity may occur alone. ECHO virus type 20 can be transmitted by the respiratory route, resulting in febrile catarrh. A large proportion of individuals in any epidemic may develop fever of short duration without other distinguishing manifestations of infection. There have also been isolated reports indicating that ECHO viruses occasionally can cause influenza-like illnesses, pleurodynia, pericarditis, ocular palsies, orchitis, minor hepatic dysfunction, postinfectious arthritis, and a syndrome simulating meningococcemia.

Despite the protean nature of these disorders, the constitutional manifestations of infection with ECHO viruses often follow a pattern similar to that of poliomyelitis. The course is frequently biphasic, dividing the illness into minor and major components. Fever is common at the onset, and the temperature may occasionally reach 105°F accompanied by true rigors. Most patients complain of frontal or retroorbital headache, anorexia, nausea, and vomiting; diffuse muscle and abdominal pains are not uncommon. Members of the ECHO group also infect the respiratory tract, frequently giving rise to cough, coryza, sore throat, and photophobia. As a good illustration of this, an agent recovered from pharyngeal secretions of patients during epidemics of acute febrile respiratory disease was originally known as the JH or 2060 respiratory virus but has been reclassified as ECHO virus type 28. Generalized lymphadenopathy has been a prominent finding in different epidemics, but splenomegaly is more variable. The total duration of illness varies from a few days to several weeks. Except for rare fatalities in infants, recovery is usually uneventful.

REFERENCES

Melnick, J. L., and A. B. Sabin: The ECHO Virus Group, p. 547 in "Viral and Rickettsial Infections of Man," 3d ed., T. M. Rivers and F. L. Horsfall, Jr. (Eds.), Philadelphia, J. B. Lippincott Company, 1959.

Sabin, A. B.: Role of ECHO Viruses in Human Disease, p. 78 in "Viral Infections of Infancy and Childhood," H. M. Rose (Ed.), New York, Paul B. Hoeber, Inc., Medical Department of Harper & Brothers, 1960.

Sanford, J. P., and S. E. Sulkin: The Clinical Spectrum of ECHO-Virus Infection, New Engl. J. Med., 262:1113, 1959.

186 VIRAL GASTROENTERITIS

*Robert R. Wagner and
Ivan L. Bennett, Jr.*

Bacterial and protozoan infections account for a minor fraction of the cases of gastroenteritis in the United States. Many of the remainder are probably not infectious in origin, but a significant proportion are thought to be of viral etiology. These viruses have been much less carefully studied than those associated with acute respiratory and systemic diseases. The frequency with which known enteric viruses produce symptoms of gastroenteritis without severe systemic illness has not been accurately determined. However, during epidemics of poliomyelitis, Coxsackie A and B infections, and infectious hepatitis, diarrhea can be the sole manifestation of infection, particularly in young children. Undoubtedly, the most important etiologic agents among the enteroviruses are various members of the ECHO group. During epidemics of diarrhea in infants and children, ECHO viruses, often of one type, have been recovered from feces in as many as 50 per cent of affected individuals. Serum antibody responses to the viruses isolated have also been demonstrated. Many children with severe illnesses are also infected with pathogenic strains of *Escherichia coli* (p. 932), a finding which has led to the hypothesis that combined viral-bacterial infection accounts for some cases of infantile diarrhea. Another important class of agents associated with gastroenteritis in children is the reovirus group (respiratory-enteric viruses), originally classified as ECHO virus type 10. As indicated by their name, infections with reoviruses may take the form of acute respiratory or gastrointestinal disease, or both. Other respiratory viruses can produce symptoms of gastroenteritis. Certain adenoviruses (p. 1116) appear to be particularly prone to cause vomiting and diarrhea, the incidence in some winter epidemics

ranging as high as 40 per cent of those individuals with respiratory symptoms. Although popularly called "intestinal flu," there is no evidence that winter gastrointestinal disorders are attributable to infection with influenza viruses.

Less is known about the viruses that cause gastrointestinal disorders in adults. Conventional laboratory methods have failed to disclose the etiology of most epidemics of nonbacterial gastroenteritis, although many of these studies were made before the availability of modern tissue culture methods. Gordon and his associates have shown that two filterable agents, presumably viruses, can be transmitted to volunteers by the oral but not by the respiratory route. Immunity to one agent persisted for at least 15 months in individuals who were fully susceptible to the other. Although the clinical and epidemiologic features of these two forms of gastroenteritis overlap considerably, it is convenient to classify them as *afebrile* and *febrile* types.

Afebrile Nonbacterial Gastroenteritis (Viral Dysentery). The incubation period is usually 2 to 3 days but varies from 1 to 5 days. The onset is often abrupt but may be gradual and preceded by malaise, anorexia, and nausea, which almost invariably persist throughout the illness. Vomiting can occur on the first day but is not prominent thereafter. Crampy abdominal pains of mild or moderate severity may be the first symptom. The most characteristic feature is persistent watery diarrhea without blood, mucus, or pus in the stools. Tenesmus is uncommon, although many patients have more than 20 bowel movements a day. Mild headache and fever with temperatures up to 101°F, a day or two after onset of gastrointestinal symptoms, are sometimes present. The usual duration of illness is 3 to 4 days but may be as long as a week.

Adults recover uneventfully without complications or sequelae. Young children can become severely dehydrated, requiring parenteral replacement of fluid and electrolyte losses. Symptomatic relief of diarrhea is best achieved with tincture of opium (paregoric) given after every bowel movement or every few hours.

Febrile Nonbacterial Gastroenteritis. The incubation period is 20 to 30 hr. The onset is usually abrupt and characterized by moderately severe colic, abdominal pain, and vomiting. Diarrhea is infrequent, although there may be an increased number of formed or soft stools. Chilliness and cold sweats may be present at the onset, and a temperature of 101 to 103°F, headache, malaise, and prostration are prominent features. The illness rarely lasts longer than 48 hr. Specific treatment is not available, but atropine may relieve the abdominal pain and vomiting.

A disorder known as "winter vomiting disease" appears to be similar in onset, duration, and clinical manifestations but is more frequently associated with diarrhea. It is only mildly contagious and has not been transmitted to volunteers.

Diarrheal Diseases Caused by ECHO Viruses. These disorders occur predominantly in children during the summer and autumn and may assume epidemic proportions. The incidence in adults is not known, but laboratory-acquired infections with ECHO virus type 11 resulted in an illness of abrupt onset and brief duration with watery diarrhea, severe vomiting, abdominal cramps, and chilliness. Intestinal infections with ECHO viruses are most severe in infants, who may require hospitalization for treatment of dehydration. Profuse diarrhea is almost invariable, and the stools frequently contain mucus or blood. Bulky and foamy stools have also been described. Vomiting occurs in the majority of cases but may be absent. Fever is generally present from the outset, but unless the illness is prolonged or complicated by severe dehydration, it is usually not prominent.

Differential Diagnosis. Dietary indiscretions, excessive ingestion of alcohol, and psychologic stress can precipitate vomiting and diarrhea that closely simulate acute viral gastroenteritis. Staphylococcal food poisoning (p. 898) invariably has a precipitous onset of severe vomiting and retching, ordinarily without fever or diarrhea, 1 to 6 hr after ingestion of the incriminated food. Salmonella gastroenteritis (p. 947) usually has a 12- to 48-hr incubation period and is often associated with systemic manifestations, fever, and leukocytosis. Outbreaks of food poisoning are characterized by explosive and simultaneous occurrence of symptoms in affected individuals without late secondary cases, whereas epidemics of "viral" gastroenteritis begin insidiously, usually continue for several weeks, and cannot be traced to food or water supplies. Mild shigellosis (p. 949) may be difficult to differentiate from "viral" gastroenteritis, but outbreaks usually result in cases with sustained fever, tenesmus, and bloody, purulent stools that contain dysentery bacilli.

REFERENCES

Dingle, J. H. et al.: A Study of Illness in a Group of Cleveland Families: XI. The Occurrence of Gastrointestinal Symptoms; XII. The Association of Respiratory and Gastrointestinal Symptoms, and Estimation of the Magnitude and Time Relations of the Association; XIII. Clinical Description of Nonbacterial Gastroenteritis; XIV. The Association of Respiratory and Gastrointestinal Symptoms; and Estimation of the Specific Symptomatology, Am. J. Hyg., 64:349, 357, 368, 376, 1956.

Eichenwald, H. F., et al: Epidemic Diarrhea in Premature and Older Infants Caused by ECHO Virus Type 18, J.A.M.A., 166:1563, 1958.

Gordon, I.: The Nonamebic Nonbacterial Diarrheal Disorders, Am. J. Trop. Med. Hyg., 4:739, 1955.

Jordan, W. S., Jr., I. Gordon, and W. R. Dorrance: A Study of Illness in a Group of Cleveland Families: VII. Transmission of Acute Nonbacterial Gastroenteritis to Volunteers: Evidence for Two Different Etiologic Agents, J. Exptl. Med., 98:461, 1953.

Ramos-Alvarez, M., and A. B. Sabin: Role of Enteropathogenic Viruses and Bacteria in Summer Diarrheal Diseases of Infancy and Early Childhood, J.A.M.A., 167:147, 1958.

Section 16: Viral Diseases of the Central Nervous System

187 VIRAL MENINGITIS AND THE SYNDROME OF ASEPTIC MENINGITIS

Ivan L. Bennett, Jr., and
Raymond D. Adams

More than 40 viruses are known to be capable of producing symptomatic injury to the human central nervous system although the frequency and severity of neurologic involvement vary widely for infection by different viruses or by different strains of a single virus. When neurologic manifestations appear during the course of a recognizable clinical entity of viral etiology such as mumps, chickenpox, or pleurodynia, diagnosis is usually easy. However, in illnesses where the overt evidences of organ involvement are confined to the nervous system, identification of the causative virus is a laborious and complicated procedure and even the most experienced laboratories fail to establish the etiology of 30 to 50 per cent of cases.

Despite the large number of viruses which are frequently or occasionally neurotropic, only three major constellations of symptoms and signs are elicited with regularity: (1) the syndrome of *poliomyelitis*, almost invariably a result of infection by one of the polioviruses, discussed in the next chapter (p. 1139); (2) the syndrome of *encephalitis* or *meningoencephalitis*, the manifestations and diverse etiologies of which are discussed beginning on p. 1152; and (3) the syndrome of *aseptic* or *nonsuppurative meningitis*, discussed in this chapter.

While the clinician is justified in suspecting a viral infection whenever one of these syndromes appears during a febrile illness, *other infective agents or inflammatory mechanisms can cause similar clinical pictures*. In most instances, the identification of a virus is achieved only after a patient is convalescent, and the information is useful in prognosis, in epidemiologic studies, or in planning prophylactic programs rather than as a guide to treatment. However, because several of the other disorders that can produce these syndromes are amenable to specific therapy, it is imperative to consider nonviral etiologic possibilities in every patient.

ASEPTIC MENINGITIS

Definition. The term *aseptic meningitis*, first used by Wallgren in 1925 to designate what was thought to be a specific disease, is now applied to a symptom complex that can be produced by many different agents. The syndrome consists of *fever, signs of meningeal irritation* (headache, stiff neck), and an *abnormal cerebrospinal fluid*. As a rule, frank signs of motor or sensory impairment are absent although drowsiness, confusion, and, rarely, convulsions or coma may appear.

The *cerebrospinal fluid findings* consist of *pleocytosis* (mainly mononuclear except in the initial stage) and *bacteriologic sterility*. The protein level is usually normal or slightly elevated. The concentration of glucose in the spinal fluid is extremely important; with rare exceptions, it is normal in viral infections. The findings of pleocytosis and low glucose in a spinal fluid that is bacteriologically sterile suggest *tuberculous meningitis* (p. 1016), *mycotic meningitis* (cryptococcal, p. 1053), or rare instances of meningeal involvement by *sarcoid, lymphoma*, or *metastatic carcinoma*. Because the spinal fluid glucose can be normal in the early stages of tuberculosis or cryptococcosis, this determination should be repeated at intervals until a diagnosis has been established or the patient is definitely convalescent.

In aseptic meningitis of viral origin, febrile illness seldom exceeds 10 days and recovery is complete without residual symptoms.

Viral Infections. The vast majority of cases of aseptic meningitis are accounted for by nonparalytic poliomyelitis (p. 1141), Coxsackie viruses (pp. 1130

and 1131), ECHO viruses (p. 1133), mumps (p. 1180), and lymphocytic choriomeningitis (see below). Indeed, these viral infections along with leptospirosis comprise more than 95 per cent of all cases of aseptic meningitis of established etiology.

In their milder forms, postvaccinal meningoencephalitis (p. 1165), or the central nervous system complications of measles (p. 1158), rubella (p. 1160), chickenpox (p. 1166), and rabies prophylaxis (p. 1149) produce aseptic meningitis. The diagnosis is usually made on the basis of recent illness or inoculation.

Herpes simplex (p. 1170) and the arthropodborne (arbor) encephalitis viruses (p. 1152) are responsible for a small proportion of cases of aseptic meningitis. Infections by the arbor viruses are likely to be encountered in epidemics along with cases of frank encephalitis and tend to occur in certain geographic areas, facilitating early clinical recognition although specific identification of the virus involved may be quite difficult.

Neurologic manifestations, including the syndrome of aseptic meningitis, appear occasionally in the course of influenza (p. 1123), psittacosis (p. 1126), lymphogranuloma venereum (p. 1177), Colorado tick fever (p. 1190), herpes zoster (p. 1168), West Nile fever (p. 1191), Rift Valley fever and encephalomyocarditis (p. 1195), and others of the "exotic" agents mentioned in Chap. 210 (p. 1192).

The icteric stage of infectious hepatitis (p. 1670) rarely is preceded by mild meningitis, the nature of which is readily evident when jaundice appears. Among diseases of possible or probable viral etiology, infectious mononucleosis (p. 1248) sometimes produces what appears to be a primary meningitis, and rarely, primary atypical pneumonia (p. 1120) is complicated by aseptic meningitis or other neurologic disorders.

Lymphocytic Choriomeningitis (LCM). This viral disease is responsible for 3 to 10 per cent of sporadic cases of aseptic meningitis throughout the world. The reservoir of infection is in lower animals of which mice are by far the most important. Mice acquire infection at or near birth, and despite the development of antibody, virus persists in urine and other excreta for life. Surveys have shown that as many as 20 per cent of wild mice are carriers, and infection is also endemic in many colonies of laboratory mice. Man acquires infection by direct exposure to animals or by inhalation of infected excreta in dust. Transmission among animals or from animals to man by arthropod vectors or by "superinfected" adult and larval forms of *Trichinella spiralis* have been shown to be feasible, but neither has been proved to occur naturally. Man-to-man transmission is extremely rare if, indeed, it occurs at all.

The *manifestations* of infection by the LCM virus

in man form a spectrum reminiscent of infection by the polioviruses (p. 1139). Serologic surveys indicate that inapparent or unrecognized infection is common in the population. It is also clear that symptomatic infection in man ordinarily consists of a clinically nonspecific, grippe-like, respiratory illness and that meningeal involvement is by no means a regular occurrence. Rather, neurologic manifestations appear only occasionally and as a late "complication," usually following a short remission of the initial symptoms.

The exact *incubation period* is not known but it is probably only a few days. There are remittent fever (sometimes with rigors), anorexia, malaise, generalized aching, headache, and respiratory manifestations ranging from pharyngitis, cough, and bronchitis, to frank pneumonia. Fever and discomfort often vary in their intensity, abating somewhat and then recurring over a period of 1 to 3 weeks. Many patients then recover completely. In others, however, apparent convalescence is interrupted by a recurrence of fever and the abrupt onset of headache, photophobia, and signs of meningeal irritation. This second stage of the disease ordinarily lasts 7 to 10 days and prompt recovery is the rule, but relapses or recurrences of meningeal symptoms are seen occasionally. A few patients exhibit transient erythematous or papular rashes during the meningeal phase. About 50 per cent of patients with aseptic meningitis caused by the LCM virus have radiologically demonstrable pulmonary infiltrates.

There is a mild leukopenia during the respiratory phase, but the peripheral leukocyte count is normal by the time of the onset of meningitis. The cerebrospinal fluid pressure may be increased; protein is normal or slightly elevated, and glucose is normal in the vast majority of cases. The cell count usually ranges from 100 to 3,000 mononuclears per cu mm, but counts of more than 30,000 have been noted.

The virus is present in the blood, nasopharynx, and urine during the respiratory illness and in the spinal fluid during meningitis. It can be isolated by intracerebral inoculation of mice or hamsters from *uninfected* colonies. Subcutaneous or intraperitoneal inoculation of guinea pigs is less satisfactory.

Specific serologic diagnosis depends upon demonstrating a rise in serum complement-fixing (after 2 weeks) or neutralizing (6 to 8 weeks) antibodies.

Rare fatalities during the initial illness have been reported. These patients showed high fever and leukocytosis, and at autopsy extensive hepatic necrosis and interstitial pneumonia were found. Also unusual is the occurrence of true encephalitis which can lead to death.

Other Causes. The isolation and characterization of newly discovered viruses will undoubtedly continue to reduce the proportion of cases of aseptic meningitis that remain undiagnosed even after complete laboratory study.

The most important nonviral cause of aseptic meningitis is *leptospirosis* (p. 1084). While the incidence of this infection varies, as many as 10 per cent of the cases in some areas are leptospiral in origin.

Acute syphilitic meningitis, usually a neurorelapse resulting from inadequate arsenotherapy in early syphilis, has virtually disappeared. Papilledema is frequent in this disease and this finding in a patient with aseptic meningitis should arouse immediate suspicion of syphilis. Occasionally, when lumbar puncture is performed on a patient with a febrile illness accompanied by headache, there will be found pleocytosis and elevated spinal fluid protein. This can lead to considerable confusion in establishing a correct diagnosis until it is realized that the spinal fluid abnormality is unrelated to the acute illness and that one is dealing with the coincidence of influenza or some similar disease in a patient with *asymptomatic neurosyphilis.*

Contiguous suppurative infection (mastoiditis, sinusitis, or brain abscess) can produce pleocytosis and elevation of spinal fluid protein (p. 1047). The spinal fluid glucose is normal and the fluid contains no microorganisms on smear or culture. The therapeutic importance of recognizing the nonviral etiology of this type of aseptic meningitis is self-evident.

Children with *scarlet fever* or *streptococcal pharyngitis* rarely develop meningeal signs and pleocytosis, the result of a sterile, "serous" inflammation that does not involve actual bacterial invasion of the meninges. Many patients with serum sickness (p. 1268) have abnormal spinal fluid and a few have frank signs of meningitis without evidence of serum neuropathy.

Headache, meningeal signs, and pleocytosis sometimes occur in the course of *systemic lupus erythematosus* (p. 1892).

Parasitic diseases in which involvement of the central nervous system occasionally takes the form of an aseptic meningitis (although it is more often a frank encephalitis) include *toxoplasmosis* (p. 1208), *schistosomiasis* (p. 1225), and *trichinosis* (p. 1221).

Finally, attention must be drawn to a clinical situation that is all too frequently seen. *Patients with pyogenic meningitis who are given antibiotics in inadequate dosage without examination of the spinal fluid* may be seen at a time when infection has been suppressed to the point that mononuclear cells predominate, glucose is normal, and organisms are not detectable in the spinal fluid. A mistaken diagnosis of aseptic meningitis is often made when the spinal fluid is first examined; the true state of affairs becomes evident only when the patient worsens and bacteria again appear. Careful attention to a history of recent antimicrobial therapy sometimes permits recognition of these cases before serious symptoms recur.

Diagnosis. In any patient suspected of viral meningitis, serum should be stored for future serologic comparison with convalescent specimens, and if viral isolation is to be attempted, properly collected specimens of stool, nasopharyngeal secretions, blood, cerebrospinal fluid, and urine should be transmitted to the laboratory.

Clinical distinctions between the many different forms of aseptic meningitis cannot be made with a high degree of reliability, but useful leads can be obtained by careful attention to certain details of history and physical examination.

The *season* during which illness occurs may be helpful. Enteroviral infections (poliomyelitis, Coxsackie, ECHO) are diseases of midsummer and early fall, August and September usually being peak months. The arthropod-borne diseases also occur in summer and fall (coinciding with the population of insect vectors), and while leptospirosis may occur at any season, its incidence in the United States shows a striking peak in August. Mumps and infectious mononucleosis occur in late winter and spring. Lymphocytic choriomeningitis is particularly common in late fall and winter, presumably because field mice enter dwellings at this time.

A definite past history of mumps aids in excluding this disease, second attacks being very unusual. A history of syphilis should be inquired about carefully. Preceding upper respiratory infection of long duration suggests lymphocytic choriomeningitis. Sore throat, lymphadenopathy, or rash point to infectious mononucleosis or ECHO infection.

Severe back and leg pain occur in poliomyelitis, leptospirosis, and trichinosis. Aseptic meningitis during pregnancy is likely to be poliomyelitis. Exposure to animals such as mice (LCM), dogs, rats, or swine (leptospirosis) may give a hint in diagnosis. Swimming in stagnant water, or an occupation such as veterinary medicine, poultry or fish dressing, and sewer work suggests leptospirosis.

Leptospirosis is predominantly a disease of males; in some series more than 90 per cent of patients are men, a disproportion not accounted for entirely by occupational exposure. Leptospirosis is unusual in children; the reasons for this are unknown. Mumps meningitis is at least five times more common in males than in females.

The presence of any condition which is known to predispose to brain abscess constitutes important information. These include recent pneumonia, chronic pulmonary suppuration, empyema, bacterial endocarditis, congenital heart disease, otitis, and sinusitis.

Careful search for *rash* must be made in considering infectious mononucleosis, ECHO viral infection, and leptospirosis (often a transient, blotchy erythema). *Icterus* suggests infectious mononucleosis or viral hepatitis; it is not present in pure meningeal leptospirosis. *Conjunctival suffusion* is common in leptospirosis and may be seen in trichinosis. The *salivary glands* and *testes* should be examined with special care; minimal involvement may be the only indication of mumps. The presence of *pulmonary infiltrates* suggests LCM, leptospirosis, infectious mononucleosis, or psittacosis.

Few laboratory tests are helpful. The peripheral leukocyte count is often normal, but leukopenia can accompany so many of the diseases responsible for aseptic meningitis (infectious mononucleosis, Colorado tick fever, LCM, lupus erythematosus, etc.) that it is rarely a useful finding. Eosinophilia should suggest a parasitic infestation, leukocytosis may accompany brain abscess, and occasionally, infectious mononucleosis will first be recognized by the blood smear. LCM produces the highest pleocytosis, and aseptic meningitis with spinal fluid cell counts of 3,000 or more mononuclears is almost surely this disease. Serologic tests for syphilis performed on spinal fluid in meningitis must be interpreted with caution because inflammation of many types can produce a false positive reaction. Infectious mononucleosis and lupus erythematosus can elicit biologic false positive serum tests for syphilis. Liver function tests are abnormal in many patients with infectious mononucleosis and in anicteric hepatitis; hepatic abnormalities are not regularly present in the other entities under consideration.

In summary, while clinical findings, seasonal occurrence, and laboratory tests can sometimes enable the physician to direct further diagnostic efforts along specific lines, they are rarely conclusive. Most important is constant attention to the possible presence of tuberculosis, cryptococcosis, syphilis, brain abscess, or inadequately treated pyogenic meningitis masquerading temporarily as the syndrome of aseptic meningitis.

REFERENCES

Adair, C. V., R. L. Gould, and J. E. Smadel: Aseptic Meningitis, A Disease of Diverse Etiology: Clinical and Etiologic Studies on 854 Cases, Ann. Internal Med., 39:675, 1953.

Beeson, P. B., and D. H. Hankey: Leptospiral Meningitis, A.M.A. Arch. Internal Med., 89:575, 1952.

Heyman, A.: Acute Syphilitic Meningitis: A Discussion of the Problems Encountered in the Diagnosis, Am. J. Med. Sci., 209:664, 1945.

Janeway, C. H., and T. W. Farmer: Infections with the Virus of Lymphocytic Choriomeningitis, Medicine, 21:1, 1942.

Meyer, H. M. et al.: Central Nervous System Syndromes of "Viral" Etiology, Am. J. Med., 29:334, 1960.

Weinstein, L.: Neurologic Complications of Infectious Diseases, G. P., vol. VI, No. 4, p. 67, October, 1952.

Wallgren, A.: Une nouvelle maladie infectieuse du systeme nerveux central?, Acta Paediat., 4:158, 1925.

Walsh, J. W.: Peripheral Neuropathy and Serous Meningitis Due to Horse Serum, New Engl. J. Med., 247:88, 1952.

Warren, J.: Lymphocytic Choriomeningitis, in "Viral and Rickettsial Infections of Man," 3d ed., pp. 900–903, T. M. Rivers and F. L. Horsfall, Jr., (Eds.) Philadelphia, Lippincott, 1956.

188 POLIOMYELITIS

Louis Weinstein

Definition. Poliomyelitis is a common acute viral infection which occurs naturally only in man and produces a wide variety of clinical manifestations. In its most severe form, it involves parts of the central nervous system. In most instances, the nervous system is not invaded; infection may take place without apparent illness, or it may result in the production of nonspecific syndromes or in invasion of the nervous system with or without the development of dysfunction.

Etiology. The causative agent of poliomyelitis is a virus ranging from 8 to 30 mμ in diameter, pathogenic for man, monkeys, and chimpanzees. Three antigenically distinct types have been defined: type I (Brunhilde), type II (Lansing), and type III (Leon). Although some degree of cross neutralization is demonstrable in highly immunized experimental animals, infection in man with one type does not protect against invasion by another. Poliomyelitis virus grows well in tissue culture.

The viruses of poliomyelitis may remain viable in water or sewage, under proper conditions, for as long as 4 months. They are not killed by ether, Merthiolate, tincture of Zephiran, ethyl alcohol, or low concentrations of phenol, but are inactivated by heat, bichloride of mercury, oxidizing agents, 2 per cent tincture of iodine, ultraviolet light, and 10-min exposure to a chlorine concentration of 0.05 ppm.

Epidemiology. Poliomyelitis is world-wide, but epidemics have been limited to a relatively small number of areas. That the disease is much more prevalent than is suggested by the number of clinically recognized cases is proved by the widespread distribution of neutralizing antibody to the virus in population groups in which it was thought to be rare. In areas where infection without involvement of the nervous system occurs, about 95 per cent of the disease is clinically unapparent. Polio-

myelitis occurs mainly in the warm months of the year, with the highest frequency from July through September in the North Temperate Zone, although it may appear as early as April or as late as December. In tropical or subtropical regions, the "season" may be prolonged.

Certain environmental factors are of importance in determining the risk of exposure to poliomyelitis virus and the development of infection. In areas of poor sanitation, most individuals develop neutralizing antibodies in early childhood, whereas in localities where sanitation is good, the peak of population immunity is not reached until fifteen years of age or older. Urban dwellers become immune earlier than those who live in rural areas. In lower-income groups, evidence of contact with poliomyelitis virus appears at a younger age than in individuals whose financial status is good; this may only reflect differences in crowding and sanitation. In some parts of the world, certain racial groups appear to be more susceptible than others, but this is not constant for a particular race in a different area.

Poliomyelitis was most common in the preschool child until about 25 years ago. In the past quarter of a century, however, it has been increasing in older age groups; in some recent epidemics, 25 to 30 per cent of patients have been older than fifteen years of age. The increase in adult cases is not due merely to aging of the population or increased reporting of paralytic and nonparalytic cases. Young children are still affected more often than adults. Paralytic disease has been described in the neonatal period and late in the sixth decade of life but is very uncommon at these age extremes.

Pathogenesis. Man is the sole reservoir of poliomyelitis virus. Human carriers, especially those with unapparent infection, are most important in transmission of the virus to susceptible contacts; history of contact with recognized cases is uncommon. Milk has been incriminated as the source of infection in one epidemic.

Virus is present in the stool and oropharynx of patients with poliomyelitis regardless of the clinical type of disease. It is recoverable from pharyngeal secretions for only a few days but is demonstrable in the feces for several weeks. The weight of opinion favors the intestinal tract as the main source from which virus is disseminated. The mode of infection is, therefore, fecal-oral, the same as that in salmonellosis, shigellosis, and other enteric infections. Very small quantities of stool contain thousands of infective doses of poliomyelitis virus. Large quantities of virus are present in sewage drained from areas in which the infection is present. The role of the fly in the transmission of poliomyelitis is not settled. Flies trapped in areas close to cases of poliomyelitis may carry the virus. Food exposed to flies from homes in which poliomyelitis was present has produced the disease in monkeys to whom it was fed. Attempts to reduce the spread of disease in epidemics by eradication of the fly population, however, has not been successful. Poliomyelitis is as highly communicable as measles or varicella; in individuals under fifteen years of age, infection, with or without clinical manifestations, occurs in 100 per cent of household and 87 per cent of daily contacts.

The theory that poliomyelitis virus multiplies only in nervous tissue and reaches the central nervous system only by way of peripheral nerves from the pharynx or intestinal tract has been seriously questioned because of the demonstration of viremia prior to the onset of clinical manifestations. Although the exact mechanism still remains to be proved, the following sequence of events has been postulated on the basis of experimental and clinical observations: (1) The virus enters by way of the mouth and begins to multiply in the oropharynx and lower intestinal tract. It escapes from either area; there is no conclusive evidence as to which is more important in transmission. The site of viral growth is probably extraneural. Virus is present in pharyngeal secretions and stool during the incubation period; it has been demonstrated in the feces as long as 19 days prior to onset of the disease. (2) The phase of "minor illness" (described below) develops in association with the presence of the virus in the blood, throat, and feces, the viremia persisting for only a few days until antibodies make their appearance. The following migration of the infectious agent has been suggested: Virus in the intestinal tract penetrates the lymphatic channels and enters the blood stream, from which it is disseminated into the interstitial tissue spaces and then reaches the lymph nodes, where it may be detected for a period after the stage of viremia. There is still some question whether viremia is primary and is followed by invasion of the nervous system, or whether it is merely a manifestation of spill-over from already infected neural tissues. (3) The final stage in the pathogenesis of poliomyelitis is invasion of the nervous system. This is thought to follow the viremic stage, during which the agent gains a foothold in the nervous system, in which it multiplies. It has been suggested that the virus enters the nervous system from the blood at one point, perhaps the area postrema in the medulla oblongata, because this is more penetrable than other parts of the brain to dyes injected intravascularly; it has also been postulated, however, that viral invasion of the nervous system occurs at many points by direct passage of virus from capillaries to neurones. Once the infectious agent has reached the nervous system, it spreads along nerve fibers.

Central nervous system invasion in poliomyelitis results from the simultaneous operation of two groups of factors: (1) those associated with the virus and (2) those related to the host. Strains of poliomyelitis virus vary greatly in their ability to invade nervous tissue from the blood or intestinal tract and to destroy neurones. Repeated passage in animals or tissue cultures induces changes in invasive capacity without affecting the basic antigenic character of the agent. One of the host factors important in determining susceptibility to disease of the nervous system is type-specific neutralizing antibody, which is present even before the onset of symptoms. The early presence of detectable immunity is in favor of multiplication of virus in nonnervous tissue, and accounts for the short persistence of virus in the pharynx and blood, sites in which antibody is demonstrable. The persistence of virus in the nervous system and intestine is probably due to the difficulty which antibody has in reaching these areas.

The most important determinant of human susceptibility to poliomyelitis is *serum antibody*. Previous inapparent infection and illness without invasion of the nervous system are common in areas where the paralytic form of the disease occurs; these produce resistance to reinvasion. Many children and most adults possess neutralizing antibody for all three types of virus; this probably accounts for the relative infrequency of the disease in older age groups. Infants under six months old rarely get poliomyelitis because immunity is passively transferred from the mother. Babies born to women in the acute phase of poliomyelitis can develop the disease shortly after birth. The *sex* of patients plays a role in determining susceptibility. Among children, males are affected more often than females; the opposite is true in adults. *Pregnancy* increases the risk of clinically apparent poliomyelitis. Multiparous females are more susceptible than primiparas. The disease is somewhat more frequent in the second than in the first or third trimesters. *Menstruation* or *ovulation* appears to heighten susceptibility. *Absence of the tonsils and adenoids,* regardless of the time of their removal, is associated with a marked increase in incidence of bulbar poliomyelitis. *Chilling or physical exertion* after invasion by the virus leads to more frequent development of paralytic poliomyelitis, especially in adults.

CLINICAL MANIFESTATIONS

The incubation period of poliomyelitis varies from 3 to 35 days; about 80 per cent of cases occur within 6 to 20 days after contact with the virus. The disease may assume one of four forms: (1) unapparent infection, (2) "minor illness," (3) nonparalytic poliomyelitis, (4) paralytic poliomyelitis.

Unapparent Infection

In families in which a clinically recognized case of poliomyelitis is present, other susceptible members usually develop unapparent infection. The bulk of infection with the virus of poliomyelitis (95 per cent) occurs in this form. There are no symptoms, but the virus is present in the pharynx and intestine. It is probably also present in the blood. Type-specific neutralizing antibody usually develops.

"Minor Illness"

The entire course of poliomyelitis may consist of a nonspecific illness without clinical or laboratory evidence of central nervous system invasion; this is "abortive" poliomyelitis. Three syndromes have been observed: (1) upper respiratory manifestations, consisting of fever of varying degree, pharyngeal discomfort, with or without coryza, and reddening and swelling of the lymphoid tissues of the throat; (2) gastrointestinal disturbances, with nausea, vomiting, diarrhea, or constipation, and abdominal discomfort, accompanied by moderate fever; (3) grippelike disease with fever and generalized aching of muscle, bones, and joints, resembling influenza. Virus can be demonstrated in the pharynx, feces, and blood in the early stages of these "minor" illnesses. Type-specific neutralizing and complement-fixing antibodies develop during convalescence.

Nonparalytic Poliomyelitis

Nonparalytic poliomyelitis consists of prodromal manifestations, signs of meningeal irritation, and abnormalities of the spinal fluid. The prodrome is similar to that of the "minor" illnesses and is usually present for several days before the onset of other signs; it may be entirely absent. Stiffness of the neck and back, positive Kernig's signs, and, with severe meningeal irritation, leg and neck Brudzinski's signs are present. The tripod (patient extends arms behind back with hands on bed for support when sitting up) and Hoyne's signs (head falls back when, with patient in supine position, shoulders are elevated) can be elicited in paralytic or nonparalytic poliomyelitis but are not pathognomonic. The spinal fluid usually contains between 25 and 500 cells, rarely as many as 1,000 to 2,000. Very early in the disease, there is often a preponderance of neutrophils (up to 80 per cent); within a few days, however, mononuclear cells predominate. The protein is normal or slightly elevated at the beginning of the illness but may increase to between 50 and 100 mg per 100 ml. The sugar content is normal or moderately elevated. These findings indicate an inflammatory reaction of the meninges but are not diagnostic of poliomyelitis. They are also present in healing bacterial meningitis, tuberculous

meningitis, focal embolic encephalomyelitis (subacute bacterial endocarditis), scarlet fever, pertussis encephalopathy, leptospiral meningitis, syphilis, mumps meningitis, Coxsackie virus infections, herpes simplex meningitis, infectious mononucleosis, trichinella meningitis, brain abscess, multiple sclerosis, tumors of the brain or spinal cord, allergic reactions involving the nervous system, postinfectious encephalitides, "infectious" polyneuritis, and lymphocytic choriomeningitis. The diagnosis of nonparalytic poliomyelitis on clinical grounds alone is impossible, because the signs, symptoms, and laboratory findings are completely nonspecific. Viral and immunologic studies suggest that less than 40 per cent of cases of "nonparalytic poliomyelitis" are actually this disease; mumps meningitis without salivary gland involvement (p. 1180) and Coxsackie vrius disease (p. 1131) are the two most common differential diagnoses.

The course of nonparalytic poliomyelitis is benign. Defervescence usually occurs in 3 to 5 days, but meningeal irritation may persist for as long as 2 weeks. No changes in reflexes or in muscle and cranial nerve function are detectable. The white blood count may be as high as 15,000 in the early stage of the disease but is usually normal within 1 week. The spinal fluid often shows mononuclear pleocytosis and elevated protein for 2 to 3 weeks after the onset of the disease.

Paralytic Poliomyelitis

The syndrome of paralytic poliomyelitis consists of prodromal manifestations ("minor" illness), signs of meningeal irritation, abnormal spinal fluid, and signs of involvement of motor nerve cells in the spinal cord, brain, or cranial nerve nuclei, resulting in paresis or paralysis of various muscles. Lesions may also be present in parts of the nervous system other than anterior horn cells; the precentral gyrus, the reticular formation in the medulla, the roof nuclei and vermis of the cerebellum, Auerbach's and Meissner's plexuses, and sympathetic ganglions are usually found to be involved in fatal cases. Seldom, however, are there clinical signs pointing to disease of these parts. "Skip" areas are common in spinal paralytic disease; e.g., involvement of the cervical and lumbar cords is often present with no dysfunction of the thoracic portion.

Paralytic poliomyelitis may be subdivided into the following types:

I. Spinal
   A. Cervical
   B. Thoracic
   C. Lumbar
   D. Any combination of A, B, and C
II. Bulbar
   A. Upper cranial nerve involvement—III,IV,V,VI, VII,VIII

B. Lower cranial nerve involvement—IX,X,XI,XII
C. Involvement of cardiorespiratory centers
III. Bulbospinal
IV. Polioencephalitis—paralytic or nonparalytic
   A. Diffuse encephalitis
   B. Focal encephalitis
   C. Cerebellar involvement (?)
   D. Bulboencephalitic disease
   E. Spinalencephalitic disease

Prodromal manifestations are often absent in paralytic poliomyelitis. In some cases, the illness is biphasic in character. In these cases, the disease starts with fever and manifestations of one of the "minor" illnesses. After several days, all symptoms disappear; in 5 or 10 days, there is recrudescence of fever, the development of signs of meningeal irritation, and the appearance of paralysis. The commonest prodromal symptoms in adults are generalized muscle and bone discomfort. In children, upper respiratory tract syndromes are most frequent. The spinal fluid findings in paralytic poliomyelitis are the same as those in the nonparalytic disease and bear no relationship to the severity of involvement or prognosis. It has been stated that the spinal fluid is completely normal in about 10 per cent of cases of poliomyelitis. This incidence is too high because of the inclusion of cases of "nonparalytic poliomyelitis," many of which, as pointed out above, are instances of some other disease. In the author's experience, paralytic poliomyelitis may be accompanied by a completely normal spinal fluid throughout its entire course, but this occurs in no more than 0.5 per cent of cases. In some patients, decrease in number of cells in the spinal fluid is accompanied by a progressive rise in protein, which may reach levels high enough to cause confusion with the cytoalbuminologic dissociation observed in "infectious" polyneuritis.

Spinal Paralytic Poliomyelitis. In the early stages of spinal paralytic poliomyelitis, cramping pain in the muscles innervated by the affected neurones and hyperesthesia of the overlying skin are present. The discomfort may be very severe; muscle "spasm," the exact mechanism of which is not clear, is usually detectable. Paralysis may not appear for some time after the onset of symptoms. In some instances, increase in muscle weakness is very slow; in others, it becomes widespread within 48 hr. Rarely, a rapidly ascending paralysis of the Landry type is observed. Age is one factor in determining the extent of involvement. In children less than five years old, paresis of one leg is most common. In patients between five and fifteen years of age, weakness of one arm, or paraplegia, is most frequent, while in adults (sixteen to sixty-five years old), quadriplegia is observed most often. Dysfunction of the urinary bladder is at least ten times more frequent in adults than in children. Paralysis of the

muscles of respiration is most common in those older than sixteen years of age. Infants younger than one year are subject to very extensive involvement. Among adults, men develop quadriplegia, respiratory paralysis, and loss of bladder function more frequently than do women. Pregnancy does not increase the severity of the disease unless parturition takes place during the acute phase. There is a definite association of inoculation of antigenic materials ("triple vaccine," for example) with an increased risk of involvement of the muscles around the site of injection.

The location of muscle weakness depends on the portion of the spinal cord affected. Isolated infection of the cervical, thoracic, or lumbar areas may be present, or two or more parts of the cord may be involved simultaneously. The lumbar area is the one most frequently damaged.

When the cervical portion of the spinal cord is involved, there is paresis or paralysis of the muscles of the shoulders, arms, neck, and diaphragm. Very early in the disease, the reflexes in the arms remain lively; they diminish rapidly, however, and are usually absent by the time paralysis has become established. Coarse twitching of the affected shoulder or arm muscles is common. With cervical cord disease, there is always danger of respiratory paralysis due to spread of the infection to the motor nuclei of the phrenic nerves and medulla.

Weakness of the muscles of the chest, upper portion of the abdomen, and spine follows involvement of the thoracic portion of the spinal cord. Difficulty in breathing results from dysfunction of the intercostal and other thoracic muscles. The chest wall may be in "spasm" and may appear rigid despite the presence of only a minor degree of paresis. Twitching of the thoracic, abdominal, or spine-supporting muscles may sometimes be noted.

Disease of the lumbar portion of the spinal cord produces weakness of the muscles of the legs and inferior portions of the abdomen and back. Again, pain, tenderness, "spasm," and twitching herald the oncoming paralysis, and the reflexes are abolished with the development of flaccid paralysis. Dysfunction of the iliopsoas muscles, indicated by inability to sit up from a lying position, the hip muscles, quadriceps femoris, hamstring, and gastrocnemii, peroneals, anterior tibials, tensor fasciae latae, glutei, and sartorius may occur in various combinations. In adults, complete paraplegia is not infrequent. Paralysis of the urinary bladder, usually temporary, occurs in about one-third of patients over sixteen years of age and is rarely observed in the absence of weakness of the legs.

The abdominal and cremasteric reflexes usually disappear before muscle weakness is marked in paralytic poliomyelitis and may be absent during the entire course of the disease. An extensor plantar response (positive Babinski) has been elicited in a few cases during the first 1 or 2 days but is a rare finding; its persistence or late development is incompatible with poliomyelitis. Hyperesthesia of the skin is frequent. Sensory loss does not occur. Constipation, abdominal cramps, and meteorism are common in spinal paralytic poliomyelitis and are due to partial ileus resulting from involvement of the autonomic nervous system and weakness of the abdominal muscles. When the disease is severe, sympathetic nervous system disturbances, with tachycardia, hypertension, abnormal sweating, and cyanosis and coldness of the involved extremities, not due to superficial vasospasm, are present.

Fever in spinal paralytic poliomyelitis is usually present for the first few days of the disease and disappears by lysis. In about 90 per cent of cases, there is little or no extension of paralysis after defervescence has been established for about 48 hr. In about 10 per cent, however, progression of weakness may continue for as long as a week or more and may be of notable degree.

Bulbar Poliomyelitis. The incidence of bulbar poliomyelitis differs from one epidemic to another and varies between 6 and 25 per cent. In patients subjected to tonsilloadenoidectomy within 30 days of onset of the disease and in those in whom the operation was carried out years before, the bulbar form of infection is present in about 85 per cent of cases. Pure bulbar involvement (without any signs of spinal cord involvement) is commonest in children; adults with bulbar disturbances usually have associated spinal paralyses. The prodromal manifestations of bulbar poliomyelitis are often the same as in the spinal form. The syndromes which develop depend on the area of the brain stem involved, and result from damage to the medulla, pons, and midbrain. Signs and symptoms are produced by (1) dysfunction of the upper cranial nerve nuclei, (2) damage to the lower cranial nerve nuclei, and (3) disturbances of the respiratory and vasomotor regulating centers in the medulla. Combined bulbar and diffuse or focal encephalitis or spinal involvement may occur.

Upper Cranial Nerve Nuclei—III, IV, V, VI, VII, VIII. Isolated ocular nerve palsies, total external ophthalmoplegia, pupillary disorders, and Horner's syndrome occur. There may be unilateral or bilateral involvement of the fifth nerve, with difficulty in chewing and closing the mouth, as well as deviation of the jaws. Paralysis of the seventh cranial nerve is common and usually unilateral; the entire face or only the upper or lower parts may be affected. Disturbances of vestibular function and deafness resulting from damage to the nucleus of the eighth nerve occur infrequently.

Lower Cranial Nerve Nuclei—IX, X, XI, XII. Life may be endangered when the muscles of de-

glutition are paralyzed because of involvement of the nucleus ambiguus in the medulla. With involvement of these nerves, the voice has a nasal quality and movement of one or both halves of the soft palate is decreased or absent. Saliva collects in the hypopharynx because of difficulty in swallowing and not because of excessive secretion. Hoarseness and laryngeal stridor follow weakness or paralysis of the vocal cords. Unilateral or bilateral weakness of the tongue, sternocleidomastoid, and trapezius muscles may be present. Inability to swallow results in pooling of saliva and food in the pharynx, with obstruction to the airway. Aspiration of fluid into the larynx, reflex spasm of the glottis, and abductor paralysis of the vocal cords constitute very serious threats to life. Minor or major pareses of the soft palate and pharyngeal muscles are detectable by a nasal quality of the voice.

Disease of the medullary respiratory center produces irregularity of the rhythm, depth, and rate of breathing. Respirations are shallow and, as the disease progresses, are interrupted by longer and longer periods of apnea until breathing stops completely. The thoracic muscles and diaphragm are not weak, unless spinal involvement is present. Hiccoughing is frequent in the early phase of respiratory center dysfunction. Hypoxia, without visible cyanosis, is common and contributes to the intensity of the manifestations. In the late stages, cyanosis, unresponsive to oxygen administration, is commonly present, and the temperature, pulse rate, and blood pressure are elevated. The final event is usually shock, which, in the majority of cases, is irreversible despite heroic measures.

The manifestations of involvement of the circulatory regulating center are a deep cherry-red color of the lips, flushed florid appearance of the skin, a very rapid, irregular pulse, small pulse pressure when the blood pressure is normal, and moderate to severe hypotension. Hyperthermia, cold, mottled, clammy skin, shallow respiration, and anxiety, restlessness, and confusion appear as the circulatory mechanism becomes progressively more impaired and irreversible shock develops.

Polioencephalitis. Encephalitic symptoms occur as isolated syndromes or together with bulbar or spinal poliomyelitis. The incidence of polioencephalitis is variable; one small epidemic in which most of the patients had this type of disease has been described. Symptoms of diffuse or focal involvement of the brain may be present. The diffuse form is characterized by confusion, agitation, anxiety with a feeling of impending doom, or somnolence. Quivering, trembling, twitching, and jerking of the facial muscles and extremities, flushing of the face, tremor of the hands, and restless movements occur. Insomnia may be severe. In fatal cases, the confusion is marked and progresses to lethargy and death.

In focal polioencephalitis, there may be clinical evidence of brain damage, or the lesions may be silent and demonstrable only at necropsy. Visual-verbal agnosia, myoclonic jerks, grand mal convulsions, which occasionally persist for a long time after recovery, spastic hemiparesis, ataxia of one arm or leg, and hydrocephalus have been described.

The diagnosis of paralytic poliomyelitis can usually be made on clinical grounds. The outstanding manifestations are a lower motor neurone lesion of rapid development with flaccid weakness and hypo- or areflexia. Signs of upper motor neurone disease or decreased sensation are not compatible with poliomyelitis. Among the diseases which may cause confusion, especially in their early stages, are toxic, "infectious," or idiopathic polyneuritis, the post-infectious encephalitides, viral encephalitides, trichinosis, acute rheumatic fever, cerebrovascular accidents with paralysis, acute syphilitic meningitis (frequent cranial nerve palsies), meningomyelo-encephalitis resulting from sensitization to foreign protein (horse serum, rabies vaccine, pertussis vaccine), osteomyelitis, scurvy, acute multiple sclerosis, pseudobulbar palsy, myalgic meningoencephalitis (Iceland, Tallahassee, or Coventry disease), spinal epidural abscess or tumor, neoplasms of the brain and spinal cord, Coxsackie virus infection, the encephalitis of the preicteric phase of infectious hepatitis, infectious mononucleosis with neurologic involvement, infections due to the enteric cytopathogenic human "orphan" (ECHO) viruses, focal embolic encephalitis associated with subacute bacterial endocarditis, tuberculous meningitis with hemiplegia or cranial nerve (especially the sixth) palsies, and brain abscess. Study of these diseases over a period of a few days to a week after onset clarifies the situation in most instances. The only positive method of establishing the diagnosis of paralytic poliomyelitis is the isolation of the virus from the stool or pharyngeal secretions (spinal cord or brain at necropsy) and the demonstration of a rise in the level of neutralizing antibody to the isolated strain in acute- and convalescent-phase serums. If virus cannot be isolated, the three type strains maintained in tissue culture may be used; a significant rise in titer of neutralizing antibody against a specific serotype is diagnostic.

Medical Complications. Paralytic poliomyelitis, especially in adults, often presents a number of serious and potentially lethal complications. These complications occur most frequently when the respiratory muscles are involved because of involvement of spinal or bulbar motor neurones; they are, at times, the direct cause of death. Disturbances in water and electrolyte balance are common in patients receiving continuous artificial respiration. Fever and the sweating which follows enclosure in a tank during the summer months, together with vomiting, diarrhea, inability to take food, and disturbances in carbon dioxide related to improperly regulated ventilation, produce a series of chemical disturbances, the repair of which taxes the ingenuity of the physician. Edema and low electrolyte levels often follow overenthusiastic hydration and have been misinterpreted as evidence of a salt-wasting syndrome. Myocarditis is not uncommon in poliomyelitis; it is probably due to direct viral invasion. ECG changes, mainly T, and ST-T and P-R abnormalities, are present in from 10 to 20 per cent of cases. Interstitial infiltration of the myocardium with round cells and mild muscle changes are not infrequent and occurs in a few cases along with degenerative changes in muscle fibers. Verrucous endocarditis involving the mitral valve has been described. Severe myocardopathy has been thought to be responsible for death in some cases. Hypertension may develop and is produced by two mechanisms: (1) transient elevation of blood pressure due to hypoxia, and (2) persistent hypertension secondary to *hypothalamic involvement,* which may become "malignant" and lead to severe retinopathy, convulsions, and mental deterioration, unless treated.

Pulmonary edema and shock, the exact pathogenesis of which is not known, are usually the terminal events in fatal cases of poliomyelitis. Although relatively young adults are involved, phlebothrombosis of the legs with or without pulmonary embolism is not uncommon. All methods of artificial respiration produce hemodynamic disturbances, which are countered by reflex mechanisms acting to maintain normal blood pressure and cardiac output. When patients are placed in respirators under negative tank pressure (positive intratracheal pressure) after hypotension and impending shock are already present, the peripheral vascular collapse often is made worse. Acute and marked dilatation of the stomach and large bowel, perforation of the cecum, acute ulceration of the duodenum, stomach, and esophagus, the formation of multiple erosions of the entire gastrointestinal tract with considerable bleeding and paralytic ileus have been observed. Marked depression of prothrombin, with massive spontaneous hemorrhage, occurs in individuals with severe poliomyelitis, especially if they are receiving large doses of broad-spectrum antibiotics orally. Severe bulbar (ninth and tenth cranial nerves) or bulbospinal disease with paralysis of the breathing muscles is accompanied by the risk of major pulmonary atelectases. Bacterial infection is one of the most dangerous complications of paralytic poliomyelitis. Pneumonia is quite common in patients with paralysis of the muscles of respiration or deglutition. The incidence of pulmonary infection is greatly increased by tracheostomy and is highest in the respirator case subjected to this oper-

The impact of paralytic poliomyelitis on the social and economic status of adults is often very severe. Every effort must be made to enlist the cooperation of social service agencies to minimize the disruptive effects of the disease. Many patients require occupational rehabilitation because of inability to perform the work in which they were engaged prior to being crippled. For others, the use of devices, such as movable splints, hooks, etc., is very helpful in physical rehabilitation, if this cannot be accomplished surgically.

Prognosis

The over-all mortality rate for poliomyelitis is about 5 per cent. Patients with the "abortive" and nonparalytic types of the disease recover completely. About 2 to 5 per cent of children and 15 to 30 per cent of adults (increasing with age) with paralyzing infection die. When bulbospinal involvement, especially with medullary or phrenic and intercostal nerve dysfunction, is present, the fatality rate varies between 25 and 75 per cent; in these cases, it is greatly influenced by age and the presence of shock, pulmonary edema, superimposed infection, or other medical complications.

Many persons with paralytic poliomyelitis recover completely. In a considerable number, there is return of muscle function to some degree. Only a few remain totally paralyzed. It is striking, though paradoxical, that the more life-threatening the disease in the acute stage, the more frequent is complete functional recovery, if the patient survives. Thus, paralysis of the respiratory center usually disappears completely. Dysfunction of the ninth and tenth cranial nerves is followed by total recovery in most instances, although mild palatopharyngeal weakness may occasionally persist for life. Paralysis of the muscles of respiration often disappears completely. In some cases, the final vital capacity, although reduced, is adequate to maintain ventilation, even with moderate physical exertion. In very few instances is chronic respirator care necessary. Weak extremities regain about 60 per cent of the total strength that they will ever recover in 3 months, and 80 per cent within 6 months. Improvement may continue for as long as 2 years. The final degree of functional return depends on the number of neurones totally destroyed; it varies from as low as none to 10 per cent to as high as 100 per cent.

Prevention

Because 90 to 95 per cent of cases of poliomyelitis are unapparent, or "minor," infections and are not diagnosed, the prevention of the disease by isolation is very difficult. The common practice of isolating clinically evident cases is of much greater individual than public health benefit. The usual period of isolation is about 2 weeks, although virus may be present in the feces for a much longer period. Contact with known cases should be avoided. Restriction of community activities such as swimming, gathering of people, etc., is not necessary except with large epidemics, when it is more effective in allaying panic than in reducing infection. Pregnant women should take special precaution because of the increased susceptibility to the disease during pregnancy. Tonsillectomy is contraindicated in areas where poliomyelitis is present. All individuals with "minor" illnesses during the poliomyelitis season should limit their physical activity and avoid chilling until all symptoms have disappeared.

The use of γ-globulin prepared from pools of normal human plasma has not been strikingly effective as a prophylactic measure in either family or outside contacts. However, in persons peculiarly susceptible or in a vulnerable position, such as pregnant women, campers, and physicians or nurses accidentally in contact with virus-containing materials, the administration of γ-globulin may be worthwhile. The dose is 0.15 ml per lb body weight; the total quantity for adults is 20 ml.

Active immunization against paralytic poliomyelitis has been successfully produced by parenteral administration of formalin-inactivated strains of the three viral serotypes grown in monkey kidney tissue culture. The vaccine is said to be about 60 to 70 per cent effective against type 1 and 85 to 90 per cent against types 2 and 3. All individuals should receive a fourth dose 1 to 2 years after the third. The necessity for this is suggested by the observation that 928 of the 5,000 cases of poliomyelitis reported in the United States in 1959 had received three or more injections of Salk vaccine. In some areas of the country in that year, the vaccine appeared to be relatively ineffective; for example, 45 per cent of the cases of paralytic poliomyelitis in Massachusetts, 40 per cent of those in Dade County, Florida, 22 per cent of those in Minnesota, and 25 per cent of those in Newfoundland had been given at least three doses of vaccine. This apparent relative inefficiency of immunization does not indicate a lack of value of the vaccine but is probably due to the relatively low antigenic potency of lots of vaccine which these individuals had received. The commercial vaccines presently available have been improved in quality so that the expected high level of protection can probably now be attained.

No antibody is demonstrable in about 20 per cent of patients after the first injection of vaccine. In most individuals without antibody prior to vaccination, neutralizing capacity of low degree appears in about 4 to 6 weeks after the first dose of vaccine but falls gradually over the next few months. The "booster" injections 7 months later and the fourth dose subsequent to this produce a rapid rise in antibody. Persons immune to a single serotype, when first inoculated, develop a rapid increase in antibody to all three types of virus.

The vaccine does not appear to decrease the incidence of nonparalytic poliomyelitis. It has no effect on the intestinal phase of the disease and fails, therefore, to interrupt the spread of virus from one vaccinated person to another. Another drawback of the formalin-inactivated vaccine is the necessity of "booster" doses for the maintenance of a protective level of antibody. While four doses are presently recommended, the necessity for more injections beyond this has not yet been determined. Reactions to the vaccine are uncommon; headache, stiffness of the neck, arms, and legs which may be accompanied by pain, skin hypersensitivity, fever, sore throat, vomiting, and pain at the site of injection have been noted. Reactions to the antibiotics contained in the vaccine have been observed and may be severe.

Experimental studies and field trials in man suggest that immunization with orally administered living poliomyelitis virus produces neutralizing antibodies and protection against infection. The virus strains are prepared by isolation of a single virus particle which has low virulence and high antigenicity. The vaccine may be given in a capsule, in milk, in candy, or by medicine dropper. It is stable in a deep-freeze icebox for many months, in an ordinary refrigerator for 1 month, and at room temperature for 3 to 5 days. Vaccine virus, after feeding, multiplies in the intestinal tract and remains at this site. Viremia occurs very rarely, and then only with some strains. Live vaccine virus spreads and infects contacts of vaccinated individuals. The incidence of spread is lowest in high-income groups (about 9 per cent), higher in families living under relatively poor conditions (about 53 per cent), and highest (40 to 80 per cent) following feeding of infants. The widespread use of this type of immunization in the presence of epidemic poliomyelitis may lead to replacement of the "wild" paralytogenic strain by the one in the vaccine.

The degree of antibody response varies, to some extent, with the strains in the "live" vaccine. Ingestion of the Sabin "triple" vaccine, for example, produces a good response to type 2 and a relatively poor one to types 1 and 3. The serologic response depends on whether single types are given separately or are administered simultaneously. In general, the effect is best with feeding of monovalent vaccine; it is less with divalent and least with trivalent preparations. An adequate antibody response is produced, however, by giving "triple" vaccine twice. Significant levels of antibody develop in 90 to 100 per cent of persons receiving "live

virus" vaccine; they develop more rapidly and persist longer than those which follow the use of formalinized vaccines. Intestinal immunity is present after feeding of the "live" preparations so that minimal or no multiplication in the bowel occurs on exposure to "wild" strains of virus. Because both intestinal immunity and circulating neutralizing antibody are present after immunization with the "live virus" vaccine, the degree of protection against infection appears to be superior to that produced by the parenteral administration of formalinized virus vaccine.

Field trials of live virus vaccines involving over 70 million persons indicate a high degree of protection (over 90 per cent) against paralytic poliomyelitis and a tendency for the epidemic strains to be replaced by the ones in the vaccine. In general, the results of such studies have proved that this type of vaccine is safe and effective in controlling poliomyelitic infection and preventing paralysis. The development of disease in some vaccinated persons has suggested the probable necessity of additional vaccine feedings to ensure a higher degree of immunity in a population.

No untoward effects have thus far followed the use of live virus vaccine. While passage of vaccine virus from one individual to another leads to an increase of pathogenicity as determined by assessment of neurovirulence in monkeys, the heightened invasive capacity quickly reaches a plateau and becomes stabilized at a level below that thought to be dangerous for man. There is presently no evidence that viral agents which may be present in the monkey kidney tissue, which is the culture medium used to grow vaccine virus, will infect man when given orally. The presence of other enteroviruses in the intestinal tracts of vaccinated subjects may "interfere" with implantation of the vaccine strains and lead to failure of immunization. That this is so has been demonstrated in field trials in the tropics where many persons carry enteroviruses and where the rate of successful immunization has been of the order of 60 per cent. This suggests that immunization with live poliomyelitis virus be carried out in the cooler months of the year when the incidence of intestinal carriage of enteroviruses is the lowest. The available data indicate that live virus vaccines offer great promise in the prevention of poliomyelitis. The relative merits of "live" and "dead" vaccine still remain to be determined.

REFERENCES

Enders, J. F., T. H. Weller, and F. C. Robbins: Cultivation of the Lansing Strain of Poliomyelitis in Cultures of Various Human Embryonic Tissues, Science, 109:85, 1949.

Grulee, C. G.: Differential Diagnosis of Poliomyelitis, J.A.M.A., 152:1587, 1953.

Hodes, J. L.: Treatment of Respiratory Difficulty in Poliomyelitis, in "Poliomyelitis, Papers and Discussions Presented at the Third International Poliomyelitis Conference," Philadelphia, J. B. Lippincott Company, 1955.

Horstmann, D. M.: The Epidemiology and Pathogenesis of Poliomyelitis, Bull. N.Y. Acad. Med., 29: 909, 1953.

—— M. D. McCollum, and A. D. Mascola: The Incidence of Infection among Contacts of Poliomyelitis Cases, J. Clin. Invest., 34:1573, 1955.

——, —— and ——: Viremia in Human Poliomyelitis, J. Exptl. Med., 99:355, 1954.

Paul, J. R. (Ed.): Symposium on Poliomyelitis, Am. J. Med., 6:535, 1949.

Second International Conference on Live Poliovirus Vaccines: Scientific Publication No. 50, Pan American Health Organization, World Health Organization, Washington, D.C., 1960.

Symposium on Poliomyelitis, Pediatric Clin. N.A., 1:1, 1953.

Symposium on Poliomyelitis Vaccination, J.A.M.A., 158:1239, 1955.

Weinstein, L.: Diagnosis and Treatment of Poliomyelitis, Med. Clin. N.A., September:1377, 1948.

——: The Influence of Muscular Fatigue, Tonsilladenoidectomy and Antigen Injections on the Clinical Course of Poliomyelitis, Boston Med. Quart., 3:11, 1952.

——: Influence of Age and Sex on Susceptibility and Clinical Manifestations in Poliomyelitis, New Engl. J. Med., 257:47, 1957.

——: Cardiovascular Disturbances in Poliomyelitis, Circulation, 15:735, 1957.

Weller, T. H.: The Application of Tissue Culture Methods to the Study of Poliomyelitis, New Engl. J. Med., 249:186, 1953.

189 RABIES
Robert R. Wagner

Definition. Rabies (hydrophobia, lyssa) is a fatal viral infection of the nervous system transmitted in saliva of rabid animals.

History. Some of the earliest extant writings contain suggestive references to mad dogs. Aristotle (*c.* 335 B.C.) described the transmission of rabies from dogs to other animals, and Celsus (*c.* A.D. 100) recognized that hydrophobia in man was caused by the bite of a rabid dog. The prevalence of the disease in man increased markedly in the eighteenth century following a European epizootic of canine rabies. The first effective control measures were instituted in Scandinavia, resulting in elimination of the disease there by 1826. Galtier's report in 1879

of transmission of rabies to laboratory rabbits led to the classical studies by Pasteur and his associates of "fixed" virus for vaccine production. Histologic diagnosis of infection became possible after Negri in 1903 described the characteristic cellular inclusion bodies of the disease.

Etiology. Rabies virus is infectious for nervous tissue of all warm-blooded animals and can also be grown in tissue culture and chick embryos. It is rapidly destroyed by heat, drying, and formalin but can be preserved in glycerol or by freezing. The term *street virus* is used to designate the agent of the naturally occurring disease. *Fixed viruses* are rapidly multiplying strains used in vaccine production which have lost their infectivity for salivary gland tissue after passage in laboratory animals. There is only one antigenic type of the virus.

Epidemiology. All mammals are potential vectors, but carnivores are responsible for most cases in man and animals. Virus is present in saliva for several days before symptoms develop and persists until the time of death. Rabies is usually contracted from bites, occasionally from scratches or abrasions contaminated with infected saliva, or rarely by penetration of mucous membranes. The principal source of infection in man is the dog, but 5 to 15 per cent of human cases are caused by cats or other animals. The usual form of the disease in dogs, called *furious rabies*, is characterized by progressive agitation, aimless wandering, difficulty in swallowing, frothing at the mouth, labored respirations, feeble bark, ataxia, convulsions, and vicious, indiscriminate attacks on all creatures and inanimate objects. Paralysis and stupor usually develop 2 to 3 days before death and are the sole manifestations (*dumb rabies*) in about one-fifth of infected dogs.

Although quarantine, killing of stray animals, and vaccination are effective in controlling canine rabies, large reservoirs of infection exist in wild animals, such as the wolf in Eastern Europe and Western Asia, the jackal in India and North Africa, and the mongoose in South Africa. Human and canine rabies caused by bites of rabid foxes is not unusual in the United States, and the disease is also found in skunks, raccoons, coyotes, squirrels, bobcats, mountain lions, and other mammals. Vigorous control measures have eliminated all foci of rabies in domestic and wild animals of Scandinavia and the British Isles and prevented importation of the disease into Hawaii and Australia.

The vampire bat transmits a paralytic form of the disease to cattle and horses and constitutes an important reservoir of rabies in South and Central America, Mexico, and the West Indies. Vampire bats are occasionally nocturnal predators of man, attacking silently to take their blood meal without the sleeping victim's knowledge. Human rabies acquired from bites of common bats was first recognized in the United States in 1951 to 1953, and subsequent surveys have revealed that the disease occurs in many insectivorous and herbivorous species. There is evidence to suggest that bats are the original hosts and constitute the largest reservoir of rabies.

Rabies is almost invariably a rapidly fatal infection in all mammals except vampire and insectivorous bats, which can continue to transmit the disease for many months. Sudden, unprovoked attacks by any animals are rare and should be considered presumptive evidence of exposure to rabies.

Pathogenesis. Rabies virus spreads from the site of inoculation along sensory nerve pathways to the posterior columns of the spinal cord, if the bite is on the extremities or trunk, or by cranial nerves to the brain stem from face wounds. The salivary glands, intestine, pancreas, renal tubules, and adrenal medulla are involved by extension along the autonomic nerves. Viremia may occur. Focal inflammation, neuronophagia, demyelinization, hemorrhages, and perivascular infiltration by mononuclear cells occur throughout the nervous system, but these changes are most marked in the basal ganglions, subcortical areas, and spinal cord. Rabies can be distinguished from other viral encephalitides only if the pathognomonic Negri bodies are found. These are eosinophilic inclusion bodies, 0.5 to 10 μ in diameter, demonstrable in the cytoplasm of nerve cells by special stains. In all animals, including man, they are found in greatest abundance in Ammon's horn of the hippocampus and to a lesser extent in pyramidal cells of the cerebral cortex, Purkinje cells of the cerebellum, and nuclei of the basal ganglions.

Manifestations. The *incidence* of rabies in unvaccinated individuals bitten by rabid animals is about 15 per cent, but varies from 5 to 70 per cent, depending on the amount of virus in the saliva and the location and depth of the wounds. It may be difficult to obtain a history of animal exposure if the disease is acquired from minor bites or scratches. The *incubation period* is usually 30 to 70 days but can be as short as 10 days or, rarely, more than a year. Short incubation periods occur after face or arm bites, multiple wounds, or wolf bites. Prodromal symptoms of fever with temperatures of 100 to 102°F, headache, malaise, nausea, vomiting, sore throat, and persistent loose cough are often present for 1 to 4 days. The most significant early manifestations, in about 80 per cent of cases, are tingling, paresthesias, and dull or stabbing pain at the site of the bite, often radiating to the hip, shoulder, or neck, and to distal parts of the involved extremity. The wound may be inflamed and excoriated by the patient's scratching. The first, or *excitement*, phase of the disease is characterized by increasing agitation, marked restlessness, excessive

motor activity, aimless pacing, dysarthria, and occasionally, visual or auditory hallucinations. Episodes of unreasoning fear and rage alternate with profound depression. The patient may become destructive, wildly apprehensive, and combative if restrained but usually does not attack his attendants. Spasmodic gross muscle contractions and generalized clonic or tonic convulsions with opisthotonos develop shortly after the onset, often precipitated by loud noises, bright lights, touch, or even drafts. Respirations become shallow and irregular, the pulse becomes rapid and thready, and the temperature usually exceeds 103°F. There may be involvement of the autonomic nervous system manifested by dilated, irregular pupils, excessive lacrimation, sweating, and salivation. Many patients also exhibit vertigo, nystagmus, optic neuritis with central blindness, diplopia, strabismus, or facial palsy. Paralysis of the vocal cords results in hoarseness or aphonia. Hyperactive deep tendon reflexes, Babinski signs, and nuchal rigidity are often present.

The most characteristic feature of the disease is severe, painful *contractions of the pharyngeal muscles,* initially precipitated by attempts to swallow fluids. This usually develops 1 to 3 days after onset and progresses until the mere sight, sound, mention, or even thought of water cause reflex spasms of the muscles of deglutition and respiration, leading to bouts of apnea, cyanosis, and generalized convulsions. Most patients manifest a *fear of water (hydrophobia)* and to avoid swallowing allow frothy saliva to drool from the mouth. Death usually follows a generalized convulsion with prolonged apnea.

Patients who survive the excitement stage of the disease develop *generalized flaccid paralysis,* often evident at first in the bitten extremity. Muscle spasms and pharyngeal contractions cease, and agitation gives way to depression, apathy, hyporeflexia, and coma. The ability to swallow may return temporarily, and there is often transient slowing of the pulse and respirations. The bladder usually becomes atonic. Generalized paralysis, resembling the Guillain-Barré syndrome, is occasionally the only neurologic manifestation. Rabies acquired from vampire bats, which frequently bite the toes, usually takes the form of Landry's ascending paralysis without excitation or pharyngeal spasm. Death usually occurs 2 to 3 days after onset of paralytic rabies but may be delayed for several weeks.

Laboratory Findings. The blood leukocyte count may be elevated, occasionally to 30,000 cells per cu mm, with an increased number of polymorphonuclear and large mononuclear cells. Glycosuria, acetonuria, proteinuria, and oliguria are present in most cases. The cerebrospinal fluid is usually normal but may contain slightly increased amounts of protein and as many as 100 mononuclear cells per cu mm. Virus may be present in saliva or, rarely, in cerebrospinal fluid. Serum antibodies can be determined by neutralization or complement fixation tests, but serologic studies are of little value for retrospective diagnosis, because almost all surviving patients have received vaccine or immune serum. Definitive diagnosis is usually made at autopsy by demonstrating Negri bodies or by isolation of rabies virus from the brain. The histochemical technique of staining brain or parotid tissue with fluorescent antibody has proved to be an accurate and rapid method of diagnosis.

Differential Diagnosis. *Hysterical reactions* to dog bites and *allergic encephalomyelitis* caused by rabies vaccine are sometimes difficult at first to differentiate from rabies. Paralytic rabies may be confused with poliomyelitis or the *Guillain-Barré syndrome,* particularly when a history of animal bite cannot be obtained or the incubation period exceeds 3 months. Many of the manifestations of *tetanus,* except trismus, resemble those of rabies. *Delirium tremens* and *intoxication with belladonna alkaloids* occasionally simulate rabies.

Treatment. There are about 5,000 cases of rabies in animals reported annually in the United States, and 5 to 10 cases are recognized in man. However, approximately 50,000 persons each year are considered to be exposed to rabies and receive vaccine treatment. The basic principle in the treatment of individuals exposed to rabies is to furnish sufficient antibody to prevent the virus from involving the central nervous system. Semple's vaccine, prepared from fixed virus grown in rabbit brain and inactivated with phenol, has been commonly used for this purpose in the United States. A course of 14 daily inoculations is recommended. A potent vaccine, free of brain tissue, can be prepared in chick embryos from the Flury strain of rabies virus, and a vaccine prepared in duck embryos has been licensed for human use in the United States. These avian vaccines induce high antibody titers in man and have proved to be effective for vaccination of dogs and cattle. Passive immunization with anti-rabies horse serum, used as an adjunct to vaccination, appears to afford enhanced resistance to infection, particularly in heavily exposed individuals. The local treatment of bites consists of thorough cleaning with strong soap or detergent solutions and infiltration of the area with immune serum. Cauterization or debridement of the wound is no longer recommended.

The chief hazards of Semple's vaccine are *hypersensitivity reactions* with severe local erythema, often accompanied by fever and arthralgia, in about 5 per cent of cases and *peripheral neuritis* or *allergic encephalomyelitis* caused by the rabbit brain tissue in 1 of 600 to 10,000 vaccinated individuals.

Encephalomyelitis usually occurs 1 to 3 weeks after the first injection of vaccine and is characterized by the sudden onset of chills, fever, headache, and vomiting, followed by disorientation, dysarthria, ataxia, paresthesias, cranial nerve palsies, visual disturbances, and, frequently, hemiparesis or paraplegia. Increased concentrations of protein in the cerebrospinal fluid and mononuclear pleocytosis are noted in the majority of cases. The mortality rate varies from 0 to 25 per cent, and about one-third of patients who recover from allergic encephalomyelitis have residual neurologic disorders.

The decision to proceed with antirabies treatment must depend on the risk of exposure in individual cases. Vaccine should be administered promptly if a person is bitten by an animal that escapes, is clinically rabid, or shows histologic evidence of infection. However, Negri bodies are not demonstrable in 12 per cent of animals with rabies proved by virus isolation. Healthy dogs or cats that inflict minor bites or scratches contaminated with saliva should be impounded and observed for 7 days. No treatment is required if the animal remains healthy. Immune serum should be administered within 24 hr to all individuals who incur severe or multiple bites, regardless of whether the animal shows signs of rabies at the time. Every bat bite should be considered to be an exposure to rabies.

Prophylactic vaccination is advisable for a small, but selected, "high-risk" segment of the population of the United States, including veterinarians, dog catchers, and postmen. After a primary course of avian vaccine, a single booster injection induces a prompt antibody response. Semple rabbit-brain vaccine should not be used for repeated revaccination because of the increased risk of allergic encephalomyelitis in individuals sensitized to rabbit brain tissue.

No specific treatment is available if clinical manifestations develop. The patient should be kept in a quiet, darkened, draftless room and disturbed as little as possible. Large doses of barbiturates are more effective than opiates in lessening anxiety, delirium, and the frequency of pharyngeal spasms and convulsions. Parenteral administration of fluids is often required.

Prognosis. Thus far, rabies has been an invariably fatal disease in man. However, every patient should receive all possible supportive treatment in the hope that the diagnosis is in error.

REFERENCES

Applebaum, E., M. Greenberg, and J. Nelson: Neurological Complications following Antirabies Vaccination, J.A.M.A., 151:188, 1953.

Enright, J. B.: Bats and Their Relation to Rabies, Ann. Rev. Microbiol., 10:369, 1956.

Fox, J. P.: Prophylaxis against Rabies in Humans, Ann. N.Y. Acad. Sci., 70:480, 1958.

Johnson, H. N.: Rabies, pp. 599–630 in "Oxford Loose-leaf Medicine," vol. 5, part 2, New York, Oxford University Press, 1943.

——: Rabies, pp. 405–431 in "Viral and Rickettsial Infections of Man," 3d ed., T. M. Rivers and F. L. Horsfall, Jr. (Eds.), Philadelphia, J. B. Lippincott Company, 1959.

Koprowski, H.: Rabies, Pediat. Clin. N.Am., p. 55, February, 1955.

Laboratory Techniques in Rabies, World Health Organization Monograph Series, No. 23, 1954.

Roueché, B.: The Incurable Wound, pp. 36–67 in "The Incurable Wound and Further Narratives of Medical Detection," Boston, Little, Brown & Company, 1958.

190 VIRAL ENCEPHALITIS

Ivan L. Bennett, Jr.,
and Raymond D. Adams

Encephalitis is much more varied in its mode of presentation than are aseptic meningitis (p. 1135) and paralytic poliomyelitis (p. 1139). As in the diagnosis of aseptic meningitis, there is a diversity of etiologic agents, infectious and noninfectious, to be considered in addition to viruses. Despite a considerable overlapping of manifestations, however, several of the encephalitis viruses produce relatively characteristic clinical pictures.

Within rather narrow limits, acute damage to a specific area of the brain, no matter what its cause, produces the same clinical manifestations. The histologic responses to injury in the central nervous system consist of various degrees and combinations of neuronal degeneration, microglial proliferation, neuronophagia, tissue necrosis, perivascular cuffing, and meningeal infiltration with lymphocytes and mononuclear cells. So nonspecific are these that the anatomic distribution of damage throughout the neuraxis is often of far more importance to the neuropathologist in his attempt to establish an etiologic diagnosis than are the microscopic details of the lesions. Because the neurologic deficit exhibited by a patient with encephalitis is also more dependent upon the location of the lesions than upon their exact nature, a fairly typical cluster of symptoms and signs is elicited by many infectious agents that affect the brain.

THE SYNDROME OF ENCEPHALITIS

The distinction between meningitis and encephalitis on clinical grounds alone is far from exact. Stupor, coma, and convulsions can occur in either meningitis or encephalitis, though they are more frequent in the latter, and do not constitute a reliable basis for separation. In addition, most viruses which ordinarily cause aseptic meningitis can produce, on occasion, the clinical picture classed as encephalitis, and the encephalitis viruses elicit no more than a meningitis in many patients. These facts make it difficult to place complete reliance upon statistical data on the relative incidence of encephalitis collected in surveys from various virus laboratories. For example, it is our impression that most cases of mumps and lymphocytic choriomeningitis classed as encephalitis or "meningoencephalitis" are little more than examples of intense meningitis. They rarely cause death with postmortem demonstration of cerebral lesions, and surviving cases seldom have residual signs.

In general, the clinical syndrome of encephalitis consists of an *acute febrile illness* with meningeal symptoms to which are added various combinations of *stupor, confusion, hallucinations, coma, hemiparesis, sensory changes, pathologic reflexes, tremor, ataxia,* and *disordered ocular movements.* The most reliable signs of encephalitis are evidence of pyramidal tract disease (flaccid paralysis and reflex changes), found in about 25 per cent of all cases, mental changes, aphasia, and disordered cranial nerve function. The illnesses produced by the many agents causing encephalitis vary in duration but are usually measured in weeks. Death occurs in 5 to 20 per cent of patients with viral encephalitis. Residual signs such as mental deterioration, amnesic defect, personality change, and paresis (usually spastic) are seen in about 20 per cent of patients who recover from all forms of viral encephalitis. This over-all figure fails to reflect, however, the wide variation in the incidence of late changes that follow infection by different viruses. For example, residual defects occur in as many as 80 to 90 per cent of patients with eastern equine encephalitis while the incidence in western equine infections is only 5 to 10 per cent.

Finally, it should be noted that paralysis without sensory changes or signs of cerebral deficit nearly always signifies paralytic poliomyelitis.

Etiology. Numerous noxious agents qualify as frequent, occasional, or rare causes of encephalitis or meningoencephalitis. Indeed for almost every malady of bacterial or viral origin, "encephalitis" has been reported as a complication although many such descriptions lack substantiation.

Table 190-1 lists most of the viruses and viral diseases that are known to be associated with encephalitis. In addition to the viruses that commonly manifest themselves by their effects on the central nervous system, there is a large group of viral diseases in which cerebral involvement is an unusual complication in the course of a well-defined clinical illness. These diseases are fully described in the other chapters of the book referred to in the table.

In most of these diseases, the pathologic findings are those of neuronal damage and inflammation; it is probable that encephalitis results from direct involvement of nervous tissue by the virus. However, the cerebral involvement which complicates vaccination against smallpox or rabies and the encephalitis which appears during convalescence from several common viral diseases seem to involve some different mechanism, possibly some form of hypersensitivity. The cerebral lesion in these cases consists of extensive perivascular demyelination, a type of damage that is not characteristic of other viral encephalitides. Demyelinating diseases are discussed in detail on p. 1829, and Table 190-1 gives references to descriptions of the specific encephalitides of this type that appear in other chapters of this book.

Other Causes of Encephalitis. The most important nonviral diagnostic possibilities to be considered in a patient with the syndrome of encephalitis are syphilis (p. 1073), pertussis (p. 956), leptospirosis (p. 1084), relapsing fever (p. 1088), epidemic typhus (p. 1105), scrub typhus (p. 1106), Rocky Mountain spotted fever (p. 1095), trypanosomiasis (p. 1205), toxoplasmosis (p. 1208), cerebral malaria (p. 1200), trichinosis (p. 1221), schistosomiasis (p. 1225), and cysticercosis (p. 1234).

Among other conditions that may be confused initially with viral encephalitis, although the subsequent course usually clarifies the picture, are tuberculous meningitis (p. 1016), brain abscess (p. 1047), subdural empyema (p. 1046), hypertensive encephalopathy (p. 1354), acute glomerulonephritis (p. 919), cerebral involvement in systemic lupus erythematosus (p. 1892), brain tumor (p. 1811), hyperparathyroidism (p. 604), Wernicke's disease (p. 1839), acute necrotizing hemorrhagic encephalopathy (p. 1832), the neuromyelitis optica syndrome (p. 1836), the acute "cerebral" type of multiple sclerosis (p. 1835), and Schilder's disease (p. 1837) or Tay-Sachs disease (p. 1859) in which there is an abrupt onset of symptoms.

Encephalitis Lethargica (Von Economo's Disease, Sleeping Sickness)

This disorder has not occurred in epidemic form since 1926 and is primarily of historical interest as the first type of epidemic encephalitis recognized clinically and subjected to extensive study in modern times. The first outbreak occurred in Rumania in 1915, and epidemics appeared in France within a year, spread over Europe, reached the United States by 1918, and continued in various parts of the world until 1926. Von Economo's careful studies were carried out in Vienna in 1917.

Table 190-1. VIRAL CAUSES OF ENCEPHALITIS

Disease	Page reference
Eastern equine	1155
Western equine	1155
Venezuelan equine (rare)	1193
St. Louis	1155
Japanese B	1155
Murray Valley (Australian X disease)	1155
Ilheus	1194
Russian tick-borne complex:	
Russian spring-summer	1156
Louping ill (rare)	1194
Kyasanur Forest disease (rare)	1193
Central European	1193
Diphasic milk fever	1194
West Nile fever (rare)	1191
Colorado tick fever (rare)	1190
Encephalitis lethargica (Von Economo)	1153
Rabies	1149
Polioencephalitis	1143
Coxsackie (rare)	1130
Herpes simplex	1170
Lymphocytic choriomeningitis (rare)	1136
Mumps (rare)	1180
Cat-scratch disease (rare)	1178
Psittacosis (rare)	1127
Influenza (rare)	1123
Lymphogranuloma venereum (rare)	1177
Primary atypical pneumonia (rare)	1120
Infectious hepatitis (rare)	1670
Encephalomyocarditis (Columbia-SK; Mengo, etc.)	1195
Postinfectious or postvaccinal demyelinating encephalitis:	
Vaccinia	1165
Rabies	1149
Varicella	1166
Rubeola	1158
Rubella	1160
Exanthem subitum	1161
Smallpox	1163
Dengue	1188
Yellow fever	1184

A viral etiology was never established for the disease, but adequate bacteriologic studies were negative and its infectious origin seems almost certain. Reports of sporadic cases occurring since 1926 are based, of necessity, upon clinical findings only and cannot, therefore, be accepted unequivocally as indicating persistence of the disease.

Epidemiologic evidence indicates an incubation period of 1 to 2 weeks, and the definite seasonal incidence in winter and early spring argues for spread by contact rather than by an arthropod vector. The majority of patients were under the age of 40 years and at least 25 per cent were in the 10- to 20-year age group. While many atypical or inapparent cases occurred (as evidenced by appearance of late sequelae), the mortality rate in patients with definite clinical illness was about 30 per cent, and residual disability affected about 20 per cent of survivors.

The signs and symptoms of encephalitis lethargica were extremely varied; for a detailed description, the reader is referred to the monograph by Neal listed at the end of this chapter. Generally, the disease is described as evolving through three stages. Initially, there were fever, meningeal signs, sleepiness, and ophthalmoplegias followed soon by the onset of other signs of cerebral disease. The two most characteristic syndromes were the so-called *somnolent-ophthalmoplegic* and the *irritative,* or *hyperkinetic,* in which choreiform and myoclonic movements predominated. However, almost every neurologic disorder from epilepsy to poliomyelitis was observed. The second stage lasted for months or years and was referred to as *pseudopsychoneurotic* as patients complained of headache, tinnitus, insomnia, fatigue, etc. The final stage sometimes blended with the first but more often appeared months or years later as parkinsonism, oculogyric crises, behavioral abnormalities (especially in children), and a variety of peculiar involuntary motor syndromes and vegetative disorders such as obesity and somnolence. It is of interest that much of our present understanding of the function of the basal ganglia derives from clinicopathologic correlations in the study of victims of this disease.

EPIDEMIC VIRAL ENCEPHALITIS

All of the diseases described here are produced by members of the large (and ever-growing) group of arthropod-borne, or *arbor,* viruses. Encephalitis is by no means the most frequent manifestation of human infection by arbor viruses, and only a minority of the members of the group are significantly encephalitogenic. Table 210-1, p. 1193, lists the most important arbor viruses and indicates the types of illness which each produces in man, the geographic distribution of infection, and the arthropod vectors responsible for transmission.

There are six arbor viruses to be considered in a discussion of epidemic encephalitis: eastern equine (EEE), western equine (WEE), St. Louis, Japanese B, Murray Valley, and the closely related viruses referred to as the Russian tick-borne complex. All are small viruses (15 to 40 mμ), and their reservoir in nature is probably persistent, inapparent infection in mammals, birds, or arthropods. EEE and WEE cause epidemics of fatal encephalitis in horses, and the Russian viruses elicit a similar disease (louping ill) in sheep. Another arbor virus, Venezuelan equine (VEE), is a cause of epidemic encephalitis in equines but very rarely produces anything more than a grippelike illness in man (p.

1193). Despite its name, then, VEE is not properly regarded as a cause of epidemic encephalitis in man.

The usual route of human infection is through the bite of an infected arthropod. However, infections among laboratory workers have been numerous, and the viruses of this group rank among the agents that carry the greatest risk in the laboratory. This danger, together with the difficulty of isolating virus from many patients, should preclude any attempt at isolation of a specific agent in cases of encephalitis except by experienced personnel in properly equipped institutions. Virus has been isolated from both blood and spinal fluid in Russian and Japanese B encephalitis rather frequently. While WEE virus, on very rare occasions, has been recovered from blood or spinal fluid, it can be found regularly only in central nervous system tissue. Similarly EEE and St. Louis viruses have been found in central nervous system tissue, but neither has ever been isolated from spinal fluid. St. Louis virus has been isolated from the blood in occasional instances, but there is on record only a single isolation of EEE virus from the blood. *Serologic diagnosis* by demonstrating a rise in neutralizing or complement-fixing antibody is quite adequate for clinical purposes. Paired serums taken early in the illness and at 3 weeks should be tested simultaneously. It is important to separate serum as soon as clot retraction occurs and to keep it frozen until testing.

Pathogenesis. Following a stage of transient viremia, the virus attacks the meninges and the gray and white matter, principally of the cerebrum and cerebellum. The lesions elicited by different arbor viruses resemble each other closely. Small hemorrhages and endarteritis appear in the cerebrum and meninges; exudation of small mononuclear cells is prominent, particularly in the perivascular spaces ("cuffing"). Neuronal degeneration and necrosis are prominent, and in Japanese B and Murray Valley infections, there is extensive destruction of the Purkinje cells. Focal encephalomalacia and demyelination are frequent, but the demyelinating process is not confined to the perivascular regions as it is in postinfectious or postvaccinal encephalitis (p. 1165), and it tends also to destroy axis cylinders.

Diagnostic Considerations. Rarely will the symptoms and signs of viral encephalitis described in the following sections permit firm diagnosis on clinical grounds alone. Serologic confirmation is always desirable. While the geographic distribution of these diseases (see Table 210-1, p. 1193) will often narrow the possibilities, today's rapid transportation has already resulted in the appearance of Japanese B encephalitis in patients in the United States. These are all diseases of warm weather, corresponding to the population of arthropod vectors, but slight differences in seasonal incidence are apparent. In the United States, St. Louis infections occur in spring and early summer while WEE and EEE infections are summer diseases. Russian infections come in spring and summer while Japanese B and Murray Valley infections reach a peak in late summer and autumn. Obviously, recognition is more difficult in sporadic cases than it is in a clearcut outbreak of encephalitis.

Western Equine Encephalitis

Serologic surveys indicate that 5 to 10 per cent of residents in endemic areas acquire subclinical infection by WEE virus. In symptomatic cases, the severity of illness varies a great deal. The incubation period ranges from 5 to 21 days but is usually less than 10 days. After a systemic illness with headache, fever, nausea, diarrhea, and lethargy, there may be complete recovery, but in severe cases there is sudden recrudescence of fever followed by severe headache, myalgia, and such neurologic disturbances as dysarthria, ataxia, nystagmus, confusion, coma, or convulsions. Frank paralysis is relatively unusual, occurring in about 15 per cent of patients; ophthalmoplegia is rare. Recovery begins after 7 to 10 days and is ordinarily complete. There is usually a peripheral polymorphonuclear leukocytosis up to 15,000 per cu mm and the cerebrospinal fluid contains 10 to 500 cells with mononuclear cells predominating after the third day. Protein is elevated and glucose is normal.

Mortality rarely exceeds 10 per cent and residual symptoms are very unusual.

Eastern Equine Encephalitis

This disease is far more severe than the western type, and while some evidence of subclinical infection in man has been encountered, it is apparently an infrequent occurrence. The onset is abrupt with fever, headache, and vomiting for a day or two. Following a short remission, there are high fever (often more than 105°F), convulsions, coma, opisthotonos, paralysis, and peculiar edema of the face and extremities. Cyanosis is frequent. Peripheral polymorphonuclear leukocytosis as high as 50,000 to 60,000 cells per cu mm is not rare. The illness lasts about 3 weeks and mortality ranges from 50 to 75 per cent. A majority of survivors show serious residual effects such as paralysis or mental deterioration.

The cerebrospinal fluid pressure is high, protein concentration is elevated, and an initial polymorphonuclear pleocytosis of 1,000 or greater gives way to a predominance of mononuclear cells after a few days.

St. Louis Encephalitis

Inapparent infection is frequent; serologic surveys indicate that the incidence may be as high as 70 per cent in endemic areas. Most symptomatic infections consist of a brief febrile illness without neurologic signs. In severe cases, there is abrupt onset with chills, fever, occipital headache, vomiting, and meningeal irritation. Convulsions are more frequent in children, lethargy and disorientation predominate in adults. Tremors, dysarthria, weakness, photophobia, and myalgia are also common. Dramatic improvement after 3 to 10 days is usual although convalescence is usually prolonged by weakness, malaise, and mental dullness. Convulsions generally signify poor prognosis. Mortality ranges from 5 per cent in young adults to 30 per cent in infants and the aged. The peripheral leukocyte count is often slightly low, but a mild leukocytosis is the rule. Cerebrospinal fluid pressure is rarely elevated, and the fluid contains up to 250 cells with an early polymorphonuclear predominance. Pleocytosis of 500 or more is seen in children. Protein is slightly increased. Sequelae of mental deterioration or paralysis are rare in adults but occur in as many as 25 per cent of infant survivors. Postencephalitic parkinsonism has not been noted following St. Louis infections.

Japanese B and Murray Valley (Australian X Disease) Encephalitis

These diseases are produced by closely related but distinctly different viruses. The geographic distribution of infection, however, is quite different (see Table 210-1, p. 1193) with Murray Valley virus being confined to Australia and New Guinea. However, clinical and pathologic manifestations of infection in man by these two viruses are so nearly identical that a single description suffices for both.

Inapparent human infection is the rule. It is reliably estimated that subclinical infections in man by Japanese B and Murray Valley viruses are five hundred to one thousand times more frequent than symptomatic cases. While the attack rate in different age groups has varied in some outbreaks of Japanese B infection, the majority of patients in epidemics of both diseases have been children, and sporadic cases tend to occur either in children or in adults entering an endemic area for the first time. This pattern is a reflection of the high rates of inapparent infection and consequent immunity in endemic populations, leaving children and recent immigrants as the only susceptible persons.

In terms of the overwhelming preponderance of asymptomatic cases, *infection* by these viruses carries a low mortality. However, among those individuals who develop *clinical disease*, fatalities are very common. In various epidemics of Japanese B infection, as many as 80 per cent of older patients have died and an over-all mortality of 35 to 50 per cent is the rule. In American military forces fatalities have occurred in 10 to 30 per cent of cases despite the favorable age of patients and excellent medical care. The mortality in Murray Valley epidemics has ranged from 40 to 60 per cent.

Occasionally, instances of fever, headache, and malaise with complete recovery after a few days have been noted in epidemics, but abortive cases of this type are not commonly seen. Encephalitis sometimes develops gradually after several days of low-grade fever and grippelike symptoms, but in both diseases the onset is usually abrupt, and prostration comes on rapidly. High fever with rigors in adults and convulsions in children are accompanied by headache, meningeal signs, myalgia, gastrointestinal disturbances, flushing of the face, and sensorial changes including lethargy, confusion, and coma. Tremors, nystagmus, spasticity, and various abnormal reflexes are frequent. Isolated facial paralysis or monoplegia is likely to be seen in children, but symmetrical spastic paresis without paralysis is the rule in adults. Sustained high fever with relative bradycardia begins to subside by lysis on the third or fourth day, and striking subjective improvement is usually apparent when patients become afebrile a few days later. However, convalescence is long and slow; lethargy, weakness, tremors, and anorexia may persist for weeks. Extensive weight loss is frequent, and a large proportion of patients show impairment of mentation, personality change, or paralyses which persist, although slow improvement may continue for months or years. More unusual residuals are aphasia, psychosis, cerebellar dysfunction, and decereberate rigidity.

Polymorphonuclear leukocytosis as high as 30,000 per cu mm in the peripheral blood subsides as defervescence occurs. Cerebrospinal fluid is rarely under increased pressure but shows elevated protein, normal glucose, and a mononuclear pleocytosis of 10 to 500, although higher counts can occur. Cases in which the spinal fluid shows no increase in cells are not unusual. Both protein and cell count in the spinal fluid tend to remain elevated well into the period of convalescence.

Russian Tick-borne Complex

The several viruses in this group are believed by many virologists to represent different strains of the same agent. All are transmitted by ticks, and while encephalitis is a prominent feature of human infection by the virus in central Europe and in the Soviet Union, including European Russia and Siberia, other clinical syndromes are also elicited. These include Omsk hemorrhagic fever (p. 1193) in Siberia and Kyasanur Forest disease (p. 1193), a similar hemorrhagic illness in south India.

While transmission of the virus to man usually occurs by the bite of a tick belonging to the family Ixodidae, transmission by ingestion of raw milk from goats bearing infected ticks has been observed in Russia and probably occurs in Austria as well (so-called diphasic or biundulant milk fever).

The disease produced in man by the encephalitogenic strains of this virus is strikingly biphasic. After an incubation period of 7 to 10 days, there is an abrupt onset of a febrile, grippelike illness, with headache, malaise, myalgia, and anorexia. There is a mild peripheral leukopenia at this stage. Within 5 to 10 days, fever and other symptoms abate, and patients may recover completely without further illness. However, in an unknown proportion of patients, a remission of 4 to 10 days is followed by fever, severe headache, and neurologic manifestations. The blood shows a mild leukocytosis during this second stage. Neurologic involvement is often limited to aseptic meningitis, but nystagmus, lethargy, disorientation, pareses, and flaccid paralysis signify central nervous system involvement in many patients. The spinal fluid shows mononuclear pleocytosis and elevation of protein. Defervescence usually occurs after 10 to 12 days, and convalescence, although prolonged by headache and asthenia, usually ends in complete recovery. Mortality rates in various epidemics have ranged from 0 to nearly 30 per cent. Residual disability occurs in 3 to 5 per cent of survivors and consists of paralysis, psychoses, and a peculiar syndrome called Kozhevnikov's epilepsy in which localized clonic muscle spasms are constantly present and occasionally intensify to the degree that an epileptic seizure occurs. The disease acquired from milk tends to be milder than the tick-borne disease in Europe, and the severest encephalitis has occurred in eastern Russia. The diseases produced by encephalitogenic strains of the virus are referred to by various names, including Central European, Czechoslovakian, or Russian tick-borne encephalitis, Russian spring-summer encephalitis, Russian Far Eastern encephalitis, and biundulant meningoencephalitis.

Prevention. Other than attempts to control vectors in local areas and the use of screening, protective clothing, and repellents for individuals entering endemic zones of infection, specific immunization is the only approach that offers hope. Formolized vaccine prepared from infected mouse brain are said to have been effective in Russia for the tick-borne complex. There is no vaccine for Murray Valley virus, and no reliable preparation for immunization against Japanese B virus is yet available despite much work on the problem. No vaccine is available for St. Louis encephalitis, and while vaccines for both WEE and EEE viruses are used to protect laboratory workers, no large-scale demonstration of their effectiveness in preventing natural infection in man has yet been attempted.

REFERENCES

Dickerson, R. B., J. R. Newton, and J. E. Hansen: Diagnosis and Immediate Prognosis of Japanese B Encephalitis, Am. J. Med., 12:277, 1952.

Kunin, C. M., and T. D. Y. Chin: St. Louis Encephalitis in Hidalgo County, Texas: Clinical and Pathological Features, Public Health Repts., 72:519, 1957.

Neal, J. B. et al.: "Encephalitis: A Clinical Study," New York, Grune & Stratton, Inc., 1942.

Olitsky, P. K., and J. Casals: Arthropod-borne Group A Virus Infections of Man, in "Viral and Rickettsial Infections of Man," T. M. Rivers and F. L. Horsfall, Jr. (Eds.), 3d ed., pp. 286–304, Philadelphia, J. B. Lippincott Company, 1959.

—— and D. H. Clarke: Arthropod-borne Group B Virus Infections of Man, in "Viral and Rickettsial Infections of Man," T. M. Rivers and F. L. Horsfall, Jr. (Eds.), 3d ed., pp. 305–342, Philadelphia, J. B. Lippincott Company, 1959.

Robertson, E. G.: Murray Valley Encephalitis: Pathological Aspects, Med. J. Australia, 1:107, 1952.

—— and H. McLorinan: Murray Valley Encephalitis: Clinical Aspects, Med. J. Australia, 1:103, 1952.

Sabin, A. B. et al.: Sequelae of the Arthropod-borne Encephalitides: Epidemiology of Japanese B Encephalitis, Neurology, 8:878, 1958.

Wolstenhölme, E. W. and M. P. Cameron (Eds.): Virus Meningo-Encephalitis, Ciba Foundation Study Group No. 7, Boston, Little, Brown & Company, 1960.

Section 17: Viral Diseases with Lesions of Skin or Mucous Membranes

191 MEASLES (Rubeola, Morbilli)

Robert R. Wagner

Definition. Measles is a highly contagious viral disease characterized by prodromal respiratory symptoms and enanthemas (Koplik spots), followed by a typical morbilliform rash.

History. At one time all epidemic eruptions (including typhus fever and scarlet fever) were considered to be variants of smallpox. Measles was probably first recognized by Rhazes, a tenth-century Arabian physician, and its identity as a specific disease was finally established by Sydenham in the seventeenth century. The description by Koplik in 1896 of buccal mucosal lesions firmly established the measles enanthem as a definite clinical basis for differentiating measles from rubella and other minor exanthematous diseases. It was not until 1954 that Enders and Peebles succeeded unequivocally in cultivating measles virus in the laboratory, thus providing reliable procedures for diagnosis and for preparation of vaccines.

Etiology. Measles virus readily infects tissue cultures of monkey or human origin and can be adapted to grow in chick embryos. However, even under the most favorable conditions the virus multiplies to relatively low titer in tissue culture and infection can be demonstrated by staining with fluorescent antibody in only a small proportion of cells.

Spread of measles virus in tissue culture occurs by fusion of cytoplasmic membranes of adjacent cells which then form multinucleated syncytiums, the characteristic cytopathology in all forms of infection with this virus. Monkeys in captivity commonly acquire the disease from man and from each other, and the virus is frequently present in a latent form in monkey renal epithelium. There is only one antigenic type of measles virus, but serologic cross reaction occurs with the virus of canine distemper. Reports that distemper vaccine could induce immunity to measles were probably premature.

Epidemiology. Measles is transmitted by the respiratory route during the prodromal and early eruptive stage of the disease. Sporadic cases occur throughout the year in all civilized countries, but epidemics are most frequent during the late winter and early spring. Measles is probably the most contagious of all diseases. An isolated community in Greenland, where measles was formerly unknown, suffered an epidemic in 1951 in which the attack rate was virtually 100 per cent at all ages. Epidemics in heavily populated areas are far less dramatic, because 95 per cent of individuals above fifteen years of age have been infected previously and are immune. The peak incidence is in young school children, and epidemics recur at intervals of 2 to 4 years as new groups of susceptible children reach school age.

Pathogenesis. The virus initially infects the mucosa and lymphoid tissue of the nasopharynx and spreads to draining lymph nodes. Viremia occurs during the prodromal stage, resulting in dissemination of virus to all internal organs as well as the skin. Histologic examination of the early macular eruption reveals nonspecific focal necrosis of epithelial cells, proliferation of capillary endothelium, and subepidermal transudation of serosanguinous fluid. The lesions in all infected tissues, with the exception of brain, are characterized by progressive formation and enlargement of syncytial giant cells, some of which may eventually contain as many as 100 nuclei. Eosinophilic inclusion bodies, composed of dense aggregates of viral antigen, are usually present within the nuclei of the giant cells. Pulmonary infection results in desquamation and squamous metaplasia of bronchial epithelium, hemorrhages, and alveolar infiltrations by giant cells. The characteristic lesions of measles encephalitis are demyelinization of the type seen in allergic encephalomyelitis, accompanied by vascular engorgement, perivascular hemorrhages, inflammation, and neuronophagia.

Manifestations. The clinical course of uncomplicated measles can be divided into three stages: the *prodrome*, the *eruption*, and *recovery*. The *prodrome* usually precedes the rash by 4 days, but sometimes by a week or longer, and is characterized by symptoms of increasing fever, coryza, conjunctivitis, photophobia, hoarseness, and cough. The *cough* is deep-seated, hacking, frequently painful, and may persist throughout the entire illness. The pathognomonic *Koplik spots* can be found in approximately 95 per cent of cases at the end of the prodromal stage and can persist for a day or two after the onset of rash. They are tiny white or bluish-white areas on a bright red base, characteristically grouped around the orifice of the parotid duct opposite the premolar teeth. Occasionally Koplik spots cover the entire buccal mucosa; they can also be present on the palpebral conjunctiva and vaginal mucosa. A prodromal rash, consisting of transient blotchy erythema, may precede the true rash.

The *incubation period* of measles, including the prodrome, is regularly 12 to 14 days and terminates in the appearance of a *morbilliform rash*. At this time, fever increases, cough worsens, the face and lips become puffy, and the patient appears lethargic, irritable, and acutely uncomfortable. Headache, retroorbital pain, itching and burning of the eyes, marked photophobia, and myalgia are common. Generalized lymph node enlargement can occur but is less striking than in rubella. Splenomegaly is occasionally present. The rash is first noted on the forehead and behind the ears and soon thereafter on the face and neck. Classically, it spreads downward in 1 to 2 days to involve the chest, back, abdomen,

and limbs, including the palms and soles. In the early stages the skin lesions are pink, discrete macules, with slightly raised irregular borders that partially blanch on pressure. Later the rash becomes confluent, particularly on the face and back, and assumes a dusky red or violaceous hue. Rarely, it is hemorrhagic (black measles) and associated with bleeding from the body orifices, often attributable to thrombocytopenia. The eruptive phase generally lasts for 3 to 5 days, terminating abruptly with fall in temperature and marked alleviation of all symptoms. *Recovery* is usually uneventful. The rash fades rapidly, leaving a brownish, blotchy discoloration of the skin and areas of superficial desquamation.

Complications. Measles may be complicated by inflammation of internal organs, caused by the virus itself or by secondary bacterial infection. *Viral bronchitis* and *peribronchial pneumonitis* are quite common and are often mistaken for bacterial bronchitis and bronchopneumonia. Abdominal pain and diarrhea may be manifestations of invasion of *intestinal mucosa* and *mesenteric lymph* nodes by measles virus. True viral *appendicitis* is an uncommon cause of abdominal complaints. Gangrene of the face and lips, or *noma*, has become very rare. Slight aberration of *liver function* has been observed, but jaundice and hepatomegaly are uncommon. Clinical and electrocardiographic evidence of *myocarditis* and *pericarditis* have been reported, but their true incidence is unknown. Superficial keratitis and *corneal ulcerations* are often found if looked for carefully; these areas usually heal without scarring, but severe bacterial keratitis and blindness sometimes occur. Unlike rubella, there is no conclusive evidence that measles in pregnancy is a cause of fetal abnormalities, but abortions may occur.

Measles virus has been shown to cause *giant-cell pneumonia* in children. The clinical manifestations are similar to those of other viral interstitial pneumonias. In addition to necrotizing bronchitis and bronchiolitis, the disease is characterized by diffuse, nodular infiltrations of the lungs, often leading to pulmonary insufficiency and death. Most of the cases have been reported in children with leukemia, mucoviscidosis, or other debilitating diseases, and several have occurred in the absence of rash or other manifestations of measles. Unusual features of measles giant-cell pneumonia are prolonged persistence of virus in pharyngeal and respiratory epithelium and absence of antibody response.

Another serious viral complication is *measles encephalitis*, encountered in about one case in every 1,000. It is usually heralded by high fever, drowsiness, excitability, and convulsions occurring at any stage of the illness from the prodrome to a week or more after the onset of rash. The mortality rate of measles encephalitis ranges from 10 to 30 per cent in different epidemics; approximately 40 per cent of survivors show permanent sequelae of mental retardation, personality changes, and behavioral disorders. In addition, electroencephalographic abnormalities have been noted in 50 per cent of children with measles who have no clinical signs of encephalitis.

Secondary bacterial infections generally develop in the late eruptive stage and, although infrequent, are the major causes of death in measles. The most serious pyogenic complication of measles is *bronchopneumonia,* which is associated with a high incidence of delayed resolution, empyema, lung abscess, and bronchiectasis. Purulent *otitis media* is occasionally encountered but usually does not lead to mastoiditis. Rarely, *bacteremia* followed by metastatic abscess formation, meningitis, or endocarditis may occur, particularly in infants or debilitated children. Paradoxically, children with *nephrosis* often undergo a prolonged remission after an attack of measles. Positive tuberculin reactions may revert temporarily to negative, and exacerbations of latent *tuberculosis* can follow an attack of measles.

Laboratory Findings. Measles virus can be isolated by inoculating human or monkey cell cultures with pharyngeal secretions or blood obtained from patients during the prodromal and early exanthematous phases of the disease. Complement-fixing and neutralizing antibodies develop in convalescence. A simple laboratory procedure is the microscopic examination of Wright's stained smears of nasal curettings or sputum for the characteristic multinucleated giant cells of measles (Warthin-Finkeldey cells). These cells are most readily found during the late prodromal and early eruptive stages. The white blood cell count may be low in the prodromal stage but is usually normal during the rash. Leukocytosis occurs in secondary bacterial infections and occasionally in measles encephalitis. The cerebrospinal fluid in measles encephalitis contains 0 to 500 cells per cu mm, mostly mononuclear cells, and a slightly increased amount of protein.

Differential Diagnosis. In measles, the rash, cough, and systemic manifestations are more pronounced than in rubella and exanthem subitum. A problem of ever-increasing importance is the differentiation of measles from drug eruptions, particularly sensitivity reactions to Dilantin. It is sometimes difficult to distinguish the early cutaneous lesions of secondary syphilis from measles rash; occasional patients with measles may also develop a false positive serologic test for syphilis.

Treatment. The treatment of uncomplicated measles is entirely symptomatic. A quiet, darkened room is much appreciated by the patient with irritability and photophobia. Nonproductive, debilitating cough is best suppressed by codeine. Antibiotics should be administered *only* if secondary bacterial complications develop.

Prophylaxis. Immune serum is probably of greater benefit in the prevention or attenuation of measles than of any other disease. The γ-globulin prepared from adult human serum always contains measles antibody, produces few untoward reactions, and is invariably free of serum hepatitis virus. The dose of γ-globulin for prevention of measles is 0.1 ml per lb body weight given on the third to eighth day of the incubation period. If attenuation is desired, 0.02 ml per lb should be given during the first week or larger doses later in the incubation period. Doses affording complete protection are advisable for infants or chronically ill children. Modified measles usually results in permanent immunity, but the aborted disease may not. No benefit can be expected from passive immunization in the prodromal or eruptive stage. The γ-globulin does not reduce the incidence or severity of measles encephalitis developing in partially protected children.

The efficacy of vaccination with infectious, attenuated measles virus grown in chick embryo tissue culture is being evaluated in the United States and elsewhere. Parenteral administration of this vaccine has been found to induce a serologic response in 95 per cent of children who had no demonstrable antibodies at the time of vaccination. Unfortunately, the incidence of untoward reactions has been disappointingly high. Most of the children exhibited moderate fever about 8 days after vaccination and a modified measles rash 3 days later, but otherwise felt well. Relatively few developed respiratory manifestations, enanthems, or viremia; encephalitis and cross infection of unvaccinated contacts have not been noted during vaccine trials. Preliminary observations also indicate that successful vaccination induces solid immunity to measles. Further studies of mass production methods and standardization of vaccines and the incidence of untoward reactions will probably be required before attenuated measles vaccines are licensed for general use.

REFERENCES

Babbott, F. L., Jr., and J. E. Gordon: Modern Measles, Am. J. Med. Sci., 228:334, 1954.

Christensen, P. E., H. Schmidt, O. Jensen, H. Bang, V. Anderson, and B. Jordal: An Epidemic of Measles in Southern Greenland, 1951: Measles in Virgin Soil, Acta Med. Scand., 144:313, 430, 480, 1952.

Enders, J. F., A. Mitus, et al.: Isolation of Measles Virus at Autopsy in Cases of Giant-cell Pneumonia without Rash; Persistence of Measles Virus and Depression of Antibody Formation in Patients with Giant-cell Pneumonia after Measles, New Engl. J. Med., 261:875 and 882, 1959.

—— and Collaborating Clinics and Laboratories: Studies on an Attenuated Measles-virus Vaccine, I–VIII, New Engl. J. Med., 263:153, 1960.

Tompkins, V., and J. F. Macaulay: A Characteristic Cell in Nasal Secretions during Prodromal Measles, J.A.M.A., 157:711, 1955.

Tyler, H. R.: Neurological Complications of Rubeola (Measles), Medicine, 36:147, 1957.

192 RUBELLA (German Measles)
Robert R. Wagner

Definition. This is a benign contagious disease of viral etiology, characterized by fever, lymphadenopathy, and morbilliform rash. Rubella is most important because of the high incidence of congenital malformations following maternal infection in the first half of pregnancy.

Etiology and Epidemiology. Rubella virus has not been cultivated in tissue culture or experimental animals, but the disease can be transmitted to volunteers by inoculation of blood or nasopharyngeal secretions obtained from infected individuals. The rarity of second attacks is evidence of the existence of only one antigenic type of rubella virus. The relatively high incidence in adults suggests that rubella is far less contagious than measles. The preeruptive stage of the disease is the period of greatest communicability, and the infection is acquired by the respiratory route. Most epidemics occur in the early spring and are rarely extensive in the community at large, but institutional outbreaks may assume major proportions. The incidence of asymptomatic, or unrecognized, infection is unknown but probably quite high.

Manifestations and Diagnosis. The *incubation period* of rubella is usually 18 days, with a range of 14 to 23 days. A distinct prodromal period is not characteristic of the disease in children, although mild fever, vomiting, and irritability may antedate the rash. In contrast to measles, rubella usually produces minimal respiratory manifestations. Many patients complain of sore gums, but there is little objective evidence of gingivitis. An enanthem, consisting of a circumscribed patch of small, dark-red macules resembling petechiae, located at the junction of the hard and soft palates, is present in many patients (*Forchheimer spots*) but is not so constant as Koplik spots in measles. In adults, systemic manifestations such as chills, fever with temperature to 105°F, headache, pain behind the eyes, diffuse muscular aches, and lymph node enlargement are often prominent, but even severe rubella rarely causes as much discomfort or prostration as does measles. The bulbar conjunctiva may be reddened, but palpebral conjunctivitis and photophobia are rare. The rash first appears on the neck and face as small pink macules, which darken and spread downward over the trunk and extremities within 24 hr. The lesions tend to remain discrete but may coalesce over the back and buttocks. The palms and soles are usually not involved. The rash rarely persists beyond the fourth day. Fine desquamation and light-brown staining of the skin sometimes occur. The most characteristic manifestation of rubella is *enlargement and tenderness* of the suboccipital and postauricular lymph nodes, which sometimes attain a diameter of 2 cm and are easily visible as well as palpable. Mild generalized lymphadenopathy is common, and splenomegaly is infrequently found.

Complications are rare. There is no definite predisposition to secondary bacterial infections. Some patients complain of mild joint pain and swelling that may continue for several weeks after rash and fever subside. *Thrombocytopenic purpura* associated with skin and mucous membrane hemorrhages has been described. *Meningoencephalitis* due to the rubella virus is uncommon and not so severe as measles encephalitis. It usually takes the form of a benign aseptic meningitis, but fatal encephalitis can occur. Peripheral neuritis and retrobulbar neuritis have also been described.

The only significant *laboratory findings* are inconstant leukopenia in the preeruptive phase and lymphocytosis, sometimes with abnormal lymphocytes, in the stage of rash.

There is no specific *treatment*, and the vast majority of cases recover uneventfully. Rarely, relapses, similar in all respects to the initial attack, occur several weeks after apparent recovery.

Congenital Rubella. Children born to women who contract rubella in the first 4 months of pregnancy are frequently malformed. Maternal rubella also results in abortion or miscarriage. The principal fetal organs involved are the eye, ear, brain, and heart, singly or in combination. Eye disorders consist of cataracts, glaucoma, microphthalmos, and retinitis pigmentosa. Malformations of the inner ear result in deaf-mutism. A variety of cerebral anomalies have been described, including microcephaly and mental retardation. Common congenital cardiac lesions are patent ductus arteriosus and interventricular septal defect.

Congenital malformations following maternal rubella were originally reported to occur with a frequency as high as 90 per cent. More discriminating prospective studies indicate that the true incidence is 10 to 15 per cent, or approximately six times the incidence of congenital malformations in pregnancies uncomplicated by rubella. Many physicians continue to advocate therapeutic abortion, particularly if rubella can be diagnosed with certainty during the first 2 months of pregnancy.

Differential Diagnosis. In addition to mild measles, rubella may simulate scarlet fever and exanthem subitum. Early differentiation of rubella and infectious mononucleosis is difficult at times owing to the similarity in rash, adenopathy, and early blood leukocyte changes.

Prophylaxis. Girls should be exposed to rubella before they reach the child-bearing age. Although opinions vary as to its efficacy, pooled human γ-globulin has been demonstrated to neutralize rubella virus. Therefore, it is advocated that all women exposed to rubella during the first half of pregnancy should receive intramuscular injections of γ-globulin in doses not less than 20 ml.

REFERENCES

Ackroyd, J. F.: Three Cases of Thrombocytopenic Purpura Occurring after Rubella, with a Review of Purpura Associated with Infections, Quart. J. Med., 18:299, 1949.

Johnson, R. E., and A. P. Hall: Rubella Arthritis, New Engl. J. Med., 258:743, 1958.

Krugman, S., and R. Ward: The Rubella Problem: Clinical Aspects, Risk of Fetal Abnormality, and Methods of Prevention, J. Pediat., 44:489, 1954.

——: Rubella, Demonstration of Neutralizing Antibody in Gamma Globulin and Re-evaluation of the Rubella Problem, New Engl. J. Med., 259:16, 1958.

Manson, M. M., W. P. D. Logan, and R. M. Loy: Rubella and Other Virus Infections during Pregnancy, "Ministry of Health Reports on Public Health and Medical Subjects No. 101," London, Her Majesty's Stationery Office, 1960.

193 OTHER EXANTHEMATOUS VIRAL DISEASES

Robert R. Wagner

It has long been known that macular or vesicular rashes occur as the cardinal manifestations of viral diseases other than measles, rubella, and chickenpox. *Erythema infectiosum* was described as a form of rubella in 1889 and acquired its name and separate status in 1899. *Exanthem subitum* (roseola infantum) also masqueraded as a variant of rubella until Zahorsky's classic description in 1910 established it as a different disease. In succeeding years, many reports of atypical rubelliform eruptions

found their way into the medical literature under such names as fourth disease or Duke's disease, but none has survived as a distinct nosologic entity. The term *Boston exanthem*, which dates to 1956, still has some generic validity, but only as one of the exanthematous diseases caused by enteroviruses.

Since 1957, there has been increasing awareness that Coxsackie A, Coxsackie B, and ECHO viruses are important etiologic agents of febrile diseases with rubelliform or vesicular eruptions. Rashes have also been described in occasional cases of poliomyelitis in adults. Descriptions of these enteroviruses, other diseases caused by them, and their pathogenetic and epidemiologic characteristics are presented alsewhere (p. 1130).

Reports claiming that the viruses of exanthem subitum and erythema infectiosum can be cultivated in tissue culture require supporting data. It would not be surprising, however, if the etiologic agents of these diseases also proved to be enteroviruses. Certain epidemiologic features of exanthem subitum and erythema infectiosum suggest that the respiratory tract is not the main portal of entry. Unlike measles and chickenpox, the respiratory manifestations of these diseases are absent or minimal, they have a relatively low degree of contagiousness, and cases do not occur predominantly in the winter months.

EXANTHEM SUBITUM (Roseola Infantum)

Exanthem subitum is a sporadic infectious disease of infants and children characterized by a typical sequence of fever, defervescence, and rash. The vast majority of cases occurs between six and eighteen months of age, and the disease is rare above the age of eight, although a few instances of typical roseola have been reported in young adults. Exanthem subitum seldom attacks more than one child in a family and almost never reaches epidemic proportions.

The incubation period is about 10 days but may be longer. Onset is abrupt, with high fever, the temperature frequently reaching 105 to 106°F in a few hours. Convulsions are common with hyperpyrexia, but in other respects the patient appears surprisingly well. There are usually no respiratory manifestations other than slight pharyngeal injection. The lymph nodes are somewhat enlarged, particularly in the suboccipital and posterior cervical areas. Many a physician's reputation has been established by making a correct diagnosis in the pre-eruptive phase. Constant or remittent fever persists for 3 to 5 days and then subsides completely. The rash appears suddenly (hence the name exanthem subitum) at the time the fever disappears or as much as 36 hr later. It consists of small, scattered rose-pink macules that blanch on pressure. The eruption is largely confined to the neck and trunk but can involve the face and arms. It usually persists for 48 hr and fades rapidly without pigmentation or desquamation. A faint enanthem may be present on the soft palate. The prognosis for complete recovery without sequelae is excellent. Secondary bacterial infections and other complications are extremely uncommon, but encephalitic manifestations and postconvulsive hemiplegia have occasionally been reported.

There are no specific laboratory tests available to aid in diagnosis. Leukocytosis during the febrile phase is followed by leukopenia during the eruptive stage.

ERYTHEMA INFECTIOSUM (Fifth Disease)

This is an uncommonly recognized contagious disease characterized by lack of systemic manifestations and a typical macular rash. It tends to occur in localized outbreaks, particularly in elementary schools, with sporadic secondary cases in family groups. It has been observed at ages from eight months to forty-five years, but most cases are found in children from six to ten years old. The incubation period varies from 4 to 14 days. No definite prodrome occurs, and the temperature is usually normal or at most transiently elevated to 100 to 102°F. Respiratory and gastrointestinal symptoms are conspicuous by their absence. A few patients may show slight conjunctival injection, pharyngeal erythema, or herpes labialis. There is no enanthem or lymphadenopathy. The disease is readily recognized by the rash, which is the only constant manifestation. It begins on the cheeks as brilliant rose-red spots with well-defined raised margins that rapidly become confluent. At this stage, the rash often resembles erysipelas, and vesicles may form within the lesions. The bridge of the nose is invariably spared; sparse discrete lesions extend from the cheeks to the forehead and neck. Circumoral pallor is often prominent. The rash spreads downward in 2 or 3 days to involve the extremities and, to a much lesser extent, the trunk. The most characteristic lesions are seen on the extensor surfaces of the arms and legs and on the buttocks, where large red macules separated by narrow rims of normal skin produce a reticular pattern. The spots fade from the center outward, leaving a lacy network of red lines. In the late stages, this network may resemble cyanotic marbling (*cutis marmorata*). The rash fades completely in 2 to 24 days without desquamation or residual pigmentation, but recrudescence may occur, particularly if the skin is irritated. The blood leukocyte count is normal except for slight eosinophilia in some cases.

ENTEROVIRAL EXANTHEMS

The exanthematous diseases caused by different enteroviruses are not sufficiently distinctive to permit etiologic subdivision into exanthems caused by Coxsackie A, Coxsackie B, and ECHO viruses. Classification of these viruses as three separate groups is in itself somewhat artificial (see p. 1128). In general, the enteroviral exanthems fall into two main clinical categories based on whether the cutaneous lesions are vesicular or rubelliform in appearance.

Enteroviral Infections with Vesicular Rash. The best authenticated epidemics of enteroviral infection characterized by vesicular rash have been caused by Coxsackie A virus either type 9 or type 16. Coxsackie B and ECHO viruses have been implicated in some outbreaks. Multiple cases occur in families during the summer and early autumn; the most seriously affected members are young children. There is no distinct prodrome, but a common manifestation is fever, with temperatures of 100 to 106°F. The illness is sometimes accompanied by gastrointestinal symptoms of abdominal pain, anorexia, nausea, vomiting, and diarrhea. Many patients complain of sore throat, and a few experience cough, chest pain, eye pain, and photophobia. A frequent occurrence is the development of an oropharyngeal and faucial enanthem consisting of vesicles 1 to 5 mm in diameter on an erythematous base that ulcerate in several days. The exanthem usually begins as discrete macules and papules which soon vesiculate. The vesicles may be concentrated on the extremities and become bullous in character, or they may predominate on the trunk and remain small. Meningitis and severe pneumonitis can occur as complications of disseminated infection with Coxsackie A virus. Among the diseases that must be considered in *differential diagnosis* are chickenpox (p. 1166), primary herpes simplex (p. 1170), and erythema multiforme (Stevens-Johnson syndrome) (p. 1924). If cutaneous lesions are absent or sparse the disease might well be called herpangina (p. 1173).

Enteroviral Infections with Rubelliform Rash. Febrile exanthems that may be difficult to differentiate from rubella or mild measles can be caused by at least seven different types of ECHO virus and two types of Coxsackie B virus. In some epidemics, meningitis is a frequent concomitant, but in others, rash is the sole distinguishing clinical characteristic. Sporadic infections occurring in infants may run a course identical to that of exanthem subitum. However, in contrast to exanthem subitum, epidemics of enteroviral exanthems also involve older children and adults. In outbreaks of infection with ECHO virus type 9, the fever and rash make their appearance simultaneously. Occasionally, the eruption in infants is petechial and can be readily confused with meningococcemia, particularly if meningitis is present. The exanthematous disease caused by ECHO virus type 18 has been shown to be associated with viremia.

Boston exanthem is perhaps the most readily recognized enteroviral infection with rubelliform rash and can serve as the prototype of these diseases. It is an acute illness of children and their parents that is now known to be caused by ECHO virus type 16 and probably other types. The incubation period varies from 3 to 8 days. Fever and systemic manifestations are more marked in adults, and the rash is more intense in children. In adults, the illness usually starts abruptly, with shaking chills, temperature to 104°F, headache, muscle pains, prostration, and, occasionally, abdominal cramps or sore throat. The usual findings in children are low-grade fever, irritability, listlessness, and anorexia, but more often, there are no prodromal symptoms. A variety of lesions, including vesicles, small punched-out ulcerations, raised reddened areas, or tiny yellowish plaques, occur in the pharynx. There is no significant lymph node enlargement. The febrile, or prodromal, phase of the disease lasts about 48 hr. The rash ordinarily appears during the 24 hr after fever subsides and consists of salmon-pink macules about 2 mm in diameter with indistinct borders. The lesions tend to remain discrete, although they can coalesce and take on a blotchy appearance. The eruption predominates over the face and upper chest but frequently extends to the arms, buttocks, and legs. Occasionally, the palms and soles are involved. The rash subsides after 72 hr, and recovery is always uneventful; no complications or sequelae have been noted. Boston exanthem is most commonly confused with German measles, exanthem subitum, and "heat rash."

REFERENCES

Kempe, C. H., E. B. Shaw, J. R. Jackson, and H. Silver: Studies on the Etiology of Exanthem Subitum (Roseola Infantum), J. Pediat., 37:561, 1950.

Krugman, S., and R. Ward: "Infectious Diseases of Children," 2d ed., St. Louis, The C. V. Mosby Company, 1960.

Lawton, A. L., and R. E. Smith: Erythema Infectiosum: A Clinical Study of an Epidemic in Branford, Conn., Arch. Internal Med., 47:28, 1931.

Magoffin, R. L., E. W. Jackson, and E. H. Lennette: Vesicular Stomatitis and Exanthem—A Syndrome Associated with Coxsackie Virus, Type A16, J.A.M.A., 175:441, 1961.

Medearis, D. N., Jr., and R. A. Kramer: Exanthem Associated with ECHO Virus Type 18 Viremia, J. Pediat., 55:367, 1959.

Neva, F. A.: Second Outbreak of Boston Exanthem Disease in Pittsburgh during 1954, New Engl. J. Med., 254:838, 1956.

Robinson, C. R., F. W. Doane, and A. J. Rhodes: Report of Outbreak of Febrile Illness with Pharyngeal Lesions and Exanthem: Toronto, Summer 1957—Isolation of Group A Coxsackie Viruses, Can. Med. Assoc. J., 79:615, 1958.

194 SMALLPOX, VACCINIA, AND COWPOX

Robert R. Wagner

Smallpox virus is the human representative of a large family of viruses that infect many mammalian and avian species. Poxviruses are characterized by their comparatively large size (220 to 280 mμ), brick-shaped appearance by electron microscopy, complex chemical and antigenic structure, and high content of deoxyribonucleic acid. The viruses of smallpox (*Poxvirus variolae*), vaccinia (*P. officinale*), and cowpox (*P. bovis*) are closely related antigenically but differ markedly in their virulence for man. Each is capable of producing either local or generalized infection, depending on the route of exposure and the state of host resistance. Smallpox acquired by intradermal inoculation of virus is usually a far milder disease than naturally acquired smallpox. This method of producing immunity, known as variolation, antedates vaccination by several centuries. The classical studies of Jenner, published in 1798, popularized the use of "cowpox" pus for active immunization against smallpox. The virus used at present (vaccinia) differs slightly from cowpox virus, owing either to mutation by human passage or to accidental contamination with attenuated smallpox virus. Jenner's original vaccinia virus, rather than cowpox, is still used for smallpox immunization.

SMALLPOX (Variola)

Definition. Smallpox is a highly contagious viral disease characterized by a diphasic febrile illness and a vesicular and pustular eruption.

Epidemiology. Smallpox epidemics have ravaged large areas of the world for the last millennium and probably longer. Major epidemics still occur in Asia, Africa, and South America, and small outbreaks with high mortality are not unusual in Great Britain and other countries in which vaccination of children is not compulsory. The respiratory tract is the commonest portal of entry of smallpox virus, but in contrast to measles and chickenpox, the period of contagiousness persists throughout the eruptive phase. One of the greatest dangers is dissemination of smallpox by partially immune individuals with only minor manifestations of infection. The virus is quite resistant to inactivation by heat and can be transmitted by contact with clothing or other personal effects of infected individuals, as well as by the air-borne route. Stringent isolation precautions until the last skin crust has separated are essential in preventing epidemic spread of the disease.

Pathogenesis. The classical studies of Fenner on mousepox (infectious ectromelia), an endemic disease of mice, serve as a model for the pathogenesis of smallpox. In mousepox and probably in smallpox (Downie), virus localizes and multiplies at the site of penetration and in adjacent lymph nodes. The liver and spleen are also infected in the early stages. After a definite interval of time, which corresponds to the incubation period, virus enters the blood stream from the lymph nodes, liver, and spleen and is widely distributed to the skin and mucous membranes. This stage of viremia coincides with the prodromal symptoms. During the next few days, antibody is formed and virus disappears from the blood but continues to multiply in the skin, mucous membranes, and in certain instances, the lung and brain. This coincides with the stage of major illness, characterized by skin eruption and parenchymal lesions of internal organs. The cutaneous lesions of smallpox evolve in a regular pattern. The earliest changes are capillary dilatation and epidermal necrosis, followed by proliferation and thickening of epidermis, vacuolization, formation of septate vesicles, and finally, pustulation produced by polymorphonuclear leukocytes that invade the vesicles from the corium. Cytoplasmic inclusions (Guarnieri bodies), composed of dense masses of virus particles, characterize the lesions of smallpox and vaccinia.

Manifestations. In its classical form (*variola major*) smallpox can be divided into a *prodromal phase*, an *afebrile period* of early rash, and a stage of *vesicular* and *pustular rash*. The *incubation period* is usually 12 days but varies from 10 to 14 days or longer. The *prodrome* starts abruptly, with shaking chills, fever with a temperature of 104 to 106°F, restlessness, irritability, headache, excruciating backache, vomiting, and prostration. A prodromal rash of faint irregular macules may be noted, particularly in the axillary and inguinal areas. An easily visible eruption at this stage usually portends a severe illness. Rarely, the prodromal rash is widespread and purpuric, an invariably fatal form of the disease known as *black smallpox* (*purpura variolosa*). Mucous membrane hemorrhages, bone marrow depression, shock, and coma accompany this fulminant illness, and death occurs before the vesicular eruption develops.

In most cases the initial fever subsides rapidly after 2 to 4 days, and the patient seems much improved. At this time a macular (followed by a papular) rash appears, with individual lesions which gradually enlarge to about 0.5 cm in diameter. Over a period of 6 to 10 days the papules progress to become firm, multiloculated vesicles and, finally, painful and pruritic pustules. With the appearance of pustular lesions, fever and systemic manifestations recur. Characteristically, the rash of smallpox is concentrated on the face, extremities, and particularly the palms and soles. However, in severe infections the eruption is diffuse, confluent, and hemorrhagic (*variola haemorrhagica*). Ulcerative lesions often occur on the mucous membranes of the oropharynx, conjunctivas, larynx, trachea, and genitalia. The individual lesions evolve in a regular sequence from papules to vesicles and finally to pustules, and at each stage all the lesions have the same appearance. The deep layers of skin are involved, resulting in typical firm, shotty nodules. During the recovery phase the pustules become umbilicated and crusted; as they heal, the deeply situated pustules leave pitted scars. In mild smallpox the lesions are sparser, located in the superficial epidermis, and heal without scarring; they are soft, friable, surrounded by a red areola, and may resemble closely the individual lesions of chickenpox.

The *complications* of smallpox are chiefly the result of systemic reactions to the virus. *Encephalitis, interstitial pneumonia,* and *myocarditis* occur rarely and are similar in many respects to infection of the brain, lung, or heart with measles or chickenpox virus. Viral osteomyelitis is said to occur in 2 to 5 per cent of children with smallpox. *Superinfections with bacteria,* particularly staphylococci and streptococci, are seen occasionally in the late pustular stage. These infections take the form of severe, often fatal, pyoderma or pneumonia.

Benign forms of smallpox occur in certain epidemics, particularly in Asia, and in partially immune individuals. *Alastrim (variola minor)* is characterized by low-grade fever, sparse rash, and almost no fatalities. It is caused by a virus identical to smallpox virus except for its reduced virulence. *Modified smallpox (varioloid)* is a mild form of the disease in vaccinated individuals infected with virulent virus. Under these circumstances temperature elevation is minimal and the rash is less marked, evolves more rapidly, or may be absent. A patient with smallpox modified by vaccination may transmit a fatal infection to a susceptible individual; alastrim, however, is invariably mild.

Laboratory Findings. Smallpox virus can be isolated from the lesions of the skin and mucous membranes by inoculation of chick embryos, mice, or rabbits. The virus is also present in the blood 1 to 6 days after onset. Serum antibodies can often be detected as early as the fifth day of the disease by complement fixation, hemagglutination-inhibition, and neutralization tests. The leukocyte count is low in the prodromal phase; leukocytosis is usual during the stage of pustular rash, even in the absence of secondary bacterial infection.

Differential Diagnosis. Smallpox is most often confused with severe chickenpox, particularly in adults. In smallpox, the lesions are situated in the deep layers of the skin, are homogeneous, and are distributed centrifugally. The rash of chickenpox is superficial, appears in successive crops, and is located mainly on the trunk. Pustular drug eruptions and erythema multiforme bullosum occasionally mimic smallpox.

Treatment. No specific treatment is available for the primary viral infection. Although success has been reported in prevention of secondary bacterial infections with antibiotics, other reports state that antibacterial therapy has not greatly reduced mortality. All individuals in contact with a suspected case of smallpox should be vaccinated forthwith regardless of previous immunization. Revaccination of exposed individuals usually induces a prompt anamnestic antibody response that affords complete protection. Primary vaccination during the incubation period does not result in sufficient immunity to prevent smallpox but may attenuate the disease.

VACCINIA

Definition. Vaccinia is a skin infection occurring in the course of vaccination against smallpox with living vaccinia virus. Generalized vaccinia and postvaccinal encephalitis are rare complications of intentional or accidental vaccination.

Vaccination. It is customary in the United States to prepare smallpox vaccine by dermal inoculation of vaccinia virus into calves. The fluid from the resulting pocks (vaccine lymph) is scraped from the skin, processed, and dispensed in sealed capillary tubes. It can be kept at refrigerator temperature for several months without deterioration. An equally effective vaccine prepared in embryonated hen's eggs (Smallpox Vaccine, Avianized) is less likely to be contaminated with bacteria and should eventually replace the standard calf-lymph vaccine. An ideal preparation, particularly for underdeveloped areas of the world, would be one that could be lyophilized and stored for prolonged periods without refrigeration.

Vaccination is usually performed in the United States by the multiple-pressure method. When this is properly done, the inoculation site is bloodless and confined to an area 1 to 2 mm in diameter. Ideally, vaccination should be carried out initially at four to six months of age and should be repeated on entering school and at 5- to 10-year intervals thereafter, or at any time that exposure to smallpox is suspected.

Three types of reaction to vaccination are distinguishable, depending on the degree of host susceptibility. A *primary reaction,* or *take,* occurs in previously unvaccinated individuals or when the level of immunity is low. It is characterized by the appearance of an erythematous papule at the local site 3 to 5 days after inoculation. The papule enlarges into a multiloculated vesicle, which pustulates on about the ninth day. Constitutional symptoms of fever, malaise, and irritability, as well as local pain and itching, are common at this time, particularly in children. The pustule hardens and dries, and a crust is formed, which usually separates at the end of the third week, leaving a rough pitted scar.

Partially immune individuals exhibit an *accelerated (vaccinoid) reaction* consisting of a less prominent and more rapidly evolving lesion. An *immune reaction* reaches its peak in 2 or 3 days and never progresses beyond the stage of erythema and papule. Failure to develop any lesion at all after vaccination is *not* indication of immunity and calls for revaccination with a fresh batch of vaccine.

Complications. A variety of untoward reactions can occur following vaccination. Groups of *satellite lesions* may surround the original inoculation site, usually as a result of scratching or careless application of vaccine. Accidental *autovaccination* of distant areas may occur from an early primary lesion, a particular hazard being conjunctival infection. Vaccination sites can undergo secondary bacterial infection. Tetanus and syphilis were at one time hazards of vaccination but are now almost completely unknown. A *false positive serologic test for syphilis,* which may persist for several months, sometimes follows vaccination.

It is likely that vaccinia virus enters the blood stream after any primary "take." However, it is only under unusual circumstances that this results in generalized infection. A transient morbilliform rash (*roseola vaccinatum*) is occasionally seen 1 to 2 weeks after vaccination; this probably represents abortive disseminated vaccinia. Urticarial rashes which may appear at this time have been attributed to allergy to nonviral protein in the vaccine. A more serious, although uncommon, complication is generalized vaccinia, or Kaposi's varicelliform eruption. This disorder has been described for the most part in infants and young children but in rare instances has been seen in adults. Unfortunate confusion has arisen from the application of this eponym to the disseminated dermal infections produced by herpes simplex virus in children (see p. 1170). The skin lesions of generalized vaccinia are thin-walled, hemorrhagic bullae that are superficial and heal without scarring. The disease is associated with fever, prostration, and high mortality. More than 90 per cent of cases of generalized vaccinia have occurred in children with preexisting skin diseases such as eczema or impetigo. The virus is often transmitted accidentally from a recently vaccinated sibling. Therefore, children with chronic skin disease should be guarded from contact with vaccinia virus. An exceedingly rare but often fatal complication of vaccination is chronic *gangrenous vaccinia* (*vaccinia gangrenosa*) which occurs in children with impaired mechanisms of antibody formation, such as agammaglobulinemia. In this disorder necrotizing and pustular lesions extend from the original site of vaccination and continue to develop over a period of weeks or months. Vaccination during pregnancy sometimes results in *congenital vaccinia* and is possibly associated with an increased incidence of abortions.

Other extremely rare complications of smallpox vaccination that have been reported are pericarditis, orchitis, osteomyelitis, thrombocytopenic purpura, and the Guillain-Barré syndrome.

The exact incidence of *postvaccinal encephalitis* is unknown but is variously estimated at one case in 5,000 to 100,000 vaccinations. The mean incubation period is 10 to 12 days, with a range of 1 to 28 days. The disease starts abruptly, with high fever, headache, vomiting, and confusion. The neurologic manifestations of postvaccinal encephalitis may be limited to transient dizziness, irritability, and ataxia, but disorientation, aphasia, delirium, convulsions, stupor, and coma are seen in severe cases. Nuchal rigidity is common, and the cerebrospinal fluid usually shows a moderate increase in mononuclear cells and protein. The mortality rate is about 40 per cent, but patients who recover are usually free of sequelae. Because the characteristic pathologic process is demyelinization, the sobriquet of "allergic" encephalitis has been applied to this disease. This complication is rare in infants, making it advisable to vaccinate all children before the age of one year.

Treatment. No treatment is available for viral complications of vaccinia other than the use of human γ-globulin in chronic gangrenous vaccinia. Secondary bacterial infections should be treated with appropriate antibiotics. Loose, dry dressings covering the vaccination site will reduce the number of suppurative complications more effectively than impregnated occlusive bandages.

COWPOX

Cowpox is an endemic disease of cattle which is transmitted to man by contact with infected cows. Human disease is characterized by the appearance of single or multiple papules on the hand or other exposed skin areas. These gradually enlarge into firm nodules which evolve into deep-seated vesicles and pustules. Inflammation and brawny edema in the surrounding tissues are frequent and painful. Lymphangitis and enlargement of the lymph nodes draining the infected area are also common. The disease is sometimes accompanied by fever and a generalized vesicular rash which heals without scarring. The local lesion is likely to ulcerate and drain purulent material for a month or longer. Serious complications such as encephalitis are exceedingly rare.

REFERENCES

Blank, H. and G. Rake: "Viral and Rickettsial Diseases of the Skin, Eye and Mucous Membranes of Man," Boston, Little, Brown & Company, 1955.

Cabasso, V. J., J. M. Ruegsegger, and I. F. Moore: Further Clinical Studies with Smallpox Vaccine of Chick-embryo Origin, Am. J. Hyg., 68:251, 1958.

Cockshott, P. and M. McGregor: Osteomyelitis Variolosa, Quart. J. Med., 27:369, 1958.

Downie, A. W.: Smallpox, Cowpox and Vaccinia, in "Viral and Rickettsial Infections of Man," 3d ed., T. M. Rivers, and F. L. Horsfall, Jr. (Eds.), Philadelphia, J. B. Lippincott Company, 1959.

Fenner, F.: Mouse-pox (Infectious Ectromelia of Mice), a Review, J. Immunol., 63:341, 1949.

Kempe, H. C., T. Berge, and B. England: Hyperimmune Vaccine Gamma Globulin: Source, Evaluation and Use in Prophylaxis and Therapy, Pediatrics, 18:177, 1956.

Marsden, J. P.: Smallpox, in "Modern Practice of Infectious Fevers," H. S. Banks (Ed.), New York, Paul B. Hoeber, Inc., Medical Book Department of Harper & Brothers, 1951.

Reynolds, A. H. and H. A. Joos: Eczema Vaccinatum, Pediatrics, 22:259, 1958.

195 CHICKENPOX (Varicella)
Robert R. Wagner

Definition. Chickenpox is a highly contagious viral disease characterized by a vesicular rash. Chickenpox and herpes zoster (see p. 1168) are caused by the same virus and can be considered as two phases of a single disease.

Etiology. Varicella virus has been successfully cultivated in the laboratory only in cells of primate origin. Virus is not released by the cells and can be transmitted serially in tissue culture only by passage of infected cells. In tissue culture the virus spreads to contiguous cells which fuse and form a syncytium of multinucleated giant cells. Each nucleus in an infected giant cell contains a large eosinophilic inclusion body, a microscopic finding which characterizes all lesions caused by active infection with this virus. There is only one antigenic type of varicella virus, and this is indistinguishable from the virus that causes herpes zoster. The binomial designation *Herpesvirus varicellae* has been suggested for the varicella-zoster virus because of its biologic and physical similarity to herpes simplex virus.

Epidemiology. The disease can be contracted from a patient with chickenpox or herpes zoster. Chickenpox is transmitted by the respiratory route and is almost as highly contagious as measles. In common with other respiratory exanthematous diseases, epidemics of chickenpox usually recur in the late winter and early spring at intervals of 2 to 4 years. The disease occurs predominantly in school and preschool children, but sharp outbreaks have been reported in military installations. Authorities disagree on whether inapparent infections occur, but it would be surprising if they did not in view of the frequency with which very mild cases are recognized.

Manifestations. Chickenpox in children is ordinarily a mild illness. An *incubation period* of 14 to 16 days is regularly observed, although a range of 9 to 23 days has been reported. Mild prodromal symptoms such as fever, malaise, anorexia, headache, and myalgia may be present for 2 or 3 days. Children sometimes complain of severe abdominal pain at the onset of chickenpox, which may lead to an erroneous diagnosis of appendicitis. However, in most instances, the initial evidence of illness is rash. High fever, severe myalgia, prostration, and occasionally delirium and stupor can occur in adults when the eruption is at its height. A macular and erythematous prodromal rash occasionally precedes the true exanthem.

The eruption of chickenpox begins on the upper trunk as small macules and papules, which vesiculate almost immediately. The vesicles are superficial and thin walled, contain clear fluid, and are surrounded by a broad zone of erythema. Pruritus is often intense. Slight pressure causes some of the lesions to rupture, but the majority become pustular and encrusted within 48 hr. Crops of vesicles continue to appear for 2 to 5 days, producing the characteristic finding of lesions in different stages of development. The rash is most extensive on the trunk, with relatively few lesions on the face and extremities; the scalp is usually involved. Occasionally, the lesions are extensive, confluent, umbilicated, hemorrhagic, or even gangrenous, making differentiation from smallpox by inspection alone difficult. The skin lesions heal rapidly without scarring, unless secondarily infected with bacteria.

Small superficial ulcers and vesicles on an erythematous base are frequent on the mucous membranes of the mouth and genitalia. Involvement of the larynx and trachea is rare. Lesions of the conjunctiva and cornea sometimes lead to scarring and impaired vision. Iritis is uncommon. Mild lymphadenopathy is frequent; swelling of the suboccipital and posterior cervical nodes is striking when scalp involvement is extensive.

Complications. *Secondary bacterial infections* of the skin and scalp are common. Bacterial infections of the respiratory tract usually occur in children after subsidence of fever and the acute stage of the exanthem. Although fewer than 1 per cent of patients develop *bacterial pneumonia,* the incidence of suppurative bronchitis is somewhat higher.

Primary varicella pneumonia, predominantly a disease of adults, is being recognized with increasing frequency. Invasion of the lungs by the virus produces an interstitial pneumonia characterized by edema and necrosis of alveolar walls, hemorrhage, perivasculitis, and a mononuclear inflammatory response. Typical intranuclear inclusion bodies have been described in macrophages and in alveolar and pleural cells. Pulmonary lesions are more likely to occur in patients with extensive or hemorrhagic eruptions. The onset of pneumonitis is usually abrupt, with air hunger, tachypnea, and cyanosis developing soon after the appearance of rash. Dry, hacking cough is frequent, and about one-third of the patients produce sputum streaked with blood. Chest pain occurs in half the cases and is often pleuritic. Examination of the lungs is entirely negative or reveals only scattered fine rales or rhonchi. The temperature is moderately elevated or normal, but the pulse rate is invariably rapid. Arterial hypotension or failure of the right heart may supervene. X-ray of the chest reveals fine miliary or nodular densities diffusely distributed throughout the lungs. The duration and course of the disease are extremely variable; most patients improve markedly within 72 hr, but in a few patients, respiratory insufficiency and roentgenographic changes persist for weeks. The mortality rate in recognized cases of varicella pneumonia has been less than 15 per cent.

Chickenpox meningoencephalitis is primarily a disease of children that resembles measles encephalitis. It usually appears on about the fourth day, but the time of onset varies from the first to the twenty-first day. Headache, vomiting, convulsions, and stupor often occur with dramatic suddenness, but the temperature rarely rises above 104°F and is frequently normal. Ataxia and other signs of cerebellar disease are often conspicuous. Meningismus, cranial nerve palsies, spastic or flaccid paralyses, and hemiplegia may also be present. The mortality rate is approximately 5 per cent; permanent paralysis, ataxia, and mental retardation occur in 15 per cent of surviving cases.

Other viral complications that have been described are myocarditis, pericarditis, orchitis, and thrombocytopenic purpura. Chickenpox in pregnancy may result in mild infection of the newborn infant or intrauterine death. Typical herpes zoster (see below) occasionally occurs in individuals exposed to chickenpox, and both diseases may be present simultaneously in the same patient.

Laboratory Findings. Fluid aspirated from the vesicles often contains multinucleated giant cells and epithelial cells with eosinophilic intranuclear inclusion bodies. Although virus isolation and serologic techniques have been devised, these procedures are not sufficiently standardized for routine use. The blood leukocyte count in all forms of chickenpox is normal or slightly elevated unless secondary bacterial infection supervenes. The cerebrospinal fluid in the encephalitic form of the disease may be normal or may contain up to 3,000 cells per cu mm, most of them mononuclear.

Differential Diagnosis. Chickenpox is readily recognizable in the vast majority of cases by the history of exposure and the clinical picture. Confusion with smallpox arises, particularly in adults, if the eruption is widespread and hemorrhagic. *Primary herpes simplex* infection of the skin (see p. 1168) and *generalized vaccinia* (see p. 1165) often produce recurrent crops of varicelliform lesions; diagnosis of these diseases depends on a history of preexisting eczema and isolation of the specific virus. *Rickettsialpox* can usually be differentiated from chickenpox by the characteristic primary eschar, severe headache, and specific complement-fixing antibody response (see p. 1101).

Treatment. None of the chemotherapeutic agents is effective in chickenpox or its viral complications. Local application of calamine lotion or systemic administration of antihistamines is helpful for pruritus. Secondary bacterial infections of the skin and respiratory tract should be treated with appropriate antibiotics. The use of cortisone or ACTH is probably warranted in the treatment of varicella pneumonia and encephalitis, although adequate clinical trials have not yet been reported. However, fatal disseminated varicella has developed in children being treated with cortisone for other disorders.

REFERENCES

Applebaum, E., M. H. Rachelson, and V. B. Dolgopol: Varicella Encephalitis, Am. J. Med., 15:223, 1953.
Griffin, W. P., and C. W. Searle: Ocular Manifestations of Varicella, Lancet, 2:168, 1953.
Henderson, A. T., and D. C. Young: Herpes Zoster Concurrent with Varicelliform Eruption: Report of Five Cases, U.S. Armed Forces Med. J., 1:1499, 1950.
Weinstein, L., and R. H. Meade: Respiratory Manifestations of Chickenpox, A.M.A. Arch. Internal Med., 98:91, 1956.
Weller, T. H., H. Witton, and E. J. Bell: Etiologic Agents of Varicella and Herpes Zoster, J. Exptl. Med., 108:843 and 869, 1958.

196 HERPES ZOSTER
Lewis L. Coriell

Definition. Herpes zoster, also called shingles or zona, is an acute infectious disease of man. It is caused by a virus and characterized by unilateral, segmental inflammation of the posterior root ganglions or extramedullary ganglions of cranial nerves and by a painful vesicular eruption of the skin along the peripheral distribution of the involved nerve.

History. The disease was called zona (a girdle) by the Greeks, because of the bandlike distribution of the eruption about the trunk. Bokay (1888) suggested a possible etiologic relationship between zoster and varicella, and Lipschutz (1921) defined the specific histopathology of the skin lesions. Successful transfer by inoculation of vesicle fluid into human subjects was first reported by Kundratitz (1925). Serial cultivation of the virus in tissue culture of human fibroblasts (1953) permitted Weller to show the serologic identity of virus from varicella and herpes zoster.

Etiology. The virus of herpes zoster is a relatively large virus (204 by 240 μ). It is strictly a parasite of man. Electron micrographs of vesicle fluid have shown the virus to be similar in size and shape to the virus of varicella. The virus may be plentiful in early vesicles but is typically scanty after 24 hr. Zoster is considered to be a reactivation of a latent varicella virus in a partially immune individual—although the mechanism is not clear.

Epidemiology. Infection is rare in children but increases in frequency, severity, and duration with advancing age. It occurs at all seasons of the year and is slightly more frequent in males than in females. In the United States the majority of, but not all, patients with herpes zoster give a history of a previous attack of varicella in childhood. Epidemics have occurred in schools and barracks but are not common. Outbreaks of herpes zoster have occurred in contacts of a patient with varicella, and vice versa. The grouping of these secondary infections suggests that zoster is infectious only during the first 2 or 3 days after appearance of the eruption. Secondary zoster following trauma such as spinal puncture, administration of arsenic or bismuth, spinal cord tumor, tabes, and lymphatic leukemia have suggested the possibility that the virus may remain dormant in the tissues over long periods of time. The disease is more common in persons who are overworked or ill. The viruses of herpes zoster and varicella are closely related, if not identical, and the various clinical manifestations can best be explained by postulating one virus which causes different diseases in the susceptible and the partially immune subject.

Pathogenesis. Whether the virus enters the skin and travels up the sensory nerve or extends peripherally is purely a matter for conjecture at the present time. The virus has been demonstrated only in the skin lesions, although an inflammatory reaction is a constant finding in the segmental nerve, its sensory ganglion, and the posterior horn of the spinal column (posterior poliomyelitis). The regional lymph nodes show an acute inflammatory reaction. The anterior horn, the meninges, and the brain may be involved. The histologic central nervous system lesions are infiltration with small round cells, hemorrhage, destruction of ganglionic nerve cells, and secondary gliosis.

The skin vesicle is confined to the epidermis, while the corium is congested and infiltrated with inflammatory cells. In the margin of the vesicle are epithelial cells undergoing balloon degeneration, some of which contain eosinophilic intranuclear inclusion bodies which displace the basichromatin to the periphery of the enlarged nucleus. Multinucleated giant cells may be present, each nucleus containing an inclusion body. Within 2 or 3 days, inflammatory cells fill the vesicle, and healing progresses from below, frequently with slight scarring.

Manifestations. The incubation period varies from 7 to 21 days. A preeruptive and posteruptive stage are distinguished. The preeruptive stage consists of fever and constitutional symptoms, with pain, paresthesias, or hyperesthesia over the segmental distribution of the involved nerve for 2 to 4 days. Following this, an erythematous dermatitis appears which quickly becomes papular and vesiculates, with large or small grouped vesicles on an erythematous base. The vesicles, at first clear, become cloudy within 2 to 3 days, then crust and dry after 5 to 10 days. The eruption may appear first near the spinal column, with successive crops over the distal distribution of the nerve. The pain and the vesicular band, following radicular lines, run transversely around the trunk and vertically over the arm and leg. The lesions are almost always unilateral. Headache and meningismus are not uncommon. Pain is frequently slight or absent in young children but may be intense and not completely controlled by analgesic drugs in adults. It is variously described as aching, soreness, burning, gnawing, shooting, stabbing, or neuralgic.

The regional lymph nodes are enlarged and tender. Secondary bacterial infection of the ruptured vesicles is common. Over 75 per cent of cases occur between the second dorsal and second lumbar vertebras and rarely below the elbow or knee. Involvement of the fifth cranial nerve is next in frequency, and in 50 per cent the globe of the eye is affected. When the nasociliary branch of the Gasserian ganglion is involved, the cornea, sclera, or ciliary body may be permanently damaged; the first branch of the fifth nerve is affected more frequently than the second or third. Disease of the geniculate ganglion may lead to zoster of the concha of the ear or the external auditory canal, the soft palate, and loss of taste (Hunt's syndrome); this is often accompanied by paralysis of the seventh nerve. Paralysis is not uncommon in cephalic and cervical zoster but is rare in zoster of the trunk, only 44 cases having been reported up to 1943. Second attacks are exceedingly rare and should suggest an alternate diagnosis of localized herpes simplex. In some patients, a generalized vesicular eruption simulating varicella appears shortly after the appearance of the localized lesion (zoster generalisata).

The total course of the disease from onset to complete recovery is 10 days to 5 weeks. Burgoon observed that in the age group up to nineteen years, 90 per cent cleared within 14 days, while in the forty- to fifty-nine-year age group, only 45 per cent cleared in this interval. If the vesicles all appeared within 24 hr, the total illness was short, and if crops of vesicles appeared up to 7 days, then the total duration was progressively longer.

A serious complication is the syndrome of *postherpetic neuralgia*, which is limited to the aged with arteriosclerosis. It usually involves only the trunk or the ophthalmic division of the trigeminal nerve. Frequently there is an interval between the acute phase and full unfolding of severe pain, which may be described in various ways by individual patients but is of such persistence and intensity that the patient cannot rest or sleep. Pain may persist for weeks or months.

Laboratory Findings. The fluid from unruptured vesicles is sterile bacteriologically. The cerebrospinal fluid is abnormal in 40 per cent of cases; pressure may be increased, and a pleocytosis of up to 300 mononuclear cells has been observed.

Differential Diagnosis. In the preeruptive stage, the diagnosis is difficult, and the disease is usually confused with many other more common causes of pain, such as pleurisy, appendicitis, "lumbago," pleurodynia, or collapsed intervertebral disk. After the unilateral eruption appears, the clinical features are so characteristic that diagnosis is simple. Occasionally, localized herpes simplex along the distribution of a segmental nerve may simulate zoster, including the localized pain and tenderness. Herpes simplex infection can be confirmed in the laboratory (see p. 1170).

Treatment. Treatment is directed at increasing the patient's comfort and preventing secondary infection. The average case of herpes zoster is self-limited and presents no serious complications. The two unsolved problems are the syndrome of post-herpetic neuralgia and ophthalmic zoster. In the acute phase, pain is usually controlled by aspirin and codeine, combined with mild sedation; local anesthetic ointments are not very effective. A petrolatum gauze pad bandage to prevent painful trauma by clothing may be helpful. The skin lesions are adequately managed with applications of calamine lotion in most cases. *Application of adhesive tape strapping for the preeruptive pain of herpes zoster should be avoided, as it will lead to extensive loss of epidermis upon removal of the tape.* Antibiotics have no effect on the virus but may be indicated to control secondary infection, particularly in ophthalmic zoster or severe spinal involvement with secondary infection. In ophthalmic involvement both oral and local antibiotics have been recommended, but the choice of antibiotic in this serious complication should be guided by bacterial cultures and sensitivity tests. Local treatment of lesions of the globe of the eye should be supervised by an ophthalmologist, and early relief of pain and inflammation follows the use of cortisone and corticotropin in these cases. Transfusions of whole blood from persons who have recently recovered from herpes zoster has been abandoned in most clinics. In this self-limited disease therapeutic regimens based on a small number of observations are apt to be unreliable.

Severe postherpetic pain may be resistant to all types of management. One theory advanced to explain this is the activation of self-contained pain circuits in and above the thalamus. The following procedures are based on the supposition that the defect is central: injection of dorsal root ganglion with alcohol or irradiation with x-ray, dorsal rhizotomy, cordotomy, and lobotomy. On the theory of peripheral nerve abnormality are based vitamin B therapy, procainization or excision of skin, surgical pituitrin, paravertebral block, intravenous tetraethylammonium chloride, and sympathetic ganglionectomy. Other empirical procedures which have also been helpful in certain cases include autohemotherapy, sodium iodide, moccasin venom, and Protamide. The multiplicity of recommended procedures is eloquent evidence that none is entirely satisfactory.

Prognosis. It is very unusual for serious complications to follow inflammation of the spinal ganglions. Partial paralysis of the third, fourth, sixth, and seventh cranial nerves, or hypesthesia, may persist for some time. Significant impairment of vision occurs in a high percentage of cases of zoster ophthalmicus.

REFERENCES

Bailey, P.: Herpes Zoster, Postgrad. Med., 12:127, 1952.

Blank, H., L. L. Coriell, and T. F. McN. Scott: Human Skin Grafted upon the Chorioallantois of the Chick Embryo for Virus Cultivation, Proc. Soc. Exptl. Biol. Med., 69:341, 1948.

Rake, G., H. Blank, L. L. Coriell, F. P. O. Nagler, and T. F. McN. Scott: The Relationships of Varicella and Herpes Zoster: Electron Microscope Studies, J. Bacteriol., 56:293, 1948.

Scheie, H. G., and M. C. Alper: Treatment of Herpes Zoster Ophthalmicus with Cortisone or Corticotropin, A.M.A. Arch. Ophthalmol., 53:38, 1955.

Stokes, J., Jr.: Varicella and Herpes Zoster, in "Viral and Rickettsial Infections of Man," 2d ed., Philadelphia, J. B. Lippincott Company, 1952.

Weller, T. H.: Observations on the Behavior of Certain Viruses That Produce Intracellular Inclusion Bodies in Man, Harvey Lecture, 52:228, 1956–57.

197 HERPES SIMPLEX
Lewis L. Coriell

Definition. Herpes simplex is an infectious disease, caused by a virus. Classically, it appears in recurrent attacks as clusters of grouped vesicles on an erythematous base, having a predilection for the face, lips, and mucocutaneous junctions. The initial infection in some individuals may be serious or even fatal. Infection of the central nervous system, the eye, the skin in eczematous patients, the viscera, or the mouth and throat in gingivostomatitis are the common forms of "primary" herpes simplex.

History. Gruter, in 1914, first transferred infection from the cornea of a patient to the cornea of a rabbit and, subsequently, back to the cornea of a blind man, reproducing a typical dendritic ulceration of the cornea. In 1938 Dodd, Buddingh, and Johnston isolated herpes simplex virus from the mouths of children suffering with febrile ulcerative stomatitis (acute herpetic gingivostomatitis).

Etiology. The virus of herpes simplex passes ordinary bacterial filters quite readily and measures 125 to 150 mμ in diameter. It is present in early vesicles. It may be propagated on the cornea or in the brain of several laboratory animals, on the chorioallantoic membrane of embryonated eggs, or in tissue culture.

Epidemiology. The serums of most adults (70 to 90 per cent) contain neutralizing antibodies against herpes simplex; many of these individuals experience recurrent manifestations of disease under suitable stimuli. Fever, whether due to infectious diseases or artificially induced ("fever blister"), and the common cold ("cold sore") are probably the most frequent precipitants of recurrent herpes, while emotional disturbance, physical fatigue, sunburn, menstruation, and food allergy are a few of the less common incitants. The virus remains latent in the tissues between attacks but is sufficiently active to stimulate antibody production. Virus has frequently been found in the saliva when there was no clinical evidence of disease. Adults who have never been infected may contract a primary infection, if suitably exposed. Full-term newborn infants are immune by virtue of transplacental transfer of antibodies, which they gradually lose after the first few months of life. However, by the fifth year, the percentage of children with specific neutralizing antibodies approaches that observed in adults, indicating a high infection rate during infancy. The clinical syndromes recognized as primary infection in this age group account for only 15 per cent of serologic infections. Herpes simplex has evolved an unusually successful host-parasite relationship with man. Most individuals harbor the virus from infancy to old age with little inconvenience to themselves, and even the primary contact in infancy is usually not accompanied by manifest clinical disease.

Pathogenesis. It is probable that during latent periods the virus lives within the cells, since the body fluids contain sufficient neutralizing antibody to inactivate the virus. The various precipitating factors which induce recurrent disease may have a common denominator in altered physiology of the host cell which permits the virus to multiply, but little specific information is available on this point. Skin biopsies taken during the early vesicular stage show congestion of the dermis, with swelling and ballooning degeneration of prickle cells of the epidermis. In some of these, the nuclear basichromatin is collected at the periphery, and the entire central area of the enlarged nucleus is filled with a homogeneous mass which at first stains blue and later red with hematoxylin and eosin. This is the type A inclusion body, found wherever there is active herpes simplex infection. Multinucleated giant cells, with each nucleus containing an inclusion body, are frequently seen in biopsies of infected human skin.

The intraepidermal vesicle does not extend below the basement membrane and hence does not cause scarring, although depigmentation may persist for some time in dark-skinned people. In the healing phase, the vesicle and corium are densely infiltrated with inflammatory cells.

Manifestations. *Recurrent herpes simplex* is a circumscribed eruption, consisting of closely grouped, thin-walled vesicles on an erythematous base, which tends to recur repeatedly in the same area of the skin, particularly at mucocutaneous junctions. It begins as a mild itching or burning; lesions appear which rapidly become papular and vesiculate, and then pass successively through crusting, scab formation, and desiccation, the whole process taking 3 to 14 days. It is typically accompanied by no fever, regional lymphadenopathy, or other signs of systemic illness. The disease is self-limited and is commonly identified with its anatomic location—herpes facialis, labialis, nasalis, progenitalis, or vulvovaginalis.

Herpetic keratoconjunctivitis is characterized usually by swelling and congestion of the conjunctiva, with superficial opacities in the cornea and a palpable preauricular lymph node. Bacterial cultures are sterile; hypesthesia is a prominent sign. The presence of typical herpetic vesicles on the eyelids may aid in the diagnosis; however, the recurrent attacks are frequently confined to the cornea in the form of dendritic ulcers or, less often, as punctate, marginate, or discoform ulcers. The corneal ulcerations may persist for several weeks and respond poorly to local therapy; they are superficial, but the occurrence of repeated attacks poses a threat to vision.

Traumatic herpes designates those cases where the primary infection occurs at the site of a skin abrasion on the hand, elbow, finger, or other skin area not commonly associated with the disease. Repeated recurrences have been observed at the same site over a period of many years.

Acute herpetic gingivostomatitis is the commonest form of primary infection and is seen most frequently in children one to four years of age, less often in adults. It is characterized by gradual or sudden onset with fever, malaise, sore mouth and throat, and extreme irritability, sometimes alternating with lethargy. The temperature may reach 104°F, but is usually 101 to 103°F. Physical examination reveals multiple painful shallow aphthous ulcers on a red base scattered over the buccal mucous membranes, tongue, and oropharynx. The gums are swollen, bleed easily on manipulation, and are typically most inflamed at the gingival margin. The regional lymph nodes are large and tender. Fever and pain usually persist for 6 to 8 days, followed by gradual healing of the ulcers during the following week. The ulcers may be confined to, or appear first in, the pharynx (herpetic pharyngitis), and in such cases the diagnosis is commonly missed.

Eczema herpeticum (Kaposi's varicelliform eruption) is a rarer manifestation of primary infection which occurs in persons with eczema or neurodermatitis. Large areas of abnormal skin are involved, the grouped vesicles usually appearing in crops over a period of several days, hence the similarity to varicella. The temperature may reach 106°F, and marked prostration is not uncommon. The fever subsides during the second week, coincident with the crusting and healing of the skin lesions.

Meningoencephalitis was formerly thought to be a rare form of primary herpes in man, but complement fixation tests indicate that 5 to 7 per cent of cases of aseptic meningitis may be due to this virus. It is accompanied by fever, headache, gastrointestinal symptoms, and signs of meningeal irritation and encephalitis.

In addition to the syndromes described above, herpes simplex has been known to occur in segmental nerve distribution simulating herpes zoster. The occurrence of repeated attacks in the same area is diagnostic.

Visceral disease, characterized by fulminating generalized infection with fever, viremia, and necrotic lesions in the liver and other viscera, and frequently terminating in death, has been recently recognized as a clinical entity in newborn infants. Skin lesions are not present in all infants. Most cases have been in premature infants, or when the mother was undergoing a primary herpetic infection herself. In several cases the mother was known to have had repeated herpes vulvovaginitis, and presumably the infant was infected in traversing the birth canal.

Laboratory Findings. The total leukocyte count is usually normal or only slightly increased, with a normal differential index. The diagnosis can be confirmed in the laboratory by (1) isolation and identification of the virus, (2) demonstration of typical eosinophilic intranuclear inclusions in tissue sections or vesicle fluid, or (3) in primary infections, a rising titer of specific neutralizing antibodies. The acute phase serum should be collected before the fifth day of illness, as antibodies appear early. In central nervous system infection, the spinal fluid pressure and protein are slightly increased, and a pleocytosis up to 500 cells is observed, with many polymorphonuclear leukocytes early, changing later to mononuclears.

Differential Diagnosis. The history and clinical appearance of the recurrent skin and eye manifestations are usually sufficient to establish the diagnosis.

The laboratory tests enumerated above are confirmatory in doubtful cases and are essential for absolute diagnosis in the primary manifestations. The condition is often confused with Vincent's angina, or trench mouth, which responds dramatically to parenteral penicillin. Recurrent solitary aphthous ulcers in the mouth are not caused by herpes simplex.

In herpangina, caused by group A Coxsackie virus, the vesicles are confined to the posterior part of the mouth, and the disease occurs in epidemics.

Large bullae, recurrent attacks, and normal lymph nodes are seen in erythema multiforme.

Eczema herpeticum may be easily confused with secondary bacterial infection of eczema. Extensive weeping and crusting may obscure the grouped vesicular nature of the lesion before the crusts are removed with wet dressings. Eczema vaccinatum (generalized vaccinia) usually presents larger vesicles with a central indentation, but this characteristic is not constant. Herpetic meningoencephalitis must be differentiated from bacterial and viral encephalitides, particularly enterovirus encephalitis, poliomyelitis, lymphocytic choriomeningitis, and postinfectious encephalitis.

Treatment. No specific treatment is available. Repeated vaccination with calf lymph vaccinia virus is currently in vogue, but the apparent successes can probably be explained by coincidence. Laboratory studies reveal no cross protection or interference between these two viruses. It is desirable to have the local treatment of eye lesions supervised by an ophthalmologist. Adrenal steroids are strictly contraindicated in corneal infections with herpes simplex virus because of the possibility of perforation of the globe.

Penicillin and other antibiotics may be helpful in controlling secondary bacterial infection. In acute gingivostomatitis, the maintenance of adequate hydration and nutrition are aided by the local application, before meals, of 1 per cent Pontocaine. A detergent mouthwash such as 1:1,000 Zephiran helps to maintain oral hygiene and inhibit bacterial proliferation. In eczema herpeticum and visceral disease, supportive therapy, fluid replacement, blood transfusions, and appropriate antibacterial measures are indicated. Convalescent serum and γ-globulin have not been beneficial.

Prognosis. Except for complications following infection of the cornea, recurrent herpes has high nuisance value but few sequelae. The primary manifestations run a self-limited course except for meningoencephalitis and visceral disease, which are sometimes fatal, and eczema herpeticum, in which the mortality rate may be 20 per cent.

REFERENCES

Burnet, F. M., and S. W. Williams: A New Point of View, Med. J. Australia, 1:637, 1939.

Dodd, K., J. Buddingh, and L. Johnston: Herpetic Stomatitis, Am. J. Diseases Children, 58:907, 1939.

Lynch, F. W., C. A. Evans, V. S. Bolin, and R. J. Steves: Kaposi's Varicelliform Eruption: Extensive Herpes Simplex as a Complication of Eczema, Arch. Dermatol. Syphilol., 51:129, 1945.

Quilligan, J. J., Jr., and J. L. Wilson: Fatal Herpes

Simplex, in "Viral and Rickettsial Infections of Man," 2d ed., Philadelphia, J. B. Lippincott Company, 1952.

——, A. J. Steigman, and J. H. Convey: Acute Infectious Gingivostomatitis, J.A.M.A., 117:999, 1941.

Scott, T. F. McN.: Infection with the Virus of Herpes Simplex, New Engl. J. Med., 250:183, 1954.

Von Seidenberg, S.: Zur Atiologie der pustulosis vaccini formis acuta, Schweiz. Z. Pathol. u. Bakteriol., 4:398, 1941.

Whitman, L., M. J. Wall, and J. Warren: Herpes Simplex Encephalitis: A Report of Two Fatal Cases, J.A.M.A., 131:1408, 1952.

Zuelzer, W., and C. Stulberg: Herpes Simplex Virus as the Cause of Fulminating Visceral Disease and Hepatitis in Infancy, A.M.A. J. Diseases Children, 83:421, 1952.

198 MINOR VIRAL DISEASES OF THE SKIN AND MUCOSAL SURFACES

Robert R. Wagner

HERPANGINA

This is a benign infectious disease characterized by sudden onset, fever, sore throat, and oropharyngeal vesicles. Almost all epidemics of herpangina occur in the summer and can be traced to infection with Coxsackie A viruses (see p. 1130), but similar disorders are probably caused by Coxsackie B and ECHO viruses. Children under four years of age are most susceptible, but the disease has affected older children and young adults. The incubation period is usually 4 days, varying from 2 to 9 days. Prodromal symptoms are uncommon, and the onset is usually abrupt, with a temperature of 100 to 105°F. Anorexia, vomiting, abdominal pain, and diarrhea may be present. The most frequent complaint is sore throat, often accompanied by dysphagia and salivation. Other respiratory symptoms are conspicuously absent, and headache and myalgia are rare. The only noteworthy physical findings are diffuse pharyngeal injection without exudate and the presence of 2 to 20 small vesicles on the anterior faucial pillars, soft palate, uvula, pharynx, and, rarely, on the tongue, mouth, or tonsils. The lesions measure 1 to 2 mm and are grayish white, surrounded by a bright red areola. They gradually enlarge to 3 to 4 mm and rupture, leaving clean, superficial ulcers. Typical vesicles containing virus have also been described on the vaginal mucosa. The cervical lymph nodes may be slightly enlarged and tender. Parotitis and aseptic meningitis have been reported as complications in a few cases. Oro-pharyngeal lesions similar to those of herpangina can also occur in infections with Coxsackie A virus that are associated with vesicular exanthems (see p. 1162).

Fever persists for 1 to 4 days, and *recovery* is always uneventful. No *treatment* is required other than mild local anesthetics such as butacaine troches. The only *laboratory findings* of diagnostic significance are demonstration of Coxsackie A virus in the feces or pharynx and a rising antibody titer in convalescence. *Differential diagnosis* should include consideration of primary herpetic stomatitis caused by herpes simplex virus (p. 1170) which also may involve the oropharynx. However, unlike herpangina, infections with herpes simplex virus do not occur in epidemics and lesions are more common on the gums and in the anterior part of the mouth. The enanthems of measles and chickenpox, aphthous stomatitis, and bacterial pharyngitis may be confused with herpangina at first, but they can be readily differentiated by their subsequent course.

FOOT-AND-MOUTH DISEASE

This is a highly contagious disease of cattle and other domestic animals, caused by the smallest virus known to infect animals. There is some question about the actual occurrence of human infection by this virus. In the United States rigid quarantine and slaughter of infected animals have confined the disease to a few outbreaks near the Mexican border. The rare instances of probable human infection seem to have resulted from ingestion of meat or dairy products or from exposure to excreta, hides, or entrails of sick animals. In man, the illness starts abruptly with fever, malaise, and headache after an incubation period of 2 to 18 days. Initially, there is extreme dryness of the mouth, followed shortly by excessive salivation and generalized pruritus. After several days, large, clear vesicles appear in the mouth and pharynx and over the palms and soles. Rarely, the skin is affected elsewhere. The lesions of the mucous membranes and skin are painful and soon become shallow ulcers that bleed easily. These heal spontaneously within 2 to 3 weeks, leaving no scars. The virus can be isolated in tissue culture, chick embryos, or guinea pigs. A complement fixation test is available for detecting specific serum antibodies in convalescence.

VESICULAR STOMATITIS

Vesicular stomatitis is a contagious viral disease of horses, mules, cattle, and swine. Human infection occurs rarely in veterinarians, farmers, and virologists after an incubation period of 24 to 48 hr. In man, the disease is characterized by sudden onset with shaking chills, high fever, headache, and prostration. The fever and symptoms subside completely after 24 to 48 hr, but may recur 3 to 4 days later. This second phase of the disease usually lasts a week and is accompanied by the appearance of papular and vesicular lesions in the oropharynx that form superficial ulcers. The cervical lymph nodes are often swollen and tender. The diagnosis can be confirmed by virus isolation or serologic studies.

ORF (Ecthyma Infectiosum)

Orf is a viral disease of sheep and goats in which it takes the form of a benign but lingering infection of the mouth and lips. The disease in man usually occurs in herdsmen who contract the infection while force-feeding sick lambs. Lesions appear on the hands or other exposed areas and consist of papules which rapidly vesiculate and enlarge into hemorrhagic bullae. Itching is frequently intense; the lesions soon rupture and become encrusted and umbilicated. Mild regional lymphadenopathy is usually present, but systemic manifestations are rare. The lesions subside spontaneously within 2 to 3 weeks unless secondarily infected. Scarring does not occur, and a single attack confers permanent immunity. The only diagnostic test is isolation of the virus by inoculation of vesicular fluid into susceptible sheep. The appearance of the lesions and a history of contact with lambs should suggest the correct diagnosis, but orf is often confused with anthrax, sporotrichosis, tularemia, milker's nodules, inoculation tuberculosis, and various forms of contact dermatitis.

MILKER'S NODULES

This is a benign infectious disease of dairy farmers contracted from infected cows. It is presumed to be of viral etiology, although the agent has not thus far been transmitted experimentally. The disease in dairy cattle is world-wide and is characterized by indolent ulcers and granulomas of the udder. In man, lesions appear 5 to 7 days after milking an infected cow; they occur mainly on the hands, but are occasionally seen on other exposed areas. The lesions are often multiple and begin as dark papules, which gradually enlarge into firm brownish-red or purple nodules 1 to 2 cm in diameter. They are rarely painful or tender and contain no fluid or pus. A gray, depressed eschar gradually forms on the surface of a red base of granulation tissue, and the lesions heal slowly after several weeks, leaving no scar. The lymph nodes draining the site of infection may enlarge, but there are no other local or systemic manifestations. Milker's

nodules are often confused with cowpox, which is caused by an entirely different virus (see p. 1166). No specific treatment is available or required.

WARTS (Verrucae)

Warts are specific infectious lesions of the skin and mucous membranes caused by a virus or group of viruses. The disease has been transmitted to volunteers by cutaneous inoculation of ground suspensions of warts. Virus particles and inclusion bodies can be seen in histologic sections examined under the electron microscope. The disease is only mildly contagious, but minor epidemics have been reported. Individual susceptibility seems to vary considerably with age and trauma. The lesions are classified clinically by their appearance and location. *Flat warts* are small round lesions usually found on the back of the hands and on the face of children. *Filiform warts* occur mostly on the face, eyelids, and lips of adults and have numerous small fingerlike projections. The *common wart* (*verruca vulgaris*) usually appears on the hands or under the fingernails as multiple raised papules with rough horny surfaces. *Plantar* and *palmar warts* are deep, painful, flat lesions of the soles and palms covered by a thick layer of cornified epithelium. *Condylomata acuminata* (moist warts) occur on the external genitalia and perianal region after sexual intercourse or other contact. They appear as multiple grapelike clusters that are readily differentiated from the flat condylomata lata of secondary syphilis (see p. 1071). The disease occurs in both sexes but is most prevalent among young women and may be markedly exacerbated by pregnancy.

All forms of warts tend to recur after removal. Various methods of eradication have been employed, including surgery, electrodesiccation, x-ray, freezing with solid carbon dioxide, and application of caustic chemicals such as phenol, salicylic acid, or silver nitrate. Local application of podophyllum resin is effective for condylomata acuminata.

MOLLUSCUM CONTAGIOSUM

Molluscum contagiosum is a benign infectious disease of the skin caused by a large virus of the pox group. The natural mode of transmission is unknown, but the disease has been produced in man by cutaneous inoculation of molluscum particles. After an incubation period of 15 to 50 days, individual lesions begin as tiny papules which gradually enlarge over a period of months to a size of 1 cm or greater. The fully formed lesion is a round, pink, waxy nodule with a centrally depressed crown. Older lesions become pedunculated and inflamed but rarely cause pain or discomfort. The papules are usually multiple and occur on any portion of the skin except the palms and soles. The only treatment is surgical removal; local recurrence is less frequent than it is with warts.

REFERENCES

Blank, H., and G. Rake: "Viral and Rickettsial Diseases of the Skin, Eye and Mucous Membranes of Man," Boston, Little, Brown & Company, 1955.

Flaum, A.: Foot and Mouth Disease in Man, Acta Pathol. Microbiol. Scand., 16:197, 1939.

Hanson, R. P., A. F. Rasmussen, C. A. Brandly, and

J. W. Brown: Human Infection with the Virus of Vesicular Stomatitis, J. Lab. Clin. Med., 36:754, 1950.

Melnick, J. L., H. Bunting, W. G. Banfield, M. J. Strauss, and W. H. Gaylord: Electron Microscopy of Viruses of Human Papilloma, Molluscum Contagiosum, and Vaccinia, Including Observations on the Formation of Virus within the Cell, Ann. N.Y. Acad. Sci., 54:1214, 1952.

Rasmussen, K. A.: Verrucae Plantares: Symptomatology and Epidemiology, Acta Dermat.-Venereol., 38:Suppl. 39, 1958.

Section 18: Viral Diseases of the Eye

199 VIRAL INFECTIONS OF THE EYE

Robert R. Wagner

The eye and its adnexal tissues may be secondarily infected during the course of many cutaneous and systemic viral diseases. Sometimes, these infections lead only to minor disturbances, examples of which are transient loss of pupillary accommodation in dengue, and inflammatory lesions of the eyelid and conjunctiva in chickenpox, pharyngoconjunctival fever, molluscum contagiosum, and orf. However, serious and permanent visual disorders can result if the cornea is infected with viruses such as herpes simplex, herpes zoster, vaccinia, smallpox, mumps, or lymphogranuloma venereum. In addition, congenital rubella is an important cause of cataracts and microphthalmos, and cytomegalic inclusion disease may involve the retina and other ocular tissues.

The diseases described in this chapter are caused by viruses that characteristically produce localized eye lesions without infecting other tissues. Although they are mainly of concern to ophthalmologists, they sometimes enter into the differential diagnosis of systemic disorders that involve the eye. A history of exposure and awareness of variation in host susceptibility will aid in their recognition.

TRACHOMA

Trachoma is an infection of the eye caused by a large virus that is related to the agents of lymphogranuloma venereum and psittacosis. Until 1957, when T'ang and his colleagues in China successfully cultivated trachoma viruses in the yolk sac of embryonated hen's eggs, experimental infections had been produced only in man, apes, and mon-

keys. The disease is probably transmitted by fingers, fomites, and flies and is endemic in areas with poor sanitary conditions and low standards of living. After an incubation period of 5 to 7 days, trachoma begins insidiously or acutely with follicular conjunctivitis, epithelial keratitis, subepithelial follicles, abundant purulent discharge, swelling of the lids, and enlargement of the lacrimal glands and preauricular lymph nodes. This acute stage may last for several weeks before giving way to a subacute phase that is characterized by marked edema of the lids, the formation of conjunctival blebs, and progressive corneal involvement. In the final stage of the disease, scarring and contractures occur, the lids frequently become everted, and the cornea is invaded by dense fibrous tissue and blood vessels (pannus). Recurrent irritation, corneal ulceration, lacrimal dysfunction, and secondary bacterial infection commonly lead to blindness. The diagnosis is most easily established in the acute stage of the disease by virus isolation or by demonstrating typical inclusion bodies in smears of conjunctival scrapings stained with iodine or by the Giemsa method. Acute trachoma can be successfully treated with oral and local tetracyclines or chloramphenicol; sulfonamides and penicillin have been reported to be effective in some cases. However, newly isolated strains of trachoma virus are beginning to vary considerably in their susceptibility to antibiotics, a finding which suggests that emergence of antibiotic-resistant mutants may become a serious problem. Surgery is required for removal of scar tissue in the advanced stages of the disease.

INCLUSION CONJUNCTIVITIS (Inclusion Blennorrhea)

This is an acute infectious eye disease of newborn infants, children, and adults. It is caused by a virus, similar to that of trachoma, which resides in the genitourinary tract and is transmitted by sexual intercourse. Genitourinary infection is usually asymptomatic or limited to mild cervicitis and urethritis. The eyes of infants are infected during passage through the birth canal; ocular infection can also be contracted in swimming pools and nurseries. The disease in babies is characterized by follicular conjunctivitis, profuse mucopurulent exudate, and pseudomembrane formation 5 to 12 days after birth. The acute illness usually runs its course in several weeks, but low-grade conjunctivitis sometimes persists for many months. Unlike trachoma, scarring and pannus formation do not occur. Inclusion conjunctivitis in adults is an invariably mild, afebrile infection, usually confined to the palpebral conjunctiva of the lower lid. The virus of inclusion conjunctivitis can be cultivated in the yolk sac of embryonated hen's eggs, and smears of conjunctival scrapings reveal inclusion bodies identical with those of trachoma; the two diseases can be differentiated only by the clinical picture and course. Oral or local treatment with tetracycline compounds is highly effective. Inclusion conjunctivitis of the newborn should not be confused with gonococcal ophthalmia, which invariably begins 24 to 72 hr after birth and is now exceedingly rare.

EPIDEMIC KERATOCONJUNCTIVITIS
(Shipyard Conjunctivitis)

This is an acute infectious disease of the conjunctiva and cornea that was unknown in the continental United States until its introduction from Hawaii during the Second World War. The etiologic agent is adenovirus type 8, which often produces far more serious ocular damage than the adenoviruses that cause pharyngoconjunctival fever (see p. 1116). Epidemic keratoconjunctivitis in the United States occurs mainly in localized outbreaks in factories, shipyards, and eye clinics. Milder infections have been recognized among family contacts of affected individuals, but the incidence of secondary cases is generally low. The incubation period varies from 5 to 10 days. The disease begins unilaterally with mild or severe conjunctivitis that tends to be follicular in type and is sometimes associated with pseudomembrane formation, iritis, and subconjunctival hemorrhages. Transient fever, headache, and malaise are the only systemic manifestations. The preauricular lymph node is usually enlarged on the affected side. Within a few days, the cornea becomes inflamed, with resultant pain, lacrimation, photophobia, and blurred vision. The other eye is involved several days after the first in about 50 per cent of cases. Subepithelial corneal opacities without ulceration appear 1 to 3 weeks after onset and can persist for years, resulting in impairment of visual acuity. Specific chemotherapy is not available, but local hydrocortisone may suppress the inflammatory reaction. Epidemics can be limited by restricting contact with objects handled by known cases. Infections that must be differentiated from epidemic keratoconjunctivitis include Newcastle disease, herpes simplex (p. 1170), leptospirosis (p. 1086), and cat-scratch disease (p. 1178).

NEWCASTLE DISEASE

This is a common and economically important disease of poultry caused by a virus of the myxovirus (influenza) group. The infection in birds may be acute or chronic and is characterized by severe respiratory, gastrointestinal, and central nervous system damage. Human infection occurs mainly in poultry workers and virologists. In man, accidental introduction of contaminated material into the eye is followed in 24 to 72 hr by conjunctivitis, edema of the lids, and profuse lacrimation. The cornea is not involved, and photophobia is unusual. Constitutional symptoms are absent or mild. The preauricular lymph node on the affected side is swollen and tender in about half the cases. Recovery is complete in 10 to 14 days, and no permanent damage results. The diagnosis can be suspected from the patient's occupation and confirmed by isolation of the virus in embryonated eggs. The antibody response to conjunctival infection is weak, and serologic tests are generally unsatisfactory. No treatment is available or required.

REFERENCES

Blank, H., and G. Rake: "Viral and Rickettsial Diseases of the Skin, Eye, and Mucous Membranes of Man," Boston, Little, Brown & Company, 1955.

Freymann, M. W., and F. B. Bang: Human Conjunctivitis Due to Newcastle Disease Virus in the U.S.A., Bull. Johns Hopkins Hosp., 84:409, 1949.

Jawetz, E.: The Story of Shipyard Eye, Brit. Med. J., 1:873, 1959.

Murray, E. S., et al.: Studies on Trachoma: I. Isolation and Identification of Strains of Elementary Bodies from Saudi Arabia and Egypt, Am. J. Trop. Med. Hyg., 9:116, 1960.

Nelson, C. B., B. S. Pomeroy, K. Schrall, W. E. Park, and R. J. Lindeman: Outbreak of Conjunctivitis Due to Newcastle Disease Virus (NDV) Occurring in Poultry Workers, Am. J. Pub. Health, 42:672, 1952.

Thygeson, P.: Trachoma and Inclusion Conjunctivitis, p. 729 in "Viral and Rickettsial Infections of Man," 3d ed., T. M. Rivers and F. L. Horsfall, Jr. (Eds.), Philadelphia, J. B. Lippincott Company, 1959.

——: Ocular Viral Diseases, Med. Clin. N. Am., 43: 1419, 1959.

Section 19: Viral Diseases Affecting Lymphoid Tissue

200 LYMPHOGRANULOMA VENEREUM

Albert Heyman

Definition. Lymphogranuloma venereum is a virus disease usually transmitted by sexual contact and characterized by a small primary lesion, regional lymphadenitis, and constitutional symptoms. The disease is known by a variety of names, such as *lymphogranuloma inguinale, lymphopathia venereum,* and *climatic bubo,* but the name generally preferred is *lymphogranuloma venereum.* This disease should not be confused with granuloma inguinale, an ulcerative infection of the skin caused by the Donovan body (p. 977).

Etiology. The etiologic agent of lymphogranuloma venereum is a comparatively large virus. When stained by special methods, the organisms can be seen with the ordinary microscope as small spherical granules or elementary bodies. The virus is also distinctive in that it is susceptible to sulfonamide therapy. It produces meningoencephalitis in mice and monkeys and can be cultured in the yolk sac of the chick embryo. Infected yolk sac tissues are used as diagnostic antigens for intradermal (Frei) tests and complement fixation reactions. There are serologic cross reactions, however, with psittacosis and certain other viruses (meningopneumonitis, feline pneumonitis).

Incidence. Lymphogranuloma venereum exists in almost every part of the world but is especially prevalent in tropical and subtropical countries. It is frequently seen in the southeastern portion of the United States, particularly among Negroes. There is no accurate information regarding the incidence of the disease. Only 485 new cases were reported in the United States in 1959, but it is likely that the incidence is much higher.

Pathogenesis. Lymphogranuloma venereum is nearly always transmitted by sexual contact. The incubation period varies from 2 to 30 days. A small evanescent lesion may appear at the site of inoculation, but more often the first sign of the infection is inflammation and suppuration of the inguinal lymph nodes. The virus is apparently disseminated throughout the body by way of the blood stream; it has been isolated from the primary lesion, the regional lymph nodes, the blood, and the spinal fluid. Severe systemic manifestations, such as meningoencephalitis, keratitis, cutaneous lesions, and arthritis may occur. Specific evidence of immunity to the virus, including skin sensitivity of the tuberculin type, and complement-fixing humoral antibodies, can be demonstrated in almost every patient shortly after the onset of the disease. Positive skin and complement fixation reactions persist for several years. Patients with lymphogranuloma venereum frequently have an increase in the globulin fraction of the blood. Following the initial infection, the patient may remain asymptomatic for a long period of time but may eventually develop late manifestations of the disease, such as rectal strictures or elephantiasis of the genitalia.

The early histologic lesion of lymphogranuloma venereum consists of a granuloma forming about a small blood vessel and composed of large mononuclear cells. The vessel is eventually compressed and obliterated, and necrosis occurs in the center of the granuloma. The "stellate" abscesses which are thus formed are characteristic of the fully developed acute lesions of this disease.

Clinical Manifestations. The initial lesion of lymphogranuloma venereum is seldom noted, since it is transitory and inconspicuous. Those which are observed consist of single, small, shallow ulcerations on the external genitalia. Shortly after the appearance of the initial lesion there are enlargement and suppuration of the regional lymph nodes. The usual site is the inguinal or femoral region, and this lymphadenitis is called the *bubo.* The typical lymphogranuloma bubo develops slowly, is bilateral, and forms an ill-defined, lobulated mass. Suppuration usually follows, producing multilocular areas of fluctuation which may rupture spontaneously, forming one or more draining fistulas.

The majority of patients with buboes show constitutional reactions: headache, malaise, fever, and anorexia. Occasionally the virus causes inflammation of distant areas, and "aseptic meningitis," pericarditis, and conjunctivitis have been observed. Generalized skin eruptions and arthritis have also been described; these apparently have been provoked occasionally by the performance of skin tests for the disease.

Many years after the onset of the infection, the patient may develop a proctitis associated with rectal bleeding and a purulent discharge. Eventually there is scar formation, and a complete fibrous ring may develop, producing a *rectal stricture,* which may necessitate colostomy. Rectal lesions are found predominantly in women and are the result of the lymphatic drainage from the posterior part of the vulva and the vagina into the perirectal and retroperitoneal lymph nodes. In the male the lymph vessels drain from the penis to the inguinal area and thence to the deep iliac nodes.

Another late complication of lymphogranuloma venereum is elephantiasis of the external genitalia. This is known as *esthiomene* and is caused by interference with lymphatic drainage. Ulceration is frequent, and secondary infection may cause marked destruction of the genitalia.

Diagnosis. Isolation of the virus is the most accurate means of diagnosis, but it is too laborious for general use. The diagnosis is usually based upon the clinical findings, together with a positive intradermal test and complement fixation reaction. Commercial antigens are available for these. A positive skin (Frei) test is of limited value, as it merely indicates that the patient has been infected with the virus at some previous time. In a recently acquired infection, the complement fixation test will usually be positive in a high titer (1:80 to 1:640). Furthermore, a change in the titer of circulating antibodies may be found in successive tests. Biopsy of the primary lesion or of a lymph node should be done whenever feasible, since the histologic picture is sufficiently characteristic to permit a diagnosis and to differentiate this disease from other venereal infections.

Treatment. Sulfonamide therapy has been the standard treatment of the early manifestations of lymphogranuloma venereum. Sulfadiazine, in doses of 4 Gm a day, usually results in disappearance of symptoms and lesions within 1 to 2 weeks. Chloramphenicol and the tetracyclines have also been found to be of some value in the treatment of buboes, draining sinuses, and early proctitis, and seem to be as effective as the sulfonamides. There is evidence to suggest that sulfonamide therapy may not destroy the virus completely and that it may persist in the body after the acute infection has subsided. The late manifestations of the disease, such as rectal stricture and elephantiasis, do not usually respond to any form of medication, and treatment is chiefly surgical. Buboes which have become fluctuant should be aspirated to prevent spontaneous rupture and subsequent sinus formation.

REFERENCES

Coutts, W. E.: Lymphogranuloma Venereum: A General Review, Bull. World Health Organization, 2:545, 1950.

Favre, M., and S. Hellerstrom: The Epidemiology, Aetiology and Prophylaxis of Lymphogranuloma Inguinale, Acta Dermato-Venereol., 34-Suppl., 30:1, 1954.

Heyman, A.: The Clinical and Laboratory Differentiation between Chancroid and Lymphogranuloma Venereum, Am. J. Syphilis, Gonorrhea, Venereal Diseases, 30:279, 1946.

Koteen, H.: Lymphogranuloma Venereum, Medicine, 24:1, 1945.

Sheldon, W. H., and A. Heyman: Lymphogranuloma Venereum: A Histologic Study of the Primary Lesion, Bubonulus and Lymph Nodes in Cases Proved by Isolation of the Virus, Am. J. Pathol., 23:653, 1947.

201 CAT-SCRATCH DISEASE
Ivan L. Bennett, Jr.

Definition and Etiology. Cat-scratch disease is a specific infection characterized by indolent, occasionally suppurative, regional lymphadenitis, secondary to a primary cutaneous lesion at the site of inoculation, usually a minor trauma. Because more than half of the reported cases have originated from cat scratches and a history of close contact with cats is often elicited, the name *cat-scratch disease* has become popular. However, the disorder has been acquired from splinters, thorns, beef-bone fragments, etc., and in a fair percentage of patients no inciting trauma is recalled. Other names such as *nonbacterial regional lymphadenitis* or *benign inoculation reticulosis* have been suggested but have not been widely used.

A specific etiologic agent has not been identified. Bacterial cultures of involved nodes are uniformly negative. The disease has been transmitted by inoculation of pus from suppurating nodes into monkeys and man, but numerous attempts to isolate a virus have failed. Intranuclear and intracytoplasmic inclusions are occasionally seen in histologic preparations of infected nodes; furthermore, complement-fixing antibodies for lymphogranuloma venereum antigen are occasionally demonstrated in sera of patients with this disease. These suggest that a virus related to the lymphogranuloma-psittacosis group may be the causative agent. Photochromogenic acid fast bacilli have been reported to cause suppurative lymphadenitis in children, and it may well be that anonymous mycobacteria are responsible for some cases of cat-scratch disease (see p. 1025).

Careful observation of cats thought to be responsible for the disease has revealed no evidence of illness; these animals do not react to intradermal injection of antigen. These facts, together with the evidence that other forms of trauma transmit the disease, may indicate that the infecting agent is simply transmitted passively by the cat's claws.

Manifestations. Systemic symptoms are usually mild, consisting of headache, fever, and malaise, which subside within a few days. Shaking chills and fever with temperatures as high as 104°F can occur but are unusual. A transient macular or vesicular rash which subsides within 48 hr is rarely present during the early stages. Erythema nodosum has been reported.

In a typical case the *primary* lesion consists of a raised, slightly tender papule crowned by a small vesicle or eschar; it often resembles an indolent furuncle or insect bite. Multiple primary lesions have been described. Some patients do not exhibit a lesion.

Regional adenopathy becomes evident in a few days to as long as 6 weeks after infection. The axillary and epitrochlear, femoral, or (most commonly) the cervical nodes on one side become visibly swollen and tender, often with redness of the overlying skin. The nodes occasionally suppurate, soften, and drain spontaneously; fistulas always heal completely with only slight scarring. Usually the tenderness subsides gradually, and nontender, firm, enlarged nodes remain palpable for some weeks or even months. There is no generalized glandular enlargement, and the spleen is not palpable.

It seems probable that clinical forms of this infectious disease other than that described above may be delineated. A few cases of *encephalitis* associated with localized adenopathy and a positive skin test have been reported. European authors have suggested that *nonspecific mesenteric lymphadenitis* in children is an abdominal form of cat-scratch disease, and in at least one reported case a previously negative skin test became positive after an illness diagnosed at laparotomy as mesenteric adenitis. A number of cases of so-called *Parinaud's oculoglandular syndrome*, characterized by conjunctivitis and regional lymphadenopathy and previously thought to be due to infection by *Leptothrix*, have been reported to show positive skin tests for cat-scratch disease. Evidence for a primary *pulmonary* form is scant but suggestive, and at least two cases of possible bone involvement in the form of osteolytic foci have been described. Specific diagnosis is made by means of a skin test. Antigen for this is prepared from pus aspirated from infected nodes; it is inactivated by heating at 60°C for 2 hr. A positive reaction is of the delayed, tuberculin type, appearing in 24 to 48 hr. Patients in this country have reacted to antigens prepared from

European countries, and vice versa—evidence that the disease is widespread and that strain differences in skin-test antigens are not significant. Skin reactivity to the antigen persists for at least 4 years after the disease. The Frei test is negative. The leukocyte count is usually normal, occasionally reaching 13,000. There may be some increase in eosinophils, but this is not prominent. The erythrocyte sedimentation rate is usually elevated. In one reported case, serum globulin was elevated early in the disease, decreasing with convalescence (reminiscent of lymphogranuloma venereum), and in another a biologic false positive serologic test for syphilis was noted. The histologic picture in excised nodes is that of a granuloma with microabscess formation; although not diagnostic, the pathologic findings are characteristic enough to suggest the possibility of the disease.

Cat-scratch disease is a benign illness, and the prognosis is uniformly good. Its main clinical importance lies in its possible confusion with other more serious diseases of the lymphatics. Diseases to be considered are tularemia, lymphatic tuberculosis, sporotrichosis, lymphogranuloma venereum, and bacterial adenitis. Because of the indolent character of the adenopathy, Hodgkin's disease or other lymphomas may be suspected. Appropriate serologic and cultural tests serve to rule out other infections; biopsy may be needed to exclude tumor, but a positive skin test with cat-scratch antigen effectively rules out the necessity for such procedures.

Treatment. In instances of node suppuration, aspiration of accumulated pus affords relief of pain (and, incidentally, serves as a source of material for the preparation of skin-test antigen). Penicillin and streptomycin are ineffective. Tetracycline drugs appear to shorten the course of the disease appreciably, but their effect is usually not dramatic.

REFERENCES

Boyd, G. L., and G. Craig: Etiology of Cat-scratch Fever, J. Pediat., 59:313, 1961.

Collins, P. J., and R. Koch: Cat-scratch Fever Associated with an Osteolytic Lesion, New Engl. J. Med., 260:278, 1959.

Daniels, W. B., and F. G. MacMurray: Cat-scratch Disease: Report of 160 Cases, J.A.M.A., 154:1247, 1954.

Margileth, A. M.: Cat-scratch Disease as a Cause of Aculoglandular Syndrome of Parinaud, Pediatrics, 20:1000, 1957.

Stevens, H.: Cat-scratch Fever Encephalitis, A.M.A. J. Diseases Children, 84:218, 1952.

Section 20: Other Systemic Viral Diseases

202 MUMPS (Epidemic Parotitis)

Robert G. Petersdorf and
Ivan L. Bennett, Jr.

Definition. Mumps is an acute communicable disease of viral etiology characterized by painful enlargement of the salivary glands and, sometimes, involvement of the gonads, meninges, and pancreas.

History. Epidemic parotitis was described by Hippocrates. The disease was produced experimentally in cats by Wollstein in 1918, but it was not until 1934 that its viral etiology was established by Johnson and Goodpasture. Habel found in 1945 that the virus could be propagated in the chick embryo, and Enders demonstrated complement-fixing antibody in the serum of patients convalescent from mumps.

Etiology. The causative agent of mumps is a virus of intermediate size which has been classified among the myxoviruses; serologic cross-reactions have been demonstrated between it and other members of the group, notably Newcastle disease virus and influenza D virus. The virus of mumps causes agglutination of erythrocytes of certain species, produces hemolysis, and fixes complement in the presence of specific antibody. It elicits a delayed allergic reaction in human beings affected with it. The virus can be cultivated in the chick embryo and propagated in tissue cultures of HeLa cells and monkey kidney cells.

Epidemiology. Mumps is world-wide. It is endemic in urban communities, although small epidemics occur in closed environments such as schools, camps, and barracks. The infection is present throughout the year, but there is a high seasonal incidence in the winter and spring. Both sexes are equally affected. Mumps is much more common among urbanites, 90 per cent of whom have been infected, than in the rural population, only 10 per cent of whom have had mumps. Although it is predominantly a disease of children, adults who have not had the disease are frequently affected. Data gathered from complement fixation and skin tests indicate that at least 40 per cent of human infections are inapparent. The isolation of mumps virus from urine suggests this as a possible mode of transmission. The virus is present in the blood and salivary secretions for several days before the appearance of symptoms and may persist in the saliva for 10 days after onset of parotitis. From a practical point of view, therefore, patients should be isolated until parotid swelling has subsided.

One attack of mumps confers lasting immunity, and second attacks are most unusual. The protection afforded by unilateral parotitis is just as effective as after bilateral involvement.

Pathogenesis. The virus enters via the respiratory tract and multiplies. After an incubation period of 8 to 28 days, averaging 18 days, the virus is widely disseminated to involve the salivary glands, meninges, testes, pancreas and, more rarely, the ovaries, breasts, thyroid, thymus, heart, liver, and cranial nerves.

Manifestations. *Salivary Adenitis.* Mumps parotitis may be preceded by a prodromal period of malaise, anorexia, chilly sensations, feverishness, and sore throat. Early findings suggesting the diagnosis are tenderness when upward pressure is exerted on the angle of the jaw, reddening and pouting of the orifice of Stensen's duct, and marked discomfort on tasting acid substances. In many cases, however, the first indication of illness is parotid swelling. Usually, swelling of one gland is followed in 4 to 5 days by involvement of the other. In about one-third of cases parotitis remains unilateral. Swelling of the submaxillary and sublingual glands is common but often overlooked. The swollen parotid extends from below the ear to the lower portion of the ramus of the mandible and to the inferior portion of the zygomatic arch. The skin over the gland may be red, hot, and taut. Considerable pain and tenderness are present, and eating, swallowing, and talking cause marked discomfort. There is edema and erythema of the orifice of Stensen's duct, but no purulent discharge is expressible. Sublingual and submaxillary adenitis sometimes produce presternal edema. Swelling of the glottis occurs rarely and may necessitate tracheostomy.

Swelling of the salivary glands reaches its peak within 2 to 3 days and then subsides during the ensuing week. It is usually associated with malaise, headache, anorexia, and fever with temperature ranging from 100 to 103°F. However, systemic manifestations may be very mild, particularly in children.

Orchitis. Mumps is complicated by orchitis in 18 to 20 per cent of postpuberal males. Testicular involvement usually appears 7 to 10 days after onset of parotitis, although it may precede it or appear simultaneously. Occasionally, orchitis occurs in the absence of parotitis. Gonadal involvement is unilateral in approximately 75 per cent of patients.

Orchitis is heralded by recrudescence of malaise and appearance of chilly sensations, headache, nausea, and vomiting. Shaking chills and high fevers with temperatures between 103 and 106°F are frequent. The testicle becomes greatly swollen and exquisitely painful. The epididymis is often palpable as a swollen tender cord; prostatitis and seminal vesiculitis are common. Swelling, pain, and tenderness persist for 3 to 7 days and gradually subside; lysis of fever usually parallels abatement of swelling. Occasionally, the temperature falls by crisis. Mumps orchitis is followed by atrophy of the testicle in one-half the cases. Even after bilateral orchitis, however, sterility is extremely unusual.

Pulmonary infarction has been noted to follow mumps orchitis. This may be the result of thrombosis of the veins in the prostatic and pelvic plexuses in association with the testicular inflammation. The incidence of testicular tumors following remotely upon mumps orchitis has been said to be increased. This observation needs further validation.

Pancreatitis. Involvement of the pancreas is a potentially serious complication which should be suspected in patients with abdominal pain and clinical or epidemiologic evidence of mumps. Abdominal tenderness, nausea, vomiting, and constipation are other symptoms sometimes found in pancreatitis. Occasionally, a mass can be palpated in the epigastrium or left upper quadrant. Shock is unusual but when present is an ominous sign. Serum and urinary amylase are elevated in pancreatitis but are of little significance as long as parotid swelling, which may also give rise to hyperamylasemia, is present. Transient hyperglycemia, glucosuria, and steatorrhea are frequent, but chronic diabetes mellitus and pancreatic insufficiency are rare.

Central Nervous System Involvement. Nearly 50 per cent of patients with mumps have cerebrospinal fluid pleocytosis although symptoms and signs of meningoencephalitis—headache, nuchal rigidity, and drowsiness—occur in only one patient in ten. Occasionally, mumps meningoencephalitis presents with coma, delirium, and convulsions. Muscle pain and slight to moderate weakness of several muscle groups may simulate paralytic poliomyelitis from which mumps can be differentiated by appropriate serologic tests. Paralysis of cranial nerves is rare.

Meningeal involvement is usually preceded by parotitis but can be the first, or the only, manifestation of infection by mumps virus. Serologic studies indicate that 10 to 15 per cent of cases of "aseptic meningitis" in this country are caused by mumps virus, and in one series of 713 cases, 91 were due to mumps. For some unexplained reason, sympto-

matic involvement of the central nervous system is more common in males than females.

The cerebrospinal fluid is clear and under slightly increased pressure. There is a moderate elevation in protein content, but glucose and chloride are generally normal.

Usually the disease runs its course within a week and leaves the patient with no residual disability. Fortunately, the commonest serious complication, nerve deafness, is rare and is likely to be unilateral.

Rarer Manifestations. Mumps virus tends to involve glandular tissues, and inflammation of the lacrimal glands, thymus, thyroid, breasts, and ovaries occurs occasionally. *Oophoritis* may be recognized by persistence of lower abdominal pain and fever. It does not result in sterility, however. Mumps virus has been implicated in the etiology of subacute *thyroiditis*, and 10 of 11 patients who acquired this illness at a time when the incidence of mumps was high, gave serologic evidence of infection with mumps virus. Furthermore, two of these patients had mumps virus isolated from the thyroid gland.

Vulvovaginitis, uveitis, and iridocyclitis have been reported in mumps, but it is difficult to be certain that they are caused by the virus.

Mumps *myocarditis* is evidenced primarily by transient abnormalities in the electrocardiogram but does not produce symptomatic disease or impair cardiac function. Similarly, *hepatic* involvement is manifested in a number of patients by mild abnormalities in liver function, but icterus and other clinical signs of hepatic decompensation do not occur.

Blood dyscrasias in connection with mumps are most unusual, and despite the association of a hemolysin with the virus, hemolytic anemia does not present a problem. Thrombocytopenic purpura as a complication of mumps has been described. It seems possible that the platelet disorder existed coincidentally with mumps infection.

A rare but interesting late complication of mumps is *polyarthritis*. Joint symptoms begin 1 to 2 weeks after subsidence of parotitis. The illness usually lasts 6 weeks, and complete recovery without residual joint damage is the rule.

Laboratory Findings. In uncomplicated parotitis, the blood leukocyte count is normal, although there may be mild leukopenia with relative lymphocytosis. Patients with mumps orchitis, however, tend to have a marked leukocytosis with a shift to the left. In meningoencephalitis, the white blood cell count is usually within normal limits. The erythrocyte sedimentation rate is usually normal but may rise with testicular or pancreatic involvement. The serum amylase is elevated both in pancreatitis and salivary adenitis. It may also be elevated in some patients in whom the sole evidence of mumps is meningoencephalitis. In these instances it probably reflects subclinical involvement of the salivary glands and may be of help in distinguishing mumps meningoencephalitis from other aseptic meningitides. In contrast to the amylase, serum lipase is elevated only in pancreatitis, which can also be accompanied by hyperglycemia and glucosuria. The cerebrospinal fluid contains 0 to 2,000 cells per cu mm, almost all of which are mononuclears, and there is no relationship between the degree of pleocytosis and the severity of central nervous system symptoms.

The serum complement fixation test becomes positive during the second week of disease and remains so for about 6 weeks. The hemagglutination inhibition reaction is demonstrable somewhat later and persists for several months. These serologic tests are indicated only in atypical cases or to ascertain the cause of "aseptic meningitis." The intradermal injection of killed mumps virus produces a delayed reaction of the tuberculin type in immune individuals. The skin test becomes positive several days after the onset of the disease, and a positive skin test early in the illness is an argument against the diagnosis of mumps. The skin test is rarely of value in the diagnosis of acute mumps infection, and because it may elevate the titer of complement-fixing antibodies should not be used in this situation. The test is of value in selecting susceptible individuals for vaccination. Skin tests are contraindicated in patients giving a history of hypersensitivity.

Diagnosis. The diagnosis of mumps during an epidemic is usually obvious. Sporadic cases, however, must be distinguished from other causes of parotid enlargement. *Bacterial parotitis* usually occurs in debilitated patients with severe underlying diseases such as uncontrolled diabetes mellitus, cerebrovascular accidents, or uremia. It may also follow operations. The parotid glands are swollen and tender, and pus can be expressed from the orifices of Stensen's ducts. Marked polymorphonuclear leukocytosis is present. The disease is usually acquired in the hospital, and *Staphylococcus aureus* is the causative organism. Dehydration followed by inspissation of secretions in the salivary ducts is probably an important predisposing factor. *Calculus* in a salivary duct, usually detectable by palpation, may cause painful swelling of the gland. *Drug reactions* can produce tender swellings of the parotid and other salivary glands. "Iodine mumps" is the commonest type; mercurialism can also produce this picture. The antihypertensive agent guanethidine may cause parotid enlargement and tenderness. Careful history usually serves to clarify the etiology of these reactions. Cervical adenitis caused by streptococci, bull-neck diphtheria, infectious mononucleosis, cat-scratch disease, sublingual

cellulitis (Ludwig's angina), and cellulitis of the external auditory canal are usually easy to distinguish from mumps by careful examination. Parotid tumors tend to follow a more indolent course, with swelling of relatively long duration. The common "mixed tumor" of the parotid is well circumscribed, nontender, and very firm, almost cartilaginous on palpation. Parotid swelling and fever, often accompanied by lacrimal adenitis and uveitis (Mikulicz's syndrome), can occur in tuberculosis, leukemia, Hodgkin's disease, and lupus erythematosus. The onset may be sudden, but the process is usually painless and of long duration. "Uveoparotid fever" of similar type may be the first manifestation of sarcoidosis; in this disease parotid swelling is frequently accompanied by single or multiple palsies of cranial nerves—in particular, the facial—and is referred to as Heerfordt's syndrome. Bilateral painless parotid swelling unassociated with fever is found in patients with Laennec's cirrhosis, chronic alcoholism, and malnutrition. Parotid swelling may also occur during rapid refeeding of undernourished individuals. Finally, there is a type of chronic inflammation of the parotid and other salivary glands which is often associated with atrophy of the lacrimal glands and occurs most commonly in women past the menopause. With cessation of lacrimal and salivary function, there may be striking dryness of the conjunctiva, cornea (keratoconjunctivitis sicca), and mouth (xerostomia). These patients may also have a variety of systemic manifestations, including arthritis of the rheumatoid type, splenomegaly, leukopenia, and hemolytic anemia. When dryness of the mucosal surfaces is a prominent feature, the name Sjogren's syndrome is often applied although some insist Mikulicz's disease (as opposed to the syndrome accompanying other diseases) is the proper term. The chronicity of the process and its occurrence in elderly women make confusion with mumps unlikely.

The causes of aseptic meningitis are listed on p. 1136.

Orchitis occurring in the absence of parotitis is likely to remain undiagnosed. Serologic testing may later confirm the diagnosis of mumps. Orchitis may occur in association with acute bacterial prostatitis and seminal vesiculitis. It is a rare complication of gonorrhea. Occasionally testicular inflammation accompanies pleurodynia, leptospirosis, melioidosis, relapsing fever, and chickenpox. In any patient with fever and orchitis, brucellosis should be ruled out by appropriate cultures and serologic tests.

Treatment. There is no specific treatment for infections with the mumps virus. Patients with parotitis should receive mouth care, analgesics, and a bland diet. Bed rest is advisable only as long as the patient is febrile; contrary to popular belief, physical activity has no influence upon the development of orchitis or other complications. Patients with epididymoorchitis may be acutely ill and in great pain. Many advocated forms of treatment including surgical decompression of the testicle, estrogens, convalescent serum and broad-spectrum antibiotics have not been regularly effective. The administration of adrenal steroids in a dosage corresponding to 300 mg cortisone or 60 mg prednisone initially, followed by a schedule of decreasing dosage for 7 to 10 days, has been markedly effective in decreasing testicular pain and swelling, damping the febrile response, and improving the patient's sense of well-being. It is important to administer adrenal hormones in large dosage initially; when smaller doses have been employed, these drugs have not been regularly effective. Adrenal steroids have not exerted an adverse effect on concomitant pancreatitis or meningitis. They have been tried specifically for the latter complication of mumps and, while effective in reducing fever and headache, their withdrawal was invariably accompanied by a sharp recrudescence of symptoms. Adrenal steroids have not prevented the appearance of parotid involvement on the contralateral side.

The management of pancreatitis is described on p. 1663. Mumps arthritis has been relieved symptomatically by adrenal steroids. Mumps thyroiditis also responded to these hormones with decrease in swelling and fever within 72 hr.

Prophylaxis. After exposure to the virus, the administration of γ-globulin is relatively ineffective in preventing or modifying mumps parotitis. Inactivated mumps virus vaccine does not abort clinical cases of mumps if given after exposure. It confers temporary immunity and may prevent orchitis or meningoencephalitis. Vaccination is rarely justified in children in whom the disease tends to be benign. However, vaccination of exposed adults who show no reaction to skin tests with mumps antigen is probably worthwhile. Because the vaccine contains small amounts of foreign protein, it should not be given to hypersensitive individuals.

Diethylstilbestrol in dosage of 1 mg daily for 1 week reduces the incidence of orchitis. A more effective regimen is the administration of 20 ml γ-globulin prepared from mumps convalescent serum.

Prognosis. As a rule, recovery from mumps and its sequelae is complete. Prognosis for life is good except for rare deaths occurring in cases of fulminating encephalitis. Deafness after meningoencephalitis, permanent diabetes following pancreatitis, or sterility subsequent to gonadal involvement is rare.

REFERENCES

Applebaum, E., J. Kohn, R. E. Steinman, and N. A. Shern: Mumps Arthritis, A.M.A. Arch. Internal Med., 90:217, 1952.

Candel, S.: Epididymitis in Mumps, Including Orchitis: Further Clinical Studies and Comments, Ann. Internal Med., 34:20, 1951.

Eylan, E., R. Zuweky, and C. Shaba: Mumps Virus and Subacute Thyroiditis: Evidence of a Causal Association, Lancet, 1:1062, 1957.

Horton, G. E.: Mumps Myocarditis, Ann. Internal Med., 49:1228, 1958.

Kolars, C. P., and W. W. Spink: Thrombopenic Purpura as a Complication of Mumps, J.A.M.A., 168: 2213, 1958.

Lennette, E. H., G. E. Caplan, and R. L. Magoffin: Mumps Virus Infection Simulating Paralytic Poliomyelitis, Pediatrics, 25:788, 1960.

Morgan, W. S.: The Probable Systemic Nature of Mikulicz's Disease and Its Relation to Sjoegren's Syndrome, New Engl. J. Med., 251:5, 1954.

Petersdorf, R. G., and I. L. Bennett, Jr.: Treatment of Mumps Orchitis with Adrenal Hormones: Report of 23 Cases with a Note on the Hepatic Involvement in Mumps, A.M.A. Arch. Internal Med., 99: 222, 1957.

—— B. L. Forsythe, and A. D. Beranke: Staphylococcal Parotitis, New Engl. J. Med., 259:1250, 1958.

Spitznagel, J. K.: Effect of Cortisone and ACTH in Mumps Meningoencephalitis, Ann. Internal Med., 49:61, 1958.

Wolfe, S. J., W. H. J. Summerskill, and C. S. Davidson: Parotid Swelling, Alcoholism and Cirrhosis, New Engl. J. Med., 256:491, 1957.

Young, L. J., and R. G. Cowley: Pulmonary Infarction Complicating Mumps, A.M.A. Arch. Internal Med., 97:249, 1956.

203 CYTOMEGALIC INCLUSION DISEASE (Salivary Gland Virus Disease)

Ivan L. Bennett, Jr.

Definition. This is a virus infection that is easily recognized by striking enlargement of epithelial cells of the salivary gland and other organs and the occurrence of prominent eosinophilic inclusions within the nuclei of affected cells. Related viruses eliciting similar tissue reactions have been isolated from lower animals, but these are apparently species-specific and do not infect man.

The vast majority of human infections are asymptomatic; the virus is frequently isolated from the adenoids or urine of well individuals, and most adults possess serum antibody against the virus. However, transplacental infection in infants can produce a fatal illness, and there is increasing evidence indicating that subclinical infection may be activated and illness may occur under a variety of conditions in older children or adults.

Manifestations. In infants, the disease is manifested as a hemolytic anemia with prominent hepatosplenomegaly and a hemorrhagic tendency. In other children, there are diarrhea, pneumonia, chorioretinitis, and signs of severe damage to liver, kidneys, and brain.

The presence of extensive lesions showing typical inclusions in the tissues of patients with other debilitating illnesses (mucoviscidosis, pertussis, chronic renal failure) is being noted with increasing frequency, supporting the idea that a lowering of resistance can activate subclinical infection.

Diagnosis. The disease should be suspected in any infant with jaundice, especially when erythroblastosis has been ruled out. Liver biopsy or the finding of epithelial cells with intranuclear inclusions in urine will confirm the diagnosis. Isolation of virus requires the use of tissue culture, but complement fixation tests on acute and convalescent serum are reliable and easy.

Treatment. Treatment is entirely symptomatic.

REFERENCES

Medearis, D. N.: Cytomegalic Inclusion Disease, Pediatrics, 19:467, 1957.

Rowe, W. P., et al.: Cytopathogenic Agent Resembling Human Salivary Gland Virus Recovered from Tissue Cultures of Human Adenoids, Proc. Soc. Exptl. Biol. and Med., 92:418, 1956.

Smith, M. G., and F. Vellios: Inclusion Disease or Generalized Salivary Gland Virus Infection, Arch. Pathol., 50:862, 1950.

Weller, T. H., J. C. Macauley, J. M. Craig, and P. Wirth: Isolation of Intranuclear Inclusion Producing Agents from Infants after Illnesses Resembling Cytomegalic Inclusion Disease, Proc. Soc. Exptl. Biol. Med., 94:4, 1957.

204 YELLOW FEVER
Ivan L. Bennett, Jr.

Definition. Yellow fever is an acute viral disease transmitted to man by mosquitoes and characterized by fever, icterus, bradycardia, proteinuria, and a bleeding tendency. The infection can be almost asymptomatic or rapidly fatal. Two types of the disease are now recognized: *urban yellow fever*, transmitted from man to man by the bite of the mosquito *Aedes aegypti;* and *sylvan* or *jungle yellow fever*, transmitted to man from monkeys by forest mosquitoes.

Etiology. The virus of yellow fever is small, its size being estimated at 17 to 28 mμ. It is inactivated by heat and ordinary antiseptics but can be preserved for months in 50 per cent glycerin and for years in the desiccated, refrigerated state. Two general types are recognized: the *viscerotropic*, which involves the liver, kidneys, and heart; and the *neurotropic*, which attacks nerve tissue. In nature, the virus possesses both affinities and is said to be *pantropic*. The various strains isolated in different parts of the world appear to be antigenically identical.

History and Epidemiology. Yellow fever occurs in large areas of South America and Africa. Since 1948 an epidemic of sylvan yellow fever has been spreading northward through Central America and in the Caribbean area. Much circumstantial evidence points to Africa as the place of origin of the disease, but the first reported epidemic was in Yucatán in 1648. From that time until the twentieth century many outbreaks occurred in the coastal regions along the trade routes of the Atlantic. The disease showed a seasonal incidence, being common during the warmer weather and subsiding with the cold weather.

Little was known of the method of transmission until Carlos Finley in 1881 incriminated the mosquito now known as *A. aegypti* as the vector. Because of the high incidence among American troops during the Spanish-American War, the Yellow Fever Commission was established under the direction of Major Walter Reed. In 1900 and 1901, through experiments on volunteers in Cuba, Reed, Carroll, Agramonte, and Lazear proved the method of transmission by mosquitoes and showed that the causative agent could pass through a Berkefeld filter, thus establishing the viral etiology of the disease. Control and suppression of yellow fever followed mosquito eradication.

From evidence that one attack of the infection produced a lifelong immunity, Carter reasoned that two factors were necessary to keep yellow fever in a community: (1) a population of nonimmune human beings and (2) a population of mosquitoes to act as vectors. Epidemiologists surveyed the key centers, and a tremendous control program was launched under the auspices of The Rockefeller Foundation, with the optimistic belief that yellow fever could be eradicated from the Americas and eventually from the world. The campaign appeared to be successful, and the disease seemed to be disappearing from South America until a mysterious epidemic broke out in Rio de Janeiro in 1928.

Extensive surveys employing serologic tests and postmortem "biopsy" studies (viscerotomy service) demonstrated that, in the forests of large areas of South America, Central America, and Africa, the disease is present in the monkey population and is transmitted by "forest-loving" mosquitoes, particularly species of *Haemagogus*. This reservoir is a potential source of danger to the native inhabitants and to rural workers who have to go into these areas. With increasing air travel and closer communication with all parts of the world, the danger of further widespread outbreaks is great, particularly in Mexico and along the Gulf of Mexico. Eradication of infection by antimosquito measures alone is no longer feasible.

Pathogenesis and Pathology. The mode of spread and multiplication of the virus has been studied in rhesus monkeys; it presumably follows the same course in man. When inoculated intradermally, the virus spreads immediately to the local lymph nodes, from which it enters the blood stream and invades the liver, spleen, kidneys, and bone marrow. The largest amounts of virus are found in the liver and serum. The organs which show the chief signs of degeneration in fatal cases are the liver, kidneys, and heart. Hemorrhages and jaundice are present in the skin and mucous membranes.

Microscopic changes are most apparent in the liver, where there is midzone necrosis with fatty degeneration. In severe cases, entire lobules may show necrosis. There is absence of inflammatory reaction, and eosinophilic Councilman bodies are numerous.

The lesions in the kidney are most evident in the tubules, chiefly the convoluted portion, where cloudy and fatty degeneration is present.

Early in the experimental disease, there is prominent necrosis of Kupffer cells. This is very characteristic, and it is probable that liver biopsy will turn out to be the most efficient method for early diagnosis in sporadic cases of human infection.

Manifestations. After an *incubation period* of 3 to 6 days, onset is usually sudden, sometimes with a chill, but it may be insidious. During the first 2 days of illness the chief symptoms are fever, headache, and backache. *Active congestion* follows, characterized by flushed face and injected conjunctivas and scleras. Nausea and vomiting are common.

As the fever increases, the pulse slows. Jaundice and evidence of hemorrhage occur on the fourth or fifth day of illness. Jaundice, even in severe cases, is not intense. Petechiae and gingival bleeding are common. Hemorrhages may occur in the stomach and intestine, giving rise to "black vomit" and melena. After 3 or 4 days, the temperature falls and there is a short remission of symptoms, followed by a recurrence of fever. Proteinuria and oliguria occur early. Recovery begins about the seventh day; it is rapid and usually without complications.

There is wide variation in the severity of the disease. The mortality is estimated at 5 per cent, most deaths occurring on the sixth or seventh day. The characteristic signs, whether in mild or severe cases, are the rise and remission of fever, the slow pulse in relation to the temperature (Faget's sign), and leukopenia.

Laboratory Findings. Proteinuria is marked in severe cases but is often absent in mild infections. A terminal anuria may occur. The leukocyte count falls steadily from the onset of infection, leukopenia being most marked on the fifth or sixth day. There is a decrease in both polymorphonuclear leukocytes and lymphocytes. As reflected in liver function tests, the liver is the organ most extensively damaged by the virus.

Three laboratory procedures are available to establish a positive diagnosis: isolation of the virus, serologic tests which demonstrate development of specific antibodies during an infection, and histologic examination of biopsies of the liver. Isolation of the virus is possible by intracerebral inoculation of mice with serum from patients up to the fifth day of the disease. Serum from patients may show positive protection tests in mice during convalescence.

Liver sections may be obtained by biopsy or, in fatal cases in countries where the disease is endemic, by the viscerotome. This is a simple instrument which permits removal of small specimens of liver after death. In South American countries where jungle yellow fever occurs over a large area, the study of liver sections of any fatal febrile case of less than 10 days' duration is a very important function of the Yellow Fever Service.

Treatment. No specific treatment is available. Bed rest, good nursing care, and supportive therapy consisting of soft diet, adequate fluids, and saline and glucose infusions are the general therapeutic measures usually employed. For high fever and headache, tepid sponges and ice caps are recommended.

Prevention. Prophylaxis consists of vaccination and the eradication of *A. aegypti* mosquitoes. Two strains of attenuated yellow fever virus are available for the preparation of vaccines: the French neurotropic and the 17D strain. The vaccine prepared from the 17D strain consists of frozen, dried extract of infected chick embryos sealed in ampuls. For use, the virus is reconstituted by the addition of sterile physiologic saline solution. One subcutaneous injection of 0.5 ml will produce immunity in man. In rural areas, mass vaccination is the only effective protection against jungle yellow fever. The use of DDT spray on the walls of houses is effective in controlling mosquitoes, but presently no method is available for eradicating jungle yellow fever.

REFERENCES

Carter, H. R.: "Yellow Fever: An Epidemiological and Historical Study of Its Place of Origin," Baltimore, The Williams & Wilkins Company, 1931.

Elton, N. W.: Progress of Sylvan Yellow Fever Wave in Central America, Nicaragua and Honduras, Am. J. Pub. Health, 42:1527, 1952.

Galindo, P., E. DeRodaniche, and H. Trapido: Experimental Transmission of Yellow Fever by Central American Species of *Haemogogus* and *Sabethes chloropterus*, Am. J. Trop. Med. Hyg., 5:1022, 1956.

Smithburn, K. C. (Ed.): "Yellow Fever Vaccination," World Health Organization Monograph Series No. 30, Geneva, 1956.

Strode, G. K. (Ed.): "Yellow Fever," New York, McGraw-Hill Book Company, Inc., 1951.

Theiler, M.: Yellow Fever, p. 343 in "Viral and Rickettsial Infections of Man," 3d ed., T. M. Rivers and F. L. Horsfall, Jr. (Eds.), Philadelphia, J. B. Lippincott Company, 1959.

Tigertt, W. D., et al.: Experimental Yellow Fever, Trans. N.Y. Acad. Sci., 22:323, 1960.

Yellow Fever Conference, Dec. 21–22, 1954, Am. J. Trop. Med. Hyg., 4:571, 1955.

205 EPIDEMIC HEMORRHAGIC FEVER

J. E. Smadel

Definition. Epidemic hemorrhagic fever is an acute illness characterized by fever of 5 days' duration accompanied by prostration, anorexia, and vomiting. Capillary abnormalities appear early in the illness; they are intensified about the fourth day, when petechial hemorrhages become prominent and increased capillary permeability results in marked proteinuria and transudation of plasma constituents into some soft tissues. With the termination of fever, some patients proceed to recovery, but about 20 per cent develop hypotensive shock and renal insufficiency. The mortality rate is about 5 per cent. No specific laboratory test is available; hence the diagnosis is based on the typical clinical or pathologic picture. Treatment consists of supportive and corrective measures. A number of other infectious diseases with hemorrhagic manifestations exist in Asia, Europe, and the Americas. These are mentioned elsewhere in this chapter.

History, Etiology, and Epidemiology. Epidemic hemorrhagic fever was first recognized in Manchuria and Siberia by the Japanese and Russians about two decades ago. During the Korean War the disease occurred in United Nation troops and was extensively investigated by Americans. The identical disease was subsequently described in the Yaroslavl area of the Volga River Basin. It now is known to be widespread in European Russia and to extend westward in Europe as far as Hungary and Czechoslovakia.

Both the Russian and the Japanese investigators who studied epidemic hemorrhagic fever in the Far East were able to transmit the disease to human beings by injecting them with urine or blood taken from patients during the first few days of disease. Moreover, each group found that the causative agent passed through filters which retained microbiologic agents larger than viruses. Neither these workers nor the Americans who investigated the Korean malady were able to establish the agent in a laboratory host. Recent studies on this type of hemorrhagic fever in the Yaroslavl area have given identical results, i.e., successful experimental transmission to man but not to laboratory animals.

Two seasonal peaks of disease incidence are characteristic of epidemic hemorrhagic fever, but sporadic cases are encountered each month of the year. Most of the 1,000 patients seen annually in Korea from 1951 to 1953 became ill between mid-April and early July and during October and November. The disease in Korea was limited essentially to military personnel stationed in rural areas north of a line drawn across the peninsula at the level of Seoul. However, a few civilians of all ages contracted the disease on returning to neglected farms in this area after the armistice. In contrast, in Europe the malady affects civilians working in rural and forested areas, with at least a thousand cases being reported annually in European Russia in recent years.

Intensive studies indicated that the majority of cases in Korea were isolated and widely spaced in time and place. In the small outbreaks (1) there was no person-to-person spread of infection, (2) food and water were unimportant in the epidemiology of the disease, and (3) the cases in a given outbreak acquired their infection over a period of a day or so during exposure in a sharply localized area of abandoned farmland or scrub-covered terrain. Although definitive proof was lacking, the Americans assumed that trombiculid mites served as the vector to man for the agent of epidemic hemorrhagic fever and that small wild rodents provided the reservoir. Russian investigators also assumed that small rodents served as the reservoir and that mites were involved in the cycle of infection. Precise information on the ecology of the agent must await the discovery of a susceptible laboratory host for use in definitive studies.

Epidemic hemorrhagic fever is distinct from Crimean hemorrhagic fever which extends from the Balkans eastward across the southern part of the USSR. The latter disease is milder and without the typical renal changes of the former. Moreover, its virus is transmitted to man by *Hyalomma* ticks during the spring-summer season. Two other hemorrhagic fevers, which are related to each other but different from the two just mentioned, are Omsk hemorrhagic fever and Kyasanur Forest disease. The former occurs in western Siberia and the latter in central India. Both are caused by members of the Russian spring-summer group of viruses and are transmitted to man by *Dermacentor* ticks which also serve as vectors in the natural cycle involving wild animals. Febrile diseases associated with hemorrhagic manifestations have been described recently in the Philippines and Thailand. These are mosquito-borne infections caused by members of the dengue group of viruses. Finally, a viral disease with a hemorrhagic diathesis has been recognized recently in Argentina.

Manifestations. Following an incubation period of about 2 weeks (with extremes of 9 to 36 days), the illness usually begins abruptly, with frontal headache, chills, high fever, anorexia, and backache. Physical findings during the first few days of fever and prostration are essentially limited to cutaneous flush, especially about the face and neck, and injection of the conjunctivas. About the third day petechiae generally appear on the soft palate and in the conjunctivas, the axillary folds, and cutaneous areas subjected to mild trauma. Increased capillary permeability becomes evident about the fourth day with the appearance of pathognomonic severe proteinuria and edema of loose tissue; edema of conjunctivas and periorbital tissue is visible on physical examination. Edema in the lumbar gutters and mesentery contributes to the abdominal and back pain, but it can be seen only at autopsy.

Fever disappears about the fifth day, but even in the moderately affected patient the disease continues, progressing through a series of phases, i.e., hypotensive, oliguric, diuretic, and convalescent. Manifestations of capillary leakage, among them a rising hematocrit, increase during the hypotensive phase but begin to abate after several days, when the oliguric phase is ushered in, with its associated mounting blood urea and creatinine levels. With the beginning of diuresis on about the tenth day, symptoms and abnormal physiologic findings generally disappear quickly. However, renal tubular function is restored slowly, and normal concentrating capacity usually does not return until the fourth to sixth week after onset of the disease. Body weight, which may have decreased as much as 20 lb in the average individual during the acute illness, is slowly restored to pre-onset levels.

Those patients in whom the disease takes a severe course display either hypotensive shock during the fifth to seventh day after onset, or progressive renal failure during the second week, or both. The acute renal failure is in no way unique in regard to its clinical manifestations; hence this phase needs no further discussion here (see p. 1496). The physical findings in the shock phase are those of peripheral vascular collapse. In spite of the marked lowering of blood pressure, the skin is warm and flushed. The loss of plasma through damaged capillaries and pooling of blood in dilated peripheral and visceral capillaries result in reduced circulating blood volume. All these abnormalities contribute to the profound dysfunction of selected organs such as the kidney.

Laboratory Findings and Pathology. Clinical laboratory data other than those already mentioned consist of (1) leukocytosis of 10,000 to 20,000 per cu mm, with many immature granulocytes by the end of the first week, (2) thrombocytopenia which reaches levels below 100,000 in half the patients, (3) disturbances of electrolyte balance, and (4) entirely negative results in various types of tests for the ordinary microbial agents.

The characteristic lesions observed at autopsy are found in the kidney, right auricle, and pituitary gland. The renal cortex is pale, while the pyramids are dark red, almost hemorrhagic in appearance. Hemorrhages occur in the auricle and pituitary gland. If death ensues during the hypotensive phase, gelatinous edema fluid is found in the retroperitoneal tissues and mesentery; if death occurs during the late oliguric phase, these tissues are usually dry. Microscopic changes other than those concerned with the lesions observed grossly are rather meager and consist of scattered small focal areas of necrosis and hemorrhage in visceral organs. Inflammatory lesions of the small vessels are conspicuously lacking, but intense capillary congestion is characteristic. Indeed, many of the areas which appear hemorrhagic at autopsy, such as the renal pyramids, actually represent sites where the capillaries are extremely dilated.

Differential Diagnosis. During the first few days of illness the disease may be confused with leptospirosis, the typhus fevers, hemorrhagic smallpox, idiopathic thrombocytopenic purpura, leukemia, or even influenza. A history of exposure in the endemic area—particularly during a seasonal epidemic—and the appearance of marked proteinuria on the fourth day and the subsequent progression of the illness through the typical hypotensive, oliguric, and diuretic stages eliminate other diseases and warrant the diagnosis "epidemic hemorrhagic fever, confirmed."

Treatment and Prevention. The treatment of hemorrhagic fever is limited at present to supportive measures; none of the chemotherapeutic or antibiotic agents has proved of value. Treatment begins with early diagnosis and prompt transfer to a hospital equipped to cope with a disease characterized by such extensive and varied physiologic disturbances.

During the febrile phase, complete bed rest, mild sedation, maintenance of reasonably normal water balance (overhydration is to be avoided), and an adequate but light diet are essential. The majority of patients in the hypotensive and oliguric phases do well on a continuation of the same regimen, but the severely ill require constant attention and often markedly different therapeutic measures within short periods of time. Shock may develop rapidly and require prompt and active measures.

Once diuresis is established, special attention must be paid to adequate intake of fluid and electrolytes, since 3 to 6 liters of urine may be excreted daily. The principal therapeutic measure during convalescence is concerned with exercise; the amount is increased *pari passu* with the recovery of concentrating capacity of the kidney.

Preventive measures against hemorrhagic fever are based on avoidance of trombiculid mites, which are assumed to be the vectors of the disease. These measures are concerned with (1) the use of insect repellents for impregnation of clothes (benzyl benzoate) and application to exposed skin surfaces (dimethyl phthalate), (2) clearing of all vegetation from camp sites (bulldozing) and treatment of the area with residual insecticides such as lindane, and (3) rodent control in and about camps by means of rodenticides.

Prognosis. The disease varies greatly in severity. In some patients it is so mild as to make the diagnosis difficult; indeed, many suspected cases are not confirmed because they fail to develop the typical renal manifestations; yet some of the patients with such cases undoubtedly are infected with the agent of epidemic hemorrhagic fever. About 20 per cent of the patients in whom the disease is diagnosed become critically ill. The following factors contribute to the severity and influence the prognosis unfavorably: delayed initiation of medical care, prolonged high fever, excessive fluid intake, prolonged or recurrent shock, persistent hemoconcentration, anuria, and progressive severe electrolyte disturbances. The fatality rate in cases among American soldiers in Korea was between 5 and 7 per cent.

REFERENCES

Chumakov, M. P.: Etiology, Epidemiology and Prophylaxis of Hemorrhagic Fevers, Pub. Health Monograph No. 50, pp. 19–25, Public Health Service, U.S. Government Printing Office, Washington, D.C., 1957.

Department of the Army Technical Bulletin TB Med. No. 240, Epidemic Hemorrhagic Fever, May, 1953.

Earle, D. P. (Ed.): Symposium on Epidemic Hemorrhagic Fever, Am. J. Med., 16:617, 1954.

Gajdusek, D. C.: "Acute Infectious Hemorrhagic Fevers and Mycotoxicoses in the Union of Soviet Socialist Republics," Med. Sci. Pub. No. 2, pp. 1–140, Army Medical Service Graduate School, U.S. Government Printing Office, Washington, D.C., 1953.

Gauld, R. L., and J. P. Craig: Epidemiological Pattern of Localized Outbreaks of Epidemic Hemorrhagic Fever, Am. J. Hyg., 59:32, 1954.

Greenway, D. J., H. R. Rugiero, A. S. Parodi, M. Figerio, E. Rivero, J. M. de la Barrera, F. Garzon, M. Boxaca, N. Mettler, L. B. de Guerrero, and N. Nota: Epidemic Hemorrhagic Fever in Argentina, Pub. Health Repts., 74:1011, 1959.

Hammon, W. McD., A. Rudnick, and G. E. Sather: Viruses Associated with Epidemic Hemorrhagic Fevers of the Philippines and Thailand, Science, 131:1102, 1960.

Hullinghorst, R. L., and A. Steer: Pathology of Epidemic Hemorrhagic Fever, Ann. Internal Med., 38:77, 1953.

Ormay, L., M. P. Aradi, I. Nikodemusz, and G. Losonczy: An Evaluation of the Results of Focus Research of the Hemorrhagic Nephroso-Nephritis in Hungary, Zentr. Bakteriol. (Orig.), 178:279, 1960.

Sizemova, G. A.: Hemorrhagic Syndrome in Patients with Omsk Fever, Sovet. Med., 23(5):81, 1959.

Smorodintsev, A. A., V. G. Chudakov, and A. V. Churilov: "Hemorrhagic Nephroso-Nephritis," pp. 1–124, New York, Pergamon Press, Inc., 1959.

Traub, R., M. Hertig, W. H. Lawrence, and T. T. Harriss: Potential Vectors and Reservoirs of Hemorrhagic Fever in Korea, Am. J. Hyg., 59:291, 1954.

Work, T. H., F. R. Roderiguez, and P. N. Bhatt: Virological Epidemiology of the 1958 Epidemic of Kyasanur Forest Disease, Am. J. Pub. Health, 49:869, 1959.

206 DENGUE
Robert R. Wagner

Definition. Dengue is an acute viral disease characterized by a diphasic course, fever, myalgia, morbilliform rash, transient personality changes, and leukopenia.

Epidemiology. The infection is transmitted by *Aedes aegypti* and other species of *Aedes* mosquitoes, which harbor the virus throughout their lives but do not pass it on to their offspring. Man and monkeys constitute the only known reservoirs of infection. Dengue is endemic in tropical and subtropical areas where mosquitoes survive throughout the year. Summer epidemics have occurred in the United States, particularly in port cities, but the climate of this country is not favorable for the establishment of endemic foci. The epidemiologic characteristics of dengue closely resemble those of yellow fever; the two diseases also have a similar geographic distribution, except in southeast Asia, where dengue is prevalent but yellow fever is unknown.

Etiology. Large quantities of virus are present in the blood during the early phase of the disease.

Although little is known of the pathogenesis of the disease or the site of virus multiplication, microscopic examination of skin biopsies suggests involvement of capillary endothelium in the infectious process. Virus isolated directly from man or mosquitoes is infectious for volunteers but is not pathogenic for laboratory animals and produces no inclusion bodies or other recognizable lesions. During the Second World War, Sabin and Schlesinger demonstrated that dengue virus produces fatal encephalitis in suckling and adult mice after repeated brain passages. Mouse-adapted virus has been cultivated in tissue cultures of monkey kidney epithelium. Four related antigenic types of dengue virus have been described, of which type 1 (Hawaiian strain prototype) and type 2 (New Guinea "C" strain prototype) appear to be the most prevalent. Dengue virus is classified with the group B arbor (arthropod-borne) viruses because of its biologic and antigenic similarity to the viruses of yellow fever and Japanese, West Nile, and St. Louis encephalitis.

Manifestations. The incubation period is usually 5 to 9 days, with a range of 3 to 15 days. About half the cases have a sudden and dramatic onset, with chills or chilly sensations, profuse diaphoresis, and temperature elevation of 102 to 106°F. Prodromal symptoms of malaise, anorexia, and lethargy precede the fever in milder forms of the disease. Severe frontal headache, retroorbital pain, and excruciating low backache are almost invariably present. Dengue is popularly known as "breakbone fever," because of incapacitating pains in the muscles and periarticular tissues of the extremities in more than half the cases. The majority of patients experience nausea, constipation, and disturbances of taste and smell in the early phases; diarrhea may be present late in the course. Agitation and insomnia alternate with depression and fitful sleep. A primary rash, consisting of blotchy erythema or flushing of the face, accompanies the initial temperature elevation in about a third of the patients. Moderate conjunctival and pharyngeal reddening may also be noted. The symptoms persist for 3 or 4 days, following which the temperature falls by crisis or rapid lysis. A bright red morbilliform or punctate rash appears in three-fourths of the patients on the third to sixth day of illness; the eruption starts on the dorsal surfaces of the hands and feet and rapidly extends over the trunk and face. Generalized lymph node enlargement is commonly encountered, but the spleen is rarely palpable.

Many patients develop a *secondary rise in temperature* 12 to 72 hr after subsidence of the initial episode, producing the typical saddleback fever curve of dengue. All the symptoms return with increased intensity; delirium and depression may be particularly marked. Cold, mottled extremities, hypotension, bradycardia, and a dicrotic pulse may be noted during the second phase of the disease. The total duration of acute illness is usually 6 to 9 days, but convalescence is often prolonged for several weeks by marked weakness, apathy, radicular pains, aching legs and back, and marked personality changes. A rare disturbance is transient loss of pupillary accommodation owing to paralysis of the ciliary muscle of the eye.

The incidence of *complications* varies in different epidemics. Jaundice occurs in less than 1 case in 100. Herpes labialis, otitis media, and bronchopneumonia are uncommon. Bleeding tendencies are occasionally noted as manifested by purpura, petechial rashes, epistaxes, and hemorrhages from the intestine and vagina. Dengue viruses, particularly types 3 and 4, have been implicated as causative agents of epidemic hemorrhagic fevers of the Philippines and Thailand, which occur almost exclusively in children under six years of age. The mortality rate in hemorrhagic forms of the disease has been recorded as 10 per cent, but is consistently low in the absence of complications.

Laboratory Findings. Complement-fixing and neutralizing antibodies appear in the serum after the seventh day of disease. Leukopenia with counts of 2,000 to 5,000 cells per cu mm and "toxic" granulation of the polymorphonuclear leukocytes are constant features of the early phase of the disease. Moderate leukocytosis often occurs during convalescence. Oliguria and proteinuria are common with high fever.

Differential Diagnosis. The sudden onset of chilliness, fever, and myalgia may simulate influenza, malaria, sandfly fever, and leptospirosis, but rash is uncommon in these diseases. Exanthematous viral infections, such as measles, can usually be differentiated by their clinical course and epidemiology. Hemorrhagic dengue occurs in different geographic areas and affects a younger age group than the epidemic hemorrhagic fevers of Northern Asia, Omsk hemorrhagic fever, and Kyasanur Forest disease (see p. 1186).

Treatment. No specific treatment is available, but analgesics and sedatives afford symptomatic relief of pain and anxiety. Control of mosquitoes by sanitation and insecticides decreases the incidence of dengue in endemic areas. Dengue virus cultivated in mouse brain has been used as a living attenuated vaccine; unfortunately, it causes mild dengue.

REFERENCES

Hammon, W. McD., A. Rudnick, and G. E. Sather: Viruses Associated with Epidemic Hemorrhagic Fevers of the Philippines and Thailand, Science, 131:1102, 1960.

Rifkin, H.: Dengue Fever (Breakbone Fever), pp.
    119–123 in "When Doctors Are Patients," M.
    Pinner and B. F. Miller (Eds.), New York, W. W.
    Norton & Company, Inc., 1952.

Sabin, A. B.: Dengue, pp. 361–373 in "Viral and
    Rickettsial Infections of Man," 3d ed., T. M.
    Rivers and F. L. Horsfall, Jr. (Eds.), Philadelphia,
    J. B. Lippincott Company, 1959.

Rosen, L.: Observations on the Epidemiology of
    Dengue in Panama, Am. J. Hygiene, 68:45, 1958.

Stewart, F. H.: Dengue: Analysis of the Clinical
    Syndrome at a South Pacific Advanced Base,
    U.S. Naval Med. Bull., 42:1233, 1944.

207 COLORADO TICK FEVER
Ivan L. Bennett, Jr.

Definition. Colorado tick fever (mountain fever, mountain tick fever) is an acute viral disease transmitted to man by the bite of the tick, *Dermacentor andersoni.*

Etiology. The etiologic virus measures 35 to 50 $m\mu$, will survive for several days in unrefrigerated blood, and is lethal for suckling mice and for hamsters. In the laboratory, it has been adapted to adult mice and chick embryos.

Epidemiology. Although virus has occasionally been isolated from several species of ticks, the geographic distribution of the disease is that of *D. andersoni,* the only tick known to transmit the disease to man. All recognized cases have originated in California, Colorado, Idaho, Montana, Nevada, Oregon, Utah, Washington, or Wyoming. The seasonal incidence corresponds to that of the tick population from March to July, with a peak in late May or early June. An animal reservoir is suggested by the finding of antibodies against the virus in the serum of jack rabbits. Recovery in man is followed by lifelong immunity. The disease occurs in tourists in the endemic area with annoying frequency, and in view of the incubation period of 3 to 6 days and the speed of modern travel, the disease can be expected to appear in any part of the United States.

Manifestations. A history of exposure to ticks is almost invariable. After 3 to 6 days there is the abrupt onset of fever, occasionally with a rigor, myalgia, photophobia, intense headache, and prostrating weakness. Anorexia, nausea, and vomiting are the rule. Sustained fever with temperatures of 102 to 104°F continues for 3 days, when a remission of 2 or 3 days occurs. During this remission, body temperature is likely to be subnormal and patients are very weak and listless. In about 90 per cent of cases, there is a second bout of high fever lasting 3 to 4 days, usually even more severe than the initial illness. Monophasic attacks occur and, rarely, three bouts of fever have been noted. Recovery is usually uncomplicated, although persistent asthenia is often a problem. Rash, splenomegaly, and lymphadenopathy are not a part of this disease.

In children, the disease has been accompanied by encephalitis, occasionally very severe, and a variety of transient neurologic abnormalities including the picture of "aseptic meningitis" can occur but none is common.

There is serologic evidence that subclinical infection occurs in man. It has been reported that peculiar ulceration that is slow to heal can occur at the site of the infected tick bite, but this is not invariable and, conceivably, has nothing to do with the disease.

Laboratory Findings. The peripheral leukocyte count falls to levels of 2,000 or 3,000, being lowest during the relapse. Although the proportion of polymorphonuclear cells is low, there is a shift to the left. Virus is present in the blood throughout the illness, including the remission. Antibody may not appear for several weeks, but usually a serologic confirmation of the diagnosis can be obtained within 2 weeks.

Diagnosis. A history of exposure to ticks in the geographic areas mentioned, biphasic fever, and severe leukopenia make the diagnosis evident as illness progresses. Initially, Rocky Mountain spotted fever, influenza, psittacosis, and several other diseases may be suspected. Despite its resemblance to dengue, the absence of rash and the completely different distribution of the disease make the differentiation a rare problem.

Treatment. There is no treatment other than sedation and the use of analgesics. In the rare instances of encephalitis, appropriate supportive therapy is, of course, indicated.

Prognosis. Recovery is complete although it may be prolonged by asthenia. With the possible exception of one reported case of encephalitis in a child, no deaths have occurred.

REFERENCES

Cox, H. R.: Colorado Tick Fever, p. 348 in "Viral and
    Rickettsial Diseases of Man," 3d ed., T. M.
    Rivers and F. L. Horsfall, Jr. (Eds.), Philadelphia,
    J. B. Lippincott Company, 1959.

Ecklund, C. M., G. M. Kohls, and J. M. Brennan:
    Distribution of Colorado Tick Fever and Virus-
    carrying Ticks, J.A.M.A., 157:335, 1955.

Florio, L., E. R. Mugrage, and M. O. Stewart: Colo-
    rado Tick Fever, Ann. Internal Med. 25:466,
    1946.

Lloyd, L. W.: Colorado Tick Fever, Med. Clin. N.
    Am., 35:587, 1951.

208 PHLEBOTOMUS FEVER
Ivan L. Bennett, Jr.

Definition. Phlebotomus fever (sandfly, pappataci, or 3-day fever) is an acute viral infection characterized by fever, severe headache, conjunctivitis, general malaise, and leukopenia transmitted to man by the sandfly, *Phlebotomus papatasii*.

Etiology. The size of the virus is estimated at 40 to 60 mμ. In frozen or lyophilized states the virus has been preserved for many years. Several strains have been isolated and appear to be immunologically different, as evidenced by lack of cross immunity in inoculated volunteers.

Epidemiology. The disease is endemic in those parts of Europe, Africa, and Asia between 20 and 45° north latitude where the vector *P. papatasii* propagates. It occurs during infancy and childhood as a mild febrile illness and is usually not recognized as a distinct clinical entity. However, outbreaks among military personnel and other immigrants who move into endemic areas occur with disturbing severity. Patients are infectious for the sandfly 1 day before the onset of fever and 2 days after the onset. The reservoir of the virus during the winter is not known.

Manifestations. After an incubation period of 2 to 6 days, there is sudden onset of malaise, giddiness, pains in the back and extremities, severe headache (usually frontal), and pain in the eyes. Fever is always present and lasts for 2 to 4 days. The temperature may rise to 104.5°F within the first 24 hr and then gradually subsides. The pulse rate is fast at first but returns to normal more rapidly than the temperature, and a bradycardia often occurs during convalescence. An erythema occurs on the face and exposed parts of the neck and chest, but no true rash develops. The conjunctivas are injected, and the eyeballs are tender. The conjunctival injection is sometimes limited to the exposed portion of the eyeball, so-called Pick's sign. Convalescence is characterized by prostration and occasionally by mental depression, diarrhea, and epistaxis. Splenomegaly and lymphadenopathy are not observed.

Laboratory Findings. A leukopenia with a predominance of neutrophilic leukocytes, many of which are immature, is present, and there is a decrease in lymphocytes. The greatest drop in the leukocyte count occurs at the end of the febrile period. The urine is normal, and there is no laboratory evidence of liver damage. The cerebrospinal fluid is normal.

Differential Diagnosis. The diagnosis usually is made on clinical and epidemiologic grounds and is suggested by the occurrence of fever of short duration during the hot, dry season in countries known to harbor the vector. Phlebotomus fever is sometimes confused with dengue, influenza, infectious hepatitis, and malaria. It differs from dengue in the short duration of the fever and the absence of rash and lymphadenopathy; from influenza by its seasonal incidence and the absence of catarrhal symptoms; from infectious hepatitis by the absence of jaundice and by normal liver function tests. Cases are often misdiagnosed as malaria, but no chills occur, and blood films are negative for parasites.

Treatment. No specific therapy is known. Control measures consist of eradicating the vector within 100 to 200 m of living quarters. DDT residual spray is successful in killing *P. papatasii* at its breeding site and within habitations.

REFERENCES

Fleming, J., J. R. Bignoll, and A. N. Blades: Sandfly Fever: Review of 664 Cases, Lancet, 1947, I:433.
Sabin, A. B.: Phlebotomus Fever, p. 374 in "Viral and Rickettsial Diseases of Man," 3d ed., T. M. Rivers and F. L. Horsfall, Jr. (Eds.), Philadelphia, J. B. Lippincott Company, 1959.

209 WEST NILE FEVER
Robert R. Wagner and
Ivan L. Bennett, Jr.

Definition. This acute febrile illness closely resembles dengue in its clinical manifestations and is caused by a group B arthropod-borne (arbor) virus.

Etiology. West Nile virus is one member of the large family of group B arbor viruses (see p. 1194). Its biologic and immunologic similarities to the viruses of Japanese, St. Louis, and Murray Valley encephalitis suggest that all these agents are descended from a common ancestor.

Epidemiology. The geographic distribution of West Nile virus includes Africa, the Near East, and parts of India. The endemic focus probably centers around Egypt, which was the site of the first isolation of this virus in 1937, but the most widespread epidemics have occurred in Israel since 1950. The best available evidence on the ecology of West Nile virus implicates birds as the reservoir of infection and culicine mosquitoes as the vectors. Although human infection is characterized by viremia, mosquitoes probably transmit the disease only from birds to man rather than from man to man. West Nile virus is said to be responsible for almost three-fourths of all summer febrile illnesses among children and young adults in Israel. Large-scale epidemics are less common in Egypt because a major segment of the population has acquired immunity through infection in early childhood. Many of these infections are asymptomatic even when viremia is demonstrable.

Manifestations. After an incubation period of 2 to 6 days, the disease usually starts abruptly with fever and a temperature that reaches 101 to 105°F. Approximately one-third of adult patients experience shaking chills. Pronounced weakness and fatigue are almost invariable from the onset, and some patients may exhibit profound prostration. Frequent early complaints are severe frontal headache and retroorbital pain accentuated by eye movements. Generalized myalgia, backache, and abdominal pain also occur in varying degrees and combinations. In some outbreaks, gastrointestinal symptoms of anorexia, nausea, vomiting, and diarrhea are quite prominent, whereas respiratory symptoms of mild sore throat and cough are less usual. Physical examination often reveals a flushed face and conjunctival and pharyngeal injection. Rash appears 2 to 5 days after onset in about half of the proved cases and disappears without desquamation or residual skin discoloration in several hours or several days. The rash is usually confined to the upper trunk and consists of pink discrete macules or diffuse erythematous mottling. One of the most prominent findings is generalized lymphadenopathy that persists for weeks after convalescence. Splenic and hepatic enlargement may also occur but are much less common.

In 3 to 5 days after onset, rarely as long as 2 weeks, the symptoms abate and defervescence occurs by crisis or lysis. Occasionally, the course is biphasic with recrudescence of acute symptoms after a brief afebrile period. *Recovery* has invariably been complete except for persistent weakness in some cases. The only noteworthy *complications* have been the rare occurrence of aseptic meningitis in the naturally acquired disease and severe encephalitis in patients with advanced cancers undergoing therapeutic trial of artificially induced West Nile fever.

Laboratory Findings. West Nile virus can often be isolated from blood during the first day or two of illness. Complement-fixing and neutralizing antibodies appear in the serum within 2 weeks. In common with infections caused by other arbor viruses, leukopenia is a usual finding during the acute phase of West Nile fever.

Differential Diagnosis. Only knowledge of its geographic distribution serves to differentiate West Nile fever from denguelike infections caused by other arbor viruses (see p. below).

REFERENCES

Goldblum, N., et al.: The Natural History of West Nile Fever. II. Virological Findings and the Development of Homologous and Heterologous Antibodies in West Nile Infection in Man, Am. J. Hyg., 66:363, 1957.

Marburg, K., et al.: The Natural History of West Nile Fever: I. Clinical Observations during an Epidemic in Israel, Am. J. Hyg., 64:259, 1956.

Taylor, R. M., et al.: A Study of the Ecology of West Nile Virus in Egypt, Am. J. Trop. Med. Hyg., 5:597, 1956.

210 EXOTIC VIRAL FEVERS

*Ivan L. Bennett, Jr., and
Robert R. Wagner*

Most viral infections of man are asymptomatic. This epidemiologic observation has been called the "iceberg phenomenon," an analogy to the small number of clinically apparent cases and the submerged or inapparent majority. An extreme example of this dichotomy has been reported in epidemics of St. Louis and Japanese B encephalitis in which neurologic disorders occur approximately once in every 500 serologically proved infections.

By far the commonest manifestation of viral infection is a grippelike syndrome that is virtually indistinguishable from influenza, dengue, or nonparalytic poliomyelitis. The enteroviruses and arbor viruses, in particular, often cause brief, nondescript, febrile illnesses, some of which tend to be biphasic. The first, or minor, phases are usually similar and coincide with the stage of viremia. The second, or major, phases are sometimes associated with severe damage to tissues, especially the central nervous system, but such serious illness is the rare exception rather than the rule. Poliomyelitis and other enteroviral infections are described in other chapters, as are the more widely recognized diseases caused by arbor viruses. The purpose of this chapter is to direct attention to the discovery of an ever-expanding list of viruses that produce febrile diseases. Some appear to be world-wide and others are found in restricted tropical locales. Mention can be made only of those which have aroused special interest and seem to be of the greatest potential significance. Table 210-1 lists some selected arbor viruses under the disease syndromes with which they are usually associated.

GROUP A ARBOR VIRUSES

The viruses of *eastern* and *western equine encephalomyelitis* are indigenous to the United States

Table 210-1. SYNDROMES PRODUCED BY HUMAN INFECTION WITH ARTHROPOD-BORNE (ARBOR) VIRUSES
(X signifies those serologically unclassified as A, B, or C)

Syndrome	Virus	Serologic group	Locality	Vector
Fever, prostration, headache, local and general myalgia	Venezuelan equine	A	Trinidad, South America	Mosquito
	Mayaro	A	Trinidad, South America	Mosquito
	Uruma	A	Bolivia	?
	Wesselsbron	B	South Africa	Mosquito
	Zika	B	Nigeria, Uganda	Mosquito
	Oriboca, Marituba, Apeú, Itaqui	C	Brazil	Mosquito
	Bunyamwera	X	Africa, South America	Mosquito
	Bwamba	X	Africa	?
	Guama	X	Brazil	Mosquito
	Phlebotomus	X	Mediterranean	Sandfly
	Colorado tick fever	X	Western United States	Tick
Fever, prostration, headache, *joint pains, rash*	Chikungunya	A	Africa	Mosquito
	O'nyong-nyong	A	Africa	Mosquito
Fever, prostration, headache, local and general myalgia, *rash, lymphadenopathy*	Dengue 1 and 2	B	World-wide (tropics)	Mosquito
	West Nile	B	Africa, Near East, India	Mosquito
Fever, prostration, headache, local and general myalgia, *hemorrhage*	Chikungunya (?)	A	Thailand	Mosquito
	Dengue 3 and 4	B	Thailand, Philippines	Mosquito
	Kyasanur Forest disease	B	India	Tick
	Omsk hemorrhagic fever	B	Siberia	Tick
	Argentinian hemorrhagic fever	X	Argentina	Mite (?)
	Crimean hemorrhagic fever	X	South Russia	Tick
Encephalitis and meningo-encephalitis	Eastern equine	A	North and South America, Philippines	Mosquito
	Western equine	A	North and South America	Mosquito
	Venezuelan equine A (rare)	A	Trinidad, South America	Mosquito
	Japanese B	B	Asia, Australia, Indonesia	Mosquito
	Murray Valley	B	Australia, New Guinea	Mosquito
	St. Louis	B	United States, South America, West Indies	Mosquito
	Ilheus	B	South and Central America, Trinidad	Mosquito
	Pawassan	B	Canada	Tick
	Russian spring-summer	B	Russia	Tick
	Central European encephalitis	B	Central Europe	Tick
	Diphasic meningoencephalitis	B	Russia	Tick (milk)
Hepatitis, nephritis, etc.	Yellow fever	B	South America and Africa	Mosquito
	Rift Valley fever	X	Africa	Mosquito

SOURCE: Adapted from World Health Organization, Technical Report No. 219, 1961.

but are also found in the West Indies and South America. Most infections with the eastern virus result in a severe, often fatal, encephalitis. The western virus may cause a similar disease, but infections are more frequently asymptomatic or are manifested by febrile illness without involvement of the central nervous system.

Venezuelan equine encephalomyelitis is a related virus of northern South America and the West Indies which is transmitted to horses and man by mosquitoes. It is also the most infectious of all known viruses by the respiratory route when artificial aerosols are created in the laboratory. Despite its name, the Venezuelan virus usually causes an acute febrile illness without overt meningoencephalitis in man. The onset of the disease is invariably abrupt with severe headache and temperature that may reach 105°F. Shaking chills, generalized myalgia, lethargy, and prostration are very common manifestations. Nausea, vomiting, and diarrhea occur less frequently. A few patients exhibit blurred vision and somnolence. Important laboratory findings are viremia and marked leukopenia with relative lymphocytosis. Accidentally infected laboratory workers have all recovered uneventfully, but a few deaths from encephalitis have occurred during epidemics of the naturally acquired disease.

Semliki Forest virus, which was first isolated in 1944 from mosquitoes in East Africa, is the prototype of another subgroup of arbor A viruses. An important related virus is the causative agent of *Chikungunya fever* which is responsible for major epidemics in East and South Africa. This disease begins very abruptly without prodromal symptoms and reaches its peak severity within minutes or hours. The temperature ranges from 102 to 105°F and is often accompanied by true rigors. The most prominent manifestation is excruciating pain in the back and in the joints of the extremities which forces the patient to assume a jackknifed, immobilized position. Chikungunya means "doubled-up" in an African dialect. Anorexia, nausea, vomiting, diarrhea, and abdominal pain occur in some patients, but, surprisingly, headache and eye pain are absent or mild. The initial symptoms last 1 to 6 days and are followed by a brief afebrile period. In most cases there is milder recrudescence with fever and a maculopapular, pruritic rash which is characteristic of the second phase of the disease. All patients have recovered, but some experience recurrent, crippling joint pains for several months.

O'nyong-nyong fever is a similar viral disease which was first reported in 1960 to have affected almost one million persons in Uganda and other parts of East Africa. The causative virus is more closely related to Semliki Forest than to Chikungunya and is transmitted by various species of *Anopheles* mosquitoes. O'nyong-nyong fever is a nonfatal illness of short duration characterized by fever, headache, agonizing joint and back pains, itching rash, and lymphadenopathy.

The South American representative of the Semliki Forest–Chikungunya subgroup of group A arbor viruses is *Mayaro virus,* which has been isolated in the British West Indies, northeast Brazil, Colombia, and Bolivia. This virus causes an illness which lasts 2 to 6 days and is characterized by fever with a temperature to 103°F, severe frontal headache, backache, arthralgia, nausea, vertigo, and occasionally, fleeting jaundice.

GROUP B ARBOR VIRUSES

The most common and widespread of the insect-transmitted viral infections of man are caused by arbor viruses of group B. All produce relatively benign febrile diseases. However, most clinically apparent infections with viruses of the *Japanese B–St. Louis–Murray Valley* subgroup are associated with manifestations of encephalitis. The denguelike illness caused by the related *West Nile virus* is considered on p. 1191. *Dengue* viruses themselves are also classified in group B but are more closely related to *yellow fever* virus. Group B viruses of the tick-borne complex, the prototype of which is *Russian spring-summer encephalitis,* are usually associated with hemorrhagic fevers or encephalitis and are described elsewhere (see p. 1156). However, each of these latter agents can also cause illnesses that resemble influenza or dengue. In particular, *louping ill,* an infection of sheep in Scotland, and *biundulant milk fever,* which is contracted in the Soviet Union by drinking milk of infected goats, tend to produce less severe human illness manifested, primarily, by monophasic or biphasic fever and myalgia. Many other group B viruses have been reported to be responsible for short-term fevers and are potentially important human pathogens; these include *Zika* and *Ntaya* viruses of Uganda, *Wesselsbron* virus of South Africa, which also causes abortion in sheep, and *Ilheus* virus of South and Central America.

MISCELLANEOUS ARBOR VIRUSES INCLUDING GROUP C

Since 1955 there have been increasing numbers of reports indicating that sporadic febrile diseases among inhabitants of the Brazilian jungles bordering the Amazon and Para Rivers are caused by related arbor viruses now classified as *group C.* These agents represent four serotypes named for the localities in which they were first isolated: Oriboca, Marituba, Apeú, and Itaqui viruses.

Symptoms of infection with group C viruses usually last only 2 or 3 days. The most prominent manifestations are temperature of 102 to 105°F, headache, joint and muscle pain, conjunctivitis, photophobia, vertigo, nausea, and vomiting.

Other arbor viruses that are unrelated immunologically to groups A, B, or C are also etiologic agents of febrile disease in man. Among this unclassified group are the viruses of *phlebotomus fever* (p. 1191) and *Colorado tick fever* (p. 1190). Another important arthropod-borne viral infection of East Africa is *Rift Valley fever,* or enzootic hepatitis of sheep and cattle. The Rift Valley virus also infects man and can cause a severe, but usually nonfatal, biphasic illness of a few days' duration. It is characterized by high fever, chills, prostration, incapacitating joint and muscle pain, gastrointestinal symptoms of vomiting and abdominal pain, and marked leukopenia. Unusual complications of Rift Valley fever are hemorrhagic retinopathy and macular edema which come on days or weeks after fever has subsided and can lead to permanent visual impairment.

Serologic surveys indicate that other unclassified arbor viruses are widespread throughout East and West Africa, including the unrelated viruses of *Bwamba fever* and the *Bunyamwera group.* The few human cases proved by virus isolation exhibited sudden onset and short duration of fever, headache, and backache. The *Guama* viruses of Brazil also form a separate group and are causative agents of a similar influenzalike illness.

VIRUSES OF THE ENCEPHALOMYOCARDITIS GROUP

These agents are not classified as arthropod-borne viruses, although their biologic and physical properties are similar, and one of them has been isolated from mosquitoes. The viruses that comprise the encephalomyocarditis group include *encephalomyocarditis, Columbia-SK, MM,* and *Mengo;* all four are identical immunologically and differ only slightly in their pathogenicity for laboratory animals. Serologic surveys indicate that asymptomatic human infection occurs in approximately 3 per cent of persons in some regions of the United States and other countries. The reservoir and mode of transmission are unknown, but these viruses have been isolated from the mongoose, chimpanzee, monkey, squirrel, and cotton rat. The few serious or fatal human infections proved by virus isolation have been diagnosed clinically as meningoencephalitis, poliomyelitis, and the Guillain-Barré syndrome. Myocarditis has not been described in man. Encephalomyocarditis virus was implicated as the causative agent of an epidemic among American troops in the Philippines which took the form of a relatively benign disease known as "3-day fever." Some of these patients presented with a denguelike illness characterized by sudden onset of fever with temperatures to 104°F, severe headache, myalgia, and pharyngitis. Others exhibited aseptic meningitis with lymphocytic pleocytosis.

REFERENCES

Casals, J.: The Arthropod-borne Group of Animal Viruses, Trans. N.Y. Acad. Sci. (ser. 2), 19:219, 1957.

Causey, O. R., and O. Maroja: Mayaro Virus: A New Human Disease Agent. III. Investigation of an Epidemic of Acute Febrile Illnesses on the River Guama in Para, Brazil, and Isolation of Mayaro Virus as Causative Agent, Am. J. Trop. Med. Hyg., 6:1017, 1957.

Olitsky, P. K., and J. Casals: Arthropod-borne Group A Virus Infections of Man, p. 286 in "Viral and Rickettsial Infections of Man," 3d ed., T. M. Rivers and F. L. Horsfall, Jr. (Eds.), Philadelphia, J. B. Lippincott Company, 1959.

Robinson, M. C.: An Epidemic of Virus Disease in Southern Province, Tanganyika Territory, in 1952–53: I. Clinical Features, Trans. Roy. Soc. Trop. Med. Hyg., 49:28, 1955.

Shore, H.: O'nyong-nyong Fever: An Epidemic Virus Disease in East Africa: III. Clinical Manifestations, Trans. Roy. Soc. Trop. Med. Hyg., 55:361, 1961.

Sutton, L. S., and C. C. Brooke: Venezuelan Equine Encephalomyelitis Due to Vaccination in Man, J.A.M.A., 155:1473, 1954.

Theiler, M., and D. H. Clarke: Arthropod-borne Group B Virus Infections of Man, p. 305 in "Viral and Rickettsial Infections of Man," 3d ed., T. M. Rivers and F. L. Horsfall, Jr. (Eds.), Philadelphia, J. B. Lippincott Company, 1959.

Warren, J.: Encephalomyocarditis, p. 903 in "Viral and Rickettsial Infections of Man," 3d ed., T. M. Rivers and F. L. Horsfall, Jr. (Eds.), Philadelphia, J. B. Lippincott Company, 1959.

WHO Technical Report 219, Report of a Study Group: "Arthropod-borne Viruses," Geneva, World Health Organization, 1961.

Section 21: Diseases Produced by Protozoa

211 AMEBIASIS
Ivan L. Bennett, Jr.

Definition. Amebiasis in an infection of the large intestine produced by *Endamoeba histolytica*. The infection is an asymptomatic carrier state in most individuals, but disease ranging from chronic, mild diarrhea to fulminant dysentery is frequently produced. Among extraintestinal complications, the commonest is hepatic abscess, which may rupture into peritoneum, pleura, lung, or pericardium.

Etiology. There are at least six different species of ameba that parasitize the mouth and intestine of man. Of these, *E. histolytica* is the only one that causes disease and *E. coli* is the species with which it is most likely to be confused in examination of stools.

Endamoeba histolytica exists in the colon as the motile trophozoite and nonmotile cyst. The stools of symptomatic amebiasis contain trophozoites; cysts predominate in stools of the carrier state. The important distinguishing features of *E. histolytica* trophozoites are their very active motility, their ingestion of erythrocytes, and the sparsity of vacuoles and ingested bacteria within them. The cysts of pathogenic amebas possess thin walls and contain two thick chromatoid bodies; those of *E. coli* are thick-walled and the chromatoid bodies are thin and pointed.

Endamoeba histolytica strains have been classified into large and small races, depending upon whether they form cysts measuring more or less than 10 μ in diameter. While it is possible that small strains (sometimes called *E. hartmanni*) are somewhat less likely to produce symptoms than are the large strains, cyst size is apparently unstable and the often-heard statement that small strains are nonpathogenic for man is not justified.

Endamoeba histolytica occurs normally in the intestines of a few dogs, monkeys, and rats; these animals, rabbits, and kittens can also be infected experimentally. Amebas can be cultivated in artificial media, a procedure that is occasionally useful in diagnosis. With rare exceptions, the presence of bacteria in the culture medium is a prerequisite to multiplication of the protozoa.

Epidemiology. Because trophozoites die rapidly after leaving the intestine, the infection is acquired in the vast majority of instances by ingestion of the more resistant cysts. Cases of amebic dysentery, therefore, are quite unimportant in transmission of the disease, asymptomatic cyst passers being the source of new infections. Amebic infection is worldwide, although both symptomatic and subclinical infection are somewhat more frequent in tropical areas. Figures obtained from local and admittedly incomplete surveys indicate that the average incidence of asymptomatic carriers is 10 per cent in Europe and the United States, 16 per cent in Asia, and 17 per cent in Africa, with great variation, particularly in the tropics. Cyst passers are more frequent among children and the inmates of institutions.

Cases of amebic dysentery are usually sporadic but epidemics, usually water-borne, have occurred. Outbreaks of amebiasis are never explosive, as are those produced by pathogenic intestinal bacteria, and may not be recognized for several weeks. The cysts are often transmitted by vegetables in countries where human excreta is used as fertilizer, and flies are capable of contaminating foodstuffs.

Symptomatic amebiasis is unusual below the age of 10 years in temperate climates, and both intestinal and hepatic lesions predominate in adult males to an extent that is not explainable solely on the basis of different rates of exposure to infection.

Pathogenesis and Anatomic Changes. After ingestion, cysts pass through the stomach unchanged. In the ileum, the cyst wall disintegrates and, eventually, eight trophozoites result. These immature amebas pass to the colon, where they attack the mucosa and divide by binary fission. Mucosal lesions too tiny to be detected probably occur in all infections. The sites of involvement in order of frequency are cecum and ascending colon, rectum, sigmoid, appendix, and terminal ileum.

The factors responsible for the development of ulceration extensive enough to cause symptoms in some individuals are not understood. Obviously, the virulence of the infecting strain is important, but this alone is insufficient to explain the occurrence of disease in only a small percentage of subjects exposed naturally to the same strain or in a minority of volunteers fed cysts from a single source. Certain experimental findings suggest strongly that the bacterial flora of the intestine may be a major determinant of the extent of amebic disease. The symbiosis between bacteria and amebas in artificial media has been mentioned. When 200 strains were cultured and tested for virulence in rabbits, disease was produced by only 4 per cent grown without bacteria, by 35 per cent grown with a single bacterial species, and by 85 per cent grown with a mixed culture of several different bacteria. Germ-free animals cannot be infected with E. histolytica but become susceptible if the intestine is first allowed to acquire a normal complement of bacteria.

Amebic ulceration of the intestinal wall is quite characteristic. A relatively small mucosal defect overlies a much larger, burrowing area of necrosis in the submucosa and muscularis, producing a bottle-shaped lesion. There is little or no acute inflammatory response to the damage, and, in contrast to the picture in bacillary dysentery, the mucosa between ulcers is normal, without hyperemia. In the cecum and sometimes elsewhere, chronic infection leads to the formation of large masses of granulation tissue. Amebas can enter the portal circulation and lodge in venules; liquefaction necrosis of liver tissue leads to the formation of an abscess cavity. Rarely, embolization results in lung, brain or splenic abscess.

Because trophozoites in histologic sections of liver or intestine are usually seen lying free in small spaces, it is often postulated that E. histolytica destroys tissue through the elaboration of a "cytolytic ferment." Not only is there no evidence whatsoever that such a cytolytic substance exists, but the histologic appearance is simply a shrinkage artefact that occurs with fixation.

Chronic Amebic Dysentery. Most patients with this commonest type of amebic disease cannot date the onset of illness accurately. There is usually intermittent diarrhea consisting of from one to four foul-smelling stools daily, sometimes containing mucus and blood, alternating with periods of relative normality for months or years. Vague abdominal cramping, weight loss, and mild fever are frequent. In such cases of "walking dysentery" the only findings are wasting, occasional mild hepatomegaly with some tenderness (not indicative of hepatic abscess), and slight pain when the cecum and ascending colon are palpated. Sigmoidoscopy sometimes reveals typical ulcerations with normal intervening mucosa, or mucosal defects may be demonstrated radiologically in the right colon. Specific diagnosis depends upon finding the organisms in the feces.

Acute Amebic Dysentery. This type of amebiasis is unusual but was observed in several patients during the large epidemic in a Chicago hotel in 1933 when massive contamination of the water supply occurred through defective plumbing; it is more likely to be seen sporadically in tropical areas. The onset is abrupt, with high fever (104 to 105°F), severe abdominal cramps, and profuse, bloody diarrhea with tenesmus. There is diffuse abdominal tenderness, often so severe that peritonitis is suspected, tender hepatomegaly is very frequent, and sigmoidoscopy almost always demonstrates extensive rectosigmoid ulceration. Trophozoites are numerous in stools and in material obtained directly from the ulcers.

Ameboma (Amebic Granuloma). Chronic infection can lead to the production of large masses of granulation tissue in the colon. When the entire circumference of the intestine is involved, there may be partial obstruction and a tender, sausage-shaped mass is often palpable. Granulomas are most frequent in the cecum, where a palpable mass and radiologic demonstration of a ragged encroachment upon the lumen have often led to a mistaken diagnosis of adenocarcinoma. A history of diarrhea with blood and mucus may be elicited, but this is compatible with the diagnosis of cancer also. The importance of searching for amebas in the feces of any patient with these findings is very great because surgical intervention in untreated ameboma can lead to fatal peritonitis or to perforation, pericecal abscess, and, eventually sinus formation with drainage of feculent material through the abdominal wall. In addition to cancer, these lesions are likely to be confused with tuberculosis or actinomycosis.

In the tropics, amebic ulceration of the appendix is responsible for a significant proportion of cases of appendicitis. Again, operative intervention is contraindicated before specific treatment. The majority of deaths among tourists infected during the 1933 Chicago epidemic were a direct result of laparotomy carried out for symptoms of appendicitis. The operations were performed in many different towns and cities after patients had returned home and before the significance of exposure to amebic infection at the Chicago hotel had been widely appreciated.

Hepatic Amebiasis. The parasites usually reach the liver through the portal vein; rarely, they may traverse the lymphatic vessels. It was long believed that the amebas which lodged in the liver could produce a diffuse hepatitis which, if enough necrosis occurred, would lead to frank abscess formation. Careful postmortem and biopsy studies indicate that the syndrome of tender hepatomegaly, right upper quadrant pain, fever, and leukocytosis in patients with amebic colitis is not a result of the presence of amebas in hepatic tissues, is accompanied by nonspecific periportal inflammation, and is rarely, if ever, a prelude to hepatic abscess. It is evident, then, that these manifestations are best regarded as an accompaniment of colitis and do not merit a separate diagnosis of "diffuse amebic hepatitis."

Hepatic abscess may develop insidiously, with fever, sweats, weight loss, and no local signs other than painless or slightly tender hepatomegaly. In other patients, there is abrupt onset, with chills, fever to 105°F, nausea, vomiting, severe upper abdominal pain, and polymorphonuclear leukocytosis. Initially, cholecystitis, perforated ulcer, or acute pancreatitis may be suspected.

Almost invariably, amebic abscess is localized in the posterior portion of the right lobe of the liver, because this lobe receives most of the blood draining the right colon through the "streaming" effect in portal vein flow. This location is responsible for several features that aid in diagnosis. *Point tenderness* in the posterolateral portion of a lower right intercostal space is frequent even in the absence of diffuse liver pain. Most abscesses enlarge upward, producing a bulge in the diaphragmatic dome, obliteration of the costophrenic gutter, small hydrothorax, basilar atelectasis, and pain referred to the right shoulder. Radiologically, unruptured abscesses do not show a fluid level and calcification of the liver parenchyma is very rare.

Needle puncture results in the withdrawal of "pus" which is nothing more than liquefied, necrotic liver, the classic "chocolate syrup" or "anchovy paste" exudate; the pus contains no polymorphonuclear leukocytes (barring secondary bacterial infection) and, usually, no amebas (the parasites are localized in the cyst wall).

Hepatic abscess complicates asymptomatic infection of the colon more often than symptomatic intestinal disease, another factor making recognition difficult. Trophozoites or cysts are demonstrable in the feces of only about one-eighth of patients with abscess, and fewer than one-half will recall significant diarrheal illness.

Pleuropulmonary Amebiasis. The right pleural cavity and lung are involved by direct extension from the liver in 10 to 20 per cent of patients with liver abscess. Rarely, amebic lung abscess has resulted from embolization rather than from direct extension.

Manifestations are those of massive pleural effusion; aspiration of chocolate fluid is diagnostic, or if the lung parenchyma is involved and perforation into a bronchus occurs, patients expectorate large amounts of the typical exudate, some patients even commenting that the sputum "tastes like liver." Cough, pleural pain, fever, and leukocytosis are the rule, and secondary bacterial infection is frequent. The trophozoites are rarely demonstrated in pleural fluid or sputum.

Other Extraintestinal Lesions. Rupture of liver abscess into the *pericardium* has occurred; these patients are usually thought to have tuberculous pericarditis. *Peritonitis* is a result of perforation of colonic ulcer or rupture of liver abscess. Painful ulcers of the genitalia, perianal skin, or abdominal wall (draining sinuses), vaginitis, urethritis, and prostatitis are unusual complications resulting from extension of intestinal disease. Metastatic brain abscess is rare and an etiologic diagnosis is seldom

made clinically. Splenic abscess has been reported but is very unusual.

Diagnosis. In amebic dysentery, the demonstration of trophozoites in feces can usually be accomplished if specimens are collected properly and repeated examinations are performed. Fresh specimens should be examined in saline solution using a warm stage. Fixation in polyvinyl alcohol and staining with iron hematoxylin constitute an even more accurate method, which permits detailed study in permanently mounted slides.

Sigmoidoscopy, radiography, and above all, the recognition of the possibility of amebic etiology in patients with colitis or liver disease have already been emphasized.

A most important diagnostic procedure in suspected liver abscess is a therapeutic trial of antiamebic drugs. Response is often dramatic within 3 days; in view of the difficulty of demonstrating parasites in this condition, a trial of treatment should be instituted without hesitation.

Cultivation of amebas from feces or pus is possible but it is not practical in most laboratories. Serologic tests, including the much-discussed complement fixation reaction, are still not reliable enough to be depended upon in diagnosis.

Treatment. In patients with acute amebic dysentery, replacement of fluid, electrolyte, and blood losses, bed rest, and relief of pain and tenesmus with opiates are all important. There is nothing specifically beneficial about components of diet per se in acute or chronic amebiasis and patients should be allowed to eat whatever is tolerated.

The numerous specific antiamebic drugs indicate the lack of a single ideal agent. While a vast majority of patients are eventually cured, initial improvement is followed by relapse so frequently that combinations of drugs and retreatment are necessary to attain many cures, especially in chronic infections. The following drugs are the most useful of those available: *Diodoquin,* an iodinated hydroxyquinoline (1.9 Gm daily in three doses for 21 days); *Milibis,* an arsenical (0.5 Gm three times daily for a week); *emetine,* a somewhat toxic ipecac derivative which kills trophozoites only (65 mg daily by intramuscular injection for no more than 10 days); *chloroquine diphosphate* (Aralen), which is effective only in hepatic disease, by virtue of its high concentration in the liver (1.0 Gm daily for 2 days, then 0.5 daily for 3 weeks); and *Terramycin,* the most effective of the antibiotics (2.0 Gm daily for 10 days).

For *acute dysentery* a combination of Diodoquin or Milibis with Terramycin gives good results. Emetine will give rapid symptomatic relief and may be given for a few days initially; it should never be relied upon to eradicate infection of the bowel.

In *chronic dysentery,* emetine has no usefulness. A combination of Diodoquin or Milibis and Terramycin should be given initially. In tropical areas, this is often followed by a course of Diodoquin and Milibis (or carbarsone, a somewhat more toxic arsenical), given in alternating weeks for 16 weeks to minimize relapse. Relapse should be expected, and monthly examination of stools should be carried out for at least a year. Relapse should be treated with a combination of Terramycin and another drug, just as they are given initially.

Symptomatic response in intestinal disease is usually evident within 3 days or even sooner with emetine. However, the goal is elimination of both trophozoites and cysts from the feces, and whether it has been reached can be determined only by examination. Diodoquin, Milibis, carbarsone, and Terramycin can all cause abdominal discomfort, cramps, or diarrhea, sometimes complicating evaluation of treatment. Milibis and carbarsone are contraindicated in persons known to be sensitive to arsenic or to have renal or hepatic insufficiency.

For *hepatic* or *pulmonary* amebiasis chloroquine is distinctly the drug of choice, giving symptomatic relief within 48 to 72 hr and producing subsidence of surprisingly large abscesses. Terramycin is often given concomitantly. Emetine is less effective than chloroquine but is sometimes useful, particularly for therapeutic trials. Failure to obtain a response calls for needling and drainage of the abscess, a procedure that will sometimes lead to subsidence. Surgical drainage is now infrequent but it should be resorted to if drugs and needle aspiration fail. The greatest hazard of needling or of open drainage is secondary bacterial infection, which, in spite of antibiotics, still leads to death in many instances.

Emetine possesses considerable toxicity, producing gastrointestinal discomfort, tremor and weakness, electrocardiographic abnormalities, and, with regularity, orthostatic hypotension. In patients with renal or cardiac disease, during pregnancy, and in children, it should be used only when all other drugs have failed.

Prognosis. Complete cure of intestinal amebiasis occurs in 75 to 95 per cent of cases with repeated courses of therapy. The relapse rate is as high as 35 per cent after a single course. The fatality rate is less than 5 per cent.

Hepatic and pulmonary amebiasis are still attended by appreciable mortality, but no reliable estimate of the percentage of deaths is available.

Prevention. For the individual, avoidance of contaminated food and water, scalding of vegetables, and the use of iodine-releasing tablets in drinking water (chlorine, in the form of Halazone, is ineffective) are important measures. Globaline tablets, containing tetraglycine hydroperiodide, are convenient and effective.

Improvements in general sanitation and the detection of cyst passers and their removal from food-handling duties are general measures in prophylaxis, but such segregation of carriers is rarely practiced.

REFERENCES

Belding, D. L.: "Basic Clinical Parasitology," New York, Appleton-Century-Crofts, Inc., 1958.
Faust, E. C.: "Amebiasis," American Lecture Series, Springfield, Ill., Charles C Thomas, Publisher, 1954.
Lamont, N. McE., and N. R. Pooler: Hepatic Amoebiasis, Quart. J. Med., 27:389, 1958.
Manson-Bahr, P.: "Manson's Tropical Diseases," 15th ed., London, Cassell & Co., Ltd., 1960.
Powell, S. J., A. L. Wilmott, and R. Elsdon-Dew: Hepatic Amoebiasis, Trans. Roy. Soc. Trop. Med. Hyg., 53:190, 1959.

212   MALARIA
Ivan L. Bennett, Jr.

Definition. Malaria is a protozoan disease transmitted to man by the bite of *Anopheles* mosquitoes. Although it is now rare in the United States, it remains one of the most prevalent infectious diseases throughout the world. Malaria is characterized by rigors, fever, splenomegaly, anemia, and a chronic, relapsing course.

Etiology. The causative organisms are protozoa of the genus *Plasmodium.* The four species known to infect man do not produce disease in lower animals, although many other species affecting animals and birds are known. *Plasmodium vivax* causes tertian malaria; *P. malariae* causes quartan malaria; *P. falciparum* causes malignant tertian (estivo-autumnal) malaria; *P. ovale* causes ovale tertian malaria, a relatively rare and mild illness.

Man is the intermediate host and the mosquito the definitive host. In man, after a stage of exo-erythrocytic development, the parasites reproduce asexually in circulating erythrocytes. They first appear in the red cells as *ring forms;* after several divisions, daughter cells (*merozoites*) fill the corpuscle, which ruptures and releases them to parasitize additional erythrocytes. With repetition of this cycle, some of the red cells become filled with sexual forms (*gametocytes*); these do not induce cell lysis and are unable to undergo further development unless ingested by an appropriate mosquito during a blood meal. In the stomach of the mosquito fertilization occurs, and the resulting *ookinete* encysts on the outer surface of the stomach and releases myriads of *sporozoites*. These migrate to the salivary glands and, if inoculated into a human subject, lead to repetition of asexual multiplication. There is variation in this cycle among different species, and several intermediate developmental stages occur.

The asexual cycle in the erythrocyte requires 36 to 48 hr for *P. falciparum*, 48 hr for *P. vivax* and *P. ovale*, and 72 hr for *P. malariae*. The periodicity of febrile paroxysms in infections by the different species coincides with the cyclic discharge of merozoites and infestation of new cells.

The incubation period between bite of an infected mosquito and onset of symptoms is 10 to 14 days in vivax and falciparum malaria and 18 days to 6 weeks in quartan infections.

There is good evidence for the existence of several strains of each species of human malarial *Plasmodium,* and greater virulence of some strains is suggested by the consistent severity of the clinical illnesses which they produce.

Epidemiology. Malaria survives only in areas where the mosquito and the infected human populations remain above a *critical density* for each. These critical densities are interdependent, but either may fluctuate in a given area. Control measures are directed toward reducing both populations to levels that are too low for the infection to survive. Important procedures include drainage or filling of breeding areas, use of residual insecticide sprays (this has largely replaced the use of oil or other antilarval measures), screening, use of skin repellents, effective treatment of cases, and large-scale suppressive drug programs in some human populations.

The disease remains highly prevalent in many parts of the world, and it is estimated that more than 200 million cases occur annually. An active international cooperative program of malaria control has resulted in a significant decline in the incidence of the disease since 1945, and, despite the enormity of the remaining problem, many areas in South America, southern Europe, and Asia are now almost free of the infection.

Manifestations. General. There is some variation in the clinical diseases produced by the different plasmodia, but in all, chills, fever, excruciating headache, muscle pains, splenomegaly, and anemia are common. Herpes labialis is very frequent but usually appears only after the infection is well established. Hepatomegaly and mild icterus are often observed, especially in estivo-autumnal infections.

The hallmark of the disease is the malarial *paroxysm* which recurs at regular intervals in all but falciparum infections. The typical paroxysm begins

with a rigor that lasts 20 to 60 min ("cold stage") followed by a "hot stage" of 3 to 8 hr with temperature of 104 to 107°F. The "wet stage" consists of defervescence with profuse diaphoresis, which leaves the patient weak and exhausted.

First attacks of malaria are often severe, but with repeated episodes symptoms become milder, although debilitation may be progressive. There is good evidence for the development of immunity to malaria, but it is of a low order in so far as protection against reinfection is concerned. Negroes are peculiarly insusceptible to *P. vivax* infections.

Tertian Malaria (*P. vivax* or *P. ovale*). This infection is rarely fatal, although relapses are common and it is the most difficult to cure. A prodrome of myalgia, headache, chilliness, and low-grade fever for 48 to 72 hr heralds the onset of the typical paroxysms. Transient urticaria sometimes precedes each of the paroxysms which occur on alternate days, unless there has been double infection with two maturation cycles, in which case daily chills can occur. Such double infections usually "synchronize" within a week, and paroxysms then follow the classic tertian pattern.

Quartan Malaria (*P. malariae*). In this infection, paroxysms occur every third day, unless multiple infection alters the cycle initially and chills occur on 2 out of 3 days or even daily until the cycles synchronize. Quartan malaria is usually a more disabling infection than tertian but responds well to treatment. Edema, albuminuria, and hematuria (not hemoglobinuria), a clinical state similar to acute hemorrhagic nephritis, occasionally appear during the course. This complication should not be confused with *blackwater fever*.

Estivo-Autumnal Malaria (*P. falciparum*). This is a severe disease. The organisms are present in enormous numbers, and there is a striking tendency for agglutinated masses of parasitized erythrocytes to block capillaries throughout the body, producing localizing signs that mimic many other diseases. There is often "asynchronization" of the cycle of multiplication; typical malarial paroxysms occur, but continuous, remittent, or irregular fever is present in many cases, and illness can be constant.

The course of uncomplicated estivo-autumnal malaria is ordinarily milder than that of tertian or quartan infections. However, capillary blockage by the parasites can give rise to serious, even fatal, complications and it is this feature of *P. falciparum* infections that accounts for the protean manifestations of estivo-autumnal malaria, and the relatively high morbidity and mortality associated with it. Depending upon the organ system involved, several so-called *pernicious syndromes* are seen. *Cerebral malaria* can lead to hemiplegia, convulsions, delirium, hyperpyrexia, coma, and rapid death. When the *pulmonary* circulation is involved, there may be cough and blood-streaked sputum, leading to confusion with many other diseases of the lung. The splanchnic capillaries can be obstructed, with consequent vomiting, abdominal pain simulating appendicitis, severe diarrhea, or melena. Such patients are sometimes thought to have bacillary dysentery or cholera. Fever in these disorders may be low or absent. Indeed, in patients with predominantly gastrointestinal manifestations, there are usually cold clammy skin, hypotension, profound weakness, and repeated syncopal attacks, so-called *algid malaria*.

Blackwater Fever. This is a disorder that occurs in association with malaria, particularly and perhaps only with *P. falciparum* infections. The usual attack begins with a rigor and fever followed by massive intravascular hemolysis, icterus, hemoglobinuria, collapse, and often acute renal failure and uremia. The pathologic findings in the kidney are typical of "lower nephron nephrosis" with necrosis of tubules and hemoglobin casts. The mortality is 20 to 30 per cent, and survivors are very likely to experience hemolytic episodes with subsequent malarial infections.

Although blackwater fever is often classified as one of the "pernicious" complications of estivo-autumnal malaria, its etiology is obscure. There is nothing to suggest that capillary blockage by the parasites produces the renal disturbance; *P. falciparum* has not been shown to elaborate a hemolysin, and, in many patients with blackwater fever, parasitemia is absent. Conflicting evidence suggests a possible role of therapy with quinine in the hemolysis; there are good observations to the effect that antimalarial drugs in general neither speed recovery from an attack nor influence the outcome. Tender splenomegaly is a constant finding, and this has led to the suggestion that the hemolysis is a result of hypersplenism. In the past, cardiac decompensation has been the usual cause of death in patients with blackwater fever. It is probable that the heart failure resulted from overhydration in ill-advised attempts to "flush" the kidneys of oliguric patients. The institution of an appropriate regimen for acute renal failure (see p. 1496) will reduce the fatality rate considerably.

Complications. In addition to the several complications already mentioned, others deserve comment. Rupture of the spleen is relatively rare, but malaria is by far the commonest cause of spontaneous rupture and predisposes to traumatic rupture of this organ.

Chronic malaria or repeated infection in an endemic area leads to anemia, debility, and cachexia. Secondary bacterial infection is often the immediate cause of death in such patients. Bacillary dysentery, cholera, and pyogenic pneumonia are common. Tuberculous foci often extend in malarial patients, and miliary tuberculosis is occasionally observed.

Laboratory Findings. The blood leukocyte count is usually low but may be normal. The erythrocyte sedimentation rate is elevated. Plasmodia are demonstrable in smears of peripheral blood from the vast majority of patients with symptomatic malaria. When the disease is suspected, appropriately stained blood films should be examined diligently. For the inexperienced examiner, a thin smear of finger-tip blood on a clean glass slide should be stained with Wright, Giemsa, or Hastings stain. Parasitized erythrocytes are most frequent at the edges of a smear; extracellular parasites are not found. Thick smears should be thoroughly dried and stained with diluted Giemsa or Field stain. This method has the advantage of concentrating the parasites, but artefacts are numerous, and correct interpretation of these preparations requires much experience.

The morphology of the four species of plasmodia that infect man is specific enough to allow identification in blood smears. The details of this morphology are available in textbooks of parasitology. The parasitized erythrocytes in *P. vivax* infections are usually enlarged and hypochromic, in *P. malariae* infections they are small and hyperchromic, and in *P. ovale* infections the red cells containing parasites are oval.

There is no advantage over blood of material obtained by splenic or sternal puncture. The administration of epinephrine with the idea of dislodging parasites by producing contraction of the spleen has been advocated, but results are irregular. There are no reliable diagnostic serologic tests.

Diagnosis. The most important diagnostic test is the search for parasites in peripheral blood. History of residence in an endemic area, previous attacks of malaria, typical malarial paroxysms, or some artificial exposure (blood transfusion, narcotic injections in an addict) should suggest the disease. Splenomegaly is an almost invariable finding; its absence is strong evidence against malaria. Leukocytosis is not a feature of malaria.

The confusion of *P. falciparum* malaria with various disorders of the brain, lung, or intestine has been mentioned.

While final cure of malaria may be difficult, particularly in *P. vivax* infections, almost all cases will respond symptomatically to quinine or one of the newer antimalarial drugs, and failure of response to a therapeutic trial argues strongly against the diagnosis.

Treatment. The use of appropriate chemotherapy can suppress symptoms in individuals exposed in endemic areas or cure malarial infection completely. The development of new antimalarial drugs has led to replacement of quinine and Atabrine (quinacrine) as the agents of choice, although both will undoubtedly continue to be used for many years. A good dosage schedule for quinine sulfate is 1.0 Gm orally t.i.d. for 2 days and 0.6 Gm daily for 1 week. Quinine dihydrochloride can be given intravenously (*not* intramuscularly) in a dose of 10 ml of a 3 per cent solution every 4 hr until oral medication can be taken.

The oral dosage of Atabrine is 0.2 Gm every 6 hr for five doses and 0.1 Gm t.i.d. for 6 days. Quinacrine dihydrochloride can be given intramuscularly (*not* intravenously) in a dose of 0.2 Gm every 6 hr until oral therapy can be tolerated.

The initial administration of 1.0 Gm of chloroquine diphosphate (Aralen), followed by 0.5 Gm 6 hr later, and then 0.5 Gm daily for 2 days usually produces complete subsidence of *P. falciparum* and *P. ovale* infections. For *P. vivax* and *P. malariae* infections, another drug should be combined with chloroquine to avoid relapse, common in both types. Primaquine base 15 mg by mouth daily for 14 days is the best regimen; relapse after treatment by this combination is extremely rare.

The suppressive dose of chloroquine is 0.5 Gm once weekly. A dose of 0.4 to 0.6 Gm of amodiaquin (Camoquin) once weekly is very effective in suppression of malaria in endemic areas. General supportive measures, fluids, good diet, symptomatic relief of headache or other pains, and, occasionally, blood transfusions are all important.

Specific antimalarial drugs should be withdrawn in patients with blackwater fever.

Overdosage of quinine produces cinchonism with tinnitus as an early manifestation. Occasional instances of mild hemolysis attributable to it have occurred, and it is a cause of allergic purpura (nonthrombocytopenic) and drug fever.

Atabrine causes a yellow staining of the skin. Given intravenously, it usually produces circulatory collapse. Primaquine produces hemolytic anemia in many Negroes, apparently because of an inborn error of erythrocyte metabolic activity (see p. 1291). Chloroquine rarely causes any reaction other than that of occasional mild desquamation and itching.

REFERENCES

Boyd, M. F. (Ed.): "Malariology," vols. 1 and 2, Philadelphia, W. B. Saunders Company, 1949.

Coggeshall, L. T.: Immunity in Malaria, Medicine, 22: 87, 1943.

Garrison, P. L., et al.: Cure of Korean Vivax Malaria with Pamaquine and Primaquine, J.A.M.A., 149: 1562, 1952.

Moulton, F. R. (Ed.): Human Malaria, Am. Assoc. Advance. Sci. Publ. No. 15, 1941.

213 LEISHMANIASIS
Ivan L. Bennett, Jr.

Definition. Leishmaniasis designates three separate disorders of man that are produced by protozoa of the genus *Leishmania*. All are transmitted by the bite of sand flies (*Phlebotomus*).

Etiology. *Leishmania tropica* is the cause of cutaneous leishmaniasis, or oriental sore, also known variously as Delhi boil, Bagdad boil, Aleppo button, Salek, and Pendeh sore.

American mucocutaneous leishmaniasis is caused by *L. brasiliensis* and is referred to in various areas as *espundia*, *uta*, forest yaws, bay sore, and *enfermedad de los chicleros*.

Leishmania donovani is the cause of kala-azar, the visceral form of leishmaniasis (Dum-dum fever, tropical splenomegaly, Burdwan fever, Sirkari disease, *Ponos, Mard el Bicha*).

In the sand fly, the parasites assume the flagellated leptomonas form, but in man, the organisms lose their flagella, enter mononuclear phagocytes, and multiply as small, rounded leishmanial forms 2 to 3 μ in diameter, the pathognomonic "Leishman-Donovan bodies." Infection may remain localized at the inoculation site or it may spread systemically.

The geographic distribution, epidemiology, and animal reservoirs for each form of leishmaniasis are discussed separately below.

KALA-AZAR

Distribution and Epidemiology. Kala-azar occurs in China, Russia, India, Egypt, Sudan, East Africa, several Mediterranean countries, including Greece, Crete, and Malta, and a few areas of South and Central America. While the manifestations of the disease throughout this area, which touches all continents but Australia, are basically similar, certain definite peculiarities in its behavior justify classification of visceral leishmaniasis into at least three main types. These differences are attributed to variations in the strains of *L. donovani* in a given area and, perhaps more important, to the length of time that the disease has been endemic in a population. It is believed that kala-azar (and also infection by *L. tropica*, p. 1204) is introduced into a new area from animal reservoirs and that this "primitive" or zoonotic infection is likely to result in many cases of acute, rapidly fatal illness among the population coming into contact with the parasites for the first time. After generations, kala-azar becomes endemic, the disease assumes a more chronic form, and the main or only reservoir of infection, especially in urban areas, is man.

Mediterranean, or *infantile*, *kala-azar* is primarily

a disease of children under the age of two years and has its reservoir in dogs, jackals, and foxes. Adults are by no means spared, but the preceding sentence describes the predominant pattern of the disorder as it occurs in the Mediterranean area, China, Russia, and Latin America.

Indian kala-azar shows no special predilection for infants and has never been found in dogs or other animals in India, indicating that the human reservoir is responsible for perpetuation of the disease.

Sudanese, or *Egyptian*, *kala-azar* shows no predilection for children, is endemic in gerbils and other rodents in many areas, and is far more resistant to therapy with antimony compounds than that found in the rest of the world.

Manifestations. The incubation period varies from 10 days to 1 year but is usually about 3 months. No lesion appears at the site of the infecting bite in most cases, but a primary "chancre" which heals with scarring before the onset of systemic symptoms is commonly noted in the African disease. The organisms multiply extensively in the macrophages of spleen, liver, bone marrow, and lymph nodes, accounting for many of the manifestations of the disease.

There are gradual or abrupt onset of fever (often characterized by two daily spikes) and progressive weakness, pallor, weight loss, and tachycardia. Gastrointestinal disturbances are frequent in Indian cases. Physical findings include enormous splenomegaly, lymphadenopathy, hepatomegaly, and, often, edema, which tends to conceal the extent of the wasting. The proliferation of parasite-loaded histiocytes in the bone marrow makes anemia the rule, and thrombocytopenia with gingival and other mucosal bleeding is common. The peripheral leukocyte count is low (usually less than 4,000 per cu mm); in children, agranulocytosis with cancrum oris and secondary pulmonary or intestinal infections contribute to the high mortality.

Hyperglobulinemia, demonstrable by flocculation when distilled water is added to plasma or by the formol-gel test, is universally present; these tests are useful in screening populations for the disease. Proteinuria and hematuria are frequent in the course of kala-azar, and symptoms of heart failure can occur terminally; uremia due to renal amyloidosis can complicate chronic cases.

Diagnosis. The diagnosis is made by finding leishmania in stained preparations of blood (often possible in Indian but rarely so in Sudanese kala-azar), bone marrow, lymph nodes, or material obtained by hepatic or splenic puncture. The last is the best source of organisms, but the spleen should be needled only by an expert. The organisms will grow out as flagellated forms in simple media containing blood incubated at 28°C.

A complement fixation test using an antigen from *Mycobacterium phlei* gives positive results in 95 per cent of patients with kala-azar, but tuberculosis gives positive test results also.

Treatment. Rest, good diet, transfusions, and treatment of complicating infections, of which tuberculosis, bacterial pneumonia, amebiasis, and bacillary dysentery are the more important, must supplement or precede specific therapy. Pentavalent antimony compounds are highly effective against the parasites. Neostibosan, as a 25 per cent solution, can be given intravenously or intramuscularly on alternate days. A total of 3 to 4 Gm in 10 injections is needed. Urea stibamine is popular in India. Solustibosan, neostam, and Pentostam are effective antimony compounds that come as permanently stable solutions in ampuls for injection.

Antimony toxicity is discussed on p. 812. More than 90 per cent of cases respond promptly to antimony except in Africa, where the cure rate is as low as 70 per cent. Resistant cases should be treated with 2 per cent pentamidine (two courses of 5 to 10 intravenous or intramuscular injections each of 4 mg per kg on alternate days) or with the more effective and also more toxic 1 per cent stilbamidine given intravenously as 10 daily injections of a fresh solution, the doses beginning with 2.5 ml and increasing by 1.0 ml daily until a total of about 70 ml is reached. Treatment with pentamidine or stilbamidine should not be repeated in less than 1 month.

Post-kala-azar Dermal Leishmaniasis. Patients treated successfully with antimony compounds for kala-azar may later develop cutaneous lesions called "leishmanoids," in which *Leishmania* are demonstrable. These are very rare in Mediterranean or Chinese kala-azar. They occur after a latent period of 1 to 2 years in as many as 10 per cent of Indian cases, and in 30 per cent of Sudanese cases, they occur almost immediately after systemic symptoms subside. The lesions range from patchy areas of depigmentation to erythematous papules and confluent nodules which may involve the ears and mucous membranes and have been mistaken for leprosy.

Antimony will cure these dermal leishmanoids but the response is slow. Large doses of potassium iodide are said to cause the nodules to ulcerate and render them more susceptible to clearing with urea stibamine.

Prognosis and Control. The mortality in untreated kala-azar is 95 per cent in adults and 80 per cent in children. This has been greatly reduced by treatment with antimony and the aromatic diamidines.

The treatment of the disease in man, the elimination of diseased dogs, and the use of DDT residual sprays against sand flies are the important preventive measures. Incidence of the disease has diminished greatly in many areas where DDT has been used to eradicate malaria—an unexpected added benefit of this program.

AMERICAN MUCOCUTANEOUS LEISHMANIASIS

This disease occurs in every country of Central and South America except Chile. In some areas, 10 to 20 per cent of the population is infected. The causative organism, *L. brasiliensis,* is present in several wild animals, but of these only the agouti is believed to be an important reservoir host. The infection is particularly common in men who work in forests, but children and women are not spared. There are three general types of the disease, all of which begin with a local lesion at the site of the infecting sandfly bite after incubation of from 10 days to 3 months. The so-called *Mexican* type of infection is characterized by lesions on the ear which are chronic, show little ulceration, and lead to deformities through scarring, producing the so-called *oreja de chicleros,* so named because it is common in chicle harvesters. Spontaneous healing is the rule and parasites are never numerous in the lesions. Mucosal ulceration does not occur.

The *uta* type, which, along with the Mexican, occurs in cooler climates and at altitudes of more than 2,000 ft, consists of single or multiple skin ulcers in which parasites are readily demonstrable. Spontaneous healing within 3 months to a year is the rule and mucosal spread is unusual.

In tropical Latin America the disease takes the better-known and more serious *espundia* form. The initial skin lesion enlarges progressively and secondary bacterial infection is frequent. There is little tendency to heal, and in 75 per cent of patients with chronic skin ulceration, the disease spreads by direct extension or by lymphatics to the mucosal surfaces of the mouth and nose, where painful, destructive, and mutilating erosions occur with extensive scarring and distortion of the involved structures. Fever, anemia, and weight loss accompany these mucosal complications. Destruction of the nasal septum produces a characteristic deformity called "tapir nose" or "camel nose." The hard palate may be destroyed, and laryngeal erosion can lead to aphonia. In Negroes, the lesion is often hypertrophic and large polypoid masses deform the lips and cheeks, perhaps representing a type of keloid reaction. This can be mistaken for South American blastomycosis (see p. 1067). Secondary bacterial infection, inanition, and respiratory obstruction lead to death.

The diagnosis is made by finding the organisms in scrapings or by culture. The Montenegro skin test is specific and highly useful. Treatment consists of antibiotics for bacterial infections and antimonials, preferably sodium antimony tartrate, which is given intravenously as a 1 or 2 per cent solution, the dose being increased on alternate days from 0.04 Gm initially to a maximum of 0.28 Gm, until a total of 2.2 Gm has been given.

The early lesions respond well but even with repeated courses of antimony, the mucosal complications of the *espundia* type heal slowly; in advanced cases, the prognosis is very poor.

CUTANEOUS LEISHMANIASIS; ORIENTAL SORE

This, the least serious form of human leishmaniasis, consists of localized cutaneous ulceration which heals spontaneously and is endemic in the European countries bordering the eastern Mediterranean, in North Africa, Asia Minor, Southwest Asia, and India. Two major strains of the causative organism, *L. tropica,* produce similar but distinctive clinical syndromes. Although homologous immunity after recovery from infection by either strain is solid and lifelong, there is no cross immunity between the two.

The *rural,* or *moist,* type has its reservoir in gerbils and other small rodents; the ulcers usually appear on the extremities 2 to 6 weeks after the bite of the sand fly and are accompanied by regional lymphadenopathy in a majority of cases. Spontaneous healing occurs within 3 to 6 months, leaving a depigmented, pitted scar.

The incubation period in the *urban,* or *dry,* type ranges from 2 months to more than a year. The lesion is usually facial and begins as a pruritic, purplish nodule (the "Aleppo button"), which slowly enlarges and finally breaks down after 3 or 4 months. Healing of the indolent, granulomatous ulcer may require a year or more; lymphatic involvement is uncommon. Man is the only known reservoir of infection.

The typical oriental sore is a sharply punched-out, ragged ulcer about 1 in. in diameter, surrounded by an erythematous rim. Satellite lesions which fuse with the original are not rare. The center of the granulating base of the ulcer frequently contains a hard excrescence called the "Montpellier sign" or the "rake," beneath which the parasites are most likely to be found when scrapings are examined.

The wet and dry types occur together in Asia Minor; indeed, it is not rare to find simultaneous infections in the same patient. In Africa, Southeastern Europe, and India, only the dry type is prevalent.

Diagnosis is usually made on clinical grounds and is confirmed by finding the parasites, which occur both intra- and extracellularly. Pyogenic infection makes direct visualization difficult, but *L. tropica* can be cultured in blood-containing broth incubated at 28°C, and a skin test using *L. tropica* antigen becomes positive in the vast majority of patients with the disease.

Treatment should include vigorous measures for bacterial infection, such as hot soaks and appropriate systemic antibiotics. Local infiltration with 10 to 15 per cent Atabrine is very effective in early lesions, but nothing seems to speed the subsidence of established ulcers except control of secondary infection. Systemic antimonials may be required where ulceration is extensive or multiple. In endemic areas the custom is to withhold treatment directed against the parasite until the initial nodule ulcerates, to assure the development of immunity against reinfection.

Prevention consists of use of insect repellents on exposed parts of the body, residual DDT sprays, and fine-mesh screening for dwellings. The lesions should be covered to prevent infection of vectors and, of course, contact with the lesion or its discharges should be avoided.

In Asia Minor, a relapsing form known as *leishmaniasis recidiva* is common. Nodules appear at the periphery of the scarred area and mimic lupus vulgaris so closely that errors in diagnosis are very frequent.

REFERENCES

Belding, D. L.: "Basic Clinical Parasitology," New York, Appleton-Century-Crofts, Inc., 1958.

Manson-Bahr, P.: "Manson's Tropical Diseases," 15th ed., London, Cassell & Co., Ltd., 1960.

214 TRYPANOSOMIASIS
Ivan L. Bennett, Jr.

Definition. Trypanosomiasis designates infection produced by protozoans of the genus *Trypanosoma*. These organisms are responsible for numerous diseases in animals and for three separate disorders in man, Gambian or mid-African sleeping sickness, Rhodesian or East African sleeping sickness, and Chagas disease in Central and South America.

Etiology. Trypanosomes are fusiform organisms, recognized by an undulating membrane which extends along the length of the cell and terminates in an anterior flagellum. The morphology of many species is so nearly identical that they are distinguishable only by their pathogenicity for certain animals, differences in biochemical requirements, and ability to multiply in insects.

Most species are transmitted to vertebrate hosts by insects and undergo a part of their life cycle in the vector, but direct transmission between warm-blooded hosts is the rule for others. *Trypanosoma gambiense*, the cause of mid-African sleeping sickness, is transmitted to man by riverine tsetse flies (*Glossina*), and *T. rhodesiense* (East African) by woodland tsetse flies. *Trypanosoma cruzi*, the agent of Chagas disease, is carried by reduviid ("assassin" or "kissing") bugs, primarily those of the genus *Triatoma*. Transmission of the trypanosomes of sleeping sickness occurs by what is referred to as the "anterior station"; after multiplication in the intestine of the tsetse fly, the parasites migrate to the salivary glands and are discharged when a host is bitten. The agent of Chagas disease, however, multiplies only in the gut of the vector and is discharged in the feces, infection of man occurring through contamination of the bite wound; this is transmission by the "posterior station."

Trypanosomiasis in animals is a great economic problem in many parts of the world. Indeed, it is said that an area of approximately 4 million square miles in Africa is now essentially unpopulated because of the impossibility of keeping domestic animals in these areas where tsetse flies are infected with *T. brucei*, the cause of *nagana*, a fatal disease of cattle and horses. Among the more important trypanosomal diseases of animals are *dourine* in horses and donkeys, caused by *T. equiperdum*, which is transmitted by sexual intercourse and is world-wide; *souma*, caused by *T. vivax* in horses and cattle (Africa); *surra*, caused by *T. evansi* in horses, cattle, and dogs (Asia, Australia, Madagascar); *mal de caderas*, caused by *T. equinum* in horses and cattle (South America); and *murina de caderas*, caused by *T. hippicum* in horses and mules (Central America). The epidemiology of each of the three trypanosomiases of man is discussed separately below.

Gambian Sleeping Sickness. This disease occurs in tropical west and central Africa, especially along the Congo River and its tributaries. While swine and goats are suspected of harboring *T. gambiense*, man is the only known reservoir. The vectors are tsetse flies that live near water, and the highest incidence of the disease is in young men, a result of increased exposure to the flies. It is interesting that less than 5 per cent of flies are infected, even in the most notorious endemic foci.

The disease in man has customarily been described as proceeding through several classic "stages" interspersed with periods of remission or quiescence. Actually, there is tremendous variation in the severity, symptomatology, duration, and outcome of the disease, all apparently dependent upon the resistance of the host, and the many so-called types or stages of trypanosomiasis are better understood in these terms than on the basis of duration of infection alone.

The *incubation period* is about 2 weeks. In many

cases, the infecting bite shows an erythematous nodule with a pale halo, the *trypanosomal chancre*, which subsides gradually. Whether a lesion is visible or not, the parasites multiply locally, enter lymphatics, and appear in the blood about 3 weeks after the bite of the tsetse fly. In the usual case, the patient experiences irregularly recurrent paroxysms of fever for months. The temperature can exceed 106°F, and during these episodes of illness, skin rashes of various types are common. These may be generalized, pruritic papular eruptions or erythema nodosum. In Caucasians, a characteristic circinate erythema resembling erythema marginatum is frequently noted. Severe headache and tachycardia accompany fever and, as the illness progresses, weight loss and progressive debilitation ensue. Tender lymphadenopathy, with gradual induration of the nodes, and splenomegaly are almost invariably present. The lymph nodes of the posterior cervical triangles are especially prominent; this is referred to as *Winterbottom's sign*. Insomnia, inability to concentrate, paresthesias, and formication are frequent, and most patients demonstrate a peculiar delayed sensation to pain combined with deep, aching hyperesthesia that can be elicited by a light blow with any hard object, known as *Kerandel's sign*. The illness can terminate spontaneously after weeks or months or can drag on intermittently for years. Death from intercurrent infections, of which bacillary and amebic dysentery, malaria, and bacterial (often pneumococcal) pneumonia are the most important, is frequent.

Eventually, the parasites enter the central nervous system, usually about 2 years after the onset of illness although it may occur much earlier or may be delayed for as long as 8 years. Cerebral trypanosomiasis can be explosive, causing repeated convulsions or deep coma and death within a few days. However, most patients show gradual progression to the classic picture of *sleeping sickness*. While spontaneous recovery is not rare in early trypanosomiasis, untreated *sleeping sickness* is almost invariably fatal within 4 to 8 months. The patient develops a vacant expression, the eyelids droop, the lower lip hangs loosely, and it becomes more and more difficult to gain his attention or prod him to any activity. Patients will eat when offered food, but they never ask for it or engage in spontaneous conversation, and speech gradually becomes blurred and indistinct. Tremors of the hands and tongue, choreiform movements, seizures with transient paralysis, loss of sphincter control, ophthalmoplegia, extensor plantar responses, and finally death in coma, status epilepticus, or from hyperpyrexia follow inexorably.

The over-all mortality of Gambian trypanosomiasis is 25 to 50 per cent; with chemotherapy, this can be reduced to 5 or 10 per cent.

Anemia and *hyperglobulinemia* (demonstrable in surveys by the formol-gel reaction) are invariably present, and spontaneous clumping of erythrocytes in blood specimens is grossly evident in many cases. The sedimentation rate is rapid, and peripheral monocytosis is frequent.

The *cerebrospinal fluid* shows mononuclear pleocytosis and increased protein content in sleeping sickness. The colloidal gold curve is tabetic. The protein content is a better index of severity of disease and therapeutic response than is the number of cells.

The trypanosomes can sometimes be found in thick blood films; examination of the sediment after centrifugation of 20 ml of hemolyzed (distilled water) blood at 3,000 rpm for 10 min is more likely to give positive results. Bone marrow and material aspirated from lymph nodes are occasionally found to contain the organisms, and they are also demonstrable in cerebrospinal fluid. A specific complement fixation test is available but it has not been used extensively in diagnosis.

Fever, lymphadenopathy, Winterbottom's and Kerandel's signs, splenomegaly, and anemia in a resident of an endemic area make the clinical diagnosis relatively easy. Hyperglobulinemia and the finding of trypanosomes are confirmatory. *Irregular fever, lymphadenopathy, and especially circinate erythema in any Caucasian who has resided in Africa within 7 years should arouse suspicion of trypanosomiasis.* While malaria, kala-azar, Hodgkin's disease, and leprosy are sometimes confused with early trypanosomiasis, the proper diagnosis usually becomes evident within a short time.

Antrypol (Bayer 205, suramin) is the most effective agent before central nervous system involvement has occurred. Ten injections at intervals of 4 to 7 days should be given, each dose consisting of 10 ml of a fresh 10 per cent solution. Albumin and casts appear in the urine of most patients after the first few injections, but the urine clears about 6 weeks after completion of the injections. *Mel B (Arsobal)*, an arsenical derivative of BAL, is sometimes effective in both early and late cases. It can be given intravenously or, with procaine, intramuscularly. The dosage is 3.6 mg per kg daily for 4 days, to be followed by four more daily injections after an interval of 1 week.

For cerebral trypanosomiasis, the most effective drug is *tryparsamide*, given intravenously as a fresh 20 per cent solution once weekly for 8 to 15 weeks. The first dose should be 5 ml, and this should be increased gradually to 15 ml (3 Gm) weekly. A course of injections may be repeated after a rest of 1 month. Arsenical hepatitis or dermatitis, abdominal cramps, and, most important, optic atrophy can result from tryparsamide; ocular symptoms make cessation of the drug mandatory. Recovery rates as high as 50 per cent have followed intensive tryparsamide therapy in sleeping sickness.

The other effective drug for early disease is *pentamidine,* given as a 2 per cent solution intramuscularly on alternate days for 5 to 10 injections; the course is repeated 1 week later. The dose for each injection is 4 mg per kg.

Prevention includes use of repellents and protective clothing (gloves, head nets) in endemic areas and chemoprophylaxis, using an injection of 5 mg per kg of pentamidine for each member of the population every 6 months. Elimination of the vector is almost a hopeless undertaking in many areas at present; indeed it has been easier to move whole villages out of infested areas than to eradicate the tsetse fly population.

Rhodesian Sleeping Sickness. This disease is found in tropical east Africa where the etiologic agent, *T. rhodesiense,* is transmitted by woodland species of tsetse flies. Antelopes are known reservoirs, and other wild animals are also suspected of harboring the parasite. More than 60 per cent of human infections occur in adult males. Rhodesian trypanosomiasis is a more acute and severe disease than the Gambian form, usually terminating fatally within a year. Fever is higher, emaciation more rapid, and lymphatic involvement is less evident. Death from intercurrent infection, myocarditis, or "toxemia" usually occurs before there is appreciable central nervous system involvement; although lethargy and somnolence are seen, the typical sleeping sickness syndrome is rare.

Rhodesian trypanosomiasis is more resistant to treatment than the Gambian disease. *Antrypol* is effective only if given within 3 weeks of the onset of symptoms; *Mel B* can be used in cases discovered too late for treatment with Antrypol, and *tryparsamide* should be given immediately if there is any evidence of neurologic disease. No drug is really effective in advanced cases.

Prevention is extremely complicated because of the much greater problems of eradicating woodland tsetse flies than the riverine and the need to shift populations into noninfected areas. While chronic human cases are relatively rare, the existence of animal reservoirs makes it impossible to prevent continuing infection of the vectors. Chemoprophylaxis requires the use of pentamidine in a dose of 5 mg per kg every 2 months. Individual protection with repellents, netting, etc., is, of course, important.

The disease is almost invariably fatal if untreated. Intensive treatment results in cure of about 50 per cent of early cases, but this falls to 15 per cent in advanced disease.

Chagas Disease (American Trypanosomiasis). This infection occurs from Argentina and Chile to southern Mexico. The etiologic agent, *T. cruzi,* is plentiful in "assassin" and "kissing" bugs as far north as Texas, but only one authenticated case is known in which the disease was acquired in the United States. Infection in man usually begins with acute systemic symptoms and then becomes chronic, resembling kala-azar more than the sleeping sickness of Africa. The parasites multiply intracellularly in a leishmania form, morphologically indistinguishable from the Leishman-Donovan bodies of kala-azar, but they assume the trypanosomal form in the blood stream.

The vector attacks man at night, usually biting the face at a mucocutaneous junction (hence the name "kissing" bug), most frequently the lip or outer canthus of the eye. An erythematous nodule, the *chagoma,* appears within a few days at the initial site where the parasites have gained entrance from the infected feces of the vector. Secondary nodules are sometimes seen along draining lymphatics. After an *incubation period* of 2 weeks, there is the onset of *fever* (coincident with the appearance of parasitemia, which lasts for about 30 days) and a morbilliform or urticarial *skin eruption,* which subsides after a few days. Painless *unilateral palpebral edema and conjunctivitis,* known as *Romaña's sign,* usually come on during the first febrile week. The fever sometimes shows two daily spikes, local lymphadenopathy and splenomegaly appear, and in severely affected young children, there may be a fatal outcome within weeks although the usual tendency is for symptoms to subside as the infection becomes chronic. The parasites spread systemically, showing a predilection for histiocytes, skeletal muscle, heart muscle, and the central nervous system. When meningoencephalitis complicates the acute illness in children, the mortality is 40 per cent. Myositis is attended by extensive gelatinous edema (*pseudomyxedema*) of the face and trunk, and the differentiation of Chagas disease from cretinism and endemic goiter is sometimes surprisingly difficult. Chronic *neurologic* manifestations include sporadic convulsions, various paralyses, and intention tremor. An extensive acute myocarditis is sometimes accompanied by pericardial effusion and can result in rapidly fatal heart failure. However, the process usually becomes chronic and slowly progressive and is a leading cause of cardiac disease in individuals under the age of forty in Central and South America. Manifestations range from arrhythmias and heart block to chronic congestive heart failure; differentiation from rheumatic heart disease is often a great problem.

The diagnosis can be made in chronic cases by the use of a complement fixation reaction (Machado-Guerreiro test), but this is positive in only about 50 per cent of acute cases. Trypanosomes can sometimes be found in the sediment of centrifuged, hemolyzed blood during the acute stages, and biopsy of lymph node or liver reveals the leish-mania forms. *Trypanosoma cruzi* is easily grown in blood broth incubated at 28°C. The technique of *xenodiagnosis* is often used in endemic areas; a laboratory-reared vector, known to be parasite-free, is allowed to feed on suspected cases, and 2 weeks later, the insect's intestinal contents are examined for parasites. Confusion sometimes arises from the finding of trypanosomes in blood. Many children in Venezuela and other South American countries are infected with a harmless species, *T. rangeli,* which produces no symptoms but can be present in the blood for many months.

There is *no specific treatment* for Chagas disease. Prevention consists of using residual insecticide sprays—of which benzene hexachloride (BHC) is the most effective—on the walls of houses, the main habitat of the vectors.

Because Chagas disease can be transmitted by blood transfusion, treatment of blood for 24 hr with 1:4,000 gentian violet is recommended in endemic areas.

REFERENCES

Ashcroft, M. T.: A Critical Review of the Epidemiology of Human Trypanosomiasis in Africa, Trop. Diseases Bull., 56:1073, 1959.

Belding, D. L.: "Basic Clinical Parasitology," New York, Appleton-Century-Crofts, Inc., 1958.

Clark, H. C., and L. H. Dunn: Experimental Studies on Chagas' Disease in Panama, Am. J. Trop. Med., 12: 49, 1932.

Duggan, A. J.: An Appraisal of the Clinical Problems of Gambian Sleeping Sickness, J. Trop. Med. Hyg., 67:268, 1959.

Manson-Bahr, P.: "Manson's Tropical Diseases," 15th ed., London, Cassell & Co., Ltd., 1960.

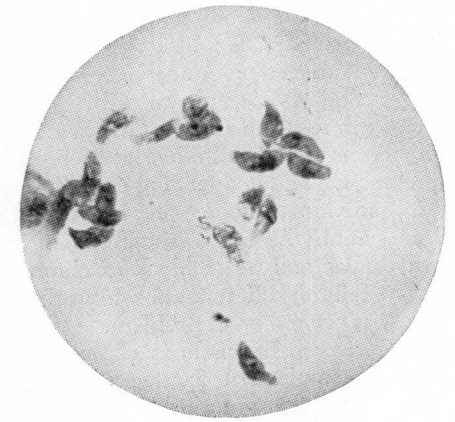

Fig. 215-1. Toxoplasma in Wright-stained impression film (×1200).

215 TOXOPLASMOSIS
Harry A. Feldman

Definition. Toxoplasmosis, a disease of increasing importance, results from infection with an obligate intracellular protozoan parasite, *Toxoplasma gondii,* which is widely distributed among mammals and birds. In man it may produce acquired (often inapparent) or congenital illness.

History. First demonstrated in 1908 by Nicolle and Manceaux in a North African rodent, the gondi, and in the same year by Splendore in Brazil, *Toxoplasma* was not definitely related to human disease until 1939, when Wolfe, Cowen, and Paige described infantile cases of encephalomyelitis which had resulted from congenital infections with the parasite. The disease-producing capabilities of the parasite have become more evident as the result of the almost simultaneous descriptions of skin, complement fixation, and dye tests. These have been utilized extensively, and it is now apparent that toxoplasma frequently infects man and animals and that congenital toxoplasmosis is only one aspect of a broad disease spectrum.

Etiology. *Toxoplasma gondii* is considered to be a protozoan. All strains, regardless of source, are antigenically similar and of the same species. The organism measures about 3.0 by 6.0 μ and may appear crescentic, oval, or round (Fig. 215-1). It divides by binary fission and is best stained with either Wright or Giemsa stain. Toxoplasma is unique in that it may infect any mammalian or avian cell, except nonnucleated erythrocytes. It can be maintained in tissue culture or embryonated eggs but does not multiply in the absence of living cells. The parasite is readily sedimented by centrifugation. Under special conditions it may be stored in the frozen state, but is killed by ordinary freezing. The parasite seems to persist in cysts which may be found in any tissue.

Laboratory Diagnosis. A specific diagnosis may be made by the application of serologic methods, by demonstrating the organism in smears, or by isolating it in mice. Toxoplasmas may be seen in Wright or Giemsa stains of the sediment of cerebrospinal fluid, or occasionally in H and E stained histologic sections of lymph node or muscle during the active phase of the illness. The laboratory mouse is the animal of choice for attempting isolations and may be inoculated with spinal fluid sediment (when acute central nervous system signs are present) or emulsions of fresh tissue.

Serum antibodies may be detected by the dye, complement fixation, or hemagglutination tests. Results are most meaningful when a rising titer is demonstrated. Dye-test antibodies seem to develop early and persist for many years, possibly for life.

Complement-fixing antibodies develop more slowly and disappear more rapidly. Thus if a high dye-test titer (1:256 or more) and a negative complement fixation reaction are encountered, one may be dealing with either an early infection or the residual serologic status of past infection. Hemagglutinating antibodies seem to behave like dye test antibodies but apparently develop at a slightly slower rate.

A positive dye reaction requires the presence of a heat-labile serum factor which now has been demonstrated to be in the properdin system. This is the first instance when presence of the properdin system has been shown to be necessary for the action of a specific antibody.

A skin test is available and may be performed with antigen prepared from mouse peritoneal fluid or embryonated eggs. The reaction is of the delayed type, and cross-reacting antigens have not been identified. The egg antigen is preferable, because suitable control material is available. There are three drawbacks which limit the value of the test as a diagnostic aid in an individual case: (1) the number of reactors in the general population is large; (2) serum antibodies have been demonstrated in nonreactors; (3) the antigen has not been standardized satisfactorily.

Epidemiology. Surveys performed with the skin, dye, and hemagglutination tests indicate that toxoplasma infections are widespread. The dye test is, perhaps, the most sensitive indicator of antibody. With this, it has been determined that approximately 33 per cent of the populations of a number of American cities and Haiti, 63 per cent of Hondurans, and 70 per cent of Tahitian natives are positive. In contrast, only 4 per cent of Navajo Indians and 11 per cent of a group of Icelanders had significant amounts of antibody. Similar studies have been conducted among various animal species; antibodies are especially frequent among dogs, cats, swine, sheep, goats, guinea pigs, and to a lesser extent, rabbits and pigeons. Although the full significance of these findings remains to be determined, it is clear that serologic evidence indicates that infection with toxoplasma may be abundant in man and many of his animal associates. The mode of transfer of parasites from animal to animal or to man is unknown; there is no evidence for human-to-human transfer. Human infection, apparently, may be contracted in any season and with equal frequency by the two sexes.

Clinical Manifestations. Human infections with toxoplasma may be either congenital or acquired. An infant *congenitally infected* with toxoplasma may be born prematurely or at term as a stillbirth or with an active infection manifested by various combinations of fever, icterus, rash, hepatomegaly, splenomegaly, chorioretinitis, convulsions, and xanthochromic spinal fluid. The newborn infant may have none of these signs, but some time later hydrocephaly or microcephaly, chorioretinitis, convulsions, psychomotor retardation, and cerebral calcifications may be noted either singly or in combination. A fatality rate of 11 per cent was noted in one series of 141 cases of congenital toxoplasmosis. Among the more important evidences of disease in these children, chorioretinitis was present in 94 per cent, while 59 per cent had cerebral calcifications, 45 per cent had psychomotor retardation, and approximately half had either hydro- or microcephaly; 39 per cent had convulsive episodes. The mothers of congenitally damaged offspring ordinarily are unaware of having had any specific illnesses during the pregnancy. These women may undertake future pregnancies without fear of a recurrence in another child.

In the proved cases of *acquired toxoplasmosis* the clinical features have shown considerable variation, but certain manifestations are being recognized as suggestive of this disease. Maculopapular rashes are not infrequent soon after the clinical onset of the illness and tend to disappear in 3 or 4 days. Lymphadenopathy is common, and local nodes may be so prominent as to suggest the possibility of Hodgkin's disease. Encephalitis may be present alone or in combination with other manifestations. Myalgias, arthralgias, myocarditis, and pneumonitis also have been noted. Siim has described a syndrome which resembles infectious mononucleosis in that lymphadenopathy and lymphocytosis with atypical lymphocytes may be present; Paul-Bunnell reactions are negative. Parasites can be demonstrated in lymph nodes removed from such patients, some of whom have afebrile courses.

Toxoplasmas now have been isolated from cases of granulomatous uveitis in adults, presumably the result of acquired infections. The proportion of such cases which is caused by toxoplasmas remains to be determined and is the subject of considerable investigation.

There is no reliable information concerning the incubation period, recovery and mortality rates, average duration of illness, or residual defects resulting from acquired toxoplasmosis. Cerebral calcifications do not appear to follow this form.

Treatment. There is good evidence from experimental infections that a combination of sulfonamide and pyrimethamine (Daraprim) is somewhat better than sulfonamides alone. Combinations of sulfadiazine or triple sulfonamides and Daraprim have been reported to yield excellent results in some cases of uveitis and to have affected others not at all. The data on the effectiveness of this treatment in systemic toxoplasmosis are inadequate. It does seem to benefit the acute symptoms but does not eradicate encysted organisms. The combination is not specific for toxoplasmosis, and the patient's response cannot be interpreted as proving or disproving a particular diagnosis. The sulfonamide should be administered in the usual dosage along with 50 mg Daraprim daily. The dose of Daraprim probably ought to be decreased after 2 weeks to 25 mg. One month of treatment constitutes an adequate trial. The leukopenia and thrombocytopenia which may result from Daraprim administration have been corrected by the simultaneous administration of citrovorum factor (Leucovorin calcium) and yeast cakes without interfering with its *anti-toxoplasmic* effect.

REFERENCES

Feldman, H. A.: Toxoplasmosis: A Review, Pediatrics, 22:559, 1958.

———: Human Toxoplasmosis, J. Chronic Diseases, 10: 488, 1959.

Remington, J. S., L. Jacobs, and H. E. Kaufman: Toxoplasmosis in the Adult, New Engl. J. Med., 262: 180 and 237, 1960.

Siim, J. Chr.: "Human Toxoplasmosis," Baltimore, The Williams & Wilkins Company, 1960.

216 PNEUMOCYSTIS PNEUMONIA (Interstitial Plasma Cell Pneumonia)

Ivan L. Bennett, Jr.

Definition. Pneumocystis pneumonia is an acute to subacute disease characterized by progressive interstitial inflammation of the lungs. The presumed etiologic agent is *Pneumocystis carinii,* a protozoan. Although adults and older children are affected only rarely, the disease is relatively common in infants in Europe and is increasing in frequency in the United States. The manifestations are progressive dyspnea and cyanosis, with death from respiratory failure in a large number of the cases after 6 to 10 weeks of illness.

Etiology. The etiologic significance of *P. carinii* in this disease is supported by the consistent finding of myriads of the organisms in histologic sections and impression smears of lungs from fatal cases. The organism has never been cultivated on artificial media, and serologic evidence of its role in the disease is equivocal, the main difficulty being lack of a reliable preparation of antigen.

Pneumocystis carinii was first identified as a parasite present in the lungs of guinea pigs, and it is now known that small numbers of the parasite also occur in the normal pulmonary tissues of rats, rabbits, monkeys, dogs, and man. While most ob-

servers believe that *P. carinii* is properly classified as a protozoan, a few are convinced that it is a fungus. The organism cannot be seen in hematoxylin and eosin preparations but is easily visualized in sections or smears stained by the Giemsa, Schiff, or silver-impregnation methods. Two forms occur: (1) the oval or elongated free (ameboid) form measures 2 to 4 mμ and contains a single nucleus; (2) the more easily recognized cysts are round, about 10 mμ in diameter and contain two to eight distinct nuclei.

Pathogenesis and Pathologic Findings. The fact that small numbers of *P. carinii* occur in the lungs of many individuals suggests, of course, that infection by this organism is often latent or subclinical and that the appearance of overt disease is dependent upon an increase in host susceptibility. There is much evidence to support this concept of the pathogenesis of interstitial plasma cell pneumonia. Serious infections by *P. carinii* are far more frequent under the age of one year, and it has been noted repeatedly that they have a distinct predilection for premature or otherwise debilitated infants. Furthermore, many children who die with *P. carinii* pneumonia are found at autopsy to have extensive lesions of cytomegalic inclusion disease also, a viral infection that is usually subclinical or latent until activated by some impairment of host resistance (see p. 1183). The administration of large doses of cortisone to otherwise normal rabbits will often induce the appearance of extensive *P. carinii* interstitial pneumonitis, highly suggestive of activation of latent disease. Finally, although fatal pneumocystis pneumonia is rare in adults, of the 13 cases reported up until 1961, 12 occurred in individuals with lymphoma, leukemia, or some other serious disorder. Also among the 12 adults at autopsy, there were 6 instances of concomitant cytomegalic inclusion disease, 2 of tuberculosis, and 2 of cryptococcosis. Therefore, although the mode of entry of *P. carinii* is still unknown, it appears that serious disease occurs as a result of lighting up of latent infection and that subclinical infection with this organism is very frequent.

The histologic changes consist of extensive mononuclear infiltration of the pulmonary alveolar septums with encroachment upon the air spaces and alveolar ducts. The exudate was originally thought to consist of plasma cells, and it is from this microscopic feature that the term interstitial plasma cell pneumonia originated. The alveoli are filled with a vacuolated, foamy exudate which is almost pathognomonic in its appearance in hematoxylin and eosin preparations. With appropriate stains, the foamy appearance of the exudate is seen to be attributable to the presence of huge masses of organisms. Fibrosis and scarring are not a feature of the histologic alterations, and the inflammation is completely reversible in patients who recover from the disease. It cannot be emphasized too strongly that *P. carinii* will be missed if hematoxylin and eosin sections only are examined and that the small size of the organisms makes them difficult to identify unless oil-immersion objectives are used. There is no doubt about the fact that the pneumonia has been misdiagnosed at autopsy on many occasions in the United States; it is now a common experience for a review of the histologic sections of past autopsies to reveal the presence of *P. carinii* in lungs of infantile pneumonia.

Manifestations. The onset is insidious, with tachypnea and poor feeding in infants. Within 2 weeks, x-ray of the lungs shows diffuse infiltration. There is little or no fever; cough and coryza are rare. Dyspnea and cyanosis are relentlessly progressive in fatal cases, and death comes during the sixth to tenth week. In survivors, there is gradual subsidence of respiratory symptoms and complete clearing of the x-ray findings. The typical course is easily recognizable in infants. In adults, the association of the disease with lymphoma, leukemia, etc., and with other infections likely to complicate debilitating illness (tuberculosis, mycoses, cytomegalic inclusion disease) might make antemortem diagnosis possible.

There are no laboratory tests other than lung biopsy that will confirm the diagnosis. It is possible that *P. carinii* might be identified in bronchial washings (this has been done retrospectively in one case). No reliable serologic test is available.

Treatment and Prognosis. The only treatment is supportive, with administration of oxygen and attention to nutrition. Any accompanying disease such as lymphoma should be managed appropriately.

Antibiotics, sulfonamides, adrenal steroids, γ-globulin, x-ray, diathermy, arsenicals, antimalarials, antifungal drugs, and a host of antiprotozoan drugs have been tried extensively without appreciable effect.

The mortality among infants is about 25 to 40 per cent.

REFERENCES

Gajdusek, D. C.: *Pneumocystis carinii*—Etiologic Agent of Interstitial Plasma Cell Pneumonia of Premature and Young Infants, Pediatrics, 19:543, 1957.

Hennigar, G. R., et al.: *Pneumocystis carinii* Pneumonia in an Adult, Am. J. Clin. Pathol., 35:353, 1961.

Rubin, E., and F. G. Zak: *Pneumocystis carinii* Pneumonia in the Adult, New Engl. J. Med., 262:1315, 1960.

Sheldon, W. H.: Experimental Pulmonary *Pneumocystis carinii* Infection in Rabbits, J. Exptl. Med., 110:147, 1959.

217 MINOR PROTOZOAN DISEASES

Ivan L. Bennett, Jr.

TRICHOMONIASIS

Of the many members of the genus *Trichomonas*, three are parasites of man: *T. hominis* in the intestine, *T. tenax* in the oral cavity, and *T. vaginalis*, the only one capable of producing disease, in the vagina and urethra. All three possess four anterior flagella, and their morphology is quite similar; *T. vaginalis* is the largest, however, and confusion in diagnosis is rare because of the anatomic specificity of their habitats.

Trichomonas vaginalis, despite some question about its role as a primary pathogen, is associated with persistent vaginitis in about 20 per cent of parasitized women. Manifestations include itching, burning, and profuse, creamy, yellow, frothy leukorrhea. Examination shows inflammation ranging from mild hyperemia of the vaginal vault to extensive erosion, petechial hemorrhages, and perineal intertrigo.

The diagnosis is made by examining a fresh unstained drop of the discharge which will be found to contain numerous motile trichomonads. The organisms are often present in urine. In males, a mild, usually asymptomatic urethritis is produced. The importance of the disease in males has to do with the transmission of infection by sexual contact, although the disease is also spread by toilet articles, fomites, etc.

Trichomoniasis is sometimes responsible for confusing changes in the cytologic pattern of exfoliated vaginal cells. However, ordinary Papanicolaou preparations are not well-suited to establishing the diagnosis of this infection, and when it is suspected, fresh material should be looked at immediately.

Treatment consists of attention to personal hygiene, the local application of Floroquin or acetarsone as insufflated powders or suppositories, and acid douches. Oral Diodoquin and tetracyclines are effective but rarely required, and antibiotics will favor the development of vaginal moniliasis. The infection in males rarely requires therapy; local treatment is not effective and Diodoquin or tetracycline should be given.

GIARDIASIS (Lambliasis)

Giardia lamblia is a pear-shaped, multiflagellar, protozoan parasite of the human duodenum. It possesses two large nuclei which give the organism the appearance of a face with two large eyes viewed under the microscope. In children, who are three times more likely than adults to be parasitized, there may be intermittent diarrhea, epigastric pain, and distention. Discomfort is rare in adults, and transmission to volunteers produces no symptoms. Occasionally, fulminating and extensive duodenal ulceration has been described. Radiologically, many asymptomatic carriers will demonstrate "irritability" of the duodenal bulb.

The diagnosis is made by finding the parasites in duodenal washings or diarrheal stools. Cyst forms are often passed; they contain two to four nuclei and are readily identified when stained with iodine.

Treatment consists of the administration of 0.1 Gm Atabrine hydrochloride three times daily for 3 days, a regimen which eliminates the organisms in 90 per cent of the cases. Chloroquine diphosphate (Aralen) 0.5 Gm daily for 5 days is about 75 per cent effective. Treatment is necessary only in symptomatic cases. The frequency of infestation in children bears out transmission by the fecal-oral route, and reinfection will occur unless appropriate measures are taken.

COCCIDIOSIS

This is a relatively unusual disease characterized by fever, abdominal pain, and diarrhea, which results from ingestion of the oocysts or spores of *Isospora belli* or *I. hominis*. Volunteers develop symptoms about 1 week after ingestion, and the disease subsides spontaneously after 1 to 4 weeks. Infection is much commoner in children and is worldwide in distribution, especially in tropical areas. The diagnosis is made by finding oocysts of the organisms in zinc sulfate concentrates of feces. *Isospora* species occur in many lower animals, but only the dog is suspected of playing any part as a reservoir of the species that are pathogenic for man.

Diagnosis can be confused if oocysts of other members of the order Coccidia are ingested in fish or meat and appear in the feces without undergoing any change in the intestinal tract.

No treatment other than symptomatic is needed as the infection is self-limited.

BALANTIDIASIS

Balantidium coli is the largest protozoan of man and inhabits the large intestine where, in addition to an asymptomatic carrier state, it elicits disease ranging from mild recurrent diarrhea to fulminant ulceration with perforation and death. In many respects the disease is similar to amebiasis in its range of manifestations, exclusive of spread to the liver.

The illness has been reproduced by feeding the organism to volunteers. The diagnosis is made by finding the parasites in the stool, but repeated examinations may be required because shedding of balantidium is intermittent. The disease is more likely to occur in tropical areas, but at least 60 cases have been reported in the United States. Swine are frequent carriers of *B. coli*, but there is great doubt about their role in the spread of the disease to man.

The tetracyclines are highly effective in treatment as is Diodoquin in a dosage of 0.65 Gm three times daily for 3 weeks.

REFERENCES

GENERAL

Belding, D. L.: "Basic Clinical Parasitology," New York, Appleton-Century-Crofts, Inc., 1958.

TRICHOMONIASIS

Novak, E., and E. R. Novak: "Gynecologic and Obstetric Pathology," 4th ed., p. 616, Philadelphia, W. B. Saunders Company, 1958.
Trussel, R. E.: "*Trichomonas vaginalis* and Trichomoniasis," Springfield, Ill., Charles C Thomas, Publisher, 1947.

GIARDIASIS

Rendtorff, R. C.: Experimental Transmission of Human Intestinal Protozoan Parasites; *Giardia lamblia* Cysts Given in Capsules, Am. J. Hyg., 59:209, 1954.

COCCIDIOSIS

Matsubayashi, H., and F. Nozawa: Experimental Infection of *Isospora hominis* in Man, Am. J. Trop. Med., 28:633, 1948.
Routh, C. F., J. E. McCroan, Jr., and C. G. Hames: Three Cases of Human Infection with Isospora in Georgia, Am. J. Trop. Med. Hyg., 4:1, 1955.

BALANTIDIASIS

Shookhoff, H. B.: *Balantidium coli* Infection with Special Reference to Treatment, Am. J. Trop. Med., 34:442, 1951.
Swartzwelder, J. C.: Balantidiasis, Am. J. Digest. Diseases, 17:173, 1950.

Section 22: Diseases Produced by Worms

INTRODUCTION

Gustave J. Dammin

Many readers of these chapters are likely to be physicians or medical students confronted with a clinical problem as it is presented by the patient who (1) has come from a tropical country where the cause of the patient's illness has not been determined, (2) now resides in this country but has his origin in an area in which parasitic diseases occur, or (3) has traveled recently in areas where he might have been exposed to parasitic diseases. For such readers these chapters need not discuss in detail the problems which abound in areas where parasitic diseases are endemic. One should be aware, however, that in these areas the major causes of death are diseases over which we have gained some control, namely, the acute respiratory and gastrointestinal infections, tuberculosis, and tetanus. These diseases occur along with the parasitic diseases in countries which are hampered by poor economic, social, and political development. We are determined, in carrying out the national policy, to assist the developing countries which are deficient in these ways. Such assistance must emphasize preventive medicine (Weller), whereas in these chapters, the emphasis will be on the diagnosis and treatment as it pertains to an individual patient. For those desiring more information about the clinical and therapeutic aspects of the helminthic diseases than space here permits, reference may be made to selected readings listed at the end of this Introduction.

For the many reasons cited by Lenczner and Owen, we may expect to encounter more instances of so-called tropical diseases in nonendemic areas. In their clinic in Toronto, cases of filariasis, schistosomiasis, clonorchiasis, hookworm infection, hydatid disease, and cysticerosis were identified. These observations raise the question of the gravity of the helminthic infection observed in a recent traveler to an endemic area, as compared with the infection as seen in the adult individual who resides in an endemic area. The clinical picture in the initially exposed is generally more severe, but the immunologic basis for differences from the clinical picture seen in the endemic area can only be inferred at the present time. It is plain from surveys made in endemic areas that the identification of helminthic infection is not necessarily indicative of helminthic disease. In the initially exposed, however, a positive laboratory finding is likely to be of much greater import.

The clinical picture presented by helminthic infection is seldom such that more than a presumptive diagnosis can be attained. Knowledge of the patient's travel is important, but the definitive diagnosis must depend upon the laboratory. Should a diagnosis of helminthic infection be made in the laboratory, it is still the clinician's responsibility to determine whether such an infection may be the basis for the entire clinical picture presented.

Brief mention should be made of the manner in which helminthic infections differ from and also resemble those produced by bacterial and other microbial agents. As adults, helminths do not multiply in the human host, and in this sense, these infections are self-limited. In their adult form, helminths make their presence known by effects which are primarily mechanical. The lumen of a hollow viscus or a duct system may be occluded (e.g., ascariasis, fascioliasis), penetration of the intestinal wall to obtain a blood meal may lead to extensive blood loss (e.g., hookworm), or residence in the wall of a hollow viscus, intra- or extravascularly, may lead to ulceration and blood loss (strongyloidiasis, schistosomiasis). As larval forms, helminths may produce symptoms during penetration of the skin (e.g., schistosomiasis) or during migration to their site of definitive development (trichinosis). Because of the self-limited aspects of these infections, therapeutic agents may be used which might not be employed if the infection were to have a prolonged course. This applies particularly to the use of the steroid hormones in the management of trichinosis in which striking symptomatic relief has followed such treatment. There is a similarity between helminthic and microbial infections with reference to the immunologic response of the host. In both, precipitins, complement-fixing, skin-sensitizing, and neutralizing antibodies have been demonstrated. Tests for immunologic response have diagnostic value in trichinosis, echinococcus disease, filariasis, and schistosomiasis.

The knowledge that immunity can be developed against metazoan parasites has been known for over 40 years. It is difficult to explain however why this observation was not used in the development of measures to control helminthic infections. Protection conferred by an initial infection against serious subsequent infections was observed in taeniasis, trichinosis, schistosomiasis, and infections with *Hymenolepis fraterna*. Recently, with improved methods of axenic culture of helminths, the prospects for development of parenteral vaccines have also improved (Soulsby). Also worthy of further study as ingredients of vaccines are related forms of pathogenic helminths, which themselves are not pathogenic but may induce immunity. The use of irradiated larvae which do not infect, but protect against subsequent challenge, shows promise. When one considers how ineffective field control, the control of vectors, and individual prophylaxis have been in our attempts to control the helminthic infections, these advances through vaccination are most welcome (Stoll).

Interest in the helminthic and other parasitic diseases has been revived, because as mentioned above, we are determined as a nation to aid the underprivileged countries, since this is believed to be a prerequisite for retaining our own eminent position internationally and therefore hopefully assuring peace in the world. However, we have not prepared ourselves properly for this task, in the sense that our teaching of tropical diseases and research in the characteristically tropical diseases have been deficient. For too long have we given these diseases an importance in the curriculum in relationship to the importance they have in this country.

REFERENCES

Chandler, A. C., and C. P. Read: "Introduction to Parasitology," 10th ed., New York, John Wiley & Sons, Inc., 1961.

Hunter, G. W., III, W. W. Frye, and J. C. Swartzwelder: "A Manual of Tropical Medicine," 3d ed., Philadelphia, W. B. Saunders Company, 1960.

Lenczner, M., and T. Owen: The Impact of Tropical and Parasitic Diseases in a Non-endemic Area, Can. Med. Assoc. J., 82:805, 1960.

Manson-Bahr, P.: "Manson's Tropical Diseases," 15th ed., London, Cassell and Co., Ltd., 1960.

Soulsby, E. J. L.: Immunity to Helminths—Recent Advances, Vet. Record, 72:322, 1960.

Stoll, N. R.: The Worms—Can We Vaccinate against Them? Am. J. Trop. Med. Hyg., 10:293, 1961.

Weller, T. H.: Tropical Medicine Today, New Engl. J. Med., 264:911, 1961.

218 INTESTINAL NEMATODES

Gustave J. Dammin

HOOKWORM DISEASE

Definition. Hookworm disease is a symptomatic infection caused by *Ancylostoma duodenale* and/or *Necator americanus*. Asymptomatic infection may be simply termed *hookworm infection*, and the individual with such infection a *carrier*.

Etiology. *Ancylostoma duodenale*, also known as the "Old World" hookworm, possesses four prominent hooklike teeth in its adult stage. The male measures about 1 cm in length and presents a characteristic copulatory bursa. The adults inhabit the upper small intestine of man. They attach to the mucosa by means of the mouth parts and suck blood. Each adult daily extracts about 0.5 ml of blood. The adults migrate within the small intestine, and each site of attachment persists temporarily as a bleeding point. Following fertilization, the female liberates eggs which measure about 40 by 60 μ and are usually in the two- to four-celled stage when discharged in the feces.

Necator americanus, the "New World" hookworm, has a buccal capsule containing dorsal and ventral plates rather than teeth.

The life cycles of these hookworms are similar. Following development to the filariform or infective stage, the larvae are capable of penetrating the skin to enter vessels which carry them to the lungs. The larvae leave the alveolar capillaries and enter the alveoli. They ascend the respiratory tree, enter the pharynx, and are swallowed. They reach the intestine about 1 week after penetration of the skin and 3 or 4 weeks later are mature. The adults have been known to survive in the human intestine for 5 years.

Epidemiology. Environmental conditions conducive to the development of the hookworm egg into the infective filariform larval stage are found in tropical and semitropical regions in which adequate rainfall occurs. Given the appropriate environmental conditions, hookworm infection will occur where there is opportunity for contact of the skin with contaminated soil. Infection can be acquired by ingestion of filariform larvae, but this mode of transmission is of little importance. That development of hookworm eggs into the filariform larval stage can occur in contaminated bedclothes has been shown, and also that fomites-borne hookworm infection may be of importance.

The white race is more susceptible to symptomatic infection than the Negro, the latter still constituting, however, an important reservoir of infection. Probably because of greater exposure, males show a higher incidence of infection than is found in females.

Regarding the relative importance of the two hookworms, it has been stated that "*Ancylostoma* presents a greater public health problem than *Necator americanus*, the species now established in the southern United States, because it is more harmful to the host, is less amenable to treatment, and its free-living stages are more resistant to climatic conditions" (McCoy).

Pathogenesis and Clinical Manifestations. The nature and severity of the clinical manifestations are determined by the stage and intensity of the infection. During the invasion of the exposed skin by the larvae, the affected parts become erythematous and edematous, and there is severe pruritus. These manifestations are more marked in *N. americanus* infection than in *A. duodenale* infection. The lesions are commonest about the feet, particularly between the toes, and have been termed "ground itch."

During passage of the larvae through the lungs, cough and, in severe infections, fever are observed. The pulmonary symptoms were particularly troublesome to soldiers engaged in close combat in the Asiatic campaign in the Second World War.

Epigastric pain, abdominal tenderness, and occasionally vomiting and diarrhea can be prominent symptoms during the establishment and migration of the hookworms in the small intestine. Roentgenographic studies at this stage may reveal a "cogwheel" pattern of the upper small intestine, presumably produced by the mucosal involvement. As hookworm disease was observed in American troops in northern India and Burma, where *A. duodenale* infection predominates, it was during this phase of the disease that medical aid was sought. Eosinophilic leukocytosis was present, but anemia was not, nor did it develop, presumably because of the short duration of the infection and early treatment. Judging from the number of adult hookworms collected from posttreatment fecal specimens, these were relatively light infections. They were predominantly *A. duodenale* infections, which are generally accepted as being more severe than those caused by *N. americanus*. Clinical observations on induced *A. duodenale* infections have been reported by Brumpt.

The clinical picture which has been described as classic occurs in residents of endemic areas and differs from the above in that anemia with symptoms and visceral changes incident to the anemia are dominant. The severity of the disease and the prognosis are dependent upon such factors as the age of the patient, the magnitude of the worm burden, the duration of the disease, and diet. Young children more often manifest the extreme anemia with cardiac insufficiency and anasarca. The anemia usually develops slowly and results from loss of blood—that which the hookworm sucks and ingests, and that which oozes into the intestinal lumen after the hookworm has left the site of mucosal attachment. Patients may have a depraved appetite with a desire to eat coarse or gritty materials. Those who survive to puberty show a retarded physical, mental, and sexual development. Milder degrees of the disease, as seen in older children and adults, are characterized by lassitude, dyspnea, palpitation,

tachycardia, and constipation, in addition to the pallor of the skin and mucous membranes. In most areas in which hookworm disease is common, dietary deficiencies are also common. Poor diet influences unfavorably the course of hookworm disease. Study of hookworm infection in the dog has shown that host control of infection depends largely upon the development of immunity, and that immunity does not develop or may be lost in the presence of malnutrition, avitaminosis, and anemia. In man, considerable clinical improvement can result from institution of a balanced high protein diet, and in the treatment of severe infection it is essential that the utmost improvement from proper diet be attained before drug therapy is begun.

Asymptomatic infection, or the carrier state, is common in endemic areas, where asymptomatic outnumber symptomatic infections, considering all age groups, 20 to 40 times. The worm burden is small, and in these areas the carrier state is probably indicative of some degree of acquired host resistance.

Laboratory Findings. In symptomatic infection, hookworm eggs are usually numerous enough to be detected by microscopic examination of a direct fecal smear. Abdominal and pulmonary symptoms appear before eggs are discharged, although a presumptive diagnosis may be made on the basis of the clinical history and the eosinophilic leukocytosis.

The feces seldom contain gross blood in hookworm disease, although usually positive for occult blood. Charcot-Leyden crystals are found in the feces in one-half to two-thirds of the cases.

Trichostrongylus eggs must be distinguished from hookworm eggs. The former are larger and in a later stage of maturation when observed in a fresh fecal specimen.

Generally, the leukocyte count is normal or slightly elevated, and the percentage of eosinophils increased to 15 or 30 per cent. However, in some early cases, the leukocytosis may be marked and the eosinophil percentage as high as 70 or 80 per cent. In such cases, a diagnosis of eosinophilic leukemia has been entertained. In general, the more marked the anemia, the lower the percentage of eosinophils. The anemia is characteristically of the hypochromic, microcytic variety.

Differential Diagnosis. Since hookworm disease occurs in areas in which beriberi and malaria in their cachectic forms are also more common, these must be differentiated from hookworm disease, or their coexistence established.

Treatment. Specific therapy for the infection and that directed toward improvement of the nutrition and anemia should be considered simultaneously. In the usual case with slight to moderate anemia, anthelmintics can be administered followed by iron therapy and a high protein diet. The current drug of choice is tetrachlorethylene administered as a single-dose oral treatment. For adults, 3 ml usually suffices, and for children, 0.2 ml is given for each year of age. The night before treatment, the patient is permitted a light, fat-free meal. The following morning, breakfast is omitted and the drug administered. No food is permitted for 4 hr and no alcohol for 24 hr. Purgation following administration of the drug is no longer recommended.

When ascariasis also is present, one of two alternative courses may be chosen. The ascariasis may be treated first with piperazine citrate (see Ascariasis, below), followed by tetrachlorethylene, or biphenium hydroxynaphthoate (Alcopar), which is effective against both nematodes, may be prescribed. A single dose of 5 Gm of biphenium hydroxynaphthoate is dispersed in water and ingested in the morning on an empty stomach. No food is permitted for 2 hr, and no purgation is recommended.

The aim in treatment is reduction of the worm burden to an asymptomatic level. Complete eradication may be difficult, especially in ancylostoma infection, which usually requires several courses of treatment.

When anemia is severe and there is malnutrition with anasarca, blood transfusions and a high-protein diet should be given before drug treatment is begun. In such cases the blood should be given in small increments and in a total amount sufficient to raise the hemoglobin level to 9 to 10 Gm per 100 ml. In advanced cases it may be necessary to delay drug treatment for 2 to 3 weeks.

Prognosis. Generally, the immediate prognosis is good. When opportunity for reinfection persists and nutrition cannot be maintained, a state of chronic debility develops. In children development is impaired, and in adults intercurrent disease proves serious.

Prevention. Many of the measures required are obvious but difficult to apply on a large scale. Even if facilities for proper disposal of feces are provided, it is no simple matter to educate the population in their use. Soil pollution must be eliminated, and until this is accomplished, avoidance of direct skin contact with the soil (as by wearing of shoes) should be encouraged. Periodic mass treatment of the population has been used in some hookworm control programs.

CREEPING ERUPTION (Cutaneous Larva Migrans)

Definition. Creeping eruption is an infection of the skin in man caused by the larvae of the dog and cat hookworm, *Ancylostoma brasiliense*. The other dog hookworms, *A. caninum* and *Uncinaria steno-*

cephala, and the horse botfly, *Gasterophilus,* in their larval stage may produce a similar cutaneous infection.

Etiology. The adult stage of *A. brasiliense* occurs regularly only in the dog and cat. The larvae emerging from eggs discharged in the feces develop to the filariform stage and then are capable of penetrating the skin. In man, the larvae usually remain in the skin and migrate, producing an irregular erythematous tunnel visible on the skin surface.

Epidemiology and Distribution. Dogs and cats constitute the reservoir of infection for man. Transmission among animals and to man requires environmental temperature and humidity appropriate for development of the egg to the infective filariform larva stage. Such conditions are found in the southeastern United States, coastal areas of Central America, northern South America, northern and southern Africa, and some areas of the Far East. Beaches and other moist, sandy areas are hazardous, because animals choose such areas for defecation, and the *A. brasiliense* eggs develop well in such soil.

Pathogenesis and Clinical Manifestations. The site of penetration of the skin by the larva becomes apparent in a few hours. The hands, feet, and legs are most frequently involved. The migration of the larva in the skin is accompanied by severe itching. Scratching may lead to bacterial infection. In the course of 1 week the initial red papule develops into an irregular, erythematous, linear lesion which may attain a length of 15 to 20 cm. Development of *A. brasiliense* to the adult stage occurs rarely in man.

Wright and Gold have observed Loeffler's syndrome in 26 of 52 cases of creeping eruption. Transient, migratory pulmonary infiltrations were associated with an increase in eosinophils in the blood and sputum. The lesions have been interpreted as an allergic reaction to the helminthic infection.

Laboratory Findings. Eosinophils occur in the lesion, but eosinophilic leukocytosis is slight, except when Loeffler's syndrome appears. The percentage of eosinophils in the blood may then rise to 50 per cent, and in the sputum to 90 per cent.

Treatment. Carbon dioxide snow or ethyl chloride may be applied to the advancing portion of the lesion. This is effective and also practical, when the lesions are few in number. Superficial bacterial infections are improved by the application of wet dressings and elevation of the extremity. For intense itching, antipruritic lotions should be applied locally and antihistaminics taken orally.

Prognosis. Untreated infections may last several months. Treatment is usually sought because of severe pruritus and moderate incapacitation. The above treatment is usually successful.

Prevention. Dogs and cats should be prevented from contaminating recreation areas. Contact of the skin with the soil should be avoided in areas suspected of being contaminated.

STRONGYLOIDIASIS

Definition. Strongyloidiasis is an intestinal infection of man and other higher mammals, caused by *Strongyloides stercoralis*.

Etiology. The adult female resides in the mucosa of the upper small intestine. The embryonated eggs soon develop into the rhabditiform larvae, in which form they are observed in the feces. Further larval development may take one of several courses: (1) In a suitable external environment, the indirect, or sexual, cycle occurs. (2) Under less suitable external circumstances, the rhabditiform larvae develop into the infective filariform stage (direct, or asexual, cycle). (3) Development to the infective stage is presumed to occur as well in the lower intestine, the filariform larvae then entering the body through the skin of the perineum, or through the intestinal wall. Mechanisms such as those mentioned in (3), above, may explain the long periods of infection observed (20 to 30 years) in those who have left endemic areas.

The course of the filariform larvae of S. *stercoralis* after entering the skin, the oral mucosa, or the intestinal mucosa resembles that of the hookworm larvae. In the intestine the females burrow into the mucosa, from which site embryonated eggs are discharged.

Epidemiology and Distribution. The usual mode of infection is the penetration of the skin by larvae present in contaminated soil. Some infections may result from ingestion of contaminated food and drink, and some are believed to be transmitted by contact.

Endemic areas are found primarily in the tropics, although sporadic cases have appeared in temperate regions.

Pathogenesis and Clinical Manifestations. Erythema with petechiae and pruritus characterizes the site of cutaneous penetration by the larvae. Cough, occasionally with dyspnea and hemoptysis, accompanies the stage of migration through the lungs. X-rays may exhibit pulmonary infiltration at this stage.

Epigastric pain and tenderness, nausea, flatulence, and vomiting, as well as diarrhea alternating with constipation, may be observed during the intestinal phase of development. The diarrhea may persist for long periods, causing excessive loss of fluid. Intestinal ulceration and sloughing are noted in severe cases. As with hookworm infection, many asymptomatic infections occur, and most symptomatic infections occasion only vague complaints.

In massive infection, there may be serious complications. The extensive involvement possible is illustrated by the fatal case described by Kyle et al., in which extensive pulmonary hemorrhage and edema were observed. Larvae were found in the myocardium, lungs, trachea, liver, and gallbladder, in addition to the intestine. In other fatal cases, intestinal perforation and peritonitis have been encountered.

Laboratory Findings. Although the nature of the clinical findings may be suggestive, the definitive diagnosis must be made in the laboratory. Fresh fecal specimens should be examined to avoid confusion with hookworm infection; generally, fresh specimens contain larvae in strongyloidiasis infections, while in hookworm infection they contain eggs. When pulmonary involvement is present, the sputum should be examined for larvae. Microscopic examination of the duodenal washings may readily establish the diagnosis. It should be performed when other studies are negative, and in determining the efficacy of treatment.

Eosinophilic leukocytosis is common, except in very severe cases in which eosinophilic leukocytes may be entirely absent.

Treatment. Dithiazanine iodide has emerged recently as the only chemotherapeutic agent of promise for this infection. Cure rates as high as 85 per cent have been achieved. For the adult, 100 mg in the form of coated tablets is given three times daily for 10 to 14 days. This dosage may be repeated after an interval of 2 weeks if eradication is not accomplished by the first course of treatment. For children, proportionately smaller doses are given and continued over a period of 14 to 21 days. Should gastrointestinal disturbance follow the initial doses, then succeeding doses should be reduced. Dithiazanine iodide should not be given to patients who have severe renal insufficiency and must be given with caution in the presence of fluid and electrolyte disorders.

Prognosis. In the usual case, the prognosis is good. Since the occurrence of hyperinfection is unpredictable, every effort should be made to eradicate the infection in each case. In severe cases with hyperinfection, the prognosis is poor.

Prevention. In general, the measures are those for the control of hookworm infection. In addition, it is well to remember that infection may be contracted by ingestion of contaminated food (especially uncooked vegetables) or of contaminated drinking water and by contact.

ASCARIASIS

Definition. Ascariasis is an infection of man caused by *Ascaris lumbricoides* and characterized by an early transient pulmonary phase related to larval migration and a later prolonged phase during which the adult ascarids inhabit the lumen of the intestine.

Etiology. The adult ascarids are large (20 to 40 cm in length) and cylindric in shape, with each extremity tapering to a blunt point. Their usual habitat is the small intestine, but they are prone to migration. The eggs are elliptic (30 to 40 μ by 50 to 60 μ) and have an irregular, dense outer shell and a regular, translucent inner shell. They are not infective upon discharge from the body. Under proper conditions of warmth and moisture the ovum develops to the infective larval stage in about 4 to 5 weeks. Upon ingestion of the egg at this stage, the larva is liberated in the small intestine. It migrates through the wall and ultimately reaches the lungs. After about 10 days in the pulmonary capillaries and alveoli, the larvae pass in turn to the bronchioles, bronchi, trachea, and epiglottis, are swallowed, and develop into male and female adults in the small intestine.

Epidemiology and Distribution. Infection follows the ingestion of the embryonated egg contained in contaminated food, or, more commonly, the introduction of the eggs into the mouth by the hands after contact with contaminated soil. Since the eggs are resistant to desiccation and wide variations in temperature, the disease is world-wide.

Pathogenesis and Clinical Manifestations. Because of the extensive migration of which both the larvae and adults are capable, clinical manifestations may be unusually diverse. In heavy infections, severe bronchopneumonia, occasionally fatal in children, can occur during the migration of the larvae through the lungs. Light infections assume importance when single or several adult ascarids obstruct the appendix, the bile, the pancreatic ducts, or other hollow structures of the upper intestinal or respiratory tracts.

Laboratory Findings. The diagnosis is usually made by finding the ova in the feces. The intact ova are characteristic and not easily confused with other ova.

Symptomatic infection, especially during the phase of larval migration through the lung, is usually accompanied by fever and eosinophilic leukocytosis.

Treatment. Only symptomatic treatment can be used during the period of pulmonary involvement by the migrating larvae. For removal of the adult worms from the intestines, piperazine citrate, as a flavored sirup administered in a single dose after breakfast on two successive days, will cure 94 per cent of cases (Brown). For younger children (30 to 50 lb), 2 Gm piperazine equivalent contained in 20 ml sirup constitutes each dose; for older children and adults, 3 to 3.5 Gm is given. No particular dietary regulation is necessary. The drug must be administered with caution when renal insufficiency is present, since impaired elimination may produce neurotoxic signs.

Piperazine citrate is the treatment of choice, but dithiazanine iodide (see Strongyloidiasis) or biphenium hydroxynaphtholate (see Hookworm Disease) may be used. When both ascariasis and trichuriasis are present, treatment with dithiazinine iodide is preferred When both ascariasis and infection with *Ancylostoma duodenale* are present, treatment with biphenium hydroxynaphthoate is recommended.

Prognosis. The prognosis in intestinal infection is generally good. When acute or chronic obstruction of ducts or hollow viscera has occurred, the immediate prognosis is determined by the promptness of diagnosis and treatment.

Prevention. Ascariasis is primarily a household infection of rural areas. All infections should be treated, personal hygiene stressed, and adequate toilet facilities provided.

VISCERAL LARVA MIGRANS

This is a clinical syndrome usually observed in children and characterized by hepatosplenomegaly, skin rash, and recurrent pneumonitis with wheezing respiratory distress. There is generally a history of dirt eating and contact with dogs or cats in or near the household. Ocular involvement and convulsions may also be observed.

Leukocytosis with eosinophilia to high levels (over 60 per cent) and hypergammaglobulinemia are common. The eosinophilic leukocytes are unusual in that they are large and have vacuolated cytoplasm containing granules which vary in size and are present in smaller than normal numbers.

This syndrome, with various degrees of clinical severity, follows the ingestion of the infective eggs of nematodes whose life cycle is not completed in man. It is caused most often by nematodes whose life cycle is completed in the dog (*Toxocara canis*) or in the cat (*Toxocara cati*). Larvae of the *Toxocara* become widely disseminated in the body and incite a granulomatous reaction. Lesions are prominent in the liver, lungs, skeletal muscle, and brain. Larvae with eosinophilic leukocytic and granulomatous reactions have been noted in liver biopsies.

The clinical diagnosis may be made on the basis of the findings described. A hemagglutination test employing ascaris and toxocara antigens has been demonstrated by Jung and Pacheco to be a valuable aid in the laboratory diagnosis of visceral larva migrans. This is another variety of helminthic infection capable of causing Loeffler's syndrome. When the respiratory difficulty is pronounced, ACTH or adrenal cortical steroids may prove helpful. There is no particular treatment for the other lesions.

In control, measures are directed toward preventing ingestion of the toxocara eggs. Removal or repeated treatment of infected cats and dogs must be considered, as well as modifying the diet to reduce the temptation to ingest contaminated materials.

ENTEROBIASIS

Definition. Enterobiasis (pinworm, seatworm, or threadworm infection; oxyuriasis) is an intestinal infection of man caused by *Enterobius vermicularis* and characterized by perianal pruritus.

Etiology. The adults are small fusiform worms usually inhabiting the cecum and colon, attached to the mucosa. The female averages 10 mm in length, the male 3 mm. The eggs are deposited by the female on the perineal skin, the migration generally occurring at night. Each egg contains an embryo which, a few hours after being deposited, develops into the infective larva. After ingestion of the egg, the larva is released in the small intestine. The adult stage is soon reached and, in less than 1 month from the time of ingestion, newly developed gravid females are again discharging eggs. They are planoconvex and measure approximately 20 by 50 μ. The shell is clear and doubly contoured.

Epidemiology and Distribution. The eggs usually reach the mouth of the human host by way of contaminated hands, food, or drink, although airborne transmission may also occur. They are relatively resistant to desiccation, and because they are infective soon after discharge from the body, transmission within family and children's groups occurs readily. Enterobiasis is found in all climates and is probably the commonest helminthic infection of man. Its low incidence in some tropical areas, however, defies explanation.

Clinical Manifestations. The commonest symptom is pruritus ani, which is most troublesome at night, being related to the migration of the gravid female worms. Scratching may lead to perineal eczema or pyogenic infection.

Laboratory Findings. Examination of material obtained from the perineal skin for ova by means of a cellophane or Scotch tape swab is essential for the detection of enterobiasis. Less than 5 per cent of infections are diagnosed by searching for ova in the feces. Scrapings from under the nails may reveal ova. The diagnosis can be made by examining the feces for adult worms following a laxative or an enema. Eosinophilic leukocytosis is inconstant.

Treatment. All infected individuals in an affected communal group should be treated simultaneously. The aim in drug treatment is reduction of the worm burden. Drug treatment combined with such measures as (1) providing a sleeping garment which prevents contamination of the fingers with ova from the perianal region, (2) instituting a morning shower, (3) lukewarm water enemas, and (4) local antipruritic ointments is directed toward producing asymptomatic infection, with eradication or cure not the immediate objective.

The preferred therapeutic agent is piperazine citrate, which has been found effective in as high as 97 per cent of cases when prescribed in a single course of 7 days. It is given in sirup form each day before breakfast, with a total daily dose of 250 mg for children weighing up to 15 lb, 500 mg for those weighing between 16 and 30 lb, 1 Gm for those between 31 and 60 lb, and 2 Gm for those over 60 lb (Brown). When renal insufficiency is present, the piperazine should be given in smaller dosage to avoid neurotoxicity.

Although piperazine citrate is the drug of choice, it should be mentioned that dithiazanine iodide and pyrvinium chloride have been demonstrated to be efficacious in enterobiasis. However, piperazine citrate is better tolerated and longer established as an effective drug.

Prognosis. The prognosis with reference to the duration of infection is good, particularly when the other measures mentioned are carried out in addition to drug treatment.

Prevention. Methods of preventing autoinfection and dissemination within a group involving children are difficult to apply. Personal and environmental hygiene should be stressed and anthelmintic and symptomatic treatment of pruritus ani instituted. To control infection within a group, simultaneous treatment of all cases must be carried out.

TRICHURIASIS

Definition. Trichuriasis (whipworm infection, trichocephaliasis) is an intestinal infection of man caused by *Trichuris trichiura* and is characterized by invasion of the colonic mucosa by the adult trichuris.

Etiology. The adult whipworms possess a threadlike anterior two-thirds and a stouter posterior third, giving them a whiplike structure. The eggs are characteristic, being barrel-shaped, brown, and translucent and having knoblike extremities.

Epidemiology. The mode of spread resembles that of ascariasis, the eggs generally being introduced into the mouth by contaminated fingers.

Pathogenesis and Clinical Manifestations. Symptomatic infection generally requires the presence of large numbers of adult whipworms and may be correlated in part with the degree of mucosal involvement. Heavy infections usually occur only in children and may be accompanied by nausea, abdominal pain, and diarrhea.

Laboratory Findings. In symptomatic infection, large numbers of eggs are present in the feces. Eosinophilic leukocytosis and anemia may accompany such infections.

Treatment. Dithiazanine iodide is now the drug recommended for trichuriasis, irrespective of the gravity of the infection. With the more severe infections, as those characterized by nausea and diarrhea, it should be remembered that dithiazanine may exaggerate such symptoms temporarily. Should marked gastrointestinal symptoms persist, the dosage should be reduced but administration of the drug continued for 10 to 14 days. Initial dosage, and one usually effective, for adults, is 100 mg three times per day for the first day, and for the subsequent 4 days, 200 mg three times per day. For children correspondingly smaller doses are administered.

If infection persists, a second course of treatment may be given after an interval of 2 weeks. Should toxicity of major import become apparent, then piperazine citrate, as recommended for enterobiasis may be given.

Prognosis. Whipworm infection, unless characterized by severe diarrhea, blood loss, and systemic reaction, usually responds well to treatment with dithiazanine. Serious infections do occur (Getz) and may require supportive treatment as well as chemotherapy.

Prevention. Measures recommended for ascariasis apply also to trichuriasis.

TRICHOSTRONGYLIASIS

Definition. Trichostrongyliasis is an intestinal infection of man and other mammalian hosts, including sheep, goats, and cattle.

Etiology. Almost a dozen species of *Trichostrongylus* are known to have infected man. Few human infections have been reported in the United States. In view of the high frequency of animal infections here, the low incidence of human infections is difficult to understand. The possibility exists that some may be diagnosed as hookworm infection.

The ova resemble those of the hookworm but are larger and, when observed in a fresh fecal specimen, show a more advanced stage of segmentation (16- to 32-celled stage).

Pathogenesis. Infection is acquired by ingestion of the larvae, rather than by their penetration of the skin. The adult maintains residence in the intestine for long periods. Sandground, who infected himself, observed infection to last more than 8 years.

Manifestations. Diarrhea is observed occasionally when infection is massive, but most infections are asymptomatic. The parasite owes its importance

primarily to the resemblance of its ova to those of the hookworms. Moreover, because the trichostrongylidae do not respond to anthelmintics effective in hookworm infection, it may be assumed incorrectly that one is dealing with refractory hookworm infection.

Laboratory Diagnosis. The diagnosis depends upon the finding of the ova in the feces. Since they are few in number, they are usually found only when a concentration method is used. In symptomatic infections, there may be leukocytosis with marked eosinophilia (e.g., 80 per cent).

Treatment. These infections do not respond to tetrachlorethylene treatment. However, good results have been obtained with dithiazanine iodide as recommended for trichuris infection, and with piperazine citrate as used in enterobius infection.

Prevention. Contamination of the hands and food grown in contaminated soil are to be avoided.

REFERENCES

Beaver, P. C.: Larva Migrans, Exptl. Parasitol., 5: 587, 1956.

Brown, H. W., K. Chan, and K. L. Hussey: Treatment of Enterobiasis and Ascariasis with Piperazine, J.A.M.A., 161:515, 1956.

Dent, J. H., R. L. Nichols, P. C. Beaver, G. M. Carrera, and R. J. Staggers: Visceral Larva Migrans: With a Case Report, Am. J. Pathol., 32:777, 1956.

Dexter, M. W., H. L. T. Dexter, and A. H. Lawton: A Note on Psychoses and Loeffler's Syndrome Complicating Creeping Eruption, Am. J. Trop. Med. Hyg., 9:297, 1960.

Getz, L.: Massive Infection with *Trichuris trichiura* in Children, Am. J. Diseases Children, 70:19, 1945.

Heiner, D. C., and S. V. Kevy: Visceral Larva Migrans: Report of the Syndrome in Three Siblings, New Engl. J. Med., 254:629, 1956.

Hoekenga, M. T.: Experiments in the Therapy of Human Trichuriasis and Hookworm Disease, Am. J. Trop. Med. Hyg., 5:529, 1956.

Hsieh, H.-C., H. W. Brown, M. Fite, L.-P. Chow, C.-S. Cheng, and C.-C. Hsu: The Treatment of Hookworm, *Ascaris* and *Trichuris* Infections with Bephenium Hydroxynaphthoate, Am. J. Trop. Med. Hyg., 9:496, 1960.

Jung, R. C., and G. Pacheco: Use of a Hemagglutination Test in Visceral Larva Migrans, Am. J. Trop. Med. Hyg., 9:185, 1960.

Karpinski, F. E., E. A. Everts-Suarez, and W. G. Sawitz: Larval Granulomatosis (Visceral Larva Migrans), A.M.A. J. Diseases Children, 92: 34, 1956.

Kirby-Smith, J. L.: The Treatment of Creeping Eruption, Southern Med. J., 28:999, 1935.

Kyle, L. H., D. G. McKay, and H. J. Sparling: Strongyloidiasis, Ann. Internal Med., 29:1014, 1948.

Loughlin, E. H., and N. R. Stoll: Fomite-borne Ancylostomiasis, Am. J. Hyg., 45:191, 1947.

McCoy, O. R.: Precautions by the Army to Prevent the Introduction of Tropical Diseases, Am. J. Trop. Med., 26:351, 1946.

Most, H.: Current Concepts in Therapy: Anthelminthic Therapy, I and II, New Engl. J. Med., 259:351, 441, 1958.

Nichols, R. L.: The Etiology of Visceral Larva Migrans: I. Diagnostic Morphology of Infective Second-stage *Toxocara* Larvae; II. Comparative Larvae Morphology of *A. lumbricoides, N. americanus, S. stercoralis* and *A. caninum,* J. Parasitol., 42:349, 1956.

Ochsner, A., E. G. DeBakey, and J. L. Dixon: Complications of Ascariasis Requiring Surgical Treatment, Am. J. Diseases Children, 77:389, 1949.

Rogers, A. M., and G. J. Dammin: Hookworm Infection in American Troops in Assam and Burma, Am. J. Med. Sci., 211:531, 1946.

Schneider, J.: Trials of Dithiazanine in the Treatment of Strongyloidiasis, Therapie, 15:685, 1960.

Strang, C., and C. K. Warrick: Radiological Demonstration of *Ascaris* Infestation, Brit. J. Radiol., 21:575, 1948.

Swartzwelder, J. C.: Clinical *Trichocephalus trichuris* Infection, Am. J. Trop. Med., 19:473, 1939.

———, J. P. Muhleisen, S. H. Abadie, W. W. Frye, C. A. Jones, P. E. Robertson, and J. F. Hebert: Therapy of Strongyloidiasis with Dithiazanine, A.M.A. Arch. Internal Med., 101:658, 1958.

Tsuchiya, H., and H. Reller: Case of *Trichostrongylus* Infection with Notes on Identification of Ova, J. Lab. Clin. Med., 30:262, 1945.

Wallace, L., R. Henkin, and A. W. Mathies: *Trichostrongylus* Infestation with Profound Eosinophilia, Ann. Internal Med., 45:146, 1956.

Watson, J. M.: Human Trichostrongylosis and Its Relationship to Ancylostomiasis in Southern Iraq, with Comments on World Incidence, J. Parasitol., 43:102, 1953.

Wright, D. O., and E. M. Gold: Loeffler's Syndrome Associated with Creeping Eruption, Arch. Internal Med., 78:303, 1946.

219 TRICHINOSIS
Gustave J. Dammin

Definition. Trichinosis is caused by the intestinal nematode *Trichinella spiralis*. As a clinical infection, it is characterized by diarrhea during the development of the adults in the intestine and by myositis with systemic reaction during the larval migration and invasion of the skeletal muscles.

Etiology and Epidemiology. Infection is contracted following ingestion of meat containing the encysted larvae of *T. spiralis*. There are no intermediate hosts, both the adult and larval stages developing in the same host. *Trichinella spiralis* exhibits little host specificity, infection having been produced or observed in the bear, wild boar, horse, cow, dog, cat, rabbit, guinea pig, mouse, and marine mammals in addition to the rat and the pig. Man is particularly susceptible; most fowl are resistant. Among pigs, infection is contracted following feeding of uncooked pork scraps, less often by eating infected rats. Rats also feed on uncooked pork scraps and, in addition, maintain a high incidence of infection by their cannibalism.

Soon after liberation of the larvae from their cysts, they migrate into the mucosa, and within a week the viviparous female is discharging larvae (100 by 6 μ), which enter vascular channels and are distributed throughout the body. Larviposition continues for about 4 to 6 weeks. The larvae enter skeletal muscle and encyst (Fig. 219-1). The muscles of the diaphragm, tongue, and eye, the deltoid, pectoral, and intercostal muscles are most often affected. Larvae carried to sites other than skeletal muscles do not encyst but disintegrate. The life cycle can be carried further only if a new host ingests the encysted larvae.

Geographic Distribution. Trichinosis is common in Europe and North America and uncommon in other parts of the world. In the United States, where the incidence is between 15 and 20 per cent, there

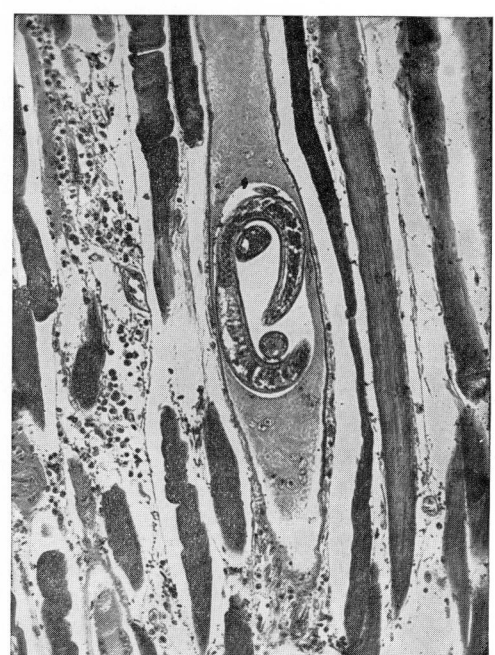

FIG. 219-1. *Trichinella spiralis.* Larva encysting within a skeletal muscle fiber. At this stage, myositis and edema have partially subsided.

is "more than three times as much trichinosis as is known in all of the rest of the world put together." Studies show that this high incidence has continued. The ratio of asymptomatic to symptomatic infection is high.

Pathogenesis and Clinical Manifestations. The course and symptomatology vary remarkably. The clinical diagnosis in the sporadic case may be difficult. Diarrhea is an early manifestation related to the development of the adults in the intestinal mucosa and is observed in about half the cases. It usually appears within 24 hr after ingestion of the uncooked or undercooked meat containing the encysted larvae. The next stage, that of muscular invasion, begins about the end of the first week and may last for as long as 6 weeks. Most of the clinical manifestations are related to the invasion and encystment of the larvae in skeletal muscles. A myositis is produced, with basophilic granular degeneration of the invaded muscle fiber. Adjacent fibers exhibit hyaline or hydropic degeneration, and the focus becomes infiltrated with neutrophilic and eosinophilic leukocytes, some lymphocytes, and mononuclear macrophages. Hyperemia, edema, and hemorrhages are constant features.

Larvae do not encyst in cardiac muscle, nor can they be found readily there. Despite this, an intense myocarditis has been observed and may be of significance in fatal cases.

Larvae have been observed in association with less severe focal lesions in the lungs and brain, and in other viscera, with no associated inflammatory reaction.

The significant clinical manifestations are noted during the period of migration and muscle invasion. Fever is probably the commonest manifestation. Ocular manifestations may be among the most striking. The edema of the eyelids, often accompanied by conjunctivitis and chemosis, is difficult to explain, but may be related to larval invasion of the eye muscles and possibly other retrobulbar tissues. Also a constant manifestation is the muscular pain and tenderness. Electromyograms have disclosed extensive fibrillation. Manifestations in the skin and appendages include (1) a maculopapular rash, which usually lasts for several days, and (2) subungual "splinter hemorrhages."

Laboratory Findings. The most constant finding, and one of significance early in the course of the disease, is the eosinophilic leukocytosis (over 500 eosinophilic leukocytes per cubic millimeter). It appears generally before the end of the second week and rises. In cases of moderate severity the percentage of eosinophilic leukocytes ranges between 15 and 50 per cent. In severe cases, particularly terminally, the eosinophilic leukocytes may disappear entirely.

The skin test becomes positive early in the third week of infection. The antigen is prepared from larvae and used in a dilution of about 1:10,000. One one-hundredth of a millimeter is injected intradermally, and immediate and delayed reactions are looked for. The usual positive response is immediate, a wheal of 5 mm or more appearing within 30 min. Nonspecific reactions may be related to the ingestion of meat containing nonviable trichinas.

The precipitin reaction becomes positive after the third week. Its value in diagnosis is increased if the reaction is initially negative and becomes positive, or if the titer rises during the course of the disease. It remains positive for about a year.

In attempting to arrive at a definitive diagnosis, examination of the feces for the adult worms is of little help. Examination of the blood, cerebrospinal fluid, or muscle biopsy is more rewarding. Microscopic study of laked venous, capillary, or arterial blood is the simplest test which may make a definitive diagnosis possible. Larvae have been found in the peripheral blood as early as the fifth day in experimental infections. Larvae may be present in the cerebrospinal fluid in the absence of clinical central nervous system involvement. Biopsied muscle is best studied by use of a compressor which permits examination of the entire specimen. Maceration and digestion methods are used in survey studies of diaphragms obtained at autopsy and for biopsy specimens as well.

Differential Diagnosis. Trichinosis must be distinguished from acute glomerulonephritis, typhoid fever, meningitis, rheumatic fever, rheumatoid arthritis, eosinophilic leukemia, dermatomyositis, and periarteritis nodosa.

Treatment. There is, as yet, no specific treatment for trichinosis. Symptomatic treatment is directed toward the relief of pain, maintenance of an adequate caloric and fluid intake, and assuring the patient of adequate sleep by use of sedatives. ACTH is reported to have controlled the systemic reaction in severe infection and is recommended for such cases. However, in experimental infections, cortisone administration results in more prolonged persistence of the adult worms in the intestine, increased numbers of larvae in the musculature, and partial suppression of the immune response.

Piperazine citrate has been found effective in removing the adults from the intestine in experimental infections. It would seem advisable to use piperazine citrate (as prescribed for enterobiasis) during the early phases when adult trichinas are suspected of being in the intestine. This would apply when diarrhea and other abdominal symptoms have developed subsequent to the ingestion of undercooked meat and also later when fever and eosinophilia have appeared, since treatment may reduce the period of larviposition and thereby shorten the clinical course.

Prognosis. The prognosis in children is usually better than in adults. If there is no serious involvement of the myocardium or respiratory muscles, the prognosis is generally good. The longer the appearance of symptoms is delayed, the better the prognosis. Diarrhea early in the course is a favorable sign. Analysis of larger series of sporadic and epidemic cases shows the mortality rate to be about 5 per cent.

Prevention. The responsibility for control rests with the consumer. Adequate cooking of pork involves heating all portions of the meat to 55°C. Freezing procedures to kill the larvae require a temperature of −15°C for 20 days or −18°C for 24 hr. Proper smoking and pickling will also destroy the larvae. Important in control is the cooking of garbage fed to hogs. There is at present no practical method of inspection which will detect trichinous pork.

REFERENCES

Carter, J. R.: Plasma Cell Hyperplasia and Hyperglobulinemia in Trichinosis: The Duration of Larviposition, Am. J. Pathol., 25:309, 1949.

Coker, C. M.: Effects of Cortisone on *Trichinella spiralis* Infections in Nonimmunized Mice, J. Parasitol., 41:498, 1955.

Dammin, G. J.: Trichinosis: Report of a Case with Demonstration of Larvae in the Arterial Blood, New Engl. J. Med., 224:357, 1941.

Davis, W. M., and H. Most: Trichinosis: Case Report with Observations on the Effect of ACTH, Am. J. Med., 11:639, 1951.

Gould, S. E.: "Trichinosis," Springfield, Ill., Charles C Thomas, Publisher, 1945.

Kagan, I. G.: Trichinosis: A Review of Biologic, Serologic and Immunologic Aspects, J. Infectious Diseases, 107:65, 1960.

Kimsey, L. S., and S. L. Adams: *Trichinella spiralis* in the Diaphragms of Humans and Swine, Public Health Repts. (U.S.), 70, 1001, 1955.

Marcus, S., and R. V. Miller, Jr.: An Atypical Case of Trichinosis with Report on Electromyographic Findings, Ann. Internal Med., 43:615, 1955.

Phillipson, R. F., and W. E. Kershaw: The Production, Deposition and Growth of the Larvae of *Trichinella spiralis,* and Their Significance in the Chemotherapy of the Infection, Ann. Trop. Med. Parasitol., 54:250, 1960.

Stoll, N. R.: This Wormy World, J. Parasitol., 33:1, 1947.

220 FILARIASIS
Ivan L. Bennett, Jr.

Definition. Filariasis is a group of disorders produced by infection with nematodes of the super-family Filarioidea. These worms invade the subcutaneous tissues and lymphatics of man, producing reactions ranging from acute inflammation to chronic scarring. The clinical pictures produced by different species in this group are more or less specific. The term *filariasis* is commonly used to designate the disease produced by *Wuchereria bancrofti* or *W. malayi,* the organisms responsible for elephantiasis. The disorders associated with infection by *Loa loa* or *Onchocerca volvulus* are usually referred to as *loiasis* and *onchocerciasis.*

Filariasis (Wuchereriasis)

Etiology and Epidemiology. Adult worms live only in the lymphatics of human beings, the male measuring 35 mm and the female, 50 to 100 mm. Gravid females release microfilariae in large numbers into the lymph and blood. These embryos develop further only if ingested by a proper mosquito vector, usually *Culex fatigans,* although many *Culex, Aëdes,* and *Mansonia* species are good hosts. After further development in the vector, larvae migrate to the mouth parts and, if inoculated into a human host, reach maturity in about a year. In the absence of reinfection, man harbors microfilariae for 5 to 10 years, the reproductive life of the adult worms. The release of microfilariae into the blood is strikingly periodic in *W. bancrofti* infections, peak concentrations being between 9 P.M. and 2 A.M. *Wuchereria malayi* is similarly but less regularly periodic. In many western Pacific islands, including Samoa and Fiji, *W. bancrofti* is nonperiodic; the reason for this is entirely unknown. The danger of infection in the *periodic* disease is nocturnal, but the nonperiodic form is often transmitted by sylvan mosquitoes in natural cover during the day.

Wuchereria bancrofti infection is endemic between latitudes 41°N and 30°S. Distribution is irregular, and there are many peculiar "skip areas" in this geographic pattern, presumably because the endemic disease can be maintained only where human infection and mosquitoes are prevalent. *Wuchereria malayi* infection is confined to the Far East, including India, Malaya, East China, and the Philippines. There were approximately 15,000 *W. bancrofti* infections among American military personnel in the Second World War (Wartman).

A small endemic focus of *W. bancrofti* once existed near Charleston, S.C., but no new cases have been observed in several years.

Pathogenesis. As larvae migrate to the lymphatics, they produce irritation, whether by some secretion or entirely by hypersensitivity responses of the host being unknown. The larvae reach maturity in lymph nodes and incite hypertrophy, granulomatous inflammation, and obstruction, often with retrograde lymphangitis. Repetition of this process for many years can lead to permanent blockage, scarring, and elephantiasis. Secondary bacterial infection is thought by some to be important in the etiology of elephantiasis, but this has not been established. Elephantiasis is actually a relatively unusual complication of filarial infections. If repeated reinfections do not occur, the disease is self-limited.

Manifestations. Acute filariasis manifests itself as a series of brief attacks over a period of weeks. Symptoms vary greatly in severity and include headache, fatigability, vertigo, photophobia, and muscle pain. Fever is low-grade and chills are rare in the early stages. Examination shows lymphadenopathy, streaks of lymphadenitis and, sometimes, circumscribed, reddish swellings of the extremities. The male genitalia are frequently involved with epididymitis, orchitis, hydrocele, or scrotal edema. Conjunctivitis is common; pleural friction rubs have been described. Urticaria is rare. Such an attack, frequently referred to by the Samoan term *mumu,* ordinarily subsides in 12 to 24 hr, but recurrences are common, particularly after strenuous exercise. Secondary bacterial infection has been found to play no part in these acute episodes, nor is mechanical blockage of lymphatics by the worms responsible for the swellings. It is probable that hypersensitivity to the parasite or its products is the underlying mechanism of *mumu,* but conclusive evidence on this point is lacking.

With repeated exposures, infected individuals show palpable thickening of lymphatic channels (often first noted in the spermatic cords), rubbery adenopathy, and in a small percentage of cases elephantiasis develops; this complication is rare below the age of twenty even in natives of heavily infested areas. The chronic stage of the disease is often punctuated by acute bouts of "filarial fever" with chills, fever, headache, tender lymphadenopathy, localized areas of erythema and edema, and severe muscle pain. These are thought to be hypersensitivity reactions induced by release of filarial antigen when adults or microfilariae die or a new infection occurs. This concept is supported by the frequent occurrence of filarial fever after institution of chemotherapy and by the fact that an attack can sometimes be produced by intracutaneous injection of the specific antigen in skin testing.

Chyloria and hematuria may occur intermittently for many years in patients in endemic areas.

Laboratory Findings. Eosinophilia accompanies *mumu* in about two-thirds of the cases and is also common during attacks of filarial fever in the later stages of the disease. Although adult worms are often demonstrable in biopsied lymph nodes, this procedure is not often used, and excision of nodes often induces a symptomatic flare-up of the disease. Complement fixation and skin tests are available, but neither is reliable in the individual case. Diagnosis is best established by demonstration of micro-filariae in Giemsa or Wright stains of peripheral blood. Microfilariae are motile and can also be found in wet smears. When the periodic form of the disease predominates, specimens should be collected at night.

Treatment. Drugs effective against the microfilariae may not influence the adult worms, which will continue to reproduce for years. Probably the most effective agent against the adult worms is thiacetarsamide (Caparsolate sodium) given intravenously in a dosage of 1.0 mg per kg daily for 15 days. Diarrhea is a frequent accompaniment of administration of this drug. Microfilariae may be demonstrable in blood smears after a course of thiacetarsamide; they soon disappear and relapse is rare.

Hetrazan (diethylcarbamazine) in an oral dosage of 2.0 mg per kg t.i.d. for 3 or 4 weeks is an effective microfilaricide. Indeed, a dosage of 2.5 mg per kg once daily for 5 days has been effective in mass trials in endemic areas. The initiation of treatment with this drug may be followed by a bout of filarial fever that usually subsides within 72 hr. Further experience with Hetrazan indicates that it probably injures the adult worms also and impairs their ability to reproduce, resulting in permanent clearing of microfilariae from the blood in many patients. At present, Hetrazan would appear to be the drug of choice and thiacetarsamide can be used for cases that relapse or fail to respond.

Antimony compounds have no place in treatment of filariasis.

Reassurance of the patient is very important in this disease. Vaccines and antiserums are valueless. Pressure bandages and surgery sometimes benefit elephantiasis. The prognosis for life is excellent, particularly if infected individuals leave endemic areas or otherwise avoid reinfections.

Onchocerciasis

This infection is produced by *Onchocerca volvulus* and is transmitted by flies of the genus *Simulium.* The disease is widespread in southern Mexico and Guatemala and is common in Central Africa. The characteristic lesions of onchocerciasis are subcutaneous nodules that tend to occur in the region of the head, although, in Africa, they are said to be common on the trunk. The aspirated contents of the nodules contain adult worms and microfilariae.

Treatment consists of surgical excision of the nodules and administration of Hetrazan. Except for occasional invasion of the eye, the disease has a favorable prognosis unless the number of nodules exceeds 50 in the individual patient.

Loiasis

This form of filariasis is produced by *Loa loa* and is prevalent in West and Central Africa. The infection is transmitted by flies of the genus *Chrysops*. Localized areas of allergic inflammation in the subcutaneous tissues known as *Calabar swellings* are the hallmark of the disease, although infestation may be completely asymptomatic. The adult worms are sometimes visible beneath the conjunctiva, and *Loa loa* is often called the *eye worm*. Diagnosis can be made by finding the adult worm or demonstration of microfilariae in contents of Calabar swellings or in blood smears. Treatment is symptomatic, and the prognosis is good.

REFERENCES

Coggeshall, L. T.: Filariasis, Ann. N.Y. Acad. Sci., 50: 21, 1948.

Filariasis (Wuchereria) with Special Reference to Early Stages, Dept. of the Army Tech. Bull., TB Med. 142, Mar. 28, 1956.

Manson-Bahr, P.: The Story of *Filaria bancrofti,* a Critical Review, J. Trop. Med. Hyg., 62:53, 85, 106, 138, 160, 1959. (A very complete summary.)

McGregor, I. A., and H. M. Gilles: Further Studies on the Control of Bancroftian Filariasis in West Africa by Means of Diethylcarbamazine, Ann. Trop. Med. Parasitol., 54:415, 1960.

Wartman, W. B.: Filariasis in American Armed Forces in World War II, Medicine, 26:333, 1947.

221 SCHISTOSOMIASIS (Bilharziasis)

Rafael Rodriguez-Molina

Definition. Schistosomiasis (bilharziasis) is a general term employed to describe a group of disease entities produced in man and animals by three closely related species of digenetic trematodes, or blood flukes, belonging to the family Schistosomatidae. These worms are *Schistosoma mansoni,* S. *haematobium,* and S. *japonicum.* They inhabit the circulatory system of man and animals living in tropical and subtropical countries. The organs and tissues most frequently affected are the colon, urinary bladder, liver, spleen, rectum, genitalia, lungs, mesentery, and peritoneum.

History. Bilharz in 1851 first demonstrated the role of S. *haematobium* in the prevailing hematuria and dysentery among the native population of Egypt. The presence of two types of spined ova and of two clinical forms of the disease, the vesical and the intestinal, caused confusion, until Sambon in 1907 demonstrated the existence of two species, S. *haematobium* and S. *mansoni.* The presence of schistosomiasis in Egyptian mummies indicates that it is an ancient disease. It was in Puerto Rico in 1904 that the ova of *Schistosoma mansoni* were first discovered among the indigenous population of the Western Hemisphere, by Gonzalez Martinez. Katsurada, in Japan in 1904, found the eggs in the stools of patients affected with Katayama disease. Other Japanese investigators demonstrated that dogs, cats, horses, cattle, and wild rats were natural hosts or reservoirs of infection.

Epidemiology and Control. Schistosomiasis is probably the most important of the parasitic diseases affecting man, not only because of the extensive pathologic changes produced by the parasites but also because of its world-wide distribution and the number of individuals affected. It is believed that about 150 million persons are affected by this condition. Control measures have not turned out to be so effective as those for malaria. It is practically impossible to prevent children from bathing in brooks and rivers, and pollution of rivers with human excrement is difficult to control. The control and eradication of schistosomiasis are a challenge to the public health officer, the sanitary engineer, the malacologist, the zoologist, and the physician.

The continuing prevalence of schistosomiasis depends upon the disposal of human excrement into fresh water, the presence of suitable snail hosts, and the exposure of persons to water infested with cercarias. Promiscuous defecation, latrine drainage, and unsanitary sewage disposal are the more important sources of pollution of streams and rivers. The disease is contracted by persons washing clothes, bathing, wading, or working in contaminated water.

Schistosomiasis is more frequently encountered in rural than in urban communities and is associated with agricultural endeavors such as the irrigation of land. It is more prevalent among low-income groups.

Of the three disease-producing blood flukes of man, S. *mansoni* is by far the most common in the Western Hemisphere. It was brought to the Caribbean area and South America by African slaves. In South America, Venezuela, Dutch Guiana, and Brazil are the areas in which it is present. In Africa it occurs in the Nile Delta, Sudan, Zanzibar, Madagascar, and Central Africa.

Schistosoma japonicum affects the population engaged in agriculture. In Japan, China, and the Philippines, men are more frequently infected than women. An important source of infection in the Orient is the use of human excreta as a fertilizer in vegetable gardens.

Schistosoma haematobium is distributed widely throughout the African continent, and to a much less extent is found in Spain, Portugal, Cyprus, and Greece. In Africa, it is highly prevalent among the indigent agricultural population of the Nile Valley.

The best attack on schistosomiasis is preventive. Public health measures, including proper disposal of human excrement and anthelmintic therapy, should be carried out in endemic areas. Extermination of the mollusk intermediate host by chemical agents in areas where the infestation rate is high is mandatory. Sodium pentachlorophenate has been tried against the snails *Australorbis glabratus* and *Oncomelania nosophora* with promising results.

Another efficient molluscacide is 2-cyclohexyl-4, 6-dinitrophenol.

SCHISTOSOMIASIS MANSONI (Intestinal Bilharziasis, Schistosomal Dysentery)

Etiology and Life Cycle. The male worm measures about 1 cm in length and has a breadth of about 0.13 cm. The female is long, slender, and cylindroid, its average length being 1.4 cm and its breadth about 0.016 cm. The male has a central trough, the gynecophoral canal, that enfolds the female during copulation. The eggs are bluntly oval, have a lateral spine, and measure about 140 μ by about 60 μ. They are passed in the feces, rarely in the urine, and can infect only the proper snail which serves as the intermediate host. The ova must reach fresh water if the parasite's life cycle is to be completed. As stated by Belding, the life cycle includes the passing of the ova from the definitive host, or man, its hatching in water, the liberation of a free-swimming *miracidium,* the penetration of a proper species of snail by the miracidium, the metamorphosis of the larvae into *cercarias* (the infective form of the schistosome), their return to water, the penetration of the skin of man, and, finally, the migration and growth of the worms in the blood vessels of man and the laying of eggs by the female. Adult worms live in the inferior and superior mesenteric veins and the hemorrhoidal plexus.

Pathology. Schistosomiasis mansoni is divisible into three stages: (1) an early stage of migration during which the cercarias are being carried by the blood to the liver, maturing into adult parasites within intrahepatic portal veins; (2) an intermediate stage during which ova are accumulating in various viscera; and (3) a late stage characterized by serious and permanent damage to organs, mainly through fibrosis.

The greatest damage to man's tissues is caused by the eggs. However, the secretions, metabolic products, and toxins of the adult worms are believed by some to play an important role. As long as they are living, the adult parasites apparently produce no reaction, but when they die, numerous eosinophils gather about them.

Histologically, the predominant lesion is the pseudotubercle—a lesion incited by the ova retained in the tissues.

In the colon, ulceration is rare, and the distal parts are more frequently and seriously involved. Congestion of the mucosa, punctate hemorrhages, and thickening of the wall due to edema and fibrosis of the submucosa are the main findings. In Egypt, pedunculated or sessile polyps are commonly found in the rectum. Changes in the liver are largely portal. Ova transported from the colon by venous blood are retained in the portal spaces. Pseudotubercles form around them, accompanied by eosinophils. Grossly, the organ is enlarged during the intermediate stage but later contracts as scarring increases. On section the characteristic feature is a periportal fibrosis. The larger portal veins are surrounded by collars of fibrous tissue, constituting the characteristic pipe-stem cirrhosis of Symmers. The spleen frequently becomes enlarged, sometimes weighing more than 1,500 Gm. Ova and pseudotubercles in the spleen are more frequently encountered in Egypt than in America. In the lungs, small grayish nodules averaging 1 mm in diameter are visible or palpable throughout the pulmonary tissue. These are made up of pseudotubercles around the eggs that have been carried by the blood. In some cases the gross appearance of the lung resembles miliary tuberculosis. Microscopically, there are pseudotubercles, patches of marked eosinophilic infiltration, and, occasionally, hemorrhages. The eggs arriving in the lungs as emboli obstruct the small arteries, and the intima becomes thickened by fibrosis. In time, the right side of the heart undergoes hypertrophy, and failure ensues.

Manifestations. The clinical manifestations of schistosomiasis may be correlated with anatomic changes resulting from the reaction of tissues to the parasites and their ova. The finding of schistosome ova in the stools of apparently healthy individuals is a relatively frequent occurrence in endemic areas. Unlike the bacterial infections, the parasites do not multiply within the human host. Thus the symptomatic disease is dependent upon the continued exposure to infection.

Itching may or may not occur shortly after exposure, and urticaria is variable. Mild pyrexia may accompany urticaria. Anorexia, headache, generalized aches and pains, and diarrhea accompanied by abdominal discomfort soon follow and last 1 to 2 weeks. These symptoms occur after invasion of the parasite and during the periods of migration of the larvae or cercarias. From 30 to 70 days following exposure, when the cercarias have become adult males and females and oviposition has occurred, more severe symptoms appear. In some cases there is high fever (temperatures of 39 to 40°C) with chills and abdominal discomfort. Diarrhea and melena are common. A persistent dry cough is present, and scattered fine or coarse rales can be heard over the chest. The peripheral blood shows an eosinophilic leukocytosis, and ova are usually found in the stools. The findings in the peripheral blood excepted, the clinical picture resembles typhoid fever or paratyphoid fever. This acute illness usually lasts 1 to 3 months and subsides by lysis. When the initial infection is not severe or when anthelmintic treatment is given, the patient may recover rapidly, but should the infection remain untreated, intermittent bloody diarrhea frequently lasts several months. The severity and duration of these symptoms depend upon the extent of the initial infection. In untreated cases, however, several years may pass without signs of visceral disease. Should reinfection occur, fever and severe gastrointestinal symptoms again ensue. Anemia, at times severe enough to cause invalidism, may be present as the result of chronic blood loss. In many cases the liver and the spleen become enlarged.

The late stage of the disease frequently gives rise to a new clinical picture. The manifestations at this time resemble Banti's syndrome, with emaciation, hepatosplenomegaly, ascites, and other evidences of hepatic cirrhosis and portal hypertension. Some patients develop leukopenia, thrombocytopenia, and macrocytic anemia. However, the bone marrow shows no megaloblastic arrest. Liver function tests are frequently abnormal. Massive hematemesis from ruptured gastroesophageal varices is a frequent cause of death, and hepatic insufficiency is not uncommon. In Egypt, rectal and colonic polyposis, prolapse of the rectum, and intestinal obstruction are common late manifestations of the disease.

In some patients, particularly adolescents in whom irreversible vascular changes have occurred in the lungs, pulmonary hypertension associated with chronic cor pulmonale dominate the clinical picture, and a form of Ayerza's disease ensues. This may overshadow the already present hepatic cirrhosis and portal hypertension.

Diagnosis and Laboratory Findings. Diagnosis of the condition must be made by finding the ova in the stools, in the rectal mucosa, or rarely, in the urine. Various techniques of stool concentration are available, and the reader is referred to texts on clinical parasitology for technical details. By the use of such methods greater numbers of eggs are picked up from a given specimen, and a larger number of cases may be detected. The intradermal skin test, employing cercaria or worm extract, possesses diagnostic value in suspected cases where no ova can be found in the stools or in the rectal biopsy. Serodiagnosis, particularly the circumoval precipitin reaction, shows promising results. However, the role of the precipitin and complement fixation reactions as indicators of improvement or cure of the disease is not yet known.

By means of a Jackson's laryngoscopic forceps 35 cm long, a piece of mucosa 2 to 3 mm in diameter can be readily obtained through a proctoscope. When this unstained tissue is compressed between two glass slides, the ova can be recognized easily under the low-power lens of a microscope. It is believed by many investigators that rectal biopsy is the most reliable method of diagnosis; a very small piece of tissue may contain up to several hundred ova. In many cases in which repeated stool examinations have been negative, rectal biopsy has shown living or dead ova. Occasionally, however, stools contain ova when biopsy is negative.

Bilirubinemia and jaundice are seen rarely, even in the presence of advanced cirrhosis.

Treatment. Certain trivalent antimony compounds have been found effective against S. *mansoni*. These are tartar emetic (antimony potassium tartrate), stibophen (Fuadin) and Anthiomaline. Tartar emetic is one of the more toxic antimony compounds. It is administered intravenously in a freshly prepared solution in initial dose of 0.06 Gm, increasing to a maximum of 0.12 Gm by the third dose, and continued every other day until a total of 2.2 Gm has been given. A second course may be given after 1 month. Antimony sodium tartrate —less toxic than the potassium salt—is being employed with great success. Fuadin is antimony pyrocatechin sodium sulfonate and contains 1.3 per cent trivalent antimony. It has the advantage of intramuscular administration. It is well tolerated, and produces a minimum of toxic reactions when given in courses of not over 50 to 60 ml each. Daily injections of 1.5, 3.5, and 5 ml are given for the first 3 days, to be continued every other day with 5 ml doses until a complete course has been administered. The effectiveness of Fuadin as an anthelmintic is believed to be not greater than 50 to 60 per cent. Antimony lithium thiomalate (Anthiomaline) is administered intramuscularly in 2- to 3- ml doses every other day, until a total of 30 to 40 ml is given, comprising one course. Lucanthone hydrochloride (Miracil D) has been employed with promising results. This drug has the advantage of being active by the oral route.

The disappearance of eggs from the stools and improvement in symptomatology constitute the criteria for evaluation of anthelmintic therapy. Experience has shown that, for a period of about 1 month following administration of either Fuadin or Anthiomaline, stool examination and rectal biopsy may give negative results which are misleading. It is preferable to give several Fuadin courses (50 to 60 ml) a year, if the tolerance of the patient permits. Toxic manifestations occur in 20 to 30 per cent of the patients. Pain at the site of the injection and generalized arthralgia are common; however, hepatitis, acute nephritis, hemolytic anemia, and thrombocytopenic purpura have been observed. Triostam (sodium antimonyl gluconate) has been used with success. It is well tolerated, and toxic reactions are rare. One disadvantage is that the drug must be administered intravenously. In the late stages of the disease, these therapeutic measures are palliative, since the patient is suffering from cirrhosis of the liver, portal hypertension, or hypersplenism. The indications for surgical procedures are the same as for the other forms of portal hypertension (p. 1689).

Prognosis. The prognosis is good in infections where the symptomatology is mainly secondary to colitis, but when the liver, spleen, and lungs are involved, the prognosis is poor.

SCHISTOSOMIASIS JAPONICA (Eastern Schistosomiasis, Katayama Disease)

Etiology and Life Cycle. The male worm has an average length of about 1.5 cm and a breadth of 0.05 cm. The female is long and slender, averaging 1.9 cm in length and 0.03 in breadth. The eggs are slightly oval and are shorter, wider, and distinctly smaller than those of the other two species, measuring about 90 by 70 μ. Mature eggs have a minute hook, or spine, laterally situated and smaller than that of S. *mansoni*. The ova are passed in the feces only. The life cycle is similar to that of S. *mansoni*, but various species of *Oncomelania* and *Katayama* snails are utilized as intermediate hosts. *Schistosoma japonicum* lives in the inferior mesenteric venules but frequently migrates into the venules draining the large intestine and oviposits there.

Pathology. *Schistosoma japonicum* resembles the mansoni type, but because of the much greater number of ova deposited by the female worms in the former disease, the manifestations are frequently more severe. Cirrhosis of the liver develops earlier, and the duration of the disease is shorter—death often ensuing in 2 to 5 years. In advanced cases the gross postmortem findings are emaciation and pallor; large or contracted liver with periportal fibrosis; splenomegaly, with fibrosis of pulp; ascites; fibrotic nodules over the colonic peritoneum; fibrous thickening and rigidity of the colon, with small polyps projecting from the mucosa; and thickening and fibrosis of the omentum. Microscopically, the tissue changes are similar to those of schistosomiasis mansoni.

Manifestations. Following penetration of cercarias through the skin, allergic manifestations such as urticaria, itching, localized dermatitis, cough, and angioneurotic edema accompanied by fever and diarrhea may appear. From 4 to 6 weeks after exposure gastrointestinal symptoms are evident, a result of ulcerations produced in the intestinal walls by the large number of eggs. Bloody mucoid stools, or periods of bloody diarrhea accompanied by abdominal pain, may be present. If untreated, symptoms may last for several months. The liver enlarges and becomes tender, and splenomegaly develops. Dwarfism may occur; the probable cause is depression of the activity of certain endocrine glands. Antimony treatment may improve the condition.

As the disease progresses, the spleen becomes larger and the size of the liver decreases. Signs of portal obstruction such as engorgement of superficial abdominal veins, ascites, etc., appear. The patient may succumb from hemorrhage due to rupture of esophageal varices. Some individuals present marked splenomegaly, a small contracted liver, profound anemia, leukopenia, and thrombocytopenia associated with severe malnutrition and hypoproteinemia. The majority of individuals suffering from schistosomiasis japonica die of cirrhosis and cachexia, massive hemorrhage from rupture of esophageal varices, or intercurrent infections.

Diagnosis and Laboratory Findings. The characteristic ova must be found in the stools in order to establish the diagnosis. In established cases ova are more difficult to demonstrate in the stools or in rectal biopsy, and the intradermal skin test is of value. Aqueous extracts of cercarias or of adult worms are employed. The cercaria membrane reaction has been positive in 94 per cent of serums from patients infected with S. *japonicum* and is considered more valuable than skin tests.

Treatment. Tartar emetic and Fuadin have been employed in doses somewhat higher than those used in schistosomiasis mansoni. Oral tartar emetic has been used with success. In general, S. *japonicum* infections are more difficult to treat, and relapses are more frequent. Miracil D (Nilodin, lucanthone hydrochloride), a synthetic nonmetallic compound containing a xanthone nucleus, has been employed by the oral route. It is absorbed rapidly, and 60 mg per kg daily in divided doses, given for a period of 3 to 6 days, is the recommended dosage. Mild toxic reactions such as abdominal pain, weakness, nausea, and vomiting have occurred, and results have not been very successful.

Prognosis. If the condition is not treated early, prognosis is poor in the majority of cases encountered in endemic communities.

SCHISTOSOMIASIS HAEMATOBIA (Genitourinary Schistosomiasis, Endemic Hematuria)

Etiology and Life Cycle. The male worm has an average length of 1.3 cm and a breadth of 0.09 cm. The female is long and slender, averaging 2.0 cm in length and 0.025 cm in breadth. The eggs are compact, elongated spindles, dilated in the middle and measuring about 140 μ by about 50 μ. At one pole they present a short, stout terminal spine. The ova are passed in the urine, and occasionally in the feces. The life cycle is similar to that of *S. mansoni.* The adult worms live in the hemorrhoidal plexus of veins, some going to the rectum for oviposition but most of them passing on to the vesical plexus. The intermediate hosts are snails of the genera *Bulinus, Physopsis,* and *Lymnaea.*

Pathology. In the urinary bladder, large numbers of ova are deposited in the submucosa and give rise to dense infiltration with eosinophils, lymphocytes, and plasma cells. These foci, or "pseudoabscesses," apparently represent an allergic reaction to the eggs, but even though many of the eosinophils undergo necrosis and fragmentation, the lesion is not a true abscess. The mucosa becomes thickened and ulcerated. The trigone is involved at first, but soon the entire bladder is affected. In chronic infections the other coats become scarred and the muscularis hypertrophies. Pedunculated papillomas often develop at the trigone and about the urethral orifices. The bladder capacity becomes greatly reduced as the organ loses its contractility. Lesions occur in the distal third of the ureters in many cases, causing obstruction and hydronephrosis. Bacterial pyelonephritis may occur. In about 10 per cent of cases, calculi develop in the bladder, renal pelvis, or ureters. Fistulas between the urogenital tract and intestines may develop. The prostate and seminal vesicles may be affected, and lymph blockage may produce an elephantoid condition of the genitalia. The cervix and vagina can be infected by extension from the bladder. Carcinoma of the bladder is a frequent late complication.

Manifestations. Painful micturition, frequency, and hematuria are the leading symptoms. Secondary bacterial infection of the urinary tract is frequent, and repeated hemorrhages from the bladder produce severe anemia.

Diagnosis and Laboratory Findings. As in the other types of schistosomiasis, diagnosis is made by finding the characteristic ova in the urinary sediment, in tissues obtained from vesical mucosa, or, less frequently, in the stools.

Treatment. Chemotherapy is effective early in the disease but is contraindicated when urinary obstruction and infection have supervened. Lucanthone hydrochloride (Miracil D) appears to be more efficient (80 to 85 per cent) than Fuadin and nearly as effective as intensive treatment with intravenous antimony sodium tartrate. Triostam (sodium antimonyl gluconate) has been found to be effective against infection with *S. haematobium.* Antimony dimercaptosuccinate, an apparently nontoxic remedy, and paraaminophemoxy-1-phthalimido-5-pentane have been used with some success. Surgery may be required for abscesses, fistulas, strictures, papillomas, and various other complications involving the bladder. Chemotherapy is indi-

cated for secondary bacterial infections of the urinary tract. The criteria of cure are the absence of ova in the urine and bladder wall and the disappearance of ulcerative and granulomatous lesions, as revealed by cystoscopic examination.

Prognosis. Provided treatment is given early, prognosis is good in recent infection, fair when damage to the bladder and urinary infection have already occurred, and very poor in chronic, late infections. After age forty-five the mortality rate increases fourfold. The frequent coexistence of infection with *S. mansoni* aggravates prognosis and the clinical picture.

SCHISTOSOME DERMATITIS

Definition and Geographic Distributions. Cort demonstrated that certain nonhuman schistosome cercarias may penetrate the skin of man and cause a dermatitis. This condition is known as *schistosome dermatitis,* or "swimmer's itch," and is common in many parts of the world. The condition apparently does not develop after a single contact with cercarias, but it ensues following multiple exposures. Definitive hosts of some of the schistosomes producing dermatitis are the muskrat and migratory birds. Again, snails are intermediate hosts.

Schistosome dermatitis has been reported from the fresh-water areas of north central United States, Canada, Oregon, Central America, Western Europe (particularly Switzerland), and the Far East.

A sea-water dermatitis believed to be produced by nonhuman schistosome cercarias has been reported in New York, Rhode Island, California, Hawaii, and Florida.

Pathogenesis and Clinical Manifestations. Because the dermatitis develops only after multiple exposures, the condition is believed to represent an allergic reaction, the nonhuman cercarias being the sensitizing agents. Exposed individuals show positive intradermal reaction when tested with cercarial antigen.

Treatment. Local application of antipruritic lotions such as calamine with menthol or phenol is used to allay itching and thereby reduce the likelihood of secondary infection. Local treatment with antihistaminic drugs will relieve the pruritus.

Prevention. Immediate drying of the skin after swimming has been recommended as a prophylactic measure. This will not completely prevent lesions, since some penetration occurs during immersion. Dimethyl phthalate cream has been reported as an effective cercarial repellent.

In some areas, control has been effected by destruction of snails. Copper sulfate and copper carbonate have been used for this purpose. Treatment of shallow waters where snails are abundant has been moderately effective.

REFERENCES

Blair, D. M., et al.: Miracil: Clinical Trials on Patients Infected with *S. haematobium* and *S. mansoni*, Brit. J. Pharmacol., 4:68, 1949.

Diaz-Rivera, F. Ramos-Morales, E. Koppish, M. R. Garcia Palmieri, A. A. Cintron-Rivera, E. J. Marchand, O. Gonzalez, and M. W. Torregrosa: Acute Manson's Schistosomiasis, Am. J. Med., 21, (6): 918, 1956.

Ferreira, J. M.: Endocrine Disturbances in the Hepatosplenic Form of Mansonian Schistosomiasis, São Paulo, Thesis, 1733, 1957.

Friedheim, E. A. H., H. H. Salem, and A. F. El Sherif: Antimony Dimercaptosuccinate in Urinary Bilharziasis, (Correspondence), Lancet, Sept. 19, 1959, p. 410.

Hernandez, F., and J. F. Maldonado: The Diagnosis of *S. mansoni* by a Rectal Biopsy Technique, Am. J. Trop. Med., 26:811, 1946.

McFarlane, W. V.: Schistosome Dermatitis in New Zealand, Am. J. Hyg., 50:143, 1949.

Most, H., C. A. Kane, P. H. Lavietes, E. F. Schroeder, A. Behn, L. Blum, B. Katzin, and J. M. Hayman, Jr.: Schistosomiasis Japonica in American Military Personnel: Clinical Studies of 600 Cases during the First Year after Infection, Am. J. Trop. Med., 30: 239, 1950.

Oliver-Gonzalez, J., P. M. Bauman, and A. S. Benenson: Immunological Aspects of Infections with *Schistosoma mansoni*, Am. J. Trop. Med. Hyg., vol. 4, no. 3, May, 1955.

Orris, L., and F. C. Combes: Clam Digger's Dermatitis: Schistosome Dermatitis from Sea Water, A.M.A. Arch. Dermatol. Syphilol., 66:367, 1952.

Rodriguez-Molina, R., and H. Shwachman: Fuadin Therapy in 150 Cases of Schistosomiasis mansoni with a Follow-up Study of 70 Cases, Am. J. Trop. Med., 27:117, 1947.

T'ao, Shou-Ch'i: Cardiac Manifestations of the Toxic Action of Potassium Antimony Tartrate in Schistosomiasis Patients, Chinese Med. J. Peking, 75(5): 335, 1957.

T'ang, Sheng-Ts'ai, and Jih-Hsin Ch'en: 3-Day Tartar Emetic Treatment of Schistosomiasis japonica in Children, Chinese Med. J. Peking, 79(2):124, 1959.

222 OTHER TREMATODES OR FLUKES

Gustave J. Dammin

Paragonimiasis

Paragonimiasis, also known as *endemic hemoptysis*, is an infection, primarily of the lung, caused by the trematode, *Paragonimus westermani*. In addition to man, the dog, cat, pig, rat, and some wild carnivores serve as definitive hosts. The characteristic cystlike pulmonary lesions measure up to about 1 cm in diameter and, when of long standing, have a stout wall composed of fibrous connective tissue. Other smaller lesions may be in the form of nodules representing reaction around deposited eggs. Eggs appear in the feces when sputum from pulmonary lesions is swallowed. In heavy infections, lesions may also be found in the liver, mesentery, skeletal muscle, and brain. According to the sites of predominant involvement, cases may be classified as pulmonary, abdominal, or cerebral. In the pulmonary type, abundant brownish sputum is produced and bouts of hemoptysis occur. Abdominal pain and dysentery characterize the abdominal type. Various types of paralysis and epilepsy are observed with cerebral involvement. Eosinophilia is rather constant in all varieties of paragonimiasis. Eggs should be searched for in the sputum and feces, in attempting to establish the diagnosis. By using an antigen prepared from the adult trematodes, complement-fixing antibodies can be demonstrated. This may be helpful in identifying occult abdominal and cerebral infections.

Treatment with emetine hydrochloride as prescribed for fascioliasis (see p. 1231) affords symptomatic relief. When given in early cases, Sadun and Buck obtained moderately good results from treatment with chloroquine. However, there is no specific effective therapeutic agent. Prevention of superimposed infections is important, since the infection is, in a sense, self-limiting.

Paragonimiasis has probably the widest geographic distribution of any of the diseases produced by the hermaphroditic trematodes. It is endemic in many parts of the Far East and has been reported from parts of Africa and northern South America.

The most practicable control measure is the adequate cooking of all shellfish to be used as food, since infection is acquired by ingestion of cysts in the second intermediate host, such as a crab, crayfish, or mollusk.

Clonorchiasis

Definition. Clonorchiasis is an infection caused by *Clonorchis sinensis* and is characterized by hepatic lesions produced by the adult worms in the biliary passages.

Etiology. *Clonorchis sinensis*, the most important liver fluke in man, is a hermaphroditic worm measuring about 15 by 5 mm. Infection of man follows ingestion of raw fish containing the larval clonorchis. Many fish-eating mammals can serve as definitive hosts (dog, cat, pig, badger, guinea pig, and others). The encysted larva is released and migrates from the duodenum into the biliary tract, where it develops into the adult form. Judging from studies on individuals who have left the Far East, the major endemic area, the adult clonorchis is capable of living as long as 25 years.

Clinical Manifestations. The percentage of asymptomatic infections is probably high. The bile ducts become thickened and dilated, and there is chronic pericholangitis and atrophy of parenchyma, but cirrhosis with the usual clinical manifestations is uncommon.

Laboratory Diagnosis. The diagnosis usually depends on the demonstration of the eggs in the feces or the duodenal contents. Using a new method of extraction of the adult clonorchis, an antigen has been prepared by Wykoff, which can be used in a complement fixation test for the detection of the host's antibody response.

Treatment. No method of treatment has been consistently successful, but some success has been noted with gentian violet and chloroquine diphosphate. Gentian violet may be given as for strongyloidiasis. Chloroquine is prescribed in a dose of 0.25 Gm twice daily for 28 days. Most infections will respond to this dosage; those which do not should be treated for an additional 2- to 3-week period.

Prevention. Adequate cooking of fresh-water fish will prevent infection.

Opisthorchiasis

Opisthorchiasis is caused by *Opisthorchis felineus* and is characterized by hepatic lesions occasioned by the presence of the adult worms in the larger bile ducts. The life cycle resembles that of *Clonorchis sinensis,* with lesions and clinical manifestations like those produced by *C. sinensis.* The geographic distribution differs in that it is endemic in Eastern and Central Europe and in Siberia and occurs in some parts of Asia. The diagnosis usually is based on the finding of the eggs in the feces or duodenal contents. Treatment as recommended for chlonorchiasis may be used. Infection can be prevented by eating only well-cooked fish.

Fascioliasis

Fascioliasis is caused by the hermaphroditic leaf-shaped fluke *Fasciola hepatica,* which inhabits the bile ducts of the definitive host. When fully matured, the adult measures about 3 by 1 cm and discharges large operculate eggs 140 by 70 mm.

Fascioliasis produces so-called "liver rot" in the sheep, the principal definitive host. The disease is most common in sheep- and cattle-raising countries but has been reported from many parts of the world. In North America it occurs in the southern and western United States, Central America, and in the Caribbean Islands.

Infection is contracted by ingestion of the encysted form attached to edible aquatic plants such as watercress.

Early clinical manifestations are related to the migration of the larval form to and within the liver. Epigastric pain, fever, diarrhea, jaundice, urticaria, pruritis, arthralgia, and eosinophilia may be observed during this stage. Cirrhosis of the liver of the variety found in clonorchiasis may be a late manifestation, appearing only after prolonged residence of many adult worms in the bile ducts. A pharyngeal form of the disease may follow the ingestion of infected raw liver, the young adults attaching themselves to the pharyngeal mucosa, occasionally interfering with respiration.

The diagnosis usually is based on the finding of the eggs in the feces or in the duodenal contents. It is difficult to distinguish the eggs from those of *Fasciolopsis buski.*

The therapeutic agent by choice is emetine hydrochloride given intramuscularly. The dose should not exceed 1 mg per kg body weight or a total daily dose of 60 mg; in these amounts it should not be given for more than 6 to 7 days. As much as 30 mg per day has been given for as long as 18 days with good results. It should be given only when there is ample opportunity for rest in bed. It should not be given to patients with chronic cardiac or renal disease or to children.

To prevent infection in man, aquatic plants such as watercress should not be eaten, vegetables grown in fields irrigated with polluted water should be boiled, and safe drinking water should be provided.

Fasciolopsiasis

Fasciolopsiasis is caused by the large intestinal fluke *Fasciolopsis buski,* which inhabits the upper intestine of its definitive host. The principal definitive host is the pig. In parts of China, India, and other parts of the Far East infection of man is common. Infection is contracted following ingestion, or peeling with the teeth, of water chestnuts and other edible aquatic plants. The large adults attach themselves to the intestinal mucosa, and these sites may later ulcerate. Diarrhea and abdominal pain appear early. Later, if heavy infection continues, asthenia with ascites and anasarca occurs. Diagnosis is based upon the history and the finding of eggs in the feces. The eggs resemble those of *Fasciola hepatica.* The prognosis in untreated heavy infections, especially in children, is poor. Hexylresorcinol administered as for trichuriasis is the preferred therapeutic agent and can be expected to cure or markedly reduce the worm burden in the majority of cases. The most practicable control measure is the brief immersion of all edible aquatic plants in boiling water.

REFERENCES

Busch, E., and M. Cooper: Paragonimiasis: A Case with Metastasis to the Brain: Surgical Removal, Acta Med. Scand., 142: Suppl. 266, 343, 1952.

Edelman, M. H., and C. L. Spingarn: Clonorchiasis in the United States, J.A.M.A., 140:1147, 1949.

Koenigstein, R. P.: Observations on the Epidemiology of Infections with *Clonorchis sinensis*, Trans. Roy. Soc. Trop. Med. Hyg., 42:503, 1949.

McCoy, O. R., and T. Chu: *Fasciolopsis buski* Infection among Schoolchildren in Shoohsing and Treatment with Hexylresorcinol, Chinese Med. J., 51:937, 1937.

Neghme, A., and M. Ossandon: Ectopic and Hepatic Human Fascioliasis, Am. J. Trop. Med., 23:545, 1943.

Olsen, O. W.: Wild Rabbits as Reservoir Hosts of the Common Liver Fluke, *Fasciola hepatica*, in Southern Texas, J. Parasitol., 34:119, 1948.

Ross, J. A., W. E. Kershaw, and A. L. Kurowski: The Radiological Diagnosis of Paragonimiasis with Report of a Case, Brit. J. Radiol., 25:579, 1952.

Sadun, E. H., and A. A. Buck: Paragonimiasis in South Korea—Immunodiagnostic, Epidemiologic, Clinical, Roentgenologic and Therapeutic Studies, Am. J. Trop. Med. Hyg., 9:562, 1960.

Tillman, A. J. B., and H. S. Phillips: Pulmonary Paragonimiasis, Am. J. Med., 5:167, 1948.

Wykoff, D. E.: Studies on *Clonorchis sinensis*, Exptl. Parasitol., 8:51, 1959.

223 CESTODES OR TAPEWORMS

Gustave J. Dammin

Diphyllobothriasis Latum

Definition. *Diphyllobothrium latum*, the fish tapeworm or broad tapeworm, produces in man and its other definitive hosts infection characterized by the presence of the hermaphroditic adult worm in the intestinal lumen.

Etiology. The adult worm may measure 5 to 10 m and possess between 3,000 and 4,000 proglottids (Fig. 223-1). The mature proglottids measure

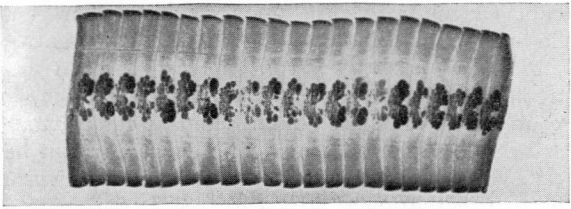

FIG. 223-1. Gravid proglottids of *Diphyllobothrium latum* (×2).

about 3 to 5 mm by 10 to 15 mm. The stage in the tissues of infected fresh-water fish, the host from which man acquires infection, is known as the *plerocercoid larva*, or *Sparganum*.

Pathogenesis. Ingestion of infected fish in the uncooked state by man, the dog, the cat, or the bear results in infection. The larva develops into the adult form in the intestine in about 3 weeks and is then capable of discharging eggs. The adults of *D. latum* have been known to survive for periods of 5 to 10 years.

Distribution. Fish tapeworm infection is common in the Baltic and Scandinavian countries, Switzerland, Italy, Russia, Japan, Chile, and Central Africa. It also occurs in the north central United States, south central Canada, and Florida.

Clinical Manifestations. Most infections are asymptomatic or produce slight transient abdominal discomfort. Infrequently, severe cramping abdominal pain, vomiting, weakness, and loss of weight are noted.

Pernicious tapeworm *anemia*, with erythrocyte counts ranging from half a million to two million, has many features in common with Addisonian pernicious anemia, including central nervous system involvement. It differs from the latter in that patients produce intrinsic factor but do not respond when given beef extract (extrinsic factor) and normal gastric juice (intrinsic factor) while the tapeworm is still present. Removal of the tapeworm and the administration of extrinsic factor lead to clinical and hematologic improvement. The position of the tapeworm in the intestine is important, anemia occurring only when the tapeworm is in the proximal small intestine. Large amounts of vitamin B_{12} have been demonstrated in the tapeworm, presumably absorbed from the host's intestine. *Taenia saginata*, which does not produce pernicious tapeworm anemia, contains about 2 per cent as much vitamin B_{12} as *D. latum*. The appearance of pernicious tapeworm anemia is related to vitamin B_{12} absorption and possibly also to a decreased production of intrinsic factor and decreased supply of extrinsic factor. It is apparent, however, that the tapeworm and the host compete for vitamin B_{12}. There may be ethnic and geographic factors involved, since most cases are reported from the Baltic countries; none to date has been reported in this country.

Treatment. Atabrine has supplanted oleoresin of aspidium and carbon tetrachloride. If prescribed as for taeniasis saginata, Atabrine can be expected to cure most infections. In the presence of severe macrocytic anemia, an adequate response to parenteral vitamin B_{12} should be obtained before an anthelmintic is used.

Prevention. The most practical control measure is the thorough cooking of all fresh-water fish. Children should not be permitted access to fish markets or to kitchens when fresh-water fish is being prepared, because of the possibility that some larvae may be ingested. To reduce contamination of waterways, dogs and cats should not be fed raw fresh-water fish.

Sparganosis

The *Sparganum*, or plerocercoid larva, of *Diphyllobothrium mansoni* will develop in man following ingestion (usually in drinking water) of a *Cyclops* bearing the procercoid larva. Sparganosis also follows application of infected fresh frog flesh used as a poultice. The frog tissues contain the *Sparganum*, which is capable of invading human tissues. The dog and cat are definitive hosts for *D. mansoni*. The location of the larvae determines the prognosis of the infection in man. Surgery and local alcohol injection are the only methods of treatment.

Sparganum proliferum, the adult stage of which is unknown, produces a more severe infection because of its unusual multiplication in the human host. Nodules containing the larvae form in the skin, lungs, intestine, brain, and other sites. The prognosis is poor in severe infections.

Sparganum mansonoides probably accounts for most of the cases of sparganosis observed in the United States.

Taeniasis Saginata

Definition. *Taenia saginata,* the beef tapeworm, is a hermaphroditic cestode which inhabits the intestinal tract of man, its only definitive host.

Etiology and Pathogenesis. In its adult stage, the *T. saginata* measures 5 to 10 m in length and possesses about a thousand proglottids. The gravid proglottid (Fig. 223-2) measures about 5 by 20 mm. It possesses 15 to 30 lateral uterine branches, thus distinguishing it from *T. solium,* which has 8 to 12. The proglottids may show independent motion for long periods after discharge with the feces. The head, or scolex, measures 1 to 2 mm in diameter and possesses prominent suckers but no hooks. The eggs are ovoid, 30 by 40 μ, and are indistinguishable from those of *T. solium.* When the eggs are ingested by cattle, the embryo is released in the intestine, invades the intestinal wall, and is carried by vascular channels to striated muscle in the hind limbs, diaphragm, and tongue, the common sites for formation of the cysticercus stage (*Cysticercus bovis*). *Cysticercus bovis* measures about 5 by 10 mm, and consists of a scolex held in a cystlike structure. When *C. bovis* is ingested in raw or undercooked beef by man, the adult tapeworm develops in the intestine in about 2 months.

Distribution. Taeniasis saginata occurs in countries in which it is the custom to eat raw or undercooked beef. It has been estimated that in the USSR alone there are about 18 million infections, and in

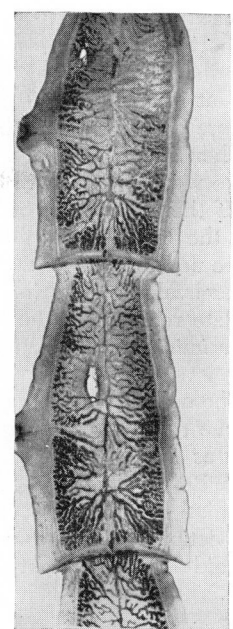

FIG. 223-2. Gravid proglottids of *Taenia saginata* ($\times 2$).

the world's population almost 40 million. Although not common in the United States, beef tapeworm infection is the most prevalent tapeworm infection observed in the northern half of this country.

Clinical Manifestations. Symptoms usually consist of mild epigastric pain, diarrhea, hunger sensations, weight loss, irritability, nausea, and, rarely, an increase in appetite. Movements of the worm may be apparent to the host. Rarely, segments may become impacted in the vermiform appendix with almost simultaneous development of appendicitis. Approximately one-fourth of the infections are asymptomatic.

Laboratory Findings. The diagnosis is usually made by the finding of proglottids in the feces. When the history suggests that proglottids may have been passed, but none are immediately available for examination, the perianal region should be examined as for pinworm infection, using the Scotch tape swab. By this method 85 to 95 per cent of infections may be detected, whereas by stool examination only 50 to 75 per cent can be recognized. When the scolex is obtained, it may be examined for suckers and the absence of rostellum and hooks, to identify it as *T. saginata.* The above study is necessary, since the ova observed in the feces cannot be distinguished from those of *T. solium.* A slight eosinophilia may accompany this infection.

Treatment. Experience with Atabrine has shown it to be a highly efficacious agent which has the advantage of ease of administration. The evening before the Atabrine is to be administered the patient takes 30 Gm of sodium sulfate in a glass of water. The following morning while still fasting, he takes 0.9 Gm of Atabrine. This is taken as three tablets of 0.1 Gm each at intervals of 30 min. Then 2 hr later a second dose of sodium sulfate similar to the first is taken. When successful, such treatment will remove the entire worm, which will be found to be stained yellow. If the scolex has not been removed, regeneration of the tapeworm will occur and re-treatment may be necessary after 2 or 3 months.

Incomplete removal by Atabrine has been followed by complete removal of the tapeworm subsequent to the administration of Benadryl in Emplet form.

Prevention. The only practical means of preventing infection is the thorough cooking of beef. Temperatures as low as 71°C for as little as 5 min will destroy *C. bovis*. Refrigeration and salting for prolonged periods also destroy the cysticercus. Adequate meat inspection and disposal of human excreta will also aid in control but are costly and seldom practical.

Taeniasis Solium

Definition. *Taenia solium*, the pork tapeworm, usually manifests itself as a parasite of man by inhabiting the intestinal lumen. Man is the only definitive host but under some circumstances may act also as the intermediate host harboring the larval stage, *Cysticercus cellulosae*. The usual intermediate host is the hog.

Distribution. Taeniasis solium has a world-wide distribution, but is commonest in the USSR, Asia, and Africa.

Etiology and Pathogenesis. The hermaphroditic adult tapeworm measures about 3 m in length and possesses a globular scolex containing a rostellum with about two dozen hooklets. There are seldom more than a thousand proglottids. The gravid proglottid measures about 6 by 12 mm and contains a uterus with 8 to 12 lateral branchings. The eggs resemble those of *T. saginata*. When ingested by the hog, the embryo is released from the egg, penetrates the intestinal wall, and is carried by vascular channels to all parts of the body. Localization with development to the encysted larval stage, *C. cellulosae* ("bladder worm"), occurs predominantly in striated muscle, particularly that of the tongue, neck, and girdle muscles. The cysticerci are ovoid, gray-white, opalescent structures about 1 cm in diameter. An opaque white spot denotes the site of the scolex. Man becomes infected following ingestion of undercooked pork containing cysticerci. The scolex is freed and attaches itself to the intestinal mucosa, and development to the adult stage begins at this time.

Clinical Manifestations. Clinical manifestations resemble those associated with *T. saginata*. The manifestations differ when man serves as the intermediate host. This may occur following ingestion of the eggs or the return of gravid segments to the stomach by reverse peristalsis. The released embryo bores into the intestinal wall and is distributed by vascular channels to various parts of the body. Cysticerci develop in the subcutaneous tissues, in muscles, in viscera, and—of most significance—in the eye and brain. Only moderate tissue reaction occurs while the scolex is viable. The dead larva, however, behaves like a foreign body and provokes a marked tissue response. Symptoms are related to active larval encystment only in heavy infections. Muscular pains, weakness, and slight fever may be observed. The involvement in the brain may be in the form of a meningoencephalitis when the cysticerci are widely distributed. However, epilepsy, brain tumor, encephalitis, and other types of neurologic disorder may be simulated. Eosinophilic leukocytosis of the blood and spinal fluid accompanying such clinical manifestations suggests cerebral cysticercosis. Degenerate cysticerci ultimately calcify.

As in other tapeworm infections, a slight to moderate eosinophilia is a fairly constant finding. The finding of eggs in perianal scrapings or in the feces will identify the infection as taeniasis. For a specific diagnosis, proglottids or the scolex must be examined. As in beef tapeworm infection, the diagnosis is usually made by finding proglottids in the feces. Roentgenographic demonstration of calcified foci may aid in diagnosis of cysticercosis. The prognosis is in large part determined by the stage and location of the parasite. Surgery may be indicated in cerebral and ocular cysticercosis.

Treatment. For removal of the worm in the adult stage, see Taeniasis Saginata. It is well to administer an antiemetic before giving the Atabrine to prevent reverse peristalsis, with return of the eggs to the stomach and release of the embryos.

Prevention. The simplest and most effective preventive measure is the thorough cooking of pork. Treatment of recognized cases will reduce the hazard of larval stage development as well as the spread of the infection.

Echinococciasis

Definition. Echinococciasis may be caused by the larval stage of *Echinococcus granulosus* or *E. multilocularis*. These species of echinococcus are distinct morphologically and biologically. In man, *E. granulosus* produces cystic, expanding lesions, involving the liver and lungs primarily, whereas the lesions of *E. multilocularis* are destructive because of their invasive character.

Etiology. *Echinococcus granulosus* infection in man, cattle, sheep, horses, and hogs, the principal intermediate hosts, is contracted by ingestion of the eggs present in the feces of the dog, the principal definitive host. Following ingestion, the embryos escape from the eggs, penetrate the intestinal mucosa, and enter venous and lymphatic channels. Some soon arrive in the liver and may form hydatid cysts there, and those entering the lymphatics are carried ultimately to the lungs. There is no exogenous budding from the wall of the cyst, only endogenous. Transmission to the definitive host occurs following ingestion of the hydatid cysts which contain scolices. An adult worm may develop from each scolex in the intestine of the dog, wolf, coyote, and other of the Canidae. The adult is small, measuring about 5 mm in length, and consists of no more than 5 or 6 segments. *Echinococcus multilocularis* infection is manifested by the same type of invasive larval-produced lesion as is observed in the natural intermediate host for this stage, the microtine rodents. The adult, or tapeworm, stage is found in the dog and fox.

Distribution. Echinococciasis caused by *E. granulosus* has its highest incidence in sheep- and cattle-raising countries, particularly in North and South Africa, Australia, Central Europe, and South America. In Iceland, a high incidence of infection in man and the dog has been markedly reduced by control measures. In the southern, western, and southwestern areas of the United States, the infection is established, and a small number of cases reported each year. *Echinococcus multilocularis* has been identified in Eurasia, Alaska, and the Kuriles and adjacent islands.

Pathogenesis and Clinical Manifestations. Two principal types of lesions develop in the intermediate host: the unilocular type of *E. granulosus* and the alveolar type of *E. multilocularis*. The former is more common, grows slowly, and consists of an external laminated cuticula and an inner germinal layer. Fluid fills and distends the cyst. Daughter cysts (Fig. 223-3) and brood capsules (Fig. 223-4)

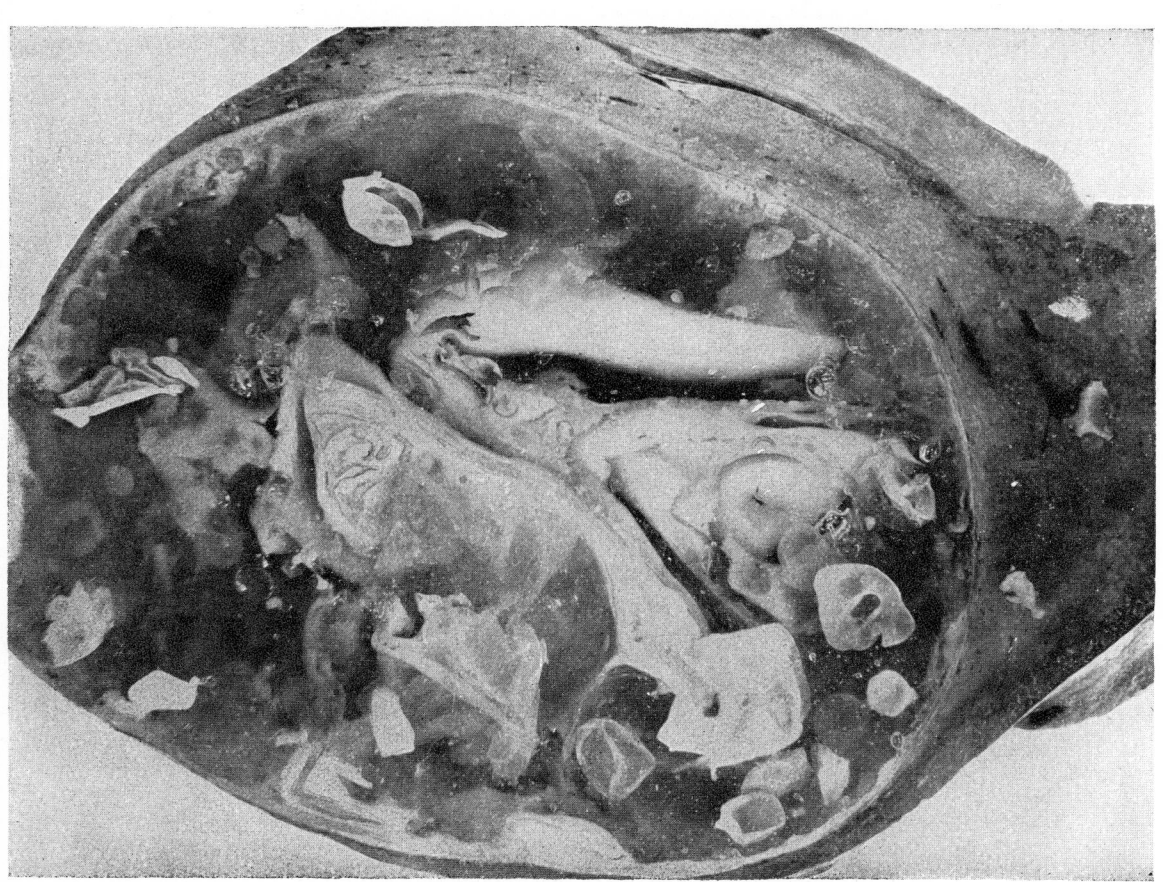

FIG. 223-3. Daughter cysts occur frequently in large old unilocular hydatid cysts. They are thin-walled balloons formed by herniations of the wall of the mother cyst and lie free in the cyst fluid. Free hooklets are also found floating in this fluid. (*Ash and Spitz: "Pathology of Tropical Diseases," Philadelphia, W. B. Saunders Company, 1945.*)

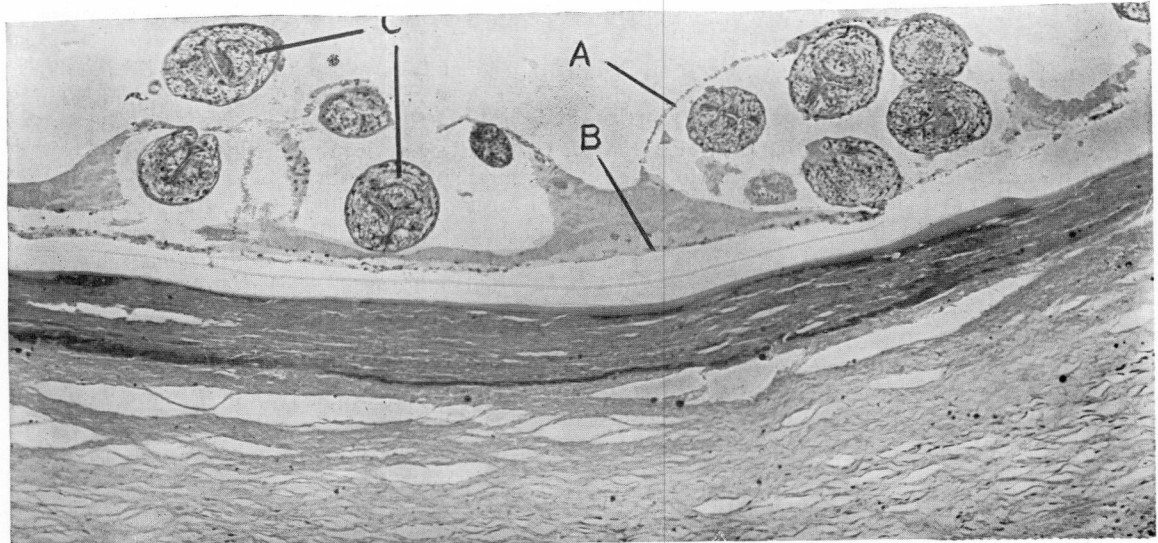

FIG. 223-4. Brood capsules are vesicles of single-cell layer (A) which arise from the germinal membrane (B). Invaginated scolices (C) arise as buds from the inner surface of the brood capsule. (*Ash and Spitz: "Pathology of Tropical Diseases," Philadelphia, W. B. Saunders Company, 1945.*)

develop from the germinal layer, representing endogenous development. "Hydatid sand" found in the cyst consists of scolices liberated from ruptured brood capsules. Exogenous development results from evagination of the cyst wall and ultimately produces the multilocular or alveolar type of lesion. Metastatic lesions occur when growth extends into vessels.

Symptoms produced depend upon the size attained by the cystic lesion and the amount of tissue destroyed. Unilocular lesions may become barren following resolution of secondary bacterial infection. Rupture into the peritoneal or pleural cavities may produce an anaphylactoid reaction, which occasionally is fatal. The unilocular type of hepatic lesion progresses slowly and is most amenable to surgical treatment. The alveolar type progresses more rapidly, with metastatic lesions developing in the bones, brain, and other sites. Pathologic fractures occur, and cerebral involvement may be manifested by epilepsy.

Diagnosis and Treatment. Clinical manifestations seldom are characteristic enough to suggest the diagnosis, but roentgenographic appearance of the lesion, especially when calcification is present, is often helpful (Schlanger and Schlanger). Eosinophilia is suggestive, although seldom present. Inquiry should be made concerning residence in an endemic area, and skin (Casoni or substitute antigen) and/or serologic tests performed, before exploration is considered. Exploration may be required as both a diagnostic and a therapeutic measure. Because of serious reactions to the leakage of cyst fluid into the tissues and body cavities, aspiration

should be attempted only during exploration. Aspirated cyst fluid should be examined carefully for scolices, hooklets, and laminated cyst wall. The size of the lesion will determine whether excision or marsupialization is the procedure of choice. Surgical treatment offers the only hope of cure.

Prevention. In prevention, (1) contact with infected dogs should be avoided, particularly fecal contamination of the hands and food; (2) infected carcasses and offal should be burned or buried, in order to prevent access of dogs to material containing scolices; and (3) dogs should be treated if found to be infected. The reduction of the incidence of echinococciasis in Iceland is an example of the efficacy of control measures.

Hymenolepiasis Nana

Definition. Hymenolepiasis nana is an intestinal infection of man caused by *Hymenolepis nana*, the dwarf tapeworm.

Etiology. The life cycle is unique in that both the larval and adult phases of development occur in the same host. Man, mice, and rats readily contract infection upon ingestion of the eggs. The adult measures about 2 cm in length and may possess over a hundred proglottids.

Distribution. The presence of dwarf tapeworm infection has been reported in temperate and tropical regions around the globe. It is the commonest tapeworm found in the United States, most of the infections occurring in the Southern states.

Clinical Manifestations. This tapeworm infection is characterized by the presence of many adult worms in the host's intestine. When infection is massive, diarrhea and abdominal pain occur.

Treatment. Atabrine, as prescribed for taeniasis saginata, is moderately effective. Because various stages of the helminth are present simultaneously, it is necessary to repeat the course of Atabrine at least once, after an interval of 2 weeks.

Prevention. This is a difficult problem, similar to that encountered in enterobiasis. Only a single host is involved, and the eggs are immediately infective. Personal hygiene should be stressed. The contamination of food by rats and mice should be prevented.

REFERENCES

Beaver, P. C., and W. A. Sodeman: Treatment of *Hymenolepiasis nana* Infection with Atabrine, J. Trop. Med. Hyg., 55:97, 1952.

Birkeland, I. W.: "*Bothriocephalus* Anemia," *Diphyllobothrium latum* and Pernicious Anemia, Medicine, 11:1, 1932.

Bonne, C.: Researches on Sparganosis in the Netherlands East Indies, Am. J. Trop. Med., 22:643, 1942.

Brooks, T. J., Jr., W. F. Hutchison, T. J. Safley, T. G. Ross: Human Sparganosis in Mississippi: Report of Two Cases, Am. J. Trop. Med. Hyg., 9:192, 1960.

Dixon, H. B. F., and D. W. Smithers: Epilepsy in Cysticercosis, Quart. J. Med., 3:603, 1934.

Dungal, N.: Echinococcosis in Iceland, Am. J. Med. Sci., 212:12, 1946.

Godfrey, M. F.: Hydatid Disease, Arch. Internal Med., 60:783, 1937.

Halawani, A., et al.: Treatment of Tapeworms with Atabrine, J. Roy. Egypt. Med. Assoc., 31:956, 1948.

Hornbostel, H., and H. Dorken: Trial of the Efficacy of Atabrine, Deut. med. Wochschr., 77:339, 1952.

Hutchison, W. F., and M. W. Bryan: Studies on the Hydatid Worm *Echinococcus granulosus*, I and II, Am. J. Trop. Med. Hyg., 9:606, 612, 1960.

Most, H.: Current Concepts in Therapy: Anthelminthic Therapy, I and II, New Engl. J. Med., 259:341, 441, 1958.

Newman, C. M., and B. S. Aron: Roentgen Diagnosis of Tapeworm Infestation, J. Mt. Sinai Hosp., 28: 91, 1961.

Newton, W. L., H. J. Bennett, and W. B. Figgat: Observations on the Effects of Various Sewage Treatment Processes upon Eggs of *Taenia saginata*, Am. J. Hyg., 49:166, 1949.

Obrador, S.: Clinical Aspects of Cerebral Cysticercosis, Arch. Neurol. Psychiat., 59:457, 1948.

Rausch, R.: Studies on the Helminth Fauna of Alaska: XXX. The Occurrence of *Echinococcus multilocularis* Leuckart, 1863, on the Mainland of Alaska, Am. J. Trop. Med. Hyg., 5:1086, 1956.

Read, C. P.: Human Sparganosis in South Texas, J. Parasitol., 38:27, 1952.

Schlanger, P. M., and H. Schlanger: Hydatid Disease and Its Roengten Picture, Am. J. Roentgenol., 60:331, 1948.

Stoll, N. R.: This Wormy World, J. Parasitol., 33:1, 1947.

Von Bonsdorff, B.: *Diphyllobothrium latum* as a Cause of Pernicious Anemia, Exptl. Parasitol., 5:207, 1956.

—— and R. Gordin: Treatment of Pernicious Anemia with Intramuscular Injections of Tapeworm Extracts, Acta Med. Scand., 144:263, 1953.

——, W. Nyberg, and R. Grasbeck: Vitamin B_{12} Deficiency in Carriers of the Fish Tapeworm, *Diphyllobothrium latum,* Acta Haematol., 24:15, 1960.

224 HIRUDINIASIS
Ivan L. Bennett, Jr.

Definition and Etiology. Human hirudiniasis results from the attachment of *Hirudinea* or leeches to the skin or, rarely, to internal mucosal surfaces. Leeches are found in lakes, ponds, and tropical forests and vary in size from a few millimeters to several centimeters in length. They attach themselves firmly to a host and suck blood. Because their salivary secretion contains an anticoagulant, the puncture wounds at the attachment site may continue to bleed freely after the dislodgment of the parasite.

Land leeches are found on bushes in tropical areas of Asia and South America, and man is infected by contact with the foliage. Attachment of aquatic species occurs during swimming or wading in infested waters. Rarely, young leeches may be ingested in drinking water, an event that can lead to serious illness.

Manifestations. *External* hirudiniasis is painless and is called to the victim's attention by finding the parasites or the bleeding puncture wounds left when the engorged leeches detach. With heavy infestations, significant amounts of blood can be lost.

Internal hirudiniasis results from the attachment of small leeches to the mucosa of the upper respiratory tract, larynx, trachea, or esophagus. Infestation of the vagina, bladder, or urethra has occurred in swimmers. As the leeches engorge and grow, they produce symptoms of obstruction, often with bleeding. Hoarseness, cough, nasal obstruction, dysphagia, nausea, and dysuria are frequent, as are hemoptysis, hematemesis, melena, and hematuria. Anemia may be severe, and death has occurred from obstruction of the epiglottis.

Treatment. Leeches must be removed with care to avoid leaving mouth parts in the wound. Application of a lighted cigarette or vinegar will help with complete removal. Skin wounds should be cleaned and covered; secondary infection is the only complication.

Removal of leeches from the genitourinary tract is facilitated by irrigation. In the respiratory tract, endoscopy and removal are necessary, using topical anesthesia.

Prevention. Use of chemical repellents on skin and clothing and boiling of water are the only measures needed to avoid hirudiniasis.

REFERENCES

Chin, T. H.: Further Note on Leech Infestation of Man, J. Parasitol., 35:215, 1949.

Masterson, E. W. G.: Hirudinea as a Human Parasite in Palestine, Parasitology, 1:182, 1908.

Section 23: Disorders Caused by Venoms, Bites, and Stings

225 SNAKES AND LIZARDS

Ivan L. Bennett, Jr.

Fewer than one-tenth of the nearly 2,500 known species of snakes are venomous. These poisonous varieties belong to five families or subfamilies: Elapidae (cobras, kraits, coral snakes), found in all parts of the world but Europe; Viperidae (true vipers), found in all parts of the world but the Americas; Hydrophidae (sea snakes); Crotalidae (pit vipers), found in Asia and the Americas; and Colubridae, represented by a few rear-fanged species of Africa. The poisonous varieties of the United States, with the single exception of the coral snake of the Elapidae, are pit vipers and include the rattlesnakes, the water moccasin, and the copperhead. This discussion will center around these species, but the therapeutic measures outlined are applicable to snake bites in all parts of the world.

The number of individuals bitten by poisonous snakes in the United States is estimated at 2,000 to 3,000 per year; deaths are not reported separately but are undoubtedly rare, numbering fewer than 20 per year. In many European countries, deaths from snake bite have averaged only one every 3 to 5 years for the last half-century. In contrast, the estimate of annual deaths from snake bite in Brazil is 2,000 (4 per 100,000 population), and 2,000 in Burma (15.4 per 100,000).

Etiology. The coral snake is found in the Southern states from Florida to Arizona. It is marked by alternating red and black bands separated by yellow rings. Coral snakes are nocturnal and placid and rarely bite man. The fangs are short and permanently erect; the highly toxic venom is injected into multiple puncture wounds produced by a series of chewing movements.

The pit vipers are so named because of a small pit between the eye and the nostril. Large venom glands in the temporal region give the head a triangular appearance. They are generally aggressive and likely to strike if disturbed. The fangs are long and hinged, folding posteriorly when the mouth is closed. Pit vipers strike suddenly with a forward thrust of the head, and the instant that the erect fangs make contact, venom is expressed by sudden muscular contraction.

The rattlesnakes, recognized by the horny rattle on the tail which buzzes when the snake is disturbed, are widely distributed. The diamondbacks (*Crotalus adamanteus* in the Southeast and *C. atrox* in the Southwest) are the largest and most dangerous snakes in this country. Others include the prairie rattler (*C. confluentus*), the timber rattler (*C. horridus*), and the pigmy rattlers.

The water moccasin, or cottonmouth (*Agkistrodon piscivorus*), is found in swampy areas or along the banks of streams. It is a strong swimmer and can bite under water. This snake is notorious for inflicting severe facial bites when disturbed in the branches of small trees. The copperhead, or highland moccasin (*A. mokasen*), is a closely related species. Its bite is painful but rarely fatal.

Pathogenesis. *Snake Venoms.* The venoms of many species have been analyzed; invariably each proves to be a mixture of several toxic proteins and enzymes. As an example, the venom of the Indian cobra (*Naja naja*) contains these distinct and separate substances: a neurotoxin, a hemolysin, a cardiotoxin, a cholinesterase, at least three phosphatases, a nucleotidase, and a potent inhibitor of cytochrome oxidase. Several venoms, including those of the pit vipers, contain hyaluronidase and numerous proteolytic enzymes. Although opinions differ about the exact role of these components in toxicity, the action of the venom of a given species is usually predominantly *neurotoxic* or *necrotizing;* frequently associated changes are hemolysis and changes in blood coagulation. The venom of elapids, including the coral snake, is neurotoxic, and death results from respiratory paralysis, probably caused by damage to brain centers, and a curariform interference with transmission at the neuromuscular junction. The venom of crotalid snakes produces local tissue injury, hemorrhage, and hemolysis; death is preceded by circulatory collapse, the mechanism of which is poorly understood. Systemic absorption of venom occurs through lymphatics, and therapeutic measures designed to reduce lymphatic function are helpful in controlling symptoms. On rare occasions, when venom is discharged directly into a blood vessel, death occurs in less than 10 min.

Factors Affecting Severity. Several factors affect the outcome of snake bite:

1. The age, size, and health of the patient. Envenomation in children is usually serious and a fatal outcome more likely.

2. Bites on extremities or into adipose tissues are less dangerous than those on the trunk or face or penetrating a vessel. A direct stroke of the fangs is more dangerous than a scratch, a glancing blow, or one hitting a bone. The discharge orifice of the fang is well above its tip, and the point of the fang can penetrate the skin without envenomation. Even a thin layer of clothing may afford great protection.

3. The size of the snake, the extent of its anger or fear (if hurt it may inject a large dose of venom), the condition of the venom glands (recently discharged or full), and the condition of the fangs (broken, recently renewed) are all important.

4. The presence of various bacteria in the mouth of the snake or on the skin of the victim (especially clostridia) may lead to serious infection in the necrotic tissues at the local site.

5. Exercise or exertion, such as running, immediately after the bite speeds systemic absorption of toxin.

Manifestations. The bite of a pit viper produces severe pain at the local site within a few minutes. There is rapid swelling; ecchymoses and bullae appear over the involved areas, and as the edema spreads, serosanguineous fluid oozes from the puncture wounds. Systemic effects include circulatory collapse with hypotension, clammy skin, tachycardia, intense thirst, nausea, hematemesis, bloody diarrhea, icterus (rarely intense), hemorrhages from the nose and into the skin, and convulsions. Death may occur after 6 to 48 hr. Survival may be attended by massive local tissue loss from gangrene

and secondary infection; amputation of an extremity is sometimes necessary. Fever with a temperature of 101 to 104°F, polymorphonuclear leukocytosis of 20,000 to 30,000, and albuminuria appear within a few hours in severe cases.

The bite of an elapine snake causes little pain, and local swelling is slight. There are usually multiple fang marks. Numbness and weakness begin in the region of the bite within 10 to 15 min and are followed by ataxia, ptosis, pupillary dilatation and loss of reaction to light and accommodation, palatal and pharyngeal palsies, slurring of speech, salivation, and occasionally, nausea and vomiting. The patient becomes comatose, respirations falter, there are convulsions, and death occurs within 8 to 72 hr.

Treatment. An attempt should be made to determine with certainty that the patient has been bitten by a poisonous snake. Absence of distinct fang punctures and failure of local pain, edema, numbness, or weakness to appear within 20 min are strong evidence against a bite's having been inflicted by a venomous species.

Treatment consists of immobilization, application of a tourniquet, incision and suction, antivenin, refrigeration, measures to combat infection, and general support. All patients should be transported to a hospital as quickly as possible.

Local Measures. A tourniquet should be placed a few centimeters above the bite (if anatomically feasible) and made tight enough to allow one finger to pass beneath it with difficulty. The purpose is to impede lymph flow, and it is not necessary to obstruct venous return; the tourniquet should be loosened and moved proximally when local swelling causes it to tighten. Using whatever antisepsis is available, 1 cm cruciate incisions about 0.5 cm deep should be made through each fang mark and suction applied for at least 30 min. A rubber bulb for this purpose is contained in first-aid kits, but a breast pump, funnel attached to a vacuum line, or heated jar can be used. Mouth suction is permissible if no oral lesions are present. Suction should be carried out for 15 min every hr, then every 2 hr, as long as fluid is obtainable. As the swelling progresses, successive rings of radiating, linear, shallow incisions at the advancing edge of the edema are useful; such cuts will be expanded by the progressive swelling. Once a patient has been hospitalized, a pavex boot is a convenient means of applying suction to an extremity. Extensive or deep slashes over the area are unnecessary. Incision and suction are extremely important and should be carried out diligently in every poisonous snake bite. Antivenin is not a substitute for them and should not be relied on alone.

Immobilization of the affected part during transportation is important in controlling lymph flow; splinting is useful in achieving this. The application of ice packs to the affected area reduces inflammation and swelling, slows drainage by lymphatics, relieves pain, and curtails local necrosis. Care should be taken to avoid freezing the tissues.

Antivenin. Many of the components of venom are antigenic, and effective antiserum can be prepared by inoculation of horses with graded doses. In this country, the only commercially available antivenin is Antivenin Crotalidae Polyvalent (North and South American Antisnakebite Serum) prepared by Wyeth Laboratories; it is effective against all pit vipers. Kits containing lyophilized antivenin (reconstituted with distilled water to 10 ml per ampul), syringe, normal horse serum for prior sensitivity testing of the patient, and detailed instructions are available. The initial dose for a serious bite should be 5 ampuls intramuscularly and, if antivenin is given within 2 hr after the bite, 10 ml of this can be infiltrated locally. Further antivenin can be given as indicated by progression of swelling or systemic symptoms.

No antivenin for coral snakes is manufactured in the United States, although antiserum is sometimes kept on hand in large zoos. Soro-Anti-Elapidico is the commercial name of an effective serum against coral snake venom that is available from the Instituto Butantan, Caixa Postal 65, São Paulo, Brazil.

The American Association for the Advancement of Science, Symposium on Venoms, listed among the references at the end of this chapter, contains a complete listing of antivenin preparations and their sources throughout the world.

Other Measures. The maintenance of respiration by manual or mechanical aids is important in patients bitten by the elapine snakes. It has been suggested that the cholinesterase of cobra and coral venom is responsible for much of the neurotoxicity and that neostigmine and atropine given as for myasthenia gravis might help. This has not been tested clinically.

Tetanus toxoid or antiserum should be given. If pyogenic infection develops, antibiotics should be used.

Alcohol has no place in the treatment of snake bite. Opiates are contraindicated. Relief of pain with salicylates or Demerol, sedation, maintenance of fluid intake, measures to combat shock, and appropriate management of coma or convulsions are all important.

Limited trials of ACTH and adrenal steroids have not shown any great usefulness of these hormones in lessening local necrosis or systemic intoxication.

Prevention. In snake-infested regions, long trousers, high shoes, boots or leggings, and gloves should be worn. Most important of all is to look where one steps or reaches. A sharp knife or lancet, tourniquet, suction bulb, and antiseptic suffice for an emergency kit, and in inaccessible areas, antivenin also should be carried.

Gila Monster Bite

The Gila monsters include the large orange and black lizard (*Heloderma suspectum*) of the arid Southwest and *H. horridum,* a closely related Mexican species. These reptiles are not aggressive, and virtually every instance of their attacking man has involved teasing or handling the animals in captivity. The venom is elaborated in eight glands in the floor of the mouth and secreted directly into the oral cavity, where it bathes the teeth which are grooved posteriorly. The lizard clings tenaciously and is often dislodged only after considerable effort; envenomation occurs by contamination of the wound. The venom contains a potent neurotoxin which is undoubtedly responsible for its lethal effect in experimental animals. Death in man has been reported as occurring within a few hours (in one case, 30 min) after a bite. The venom also produces local tissue injury, excruciating pain, massive edema, and patchy erythema. In recovered cases, acute symptoms have lasted for 3 to 4 days and include nausea, vomiting, hematemesis, blurred vision, dyspnea, dysphonia, and profound weakness. Intense hyperesthesia of the bitten extremity can persist for several weeks. There is no antivenin available. Treatment should consist of tourniquet, incision, suction, measures to prevent or combat infection, including tetanus, and supportive measures. Because Demerol has been shown to potentiate the venom's action in animals, some other analgesic should be used to relieve pain.

REFERENCES

Buckley, E. E., and N. Porges (Eds.): Symposium on Venoms, Am. Assoc. Advance. Sci., Publ. No. 44, Washington, D.C., 1956.

Essex, H. E.: Animal Venoms and Their Physiologic Action, Physiol. Revs., 25:156, 1945.

Jackson, D.: Treatment of Snake Bite, Southern Med. J., 22:605, 1939.

Kellaway, C. H.: Animal Poisons, Ann. Rev. Biochem., 8:545, 1939.

Klauber, L. M.: "Rattlesnakes, Their Habits, Life History and Influence on Mankind," vol. 2, Berkeley, University of California Press, 1956.

Shannon, F. A.: Case Reports of Two Gila Monster Bites, Herpetology, 9:127, 1953.

Storer, T. I.: *Heloderma* Poisoning in Man, Bull. Antivenin Inst. Am., 5:12, 1917.

Tinkham, E. R.: The Deadly Nature of Gila Monster Venom, p. 59 in Symposium on Venoms, American Association for the Advancement of Science, Washington, D.C., 1956.

226 SPIDERS, SCORPIONS, INSECTS, AND OTHER ARTHROPODS

Ivan L. Bennett, Jr.

The bite of many spiders is locally irritating, and several species can cause severe, even fatal systemic poisoning in man. The most numerous and important of the venomous spiders are the members of the genus *Latrodectus*, widely distributed throughout the world. In the United States and Canada, *L. mactans*, the black widow or "shoe-button" spider, causes nearly all clinically significant arachnidism. In Florida, *L. bishopi*, the red-legged widow spider, has been reported to produce human poisoning resembling mild black widow bite.

The symptomatology and mortality from bites of large, hairy spiders, the tarantulas, such as *Lycosa raptoria* and *Phoneutria fera* in Brazil, *Glyptocranium gastereanthoides* in Peru, and *Loxosceles laeta* in Chile, differ in no important respects from those produced by *Latrodectus* except that there are also likely to be severe necrosis and ulceration locally and hemolysis sometimes occurs.

It is the female *Latrodectus mactans*, the black widow, that bites man. She is glossy black with a body 1 cm in diameter and a leg span of 5 cm. There is a characteristic red "hourglass" mark on the ventral abdomen. She spins her web in woodpiles, sheds, basements, or outdoor privies, is very aggressive, and will bite on slight provocation. The venom is said to be about fifteen times as potent as that of the rattlesnake on a weight-for-weight basis. It produces diffuse central and peripheral nervous excitement, autonomic activity, muscle spasm, hypertension, and vasoconstriction.

In the United States, most spider bites occur between April and October, and many patients are males bitten on the genitalia or buttocks while using a privy. After a momentary sharp pain at the site, there is cramping pain that begins locally within 15 to 60 min and gradually spreads. It can involve all extremities and the trunk. The abdomen is boardlike, and the waves of pain become excruciating, causing the patient to turn, toss, and cry out. Respirations are often labored and grunting. There are also nausea, vomiting, headache, sweating, salivation, hyperactive reflexes, twitching, tremor, paresthesias of hands and feet, and occasionally, systolic hypertension. A mild polymorphonuclear leukocytosis is usual, and many patients have a temperature up to 100°F. After several hours, the pains subside, although mild recurrences for 2 or 3 days are common. It may be a week before well-being is restored. Deaths have occurred, mostly in children and the aged. In an analysis of nearly 1,300 cases from the United States and Canada, the mortality varied from 2.4 to 6.0 per cent. This is higher than is usually stated.

Because the bite itself is not prominent, patients are often thought to have some abdominal catastrophe such as perforated ulcer, pancreatitis, or volvulus. Renal colic, coronary occlusion, tetanus, strychnine poisoning, tabetic crisis, lead colic, and porphyria are other conditions to be ruled out. The abdomen is not tender to palpation in arachnidism, and pains in the extremities are not typical of most of these other disorders.

Treatment. This consists of antiserum and measures to relieve pain. The antiserum is produced in horses by Merck Sharp and Dohme, and a single intramuscular injection of one ampul (2.5 ml) of reconstituted material is all that is needed in most cases; relief is gradual. Hot baths alleviate pain temporarily, and intravenous calcium gluconate or magnesium sulfate will produce dramatic, but usually transient, cessation of cramps. Opiates are sometimes effective. Neostigmine, epinephrine, ACTH, and adrenal steroids have all been reported to give relief in isolated cases and are worth trying.

Scorpion Sting

Scorpions are eight-legged arthropods. Adults are 2 to 20 cm in length. Glands in the terminal segment produce venom, which is injected into the victim by a stinger located on the tip of the tail. Scorpions often enter dwellings. During the day they retreat into crevices; emerging at night, they often get into shoes and clothing and even into bedding. They do not deliberately attack man, but accidental contact results in a sting.

Of about 650 species, roughly 40 occur in the United States, distributed over three-fourths of the nation. They are most numerous in the South from Florida to California, but the only two lethal species, *Centruroides sculpturatus* and *C. gertschi*, are limited to Arizona and portions of neighboring states. In general, scorpions are not encountered in New England and the Great Lakes area.

The venom is neurotoxic. It acts locally upon sensory nerves and centrally upon the medulla and involuntary nervous system causing circulatory, respiratory, and widespread autonomic disturbances.

Dangerous species found in the United States, *C. sculpturatus* and *C. gertschi*, reach a maximal length of about 7 cm. Their sting may be fatal to young children or old people, but seldom to a healthy adult. In the years 1929 to 1948, there were 68 deaths from scorpion sting reported from the state of Arizona.

Most of the nonlethal species of scorpions in the United States cause only minor reactions, like a bee sting. Some in the Southwest, however, produce local edema and ecchymosis, with burning pain. In contrast, many species whose venom has potentially dangerous systemic effects, including the Arizona *Centruroides,* evoke little or no visible reaction at the site of the sting. There is an immediate burning sensation followed by local paresthesia ("pins and needles"), hyperesthesia, or numbness. These spread to involve the whole extremity, and within an hour or two, malaise, restlessness, lacrimation, rhinorrhea, salivation, perspiration, nausea, and vomiting appear. The emeses may contain blood. Transient hypertension, glucosuria, and premature ventricular contractions have been recorded. In fatal cases, dyspnea may occur without cyanosis. Tachycardia with muffled heart sounds and feeble pulse may be noted, or there may be bradycardia and respiratory depression, with irregular or Cheyne-Stokes breathing. Pulmonary edema develops terminally. The patient passes from an agitated state with hyperactive reflexes into coma; convulsions follow. Death usually occurs within 12 hr, but sometimes as late as 2 days after the sting.

Treatment. This consists of immediately placing a tight ligature on the extremity just proximal to the sting, followed by application of ice and, as soon as possible, immersion of the involved member above the ligature in ice water. The ligature must be removed in 5 to 10 min, but the limb is kept refrigerated for at least 2 hr. After this time, if treatment has been applied promptly, it is said that no serious effects are experienced following the sting of *C. sculpturatus* or *C. gertschi.* If the sting is on the head, trunk, or genitalia, of course, the ligature cannot be used, but the area may be chilled with an ice pack.

Other authors recommend tourniquet, incision, and suction as in the treatment of snake bite. However, the amount of venom is minute; it produces no local necrotizing effect and is absorbed so rapidly that unless these procedures are carried out very promptly they are of doubtful value.

Supportive therapy is directed at combating shock and dehydration. Barbiturates in large doses are useful in reducing restlessness.

Prevention. This depends upon alertness in avoiding contact with scorpions in infested areas. Clothing and shoes should be well shaken before being put on in the morning. Towels and bedclothes should be inspected. A house infested with scorpions can in time be rid of them by closing all obvious ways of ingress; picking up debris in the environment, such as piles of brush, logs, stones; introducing a mixture of fuel oil or kerosene, containing a small amount of creosote, between the earth and the house foundation; and spraying with a mixture of 2 per cent chlordane, 10 per cent DDT, and 0.2 per cent pyrethrins in an oil spray base. The spray is applied in a band 3 ft wide to the outer walls, to the undersurface of the house, also to screens and crevices around windows and

plumbing, and under the eaves. Inside the house, the attic, woodwork, plumbing, cupboard, and closet interiors are similarly coated with the residual spray, which under protected conditions has proved effective for as long as 6 months.

Bees, Wasps, and Ants

Bee or wasp venom is hemolytic and neurotoxic and has a histamine-like action. Multiple stings in man cause pain and discomfort, but only in enormous numbers (500 to 1,000) can they cause death. Apiarists become immune to the venom and can sustain many stings without effect.

The usual reaction to a single bee or wasp sting is sharp pain, local wheal and erythema, intense itching, and, in loose tissues such as the eyelid or genitalia, considerable local edema. This subsides in a few hours. Only in the rare case when a bee is inhaled or swallowed and edema of the laryngopharynx or glottis develops is there danger. A sting directly into a peripheral nerve may destroy its function for a time, much as does an injection of alcohol. There have, for example, been cases of Bell's palsy following sting into the trunk of the facial nerve.

In hypersensitive individuals, a single sting may produce serious anaphylaxis with urticaria, nausea, abdominal cramps, asthma, massive edema of the face and glottis, dyspnea, cyanosis, hypotension, coma, and death. Sensitization is usually a result of previous stings; beekeepers sometimes develop allergic rhinitis followed by asthma when near bees or objects that have been in contact with bees. These individuals are likely to have serious reactions to a sting.

Many ants can produce stinging bites with local redness and swelling, including the notorious "fire ant" whose bite can result in vesiculation.

The usual sting is treated by local cool applications and antipruritic lotions or oral antihistaminics. Epinephrine, 0.3 to 0.5 ml of 1:1,000 aqueous solution subcutaneously, repeated every 20 to 30 min, may be lifesaving in patients allergic to bees and/or wasps. This drug can be given as 1:100 solution in oil intramuscularly. Oxygen, antihistaminic drugs, and other supportive measures should be used. Desensitization by injections of extracts of whole bees and wasps has been reported but if this is not practical, contact with these insects should be avoided and, if exposure seems likely, epinephrine or sublingual Isuprel tablets should be kept on hand.

Tick Bite and Tick Paralysis

The local reaction to the bite of a tick may be nothing more than an itching papule which subsides within a few days unless there is secondary bacterial infection. However, incomplete removal of a tick, with retention of the mouth parts can result in the local formation of a nodule which continues to grow and is sometimes annoyingly pruritic. The definitive treatment is surgical excision of the nodule. Histologically, the nodule is a granuloma, but the inflammatory response is sometimes so bizarre and changes in the overlying epithelium so striking that, in the absence of a history of tick bite, a mistaken diagnosis of malignant tumor has been made.

Removal of a tick by steady pulling is preferable to crushing. Touching with a glowing cigarette, freezing, or application of a drop of oil facilitates removal without leaving embedded remnants.

Tick Paralysis. Tick paralysis is a reversible disorder of the nervous system which sometimes develops in the host while a tick is engorging. It may occur in man or animals. The disease has been reported from many countries. It has long been recognized in the northwestern United States and western Canada, where the wood tick, *Dermacentor andersoni* Stiles, is responsible. More recently the dog tick, *D. variabilis* Say, has been identified in a number of cases occurring in the Eastern states. *Amblyomma americanum*, the lone star tick, and *A. maculatum*, the Gulf Coast tick, have also been incriminated.

While engorging, the tick apparently injects a neurotoxin which acts upon the spinal cord and bulbar nuclei, causing incoordination, weakness, and paralysis. It has been shown in animals that there is failure of neuromuscular transmission and striking impairment of stretch reflexes. The toxin is rapidly destroyed or excreted, for when the tick is removed the nerve cells soon regain normal function.

Tick paralysis has been produced in experimental animals only with gravid female ticks, suggesting that the toxin might be elaborated by the ova. However, injection of extracts prepared from tick eggs has failed to reproduce the clinical picture in convincing fashion.

The tick must feed for several days before symptoms develop. Female ticks commonly remain attached for 7 to 9 days or longer. Paralysis is seen in experimental animals after 5 to 7 days of engorgement. Male ticks feed for a shorter period, a fact which may explain why they are less likely to cause paralysis.

Experimental confirmation of the theory that the toxin is produced in tick salivary glands is also lacking. It has been found that not all gravid female ticks of incriminated species cause paralysis. The nature, site of production, and mode of action of the toxin have not been established.

Most human cases occur in children, generally in young girls. The tick is usually attached to the scalp and hidden by the hair, but may be found on any part of the body, especially the ear, axilla, groin, vulva, or popliteal region. Both white and Negro races are susceptible.

The patient may be irritable for 24 hr before motor involvement appears. Mild diarrhea may occur. There is weakness and poor control of the legs. The tendon reflexes in the legs are diminished or absent, and the Romberg sign is positive. Temporary improvement may occur, and if the tick is removed at this stage, true paralysis may never develop. Otherwise the symptoms recur within 24 hr, with flaccid paralysis which extends in one or more days to involve the trunk, arms, neck, tongue, and pharynx. Sensory changes are usually absent, but there may be paresthesia and hyperesthesia in the affected extremities. Nystagmus, strabismus, and facial paralysis are sometimes noted. The respirations become shallow, rapid, and finally irregular. The patient sinks into stupor, cyanosis appears, and death results from respiratory paralysis or from obstruction of the airway by aspirated material.

There is little or no fever unless a secondary infection is present. The leukocyte count is usually not elevated, but moderate leukocytosis may occur. The spinal fluid is almost always normal.

Tick paralysis is apt to be confused with poliomyelitis, the more so because ticks are active in warm weather when poliomyelitis is most prevalent. In tick paralysis, however, there is usually no fever and the spinal fluid is normal. Muscle spasm and stiffness of the neck and back are minimal or absent. Ataxia, sometimes with paresthesia, often precedes paralysis by hours or days, first in the legs, then in the arms. Ascending involvement is characteristic, whereas progression of paralysis without fever is exceptional in poliomyelitis.

Among other diseases which might be considered in differential diagnosis are polyneuritis, transverse myelitis, infectious neuronitis (Guillain-Barré syndrome), syringomyelia, and spinal cord tumor.

Definitive treatment is removal of the tick. Mouth parts retained in the skin should be promptly excised. The patient's body should be searched for other ticks. There is striking improvement within a few hours after removal.

If the tick is removed before bulbar involvement develops, the paralysis subsides, and recovery is complete in a few days, sometimes within 24 hr. The patient should be observed until the recovery trend is established, because if other ticks or retained mouth parts have been overlooked, the paralysis may progress. When bulbar or respiratory paralysis is present, death may occur if the tick is not removed in time. Other treatment is supportive.

Other Arthropods

Flea Bite. There are many fleas that attack man, including *Pulex irritans*, and chicken fleas. In sensitive individuals, the salivary secretion of these bloodsuckers produces large, itching papules. Treatment is symptomatic only. Elimination of fleas in an environment may be very difficult, but persistent treatment of animals and of premises with appropriate insecticides is usually successful.

Centipede Bite. Local irritation is the usual reaction to centipede venom, although extensive necrosis and systemic illness have followed severe poisoning by tropical species. Treatment is purely symptomatic.

Caterpillar Urticaria. Contact with hairy caterpillars of many species produces irritation of skin or mucous membranes. The type of venom involved is not known but severe pain, erythema, urticaria, and even blister formation can come on rapidly after direct contact with caterpillars, after handling cocoons, or on being exposed to windblown fuzz. There is often a regional lymphangitis and transient eosinophilic leukocytosis. The discomfort subsides within 24 hr, but local soaks, oral antihistaminics, and where pain is severe, oral codeine are often indicated.

Bedbug Bite. Members of the genus *Cimex* inflict bites that leave reactions varying from a simple puncture to large urticarial lesions, apparently depending upon the sensitivity of the bitten individual. There is no specific treatment.

Chiggers or Redbugs. These are tiny mites which are commonly found in foliage, grass, etc., in many parts of the world. In the United States, the larval form of *Eutrobicula alfreddugesi* attacks the skin by secreting a substance which digests tissue, creating a red papule that itches intensely. The tiny reddish larva can be seen in the center of the lesion. Treatment is palliative with antipruritic applications. There is no better example of the virtues of prevention than this annoying affliction. The use of insect repellents, appropriate protective clothing, and prompt bathing after exposure reduce the risk of infestation considerably.

Myiasis. There are, generally speaking, three ways in which human tissues may become infested by maggots. Species of flies which usually deposit eggs in carrion, feces, or garbage may lay eggs in an open wound or ulcer, usually a lesion that is necrotic and suppurating. When the larvae hatch, they feed upon the dead tissue, and despite the unesthetic aspects, the deliberate introduction of maggots has been used to supplement surgical debridement.

Occasionally, food containing fly eggs will be ingested, and when the larvae hatch, *intestinal myiasis* can result in nausea, cramps, and diarrhea. The larvae are passed in the feces.

Finally the larvae of many flies, including the sheep fly and horse fly, will attack living, viable tissue. If eggs are laid in the eyes, nose, ears, mouth, or vagina, an event that usually occurs in sleeping infants, the larvae hatch out and can produce extensive destructive lesions; indeed fatalities have been reported.

The treatment for maggot infestation is surgical removal by irrigation and mechanical extraction. Obviously, control of fly populations by appropriate sanitary precautions is the important step in prevention. Protection of infants by screening and of wounds by bandaging is indicated in infested areas.

REFERENCES

BEE STING

Helm, S.: Severe Anaphylactic Reaction to a Bee or Wasp Sting, Military Surgeon, 92:64, 1943.
Perlman, F.: Desensitization to Wasp Sting, J.A.M.A., 156:1470, 1954.

CATERPILLAR URTICARIA

Randel, H. W., and G. B. Doan: Caterpillar Urticaria in the Panama Canal Zone: Report of Five Cases, p. 111 in Symposium on Venoms, American Association for the Advancement of Science, Washington, D.C., 1956.

SCORPION STING

Balozet, L.: Scorpion Venoms and Antiscorpion Serum, p. 141 in Symposium on Venoms, American Association for the Advancement of Science, Washington, D.C., 1956.
De Magalhaes, O.: Scorpionism, J. Trop. Med. Hyg., 41:393, 1938.
Essex, H. E.: Animal Venoms and Their Physiologic Action, Physiol. Revs., 25:150, 1945.
Waterman, J. A.: Some Notes on Scorpion Poisoning in Trinidad, Trans. Roy. Soc. Trop. Med. Hyg., 31:607, 1938.

SPIDER BITE

Bogen, E.: The Treatment of Spider Bite Poisoning, p. 101 in Symposium on Venoms, American Association for the Advancement of Science, Washington, D.C., 1956.
Sampayo, R. R. L.: Pharmacological Action of the Venom of *Latrodectus mactans* and Other *Latrodectus* Spiders, J. Pharmacol. Exptl. Therap., 80:309, 1944.
Thorpe, R. W., and W. D. Woodson: "The Black Widow: America's Most Poisonous Spider," Chapel Hill, N.C., University of North Carolina Press, 1945.

TICK PARALYSIS

Esplin, D. W., C. B. Philip, and L. E. Hughes: Impairment of Muscle Stretch Reflexes in Tick Paralysis, Science, 132:958, 1960.

Ransmeier, J. C.: Tick Paralysis in the Eastern United States, J. Pediat., 34:299, 1949.

Stanbury, J. B., and J. H. Huyck: Tick Paralysis: A Critical Review, Medicine, 24:219, 1945.

227 MARINE ANIMALS
Ivan L. Bennett, Jr.

The elaboration of substances that are poisonous for man is by no means an exclusive property of reptiles and arthropods. Several plant and animal products that are toxic when ingested are described in Chap. 103 (p. 815). In this chapter, discussion will center around venoms of marine animals known definitely to cause illness in man after injection or inoculation under naturally occurring conditions. Information about these toxins is limited, a few isolated clinical observations being the only data available about some of them. An excellent compilation and bibliography will be found in the review by Halstead listed at the end of the chapter.

Sea Anemone Sting (Sponge Diver's Disease). Contact with certain sea anemones (especially *Sargatia elegans*) in Mediterranean and African waters produces extensive dermatitis with chronic ulceration. Occasionally, especially during August and September, systemic symptoms of headache, sneezing, nausea, chills, fever, and collapse are noted. Rare fatalities have occurred. No specific therapy is known; the skin lesions have been thought to benefit from local x-ray irradiation. The disease confers no immunity.

Sponge Poisoning. Direct contact with several species of sponge results in a painful dermatitis. It is known that extracts of the sponges are lethal for mice. Dilute acetic acid ameliorates local pain strikingly and alkali will intensify it. The lesions are self-limited.

Portuguese Man-o-War and Jellyfish Stings. The burning discomfort induced by contact with "sea nettles" or jellyfish is familiar to most surf bathers. Contact with the tentacles of the colorful Portuguese man-o-war (*Physalia* species) or more toxic jellyfish (*Chiropsalmus* of the Indian Ocean and *Rhizostoma* of the Atlantic) is followed by severe pain, swelling, and erythema. Muscle pain, weakness, abdominal cramps, nausea, dyspnea, cyanosis, and collapse may persist for several days, and fatalities have occurred, sometimes within hours after contact.

Treatment consists of local application of ammonia, alcohol, or calamine, oral or parenteral antihistaminics, and systemic support. Cortisone has been thought to help in a few cases.

Cone Shell Poisoning. The colorful cone shells are highly prized by collectors. Many species in the Pacific are venomous, a great danger to unwary hobbyists who pick them up. The poison is delivered into a wound inflicted by pointed hollow teeth resembling darts in the long proboscis of the animal. Local manifestations include sudden intense pain, swelling, and cyanosis followed by numbness. The venom is apparently a neurotoxin and produces muscular incoordination, weakness, confusion, tachycardia, and dyspnea. Death can occur within 3 to 5 hr, but recovery within 24 hr is the rule. Recommended treatment is the use of tourniquet, incision, and suction (as for snake bite) and supportive measures which may include artificial respiration and oxygen.

Sea Urchin Sting. Contact with the spines of some species of sea urchin results in painful erythema and ulceration with or without neurotoxic symptoms of weakness and frank paralysis of lips, tongue, and face lasting for several hours. Treatment is purely symptomatic and supportive. The toxins isolated from sea urchins have produced paralysis in animals and are notably resistant to heat. Deaths from paralysis and drowning have been reported.

Fish Stings. The dorsal fins or spines of bullhead sharks, dogfish (the familiar *Squalus acanthias* of biology classes), and ratfish and the dorsal and other fins of the scorpion fish, weeverfish, toadfish, and catfish are grooved and at their bases are found venom glands. Injury by these spines results in severe pain and swelling and, in some instances, neurotoxic manifestations. Local gangrene with extensive tissue loss is a complication of catfish stings that may prolong convalescence. Little or nothing is known of the venoms involved. Suction and hot applications are advocated immediately after injury. Tetanus toxoid or antitoxin should be given also. Narcotics are often required to control the pain. Secondary pyogenic infection is a frequent complication to be watched for and managed appropriately.

Probably the most frequent type of venomous fish injury in this country is that produced by the lashing tail of the stingray of the California coast (*Urobatis halleri*). The bony spine is encased in a sheath of epithelial cells containing venom which is expressed into the puncture wound. The wound may be several centimeters deep, portions of the bony spine may break off in it or, more often, the integumentary sheath remains in the wound.

The venom is a circulatory depressant in animals, but local injury predominates in man. There is immediately severe pain and cyanosis followed by erythema and edema. Weakness, rarely, convulsions, and death can ensue. Treatment consists of application of a tourniquet (the vast majority of these injuries occur on the legs) and copious syringing of the wound with salt water to remove fragments of sheath followed by immersion in water as hot as the patient can stand for 1 hr. The venom is heat-labile, and extensive trials have indicated the usefulness of this last procedure. Tetanus toxoid or antiserum is indicated and, as with other fish stings, pyogenic infection is a frequent complication.

REFERENCES

Halstead, B. W.: Animal Phyla Known to Contain Poisonous Marine Animals, p. 9 in Symposium on Venoms, American Association for the Advancement of Science, Washington, D.C., 1956.

Russell, F. E., and R. D. Lewis: Evaluation of Current Status of Therapy for Stingray Injuries, p. 43 in Symposium on Venoms, American Association for the Advancement of Science, Washington, D.C., 1956.

Section 24: Diseases of Uncertain Etiology

228 SARCOIDOSIS
Ivan L. Bennett, Jr.

Definition. Sarcoidosis (Besnier-Beck-Schaumann disease) is a granulomatous inflammatory disease of uncertain etiology. The typical lesions, so-called hard tubercles, are distributed systemically, involving particularly lymph nodes, lungs, skin, liver, spleen, bones, eyes, heart, and skeletal muscle. Other manifestations include hyperglobulinemia, cutaneous anergy, and hypercalcuria, the last associated in many cases with renal insufficiency. The course may be chronic with intermittent disability depending upon the organs involved, there may be eventual complete clearing, or the disease may progress steadily to a fatal outcome.

Etiology. The etiology of sarcoidosis is a complete mystery. Suggestions have included atypical tuberculosis, infection by various viruses and fungi, exposure to beryllium, silica, etc., and sensitization to pine pollen. None of these is supported by firm evidence. The histologic similarity of sarcoid and several other specific or nonspecific granulomatous diseases has given rise to the suggestion that sarcoidosis is a tissue reaction that can be evoked by noxious stimuli of several types. This is nothing more than speculation.

Epidemiology. Sarcoidosis occurs all over the world, but the vast majority of cases have been observed in Great Britain, Scandinavia, Germany, Switzerland, France, and the United States, a situation that may change as the disease is recognized elsewhere. The peak incidence comes between twenty and forty years of age, and there is no sex predominance. Careful epidemiologic studies have shown a clear predilection for rural dwellers, and most striking of all, the disease is at least fifteen times as common in Negroes as it is in whites in the United States. Although sarcoidosis has been observed occasionally in identical twins and in siblings, there is little to indicate that it is transmitted from patient to patient by contact.

Pathology. The characteristic lesion is the hard tubercle consisting of compact clusters of epithelioid cells. These heal by fibrosis, leaving hyaline scars. Tubercles often coalesce, and giant cells are usually evident. These cells are frequently seen to contain laminated "Schaumann" bodies or stellate "asteroid" bodies, inclusions that are by no means pathognomonic of sarcoidosis although they are far more frequent in the lesions of this disease than any other. It is most unusual to see lymphocytes in appreciable numbers associated with hard tubercles, and caseation is not a feature of sarcoidosis. Fibrinoid necrosis of the centers of hard tubercles is sometimes observed, but this is never extensive and it incites little or no secondary inflammatory response.

It must be emphasized that these histologic changes are not pathognomonic of sarcoidosis although they are characteristic enough that biopsy examination will confirm the diagnosis in the presence of appropriate clinical findings. Exposure to beryllium and silica and the presence in the lesion of tubercle bacilli or fungi must always be excluded.

Active lesions produce symptoms by displacement of or encroachment upon normal structures, and with healing there may be permanent distortion by scars.

Manifestations. Because sarcoidosis can involve almost any tissue, the symptoms and signs are extremely variable. Constitutional symptoms of mild fever, weight loss, etc., are present in many cases and progress insidiously without localizing complaints or signs.

The *lungs* are very frequently involved. Often, the first indication of the disease is the detection of pulmonary lesions by routine chest x-ray. The changes are extremely variable, including diffuse reticular or miliary infiltrates, large nodules, or multiple "soft" lesions; bilateral symmetry is the rule. Mediastinal lymphadenopathy is frequent and sometimes massive, so-called "potato nodes" are seen. Enlargement of the right paratracheal nodes is very common, but this finding is by no means so characteristic of sarcoidosis as has been stated in the past.

Dyspnea with progressive disability is sometimes a presenting complaint, but generally, symptoms are milder than would be expected from the extent of x-ray changes. The functional alterations produced by pulmonary sarcoidosis are discussed in detail on p. 1527.

In a few patients, sarcoidosis begins abruptly with the onset of *uveoparotid fever* (Heerfordt's syndrome). There are high fever, swelling of the parotid and lacrimal glands (usually painless), granulomatous uveitis (see p. 423), and cranial nerve palsies, the facial nerve being by far the most frequently involved. This illness subsides spontaneously after a few weeks; the only residual is occasional incomplete clearing of the ocular lesion.

Generalized *lymphadenopathy* is common. However, tubercles are found with great frequency in nodes that are only slightly enlarged, and in seeking to confirm the diagnosis, biopsy examination of any palpable lymph node is well worthwhile.

From 20 to 40 per cent of patients develop *cutaneous nodules, papules,* or *plaques* containing hard tubercles. Because the skin lesions are so variable in their gross appearance, biopsy of any dermatologic abnormality should be carried out when sarcoidosis is suspected. *Erythema nodosum* with arthralgia, fever, and hilar adenopathy is particularly common in females at the onset of sarcoidosis. Usually, these patients do not go on to chronic disability and become free of the disease within 2 years. Interestingly enough, patients who show hilar adenopathy without erythema nodosum are far more likely to develop chronic, progressive sarcoidosis.

Granulomatous uveitis, usually bilateral, occurs in many patients with sarcoidosis and may leave residual visual impairment because of corneal or lenticular opacities or glaucoma. Chronic enlargement of the lacrimal glands is seen with considerable frequency.

The *heart* is sometimes involved by sarcoid tubercles, leading to arrhythmias, conduction defects, or very rarely, myocardial insufficiency with congestive heart failure.

The *liver* contains hard tubercles in about three-fourths of all cases, although it is unusual for this to result in any symptoms. Hepatomegaly is detectable in 25 per cent of patients, but jaundice or significant alterations of liver function are exceptional.

Splenomegaly is frequent at autopsy, and the spleen can be palpated in about 25 per cent of cases. Occasionally, sarcoidosis is accompanied by *thrombocytopenic purpura* or *hemolytic anemia,* disorders that are usually alleviated by splenectomy.

Bone involvement occurs most frequently in patients with cutaneous sarcoidosis. Radiologically, punched-out lesions of the terminal phalanges or more diffuse resorption of medullary bone with trabecular reticulation are the two most typical patterns observed.

It is often stated that sarcoidosis does not involve the joints. However, several instances of *acute polyarthritis* as a presenting manifestation of the disease are on record, and the presence of hard tubercles in the synovial tissues has been confirmed by biopsy. Some of these patients were thought initially to have rheumatoid arthritis.

The *nervous system* is affected in occasional patients. The cranial palsies associated with uveoparotid fever have been mentioned. Encephalitis, meningism, convulsions, diabetes insipidus, and expanding lesions of the spinal cord are rare, but all have been observed and confirmed as resulting from sarcoidosis.

Renal failure is rarely a result of direct involvement of the kidneys by hard tubercles. However, many patients with sarcoidosis have hypercalcuria with or without hypercalcemia, and this results in impairment of kidney function, nephrocalcinosis, or the formation of renal calculi. There is increased absorption of calcium from the intestine in these cases, resembling increased sensitivity to vitamin D or the activity of some endogenous substance with activity similar to that of vitamin D.

Laboratory Findings. Mild anemia is frequent, and the sedimentation rate is usually elevated. Hemolytic anemia and thrombocytopenia have been mentioned elsewhere. A few patients show mild eosinophilia, but this is not helpful in diagnosis. Hypercalcemia and hypercalcuria have already been discussed. Serum phosphorus is usually normal. Hyperglobulinemia is present in a majority of patients, usually a result of increase in γ and α_2 fractions. Occasionally, the serum alkaline phosphatase will be strikingly elevated in the absence of demonstrable bony involvement.

X-ray changes in the lungs and phalanges have been described already, and the electrocardiogram will sometimes show arrhythmias, conduction defects, or the changes of cor pulmonale.

About 85 per cent of patients with sarcoidosis fail to react to intracutaneous tuberculin. However, this anergy extends to other protein antigens and is in no way diagnostic.

The so-called Kveim reaction is elicited by intracutaneous injection of a 10 per cent suspension of lymph node tissue obtained from a patient with sarcoidosis. After 1 month or more, a small nodule will appear at the injection site. If, on biopsy, this contains hard tubercles, the test is positive. Despite lack of a standard antigen and occasional difficulties in interpreting the test, the Kveim reaction is a valuable diagnostic aid. It is positive in 60 to 80 per cent of cases of sarcoidosis.

Diagnosis. In the presence of pulmonary lesions, hilar and general lymphadenopathy, uveoparotid fever, skin lesions, hypercalcemia, erythema nodosum, rheumatoid-like arthritis, granulomatous uveitis, or combinations of these manifestations, sarcoidosis should be suspected. Confirmation by biopsy of lung (rarely indicated), scalene or other lymph node, skin, liver, skeletal muscle (a surprisingly frequent source of hard tubercles) or synovium should be attempted.

Other situations in which sarcoidosis should be considered are thrombocytopenic purpura, hemolytic anemia, diabetes insipidus, unexplained renal failure, arrhythmias or heart block, and unexplained myocardial insufficiency.

Complications. Other than the many types of functional impairment already mentioned, infection is the only significant complication. *Tuberculosis* and *cryptococcosis* are more likely to occur in patients with sarcoidosis than in the general population and should be watched for carefully.

Treatment. Many patients with sarcoidosis are asymptomatic and require no therapy at all. The only agents that have any effect upon the lesions are the adrenal steroids and ACTH. Steroid therapy is indicated in patients with pulmonary, cardiac, or renal insufficiency, nervous system involvement, hypercalcuria, and active ocular disease as well as rapidly spreading lesions in the absence of specific disability.

A dose of 25 to 40 mg prednisolone daily or the equivalent of another steroid should be given. Response is slow and may not be evident for 3 to 6 weeks. Steroids should not be abandoned as ineffective until a trial of at least 8 to 12 weeks has been completed. If symptoms subside, dosage should be reduced gradually until a maintenance level is found. Patients should be continued on steroids indefinitely, with periodic attempts to reduce dosage or to discontinue the drug entirely.

Prognosis. The mortality in sarcoidosis is low, probably about 5 per cent. Residual disability is entirely dependent upon the sites involved and the amount of irreversible functional loss attributable to fibrosis. The most frequent cause of death is cor pulmonale secondary to pulmonary insufficiency.

With steroid therapy, patients are certainly better assured of comfort and activity, but it cannot yet be said that mortality or length of life have been affected by hormonal treatment.

REFERENCES

Cummings, M.M., and M. Michael, Jr.: "Sarcoidosis," Disease-a-Month Series, Chicago, Year Book Publishers, May, 1960.

James, D. G., and A. D. Thompson: The Course of Sarcoidosis and Its Modification by Treatment, Lancet, 2:1057, 1959.

Lofgren, S.: Primary Pulmonary Sarcoidosis, Acta Med. Scand., 145:424, 1953.

Longcope, W. T., and D. G. Freiman: A Study of Sarcoidosis, Medicine, 31:1, 1952.

Michael, M., Jr.: Epidemiology of Sarcoidosis, Ann. Internal Med., 45:151, 1956.

Scholz, D. A., and F. R. Keating, Jr.: Renal Insufficiency: Renal Calculi and Nephrocalcinosis in Sarcoidosis, Am. J. Med., 21:75, 1956.

Siltzbach, L. E., and J. C. Ehrlich: The Nickerson-Kveim Reaction in Sarcoidosis, Am. J. Med., 16:790, 1954.

229 INFECTIOUS MONONUCLEOSIS
M. M. Wintrobe

Definition. This disorder is of unknown etiology, usually benign and probably of infectious origin, which is characterized by irregular fever, sore throat, lymphadenopathy, and enlargement of the spleen, as well as by an absolute lymphocytosis made up of cells of a peculiar type. High concentrations of antibodies against sheep erythrocytes are demonstrable in the blood serum.

History. Since the designation "infectious mononucleosis" was first proposed by Sprunt and Evans in 1920, an ever-increasing number of cases has been observed and reported, especially since 1935. This is due, at least in part, to better recognition of the disease. Prior to 1920 a few sporadic cases had been observed. The relationship of epidemics in children and in adults described under the title of "glandular fever" to infectious mononucleosis is in doubt because in most instances appropriate serologic techniques were not used, and when they were, the results were indefinite and irregular.

Etiology and Pathogenesis. This is a disease of young people, including children, which has now been observed practically throughout the world. In the United States, infectious mononucleosis has been less frequent in Negroes than in white persons. It is a relatively common condition in interns, medical students, and nurses, but many cases among other persons undoubtedly pass unnoticed. The mild or nonspecific character of many of the symptoms may be responsible, or the fact that appropriate blood examinations have not been made. With increasing frequency, sporadic cases have been observed wherever young people live together, as in boarding schools, colleges, and military groups. Infectious mononucleosis is quite uncommon over the age of forty but has been encountered occasionally.

The etiology is unknown, although it is generally believed that the disease is infectious in nature. It is likely that individual susceptibility is low and that the causative agent is extremely labile. It has been stated that it is acquired by the intimate oral exchange of saliva. No clear instances of successful experimental transmission to human subjects have been reported and, in the main, experiments both in man and in animals have yielded little knowledge as to the nature of the causative agent.

Clinical Picture. In the absence of a demonstrable etiologic agent, some have assumed that the clinical manifestations of infectious mononucleosis are protean and have been willing to include under this diagnosis many cases of otherwise unexplained, self-limited febrile disorders with clinical and hematologic features somewhat resembling those of infectious mononucleosis, especially when occurring in young persons. Such a comprehensive approach does not seem to be justified. For the present, at least, it would seem better to restrict the diagnosis to cases in which the lymphocytes constitute more than 50 per cent of the leukocytes, "atypical" lymphocytes are present, and both of these features have been present for a period of at least 10 days. In addition, the titer of heterophil antibodies, after guinea pig absorption, should be at least 1:28. The clinical picture of the disorder, so defined, is quite a consistent one.

Three clinical stages can be identified, namely, (1) a prodromal period of 3 to 6 days, characterized by nonspecific features similar to those of other infections and during which diagnosis may be difficult; (2) a mid-stage of 4 to 20 days during which the full-blown disease presents itself; and (3) the stage of convalescence.

The incubation period is uncertain and may be as long as 4 to 7 weeks. The onset is gradual, but ultimately bilateral *lymph node enlargement* develops in practically all cases. The cervical glands are always affected, the axillary and inguinal frequently but not invariably. The glands are affected singly or in groups. Local heat, redness, or marked tenderness of the glands are conspicuously absent. The spleen is enlarged in at least 50 per cent of cases.

The most common *syndrome* is the *pharyngeal* (80 per cent of cases). Pharyngeal inflammation varies in intensity, but hyperplasia of pharyngeal lymphoid tissue is almost always present. The palatal arch and uvula often have a gelatinous appearance, but significant edema of the uvula is unusual. In some cases the throat presents the typical picture of follicular tonsillitis or that of Vincent's angina or of diphtheria. Stomatitis may be present.

The *fever* is of no characteristic type. It may be transient in degree, but in one-sixth to one-third of cases the temperature reaches a peak of 103 to 104° F, only occasionally higher. The temperature may rise in a remittent manner in the course of 4 to 8 days. A secondary rise after an initial drop to normal may accompany the onset of glandular swelling or sore throat.

A *typhoidal syndrome,* with fever, malaise, and headache predominating, is seen in 12 per cent of cases. The headache may be so severe as to suggest meningitis. Gastrointestinal symptoms are rare.

In about 8 per cent of cases *icterus* occurs and the picture of hepatitis is found. In the majority of cases, however, hepatitis without jaundice is present, as judged by liver function tests. The hepatic disease is usually mild.

Edema of the eyelids has been described in a third of the cases and a palatal enanthem in almost as many. The latter consists of 5 to 20 pinhead-sized red spots, usually at the junction of the soft and hard palates, which appear in crops, darken in about 48 hr, and disappear after 3 or 4 days. Cutaneous lesions are unusual except for faint erythema or, rarely, a maculopapular eruption. Petechial hemorrhages and purpura are encountered sometimes, and other hemorrhagic manifestations, such as epistaxis, may occur.

Other manifestations are rare. These include abdominal pain of a type to suggest acute appendicitis, possibly due to swelling of mesenteric nodes; cardiac and pulmonary manifestations, such as tachycardia, cyanosis, signs of pericarditis, transient T wave changes, and enlargement of mediastinal lymph nodes or pulmonary parenchymal changes; and a variety of neurologic manifestations. The last include headache, blurring of vision, even convulsions, stupor, coma, bradycardia, stiff neck, the Guillain-Barré syndrome, and encephalitis.

Convalescence is sometimes slow and may be associated with marked prostration. Recrudescences are very common. Relapse has occurred in about 6 per cent of cases. Recovery is the rule, but death has been observed in a few instances from such complications as rupture of the spleen, respiratory paralysis in association with nervous system involvement, pneumonia, edema of the glottis, and hemorrhage from a deep tonsillar ulceration.

Blood Picture. The leukocyte count is usually increased but, in the first week especially, there may be leukopenia due to granulocytopenia. The leukocytosis is usually moderate (10,000 to 15,000 cells per cu mm), but it may sometimes be very marked. It is due to an increase in lymphocytes, and these, in the main, are of a peculiar type: their nucleus may be oval, kidney-shaped, or slightly lobulated, and the cytoplasm is often somewhat basophilic and may be vacuolated or foamy in appearance. The nuclear chromatin is usually coarse and irregular, and nucleoli are rarely seen. These cells make up 60 per cent or more of all the leukocytes.

The characteristic changes in the leukocytes may appear as early as the second day of illness or as late as the twelfth day. They attain a peak by the seventh to tenth day and persist usually for 1 to 2 months.

Anemia is extremely rare, but several instances of hemolytic anemia complicating infectious mononucleosis have been reported. Thrombocytopenia is rare, but in a few cases the clinical picture resembled that of idiopathic thrombocytopenic purpura. The bone marrow reveals a slight myeloid hyperplasia and immaturity; there may be an increase in lymphocytes.

The serum characteristically contains agglutinins against sheep red cells in high titer (heterophil antibodies, Paul-Bunnell test, see Chap. 110). This has been observed, in different series and according to the diagnostic criteria of the authors, in 60 to 100 per cent of cases. The Paul-Bunnell test is actually nonspecific. Anti-sheep agglutinins are present in titers up to 1:28 in most normal persons and occasionally even in a titer of 1:56. In various infections a titer of 1:112 and occasionally of 1:224 may be seen. Persons receiving injections of horse serum and horse immune serum may develop titers as high as any seen in infectious mononucleosis. For these reasons it is generally considered that, in the presence of clinical and hematologic findings suggestive of infectious mononucleosis, only a titer of 1:224 or higher can be interpreted as confirming the diagnosis. When there is doubt, a differential test is required. This is based on the observation that heterophil antibodies in normal serum, in horse serum sensitization, and in a variety of infections can be absorbed completely by guinea pig kidney. On the other hand, anti-sheep agglutinins in infectious mononucleosis are never completely removed by treating the serum with guinea pig kidney although they are, as a rule, completely removed by beef red cells. The differential test is carried out by absorbing a portion of the patient's serum with guinea pig kidney and another portion with beef red cells. After this the absorbed specimens are tested for sheep red-cell agglutination.

In infectious mononucleosis, highest heterophil antibody titers are found usually during the second and third weeks of illness and, as a rule, positive reactions last 4 to 8 weeks. The titer bears no relation to the severity of the disease or the degree of lymphocytosis. The serologic test for syphilis may become transiently positive.

Renal function is rarely impaired, but albumin and red cells may be found in the *urine*. The *cerebrospinal fluid* pressure may be moderately elevated, and pleocytosis due to lymphocytes may be found.

Diagnosis. Glandular enlargement, sore throat, fever, the characteristic cells in the blood, and an increased titer of heterophil antibodies are a combination of findings which makes recognition of infectious mononucleosis easy in most instances. However, as discussed earlier, some have been willing to define infectious mononucleosis quite broadly. It can be admitted that, in the absence of an identifiable specific etiologic agent, there is room for differences of opinion regarding the diagnostic criteria upon which one should insist. However, it seems reasonable to require a minimum of 20 per cent lymphocytes of the characteristic type at the time of the fever peak and a positive heterophil antibody reaction. In the absence of a positive heterophil antibody test, it is difficult to maintain this diagnosis. The paradox of a positive heterophil antibody test unaccompanied by characteristic clinical and hematologic features of infectious mononucleosis can be explained by persistence of the antibodies from an earlier unrecognized attack and, in rare instances, by a resurgence of heterophil antibodies with another illness.

The above criteria should help to differentiate infectious mononucleosis from other infectious disorders. It may be added that certain symptoms are so unusual in infectious mononucleosis that their presence militates against the diagnosis, namely, nasal discharge or congestion, paroxysmal harassing cough, sputum, chest pain, joint pains, painful or extremely tender lymph nodes, watery diarrhea, and hematuria or dysuria.

Lymphocytosis, relative or absolute, may be encountered regularly or occasionally in a number of the diseases with which infectious mononucleosis may be confused on clinical grounds. Marked leukocytosis (40,000 cells per cu mm or even higher), chiefly due to the presence of small lymphocytes of normal appearance, characterizes a benign disorder, *acute infectious lymphocytosis,* which has been observed chiefly in children and is accompanied by only mild constitutional manifestations and no lymphadenopathy, splenomegaly, or positive heterophil agglutination reactions.

The clinical picture may be like that of serum sickness, a condition in which lymphocytes quite similar to those seen in infectious mononucleosis may be found and a positive heterophil antibody test may be obtained. The differential test is required to distinguish between the antibody reactions in infectious mononucleosis and the rise in titer produced by horse serum.

It is not rare for infectious mononucleosis to be confused with acute leukemia. Differentiation of the latter depends on the demonstration of very immature leukocytes ("blasts") in the blood or the bone marrow and the presence of anemia and thrombocytopenia, both of which are rare in infectious mononucleosis. The heterophil antibody test will be negative.

Treatment. There is no specific therapy. Sodium perborate mouth washes are recommended since Vincent's infection is frequently associated with infectious mononucleosis. From time to time many agents have been advocated, such as arsenicals, penicillin, the tetracyclines, chloroquine, and adrenocorticosteroid therapy, but such claims are difficult to evaluate. As a rule, without treatment, the irregular fever persists for 1 to 3 weeks, and subjective symptoms disappear in 2 to 4 weeks. *Relapses* are not uncommon and may be late, but recurrences are very rare. The positive heterophil antibody reaction may persist for as long as 5 or 6 months, rarely longer. In the rare instances of more than average severity, the corticosteroids may give symptomatic relief without harm resulting, provided that treatment is continued for only 5 to 10 days.

REFERENCES

Custer, R. P., and E. B. Smith: The Pathology of Infectious Mononucleosis, Blood, 3:830, 1948.

Davidsohn, I., K. Stern, and C. Kashiwagi: The Differential Test for Infectious Mononucleosis, Am. J. Clin. Pathol., 21:1101, 1951; J. Lab. Clin. Med., 45:561, 1955.

Gardner, H. T., and J. R. Paul: Infectious Mononucleosis at the New Haven Hospital, 1921–1946, Yale J. Biol. and Med., 19:839, 1947.

Hoagland, R. J.: Infectious Mononucleosis, Am. J. Med., 13:158, 1952; Ann. Internal Med., 43:1019, 1955; Am. J. Med. Sci., 232:252, 1956; *ibid.*, 240:21, 1960; Blood, 16:1045, 1960.

Wintrobe, M. M.: "Clinical Hematology," 5th ed., Philadelphia, Lea & Febiger, 1961.

230 FAMILIAL MEDITERRANEAN FEVER

Robert G. Petersdorf and Ivan L. Bennett, Jr.

Definition. Familial Mediterranean fever is an inherited disorder of unknown etiology characterized by recurrent episodes of fever, abdominal pain, chest pain, arthralgia, and rash, terminating in some instances in chronic renal failure secondary to amyloidosis. The illness has also been termed "benign paroxysmal peritonitis" and "periodic disease."

Epidemiology. Familial Mediterranean fever (FMF) occurs almost entirely in peoples originating in countries bordering on the coast of the Mediterranean—North Africa, Libya, Syria, Iraq, Iran, Armenia, Turkey, Spain, Italy, and Israel. Most patients have been Sephardic and Iraqui Jews (Jews who originated in this area, as opposed to Ashkenazi Jews most of whom stem from Eastern Europe) and Armenians. In the United States, the disease has been described in individuals of similar racial origin. The disease is frequent among siblings and rare among their antecedents. Consanguinity between parents of those affected is much higher than in the general population. These data indicate that the gene of FMF is inherited as a typical autosomal recessive trait. The ratio of affected males to females is approximately 3:2.

Etiology. The cause of FMF is not known. It is a genetically determined inborn error similar to Mediterranean anemia, sickle-cell disease, or congenital spherocytosis. No abnormal hemoglobins have been demonstrated. There is no evidence that FMF is an autoimmune or lipid storage disorder. Abnormal excretion of the amino acid, histidine, has been found in some patients. However, this has not been a consistent finding. Etiocholanolone (3α-hydroxyetiocholane-17-one), a steroid hormone metabolite which has been found to be pyrogenic for man, may be implicated in the pathogenesis of FMF (see below).

Pathology. Biopsy of liver, spleen, bone marrow, lymph node, skin, and muscle have not revealed any lesions. Patients dying from renal failure have had amyloidosis involving the kidneys and other viscera.

Manifestations. Familial Mediterranean fever begins prior to the age of ten in 70 per cent of patients, and 95 per cent have their first attack before they are twenty years old. Episodes of fever, abdominal pain, chest pain, arthralgia, and erysipeloid rashes comprise the syndrome. An attack lasts 12 hr to 3 days; occasionally symptoms persist for 7 to 10 days. They recur at varying intervals; some patients are free of symptoms as long as a year, others have attacks once a week.

Fever. Fever is present in 100 per cent of patients and is the *sine qua non* for the diagnosis. The temperature ranges between 100.4 and 104°F, rises steeply, and usually falls abruptly. Pyrexia generally lasts 12 to 24 hr. In most instances the temperature is normal between attacks, but a few patients, particularly those with joint involvement, maintain low-grade pyrexia.

Abdominal Pain. Attacks of abdominal pain occur in 90 per cent of patients and are the presenting symptom in 40 per cent. The pain may be anywhere in the abdomen and may radiate to the shoulders, chest, or back. The abdominal wall may be doughy or rigid, with rebound tenderness, guarding, and absent bowel sounds—the hallmarks of acute peritonitis. It is not surprising, therefore, that many of these patients have been subjected to laparotomy. Vomiting frequently accompanies the attacks, but disturbances in lower bowel function are unusual.

Chest Pain. Some 80 per cent of patients have chest pain with or without concomitant abdominal pain. The pain is stabbing, knifelike, and pleuritic in character. It often radiates to the shoulder. Tachypnea is common, but dyspnea and cyanosis do not occur. Chest x-rays are normal except for occasional small accumulations of fluid in the costophrenic angles.

Arthralgia. Four-fifths of patients with FMF have involvement of the joints. Attacks of arthralgia vary widely in duration, intensity, and location. The ankle is most frequently involved, with other joints of the lower extremities next in importance. The joints are tender, and there is redness and swelling. As a rule, several joints are affected. Each episode lasts 1 to 3 days, and it is not unusual to observe mild fever between attacks. Most patients have no lasting functional impairment although, rarely, chronic deformities develop.

Cutaneous Manifestations. Almost 50 per cent of patients have some type of rash in association with the febrile attack. Usually this takes the form of well-demarcated, slightly raised, erythematous patches over the ankle joints, dorsums of the feet, and calves. As with the other components of FMF, the rash is evanescent.

Renal Involvement. About one-third of patients with FMF have proteinuria, and in about one-half of these excretion of protein in the urine exceeds 2.0 Gm per day. Several patients have developed the full-blown nephrotic syndrome—edema, hypoalbuminemia, and hypercholesterolemia—and at necropsy have shown classical amyloidosis.

The cardiovascular, central nervous, endocrine, and reticuloendothelial systems remain normal in FMF. Splenomegaly occurs in some patients, but since the majority also live in areas with a high prevalence of malaria and thalassemia, the significance of splenic enlargement is difficult to assess.

Laboratory Findings. Since the cause of FMF remains an enigma, it is not surprising that the patients have been subjected to extensive laboratory investigation. Aside from marked elevation in the sedimentation rate, leukocytosis with counts ranging between 10,000 and 20,000 cells per cu mm during attacks (but not during asymptomatic intervals), hyperfibrinogenemia, a questionable increase in uroporphyrins, and sporadic increase in spherocytes in the blood, laboratory data are entirely normal. These include the hemogram, platelets, liver function tests, serum proteins and lipids, circulating hormone levels, and amino acid excretion patterns, except for histidine. Red cell fragility is normal, Coombs test is negative, and porphobilinogen absent. As has been mentioned, there are no significant microscopic lesions in any organ referable to FMF per se.

Diagnosis. The diagnosis of FMF is not difficult in the classical case occurring in an Armenian or a Jew with a positive family history and with recurrent attacks and relative well-being in the intervals between febrile episodes. The most difficult problem is presented by patients with signs of acute peritonitis, and many have had repeated exploratory operations. It is not uncommon for some of these patients who are familiar with their symptom complex to refuse surgical intervention. The differential diagnosis of fever should include malaria, relapsing fever, brucellosis, Hodgkin's disease and other lymphomas, and collagen-vascular diseases. However, the marked chronicity of FMF and lack of symptoms between bouts of pyrexia should distinguish FMF from other subacute and chronic febrile illnesses.

Articular involvement raises the question of rheumatoid disease, which can be ruled out by absence of positive sheep cell, latex, or bentonite flocculation tests and synovial biopsy.

The relationship of FMF to two other entities, "periodic disease" and "etiocholanolone fever," is of interest.

Periodic Disease. In 1946 Reimann described a group of disorders characterized by short, regular episodes of a symptom complex which recurred over many years without affecting the patients' general health. He named these according to their outstanding clinical features such as periodic fever, periodic abdominalgia, periodic arthralgia, periodic neutropenia, periodic purpura, and periodic edema. The emphasis on the regular occurrence of these attacks is unfortunate because, in actuality, the majority of episodes in Reimann's patients occurred at irregular intervals, much like those in FMF. Furthermore, many patients described as having "periodic disease" clearly have had FMF. Others have had angioneurotic edema, Henoch-Schönlein (anaphylactoid) purpura, and a peculiar disorder, cyclic granulocytopenia, characterized by regularly recurring neutrophilic granulocytopenia, accompanied by anorexia, malaise, fever, and secondary infections such as stomatitis, pharyngitis, and pneumonitis. The last three disorders appear to be far removed clinically from the well-defined picture of FMF. The various periodic disorders were ascribed to some underlying occult rhythm, perhaps a neurovascular disturbance. Since the cognomen "periodic disease" obviously represents several nosologic entities, there seems little to be gained by its use. "Benign paroxysmal peritonitis" merely refers to the abdominal aspects of FMF. Since it is not a benign process, the term is inaccurate and should be discarded.

Etiocholanolone Fever. In 1958 Bondy and his colleagues reported two patients with recurrent attacks of fever, abdominal pain, arthralgia, and leukocytosis whose main urinary steroid breakdown product during the febrile attack was etiocholanolone and who, at the same time, had unconjugated etiocholanolone in the plasma. This observation was of particular interest since it had previously been shown that a few specific steroids, notably etiocholanolone, were capable of producing fever when injected into man. It is postulated that these patients have one or several abnormal pathways for the metabolic breakdown of endogenous steroid products. This results in the intermittent appearance of etiocholanolone in the bloodstream followed by elevation in temperature. In contrast to etiocholanolone fever, patients with FMF have not been found to have abnormalities in steroid metabolism. Furthermore, the racial predisposition, amyloidosis, and histidinuria found in FMF are absent in etiocholanolone fever. Finally, some patients with this illness improve following administration of cortisone, which has been consistently ineffective in FMF. Despite these differences, some patients with etiocholanolone fever were of Jewish extraction, and one had a family history which was positive for similar febrile attacks. The relationship of etiocholanolone to FMF needs further clarification.

Treatment. A plethora of therapeutic regimens including antibiotics, arsenicals, and adrenal steroids has been tried in the treatment of FMF without avail. There is some indication that ACTH and cortisone enhance the deposition of amyloid and are contraindicated. A striking reduction in the number of attacks of FMF has been described following institution of a low-fat diet and exacerbations followed dietary indiscretions, particularly ingestion of foods high in fat. Whether fat per se or some other chemical moieties in fatty foods are responsible is not known at present.

Prognosis. Familial Mediterranean fever is a chronic disease, persisting throughout life. The only known ameliorating factor is pregnancy, and complete remissions are seen in gravid women. Since the disease appears predominantly in the young and middle-aged, it is conceivable that recovery takes place with advancing age. It is more likely, however, that the majority of patients die of renal failure and that the migratory habits of many patients with this disease have prevented adequate follow-up studies.

REFERENCES

Bondy, P. K., G. L. Cohn, W. Hermann, and K. Crispell: The Possible Relationship of Etiocholanolone to Periodic Fever, Yale J. Biol. Med., 30:395, 1958.

——, —— and C. Castiglione: Etiocholanolone Fever: A Clinical Entity, Trans. Assoc. Am. Physicians, 73:186, 1960.

Heller, H., E. Sohar, and L. Sherf: Familial Mediterranean Fever, A.M.A. Arch. Internal Med., 102: 50, 1958.

——, et al.: Amyloidosis in Familial Mediterranean Fever, A.M.A. Arch. Int. Med., 107:539, 1961.

Kappas, A., L. Hellman, D. K. Fukushima, and T. F. Gallagher: The Pyrogenic Effect of Etiocholanolone, J. Clin. Endocrinol. and Metabolism, 17: 451, 1957.

Lawrence, J. S., and S. M. Mellinkoff: Familial Mediterranean Fever, Trans. Assoc. Am. Physicians, 72:111, 1959.

Mellinkoff, S. M., A. D. Schwable, and J. S. Lawrence: A Dietary Treatment for Familial Mediterranean Fever, Trans. Assoc. Am. Physicians, 73: 197, 1960.

Reimann, H. A.: Periodic Disease, Arch. Internal Med., 92:494, 1943.

Sohar, E., et al.: Genetics of Familial Mediterranean Fever (FMF), A.M.A. Arch. Int. Med., 107:529, 1961.

231 MIDLINE GRANULOMA
Lawrence E. Shulman

Definition. This peculiar condition, also known as *lethal midline granuloma* or *granuloma gangraenescens*, is characterized by progressive destruction of the soft tissues and bony structures of the face, terminating almost invariably in death after several months or a few years of illness. It occurs in young adults and the middle-aged and seems to be more common in men. The first case was described by McBride in 1897 and since then more than 100 cases have been reported, mostly in the otolaryngologic literature.

Etiology and Pathology. Not only is the etiology of midline granuloma unknown, but the category of disease in which it belongs is uncertain. There is disagreement as to whether it is primarily (1) infectious, (2) vascular or allergic, or (3) neoplastic. Only a few complete autopsy studies have been reported. In half of them, lesions have been found in skin, lungs, and mesenteric lymph nodes as well as the face.

Histologically, the lesions of midline granuloma vary from case to case and also from one area to another in the individual case. The most common finding in the facial lesion is chronic inflammation. In the face and elsewhere there are focal areas of necrosis and necrotic small blood vessels, often containing granular thrombi, suggesting that the process is primarily vascular. The vascular lesions, however, differ from those of polyarteritis nodosa in that the characteristic inflammatory reaction of a true vasculitis is absent. Some areas contain large numbers of cells of varying sizes with large, pale, multilobulated nuclei, simulating Hodgkin's disease and mycosis fungoides. In other areas, hyperchromatic nuclei and numerous mitotic figures resemble those seen in undifferentiated tumors.

Clinical Features. Midline granuloma begins with a prodromal period of months to years of nasal obstruction and discharge, at first mucoid and later purulent. During this time, the patient is usually thought to have allergic rhinitis or sinusitis. Progressive inflammation and ulceration follow. The first ulcerations are found in the nasal septum, the mucosa or skin of the alae nasi, or the center of the palate. The lesions invade underlying cartilage and bone, giving rise to septal or palatal perforations. The condition spreads by local extension to involve the rest of the nose, paranasal sinuses, eyes, mouth, pharynx, and larynx. Eventually, the structures of the midface are totally destroyed by erosion. Gradually, the functions of sight, speech, and ventilation are impaired or lost. The end result is the formation of a large cavity, bounded above by the frontal bone and superior aspect of the orbits and below by the mandible, which is never affected.

During periods of activity, and especially preterminally, the patient becomes febrile. Usually the fever does not respond to appropriate chemotherapy for the secondary bacterial infection which is almost always present. Moreover, even in the presence of obvious pyogenic infection, the patient often fails to develop leukocytosis and during the later stages may become chronically leukopenic. Another curious feature is the absence of cervical lymphadenopathy during periods of active inflammation and progression of the disease. A few patients show red, raised, indurated areas on the skin of the legs and abdomen, resembling those of erythema nodosum clinically and histologically. There is no anemia, and the bone marrow and serum proteins are normal. Microbiologic investigations have failed consistently to detect a specific virus, bacterium, or fungus.

The course of the disease varies greatly; some cases last for more than a decade with long periods of quiescence and others are fulminant, ending fatally after a few months. Death usually results from meningitis, pneumonia, inanition, or massive hemorrhage.

Diagnosis. During the early phases of midline granuloma it is important to rule out several specific nasal and facial conditions, many of which are treatable. These include: leprosy, syphilis, yaws (gangosa), tuberculosis (lupus vulgaris), glanders, leishmaniasis, blastomycosis, and coccidioidomycosis, chromate poisoning; lupus erythematosus; also lymphomas, mycosis fungoides, and other malignant tumors. Midline granuloma is differentiated from Wegener's granulomatosis (p. 1900) by the absence of generalized polyarteritis nodosa and glomerulonephritis. Noma is readily distinguished by its being largely restricted to children, involving the cheeks and mouth, but not the nose.

Treatment. No effective therapy for midline granuloma has yet been found. The basic disease progresses despite administration of antibiotics or adrenocortical steroids. A few early reports of benefit following radiotherapy have not been substantiated by further experience, and nitrogen mustards have failed. Radical surgical excision is no more effective than conservative debridement. Various prostheses designed to maintain the integrity of the normal facial passages are helpful both functionally and cosmetically.

REFERENCES

Edgerton, M. T., and J. D. Desprez: Lethal Midline Granuloma of the Face, Brit. J. Plastic Surg., 9: 200, 1956.

McBride, P.: Photographs of a Case of Rapid Destruction of the Nose and Face, J. Laryngol. and Otol., 12:64, 1897.

Pardo-Castello, V., F. L. Blanco, and R. Rivera del Sol: Granuloma Gangraenescens, Southern Med. J., 46:149, 1953.

Spear, G. S., and W. G. Walker, Jr.: Lethal Midline Granuloma (Granuloma Gangraenescens) at Autopsy, Bull. Johns Hopkins Hosp. 99:313, 1956.

Stewart, P.: Progressive Lethal Granulomatous Destruction of the Nose, J. Laryngol. and Otol., 48:657, 1933.

PART SEVEN

Reactions to Antigens and Other Foreign Substances

Section 1: Reactions to Antigens and Other Foreign Substances

232 ALLERGY AND ITS MANIFESTATIONS IN MAN

Leighton E. Cluff

Definition. Allergy designates the adverse reactions, and immunity designates the protective reactions, observed upon exposure to a foreign substance (antigen) following an initial sensitizing or immunizing contact.

History. Acceleration of the local reaction to cowpox vaccination in immune persons was described by Jenner in 1801, and this was the first recognized immunologic reaction in man. Koch described the hypersensitivity reaction to tuberculin in individuals with tuberculosis in 1890. Severe systemic reactions, occasionally leading to death, following repeated intravenous inoculations of foreign protein into animals were described by Portier and Richet and by Theobald Smith in 1902. This phenomenon was called *anaphylaxis*, the antithesis of prophylaxis or protection. Rosenau and Anderson showed that anaphylaxis was elicited only by the specific *antigen* to which an animal had been sensitized. Von Pirquet coined the term allergy in 1907 to describe the altered reaction and clinical manifestations observed following exposure of human beings to foreign proteins.

Etiology and Pathogenesis. Allergy in man and in experimental animals may be of two types: (1) reactions associated with serum antibody, and (2) reactions unrelated to serum antibody. The allergic reaction unassociated with serum antibody is often referred to as *delayed hypersensitivity,* while the reaction related to serum antibody is referred to as *immediate hypersensitivity.*

Allergic reactions in man attributed to serum antibody primarily involve smooth muscle and blood vessels, as illustrated by hay fever, asthma, anaphylaxis, urticaria, and periarteritis nodosa, resulting in increased vascular permeability, edema, vasculitis, and probably smooth muscle contraction. Anaphylaxis, serum sickness, arteritis, and glomerulonephritis can be induced in experimental animals by injection of foreign protein or serum. These allergic reactions appear when antigen is in excess of serum antibody and soluble antigen-antibody complexes are present in the circulation, illustrating the important quantitative relationship between antigen and antibody in the production of disease.

Delayed hypersensitivity reactions not related to serum antibody may not be primarily associated with vascular lesions, but are characterized by perivenous inflammation with mononuclear cells, and tissue injury possibly results from effects other than vasculitis and smooth muscle contraction. Allergic reactions to bacterial antigens following infection, such as the tuberculin reaction, contact dermatitis, and possibly others are attributed to delayed hypersensitivity.

The relationship of immediate hypersensitivity reactions to serum antibody is illustrated by passive transfer of the allergic state with serum. Delayed hypersensitivity reactions, on the other hand, can be transferred only with mononuclear cells from the allergic individual.

Most antigens of organic substances, including pollen, dust, and dander which are common causes of allergy in man, are proteins. Other substances capable of inducing an immunologic response, however, may be polysaccharides, chemicals such as drugs, and possibly lipids. From the classical studies of Landsteiner, Chase, and others, it is likely that chemicals or drugs, and frequently polysaccharides, become antigenic only when complexed to protein. In this way the chemical or polysaccharide serves as an antigenic determinant or *hapten.*

Although the character of an antigen may condition the type of immunologic response induced, the route of inoculation and the conjugated state of the hapten are of greater importance. For example, injection intradermally of a chemical such as picryl chloride into man or experimental animals results in the development of nonantibody-mediated or delayed hypersensitivity, whereas, injection of the same chemical intravenously results in development of antibody-mediated or immediate hypersensitivity.

Antibodies specifically associated with certain allergic diseases in man, such as hay fever, have features which distinguish them from antibodies of other types and frequently are referred to as *reagins.* Reagins are not detectable by the usual in vitro immunologic procedures (precipitation and complement fixation with antigen), they are less resistant to heat than other antibodies, and they are firmly fixed in the skin at the site of inoculation. The presence of a reagin in serum correlates with the wheal and erythema elicited by intracutaneous injection of antigen, but bears no constant relationship to the presence or the severity of clinically significant allergic disease. Certain individuals have a particular propensity for developing reaginic antibodies, and as illustrated by immunization with diphtheria toxoid, individuals with a personal or family history of allergic disease, such as hay fever, urticaria, and asthma, develop "skin sensitizing" or reagin antibodies to diphtheria toxoid with greater frequency than persons without such a history.

There are important quantitative relationships between antigen and antibody that are required for the elicitation of a hypersensitivity reaction. For example, an Arthus skin reaction, characterized by acute inflammation and hemorrhagic necrosis, regularly can be induced only when the intracutaneous dose of antigen is specifically related to the amount of antibody an animal possesses. Furthermore, as mentioned previously, anaphylaxis and serum sickness are elicitable most readily only when antigen is in excess of the available specific antibody.

Serum complement often is involved in the interaction of antigen and serum antibody, and it is probable that complement plays an essential role in some allergic reactions. Allergic reactions associated with serum antibody are commonly characterized by the elaboration of histamine, proteolytic enzyme activity, and changes in blood potassium, adenosine, serotonin, heparin, "slow reacting substances," and other substances. None of these biochemical changes has led to a satisfactory understanding of the mechanisms of allergic disease in human beings, but the liberation of histamine probably accounts for the wheal and flare reaction of reaginic skin reactions and may account for some of the effects of hay fever, as these reactions can be reproduced with histamine and are alleviated with histamine inhibitors.

The ability to produce reagin, as indicated above, is probably genetically determined, although this has not been satisfactorily defined. In addition, selective animal breeding can result in evolution of strains with varying immunologic responsiveness. Congenital agammaglobulinemia characterized by a defect in serum antibody synthesis is a gross example of varying immunologic responsiveness in the human being. There are, in addition, acquired diseases that may significantly alter immunologic responsiveness, illustrated by the failure to develop delayed hypersensitivity in sarcoidosis and Hodgkin's disease. Furthermore, patients with lymphatic leukemia are often defective in the ability to produce serum antibody, as also are patients with multiple myeloma. Experimentally, it has been shown that exposure to ionizing radiation can impair immunologic responsiveness.

Allergy, itself, is not inherited, but the existence of a *familial predisposition* to its development seems firmly established, and familial allergic disease is commonly called *atopic*. About 50 per cent of patients with hay fever or asthma will have a family history of allergic disease, as opposed to only 15 per cent of the remaining population.

The characteristics of antigen, antibodies, and the immunologic mechanisms probably associated with certain allergic diseases of man are listed in Table 232-1.

Hyposensitization or *desensitization* has been the principal means of specific treatment in allergic disease of man. The immunologic mechanisms involved in specific reduction of hypersensitivity reactions have been extensively studied but still are poorly understood. In experimental animals and in the human being, desensitization can be accomplished by two principal methods of antigen administration: (1) by repeated and frequent injection of small but increasing doses of antigen over an extended period of time, and (2) by injection of a large dose of antigen in one inoculation or several doses over a short period of time. The first method is the one commonly used in desensitization of patients with allergic diseases such as hay fever and asthma, while the second is usually employed in desensitization of patients to horse serum.

Injection of a large but sublethal dose of antigen into the sensitive individual is followed by decrease or disappearance of specific serum antibody, and the accompanying desensitization persists as long as the serum antibody is suppressed. When the serum antibody reappears, however, sensitivity to the antigen reappears.

Repeated and frequent injection of antigen into the sensitive individual may not result in a decrease but may result in a rise in serum antibody levels. It has been suggested that one possible explanation for desensitization accomplished in this way is a change in the quantitative relationships between level of antibody and dose of antigen required to elicit a hypersensitive reaction. In other words, as the antibody titer rises, larger amounts of antigen would be required to elicit a hypersensitivity reaction, and there is decreasing reactivity to doses of antigen that were previously harmful.

From the studies of Cooke and Loveless it seems clear that in atopic or reaginic disease there may be an alternative explanation for desensitization in man accomplished by repeated injections of small doses of antigen. Following *parenteral* injections of pollen antigens into the sensitive or normal person, an antibody (*blocking antibody*) may develop that can block the reaction of antigen with reagin. The

Table 232-1. IMMUNOLOGIC MECHANISMS OF ALLERGIC REACTIONS

	Serum antibody		No serum antibody
	I ("Classical")	II (Reagin)	III
Clinical types:			
Serum sickness	+	0	0
Anaphylaxis (insect, drug infection)	+	+	0
Hay fever	0	+	0
Asthma	±	+	?
Urticaria	±	+	0
Contact dermatitis	0	0	+
Immunologic (drug) thrombopenia	+	0	0
Immunologic (drug) leukopenia	+	0	0
Immunologic (drug) hemolytic anemia	+	0	0
Chronic (Hashimoto's) thyroiditis	±	0	±
Sympathetic ophthalmia	?	0	±
Lenticular phacoanaphylactica	±	0	±
Homograft rejection	±	0	+
Allergic encephalomyelitis	0	0	+
Periarteritis nodosa	+?	0	0
Systemic lupus erythematosus	±	0	±
Usual requirements for sensitization:			
Infection, skin contact	0	0	+
Parenteral contact (not bacteria)	+	±	0
Inhalation (not bacteria)	+	+	0
Characteristics of serum antibody:			
Complement fixation	+	0	
Heat labile	0	+	
Skin fixation	0	+	
Placental transfer	+	0	
Familial	0?	+	
Transferable with serum	+	+	
Precipitating with antigen	+	0	
Nonprecipitating with antigen	+	+	
Passive transfer with cells (mononuclear)	±	?	+
Reaction site:			
Blood vessels	+	+	0
Smooth muscles	+	+	0
Extravascular cells	0	0	+

±—inconclusive evidence; ?—unknown.

"blocking" antibody is heat stable and does not become fixed in the skin at the site of injection, distinguishing it from reagin. Reduction in sensitivity by repeated injection of small doses of antigens, whether attributable to increased levels of serum antibody or appearance of blocking antibody, may persist for a very limited period of time.

Nonspecific desensitization or suppression of allergic reactions can be accomplished with a variety of drugs and other substances. For example, adrenal cortical steroids can suppress the inflammation associated with cellular hypersensitivity but are less effective in suppressing most reactions in experimental animals mediated by serum antibody. In this respect, it is of interest that adrenal steroids have such a profound effect in suppressing the symptoms of hay fever, urticaria, and serum sickness which are probably mediated by serum antibody. Antihistamines, bacterial endotoxin, and many other substances also will reduce many experimental and clinical allergic reactions.

HAY FEVER

Definition. *Hay fever* is characterized by sneezing, rhinorrhea, itching of the eyes, and lacrimation. It is most commonly attributed to pollen antigens in the air and, therefore, occurs during particular seasons of the year. *Allergic rhinitis* is not necessarily seasonal and can develop upon exposure to airborne antigens other than pollen. *Vasomotor rhinitis* designates perennial allergic rhinitis as well as other nasal diseases that may not be allergic but are characterized by symptoms resembling hay fever.

Etiology. The immunologic mechanisms associated with hay fever, characterized by the presence of serum reagin, familial history of allergic disease, and wheal and erythema reactions in the skin following injection of specific antigen, have been described. Of particular importance and interest in hay fever are the pollens which serve to induce the immunologic response and elicit the hypersensitivity reaction responsible for producing rhinitis. Plants which depend on the wind for cross-pollination are common sources of antigens responsible for hay fever. Plants that are pollinated by insects, including most flowering plants such as roses and goldenrod, are not important causes of hay fever.

Ragweed pollen is the principal offender responsible for hay fever in the United States. It is prevalent in the central, eastern, and southeastern part of the country, virtually absent in the northwest, and west of the Rocky Mountain states, and of little importance in the southwest. Ordinarily, ragweed pollinates between the first of August and the end of October, and early fall is the most likely season for a patient to experience symptoms of ragweed hay fever.

Grass, weed, and tree pollens also are important causes of hay fever in this country. In the northern half of the country, grasses pollinate from May to July, while in the south, grass may pollinate throughout the year.

Although the time of year when trees pollinate may vary, they ordinarily do so in early spring, and earlier in the south than in the north.

Most pollen particles are about 25 to 40 μ in diameter and, therefore, settle promptly from the air, varying, of course, with wind velocity. The settling properties of airborne pollen are used for crude estimations of the "pollen count" in the air by collecting and enumerating particles on a greased glass slide. There is an approximate but regular correlation between the pollen count and the frequency of occurrence and severity of hay fever in the exposed population.

The relatively large size of pollen particles is of importance in considering the pathogenesis of hay fever. Most particles the size of pollen suspended in the air will be impinged and deposited within the nose during inhalation. Very few if any of the particles would be expected to reach the terminal bronchioles.

Wind velocity, humidity, temperature, time of day, and other meteorologic conditions undoubtedly influence the aerodynamics of pollen and are of importance in explaining the variations in severity of hay fever with changing climatic conditions. For example, rain causes a sharp decrease in the concentration of large particles, including pollen, in the air, although it may not affect the concentration of airborne particles less than 5 μ in size.

Pollen particles from plants, grasses, or trees of varying types can be differentiated by microscopic examination, enabling one to define precisely the airborne pollens likely to be responsible for hay fever.

Other airborne antigenic particles have been incriminated in the etiology of perennial allergic rhinitis, including material from feathers, dust, animal danders, facial powders, fungus or molds, clothing, and food particles disseminated during cooking.

The specific antigenic determinants in pollen, dust, and other airborne particles responsible for allergic rhinitis have not been precisely characterized.

There is evidence suggesting that the nasal mucosa of the patient with hay fever or allergic rhinitis is more susceptible to the inflammatory effects of inhaled irritants than is the nasal mucosa of normal persons. Furthermore, recent studies in volunteers indicate that persons with allergic rhinitis are more susceptible to infection by respiratory viruses than are normal persons. This enhanced reactivity of the nasal mucosa to a variety of stimuli also may explain the effects of emotional disturbances in exaggerating and possibly initiating symptoms of rhinitis in the allergic individual.

Manifestations. Pruritus about the eyes, nose, throat, and mouth, nasal discharge, sneezing, and lacrimation are the characteristic features of hay fever or allergic rhinitis. Particularly troublesome to the patient is occlusion of the nasal airway, making breathing difficult and often causing insomnia. Symptoms vary in severity from day to day and from one patient to another. This variability in the symptoms of hay fever can be explained partly by changing concentration of airborne antigens, but the variability between patients is not always easily understood.

The nasal mucosa usually is pale and edematous, but may appear hyperemic if the disease persists. The conjunctiva and the skin about the eyes, nose, and occasionally the mouth often are reddened. Microscopic examination of the nasal secretions may show many eosinophils.

Occlusion of the nasal passages by swelling of the turbinates and mucous membranes may result in obstruction of the sinus ostia or the Eustachian tube, and infection of the sinuses and middle ear is a relatively common complication of perennial allergic rhinitis but uncommon in seasonal hay fever. In addition, infection of the sinuses or nose in patients with allergic rhinitis results in formation of *polyps* of the nasal mucosa. These polyps can further obstruct the nasal passages and cause more severe symptoms and exaggerate infection. It is unusual to observe nasal polyps in the absence of nasal or paranasal infection. When sinusitis develops in the patient with allergic rhinitis, polyps may form also in the sinuses; these are recognizable radiologically.

Many persons with hay fever or allergic rhinitis subsequently may develop asthma. Retrobulbar neuritis, laryngeal edema with hoarseness, angioedema, urticaria, and other allergic illnesses occasionally accompany allergic rhinitis.

Diagnosis. Symptoms resembling those of allergic rhinitis or hay fever can occur in other situations where allergy cannot be incriminated. It is a common experience, for example, to develop sneezing, watery nasal discharge, and lacrimation upon exposure to an atmosphere heavily contaminated with smoke, dust, or other irritants. Similarly, these same symptoms often herald the onset of a viral upper respiratory tract infection. It is important to remember that the symptoms of hay fever are attributable to nonsuppurative inflammation of the nasal mucosa, and any situation resulting in inflammation of the nose can produce an illness often indistinguishable from allergic rhinitis. In addition, the nasal mucosa of the patient with allergic rhinitis is much more susceptible to the inflammatory effects of irritants, and exposure to irritants can result in nasal symptoms that ordinarily would not occur in normal persons. Ingestion of alcoholic beverages and emotional stimuli may also produce hyperemia of the nasal mucous membranes, exaggerating the symptoms of allergic rhinitis. *Polycythemia vera* may occasionally be recognized initially because of nasal and conjunctival hyperemia, resulting in symptoms resembling hay fever.

The pale and edematous appearance of the nasal mucosa often is helpful in distinguishing allergic rhinitis or hay fever from other conditions. In addition, the presence of nasal polyps is characteristic of allergic nasal disease, although indicative of coexistent infection in the nose or sinuses.

Of great importance in the diagnosis of hay fever is its seasonal occurrence, coinciding with pollination of weeds, grasses, or trees. The nonseasonal character of perennial allergic rhinitis makes it less readily recognizable. Examination of nasal secretions for eosinophils, however, is often helpful. Blood eosinophilia is also occasionally found in patients with allergic rhinitis.

Skin Tests. Approximately 25 per cent of the normal population will have wheal and erythema skin reactions when tests are made by the intracutaneous inoculation of common airborne antigens. Not all these persons with positive skin test reactions, however, have allergic rhinitis or hay fever. Nevertheless, individuals with serum reagin de-monstrable by skin testing are more likely to develop allergic respiratory disease than are persons without such positive reactions. Commonly, it is found that the allergic patient will have positive skin reactions to many antigens even though it may not be possible specifically to incriminate any one of them as responsible for the production of symptoms of allergic disease. Therefore, skin tests with antigens potentially capable of causing allergic rhinitis or hay fever are of greatest value in detecting the presence of an allergic propensity rather than detection of the specific antigen responsible for the patient's symptoms. Only by careful correlation of the skin test reactivity with the environmental circumstances when the patient develops symptoms of rhinitis is it possible to delineate the incriminated antigen. Therefore, antigens for skin testing should be selected from those probably responsible as determined by a careful historical analysis of the situations when the patient experiences his symptoms.

Skin tests usually are performed with crude aqueous extracts of dried pollen, dust, foods, animal fur, insects, and other substances considered potentially capable of causing allergies. These antigen extracts are commercially available. The potency of the extracts may vary considerably, and a number of criteria have been devised for standardization. None of these methods of standardization, however, is very reliable, as the extracts are crude and the measurement of specific antigen in the extracts at present is impossible. The techniques for standardization are: (1) the pollen unit of Noon, representing the extract from 1 μg of pollen; (2) weight by volume and dilution method, representing dilutions of a concentrated extract; (3) protein nitrogen unit, 1 unit representing 0.01 μg of chemically determined protein nitrogen in the extract. None of these systems is satisfactory but may facilitate standardization of extract potency in use in a single clinic or from a single source.

Skin tests are done by application of a drop of antigen to a skin scratch or by intradermal inoculation of 0.01 to 0.02 ml to produce a small welt in the skin. In the beginning, very dilute extract should be used for skin testing as large amounts of antigen may produce severe systemic reactions in the allergic patient. The concentration of antigen may be gradually increased until one is satisfied that the patient has a negative reaction. Ordinarily, it is unwise repeatedly to test a patient on the same day or to test with a large number of extracts at one time. Positive reactions to extracts of antigens responsible for hay fever or allergic rhinitis usually are apparent within 15 to 20 min and are characterized by wheal and erythema and by local pruritis. When large doses of extract are given, symptoms of hay fever or even a generalized reaction may be produced. Occasionally, reactions may be delayed and result in erythema and induration at the site of injection at 24 hr. The importance of such reactions in diagnosis of allergic respiratory disease is not clear. The scratch skin test ordinarily is safer than the intradermal injection of antigen, although the latter is more reliable and reproducible.

Extracts of foods are available for skin testing, but their use should be limited as it is preferable to diagnose allergy to foods by anamnesis and by elimination diets.

Extracts of bacteria and killed bacterial vaccines for skin testing are useful, of course, in the diagnosis of certain types of infection, but the relationship of hypersensitivity to respiratory microorganisms in the production of allergic rhinitis is far from clear. Until this relationship is better defined, it is impossible to place any diagnostic significance upon positive reactions in the diagnosis of allergic respiratory disease. Cultural identification of bacteria in the respiratory tract potentially responsible for infection is of greater use than skin testing.

When it is undesirable to perform skin tests in a patient, such as in young children or persons with generalized skin disease, passive transfer of the patient's serum to normal recipients may be performed (Prausnitz-Küstner or P-K). Ordinarily, 0.05 to 0.1 ml of the patient's serum is injected intradermally into the recipient, and 24 hr later normal skin and sites injected with serum are tested with the antigenic extracts.

Epinephrine and ephedrine greatly reduce the wheal and erythema response to intradermally injected antigen, as do large doses of antihistamines. These drugs should not be administered to the patient, therefore, prior to skin testing. Adrenal cortical steroids have little effect upon these reactions.

Although diagnostic testing with antigen extracts of patients with allergic disease is useful in determining the degree of skin hypersensitivity and the variety of antigens to which the patient may have demonstrable serum reagin, *this technique is not adequate by itself for identifying the agent responsible for allergic symptoms.* Skin testing is only one aspect of the diagnostic methodology and must be weighed in relationship to information derived from history, physical examination, and a careful definition of the environmental circumstances associated with development of symptoms of illness.

Therapy. *Specific Treatment.* Elimination of the offending antigen from the patient's environment is the most effective means of controlling allergic disease. This is not always easy, even when the antigen is known. If it is determined that dander from dogs or cats is responsible, for example, then animals should be avoided. When feathers are found to be responsible for allergic symptoms, a feather pillow should be replaced by one of foam rubber. Air filtration is often useful in controlling symptoms due to airborne pollens, but occasionally it may be necessary to advise the patient to live in a pollen-free area during the season of the year when he experiences hay fever. Mechanical obstruction of the nasal airway, which may aggravate the symptoms of rhinitis, should be corrected. Infection, if present, should be treated with an antibacterial drug capable of eradicating the specific microorganism. Alleviation of emotional disturbances by the use of drugs, correction of the environment, or psychiatric guidance occasionally will assist materially in alleviating the symptoms of allergy.

Desensitization, hyposensitization, or *immunization* with the antigens recognized as specifically responsible for allergic respiratory disease is effective. Controlled studies of desensitization in patients with hay fever due to ragweed pollen have shown that approximately 80 per cent of patients are relieved of their symptoms, whereas about 25 per cent of patients given placebo are improved. The possible mechanisms involved in alleviation of the manifestations of allergy accompanying the injection of antigen for desensitization were discussed before.

Treatment by desensitization may be perennial, coseasonal, or preseasonal. Continued therapy throughout the year probably is preferable to discontinuous treatment, but the dose of antigen in some patients must be reduced considerably during the season of the year when the patient's symptoms are expected to occur.

In some instances, the beneficial effects of desensitization may persist after the inoculations are discontinued, but more often, the allergic symptoms recur. Recently, the beneficial effects of desensitization have been obtained by injection of antigens in adjuvant containing mineral oil and an emulsifier. One injection given prior to the season when symptoms will appear has produced results equivalent to desensitization by repeated injection of the aqueous extract. Ordinarily, 100 to 3,000 protein nitrogen units of ragweed pollen extract is incorporated into the adjuvant for desensitization. Some individuals given such injections have developed sterile cysts at the site of inoculation. Although this method of desensitization holds great promise, it cannot yet be generally recommended.

Bacterial vaccines have been employed in desensitization of patients with allergic rhinitis. The lack of evidence for bacterial hypersensitivity as a cause of allergic respiratory disease and the lack of conclusive evidence for the effectiveness of such treatment in allergic rhinitis indicate that it cannot be generally recommended.

Nonspecific Treatment. If treatment of hay fever is begun when symptoms are present, only measures to relieve manifestations of the disease should be employed. Furthermore, many patients can be relieved of their complaints with symptomatic remedies alone. The severity, recurrence, and refractoriness to symptomatic treatment of the illness will determine whether or not specific desensitization should be attempted. *Antihistamines* such as Pyribenzamine (50 mg), Benadryl (50 mg), Chlortrimeton (4 mg), and many others often are effective in controlling hay fever. Repeated use, however, frequently is associated with a gradually decreasing effectiveness of the drugs, but when one fails another may be effective. In addition, they may produce drowsiness and reduce physical and mental dexterity in 10 per cent of patients depending, of course, on dosage. Although very useful therapeutic agents, therefore, they have certain features limiting their application.

Adrenal cortical steroids given orally are extraordinarily effective in relieving the symptoms of most patients with allergic respiratory disease and were it not for their side effects could be generally recommended as drugs of choice in hay fever. Nevertheless, they can be used in the management of acute symptoms, and in some patients very small doses will completely suppress the symptoms during an entire season when administered daily. Hydrocortisone in dosage of 25 to 100 mg each day is usually quite effective. In addition, prednisone in a dosage of 5 to 20 mg and methylprednisone in a dosage of 4 to 12 mg will serve equally as well as hydrocortisone in the treatment of hay fever. This form of therapy cannot be generally recommended. Adrenal steroids can cause a remarkable disappearance of nasal polyps when used in patients with rhinitis and hay fever.

A variety of agents are available for shrinking the nasal mucous membrane to relieve obstruction of the nasal airway in rhinitis. Aqueous Neosynephrine (¼ or ½ per cent) is an effective nasal decongestant that can be useful in patients very uncomfortable from hay fever or allergic rhinitis until other remedies can correct the underlying disease. Repeated use of the drug, however, can cause reactive hyperemia of the nasal mucosa, further exaggerating the symptoms of rhinitis. Orally administered ephedrine (15 mg) or Propadrine hydrochloride may also be used to shrink nasal mucous membranes, but they have limited effectiveness.

ASTHMA

Definition. Asthma is characterized by expiratory dyspnea, cough, overinflation of the lungs, expiratory wheezing, and rhonchi. It is attributed to partial bronchial airway obstruction and often is caused by allergy to inhaled antigens. The symptoms frequently are episodic and may develop during particular seasons of the year. Respiratory infection and other conditions occasionally associated with partial bronchial airway obstruction may produce symptoms indistinguishable from allergic asthma.

Etiology. Asthma commonly is attributable to: (1) allergy to inhaled antigens when symptoms may be seasonal or perennial; (2) respiratory infection, when symptoms may be intermittent or chronic; and (3) a combination of infection and allergy to inhaled antigens, when symptoms may be seasonal, intermittent, and chronic.

Airborne antigens such as plant pollen, animal dander, dust, molds, or fungi and other substances may be the cause of asthmatic symptoms as well as hay fever and allergic rhinitis. In addition, the immunologic relationships probably are alike in hay fever and allergic asthma.

Bronchial airway obstruction associated with asthma invariably is generalized and may be produced by accumulation of secretions in the bronchial lumina, edema of the bronchial mucosa, hypertrophy of the bronchial wall, contraction of bronchial smooth muscle, dilatation of the bronchial and pulmonary blood vessels, or a combination of these. In allergic asthma, it is probable that mucosal edema, bronchial secretions, and bronchospasm are the principal mechanisms producing airway obstruction. It is likely that the small bronchioles initiate the reaction, although the entire respiratory mucosa may be involved.

The bronchial lumina increase in diameter upon inspiration and become narrower upon expiration, resulting in airway obstruction most pronounced during exhalation and producing high-pitched wheezing or whistling sounds in the chest. Expiratory dyspnea requires the use of accessory muscles to deflate the lung, increasing the intrathoracic pressure. During inspiration, the negative intrathoracic pressure often is noticeable by retraction of the intercostal, suprasternal, and supraclavicular spaces. The expiratory airway obstruction in asthma leads to hyperinflation or emphysema of the lungs. The emphysema accompanying episodic allergic asthma, however, is reversible (see p. 1514).

The precise mechanism producing *dyspnea* in asthma is not known, but this symptom probably results from several events, including a conscious recognition of obstruction to breathing, hyperinflation of the lungs, changes in intrapleural pressure, and the increased work involved in respiration. A consequence of the airway obstruction is an increase in residual air in the lung, with a corresponding decrease in breathing reserve. To maintain air exchange additional effort is required, leading to fatigue, which can further exaggerate dyspnea.

Orthopnea is a common feature of asthma but

undoubtedly is attributable to an entirely different mechanism than the orthopnea of cardiac failure. Elevation of the diaphragm while in the horizontal position reduces the respiratory reserve, making the asthmatic patient more dyspneic. The sitting posture, leaning forward to reduce the intraabdominal pressure and to allow the viscera to move downward and forward, probably improves the breathing reserve and the dyspnea.

During the early and less severe stages of asthma there may be *hyperpnea,* in excess of that required for gas exchange, and the blood CO_2 may fall below normal. When the disease is severe, and particularly when protracted, however, there often is oxygen unsaturation and increased CO_2 in the blood. Frequently, in this stage, and possibly attributable to fatigue, the patient's respiratory rate may be slowed, exaggerating the impaired ventilation caused by airway obstruction.

Anoxemia in asthma may lead to an increase in pulmonary vascular resistance and pulmonary blood pressure. Little is known, however, of the vascular abnormalities that accompany asthma, although the development of right ventricular hypertrophy and heart failure may be late complications of the disease.

The physical properties of the *bronchial secretions* undoubtedly influence the manifestations of asthma, but very little is known of the changes that may occur in sputum viscosity, elasticity, and stickiness. The ease with which sputum can be evacuated from the bronchi, however, obviously is an important factor in the severity of airway obstruction.

It has long been suspected that the *autonomic nervous system* is incriminated in the pathogenesis of asthma. The administration of acetylcholine, mecholyl, or cholinesterase inhibitors will induce symptoms of partial airway obstruction which can be alleviated by atropine. There is no clear evidence, however, indicating the importance of parasympathetic activity, and atropine usually is of no value and may have a deleterious effect in allergic asthma. Drying of bronchial secretions following administration of atropine may decrease the fluidity of bronchial mucus, however, and be responsible for its ineffectiveness.

Similarly, *histamine* has been incriminated in the pathogenesis of asthma, as administration of this drug can produce bronchoconstriction and expiratory dyspnea in man and experimental animals. This effect of histamine, however, can be nullified with antihistaminic drugs, whereas, these drugs have little effect upon asthma. In addition, *serotonin* has been shown to produce asthma-like symptoms, but its relation to allergic asthma has not been shown conclusively.

Parasympathomimetic drugs, histamine, and sero-tonin will induce expiratory dyspnea in patients with a propensity to asthma, in doses ordinarily incapable of inducing such a reaction in normal persons. This increased reactivity in asthmatic patients is not confined to their response to drugs as they also may have an increase in bronchial airway resistance during respiratory infection and upon the inhalation of irritants, but this peculiar responsiveness is unexplained.

Besides the increased reactivity of the bronchial tree to drugs, inhaled irritants, and infection, it is clear that *emotional disturbances* may exaggerate or precipitate asthma. The mechanisms involved are not known, but may resemble those in animals in which it has been possible to produce manifestations of anaphylaxis by stimuli, such as bell ringing, inducing a conditioned response.

Manifestations. Expiratory wheezing, dyspnea, and cough, occurring spasmodically, are the characteristic features of asthma. These symptoms are worse during effort, are exaggerated by anxiety which almost invariably accompanies each attack, and may be most severe at night. During a paroxysm there is orthopnea, and the patient is most comfortable in a sitting position with the trunk bent forward and the arms elevated to rest at shoulder level. Dyspnea is most pronounced, and wheezing and rhonchi are audible, during expiration. There is prolongation of the expiratory phase of respiration, and inspiration characteristically is not so difficult as expiration. The wheezing and rhonchi are heard *throughout the chest* in asthma, and *localized wheezing* is indicative of some other cause of bronchial obstruction (see p. 1552).

Cough frequently becomes more severe during recovery from an asthmatic attack, when sputum seems more liquid and is produced in larger quantities. Occasionally, cough is so severe as to make the patient vomit. The sputum produced during paroxysm usually is white and mucoid, containing no blood or pus. Occasionally, however, if cough is severe or if the attack is protracted (*status asthmaticus*), the sputum may contain traces of blood. Microscopic examination of the sputum may show large numbers of eosinophils and occasionally crystals (Curschmann's spirals). In addition, as an asthmatic attack subsides, mucus casts of the bronchi or bronchioles may be seen in the sputum (Laennec's perles). Purulent sputum is indicative of bronchial or pulmonary infection as a cause of the asthma or as a complication of allergic asthma.

Hay fever and urticaria sometimes precede development of asthma, or occur simultaneously, and suggest that the asthma is attributed to inhaled or ingested antigen and reaginic or atopic allergy. This type of asthma is observed most commonly in young persons and usually is seasonal (*extrinsic asthma*). Nonseasonal asthma may also be attributed to allergy to inhaled antigens such as dust, feathers, animal dander and to ingested foods or drugs. Older persons, however, most often have nonseasonal asthma which characteristically is associated with respiratory infection such as sinusitis, bronchitis, or pneumonia (*intrinsic asthma*), but may have symptoms more commonly in winter. Airborne or ingested antigens are not always associated with chronic asthma in adults, but may complicate the symptoms attributed to recurrent infection. Inhaled molds and fungus spores have been related to asthma in young and old individuals, particularly when the person is exposed to a damp or wet environment.

During severe attacks, hypoxia may lead to cyanosis, but rarely does this result in coma and death. Status asthmaticus, however, usually is accompanied by fatigue and exhaustion. In addition, if the patient does not drink, dehydration may develop, and failure to eat can further exaggerate the fatigue and exhaustion. Dehydration is associated with drying of the bronchial mucus, and this can make the patient's asthmatic symptoms more severe.

There is no fever unless asthma is caused by or associated with infection. After a prolonged attack the patient may complain of soreness in the chest or abdomen as well as tiredness, but otherwise there usually are no systemic manifestations of the disease. Examination of blood often shows eosinophilia but no leukocytosis, and the urine is normal.

Spontaneous pneumothorax and *mediastinal emphysema* rarely are complications of an asthmatic attack. Ordinarily, asthma does not affect cardiac function unless protracted or accompanied by irreversible emphysema, when cor pulmonale may develop. Usually, episodic asthma is benign and does not result in death. Patients may be crippled by their disease, however, because of intractable or frequently occurring paroxysms. With these qualifications, the prognosis is good.

Diagnosis. A history of allergic disease in the family, seasonal attacks of nasal or bronchial symptoms, and manifestations such as urticaria or hay fever are helpful in recognition of allergic asthma. Furthermore, asthma occurring during particular seasons or under certain environmental circumstances facilitates detection of the offending antigen.

As previously mentioned, localized wheezing in the lungs is not a manifestation of asthma but is indicative of endobronchial disease, such as foreign body aspiration, neoplasm, or stenosis. In contrast to these conditions, the lungs are usually normal between paroxysms of uncomplicated asthma. Generalized wheezing predominantly occurs during expiration, whereas in bronchiectasis, acute pulmonary edema, or pneumonia there are inspiratory rales as well. Of course, asthma complicated by

pneumonia may be associated with signs of parenchymal lung disease. The presence of inspiratory moist rales, bloody sputum, and cardiomegaly in acute pulmonary edema or "cardiac asthma" usually enables its differentiation from paroxysmal asthma.

Asthma occasionally is a presenting manifestation of polyarteritis nodosa (p. 1889). Drug reaction, particularly with aspirin, is an occasional cause of severe asthma in patients with respiratory allergy attributed to other causes. Loeffler's allergic pneumonitis, occasionally due to parasitic infestation of the lungs, is often accompanied by asthma (p. 1556).

Poisoning with cholinergic drugs or insecticides may induce bronchoconstriction and expiratory dyspnea which can be specifically relieved with atropine. Carcinoid tumors elaborating serotonin may be associated with asthma. In addition, traumatic cerebral disease may result in asthmatic symptoms. There are examples of outbreaks of asthma in a large population or in individuals exposed to irritants in polluted air. Furthermore, silofiller's disease and farmer's lung disease may be associated with asthma attributed to inhalation of nitrogen dioxide or microorganisms which cause inflammation in the bronchial tree (pp. 1532 and 1533).

Skin tests used for the diagnosis of asthma are no different from those used for the diagnosis of hay fever and were described previously. There are no specific laboratory tests that will define the allergic etiology, but measurements of pulmonary function will demonstrate the presence of increased airway resistance. The finding of increased numbers of eosinophils in sputum and blood, however, occasionally will suggest an allergic cause of asthma.

Therapy. *Specific Treatment.* Elimination of the offending antigen from the patient's environment is the most successful means of preventing and treating allergic asthma, as in hay fever. Similarly, mechanical obstruction of the tracheobronchial tree should be corrected, and infection of the sinuses should be treated.

Specific desensitization or hyposensitization of the patient with asthma due to inhaled antigens can be done as in hay fever but may be less effective, and improvement usually does not persist when desensitization is discontinued.

The frequent occurrence of bronchial infection in adults with nonseasonal or chronic asthma necessitates special consideration. The pneumococcus and *Hemophilus influenzae* are the microorganisms most often isolated from the bronchi and sputum of patients with asthmatic or chronic bronchitis, and exacerbations of symptoms with cough and dyspnea may be associated with an increase in number of these bacteria. Treatment of these patients with tetracycline (0.5 to 1.0 Gm per day) continuously, during winter months or upon the appearance of increasing symptoms, will decrease significantly the severity and frequency of exacerbations of their symptoms. Such treatment frequently is associated with a decrease in number of pneumococci and hemophili in sputum. Untoward consequences of this treatment in these patients are rare.

Chronic asthma with or without bronchitis may be complicated by acute infection by pneumococci, *Klebsiella pneumoniae,* or staphylococci, and when these infections appear they should be treated specifically with an appropriate antibiotic.

Nonspecific Treatment. Treatment of acute asthma is most effective when begun soon after onset of the paroxysm. Prompt relief can usually be achieved by subcutaneous injection of epinephrine, 0.2 to 1.0 ml of a 1:1,000 solution, repeated as needed, but no oftener than every 30 min. It is advisable to administer a sedative, such as phenobarbital, 60 to 90 mg, with epinephrine to allay agitation and to relieve the anxiety accompanying an attack of asthma. Epinephrine may become ineffective after repeated use. It may be used in oil, 1.0 ml of a 1:100 solution and injected intramuscularly for prolonged effect, and may be vaporized as a 1:100 aqueous solution for inhalation. Nebulized epinephrine analogues can be administered by the patient, but, if used repeatedly, irritate the respiratory mucosa. Aminophylline is an active bronchodilator which is beneficial in the person refractory to the action of epinephrine. It may be used occasionally in preference to, or in addition to, epinephrine, and may be given intravenously, rectally, or orally in decreasing order of effectiveness. The dosage is 0.25 to 0.5 Gm. When given intravenously, the drug must be given slowly. Rectal administration as a suppository or in water or oil is effective. If the patient is cyanotic, oxygen may be given but should be used intermittently, particularly if chronic diffuse lung disease is present. Ether administered rectally or as a general anesthetic occasionally may be successful in halting a severe attack of asthma. Adrenal cortical steroids may be given in severe or intractable paroxysms in the same dosage as described for hay fever, but are not always effective. Continuous administration of adrenal cortical steroids to the patient with chronic asthma or asthmatic bronchitis has been shown to be an effective and safe means of preventing patients from becoming crippled by this disease. This treatment has been continued for several years without serious side effects or complications. In fact, patients with severe asthma and infection have fewer episodes of infection while receiving adrenal steroids continuously. Steroid dosage may be increased if exacerbations occur while the patient is receiving the drug continuously.

If an asthmatic episode is unresponsive to the use of epinephrine and aminophylline, or recurs promptly, it may be advisable to give an intravenous infusion of 1 liter of 5 per cent glucose containing 0.25 to 0.5 Gm aminophylline. *Morphine should never be given to the patient with acute asthma,* but Demerol, 50 to 100 mg, is useful as a sedative and antispasmodic. Hydration should be maintained to prevent inspissation of bronchial mucus.

Prophylactic management of the asthmatic patient involves the use of drugs with which the patient can abort paroxysms and institution of measures directed to improve general health. Oral ephedrine (25 to 50 mg) and phenobarbital (30 to 60 mg) are commonly used to abort an asthmatic attack, but this combination is less effective in management of a fully developed asthmatic paroxysm. Aminophylline (0.25 to 0.5 Gm) may be added to the combination of ephedrine and phenobarbital. During a period of time when the patient is most likely to develop asthma, ephedrine, phenobarbital, and aminophylline (APE) may be given three or four times a day.

Smoking is undesirable in asthmatics, as are obesity, excessive exertion, fatigue, and dietary indiscretion.

ALLERGIC SKIN DISEASE

There are many dermatologic manifestations of allergic reactions, including urticaria, angioedema, contact dermatitis, erythematous rashes, eczematous eruptions, and others. These lesions, when attributable to immunologic processes, are divisible into those related to delayed hypersensitivity and to immediate hypersensitivity, as discussed previously. Urticaria, angioedema, and many erythematous lesions usually are attributable to immediate hypersensitivity reactions, whereas contact dermatitis and possibly many instances of eczematous dermatitis are attributable to delayed hypersensitivity reactions. Histopathologic examination of allergic skin lesions generally reveals findings which may differentiate reactions associated with immediate or delayed hypersensitivity. Vasculitis, edema, and polymorphonuclear or eosinophilic cellular response are most characteristic of urticaria and erythematous lesions, whereas mononuclear cells predominate in lesions such as contact dermatitis.

At times an antigen may induce and elicit both immediate and delayed hypersensitivity, and upon contact, ingestion, or injection of the antigen the allergic person may experience urticaria and eczematous dermatitis.

Urticaria, angioedema, contact dermatitis, and erythematous rashes are the principal forms of allergic reactions in which the skin may be the major or only site of involvement. Many other types of skin lesions, however, are attributable to systemic allergic disease, as illustrated by those seen during drug reactions. Erythema nodosum, erythema multiforme and its variants, exfoliation, bullae, purpura, "fixed" drug eruptions, photosensitivity, necrosis, and other types of skin lesions are seen in which an allergic reaction has been found or is thought to be responsible. Petechiae, erythema nodosum, erythema multiforme, and urticaria are observed in patients with infection and have been related to hypersensitivity reactions to microbial antigens. Certain types of supposed systemic immunologic disease such as systemic lupus erythematosus, dermatomyositis, rheumatic fever, and scleroderma also are characterized by skin lesions thought to be allergic. These special types of systemic disease associated with probable allergic skin reactions are discussed separately elsewhere.

Contact Dermatitis. See p. 1926.

Urticaria. Urticaria (hives) is characterized by white or red evanescent wheals, papules, or macules that are usually surrounded by erythema and are pruritic. They may be localized or generalized, but commonly appear in areas of skin covered by clothing. Urticaria also may occur in mucous membranes such as stomach and mouth, and frequently is accompanied by eosinophilia. Immediate hypersensitivity is the principal immunologic mechanism responsible for urticaria, as illustrated by the frequent occurrence of hives in serum sickness. In addition, urticaria often occurs in combination with hay fever and allergic asthma. Emotional tension, increased heat, and physical exercise may exaggerate the urticarial reaction.

Urticaria can be induced by histamine and acetylcholine, and there is good evidence indicating that liberation of histamine during an allergic reaction is responsible for hives.

Urticaria may occur from ingestion, inhalation, injection, or contact with the offending antigen by the allergic person. Foods and drugs frequently are responsible, but hives also have been related to a great variety of inhalants and contactants, such as pollen, dander, dust, feathers, and wool. The responsible antigen may be detected as in other allergic diseases by a historical dissection of the occasions when symptoms occur, by skin test, or by elimination diets.

Many instances of urticaria are chronic and cannot be related to a recognizable antigen. Occasionally parasitic infestation, such as trichinosis and echinococcosis, or bacterial infection can be associated with hives, but more often the cause of chronic urticaria will remain undetermined. Chronic idiopathic urticaria has been attributed to nervous tension or neurosis, and this may explain some cases but other causes should be examined. A relationship has been shown occasionally between thyroid and other endocrine disorders and urticaria, but this association remains somewhat vague.

If a specific cause of urticaria is detected, it should be corrected or the antigen eliminated from the patient's environment. Acute symptoms usually can be relieved with antihistamine drugs, but occasionally adrenal cortical steroids may be needed. Intramuscular epinephrine (0.2 to 1.0 ml of a 1:1,000 aqueous solution) can provide prompt relief of symptoms in most instances. Chronic urticaria of undetermined cause ordinarily is quite refractory to treatment, and many of these patients may require psychiatric assistance. Prolonged use of adrenal cortical steroids in chronic urticaria is undesirable.

Angioedema is characterized by edema of the eyelids, lips, external genitalia, and the mucous membranes of the mouth, tongue, or gastrointestinal tract. The swellings may be localized to one area or may be diffuse, and commonly are accompanied by urticaria elsewhere. When the respiratory tract is involved the patient may have laryngeal edema with hoarseness, stridor, cyanosis, and, rarely, death.

Generally, angioedema is attributed to allergy to foods, and shellfish very commonly are incriminated. In addition, the reaction may occur from the many antigens responsible for urticaria. A rare form of angioedema is familial.

The treatment of angioedema is the same as for urticaria. If respiratory tract obstruction occurs, tracheotomy may prove lifesaving.

REFERENCES

Alexander, H. L.: "Reactions to Drug Therapy," Philadelphia, W. B. Saunders Company, 1955.

Gay, L. N.: The Pathology of Asthma, Clinics, 5:347, 1946.

Lawrence, H. S.: Delayed Type Allergic Inflammatory Response, Am. J. Med., 20:428, 1956.

——: "Cellular and Humoral Mechanisms of the Hypersensitive States," New York, Paul B. Hoeber, Inc., Medical Department of Harper & Brothers, 1959.

Lowell, F. C.: Bronchial Asthma, Am. J. Med., 20:778, 1956.

Samter, M., and O. C. Durham: "Regional Allergy," Springfield, Ill., Charles C Thomas, Publisher, 1955.

Sherman, W. B.: Diagnostic Methods for Allergic Disease, Am. J. Med., 20:603, 1956.

233 SERUM SICKNESS AND RELATED DISORDERS

Ivan L. Bennett, Jr.

Definition. Serum sickness is a systemic illness which occurs in certain susceptible individuals as a reaction to the administration of foreign serum or serum products. Common manifestations are fever, skin eruptions, lymphadenopathy, edema, and arthralgias. An indistinguishable clinical picture can result from drug hypersensitivity; indeed the syndrome is now caused more frequently by drugs than by serum products.

Etiology and Pathogenesis. Serum sickness was first recognized when the use of immune horse serum for prophylaxis and therapy of diphtheria became widespread. With advances in chemotherapy, serum is used less and less frequently, being limited for the most part to diphtheria, tetanus, gas gangrene, envenenation by reptiles, and rabies. For reasons not entirely clear, transfusion of blood is occasionally followed by serum sickness. While "raw" or whole serum is more likely to elicit a reaction, purified fractions are also capable of producing illness. The incidence and severity of serum sickness increase with dosage of the antigen.

The development of serum sickness is dependent upon an antigen-antibody reaction. An individual given an initial injection of serum will develop antibody within about 1 week and, presumably, the reaction (precipitation) of antibody and the remaining antigen leads to the illness. The onset of symptoms coincides with the appearance of antibody, disappearance of circulating antigen, and a sharp fall in serum complement. An individual previously exposed to an antigen develops antibody sooner (anamnestic or booster response) and illness is earlier in onset. Depending upon the degree of prior sensitization, a severe reaction may occur within minutes or hours.

Apparent relapses or recurrences of serum sickness are not unusual. When it is remembered that serum is not a single antigenic substance, it is clear that such a course results from a series of reactions to different antigenic components of the injected material.

The questions of the mode of injury to tissue, the release of histamine, serotonin, acetylcholine, etc., by antigen-antibody union are discussed on p. 1258. The elicitation of illness by nonprotein drugs undoubtedly involves immunologic mechanisms also. These are discussed on p. 1270.

Pathology. Serum sickness is rarely fatal. However, examination of tissues of patients dying of other causes during or shortly after an episode of serum sickness often shows lesions indistinguishable from those of polyarteritis nodosa. Similar lesions are readily produced in rabbits by injection of foreign protein. This experimental finding is one of the several factors that have led to the idea that hypersensitivity may be important in the etiology of polyarteritis nodosa, rheumatic fever, systemic lupus erythematosus, and other diseases characterized by vascular damage.

Manifestations. After an incubation period of 4 to 10 days (it may be much shorter in sensitized individuals or can be as long as 21 days in others) there is the onset of *pruritus* followed shortly by *rash*. The rash may be any form of erythematous, morbilliform, or petechial eruption, but by far the commonest is urticaria. Often, the skin lesions appear at the local site of injection of the serum several hours before the rash becomes generalized. *Lymphadenopathy*, most prominent in the area draining the injection site, is usual as is *edema* of the face, lips, eyelids, or, rarely, the glottis. There are *fever, myalgia,* mild or severe *arthralgias, headache, nausea,* and *vomiting.* Other manifestations include abdominal pain, diarrhea, and cardiac arrhythmias.

The most disabling complications of serum sickness are neurologic disorders which occur in a minority of cases. The usual syndrome observed is a unilateral mononeuritis involving the shoulder girdle or arm with weakness and sensory deficit. Isolated facial palsy occurs and, occasionally, there may be extensive polyneuritis or meningoencephalitis, but these are rare.

Laboratory Findings. There is usually a mild peripheral polymorphonuclear leukocytosis, and the bone marrow shows an increase in plasma cells. Eosinophilia is not a feature of classical serum sickness, but it occasionally accompanies the drug-induced syndrome. The urine may contain protein, casts, and erythrocytes. Electrocardiograms sometimes show transient conduction defects. Slight pleocytosis in the cerebrospinal fluid is frequent even in the absence of demonstrable neurologic dysfunction.

Course. Serum sickness is a benign, self-limited disease which subsides within 1 to 3 weeks. In patients with neuropathy, residual weakness may require several weeks to abate, but complete restoration of function is the rule. Rare deaths from edema of the glottis are recorded, but a fatal outcome is more often a result of the intercurrent disease of the patient.

Treatment. Urticaria usually responds to small doses of epinephrine and can be controlled with ephedrine and antihistaminics. Local application of calamine is permissible but usually unnecessary. Contrary to early statements, joint pains are usually relieved promptly by aspirin or other salicylates.

For severely ill and uncomfortable patients, adrenal steroids offer prompt relief, and the great efficacy of these compounds has led to their increasing use for symptomatic relief. They need to be given for only 4 to 7 days in most patients. Tracheostomy is sometimes needed for sudden respiratory obstruction by edema, and equipment for this procedure should be at hand during the early stages of the disease. Adrenal steroids relieve incipient obstruction promptly.

In patients who have developed serum sickness as a result of prophylactic administration of tetanus or diphtheria antiserum, active immunization with toxoid should be initiated before release from medical care to avoid later recurrence of the same problem.

Anaphylaxis. Occasional patients given an injection of serum, of skin-test antigen, or a drug will become profoundly ill and may collapse and die within minutes. There is often asthmatic wheezing and cyanosis at the onset of illness. This type of severe reaction closely resembles and, very probably, is the human counterpart of anaphylactic shock in lower animals. Because it can occur in individuals with no prior history of hypersensitivity and because fatalities have followed the injection of tiny amounts of serum for the purpose of determining a patient's state of sensitization, prevention is a very difficult matter. Perhaps the most important step in reducing the incidence of this tragic disorder is for the physician to remember that no serum product or drug should be given to any patient without clear indications. While most severe reactions occur after parenteral administration of the antigen or drug, fatalities have also been reported after oral ingestion.

Treatment consists of the intravenous or intracardiac administration of epinephrine and vigorous support of respiration and circulation. Adrenal steroids can be given parenterally but are no substitute for vasopressors, positive pressure oxygen, etc. When the injection site permits, a tourniquet may be applied to slow absorption.

Arthus Reaction. When experimental animals are sensitized to foreign serum or other proteins, reinjection of antigen into the skin often elicits transient erythema and edema, similar to a "positive" skin test in man. If animals are highly sensitive or if the dose of antigen is large, the skin lesion may progress to hemorrhage and necrosis with eventual ulceration and scarring. This irreversible tissue damage after local application of antigen in a sensitive animal is the classic *Arthus phenomenon*. Rarely, a similar type of hemorrhagic necrosis occurs at sites of injection of serum or drugs in man. These Arthus-like reactions are unusual, however, and are far outnumbered by inflammations at injection sites attributable to the intrinsic irritating properties of a drug, to hemorrhage in patients with hemophilia,

thrombocytopenia, or drug-induced coagulation defects, or to secondary pyogenic infection. Until these disorders have been ruled out, an Arthus reaction should not be invoked as the cause of tissue damage at the point of inoculation.

Shwartzman Reaction. Appropriately timed intradermal injections of bacterial endotoxins (see p. 925) or endotoxins in combination with various other substances can elicit in rabbit skin a type of hemorrhagic necrosis that resembles the Arthus reaction. However, this so-called *Shwartzman reaction* is independent of antigen-antibody union. The mechanism of the reaction is not clear, but it is not, in the immunologic sense, an allergic or hypersensitivity phenomenon although it is sometimes erroneously so classified. Numerous attempts have been made to demonstrate the importance of this reaction in the pathogenesis of human diseases including peptic ulcer, acute pancreatitis, and focal reactions in tuberculosis, but it remains, for the most part, a dramatic laboratory phenomenon. The confluent purpura of meningococcemia comes closest to being a human counterpart of the Shwartzman reaction.

REFERENCES

Bennett, I. L., Jr., M. Berthrong, and A. R. Rich: A Further Study of the Effect of Adrenocorticotrophic Hormone (ACTH) upon the Experimental Cardiovascular Lesions Produced by Anaphylactic Hypersensitivity, Bull. Johns Hopkins Hosp., 88:197, 1951.

Germuth, F. G., Jr.: A Comparative Histologic and Immunologic Study in Rabbits of Induced Hypersensitivity of the Serum Sickness Type, J. Exptl. Med., 97:257, 1953.

Kojis, F. G.: Serum Sickness and Anaphylaxis, Am. J. Diseases Children, 64:93,313, 1942.

Longcope, W. T.: Serum Sickness and Analogous Reactions from Certain Drugs, Particularly the Sulfonamides, Medicine, 22:251, 1943.

Rich, A. R.: Hypersensitivity in Disease, Harvey Lectures, 42:106, 1946.

234 REACTIONS TO DRUGS
Leighton E. Cluff

The increase in allergy to drugs parallels the growing use of pharmaceutic agents in the management of disease. With the continual introduction of new drugs, this problem can be expected to become even more serious.

Definition. Classification of a drug reaction is not always easy, but undesired responses to therapeutic agents have certain specific features which facilitate their characterization. Nearly all drugs can elicit pharmacologic effects other than those for which they are administered, and when these appear they are referred to as *side effects* or *toxic effects*. Some patients exhibit unusual susceptibility to the pharmacologic actions of a drug and are said to have an *idiosyncrasy*. In addition, reactions not explained by the pharmacologic properties of a drug and, therefore, indicative of altered reactivity of the patient are termed *allergic*. Side effects, as a rule, are intensified by increasing dosage or cumulative action, and readministration is not associated with increased reactivity of the patient. For example, nausea, hyperpnea, and tinnitus in a person given large doses of aspirin are side effects, and reduction in dosage will usually alleviate the situation. The occasional patient who displays these symptoms after taking a small amount of aspirin has an idiosyncrasy to the drug. However, if ingestion of aspirin is followed by bronchial asthma or urticaria, reactions not explainable by the drug's pharmacologic action, the patient is allergic to it. This type of reaction is likely to be associated with symptoms commonly ascribed to hypersensitivity (rash, asthma, pruritus, arthritis, fever, leukopenia, etc.), frequently recurs promptly on readministration of the drug, and is not closely dependent on dosage or cumulative action.

The clinical importance of differentiating side effects, idiosyncrasy, and allergy relates, of course, to the hazard of readministration of a drug or its probable safety in lower dosage.

Etiology. Allergy to drugs may be attributed to immediate or delayed hypersensitivity reactions. Most pharmacologic agents, however, are incapable of initiating an immunologic response by themselves, and it is thought that the actual antigen is a conjugate of the drug or its derivatives with serum or tissue proteins. Under such circumstances, the drug would act as a hapten, nonantigenic by itself, but conferring antigenic specificity to the protein, and capable of combining with the antibody or reacting with cells of the sensitized person in response to the drug protein conjugate. Many drugs are bound by body proteins, and there is experimental evidence that the ability of chemical compounds to elicit allergic contact dermatitis can be correlated with their affinity for sulfhydryl containing proteins of skin. Practically all drugs bind to serum protein, particularly albumin, following absorption, but there is little to suggest that such protein-drug conjugates are important in drug allergy. Other tissue proteins also may bind drugs, but those specifically responsible for rendering a chemical antigenic are not known. Furthermore, the administered drug may be of less importance in inducing an immunologic response than its degrada-

tion products. For example, recent observations show that penicillenic acid and penicilloic acid, degradation products of penicillin, may be responsible for most instances of penicillin allergy.

Serum antibody has been demonstrated in some persons with drug allergy involving cellular elements of blood, such as in agranulocytosis, hemolytic anemia, and thrombocytopenia. In other types of drug hypersensitivity, however, the usual techniques for demonstrating antibody ordinarily yield negative findings. Precipitation, hemagglutination, or complement fixation tests with a patient's serum may be negative, and direct intradermal or passive transfer tests of the Prausnitz-Küstner type are often unrevealing. In addition, demonstration of agglutination by serum of erythrocytes sensitized with a drug such as penicillin may fail to differentiate the allergic from the nonallergic individual. These results, however, are more indicative of the inadequacy of present methods of testing than an argument against an immunologic basis for hypersensitivity to drugs. The lack of consistently effective testing methods, of course, is a great handicap to clinical investigations of drug reactions.

Most types of allergic reactions to drugs do not appear to be familial; however, it has been suggested that anaphylaxis may occur more commonly in persons with other allergic disease such as hay fever, asthma, or urticaria. Certain types of underlying disease, however, may possibly predispose to the development of drug allergy. For example, patients with systemic lupus erythematosus probably experience more drug allergic reactions than do normal individuals. Similarly, patients with severe infection such as pneumonia and septicemia have allergic reactions to drugs more commonly than persons with less intense infection such as latent or primary syphilis. Furthermore, the patient acquiring an allergic reaction to one drug often will develop at the same time allergic reactions to other drugs he is receiving, but the manifestations of the reactions may differ.

Manifestations. The commonest manifestations of allergy to drugs are no different from hypersensitivity reactions of other types, and include rashes, asthma, and the symptoms of serum sickness (see Table 234-1). These are easily recognized clinically as allergic in origin. Other features of drug allergy are sometimes less easily characterized, however. The tabulation (see Table 234-1) of common drugs and reactions which they may elicit includes some effects that may not be allergic at all. A few examples of allergic drug reactions will illustrate the variations seen with different pharmacologic agents.

Skin. Morbilliform, urticarial, and maculopapular rashes are the most common skin reactions, but many others are observed, including vesicular, bullous, exfoliative, eczematous, and purpuric eruptions. Pruritus is frequent. Although the type of skin lesion usually will not aid in identifying the causative drug, there are certain skin reactions which are somewhat specific. Erythema multiforme or nodosum is particularly seen in allergy to Dilantin, bromides, iodides, trimethadione, and sulfonamides. "Fixed" drug eruptions are most frequently due to amidopyrine, phenolphthalein, or Atabrine. Photosensitization during drug therapy occurs characteristically with chlorpromazine, phenothiazine, sulfonamides, and tetracycline derivatives.

Fever. Fever may be an isolated manifestation of drug allergy, and at least 35 pharmaceuticals in common use can produce a febrile reaction, including most antibiotics and chemotherapeutic agents. However, the tetracycline derivatives are uncommon causes of drug fever, and digitalis has rarely, if ever, been incriminated as the cause of a pyrogenic reaction. Elevation of temperature can appear abruptly after initiation of treatment or develop in a stepwise fashion during or after the second week of drug administration. Drug fever is often associated with chills and constitutional symptoms and can be accompanied by leukocytosis. Discontinuance of therapy usually results in defervescence within a very few hours, although several days may be required for return of temperature to normal.

Blood. Changes in the formed elements of the blood are rather common during drug allergy and may have no specificity. Some drugs have been found to have limited or no effects on the blood, while others produce specific abnormalities. For example, penicillin has never been incriminated as a cause of serious hematologic abnormalities. In therapeutic doses, acetanilid is probably not a cause of anemia, agranulocytosis, thrombocytopenia, or aplastic anemia; in high dosage, however, it may produce leukocytosis, methemoglobinemia, and acute hemolysis. Methemoglobinemia also occurs with antipyrine, nitrites, sulfonamides, primaquine, and pamaquine, but this reaction is probably not allergic in origin. Barbiturates, salicylates, and paraaminosalicylic acid rarely, if ever, produce agranulocytosis. Eosinophilia can accompany allergic reactions of many types, but occurs with such frequency as an isolated finding during therapy with streptomycin or nirvanol that it has no significance in these instances. Lymphocytosis is common in patients receiving Dilantin and nirvanol, but polymorphonuclear leukocytosis may be found in individuals taking Dilantin or atropine. Recent studies of the erythrocyte abnormality responsible for the acute hemolytic anemia induced by primaquine, sulfonamides, and nitrofurans in certain individuals indicates that what was thought to be drug allergy is actually a genetically determined idiosyncrasy

(see p. 1291). Jaundice and acquired hemolytic anemia due to pharmaceutic agents are discussed elsewhere (p. 1289).

Nervous System. A variety of neurologic manifestations may appear during drug therapy, but in the majority of instances there is little evidence to incriminate allergy as a cause. The commonest reaction, by far, is delirium, seen particularly with digitalis, atropine, thiocyanates, and sedatives. Other drugs which produce adverse effects upon the nervous system (ranging from paresthesias and peripheral neuritis to deafness) are streptomycin, hydralazine, chlorpromazine, Diamox, isoniazid, polymyxin, and neomycin.

Others. Nausea, *vomiting,* and *diarrhea* are exceedingly common drug reactions. In addition, *abdominal pain* in the absence of other symptoms may be produced by quinidine, chlorpromazine, and primaquine. *Albuminuria* and *cylindruria* occur particularly with heavy metals, bacitracin, and polymyxin. Dilantin, chloral hydrate, sulfonamides, trimethadione, Phenurone, colchicine, and thiocyanate occasionally produce renal dysfunction, probably by direct toxic action. Hypersensitivity to sulfonamides has resulted in acute hemorrhagic nephritis.

Histologic lesions indistinguishable from those of *polyarteritis nodosa* have been found in the tissues of patients who have experienced allergic reactions to iodides, Dilantin, sulfonamides, and penicillin. Manifestations of systemic lupus erythematosus have appeared during therapy with gold or hydralazine.

Anaphylaxis may follow the parenteral administration of a variety of drugs, but the agent most seriously incriminated at present is penicillin. Development of anaphylaxis has been reported after oral ingestion of the drug, but this is exceedingly rare.

The incidence of drug allergy is not high and is particularly related to the frequency with which a pharmacologic agent is used clinically. For this reason, probably, these reactions are now often observed with antibiotics. However, the incidence of allergic reaction also varies with the agent, and with some drugs may be as high as 10 per cent.

Treatment and Prophylaxis. Allergic reactions to drugs usually subside promptly when the agent is discontinued. For reasons that are not understood, however, the reaction occasionally persists for prolonged periods in spite of withdrawal; recurrent urticaria for many months after a penicillin reaction is a common example. The management of serum sickness is described elsewhere. In the event of persistent or severe manifestations of drug allergy, the use of adrenocortical steroids is indicated. Adrenal steroids, antihistamines, and epinephrine are usually ineffective in alleviating reactions due

Table 234-1. COMMON DRUG REACTIONS

Drug	Anemia	Agranulocytosis	Eosinophilia	Hemolysis	Thrombopenia	Aplastic anemia	Lymphocytosis	Leukocytosis	Rash	Bullae and vesicles	Exfoliation	Urticaria	Erythema multiforme	Eczema	Purpura	"Fixed" eruption	Photosensitization	Contact dermatitis	Fever	Serum sickness (anaphylaxis, asthma, etc.)	Jaundice	Delirium	Orthostatic hypotension	Peripheral neuritis	VIII nerve palsy	Paresthesia	Parkinsonism	Ascending paralysis	Nausea-vomiting	Abdominal pain	Diarrhea	Renal disorders	Periarteritis nodosa	Systemic lupus erythematosus
Acetanilid	0	0		+*	0	0		+	+			+				+			+															
Amidopyrine									+							+			+	+														
Aminopyrine		+							+							+			+	+														
Amphetamine (Benzedrine)									+													+												
Antihistamines		+							+				+						+	+														
Arsenicals		+		+	+	+			+	+	+				+				+	+	+	+		+								+		
Atropine								+	+			+							+	+		+												
Bacitracin																																+		
BAL (dimercaprol)									+									+	+															
Banthine									+			+																						
Barbiturates	+	0							+	+	+	+							+			+												
Bismuth									+		+								+		+			+								+	+	
Boric acid									+									+											+					
Bromides										+			+						+			+							+			+		
Carbarsone									+		+								+			+												
Chloral hydrate									+				+		+				+										+			+		
Chloramphenicol		+			+	+			+										R	+	+								+					
Chloroquine									+																				+					
Chlorpromazine (Thorazine)													+				+	+	+		+						+	+						
Cocaine (derivatives)															+				+	+														
Codeine										+	+																		+					
Colchicine																												+	+	+	+	+	+	
DDT		+							+																								+	
Dextran												+								+														
Diethylstilbestrol						+			+																									
Digitalis			+				+		+				+									0	+		+	+								
Dilantin			+				+	+	+		+		+						+					+									+	+
Diodoquin									+	+									+															
Emetine												+			+	+								+										
Ephedrine																				+														
Ergot alkaloids																										+			+					
Formaldehyde														+				+																
Gold		+			+				+		+										+											+	+	+
Heparin												+							+	+														
Hydralazine	+					+			+			+							+					+					+		+			+
Insulin									+			+								+														
Iodides										+	+				+				+	+												+	+	
Iproniazid																						+												

0 = reaction never reported with this drug; * = related to dose; † = genetic idiosyncrasy; R = rare.

Table 234-1. COMMON DRUG REACTIONS (Continued)

Drug	Blood								Skin										Fever	Serum sickness (anaphylaxis, asthma, etc.)	Jaundice	Delirium	Neurologic						Gastro-intestinal			Renal disorders	Periarteritis nodosa	Systemic lupus erythematosus
	Anemia	Agranulocytosis	Eosinophilia	Hemolysis	Thrombopenia	Aplastic anemia	Lymphocytosis	Leukocytosis	Rash	Bullae and vesicles	Exfoliation	Urticaria	Erythema multiforme	Eczema	Purpura	"Fixed" eruption	Photosensitization	Contact dermatitis					Orthostatic hypotension	Peripheral neuritis	VIII nerve palsy	Paresthesia	Parkinsonism	Ascending paralysis	Nausea-vomiting	Abdominal pain	Diarrhea			
Isoniazid		+	+												+						+	+												
Khellin									+																									
Liver extract												+							+	+														
Mandelic acid									+			+														+								
Meperidine (Demerol)																			+															
Mercurials		+							+	+	+	+							+	+									+			+		
Mesantoin		+		+	+	+															+													
Methyltestosterone																					+													
Morphine												+								+		+												
Neomycin or kanamycin																									+									
Nirvanol		+	+				+		+			+							+	+														
Nitrofurantoin (Furadantin)			+	†															+										+					
Pamaquine			+	†																														
p-Aminosalicylic acid		0							+										+															
Penicillin	0	0	0	0	0	0			+	+	+	+	+						+	+	+								+					+
Phenolphthalein									+	+						+																		
Phenurone		+			+				+			+							+					+					+			+		
Phenylbutazone (Butazolidin)		+			+	+			+										+															
Piperazine (Antepar)															+																			
Polymyxin																																+		
Primaquine				†																			+	+					+	+				
Probenecid (Benemid)									+																				+					
Procaine amide (Pronestyl)		+							+			+							+	+			+						+		+			+
Quinacrine (Atabrine)	+								+			+			+				+	+			+	+					+					
Quinidine					+				+			+							+	+			+			+			+	+	+			
Quinine		+		+					+										+	+				+								+		
Rauwolfia												+																	+	+				
Salicylates (aspirin)		0		+					+	+	+	+			+	+			+	+									+					
Scopolamine									+			+							+	+			+											
Streptomycin			+		†	+			+			+	+						+	+			+		+	+			+					
Sulfonamides		+	+	+	†	+			+	+	+	+	+				+		+	+			+	+									+	+
Tetracycline (derivatives)									+			+	+					+	R		+								+		+			
Thiocyanate	+	+							+			+			+				+				+	+	+				+			+	+	
Thiouracil									+										+															
Trimethadione (Tridione)				+	+				+				+		+						+										+			
Veratrum alkaloids																							+			+								

0 = reaction never reported with this drug; * = related to dose; † = genetic idiosyncrasy; R = rare.

to idiosyncrasy or side effects of a drug. Reactions of this type are best managed by administration of other drugs with appropriate pharmacologic actions, i.e., sedatives for excitability, stimulants for depression, etc., and by withdrawal of the offending drug.

Although it is not possible to predict the occurrence of drug allergy in a patient, the fact that hypersensitivity to drugs may be commoner in individuals with other allergic reactions makes it reasonable to inquire about this before initiation of treatment with any agent. A specific history of hypersensitivity to a given drug contraindicates its readministration unless the clinical situation is serious. In a number of instances where it has been judged necessary to prescribe a drug to which a patient is known to be allergic (e.g., penicillin for bacterial endocarditis), the concomitant administration of adrenal steroids has completely suppressed the manifestations of hypersensitivity.

Although it is commonly said that sensitivity to a drug will subside if its administration is continued, this is not a regular occurrence and should not be accepted as a basis for further therapy with the incriminated agent.

REFERENCES

Alexander, H. L.: "Reactions to Drug Therapy," Philadelphia, W. B. Saunders Company, 1956.

Carr, E. A., Jr.: Drug Allergy, Pharmacol. Rev., 6: 365, 1954.

Landsteiner, K.: "The Specificity of Serological Reactions," Cambridge, Mass., Harvard University Press, 1945.

Eisen, H. N.: Hypersensitivity to Simple Chemicals, in "Cellular and Humoral Aspects of Hypersensitivity," New York, Paul B. Hoeber, Inc., Medical Department of Harper & Brothers, 1959.

PART EIGHT
Diseases of Organ Systems

Section 1: The Hematopoietic System

INTRODUCTION

M. M. Wintrobe

The hematopoietic system includes the circulating blood, the bone marrow, the spleen, and the lymph nodes, supplemented by the reticuloendothelial cells scattered about the body. The liver, through the presence there of reticuloendothelial cells, as well as by reason of other functions, is also intimately concerned in blood formation and destruction. Since the function of the red corpuscles is to hold in nondiffusible form the pigment, hemoglobin, essential for the transport of oxygen, any alteration in the quantity of red corpuscles or in their hemoglobin content affects the function of all the organs of the body. An important function of the leukocytes is to take part in the reaction to injury, particularly in the defense against infection. The blood platelets are concerned in maintaining the integrity of the vascular endothelium and in the clotting of blood. The blood plasma, which carries these three types of corpuscles, is also the medium for the transport of many substances concerned in the metabolism of the organism.

Since the blood and its constituents are so intimately related to the body as a whole, much will be found concerning the blood in various chapters in this book and particularly in those in Part Two. In regard to the red blood corpuscles, attention should be called especially to Chap. 23 (Pallor and Anemia), where the synthesis and the destruction of hemoglobin and the classification, pathogenesis, and management of anemia are considered, as well as the symptomatology and methods of study of a patient with anemia. The platelets, the phenomenon of coagulation, and the various ways in which bleeding is produced receive attention in Chap. 24 (Bleeding).

In the present section, disorders of the hematopoietic system will be considered. It is evident that such disorders make themselves known in a variety of ways. These may be such that discovering their cause may tax the acumen of even the most discerning physician. In the main, however, they are characterized in part or whole by symptoms and signs such as pallor, cyanosis, jaundice, bleeding, or enlargement of the lymph nodes or spleen. A thorough understanding of these manifestations of disease is a prerequisite to the correct differentiation as well as the effective treatment of the disorders of the hematopoietic system.

The *approach* to the patient suspected of having a hematopoietic disorder is discussed, therefore, in Part Two under headings such as Pallor and Anemia, Bleeding, and Enlargement of Lymph Nodes and Spleen. Although, in the subsequent pages, descriptions of the various recognized disorders of the hematopoietic system will be found and their treatment discussed, it is urged that the reader confronted with a problem, for example, of anemia, first study Chap. 23, because he will find there a discussion of anemias in general and he will thereby make his way more readily through the pages that follow or, for that matter, through other sections in this textbook. The same is true, in principle, if the problem is one of bleeding or lymph node enlargement or splenomegaly.

235 THE ANEMIAS
M. M. Wintrobe

POSTHEMORRHAGIC ANEMIA

Anemia resulting from blood loss may have developed suddenly because of the rapid loss of a large quantity of blood, or it may have come about very gradually over a period of many months or even years. Obviously there are also many possible variations between these two extremes. The causes of posthemorrhagic anemia are numerous and the manifestations differ widely, the latter depending in part on the nature of the underlying disorder and in part on the quantity and speed of the blood loss. It is convenient to consider acute and chronic posthemorrhagic anemias separately because their manifestations and, in certain respects, their treatment differ so greatly. It should be realized, however, that these two syndromes represent two extremes depending, in the main, on the same underlying defect, and that in practice variations will be encountered which represent all stages between these extremes.

Acute Posthemorrhagic Anemia

Etiology. Trauma, the rupture of a peptic ulcer or an ectopic pregnancy, and bleeding in connection with hemophilia or purpura hemorrhagica are examples of the widely varied possible causes of acute blood loss. They indicate that the blood loss may be external and recognizable at once, or internal and, consequently, sometimes not readily discovered.

Symptomatology. The rapid loss of blood leads to reduction in blood volume, and the clinical manifestations are mainly circulatory. If the blood loss is great, "acute posthemorrhagic shock" develops (see Chap. 13). If the hemorrhage is visible to the patient, whether the amount of blood lost is great or small, symptoms may arise from the psychic effect of such bleeding. Generally speaking, symptoms are likely to appear sooner and are more pronounced in relation to the amount of blood lost when the bleeding is external than when it is not recognizable by the patient. The manifestations of anemia in general have been discussed already (p. 207). In addition, the symptoms of the underlying disorder may be present as well.

Blood Picture. Polymorphonuclear leukocytosis with the appearance of immature forms ("shift to the left") is the first discernible change. An increase in platelets often takes place as well. The anemia may not be apparent at once since, at first, plasma is lost as well as red corpuscles, so that the ratio of cells to plasma remains the same. As fluid is drawn from the tissues to restore the blood volume, anemia becomes apparent. This is normocytic at first. Blood loss in an otherwise healthy organism, however, profoundly stimulates the bone marrow. This becomes hyperplastic, and immature corpuscles are liberated in larger numbers than usual. Reticulocytosis ensues, polychromatophilia is found, and even nucleated red corpuscles find their way into the blood. At this stage the anemia may be macrocytic since the immature cells are larger than the older forms. Reticulocytes begin to appear within 48 hr following a brisk hemorrhage and may continue to increase for several more days. A persistent reticulocytosis, forming a plateaulike curve, suggests that bleeding is continuing, for cessation of hemorrhage is marked by quick restoration of physiologic balance with rapid regression of the signs of stimulated hematopoiesis. If the iron stores of the body are good and the blood loss has not been extreme, iron deficiency does not occur and hypochromia is slight or absent. When the drain on iron is greater than can be readily replenished, iron deficiency begins.

When the acute hemorrhage is internal, destruction of the blood and absorption of the products may lead to an increased excretion of urobilinogen in the urine and stools, and, rarely, even slight bilirubinemia may be found. Bowel hemorrhage is often associated with an increase in the blood urea nitrogen level.

Diagnosis. When acute hemorrhage is not evident, such signs as pallor, faintness, restlessness, sweating, and palpitation should lead to a search for hemorrhage. If the subject is recumbent, much blood may be lost before these signs appear. They can be brought out by tilting the patient to the erect position. Late signs of acute blood loss are air hunger, thirst, and a falling blood pressure.

Prognosis. The amount and rapidity of the blood loss, the acuteness of the physician in discovering it, the availability of blood for transfusion, and the accessibility of the site of bleeding are the important considerations.

Treatment. Stopping of the hemorrhage and restoration of the blood volume to normal, preferably by transfusions of whole blood, otherwise by administration of plasma or other fluids, are the essentials. Speed in restoration of blood volume is more important than whether plasma or whole blood is used. If the blood loss has been great and the blood volume is profoundly reduced, multiple portals should be used for administration of blood, and even intraarterial administration may be advisable. Fluids by mouth (unless the bleeding is from the upper portion of the alimentary tract) and by hypodermoclysis are valuable adjuncts, as are rest and quiet, induced by morphine if necessary. Following the acute phase, a good diet containing meat, fruit, and vegetables affords the proteins and vitamins needed for erythropoiesis. Iron can be given in the form of ferrous sulfate (0.2 to 0.4 Gm t.i.d.) but is not needed in previously normal individuals unless blood loss has been great.

Chronic Posthemorrhagic Anemia

This refers to that state in which blood loss has produced a chronic anemia, and a deficiency of substances necessary for blood formation has developed. Although the factors essential for erythropoiesis are many, the chief deficiency resulting from chronic blood loss is that of iron. The manifestations of chronic posthemorrhagic anemia can therefore be discussed in the section which follows.

IRON-DEFICIENCY ANEMIA (Hypochromic Microcytic Anemia; Idiopathic, Chronic, or Nutritional Hypochromic Anemia; Chlorosis, Chlorotic Anemia, Chloranemia)

Etiology. Iron is normally obtained by digestion of food and is absorbed chiefly in the upper portion of the gastrointestinal tract. This is aided by the acid secretion of the stomach. The absorbed iron is utilized for hemoglobin formation, as well as for the production of myoglobin and other enzymes. Normally a large reserve is stored in the liver, spleen, and other tissues. The total iron store in man which is available for blood formation has been estimated to amount to 1.2 or 1.5 Gm. Once absorbed, iron is conserved tenaciously. The amount lost per day by the normal adult male has been estimated as approximately 1 mg.

Any circumstance which leads to a greater demand on the iron stores of the body than can be supplied results in iron deficiency. In logical order, the possible factors leading to iron deficiency are (1) insufficient iron in the diet, (2) impaired absorption, (3) increased requirements, and (4) loss of blood. Of these, the *chronic loss of blood* by hemorrhage is by far the most common factor in the development of iron deficiency. Excessive menstruation and occult bleeding from the gastrointestinal tract (peptic ulcer, esophageal varices, hookworm infection, etc.) are the most common types of bleeding which may result in iron deficiency, since the former is but an exaggeration of a physiologic process and may thus receive little attention, while the latter may pass unnoticed for a long time.

Impaired absorption of iron is rarely an important factor in the development of iron deficiency, even though various influences favor or inhibit the availability and absorption of iron. Thus, a high level of calcium in the diet diminishes the formation of insoluble iron phosphates and favors absorption of iron, but excess calcium inhibits iron assimilation. Ascorbic acid favors iron assimilation, probably by promoting the reduction of ferric iron in food to the ferrous form. Although the gastric hydrochloric acid favors ionization and thus absorption, many persons are encountered in whom achlorhydria has existed for years without iron deficiency developing. Chronic diarrhea, however, is of more importance. Certainly iron deficiency may be encountered in sprue.

Deficiency of iron in the diet alone is rarely a cause of iron deficiency except in infants receiving a milk diet exclusively, and occasionally in elderly people who, although they have had no blood loss for many years, have depleted their stores by consuming a diet very low in iron.

In children and adolescents the iron needs for *growth* are very important, and it is largely because of the demands made by the ever-expanding blood volume that infants receiving an unsupplemented diet of milk develop iron deficiency. In older children and adolescents, poverty or faulty habits may contribute to the mounting deficiency by causing consumption of a diet too low in iron to supply the needs. In girls, the menstrual loss of blood accentuates this deficiency. Normal menstruation results in an average loss of 0.5 to 1.0 mg iron per day. *Chlorosis,* the "green sickness" of the last century and before, was probably no more than iron deficiency in adolescent girls in whom low dietary iron was insufficient to meet the needs. In adult women the iron requirements during *pregnancy* and *lactation* are factors which may lead to the development of iron-deficiency anemia. Pregnancy results in a net deficit of iron of approxi-mately 1 mg per day, lactation about 0.5 mg per day. Often these circumstances are superimposed on a state of gradually increasing iron depletion which may have had its beginning in adolescence. The ultimate combined effect of chronic loss of blood, increased demands, and faulty diet may not become clearly manifest until thirty to forty-five years of age, the period in which the *chronic hypochromic anemia* of women is most often seen. It is of interest that in such individuals certain *constitutional features* similar to those encountered in pernicious anemia may be observed, such as early graying of the hair and achlorhydria.

Since so little iron is excreted normally, iron deficiency develops *in the adult male* only from loss of blood or, rarely, from dietary deficiency or impaired absorption which has existed over a period of many years. In the male, ulcerative lesions in the gastrointestinal tract are by far the most likely causes of long-continued, undetected loss of blood.

Symptomatology. The symptoms are those common to all chronic anemias and may include a variety of vague gastrointestinal complaints, such as anorexia, capricious appetite, or heartburn and, more rarely, sore tongue, sore mouth, and dysphagia (Plummer-Vinson syndrome); or palpitation, dyspnea, and edema about the ankles; or neuralgic pains, vasomotor disturbances, or numbness and tingling. Menstrual disturbances are common—menorrhagia, irregularity of flow, or even phases of amenorrhea.

A tired, lifeless appearance; pallor; inelastic and often dry and wrinkled skin, sometimes with a brownish hue; dry and often scanty hair; and blue scleras are found in cases of long standing. In many, some degree of papillary atrophy of the tongue, slight cardiac enlargement, functional systolic murmurs, and a palpable spleen are discernible. When the deficiency is severe, the nails may be flattened, longitudinally ridged, or even concave (koilonychia), and may break easily. The sore tongue, dysphagia, and changes in the hair, nails, and skin may occur in iron deficiency prior to the development of anemia.

Blood Picture. A good blood smear will reveal thin, pale red corpuscles poorly filled with hemoglobin. In some cases these may be mere rings. Tiny microcytes, "target-like" cells, elliptic cells, and bizarre poikilocytes are also found, as well as a certain proportion of normally filled corpuscles. The anemia is hypochromic and microcytic. Only in this type of anemia is a substantially reduced mean corpuscular hemoglobin concentration (MCHC) encountered (less than 30 per cent). This hypochromia is more significant than the microcytosis, although the latter may be extreme (mean corpuscular volume 55 to 75 cuμ). The red corpuscle count may be normal or nearly so, or even greater than normal, while the hemoglobin and volume of packed red corpuscles are greatly reduced. The leukocyte count is normal or slightly reduced, and a slight thrombocytopenia may exist.

The *bone marrow* is hyperplastic and contains an excessive number of normoblasts.

Diagnosis. The symptoms are naturally varied, since iron deficiency may result from a large variety of causes. When iron depletion is only moderate in degree, the changes in the blood may not be striking. In more advanced cases, adequate examination of the blood should make it clear that hypochromic microcytic anemia exists. This type of anemia is most often due to lack of iron. Experimentally a similar anemia is observed in copper and in pyridoxine deficiency, but in man such deficiencies are exceedingly rare, if they occur at all. Metabolic disorders involving these substances have been described, however. Thus, there is a syndrome in infants and young children in which low serum copper values and hypoproteinemia accompany a hypochromic microcytic anemia which responds to iron therapy. Again, a refractory, microcytic hypochromic anemia accompanied by hyperferremia and, in a few instances, by splenomegaly and hepatomegaly has been observed in eight cases which responded to the administration of pyridoxine in large quantities. Other instances of refractory hypochromic microcytic anemia have been described, such as "hereditary, sex-linked (?) anemia," which may be related to the pyridoxine-responsive type, but these are all exceedingly rare. The only form of hypochromic microcytic anemia which is not extremely rare and which may be mistaken for that due to iron deficiency is thalassemia (p. 1301). Consequently, the discovery of hypochromic microcytic anemia usually calls for a search for causes of iron deficiency and, in particular, requires a thorough search for sources of blood loss.

Prognosis. This is excellent in so far as the possibility of relieving the anemia is concerned. The prognosis otherwise depends on the character of the contributory causes.

Treatment. Only in iron-deficiency anemia is iron therapy of value. Here the administration of *ferrous sulfate* or *ferrous gluconate* is followed by a reticulocyte response, and subsequently rapid red corpuscle regeneration occurs. Gastric irritation is less likely to occur if tablets of 0.2 Gm are taken on a full stomach. To allow the patient to become accustomed to it, at first a total of 0.4 Gm is given per day, but this may be increased to 1 Gm. In addition to iron therapy, a good diet containing meat, fruit, and vegetables is to be recommended, and any underlying or associated disorder should be corrected. Transfusion of blood is rarely if ever needed, even in the most anemic patient, and free hydrochloric acid is not required even if achlorhydria is present. Failure to respond to oral iron ther-

apy, necessitating intravenous administration, has been described but is exceedingly rare.

MACROCYTIC ANEMIAS

Elucidation of the pathogenesis of pernicious anemia, even though still incomplete, has made it clear that there are a number of closely related disorders which have in common a characteristic type of anemia, megaloblastic hyperplasia of the bone marrow, and the capacity to respond to liver therapy, yeast, pteroylglutamic acid, vitamin B_{12}, or related substances. These conditions, the *megaloblastic macrocytic anemias,* must be differentiated from those instances of macrocytosis which represent increases in mean corpuscular volume from other causes, usually from the presence in the circulation of a relatively large number of immature red corpuscles appearing in response to such hematopoietic stimulants as severe hemorrhage or acute blood destruction (Table 235-1). In this second type of macrocytic anemia the bone marrow is not megaloblastic and liver, vitamin B_{12}, or folic acid therapy has no value. The clinical differentiation is usually easy.

Pernicious Anemia (Addisonian Pernicious Anemia, Addison's or Biermer's Anemia, Primary Anemia)

Definition. Pernicious anemia is a chronic disorder characterized by macrocytic anemia, megaloblastic hyperplasia of the bone marrow, gastric achlorhydria, and often glossitis and changes in the nervous system. This disorder appears to be the consequence of a permanent gastric secretory defect associated with atrophy which results in a deficiency in the body of a substance derived from food. The deficiency can be corrected by supplying a substance present in certain liver extracts which appears to be identical with vitamin B_{12}.

History. Although the disorder was described at least as early as 1823 by Combe, it was the picture given by Thomas Addison in 1855 and the comprehensive description by Biermer in 1872 which drew attention to this ultimately fatal (therefore "pernicious") anemia. The discovery of the value of liver therapy by Minot and Murphy in 1926 and the elucidation of the role of the stomach in the pathogenesis of the disorder by Castle in 1929 completely changed the prognosis of the condition and profoundly stimulated hematologic research in general.

Etiology. This disorder is very rare in persons under the age of thirty and is encountered much more frequently in light-haired, blue-eyed individuals than in the darker races or in Orientals. It is

Table 235-1. CLASSIFICATION OF MACROCYTIC ANEMIAS

I. Megaloblastic macrocytic anemias
  A. Conditions responding to administration of both vitamin B_{12} (liver extract) and folic acid

Condition	Probable pathogenesis
1. Pernicious anemia*	Deficiency of gastric intrinsic factor
2. Total gastrectomy	Removal of source of intrinsic factor
3. Nutritional macrocytic anemia	Dietary deficiency
4. Sprue, idiopathic steatorrhea	Impaired absorption
5. Resection of small intestine	Impaired absorption
6. Intestinal strictures and anastomoses	Diversion of vitamin B_{12} and folic acid from host
7. Fish tapeworm anemia	Diversion of vitamin B_{12} and folic acid from host

  B. Conditions responding only, or usually, to folic acid, rather than to vitamin B_{12}

8. Megaloblastic anemia of pregnancy	Metabolic disturbance? Increased requirements?
9. Megaloblastic anemia of infancy	Deficiency of folic acid *and* ascorbic acid
10. "Achrestic" anemia and "refractory megaloblastic" anemia	Metabolic disturbance? Complex or unusual deficiencies?
11. Anticonvulsant drugs	Metabolic antagonists
12. Amethopterin or 6MP therapy	Metabolic antagonists
13. Unusually vigorous erythropoiesis	Increased demands, low stores

II. Nonmegaloblastic macrocytic anemias

A. Acute posthemorrhagic anemia	Presence in blood of many immature erythrocytes
B. Hemolytic anemia	Presence in blood of many immature erythrocytes
C. Aplastic anemia	Unknown
D. Hypothyroidism	Unknown
E. Liver disease	Unknown

* Pernicious anemia is distinguished from the other conditions listed in that achlorhydria is always present and neurologic changes may occur.

N.B. In practice, the most common cause of what appears to be macrocytic anemia is laboratory error, most often in red corpuscle counting.

seen especially in natives of the British Isles, the Scandinavian countries, and other more northern regions, as well as in their offspring in other parts of the world. Nevertheless, although less common, pernicious anemia is seen in Negroes.

A familial incidence is not unusual. Those affected often have turned gray prematurely, and they may have broad faces and large, bony frames. Males and females are affected about equally.

That a gastric secretory defect is a fundamental factor in the pathogenesis of pernicious anemia was suspected almost as early as the disease was recognized. It was shown later that absence of hydrochloric acid in the gastric secretion and a greatly reduced total gastric secretion (achylia) precede the development of the anemia by many years. It has also been shown that such achylia is a defect which persists in spite of successful antianemic therapy. Castle demonstrated that the significant abnormality in gastric secretion is not lack of hydrochloric acid but absence of an "intrinsic factor" which normally acts upon an "extrinsic factor" derived from food. The material so produced was regarded as leading to the formation of a substance stored in the liver without which normal hematopoiesis cannot take place. The gastric factor is thermolabile. It seems to be contained in or adsorbed to the glandular mucoprotein of the stomach. The thermostable food factor is present in meat, eggs, cereals, and other natural sources of the vitamin-B complex and is also present in liver. Desiccated hog's stomach given orally has the same hematopoietic effect in pernicious anemia as liver, and its effectiveness was assumed to be due to the interaction of the intrinsic and extrinsic factors in gastric tissue.

The discovery of vitamin B_{12} (cyanocobalamin), a red pigment containing cobalt, and the demonstration of its therapeutic effectiveness in pernicious anemia on parenteral administration in amounts as small as 1 μg have clarified some of the puzzling aspects of the pathogenesis of this disease. Vitamin B_{12} is also active orally if given in very large amounts (100 to 150 μg), but its hematopoietic effectiveness is greatly increased by normal human gastric juice. Vitamin B_{12} is apparently the extrinsic factor as well as the liver factor or "antiperniciousanemia principle." The role of the gastric or intrinsic factor is simply to promote the absorption of vitamin B_{12} from the alimentary tract, possibly by binding with vitamin B_{12} and, in turn, being bound by receptors in the intestinal wall. Because of the absence of intrinsic factor in patients with pernicious anemia, the absorption of vitamin B_{12} is impaired and the effects of deficiency ultimately develop.

The vitamin pteroylglutamic acid (folic acid) has been shown to produce a hematopoietic response in pernicious anemia when given orally or parenterally. It is neither Castle's intrinsic factor nor the extrinsic factor. In nature it is found in conjugated form, as the heptaglutamate (yeast) or as triglutamate. An observation of great practical importance is that whereas the administration of liver extract or vitamin B_{12} prevents the development or advancement of the neural manifestations of pernicious anemia, these may appear in spite of folic acid therapy.

The metabolic functions of vitamin B_{12} and folic acid are, in the main, closely related but they are by no means fully understood. They are both concerned in the metabolic reactions which involve one-carbon fragments and thereby are important in the biosynthesis of purines, pyrimidines, and certain amino acids. Vitamin B_{12} is also involved in the incorporation of amino acids in protein and influences folic acid metabolism in several ways. The close metabolic relationship of the two substances appears to be the reason why a deficiency of either or both results in a number of abnormalities, of which megaloblastic bone marrow is the most readily recognized. Reasons have been offered for the progress of the neural changes observed in some patients with pernicious anemia receiving folic acid therapy, but none has found adequate support.

The red corpuscles of patients with untreated pernicious anemia appear to have a shortened survival time. Thus the bilirubinemia and urobilinogenuria so characteristic of pernicious anemia would seem to be manifestations of a more rapid blood destruction, which may be the consequence of imperfect construction of the red corpuscles resulting from a deficiency of building materials. That this is not the sole explanation of the disturbance in pigment metabolism in pernicious anemia, however, is suggested by the observation that 40 per cent or more of labeled stool urobilin in pernicious anemia is not derived from circulating red corpuscles. Some of the pigment apparently comes from heme or hematin which has not been used for hemoglobin synthesis.

Pathology. The significant findings are in the alimentary tract, the bone marrow, and the nervous system. The tongue usually appears smooth and the papillae may be absent. Atrophy of the mucous membrane may be striking in the tongue and in the stomach. The changes in the stomach have been observed particularly in the fundic zone, where the parietal and chief cells are usually absent.

Appropriate staining reveals the liver as well as the spleen and kidneys to be abnormally laden with iron. In the liver this is found in the periphery of the lobules and in the Kupffer cells. There may also be fatty degeneration in the central cells of the lobules of the liver. The heavy deposit of iron is the consequence of the fault in red corpuscle formation which leads to the development of anemia;

when active blood regeneration follows therapy, the iron is used in blood formation.

The *bone marrow* is red and is found to be crowded with cells. Cells of the red series make up 30 to 50 per cent, rather than about 20 per cent of the cells of the marrow. The degree of hyperplasia and the degree of immaturity of the cells are roughly proportional to the severity of the anemia. The nucleated red corpuscles ("megaloblasts") differ from those found in other types of anemia in several respects. They are exceptionally large and, more significantly, the nuclear chromatin is fine and sievelike, unlike the relatively coarse and "lumpy" material seen in normoblasts. The cytoplasm of these cells may be polychromatophilic or orthochromatic, and in a few is basophilic. Many abnormal mitotic figures may be present. At the same time, extraordinarily large leukocytes may be found in the marrow; in particular, large metamyelocytes can be seen with bizarre-shaped nuclei and peculiarly staining or vacuolated cytoplasm. Megakaryocytes may be reduced in number and may be morphologically abnormal. In spite of the evidence of cellular activity, hematopoiesis is inefficient and anemia develops.

In the nervous system, degenerative changes may be found in the dorsal and lateral tracts of the cord, in the dorsal root ganglions, and in the peripheral nerves. Myelin degeneration and loss of nerve fibers occur. More rarely, changes are encountered in the brain.

Symptomatology. The onset of the disease is generally insidious. In many instances at least two of the diagnostic triad of symptoms are encountered; namely, weakness, sore tongue, and numbness and tingling in the extremities. However, other complaints may overshadow these, and the presenting clinical picture may suggest some disorder of the digestive tract because of anorexia, diarrhea, and various other gastrointestinal symptoms; it may simulate cardiac dysfunction of the anginal or the congestive failure type; or one may be led to search for some malignant neoplasm or an obscure infection. In some instances the neural involvement is so pronounced that a primary neurologic disease is considered. Even renal or genitourinary disease or a mental disorder may be simulated.

The degree of soreness of the tongue varies greatly and the involvement may be complete or patchy. The tongue may be "beefy" red when the symptoms are pronounced and is less red and smooth when they subside. The gastrointestinal symptoms vary greatly. However, one consistently found in relapse is anorexia. Symptoms referable to the circulatory system include dyspnea, palpitation, sensations of extra beats, weakness, vertigo, tinnitus, and precordial pain. Since pernicious anemia often appears for the first time in the older age groups, it may be difficult to determine to what extent anemia or the degenerative changes of old age have contributed to the development of heart failure.

Pallor; a flabby rather than wasted appearance; a slight or pronounced yellowish color of the skin together with faint icterus of the scleras; a tongue which is often glazed in appearance and sometimes is red and sore; a rapid pulse with slight cardiac enlargement and often precordial hemic murmurs; in many, a spleen which is just palpable; and often a slightly enlarged liver are the chief findings outside the nervous system. In the nervous system, loss of vibratory sense in the lower extremities (not necessarily symmetric), incoordination of the lower extremities, loss of finer coordination of the fingers, signs suggestive of lateral as well as posterior spinal cord involvement, and evidence of peripheral nerve degeneration are the most common findings and may be present in all degrees from slight or none to extensive involvement. Positive Babinski response, positive Romberg's sign, disturbed position sense, spasticity, increased or diminished reflexes, and sphincter disturbances may be encountered. Minor mental disturbances (irritability, memory disturbances, mild depression) or more serious mental symptoms may develop.

Laboratory Findings. *Blood.* The anemia is usually more severe than the complaints and physical examination would lead one to suspect. In the blood smear, macrocytes, often oval in shape, are characteristically seen (Fig. 235-1), but there is actually a great range in the size of the cells, and in addition, many bizarre-shaped corpuscles are found (poikilocytosis). Since the abnormally large cells predominate, the mean corpuscular volume is found to be greater than normal and ranges between 100 and 160 μ (Fig. 235-2). There is a corresponding increase in the hemoglobin content of the red corpuscles (mean corpuscular hemoglobin), so that the concentration of hemoglobin in the corpuscles (mean corpuscular hemoglobin concentration) is normal. The red corpuscles in pernicious anemia and in other macrocytic anemias are not "hyperchromic," but, being thicker as well as larger in diameter than normal corpuscles, they appear to be supersaturated with hemoglobin, as one looks at them through a microscope. Some degree of diffuse polychromatophilia as well as basophilic stippling is found, and occasional nucleated red corpuscles may be encountered. The most striking changes, described in classic cases, are observed only when the anemia is very severe. Since the anemia is macrocytic, the red corpuscle count is reduced more than proportionately as compared with the hemoglobin or the volume of packed red

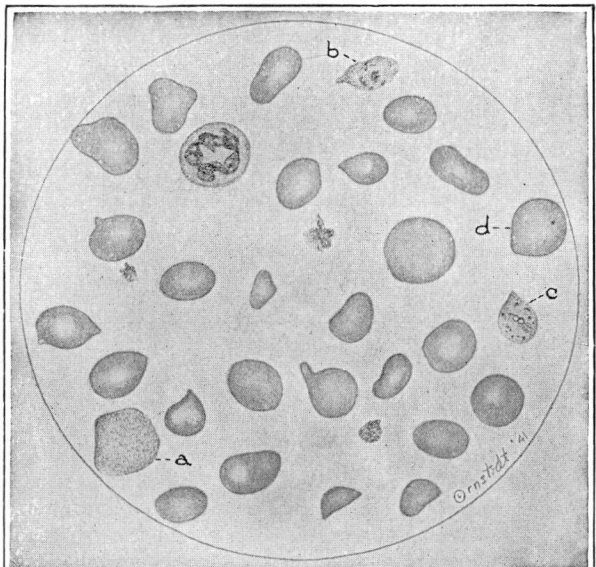

FIG. 235-1. Drawing of a blood smear from a case of pernicious anemia in relapse. From a preparation stained with Wright's and magnified ×960. Note the extreme variation in the size and shape of the red corpuscles, the large polychromatophilic red corpuscle (*a*), the cells containing nuclear remnants and Howell-Jolly bodies (*b, c*) and a Cabot ring (*c*), the granular red corpuscle (*d*), and the multisegmented polymorphonuclear leukocyte. (*Wintrobe: "Clinical Hematology," 5th ed., Philadelphia, Lea & Febiger, 1961.*)

corpuscles. Reticulocytes are usually within normal limits in untreated patients or, at most, do not run higher than 3 or 4 per cent.

The leukocyte count is usually lower than normal, chiefly because of a granulocytopenia. Thus, there is relative lymphocytosis. The polymorphonuclear neutrophilic leukocytes often show an unusual number of segments and may be exceptionally large. An occasional myelocyte is present in many cases. Sometimes some degree of eosinophilia is encountered. The platelets are generally reduced in number, sometimes to levels below 100,000 per cu mm, and bizarre forms, including giant platelets, may be found. When there is thrombocytopenia, the bleeding time may be prolonged, the blood clot retracts poorly, and purpura may develop.

The resistance of the red corpuscles to hypotonic saline solutions is not significantly altered. The icterus index usually ranges between 8 and 15; sometimes it is as high as 20 or 25. The average plasma bilirubin content is 1 mg per 100 ml but often is higher, and the van den Bergh reaction is "indirect."

Other Laboratory Findings. With extremely rare exceptions, there is, in cases of pernicious anemia,

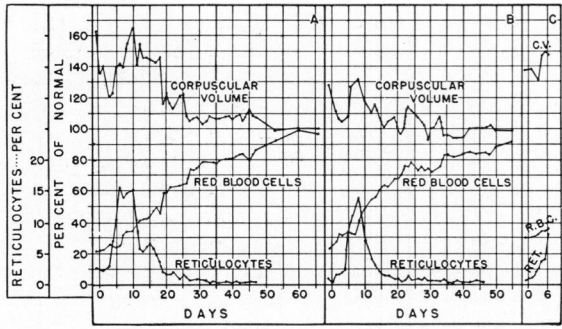

FIG. 235-2. Variations in mean volume of red corpuscles compared with reticulocyte count in three cases of pernicious anemia. The mean corpuscular volume (CV) and the red cell count (RBC) are represented as percentages of their respective average normal values. By this method the red cell count and mean corpuscular volume of a hypothetic normal individual would fall on the line at 100 per cent. Reticulocytes are recorded directly. The abscissa records number of days following the commencement of liver therapy. (*Wintrobe: Relation of Variations in Mean Corpuscular Volume to Number of Reticulocytes in Pernicious Anemia, J. Clin. Invest.,* 13:669, 1934.)

persistent failure to secrete hydrochloric acid in the stomach even following the injection of histamine. Furthermore, in the great majority of cases, the enzymes are deficient as well, and only a small amount of mucus rewards the gastric extraction.

In addition to the bilirubinemia, already mentioned, the urobilinogen content of the urine and stools is increased. Detailed examinations reveal many other evidences of metabolic disturbance involving, especially, protein and uric acid as well as fat metabolism.

Diagnosis. When the combination of the classic symptoms—weakness, sore tongue, and numbness and tingling—together with macrocytic anemia and achlorhydria is found, there need be no difficulty in diagnosis. Confusion may arise if the symptoms have led one to suspect some other condition and the blood examination has not been appropriate to demonstrate the existence of a macrocytic anemia. Confusion may also arise when symptoms referable to the nervous system are prominent and anemia is only moderate or slight in degree. For all practical purposes, since achlorhydria is so characteristic a feature of pernicious anemia, a diagnosis of pernicious anemia should never be made without demonstrating a failure to secrete hydrochloric acid following the injection of histamine. The existence of a macrocytic anemia, as indicated by calculation of red corpuscle size, should, furthermore, be confirmed by examination of the blood smear. In practically all cases such anemia is found to be associated with evidences of altered pigment metabolism

such as some increase in plasma bilirubin and an increased output of urobilinogen in the urine and stools. Where anemia is slight in degree, the combination of achlorhydria, slight macrocytosis as indicated by calculation of mean corpuscular volume and by the presence of macrocytes in the blood smear, together with a slight degree of bilirubinemia, makes pernicious anemia highly likely.

It must be kept in mind that the demonstration of macrocytic anemia is not in itself diagnostic of pernicious anemia, for, as already indicated, macrocytic anemia may appear under a variety of circumstances. When the macrocytic anemia is part of another disorder such as "aplastic" anemia, "aleukemic" leukemia, or some type of hemolytic anemia, differentiation is important, for vitamin B_{12} or folic acid therapy is then valueless. In aplastic anemia, achlorhydria is only sometimes present, glossitis is rare, and signs of involvement of the nervous system, such as loss of vibratory sense, are unusual. In aleukemic leukemia, sternal marrow examination should reveal a characteristic picture quite different from that of pernicious anemia, and in hemolytic anemia the marrow is normoblastic, not megaloblastic. Even when the macrocytic anemia is accompanied by megaloblastic bone marrow, differentiation is important, since some forms, unlike pernicious anemia, are not permanent in character and do not require treatment for the remainder of the patient's life. Certain rare megaloblastic macrocytic anemias, furthermore, do not respond to the administration of vitamin B_{12}. Some of these conditions are described briefly below.

It is important that diagnosis be established accurately before treatment is initiated, since, as already indicated, a diagnosis of pernicious anemia implies the need for therapy for the rest of the patient's life. In doubtful cases, a therapeutic test, if properly performed, can be very helpful. It is important, however, that the test be made with vitamin B_{12} alone and not with some agent containing iron or other substances in addition, and that the reticulocyte response be observed daily for 7 to 10 days until a positive or negative result has been obtained.

The discovery of vitamin B_{12} and the fact that the cobalt contained therein can be labeled radioactively have provided a method whereby the absorption of this vitamin can be measured. This offers a means by which defective absorption of the vitamin from the gastrointestinal tract can be demonstrated even in the absence of anemia, as in treated cases of pernicious anemia, and to some extent megaloblastic macrocytic anemias other than pernicious anemia can be differentiated from that condition. Several different techniques are available, but the most commonly used one, the *Schilling test,* depends on measurement of the excretion of the administered radioactive material in the urine. When radioactive vitamin B_{12} is given by mouth to persons who can absorb it, radioactivity will appear in the urine if the person is "flooded" with an intramuscular injection of nonradioactive vitamin B_{12}. Normal individuals have been found to excrete 11 to 26 per cent of the orally administered radioactivity in the urine in the next 24 hr, depending on the size of the dose (0.5 to 2.0 μg). Patients with pernicious anemia have been observed to excrete only 0 to 7.0 per cent under these conditions. In them the simultaneous administration of intrinsic factor and radioactive vitamin results in increased excretion (3.1 to 30, average 9.8 per cent).

Prognosis. With appropriate therapy it is now possible to restore the blood to normal and to promote a return of the general nutrition to normal. If changes are present in the nervous system, their advance can at least be halted, and in some cases improvement may take place. The danger in pernicious anemia arises from failure to continue therapy and from complications and intercurrent conditions. In a chronic ailment like pernicious anemia, other diseases develop in the course of time. Among these, carcinoma of the stomach is particularly noteworthy, since the incidence of this disease in patients with pernicious anemia is more than three times as great as in other individuals. When changes in the nervous system exist, particularly if they involve the urinary sphincter, infection may occur. The existence of infection at the time of relapse may seriously interfere with the response to therapy.

Treatment. Treatment, in so far as the blood changes are concerned, is extremely simple. The administration of an adequate amount of vitamin B_{12} is followed by a reticulocyte response which reaches its maximum 5 to 7 or 8 days following initiation of therapy. This is succeeded, as the reticulocyte count falls to normal, by a rapid disappearance of anemia and by the production of cells of normal size and shape. The leukocyte and the platelet counts likewise return to normal, bilirubinemia disappears, and the increased quantities of urobilinogen in the urine and stools are reduced to the normal range. The gastric achlorhydria persists.

Effective treatment may produce subjective improvement within 48 hr, and evidence of a change is often noted by the patient before the reticulocytes increase. There is a gain in appetite and a sense of well-being. Tongue symptoms, if present, disappear promptly. On the other hand, neural symptoms do not change quickly. Although in the course of 2 months from the beginning of treatment the patient usually attains a normal blood, the neurologic symptoms may still be present. However, those of milder intensity are likely to decrease or disappear.

The most efficient means of treatment is by the intramuscular injection of vitamin B_{12}. The effects of the administration of vitamin B_{12} in pernicious anemia appear to be in every way similar to those produced by liver extract and, like the latter, are very much more pronounced when the vitamin is given parenterally than when it is taken orally (60 to 100 times). The minimal effective intramuscular dose of vitamin B_{12} is 1 μg, and good hematopoietic responses may be expected from doses of 10 μg daily. Larger amounts up to 80 μg or more daily produce greater effects, the mean response being roughly proportional to the logarithm of the dose. As larger doses are given, however, a greater proportion is promptly excreted.

For a patient in relapse, between 1,000 and 5,000 μg vitamin B_{12} is given, since the substance is needed not only to produce a remission but to replenish the greatly depleted body stores. However, this is best administered in divided doses in the course of the first 2 weeks or more of therapy; otherwise, much of the vitamin will be excreted before it can be used or stored, as already indicated. An injection of 100 μg is a satisfactory amount to be given at one time. If possible, reticulocytes should be counted daily in order that the effectiveness of therapy, or lack of response, may be demonstrated early. An increased quantity of red cells as measured by the volume of packed red cells is not usually detectable before 10 days.

Maintenance therapy may be calculated on the basis of approximately 2 μg vitamin B_{12} for each day, but this does not need to be given at intervals shorter than a month or two; i.e., 60 μg is injected intramuscularly every 30 days or 120 μg every 60 days.

Intravenous therapy is unnecessary. Oral therapy with liver extract or B_{12}–intrinsic factor combinations is inconvenient, since daily intake is necessary. Only where some idiosyncrasy on the part of the patient exists, or where sensitivity to the parenteral administration of vitamin B_{12} cannot be overcome otherwise, is oral therapy justified. Then 1,000 μg vitamin B_{12} orally each day is preferable to the use of vitamin B_{12}–intrinsic factor combinations or liver extracts. Folic acid should not be used.

The diet should be such as to restore the patient to a state of normal nutrition and to maintain him so, but need not contain any unusual foods, except perhaps where neurologic changes are present. In such cases, it may be wise to recommend the consumption of, say, a half pound or more of cooked liver per week. This recommendation is made since information is still lacking as to the exact nature of the deficiency which leads to the development of changes in the nervous system. By the consumption of whole liver the patient possibly obtains substances of value in addition to the antianemic factor.

Transfusion is rarely, if ever, required in pernicious anemia, since a physiologic response can be achieved in 48 to 72 hr if vitamin B_{12} is given parenterally. Since the patient's anemia has developed gradually, he has become adjusted to it. Where the cardiovascular system is imperfect, transfusion, by producing a sudden increase in blood volume, may sometimes be harmful and may precipitate acute cardiac failure with pulmonary edema. Iron is not needed as an adjunct except where iron deficiency exists as well. Supplementary therapy with various vitamins is likewise unnecessary. These can be and should be furnished in the diet in the form of food. The administration of dilute hydrochloric acid (USP), in amounts of 4 to 8 ml t.i.d. with meals, is sometimes of value when gastrointestinal complaints persist, particularly eructations or frequent bowel movements. In the absence of such complaints hydrochloric acid is unnecessary.

Particularly where changes in the nervous system exist, confinement to bed should be as brief as possible, and the patient should be encouraged to use the limbs even when lying in bed. In addition, passive movement, massage, and dry heat are valuable for improving the tone of the muscles. Physiotherapy may permit adjustment to permanent damage resulting from the neurologic changes.

The development of an intercurrent disease, particularly infection, calls for an increase in the amount of vitamin B_{12} therapy, since requirements under such conditions seem to be increased.

Vitamin B_{12} therapy has now replaced treatment with liver extract. Even when "refined" liver extracts were used, sensitivity was sometimes observed to develop in the form of severe flushing, dizziness, a sense of oppression, or urticaria following its intramuscular administration. Sometimes even peripheral vascular collapse occurred. Sensitivity to the crystalline vitamin B_{12} is extremely rare.

Megaloblastic Macrocytic Anemias Other than Pernicious Anemia (Table 235-1)

Nutritional Macrocytic Anemia. This term refers to macrocytic anemia arising from dietary deficiency, as distinguished from deficiency resulting from lack of intrinsic factor or from faulty absorption. Since such anemia has been seen most often in the tropics, *tropical macrocytic anemia* is another synonym. The condition is particularly common in pregnant women. Weakness, shortness of breath, sore mouth, sore tongue, diarrhea, and edema are common complaints. In contrast to pernicious anemia, in nutritional macrocytic anemia achlorhydria is no more common than in the population in general, and degenerative changes in the nervous system are practically never found. The blood picture

and bone marrow are indistinguishable from those of pernicious anemia. Tropical macrocytic anemia probably is not a single clinical entity. In many cases the anemia has been relieved by the administration of yeast, Marmite (autolyzed yeast), or liver. In some cases a good hematopoietic response has followed the administration of pteroylglutamic acid, and in a few, a good response to vitamin B_{12} and even to oral penicillin has been reported. In certain cases, however, these agents have not been effective, and the need for still another factor (Wills's factor) has been postulated. That some form of dietary deficiency is the cause of this disorder is indicated by the observation that it does not recur if the diet is satisfactory.

Nutritional macrocytic anemia is uncommon in the Temperate Zones. Few of the instances of macrocytic anemia seen in *pellagra* can be accounted for by a lack of extrinsic factor in the diet. In other cases faulty absorption is important, and in many both mechanisms play a role. In *sprue* and in *idiopathic steatorrhea*, as described elsewhere (p. 557), inadequate absorption is the main cause for the development of macrocytic anemia. In Great Britain in particular, occult idiopathic steatorrhea with insignificant alimentary symptoms but accompanied by megaloblastic macrocytic anemia is not uncommon. This usually responds much better to the administration of pteroylglutamic acid than to vitamin B_{12}.

Patients described at one time as having "achrestic anemia" and "refractory megaloblastic anemia," because they failed to respond to liver therapy, may have impaired metabolism of folic acid or complex deficiencies of folic acid, ascorbic acid, choline, or perhaps other substances essential for the metabolic steps which result in normal erythropoiesis.

In Pregnancy. In addition to megaloblastic anemia in pregnancy which may be regarded as nutritional macrocytic anemia, as mentioned above, such anemia is sometimes seen in the absence of dietary deficiency. Although this type of anemia is often refractory to liver extract or vitamin B_{12}, most patients have responded to folic acid; the prognosis, which was very poor at one time, has thus been improved. The pathogenesis of this form of megaloblastic anemia is obscure. Increased demands as the result of the needs of the fetus, defective utilization, or some other metabolic abnormality are possibilities which have not been excluded.

Following Surgery. Following *total gastrectomy*, megaloblastic anemia may develop because the source of intrinsic factor has been removed. The absorption of orally administered vitamin B_{12} has been shown to be impaired. Following *partial gastrectomy* the incidence of megaloblastic anemia is very much lower than after total gastrectomy, although iron-deficiency anemia is relatively common.

The macrocytic anemia seen in association with *intestinal strictures* and *anastomoses* has been attributed to impaired absorption, but as good hematopoietic responses have been observed when tetracyclines were given, it seems plausible that the anemia is caused by the colonization of the small intestine by abnormal bacteria which in some way divert folic acid or vitamin B_{12} from the host.

In Liver Disease. Macrocytic anemia occurs in a variable number of cases of chronic liver disease and it is megaloblastic in a few. No wholly satisfactory explanation for the latter has been found. It is conceivable that the requirements for folic acid and vitamin B_{12} may be increased or their storage or utilization impaired, or that other factors are involved.

In Hypothyroidism. Macrocytic anemia is sometimes seen in hypothyroidism, but the bone marrow is usually hypoplastic and normoblastic, and desiccated thyroid, not liver extract, vitamin B_{12}, or pteroylglutamic acid, is effective in relieving the anemia. Defective intestinal absorption of vitamin B_{12}, uninfluenced by intrinsic factor, has been demonstrated in some cases.

In Fish Tapeworm Infestation. True megaloblastic macrocytic anemia is seen, in Finland especially, in persons harboring the tapeworm, *Diphyllobothrium latum.* The anemia is attributable to competition with the host by the worm for vitamin B_{12}. How this interference is accomplished is unclear; perhaps by utilization of the vitamin, breakdown of its interaction with intrinsic factor, or prevention of its absorption through the intestinal wall.

During Administration of Antimetabolites. One of the toxic effects of amethopterin and 6-mercaptopurine, used in the treatment of leukemia, is the production of megaloblastic anemia. Interference with the metabolism of folic acid appears to be the explanation for the development of such anemia in a small proportion of patients receiving *anticonvulsant* drugs, such as diphenylhydantoin sodium, primidone, and barbital derivatives, although the possible coexistence in the individuals affected of some degree of folic acid deficiency must be considered to be likely.

In Cases of Excessive Demands. In rare instances of very active hematopoiesis, especially in hemolytic anemias, megaloblastic anemia has been observed, presumably because the demands for building materials exceeded those available in persons whose stores of these substances were marginal.

Review of the conditions in which megaloblastic anemia may be encountered thus reveals that under certain circumstances dietary deficiency of folic acid may develop and result in nutritional macrocytic anemia. In other patients there may be defective absorption of folic acid (sprue, idiopathic stea-

torrhea), but in some such patients the absorption of vitamin B_{12} may be impaired as well. In still other cases, alterations in the gastrointestinal tract may lead to consumption or destruction of one or both of these substances, or an antimetabolite may be produced there (fish tapeworm anemia, intestinal strictures and anastomoses). Only following total gastrectomy is absorption of vitamin B_{12} impaired in a manner corresponding to that encountered in pernicious anemia; i.e., as the result of lack of intrinsic factor. Various combinations of defects in dietary content, absorption, consumption, destruction, or antagonism may result in various degrees of deficiency of vitamin B_{12} or folic acid or both. In addition, it has been postulated that vitamin B_{12} in some manner influences the storage, absorption, and utilization of folic acid and that when vitamin B_{12} is lacking, these functions are impaired.

HEMOLYTIC ANEMIAS

Manifestations. Under the heading of hemolytic anemias a number of conditions may be included which differ widely in etiology, symptomatology, severity, and course. The symptoms depend upon the rapidity and extent of hemolysis, its duration, and whether or not it is taking place in the blood stream or in the reticuloendothelial system. Jaundice is a sign common to all, but its degree may be such as to be barely perceptible (when it is often overlooked) or so great as to be very striking. Other symptoms may be entirely absent. Thus patients with hereditary spherocytosis are "more yellow than sick" except when a hemolytic crisis occurs. In other cases there may be slowly progressive anemia and gradually increasing jaundice. The anemia may become profound and yet there may be few manifestations, since in such cases there is time for cardiovascular adjustments (p. 208) to be made. In chronic hemolytic anemia, splenomegaly is common and the liver may be enlarged. Complications such as gallbladder disease or chronic leg ulcers may develop.

On the other hand, the onset of hemolytic anemia may be heralded by a severe, shaking chill followed by high fever, malaise, headache, and pain in the back, abdomen, or limbs. The abdominal pain may be so severe and may be accompanied by such marked muscular rigidity and spasm as to simulate an acute surgical condition. If the hemolysis is rapid and severe enough, profound prostration and shock, accompanied by anuria and oliguria, may ensue. When urine is passed, it is found to be very dark. Jaundice develops rapidly. As anemia ensues, weakness, palpitation, dyspnea, tachycardia, cyanosis, cardiac enlargement, hemic murmurs, vertigo, faintness, and other manifestations of rapidly developing anemia (Chap. 23) make their appearance. In certain types of acute hemolytic reactions, urticaria, vascular disturbances suggesting Raynaud's phenomenon, and thrombosis and gangrene may develop.

All grades, from such acute fulminating disorders of several days' duration to extremely benign conditions of many years' standing, may be encountered. A chronic, congenital process may be interrupted by acute exacerbations.

Hematologic Manifestations. The hematologic manifestations which accompany acute blood destruction consist of an initial phase of rapid destruction of red corpuscles and a second phase of rapid blood regeneration. These two phases usually overlap, especially when the hemolytic agent acts over a prolonged period of time.

The anemia may be mild or severe, depending upon the intensity and duration of the hemolytic process. It is usually normocytic but may be macrocytic, especially during the stage of rapid regeneration when many relatively immature and reticulated cells are present. It is not uncommon to find 10 to 25 per cent reticulocytes in chronic cases, and as many as 60 per cent or even more in acute cases. Polychromatophilia, nucleated red blood corpuscles, and Howell-Jolly bodies are usually present. There generally is marked variation in the size of the cells (anisocytosis) and usually little variation in their shape (poikilocytosis), except in patients with sickle-cell anemia. Spherocytes may be numerous.

Marked stimulation of the leukopoietic tissues, manifested by leukocytosis and a "shift to the left," with myelocytes and even rare myeloblasts, accompanies the red corpuscle regeneration. Platelets may increase in number, and large, bizarre forms may make their appearance. In certain cases, however, and especially in paroxysmal nocturnal hemoglobinuria, leukopenia and thrombocytopenia may be present.

The *bone marrow* is hyperplastic. There is a great increase in normoblasts and a consequent reduction in the myeloid leukocyte/erythrocyte ratio from the normal of 4 or 5:1 to about 1:1 or even less. The normoblasts are chiefly polychromatophilic and orthochromatic forms; as a rule there are not many pronormoblasts or basophilic normoblasts. Megaloblasts, so characteristic of pernicious anemia and related macrocytic anemias, are not present.

Pigment Metabolism. When the degree and rate of blood destruction are very great, hemoglobin is liberated into the plasma and, if the hemoglobin-binding capacity of the plasma (haptoglobin, p. 203) is exceeded, free hemoglobin is excreted by the kidneys and hemoglobinuria results. However, the finding of red urine must not be assumed to be necessarily indicative of hemoglobinuria. The color may also be produced by intact red corpuscles,

porphyrin, or myoglobin. Microscopic and spectroscopic examination of the urine will reveal the cause of the abnormal color. Under certain circumstances hematin (p. 204) may be released.

More often, blood destruction is less rapid. In such cases hemoglobinemia and hemoglobinuria are not found and there is only an increase in the icterus index, serum bilirubin, and urobilinogen excretion in the urine and feces. The stools assume a dark color, and from 300 to 4,000 mg urobilinogen may be found in a 24-hr stool, as compared with the normal of 40 to 280 mg. The 24-hr urine may contain 5 to 200 mg urobilinogen (normal, 0 to 3.5 mg). The fecal urobilinogen may be increased when the urine urobilinogen and the bilirubin in the blood are not significantly greater than normal.

The quantity of bilirubin in the plasma may rise as high as 10 mg per 100 ml. The reaction is indirect but some increase in direct or "one-minute" bilirubin (bilirubin glucuronide) may also occur. The intensity of the bilirubinemia depends not only on the extent of the blood destruction but also on the capacity of the liver to remove the pigment from the blood stream and excrete it in the bile. A normally functioning liver is capable of excreting large quantities of bilirubin, but it is assumed that as anemia and consequent hypoxemia develop, its functional capacity becomes impaired and bilirubin accumulates in the blood stream.

Classification

The hemolytic disorders may be classified in various ways, none of which is entirely satisfactory. A clinical classification based on the severity of the manifestations may be confusing, since a chronic process may come to notice only during an acute exacerbation. Differentiation of congenital and acquired forms is useful. Better still, however, is classification on the basis of pathogenesis, even though understanding of the pathogenesis of the hemolytic anemias is still incomplete.

By transfusing corpuscles which differ from those of the recipient with respect to their MN or Rh type or by giving group O corpuscles to recipients belonging to one of the other three major blood groups, it has been shown that when normal corpuscles are transfused to patients in whom there is an extracorpuscular cause for hemolysis, the donated corpuscles are destroyed as rapidly as the patient's own corpuscles. If, on the other hand, the patient's corpuscles are removed from their abnormal environment and transfused to a normal recipient, their survival time is normal. Hemolytic anemias which have been shown to be or are thought to be of this type are listed in group I of Table 235-2. Group II includes disorders in which hemolysis is the result of a defect in the patient's own

Table 235-2. CLASSIFICATION OF HEMOLYTIC DISORDERS

I. Extracorpuscular causes
  A. Acute hemolytic anemias due to immune body reaction
    1. Isoagglutinins anti-A, anti-B (transfusion reactions)
    2. Isoagglutinins anti-Rh, Kell, Duffy, etc. (hemolytic disease of the newborn, "intra-group" transfusion reactions)
    3. Cold hemolysins (paroxysmal cold hemoglobinuria)
  B. Idiopathic acquired hemolytic anemias
  C. Secondary, or symptomatic, hemolytic anemias
    1. Hodgkin's disease
    2. Chronic lymphocytic leukemia, lymphosarcoma
    3. Disseminated lupus erythematosus
    4. Metastatic carcinomatosis
    5. Sarcoidosis, myelofibrosis
    6. Liver disease, ovarian tumors
    7. Thrombotic thrombocytopenic purpura
  D. Infectious agents
    1. Malaria
    2. *Bartonella* (Oroya fever)
    3. Septicemia: *Clostridium welchii, Vibrio comma* (cholera), rarely others
    4. Viruses (atypical pneumonia, infectious mononucleosis)
  E. Chemical agents
    1. Related to size of dose
      a. Phenylhydrazine   *f.* Phenacetin
      b. Toluene   *g.* Aniline
      c. Trinitrotoluene   *h.* Methyl chloride
      d. Benzene   *i.* Arsine
      e. Acetanilid   *j.* Lead
    2. Depending on hypersensitivity
      a. Sulfonamides   *h.* Para-phenylenediamine
      b. Quinine, quinidine
      c. Pamaquine   *i.* Naphthalene
      d. Primaquine   *j.* Sulfones
      e. Para-aminosalicylic acid *k.* Nitrofurantoin
                      l. Phenothiazine
      f. Benzedrine   *m.* Vitamin K substitutes
      g. Mesantoin
  F. Physical agents (heat—severe thermal burns)
  G. Vegetable and animal poisons
    1. Vegetable poisons
      a. Fava bean (*Vicia faba*)
      b. Castor bean (ricin)
    2. Animal poisons
      a. Snake venoms
II. Intracorpuscular defects
  A. Hereditary spherocytosis (familial or congenital hemolytic jaundice)
  B. Hereditary elliptocytosis
  C. Hereditary nonspherocytic hemolytic anemias
  D. Hereditary leptocytosis (thalassemia, Mediterranean anemia)
  E. Sickle-cell disease
  F. Other hereditary hemoglobinopathies (C, E)

Table 235-2. CLASSIFICATION OF HEMOLYTIC DISORDERS
(*continued*)

  G. Combinations of thalassemia and sickle-cell disease or other hemoglobinopathies
  H. Paroxysmal nocturnal hemoglobinuria
  I. Miscellaneous congenital hemolytic anemias ("inclusion body," "Heinz body," "Pappenheimer body")

red corpuscles. The patient's corpuscles, when given to a normal recipient, can be shown to be disposed of more rapidly than those of the recipient, while the latter's corpuscles, if transfused into the patient, maintain a normal "life span." It may be noted that, in the main, hemolytic anemias due to intracorpuscular defects are familial and hereditary; those produced by extracorpuscular factors are "acquired."

Acute Hemolytic Anemias Due to Immune Body Reactions. The naturally occurring agglutinins α and β cause hemolysis when incompatible blood is given by transfusion. When hemolytic transfusion reactions take place in spite of A, B, and O blood-group compatibility, they are attributable in most instances to the development of anti-Rh (D) agglutinins. Next in frequency are the Kell antigen and antibody. Other blood groups are only rarely involved (p. 440). Such agglutinins are also responsible for the development of hemolytic disease of the newborn (*erythroblastosis fetalis*), a condition in which the red corpuscles of an Rh-positive fetus are destroyed as the result of the action of antibodies produced in the Rh-negative woman carrying the fetus.

Although the number of possible causes of hemolytic anemia is large, as Table 235-2 indicates, in a very significant number of cases of acquired hemolytic anemia no cause is found and no associated disease is recognized. *Idiopathic cases* have been observed at all ages, from five months to seventy-eight years, but females are more often affected than males. The clinical manifestations range in the extreme. The course may be acute, severe, and fulminating, or the illness may be insidious in onset and chronic in course. In the latter instances, repeated attacks of greatly exaggerated blood destruction may punctuate the course and may be followed by spontaneous remissions. By and large the manifestations are rarely as mild as they may be in hereditary spherocytosis. The hematologic features are similar to those of other hemolytic anemias, varying according to the severity of the condition. In most instances, however, certain immunologic manifestations may be demonstrated if they are looked for. The introduction of serologic methods like the Coombs test has made possible the demonstration of antibodies in the majority of cases of idiopathic acquired hemolytic anemia.

There appear to be several varieties of idiopathic acquired hemolytic anemia. They are, in part, associated with differences in the type of antibody which is found. In the majority a "warm" antibody is present; i.e., the antibody reacts well at 37°C and is not potentiated at lower temperatures. The most common warm antibodies are "incomplete"; that is, they sensitize normal erythrocytes to antiglobulin serum but do not cause agglutination in a saline medium. The sensitization is not inhibited by previous heat inactivation of the patient's serum at 56°C and it is increased only slightly by acidification of the serum to pH 6.5 or 7. Typically, these warm antibodies cause agglutination and not hemolysis. The sensitizing antibodies usually are γ-globulins.

"Cold" antibodies are markedly potentiated by reducing the temperature below 37°C. These antibodies are "incomplete," but they may also act as "complete" agglutinating antibodies and under certain circumstances may also bring about hemolysis. Two main forms of cold antibodies have been demonstrated in acquired hemolytic anemias. The common, typical type is a powerful antigen; the rare variety is similar to the Donath-Landsteiner antibody of paroxysmal cold hemoglobinuria. In cases of acquired hemolytic anemia associated with the presence of cold antibodies, cyanosis and Raynaud's phenomenon on exposure to cold as well as hemoglobinuria may be noted. Spherocytes are not conspicuous and osmotic fragility may be normal. The course of these cases is generally chronic and often is relatively mild. They most commonly occur in elderly persons.

In addition to these warm and cold autoantibodies, it is not uncommon to find other manifestations of abnormal protein formation in patients with acquired hemolytic anemia. Thus, antibodies against lipoid antigens may be present and may give rise to false positive Wassermann and Kahn reactions. This is especially frequent in disseminated lupus erythematosus. Again, serum complement may be reduced and hypergammaglobulinemia and cryoglobulins may develop.

It was assumed at first that the autoantibodies found in acquired hemolytic anemia were nonspecific; i.e., that they reacted with all types of human red cells without relation to any known blood group antigens. In some cases, however, the autoantibodies have been found to be specific and were directed against various Rh antigens and, more rarely, against other blood groups, such as Kell, B, and O. The serology of the acquired hemolytic anemias is complicated, however. Autoantibodies without apparent specificity have been observed in the same blood as those in which specific antibodies were discovered. Furthermore, it has been observed that the antibodies of one patient often differ considerably from those of another in temperature requirements, specificity, chemical nature, and in their reactions in vitro. A few cases have been described in which the patients' serums contained a potent agglutinin for enzyme-treated cells, but this was not associated with a positive direct Coombs test. In cases in which cold antibodies have been demonstrated, there has not been a clear correlation between their titer and hemolysis, nor has there been such exposure to cold as might be expected to lead to agglutination and subsequent mechanical destruction of the red corpuscles.

Certain features serve to distinguish chronic hemolytic anemia with erythrocyte-bound antibody from other types of hemolytic anemia. As already indicated, warm or cold hemagglutinins are present and the Coombs test (p. 1293) is positive. Spherocytosis is usually marked when the disease is active, and at such times the osmotic fragility of the red corpuscles is irregularly increased and their mechanical fragility is also increased. Even normal transfused cells become spherical, their fragility becomes increased, and they are rapidly destroyed. In quiescent stages, however, the spherocytosis may be absent, and osmotic and mechanical fragility may be normal.

It has been pointed out that oxalated blood from patients with hemolytic anemia associated with immune bodies may have a granular appearance when examined with a hand lens as the blood is allowed to flow in a thin layer along the side of a glass container. In rare cases this may even be seen with the naked eye. The phenomenon is attributable to the agglutination of the red corpuscles in the plasma.

Other Hemolytic Anemias, Presumably Due to Extracorpuscular Causes. The clinical manifestations of the hemolytic anemias associated with various disorders ("symptomatic" hemolytic anemias) are similar to those in cases of the idiopathic variety except for the presence of manifestations of the underlying disease. The latter, however, are sometimes not apparent and must be sought out carefully. Although it was at first thought that erythrocyte-bound antibodies do not develop in cases of symptomatic hemolytic anemia, with the introduction of appropriate serologic techniques it is becoming clear that at least a great proportion of these cases are of the immune body type.

Table 235-2 lists the large variety of infectious, chemical, and physical agents which may be associated with the development of hemolytic anemia. Hemolytic anemia associated with exposure to chemical agents can develop in a number of different ways. Some chemical agents cause anemia which is related in its severity to the quantity of the chemical absorbed. Other chemicals, such as benzene and trinitrotoluene, may have an earlier hemolytic effect which is followed by a toxic, inhibitory action on the bone marrow, with aplastic anemia as the ultimate result. Another group are the derivatives of aniline and the nitro compounds, which more regularly cause methemoglobinemia but may also cause blood destruction. Plumbism represents still another category.

In addition to these, there are chemical agents which cause hemolytic anemia only in a small proportion of exposed individuals. Even a small dose may precipitate the reaction. Because the nature of one form of such drug sensitivity was first disclosed in the course of a study of sensitivity to the antimalarial compound primaquine, it has come to be designated as the *primaquine-sensitive type of hemolytic anemia*. It has been shown that in such sensitive persons the glucose 6-phosphate dehydrogenase (G6PD) activity of the red blood corpuscles is substantially reduced below the normal. This enzyme is concerned with the regeneration of reduced triphosphopyridine nucleotide (TPNH), which, in turn, is required in the reduction of oxidized glutathione. It was observed that the reduced glutathione (GSH) level of sensitive erythrocytes was consistently lower than that of nonsensitive cells and that a rapid fall in red cell GSH occurred when primaquine was administered to sensitive individuals. This phenomenon can also be demonstrated in vitro by incubating sensitive cells with acetyl phenylhydrazine. Various tests have been devised whereby "primaquine sensitivity" can be demonstrated. Hemolytic anemia associated with a large number of drugs, some of which are listed in Table 235-2, is of this type. It is not known whether the fundamental abnormality in erythrocyte metabolism is GSH depletion or whether this is only a convenient indicator of other important changes. It has been shown that the abnormality is an inherited trait which appears to be transmitted as a sex-linked, incompletely dominant gene of intermediate penetrance. Males are affected, but in the heterozygous female the defect may range from full expression to nonpenetrance. The abnormality is present in about 7 per cent of American Negroes and in Caucasians of Italian and Greek extraction as well as in other Mediterranean peoples. The hemolytic anemia associated with exposure to the fava bean may depend on the same mechanism or a similar one. An important distinction between the red cell abnormality in these sensitive persons and that seen in disorders classified in Table 235-2 under the general heading of Intracorpuscular Defects, such as hereditary spherocytosis, is that the red cell abnormality of sensitive persons has no known deleterious effect on the individual or on the red cell life span in the absence of the offending chemical agent.

Hemolytic reactions to all drugs cannot be explained by the heritable enzymatic mechanism described above. However, nothing is known concerning the pathogenesis of other forms of drug idiosyncrasy.

Intracorpuscular Defects. A number of the disorders coming under this head are described separately below.

Mechanisms of Hemolysis. Various processes condition or cause the destruction of red corpuscles: phagocytosis, agglutinins and hemolysins, osmotic lysis, mechanical factors, and sequestration with erythrostasis. The importance of phagocytosis is not clear. Some regard it as a primary and important factor, while others relegate it to an accessory role dependent on other mechanisms of red corpuscle destruction. Various types of hemagglutinins and hemolysins have been described, as already mentioned. Immune hemolysins are not found free in the serum except in disorders which require special conditions for their maximum operation. Thus in paroxysmal cold hemoglobinuria a fall in temperature is required for maximum activity of the hemolytic system, while in paroxysmal nocturnal hemoglobinuria a fall in the pH of the blood is necessary. In most instances immune hemagglutinins remain attached to the red corpuscle. The Coombs or "developing" test serves to demonstrate such factors (p. 1293).

The role of mechanical factors is indicated by the fact that the osmotic and mechanical fragilities of the red corpuscles increase when the corpuscles are placed in natural or artificial immune serums in which hemolysins and agglutinins are present. Similar changes in fragility have been observed in association with the action of hemolytic agents, such as saponin, or physical factors, such as heat. Osmotic lysis, usually determined by the familiar hypotonic saline fragility test, probably does not operate in vivo except perhaps in the spleen under certain conditions. It is a plausible hypothesis that mechanical trauma is the ultimate mechanism whereby cell destruction occurs under normal circumstances and in many varieties of hemolytic anemia. It has been shown that nearly spherical cells, strongly agglutinated cells, and those with weakened cell membranes are abnormally susceptible to mechanical destruction. In certain cases of acquired hemolytic anemia, increased mechanical fragility has been observed when osmotic fragility was normal. It was found that such cells did not survive normally in the circulation of normal individuals. The increased mechanical fragility of sickled masses of erythrocytes may explain the increased red corpuscle destruction in sickle-cell anemia.

The term *erythrostasis* has been applied to the processes to which red corpuscles are subjected when denied free access to fresh plasma. The spleen appears to have the property of selectively removing and concentrating spheroidal cells. Erythrostasis may lead to increased osmotic and mechanical fragility of the red corpuscles and thereby favor their destruction. It has been suggested that the spleen is of importance in hereditary spherocytosis because of the inherently abnormal susceptibility of the red corpuscles to the effects of erythrostasis. It was demonstrated that in a patient with this disease who had received transfusions of identifiable normal corpuscles, the spleen, removed at operation, had selectively retained the patient's own corpuscles. Perfusion experiments have shown that even the spleen from a case of purpura hemorrhagica, where no hemolytic process existed, likewise selectively removed transfused red corpuscles from cases of hereditary spherocytosis but did not retain normal corpuscles.

Sequestration in the spleen and also in the liver plays an important role in acquired hemolytic anemias. In sequestering sensitized red corpuscles from the circulation the spleen behaves as a highly proficient, passive filter. Thus, it has been shown that when sensitized red corpuscles are injected in the circulation of normal subjects, they are agglutinated by the plasma globulins, following which they are sequestered in the spleen and are hemolyzed within a few minutes. The speed of the hemolysis is such as to suggest the presence of a preformed lysin; leukocytes may be involved in this lytic process. However, in contrast to the fate of these sensitized corpuscles coated with "incomplete" antibodies, in reactions involving "complete" antibodies, as when red corpuscles are injected into normal subjects hyperimmunized against them, sequestration and destruction occur in the liver to a greater extent than in the spleen.

Studies of spontaneous hemolysis of red corpuscles in vitro (autohemolysis) have led to the recognition of a metabolic defect in the red corpuscles of hereditary spherocytosis. The continued presence of glucose during incubation of the red corpuscles was observed to retard markedly the potassium loss and the increase in osmotic fragility of the cells. It was possible to demonstrate that abnormalities in the dynamics of intracellular carbohydrate metabolism exist. Thus, using radioactive phosphorus as a tracer, it was found that in cells from patients with hereditary spherocytosis there is a smaller flux of P^{32} into adenosinetriphosphate and 2,3-diphosphoglyceric acid than in normal cells and a concurrent increase in the flux into orthophosphate. It was shown also that in many instances the metabolic lesion could be reversed with adenosine and glucose. Thus, some of the deleterious effects of erythrostasis can be explained. An adequate rate of supply of energy-rich phosphate bonds is necessary for the maintenance of the biconcave shape of the red corpuscle. Energy production may be defective as the result of genetically controlled enzyme deficiencies or functional inadequacies. Such red corpuscles are less well able to maintain their integrity than normal ones.

Study of a Patient with a Hemolytic Disorder

Hemolytic anemia can be recognized by the development of certain symptoms and signs, certain changes in the blood and bone marrow, and characteristic alterations in pigment metabolism, as already outlined. The differentiation of the various hemolytic disorders is important since treatment depends on their nature. The history alone may suffice to reveal an etiologic agent or may indicate that one is dealing with one of the familial or hereditary disorders. Physical examination may reveal one of the conditions of which hemolytic anemia can be symptomatic. In addition, certain simple tests have been devised which give some clue to the nature of the disorder.

Osmotic Fragility Test. In certain cases of hemolytic anemia one demonstrates, by this test, the susceptibility of red corpuscles to hemolysis in concentrations of salt which fail to cause rupture of normal corpuscles. Such osmotic fragility is characteristic of corpuscles which are more nearly spherical than normal corpuscles. The test is generally positive in hereditary spherocytosis and negative in acquired forms. Unfortunately, however, there are exceptions to this statement. Spherocytosis and increased osmotic fragility are encountered in certain acquired cases, especially in an acute phase. The sensitivity of the test can be increased by first incubating the corpuscles to be tested in vitro at body temperature for 24 hr. Under such conditions the fragility of normal corpuscles is increased slightly; that of corpuscles from cases of hereditary spherocytosis is increased markedly and symmetrically.

Mechanical Fragility Test. A small amount of oxalated or defibrinated blood is placed in an Erlenmeyer flask containing glass beads and rotated, following which the hemoglobin liberated from the cells is measured and compared with controls. Increased mechanical fragility has been observed in congenital hemolytic jaundice, in sickle-cell anemia, and in the presence of cold agglutinins and isoagglutinins after agglutination of the cells in the cold, as well as in a few cases of atypical hemolytic anemia in which osmotic fragility was normal or decreased.

Autohemolysis. This test depends on the incubation of sterile defibrinated blood at 37°C for 24 and 48 hr and measurement of the amount of spontaneous hemolysis which occurs. Normally 0 to 0.5 per cent hemolysis takes place in 24 hr, 0.4 to 3.5 per cent in 48 hr. In general, autohemolysis is increased when osmotic fragility is increased and when there is hemolysis in vivo. The procedure may have some value in differentiating certain forms of nonspherocytic hemolytic anemia from hereditary spherocytosis.

Serologic Tests. A simple presumptive test is performed by placing washed red corpuscles from fresh defibrinated blood in each of three test tubes. The first is incubated for 1 to 2 hr at body temperature and then centrifuged. If hemoglobin is present in the supernatant serum, the presence of a *warm hemolysin* is suggested. The second tube is chilled for 20 min in cracked ice, then incubated for 1 hr and centrifuged. If the result is positive, the presence of a *cold hemolysin* is indicated. The test tube should be examined before it has been warmed. If only *cold agglutinins* are present and no hemolysins, it will be seen that the red corpuscles agglutinate in the cold but fail to hemolyze when the tube is warmed, the clumps disappearing instead. When cold agglutinins are present, one must be careful not to shake the cells too much while they are agglutinated in the cold, since they may hemolyze and give a false cold hemolysin test. The blood placed in the third tube is acidified with carbon dioxide. If hemolysis is apparent after incubation for 1 hr and subsequent centrifugation, *increased acid hemolysis* is suggested. This test is positive in paroxysmal nocturnal hemoglobinuria.

When positive results are obtained in any one of these tubes, the test should be repeated with adequate controls and by the more complete procedures which are available. Thus, if a cold hemolysin appears to be present, the Donath-Landsteiner test should be carried out.

The *Coombs antiglobulin test,* as already indicated, has proved to be very valuable in helping to clarify the heterogeneous group of acquired hemolytic anemias. The *"direct" Coombs test* is carried out simply by mixing the patient's washed red cells with serum from rabbits immunized to human γ-globulin and examining the mixture for agglutination. It serves to demonstrate the presence of "incomplete" antibodies; i.e., those which are attached at some points on the surface of the red corpuscles and require a completing substance, such as antihuman globulin, to cause an agglutination reaction to take place. A positive result has been observed in cases of idiopathic acquired hemolytic anemia, in that type of paroxysmal cold hemoglobinuria which is associated with syphilis, and in many instances of "symptomatic" hemolytic anemia. The test has been negative in most cases of hereditary spherocytosis and is generally negative in sickle-cell anemia and in paroxysmal nocturnal hemoglobinuria, but in hemolytic anemia, because of various physical or chemical agents, it has sometimes been positive.

A positive direct Coombs test is also observed when isoimmunization to known immune bodies has occurred, as in hemolytic disease of the newborn and in sensitization following transfusion. The "indirect" test detects antibodies in the patient's serum. In the indirect test antihuman globulin serum is mixed with normal group O, Rh-positive, and Rh-negative red corpuscles which have been incubated in the patient's serum. The resulting reactions are shown in Table 235-3. If agglutination occurs with both Rh-positive and Rh-negative cells, Rh antibodies can be excluded and the conclusion drawn that circulatory antibodies are present.

In performing the Coombs test it is important that potent antiserum be used and adequate controls

Table 235-3. COOMBS TEST

Hemolytic disorder	Antihuman globulin serum mixed with patient's RBCs (*direct*)	Antihuman globulin serum mixed with normal RBCs after incubation in patient's serum (*indirect*)	
		RH +	RH −
Acquired hemolytic anemia:			
With circulating antibodies	+	+	+
Without circulating antibodies	+	−	−
Due to Rh antibodies in Rh + infant (erythroblastosis fetalis)	+	+	−
Due to physical or chemical agents	±	−	−
Congenital hemolytic anemia (hereditary spherocytosis)*	−	−	−
Sickle-cell anemia	−	−	−
Paroxysmal nocturnal hemoglobinuria	−	−	−
Paroxysmal cold hemoglobinuria (type associated with syphilis)	+	−	−

* The occasional finding of a positive reaction to the Coombs test in this and in other hemolytic anemias where the test result is usually negative is explained by superimposed, frequently transient episodes of acquired hemolytic anemia.

carried out. False negative results may occur if the red corpuscles have not been washed sufficiently or as a result of a prozone reaction due to inadequate dilution of the serum. Cold hemagglutinins may cause a false positive reaction.

The detailed elucidation of a case of hemolytic anemia of the antibody type will often require the use of still other procedures, but these, in the main, are quite simple. They include (1) the setting up of agglutination tests at various temperatures and in several media, such as isotonic sodium chloride solution and bovine albumin solution, which are helpful in demonstrating and characterizing the agglutinin, and (2) the treatment of the red corpuscles with proteolytic enzymes, such as papain and trypsin, which renders them more susceptible to the demonstration of antibodies. For the antibody tests it is necessary in some instances to use the patient's own red corpuscles rather than any available group O red corpuscles, as is often the practice.

Heinz Bodies. These are intracorpuscular structures which probably represent denatured globin derived from hemoglobin in the course of an irreversible reaction with a toxic substance. They appear as refractile, irregularly shaped bodies often lying at or close to the periphery of the red cells, sometimes attached to the outer surface of the cell. They range in size from minute particles to bodies up to 3 μ in size. Several bodies may be present in the same cell but the largest ones usually appear singly. They are not visible in blood films fixed in methanol and stained with Romanowsky dyes since the bodies and the surrounding hemoglobin stain the same pink color, but they can be stained supravitally by mixing a drop of blood with 4 drops of 0.5 per cent methyl violet in saline solution or by using a saline solution of brilliant cresyl blue and examining the preparation, after ringing it with petroleum jelly, under the oil immersion lens of the microscope. In methyl violet Heinz bodies stain deep purple; Howell-Jolly bodies, which are always round, and Pappenheimer bodies stain darkly, almost black with a bluish tinge. The reticulofilamentous material of reticulocytes stains a pale blue. In brilliant cresyl blue Heinz bodies stain a distinctly lighter shade of blue than the reticulocyte substance. Heinz bodies can be produced in normal blood by mixing it with acetylphenylhydrazine, but a great many more develop in "primaquine-sensitive" (p. 1291) red cells. In addition, a wide range of aromatic nitrogen compounds of the nitrobenzene series and those related to aniline are capable of producing Heinz bodies. They have also been observed in an obscure type of hemolytic anemia unrelated to exposure to recognized toxic agents ("inclusion body" anemia).

Erythrokinetic Studies. These techniques provide a means whereby erythrocyte production and destruction can be quantitated. They also can be used to demonstrate whether the increased blood destruction is due to intracorpuscular or extracorpuscular causes and to determine if the increased breakdown is occurring mainly in the spleen or elsewhere. As a rule, however, such measurements are not required to arrive at a diagnosis.

Prognosis and Treatment. Prognosis and treatment depend on the nature and cause of the hemolytic disorder. The causative agent, such as a parasite or chemical, if discovered, must be removed. An acute attack of hemolysis requires rest, maintenance of fluid balance, and relief of pain. Blood transfusion may be dangerous if the cause of the hemolysis is extracorpuscular and still operating, for then the introduced blood may also be destroyed. Yet, when blood destruction is so acute that hemoglobinemia and hemoglobinuria are present, the possibility of death from circulatory collapse is so great that frequent and sometimes massive blood transfusions must be given.

An important advance in the management of many cases of acquired hemolytic anemia is the discovery that the administration of adrenocorticotropic hormone (ACTH) or of prednisone or other adrenocorticosteroids will control the hemolytic manifestations. The latter are preferable since they can be given orally. As much as 60 to 100 mg prednisone per 24 hr may be required. In some instances transfusion can be withheld entirely, while in other cases, where the anemia is so severe that transfusion is necessary, blood can be given with much less chance of a reaction if steroid therapy has been started. As in the treatment of other disorders, the usual precautions, such as salt restriction and administration of potassium chloride, should be taken when these agents are used in the treatment of hemolytic anemia.

Splenectomy, while almost invariably beneficial in hereditary spherocytosis, is much less successful in the acquired forms. Furthermore, if carried out in an acute hemolytic phase, the operative mortality is high. In idiopathic acquired hemolytic anemia, therefore, the hormones should be used first, at least in preparation for operation. Unfortunately, neither splenectomy nor hormone therapy is permanently helpful in all cases; in many the evidence of hemolysis returns when hormone therapy is interrupted.

In some cases of "symptomatic hemolytic anemia" treatment of the underlying disorder, when possible, relieves the hemolytic anemia as well. When this does not occur, a trial of steroid therapy is justified. In certain instances splenectomy may be helpful, especially if leukopenia and thrombocytopenia are also present and the picture is that of "hypersplenism."

Splenectomy is of no value in sickle-cell anemia,

thalassemia, or paroxysmal nocturnal hemoglobinuria.

Paroxysmal Cold Hemoglobinuria

This is an uncommon disorder characterized by the sudden passage of hemoglobin in the urine, following local or general exposure to cold. Aching and pain in the back, legs, or abdomen, and other symptoms of acute hemolysis, such as a chill, fever, and malaise, are associated with the passage of dark brownish urine. Other findings are those characteristic of acute hemolytic anemia. Symptoms may appear at any time from a few minutes to 7 or 8 hr following exposure.

Donath and Landsteiner showed that the hemoglobinuria is due to the sudden intravascular hemolysis of blood as the result of the action of an autohemolysin contained in the patient's blood. The hemolysin unites with the red corpuscles only at a low temperature, but destruction of the corpuscles occurs only after the temperature of the blood has returned to body temperature. Appropriate tests have been devised to demonstrate such a cold hemolysin. At the time of hemolytic attacks produced by chilling, strongly positive direct antiglobulin (Coombs) reactions have been observed, but they become negative after the attacks. The typical condition is a manifestation of syphilis, the congenital form particularly, and thorough antisyphilitic therapy ends the clinical manifestations.

A number of cases have been described, however, in which indications of syphilis were lacking even though, in some of the cases, the Wassermann reaction was positive. Since false positive Wassermann and Kahn reactions are not uncommon in acquired hemolytic anemia of the autoantibody type, it has been suggested that paroxysmal cold hemoglobinuria is not exclusively a manifestation of syphilis and that some of the cases regarded as the typical condition of syphilitic origin may well have been examples of autoimmune hemolytic disease of the cold antibody type.

Chronic Hemolytic Anemia with Paroxysmal Nocturnal Hemoglobinuria (Marchiafava-Micheli Syndrome)

This is a rare disorder of insidious onset which is characterized by signs of hemolytic anemia and is marked by attacks of hemoglobinuria which occur chiefly at night. The symptoms are those of long-standing anemia, but there may be abdominal, lumbar, or substernal pain, which often ushers in an attack of hemoglobinuria. The findings are similar to those in other hemolytic anemias and include splenomegaly and well-marked anemia. The osmotic fragility of the red corpuscles is normal and sphero-

cytosis is not characteristic. There may be hemoglobinemia even when there is no hemoglobinuria. Leukopenia is usual and may be marked, and there may be thrombocytopenia; the pancytopenia may, in fact, lead to an erroneous diagnosis of aplastic anemia. The urine contains increased amounts of urobilinogen as well as hemoglobin. Hemosiderin can often be demonstrated in the leukocytes or epithelial cells of the urine.

The fault appears to reside in the red corpuscles, which are unusually susceptible to acid hemolysis. A simple test for this has been described already (p. 1293). It has been suggested that the destruction of the cells is promoted by the accumulation of carbon dioxide during sleep, an optimum acid pH being required for hemolysis to take place. The latter has been shown to be brought about by the action of the *properdin system*. The components of this system are properdin (a protein), Mg^{++}, and cofactors resembling complement, all of which are normal constituents of plasma. Normal human red cells are not damaged by this system. The defect in PNH (paroxysmal nocturnal hemoglobinuria) red corpuscles which renders them susceptible to the properdin system may possibly reside in the lipid pattern of the lipoproteins of their stroma.

This disorder does not appear to be hereditary. Treatment is purely symptomatic. Splenectomy is of no value. The intensity of the hemolytic process varies; crises of severe anemia may occur. Transfusion of plasma usually precipitates hemolytic crises, but saline-washed red corpuscles can be given with impunity. Although thrombocytopenia is common, purpuric or hemorrhagic manifestations are unusual; in fact, thrombotic complications are not infrequent. It has been found that the anticoagulant dicoumarin (Dicumarol) impedes hemolytic activity in this disease, but this drug is chiefly of importance in order to prevent thrombotic complications. Infections are frequent in these patients, partly, perhaps, because of the associated leukopenia. Prognosis varies greatly. Although a fatal termination may ensue in several years, in some cases the disorder has been compatible with life for many years.

Hereditary Spherocytosis (Chronic Acholuric Jaundice, Spherocytic Anemia, Chronic Familial Icterus, Congenital Hemolytic Jaundice)

Definition. This is a familial and hereditary disorder characterized by spherocytosis, increased osmotic fragility of the red corpuscles, splenomegaly, and a variable degree of hemolytic anemia.

History. Chiefly as the result of the observations of the French school, during the early part of the present century this familial disorder was clearly defined, becoming known as the type of Chauffard and Minkowski. It was distinguished from the acquired form of hemolytic anemia of Hayem and Widal.

Etiology. Transmitted as a mendelian dominant trait by either parent, this disorder is due to an inherited defect of the red corpuscles, which tend to be more spheroid than normal and thus are more subject to destruction. The significance of spheroidicity of the red corpuscles and of increased osmotic fragility and the role of the spleen have been discussed already (p. 1292).

Morbid Anatomy. The spleen is greatly enlarged, often weighing 1,000 to 1,500 Gm. The pulp and, to a lesser extent, the sinuses are greatly congested. Depending on the degree of anemia and the extent of blood destruction, hyperplasia and even metaplasia of the bone marrow occur, and deposits of iron pigment are found in the liver, kidneys, and even lymph nodes.

Symptoms. Jaundice and splenomegaly are the most common manifestations and may pass unnoticed for many years. A persistent sallow appearance rather than obvious jaundice may be present. Symptoms of anemia are usually absent or mild. At any time from birth to late adult life, attention may be drawn to the disorder by the *crise de déglobulisation,* which is characterized by fever, lassitude, palpitation, and shortness of breath or even violent abdominal pain, vomiting, and anorexia. Rather than being episodes of increased blood destruction, as has always been assumed, these crises have been observed by several investigators to be associated with sudden temporary cessation of blood formation. Since the life span of the red corpuscles of congenital hemolytic icterus is very brief, anemia develops rapidly under these circumstances. It remains to be shown how often such a mechanism, rather than hemolysis, is the cause of the crises which occur in this disease.

The liver may or may not be enlarged. Developmental anomalies are often present. A chronic leg ulcer may be found. Cholelithiasis is a frequent complication, and symptoms due to this cause may first bring the patient to the physician.

The anemia is usually moderate in degree, but may be very mild or severe. It is normocytic or simple microcytic in type but, when severe and associated with marked reticulocytosis, it can be macrocytic. There is little poikilocytosis, but small, bright, deeply staining red corpuscles (spherocytes) are often seen scattered among the cells of normal size. Reticulocytes are characteristically increased in number, most often numbering 5 to 20 per cent. Polychromatophilia and normoblasts may be seen in the blood smear. The leukocytes are usually normal in number or slightly increased. The platelet count is generally normal.

Increased osmotic fragility of the red corpuscles

is characteristic. Hemolysis beginning at 0.64 per cent saline solution is not unusual and may be complete at the point where hemolysis normally begins.

Bilirubinemia of the "indirect" type and increased quantities of urobilinogen in the urine and stools, without bile in the urine (acholuric), are the characteristic changes in pigment metabolism.

Diagnosis. Splenomegaly, icterus of the hemolytic type, reticulocytosis, increased osmotic fragility, and presence of the anomaly in other members of the family are the characteristic findings. The Coombs test is negative except in occasional cases. In these it is likely that a superimposed acquired immunohemolytic process has developed. When the picture is not entirely typical, a careful study to rule out other types of hemolytic anemia must be made, as outlined previously.

It is especially important to distinguish cases of *congenital nonspherocytic hemolytic anemia,* because they have not been benefited by splenectomy. Although such cases resemble hereditary spherocytosis in their mode of inheritance, they differ in that the anemia is generally macrocytic, there is often a moderate degree of ovalocytosis, and sometimes there is conspicuous punctate basophilia. Spherocytes are not found, and osmotic fragility is normal. The reported cases have not been identical in all respects, however, and probably represent several different disorders. This statement is based on observation of morphologic differences, such as the presence of crenated and irregularly contracted corpuscles in some cases, Pappenheimer bodies in others, extreme variation in red cell size and shape in still others, and even increased resistance to saline hemolysis and the presence of target cells, as found in certain abnormal hemoglobin disorders. It has been shown that the reversibility of the metabolic lesion by adenosine, observed in certain cases of hereditary spherocytosis, did not occur in congenital nonspherocytic hemolytic anemia. Studies of autohemolysis have revealed at least two forms of the nonspherocytic disorder.

Treatment. This is the one disorder in which splenectomy is associated with consistently satisfactory results. The operation is indicated in every patient in whom clinical manifestations are present. Although remissions develop and latent periods of many years' duration may occur, spontaneous recovery does not take place. At operation, a careful search should be made for accessory spleens, and they should be removed if found. Following operation, anemia, jaundice, and reticulocytosis disappear. The osmotic fragility of the red corpuscles, however, as well as the spherocytosis, may persist.

During a crisis, repeated blood transfusions must be given.

SICKLE-CELL ANEMIA AND OTHER ABNORMAL HEMOGLOBIN SYNDROMES

Definition. Sickle-cell anemia is a hereditary and familial hemolytic anemia, essentially peculiar to Negroes and characterized by the presence of red corpuscles which, under appropriate conditions, assume sickle-shaped or oat-shaped forms.

Etiology. Just as hereditary spherocytosis is rare in the Negro, sickle-cell anemia is extremely rare except in Negroes or when mixture with Negro blood has occurred. The anomaly appears to be inherited as a mendelian dominant characteristic. Inheritance of the abnormality from only one parent, the heterozygous state, is represented by the sickle-cell trait, in which sickling of the red corpuscles can be demonstrated but is not accompanied by symptoms of anemia. Sickle-cell anemia is the homozygous state in which one abnormal gene has been inherited from each parent. Sickle-cell anemia possesses all the characteristics of a chronic hemolytic anemia with certain special features as well.

From time to time exception has been taken to the heterozygous-homozygous theory described above because of certain family studies which failed to demonstrate the sickle-cell trait in both parents of children with sickle-cell anemia and also because certain cases were observed which seemed to be intermediate in their clinical manifestations between those of the severe hemolytic anemia of sickle-cell anemia and the asymptomatic state, the sickle-cell trait. The discovery of abnormal hemoglobins other than sickle-cell hemoglobin has offered a reasonable explanation for these seeming exceptions.

The discovery by Pauling and his associates that the electrophoretic mobilities of sickle-cell anemia (S) and normal hemoglobin (A) differ led to establishment of the principle that a molecular abnormality in a single protein may cause a sequence of events such as that which characterizes the complex disease, sickle-cell anemia. It was shown that in a buffer of suitable pH, the two components of a mixture of normal and sickle-cell hemoglobin migrate in opposite directions. Since the heme moiety is the same in sickle-cell and in normal hemoglobin, the electrophoretic differences were attributed to differences in the globin portion.

These investigations were the first of an ingenious series of studies carried out with the aid of paper, starch gel, and other techniques for electrophoresis, and by means of ion exchange chromatography and various procedures for the study of protein structure. As a result it has been learned that the globin of normal adult hemoglobin is made up of two pairs of polypeptide chains, each containing about 150 amino acids, now termed the alpha and beta chains.

Fetal hemoglobin is composed of two alpha chains and two different chains, termed gamma chains. A very small quantity of the latter persists, even in adult life. Still another polypeptide chain is found, in small quantity, in normal adult hemoglobin. This has been designated the delta chain: two alpha and two delta chains make up the so-called normal A_2 hemoglobin.

The application of the above techniques has uncovered a large number of "abnormal" hemoglobins which differ from normal hemoglobin in one or more of several ways; namely (1) replacement of one amino acid by another in the normal amino acid sequence of one of the peptides separated from the α or β polypeptide chains; (2) replacement of certain normal chains by other apparently normal chains; (3) absence of certain peptides.

Thus, hemoglobin S differs from hemoglobin A in that valine replaces a glutamic acid in peptide 4 of the β chain. In hemoglobin C, lysine rather than valine replaces the same glutamic acid. In the type of hemoglobin G first found in San José, glycine replaces a different glutamic acid in the same peptide. Hemoglobin E differs from hemoglobin A in that lysine replaces a glutamic acid in peptide 26 of the β chain. In hemoglobin I glutamic acid replaces lysine in peptide 23 of the α chain. Hemoglobin H differs from all others in that it is composed of four β chains. Hemoglobin Bart's, on the other hand, is made up entirely of γ chains. In one form of hemoglobin D, peptide 26 of the β chain is absent. Other examples could be cited.

The number of abnormal hemoglobins is constantly increasing. In addition, various combinations of normal and abnormal polypeptide chains, or combinations of two or more abnormal polypeptide chains may occur, as well as combinations of various abnormal hemoglobins with the thalassemia trait (p. 1302). These discoveries are of great interest and importance in human genetics and anthropology. However, only a limited number of abnormal hemoglobins are associated with clinical manifestations. Some of these are presented in Table 235-4.

It is natural that problems should have arisen in developing a suitable *terminology* for the abnormal hemoglobins. To distinguish it from normal adult hemoglobin (A) and from sickle-cell hemoglobin (S), the third type of adult hemoglobin which was found was named C. The succeeding letters of the alphabet were given to other hemoglobins, as they were uncovered, except for F, the letter reserved for fetal hemoglobin. However, as abnormal hemoglobins have been discovered in different parts of the world, the same letter has been given to more than one hemoglobin. This has led to the practice

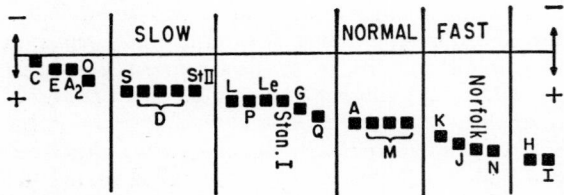

FIG. 235-3. Relative mobilities of normal and abnormal hemoglobins on paper electrophoresis at pH 8.6. The mobility of hemoglobin M (Chap. 237) is similar to that of normal hemoglobin (hemoglobin A). Other hemoglobins can be classified as *slow* (e.g., hemoglobin S; this group includes the D hemoglobins and Stanleyville II), *very slow* (e.g., hemoglobin C; this group includes the normal hemoglobin A₂ as well as the abnormal hemoglobins E and O), or *moderately slow* (e.g., the G hemoglobins; this includes L, P, Q, Lepore (Le), and Stanleyville I). In addition, there are *fast* hemoglobins with electrophoretic mobilities faster than that of hemoglobin A. These include H, I, J, K, N, Norfolk, and Hopkins-1 and Hopkins-2. (*Wintrobe: "Clinical Hematology," 5th ed., Philadelphia, Lea & Febiger, 1961.*)

of designating the abnormal hemoglobin according to the geographic area where it was first discovered, as well as by a letter; for example, $G_{San\ José}$, G_{Ibadan}. With advances in knowledge concerning the chemical constitution of the various hemoglobins, more exact terminology will undoubtedly be adopted; e.g., $\alpha_2^A \beta_2^S$ for that found in sickle-cell blood to indicate the polypeptide chain in which the abnormality resides. Quite possibly, even more specific designation will be adopted. For the purposes of the following discussion, however, these details are not essential.

Sickle-cell anemia was first described in Negroes in North America. In Africa a broad belt with high incidence of the sickling trait extends roughly across the middle third of the continent, the highest figures being in eastern and central Africa. The sickling trait, however, does not seem to be present exclusively in the Negroes of Africa or in Negroes of African origin. It has been discovered in certain aborigines in southern India and southern Arabia as well as in Greece and southern Turkey. Instances of "sickle-cell anemia" described so far in white persons have been mainly in those of Greek or Italian stock. These cases, it now appears, are examples of admixture of the sickling and the thalassemia traits, not of homozygous sickle-cell disease.

The incidence of hemoglobin C is highest in West Africa. Surveys of randomly selected Negroes in the United States have yielded values of 2 to 3 per cent, as compared with 8.5 per cent for hemoglobin S. Hemoglobin D has been found in, at most, 0.4 per cent of American Negroes and may well have originated in non-Negroes. Actually nine types

of hemoglobin D have been found. Hemoglobin E is present in large numbers of Thais (13.6 per cent) and Cambodians (35 per cent) and appears to be a characteristic of the peoples of southeast Asia. It has been encountered frequently in association with the gene for thalassemia. Nine hemoglobins G have been described; all are rare. Hemoglobin H is the first of a series of "fast" hemoglobins, so called because their anodal mobility in paper electrophoresis at pH 8.6 is faster than that of normal hemoglobin. Other "fast" hemoglobins include I, J, K, and N. Still other abnormal hemoglobins have been described: hemoglobins L, O, P, Q, Lepore, Stanleyville I and II, Hopkins-1 and -2, Norfolk, F and P or Singapore-Bristol, Bart's, and Alexandra. The electrophoretic mobilities of a number of the abnormal hemoglobins are illustrated diagrammatically in Fig. 235-3.

Pathology. In sickle-cell anemia, in addition to the signs of a chronic hemolytic anemia (normoblastic hyperplasia of the bone marrow, hemosiderosis), evidence of thrombosis, infarction, necrosis, or hemorrhage may be present, especially in the lungs, spleen, and nervous system. The spleen may be shrunk to a tiny, wrinkled mass.

Symptoms. In sickle-cell anemia, jaundice and a chronic anemia with few or no complaints are interrupted by periods of increased weakness, episodes of aching pain in the joints or elsewhere in the extremities, or sudden attacks of severe abdominal pain which have often been mistaken for ruptured peptic ulcer, intestinal obstruction, or some other abdominal emergency.

The victims of sickle-cell anemia are often poorly developed, and bony deformities of various types may be discovered. The scleras are icteric, and there may be slight general glandular enlargement, but splenomegaly is encountered in only about 15 to 20 per cent of cases. The heart may be enlarged, and the physical signs may closely simulate those of mitral stenosis due to rheumatic fever. Hyposthenuria is common. In many instances chronic leg ulcers are found over the internal or external malleoli. Roentgenograms may reveal radial striation in the skull, osteoporosis in the vertebral bodies, or other changes in the long bones. Osteomyelitis is a not-infrequent complication.

The anemia is usually surprisingly severe, erythrocyte counts below 2.5 million being common. The anemia may be normocytic or macrocytic. Oval, cigar-shaped, or other bizarre forms of red corpuscles may be seen in the stained blood smear. The sickling is brought out clearly in wet films of blood which have been fixed under a cover glass and sealed with paraffin. In cases with sickle-cell anemia the typical sickled and oat-shaped forms with elongated, pointed filaments appear within a few hours. When only the sickle-cell trait exists, 24 hr is often required to produce this change and only a proportion rather than practically all of the cells are affected. By the use of reducing agents such as sodium bisulfite, sickling can be hastened and the characteristic forms appear promptly.

In sickle-cell anemia, reticulocytosis, polychromatophilia, normoblasts, leukocytosis with "shift to the left" in the myeloid series, and an increase in platelets are found as well as hyperbilirubinemia and increased urobilinogen in the urine and stools. Osmotic fragility is decreased, not increased. The bone marrow shows striking normoblastic hyperplasia.

Carriers of hemoglobin C are asymptomatic, but target corpuscles are found characteristically in their blood. The homozygous state, hemoglobin C disease, is associated with symptoms similar to those of sickle-cell anemia but in general much milder. Anemia is common but usually of moderate degree, normocytic or microcytic in type, and accompanied by slight bilirubinemia. Under conditions which permit partial drying and partial hemolysis, crystallization of hemoglobin C occurs in vitro when the concentration of the abnormal hemoglobin in the red cells is sufficiently great.

A number of instances have been discovered in which both S and C hemoglobin were demonstrated. The combination of hemoglobin C with S hemoglobin is accompanied by sickling of the red corpuscles as well as by a hemolytic syndrome similar to sickle-cell anemia but differing in that the hemolytic anemia is milder, target cells are more plentiful in the blood, and there is slowly progressive splenomegaly. It is very probable that most of the cases formerly reported as forms of sickle-cell anemia intermediate between the asymptomatic carrier state and the homozygous classical disease were actually cases simultaneously heterozygous for S and C hemoglobin.

Of the other abnormal hemoglobin syndromes, as outlined in Table 235-4, few are associated with clinical manifestations unless they occur in combination with hemoglobin S or the thalassemia gene. Hemoglobin E disease, the homozygous EE state, is characterized as a rule by mild microcytic, normochromic anemia and minimal signs of hemolytic anemia. Target cells are plentiful. The size of the spleen is normal or only slightly enlarged. Hemoglobin H is unique in that it has been demonstrable only when it was accompanied in the same individual by another genetic anomaly of hemoglobin formation, the thalassemia gene or a closely related disorder. Clinical manifestations suggest thalassemia but spontaneous denaturation of hemoglobin H within intact erythrocytes in vitro results in formation of multiple inclusion bodies.

Diagnosis. Sickle-cell anemia is often mistaken for some other disease. Rheumatic fever, peptic ulcer, renal or biliary calculus, osteomyelitis, and various neurologic disorders may be simulated. Recognition depends on the demonstration of sickling and the finding of anemia of the hemolytic type.

In distinguishing persons with the sickle-cell trait who may have some disorder accompanied by anemia from those who have sickle-cell anemia, it must be kept in mind that the former may develop any type of anemia, while in the latter the anemia is always hemolytic in type.

Some of the distinguishing features of the other hemoglobinopathies and of disorders resulting from combinations of the sickle-cell gene with the genes for other abnormal hemoglobins or with the thalassemia gene have been discussed already and are summarized in Table 235-4. The proportions of target cells present, the finding of intraerythrocytic crystals, or the demonstration of inclusion bodies in the red corpuscles gives clues concerning the nature of the disorder in question. Paper electrophoresis (Fig. 235-3) and the alkali denaturation procedure for the demonstration of hemoglobin F are simple and essential additional procedures which should be employed. For the elucidation of the more unusual syndromes, the cooperation of a laboratory is needed where special techniques for the study of the abnormal hemoglobinopathies are available.

Treatment and Prognosis. Since these abnormal hemoglobin syndromes represent inherited anomalies of hemoglobin formation, it is apparent that no treatment other than symptomatic therapy can be provided. No method is known whereby the abnormal state can be altered. Fortunately a number of these conditions are asymptomatic. Sickle-cell anemia, however, is a serious disease which is ultimately fatal, often before the age of thirty. Death may result from intercurrent infection, renal or cardiac failure, thrombosis or hemorrhage involving vital tissues, or it may follow one of the abdominal crises. Blood transfusions are of little value except in the abdominal crisis if shock is present. Antianemic agents are of no value and splenectomy also has no place in therapy.

The prognosis of hemoglobin C disease is good but that of sickle-cell–hemoglobin C disease is less favorable, although usually much better than that of sickle-cell anemia. As in that disease, acute infarction of the bone marrow and fat embolization play an important role in the pathogenesis of many of the acute manifestations of the disorder. Aseptic necrosis of the femoral heads is a curious complication. The morbidity and mortality during pregnancy are usually great in hemoglobin S-C disease.

Pathogenesis. The ratio of sickle-cell hemoglobin to normal hemoglobin in the blood of individuals with the sickle-cell trait has been found to vary

Table 235-4. SUMMARY OF USUAL FINDINGS IN ABNORMAL HEMOGLOBINOPATHIES AND THALASSEMIA

Condition	Hb types[1]	Sickling	Micro-cytosis	Hypo-chromia	Target cells[2], %	Hemolytic anemia[3]	Spleno-megaly
None—adult	AA	0	0	0	0	0	0
None—newborn	AF	0	0	0	0	0	0
Traits[11]:							
Sickle-cell[4]	AS	+	0	0	4	0	0
Hb C[4]	AC	0	0	+	1–100	0	0
Hb D	AD	0	0	0	0	0	0
Hb E	AE	0	0	0	0	0	0
Hb G[4]	AG	0	0	0	0	0	0
Hb I	AI	0	0	0	<2	0	0
Diseases:							
Sickle-cell anemia[4]	SS	++	0	0, +	5–30	++++	0
Homozygous Hb C[4,9]	CC	0	±	+	30–100	++	++
Homozygous Hb E	EE	0	++	0	25–60	+[7]	±
Homozygous Hb G[4]	GG	0	0	0	0	0	0
Sickle-cell–Hb C[4,5]	SC	+	±	+	20–85	++	++
Sickle-cell–Hb D[6]	SD	+	+	++	+	++	++
Sickle-cell–Hb G	SG	+	0	0	0	0	0
Thalassemia minor	AA$_2$[8]	0	+	+*	+	+[7]	±
Thalassemia major	AF	0	++	++*	10–35	+++	++++
Sickle-cell–thalassemia[6]	SF	+	+	+*	20–40	++	++
Hb C–thalassemia[4]	CA	0	+	+*	+++	+	0
Hb E–thalassemia	EF	0	++	++*	10–40	++	+++
Hb G–thalassemia (?)	GF	0	+	+	+	+	0
Hb H–thalassemia[10]	AH	0	++	++	++	++	±
Sickle-cell–hereditary spherocytosis	SA	+	+	0	+	++	++

[1] The major hemoglobin component is shown first. In sickle-cell anemia especially, there may also be a substantial proportion of Hb F.

[2] Osmotic fragility is reduced more or less proportionately to the number of target cells.

[3] Mechanical fragility and RBC survival correspond *as a rule* to the presence and degree of hemolytic anemia.

[4] Chiefly in Negroes.

[5] Cases of sickle-cell anemia intermediate in severity between sickle-cell trait and sickle-cell anemia.

[6] Sickle-cell disease in Caucasians.

[7] Or polycythemia with microcytosis.

[8] In the majority of cases.

[9] Partial drying and partial hemolysis are associated with crystallization of hemoglobin. Rod-shaped erythrocytes with squared corners are seen in blood smear.

[10] Inclusion bodies demonstrable in red corpuscles.

[11] No clearly defined hematologic abnormalities have been reported to be associated with the inheritance of the following traits: J, K, L, N, O, P, Q. The manifestations of the Lepore trait are like those of thalassemia minor; when Lepore is associated with the thalassemia trait, the clinical picture is that of thalassemia major.

* Basophilic stippling of the red corpuscles.

SOURCE: Wintrobe, M. M., "Clinical Hematology," 5th ed., Philadelphia, Lea & Febiger, 1961.

from 22 to 45 per cent, while the amount in the blood of those with sickle-cell anemia has ranged from 76 to 100 per cent. The variations in the amount of sickle-cell hemoglobin have been explained on the ground that the expression of the S gene may be under the modifying influence of other genetic factors; the lower and higher proportions of S hemoglobin are a familial characteristic.

Hemoglobin S is relatively insoluble. The sickling process seems to be best explained on the assumption that in the oxygen-unsaturated state the S hemoglobin molecule undergoes orderly orientation, forming, by specific linkage of the individual molecules, long chains of hemoglobin elements. Subsequent parallel alignment of these elements results in birefringent tactoids, the sickled cell being a hemoglobin tactoid, thinly veiled and somewhat distorted by the cell membrane. The clinical and hematologic manifestations and the pathologic changes found in sickle-cell anemia can be explained by the peculiar physical properties of the sickle cell. The intracellular molecular orientation produces the sickled form of the erythrocyte. At decreased oxygen tensions the viscosity of the whole blood and the mechanical fragility of the erythrocytes are significantly increased, owing to the assumption of the sickled form. With the increase in viscosity, a cycle is initiated in which the factors of stasis, lowered pH, and continuing oxygen uptake combine to augment the number of sickled cells and prolong the stasis. Plugs or masses of sickled erythrocytes become solid enough to occlude vessels, resulting in the "thrombotic" episodes associated with pain which are characteristic of the disease. Erythrostasis limits access to cell-maintaining energy and also favors the sickled state. When red cells after stasis are released into free circulation, a certain proportion, having been fixed in irreversible sickled form, have also become more fragile in terms of mechanical trauma. Consequently, they are more than normally susceptible to the trauma associated with circulation. Increased blood destruction is the result. The development of these changes depends on the quantity of abnormal hemoglobin present; it is assumed that in the homozygous state the erythrocytes contain sufficient abnormal hemoglobin to result in sickling within the physiologic range of oxygen tensions. It is noteworthy that, although the heterozygous state is ordinarily benign, splenic infarction has been observed in a number of persons with the sickle-cell trait who were subjected to conditions of greatly reduced oxygen tension.

Many of the clinical manifestations of sickle-cell anemia can be explained on the basis of obstruction of vascular channels by tangles of sickled erythrocytes. Thus, the picture of shock presented by patients with the abdominal crisis of sickle-cell anemia may be due to the packing of sickled erythrocytes in small capillaries, thus removing them from a functional status and adding to the anemia already present. The capillary hypoxemia would result in plasma loss, hemoconcentration, and further stagnation. Bone pain may be due to distention of the intramedullary cavity of the bones by the vascular engorgement. In some cases there may be focal infarction of bone marrow. It is possible that the irregular sclerosis visible in roentgenograms of the long bones is due to healing of such infarcted areas with scarring and subsequent osteoid deposition. Other changes in the bones may perhaps be the result of hyperplasia compensatory to the increased blood destruction.

THALASSEMIA (Cooley's Anemia, Erythroblastic Anemia, Mediterranean Anemia, Target-cell Anemia, Familial Microcytic Anemia)

Definition. An inherited disorder originally seen, in particular, in individuals living in countries bordering the Mediterranean or in their offspring elsewhere, which is characterized by the presence of unusually thin red corpuscles, microcytosis, various degrees of anemia, and, when the anemia is severe, numerous nucleated red corpuscles. This concept of thalassemia has now been broadened, as will be described below.

History. Cooley and Lee (1925) described a chronic progressive anemia commencing early in life, which was associated with a characteristic facies, splenomegaly, and a familial and racial incidence. Later it became clear that this was the severe and fatal form of a disorder which in milder form is seen in adolescents and in adults.

Etiology. Those first discovered to be affected were chiefly of Italian, Greek, Syrian, or Armenian parentage. In certain communities of Italians, the anomaly has been observed in as many as 20 per cent of those examined. The disorder is presumed to be due to the inheritance of a factor which leads to an anomaly of red corpuscle production. While there is in this condition a disturbance in iron metabolism, the primary defect appears to be in hemoglobin synthesis. It was found that the red corpuscles in this disorder contain a variable and often large proportion of fetal hemoglobin, as indicated by the high resistance of the hemoglobin to denaturation in aqueous alkaline solutions as well as by other physical properties. In the severe form of the disease, the electrophoretic pattern of the hemoglobin resembles a mixture of normal and fetal hemoglobin. This led to the suggestion that the gene governing this disorder blocks the production of normal hemoglobin and causes the production of fetal hemoglobin as a compensatory phenomenon. The mode of inheritance is that of a recessive trait. In the heterozygous state, when only one allele is inherited (thalassemia minor), the interference with hemoglobin synthesis is not serious. In the homozygous condition, when two alleles are inherited, one from each parent (thalassemia major), there is a drastic reduction in normal hemoglobin production.

Subsequent studies showed that thalassemia affects many of the peoples of the Eastern Hemisphere and that a whole spectrum of disorders can be included under this heading. Not only is this trait encountered in the Mediterranean basin, but a high incidence occurs in Thailand and elsewhere in the Far East. Furthermore, the range of severity is much broader than defined by the above two categories, thalassemia minor and thalassemia major.

Three observations have proved of great importance in the elucidation of the thalassemia states. First is the demonstration by starch block electrophoresis of a component of normal hemoglobin, A_2, which moves more slowly than the major component of normal adult hemoglobin. This is thought to be composed of two α polypeptide chains and a pair of distinctive chains, termed δ chains. In the majority of persons with the thalassemia trait the quantity of hemoglobin A_2 is greater than normal (i.e., above 2.54 ± 0.35 per cent). However, a minority are found without such an increase. In some individuals with normal or low hemoglobin A_2 there has been evidence of double heterozygosity for thalassemia and hemoglobin H, hemoglobin I, or some other, unidentified abnormal hemoglobin.

It has been noted, in addition, that in some instances of thalassemia major, the production of normal adult hemoglobin is suppressed. Again, as already mentioned, fetal hemoglobin is found in increased amounts. However, in thalassemia minor, the amount of hemoglobin F is normal or minimally elevated as a rule; yet, in several instances, large amounts of hemoglobin F have been demonstrated. In these and other observations support is found for the concept that there are several varieties of thalassemia. In addition, there are the cases in which the thalassemia trait is clearly associated with one of the abnormal hemoglobins, such as S, C, E, and H. It is possible that hemoglobin A_2 is inherited as an independent system, and this may be true also of hemoglobin F. A specific thalassemia hemoglobin abnormality has not been identified, but it is conceivable, at least, that such an abnormality exists but has remained in hiding because the aberrant amino acid sequence may be of such a nature that the hemoglobin produced is electrophoretically normal. In essence, then, the spectrum of disorders which has been included under the designation of thalassemia, as recognized clinically, may represent a great variety of inherited abnormalities, joined in various combinations.

Symptomatology. The full-blown disorder (*thalassemia major, Cooley's anemia*) develops insidiously within the first year or two of life, perhaps at birth, and is marked by pallor and great enlargement of the spleen and even the liver. The appearance of the child is often mongoloid. Roentgenograms reveal great thickening of the diploë of the skull with perpendicular striation, increase in the medullary portion of the long bones with thinning of the cortex, and other changes attributable to the extreme hyperplasia of the bone marrow. Anemia is severe, hypochromic and microcytic in type, and the red corpuscles contain so little pigment and are so thin that their "buckling" produces forms which have the appearance of targets. Fragility tests in hypotonic saline solutions reveal that the corpuscles are unusually resistant to hemolysis by this means. Normoblasts and microblasts, as well as polychromatophilia, basophilic stippling, Howell-Jolly bodies, and moderate reticulocytosis, in addition to

leukocytosis (19,000 to 25,000 per cu mm) with "shift to the left," reflect the myeloid hyperactivity. There is usually slight or moderate bilirubinemia, with a corresponding increase in the urobilinogen content of the urine and stools.

Thalassemia minor may pass entirely unnoticed; painstaking examination may be necessary to reveal any abnormality. Slight anemia, splenic enlargement, microcytosis and hypochromia, target cells, poikilocytosis out of proportion to the existent anemia, decreased hypotonic saline fragility, basophilic stippling of the red corpuscles, and bilirubinemia are some of the signs which, singly or in various combinations, mark this disorder. Roentgenographic changes in the bones similar to, though less pronounced than, those found in the severe form may be observed.

The term *thalassemia minima* has been applied to instances in which manifestations are very slight. Additional designations and clinical subdivisions have been proposed for other variations of the clinical picture, since such a wide range is observed. Little is to be gained from such a classification, however. *Microdrepanocytic disease* is the name given to the combination of sickle-cell and thalassemia genes which results in a chronic hemolytic anemia with some of the characteristics of both sickle-cell disease and thalassemia.

Diagnosis. The various forms of congenital hemolytic anemia, as well as plumbism and other acquired forms of "refractory" anemia, must be distinguished from thalassemia. The clinical and hematologic manifestations of some of the hemoglobinopathies which may be associated with thalassemia are presented in Table 235-4. Thalassemia minor and minima have occasionally been confused with polycythemia vera because the erythrocyte count may be greater than normal. However, in such cases the hemoglobin and volume of packed red cells are usually slightly below the average normal values since the red corpuscles are microcytic and hypochromic.

Prognosis. The severe form is fatal. Prognosis is more grave the earlier the disease becomes manifest. Less severe forms are compatible with life, and the mildest forms may even have no influence whatever on life span.

Treatment. With the exception of the rare forms of hypochromic, microcytic anemia which were discussed earlier (p. 1280), this is the only form of hypochromic microcytic anemia in man which does not respond to iron therapy. Splenectomy is of no value, as a rule, nor are any other measures now known.

Pathology. Evidences of pronounced myeloid hyperplasia, both medullary and extramedullary, the effects of such changes on the bones, and deposits of iron-containing pigment in the liver, pancreas, and other tissues are the most significant findings.

ANEMIAS ASSOCIATED WITH INFECTIONS AND VARIOUS OTHER DISORDERS, CHIEFLY CHRONIC

In the preceding sections, anemia resulting from blood loss, as well as anemias due to excessive blood destruction and those associated with deficiency of certain factors concerned in erythropoiesis, were discussed. The characteristics of these anemias are, in the main, well defined, and much has been learned in recent years about their pathogenesis. The hemolytic anemias and the specific nutritional deficiency anemias are, however, relatively uncommon. Far more frequent in occurrence and yet much less well understood are the anemias associated with various chronic disorders and with infection. Such anemia is usually only moderate in degree: hemoglobin values of 13 to 10 Gm per 100 ml of blood are seen more frequently than lower values. The anemia is usually normocytic, and in the smear the red corpuscles generally show little abnormality in size or shape, a monotonous picture unaccompanied by polychromatophilia, basophilic stippling, or nucleated red corpuscles. Exceptions are found in *lead poisoning*, where basophilic stippling is characteristically seen; in the so-called *myelophthisic anemias*, such as those associated with metastases to the bone marrow, leukemia, multiple myeloma, or myelosclerosis; and in severe *renal disease*. There, often corresponding rather closely to the gravity of the renal disorder, as manifested by the degree of retention of nitrogenous and other waste products, hemoglobin values as low as 5 Gm per 100 ml are found; and the blood smear may reveal normoblasts, stippling, and moderate anisocytosis and poikilocytosis. The anemia may be somewhat microcytic or hypochromic, and occasionally is macrocytic. If the renal disease has been insidious in onset and is chronic in type, the clinical manifestations and the anemia may be quite confusing unless one is aware that striking degrees of anemia may be encountered in the absence of impressive signs of renal disorder.

The *bone marrow* in these conditions shows nothing characteristic. The nucleated red corpuscles are of the normoblastic type. The marrow may appear hyperplastic, normal, or hypoplastic. Hyperplasia of the leukopoietic tissue is found if the disorder is one which calls forth a leukocytic response.

The *pathogenesis* of the anemia in these conditions has been discussed elsewhere (p. 206). It seems likely that some fault in the construction of red corpuscles is an important underlying mechanism in their development. In any event, the impact of infection on erythropoiesis is such that no form of antianemic therapy, such as the administration of vitamin B_{12} or of iron, has any influence. The anemia disappears spontaneously if the infection is successfully treated, or subsides as the result of the defense reactions of the host. Similarly the anemia of renal insufficiency is closely tied with the underlying disorder and is generally not influenced by measures other than those which affect renal function.

It is both interesting and curious, therefore, that the oral administration of *cobaltous chloride*, in doses ranging from 20 to 160 mg per day, generally in the form of 20-mg-size, enteric-coated tablets taken with meals, has been observed to produce a modest reticulocytosis and a significant moderation in the degree of anemia both in cases of anemia accompanying chronic infection and in that associated with renal disease. In the latter, appetite may improve and there may be increased tolerance for the medications necessary to correct electrolyte abnormalities. There is no evidence that cobalt therapy alters the course of renal disease, and the hemoglobin has been found to return to pretreatment levels after cobalt administration has been discontinued. The mode of action of cobalt is obscure, but it is generally assumed that it serves as a nonspecific erythropoietic stimulant rather than as a specific nutritional component required for red cell or hemoglobin production.

Malignant disease is not necessarily accompanied by anemia. Anemia accompanies malignancy in the alimentary tract more often than elsewhere. In such cases nutritional deficiency may play an important role in the pathogenesis of the anemia, and in many cases blood loss is also a contributory factor. Malignant disease of the kidneys, breast, prostate, thyroid, and lungs, in particular, may metastasize to bones, and in such an event *"myelophthisic" anemia* may develop. The picture then may be that of a pancytopenia (see p. 1325), or a leukemoid picture may result. The latter is marked by leukocytosis together with a moderate "shift to the left" in the leukocytic formula, and normocytic anemia. When a number of nucleated red corpuscles also appear in the peripheral blood, as they sometimes do, the term *leukoerythroblastic* anemia appropriately describes what is found. The pathogenesis of myelophthisic anemia was discussed briefly elsewhere (p. 207).

Endocrine insufficiency may be associated with anemia. Hypothyroidism is often accompanied by anemia of moderate degree. This is usually normocytic but can be macrocytic (p. 214). Slight or moderate anemia, usually normocytic, is found in Addison's disease and in pituitary insufficiency (Simmonds' disease).

As already described, the anemia of *iron deficiency* is hypochromic microcytic in type, and that due to lack of anti-pernicious-anemia principle and related substances is macrocytic. *Protein deficiency* is characterized by the presence of normocytic anemia. Deficiencies of the various B vitamins are rarely encountered in man in pure form. Multiple nutritional deficiencies are associated, as a rule, with only moderate anemia, usually normocytic in type.

BLOOD TRANSFUSION

Uses of Blood Transfusion. By far the most important and most frequent uses of *whole blood transfusion* are to restore blood volume after hemorrhage, trauma, or burns and to maintain the concentration of circulating hemoglobin at an adequate level in those types of anemia which cannot be relieved by specific measures such as liver or iron therapy.

The extent to which blood may be lost when hemorrhage occurs within a viscus or a muscle mass is frequently underestimated. Likewise it is not easy to judge the degree to which plasma has been depleted by leakage or how many red cells have been lost by hemolysis after a severe burn. Severe arterial hypotension following a traumatic injury or an event suggesting the possibility of a concealed hemorrhage, in the absence of evidence of other causes, is indicative of a blood volume deficit exceeding 30 per cent, i.e., 1,500 ml or more. When the blood volume deficit is 20 per cent or less, patients are unlikely to exhibit marked hypotension as long as they remain in the horizontal position. In general it may be said that it is more common to underestimate than to overestimate the amount of blood needed in the management of shock and to restore blood which has been lost.

Blood Substitutes. It should be emphasized that no substitute for whole blood has been found which is in any way comparable to the value of the red corpuscles and plasma. However, if whole blood is not available to restore blood volume, substitutes must be employed in emergencies. Of these, blood plasma is the best and in the dry form can be transported easily and kept ready at hand, but the danger of transmitting the virus of homologous serum hepatitis is so great that the use of pooled plasma cannot be recommended. Next in order of effectiveness is serum albumin, which has a physiologic effect closely approaching that of plasma. However, it is very expensive. For this and other reasons much attention has been given to the development of "plasma expanders," substances of such physicochemical properties that they will overcome the disparity between the capacity of the circulatory system and the circulating blood volume that exists in shock. Of these the gelatins possess the fewest disadvantages, but dextran, a biosynthetic polysaccharide, has been found to be very effective and is being used more and more. It should be borne in mind that the plasma expanders should be employed only for the immediate emergency rather than repeatedly.

When shock is clearly not due to blood loss, transfusions are often withheld on the ground that such treatment is futile and may be dangerous. Nevertheless, where doubt exists concerning the nature of the shock, whether oligemic or nonoligemic, the administration of whole blood, plasma, or packed cells is justified and is not likely to be harmful. In nonoligemic shock pressor amines, such as norepinephrine, have been found useful, but such agents have been effective as interim therapy even in oligemic shock until whole blood could be obtained.

In the management of anemia other than that due to the acute loss of blood, blood transfusions are commonly used more generously than is necessary or desirable. The discovery of such anemia calls for careful study to determine its cause, rather than the blind administration of blood. Thus there is no justification for blood transfusion in iron-deficiency anemias or in the macrocytic anemias with megaloblastic bone marrow unless the anemia is extremely severe or unless surgical measures must be carried out at once. The patient who has such anemia has become adjusted to it, and the sudden change produced by transfusion is unnecessary. A physiologic response can be achieved by oral iron therapy or vitamin B_{12} or folic acid administration, according to the nature of the deficiency. Again, in anemia associated with infection or in the management of the anemia of leukemia, Hodgkin's disease, or other disorders, the treatment of the underlying condition, whenever possible, is preferable to blood transfusion. Even in the management of aplastic anemia or other forms of anemia for which no specific therapy is available, it is better to give only enough transfusions to maintain the hemoglobin at a level consistent with reasonable activity rather than to attempt to maintain a normal level. Thereby the risk which each transfusion presents is reduced and the accumulation of iron in the tissues is less. Such patients are often maintained quite satisfactorily at hematocrit levels between 35 and 40 ml per 100 ml blood.

Whole blood, plasma, or albumin can be used to restore the colloid osmotic pressure of plasma to physiologic levels in cases of hypoproteinemia. Intravenous injections of salt-poor human serum albumin are particularly valuable in certain patients with hepatic cirrhosis and ascites, the nephrotic syndrome, idiopathic hypoproteinemia, and the edema of malnutrition.

As a means for providing protein nutrients in patients restricted to parenteral feeding, other than as a temporary measure, intravenous injections of whole plasma or of serum albumin are impractical. This is because of their colloid osmotic activity and the consequent expansion of the recipient's plasma volume. Whole blood is even less valuable as a protein nutrient, in spite of its high protein content. This is not only because of the expansion of the patient's plasma volume thereby, but also because the contribution of the protein in the red corpuscles to the protein metabolic pool must await the natural destruction of the red corpuscles.

There is no sound basis for the use of transfusions in the management of the great majority of infections. It is true that blood transfusions have been employed effectively for the transfer of specific immune antibodies from convalescent donors to susceptible contacts where measles, mumps, and yellow fever have been present in epidemic form, and immune transfusions have been considered to be of value in treating certain infections, notably herpes ophthalmia and scarlet fever. However, other methods are now available for the management of most of these conditions.

Whole blood transfusions, plasma, or plasma fractions also can provide specific clotting factors which may be lacking in certain patients, such as antihemophilic globulin (fraction I), prothrombin, factors V (Ac-globulin) and VII (spca), and fibrinogen. Fresh normal plasma is capable of restoring all clotting factors and is particularly necessary for supplying factor V and the antihemophilic factor. Stored plasma can be depended on only for prothrombin, factor VII, factor IX (the plasma thromboplastin component, PTC), and fibrinogen. When equipment constructed entirely of plastic or coated material is used, fresh blood transfusions may also serve temporarily for the successful transference of blood platelets from one person to another. As a method of treating conditions where leukocytes are needed, this procedure is as yet neither practical nor very successful.

Finally, the removal of blood possessing pathogenic properties and its replacement with normal blood (exchange transfusion) is a valuable procedure in special circumstances as, for example, in certain cases of hemolytic disease of the newborn (erythroblastosis fetalis).

Although additional therapeutic benefits have been ascribed to blood transfusions, their value and therapeutic rationale remain unproved. Their use to "pep up" a patient who is not anemic and whose blood volume is normal is certainly unwarranted.

Risks Inherent in Blood Transfusion. The *risk inherent in blood transfusion* is not inconsiderable. In spite of the general knowledge of the danger of a hemolytic transfusion reaction resulting from mismatching of the major blood group antigens A, B, and D (Rh), and notwithstanding the care taken to avoid such errors, the incidence of hemolytic reactions to blood transfusions is substantial (Table 235-5). The mortality of hemolytic transfusion reactions is approximately 50 per cent. Furthermore, as discussed earlier (Chap. 47), there is a good chance of immunizing a recipient to one or more of the blood group antigens not tested for in the routine preparation for transfusion. It is noteworthy that the risk from sensitization is increased if a woman is transfused with blood from her husband or one of his relatives because of the possibility of her having been previously sensitized during pregnancy to a blood group substance foreign to her but inherent in the fetus. There is also the risk of erythroblastosis fetalis in subsequent pregnancies if sensitization occurs as a result of the transfusion.

In addition to hemolytic transfusion reactions, febrile or pyrogenic, anaphylactic, and infectious reactions may occur. Pyrogenic and urticarial reactions are usually mild and may be induced by small thrombi in the transfused blood, soluble toxic substances in new rubber tubing, improperly cleaned tubing, or insufficiently sterilized solutions which may contain small amounts of bacterial pyrogen. Of great seriousness are reactions due to the administration of blood heavily laden with dead or viable bacteria which have gained access to the blood by accident. Serum hepatitis is another serious and not completely avoidable complication of blood transfusion. There is also the possibility of transmission of malaria or of syphilis, but this can

Table 235-5. TRANSFUSION REACTIONS

Type	Cause	Incidence, %
Pyrogenic	Bacterial pyrogens	1.8–2.9
Febrile	Leukoagglutinins	
Urticarial	Sensitivity (?)	0.8–1.1
Serum sickness	Unknown	Rare
Hemolytic	Mismatching of blood	0.1–0.5
Isosensitization	Repeated transfusions and in pregnancy	Not rare
Circulatory overload	Injudicious augmentation of blood volume	Not rare
Infectious	Grossly contaminated blood	Rare
Transmission of disease	Homologous serum jaundice, syphilis, malaria	0.45–1.0
Air embolism	Entry of air into vein via tubing	Rare
"Cold reaction"	Cold agglutinins (?)	Not rare
Hypocalcemia	Exchange transfusions	Not rare
Hemorrhagic diathesis	Massive transfusions, etc.	Rare (?)
Fat embolism	Transfusion via bone marrow	Rare
Plasma sensitivity	Heat-labile plasma factor	In PNH

usually be avoided by appropriate inquiry and examination of the donor.

Before subjecting a patient to blood transfusion, thought should be given to his cardiovascular status. In all persons with impaired cardiac function the administration of whole blood or other osmotically active solutions must be made cautiously and slowly, since an increase in venous pressure and pulmonary edema is easily produced. Particular care should be used in regard to concentrated serum albumin because of its capacity to withdraw fluid from the tissues into the circulation. Such patients, furthermore, should be propped in a sitting position during the transfusion. The so-called "speed reaction" is the result of circulatory overloading, and its manifestations are those of right-sided heart failure. It is produced by overrapid infusion in relation to the cardiovascular reserve of the patient and can be prevented by slow administration of blood. If the purpose of transfusion is to raise the concentration of circulating hemoglobin rather than to increase the total blood volume, red cell suspensions are as effective as are whole blood transfusions and offer the advantage that the volume of injected material is relatively small. When it is not convenient to prepare red cell suspensions, 60 to 80 per cent of the plasma can be withdrawn from the blood after spontaneous or mechanical sedimentation of the red cells, thereby reducing the volume of injected material as well as its salt content.

Patients who have received many transfusions may develop cold agglutinins and may react with a chill if blood is given without being warmed. Sometimes allowing the blood to stand at room temperature is adequate, but in many instances it is necessary to have some of the transfusion tubing rest in a water bath maintained at body temperature, thus allowing the blood to be warmed before it enters the patient's vein. Other complications which may develop in those subjected to repeated transfusions are febrile reactions due to leukoagglutinins and, especially in paroxysmal nocturnal hemoglobinuria, sensitivity to a heat-labile constituent of fresh normal plasma. In such patients only well-washed red cells can be used in transfusion.

Except in emergency, it is always wise to give the first 50 ml of blood slowly and under the scrutiny of a doctor or nurse. In addition it is well, whenever possible, to wait 30 min in order to determine whether a reaction will occur. Fatal transfusion reactions have occurred only when more than 300 ml of blood has been given. It is unwise to use blood for transfusion which has been brought to room temperature, cooled, and then rewarmed, since the likelihood of an infectious reaction is thereby increased.

Universal Donor. While the use of group O blood (universal donor) for general transfusion purposes is undesirable, in certain types of hospitals which use transfusion therapy almost exclusively on an emergency basis, the practice is followed. In such situations the two chief hazards should be kept in mind. One is the danger of mistyping A_2 donors as group O, an error which can be eliminated by serum or "back typing." The second danger, that of the group O person whose serum contains high titers of anti-A and anti-B or both, is met in part by attempting to discover and screen out such donors, and in part by adding A and B substances to the group O blood.

REFERENCES

GENERAL

Wintrobe, M. M.: "Clinical Hematology," 5th ed., Philadelphia, Lea & Febiger, 1961.

HEMOLYTIC ANEMIAS

Beutler, E.: The Hemolytic Effect of Primaquine and Related Compounds, Blood, 14:103, 1959.

Crosby, W. H., and J. H. Akeroyd: The Limit of Hemoglobin Synthesis in Hereditary Hemolytic Anemia: Its Relation to the Excretion of Bile Pigment, Am. J. Med., 13:273, 1952.

Dacie, J. V.: "The Haemolytic Anaemias," 2d ed., part I, New York, Grune & Stratton, Inc., 1960.

Jandl, J. H., A. R. Jones, and W. B. Castle: The Destruction of Red Cells by Antibodies in Man: I. Observations on the Sequestration and Lysis of Red Cells Altered by Immune Mechanisms, J. Clin. Invest., 36:1428, 1957.

Szeinberg, A., Y. Asher, and Ch. Sheba: Studies on Glutathione Stability in Erythrocytes of Cases with Past History of Favism or Sulfa-drug-induced Hemolysis, Blood, 13:348, 1958.

Paroxysmal Nocturnal Hemoglobinuria

Hartmann, R. C., and J. V. Auditore: Paroxysmal Nocturnal Hemoglobinuria, Am. J. Med., 27:389, 1959; J. Clin. Invest., 38:702, 1959; J. Appl. Physiol., 14:589, 1959.

Congenital Hemolytic Anemias

Prankerd, T. A. J., K. I. Altman, and L. E. Young: Abnormalities of Carbohydrate Metabolism of Red Cells in Hereditary Spherocytosis, J. Clin. Invest., 34:1268, 1955; Am. J. Med., 22:724, 1957; Quart. J. Med., 29:199, 1960.

Shahidi, N. T., and L. K. Diamond: Enzyme Deficiency in Erythrocytes in Congenital Nonspherocytic Hemolytic Anemia, Pediatrics, 24:245, 1959.

Zinkham, W. H., and R. E. Lenhard, Jr.: Metabolic Abnormalities of Erythrocytes from Patients with Congenital Nonspherocytic Hemolytic Anemia, J. Pediatrics, 55:319, 1959.

Paroxysmal Cold Hemoglobinuria

Jordan, W. S., Jr., R. L. Prouty, R. W. Heinle, and J. H. Dingle: The Mechanism of Hemolysis in Paroxysmal Cold Hemoglobinuria: III. Erythrophagocytosis and Leukopenia, Blood, 7:387, 1952.

Parish, D. J., and J. R. A. Mitchell: Syphilitic Paroxysmal Cold Haemoglobinuria, J. Clin. Pathol., 13:237, 1960.

Sickle-cell Anemia and Other Abnormal Hemoglobinopathies

Greenberg, M. S., E. H. Kass, and W. B. Castle: Factors Influencing the Role of S Hemoglobin in the Pathologic Physiology of Sickle Cell Anemia and Related Disorders, J. Clin. Invest., 36:833, 1957.

Myerson, R. M., Esther Harrison, and H. W. Lohmuller: Incidence and Significance of Abnormal Hemoglobins, Am. J. Med., 26:543, 1959.

IRON-DEFICIENCY ANEMIA

Heath, C. W., and A. J. Patek, Jr.: The Anemia of Iron Deficiency, Medicine, 16:267, 1937 (Bibliography).

Wintrobe, M. M., and R. T. Beebe: Idiopathic Hypochromic Anemia, Medicine, 12:187, 1933 (Bibliography).

MACROCYTIC ANEMIAS

Castle, W. B.: Development of Knowledge Concerning the Gastric Intrinsic Factor and Its Relation to Pernicious Anemia, New Engl. J. Med., 249:603, 1953.

Gatenby, P. B. B., and E. W. Lillie: Clinical Analysis of 100 Cases of Severe Megaloblastic Anaemia of Pregnancy, Brit. Med. J., 2:1111, 1960.

Hawkins, C. F., and M. J. Meynell: Macrocytosis and Macrocytic Anaemia Caused by Anticonvulsant Drugs, Quart. J. Med., 27:45, 1958.

Nyberg, W.: Absorption and Excretion of Vitamin B_{12} in Subjects Infected with *Diphyllobothrium latum* and in Non-infected Subjects Following Oral Administration of Radioactive B_{12}, Acta haematol., 19:90, 1958; New Engl. J. Med., 259:216, 1958.

Reisner, E. H., Jr., J. P. Gilbert, C. Rosenblum, and M. C. Morgan: Applications of the Urinary Tracer Test (of Schilling) as an Index of Vitamin B_{12} Absorption, Am. J. Clin. Nutrition, 4:134, 1956.

Schilling, R. F.: The Effect of Gastric Juice on the Urinary Excretion of Radioactivity after the Oral Administration of Radioactive Vitamin B_{12}, J. Lab. & Clin. Med., 42:860, 1953; *ibid.*, 45:926, 1955.

Thompson, R. B., and C. C. Ungley: Megaloblastic Anemia Associated with Anatomic Lesions in the Small Intestine, Blood, 10:771, 1955.

Wills, Lucy: Pernicious Anemia, Nutritional Macrocytic Anemia, and Tropical Sprue, Blood, 3:36, 1948.

THALASSEMIA

Chernoff, A. I.: The Distribution of the Thalassemia Gene: A Historical Review, Blood, 14:899, 1959.

236 ERYTHREMIA (Polycythemia Rubra Vera)

M. M. Wintrobe

Definition. Erythremia, also known as Vaquez' or Osler's disease or splenomegalic polycythemia, is a disease of unknown etiology and of insidious onset and slow, chronic course. It is characterized by a striking absolute increase in the quantity of circulating red corpuscles and, often, by evidence of increased production of myeloid leukocytes and even of platelets. Splenomegaly and a red "cyanosis" of the skin, as well as increase in the viscosity of the blood and in the total volume of the blood, are additional features of this disorder.

History. Vaquez in 1892 described a case of polycythemia which he had originally attributed to congenital heart disease. Osler gave a more complete description in 1903.

Etiology and Pathogenesis. The term *polycythemia* signifies an increase above the normal in the number of red corpuscles in the circulating blood. This increase usually, though not always, is accompanied by a corresponding increase in the quantity of hemoglobin and in the volume of packed red corpuscles. The increase may or may not be associated with an increase in the total quantity of red cells in the body. It is important to distinguish between *absolute* polycythemia (an increase in the total red corpuscle mass) and *relative* polycythemia, which occurs when, through loss of blood plasma, the concentration of the red corpuscles becomes greater than normal in the circulating blood. This may be the consequence of abnormally lowered fluid intake or of marked loss of body fluids, such as occurs in persistent vomiting, severe diarrhea, copious sweating, or acidosis (Chaps. 13, 50). Loss of electrolyte from the extracellular compartment, when not accompanied by corresponding loss of water, leads to a decline of osmolar concentration in the extracellular fluid. The resulting shift of water into the tissue cells may produce relative polycythemia, sometimes of high grade. In certain types of peripheral circulatory failure there is a loss of plasma into the interstitial fluid. Such a shift takes place largely in the periphery, with the result that the polycythemia may be more marked in capillary blood than in that from central blood vessels.

Because the term *polycythemia* is loosely used to refer to all varieties of increase in the number of red corpuscles, the terms *erythrocytosis* and *erythremia* are preferred in referring to two forms of absolute polycythemia. *Erythrocytosis* denotes absolute polycythemia which occurs in response to some known stimulus; *erythremia* refers to the disease of unknown etiology which is the main subject of this chapter.

Erythrocytosis develops as a consequence of a variety of factors and represents a physiologic response to conditions of hypoxia. Sojourn at high altitudes leads to defective saturation of arterial blood with oxygen and stimulates the production of more red corpuscles. Immediately on ascent to a high altitude, symptoms such as fatigue, dizziness, headache, nausea, vomiting, ringing in the ears, and prostration may appear. In most persons adaptation soon occurs, with the development of polycythemia and other compensatory adjustments. However, a disorder may set in insidiously a few years later, or even as long as 20 years after continued residence at high altitudes, leading to the development of a condition known as *chronic mountain sickness* or *seroche* (*Monge's disease*).

Emphysema is the most common of the chronic pulmonary conditions which may lead to erythrocytosis. Silicosis, with extensive pulmonary fibrosis, is another. Pulmonary arteriovenous fistula may lead to impaired saturation of arterial blood with oxygen, with the consequent development of erythrocytosis and of a clinical picture resembling closely that of certain types of congenital heart disease. Cavernous hemangioma of the lung may be associated with polycythemia. Hypertension of the lesser circulation, with pulmonary arterial and arteriolar sclerosis, may be accompanied by a train of symptoms such as asthma, bronchitis, dyspnea, and cyanosis, as well as erythrocytosis—a syndrome known as *Ayerza's syndrome,* or *cardiaco negro.*

Under the mechanical conditions existing in obese patients, periods of shallow breathing may develop and result in alveolar hypoventilation and erythrocytosis. The fat, somnolent, red-faced boy of Dickens' "The Pickwick Papers" may well have been an example of this disorder. The claim that abnormal function of the respiratory center may be the cause of hypoxemia and absolute polycythemia requires substantiation.

The partial shunting of blood from the pulmonary circuit, such as occurs in congenital heart disease, is the cause of the most striking erythrocytosis resulting from abnormality in the circulation. Erythrocyte counts as high as 13 million, which are possible only when the red corpuscles are smaller than normal, have been observed in such cases, with volumes of packed red cells even as high as 86 ml per 100 ml of blood. The most common defects producing such polycythemia are pulmonary stenosis, usually with defective ventricular or auricular septum, patent foramen ovale, or patent ductus arteriosus; complete transposition of arterial trunks; and tetralogy of Fallot. Erythrocytosis does not usually occur in patients with acquired heart disease

but occasionally is seen in persons with mitral stenosis.

The excessive use of coal-tar derivatives and other forms of chronic poisoning, by producing abnormal hemoglobin pigments such as methemoglobin and sulfhemoglobin (Chap. 237), may cause erythrocytosis. Another chemical agent, cobalt, has produced erythrocytosis in experimental animals but the mechanism is obscure.

Erythrocytosis is found in Cushing's syndrome and can be produced by the administration of large amounts of adrenocorticosteroids. In many ways most curious of all are the instances of polycythemia observed in association with various tumors. These have been chiefly of two varieties, infratentorial and renal. The tumors in the posterior fossa of the skull have usually been vascular, and their removal has frequently been associated with a return to normal hemoglobin levels. This response has also been noted in many of the cases of hypernephroma, polycystic disease of the kidneys, and hydronephrosis which were accompanied by polycythemia. The frequency of the association of polycythemia with the above-mentioned renal disorders has ranged from 0.3 to 2.6 per cent of cases in different series.

The term *stress erythrocytosis* has been applied to the polycythemia seen occasionally in very active, hard-working persons in a state of anxiety, who appear florid but who have none of the characteristic signs of erythremia—no splenomegaly or marked leukocytosis with immature cells in the blood. In such individuals the total red cell mass is normal and the plasma volume is below normal.

In essence, then, erythrocytosis is known to develop when there is

1. Defective saturation of arterial blood with oxygen, resulting from (*a*) decreased atmospheric pressure, and (*b*) impaired pulmonary ventilation

2. Abnormality in circulation, due to (*a*) shunting (congenital heart disease), and possibly (*b*) diminished blood supply to the bone marrow (in certain patients with chronic cardiac disease)

3. Defect in circulating blood pigment

It is clear, however, that in addition to these long-recognized mechanisms, some instances of erythrocytosis cannot be explained on these grounds.

4. The adrenocortical secretions may produce polycythemia

5. Humoral mechanisms of less well-defined nature may play a role. Considerable evidence supports the view that a humoral factor, "erythropoietin," plays a significant role in erythropoiesis and also indicates that this factor may arise in the kidneys. In fact, even the effect of anoxia on the bone marrow may not be direct but may be medi-

ated by a humoral mechanism. Thus, in a case of patent ductus arteriosus occurring distal to the origin of the subclavian artery, it was shown that the sternal marrow manifested the same pronounced normoblastic hyperplasia as the iliac marrow even though the oxygen saturation of the latter was markedly decreased as compared with the normal saturation of the sternal marrow.

In the disease *erythremia*, however, the above mechanisms have not been found to be involved. The most common form of erythremia appears in middle or late life, it is often accompanied by splenomegaly, and often the increase in number of red corpuscles is but a part of a generalized myeloid hyperplasia which may be manifested in elevated leukocyte counts and an increase in the number of platelets. A close relationship to chronic myelocytic leukemia is suggested by such cases.

Polycythemia of unknown cause has also been seen in children, in rare instances, and occasionally appears as a familial disorder. Such cases may well be unrelated to the classical disorder described by Vaquez and Osler.

Pathology. The striking changes are those related to the increase in total blood volume. All the organs are engorged with blood, the veins stand out like "bunches of thick worms," and there may be thromboses or anemic infarcts. The *bone marrow* is dark red in color and very cellular. Microscopically, this is found in most instances to be due to hyperplasia of all the marrow elements. In some cases the percentage of normoblasts is increased, in others the proportions of myelocytes and myeloblasts or of basophilic and eosinophilic cells may be greater than normal.

The *spleen* is enlarged, chiefly from hyperplasia of the pulp and distention with blood. Infarcts are common. There may be foci of extramedullary blood formation in the spleen, the liver, and occasionally elsewhere as well. Cirrhosis of the liver has been observed in a number of instances.

Symptomatology. The onset is insidious and the progress gradual. Headache, dizziness, ringing in the ears, or visual disturbances; dyspnea, lassitude, or weakness; skin or mucous membrane hemorrhages; a sense of weight in the abdomen due to the enlargement of the spleen; or irritability, depression, forgetfulness, or vague symptoms suggesting neurasthenia are complaints encountered in many cases. Various gastrointestinal symptoms such as fullness, belching, or constipation may be present, or symptoms of peptic ulcer may be found. Sometimes the symptoms are those attributable to increased metabolism: lassitude, increased sweating, and loss of weight. Swelling and pain in the extremities may be very troublesome. In still other cases the symptoms are so insignificant that the polycythemia is discovered only accidentally.

The face is a deep red rather than truly cyanotic. The color is most noticeable in the lips, cheeks, tip of the nose, ears, and neck. The distal portions of the extremities may be more truly cyanotic, since the highly viscous blood circulates more sluggishly there than is normal. Ecchymoses are common, and epistaxis and bleeding of the gums are frequently encountered. Cardiac abnormality is unusual, but vascular disturbances are common. These include venous thromboses, coronary thrombosis, and cerebrovascular accidents. The blood pressure is more often normal than elevated. Enlargement of the liver is frequent, and splenomegaly is found in at least 75 per cent of cases. The spleen may be just palpable or it may extend even to the pelvic brim.

Blood. Erythrocyte counts of 7 to 10 million cells per cu mm are common. Unless hemorrhage has occurred or venesections have been performed, there is a corresponding increase in hemoglobin and in volume of packed red corpuscles. The individual red corpuscles appear normal, although occasional polychromatophilia or basophilic stippling may be noted. The finding of nucleated red corpuscles and the appearance of small numbers of myelocytes and even earlier forms in the blood give a clue to the hyperplastic state of the bone marrow; leukocytosis, sometimes of marked degree (60,000 per cu mm), due to an increase of the granulocytes, and high platelet counts, when present, give further evidence of overactivity. The percentage of reticulocytes is not increased unless there has been recent bleeding. The osmotic fragility of the red corpuscles is not significantly altered. There may be some evidence of increased blood destruction, in the form of slight bilirubinemia and increased excretion of urobilinogen. The viscosity of the blood is greatly increased, even five- to tenfold. The thick, sticky blood may be slow to coagulate and the clot may not retract. Bleeding and clotting times are usually normal, however.

The total blood volume is substantially increased (150 to 300 per cent of normal), entirely because of an increase in red corpuscle mass.

Other Laboratory Findings. These include increased basal metabolic rate in many cases; normal, increased, or reduced gastric secretion, even achlorhydria; occasionally, increased serum uric acid level and, sometimes, increased endogenous uric acid excretion; and normal urine or slight proteinuria.

Diagnosis. The symptoms of erythremia alone may suggest a variety of disorders, but once the blood has been examined, the problem is to differentiate secondary forms of polycythemia (erythrocytosis) from the "primary" disorder. Failure to discover a cause for the polycythemia, and the presence of a reddish rather than bluish cyanosis favor the diagnosis of erythremia. Splenomegaly is very unusual in erythrocytosis, even when the erythrocyte count is very much increased. What is more, in the latter condition, leukocytosis, immature leukocytes, and an increase in the platelet count are hardly ever found and normoblasts are much more uncommon in the blood than in erythremia.

An absolute increase in red corpuscle mass is found in erythrocytosis as well as in erythremia. Measurement of blood volume, therefore, does not aid in differentiating "secondary" polycythemia, but because of variations in plasma volume it is a truer index of the degree of polycythemia than the hematocrit level. It is also helpful in the occasional patient, often a heavily built, middle-aged, and sometimes hypertensive male, in whom there is only relative polycythemia ("stress erythrocytosis"). Measurement of arterial oxygen saturation is useful in differentiating erythrocytosis due to cardiac or pulmonary disease, for in the latter, oxygen saturation is reduced more or less in inverse proportion to the degree of polycythemia, whereas in erythremia it is normal or nearly normal.

Course and Complications. Barring the development of serious complications, the course of erythremia, adequately treated, is chronic and the disorder is often compatible with many years of life. The most dangerous complications are vascular: thrombosis or hemorrhage. Therapy, by keeping the red corpuscle mass at a nearly normal level, can effectively reduce blood viscosity and thus serves to reduce the likelihood of such vascular accidents. Intercurrent infections, especially of the respiratory tract, may be troublesome, and bronchitis and emphysema may develop. Peptic ulcer and hypertension are frequent complications; less often, gout and cirrhosis of the liver occur. The development of typical chronic myelocytic leukemia in a number of cases of erythremia has given support to the view that there may be a close relationship between these two disorders.

Treatment. Treatment is symptomatic, since the cause of erythremia is unknown. Symptomatic relief is best achieved by reducing the red corpuscle mass to something approaching normal. This is most quickly achieved by *venesection*. Approximately a pint of blood is removed twice a week or even more often, until the volume of packed red corpuscles approaches normal. Then the procedure may need to be repeated only once a month or less often. *Phenylhydrazine hydrochloride*, though now rarely used, is effective in destroying the red corpuscles, but it is best first to use venesection to lower the blood level to normal, subsequently giving only enough of the hemolytic agent to maintain the blood at normal. For this purpose 0.1 Gm. in capsules, once a day, every other day, or every third day should be adequate. The use of such small doses will avoid complications of phenylhydrazine

therapy such as thrombosis and acute hemolytic anemia. This drug should not be used for bedridden patients or for those who have thrombosis already.

Instead of removing or destroying the excessive red corpuscles, hematopoiesis may be inhibited by irradiation or by chemotherapy. The effects of *irradiation* are slow to appear, however, and consequently venesection must be used at the same time initially. The intravenous injection of radioactive phosphorus (P^{32}) is more satisfactory than roentgen therapy. The procedure depends on the fact that the radioactive phosphorus passes to tissues which have a high phosphorus content. The concentration of P^{32} in the bones places this agent in a strategic position. Usually 3 to 5 millicuries of P^{32} is given. After 10 to 12 weeks, if symptomatic and hematologic improvement are inadequate, a second dose is administered. Subsequent therapy is "titrated" according to need, but intervals between injections should not be shorter than 10 weeks, and leukocyte and platelet counts should be included in the blood examinations as guides in avoiding marrow aplasia from overdosage. Remissions of 6 to 10 months are common, but much longer ones are not unusual.

Although agents such as triethylenemelamine and busulfan have been shown to be effective in the treatment of erythremia, they offer no advantages over radioactive phosphorus.

REFERENCES

Burwell, C. S., E. D. Robin, R. D. Whaley, and A. G. Bickelmann: Extreme Obesity Associated with Alveolar Hypoventilation: A Pickwickian Syndrome, Am. J. Med., 21:811, 1956.

Hurtado, A.: Some Clinical Aspects of Life at High Altitudes, Ann. Internal Med., 53:247, 1960.

Lawrence, J. H., N. I. Berlin, and R. L. Huff: The Nature and Treatment of Polycythemia, Medicine, 32:323, 1953; Am. J. Med. Sci., 233:268, 1957.

Ways, P., J. W. Huff, C. H. Kosmaler, and L. E. Young: Polycythemia and Histologically Proven Renal Disease, A.M.A. Arch. Internal Med., 107:154, 1961.

Wintrobe, M. M.: "Clinical Hematology," 5th ed., Philadelphia, Lea & Febiger, 1961.

237 METHEMOGLOBINEMIA, SULFHEMOGLOBINEMIA

George E. Cartwright

METHEMOGLOBINEMIA

Methemoglobin is an oxidation product of hemoglobin in which the iron is in the ferric state. Methemoglobin cannot bind oxygen or carbon dioxide. Within the erythrocyte, about 99 per cent of the hemoglobin is in the reduced state ($HbFe^{++}$) and 1 per cent is in the oxidized state ($HbFe^{3+}$). Under normal circumstances these two forms of hemoglobin are in equilibrium.

The system in the red cell for reduction of methemoglobin employs reduced diphosphopyridine nucleotide (DPNH), formed from the oxidation of glucose, as the electron donor. Reduced DPN does not react directly with methemoglobin. The enzyme, DPN diaphorase, is required for the reduction. This was originally referred to as the "methemoglobin reductase a" system.

$$\tfrac{1}{2} \text{ glucose} + \text{DPN} \longrightarrow \text{pyruvate} + \text{DPNH}$$

$$\text{DPNH} + HbFe^{3+} \xrightarrow[\text{enzyme}]{\text{diaphorase}} \text{DPN} + HbFe^{++}$$

Etiology. Methemoglobinemia may be either inherited or acquired. Two distinct types of *hereditary methemoglobinemia* have been described. A number of cases of hereditary methemoglobinemia have been observed in Greece but have not yet been classified as to the type of biochemical abnormality.

Hereditary methemoglobinemia due to a deficiency of the enzyme DPN diaphorase has been described in Alaskan Eskimos and Athabaskan Indians. The disease is transmitted as an autosomal recessive trait. Individuals heterozygous for the trait have about half the normal level of the diaphorase enzyme and are asymptomatic; 98 to 99 per cent of the hemoglobin is in the reduced state. Individuals homozygous for the trait have a complete lack of the erythrocyte enzyme and are cyanotic from birth; 5 to 60 per cent of the hemoglobin is present as methemoglobin. The rate at which methemoglobin is reduced is greatly impaired. The disease has been described in infants and children. The failure to observe the disease state in adults suggests that the disease is associated with early mortality or that this form of methemoglobinemia disappears with age.

Hereditary methemoglobinemia associated with an abnormal hemoglobin (hemoglobin M) has been described in families of German, Greek, Swiss, and Italian descent. The disease is transmitted as a non-sex-linked dominant trait. The fundamental defect exists in the structure of the globin. The formation of methemoglobin is due to increased sensitivity of hemoglobin M to oxidation and not to a slow rate of methemoglobin reduction. On the basis of absorption spectra at least three different M hemoglobins have been described. These have been designated hemoglobins M_B, M_S, and M_M after the cities (Boston, Saskatoon, and Milwaukee) where they were described. Cyanosis is the only clinical manifestation described. Cyanosis is usu-

ally absent at birth and first appears 6 weeks to 6 months after birth. Hemoglobin M, unlike most of the other hemoglobinopathies, is not associated with hemolytic anemia.

A number of patients with *congenital methemoglobinemia* have been reported without a familial history of the disease, and a few patients with *idiopathic methemoglobinemia* have been observed in whom the congenital nature of the disease was not clearly demonstrated.

Acquired (secondary) methemoglobinemia is more common than hereditary methemoglobinemia and is caused by contact with drugs containing amino or nitro groups (Table 237-1). These drugs preferentially oxidize hemoglobin and, in sufficient amounts, overcome the normal reducing mechanism of the *erythrocytes*. When exposure to the offending drug ceases, the methemoglobin is rapidly converted to the reduced compound and the cyanosis disappears. Nitrates after ingestion may be converted to nitrites by intestinal bacteria, and after absorption from the intestine produce methemoglobin. Cases of methemoglobinemia due to nitrates or nitrites have been reported following the use of bismuth subnitrates or of ammonia or potassium nitrate, from the therapeutic use of amyl nitrite or nitroglycerin, from food high in nitrates, in infants drinking well water high in nitrates, from the inhalation of nitrous gases by arc welders, and from the ingestion of corning syrup. Aniline dyes may produce methemoglobinemia by penetration of the intact skin. Contact with dyed blankets, laundry marks on diapers, and freshly dyed shoes have produced methemoglobinemia. The ingestion by children of certain red wax crayons containing *p*-nitroaniline has resulted in methemoglobinemia. The commonly dispensed analgesic and antipyretic drugs, acetanilid and phenacetin, are aniline derivatives and have frequently been found responsible for methemoglobinemia. Certain sulfonamides, such as sulfanilamide, Prontosil, sulfathiazole, and sulfapyridine, but not sulfadiazine or sulfamerazine, produce the condition.

Enterogenous cyanosis is a term used to refer to a clinical syndrome characterized by attacks of cyanosis, headache, abdominal pain with either diarrhea or constipation, dyspnea, dizziness, collapse, and syncope. Many of the patients reported were taking aniline derivatives for headache. It has been suggested that because of the gastrointestinal disease there was an abnormal production and absorption of nitrites. Sulfhemoglobinemia has been present frequently, together with methemoglobinemia, in the blood of these patients.

In addition to the above types of methemoglobinemia, rare cases of acquired hemolytic anemia with paroxysmal methemoglobinemia have been reported.

Clinical Manifestations. When as little as 1.5 Gm of methemoglobin is present in 100 ml of blood, recognizable cyanosis results. In contrast, about 5 Gm of reduced hemoglobin must be present before a comparable degree of cyanosis occurs. Since methemoglobin is incapable of combining with oxygen, the symptoms of methemoglobinemia are attributable to the hypoxia produced by the lowered oxygen capacity of the blood. The severity of the symptoms is related to the quantity of methemoglobin present, the rapidity with which the methemoglobinemia develops, and the capacity of the individual's cardiorespiratory and hematopoietic systems to adjust to the hypoxia. In general, levels of less than 20 per cent methemoglobin are usually not associated with symptoms. At levels of 20 to 50 per cent, fatigue, weakness, dyspnea, tachycardia, headaches, and dizziness may occur. Only rarely is enough methemoglobin present to cause coma and death.

Diagnosis. Methemoglobinemia should be suspected in any patient with intense cyanosis, especially if physical examination fails to reveal evidences of cardiovascular or pulmonary disease and if the cyanosis is unrelieved by oxygen therapy. If blood withdrawn from a vein shows the characteristic chocolate-brown coloration, the diagnosis of an abnormal blood pigment is almost certain. If the pigment is not in the plasma but in the erythrocytes, and if the chocolate-brown color remains after shaking the blood in air for 15 min, there is additional presumptive evidence for the presence of either methemoglobinemia or sulfhemoglobinemia.

A family history of cyanosis helps to delineate the hereditary forms of the disease. A negative family history of cyanosis and a recent history of drug ingestion (Table 237-1) suggest the acquired form of the disease. The hereditary form of the disease, which is due to a deficiency of the diaphorase enzyme, can be recognized with certainty only by determination of erythrocyte diaphorase activity. The diagnosis of the hemoglobin M disorders can be established by starch block electrophoresis (pH 7.0 to 7.2) of hemolysates and by a spectrophotometric absorption analysis of the patient's hemoglobin.

Methemoglobin (other than M hemoglobins) may be differentiated from sulfhemoglobin by examining a 1:10 or 1:100 aqueous dilution of blood in a hand spectroscope. The absorption band of methemoglobin (630 mμ) may be confused with that of sulfhemoglobin (618 mμ), but on the addition of 2 or 3 drops of 5 per cent potassium cyanide the band due to methemoglobin disappears, whereas the sulfhemoglobin band is unchanged. The addition of hydrogen peroxide causes dissolution of the sulfhemoglobin band, but not of the methemoglobin band.

Table 237-1. AMINO AND NITRO COMPOUNDS PRODUCING METHEMOGLOBINEMIA

Aromatic drugs	Aliphatic and inorganic drugs
Aniline	Sodium nitrite
Anilinoethanol	Hydroxylamine
Phenacetin	Dimethylamine
Acetanilid	Nitroglycerin
Methylacetanilide	Amyl nitrite
Hydroxylacetanilide	Ethyl nitrite
Prontosil	Bismuth subnitrate
Sulfanilamide	Ammonium nitrate
Sulfathiazole	Potassium nitrate
Sulfapyridine	
Phenylenediamine	
Aminophenol	
Toluenediamine	
Alpha-naphthylamine	
Para-aminopropiophenone	
Phenylhydroxylamine	
Tolylhydroxylamine	
Nitrobenzene	
Dinitrobenzene	
Trinitrotoluene	
Nitrosobenzene	
Para-nitroaniline	

SOURCE: C. A. Finch: Methemoglobinemia and Sulfhemoglobinemia, New Engl. J. Med., 239:470, 1948.

Treatment. In patients with hereditary methemoglobinemia due to deficiency of DPN diaphorase, the reducing agent ascorbic acid may be given daily by mouth in an amount of 100 to 500 mg. Methylene blue accelerates the reduction of methemoglobin and is effective in a daily dose of 100 to 300 mg by mouth.

Ascorbic acid and methylene blue are of little or no value in alleviating the cyanosis due to hemoglobin M.

In patients with mild drug-induced methemoglobinemia no therapy is necessary other than removal of the offending agent, since reduction of the methemoglobin occurs rapidly as a result of the intact normal reconversion mechanism. In those patients in whom therapy is necessary, methylene blue, 1 to 2 mg per kg body weight given intravenously over a 5-min period in a 1 per cent solution, is the agent of choice. If cyanosis has not disappeared within an hour, a second dose of 2 mg per kg body weight should be given. Dosages should not exceed 7 mg per kg since toxic effects such as dyspnea, precordial pain, restlessness, apprehension, a sense of oppression, and fibrillar tremors may occur.

SULFHEMOGLOBINEMIA

Sulfhemoglobin is a sulfur-containing hemoglobin derivative. The exact mode of linkage of the sulfur to the hemoglobin is unknown. Sulfhemoglobin is not found in erythrocytes under normal circumstances. Once it has been formed it is not reversible to hemoglobin, the abnormal derivative remaining in the erythrocytes until they are destroyed.

Sulfhemoglobinemia may result when one of the oxidizing drugs listed in Table 237-1 has been taken.

Phenacetin (A.P.C., Empirin Compound, Anacin, Stanback) and acetanilid (Bromoseltzer) are the drugs found most frequently to be the causative agents. Constipation is present in at least half the patients, and it has been suggested, without documentary proof, that this contributes to the development of the condition by enhancing the production of hydrogen sulfide in the bowel.

Sulfhemoglobin is inert as an oxygen carrier, and when it is present intense cyanosis results. Somewhat less than 0.5 Gm sulfhemoglobin per 100 ml blood causes a degree of cyanosis equal to that of 1.5 Gm methemoglobin or 5 Gm reduced hemoglobin. Although the concentration of sulfhemoglobin may be found to be as high as 10 Gm per 100 ml, the life of the patient is not endangered and symptoms which can be attributed to the sulfhemoglobinemia are rarely present. Since many of the patients in whom sulfhemoglobinemia develops are neurotic or are taking drugs for a chronic headache or constipation, the symptoms which can be elicited are probably not attributable to the sulfhemoglobinemia. Symptoms of bromide intoxication frequently complicate the clinical picture in those ingesting Bromoseltzer. Once formed, there is no way of removing the sulfhemoglobin except by phlebotomy. In time the affected red corpuscles wear out and are destroyed. Treatment requires interdiction of the offending drug and correction of the intestinal conditions causing the disorder.

Enterogenous sulfhemoglobinemia is a term used to refer to the syndrome of sulfhemoglobinemia, cyanosis, and constipation or other evidence of disturbed bowel function without the history of the ingestion of an oxidizing or sulfur-containing drug. Rare cases of acquired hemolytic anemia with paroxysmal sulfhemoglobinemia and methemoglobinemia have been reported.

REFERENCES

Codounis, A.: Hereditary Methemoglobinemic Cyanosis, Brit. Med. J., 2:368, 1952.

Finch, C. A.: Methemoglobinemia and Sulfhemoglobinemia, New Engl. J. Med., 42:582, 1951.

Gerald, P. S., and P. George: Second Spectroscopically Abnormal Methemoglobin Associated with Hereditary Cyanosis, Science, 129:393, 1959.

Pisciotta, A. V., S. N. Ebbe, and J. E. Hinz: Clinical and Laboratory Features of Two Variants of Methemoglobin M Disease, J. Lab. Clin. Med.,

54:73, 1959.

Scott, E. M.: The Relation of Diaphorase of Human Erythrocytes to Inheritance of Methemoglobinemia, J. Clin. Invest., 39:1176, 1960.

Scott, E. M., and D. D. Hoskins: Hereditary Methemoglobinemia in Alaskan Eskimos and Indians, Blood, 13:795, 1958.

238 THE PURPURAS
M. M. Wintrobe

Definition. The term *purpura* refers to extravasations of blood into the skin or mucous membranes. They may vary from the size of a pin point or slightly bigger (petechiae) to much larger areas (ecchymoses). Purpura is but one manifestation of abnormal bleeding, already discussed (p. 217).

THROMBOCYTOPENIC PURPURA

Definition. This term refers to purpura which is accompanied by a significant reduction in the platelet count. There is at the same time prolongation of bleeding time, a positive tourniquet test result, and poor clot retraction, but the coagulation time and prothrombin time are normal. The purpura may be *idiopathic*, this also being known as *purpura hemorrhagica* or *Werlhof's disease;* or it may be symptomatic: the effect of various chemical, vegetable, animal, or physical agents, the accompaniment of certain infections, or a part of the picture of various blood disorders.

History. Werlhof, in 1735, distinguished purpura hemorrhagica as an entity distinct from the purpuric manifestations of various pestilential fevers and differing from other hemorrhagic disorders. Denys noted the thrombocytopenia in 1887, while Kaznelson proposed treatment by splenectomy in 1916.

Etiology and Pathogenesis. Purpura hemorrhagica occurs most frequently in children and in young adults, and is somewhat more common in the female than in males. No more than 10 per cent of cases begin after the age of forty. Not infrequently there is a family history of excessive bleeding. The condition is rare in Negroes.

In the bone marrow the number of megakaryocytes is normal or may even be increased. However, in contrast to the normal picture, few or no platelets are found about their margins. It is also significant that splenectomy is often followed by striking improvement. These observations have led to the assumption that this disorder is caused by

(1) a decreased rate of formation of platelets from megakaryocytes as the consequence of splenic inhibition, (2) platelet destruction by the spleen, or (3) a combination of damage to both megakaryocytes and circulating platelets, perhaps through the action of a humoral factor in the plasma. That the last is true in many cases, probably as the result of an immunologic mechanism, is indicated by studies in which platelet agglutinins were shown to be present in the plasma of patients with essential thrombocytopenic purpura. It was also demonstrated that the injection of plasma from patients with this disease into normal recipients was associated with thrombocytopenia, bleeding phenomena, and alterations in the megakaryocytes. Furthermore, transfused platelets disappear with extraordinary rapidity from the circulation of patients with acute idiopathic thrombocytopenic purpura. It is plausible to assume that the spleen removes sensitized platelets and may also produce some of the platelet agglutinin.

Platelet agglutinins were first described in patients with thrombocytopenic purpura due to Sedormid. In these cases it was shown that the drug forms an antigenic complex with the platelets, to which an antibody is formed. It is possible that in "idiopathic" thrombocytopenic purpura an unidentified toxin affects both platelets and capillary endothelium, which are antigenically similar, and that an antibody to these damaged tissues is produced.

That there is, in addition to thrombocytopenia, a defect in the capillary endothelium is suggested by the fact that hemorrhage in this disease is not always closely correlated to the degree of platelet reduction. It has been proposed that the capillaries are unusually permeable or that they are incapable of adequate contraction. For the latter hypothesis, evidence has been presented which is based on direct observation.

The *prolonged bleeding time* is explained by a failure of the capillaries to retract as well as by the lack of sufficient platelets to plug the opening of a bleeding vessel. The intracutaneous oozing of blood when capillary pressure is increased (tourniquet test) is explained in the same way. Coagulation time is normal because few platelets are needed to initiate clotting. The clot, however, is loose and retracts poorly because a large number of platelets are needed for syneresis.

There is much to suggest that idiopathic thrombocytopenic purpura is a syndrome which may arise in a number of different ways. Although an immunologic mechanism is probably important in many cases, it seems likely that in other instances the underlying cause may be splenic dysfunction which leads to suppression of platelet formation, or metabolic aberrations leading to deficiency of factors necessary for platelet production, or still other mechanisms or etiologic factors as yet unrecognized.

Symptomatology. Purpura hemorrhagica may begin abruptly and disappear spontaneously just as suddenly; or its manifestations may seem to have been present a long time, occasionally so long that they might appear to be characteristic of the individual concerned. The bleeding may be mild with perhaps only inconspicuous purpuric spots in the skin; or it may be severe and not only may lead to serious loss of blood but also may occur into vital areas such as the cranium or the diaphragm. All variations between these extremes may be encountered, and the disorder may wax and wane in intensity. Acute and chronic forms of the disorder have been described, and by some investigators are regarded as different entities. It is not unusual for symptoms first to become apparent following an acute infection.

The lesions in the skin usually consist of minute, red hemorrhages which differ from telangiectases in that they do not blanch on pressure. Often ecchymoses are found as well. Mucous membrane hemorrhages are common, bleeding from the nose, mouth, or uterus being particularly frequent and sometimes severe. Not rare are instances in which menorrhagia is the chief complaint, and this often is the only prominent clinical sign other than the abnormalities in the blood. Bleeding, however, may occur into any tissue and from any orifice. Frequently, also, excessive bleeding may be noted following tooth extraction, tonsillectomy, operations, or injuries.

Fever of mild degree may be present in acute cases. The spleen may extend a fingerbreadth below the costal margin. There is no general glandular enlargement, sternal tenderness, or other physical sign other than those attributable to hemorrhage or anemia.

Blood and Bone Marrow Findings. These have, in the main, been mentioned already. What platelets may be seen in the blood smear are often unusual in appearance: giant or minute forms, or deeply stained ones. The bleeding time may be slightly, moderately, or greatly prolonged (8 to 60 min or more). Anemia, if present, is proportional to the amount of blood lost. If there has been much bleeding, signs of stimulated erythropoiesis will be found: reticulocytosis, polychromatophilia, even occasional normoblasts. The leukocyte count may be normal, but if acute blood loss has taken place there may be a moderate leukocytosis with slight "shift to the left." In some chronic cases lymphocytosis has been observed.

Diagnosis. Hemorrhage not due to obvious cause, if associated with thrombocytopenia, prolonged bleeding time, poor clot retraction, and positive tourniquet test can be attributed to thrombocytopenic purpura. Prolonged bleeding time is characteristic of von Willebrand's disease (p. 1317) and may be found, though rarely, in a number of conditions in which coagulation time is prolonged, provided the blood and tissues are severely impoverished in coagulation factors (see Table 24-4, Chap. 24, p. 228). These include hemophilia and hypoprothrombinemia. A positive tourniquet test is found in many circumstances other than thrombocytopenic purpura (p. 227). Poor retraction of the clot is found, with rare exceptions, only when the platelets are reduced in number. The combination of these abnormalities is characteristic of thrombocytopenic purpura.

Before a diagnosis of purpura hemorrhagica can be made, however, the recognized causes of thrombocytopenic purpura must be excluded. They are listed in Table 238-1. The history and physical examination will serve to rule out many of these conditions. Adenopathy and sternal tenderness, as well as anemia out of proportion to the blood loss, even in the absence of striking changes in the leukocytes, should suggest leukemia. Persistent leukopenia suggests leukemia, aplastic anemia, disseminated lupus erythematosus, or one of the splenic disorders.

Treatment and Prognosis. The first principles in the therapy of thrombocytopenic purpura are expectant management and a search for possible etiologic factors. If one is found or suspected, further exposure should be stopped. Expectant therapy, in addition to appropriate rest, nursing, and diet, includes iron if there has been blood loss, and blood transfusion if this loss has been severe. The use of siliconized apparatus or plastic equipment in transfusion or the use of platelet-rich blood, or both, is helpful as a temporary measure, but it is noteworthy that platelet transfusions have limited value, since platelet survival tends to decrease progressively when repeated transfusions are given.

These measures are recommended because spontaneous remissions are common, especially in children. They can be complete and permanent. Remissions are particularly likely to occur if the onset has been acute and there is no history of previous hemorrhagic manifestations. Unfortunately the danger of bleeding into a vital organ such as the brain makes the waiting period a trying one. Recurrences are twice as common in females as in males. A more or less chronic course, punctuated perhaps by more acute phases, is more often seen in adolescents and adults but occurs at all ages.

The use of adrenocorticotropic hormone, cortisone, or prednisone is often associated with a decrease of bleeding phenomena and the thrombocytopenia may decrease or disappear, but these effects are temporary. These hormones are useful chiefly, therefore, in the management of hemorrhagic emergencies and in the preoperative preparation of patients for splenectomy. Those which can

Table 238-1. CLASSIFICATION OF THROMBOCYTOPENIC PURPURAS

I. "Essential" or "primary" purpura hemorrhagica; idiopathic thrombocytopenic purpura (ITP)
II. Symptomatic purpuras
    A. Chemical, vegetable, animal, and physical agents
        1. Chemical
            a. Myelosuppressive agents: nitrogen mustards, TEM, busulfan, urethan, antimetabolites, benzol
            b. Agents which in therapeutic doses produce purpura mainly because of individual sensitivity: organic arsenicals, Sedormid, quinidine, quinine, sulfonamides, gold salts, chlorothiazide (Diuril), hydrochlorothiazide, butobarbitone; and possibly also acetazolamide (Diamox), chloramphenicol, penicillin, chlorophenothane (DDT), meprobamate (Equanil, Miltown), stibophen, oxytetracycline, para-aminosalicylic acid, streptomycin, phenylbutazone, antipyrine, sodium salicylate, tridione, meparfynol, phenobarbital, allyl-isopropylbarbituric acid, thiourea, dinitrophenol, digitoxin, mercurials, potassium iodide, bismuth, ergot, organic hair dyes, estrogens, tolbutamide (Orinase), chlorpropamide (Diabenese)
        2. Vegetable: Foods, orris root
        3. Animal: Snake venoms, pertussis vaccine, insect bite
        4. Physical: X-rays and other forms of ionizing radiation, heat stroke, extensive burns
    B. Blood disorders
        1. Leukemias: Acute, or late stages of chronic
        2. Anemias
            a. Aplastic—idiopathic or due to physical or chemical agents
            b. Myelophthisic (tumors in bone marrow, osteosclerosis, etc.)
            c. Pernicious anemia
            d. Acquired hemolytic anemias of immune body type
        3. Splenic disorders: Congestive splenomegaly, Gaucher's disease, Felty's syndrome, rarely Hodgkin's disease
        4. Miscellaneous: Acute purpura with platelet thrombi in capillaries ("thrombotic thrombocytopenic purpura")
    C. Infections and other conditions: Septicemia, subacute bacterial endocarditis, typhus, measles, vaccinia, infectious mononucleosis, etc.; lupus erythematosus, sarcoidosis, hemangioendothelioma, massive blood transfusions

SOURCE: Adapted from M. M. Wintrobe: "Clinical Hematology," 5th ed., Philadelphia, Lea & Febiger, 1961.

be given orally are preferred. In general 75 to 250 mg cortisone or 20 to 60 mg prednisone is given per day, in divided doses.

Splenectomy results in "cure" in approximately two-thirds of patients. Following splenectomy the platelet count may increase rapidly and to abnormally high levels or, more often, it may rise gradually. Bleeding often ceases even though the platelet count may not have increased greatly, an effect which suggests an influence of the spleen on capillary function. In the bone marrow the previously abnormal megakaryocytes in most instances soon appear to be quite normal again and are seen to be surrounded by platelets. Even when splenectomy is not followed by complete recovery, considerable improvement can be expected.

Splenectomy is *indicated* (1) in those cases of idiopathic thrombocytopenic purpura in which spontaneous remission has not occurred after six or more months' observation and the clinical manifestations are moderate or severe; (2) in patients who appear to respond to steroid therapy but require relatively large doses to maintain a clinical state devoid of serious hemorrhage and who have shown no tendency to spontaneous remission in 6 to 12 months of observation; (3) in the rare patient whose growth and development or social or economic status is seriously impaired by recurrences; (4) in a woman in the later stages of pregnancy, if the condition is severe and if other measures have failed; (5) in secondary forms of thrombocytopenic purpura in which the cause cannot be treated or removed and yet the bleeding manifestations are severe (e.g., some cases of Gaucher's disease). The operation is *not indicated* (1) early in the first episode, especially in children, since spontaneous recovery is much more common than the reverse; (2) in most cases of symptomatic purpura; (3) in neonatal purpura, since recovery takes place naturally; (4) in cases in which the diagnosis has not been established clearly; and, some would add, (5) in acute fulminating cases since mortality then is high. However, others consider this to be an indication for emergency splenectomy, and the question must be considered unsettled. Claims that splenectomy causes "dissemination" of unrecognized lupus erythematosus and increases the hazard of infection have not been substantiated convincingly.

In patients with idiopathic thrombocytopenic purpura other operations should not be carried out before splenectomy has been done, since the bleeding may be severe and serious.

NONTHROMBOCYTOPENIC PURPURAS

A number of types of purpura are not accompanied by thrombocytopenia.

Some of these purpuras have been discussed already (p. 223), but allergic purpura and certain other rare purpuric disorders deserve more complete consideration.

Allergic Purpura

In this form of purpura there is found one or more of the common symptoms of allergy such as erythema, urticaria, or effusions of serum into subcutaneous or submucous tissues or viscera. There may be concomitant articular symptoms (*Schönlein's purpura, peliosis rheumatica*), crises of abdominal pain (*Henoch's purpura*), or no localized signs (*purpura simplex*). Constitutional symptoms such as fever and malaise may be present. The manifestations may wax and wane in intensity, extent, and nature. In various combinations, erythema (multiforme, bullosum, vesiculosum, nodosum), urticaria, and edema may be encountered. Necrotic areas may develop, to be followed by the formation of bullae or ulcers. The skin lesions may appear in crops and may be accompanied by itching or paresthesias. There may be hemorrhage from the visible mucous membranes. Kidney lesions similar in nature to those found in the skin may develop and cause hematuria, proteinuria, and profound though temporary disturbance of renal function.

Etiology and Pathogenesis. These purpuras are more common in children and young adults than in older age groups. The true nature of these purpuras is unknown. The resemblance to serum sickness suggests an allergic basis, but only in a minority has an allergic cause been demonstrated. In some cases the exciting agent appears to have been bacterial (streptococcus, antityphoid vaccine) or an article of food (milk, eggs, pork, strawberries, etc.). In others, hypersensitivity to cold has appeared to be the factor. Comparison of the sex ratio, age of onset, seasonal trends, and incidence of previous upper respiratory tract infections, particularly those associated with a hemolytic streptococcus, and similarities in the latent period before the onset of symptoms suggest a close relationship between the Henoch-Schönlein syndrome and acute nephritis.

It is likely that an antigen-antibody reaction occurs which takes place especially in the endothelium of certain blood vessels. As a result, there is an alteration in the permeability of the small blood vessels. Perivascular inflammation has been observed about the small vessels of the corium of the skin. The various manifestations arise from extravasations of varying proportions of plasma and formed elements of the blood. Mechanical factors may possibly influence the localization of the lesions in addition to the local vascular changes. In Henoch's purpura, an urticarial, serohemorrhagic effusion into the intestinal wall is the cause of the colicky pain and sometimes even leads to intussusception.

Diagnosis. Diagnosis is most difficult when purpura is not present or not obvious. In Henoch's

Table 238-2. CLASSIFICATION OF NONTHROMBOCYTOPENIC
PURPURAS

I. Allergic purpura: Purpuras of Henoch and Schönlein, erythemas of Osler
II. Symptomatic purpura
    A. Infections: Subacute bacterial endocarditis, meningococcemia, staphylococcemia, typhoid fever, rheumatic fever, scarlet fever, smallpox, measles, diphtheria, Rocky Mountain spotted fever
    B. Chemical and animal agents: Iodides, belladonna, atropine, quinine, procaine penicillin, bismuth, mercury, copaiba, phenacetin, salicylic acid, merbaphen, chloral hydrate and other hypnotics; snake venoms
    C. Avitaminosis: scurvy
    D. Certain skin diseases: Ehlers-Danlos syndrome, annular telangiectatic purpura, etc.
    E. Chronic diseases: renal, cardiac, hepatic; hemochromatosis, Cushing's syndrome, polycythemia vera; generalized amyloidosis, blood-borne carcinoma emboli
    F. Various forms of dysglobulinemia: multiple myeloma, cryoglobulinemia, hyperglobulinemia, macroglobulinemia; purpura hyperglobulinemica
III. Purpuric disorders associated with qualitative abnormalities of platelets. Thrombocytopathic purpuras
    A. Prolonged bleeding time: von Willebrand's disease. Constitutional thrombopathy
    B. Other thrombocytopathies, congenital and acquired
    C. Defective clot retraction. Glanzmann's thrombasthenia
    D. Unclassified varieties
IV. Purpura associated with increased capillary fragility
    A. Hereditary familial purpura simplex
    B. Unclassified varieties
V. Purpura associated with increased number of platelets. Hemorrhagic thrombocythemia
VI. Miscellaneous forms of purpura
    A. Purpura simplex, purpura senilis, purpura cachectica, mechanical purpura, orthostatic purpura
    B. Purpura fulminans
    C. Purpura in women. Vicarious bleeding. Autoerythrocyte sensitization

SOURCE: Adapted from M. M. Wintrobe: "Clinical Hematology," 5th ed., Philadelphia, Lea & Febiger, 1961.

purpura, crises of pain may develop which, in the absence of purpura and accompanied as they may be by leukocytosis, cannot be clearly distinguished from acute abdominal conditions which call for operative intervention. Eosinophilia may be present, and then an allergic rather than an inflammatory reaction may be suspected. Acute nephritis may be simulated when the kidney is involved. Hematuria may be a prominent symptom in such cases, just as melena may occur in Henoch's purpura. The Schönlein type may be mistaken for rheumatic fever.

When purpura is discovered and there are exudative skin lesions at the same time, diagnosis is much easier, since these lesions are not encountered in other forms of purpura as a rule. Various chemical agents (e.g., quinine) may also produce nonthrombocytopenic purpura (Table 238-2). Furthermore, this may be a symptom of a variety of diseases, already discussed (p. 223).

Treatment and Prognosis. Treatment is purely symptomatic. Naturally, if an etiologic agent is discovered or suspected, further exposure should be eliminated. Desensitization may be attempted if the exciting agent is protein in nature. Allergic purpura is rarely fatal. Individual attacks last from 1 to 6 weeks. Recurrences at intervals of months or years are not unusual, however, and in some cases glomerulonephritis has developed in association with or in the wake of the purpuric disorder, with the consequences usual in that condition. Results of hormone therapy (ACTH, adrenocorticosteroids) have been equivocal or disappointing.

Other Hemorrhagic (Purpuric) Disorders

A variety of hemorrhagic disorders characterized in the main by spontaneous bleeding from the mucous membranes and from the internal surfaces of the body, and often by petechiae and ecchymoses as well, have been described which cannot be fitted into the categories already discussed. Posttraumatic and postoperative bleeding is not unusual in these cases. Of these conditions, von Willebrand's disease and Glanzmann's thrombasthenia are becoming better defined as entities.

Von Willebrand's disease, a hemorrhagic diathesis inherited as a simple mendelian dominant trait and affecting both sexes, is characterized by prolonged bleeding time, normal platelet count, normal coagulation time, and normal clot retraction. The tourniquet test may or may not be positive. The tendency to bleed appears early in childhood and takes the form of epistaxis, bleeding from the gums, or from the female genitalia. Hemorrhage from the gastrointestinal or urinary tract may occur, and there may be prolonged bleeding from injuries and operation sites.

The discovery that similar cases might be associated with a deficiency of factor VIII, the antihemophilic globulin, led to the introduction of the terms *vascular hemophilia* and *angiohemophilia.* It is possible that von Willebrand's disease and angiohemophilia represent a single entity with variable expressivity. The underlying heritable defect is obscure. Cases have been described with morphologic defects in the platelets, or functional abnormality, or distorted and bizarre capillaries which fail to contract following injury.

The term *thrombocytopathy* has been applied to disorders characterized by deficient platelet functional activity. The platelet abnormality is *qualitative* rather than quantitative, as in the thrombocytopenias. Von Willebrand's disease is thought to represent one form of constitutional thrombocytopathy. Faulty platelet function may also develop in association with various clinical states, such as uremia ("acquired thrombocytopathy").

Glanzmann's thrombasthenia, another form of constitutional thrombocytopathy, refers to excessive hemorrhage in which the bleeding time, platelet count, and coagulation time are normal but clot retraction is poor and the morphology of the platelets is abnormal. Several varieties have been described. Thus, in the so-called *Glanzmann-Naegeli* type of thrombasthenia, small round platelets, normal or increased in number but with impaired adhesiveness and agglutinability have been described. By electron microscopy it has been observed that the platelets are unable to form pseudopods or to spread in contact with a wettable surface. Enzymatic deficiencies and reduced levels of adenosine triphosphate (ATP) have been demonstrated in the platelets in one group of cases; evidence has been given of defective utilization of ATP in other cases.

Surgical procedures in cases such as these should be avoided. Bleeding is managed by pressure, the application of thrombin-fibrin foam, and blood transfusion, when necessary.

Hemorrhagic thrombocythemia is a strange and rare disorder in which hemorrhagic phenomena occur in spite of the presence of greatly excessive numbers of platelets. The spleen may be enlarged and leukocytosis of marked degree may also be present.

REFERENCES

NONTHROMBOCYTOPENIC PURPURAS

Allergic Purpura

Allen, D. M., L. K. Diamond, and Doris A. Howell: Anaphylactoid Purpura in Children (Schönlein-Henoch Syndrome), A.M.A. J. Diseases Children, 99:833, 1960.

Gairdner, D.: The Schönlein-Henoch Syndrome (Anaphylactoid Purpura), Quart. J. Med., 17:95, 1948.

Sterky, G., and A. Thilén: A Study on the Onset and Prognosis of Acute Vascular Purpura (the Schönlein-Henoch Syndrome) in Children, Acta paediat., 49:217, 1960.

Vernier, R. L., H. G. Worthen, R. D. Peterson, Eleanor Colle, and R. A. Good: Anaphylactoid Purpura. I. Pathology of the Skin and Kidney and Frequency of Streptococcal Infection, Pediatrics, 27:181, 1961.

Miscellaneous Purpuras

Achenbach, W.: Angiohämophilie, Ergeb. inn. Med. u. Kinderheilk., 14:68, 1960.

Gross, R., W. Gerok, G. W. Loehr, W. Vogell, H. D. Waller, and W. Theobold: Über die Natur der Thrombasthenie, Klin. Wochschr., 38:193, 1960.

Shuster, S., and H. Scarborough: Senile Purpura, Quart. J. Med., 30:33, 1961.

Soulier, J. P., and M. J. Larrieu: Syndrome de Willebrand-Jürgens et thrombopathies, Rev. d'hématol., 9:77, 1954.

THROMBOCYTOPENIC PURPURA

Ackroyd, J. F.: The Pathogenesis of Thrombocytopenic Purpura Due to Hypersensitivity to Sedormid, Clin. Sci., 7:249, 1949; *ibid.*, 8:235, 269, 1949.

Carpenter, A. F., M. M. Wintrobe, E. A. Fuller, A. Haut, and G. E. Cartwright: Treatment of Idiopathic Thrombocytopenic Purpura, J.A.M.A., 171:1911, 1959.

Harrington, W. J.: Therapy of the Purpuras, J. Chron. Dis., 6:365, 1957.

Krevans, J. R., and D. P. Jackson: Hemorrhagic Disorder Following Massive Whole Blood Transfusions, J.A.M.A., 159:171, 1955.

239 HEMOPHILIA AND RELATED DISORDERS

M. M. Wintrobe

HEMOPHILIA

Definition. Hemophilia is a constitutional anomaly of blood coagulation which depends on the inheritance of a sex-linked, recessive mendelian trait transmitted by the female and affecting only males. It is characterized by a lifelong tendency to excessive bleeding. The coagulation time is prolonged.

History. A clear description of this disorder was published in 1803 by Otto of Philadelphia. However, it is apparent from passages in the Talmud that the condition was known to the ancient Jews, who even proscribed circumcision in those whose family history suggested this disorder.

Etiology and Pathogenesis. The factor or gene responsible for the development of hemophilia appears to be carried in the X chromosome of the reproductive cells. The disease is limited to the male and is transmitted from the male through an unaffected daughter to her son. The daughters of an affected male transmit the trait as an evident defect to half their sons and as a hidden (recessive) characteristic to half their daughters. The occurrence of hemophilia in the female would require the marriage of a hemophiliac male with a carrier female. Such cases have been described, but they are exceedingly rare. Sporadic cases of hemophilia have been observed in which the family history was negative. These can sometimes be explained by long inheritance through females with the males being, by chance, unaffected. Illegitimacy may be responsible for other instances, while still others may represent the disease arising *de novo*.

It is generally accepted that the abnormality in hemophilia is due to the absence or reduction in the blood of a component essential for the formation of plasma thromboplastin (factor VIII, antihemophilic globulin). The role which this substance plays in the process of coagulation was discussed earlier (Chap. 24).

Symptomatology. Hemorrhage, usually following trauma but sometimes spontaneous, is the essential symptom. The bleeding is in the nature of a persistent, slow oozing which is out of all proportion to the extent of the injury. This tendency to prolonged bleeding usually appears in early childhood, even in infancy. The bleeding may last not only hours but days and even weeks, and may lead to profound anemia. Subcutaneous and intramuscular hemorrhages are common. Petechiae are very rare. Hematomas may be large. There may be severe bleeding from the mouth, gums, lips, tongue, or gastrointestinal tract. Epistaxis is a common symptom. The eruption and loss of teeth may be accompanied by severe bleeding. Hematuria is relatively common and hemorrhage into joints is characteristic. Recurrences are the rule, and ultimately a permanently swollen joint with local deformity, contractures, and muscular atrophy are produced.

The *blood* in typical cases is normal except for the prolonged coagulation time and the manifestations which hemorrhage produces (p. 1278). Curiously, the degree of prolongation of coagulation time, like the symptoms of this disorder, varies from time to time. Platelets are normal in number. Only rarely is bleeding time prolonged.

It has been shown that cases of hemophilia occur which are less severe than the classic type just described. Assays of plasma antihemophilic globulin (AHG) have shown a great range in the quantity of this essential substance. Four grades of hemophilia have been distinguished, viz., classical hemophilia, in which the plasma AHG is 0 per cent; moderate hemophilia, characterized by the occurrence of subcutaneous hematomas and postoperative hemorrhages, essentially normal coagulation time, normal prothrombin consumption, and less than 3 per cent AHG; mild hemophilia, in which coagulation time and prothrombin consumption are normal and the plasma AHG is approximately 16 per cent; and subhemophilia, in which there may only be a history of prolonged postoperative oozing. The plasma AHG is in the neighborhood of 33 per cent, as compared with the normal value of 65

to 136 per cent. Frequently the severity of the disorder is constant in a given family, as if not only the defect but also its degree were an inherited characteristic.

The *bone marrow* is normal except for normoblastic hyperplasia when hemorrhage has been severe.

Diagnosis. Although hemophilia and purpura hemorrhagica are often confused with each other, differentiation is easy as a rule, for the latter condition involves thrombocytopenia, prolonged bleeding time, poor clot retraction, and a positive tourniquet test. In hemophilia the patient is normal in these respects and, in the classical disorder, coagulation time is prolonged. There is, in addition, the history of repeated, protracted hemorrhage, usually first manifested in early childhood, as well as the characteristic family history. Occasionally difficulty in diagnosis may arise if attention is attracted only to the joint manifestations or to a swelling not recognized as a hematoma. In a similar manner, the bleeding may suggest kidney disease, pulmonary disease, or peptic ulcer.

Other Disorders of Coagulation. The development of more precise methods of laboratory examination has resulted in the discovery of new entities, hitherto confused with classic hemophilia and the purpuras, in addition to recognition of the fact that mild forms of hemophilia exist. Many of these disorders were mentioned earlier (Chap. 24). The results of various laboratory tests in a number of these conditions are presented in Table 239-1.

In cases of hemophilia with normal or only slightly impaired coagulation time, the prothrombin consumption test will be found reliable and sensitive, although it is not specific; reduced prothrombin consumption is found also in various disorders associated with thrombocytopenia, as well as in patients with hemorrhagic manifestations due to anticoagulants affecting thromboplastic activity. The absence of a circulating anticoagulant can be demonstrated by adding the patient's blood in varying proportions to normal blood. The clotting of normal blood is not delayed by the addition of even 50 per cent of hemophilic blood.

The one-stage prothrombin time separates hemophilia from conditions associated with true prothrombin, factor V, factor VII, and factor X deficiencies, and also from many cases in which there is a circulating anticoagulant. In hemophilia, in contrast to these conditions, prothrombin time is normal. The deficiency in hemophilic blood can be corrected by the addition of a small proportion of normal plasma. The degree of reduction in antihemophilic globulin content can be assayed roughly by this means.

It was pointed out earlier that assays for antihemophilic globulin have revealed a *mild* form of

Table 239-1. BLEEDING AND COAGULATION TESTS IN SOME OF THE HEMORRHAGIC DISORDERS

Disease or condition	Thrombocytopenia	Bleeding time prolonged	Clot retraction poor	Tourniquet test positive	Coagulation time prolonged	Prothrombin time (one-stage) prolonged	Prothrombin consumption impaired and thromboplastic generation reduced
Purpura, thrombocytopenic....	+	+	+	+	−*	−	+
Purpura, nonthrombocytopenic.	−	−	−	±	−	−	−
Hemophilia (hemophilia A)....	−	−*	−	−	+†	−	+†
PTC deficiency (hemophilia B).	−	−*	−	−	+†	−	+†
Dicoumarin excess............	−	−*	−	−*	−*	+	−
Factor V deficiency...........	−	−	−	−	+†	+	+
Factor VII deficiency.........	−	−	−	−	+†	+	−
Hypoprothrombinemia........	−	−	−	−	+	+	−
Afibrinogenemia..............	−	+†	−	−	+	+	−
Anticoagulant excess..........	−	−*	−	−	+	±	±
von Willebrand's disease.......	−	+	−	±	−	−	−

* May be prolonged if condition is severe.

† May be normal if condition is mild.

hemophilia in which even prothrombin consumption is normal or equivocal. An additional observation of interest is that, unlike classic hemophilia, some of the heterozygotes show a diminution in antihemophilic globulin, a finding which suggests that the gene is not completely recessive, as it is in classical hemophilia, and for this reason the condition has been attributed to an allelic mutant of the hemophilia gene.

The unequivocal identification of *female carriers* of hemophilia cannot be made by present methods, but low levels of antihemophilic globulin have been demonstrated in a number of female carriers. Furthermore, some female carriers have an unusual tendency to bleed.

A number of disorders are now recognized which involve the first stage of coagulation. To distinguish these from one another the thromboplastin generation test is especially useful. Thus *factor IX deficiency [plasma thromboplastin component (PTC) deficiency, Christmas disease]* is clinically indistinguishable from classic hemophilia. This disorder is due to the lack or deficiency of a coagulation factor necessary for the formation of thromboplastin which is present in normal and in hemophilic plasma. Both severe and mild forms of the disorder have been encountered. The coagulation time is usually prolonged, and prothrombin consumption is impaired, but cases with normal values have also been observed. The missing coagulation factor is most readily obtained from serum. Since

this condition resembles hemophilia in its clinical manifestations and mode of inheritance, it has been called *hemophilia B*, the letter *A* being used to refer to the classic condition. The two types of hemophilia can be distinguished in vitro by the correction of the coagulation defect of the one by the other, and of both by the addition of normal plasma. Another simple test consists in the correction of the clotting defect in PTC deficiency by the addition of normal serum and the failure of such correction in classical hemophilia.

Still other disorders resembling hemophilia have been described. They include *plasma thromboplastin antecedent (PTA) deficiency*, which differs from hemophilia and PTC deficiency in that the manifestations occur in *either sex*. The condition appears to be transmitted as an autosomal dominant trait with a high degree of penetrance but variable expression. Spontaneous bleeding is rare; bleeding has occurred usually following trauma or a surgical procedure, including tooth extraction. Various degrees of severity have been observed, ranging from a severe form with prolonged coagulation time and markedly abnormal prothrombin consumption, to a mild form with normal coagulation time and only slightly impaired prothrombin consumption. Thromboplastin generation is markedly impaired. The deficiency in this disorder is corrected both by plasma absorbed with $BaSO_4$, which corrects factor VIII (AHG) deficiency, and by serum, which corrects factor IX (PTC) deficiency. PTA is a globulin which is stable on storage and is present in normal serum, where it is localized in the β_2-globulin fraction. Studies of the relative incidence of hemophilia, PTC, and PTA deficiencies have yielded ratios of approximately 10:2:1.

Course and Prognosis. The tendency to bleed varies from time to time and differs in degree from one family to another. The typical hemophiliac patient rarely survives to adulthood without suffering some disabling deformity of the joints. The prognosis differs, however, in accordance with the severity of the deficiency. Death may occur from exsanguination following surgical procedures or accidental cuts. Less often it is due to internal hemorrhage.

Treatment. The prevention of hemophilia, whether due to factor VIII or factor IX deficiency, depends on appropriate restriction of marriage or at least of propagation. Only unaffected males can marry with any assurance that the hemorrhagic tendency will not be transmitted.

Affected individuals and male children of tainted stock must be guarded against trauma, and surgical measures, even the most minor ones, should be avoided whenever possible. If some procedure which may entail bleeding is absolutely necessary, it should be done only in a hospital and with plentiful amounts of fresh blood and plasma available. Normal plasma, kept solid or dried lyophilically within a few hours of its withdrawal from the body, will retain its antihemophilic effect almost indefinitely. Although as little as 50 ml fresh plasma will maintain the coagulation time of a hemophiliac of moderate severity within normal limits for about 24 hr, in practice it is wise to use much larger amounts. Therapeutic failures are almost always attributable to the administration of too little blood or plasma, to the too wide spacing of transfusions (intervals longer than 6 hr), and to the too early interruption of therapy. The administration of blood should be continued for several days after bleeding seems to have ceased. Unfortunately no satisfactory source of antihemophilic factors is readily available other than whole blood or plasma. When internal bleeding occurs, transfusions of blood and plasma are the only measures of value and carry the minimum of risk. Surgery is contraindicated. Prior to any surgical measure, such as tooth extraction, at least 500 ml fresh plasma should be given. In contrast to its effectiveness in PTC deficiency, serum is devoid of activity in classic hemophilia.

An essential in the local management of bleeding in hemophilia is the avoidance of tissue injury. The existence of damaged or devitalized tissue merely prolongs the period of subsequent hemorrhage. Thus, for example, in dental extraction, gum margins should not be sewn together. When there is free bleeding, pressure must naturally be applied, but it should be temporary and gentle and should be supplemented by the use of coagulants such as Russell's viper venom or thrombin ("hemostatic globulin"). These measures may be followed by the application of absorbable hemostatic dressings such as human fibrin, fibrin foam, gelatin sponge, or oxidized cellulose. Following tooth extraction, a previously made dental splint will keep the dressing in place with a minimum of movement.

Unfortunately, in some patients with hemophilia antibodies with an anticoagulant action have developed following repeated transfusions. This appears to be due to immunization against the antihemophilic factor.

HEREDITARY HEMORRHAGIC TELANGIECTASIA

Definition. This is a vascular anomaly characterized by multiple dilatations of capillaries and venules in the skin and mucous membranes. The anomaly is transmitted as a simple dominant trait by both sexes.

Etiology. The telangiectases may be found in childhood, but they increase in number as age advances. Bleeding may not commence until adult life has been reached.

Symptomatology. Epistaxis is especially common, but bleeding may come from telangiectases wherever they are: the face, tongue, lips, or gastrointestinal, respiratory, or genitourinary tracts. Those on the skin are less likely to bleed than are telangiectases on mucous membranes. The telangiectases range from pin point to about 3 mm in diameter, are bright red or violaceous in color, and characteristically blanch on pressure. Sometimes they form nodular vascular tumors the size of a split pea; such lesions resemble those of a very rare, probably systemic condition, angiokeratoma corporis diffusum (Fabry), which may be due to a hereditary defect in lipid metabolism and in which there is widespread involvement of the media of the blood vessels, with manifestations in the renal, pulmonary, and other systems of the body. In elderly patients some of the lesions of hereditary telangiectasia may become spiderlike, resembling those associated with hepatic insufficiency. Trivial trauma sustained by these abnormal, relatively exposed vessels results in an unusual amount of bleeding. The blood is normal except for the effects hemorrhage may have produced. The tourniquet test is negative.

Diagnosis. This depends on recognition of the vascular anomalies, which are easily overlooked. Purpuric spots do not fade on pressure.

In a number of cases of this disorder pulmonary arteriovenous fistula has been observed.

Treatment. The telangiectatic vessels are excessively fragile, but oxidized cellulose (Oxycel), Gelfoam, or similar hemostatic agents usually suffice to control an existing hemorrhage if they are applied carefully. Although the primary bleeding site can be cauterized or destroyed by electrocoagulation, satellite lesions soon form nearby. Prophylaxis is unsatisfactory. Many procedures have been tried, including estrogen and androgen therapy, with doubtful effect.

REFERENCES

HEMOPHILIA AND RELATED DISORDERS

Aggeler, P. M., M. Silvija Hoag, R. O. Wallerstein, and Dorothy Whissell: The Mild Hemophilias. Occult Deficiencies of AHF, PTC and PTA Frequently Responsible for Unexpected Surgical Bleeding, Am. J. Med., 30:84, 1961.

Graham, J. B., W. W. McLendon, and K. M. Brinkhous: Mild Hemophilia: An Allelic Form of the Disease, Am. J. Med. Sci., 225:46, 1953.

Howell, W. H.: Hemophilia, Bull. N.Y. Acad. Med., 15:3, 1939.

Jordan, H. H.: "Hemophilic Arthropathies," Springfield, Ill., Charles C Thomas, Publisher, 1958.

Margolius, A., Jr., D. P. Jackson, and O. D. Ratnoff: Circulating Anticoagulants: A Study of 40 Cases and a Review of the Literature, Medicine, 40:145, 1961.

Wintrobe, M. M.: "Clinical Hematology," 5th ed., Philadelphia, Lea & Febiger, 1961.

HEREDITARY HEMORRHAGIC TELANGIECTASIA

Dolowitz, D. A., O. N. Rambo, and F. E. Stephens: Hereditary Hemorrhagic Telangiectasia, Ann. Otol. Rhinol. & Laryngol., 62:642, 1953.

Tobin, J. R., and T. C. Wilder: Pulmonary Arteriovenous Fistula Associated with Hereditary Hemorrhagic Telangiectasia: A Report of Their Occurrence in a Father and Son, Ann. Internal Med., 38:868, 1953.

240 AGRANULOCYTOSIS AND THE PANCYTOPENIAS

M. M. Wintrobe

AGRANULOCYTOSIS

Definition. Agranulocytosis (agranulocytic angina) is a disorder characterized by severe sore throat, marked prostration, and extreme reduction or even complete disappearance of the granulocytes from the blood. This clinical picture, first recognized by Schultz in 1922, was observed most frequently in women of middle age and often ended in sepsis and death. An etiologic relationship to the taking of certain drugs has been demonstrated.

Etiology and Pathogenesis. In 1931 Kracke pointed out that the sudden appearance of this syndrome corresponded with the introduction of certain coal-tar derivatives as therapeutic agents. This was borne out by considerable circumstantial evidence which incriminated, in particular, the antipyretic, aminopyrine (Pyramidon). The course of events in affected individuals would seem to be (1) granulocytopenia as the result of some effect induced by the drug; (2) loss of resistance to infection, development of sore throat; (3) overwhelming sepsis and death. That some form of tissue injury, in addition to leukopenia, may be a factor in the pathogenesis of this syndrome is suggested by the frequency with which one may encounter leukopenia, even of severe degree, following nitrogen mustard therapy without sepsis developing.

The most striking change observed in the bone marrow is a lack of juvenile and segmented neutrophilic leukocytes, less mature forms being plentiful. This picture has been referred to as "maturation arrest," but it could as readily result from abnormal peripheral destruction of the leukocytes or their segregation somewhere.

Drugs producing leukopenia may be divided into two main groups—namely, those which produce this effect in all individuals if given in sufficient amounts, and those which cause leukopenia only in certain "sensitive" persons (Table 240-1). Various data suggest that between 0.5 and 4 per cent of patients taking the second group of drugs develop granulocytopenia. In group III are listed drugs which have been incriminated in a few case reports but which cannot be regarded as well-established causes of leukopenia.

It is likely that granulocytopenia develops by more than one mechanism. Some cases are encountered in which no drug seems to be incriminated. Those drugs which produce granulocytopenia in all persons when given in sufficient amounts probably do so through their toxic effects. Agents such as aminopyrine probably require a peculiar sensitivity or idiosyncrasy on the part of the patient. Rarely other manifestations of sensitivity, such as rash, urticaria, and edema, may be present or may have occurred on other occasions. Furthermore, in patients who have recovered from aminopyrine-induced agranulocytosis, the administration of small amounts (0.2 Gm) of the drug may be followed within 6 to 10 hr by disappearance of all the neutrophils from the blood. It has also been shown that the blood of such a person, withdrawn 3 hr following ingestion of the drug, produces outspoken granulocytopenia within 20 to 40 min after its transfusion into normal persons. In the plasma and serum of the sensitive patient a sub-

Table 240-1. LEUKOPENIA-PRODUCING DRUGS

Group I—regularly produce leukopenia if given in sufficient amounts
  Mustards (sulfur and nitrogen mustards, TEM, etc.)
  Urethan, busulfan, Demecolcin
  Antimetabolites (antifolic acid compounds, 6-mercaptopurine, etc.)
  Benzene
Group II—produce leukopenia in "sensitive" persons only
  Analgesics (aminopyrine, phenylbutazone, etc.)
  Antithyroid drugs (thiouracil, methimazole, etc.)
  Anticonvulsants (trimethadione, phethenylate, etc.)
  Sulfonamides [sulfanilamide, sulfisoxazole (Gantrisin), etc.]
  Antihistamines (Pyribenzamine, phenothiazine, etc.)
  Antimicrobial agents (organic arsenicals, chloramphenicol)
  Tranquilizers (chlorpromazine, etc.)
  Miscellaneous (dinitrophenol, tolbutamide, gold salts, etc.)
Group III—very rarely cause leukopenia, if at all
  Barbiturates (acetanilid, acetophenetidin)
  Quinine
  Cinchophen, etc.

stance has been found at the height of the aminopyrine granulocytopenia which produces agglutination of homologous and heterologous leukocytes. If, as seems likely, an immune mechanism is involved in the pathogenesis of this type of granulocytopenia, removal of the agglutinated leukocytes from the circulating blood may be postulated, with resulting depletion of the more mature forms from the bone marrow.

Symptomatology. The condition described by Schultz was an *acute, fulminating disorder.* In such cases there may be a prodromal period, marked only by malaise or moderate fever, which often is overlooked. If the granulocytopenia is recognized at this stage, and sepsis is prevented or does not develop, no other manifestations may appear. If infection supervenes or if the condition is first recognized at this stage, the onset appears to be sudden and is marked by a chill, high fever, and often sore throat. Prostration is extreme. Gangrenous ulceration may be found on the gums, tonsils, soft palate, lips, pharynx, or buccal mucous membranes. Regional adenopathy may be present, but generalized adenopathy and sternal tenderness are not found, and splenomegaly, when present, is minimal. Brawny edema of the neck can become extreme. Necrosis of the gastrointestinal tract may occur. Jaundice has been described in some cases. In fatal cases the duration of the illness is 3 to 9 days.

In the *blood,* granulocytopenia is the outstanding finding. Since the leukocyte count is usually under 3,000 per cu mm and often is as low as 500, a reduction in the absolute number of all cells actually takes place. Of the leukocytes which remain, 95 to 100 per cent may be lymphocytes. Anemia and thrombocytopenia are not found; if they are present, another cause should be suspected.

The *bone marrow* is normal except for the "maturation arrest" described already.

In addition to the acute form, described above, *chronic, cyclic,* and *recurrent* forms of granulocytopenia, as well as *familial, transitory neonatal, childhood,* and other rare varieties, have been observed. They may or may not be related to the acute disorder. In the chronic cases the course is prolonged, and infections which often are relatively resistant to therapy, especially in the skin and oral cavity, occur repeatedly. Hypoplasia of granulocytic precursors in the bone marrow, slight splenomegaly, and absolute lymphocytosis and monocytosis have been described. In other instances there is a cyclic or recurrent periodicity of attacks at intervals of weeks or months, with more or less normal leukocyte counts in the symptom-free period. Unexplained fatigue is a common complaint. In some cases the leukopenia has been observed to occur in remarkably regular, 3-week cycles (*periodic neutropenia*).

Primary splenic neutropenia is a name applied to a clinical picture characterized by fever, pain over the splenic region and splenic enlargement, granulocytopenia, and essentially normal or somewhat hyperplastic bone marrow. The manifestations may be acute, subacute, or chronic and have been attributed to excessive lysis of neutrophils by the spleen. Splenectomy is reported as bringing complete relief, and excessive phagocytosis of leukocytes has been described in the spleen. The disorder is very rare.

Diagnosis. The clinical picture may suggest a variety of buccal and pharyngeal infections. The great majority of these infections, however, are accompanied by leukocytosis. Infections characteristically accompanied by leukopenia, such as measles, undulant fever, and typhoid, should rarely give difficulty, although influenza may. "Aleukemic" leukemia may present a similar clinical picture, but sternal tenderness, general glandular enlargement, and splenomegaly, as well as anemia, thrombocytopenia, and, usually, very immature leukocytes in the blood, make differentiation no serious problem. Aplastic anemia is recognized by evidence of involvement of red corpuscles and platelets as well as leukocytes.

Treatment and Prognosis. The offending drug must be searched for and its further use prohibited. Of equal importance is the administration of chemotherapeutic agents, such as penicillin, which will hold the infection in abeyance until leukocyte formation becomes normal and is able to cope with the offending organisms. There is no conclusive evidence that various agents which have been proposed as stimulants of leukocyte recovery, including one which was at one time very popular, Pentnucleotide, are of any value. Before the sulfonamides and penicillin were available, the prognosis was very poor. Mortality was as high as 70 to 90 per cent. With modern chemotherapy, only a small proportion of patients fail to recover. During recovery, with the reappearance of leukocytes, abscesses may develop which will require appropriate therapy.

Splenectomy has been associated with considerable improvement or even recovery in some cases of the chronic, recurrent, and cyclic varieties, but this result is unpredictable. The steroid hormones may be of temporary value, perhaps in the cases most likely to respond to splenectomy, but they are difficult to evaluate in disorders of this type. In the chronic cases with *hypoplastic* bone marrow, splenectomy has not been found to be helpful.

THE PANCYTOPENIAS

Definition. The term *pancytopenia* refers to a reduction in the number of all three formed elements of the blood: the red corpuscles, the leukocytes, and the platelets. This is not a disease entity but a triad which is encountered under a widely differing group of circumstances.

Classification. This triad may be encountered in "aplastic" or "hypoplastic" anemia, in "aleukemic" or subleukemic leukemia, in myelosclerosis and in myelophthisic anemias, in pernicious anemia, and in association with a number of disorders of the spleen (Table 240-2). Under this heading "agnogenic myeloid metaplasia" and "primary splenic panhematopenia" must also be considered.

Aplastic Anemia

This term, in its strict sense, refers to a condition in which signs of hematopoiesis are lacking in the bone marrow, fat having replaced the bloodforming tissue. At the same time, there are anemia, granulocytopenia, and thrombocytopenia. There are no signs of blood regeneration. The reticulocyte count is very low or zero, there is no polychromatophilia or basophilic stippling, and nucleated red corpuscles and immature leukocytes of all types are absent. The anemia is usually normocytic, sometimes macrocytic; the red corpuscles vary little in size and not at all in shape. Bleeding time is usually moderately prolonged, the clot retracts poorly, and the tourniquet test is positive. Coagulation time is normal.

The onset of the disorder is insidious. The symptoms may be those attributable to anemia, or the effects of thrombocytopenia or of granulocytopenia may dominate the clinical picture. There is striking, often "waxy" pallor, but weight loss is unusual.

Table 240-2. CAUSES OF PANCYTOPENIA

I. "Aleukemic," leukopenic, or subleukemic leukemia
II. "Primary" refractory anemias
    A. Aplastic anemias due to chemical or physical agents
    B. "Idiopathic" aplastic anemia, including the familial type ("Fanconi syndrome")
III. Myelophthisic anemias
    A. Metastatic carcinoma in bone marrow
    B. Multiple myeloma
    C. Myelofibrosis, "agnogenic myeloid metaplasia," etc.
    D. Marble bone disease (osteopetrosis)
IV. Disorders involving the spleen—"hypersplenism"
    A. Congestive splenomegaly
    B. Lymph node disorders: lymphosarcoma, reticulum cell sarcoma, Hodgkin's disease, giant follicular lymphoma
    C. Infiltrative disorders: Gaucher's disease, Niemann-Pick disease, Letterer-Siwe disease
    D. Infectious diseases: kala-azar, miliary tuberculosis, sarcoid, syphilis
    E. "Primary splenic panhematopenia"
V. Deficiency anemias: pernicious anemia and other megaloblastic macrocytic anemias
VI. Paroxysmal nocturnal hemoglobinuria (rarely)

SOURCE: Adapted from M. M. Wintrobe: "Clinical Hematology," 5th ed., Philadelphia, Lea & Febiger, 1961.

There may be bleeding from the nose, mouth, vagina, or elsewhere. Hemorrhages may be found in the eye grounds or skin. Ulceration in the mouth and pharynx or other evidence of infection may be encountered. There is no sternal tenderness, splenomegaly, or hepatomegaly, and lymph node enlargement, if present, is found only in relation to local infection.

This picture may follow exposure to a variety of *chemical and physical agents.* As with the causes of granulocytopenia, the agents associated with the occurrence of aplastic anemia may be divided into two groups; viz., (1) those which regularly produce marrow hypoplasia and aplasia if a sufficient dose is given, and (2) those which are only occasionally associated with such a change and presumably depend on idiosyncrasy. In the former category may be included ionizing radiation (roentgen rays, radioactive phosphorus, etc.), the mustards (sulfur and nitrogen mustards, TEM, etc.), urethan, busulfan, benzol, and the antimetabolites (antifolic acid compounds, 6-mercaptopurine, etc.). It will be noted that these agents have been or are used in the treatment of leukemia, Hodgkin's disease, and related disorders. Excessive dosage will result in the production of marrow aplasia. Benzene (benzol) is no longer used in the treatment of leukemia, but it is employed in many industries (leather, enamel, rubber, lacquer, electroplating, airplanes, linoleum, celluloid, etc.) and must thus be kept in mind when aplastic anemia is encountered in a person working in one of these industries. Of the agents occasionally associated with hypoplasia or aplasia of the bone marrow, the following should be mentioned in particular: antimicrobial agents (arsenobenzols, chloramphenicol), anticonvulsants (Mesantoin), antithyroid drugs, antihistamines, insecticides, and various miscellaneous agents such as gold preparations and trinitrotoluene. Although the evidence incriminating these drugs is only circumstantial, a sufficient number of cases have been reported to make it seem very likely that development of aplastic anemia following exposure to the drugs named is more than a coincidence. Less convincing is the evidence that other drugs are the cause of aplastic anemia, since there are only single or very few reports incriminating them. In this last group may be mentioned the sulfonamides, oxytetracycline, chlortetracycline, Tridione, Nuvarone, Carbimazole, Tapazole, quinacrine, phenylbutazone, chlorpromazine, and various hair dyes and volatile insecticides.

"Idiopathic" cases have also been described in which exposure to an offending agent could not be discovered. Such cases have been observed most frequently in young adults or adolescents. Still another form of pancytopenia with hypoplastic bone marrow has been observed, usually at an even younger age, which may be familial and is associated with a variety of congenital defects (bone abnormalities, particularly of the forearms and thumbs, microcephaly, hypogenitalia, genitourinary tract abnormalities) and a generalized olive-brown pigmentation of the skin (*Fanconi syndrome*).

In addition to such cases of classic aplastic anemia, a very similar clinical and hematologic picture can be observed together with cellular or even hyperplastic bone marrow. In still other cases little or no reduction was present in the leukocyte or platelet count. Such *pure erythrocyte hypoplasia* has been observed as a congenital disorder, but rarely it appears also to be acquired. In a number of cases benign thymoma was associated. In some cases occasional nucleated red corpuscles, polychromatophilia, stippling, and immature white cells have been found in the blood, and splenic and hepatic enlargement and even general lymphadenopathy have been described. Whether all these cases should be classed with the true aplastic anemias under one category of "refractory anemias" cannot be settled until their pathogenesis is clear. That these various pictures may be variants of the same fundamental process is suggested by the observation that benzene poisoning not only may produce aplastic anemia but also can be associated with a regenerative blood picture, including even a leukemoid reaction, and the bone marrow may be hyperplastic rather than

acellular. Again, *internal irradiation* produced by the ingestion of radium by watch-dial workers was found to be characterized by macrocytic anemia with nucleated red corpuscles in the blood, and bone marrow with primitive red corpuscle and leukocyte hyperplasia.

Under the title of *"sideroblastic" refractory anemias* still another group of cases has been recognized which must be distinguished from "idiopathic" aplastic anemia and can be separated from thalassemia and the hemoglobinopathies (Chap. 235), from pyridoxine-responsive anemia, and from inclusion body anemias. Anemia refractory to all known forms of therapy, hyperplastic bone marrow, and signs of impaired iron utilization (sideroblasts, hemosiderosis) characterize these cases. Some appear to have begun in childhood, others have appeared in older patients. Their nature awaits clarification.

Myelophthisic Anemia

This term is applied to the type of anemia associated with space-occupying disorders of the bone marrow. Metastatic carcinoma (e.g., that arising from malignancy of the breast, prostate, lung, kidney, adrenal or thyroid gland), leukemia, multiple myeloma, and a disorder known as myelofibrosis or myelosclerosis are conditions which produce myelophthisic anemia. In *myelofibrosis* there is an irregular increase of fibrous or bony tissue in the bone marrow which is often associated with progressive anemia. The outstanding symptom is splenomegaly. The course is very slow. Bone marrow involvement may also occur in Hodgkin's disease and in the primary xanthomatoses (Gaucher's disease, Niemann-Pick disease, Schüller-Christian disease).

Agnogenic Myeloid Metaplasia

The term agnogenic myeloid metaplasia has been applied to cases in which the spleen showed marked myeloid metaplasia, apparently as the result of a compensatory reaction. This does not seem to be a disease entity. The bone marrow has been variously fibrotic, hyperplastic, aplastic, or normal. The blood picture has varied, like that described under Myelophthisic Anemia above. In some cases jaundice was present. In a number of instances a history of exposure to certain industrial solvents, including benzene and carbon tetrachloride, was obtained.

Primary Splenic Panhematopenia

Primary splenic panhematopenia is the term which has been applied to cases associated with splenomegaly in which all three formed elements of the blood have been reduced in number, and where excessive phagocytosis of these elements by the splenic macrophages has been conceived as being the fundamental disorder. Splenectomy is described as producing dramatic improvement. In these cases little or no evidence of increased blood destruction has been observed, the reticulocyte percentage has been slightly or greatly increased, polychromatophilia has been noted, and the bone marrow picture has been one of hyperplasia. As will be pointed out in the next section, many splenic disorders are accompanied by pancytopenia.

Diagnosis and Treatment. It is evident from this outline that pancytopenia may be due to a number of causes of greatly varying nature. The recognition of the underlying disorder will depend on thorough study, which includes a painstaking history with careful inquiry about possible exposure to toxic agents, thorough physical examination and bone marrow examination, in addition to a complete survey of the blood.

While the *blood picture* in these conditions may be that of a pancytopenia and may appear "aplastic," as described above, it is necessary to stress that this is not always the case. Anemia is variable in degree. It may be normocytic or macrocytic, and nucleated red corpuscles may be seen in the blood even when there is little anemia. Reticulocytes may be increased and polychromatophilia and stippling, as well as "teardrop" poikilocytes, may be present. Such poikilocytes have been thought to be characteristic of myelofibrosis. The leukocyte count may be normal, reduced, or increased. If there is leukopenia there may be a uniform reduction in all the cells. The blood may contain myelocytes and myeloblasts. The platelet count may be normal or moderately reduced.

However, bone marrow punctures in various sites (sternum, pelvic crest, spinous processes) may be required before tumor cells are discovered. Roentgenograms, especially of the bones, may be helpful, and trephine biopsy of the marrow may be necessary. If an enlarged lymph node is accessible, it may be advisable to examine this microscopically, and other procedures may need to be carried out in the search for malignancy. A diagnosis of "idiopathic" aplastic anemia or of "primary splenic panhematopenia" should be one of exclusion.

Treatment will depend on the nature of the underlying disorder. Blood transfusions are of temporary value in all the conditions which may produce this picture. Ultimately, if many transfusions are given, hemochromatosis is produced, since the iron from the transfused cells cannot be excreted. Liver extract, vitamin B_{12}, folic acid, and iron are of no value. The temptation to remove an enlarged spleen must be tempered with good judgment. This is especially important in those cases in which the spleen has assumed the function of the bone marrow, for in such cases splenectomy can be harmful and at least is often of little or no value. Neverthe-

less, occasional patients derive definite benefit from splenectomy, particularly when there is severe thrombocytopenia or increased blood destruction. In cases in which large numbers of leukocytes in the circulating blood have been present, roentgen therapy or chemotherapy such as that used in the treatment of chronic leukemia has been helpful.

REFERENCES

AGRANULOCYTOSIS

Kracke, R. R.: Relation of Drug Therapy to Neutropenic States, J.A.M.A., 111:1255, 1938.

Moeschlin, S., and K. Wagner: Agranulocytosis Due to the Occurrence of Leukocyte-agglutinins, Acta Haematol., 8:29, 1952; Rev. hematol., 8:249, 1953.

Rieman, H. A., and C. T. de Berardinis: Periodic (Cyclic) Neutropenia: An Entity, Blood, 4:1109, 1949; A.M.A. Arch. Internal Med., 92:494, 1953.

Spaet, T. H., and W. Dameshek: Chronic Hypoplastic Neutropenia, Am. J. Med., 12:35, 1952.

Wiseman, B. K., and C. A. Doan: A Newly Recognized Granulopenic Syndrome Caused by Excessive Splenic Leukolysis and Successfully Treated by Splenectomy, J. Clin. Invest., 18:473, 1939; Ann. Internal Med., 16:1097, 1942.

THE PANCYTOPENIAS

Bomford, H. R., and C. P. Rhoads: Refractory Anaemia, Quart. J. Med., 10:175, 1941.

Dacie, J. V., Mary D. Smith, J. C. White, and D. L. Mollin: Refractory Normoblastic Anaemia, Brit. J. Haematol., 5:56, 1959.

Doan, C. A., and C. S. Wright: Primary Congenital and Secondary Acquired Splenic Panhematopenia, Blood, 1:10, 1946.

Green, T. W., C. L. Conley, L. L. Ashburn, and H. R. Peters: Splenectomy for Myeloid Metaplasia of the Spleen, New Engl. J. Med., 248:211, 1953.

Heilmeyer, L., W. Keiderling, R. Bilger, and H. Bernauer: Über chronische refraktäre Anämien mit sideroblastischem Knochenmark (Anaemia refractoria sideroblastica), Folia Haematol., 2:49, 61, 1958; Deut. med. Wochschr., 84:1761, 1959; Schweiz. med. Wochschr., 90:934, 1960.

Jackson, H., Jr., F. Parker, Jr., and H. M. Lemon: Agnogenic Myeloid Metaplasia of the Spleen, New Engl. J. Med., 222:985, 1940; Science, 93:541, 1941.

Loeb, V., C. V. Moore, and R. Dubach: The Physiologic Evaluation and Management of Chronic Bone Marrow Failure, Am. J. Med., 15:499, 1953.

McDonald, R., and B. Goldschmidt: Pancytopenia with Congenital Defects (Fanconi's Anaemia), Arch. Disease Childhood, 35:367, 1960.

Rubin, D., A. S. Weisberger, R. E. Botti, and J. P. Storaasli: Changes in Iron Metabolism in Early Chloramphenicol Toxicity, J. Clin. Invest., 37:1286, 1958; J. Lab. Clin. Med., 56:453, 1960.

Scott, J. L., G. E. Cartwright, and M. M. Wintrobe: Acquired Aplastic Anemia: An Analysis of Thirty-nine Cases and Review of the Pertinent Literature, Medicine, 38:119, 1959.

Wintrobe, M. M.: "Clinical Hematology," 5th ed., Philadelphia, Lea & Febiger, 1961.

241 THE LEUKEMIAS
M. M. Wintrobe

Definition. Leukemia, probably a neoplastic disease, is characterized by widespread and abnormal proliferation of the leukocytes and their precursors throughout the body, particularly in the bone marrow, spleen, and lymph nodes. There are various types of leukemia, differentiated mainly according to the predominant abnormal cell forms. The morbidity of the process ranges from an acute disorder of but a few weeks' duration to a chronic one compatible with life even for many years. The termination, however, is always fatal.

History. Knowledge of leukemia can be traced back to the period from 1839 to 1845 when Donné made the first microscopic observations and Craigie, Bennett, and Virchow distinguished the clinical entity. Virchow recognized the cells as being leukocytes, not pus cells, and distinguished a lymphatic and a splenic type of leukemia. With the development of Ehrlich's blood-staining methods in 1891, Neumann's myelogenous form was recognized as being the same as Virchow's splenomegalic type. Acute leukemia was recognized by von Friedreich in 1857 and by Ebstein in 1889, and the myeloblastic form was separated from the lymphoblastic type when Naegeli described the myeloblast in 1900. Reschad and Schilling-Torgau described monocytic leukemia in 1913. Since then variations from the classic pictures have been recognized and methods for palliative management have been developed, but little advance has been made in gaining an understanding of the actual cause of this invariably fatal process, or in its prevention or specific treatment.

Varieties of Leukemia and Incidence of Various Types. Acute and chronic forms of leukemia can be distinguished on clinical grounds as well as on the basis of the predominant abnormal cell types. Without treatment, acute leukemia usually is fatal within 6 *months;* the duration of life in chronic leukemia may be several *years*—usually 3 to 5, sometimes 1 or 2, and in other cases 10 or more. "Subacute" leukemia is not truly intermediate between acute and chronic leukemia. The course and the clinical and hematologic pictures resemble those of the acute form, but the progress of the disease is slower than in acute leukemia. Since myeloblasts, lymphoblasts, myelocytes, lymphocytes, or monocytes are the predominant cells in the great majority of cases of leukemia, the terms *acute* or *chronic* (and, if one wishes, *subacute*), qualified by the name of the predominant cell type, appear to be the most satisfactory designations for the different varieties of leukemia.

Leukocytosis is found in the majority of cases of leukemia. "Aleukemic" or, more correctly, subleukemic leukemia refers to cases in which leukocytosis is absent. Such cases are more often acute than chronic.

Leukemia is as common a cause of death as diphtheria or measles. Deaths from leukemia represent about 3.6 per cent of those due to cancer. There was a steady increase in the number of deaths from leukemia until 1940 or 1950 but the rate of increase has declined since then. Contrary to earlier statistics, it appears now that the proportions of cases of chronic myelocytic and chronic lymphocytic leukemia are approximately equal. Chronic leukemia is perhaps twice as common as the acute variety. The incidence of the various types of acute leukemia, including monocytic leukemia, is difficult to determine because conclusions must necessarily be influenced by differences in interpretation of the cell morphology. In various series, 11 to 21 per cent of the cases were subleukemic.

Etiology and Pathogenesis. While any variety of leukemia may occur at any *age*, it is nevertheless true that acute leukemia is much more common before the age of twenty-five than later, and is especially frequent under five years of age; chronic myelocytic leukemia has its highest incidence between the ages of twenty-five and forty-five, and chronic lymphocytic leukemia is seen especially after the age of forty-five or fifty. A difference in the *sex* incidence of leukemia becomes perceptible as age advances, there being essentially no difference in the occurrence of acute leukemia in male and female children and young adults, a slight preponderance of chronic myelocytic leukemia in males, and a distinct preponderance of chronic lymphocytic leukemia in males (3:1).

On the basis of past experience it can be stated that the probability that leukemia will occur more than once in a family is very small. This seems strange when one considers that susceptibility to experimental leukemia and the transmission of the spontaneous disease in experimental animals follow definite genetic laws. The explanation probably lies in the fact that, although hereditary factors do exert an influence on the etiology of human leukemia, as exemplified by familial cases of chronic lymphocytic leukemia especially, their effect is modified by external influences and by other genes. External factors include the effects of irradiation and perhaps also of chemical agents and of trauma. Leukemia has been described so much more often in persons exposed to radiation (such as roentgenologists and those who were exposed to the atom bomb in Japan as well as in patients with ankylosing spondylitis who received roentgen therapy) than in those not so exposed that this agent cannot be overlooked in a consideration of etiologic factors. Not so well documented, but nevertheless deserving serious consideration, as causes of leukemia are trauma, especially to bones, and exposure to certain chemical agents, especially benzol.

The febrile character of acute leukemia and the evidences of infection, about the mouth especially, which can be seen in many cases have led some to hold the opinion that the disease is caused by an infectious agent. Such a concept is difficult to accept, as none of the other customary evidences of infection has been observed, such as transmission from man to man or from mother to fetus. Experimental fowl leukemia, it is true, is carried by a filtrable agent, but this is so also with certain other types of neoplasms. Newer knowledge is developing concerning the existence of transmissible cytoplasmic agents which determine the character of cells. The role of viral agents in the etiology of human leukemia is under active investigation.

The essential change in this disease is thought to reside in the leukemic cell and is believed to consist of an acquired inability of these leukocytes to respond to forces which normally regulate their proliferation and maturation. The end result is a new type of cell with certain fixed abnormalities in appearance and behavior. Peculiarities have been observed in leukemic cells which are like those of neoplastic cells, including abnormal size and number of nucleoli and atypical as well as abnormal mitoses. In some leukemic leukocytes chromosomal changes have been observed. The causes of this change may be manifold; perhaps in a given case the development of the disease depends on the interplay of a variety of factors, including genetic constitution and external influences, such as irradiation, chemical agents, and cytoplasmic particles.

Pathology. The fundamental change in leukemia is widespread proliferation in the tissues, and usually also in the blood stream, of cells of a particular type. In chronic myelocytic leukemia the bone marrow and spleen are chiefly involved, but the lymph nodes, liver, kidneys, lungs, skin, and other organs are also infiltrated. The splenic pulp is full of myeloid cells, and infarcts are commonly present. In the chronic lymphocytic variety the lymphoid organs in particular show striking hyperplasia with disturbance of architecture, and the liver, bone marrow, and other tissues are affected as well. In acute leukemia the changes are similar and are ac-

companied by evidences of hemorrhage, the result of the accompanying thrombocytopenia.

Clinical Manifestations. The clinical manifestations of the chronic and the acute leukemias differ from one another a great deal, but there is comparatively little difference in the symptomatology of the various types of chronic leukemia, and essentially no difference in the clinical pictures of the different forms of acute leukemia.

Chronic Myelocytic Leukemia. The onset is insidious, and complaints may not develop until the disease has been in progress for a long time, perhaps a year or two. The most common symptoms are those of anemia (weakness, pallor, palpitation, or dyspnea); or a dragging sensation or swelling in the left side of the abdomen, due to the splenic enlargement; or complaints attributable to the increased metabolic rate which develops as the disease progresses (loss of weight, weakness, nervousness, cachexia, etc.). There may be slight fever, rising as high as 101°F, rarely higher. As the disease advances, the clinical picture may become more "acute" in that chills and fever may develop, weight loss may become excessive, and an abnormal tendency to bleed may become manifest.

The appearance of the patient ranges from that of seeming perfect health to one of extreme cachexia with marked pallor. Splenomegaly is often the first physical sign of the disease. The spleen may be just palpable or it may be huge, the abdomen, protuberant from this cause, standing out in striking contrast to the general emaciation. Lymph node enlargement is rarely significant, but tenderness, elicited on pressure over the lower portion of the sternum, is a moderately early sign.

Other symptoms and signs are less common, but any system of the body can be affected. The *liver* is often enlarged, sometimes greatly, and, like the spleen, is firm and not tender. The *skin* may show small, bluish-gray, elevated nodules, due to specific infiltration. The *retinas* may show hemorrhages and leukemic infiltrations. There may be subperiosteal infiltration and even destructive lesions of *bone* leading to pathologic fractures. Deafness, from infiltration in the middle or inner ears, or from hemorrhage; evidences of nervous system involvement due to the same causes; hematuria in association with infiltration of the kidney; or other still less common manifestations may be observed. Pain may develop from perisplenitis, or in some cases pleural effusion may occur.

The *blood picture* depends on the stage of the disease. The earliest manifestation is leukocytosis, due to an increase in the myeloid series of cells. Early in the disease the "shift to the left" is usually orderly with fewer metamyelocytes than segmented neutrophils, fewer myelocytes than older forms, and often few or no myeloblasts. Later the myelocytes,

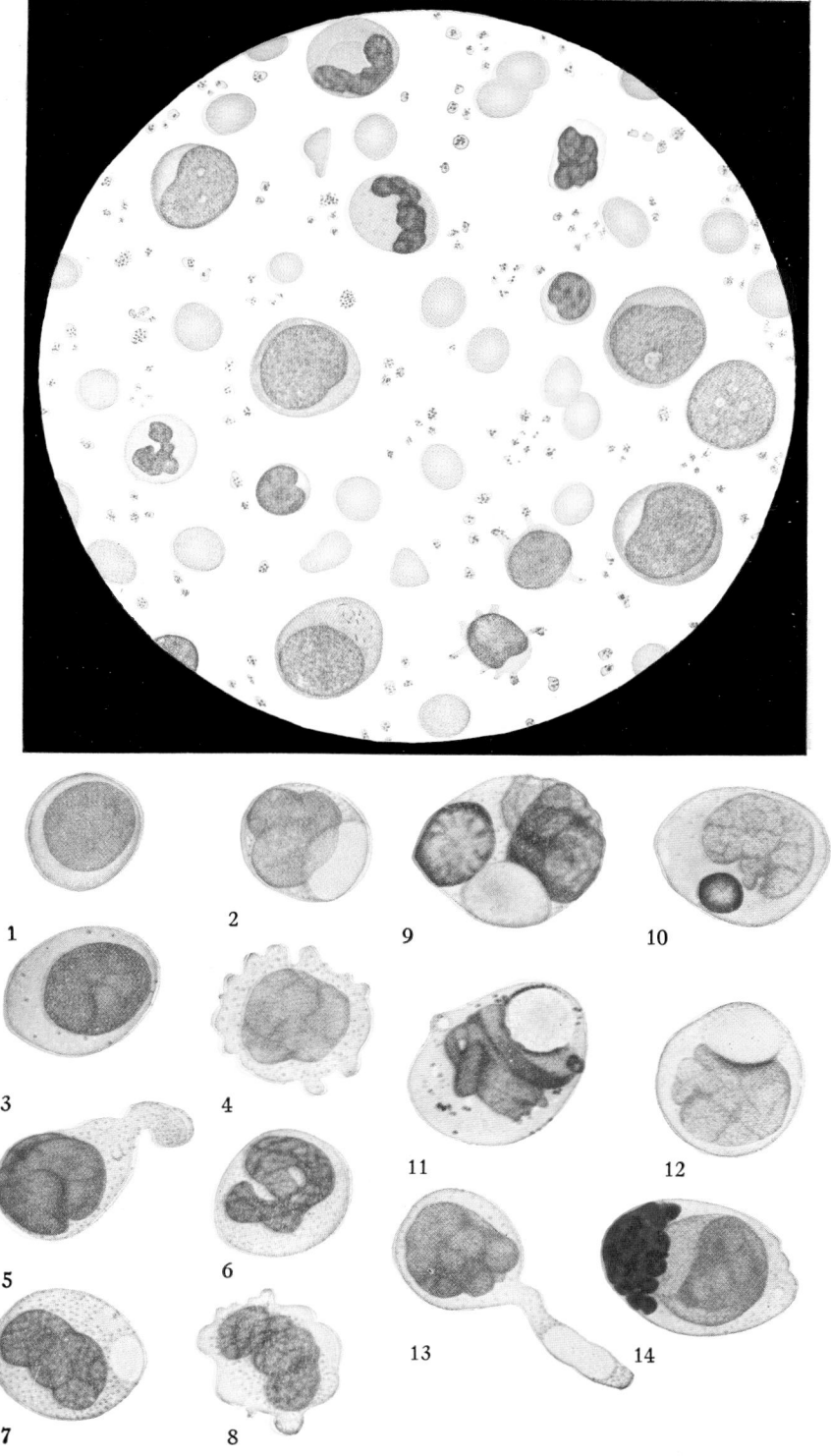

PLATE II

(*Top*) Acute leukopenic myelogenous leukemia. (WBC 3,000.) Film from buffy coat. Actual field. Five myelo-blasts, several showing nucleoli. (*Lower left*) Promyelocyte. Three nonsegmented neutrophils, practically desti-tute of granules (toxic-degenerative changes). (*Lower right*) Two megakaryocyte nuclei with shreds of platelet material attached. (*Bottom*) Cells from case of acute monocytic leukemia. (1 to 14) Monocytes. (1 and 3) Monoblasts. (*Stitt, Clough, and Branham: "Practical Bacteriology, Hematology, and Parasitology," 10th ed., New York, The Blakiston Division, McGraw-Hill Book Company, Inc., 1952.*)

including the earlier forms, tend to dominate the picture, especially in the most advanced and more "acute" stages. Eosinophils and basophilic leukocytes are likely to be found, sometimes in substantial numbers. If they are very numerous, the terms *eosinophilic leukemia* and *basophilic leukemia* are appropriate. The leukocyte count most often ranges between 100,000 and 500,000 cells per cu mm when the disease is first discovered, but values as great as 1,000,000 are sometimes seen. Monocytes are present in normal or slightly increased numbers, whereas lymphocytes, though reduced in percentage, maintain about a normal absolute value.

The degree of anemia is a good index of the extent of the leukemic process. In the earliest stages there is no anemia; in far advanced cases it is profound. The manner in which anemia is relieved when therapy reduces the extent of myeloid infiltration or becomes more severe as the disease advances gives support to the view that its cause is related to encroachment on the erythrocyte-forming elements by the leukemic cells. The anemia is usually normocytic in type. A few normoblasts are likely to be seen in the blood smear, as well as slight polychromatophilia and occasional stippling.

The platelets are normal in number or increased, except in the terminal stages of the disease when infiltration is extensive. Then hemorrhagic manifestations, prolonged bleeding time, and other signs of secondary thrombocytopenic purpura are found. In rare cases the platelet count may be extremely high, and even megakaryocytes or fragments thereof may be found in the circulating blood.

Chronic Lymphocytic Leukemia. The onset is insidious, as in the myelocytic form, but the first symptom is likely to be painless enlargement of lymph nodes in the neck, axilla, or groin. In other instances manifestations of anemia may dominate the picture, and less commonly splenic enlargement or hemorrhagic manifestations may be the presenting complaints. The skin is more often involved in the lymphocytic form than in the myelocytic, as are also the gastrointestinal tract and the mediastinum. There may be itching and burning, with yellowish-brown, red, bluish-red, or purple, nodular skin lesions. Bone tenderness is less frequent than in myelocytic leukemia. The lymph nodes vary in size from that of a pea to that of a hen's egg; though they are discrete, several lying together may produce a huge mass. They are moderately firm and smooth. Other manifestations are similar to those encountered in chronic myelocytic leukemia.

The *blood picture* is that of a monotonous collection of small lymphocytes each looking just like its fellow, contrasting strikingly with the colorful picture of myelocytic leukemia. The leukocyte count more often ranges between 50,000 and 250,000 per cu mm than at higher levels, and 90

per cent or more of these cells are lymphocytes. They often possess only a narrow rim of cytoplasm and may even appear to have none. Larger lymphocytes may be seen, but true "blast" forms with clearly defined nucleoli are unusual.

As in myelocytic leukemia, the presence or absence of anemia and its degree are good indexes of the extent of infiltration. The anemia is normocytic, and there may be occasional immature red cell forms in the blood smear. Early, the platelet count is normal; as the disease advances, it becomes greatly reduced and hemorrhagic manifestations may develop.

Acute Leukemia. The onset of acute leukemia is frequently rather abrupt, and, depending on the location and nature of the initial disturbance, a great variety of clinical pictures may be encountered. The initial symptoms may arise from leukemic infiltrations and glandular enlargement, from hemorrhages, or as the result of the systemic effects of the disease, including those associated with anemia. Sore throat, abnormal bleeding from the mucous membranes or petechiae or ecchymoses in the skin, cough or dyspnea resulting from enlargement of the thymus or mediastinal lymph nodes, rheumatoid pains, and a variety of neurologic complaints are among the manifestations which may be encountered. Excessive bleeding following the extracting of a tooth or from minor injuries may be the first evidence of the disease. Fever, headache, and general malaise may be soon followed by marked prostration, and the onset of some severe, malignantly virulent form of sepsis may be suspected.

Lymph node enlargement is usually less conspicuous than in chronic leukemia, but a systematic search will frequently reveal more or less generalized involvement of the lymph nodes. The spleen is usually palpable but is rarely very large. The liver is often enlarged. The gums may be swollen and purplish in color, and there may be ulceration in the mouth. Sternal tenderness is present in the great majority of cases.

Differentiation of the various types of acute leukemia cannot be made on clinical grounds and is often difficult even from the *blood examination.* Anemia is practically always present when the disease is first discovered; often it is severe. The anemia is usually normocytic, sometimes macrocytic. Polychromatophilia, as well as normoblasts, are often found. The platelet count is usually decreased, at least to some degree, even when the disease is first discovered. The bleeding time then is prolonged, the clot retracts poorly, and the tourniquet test is positive.

The leukocyte count rarely attains levels higher than 100,000 per cu mm; not infrequently it is below normal, even below 1,000. At first glance the predominant cells are likely to be mistaken for lymphocytes. Well-stained, thin smears are needed to demonstrate that the cells are abnormal and contain nucleoli. When they are lymphoblasts or myeloblasts or even more immature forms (stem cells) they are difficult to distinguish from one another. The nuclear differences are not easily recognized even by those with considerable experience, and their cytoplasm is scanty and nongranular. However, in *acute myeloblastic leukemia* a small proportion of cells of slightly later development will often be found which will be seen to contain peroxidase-positive granules. Since such cells are lacking in *acute lymphoblastic leukemia*, differentiation can sometimes be made on this basis. *Acute monocytic leukemia* can be distinguished more easily, however. The "pure" and rarer form, the *Schilling type*, is characterized by the presence of large cells with lacy chromatin, irregular nuclei, inconspicuous nucleoli, and irregular cell borders. The cytoplasm contains innumerable very fine, dustlike granules. At the same time a few nongranular, "blastlike" cells with nucleoli are found, probably "monoblasts." In the *Naegeli type* of monocytic leukemia, myelocytes are found in relatively large numbers, in addition to cells resembling monocytes.

Less Common Types of Leukemia. SUBLEUKEMIC (ALEUKEMIC) LEUKEMIA. This term refers to leukemia of any type in which the leukocyte count is only slightly elevated, normal, or less than normal. In such cases the abnormal cells may not predominate in the blood smear; in fact, they may be scarce and may not be readily discovered. In most instances in which leukemic cells are stated to be absent, however, a good smear and stain and careful scrutiny by a person with some experience will usually reveal at least a few. In any event, the bone marrow contains a large number of the abnormal cells, although sometimes they may be held together so firmly that they are not readily aspirated. A normal or subnormal leukocyte count may be encountered at some stage of chronic or acute leukemia, especially the latter. This may be followed by a phase of leukocytosis or, more often, leukocytosis may be only a terminal event. Sometimes leukocytosis never develops.

CHLOROMA. This term refers to a variant of acute leukemia which is characterized by the presence of greenish localized tumors, connected particularly with the periosteum and ligamentous structures of the skull, paranasal sinuses, orbits, spine, ribs, and sacrum. Protrusion of an eyeball, with diplopia and loss of vision, pain, deafness, and signs of various cranial nerve palsies, or other effects of pressure or infiltrative growth in a case otherwise consistent with a diagnosis of acute myeloblastic leukemia should lead to suspicion of chloroma.

CHRONIC MONOCYTIC LEUKEMIA. The great majority of cases of monocytic leukemia are acute or sub-

acute, as already described. A small number are slower in their course. Relatively low or subnormal leukocyte counts, bone pain, and cutaneous manifestations have characterized these cases.

LYMPHOSARCOMA CELL LEUKEMIA. The "lymphosarcoma cell" is about 9 to 14 μ in diameter, has a sparse but deeply basophilic cytoplasm, an oval, oblong, or kidney-shaped nucleus with coarsely reticular, spongy chromatin, and a single, prominent nucleolus. Such cells are seen in cases fitting the category of "leukosarcoma," proposed by Sternberg. Enlargement of lymph nodes in any one of many sites, but especially in the anterior mediastinum, or symptoms referable to anemia, may for months or even years precede the appearance of these cells in the blood. The leukocyte count may remain normal or low for a long time or even throughout the illness, even though 30 to 98 per cent of the cells may ultimately be of the lymphosarcoma cell type.

PLASMA CELL LEUKEMIA. This term is applied to rare cases in which plasma cells have been found in the blood but which in other respects resemble leukemia—i.e., there are leukocytosis, anemia, and splenic and frequently lymph node and hepatic enlargement. This disorder is perhaps but a variant of plasma cell myeloma, but in contrast to typical multiple myeloma (Chap. 244), bone involvement and hyperproteinemia may not be present. There may be extraosseous plasmacytomas in the upper respiratory passages, the cornea, the pleura, and elsewhere.

A number of other, still more rare forms of leukemia have been described. They include so-called "megakaryocytic" and "acute megakaryoblastic" leukemia, eosinophilic leukemia, and basophilic, or mast cell, leukemia. The clinical course of some cases of eosinophilic leukemia is so unlike that of myelocytic leukemia that in some instances one wonders whether they represent true leukemia. *Acute and chronic erythremic myelosis* (di Guglielmo syndrome) refers to a disorder in which the erythropoietic tissue, rather than the leukopoietic tissue, seems to be involved in a neoplastic process. The blood contains numerous erythroblasts in all stages of maturation, but the most immature forms are found in disproportionately large numbers. Other manifestations are similar to those seen in leukemia. The term *erythroleukemia* refers to a very rare disorder in which there appears to be a combined neoplastic hyperplasia of both erythroblastic and leukoblastic tissues. Cases such as these and lymphosarcoma cell leukemia, plasma cell leukemia, and cases of lymphocytic leukemia with only minor changes in the blood give support to the view, now widely held, that these conditions and those chiefly affecting lymph nodes, such as lymphosarcoma, as well as multiple myeloma, are very closely related disorders or simply variations of a single abnormal process.

Diagnosis. The diagnosis of leukemia is not difficult in most cases. Confusion may arise when the blood has not been examined thoroughly, when the question of a leukemoid reaction arises, or when the blood is subleukemic.

Instances of chronic leukemia, because of lymph node or splenic enlargement, may suggest one of the various disorders affecting lymph nodes or the spleen (Chaps. 242 and 243), or if the chief symptoms draw attention to other systems of the body, a very great variety of conditions may be simulated. Acute leukemia, as already mentioned, may suggest acute inflammatory conditions of various kinds, purpura hemorrhagica, or other disorders.

Hematopoietic responses which suggest leukemia (*leukemoid pictures*) may be observed under a variety of circumstances:

1. In association with *infections*. A picture resembling myelogenous leukemia is sometimes associated with pneumococcal and meningococcal infections and rarely is seen in diphtheria and tuberculosis. Lymphocytic leukemia may be suggested by the leukocytic reaction in whooping cough, infectious mononucleosis, and infectious lymphocytosis, in particular, and sometimes in chickenpox.

2. *Intoxications.* In rare instances of eclampsia, severe burns, diabetic acidosis, and mercury poisoning, leukemoid pictures have been observed.

3. *Malignancy,* especially with bone metastases, as well as in multiple myeloma, myelosclerosis, and Hodgkin's disease.

4. Following *severe hemorrhage or the rapid destruction of blood,* when the profound stimulus to the bone marrow may bring forth a marked leukocytosis as well as immature forms of the nucleated red corpuscle series.

The essential findings in the blood which favor leukemia rather than a leukemoid reaction are (1) pronounced immaturity of the leukocytes, which is more significant than their number; and (2) evidence of other hematopoietic disturbances, which includes (*a*) anemia; (*b*) the presence of immature red corpuscle forms in the blood, such as nucleated red corpuscles and polychromatophilia; and (*c*) platelet abnormalities, especially thrombocytopenia. Only in the early stages of chronic leukemia are anemia and other signs of disturbed hematopoiesis lacking. In leukemia the immaturity of the leukocytes often is not orderly as in the case of a physiologic response, where there are successively fewer numbers of the various immature forms, with at most but a small number of myelocytes and but 1 or 2 per cent of myeloblasts.

These criteria usually suffice to distinguish leukemia from a leukemoid reaction. In addition, the clinical findings, such as splenomegaly, lymphad-enopathy, and sternal tenderness, make it apparent that one is dealing with leukemia. On rare occasions, however, differentiation is quite difficult, for the disease simulating leukemia may be accompanied by some of these physical signs, and even immature forms of the red corpuscle series may find their way into the blood.

In subleukemic leukemia especially, and in the less clear instances where leukocytosis is present, the *bone marrow* examination is very helpful, for there abnormalities will usually be found which are well beyond the normal variations. Only in the early stages of chronic lymphocytic leukemia or in the rare cases in which the marrow involvement is not diffuse, is the sternal puncture likely to be disappointing. In chronic myelocytic leukemia the cells in the bone marrow may be at a slightly less mature level than in the blood. In acute myeloblastic leukemia, even when there are few immature forms in the blood, the marrow is crowded with myeloblasts. In other types of acute leukemia the corresponding cells or their precursors will be found in large numbers in the marrow (see p. 213).

Other examinations which may be helpful in reaching a diagnosis include *roentgenography* of the bones, which may reveal subperiosteal infiltration, osteolytic or tumorlike changes; measurement of the *basal metabolic rate,* which is increased in many cases of leukemia; and sometimes lymph node biopsy.

Course and Prognosis. With the possible exception of two or three instances, there are no authentic reports of cure of leukemia. In chronic leukemia the course is rarely interrupted by spontaneous remissions. In acute leukemia such remissions are observed occasionally, especially following infections, and may last for several weeks. The duration of life in cases of chronic leukemia varies greatly. In some, death ensues in a year or two after symptoms first appear; in others, the course may be extremely protracted, extending over 10 or 15 years and, very rarely, even longer. In certain cases such apparent long or short duration depends respectively upon early diagnosis or late discovery of the disease. In most instances the essential factor probably consists in different intensities of the pathologic process. The average duration of life in chronic myelocytic leukemia is 3.2 years; in the lymphocytic variety, 5.4 years. It is thought that about 20 per cent of patients survive more than 5 years. For acute leukemia, available statistics vary, but in the largest series which has been studied, the mean survival time from the onset of symptoms was 4.7 months in patients treated only with transfusions and antibiotics. The longest was 58 weeks, but 50 per cent of the patients were dead within 17 weeks, 90 per cent within 36 weeks.

In chronic leukemia, treatment, even though it

may not increase survival time by more than 6 months or a year, can for much of the time make the difference between a state of chronic invalidism and a condition of well-being which may approach normality. In acute leukemia the newer methods of treatment have made it possible in many instances to bring about and maintain remission in children for significant periods of time and perhaps also to prolong life. In adults the results of treatment in most cases have been much less satisfactory.

Prognosis in chronic leukemia can be judged more from the degree of anemia and the extent of weight loss than from the magnitude of the leukocyte count, especially if these fail to respond following therapy. Thrombocytopenia is also an unfavorable sign, for, except in occasional cases of chronic myelocytic leukemia, this indicates extensive infiltration of a degree not likely to be greatly influenced by treatment.

Treatment. Although cure of leukemia has not been achieved as yet, present-day methods of therapy provide considerable improvement, reduce morbidity, and may even prolong life, as outlined above. In addition to irradiation and chemotherapy, which will be considered below, *general measures* of management are important. These include blood transfusions, when necessary, and antibiotics. The latter are often not needed if only leukopenia is present; they are better reserved for prompt use at the first sign of infection. Good oral hygiene is important, as well as a well-balanced, nourishing diet. Advice concerning rest and activity should be guided by the make-up of the patient. In general, patients with leukemia should be encouraged to maintain their normal activities in so far as possible, treatment should be provided with the object of reducing morbidity, and hospitalization should be reduced to a minimum.

Irradiation. This is of value in chronic leukemia and may be given by means of roentgen rays, radioactive phosphorus (P^{32}), radium, thorium X, or mesothorium. Only the first two are now used. Increasing anemia, loss of weight, pressure symptoms, invasion of tissues with production of pain, or disfiguring or uncomfortable glandular enlargement are indications for treatment. These are of more importance than a high or rising leukocyte count. While hemorrhagic manifestations and thrombocytopenia, like anemia, may be due to marrow infiltration by leukemic cells and thus may be alleviated by treatment, more often they are part of the terminal picture of chronic leukemia and indicate that treatment is likely to be ineffective. Acute leukemia is another contraindication to irradiation. Such treatment is not only of little or no value but may be harmful.

Although roentgen therapy has been the gen-erally accepted form of radiation therapy, the choice between this and treatment with P^{32} is mainly a matter of availability and convenience. The details of dosage are matters for the specialist. Serial daily doses of 100 to 200 r or as little as 25 to 50 r, appropriately filtered and over specified areas, are used by various workers. Treatment is stopped when the leukocyte count has fallen to approximately 25,000 per cu mm, but this is not an absolute criterion since irradiation, given cautiously, may prove effective even in cases with leukopenia.

Treatment with phosphorus made radioactive (P^{32}) offers the advantage that the radioactive material is concentrated in the position where it is especially required—that is, in those tissues which have a high phosphorus content and metabolize phosphorus rapidly: the liver, spleen, kidneys, and bone marrow. The material can be given orally or intravenously and, unlike roentgen irradiation, it does not result in radiation sickness.

There is good evidence that life can be prolonged with regularly spaced irradiation designed to keep the patient in a good state of health and at his normal occupation. There are few now who hold to the view that irradiation therapy, or chemotherapy for that matter, should be reserved for use only in well-established relapse or when symptoms are prominent.

Chemotherapy. Chemotherapy, besides being less expensive than roentgen-ray therapy as a rule, makes management practical for those patients who do not reside where roentgen therapy apparatus is available. Many roentgenologists employ daily treatments for 2 to 3 weeks, which may be inconvenient as well as expensive in some cases. A variety of chemotherapeutic agents is now available which can be taken orally. Observations on patients treated with such agents may be spaced at intervals of one to several weeks, thus permitting a return to normal activities and reducing cost. In the last analysis, however, treatment must be designed to suit the individual needs of the patient, and often both irradiation and chemotherapy are required at different times in the same person. Thus, disfiguring and uncomfortable adenopathy or great splenomegaly may call for local roentgen therapy, whereas systemic manifestations are well handled by chemotherapy or radioactive phosphorus.

In general, the chemotherapeutic agents useful in the treatment of chronic leukemia differ from those valuable in acute leukemia (Table 241-1).

CHRONIC LEUKEMIA. Chemotherapeutic agents include busulfan (a sulfonic acid ester, 1:4-dimethanesulfonyloxybutane), demecolcin (desacetylmethylcolchicine), chlorambucil [*p*-(di-2-chloroethyl) aminophenylbutyric acid], and triethylenemelamine.

Table 241-1. RELATIVE VALUE OF DIFFERENT AGENTS IN TREATMENT OF LEUKEMIAS AND LYMPHOMAS

	Chronic leukemia		Acute leukemia			Hodgkin's disease	Lympho-sarcoma
	Myelo-cytic	Lympho-cytic	Myelo-blastic	Mono-blastic	Lympho-blastic		
Irradiation:							
Roentgen ray	++++	++++	0	0	0	++++	++++
Radioactive phosphorus	++++	+++	0	0	0	+	++
Chemotherapy:							
Nitrogen mustard	+	+	0	0	0	++++	++
Triethylenemelamine	+	++	0	0	0	++	+
Chlorambucil	+	+++	0	0	0	+++	++
Demecolcin	++	0	0	0	0	0	0
Busulfan	++++	+	0	0	0	0	0
Antifolic acid compounds	0	0	++	+	+++	0	0
Cortisone, prednisone	0	++	0	0	++++	+	++
6-Mercaptopurine	+	0	+++	++	+++	0	0

Although the nausea and vomiting associated with *nitrogen mustard* therapy (p. 1341) can be allayed considerably by sedatives or an antiemetic such as chlorpromazine, the discovery of other agents equally or more effective without such unpleasant action makes it unnecessary to use this drug. Similar to nitrogen mustard in pharmacologic effects is *triethylenemelamine,* which can be given orally and rarely causes gastrointestinal symptoms. This agent is a potent hematopoietic depressant and must be used with great caution. It is most useful in chronic lymphocytic leukemia. For the myelocytic variety other less toxic agents are available. Daily administration for a week or more seems unwise, since the depressant effect is cumulative. It is better to give the agent over a period of 1 to 3 days, waiting then for 2 or 3 weeks before more is given so that its full effect can be determined. As little as 1 or 2 mg may produce a fall in the leukocyte count and reduction in lymphadenopathy in chronic lymphocytic leukemia, but in other cases 5 mg and, rarely, even 10 mg may be required. The drug is usually given when the patient awakens in the morning together with 2 Gm sodium bicarbonate. Breakfast may be taken 2 hr later.

Even more useful in the treatment of chronic lymphocytic leukemia because it is somewhat less toxic is *chlorambucil,* an aromatic mustard. The usual dose is 0.1 mg/kg/day by mouth.

Busulfan (Myleran) is the most useful of the chemotherapeutic agents for chronic myelocytic leukemia. In oral doses of 4 to 6 mg daily, its use is associated with a reduction in the leukocyte count in the course of several weeks and a rise in hemoglobin, together with corresponding clinical improvement. Thrombocytopenia and purpura are the chief toxic manifestations, but these are uncommon.

Only rarely is there any gastric discomfort. When the leukocyte count has decreased to approximately 10,000 per cu mm, treatment is stopped. Remissions measured in months have been observed. Demecolcin (Colcemide, an alkaloid isolated from colchicum), also is effective in chronic myelocytic leukemia. The oral dose is 4 to 6 mg daily. However, relapse occurs promptly unless the drug is continued. Urethan is no longer used.

These agents, as already indicated, will bring symptomatic relief in many cases of chronic leukemia: lymph nodes will decrease in size, the spleen will become smaller, anemia will decrease or disappear, weight will be gained, and a sense of wellbeing will return, to remain for variable lengths of time. For the treatment of chronic lymphocytic leukemia, chlorambucil is perhaps the best of the chemotherapeutic agents available at present. For chronic myelocytic leukemia, busulfan is the most satisfactory drug, but demecolcin is sometimes effective when busulfan fails. They have little value in the lymphocytic form.

Splenectomy has been helpful in occasional cases of chronic lymphocytic leukemia when there was severe anemia associated with a reduced survival time of transfused red corpuscles, even in the absence of frank signs of hemolytic anemia. In such cases the steroid hormones, cortisone and prednisone, and adrenocorticotropic hormone have also been useful, and they should therefore be given a trial before splenectomy is considered.

ACUTE LEUKEMIA. In acute leukemia, roentgen therapy is of no value, radioactive phosphorus has limited application, and the above-mentioned chemotherapeutic agents are of no benefit. Nitrogen mustard will reduce the leukocyte count and may relieve bone pain but offers nothing more. On the other hand, the steroid hormones, the folic acid antagonists, and other agents, such as 6-mercaptopurine, are valuable in many cases.

The steroid hormones, of which *prednisone* and similar compounds are preferable since they can be administered by mouth, have been found to bring about a remission in at least two-thirds of the cases of acute lymphoblastic leukemia in children and perhaps in half this proportion of adults. To achieve these results, usually a dose must be given which is large enough to produce signs of hypercorticism, generally 40 mg prednisone daily. Such treatment rarely needs to be supplemented by potassium chloride (2 to 6 Gm daily), and the diet need not be salt-free. A similar beneficial effect is rarely observed in myeloblastic or monocytic leukemia; in fact, these types may even be made worse. Once a remission has been attained, steroid therapy is stopped. The remission may last several weeks or sometimes months. One may attempt to prolong the remission by the administration of one of the antagonists. Re-treatment with steroid hormones may produce a second remission, but this is usually less complete than the first.

A variety of folic acid antagonists is available, but *amethopterin* (methotrexate, 4-amino-N^{10}-methylpteroylglutamic acid) is more generally employed. The daily oral dose range of amethopterin is 1.25 to 5.0 mg, rarely more. The drug is given until a remission has been produced or severe toxic symptoms occur: oral ulceration, anorexia, nausea, vomiting and diarrhea, leukopenia, increasing thrombocytopenia and hemorrhage, and increasing anemia, alopecia, and skin rash. Sometimes it is very difficult to distinguish between toxic effects and an increase in the signs of leukemia. When given in large enough doses the antagonists will lead to the appearance of megaloblasts in the bone marrow. In children, with amethopterin as with steroids, remissions have been observed in approximately 60 per cent of those treated; in adults these agents are much less successful. Ultimately resistance develops in all cases and the drugs become no longer effective.

Of the other analogues of folic acid, purines, pyrimidines, and amino acids which have been studied with the object of discovering additional antileukemic agents, *6-mercaptopurine* (6MP, Purinethol) is the most clearly useful agent. Good clinical and hematologic remissions have been observed in somewhat less than 50 per cent of children with acute leukemia and in about 25 per cent of adults. Remissions have lasted from 1 to 10 months and have been observed even in patients who had become resistant to folic acid antagonists or to the steroids. The usual therapeutic dose is 2.5 mg per kg body weight per day by mouth. Sometimes twice

this amount is given for a short time, but in such cases the danger of producing marrow hypoplasia must be kept in mind. This drug has also been found to produce improvement in early chronic myelocytic leukemia, and occasional beneficial effects have been observed in the terminal "acute" stage of chronic myelocytic leukemia. Such remissions, however, have usually been of short duration.

The most effective method for the treatment of acute leukemia is to use one agent at a time and to follow this with another one of the agents which has been shown to be effective. Thus, in the management of a case of acute lymphoblastic leukemia, one might initiate treatment with steroids, this being continued until a remission has been produced. Therapy is then interrupted, and the patient is observed at weekly or fortnightly intervals until the first suggestion of relapse appears. When beginning anemia, thrombocytopenia, fever, sternal tenderness, an occasional immature leukocyte in the blood, or any other evidence of beginning relapse appears, either a folic acid antagonist or 6MP is administered until a new remission has been achieved. If the remission is complete, treatment may be again interrupted and is resumed when evidence of relapse once again begins to appear, this time the third agent, either amethopterin or 6MP being used. Later still, any one of these agents may be tried again. By such a plan of alternating use of drugs, the development of "resistance" to one of these agents may possibly be delayed and it may be possible to prolong the life of the patient. In cases of acute myeloblastic or monocytic leukemia, the steroid hormones are of little or no value, as already mentioned, and treatment must depend on the antifolic acid compounds and 6MP.

A more common practice than the above method of interrupted therapy is to give *maintenance therapy*. Thus, when a remission has been brought about in a case of acute lymphoblastic leukemia with steroid therapy, usually after 5 to 6 weeks of such treatment, steroid administration is reduced and in the course of about 2 weeks it is stopped. Instead, 6MP is given, in doses of 2.5 mg per kg body weight per day. This is continued until signs of relapse, or of toxicity, appear. Remission may be maintained for many months in this way. If toxic symptoms develop, interruption of therapy for a week or two should suffice to eliminate them and treatment is then resumed, usually at a lower dose. When 6MP ultimately fails, a course of steroid therapy may be given again, to be followed by amethopterin maintenance therapy. Although it has not been proved that maintenance therapy permits longer survival than interrupted therapy, it is clear that long survivals can be achieved in this way. The use of a single agent at one time is important not only because this permits other drugs to be held in reserve for use when relapse occurs but also because the interpretation of clinical and hematologic changes which occur during therapy is simpler and the differentiation of toxic effects from the signs of disease is easier.

Many other chemical compounds have been tested in the treatment of leukemia, but as yet none has been shown clearly to offer any advantages over the drugs discussed above.

Attempts to *transplant human bone marrow* in patients with leukemia who have been given heavy irradiation or chemotherapy with the object of destroying all the leukemic tissue have not met with success. The concept is intriguing but its value remains to be demonstrated.

REFERENCES

Burchenal, J. H., M. L. Murphy, R. R. Ellison, M. P. Sykes, T. C. Tan, L. A. Leone, D. A. Karnofsky, L. F. Craver, H. W. Dargeon, and C. P. Rhoads: Clinical Evaluation of a New Antimetabolite, 6-Mercaptopurine, in the Treatment of Leukemia and Allied Diseases, Blood, 8:965, 1953; Am. J. Med. Sci., 228:371, 1954.

Burnet, M.: Leukaemia as a Problem in Preventive Medicine, New Engl. J. Med., 259:423, 1958.

Court-Brown, W. M.: Radiation-induced Leukemia in Man, J. Chron. Dis., 8:113, 1958.

Farber, S.: Some Observations on the Effects of Folic Acid Antagonists on Acute Leukemia and Other Forms of Incurable Cancer, Blood, 4:160, 1949.

Ferrebee, J. W., and E. D. Thomas: Transplantation of Marrow in Man, A.M.A. Arch. Internal Med., 106:523, 1960.

Haut, A., W. S. Abbott, M. M. Wintrobe, and G. E. Cartwright: Busulfan in the Treatment of Chronic Myelocytic Leukemia. The Effect of Long Term Intermittent Therapy, Blood, 17:1, 1961.

Haut, A., M. M. Wintrobe, and G. E. Cartwright: The Clinical Management of Leukemia, Am. J. Med., 28:777, 1960.

Miller, D. G., H. D. Diamond, and L. F. Craver: Clinical Use of Chlorambucil, New Engl. J. Med., 261:525, 1959.

Osgood, E. E., and A. J. Seaman: Treatment of Chronic Leukemias: Results of Therapy by Titrated, Regularly Spaced Total Body Radioactive Phosphorus, or Roentgen Irradiation, J.A.M.A., 150:1372, 1952; Blood, 16:1104, 1960.

Reinhard, E. H., C. V. Moore, O. S. Bierbaum, and S. Moore: Radioactive Phosphorus as a Therapeutic Agent, J. Lab. Clin. Med., 31:107, 1946; Ann. Internal Med., 50:942, 1959.

Wintrobe, M. M.: "Clinical Hematology," 5th ed., Philadelphia, Lea & Febiger, 1961.

242 DISEASES OF THE SPLEEN AND RETICULOENDOTHELIAL SYSTEM

M. M. Wintrobe

The functions of the spleen were outlined in an earlier chapter (p. 232). Disorders of the spleen most frequently produce enlargement of this organ. The significance of splenic enlargement has been considered already, and the differential diagnosis of splenomegaly was discussed there (p. 233). Here several of the disorders which involve the spleen, in particular, will be described.

Disorders of the spleen not hitherto considered include congenital anomalies, rupture, and infarction. *Congenital anomalies* may take various forms. Instead of being a single organ, the spleen may be subdivided into numerous small spleens, or a spleen of normal size and shape may be accompanied by one or more accessory spleens. Rarely, the spleen assumes a retroperitoneal position and may force the left kidney downward. A *movable* spleen may be found in any part of the abdomen. If its pedicle becomes twisted, there may be sudden pain, enlargement, and signs of shock, as well as fever and vomiting if the torsion has developed acutely. Less severe symptoms occur if the process is more gradual.

Rupture of the spleen may occur following trauma, particularly if the spleen is diseased. Malaria, typhoid fever, and infectious mononucleosis are among the diseases in which this has been observed. Agonizing abdominal pain or pain in the left scapular region, together with signs of internal hemorrhage, characterizes this catastrophe. Anemia develops rapidly and leukocytosis occurs. Prompt surgical treatment is imperative. After traumatic rupture autotransplantation of splenic tissue (*splenosis*) sometimes occurs.

Infarction of the spleen may be sterile, in which event it is followed eventually by fibrosis and shrinkage. This has been observed as a complication of leukemia. A septic infarct may terminate with the formation of an abscess. The most common symptom of infarction is pain. Careful examination will reveal a friction rub. Unless an abscess forms, necessitating surgical intervention, sedation and abdominal support to impair movement of the spleen suffice.

Congenital absence of the spleen may be suspected when Howell-Jolly bodies, occasional nucleated red cells, target cells, decreased osmotic fragility, siderocytosis, leukocytosis, and a variable degree of thrombocytosis are found in the absence of a discoverable cause and particularly when there is associated congenital heart or intestinal malformation.

CHRONIC CONGESTIVE SPLENOMEGALY

Definition. This syndrome, also called *Banti's syndrome* or *splenic anemia*, is characterized by splenic enlargement, leukopenia, anemia and often thrombocytopenia, a tendency to gastric hemorrhage, and, in many cases, cirrhotic changes in the liver.

History. The term *splenic anemia* was originally used (1866) to refer to cases of anemia with splenomegaly which were not frank leukemia. Banti, in 1882 and subsequently, described a form of splenomegaly of unknown etiology associated in its earliest stages with leukopenia, asthenia, and occasional hemorrhagic episodes. In the intermediary stage, hepatic enlargement occurred, as well as urobilinuria and a dirty-brownish discoloration of the skin. The final stage consisted of liver atrophy and ascites.

Etiology. Banti described the spleen as being characterized by conspicuous thickening of the fibrillar reticulum in the Malpighian corpuscles and red pulp ("fibro-adenie"). These changes originated around the central artery of the follicle. In his opinion, the spleen was the primary seat of the disease. Later work showed that these changes are not specific and can be encountered particularly when there is increased venous pressure in the portal bed. Thus the designation *chronic congestive splenomegaly* has arisen. Cirrhosis of the liver, cavernous transformation of the portal vein, portal vein and splenic vein thrombosis, or variants in the anatomy of the venous pattern have been found in as many as 60 per cent of the cases. Active congestion in the spleen in the absence of venous obstruction has also been proposed as a cause of this syndrome. This concept depends on the hypothesis that disease of the splenic arteries is the primary fault, with the result that they fail to control the amount of blood entering the spleen, thus permitting congestion to develop.

The hematologic changes observed in the Banti syndrome are attributable to the unequal distribution of the cells of the blood in the splenic vascular bed and the remaining parts of the circulation resulting from stasis of the portal circulation. Following splenectomy the blood values usually have returned to normal.

Pathology. The spleen weighs 600 to 1,200 Gm as a rule, but may weigh as much as 5,000 Gm. At first one finds an increase in the reticulum, cellular hyperplastic pulp, degenerative changes in the follicular arterioles, and congestion. Later the follicles become smaller, while fibrosis of the reticulum, trabeculae, and capsule increases. Periarterial hemorrhages, and siderotic nodules deposited in the fibrous tissue around the arterioles are found in many instances.

Symptoms. Young adults are most frequently affected, but the disease may come on in childhood. The onset is usually insidious. The condition may ultimately attract attention in a variety of ways. There may be gastrointestinal complaints of vague character, probably attributable to the large mass in the left upper quadrant; the mass itself may be noticed accidentally; symptoms of anemia may become prominent; or the disorder may be announced explosively by the occurrence of a gastric hemorrhage. The spleen may extend to the pelvic brim. Ultimately the symptoms and signs of cirrhosis of the liver may appear. Obstruction of mesenteric veins may lead to the development of hemorrhoids; occlusion of the portal vein is followed by the appearance of signs of collateral circulation.

The anemia is normocytic and moderate in degree unless hemorrhage has occurred, when it may be microcytic hypochromic in type. In cases with long-standing and severe liver disease the anemia may be macrocytic. Leukopenia is found consistently, and thrombocytopenia is observed frequently. The bone marrow may show no abnormality, or slight myeloid hyperplasia may be present.

Diagnosis. Other conditions leading to pancytopenia (p. 1324) must be excluded, as well as the various causes of splenomegaly (p. 233). Even when gastrointestinal hemorrhage has occurred, the diagnosis should be made only after other possibilities have been excluded. Thus, a "silent" peptic ulcer may produce hypochromic microcytic anemia with slight splenic enlargement. Hookworm infection may produce chronic hypochromic anemia with moderate splenomegaly. Liver function should be studied in suspected cases, and esophageal varices looked for. If liver function is good and other conditions have been excluded, portal or splenic vein thrombosis should be suspected. Congestive splenomegaly due to extrahepatic causes is more likely to be found in patients below the age of eighteen than in older patients.

Prognosis and Treatment. Unless serious hemorrhage ensues, the course of the disease is slow as a rule and relatively benign. Patients may live for 10 years or longer. The chief nonsurgical procedures are administration of a diet rich in protein and otherwise complete as well; administration of iron if there has been hemorrhage; and blood transfusion if bleeding has occurred recently. If there is gastroesophageal bleeding, abdominal exploration is advisable, since some cause for congestion in the portal bed may be discovered and treated. At one time splenectomy was the sole surgical measure employed. However, although this procedure is likely to relieve the leukopenia—and thrombocytopenia if it is present—it is of little value in relieving the portal hypertension. Now, therefore, it is considered that a surgeon should not perform splenectomy in congestive splenomegaly unless he is prepared to form a venovenous anastomosis with the object of reducing the increased pressure in the portal bed. Portacaval shunt is usually preferred because of the large size of the vessels involved. If a large-caliber splenic vein is available or when the portal vein is obliterated, splenectomy and splenorenal shunts are recommended. When an adequate shunt cannot be made, esophagogastrectomy is employed. Following removal of the spleen, the leukopenia disappears, the anemia is relieved in whole or in part, and the platelet count is also likely to be restored to normal. The risks of surgery in these patients are substantial, however, and surgical intervention is advocated only (1) in cases in which there is severe upper intestinal bleeding and in which the portal hypertension is due to extrahepatic block; and (2) in cases of portal hypertension associated with cirrhosis of the liver where ascites and icterus are minimal or absent and there is a reasonable degree of hepatic reserve.

GAUCHER'S DISEASE

Definition. This is a rare, chronic familial disorder characterized by marked splenomegaly and often also by skin pigmentation, pingueculae of the scleras, and bone lesions.

Etiology, Morbid Anatomy, and Pathogenesis. The disorder usually is apparent early in life. It has a predilection for females, and the condition has been observed most often in Jewish families. Its mode of inheritance is uncertain. The characteristic finding is widespread reticulum cell hyperplasia, these cells being filled with lipid, mainly sphingolipids, as discussed elsewhere (Chap. 95). Consequently, Gaucher's disease is classed as a disturbance of lipid metabolism. The cause is unknown. The cells are distinctive, being 20 to 80 μ in diameter, round, oval, or spindle-shaped, and possessing one or more small, eccentrically placed nuclei. Appropriately stained, the cytoplasm shows numerous wavy fibrillae. These cells are found in the spleen, bone marrow, lymph nodes, and liver. The spleen may weigh as much as several thousand grams.

Symptoms. There is considerable variation in the age of onset and in the rate of progression of symptoms. As a rule, the earlier the onset the more rapid the course. The enlargement of the spleen is usually the outstanding manifestation, sometimes the only one. There may be a dragging sensation or pain due to infarction. Pain in the limbs, due to bone involvement, may develop. The liver may be enlarged, but the lymph nodes usually are not palpable. Roentgenograms may reveal osseous changes. Hemorrhage from the nose or gums is relatively common. Light yellowish-brown discolorations on the conjunctivas on either side of the cornea, and an ocher-to-brown hue of the skin, may be present.

As in other splenic disorders, moderate anemia, leukopenia, and thrombocytopenia are the usual blood findings.

Diagnosis. Diagnosis can be made by sternal or splenic puncture, which will reveal the characteristic cells. The plasma acid phosphatase activity is increased (p. 780).

Treatment and Prognosis. Although the disease coincidentally involves other parts of the reticuloendothelial system, splenectomy is worthwhile if the spleen is very large and thereby causes discomfort, or if there are serious symptoms attributable to the blood changes. In infants the prognosis is not good, but those who have survived to adolescence may live for many years even if splenectomy is not performed.

NIEMANN-PICK DISEASE

This is a lipid disorder of the reticuloendothelial system very similar to Gaucher's disease except that the condition has been observed only in infancy and its course is much more acute, death occurring within a few months after birth. The characteristic cells are filled with small, round, hyaline droplets, grouped in clusters and giving the appearance of a honeycomb. The stored material is a phospholipid, perhaps sphingomyelin (see Chap. 95).

HAND-SCHÜLLER-CHRISTIAN DISEASE

Exophthalmos, diabetes insipidus, and defects in the membranous bones form the triad which characterizes Hand-Schüller-Christian disease. At one time the manifestations of this disorder were considered to be produced by the growth of a characteristic type of granulation tissue with cells containing cholesterol and its esters. The present tendency is to regard Schüller-Christian disease as being closely related to Letterer-Siwe disease and to eosinophilic granuloma. *Eosinophilic granuloma* is a disorder localized to bone, consisting of solitary or multiple osteolytic lesions, but with no discernible visceral involvement. It is found in infants, children, and young adults, and occasionally at a later age, and is treated satisfactorily by curettement or roentgen therapy. *Letterer-Siwe disease* has been observed most often in infants and young children, is variable in duration (a few weeks to several years), and has often proved fatal. There is evidence of a wasting disorder, with enlargement of the spleen and liver, generalized lymphadenopathy, a hemorrhagic diathesis, especially petechiae and purpura, skeletal lesions, progressive anemia, and cutaneous manifestations. The last consists of discrete, yellowish-brown maculopapular lesions, or papules with a red border and yellow center. They are scattered over the face and trunk particularly, but may be found in the scalp and elsewhere. Whitish macules over the palate and tongue and weeping erosions in the axillas and other moist areas may develop. The three conditions possess as a common denominator a distinctive, inflammatory histiocytosis. Some regard Letterer-Siwe disease as the acute or subacute form of a disorder of which the Schüller-Christian picture is the chronic counterpart. The onset of the latter is in children and in young adults. The histiocytosis or granulomatosis may or may not be accompanied by intense eosinophilic reaction; the characteristic lipogranuloma is now thought to be the late phase in the evolution of the histiocytic lesion. Unlike Gaucher's disease and Niemann-Pick disease, there is no family predilection, and splenomegaly and hepatomegaly do not always occur and are never conspicuous. The blood may show pancytopenia. Death may not ensue for many years, but considerable disability may occur in the interval.

REFERENCES

Avery, Mary Ellen, J. G. McAfee, and Harriet G. Guild: The Course and Prognosis of Reticuloendotheliosis (Eosinophilic Granuloma, Schüller-Christian Disease and Letterer-Siwe Disease), Am. J. Med., 22:636, 1957.

Crocker, A. C., and S. Farber: Niemann-Pick Disease, Medicine, 37:1, 1958; Am. J. Clin. Nutrition, 9:63, 1961.

Lichtenstein, L.: Histiocytosis: X. Integration of Eosinophilic Granuloma of Bone, "Letterer-Siwe Disease," and "Schüller-Christian Disease" as Related Manifestations of a Single Nosologic Entity, A.M.A. Arch. Pathol., 56:84, 1953.

Macpherson, A. I. S.: Assessment of the Results of Surgical Treatment in Portal Hypertension, Gastroenterology, 38:142, 1960.

Rousselot, L. M., A. H. Moreno, and W. F. Panke: Studies on Portal Hypertension. IV. The Clinical and Physiopathologic Significance of Self-established (Nonsurgical) Portal Systemic Venous Shunts, Ann. Surg., 150:384, 1959.

Trams, E. G., and R. O. Brady: Cerebroside Synthesis in Gaucher's Disease, J. Clin. Invest., 39:1546, 1960.

243 HODGKIN'S DISEASE AND OTHER "LYMPHOMAS"

M. M. Wintrobe

In an earlier chapter (p. 231) the causes of lymph node enlargement were discussed and their differential diagnosis was considered. In this section the clinical manifestations of Hodgkin's disease and of other conditions chiefly affecting lymph nodes, such as lymphosarcoma, will be described. These disorders will be considered under one heading because their clinical manifestations are very similar.

Definition. Hodgkin's disease, lymphosarcoma, giant follicular lymphoblastoma (lymphoma), and reticulum cell sarcoma are included in this group. They are characterized by painless, progressive enlargement of lymphoid tissue. Lymphadenopathy is a characteristic feature, and the spleen is frequently enlarged. Cachexia, anemia, and, in many instances, fever usually are late symptoms.

History. A disorder affecting the "absorbent glands and spleen" was described by Hodgkin in 1832. *Lymphoblastoma, malignant lymphogranuloma,* and many other terms were used in referring to the disease in subsequent descriptions. Jackson and Parker attempted to classify the disorder in three categories—paragranuloma, granuloma, and Hodgkin's sarcoma. The picture of lymphosarcoma was described by Kundrat in 1893; Brill, Baehr, and Rosenthal differentiated giant follicular lymphoblastoma in 1925. Roulet (1932) separated reticulum cell sarcoma from the general group of malignant diseases of lymphoid tissue. Some pathologists differentiate still other groups or call these by other names; others seek to avoid fine separations.

Classification. Clinically these disorders vary considerably in severity. Histologically they show marked differences, but these are not well correlated with the clinical picture. They have been classified in various ways on histologic grounds. One of the most simple is that which differentiates those conditions with a simple histologic pattern from those with more complex patterns. In the first category are reticulum cell sarcoma and lymphosarcoma. The proliferating cells tend to encroach upon, obscure, and finally replace the architecture of the lymph node. The histologic pattern of Hodgkin's disease is more complex. Lymphocytes, plasma cells, granulocytes (eosinophilic and neutrophilic), monocytes, fibroblasts, and giant cells make up the picture. The giant Reed-Sternberg cells, 10 to 40 μ in diameter, are possessed of abundant cytoplasm, a multilobed nucleus or multiple nuclei, and prominent nucleoli. A variable amount of fibrosis may be present, and the lymph node architecture is often lost. In giant follicular lymphoma the histologic pattern is also somewhat complex, but the striking feature is the presence of multiple, follicle-like nodules of various sizes. Other types of "lymphoma," difficult to classify, are observed from time to time.

Etiology. Hodgkin's disease forms about one-third to one-half of all cases of this group. It affects a younger age group than the other conditions, being most common in the second and third decades. However, no age is immune. Males are more frequently affected than females.

The cause of these disorders is unknown. There may not even be the common denominator of neoplastic growth to unite them, for many investigators consider Hodgkin's disease to be an infectious granuloma. Efforts to transmit the disease to animals have failed, however, and attempts to incriminate various organisms, including the tubercle bacillus (human and avian), diphtheroid bacilli, and *Brucella* organisms, have not succeeded. An agent in the lymph nodes found to produce encephalitis on inoculation into animals appears to be a nonspecific chemical substance derived most probably from eosinophilic leukocytes. The other disorders in this group are assumed generally to be true neoplasms. This applies even to giant follicular lymphoma, which at first was considered a benign disease.

Symptoms. In most cases lymph node enlargement, usually cervical, is the first symptom to attract attention. This may be bilateral but is more often unilateral at first. More rarely the axillary or the inguinal nodes are the first to enlarge. The nodes are discrete and movable at first; only later do they become matted together and fixed. As a rule, they are painless and not tender, and the overlying skin is normal. However, when they have developed rapidly or when nerves are infiltrated as well, they may be painful. This is true in Hodgkin's disease especially. The size of the nodes ranges from that of a pea to that of a large orange. There is a resilient firmness in most instances, but the growth of connective tissue may make the nodes of Hodgkin's disease harder in the course of time. Occasionally the nodes in the axillary or inguinal regions may become secondarily inflamed and even break down.

After an interval varying from months to years, evidence appears of lymph node involvement elsewhere. This may affect other superficial nodes: supraclavicular, axillary, inguinal, subpectoral, brachial, or femoral. A common site, also, is the mediastinum, to which such symptoms as cough, dyspnea, stridor, or dysphagia should attract attention. Splenomegaly develops in more than half the cases of Hodgkin's disease and of giant follicular lymphoma; less frequently in the other forms. The liver is often palpable. Ultimately cachexia develops and weight loss occurs.

The mode of onset of these disorders may vary greatly, however. The manifestations may arise first in the mediastinum, the lungs, the digestive tract, the genitourinary tract, the bones, and, rarely, the nervous system. Infiltration of the lungs, atelectasis, or pleural effusion may occur. In the gastrointestinal tract the tumor may be far advanced before it is first discovered. Colicky pain, loss of weight, anemia, a palpable tumor, and obstruction are signs produced by lymphosarcoma of the small intestine. When the retroperitoneal nodes are the chief ones to enlarge, the diagnosis may be very difficult to make and the chief symptoms may be fever, pain, and loss of weight. Hematuria, pyuria, or pain is found when the genitourinary tract is involved. Localized pain and tenderness, spontaneous fractures, and neurologic changes due to extension into the spinal canal from vertebral lesions are the most common manifestations of bone involvement. Areas of rarefaction may be demonstrable in roentgenograms, although symptoms may be present long before roentgenographic signs become evident. Subperiosteal infiltration may occur, or the bone marrow involvement may be extensive. Of cutaneous manifestations, pruritus is the most frequent; it is encountered particularly in Hodgkin's disease. Brownish skin pigmentation, herpes zoster, and nodules produced by infiltration by the specific cells are among other skin manifestations which may be encountered. Symptoms and signs may also develop which are secondary to swellings producing pressure in various areas.

Constitutional symptoms may appear early in Hodgkin's disease, but they occur late in the other lymph node disorders. Hodgkin's disease, in particular, may produce a great variety of manifestations, so that, in addition to the localized form, which is much the most common, a generalized type, an acute type with death in a few weeks or months, a "larval" or abdominal form, and a splenomegalic type have been described.

Fever is common in Hodgkin's disease, although the well-known Pel-Ebstein type of fever is actually uncommon, appearing no oftener than in 16 per cent of cases. This form of fever consists of febrile periods of several days' to several weeks' duration in which the temperature remains at levels of approximately 102 to 104°F, alternating with periods of weeks to even months during which there is no fever whatever.

Blood Picture. The greatest degree of variation is found in the blood picture associated with these disorders. There may be no changes whatever. On the other hand, there may be profound anemia as well as striking changes in the leukocytes and platelets. In Hodgkin's disease, changes in the blood occur relatively early. The anemia in Hodgkin's disease is usually only moderate in degree and normocytic in type; very occasionally, hemolytic anemia develops. The total leukocyte count in Hodgkin's disease may be slightly or moderately increased, it may be normal, or there may be leukopenia. Sometimes the leukocyte count may exceed 25,000 per cu mm. The differential count may show neutrophilia, relative and absolute lymphocytopenia, monocytosis, or eosinophilia. All these changes may be present at the same time, or none of them. Eosinophilia, which is mentioned frequently as characteristic of Hodgkin's disease and which may sometimes be very pronounced, is found only in about 20 per cent of cases. An absolute increase in the number of lymphocytes suggests some disease other than Hodgkin's. Neutropenia suggests extensive bone marrow or splenic involvement.

The leukocyte picture in the other forms of disease chiefly affecting lymph nodes is more frequently normal than in Hodgkin's disease. Relative and even absolute lymphocytosis may be seen. The lymphocytes may be of normal types, but unusual forms and "tumor cells" (p. 1330) have been described. Monocytes may be increased in number and young forms may be seen, but a consistent and characteristic picture has not been described.

The platelet count may be increased in Hodgkin's disease, and large, bizarre forms may be seen. It is more common, however, to find the platelet count normal. In some instances thrombocytopenia is present; this usually occurs when leukopenia is found as well. The presence of thrombocytopenia suggests extensive bone marrow or splenic involvement and is usually, although not necessarily, a grave sign.

Bone Marrow Picture. As would be expected from this description of the blood findings, changes in the bone marrow are not characteristic and are seldom helpful except in rare cases of so-called "bone marrow Hodgkin's," in which there is extensive involvement of the bone marrow. Reed-Sternberg cells have been demonstrated in the bone marrow in a few cases of Hodgkin's disease. Lymphocytosis may be found in the bone marrow in some cases of lymphosarcoma and of giant follicular lymphoma. Such cases raise serious doubt as to whether there is any true difference between them and chronic lymphocytic leukemia.

Diagnosis. The differential diagnosis of lymph node enlargement was discussed in an earlier chapter (p. 231). Cases in which there is little or no enlargement of the superficial lymph nodes present the most difficult problem in diagnosis, for then a variety of inflammatory and neoplastic disorders of the mediastinum, lungs, gastrointestinal tract, or liver must be considered, and the possible presence of chronic infections such as brucellosis must be ruled out. Hodgkin's disease, in particular, may produce such varied manifestations that this disorder must be kept in mind almost whenever diagnosis is obscure. This disease is particularly suggested by such symptoms as relapsing fever, loss of weight, and splenic or hepatic enlargement, together with anemia and leukocytosis or leukopenia.

Treatment. Surgical excision, irradiation, and chemotherapy all have their place in the treatment of these disorders. Surgery is useful when the condition is definitely localized, irradiation is effective in the treatment of local manifestations and when the disease is generalized, and chemotherapy is particularly indicated when the disorder is widespread. Sometimes all three forms of therapy can be employed, and frequently there are advantages in using both irradiation and chemotherapy.

Since these conditions, in many instances, appear to arise locally and only disseminate later, *surgical excision* should be an excellent form of therapy. Unfortunately, correct diagnosis is not often made early. Furthermore, in many instances in which the disease seems to be local, dissemination has already occurred or has been present from the beginning. Nevertheless, this form of therapy, when appropriately applied, offers the only chance of cure. Surgical excision, if undertaken, must be radical and should be followed by irradiation or chemotherapy or both. Surgery, in the form of splenectomy, should also be considered when signs of "hypersplenism" are present: severe anemia with shortened life span of transfused red corpuscles, leukopenia, and thrombocytopenia.

Roentgen rays represent the preferred method of *irradiation,* apparently being somewhat superior to the use of radioactive phosphorus and more effective than radium. Generally speaking, segmental or localized irradiation is used rather than total irradiation, except when generalization has taken place. Various areas are treated in succession. The decision as to dosage is the problem of the radiotherapist. The total amount depends on the response of the lesions to therapy, the general effects on the patient, and the effect on the blood. The effect of irradiation may be dramatic, large masses melting away in the course of a week. Pressure symptoms may disappear; fever and pruritus, if present, may be relieved; and pain caused by bone involvement may be alleviated. Pulmonary lesions may decrease in size and pleural effusions may clear. Anemia may disappear and the leukocyte count, if elevated, may drop to normal. In other cases, irradiation is less effective, in some instances being of scarcely any benefit. Prediction in advance as to the likelihood of benefit from therapy is often difficult. In general, the more chronic and slowly growing forms respond best to therapy. Remission following treatment may last but a few weeks or may persist a year or longer. In some cases such improvement can be reproduced many times by additional therapy.

The action of *nitrogen mustard* in these disorders is similar to that of irradiation, but in certain cases of Hodgkin's disease this drug seems to be more effective than irradiation. It has been found that in some cases previously given roentgen therapy and no longer responding to such treatment, nitrogen mustard therapy has been distinctly beneficial. Other cases treated with nitrogen mustard from the beginning have responded well and, in general, in a manner similar to that already described under roentgen therapy. Fever often disappears promptly, and anemia, if present, also is alleviated. Abnormalities in the leukocytes may revert toward normal although the immediate effect, noticeable within 5 to 14 days following the first dose of nitrogen mustard, may be leukopenia and an increase of anemia. Thrombocytopenia, if present at the initiation of therapy, is less likely to be relieved by treatment.

Nitrogen mustard [methyl-bis(β-chloroethyl)-amine hydrochloride, HN2] is given intravenously in doses ranging from 0.1 to 0.3 mg per kg body weight per injection each day. As much as 0.8 mg per kg has been given in a course of therapy, but the usual amount is 0.4 to 0.6 mg. The drug is available in vials containing 10 mg. To prevent thrombosis, an intravenous infusion of normal saline solution is first introduced, and when this is flowing freely, 10 ml saline solution is added to the vial containing the mustard. The drug dissolves readily. The appropriate dose is then withdrawn and injected through the rubber tubing of the saline infusion. Nausea and even vomiting may follow several hours after injection of the drug, but are usually of shorter duration, even though sometimes more intense, than in irradiation sickness. The nausea and vomiting can be allayed or prevented by giving chlorpromazine in three 20- to 30-mg doses, 6 and 4 hr before and at the time of the injection.

The discovery of other chemotherapeutic agents has reduced the comparative importance of nitrogen mustard in the treatment of the various forms of leukemia and the lymphomas, with the exception of Hodgkin's disease. *Triethylenemelamine* (p. 1333) appeared at first to be very promising because it has the advantages, as compared with nitrogen mustard, that it can be given by mouth and produces little or no nausea and vomiting. In Hodgkin's disease 10 to 15 mg may be given in a course, and maintenance doses of 5 to 10 mg per month have been employed. Lymphosarcoma, like chronic lymphocytic leukemia, is more sensitive, and 2 to 5 mg may produce an effect. Other lymph node disorders may require amounts intermediate between these quantities. However, the potential hematopoietic depressant action limits its usefulness.

Chlorambucil, an aromatic mustard which can be taken by mouth, has proved to be useful in the treatment of these disorders because its absorption is more consistent than that of TEM and the effect on the bone marrow is more easily controlled. Since its action is slow, beneficial effects not appearing before 3 weeks as a rule, chlorambucil is especially useful when remission following nitrogen mustard therapy is short-lived and maintenance therapy is required or when intravenous therapy is not practicable. The usual dose is 0.1 mg per kg body weight per day, but in Hodgkin's disease, larger doses may be tolerated. As with other agents of potential hematopoietic toxicity, measurements of hemoglobin, leukocytes, and platelets should be made at regular intervals to avoid serious hematopoietic depression.

Urethan, busulfan, and the folic acid antagonists offer little or nothing in the treatment of the lymph node disorders under discussion, and the steroid hormones are only occasionally and transiently useful. The effects of irradiation and various chemotherapeutic agents are compared in Table 241-1 (p. 1333).

In addition to these measures, general supportive and symptomatic therapy will be required in individual cases.

Prognosis. The most important factor which seems to determine the course of these disorders is their inherent character. Cases of Hodgkin's disease and of lymphosarcoma are known to have run a chronic course for many years. In other instances the course is rapid and progression occurs in spite of therapy. In general, cases with the most favorable outlook are those in which only one accessible lymph node group is affected and where evidences of systemic involvement such as fever, loss of weight, increased sedimentation rate, and changes in the blood are lacking. In the last analysis, a therapeutic trial should be attempted, for a prolonged remission may sometimes be encountered even in cases in which the general examination suggests a hopeless prognosis.

REFERENCES

Jackson, H., Jr., and F. Parker, Jr.: "Hodgkin's Disease and Allied Disorders," New York, Oxford University Press, 1947.

Kaplan, H. S., and D. W. Smithers: Auto-Immunity in Man and Homologous Disease in Mice in Relation to the Malignant Lymphomas, Lancet, 2:1, 1959.

Rosenberg, S. A., H. D. Diamond, and L. F. Craver: Lymphosarcoma: The Effects of Therapy and Survival in 1269 Patients in a Review of 30 Years' Experience, Ann. Internal Med., 53:877, 1960; Medicine, 40:31, 1961.

Wintrobe, M. M.: "Clinical Hematology," 5th ed., Philadelphia, Lea & Febiger, 1961.

244 MULTIPLE MYELOMA, CRYOGLOBULINEMIA, AND MACROGLOBULINEMIA

M. M. Wintrobe

MULTIPLE MYELOMA

Definition. Multiple myeloma is characterized by the development of multiple tumors of bone which produce pain, pathologic fractures, and anemia. There may be diffuse involvement of the bone marrow, and in the urine or blood a peculiar protein is usually found. Rarely, a localized tumor is the only manifestation. Tumors composed of other types of cells have been described, but the evidence is all in favor of a single type ("myeloma" or plasma cell).

Etiology. The disease appears most commonly after the age of forty and is twice as frequent in males as in females. The cause is unknown. The true nature of the peculiar protein is not clear. It is presumed that the myeloma cell is responsible for the protein anomalies of multiple myeloma. This cell has the cytochemical characteristics of an intensely protein-producing cell, as judged by ultraviolet microscopy. Protein with ultracentrifugal and electrophoretic properties similar to those of the abnormal components present in the plasma in this disease has been extracted from myeloma tumor tissue. Myeloma proteins of various electrophoretic mobilities appear to be related to one another but are not identical; they differ from those of normal serum. Thus the myeloma globulins were found to lack antigenic determinants that are present in the γ-globulins of normal serum. Likewise investigation of amino acid composition, of N-terminal groups, and of the peptides derived by tryptic hydrolysis has provided evidence that the tumor produces a new type of globulin that differs structurally from normal γ-globulin. The urinary Bence-Jones proteins are not derived by renal cleavage of the myeloma globulins but, in fact, may be their precursors. The paramyloidosis (see below) has been attributed to the production of proteins of such low molecular weight that they are capable of diffusing through the capillary beds of many, if not all, tissues. When these proteins find complementary polysaccharides which they can bind, insoluble complexes are formed and the proteins remain.

Symptoms. Pain is the most frequent complaint and is produced by the tumors which, according to their location, may or may not be discoverable on physical examination. The tumors range from the size of a pea to that of a hazelnut. They are confined, for the most part, to the sites of the red marrow: the ribs, sternum, spine, clavicles, skull, or the extremities about the shoulder or pelvic girdle. Roentgenograms reveal discrete, punched-out lesions and pathologic fractures. However, in 13 per cent of cases, or more, no significant osseous lesions are found, or only diffuse osteoporosis may be seen. Paraplegia due to compression of the spinal cord is the most common symptom referable to the nervous system, but intercostal neuralgia, radiculitis, diplopia, anisocoria and failing vision, or neuropathy from direct infiltration of nerve roots and peripheral nerves may occur. Anemia, abnormal bleeding, or symptoms suggesting nephritis sometimes dominate the clinical picture. Recurrent bouts of bacterial pneumonia are common. Extraosseous involvement of lymph nodes, spleen, tonsils, liver, and other tissues has been described.

Laboratory Findings. Anemia is moderate in degree, as a rule, and normocytic, but sometimes it is severe and macrocytic. Enumeration of the cells may be difficult because of clumping, a peculiarity often related to the great quantity of globulin in the plasma. In blood smears there may be a marked tendency to rouleaux formation. Polychromatophilia, stippling, and even normoblasts may be found in the blood smear. The leukocyte count may be normal, slightly increased, or low. Myeloma cells like those seen in the bone marrow may be found. The platelet count is usually normal.

Hyperproteinemia may be present (50 to 65 per cent of cases), and sometimes extremely high values are found. The increase is due to the globulin fraction. Sometimes the protein precipitates or coagulates spontaneously when the plasma is exposed to low temperatures (cryoglobulin, see below). Its presence may be associated with a variety of symptoms, especially those suggesting the Raynaud syndrome. Detailed studies have revealed that the predominant type of protein differs from one case to another. In the majority of cases, γ-globulin is increased; in others it is β-globulin, and in the minority the substance is an α-globulin. The diagnostic patterns in multiple myeloma as measured by the Tiselius electrophoretic technique are characterized by tall, narrow, sharply defined peaks owing to the presence of large amounts of a relatively homogeneous abnormal protein (Fig. 244-1 *B* and *D*).

When the *urine* is heated, a white cloudy precipitate appears at temperatures of 50 to 60°C, but when the temperature is raised to near the boiling point the precipitate redissolves. Such Bence-Jones protein has been observed in 40 to 50 per cent of cases. As judged by various physicochemical determinations, Bence-Jones proteins are related neither to normal serum proteins nor to the abnormal serum proteins. As judged by serologic reactions, however, they appear to be related to normal serum proteins. Bence-Jones protein can be synthesized readily from free amino acids rather than from tissue protein precursors. There is evi-

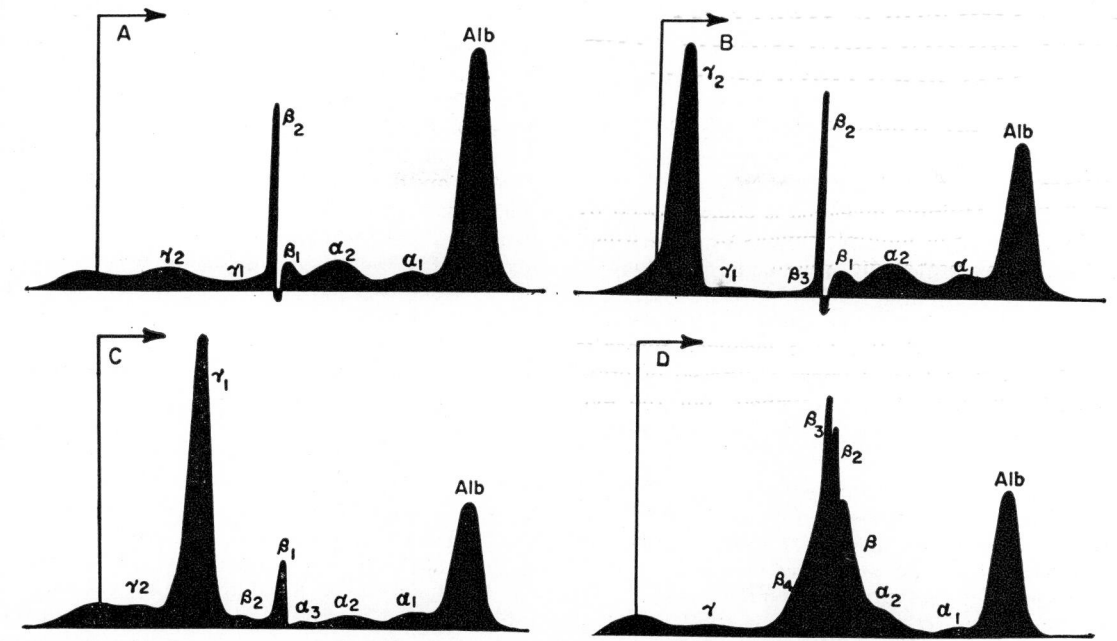

FIG. 244-1. Descending patterns (after 250 min) of pooled normal serum (*A*), and serum from two patients with multiple myeloma (*B* and *D*) and one patient with macroglobulinemia (*C*), determined by electrophoretic analysis at 1°C in 0.1 ionic strength. Veronal buffer at pH 8.4 to 8.5. Note the large γ-globulin component (γ₂) in (*B*) and the β-globulins in (*D*), as well as the γ-globulin (γ₁) in the case of macroglobulinemia (*C*). The very narrow β₂ peaks in (*A*) and (*B*) are anomalies, probably due to lipoproteins, and are not unusual in serums from nonfasting subjects. (*Courtesy, Drs. Emil L. Smith and B. V. Jager and Mr. Douglas M. Brown.*)

dence that myeloma serum globulins may be conjugated glycoproteins containing a significant quantity of carbohydrate bound to the protein component. In contrast, the urine myeloma proteins seem to be devoid of any significant carbohydrate component.

In addition to the hyperproteinemia and the Bence-Jones proteinuria, a third form of protein abnormality may be observed in multiple myeloma. This is the deposition of a peculiar protein in the tissues, producing atypical amyloidosis or *paramyloidosis*. This has been observed upon histologic examination in 6 to 10 per cent of cases of multiple myeloma.

Not infrequently, certain chemical changes are found in the blood. *Hypercalcemia* has been observed in 20 to 53 per cent of cases, values of 12 to 16 mg per 100 ml being not unusual. With progression of the disease the hypercalcemia may increase. The high serum calcium levels have been attributed to the resorption of bone which takes place, but they are further increased by secondary hyperplasia of the parathyroids caused by renal impairment. As a rule, the hypercalcemia is not accompanied by a decrease in the inorganic serum phosphorus or by much increase in alkaline phosphatase, thus differing from the changes found in primary hyperparathyroidism.

The serum uric acid concentration is not infrequently increased, and nitrogen retention has been noted in many cases. Both these changes can be ascribed to the renal damage associated with the deposits of Bence-Jones protein which are found not only in the distal tubules but in the entire nephron up to the proximal convoluted tubules. The resulting distention and obstruction to renal flow lead to glomerular atrophy and ultimate renal failure ("myeloma kidney"). It is thus not unusual in multiple myeloma to find albumin, casts, and renal epithelial cells in the urine, and evidence of renal functional impairment as well as nitrogen retention often develop.

The *bone marrow* frequently contains the tumor cells, although their number may range from 3 to 96 per cent. The myeloma cell is moderately large (15 to 30 μ), and round or ovoid, and contains a round, eccentrically placed nucleus which may contain one or two nucleoli. The chromatin is moderately coarse. The cytoplasm is bright blue. Attempts have been made to classify myeloma cells according to their maturity and to establish some correlation to the clinical manifestations of the disease. Some tendency for patients with the more mature cell types to live longer and for those with greater percentages of immature cells to manifest renal involvement has been observed, but extreme variations have been encountered in individual cases, and no consistent correlation between cell type and extent of bone involvement, hyperglobulinemia, Bence-Jones proteinuria, or the electrophoretic distribution of the various globulin fractions has been established.

Diagnosis. The multiple bone lesions, the excretion of Bence-Jones protein, the hyperproteinemia, and the characteristic cells in the bone marrow form a combination of findings which makes the diagnosis evident. Difficulty arises when back pain, obscure anemia, or some complaint of nonspecific character has failed to suggest this disease and the appropriate examinations have not been made; or when extraosseous tumors exist. Sometimes the picture may closely simulate hyperparathyroidism (see p. 604). Paper electrophoresis of serum and urine now provides a means for the ready detection of the protein abnormalities characteristic of multiple myeloma. When both serum and urine have been examined, a significant abnormality has been detected in 97 per cent of cases. The distinctive feature is the tall, narrow, sharply defined peak due to the presence of large amounts of a relatively homogeneous abnormal protein.

Prognosis and Treatment. The prognosis is unfavorable. The average duration is 2 to 3 years. Great variations occur, however, and some patients live for many years. Local irradiation is often helpful and may be strikingly so if there is a single bone lesion. The effects of irradiation on myeloma are rather unpredictable, however. Urethan is perhaps the best therapeutic agent currently available but even its value is limited. Although subjective improvement is associated with its administration in about half the cases, objective improvement has been observed in only about 20 per cent. To achieve any benefit, doses of 2 to 5 Gm daily have to be given for periods of 6 to 10 weeks. With these doses nausea and vomiting may develop and may necessitate withholding the drug. Other chemotherapeutic agents, including stilbamidine, nitrogen mustard, and triethylene melamine, are of even less value. The steroid hormones may sometimes be helpful but often have been disappointing.

CRYOGLOBULINEMIA AND MACROGLOBULINEMIA

History, Definitions, and Clinical Syndromes. Although multiple myeloma and Bence-Jones proteinuria were recognized in 1845, the presence of a cold-precipitable protein in the serum of a patient with this disease (*cryoglobulin*) was not described until almost a century later (Wintrobe and Buell, 1933). *Macroglobulins,* high molecular weight proteins demonstrable only by ultracentrifugation, and a syndrome associated with macroglobulinemia were described in 1944 (Waldenström). Since that time, with the exploitation of electrophoretic, ultracentrifuge, and serologic techniques, considerable attention has been attracted to the occurrence of aberrations in protein metabolism in association with various diseases and, sometimes, in the absence of any associated disorder. In some instances it appears that the unusual findings represent only increases of normally occurring protein molecules (*dysproteinemias,* Chap. 89), whereas other studies suggest that they denote aberrant protein synthesis (*paraproteinemia*).

Cryoglobulinemia of minor degree (less than 25 mg per 100 ml) may be encountered in a large variety of disorders, including systemic lupus erythematosus, rheumatoid arthritis, periarteritis nodosa, chronic lymphocytic leukemia, lymphosarcoma, polycythemia rubra vera, kala-azar, subacute bacterial endocarditis, coronary artery disease, hepatic cirrhosis, and numerous other diseases. Rarely, the cold-precipitable protein is present in large amounts and is associated with atypical Raynaud phenomena, purpura, bleeding from nose and mouth, retinal hemorrhages, cold sensitivity, cyanosis, mottling, and even gangrene of the lower extremities. Multiple arterial and venous occlusions may occur. Rouleaux formation, pseudoagglutination of the red cells, and an elevated erythrocyte sedimentation rate are likely to be found as well. In most instances of this sort, multiple myeloma has been demonstrated and, rarely, other disorders, such as chronic lymphocytic leukemia. In a few instances no underlying disease entity could be demonstrated (*essential cryoglobulinemia*).

The concentration of cryoglobulin in plasma or serum has ranged from trace amounts to 10 Gm per 100 ml. The amount may vary over the course of the illness in the same patient. The minimum concentration of cryoproteins required for massive reversible precipitation is about 1 Gm per 100 ml. The precipitation of the plasma protein is due to its decreased solubility in the blood and can be demonstrated in vitro. The most commonly occurring cryoglobulins have been found in the gamma fraction, but globulins in the alpha fraction, in the beta fraction, and between the beta and gamma peaks have also shown this property. Molecular weights have ranged from 165,000 to 600,000.

Macroglobulinemia is detectable with certainty only by ultracentrifugal analysis. The molecular weight of the macroglobulins is greater than 1 million. Trace amounts of macroglobulins are present in normal serums. The term *macroglobulinemia* is applied to serums containing more than 5 to 10 per cent of components sedimenting with a Svedberg constant greater than 15. Pathologic macroglobulin molecules have the electrophoretic mobility of β-

or γ-globulins or are intermediate between these two. Occasionally an abnormal plasma protein may be both a cryoglobulin and a macroglobulin.

Macroglobulinemia has been observed in neoplastic diseases, collagen disorders, chronic infections, amyloidosis, and cirrhosis. Serums of multiple myeloma have seldom been reported to show abnormal high molecular weight components. In the syndrome described by Waldenström, *primary macroglobulinemia,* in contrast to multiple myeloma, focal bone lesions are not found, there being at most a diffuse osteoporosis, but slight to moderate lymphadenopathy and hepatosplenomegaly are characteristically encountered. Bone pain is conspicuously absent. In clinical features, primary macroglobulinemia thus resembles lymphosarcoma rather than multiple myeloma. Symptoms and signs of vague ill health, some weight loss, lassitude, dyspnea, and recurrent infections are common, as well as pallor and edema. Sjögren's syndrome (dryness of mucous membranes in eye, nose, mouth, and vagina) has been described in association with macroglobulinemia. Epistaxis and mucosal bleeding are frequent. Anemia, usually normocytic, is present; leukopenia, relative lymphocytosis, sometimes eosinophilia or monocytosis, as well as thrombocytopenia, hemolytic anemia, and pancytopenia have been observed. Bence-Jones proteinuria and paramyloidosis such as are seen in multiple myeloma have been reported. The bone marrow characteristically shows large numbers (40 to 80 per cent) of small, atypical "lymphocytic" cells with protoplasmic shedding and "naked nuclei." The erythrocyte sedimentation rate is markedly elevated. Bleeding time, coagulation time, and prothrombin time may be prolonged, and prothrombin consumption may be impaired. On paper electrophoresis, a symmetric gradient with a narrow, sharp, and high peak in the globulin fraction is found, most often in the γ position. In the latter instances the Sia or water test (see below) is positive.

Pathology and Pathogenesis. In the secondary forms of dysproteinemia and paraproteinemia the pathologic findings are those of the underlying disorder. In the "primary" disorders no specific changes have been noted except for the signs of reticuloendothelial hyperplasia and the bone marrow and lymph node infiltration with small atypical lymphocytes which have been observed in primary macroglobulinemia. When cryoglobulinemia has been present, pulmonary arteriolar obstruction has been described, as well as vascular occlusion elsewhere (kidneys, etc.). Symptoms associated with cryoglobulinemia have been attributed to precipitation of cryoprotein in peripheral blood vessels as well as to cold agglutination of red cells by this protein in vivo. The bleeding tendency has been attributed to intravascular precipitations with secondary capillary damage and, in some cases, to defects in platelet function.

No uniformity in the physicochemical characteristics of macroglobulins has been demonstrated. Macroglobulin peaks in the electrophoretic diagram are sharp and cannot be differentiated from myeloma proteins (Fig. 244-1,*C*). Macroglobulins frequently sediment in the ultracentrifuge as multiple components. Studies of their amino acid composition have shown variations from patient to patient. It is uncertain from immunologic studies whether the macroglobulins and cryoglobulins represent increases of normally occurring protein molecules or denote aberrant protein synthesis.

Plasma cells are thought to be the source of cryoglobulins and atypical lymphocytic cells the source of macroglobulins, but more primitive or more malignant precursors of these cell types are also thought to produce these unusual plasma proteins.

Diagnosis. Hyperproteinemia is found in most cases and is generally attributable to a great increase of globulin, usually γ-globulin. In most instances the globulin fraction amounts to 4 to 8 Gm per cent. The Sia test, which involves mixture of the patient's blood with distilled water and observation of the formation of a precipitate when positive, has not been found to be a reliable screening test for macroglobulinemia. The electrophoretic pattern of severe macroglobulinemia is indistinguishable from that of multiple myeloma. Immunologic diagnosis with antimacroglobulin serum has been successful in most cases studied, but ultracentrifugation should be carried out in suspected cases since it yields the critical evidence.

The diagnosis of cryoglobulinemia offers no particular difficulty, but since cryoglobulins have a wide thermal amplitude, blood for these studies should be drawn into warm syringes and separation of serum or plasma carried out at 37°C. Cold precipitation reversible on warming is characteristic. The differential diagnosis of cryoglobulinemia should include consideration of cryofibrinogens and cold agglutinins.

Macroglobulinemia should be distinguished from *purpura hyperglobulinemica,* characterized by dependent purpura and hypergammaglobulinemia. The characteristic electrophoretic γ-globulin peak in this syndrome is a broad hump, in contrast to the sharp peak of macroglobulinemia.

Prognosis and Treatment. The prognosis in the secondary forms depends upon the nature of the underlying disease process. The primary disorders are compatible with survival for several years. If death occurs it is usually due to severe anemia, complicating infections, or the hemorrhagic diathesis. ACTH or adrenocorticosteroid therapy has sometimes seemed to be helpful.

REFERENCES

Farmer, R. G., T. Cooper, and C. A. Pascuzzi: Cryoglob-
ulinemia, A.M.A. Arch. Internal Med., 106:483,
1960.
Mackay, I. R., N. Eriksen, A. G. Motulsky, and W.
Volwiler: Cryo- and Macroglobulinemia, Am. J.
Med., 20:564, 1956.
Osserman, E. F.: Plasma-cell Myeloma, New Engl. J.
Med., 261:952 and 1006, 1959.

Putnam, F. W.: Plasma-cell Myeloma and Macroglob-
ulinemia, New Engl. J. Med., 261:902, 1959.
Ritzmann, S. E., R. H. Thurm, W. E. Truax, and W. C.
Levin: The Syndrome of Macroglobulinemia,
A.M.A. Arch. Internal Med., 105:939, 1960.
Zinneman, H. H., H. Glenchur, and D. F. Gleason: The
Significance of Urine Electrophoresis in Patients
with Multiple Myeloma, A.M.A. Arch. Internal
Med., 106:172, 1960.

Section 2: The Cardiovascular System

A. DISEASES OF THE VASCULAR SYSTEM

245 HYPERTENSIVE VASCULAR DISEASE

John P. Merrill

Arterial hypertension in man may be arbitrarily divided into two categories: pulmonary hypertension and systemic hypertension (Table 245-1). The more important problems related to pulmonary hypertension are considered in Chap. 262.

Systemic hypertension is the manifestation of an abnormal state of the circulation, just as fever is a sign of altered temperature regulation. The word *hypertension* in itself implies nothing as to the associated prognosis or organic vascular or renal disease. Indeed, the role of elevated blood pressure in the production of aggravation of vascular disease is a disputed but important association which will be discussed separately. As a clinical phenomenon, hypertension may be diagnosed if on repeated examinations the blood pressure is found to be above that considered normal for adolescents of similar racial and environmental background. In North American adults, 140/90 may be regarded as abnormally high arterial pressure; for coolies in Peiping, 125/80 might have a similar significance.

It is now apparent that the hypertensive syndrome has no single clear-cut etiology. Many factors are involved, some of which may be thought of as mere exaggerations of the physiologic mechanisms by which normal arterial pressure is maintained. Others are obviously abnormal in the sense that they play little or no role in normal circulatory regulation and are prominent only in disease states. Any or all of these factors may be involved in any given case of hypertension. It is not surprising, therefore, that in spite of a vast amount of interest and work no single therapeutic agent for the treatment of hypertension has come to light. The physician or student who undertakes to study or treat hypertension must seek to understand the various mechanisms which may be involved when he attempts to evaluate their importance in the individual problem.

FACTORS DETERMINING BLOOD PRESSURE

Blood flow through the normal vascular bed may be thought of as a system in which pulsatile flow occurs in a series of elastic tubes. The larger tubes, represented by the arteries, gradually decrease in caliber through the arterioles to the capillaries and similarly decrease the magnitude of each pulsation until in the capillaries the flow becomes steady. In this system the pulsating force is provided by the contraction of the left ventricle, the elasticity by the walls of the arteries, and the major portion of the resistance to flow by the arteriolar bed. The pressure produced at the peak of ventricular contraction in this elastic system is represented by the systolic blood pressure, and the total resting resistance of the system in ventricular diastole by the diastolic pressure. The difference between these two values is the pulse pressure. The mean arterial pressure is usually thought of as one-half the sum of the systolic and diastolic pressures. However, the true mean pressure, which is the average pressure throughout the cardiac cycle, is not faithfully reflected by this value, since the fall in pressure from the systolic to the diastolic level is not a decline over a steady slope. In measuring the arterial blood pressure, the observer is assessing a

* Any of the conditions associated with diastolic hypertension may become rapidly progressive (malignant).

value which is determined by a number of factors not ordinarily measured directly.

We may consider these factors in order:

1. Since increasing resistance to flow is developed by increasing viscosity, *blood viscosity* is one factor altering blood pressure. Blood viscosity is influenced chiefly by the concentration of the plasma proteins and of the white and red corpuscles suspended in it. Marked polycythemia may thus give rise to hypertension both by reason of increased blood viscosity and by the increased whole blood volume.

2. *The amount of whole blood or plasma in the intravascular compartment* contributes also to the arterial pressure. Since the intravascular fluid except for the blood proteins is continuous across the capillary walls with extracellular fluid in general, the volume of this latter compartment also contributes to arterial blood pressure. Thus severe de-

pletion of either or both compartments by bleeding or acute dehydration will produce hypotension; increase of the volume of either may result in hypertension. An increase in intravascular volume alone, however, may give rise to an increase in neither blood pressure nor cardiac output if the ability of the autonomic nervous system to prevent such change is not exceeded. Failure of the cardiac output to respond to increased intravascular volume may also prevent increase in blood pressure. Possibly for this reason patients with cyanosis and congenital heart disease who have increased blood volumes fail to show hypertension as do many patients with other forms of heart failure who have an increase in blood volume but no increase in blood pressure. Thus modification of one of the factors by another or all of the others may influence the alteration in blood pressure.

3. In a sense, *the rebound of the elastic arterial walls in ventricular diastole* serves to maintain the propelling force of the blood in the interval between systolic contractions. It thus serves, together with the peripheral resistance to flow in the arteriolar bed, to maintain the resting or diastolic pressure in the vascular system. The effect of decreasing elasticity of the large vessel walls may be seen particularly in the elderly arteriosclerotic patient. Here, failure of the rigid vessel wall to distend with the systolic thrust of the heart results in a sudden increase in pressure in the system, producing a high systolic pressure. Similarly, lack of elastic "recoil" results in a rapid drop of pressure in diastole, and this failure to maintain the resting pressure in the vascular bed may be recorded as a low diastolic pressure.

4. An increase in *cardiac output*, such as is mediated through exercise, fever, or thyrotoxicosis, may cause increases in blood pressure by increasing the amount of blood pumped into the vascular system per unit of time. Since the effect is primarily a result of the ventricular contraction, the predominant effect upon blood pressure is an increase of the systolic phase. As a clinical phenomenon, this has much less significance for the hypertensive syndrome than does elevation of the diastolic blood pressure. Decrease in cardiac output secondary to severe myocardial damage results in hypotension. If compensatory vasoconstriction occurs, the diastolic pressure may be relatively well maintained, and the hypotension is characterized by a low systolic and a narrow pulse pressure.

5. The single most important factor in the production of the type of arterial hypertension with which the physician is usually concerned is an *increase in peripheral resistance*. The greatest part of this increase is contributed by the arteriolar segments. Relatively small changes in caliber cause marked changes in resistance, which varies inversely

as the fourth power of the radius of the lumen. Thus a decrease of 10 per cent in the average arteriolar lumen will lead to a rise of 30 per cent in mean arteriolar resistance. The diastolic pressure, which represents the residual resistance in the peripheral vascular bed after systole, more closely reflects the factor of peripheral resistance. As reflecting this factor, elevation of the diastolic pressure is of crucial importance in the syndrome concerned in a study of hypertension in man, though systolic hypertension alone, which may result from several causes of increased stroke volume, may have little bearing in itself. *Decrease* in arteriolar tone secondary to toxins, nervous influence, or drugs results in increase in caliber and may produce *hypo*tension.

Alterations in blood pressure, in either direction, produced by changes in any of the five factors previously mentioned are modified by reflex arcs of the autonomic nervous system. Through vasoconstrictor or vasodilator fibers, these arcs change arteriolar tone and lumen following appropriate stimulation of receptors on the afferent side of the arc. Similar reflex arcs modify the cardiac output. Medullary centers exist for control of cardiac rate as well as for vasoconstrictor and vasodilator effects. These medullary centers in turn may be influenced by higher vasomotor centers situated in the hypothalamus and possibly even in the cerebral cortex. Stimulation of vagal afferent fibers located in the aortic arch and the heart may result in alteration in caliber of the blood vessels through impulses transmitted via these vasomotor centers over efferent fibers to the vasculature. A rise in blood pressure, by stretching special proprioceptors in the aortic wall, is thought to be the stimulus for the resultant depressor response. Similar receptors are located in the carotid sinus. Stimulation of these by increase in pressure may lead to vasodilator responses, whereas decrease in pressure may produce a vasoconstrictor reflex through the afferent limb of the reflex arc. The sinus and aortic nerves are the so-called "buffer nerves" and together make up an important mechanism for controlling arterial blood pressure. The rise in diastolic pressure which occurs when the upright position is assumed is one of the many important manifestations of this control.

INCREASES IN BLOOD PRESSURE SECONDARY TO CHANGES IN ARTERIOLAR CALIBER

From the foregoing, it would appear that factors which influence arteriolar tone and caliber play an important role both in maintaining normal blood pressure and in producing hypertension. The following factors have been thought to be of importance in influencing arteriolar tone.

Decrease in Vasodilator Tone. Some authorities hold that the kidney elaborates a vasodilator substance whose production is impaired in renal disease or nephrectomy. Practical applications of this theory are lacking in the clinical hypertensive syndrome.

Humoral Agents Which Raise Smooth Muscle Tone. For more than half a century, workers in the field of hypertension have been interested in circulating humoral substances whose primary action is to increase arterial tone. Some of these substances have been thought to arise in the central nervous system, but the greatest interest has centered around the release by a kidney, whose blood supply has been compromised (though not made anoxic), of a substance (renin) which, by interaction with a serum globulin, is capable of causing an increase in smooth muscle tone in arterioles. The resultant pressor substance (angiotensin) has been investigated, and in some cases antiserums to renin, which will prevent its action in animals, have been prepared. Serotonin, which causes a variable pressor response, is among many other substances found in the plasma of hypertensive animals. Investigators have isolated from dogs a pressor substance, released from the central nervous system on centripetal vagal stimulation, which has common properties with serotonin and has been postulated as an explanation for the failure of so-called "neurogenic" hypertension to respond to sympathectomy. To the great misfortune of the hypertensive population, the role of all these substances in chronic hypertension in man is still obscure. The hormones of the adrenal medulla, however, are humoral agents which can and do play a well-defined role in some instances of human hypertension. Primarily implicated are epinephrine and its demethylated analogue, norepinephrine. From the physiologic viewpoint, norepinephrine appears more closely associated with the human hypertensive syndrome. Its action is characterized by an increase in peripheral resistance (primarily because of increased small vessel tone) with no increase, or an actual fall, in cardiac output. Functioning tumors of the adrenal medulla and chromaffin tissue elsewhere can closely mimic the clinical picture of hypertensive disease, although in "essential" hypertension blood levels of norepinephrine are not elevated.

Humoral Agents Which Potentiate either Neurotonic or Humoral Tonic Effects. It has been suggested that the kidney may be the site of a vasoexciter material (VEM) which potentiates (in the experimental animal) the response of small arterioles to topical application of epinephrine. Of much greater significance, however, is recent evidence both in the experimental animal and in human beings that the kidney's role in renal hypertension may be its failure to excrete or to metabolize a circulating pressor substance similar to, or identical with, norepinephrine. It has been known for some time that the synthetic analogue of the sodium retaining hormone of the adrenal cortex (DOCA) may potentiate the rise in blood pressure caused by pressor agents. Recent studies on the naturally occurring hormone, aldosterone, have great pertinence for the understanding and therapy of hypertension. Patients with adrenal cortical adenomas secreting excess aldosterone may have hypertension. With bilateral adrenal hyperplasia and excess aldosterone production, *malignant hypertension* is frequent. In these instances not only is the blood pressure markedly elevated but there is coexistent vasculitis. The effect appears not to be due simply to sodium retention since such patients show high urinary sodium excretions and have no increase in blood volume. Patients with malignant hypertension from any cause may show a striking increase in aldosterone excretion. Since such patients invariably have renal vascular involvement, and since the injection of purified angiotensin causes a rise in aldosterone, excretion of the latter may be a secondary result of renal origin.

Nervous Constrictor Influence. As an explanation for the increased peripheral resistance which appears to be common to the hypertensive syndrome almost independent of its etiology, it is natural to inquire into the role of increased vasomotor tone. Increased vasomotor tone and augmented spontaneous vasomotor activity have been observed experimentally under the microscope, and are well known to occur in many hypertensive and prehypertensive patients. Many factors which block or reduce sympathetic tone at cortical levels, such as psychotherapy and sedation, and sympathectomy and sympatholytic drugs at a more peripheral mechanism, tend to decrease blood pressure, Similarly, factors known to augment constrictor nervous influence, such as emotion and chilling, tend to increase blood pressure. The hypertensive individual tends to have an increased pressor response to the infusion of norepinephrine, to cold stimuli (cold pressor test), and to the augmented blood pressure that follows termination of the Valsalva maneuver (Valsalva overshoot). Possibly in some cases the central nervous system participates by elaboration of the humoral agent. It should be remembered, also, that the adrenal medulla is under the influence of nervous stimulation. When the autonomic pathways are interrupted by chemical blockade of the sympathetic ganglions, it has been found that in both normo- and hypertensive patients blood pressure falls are greater when the initial blood pressure is high. In both normo- and hypertensive patients, however, elevation of the blood pressure by the administration of norepinephrine leads to a decrease in the extent of the blood pressure fall which may

be obtained by ganglionic blockade. In spite of the fact that vasomotor activity is not always increased in essential hypertension, it is reasonable to conclude that neurogenic mechanisms play prominent contributory roles. In established hypertension, the vasomotor centers continue to regulate blood pressure levels in response to both pressor and depressor stimuli. In hypertensive individuals, however, the "set" of the regulatory mechanism is at higher levels of blood pressure. Thus, although "fixed" hypertension is rare, nervous influences, however, play a lesser role in well-established or malignant hypertension because of the increased participation of humoral factors, or because of decreased reactivity of the blood vessels secondary to pathologic change.

CONSTITUTIONAL FACTORS IN HYPERTENSION

In attempting to assay the significance of alterations in blood pressure in the light of the various factors which have been delineated, it is most important to remember that range of blood pressure compatible with normal activity and good prognosis may be extremely wide when compared with the range of such parameters as body temperature. This is truer, perhaps, of the systolic than of the diastolic variation, but it is to be emphasized that daily or even hourly fluctuations in blood pressure per se may be without real prognostic significance.

In infancy, arterial pressure may be 70/45. It then rises in late infancy and early childhood to values approximating 80/55, and by adolescence reaches levels of 95 to 110 systolic and 65 to 80 diastolic. The upper limit arbitrarily chosen by many for the "normal" blood pressure in the adult is 140/90. All values cited above are approximations, and fluctuations in either direction may occur without true prognostic significance. Lower values are often diagnosed and treated as "low" blood pressure because of the well-perpetuated myth that "normal" systolic blood pressure should equal the sum of 100 plus chronologic age. Levels based on this formula, however, should be regarded as a statistically common misfortune rather than the ideal concomitant of advancing years. In the absence of obvious causes for true hypotension, values below that proposed by such a formula are, in fact, likely to be correlated with longevity. In more than a third of the population, however, arterial *hypertension*, as manifested by resting blood pressures of 150/90 or above, may be noted as a transient phenomenon in early adult life, and as the usual finding beyond the age of sixty. Although in themselves such increases in blood pressure may be of little significance in any one individual, statistics based on hundreds of thousands can leave no doubt that even occasional rises in resting levels of pulse and blood pressure are associated with a shortening of the life span.

Factors of importance in alterations of arterial blood pressure may also be found in a consideration of race, environment, individual heritage, and state of activity. Thus, hypertension occurs earlier and in a higher percentage of Negroes, both in the United States and in tropical Panama, than in white or Indian populations. Evidence from such surveys suggests that the increased incidence of hypertension may be correlated with an increased incidence of subclinical pyelonephritis. Women develop hypertension slightly more frequently than men but appear to tolerate it better. The basal pressures determined on awakening, before morning activity begins, are lower than during the day: 90/60 in many healthy whites, and 80/50 or less in many natives of the tropics and of Asia. Sitting or standing normally raises the diastolic levels 5 to 10 mm Hg; exercise and hypoxia, or marked anemia, lower the diastolic and raise the systolic level.

Recent statistical studies indicate that, although blood pressure tends to rise with age in the relatives of both hypertensive and nonhypertensive individuals, blood pressure elevations are found earlier in the relatives of the hypertensive population, and tend to remain higher throughout their life span. Similarly, hypertension frequently develops earlier and with greater severity in successive generations with hypertensive predecessors. Whether this predisposition represents an accentuated tendency for blood pressure elevation in hypertensive individuals and their relatives or whether one may interpret such data as an overlapping of two population groups, hypertensive and nonhypertensive, is not at present clear. In those with the hypertensive predisposition, inherited or not, a rise in systolic and diastolic pressures may be caused by chilling, anger, frustration, anxiety, or even pleasant anticipation of an exciting event; whereas others with no predisposition may show no rise, even with the most intense emotional stimuli. The value obtained with the sphygmomanometer is thus only one of the many factors whose importance must be assessed in considering the significance of alterations in blood pressure.

CLASSIFICATION OF HYPERTENSION

A system of classification of hypertension is presented in Table 245-2. It should be noted that systemic hypertension may be differentiated by reason of the phase in which the elevation occurs. Marked elevation of systolic pressure with little or no elevation of diastolic pressure has a different etiologic connotation and, even more important, an entirely

Table 245-2. CURABLE HYPERTENSION

Systolic hypertension only	Combined systolic and diastolic hypertension
Thyrotoxicosis	Brain tumor
Arteriovenous fistula	Unilateral renal disease
Anemia	Adrenal cortical hyperfunction
	Aldosteronism
	Cushing's syndrome
	Pheochromocytoma
	Pituitary tumors
	Coarctation of the aorta
	Increased intravascular volume
	Eclampsia
	Polycythemia

different prognostic significance than does elevation of the diastolic phase. As has been pointed out previously, predominance of systolic elevation depends more upon the factor of cardiac output. Predominance of diastolic elevation is a manifestation of increased residual resistance in the peripheral vascular bed after systole and, as such, more closely represents the clinically significant abnormality in the hypertensive syndrome. The term *essential hypertension* has been employed to indicate those cases of hypertension for which a specific endocrine or renal basis cannot be found, and in which the neural element may be only a mediator of other influences. Since even this latter relationship is not entirely clear, it is more properly listed for the moment in the category of unknown etiology. The term essential hypertension defines simply by failing to define; hence it is of limited use except as an expression of our inability to understand adequately the forces at work. Nevertheless, the bulk of patients with significant and persistent elevation of diastolic pressure form a fairly uniform group for which no well-defined etiologic process has been delineated. From the standpoint of wide acceptance, the term probably should be retained. Unquestionably, cases of essential hypertension in the progressive form may develop a renal component which perpetuates this syndrome as a result of development of vascular lesions in the kidney. The development of vascular lesions here and elsewhere has served for some authors to differentiate *hypertensive disease* from *hypertension,* which latter term connotes only elevation of blood pressure without associated vascular lesions. The prognostic significance of this division is obvious, but the dividing line is often difficult to draw. Essential hypertension may be further subdivided into two types, *benign* and *malignant.* These terms should be employed only as relating to the rapidity and severity of the vascular disease accompanying increased blood pressure levels. The malignant type may be superimposed upon the benign type; occasionally, however, it may be so rapid in onset and so severe in its course as to appear a separate entity. In addition, the severity and rapid progress of vascular disease associated with hypertension primarily renal in origin may justify the term *malignant hypertension*.

Many factors involved in the hypertensive syndrome have now been delineated. It may be permissible to attempt to integrate them in a theoretic case of human "essential" hypertension in a fashion which lays much stress upon the primary role of nervous vasoconstrictor influences. In this idealized view an individual, by reason of inherited traits, including race and sex, may be particularly susceptible to vasomotor reactions resulting from a stressful environment. Specific reasons for this susceptibility might include emotional instability, a labile vasomotor apparatus, possibly including the vasomotor center in the medulla, and a peripheral vasculature which hyperreacts to nervous constrictor stimuli. Such an individual would manifest early in life greater rises in blood pressure in response to environmental stimuli than his fellow born without these genetic traits. Such abnormal responses might be elicited by the cold pressor test and Valsalva maneuver. During early adult life these rises would be more frequent, reach higher levels, and tend less and less to return to so-called "normal" values. The continued stress of pressure upon a genetically sensitive vasculature might then result in small blood vessel changes which would be manifest in the optic fundi and kidneys. With the involvement of the kidneys and possibly the adrenals, a second, humoral mechanism might originate which could then overlay and finally completely dominate the original neurogenic origin. At this point, although the labile vasomotor response might still be elicited, its importance from an etiologic and therapeutic standpoint would be secondary. Such a formulation is admittedly speculative. It does, however, fit many of the observed facts. Although many doubt that increased pressure per se may cause vascular disease, in the author's view, the statistical correlation in mortality tables is too impressive to neglect. By analogy, too, the pulmonary vascular disease that may result from prolonged increased pulmonary arterial pressure with mitral stenosis suggests very strongly that this relationship may obtain.

A second and possibly more important classification has been constructed in Table 245-2. Such a table emphasizes the fact that the physician confronted with the problem of hypertension must think first of those situations in which the hypertension may be associated with a specific defect which may be amenable to specific therapy. A causal relationship of this type may be difficult to establish and may be defined only by the resultant success or failure of therapy. Nevertheless, the opportunity to "cure" hypertension must be sought diligently in each hypertensive patient.

The diagnosis and treatment of *thyrotoxicosis* have been discussed in Chap. 66. The presence of an *arteriovenous fistula* may be manifested by systolic hypertension and a wide pulse pressure, and may be diagnosed by the presence of a murmur or thrill over the site of the abnormal communication. This may be over the peripheral vessels where involved, or a typical "machinery murmur" may be heard over the left precordium in the case of patent ductus arteriosus. Both of these conditions may be amenable to surgical correction.

Adrenal cortical hyperfunction may be manifest by hypertension as well as the other signs of Cushing's syndrome (Chap. 68). Osteoporosis, hirsutism, "buffalo hump," striae, and disorders of glucose metabolism are typical. Hypersecretion of aldosterone and its relation to hypertension are discussed elsewhere in this chapter and in Chap. 68. Patients with hypertension with hypopotassemic alkalosis should be evaluated carefully for this syndrome. Two factors may confuse the diagnosis. The common administration to hypertensive patients of thiazide diuretics may cause potassium depletion. The administration of diets low in sodium may prevent hypopotassemia in hypertensive patients and alkalosis in patients with full-blown hyperaldosteronism.

Pheochromocytoma, though rare, produces a completely curable form of hypertension when surgery is performed before the vascular disease has become irreversible. In spite of such diagnostic techniques as perirenal air injection and retroperitoneal insufflations with oxygen, the newer pharmacologic agents for provocative and blocking tests, the assay of urinary pressor amines and their metabolites (VMA), the diagnosis remains extremely difficult and may be established only by exploration. Pheochromocytoma, in addition to the typical intermittent attacks, may produce a steady hypertension. The problem is discussed further in Chap. 69.

The diagnosis of *coarctation of the aorta*, if considered, will usually be made by comparison of blood pressure in the arm and leg, and appropriate x-rays of the chest may show the typical notching of the ribs.

The problem of unilateral renal disease as a cause of hypertension has received increasing attention with the advent of newer diagnostic methods and forms of surgical therapy. Occlusion of a renal artery or one of its branches should be suspected when malignant hypertension appears suddenly in patients with no previous history. A strong family background of hypertension in a patient with long-standing disease may make the coexistence of a renal lesion and hypertension coincident rather than causal. A marked discrepancy in renal size as indicated by intravenous pyelography is an important clue. If enough functioning parenchyma remains, increased concentration of contrast medium may be evident on the side with the vascular lesion. Obstruction of renal arterial flow may cause hypertension even when intravenous pyelography reveals no difference between the two kidneys. The measurement of the uptake and excretion of radioactive iodopyracet (Diodrast) or iodohippurate sodium (Hippuran) may be made by counters placed over the renal area, following the intravenous injection of the isotope. This has proved an innocuous and frequently helpful screening test. Simultaneous comparison of the function of the two kidneys by samples obtained from each ureter may yield important information, particularly when there is no discrepancy in over-all function as measured by the intravenous pyelogram. Characteristically, the kidney whose arterial inflow is impaired shows a smaller volume of urine with a higher osmolality and creatinine concentration and a lower sodium concentration than on the contralateral side. Translumbar aortography or renal arteriograms made by the injection of contrast media directly into the renal arteries by a catheter passed percutaneously up the femoral artery may directly visualize the affected vessel. None of these tests, however, is infallible, and the data from all of them should be compared before surgical intervention is decided upon. If, at exploration, obstruction of one renal artery is found, with a marked pressure drop across the area of obstruction, and if the contralateral kidney is normal, removal of the affected kidney or the placing of an arterial graft may be curative. Involvement of the contralateral side by vascular disease, however, may militate against surgical cure, even when the obstruction is relieved. With correction of the obstruction, however, hypertension due to mild vascular change on the contralateral side may respond to medical therapy. It is the duty of the internist to keep in mind that mild to moderate hypertensive disease may respond to medical therapy, even when conclusively due to unilateral renal disease. This fact must be weighed carefully against the morbidity and mortality of renal vascular surgery.

Polycythemia, as a cause of increased intravascular volume, may be diagnosed upon estimation of the hematocrit and erythrocyte count. Phlebotomy, the administration of phenylhydrazine hydrochloride, radioactive phosphorus, and irradiation have been used successfully in treatment.

Pituitary tumors, accompanied by hypertension, may be associated with the picture of hyperadrenalism or with that of acromegaly, in which case the characteristic facies, increase in head, hand, and foot size, as well as x-rays of the extremities and sella turcica, may confirm the diagnosis. The therapy of choice is irradiation.

TOXEMIAS OF PREGNANCY

The toxemias of pregnancy are arbitrarily divided into preeclampsia and eclampsia. Eclampsia is characterized by a more severe course and more diffuse lesions; it differs from preeclampsia by the presence of convulsions and coma. The syndrome is manifested by hypertension, proteinuria, and retention of fluid. Common symptoms are headache, visual disturbances, and epigastric pain. In the past the incidence of eclampsia has varied from 0.2 to 1.5 per cent. With better prenatal care, however, this incidence has markedly decreased in recent years. The disease is more common in primiparas than in multiparas, though this may reflect only the decreased tendency of toxemic primiparas to become pregnant again. Diabetes, multiple births, and hydatidiform moles are all reported as increasing the incidence of toxemias. The primary pathologic lesions are seen in the kidneys, and consist of thickening of the walls of the glomerular capillaries and the capillary basement membrane. In the more severe cases, petechial hemorrhages and small areas of necrosis are found in the brain. In severe eclampsia, the liver shows characteristic lesions consisting of irregular areas of hemorrhage and necrosis. This may occasionally be severe enough to produce jaundice. Bilateral symmetric necrosis of the cortices of the kidney occurs most often at the onset of eclampsia. The etiology is still obscure. Many of the reported cases of eclampsia may be simply the aggravation, by the pregnant state, of preexisting essential hypertension or of glomerular nephritis. When these can be shown to be absent in the first 5 months of pregnancy, it is postulated that a toxic or pressor substance formed in the placenta, possibly at the site of placental infarction, may be implicated in the production of the profuse vascular lesions.

Course. True eclampsia or preeclampsia rarely manifests itself before the sixth month of pregnancy. In the cases which are carefully followed, the earliest clues may be headache, anorexia, proteinuria, elevations of blood pressure, and excessive gain in weight. There is frequently some degree of oliguria in eclampsia, and in severe cases, frank renal failure with anuria may supervene. Marked hematuria is not usually seen except in association with cortical necrosis. In the absence of frank renal failure, renal blood flow is usually normal, but there is characteristically a depressed filtration rate. In the severe cases, convulsions are characteristic and may be the cause of death. Termination of pregnancy is usually accompanied by marked improvement, although symptoms may continue for as long as 24 to 36 hr after delivery. The recovery stage is usually characterized by a drop in blood pressure and a profuse diuresis with loss of edema. The prognosis is good in carefully managed patients without severe renal lesions. The internist must concern himself with the possibility of the development of permanent renal disease or hypertension following eclampsia. Unfortunately, there is no agreement on the frequency with which this occurs. In most of the reported series, some renal disease and hypertension persist following eclampsia, but it is not clear whether this is due to aggravation of preexisting renal disease and hypertension, or whether it dates specifically from the eclampsia. Severe previous eclampsia in women over thirty-five contraindicates a further pregnancy. In the presence of slight hypertension or minimal urinary findings, the patient may be allowed to become pregnant and should be carefully followed during her pregnancy, with the possibility of electively terminating it when signs of eclampsia appear. There is no good evidence that normal, well-conducted pregnancy aggravates mild "essential" hypertension if toxemia does not supervene. Patients with preexisting renal disease, however, may do poorly, particularly if functional impairment exists.

The *treatment of toxemia* should be divided into prophylactic and therapeutic measures. Prophylaxis consists of careful surveillance with restriction of sodium to less than 2 Gm per day if edema appears. The treatment of severe eclampsia is the termination of pregnancy. Medical measures are similar to those outlined for the treatment of hypertensive encephalopathy. Magnesium sulfate, as well as protoveratrine and reserpine, have been used with good results. It has been reported that the use of hydralazine (Apresoline) in the hypertensive disease of toxemia of pregnancy is more specific than for other forms of hypertension. Massive doses of penicillin, which appear to exert some antitoxic action, have been used with some success, and good results have been reported from the prophylactic use of stilbestrol.

SYSTEMIC HYPERTENSION

Signs and Symptoms. The signs and symptoms of hypertension can rarely be attributed to the elevated blood pressure itself. A large number of patients with elevated blood pressure may have no symptoms or signs whatever. In the more advanced stages of hypertensive disease, signs and symptoms depend upon the organ involved by the vascular disease accompanying the hypertensive process. These include, of course, cerebral arterial and arteriolar disease, coronary artery disease, congestive

heart failure, and renal failure, which will be discussed in separate chapters. A not infrequent early symptom is the presence of headache. This may take any form but classically is a dull, pounding occipital headache, which is present upon awakening in the morning and tends to wear off during the day. Many patients with hypertension complain of nonspecific difficulties such as weakness, nervousness, flatulence, palpitation, and dizziness. Since hypertensive patients are prone to emotional and psychic difficulties, it is frequently difficult to evaluate these symptoms.

Epistaxis may occur, as well as microscopic and even gross intermittent hematuria accompanied by moderate proteinuria. The latter findings may signify vascular involvement of the kidney, but should alert the physician to the possibility of preexisting renal disease. An important physical finding, which may give some clue to prognosis and progress of the vascular disease, is the change in the vessels of the optic fundi. The damage caused by hypertensive disease is better recognized by a careful study of the retina than by any other means. These changes deserve careful attention and should be accurately described in the patient's record. The physician should note exactly what he sees in the retina and not use one of the grades or classifications currently employed. The grading method is useful for statistical studies by one person or group, but a subsequent examiner cannot be sure that he and the previous examiner understood exactly the same changes implied by a numerical grade. If possible, the lesions when seen should be described as to character and location and, even better, drawn. Early changes in the retinal vessels include diminution in the caliber of the smaller vessels most distal from the disk. A convenient standard of reference is to relate the arteriolar diameter to that of the vein. Generalized constriction or "spasm" of the arterioles may be seen in severe toxemia of pregnancy. A more specific lesion, however, is segmental constriction of the arterioles. This is a permanent lesion and characteristic of significant diastolic hypertension. Tortuosity of the larger vessels close to the disk appears in hypertensive disease, but may also be seen in arteriosclerosis without hypertension, and is of little significance to the hypertensive process itself. Arteriovenous nicking is characteristic of chronic moderate hypertension but may also be seen in those patients with severe elevation of diastolic blood pressure. True arteriovenous nicking requires the presence of an open space between artery and vein on both sides of the artery (Fig. 245-1). Frequently, a darker red area in that portion of the vein just peripheral to the crossing may be seen, representing stasis of venous flow at that point. Since both segmental constriction and arterio-

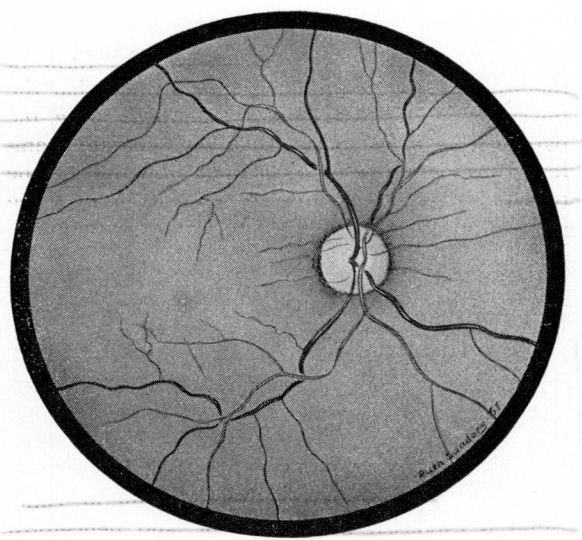

FIG. 245-1. Retinal changes of hypertension—arteriovenous compression and segmental constriction of the arterioles. (*S. A. Shelburne: Ann. Internal Med., 1957.*)

venous nicking are permanent changes, they represent evidence of a preexisting hypertensive state. As such, they may have important diagnostic importance in a patient who at the time of examination has a drop in blood pressure secondary to myocardial infarction or hemorrhage.

An increased light reflex signifies thickening of the vessel wall. With advancing changes, small flame-shaped hemorrhages and glistening white exudates may make their appearance. A serious prognostic sign, indicative of advanced disease, is papilledema, manifested by blurring of the disk margins. This should be particularly evaluated at the temporal margin, since some degree of blurring of the nasal margin may be physiologic. Separation of the retina has been observed in the acute hypertensive episodes of eclampsia. Although somewhat unusual, there may be marked differences in the degree of involvement of the retinas. The visual symptoms usually depend upon the degree of involvement and the location of the lesions.

Patients with hypertensive disease occasionally suffer from acute episodes characterized by marked rise in blood pressure above the previous level, and by disorders of the nervous system which last for minutes, hours, or days, and then disappear without clinical evidence of lasting damage. Such episodes, described as *hypertensive encephalopathy,* are not limited to any single etiologic type of hypertensive disease but are particularly common in association with renal disease, especially where a common factor, such as acute glomerulonephritis or disseminated lupus erythematosus, has produced both vas-

cular lesions and hypertension. Spasm of cerebral vessels is generally thought to be the cause of these attacks, although adequate demonstration of this has yet to be made. Small thrombi and edema play a role in some cases. This syndrome may frequently simulate the hypertensive crises of pheochromocytoma or mimic brain tumor. The clinical syndrome appears in two forms, depending upon whether the disturbances in the nervous system are chiefly of generalized or of focal nature.

The general form usually appears in individuals without previous long-standing hypertension. It may occur in women with eclampsia and in children and young adults with acute glomerulonephritis. Rapidly progressing malignant hypertension is frequently accompanied by hypertensive encephalopathy. Aside from a rapidly rising blood pressure, the attacks are characterized by headache, visual disturbances which may progress to blindness, papilledema, vomiting, stupor, coma, stertorous breathing, psychoses, and convulsions. All these manifestations may be hastened and enhanced by the administration of excessive amounts of fluid.

The focal type of hypertensive encephalopathy may appear in any individual with chronic hypertension, but is especially frequent in older individuals and in the malignant form of the disease. Loss of consciousness, convulsions, and paralysis involving one-half of the body are especially common, and the clinical picture, though reversible, may exactly resemble cerebral vascular accident due to hemorrhage, thrombosis, or embolism, at the beginning. The differentiation may be impossible until the patient has been observed for a number of hours or even for several days.

Prognosis in Hypertension. Few problems in clinical medicine are as difficult or as controversial as the evaluation of the prognosis for any individual patient with early but marked hypertension. Although the statistics of the insurance companies clearly indicate that, in general, the mortality experience is increasingly unfavorable with progressive elevation of the blood pressure, individual variation in tolerance to hypertension and hypertensive disease is marked. A few of the factors affecting prognosis have already been mentioned. In Table 245-3 are listed factors which are known to affect adversely the prognosis in patients with hypertension. These are listed in order of increasing gravity. Systems of classification of hypertension, characterizing the disease in varying grades of severity and with varying prognoses, have been devised on the basis of (1) retinal changes and (2) a combination of the factors listed in Table 245-3, plus phenolsulfonphthalein excretion and response to sedation. It can be concluded that young male patients of racial origins known to be susceptible to hypertensive disease, with high, relatively fixed

Table 245-3. FACTORS INDICATING AN ADVERSE
PROGNOSIS IN HYPERTENSION

Negro origin
Youth and male sex
Persistent diastolic pressure > 110
Marked cardiac enlargement
ECG changes of ischemia or left ventricular strain
Renal functional impairment
Retinal hemorrhages and exudates
Angina pectoris
Myocardial infarction
Cerebrovascular accident
Congestive heart failure
Marked retinal arteriolar sclerosis
Nitrogen retention*
Papilledema

* Nitrogen retention, when due to vascular disease of
the kidney, indicates a very grave prognosis. Its occurrence in primary renal disease with only mild hypertension may be less important.

diastolic pressures, are apt to do badly. On the
other hand, women apparently tolerate elevated
blood pressure and even hypertensive vascular diseases better than do men. Every physician interested in hypertensive disease has followed women
and an occasional man through many years of relatively good health with persistent diastolic pressures of 120 mm or more. The degree of retinopathy may give some clue as to the prognosis, although this, in general, is a better guide to the
progress than to the ultimate prognosis, since even
severe retinopathy may be reversed occasionally by
appropriate therapy, and rarely improves spontaneously. Papilledema and renal insufficiency are extremely grave prognostic signs in every instance.
The occurrence in the hypertensive patient of myocardial infarction, congestive heart failure, or cerebral vascular accident signifies a poor prognosis,
although, again, every hypertensive clinic has its
share of patients constituting exceptions to this general rule. Emotional instability, while making the
treatment somewhat more difficult, does not otherwise affect prognosis itself. Poor response to adequate treatment of any sort, including failure to
correct obesity, frequently indicates impaired prognosis.

Diagnosis. The diagnosis of hypertension may be
made with a blood pressure cuff, and the diagnosis
of hypertensive vascular disease by the usual methods for evaluating the cardiovascular system, kidneys, and optic fundi. The differential diagnosis
should, from the very first, include disease states
giving rise to hypertension for which more specific
therapy exists. A list of these, which should be
considered during the first evaluation of any hypertensive problem, is given in Table 245-2.

Treatment

Principles of Therapy. Whatever the form of
therapy selected, it must not be forgotten that the
physician who treats hypertension is treating the
patient as a whole rather than the separate manifestations of a disease. The first principle of the
therapy of hypertension is the knowledge of when
to treat and when not to treat. Two essentially opposing viewpoints are maintained in this regard,
with various shades of opinion in between. Both
agree that the accelerated phase of hypertension
with a high diastolic pressure, and rapid progress of
vascular lesions in the retinas, heart, and kidneys,
markedly affects the prognosis and justifies any form
of treatment aimed at lowering the blood pressure,
except in the presence of marked nitrogen retention. The differences are sketched in Table 245-4.

The viewpoint indicated on the right in Table
245-4 is espoused by the author, and henceforth
the discussion of therapy will be oriented from this
point of view.

Selection of Patients for Therapy. In the decision
to institute treatment, the factors delineated in the
paragraph on prognosis must bear considerable
weight. Factors of increasing gravity, shown in
Table 245-3, are increasingly important indications
for specific therapy. Frank nitrogen retention, however, may contraindicate and obviate any specific
form of depressor therapy. Sudden, marked, and
persistent elevation of diastolic pressure may precede signs and symptoms and, as such, indicates
need for therapy. A knowledge of when to withhold specific treatment is equally important. A
woman who has tolerated her diastolic pressure of
120 for 10 years without symptoms or deterioration
does not need immediate specific treatment for
hypertension. Marked elevation of systolic pressure,
with little or no rise in diastolic, does not constitute
an indication for depressor therapy. This is particularly true in the elderly or arteriosclerotic patient,
even though the diastolic pressure may also be
moderately elevated. A trial of mild forms of therapy, including psychotherapy, reducing diets, sedation, or mild depressor agents, which fails to
improve signs or symptoms, may justify more intensive forms of therapy. The physician must, however, carefully weigh the value of making his patient "blood pressure conscious" by a specific regimen and regular follow-up, against real need for
any particular form of therapy. Above all, in treatment or prognostication, he must avoid engendering
in the patient a fear of the disease which may be
unwarranted in our present state of knowledge.
Promising therapies are available, however, and it
should be remembered that the forms of treatment
are not mutually exclusive. Particularly, it should
be remembered that the confidence, patience, and

Table 245-4. OPPOSITE VIEWPOINTS ON THERAPY OF HYPERTENSION

The exact level of the blood pressure may have little clinical significance, since it correlates poorly with the incidence of vascular disease and with mortality figures. Treatment of hypertension per se is unjustified.

Spontaneous remissions of hypertensive vascular disease, tolerance of it, and response to nonspecific therapy make results of specific hypotensive therapy difficult to evaluate. In a few cases vascular disease has progressed in hypertensive individuals in spite of the fact that adequate lowering of the blood pressure has been obtained with hypotensive agents.

The dangers and side effects of "specific" therapy may be worse than the natural course of the disease.

The level of diastolic pressure may not correlate with vascular disease or mortality in the individual, but in a large series it can be statistically shown to shorten the life span.

In spite of the variables, irreversible fatal vascular disease may result from essential hypertension. There is reason to believe that elevation of the diastolic pressure contributes to this, and in the absence of knowledge of other factors and with the ability to lower blood pressure with specific therapy, attempts to lower pressure seem justified in properly selected cases.

Various effective forms of hypotensive therapy exist, including psychotherapy. It is justifiable to apply mild therapy to mild forms of hypertension, and since the problems and dangers of therapeutic methods increase with increasing order of efficacy, they may be justified in severe forms of the disease. In experienced hands specific forms of therapy, even though dangerous, need not be delayed until irreversible changes have taken place.

enthusiasm of the physician are important ingredients in any form of therapy. The hypertensive process being what it is, this factor undoubtedly accounts in large part for the varying degrees of success achieved by different investigators with the same therapeutic program.

Symptomatic Therapy. Improvement in symptoms, as well as blood pressure levels, frequently results from adequate psychotherapy (see below). For the relief of hypertensive headache, elevation of the head of the bed during the night is usually beneficial. Thiocyanate salts have been used with some success, although the necessity for carefully checking blood levels of this drug to prevent toxicity has greatly decreased its usefulness. Not infrequently a cup of black coffee or the administration of 200 to 400 mg caffeine as the citrate or sodium benzoate salt, given on arising, may help the hypertensive headache. Periodic venesection has met with occasional success in alleviating headache and dizzy spells. Small amounts of sedation in properly selected patients may be of some value. They should be carefully evaluated after preliminary therapeutic trial for the undesirable side effects. With renal failure, the short-acting barbiturates Seconal and Amytal are preferable to phenobarbital, since they do not require the renal route for their excretion. Because sedation may play a more fundamental role in hypertension than that of symptomatic therapy, its use becomes a highly individualized problem. The administration of 30 mg phenobarbital three to four times a day to one patient may well dull the knife-edge of anxiety and result in improvement. In other individuals, the mental confusion that may result, as well as the necessity for taking medica-

tion continually, may do more harm than good. The conscientious executive, faced with a problem which he is capable of solving with a clear head, does not benefit his hypertensive disease by grappling with his problem under the influence of sedatives which cloud his thinking. Such situations must be carefully assessed on their individual merits. The tranquilizing agents (Miltown, Equanil) may be useful in allaying anxiety and tension without impairing critical faculties.

Psychotherapy. A majority of patients with essential hypertension have disorders of personality which may be aggravated by environmental or emotional stress resulting in conflicts and anxiety which may be correlated with fluctuations in blood pressure. Although there is little agreement on the specific personality patterns involved, such emotional contributions may be recognized frequently; they are particularly evidenced in the tense, anxious individual with marked fluctuations in blood pressure. In such cases, psychotherapy alone has produced results equal to the best of other forms of therapy. It is, moreover, an indispensable adjunct to them. Intensive psychotherapy may not be necessary and, indeed, should not be undertaken unless it can be followed to completion, since the early part of the exhaustive psychiatric approach may often be followed by exacerbation of hypertension. One should not underestimate the value of the psychotherapy resulting from a good physician-patient relationship. It is probable that just this resulted in the improvement in hypertension attributed to nostrums such as watermelon seed and garlic. It follows from this example, however, that an emotionally labile patient, with numerous emotional problems and psychosomatic complaints, cannot always be told—because of the absence of vascular or renal disease—simply to forget his problems. In the vast majority of instances, a discussion of the problem with reassurances fortified by mild medication and follow-up visits at infrequent but regular intervals will do more good.

Dietary Management. Obesity is frequently a sign as well as a complication of the hypertensive personality. Since it has an undoubted adverse effect upon prognosis and progress of the disease, it should be specifically treated by an adequate weight-reducing regimen, such as has been outlined in Chap. 22. The patient should fully understand the necessity for this regimen without being frightened by it.

There can be no question but that, in the hands of certain workers, diets low in sodium and in protein have resulted in striking amelioration of hypertensive vascular disease. Of these, the so-called "rice diet," containing 200 mg sodium, 25 Gm protein, and approximately 2000 nonprotein calories, is an example. Recent work has indicated that it is the low sodium content rather than the protein deficiency that is responsible for the beneficial results. The true rice diet probably does not maintain nitrogen balance, and it must be strictly adhered to for at least 6 to 8 weeks, during which time most patients find it extremely unpalatable. More palatable diets may be planned which contain less than 600 mg sodium chloride per 24 hr, and among several excellent booklets on this subject, one is prepared for the patient by the American Heart Association. For the treatment of hypertension per se, 0.5 Gm sodium chloride constitutes a maximal dietary salt intake, although congestive heart failure and edema per se may respond at slightly higher levels. Cation exchange resins, which prevent absorption of dietary sodium, have been used with success to effect decreased sodium absorption from diets containing more than 1 Gm ingested sodium chloride, and the thiazide diuretics are an additional adjunct. Such programs may make meals more palatable for many patients, particularly with the judicious use of one of the salt substitutes. The usual precautions should be observed with the ingestion of cation exchange resins. A low sodium intake may effectively potentiate the effect of other forms of treatment, both surgical and pharmacologic.

Drug Therapy. The rationale for the use of drugs which lower blood pressure is based on the belief that prolonged, marked elevation of systemic arterial pressure is in itself harmful, and may contribute to and hasten the vascular lesions. While this view is regarded with skepticism by some, there can be no question but that there are well-documented cases in which the use of depressor drugs

has aborted or reversed progressive changes of malignant hypertension. Furthermore, there is evidence that patients with severe hypertension whose blood pressure has been effectively lowered by drug therapy over a period of 3 to 4 years may then be maintained on gradually decreasing doses and eventually no drug at all. Since peripheral resistance is the most important of the factors which determine the level of the blood pressure, hypotensive agents, to be effective therapeutically, should act by decreasing resistance rather than by decreasing cardiac output or flow. The introduction of hypotensive agents with varying sites of action has provided the physician with a new approach to medical therapy of hypertension. These drugs, although effective, require of the physician a thorough knowledge of the disease as well as of the agent employed. In Table 245-5 are listed in some detail the important properties of currently available hypotensive agents which the author believes to be worthy of trial when hypotensive therapy is indicated. The use of sodium thiocyanate and nitroprusside, whose actions are similar, has been found by some to be effective in the treatment of hypertensive headache and in lowering of arterial pressure. Because of the necessity for controlling blood levels, however, their use is not widespread.

Of the agents listed in Table 245-5, the ganglionic blocking agents are of extreme and unquestioned potency. Their side effects, however, as well as the need for careful control by frequent blood pressure readings suggest that their use should be relegated to the severer forms of hypertensive vascular disease. The uncertain absorption from the gastrointestinal tract of some of the blocking agents listed in the table constitutes an additional difficulty, although this particular objection appears to be overcome by mecamylamine (Inversine), which is completely absorbed. A significant advance in therapy is represented by the introduction of two agents, *guanethidine* and *bretylium tosylate,* whose action is apparently specific for the postganglionic nerve terminals. In effect, the sympathetic impulses are blocked, leaving unopposed parasympathetic action, thus minimizing those undesirable side effects of the ganglionic blockers which are specifically related to parasympathetic blockade. Of these two agents, guanethidine appears to be somewhat preferable because of its more gradual and prolonged action. The widespread use of the thiazide diuretics to potentiate the action of other hypotensive agents is another significant advance. There appears to be little difference between the various substituted thiazides except in the dosage required. One exception to this is the drug *chlorthalidone* (Hygrotron), whose action appears to be more gradual and prolonged than the other thiazides. Sympathetic blockade usually results in a decrease

Table 245-5. DRUGS USED IN THERAPY OF HYPERTENSION

Drug	Site of action	Pharmaco-dynamics	Dosage*	Special indications	Contra-indications	Side effects
Hydralazine (Apresoline)	Central vasodilator + Adrenergic blockade	Vasodilation. Increased cardiac output Increased renal blood flow ($\pm$) Tachycardia	Oral: 10–200 mg 4 i.d. Tolerance ++	As an adjunct with methonium compounds and protoveratrine	Coronary artery disease Peptic ulcer (?)	(1) Arthritis, lupus (2) Headache, edema, nausea, tachycardia (3) Unopposed cholinergic hyperacidity *Rx: (1) Stop drug, (2) antihistaminics, (3) aluminum hydroxide gels*
Ganglionic blocking agents:	Blocks autonomic transmission at ganglion	Sympathetic and parasympathetic inhibition (orthostatic hypotension with compensatory tachycardia, decreased intestinal motility, etc.)	. . . .	In moderate to severe hypertension As medical sympathectomy (?)	Coronary artery disease Arteriosclerosis Diabetes Glaucoma Prostatism	(1) Constipation, visual symptoms (2) Urinary retention (3) Impotence *Rx: Decrease dose, (1) cathartics, (2) bethanechol (Urecholine)*
Pentolinium (Ansolysen)		Variable absorption from GI tract	Oral: 10–70 mg q. 6–8 hr SC: 2–10 mg q. 4–8 hr			
Chlorisondamine (Ecolid)	. . . .	. . . .	Oral: 25–100 mg q. 12 hr SC: 2–10 mg q. 8 hr			
Mecamylamine (Inversine)	. . . .	Complete absorption	SC: 2–10 mg q. 8–12 hr			Tremor
Protoveratrine	Stimulates afferent side of vagal reflex	Fall in BP Bradycardia Cerebral resistance Renal resistance Cardiac output unchanged	Oral: 0.5–1.5 mg p.c. breakfast plus 0.5 mg p.c. lunch and supper IV: 1.5–1.9 µg/kg IM: 4–6 µg/kg q. 6–8 hr	Hypertensive encephalopathy Hypertensive pulmonary edema	Intolerance Coronary artery disease (?)	(1) Epigastric oppression, nausea, vomiting, salivation (2) Angina (?) (3) Arrhythmias *Rx: Decrease dose, (1) atropine, chlorpromazine (Thorezine), (2) ephedrine for hypotension*
Reserpine (Serpasil) (crystalline alkaloid of *Rauwolfia serpentina*)	Central sedative effect Central inhibition of pressor reflexes Direct peripheral vascular action (?)	Central sedation Mild hypotension Increased intestinal motility Miosis Full action requires 3–6 days	Oral: 0.1–0.5 mg t.i.d. Tolerance $\pm$	As adjunct to other drugs Alone, in labile neurotic hypertensives 2–5 mg daily in hypertensives with renal failure	Elderly depressed patients	(1) Sedation (2) Diarrhea (3) Bradycardia (4) Nightmares (5) Nasal congestion (6) Weight gain, increased appetite (7) Depression *Rx: Decrease dose*
Phenoxybenzamine (Dibenzyline)	Adrenergic blockade Blocks circulating catechol amines (epinephrine, norepinephrine)	Prevents action of adrenergic mediators (epinephrine, norepinephrine) Miosis Orthostatic hypotension	Oral: 20–120 mg q.i.d. Tolerance ++	As adjunct In hypertension with renal failure	Angina pectoris	(1) Miosis (2) Dry mouth (3) Nasal congestion (4) Impotence (5) Tachycardia *Rx: Decrease dose*
Bretylium tosylate (Darenthin)	Blocks postganglionic sympathetic fibers	Sympathetic inhibition (orthostatic hypotension) Parasympathetics intact	Oral: 0.25–2.0 Gm q.i.d. IV 0.5 mg/kg	Moderate to severe hypertension	Coronary disease Glaucoma Arteriosclerosis Pheochromocytoma	Facial pain, parotitis, impairment of ejaculation, abdominal pain, visual blurring
Guanethidine (Ismelin)	Blocks postganglionic sympathetic fibers	Sympathetic inhibition (orthostatic hypotension) Parasympathetics intact Prolonged effect	Oral: 10–80 mg per day IV 0.5 mg/kg	Moderate to severe hypertension	Coronary disease Glaucoma Arteriosclerosis Pheochromocytoma	Facial pain, parotitis, impairment of ejaculation, abdominal pain, visual blurring
Monamine oxidase inhibitors (iproniazid, carboxazid)	Blocks destruction of monamines	Orthostatic hypotension	Oral: iproniazid 50–150 mg per day	Coronary disease	Coronary disease Glaucoma Arteriosclerosis Pheochromocytoma	Flushing, dizziness, confusion
α-Methyl DOPA	Inhibits decarboxylation of aromatic amino acids	Reduction of amine Biosynthesis	Oral: 0.25–2.0 Gm t.i.d.	?	?	Sedation, fatigue

* Tolerance ++ indicates a strong likelihood that the dose will eventually need to be increased in order to maintain a given effect.

in peripheral resistance, with decreases in cerebral and renal blood flow. Frequently, the cardiac output may fall. For this reason, these agents may be hazardous in cerebral, renal, and coronary vascular disease. Since the blood pressure fall produced by these agents is most marked in the upright position, it may be of value to test their effects upon the electroencephalogram and the electrocardiogram, when the desired fall in blood pressure is achieved by gradual assumption of the upright posture on a tilt table. Decreased sensitivity or tolerance to all these agents has been reported. Because of its effect in increasing renal blood flow, Apresoline may be an important adjunct to the use of the blocking agent. The increase in renal blood flow which occurs with Apresoline, however, is not entirely consistent and results in part from increased cardiac output, in which the renal share of the cardiac output may be actually increased. The production of a syndrome resembling rheumatoid arthritis and disseminated lupus erythematosus with the prolonged use of Apresoline is now well documented. Although, usually, this syndrome is reversible with cessation of therapy, in a few instances persistence of the disease has occurred following cessation of the drug.

The thiazide diuretics potentiate the action of other antihypertensive drugs through their natruretic action and, possibly, through some direct action on the vasculature. The various substituted thiazides differ in dosage, but are essentially similar in their mode of action. The one exception is chlorthalidone, whose action is more prolonged, requiring only a single daily dose, varying from 100 to 600 mg.

Dramatic and unquestioned therapeutic results have been obtained with the use of these substances. They are toxic and dangerous in excessive dosage, however, and the margin between the toxic and the therapeutic dose is relatively narrow; hence, all such therapy should be begun in the hospital. The hypotensive agents selected should be administered initially in less than effective dosage and increased slowly, until either the desired therapeutic effect or toxicity supervenes. As with insulin therapy it may be wise, under controlled conditions in the hospital, to familiarize the patient with mild toxic effects so that they can be recognized. Alternate dosage with the initial agent and one of the others, or preferably the potentiation of the depressor effect of the initial agent by the addition of small doses of another drug, may increase the depressor effect while decreasing the side effects inherent in both. Such a combination, too, may minimize the effect of tolerance to either agent. Experience suggests that the concurrent use of two or three of these agents with different sites of action

may be the method of choice. When the patient's dosage has been established in the hospital, he may be seen at less frequent intervals on the outside, and the therapeutic effects may be increased without increasing toxic effects by the addition of a third agent or by the substitution of a new agent for one of the two when tolerance becomes apparent. Potentiation of depressor effect can be achieved also by decreasing the sodium content in the diet. Cessation of therapy should never be abrupt, since dangerous hypertensive rebounds may result. The necessity for carefully controlling the use of these agents carries with it the disadvantage of making the patient drug conscious and blood pressure conscious. Once he has become familiar with the drugs, however, and confident of their therapeutic benefits he may learn to regulate them by taking his own blood pressure in the same manner that an intelligent diabetic regulates his insulin by testing his urine.

The presence of advanced renal failure contraindicates the use of the drugs listed here with the possible exception of small doses of Dibenzyline (10 to 20 mg t.i.d.). This appears to be useful in hypertension with renal failure, possibly through its action on unexcreted pressor amines. In mild renal failure, large doses of reserpine (2 to 5 mg per day) or the combined use of ganglion block and Apresoline may be of value. In properly selected cases, an initial increase in nitrogen retention may be followed later by improvement in renal function, although at considerably decreased blood pressure levels. The sites of action of the various depressor agents are shown schematically in Fig. 245-2.

Surgical Therapy. In the past, interruption of the autonomic pathways by sympathectomy, particularly by the lumbodorsal technique of Smithwick, has produced a convincing decrease in mortality in some severe cases of hypertensive vascular disease. This treatment should probably be reserved until after drug and/or dietary treatment has been tried and failed or been rejected. In this sense, its value has the same relationship to medical therapy as does the surgical treatment of peptic ulcer. Undesirable side effects of sympathectomy are postural hypotension and disturbance of sexual function in the male. Renal failure, cerebral vascular accidents, and congestive heart failure are contraindications. Bilateral total adrenalectomy as a treatment for hypertension is still in the process of evaluation, but may be of value in intractable congestive heart failure with minimal renal functional impairment.

Pyrogens. It has been reported that a prolonged course of high fever induced by the intravenous administration of pyrogens may be effective in some cases of malignant hypertension. This is drastic

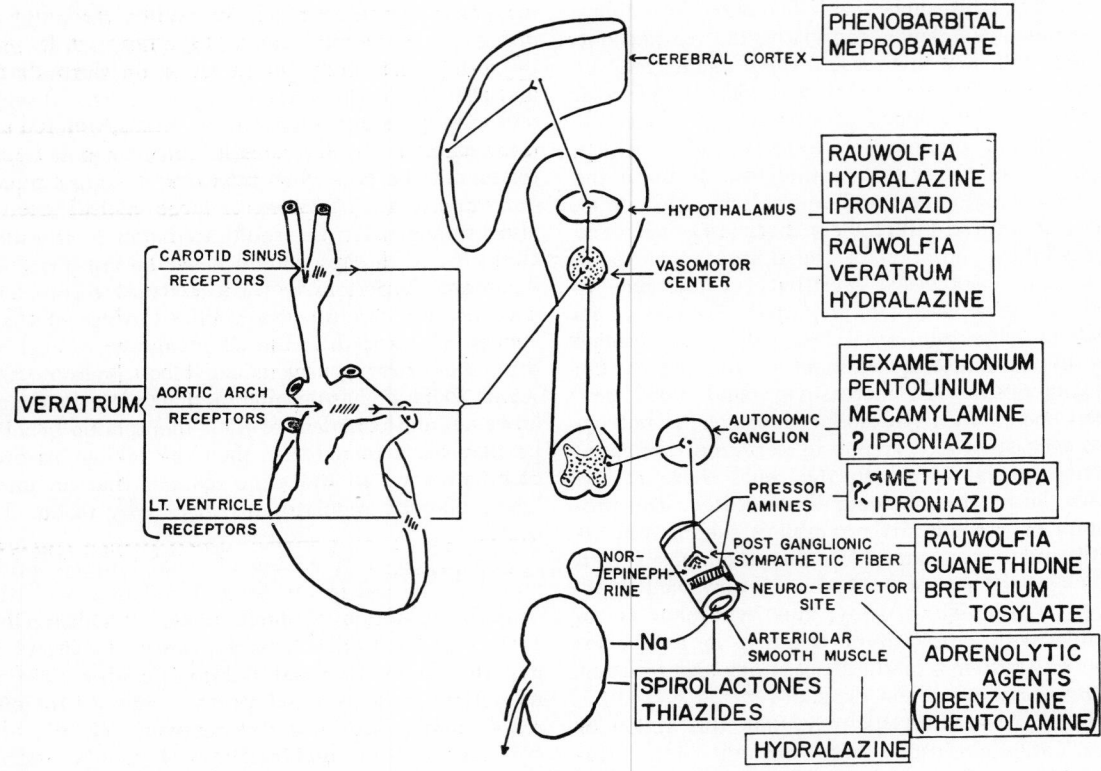

FIG. 245-2. Sites of action of the antihypertensive drugs.

treatment for a drastic disease state, and should be carried out only under the supervision of those with some degree of experience in this technique.

Treatment of Hypertensive Encephalopathy. The incidence and clinical picture of hypertensive encephalopathy have been described earlier in this chapter. Although in certain cases hypervolemia may contribute greatly to the abnormality, the common denominator is hypertension due largely to generalized vasospasm. It is rational, therefore, to attempt to lower the diastolic blood pressure by pharmacologic means. This may be done effectively in children, and in a small percentage of young adults, by the intramuscular injection of a 50 per cent solution of magnesium sulfate, in doses of 0.2 ml per kg body weight. This may have to be repeated several times at 4-hr intervals, to keep pressure at satisfactory levels, following which the oral administration of 13 to 30 ml of 50 per cent magnesium sulfate two to three times a day may satisfactorily control the blood pressure. If intravenous injection is necessary, a 3 per cent solution of hydrated magnesium sulfate may be given slowly; 150 mg of the salt per kg of body weight is given over a period of 1 hr. The effects of overdosage (somnolence, respiratory difficulty) may be counteracted by the administration of a 10 per cent so-

lution of calcium gluconate by vein. Oxygen therapy, sedatives, and occasionally, venesection and spinal tap may be useful. Dramatic results have been observed with the use of intravenous or intramuscular protoveratrine or with large doses (2 to 5 mg of parenteral reserpine), and with the continuous drip of an aqueous solution of trimethaphan (Arfonad), a rapidly acting, short-lived ganglionic blocking agent whose effect by this route can be easily controlled by the rate of the drip.

REFERENCES

Brown, J. J., K. Owen, W. S. Peart, J. I. Robertson, and D. Sutton: The Diagnosis and Treatment of Renal-artery Stenosis, Brit. Med. J., 2:347, 1960.

Connor, T. B., W. C. Thomas, L. Maddock, and J. E. Howard: Unilateral Renal Disease as Cause of Hypertension: Its Detection by Ureteral Catheterization Studies, Ann. Internal Med., 52:544, 1960.

Laragh, J. H. M.: The Role of Aldosterone in Man, J.A.M.A., 174:293, 1960.

Moyer, S. H. (Ed.): "First Hahnemann Symposium on Hypertensive Disease," Philadelphia, W. B. Saunders Company, 1959.

New Diuretics and Antihypertensive Agents: Symposium, Ann. N.Y. Acad. Sci., 88:771, 1960.

Page, I. M., H. B. Dustan, and E. F. Poutasse: Diagnosis and Treatment of Hypertension of Renal Vascular Origin, Ann. Internal Med., 51:196, 1959.

Shelburne, S. A.: The Retina in Hypertensive Disease, Ann. Internal Med., 47:1154, 1957.

246 ARTERIOSCLEROSIS
William Dock

The pathologist recognizes many types of arteriosclerosis, but clinical disorders due to noninfectious, noninflammatory arterial disease result mainly from atherosclerosis. Even with this condition, pathologic lesions may be widespread and the x-ray may reveal chalk in the aortic knob, the coronary arteries, or the abdominal aorta and its main branches, with not the slightest impairment of bodily function.

The media of the arteries of men and animals show varying degrees of loss of muscular and elastic elements as age advances, and with this the vessels become tortuous and dilated. This change, affecting temporal and splenic arteries and the aorta, may be well advanced by the fourth decade of life. A similar change in the walls of the veins predisposes them to varicosity and to formation of hemorrhoids. But in the arteries neither this medial change nor medial calcification, which is less frequent and occurs later in life, leads to occlusion of the lumen or rupture of the wall. The involutional changes in the media have few or no clinical sequelae.

When age or involution of parenchymal or muscular organs leads to atrophy or, in the brain, to progressive loss of neurones, the vascular bed atrophies and the intima proliferates. A lumen adequate for the needs of the shrunken organ remains, but intimal thickening, free of lipid and physiologically harmless, may lead the unwary pathologist to ascribe atrophy to arteriosclerosis. This is most often said of the cerebrum; in the uterus or ovaries atrophy is accepted as a "normal" concomitant of aging and not blamed on intimal thickening, which is secondary to disuse.

All the changes mentioned above are seen in aged mammals; they are usually bilaterally symmetrical and widely disseminated or diffuse. This contrasts strikingly with the patchy atheromas, lipid-rich intimal thickenings, which occur very rarely in aged wild or domestic animals or even in primitive or very poor populations but are apparent by the age of forty in the bodies of most prosperous people, on the diets usual in North America and Western Europe. As noted by Lober, the process of lipid deposition in the intima of coronary arteries begins with suckling and in our culture continues throughout life. In rabbits, and in most human populations, lipid deposition ends with weaning, and the deposits are reabsorbed during growth.

Many species of birds and mammals, well fed and growing old in the crowded zoos, have atheromatous arteries, and wild omnivorous baboons have similar lesions. Occlusion of large critical arteries, such as the coronaries and cerebrals, is extremely rare in such instances. In India and in Morocco coronary disease, uncommon even in the prosperous, is very rare in the mass of undernourished people. These differences in incidence in the rich and poor were striking in America before 1920, and also in Russia, where they led Ignatovsky to feed rabbits eggs and butter, and thus initiate the experimental production of atheroma by dietary manipulation, in 1907.

DIET, PLASMA LIPIDS, ATHEROSCLEROSIS, AND THROMBOGENESIS

In the past two decades it has become evident that diets rich in saturated fats (beef, butter, coconut oil) cause an elevation in plasma lipids, including phospholipids, triglycerides, and cholesterol. Unsaturated fats (corn or cottonseed oil, fish oils) and low-fat diets barely adequate to meet caloric needs cause a fall in these lipids. Human populations, shifted from diets rich in saturated fats to those low in these items, show a fall in rate of postoperative thromboembolism and in myocardial infarction. Negroes living on low-fat diets in Uganda and coming to necropsy at ages over forty, had less than 10 per cent the incidence of myocardial scars and infarcts or thrombi in veins and lungs as Negroes of the same age in Missouri, living on American diets rich in pork, butter, and eggs. Rats on atherogenic diets (added cholesterol, bile salt, thiouracil) developed a high rate of coronary and renal artery thrombosis if the dietary fat was butter, a very low incidence if fed the same amount of corn oil.

Diets rich in saturated fat cause the liver to excrete relatively little bile salt, a degradation product derived from cholesterol, and abundant cholesterol, while diets rich in unsaturated fats have the reverse effect. Cholesterol is constantly synthesized by vertebrates, but the amount secreted in bile and reabsorbed from the gut has a large influence on the plasma lipid level. Because diets low in animal fat, rich in vegetable oil lead to secretion of abundant cholate, which has a detergent-like action and renders cholesterol more soluble, cholesterol stones rarely form in those adhering to such diets. In populations living on diets rich in animal fat, as in North America, there is a variation in plasma cholesterol, in healthy adults, from 150 mg per 100 ml to above 600. Levels over 300 usually indicate familial hyperlipemia, with high triglyceride levels in most cases, or pure familial hypercholesterolemia. Such patients, on low-fat cholesterol-free diets, have daily biliary excretion of cholesterol higher than those with plasma cholesterol levels under 250 mg per 100 ml. Fortunately, many of the hyperlipemics show a striking drop in all lipid fractions on diets with a liberal intake of polyunsaturated fatty acids.

Cholesterol added to diets merely augments the effect of the saturated fats in some species, but in rabbits and chicks cholesterol alone, added to a diet rich in unsaturated fat, raises plasma lipid and causes rapid atherogenesis. Since most of the cholesterol-rich foods (brain, egg yolk, butter) also are rich in saturated fats, the "low cholesterol diet" emphasized by some physicians before 1950 was also a diet low in saturated fat and in many patients did actually reduce plasma lipid levels. Today, substitution of corn or cottonseed oil for butter, and fish for beef and pork, is usually recommended and has proved more effective than low-fat diets.

While diet and elevated levels of cholesterol and triglyceride are of established importance both in atherogenesis and thrombogenesis, many remarkable deviations from a simple diet → plasma lipid → vascular disease pattern remain unexplained. Thus baboons develop atheromas with blood cholesterol levels of 40 to 100 mg per 100 ml, rabbits only when the level is over 150, dogs only when it is over 400 mg per 100 ml. The α-lipoproteins of the plasma stabilize or hold in solution triglyceride while β-lipoproteins, poorer in lecithin and phosphorus, appear to form atheromas. Dog plasma has a relatively low ratio of β- to α-lipoprotein. In man atheromas form slowly or not at all at levels under 160 mg per 100 ml, but they form more rapidly in infants and in adolescent boys, and in Negro but not in white girls, than in senescent people whose blood cholesterol levels are higher. Thrombogenesis is, of course, very rare in infants and adolescents, but common in mature people living on diets rich in animal fat. Hyperlipemia accelerates clotting, but only to a very slight degree. It does, however, significantly retard fibrinolysis, and its effect in thrombogenesis, in veins or diseased arteries, seems mainly based on interference with clot lysis.

Other known factors in raising plasma lipids are intense emotion, adrenal corticosteroid, ACTH, and fat mobilizing hormone of hypophyseal origin. Epinephrine also acts, in part through stimulating release of these factors, to raise levels of unesterified fatty acid, triglyceride, and cholesterol in the blood. Osler and others emphasized the effect of "lives of high tension" in hastening vascular disease. The effects of intense emotion in raising plasma cholesterol were reported from Walter Cannon's labora-

tory in 1930, and recent workers have demonstrated that emotional burden or response to competition raises plasma lipid and shortens clotting time. On the other hand, muscular exercise greatly increases fat combustion and lowers plasma lipid levels as do elevated levels of thyroid hormone, although the latter augments epinephrine action and emotional response to the environment.

Heparin activates or liberates lipoprotein lipase and hastens the solution of the chylomicra which make plasma hazy after a high-fat meal. Lipoprotein lipase levels, and plasma heparin levels, are reported to decline in the aging human, and to be lower in those with coronary disease than in control subjects of the same age. Albumin serves as carrier for the fats released by lipase, and in hypoalbuminemia this mechanism breaks down, leading to hyperlipemia and hypercholesterolemia. In obstructive jaundice, plasma lipids rise to extremely high levels, but the plasma is clear because of the high level of α-lipoprotein, rich in lecithin. The clear icteric plasma becomes cloudy with fat droplets if lecithinase is added. Neither atherogenesis nor thrombogenesis is initiated by the intense hyperlipemia caused by obstructive jaundice, but many xanthomas may appear in the skin.

Diabetes includes several types of disturbed metabolism. Pancreatic insufficiency, in rabbits and probably in men, does not greatly alter atherogenesis. But the more common type of diabetes, with intact or hypertrophied pancreatic islets, does cause hyperlipemia. Even when subclinical in severity, it may lead to precocious atherosclerosis, and many cases, well-controlled by insulin, develop remarkable arteriolar atheromas, in the kidney and retina, as well as clinical evidence of coronary disease or impaired circulation in the legs. These lesions developed rapidly when diets rich in animal fat were used in juvenile diabetics. They can be arrested or reversed by diets low in animal fat.

White men are far more prone to coronary occlusion before the age of sixty than white women, and white boys show far more rapid lipid disposition in the coronary arteries and aorta during adolescence than do white girls. In American Negroes there is no such sex difference. The ratio of β- to α-lipoprotein in white males is higher than in females, and can be reduced by estrogen therapy. This does not occur in myxedematous patients, and the effects of androgens, estrogens, and thyroid hormone seem interrelated. It is also known that adolescent white boys in America greatly increase their intake of animal fat during adolescence, while girls do not. Finally, there are anatomic differences in the intima of the coronary arteries of white males and females, even at birth, which may contribute to the more rapid evolution of obstructive disease in young men.

HYDRAULIC AND ANATOMIC FACTORS IN ATHEROGENESIS

One of the most striking features of atherosclerosis is the spotty distribution of lesions and the variation in severity in different vessels in different bodies. One person may have extensive, almost xanthoma-like disease of the coronary arteries in the epicardial fat, with none in deeper muscular branches, and only a few small plaques in the abdominal aorta. Another may have severe ulcerated, thrombus-covered plaques in the abdominal aorta and iliac artery, with rare and small coronary lesions. Or the favored site may be the internal carotids, the basilar and cerebral arteries, or the leg vessels below the popliteals. The rarity of pulmonary arterial lesions, except with pulmonic hypertension, and of disease of branches of the brachial arteries, as compared with that in femoral branches indicates that high intraarterial pressure as well as hydraulic stresses at bifurcations favor plaque formation. In animals and man, hypertension accelerates atherogenesis. Vessels damaged by syphilis, tuberculous meningitis, or pericarditis also develop severe lesions in Americans, but not in poor Chinese on diets of millet and soybeans. The intimal struts of loose connective tissue with longitudinal muscle fibers, peculiar to the coronary arteries and larger in males than females, seem to be particularly important in predisposing these vessels to atheroma. Because these struts or cushions of thick intima vary greatly in individuals, it is not surprising that some of us die of coronary disease with few other lesions, while others, with marked hypercholesterolemia, only show aortic lesions at seventy or eighty. It is for this reason that "coronary indices," based on plasma lipid levels, are of little value in individual cases, while family histories of frequent cerebral or coronary accidents correlate well with higher risk of similar lesions in the offspring.

One may summarize the human problem of pathogenesis by saying that, in countries with undernourished populations, atherosclerosis is a disease of the rich and well-fed; in well-nourished countries, it favors men and women competing most fiercely for status. Yet, in some fields of business (telephone, insurance), coronary rates are lowest in executives, highest among the clerks.

Tobacco, which acts much like epinephrine, accelerates atherosclerosis, but part of the higher death rate from coronary disease among smokers may be due to the fact that tense competitive people seek sedation from smoking. Malnutrition plus constant alcoholic intake damages cholesterol synthesis and spares the arteries, but acute alcoholism or even the daily intake of one or two ounces of alcohol increases hepatic synthesis and raises plasma levels of cholesterol and fat. When it is recalled that eggs and milk, like alcohol and nicotine, are not biologically normal foods for weaned mammals, it can be seen that our present knowledge confirms Osler's statement: "Angiosclerosis is the Nemesis through which Nature exacts retributive justice for the transgression of her laws."

RECOGNITION AND MANAGEMENT OF ARTERIOSCLEROSIS

Necropsy showed that 50 per cent of American soldiers, dying of wounds at an average age of twenty-two years, had grossly apparent atherosclerosis. By age fifty this rises to over ninety per cent, and nearly 50 per cent have marked narrowing of one or more main coronary arteries. The physician's problem is not to diagnose or exclude arteriosclerosis but to determine which patients have experienced or are seriously threatened by occlusion of vessels capable of causing disability or death.

When this disease was regarded as a relentlessly advancing degeneration, for which there was no remedy, the diagnosis merely added a new emotional burden of frustration and fear. This accelerated the progress of the disease. Now that many physicians and laymen accept the idea that atherosclerosis and thrombogenesis may be halted by change in way of life, by drugs that alter plasma lipids and by others that retard intravascular clotting, the diagnosis carries a different meaning. Because many public figures are known to be active and effective years after serious vascular accidents, the need for reassurance is lessened and the effectiveness of sound medical advice is much greater than it was in 1955, when most physicians and textbooks began to reflect the knowledge gained since Ignatovsky's experiments in 1907.

Significant arteriosclerosis is diagnosed by excluding embolic, arteritic, or congenital vascular lesions in patients with such disorders as angina pectoris, myocardial infarction, hemiplegia, intermittent claudication, and other focal evidence of tissue ischemia, or by observing retinal hemorrhage or exudate without embolic or hematologic basis. Roentgen study may reveal chalk, or palpation of peripheral vessels may demonstrate calcification in arteries when none of the above disorders exists. Diabetes, hypertension, or very high plasma lipid levels without jaundice may indicate unusual risk of vascular occlusion in individuals with faultless organic function. Present-day roentgen angiography, with contrast media, permits accurate study of the extent and severity of vascular lesions due to arteriosclerosis and has proved invaluable in the study of cerebral disease, aortic or renal arterial obstruction, and coronary sclerosis. These studies carry some risk, they are expensive and uncomfortable, so that they are used only when clinical findings suggest that surgical intervention to improve function should be considered.

Renal arterial obstruction causing hypertension, like coronary disease, may be the only significant arterial lesion. Such lesions may be due to trauma, but most of them comprise atheromas. Careful abdominal auscultation in a very quiet room may reveal bruits arising in renal stenosis, and separate functional study of both kidneys may indicate unilateral renal disease, probably vascular. Angiography is usually of critical value in identifying these lesions.

Some pathologists believe that renal arteriolar lesions precede and cause arterial hypertension in most cases now called essential or familial hypertension. This is difficult to accept in those persons whose hypertension remains benign, with no retinal or renal damage, after decades. Unexplained heart failure should not be diagnosed as coronary disease or "arteriosclerotic heart," nor unexplained hypertension labeled "renal arteriosclerosis," nor loss of memory or personality change accepted as "cerebral arteriosclerosis." Other causes must be carefully excluded before arterial obstruction is blamed, and in doubtful cases roentgen study may be necessary to confirm this impression, in cases where endarterectomy offers possible relief of ischemic pain, recurrent paralysis, or renal hypertension.

Medical management, aimed to establish collateral circulation to the legs or the myocardium, and to retard or reverse occlusive disease, includes regular quiet exercise as well as diets low in animal fat, drugs such as nicotinic acid, and the newer synthetic drugs which impair cholesterol synthesis, heparin which affects both lipid levels and coagulation, and agents which impair prothrombin production. Because of expense and inconvenience, heparin is rarely used over long periods, but coumarin analogues in doses adequate to hold prothrombin at one-quarter or less of its normal level have been widely used for years. Claims for its value often cite "control" death rates in angina or healed myocardial infarction which are much higher than those reported in large series of untreated patients in most clinics. Controlled studies, in Norway and England, indicate very modest success for such a preventive antiprothrombin regimen. Patients are greatly reassured and anxiety is reduced when physicians treat them with confidence, with either drugs or diet; so it is unwise to advise discontinuing such a regimen when a patient has accepted it.

The conservative, or Hippocratic, management is to persuade patients to accept a sane diet and way of life, with minimal use of tobacco, alcohol, dairy fat, eggs, and stall-fed beef or pork, and

minimal use of drugs. Page's experience indicates that, in most men, vegetable oil diets are more effective than low-fat diets in lowering triglyceride levels, but in women this is less often the case. For those who prefer expensive substitutes for familiar foods, one may obtain in England all sorts of dairy foods made from skim milk and corn oil; presumably the larger American market will eventually be supplied by the less enterprising dairy industry here. Margarines are now marketed with corn or cottonseed oil base. There is so little difference in the hydrogenated fat added to solidify various margarines advertised for lowering cholesterol, that taste and cost rather than relative unsaturation should determine the choice of these.

When cholesterol levels remain over 200 mg per 100 ml on such a regimen, 2 to 6 Gm of nicotinic acid daily, the cholesterol depressant triparanol (MER-29), 200 mg daily, dextrothyroxin, 2 to 8 mg or USP thyroid extract, 60 to 180 mg daily, may prove effective. All the drugs have maximal effect when a proper diet is used, but all may be of value in those who cannot or will not diet. Often combinations prove effective, using two agents, each in doses below levels which evoke unwanted effects. As therapy may be needed for years or decades, the physician must determine by trial in each patient which effective drug or combination is least troublesome and least expensive. The flush due to nicotinic acid at the start of treatment is accepted when patients feel that this is good to maintain a youthful skin, but peptic ulcer, gout, and glycosuria, though rare, may bar use of this agent, which lowers triglycerides as well as cholesterol. Triparanol may cause indigestion or other unacceptable symptoms. Thyroid extract and, even more often, dextrothyroxin may be very effective in altering lipid levels at doses which cause no rise in heat production and no angina even in coronary disease. Both cause more symptoms at high dosage in myxedematous than in euthyroid subjects.

With no change in way of life, such famous physicians as John Hunter, James MacKenzie, and Frank N. Wilson lived active lives for nearly two decades after myocardial infarction, so that one hesitates to start on perennial therapy bold patients who are more stressed by restrictions or drugs than by the risk of the untreated disorder. Some men, who are intolerant of the brief "sun-burned" feeling which occurs at the start of nicotinic acid therapy, unhesitatingly face the pain of thoracotomy and the relatively high mortality (over 25 per cent) of the pioneer coronary endarterectomies. Many other patients are delighted to accept any inconvenience in order to diminish the risk of progressive vascular disease, so long as they can avoid operation. Osler's dictum, "It is often more important to know what sort of patient has a disease than to know what sort of disease a patient has," applies with unusual force to the management of patients with significant arteriosclerotic lesions.

REFERENCES

Brown, H. P., and I. H. Page: Variable Responses of Hyperlipemic Patients to Altered Food Patterns, J.A.M.A., 173:248, 1960.

Dock, W.: Why Are Men's Coronary Arteries So Sclerotic? J.A.M.A., 170:152, 1959.

Hardy, R. W. F., et al.: Biosynthesis of Sterols and Fatty Acids as Affected by Nicotinic Acid and Related Compounds, J. Nutrition, 71:159, 1960.

Kountz, W. B., et al.: Conference on MER/29, Progr. Cardiovascular Diseases, 2:541, 1960.

Kritchevsky, D., et al.: Regulation of Cholesterol Biosynthesis, Am. J. Clin. Nutrition, 8:411, 1960.

Little, A., et al.: Relationship between Changes in Coagulation and Blood Lipids during Alimentary Lipemia, Circulation, 20:987, 1959.

Morgan, A. D.: "The Pathogenesis of Coronary Occlusion," Springfield, Ill., Charles C Thomas, Publisher, 1957.

Peterson, J. E., et al.: Hourly Variations in Total Serum Cholesterol, Circulation, 22:247, 1960.

Starr, P., et al.: Reduction of Serum Cholesterol by Sodium Dextro-Thyroxine, A.M.A. Arch. Internal Med., 105:831, 1960.

Thomas, W. A., et al.: Modification of Diets Responsible for Induction of Coronary Thrombosis and Myocardial Infarcts in Rats, J. Nutrition, 69:325, 1959.

247 DISEASES OF THE AORTA
Victor A. McKusick

DISSECTING ANEURYSM OF THE AORTA

Cystic Medial Necrosis. This is the most frequent morphologic substrate of dissecting aneurysm. It is not the only structural change which can lead to dissection, and conversely it can produce clinical manifestations in the absence of dissection. Cystic medial necrosis appears to be a nonspecific change in the aorta in response to hemodynamic stresses. The frequency with which it is found at autopsy increases with the age of the group studied. (The age distribution of cases of dissecting aneurysm is similar.) Its anatomic distribution is also characteristic, being most marked in the ascending aorta and decreasing progressively as one passes farther from the aortic valve, especially beyond the vessels which branch at the aortic arch. Hypertension accelerates the development of cystic medial necrosis. Furthermore, cystic medial necrosis and dissecting aneurysm are rather frequent complications of coarcta-

tion of the aorta. The hemodynamic changes produced by aortic stenosis and regurgitation accelerate the development of cystic medial necrosis in the ascending aorta. In the genetically defective aorta—that of the Marfan syndrome (p. 1884) is the only clear example one can cite—the ordinary hemodynamic stresses lead to early development of cystic medial necrosis, especially in the ascending aorta, with progressive dilation and/or dissecting aneurysm. (In all dissecting aneurysm, the intimal rent occurs most often in the ascending aorta.) All these features suggest that cystic medial necrosis is a relatively nonspecific morphologic expression of "wearing-out" of the aorta in response to hemodynamic stress. The stress to which the ascending aorta is particularly subject is repetitive expansile pulsation. With each heart beat the ascending aorta is subjected to greater expansile pulsation than any other part of the aorta, especially more than that beyond the aortic arch.

Syphilitic aortitis does not lead to dissection nor does atherosclerosis per se.

Dissecting aneurysm occurs more commonly in men. Under the age of forty years, approximately half the instances of dissecting aneurysm in women occur in relation to pregnancy. Hormonal changes associated with pregnancy seem to be responsible for effects on connective tissues, including those of the aorta.

Usually from an intimal rent in the ascending aorta, dissection extends proximally to the aortic ring and distally for a variable distance. (Occasionally an intimal rent is absent. Bleeding into the media from vasa vasorum is obviously important in such cases and probably is important in the initiation of most cases. Hence the synonyms for dissecting aneurysm: medial hematoma and dissecting hematoma of the aorta.) "Reentry" may take place at some site, such as just beyond the left subclavian orifice or in the abdominal aorta, with creation of a "double barrel aorta." Prognosis is better in such cases. The dissection may extend for a considerable distance into one or several of the branches of the aorta, from the coronary arteries to the iliac arteries. The proximal dissection may distort the aortic ring and result in aortic regurgitation. (Cystic medial necrosis antedating the dissection may have resulted in dilation of the sinuses of Valsalva and aortic regurgitation.) Rupture of the aorta into the pericardial or pleural cavity occurs in a majority of cases, although other sites of rupture such as the transverse portion of the duodenum are occasionally observed. Rupture into the pericardial sac is not surprising since the pericardial deflections extend high on the ascending aorta in many persons.

The clinical manifestations of dissecting aneurysm can be classified as follows:

1. Pain

2. Aortic regurgitation

3. Interference with the blood supply through branches of the aorta

4. X-ray evidence of progressive widening of the aorta

5. Rupture of the aorta

In addition, tissue destruction may be of sufficient proportions to produce mild fever, leukocytosis, and elevation of sedimentation rate.

The pain of dissecting aneurysm is sometimes described as tearing in quality. It is questionable that its quality is truly different from that of coronary occlusion. Characteristically it attains peak intensity very shortly after onset. It may involve the anterior chest, back, lumbar area, or abdomen, sometimes in a progression. Dissecting aneurysm may occur, however, with little or nothing the patient describes as pain. The blood pressure may drop precipitously during the dissection, but maintenance of hypertension or increased blood pressure in response to the pain is often the finding.

The most frequently observed evidence of disturbance at the orifices of the branches is discrepancy in the pulses and blood pressure readings in the arms. Asymmetrical diminution in these may occur. The same observations may be made in the carotid and femoral vessels. Myocardial infarction or changes of myocardial ischemia, neurologic signs from interference with cerebral and/or spinal blood flow, intestinal symptoms, and hematuria may occur.

Rupture of the aorta is, of course, usually fatal. However, in rare instances leakage into the pericardial cavity may be interrupted and the patient survive for months or even years. The chest pain, together with a pericardial friction rub, can indicate the presence of leaking dissecting aneurysm hours before the leak proceeds to the point of producing cardiac tamponade.

In the differential diagnosis of dissecting aneurysm, myocardial infarction and pulmonary embolus present the greatest problems. Pain reaching a rapid peak of intensity, especially if followed within minutes or hours by signs of arterial occlusion, favors the diagnosis of dissecting aneurysm. Unconsciousness may result from involvement of the cephalic trunks in the dissection and is unusual in myocardial infarction in the absence of severe hypotension or arrhythmia. The maintenance of arterial hypertension favors dissecting aneurysm, although profound hypotension can occur in both dissection and myocardial infarction.

Only a few cases survive more than a few days after an acute dissection. Most of the survivors succumb to rupture of the aorta or other complications within a year. Surgical treatment is in its infancy. The ingenuity of the surgeon will undoubtedly permit, in the future, correction of the aortic lesion in a larger proportion of cases. Pharmacologic hypotension in those cases with maintained hypertension during the acute dissection has a rational place in treatment of the early stages.

Cystic medial necrosis sometimes results in aneurysm, usually of the ascending aorta, without dissection. The clinical behavior resembles syphilitic aneurysm in many respects. In other cases, aortic regurgitation is the main and presenting problem. Surgical treatment has been successful in some of these instances.

SYPHILITIC AORTITIS

Syphilitic involvement is limited largely to the thoracic aorta, particularly the ascending aorta. Syphilitic cardiovascular disease rarely occurs in persons who have had syphilis for less than 10 years or in those who received even a moderate amount of antisyphilitic treatment in the early stage of the infection. On the other hand, so great is the predilection of *Treponema pallidum* for the aorta that a majority of untreated cases have involvement of that vessel. Fortunately, the frequency of syphilitic cardiovascular disease has decreased markedly in the last decade.

The predominant localization of syphilitic change to the ascending aorta may be the result of the combination of the particular hemodynamic stress (see Cystic Medial Necrosis, p. 1365) with the medial damage by the treponemal infection. Other explanations are probably less satisfactory.

Aortic regurgitation, fusiform aneurysm, or saccular aneurysm can result. Syphilitic aortitis uncomplicated by any one of these three may betray its presence by a change in the quality of the aortic second sound usually referred to as "tambouric" (scarcely a pathognomonic sign, however) and by the presence of intimal, shell-like calcification in the first part of the ascending aorta. In some cases this calcification even extends proximally to outline the sinuses of Valsalva. Atherosclerosis alone usually does not produce calcification in the first part of the ascending aorta. The primary lesion of syphilitic aortitis is medial, but intimal atherosclerosis is accelerated by the damage to the media. Occlusive change in the ostia of branch arteries, such as the coronaries with production of angina pectoris or the aortic arch vessels with production of the aortic arch syndrome (p. 1367), occurs by a similar mechanism.

Syphilitic aneurysms occur with diminishing frequency from the ascending aorta distally toward the abdominal aorta. They may be single or multiple, diffuse or sharply localized, fusiform or saccular, smooth-walled or thrombus-filled. Symptoms are likely to be due to compression (e.g., of the trachea, pulmonary artery, or superior vena cava) or erosion (e.g., of the sternum or vertebral column). Rupture into the superior vena cava or pulmonary artery may occur and the patient survive for some time, with dramatic physical findings. Sudden death may result from external rupture or rupture into the tracheobronchial tree, pericardium, esophagus, etc. Happily, with improved public health control of syphilis and with better treatment, syphilitic aneurysm may soon become a matter of no particular concern to the clinician.

There has never been convincing evidence that specific treatment given after the development of clinical signs of cardiovascular syphilis prolongs life. There is evidence that aortic regurgitation is more frequent in syphilitic aortitis than previously thought; however, the prognosis in these patients is better than previously realized.

Herxheimer reactions following closely after the administration of penicillin have been observed in early syphilis in which fever may occur and in central nervous system syphilis in which fever and aggravation of mental disturbances may be seen. Although the occurrence (after penicillin treatment) of Herxheimer reactions involving the coronary ostia remains to be established, it is probably wise in a patient with cardiovascular syphilis and angina pectoris or electrocardiographic signs of myocardial ischemia to improve the myocardial status as much as possible before antisyphilitic therapy and to institute such therapy only under conditions of optimal rest and observation.

Surgical therapy for syphilitic aneurysms has made outstanding advances.

ARTERIOSCLEROTIC ANEURYSMS

Arteriosclerotic aneurysms occur most frequently, although not exclusively, in the abdominal aorta, especially in that portion between the ostia of the renal arteries and the bifurcation. The patients are usually men in the sixth and seventh decade of life or older. Both dilatation and buckling of the aorta are usually involved, and the buckling is usually predominantly to the left.

Manifestations include primarily pain in the back or anterior abdomen and a pulsatile abdominal mass which usually presents in the epigastrium. (As projected on the anterior abdominal wall, the bifurcation lies at approximately the level of the umbilicus.) The patient may discover that the knee-elbow position relieves the pain. The diagnosis may be obvious from ordinary x-ray films of the abdomen if an eggshell-like or other calcification outlines the aneurysm. Aortograms can make the definitive anatomic diagnosis.

Rupture of arteriosclerotic aneurysms is frequently the mechanism of death. Rupture is likely to begin in the ulceration of an atheromatous plaque. There is usually no more than short medial dissection. Rupture may result in the rapid development of a mass in the left flank. The hematoma may dissect retroperitoneally into the groin and produce manifestations simulating incarcerated inguinal hernia. Rupture into the duodenum, another indication of the high location of these aneurysms, may occur.

Arteriosclerotic aneurysm of the abdominal aorta has been treated surgically with success. Resection of the affected portion and replacement with aortic homograft or a synthetic prosthesis has been performed. In the minority of cases in which the renal arteries and higher branches of the aorta are involved in the wall of the aneurysm, modifications of the basic procedure are necessary.

AORTIC ARCH SYNDROMES
(**Pulseless Disease, Young Female Syndrome, Takayasu Syndrome, Reverse Coarctation**)

Slowly progressive change can lead to partial or total obliteration of the major branches of the aortic arch. Intimal atherosclerosis alone can produce at least a partial aortic arch syndrome, and it often collaborates with other factors such as syphilis and trauma in producing obliteration. Severe trauma to the upper chest, especially if the neck is extended, may rupture elements of the media in the region of the ostia of the arch branches and thus lay the groundwork for progressive intimal atherosclerosis at these sites. An inadequately understood progressive disorder occurs especially in young females for which reason the designation *young female syndrome* has been used. Histopathologically these cases have been characterized by collections of chronic inflammatory cells, including giant cells. In this disorder the obliteration of major branches is especially likely to be complete, and the designation *pulseless disease* is particularly appropriate. Because of the absence of pulses in the upper part of the body with normal femoral pulses, the term *reverse coarctation* has also been applied to this group of conditions.

In addition to the loss of palpable pulses, clinical manifestations include easy fatigability of the arms, atrophy of the muscles and other soft tissues of the face, necrosis of the cartilaginous nasal septum, and cataract. Systolic murmurs may be heard just above and below the clavicles if the occlusion is partial. If the pressure proximal to the obstruction is at all times in the cardiac cycle higher than that distal to the obstruction, a continuous murmur simulating that of patent ductus arteriosus may be heard in the same area. Syncopal attacks, especially with quiet standing after exercise, also occur.

Surgical replacement of the aortic arch has been performed in a few cases and will undoubtedly become increasingly feasible in the future.

THROMBOTIC OBLITERATION OF THE BIFURCATION OF THE AORTA
(Leriche Syndrome)

The bifurcation of the aorta is, like the bifurcation of the common carotid artery and the coronary arteries, an Achilles heel of the arterial tree as far as the development of atherosclerosis is concerned. Slowly progressive thrombosis at the bifurcation can result in complete obliteration of the aorta. The patients are usually men and may be as young as the fourth decade. Some of the patients have hypercholesterolemia. The same clinical picture can result from saddle embolism of the bifurcation, as in mitral valve disease or myocardial infarction, if the patient survives the acute episode and is not operated on early.

The clinical manifestations of the Leriche syndrome are (1) intermittent claudication, with pain in the low back or *gluteal area* which may be mistaken for "sciatica"; (2) loss of the ability to maintain a stable erection, because of the poor blood supply to the penis; (3) globose, that is, symmetrical, atrophy of the legs, which may be difficult to appreciate because of its symmetry; and (4) absence of both femoral pulses. Most of the patients have manifestations of atherosclerosis elsewhere—cerebral, coronary, aortic arch ostia—and hypertension is frequent. Differentiation from coarctation of the aorta is afforded by feeling an aortic pulse in the epigastrium and by the absence of certain other signs of coarctation such as notching of the ribs and dilated collateral vessels over the thorax. Lateral x-ray views of the lumbar spine may reveal basketlike or other calcification in the region of the bifurcation. Aortograms can make the diagnosis definite.

Surgical replacement of the aortic bifurcation with homograft or synthetic prosthesis has been attended with considerable success.

TRAUMA OF THE AORTA

Penetrating wounds of the chest may be rapidly fatal because of puncture of the aorta. Nonpenetrating trauma to the chest, most commonly the steering wheel injuries in automobile accidents, may lead to rupture of the aorta. In over one-third of cases such rupture is just beyond the mouth of the left subclavian artery. If the victim survives the acute tear, a false aneurysm may result at this site. Such aneurysms are susceptible to surgical resection. As mentioned elsewhere (p. 1367), progressive obliteration of ostia at the aortic arch with production of the aortic arch syndrome may be a late complication of trauma of particular type.

AORTIC SINUS ANEURYSM

Aneurysms may occur in the sinuses of Valsalva from syphilis, idiopathic cystic medial necrosis, or a presumably congenital (ill-understood) basis. Rupture into the right atrium or right ventricle may occur. Successful surgical closure has been effected in such cases. Aneurysm of the aortic sinuses usually with symmetric involvement of all three sinuses occurs as a characteristic feature of the Marfan syndrome. Such aneurysms rarely if ever rupture into the right heart.

UNUSUAL FORMS OF AORTITIS

Unusual forms of aortitis include mycotic aneurysm, such as that produced by aortic tuberculosis, temporal arteritis with aortic involvement, and granulomatous aortitis of the proximal few centimeters in ankylosing spondylitis.

Coarctation and other congenital anomalies of the aorta are discussed elsewhere (pp. 1430 and 1432).

REFERENCES

Boyer, S. H., IV, and V. A. McKusick: Diseases of the Aorta, Ann. Rev. Med., 9:85, 1958.

Leriche, R., and A. Morel: The Syndrome of Thrombotic Obliteration of the Aortic Bifurcation, Ann. Surg., 127:193, 1948.

Ross, R. S., and V. A. McKusick: Aortic Arch Syndromes, A.M.A. Arch. Internal Med., 92:701, 1953.

Shennan, T.: "Dissecting Aneurysms," Medical Research Council, Special Report, Ser. 193, London, His Majesty's Stationery Office, 1934.

248 VASCULAR DISEASE OF THE EXTREMITIES
Eugene A. Stead, Jr.

SYMPTOMS AND SIGNS

One should suspect peripheral vascular disease in a patient with the following symptoms and signs:

1. Pain in an extremity which is induced by exercise and relieved by rest; pain which is influenced by posture, is localized to one digit, is unilateral, or is paroxysmal

2. Impaired pulsations of peripheral arteries

3. Abnormal color of the skin, particularly when affected by raising or lowering of the part

4. Gangrene, ulceration, impaired nail growth, scleroderma, excessive calluses, or paronychial infections

5. Abnormal pulsations, enlarged veins, or edema

6. Unusual warmth or coldness

7. Swelling, atrophy, or difference in length of extremities

8. Auscultatory evidence of arteriovenous fistula

9. Localized systolic murmur over a large peripheral artery

10. Cyanosis of digits when immersed in cold water

11. Peripheral neuritis

If the above signs and symptoms are absent, peripheral vascular disease need not be considered.

The arteries, capillaries, veins, and lymph vessels may be involved separately or in varying combinations. The disturbances may be due to organic disease of the vessels or abnormal constriction or dilatation caused by dysfunction of the autonomic nervous system.

DISTURBANCES IN ARTERIAL FUNCTION

Special Points in History and Physical Examination. Arterial insufficiency causes disturbances in nutrition to the part. The following points in the history and examination are to be noted:

Sensitivity to Cold with Blanching or Cyanosis of Digits. On examination, the part with arterial insufficiency may be colder than the corresponding part of the opposite extremity.

Muscle and Nerve Ischemia. Pain which develops in the muscles of the foot or calf on walking and which disappears on rest is called *intermittent claudication.* If exercise is continued after the pain appears, the muscles may become tender. In more severe ischemia of the leg, pain may occur at rest and be relieved by dependency. The pain of ischemic neuritis is severe and diffuse, with severe exacerbations. Sharp shooting pains may dart through the entire extremity. The acute paroxysms are apt to occur at night.

State of Peripheral Vessels. Presence or absence of femoral, popliteal, dorsalis pedis, and posterior tibial pulses is noted. Gangrene of the digits may occur without disturbances in these pulses. In the absence of a palpable pulse, the skin may show no evidence of malnutrition.

Murmurs over Peripheral Vessels. Pistol shot sounds are heard over the major vessels when the diastolic pressure is low and the stroke output high. Localized systolic murmurs are heard over areas of narrowing produced either by disease of the blood vessel or by external pressure. When the vessel is narrowed, the local points of stenosis produce a murmur similar to that heard in aortic stenosis. If the diastolic pressure below the point of narrowing is low, either because of poor collateral circulation or because of wide vasodilatation produced by exercise, a continuous murmur may be heard. With this exception and that of venous hums, continuous murmurs are commonly the result of an arteriovenous communication.

Blanching on Elevation; Redness and Cyanosis on Dependency. On elevation to a 90° angle, the part becomes pale and at times white. The extent of the pallor indicates the extent of the arterial insufficiency. If only the toes or a part of a toe is involved, the pallor is limited to the ischemic area. The color returns slowly on lowering the part to *heart level.* The pallor occurs on elevation because the blood in the capillaries and venules drains out of the part by gravity, and because the effective arterial pressure is lowered by having to overcome the hydrostatic force of a column of blood extending from the heart level to the elevated part. Some pallor on elevation will occur in a normal foot, but the pallor of arterial insufficiency is much more marked.

When the part hangs down, the blood flow is increased temporarily over the horizontal position because the hydrostatic pressure is added to the pressure created by the heart. The increase in arterial pressure is effective until the veins fill. Then it is opposed by an equal column of blood on the venous side, and the pressure differential between artery and vein returns approximately to the differential present in the horizontal position. The minute vessels of the part, being in a state of chronic injury because of an inadequate circulation, are dilated. When these vessels first fill, they are red. Varying degrees of cyanosis gradually develop because of the slow blood flow.

Atrophic Changes in Skin and Edema. The skin becomes thin and atrophic. Slight edema with loss of normal wrinkles is common. If the patient keeps the foot dependent day and night to relieve pain, pitting edema may develop from the combination of a high capillary pressure from dependency and the damaged state of the capillaries caused by ischemia.

Gangrene

Infection. Devitalized tissue offers a good place for infection to spread. When peripheral neuritis is present, infection may be more prominent than ischemia. Osteomyelitis may occur.

Neurologic Findings. Peripheral neuritis is a common complication of diabetes. Periarteritis nodosa and arteriosclerosis may cause neuritis because of the interference with the blood supply to the nerves. In periarteritis, motor paralysis as well as sensory loss and pain is common.

Occupation. There may be a history of unusual exposure to cold and dampness. Use of the pneumatic hammer has been said to cause Raynaud's phenomenon.

Determination of Cause of Arterial Circulatory Insufficiency. If the findings are those of arterial circulatory insufficiency, it must be determined whether the insufficiency results (1) from occlusive disease entirely, (2) from overactivity of the sympathetic nervous system, (3) from abnormal reaction of the blood vessels to cold, (4) from the effect of cold agglutinins or cryoglobulins on the physical state of the blood, or (5) from a combination of mechanisms.

The constrictor effect of the autonomic nervous system may be removed by paravertebral block of the appropriate sympathetic ganglion with procaine or by release of vasoconstrictor tone by body heating. In either method, the patient, with body exposed, is placed in a cool room (temperature 18 to 20°C). The body temperature may be raised by enclosing the trunk in a heating cabinet or by immersing two uninvolved limbs in water baths at 43°C for 40 min. When vasodilatation is produced in the upper extremities by body warming or by blocking of the sympathetic ganglion, the temperature of the digits rises rapidly to between 30.5 and 33°C. If the temperature rises to between 27 and 29°C, there is moderate organic vascular disease. If no rise occurs or if the temperature falls, advanced local arterial disease is present. Body warming is the simplest and most effective method of relieving vasoconstrictor tone in the upper extremities. It fails occasionally in the lower extremities. Therefore, if full vasodilatation does not occur, paravertebral block is indicated in the lower extremities.

ORGANIC OBSTRUCTION

Balance between Vessel Obstruction and Vessel Formation. Obstruction of a large artery is a strong stimulus for new vessel formation and collateral circulation. The symptoms produced represent the result of the balance between these two processes. Complete obstruction of the aorta below the renal vessels which occurs slowly may produce no symptoms or the picture of impotence and thigh claudication. The extremities may appear normally nourished. When skin involvement becomes marked, little blood vessels are usually thrombosed. This may be primary small vessel endarteritis as in diabetes, or it may be secondary small vessel thrombosis secondary to occlusions higher up. Gangrene with normal pedal pulses indicates small vessel disease. Intermittent claudication with normal appearing vessels and absent popliteal or femoral pulses suggests larger vessel obstruction, which is frequently segmental.

Peripheral Arteriosclerosis. The etiology and pathology of peripheral arteriosclerosis have been discussed in Chap. 246. The history and physical findings are those of arterial insufficiency. The diagnosis is based on the following factors:

1. Age of the patient. It usually occurs after fifty years of age.
2. Sex. Males are more commonly affected than females.
3. Diabetes. The incidence of arteriosclerosis is increased in patients with diabetes.
4. Evidence of arteriosclerosis is usually present bilaterally, although the symptoms may be unilateral.
5. There are no symptoms of arterial disease in the upper extremities.
6. The arteries, as seen by x-ray, are frequently calcified.
7. In patients with diabetes, the small vessels may be occluded, although the larger vessels are only moderately diseased. Local gangrene of the skin of the toes may occur, even though the rest of the foot is warm.
8. In patients with diabetes, neuropathy is common.

Thromboangiitis Obliterans. This condition was described by Buerger in 1908 as an obliterative vascular disease affecting chiefly the peripheral arteries and veins of Jewish males in early adult life. The disease involved primarily the blood vessels of the extremities, beginning in medium- and small-sized arteries. Veins were involved less commonly. The lesion was a nonsuppurative panarteritis or panphlebitis and was segmental, leaving normal vessels between diseased segments. The lesions came in crops, producing complete and usually permanent obstruction, followed by the development of extensive collateral circulation. The history and physical findings were those of arterial insufficiency or superficial phlebitis. The diagnosis was based on these considerations:

1. Age. Onset was usually between twenty and forty-five years.
2. Sex. Males predominate in a ratio of 75:1.
3. Race. Half the patients were Jewish.
4. Migratory phlebitis preceding or accompanying arterial disease.
5. Severe pain at rest from ulceration or from ischemic neuritis.
6. Absence of calcification as seen by x-ray.
7. Small vessels of the hands might be involved. Thrombosis of mesenteric, coronary, cerebral, or renal arteries was not uncommon.

Atherosclerosis in young men is now a well-known entity. It is a segmental disease. Thrombosis in the arteries is frequently associated with thrombosis in the veins. The arteries and veins respond to thrombosis with an inflammatory reaction, followed by various degrees of recanalization. There is reasonable doubt that thromboangiitis obliterans is a distinct clinical entity. It is certain that the diagnosis is now made much less frequently than in past years.

Thrombosis. Thrombosis of the larger arteries of the lower extremities is common in the natural course of arteriosclerosis. Whether or not dramatic symptoms of acute arterial insufficiency appear will depend on the degree of collateral circulation which has developed. Gradual narrowing of a major vessel may progress unnoticed to complete occlusion, because the symptoms of arterial insufficiency may not develop until the collateral channels begin to thrombose.

Embolus. Emboli are usually fragments from more centrally placed thrombi. The occurrence of sudden arterial insufficiency without physical findings of marked peripheral vascular disease generally indicates an embolus. The common sources are:

1. Mural thrombus from the left atrium of a patient with chronic atrial fibrillation

2. Mural thrombus from the left atrium of a patient with mitral stenosis and commonly, but not necessarily, with atrial fibrillation

3. Mural thrombus from myocardial infarction of the left ventricle or, more rarely, from acute or subacute myocarditis

4. Thrombi on valves from subacute or acute bacterial endocarditis

Less common sources are:

1. Thrombi in the aorta or its large branches

2. Venous thrombosis in patients with a right-left shunt from congenital heart disease

3. Venous thrombosis causing pulmonary embolization, right heart failure, and the passage of a clot through the patent foramen ovale

4. Myxoma of the left atrium

Emboli are likely to lodge at the bifurcation of large vessels. A saddle embolus riding on the bifurcation of the aorta may cause circulatory insufficiency in both lower extremities. The signs of circulatory insufficiency are usually considerably distal to the embolus because of the effectiveness of collateral circulation. The degree of circulatory impairment caused by arterial obstruction and that caused by secondary arterial spasm cannot be determined on inspection. The effects of paravertebral block must decide this question. The local examination reveals the symptoms and signs of arterial insufficiency. Loss of motion and of sensation may occur rapidly. Pain has been discussed on p. 58. At first there is no pain at the site of the embolus, but tenderness may develop after a few hours, as the embolus sets up a local inflammatory reaction in the vessel.

Exposure to Cold; Trench Foot. Extremities with normal blood vessels are injured by prolonged exposure to cold. Dependency and wetness combined with cold cause tissue damage even though actual freezing of the tissues does not occur. On warming, the injury results in extreme vasodilatation with swelling of the part because the capillaries have been damaged. Later, true capillary flow in the skin may cease because of capillary stasis and thrombosis although flow continues through small arteriovenous communications. This gives the clinical picture of superficial gangrene in a warm part. Whether complete recovery or gangrene occurs depends upon the extent of the injury. Persistent tenderness because of fibrosis and ischemic neuritis may develop.

Obstruction of Main Arterial Trunks. Broad insertion of the scalenus anticus muscle with or without cervical rib is a rare cause of Raynaud's phenomenon or organic arterial occlusion. The vascular disturbances may be reflex from compression of a portion of the brachial plexus. At times, trauma from compression of the artery causes thrombus formation with or without embolic phenomena distal to the area of injury.

Persons who sleep with their arms hyperabducted above the head or whose occupation causes them to work with their arms hyperabducted may develop numbness and tingling from occlusion of the subclavian axillary vessels. Usually discomfort causes the arms to be moved to a different position, but gangrene of the fingers has been reported in some cases.

Syphilitic aneurysm or dissecting aneurysm may cause obstruction to the main artery supplying the limb.

Obstruction of Aorta below the Renal Vessels and Obstruction of the Vessels Arising from the Arch of the Aorta. These disorders have been considered in the preceding chapter.

Obstructive Disease of the Small Vessels. Inflammatory involvement of the smaller divisions of the vascular tree may cause local areas of gangrene. In time, thrombosis may occur in larger vessels. The cause of the arteritis is usually unknown, but occasionally it occurs as the result of a reaction to a specific agent. Occasionally, cigarette smoking is the cause and complete abstinence the cure.

SPASM OF ARTERIES AND ARTERIOLES

Raynaud's Disease and Raynaud's Phenomenon. Raynaud's disease is an idiopathic bilateral paroxysmal contraction of the arteries and arterioles of the digits, usually without local gangrene. The primary fault seems to be a local sensitivity of the digital vessels to cold. The attacks are precipitated by cold or emotion and are relieved by warming. Raynaud's phenomenon consists of paroxysmal attacks of ischemia of the digits occurring in the course of other diseases, such as scleroderma, thromboangiitis obliterans, cervical rib, arteriosclerosis, crutch paralysis, and pneumatic hammer disease.

Diagnosis of Raynaud's disease from the history

and examination is made from the following points:

1. Sex. Females are affected much more often than males.

2. Age. It is less common before puberty and after forty, although it may occur at any age.

3. Bilateral and symmetric involvement of digits. It is more common in the hands than in the feet.

4. Attacks of cyanosis can be reproduced by immersion of the hands in cold water or by cooling the body rapidly by a cool shower. The digital arteries and arterioles contract. The fingers become blue if the minute vessels remain dilated, pale if they contract. On rewarming, reactive hyperemia occurs.

5. If the disease is of many years' duration, small superficial areas of gangrene may occasionally be present.

Diagnosis of Raynaud's phenomenon is made if the above findings are noted in conjunction with organic arterial disease, scleroderma, cervical rib, or history of the use of a pneumatic hammer. In the beginning, it is frequently impossible to differentiate between benign Raynaud's disease and progressive scleroderma with Raynaud's phenomenon.

Scleroderma. This is a diffuse disease of the collagenous system with skin and visceral manifestations. The etiology is unknown. Raynaud's phenomenon is frequently seen before the characteristic skin changes occur. In many instances the skin changes are localized to the distal portions of the extremities (acroscleroderma). The skin becomes boardlike and is bound down to the underlying tissues. Decreased sweating, increased pigmentation, and calcification of the skin occur. Gangrene of the digits, with marked shortening of the phalanges, is not uncommon (sclerodactylia). Involvement of the esophagus, heart, and lungs may occur early or late in the disease (Chap. 299).

Ergotism. Spasm of the arterioles with thrombosis and gangrene is produced by ergot poisoning. In the past, it was seen in epidemic form as the result of the contamination of rye with ergot fungus (*Claviceps purpurea*). It is occasionally seen after the repeated use of ergot to induce abortion or after the use of ergotamine tartrate for pruritus.

Reflex Spasm. Any painful area in the extremities may cause symptoms and signs of ischemia from stimulation of the autonomic nervous system. The ischemia of embolus or thrombus is intensified by reflex activity. Ischemia from organic disease of the vessels, from arteriosclerosis, or from thromboangiitis obliterans may be intensified by active vasoconstriction mediated through the autonomic nerves.

Disturbances in Small Vessels from Changes in Blood

Changes in the physical state of the blood may cause small vessel obstruction. Patients with sickle-cell anemia are prone to multiple thromboses. The leg ulcers seen in this disease are probably an example of small vessel thrombosis on the basis of mechanical obstruction caused by the sickled cells. When the titer of cold agglutinins is high, exposure to cold may cause Raynaud's phenomenon. The development of globulins which precipitate in the cold (cryoglobulins) in patients with leukemia or myeloma may also cause Raynaud's phenomenon.

PROGNOSIS IN DISEASE OF THE ARTERIES

The prognosis depends upon the age of the patient, the rate of progression of the primary disease, the degree of the development of the collateral circulation, and the amount of involvement of the cerebral coronary and visceral vessels. The clinical course is very variable. Fingers are occasionally lost, the hand almost never. One or both lower limbs are more frequently lost. The mortality and development of gangrene in embolus and thrombosis are approximately the same.

In *Raynaud's disease,* as defined in this discussion, the prognosis is good by definition. Complications are rare, and the digits are not lost. In *Raynaud's phenomenon* accompanying other disease, the prognosis is that of the primary disease. Thus, in scleroderma associated with Raynaud's phenomenon, the outlook depends on the extent and rate of progression of the scleroderma. This is true whether the sclerodermatous changes are generalized or are still localized to the extremities.

TREATMENT OF ARTERIAL INSUFFICIENCY

Chronic Arterial Insufficiency. Since the etiology of arteriosclerosis is not known, treatment directed toward prevention or removal of the primary factors is not possible. In segmental obstruction of the femoral and iliac arteries, intimal stripping and grafting offer new hope for improving the circulation.

General Care. The *reduction of blood cholesterol* by dietary management and by drugs has been considered in Chap. 246. Because of the *frequency of diabetes* in persons with vascular disease, fasting and postprandial blood sugars should be measured routinely in all such patients. *Complete abstinence from tobacco* should be advised.

Care of Local Areas. The care of the local area with circulatory impairment from arteriosclerosis, thromboangiitis, or damage from exposure to cold is similar. The greatest danger is gangrene in the toes. This is usually precipitated by *trauma, infection,* or *burns,* all of which can ordinarily be prevented by good foot care. Care of the feet means careful washing in tepid water at night; keeping the skin pliable with lanolin; use of a bland dusting powder to absorb perspiration; use of warm, finely woven woolen socks in winter; careful cutting of the nails, with the ends cut straight across to avoid ingrowing nails. Epidermophytosis must be treated when present, but strong ointments or solutions are to be avoided. Soaking twice daily in 1:8,000 potassium permanganate solution is satisfactory. Dry heat is contraindicated. Remember that sensation may be impaired because of peripheral nerve involvement. Heat above the temperature of the blood raises the temperature of a part with impaired blood supply much more rapidly than that of a normal part. In this situation, the blood acts as a cooling system to lower the temperature of the tissues; if this cooling system does not function efficiently, burns occur. Heating the part by reflex vasodilatation is safe; local heat may raise the metabolism, without a corresponding increase in blood supply, and precipitate gangrene. The shoes should fit perfectly and should be broken in gradually. If any break in the skin or blister occurs from any cause, the patient should go to bed and call his physician. Reflex vasoconstriction is to be minimized. In the winter, there is need not only for adequate protection for the part itself but also for attention to preserving the warmth of the body. No local protection will keep the extremities warm if the trunk is cool and the body is attempting to preserve heat.

Reflex vasoconstriction may accompany organic occlusive vascular disease. If body warming or paravertebral block demonstrates release of reflex tone, improvement of the circulation to the extremity by sympathectomy is indicated. Some observers have reported improvement after sympathectomy even though paravertebral block caused no rise in temperature. Sympathectomy may be followed by gangrene in advanced disease because it may divert the greatly limited supply of blood from the severely ischemic tissues to the more normal tissues of the part.

Sympathectomy does not increase the flow of blood through muscles and has no direct effect on intermittent claudication. If sympathectomy is performed in patients with intermittent claudication, it should be more extensive than is necessary to release the vasoconstrictor tone of the vessels of the skin of the leg and foot. A higher sympathectomy may be effective in increasing the circulation in collateral vessels.

Buerger's exercises are useful. They have the disadvantage of being too tiresome to continue for a long period of time. They help because, when the foot is dependent, the effective arterial pressure is increased until the pressure from gravity is counteracted by an equal column of blood in the veins. The foot is emptied by raising it just far enough above heart level to produce collapse of the veins

and slight pallor. It is then returned to the dependent position. The ideal conditions are (1) maximal lowering of the foot below heart level and leaving it there until the veins are full and (2) the least elevation for the shortest period of time which will suffice to empty the foot. When the valves of the veins of the legs are competent, walking slowly is an effective form of Buerger's exercises. In many patients it appears that frequent short walks constitute the most effective of all methods of treatment. The contraction of the muscles forces blood up the deep veins, the venous pressure falls sharply as the muscles relax, and the high arterial pressure produced by gravity is effective until the veins fill.

Pyogenic infections of the feet and toes are common in patients with impaired blood supply. This is particularly true if peripheral neuritis is present. If an apparently gangrenous part is warm, infection is playing an important role, and intensive penicillin therapy may greatly change the picture. Each time the physician must ask himself: Is infection or ischemia the primary cause of the acute episode?

Acute Arterial Insufficiency. In the acute circulatory insufficiency caused by thrombosis or embolism, there are four considerations: (1) mechanical removal or bypassing of the obstruction if the occlusion is in a major vessel, (2) sympathetic blockade by paravertebral or spinal anesthesia, (3) enhancing fibrinolysis by the intravenous administration of either purified streptokinase or human fibrinolysin, followed by (4) routine anticoagulant therapy with heparin and the coumarin drugs. Operative removal of an embolus in a major vessel is usually beneficial in the first 8 to 10 hr. Thrombectomy, thromboendarterectomy, or bypass grafting is worthwhile if the occlusion is localized but is to no avail in diffuse obstructions.

Sympathetic blockade should always precede the administration of fibrinolytic and anticoagulant drugs to avoid hematomas. The type and dosage of human fibrinolytic agents are currently under investigation; they are optimal for thromboses of less than 48-hr duration.

For anticoagulant therapy, the preferred method of heparin administration is to give the initial dose intravenously and to maintain the patient thereafter on subcutaneous heparin every 4 hr. Concomitantly, one of the coumarin drugs may be administered by mouth after determining the prothrombin time; when the prothrombin level is lowered to below 30 per cent of normal, the heparin therapy is discontinued and the patient maintained on the coumarin drug exclusively. If the arterial insufficiency is the result of an embolus, effective anticoagulant therapy is usually continued for approximately three weeks until there has been time for the site of the embolus to be covered with endothelium.

Maintaining the affected part in the dependent

position may help the gravitational flow in collateral channels. Local heat is detrimental since it would increase the metabolic requirement in an area of limited arterial inflow.

Raynaud's Disease. The body should be dressed warmly so that the vessels in the hands and feet will dilate to help dispose of body heat. The hands and feet should be protected with warm socks and gloves. Minor episodes of "dead fingers" should not occasion alarm. If these measures are not adequate, Priscol given orally in doses of 25 to 75 mg every 3 or 4 hr is frequently helpful.

Raynaud's Phenomenon. Adequate heat to the body and protection of the extremities from cold and trauma are important. The response of the underlying disease to therapy is more important than the treatment of the vasospasm. When associated with scleroderma, the prognosis is guarded. Priscol has been reported to be effective in controlling the vasospasm. Sympathectomy may be tried, but the effect is usually temporary. Testosterone has been reported to have a favorable effect in scleroderma when given for several months.

Amputation. The indications for amputation are (1) gangrene, (2) uncontrollable infection, (3) intractable pain, and (4) such complete loss of function from deformity or contracture that the limb is a burden. Amputation is a last resort, and conservative therapy has saved many limbs. The site of amputation must be at a level where tissue nutrition is good. In the last analysis, the amount of bleeding at operation and the appearance of the tissues after incision determine whether the stump will be viable. Usually, clinical observation determines the level of the trial incision, but special tests such as the appearance time of intravenous fluorescein and the effect of intradermal histamine may be helpful.

DISTURBANCE IN VENOUS FUNCTION

Varicose Veins. Dilatation and tortuosity of the superficial veins of the lower extremities result from constitutionally defective valves affected by postural strain or from the enlargement of the superficial circulation to compensate for obstruction of the deep circulation. The obstruction of the deep circulation usually results from deep thrombophlebitis. Increased blood flow from an acquired or congenital arteriovenous fistula is a rare cause of varicosities. The varicosities caused by defective valves are easily treated surgically. Those resulting from deep vein obstruction are compensatory, and the extremities are not helped by ligation and vein stripping.

In a normal person who stands motionless for a short time, the hydrostatic pressure in the leg veins is equal to the height of a column of blood extending from the fourth rib to the level of the vein. In a man 6 ft in height, the pressure at the ankle is about 105 mm Hg. Blood from the foot is returned by the force of the heartbeat, and all the valves are open. These pressure relations are the same, therefore, in valved and nonvalved veins. On contracting the muscles of the leg and thigh, blood is forced up the extremity by the high intramuscular tension. With normal valves, it cannot be forced downward or outward into the superficial circulation through the communicating veins. The blood in the superficial veins of the leg is not forced upward by the contraction because the skin tension does not exceed the hydrostatic pressure. When the extremity is relaxed, blood does not flow downward into the muscles because the valves control it. Blood enters the veins in the muscles from the arteries and from the superficial veins by way of the communicating veins. Backflow from the cava is prevented by valves, and the runoff through the communicating veins lowers the pressure in the superficial veins effectively. The fall in hydrostatic pressure in the venous system lowers capillary pressure effectively and prevents edema. When the valves of the veins are destroyed, the venous and capillary pressures are not lowered by exercise. Chronic edema, petechial hemorrhage, poor drainage, and infection frequently result.

Varicose veins fall into the following groups. (1) Simple dilatation of the veins with competent valves. The lowering of capillary pressure by exercise is maintained, and edema does not result. Superficial venous thrombosis in the dilated, tortuous vessels may be troublesome. (2) Varicose veins with incompetent valves in the superficial veins, but competent perforating and deep valves. On walking, the venous pressure is not lowered unless the superficial veins are prevented from filling from above by local pressure. When the superficial veins are correctly obstructed by a tourniquet, exercise effectively lowers the venous pressure. (3) Varicose veins secondary to occlusion of the deep femoral veins. The varicosities have resulted from thrombophlebitis of the deep veins, and the valves of the deep veins are destroyed. Exercise has no effect in lowering the venous pressure when walking. Brawny edema may mask the superficial varicosities, and their extent is rarely realized until the venous tree is visualized by the use of Hypaque. Intractable chronic ulcers are common.

Treatment. The treatment of the first two groups by the combination of high ligation and injection of sclerosing solutions, or removal by vein stripping, is satisfactory. The treatment of the last group is unsatisfactory, and prevention by more intensive treatment of the deep vein thrombophlebitis is the most satisfactory answer. Once the condition is present, it is beneficial to prevent edema formation by application of external force to counteract the effect of gravity. Bed rest with elevation of the parts allows healing. The application of pressure bandages or of a jelly boot prevents the breakdown of the healed lesion when the patient is up. One should remember the magnitude of the hydrostatic force that one must counteract when the patient stands. Ace bandages are rarely adequate; a pure rubber roller bandage 3 in. wide and 15 ft long is much more effective.

Thrombophlebitis. Thrombus formation in veins is common. Dilated, tortuous superficial varicose veins frequently become tender and hard, with redness of the overlying skin. The inflammatory reaction usually subsides uneventfully, and embolic complications are unusual. Recurrent superficial or deep venous thrombosis is a common occurrence in the natural history of obliterative arterial disease. Local trauma from the administration of various solutions and medications is a not uncommon cause of superficial thrombophlebitis. Again, embolic phenomena are rare.

Thrombus formation in veins occurs at times in all acute and chronic infections, after operations, and after childbirth. It is common in patients with chronic debilitation, heart failure, or carcinomatosis, and occasionally occurs in apparently normal persons. Venous thrombosis is apt to occur contiguous to areas of local infection or trauma. It is seen in the pelvis in puerperal infection and in the prostatic veins after prostatectomy. In the majority of instances, the thrombus begins in the deep veins of the calf and extends proximally. The process may cause very little reaction in the vein wall (phlebothrombosis), and if this is the case, the thrombus is particularly prone to break loose and lodge in the pulmonary tree. On the other hand, the reaction may involve the veins of the entire extremity, with the inflammatory reactions extending into surrounding lymph channels (thrombophlebitis). With an extensive reaction, the clot adheres tightly to the vein wall, and then embolic phenomena are less common.

The precise etiology of thrombophlebitis is unknown. Slowing of the blood stream seems to be an important factor in thrombus formation. Acceleration of the clotting time probably plays a part. The role of changes in the vein walls has not been determined. In spite of the severe systemic reaction and the evidence of the reaction of inflammation in the extremity in the more fulminating cases, no infectious agent has been found.

Local symptoms may be absent. A rise in pulse rate or an unexplained slight fever in a patient in bed may be the only sign of phlebothrombosis, and the condition may not be recognized until an embolus has lodged in the pulmonary artery. Several days later, tenderness in one or both calves

may occur. Tenderness in the calf and pain in the calf on dorsiflexion of the foot may be the only sign. If the foot is dependent, slight edema and cyanosis may be observed. Other findings may include a measurable, although not always visible, increase in the circumference of the calf as compared to the opposite leg, slight prominence of the veins, increased local warmth or diminished pulsation on the affected side, and local pain on compression with a blood pressure cuff at a pressure of 80 to 120 mm Hg.

At the other extreme is the painful, swollen, cyanotic leg of acute thrombophlebitis. In this condition, the arteries are not involved directly; intense reflex vasoconstriction may occur, however, and at times the arterial pulse is felt with difficulty. Fever and leukocytosis are present.

Treatment. The treatment is divided into three parts:

1. Prevention of clot formation in the leg veins by early ambulation or by bandaging of lower extremities when the patient is confined to bed, and by the use of heparin and bishydroxycoumarin (Dicumarol).

2. Prevention of pulmonary emboli after leg veins are involved. Anticoagulant therapy is usually successful. Pulmonary emboli continue in an occasional patient, and ligation of both common femoral veins or the vena cava becomes necessary. (Embolism and infarction of the lungs are discussed in Chap. 262.)

3. Prevention of destruction of lymphatic vessels and veins which leads to persistent edema and chronic ulcers. Pain is relieved and edema clears more quickly when the sympathetic tone is released by repeated paravertebral blocks. Anticoagulant therapy may reduce the number of vessels permanently thrombosed. Elevation and proper bandaging will minimize the edema. Particular attention to bandaging should be given when the patient is allowed to be up.

DISORDERS OF PERIPHERAL LYMPHATIC VESSELS

Water and electrolytes which leave the capillaries can reenter the capillaries without difficulty. Protein and various forms of particulate matter pass into the lymphatic capillaries. If the lymphatic drainage to a part is blocked, the extracellular fluid will gradually assume a high protein content. The capillary filtrate may contain very small amounts of protein, but as the water can be reabsorbed by the blood capillaries and the protein cannot, an effective concentrating mechanism is present. When the lymph vessels are normal, lymph flow depends on muscular contraction, respiratory movements, transmitted movements from arterial pulsations, and to a certain extent, on gravity. Complete immobilization of the lower extremity in a patient sitting in a chair leads to physiologic lymphatic obstruction.

Acute Lymphangitis. When bacterial infection in an extremity is not localized, the inflammatory products pass proximally along the lymphatic channels. The material carried in the lymph channels causes dilatation of the small blood vessels about the lymph vessels, and their courses are outlined by one or more red streaks. Before chemotherapy was available, lymphangitis always carried a serious prognosis because it is a sign of uncontrolled, spreading infection. Immobilization of the part greatly reduces the rate of spread of the infection by reducing the rate of lymph flow. With chemotherapy, fear of lymphangitis and the surgery necessary with lymphangitis has largely disappeared.

Chronic Lymphatic Obstruction. Widespread obstruction of the lymph vessels may result from congenital or familial disorders of the lymph vessels. The lymphedema of the familial type is called Milroy's disease. Acquired chronic lymphedema results from obstruction of the lymph channels by neoplasm, scar, operative removal of lymph nodes, and fibrosis caused by x-ray therapy. It may follow low-grade lymphangitis from filariasis, from lymphogranuloma venereum, and from repeated streptococcal infections. It may be a complicating factor in certain instances of severe edema following thrombophlebitis.

In its early stages, lymphedema cannot be distinguished physically from any other form of soft pitting edema. On laboratory examination, the high protein concentration separates it from cardiac and nephritic edema but not from the fluid of myxedema. Lymphedema causes fibrosis in the tissues, and in time the tissue becomes hard and brawny. The skin may be thick and folded with indolent ulcerations.

Treatment of Chronic Lymphedema. Early and persistent therapy is important. If marked edema is prevented by postural drainage, by effective bandaging, and by limiting upright activity to periods short of edema formation, much of the fibrosis and recurrent infection will be prevented. This program calls for persistence on the part of both physician and patient. Acute attacks of lymphangitis can be controlled by appropriate chemotherapy.

LEG ULCERS IN PATIENTS WITHOUT PERIPHERAL VASCULAR DISEASE

In a normal person, an injury to the skin of the foot or ankle is much more serious than one to the hand or wrist. In the ambulatory patient, lesions on the lower leg and foot may heal slowly. If healing does not occur promptly, the patient should be put to bed and the part elevated. If the lesion is allowed to become chronic, low-grade local phlebitis, lymphangitis, and arteritis develop. Even if the main vessels to the part are unaffected, these local changes cause poor tissue drainage and there is a tendency to recurrent infection and ulceration. A nonhealing, nontraumatic ulcer of the lower leg is an emergency and requires bed rest until healing occurs.

SPECIAL DIAGNOSTIC TESTS

The history and physical examination will establish the presence or absence of arterial insufficiency. When the circulation is normal, no instruments are necessary to demonstrate the fact. The skin shows no trophic changes and does not blanch abnormally on elevation. The arterial pulses are palpable. If the main artery is occluded by pressure for several minutes, release of pressure will cause bright-red reactive hyperemia. Heating of the body causes the extremities to warm, and immersion of the part in hot water brings out the capillary pulse. Histamine pricked into the skin produces a typical wheal and erythema. When there is obvious arterial insufficiency, these findings are changed as outlined under Special Points in History and Physical Examination. When other signs of arterial insufficiency are present, it is not safe to attempt to demonstrate the capillary pulse by placing the involved extremity in hot water.

Special tests have been of value in understanding the normal physiology of the peripheral circulation. They have been of use in quantitating the degree of damage caused by pathologic processes and have aided our understanding of the development of collateral circulation. They have been useful in determining, in at least a semiquantitative way, the effects of therapy in occlusive vascular disease.

The following tests are useful at times:

1. Measurement of skin temperatures in a cool room (18 to 20°C) before and after release of sympathetic tone. When the blood supply is decreased by occlusive arterial disease or by reflex vasoconstriction, or by both, the extremities cool. Release of sympathetic tone is accomplished by paravertebral block, by spinal anesthesia, or by raising the rectal temperature by body warming. If the skin temperature does not rise, the decrease in blood flow is the result of occlusive vascular disease. A rapid rise to 30.5 to 33°C indicates normal blood supply. An intermediate rise indicates both reflex sympathetic constriction and occlusive vascular disease. This test has the virtue of simplicity and has proved to be of clinical use.

2. Arteriography and venography. The arterial tree is visualized by x-ray after the intraarterial in-

jection of 50 per cent Hypaque or other contrast media. When the femoral pulses are absent, injection is made into the aorta. The exact point of arterial obstruction and the pattern of the collateral circulation can be determined. It is helpful in showing segmental occlusion in the iliac and femoral vessels. These lesions can now be approached surgically. Visualization of the veins by the injection of Hypaque is occasionally useful.

3. Circulation time to the extremities. Several methods are available. The fluorescein test is the most objective. For this, 3 ml of a 20 per cent aqueous solution of fluorescein is injected quickly into the antecubital vein, and the time of appearance of a greenish-yellow glow in various parts of the body is observed. When arterial insufficiency is present, the appearance time of the fluorescein is prolonged. In severe ischemia no fluorescein may appear.

4. Oscillometer. This is a volume recorder which magnifies the changes in volume which normally occur with each cardiac systole. The ordinary blood pressure recording apparatus may be used as a crude oscillometer. Refinements of the oscillometer have not increased its clinical usefulness.

5. Histamine wheal test. If the arterial circulation is inadequate, histamine pricked into the skin gives a subnormal or absent reaction.

6. Measurement of blood flow by plethysmographic techniques has advanced our knowledge of the circulation, but the method is not suitable for routine clinical use.

REFERENCES

Allen, E. V., W. Barker, and E. A. Hines: "Peripheral Vascular Disease," Philadelphia, W. B. Saunders Company, 1946.

Izzo, P. A., R. C. Stevens, A. J. Tomsykoski, and C. E. Rodriguez: Hemopericardium Associated with Anticoagulant Therapy, A.M.A. Arch. Internal Med., 92:350, 1953.

Lewis, T.: "Vascular Disorders of the Limbs," London, Macmillan & Co., Ltd., 1946.

Lowenberg, R. I.: Early Diagnosis of Phlebothrombosis with Aid of a New Clinical Test, J.A.M.A., 155:1566, 1954.

Wesler, Stanford: Intermittent Claudication, Circulation, 11:806, 1955.

Wilkins, R. W., and J. R. Stanton: Elastic Stockings in Prevention of Pulmonary Embolism, New Engl. J. Med., 248:1087, 1953.

Wright, I. S.: "Vascular Diseases in Clinical Practice," Chicago, Year Book Publishers, Inc., 1948.

Wylie, E. J.: Thromboendarterectomy for Arteriosclerotic Thrombosis of Major Arteries, Surgery, 32: 275, 1952.

B. DISEASES OF THE HEART

INTRODUCTION

William H. Resnik and
T. R. Harrison

In previous chapters the basic mechanisms underlying the important manifestations of disorders of the heart have been described. In the succeeding chapters, the clinical aspects of heart disease are presented.

"Curable" Heart Disease. The term "curable" requires definition. The patient whose heart disease stems solely from a patent ductus that has been closed may be considered cured in the strictest sense. The patient with valvular heart disease whose intractable heart failure has been eliminated by the adequate treatment of an associated thyrotoxicosis is not "cured" in the sense that the heart has been restored to structural normality. Nevertheless, he has been cured of heart failure in that it may now be possible for him to lead a practically unrestricted life. In other words, we mean by curable a form of heart disease that is amenable to specific treatment, even though an anatomic lesion may continue to exist.

The introduction of the important differentiation between low-output and high-output failure (p. 99) not only has clarified vexing and disputed points of view regarding the nature of heart failure, but it has brought into focus a group of disorders with high-output failure that are susceptible to cure. In addition, the spectacular advances in cardiac surgery and the development of potent antibiotics have completely altered the previous hopeless outlook of persons afflicted with many forms of congenital and acquired heart disease. As a consequence, we can no longer be content with the mere recognition that heart disease exists. *We must be constantly mindful that the patient may have a curable form of heart disease.* Overlooking such a disorder constitutes a far graver error than diagnosing incorrectly a form of heart disease that could not have been better treated even if it had been precisely recognized. The restoration of a patient to a normal life of useful activity by the discovery and appropriate treatment of bacterial endocarditis constitutes a far greater triumph than the lucky speculation at the clinical pathologic conference that the patient with the typical history of ischemic pain has suffered from endocardial fibroelastosis and not from coronary obstruction.

Moreover, the proper management of heart disease and of heart failure is based on something more than recognizing a "cause," e.g., rheumatic heart disease with mitral stenosis, and administering the standard procedures for the control of congestive failure. In all cases, *every possible contributing factor should be considered and treated if present*: infection and emotional stress, excessive activity and ingestion of salt, anemia, hyperthyroidism, thiamine deficiency, electrolyte imbalance, etc.

Cardiac Reserve. Cardiac reserve is the capacity of the heart to respond to increasing burdens without displaying manifestations of failure. In practice, the reserve is ordinarily estimated by observing the patient's response to varying degrees of activity. When more accurate information is required, hemodynamic measurements before and after exercise or after the administration of digitalis are necessary. In a previous chapter (p. 93) the question of cardiac reserve and the physiologic problems associated with it have been discussed in detail. Suffice it to repeat here that any increased work that is imposed on the heart, whether by augmenting its output, or the pressure that it must eject against, or its rate of beating, diminishes the cardiac reserve; and the loss of cardiac reserve is proportional to the increased energy requirements demanded by the added load. Experimental observations demonstrate that, for a given increase of work, increased volume (cardiac output) is least costly in terms of cardiac reserve, whereas increased heart rate is most costly and hence most destructive of cardiac reserve.

These experimental observations conform with clinical experience. *The failing myocardium is always overloaded in relation to its contractile strength. Anything that is responsible for a rapid heart rate constitutes a deleterious influence on an already overloaded heart,* and this explains why, for example, ectopic tachycardias are so harmful in myocardial infarction. The experimental observations explain why patent interventricular septum is usually so much more serious than patent interatrial septum, since in the latter lesion the primary load is a volume load, the least serious, whereas in the former there is in addition to the volume load a further pressure load, far more serious. Aside from the administration of digitalis which increases the efficiency of the myocardium, everything that the physician utilizes is designed to diminish the load of the already overburdened heart.

The Senile Heart (Presbycardia, the Aging Heart). Clinicians have long been familiar with the progressive loss of cardiac reserve with advancing years. The most thoughtful and lucid expression of the concept was given by William Dock. We consider its appreciation essential in understanding many otherwise perplexing problems of heart disease. The reserve capacity of the youthful heart is very great, and it is a matter of common experience that *the young person will tolerate without difficulty a burden such as a severe thyrotoxicosis or a paroxysmal tachycardia of long duration whereas an older person will develop congestive failure with the same disorders,* even when of milder intensity and briefer duration. The explanation for the effect of age on the adaptive capacity has never been clearly understood, chiefly because no histologic lesion in the aging myocardial fibers is visible that could account for the loss of efficiency. One widely accepted view has held that the diminished cardiac reserve in the aging individual is caused by an ischemia that increases with age, either because of the development of diffuse arteriolar disease in the coronary bed or because of the inadequate growth of capillaries to the myocardial fibers. Dock's perfusion studies have clearly indicated that ischemia is not the basis of myocardial failure in the aged, when there is no gross atheromatous involvement of the epicardial portions of the coronary arteries. Since the biochemical defect is as yet unknown, Dock ascribes the loss of cardiac reserve to normal aging or involutionary processes. The extent to which involution impairs myocardial efficiency varies from individual to individual at the same age, just as physical fitness and mental alertness are differently affected in aging persons. This explains why one person may tolerate a very high arterial pressure, for example, whereas another person of the same age suffers from congestive failure caused by an elevated pressure of much more moderate degree, when meticulous clinical as well as autopsy studies reveal no reason for the difference.

There can hardly be any dispute about the influence of presbycardia on the heart that has already sustained an impairment of cardiac reserve. The valvular lesion that caused no symptoms whatsoever at twenty may lead to severe disability at fifty, or the hypervolemia due to a saline infusion which is easily tolerated by the young adult may precipitate congestive failure in the elderly subject. There has been far more skepticism about the ability of age alone, pure presbycardia without any additional load, to cause failure of the myocardium. One is necessarily uncertain about the relative contributions of involution and coronary sclerosis to the development of failure in the aged, especially when the atheromatosis of the coronaries is of very moderate degree and has given rise to no clinical or anatomic manifestations of ischemia. But *there are occasional instances of heart failure in the elderly, carefully observed during life and at autopsy, when coronary disease, hypertension, valvular disease, anemia, thyrotoxicosis, etc., have been excluded and histologic examination reveals no structural myocardial disease. We believe that these represent myocardial failure caused by senile heart disease alone.* We do not mean to imply that the diagnosis "senile heart disease" should become a scrap basket for all forms of heart failure in individuals over the age of forty-five or fifty, although the scrap-basket diagnosis of "arteriosclerotic heart disease," for which there is little or no evidence when there is no gross atheromatous disease of the coronaries, seems to be accepted without protest by those who demur at the diagnosis "presbycardia or senile heart disease."

It would be preferable if we conceded frankly that the diagnosis should be: "heart disease and failure of undetermined origin"; that some degree of coronary disease will probably be found in a high percentage of cases, although the relationship of the coronary disease to the failure may be in doubt when there is no clear evidence that it has led to a critical diminution of coronary flow; but in a small percentage of cases, no physiologic or biochemical or anatomic cause for the failure will be demonstrated. The frequency with which this latter occurs is a matter of dispute; certainly, it is not common. Nevertheless, we do not believe that the *concept* of the aging myocardium, presbycardia, can be in doubt.

The Scope of "Heart Failure." Some believe that this term should be applied only to myocardial failure and should even be still further limited to failure of the ventricular myocardium. This concept holds that the congestive syndromes resulting from stenosis of the atrioventricular valves or from pericardial disease are not heart failure. In our opinion "heart failure" should include all disorders in which congestive phenomena occur as the result of the *inability of the heart to receive and propel the blood which is offered to it.* The *principle* involved is the same whether heart failure is due to aortic stenosis or to mitral stenosis, even though in the one case it is inadequacy of the thick left ventricle and in the other incompetence of the thin atrium. In these instances and in patients with endocardial fibrosis or with constrictive pericarditis, *congestive phenomena due to structural disease of the heart* are observed and the restriction of the term "heart failure" to those disorders in which the ventricular myocardium is at fault can lead only to confusion.

The concept that *heart failure occurs when cardiac output is inadequate in relation to filling load* (p. 100) is also of importance in comprehending the significance of the high-output disorders which, as already mentioned, are likely to be curable. In the case of most of these, such as thyrotoxicosis and anemia, the presence of congestive phenomena indicates heart failure. However, when there is a *primary* increase in blood volume (as contrasted to hypervolemia secondary to heart failure), such as may occur in the oliguric states induced by acute renal necrosis or by glomerulonephritis or following administration of intravenous fluid in excessive quantities to elderly patients, a true state of "noncardiac circulatory congestion" may exist. Under such circumstances, slight elevations of venous pressure and even of ventricular end-diastolic pressure may be present without heart failure. Since in the case of the young normal heart the output may increase severalfold without significant rise in pulmonary pressures, it is not likely that pulmonary capillary pressure can increase so much as to exceed oncotic pressure as the result of hypervolemia alone. The degree of hypervolemia and hence of filling load required to produce such a marked elevation of the pulmonary pressure will necessarily depend on the myocardial reserve. This explains why the state of "noncardiac circulatory congestion," induced by intravenous fluids, rarely leads to true heart failure in young persons but frequently does so in elderly subjects with previously asymptomatic presbycardia. In any patient with an elevated filling load, the presence of rales constitutes strong evidence that true heart failure is present. The differentiation between the rare disorder "noncardiac circulatory congestion" and heart failure thus depends largely on the presence of rales, gallop, and especially on the demonstration that digitalis administration produces improvement.

The Total Picture. The physician should constantly bear in mind that a single laboratory or instrumental report should rarely be the sole basis on which a clinical judgment is based. If we emphasize the electrocardiogram in the following chapters, it is only because this particular form of evidence pertaining to the heart is so widely employed and one to which so much deference is paid. The clinician should never forget that the electrocardiogram is a very precise instrument but the information that it affords us is limited. Technical errors may lead to confusion. The person who interprets the tracings is not infallible, and the most experienced and authoritative electrocardiographers may disagree about the reading of a record. The physician would do well to be wary about being misled by a purposefully and even necessarily ambiguous report: "consistent with myocardial ischemia." Practically any type of tracing is consistent with myocardial ischemia, even a perfectly normal record, let alone one displaying minor S-T or T-wave alterations. We do not mean to imply that the electrocardiogram is to be ignored. We do mean to emphasize that the physician must not relinquish his responsibility, which is to integrate the total picture: history, physical examination, as well as data obtained by instrumental and laboratory procedures. He should not permit his judgment to become paralyzed by a report dictated in a distant office by a person who has available only a fraction of the information necessary for a valid decision about the condition of a patient. Above all, he should avoid the fallacy of treating the electrocardiogram and of creating an iatrogenic invalid. Negative T waves do not constitute a disease. Exactly the same admonitions apply to murmurs, irregularities of the heart, and other deviations from the norm. Each must be interpreted in the context of the total picture. *The clinician must remain a clinician and not become a mere recipient and slave of reports; that is, he must never cease exercising judgment in his management of a clinical problem.* Finally, in his assessment of the total picture, he must constantly bear in mind that even the person with unquestionable organic heart disease may be suffering from symptoms of psychogenic origin and that these may be responsible for more concern and apprehension than may be caused by structural disease.

REFERENCES

Davies, L. G.: Observer Variation in Reports on Electrocardiograms, Brit. Heart J., 20:153, 1958.

Dock, W.: The Capacity of the Coronary Bed in Cardiac Hypertrophy, J. Exptl. Med., 74:177, 1941.

———: Presbycardia or Aging of the Myocardium, N.Y. State J. Med., 45:983, 1945.

Eichna, L. W.: Circulatory Congestion and Heart Failure, Circulation, 22:864, 1960.

McMichael, J.: Changing Views on Heart Failure, Ann. Internal Med., 51:635, 1959.

Rose, G. A., and R. R. Wilson: Unexplained Heart Failure in the Aged, Brit. Heart J., 21:511, 1959.

249 CONGESTIVE HEART FAILURE

*T. R. Harrison and
William H. Resnik*

The patient with cardiac disease may face any one of four major hazards or a combination of them. These are (1) inadequate coronary circulation, (2) bacterial endocarditis, (3) embolic complications, and (4) congestive failure. The first three of these

hazards are dealt with in Chaps. 254, 151, and 262, respectively, and the present chapter is limited to the subject of congestive failure. This may be defined as that disorder in which the response of the heart is inadequate in relation to the blood which is offered to it (p. 100).

NATURAL HISTORY

The concept of the senile heart (Dock's presbycardia) is fundamental for the understanding of the pathogenesis of many instances of heart failure. It explains why loads which are readily tolerated by young persons may lead to severe and even fatal failure in elderly individuals (p. 1378).

Heart Failure with Effort. *Manifestations and Diagnosis.* The early symptoms of heart failure are undue dyspnea and fatigue during muscular exercise. Since ready fatigability occurs in so many diseases it has little diagnostic import, and when due to cardiac disease it is often masked by the discomfort of breathlessness. Thus the recognition of incipient heart failure depends, in the main, on the evaluation of dyspnea.

The patient's age, weight in relation to height, and exercise habits must be evaluated before it is decided that the shortness of breath is anything other than a normal physiologic phenomenon. Likewise, the emotional status must be considered. Worry about the presence of a minor valve lesion may lead to a sensation of smothering, with the typical sighing which is so characteristic of the anxiety state (p. 391).

Even when an individual's shortness of breath is known to be beyond the physiologic limits, it does not necessarily follow that cardiac disease is the cause. Frequently, emphysema, advanced bronchitis, or other pulmonary disorders are responsible. Less commonly, anemia or even muscular weakness consequent to any grave constitutional disorder may lead to some shortness of breath. The differential diagnosis of dyspnea has been discussed in some detail in Chap. 14, but three points merit emphasis here: (1) In deciding whether dyspnea is of cardiac origin, the presence of clinical, electrocardiographic, or radiologic evidence of organic cardiac disease is important but not necessarily conclusive. (2) The measurement of circulation time is a simple and valuable procedure. With the exception of those disorders associated with increased cardiac output (Chap. 13), cardiac dyspnea of significant degree is associated with prolongation of the circulation time through the lungs. On the contrary, noncardiac dyspnea is usually associated with normal values. (3) In most borderline situations the response to a therapeutic test will supply conclusive information. If the dyspnea is of cardiac origin, the administration of digitalis and of a mercurial diuretic, plus the ingestion of a salt-poor diet, will usually produce decisive benefit within 3 or 4 days. The patient's subjective impression concerning his dyspnea should be supplemented by observation of the breathing after a given exercise and, in doubtful instances, by measurements of circulation time before and after the therapeutic test.

Heart Failure at Rest. *Manifestations and Diagnosis.* After a period of months or years, the patient with cardiac dyspnea tends to progress into a state of frank congestive heart failure (advanced heart failure). At this time symptoms begin to be present at rest. In some instances these symptoms are related to congestion of the lungs alone, and there is no evidence of systemic congestion. The patient then has shortness of breath in the recumbent posture and frequently suffers from paroxysms of dyspnea (see discussion below, under Acute Failure of the Left Side of the Heart). The evidences of cardiac enlargement are likely to be clearly apparent, and gallop rhythm is the rule. Rales at the lung bases will usually be found, but their absence does not exclude the presence of left-sided heart failure associated with congestion but without edema of the lungs. Some patients display hydrothorax at this time, but in most instances this complication occurs later as general anasarca begins to appear.

The clinical picture of left-sided failure is usually so distinctive as to offer little problem in diagnosis. In doubtful instances, measurement of the circulation time and observation of the response to digitalis will usually remove all doubt.

Eventually, the pattern of right-sided heart failure develops. In some instances this does not appear until the patient has already experienced the phenomena of left-sided failure for some weeks or months. However, occasionally the two sides of the heart appear to fail at about the same time. The usual signs of right-sided failure are distention of the veins associated with increased venous pressure, the presence of an enlarged, tender, and often painful liver, edema, albuminuria, and frequently cyanosis. Hydrothorax is usually present when there is failure of both sides of the heart, and is of great practical importance because of the relief that frequently follows removal of fluid. The right pleural cavity is affected somewhat more frequently than the left. This is possibly related to the tendency of some patients with heart failure to lie on the right side more than on the left.

Ascites is present in almost all instances of advanced right-sided failure and, under certain circumstances, may be out of proportion to the fluid accumulation elsewhere. This is seen frequently in children, in patients with constrictive pericarditis, and in patients with rheumatic disease affecting the tricuspid valve. Patients with mitral stenosis may also exhibit prominent ascites with only slight edema of the legs. This is probably to be ascribed to anatomic changes in the pulmonary arterial branches, with secondary mechanical limitation of congestion and edema of the lungs. Thus orthopnea is minimal, and the effect of gravity on the distribution of dropsical fluid is less pronounced than in most instances of congestive failure.

The clinical picture of a patient with right-sided failure or with combined failure of the left and right sides of the heart is so characteristic that ordinarily there will be no difficulty in recognizing it. Other disorders such as cirrhosis of the liver and thrombosis of the hepatic veins (Chiari's syndrome), which may produce enlargement of the liver and ascites, are not associated with elevation of venous pressure in the arms unless congestive failure is also present. Obstruction of the superior cava may lead to striking distention of the veins of the neck and chest, with edema of the upper part of the body. However, the evidences of collateral circulation are usually outspoken. Edema due to renal disease, to hepatic disorders, or to rarer causes can usually be readily differentiated from the edema due to heart failure, by the absence of venous distention, of rales in the lung bases, of orthopnea, etc.

In a few patients the pain consequent to hepatic congestion may lead to confusion with primary intraabdominal disorders. This error can be avoided by a thorough examination of the circulatory system as well as of the abdomen.

Many patients without cardiac failure display prominence of the cervical veins when recumbent. Distention of these veins is indicative of increased venous pressure only when it is present in the sitting or semisitting position. In doubtful instances the demonstration that compression of the upper abdomen causes marked distention of the cervical veins may be helpful. Patients who are recovering from cardiac failure may not have elevation of venous pressure. Likewise, individuals in whom heart failure develops very suddenly, without sufficient time for compensatory elevation of blood volume, may have no measurable increase of venous pressure despite marked edema of the lungs. In other patients with rapidly developing failure there may be distention of the central and cervical veins, with collapse (or constriction) of the peripheral veins. As a rule, however, this function is elevated in individuals with failure of the right side of the heart.

The distinction of heart failure from hypervolemic states and the relationship of "noncardiac circulatory congestion" to heart failure have been discussed on p. 1379.

Progression of Heart Failure. The advance from the early stage, with dyspnea only on effort, to the full-blown picture of combined left- and right-sided failure may occur gradually over a period of years, even though there is no evidence of increasing load. In such an instance, either progressive myocardial disease or loss of myocardial reserve as the result of the aging process is probably responsible. More commonly, however, progression tends to occur in a jerky, stepwise fashion rather than in a slow continuous evolution. Anything which accelerates the heart rate or increases cardiac output is likely to precipitate the next stage of heart failure. Thus any ectopic tachycardia may precipitate grave heart failure in a person with diminished cardiac reserve due to disease or age. Also important are other causes of tachycardia, such as fever from any cause, respiratory infections with severe coughing, excessive physical exertion, prolonged and severe emotional stress, anemia consequent to concurrent disease in other areas, pregnancy, and especially, pulmonary infarction. Another frequent aggravating cause of heart failure is the excessive ingestion of salt.

COMMON CLINICAL FINDINGS

There are a number of situations in which the heart fails suddenly. They include myocardial infarction, fulminant myocarditis, certain ectopic tachycardias, and various rarer disorders. These several types of acute cardiac failure are associated with evidence of minimal systemic congestion, because they set in so rapidly that there is not time for compensatory increase in blood volume to occur. Hence these conditions are likely to be characterized by a shift of blood from one portion of the circulation to another, and in most instances, the clinical picture mimics that of peripheral circulatory failure or shock, the manifestations of congestion being limited to the pulmonary vascular bed. This type of sudden cardiac failure is discussed in Chap. 13 and need not be considered further here. However, there is one form of acute heart failure which merits detailed discussion because of its frequency and of its response to therapy. This is the condition known as *cardiac asthma* or *acute pulmonary edema*.

Acute Failure of the Left Side of the Heart (Paroxysmal Dyspnea, Cardiac Asthma, and Acute Pulmonary Edema). Patients with hypertension, with lesions of the aortic valve, and with coronary sclerosis frequently are awakened by seizures of dyspnea. Similar attacks may occur in patients with mitral stenosis when marked tachycardia, due to exercise or an ectopic rhythm, reduces the diastolic filling period. Various names have been applied to these episodes. The severe and fatal instances are characterized by acute edema of the lungs. In many of the patients the moist rales are limited to the bases, and the physical signs are chiefly those of

bronchial obstruction, with wheezes and rhonchi. It is probable that edema of the bronchial walls is especially important here, although some believe bronchospasm to be concerned. When the number of moist rales is limited in relation to the wheezes and squeaks, the condition may be confused with bronchial asthma or with other causes of wheezing. Since the episodes usually occur at night, the term *paroxysmal nocturnal dyspnea* has been widely employed, but it has the disadvantage that similar episodes may occur during the day and that other diseases, such as bronchial asthma, occasionally cause paroxysmal dyspnea at night. From the standpoint of tradition there is some advantage in retaining these several terms, provided it is clearly understood that they all refer to one fundamental disorder—acute failure of the left side of the heart.

Acute left ventricular failure may be induced either by abrupt decrease in strength or by sudden increase in load. In the former instance, which is usually the result of acute myocardial infarction, there is no time for compensatory increase in total blood volume to occur and the combination of sudden trapping of blood in the pulmonary circuit with decline in cardiac output produces decrease in blood pressure and the picture of oligemic shock in the systemic vessels.

More commonly, these seizures are precipitated by an elevated filling load. This is usually caused by a temporary increase in total blood volume consequent to the recumbent posture, with reabsorption of extracellular fluid from the dependent parts of the body. Under these circumstances there is no deficiency of blood in the systemic area, the cardiac output and blood pressure are well sustained, and the shocklike state is minimal or absent. Less important causes of increased venous return and filling load are cough, nightmares, excessive warmth, and possibly abdominal distention. Ordinarily, they represent the final straws which may awaken the patient or exaggerate the effects of the reabsorbed fluid.

In a typical instance the patient, who has previously had some shortness of breath on effort but no symptoms at rest, retires for sleep in his usual state of health. After an hour or more he is awakened with a sense of suffocation, sits up, and may seek an open window. At the same time there is some coughing, and examination of the lungs at this period will reveal a few moist rales at the bases and scattered squeaks over the lung fields. In most instances the attack subsides after a few minutes of panting and coughing in the upright position. However, in the more severe attacks the dyspnea becomes progressively worse, the cough more severe, and there is expectoration of copious frothy sputum tinged with blood. Examination reveals scattered wheezes and squeaks and, in addition, moist rales all over both lung fields. This is acute pulmonary edema, which may be fatal within an hour or two unless appropriate therapy is promptly instituted.

The gravity of the attacks is related to the degree of transudation from the pulmonary capillaries. This depends on the balance between the oncotic and mechanical pressures. Because of the low pressure (8 to 10 mm Hg) normally present in the pulmonary capillary bed, there is a wide margin of safety. Increments up to a value of about 25 mm Hg lead to *congestion* of the lungs and relatively mild dyspnea. At higher levels the oncotic pressure is exceeded and the rapidly developing pulmonary *edema* causes the more severe attacks.

Typically, these seizures occur in patients with left ventricular failure due to hypertension, lesions of the aortic valve, or myocardial disease. The first episode may be initiated by a myocardial infarction, which may be painless.

Attacks of dyspnea which awaken the patient from sleep are rather uncommon in patients with mitral stenosis, except when precipitated by atrial fibrillation or pulmonary infarction. However, persons with mitral stenosis may suffer from acute pulmonary edema precipitated by exertion or even by recumbency. In the latter instances the attacks usually begin before the onset of sleep.

Diagnosis. Disorders other than left-sided heart failure may cause acute pulmonary edema. It may occur in patients with inspiratory obstruction or be caused by inhalation of irritating gases or particulate matter.

Acute pulmonary edema may develop following severe brain injury, e.g., in massive intracerebral or intraventricular hemorrhage or in bulbar poliomyelitis. Although acute hypertension may be present, the precise mechanism is disputed and little can be done to alleviate the situation.

Gravely ill, comatose patients often exhibit coarse and rattling respiration. This does not represent true pulmonary edema but instead is due to accumulation of mucus in the bronchi because of muscular weakness and depression of cough reflexes.

Treatment. The initial step should be the administration of morphine or an allied drug. The benefit resulting from respiratory depressants is probably due to the effect of these drugs in breaking the vicious cycle whereby dyspnea, itself a result of congestion of the lungs, leads to reduction of mean intrathoracic pressure, which causes greater inflow into the right ventricle and increase in the severity of the congestion when the left ventricle is less able to propel the blood offered to it. Thus dyspnea causes more congestion, which causes more dyspnea, and so the vicious cycle proceeds until the respiration is depressed by a drug of the morphine group.

Reduction of venous return to the right side of the heart can be accomplished to some extent by venostasis, which consists in applying tourniquets to three extremities. Every few minutes a tourniquet is placed on the fourth extremity and one of the others is released. Thus the danger of thrombosis is minimized. In the severer instances venesection should be employed, and one should not hesitate to withdraw as much as a liter of blood in successive bleedings of 500, 300, and 200 ml.

Oxygen is urgently needed in patients with acute pulmonary edema. Details concerning its administration are presented in Chap. 268.

When patients who have not received digitalis develop acute pulmonary edema, the rapid-acting digitalis preparations must be administered immediately. Lanatoside C (Cedilanid) should be given intravenously. The total dose for a patient not previously receiving digitalis is usually 1.2 to 2.0 mg, which may be given over a period of 2 hr, or less, in urgent instances. The initial dose should be 0.8 mg, and subsequent doses of 0.4 mg may be given at half-hourly intervals.

When a patient has already been receiving digitalis the problem is more difficult. Once it has been determined that the patient is only partially digitalized, then lanatoside C should be used with caution in an initial dose of 0.4 mg, followed by 0.2 mg at half-hourly intervals, until improvement occurs or evidence of digitalis intoxication appears.

In the *prevention* of attacks of acute pulmonary edema the following principles of therapy are important: (1) The maintenance of adequate digitalization. (2) The treatment of extracellular fluid excess, even though there may be no detectable pitting edema. This involves the utilization of diuretics and restriction of sodium chloride. (3) Every attempt should be made to avoid the precipitating factors. A patient who has been having attacks of acute pulmonary edema should sleep in the semisitting position and should have a special bed when this is available. Mild sedatives should be administered to minimize disturbing dreams. Cough and emotional stresses should be controlled so far as possible. The evening meal should be small, in order to minimize cardiac work. When the condition occurs repeatedly, a responsible member of the family should be instructed in the administration of morphine or an allied drug as soon as the attack begins. Otherwise, the patient may succumb before the physician can reach the bedside.

To summarize, attacks of pulmonary edema can be best prevented by vigilant and vigorous application of those therapeutic principles which are used to treat heart failure in general, and which are discussed later in more detail.

Periodic Breathing. In elderly persons with failure of the left side of the heart, periodic breathing

(Cheyne-Stokes respiration) may be accompanied by recurrent brief episodes of dyspnea. The same patient may have this periodic dyspnea as he dozes off to sleep and then be awakened by acute pulmonary edema. More commonly, a patient has only one of these syndromes. The treatment of nocturnal dyspnea due to Cheyne-Stokes respiration is essentially that of heart failure in general. However, opiates should be used sparingly, and the milder sedatives are often efficacious. This type of dyspnea usually indicates a poor prognosis but, unlike acute pulmonary edema, does not constitute a grave emergency.

Chronic Congestive Heart Failure. The majority of patients who have chronic heart failure have involvement of both sides of the heart. All the manifestations of both right- and left-sided failure are present in many patients, but some of them present only a portion of these manifestations, such as edema without detectable hepatic enlargement, or the reverse situation. Other patients will have right-sided hydrothorax with no other evidences of failure of the right ventricle. In such instances it is uncertain whether the accumulation of fluid in the pleural cavity comes from the visceral pleura and is a manifestation of left-sided weakness, or whether it arises from the parietal pleura and is the result of early right-sided failure. The rarity of hydrothorax in patients with involvement of one side of the heart only and its frequency when left and right failure coexist suggest that congestion of both parietal and visceral pleura may be necessary for its development.

It should be emphasized that slight pitting of the ankles at the end of the day occurs in many healthy persons. Individuals who have lost weight frequently have a palpable liver. Elderly persons who are leading a sedentary life are often short of breath on exertion. Emotional disturbances may rarely cause episodes of shortness of breath (usually described as "smothering") at night. Thus there may be some doubt in a borderline situation as to whether a patient does or does not have cardiac failure. In such an instance observation of the response to a diuretic and to digitalization will usually supply conclusive evidence. When the symptoms mentioned are not due to cardiac disease, little or no improvement will be noted, and even this will be mainly the result of suggestion. When, however, such apparently minor symptoms are in reality the earliest indication of myocardial failure, the administration of digitalis to a patient who has not previously received it, and of diuretics, will usually result in such striking improvement as to remove all doubt from the physician's mind. Actually, in most instances such a therapeutic test is not necessary because the presence of a diastolic gallop will often settle the question conclusively.

However, one should remember that the presence of objective evidence of cardiac disease, such as an organic murmur or an unquestionable abnormality of the electrocardiogram, does not necessarily mean that the symptoms are the result of cardiac disease. Individuals with such minor cardiac abnormalities may have symptoms which are the result of coexistent emotional or physical disorders. In such persons impressive responses to digitalis and diuretics will not be observed.

It should be emphasized again that the diagnosis of congestive failure must not be based on any one manifestation but rather on a combination of them. Thus enlargement of the liver and ascites may be the result of cirrhosis, and an almost identical picture may be caused by constrictive pericarditis. In the latter instance there will be increased pressure in the cervical veins and in those of the upper extremities, such manifestations being absent in patients with cirrhosis. Likewise, mediastinal tumors may be associated with increased pressure in the veins of the neck and of the arms, but evidence of congestion in the lower part of the body will be absent.

Edema due to renal disease is associated with characteristic changes in the urine. The findings are either those of the nephrotic syndrome, with massive albuminuria, or of acute glomerular nephritis, with hematuria and cellular casts. Hypoalbuminemia is frequently present in minimal degree in patients with chronic cardiac edema but rarely approaches the low values observed in persons with nephrosis and cirrhosis. Patients with acute glomerulonephritis often have both cardiac and renal factors present and operative in the causation of edema. The presence of dyspnea, hypertension, cardiac enlargement, a diastolic gallop and, especially, of improvement following digitalization will usually be sufficient to indict the heart as one factor in the production of edema.

Prognosis is uncertain in patients with chronic cardiac failure. One cannot predict when massive pulmonary infarction, a severe intercurrent infection, or cerebral vascular complications will occur. Despite such uncertainties, several factors are of particular importance in prognosis. The first is the *response to treatment*. The failure of impressive improvement to set in within a few days following vigorous therapy is likely to indicate a grave outlook.

The second factor is *the type of underlying cardiac disease*. When the congestive failure is basically the result of a mechanical lesion such as tricuspid stenosis, mitral stenosis, or constrictive pericarditis, the prognosis is likely to be much better than when the clinical manifestations are the result of a failing myocardium. It is the latter which is responsible for heart failure in patients with coronary artery disease and in those with hypertension and aortic valvular disease. Although these latter individuals have a mechanical burden, symptoms do not occur until the left ventricular myocardium has lost its reserve. On the other hand, the pulmonary manifestations of mitral stenosis are dependent on a purely mechanical disorder, as are the systemic congestive manifestations of tricuspid stenosis. Therefore, patients with heart failure due to stenosis of the atrioventricular valves may live for many years in a state of semi-invalidism. This is rarely the case when, as the result of disease or of the mechanical load, the myocardium has to become defective before heart failure develops.

A third important factor in prognosis is the *evaluation of the circumstances under which heart failure develops.* When it has occurred as the result of some circumstance that is particularly amenable to treatment or correction, such as atrial fibrillation with a rapid rate, or respiratory infection, or undue exertion, or the excessive ingestion of salt, the prognosis is likely to be much better than when heart failure has developed in the absence of any such additional stress.

As a general rule, marked cardiac enlargement indicates a gloomy outlook, provided it is mainly due to ventricular enlargement and not to atrial dilatation or pericardial effusion. In the final analysis, however, *the response to treatment is the single most important point in prognosis.*

TREATMENT OF CHRONIC CONGESTIVE HEART FAILURE

Prevention and Management of Aggravating Factors. The clinical state of patients with chronic cardiac disease does not progress steadily downward but tends to remain stationary or improve slightly for long periods of time, with sudden worsening as the result of various complications. Most of these complications are conditions which cause acceleration of the heart rate and/or increased output. Ectopic tachycardias, with extremely rapid rates, may precipitate failure in individuals with previously good myocardial reserve. However, when the reserve power of the heart is much diminished, even slight degrees of sinus tachycardia may exert deleterious effects. Respiratory infections with the associated distressing cough, physical exertion beyond that which produces dyspnea, fever due to any cause, emotional stress, and anemia are particularly important in this respect. The therapeutic implications are obvious.

Pulmonary infarction, discussed in Chap. 262, is one of the commonest complications. Its likelihood can be reduced by avoiding excessive rest in bed, by permitting some slow walking, by elastic bandages, by alertness in the detection of phlebothrom-

bosis, and by the use of anticoagulants in appropriate instances.

In patients with cardiac disease, *pregnancy* involves a number of special problems, which are discussed later.

Rest and Activity. The initial consideration in the management of the patient with congestive failure is that of placing him in a position in which dyspnea and the consequent metabolic demands of labored breathing on the heart are minimal. In most patients the semirecumbent position in bed meets these requirements. The upright posture favors edema formation in the dependent portions of the body but tends to diminish pulmonary edema, a far more serious condition than peripheral edema.

Ordinarily, the patient with congestive failure should be allowed to get out of bed and walk to a nearby commode for bowel movements. This procedure has the additional advantage of tending to exercise the leg muscles and thereby reduce the likelihood of phlebothrombosis and pulmonary infarction. When for any reason the patient's strength does not permit being out of bed and walking a little each day, anticoagulant drugs, elastic stockings, and passive exercises of the legs plus massage are indicated.

The advantages of the recumbent position are its favorable effects on peripheral edema and on fatigue. On the other hand, this position encourages reabsorption of fluid and thus tends to induce paroxysmal dyspnea. There is some advantage in attempting to induce diuresis by having the patient assume the horizontal position for several hours a day, preferably in the late afternoon provided dyspnea is not induced. When this daily rest period induces diuresis, it should be carried out indefinitely, as long as the activities of the day in the upright position result in the development of more than a slight amount of edema of the lower extremities.

Diet and Fluids. All patients with heart failure should be placed on a low-sodium diet, the extent of the sodium restriction depending on the severity of the cardiac failure. With the elimination of salted foods, the use of sodium-free milk, bread, and butter, and the avoidance of canned vegetables and prepared condiments, diets containing not more than 200 to 400 mg sodium per day can be administered. At the same time it is important to be certain that the water ingested (especially if it is water that has been softened) is poor in sodium and that drugs containing sodium are avoided. This extremely unpalatable type of diet is necessary only for patients with advanced heart failure. In milder instances diets containing 1.0 to 2.0 Gm sodium (2.5 to 5.0 in salt) may be permitted.

When the patient with congestive failure is first seen, anorexia may be so severe as to preclude a reasonably well-balanced diet. Under these circumstances sodium-free milk (Lanolac) or fruit juices and bananas, containing only minute quantities of sodium, are preferable to the traditional Karell diet (800 ml milk per day, containing about 400 mg sodium) for the first 2 or 3 days. At the end of this time, and as the result of this regime and other therapeutic measures simultaneously instituted, it is usually possible to administer a balanced diet containing not more than 200 to 400 mg sodium (equivalent to about 0.5 to 1 Gm sodium chloride). When compensation is fully restored or when the maximal therapeutic effect has been achieved, some of the dietary restrictions may be lifted. However, it is preferable to insist that the patient remain permanently on a diet containing not more than 1.0 to 2.0 Gm sodium, and considerably less in the case of those individuals whose myocardial efficiency is markedly impaired. The less the sodium intake, the less the tendency for outspoken congestive failure to recur, and the less the need for diuretics.

The various commercial sodium-free substitutes for table salt are considered to be palatable by a few patients. Others prefer vinegar, onion, or lemon juice to overcome the insipid taste of a sodium-poor diet.

The intake of water should usually be regulated by the desire of the patient.

Weight reduction is desirable for obese patients, and thiamine is indicated when there is protracted anorexia even of mild degree. The other vitamins may be given also when the anorexia is both prolonged and severe.

Digitalis. Since this drug constitutes one of the cornerstones of management, it will be discussed in some detail.

Mode of Action. The main effect of digitalis appears to be strengthening of the cardiac muscle with increase in ventricular emptying. Thus the drug tends to overcome the cardinal hemodynamic defect of myocardial failure, which is defective emptying of the ventricles (Chap. 13). In patients with atrial fibrillation, digitalis causes additional benefit by producing pronounced slowing of the ventricular rate by reducing the responsiveness of the junctional tissues to the barrage of impulses arising in the atrium. The slowing of the rate is slight in patients with regular rhythm and appears to be of vagal origin.

Indications. Atrial fibrillation with a rapid ventricular rate constitutes one of the chief indications for digitalis. When the drug is given intravenously as lanatoside C, and when the arrhythmia is of the paroxysmal type and of short duration, normal rate and rhythm are restored in some patients. However, this happens more frequently in patients with paroxysmal tachycardia. *In chronic atrial fibrillation*

the drug slows the rate without abolishing the abnormal atrial rhythm. Digitalis frequently converts atrial flutter into atrial fibrillation. Therapeutic doses will abolish premature beats in many patients with cardiac failure. Toxic doses produce premature beats, often in the form of bigeminal rhythm or, less frequently, paroxysmal atrial tachycardia with block, ventricular tachycardia, or nodal rhythm. These grave toxic effects usually occur in patients who, because of diuretics or anorexia, are depleted of potassium (p. 1390). Further details concerning digitalis and arrhythmias will be found in Chap. 250.

The most common indication for digitalis is the presence of congestive heart failure, even when the rhythm is regular. When failure is severe, the drug alone is often ineffective, and other measures such as diuretics are needed. However, in the earlier instances, and especially in patients having attacks of paroxysmal nocturnal dyspnea, digitalis alone is usually efficacious in treating and preventing the seizures.

The drug should be used in patients with early failure when the cardiac reserve is diminishing, as indicated by increasing dyspnea for a given effort or by diastolic gallop.

In doubtful instances the value of the drug can be tested by clinical observation of the response, supplemented at times by measurement of vital capacity and circulation time, before and after digitalization. This procedure is occasionally of value in differentiating dyspnea due to cardiac disease from that due to emphysema and other pulmonary disorders. As a rule, a patient should be given digitalis when the exertion incidental to a reasonably active life begins to induce dyspnea.

Once digitalis has been administered for congestive failure, the patient will usually need it either continuously or for long intervals throughout most of his life. The practice, frequently followed, of discontinuing the drug as soon as the overt manifestations of congestive failure have disappeared is not sound.

In some patients with paroxysmal atrial tachycardia, the seizures are prevented by the daily administration of digitalis; in other instances, this procedure is ineffective.

Contraindications. This drug, like any other, is contraindicated under conditions where there is no clear indication for its use. Neither enlargement nor murmurs constitute an indication unless there is dyspnea or edema. It should not be given to patients with sinus tachycardia, except when clear evidence of congestive failure, either actual or imminent, is present.

Digitalis may cause nodal or ventricular tachycardia, or atrial tachycardia with block (p. 1400), and most instances of fatal digitalis intoxication arise from the mistaken assumption that the presence of the rapid rate in such patients constitutes an indication for larger doses. Bradycardia of moderate degree is often a desirable effect, and the common practice of discontinuing the drug when the heart rate is less than 70 per minute is unsound. In some patients maximal benefit is achieved at resting rates between 50 and 60. In persons with atrial fibrillation it is desirable to administer enough of the drug so that the heart rate after mild exercise also remains within the normal range.

Preparation and Dosage. If one form of digitalis, administered properly, fails to produce improvement, it is unlikely that significant benefit will be obtained by a different preparation. The best results will usually be achieved by the physician who familiarizes himself thoroughly with only two preparations, one a rapid-acting type for emergencies and the other an intermediate or long-acting product for long-term digitalization.

The idea that all patients require about the same dosage of digitalis is mistaken. Actually, there are wide variations. The powdered leaf, about 1.2 to 1.6 Gm in 48 hr, and gitalin (Gitaligin), about 5 to 7 mg in 48 hr, are excellent preparations for most patients who have not been previously receiving the drug. When there is no emergency, the best procedure is to give a patient about two-thirds of the minimal digitalization dose in the first 24 hr. If such a dose causes no improvement, it is unlikely that digitalis will be of much value. If the expected benefit has been achieved, the maintenance dose may be instituted without proceeding to "full" digitalization. If the degree of improvement is less than anticipated, the average maintenance dose may be given three times daily after meals for several days, and then twice daily after meals. The patient should be instructed not to take the drug unless the meal has been eaten and enjoyed. In this way the onset of anorexia, which is usually the initial manifestation of toxic effects, tends to limit the dosage of the drug. The usual maintenance dose is about 0.5 mg gitalin, 0.1 mg digitoxin, or 0.1 Gm powdered leaf.

Many physicians prefer to use digitoxin because the available knowledge concerning its absorption, excretion, and destruction appears to be more precise than in the case of other preparations. Such knowledge indicates that about one-half the daily administered dose is excreted daily and that the destruction is largely independent of dosage and proceeds at a fixed rate for a given patient. If the sum of excretion and destruction is greater or less than the daily intake, the patient will eventually lose the digitalis effect or develop digitalis intoxication. It is probable that the same principles apply to other digitalis preparations, and if so, it is *theoretically impossible to maintain a patient in a properly digitalized state on a constant daily main-*

tenance dose unless it is almost exactly equal to the sum of the daily excretion and destruction. This dilemma may be avoided by routinely utilizing the average maintenance dose, or slightly less of one of the intermediate preparations (digoxin or gitalin), and giving *augmentation doses* for a few days every 2 or 3 weeks. The patient is instructed to take the previous daily maintenance dose three times daily after meals and only provided the appetite has not suddenly declined. This procedure is continued until (1) anorexia and/or nausea develops, (2) the physician, who should see the patient daily during this period of augmented dosage, detects frequent premature beats or sudden increase in heart rate, or (3) the desired clinical improvement occurs. In the latter instance, there is no need to continue to the point of toxic effects. Many patients do not require complete digitalization and will improve on this plan without untoward effects.

This third phase of digitalis therapy, i.e., periodic augmentation in addition to the traditional phases of initial digitalization and daily maintenance dosage is of great practical value in preventing the loss of effectiveness of the drug and the consequent worsening of heart failure which otherwise occurs in most patients who are kept on a constant daily dose for a long period of time. However, the procedure is hazardous unless certain precautions are observed. One of these is the concomitant administration of 1 Gm potassium chloride after each meal. This may be given either as tablets or as a 25 per cent solution, 4 ml being added to a *large* glass of orange juice. The likelihood that serious arrhythmias will precede the annoying but much less dangerous anorexia is thereby sharply reduced. When anorexia and nausea develop it is essential to decide whether these symptoms are due to digitalis or to some other cause such as potassium salts, ammonium chloride, or opiates. Another precaution implies daily observation by the physician during the period of augmented dosage, in order that the exceptional situation in which, despite potassium therapy, the digitalis induced arrhythmias appear first may be detected. A third precaution involves the use of those preparations (gitalin and digoxin) which, while effective by the oral route, have a relatively brief duration of action. They are preferable both for maintenance and for augmentation, because intoxication of mild degree frequently occurs during the periods of augmentation, and the duration of such intoxication is less than when digitoxin or powdered leaf is employed.

When a rapidly acting digitalis is desired, or when one is uncertain as to whether or not the drug should be given and wishes to use a preparation the effect of which will wear off within a few days, *Digitalis lanata* may be administered intravenously. The most satisfactory preparation of

Digitalis lanata is lanatoside C. Its quick onset of action makes it especially valuable in the management of such emergencies as acute pulmonary edema. Its rapid disappearance from the body makes it useful in patients who need digitalis but who are particularly susceptible to its untoward effects. Hence, in a person with myocardial infarction and increasing congestive failure, in whom digitalization may precipitate a serious disturbance of rhythm, this drug is preferable to others of the digitalis group. On the other hand, the rapidity of elimination makes it less desirable for use in the management of the usual patient with congestive failure. The usual total dose of lanatoside C required for digitalization is 1 to 2 mg for adults. This is administered intravenously in divided doses over a period of 4 to 8 hr. When good response is obtained, a longer-acting preparation should be used to maintain the effect. Since lanatoside C is rapidly dissipated, this can be accomplished by giving gitalin 0.5 mg three times daily after meals for about 5 days, and then 0.5 mg once daily indefinitely. The drug is temporarily discontinued if the appetite is lost or nausea develops. In the above plan one may substitute 0.1 mg digitoxin, or 0.1 Gm powdered leaf for 0.5 mg gitalin. The administration of the longer acting preparation is begun about 8 to 12 hr after the final dose of lanatoside C.

In patients who have been receiving digitalis and who have nausea and vomiting, it may be difficult to decide whether these symptoms are the result of abdominal congestion and constitute an indication for additional digitalis, or whether they represent toxic effects from overdosage. Under such circumstances the use of acetylstrophanthidin has been proposed. However, this is a hazardous procedure. In the usual patient the same information can be obtained by stopping digitalis therapy for a few days and noting whether the clinical state improves, as will occur if digitalis intoxication has been present.

Manifestations of Digitalis Intoxication. The most important of these include gastrointestinal disturbances—i.e., anorexia, nausea, and vomiting, developing in that order—and disturbances of the cardiac rhythm, of which the frequent premature beat, usually in the form of bigeminal rhythm, and atrial tachycardia with block are the most common. Inversion of the T waves and slight increase in the P-R interval are normal effects of the drug. Severe degrees of heart block due to digitalis intoxication occur frequently in animals but are very rare in man unless there is preexisting conduction impairment. In an occasional patient the drug converts sinus rhythm into atrial fibrillation. The reverse effect—conversion of atrial fibrillation to normal rhythm—may occur when the arrhythmia is of recent onset. Nodal rhythm with moderate to marked

tachycardia occasionally appears, and ventricular tachycardia may develop, with danger of ventricular fibrillation if the administration is continued. Less common toxic effects include diarrhea and xanthopsia (yellow vision).

When doses within the therapeutic range are employed and potassium depletion is avoided, the only common toxic effects are anorexia, nausea, and bigeminal rhythm, all of which disappear within a few days after withdrawal of the drug. Since it is often desirable that the drug be pushed to the onset of the minor toxic effects, it is well to warn the patient that vomiting may occur. Such warning not only will alleviate anxiety if vomiting does appear, but will make the patient more alert to report the onset of anorexia, which is usually the initial and the most benign indication that the toxic effect has developed. However, it is important to remember that the more serious toxic effects may supervene without the preliminary appearance of the usual warning signals in the form of the milder manifestations of toxic action.

Premature beats, or other arrhythmias, when induced by digitalis, may be improved by the oral administration of potassium salts (Chap. 250). Such arrhythmias are especially likely to be caused by digitalis when there is potassium depletion as the result of the frequent use of diuretics. Since glucose ingestion causes decline in plasma potassium, the toxic arrhythmias due to digitalis should be sought especially carefully during the period of 30 to 60 min after a carbohydrate-rich meal. When digitalis intoxication is present or imminent, protein-rich, carbohydrate-poor meals are indicated, and potassium chloride (1 Gm three to six times daily) should be administered orally unless renal insufficiency is present.

The most important principle of digitalis therapy is to push the drug until the patient exhibits either the desired therapeutic action or definite evidence of toxic effects. This is only another way of saying what William Withering, who introduced the drug into medical practice, stated so clearly: "Let the medicine . . . be continued until it either acts on the kidneys, the stomach, the pulse, or the bowels; let it be stopped upon the first appearance of any of these effects."

Diuretic Drugs. The rational use of these valuable agents depends upon an understanding of their effects on the disturbances of renal function responsible for the retention of sodium and of water. Although knowledge of these disturbances is still incomplete, it would appear that there are at least three different but related mechanisms which call for different treatment. One of these is the increased reabsorption of water and sodium in the *proximal tubules,* which appears to be dependent in some measure on hemodynamic factors and, especially, on the high filtration fraction which produces an abnormally high oncotic pressure in the blood of the peritubular capillaries. Unknown enzymatic reactions are probably also concerned. The commonly employed diuretic drugs such as chlorothiazide and the mercurials tend to block the proximal reabsorption not only of sodium and of chloride but also of potassium. They, therefore, cause diuresis but also often lead to *potassium depletion which is not necessarily reflected in the plasma potassium level.*

Another mechanism responsible for increased reabsorption of sodium and water is the excessive formation of aldosterone, which is believed by some to act chiefly on the *distal tubules.* Spironolactone (Aldactone), which is an aldosterone antagonist, blocks this action. However, if its main action is distal, it can be effective only when significant quantities of sodium are delivered to the distal tubule. Thus if most of the sodium should be reabsorbed in the proximal portion, spironolactone would be of little value. This is a possible explanation for its frequent ineffectiveness. However, it may be useful as an adjuvant to the conventional diuretics which block proximal reabsorption. Actually, because of its expense, this drug should be reserved for patients who display an inadequate response to other diuretic measures. Spironolactone, unlike chlorothiazide and mercurials, does not tend to induce potassium deficit.

A third and probably less common renal mechanism is the retention of excessive quantities of water in response to the antidiuretic hormone or to some substance having a similar action. This is probably one factor in the production of the serious "dilution syndrome," which is considered later.

All patients who have ever suffered from edema of cardiac origin and who have a tendency toward recurrence should weigh themselves each day under standard conditions. As a rule this means weighing in the morning immediately after rising and emptying the bladder, without clothing other than slippers and pajamas. The written record of such daily weighings constitutes the guide to therapy by diuretic drugs.

The most generally useful diuretics are those of the chlorothiazide group. They are indicated when the weight record shows a rapid increase. Since anorexia is common in patients with congestive failure, the effects on body weight of expansion of extracellular fluid volume may be masked by concomitant loss of flesh. Therefore, even though the patient's weight is stationary, chlorothiazide is needed when there is progressive swelling of the ankles, or whenever there is a sharp increase in the degree of dyspnea.

A generally suitable plan is to administer 250- to 500-mg doses of chlorothiazide two to four times daily for five successive days out of each week, as long as the above-mentioned indications exist. Because of the strong tendency for potassium depletion to occur, potassium chloride should be also administered, as already described (p. 1388). This is especially important when the normal dietary intake of potassium is limited because of anorexia. When there is persistent oliguria or grave impairment of renal function, potassium administration may be hazardous and should be controlled by repeated measurement of the plasma level.

Since the advent of the chlorothiazide group of drugs the mercurial diuretics are needed much less frequently than formerly. They should be reserved for patients with massive edema, in whom especially profuse diuresis appears desirable, or for persons who fail to respond well to chlorothiazide.

Convincing evidence that any one of the currently available mercurial preparations is superior to the others is lacking. The initial dose should be 1 ml intramuscularly. If a satisfactory diuresis is not produced, 2 ml is given, and this dose may be repeated after several days. Unless renal function is seriously impaired, it is well to administer potassium chloride (3 to 4 Gm per day) routinely, and to add ammonium chloride for 3 days when a mercurial diuretic is to be administered. The effectiveness of the latter is sometimes enhanced by the prior injection of aminophylline intravenously.

When these measures fail, spironolactone may be used in conjunction with chlorothiazide or mercurial diuretics. It is likely to be ineffective if administered alone (see above), is expensive, and is only rarely needed.

The untoward effects of diuretics fall into several categories, the most important being those related to *electrolyte depletion* of different types. These electrolyte disturbances are likely to occur in persons whose salt intake has been severely restricted and who have received vigorous mercurial therapy with massive diuresis. Aside from refractoriness to diuretic drugs, there may be no symptoms, or there may be a group of symptoms common to all, regardless of the electrolyte patterns; lassitude, apathy, mental confusion, anorexia, decrease in urine volume, and azotemia. When adequate facilities are available, frequent measurement of the serum levels of sodium, potassium, chloride, and carbon dioxide as well as of urea should be carried out, especially when congestive failure does not respond to adequate therapy.

When water, chloride, and sodium are excreted in excessive quantities but in ratios similar to those present in normal serum, a state of *absolute extracellular fluid deficit* with dehydration may occur. A somewhat analogous disorder is the *distributional disturbance of extracellular fluid.* This occasionally appears in individuals who continue to have edema of the legs because of the orthopneic position but who, as the result of diuretic drugs, have a deficiency of extracellular fluid in the upper parts of the body. In such patients the diagnosis rests on the clinical manifestations of dehydration (p. 459) in the affected areas. Measurements of plasma electrolytes yield normal values, but urea nitrogen is usually elevated. The treatment consists of the administration of salt-enriched foods. Only rarely is parenteral administration of sodium chloride solution necessary.

More common and more serious are those disorders characterized by lowered concentration of sodium and chloride in the plasma. These may be induced by (1) disproportionate urinary loss of electrolytes as compared to water during diuresis; (2) retention of excessive volume of water by the kidneys, probably as the result of the action of the antidiuretic hormone or of related substances; or (3) a shift of chloride and sodium from the extracellular to the intracellular fluid. Two entirely different disturbances may occur, and their distinction is of practical importance in treatment.

The *salt depletion syndrome* is closely related to the disorders of extracellular volume which have been mentioned above, but differs from them in exhibiting low values for the plasma sodium and chloride. It usually is seen when edema is absent or minimal; evidence of extracellular fluid deficit is commonly observed in the upper part of the body. The ingestion of salt-enriched food or the cautious daily intravenous infusion of 200 to 300 ml of 5 per cent sodium chloride will overcome the symptoms within a few days.

The *salt dilution syndrome* presents the same electrolyte pattern, with low sodium and chloride levels, but this condition is more grave and appears to develop through a different mechanism. It is usually encountered in markedly edematous patients during the late stages of heart failure as well as in a variety of other unrelated terminal illnesses, even when there have been no unusual losses of salt. Hypertonic sodium chloride is rarely of benefit in these patients, and although the plasma electrolyte pattern may be temporarily corrected, thirst is aroused, further excesses of water are retained, the serum sodium and chloride levels fall to their previous levels, and the net result is an increase in the extracellular fluid volume with further increase in edema. The proper treatment is marked restriction of water intake, thus allowing the insensible water loss to repair, in time, the relative electrolyte deficit.

Another important electrolyte disturbance, stemming primarily from diuresis, is *hypochloremic alkalosis* due to the disproportionate loss of chloride and of potassium. Body stores of potassium are usually depleted even though serum potassium may be normal. Serum chloride is abnormally low, bi-carbonate is correspondingly elevated, and sodium remains normal or at near-normal levels. Exactly the same chemical findings occur in respiratory acidosis, and differentiation between the two must be made on clinical grounds unless means for accurate measurement of the plasma pH are available. Respiratory acidosis occurs when the primary cause of the difficulty is a pulmonary disorder such as obstructive emphysema, interfering with O_2 and CO_2 exchange, or a depression of ventilation (e.g., morphine or sedatives) acting in essentially the same way. The treatment of hypochloremic alkalosis consists of the administration of ammonium chloride, 4.0 to 6.0 Gm per day in divided doses or, when oral administration is not possible, by the slow intravenous infusion of a 1 per cent solution of ammonium chloride, at a rate not greater than 100 ml per hr. A total of 500 ml may be given on one day and repeated the next, if necessary. The effect of acetazoleamide (Diamox) is very similar to that of ammonium chloride, and the combined effect of acetazoleamide, 250 mg t.i.d., and ammonium chloride, 4.0 Gm per day, may bring about a fairly rapid restoration of chloride to normal levels. Potassium chloride, 1.0 Gm four times daily, should be given orally, since a potassium deficit practically always accompanies hypochloremic alkalosis.

Potassium deficiency in the absence of alkalosis may occur following the prolonged use of diuretics, particularly when there have been additional losses of potassium by vomiting or diarrhea, and when anorexia has limited the supply of food. The chief manifestations, in addition to those described above as being common to all electrolyte disturbances, are unusual muscular weakness, abdominal distention due to intestinal atony, and electrocardiographic alterations: progressive depression of the S-T segment and rounding, lowering, and inversion of the T wave; increasing amplitude of the U wave in the left precordial leads. It is important to bear in mind that serious potassium deficits may exist even though the serum potassium level may be normal, and such a deficiency should be presumed to exist when ammonium chloride or acetazoleamide has been administered, when hypochloremic alkalosis occurs, and particularly when unexpected digitalis intoxication develops.

Refractoriness to diuretics represents a grave situation. Potassium deficit is probably the commonest cause. When such refractoriness is not responsive to potassium salts alone, it can often be overcome by the production of hyperchloremic acidosis. For this purpose ammonium chloride (8 Gm daily in divided doses) is given for 5 days. Unless the patient is eating normally, potassium chloride (4 to 6 Gm daily) should likewise be prescribed. During the first 3 days of the regime, acetazoleamide is administered in doses of 250 mg twice daily. On the fifth and several subsequent days, mercurial diuretics are administered. In doubtful instances blood chloride and carbon dioxide combining power should be measured daily and the acetazoleamide and ammonium chloride administration continued until the respective values are significantly altered. In some patients it appears to be necessary to achieve levels of 120 mEq per liter or more for chloride and 20 mEq per liter or less for bicarbonate, before the refractoriness can be overcome.

Other Therapeutic Measures. *Sedatives.* The judicious administration of sedatives is helpful, especially in the early days of severe congestive failure. For dyspnea, morphine (10 to 20 mg) or Pantopon (10 to 20 mg), administered parenterally, is usually effective in affording some degree of comfort and in ensuring sleep. They are best given in the evening and, after 4 hr or more, repeated once during the night if necessary, but always with due regard for the caution necessary in the use of these drugs in the aged, and for the dangers of habituation if they are used for more than a few days. Aside from promoting sleep, opiates are valuable because they reduce the strenuous work of the respiratory muscles. They also enable the patient to assume the recumbent position, which often initiates diuresis. After the first few days, when congestive failure has been considerably alleviated, moderate amounts of barbiturates may be substituted. During the day the meprobamate tranquilizing drugs or small doses of phenobarbital (15 to 30 mg), two or three times daily, may diminish undue restlessness and apprehension. *It is most important, however, that one be particularly careful to avoid excessive sedation* because of the possibility of rendering the patient so lethargic that he is unwilling or unable to participate in sufficient activity to minimize the danger of phlebothrombosis, and because of the undesirability of excessive respiratory depression in a patient with lowered vital capacity.

Venesection. Seizures of acute pulmonary edema constitute the most important indication for venesection, which is a rapidly effective and often a lifesaving procedure under these circumstances (p. 1383). Venesection is usually beneficial in patients with chronic cor pulmonale who have hematocrit values of 50 per cent or more. Painful congestion of the liver may likewise be benefited. Venesection may be employed in all patients with intractable heart failure, but under such circumstances lasting benefit is rarely produced. Ordinarily, the amount of blood removed should be 300 to 400 ml for an adult patient of average size without anemia.

Oxygen. Administration of oxygen is indicated (1) in any patient with evidence of outspoken arterial hypoxia, (2) when dyspnea is severe, and (3) possibly in patients with intractable congestive failure. When oxygen is needed for several days, a tent is the most useful method of administration; for periods of a few hours, a mask is convenient, effective, and relatively inexpensive (Chap. 268).

Thoracentesis. This is a valuable procedure in many patients with congestive failure. It should be employed in all severely dyspneic patients who present evidence of hydrothorax. *Abdominal paracentesis* is indicated whenever ascites is prominent and fails to respond promptly to sodium restriction and diuretics.

Puncture of the Legs. In those few patients who respond poorly to properly used diuretic measures, edema may be overcome by puncturing the skin of each leg 10 or more times with an 18-gauge needle. The patient should then remain in the sitting position for 12 hr or more and should be given appropriate antibiotics, usually penicillin, to prevent infection.

Special Problems in the Management of Heart Failure

Pregnancy. The physiologic adjustments that normally take place during pregnancy, the increase in heart rate, cardiac output, and blood volume place a burden on the cardiovascular system. This burden, unlike that due to muscular effort, is present continually, both night and day. It reaches its peak at about the seventh or eighth month of pregnancy. Thereafter, these functions decline and tend to approach normality up to the time of labor. This hyperkinetic state of the circulation acts to diminish the cardiac reserve, a reduction of which is well tolerated by the pregnant woman with the normal heart, but is tolerated with varying degrees of success by the woman with organic heart disease, depending on the extent to which her cardiac reserve has already been diminished by the structural lesion of the heart. *The greatest danger of congestive failure to the woman with heart disease occurs at the seventh or eighth month of pregnancy.*

The increase in blood flow through the heart is frequently responsible for the appearance in normal persons of functional systolic murmurs which, with the edema of the ankles, that is also not uncommon, and the displacement of the cardiac impulse by the elevated diaphragm and the resulting mistaken impression that there is cardiac enlargement, sometimes may give rise to the erroneous idea that heart disease is present. The increased blood flow also tends to accentuate murmurs in those who do have organic heart disease, thus occasionally revealing for the first time a hitherto undetected lesion such as mitral stenosis. Though there is no diminution in vital capacity, ventilation increases and the respiratory reserve is curtailed, thus facilitating the appearance of dyspnea with any given effort.

The chief practical problems presented by pregnancy in relation to heart disease are as follows: (1) Should the woman with cardiac disease become pregnant? (2) What should be done about a woman already pregnant who presents evidence of cardiac disease? In general, these questions are answered by an assessment of the patient's functional capacity, and this, in turn, is best determined by estimation of the symptoms caused by varying degrees of activity. The patient who is asymptomatic or whose dyspnea is minimal even with strenuous exertion can undertake pregnancy with practically no more risk than can the woman with a normal heart. On the other hand, the presence of relatively severe symptoms with ordinary activity, a history of hemoptysis (indicating the probability of an already significantly elevated left atrial and mean pulmonary capillary pressure), or a previous history of congestive failure makes it inadvisable that pregnancy be undertaken and may indicate that the pregnancy should be terminated. The same advice should be given if atrial fibrillation is present, not because of the deleterious effects of the abnormal rhythm, but rather because its presence indicates that an advanced stage of rheumatic heart disease is already present. Nevertheless, even atrial fibrillation is not an absolute contraindication to pregnancy or its continuation to term, provided the functional capacity of the heart is deemed to be reasonably good, the desire for the child great, and the risks understood by the parents. It is the intermediate group of patients, those with symptoms on moderate activity, who present the most difficult problem, the decision depending on a multitude of factors aside from the status of the heart: the number of children in the family, the economic circumstances, the opportunity for restriction of activity, the likelihood that the patient will cooperate in reducing the preventable stresses on the heart, the willingness to accept a calculated risk, etc.

Since the patient with heart disease starts out with the handicap of a diminished cardiac reserve which is still further lessened by the normal physiologic adjustments of pregnancy, all other stresses that confer additional burdens on the heart and circulation require meticulous attention: avoidance of overexertion and emotional tension, correction of anemia, careful supervision of even minor infections, correction of obesity, restriction of salt intake, prompt treatment of abnormal rhythms—especially tachycardias—and frequent search by the physician for early signs of pulmonary congestion.

Termination of Pregnancy. If the patient is already pregnant and falls into one of the unfavorable categories, or if manifestations of congestive failure

appear early, termination by the vaginal route should be carried out during the first trimester. After this time, disposition of the patient is a matter of judgment and always entails uncertainty and risk. If the symptoms are mild or moderate, the patient may with careful medical supervision be carried beyond the critical seventh or eighth month, after which the danger diminishes. On the other hand, if the symptoms are severe, termination of the pregnancy may be considered imperative, the method being left to the obstetrician.

Once a patient has arrived at term, the route of delivery should be decided by the obstetrician on obstetric grounds. Usually, spontaneous delivery aided by low forceps is preferable. Resort to cesarean section as a routine measure is no longer considered desirable, this mode of delivery being reserved only for women who are expected to face a difficult and exhausting labor.

The above comments are applicable in a general way to all women with heart disease, but they refer particularly to women with rheumatic heart disease and mitral stenosis, since they constitute the bulk of those with heart disease in pregnancy. Mitral commissurotomy has been successfully employed in some women in whom threatening symptoms have appeared during pregnancy. It is generally believed, however, that medical supervision alone or termination of the pregnancy is preferable, operative dilatation of the valve being reserved for a later time when the patient is not pregnant.

Patients with the cyanotic types of congenital heart disease usually do not survive until the childbearing age. When they do become pregnant, the hazard is high and early termination is likely to be indicated. Usually, pregnancy in the patient with acyanotic congenital heart disease is well tolerated. Repair of coarctation of the aorta should be done prior to pregnancy. The occasional development of dissecting aneurysm during pregnancy or of a cerebral vascular accident during delivery makes this condition somewhat more hazardous than other asymptomatic cardiac disorders. Advice regarding future pregnancies will depend on the course of the preceding ones and on the state of the heart at the time the next pregnancy is contemplated.

Intractable Heart Failure. From time to time physicians encounter patients with cardiac failure who either do not show a satisfactory initial response to therapy or who, having previously responded well, become progressively more refractory to management. Under these circumstances the physician will do well to ask himself the following questions: (1) Is the therapy adequate? (2) Is there in this patient an unrecognized etiologic factor which might be treated successfully? (3) Is some complication making the patient respond so poorly? (4) Is the intractable heart failure due to extreme myocardial impairment? These questions will now be considered in some detail.

1. *Has the patient received adequate therapy for congestive heart failure?* Is the dose of digitalis properly adjusted? If the patient has been receiving a constant maintenance dose of any digitalis preparation, there is a definite possibility that he has escaped digitalization because the combined effects of excretion and destruction of the drug have exceeded the daily maintenance dose. Under these circumstances it is frequently desirable to administer for a few days one of the intermediate drugs, such as gitalin or digoxin, in a dose equal to two or three times the average maintenance of such a preparation (p. 1387).

Digitalis intoxication is likewise a common cause of what may appear to be intractable heart failure. The presence of undoubted signs of such intoxication in an individual who has been receiving a relatively small maintenance dose makes it highly probable that potassium deficit has occurred as the result of anorexia and the frequent administration of thiazide diuretics. Under such circumstances rapid improvement may follow the administration of potassium chloride, 3 to 6 Gm daily in divided doses, for a few days. If the maintenance dose of digitalis has been relatively large, then the patient may be suffering from digitalis intoxication, even though there is no potassium deficit. Careful inquiry should be made concerning the presence of anorexia, nausea, and arrhythmias due to digitalis, and the less frequent and less obvious manifestations of digitalis intoxication such as diarrhea, blurring of vision, and xanthopsia should be sought. If the patient has been receiving one of the intermediate drugs, the manifestations of digitalis intoxication will disappear within 3 to 6 days after withholding it. If powdered leaf or digitoxin has been employed, improvement may be delayed for as long as 1 to 2 weeks after discontinuing digitalis.

Defective restriction of sodium is another common cause of apparent intractability. A patient may religiously refrain from adding salt at the table or during cooking and yet fail to realize that the bread he eats and the water he drinks may be excessively rich in sodium. The physician should be familiar with the sodium content of the tap water in his community and should prescribe distilled water whenever necessary. Sodium-free bread and butter are now available at most large grocery stores.

2. *Is there an unrecognized etiologic factor which might be successfully treated?* One thinks first of all of masked thyrotoxicosis. This condition may present none of its usual clinical manifestations when occurring in an elderly patient with congestive heart failure. The physician should entertain a high degree of suspicion toward such physical signs as unusual softness of the skin, excessive sweating, frequent bowel movements, heat intolerance, unexplained tachycardia, etc. Even with a high index of clinical suspicion, patients with thyrotoxicosis will be overlooked unless one makes it a rule to determine the protein-bound iodine of the serum in all patients with congestive failure, and particularly in those with atrial fibrillation.

Chronic arterial hypoxia due to primary disorders of the lung is frequently complicated by congestive heart failure and may be strikingly benefited by oxygen therapy properly administered. Anemia of clinically significant degree is usually obvious upon inspection of the patient's skin and mucous membranes, but it may be overlooked. The possibility of thiamine deficiency due to the long-standing anorexia induced by abdominal congestion should be considered in every patient with congestive heart failure. The suspicion should be particularly strong when treating elderly men who live alone or individuals who partake freely of alcohol. In the younger group of patients with valvular disease the possibility that smoldering rheumatic myocarditis or bacterial endocarditis is present should be kept constantly in mind.

It is perhaps even more important to look for evidences of those types of cardiac disease which are particularly amenable to surgical management. Mitral stenosis may be readily overlooked in a middle-aged or elderly patient with atrial fibrillation. The presence of obvious congestive failure may keep the physician from a careful search for such congenital disorders as coarctation of the aorta and patent ductus with a systolic murmur only. Constrictive pericarditis is especially likely to be missed unless constantly kept in mind.

3. *Is there a hitherto unsuspected complication?* In patients who have been subjected to repeated diuretics plus a long-standing low-salt diet, and more particularly, if anorexia has been an important symptom, one should be on constant watch for those electrolyte disturbances already discussed. They are likely to manifest themselves by the relatively rapid onset of refractoriness to diuretics and by the simultaneous appearance of marked lassitude and apathy. In the absence of some serious primary disease of the kidney or of some obvious grave intercurrent disorder, the presence of refractoriness to diuretics constitutes strong evidence for the presence of one of these electrolyte disturbances.

Advanced renal disease frequently is present in patients with congestive failure and especially in those who have either hypertension or bacterial endocarditis. During the initial phase of management the manifestations of congestive failure may overshadow those of the less obvious but often more serious renal disease. The coexistence of nitrogen retention and of a urine of low specific gravity, despite a small urine volume, makes it highly probable that there is grave functional impairment of the kidneys and that the management of the cardiac failure and, more particularly, of electrolyte disturbances will be relatively unsuccessful.

Pulmonary infarction, discussed in Chap. 262, is one of the commonest causes of intractable heart failure. If this complication is recognized and vigorously treated either with anticoagulants or, in suitable cases, by venous ligation, the heart may again respond to treatment after a period of days or weeks has elapsed. In many instances the expected manifestations (pleural pain, hemoptysis, and changes in the x-ray) will be absent and the sole clues to pulmonary infarction may be unexplained elevations of temperature, leukocyte count, or sedimentation rate, plus aggravation of the cardiac status and, at times, an evanescent increase in the serum bilirubin values or frank jaundice.

4. *Is the intractable heart failure due to extreme myocardial impairment?* This suspicion should be entertained seriously only after the problem has been approached from the standpoint of the questions above. Once one is satisfied that the therapy is entirely adequate, that there is no complicating unrecognized etiologic factor and no serious complication, one is justified in entertaining the question of myocardial disease so advanced that the heart failure has become and will remain intractable.

REFERENCES

Bartter, Frederic C.: "The Clinical Use of Aldosterone Antagonists," Springfield, Ill., Charles C Thomas, Publisher, 1960.

Blackard, Embree, and T. R. Harrison: Augmentation: A Third Stage of Digitalis Therapy, A.M.A. Arch. Internal Med., 103:543, 1959.

Burwell, Charles Sidney: "Heart Disease and Pregnancy; Physiology and Management," 1st ed., Boston, Little, Brown & Company, 1958.

Dock, W.: Aging of the Myocardium, Bull. N.Y. Acad. Med., 32:175, 1956.

Friedman, Meyer: Digitalis Therapy and Intoxication, Modern Concepts Cardiovascular Disease, 25:311, 1956.

Lown, Bernard, and Samuel A. Levine: "Current Concepts in Digitalis Therapy," 1st ed., Boston, Little, Brown & Company, 1954.

Luckey, E. Hugh, and Albert L. Rubin: The Correction of Hyponatremia in Congestive Heart Failure, Circulation, 21:229, 1960.

McMichael, John: Changing Views of Heart Failure, Ann. Internal Med., 51:635, 1959.

Moyer, J. M., and M. Fuchs: "Edema: Mechanisms and Management," Philadelphia, W. B. Saunders Company, 1960.

Symposium on Congestive Heart Failure, Circulation, 21: January, February, March, 1960.

Symposium on Congestive Heart Failure, J. Chronic Diseases, May, 1959.

Symposium on Salt and Water Metabolism, Circulation, 21:806, 1960.

250 ARRHYTHMIAS
William H. Resnik and
T. R. Harrison

The normal stimulus for the heartbeat arises in the sinoatrial node, spreads through the atrial musculature, traverses the AV node (node of Tawara), the AV bundle (bundle of His), through the Purkinje fibers of the left and right bundle branches, and finally through the ventricular musculature. When this orderly and regular sequence is disturbed, or when the rate of conduction of the impulse is abnormal, a variety of disorders of the heartbeat may follow, the most common and important of which are discussed here. Almost all of these disorders may be the result of structural disease of the heart, but most of them may also be encountered in normal, healthy persons in whom no evidence of organic heart disease is ever discovered or who reveal no abnormalities by histologic examination at autopsy. The most precise method of diagnosis of the various arrhythmias is by electrocardiographic examination. However, the physician who has regularly correlated his observations by simple examination with electrocardiographic tracings can usually recognize most of the arrhythmias by auscultation alone.

Mechanism of Arrhythmias. The hypotheses so widely accepted but a short time ago regarding the pathogenesis of the various arrhythmias are no longer considered as established beyond question. For example, for a number of years the circus movement as the explanation for atrial flutter and fibrillation seemed to have been indisputable, only to be replaced by the concept that these ectopic rhythms were the result of very rapid and irregular stimuli being discharged from a single focus. Actually, this latter view was simply an elaboration, based on rather extensive experimental work, of a hypothesis that had preceded that of the circus movement. At the present time, there is abundant evidence in favor of and in refutation of both concepts, and it is probable that neither is strictly true. Moreover, it is likely that from the newer studies on alterations of the myocardial cell, cell membrane, and cellular environment and the abnormalities of electrical potential, conduction, and excitability resulting from these ionic disequilibria and disturbances in myocardial cellular metabolism, will come a truer knowledge of the mechanisms of the various arrhythmias and of the manner in which they are influenced by drugs and other procedures.

The value of the electrocardiographic tracings in the differential diagnosis of the tachycardias is obvious. Since registration of atrial activity is particularly desirable, records should be obtained from the right of the sternum, and in many instances while carotid sinus pressure is being applied. At times, the use of esophageal leads may demonstrate P waves not clearly seen in conventional leads, and thus clarify the nature of the tachycardia.

Harmful Effects of the Arrhythmias. The influence of changes of rate on coronary flow and the cardiac output has been described in some detail in a previous chapter (p. 33). It will suffice here to state that, when the heart rate is 30 or more, the bradycardias cause no significant alterations in coronary flow or cardiac output. The danger of a bradycardia exists when it is due to a high-grade partial or to a complete AV block caused by a lesion affecting the AV node or bundle. The ventricular rate may suddenly diminish to 5 to 10 per minute or may come to a complete standstill for 15 sec or more; or ventricular fibrillation may develop, the effect being essentially the same as that of ventricular standstill; circulation to the brain becomes inadequate, syncope of varying degree occurs, and when effective circulation halts for 15 sec or longer, convulsions appear. These attacks are known as Stokes-Adams attacks, and a person subject to them is always in danger of sudden death.

Because diastole is abbreviated to a greater extent than is systole in a tachycardia, the effect of a rapid increase in rate is to increase oxygen consumption of the heart and to diminish coronary flow. When the rate of an ectopic tachycardia is 160 or more, and there is no concomitant increase in cardiac output such as would occur if strenuous exercise induced a heart rate of this magnitude, the efficiency of the heart is reduced, cardiac output declines from its previous normal level at rest, and cerebral blood flow diminishes. In brief attacks, this may result only in a sense of fluttering in the chest or neck, or the patient may be quite unaware of the ectopic rhythm, or he may experience a sense of faintness in the upright position. In longer attacks, depending on the age of the patient, on the presence or absence of some other form of structural disease of the heart, and on the ventricular rate, cardiac output may fall to a level where the characteristic features of forward failure appear with cool, moist, pallid skin and diminished pulse pressure; or cardiac reserve may be reduced and failure

may appear; or angina or myocardial infarction may develop, if the patient has a condition that predisposes to myocardial ischemia. Occasionally, fever may occur with the tachycardia, owing to the disturbed dissipation of heat caused by the peripheral vasoconstriction, and when this is associated with leukocytosis, angina, and infarction-like T waves which may persist for many days following the cessation of the attack, confusion with myocardial infarction is a possibility. *The harmful effect of tachycardia is most strikingly apparent when the heart is already badly damaged, as in acute myocardial infarction, and there should be no delay in instituting the most effective measures of therapy.* Even extrasystoles, when they are frequent enough, may exert the same harmful effects as tachycardia, though to a lesser degree. Moreover, there is evidence that a paroxysmal ventricular tachycardia magnifies the harmful effects of rapid heart rate because the ventricular impulse, pursuing an abnormal course, gives rise to a relatively ineffective contraction.

Drugs in Arrhythmias. Since the same agents are employed in many of the arrhythmias, their description will be given here to avoid repetitiousness.

Pressor Amines. When an ectopic tachycardia is associated with hypotension and the usual antiarrhythmic agent is ineffective, the additional administration of a pressor amine, such as *phenylephrine* (*Neo-synephrine*), 0.5 to 1.0 mg diluted in 10 ml saline and given slowly intravenously, may terminate the tachycardia. Such treatment alone is frequently effective in *paroxysmal atrial tachycardia,* especially when the blood pressure has fallen appreciably as a result of the tachycardia. Blood pressure observations are made while the drug is being given, and one endeavors to increase the pressure to about 160, not more, an admonition that is important in older persons. Control of hypotension is especially urgent when an ectopic rhythm complicates acute myocardial infarction with shock, an extremely critical condition. All the pressor amines tend to induce ectopic rhythms, but experience appears to indicate that this tendency is not great and that their advantages outweigh the disadvantages.

LEVARTERENOL (LEVOPHED). When an ectopic rhythm occurs in *myocardial infarction* with shock or in any other disorder with profound hypotension, levarterenol is the pressor amine most commonly employed, because it is the most potent and its action is prompt and evanescent. Consequently, its effect can be accurately titrated by the rapidity of administration. It must be given by intravenous drip (4 to 8 mg per liter 5 per cent glucose), the blood pressure frequently observed, and care taken to prevent extravasation into the subcutaneous tissues. Should extravasation occur, 5 mg phentolamine (Regitine) diluted in 20 ml water and infiltrated throughout the involved tissues will prevent necrosis. If some other antiarrhythmic agent must be given simultaneously (e.g., procaine amide, Pronestyl), the flask containing the latter can be connected with a Y tube to the levarterenol infusion, and each drug can be given at its own rate independent of the other. This leaves the other arm free for blood pressure determinations, and electrocardiographic monitoring can be carried out at the same time. One endeavors to maintain the systolic level at 100 to 120 in a normotensive person and 120 to 160 in a person previously hypertensive. Metaraminol (Aramine) and mephentermine (Wyamine) may be given subcutaneously or intramuscularly, 3 to 15 mg, the exact dose and frequency depending on the behavior of the blood pressure. Acidosis renders the vasculature less responsive to the pressor amines, and this should be corrected with molar sodium lactate (p. 471).

Sympathomimetic Drugs. The pressor amines are also sympathomimetic drugs, but those mentioned in the previous paragraph are given primarily for the purpose of elevating the blood pressure. The agents now to be discussed are used primarily to increase the rhythmic activity of the myocardial cells, and they are the mainstay of the management of the patient with *heart block* and *Stokes-Adams attacks. Isopropylnorepinephrine (isoproterenol, Isuprel)* is the most widely used since it is considered least likely to provoke a serious ectopic rhythm, its predominant effect being the stimulation of the higher ventricular and nodal tissues rather than the excitation of lower ventricular foci. When the exact mechanism of the Stokes-Adams attack is uncertain, isoproterenol is considered the safest drug available. This may be given intravenously, 4 mg per liter 5 per cent glucose, and the dosage titrated to give a ventricular rate of about 50. It may also be given subcutaneously 0.2 mg every 1 to 2 hr, or sublingually, 10 to 15 mg several times a day. The mode and frequency of administration will depend on the particular circumstances of the illness. *Epinephrine,* aqueous (0.3 ml of 1:1,000 solution every hour) or suspended in oil for a more prolonged effect (2.0 mg three to four times daily) may be used. A convenient oral preparation is a capsule containing *ephedrine* 0.025 Gm and Amytal 0.05 Gm which is given several times a day.

Digitalis. Lanatoside C (Cedilanid) is a satisfactory preparation for the treatment of any of the *supraventricular paroxysmal tachycardias* excepting, of course, paroxysmal atrial tachycardia with block, usually caused by digitalis intoxication. This may be given intramuscularly or intravenously, 0.8 to 1.2 mg with additional doses of 0.4 mg at half-hourly intervals until the desired result is obtained and not exceeding a total of 2 mg. These amounts are based on the presumption that the patient has had no

digitalis during the preceding 2 weeks. For the control of *established flutter* and *fibrillation,* digitalis is employed in the usual manner (p. 1387).

Quinidine. This drug has a place in the management of practically *all ectopic arrhythmias* that require treatment, although it is not necessarily the first choice except in the *ventricular arrhythmias. Quinidine should never be employed in the presence of high-grade block.* In all persons, the use of quinidine introduces a small risk of sudden death, the mechanism of which is unknown, for autopsy investigation has never revealed any structural lesion that could account for the fatality. It is our conjecture that the mechanism of sudden death is similar to that in myocardial infarction and probably due to ventricular fibrillation or standstill. The risk of embolism is about $\frac{1}{2}$ per cent in patients with atrial fibrillation. There is still a difference of opinion regarding the hazards of quinidine therapy when the patient has a bundle branch block. The appearance of syncope is an indication for the prompt discontinuation of the drug since the mechanism of the syncope is probably intimately allied or identical with that responsible for sudden death. Nausea, vomiting, diarrhea, allergic skin rashes, purpura are other untoward manifestations that may necessitate cessation of the use of the drug. It is essential to bear in mind that quinidine is a myocardial depressant, that intravenous administration should be employed only under the gravest circumstances, and that intramuscular therapy, too, should be given cautiously. It is customary to give a preliminary dose of 0.2 Gm to determine the presence of hypersensitivity. Quinidine sulfate 0.2 Gm is given four times a day as a maintenance dose or for the control of *premature beats;* or the long-acting quinidine gluconate (Quinaglute Dura-Tab) 0.3 Gm may suffice in only two or three doses per day. For a more intensive course of therapy, as in the attempted conversion of *chronic atrial fibrillation,* the patient is first fully digitalized, and quinidine 0.2 Gm every 2 hr for five doses is given on the first day. If, by the following morning, fibrillation persists, 0.4 Gm is administered in the same way and, if necessary, 0.6 Gm on the next. When 0.4 or 0.6 Gm is given, electrocardiograms should be taken prior to each dose of the drug. Quinidine is discontinued if the QRS increases by 50 per cent over the control or if numerous ventricular premature beats occur and, obviously, if ventricular tachycardia develops. Intramuscular quinidine, the hydrochloride or gluconate or lactate, may be given according to these schedules, if one deals with a more urgent problem such as *ventricular tachycardia.* These preparations, 1.0 Gm diluted in 100 ml 5 per cent glucose, may be used intravenously. If quinidine intoxication develops, the most effective therapy is molar sodium lactate given intravenously, 100 ml followed by 50 ml every 30 min until the signs of toxicity disappear, more than 300 to 500 ml rarely being required.

Procaine Amide (Pronestyl). This drug has essentially the same effect as quinidine, the indications for its use are the same, and there have been no well-controlled studies that clearly demonstrate the superiority of one over the other. It is convenient to have an alternative, if the patient happens to be hypersensitive to the other. Orally, procaine amide 0.25 to 1.0 Gm is given two to four times daily, and the same doses may be administered intramuscularly. Its most important use is in the treatment of *ventricular tachycardia* for it can be given intravenously with reasonable safety. Since hypotension may be present as a result of the ventricular tachycardia or the myocardial infarction or may be caused by the procaine amide, a flask containing levarterenol and a flask containing procaine amide (2.0 Gm diluted in 250 ml 5 per cent glucose) are joined by a Y tube as described in the discussion of the pressor amines. If hypotension is already present, levarterenol should be allowed to flow in until the desired blood pressure level is attained. If this does not terminate the tachycardia, procaine amide is then given at a rate of 1.0 Gm in 1 hr. Blood pressure observations are made from the other arm and very frequent electrocardiographic tracings taken. If the blood pressure falls appreciably, procaine amide is stopped temporarily and levarterenol given. If the ectopic rhythm is converted to a normal sinus rhythm during the flow of the procaine amide solution, as is usually the case, the infusion is discontinued. If conversion does not take place, the second gram in the remaining 125 ml solution is given after waiting 1 hr. If the ectopic rhythm is abolished, the patient is then given a maintenance dose of procaine amide or quinidine for about 4 weeks.

Potassium. The chief use of potassium is in the treatment of *arrhythmias caused by digitalis intoxication,* and especially where there is reason to believe that potassium depletion has occurred, as through vigorous diuretic therapy, vomiting, or diarrhea. When the patient does not appear to be critically ill, 1.0 Gm of a potassium salt (4 ml of 25 per cent solution of potassium chloride or a similar amount of elixir potassium triplex) well diluted is given orally every hour for five doses. If the patient's condition demands more aggressive action, 5.0 Gm of the potassium salt is given orally and if, at the end of 2 hr, the manifestations of toxicity have not appeared, an additional 2.5 Gm dose is given. If the patient appears to be critically ill, 40 mEq potassium dissolved in 500 ml 5 per cent glucose in water is administered over a period of 2 hr. A similar amount may be repeated if necessary. Electrocardiographic control is essential when large amounts of potassium are given, especially during the period of intravenous administration.

Other Drugs. Corticosteroids, such as dexamethasone 0.75 mg or prednisone 5 mg (4 to 8 tablets per day of either), are frequently effective in *heart block with Stokes-Adams attacks.* Chloroquine 0.25 Gm four times a day, diphenylhydantoin sodium (Dilantin) 250 mg in 1 liter glucose in water given intravenously, reserpine and other tranquilizers, 10 ml of 20 per cent magnesium sulfate given intravenously—all these have been reported as having been successful in serious arrhythmias, such as *ventricular tachycardia,* when procaine amide or quinidine have been ineffective. More studies with each of these are required before we can judge of their place in the management of the various arrhythmias.

Sinus Arrhythmia. This type of irregularity is observed in most healthy young persons at rest, and consists of a quickening of the heart during inspiration and slowing during expiration. It tends to be intensified by deep breathing and to disappear when the breath is held or when the heart rate is increased by exercise or fever. This arrhythmia has no significance.

Premature Beats. These may arise in the atrium, the junctional tissues, or much more frequently, in the ventricle. They are relatively more frequent in patients with structural cardiac disease than in healthy persons, but *they are so common in the healthy that their presence has no diagnostic significance* unless they appear only or increase in frequency markedly after exercise; or when numerous premature beats occur, about 8 to 12 or more per minute. In the latter case, atrial extrasystoles may be a forerunner of atrial fibrillation, or ventricular premature beats, particularly when of variable form, may indicate a more or less serious disturbance of ventricular function. Occurring in the absence of organic heart disease, premature beats may be due to excessive use of tobacco, coffee, tea, and occasionally alcohol or to reflexes from the gastrointestinal tract; often they are caused by emotional stress, or no definite factor can be ascertained. The premature beat is usually recognized with ease because it consists of a contraction appearing before the next beat would ordinarily occur and is usually followed by a pause longer than the usual interval. The patient may or may not be conscious of the premature beat (p. 90). When the extrasystoles are frequent, there may be confusion with atrial fibrillation, an error that can be avoided by noting that the rhythm becomes regular when the heart is accelerated by exercise.

There is still uncertainty whether the premature beat is caused by an irritable focus or by reentry, the available evidence favoring the former view.

The *bigeminal rhythm,* a state in which every alternate beat is premature, is usually the result of digitalis overdosage and disappears within a few days after the drug has been withheld. It should not be confused with *pulsus alternans* or with the *paradoxic pulse* (p. 1468); in the latter two, the rhythm remains regular. Bigeminy not due to digitalis is usually, though not always, associated with structural heart disease.

The treatment of premature beats depends on the circumstances. When they occur only occasionally, and evidence of cardiac disease is lacking, no treatment is necessary. When there is reason to believe that tobacco or coffee is responsible, its use should be discontinued or curtailed. In excitable patients, extrasystoles may disappear following the administration of a mild sedative: barbiturates, reserpine, or other tranquilizers. In fully digitalized patients, premature beats, if caused by the digitalis, will disappear if the drug is withdrawn; or, if the irregularity occurs after the ingestion of a high carbohydrate meal, it will be abolished by the administration of potassium. It should also be mentioned that the occurrence of extrasystoles not caused by digitalis does not constitute a contraindication to the use of digitalis if the patient suffers from congestive failure. Often with the restoration of myocardial function, the irregularity will disappear. Quinidine, procaine amide, and digitalis are all effective in the treatment of extrasystoles, the relative efficacy of each drug varying in different patients.

While premature beats may ordinarily be considered a benign form of irregularity, the occurrence of numerous such beats may diminish the efficiency of the heart whose reserve is already impaired. Moreover, the appearance of ventricular extrasystoles following an acute myocardial infarction should not be viewed with complacency, since they may then herald the onset of ventricular tachycardia; or an isolated ventricular beat, occurring in the "vulnerable" period, at the end of the previous systole, may initiate ventricular fibrillation and sudden death. It is for this reason that some believe that quinidine, in the form of the long-acting gluconate, 0.3 Gm two times daily should be administered in all patients with acute ischemic heart disease, although this policy is not accepted by others.

Atrial Fibrillation. The effect of atrial fibrillation is to obliterate the effective contraction of the atria and to bombard the atrioventricular node and the ventricles with a very rapid and irregular series of stimuli. Many of these impulses are blocked at the AV node, but many are passed through, so that the ventricular contractions in the untreated patient are usually rapid and completely irregular.

The untoward effects of atrial fibrillation depend on the rapidity of the ventricular rate and the extent of the pulse deficit (i.e., on the proportion of ineffective and wasted ventricular beats), on the prior state of the affected heart, on the duration of the arrhythmia, and on the virtual paralysis of effective atrial contraction. Cardiac output may be diminished as a result of the reduction of total diastolic filling time and also because coordinated atrial contraction may be essential for adequate ventricular filling: the net result may be myocardial failure. Stagnation of blood in the essentially paralyzed atria tends to predispose to the development of thrombi and embolism in both pulmonary and systemic circulations. Finally, the cardiac irregularity, if uncontrolled, gives rise to an unpleasant consciousness of palpitation.

When the rate is rapid, 120 or more, the diagnosis is readily made, because atrial fibrillation is the only common condition in which one observes the combination of a well-marked tachycardia with a gross irregularity. When the rate is normal or only slightly increased, as in digitalized patients, the diagnosis is less apparent. The distinction from numerous extrasystoles can be made by noting that it is only in atrial fibrillation that abnormally long pauses occur in groups of two or more. Moreover, exercise tends to abolish the extrasystolic arrhythmia, whereas it exaggerates the irregularity of atrial fibrillation. More difficult, and frequently impossible, is the differentiation of fibrillation from atrial flutter with varying block, and from a shifting pacemaker associated with multiple atrial ectopic beats.

Atrial fibrillation may be paroxysmal or persistent. Occasionally the paroxysmal form occurs in healthy persons in whom no evidence of structural cardiac disease can be found. It is also encountered in individuals who, otherwise normal, suffer from acute infections such as pneumonia, or in patients with rheumatic heart disease or acute myocardial infarction. Rarely, paroxysmal atrial fibrillation may be the consequence of anesthesia, potassium deficiency, digitalis intoxication, or other forms of poisoning. Most frequently, however, paroxysmal atrial fibrillation is seen in thyrotoxicosis, mitral stenosis, or in senile heart disease, usually associated with coronary disease. In the latter group, the paroxysmal attacks frequently occur before the arrhythmia is permanently established. The paroxysmal bouts may last for a few seconds to a few days, and as is true in all types of paroxysmal rapid heart action, the onset and offset are sudden. Unless the patient happens to be observed in the midst of an attack, the nature of the episode will depend on the observation of the patient that the heart action is highly irregular during the attack.

The permanent form of atrial fibrillation is confined almost exclusively to patients with senile heart disease, mitral stenosis, or thyrotoxicosis. In elderly patients the usual signs of thyrotoxicosis may be absent and the arrhythmia may be the only feature suggesting the possibility of thyroid disease. Rarely, chronic atrial fibrillation may be the sole cause of congestive failure that persists despite full digitalization, and in such instances reversion to normal rhythm is a curative procedure. When the ventricular rate fails to slow in the usual fashion after full doses of digitalis, the presence of thyrotoxicosis, a recent silent coronary occlusion, multiple pulmonary infarcts, or acute rheumatic carditis should be suspected. The onset of the ectopic rhythm in a person who has received therapeutic doses of digitalis and of diuretic drugs, such as mercurials or chlorothiazide, may be a manifestation of potassium deficiency and an indication for potassium therapy.

In a person with atrial fibrillation, one faces the choice between two plans of therapy: that of attempting to control the ventricular rate with digitalis, the rhythm remaining irregular; and that of abolishing the arrhythmia by quinidine or other antiarrhythmic drugs. In patients with mitral stenosis, or with marked cardiac enlargement with failure, quinidine is rarely successful in permanently restoring a normal sinus rhythm, and in these patients, the drug appears to be especially hazardous. In other patients with chronic atrial fibrillation, a normal rhythm can be restored if one administers large enough doses of quinidine, often bordering on toxic ranges, but usually the normal sinus rhythm can be maintained only by permanent maintenance doses of quinidine and even so but for a variable period of time before the arrhythmia reasserts itself. In general, patients with chronic atrial fibrillation can be well controlled with digitalis, and little is gained by the conversion of the arrhythmia to a normal sinus mechanism. Hence, quinidine is likely to be of greatest value in patients with fibrillation of recent development who are known to have had no evidences of congestive failure prior to the onset of the arrhythmia. It should also be given when the ventricular rate is not well controlled by digitalis; and it may be given in intractable failure provided one recognizes the risks inherent in quinidine therapy under these circumstances. In all cases of atrial fibrillation, therapeutic doses of digitalis should be administered before quinidine is given. Following acute myocardial infarction with atrial fibrillation, it is particularly important that one's first and most important objective be the slowing of the ventricular rate with digitalis. For the treatment of paroxysmal atrial fibrillation, a rapid-acting digitalis such as lanatoside C is preferable, while for the control of the established fibrillation, one of the slower-acting digitalis preparations should be used (p. 1396). The details of quinidine therapy are described above (p. 1396).

One point needs emphasis: although there are many instances of transient atrial fibrillation in which the administration of digitalis is followed by the disappearance of the arrhythmia, when atrial fibrillation is of long duration, digitalis rarely abolishes the ectopic rhythm. Under these latter circumstances, the ventricular rate slows and becomes less obviously irregular unless a complete AV block and a regular idioventricular rhythm develops; but electrocardiographic tracings reveal that the atria continue to fibrillate.

Thromboembolism is common in patients with atrial fibrillation, particularly the chronic form, and is especially frequent in patients who also have mitral stenosis, being responsible for about 20 per cent of the deaths in the latter. To prevent such catastrophes, long-term anticoagulant therapy has been advocated, especially important in patients who have already experienced one or more episodes of embolism.

Regular Tachycardias. Given a patient with well-marked increase in the heart rate, or with a history of such attacks, the first decision to be made is whether one is dealing with sinus tachycardia or with one of the ectopic tachycardias. The latter group will usually respond to therapy aimed directly at the heart, while in the case of sinus tachycardia, the treatment of the rapid rate depends on the management of the underlying condition. If one can obtain a reliable history of sudden onset and offset, one knows immediately that the attack represents an ectopic tachycardia of some type. However, the patient is often unable to state whether the onset is absolutely sudden, and even when a paroxysmal tachycardia has actually taken place, still less often is he certain that the ending was abrupt. When the rate is less than 140 per minute, the chances are strong that one is dealing with sinus tachycardia, but one must bear in mind the occasional patient with atrial flutter with a ventricular rate below 140, and above all, that form of serious digitalis intoxication known as paroxysmal tachycardia with AV block (p. 1400). Rates of 170 or more per minute are almost invariably the result of ectopic rhythms, and the difficulty comes chiefly in the group of patients with heart rates between 140 and 170. The response to carotid sinus pressure is important in the differentiation; often, the definitive diagnosis is made only by electrocardiography.

Extreme Sinus Tachycardia. The chief causes of extreme sinus tachycardia are marked elevation of body temperature, severe thyrotoxicosis, any condition that produces profound circulatory collapse, and occasionally an anxiety attack or acute myocardial injury due to infection or infarction. In most instances, however, sinus tachycardia of severe degree is due to extracardiac causes. Sinus tachycardia usually responds little or not at all to carotid sinus pressure, in the latter case resembling ventricular tachycardia. If there is a slight response, neither the slowing nor subsequent acceleration occurs with the abruptness observed in patients with atrial flutter or paroxysmal tachycardia with AV block. In the absence of marked hyperthermia, severe thyrotoxicosis, or anxiety state, a patient with outspoken sinus tachycardia will usually display manifestations of forward failure (p. 101). Digitalis or other cardiac therapy has no value in normal sinus tachycardia unless there are manifestations of congestive failure. The problem is discovering the basic cause and correcting it.

Paroxysmal Atrial Tachycardia. This is the most common of the ectopic tachycardias aside from atrial fibrillation. It is generally attributed to rapid discharges from an irritable focus. Usually it appears first in youth, and attacks may recur throughout life. The majority of patients with this disorder display no evidence of any other cardiac abnormality, and *in the absence of structural disease, atrial tachycardia should be considered a benign affection* except under circumstances described above (p. 1395). They may, however, produce great anxiety on the part of the patient and his family. When a patient is seen during an attack, the heart is found to be perfectly regular and the rate is 160 to 170 or more. Procedures such as carotid sinus pressure or other types of vagal stimulation will have no effect or will terminate the attack abruptly. Atrial tachycardia may be accompanied by such an aberration of the QRS complex that an erroneous diagnosis of ventricular tachycardia may be made and sometimes the differentiation may be impossible.

The causes of atrial tachycardia are not known since most patients exhibit no signs of organic disease. Prognosis is excellent unless the attack brings on congestive failure or myocardial ischemia. The keystone of therapy is reassurance coupled with attempts to prevent the seizures and to terminate the disorder when it occurs. For many patients digitalis is the most effective drug for the prevention of the attacks; in others, quinidine is more useful. Certain patients notice that the attacks are regularly precipitated by certain trigger factors, such as anxiety or digestive disturbances, and avoidance of these will have a salutary effect. In many, the attacks occur at such long intervals that the patient himself will prefer to treat the disorder only when it transpires rather than to take a drug indefinitely to prevent the ectopic rhythm.

For the treatment of paroxysmal atrial tachycardia, the patient should assume the recumbent position and be given a sedative, such as sodium pentobarbital or secobarbital, 0.2 Gm given intramuscularly. If significant hypotension is present, 90 mm systolic or less, slightly higher if the patient has previously been hypertensive, elevation of the blood pressure by phenylephrine to not more than 160 systolic may suffice to restore a normal rhythm

or to make the heart more responsive to other measures (p. 1396). The carotid sinuses should be massaged for about 15 to 20 sec, each one separately, while listening to the heart, discontinuing the massage if the rate slows abruptly. If the ectopic rhythm persists, lanatoside C, 0.8 to 1.2 mg, should be given intramuscularly or very slowly intravenously, provided, of course, that the patient has not received digitalis during the preceding 2 weeks. The digitalis acts as a vagal stimulant. If after 1 hr the tachycardia continues, carotid sinus pressure should again be attempted, and if this fails, neostigmine (Prostigmine) 0.5 to 1.0 mg, a cholinesterase antagonist, may be administered intramuscularly, followed again by carotid sinus massage. If all these measures fail, morphine sulfate 10 to 15 mg subcutaneously is given, and during the ensuing sleep the attack will usually cease.

Almost invariably one or more of these procedures will be effective and methacholine (Mecholyl), a very powerful vagal stimulant and likely to produce alarming reactions, is practically never required. Quinidine may be given by mouth or parenterally, but it is not often needed.

The treatment outlined above refers to the measures taken by the physician. Often, however, the patient has previously learned how to terminate the attack by utilizing carotid sinus pressure, or by inducing gagging and vomiting, or by the Valsalva maneuver (attempting to expire against a closed glottis). Naturally, these simple methods can also be employed by the physician before carotid sinus massage or drug therapy is instituted.

Paroxysmal Atrial Tachycardia with Block. It is primarily through the investigations of Lown and his associates that the importance and significance of this disorder have been recognized. The arrhythmia has certain characteristics of flutter in that the responses to vagal stimulation are similar; in other respects, it resembles atrial tachycardia in that the atrial rate usually lies between 150 and 250. It is generally considered to be a variant of flutter, and the exact mechanism is not known. Digitalis intoxication is the usual cause, and on this account, this ectopic rhythm requires separate discussion because the treatment is altogether different from that of atrial tachycardia or flutter. Sensitivity to digitalis increases with the severity of heart failure, age, and particularly with potassium depletion, usually resulting from excessive diuretic therapy or vomiting or diarrhea, in a patient on a low-sodium diet. Thus, under these circumstances, serious digitalis intoxication may ensue with doses that would ordinarily be considered physiologic.

Paroxysmal atrial tachycardia with block should be sought for in any digitalized patient who displays other symptoms of intoxication such as nausea and vomiting, or who has received vigorous diuretic treatment or who may otherwise have lost potassium as a result of vomiting or diarrhea, or whose heart rate increases after having received full doses of digitalis. The diagnosis is established by obtaining an electrocardiographic tracing displaying an atrial rate of 150 to 250, an isoelectric line between P waves in all leads, and AV block more pronounced than mere prolongation of the P-R interval.

The earliest stage is an alteration in the form of the P wave and an increase in the atrial rate, usually with a 1:1 ventricular response. Thus, the rate may increase to 120 to 140 and still resemble a normal sinus rhythm, the impaired AV conduction inapparent except when carotid sinus pressure is applied. At higher atrial rates, a 2:1 block usually appears. *The danger of this abnormal rhythm comes from the fact that it is a manifestation of serious digitalis poisoning, is likely to be confused with a sinus tachycardia or flutter, and because of the presence of congestive failure, digitalis may be pushed even more vigorously.* The proper treatment is prompt cessation of digitalis and of diuretic drugs and the administration of potassium by mouth or parenterally (p. 1397), depending on the urgency. *The serum potassium level must not be relied on as a criterion of diagnosis;* most patients with this form of disturbed heart action have little or no diminution in the level of serum potassium.

In about 20 per cent of patients, the arrhythmia is unrelated to digitalis intoxication and potassium depletion. Procaine amide is then employed. If there is doubt about the role of potassium depletion and there is no uremia that could cause a hyperkalemia, and there is no electrocardiographic evidence of excessive serum potassium, potassium therapy may be tried. If this is ineffective, procaine amide should be given.

Atrial Flutter. This arrhythmia is much less common than fibrillation, but it is very closely allied and the mechanism must be similar. As a rule, the atria beat at a rate of approximately 300 and a 2:1, 3:1, 4:1 AV block exists, the corresponding ventricular rates being 150, 100, or 75. When the block is constant and of high degree, the condition will usually not be suspected; but if it is suspected, its presence can be confirmed by the fact that exercise increases the rate suddenly rather than gradually, and in the postexercise period slowing occurs suddenly, not gradually. This behavior arises from the fact that exercise and flutter have no influence on the atrial rate, but the decrease in vagal tone reduces the degree of block, a 4:1 giving way to a 2:1 block, for example, and the acceleration occurs within one beat; the reverse takes place as vagal tone is restored in the postexercise period. Usually, a 2:1 block is present when the patient is seen and the ventricular rate lies between 140 to 160. This fact alone should make one suspect the

presence of flutter, because other types of ectopic tachycardia are likely to be associated with faster rates. Carotid sinus pressure slows the ventricular rate in flutter by increasing vagal tone and hence the degree of AV block. The slowing is maintained only for the brief period of pressure, and both the slowing and quickening occur instantly rather than gradually, as would be the case with sinus tachycardia if there were any response at all. Occasionally, the block is so variable that the ventricular irregularity is virtually identical with that observed in fibrillation. However, after exercise, the irregularity of flutter tends to disappear whereas in fibrillation it is enhanced.

Careful auscultation will frequently reveal an appreciable difference in the intensity of the first sound in flutter, due to slight variations in timing of the ventricular contraction in relation to the preceding atrial contraction (p. 89). This variation in the loudness of the first sound is never present in sinus tachycardia or paroxysmal atrial tachycardia, but it occurs frequently in ventricular tachycardia and thus serves to limit the diagnostic possibilities when a tachycardia is first encountered.

Flutter is caused by essentially the same conditions that cause fibrillation, has essentially the same prognosis, and is treated in a somewhat similar manner. The usual method of treatment is to give digitalis, which slows the ventricular rate by increasing the degree of AV block, and commonly converts flutter to fibrillation. When the drug is withdrawn, these patients will frequently revert spontaneously to normal rhythm; if this does not occur, quinidine may be employed. If the abnormal atrial rhythm cannot be abolished, digitalis is given in doses sufficient to maintain the ventricular rate at a relatively normal level.

Quinidine sometimes converts atrial fibrillation to flutter and the flutter may persist, the atrial rate decreasing from about 300 to 200. Under these circumstances, the ventricular rate may suddenly increase, the previous 2:1 ratio being replaced by a 1:1 response. Quinidine should be discontinued and digitalis administered even though fibrillation will probably be reestablished.

Paroxysmal Ventricular Tachycardia. This is much less frequent and far more serious than paroxysmal atrial tachycardia. The commonest cause is coronary disease, and this arrhythmia frequently occurs within a few days following the development of an acute myocardial infarction. Less commonly, it is induced by digitalis or quinidine intoxication, and very rarely the arrhythmia appears spontaneously in healthy persons without any evidence of cardiac disease. The diagnosis should be suspected when the following clinical features are observed: (1) The patient has evidence of coronary disease or has been receiving digitalis or quinidine in large doses. (2) As a rule, there is no history of numerous previous attacks. (3) During the attack, the ventricular rate is usually between 160 and 210, and although it is essentially regular, there are often slight variations in the regularity of the rhythm and in the intensity of the first sound from beat to beat because the relationship between the atrial and ventricular contractions is somewhat variable. (4) Carotid sinus stimulation has no effect on the rate.

Although these clues are very important, the clinical impression should be confirmed by an electrocardiogram, but even here the interpretation may be rendered difficult because atrial tachycardia may be associated with ventricular conduction defects (aberrant QRS complexes) which cause the tracing to resemble that of ventricular tachycardia. In other words, the electrocardiographic diagnosis cannot be made with certainty on the sole basis of the abnormal complexes. In addition, it is necessary that the P waves be shown to occur at a rate independent of the ventricular rate, or that there be demonstrated, in the intervals between attacks, ventricular premature beats identical in form with the complexes seen during the paroxysm.

Since it is but one step removed from the almost invariably fatal ventricular fibrillation, ventricular tachycardia is the most serious of the ectopic tachycardias. If the attack occurs during a bout of acute myocardial infarction, quinidine or procaine amide (p. 1397) may be effective in terminating it; but one should not adopt an attitude of complacency, for there is a strong probability that another episode will soon recur. Hence, a maintenance dose of the successful drug should be continued until the healing of the infarct is complete.

When heart failure occurs in an undigitalized patient with ventricular tachycardia, digitalis should be administered since the drug is not especially hazardous in such patients, as was formerly believed.

Some patients with ventricular tachycardia who are receiving large doses of quinidine or of procaine amide fail to revert to the normal mechanism but do exhibit marked slowing—to 120 per minute or less—of the ectopic rhythm. Under these circumstances the administration of large doses of atropine (up to 2 mg intravenously) may increase the atrial rate to a level above that of the ectopic rhythm and so permit the sinoatrial node to resume its normal role as pacemaker and thus restore the normal sinus mechanism.

When all these measures fail and the patient's condition remains critical, external countershock (250 to 400 volts) may be employed. This procedure requires general anesthesia.

Ventricular Fibrillation. This arrhythmia may occur in very brief bursts, lasting for a few seconds, then subsiding spontaneously, following which the rhythm previously present is resumed. These episodes are responsible for some of the Stokes-Adams attacks that characterize high-grade AV block. Usually, however, ventricular fibrillation is synonymous with practically instantaneous death, since effective ventricular contraction and circulation cease. Aside from AV block, ischemic heart disease is the most common cause of the arrhythmia, particularly during attacks of acute myocardial infarction. There had been no treatment for this calamitous disorder until the introduction of externally applied countershock. Needless to say, this form of therapy must be applied promptly, for cessation of the circulation beyond 2 to 4 min leads to irreversible damage in the brain and heart. This means that a candidate for the arrhythmia, whether he is suffering an acute myocardial infarction or has sustained a series of Stokes-Adams attacks, must be under constant observation, and there must be constant readiness to apply countershock. This incessant watch may be required for weeks, until the patient has been free of attacks for at least a few weeks. In the absence of this special equipment, vigorous pounding of the precordium, coupled with artificial respiration, preferably mouth-to-mouth, may be attempted. If the heartbeat does not return immediately, the procedure of closed-chest cardiac massage should be employed. This involves manual rhythmic compression of the sternum once per second, plus mouth-to-mouth respiration. Thus it may be possible to sustain life during the crucial time required to secure and apply the apparatus needed for countershock.

Wolff-Parkinson-White Syndrome (Anomalous Atrioventricular Excitation). This is a congenital disorder characterized by the presence of normal P waves, a P-R interval of 0.1 sec or less, an increased QRS interval, a slur on the initial phase of the QRS complex (delta wave), and a pronounced tendency for the occurrence of paroxysmal tachycardia: either atrial tachycardia or atrial flutter or fibrillation. It is thought by some that the entire picture is based on the presence of an accessory neuromuscular tract (the bundle of Kent) connecting the atria with the ventricles over which impulses bring about premature activation of a portion of the ventricular musculature. There is other evidence that the disorder is caused by accelerated conduction through some of the fibers in the AV node or bundle.

The electrocardiogram shifts between the abnormal (W-P-W type) and the "normal," although this latter may now reveal abnormalities that have been masked by the W-P-W form. Since the latter displays a Q in leads II, III, and F, it is not infrequently mistaken for the tracing of a myocardial infarction, especially when the patient is in the midst of an attack of paroxysmal tachycardia, which occurs in about 75 per cent of the patients with this anomaly. The shift to the anomalous conduction can be induced by vagal stimulation as by carotid sinus pressure or by digitalis given intravenously. The normal type of conduction can be brought on by vagal inhibition as by atropine or exercise, also by quinidine and procaine amide.

The condition should be suspected in any person subject to paroxysms of tachycardia, particularly when they have occurred from youth. The diagnosis is established by careful scrutiny of the electrocardiographic tracings for the criteria enumerated above. Since digitalis appears to be less effective than usual in the treatment of the paroxysms of rapid heart action, quinidine or procaine amide should be employed for such attacks. A few instances of sudden death during an attack have been reported. Hence, with a history of frequent bouts of paroxysmal tachycardia, maintenance doses of either quinidine or procaine amide should be given indefinitely.

Sinus Bradycardia. This is a condition in which excitation of the heart proceeds in the normal fashion, although the sinoatrial pacemaker discharges at the unusually slow rate of about 40 to 50. It is occasionally seen in normal persons, particularly trained athletes. It may also be encountered in patients with increased intracranial pressure, in convalescence after febrile illnesses, in obstructive jaundice and myxedema. Practically never does the slow heart alone cause symptoms, for cardiac output is maintained at a normal level through a corresponding increase in stroke volume. Differentiation from complete AV block is readily made by electrocardiogram and also by the quickening of the heart rate with atropine and exercise, and the failure of these measures to bring about an appreciable increase in ventricular rate in complete AV block.

Heart Block. This term refers to a condition in which the wave of excitation from the atria is delayed or blocked at the junctional tissues (AV node and common bundle). The P-R interval represents the time required for the impulse to traverse the AV node and bundle, and 0.20 to 0.21 sec is generally accepted as the upper limit of normal. When the P-R interval exceeds this period of time and all the atrial beats are followed by ventricular beats, the state is called *first degree block*. A more advanced disturbance in the conduction system, *second degree block*, is present when from time to time the atrial impulses are incapable of penetrating the conduction system and of exciting the ventricles. *Third degree* or *complete heart block* describes the condition in which the conduction system is so altered that no atrial impulses reach the ventricles, and the atria and ventricles maintain separate and independent rhythms.

First Degree Block. This may be due to increased vagal tone in a healthy, normal person. We have seen an Olympic champion whose P-R interval is regularly 0.26 to 0.28 sec. Prolongation may be caused by impairment of the conduction system as a result of digitalis or any of the inflammatory, toxic, degenerative, or vascular processes that may affect the heart. Prolongation of the P-R interval, as may occur in rheumatic fever, may be suspected when the intensity of the first heart sound suddenly declines in intensity without any other change in the clinical picture and without evidence of fluid in the pericardium, or when a presystolic murmur becomes middiastolic in the absence of atrial fibrillation.

In the absence of any other criteria to indict the heart, this one electrocardiographic deviation from an arbitrary norm should not be construed as evidence of organic heart disease, and it requires no treatment.

Second Degree or Partial Heart Block. The careful and extensive studies of Gilchrist have illuminated important aspects of partial heart block that have not previously been widely appreciated. We draw on his observations freely in this discussion. Second degree block may be divided into two groups. In the benign form, type I, the P-R interval increases progressively until finally an atrial beat is completely blocked, the corresponding ventricular beat dropping out (Wenckebach pause). The P-R interval after the pause shortens to within the normal range but each successive one lengthens, and the cycle is repeated. The dropped beat may occur after six to eight conducted beats, or it may take place after every second atrial impulse, thus giving rise to a 2:1 AV block and becoming indistinguishable at first glance from the more serious 2:1 block to be described below. However, the differentiation can be readily made by inhibition of vagal tone, as by intravenous injection of atropine (1 to 2 mg) or exercise. In the benign type I, the block diminishes or disappears with such a procedure, whereas it increases with type II partial block and may promptly develop into a complete, though temporary, AV block. Type I second degree block is usually due to increased vagal tone, occurring spontaneously or after carotid sinus pressure or following digitalis therapy. It is almost always a transitory phenomenon and requires no treatment.

Type II, a far more serious disorder, appears as a 2:1, 3:1, or 4:1 block, the P-R interval being either normal or increased, but always fixed and unvarying. This form of heart block may be caused acutely by a posterior myocardial infarction or by diphtheria, usually a transient block with the former, almost always with the latter. It may also result from coronary sclerosis in the absence of an acute episode of infarction, calcification of the mitral annulus, extension of the lesion of aortic stenosis into the septum, any of the diffuse disorders of the myocardium (p. 1464), or congenital heart disease, usually a patent ventricular septum.

Syncopal attacks are common in type II block, and they display the characteristics of all such syncopal attacks as are due to a sudden cessation of circulation (p. 305). The attacks occur suddenly and without warning and in both the upright and recumbent postures, in contrast to the premonitory lightheadedness, faintness, "blacking out" that always precede the simple vasodepressor syncope which always develops in the upright position and is relieved by the recumbent posture. If patients with type II 2:1 block, for example, are carefully observed during or shortly after the lapse of consciousness, ventricular standstill or fibrillation will be recorded during the syncopal period, followed by complete block in the early recovery state, a 2:1 block being restored after a few hours or days. When a person with a slow heart rate or with an electrocardiographic tracing of partial block develops a syncopal attack with the characteristics described above, the diagnosis should be simple. However, in a number of patients, syncopal attacks may appear at relatively long intervals over a number of years, during which time the electrocardiogram may be perfectly normal and the P-R interval well within the normal range. Nevertheless, intravenous atropine in such persons will usually unmask a concealed block. *The important lesson to be drawn is that, when a middle-aged or elderly person gives a history of syncopal attacks that develop without warning, one should suspect a Stokes-Adams attack even if the electrocardiogram at the time of the examination is normal in all respects.* Eventually, most of the persons with type II block, whether of the overt or concealed form, will develop complete block, if prior to this eventuality, they have not succumbed in a Stokes-Adams attack or to some other disease. One condition, less serious, that may cause identical syncopal attacks, is a hypersensitive carotid sinus that is responsible for fainting attacks of the cardioinhibitory type.

Complete or Third Degree Block. This condition is caused by any of the disorders responsible for type II partial block. Occasionally, one encounters an otherwise normal person with congenital block, and rarely a patient with persistent complete block will be found at autopsy to display no demonstrable microscopic lesion in the conduction system. A transitory form, lasting a few seconds, may follow carotid sinus pressure, and it may also be a consequence of digitalis intoxication, disappearing a week or two after the drug is withdrawn. The ventricular rate is 45 or less, although following an acute posterior infarction or digitalis intoxication, the rate may be as rapid as 65. The rhythm is regular, and

the rate increases slightly after exercise. Paradoxically, the rate may increase after atropine. The intensity of the first heart sound varies from beat to beat, sometimes being almost inaudible and at other times so loud as to merit the term *bruit de canon* (p. 89). Faint atrial contractions can also be heard, and if atrial contraction occurs during an early ventricular filling period, a short blowing mitral diastolic murmur may be heard and recorded (Rytand murmur).

The *prognosis* of first and second degree, type I, block is favorable. The outlook for high grades of block (type II, partial or complete AV block) is always uncertain since the patient is constantly subject to the risk of Stokes-Adams attacks, any of which may be fatal. When such attacks occur frequently in patients with complete block and are uncontrolled, death usually occurs within a year. During this period the patient who is having numerous and prolonged attacks seems, like Castor and Pollux, to alternate between the realm of the living and the kingdom of the dead. In acute myocardial infarction, the presence of high-grade block doubles the risk during the first 2 to 3 weeks.

Treatment of Heart Block. The important problem is the management of the Stokes-Adams attacks. The most generally effective drugs are the sympathomimetic agents, such as isoproterenol, epinephrine (aqueous or suspended in oil), and ephedrine. In acute myocardial infarction they may also be employed but all these drugs, including isoproterenol, the one most favored, increase myocardial metabolism and, hence, tend to cause hypoxia and occasionally prolonged anginal attacks. Should these occur, the drugs should be discontinued promptly. Corticotropin and corticosteroids sometimes are efficacious when the sympathomimetic drugs are not helpful or cannot be continued; the mechanism of their beneficial effect is not certain. Because potassium depletion accelerates conduction, chlorthiazide, 500 to 750 mg combined with sodium bicarbonate 10 Gm given throughout the day, has been found to exert a favorable effect in partial heart block. In life-threatening situations where syncopal attacks are frequent and uncontrolled, the application of the external pacemakers under constant observation may be used for ventricular standstill and external countershock for ventricular fibrillation, and these measures may tide the patient over a very stormy period. During the minutes required to initiate these procedures, life may be sustained by the method of closed-chest cardiac massage, as discussed on p. 1402. For congestive failure in conjunction with complete block, digitalis may be used without reservation. With partial block, digitalis therapy may either improve or worsen the degree of block. Hence the drug should be withheld unless congestive failure fails to respond to other measures. *Under no circumstances should quinidine or procaine amide ever be used in the presence of high-grade block*, regardless of what other indications may exist, since in these patients the fibrillatory action of these drugs predominates over the antifibrillatory effect.

When, despite drug therapy, syncopal attacks continue at frequent intervals, an internal pacemaker may be inserted surgically.

Bundle Branch Block. These disorders, which are not arrhythmias in the strictest sense, may be conveniently mentioned at this point. When the duration of the QRS complex is 0.13 sec or more, and when the main deflection is positive in leads I and V_6 and negative in leads III and V_1, left bundle branch block is said to be present. Similar prolongation but with the opposite directional deflections in the leads mentioned, is characteristic of right bundle branch block. Lesser degrees of QRS lengthening with an RST pattern are often designated as incomplete left or right bundle branch block. In some instances there may be marked prolongation of the ventricular complex without the above-mentioned characteristic reciprocal changes in the opposite leads. These are usually considered interventricular block.

These several disorders are all related to delayed spread of ventricular excitation. The commonest causes are coronary disease, inflammatory or infiltrative disease of the myocardium, and marked univentricular hypertrophy, producing delay in the spread of the impulse through the thickened chamber.

None of the rather numerous physical signs which have been attributed to bundle branch block are wholly reliable. The electrocardiogram remains the only consistently accurate method of diagnosis.

These disturbances of conduction are usually encountered in persons with advanced myocardial disease or severe pressure loads but may be seen in association with volume loads, atrial septal defect being the classic example. It is probable that the abnormal sequence of contraction consequent to the disordered excitation impairs further the effectiveness of ventricular systole. *In a patient with heart failure, marked prolongation of the QRS adds to the gravity of the prognosis. However, when right bundle branch block is encountered in an asymptomatic person under the age of 40 who lacks all other objective evidence of cardiac disease, the outlook is excellent.* In asymptomatic patients of any age with left bundle branch block, and in those with the right bundle disorder who are older than 40, the prognosis is less certain because there is always the possibility that the conduction disorder may be the sole manifestation of

coronary disease. Even so, any activity which causes no symptoms should be permitted.

It is probable that contusion of the heart (steering-wheel injury, boxing, football, etc.) is a frequent cause of the benign varieties of bundle branch block. However, a history of injury is not always obtainable, and the cause of these benign instances often remains uncertain.

The treatment of bundle branch block is that of the associated disorder. No therapy except judicious reassurance is indicated for those persons who lack symptoms and present no objective abnormalities other than the prolonged intraventricular conduction. It should be repeated that one treats patients—not electrocardiograms.

REFERENCES

Burn, J. H.: Pharmacology of Cardiac Failure, Proc. Roy. Soc. Med., 52:1057, 1959.

Gilchrist, A. R.: Clinical Aspects of High-grade Heartblock, Scottish Med. J., 3:53, 1958.

Kouwenhoven, W. B., J. R. Jude, and G. G. Knickerbocker: Closed-chest Cardiac Massage, J.A.M.A., 173:1064, 1960.

Lown, B., N. F. Wyatt, and H. D. Levine: Paroxysmal Atrial Tachycardia with Block, Circulation, 21:129, 1960.

Thompson, G. W.: Quinidine as a Cause of Death, Circulation, 14:757, 1958.

Wolff, L.: Diagnostic Clues in the Wolff-Parkinson-White Syndrome, New Engl. J. Med., 261:637, 1959.

Zoll, P. M., A. J. Lilenthal, and M. D. Phelps, Jr.: Termination of Refractory Tachycardia by External Electric Countershock (P), Circulation, 24: (part II) 1078, 1961 (Abstract).

In Progress in Cardiovascular Disease, vol. II, 1960, there are a number of authoritative reviews on practically all aspects of the arrhythmias.

251 PRINCIPLES OF PHYSICAL SIGNS REFERABLE TO THE HEART

T. R. Harrison and
William H. Resnik

Dyspnea and ischemic pain, which are the most important *subjective* manifestations of structural disease of the heart, have been discussed in earlier chapters (pp. 104 and 32). The *objective* signs fall into two general groups: those which are related to cardiac *failure* (Chap. 249) and which are found mainly in organs other than the heart, and those which are due to cardiac *disease* and which are detected by examination of the heart itself. It is with the latter phenomena that this chapter is concerned. It should be emphasized that, while these objective signs of abnormality are almost invariably concomitants of heart disease in young persons, they are often absent in older patients, despite the presence of a serious disorder.

CARDIAC ENLARGEMENT

Increase in the size of the cardiac *shadow* due to pericardial effusion, which may exist in the absence of any enlargement of the heart itself, is considered in Chap. 256, Pericarditis. Aside from these effusions, the x-ray is of particular value in regard to dilatation but often fails to detect hypertrophy which, when marked, usually produces characteristic alterations in the electrocardiogram. A very slight degree of hypertrophy may elude recognition by all methods, including autopsy, but moderate degrees are frequently best found by palpation.

The normal apex tap is mainly due to recoil of the ventricles as ejection starts. Left ventricular hypertrophy usually produces an exaggerated apical thrust which is felt over a larger area and is longer sustained than the normal sharply localized brief tap. Similar changes may occur following apical infarction, and the differentiation between the two causes will depend on the associated findings. Less frequently, a striking but temporary exaggeration of the apex thrust appears during anginal attacks and vanishes as the pain subsides. The anginal and postinfarctional apical bulges are apparently caused by ballooning of feebly contracting ischemic areas, as the remaining healthy muscle undergoes vigorous contraction.

In the case of left ventricular enlargement the exaggerated thrust is probably due to one of two mechanisms, or a combination of them.

Since the base is normally thicker than the apex, an equal *relative* degree of hypertrophy will mean greater *absolute* thickening at the base and relative weakness of the apex. Thus the exaggerated apical thrusts due to ischemia and to hypertrophy are probably both related to an increase in the base/apex contractile ratio.

The mechanism of the exaggerated apex thrust seen with acute dilatation, in the absence of hypertrophy, is probably different. Here, the apex becomes rounded, with loss of the normal conical shape of the left ventricular cavity. Thus, since tension = pressure × radius, the thinner apex is now subjected to the same tension as the thicker base, and this causes apical systolic ballooning. In the normal heart this does not occur because the smaller apical radius reduces the tension in that region.

Right ventricular hypertrophy usually produces a diffuse precordial systolic lift which is more marked in the left parasternal than in the apical region. It is uncertain whether this is caused by exaggeration of the rightward-forward twist, which was first described by William Harvey, or by a change in shape of the right ventricle due to increased pull of the tricuspid ring toward the apex.

Elevated cardiac output, whether due to exercise, excitement, or such conditions as thyrotoxicosis or anemia, may also cause a diffuse precordial impulse. This is likewise often observed in patients with congestive heart failure, and in some persons with infarction of the interventricular septum, which apparently bulges toward the right ventricle when its contractile power is reduced. Similar but temporary changes may occur during anginal attacks. Patients with emphysema and low diaphragms often exhibit a pronounced systolic footward-forward thrust of the inferior cardiac border. This can be readily felt in the epigastrium, but must be distinguished from the forward pulsation of the abdominal aorta and the right subcostal systolic movement of the liver in patients with tricuspid insufficiency.

When hypertrophy is marked, the palpatory findings may be confusing because extreme hypertrophy of either ventricle may cause exaggeration of both the apical and parasternal motions. In this circumstance the electrocardiogram is more reliable. However, when hypertrophy is of moderate degree, simple palpation is usually more trustworthy than instrumental methods, provided the other conditions which have been cited can be excluded.

The x-ray sometimes supplies indirect information concerning hypertrophy by demonstrating valvular calcification. More commonly, it detects enlargement but does not distinguish between dilatation and hypertrophy. Since, in the absence of pericardial effusion, marked enlargement of the cardiac shadow is mainly due to dilatation, the x-ray is especially useful in detecting the latter process. It is also the most reliable method for recognition of atrial enlargement, although the electrocardiogram is sometimes valuable in this respect. Thus broad notched P waves and narrow tall P waves point toward hypertrophy of the left and right atria, respectively. Because the congenital lesions often produce bizarre and sometimes characteristic changes in the shape of the cardiac chambers or of the great vessels, the fluoroscopic and, especially, angiographic methods are particularly useful in these conditions (Chap. 252).

ALTERATIONS IN HEART SOUNDS

Improved methods for recording heart sounds have extended the information which can be obtained by auscultation. The following discussion, which is based largely on the work of Leatham, deals mainly with such aspects of heart sounds and murmurs as can, with some practice, be elicited at the bedside. Phenomena which can be recorded but not readily heard will be mentioned only when they illustrate general principles.

The observer who desires to obtain maximal information from auscultation of the heart should keep two points constantly in mind: (1) In order to hear a faint sound or murmur it is necessary to listen specifically for it, i.e., to focus one's attention on that phase of the cycle during which the manifestation in question may be expected to occur. (2) The accurate timing (which is essential for correct interpretation) of a phenomenon necessarily involves relating it to known events. Frequently, the relationship to the first or second sound will suffice, but in many instances the clarification will come from simultaneous auscultation and inspection or palpation of the jugular pulse, the carotid upstroke, the apical thrust, or the precordial heave.

The low-pitched sounds and murmurs are best heard with gentle pressure, using the bell-shaped stethoscopic endpiece. However, high-pitched sounds, such as diastolic blows, are better heard with the diaphragm stethoscope, or with firm pressure if the bell is used. The tense skin then acts like a diaphragm and tends to transmit high-frequency vibrations.

The interventricular septum often inhibits the transmission of the left-sided phenomena to the anterior precordium. Hence the signs arising at the mitral valve are best heard at the apex, which is normally part of the left ventricle. Likewise, the second sound at the apex, as well as in the right second space, is mainly due to aortic closure. The tricuspid first sound is best heard in the fourth or fifth interspace just to the left of the sternum, while the pulmonic second is usually maximal in the second or third space. However, the blow of aortic insufficiency and the opening snap of mitral stenosis are exceptions; both these phenomena are often best heard in the tricuspid area.

There is still some dispute concerning the relative significance of valvular, muscular, vascular, and pericardial vibrations in the production of the heart sounds. In our opinion, the evidence indicates that abrupt change in tension of the valve cusps is the sole factor in the production of the *audible components* of the three normal sounds. Under abnormal conditions, the great vessels or the pericardium may produce sounds, but there is no convincing evidence that these ever arise in the myocardium.

Intensity. The chief factors which influence the intensity of the first sound are (1) the position of the valves at the onset of ventricular systole, which is usually determined by the length of time elapsing between atrial and ventricular contraction (p.

89); (2) the rate of rise of ventricular pressure; (3) the presence or absence of structural disease of the mitral valve; and (4) the amount of tissue, air, or fluid between the heart and the surface. Loudness of the first sound is favored by short conduction time, high cardiac output, mitral stenosis, and thinness. The reverse of these conditions tends to be associated with faintness of the first sound.

Aside from such extracardiac factors as obesity, emphysema, and effusions in the chest, the intensity and to some extent the quality of the second heart sound may be influenced by alterations in the character of the vessel walls. Accentuation of the aortic second sound is a normal phenomenon with age and occurs in such conditions as arteriosclerosis or syphilitic aortitis, which may cause diffuse change in the physical properties of the wall of the aorta. The other conditions which affect the intensity of the second sound are primarily those which alter pressures in the aorta and pulmonary artery, an increase in pressure tending to be associated with accentuation of the corresponding sounds.

The loud first sound of mitral stenosis is probably related not only to the thickening of the cusps but to the delay in onset of the mitral component because of the elevated left atrial pressure. Thus the normal splitting due to earlier mitral closure is absent, the mitral and tricuspid components are fused, and the first sound tends to be louder but briefer than normal. When the period elapsing between the start of excitation and mitral closure ($Q-S^1$ time) exceeds 0.07 sec, mitral stenosis is probable and the degree of prolongation bears a general relationship to the height of left atrial pressure and hence to the degree of stenosis.

Quality. Judgments concerning the state of the heart on the basis of the "quality" of the first sound are likely to be fallacious. The tic rhythm (embryocardia) of shock is a reflection of tachycardia and defective venous return. The diminished intensity which is so common in older persons is usually the result either of such extracardiac factors as emphysema or obesity or of a relatively long P-R interval caused by vagal tone. The *functional integrity of the myocardium cannot be assessed by the intensity or pitch of the first heart sound*. Other criteria should be utilized (Chap. 249).

Three-sound Rhythms. These fall into several general groups (Fig. 251-1). The additional sound may be heard in close approximation to the normal first or second sound, or in midsystole, or in middiastole.

Splitting of the First Sound. This is a normal phenomenon because closure of the mitral valve precedes that of the tricuspid by 0.01 to 0.02 sec. This splitting is usually best heard at the tricuspid area where the second and fainter component is loudest. It may be heard in a considerable propor-

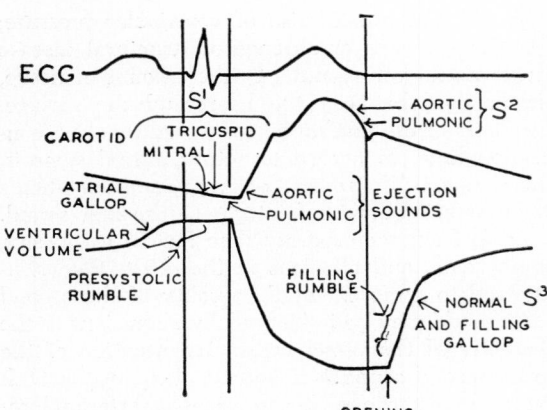

FIG. 251-1. The middiastolic sounds due to a prolonged P-R interval or to a one-sound ventricular premature beat (see text) are not shown because their times are inconstant in relation to the cardiac cycle. The midsystolic extracardiac noises are likewise not indicated.

Because of their close temporal approximation, the ejection clicks cannot be separated from splitting of the first sound by auscultation. The presystolic rumble, when very brief, may be confused with an atrial gallop, but both may usually be distinguished from the other phenomena.

During relaxation and early filling, the split second sound may be confused with the opening snap, the normal third sound, the filling (protodiastolic) gallop, or with a filling rumble of unusually brief duration. The distinction between these several phenomena, while often possible by auscultation alone, sometimes requires simultaneous phonocardiograms, electrocardiograms, pulse tracings, and records of precordial movement.

tion of healthy persons. The distinction from the less frequent *ejection sound* usually requires graphic methods. The latter phenomenon is apparently due either to semilunar opening or to the sudden expansion of the great vessels and is usually best heard at the pulmonary area in persons with pulmonary hypertension. It may be recorded by sensitive techniques at the aortic or mitral areas in many normal persons but is rarely audible and has little practical significance.

When the P-R interval is normal, the very small vibrations of the atrioventricular cusps related to atrial activity are blended with the larger forces of the first heart sound and are usually inaudible. When, as occurs in the several types of heart block, this interval is abnormally long, the atrial sounds may be heard (see below). In patients with heart failure and regular rhythm, the force of atrial contraction is nearly always increased and, even though the P-R interval is normal, an audible sound—the *presystolic* or *atrial gallop*—is commonly noted. This phenomenon, although occasionally audible in the absence of heart failure, usually signifies that

failure is present or imminent and is, therefore, of practical importance. Just prior to atrial contraction, the atrial pressure is equal to that in the corresponding ventricle. A slight elevation of ventricular diastolic pressure causes relatively great stretch of the thin-walled and highly distensible atrium. Thus, in accordance with Starling's law, the changes in pressure as the atrium contracts and then relaxes are greater than normal. The resulting exaggerated tensing of the cusps is apparently responsible for the atrial sound.

The presystolic gallop may usually be distinguished from a split first sound by the longer interval (ta-lubb—dup, rather than t'lubb—dup). The differentiation from an exceptionally brief presystolic rumble, a rare source of confusion, can be made by listening after exercise, which increases the duration of the latter.

The *third sounds occurring during midsystole* are nearly always of extracardiac origin. They commonly arise from bubbles of air in the neighboring alimentary organs but may be due to pneumothorax or to mediastinal emphysema. In some instances, their site and mechanism are unknown, but they have no significance as regards the heart.

Splitting of the second sound is a normal phenomenon during inspiration, when the greater inflow into the right ventricle produces some prolongation of its ejection. The delay in pulmonic closure due to the lower pressure as compared with that in the aorta is normally very slight during expiration, and can be demonstrated only by graphic methods. *Audible expiratory splitting*, which is best heard in the tricuspid or pulmonary areas, is probably always abnormal when it is present in the sitting or standing position. It is usually but not invariably abnormal in the recumbent position. Such splitting may be due to delayed pulmonary closure because of an increased flow load involving the right ventricle only (interatrial defect or anomalous venous drainage with one or more pulmonary veins emptying into the right atrium) or, more rarely, to an increased pressure load from pulmonic stenosis. Although phonocardiograms may display the same phenomenon with right bundle branch block, the change is rarely so pronounced as to be of bedside diagnostic value in the latter condition. Unusually early aortic closure, such as occurs with mitral insufficiency, may also produce audible expiratory splitting.

In patients with large interatrial defects, the filling of the right atrium from the left may exceed that from the cavae. Hence the volume and duration of right ventricular ejection are not significantly increased by inspiration. Therefore, there is no inspiratory exaggeration of the splitting of the second sound. This phenomenon is of diagnostic value, i.e., a pronounced expiratory split which is not audibly greater during inspiration is suggestive evidence for the presence of an interatrial defect.

The *opening snap* is occasionally due to tricuspid stenosis. Much more commonly, it is an important sign of mitral stenosis. Its time of onset after the second heart sound is inversely related to the height of the left atrial pressure. Thus a very short S^2-OS time, like a very long Q-S^1 time, speaks for a high degree of mitral stenosis.

The opening snap is of brief duration, high-pitched, and usually best heard in the fourth or fifth space between the left sternal margin and the apex. These features will usually distinguish it from the split second sound which occurs somewhat earlier and is likely to be better heard at the pulmonic or apical regions.

Three sounds may be noted during the phase of rapid filling. Two of these, the *physiologic third sound* and the *protodiastolic (filling) gallop*, are apparently both due to a rapid equalization of pressure between atrium and ventricle, with headward rebound of the atrioventricular cusps. Although they occur at the same time, have the same low pitch, and are heard in the same (mitral or tricuspid) areas, they are not likely to be confused with each other. The physiologic third sound occurs in young persons and probably signifies rather complete ventricular emptying. In the case of the protodiastolic gallop, the rapid filling is due not to unusually low pressure in the ventricle but to elevation in the atrium and possibly also to some dilatation of the atrioventricular orifice. Thus we have the paradox of a somewhat similar phenomenon indicating either a vigorous or an impaired heart. The distinction is based on such associated findings as age, heart size, and the history of exercise tolerance. Furthermore, the normal third sound is usually best heard when the rate is slow, while moderate tachycardia is the rule in patients with the filling gallop. Because of this, the cadence resembling that of a cantering horse is usually present only with the latter condition.

Confusion between these two phenomena and a very brief *filling rumble* is rare and can usually be settled by exercise, which tends to prolong the latter phenomenon.

The filling gallop is of great practical importance. It is often the sole *cardiac* sign of heart failure, the other manifestations being found in the lungs or elsewhere. It may also be the earliest sign, preceding the congestive phenomena by months or even years. When, as is commonly true, it arises on the left side, it is best heard at the apex and is louder during expiration. However, right ventricular gallops occasionally occur. They are likely to be equally or more loud during inspiration and are best heard in the lower parasternal region or, when emphysema is present, in the epigastrium.

These several phenomena, which occur during early filling, may usually be separated from the split second sound and from the opening snap by their lower pitch and by their point of maximal intensity, which is ordinarily in a more inferior interspace. However, doubt may occur in a patient presenting signs of both stenosis and insufficiency of the mitral valve. Here, the distinction assumes great practical significance in relation to cardiac surgery. An opening snap speaks strongly for predominant stenosis, while a left ventricular filling gallop precludes marked narrowing of the valve because pronounced stenosis prevents the rapid pressure equalization which produces the gallop. Under this circumstance it may be necessary to make simultaneous recordings of heart sounds and of precordial motions, in order to learn whether the sound in question precedes the onset of filling (split sound), coincides exactly with it (opening snap), or appears 0.04 to 0.06 sec later (filling gallop). Even so, caution must be exercised to avoid confusion between (1) mitral insufficiency with both a rumble due to rapid filling and a left-sided filling gallop; and (2) mitral stenosis, as the cause of the rumble, associated with a right ventricular filling gallop (pp. 1412 and 1440).

The pansystolic murmur of mitral insufficiency may continue during relaxation and thus mask the second sound at the apex. Under this circumstance the filling gallop may be mistaken for the second sound.

Being low-pitched, the protodiastolic gallop is best heard with a bell-type stethoscope, using gentle pressure. It is ordinarily the faintest of the three sounds but may be the loudest. This confusing sign is especially common when the rate is rapid, diastole short, and the atrial and filling gallops are superimposed during rapid filling (summation gallop).

Although rubs, murmurs, or even extracardiac noises may be heard during middiastole, true heart sounds are rare at this time of the cycle. When the P-R interval is long, the faint vibrations of the valves induced by atrial activity may produce a low-pitched and faint but audible sound. It is important to separate this from the single sound caused by a very premature ventricular beat which is too feeble to open the semilunar valves and hence causes no second sound. Either phenomenon may occur in middiastole. In most instances, the premature beat has a higher pitch. However, the differentiation may be impossible by auscultation. This is almost the only situation in which the electrocardiogram will supply crucial information concerning the exact nature of heart sounds. Such a tracing should always be made because both conditions—heart block and frequent premature beats—may require treatment and the drug which is indicated

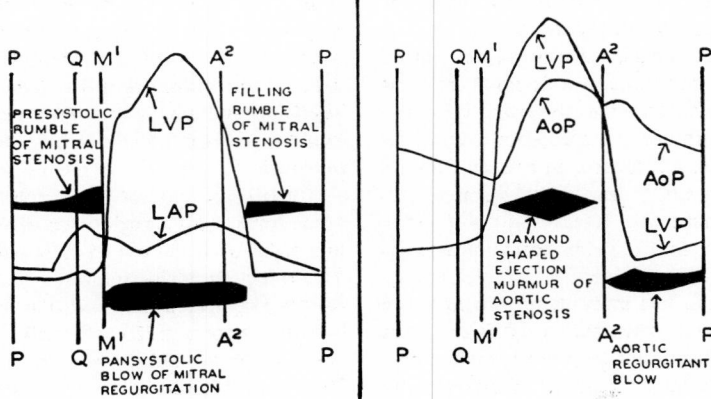

Fig. 251-2. The onset, offset, and "shape" (*crescendo, diminuendo,* or *diamond*) of murmurs in relation to the pressure differences between adjacent areas are illustrated. *P* and *Q* indicate the onset of atrial and ventricular excitation, respectively.

Note that the murmur of mitral insufficiency starts with the beginning of the first sound (M^1), and endures beyond the second, or until the pressure in the left ventricle (*LVP*) falls below that in the left atrium (*LAP*). In contrast, the "diamond" murmur of aortic stenosis starts later, as ejection begins. It increases and then decreases in intensity, according to the pressure gradient between the left ventricle and the aorta (*AoP*), and ceases just before the aortic second sound (A^2) as these pressures become equalized.

The murmur of aortic insufficiency starts with the second sound because the left ventricular pressure falls below the aortic at this time. The filling rumble of mitral stenosis begins later as the ventricular pressure descends below the atrial. The presystolic accentuation of the stenotic murmurs occurs as the left atrium contracts.

for one of them may be seriously hazardous for the other (p. 1405).

MURMURS

The discussion to follow is concerned primarily with murmurs arising in the heart, and only incidentally with those in other areas. It deals with the mechanisms and types of murmurs and their general significance but not with the specific causative lesions, which are considered in the next two chapters.

Most murmurs are limited to systole or diastole; a few are continuous. Diastolic murmurs always mean organic disease, and the main problem is that of hearing them. Systolic murmurs are more readily heard, may or may not signify a structural disorder, and the chief question is that of interpretation. In this regard a rheumatic history, an associated thrill, or the demonstration of a calcified valve may be of crucial importance.

The precise time of onset and of offset of murmurs depends on the point of the cardiac cycle at which an adequate pressure difference between two chambers appears and disappears. This general principle, which is considered in some detail in subsequent pages, is illustrated in Fig. 251-2. Inspection of this diagram will reveal the reasons why murmurs are called *pansystolic, ejection, late systolic, regurgitant, early filling,* and *presystolic.*

The accentuation of a murmur during inspiration

means that it is almost certainly arising on the right side of the heart, the effect of the augmented venous return predominating over the damping tendency of lung expansion. Expiratory exaggeration has less significance. It is the rule with left-sided murmurs but may also occur with those arising in the right chambers if the intensifying result of reduced lung volume predominates over the hemodynamic effect of reduced venous return.

There is no simple relation between the loudness of a murmur and the severity of the responsible lesion. Thus in the advanced stages of mitral stenosis the diastolic rumble may actually decrease because of diminished flow through the orifice. Similarly, in patent ductus arteriosus the development of secondary pulmonary hypertension, with aggravation of the patient's symptoms, may be associated with reduced intensity of the murmur as the left-to-right shunt diminishes.

The murmurs of aortic and pulmonic stenosis are low-pitched and "rough" because they are related to the low-frequency vibrations of the semilunar cusps. However, the insufficiency murmurs, being due to vibrations (eddies) of blood, are higher pitched and resemble the swishing sound of a mountain stream.

Murmurs and Turbulence. When a liquid or a gas moves, not in smooth straight lines but in constantly changing directions and velocities, the flow is said to be turbulent. Murmurs, wheezes, and the sounds of mountain streams are the results of turbulence, which tends to be produced by rapid velocity, by irregularity or increase in stream-bed diameter, and by high density of the flowing fluid. The latter influence presumably accounts for the beneficial effect on wheezing of helium, which is much lighter than nitrogen. Turbulence varies inversely with viscosity. Therefore, murmurs tend to occur in anemic patients, even if the volume and velocity of flow remain constant. Actually, they usually increase, and this also favors the production of murmurs.

These considerations explain many aspects of murmurs: their frequent occurrence during systole in vigorous young hearts (high velocity of flow), their appearance even in diastole when flow is sufficiently rapid (the "pseudostenotic atrioventricular rumbles" in patients with atrial septal defect, patent ductus, or even with uncomplicated mitral insufficiency); their presence with stenotic lesions (for a given total flow the velocity is inversely proportional to the square of the orifice size). Insufficiency murmurs are related not only to the high velocity because of the large pressure difference between the respective chambers, but also to the additional turbulence caused by the convergence of two streams of blood.

The bruits heard over aneurysms are related to the increase in diameter. The murmur caused by the increase in velocity at the site of a narrowed vessel is usually systolic only because collateral circulation above the constriction reduces the diastolic pressure gradient; when collaterals are absent, partial occlusion may cause a continuous murmur.

The energy (pressure gradient) necessary to produce a given volume flow is proportional to V (velocity) when the flow is laminar but to V^2 when it is turbulent. Thus a stenotic lesion exerts two harmful mechanical effects—that due to the narrowing per se and that due to the turbulence secondary to the narrowing. As the velocity of flow increases with exercise, the second effect becomes progressively more important, as shown by increasing loudness of the murmur.

Systolic Murmurs. These may be divided into three groups in relation to their time.

Pansystolic Murmurs. This group includes those murmurs involving two chambers which have widely different systolic pressures, such as the left ventricle and either the left atrium or the right ventricle. The pressure gradient is established very early in contraction and lasts until relaxation is almost complete. Thus such murmurs begin during isometric contraction and at the area of maximal intensity tend to mask both heart sounds because they begin with the first and cease after the second. The pansystolic murmurs due to ventriculoatrial regurgitation may be dependent either on deformity of the cusps ("organic") or on dilatation of the

rings ("relative"). The latter murmurs are associated with well-marked cardiac enlargement and become fainter with improvement of heart failure. The organic regurgitant murmurs may occur in hearts of any size and, when accompanied by congestive failure, are likely to become louder as improvement occurs.

Pansystolic murmurs are not found in patients with interatrial defects unless there is atrioventricular regurgitation due to associated deformities of the mitral or tricuspid valves. In the case of those interventricular shunts which are accompanied by a large pressure gradient between the two ventricles, these murmurs do occur. Large openings in the interventricular septum usually lead to early pulmonary hypertension, which raises the right ventricular systolic pressure and thus tends to reduce the shunt. Furthermore, the turbulence is related to the velocity of flow which, if pressures are constant, is inversely proportional to the square of the size of the orifice. A high pressure gradient is likely to be associated with a high-pitched murmur. These considerations explain why the small and relatively innocent defects of the muscular part of the septum are likely to be associated with louder murmurs of higher pitch than the larger and more serious shunts which are situated higher and involve the membranous portion. In the latter circumstances the faint pansystolic murmur may be overshadowed by the louder ejection blow caused by the relative stenosis consequent to increased flow through the dilated pulmonary artery.

Ejection Murmurs. These are related to a disproportion between the flow and the size of the orifice. Even though the semilunar valves are normal, a large flow or dilated vessel may be responsible. Narrowing of the outflow tract or of the valves may cause such a murmur, the intensity being related to the flow. Thus the murmur of aortic stenosis becomes faint and may disappear during heart failure and return with great intensity following digitalization.

The ejection murmurs start shortly after the first sound and do not actually replace it, although this may seem to be the case by auscultation. As the ventricular pressure rises and declines during ejection, the murmur becomes louder and then fainter. This "diamond shape" is readily seen in phonocardiograms but may not be apparent to the ear. The second heart sound may be exaggerated or normal and is not obscured by the murmur, which ceases before semilunar closure occurs. However, when stenosis of one of the valves is responsible, the corresponding second sound may be faint or absent because the cusps are no longer pliable.

The age of the patient and the area of maximal intensity are of great importance in determining the significance of ejection murmurs. Thus in a young adult with vigorous contraction and a high ejection velocity, a faint or moderate ejection blow heard only in the pulmonary area is usually without significance, while a similar murmur in the aortic area is likely to indicate stenosis of the valve or some congenital abnormality. In elderly persons, functional pulmonic blows are rare, while aortic systolic murmurs may be due to dilatation or roughening of the aorta, to left ventricular hypertrophy with vigorous contraction and functional stenosis of the left ventricular outflow tract, to an important degree of aortic stenosis, or to slight narrowing of the valve. The latter condition, when associated with a high level of cardiac output, may produce a loud murmur even though the stenosis is of no hemodynamic importance, as shown by the lack of a significant pressure gradient between the left ventricle and the aorta.

The most common ejection murmur is that heard at the pulmonary area in healthy young persons with small and vigorous hearts. It is probably due to the combination of a high velocity of flow and a thin chest wall. When it is faint (grade I or II), blowing, and unassociated with evidence of disease, the diagnosis of an innocent functional murmur will be apparent. Less frequently, the quality is rough and the intensity may be grade III or IV. Such patients, who are called "paranormals," are frequently anxious and may have multiple cardiovascular complaints. Under these exceptional circumstances, cardiac catheterization may be necessary in order to separate such an exaggerated functional murmur from one due to a slight congenital deformity. However, careful attention to the second heart sound may yield an important clue (p. 1408). Audible *expiratory* splitting indicates that the duration of right ventricular ejection remains long and its stroke volume large, despite the diminished systemic venous return during expiration. This suggests that a large fraction of the blood entering the right ventricle is coming from intrathoracic structures. Pronounced and audible expiratory splitting of the second sound in a person with an ejection murmur, therefore, points toward a defect of the interatrial septum or anomalous drainage of one or more pulmonary veins into the right atrium. Inspiratory splitting, a normal phenomenon, has no diagnostic significance.

Late Systolic Murmurs. Many patients with coronary disease present faint or moderate (rarely loud) blowing apical systolic murmurs which seem to start well after ejection and do not mask either sound. The exact mechanism responsible for them has not been clarified. Since they may be much louder or heard only during anginal attacks, it is probable that they are related to ischemia of the papillary muscles or, possibly, to distortion of these structures by the ischemic bulges (functional aneu-

rysms), which so commonly occur following infarction or during anginal episodes (p. 35).

The late systolic murmurs which occasionally occur in young subjects are usually musical or "whistling." Their mechanism is not known. In most instances, there is no evidence of cardiac disease and the murmurs are without significance. Rarely, such a musical or squeaking late systolic murmur is seen in a young person with undoubted rheumatic heart disease. In such an instance, the differentiation from the similar innocent murmur will depend on the associated findings.

Diastolic Murmurs. These also include three main types.

Regurgitant Murmurs. The *regurgitant* diastolic murmurs begin with or shortly after the second heart sound, or as soon as the corresponding ventricular pressure falls sufficiently below that in the aorta or pulmonary artery. Since they are mainly due to eddies of blood rather than to vibrations of valve cusps, they have a high-pitched swishing quality resembling breath sounds. They are best heard during held forced expiration, with the patient leaning forward or on his hands and knees. The high-frequency vibrations are best detected by a diaphragm stethoscope or by firm pressure, if a bell is used.

Regurgitation through the aortic valve is usually due to deformity of the cusps rather than to dilatation of the annulus. The reverse is true of pulmonic insufficiency. The differentiation of these conditions is discussed in a later chapter (p. 1442).

Filling Murmurs. Diastolic murmurs during early filling are, like ejection blows, due to disproportion between orifice size and flow rate. Thus mitral and tricuspid stenosis are associated with rumbles which start soon but at an appreciable interval after the second sound. With normal or high flow, such murmurs may be loud when stenosis is slight. Conversely, a high degree of obstruction may cause a very faint or even no rumble if cardiac output is sufficiently reduced. When stenosis is marked, ventricular filling is inevitably prolonged. *Thus the duration of the murmur is more reliable than the intensity as an index of the degree of narrowing.*

Despite normal mitral cusps, patients with aortic insufficiency may have a diastolic mitral rumble (the Austin-Flint murmur). This is probably due to vibration of the aortic cusp of the mitral valve between the normal and abnormal streams of blood into the ventricle.

A faint diastolic murmur heard in a patient with acute rheumatic fever may sometimes disappear. In such an instance (Coombs's murmur) edema of the mitral cusps is probably responsible.

Very high rates of flow may cause loud but brief filling rumbles, despite normal cusps, at either atrioventricular orifice. In the case of the tricuspid valve, the usual cause is a large interatrial defect. Such "relative stenosis" of the mitral valve is seen in patients with patent ductus and is particularly confusing when mitral insufficiency with minimal or no stenosis is the cause. Aside from the duration of the rumble, the intensity of the first sound, the presence or absence of a well-marked opening snap, and the type of hypertrophy are important guides to the predominant lesion (p. 1439).

Presystolic Murmurs. The *presystolic* or atrial systolic murmur is usually due to mitral (rarely tricuspid) stenosis. It has the same quality as the filling rumble but is usually crescendo rather than decrescendo. Because of its short duration it may be confused with an atrial gallop or a split first sound. Its accentuation and prolongation, due to fusion with the filling rumble, by exercise will usually make the distinction.

When these filling rumbles, whether early or presystolic, arise at the mitral orifice, they are best heard with a bell stethoscope at the exact point of the apex, while the patient lies on the left side and during expiration. Occasionally, they are audible only after exercise. The tricuspid rumbles, which are much less common, are heard in the left parasternal region and are sometimes louder during inspiration.

Continuous Murmurs. These signify continuous flow due to a communication between a high-pressure and a low-pressure area, without an intervening valve. The commonest cause is patent ductus arteriosus, which causes a continuous murmur as long as the pressure in the pulmonary artery is much below that in the aorta. When pulmonary hypertension due to left-sided failure or to arteriolar changes in the lungs supervenes, the duration of the murmur lessens and it may eventually disappear or persist only during systole.

Less common causes of continuous murmurs include systemic or pulmonary arteriovenous fistula, the development of marked bronchial collateral circulation in patients with pulmonary stenosis, rupture of an aortic aneurysm into the pulmonary artery, and a congenital window between the roots of the aorta and pulmonary artery. Coarctation of the aorta and stenosis of a main pulmonary artery usually cause systolic murmurs only, but when because of poor collaterals proximal to the obstruction the pressure gradient remains large throughout diastole, this murmur may be continuous.

Rupture of a sinus of Valsalva into the right atrium or ventricle is a rare but surgically curable cause of a continuous murmur which, under this circumstance, may be loudest in the lower sternal region.

The cervical venous hum or *bruit de diable* is a faint continuous musical murmur at the base of the neck. Gentle pressure by the stethoscope causes it to disappear. It has no significance.

Significance of Murmurs. All diastolic murmurs and, with the exception of the cervical venous hum, all continuous murmurs indicate structural disease. The systolic bruit, when very loud or associated with a thrill, has the same significance. The problem of interpretation arises with the moderately loud systolic blow, which usually is due to an organic lesion and, especially, with the faint (grade I or II) systolic murmur. Here, the decision will depend on consideration of all the evidence and will sometimes be in doubt, even after cardiac catheterization. Small left-to-right shunts may be overlooked unless the newer methods, such as the hydrogen electrode, are utilized. In borderline instances, a faint systolic murmur, loudest at the base, should be considered innocent until proved otherwise. A similar murmur heard only at the apex is more likely to be of structural origin. Even so, if there are no other signs of organic heart disease, the only therapeutic considerations are those of prophylaxis against rheumatic fever and bacterial endocarditis (pp. 918 and 1043).

Thrills. In the region of the apex, thrills are of limited diagnostic import because they may be confused with vibrations set up by a vigorously beating heart. On the other hand, the presence of a thrill at the base of the heart or along the left sternal border constitutes practically conclusive evidence that the accompanying murmur is of the organic type. It is true that thrills are simply the tactile equivalent of the auditory basis of the murmur and hence have no greater significance than the murmur itself. It happens, however, that the kind of murmur which gives rise to vibrations that can be felt as a thrill is almost invariably of organic origin. Such thrills are of especial importance in the diagnosis of aortic stenosis.

The *pericardial friction rub* may occasionally be confused with a harsh systolic murmur or with an insignificant adventitious sound ("sternal crunch"). Such uncertainty, which arises when the rub is only systolic, will be solved by consideration of the total clinical picture. The characteristic to-and-fro squeaking sound signifies pericarditis and is nearly always accompanied by other findings of this disorder (p. 1467).

ELECTROCARDIOGRAPHY IN THE DIAGNOSIS OF CARDIAC DISEASE

In patients with arrhythmias, the electrocardiogram usually supplies precise information. Under other circumstances, the records are likely to lead to erroneous conclusions unless evaluated in relation to the total picture. Variations in the placement of precordial electrodes during successive tracings may lead to an erroneous conclusion that an acute myocardial disorder is present because of "changes" in the record. Similarly, a chest deformity or an unusually low diaphragm, with a vertical position of the heart, may be associated with an "abnormal" record when the precordial electrode is placed in the usual positions. Such errors may be avoided by securing each V lead from multiple interspaces. Certain innocent electrocardiographic findings which are likely to be misinterpreted are illustrated on p. 1446.

Abnormalities in the form of the ventricular complex are often erroneously evaluated. There is strong evidence that the Q-R-S-T sequence is mainly dependent on the subepicardial portions of the ventricle and that the subendocardial fibers are electrically silent. Therefore, subepicardial fibrosis due to such innocent causes as healed focal pericarditis or remote contusions of the heart may cause impressive changes in the electrocardiogram, while an extensive recent subendocardial infarction may show no significant change. T waves are especially labile and may be altered by electrolyte shifts, emotion, tachycardia, pressure on the ventricle, ingestion of iced drinks, or even by a carbohydrate-rich meal. The QRS complex is less unstable, and the presence of Q waves of 0.04 sec or longer duration has greater or lesser significance as a sign of focal myocardial disease, depending on the leads in which the Q waves occur. However, there is no necessary parallelism between such a change and the gravity of the clinical picture, or even the nature of the underlying disease process. It so happens that coronary disease is the commonest cause of focal myocardial disease, but identical changes may be induced by other localized disorders such as abscess or tumor. Thus, except in patients with arrhythmias, therapy should be based on the clinical picture. Diagnosis is based on evaluation of *all* the evidence, with emphasis in most instances on that derived from the clinical study.

OTHER DIAGNOSTIC PROCEDURES

The importance of the fluoroscopic examination has already been mentioned. Certain methods, such as cardiac catheterization, angiocardiography, and oximetry, which are widely used in the study of congenital lesions, are considered in Chap. 252, which deals with those disorders.

In the hands of those who are experienced with them, the ballistocardiographic, electrokymographic, and kinetocardiographic techniques yield certain information of practical value. Their main present value, however, is in the field of research.

For a more detailed consideration of physical signs in relation to specific congenital and acquired lesions, the reader is referred to the two succeeding chapters.

REFERENCES

Harrison, T. R.: Palpation of the Precordial Impulses, Stanford Med. Bull., 13:385, 1954.

Jeffries, J. L.: Kinetocardiographic Tracings as an Aid in the Differentiation of Three-sound Rhythms, Am. Heart J., 57:904, 1959.

Leatham, A.: The Place of Phonocardiography in Clinical Cardiology, Prog. in Cardiovasc. Diseases, 2:76, 1959.

——: Auscultation of the Heart: First Goulstonian Lecture, Lancet, 2:703, 1958.

Vakil, R. J.: Ventricular Aneurysm of the Heart: Preliminary Report on Some New Clinical Signs, Am. Heart J., 49:934, 1955.

Warren, J. V., J. J. Leonard, and A. M. Weissler: Gallop Rhythm, Ann. Internal Med., 48:580, 1958.

252 CONGENITAL HEART DISEASE

William R. Milnor and Henry T. Bahnson

The demonstration that many congenital malformations of the heart can be treated successfully by surgery has radically changed the physician's approach to congenital heart disease. Not long ago the nonspecific clinical diagnosis of *congenital heart disease* was regarded as all that was possible or necessary in many cases. Today, the accurate recognition of specific lesions and a quantitative estimate of the burden they impose on the heart in each case is of great practical importance.

Incidence. Congenital heart disease occurs in approximately 0.3 per cent of all live births, and congenital malformations constitute 1 to 5 per cent of all cases of recognized heart disease after infancy.

Etiology. Many abnormalities of the heart and great vessels can be explained by failure to progress beyond an early stage of embryologic development, while others seem to represent aberrant development of a normal structure. The cause of these embryologic misadventures is unknown in most cases, but various theories involving fetal hypoxia, fetal endocarditis, immunologic abnormalities, vitamin deficiencies, and specific genetic abnormalities have been proposed.

In some cases a clear relation between maternal rubella during gestation and congenital malformations of the heart has been demonstrated. It appears that maternal rubella during the first 2 months of pregnancy will lead to congenital malformations of the heart, cataracts, deaf-mutism, or other anomalies in almost all cases. The later in gestation the rubella occurs, the lower the incidence of congenital abnormalities, but cases of congenital heart disease have occurred following rubella in the sixth month of pregnancy. In clinical practice, however, relatively few cases of congenital heart disease—probably less than 2 per cent—can be attributed to this cause, and in most instances no significant environmental factor during fetal development can be elicited by history.

Inheritance. With few exceptions, patients with congenital heart disease have a negative familial history for congenital malformations. There are, nevertheless, well-documented exceptions, including families in which the same malformation has recurred in two or three successive generations. Patent ductus arteriosus is the commonest lesion thus reported, but this may simply reflect the relatively benign course of this anomaly.

The birth of one child with a congenital malformation of the heart does not in itself contraindicate future pregnancies, since the risk that subsequent siblings will have congenital malformations is extremely small.

There is good evidence that factors concerned with some congenital malformations can be transmitted as mendelian recessive traits, while others may arise as a result of mutation *de novo*. In at least one heritable disorder of connective tissue (Marfan's syndrome, p. 1884) cardiovascular manifestations are a prominent feature.

The incidence of some congenital malformations of the heart shows clear sex differences, which may be attributed to either sex-linked inheritance or environmental factors in utero. Defects of the atrial septum and persistent patency of the ductus arteriosus are much more common in females than in males; pulmonic stenosis and ventricular septal defect show little or no sex difference; coarctation of the aorta and congenital aortic stenosis affect males predominantly.

PHYSIOLOGIC EFFECTS

Shunts

A cardiovascular shunt may be broadly defined as blood flow through an abnormal pathway. It requires an open communication (or one potentially open, such as a patent foramen ovale) between the pulmonic and systemic circulations. The direction and degree of blood flow are determined by the dimensions of the opening and the pressures existing on either side of it. Such communications usually represent persistence of an embryonic stage of development into postnatal life.

In some cases changing pressure gradients during the heart cycle will produce shunts that vary in direction. In other instances the existence of roughly equivalent pressures on opposite sides of a defect may prevent shunting of blood, even if the defect is large. Streamlining of flow is an important factor in some instances and may produce shunting in the absence of measurable pressure gradients.

Left-to-Right Shunts. In this situation, a portion of the blood which flows through the lungs is diverted before reaching the systemic capillaries and is recirculated through the pulmonary bed. The volume of blood pumped through the pulmonary capillaries therefore exceeds the systemic flow per minute, unless complicating shunts in the opposite direction are also present. Pulmonic blood flows of 12 to 15 liters per min, with systemic flows of 4 to 5 liters per min, are common, and the ratio of pulmonic/systemic flow may reach 20 or more. In the latter situation, however, the difference in oxygen saturation between arterial and venous blood is so small that accurate calculation of pulmonary flow by the usual methods of cardiac catheterization is impossible.

With left-to-right shunts at the atrial or ventricular level, the right ventricle is required to pump an increased volume of blood per minute, at pressures which may or may not be higher than normal. This results in right ventricular dilatation and hypertrophy, the degree of hypertrophy being roughly proportional to the degree and duration of pulmonary hypertension. When the shunt is at the level of the pulmonary artery, as in patent ductus arteriosus uncomplicated by pulmonary hypertension, only the left ventricle hypertrophies; when pulmonary hypertension appears, right ventricular hypertrophy is superimposed.

Left ventricular work is increased if the site of the shunt is in the ventricular septum or distal to the left ventricle. Left ventricular hypertrophy and dilatation result but may be overshadowed by simultaneous right ventricular hypertrophy.

Arterial unsaturation does not occur with pure left-to-right shunts, but clinical cyanosis may occasionally be present as a result of decreased systemic flow or inadequate oxygenation in the lung. The latter is rare.

Auscultatory findings with left-to-right shunts depend on the specific malformations. When the shunt is distal to the mitral valve, an apical mid- or late diastolic murmur is often present, presumably because the greatly increased blood flow across a normal mitral orifice is equivalent to relative mitral stenosis. A similar diastolic murmur is sometimes present in cases of atrial septal defect, and may be due to relative tricuspid stenosis.

Right-to-Left Shunts. In this condition systemic venous blood returning to the heart enters the left heart chambers or systemic arterial circuit without passing through the pulmonary capillary bed.

The major signs and symptoms accompanying right-to-left shunts result not only from the diversion of blood through abnormal pathways but also from the obstruction to blood flow through normal pathways (e.g., pulmonic stenosis) which is often present. The functional effect of these abnormalities is to reduce the partial pressure of oxygen in arterial blood and to burden one or both ventricles with extra work. Some of the resulting signs and symptoms are common to many different malformations and will be discussed individually.

Cyanosis. Cyanosis, or the appearance of clinically recognizable blueness in the systemic capillaries, is usually a direct result of lowered arterial oxygen saturation. Slowed peripheral blood flow and inadequate saturation in the lungs can also cause cyanosis, but these factors are of secondary importance in cyanotic congenital heart disease. The oxygen saturation of the blood leaving the lungs is usually normal, but the admixture of venous blood distal to the site of the right-to-left shunt reduces the arterial saturation. The degree of arterial unsaturation varies directly with the volume of the venous-arterial shunt, and inversely with the volume of pulmonary blood flow.

Cyanosis is best observed in the nail beds, buccal mucous membranes, and lips. It becomes evident clinically only when the equivalent of approximately 5 Gm per 100 ml unsaturated hemoglobin is present in arterial blood; hence patients with anemia may not show clinical cyanosis even though the oxygen saturation of arterial blood is well below normal, while polycythemia accentuates cyanosis with even minimal degrees of arterial unsaturation.

In congenital heart disease, cyanosis usually implies the existence of an abnormal communication between the venous and arterial sides of the circulation, which may be a patent foramen ovale, defect of the interatrial or interventricular septum, transposed great vessels, patent ductus arteriosus or other communication between the aorta and pulmonary artery, or (rarely) direct entry of systemic veins into the left atrium. In addition to the abnormal communication, hemodynamic conditions must be such that blood flows through the opening from "right to left," producing a venous-arterial shunt; this usually requires elevation of right atrial, right ventricular, or pulmonary artery pressure above normal levels. An extreme example of a structural anomaly which produces a right-to-left shunt is seen in complete transposition of the great vessels, in which the right ventricular outflow enters the aorta instead of the pulmonary artery. In occasional cases, clinical cyanosis may be due to diminished peripheral flow or other factors, as in the normal vigorously crying child. It is almost never due to inadequate pulmonary oxygenation.

Polycythemia. Polycythemia with red cell counts of 6 to 9 million per cu mm, and hematocrits as high as 80, develops in response to the lowered arterial oxygen tension. The oxygen-carrying capacity of the blood is thereby increased, partially compensating for the decreased oxygen saturation. In many cases the increase of circulating hemoglobin is such that the oxygen content of the arterial blood is actually higher than normal.

The polycythemia is absolute rather than relative, i.e., the total red cell mass is increased. The plasma volume is usually decreased, but the red cell volume increase is of such magnitude that total blood volume is greater than normal.

This adaptative response is not entirely beneficial, since the blood viscosity increases as the hematocrit rises. The resulting increase in heart work is undesirable, but of even greater significance is the tendency to vascular thromboses. Hemiplegia and other cerebrovascular accidents occur frequently in polycythemic congenital heart disease. Dehydration is particularly to be avoided in these patients, since further reduction of plasma volume increases the predisposition to thromboses. In some patients with cyanotic congenital heart disease, polycythemia is accompanied by thrombocytopenia and low blood fibrinogen levels, leading to impaired clot retraction. Severe postoperative bleeding following the surgical repair of congenital cardiac defects can sometimes be attributed to this deficiency.

Clubbing. Clubbing of the fingers, and less often of the toes, is usually found in patients who have had cyanosis and polycythemia over a period of years. The pathogenesis of such clubbing is unexplained, but it may represent excessive growth of local tissue due to increased blood flow. Clinically identical clubbing may occur with pulmonary abscess or other diseases of the lung.

Impaired Growth. Impaired growth and development in children has been attributed to tissue hypoxemia in venous-arterial shunts, but it is open to question whether such a causal relationship exists. Some children with congenital heart disease are unquestionably stunted in growth and development, while others develop normally. Underdevelopment may be associated with malnutrition from inadequate feeding, or with the frequent respiratory and other infections to which these children are prone, or it may represent a concomitant congenital defect.

Squatting. Many patients with tetralogy of Fallot, and some with other lesions which obstruct blood flow to the lungs, find that squatting with the knees drawn up to the chest is the most comfortable resting position. They are uncomfortable, and often show increasing cyanosis, if made to stand quietly, or if they are tilted passively on the fluoroscope table. Their avoidance of postures in which the legs are dependent suggests that decreased venous return is the important factor in these phenomena, but the mechanism is not well understood. Squatting is also observed in many normal children, and is a habitual resting position of adults in many parts of the world. The posture is clinically significant only if it can be shown to give symptomatic relief after exertion.

Paradoxic Embolism. This condition, in which emboli arising in the systemic veins travel through a defect and lodge in a peripheral artery, is always possible with right-to-left shunts. This is probably responsible in part for the increased incidence of brain abscess in these patients.

Pulmonary Hypertension

In the normal adult the pulmonary circulation is a relatively low-pressure system. Mean pulmonary artery pressures of 15 mm Hg, or about 10 mm Hg higher than mean left atrial pressure, are sufficient to maintain adequate blood flow through the lungs at rest. When the cardiac output is increased by exertion, the normal pulmonary vascular bed is so distensible that pulmonary blood flow can be doubled with very little increase in pulmonary artery pressure.

Two different mechanisms commonly give rise to pulmonary hypertension in congenital heart disease: greatly increased pulmonary blood flow and increased pulmonary arteriolar resistance. Increased resistance to pulmonary venous outflow, as in mitral stenosis or left ventricular failure, is a third cause of pulmonary hypertension, but is more common in acquired heart disease.

The increased pulmonary blood flow accompanying large left-to-right shunts is often four to five times the normal flow, which requires increased pulmonary artery pressure even when the pulmonary vascular bed is normal. In these circumstances pulmonary vascular resistance, which is defined as the pressure drop across the pulmonary bed (mm Hg) per unit of pulmonary blood flow (liters/min/m²), remains normal or even decreases if the vessels are readily distensible. Pulmonary hypertension of this type is usually moderate in degree, with mean pulmonary artery pressures less than 40 mm Hg.

Increased pulmonary vascular resistance due to narrowing or partial obliteration of pulmonary arterioles, on the other hand, makes necessary an increased perfusion pressure to maintain even normal flow, so that pulmonary artery pressure rises without a proportionate increase in flow. In some cases this increased arteriolar resistance is predominantly due to irreversible structural changes, while in others vasoconstriction plays the dominant role. Pulmonary vascular resistance in this latter group can be temporarily lowered by inhalation of 100 per cent oxygen or by injection of acetylcholine and usually falls after successful correction of the accompanying cardiovascular defect.

Pulmonary vascular resistance is normally high at birth, and the small pulmonary arteries possess thick walls and relatively narrow lumina characteristic of the fetal circulation. After birth the arterial walls gradually become less thick and pulmonary vascular resistance falls. In patients with large communications between the ventricles or between pulmonary artery and aorta, the fetal structure of the pulmonary arteries persists into adult life; pulmonary hypertension is found in infancy and cyanosis appears early. Smaller communications between the ventricles, atria, or great vessels are usually accompanied by normal regression of pulmonary vascular resistance during infancy. The pulmonary arteries assume the normal thin-walled postnatal structure and remain normal throughout childhood or longer. In many of these cases the pulmonary vascular resistance eventually begins to rise, although the onset varies from adolescence to the fifth decade.

It seems clear that the absolute magnitude of pulmonary blood flow is not the only factor which influences the development of pulmonary hypertension. Abnormally high pulmonary artery pressures are found more often with ventricular than with atrial septal defects, and only occasionally with patent ductus arteriosus, although pulmonary blood flow is often three or more times the systemic flow in all these abnormalities.

The significance of pulmonary hypertension in each case, therefore, depends on its duration, the site and size of the cardiovascular defect, the anatomic changes in the pulmonary vessels, and the part played by active vasoconstriction. The desirability of correcting defects before irreversible pulmonary vascular changes have taken place whenever possible and the increased operative risk in patients with extremely high pulmonary vascular resistance are factors that play a large part in deciding on surgical therapy.

The most important clinical effects of pulmonary hypertension are: (1) *Right ventricular hypertrophy,* with characteristic left parasternal thrust and changes in the electrocardiogram and roentgenogram. If the strain on the right ventricle is too severe or too prolonged it may fail, with the same increased venous pressure, distention of the liver, and peripheral edema seen in right ventricular failure from other lesions. (2) *Enlargement of the pulmonary artery* and its main branches, which can be recognized by fluoroscopy or roentgenography. Precordial pain (p. 34), coming on either spontaneously or with effort, is frequently a troublesome symptom in patients with a dilated pulmonary artery and pulmonary hypertension. (3) *Cyanosis,* if the right-sided pressures rise enough to produce a right-to-left shunt through the existing defect.

The principal auscultatory signs of pulmonary hypertension are accentuation of the pulmonic component of the second sound, often with splitting, and a systolic murmur in the pulmonic area attributable to turbulence as blood is ejected into the dilated pulmonary artery. Such murmurs may be as loud as grade 4, but are not usually accompanied by a thrill. When the pulmonary artery is greatly dilated, there is sometimes an extra sound early in systole ("systolic click").

Primary pulmonary hypertension is characterized by increased pulmonary vascular resistance in the absence of cardiovascular shunts or other abnormalities that are known to produce pulmonary hypertension. A similar disease in adults (p. 1538), seen most often in women between twenty and thirty-five years, appears not to be congenital in origin, but is usually fatal within a few years after the onset of symptoms. The condition is rare, and many suspected adult cases prove to be due to multiple small pulmonary emboli or to intracardiac shunts which had not been detected clinically.

SPECIAL DIAGNOSTIC METHODS

Roentgenography. The importance of roentgenographic examination in congenital heart disease can hardly be overstated. Fluoroscopic examination should be carried out in every patient suspected of having a cardiac malformation, and full-size chest films in the posteroanterior and oblique positions, with barium in the esophagus, should be recorded. The size and position of the great vessels and heart chambers, the vascularity of the lung fields, and the pulsations observed during fluoroscopy are often the deciding clues in differential diagnosis. Characteristic configurations in some congenital anomalies of the heart are shown in Fig. 252-1.

Angiocardiography. The introduction of radiopaque solutions into the blood stream to demonstrate the course of the blood and to outline the chambers of the heart is often of great help in diagnosis. Angiocardiography is most helpful with complex malformations in which data from catheterization are inadequate or equivocal, particularly when there is some uncertainty as to how blood reaches the lungs or which ventricle communicates with the systemic circulation.

The solution may be introduced through a peripheral vein, but injection directly into the heart through a catheter (selective angiocardiography) allows the use of smaller volumes and gives a more satisfactory visualization of intracardiac structures. Motion pictures of the fluoroscopic image (cine-

angiocardiography) give an essentially continuous record of the passage of the contrast medium and may show details not readily appreciated in single films.

The mortality associated with these procedures is in the neighborhood of 0.3 per cent. As with cardiac catheterization, the hazard is greatest in the presence of pulmonary hypertension or cyanosis.

Electrocardiography. In congenital heart disease the principal contribution of electrocardiography is the determination of specific ventricular hypertrophy, and it is often more sensitive for this purpose than roentgenography. Right ventricular hypertrophy and enlargement are common with many types of congenital malformation. In the most extreme examples of right ventricular hypertrophy the QRS axis may come to point over the right shoulder, giving prominent S waves in standard lead III which may erroneously be interpreted as left axis deviation. The amplitude of the QRS complexes is as important as the QRS axis in evaluating ventricular hypertrophy. QRS changes are always more specific than T-wave abnormalities in indicating which ventricle is involved.

Prolongation of the QRS duration beyond 0.12 sec is *uncommon* in congenital heart disease. An rsR′ complex in precordial lead V, and adjacent leads occur frequently with right ventricular hypertrophy, but the duration usually ranges from 0.06 to 0.11 sec. This pattern has been termed "incomplete right bundle branch block" when the QRS duration is 0.10 to 0.12 sec, but the clinical significance in this situation is the same as with shorter QRS durations. The Wolff-Parkinson-White conduction anomaly is not common in congenital heart disease, except in Ebstein's anomaly.

Prolonged P-R intervals are particularly frequent with atrial septal defect and are found occasionally in other malformations. Complete atrioventricular block is rare. Although it is said to be common in ventricular septal defects, its incidence in this anomaly has probably been overestimated. Congenital complete heart block is a rare functional abnormality which may occur in the absence of other defects and is usually of no functional consequence.

Supraventricular arrhythmias, including atrial fibrillation and flutter, atrial and nodal tachycardia, and wandering of the pacemaker, occur with many malformations, particularly with atrial septal defect and with Ebstein's anomaly. Ventricular arrhythmias are no more frequent than in acquired heart disease.

Cardiac Catheterization. Information obtained by catheterization of the right side of the heart has been essential to the development of knowledge in the field of congenital heart disease. In many cases it gives an accurate indication of the lesions present

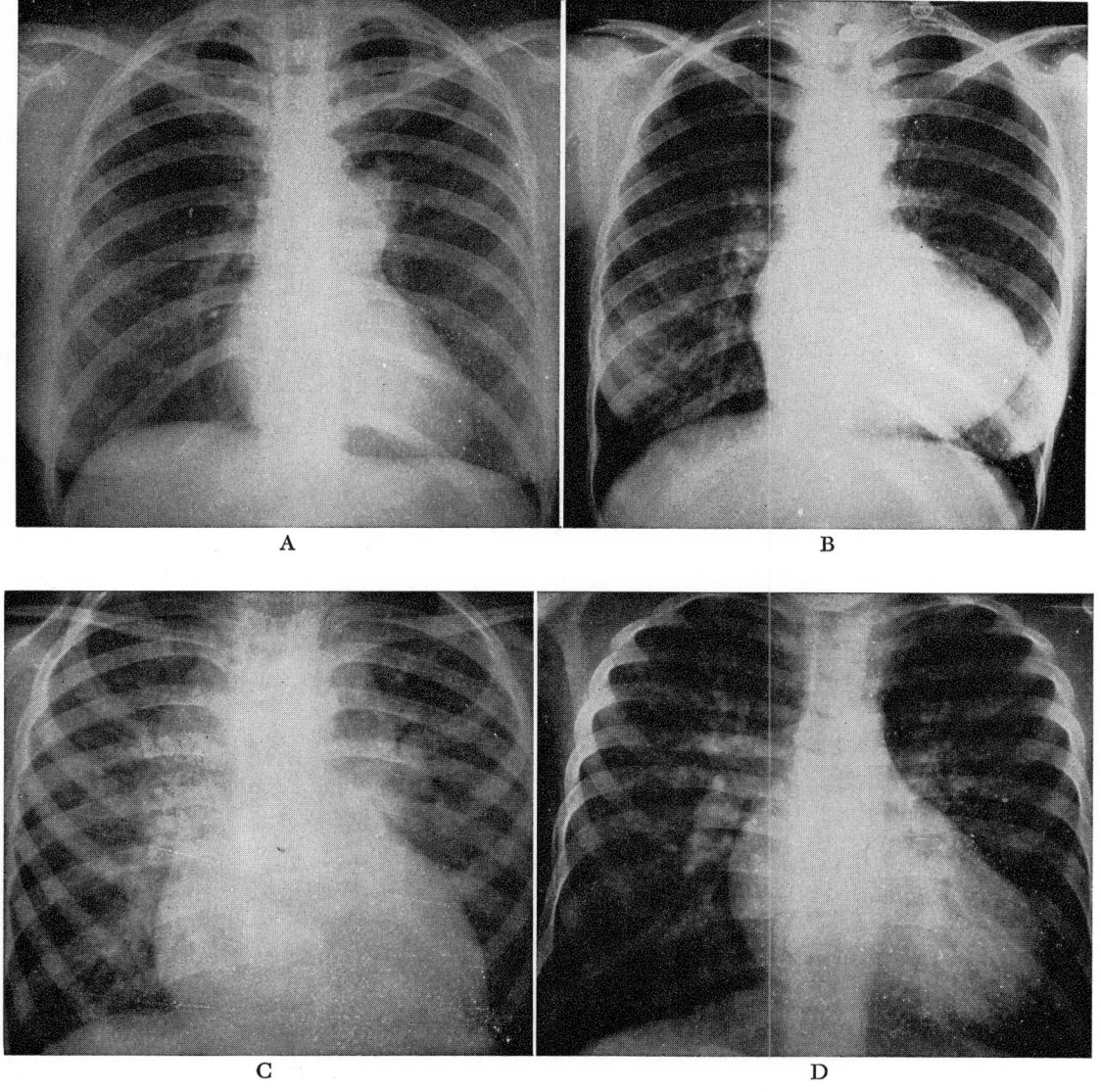

FIG. 252-1. *A.* Pure pulmonic stenosis, with prominent poststenotic dilatation of the pulmonary artery, in a 42-year-old woman. Pulmonary vascular markings in the peripheral lung fields are less prominent than normal.

B. Tetralogy of Fallot in a girl 17 years of age. Greatly increased transverse diameter, with apex of the heart "tipped up," and relatively avascular lung fields. (The three small radiopaque shadows at the upper margin of the film are artefacts.) In many cases the heart size is normal.

C. Anomalous drainage of all pulmonary veins into the left brachiocephalic (innominate) vein, with typical "figure-8" contour, in a 4-year-old boy.

D. Complete transposition of the great vessels in a 12-year-old boy. Note absence of normal pulmonary conus, with narrowing of upper mediastinal shadow in this view, prominent pulmonary vascular markings, and ventricular enlargement.

and a quantitative estimate of their functional significance.

In general, three questions can be answered by cardiac catheterization:

1. Are the pressures and pressure gradients in the heart and vessels normal? The most important deviations from normal pressure relationships to be recognized are elevation of right ventricular or pulmonary artery pressure, or an exaggerated pressure drop across a valve, indicating stenosis.

2. Is highly oxygenated blood admixed with systemic venous blood at any point? The finding of

blood which is more highly oxygenated than samples taken further upstream (a "step-up" in oxygen saturation) may indicate a left-to-right shunt through a defect, but interpretation of such measurements is sometimes difficult. As a result of incomplete mixing of the incoming streams from the superior and inferior venae cavae and from the coronary sinus, which normally has a very low oxygen content, there is a normal variation between samples from the same chamber. In the right atrium samples may differ normally by as much as 20 ml per liter (or 2 vol per cent), in the right ventricle by less than 10 ml per liter, in the pulmonary artery by less than 5 ml per liter. Differences of larger magnitude usually indicate a left-to-right shunt, and their significance is increased if confirmed by multiple samples. It follows that small left-to-right shunts amounting to less than 15 per cent of systemic blood flow will not ordinarily be detected by their effect on blood oxygen content. Right heart catheterization will not identify the site of a right-to-left shunt unless the catheter passes through a defect or indicator-dilution curves are employed.

3. Does the catheter follow an abnormal course or pass through an abnormal opening? Under the fluoroscope the catheter may sometimes pass through a congenital defect and thus provide prima facie evidence of an anomalous communication. Such observations must, however, be interpreted cautiously, for the fluoroscopic image of the catheter in a single plane does not always identify its anatomic location unequivocally. Moreover, it is not always possible to put the catheter where one wants it. In occasional patients, for example, repeated attempts to advance the catheter into the pulmonary artery will fail, even in the absence of pulmonary stenosis or other abnormality. Failure to pass the catheter through a suspected defect is therefore of limited significance.

Catheterization studies are usually done with the patient at rest, under conditions approaching as nearly as possible a steady basal state. Alterations in this steady state during the procedure, which may change the relative oxygen saturation of consecutive blood samples, are to be avoided.

In many cases, a reliable diagnosis can be reached on the basis of history, physical examination, and roentgenographic and electrocardiographic studies, and cardiac catheterization is not needed. Unnecessary catheterization is obviously to be avoided, although the risk is small. In large diagnostic laboratories the average mortality in cardiac catheterization is approximately 0.05 per cent. The risk in acyanotic patients with moderate symptoms is distinctly less than this figure, and most of the fatalities occur in severely ill patients with pulmonary hypertension and cyanosis. The procedure is particularly hazardous in patients with primary pulmonary hypertension.

Cardiac catheterization is indicated when data so obtained are essential to the management of the patient, as, for example, in deciding on surgical treatment. One hesitates to use cardiac catheterization when the diagnosis is already reasonably clear from routine examination and surgery seems not indicated, but if the diagnosis is uncertain, it is better to secure the additional information provided by cardiac catheterization than to deprive a patient of possible surgical benefit. With more malformations being added constantly to the list of those amenable to surgery, it becomes increasingly important to identify the lesions in each case of congenital heart disease, by catheterization or other appropriate methods. Table 252-1 lists typical data obtained by cardiac catheterization in some of the more common congenital anomalies.

Catheterization of the chambers of the left heart can be carried out by a number of different routes. It is most widely used to evaluate acquired abnormalities of the mitral or aortic valve, but in congenital disease combined right and left heart catheterization can be used to localize left-to-right shunts and to obtain the measurements needed to estimate pulmonary vascular resistance.

Pressure measurements by direct puncture during open thoracotomy are now routine in many surgical departments and can give valuable data concerning the lesion and the immediate results of surgery. It should be emphasized, however, that measurements obtained in the presence of the relatively low cardiac output, systemic pressure, and pulmonary artery pressure of the anesthetized patient with an open chest may be radically different from those under more normal conditions.

Indicator-dilution Curves. Rapid injection of a small amount of dye or other indicator into one of the chambers of the heart is followed by a characteristic arterial time-concentration curve in the normal circulation (Fig. 252-2). A shunt that permits the indicator to reach the artery prematurely superimposes an early curve on the normal one, while a shunt that delays some portion of the indicator gives a typically low, prolonged curve. Successive injections in the venae cavae and right heart chambers can identify the site of a right-to-left shunt, since injections distal to the shunt will produce normal arterial curves, while injections proximal to the shunt demonstrate the premature arrival of indicator that travels through the shunt. Very small shunts can be detected by this method under optimal conditions, and a rough estimate of the shunt flow can be made from the resulting curves.

Numerous diagnostic tests employing this principle have been devised. By varying the site of

Table 252-1. TYPICAL HEMODYNAMIC MEASUREMENTS IN SOME CONGENITAL CARDIOVASCULAR MALFORMATIONS

Measurements	Normal	Atrial septal defect	Ventricular septal defect	Patent ductus arteriosus	Ventricular septal defect with pulmonary hypertension	Tetralogy of Fallot	Pulmonic stenosis (valvular)
Pressures, mm Hg:							
RV...............	20/0	30/0	32/0	30/0	120/6	105/5	92/2
PA...............	20/9 (13)	30/10 (17)	32/15 (20)	30/10 (17)	120/65 (88)	15/8 (10)	17/8 (11)
FA...............	120/70 (85)	120/70 (85)	120/70 (85)	130/45 (70)	120/70 (85)	120/70 (85)	120/70 (80)
Oxygen content, ml/L:							
VC...............	152 (76%)	149 (74%)	149 (74%)	152 (76%)	148 (70%)	127 (59%)	136 (68%)
RA...............	152 (76%)	181 (90%)	149 (74%)	152 (76%)	148 (70%)	127 (59%)	136 (68%)
RV...............	152 (76%)	181 (90%)	171 (85%)	152 (76%)	173 (82%)	143 (66%)	136 (68%)
PA...............	152 (76%)	181 (90%)	171 (85%)	171 (85%)	173 (82%)	143 (66%)	136 (68%)
FA...............	190 (95%)	186 (93%)	186 (93%)	190 (95%)	185 (88%)	172 (80%)	190 (95%)
Oxygen capacity, ml/L:	200	200	200	200	210	215	200
Blood flow, L/min/m²:							
Systemic...........	3.6	3.6	3.6	3.6	3.6	3.0	2.5
Pulmonic..........	3.6	14.4	7.2	7.2	5.0	2.2	2.5
Shunt L to R.......	0	11.1	3.9	3.6	2.4	0.4	0
Shunt R to L.......	0	0.3	0.3	0	1.0	1.2	0
Pulmonary vascular resistance, R.U./m²...	1.9	0.8	1.5	1.5	16.4	1.9	2.0

The values given represent typical patients, but individual cases differ widely. Mean pressure in the left atrium is assumed to be 6.0 mm Hg, and pulmonary venous oxygen saturation 95 per cent. Mean pressures and oxygen saturation are listed in parentheses.

Symbols:

VC = average of superior and inferior vena cava samples; RA = right atrium; RV = right ventricle; PA = pulmonary artery; FA = femoral artery; R.U. = resistance units, in mm Hg/liter/min; multiply by 80 to convert to dyne/sec/cm⁵].

injection, and sampling from catheters in the heart as well as the peripheral artery, the site, direction, and approximate magnitude of most shunts can be accurately determined. Radioactive materials, inhaled gases, and substances that alter the electrical resistance or redox potential of the blood can be used as indicators, as well as nontoxic dyes. One or more of the available techniques should be available in any catheterization laboratory concerned with the diagnosis of congenital heart disease.

Phonocardiography. The graphic recording of heart sounds and murmurs has clarified the interpretation of a number of auscultatory phenomena and made possible a more intelligent use of the stethoscope. In practice, however, it is rarely necessary to record the phonocardiogram except when the precise timing of an extra sound or the duration of a murmur is in question.

COMPLICATIONS

In many types of congenital heart disease there appears to be a lowering of resistance to infections in general and to respiratory infections in particular. A history of repeated attacks of bronchitis or pneumonia is common, particularly in children and particularly with atrial septal defect. In at least some cases malnutrition and underdevelopment may be ascribed to these recurrent illnesses. Neither hypogammaglobulinemia nor deficient antibody for-

mation seems to be concerned in this lowered resistance.

Bacterial endocarditis, acute or subacute, is a common complication of congenital heart disease. About 10 per cent of all cases of subacute bacterial endocarditis occur in congenital heart disease. Patent ductus arteriosus, ventricular septal defect, coarctation of the aorta, and bicuspid aortic valve are

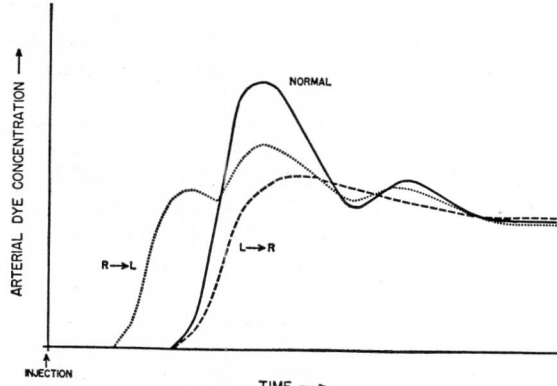

FIG. 252-2. Schematic representation of arterial indicator-dilution curve after injection of dye into right atrium: normal circulation (———); left-to-right shunt (— — —); right-to-left shunt (.......). Injections at other sites would be needed to determine whether the shunt were between the right and left atrium, the right and left ventricle, or the pulmonary artery and aorta.

the lesions most likely to become infected, while patients with atrial septal defect rarely develop this complication. It may appear at any age but is commonest in young adults. The symptoms, signs, and treatment of subacute bacterial endocarditis are the same with congenital heart disease as with other cardiac abnormalities. Subacute bacterial endocarditis in patent ductus arteriosus is in itself an indication for surgical closure, and this procedure alone will usually terminate the infection.

Because of the susceptibility of many congenital cardiovascular malformations to bacterial endocarditis, prophylactic antibiotic treatment should be carried out during procedures which may produce transient bacteremia, such as dental extractions. Continuous prophylaxis similar to that employed in rheumatic heart disease is not indicated, however.

Thromboses are common, particularly in the cerebral circulation. The high incidence in polycythemic patients, and after dehydration, suggests a relationship with blood viscosity. Fluid intake should be carefully watched in such patients, particularly in warm weather. Cerebral thromboses may present with convulsions or sudden hemiplegia, or they may be immediately fatal. Treatment of the polycythemic patient is based on use of anticoagulant drugs, venesection, and hemodilution with intravenous isotonic fluids.

Brain abscess is a serious complication of congenital heart disease which may appear any time after the first year or two of life. It is more frequent in patients with right-to-left shunts, since bacterial emboli bypass the lung filter and enter the brain. Successful treatment depends largely on early diagnosis, and the possibility of brain abscess should be considered promptly in any patient with congenital heart disease who develops unexplained fever, headaches, or other appropriate signs or symptoms.

THERAPY

Medical. Medical treatment of congenital heart disease consists mainly in the treatment of heart failure, maintenance of myocardial compensation, and prevention and treatment of complications.

Many cases of congenital heart disease are instances of "high-output failure" (see Chap. 13), in the sense that at least one ventricle is required to pump more than its normal output per minute. Digitalis is nevertheless just as effective in these cases as in the "low-output failure" of most forms of acquired heart disease.

The congestive heart failure which occurs with congenital malformations of the heart does not differ essentially from that seen in other diseases of the heart, and the principles of treatment are similar. Right ventricular failure is more common than left in congenital heart disease, and is usually a more chronic problem.

Digitalis is the keystone of therapy for establishing and maintaining cardiac compensation. The choice of a digitalis preparation is dictated by the speed of action required and the personal prejudices of the individual physician. There is no convincing evidence to show that the numerous digitalis preparations available differ in their clinical effects except in rapidity and duration of action.

In the polycythemic patient venesection serves a double purpose by decreasing blood viscosity as well as temporarily reducing total blood volume, but it must nevertheless be used cautiously.

Surgical. The list of congenital abnormalities which can be corrected or relieved by surgery is constantly growing, but the more common abnormalities which can at present be successfully treated include: patent ductus arteriosus, pulmonary valvular or infundibular stenosis (either isolated or in the tetralogy of Fallot), coarctation of the aorta, atrial septal defect, anomalous pulmonary venous drainage, aortic stenosis, ventricular septal defect, transposition of the great vessels, and congenital stenosis of the mitral and tricuspid valves. These anomalies are enumerated in approximately the order of increasing operative risk, which varies widely with the different lesions. Closure of patent ductus arteriosus, for example, has been carried out in hundreds of patients since 1939, and the present operative mortality is about 2 per cent, while open-heart surgery on transposition of the great vessels has been successful for only a short time, and complete evaluation of the risk and the results is not yet possible.

The responsibility of deciding whether surgery is to be advised in the individual case should be shared by the internist and the surgeon. The only rational basis for such a decision is accurate knowledge of the prognosis without operation in the case in question, as compared with the risk and chance of benefit from surgery. Under many conditions the factors which enter into this comparison are not completely known.

In general, patients with physical signs of congenital heart disease but without symptoms clearly related to their heart disease or signs of cardiac embarrassment should not undergo corrective surgery as prophylaxis against future difficulty. There are at least three exceptions to this generalization: patent ductus arteriosus, coarctation of the aorta, and atrial septal defect. The chances of subacute bacterial endocarditis, increasing difficulty with advancing age, or other possibly fatal complications are great enough with these three lesions and the risk of operation low enough that surgical correction should be considered in all affected patients under the age of thirty years, even in the absence of symptoms.

Patients with congenital malformations of the heart and symptoms which unmistakably limit their activity or in whom there are signs of cardiac embarrassment or symptoms of increasing severity should be carefully studied as possible candidates for surgery. The risk of correction with open-heart surgery has steadily diminished since Gibbon began the use of the pump oxygenator in 1953, and correction is possible with an operative mortality of no more than several per cent.

In estimating the severity of the burden imposed on the heart, the patient's response to such ordinary activities as walking and climbing stairs is a good guide. Dyspnea is a subjective phenomenon, however, and the patient's own estimate of his limitations may be misleading in either direction. An objective test of myocardial competence in relation to ordinary activity is badly needed. Measurement of cardiac output, shunts, and intracardiac pressure, particularly under resting conditions, does not sufficiently answer this need.

In cases with severe and prolonged pulmonary hypertension, the decision to operate is particularly difficult. In many patients, but not all, pulmonary hypertension appears to be reversible when a right-to-left shunt is corrected early in life. There is less likelihood of complete reversibility if the increased pulmonary flow has persisted for a long period or if the pulmonary vascular resistance is greatly increased. In the advanced states the shunt may reverse, producing cyanosis and a larger systemic than pulmonary flow. Unless there is reversal of the shunt, correction of the defect should be theoretically beneficial, but patients with advanced pulmonary vascular changes may not withstand the stress of operation. In brief, unless there is evidence of a significant left-to-right shunt, there is little likelihood of benefit from the operative procedure unless the patient is a young child.

SPECIFIC MALFORMATIONS

Congenital heart disease includes such a variety of anatomic lesions and so many possible combinations of lesions that some system of classification is essential. Either structural or functional abnormalities can be used as a basis for such classification, but it is difficult to reconcile the two in a single system. Most cases of ventricular septal defect with pulmonic stenosis are cyanotic, for example, and most cases of atrial septal defect are not, but exceptions are too frequent to be ignored. The classification introduced by Maude Abbott, a pioneer in this field, depends primarily on the presence or

absence of cyanosis; yet this sign is found with many lesions that have little else in common.

The compromise adopted in the section that follows is to group congenital anomalies under three major headings according to their effect on blood flow:

1. Malformations that permit shunting of blood
   a. Initial shunt left to right
   b. Initial shunt right to left
2. Malformations that obstruct blood flow
3. Malformations with no direct effect on blood flow

Malformations with Potential Shunts

Initial Left-to-Right Shunt

Atrial Septal Defect. This is the most common congenital lesion of the heart. The defects may be single or multiple and vary in size from an open foramen ovale to complete absence of the interatrial septum (cor triloculare biventriculare). Patency of the foramen ovale with an unsealed valve, which persists in 5 to 20 per cent of the adult population, does not usually permit shunting of blood, since the valve flap over the foramen prevents left-to-right flow and is held closed as long as atrial pressures remain normal.

Atrial septal defects may be divided into two general types: *persistent ostium secundum* (cephalad or midseptal in location) and *persistent ostium primum* (caudad, with one margin of the opening made up by the tissue between the atrioventricular valves). This distinction has a practical value for the surgeon, since the persistent ostium primum is technically much more difficult to repair. It also serves a clinical purpose in that the ostium primum type of defect, also called atrioventricular canal or endocardial cushion defect, is often accompanied by persistence of the atrioventricular cleft in the mitral and tricuspid leaflets, which may cause clinically recognizable insufficiency of one valve or of both.

Ostium Secundum Defects. The shunt through an atrial septal defect is predominantly from left to right, presumably because left atrial pressure is normally slightly higher than right atrial pressure and because the right ventricle presents less resistance to diastolic filling than the left. Pulmonary blood flow is usually two or three times the systemic blood flow. At the same time, streamlining of flow often produces a small right-to-left shunt, which lowers systemic arterial oxygen saturation slightly. Marked arterial unsaturation does not appear unless complications such as pulmonic stenosis or increased pulmonary vascular resistance are present.

The clinical effects of an atrial septal defect depend primarily on the size of the defect and the volume of the shunt through it. A small proportion of cases remain asymptomatic throughout adult life. In patients who develop symptoms, the earliest complaints are exertional dyspnea and fatigue. Paroxysmal atrial tachycardia with varying degrees of block is a frequent manifestation. Growth and development are essentially normal unless there is an unusually large shunt, and the "gracile habitus" shown by some children is relatively rare. Cyanosis and evidence of pulmonary hypertension are not encountered until late in the disease, if at all.

A systolic murmur in the second left intercostal space is the most prominent and constant physical finding. It begins early in systole, reaches a maximal intensity in midsystole, and diminishes rapidly to terminate before the pulmonic second sound, characteristics which suggest that it arises from ejection of a large stroke volume into the dilated pulmonary artery (p. 1411).

The aortic and pulmonic components of the second sound are clearly separated so that the second sound in the pulmonic area is split, and this splitting varies little if at all with respiration. In normal persons the second sound splits appreciably only on inspiration (p. 1408).

Fluoroscopy shows a greatly enlarged pulmonary conus and pulmonary arteries, increased pulmonary vascularity, a "hilar dance," and enlargement of the right atrium and right ventricle. The electrocardiogram shows signs of right ventricular hypertrophy in almost all symptomatic cases. It has frequently been stated that the electrocardiogram in this malformation usually shows right bundle branch block, but it is more accurate to say that an rsR' pattern is often found in VI and other right precordial leads, usually with a QRS duration less than 0.12 sec. This rsR' pattern in itself is probably an indication of right ventricular hypertrophy. Paroxysmal atrial tachycardia, atrial fibrillation, and prolongation of the P-R interval are all common.

Ostium Primum Defects. When this lesion is present symptoms almost always appear in childhood, and an apical systolic murmur, plus radiologic and electrocardiographic signs of *left* ventricular hypertrophy as well as right suggest the diagnosis. Signs of free mitral or tricuspid insufficiency also favor the diagnosis of persistent ostium primum.

Cardiac catheterization will usually establish the diagnosis, subject to the general limitations of this procedure discussed above. The differential diagnosis between atrial septal defect and anomalous pulmonary veins draining into the right atrium is often impossible.

The majority of atrial septal defects are not complicated by other congenital lesions, except for the tricuspid and mitral valve deformities mentioned. The combination of atrial septal defect and mitral stenosis (Lutembacher's syndrome) appears to be much less common than previously supposed. Modern diagnostic methods and surgical exploration have shown that an apical diastolic murmur is often present in cases of atrial septal defect when the mitral valve is entirely normal, and the diagnosis of Lutembacher's syndrome should therefore be made with considerable caution.

Ventricular Septal Defect. This is the second most frequent congenital anomaly of the heart. More than 90 per cent are defects of the membranous portion of the septum, the remainder being in the muscular portion and usually unaccompanied by other cardiac malformations. They vary in size from very small ventricular defects, which produce a loud systolic murmur but no symptoms throughout adult life (*maladie de Roger*), to complete absence of the interventricular septum (*single ventricle, cor triloculare biatriatum*).

The direction and magnitude of the shunt depend on the size of the defect and on the relative resistances to pulmonic systemic flow. In the majority of cases the shunt is predominantly from left to right, but the development of increasing pulmonary vascular resistance can reverse the direction. Patients with extremely large defects or complete absence of the interventricular septum (single ventricle) usually have increased pulmonary vascular resistance from birth.

A harsh systolic murmur, of greatest intensity in the third and fourth interspaces just left of the sternal edge, is the classic sign of ventricular septal defect; in the majority of cases it is accompanied by a thrill. It usually extends throughout systole (p. 1411) and is maximal in mid- or late systole. If the pressure gradient between the two ventricles decreases as pulmonary hypertension develops, the systolic murmur decreases in intensity as the pulmonic second sound increases. An apical diastolic murmur is present in most cases with large shunts, because of either relative mitral stenosis or pulmonary insufficiency (p. 1412, Chap. 251).

As long as the left-to-right shunt predominates, the roentgenogram shows increased pulmonary vascularity, and the electrocardiogram reflects combined ventricular hypertrophy. If the pulmonary vascular resistance increases markedly, the peripheral lung fields become relatively avascular, in contrast to the dilated main branches of the pulmonary artery, and signs of right ventricular hypertrophy predominate in the electrocardiogram.

Stenosis of the pulmonary valve or infundibulum may give a murmur similar to that of ventricular septal defect, but it is usually loudest in the second or third interspace, particularly with valvular stenosis. The decreased pulmonary vascularity seen by x-ray is the most important point in distinguishing these lesions from pure ventricular septal defect. If phonocardiograms show that the murmur is undoubtedly pansystolic and definitely starts before ejection, then this evidence speaks strongly for interventricular defect as compared to pulmonary stenosis.

The systolic murmur of atrial septal defect is occasionally quite loud and may even produce a thrill, but it too is typically higher on the chest wall than in ventricular septal defect. Moreover, with atrial septal defect left ventricular hypertrophy does not occur unless mitral incompetence is also present. In ventricular septal defect with marked pulmonary hypertension, right ventricle enlargement predominates, and differentiation from atrial septal defect by clinical means may be impossible.

Ventricular Septal Defect in Combination with Other Lesions. Approximately 9 out of every 10 patients with an interventricular septal defect have other cardiac malformations as well, the most common being pulmonary stenosis. Aortic incompetence due to an anomalous aortic cusp is an occasional complicating lesion of considerable importance, because the murmurs and wide pulse pressure may lead to an erroneous diagnosis of patent ductus arteriosus.

Eisenmenger's complex is the name sometimes applied to a condition characterized by ventricular septal defect in which cyanosis develops in adolescence or later adult life. The aortic root is normally positioned in most cases, and the clinical course is the result of gradually increasing pulmonary vascular resistance, with increasing pulmonary hypertension and eventual reversal of the shunt.

Patent Ductus Arteriosus. The ductus arteriosus, which is an essential communication between the pulmonary artery and aorta during fetal development, normally closes before the age of two years.

Persistent patency of the ductus arteriosus beyond this age is a common abnormality, representing approximately 10 per cent of all congenital malformations seen clinically. The lumen varies from 5 to 10 mm in most patients. With the normally existing pressure gradients, there is a left-to-right shunt from the aorta to the pulmonary artery, but this varies greatly in magnitude in different patients and is often well tolerated. The majority of patients with this anomaly are asymptomatic and are unaware of its existence until it is discovered on routine physical examination.

The open ductus provides a low-resistance pathway from the aorta during diastole as well as systole, and a lowering of the arterial diastolic pressure results. The arterial pulse pressure is thereby widened, just as in aortic regurgitation.

The left ventricle bears the burden of the shunt, showing hypertrophy and enlargement in cases where the shunt is large enough to cause symptoms. As in other left-to-right shunts, continued high pulmonary blood flow is sometimes followed by the development of pulmonary hypertension. This tends to decrease the left-to-right shunt, and if the pulmonary artery pressure reaches systemic levels, the flow through the ductus will be reversed, with cyanosis of the toes and the area of the body nourished by branches of the aorta distal to the ductus. In such cases, cyanosis may appear at first only with exertion, but if the patient survives, the right-to-left shunt becomes permanent, even at rest.

When the ductus enters the aorta distal to the great vessels of the aortic arch, as is customary, a venous-arterial shunt through it gives rise to the almost pathognomonic finding of cyanosis of the lower extremities with normally pink upper extremities. Once this stage has been reached the prognosis is poor, and survival for more than a few years is exceptional.

The classic machinery murmur of patency of the ductus extends through systole and diastole, as does the flow of blood through the ductus. The murmur reaches its maximal intensity about the end of systole and "overrides" the second sound, which may be completely obliterated. It may begin with the first sound or in early systole, and may extend throughout diastole, or die away in late diastole. The second left interspace at the sternal border is most often the area of maximal intensity. The systolic element may be heard over most of the precordium and above the clavicles, while the diastolic is sometimes less widely transmitted. As in other left-to-right shunts, a separate apical diastolic murmur from relative mitral stenosis is sometimes heard.

Pulmonary hypertension modifies the typical murmur just as it modifies the size and direction of the shunt. With roughly equal pressures in aorta and pulmonary artery and little or no shunt, the murmur may disappear entirely, while under other circumstances either the diastolic or the systolic component may be absent. Other causes of continuous murmurs are considered on p. 1413, Chap. 251.

Fluoroscopy may show a prominent pulmonary conus, slight right and left ventricular enlargement, slight increase in pulmonary vascularity, or no abnormality at all. The electrocardiogram may show moderate left, or combined ventricular, hypertrophy but is more often within normal limits.

Patent ductus arteriosus can occur in combination with many other malformations. In some instances, such as complete pulmonary atresia, a patent ductus performs an essential function by carrying blood to the lungs.

Differential diagnosis is relatively easy in the average patient with a typical murmur and no cyanosis. Although many other lesions produce both systolic and diastolic murmurs, the two murmurs are usually separate and do not continue through the second sound. Defects of the septum between the ascending aorta and pulmonary artery are an exception to this rule, which is not surprising since this anomaly is physiologically identical with patent ductus, except for the slightly more proximal site of the communication. Cardiac catheterization may be of help in differentiating between patent ductus arteriosus and such aortic septal defects, if the catheter passes through the defect. Retrograde aortography may establish the diagnosis.

Anomalous Pulmonary Venous Drainage. This is a relatively uncommon malformation. The most frequent sites of drainage are the superior vena cava, the right atrium, the left innominate vein, and the coronary sinus. The effects of this malformation are determined by the proportion of the blood from the lungs that is returned to the right heart. If all pulmonary veins drain into the right heart, an associated patent foramen ovale or atrial septal defect is essential for survival. Partial anomalous drainage, in which some pulmonary veins enter the right side of the heart while others enter the left atrium normally, may occur without other complicating lesions.

Partial anomalies are often well tolerated and may be entirely asymptomatic, while total anomalous drainage is a much more severe handicap; less than a fifth of patients with the latter condition survive beyond infancy.

In both situations there is a left-to-right shunt, and therefore increased pulmonary blood flow, but the size of the shunt varies greatly. In patients with total anomalous pulmonary venous drainage, there may be a history of cyanosis at birth and infancy and mild degrees of cyanosis at rest or on exertion, and even clubbing in later life.

Physical signs may be lacking in cases of partial anomalous pulmonary venous drainage, but in the total anomalies there is almost always a grade 2 to 4 systolic murmur, often with a thrill, in the second to fourth intercostal space at the left sternal border. This is probably related to an associated atrial septal defect and the accompanying dilatation of the pulmonary artery. A softer, continuous murmur is often heard in the aortic area, probably a true "venous hum" from increased flow through the anomalous veins.

Roentgenograms may be characteristic in three specific patterns of anomalous pulmonary venous drainage: (1) a common right pulmonary vein draining into the inferior vena cava, which adds a smooth semicircular shadow to the right heart border; (2) total pulmonary venous drainage into a persistent left superior vena cava, giving a "figure-8" or "snowman" contour to the whole cardiovascular silhouette (Fig. 252-1C); (3) total pulmonary venous drainage into the coronary sinus, in which

the greatly dilated coronary sinus and anomalous veins displace the esophagus posteriorly, simulating left atrial enlargement. The electrocardiographic findings are normal in most asymptomatic patients and show signs of right ventricular hypertrophy as symptoms become predominant.

Hemodynamically, the systemic flow is normal or slightly lowered, while the left-to-right shunt gives an increased pulmonary flow varying from one and one-half to five or more times the systemic flow. Peripheral arterial oxygen saturation may be normal with partial anomalies, but with totally anomalous drainage the pulmonic and systemic venous blood are mixed in the right atrium, and pulmonary arterial and aortic blood are equally unsaturated. Pulmonary artery pressure is usually normal or slightly elevated.

Cardiac catheterization can demonstrate the left-to-right shunt and "step-up" in oxygen saturation in the right atrial blood but cannot distinguish between anomalous pulmonary venous drainage into the right atrium and atrial septal defect unless the catheter actually passes out one of the pulmonary veins from the vena cava or the right atrium. Even this finding is often equivocal, since it is difficult to be sure that the catheter has not passed into normally draining pulmonary veins by way of an atrial septal defect. The situation is further complicated by the frequent association of the two anomalies. Angiocardiography can be helpful in demonstrating anomalous pulmonary veins draining into the venae cavae or coronary sinus, but it does not rule out concomitant atrial septal defect. In many cases, therefore, differential diagnosis of these two malformations can be made only at thoracotomy.

When the anomalous veins drain only one lung, a specialized application of the dye-dilution method may establish the diagnosis. Injection of dye or other indicator into first one and then the other main branch of the pulmonary artery will give a normal dilution curve in the systemic arteries after injection into the normally drained lung and a curve typical of a left-to-right shunt after injection into the anomalously drained pulmonary bed.

As has been indicated, many patients with partial anomalous pulmonary venous drainage are without symptoms, and therapy is not needed. In others, however, and particularly in the total anomalies, signs of right heart failure develop because of a large shunt or pulmonary hypertension, or both. In these patients surgical intervention should be considered, although with total anomalies and with marked pulmonary hypertension, the risk of operation is high.

Initial Right-to-Left Shunt

These are the cases of "cyanotic heart disease" in which the malformed structure of the heart and great vessels diverts all or part of the right ventricular output into the aorta from birth, so that the fetal predominance of the right ventricle persists.

The partitioning of the embryonic truncus arteriosus into pulmonic and aortic channels is a key stage in the development of the heart, and anomalies in this process underlie a number of clinical malformations, including complete transposition of the great vessels, Fallot's tetralogy, and some defects of the membranous portion of the interventricular septum. An understanding of this episode in the development of the human fetus is essential to a logical appreciation of these lesions, and the excellent reviews of Harris and Farber and Patten are recommended.

Deviations in the location of the partitioning septum can produce great variations in the relative size of the aorta and pulmonary artery. Failure of the normal twisting of the truncus may leave the aorta in direct communication with the right ventricle only, and the pulmonary artery with the left ventricle, as in complete transposition. The almost unlimited permutations and combinations of such developmental errors can lead to the most complex malformations. The caudad end of the truncus septum is contiguous with the membranous portion of the interventricular septum and with the edge of the interatrial septum which closes the ostium primum. Any abnormality of development in this relatively small area in the fetus can give rise to such apparently diverse anomalies as transposed great vessels, defects of the interatrial and interventricular septum, and anomalies of the atrioventricular valves.

Transposition of the Great Vessels. In this malformation the failure of normal torsion of the primitive truncus leaves the aortic root opening into the right ventricle and the pulmonary artery into the left. This separation of the pulmonic and systemic circulation into two independent circuits is obviously incompatible with life unless some additional anomaly provides a communication between them. Complete transposition of aorta and pulmonary artery is, therefore, not seen clinically except in combination with other anomalies such as patent foramen ovale, atrial septal defect, ventricular septal defect, or patent ductus arteriosus. The bronchial arteries provide an additional shunt pathway in many cases. The larger the communication, the better the patient's chances for survival.

In patients with these conditions the paths of blood flow are not yet fully understood, but they involve mixed shunts which may reverse their direction from systole to diastole. There is usually marked lowering of peripheral arterial saturation, with cyanosis and polycythemia.

Signs and symptoms, including cyanosis, are present from birth, and rapid cardiac enlargement during the first year of life is the rule. The malformation is occasionally seen in older children, but the majority of the infants affected die during the first year, unless compensating anomalies coexist.

A precordial bulge is frequently present, owing to the early cardiac enlargement, and the precordial pulsation is indicative of dominant right ventricular enlargement. The second pulmonic sound is greatly accentuated and not split. Systolic murmurs and thrills are usually found but are related to the associated defects rather than to the transposition itself. Some patients with a patent foramen ovale or patent ductus arteriosus have only faint systolic murmurs or none at all.

The radiologic picture is often characteristic (see Fig. 252-1D).

When the ascending aorta lies directly ventral to the pulmonary trunk, their shadows are superimposed, giving an unusually narrow upper mediastinal shadow and an absence of the usual pulmonary conus. The pulmonary arteries and smaller vessels are large and pulsate vigorously. Both ventricles, and often both atria, are enlarged. Right axis deviation and marked right ventricular hypertrophy are found in the electrocardiogram.

The diagnosis can usually be made from the history and roentgenologic features. On cardiac catheterization the catheter may enter the aorta, and the characteristically anterior origin of the aorta may be identified in the lateral view.

Surgical creation of an atrial septal defect may help patients with this condition by allowing greater mixing of pulmonary and systemic blood. More complete correction has been possible in a few instances with open-heart surgery, the most successful operations being directed at producing transposition of the pulmonary veins and venae cavae to correct for the transposed great arteries. The operation is better done in infants before pulmonary vascular changes become excessive.

A variant of this anomaly is complete transposition of the aorta with only partial transposition of the pulmonary artery, so that the pulmonary artery overrides the right ventricle, and a high ventricular septal defect (Taussig-Bing complex). Although this malformation differs developmentally from the Eisenmenger complex, the clinical pictures are similar. The single distinguishing feature is the appearance of cyanosis at birth in the Taussig-Bing complex, as contrasted with its later appearance in the Eisenmenger complex.

Persistent Truncus Arteriosus. This is a rare anomaly in which blood flows from both ventricles into a single common trunk overriding a high ventricular ventral defect. Blood reaches the lungs through pulmonary arteries branching from this trunk. There may be a right or left aortic arch.

Cyanosis is present, but its degree depends on

the relative proportions of pulmonary blood flow and venous-arterial shunt. Pulmonary blood flow exceeds normal values if there is free communication from the truncus to the lungs and no pulmonary vascular changes occur. This increased pulmonary blood flow, mixing with the systemic venous return, often results in an almost normal oxygen content of arterial blood, in spite of a large right-to-left shunt. The pulmonary arteries may be large, in which case pulmonary blood flow is apt to be high and cyanosis minimal early in life. At the other extreme there may be no connection of pulmonary arteries with the truncus, so that the bronchial arteries may provide the only pathway for blood flow to the lungs. Pulmonary blood flow is low and cyanosis is intense. Anatomically, this condition more closely resembles the tetralogy of Fallot than the usual truncus arteriosus.

In infants the roentgenogram may be diagnostic, with a sharp right angle between the shelflike upper surface of the right ventricle and the aorta in the left anterior oblique view. With increasing age this disappears, and the great right ventricular enlargement and absent pulmonary conus give a picture similar to that in Fallot's tetralogy.

Tetralogy of Fallot. The structural anomalies in Fallot's "tetralogy" are actually two in number: ventricular septal defect and pulmonic stenosis. Although overriding of the aorta was originally considered an essential feature of this syndrome, defects of the membranous portion of the ventricular septum leave the aortic root in close proximity to the right ventricular outflow tract even when the aorta is in normal position, so that the anatomic and hemodynamic findings in most cases can be explained without assuming dextroposition of the aorta. The right ventricular hypertrophy that completes the tetralogy is a consequence of the functional abnormality induced by the structural lesions.

Fallot's tetralogy is the most common combination of lesions which leads to early cyanosis yet often allows survival into adult life. The stenotic obstruction is usually in the infundibulum or right ventricular outflow tract, but may be in the valve itself, or at both sites. Dilatation of the pulmonary artery beyond the stenosis is usually not striking. In some instances, there is atresia of the pulmonary artery, and blood reaches the lung through other channels, a condition sometimes confusingly referred to as "pseudotruncus arteriosus." A large right-to-left shunt is present, with cyanosis appearing either at birth or within the first two years. Clubbing and polycythemia follow at an early date. The pulmonic stenosis produces a characteristic murmur, described below, and decreased pulmonary vascularity. The electrocardiogram shows right ventricular hypertrophy. The size of the heart radiologically is usually normal, but the normal leftward

convexity of the pulmonary conus is missing. In some cases the apex of the heart is somewhat "tipped up" in the anteroposterior view (see Fig. 252-1B). A right aortic arch occurs in about 25 per cent of patients and can be seen to displace the barium-filled esophagus to the *left* in the anteroposterior view, and *posteriorly* in the left anterior oblique view.

In rare cases there may be only moderate pulmonic stenosis and a left-to-right shunt. Such cases of "atypical" or "acyanotic" tetralogy of Fallot have normal or increased pulmonary vascularity, and diagnosis is often difficult.

In the typical case the diagnosis can usually be made clinically. These patients are more cyanotic than the usual case of uncomplicated pulmonic stenosis and do not have the greatly enlarged heart of complete transposition of the great vessels or the enlarged, pulsating pulmonary artery of Eisenmenger's complex.

Although many patients with tetralogy of Fallot reach adult life, their exercise tolerance is invariably limited, and very few survive beyond the age of thirty years. The Blalock-Taussig operation provides an increased blood flow to the lungs through an artificial ductus, relieving the cyanosis and clubbing and greatly increasing ability to exercise.

Anomalous Origin of Coronary Arteries. This is a rare malformation in which one coronary artery, usually the left, arises from the pulmonary artery. A few cases with both coronary arteries arising from the pulmonary artery have been reported. The combination of low coronary perfusion pressure and low oxygen tension seriously impairs myocardial function. Severe congestive heart failure and cardiac enlargement appear in the first few months of life. Pulmonary and peripheral edema may both develop. The electrocardiogram shows S-T and T-wave abnormalities strikingly similar to those seen in adults with acute myocardial infarction (see Fig. 252-3). Murmurs are usually absent. Differentiation from other rare causes of early cardiac enlargement without cyanosis or murmurs, discussed later in this chapter, is based principally on the characteristic electrocardiographic changes. In several reported cases retrograde flow has been present in the vessel arising from the pulmonary artery, constituting in essence an arteriovenous fistula. In such cases ligation of the anomalous artery has given relief of the myocardial ischemia.

Malformations Which Obstruct Blood Flow

Pulmonary Stenosis. This may involve either the pulmonic valve or the pulmonary infundibulum. Since it is often associated with other anomalies, the terms *pure* and *isolated* pulmonic stenosis are often used to indicate the absence of complicating lesions. Cases of valvular stenosis with normal ventricular septum are relatively common and may constitute as much as 10 per cent of all patients with congenital heart disease. The degree of stenosis varies from slight narrowing to a domelike membrane with only a pinhole opening.

The principal effects of this lesion are reduction of the pulmonary blood flow and right ventricular hypertension and hypertrophy. When the right ventricle can no longer maintain the high pressure needed to propel blood through the lungs, congestive failure supervenes, with the increased peripheral venous pressure, hepatic distention, and peripheral edema characteristic of right ventricular failure.

Shunts are not usually present in the early course of the disease or in mild cases, but right-to-left shunts may develop through an unsealed foramen ovale or concomitant atrial septal defect if right atrial pressure eventually rises.

Patients with mild degrees of pulmonary stenosis may have no symptoms and have an excellent prognosis. In more severe cases, the age of onset of symptoms—primarily exertional dyspnea or syncope—varies widely, but in the average case is during adolescence. Exertional dyspnea usually precedes the appearance of cyanosis and for some time is more striking than the cyanosis. Once cyanosis has appeared symptoms gradually become more severe, but there are striking exceptions to this rule, and occasional patients continue to exhibit cyanosis on exertion for 20 years or more, with little change. Clubbing is present in proportion to the severity and duration of cyanosis.

The most important physical signs of pulmonic stenosis are a systolic murmur with maximal intensity (usually at least grade 4) in the pulmonic area and a diminished or absent second pulmonic sound. Phonocardiograms reveal a splitting of the second sound, but only the first (or aortic) component may be audible. With infundibular stenosis the site of greatest intensity is somewhat lower, in the third to fourth interspace at the left sternal border. The murmur terminates before the second pulmonic sound. Diastolic murmurs are not usually present, a point which is helpful in differentiating this lesion from ventricular septal defect. Signs of right ventricular failure, including enlargement and sometimes pulsation of the liver, develop in the most severe instances.

Radiographic study shows a prominence or actual enlargement of the pulmonary artery and its main branches, the so-called "poststenotic dilatation" (see Fig. 252-1), with valvular stenosis but usually not with infundibular stenosis. The pulmonary arteries do not pulsate actively as a rule, but with mild stenosis slight pulsation may occur. The vascularity of the lungs is diminished, giving a relatively clear appearance to the peripheral lung fields. In mild cases the ventricles are of normal size, while in severe cases the right ventricle may be enormously enlarged. The right atrium usually enlarges along with the right ventricle.

Electrocardiographic signs of right ventricular hypertrophy are roughly proportional to the degree of obstruction. Severe degrees of pulmonic stenosis produce the greatest increase in the amplitude of the R wave over the right precordium (up to 4.0 mv) encountered clinically. Right atrial enlargement is indicated by increased P-wave amplitude, most prominently in leads II and V_1.

The most important hemodynamic finding is an increase in right ventricular pressure and the demonstration of a large pressure gradient across the site of the stenosis. Right ventricular systolic pressure in symptomatic patients is usually between 60 and 180 mm Hg, but one patient with a pressure of 270 mm Hg has been reported. The pressure drop across the stenosis is often 100 mm Hg, or more. The systemic flow is usually slightly below normal, but not so much below as one would expect from the severity of symptoms. One critical handicap in patients with this condition is their limited ability to increase pulmonary flow on exercise, even with considerable increase in right ventricular pressure. In extreme instances, exertion may lead to syncope.

Cases showing early cyanosis must be differentiated from tetralogy of Fallot, and those with late onset of cyanosis from Eisenmenger's complex. A prominent pulmonary artery, enlarged heart and right atrium, and marked dyspnea with relatively little cyanosis help to rule out tetralogy of Fallot, while clear lung fields and absence of pulmonary artery pulsation are not usually found in Eisenmenger's complex. Cardiac catheterization can furnish direct evidence of the stenosis and the degree of right ventricular hypertension. Accurate diagnosis is of particular importance because the Blalock-Taussig operation does not benefit patients with isolated pulmonic stenosis, the increased left-to-right shunt apparently being the last straw for an already overburdened right ventricle, which rapidly fails. A specific attack on the pulmonic stenosis is the treatment of choice.

Other malformations may be found in combination with pulmonic stenosis, including anomalous pulmonary veins, atrial or ventricular septal defects, and patent ductus arteriosus.

The prognosis is good in uncomplicated cases without cyanosis, cardiac enlargement, or electrocardiographic signs of right ventricular hypertrophy. When any of these findings is present, with severe or increasing symptoms, surgical relief of the stenosis should be considered. In borderline cases, the right ventricular systolic pressure is a useful guide to prognosis, and systolic pressures greater than 100 mm Hg are usually an indication for operation.

Coarctation of the Aorta. This obstructive lesion results from an abnormal obliteration of the aorta during regression of the multiple aortic arch system of the embryo. The common classifications are based largely upon the age at death (infantile and adult) and on the site of coarctation in relation to the ductus arteriosus. The infantile or preductal type occurs in the aortic arch or just proximal to the ductus arteriosus, which is usually patent. Commonly, there are other intracardiac defects which account for death at an early age. In most instances,

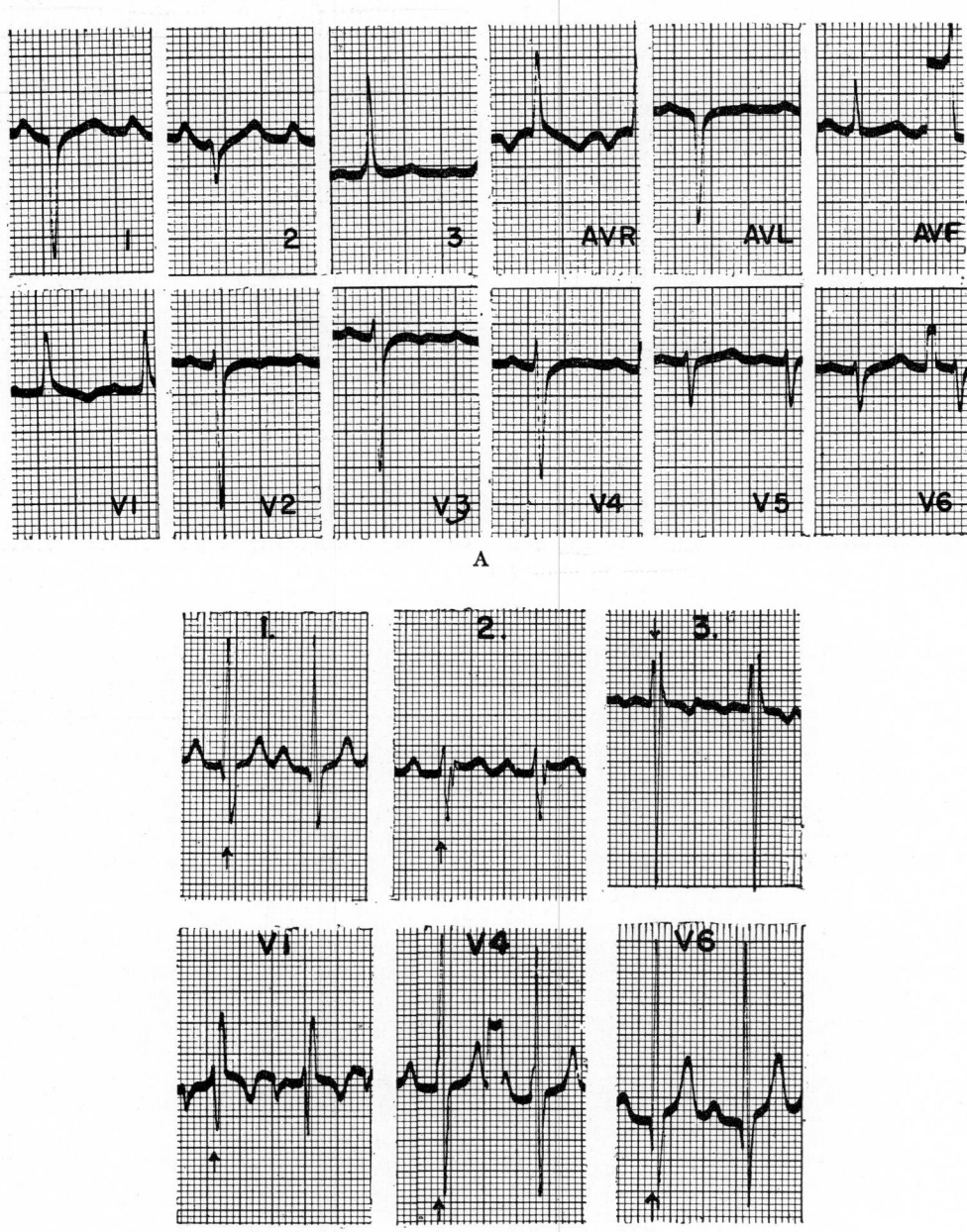

FIG. 252-3. *A.* Electrocardiogram from a 9-year-old girl with pure pulmonic stenosis. The right axis deviation in the limb leads, tall R wave in lead V₁, and reversal of the normal precordial transition indicate marked right ventricular hypertrophy. Note that precordial leads were recorded at half normal sensitivity.

B. Electrocardiogram from a 5-year-old boy with an atrial septal defect ("persistent ostium primum") and

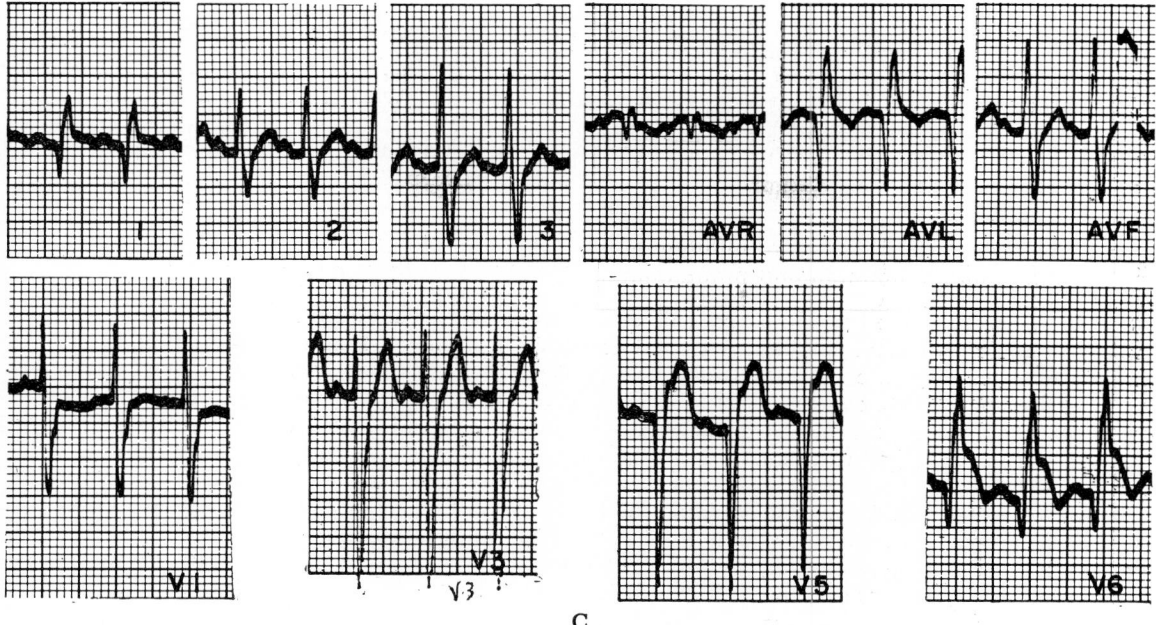

C

cleft mitral leaflet producing mitral regurgitation. Combined right and left ventricular hypertrophy is indicated by the left axis deviation, tall R'-V₁, and tall R-V₆. A double R wave is present in lead V₁, with QRS duration of 0.09 sec, and the P-R interval is prolonged. (Arrows indicate the peak of R-1 and synchronous points in other leads.)

C. Electrocardiogram from an infant boy aged 4 months with anomalous origin of the left coronary artery. The prominent Q waves and S-T elevation in leads I, V₅, and V₆ are characteristic of anterior myocardial infarction.

blood from the pulmonary artery supplies the lower half of the body (through the ductus) and the toes are cyanotic, often in contrast to the fingers.

Postductal or adult coarctation is usually located immediately distal to the left subclavian artery, and a narrowed or obliterated ductus enters the segment proximal to the coarctation. Bicuspid aortic valve is present in 25 to 40 per cent of cases, but otherwise the heart is normal. In rare instances, coarctation may be in the midthoracic aorta, at the diaphragm, or even in the abdomen.

The presenting signs are hypertension in the arms proximal to the obstruction, and hypotension or absent pulses in the legs distal to it; by these signs the diagnosis is made. In the preductal type the associated intracardiac defects are prominent and incapacitating, and the clinical picture is largely determined by these defects. Patients with a postductal coarctation characteristically are troubled either early in life or a number of years later. A few infants develop cardiac failure because of the load placed upon the left ventricle, but most patients with coarctation of the aorta weather early childhood without symptoms or diagnosis. Heart failure in an infant suggests some other lesion, notably endocardial fibroelastosis, for most infants with

coarctation develop collateral circulation, and hypertension is not striking until late childhood or adulthood. Complaints rarely arise from diminished flow to the legs.

In addition to the pathognomonic pulse and pressure gradients, there are striking pulsations in the neck and supraclavicular areas. Systolic murmurs may be heard posteriorly from the coarctation or anteriorly from an abnormal aortic valve, and diastolic murmurs may arise from collateral circulation. Enlarged collateral vessels may be felt in the interscapular and subscapular areas.

Notching of the ribs is the most characteristic radiologic observation, caused by dilatation and tortuosity of intercostal arteries carrying the collateral flow. A "three sign" may be produced in roentgenograms of the left upper mediastinum by the enlarged left subclavian artery, the constriction at the coarctation, and poststenotic dilatation distal to it.

The electrocardiogram may be normal or may show left axis deviation and signs of left ventricular hypertrophy.

In addition to cardiac failure, these patients ultimately suffer cerebral accidents, rupture of the aorta, or other complications of hypertension. Unless surgical correction is carried out, 51 per cent of patients with this condition die before the fortieth year, but a few survive to old age.

The pathologic physiology has been of considerable interest because hypertension in this disease is associated with a discrete lesion which can be surgically corrected. In addition to increased resistance from the constriction and the collateral vessels, a renal mechanism activated by the lowered renal blood flow and pressure seems to contribute to this hypertension.

Surgical correction is indicated in most children, and also in adults in whom hypertension is great or symptoms related to it are present. The segment can be excised and end-to-end suture performed in most instances, but in some cases a graft may be required to bridge the gap or to obtain a satisfactory lumen.

Stenosis or Atresia of Other Valves. Congenital stenosis of the mitral, tricuspid, or aortic valves is uncommon. Except for the relatively early appearance of signs and symptoms as compared with their counterparts in rheumatic heart disease, the effects are similar. *Tricuspid atresia* is usually associated with an underdeveloped or absent right ventricle, atrial septal defect, and atretic pulmonary artery. Blood flows from the right into the left atrium and left ventricle and reaches the lungs through a patent ductus arteriosus. The right ventricular cavity is absent or filled with blood clot, or it communicates with the left ventricle through a ventricular septal defect, but does not function. Left axis deviation in the electrocardiogram results, and this finding in a cyanotic patient suggests either tricuspid atresia or single ventricle.

Aortic atresia, extremely rare, is associated with a hypoplastic, nonfunctioning left ventricle, and frequently with *mitral atresia* as well. Blood flows from left atrium to right atrium to the lungs, and reaches the systemic circuit only through a patent ductus. Survival for more than a few weeks is rare. Congenital and acquired varieties of aortic stenosis, as well as the vigorous contractions of the aortic outflow tract, which mimic true stenosis are considered on p. 1434, Chap. 253).

Malformations without Direct Effect on Blood Flow

Dextrocardia and Situs Inversus. Dextrocardia may occur as an exact mirror-image reversal of the heart within the thorax (*true dextrocardia*) or as abnormal rotation of the heart, with twisting of the great vessels (*dextroposition* or *dextrorotation*) of the heart. Situs inversus, or reversal of all the viscera, may accompany any form of dextrocardia, or it may occur with normal heart position. Neither dextrocardia nor situs inversus is of any functional significance in itself, but additional cardiac malfor-

mations are common and may be severe. Mirror-image dextrocardia produces an almost pathognomonic electrocardiogram in the limb leads, i.e., inversion of all waves in lead I and reversal of leads II and III.

Ebstein's Anomaly. The rare anomaly of the tricuspid valve which bears this eponym consists of a congenital downward displacement of the valve into the right ventricle, with anomalous insertion of one or more valve leaflets. The malformation sometimes produces surprisingly little functional disturbance, while in other cases incompetence of the tricuspid valve and impaired function of the right ventricle produce prominent signs at an early age. Sudden death has often been reported.

Although patients with Ebstein's disease are not cyanotic in infancy, they may eventually develop right-to-left shunts through a patent foramen ovale. The right atrium and right ventricle are then greatly enlarged, and the pulmonary vascularity may be decreased. The electrocardiogram shows tall P waves but no signs of ventricular hypertrophy. Complete right bundle branch block and paroxysmal tachycardia are common. There is often a tricuspid apical systolic murmur, which is attributed to incompetence of the dislocated tricuspid valve.

Anomalies of the Aortic Arch. The multiple bilateral aortic arches of the embryo provide a background for a great variety of anomalies. One of the commonest is a *right aortic arch,* in which the ascending aorta arches toward the right instead of the left. The aorta may then continue to lie on the right in its descent, or may cross over to descend in the normal position just left of the midline. In either case, the anomaly is of no functional significance. A right aortic arch may be recognized by its indentation of the barium-filled esophagus, since it impinges on the *right* side of the esophagus in the anteroposterior view, and displaces the esophagus backward in the left anterior oblique view.

In some cases, both right and left aortic arches persist, forming a vascular ring. Such a ring, which may also result from anomalies of the subclavian or other arteries or from the ductus or ligamentum arteriosum, usually has no effect on cardiac function, but it may produce symptoms by compression of the esophagus or trachea.

Anomalies of the Great Veins. Many variations in the structure of the superior and inferior venae cavae and their major branches are possible. A persistent left superior vena cava, for example, is a fairly common anomaly. Anomalous venae cavae may drain normally into the right atrium and be of no functional significance, or they may drain into the left atrium, producing major venous-arterial shunts. The course of such anomalies can usually be clearly outlined by angiocardiography.

Congenital Cardiac Hypertrophy. On rare occasions, cardiac dilatation and hypertrophy, with congestive heart failure, develop during the first few months of life, in the absence of cyanosis, thrills, or murmurs. In a few of these cases no clear etiologic factors can be discovered, even on pathologic examination, and they are accurately termed *idiopathic congenital cardiac hypertrophy.*

The same clinical picture may be produced by a variety of causes, including endocardial fibroelastosis, von Gierke's disease, nonspecific myocarditis, and prolonged ectopic tachycardia.

Endocardial fibroelastosis is a collagenous and elastic tissue thickening of the endocardium lining the heart chambers, most frequently limited to the left ventricle. The etiology is not known; "fetal endocarditis" has been suggested as a possible cause, but the evidence is not convincing. In some cases the cardiac enlargement is predominantly left ventricular, while in others the endocardial sclerosis appears to constrict the left ventricle and lead to right ventricular hypertrophy.

Von Gierke's disease is a general metabolic disorder in which glycogenolysis is impaired and intracellular deposits of glycogen are found in the liver, kidneys, and myocardium. Hepatomegaly, fasting hypoglycemia, and ketonuria are characteristic features.

The diagnosis of *nonspecific myocarditis* is based on the microscopic finding of interstitial round-cell infiltration, often with small areas of necrosis or fibrosis, in the myocardium, in the absence of infectious or other known causes of myocarditis.

Prolonged paroxysms of tachycardia in infants have occasionally been reported as a cause of marked cardiac enlargement and death. Although prominent dilatation of the ventricles can occur under these circumstances, it is unlikely that myocardial hypertrophy can be attributed to a prolonged rapid heart rate alone.

REFERENCES

Abbott, M. E.: "Atlas of Congenital Heart Disease," New York, American Heart Association, 1936.

Allen, J. G. (Ed.): "Extracorporeal Circulation," Springfield, Ill., Charles C Thomas, Publisher, 1958.

Bahnson, H. T., S. C. Spencer, R. A. Gaertner, and D. W. Benson: Experiences with Open Heart Surgery during Cardiopulmonary Bypass in 270 Cases, Am. Surgeon, 26:227, 1960.

Blalock, A., and H. B. Taussig: The Surgical Treatment of Malformations of the Heart in Which There Is Pulmonic Stenosis or Pulmonic Atresia, J.A.M.A., 128:189, 1945.

Brotmacher, L., and Maurice Campbell: The Natural History of Ventricular Septal Defect, Brit. Heart J., 20:97, 1958.

Clowes, G. H. A., Jr.: Extracorporeal Maintenance of

Circulation and Respiration, Physiol. Rev., 40: 826, 1960.

Dexter, L.: Atrial Septal Defect, Brit. Heart J., 18: 209, 1956.

Edwards, J. E.: Functional Pathology of the Pulmonary Vascular Tree in Congenital Heart Disease, Circulation, 15:164, 1957.

Harris, J. S., and S. Farber: Transposition of the Great Cardiac Vessels, with Special Reference to the Phylogenetic Theory of Spitzer, Arch. Pathol., 28:427, 1939.

Kirklin, J. W., E. H. Wood, H. J. C. Swan, H. F. Helmholz, I. J. Fox, L. G. S. Brooker, D. W. Heseltine, H. E. Essex, H. B. Burchell, J. L. Wright, J. R. F. Penido, and N. C. Birkhead: Symposium on Diagnostic Applications of Indicator-Dilution Technics, Proc. Staff Meetings Mayo Clinic, 32:463, 1957.

McCord, M. C., J. van Elk, and S. G. Blount: Tetralogy of Fallot: Clinical and Hemodynamic Spectrum of Combined Pulmonary Stenosis and Ventricular Septal Defect, Circulation, 16:736, 1957.

Morrow, A. G., R. J. Sanders, and E. Braunwald: The Nitrous Oxide Test: An Improved Method for the Detection of Left-to-Right Shunts, Circulation, 17: 284, 1958.

Patten, B. M.: The Development of the Heart, in "Pathology of the Heart," S. E. Gould (Ed.), Springfield, Ill., Charles C Thomas, Publisher, 1953.

Spencer, S. C., and H. T. Bahnson: Intracardiac Surgery Employing Hypothermia and Coronary Perfusion Performed on 100 Patients, Surgery, 46:987, 1959.

Taussig, H. B.: "Congenital Malformations of the Heart," rev. ed., Cambridge, Mass., Harvard University Press, 1960.

Zimmerman, H. E. (Ed.): "Intravascular Catheterization," Springfield, Ill., Charles C Thomas, Publisher, 1959.

253 ACQUIRED VALVULAR DISEASE OF THE HEART

*T. R. Harrison and
William H. Resnik*

Those congenital malformations which cause valvular deformity are discussed in Chap. 252. These include almost all instances of disease of the pulmonic cusps and rare disorders of the other three valves. However, the great majority of aortic, mitral, and tricuspid lesions are not congenital but acquired and are due to rheumatic fever. Although this disorder, which has been considered in some detail in a previous chapter (p. 913), affects all parts of the heart, *its distinctive feature is valvular deformity, evidence of which is essential for the diagnosis of chronic rheumatic heart disease.* Nevertheless, all acquired valvular distortions are not of rheumatic origin, and in the following pages lesions due to the other causes are also considered.

Bacterial infection may be superimposed on any valvular lesion. It is relatively uncommon when the valve is extremely deformed or calcified and especially likely to develop upon a valve which has a slight impairment due to rheumatic fever. The simultaneous presence of murmur and fever should arouse the suspicion of bacterial endocarditis and also of an acute flare-up of the rheumatic process.

The precise identification of valvular disease has assumed increasing importance as cardiac surgery has advanced. Such evaluation depends in large measure on the proper interpretation of heart murmurs. The general principles involved have been discussed in Chap. 251. Here, we are concerned with the more practical aspects of valvular disease.

AORTIC STENOSIS

During the first two decades, this lesion is usually due to congenital abnormality of the cusps or of the outflow tract of the left ventricle. Between the ages of thirty and fifty the usual cause is rheumatic fever. In elderly persons, degenerative distortion of the valves is the major factor, although there is some evidence that minimal and clinically undetectable injury by rheumatic fever is often present and predisposes to these changes. At all ages there is a striking predominance of males.

Mechanism of Symptoms. The obstructive lesion at the aortic orifice is rarely of hemodynamic significance until the stenosis has reduced the cross-sectional area by 75 per cent. Eventually, this leads to left ventricular hypertension, with a large pressure gradient across the aortic valve. However, since the flow varies with the *fourth* power of the radius and only with the *first* power of the pressure difference, this is not an ideal compensatory mechanism. Thus there occurs an increasingly fixed cardiac output, that is, a progressive inability of the heart to elevate output in response to the metabolic needs of the body.

Syncope on exertion occurs in 10 to 20 per cent of the patients, probably due to the failure of cardiac output to increase as peripheral resistance diminishes in response to muscular exertion. This presumably leads to a sudden fall in cerebral blood flow and hence to loss of consciousness. This symptom has grave prognostic significance, and death usually occurs within 3 years.

Angina pectoris develops in about one-third of the patients. Sometimes it may be caused by the not infrequent coexistence of coronary disease, but it may occur in the absence of coronary obstruction,

and is attributable then to the incapacity of the coronaries to supply a flow of blood to the myocardium adequate to meet the demands of the hypertrophied left ventricle. Indeed, myocardial infarction may ensue even when the coronaries are relatively normal. *Sudden death* occurs in 20 to 25 per cent of cases, as it may in any ischemic heart.

Eventually, if the patient survives, congestive failure appears, becomes increasingly refractory to treatment, and death usually ensues within 2 or 3 years. A curious phenomenon, as yet unexplained, is the persistence of a normal or slightly elevated resting cardiac output even when the left ventricular end-diastolic pressure is elevated (left ventricular failure).

Signs. The classic signs of this disorder are the loud, rough systolic murmur, usually heard best in the second right interspace and transmitted into the neck; the corresponding thrill; the diminished or absent second aortic sound; the slowly rising pulse of low volume (plateau pulse); and the presence of calcification in the region of the aortic cusps as revealed by fluoroscopy. *However, departures from this idealized picture are frequent, and unsuspected aortic stenosis is frequently discovered only at the autopsy table.* The murmur may be loudest at the apex and may disappear completely during congestive failure, reappearing when compensation has been restored. The thrill may not be present, the second sound over the aortic area may be well heard, and the character of the pulse may not conform to the classic description. Finally, calcification of the valves is present in only half the patients, and even then its detection depends on the skill and experience of the fluoroscopist.

Left ventricular hypertrophy is indicated by the forceful thrust at the apex, even though definite cardiac enlargement is usually absent by x-ray. The electrocardiogram may display the characteristic signs of left ventricular hypertrophy, and when coved T waves are present and the R wave is absent in the first three precordial leads, differentiation from an old septal infarct may be difficult or impossible.

Diagnosis. The several varieties of *subaortic stenosis* may present physical signs which are identical with those of valvular obstruction, although the diminution of the aortic second sound is likely to be less pronounced. The distinction is likely to require catheterization of the left side of the heart, with careful "pull-back" observations and the demonstration that the site of the systolic pressure gradient is below rather than at the valve.

Two different types of congenital subaortic stenosis have been described. Surgical treatment may be highly successful when the hindrance is due to endocardial fibrous thickening of the outflow tract, but has little to offer when hypertrophy of the musculature (idiopathic hypertrophic subaortic stenosis) is at fault. Both conditions may be associated with similar signs, although it has been stated that the murmur of the latter disorder is more apt to be maximal to the left of the sternum and is less well transmitted to the neck. The angiocardiographic findings may be of differential value.

The acquired type of subaortic stenosis is usually seen in older persons with left ventricular hypertrophy due to any cause. It is ascribed to unusually vigorous contraction of the muscles encircling the outflow tract. In most instances the pressure gradient between aorta and left ventricle is small and the functional stenosis is of no clinical significance other than the possible confusion with true stenosis. The murmur is the only physical sign in these persons with "pseudoaortic stenosis." Occasionally, however, there may be a thrill with the peripheral signs of true obstruction. In such instances cardiac catheterization will reveal a significant systolic pressure gradient, but the "pull-back" technique (see above) will demonstrate that it is below the valve and hence that surgical intervention is not indicated.

The symptoms and management (except surgical) of subaortic stenosis are the same as those of the valvular variety.

Prognosis. The appearance of syncope on exertion or congestive failure is ominous and that of angina only slightly less so. Nevertheless, there are individuals who may present the characteristic murmur and thrill of aortic stenosis and who survive without symptoms until their seventies or eighties. This must be due to the fact that there is no necessary parallelism between the signs and the degree of obstruction.

Treatment. This consists of the usual precautionary measures against the development of subacute bacterial endocarditis and of the usual management of congestive failure or angina, should they occur. Surgical dilatation of the valve is still hazardous, although an operative mortality as low as 5 per cent has been reported in some series. The decision is difficult because the risk is altogether too great for the asymptomatic patient, and it is still greater when disability has appeared. Yet, when symptoms are present, especially early congestive failure, the over-all outlook statistically is better with surgical than with medical treatment. In facing this problem the physician may wish to recall the statement of Claudius, the stepfather of Hamlet, that,

> ". . . diseases desperate grown,
> By desperate appliance are relieved,
> Or not at all."

We do not believe that any patient should undergo so hazardous an operation unless preliminary left ventricular catheterization reveals a cross sectional orifice of 0.8 cm^2 or less, as calculated from the pressure gradient and the blood flow. Likewise, the "pull-back" procedure (see above) should be used to learn whether the valve rather than the subvalvular outflow tract is the site of the obstruction.

AORTIC INSUFFICIENCY

Occasionally, this defect may result from congenital weakness of the root of the aorta, sometimes associated with arachnodactyly or with medial necrosis. It may likewise be produced by a congenital bicuspid valve, usually in conjunction with coarctation of the aorta. In practically all other instances up to the age of thirty, the lesion is due to rheumatic fever. In the thirties and forties, the problem is usually one of differentiation of rheumatic from syphilitic aortic regurgitation, and in the late fifties and beyond from atherosclerotic disease of the aortic valves. In male patients aortic insufficiency may occur as an apparent complication of rheumatoid arthritis or rheumatoid spondylitis. Rarer causes of the valvular defect are bacterial endocarditis, the anatomic disruption of the valve being one of the chief causes of mortality in this condition even when the infection is eradicated; injury to the cusps by trauma; distortion of the valve by dissecting aneurysm; stretching of the aortic ring in severe hypertension, producing a relative regurgitation; and fenestration of the aortic cusps.

When the lesion is advanced, dilatation carries the usual disadvantage of diminished pressure for a given degree of systolic fiber tension (p. 1406) but is advantageous in that it permits filling from the low-pressure atrium despite pronounced regurgitation from the aorta. However, when the volume of this backflow is very great, the left ventricular pressure during late diastole may exceed that in the atrium and so produce diastolic closure of the mitral valve.

Symptoms and Natural History. The patient with aortic insufficiency usually remains asymptomatic for a long period. Once dyspnea on mild effort appears, seizures of paroxysmal nocturnal dyspnea are common, and from this point on congestive failure tends to progress rapidly.

Syncope and angina may occur but are much less frequent than in patients with aortic stenosis. The reduction in coronary flow during diastole because of the lowered aortic pressure is compensated for in part by increased subepicardial flow during systole (p. 33).

Diagnosis. The first problem involves the detection of the lesion; the second is concerned with the recognition of its cause. The high-pitched blowing diastolic murmur heard best at the aortic area or along the left sternal border is the cardinal sign. Sometimes it can be elicited only at the end of held expiration when the patient leans forward. Most of the patients also have systolic murmurs at the base, and many have them at the apex. The Austin Flint murmur, mimicking mitral stenosis, is frequently heard. The peripheral signs are also important: the wide pulse pressure, the water-hammer pulse, the collapsing pulse, the pistol-shot sound, the double Duroziez murmur, and the capillary pulse—all indicative of a leak from the arterial system and of a peripheral vasodilatation. The x-ray reveals the enlargement of the left ventricle, and when the lesion is pronounced the electrocardiogram displays evidence of left ventricular hypertrophy and "strain." A more reliable manifestation of moderate left ventricular hypertrophy is the exaggerated localized apical thrust.

Two conditions may be readily confused with aortic insufficiency. One of them, fortunately rare, is rupture of a sinus of Valsalva, and the other is patent ductus arteriosus. However, careful auscultation will usually enable one to distinguish between the continuous murmur of these conditions and the to-and-fro basal murmur which is commonly heard in patients with aortic regurgitation. The differentiation from pulmonic insufficiency is considered later.

The recognition of aortic insufficiency due to congenital anomalies, hypertension, or senile degeneration of the cusps will depend in large measure on the age of the patient and the associated findings. The common problem is the distinction between rheumatic fever and syphilis as the cause. Although this differentiation is impossible in some instances, certain points are likely to be of value.

Syphilitic aortic insufficiency should be suspected when a middle-aged individual, usually a male lacking a story of rheumatic fever, presents the classic manifestations of aortic regurgitation. The suspicion is strengthened when there is a history of a primary lesion or of antisyphilitic treatment in the past and when the serologic tests for syphilis are positive (they are positive in about 85 per cent of such cases). The tambour quality of the second heart sound at the aortic area is often present but is also heard in patients with aortic atheroma or hypertension. Hence it is significant only when heard in a comparatively young patient with a normal blood pressure.

Although syphilis does not produce deformity of the mitral valve, the dilatation of the mitral ring consequent to aortic regurgitation frequently causes an apical systolic murmur. Furthermore, the Austin Flint murmur ("relative mitral stenosis") is frequently heard in patients with syphilitic aortic regurgitation, and this murmur cannot be differentiated with certainty from the similar murmur of mitral stenosis. Rough basal systolic murmurs are commonly present, and rarely, a systolic thrill is

felt, but other evidence of aortic stenosis is not encountered. Hence, in an individual presenting aortic insufficiency, the differentiation between syphilitic disease involving the aortic valve only and rheumatic disease involving either the aortic valve only, or both the aortic and mitral valves, cannot be made by auscultation alone. The presence of chronic atrial fibrillation constitutes almost conclusive evidence that the lesion is rheumatic, as does the presence of peripheral signs of aortic stenosis or x-ray evidence of compression of the esophagus by an enlarged left atrium. In the absence of such differential points, the distinction between syphilitic and rheumatic disease has to be made on the basis of the history, the serologic reactions, etc.

Treatment. The management is essentially that of congestive heart failure plus the usual prophylaxis against rheumatic recurrence and against bacterial endocarditis. When syphilis is the cause, antiluetic therapy is indicated but is probably of little value once congestive failure has appeared. Surgical treatment is still experimental and is far less likely to be successful than for aortic stenosis.

MITRAL STENOSIS

This lesion is practically always the result of rheumatic fever. Thus the diagnosis of mitral stenosis automatically implies that the patient has rheumatic heart disease, even though a history of previous joint pains and fever can be elicited in only about 60 per cent of the patients.

In the typical patient, the physical signs are characteristic: the sustained right parasternal heave of right ventricular hypertrophy; the loud staccato high-pitched "snapping" first sound, the exaggerated second pulmonic sound, the short opening click, and the long diastolic rumble with presystolic intensification. The electrocardiogram displays right axis deviation, which is confirmed by fluoroscopic examination, which also indicates prominence of the left atrium with encroachment on the barium-filled esophagus.

In the early stages of the disease, the characteristic phenomenon, the diastolic rumble, may be difficult to elicit. It may be heard only after exercise when the stethoscope is placed at the exact point of the apex thrust, while the patient lies on the left side. The murmur may be very brief and audible only during the brief interval between atrial contraction and the first sound or only during the early part of diastolic filling. At this stage, all the other signs may be absent.

Difficulty may also be encountered when the lesion is advanced. Here, the advent of atrial fibrillation, which is such a common complication, causes disappearance of the rumble associated with atrial contraction, while the marked reduction in cardiac output and hence in flow through the very narrow mitral orifice reduces the intensity of the early filling murmur and, very rarely, may even cause it to disappear. However, the other characteristic signs are likely to be marked, and their presence should lead to a meticulous search for the filling rumble under the conditions already mentioned. As a general rule it is not the intensity but *the duration of the murmur which is the most reliable guide to the degree of stenosis.*

Pathophysiology. In the early phase, dyspnea on exertion due to the mechanical effect of the obstruction is the outstanding symptom. The capacity to increase the flow through the narrowed valve is limited, and the increase in venous return with exercise tends to aggravate pulmonary congestion. As the lesion becomes more advanced, two types of compensatory adjustment occur; the clinical picture depends in large measure upon which predominates.

Rise in pressure in the left atrium and in the pulmonary veins and capillaries tends to maintain cardiac output. However, the flow varies with the fourth power of the radius of the orifice and only with the first power of the pressure gradient on the two sides of the valve. Thus, in the presence of significant stenosis, a normal flow can be obtained only by means of a well-marked rise in atrial pressure, which leads to congestion of the lungs. Thus dyspnea is progressive and pulmonary edema, occasionally fatal, may occur when venous return is increased by exertion or fever or when rapid atrial fibrillation causes further impairment of ventricular filling by reducing the duration of diastole. Recurrent hemoptysis due to the development of anastomotic channels between the pulmonary and bronchial veins is common, but right-sided failure may be absent or minimal.

The second method of adjustment is by increase in pulmonary arteriolar resistance. This may be caused by structural thickening of the vessels, by anoxia resulting from pulmonary edema, and perhaps also by reflex vasoconstriction consequent to congestion of the lungs, although the latter mechanism is disputed. When this increase in pulmonary arteriolar resistance is predominant, right-sided heart failure occurs at a relatively early stage, with decline in output of the right ventricle. Thus the pulmonary capillaries are protected against excessive congestion and dyspnea may be relatively slight, despite the presence of the classic manifestations of right ventricular failure. Because of the decline in cardiac output and in flow from left atrium to left ventricle, the diastolic rumble may be faint or even absent, and the opening snap may not be heard. It is this type of patient which may be mistakenly thought to have primary pulmonary hypertension or myocarditis as the cause of the heart failure.

Both types of compensation are present in most instances, but the extent to which one or the other is predominant tends to determine the outstanding clinical features.

Natural History. Patients with mitral stenosis may survive for many years after the onset of heart failure. In this respect, the disorder resembles tricuspid stenosis but is entirely different from aortic lesions. The latter do not induce symptoms until failure of the left ventricle has occurred, but in the case of mitral stenosis the symptoms are due to the mechanical effect of the valvular narrowing. This may be nonprogressive over a period of many years.

Atrial fibrillation eventually occurs in the great majority of patients and increases markedly the hazard of peripheral or pulmonary embolism. In the absence of such complications, the arrhythmia is compatible with many years of life, provided the ventricular rate is controlled by digitalis. Even so, repeated, massive, and fatal pulmonary infarction may supervene, once right-heart failure has developed.

The frequency of hemoptysis due to collateral venous channels has been mentioned. This manifestation is likewise often the result of pulmonary infarction.

The long-standing congestion due to mitral stenosis leads to important secondary changes in the lungs. Some patients develop extensive hemosiderosis and a pulmonary state not unlike that resulting from one of the primary pneumoconioses. Much more frequently, there is chronic bronchitis with winter aggravation, the symptoms becoming severe with each minor respiratory infection. The prevention and management of such infections are among the important principles of treatment.

When pulmonary hypertension is present, severe pain may occur. This resembles that of angina in its relation to effort but is often of longer duration and responds poorly to nitroglycerin. It is probably due to reduction in the coronary flow relative to the needs of the hypertrophied right ventricle (p. 34).

The thromboembolic complications have been mentioned. The valvular obstruction predisposes to thrombosis in the left atrium, and systemic embolism may occur even in patients with normal rhythm. However, this complication is far more common in patients with long-standing atrial fibrillation. Pulmonary embolism and infarction are rare in the absence of right-sided failure but in its presence are very common. More than one-half the fatal instances display evidence of recent or old infarcts in the lungs.

Bacterial endocarditis is a rare complication of

mitral stenosis. It is more likely to affect the less severely damaged valves.

Diagnosis. The most characteristic phenomenon of mitral stenosis, the diastolic rumble, may be due to other causes. Thus the Austin Flint murmur is often encountered in patients with free aortic regurgitation, even though the mitral valve is normal. This rumble is presumably due to displacement of the aortic cusp of the mitral valve and its vibration between the forward stream of blood from the atrium and the regurgitating blood from the aorta.

When the diastolic flow through the mitral valve is greatly increased, as in patients with patent ductus arteriosus or in those with outspoken mitral insufficiency, a diastolic rumble may occur even though the cusps are normal. In such instances there is relative stenosis, in terms of the size of the valve orifice as compared to the flow through it. Relative tricuspid stenosis with a diastolic rumble may occur when, because of atrial septal defect, right ventricular filling is markedly increased. Structural tricuspid stenosis is almost always of rheumatic origin and associated with mitral stenosis. Atrial myxoma (p. 1465) is a rare cause of a diastolic rumble. Its preoperative distinction from mitral stenosis may be possible only by means of the angiocardiogram.

Those several conditions which mimic mitral stenosis by causing a diastolic rumble may be recognized by the signs of the basic disorder and, with the exception of tricuspid stenosis, by the absence of an audible opening snap. Unlike mitral stenosis, they do not cause prolongation of the time elapsing between the onset of excitation and the beginning of the first heart sound (Q-S$_1$ time).

As has been mentioned, the intensity of the mitral stenotic murmur is related not only to the degree of narrowing but also to the rate of flow through the orifice. Occasionally, when cardiac output is markedly decreased, there may be no audible rumble, despite a high degree of obstruction. The absence of a rumble has also been noted in association with large thrombi in the left atrium. Thus in a patient—usually a young woman—with a rheumatic history, severe heart failure, and no murmur, the slight hazard of left-sided cardiac catheterization, with measurement of the atrioventricular pressure gradient and of cardiac output, is justifiable. Unless this information, which allows a reasonably accurate calculation of the size of the orifice, is obtained one will occasionally overlook a surgically treatable obstruction.

The so-called primary pulmonary hypertension is, like mitral stenosis, usually a disease of young women (p. 1538). The patients may exhibit a presystolic gallop and a split first sound. These auscultatory phenomena may mimic closely the presystolic rumble of mitral stenosis. Both disorders are commonly associated with clinical and electrocardiographic evidence of right ventricular hypertrophy. However, the shape of the atrial complex is usually different, the P wave being broad and notched in patients with mitral stenosis, and narrow and spiked (P-pulmonale) in those with primary pulmonary hypertension. When doubt exists, there is indication for right-heart catheterization, with measurement of the pulmonary capillary (wedge) pressure, which remains normal in patients with pulmonary hypertension but is elevated in the presence of hemodynamically significant mitral stenosis.

Treatment. Surgical treatment will be discussed later. The medical management consists of prophylaxis against rheumatic recurrences (p. 918), the prevention of thromboembolic episodes, control of atrial fibrillation, and treatment of congestive heart failure (p. 1385). Although these conditions are discussed in detail in other chapters, certain points may be emphasized here.

The presence of a normal resting heart rate in a patient with atrial fibrillation and mitral stenosis does not invariably mean adequate digitalization. It is essential to be certain that slight exertion does not provoke undue tachycardia. Periodic augmentation of a standard maintenance dose of digitalis is usually necessary to ensure optimal digitalization (p. 1387).

The attempt to reestablish sinus rhythm is rarely permanently successful when atrial fibrillation is due to tight mitral stenosis. Following surgical widening of the valve, the likelihood of success is greater. When fibrillation persists, permanent anticoagulant therapy is desirable in order to reduce the hazard of the serious thromboembolic complications.

MITRAL INSUFFICIENCY

This lesion is occasionally of congenital origin, being associated with a low interatrial or high interventricular septal defect. Coronary disease is a not infrequent cause, and in such an instance the murmur is usually in late systole and may appear during anginal attacks and vanish as the pain subsides (p. 1412). Marked dilatation of the left ventricle from any cause may produce relative mitral insufficiency because of dilatation of the mitral ring, the murmur diminishing as improvement occurs. Bacterial endocarditis is a rare primary factor but frequently causes a previously damaged valve to become more incompetent. However, in the absence of marked left ventricular enlargement or of obvious coronary disease, rheumatic fever is by far the most frequent etiologic factor.

The following description of uncomplicated mitral insufficiency will be relatively brief, as many of the problems involved may be more appropriately considered in the subsequent discussion of combined stenosis and insufficiency.

In most instances, this lesion is associated with a faint apical first sound which may be replaced entirely by the loud blowing pansystolic murmur extending into the axilla and even to the back. No opening snap is heard. The apex beat is often of the strong localized type indicative of left ventricular hypertrophy. X-ray examination reveals enlargement of the left ventricle and of the left atrium, and the latter chamber may exhibit systolic expansion. A huge left atrium always signifies the presence of a significant degree of regurgitation. The electrocardiogram usually exhibits evidence of left ventricular hypertrophy, but this may be overshadowed by the coexisting right ventricular enlargement when, as occasionally occurs, there is a secondary marked rise in pulmonary resistance.

The distinction between mitral insufficiency and aortic stenosis, which sometimes produces a murmur loudest at the apex, may present difficulty. The demonstration by phonocardiograms that the murmur begins before ejection is conclusive evidence against aortic stenosis. The leftward transmission of the murmur will usually differentiate mitral insufficiency from interventricular septal defect, which also produces a pansystolic murmur. However, in doubtful instances this separation may require cardiac catheterization.

The recognition of mitral regurgitation due to a dilated ring (relative insufficiency) is easy when there is pronounced cardiac enlargement due to some cause other than rheumatic fever. However, in a patient with obvious rheumatic aortic insufficiency and a markedly dilated left ventricle, the distinction between the organic and relative types of mitral insufficiency may be impossible. The late systolic murmur, which is so frequent in patients with coronary disease, is probably due to mitral regurgitation resulting from distortion of ischemic papillary muscles. It will rarely be confused with the blow of rheumatic mitral insufficiency because the latter is in most instances pansystolic, obscuring the first sound and continuing until very shortly after the second.

Patients with slight incompetence of the mitral valve usually remain free of symptoms but are particularly susceptible to the development of bacterial endocarditis. As the lesion becomes more severe, dyspnea is increasingly pronounced, and once congestive failure begins, it is likely to progress rather rapidly.

The management of mitral insufficiency consists of prophylaxis against recurrences of rheumatic fever (p. 918) and of bacterial endocarditis (p. 1043) and the treatment of these disorders or of congestive heart failure when either occurs. The advent of open-heart surgery, with the bypassing pump, has made practical the attempts at plastic repair of insufficient mitral valves. However, the hazard is still high and the results are rarely gratifying.

COMBINED MITRAL STENOSIS AND INSUFFICIENCY

A large percentage of patients with rheumatic disease of the mitral valve have a combination of narrowing and regurgitation. However, marked insufficiency requires a large left ventricular output, including both the backward and forward flow, while a high degree of stenosis makes this impossible because it reduces filling. Thus one lesion or the other is predominant. The accurate evaluation of the relative significance of each is a matter of great practical importance in relation to the question of surgical treatment. Such evaluation may be very difficult by ordinary methods and may require catheterization of the left atrium and ventricle, with measurements of pressure and flow and calculation of orifice size. Observation of the effect on pulmonary capillary (wedge) pressure of drugs which alter systemic peripheral resistance may be helpful. Thus norepinephrine may increase the degree of regurgitation, the wedge pressure, and the intensity of the regurgitant murmur, while nitrites tend to have the opposite effects.

Clinical findings, although not always decisive, are often of value in estimating the relative degrees of stenosis and insufficiency.

Systolic Murmurs in Patients with Mitral Stenosis. Aside from mitral insufficiency, there are three other common causes. (1) *Concomitant aortic stenosis.* When this lesion coexists, the additional signs are similar to those of aortic stenosis alone except that the diminished flow into the left ventricle may reduce the intensity of the ejection murmur. The demonstration by phonocardiographic means, that the systolic murmur does not start until ejection, will usually separate it from that due to mitral insufficiency. (2) *Ejection murmurs into a dilated pulmonary artery* occur in most patients with mitral stenosis and may occasionally be as loud as grade IV. The absence of left ventricular hypertrophy and the observation that the intensity is greatest in the left upper interspaces will usually distinguish this murmur from others. Occasionally, the separation from aortic stenosis may require left-sided catheterization, with measurement of flow and pressure gradient and calculation of the size of the aortic orifice. (3) *The murmur of tricuspid insufficiency,* whether due to structural distortion of the valves or dilatation of the ring, resembles that of mitral insufficiency in being pansystolic. However, it is likely to be loudest in the lower left parasternal region and tends to be transmitted to the right precordial area rather than toward the left axilla.

These several features, plus evidence as to whether there is right ventricular hypertrophy only, or both right and left, will usually allow these conditions to be separated from mitral insufficiency and from each other. The presence of left ventricular hypertrophy constitutes strong evidence that a systolic murmur is due either to mitral insufficiency or to aortic stenosis and indicates that operative treatment, while not necessarily out of the question, is likely to carry a large hazard. On the other hand, the murmurs of tricuspid insufficiency or of ejection into the dilated pulmonary artery do not militate against mitral valvulotomy.

Diastolic Rumbles in Patients with Mitral Insufficiency. The blowing systolic mitral regurgitant murmur usually extends slightly beyond the second heart sound, because during the early phase of relaxation the pressure in the ventricle is above that in the atrium. Since this early diastolic blow is continuous with the systolic component, it does not cause confusion with the lower-pitched rumble of stenosis. However, there may be a short loud filling rumble when narrowing is minimal or even absent. This is produced by the increased rate of filling consequent to the elevated atrial pressure due to the systolic regurgitation. *Thus a loud filling rumble does not prove a high degree of mitral stenosis.* However, when the valve is not narrowed, early diastolic filling occurs quickly and the duration of the rumble is brief. When stenosis is marked, filling necessarily occurs at a much slower rate and the duration of the rumble is long. Hence *a faint or moderate but prolonged rumble is a more reliable sign of advanced stenosis than is a louder but briefer rumble.*

The methods used to distinguish between right and left ventricular hypertrophy have been previously discussed (p. 1406). Here, it need only be reiterated that the accurate assessment of hypertrophy is of the greatest importance in the evaluation of mitral valvular disease. The presence of any degree of left ventricular enlargement indicates that some additional disorder—usually mitral insufficiency or an aortic lesion—is present, in addition to whatever degree of mitral stenosis the patient may have. In most instances, mechanically significant mitral regurgitation is associated with detectable left ventricular hypertrophy. However, when there is marked secondary rise in pulmonary resistance, this may be masked by predominant right ventricular enlargement.

The inadequacies of the x-ray method of evaluating ventricular hypertrophy have already been mentioned (p. 1406). Some dilatation of the left atrium may occur with either insufficiency or stenosis. However, either extreme enlargement or marked systolic expansion of this chamber is nearly always associated with pronounced regurgitation.

Replacement of the first heart sound by the systolic murmur constitutes strong evidence for a well-marked degree of insufficiency; exaggeration of the first sound and the phonocardiographic demonstration of a delay (0.07 sec or more after the beginning of the QRS) of the apical S_1 both speak for stenosis. Normally, the mitral first sound begins very early—0.04 to 0.06 sec after the start of the QRS because of the low left atrial pressure. However, when this function is elevated, more time is required for the left ventricular pressure to exceed that in the left atrium and produce mitral closure.

A loud opening snap points toward mitral stenosis but must be distinguished from the filling gallop which is so common with insufficiency, and which occurs only about 0.04 sec after the opening of the mitral valve. Despite the higher pitch of the opening snap, the differentiation may be impossible by auscultation. Indeed, in some instances, this distinction cannot be made by phonocardiograms alone and requires simultaneous records of precordial motion in order that one may know when filling actually begins. The recognition of these and of other causes of three-sound rhythms has been considered on p. 1407.

Catheterization of the left side of the heart is attended by a small hazard. However, this is justifiable in doubtful instances. The measurement of the atrioventricular pressure gradient is per se not sufficient to afford an absolute distinction between predominance of stenosis or of regurgitation. However, such measurements, when coupled with determination of cardiac output, allow the calculation, with reasonable accuracy, of the size of the valve orifice. If this is greater than 1 cm², insufficiency is probably the chief lesion, while an orifice of less than 0.6 cm indicates that stenosis is the main disorder. When, as in most patients, the physical signs are conclusive, left-sided catheterization is not essential. However, when doubt exists, this procedure is more useful than catheterization of the right chambers, which even when accompanied by measurement of the wedge ("pulmonary capillary") pressure will not always distinguish clearly between insufficiency and stenosis.

THE SURGICAL TREATMENT OF MITRAL VALVE DISEASE

In the selection of patients for operation, the first problem is that of the detection of valvular disorders other than mitral stenosis. In this respect the evaluation of coexistent systolic murmurs, which has already been discussed, is of great importance. When such murmurs are of the ejection type and due to a dilated pulmonary artery, or of the pansystolic variety and caused by tricuspid insufficiency, they do not militate against surgical treatment. However, ejection murmurs of aortic stenosis or pansystolic murmurs of mitral insufficiency, while not necessarily constituting contraindications, indicate increased hazard and lesser likelihood of benefit than is the case with mitral stenosis alone.

A diastolic blow associated with the peripheral signs of aortic insufficiency is a contraindication. In the absence of the latter signs, such a blow may signify a slight degree of aortic regurgitation, which reduces the chances of a good result, or the Graham Steell murmur of relative pulmonic insufficiency, which constitutes an additional reason for the operation. If such a blow is audible to the right of the sternum, it probably indicates aortic regurgitation. However, either condition may produce a diastolic murmur, loudest in the left third or fourth interspace at the sternal margin, and in the absence of peripheral signs the distinction between the Graham Steell murmur and minimal aortic regurgitation may be impossible.

Either bacterial endocarditis or an acute rheumatic flare-up precludes operation until these complications have been thoroughly controlled. However, low-grade smoldering rheumatic activity is not necessarily a compelling reason for deferring surgical treatment.

The operation may be done at any age, but the chances of restenosis due to recurrent rheumatic fever are greater in those under the age of thirty. Thus the ideal patient for operation is aged thirty to forty-five, with progressive exertional dyspnea which is beginning to interfere with normal activity, with a prolonged diastolic rumble and no other murmurs, and with clinical, electrocardiographic, or radiologic evidence of right ventricular hypertrophy but little or no increase in the transverse diameter of the heart. If, in addition, there is a history of hemoptysis, of attacks of pulmonary edema, or of systemic embolism in such an individual, operation is almost imperative.

It should be emphasized again that in doubtful instances right-sided catheterization, with measurements of the wedge pressure, may be necessary to distinguish mitral stenosis from pulmonary hypertension consequent to disease of the lungs or to embolism. The same procedure will also identify atrial shunts as the cause of flow rumbles. Catheterization of the left chambers will occasionally be needed to evaluate the relative degrees of stenosis and insufficiency of the mitral valve and to decide whether a coexisting aortic stenosis is of any real mechanical significance.

In patients with evidence of previous systemic or pulmonary embolism, and in persons with long-standing atrial fibrillation, operation should be preceded by several weeks of anticoagulant therapy.

Neither an age beyond fifty-five nor advanced heart failure is a contraindication, provided one is satisfied that mitral stenosis is the sole or chief cause of the symptoms. However, the operative hazard is much greater in patients with severe heart failure. A previous acute pericarditis does not preclude operation, although adhesions resulting from it may add to the technical difficulty. Knowledge from long-term observation that the signs of mitral stenosis are of recent origin is a contraindication because there is a possibility that the rumble is a result of edema of the valves and that the stenotic lesion may disappear with time and with treatment of the rheumatic process.

Surgical treatment may be instituted during pregnancy but, in general, the procedure should be postponed until after delivery.

The operative hazard naturally varies with the stage of the disease. In experienced hands it is less than 1 per cent in those patients (class II) who have no symptoms except exertional dyspnea. It is relatively low even in persons (class III) who have had early congestive failure, with mild symptoms at rest. The formerly high mortality for patients with advanced failure (class IV) is steadily declining.

Opinions differ as to the long-range results. In the experience of the writers, improvement has been striking in many instances, and is sufficient to justify the procedure in most of the others. Failure to improve has usually occurred only in individuals who have presented one or more of the contraindications already discussed, in those who have had mitral insufficiency produced by the procedure, or in those in whom extensive calcification prevented adequate dilatation of the valve. Restenosis, requiring a second operation, has been very rare in patients beyond the age of thirty-five but has occasionally occurred in younger patients.

Types of Chest Pain Following Operation. The multiplicity of painful syndromes which may be observed has been a source of considerable confusion. The following clinical pictures may occur singly or in various combinations.

Nonrecurrent pain in the early postoperative period arising in the pericardium, the pleura, or the wound. This type of discomfort is regularly observed during the first few postoperative days and may endure for several weeks. It is sometimes associated with a pericardial or pleural friction rub and usually appears to be related to a sanguinous or serofibrinous reaction of these membranes to injury. Since a similar disorder of the pleura—but not of the pericardium—may follow noncardiac thoracotomies, it is clear that this syndrome is not related specifically to the heart.

Repeated episodes of fever associated with pericarditis and/or pleuritis (the "postcommissurotomy syndrome"). These attacks may recur for 6 to 18 months or, rarely, over a period of several years. An identical syndrome may follow myocardial infarction (p. 1454) or cardiac trauma, whether of the penetrating or nonpenetrating type. Therefore, the term *postcardiac injury syndrome* is perhaps the most suitable designation. This disorder, of which pericarditis is usually the outstanding manifestation, is considered in more detail in Chap. 256.

Coincidental reactivation of rheumatic fever. This is rare, and there is no proof that it is a result of the operative procedure. When it does occur, the rheumatic pericarditis, pleuritis, or possible myositis may produce a clinical picture which, except for the elevated antistreptolysin titer, is indistinguishable from the postcardiac injury syndrome. The differentiation is of prognostic import because of the greater likelihood of restenosis following rheumatic recrudescence.

Chest wall pain following injury to intercostal nerves. The anatomic relationship of these nerves to the ribs renders them especially susceptible to injury by retractors during the operation. A causalgic syndrome may result and produce troublesome pain (without fever, pleuritis, or pericarditis), which may endure for months. The occasional coexistence of this disorder with the postcardiac injury syndrome is one of the factors which has delayed the clarification of these several painful conditions.

RIGHT-SIDED VALVULAR LESIONS

Tricuspid Stenosis. This lesion occurs in 3 or 4 per cent of all instances of mitral stenosis. The diagnosis should be suspected when intractable but nonprogressive right-sided heart failure is present for years, with little or no dyspnea or orthopnea, and when the physical signs of pulmonary hypertension (precordial systolic lift, accentuated second pulmonic sound, and electrocardiographic evidence of right ventricular hypertrophy) are slight. Ascites is sometimes a prominent feature, as is also some degree of icterus due to persistent congestion and fibrosis of the liver. A diastolic or presystolic murmur, increased by inspiration (p. 1410), may be heard in the tricuspid area. X-ray reveals conspicuous dilatation of the right atrium, without enlargement of the pulmonary artery, and the lung fields are characteristically clear.

This clinical picture represents the result of a malady whose preponderant effect is an obstruction of the tricuspid orifice. However, tricuspid stenosis occurs almost invariably in conjunction with other valvular lesions, notably mitral stenosis, and the clinical phenomena of "pure" tricuspid stenosis are necessarily modified by the hemodynamic consequence of these other valvular lesions. Thus pulmonary congestion, with dyspnea on exertion, may be a prominent feature even though tricuspid stenosis is present. In practice, diagnosis of the latter lesion is difficult and frequently missed. The only certain method of establishing it is by cardiac catheterization and demonstrating a distinct diastolic pressure gradient between right atrium and ventricle. When such a finding exists in a patient with mitral stenosis, both valves may be widened at the same operation.

Tricuspid Insufficiency. This lesion may be due to congenital displacement of the tricuspid valve (Ebstein's disease, p. 1432). Organic tricuspid insufficiency may also be present when associated with a tricuspid stenosis of rheumatic origin. However, the usual cause for this valvular defect is functional: stretching of the tricuspid ring and imperfect closure of the leaflets due to right ventricular failure, commonly secondary to left-sided failure. When tricuspid stenosis can be diagnosed with assurance, a coexistent organic insufficiency of the valve may be suspected when there is pronounced systolic pulsation of the neck veins and an expansile systolic pulsation of the liver, determined by bimanual palpation.

Malignant carcinoid is a rare cause of deformity of the tricuspid valve.

Pulmonic Insufficiency. Organic disease of the pulmonary valve is practically never of rheumatic origin. However, functional pulmonary insufficiency, with a Graham Steell murmur, is common in patients with mitral stenosis and congenital heart disease, that is, in any condition characterized by a marked elevation of pressure in the pulmonary artery. The Graham Steell murmur is nearly always faint (grade 1 to 2) and is usually heard best in the left second and third interspaces. Differentiation of this murmur from the faint murmur of aortic insufficiency is difficult or impossible unless the peripheral signs of aortic insufficiency are so pronounced as to make the existence of the latter lesion certain. In the presence of aortic incompetence and a condition causing pulmonary hypertension, the coexistence of a Graham Steell murmur is impossible to ascertain and is not of much importance.

Experimental studies on dogs have shown that pulmonary insufficiency per se is well tolerated. However, the pulmonary hypertension responsible for the functional leakage through the valve is a serious disorder and, when associated with left-to-right shunts of congenital origin, adds materially to the operative hazard (p. 1417). On the other hand, pulmonary hypertension secondary to mitral stenosis is not a contraindication to operation.

Pulmonic Stenosis. Pulmonic stenosis due to rheumatic fever is also a rarity. Almost invariably this lesion is of congenital origin, except for the unusual instances in which it occurs with malignant carcinoid, practically always with liver metastases.

Certain other aspects of chronic valvular disease of the heart are considered in the chapter dealing with congenital disorders.

REFERENCES

Braunwald, E., A. G. Morrow, and W. P. Cornell: Idiopathic Hypertrophic Subaortic Stenosis; Anatomic, Hemodynamic, Clinical and Angiocardiographic Factors, Trans. Assoc. Am. Physicians, 73:297, 1960.

Dexter, L., D. E. Harken, L. A. Cobb, Jr., P. Novack, R. C. Schlant, A. O. Phinney, Jr., and F. W. Haynes: Aortic Stenosis, A.M.A. Arch. Internal Med., 101:254, 1958.

Feinstein, A. R., and M. Rodolfo: Prognostic Significance of Valvular Involvement in Acute Rheumatic Fever, New Engl. J. Med., 260:1001, 1959.

Fish, R. G., T. Takaro, and T. Crymes: Prognostic Considerations in Primary Isolated Insufficiency of the Pulmonic Valve, New Engl. J. Med., 251:739, 1959.

MacDonald, L., J. B. Dealy, M. Rabinowitz, and L. Dexter: Clinical Physiological and Pathological Findings in Mitral Stenosis and Regurgitation, Medicine, 36:237, 1957.

Morrow, A. G., and E. Braunwald: Functional Aortic Stenosis, Circulation, 20:181, 1959.

Sanger, P. W., F. Robicsek, F. H. Taylor, R. Magistro, and E. Foti: Observations on Pulmonary Vasomotor Reflexes, J. Thoracic Surg., 37:774, 1959.

254 ISCHEMIC HEART DISEASE (Angina Pectoris and Myocardial Infarction)

William H. Resnik and
T. R. Harrison

The specific and distinguishing feature of ischemic heart disease is pain due to oxygen deficiency in the myocardium (Chap. 5). The clinical picture depends on whether this deficiency is permanent, complete, and accompanied by necrosis of muscle fibers (myocardial infarction) or temporary, relative, and without concomitant evidence of such destruction (angina pectoris). Both types of myocardial hypoxia are accompanied by a tendency toward sudden death. This is due to ventricular fibrillation, which can be induced in animals by experimental procedures which cause a large oxygen gradient between adjacent normal and ischemic areas.

Congestive heart failure is a frequent but much less specific complication of ischemic heart disease. It may set in abruptly following myocardial infarction, or may appear gradually over a period of months or years. When there is a story of the typical anginal pain, coronary disease is readily identified as the cause of the heart failure. However, when pain is absent, the recognition of ischemic heart disease is likely to be difficult and may be impossible.

The problem of diagnosis in the elderly patient with nonvalvular normotensive heart disease and failure has long been a difficult one. Disregarding those rare instances due to disorders such as amyloid, scleroderma, Fiedler's myocarditis, etc., a high percentage of the remainder will be found at autopsy to have moderate to severe coronary sclerosis. However, this is often no more advanced than that seen in other elderly persons who had been free of clinical evidence of disease and have succumbed to unrelated disorders. Thus in the absence of clear evidence of a critical diminution of coronary flow, either by the presence of infarctional scars or through a previous clinical history of angina or infarction, the relationship between the coronary disease and the heart failure must be uncertain. The application of the term "arteriosclerotic heart disease" to such patients is unjustifiable. It is preferable to speak of "heart disease and failure of undetermined origin." Senile heart disease (Dock's presbycardia, p. 1378) alone, as the cause of heart failure, must be quite rare. Nevertheless, we do not believe that the *concept* of the aging myocardium as a frequent contributory cause of failure can be in doubt.

It is because of these considerations that we believe the term "arteriosclerotic heart disease" is misleading and should be discarded. "Coronary disease" is preferable but, by definition, includes the large number of insignificant atheromas found at autopsy. However, the term "ischemic heart disease," which is already widely used in Britain, is free from those objections because it implies a disturbance of function and that is what the physician can diagnose and treat.

Disease of the coronary arteries is the single most important cause of death in the United States. In men, atheroma begins in youth and occasionally produces its characteristic clinical effects in the third or fourth decades. More commonly, the process remains asymptomatic until after the age of forty in men, and until after fifty-five in women, who lose their remarkable immunity after the menopause.

The symptoms of coronary atheroma are due not to the intimal roughening but to the ischemia caused by the commonly associated narrowing. When the lumen is not compromised, the process cannot be detected. However, a roughened vessel, not previously narrow, may be the site of thrombus formation. Therefore, coronary thrombosis, myocardial infarction, and even sudden death may occasionally occur without previous symptoms. When symptoms do occur, they depend not directly on the degree of narrowing of the main arteries but rather on the balance between the progression of this narrowing and the rate at which collateral channels develop.

Etiologic Considerations. The usual cause of ischemic heart disease is atheromatous narrowing of the coronary arteries. The role of dietary and other factors in producing such changes has been discussed in some detail in Chap. 246.

Much less commonly, the coronary arteries may be compromised at their orifices by luetic aortitis or by dissecting aneurysm or affected by arteritis or embolism. The myocardial oxygen supply may also be impaired by congenital anomalies such as the origin of one main branch from the pulmonary artery or a congenital fistula between a coronary artery and a cardiac vein. However, disease of the aortic valves (p. 33), and especially stenosis, is the commonest cause, other than atheroma, of myocardial ischemia.

Conditions which impose a pressure load on the right ventricle may lead to pain which apparently arises in the wall of this chamber, as the result of its increased need for oxygen and the impairment of the normally great systolic flow to it (p. 34).

Ectopic tachycardia frequently induces anginal pain in older persons and may even do so in young patients who present no detectable evidence of structural disease of the coronary arteries.

Diffuse, nonischemic myocardial disease has occasionally been reported as being associated with anginal pain. Presumably, this is due to involvement of the sensory nerve fibers in the myocardium.

Aside from these several anatomic disorders, there are various other conditions which tend either to reduce coronary flow or to increase myocardial oxygen need. Paroxysmal tachycardia has already been mentioned. Anemia, thyrotoxicosis, and hypertension are rarely if ever primary causes of angina, but frequently aggravate it. In persons with coronary disease the attacks are often induced by emotion, eating, cold, or hypoglycemia. Physical exertion has a twofold effect. It increases cardiac work and hence is the commonest precipitating cause of attacks. However, it also tends to promote the development of collateral circulation through the smaller coronary channels. There is evidence (p. 1448) that minimal exercise which is one-half or less of that required to produce pain may actually improve the myocardial contraction, while effort sufficient to cause pain has the reverse effect. This apparent paradox, which was mentioned by William

Heberden in his initial description of angina pectoris, can be readily explained if one assumes that the milder exercise causes greater increase in coronary flow than in cardiac oxygen need, while in the presence of narrowed vessels the more strenuous effort has the reverse effect.

Many patients have attacks of angina appearing during recumbency and especially during sleep. Occasionally, these are precipitated by reabsorption of edema fluid from the legs as the result of the recumbent position, and in such an instance diuretic drugs may prevent the seizures. More commonly, the cause of the nocturnal attacks cannot be established. Various hemodynamic factors such as increased cardiac output in the horizontal position, higher recumbent blood pressure (in subjects with postural hypotension), carotid sinus effects, and in the left lateral position, the higher level of the orifice of the coronary sinus as compared to the arterial ostia have been proposed, but none has been clearly demonstrated to constitute the responsible mechanism.

ANGINA PECTORIS

Clinical Picture. The majority of patients with angina pectoris have pain that conforms closely to the classic pattern originally described so vividly and precisely by William Heberden in 1768. He pointed out that the subjects of the malady are more commonly men past their fiftieth year; that they are seized while walking, especially if uphill, and soon after eating, with a painful, strangling sensation behind the breastbone; the moment they stand still, the pain begins to subside. He also pointed out that the pain often extends into the left arm. Finally, he was familiar with the remarkable termination of the disorder: "For if no accident intervenes, but the disease go on to its height, the patients all suddenly fall down and perish immediately."

It is important to emphasize that the anginal pain is steady, and its unwavering quality is more important than the adjective that the patient uses to describe it. It is not influenced by breathing, swallowing, or twisting or turning of the body or arms.

The deviations from this pattern are frequent enough so that some of the more important ones deserve mention. The patient may insist the pain is "burning," not constrictive. It is not uncommon for anginal pain to be attributed to indigestion because it occurs after eating, but in the majority of such cases, the pain is actually precipitated by exercise which happens to be taken after a meal. In a small group of patients, it occurs after a meal, even though the patient remains completely at rest. Indeed, in some of these individuals, angina of effort may be absent. This unusual behavior is open to two interpretations. It may be that some persons are particularly susceptible to the reflex coronary constriction known to occur with the distention of abdominal viscera. On the other hand, it is possible that in such patients increased cardiac output during digestion, not attended by a decline in peripheral resistance such as occurs during exercise, may impose a load on the heart after eating that is greater than occurs during slow walking.

Some patients experience their initial attacks only on assuming the recumbent position, especially on retiring; only later does the angina of effort appear. In other patients, typical angina appears *not during* the exertion but immediately after. In some of these individuals postural hypotension is present, and the postexertional fall in mean aortic pressure may be sufficient to reduce coronary flow to the point where myocardial hypoxia and anginal pain at rest appear. This is particularly likely to happen in persons receiving ganglionic blocking drugs for the treatment of hypotension.

The location of the anginal pain may differ from the usual site and offer some difficulty of interpretation. Radiation into the neck and to the angles of the lower jaw is not uncommon, and the pain may be felt only there. In some cases, the pain may be experienced only in the back of the neck at about the level of the lower cervical vertebras, or in the interscapular space, or in the left shoulder (p. 18).

Finally, many patients do not "perish immediately."

Diagnosis. The cardinal clinical characteristics of angina are the *steady* unwavering chest pain that appears on exertion and that begins to subside promptly on resting. *When such history is obtained and, in addition, there is unquestionable and rapid relief of pain, or increased exercise tolerance, after the sublingual administration of an adequate dose of glyceryl trinitrate (nitroglycerin), the diagnosis may be considered established, regardless of the outcome of all other forms of examination.*

Diagnostic difficulties may arise from several sources. The patient may be unable to recall whether his pain was related to exertion; or he may be unable to say whether the "tightness" in his chest represents pain or dyspnea. Because the pain may not be described as constrictive or because it appears in an unusual location, the physician may not consider angina as a possibility and hence may fail to ascertain the influence of exercise.

When the patient suffers from the classic exertional angina and later experiences a similar pain at rest, there is usually no problem in recognizing the nature of the rest pain. It is when angina at rest appears as the initial symptom that the diagnosis may be obscure, for other conditions such as hiatal hernia, gallbladder disease, and esophageal spasm may simulate every feature of angina pec-

toris, aside from the characteristic relationship to exertion and the dramatic response to nitroglycerin. Careful study of these instances of angina at rest will sometimes uncover precipitating factors such as emotional strain, paroxysmal tachycardia, hypoglycemia, paroxysms of hypertension due to pheochromocytoma, or mild congestive failure with edema. Since even strenuous exertion may fail to induce an attack in an occasional patient, and since it may not be possible to secure an electrocardiogram during a bout of pain, the influence of nitroglycerin may constitute the sole evidence on which a somewhat equivocal diagnosis may be made. As is true for all such pains at rest, investigations must be made to exclude actual myocardial infarction, or hiatal hernia, gallbladder disease, etc. (p. 1454). However, the discovery of one of these abdominal disorders does not *ipso facto* prove that it was the cause of the pain.

Rarely, a skeletal pain arising in the chest wall or shoulder may seem at first glance to represent anginal pain, for the increased movements of the thoracic cage or the swinging of the arms during exertion may enhance pain arising from these structures. However, the character of the pain and the presence of tender areas in the chest wall or shoulder should clarify the nature of the pain without much difficulty.

The greatest difficulty arises with those patients who have not only angina but also some less serious cause of pain which is in the same general area and has a similar quality. At least a third of the patients with angina have one or more additional types of chest pain. The innocent cause, which is usually of skeletal origin, is then confused with the serious disease unless the patient is subjected to the most careful study (p. 37).

The physical examination is only occasionally helpful in the diagnosis of angina. The finding of aortic stenosis, or of ectopic tachycardia, or of a late systolic apical murmur (p. 1412) makes it probable but not certain that an accompanying chest pain is of anginal nature. If the patient is seen during an attack, an apical or precordial bulge may be felt in about a fifth of the subjects. However, this may be due to some other cause, such as a previous infarction, and is significant in the diagnosis of angina only if it vanishes as the pain disappears.

The common tendency to place a large emphasis on the resting electrocardiogram leads to serious errors in both directions. Misplaced precordial electrodes may give a mistaken impression that the record has changed (Fig. 254-1). Patients who, having had a myocardial infarction, have made a complete clinical recovery usually exhibit abnormal resting records and often have innocent chest pain arising in the skeletal tissues. This may be confused

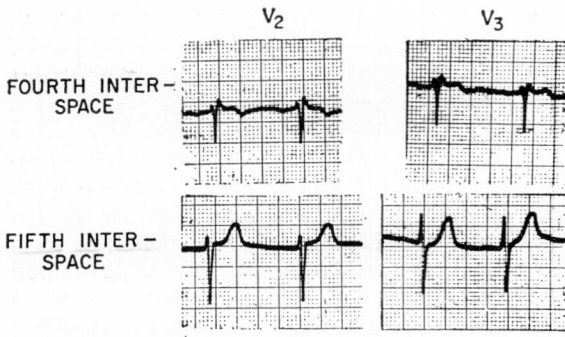

FIG. 254-1. This 65-year-old man had symptoms referable to an irritable colon but no clinical evidence of cardiovascular abnormalities. The electrocardiogram was initially thought to point toward coronary disease. X-ray revealed a low position of the diaphragm and of the heart. When the precordial tracings were repeated in a lower interspace, normal configurations were observed. Rigid adherence to rule-of-thumb techniques in recording precordial tracings, without consideration of the anatomic position of the heart, is often responsible for a false positive diagnosis of cardiac disease.

with anginal pain. Other persons who have healed pericarditis, emotional disturbances, old cardiac contusions, or postprandial hypokalemia may also present the combination of T-wave inversion at rest and insignificant chest pain (Figs. 254-2, 254-3, and 254-4). The electrocardiogram, though often normal or borderline, is sometimes invaluable in the diagnosis of angina, provided rigid criteria are utilized in interpreting those changes induced by exercise or occurring during a spontaneous attack

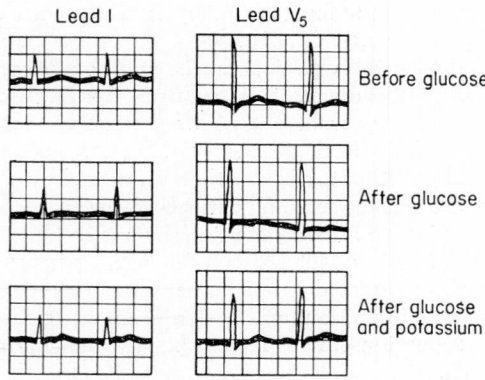

FIG. 254-2. The patient is a healthy 44-year-old man without evidence of cardiovascular disease. The T waves, which were upright in the fasting state, became inverted in V₅ and isoelectric in lead I, 40 min after the ingestion of 100 Gm glucose. When KCl was administered on the following day, the T waves remained unchanged. The record illustrates the fallacy of diagnosing coronary disease, or any type of organic heart disease, on the basis of T-wave inversion alone.

of pain, provided also that little attention is paid to those alterations found in the resting pain-free state.

We see no purpose in subjecting the patient even to the small risk of an exercise test when the story is already decisive. When, however, the history leaves doubt, as in the case of an initial bout of possible angina at rest, one may resort to an exercise test, provided one is reasonably sure that the pain had not been caused by an infarction. There is no virtue in a standardized test. The amount of exercise required to bring on anginal pain or the characteristic electrocardiographic changes is influenced little, if at all, by age, sex, or size. The history should provide the physician with a reasonably accurate idea of how vigorous and how long the exercise should be. Figure 254-5 illustrates diagrammatically the changes that occur with exertion and those which should be considered indicative of myocardial ischemia.

Anginal pain is often a more sensitive indicator than the electrocardiogram, and when exertion under the observation of the physician does induce characteristic pain and when the amount of tolerated exercise is significantly increased by prior administration of nitroglycerin, the result may be considered conclusive, regardless of the outcome of the serial electrocardiograms. If no pain is caused, but the electrocardiogram is decisive (Fig. 254-5), one can be almost equally certain that the patient does suffer from myocardial ischemia. However, a negative electrocardiographic response does not at all exonerate the patient, for in different studies 20 per cent or more of patients with unquestionable angina pectoris have failed to display the electrocardiographic abnormalities characteristic of coronary insufficiency after exercise.

Spontaneous Electrocardiographic Changes. Unless there has been a previous infarction, the electrocardiogram is usually normal during the pain-free state. A few patients continue to exhibit normal records during the attacks, but more often S-T segment depression occurs in multiple leads and vanishes as the pain subsides. This alteration has been interpreted as due to subendocardial ischemia. However, similar changes have been observed in direct epicardial leads from dogs during hemorrhagic shock and from patients with known ischemic heart disease during thoracotomy. Such tracings, indicating scattered regions of ischemia surrounded by large areas of electrically normal tissue, throw doubt on the concept of the subendocardial origin of S-T segment changes. In any case, it would appear that multiple areas of focal ischemia are responsible for the widespread S-T depression commonly seen during anginal attacks.

An occasional patient exhibits, during the seizures, marked reciprocal S-T changes, with elevation and depression in opposite leads. These temporary alterations, which are identical with those commonly observed during the early phase of myocardial infarction ("current of injury"), have been produced in dogs by the temporary occlusion of a main coronary branch. It is, therefore, probable that when seen in man these reciprocal changes indicate predominancy of a single large area of ischemia rather than the effects of multiple smaller patches.

The administration of potassium salts may be of value in the differentiation of T-wave inversions of innocent origin (anxiety, hyperventilation, carbohydrate ingestion, etc.) from somewhat similar inversions due to ischemia. Only in the former group is complete abolition of the inversion in all leads likely to occur.

It is essential to bear in mind that the physical examination and resting electrocardiogram can never establish the diagnosis of angina pectoris. All that they can do is to provide information indicating that a cardiac disorder that *could* cause myocardial ischemia is present. Except when the post-exertional electrocardiogram is characteristic or when one may secure an electrocardiographic tracing during an attack of spontaneous pain, the diagnosis of angina must rest on the history and the response to drugs. It should be reemphasized that anginal pain is practically always rapidly and completely relieved by nitroglycerin, provided the dose taken is sufficient to produce headache and/or flush. The use of old tablets which have deteriorated because of exposure to light is a common source of error. *Direct observation of the response to effort and to nitrites will usually prove to be the most valuable method of diagnosis when the story is confusing.*

Prognosis. Prognosis is more uncertain in this disorder than in any other chronic disease. Occasionally, a patient may suffer from angina for a period of time, following which the pain may disappear permanently, even with strenuous activity; presumably, completely compensatory collaterals to the previously ischemic area have developed. In others, the severity of the angina may wax and wane over periods of time, depending on the race between the growth of collaterals and the progression of obstructive lesions. Angina may disappear after an infarction; or, frequently, it becomes worse than it had been before. An important point to remember is that, even in patients with infrequent and mild attacks of angina, sudden death is always a possibility. The other extreme is illustrated by a patient we have personally observed who survived for forty-eight years after the diagnosis was made by William Osler.

There is a long tradition that angina disappears with the onset of congestive failure. This is certainly not always true and, when it occurs, is presumably due to the obligatory restriction of activity

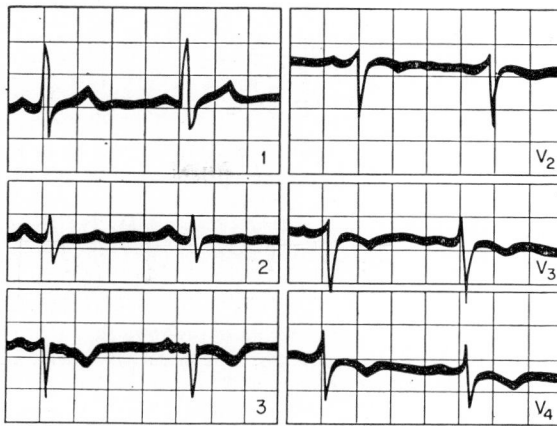

Fig. 254-3. This 32-year-old man had been rejected for insurance because of the inverted T waves in the precordial leads. These had been interpreted as evidence of coronary disease. The history, physical examination, and fluoroscopic study revealed no evidence of cardiac disease. The patient was able to perform vigorous and even violent exercise without any symptoms pointing toward cardiac disease.

Four years previously his sternum had been fractured by impact against the steering wheel in an automobile accident. The electrocardiographic changes illustrated are believed to have resulted from a contusion of the heart and are not considered to have any clinical significance. The record illustrates the fallacy of placing predominant emphasis upon the electrocardiographic rather than on the clinical findings.

and not to any inherent incompatibility between the mechanism of congestive failure and of anginal pain.

Treatment. Aside from relief of discomfort, the therapy is aimed at the promotion of collateral circulation and at prevention of further atheromatous deposit and of the common complications, which are myocardial infarction, congestive heart

S-T segment depression due to anxiety

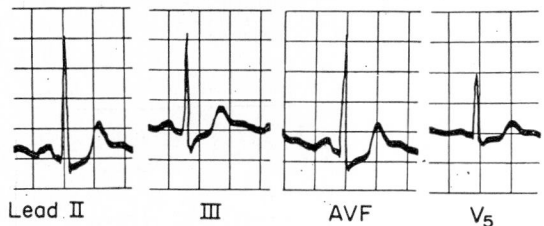

Lead II   III   AVF   V₅

Fig. 254-4. This man was rejected by the draft board because of a murmur. Since then he has suffered from a chronic anxiety state. This type of depressed S-T junction with an S-T segment rising to the base line may be seen in some healthy persons following exercise and/or tachycardia. It has no significance as an indication of coronary disease (see Fig. 254-5).

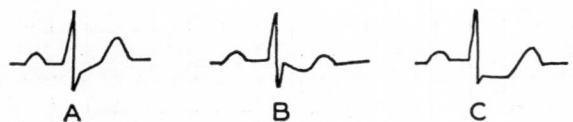

FIG. 254-5. *A.* Slight to moderate postexertional depression of the S-T junction with an upsloping S-T segment is of no significance (see Fig. 254-4).

B. Postexertional downsloping S-T segment. This may be due to digitalis therapy. Otherwise, its appearance after exercise is strong evidence of myocardial ischemia.

C. Marked depression of the entire S-T segment. This change, when occurring after exertion and disappearing within a few minutes, is conclusive evidence of ischemia, but few patients with angina exhibit such a marked alteration.

failure, and sudden death. Another aim is to detect and manage certain commonly associated conditions which are likely to aggravate angina. Of these, obesity, diabetes, hypertension, ectopic rhythms, anemia, and thyrotoxicosis are especially significant.

Physical Activity. The circumstances which induce pain should be avoided. Therefore, walking should be reduced during the first 2 hr after meals, or when there is emotional stress. Outdoor activity should be sharply curtailed during cold weather.

There is now convincing evidence that exercise of a degree considerably less than that required to induce the pain is not only harmless but likely to be positively beneficial (Fig. 254-6). It is probable but unproved that, when undertaken after a coronary dilator drug, the desirable effect of widening collateral channels is enhanced. Although the actual amount of activity prescribed will vary widely from patient to patient, according to the severity of the disorder, the general principle that *exertion which induces pain or dyspnea should be avoided, while that which does not cause these symptoms should be encouraged* is applicable to all.

Emotional Stress. All efforts should be made to curtail anxiety and worry. When, as is often true, this aim cannot be achieved, tranquilizing drugs are indicated. The relative value of meprobamate, rauwolfia—with due consideration of its tendency to cause depression in predisposed persons—and of

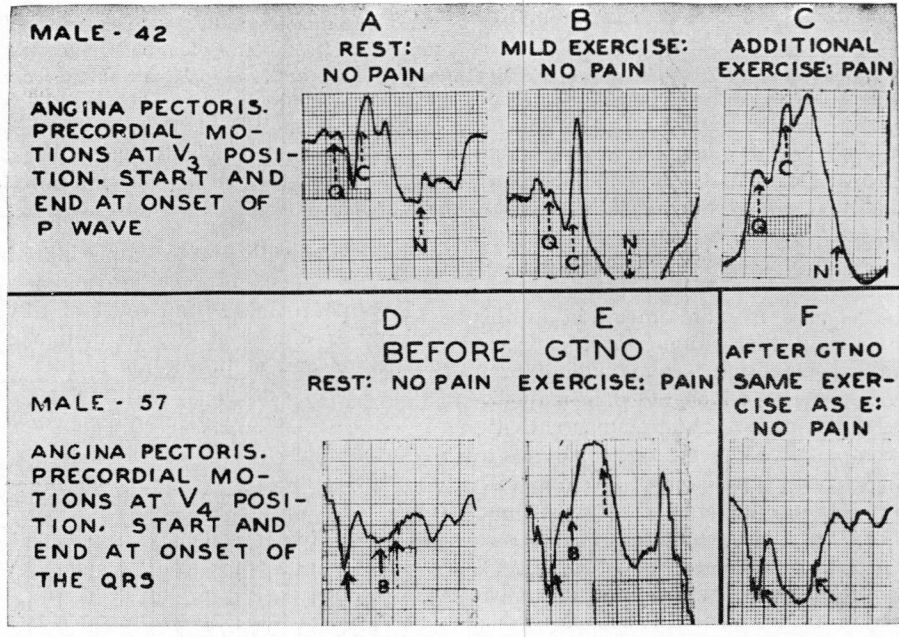

FIG. 254-6. *A, B, C:* Q, C, and N indicate, respectively, times of Q of ECG of carotid upstroke and of carotid incisura. At rest (*A*) the trace is somewhat abnormal because the downstroke of ejection is delayed. Following mild exercise the record (*B*) is entirely normal, with a large inward motion (downstroke) during systole. Additional exercise which produced anginal pain caused the record to become grossly abnormal (*C*). The systolic bulge has now returned in exaggerated form and the atrial motion (upstroke before Q) is pronounced, indicating defective ventricular emptying and increased atrial stretch.

D, E, F: The solid and dotted arrows indicate the carotid upstroke and incisura, respectively. The resting record (*D*) is borderline, showing a rather small downstroke during ejection. Exercise sufficient to produce pain caused a large outward systolic bulge (arrow *B* in *E*). The same exercise caused no such effect when undertaken 1 hr after the application of glyceryl trinitrate ointment (*F*). The precordial trace at this time is entirely normal. (Paper speed 50 mm per sec.)

barbiturates will vary from one patient to another. Anxiety about the heart which is often a major cause of emotional stress can be partially alleviated by reassurance, including the true statement that many patients with angina live for decades.

Mild physical fatigue is often the best antidote for emotional stress. Thus fishing, golf, and other recreational activities should be encouraged, provided they do not induce attacks and the patient enjoys them. The spectator sports may be harmful because they provide the undesirable effect of excitement without the benefit of mild physical exertion.

Reduction of Cholesterol. Although the problem of diet remains controversial, we believe that restriction of foods rich in saturated fatty acids is advisable. The foods to be avoided are those rich in butterfat, yolks of egg, fats of meat, hydrogenated vegetable oils, coconut, and cocoa butter. Vegetable oil containing a high percentage of unsaturated fatty acids, such as cottonseed, corn, peanut, or soybean oils, are considered beneficial if they are given in large quantities (40 per cent of total caloric intake). Further details of dietary management and of the use of such drugs as triparanol (MER/29), nicotinic acid, and thyroid derivatives are presented on p. 1364. The unpleasant side effects of nicotinic acid can be reduced either by the use of the aluminum salt, which is expensive, or by gradual increments of dosage up to 1.5 to 3 Gm after each meal. The effects of these several substances are additive, probably because the mechanism of the action of each drug differs, and the most effective results are usually obtained when two or more are employed simultaneously.

It is probable that the hypercholesterolemia, which is common in patients with angina, is secondary to distortions of the metabolism of other fats and especially of the triglycerides. The therapeutic implications of this concept are not yet entirely known.

Drugs. Sublingual nitroglycerin is indicated (1) to treat pain, (2) to prevent it, and (3) in conjunction with subthreshold exercise to promote collateral circulation (see discussion above). It should be taken prophylactically before activities, such as sexual intercourse or a tense business conference, which have been found by experience to induce attacks. When used for pain it should be repeated every 5 min until relief is obtained. If this does not occur after several pills, there is a strong possibility of myocardial infarction. The dose varies from one patient to another but in most is slightly less than that required to produce headache.

Long-acting coronary dilator drugs are rarely of striking benefit in patients with mild angina. Their use in the severer variety is discussed later.

Anticoagulants and monamine oxidase inhibitors are considered later in the discussion of the management of preinfarctional angina.

Frequent premature beats in patients with angina indicate increased likelihood of ventricular fibrillation. They should usually be treated with quinidine or procaine amide, unless there are contraindications to the use of these drugs (p. 1396).

In patients with angina and overt congestive failure, or with nocturnal attacks that are suspected of being precipitated by reabsorption of edema fluid, digitalis and sodium restriction are employed. *Diuretics must be given with great caution,* because of the possibility of potassium depletion and consequent intoxication by amounts of digitalis ordinarily well tolerated. We are familiar with several instances of sudden death occurring within a brief period after diuretics were first employed in patients with ischemic heart disease. In the opinion of some, salt restriction should be practiced by all patients with angina.

Tobacco should be prohibited when it clearly induces pain, premature beats, or pronounced increase in heart rate or blood pressure. It is possibly harmful in others, and its reduction or withdrawal will depend on the reaction of the individual. There is no evidence that alcohol in strict moderation has either harmful or beneficial effects. Coffee and tea should be allowed also unless they can be shown to cause pain, premature beats, or sleeplessness.

Certain additional therapeutic procedures which may be considered in patients with unusually severe or "intractable" angina are discussed later.

Preinfarctional Angina (*Coronary Insufficiency*)

The choice of a suitable designation for the intermediate form of coronary pain, one that does not fall into the category of effort angina of brief duration or the prolonged pain with unquestionable manifestations of myocardial necrosis, is difficult. "Coronary insufficiency" and "coronary failure" are not accurate, since any pain due to hypoxia of the myocardium, whether brief or prolonged, is due to insufficiency or failure of the coronary circulation. "Status anginosus" simply implies a prolonged pain but does not indicate whether or not infarction is present. "Prolonged angina without evidence of myocardial necrosis" appears to be the most accurate designation, but it is clumsy. The term *preinfarctional angina* is not free from objections, but since prolonged angina is actually a forerunner of infarction in many instances and since, from a physiologic standpoint, it is but one step away from the stage of myocardial necrosis, it appears to us to be the most suitable for the condition under consideration.

Occasionally, preinfarctional angina develops in a previously asymptomatic subject. Much more commonly, its onset is heralded by a sudden worsening of previous exertional angina, the attacks appearing with much less effort than before and also occurring frequently at rest.

Prolonged, frequent, and severe anginal attacks appearing at rest or with minimal exertion are likely to be observed under any of three conditions. In a few patients they may be induced by an *increased load on the heart*, such as severe emotional stress or the excessive ingestion of salt. When the cause is removed, the patient will usually return to the previous state, having only brief and milder pain with exertion.

Less frequently, severe and prolonged angina is initiated by some condition such as dehydration, hemorrhage, shock, ectopic tachycardia, or pulmonary embolism, which *reduces cardiac output* and thus causes further decline in blood flow through a coronary system already compromised by atheromatous disease. Of particular importance are those instances in which the circulatory failure induced by an initial myocardial infarction may lead to ischemic pain in other myocardial regions and thus be a threat of more extensive infarction.

More commonly, however, these prolonged and severe attacks are not associated with demonstrable increase in load or decline in output, but apparently with progression of coronary obstruction and an *increasingly unfavorable balance between narrowing of main branches and widening of collateral channels*. The patient now begins to have attacks of increasing severity and duration on less and less exertion and to be awakened frequently by seizures. Some patients may have only one such attack of prolonged pain. The electrocardiographic changes may be absent or minimal, but records during the pain will usually exhibit depression of S-T segments in multiple leads (p. 1446).

The traditional distinction between acute myocardial infarction and preinfarctional angina is a somewhat artificial one since daily measurements of transaminase over a period of 1 or 2 weeks have shown that most instances of the latter disorder are actually associated with some tissue necrosis. The area destroyed is often so small that the other signs of infarction, such as fever, leukocytosis, elevation of the sedimentation rate, overt congestive failure, and permanent electrocardiographic changes, are lacking. Thus one is not justified in an attitude of complacence when the usual signs of infarction are absent, since preinfarctional angina appears to be frequently caused by a partial or even a complete closure of a coronary branch, and the collateral blood supply to the involved area maintains a tenuous balance between supply and need. Without proper therapy, a fairly high percentage of the patients will, within a short time, develop a much more severe attack with unquestionable infarction. Thus, in one large series, about 50 per cent of

those untreated or inadequately treated developed a frank myocardial infarct, while this occurred in only 7 per cent of those properly managed.

Treatment. The patient should be hospitalized. The sedimentation rate, transaminase, and electrocardiogram must be repeated frequently. An accurate pain diary should be kept by the patient and should include meals as well as the exact time of onset and relief of the pain, the number of sublingual pills, and the time and dosage of long-acting coronary dilator drugs. In order to facilitate widening of collaterals, slow brief walks should be taken every hour when awake provided they induce no pain, which they usually do not, and also provided there is no clinical or electrocardiographic evidence of infarction. Unless a contraindication, such as an active peptic ulcer, exists, heparin should be administered for several weeks. When economic or other reasons make this impractical, one of the coumarin drugs may be employed.

There is wide difference of opinion concerning the long-acting coronary dilator drugs. Assessment of their value is made difficult by spontaneous fluctuation in the severity of angina, by the necessity for separation of psychic from pharmacologic effects, and by those subconscious preconceptions which affect all physicians. There is pressing need for the most rigidly controlled "double blind" studies on a very large series of patients. Pending such, one must rely on such sparse objective evidence as is available, plus clinical experience tempered with Osler's optimistic skepticism. Subject to these reservations, our present opinion of these drugs is that despite an occasional exception most of them are of limited value in most patients. However, nitroglycerin ointment (Nitrol) is usually effective as demonstrated not only by (1) the appearance of the typical headache, indicating a pharmacologic effect, and (2) an abrupt decrease in the number of attacks of pain, but also by (3) objective evidence of improved myocardial contraction (Fig. 254-6).

The 2 per cent nitroglycerin ointment should be applied to the skin and spread as thinly as possible without massage. The initial dose should be a 1-in. column as measured from the containing tube, and should be progressively increased until one has determined the largest dose which can be taken without unpleasant side effects (commonly, headache; rarely, postural hypotension). This will usually be $1\frac{1}{2}$ to 2 in. The ointment is applied every 4 hr, an alarm clock being used to prevent omission of the midnight dose. If the diary shows that the pain is appearing at the height of the ointment's action, 1 to 2 hr after application, the dose should be increased. The occurrence of pain as the drug's effect diminishes, 3 to 4 hr after application, calls for greater frequency of administration. Most patients respond better to this regime than to the orally or sublingually administered long-acting dilators such as erythritol tetranitrate or pentaerythritol tetranitrate. In a few the reverse seems to be true, and in some patients the alternation of one of these drugs with the ointment appears desirable.

Once the pain has been controlled, the dosage of the ointment should be slowly reduced over a period of several weeks, in order to decrease the likelihood of the patient's becoming unresponsive to nitroglycerin, which otherwise occasionally occurs.

The value of prolonged or permanent anticoagulation is disputed. There is evidence that heparin, although more expensive, is the drug of choice for this purpose.

The monamine oxidase inhibitors are being widely used in patients with angina. There is no convincing evidence that they have any direct action on the coronary flow. Such beneficial effects, occasionally striking, usually questionable, as are observed are perhaps to be ascribed to a central action, with improvement in general outlook and reduction in emotional stress, or possibly, to an effect on norepinephrine metabolism. Some of these drugs may have serious toxic effects. Pending more complete information, they should be employed with great caution and only in those rare patients who do not respond to other measures.

The remaining measures which are valuable in treating preinfarctional angina are those which have already been discussed in the management of the less severe form of the disease. These include for all patients regulation of activity and of diet, plus reduction of emotional stress. The antiarrhythmic drugs, digitalis, diuretics, and potassium salts are utilized when the aforementioned indications exist. Those additional measures which are of prime importance in the preinfarctional type of angina are (1) anticoagulation, (2) frequent minimal subthreshold exertion, and (3) long-acting coronary dilator drugs. The last two measures are aimed at the promotion of collateral circulation to the critically ischemic regions of the heart.

"Intractable" Angina

In some patients the relationship between progressive narrowing of main arteries and compensatory widening of smaller channels may remain in a state of precarious balance for months, with episodes of angina during the slightest physical or emotional stress and also during sleep. Under such circumstances various special therapeutic measures have been advocated. Among them are some, such as ligation of the internal mammary artery, which have no sound rational basis and which appear to act only by suggestion. The various other surgical procedures aimed at increasing myocardial blood supply are still to be regarded as being in the experimental stage. Interruption of afferent pathways by direct section or by alcohol injection and reduction of the demands on the heart by the administration of radioiodine are rarely if ever indicated. The so-called intractable angina is actually a chronic form of the preinfarctional type. There is no convincing evidence that any of these procedures prevent the massive infarction or the sudden death which may occur despite the most vigorous therapy. In any case, the large majority of patients survive and improve when the conservative plan of management which has been discussed is applied for several weeks. A goodly percentage of them eventually return to useful but restricted activity.

The surgical treatment of angina due to aortic stenosis is an exception to these general statements. Although the risk remains high, this procedure is entirely justified in properly selected patients (p. 1435).

ACUTE MYOCARDIAL INFARCTION

Coronary occlusion, coronary thrombosis, and *myocardial infarction* are often used synonymously, although the last term is the proper clinical designation for the condition to be discussed. Myocardial infarction is always the result of a gross discrepancy between the blood supply and needs of the myocardium, usually developing so rapidly that compensatory flow through collateral channels is inadequate to nourish the compromised area of myocardium. This may take place as a result of progressive atherosclerotic narrowing, with or without thrombosis or hemorrhage at the site of a sclerotic plaque, or of any of those circumstances responsible for increased load on the heart or diminished coronary flow described under Preinfarctional Angina (p. 1450), provided they are sufficiently severe and prolonged. Among the rarer causes are coronary embolism, occlusion of a coronary ostium by luetic aortitis, dissecting aneurysm, and polyarteritis. Right ventricular infarction is quite uncommon (about 3 per cent), the immunity of the right ventricle being due to the lesser work load and the proportionately greater coronary reserve.

The Classical Clinical Picture. In the usual case, the patient is seized with a chest pain similar to that of angina, except that it is unrelated to exertion. It is more intense and prolonged, tends to radiate more widely, and is not ordinarily influenced by nitroglycerin. The pain usually is described as having a constrictive quality, it tends to reach a peak rapidly, and it remains at this level without wavering from moment to moment; in other words, it is a *steady* pain, not affected by bodily movements or breathing or swallowing, an extremely important diagnostic feature. Shortly after the onset of the pain, the patient perspires profusely, the skin becomes pallid, cool, and moist, and there is a moderate drop in blood pressure. At the same time, dyspnea, weakness, and faintness occur; nausea and vomiting are common. The heart rate is increased somewhat, although occasionally it remains as low as 70 to 80; an early diastolic gallop rhythm is frequently heard, and fine and medium moist rales are audible at the bases of the lungs. After a variable period of time, the manifestations of shock disappear, and the pain gradually subsides, leaving behind a dull ache that may persist for a few hours or up to a day or so. Within a few hours after the beginning of pain, leukocytosis is observed, followed by fever; still later, usually between 24 and 48 hr after the onset, the sedimentation rate becomes elevated. In the more severe cases, the white blood count rises to 12,000 to 20,000 and may remain elevated up to 10 to 14 days; the fever reaches levels of 100 to 103°F, usually subsiding within 10 days; the sedimentation rate may be elevated for 3 or 4 weeks. The serum transaminase usually begins to rise in 6 to 12 hr and reaches a peak within 24 to 48 hr and then subsides to normal levels in 4 to 7 days. In about 80 per cent of the cases, characteristic electrocardiographic alterations are noted: S-T elevation followed by inversion of the T waves and the appearance of Q waves. In the remainder, the electrocardiographic abnormalities, absent in the first day or two, are observed to appear within 7 to 10 days provided daily tracings are recorded. A small percentage of patients exhibit only minor and nonspecific alterations or no abnormalities at all even in the presence of an otherwise classical clinical picture.

After the first day or two, when the pain has usually disappeared, the patient may be so free of subjective symptoms that it may be difficult to persuade him of the seriousness of the attack and of the necessity of several weeks of careful management. The gallop rhythm and the basilar rales may persist for as long as 2 to 3 weeks. Sometime during the first week, usually after the first day and before the seventh, a pericardial friction rub may be heard in about 10 to 15 per cent of cases. The pericarditis is usually asymptomatic but may rarely be associated with mild pain aggravated by breathing.

The above description applies to patients suffering an attack of moderate severity. In milder attacks, all the clinical manifestations are correspondingly reduced, some even being absent, and the evidence of myocardial necrosis (fever, elevated sedimentation rate, and leukocytosis) is minimal or absent. Practically invariably, however, the serum transaminase is slightly increased or displays variations of range greater than 12 to 15 units, even though the highest figure may be less than 40. On the other hand, in the most severe cases, shock is profound and may last for hours or even days, death being prevented only by the most vigorous therapy. Pulmonary edema and later systemic failure are more pronounced. Cardiac output may be so reduced and peripheral blood flow so impaired that cerebral infarction, gangrene of the extremities or bowel, or acute tubular necrosis of the kidneys may ensue.

The severity of the attack, which is an important guide to the immediate and distant prognosis, is judged not by the extent of the electrocardiographic alterations, but by the total clinical picture and the magnitude of those manifestations which signify myocardial necrosis. The more severe the signs of left ventricular failure (dependent, in addition, on the preexisting condition of the myocardium), the more profound the shock, the higher and longer the duration of the fever, serum transaminase, leukocytosis, and sedimentation rate, the greater has been the myocardial damage, regardless of the appearance of the electrocardiogram. The converse is also true: when all the above phenomena are minimal, the myocardial insult has been small, even in the face of an electrocardiogram that may be interpreted as revealing "massive" infarction (QS waves in all or most of the precordial leads). The electrocardiogram is invaluable in substantiating a clinical impression of acute myocardial infarction; it is of little value in informing us as to the gravity of the attack. Of all the laboratory tests, the transaminase level is the one that parallels best the actual severity of the infarction. Figures of 300 or more always indicate a large and probably fatal infarction. One must bear in mind, however, that a very high transaminase figure that is altogether inconsistent with the mildness of all other clinical signs and symptoms may be caused by central necrosis of the liver lobules, particularly prone to occur if the initial fall in blood pressure is rather severe and prolonged. There is some evidence that estimations of serum lactic dehydrogenase activity may provide more accurate information than does the serum glutamic oxalacetic transaminase activity, now almost universally employed.

Mode of Onset. Myocardial infarction may present itself in a wide variety of pictures aside from the usual and classical one depicted above. A completely painless and symptomless infarct may be discovered in an electrocardiogram taken on a presumably healthy and active person who is simply having a routine checkup. There are a number of other forms of painless infarction, and these may present themselves as acute pulmonary edema or the sudden and rapid worsening of congestive failure; development of arrhythmias, such as heart block, ventricular tachycardia, atrial flutter, or fibrillation; transitory syncope that may not appear to differ from an ordinary innocent faint were it not for the appearance of unquestionable electrocardiographic and transaminase alterations; the development of the typical picture of shock of obscure origin, again recognized only by these same diagnostic findings; focal cerebral symptoms, such as a hemiplegia, caused either by a sudden drop in blood pressure with impairment of blood flow through a sclerotic but hitherto asymptomatic cerebral vessel, or by an embolus originating in a mural thrombus overlying a painless infarct or scar. It is important to bear in mind that painless infarctions occur not uncommonly during anesthesia or postoperative narcosis or in the course of illnesses, such as diabetic acidosis, which impair consciousness.

Complications. There are a relatively limited number of serious complications that introduce special problems of management and that are responsible for most of the deaths in acute myocardial infarction.

Shock. When, at the onset of the attack, the systolic blood pressure level falls below 80 to 90 mm Hg in a previously normotensive person or below 110 to 120 mm Hg in a previously hypertensive patient and remains at these low levels for 2 hr or more, and *when this fall is associated with the clinical picture of shock*, the prognosis is extremely grave, over 90 per cent ending in death unless prompt treatment is administered. The cause of the shock is not fully understood; a major factor in most instances must be the sudden decline in cardiac output. This cannot be the whole story, however, for occasionally one sees shock as the initial manifestation when there are no signs of acute left ventricular failure (gallop rhythm, basilar rales) and almost no evidence of myocardial necrosis except a minimal elevation of the serum transaminase. There is some experimental evidence that obscure reflexes arising from the heart play a contributory role.

Acute Pulmonary Edema. In the earliest stages of a severe attack, the sudden impairment of contractile power of the left ventricle may lead to serious or fatal pulmonary edema. This is usually associated with more or less severe shock; signs of systemic congestive failure are absent. If the patient survives for more than a day or two and left ventricular contractile power fails to recover, or if he has improved and a complication supervenes that imposes an additional burden on the heart (ruptured septum, new infarction, ectopic tachycardia), the picture of systemic congestive failure appears.

Abnormal Rhythms. The appearance of an ectopic tachycardia, which can be of any type, may suddenly alter the course from one that is progressing favorably to one of grave danger. The harmful effect of the tachycardias is due to the rapid rate with its accompanying relative increase in systolic contraction time and abbreviation of diastole. The net result is increased work of the heart, diminished coronary flow and cardiac output. Heart block of either high second degree or complete block introduces the risk of ventricular standstill or fibrillation; fortunately, the block almost invariably disappears within 2 weeks, provided the patient survives.

Rupture of the Myocardium. Rupture of the free wall of the ventricle at the site of the infarction with rapid development of cardiac tamponade occurs in about 10 per cent of the fatal cases; the incidence is higher in older patients beyond seventy and is particularly likely to occur in older women. Rupture is apt to develop within the first 14 days, and death occurs so rapidly that it is rarely possible to determine which of the causes of sudden death has been responsible. Rupture of the interventricular septum is much less common. The diagnosis is suggested by the appearance of a loud systolic murmur at the lower left sternal border, often associated with a systolic thrill, the rapid increase in congestive failure, and death within a week. Rarely, a patient with this complication may live for several years. Far more uncommon than either of the above forms of rupture is the rupture of an infarcted papillary muscle, which is responsible for the sudden appearance of murmurs, loudest at the apex, and the development of a fatal pulmonary edema within a few hours. The appearance of a late systolic murmur unassociated with heart failure is not uncommon and does not signify myocardial rupture. It is probably due to a distortion of a papillary muscle by the ischemic process. If the heart enlarges markedly, the pansystolic murmur of a relative mitral insufficiency may appear.

Thromboembolism. Systemic embolism arising from left ventricular thrombi may lead to serious or fatal complications: gangrene of the legs, hemiplegia, occlusion of abdominal vessels, etc. Much more common are pulmonary emboli, sometimes due to a right ventricular mural thrombus overlying a septal infarct, but far more often due to emboli originating in the deep veins of the legs. Finally, a second myocardial infarct due to development of another coronary thrombosis may occur while the patient is recovering from the first. These various thromboembolic complications are less common at present than before the widespread employment of anticoagulant therapy.

Other Complications and Sequelae. During the past few years, increasing attention has been directed to the *post-myocardial-infarction syndrome*. This usually occurs within 2 months after the acute infarction, in about 3 to 5 per cent of the cases. Recurrences may develop up to 2 years or even later. The characteristic features are fever, leukocytosis, pleuritis and pericarditis—often with effusion—and pneumonitis; the pleural and pericardial exudates may be hemorrhagic. It is evident that the clinical picture is practically identical with that of the postcommissurotomy syndrome, and it has been postulated that both syndromes have a common basis: sensitization to antigens resulting from myocardial necrosis (p. 1468). The importance of the syndrome lies in the fact that it is generally a benign disorder but that it may be mistaken for a recurrence of myocardial infarction.

Ventricular aneurysm occurs in about 20 per cent of cases within weeks or months after the acute attack. It is more frequent in hypertensive persons, usually appearing at the apex or anterior wall of the left ventricle, and it may be recognized at the bedside by the observation of a large area of pulsation that is distinctly independent of the apical pulsation. By x-ray, abnormal bulges of the ventricular contour and a paradoxical pulsation may be witnessed. The aneurysm practically never ruptures and in most instances does not alter the prognosis.

The shoulder-hand syndrome is characterized by pain and tenderness of the shoulder, followed by pain, redness, swelling, and stiffness of the hand and fingers, occasionally terminating in atrophy of the small muscles of the hand. The cause is unknown. The syndrome occurs in 5 to 10 per cent of patients and develops any time within a year following the attack (p. 1923).

Perforation of or massive hemorrhage from a peptic ulcer may develop during an acute myocardial infarction and is possibly caused by increased adrenocortical activity.

The Problem of Acute Prolonged Chest Pain (Diagnosis of Acute Myocardial Infarction). We are here concerned with the question of acute, prolonged chest pain, steady and unwavering, persisting for 20 min or more; unprovoked and uninfluenced by exertion, breathing, swallowing, turning or twisting of chest or shoulders or by any other bodily function or activity; unrelieved by nitroglycerin; and subsiding spontaneously or only after the administration of a narcotic. One is faced not only with the problem of deciding whether the patient is suffering from infarction or preinfarctional angina (p. 1449) but also with the possibility that any one of a number of other conditions aside from acute myocardial ischemia may have given rise to this type of pain. It is simple enough to lay down rules of differentiation when each of these disorders presents itself in so classical a form that confusion, one with the others, constitutes no serious problem. But there are a number of circumstances that often interfere with the ready solution of the matter.

In acute myocardial infarction, the characteristic electrocardiographic alterations may be absent during the first few days or even throughout the entire course; or they may be obscured by electrocardiographic changes caused by previous and now completely healed infarcts or by left bundle block or left ventricular hypertrophy. The introduction of the serum transaminase test has been of great value, but quite aside from the elevations associated with necrosis of the liver or with acute pancreatitis, we must bear in mind that chest pain with an accompanying elevation in the transaminase level may be due to an *acute pulmonary embolism*, the transaminase increase being caused by involvement of skeletal muscle adjacent to the thrombophlebitis responsible for the embolus. Moreover, the characteristic electrocardiogram of acute cor pulmonale occurs too infrequently to be of much assistance. The combination of elevated lactic dehydrogenase, normal transaminase, and increased serum bilirubin is suggestive of pulmonary infarction; increase in the serum level of both enzymes with little or no elevation of bilirubin points toward myocardial infarction.

If one lays any stress on the "tearing" pain said to be characteristic of *dissecting aneurysm*, one relies on a myth that has been conjured up by writers who assume that a tear should be associated with a "tearing" pain. The chest pain of dissecting aneurysm is identical with the pain of acute myocardial infarction, and if perchance, a rare individual happens to use the term "tearing," the adjective means little or nothing: it is employed just as frequently, or more accurately, rarely, by patients who suffer from other disorders aside from dissecting aneurysm. It is often written that a distinction between the pain of dissecting aneurysm and myocardial infarction may be made on the basis that the former reaches its peak very rapidly or instantaneously. We have found this point, too, of value only occasionally, since patients suffering from a severe pain of this type are rarely able to give a clear story about the rapidity with which the peak is reached. Finally, the dissection may involve a coronary artery, in which case dissecting aneurysm no longer merely mimics but actually causes infarction.

The pain of *acute pericarditis* may for the first few hours have a steady quality indistinguishable from that of acute infarction, and it may be referred to the arms and back or jaws in identically the same manner.

In a very high percentage of cases, pain due to *hiatal hernia, gallbladder colic, acute pancreatitis, ruptured peptic ulcer* is centered at or below the level of the xiphoid, whereas the pain of acute myocardial infarction is centered above these levels; but occasionally, pain may be distributed in an atypical fashion, the former above and the latter below the xiphoid (p. 16).

The lesson to be drawn from these reflections is

that, *since by definition, the chest pain has occurred spontaneously, we cannot derive any assistance from provoking or relieving factors; and since the character and location and reference of the pain may be identical in all the disorders enumerated, one can reach a diagnosis only by consideration of corollary features, clinical and laboratory, that may be present at the onset or that may appear after a day or several days of observation.* Thus we refer, to name only some of the items, to the development of manifestations of thrombophlebitis especially in a person confined to bed and of the x-ray findings in the chest indicative of pulmonary infarction (acute pulmonary embolism); or the distribution of pain at a distance far more remote than could be attributed to infarction, inequality of arterial pulsations in upper and lower extremities, appearance of a new diastolic murmur typical of aortic insufficiency (dissecting aneurysm); or the development of fever and pericardial friction rub from the very onset of the pain or within 2 to 4 hr, the early aggravation of the pain by breathing, swallowing, or change of position (acute pericarditis); or the information contributed by the serum amylase, bilirubin, alkaline phosphatase or by x-ray studies in the diagnosis of hiatal hernia, gallbladder colic, acute pancreatitis, and perforation of peptic ulcer. Often, even if one does secure unassailable evidence of an acute pericarditis, one still remains in doubt as to whether one is dealing with an acute, benign (viral) pericarditis or the pericarditis of post-myocardial-infarction syndrome.

Finally, in the interests of completeness and accuracy, one must add that there are instances of chest pain (or high epigastric pain) in which the corollary data at the onset or acquired after observation are insufficient to permit one to arrive at a diagnosis with anything approaching certainty and in which one must concede that one can speak only in terms of relative probability or possibility.

The differentiation of the various causes of chest pain is not the only problem introduced by the question of acute myocardial infarction. We have already enumerated the syndromes that may be caused by acute painless infarction: syncope, shock, sudden dyspnea and congestive failure, cerebrovascular episodes. Each one introduces its own problems of diagnosis and, once again, the solution is not always simple and certain. There is no royal road to the diagnosis of acute myocardial infarction, not even when the road is traveled by the most astute and experienced clinician.

Prognosis. The prognosis is always uncertain. The patient apparently progressing most favorably may die suddenly and unexpectedly; another person, desperately ill, may recover to lead a useful active life. Statistics based on a large series of cases may give a general idea of what happens to large numbers of patients, but they are utterly worthless in assisting one in the prognostication of an individual patient because the outcome depends in each instance on a great many variables: the size of the infarct, the damage inflicted by previous and possibly silent infarcts, the inherent reserve of the myocardium, the presence of serious concurrent disease, the development of unpredictable disasters, such as rupture, serious arrhythmias, recurrent coronary occlusions, and other thromboembolic phenomena. In general, if the patient has surmounted the initial insult to the myocardium and has survived beyond 21 days when rupture and ectopic rhythms are most likely to have occurred, the chief risk is the development of a thromboembolic complication, now minimized by anticoagulant therapy. At no time, however, is the risk of sudden death due to ventricular standstill or fibrillation absent.

Treatment. The first principle is that the treatment should be directed at the patient rather than at the electrocardiogram. This is especially important in the decisions concerning activity and return to work.

During the first few hours, complete rest is indicated, and sufficient opiates or other analgesics should be used to relieve the pain. Food may be restricted to fruit juices for the first 24 to 48 hr, and water given in amounts of 1,000 to 1,500 ml, or more, depending on the extent of the loss by sweating. Enough fluid should be given to ensure a urinary output of at least 700 ml. The intravenous route for administration of fluids and drugs should be avoided except when imperative. If there are numerous rales in the lungs, or if cyanosis is present, oxygen is urgently needed. Even in the absence of these signs, oxygen is probably of value, as the elevation of the arterial oxygen content, although small in degree, will allow a given level of tissue oxygen tension to be achieved at a lower level of cardiac output and may, therefore, rest the heart. It has been demonstrated in animals that the oxygen content of the marginal areas around the infarct is increased by the administration of oxygen.

Despite the risk of anticoagulant therapy, such as the occurrence of bleeding, of increasing the gravity of cerebral and other embolisms, of promoting the development of hemopericardium, the benefits accruing from this form of therapy now appear definitely to outweigh the risks. Inasmuch as a serious thromboembolic episode may occur even in an individual who has sustained only a mild infarction, we believe that it is probably wise to administer anticoagulants to all persons, provided reliable laboratory control is available and the patient is cooperative. Heparin is unquestionably the best anticoagulant, and it may be given in doses of 50 to 75 mg every 6 to 8 hr intravenously, or with a small amount of procaine subcutaneously. The expense and the inconvenience of so many punctures usually persuade the physician to employ one of the oral drugs, either one of the coumarins or indandiones, after the first 2 to 3 days. Bishydroxycoumarin (Dicumarol), warfarin (Coumadin), and other derivatives and the indandiones are all reliable and effective. It is important that the physician become thoroughly familiar with the behavior of one drug and stick to it; that the prothrombin times be dependable; and that vitamin K_1 (Mephyton) always be immediately available if hemorrhage or dangerous prolongation of prothrombin time should occur; and that this type of therapy be omitted in any patient with a hemorrhagic diathesis, with known ulcerative disease of the gastrointestinal tract or any other localized bleeding lesion, or with seriously disturbed hepatic or renal function.

After the initial nausea and pain have disappeared, the patient is given a diet low in salt, saturated fatty acids, and calories and abundant in fruit juices. There should be no fixed rule regarding the duration and rigidity of restriction of activity, the program depending on the severity of the illness. When the condition of the patient permits, often after a few days, he may be allowed to sit up in a chair, use a bedside commode, or even walk a few steps to an adjoining toilet. A mild laxative may be necessary to prevent straining, a particularly harmful form of exercise. Sedatives, such as the barbiturates or reserpine, may be useful, and the latter may exert a further beneficial effect by slowing the heart rate and reducing an elevated pressure. During the period of bed rest, active movement of the legs should be encouraged to minimize the likelihood of phlebothrombosis, and elastic stockings are also useful for this purpose. If the patient's progress is satisfactory, he is permitted to walk about the room after 10 to 14 days, gradually increasing the activity until he is fully recovered.

Congestive Failure. Congestive failure usually takes the form of pulmonary edema. If dyspnea is severe and if digitalis has not been recently taken, lanatoside C (Cedilanid) 0.8 mg may be given intramuscularly or intravenously, following which another dose of 0.4 mg in 2 to 4 hr may be given once or twice. The patient should be constantly observed for the appearance of arrhythmias or nausea. Once congestive failure has been controlled, parenteral doses of the same drug 0.4 mg may be given daily for a few days; or one can change to an oral preparation such as digoxin 0.25 mg t.i.d. (to allow for the rapid excretion of lanatoside C) for 2 to 4 days, reducing to a maintenance dose of 0.25 to 0.5 mg per day. Other procedures employed in the management of congestive failure are discussed in Chap. 249.

Shock. By shock we mean not only a fall of blood pressure below 100 mg Hg, with a pulse pressure of 20 mm Hg or less, but also the accompanying cool, clammy skin, ashen color, apathy, lassitude, and diminished urinary output. Without these manifestations indicative of intense sympathetic activity and inadequate profusion pressure, blood pressures as low as 90/60 require no treatment. Shock is a grave complication, usually but not necessarily coexisting with pulmonary edema. Pressor amines (p. 1395) and oxygen by mask or nasal tube should be given, as well as digitalis (p. 1383) if signs of left ventricular failure are elicited. When pressor amines are administered, one should be particularly careful to watch for the development of arrhythmias, particularly those of ventricular origin.

Arrhythmias. The management of the arrhythmias is discussed in Chap. 250. The most serious arrhythmias are the ectopic tachycardias: uncontrolled atrial flutter and fibrillation, because of the increased work and diminished coronary flow in an already badly damaged heart; ventricular tachycardia is even more serious since it carries the additional risk of developing into ventricular fibrillation. The serious forms of heart block are dangerous because of the likelihood of ventricular standstill or fibrillation. Even when bundle block alone develops, the mortality increases, probably because the ventricular contraction becomes less efficient. Ventricular premature beats are potentially hazardous because they may be the forerunner of a dangerous or fatal tachycardia or fibrillation. While the question is still controversial and the evidence indecisive, some believe that quinidine sulfate, 0.2 Gm four times a day, should be given to all patients as a prophylactic measure and certainly should be given when ventricular premature beats occur, provided heart block is not present.

Thromboembolic Episodes. The best treatment is prophylaxis: anticoagulants, elastic bandages for the legs, permitting the patient to take a few steps each day provided he is able to make this effort, and frequent active movements of the legs when the patient is confined to bed.

Rupture of the Heart. Transmural rupture and rupture of a papillary muscle are not amenable to therapy, since death usually occurs so rapidly. Occasionally, a patient suffering from interventricular septal rupture may survive for weeks or months, in which case corrective surgery may be possible. It is advisable to administer vitamin C if there is any question about the adequacy of the patient's diet prior to the infarction.

Shoulder-Hand Syndrome. It is possible that encouragement of the use of the muscles of the shoulder girdles shortly after the onset of the infarction may have some value as a means of preventing this syndrome. For the milder forms, including those involving the pectoral muscles, only reassurance, aspirin, and heat are necessary. In the more severe forms, steroid therapy or a stellate ganglion block may be beneficial.

Post-myocardial-infarction Syndrome. Aside from symptomatic relief, nothing needs to be done unless the fever and tachycardia constitute a threat, in which case cortisone or a derivative usually confers dramatic benefit. Because of the possibility of the development of a large pericardial effusion when anticoagulants are given in the presence of an extensive pericarditis, the patient should be observed very closely for early signs of tamponade. In the latter case, the pericardium should be tapped promptly.

Anxiety States. Emphasis has been directed repeatedly at the importance of psychologic management in all cases of disorders of the heart. In none are sympathetic understanding and insight into the emotional problems of the patient more necessary than when dealing with individuals who have suffered a myocardial infarct. Most of these patients are stricken at the height of their business or professional careers and of their responsibility to family and colleagues. The ominous significance of "heart attack" and "coronary thrombosis" has attained such wide diffusion among the laity, especially through reports of the unexpected deaths of friends who but a few days before had seemed robust and well, that hardly anyone who has sustained such an attack can fail to ponder anxiously on what the future will hold for him. Aside from the immediate threat to his life, the questions of his capacity to carry on his business, job, or profession, and of the far-reaching influence this illness will have on the lives of his wife and children, must obtrude on his thoughts. It is not necessary to discuss the innumerable anxieties that inevitably attend the convalescence of the person who lies in bed or leads the restricted life following the acute attack. Suffice it to say that these ideas do preoccupy a large part of his thoughts, and recognition of their existence must not be overlooked by the physician, however impassive and philosophic the patient may seem to be. It is during these days that the physician must exert his utmost skill in restoring confidence, in explaining in simple terms the significance of the illness, and in allaying fears and anxieties. The task is not easy, for the physician cannot forget that behind the apprehensions of the patient there is a core of truth that can never be dissipated. He can, however, come to a reasonably accurate estimate as to the degree of activity in which the patient may ultimately participate; and he can, within the limitations imposed by a malady of such uncertain course, encourage a life that will often be more active and useful than the patient had imagined. He can point out the many useful and productive years that others suffering from the same disorder have experienced. The details and the intricacies of this problem will be as varied as the temperaments and the circumstances surrounding each individual patient. The administration of drugs and the supervision of strictly medical measures constitute a progressively diminishing part of the total management as the days of the acute attack recede and the days of convalescence and resumption of more or less normal life progress.

The question arises as to how soon a patient may resume his work after a myocardial infarction. The answer should never be based on the electrocardiogram alone, but rather on the total clinical picture: the severity of the attack and the rate and completeness of recovery as well as the nature of the patient's occupation. There can be no rigid rules. The individual who has sustained a mild attack may be permitted to return to work within 4 to 6 weeks, whereas the patient who has suffered a more serious attack may require many weeks or months, or may never be able to return to work again, particularly when the occupation is one in which strenuous exertion is unavoidable. The physician should never advise a change of occupation unless such a step is imperative. Searching for a new position, becoming accustomed to unfamiliar duties may impose far more stress on the heart than continuing at the old occupation.

Long-term Management. Long-term anticoagulant therapy should be employed only when the patient is intelligent and cooperative, the laboratory controls are reliable, the physician is familiar with this form of treatment, and there are no contraindications such as have been enumerated above. Even under such optimal conditions there is uncertainty concerning the value of prolonged anticoagulant treatment. Restriction of saturated fats and reduction of weight to the ideal level for the person's height are also of importance. Regular exercise, such as walking or playing golf, is beneficial, provided it does not provoke angina or dyspnea. Moderate use of alcohol, coffee, and tea is permissible, and tobacco should be discouraged, although we have seen few patients who have observed this last admonition.

REFERENCES

ANGINA PECTORIS

Albrink, M. J., J. W. Meigs, and E. B. Man: Serum Lipids, Hypertension, and Coronary Artery Disease, Am. J. Med., 31:4, 1961.

De Bakey, M. E., and W. S. Henley: Surgical Treatment of Angina Pectoris, Circulation, 23:111, 1961.

Goble, A. J., and E. N. O'Brien: Acute Myocardial Ischaemia: Significance of Plasma-transaminase Activity, Lancet, 2:873, 1958.

Gorlin, R., N. Brachfield, C. MacLeod, and P. Bopp: Effect of Nitroglycerin on the Coronary Circulation in Patients with Coronary Artery Disease or Increased Left Ventricular Work, Circulation, 19: 705, 1959.

Gregg, D. A.: "Coronary Circulation in Health and Disease," Philadelphia, Lea & Febiger, 1950.

Harrison, T. R.: Some Clinical Aspects of Angina Pectoris, Bull. Johns Hopkins Hosp., 104:275, 1959.

Heberden, Wm.: Some Account of a Disorder of the Breast, Med. Trans. Roy. Coll. Phys., London, 2:59, 1772.

Hern, H., L. E. Field, S. Dack, and A. M. Master: Acute Coronary Insufficiency: Pathological and Physiological Aspects, Am. Heart J., 40:63, 1950.

Keefer, C. S., and W. H. Resnik: Angina Pectoris: A Syndrome Caused by Anoxemia of the Myocardium, Arch. Internal Med., 41:769, 1928.

Mayer, J.: Nutrition and Heart Disease, Am. J. Pub. Health, 50:5, 1960.

Möller, O., and K. Rørvik: Haemodynamic Consequences of Coronary Heart Disease with Observations during Anginal Pain and on the Effect of Nitroglycerine, Brit. Heart J., 20:302, 1958.

Morris, J. N.: Epidemiology and Cardiovascular Disease of Middle Age: Part I, Mod. Concepts of Cardiovascular Dis., 29:625, 1960; Part II, *ibid.*, 30:633, 1961.

Nichol, E. S., W. C. Phillips, and G. G. Casten: Virtue of Prompt Anticoagulant Therapy in Impending Myocardial Infarction: Experiences with 318 Patients during a 10-Year Period, Ann. Internal Med., 50:1158, 1959.

Prinzmetal, M., A. Akmeki, H. Toyoshima, and J. K. Kwoczynski: Angina Pectoris: III. Demonstration of a Chemical Origin of S-T Deviation in Classic Angina Pectoris, Its Variant Form, Early Myocardial Infarction, and Some Noncardiac Conditions, Am. J. Cardiol., 3:276, 1959.

ACUTE MYOCARDIAL INFARCTION

Binder, M. J.: The Mechanism and Treatment of Shock in Acute Myocardial Infarction, Progr. Cardiovascular Diseases, 1:206, 1958.

Dressler, W.: The Post-Myocardial-Infarction Syndrome, A.M.A. Arch. Internal Med., 103:28, 1959.

Edeiken, J.: Shoulder-Hand Syndrome Following Myocardial Infarction with Special Reference to Prognosis, Circulation, 16:14, 1957.

Herrick, J. B.: Thrombosis of the Coronary Arteries, J.A.M.A., 72:387, 1919.

Killip, T., III, and M. A. Payne: High Serum Transaminase Activity in Heart Disease. Circulatory Failure and Hepatic Necrosis, Circulation, 21:646, 1960.

Pickering, G., W. M. Arnott, and others: An Assessment of Long-term Anticoagulant Administration after Cardiac Infarction: Report of the Working Party on Anticoagulant Therapy in Coronary Thrombosis to The Medical Research Council, Brit. Med. J., 1:803, 1959.

Wacker, W. E. C., M. Rosenthal, P. J. Snodgrass, and E. Amador: A Triad for the Diagnosis of Pulmonary Embolism and Infarction, J.A.M.A., 178:8, 1961.

Wright, I. S.: The Use of Anticoagulants in Coronary Heart Disease: Progress and Problems: 1960, Circulation, 22:608, 1960.

Zeman, F. D., and M. Rodstein: Cardiac Rupture Complicating Myocardial Infarction, A.M.A. Arch. Internal Med., 105:431, 1960.

255 MISCELLANEOUS AND RARE CAUSES OF HEART DISEASE

William H. Resnik and T. R. Harrison

HYPERTENSIVE HEART DISEASE

The problem of hypertension is examined in Chap. 245. The present discussion deals only with the heart disease resulting from hypertension. It is caused by the increased work of the left ventricle contracting against a permanently increased arteriolar resistance, leading to left ventricular hypertrophy of lesser or greater degree, in some instances so slight as to be clinically indetectable and insignificant.

Clinical Course. Following the development of hypertension, a number of years may elapse, 10 or 20 or even 30, before symptoms referable to the heart occur, if they develop at all. Since coronary sclerosis is a frequent accompaniment of hypertension, the clinical picture may be that of angina pectoris or myocardial infarction, with or without congestive failure. In others, congestive failure alone ensues, uncommon before the age of forty, becoming increasingly frequent with advancing years. The age at which the heart begins to fail depends on a number of variables: the level of the mean arterial pressure, the extent of myocardial scarring due to coronary sclerosis, and the degree of involutionary change (p. 1378) being the most important. It is not uncommon to observe individuals who have sustained levels as high as 240 systolic and 120 diastolic for many years and who have led active, unrestricted lives without ever experiencing any symptoms indicative of diminished cardiac reserve. Because the strain is primarily on the left ventricle, left-sided failure, with rise in pressure in the left atrium and consequent pulmonary engorgement, may set in suddenly and produce attacks of paroxysmal nocturnal dyspnea or of acute pulmonary edema. These attacks may seem to be the first manifestation of congestive failure; practically always, however, the patient has already experienced at least mild exertional dyspnea and may also have noted slight ankle edema at the end of the day (p. 1382). Physical examination reveals the manifestations of left ventricular hypertrophy, the most characteristic being the localized thrusting, forceful apex beat, enlargement of the heart, accentuation of the aortic second sound, and often pulsus alternans. With failure, actual or impending, a diastolic gallop rhythm is frequently heard. Eventually, provided the patient does not succumb during an attack of acute pulmonary edema, left ventricular failure progresses to the complete picture of congestive failure.

Treatment. The management of hypertensive heart disease consists essentially of the treatment of hypertension (p. 1355) plus the usual treatment of congestive failure (p. 1384) or of angina pectoris (p. 1447), according to which of these conditions exists.

SYPHILITIC HEART DISEASE

With rare exceptions, syphilitic disorders of the heart are secondary to involvement of the aorta (p. 1366), and the following discussion is concerned only with such aspects as affect the heart directly. Barring the unusual instance of gumma of the myocardium, syphilitic heart disease is primarily a problem of aortic insufficiency (p. 1435) when the luetic aortitis involves the aortic leaflets, as is usually the case. Occasionally, ischemic heart disease (p. 1444) occurs when a coronary ostium is occluded.

Clinical Course. The patient may reveal the fully developed signs of aortic insufficiency for years without suffering any symptoms, but once the latter develop, the progress of the patient is usually rather rapidly downhill. Acute left ventricular failure with paroxysmal nocturnal dyspnea is sometimes the earliest manifestation, though usually following slight but hardly noticeable exertional dyspnea and edema. When failure occurs, management is usually effective at first but often futile at the end of 1 to 3 years. When a coronary ostium closure takes place, the absence or presence of symptoms will depend on the completeness with which the compensatory collateral circulation follows. Often no symptoms develop, but when the collaterals are inadequate, angina or even myocardial infarction will ensue. Since ostial occlusion occurs so commonly in conjunction with free aortic regurgitation, which also impairs coronary flow (p. 33), it is difficult to know in any one patient how much the ischemia

is due to the regurgitation alone and how much to the coronary obstruction. Certainly one has good reason to suspect syphilitic coronary ostial occlusion when ischemic heart disease occurs in a young person with a positive serologic test for syphilis.

Treatment. The treatment of the failure is identical with that of congestive failure in general (p. 1385). Once the valvular disease is discovered, and particularly when failure has already occurred, the value of antisyphilitic therapy is dubious. In any case, such therapy should be administered with great caution, as a Herxheimer reaction causing complete occlusion of a coronary ostium may be disastrous (p. 1079).

HIGH-OUTPUT FAILURE

Diseases which alter the oxygen tension or the metabolism of the tissues, disorders which lead to arteriovenous communications, and certain hypervolemic disturbances may cause increase in the venous return to the heart and thus eventually produce "high-output failure." The pathophysiology of these conditions has been discussed in some detail (p. 99). Here we are concerned with the clinical picture. The recognition of these disorders is of great practical importance because most of them are amenable to specific treatment. Such recognition depends on the specific manifestations of each of these several diseases and also on the evaluation of these circulatory phenomena which, being directly related to the increased flow of blood, are likely to be found in all the high-output disorders.

Palpitation, fatigability, and "nervousness" are common complaints. Tachycardia is usually present and occasionally is pronounced. The pulse is full with a rapid rise and fall, and the pulse pressure is elevated. The skin is warm and usually moist.

A quick lift is usually present in the left parasternal area and may be confused with the more sustained heave of right ventricular hypertrophy. The heart sounds are usually loud but do not have the high-pitched staccato quality so characteristic of the first sound in mitral stenosis. Systolic murmurs may be heard at the mitral, aortic, and especially the pulmonic areas. They are of the ejection type and do not replace the first sound. The combination of diastolic gallops with split first or second sounds is common and may lead to a mistaken impression that an opening snap, filling rumble, or presystolic rumble is present.

It should be noted that these peripheral phenomena are similar to those of aortic insufficiency, while the cardiac findings mimic those of mitral stenosis. The presence of such a combination should always lead to the search for one of the high-output disorders. Before discussing the more common and important of these conditions, it should be emphasized that, when one of them is undoubtedly present, the diagnosis of organic disease of the mitral valve should be made with great reluctance. When one thinks that both conditions are present, it is well to defer judgment until the cause of the high-output syndrome has been found and removed. This will result in many instances in disappearance of those signs previously attributed to mitral disease.

Thyrotoxic Heart Disease

Heart disease caused by hyperthyroidism may present itself in the form of congestive failure, or angina pectoris, or atrial fibrillation, or in any combination of these disorders. It is uncommon before the age of forty, usually occurring in individuals who already suffer from some other form of heart disease but not at all infrequently in persons who, after cure of the hyperthyroidism, display no recognizable cardiac abnormalities. Moreover, autopsies on patients dying of thyrotoxic heart disease have confirmed the fact that hyperthyroidism alone may cause failure and death. Histologic examination of these hearts reveals no consistent type of lesion, in some no abnormalities being present, in others, rather insignificant fatty infiltration, myocardial necroses, or interstitial myocarditis. There is no basic difference between the influence of toxic nodular thyroid and toxic diffuse thyroid disease on the heart.

Pathologic Physiology. The fundamental derangement is the increased load imposed on the heart by the augmented bodily oxygen requirements in which the heart, itself, participates and the necessity for increased heat loss. Because of the increased skin and peripheral blood flow, peripheral resistance is diminished, arteriovenous difference is narrowed, cardiac output and heart rate are increased, the work of the heart increases because of the enhanced volume and rate loads, and the heart hypertrophies. In addition, it is possible that increased catecholamines demonstrated in the myocardium of experimentally induced hyperthyroidism in dogs may interfere with myocardial enzyme action and energy production as well as contributing to myocardial hypoxia. When failure finally ensues, the resting cardiac output falls from its previously elevated levels, increasing or not with exercise depending on the cardiac reserve; but even in failure, the cardiac output and stroke volume are often higher than the same functions in a resting euthyroid individual without failure. In other words, thyrotoxic heart disease with failure represents a typical form of high-output failure. The load resulting from the overactive thyroid is well tolerated by the young and healthy heart. It is when this load is superimposed on the heart already affected by involutionary changes (presbycardia), and par-

ticularly when cardiac reserve has been diminished by some other form of heart disease, that thyrotoxic heart disease manifests itself. Angina pectoris occurs only in those who already have a lesion predisposing to myocardial ischemia, such as coronary sclerosis or aortic stenosis, and the increased load serves merely to raise a subclinical condition to the clinical level.

Clinical Manifestations and Course. In some persons, the characteristic features of hyperthyroidism are so conspicuous even after the development of failure that the diagnosis is simple. In others, when the eye phenomena and thyroid enlargement are not striking and other classic manifestations of thyrotoxicosis are obscured and masked by the antagonistic effects of cardiac failure, it is not surprising that the basic overactivity of the thyroid is hardly discernible. Nevertheless, thyrotoxicosis should be suspected as a contributing factor in patients with cardiac disease under the following circumstances: persistent tachycardia that endures after prolonged rest and during sleep; any suggestion of high-output failure (p. 1377) in the absence of other recognizable causes; failure of the usual measures in the management of failure to bring about a satisfactory response. Attacks of paroxysmal atrial fibrillation or the presence of chronic atrial fibrillation in a person without mitral stenosis, particularly when the ventricular rate is resistant to the slowing effect of full doses of digitalis, should be especially suspected, since atrial fibrillation occurs in approximately 60 per cent of patients over the age of forty-five with hyperthyroidism.

After treatment has been instituted and thyrotoxicosis eradicated, remarkable improvement in a previously intractable form of heart disease usually follows. About one-third of those with fibrillation revert spontaneously to a normal sinus rhythm; angina and congestive failure disappear or become easily controllable.

Diagnosis. Estimations of the basal metabolic rate and of the serum cholesterol are subject to so many influences unrelated to the activity of the thyroid that they are of little value. A circulation time that is within the normal range in a person suffering from congestive failure is highly suggestive of some type of high-output failure; but the most reliable methods of diagnosis are the determinations of the protein-bound iodine of the plasma and of radioiodine studies, provided one bears in mind the sources of error even in these procedures. Finally, the diagnosis should be confirmed by a favorable response to therapy directed at the hyperthyroidism.

Treatment. The management of thyrotoxic cardiac disease is that of heart failure but primarily that aimed at eradication of the hyperthyroidism (p. 591).

The Heart in Anemia

Pathologic Physiology. In chronic anemia, when the hemoglobin falls to about 7 Gm or less, tissue hypoxia leads to a decline in peripheral resistance, increased cardiac output, and tachycardia. Since oxygen extraction in the coronary circulation is already practically maximal even in the normal person, myocardial oxygen requirements in anemia can be met only by increased coronary flow due to coronary dilatation. Pallor is usually greater than one anticipates with a given degree of anemia, and this is caused by the vasoconstriction in the skin, the blood being diverted to more important tissues. There is also a compensatory shunting of blood from the kidneys, but the glomerular filtration rate remains normal. It is the continued effect of the sustained increase in cardiac output and the inability of the coronary bed to expand beyond a certain limit that are responsible for the ultimate failure that may develop in some instances of severe anemia—another example of high-output failure. Congestive failure is especially likely to occur when cardiac reserve is already compromised by the involutionary changes of age or by concomitant heart disease. Apparently some individuals with severe and long-standing anemia are able to compensate for the impoverished blood sufficiently well so that they engage in fairly strenuous physical work, even in a tropical climate. On the other hand, there are other patients with severe anemia who display failure without tachycardia or the clinical signs of increased cardiac output. The reasons for the absence of these compensatory mechanisms are unknown.

Clinical Picture. The clinical picture is that of high-output failure with anemia. Cardiac enlargement, occasionally with hypertrophy; unusually pronounced systolic murmurs because of the combined effects of decreased viscosity, increased flow, and dilatation of the mitral ring; rarely an early diastolic rumble at the mitral area due to increased flow or an aortic diastolic blow, presumably due to dilatation of the aortic ring, may present a confusing problem of diagnosis. Thus, when slight fever is also present, subacute bacterial endocarditis may be mimicked. In patients with sickle-cell anemia with fever and joint pains, acute rheumatic fever may be suspected.

With an organic obstruction in a coronary artery, thus nullifying the compensatory increase in coronary flow that would otherwise take place in anemia, angina may appear in a person with subclinical coronary sclerosis, or anemia may aggravate an already existent angina.

Treatment. The treatment is primarily that of the anemia, which naturally depends on the cause, and of the usual means of managing congestive heart failure. If it is deemed necessary to transfuse, only red cells, free from plasma, may be given in small daily doses.

Thiamine Deficiency (Beriberi Heart Disease)

Thiamine deficiency (p. 545) leads to a derangement of carbohydrate metabolism the effects of which are similar to those caused by hypoxia, all the tissues including the myocardium being involved. This disturbance in myocardial metabolism, to which is added a further interference of fatty acid catabolism due to the deficiency of cocarboxylase, results in impaired myocardial energy production. The defect in the peripheral tissues causes a peripheral vasodilatation, increased venous return and cardiac output, and consequently an increased load on a heart already handicapped by the metabolic defect. Clinical and experimental evidence indicate that cardiac failure is more prone to occur in persons who have the least involvement of the nervous system and a greater capacity for work and, hence, a greater opportunity for increased load on the heart.

The usual clinical picture of beriberi heart disease as seen in the Orient and described by Wenckebach and by Keefer is characterized by an enlargement of the heart, absence of arrhythmia, predominant failure of the right ventricle, bounding arterial pulsations, and the classical phenomena of high-output failure. This picture is rarely encountered in the occidental countries; the more common one is that of an individual who has been on a clearly deficient diet over a long period of time (excessive consumption of alcohol is almost invariably the cause), who has heart disease of uncertain origin, failure that does not respond to the usual methods of treatment, signs of mild peripheral neuritis or of other manifestations of dietary deficiency, and whose heart failure and cardiac enlargement disappear with the administration of thiamine. The electrocardiogram reveals only nonspecific abnormalities. Not all patients respond quickly, spectacularly, and completely to thiamine treatment, and there is still disagreement as to whether thiamine deficiency can lead to irreversible myocardial changes.

It is evident that the diagnosis depends mostly on securing a good dietary history and on response to treatment. One should be particularly suspicious when high-output failure is observed. One should also bear in mind that the factor of thiamine deficiency may be playing a contributing role in all alcoholics who may have failure ostensibly due only to one of the more common forms of heart disease.

Arteriovenous Fistula

The acquired type of this disorder is usually the result of a penetrating injury, such as a knife or bullet wound. Congenital fistulas, usually multiple, also occur.

Pathologic Physiology. The initial effect of the leakage is a reduction of effective blood volume by the amount of blood that leaks into and is sequestered in the involved extremity. This promotes increase in total blood volume. The fall in blood pressure leads to an increase in heart rate and a generalized vasoconstriction. Nevertheless, despite the peripheral vasoconstriction, the total peripheral resistance is diminished because of the predominant effect of the leakage. Renal vasoconstriction causes a fall in glomerular filtration rate but an increase in filtration fraction (p. 183), and this plus increased tubular sodium reabsorption leads to an increased extracellular volume. In turn, this raises the cardiac output, mediated through a moderate tachycardia and elevated stroke volume (increased systolic emptying against a lowered peripheral resistance). Eventually, the heart fails when the myocardium is incapable of coping with the burden of the sustained elevation of cardiac output.

Symptoms and Diagnosis. The diagnosis of arteriovenous fistula is not difficult if one keeps the possibility in mind. The swelling and increased warmth in the vicinity of the fistula, the continuous murmur with systolic accentuation, usually associated with a thrill, the enlargement of the heart with the bounding pulse, the slowing of the heart when the fistula is compressed (Branham's sign) constitute a characteristic clinical picture. When myocardial failure develops, the features are those of the high-output type. Even if an arteriovenous fistula is not immediately apparent, cardiac failure with outspoken signs of aortic insufficiency without the murmur of that lesion should lead to a careful inquiry into possible injuries and wounds and the search for a fistula. Since extensive *Paget's disease* causes heart failure on essentially the same basis because of the development of innumerable arteriovenous fistulas in the abnormal bone, it should also be borne in mind under these circumstances.

Pulmonary arteriovenous fistulas may be congenital (p. 1534) or acquired. They may produce cyanosis, polycythemia, and clubbing of the fingers and thus mimic the cyanotic forms of congenital heart disease. However, the heart is usually normal or may show slight enlargement.

The Heart in Acute Nephritis

The edema and the congestive phenomena of acute glomerulonephritis probably depend on several mechanisms. The peripheral resistance may be increased, but more important is the primary retention of sodium which then causes an increase in plasma volume and a hyperkinetic (high-output) state (p. 1379). This is what has been termed "noncardiac circulatory congestion" and would account for the usually inconspicuous lengthening of the circulation time and the absence or minimal engorgement of the lungs and liver, despite the increased venous pressure. Nevertheless, one does occasionally encounter patients in whom the circulation time is definitely prolonged, the congestive phenomena resemble those of myocardial failure, and who display a prompt improvement with diuresis after digitalis. How much this failure of the myocardium depends on the increased work load of the heart and how much to an obscure effect of the disorder on the myocardium is not known.

THE HEART IN MYXEDEMA

The hypercholesterolemia associated with myxedema favors the development of coronary sclerosis and angina. In addition, myxedema may be complicated by pericardial effusion that rarely, if ever, causes tamponade. Finally, myxedema may produce electrocardiographic changes with prolonged PR conduction time and lowered voltage, although it is dubious whether myxedema ever causes actual myocardial failure. The dramatic decrease of the cardiac silhouette and the disappearance of the electrocardiographic abnormalities are usual after the administration of thyroid extract. However, it should be given with great caution in persons with myxedema because of the possibility of inducing anginal attacks or psychic disorders, when sclerotic vessels inhibit increase in blood flow parallel with the rising oxygen need of the heart and brain.

POST-PARTUM HEART DISEASE

Whether such a specific entity exists is a debatable subject. The term has been applied to cardiac disease of unknown etiology, presumably related in some way to pregnancy, for the reports in the literature indicate that symptoms usually appear 2 to 6 weeks after the termination of pregnancy, occasionally a short time before the termination. The heart enlarges, there are no characteristic murmurs or irregularities, gallop rhythm is common, as are pulmonary and systemic emboli. Response to treatment is unsatisfactory, and the prognosis has varied in different accounts. If one excludes those cases which are related to toxemia of pregnancy, to embolism (p. 1538) and to postinfectious myocarditis, one gains the impression that a specific form of heart disease, somehow related to the post-partum period, is a very rare entity, if it exists at all.

MYOCARDITIS

Almost any acute generalized infectious disease may cause inflammatory changes in the myocardium, but ordinarily significant clinical findings are not encountered. However, in certain well-defined disorders, such as rheumatic fever, diphtheria, scrub typhus, Chagas disease, the involvement of the heart may be clinically important and even fatal. There are other instances, both with an acute and also with a chronic course, in which myocardial failure seemingly develops without cause and when, in such a case, a more or less diffuse inflammatory lesion is confined to the myocardium, all other evidences of a related infection or other disorder being absent, the condition has commonly been designated *isolated* or *Fiedler's myocarditis*. Viral studies have indicated, however, that at least in some the myocarditis has been caused by strains of Coxsackie or of influenza virus. In other instances, such as primary atypical pneumonia, the coexistence of myocarditis with the pulmonary disorder constitutes indirect evidence that the same agent is responsible for both. In some of these various disorders, pericarditis has also been present. Some investigators believe that these forms of chronic myocarditis, of known or of as yet unidentified viral origin, may be responsible for "endocardial fibroelastosis," "idiopathic ventricular hypertrophy," and for some of the cases of "post-partum heart disease." The failure to recognize the relationship of the myocarditis to a respiratory infection may come from the fact that several weeks may elapse before the onset of the cardiac manifestations. The clinical picture may be that of a fulminating and rapidly fatal form of cardiac failure or of a slowly developing course, extending over a period of years and characterized by enlargement of the heart, arrhythmias, and eventually failure. When, during or shortly after a respiratory infection, clinical signs of cardiac complications are absent and the only manifestations are such electrocardiographic changes as prolongation of the P-R interval or T-wave alterations, complete recovery nearly always occurs.

TRAUMATIC HEART DISEASE

Cardiac damage may be due to both penetrating and nonpenetrating injuries, the most frequent cause of the latter being impact of the chest against the steering wheel of a motorcar. Serious injury of the heart may ensue though there is no external sign of disease.

Although the common type of injury is myocardial contusion, any structure of the heart may be affected. The valve cusps may be ruptured, and the appearance of a loud murmur in a previously healthy person is followed by rapidly progressive myocardial failure. A coronary artery may be lacerated, leading to fatal tamponade. The frequency of coronary thrombosis after coronary injury is uncertain. It is usually accepted that the relationship

between coronary thrombosis and infarction and a preceding injury is uncertain or unlikely if the former occurs more than 2 to 3 days after the trauma. Myocardial contusion may cause arrhythmias, bundle branch block, or electrocardiographic abnormalities resembling those of infarction. The most serious consequence of nonpenetrating injury is rupture of either of the atria or ventricles, which is always fatal; rarely, a patient with ruptured ventricular or auricular septum may survive. It is important to bear in mind trauma as a cause of otherwise unexplained electrocardiographic changes (Fig. 254-3). Hemopericardium with tamponade may follow tear of the myocardium or of a pericardial vessel or of a coronary artery.

Treatment for myocardial failure due to valve rupture is rarely effective. If the electrocardiographic abnormalities are those of infarction, it is impossible to distinguish between contusion and infarction secondary to coronary artery injury; in any case, treatment is the same and is that accorded the patient with infarction. Pericardial tamponade has been managed successfully by repeated taps alone. Others recommend operation when tamponade recurs rapidly or when bleeding takes place into the thoracic or abdominal cavity. Pericardial hemorrhage may be followed by permanently inverted T waves and occasionally by constrictive pericarditis.

The electrocardiographic changes that may follow myocardial contusion are of no significance unless accompanied by clinical manifestations. However, their confusion with similar changes following infarction may make it difficult or impossible for the patient to secure life insurance.

MALIGNANT CARCINOID

The cardiac manifestations of this disorder are considered in Chap. 90.

HEART DISEASE OF OBSCURE ETIOLOGY

Occasionally the physician is confronted by a form of heart disease that does not appear to belong to any of the more common categories previously described, and he is obliged to consider more unusual types of heart disease. Before embarking on a speculative voyage in search of some esoteric kind of cardiac disease, he should give thought again to the possibility that an ordinary type may actually be present. Aortic or mitral stenosis may be missed because the characteristic murmurs are absent as a result of diminished cardiac output, especially in failure. The various forms of hyperkinetic heart disease are often forgotten if one has ignored the manifestations of the overactive heart. The most frequent in this group is the thyrotoxic heart which may be so masked by congestive failure that the customary clues are largely obliterated. In a person beyond forty-five or fifty years, congenital heart disease is likely to be forgotten, and patent atrial septum, which is the one form of congenital heart disease that is most likely to go on to old age, may be ignored. In younger persons, the development of pulmonary hypertension with Eisenmenger's syndrome may abolish the gradients of pressure responsible for the typical murmurs of patent ductus, atrial and ventricular septal defect, with the result that a common form of congenital heart disease will be undetected. Chronic constrictive pericarditis and chronic pericardial effusion are other disorders that are important to keep in mind since they are often curable.

It should be evident that the question of obscure heart disease arises when the patient presents no significant murmurs, hypertension, pulmonary disease, outspoken signs of hyperkinetic heart disease, or unequivocal coronary disease (angina pectoris or myocardial infarction). When the situation arises in an older person, it is hardly ever considered a problem, since this kind of case is almost automatically labeled "arteriosclerotic heart disease." However, it has been pointed out previously that the statistical frequency of coronary disease should not exclude the consideration of other nonvalvular, normotensive forms of heart disease. Moreover, exactly the same problem appears in younger persons, although coronary disease is not so likely here to interfere with the contemplation of other possibilities. *In both young and old, one should bear in mind that many instances of heart disease of apparently obscure etiology are simply unrecognized examples of common heart disease.* If these can be reasonably excluded, one is then forced to speculate on the possibility or probability that an unusual kind of heart disease may actually be present.

Disorders Affecting the Mural Endocardium. This group of disorders of unknown etiology and pathogenesis constitutes one of the most confusing fields in cardiology. These disorders have certain superficial anatomic features in common, but careful morphologic study reveals sufficiently significant differences between them to make it likely that they represent diseases of varying origin. It is uncertain whether any of them are related to obstruction of cardiac lymphatic drainage, which has been shown to produce similar anatomic changes in dogs.

In this country and in a few reports from Europe, there has been described a condition known as *idiopathic hypertrophy of the heart* or *subendocardial fibrosis.* Because a number of these patients had been chronic alcoholics and had suffered from long-standing malnutrition, it has been suggested that the heart disease represents the end stage of

thiamine deficiency, a view that has not been generally accepted. Mural thrombosis is a characteristic finding, and the usual clinical picture is that of enlargement of the heart, systemic embolic manifestations, arrhythmias, progressive failure of the heart unresponsive to digitalis or vitamin therapy. *Endocardial fibroelastosis* occurs most frequently in infants, but adults may be afflicted. At autopsy, marked hypertrophy of the heart, more or less generalized thickening of the endocardium, chiefly of the left ventricle, and frequently mural thrombi are found. The clinical picture is similar to the one described above. In a very few instances, typical angina pectoris has been present, although coronary sclerosis has been absent at autopsy. Some very competent pathologists are convinced that this disease, in adults at least, is a result of chronic myocarditis, since transition stages between the two can be demonstrated. An identical clinical picture, with *endocardial fibrosis and subendocardial necrosis* has been described in South Africa (Becker's disease), and another variant is *endocarditis fibroplastica with eosinophilia* (Loeffler's disease), reported from Western and Central Europe and very rarely encountered in Great Britain and the United States. From Uganda and other parts of tropical Africa have come reports of *endomyocardial fibrosis,* again with somewhat similar manifestations except that mural thrombi and systemic emboli are quite infrequent whereas pericarditis is often present.

Disorders Affecting the Myocardium. The recognition of cardiac involvement by *sarcoidosis, scleroderma, hemachromatosis,* and *amyloid disease* will depend on the demonstration of these disorders elsewhere in the body by biopsy or by other precise methods. All these diffuse disorders of the myocardium, as well as an occasional instance of diffuse fibrosis secondary to coronary disease, may present the clinical and hemodynamic characteristics of chronic constrictive pericarditis. *Von Gierke's disease, Friedreich's ataxia, muscular dystrophy,* and *trichinosis* are other diseases that may be associated with myocardial involvement. *Hurler's syndrome* is frequently responsible for lesions in the valves, especially the mitral and aortic, as well as in the myocardial cells and coronary arteries. *Disseminated lupus* is very frequently complicated by pericarditis and occasionally by signs of valvular disease; *polyarteritis nodosa* is often associated with coronary involvement, myocardial disease, or pericarditis.

The combination of marked eosinophilia with clinical or electrocardiographic evidence of myocardial injury should arouse the suspicion of polyarteritis, trichiniasis, eosinophilic leukemia with infiltration of the heart, or Loeffler's fibroplastic endocarditis.

Familial cardiomegaly is a term that has been applied to cardiac disorders of undetermined origin occurring in two or more members of a family. Review of the literature indicates wide differences of age distribution, clinical characteristics such as rapidity of progression, presence or absence of endocardial thrombi, frequency of sudden death and, finally, in the histologic appearance of the myocardium. Evidently, the designation familial cardiomegaly must embrace several distinct disorders.

Neoplasms of the Heart. With the exception of myxoma of the left atrium, primary tumors of the heart (rhabdomyoma, mesothelioma of the pericardium, a variety of other benign tumors or their malignant counterparts) are medical curiosities. *Myxoma of the atrium,* usually of the left, is rare but should not really be considered in a discussion of heart disease of obscure origin, because almost invariably it, like ball valve thrombus, is usually diagnosed as mitral stenosis and recognized first at operation. Occasionally, however, attention to certain striking features may lead to correct diagnosis before operation: variability of the murmurs of mitral stenosis with change of position, syncope, paroxysms of acute pulmonary edema—all caused by sudden and intermittent obstruction of the mitral orifice.

Secondary tumors of the heart are much more frequent and have been reported as occurring in 10 to 20 per cent of cases of malignancy. The most common form is by direct extension to the pericardium of a primary carcinoma of the breast or bronchus, malignant thymoma, or lymphoma. The clinical picture is that of rapidly recurring pericardial effusion, usually bloody. Metastases to the myocardium are rarely responsible for symptoms or signs that permit recognition, although suspicion should be aroused when the development of intractable failure or a distinctly abnormal electrocardiogram takes place in a person known to harbor other metastatic lesions and previously free of heart disease.

Geographic factors are sometimes of importance in determining the cause of heart disease of obscure origin. Residents in areas where *Schistosomiasis mansoni* is endemic should bring to mind the possibility that this disease may cause cor pulmonale, while *cardiac trypanosomiasis (Chagas disease)* should be considered in persons living in northern and central South America. In the Orient, heart disease due to *scrub typhus* is encountered.

For the sake of simplicity of presentation, these various unusual diseases of the heart have been classified as involving primarily the endocardium or myocardium or pericardium. Clinically these distinctions will rarely be apparent, nor will these disorders differ very much from the heart disease and failure that occur in about 10 per cent of cases of advanced *cirrhosis of the liver* and are attributed to the increased cardiac output that has been demonstrated in this disease. When sarcoidosis or amyloidosis or cirrhosis of the liver or malignant disease of the mediastinum, to name but a few, is known to be present or strongly suspected, there is a logic in assigning cardiac disease of otherwise undetermined origin to the respective disorder. But when definite clues or biopsy proof is lacking, the diagnosis of many of these rare forms of heart disease can hardly be anything other than a lucky guess, the artificial by-product of the clinical pathologic conference atmosphere. One cannot help gaining the impression that a lengthy and seemingly scholarly differentiation under these circumstances can only be "a tale . . . full of sound and fury, signifying nothing."

Since cure or significant amelioration of certain forms of heart disease is now possible, they must always be borne in mind when an obscure form of heart disease is considered. One should never fail to search carefully for subacute bacterial endocarditis, the various hyperkinetic circulatory states, certain types of congenital and acquired valvular heart disease, constrictive pericarditis, and cor pulmonale due to thromboembolic disease.

REFERENCES

SYPHILITIC HEART DISEASE

Rich, C., Jr., and B. Webster: Natural History of Uncomplicated Syphilitic Aortitis, Am. Heart J., 43:321, 1952.

Woodruff, I. O.: Cardiovascular Syphilis, Am. J. Med., 2:248, 1948.

THYROTOXIC HEART DISEASE

Bortin, M. M., S. Silver, and S. B. Yoholen: Diagnosis of Masked Hyperthyroidism in Cardiac Patients with Auricular Fibrillation, Am. J. Med., 11:40, 1951.

Graettinger, J. S., J. J. Muenster, and others: A Correlation of Clinical and Hemodynamic Studies in Patients with Hyperthyroidism with and without Congestive Failure, J. Clin. Invest., 38:1316, 1959.

Sandler, G., and G. N. Wilson: The Nature and Prognosis of Heart Disease in Thyrotoxicosis, Quart. J. Med., 28:347, 1959.

THE HEART IN ANEMIA

Case, R. B., E. Berglund, and S. J. Sarnoff: Ventricular Function: VII. Changes in Coronary Resistance and Ventricular Function Resulting from Acutely Induced Anemia and the Effect Thereon of Coronary Stenosis, Am. J. Med., 18:397, 1955.

Porter, W. B., and G. W. James, 3: The Heart in Anemia, Circulation, 8:111, 1953.

Sharpey-Schafer, E. P.: Cardiac Output in Severe Anemia, Clin. Sci., 5:125, 1944.

Wintrobe, M. M.: Cardiovascular System in Anemia, Blood, 1:121, 1946.

THIAMINE DEFICIENCY HEART DISEASE

Blankenhorn, N. A., C. F. Vilter, and others: Occidental Beriberi Heart Disease, J.A.M.A., 131:717, 1946.

Jones, R. H., Jr.: Beriberi Heart Disease, Circulation, 19:275, 1959.

Keefer, C. S.: The Beriberi Heart, Arch. Internal Med., 45:1, 1930.

Rowlands, D. T., Jr., and C. F. Vilter: A Study of the Cardiac Stigmata in Prolonged Thiamine Deficiency, Circulation, 21:4, 1960.

Weiss, S., and R. W. Wilkins: Nature of Cardiovascular Disturbances in Vitamin Deficiency States, Trans. Assoc. Am. Physicians, 51:341, 1936.

ARTERIOVENOUS FISTULA

Muenster, J. J., J. S. Graettinger, and J. Campbel: Correlation of Clinical and Hemodynamic Findings in Patients with Systemic Arteriovenous Fistulas, Circulation, 20:1079, 1959.

Pierce, J. A., W. P. Reagan, and R. W. Kimball: Unusual Cases of Pulmonary Arteriovenous Fistulas, with a Note on Thyroid Carcinoma as a Cause, New Engl. J. Med., 260:901, 1959.

Schreiner, G. E.: The Physiology of Arteriovenous Fistulas, Med. Ann. Dist. Columbia, 24:1, 1955.

THE HEART IN ACUTE NEPHRITIS

DeFazio, V., R. C. Christensen, and others: Circulatory Changes in Acute Glomerulonephritis, Circulation, 20:190, 1959.

Eisenberg, S.: Blood Volume in Patients with Acute Glomerulonephritis as Determined by Radioactive Chromium Tagged Red Cells, Am. J. Med., 27:241, 1959.

Peters, J. P.: Edema of Acute Nephritis, Am. J. Med., 14:48, 1953.

THE HEART IN MYXEDEMA

Ellis, L. B., and R. A. Bloomfield: The Effect of Myxedema on the Cardiovascular System, Am. Heart J., 43:341, 1951.

POST-PARTUM HEART DISEASE

Benchimol, A. B., R. D. Carneiro, and P. Schlesinger: Post-partum Heart Disease, Brit. Heart J., 21:89, 1959.

Silber, E. N.: Respiratory Viruses and Heart Disease, Ann. Internal Med., 48:228, 1958.

MYOCARDITIS

Adams, C. W.: Postviral Myopericarditis Associated with the Influenza Virus: Report of 8 Cases, Am. J. Cardiol., 4:56, 1959.

Kline, I. K., and O. Saphir: Chronic Pernicious Myocarditis, Am. Heart J., 59:681, 1960.

Nikkila and R. Pelkonen: Isolated (Fiedler's) Myocarditis and Idiopathic Cardiac Hypertrophy. Related Disorders with Possible Genetic Basis? Acta Med. Scand., 162:421, 1959.

Null, F. C., Jr., and C. H. Castle: Adult Pericarditis and Myocarditis Due to Coxsackie Virus Group B, Type 5, New Engl. J. Med., 261:937, 1959.

Silber, E. N.: Respiratory Viruses and Heart Disease, Ann. Internal Med., 48:228, 1958.

TRAUMATIC HEART DISEASE

Parmley, L. F., T. W. Mattingly, and W. C. Manion: Penetrating Wounds of the Heart and Aorta, Circulation, 17:953, 1958.

——, W. C. Manion, and T. W. Mattingly: Nonpenetrating Traumatic Injury of the Heart, Circulation, 18:371, 1958.

OBSCURE HEART DISEASE

Barritt, D. W., and W. O. Brien: Heart Disease in Scleroderma, Brit. Heart J., 14:421, 1952.

Benson, R., and J. F. Smith: Cardiac Amyloidosis, Brit. Heart J., 18:529, 1956.

Bridgen, W., E. G. L. Bywaters, and others: The Heart in Systemic Lupus Erythematosus, Brit. Heart J., 22:1, 1960.

Burwell, C. S., and E. D. Robin: Diagnosis of Diffuse Myocardial Fibrosis, Circulation, 20:606, 1959.

Coe, G. C.: Primary Rhabdomyosarcoma of the Heart, Am. Heart J., 52:1124, 1960.

Davies, J. N. P.: Some Considerations Regarding Obscure Diseases Affecting the Mural Endocardium, Am. Heart J., 59:600, 1960.

Finch, S. C., and C. A. Finch: Idiopathic Hemochromatosis, and Iron Storage Disease, Medicine, 34:381, 1955.

Harvey, J. C.: Myxoma of the Left Auricle, Ann. Internal Med., 47:1067, 1957.

Murray, J. F. P., A. M. Dawson, and S. Sherlock: Circulatory Changes in Liver Disease, Am. J. Med., 24:358, 1958.

Porter, G. H.: Sarcoid Heart Disease, New Engl. J. Med., 263:1350, 1960.

Read, J. A., R. R. Porter, and others: Occlusive Auricular Thrombi, Circulation, 12:1250, 1955.

Rodman, T., J. K. Hurwitz, and others: Cyanosis, Clubbing and Arterial Oxygen Unsaturation Associated with Laennec's Cirrhosis, Am. J. Med. Sci., 238:534, 1959.

Taubenhaus, M., B. Eisenstein, and A. Pick: Cardiovascular Manifestations of Collagen Disease, Circulation, 12:903, 1955.

Van Buchem, F. S. P., A. Arends, and A. E. Schroder: Endocardial Fibroelastosis in Adolescents and Adults, Brit. Heart J., 21:229, 1959.

Walther, R. J., I. M. Madoff, and K. Zinner: Cardiomegaly of Unknown Cause Occurring in a Family; Report of Three Siblings and Review of the Literature, New Engl. J. Med., 263:1104, 1960.

256 PERICARDITIS

William H. Resnik and
T. R. Harrison

Pericarditis may be classified according to two different methods, both of practical importance.

CLASSIFICATION

I. Morphologic and clinical classification
  A. Acute
    1. Fibrinous
    2. Pericardial effusion
  B. Chronic pericardial effusion
  C. Chronic constrictive pericarditis
II. Etiologic classification
  A. Infectious
    1. Acute benign
    2. Tuberculous
    3. Pyogenic
    4. Mycotic (fungous infection)
  B. Noninfectious
    1. Ischemic (acute myocardial infarction)
    2. Uremic
    3. Neoplastic
    4. Myxedematous
    5. Traumatic
    6. Anticoagulant therapy
  C. Uncertain etiology
    1. Rheumatic
    2. Disseminated lupus erythematosus and other collagen diseases
    3. Post-cardiac-injury syndrome
      a. Post-myocardial-infarction syndrome
      b. Postpericardiotomy (postcommissurotomy) syndrome
      c. Posttraumatic syndrome

General Comments. The above classification implies that not only must one determine whether or not pericarditis is present, with or without effusion or constrictive scar, but one must also seek to determine the cause.

Pain is an important symptom in various forms of pericarditis, usually being present in the acute infectious types and also in those forms enumerated under "uncertain etiology." Pain, however, is often absent in a slowly developing tuberculous or neoplastic pericarditis, and it is usually absent in the pericarditis of myocardial infarction. Pain rarely constitutes an important complaint in uremic pericarditis, probably because of the stuporous or comatose state of the patient. The character of the pain has been described in a previous chapter (p. 36). Any one or combination of the three components of pericardial pain may occur, but *usually* the predominant one is the pleuritic type of pain. Occasionally the steady, constrictive pain, radiating into either or both arms and identical with the pain of

ischemia, may overshadow the pleuritic pain, or it may occur alone at the onset of the illness, with the result that confusion with myocardial infarction is not infrequent. This problem becomes even more perplexing when, with acute pericarditis, the serum transaminase rises to levels of about 80 units but occasionally to 125 to 135. Moreover, shock may appear, the mechanism being uncertain. Possibly in some instances it may be caused by the same obscure reflexes that play a part in the shock of myocardial infarction; in other cases, it may be brought about by tamponade caused by the rapid development of pericardial fluid, too small in amount to be detected by x-ray. The location of pericardial pain has also been described (p. 36). Suffice it to say that a pain felt either in the precordium or in one or both shoulders or trapezius ridges and aggravated by inspiration should alert one to the possibility of an acute pericarditis.

The *pericardial friction rub* is the most important physical sign, sometimes elicited only when firm pressure with the stethoscope is applied to the chest wall. The pericardial rub is likely to be inconstant and transitory, and a loud to-and-fro leathery sound may disappear within a few hours, possibly to reappear the following day.

The *electrocardiogram* usually displays elevation of the S-T segments in several leads without reciprocal depressions in others and without significant changes in the QRS complexes. Later, the T waves become inverted, and in some instances this latter change is permanent.

Pericardial effusion is usually associated with an enlargement of the cardiac silhouette, and this is especially important when it occurs rapidly under observation. There is no definitive contour to the cardiac shadow in effusion, and differentiation from enlargement of the heart may be difficult. A very important bedside clue to the presence of effusion is the increase in the area of cardiac flatness (not dullness) on percussion, extending to the third left interspace and to the right of the midline of the sternum, with loss of the normal percussion resonance over the lower sternum. The heart sounds tend to become faint, but they may remain loud; the friction rub may disappear or remain clearly audible; the apex impulse may vanish but sometimes is felt well within the left border of dullness. On fluoroscopic examination, the ventricular pulsations are usually diminished or absent. When the effusion is large, one often encounters an area of dullness and tubular breath sounds at the angle of the left scapula, probably caused by compression of the lung (Ewart's sign). The importance of this finding comes from the fact that often the signs may be interpreted as being due to a pneumonic consolidation.

When an effusion develops, the fluid nearly always has the physical characteristics of an exudate. Bloody fluid is commonly due to tuberculosis or tumor, but it may also be found in the effusion of rheumatic fever or in the post-cardiac-injury syndrome (see below). Occasionally, bloody fluid may be found in the effusion of uremic pericarditis and, of course, in the hemopericardium following infarction, especially when anticoagulants have been given.

TAMPONADE

When fluid in the pericardium accumulates in an amount sufficient to cause serious obstruction to the inflow of blood to the ventricles, *tamponade* is said to be present. The amount of fluid necessary to produce this critical state may be as small as 250 to 300 ml, when the fluid develops rapidly; or it may be over 1,000 ml in slowly developing effusions when the pericardium has had the opportunity to stretch and adapt to the increasing volume of fluid. Tamponade is usually due to tuberculosis, pyogenic infection, or tumor, but it may occur in rheumatic fever, acute benign infectious pericarditis, the post-cardiac-injury syndrome, and disseminated lupus erythematosus. The symptoms are due to the sudden fall in cardiac output and to systemic congestive failure. Orthopnea with few or no rales is prominent, the mechanism of this dyspnea not being fully understood. The heart rate increases, the blood pressure and pulse pressure decline. Distention of the neck veins and rapid enlargement of the liver occur. The fullness of the neck veins is increased during inspiration or when pressure is applied with the palm of the hand over the liver (hepatojugular reflux). This phenomenon is due to the inability of the right chambers to accommodate the increased inflow of blood from the abdomen and the consequent reflux of blood into the veins already under increased tension. A protodiastolic gallop is usually heard.

An important clue to the presence of pericardial tamponade and of constrictive pericarditis is the *paradoxic pulse.* This phenomenon consists of *two essential features: an inspiratory decrease in arterial pressure and an absence of the normal inspiratory fall in venous pressure.* Indeed, there may be an actual inspiratory rise in venous pressure (first described by Kussmaul), often visible in constrictive pericarditis, only occasionally visible in tamponade.

The mechanism of the paradoxic pulse, long a subject of controversy, seems now to be definitely settled. Normally, the inspiratory decline in intrathoracic pressure enhances right ventricular filling by virtue of the increased gradient of pressure between the extrathoracic veins and the right chambers of the heart. Right ventricular output increases,

but a fraction of the expelled blood is trapped in the disproportionately enlarged pulmonary vascular bed. A corresponding reduction of flow into the left ventricle takes place, left ventricular output decreases, and there is a normal slight inspiratory diminution in systemic arterial pressure.

In the person with tamponade or constrictive pericarditis, the inspiratory descent of the diaphragm elongates the heart, a change in shape that tends to increase intraventricular pressure. Such an increase in pressure does not take place in the normal heart because the distensibility ("compliance") of the ventricular wall is adequate to prevent a rise in pressure even with the normally increased inspiratory flow into the right ventricle. When, however, the heart is surrounded by fluid or thick unyielding scar, the distensibility of the heart is greatly impaired and the diminished spheroidicity of the ventricular cavity now causes an increased intraventricular pressure, decreased filling in diastole, and hence, a fall in output from both ventricles. The decline in left ventricular output is responsible for the greater than normal inspiratory drop in systemic arterial pressure (a difference of at least 10 mm Hg between inspiration and expiration), and the elevated right ventricular pressure in inspiration accounts for the equally important failure of the systemic venous pressure to decline in the usual manner. It is very important, then, not only to observe whether the cervical veins are distended, but also to observe whether the distention increases during inspiration.

Treatment. All patients with an acute pericarditis should be observed frequently and carefully for the possibility of a developing effusion or, if effusion is already present, for signs of tamponade. Blood pressure and heart rate should be recorded at frequent and regular intervals and serial chest films obtained. If the manifestations of tamponade appear, pericardial paracentesis should be instituted at once, since relief of the intrapericardial pressure may be lifesaving. When pericardial effusion recurs rapidly and frequently, a pleuropericardial window may be established. When the presence of effusion or thickened pericardium remains in doubt, angiocardiography is sometimes employed, but we believe exploration is preferable, since tissue or fluid can be secured for bacteriologic or histologic examination. Specific antibiotic therapy should be employed, of course, when an agent responsive to such therapy has been isolated.

POST-CARDIAC-INJURY SYNDROME

During the past few years, it has been recognized that a number of disorders, identical in their clinical manifestations, may appear under a variety of circumstances. They have one common feature: previous injury to the heart. The syndrome has been observed when the injury has been induced surgically in the course of a heart operation (postpericardiotomy syndrome or, as it was originally designated, postcommissurotomy syndrome, p. 1441). It may also follow myocardial infarction (post-myocardial-infarction syndrome), or it may develop after trauma of the heart (stab wound, nonpenetrating blow to the chest).

The symptoms usually occur after an interval of 2 weeks or more following the cardiac injury, and sometimes the symptoms may appear only after a lapse of months. Recurrences are common and may occur up to 2 years or more. Fever up to 102 to 104°F, pericarditis, pleuritis, pneumonitis are the outstanding features, the bout of illness usually subsiding in 1 or 2 weeks. The pericarditis, which appears to be the most constant lesion, may be of the fibrinous variety, or it may assume the character of a pericardial effusion, the latter often being serosanguineous and sometimes causing tamponade.

The mechanism whereby the clinical manifestations are induced is not certain, but there is a strong likelihood that they are the result of an antigen-antibody relationship. Whether the antigen originates from injured pericardial or myocardial tissue is not known, and the name *post-cardiac-injury syndrome* is tentatively suggested as an appropriate designation for this interesting group of disorders. It is meant only to imply that these various disorders have a common clinical picture and that they may have a common pathogenetic mechanism.

It is obvious that the clinical picture mimics in practically every detail the one known as "acute benign infectious pericarditis." Moreover, it is possible that the recurrences that occur so frequently in this latter condition are not always caused by an exacerbation of the original viral infection. It is conceivable that the original viral injury may now have initiated the sequence of events that culminates in the post-cardiac-injury syndrome. This concept is speculative, and further investigation is required.

"Cardiac injury" can be used in both a broad and restricted sense. We employ the term *post-cardiac-injury* broadly to include various types of heart injury: necrosis due to ischemia, the trauma of surgery, possibly the damage resulting from a viral infection of the pericardium. It also embraces the injury caused by contusions and penetrating wounds of the heart. For this last group and the identical syndrome that may follow, we have used the term "post-traumatic syndrome" in the restricted sense and imply that it is simply one form of the post-cardiac-injury syndrome.

Treatment. Often no treatment is necessary aside from analgesics for pain. The management of pericardial effusion and tamponade has already been discussed. When the illness is severe and is followed by a series of disabling recurrences, steroid therapy is usually effective.

We believe that the proper approach to the clinical problems of pericardial disease is to consider that the latter consists of three syndromes: *acute fibrinous pericarditis, pericardial effusion, constrictive heart disease.* The physician should first determine whether any of these syndromes is present; and if one of these forms of pericardial disease is found, his task is then to decide what is the etiology. To simplify the discussion and to avoid needless repetition, we have chosen to select one important example of each of the syndromes as the prototype and then to discuss the problem of etiologic diagnosis.

ACUTE BENIGN INFECTIOUS PERICARDITIS

This disorder is an important clinical entity because of its frequency and because it may be confused with other more serious affections. In some, a Coxsackie B virus has been isolated; in other instances, acute pericarditis has occurred in association with illnesses of known viral origin and, presumably, is caused by the same agent. It occurs at all ages but most frequently in young adults. Often there is a history of an antecedent respiratory infection within the preceding 2 to 3 weeks. Fever and precordial pain appear at about the same time, an important feature in the differentiation from myocardial infarction. The constitutional symptoms are usually mild to moderate, but occasionally the initial symptoms are stormy, the temperature rising to 104 to 105°F. The disease ordinarily runs its course in a few days to 2 weeks, but occasionally after the patient has presumably recovered, one or more recurrences may take place after weeks or even months. Tamponade is exceptional, and rarely constrictive pericarditis has been reported to develop. As is true in other forms of acute pericarditis, the pain is usually exaggerated by breathing, change of position, or swallowing. The T-wave alterations in the electrocardiogram are usually transitory, but they may persist for several years or indefinitely, constituting a subsequent source of confusion in persons without a clear history of pericarditis. There is no specific therapy. When repeated recurrences develop, early pericardiectomy has been found to be effective in terminating the illness.

Focal Pericarditis. One occasionally sees a patient, usually a young man, who has pericardial pain of the common pleuritic variety and who displays slight to moderate T-wave changes in only one or two leads. Serial electrocardiograms exhibit the typical evolutionary pattern of pericarditis, the

S-T segment elevation soon being replaced by inversion of T in the same lead. Slight fever and/or an evanescent friction rub may or may not be observed. This syndrome is thus similar to the more usual varieties of fibrinous pericarditis but displays the following differences. (1) The electrocardiographic findings point toward focal rather than diffuse inflammation of the pericardium. (2) The clinical course is unusually mild. (3) Pericardial effusion does not occur to a detectable degree.

Pathologists have long recognized focal patches of pericardial thickening as incidental findings at necropsy and, because of the frequency in young men, have designated them as "soldier's patches." It is tempting to speak of the clinical picture described in the preceding paragraph as the *soldier's patch syndrome*, but if this is done there should be clear recognition that such a designation is based only on a logical inference and not on any proof that the clinical disorder mentioned is in fact the analogue of the anatomic finding.

Differential Diagnosis of Acute Fibrinous Pericarditis

Since there is no specific test for acute benign infectious pericarditis, the diagnosis is primarily one of exclusion. Consequently, before concluding that one is dealing with the disorder known as acute benign infectious pericarditis, one must consider all other disorders that may be associated with an acute fibrinous pericarditis.

Acute Myocardial Infarction. When an ischemic pericarditis gives rise to a pleuritic type of pain, confusion with an infectious form of pericarditis is possible and one must rely on the time of occurrence of fever and pain, electrocardiographic abnormalities, such as the appearance of Q waves, the extent of the transaminase elevations, and the total clinical picture. More common is the error of assuming that acute benign infectious pericarditis is an acute myocardial infarction (p. 1454).

Post-Cardiac-Injury Syndrome. The two disorders in this category that are likely to be confused with acute benign infectious pericarditis are the *post-myocardial-infarction syndrome* and the pericarditis that may follow a nonpenetrating bruise to the chest. When the pericarditis occurs within a few weeks or months after the infarction or the blow to the chest, one is justified in concluding that the two are probably related. However, it is known that many individuals suffer a completely symptomless infarct. When an acute pericarditis occurs in such a person and when there is no reason to suspect a previous infarction, differentiation between the post-myocardial-infarction syndrome and acute benign infectious pericarditis is impossible on clinical grounds. Subsequently, the development of angina pectoris or acute infarction may then, in retrospect, clarify the nature of the previous illness. The conclusion to be drawn is that, in any person over the age of forty to forty-five, an apparently classical picture of acute benign infectious pericarditis may actually be the first overt manifestation of serious coronary disease. Similarly, a nonpenetrating chest-wall blow may be forgotten when the acute pericarditis develops several weeks later, and the relationship between the two may not be recognized. One must also bear in mind that the person who has sustained a myocardial infarct or a blow to the chest acquires thereby no immunity to the viruses that cause the infectious form of pericarditis and that, when we make the diagnosis of post-myocardial-infarction syndrome or pericarditis following a chest bruise, we are speaking in terms of probabilities and not certainties, until more precise methods of differentiation are available.

Pericarditis Due to Collagen Disease. Most important in the differential diagnosis is the pericarditis due to disseminated lupus, in which disease it occurs at some time in its course in over 50 per cent of the cases. Sometimes it appears as an asymptomatic effusion, but more often pain is present and very rarely tamponade may develop. When it occurs in the absence of other evidences of the underlying disorder, differentiation from acute benign infectious pericarditis or a mild form of *tuberculous pericarditis* may be made only on discovery of LE cells or by the specific methods of diagnosis of tuberculosis (p. 1007).

The pericarditis of *acute rheumatic fever* is always associated with evidences of severe pancarditis. *Pyogenic pericarditis*, usually secondary to pneumonia, is now far less common than before the advent of effective antibiotics. These conditions, as well as *uremic* or *neoplastic pericarditis*, should cause little difficulty of diagnosis.

CHRONIC TUBERCULOUS PERICARDIAL EFFUSION

Tuberculous pericarditis has been described in Chap. 146, Tuberculosis. The acute form has already been mentioned, and it needs to be stated here only that in other cases there may be no history of pain, the symptoms being those of infection in an individual with massive effusion, with or without manifestations of tuberculous involvement of other structures. It is important to bear this condition in mind when a middle-aged or elderly person with fever has what appears to be an enlarged heart of undetermined etiology, with or without congestive failure. Inasmuch as we now have effective specific methods of therapy that have reduced the mortality radically from the previous figures of 50 to 80 per cent, overlooking a pericardial effusion of tuberculous origin must be deemed a serious error. Consequently, no method of examination should be left undone to establish or rule out the diagnosis. This means chest films for pulmonary tuberculosis and a search for tuberculosis in other structures; tuberculin tests, repeated after several weeks; cultures and smears of gastric washings and of pericardial fluid. Finally, if the diagnosis is still obscure, one should resort to pericardial biopsy. If one is still unable to secure definitive evidence and one has good reason to be highly suspicious of the presence of tuberculosis, antimicrobial therapy is justified. Pericardiectomy with concomitant antituberculous therapy has been successfully employed if exploration reveals a thickened pericardium.

Differential Diagnosis of Chronic Pericardial Effusion

Cultures and smears of the pericardial fluid are so frequently negative in subsequently proved cases of tuberculous pericarditis, and a positive tuberculin test (p. 1006) so often found in persons who have no active tuberculosis, that one is sometimes faced with the dilemma of trying to decide how much emphasis to attach to each of these conflicting findings.

Myxedema may be responsible for a pericardial effusion that is sometimes massive. The other manifestations of myxedema should clarify the diagnosis, but unfortunately, even when they are present, the diagnosis is frequently overlooked. It is important, therefore, to make appropriate tests for thyroid function in every person with an enlarged cardiac outline of undetermined origin.

Neoplasms, disseminated lupus, rarely *polyarteritis nodosa, mycotic infections,* certain forms of *endomyocardial fibrosis* found in Africa, and very rarely, *severe anemia* and *scleroderma* may be the cause of a chronic pericardial effusion.

Finally, there are individuals who, without fever or other constitutional symptoms, are known to have had an "enlarged heart" for years, sometimes with, more often without, congestive failure, and who have subsequently been found to be suffering from a chronic pericardial effusion. The most exhaustive studies have failed to reveal the etiology of these effusions, but they have all been completely relieved by the establishment of a pleuropericardial window. Such disorders have been designated *chronic idiopathic pericardial effusion,* with full recognition that "idiopathic" merely signifies our present ignorance of the cause of these disorders. For example, one form of pericardial effusion, apparently "idiopathic," has been found to be caused sometimes by an *injury to the heart* following a nonpenetrating blow to the chest, the relationship between the injury and the subsequent effusion being obscured by the lapse of weeks before the effusion develops. This type of pericardial effusion is simply another form of the post-cardiac-injury syndrome.

CHRONIC CONSTRICTIVE PERICARDITIS

This disorder results when the healing of an acute fibrinous or serofibrinous pericarditis is followed by obliteration of the cavity of the sac, with the formation of granulation tissue which gradually contracts and forms a firm scar, encasing the heart and interfering with filling. The condition may be the result of tuberculous, staphylococcal, or pneumococcal infection, acute benign infectious pericarditis, traumatic pericarditis, but more often the cause is undetermined. Rarely, routine fluoroscopic examination may reveal calcification of the pericardium in an individual who is free of all symptoms referable to the heart. Usually, however, the clinical picture is characterized by dyspnea on exertion, which, however, is often relatively slight at rest, while orthopnea may be entirely absent; pronounced enlargement of the liver; distention of the cervical veins; ascites; and peripheral edema. The heart is normal in size in about half the cases; in others it is slightly to markedly enlarged. A paradoxic pulse is frequently encountered, and a protodiastolic gallop is present in most patients. Both by palpation and by x-ray, marked diminution in cardiac pulsation is noted. A very important finding is the presence of calcification of the pericardium, visible by x-ray in about one-half the cases. The spleen is sometimes palpable, and in the absence of evidence of bacterial endocarditis, splenomegaly in a patient with congestive failure should arouse suspicion of constrictive pericarditis. The electrocardiogram frequently displays low voltage and flattening or inversion of the T waves in all three limb leads. Atrial fibrillation is often present in this condition.

Congestive failure is initially the result of impaired filling of the ventricles caused by the restrictive action of the inelastic pericardium. However, the fibrotic process may extend into the myocardium, and congestive failure may then be due to the combined effects of the myocardial and the pericardial lesions. The interference with filling reduces the work of the heart, and myocardial atrophy may occur. This probably accounts for the delayed beneficial effects of operative treatment. Improvement may not become apparent until a number of months have elapsed. Presumably, the atrophy disappears when the impairment of filling is removed by resection of the pericardium. Because the filling of the right ventricle is impeded, this chamber is unable to flood the lungs with blood, acute pulmonary edema does not occur, and orthopnea is minimal.

Inasmuch as the usual physical signs of cardiac disease (murmurs, cardiac enlargement) may be inconspicuous or entirely lacking, the presence of hepatic enlargement and intractable ascites may lead to a mistaken diagnosis of cirrhosis of the liver. This error should be avoided if the neck veins are inspected carefully in all patients with ascites and hepatomegaly. *Given a clinical picture resembling cirrhosis but with the added feature of distended neck veins, careful search for calcification of the pericardium by chest films, with the patient in the oblique position, should be carried out and may disclose a curable or remediable form of heart disease.* Since calcification occurs in only about 50 per cent, exploration of the pericardium is justifiable if the clinical picture is suggestive enough.

The clinical picture described above represents the full-blown and classical disorder. It is important to bear in mind that sometimes a calcified pericardium, clearly visible by x-ray, may cause no symptoms whatsoever; or a patient may display symptoms of congestive failure without the classical features of constrictive pericarditis, and autopsy may nevertheless reveal the latter type of lesion.

Treatment. In the treatment of constrictive pericarditis, diuretic drugs and sodium restriction are useful. Digitalis, which is rarely of value in the preoperative state, may be beneficial in the prevention of heart failure when resection of the thickened pericardium permits an increased inflow into the ventricles and hence an enhanced burden on an atrophic myocardium. The benefits derived from cardiac decortication are often striking, and frequently the improvement, while slight at first, is progressive over a period of many months. The patient may be restored from a state of invalidism to something approaching normal activity.

Many instances of constrictive pericarditis are of tuberculous origin. Antituberculous therapy during the phase of effusion may prevent the development of constriction, and such specific therapy carried out before and after operation, if any tuberculous activity is present, will prevent the spread of the infection.

No treatment is required for those persons who are found to have a calcified pericardium but in whom there is no evidence of increased venous pressure.

Differential Diagnosis of Constrictive Heart Disease

There are two general problems in the diagnosis of constrictive heart disease. The first is the differentiation of the constrictive from the nonconstrictive disorders that lead to congestive failure. The second is the separation of constrictive pericarditis from other forms of constrictive heart disease. The clinical picture caused by any of the forms of constrictive heart disease may not be so fully developed as to display the classical features described above, and one may not suspect that heart failure is being caused by one of these disorders. On the other hand, a nonconstrictive type of heart disease may simulate the constrictive forms: e.g., cor pulmonale may be associated with severe systemic venous congestion and with little or no pulmonary congestion; the heart may not appear to be enlarged; a striking inspiratory fall in arterial pressure may be present. However, there is also an inspiratory fall in venous pressure, thus differentiating the phenomenon from the true paradoxic pulse (p. 1468). If it is concluded that constrictive heart disease is present, the second problem is to determine the cause.

The basic abnormality in chronic constrictive pericarditis is the inability of the ventricles to relax adequately during diastole because of the limitations imposed by the rigid, thickened pericardium. This limits diastolic filling, and stroke volume is diminished; atrial, pulmonic, and systemic venous pressures are elevated to about the same levels; congestive hepatomegaly with ascites and occasionally congestive splenomegaly as well as peripheral edema appear. The heart sounds are distant, cardiac pulsations under fluoroscopic examination are diminished, an early diastolic gallop is heard, and a paradoxic pulse can be elicited. The course of the illness is slow and progressive, and the usual medical treatment is relatively ineffective and disappointing.

This description applies to the full-blown picture, but there are lesser degrees of disability, and one may encounter persons with thickened, calcified pericardium who lead normal unrestricted lives. The same physiologic abnormalities and the same clinical picture may be induced by other forms of constrictive heart disease. *Endocardial fibrosis,* the various forms of *endomyocarditis,* extensive involvement of the myocardium by *amyloid disease, scleroderma, fibrosis secondary to myocarditis, constrictive epicarditis (Porter's syndrome)* are all capable of inducing the same hemodynamic defect leading to a disorder that is practically indistinguishable from that caused by constrictive pericarditis. It has also been shown that diffuse and severe scarring of the myocardium caused by *coronary sclerosis* that has been responsible for no pain is another disorder that mimics constrictive pericarditis.

The lesson to be learned is that when a patient has progressive, disabling, and unresponsive congestive failure, and particularly if he displays any of the phenomena of constrictive heart disease, however minimal they may be, the only decisive method of determining whether or not constrictive pericarditis is responsible is by exploration of the pericardium.

OTHER DISORDERS OF THE PERICARDIUM

Tumors of the pericardium are almost always secondary to malignant neoplasms of the mediastinum. The most common primary sources are carcinoma of the bronchus or breast, lymphoma, and occasionally other malignancies of the mediastinum, such as thymoma. Rarely, the tumor may originate in the pericardium as a mesothelioma. The usual clinical picture is that of an insidiously developing pericardial effusion, often bloody, and the chief problem is differentiation from a tuberculous effusion.

Pericardial cyst appears as a rounded or lobulated deformity of the cardiac silhouette, the most common location being at the right cardiophrenic angle. Its only clinical significance lies in the possibility of confusion with tumor.

REFERENCES

Burwell, C. S., and E. D. Robin: Diagnosis of Diffuse Myocardial Fibrosis, Circulation, 20:606, 1959.

Clark, G. M., E. Valentine, and S. G. Blount, Jr.: Endocardial Fibrosis Simulating Constrictive Pericarditis, New Engl. J. Med., 254:349, 1956.

Connolly, D. C., T. J. Dry, and others: Chronic Idiopathic Pericardial Effusion without Tamponade, Circulation, 20:1095, 1959.

Dock, W.: Inspiratory Traction on the Pericardium: The Cause of Pulsus Paradoxus in Pericardial Disease, A.M.A. Arch. Internal Med., 108:837, 1961.

Gimlette, T. M. D.: Constrictive Pericarditis, Brit. Heart J., 21:9, 1959.

Sawyer, C. G., C. S. Burwell, and others: Chronic Constrictive Pericarditis: Further Considerations of the Pathologic Physiology of the Disease, Am. Heart J., 44:207, 1952.

Weatherbee, H. R., Jr., and M. L. Pearce: Shock and Acute Abdominal Symptoms Complicating Acute Idiopathic Pericarditis, Ann. Internal Med., 49:876, 1958.

Williams, C., and L. Soutter: Pericardial Tamponade, A.M.A. Arch. Internal Med., 94:571, 1954.

Section 3: The Kidneys

INTRODUCTION

*T. R. Harrison and
Franklin H. Epstein*

The patient with renal disease may exhibit any one of a wide variety of problems. These include headache, hypertension, edema, heart failure, anemia, and coma. Less overt but no less frequent presenting symptoms are lassitude, anorexia, nausea, and unexplained fever. The common causes and the differential diagnosis of these several phenomena have been considered in previous chapters. The reader is referred particularly to Chap. 20, which deals with disordered renal function.

Few instances of clinically significant bilateral kidney disease will be overlooked if the urine is examined routinely and carefully for protein. The evaluation of the degree of renal damage rarely requires elaborate tests and can usually be based on such simple measurements as the concentrating power, the excretion of phenolsulfonphthalein, and the urea content of the blood. The rate of progression of the disease can be determined only by serial clinical observation. In this respect, laboratory tests may be misleading unless correlated with the patient's symptoms.

The physician should be continually alert to the possibility that certain curable but rare renal disorders may produce clinical pictures which are almost identical with those caused by more common but less treatable diseases. Thus he should consider the possibilities that hypertension may be due to unilateral renal disease (p. 1351) and that syphilis is a very rare but curable cause of the nephrotic syndrome. In a patient with renal insufficiency, the diagnosis of chronic uremia should not be entertained until such occasional but removable causes as obstruction, acute infection, shock, sodium or potassium depletion, congestive heart failure, tubular necrosis, or acute glomerulonephritis have been considered and excluded.

The discussion to follow is divided into two chapters. The first deals with general aspects of disorders of the kidneys and includes the treatment of chronic renal failure, which is a complication of a wide variety of different conditions. The second chapter is concerned with the specific diseases of the kidney and includes the management of acute renal failure, which has a smaller number of underlying causes. Tumors of the bladder and the treatment of stones are considered in this second chapter. The mechanisms underlying stone formation and the problems of renal and bladder infections have already been discussed in Chaps. 20 and 50, respectively.

257 GENERAL ASPECTS OF RENAL DISORDERS

Franklin H. Epstein

The Relationship between Diseases of the Kidney and Hypertension. The association of cardiac hypertrophy with contracted kidneys and albuminous urine was commented on by Richard Bright; since that time the relationship between hypertension and renal disorders has been a fruitful subject for study and speculation. It is clear that renal distortion or scarring resulting from many diseases may cause arterial hypertension and generalized vascular disease (Chap. 245). Often, however, there appears to be only the most casual relationship between the degree of encroachment upon renal excretory function and the incidence or degree of high blood pressure. For example, hypertension may be severe and rapidly progressive in a patient with unilateral constriction of a renal artery, who has a normal urea clearance and phenolsulfonphthalein excretion (and even a normal "routine urine"). On the other hand, another patient with severe chronic pyelonephritis, marked azotemia, and anemia may have a normal blood pressure throughout most of his life, only to develop a mild elevation terminally. In a third patient, small areas of scarring caused by bilateral interstitial pyelonephritis, which are themselves insufficient to produce detectable impairment of renal function, may be associated with malignant hypertension. In turn, the generalized vascular disease which accompanies hypertension may involve renal parenchyma, thus creating and reinforcing a vicious circle.

Characteristic of the natural history of many renal disorders is a *latent period* between the initial insult to the kidney and the appearance of fixed hypertension. Thus, although polycystic kidneys are undoubtedly abnormal from birth, hypertension usually does not appear until the third or fourth decade of life. Following acute glomerulonephritis, blood pressure usually returns to normal, though other signs of activity may persist. If healing is incomplete, the patient may again become hypertensive years later, this time, perhaps, with the development of progressive azotemia. A similar latent period before the appearance of hypertension may mark the course of some patients who have suffered episodes of pyelonephritis or preeclampsia.

The Relationship between Signs of Renal Failure and Functioning Renal Mass. As illustrated in Fig. 257-1, the relationship between the plasma level of urea or creatinine and the rate of glomerular filtration takes the form of a hyperbola. The shape of this curve has important implications for the clinician, for it illustrates the extent of the physiologic reserve of the kidneys. Although the concentration of urea in the blood varies inversely with the glomerular filtration rate from the very first reduction in the latter, one-half to three-quarters of both kidneys can be removed before the level of nonprotein nitrogen is necessarily elevated above "normal" limits. Conversely, if the blood urea nitrogen is persistently elevated in a patient with what appears at first glance to be only unilateral renal disease, impaired function of the opposite kidney must be suspected.

It is possible, very roughly, to generalize the relationship between functioning renal tissue and the signs and symptoms of renal failure in the same fashion, as in Fig. 257-2. The hyperbolic curve clarifies some aspects of the course of many chronic progressive renal diseases characterized by a long "latent" period and rapid terminal progression. One can visualize a slowly progressive process, relentlessly destroying renal substance, which is relatively asymptomatic for many years. When the limits of renal reserve are reached, symptoms appear in swift succession and the condition of the patient deteriorates rapidly, though there may be little actual acceleration of the rate of pathologic destruction of the kidneys.

The admittedly oversimplified curve of Fig. 257-2 provides a rationale for the treatment of patients with renal disease. The less kidney tissue there is remaining, the more difference an increment in function makes to the patient. The fragility of patients with little remaining renal function is apparent. Prolonged dehydration, the depressant effects of anesthesia, the circulatory shock of septicemia may be easily withstood by a person with normal or slightly impaired renal reserve but disastrous to a patient balanced on the knife-edge of renal decompensation. In evaluating the prognosis of a patient with renal insufficiency, the extent of damage *that is reversible* is obviously tremendously important. The goal of the physician in the treatment of advanced renal disease is the discovery and treatment of reversible disorders, no matter how insignificant they may at first appear, because for a patient on the steeply ascending portion of the curve, a small improvement in function may mean the difference between life and death.

Treatment of Chronic Renal Disease. One of the more important reversible disorders frequently contributing to uremia is *congestive heart failure*. In the presence of intrinsic renal disease, anemia, and hypoproteinemia, the contribution of heart failure to renal insufficiency can frequently be assessed only by the use of digitalis in a therapeutic trial. It is generally not necessary to reduce the daily maintenance dose of digitalis even in patients with severe renal excretory impairment. However, because of the vicious consequences of dehydration and salt depletion in such patients, casual administration of this drug to the point of toxic symptoms including nausea and vomiting should be avoided.

In many patients with renal insufficiency, *pulmonary edema* tends to be central, producing a "butterfly pattern" on the chest x-ray. Rales may be absent. Increasing agitation and restlessness, coupled with accentuation of the second pulmonic heart sound, are often the first warning to the physician of an impending explosion of paroxysmal dyspnea which may be warded off with digitalis. Diuretic drugs are generally ineffective when glomerular filtration rate is greatly restricted, i.e., when the blood urea nitrogen is over 80 to 100 mg per 100 ml. Chlorothiazide and its derivatives are probably safer under such circumstances than mercurials, which may, especially after repeated cumulative doses, cause necrosis of renal cells. Ammonium chloride and other acidifying diuretic agents are useless and may be harmful in renal insufficiency.

In every case of chronic renal insufficiency it is important to consider the possibility of lower urinary tract *obstruction*. Patients with chronic prostatic retention or urethral stricture, with overflow incontinence or infection that can be cleared only when the bladder is allowed to empty normally, may improve remarkably with drainage. Chronic partial obstruction to the flow of urine, either at the bladder outlet or at the level of the ureters (as in the syndrome of *periureteral fibrosis*), may produce azotemia without oliguria; in fact, urinary output may be increased because of the loss of concentrating power. In the bedridden and obtunded patient with chronic renal disease and advanced uremia, unrecognized functional difficulty in bladder emptying, often precipitated by sedatives, but treatable with Urecholine or Prostigmine, may be the cause of rapid and otherwise inexplicable deterioration. A delayed pattern of phenolsulfonphthalein excretion will sometimes supply the clue to the presence of bladder neck obstruction. An x-ray of the abdomen should be one of the initial studies of every patient with uremia, especially when oliguria is present, since calculi may obstruct both ureters simultaneously, or a single ureter when there is only one kidney. Failure to investigate the possibility of ureteral obstruction in such cases may be as disastrous as too vigorous instrumentation of the urinary tract in chronic nephritis.

A search for urinary *infection* should be made in

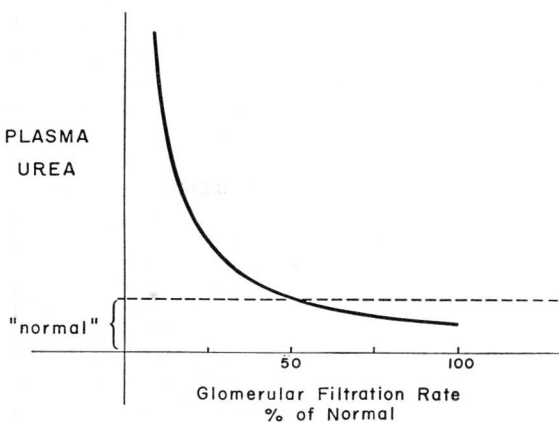

PLASMA UREA

"normal"

50   100

Glomerular Filtration Rate
% of Normal

Fig. 257-1

every patient with chronic renal disease, and treatment with the appropriate antibiotic instituted if an infecting organism is found. In this connection, unnecessary instrumentation of the urinary tract should be avoided. In particular, the use of inlying catheters should be strongly condemned except when absolutely necessary to relieve obstruction. Patients with indwelling catheters almost invariably develop an active urinary infection, even when receiving antibiotics prophylactically. The resulting necrotizing cystitis, active pyelonephritis, or bacteremia not infrequently proves fatal to the fragile patient with renal insufficiency.

Streptomycin, normally excreted by the kidney, may rapidly accumulate to toxic levels when given in usual doses to patients with impaired renal function. Tetracyclines also are excreted slowly in patients with damaged kidneys. Chloromycetin is inactivated normally, but its metabolic products are only slowly eliminated.

In azotemic patients without edema, congestive failure, or oliguria, restriction of salt is unwise as well as unnecessary. The intake of sodium by such patients should be encouraged, preferably as salty

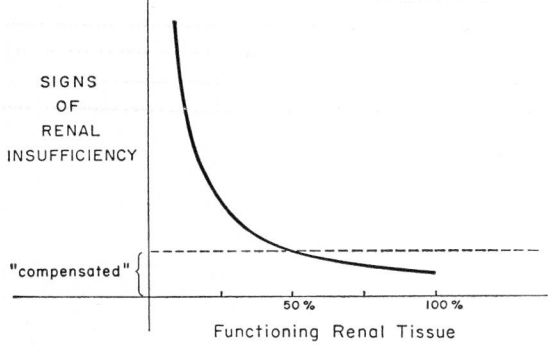

SIGNS OF RENAL INSUFFICIENCY

"compensated"

50 %   100 %

Functioning Renal Tissue

Fig. 257-2

foods and drinks, rather than pills of sodium chloride, which tend to irritate the stomach. The slight expansion of extracellular fluid induced by a diet high in sodium is often reflected in improved renal blood flow and glomerular filtration. Excretion of urea, sulfates, and phosphates is augmented, and the secretion of acid and potassium is promoted (Chap. 51). Because salt stimulates thirst, the intake of water is encouraged in a natural fashion and urinary flow is improved. The appearance of congestive failure sharply limits the extent to which an increased intake of salt can be used as a lever to improve renal function in chronic renal disease. Because of the beneficial effects of salt on renal function, an attempt should be made to control early congestive heart failure in patients with chronic renal disease with digitalis, rather than by rigid limitation of dietary sodium. Unnecessary restriction of salt and consequent salt depletion may, in fact, result in considerable further impairment of renal function in many patients with renal insufficiency who are unable to conserve sodium in the normal fashion when the intake of this ion is limited (p. 172). Salt-wasting is more common in patients with chronic pyelonephritis than chronic glomerulonephritis but may occur in renal insufficiency of any etiology; in such cases the triad of asthenia, dehydration, and hyponatremia may even suggest the diagnosis of Addison's disease. From 5 to 8 Gm sodium chloride daily may be required to prevent sodium depletion. Salt-losing may disappear or become less marked in the terminal stages of renal failure, as glomerular filtration becomes progressively compromised, congestive heart failure makes its appearance, and oliguria supervenes.

The systemic *acidosis* which accompanies chronic renal insufficiency is often responsible for mild to severe nausea, fatigue, malaise, and breathlessness on exertion, long before Kussmaul respirations are clinically apparent. Prescription of the equivalent of 4 to 6 Gm sodium bicarbonate daily (as, for example, 1 to 2 tbsp of 10 per cent sodium citrate in syrup of wild cherry, after each meal) usually suffices to maintain serum bicarbonate at 18 to 22 mEq per liter, and thereby to avoid the unpleasant side effects of acidosis. Excessive administration of alkali must be avoided, especially in the presence of hypocalcemia (p. 470), where correction of acidosis without the simultaneous administration of calcium may precipitate tetany or convulsions. Large amounts of sodium bicarbonate or lactate are also contraindicated in congestive heart failure.

Because of the obligatory polyuria evident in most patients with chronic renal insufficiency, *dehydration* may be readily produced, even by relatively brief abstention from fluids. Thirsting and purgation in preparation for x-ray studies may prove fatal in the delicately balanced patient with renal decompensation. In such patients it is usually unnecessary and unwise to withhold fluids before blood is drawn for chemical determinations in the morning. Even minor surgical procedures should be undertaken against a background of adequate hydration, by the intravenous route if necessary, both before and after operation. Overnight polyuria in many patients results in early morning thirst and a feeling of hunger on awakening which quickly turns to nausea and vomiting, thereby perpetuating the vicious circle of dehydration. This can sometimes be prevented by taking a drink of water after urinating at night or be allayed by a small preliminary feeding immediately after waking.

The treatment of *nausea* in patients with chronic renal disease should, as already indicated, include close attention to proper hydration, correction of acidosis, and treatment of sodium depletion. Anorexia is one of the first signs of a low serum sodium, and nausea is often dramatically improved when hyponatremia is corrected. The administration of one of the phenothiazine derivatives several times daily or of Benadryl, coupled with small frequent feedings, has proved helpful. The pattern of meals should be adjusted flexibly to take advantage of the patient's sometimes unpredictable periods of hunger and well-being. When vomiting is persistent, all feeding should be stopped and fluids given intravenously for 1 or 2 days. The vomiting which marks the terminal stage of nephritis may be particularly intractable; it is one of the few types that will continue after all food and fluids are withheld. Although restriction of the fluid intake is contraindicated, there is no reason to push fluids to the point of discomfort. The efficiency of the kidney in excreting urea and other solutes appears to reach a maximum at a urine volume of 2,500 to 3,000 ml; even the diseased kidney is not much more effective at higher volumes. Moreover, the ability to excrete large loads of water rapidly is impaired in most patients with azotemia. Excessive administration of water, especially when salt intake is limited, is likely, therefore, to result in hyponatremia, with its attendant symptoms of nausea, muscle cramps, and mental disturbances.

The *anemia* of renal insufficiency is unresponsive to liver and to iron. The latter may be given in a therapeutic trial, but if it is effective, it may reasonably be concluded that the anemia is not the product of uncomplicated renal failure. Reticulocytosis is reported to follow the administration of cobalt, but gastric irritation generally precludes the use of this medication in effective doses. For the treatment of the anemia of advanced renal disease, reliance must be placed on transfusions. Although the degree of tolerance to anemia varies greatly, weakness, shortness of breath, and poor appetite are likely to be improved by transfusions when the hemoglobin is below 8 Gm per 100 ml. Strenuous efforts to maintain normal or near-normal hemoglobin levels by transfusion are, however, unwise and unnecessary. Unless serum proteins are depleted, or hemostatic defects are present, in which case whole blood should be given, transfusions should ideally be of packed red cells derived from fresh blood. Transfusion should be given cautiously in the presence of congestive heart failure, but treatment of severe anemia should not be neglected because the heart is failing; in such circumstances, transfusions should be of packed red cells given slowly in small amounts, with the patient in a sitting position. If blood is given at intervals to ambulatory patients with advanced renal disease before the red blood cell count has fallen to a critical level, general well-being and strength may be greatly improved and the remaining days made happier and more useful.

When *oliguria* is present, at any stage of renal disease, it is clear that the dietary intake of *protein* should be restricted, if not eliminated. Similarly, there is general agreement that protein intake should be increased in the nephrotic syndrome. Controversy still surrounds the proper prescription of protein in the diet of the large number of patients with chronic renal disease and azotemia who have an undiminished or increased urinary output. Unfortunately, adequate studies on the long-range effect of variations in protein intake on the course of renal disease in man are almost nonexistent. It would seem reasonable that the common sense of the physician and a consideration of the nutritional needs of the whole patient should control advice about diet. Chronic nephritis is a wasting disease. Patients are frequently protein-depleted and anemic. Fatigue, anorexia, and weakness are prominent complaints. In many cases malnutrition has been intensified by unreasonable fear of protein. Too often in renal insufficiency the patient's appetite forcibly limits any theoretical discussions of the optimum diet, but when a diet adequate in calories and protein can be supplied, a positive nitrogen balance (implying previous depletion of tissue stores of protein) can almost always be demonstrated. Obesity, to be sure, should be avoided, but where appetite is present, the clinician should be grateful and allow it full scope. A hungry patient, permitted to eat a diet normal in protein (1 Gm per kg per day), may exhibit a gratifying return of strength, appetite, and well-being. The commonly encountered belief that red meat and eggs are more harmful to patients with nephritis than the protein of fish, milk, or vegetables is not valid. Alcoholic beverages, in modest amounts, are not harmful to the kidneys, and their sedative qualities should not be neglected.

The *neuromuscular disturbances* of uremia are often distressing and difficult to treat. Frank hypocalcemic tetany can be relieved by intravenous calcium salts (1 Gm calcium daily as the gluconate or chloride for 2 to 3 days), but the gross tremors, twitchings, and jactitations of uremia are generally not improved by the administration of calcium. Occasionally they disappear or improve when hyponatremia is corrected. Care must be taken not to mistake the rigidity, tremor, and occasional convulsive episodes which sometimes follow overdoses of the phenothiazine drugs for the neuromuscular deterioration of renal insufficiency. Convulsions are best controlled by the intravenous or intramuscular administration of sodium phenobarbital. Chloral hydrate (1 to 2 Gm nightly) and Benadryl (100 mg) are useful sedatives. *Itching* is an extremely variable symptom of uremia and not closely correlated with the level of blood urea. It may sometimes be controlled by daily cleansing baths, bland lubricating ointments, and the use of Benadryl or similar antihistaminic and sedative drugs. The author has occasionally observed relief when topical adrenal cortical steroids were used.

Vigorous treatment of *hypertension* with ganglionic blocking agents is often unsuccessful and may be hazardous when blood urea nitrogen reaches 60 mg per 100 ml or more. Under these circumstances small reductions in perfusion pressure and blood flow through the kidneys may precipitate renal decompensation. Cautious use of small doses of ganglionic blocking agents may be attempted when retinopathy or hypertensive heart failure is producing symptoms. Reserpine may be prescribed more freely, but is rarely completely effective. Sodium depletion with diet or diuretic agents generally is harmful to renal function. Hypertensive headaches may be treated with aspirin or phenacetin; when they occur on awakening, elevating the head of the bed often provides some measure of relief. In this phase of management, as in many others, *primum non nocere* should be the rule; the patient with chronic renal insufficiency and hypertension who is asymptomatic should in general be left alone.

The role of *artificial dialysis* in the management of chronic renal disease has not been well delineated. It seems clear that some patients with chronic renal insufficiency, especially those in whom vascular disease is not far advanced, can be helped through an otherwise fatal complication, such as an acute infection or a surgical operation, by the judicious use of dialysis. Patients with chronic glomerulonephritis in whom an attempt has been made to prolong life by repeated hemodialysis have eventually succumbed to rapidly progressive vascular complications or infection. Transplantation of a normal kidney from an identical twin has been successfully accomplished in a few patients with chronic renal disease, with disappearance of the uremic syndrome. Immunologic barriers, however, continue to prevent the successful transplantation of organs from nonidentical donors.

Approach to the Diagnosis of Asymptomatic Proteinuria. A few points in the study of the patient with asymptomatic proteinuria deserve special emphasis. Postural proteinuria (p. 173) should be ruled out, as well as the proteinuria which is normally associated with exercise or which follows certain febrile diseases. A careful history should inquire into the possibility of recent respiratory or skin infections, recurrent pyelitis, edema or hypertension during pregnancy, arthritis, rash, and drug sensitivity. A history of enuresis past the age of six may suggest congenital structural or neurologic anomalies of the urinary tract or chronic childhood pyelitis. The results of prior examinations for employment, insurance, or military service should be ascertained. The family history may be positive for renal and vascular diseases; inquiry should also be made about gout and diabetes. Blood pressure should be checked in the erect as well as supine position and retinal as well as peripheral vessels examined. Amyloidosis may be suggested by an enlarged liver or spleen; the presence of palpable masses in both upper quadrants should also raise the question of polycystic kidneys. Physical examination should not overlook the possibility of a cystocele or enlarged prostate.

A clean urine should be obtained and cultured (p. 1037). Examination of a *fresh* urine sediment *by the physician* is a most important diagnostic maneuver. The composition of casts is particularly significant. Clumps of leukocytes and white blood cell casts with or without bacteria apparent on the stained smear suggest pyelonephritis. Leukocyte casts are also sometimes seen in acute glomerulonephritis. If hematuria is accompanied by red blood cell casts, an active hemorrhagic lesion in the glomerulus is likely. Red blood cells and epithelial cells entrapped in casts, together with casts containing lipid droplets, should suggest glomerulonephritis, without distinguishing among its various etiologies. It should be emphasized that the absence of characteristic formed elements in the urinary sediment does not rule out either chronic glomerulonephritis or pyelonephritis. If more than 2 to 3 Gm of protein is excreted in the urine daily, a generalized disease primarily affecting glomeruli is likely to be present. Congestive heart failure and malignant hypertension, regardless of etiology, may also be associated with heavy proteinuria.

Blood urea, serum creatinine, and phenolsulfonphthalein excretion are useful in assessing the degree to which renal reserve has been impaired. If the blood urea nitrogen is over 20 mg per 100 ml or the serum creatinine above 2.0 mg per 100 ml, it is likely that both kidneys are involved by the disease process. A phenolsulfonphthalein excretion of less than 25 per cent in 15 min or 60 per cent in 2 hr is indicative of renal impairment; excretion which is greater during the second hour than the first may suggest hydronephrosis or incomplete bladder emptying. (Inadequate urine volumes in the 15-min sample may be avoided by starting the phenolsulfonphthalein test after the patient has been hydrated and injecting the dye only after he feels an urge to void.) Occasionally, a disproportionate elevation of blood uric acid will suggest underlying gouty nephropathy. Examination of the blood for LE cells or of the serum for antinuclear antibodies may detect early lupus erythematosus. Electrophoresis of the serum may reveal globulins characteristic of multiple myeloma.

The size and shape of the kidneys as well as the structure of calyces and ureters may be ascertained from an intravenous pyelogram. At the conclusion of this examination, a postvoiding film of the bladder may give information about residual urine without the necessity for catheterization. The size of the kidneys can be estimated in relation to the vertebral shadows on the plain film of the abdomen; normal kidneys are approximately as long as three to three and one-half lumbar vertebral bodies. When one kidney is shrunken and the other has failed to hypertrophy, disease is usually bilateral.

Percutaneous needle biopsy of the kidney has provided much useful information for the student of renal disease, but even in the most skillful hands, it is not without hazard. In the author's experience, it has not infrequently contributed helpfully to the management of the individual patient (e.g., the unexpected finding of amyloidosis or periarteritis; the detection of advanced changes of pyelonephritis in an apparently uninvolved kidney), but its greatest value has been to illuminate the still ill-defined natural history of diffuse diseases of the kidney. The accuracy of needle biopsy as a diagnostic technique is limited in focal disorders of the kidneys by the small size of the specimen and in diffuse glomerular disease by the fact that the sample obtained may contain no or few glomeruli. In most patients with proteinuria, proper use of the more conventional diagnostic methods will permit an accurate working diagnosis. Interpretation of biopsy sections must be made with proper regard to the rest of the clinical and laboratory findings and to the fact that, in this relatively new area of clinical investigation, both pathologist and clinician still have a great deal to learn.

Finally, the diagnostic maneuver of *following the patient,* in addition to being innocuous, has a great deal to recommend it. Acute or self-limited processes, even when the histologic picture is clear, can sometimes be diagnosed only in retrospect.

258 DISEASES OF THE KIDNEYS

Franklin H. Epstein

ACUTE GLOMERULONEPHRITIS

Acute glomerulonephritis is an acute, diffuse inflammation of the glomeruli of the kidneys. It represents about 0.5 per cent of all admissions to general hospitals in the United States and is found at autopsy in 0.1 to 0.2 per cent of deaths. The disease is twice as frequent in males as in females. Although it is commoner in children than adults, it may occur in adults of every age.

Etiology. Acute glomerulonephritis is best thought of as a pattern of reaction of the kidneys, rather than as a single disease with a specific etiology. Preceding infection with the group A, β-hemolytic *streptococcus* is by far the most common cause (p. 918). The infection usually arises in the upper respiratory tract, and its severity is not necessarily related to the incidence or severity of the ensuing nephritis. Streptococcal infection of the skin or of wounds may also be followed by glomerulonephritis. There is considerable evidence that only certain strains of group A streptococci are nephritogenic; these include types 12, 4, 25, and Red Lake.

Acute nephritis has been reported by Bates, Jennings, and Earle as a complication of an epidemic of acute pharyngitis, presumably of *viral origin*, in which streptococcal infection was excluded by bacteriologic and immunologic evidence. *Bacterial endocarditis* is frequently complicated by acute glomerulonephritis. Glomerulonephritis has occasionally been reported to follow *other acute infections,* but most such reports lack convincing evidence to rule out associated streptococcal infection.

Acute hemorrhagic nephritis superficially resembling the poststreptococcal variety may occur in the course of *lupus erythematosus, periarteritis,* or *erythema nodosum*. It is commonly seen as a complication of the *allergic purpuras,* associated with joint or abdominal pain. Finally, it may be a manifestation of *hypersensitivity to drugs* or other foreign agents.

Pathogenesis. Attempts to produce acute glomerulonephritis in animals by establishing an infection with streptococcus or by injecting dead or living streptococci have generally been unsuccessful. Nevertheless, it seems possible that alteration of glomerular tissue, perhaps by a blood-borne produce of the streptococcus, is the first step in the pathogenesis of most cases of acute nephritis in man. The disease is probably the result of an autoimmune reaction, in which components of the glomeruli and perhaps of small blood vessels in the kidney, injured or modified by an inciting agent, serve as antigens. The evidence for this can be summarized as follows. (1) There is invariably a latent period (which may last 1 to 4 weeks but averages 10 to 14 days) between the acute streptococcal pharyngitis and the first manifestations of acute nephritis. (2) Serum complement falls coincident with the attack of acute nephritis (presumably as a result of combination with antigen and antibody in the kidney). (3) High concentrations of gamma globulin can be detected on the basement membrane of injured glomeruli in renal biopsies from patients with acute glomerulonephritis. It is of interest in this connection that heterologous immune responses are much more easily demonstrated with components of glomerular basement membrane than with glomerular epithelial and endothelial cells and that the globulin fraction of antikidney serums prepared in animals can be shown to attach primarily to glomeruli.

Although the clinical picture as seen in man has not been exactly reproduced in animals, the most convincing experimental analogues of glomerulonephritis are those produced by injecting specific antibodies to the kidney (Masugi nephritis). Whole kidney tissue or glomeruli from one animal are injected into another species, antibodies are allowed to develop, and after an appropriate interval, serum from the second animal is injected intravenously into a new member of the original species. Proteinuria, hypertension, and nitrogen retention occur. The onset of the nephritis is generally abrupt but is sometimes (like poststreptococcal nephritis) characterized by a latent period. The lesions of the disease may heal, or they may become chronic. It is of some interest to students of the toxemias of pregnancy that antibodies to placental tissue are also nephrotoxic.

Lesions resembling glomerulonephritis are also observed in rabbits as part of the generalized anaphylactic reaction involving vascular endothelium which follows sensitization to foreign proteins. These have an obvious analogy to those cases of nephritis in human beings associated with hypersensitivity reaction.

Pathology. The kidneys may be normal in size, but as a rule are swollen. The surfaces are usually smooth and spotted with fine punctate hemorrhages; the pyramids are markedly congested. The histologic picture may vary considerably, probably as a result of differences in the duration of the process and the degree of immunologic reaction as well as in the nature and intensity of the provocative agent. All or almost all glomeruli are generally involved; yet the degree of inflammation may vary from one to another and be focal in distribution inside the glomerular tuft. In poststreptococcal nephritis, the glomeruli are usually swollen and hypercellular, with thickened glomerular loops, infiltrating polymorphonuclear leukocytes, and proliferation of endothelial and epithelial cells. Occasionally, however, especially when function is completely recovered, but while the urine sediment is still abnormal, renal biopsy will reveal glomeruli which appear normal except for occasional focal thickening of basement membranes. Red cells and red cell casts are present in the tubular lumens. Tubular cells may appear flattened or vacuolated, but pathologic changes in tubules are minimal compared with those in the glomeruli. Afferent arterioles may sometimes show focal medial necrosis with perivascular cellular infiltrates, and there may be similar lesions of the interlobular vessels.

As the disease process subsides, there may be resolution of the inflammatory process, with restoration of normal architecture. More frequently, hyalinized glomeruli, glomerular adhesions, and vascular changes persist, with wedge-shaped areas of atrophy and fibrosis separated by areas of relatively well-preserved tissue in which the remaining tubules are dilated. Even after the urine has completely cleared, focal hypercellularity and thickening of the stalks of glomerular lobules may persist. Widespread proliferation of the capsular epithelium, producing glomerular "crescents," is a characteristic finding in those patients who deteriorate rapidly, dying with hypertension and oliguria within 1 to 12 months of the onset of the disease.

Clinical Features and Pathologic Physiology. Common clinical manifestations of poststreptococcal glomerulonephritis are detailed on p. 918. The clinical picture is not infrequently dominated by one or more signs or symptoms which overshadow the rest and may initially mislead the physician who anticipates a "classical" pattern. Frequent presenting symptoms include anorexia, abdominal pain, facial edema, congestive heart failure, gross hematuria or coffee-colored urine, oliguria or anuria, and unexpected convulsions.

Fatigue and anorexia are almost universal; it is unusual for a patient with acute glomerulonephritis to feel as well as before the illness or to have a good appetite.

Pain in the loins or abdomen may be colicky or steady, and in exceptional instances, so severe as to simulate a surgical condition. *Fever* generally does not exceed 101°F and usually subsides within a few days after hospitalization; persistent fever may sometimes be caused by residual streptococcal or other infection or by a reaction to antibiotics.

Although facial *edema* is extremely common, edema of the legs without any swelling of the face is frequent, especially in older persons. Edema may be generally distributed and hence unapparent, and the only clue to its presence may be a 5- or 8-lb weight loss after the patient is put to bed and given a low-salt diet. Localization of edema about

the eyes is best explained by the low tissue turgor in this region. The absence of orthopnea, at least during the early stages of the disease, further favors accumulation of fluid in the upper half of the body during the hours of sleep.

Whether salt and water retention in acute nephritis is primarily due to renal disease per se or secondary to other circulatory disturbances which provoke even normal kidneys to retain sodium is not entirely clear. Considerable evidence suggests that disproportionate reduction in glomerular filtration rate is responsible for the initial oliguria and subsequent retention of sodium which result in excessive accumulation of extracellular fluid. Edema formation is generally associated with some decrease in the inulin clearance, and diuresis with a fall in blood urea nitrogen. Nevertheless, diuresis may be initiated in acute nephritis without any measurable improvement in a depressed filtration rate; the relationship between impaired inulin clearance and sodium retention is therefore not simple or clearcut.

Generalized capillary damage is probably *not* a cause of edema in nephritis, since the edema fluid does not contain increased amounts of protein. Although hypoalbuminemia resulting from extensive losses of plasma protein into the urine may contribute to edema in some cases, this factor cannot be the most important one in the many instances where plasma volume, by direct measurement, is increased or normal. Urinary excretion of aldosterone may be low in acute glomerulonephritis in the presence of edema, even when the patient is on a salt-free diet. As might be expected in such a situation, spironolactone does not provoke diuresis. Renal retention of sodium under these circumstances is probably a result of altered renal hemodynamics, rather than excessive secretion of salt-retaining hormone by the adrenal cortex.

Together with edema, signs and symptoms of *congestive heart failure* are often prominent, whether or not arterial hypertension is present. The sudden onset of heart failure in a previously well person may be the manifestation which brings the patient with acute nephritis to the doctor. Fatal pulmonary edema may be precipitated by convulsions. The heart is usually somewhat enlarged, and the venous pressure may be elevated. Nonspecific alterations in the electrocardiogram are common. Unlike the pattern of "low-output" cardiac failure, the circulation time is typically normal or short, and cardiac output is normal even when edema is present or increasing. Under such circumstances cardiac output does not rise further when digitalis is administered. It seems probable that, in most cases, circulatory congestion is a result of fluid retention rather than its cause.

It should be emphasized, however, that heart

failure responsive to digitalis (and associated with a prolonged circulation time) may at times complicate acute nephritis. When orthopnea is present, especially if accompanied by rales or gallop rhythm, digitalis should be prescribed. In other instances of edema and elevated venous pressure, a careful therapeutic trial of digitalis should be undertaken, with the knowledge that in many instances it will be found ineffective.

Hypertension is observed in approximately 50 per cent of adults with nephritis admitted to a general hospital. The incidence may be lower in mild cases detected in the course of a streptococcal epidemic. The onset is usually coincident with the first abnormal urinary findings, although in certain cases it may even precede and in others follow them. The elevated blood pressure is presumably caused by the release of renin, which has been detected in the peripheral blood of patients with fulminating acute nephritis.

The *optic fundi* are generally normal but may show arteriolar narrowing and in exceptional circumstances, papilledema, hemorrhages, and fluffy exudates.

When the blood pressure rises rapidly, headache, somnolence, and *convulsions* may develop, simulating in an occasional case the clinical picture of brain tumor. The differential diagnosis in such instances is not made easier by the fact that proteinuria and microscopic hematuria are often detected immediately following generalized seizures of any origin. Vomiting, dehydration, and heart failure appear to predispose to convulsions. They are not dependent on nitrogen retention but are probably the result of cerebral ischemia or tiny hemorrhages secondary to changes in the cerebral vasculature.

Mild *anemia* occurs frequently in acute glomerulonephritis, especially with edema. Total red cell volume has been found to be normal in many such patients, in whom the low hematocrit reflects dilution. In addition, depression of the bone marrow and increased destruction of red cells may contribute to anemia in certain azotemic patients. Serum albumin may be low, as a result of urinary losses and of the excessive catabolism of protein observed in many acute diseases or injuries. Serum cholesterol may be elevated, even when serum albumin is not greatly decreased. The presence of anemia and hypercholesterolemia, then, does not necessarily mean that nephritis is chronic or progressive.

Changes in renal function which occur in acute nephritis are characteristic. Glomerular filtration rate is usually depressed, and to a greater degree than renal blood flow. The latter may, indeed, be elevated, though in severe cases it falls as well. Filtration fraction is therefore reduced. Blood urea nitrogen is elevated in perhaps half of the patients with glomerulonephritis. In cases of mild or moderate severity, phenolsulfonphthalein excretion is either normal or only slightly decreased, even when the blood urea nitrogen is elevated. With more severe initial involvement, or with progression of the disease, excretion of phenolsulfonphthalein may fall. Acid urine of high specific gravity may be excreted early in the course of the illness, despite pronounced azotemia. *The combination of azotemia with well-maintained phenolsulfonphthalein excretion and high urinary specific gravity is seen in few diseases of the kidney other than acute glomerulonephritis.*

The *urine* may be grossly bloody or coffee-colored; on the other hand hematuria may be apparent only on careful inspection of the spun sediment. The identification of red cells embedded in *casts* establishes the glomerular origin of the bleeding. Granular and epithelial cell casts, especially the latter, are characteristically present. Lipid droplets and fatty casts are usually not present at the very onset of the disease, but may appear within the first few weeks, regardless of the presence or absence of hyperlipemia in the serum. Leukocytes and white blood cell casts reflect the essentially inflammatory character of the glomerular lesion. *Proteinuria* may reach impressive levels, over 6 to 8 Gm daily, but is more often below 2 Gm per day. Especially during recovery, protein may disappear from the urine while red cells and red cell casts continue to be excreted.

The disease is sometimes ushered in by a period of *oliguria* which may progress to complete anuria. Usually this lasts only a few days, but an occasional case of anuria lasting more than 10 days has been reported in acute glomerulonephritis followed by complete recovery. The oliguria which occurs at the onset of acute nephritis has a much better prognosis than that which may supervene when the disease has been active for several weeks. In contrast to patients with acute tubular necrosis, urinary sodium concentration is very low (less than 15 mEq per liter) in oliguria secondary to glomerulonephritis, and urinary osmolarity is often significantly above that of plasma.

Extrarenal *vasculitis* may be an important concomitant of acute nephritis. Its myocardial and cerebral manifestations have already been mentioned. Purpuric rashes, subungual hemorrhages, and even acute arthritis may rarely be seen in the course of severe poststreptococcal nephritis. At postmortem, necrotizing and organizing lesions of periarteritis may be found in the kidneys and elsewhere.

Finally, it should be emphasized that patients may develop acute nephritis with no symptoms and no abnormal physical or laboratory findings other than mild proteinuria and an abnormal urinary sediment.

Differential Diagnosis. Periorbital edema, occurring as an initial symptom of urticaria, trichinosis, infectious mononucleosis, or insect bites about the face, may suggest acute nephritis until the urine is examined. The finding of red cell casts and the coincidence of an elevated blood urea nitrogen with normal phenolsulfonphthalein excretion serve to exclude many other diseases of the urinary tract, in which glomeruli are not primarily affected. The nephritis associated with lupus, polyarteritis nodosa, and subacute bacterial endocarditis will often be recognized as a complication of the primary disease, but sometimes may be its only manifestation. The characteristic elevation and subsequent fall of antistreptolysin titer is excellent evidence of preceding streptococcal infection, but may not be present, especially when the infection has been treated with penicillin. Gross hematuria with lower urinary symptoms is much more likely to be due to hemorrhagic cystitis or prostatitis. In middle-aged and elderly men, azotemia and hematuria may be mistakenly ascribed to the prostate until the daily excretion of protein is found to be greater than 2 Gm, suggesting the correct diagnosis of glomerulonephritis. The presence of small kidneys or of severe anemia (less than 8 Gm of hemoglobin) suggests chronic renal disease, as do the stigmata of prolonged hypertension in heart, blood vessels, and fundi. The appearance of acute nephritis immediately following a respiratory infection, without a latent period, suggests an acute exacerbation of chronic nephritis. Persistent fever, cardiac murmurs, or a palpable spleen should spur a search for subacute bacterial endocarditis.

Course and Prognosis. The course and outlook of acute glomerulonephritis vary widely. In children or young adults who develop nephritis following streptococcal infection, the entire disease may be over within 2 to 4 weeks. Most patients recover completely, although a small number (less than 10 per cent) go rapidly downhill and die within the first few months. On the other hand, in the adult population of a general hospital, the likelihood of chronicity appears to be much greater. It has been estimated that 20 to 50 per cent of adult patients hospitalized with acute glomerulonephritis either succumb to the acute episode or go on to develop chronic desease. The latter may be quiescent for long periods and manifested only by proteinuria and an abnormal urinary sediment. The ultimate outcome bears a rough relation to the initial severity of the illness, though there are many exceptions to this rule. The most frequent duration of the disease in hospitalized adults is probably about 2 to 3 months. Blood pressure usually returns to normal before the urine clears. Heavy proteinuria lasting longer than 3 to 4 months suggests a poor prognosis, though nephritis may heal completely even after proteinuria has been present for as long as 2 years. Microscopic hematuria commonly persists for some months after proteinuria has disappeared or diminished to a faint trace. Postural dizziness, easy flushing, and other signs of autonomic instability, as well as postural proteinuria, are not infrequent during convalescence. After the urine has become completely normal on several examinations, a second attack of nephritis is extremely unlikely, probably because of the persistence of type-specific antibodies to the hemolytic streptococcus.

Acute nephritis associated with anaphylactoid purpura (Henoch-Schönlein disease) has a much worse initial prognosis and higher incidence of chronicity than the poststreptococcal variety.

Treatment. *Penicillin* should be given to eradicate residual streptococcal infection, even when this is not proved, but only suspected. It has been suggested that early treatment of streptococcal infections with penicillin may prevent nephritis, but in the only study performed to test this hypothesis the number of patients observed was too small to draw statistically valid conclusions.

During the acute stages *bed rest* is indicated, at least until the systemic manifestations of the disease have disappeared. There is no critical evidence to establish that further rest in bed appreciably modifies the course, although most studies concerned with this problem have been carried out in cases of mild nephritis in children in whom complete recovery is the rule. If proteinuria or microscopic hematuria is the only remaining sign after 6 weeks to 2 months of rest in bed, the patient may be allowed up.

In the presence of *edema*, salt should be restricted. Mercurial diuretics are contraindicated. Chlorothiazide may be employed. Treatment for congestive heart failure is discussed above and on p. 1385. During the initial stages of the disease, when urinary output is restricted, it may be wise to limit the intake of *protein* as outlined below under Acute Renal Failure (Treatment). There is no reason, however, to restrict protein during convalescence.

Hypertensive crises may be treated with 2.5 mg of reserpine intramuscularly two to four times a day or by an infusion of magnesium sulfate.

Adrenal steroids have no clear-cut beneficial effect in acute nephritis. When massive doses of steroids and of nitrogen mustards have been used in occasional instances of rapidly progressive glomerulonephritis with oliguria, they have failed to modify the course.

CHRONIC GLOMERULONEPHRITIS

Chronic glomerulonephritis is in all likelihood not a single entity but a collection of different diseases which predominantly affect the glomerular tufts, causing inflammatory changes and subsequent scarring. The course and pathologic findings vary widely, not only because of diverse etiologies, but also because of variations in the response of different patients to the same injurious agent. It may be expected that, as knowledge of the nature of renal disease expands, additional nosologic entities will emerge from the group termed "chronic glomerulonephritis" as distinctly as Kimmelstiel-Wilson disease and lupus nephritis have in the past.

Chronic glomerulonephritis affects all ages, but is most frequent in the earlier periods of life. It is more common in men than in women. Only a minority of patients have a clear-cut history of acute onset following infection or have evidence of antibodies against nephritogenic strains of streptococci. Some cases of chronic nephritis probably originate in an unapparent infection with streptococcus, following which edema or bloody urine was not noticed, but it seems likely that many instances represent a different disease from that of poststreptococcal glomerulonephritis. Occasionally a strong familial predisposition to chronic nephritis is apparent. Some characteristic patterns are considered below.

"Crescentic Glomerulonephritis." The entire course lasts only a few months, usually less than a year. Sometimes the onset is explosive, originating in acute nephritis following an infection. In other instances evidence for an infectious etiology is absent and the beginning of the disease can be dated only by the last normal examination. In any case, fatigue, anemia, and breathlessness quickly appear, hypertension is prominent even though the heart may initially not be enlarged, the urine contains large quantities of protein and red cells and may be grossly bloody. Oliguria and rapidly advancing uremia, complicated by pulmonary edema, characterize the terminal weeks. The kidneys are usually normal in size, and the glomeruli are swollen, with intense proliferation of the capsular epithelium, resulting in widespread crescent formation.

"Latent Nephritis." Abnormal urinary findings may be detected in a completely asymptomatic patient in the course of a routine physical examination. Renal biopsy may show a patchy glomerulitis, with focal thickening of glomerular loops, occasional capsular adhesions, and some completely hyalinized glomeruli. Other glomeruli may appear completely normal. Alterations in arterioles of the kidney can sometimes be detected even though blood pressure is normal.

Hypertension is often absent. The fundi are normal. The usual tests of renal function may be completely within normal limits, and serial studies over many years may show no or very slow progression of functional impairment. The character of the urinary sediment is often a poor guide to prognosis; moderate proteinuria, red cells, and red cell casts may be present intermittently or continuously for years, with a normal or only slightly elevated serum creatinine. There is reason to believe that the pathologic process is continuously active at a low level, though counterbalanced by forces of repair and renal hypertrophy. Some patients live normal lives for decades without any change, or occasionally are cured; others eventually develop severely impaired renal function and hypertension.

Pregnancy may in some cases be safely undertaken by patients in whom hypertension has not appeared and whose blood urea nitrogen is normal; in others the risk of preeclampsia or exacerbation of nephritis is greatly increased.

Nephrotic Syndrome. In the course of glomerulonephritis in some patients the disease begins insidiously with nightly swelling of the ankles and early morning puffiness of the eyes. Proteinuria is in excess of 5 Gm daily, and serum albumin is low. Hypertension may or may not be present initially but eventually makes its appearance. Renal biopsy may reveal diffuse thickening of all glomerular loops, with little or no cellular proliferation, capsular adhesions, or crescent formation, though all these changes may be present in occasional instances. In some cases interlobular thickening in the glomerular tufts is focal rather than diffuse (chronic interlobular glomerulonephritis), resulting in a pathologic picture that superficially resembles the nodular form of Kimmelstiel-Wilson disease. The rate of progression of the lesion is extremely variable, though within 6 years perhaps half of all patients will have developed the uremic syndrome. Occasional patients appear to recover completely. In many cases, edema remits as the glomerular filtering area is progressively restricted and the excretion of protein falls; in others, hypoalbuminemia and edema persist to the end.

Hypertension. Many patients with chronic glomerulonephritis seek medical attention because of complaints associated with hypertension. Sometimes high blood pressure will be found to have developed without significant impairment of renal function. Such cases may be indistinguishable in their clinical manifestations and course from benign essential hypertension, except for the fact that proteinuria, dating in occasional instances from a clear-cut attack of acute nephritis, has antedated the hypertension. In some instances "malignant hypertension," with papilledema and extremely high diastolic blood pressure, may develop and dominate the picture. In patients in whom azotemia has not become pronounced, judicious use of ganglionic blocking agents may produce a remission in the pattern of malignant hypertension without seriously damaging renal function.

Exacerbations of Chronic Nephritis. Respiratory infections, especially with the streptococcus, sometimes cause an increase in proteinuria, hematuria, and hypertension as well as a variable decrease in renal function in patients with chronic nephritis. These exacerbations may be distinguished from attacks of acute nephritis, which they resemble, by the short latent period between the onset of the infection and the exacerbation. In some patients, reversible exacerbations of vascular disease characterized by rising blood pressure, hematuria, and retinitis occur without evidence of preceding infection and subside spontaneously.

As has been emphasized above, the course and duration of chronic glomerulonephritis are highly varied and often unpredictable. While many patients fit a "classical" pattern, others partake of several. Many patients progress into the terminal stage without ever having experienced edema. An occasional patient develops clear-cut acute glomerulonephritis following respiratory infection, succeeded by a "nephrotic stage," which yields over a period of years to slowly progressive renal insufficiency and mounting hypertension. It is not usual, however, to observe this full sequence of events in one individual.

It is almost impossible, except in the most advanced cases, to offer an accurate prognosis from a single set of clinical observations and tests of renal function. Serial observations of the blood urea nitrogen or serum creatinine, phenolsulfonphthalein excretion, the degree of proteinuria and anemia, and the blood pressure may afford an estimate of the velocity and character of the process. *Probably because of the intensity of the associated vascular disease, the prognosis is much worse in glomerulonephritis with renal insufficiency than in pyelonephritis with azotemia of comparable severity.*

Although the blood in chronic glomerulonephritis may remain normal for years, *anemia* eventually develops in most patients by the time renal insufficiency makes its appearance. In patients in whom renal failure has developed only slowly, fatigue associated with anemia may be the presenting symptom. Severe anemia, recurrent after transfusions, implies a poor prognosis.

By the time azotemia has appeared, hypertension is present in most patients with glomerulonephritis, and as the disease approaches its terminus, blood pressure is elevated in all. When progression is very slow, both azotemia and mild hypertension may be borne without symptoms for years. Polyuria and nocturia may be the first signs of renal insufficiency. Loss of appetite and intractable nausea frequently bring the patient to the physician. Heart failure, anemia, and bleeding into the skin, mucous membranes, and gastrointestinal tract herald the final illness. The skin becomes dry, with a sallow tint,

the breath uriniferous. Exophthalmos may be apparent. Hemorrhages and exudates appear in the fundi. The urinary output becomes progressively restricted. Fibrinous pericarditis or pleurisy may appear within a few weeks of death. Disorientation and coma mercifully precede the end.

At postmortem the kidneys are shrunken and fibrotic. Many glomeruli are completely hyalinized; in others there is only partial eccentric fibrosis, with varying degrees of adhesion of capillary loops to each other and to Bowman's capsule. The few glomeruli which are not injured are enlarged, as if stimulated to compensatory hypertrophy.

Differential Diagnosis. In patients with renal insufficiency, the possibility of other diseases of the kidney must be kept in mind. A history of acute nephritis with edema is helpful if present, but a detailed account of the illness should be obtained because what the patient refers to as "nephritis" may have been a urinary infection. Patients with primary hypertension usually do not develop renal failure unless the diastolic pressure is very high (over 130). Multiple myeloma and amyloid disease may mimic chronic nephritis in the middle-aged and elderly. Hypercalcemia may produce polyuria, azotemia, and anemia, all of which are potentially reversible.

Heavy proteinuria (over 2 to 3 Gm daily) is present in most patients with chronic glomerulonephritis (and the various other disorders which cause the nephrotic syndrome), but in few other renal diseases unless heart failure or malignant hypertension is present. Epithelial cell casts, red cell casts, and lipid droplets in the urinary sediment are useful in distinguishing the disease from pyelonephritis or primary nephrosclerosis. The kidneys are of equal size, usually without evidence of distortion of the calyxes on pyelography and if small, are contracted symmetrically. The possibilities of lupus erythematosus, periarteritis, and bacterial endocarditis should be kept in mind. The author has seen a patient with endocarditis, without fever or murmurs, who presented as a case of chronic nephritis and died, undiagnosed, of progressive renal insufficiency.

Treatment. Restriction of activity is indicated in patients with heart failure, an acute exacerbation of nephritis with hematuria, or an intercurrent infection. Patients who feel well enough to be up and about should be permitted to do so and should be encouraged to lead normal lives. Diet should not be restricted except for the clear indications mentioned on p. 1477. Strenuous exertion leading to fatigue is probably best avoided. Since the day of Richard Bright, moving to a warm climate has been recommended to patients with nephritis by physicians living in cold climates; there is no evidence that it influences the natural history of the disease except possibly in patients in whom frequent exacerbations are clearly related to respiratory infections. Prophylactic administration of penicillin (p. 921) may have similar theoretical advantages but has not been shown to alter the course of the disease. Treatment of the nephrotic syndrome is dealt with on p. 1490 and management of renal insufficiency on p. 1475.

CHRONIC PYELONEPHRITIS

Chronic pyelonephritis is present in 6 to 8 per cent of autopsied patients and accounts for over one-third of those dying with uremia. Up to middle age it is far more frequent in women, for the reasons mentioned on p. 1037. In old age, obstruction of the bladder in males by prostatic hypertrophy restores the balance. In contrast to the preponderance of women with pyelonephritis in the clinic, the incidence of pyelonephritis at postmortem is approximately equal in men and women. This may be a reflection of the frequency of lower urinary symptoms in women or of the nonspecific nature of some of the morphologic changes usually attributed to chronic or repeated bacterial infection.

About two-thirds of patients with chronic pyelonephritis have an obstructive lesion of the upper or lower urinary tract. In a large proportion of patients, however, there is no evidence of predisposing disease, obstructive or otherwise.

Pathology. The kidneys are frequently asymmetrical in size. The parenchyma is scarred, and the surface is coarsely and irregularly pitted. In many areas glomeruli and tubules are completely replaced by connective tissue which may contain lymphocytes and plasma cells. Foci of active interstitial inflammation may be seen throughout medulla and cortex, and leukocyte casts are found in some tubules. Other tubules are dilated and contain large amounts of homogeneous eosinophilic material (colloid casts). Most glomeruli appear relatively normal in comparison with the nearby atrophic tubular and inflammatory interstitial changes. The capsule of many glomeruli is disproportionately thickened and fibrotic in contrast to the relative integrity of the malpighian tufts. Some glomerular loops may be thickened or hyalinized, probably as a result of vascular changes proximally, and there are cortical clusters of fibrotic glomeruli, especially within the wedges of atrophic areas. Often distinctive inflammatory changes in the pelvic mucosa are lacking. A proliferative endarteritis is usually present, most marked in the areas of chronic inflammation. More generalized and severe vascular changes develop with the onset of hypertension.

It should be emphasized that, even at the autopsy table, the diagnosis of chronic pyelonephritis is often not clear cut. None of the foregoing changes is pathognomonic of chronic infection of the kidneys, though when taken together, they are useful in suggesting the diagnosis. Similar morphologic features may be encountered as a result of other diseases, including the nephropathy of chronic potassium depletion, nephrocalcinosis, chronic phenacetin poisoning, and primary vascular disease of the kidneys.

Clinical Features. "Starting with a pyelitis in childhood, an infection of the urinary tract during pregnancy, or, in rare instances, an acute pyelonephritis, there may be from time to time attacks of unexplained fever, with or without slight or fairly severe pain in the lumbar regions. These attacks are often accompanied by the passage of cloudy urine. Occasionally there is a history of albuminuria of many years' duration. Often there is a story of malnutrition or sometimes of retarded growth in children, leading occasionally to rickety deformities. In some instances the progress of the disease is, for years, symptomless" (Longcope). The majority of patients fall into the last-named category. Early symptoms are particularly infrequent in the group with bilaterally atrophic, nonobstructed kidneys. A history of acute pyelitis in childhood may be especially difficult to obtain because the symptoms are mainly gastrointestinal, the physical signs are scanty, and pyuria is difficult to demonstrate; a history of persistent enuresis is sometimes the only helpful clue.

Patients often, therefore, come to the attention of the physician only when renal failure or hypertension has made its appearance, or because of the accidental discovery of proteinuria. Fatigue and lassitude associated with anemia may be the presenting complaints. If renal failure is severe, nausea and vomiting or breathlessness may be present. Edema is rare, and when it occurs it is a result of heart failure. Hypertension may be accompanied by headaches, visual disturbances, and signs of congestive failure. Splenomegaly occurs in some patients with chronic pyelonephritis; when it is associated with anemia, a primary hematologic disease may be simulated.

About two-thirds of patients with chronic pyelonephritis develop hypertension at some time in the course of their illness. It has been suggested that this is related to the contraction of scar tissue and to endarteritis obliterans with focal renal ischemia, rather than to diffuse renal damage. The blood pressure may become elevated long before there is measurable impairment of renal function, and only a persistently positive urine culture or characteristic changes in the intravenous pyelogram may distinguish the clinical picture from that of "essential" or "malignant" hypertension. The incidence of hypertension is greater in the interstitial, nonobstructive form of pyelonephritis than in the obstructive variety; in the former group rapidly progressive vascular disease occurs terminally in 15 to 20 per cent. A large proportion (estimates vary widely from 16 to 75 per cent) of all patients dying of malignant hypertension are found to have kidneys characteristic of atrophic interstitial pyelonephritis ("pyelonephritis lenta" of Saphir). Accurate estimates of the role of bacterial infection in this syndrome are limited by the nonspecific nature of many of the pathologic changes.

In general, glomerular filtration and renal blood flow decline together and proportionally as the disease progresses. As might be expected, there is usually more disparity between the function of the right and left kidneys than is generally the case in diffuse diseases of the kidney like glomerulonephritis or nephrosclerosis. Maximum concentrating ability tends to become impaired earlier in the course than in patients with chronic glomerulonephritis. Occasional patients with advanced azotemia may excrete a urine hypotonic to plasma, even when dehydrated. Many patients are unable to conserve sodium on a low-salt diet, even when only mild azotemia is present. Polyuria and nocturia are prominent in such cases. Hyperchloremic acidosis as a result of impaired renal excretion of acid and reabsorption of bicarbonate is more often a feature of chronic pyelonephritis than of glomerulonephritis. Proteinuria is usually less than 2 Gm (rarely as much as 4 to 5 Gm) daily.

Careful examination of the *urinary sediment* is often the key to diagnosis. Leukocytes may be numerous or infrequent, but the appearance of *white cell casts* should alert the physician to the possibility of chronic pyelonephritis. Bacteria may be present on the fresh stained smear but, together with pus cells, often appear intermittently or not at all in the chronic atrophic stage of the disease. It should be noted that the urine sediment may be normal and, especially with a dilute urine of fixed specific gravity, that no albuminuria, or only a trace, may be detected. Although characteristic distortion, flattening, and reduction in size of the renal pelves, frequently without ureteral changes, are usually found on pyelography (p. 1038), their absence does not rule out chronic pyelonephritis.

When pyelonephritis is not accompanied by hypertension, the course may be prolonged and compatible with comfortable and useful life even after considerable encroachment upon renal function. In perhaps no other disease of the kidneys can fluctuations in renal function be so marked or so frequent. During acute infections or episodes of dehydration, renal decompensation may progress to the stage of advanced uremia; yet the patient may be able to recover and carry on with adequate though impaired renal function for years. Nonspecific complaints of fatigue, anorexia, and weakness often remit remarkably when the urine is sterilized by an appropriate course of antibiotics and if acidosis, dehydration, and salt depletion are adequately treated.

The problem of *recurrent infections* with resistant bacteria is an important and unsolved one. An effort should be made to treat urinary tract obstruction and to improve bladder emptying, when residual urine is present. Reducing the bacterial population of bladder urine by the prolonged administration of urinary antiseptics may offer some hope for halting the indolent progression of the disease; in this connection, however, acidifying agents are likely to be ineffective and harmful in patients with azotemia.

It should be emphasized that, even in cases where one kidney appears small and the other normal in size, pyelonephritis is in most instances bilateral. Nephrectomy which is undertaken in the hope of eradicating the disease is generally doomed to failure. Excision of hydronephrotic, pus-filled renal shell will, however, sometimes permit a successful therapeutic attack on infection in the opposite kidney with a carefully chosen antibiotic given in adequate dosage for a long period of time.

NEPHROSCLEROSIS

Definition and Pathology. Although early in the course of "essential" hypertension there may be no morphologic changes in the kidney at all, structural alterations in the small arteries and the arterioles are almost always present in the kidneys of patients who die in the course of hypertensive disease. In about 10 per cent of such patients the changes are severe enough to produce marked renal insufficiency. Large and medium-sized arteries show a variable degree of intimal thickening. This change is more ubiquitous and more severe in the small arteries and arterioles. In addition, an eosinophilic hyaline thickening frequently involves the entire wall of arterioles and prearterioles. These changes may lead to mild generalized atrophy of the cortex with focal scars. Hyalinized glomeruli are a conspicuous microscopic feature.

In patients who die with rapidly progressive, "malignant" hypertension, especially after renal insufficiency has appeared, there is often intense intimal hyperplasia of the medium-sized and small arteries, so that the lumen may be substantially reduced. Necrosis of the preglomerular arterioles is present, which frequently extends into the glomerular tufts. There may be hemorrhages into Bowman's space and occasional crescent formation.

It is not generally realized that similar but less intense changes may be found at postmortem in patients without systemic hypertension. Arteriolosclerosis may be observed in the renal biopsies of a few patients with normal blood pressure and mild asymptomatic proteinuria. Definite arteriolosclerosis was described by Bell in 10.6 per cent of normotensive patients fifty to sixty years of age and increased in intensity and frequency in older age groups. It seems clear that renal arteriolosclerosis may occur in the absence of systemic hypertension, though it rarely produces symptoms or signs. Such vascular changes may account for the moderate decrease in renal reserve often observed in elderly patients.

Clinical Features. Hypertension antedates proteinuria by many years in most patients with "essential" hypertension. When proteinuria does appear it is usually minimal. The urinary sediment is usually not remarkable, although microscopic hematuria and occasionally gross urinary bleeding may occur in the accelerated phase, when the excretion of protein may also increase to more than 4 Gm daily, reflecting widespread necrosis of glomerular capillaries. The anemia associated with advanced renal insufficiency occurs in some patients with nephrosclerosis as in other renal diseases, although the appearance of hypertensive neuroretinopathy with azotemia *in the absence of anemia* should suggest primary vascular disease. The patient with hypertension and uremia whose optic fundi are normal usually has glomerulonephritis or pyelonephritis. At the inception of the hypertensive process, renal blood flow is usually depressed more than glomerular filtration rate. The opposite is true in glomerulonephritis, but the difference has no important clinical significance.

The course of nephrosclerosis is extremely variable and cannot be predicted with regularity from the height of the blood pressure. Proteinuria and even mild azotemia may be borne without symptoms for many years. The abrupt change in course which marks the onset of the malignant phase is characterized by an increase in proteinuria, hematuria, and progressive azotemia. It is of interest that most cases in which this syndrome occurs have been known to have hypertension for less than 8 years.

The term "malignant hypertension" has been used variously to indicate (1) hypertension with papilledema, (2) hypertension with rapidly progressive renal insufficiency, or (3) hypertension with necrotizing arteriolitis. These arbitrary definitions should not be confused or allowed to obscure the facts in individual cases. Papilledema, hematuria, weight loss, advancing uremia, and necrotizing arteriolitis usually coexist in hypertensive patients, but it is not unusual for any of these features to be absent in the presence of the others. Thus, 23 per cent of 68 cases studied by Goldring and Chasis with excessively high diastolic pressure and rapidly advancing uremia did not have papilledema. In some, the fundi showed only arteriolar narrowing without hemorrhages. Contrariwise, papilledema may be present in occasional patients at intervals for many months or even years without advanced renal involvement or necrotizing arteriolitis. In some patients the uremic syndrome appears over the course of a year or two, but hematuria and proteinuria remain minimal, and neuroretinopathy may never be present. Such cases are likely to have massive cellular intimal hyperplasia of the interlobular arteries with little necrotizing glomerulitis.

In addition to "primary" nephrosclerosis, the clinical syndrome of malignant hypertension may occur in the course of chronic pyelonephritis, glomerulonephritis, periarteritis nodosa, scleroderma, pheochromocytoma, and unilateral renal arterial occlusion.

NEPHROSIS

The nephrotic syndrome is not a single disease but a clinical constellation characterized by (1) massive proteinuria, (2) hypoalbuminemia, and (3) edema. Hyperlipemia is frequently but not invariably present. The term "nephrosis" is sometimes used by pathologists to indicate degenerative changes in renal tubular epithelium, but this definition should not be confused with the clinical syndrome under discussion.

Etiology. The *nephrotic syndrome* is primarily the result of diffuse injury to the *glomerulus*. In most cases the origin of the disorder is uncertain, although it presumably reflects an autoimmune reaction involving the glomerular basement membrane. It is of interest that many patients with the nephrotic syndrome have a history of allergic disease and may show striking eosinophilia. The injury may occur in the course of poststreptococcal glomerulonephritis or in association with amyloid infiltration of the glomeruli, diabetic intercapillary glomerulosclerosis, or lupus erythematosus. It may rarely be observed in allergic reactions to plant pollens, poison ivy, poison oak, or insect stings or as a manifestation of sensitivity to trimethadione or paramethadione. It may occur as a complication of secondary syphilis or malaria. The nephrotic syndrome has occasionally appeared in the course of treatment with mercurial diuretics and salts of gold and bismuth. Some of these cases may be examples of a hypersensitivity reaction; the evidence that heavy metals can cause massive albuminuria even in doses which induce tubular necrosis is not convincing. Massive proteinuria may result from the marked elevation in glomerular capillary pressure which follows thrombosis of the renal veins or constrictive pericarditis. Uncomplicated pyelonephritis or nephrosclerosis does not cause the nephrotic syndrome.

Pathology. Histologic examination of the kidneys reveals a spectrum of morphologic changes which vary in individual patients as well as from case to case. Some glomeruli may appear quite normal by light microscopy, but under the electron microscope the foot processes of glomerular endothelial cells are seen to be broadened and smudged. (There is evidence that this particular change may be a result of proteinuria, rather than its cause.) When the lesion is more advanced, definite spotty or diffuse thickening of the basement membrane is apparent by the usual histologic techniques, often with little or no cellular infiltration or endothelial proliferation, hence the term *membranous glomerulonephritis*. In other patients there is an increase in glomerular cellularity, and occasional capsular adhesions may be observed. In still other cases, the process of basement membrane thickening has gone on to fusion and simplification of the glomerular loops and to partial or complete hyalinization of some glomeruli. In all instances, the proximal tubular cells are swollen with intracytoplasmic droplets and vacuoles, some of which are doubly refractile. It is not clear whether these represent protein and lipid reabsorbed in huge quantities from the glomerular filtrate or that deposited from the blood in injured cells.

Clinical Features. The disease is commoner in children than adults and is more frequent in males, but may affect any age and either sex. Occasionally a respiratory infection may have occurred just before the onset, but it is uncommon to find evidence of preceding streptococcal infection. The patient usually presents himself because of the insidious onset of *edema*. This is often particularly noticeable in the face because of the absence of orthopnea. The edema is characteristically soft and pits easily. Ascites and pleural effusions are frequently present, but pulmonary edema does not occur without heart failure. Though edema may be the only manifestation, other symptoms may be present, vaguely suggestive of the extensive depletion of body proteins that hypoalbuminemia betokens. Loss of appetite is frequent, although not so common as in poststreptococcal glomerulonephritis. A previously active child may feel tired and rundown. Amenorrhea or some irregularity in menses is the rule in women. The course is sometimes punctuated by unexplained episodes of abdominal pain, vomiting, and diarrhea.

The blood pressure is often normal; the heart is generally not enlarged in the absence of hypertension. The fundi are normal except when diabetic glomerulosclerosis is the cause of the disorder. The skin looks puffy and pale; there may be a mild normocytic anemia, but the hematocrit is usually higher than the pasty appearance of the patient suggests. Mild generalized osteoporosis is frequently observed, especially in children.

The daily urine usually contains more than 4 to 5 Gm of protein, chiefly albumin, but significant quantities of α_1-, β-, and γ-globulins are found as well. Some nephrotics excrete as much as 20 to 30 Gm of protein each day. The serum proteins are grossly reduced, especially the albumin and, less predictably, the γ-globulin fraction. Serum γ-globulins are said to be normal in the nephrosis caused by lupus erythematosus or amyloid disease; they may also be found within normal limits, in the author's experience, in the nephrosis associated with membranous glomerulonephritis. α_2-Globulins are generally elevated, but this occurs in many chronic diseases. Serum albumin is usually below 2.0 to 2.5 Gm per 100 ml when edema is present and with massive edema is frequently below 1.0 gm per 100 ml. It should be noted that conventional salting-out techniques frequently overestimate the concentration of serum albumin at low levels of this component. The over-all increase in the lipid-carrying globulins conceals a reduction in the concentration of the smaller metal-carrying proteins, transferrin (iron) and ceruloplasmin (copper). Serum complement is decreased in membranous glomerulonephritis, although not in diabetic glomerulosclerosis. Serum calcium is low, entirely as a result of a decrease in the fraction bound to albumin. Plasma fibrinogen is elevated, and the sedimentation rate is greatly accelerated. The cholesterol, phospholipids, and triglycerides in the serum are usually elevated, and the serum is often lactescent. The low-density β-lipoproteins, to which these molecules are attached, increase in concentration. When caloric intake has been low and nutrition poor, however, serum cholesterol and triglycerides may be normal. This is frequently the case in instances of the nephrotic syndrome caused by lupus erythematosus and Kimmelstiel-Wilson disease.

The basal metabolic rate is usually low, perhaps as a result of malnutrition and, in some cases, of failing to correct for edema fluid in estimating weight. The impression of hypothyroidism may be strengthened by a puffy face and pasty appearance, by an elevated serum cholesterol, and by the decrease in serum precipitable iodine, which, however, is a consequence of the low concentration of thyroxin-binding proteins in the serum, rather than of impaired thyroid function. Treatment with thyroid produces no improvement.

The urinary sediment is filled with granular and epithelial cell casts, and casts in which highly refractile lipid droplets are embedded. Fat bodies may be seen in the urine even when the serum cholesterol is normal. Red blood cells are often absent, but many patients show some degree of continuous or intermittent microscopic hematuria.

Glomerular filtration rate is frequently normal or above normal early in the course of the nephrotic syndrome, and blood nonprotein nitrogen is not elevated. Azotemia gradually develops, together with a fall in filtration rate and filtration fraction, in patients with progressive nephritis. In others renal function may remain normal, despite edema, for years, but may be depressed transiently, particularly during or immediately following infections. Tubular functions such as concentrating ability and phenolsulfonphthalein excretion are generally normal. Occasionally aminoaciduria or renal glycosuria is observed, presumably as a result of interference with proximal tubular reabsorption.

The term "pure" or "lipoid" nephrosis has been used in the past to designate patients with the nephrotic syndrome without hematuria, hypertension, or azotemia and without discernible etiology. Although prognosis is clearly better the longer patients escape hypertension or renal insufficiency, the author believes that it serves no useful purpose to classify such patients in a separate category from others with membranous glomerulonephritis and the nephrotic syndrome, since glomerular lesions are observed in all by electron microscopy and some develop hematuria, high blood pressure, and azotemia later in their course.

Pathologic Physiology. Much evidence indicates that the glomerular basement membrane is abnormally permeable to proteins. Those of low molecular weight and small size, like albumin, are lost into the urine in greatest quantity. Although it is conceivable that failure of the renal tubular epithelium to reabsorb protein might contribute to proteinuria, the massive amounts of protein excreted by some nephrotics and the striking increase in protein excretion observed following infusions of concentrated serum albumin suggest that increased glomerular permeability is the major determinant of the nephrotic syndrome. Indeed, there is good reason to believe that tubular reabsorption of protein is increased. There is no evidence (except in nephrosis associated with multiple myeloma) that abnormal proteins appear in plasma or urine. Hypoalbuminemia is chiefly a result of the extensive urinary losses of this protein; its synthesis is normal or even increased. In addition, in some patients the rate of catabolism of albumin is accelerated in a manner similar to that observed in a variety of acute injuries or infections. Associated with the reduction of serum albumin there is usually marked wasting of tissues, which may be clinically evident only after the edema disappears. Balance studies carried out in nephrotic patients during refeeding with high-protein, high-calorie diets suggest that, for every gram of protein added to the plasma, 20 to 100 Gm of tissue protein must be incorporated in tissue.

The decrease in plasma albumin and consequent fall in the oncotic pressure of plasma results in an increased transudation of fluid from the blood stream to extravascular spaces. Plasma volume tends to fall. The reaction of the kidneys to these events is to diminish the excretion of sodium and of water, as in many other situations where the integrity of the effective circulating blood volume is threatened. The mechanism by which this is accomplished involves the greatly augmented secretion of aldosterone by the adrenal cortex, although the exact nature and pathway of the afferent stimulus for this adjustment are not yet clear. Changes in glomerular filtration rate may also be contributory in some patients. The primary role of sodium in the production of nephrotic edema is demonstrated by the fact that, when administered without salt, water may be excreted normally. When the intake of sodium is continued, it is retained by the kidneys and sequestered with water in an expanded interstitial fluid. Despite edema, plasma volume remains normal or low. If albumin is added to the blood stream in increased amounts, or its rate of loss is diminished, the sequence of events will be reversed and diuresis will ensue.

When the quantity of circulating albumin is increased in a nephrotic patient, plasma volume is expanded by dilution with extravascular edema fluid, thereby minimizing the expected rise in albumin *concentration*. For this and other reasons, diuresis and edema formation need not be correlated with the exact concentration of albumin in the serum.

The pathogenesis of the hyperlipemia associated with the nephrotic syndrome is not clear. Serum cholesterol, phospholipids, and triglycerides usually are all increased in nephrotic patients. The rise in triglycerides may be so marked that the serum is milky. At least one reason for the elevation in serum cholesterol is its increased solubility in fatty serum, though increases in serum cholesterol may also be observed in the absence of lactescent serum and even when serum triglycerides are normal. Decreases of cholesterol and lipid phosphorus frequently coincide with periods of especially severe anorexia or vomiting; increases with periods in which appetite is good. Nevertheless, the most intense lipemia may be observed in wasted patients with extreme hypoproteinemia and the most massive edema. Though hyperlipemia usually disappears when elimination of edema marks regression of or recovery from the disease, it may persist in rapidly progressive cases despite advanced azotemia and hypertension

Hyperlipemia is not secondary to increased synthesis of fat or to increased fat in the diet, but appears to be caused by a defect in fat transport. The removal of triglycerides from the blood stream normally involves their hydrolysis by lipoprotein lipase, with the liberation of free fatty acids to the circulation. Of the small quantity of unesterified fatty acids normally present in serum, most are transported bound to albumin. Infusion of albumin into patients or animals with the nephrotic syndrome produces an immediate fall in serum lipids, often but not always to normal, and in general in nephrosis, elevation of all the lipid components of serum tends to be inversely proportional to the level of serum albumin. It has been postulated that, when the concentration of albumin falls, the hydrolysis of plasma triglycerides is inhibited by the absence of adequate plasma albumin with available binding sites for fatty acids, thereby "trapping" neutral fat in the plasma. Other factors necessary for normal transport of fats may also be deficient. It is of interest that infusions of dextran, which restore the colloid osmotic pressure of serum, result in a fall in plasma lipids in patients with nephrosis. Patients who have hypoalbuminemia for other reasons may not demonstrate the marked hyperlipemia and hypercholesterolemia of nephrosis. In such disorders decreased intake or absorption of food may play a role in muting this manifestation, as it presumably does in some patients with the nephrotic syndrome.

Natural History and Prognosis. The clinical course of the nephrotic syndrome is highly variable, depending to some extent upon the nature of the underlying disease. The following discussion will be concerned with nephrosis of uncertain etiology characterized by glomeruli which appear "normal" on light microscopy or have the morphologic changes of membranous glomerulonephritis.

A distinction should be made between the course and prognosis of the disease in children and in adults, the prognosis being appreciably better in children. Before the introduction of steroid treatment, the disease was eventually cured or arrested in about 50 per cent of children, although 40 per cent died within 5 years of onset. By contrast, in only one-quarter of adults with the nephrotic syndrome was a cure or spontaneous arrest of the disease observed which lasted longer than 2 years. Spontaneous diuresis is occasionally observed to follow measles, but in other instances bacterial or viral infections appear to induce a relapse. Before antibiotics were available, deaths from infections, frequently with the pneumococcus, were common. Erysipelas, pneumonia, septicemia, and peritonitis can now be avoided or successfully treated, and as a result, early mortality has been sharply reduced. The disease is frequently remittent, with intervals in which proteinuria is decreased or absent, and cases are occasionally seen in both children and adults in whom episodes of proteinuria and edema are separated by intervals of many years. Repeated remissions and exacerbations are uncommon, on the

other hand, in the course of the nephrotic syndrome which follows in the wake of acute hemorrhagic glomerulonephritis. Persistent hypertension and azotemia are associated with a poor prognosis. Mild elevation of blood urea, intermittent hypertension, and microscopic hematuria have been observed in patients who improve spontaneously, as well as in those who develop progressive impairment of renal function. About one-quarter to one-third of children and one-half to two-thirds of adults with nephrosis develop progressive renal insufficiency and increasing hypertension and die of heart failure or uremia, generally within 2 to 5 years. In others, proteinuria is diminished but seldom disappears, renal function remains stationary at a level near normal, and the patient is asymptomatic, with or without hypertension. In patients whose dietary intake of protein is high, considerable proteinuria may be compatible with only moderate reductions of serum albumin, without edema. Edema may be precipitated by intercurrent infections which decrease appetite and promote the breakdown of protein, and may disappear when these disturbances are removed, without alterations in the urinary excretion of albumin. With the development of advancing glomerular hyalinization, proteinuria frequently diminishes in amount, serum albumin rises, and edema disappears as azotemia progresses.

Treatment. Although a few days in bed may help to mobilize edema, there is no indication for prolonged bed rest. Hospitalization is indicated at the onset of the disease to confirm the diagnosis and to obtain base-line studies but need not be prolonged.

The diet should be low in sodium and high in protein. Except in the presence of hyponatremia, water should not be restricted. Very low sodium diets (200 mg) are unpalatable, although the development of "sodium-free" milk and milk powders has made a satisfactory high-protein, low-salt diet more feasible. Sodium restriction should, however, be considered an emergency measure to control edema; it is not indicated during convalescence from the nephrotic syndrome or when edema is minimal. A high consumption of protein, together with adequate calories, leads to steady replenishment of wasted tissues. Since the goal is to restore body proteins, not simply to prevent further wastage, additional intake of protein above the normal requirement of 1 Gm per kg per day, plus urinary losses, is of importance. If the additional protein is to be utilized, sufficient calories must be given. The proportion of fat and carbohydrates is determined, as a practical matter, by the composition of the supplements of milk or milk powder. There seems to be no great advantage to restriction of fat. With such liberal intake of protein and calories, there is usually some subjective increase in feeling of well-being, and over many months a slow rise in plasma albumin. The increase in blood urea which invariably occurs on a high-protein diet reflects the additional amount of urea presented to the kidney for excretion, rather than deterioration of renal function. Proteinuria may also increase when serum albumin rises.

Adrenal steroids or ACTH produce improvement in about 75 per cent of children and a somewhat lower proportion of adults with the nephrotic syndrome. Dosage schedules vary, but a reasonable plan is to give 60 to 80 mg prednisone or 40 to 80 units zinc corticotropin suspension daily until a remission occurs or treatment has been continued for 4 weeks. Daily doses of prednisone lower than 40 mg are often insufficient to control proteinuria, while amounts higher than 80 to 100 mg are unnecessary. Remission generally requires the development of Cushing's syndrome. If no improvement is observed after a month of treatment with high doses of adrenal hormones, further prolonged treatment is not likely to produce a cure, although the patient may improve spontaneously. Diuresis sometimes occurs when steroids are discontinued, without diminution in proteinuria, but this is a nonspecific and transient response probably ascribable to temporary suppression of endogenous adrenal secretion. The earliest sign of a therapeutic effect upon the disease process is a diminution in the number of grams of protein excreted daily. This may be observed as early as 2 days after the beginning of treatment, but usually after 10 days to 2 weeks. During the initial stages of therapy, blood urea may rise because of the increased catabolism of protein induced by steroids. Glomerular filtration rate, however, usually is unchanged or increased by steroid treatment, so that serum creatinine does not rise and may even decrease. Once begun, the decrease in proteinuria proceeds rapidly, succeeded by a rise in serum albumin and loss of edema. Proteinuria may disappear completely or diminish to a constant low level. After no further improvement can be detected, the dose of steroids is gradually reduced over a period of about 4 to 6 weeks. If the drug is interrupted at this time, some patients will continue in remission indefinitely, but many relapse at varying intervals up to years following cessation of treatment. In an attempt to prevent such recurrences, it is common practice to keep patients on some maintenance schedule of steroid, administered either daily or 3 to 4 days per week, in a dose intermediate between that originally required to induce remission and that at which proteinuria occurs. Serial biopsy studies suggest that, when successful, such treatment decreases cellular proliferation in glomeruli and arrests the usual progression from thickening of capillary basement membrane to obliteration of the glomerular capillary.

Complications of steroid treatment include hypertension, muscular weakness and cramps, peptic ulcer, potassium depletion, diabetes, and osteoporosis (p. 626). Striae which break down and become infected may be most troublesome in edematous nephrotic patients. The leukocytosis which regularly accompanies administration of large doses of steroids may confuse proper evaluation of infection. Hyponatremia associated with rising serum potassium and high blood pressure may be observed in occasional unresponsive patients who have received large doses of hormone for long periods of time. The advantages of a proper dietary regimen must not be neglected in the course of treatment with steroids.

Patients with amyloid disease or the Kimmelstiel-Wilson syndrome do not respond to treatment with steroids, nor do those with the nephrotic syndrome occurring in the course of acute poststreptococcal glomerulonephritis. Treatment of nephrosis complicating lupus erythematosus is discussed under that heading.

Except for helping to rule out amyloid disease and diabetic nephropathy, renal biopsy has so far not proved helpful in predicting which patients will improve with steroid therapy. It is clear that the presence of some hyalinized glomeruli, cellular proliferation, or membranous thickening of capillary loops does not rule out the possibility of a remission with steroids. A favorable response may be observed in the presence of mild hypertension, microscopic hematuria, and even moderate azotemia.

Diuretics may be used to control edema in conjunction with sodium restriction, whether or not adrenal steroids are prescribed. Mercury is not contraindicated unless azotemia is present, but should not be administered repetitively if the initial few doses do not produce a diuresis. The action of diuretics may often be enhanced by infusions of albumin, plasma, or dextran. These agents raise the oncotic pressure of plasma and expand plasma volume temporarily but are rapidly lost into the urine through the leaky glomerular filter. Diuresis is not an end in itself; a little edema is often to be preferred to the complications of too-vigorous diuretic therapy.

Nitrogen mustard has been reported to induce transient remissions in proteinuria in patients with the nephrotic syndrome, but there is no evidence of any long-term benefit.

In the rare forms of the nephrotic syndrome caused by secondary syphilis or malaria, specific antiluetic or antimalarial treatment usually results in complete cure.

DIABETIC NEPHROPATHY– INTERCAPILLARY GLOMERULOSCLEROSIS– KIMMELSTIEL-WILSON DISEASE

Pathology. In about 25 per cent of patients with diabetes mellitus a distinctive nodular glomerular lesion is evident at autopsy, which was first described by Kimmelstiel and Wilson as *intercapillary glomerulosclerosis.* The typical ball-like hyaline, acidophilic masses are situated at the periphery of the glomerular tuft, often with an apparently intact capillary running over the surface. The mass often contains cell nuclei, but these are usually distributed around its periphery. The wall of the afferent arteriole is usually hyalinized, and hyaline change in the efferent arteriole is frequently present as well. (The latter change is said to be so characteristic of diabetes as to be almost specific.) The nodules may be sparse or frequent; they rarely involve every glomerulus but may completely obliterate some. In addition, a more diffuse hyaline thickening of the glomerular basement membrane is apparent in many cases of diabetes, even when the nodules are absent, although this change is more difficult to distinguish from similar "axial thickenings" in such diseases as benign nephrosclerosis and membranous glomerulonephritis. It has been claimed that examination of renal biopsies from patients with diabetes by the electron microscope invariably demonstrates abnormalities of the glomerular tufts, though proteinuria and hypertension are absent and conventional histologic sections appear normal. In patients with diabetes of long duration, three renal diseases are likely to be present: intercapillary glomerulosclerosis, arteriolar nephrosclerosis, and pyelonephritis.

Clinical Features. The age and sex of patients with diabetic glomerulosclerosis parallel those of patients with diabetes in general; that is, it is more frequent in women and in middle life. The incidence increases with the duration of diabetes. It is rarely evident until 5 years have elapsed with diabetes and usually not for 10 to 15 years. Nevertheless, in occasional patients, diabetes and nephropathy are discovered simultaneously, and there are scattered reports of typical nodular glomerular lesions discovered at autopsy in patients whose fasting blood sugar was normal. There is no evidence that meticulous control of the blood sugar postpones the appearance of the lesion, although the malnutrition associated with grossly inadequate diabetic control may contribute to hypoalbuminemia and accelerate the onset of edema.

Most patients have both *hypertension* and *proteinuria.* In elderly patients, systolic hypertension alone is not infrequent. The proteinuria often exceeds 5 to 8 Gm daily. Urinary losses of protein frequently result in the nephrotic syndrome. The urinary sediment is usually loaded with hyaline and granular casts and contains doubly refractile fat. Though this has been held to be characteristic for this disease, it is not unique. Hematuria is rare, the exception being in those cases with malignant hypertension.

Edema is usually present, associated with *hypoalbuminemia* which, however, rarely reaches the low levels commonly observed in the nephrotic syndrome secondary to glomerulonephritis. The frequent contribution of *congestive heart failure* to edema in the Kimmelstiel-Wilson syndrome is often overlooked. The responsibility of the physician to undertake a careful therapeutic trial of digitalis in these circumstances is apparent.

The typical changes of *diabetic retinopathy* (p. 655) are present in almost every diabetic with advanced nodular lesions of the kidney. Their absence, in a patient with diabetes and a well-marked nephrotic syndrome, should suggest another lesion than diabetic glomerulosclerosis. Capillary aneurysms and advanced retinopathy may be present in some patients, however, in whom nodular intercapillary glomerulosclerosis has not yet appeared.

There appears to be no support for the suggestion that the defect in carbohydrate metabolism is of a special type. Episodes of diabetic acidosis occur as frequently in the history of patients with the Kimmelstiel-Wilson lesion as in those of other diabetics without it, and the range of insulin requirement is similar to that of diabetics in general. In some patients the requirement for insulin appears to decrease during the terminal stages of their disease, but this is a common phenomenon in states characterized by anorexia and wasting.

After a few years of well-marked proteinuria and persistent hypertension, *azotemia* gradually develops. Few patients live 5 years after the appearance of hypertension, heavy proteinuria, and hypoproteinemia. The remainder of the course is usually characterized by renal insufficiency, congestive heart failure, and edema relatively resistant to diuretics because of the lowered rate of glomerular filtration. The renal lesion of intercapillary glomerulosclerosis is not known to be reversible. However, the striking frequency of urinary infection suggests that prompt and vigorous treatment of renal infections, as well as their prevention (for example, by avoiding unnecessary catheterizations), may prolong life and postpone the appearance of renal decompensation in some patients.

Diabetic neuropathy contributes to the pathogenesis and complicates the management of urinary infection in many instances. Inability to empty the bladder completely predisposes to chronic and recurrent infections. Such patients may be helped by cholinergic drugs, whereas inlying catheters often initiate necrotizing cystitis.

ACUTE TUBULAR NECROSIS—ACUTE RENAL FAILURE

The term *acute renal failure* has been used loosely to include all forms of acute urinary suppression, generally secondary to acute parenchymal damage. *Acute tubular necrosis* (or lower nephron nephrosis) indicates the clinical and pathologic syndrome which results when renal excretory function is temporarily lost because of renal tubular degeneration caused by renal ischemia or toxic agents.

Pathology. Microdissection studies reveal two types of lesions. When specific toxins (bichloride of mercury, carbon tetrachloride, diethylene glycol) have been administered, there is diffuse necrosis of the proximal tubular cells, while the basement membrane of the proximal tubules, from which a new lining may regenerate, is spared. The lesion caused by ischemia, on the other hand, occurs at random among nephrons and in any part of a nephron. It consists of complete destruction of limited stretches of tubular lining scattered along the course of an otherwise well-preserved nephron. The basement membrane is frequently disrupted. During recovery from both types of lesions, mitotic cells may be seen. Except in cases in which extremely severe and prolonged ischemia has produced renal cortical necrosis, the glomeruli are intact. Casts packed with degenerating epithelial cells and hemoglobin are seen in the straight tubules of the medulla. The most important inference to be drawn from the nature of the pathologic process is that, should the patient survive his other injuries, the renal lesions will be repaired.

Etiology and Pathogenesis. Acute tubular necrosis typically occurs in a setting of sudden injury or illness usually associated with shock or with intense renal vasoconstriction. Even those cases which follow the administration of known tubular toxins are generally aggravated by vascular collapse and renal ischemia. Nevertheless, perhaps because of difficulty in recognizing and quantifying the ischemic state, the etiology may go undiagnosed in as many as 25 per cent of patients. Common causes include hemolysis and hypotension following extensive burns, rapid hemorrhage or hypotension on the operating table, bacteremic shock, crushing injuries in which the toxic effects on the kidney of myoglobin are added to those of vasoconstriction and shock, and intravascular hemolysis from transfusion of mismatched blood as well as rapid infusions of distilled water (e.g., during transurethral prostatectomy). Following operations on the heart, aorta, or great vessels during which renal circulation is interrupted, some degree of acute tubular necrosis is almost invariable. Pregnancy appears in some way to predispose to ischemic renal insults; in a large proportion of most published series, acute renal failure followed placenta previa, septic abortion, post-partum hemorrhage, or eclampsia. Other conditions which have triggered tubular necrosis include sudden defervescence following salicylate administration and status epilepticus. Acute renal failure is the most important cause of death in epidemic hemorrhagic fever.

Tubular necrosis resulting from many poisons is enhanced by prior dehydration and tends to be prevented by infusions of saline if these are given before the noxious agent is presented to the kidneys. Paradoxically, healthy renal tubules may be more susceptible to certain types of injury than are poorly functioning ones. A dose of uranium nitrate that induces acute tubular necrosis in a healthy dog may not interrupt the urine flow when given again to the same animal during the diuretic phase of early recovery from renal insufficiency. The role of free pigments derived from blood and muscle in the pathogenesis of tubular necrosis is not clear. Infusions of purified hemoglobin decrease renal blood flow and may be toxic to tubular cells. In addition, intravascular hemolysis may liberate other vasoconstrictor substances which promote renal ischemia.

Pathophysiology of Anuria. The formation of casts which occlude the renal tubular lumina may play some part in the pathogenesis of oliguria. In most patients, however, casts appear to be a result of diminished urinary flow rather than its cause. An exception is the renal failure which not infrequently follows dehydration in *multiple myeloma* and which may be characterized by extensive gel formation by abnormal proteins in renal tubules.

Following the acute renal ischemia which usually initiates tubular necrosis, renal blood flow is decreased to approximately one-third to one-half normal during the first days of oliguria. It is not clear whether or not this precludes any appreciable persistence of glomerular filtration. Increased interstitial pressure secondary to edema probably reduces renal blood flow and filtration rate and collapses tubules. The presence of interstitial edema may be inferred from the increase in the weight of the kidneys during acute tubular necrosis. Experimental measurements of wedged-renal vein pressure and of pressures at the end of a fine needle inserted directly into the kidneys have, however, not shown elevation. The pressures may, nevertheless, have been sufficient to collapse renal tubules which were distended with less than the normal pressure derived from glomerular filtration and urine flow. In any case, much fluid which is filtered at the glomerulus must leak back into the substance of the kidney through the widely scattered disruptions in the denuded tubular basement membranes. As tubular repair proceeds and these leaks are mended, urinary flow improves.

Clinical Features. In the majority of cases, acute tubular necrosis is characterized by a period of oliguria and increasing clinical and chemical evidence of renal failure, lasting from a few days to as long as 3 weeks, and averaging about 10 to 14 days. This is succeeded by a period of relatively rapid return of urine flow and improvement in renal function, while water and metabolites accumulated during the oliguric phase are excreted.

During the first few days of *oliguria,* the clinical picture is dominated by the underlying illness. The urine is scanty and usually bloody. Although the specific gravity may be high owing to the presence of red cells and protein, its freezing point is close to that of plasma, and the sodium concentration is usually over 50 mEq per liter. Traces of glucose may appear in the urine. Complete anuria for more than 24 hr is infrequently encountered, though it is common to see less than 30 to 40 ml of urine for several days. If the condition is not recognized early, edema and/or hyponatremia may develop as a result of the unrestricted intake of fluids. If this pitfall is avoided and shock is successfully treated, the only symptoms during the first week may be lethargy and nausea. The latter is related partially to the development of metabolic acidosis. Fever is uncommon after the first day or two. Leukocytosis, on the other hand, is the rule, with or without infection. It should be emphasized that severe systemic symptoms during the first several days are usually *not* a result of renal failure but of associated conditions.

Serum amylase and lipase may be elevated as a result of renal failure per se, without implying active pancreatitis. Blood urea nitrogen rises at a rate influenced by the degree of tissue necrosis and endogenous protein catabolism. In a chronically ill patient who has had a mismatched transfusion, a daily rise of 20 mg per 100 ml might be expected; increments of 50 mg per 100 ml per day in blood urea nitrogen are not uncommon in previously healthy persons who have undergone severe crushing injuries or overwhelming infections. Disproportionate elevations in serum phosphate or serum creatine have been proposed as diagnostic aids in the detection of devitalized tissue.

During the second week of oliguria, nausea, weakness, and somnolence become more prominent as azotemia mounts, acidosis increases, and the serum potassium becomes elevated. Thirst is commonly present and may be severe, although the serum sodium is frequently depressed, extracellular fluid volume is expanded, and there are no clear signs of shock or heart failure.

Cardiovascular complications arise in most patients during the oliguric phase of acute renal failure. Although overhydration is perhaps the most important cause of pulmonary edema, signs of pulmonary congestion and cardiac failure may appear even in patients who have been optimally treated. Pulmonary edema may develop in the absence of hypertension and without peripheral edema. Diastolic hypertension becomes evident in about 25 per cent of patients during the second week of oliguria. The fundi, however, remain normal. In exceptional instances in which the tension is very high, arteriolar necrosis develops. Arrhythmias are frequent and are not necessarily associated with potassium intoxication or removal. Pericarditis may develop but does not have the grave prognosis attached to its appearance in chronic renal disease. It may be extremely painful and simulate intraabdominal disease. Occasional patients die of acute cardiorespiratory failure characterized by apprehension, tachypnea, inconstant respiratory wheezing, progressive cyanosis, and hypotension. At postmortem no evidence is found of pulmonary emboli, and the lungs show mild to moderate terminal congestion.

Potassium intoxication may arise because of the liberation of large amounts of potassium from injured or infected muscle, intravascular hemolysis, or hematomas. It rarely occurs in the course of renal failure following a postoperative hemorrhage or transfusion reaction, in which the rate of tissue catabolism is not increased and in which proper attention has been paid to hydration and caloric needs from the inception of the disease. The rate of rise of the serum potassium reflects the catabolic response of the patient to injury. In addition, anoxia, acidosis, and dehydration are important determinants of the rate of loss of potassium from cells. The chief dangers are cardiac arrhythmias and standstill. Electrocardiographic abnormalities rarely occur when the serum potassium is below 7 mEq per liter but are almost always present above 9 mEq per liter. As serum potassium rises, the T waves become high and peaked. The P wave disappears, the QRS complex becomes broad and slurred, bradycardia and arrhythmias ensue, and the ventricular complexes finally resemble those of ventricular tachycardia. These changes may be modified by digitalis and by correction of acidosis and hyponatremia. Susceptibility of the heart to vagal standstill is enhanced, and sudden death may occur, even in the absence of characteristic electrocardiographic changes of potassium intoxication. The electrocardiogram, though a necessary adjunct, is not an entirely satisfactory replacement for the flame photometer in evaluating such situations.

Infection is the most frequent complication of acute tubular necrosis and the most common cause of death. Sepsis may often be overlooked because of confusion with uremic symptoms. Pulmonary and blood stream infections with "hospital" organisms, particularly the staphylococcus, are frequent in exhausted, semicomatose patients. Common predisposing factors are loss of ability to cough or change position, drying of pharyngeal mucosa from constant mouth breathing, and the aspiration of inspissated mucus plugs or vomitus. Healing of surgical wounds seems to be impaired, and infection or dehiscence of incisions is common. Infection of the urinary tract, sometimes silent but often with fever, flank pain, and gram-negative septicemia, frequently results from the use of inlying catheters or repeated instrumentation of the bladder.

Neurologic manifestations are common, the two most important being coma and convulsions. Hyponatremia may be responsible for somnolence or seizures early in the course of acute renal failure and may be corrected by hypertonic saline, with proper regard for the complications of overhydration and heart failure. Hypocalcemia may also predispose to convulsions, as may too-vigorous administration of alkali without accompanying calcium in the treatment of acidosis. Seizures may be focal in nature or generalized; some presumably have a vascular basis. They sometimes appear to be triggered by vomiting, heart failure, or the rapid changes in body volume and composition which may accompany the onset of profuse diuresis.

Anemia usually appears in the second week, even without bleeding, presumably as a result of a mild increase in erythrocyte destruction and a deficiency in erythroid hyperplasia. Defects in hemostasis are commonly encountered and include thrombocytopenia, abnormal prothrombin consumption time, and other less well-defined coagulation deficiencies.

In some patients tubular necrosis is not associated with oliguria, or the period of diminished urine flow is so short as to pass unrecognized. The urine volume in such cases is, however, not flexible or responsive to body needs and may be fixed at perhaps 800 to 1,200 ml per day. The diagnosis may only be appreciated when the blood urea nitrogen is seen to rise at the rate of 15 to 20 mg per 100 ml per day and when the patient becomes edematous owing to retention of fluids in excess of the excretory capacity of the kidneys. Unlike most other edema-forming states, the urine in such cases contains sodium in a concentration higher than 20 to 30 mEq per liter and the concentration of total solutes does not differ significantly from that of plasma.

After the first few days of oliguria the urine loses its grossly bloody character and becomes clear, increasing slightly in amount every day. The *onset of tubular recovery* is usually heralded by an increase in daily urinary output to 400 ml. At this point the urine usually contains very little protein, although the sediment may still contain red cells and many large dark hematin casts. Further increases in flow are sometimes dramatic, the urine volume increasing by 50 to 100 per cent each day until polyuria exceeds 3,000 ml daily. In other patients daily urine volume only gradually approaches a liter over the course of a week or two. If brisk diuresis is never achieved, the blood urea falls only slowly or not at all, and the urine contains more than 3 to 4 Gm of protein per liter, cortical necrosis must be suspected. The blood urea *usually continues to rise* for several days after urinary output exceeds 1 liter per day, until the excretion of urea exceeds its production. In addition, during the early diuretic phase of recovery, hyperpotassemia, congestive heart failure, and convulsions may complicate the clinical picture. Pyelonephritis frequently makes its appearance at this time, and death from infection, when it occurs, is commonly during diuresis. The onset of the diuretic phase, therefore, should not cause the physician to relax his vigilance.

Diuresis is usually associated with a striking weight loss, representing fluid accumulated during the period of oliguria. The urinary concentration of sodium usually varies from 50 to 75 mEq per liter. Some of the excreted sodium is derived from edema fluid, but if the remainder is not replaced, hyponatremia and dehydration may ensue. Elevated levels of serum sodium and chloride are observed during the diuretic phase when water replacement is inadequate and the patient is allowed to dehydrate himself through the obligatory excretion of a large volume of urine containing sodium at a lower concentration than plasma. Occasionally, urinary losses of potassium so greatly exceed intake that hypopotassemia is noted. Once established, diuresis proceeds smoothly unless interrupted by urinary obstruction or shock, and azotemia regresses over the course of 1 to 3 weeks. *If diuresis is interrupted by a second period of oliguria and rising blood urea, obstruction to bladder or ureters must be seriously considered.*

After discharge from the hospital, anemia sometimes persists for weeks or months, gradually disappearing without benefit of hematinics. Muscle weakness and joint stiffness slowly improve. Chronic pyelonephritis may be a major problem. Although azotemia generally disappears and renal function may be restored, renal blood flow and glomerular filtration rate usually do not return completely to normal. Hypertension is not a sequel in those who recover from acute tubular necrosis, though it may complicate the unusual case of cortical necrosis who survives anuria.

Differential Diagnosis. The physician is frequently faced with an oliguric patient who has just passed through an episode which may have produced tubular necrosis, but in whom the diagnosis is not yet established. Vigorous treatment of shock, congestive heart failure, dehydration, or hyponatremia frequently resolves the question by promoting diuresis. Urinary osmolarity is not appreciably higher than that of plasma after the first few hours of acute tubular necrosis, whereas it may be elevated in simple dehydration and other prerenal causes of oliguria. The sodium concentration of the urine in acute tubular necrosis is usually over 30 mEq per liter; in oliguria secondary to acute glomerulonephritis or renal arterial occlusion it is usually much less than this. Low urinary sodium concentrations may, however, be observed in tubular necrosis associated with terminal hepatic and cardiac failure. Failure of blood urea to rise in a stepwise fashion makes the diagnosis of tubular necrosis unlikely, even though oliguria is present. If doubt persists, a liter of glucose in water may be infused rapidly to determine the effect upon urine flow.

Lower urinary tract *obstruction* must always be kept in mind. A plain x-ray of the abdomen should be obtained in all patients with acute renal failure to delineate the size of the kidneys and detect radiopaque stones. If the possibility of ureteral obstruction exists, gentle investigation of the patency of one ureter is indicated.

Complete anuria for more than 48 hr should suggest obstruction, bilateral renal arterial emboli or thrombosis, cortical necrosis, or acute glomerulonephritis. Atheromatous emboli to the small renal arteries sometimes produce irreversible anuria following attempts at aortic resection. Carcinomatous obstruction to the ureters and idiopathic retroperitoneal periureteral fibrosis are frequently associated with intermittent oliguria, alternating with periods of polyuria and diuresis. Occasionally, acute papillary necrosis is attended by oliguria. Uric acid crystals may obstruct both ureters temporarily in patients with leukemia or lymphoma who have received nitrogen mustards or x-ray irradiation. Similar obstruction may be caused by certain sulfonamides given to dehydrated individuals. The prolonged anuria which occasionally follows bilateral retrograde pyelography is probably a result of obstruction to the lower ureteral orifices by inflammatory edema.

Oliguria attending the terminal stage of chronic kidney disease can usually be distinguished by the history, presence of hypertension, abnormal fundi, and small size of the kidneys. During the terminal stages of hepatic failure, especially in cases complicated by hemorrhage and hypertension, a syndrome of oliguria and progressive azotemia often appears which is associated with the lesions of tubular necrosis at postmortem but differs in some respects from the course of acute tubular necrosis outlined above. The oliguria is not severe, urine flow usually exceeding 150 ml per day. Urinary osmolarity may in some instances be distinctly elevated above that of plasma, and urinary sodium concentration is low. Vigorous transfusion and the use of vasopressor agents improve urinary flow only inconstantly and transiently. Although progression of the syndrome may in rare instances be halted, a typical diuretic phase does not ensue.

Treatment. Perhaps more than in any other renal disease, the course of acute renal failure is determined by the therapy the patient receives. Treatment during the initial stages of the disease must be directed toward reversing circulatory failure, which may have initiated the ischemic episode. Although overhydration predisposes to later pulmonary edema if renal failure is established, too timid replacement of blood or saline in shocked or dehydrated patients may perpetuate oliguria and permit tubular necrosis to develop. If vasoconstrictor agents are substituted for blood in hypovolemic shock, further renal damage with ischemic coagulative necrosis of cortical tubules may result.

Having restored circulatory efficiency, only current losses should be replaced. The patient should receive enough water and salt to provide for obvious extrarenal (e.g., gastrointestinal) and urinary losses and, in addition, enough water to compensate for insensible perspiration and water in expired air. Under average conditions of environmental and body temperatures, normal hydration in an adult patient can be maintained by the daily administration of about 600 ml of water in addition to other measured losses (since some water is provided from oxidized foodstuffs and tissue breakdown). Accurate daily weights provide a reliable index of fluid balance; ideally the patient should lose $\frac{1}{4}$ to $\frac{1}{2}$ lb daily as a result of consuming his own fat calories.

At least 100 to 150 Gm of carbohydrate should be given daily, to minimize protein breakdown and prevent ketosis. Its effect in this direction is enhanced if it is administered throughout the day rather than over a short period of time. There is no evidence that high-calorie mixtures containing more carbohydrate and much fat are appreciably more efficacious in reducing protein catabolism *when the intake of protein is interdicted,* as it must be in acute renal failure. When nausea is not present, 50 Gm lactose, 25 Gm sucrose, and 25 Gm glucose may be dissolved in the daily water requirement, flavored with a little lemon and served cold, to be sipped throughout the day. Ordinary food, especially juices, should not be given, since potassium intake is undesirable. *Oral feedings should not be attempted in the presence of nausea or vomiting.* Sodium lactate, accompanied by calcium, may be given in amounts of 40 to 80 mEq per day to avoid further acidosis, when the plasma CO_2 has fallen to 16 mEq per liter. Larger amounts may be indicated, especially when overhydration is not apparent and congestive heart failure is not present.

Potassium intoxication may be prevented in many cases by proper attention to requirements for water and glucose, as well as by the prophylactic oral administration of a teaspoon of potassium-exchange sulfonic resin, sodium polystyrene sulfonate (Kayexalate, Winthrop), three times daily. Larger amounts of the latter may be used if necessary. One tablespoon four times daily by mouth or enema usually serves to reduce an elevated serum potassium by 1 or 2 mEq every 24 to 48 hr. If hyperpotassemia is associated with acidosis, it may frequently be brought under control by infusions of sodium bicarbonate or sodium lactate. Infusions of hypertonic glucose solutions, with or without insulin, have a similar but more transient effect. The deleterious action of potassium on the heart may to some extent be counteracted by infusions of calcium or by the administration of digitalis. If hyperpotassemia cannot be controlled by these measures, artificial dialysis is indicated.

Heart failure should be treated with digitalis in the usual doses. Artificial dialysis with the removal of several kilograms of edema fluid by ultrafiltration may be dramatically effective in relieving pulmonary edema. Testosterone propionate or norethandrolone, 25 to 50 mg daily, may be given during the first 2 weeks in an attempt to reduce nitrogen breakdown. Its action in this regard, however, is frequently overwhelmed by the intense catabolic reaction to acute injury.

Scrupulous care should be taken to avoid *infection.* After the diagnosis is established, an accurate estimate of the daily output may be obtained by catheterizing the patient, using sterile precautions, only once in 24 or 48 hr, thus dispensing with an inlying bladder catheter. As the urinary volume reaches a significant level, most patients will be able to void spontaneously. It is desirable for hospital personnel handling the patient to wear mask and gloves. In alert patients, deep breathing and forced coughing should be stressed to avoid atelectasis. Tracheotomy should be considered early if there is difficulty in handling bronchial secretions. Careful mouth care with prevention of crusting and ulceration is important in avoiding parotitis and aspiration of infected material. Prophylactic administration of antibiotics should be avoided.

Several procedures have been proposed to substitute for renal function during acute renal failure. Irrigation of the stomach, intestines, or peritoneum may remove significant quantities of urea and potassium, although these procedures are less effective than hemodialysis. In an artificial kidney, blood rendered incoagulable by heparin is pumped through cellophane tubing surrounded by a bath with a composition approximating normal extracellular fluid. The oncotic pressure of plasma proteins is balanced by adding glucose to the bath. With certain models, fluid can be removed from the blood by ultrafiltration. Artificial dialysis may also be used to remove exogenous toxins such as barbiturates, bromide, and salicylates. Indeed, a portion of the clinical improvement following dialysis in some patients with uremia may be related to removal of sedatives. The use of the artificial kidney requires a trained and experienced team; if this is not available, attempts at dialysis may do more harm than good.

The prime indication for *artificial dialysis* in acute renal failure is uncontrollable hyperpotassemia. Dialysis is also helpful, however, in temporarily inducing a return of appetite and mental clearing in severely azotemic patients whose serum potassium is normal; it may thus make management during the remainder of the oliguric period considerably simpler by preventing or delaying clinical deterioration. The electroencephalogram may improve even though serum electrolytes are not greatly changed. Acidosis cannot be successfully treated by measures short of dialysis without administering sodium; mounting acidosis in the presence of congestive heart failure is therefore another clear indication for dialysis. Sudden lowering of the serum potassium by dialysis may induce dangerous arrhythmias in digitalized patients. It should be emphasized that, in civilian practice, dialysis is seldom necessary if proper care is instituted from the onset of anuria. Extensive wounds, severe infection, or extremely prolonged oliguria may, of course, result in the accumulation of such quantities of potassium and other metabolites that conservative measures fail.

During the *early diuretic* phase, every effort should be made to avoid salt depletion and dehydration and to sustain diuresis by replacing the previous day's urinary losses. Daily weights and determinations of serum and urinary electrolytes serve as guides; a useful approximation for replacement is to give one-quarter of the urine volume as 0.9 per cent saline, one-quarter as $\frac{1}{6}$ M sodium lactate, and one-half as 5 per cent glucose in water in addition to replacing other losses. Equivalent quantities of sodium and water may be provided by mouth if oral feedings are tolerated. As azotemia recedes, tubular ability to reabsorb salt and water improves, and the daily provision of large volumes of fluid becomes unnecessary. In a patient who is alert, spontaneous intake of food and water may usually be trusted to prevent depletion after the blood urea nitrogen has fallen below about 80 mg per 100 ml. At this time protein may be allowed in the diet and will generally be well utilized in repleting tissue stores.

Prevention. The development of toxic or ischemic tubular necrosis in experimental and clinical situations is conditioned by the state of hydration and the concentration of the urine. Renal vasoconstriction is potentiated in dehydrated animals. Hemorrhagic or tourniquet shock is enhanced by dehydration and modified by prior infusions of saline. It would seem wise to give enough saline and glucose solution before and during surgical operations to compensate for antecedent losses as well as those anticipated during the operative procedure. Since dehydration contributes to the production of shock, it is likely that these simple measures will reduce the necessity for transfusions and therefore the likelihood of transfusion reactions.

Prognosis. Despite the fact that in most cases the damage to tubular epithelium is theoretically reparable, acute tubular necrosis is a dangerous disease with a serious prognosis. The mortality in many large series of cases is about 50 per cent, in spite of the most careful attention to details of fluid and electrolyte balance and with the aid of the artificial kidney. The result depends to a large extent upon the background of associated illness leading up to the acute episode and the outcome of infections acquired during its course.

When renal ischemia is extremely intense or prolonged, *acute cortical necrosis,* with destruction of glomeruli, may occur. Such lesions are not reversible and most patients die without emerging from anuria. Most instances of acute cortical necrosis have followed complications of pregnancy, particularly premature separation of the placenta, eclampsia, and septic abortion, although the disease is also encountered following severe shock in nonpregnant patients with preexisting vascular disease. Anuria for several days is common, followed by prolonged oliguria. The protein content of the urine is elevated. In the few patients who survive, renal calcification and contraction of the kidneys may be observed. The author has seen malignant hypertension develop after 4 months in one such patient.

PAPILLARY NECROSIS

When severe infection of the renal pyramids is present in association with vascular diseases of the kidney or urinary tract obstruction, *renal papillary necrosis* is likely to result. Patients with diabetes and vascular disease seem peculiarly susceptible to this complication. Pain in the flank or abdomen, chills, and fever are the most common presenting symptoms. Acute renal failure with oliguria or anuria is not infrequent. Rarely, sloughing of a pyramid may take place without symptoms in a patient with chronic urinary infection, and the

diagnosis is made when the tissue is passed in the urine or identified on pyelography. If renal function deteriorates suddenly in a diabetic patient, this diagnosis should be entertained, even in the absence of fever or pain.

PREECLAMPSIA AND ECLAMPSIA— TOXEMIAS OF PREGNANCY

The term *toxemia of pregnancy* is generally defined as including those disorders encountered during gestation or shortly after delivery, which are characterized by the appearance of hypertension, edema, and proteinuria (preeclampsia) and, in severe cases, convulsions and coma (eclampsia). There is no reason to believe that patients with convulsions suffer from a disease essentially different from that of patients with preeclampsia. Such a classification necessarily includes a large number of diverse diseases of the kidneys and blood vessels which may begin or be exacerbated during pregnancy and to which pregnancy may lend a distinctive coloration. There appears to be in addition, however, a specific disease affecting the kidneys and the vascular system, usually commencing in the last trimester of pregnancy, which in most cases is dramatically improved when the pregnancy is terminated.

Pathology. The most common histologic finding in the kidneys in toxemia of pregnancy is marked swelling of the endothelial and epithelial cells of the glomeruli. In severe or prolonged cases, thickening of afferent arterioles may be apparent. Generalized and focal thickening of the glomerular basement membrane and fibrinoid necrosis of glomerular tufts have been described at postmortem, but these changes are rarer in renal biopsies obtained from patients who recover. Tubular necrosis is present in almost all patients who die of acute toxemia of pregnancy. Necrosis of liver cells and hemorrhages in the periportal areas are present in some but not all fatal cases; it has been suggested that these as well as the necrotic lesions of the kidneys may be secondary to vascular spasm and shock.

Clinical Features. Toxemia occurs more often in women pregnant for the first time and in those in the age group over thirty-five. It is more common with twins than in single pregnancies. Interestingly, its incidence is especially high in mothers bearing hydatiform moles, in which albuminuria and hypertension characteristically appear early rather than late in pregnancy, suggesting that the disorder is associated with the placenta, rather than the fetus. As with most vascular disorders, its manifestations are more frequent and pronounced in the obese, though paradoxically its incidence is higher in economically underprivileged and poorly nourished segments of the population. Toxemia of pregnancy is especially frequent in patients with prior renal and vascular disease. From 35 to 50 per cent of pregnant women with preexisting hypertension can expect to have their pregnancy complicated by a toxemic episode. The incidence increases in general with the height of the diastolic blood pressure and is especially high if in previous pregnancies preeclampsia was superimposed upon chronic hypertensive vascular disease. Preceding toxemia of pregnancy appears to predispose to recurrence in 30 to 60 per cent of patients even if blood pressure and urine have been normal between pregnancies. Evidence of pyelonephritis is encountered clinically in about one-fifth of patients with preeclampsia. Patients with diabetes are not especially susceptible to the disorder unless vascular or renal disease is present.

The *onset* may be either insidious or shockingly abrupt. Although toxemia commonly appears after the twenty-fourth week of gestation and frequently only a day or two before delivery, the onset may be earlier, particularly in patients with underlying renal disease. *Hypertension* is usually an early sign. Because of the normal decline in blood pressure during the latter two-thirds of pregnancy, the physician should not ignore the significance of a *rising blood pressure,* even though it may not exceed 140/90. With hypertension, *headaches* and visual disturbances are frequent but not universal complaints. The *fundi* often show narrowing and spasm of the retinal arterioles. The retina may appear glistening or wet, but the author has not been impressed with the frequency or specificity of this sign. Exudates and hemorrhage are late occurrences in severe cases.

The appearance of *proteinuria* is usually coincident with hypertension, although it may follow (less often, precede) the rise in blood pressure by a week or so. The amounts may vary from a trace of protein to 8 or 10 Gm in 24 hr. Granular and hyaline casts are found in the urinary sediment. Unlike acute glomerulonephritis, red cells are usually not present in large numbers. Renal concentrating ability is generally unimpaired, and phenolsulfonphthalein excretion is normal except in severe cases and in patients with previously decreased renal function. The blood urea nitrogen does not often rise above 20 mg per 100 ml. Nevertheless, glomerular filtration rate is probably diminished by the disease in most cases. Even slight nitrogen retention must be interpreted with due regard to the physiologic increase in glomerular filtration rate and fall in blood urea which characterize the normal pregnancy. Blood *uric acid* is commonly though not invariably elevated, reflecting a decrease in renal clearance of urate. In fulminant cases, oliguria may be prominent and presage the acute renal failure of tubular necrosis.

The *edema* which characterizes preeclampsia resembles that of acute glomerulonephritis in its distribution and probably in its pathogenesis. Edema may be absent when the toxemia has been explosive in its onset, as with convulsions. In other cases excessive weight gain with puffiness of the face, fingers, and ankles is the earliest symptom, antedating hypertension or proteinuria. Edema is usually contributed to by hypoalbuminemia; yet the serum albumin, though diminished, is not often below 2 Gm per 100 ml, and the edema of toxemia is not so dramatically relieved by injecting serum albumin as is the edema of nephrosis.

Signs of *cardiac failure* are present in a significant proportion of cases. With the appearance of edema, orthopnea and exertional dyspnea are often exaggerated. These symptoms frequently subside with bed rest, digitalis, and diuresis. As in glomerulonephritis, the circulation time may be normal while the venous pressure is elevated.

Certain patients with severe toxemia, with or without eclamptic convulsions, may develop multiple clotting deficiencies or intravascular hemolysis, often following delivery.

Convulsions are often preceded by the development of hyperactive tendon reflexes and occasionally by epigastric pain. Though they are often associated with marked hypertension, their appearance is not necessarily correlated with the height of the blood pressure. They may occur within the first day or two following delivery, as well as before or during labor. Petechial hemorrhages are observed in the brain in most patients who die of eclampsia.

Termination of the pregnancy is usually followed by prompt improvement of the mother. Proteinuria and hypertension usually disappear by the end of 1 or 2 weeks, though occasionally they persist longer. Nevertheless, in perhaps 50 per cent of patients with preeclampsia, hypertensive vascular disease indistinguishable from essential hypertension develops later. The incidence of irreversible renal changes and of late hypertension increases significantly with the duration of the toxemia.

Treatment. The most effective treatment is prompt emptying of the uterus. Ganglionic blocking agents should not be used to treat the hypertension since they cross the placental barrier and may injure the fetus. Abrupt and severe hypotension induced by drugs may result in fetal distress and cause acute renal failure in the mother. In mild cases, hypertension may be treated by vasodilating agents like reserpine, hydralazine, veratrum, or magnesium sulfate, and edema can be eliminated with diuretics, bed rest, and a low-salt diet. When proteinuria and hypertension persist, however, it is doubtful that such treatment prevents further vascular injury to the placenta and the kidneys. In such instances attempts to prolong the pregnancy for several weeks are associated with a high fetal mortality and the risk for the mother of permanent vascular disease.

ORTHOSTATIC AND FUNCTIONAL PROTEINURIA

In perhaps three-quarters of adolescents and young adults, proteinuria may be induced by prolonged standing in the erect position. This effect is more pronounced when a lordotic posture is assumed. In some patients lordosis has been demonstrated to result in compression of the inferior vena cava by the liver, and it has been postulated that the resulting increase in pressure in the renal veins is responsible for proteinuria. It appears more likely, however, that changes in the renal circulation secondary to peripheral sequestration of blood may be involved since proteinuria can be produced in susceptible individuals by applying tourniquets in the supine position, prevented by standing upright in water, and aggravated by the peripheral vasodilatation induced by heat. Urine passed early in the morning, before arising, is free of protein although of high specific gravity. Care must be taken to have the patient empty his bladder at midnight, without getting up, so that urine formed in the erect position during the previous evening is discarded. Urine produced after the patient has been up may contain as much as 1 to 3 Gm of protein per liter, although usually less than 1 Gm of protein is excreted per day. The excretion of casts and other formed elements may also increase with the appearance of protein. Often a history of easy flushing, fainting, or other evidence of autonomic instability is obtained. It should be recalled that the erect posture may increase proteinuria in some patients with renal disease, especially in healing or "latent" nephritis. Such cases, however, make up only a small percentage of young individuals with orthostatic proteinuria, in the majority of whom the condition is entirely benign and unassociated with other clinical evidence of impaired renal function.

Strenuous physical exercise produces transient proteinuria and microscopic hematuria in most people. "Functional" proteinuria may also occur during fever, after injections of epinephrine or norepinephrine, and during severe mental or emotional stress.

RENAL ARTERIAL OCCLUSION

Arterial infarction of the kidney is usually attended by sudden sharp unremitting pain in the upper abdomen or flank. The most common cause

is embolic occlusion. Fever and moderate leukocytosis are common, especially when a major branch of the renal artery has been occluded. Gross hematuria is not unusual, and microscopic hematuria is present in more than half the cases. The blood urea nitrogen usually is not abnormal unless there is contralateral disease. Shortly after a renal infarct, the kidney may not function on intravenous pyelography, although it appears normal in size and retrograde pyelograms are normal. During the ensuing days or weeks, function is slowly regained.

When occlusion of the renal artery is *incomplete* as a result of atherosclerotic narrowing, or if a branch of the main renal artery is occluded, and viability of kidney tissue is preserved by collateral circulation, hypertension may ensue, which is often of the rapidly progressive type, though reversible by nephrectomy. In such patients intravenous pyelograms may be normal. Often the affected kidney is contracted. In a significant minority of cases, albuminuria is absent and the urinary sediment may be completely normal. The diagnosis may be made by studies of the volume and composition of urine obtained on bilateral ureteral catheterization and by aortography (p. 1352).

RENAL VEIN THROMBOSIS

Etiology. One or both kidneys may be involved by renal vein thrombosis. Occlusion of renal veins usually implies thrombosis of the inferior vena cava as well. A common cause is invasion of the veins by *hypernephroma* or compression by *malignant metastases* to retroperitoneal lymph nodes at the level of the celiac axis. *Thrombophlebitis* of the legs with extension upward, *periarteritis*, *congestive heart failure*, or severe *dehydration*, especially in children, may be etiologic factors. The venous occlusion may follow an *abdominal injury* or *operation*. In adults, renal vein thrombosis may occur as a secondary and often terminal complication of renal disease which has previously caused perinephric inflammation or reduction of renal blood flow. It is particularly likely to occur in *papillary necrosis* and in renal *amyloidosis*.

Clinical Features. Sudden complete thrombosis of a renal vein causes severe lumbar pain, enlargement of the affected kidney, hematuria, and proteinuria. If the condition is bilateral, oliguria and death from uremia usually ensue. If the occlusion is more gradual, renal function may be partially preserved by the development of collateral venous channels. In a few such cases, massive proteinuria results in a full-blown *nephrotic syndrome;* in other instances, proteinuria is not prominent and is overshadowed by hematuria. The blood pressure is usually normal, and when hypertension occurs it is not severe. The presence of collateral abdominal veins with upward blood flow, unexplained edema of the legs or lower trunk, or recurrent pulmonary emboli may suggest the diagnosis which can be established by venography of the inferior vena cava.

RENAL DISEASE IN LUPUS ERYTHEMATOSUS

Incidence. In about two-thirds of all patients with lupus erythematosus there is clinical evidence of renal involvement. Nephritis is found at postmortem in 75 per cent of these patients, the majority of whom die of renal failure. The diagnosis of lupus nephritis was made in one-third of all adult and adolescent women with the nephrotic syndrome examined at the Presbyterian Hospital of New York over the course of 20 years.

Pathology. The earliest lesion is a focal membranous glomerulonephritis involving the periphery of the glomerular tuft, usually in conjunction with small areas of endothelial proliferation. As the disease advances, the glomerular process becomes more generalized, with diffuse thickening of the basement membrane, resulting in "wire loop" formation and intense focal cellular proliferation, with capsular adhesions and epithelial crescent formation, progressing to hyalinization. Lesions are frequently seen in various stages of development. It should be emphasized that they overlap morphologically with those observed in chronic glomerulonephritis (p. 1483). Some of the morphologic differences may be expressions of the relatively rapid rate of progression of the disease. Thus, contracted kidneys with many fibrotic and hyalinized glomeruli are uncommon, while focal zones of necrosis in the glomeruli, with nuclear fragmentation, are frequent. Hematoxylin bodies, consisting of depolymerized ribonucleic acid, are occasionally observed in the glomeruli; they have not been reported in chronic glomerulonephritis.

Clinical Features. Lupus nephritis may present as acute glomerulonephritis, "latent" nephritis with asymptomatic albuminuria, nephrosis, or chronic glomerulonephritis with renal insufficiency. Its course may be fulminating, with death in uremia after only a few weeks of onset, or the patient may live for years, with proteinuria and microscopic hematuria regarded as merely subsidiary to the other vicissitudes of the disease. In its early phases, signs of renal disease may be remittent, but when massive proteinuria or azotemia has appeared, the course is generally rapidly downhill within 1 to 3 years. Hypertension is rare unless azotemia is present or the patient is being treated with steroids. The urinary sediment is characteristic of chronic active glomerulonephritis, with leukocytes, red cell casts, doubly refractile lipid granules, and broad granular casts. Other systemic signs of lupus, such as rash and arthritis, as well as the LE test, may disappear while the nephritis is active; this is especially likely with the development of the nephrotic syndrome or signs of uremia.

Treatment. Treatment with relatively small doses of adrenal steroids (e.g., 100 mg of cortisone daily), which may be enough to suppress fever and arthritis, rarely improves advanced lupus nephritis and does not prevent its development, though mild proteinuria and hematuria may show improvement. Larger doses of steroids (e.g., 60 to 80 mg of prednisone daily) plus antimalarials may produce temporary remission of proteinuria and improvement in renal function. Many patients, however, continue to progress regardless of treatment. This is especially true after azotemia and hypertension have appeared. Remission has been reported in some after treatment with nitrogen mustard.

SCLERODERMA

About one-third of patients with scleroderma die of renal failure, and in two-thirds renal changes are present at death. The characteristic lesions consist of extensive intimal thickening of the interlobular arteries, fibrinoid necrosis of the cortical arterioles, thickening of glomerular loops, and spotty ischemic cortical necrosis. These changes may be indistinguishable from those seen in malignant hypertension. Proteinuria does not generally exceed 2 Gm per day. The blood pressure is usually elevated, especially terminally. In exceptional instances, however, it may be normal, even in patients with widespread arterial and arteriolar lesions at postmortem. Minimal proteinuria may be the only sign for long periods. Once renal involvement is moderately advanced, the course is rapid, leading to death from renal insufficiency a few weeks or months after azotemia has appeared. Terminal oliguria or anuria is common. The rapid progression of renal insufficiency frequently appears to be precipitated by the use of hypotensive agents. Adrenal steroids do not prevent or ameliorate the renal disease; it has been suggested that they accelerate it, but the evidence for this is not entirely convincing.

PERIARTERITIS NODOSA— HYPERSENSITIVITY ANGIITIS

The kidney is said to be involved in approximately 80 per cent of all patients with periarteritis nodosa. It must be pointed out that precise nosology in this area is somewhat complicated by the fact that arteritic lesions may occur in the course of malignant hypertension and may occasionally appear in the course of glomerulonephritis.

Pathology. Renal lesions in periarteritis are of two types. The *first* is characterized by segmental fibrinoid necrosis of part or all of an arterial wall, with an inflammatory perivascular infiltrate. Usually, arteries of medium size are involved (arcuate arteries or larger), but arterioles and even capillaries may be attacked. Signs of organization may be evident, with fibrous replacement of the damaged media and the formation of aneurysms at weakened spots in the larger muscular arteries. Multiple infarctions and gross cortical scars are apparent in the renal parenchyma. There may be scattered focal glomerulitis of varying age and activity. The *second* type of involvement is characterized by an active, rapidly progressive glomerulonephritis, with widespread fibrinoid necrosis of glomeruli and epithelial crescent formation. Combinations of these types of lesions may occur.

Clinical Features. With lesions of the larger renal arteries, hypertension is usual and may dominate the clinical picture. Albuminuria is always present, and the urinary sediment frequently contains red cell casts and fat bodies. Episodes in which the urine is grossly bloody are common. Uremia may be noted terminally, but azotemia frequently is absent or mild, and only slowly progressive. Remissions and relapses often mark the clinical course. Persistent hypertension may be a serious sequel when the disease is no longer active.

When the clinical and pathologic features of acute glomerular nephritis are present (as in the variety of hypersensitivity angiitis commonly caused by reaction to drugs), hypertension is more often absent, even in the presence of marked azotemia. Although death from renal insufficiency usually takes place within 6 months to a year of onset, in milder cases permanent spontaneous remissions have been observed.

Periarteritis should be suspected in patients with renal failure or hypertension, especially when features suggesting glomerulonephritis are present, when other organ systems are involved, or in the presence of obscure fever or unexplained leukocytosis or eosinophilia.

Large doses of adrenal steroids produce improvement in renal function in some patients. In a few of these, the manifestations of renal involvement completely disappear and the remission persists after steroids are withdrawn. In others, maintenance on steroids is necessary to sustain the remission, and in many patients the renal lesion appears to progress in spite of treatment.

AMYLOID KIDNEY

Renal amyloidosis is most commonly encountered as a complication of a variety of chronic suppurative diseases, such as osteomyelitis, tuberculosis, tertiary syphilis and leprosy, as well as Hodgkin's disease, ulcerative colitis, and rheumatoid arthritis. As the incidence of chronic infection has declined owing to the introduction of antibiotics, the amyloid kidney of "primary amyloidosis" and amyloidosis secondary to multiple myeloma and rheumatoid arthritis have become relatively more prominent. Amyloid involvement of the kidneys, as well as of other organs, commonly occurs in the course of familial Mediterranean fever, where renal insufficiency secondary to amyloidosis is usually the cause of death. The clinical and pathologic features of the renal disease produced by "primary" and "secondary" amyloidosis are similar.

Amyloid deposition may be most prominent in the walls of blood vessels (especially the small arteries), in the glomeruli, or surrounding the collecting tubules and small blood vessels of the medulla. In all these locations its distribution often tends to be patchy rather than diffuse and uniform.

The clinical picture is influenced by the location and degree of involvement. When amyloid deposits are limited to blood vessels and to occasional focal deposits in glomeruli, mild proteinuria, sometimes with hematuria, may be the only sign. On the other hand, when glomeruli are massively infiltrated, heavy proteinuria is the rule, associated with the nephrotic syndrome. In such cases, glomerular filtration may be surprisingly well maintained despite extensive deposits of amyloid in the malpighian tufts. The rare instance of amyloidosis confined chiefly to the medulla may be marked by polyuria resistant to vasopressin. Hypertension is unusual unless the disorder has progressed to the stage of azotemia and contracted kidneys. Generalized muscular weakness, difficulty in swallowing, and postural hypotension are frequent accompaniments of primary amyloidosis. Biopsy of the liver or kidney is useful in establishing the diagnosis. The course of the disease is generally prolonged, but in some cases secondary to advanced tuberculosis, only 6 months may elapse from the first appearance of albuminuria to the development of advanced uremia. Death occurs from the primary disease, amyloid involvement of the myocardium, intercurrent infection, or renal insufficiency. The disease does not respond to steroid treatment. In those instances in which a chronic suppurative disease can be eradicated, a complete remission may be observed.

MULTIPLE MYELOMA

Impairment of renal function occurs in over 50 per cent of patients with multiple myeloma. Proteinuria is even more common. Renal damage can be related in many cases to the excretion of abnormal proteins of low molecular weight and the injurious effect of these substances on the renal tubules and ultimately the entire nephron. Impairment of renal function is not necessarily correlated, however, with the *degree* of albuminuria or Bence Jones proteinuria. In addition, hypercalcemia may produce transient or irreversible renal damage. In some cases the kidney may be infiltrated by amyloid. Rarely, deposits of myeloma cells may diffusely infiltrate the kidneys.

The major early change produced by the Bence Jones proteins is in the tubules. Proximal tubular cells are swollen and have droplet or rodlike inclusions. Large obstructing casts form along the entire length of the renal tubule, most prominently in the straight tubules of the medulla. These are often laminated and surrounded by multinucleated giant cells possibly derived from degenerating tubular epithelium. In addition, there is usually distinct thickening of the glomerular basement membrane, without cellular proliferation or crescent formation. Vascular sclerosis is not common; when it occurs it is probably coincidental.

Alteration in renal function is most frequently characterized by nitrogen retention and loss of concentrating power, without hypertension, retinitis, or edema. Proteinuria is usually present, consisting of albumin as well as certain globulins and Bence Jones proteins which may be excreted only intermittently. Anemia may seem out of proportion to the degree of azotemia. The disease may superficially resemble the chronic forms of glomerulonephritis or pyelonephritis. The nephrotic syndrome probably does not occur in multiple myeloma unless the disease is complicated by amyloidosis. In unusual instances, and before azotemia has become prominent, disturbances in renal tubular function may dominate the picture, with renal glycosuria, aminoaciduria, low levels of serum uric acid, and renal potassium wasting. Loss of concentrating power is common, and nephrogenic diabetes insipidus has been reported. Renal loss of phosphate with consequent hypophosphatemia and elevation of the serum alkaline phosphatase may, in rare cases, cause confusion with hyperparathyroidism. Because of the exceptional tendency to formation of obstructive casts, procedures which cause dehydration must be carefully avoided in the patient with multiple myeloma. Acute anuria has been observed in several instances following intravenous pyelography, probably as a result of the dehydration which is often induced in preparing for this procedure. Acute renal failure with anuria or oliguria which follows an episode of dehydration in an elderly person should suggest the possibility of myeloma kidney.

HYPERCALCEMIC NEPHROPATHY

Acute elevations of serum calcium may be associated with marked polyuria, succeeded by dehy-

dration, oliguria, and rapidly advancing azotemia. Prolonged hypercalcemia and/or hypercalcuria, as in hyperparathyroidism, vitamin D intoxication, the milk-alkali syndrome, Boeck's sarcoid, multiple myeloma, or carcinomatosis, may result in diffuse nephrocalcinosis and present as renal insufficiency, insidious in onset and only slowly progressive. In such cases, severe disturbances in renal function need not be associated with stones or with radiologic evidence of calcification in the kidneys. Impairment of urinary concentrating capacity is an early sign of calcium nephropathy, and polyuria and polydipsia are frequent, although not invariable. In more severe cases, there is a depression in filtration rate and renal blood flow, with retention of nitrogen. The urinary sediment may contain red blood cells, as well as leukocytes and white blood cell casts; in many patients, however, it is remarkably free of formed elements. Unless congestive heart failure is present, proteinuria is slight. Hypertension is common when nephrocalcinosis is established and does not disappear when the serum calcium has returned to normal, even though renal function improves. Renal insufficiency may sometimes be completely or partially reversed when hypercalcemia is eliminated. In other cases, uremia and hypertensive vascular disease progress to a fatal termination despite the disappearance of hypercalcemia. The degree of reversibility of renal impairment is related to the extent of scar formation and permanent medullary obstruction by calcium precipitates as well as to the presence of vascular disease and infection.

POLYCYSTIC KIDNEYS

In this disorder normal renal tissue is gradually replaced and encroached upon by multiple cysts of the renal parenchyma of varying size. The disease is congenital and in one-half to two-thirds of cases appears to be familial and transmitted as a dominant gene, which is probably not sex-linked, since the incidence is equal in the two sexes. The condition is bilateral, though one kidney may be involved to a greater extent than the other.

Pathology. The kidneys are enlarged to several times normal size and are filled with grapelike clusters of cysts containing clear or hemorrhagic fluid. Between the cysts islands of normal or partially fibrotic renal parenchyma persist. In infants the cysts are said to be closed and do not communicate with the renal pelvis, while in adults there is evidence that some cysts are functional. In patients with polycystic kidneys cysts of the liver may be present and, more rarely, cysts of the pancreas and spleen. These are usually asymptomatic. There is a high associated incidence of intracranial aneurysms, and death from cerebral hemorrhage occurs in about 10 per cent.

Clinical Features. The disease is found in infants, many of whom are premature and in whom it is rapidly fatal, as well as in adults in whom the course is only slowly progressive. The two diseases appear to be distinct, since families have not been reported in which both the infantile and the adult forms have appeared. The condition in the adult is commonly discovered in the fourth, fifth, and sixth decades, frequently in the course of a routine physical examination or as part of an investigation of asymptomatic hematuria, proteinuria, or hypertension. Both kidneys are usually palpable; only one can be felt in one-fifth of the cases, and occasionally no mass can be palpated. In all instances, however, intravenous or retrograde pyelography demonstrates enlarged kidneys with elongation of the pelvis, flattening of the calyxes, and indentations due to the cysts. Lumbar and abdominal ache is a frequent complaint, owing to the weight of the kidney which produces tension on the pedicle, to intracystic hemorrhages, or to pressure on other organs. The pain is often increased by exertion and relieved by lying down. Pain may also be colicky and associated with hematuria and the passage of clots or with concomitant renal calculi. Hypertension appears in the third or fourth decade, when symptoms referable to high blood pressure may predominate. After the age of forty or forty-five, the more common presenting complaints are those associated with renal insufficiency. When a patient presents with uremia and a palpable "liver" and "spleen," the diagnosis of polycystic kidneys must be considered. Polyuria is common and oliguria rare, even terminally. The average age at death is between fifty and sixty years; several patients have lived past seventy. Although the rate of progression may be extremely slow, patients generally do not live longer than 5 years after the blood urea nitrogen rises above 50 mg per 100 ml; superimposed pyelonephritis, however, occurs frequently and may induce renal decompensation which can be reversed by appropriate treatment.

Treatment. It is important to remember that polycystic kidney disease is compatible with a normal life span. Puncture or marsupialization of the cysts has not been demonstrated to prolong life and may introduce a disastrous infection. Because of the high incidence of bilateral disease, excision of one polycystic kidney is practically never indicated unless it is irretrievably infected or causing alarming hemorrhage, and then only after the other kidney has been shown to have fair function and to be only moderately involved in the cystic process. Hematuria usually responds to bed rest but should be disregarded if it is microscopic and asymptomatic. Pregnancy may be undertaken before hypertension and azotemia have appeared.

OTHER CYSTS OF THE KIDNEY

Solitary cysts usually occur at the lower pole, projecting from the surface of the kidney. They contain a serous fluid which is not urine. They may be associated with a dull, dragging pain in the side, but are most often asymptomatic unless complicated by hemorrhage of infection. Occasionally one kidney is completely replaced by *multiple congenital cysts*, while the other is uninvolved. *Multiple small retention cysts*, secondary to obstruction of tubules, are common in nephrosclerosis and pyelonephritis. *Medullary cystic disease* is a rare disorder of childhood in which the medulla is honeycombed with small cysts of uniform size, lined with epithelium. The kidneys are not enlarged. Death occurs, sometimes after many years, from renal insufficiency. *Echinococcus cysts* occur in the kidney in a small percentage of infestations.

OTHER MALFORMATIONS

Congenital malformations of the kidney are sometimes associated with malformations of the external ear. Complete *absence of one kidney* occurs about once in 500 births. *Unilateral hypoplasia* is a rarer congenital anomaly. *Horseshoe kidney* results from fusion of the renal blastemas at the eighth to tenth fetal week, generally at their lower poles. The common location is close to the region of the aortic bifurcation. The anomaly is found once in every 500 to 1,000 autopsies and in most instances is asymptomatic and compatible with long life. It may, however, be complicated by renal calculi, recurrent pyelonephritis, hematuria, and abdominal pain. A few patients have nausea and vomiting associated with abdominal pain which is accentuated by hyperextension and relieved by leaning forward (Rovsing's syndrome). In some, a mass may be palpated in the lower abdomen. In *crossed ectopia* the renal blastema becomes deviated to the opposite side where it usually lies caudal to the normal kidney, with which it may fuse. Its ureter usually crosses the midline to terminate in the normal position. Such kidneys, as well as *unilaterally fused kidneys*, are predisposed to hydronephrosis and pyelonephritis, but not to other renal lesions. Pain is the most common symptom; many patients are entirely asymptomatic.

Anomalies of the ureter include bifurcation, complete reduplication, and abnormal implantation in the bladder, as well as stricture at the ureteropelvic or ureterovesical junction. Habitual reflux from the bladder into the ureter during the act of voiding may initiate hydronephrosis and infection. *Anomalies of the vesical neck* may underlie enuresis in children, which may sometimes be treated as a behavior problem, while the kidneys are irretrievably damaged.

THE KIDNEY OF GOUT

From 30 to 50 per cent of gouty patients are said to die of renal disease. The kidney of most patients with gout contains characteristic fan-shaped clefts containing deposits of urate in the interstices of the medulla. Pyelonephritis is a frequent finding, and arteriolar sclerosis is almost always present.

Urate calculi occur in approximately 15 per cent of patients with gout and are particularly common during uricosuric therapy if a high fluid intake is not maintained. Both uric acid stones and interstitial deposits of urate crystals in the kidney may occur in patients with hyperuricemia who have never had gouty arthritis.

The most common indications of early renal damage are mild proteinuria, decreased excretion of phenolsulfonphthalein, and a reduction in concentrating ability. Slowly progressive azotemia with minimal albuminuria and little or no abnormality in the urinary sediment may characterize the course of some patients. Though hypertension may be absent, the blood pressure is commonly elevated; in fact, it has been suggested that hypertension and vascular sclerosis, especially nephrosclerosis, occur as part of a constitutional diathesis of which gout or hyperuricemia is a component part. Hyperuricemia and evidence on renal biopsy of arteriolar sclerosis may occasionally be the only positive findings in patients with asymptomatic proteinuria.

In rare instances of gouty kidney, renal function has been reported to improve slowly and urate stones to dissolve following the long-term administration of a high fluid intake and alkali, in association with uricosuric agents.

NEPHROLITHIASIS

Renal stones may vary in size from tiny particles to large staghorn calculi which fill the entire renal pelvis. They may be asymptomatic or may continue to be formed and passed for years with no deleterious effect on renal function and no discomfort except occasional renal colic. Even a large staghorn calculus may produce no symptoms save, perhaps, for occasional nagging abdominal or flank pain. Often, however, renal calculi are associated with infection and progressive encroachment on renal function. Stones passed from above are rarely retained in the bladder unless there is obstruction and residual urine.

The typical attack of renal colic is exquisitely painful, causing the patient to double up in agony. The crampy pain begins in the side or back, radiat-

ing to the lower abdomen, genitals, and inner thigh. The attack usually persists for several hours, although it may be over in a matter of minutes. Dysuria is frequently present, and even after the attack has subsided, tenderness along the course of the ureter often persists. Fever and leukocytosis signal the presence of associated infection. Hematuria and proteinuria are almost always present. Sometimes the pain is not referred in the usual manner and may simulate gallbladder disease, appendicitis, peptic ulcer, or disease of the spine. Renal colic may also be produced by blood clots or pus obstructing the ureter.

In about half of all patients with renal calculi, some predisposing causes can be found. These include *hyperparathyroidism,* excessive ingestion of *milk, alkali,* and *vitamin D, bone disease* producing hypercalcuria, *sarcoid* and *renal tubular acidosis. Idiopathic hypercalciuria* is found in a large proportion of patients with recurrent calcium stones.

Cystinuria (p. 747) is a congenital disorder characterized by decreased tubular reabsorption of cystine, arginine, ornithine, and lysine. Owing to its relative insolubility, cystine tends to precipitate in the urinary tract to form stones which are radiopaque on account of their high content of sulfur. The condition may be diagnosed from the hexagonal appearance of cystine crystals in the urine and their characteristic reaction with nitroprusside. Cystine stones may be dissolved or prevented from forming if the reaction of the urine is kept alkaline and the urine volume high. *Hereditary glycinuria* is a rare familial disorder associated with nephrolithiasis and excessive urinary excretion of glycine unaccompanied by other amino acids.

Uric acid stones are radiolucent, form most readily in acid urine, and may be prevented if the urine is kept persistently alkaline. They frequently complicate gout and may appear in a variety of hematologic diseases, notably polycythemia. More than half of all patients with urate calculi have neither hyperuricemia nor increased urinary excretion of uric acid. In this group of patients an unexplained tendency to excrete urine of pH below 5.5 may predispose to uric acid stones.

Although most patients with calcium oxalate stones do not excrete excessive amounts of oxalate, the rare condition of *primary hyperoxaluria* is characterized by progressive calcium oxalate urolithiasis and nephrocalcinosis beginning in early childhood. Finally, *primary renal infection,* especially with urea-splitting organisms and in the presence of hydronephrosis, may promote the formation of renal calculi.

Treatment must be individualized and governed by the patient's symptoms and the signs of associated renal disease. A small asymptomatic calculus entrapped in a renal calyx and unassociated with infection may be best left alone. Many stones pass spontaneously, but in the majority of instances special urologic and surgical procedures are eventually required. Daily urine volume should be kept over 2,500 ml. Special emphasis should be placed on drinking before retiring and once more during the night. Infection should be vigorously treated. Aluminum hydroxide or aluminum carbonate gel in amounts of 30 ml three or four times daily has been advocated to reduce the intestinal absorption and urinary excretion of phosphate in individuals with calcium phosphate stones.

SICKLE-CELL NEPHROPATHY

Patients with sickle-cell anemia often develop progressive changes in renal function as a result of multiple small ischemic and hemorrhagic infarcts in the kidney. In children the principal anatomic finding is congestion of blood vessels with sickled erythrocytes; in adults interstitial fibrosis and areas of cortical necrosis and hyalinization may be seen. Frequently the changes resemble those of chronic glomerulonephritis. There is early impairment of renal concentrating ability, even when blood urea nitrogen, glomerular filtration rate, and renal plasma flow are normal. This selective disturbance in renal function may be present in patients with sickle-cell trait as well as in the full-blown disease. It is said to be temporarily reversed in children by transfusion of normal blood, but this is not the case in adults. Gross and microscopic hematuria occur frequently; bleeding may come from lesions in the papillae and pelvic mucosa as well as miliary infarctions in the cortex. Hypertension is not common. Despite the high incidence of at least minimal renal changes, the sickle-cell trait does not appear to predispose to toxemia of pregnancy.

CHYLURIA

The chief cause of chyluria is filariasis (p. 1223) with obstruction between the abdominal lymphatics and the thoracic duct, producing lymph varices in the kidney which rupture into the renal tubules. The urine is milky and on standing settles into a top layer of fatty material, a middle pinkish layer, often containing a clot, and a bottom layer containing blood and debris. Hematuria is common, and pyelonephritis is almost universal. Microfilarias are usually found in the urine for about 6 weeks after an acute infection but not thereafter unless the patient is in an endemic area. The lymph and blood may coalesce into ureteral casts, causing flank pain and renal colic. Chyluria may disappear with recumbency and be aggravated by exertion. The condition may be entirely suppressed in some cases by wearing a tight abdominal corset.

RADIATION NEPHRITIS

Following the administration of large doses of x-ray (2,300 r during 5 weeks) to the kidneys in the course of therapy for abdominal carcinoma or lymph node metastases from testicular tumors, a characteristic syndrome may develop. The latent period between irradiation and the appearance of symptoms is usually at least 6 months but may be much longer. Hypertension invariably appears and may lead to congestive heart failure, retinopathy, and encephalopathy. Refractory anemia is often prominent. Uremia is usually progressive, but in some cases renal insufficiency may be reversible, improvement commencing about 6 months after the onset of symptoms. Proteinuria is present but slight; hematuria is characteristically absent. Oliguria is never observed except with heart failure. The clinical disease may mimic either benign or malignant hypertension or chronic glomerulonephritis. Histologic features include widespread fibrosis between atrophic tubules, damage to almost all the glomeruli, and fibrinoid necrotic lesions of arterioles.

MEDICAL ASPECTS OF RENAL TUMORS

Malignant tumors of the kidney occur chiefly in childhood and after forty. The incidence is considerably higher in males. The common malignant tumor of children is *Wilms's tumor*, or embryonal adenosarcoma, which constitutes 20 to 25 per cent of all malignant neoplasms of childhood and is observed before the age of seven in 90 per cent of cases. The tumor usually presents as a palpable abdominal mass and may grow to enormous size. It is the only renal neoplasm associated in a high proportion of cases with hypertension.

In adults *hypernephroma* is the most common neoplasm of the kidney. The classic triad of hematuria, flank pain, and abdominal mass is present in two-thirds of the cases, but not infrequently the first symptoms arise from metastases to lung, bone, liver, or brain. Obscure fever is a common presenting symptom, even when evidence of infection is lacking. Serum alkaline phosphatase is frequently elevated, regardless of the presence or absence of bony metastases. In rare instances, polycythemia may be observed, unaccompanied by leukocytosis, thrombocytosis, or splenomegaly. In such cases the polycythemia may be cured by removal of the tumor. Hypertension, if present, is coincidental and is not improved by nephrectomy. Extension of the tumor into the renal veins with subsequent venous thrombosis is not infrequent. About one-quarter of patients with hypernephroma survive more than 10 years.

Papillary neoplasms of the renal pelvis are often associated with similar tumors of the ureter and bladder. Hematuria is the outstanding symptom. An association with calculi and infection is frequent. Carcinoma of the renal pelvis may appear deceptively benign, and failure to find infiltration at operation does not ensure survival. The prognosis is worse than that with hypernephroma.

The most frequent symptom of *tumors of the bladder* is painless hematuria. Dysuria and frequency are also common, especially with superimposed infection. A small number of papillary bladder tumors arise from metaplasia of the epithelium of the bladder which follows long-standing cystitis. The incidence of bladder tumors is said to be increased in workers exposed to certain aniline dyes.

REFERENCES

GENERAL

Allen, A. C.: The Kidney, in "Medical and Surgical Diseases," New York, Grune & Stratton, Inc., 1951.

Bell, E. T.: "Renal Diseases," 2d ed., Philadelphia, Lea & Febiger, 1950.

Fishberg, A. M.: "Hypertension and Nephritis," 5th ed., Philadelphia, Lea & Febiger, 1954.

Lippman, R. W.: "Urine and the Urinary Sediment: A Practical Manual and Atlas," Springfield, Ill., Charles C Thomas, Publisher, 1957.

GLOMERULONEPHRITIS

Jennings, R. B., and D. P. Earle: Post-streptococcal Glomerulonephritis, J. Clin. Invest., 40:1525, 1961.

Peters, J. H., and P. Freedman: Immunologic Aspects of Renal Disease, New Engl. J. Med., 261:1166, 1959.

Symposium on Glomerulonephritis, D. P. Earle and D. Seegal (Eds.), J. Chron. Diseases, 5:1, 1957.

NEPHROTIC SYNDROME

Allen, A. C.: The Clinicopathologic Meaning of the Nephrotic Syndrome, Am. J. Med., 18:277, 1955.

Derow, H. A.: The Nephrotic Syndrome, New Engl., J. Med., 258:77, 1958.

PYELONEPHRITIS

Kleeman, C. R., W. L. Hewitt, and L. B. Guze: Pyelonephritis, Medicine, 39:3, 1960.

DIABETIC NEPHROPATHY

Rogers, J., and S. L. Robbins: Intercapillary Glomerulosclerosis: Clinical and Pathologic Study. I. Specificity of Clinical Syndrome, Am. J. Med., 12:688, 1952.

NEPHROSCLEROSIS

Kincaid-Smith, P., J. McMichael, and E. A. Murphy: The Clinical Course and Pathology of Hypertension with Papilloedema (Malignant Hypertension), Quart. J. Med. (n.s.), 27:117, 1958.

ACUTE TUBULAR NECROSIS

Swan, R. C., and J. P. Merrill: The Clinical Course of Acute Renal Failure, Medicine, 32:215, 1953.

Bluemle, L. W., Jr., G. D. Webster, Jr., and J. R. Elkinton: Acute Tubular Necrosis: Analysis of One Hundred Cases with Respect to Mortality, Complications, and Treatment with and without Dialysis, A.M.A. Arch. Internal Med., 104:180, 1959.

TOXEMIAS OF PREGNANCY

Pollak, V. E., and J. R. Nettles: The Kidney in Toxemia of Pregnancy: A Clinical and Pathological Study Based on Renal Biopsies, Medicine, 19:469, 1960.

ORTHOSTATIC AND FUNCTIONAL PROTEINURIA

Greiner, T., and J. P. Henry: Mechanism of Postural Proteinuria, J.A.M.A., 157:1371, 1955.

RENAL ARTERIAL OCCLUSION

Yendt, E. R., W. K. Kerr, D. R. Wilson, and Z. F. Jaworski: The Diagnosis and Treatment of Renal Hypertension; with Special Reference to a Case of Hypertension Due to Stenosis of Both Renal Arteries, Am. J. Med., 28:169, 1960.

RENAL VEIN THROMBOSIS

Harrison, C. V., M. D. Milne, and R. E. Steiner: Clinical Aspects of Renal Vein Thrombosis, Quart. J. Med. (n.s.), 25:285, 1956.

RENAL DISEASE IN LUPUS ERYTHEMATOSUS

Muehrcke, R. C., R. M. Kark, C. L. Pirani, and V. E. Pollak: Lupus Nephritis: A Clinical and Pathologic Study Based on Renal Biopsies, Medicine, 36:1, 1957.

SCLERODERMA

Levine, R. J., and B. R. Boshell: Renal Involvement in Progressive Systemic Sclerosis (Scleroderma), Ann. Internal Med., 52:517, 1960.

PERIARTERITIS NODOSA

Davson, J., J. Ball, and R. Platt: The Kidney in Periarteritis Nodosa, Quart. J. Med. (n.s.), 17:175, 1948.

AMYLOID KIDNEY

Altnow, H. O., C. C. Van Winkle, and S. S. Cohen:
Renal Amyloidosis: Further Study of Clinical
Course and Pathologic Lesions in 57 Cases, Arch.
Internal Med., 63:249, 1939.

HYPERCALCEMIC NEPHROPATHY

Epstein, F. H.: Calcium and the Kidney, J. Chron.
Diseases, 11:255, 1960.

POLYCYSTIC KIDNEYS

Dalgaard, O. Z.: Bilateral Polycystic Disease of the
Kidneys, Acta Med. Scand., Suppl. 328:1, 1957.

THE KIDNEY OF GOUT

Talbott, J. H., and K. L. Terplan: The Kidney in Gout,
Medicine, 19:405, 1960.

NEPHROLITHIASIS

Melick, R. A., and P. H. Henneman: Clinical and
Laboratory Studies of 207 Consecutive Patients in
a Kidney-stone Clinic, New Engl. J. Med., 259:
307, 1958.

RADIATION NEPHRITIS

Luxton, R. W.: Radiation Nephritis, Quart. J. Med.
(n.s.), 22:215, 1953.

Section 4: The Respiratory System

INTRODUCTION

Ben V. Branscomb and
T. R. Harrison

The distortions of function responsible for the
manifestations of pulmonary disorders have been
considered in a preceding section (p. 104). Here,
we are concerned with the specific diseases which
involve the respiratory system.

Presenting Problems. The patient with respiratory disease may exhibit one or more of a number
of problems. The most compelling of these is sudden severe dyspnea. Under such circumstances a
quick tentative distinction must be made between
acute failure of the left side of the heart and some
pulmonary disorder such as acute pneumothorax
or asthma. Only after immediate therapy has led to
improvement will there be opportunity for more
detailed study. When doubt exists it may be necessary to initiate procedures which are beneficial in
both cardiac and pulmonary dyspnea (pp. 1383
and 1573).

Another common situation is that of fever with
progressive dyspnea. Here, the differentiation of
pneumonia from infarction and from other disorders
will usually be apparent in young persons but may
require extensive study in older individuals (p.
891).

The problem presented by the afebrile patient
with slowly progressive exertional dyspnea is less
urgent, and the recognition of pulmonary or cardiac
disease as the cause will usually be achieved on
the basis of the office examination, supplemented
by observation of the response to therapeutic measures. Shortness of breath at rest is likely to be
more serious and, when not obviously due to

bronchial asthma or to emotional disturbance will
commonly call for an initial period of hospital
management.

Even more frequent is the syndrome of cough,
with little or no dyspnea or fever but often associated with difficulty in producing sputum. Since
the usual cause is acute bronchitis, with recovery
in a short time, a watch-and-wait period of ambulatory treatment is justified. Persistence of the symptoms should raise the question of tuberculosis or
carcinoma and call for more complete investigation.

Hemoptysis, unless minimal and obviously due
to the strain of coughing, should be regarded as
serious and as an indication for detailed study
(p. 122).

Various combinations of these presenting syndromes are often encountered. Only by the exercise
of sound judgment, based on a comprehension of
all the likely causes, will it be possible to avoid
the error of overlooking grave disorders in their
earlier stages and the opposite mistake of subjecting
every patient with minor symptoms to unnecessarily
elaborate and expensive investigation.

Another common presenting problem is that of
the patient who has minimal or no symptoms but
is found in the course of a routine x-ray of the
chest to display some unexpected change. This
may involve either the lungs or some other thoracic
structure. Thus notching of the ribs may furnish the
first clue to coarctation of the aorta, while a cervical
rib may explain an otherwise mysterious paresthesia of the arm. Similarly, the finding of an
unusual shape or of enlargement of the heart may
be the initial guide to the presence of a curable
congenital or acquired disorder. In order to avoid
the common error of confusing an apical fat pad

with cardiac enlargement, the planographic technique may be required.

Even more frequent are the unexpected radiologic changes in the lungs. Large irregular shadows are often caused by the various pneumonias, by tuberculous and fungous infections, by tumors, and by numerous other disorders. Some of the more important causes of discrete localized lesions are listed in the following table.

Simple Procedures. Acute bronchitis and acute pleuritis, the two most frequent disorders of the lower respiratory tract, cause no changes in the x-ray but are readily detected by the history and the physical examination. However, there are many disorders of the pulmonary parenchyma which produce radiologic changes prior to physical signs. Therefore, an x-ray film of the chest is to be routinely made in patients with pulmonary problems. When the dynamic functions of the thorax and lungs are involved, as in patients with emphysema or with diaphragmatic paralysis, fluoroscopy is useful, provided the undesirability of excessive radiation is remembered.

The total vital capacity is a valuable guide to

SOME OF THE CAUSES OF PUZZLING RADIOLOGIC PULMONARY SHADOWS

Disorder	Nodular lesions							Increased linear markings	Calcification
	Single				Multiple				
	Small or "coin" lesions	Large, 3 cm or more			Large	Small (miliary)			
		Sharply outlined	Irregular margins	Containing air or fluid		Acute	Subacute or chronic		
Tuberculosis	+	....	+	+	....	+	+	....	+
Fungus	+	....	+	+	....	+	+	....	+
Other granulomas	+	....	+	....	....	....	....	....	+
Carcinoma	Primary or meta-static	....	+	+	Metastatic	....	+	+	
Pleural tumors	....	+	+						
Phantom tumor (interlobar) effusion	....	+							
Infarct	....	....	+	+					
Abscess	....	....	+	+					
Arteriovenous fistula	....	+	+						
Pulmonary sequestration	....	....	+						
Cyst	....	+	....	+					
Bulla	....	....	....	+					
Pneumoconiosis	....	....	....	....	+	....	+	+	
Sarcoid	....	....	....	....	+	....	+	+	
Nonbacterial pneumonias	....	....	....	....	Loeffler's	Measles			
Rheumatic and collagen	....	....	....	....	....	....	+	+	
Congestion	....	....	....	....	....	....	....	+	
Uremia	....	....	....	....	....	....	....	+	
Miscellaneous	Pneumonia; atelectasis	....	Lipid granuloma	....	....	Viral rickettsial	Amyloid lipidoses	Interstitial fibrosis; lymphoma; hemosiderosis; scleroderma	Aneurysm

the presence of a restrictive disorder, and one of the simple respiratory flow tests may be essential for the early recognition of an obstructive disorder. Only occasionally will the more complex methods for study of respiratory function be needed (p. 107).

The x-ray will often be of particular importance in detecting the presence of pulmonary disease; the sputum in determining its cause. The history will usually be the most accurate guide to its rate of progress. Treatment will depend on sound clinical judgment based on the total information supplied by these multiple methods of study.

The Systematic Approach to Therapy. In order to avoid neglect of important methods of treatment, the following problems must be considered in all patients with respiratory disorders.

The importance of *infection* is to be evaluated. Antibiotics should usually be withheld when the evidence points toward an acute viral disorder, and their use in bacterial infections will depend in large measure on cultures and smears of the sputum.

The role of *bronchial obstruction* should be considered as a likely factor in aggravating either dyspnea or infection. The relative significance of allergy, of mechanical blockage by thickened sputum, and of bronchospasm must be assessed.

A search should be made for evidence of *failure of the right ventricle* in order that the need for digitalis, oxygen, or venesection may be determined.

In persons with chronic pulmonary disorders, the therapeutic plan will also depend on the extent to which there is *reversibility* of the functional impairment. This is always present in some measure, but the degree varies markedly from one patient to another.

Terminology and Classification. The important conceptual clarifications of the past few years have been accompanied by confusion in nomenclature. Thus the term "emphysema" is employed by some to mean any overdistended lung; others reserve it for that distention due to destruction of the walls of the respiratory bronchioles or alveoli. Some authors consider a change in shape of the thorax with increased anteroposterior diameter due to senile kyphosis as a variety of emphysema; other writers insist that such a designation is unjustified unless there is also clear evidence of expiratory obstruction. There is no general agreement concerning the inclusion or exclusion of the elderly person with a few radiologically demonstrable but asymptomatic bullae in the category of emphysema. These differences in usage have led some of the students of pulmonary disease to believe that the word "emphysema" should be reserved for the pathologist and that clinicians should utilize the more precise

(if more awkward) term "generalized obstructive lung disease," subdividing it according to its episodic and reversible (bronchial asthma) or persistent and largely irreversible (clinically significant emphysema) varieties.

"Chronic bronchitis" is used by some to signify a grave and progressive disorder, terminating in respiratory or cardiac failure, and by others to indicate a minor nuisance, with cough and expectoration in a vigorous individual. This is analogous to the use of the unqualified term "hypertension" to describe both the healthy person with minor elevation of systolic pressure and the patient with malignant nephrosclerosis.

In the strictest sense "bronchiectasis" means dilated bronchi, and some apply this term to any patient with persistent abundant purulent sputum dependent on diffuse bronchial disease (cylindrical bronchiectasis). Other writers decry the word "bronchiectasis" for the disorder which they designate as "chronic bronchitis," and would limit it to the localized saccular type which is sometimes amenable to surgical treatment. The evidence of the postmortem examination suggests that neither term (bronchitis nor diffuse bronchiectasis) is ideal because, although both conditions are present, it is the destructive bronchiolitis which is responsible for the expiratory obstruction and the trapping of air which is the major cause of the respiratory impairment. The distinction between the terms chronic bronchitis and bronchiectasis as they are employed in this book is discussed on p. 1551.

The similar confusion which existed some decades ago in the field of heart disease was partially eliminated by a classification which took cognizance of etiologic, morphologic, and physiologic relationships. The following classification is based on a somewhat similar approach. It is not intended to be all-inclusive but is presented to illustrate and clarify the chapters to follow. The third, or clinical, classification is applied only to those disorders which do not fit readily into the etiologic division.

CLASSIFICATION OF CHRONIC LUNG DISEASE

I. Etiologic
   A. Congenital
   B. Specific infective agents
   C. Allergic
   D. Physical or chemical agents
   E. Fibrotic and infiltrative (e.g., sarcoid, amyloid, collagen disease)
   F. Circulatory
   G. Neoplastic
   H. Nonspecific, mixed and unknown causes (e.g., the common varieties of chronic bronchitis and of emphysema) (see III for subgroups)

II. Physiologic
    A. Disturbances of ventilation
        1. Restrictive
        2. Obstructive
    B. Disturbances of diffusion
    C. Disturbances of perfusion

> In most instances there are various combinations of these physiologic disorders.

III. Clinical classification of chronic nonspecific lung disease and of complicating cor pulmonale
    A. Bronchial asthma (see Chap. 232)
    B. Bronchitis (including the milder type and the grave variety associated with destruction of bronchioles, the latter being usually consequent to the former)
    C. Emphysema
        1. Relatively innocent varieties (including compensatory, senile blebs without generalized obstruction, etc.)
        2. Generalized obstructive (essentially the same as advanced chronic bronchitis with bronchiolar destruction)
    D. Cor pulmonale in chronic nonspecific lung disease
        1. Right ventricular hypertrophy without failure
        2. Right ventricular hypertrophy with failure

It should be noted that the term "generalized obstructive lung disease" includes both a reversible condition (bronchial asthma) and the largely irreversible disorder generalized obstructive emphysema, which with the associated bronchitis may be designated as "chronic diffuse nonspecific lung disease."

In the following presentation, the etiologic classification will be used for those disorders which fall into clearly defined categories. However, the clinical and physiologic classifications will be employed in the discussion of chronic bronchitis, of emphysema, and of the large group of diseases which restrict ventilation and impair diffusion.

Arrangement of Chapters. Acute disorders of the respiratory tract are usually of infectious nature, and most of them have been discussed in preceding chapters dealing with illness due to specific organisms. This section of the book is, therefore, concerned mainly with chronic diseases.

Because of the importance of chronic obstructive disease (bronchitis and emphysema), this is discussed first. Then the restrictive and diffusional disorders are considered, followed by various specific conditions.

Those therapeutic procedures which are of limited scope and mainly applicable to a specific disease are considered with that disease. Those which have a wider application are placed in the last chapter, which deals with the more general treatment of pulmonary problems.

259 DISORDERS OF THE UPPER RESPIRATORY TRACT

Ivan L. Bennett, Jr.

This chapter summarizes some of the diseases that are manifested in whole or in part by structural alterations or dysfunction of the nose, nasopharynx, paranasal sinuses, and larynx. In the course of their normal function of warming, humidifying, and preliminary cleansing (by impingement of inhaled particles upon the mucosa) of inspired air, these passages are exposed to a multitude of irritants and infectious agents. Their lining membranes contain many mucous glands and deposits of lymphoid tissue; the vascular bed of the nasal mucosa is capable of such rapid and extensive alterations in response to local or systemic stimuli that it is often classified as an erectile tissue. Engorgement, hypersecretion of mucus, and hyperplasia of the adenoids and other lymphatic foci in response to irritation or infection can produce acute or chronic obstruction of the passages draining the sinuses, conjunctivas, and middle ears. This leads to initiation or aggravation of bacterial infection in these areas.

The annoying and distracting discomfort occasioned by interference with inspiration and speech, coupled with the frequency of viral and allergic disorders of this region, makes upper respiratory disease the most important transient disability that afflicts mankind.

DISEASES OF THE NOSE AND NASOPHARYNX

Hay fever, vasomotor rhinitis, and complicating nasal *polyposis* are discussed on p. 1259.

Acute *coryza* and other forms of viral rhinitis are discussed on p. 1116; the upper respiratory prodrome of *measles* is discussed on p. 1158.

Among bacterial infections, the persistent rhinitis ("Snuffles") of *congenital syphilis* (p. 1076), nasal diphtheria (p. 987), and *furunculosis* of the nares (because of the complication of *cavernous sinus thrombosis,* p. 1046) are the more important.

Clear, watery discharge characterizes *cerebrospinal rhinorrhea.* Chronic, mucoid, occasionally blood-stained discharge is frequent in children with enlarged *adenoids.*

Unilateral purulent or sanguineous discharge suggests foreign body, diphtheria, or tumor.

Perforation of the nasal septum results most commonly from habitual nose picking, but syphilis and occupational exposure to chromate are other causes to be considered. Many diseases, some of them unusual or exotic, are characterized by extensive destructive and deforming lesions of the nose and adjacent structures. These include *leprosy* (p. 1020), the *gangosa* and *goundou* lesions of yaws (p. 1082), the *espundia* type of American leishmaniasis (p. 1204), *South American blastomycosis* (p. 1067), *lethal midline granuloma* (p. 1253), and Wegener's granulomatosis (p. 1900).

In *rhinoscleroma,* chronic obstruction of the nasal passages is produced by recurrent, indurated, nonulcerating, inflammatory nodules. Rarely, sinuses or the upper trachea are involved also. The disorder occurs primarily in the Mediterranean countries, South Asia, Indonesia, and Latin America; most cases seen in the United States are in immigrants. Rhinoscleroma is probably an infection, caused by the Von Frisch bacillus, *Klebsiella rhinoscleromatis,* which is always present in the lesions, but the diagnosis is usually established by the pathognomonic histologic finding of masses of atypical plasma cells interspersed with large, foamy Mikulicz cells. Treatment is surgical excision of the recurrent nodules. Untreated, the disease can lead to enormous nasal enlargement with flared nares, the *Hebra nose.*

Rhinosporidiosis, caused by a yeastlike organism, *Rhinosporidium seeberi,* is common in India and Ceylon; sporadic cases occur in many other areas. Soft, pinkish, sessile or pedunculated polyps appear on the nasal mucosa; sometimes the conjunctivas and, rarely, other mucosal surfaces are involved. Treatment is simple excision.

Rhinophyma or *Pfundnase* is a progressive, deforming, nodular enlargement of the alae nasi due to hypertrophy of sebaceous follicles in patients with chronic, severe *acne rosacea.* There is no specific treatment; plastic repair may be necessary.

Ozena is a severe chronic rhinitis of unknown cause characterized by thick, greenish discharge, mucosal crusts, turbinate atrophy, and an offensive odor. Patients eventually become anosmic. Even when the nasal passages are widened and resistance to airflow is decreased, obstruction is a constant complaint. Cultures grow gram-negative bacilli (*Klebsiella, Pseudomonas,* etc.). Treatment with local or systemic antibiotics and large doses of vasodilators (Priscoline, nicotinic acid) will often reduce the discharge without halting the atrophy. Most important for these unfortunate patients, the odor is lessened or eliminated in many instances.

Mycosis leptothrica (so-called because infection by *Leptothrix* was thought to be its cause) is a focal hyperkeratosis of the tonsils, pharynx, and larynx that occurs in young adults. The many small, white, raised patches over the mucosa are striking and are often mistaken for exudate; removal causes no bleeding. Patients are sometimes asymptomatic but may complain of "scratchy" throat. There is no

treatment; the lesions regress after months or years.

Pharyngeal bursitis, or Tornwaldt's disease, is bacterial inflammation of a small recess in the posterior nasopharyngeal wall which sometimes persists into adulthood. Obstruction of the neck of the pouch leads to infection and abscess formation. Treatment consists of antibiotics followed by surgical *excision* of the bursa rather than simple drainage.

Recurrent, profuse epistaxes occur with hypertensive vascular disease, familial telangiectasia (p. 1321), coagulation defects (p. 1318), and tumors.

Basal cell carcinoma of the nares and *septal hemangioma* are relatively common. Carcinomas of the nasal mucosa are unusual; they occur in elderly individuals and are late to invade or metastasize.

Carcinoma of the nasopharynx (so-called *lymphoepithelioma*) occurs in young and middle-aged adults and is especially common among Chinese. These tumors metastasize very early. Large, cancerous cervical lymph nodes often result from a primary lesion so small that it is found with great difficulty. These tumors tend to occur near the orifice of a eustachian tube, and the combination of *cervical adenopathy and ipsilateral ear pain or deafness* is a signal for careful examination of the nasopharynx. These tumors are radiosensitive, and survival for several years with repeated courses of therapy is usual; complete cures are rare.

Lymphoma and *reticulum cell sarcoma* are often first detected as nasopharyngeal masses. Isolated *plasmacytomas* of the nasopharynx are found predominantly in elderly males, some of whom develop multiple myeloma (p. 1342). Two tumors of children deserve mention. A highly malignant and rapidly fatal lesion which tends to arise in the nasopharynx or soft palate is the *sarcoma botryoides* or *embryonal rhabdomyosarcoma. Juvenile angiofibroma* is a benign growth that occurs almost exclusively in young boys, arising from the base of the sphenoid and filling the nasopharynx. Sometimes the tumor will regress during puberty but excision is usually necessary. These tumors bleed spontaneously, and profuse hemorrhage is very likely to complicate surgical manipulation.

DISEASES OF THE PARANASAL SINUSES

The mucosa of the ethmoid and maxillary sinuses may become involved by the polyposis that occurs in patients with allergic rhinitis (p. 1259). While primary *tumors* of the sinus mucosa are rare, encroachment by neoplasms arising in contiguous structures is common and easily visualized by x-ray. *Osteoma of the frontal sinus* is the most frequent lesion of this type; neoplasms of the maxilla and mixed tumors of the salivary gland type arising in the palate invade the antrum.

Sinusitis. In the vast majority of cases, acute sinusitis is a bacterial infection brought on by impairment of drainage by the boggy, engorged nasal mucosa of allergic or viral rhinitis. Occasionally, pressure changes of air travel may result in an "aerosinusitis" similar to "aerotitis media"; deviations of the nasal septum are contributory.

The manifestations are local pain and tenderness, sometimes with edema of the overlying facial skin, headache, and fever. The headache is worse in the morning, when exudate has accumulated overnight, and tends to improve with upright posture and drainage during the day. If fluid has filled the frontal or maxillary sinuses, they cannot be transilluminated. Treatment consists of analgesics, appropriate antibiotics, and, most important, the establishment of adequate drainage. This last includes reduction of nasal swelling by astringents such as Neo-synephrine or ephedrine, antihistaminics in patients with allergy, and, frequently, aspiration or irrigation of the infected cavity by an otorhinolaryngologist. When coryza or allergic rhinitis runs its course, acute sinusitis usually clears up promptly.

About 10 per cent of antral infections are secondary to dental sepsis or result from fractures of the bony floor during dental extractions.

Complications of acute sinusitis are statistically rare but may be serious. Frank suppuration and abscess may lead to osteomyelitis and spread of infection to the orbit (retrobulbar abscess, cavernous sinus thrombosis), the meninges (see pneumococcal meningitis, p. 892), and brain (via the diploic veins). Surgical drainage of frontal and ethmoid abscesses is sometimes an emergency procedure. About 10 per cent of brain abscesses originate from frontal sinusitis, and infection of the frontal or sphenoid sinus precedes almost every case of subdural empyema (p. 1046). A serious complication of frontal suppuration is osteomyelitis of the skull, recognized by doughy edema of the forehead ("Pott's puffy tumor") and rapid destruction of bone.

With repeated episodes of acute infection, there may be thickening of the sinus mucosa, continual partial obstruction, and chronic inflammation that flares up with the stimulus of even slight obstruction such as that which follows smoking, ingestion of spicy foods, the use of alcohol, or chilly, damp weather. Each acute episode becomes more difficult to control, and the patient may be continuously miserable. Rigid control of exposure to allergens and extremes of temperature, correction of structural defects such as deviated septum, and intensive treatment of acute exacerbations will sometimes bring relief, but radical surgery to ensure free drainage is eventually necessary in many instances.

Chronic sinusitis is especially common in pa-tients with bronchiectasis (p. 1550), but a causal relationship between lung and sinus disease has not been shown.

Cerebral *mucormycosis* in patients with diabetic acidosis (p. 1063) usually originates as a sinusitis, invading the orbit and cranium secondarily.

It is important to remember that when a diagnosis of "sinusitis" has been made radiologically, usually distinction between acute, chronic, or inactive disease is not automatically made at the same time; this is also true of x-ray diagnosis of mastoiditis.

Finally, nasal swab cultures are *never sterile*. Choice of an antibiotic should be based upon the predominating pathogenic organism in cultures of exudate from the sinus; it is fruitless to change antimicrobial drugs as resistant organisms appear in the normal nasal flora of patients taking antibiotics.

DISEASES OF THE LARYNX

The two most important manifestations of laryngeal disease are *hoarseness* and *respiratory obstruction*. Aphasia (p. 376) and *aphonia* do not signify a lesion of the larynx. *Hoarseness that persists for more than 3 weeks* in an adult calls for intensive investigation, tumor, chronic infection (tuberculosis, mycosis), and vocal cord paralysis being the important possibilities. *Respiratory obstruction* by edema, exudate, foreign body, or bilateral cord paralysis is an acute emergency.

Angioneurotic laryngeal edema is discussed on p. 1267. Among infectious agents, the *diphtheria* bacillus (p. 984), *Hemophilus influenzae* (p. 954), the viral agents of croup and laryngotracheitis (Tables 180-1 and 180-2, p. 1115), *Treponema pallidum* (p. 1073), the *tubercle bacillus* (p. 1015), and *fungi*, especially monilia (p. 1062), are the ones most likely to attack the larynx. Laryngitis and hoarseness are *not* complications of streptococcal pharyngitis; their appearance in a patient with sore throat indicates a viral etiology or complicating diphtheria (formerly a frequent occurrence in streptococcal disease).

Laryngeal *papillomatosis* is believed by many to be a viral disease. Multiple pedunculated growths on the cords, easily excised but recurrent, are seen exclusively in children. Respiratory obstruction is rare but has occurred. The disease recedes spontaneously at puberty.

Laryngeal *acanthosis* or hyperkeratosis (*pachydermia laryngis*) causing hoarseness, may be a result of misuse of the voice, smoking, and probably of alcoholism; it is not a precancerous lesion. *Leukoplakia* of the larynx has the same significance in terms of later development of cancer that it has elsewhere and calls for local excision. It is important not to confuse *acanthosis* and *leukoplakia*.

The so-called *singers' nodule* or *amyloid nodule* is a lesion of the vocal cord that appears almost exclusively in white males over the age of thirty years who have strained or misused their voices. Treatment is excision; the lesion does not recur. Incidentally, the lesion contains no amyloid.

Carcinoma of the larynx is ten to twelve times more common in men than in women; the average age at which it appears is sixty years. Tumors arising on the vocal cords are classified as "intrinsic" and constitute 70 per cent of the lesions; those extending beyond the cords are "extrinsic." Hoarseness is an early symptom with intrinsic cancer; it is often delayed in the extrinsic type. Treatment varies, but radiation alone is recommended only for small lesions of the middle third of the cord. Laryngectomy is the treatment of choice for all other cancers; preoperative radiation and extensive removal of lymph nodes are used in many clinics.

Among the many causes of partial or complete paralysis of the vocal cords are pressure by aortic aneurysm, mediastinal tumors, metastatic esophageal cancer, postdiphtheritic neuritis (p. 985), poliomyelitis (p. 1139), and operative trauma (especially thyroidectomy). If a nerve is cut at operation, there will be sudden stridor; if stretching and edema are affecting the nerve, the onset of stridor and hoarseness will be gradual. Bilateral injury may cause sudden obstruction, necessitating tracheostomy.

260 CHRONIC BRONCHITIS AND EMPHYSEMA (Chronic Nonspecific Lung Disease)

John H. Knowles

The problem of chronic nonspecific pulmonary disease, consisting mainly of chronic bronchitis and obstructive emphysema, has become the most important one in the field of pulmonary disease from all standpoints, including prevalence, morbidity, mortality, and economic loss. Knowledge of these conditions has been incomplete and uncertain for a number of reasons. A persistent cough has been accepted as a normal phenomenon in the cigarette smoker, and rarely is the physician consulted for this complaint alone. Because of the length of time required for all the dire consequences of chronic bronchitis to unfold and because it frequently accompanies a more dramatic illness, such as bronchogenic carcinoma, pneumonia, or peptic ulcer, it has been relegated to a position of secondary importance by lay people as well as the

medical profession. Clinically, the differentiation of asthma, chronic bronchitis, and the various types of emphysema (senile, "compensatory," obstructive, for example) has been difficult because of confusion concerning the etiologic significance of the barrel chest, "smoker's cough," and wheezing respiration (the patient compounds this felony by announcing that he has "asthma"), the inadequacies of radiologic diagnosis in these conditions, and generally, the unqualified use of the word emphysema, to denote anything from the kyphotic chest deformity of old age to the hyperinflated chest of the child with acute bronchial asthma.

DEFINITIONS AND CLASSIFICATION

Chronic diffuse nonspecific lung disease refers to a condition of chronic cough with sputum production with or without paroxysmal or persistent uncomfortable shortness of breath, which cannot be attributed to localized lung disease, generalized pulmonary infection, granulomatous, fibrotic, or collagen disease of the lung, pneumoconiosis, primary cardiovascular disease, disorders of the chest wall, or psychoneurosis. It may coexist with any of these conditions and not infrequently does. In such instances two diagnoses should be made. There are two main categories of chronic diffuse nonspecific lung disease: chronic bronchitis and generalized obstructive lung disease.

Chronic bronchitis has been arbitrarily separated from recurrent acute bronchitis in epidemiologic studies as "cough with production of sputum occurring on most days for at least 3 months in the year during at least 2 years." The sputum may be mucoid or purulent. Chronic bronchitis predisposes to recurrent respiratory infection, particularly during the winter months, and eventually may lead to dyspnea by virtue of a gradual loss of ventilatory capacity due to the development of emphysema. The smoker's cough, when it conforms to the above description, is an example of chronic bronchitis.

Generalized obstructive lung disease is a condition characterized by increased airway resistance due to diffuse narrowing of the bronchial tree. This is the result of hypersecretion, smooth muscle spasm, a check-valve mechanism, bronchiolar fibrosis, or all four of these factors. *It is diagnosed simply and with certainty by finding a reduction in the timed vital capacity* (one second forced expiratory volume—F.E.V.$_{1.0}$ in British terminology) or maximal midexpiratory flow rate. The severity of dyspnea depends on the degree of obstruction.

Generalized obstructive lung disease is subdivided into reversible and irreversible forms.

Reversible obstructive lung disease is chiefly caused by bronchial asthma, which is characterized by intermittent, reversible increases in airway resistance due to excessive mucous secretion and smooth muscle spasm and is associated with paroxysmal shortness of breath and wheezing respiration. Obstruction to air flow may vary and improve spontaneously or with the use of bronchodilator drugs, including corticosteroids. Bronchial asthma is discussed on p. 1263 and the differential diagnosis of asthma and emphysema on p. 1521.

Airway obstruction caused by excessive secretions as a result of infection is the other important cause of reversible airway obstruction. Varying degrees of reversible obstructive lung disease may coexist with irreversible obstructive lung disease, chronic bronchitis, or both, and the amount may be accurately quantified by simple pulmonary function tests.

Irreversible obstructive lung disease refers to irreversible generalized narrowing of the bronchial tree and increased airway resistance which has persisted for more than 1 year, unaffected by treatment including bronchodilator drugs as well as corticosteroids. The majority of such patients will be found to have emphysema at postmortem examination. A few reveal only varying combinations of chronic bronchial asthma, chronic bronchitis, or tubular bronchiectasis. The British make a diagnosis of "irreversible obstructive lung disease," appending "with emphysema" if the clinical picture warrants the anatomic statement.

The above definition and classification of chronic nonspecific lung disease was developed by British authorities to supplant the irrational use of the terms chronic bronchitis, asthma, and emphysema. It is presented here because it stresses (1) the use of functional rather than anatomic diagnosis clinically and (2) the difficulties in the accurate diagnosis of emphysema and the various combinations of bronchitis, reversible and irreversible obstructive lung disease which may occur during life. In the discussion that follows, chronic bronchitis and obstructive emphysema will be considered as such, as is the practice in the United States.

CHRONIC BRONCHITIS

Occurrence. Chronic bronchitis marks its onset usually between the ages of thirty and sixty years. There is a preponderance in men of approximately 4:1. In England there exists an inverse relationship between the social scale and the incidence of the disease—the laboring classes being the most commonly afflicted, the professional classes least so. The death rate also rises steeply from rural to urban and highly industrialized areas, suggesting that atmospheric pollution plays an important role. It is possible that the disease is more common and more severe in England than in the United

States because of the damp, cold climate and degree of atmospheric pollution in England, both of which aggravate the symptoms. However, the only epidemiologic study carried out in the United States (Pemberton) indicated that the prevalence of uncomplicated bronchitis was similar in the two countries. The presently available figures indicate greater disability and far higher mortality from the disease in England as compared with North America. In England it is the commonest cause of death and morbidity among all respiratory diseases, including pneumonia, tuberculosis, asthma, and lung cancer.

Etiology. The disease may be insidious in onset, or it may follow a bout of acute pneumonia or bronchitis or well-established bronchial asthma. A possible etiologic relationship has been suggested for bronchiectasis and pulmonary tuberculosis because of their frequent association with chronic bronchitis. In the United States the disease is associated with a history of heavy cigarette smoking in more than 75 per cent of patients. Present evidence favors the theory that exposure to irritants (cigarette smoke, air pollutants) in the susceptible individual leads to chronic hypersecretion of mucus in the bronchial tree.

Pathology. The most important lesion in chronic bronchitis is hyperplasia and hyperactivity of the mucus-secreting glands in the trachea and bronchi and of the goblet cells of the bronchial epithelium. The bronchial wall may show varying degrees of chronic inflammation with focal scars. Many older patients with a long history of chronic bronchitis will show, in addition, the changes of emphysema at postmortem examination, even though this may not have been clinically manifest as breathlessness (associated with the symptoms of chronic bronchitis) during life.

Clinical Manifestations. The patient consults the physician because of (1) cough and expectoration, (2) an acute respiratory infection, (3) breathlessness, which usually signifies the association or onset of complicating bronchospasm (asthma) or obstructive emphysema, or (4) fear of cancer. The chronic productive cough is usually attributed to cigarette smoking or is dated from childhood or an attack of influenza. The sputum is ropy, white, and elastic and varies in amount from a few milliliters to several ounces daily. During superimposed infections ("chest colds") cough and sputum increase and the secretions become yellow or yellow-green and occasionally bloodstreaked. The symptoms are worse in the winter, in the morning on awakening, and at the end of the day; with changes in barometric pressure and humidity; on exposure to dusts, air pollution, and cigarette smoking; in crowds and after excessive talking and alcohol ingestion. Severe paroxysms of coughing may occur nocturnally or on awakening in the morning. Post-nasal drip and symptoms suggestive of chronic sinusitis are frequent. Acute chest pain may be due to rib fracture incurred during severe coughing, to pleurisy associated with a complicating pneumonia, or to muscular strain around the lower costal margins. Syncope may occur during a sudden fit of coughing (tussive syncope, p. 306). Vigor is usually well maintained, and there is no loss of appetite or weight. Dyspnea is not a feature of uncomplicated chronic bronchitis.

Physical examination is remarkable for the lack of positive findings. The nose may contain crusted purulent material, and the nasal and pharyngeal mucosa may be fiery red, raw, and dry appearing, and the uvula, slightly edematous. The patient clears his throat frequently, and deep breathing may result in a violent fit of coughing. The lungs may be clear, or there may be scattered basilar rales and transient rhonchi, frequently clearing with cough. The heart is normal. There is no clubbing of the fingers.

Blood counts and radiologic examination of the chest and paranasal sinuses are usually completely normal. Culture of sputum may yield pathogenic organisms, most commonly the pneumococcus or *Hemophilus influenzae. Staphylococcus aureus* and gram-negative organisms are found occasionally, and the hemolytic streptococcus is remarkable for its rarity. Pulmonary function may be completely normal, or there may be slight reduction in timed vital capacity (60 to 75 per cent in the first second as compared with greater than 80 per cent normally) or maximal midexpiratory flow rate (e.g., 1.5 to 2.0 liters per sec as compared with greater than 3 liters per sec normally) and maximal breathing capacity (55 to 70 liters per min in contrast to 100 liters per min or more, normally).

Bronchoscopy and bronchography may be necessary to rule out other causes of chronic cough such as tumor, bronchiectasis, and foreign body. At bronchoscopy, the tracheobronchial mucosa is usually hyperemic and redundant. Bronchography may show diverticula on the inferior surface of the main stem and primary segmental bronchi which represent the filling of the dilated ducts of mucous glands. Beading of the bronchial lumen may be observed because of excessive mucus, or there may be an accordion-like appearance due to shortening of the bronchus with heaping up of redundant mucosa. Failure of peripheral filling and dilated bronchioles presenting as peripheral "pools" of dye may be seen in long-standing cases and probably indicate coexistent emphysema. Occasionally an area of tubular bronchiectasis is found. The differentiating features of bronchitis and bronchiectasis are discussed on p. 1551. The diseases may coexist, and some observers believe that local bron-

chiectasis may lead to diffuse chronic bronchitis elsewhere in the lung. There is, however, no evidence that bronchitis has been cured by resection of localized bronchiectasis.

The *course of chronic bronchitis* is not completely known as there have been no studies of its natural history spanning more than several years. It seems clear, however, that subjects with chronic bronchitis often continue to have their symptoms for many years without further complication and die of some totally unrelated disease. Others suffer repeated respiratory tract infections and develop paroxysmal, reversible obstructive pulmonary disease (bronchial asthma). In this group as well as in a number of patients who remain noninfected and produce minimal sputum ("dry" bronchitis), there arise a certain number who ultimately develop obstructive emphysema.

EMPHYSEMA

The term emphysema is derived from the Greek and means to blow into or inflate. *Subcutaneous emphysema* occurs with soft tissue infection with gas-forming organisms such as colon and Welch bacilli. It is also seen in the area of the incision following thoracotomy or with dissection of air from mediastinal emphysema. *Interstitial emphysema* refers to the escape of air from alveoli into the interstices of the lung where it dissects along vascular sheaths into the mediastinum to give rise to *mediastinal emphysema*, which, in turn, can also result from perforation of the thoracic esophagus. *Senile emphysema* refers not to a primary disease of the lungs but to a degenerative disease of the thoracic spine occurring in elderly individuals (see below).

Pulmonary emphysema is characterized pathologically by increase in the size of the air passages distal to terminal bronchioles due to *dilatation* or *destruction* of their walls. Further subdivision includes the factor of distribution, e.g., *selective* as occurs in the focal emphysema due to dust versus *unselective* as with the dilatation of air spaces seen in pulmonary tissue adjacent to a resected area ("compensatory emphysema"). The classification adheres to the recommendations of the Ciba Guest Symposium and is slightly modified.

Emphysema Due to Dilatation Alone

Unselective Distribution—Panacinar Dilatation Emphysema. There are two main conditions in this category: (1) compensatory or overdistention emphysema and (2) emphysema secondary to partial bronchial obstruction as with foreign body or bronchogenic carcinoma. The term panacinar means that all the air spaces distal to the terminal bronchiole are affected.

Panacinar dilatation emphysema results from expansion of lung (by virtue of negative intrapleural pressure) to fill the empty space created by removal or shrinkage of lung tissue. It has been called overdistention or compensatory emphysema in the past. It is not possible to relate pulmonary disability or insufficiency to this phenomenon, nor is there any evidence that it leads to destructive or obstructive changes in the area involved, either pathologically or by pulmonary function test. Following pneumonectomy, for example, the remaining lung overdistends without the occurrence of dyspnea or disability.

Panacinar dilatation emphysema occurs distal to partial bronchial obstruction. Partial bronchial obstruction becomes complete with the normal narrowing of the bronchus in expiration and air is trapped. Pulmonary function shows chiefly obstruction to air flow, which is variable in amount depending on how early in expiration the obstruction becomes complete. The main significance of this type of panacinar dilatation emphysema is that its discovery as an area of increased radiolucency in the lung fields by x-ray may be the first sign of bronchogenic carcinoma.

Selective Distribution—Focal Emphysema. This is a disease of coal workers. Inhaled dust is deposited around the respiratory bronchiole, eliciting fibrosis and atrophy of smooth muscle. Coalworker's pneumoconiosis is the only known form of dilatation emphysema localized to the respiratory bronchiole, hence the term focal emphysema. There may be no symptoms and minimal or no change in pulmonary function. In advanced cases, however, the clinical picture of obstructive emphysema may appear. The x-ray shows diffuse bilateral nodulations. The disease is described in greater detail on p. 1547.

Aging Lung Emphysema. This third category of dilatation emphysema is added here with the presumption that aging results in loss of elasticity of pulmonary tissue, leading to dilatation of air spaces. A change in the size of air spaces with advancing age has not been demonstrated pathologically as yet; however, changes in pulmonary function as a result of aging are well established. These changes suggest a state of hyperinflation of the lung and mild obstructive emphysema. There is an increase in residual lung volume, decrease in maximal breathing capacity and mild increase in airway resistance, decrease in arterial oxyhemoglobin saturation, and mild maldistribution of inspired air. More air is contained in the aged than the youthful lung at the same intrapleural pressure, indicating loss of elasticity of the lung and presumably, therefore, dilatation of air spaces. No definite symptoms or disability can be attributed to these changes alone in the otherwise healthy elderly individual.

The term "senile emphysema" has not been used above because it should be reserved to refer to changes in the thoracic cage with age and not to pulmonary changes. Loss of water and disorganization of the cartilaginous intervertebral disks result in a kyphotic distortion of the thoracic spine, in turn resulting in rotation of the ribs so that the anterior chest is thrown out and up and assumes the barrel shape. Pulmonary function is unimpaired save for the minor changes expected as a consequence of normal aging (above), and dyspnea and disability should not be attributed to this skeletal deformity alone. The aged individual, although showing the functional changes described above, may or may not have an accompanying dorsal kyphosis.

Emphysema Due to Destruction of the Walls of Air Spaces

Unselective Distribution—Panacinar Destructive Emphysema. The word panacinar refers to uniform dilatation of all air passages distal to the terminal bronchiole. The lesions may be localized or widespread and vary in different parts of the lung.

Selective Distribution—Centrilobular Destructive Emphysema. This type of emphysema selectively affects the respiratory bronchiole, resulting in dilatation of air spaces in the proximal portion of the acinus, i.e., there exists a state of bronchiolectasis. Lesions may be local or widespread.

Irregular Distribution—Irregular Emphysema. Irregular emphysema refers to the dilatation and destruction of air spaces seen adjacent to scars or in diffuse fibrotic disease such as the Hamman-Rich syndrome. As such it may occur anywhere in the acinus and hence the term "irregular." The word focal should not be used here as it refers specifically to dilatation of respiratory bronchioles associated with coal-worker's pneumoconiosis.

Panacinar and centrilobular destructive emphysema may be seen singly or together in the same lung, and it is these pathologic forms which are demonstrated in subjects with obstructive pulmonary emphysema (see below). They cannot as yet be differentiated clinically. Blebs and bullae can be seen in any type of destructive emphysema, and therefore the term "bullous emphysema" should not be used to imply a special form of the disease.

Obstructive Pulmonary Emphysema

Obstructive pulmonary emphysema is a disease that affects predominantly men between the ages of forty-five and sixty-five years. It is usually preceded by chronic bronchitis and is characterized by dyspnea on exertion, hyperinflation of the chest, irreversible obstruction to airflow, and destruction and dilatation of the walls of air spaces.

Etiology. Because of the association of chronic bronchitis as a concomitant event or as one preceding the onset of exertional dyspnea in over 70 per cent of patients, most observers have favored this disease as the inciting factor. The cause of chronic bronchitis is unknown, but because of the high association of cigarette smoking with bronchitis and emphysema, an etiologic role has been assigned to cigarettes. This may be so, just as the cold damp weather and a dusty working or polluted urban environment may also lead to hypersecretion of mucus in the bronchial tree and ultimately obstructive emphysema. In short, the etiologic factors of chronic bronchitis apply equally well to patients with obstructive emphysema. Dyspnea in the patient with chronic bronchitis usually signifies either reversible bronchial narrowing due to secretions or bronchospasm or irreversible obstruction to airflow due to the development of destructive emphysema. It may well be that the development of obstructive emphysema results from gradual extension of chronic bronchitis into the bronchioles, perhaps accelerated by repeated bouts of secondary bacterial infection. In some this sequence of events is obvious, but in others it must be assumed that the process is subclinical and smolders over a period of many years. Obstructive emphysema is due partly to the destructive effects of chronic bronchiolitis per se and partly to the distending effect of air trapped distal to the obstructing lesions. The theory that a primary degeneration of pulmonary elastic tissue initiates the disease has been abandoned.

The etiologic role of bronchial asthma remains obscure, but the few careful studies reported indicate that it rarely progresses to obstructive emphysema. Part of the confusion on this point has arisen from the difficulties of differentiating obstructive emphysema with attacks of bronchospasm from bronchial asthma (see below).

Several investigators have pictured emphysema as an abnormal acceleration of the aging process because of the functional changes resembling a mild state of emphysema seen regularly in most elderly individuals (above).

The finding of high concentrations of sodium and chloride in the sweat of a few patients with obstructive emphysema, similar to the abnormal pattern demonstrated in childhood fibrocystic disease of the pancreas (see p. 1666), has led to the suggestion that secretion of abnormally viscid mucus in the bronchial tree with resultant obstruction and infection of the bronchioles might explain the pathogenesis of some instances of emphysema.

Regardless of one's opinion concerning the role of smoking in chronic bronchitis, there remain approximately 10 per cent of patients who deny chronic productive cough ("dry emphysema") and perhaps 20 per cent who have never smoked. In some a family history of chronic bronchitis is obtained, in others, repeated bouts of pneumonia. In some individuals, preexisting localized bronchiectasis or long-standing pulmonary tuberculosis seems to have been complicated by slow superimposition of diffuse, chronic bronchitis and obstructive emphysema.

Because of the many and diverse associated conditions and possible etiologic factors, it is important at the present time to consider obstructive emphysema to be a syndrome as well as a disease. In addition to the above conditions, a number of known disease processes can produce or be associated with a picture which is clinically and physiologically indistinguishable from the "idiopathic" disease. These include silicosis, coal-worker's pneumoconiosis, sarcoidosis, bronchogenically disseminated tuberculosis, and some cases of kyphoscoliosis. In these instances localization of the disease process at the level of the respiratory bronchiole or associated chronic bronchitis gives rise to chronic irreversible obstruction of air flow and the picture of obstructive emphysema. All these conditions must be considered in diagnosis when the patient with apparent chronic bronchitis and obstructive emphysema is seen.

Pathology. Classically the lungs are large and do not collapse when the thorax is opened. Blebs (subpleural air collections) and bullae (parenchymal emphysematous spaces with a diameter greater than 1 cm) may be noted, as well as generalized dilatation of air spaces. Nodular areas of scarring and fibrosis may be visible subpleurally. If the lung is fixed under a constant head of distending pressure, centrilobular or panacinar types of emphysema may be distinguished in nearly equal frequency. Microscopically there are seen chronic bronchiolitis and peribronchiolitis, ulceration of the epithelium, intraluminal granulation tissue, and fibrosis. Smooth muscle may be hypertrophied. The lumen of the bronchiole supplying areas of emphysema is often narrowed but may be normal or even dilated. The distal alveoli are obliterated and larger air spaces formed, presumably by confluence of alveoli and increased by air trapping due either to check-valve mechanism or collateral ventilation. Loss or degeneration of alveolar elastic tissue is seen. The number of visible capillaries is reduced because of destruction of alveolar walls. Foci of intrabronchiole mucus ("mucous plugging") and pus are seen as are occasional areas of pneumonia. Besides reduction in capillary bed, there may be marked enlargement of the bronchial venous system. The evidence is not convincing that the bronchial arterial system is diseased. Obstructive emphysema is the commonest cause of cor pulmonale (see p. 1537).

Clinical Manifestations. The typical patient gives a history of chronic bronchitis. Frequent respiratory infections have occurred, usually during the winter months, characterized by febrile episodes with increase in purulent sputum. Finally, at some point after years of bronchitic symptoms, breathlessness on exertion makes its appearance. Early in the course, dyspnea may occur only during the winter months with exacerbations of infection and is due to partially reversible ventilatory defects, i.e., bronchospasm and excessive secretions. Later, dyspnea on exertion becomes firmly established, persists the year around, and signifies the development of irreversible obstructive ventilatory defect. Of all the clinical clues, persistent breathlessness is the most reliable sign on which to establish a presumptive diagnosis of obstructive emphysema. The *clinical* diagnosis cannot be made in its absence even though many patients with chronic bronchitis and no dyspnea may be found at postmortem examination to have mild emphysema.

The *onset* may be acute, and breathlessness is dated from an episode of pneumonia or severe, acute bronchitis. In some subjects, this is the easily remembered episode in what really is a long history of slowly progressive bronchitis. In other patients, breathlessness and cough have been accepted as concomitants of "getting old" or of smoking. The disease may come to the physician's attention in a number of ways: (1) by the development of acute respiratory failure with acute bronchitis or pneumonia, or during the postoperative period following intubation, atropine, and morphine—when the retrospective history of chronic cough and dyspnea is finally obtained and its significance fully appreciated; (2) by the development of bronchogenic carcinoma; (3) by the development of inguinal hernia because of chronic cough; and (4) because of the occurrence of the symptoms or complications of peptic ulcer (see below). The disease may be so insidious in development that the diagnosis is not established until post-mortal examination.

Other complaints are frequent. Because of limitation of activity the patient may gain weight initially, but later anorexia leads to loss of weight. Vigor is lost, and sleep is difficult. As the disease becomes more severe, changes in the arterial blood gases occur and cor pulmonale develops.

Physical signs may scarcely be more notable in the early phase of the disease than those seen in the patient with uncomplicated chronic bronchitis. In the moderately ill patient who exhibits no alteration in the blood gases at rest, the following signs are likely to be noted. The patient appears dyspneic with exertion. The fingers may be tobacco stained, but are usually not clubbed. The eyes are prominent. The neck veins distend on expiration.

The chest is fixed in the hyperinflated, inspiratory position, and the flesh about the neck and supraclavicular spaces is sunken. The accessory muscles of respiration, particularly the sternomastoids, are large and active during inspiration, and the trachea descends markedly on maximal inspiration. Lower rib margins may flare outward, and the subcostal angle is wide. There is frequently a dorsal kyphosis. Prominent cutaneous venules are seen anteriorly and laterally around the lower costal margins. During inspiration, the chest moves *en bloc* instead of "unfolding" from below upward during expansion. Expiration is prolonged. Cardiac and hepatic dullness are impaired or even absent, and heart sounds are distant. The pulmonary second sound is prominent and may be split, particularly on expiration. The percussion note of the chest is hyperresonant, and the diaphragms are low with minimal or absent excursion. The breath sounds are distant or even absent and when heard have a more bronchovesicular than vesicular quality. Occasional early inspiratory ("opening") rales are heard at the bases. Expiratory wheezing during spontaneous respiration is heard only if excessive secretion or bronchospasm is present. The impulse of the heart is prominent in the epigastrium, and the sounds are best heard here. The liver is displaced downward, and the edge easily palpable. The abdominal muscles are lax. A decline in arterial pressure during inspiration may be observed, but the veins continue to display inspiratory collapse. Thus the complete picture of the paradoxic pulse (see p. 1468) is lacking.

Roentgenography is of little help in diagnosis until the disease is advanced, at which time the following picture is seen. The thoracic cage is large with low diaphragms, an apparent horizontal position of the ribs, and wide intercostal spaces. Prominent soft tissue shadows may indicate hypertrophy of the pectoralis muscles. The heart lies vertically and appears small. The mediastinal shadow is elongated. The hilar vascular shadows may be prominent, but the peripheral vessels are small and appear reduced in number. Thin-walled areas of translucency in which no vascular shadows can be seen represent blebs and bullae and are seen commonly at the apices and bases of the lungs. Nodular or linear areas of scarring and fibrosis may be seen, but generally the lung fields are notable for their radiolucency. In the lateral projection, an increase in size of the thoracic cage and a dorsal kyphosis are present. The retrosternal and retrocardiac air spaces are increased. Fluoroscopy is vital to the diagnosis, and the best radiologic sign is reduction in the excursion of the diaphragm. Air trapping is demonstrated on rapid expiration by areas of local radiolucency. Tomography may occasionally be helpful in delineating vascular changes such as prominent hilar vessels, small and fewer peripheral vessels, or absence of vessels in bullous lesions.

Blood counts and urinalysis are normal. The electrocardiogram is normal in uncomplicated cases; it may reveal a loss of the usual tendency to left axis deviation seen in older individuals. The sputum has been described. Sputum cell counts usually reveal lymphocytes or polymorphonuclear leukocytes, but occasionally eosinophiles are numerous (see below). The results and use of pulmonary function tests are described below.

Pathophysiology. Obstruction to air flow as a result of granulating and fibrosing bronchiolitis and expiratory closure of loosely supported respiratory bronchioles, coupled with degeneration of elastic tissue, result in hyperinflation of the lung. This is demonstrated by finding an increase in functional residual capacity, residual volume, and residual volume to total lung capacity ratio. The work of breathing is increased because of increased airway resistance. Timed vital capacity, maximal mid-expiratory flow rate, and maximal breathing capacity are reduced in proportion to the degree of obstruction and therefore correlate well with the severity of dyspnea. If a partially reversible ventilatory defect exists because of acute infection or bronchospasm, these tests will indicate improvement with effective therapy. Obstructing lesions vary throughout the lung, and therefore abnormalities of distribution are seen, including maldistribution of inspired air, venous admixture, and dead space effects (p. 112). Areas perfused with blood but poorly ventilated cause increased venous admixture of arterial blood ("physiological shunting"); other areas, including bullous lesions, are ventilated but not perfused, leading to dead space effect. Cardiac work is wasted in the first situation and ventilatory work in the second instance. Both pumps have to increase their work to compensate. Increased ventilation of well-perfused areas can compensate for the shunted carbon dioxide and maintain a normal CO_2 tension of arterial blood. It cannot add appreciable amounts of oxygen to the blood, however, to compensate for hypoxemia (p. 111). This is due to the difference in the shapes of the CO_2 and O_2 dissociation curves and explains the sequence of changes in arterial blood gases, beginning first with mild arterial oxygen unsaturation and normal CO_2 contents and tension. As the disease becomes more severe, hypoxemia increases, and finally alveolar hypoventilation results in CO_2 retention, with respiratory acidosis. Earlier in the disease, the increased requirements of gas exchange necessitated by exercise may result in unsaturation of blood, normally saturated at rest.

As the disease progresses and continued destruc-

tion of pulmonary capillary bed occurs, the pulmonary diffusing capacity falls and the pulmonary vascular resistance rises. Hypoxemia stimulates erythropoiesis and causes secondary polycythemia. It also leads to pulmonary vasoconstriction and an increase in arterial resistance. The work of the right heart is increased and cor pulmonale ultimately ensues, signifying the final and most advanced stage of the illness (p. 1537).

Course of the Disease. The course of the disease is extremely variable, and prognostication is difficult. At any time, superimposed pulmonary infection causes an increase in the severity of the disease due to further reduction in functioning lung tissue because of consolidation, secretions, or bronchospasm. The course may be a rapidly malignant one with death in respiratory failure in a matter of several years, or the duration from onset of dyspnea may be as much as 20 or 30 years with death due to intercurrent disease. The occurrence of hypoxemia and hypercapnia or the development of cor pulmonale are bad prognostic signs, and death usually occurs within several years of their onset. Mild hypoxemia by itself does not carry such a dire prognosis.

Respiratory failure is said to have occurred when the lung can no longer provide for normal gas exchange and CO_2 retention and arterial oxygen unsaturation are the result. As hypoxemia supervenes further weight loss may occur, and when CO_2 retention follows, headache, difficulty in concentrating, drowsiness, and confusion are common findings. In the presence of cor pulmonale with right heart failure, papilledema may be seen. There may also be a curious inability to sustain a posture (asterixis, "flapping tremor") identical with that observed in hepatic insufficiency or uremia. This is particularly common in acute respiratory failure. Respiratory failure may occur insidiously without obvious precipitating event but commonly occurs because of acute respiratory infection, administration of sedative, narcotic, or anesthetic agents, or heart failure. Administration of oxygen is absolutely necessary but may be hazardous (see p. 1575).

The association of peptic ulcer and emphysema appears to be more than fortuitous. About 20 per cent of patients with emphysema have a peptic ulcer, usually duodenal in location, and the incidence of emphysema is two to three times as common in patients with peptic ulcer as in the normal population. Whether common psychic factors, cigarette smoking, or hypoxia are important etiologic factors is unknown, but it is important to keep the relationship in mind.

Diagnosis. Obstructive pulmonary emphysema is misdiagnosed frequently. Physical signs, except in advanced cases, are notoriously misleading and unreliable. The diagnosis should not be made without demonstrating obstruction to air flow. Persistent dyspnea on exertion and depression of breath sounds are the cardinal features. Restriction of diaphragmatic motion correlates best with the severity of the process. The finding of radiolucency and a large chest does not in itself establish the diagnosis.

Once the diagnosis has been established, the degree of reversibility or irreversibility must be determined by measuring the timed vital capacity before and after the use of a suitable bronchodilator such as aerosolized isoproterenol hydrochloride. In occasional patients with chronic intrinsic bronchial asthma, intensive treatment with corticosteroids may be necessary to achieve maximal reversal of the obstructive ventilatory defect.

If the patient has bronchial asthma, certain features may suggest this diagnosis, namely, family history of allergic disease, lack of smoking because of aggravation of asthmatic symptoms, positive skin tests, peripheral blood eosinophilia and, most important, intermittency of symptoms and spontaneous reversibility to normal or near normal of abnormal pulmonary function or with the use of bronchodilators, including corticosteroids. The pulmonary diffusing capacity is normal in uncomplicated asthma and reduced in obstructive emphysema; thus differentiation is possible. The differentiation of emphysema and pulmonary congestion due to heart disease is discussed on p. 1380.

The treatment of chronic nonspecific pulmonary disease (bronchitis and emphysema) and of respiratory failure is discussed on p. 1573.

REFERENCES

Barach, A. L., and H. A. Bickerman (Eds.): "Pulmonary Emphysema," pp. 526, Baltimore, The Williams & Wilkins Company, 1956.

Fletcher, C. M.: Chronic Bronchitis: Its Prevalence, Nature and Pathogenesis, Am. Rev. Respirat. Diseases, 80:483, 1959.

Knowles, J. H.: "Respiratory Physiology and Its Clinical Application," pp. 135, 142, Cambridge, Mass., Harvard University Press, 1959.

Oswald, N. C. (Ed.): "Recent Trends in Chronic Bronchitis," p. 191, London, Lloyd-Luke, 1958.

Stuart-Harris, C. H., and T. Hanley: "Chronic Bronchitis, Emphysema and Cor Pulmonale," p. 235, Bristol, John Wright and Sons, Ltd., 1957.

Symposium on Emphysema and the Chronic Bronchitis Syndrome, Am. Rev. Respirat. Disease, 80:1, 1959 (part 2).

Terminology, Definitions and Classification of Chronic Pulmonary Emphysema and Related Conditions, Thorax, 14:286, 1959.

261 RESTRICTIVE PULMONARY DISEASES AND DISORDERS OF PULMONARY DIFFUSION

Eugene Robin

RESTRICTIVE DISEASES

Restrictive pulmonary diseases are characterized by a significant decrease in the expansibility of the lungs. Restrictive factors are important in many different kinds of pulmonary disease. This section will be devoted to a discussion of disorders in which a restrictive ventilatory defect is the major abnormality. The physiologic abnormalities characterizing such disorders are a reduction in all lung volumes without evidence of airflow obstruction or of abnormality in intrapulmonary gas mixing.

A major consequence of restrictive pulmonary disease may be the development of alveolar hypoventilation, the manifestations of which frequently dominate the clinical picture. Alveolar hypoventilation has already been discussed (p. 109). It exists when alveolar ventilation is insufficient to maintain normal alveolar gas tensions. It is therefore characterized by a low mean alveolar O_2 tension and a high alveolar CO_2 tension, resulting in corresponding abnormalities of pulmonary capillary blood, arterial blood, and ultimately of tissue gas tensions. Since the adequacy of gas exchange is based on measurements of arterial blood gases, the cornerstone of alveolar hypoventilation is an elevated arterial CO_2 tension (Pa_{CO_2}).

The physiologic and clinical consequences of alveolar hypoventilation are related to the associated hypoxia and hypercapnia. With hypoxemia of sufficient magnitude cyanosis is apparent. Hypoxic stimulation of the bone marrow produces polycythemia. The presence of hypoxia and hypercapnia may produce an increase of cerebrospinal fluid pressure with or without papilledema by unknown mechanisms. Chronic hypercapnia leads to bicarbonate retention by the kidney, resulting in an increased concentration of this anion in extracellular fluid. Chronic hypercapnia likewise leads to a depression of respiratory center sensitivity to the normal stimuli of CO_2 and pH, thus accentuating the degree of alveolar hypoventilation. Periodic breathing of the Cheyne-Stokes variety is common and likewise reflects respiratory center depression. The combination of hypoxia and hypercapnia may lead to mental symptoms. Prominent among these is somnolence, which may constitute the patient's chief complaint. There is no clear-cut relationship between the degree of hypercapnia and the degree of somnolence. There may be marked hypercapnia without somnolence or somnolence with only minor degrees of hypercapnia. With acute rises in CO_2, delirium and even coma may occur. The electro-encephalogram may show abnormalities consisting of slow-frequency, low-voltage waves. The combination of papilledema, central nervous system signs, and an abnormal electroencephalogram may lead to an erroneous diagnosis of brain tumor.

The combination of hypoxia and hypercapnia produces pulmonary hypertension and right heart failure by mechanisms discussed later (p. 1537). This form of cor pulmonale is characterized by its reversibility when blood gases are restored to normal.

The symptoms of alveolar hypoventilation are so varied that the diagnosis can be securely established only by demonstrating a significant increase of arterial or alveolar CO_2 tension.

Pulmonary restriction may result from abnormality of any segment of the respiratory apparatus. Disorders involving the respiratory center, its peripheral neural connections, the respiratory muscles, thoracic cage, pleura, mediastinum, pulmonary parenchyma (including its vasculature), and abdominal cavity may produce limitation of the respiratory stroke volume.

Restrictive Disease Associated with Neurologic, Neuromuscular, or Muscular Disorders. Restrictive disease may be produced by direct involvement of the medullary respiratory center by a number of different processes. The existence of hypoxemia, hypercapnia, and polycythemia in patients without clinical or physiologic evidence of primary respiratory or cardiac disease has been attributed to idiopathic disease of the medullary respiratory center. Such patients are capable of restoring blood gases to entirely normal values by voluntary hyperventilation. Meticulous investigation of pulmonary and cardiac function fails to reveal any abnormalities of ventilation, diffusion, or perfusion. Cardiac abnormalities, when present, are related to cor pulmonale produced by the blood gas abnormalities. Inhalations of high concentrations of CO_2 (5 to 8 per cent) in air by these patients fails to elicit the degree of hyperventilation seen in normal subjects or may even lead to depression of ventilation. For this reason, it has been suggested that the underlying mechanism is an injury involving the medullary respiratory center (such as tumor, inflammatory disease, or vascular accident) and resulting in relative insensitivity to its normal stimuli, P_{CO_2} and pH. Alveolar hypoventilation develops with resultant hypoxemia and hypercapnia. The chemical control of breathing depends to a great extent on impulses arising from the peripheral chemoreceptors located in apposition to the great vessels (carotid body, vertebral body, aortic body), which are primarily sensitive to a fall in the oxygen tension of arterial blood (hypoxemia). The volume of involuntary ventilation achieved by the patient represents a new steady state, which depends on the degree of respiratory center depression and on the degree of respiratory stimulation arising from the peripheral chemoreceptors. This steady state operates in such a manner that the patient has persistent hypoxemia and hypercapnia.

A number of inflammatory and miscellaneous diseases involving the brain often may result in alveolar hypoventilation. For example, acute bulbar poliomyelitis causes respiratory abnormalities in the absence of respiratory muscle paresis or paralysis produced by lower motor neurone lesions. Breathing becomes irregular in rate, shallow, and exceedingly slow. It is striking that such patients can breathe normally when commanded to do so by frequent and firm verbal orders. The retention of volitional control with the loss of reflex rhythmic control is presumably caused by impaired sensitivity of the respiratory center to the CO_2-pH stimulus. Not infrequently, swallowing and coughing are likewise impaired, again suggesting brain stem localization of disease. Generally this variety of respiratory disturbance is acute and transient, although the patient may then develop frank respiratory paralysis because of lower motor neurone disease.

A number of drugs are capable of producing respiratory center depression, thereby resulting in alveolar hypoventilation. Drug-induced respiratory depression is most frequently seen during administration of anesthesia. The reduction of ventilation is noted by the anesthesiologist and is treated by assisted ventilation. However, if specific measurements of alveolar or arterial CO_2 tension are not performed, significant hypoventilation, during or after the operative procedure, may be overlooked. All drugs of the morphine group and the barbiturate group may produce respiratory center depression and hypoventilation. With ordinary doses in patients without preexistent respiratory center depression, the respiratory effects of these drugs are ordinarily not of great clinical significance. However, overdosage (e.g., in attempted suicide) or the administration of even modest doses to patients with established respiratory depression may result in life-threatening alveolar hypoventilation.

An important variety of respiratory center depression is seen commonly in patients with prolonged hypercapnia, which occurs most commonly in obstructive emphysema. Such patients show a subnormal ventilatory response to the inhalation of CO_2-enriched air. At least two basic factors are involved. One factor is related to the disordered ventilatory mechanics of diffuse obstructive disease. This factor can be demonstrated by having normal subjects inhale CO_2-enriched mixtures while airway resistance is artificially increased. Under these circumstances there is a diminished ventilatory response to CO_2 inhalation. The second factor is related to the decreased sensitivity of the medullary respiratory center to the CO_2-pH stimulus following prolonged hypercapnia. This factor can be demonstrated by chronically exposing normal subjects to increased concentrations of CO_2 in the inspired air. After a period of several weeks under these conditions, there is a decrease in the ventilatory response to CO_2, even in the absence of obstruction.

The relative importance of mechanical and chemical factors in the genesis of CO_2 insensitivity in obstructive emphysema is not clear. However, it seems certain that chemical factors play an important role in some patients. This is best seen in the syndrome called "carbon dioxide narcosis," which occurs in patients with chronic hypercapnia and hypoxia. When the degree of hypoxia is decreased by the administration of high concentrations of oxygen, and without any change in respiratory mechanics, there follows the development of confusion, coma, and profound hypoventilation, occasionally to the point of apnea. The chemical control of breathing depends no longer on the CO_2-pH stimulus but on the stimulus of hypoxemia acting through the peripheral chemoreceptors. When hypoxemia is relieved, the stimulus for ventilation decreases and hypoventilation is accentuated.

The term carbon dioxide narcosis, frequently used to describe the above sequence of events, is misleading. No direct relationship exists between the absolute level of arterial CO_2 tension and either the cerebral symptoms or the hypoventilation. Severe hypoventilation may occur following oxygen administration to patients free of pulmonary disease with only modest initial elevations of CO_2 tension induced by narcotics. Also, some patients with marked elevations of CO_2 tension may show little or no central nervous system malfunction. The exact role of CO_2 in the pathogenesis of the syndrome remains to be elucidated.

Therapy of carbon dioxide narcosis should include measures which improve both the blood gas abnormalities and the mechanical abnormalities. Although oxygen administration in hypercapneic patients should be undertaken with great care, the question confronting the physician is not whether oxygen therapy is advisable but how to give oxygen without incurring additional hypoventilation. Relief of hypoxia must be a cardinal objective. If oxygen administration results in severe hypoventilation, assisted breathing is indicated. Bronchodilators, sputum liquefaction and removal, and the other measures designed to relieve pulmonary obstruction (p. 1573) are mandatory.

Abnormalities of neural or neuromuscular transmission to the respiratory muscles may result in paresis or paralysis leading to alveolar hypoventilation. Amyotrophic lateral sclerosis is an example of an upper motor neuron lesion which may produce respiratory insufficiency. Direct involvement of the anterior horn cells by poliomyelitis virus represents a lower motor neuron lesion which produces respiratory insufficiency. Infectious neuronitis (Guillain-Barré syndrome) produces flaccid paralysis by means of an inflammatory reaction involving ganglion cells and peripheral nerves. Myasthenia gravis produces respiratory failure by abnormalities involving the myoneural junction.

Direct involvement of respiratory muscles by diseases diffusely affecting skeletal muscle, like progressive muscular dystrophy and the myotonic dystrophies, may lead to restrictive disease. These diseases are commonly associated with reduction of vital capacity, total lung capacity, and maximal breathing capacity without obstructive disease.

The severity of respiratory involvement in any of the above diseases depends on the amount of anatomic involvement. Vital capacity is reduced in proportion to the degree of paresis of the respiratory muscles. There are generally an increased residual volume and a decreased air flow velocity. In moderately severe involvement, there may be alveolar hypoventilation with hypoxemia, hypercapnia, and respiratory acidosis. In very severe involvement, there may be total apnea requiring assisted ventilation for survival.

Because of ineffective coughing and the limitation of respiratory excursions, recurrent bronchial infection is frequent in the convalescing or chronically ill patient. Although none of these diseases is associated with parenchymal lung damage, per se, recurrent infections may result in permanent structural damage. In some patients, the neuromuscular or muscular disease may result in kyphoscoliosis, giving rise to additional pulmonocardiac abnormalities, as discussed below.

Recognition of pulmonary insufficiency may be difficult in the milder forms of these diseases. An awareness of the frequency of respiratory insufficiency is an important factor in formulating therapy. Quantitative serial measurements of vital capacity and blood gases are important guides as to the intensity of disease and the degree of therapy required. When relatively specific measures are available for a given disease (e.g., anticholinesterases for myasthenia gravis), they should be energetically employed. Assisted ventilation, control of secretions, and prompt therapy of infections are frequently critical aspects of the care of these patients.

Thoracic Cage Limitation. Limitation of motion of the thoracic cage may be associated with the development of severe alveolar hypoventilation. The mechanisms underlying this development may be illustrated by considering pulmonary-cardiac failure associated with kyphoscoliosis and with obesity.

Pulmonary-cardiac Failure Associated with Kyphoscoliosis. Kyphosis refers to any posterior angulation of the spine. Clinically significant kyphosis is generally associated with a marked gibbus and loss of stature. Scoliosis consists of a lateral displacement of the spine with at least one other compensatory curve in an opposite direction. Of these two processes, scoliosis appears to be the more important in the genesis of pulmonary and/or cardiac insufficiency. Approximately 80 per cent of cases of kyphoscoliosis are of unknown etiology. The sequelae of poliomyelitis or of Pott's disease account for most of the remaining 20 per cent. Although kyphoscoliosis is relatively common (in approximately 1 per cent of the United States population), a deformity severe enough to produce pulmonary or cardiac insufficiency is found in only a relatively small number of these patients.

Kyphoscoliosis is associated with marked structural abnormality of the thoracic cage, leading to abnormal positioning and functioning of the respiratory muscles. The lungs are compressed by the thoracic deformity, leading to a small lung volume. There is a high work and energy cost of breathing, primarily because of the abnormal elastic resistance of the chest and, to a lesser degree, because of increased elastic resistance of the lung. In some unknown manner, the increased elastic work leads to the development of rapid shallow breathing, which in turn leads to alveolar hypoventilation by preferential ventilation of the anatomic dead space at the expense of the alveoli. As a result hypoxemia, hypercapnia, and respiratory acidosis develop. Prolonged hypercapnia leads to a depression of respiratory center sensitivity, accentuating the degree of hypoventilation.

The thoracic deformity leads to compression of pulmonary vessels which, therefore, present an increased resistance to pulmonary blood flow. With prolonged pulmonary hypertension, there is damage to the intima of pulmonary vessels with the development of pulmonary arteriosclerosis, which further increases pulmonary vascular resistance and aggravates pulmonary hypertension. The combination of hypoxia, hypercapnia, vascular compression, and intimal changes produces high degrees of pulmonary hypertension, leading ultimately to right ventricular failure.

It should be emphasized that the physiologic processes leading to alveolar hypoventilation in kyphoscoliosis are quite distinct from those seen in obstructive emphysema. In kyphoscoliosis, lung volumes are small; there are, at most, moderate disturbances in the distribution of inspired air, and air flow resistance is normal. In chronic obstructive emphysema (p. 1520), the residual volume is abnormally large, there are marked disturbances in the distribution of inspired air, and the major defect is an abnormally high resistance to air flow.

Recurrent pulmonary infections are not uncommon in kyphoscoliosis because of abnormal cough dynamics and inadequate bronchial drainage. Such infections may lead to parenchymal pulmonary structural abnormalities and occasionally to obstructive emphysema. In such patients diffuse obstructive disease represents a complication superimposed on the fundamental physiologic abnormalities related to the thoracic deformity.

The therapy of pulmonary and cardiac failure in kyphoscoliosis should be directed toward correcting the physiologic abnormalities, since the underlying anatomic abnormality is unfortunately almost never correctible. The periodic use of mechanically assisted ventilation decreases the work cost of breathing and increases alveolar ventilation. Control of bronchial secretions and prompt therapy of pulmonary infections decrease parenchymal pulmonary destruction. Avoidance of drugs which depress ventilation prevents additional hypoxia and respiratory acidosis. Oxygen administration relieves hypoxia and tends to decrease the right ventricular work. Cardiac glycosides, diuretics, and a low sodium diet are useful in the management of congestive heart failure.

Pulmonary-cardiac Failure Associated with Obesity (Pickwickian Syndrome). The association of obesity, somnolence, polycythemia, and excessive appetite has long been recognized. A classic description of the association of these signs and symptoms was written by Charles Dickens. In "The Pickwick Papers," he described, "a fat and red-faced boy in a state of somnolency." The boy (Joe) was subsequently addressed as "Young Dropsy," "Young Opium Eater," and "Young Boa Constrictor," no doubt in reference to his obesity, his somnolence, and his excessive appetite, respectively. Because of the resemblance of Joe, the fat boy, to patients with obesity associated with pulmonary-cardiac failure, this combination has been referred to as a "Pickwickian syndrome."

In its fully developed form, the Pickwickian syndrome consists of marked obesity, somnolence, cyanosis, periodic respiration, secondary polycythemia, and right ventricular failure. Blood gas measurements reveal hypoxemia and hypercapnia, documenting the existence of alveolar hypoventilation. Measurements of lung volumes reveal a decrease of total lung capacity, a decrease of vital capacity, and a striking reduction of the expiratory reserve volume. The total energy cost of breathing in obese subjects is high. However the work cost of moving the lung is not increased. This suggests either that the excess energy is used to impart motion to extrapulmonary structures or that excess energy is required by the respiratory muscles to perform a given amount of mechanical work. Obesity, like kyphoscoliosis, is associated with an increased work cost of moving the thorax and is likewise associated with a tendency for the development of rapid, shallow breathing. A common pathogenetic mechanism responsible for the development of alveolar hypoventilation seems probable for both diseases. In the case of kyphoscoliosis, the increased work load is imposed by the thoracic deformity. In the case of the Pickwickian syndrome, the increased work load is imposed by the excessive deposition of fat. In Pickwickians, as in kyphoscoliosis, the increased work load leads to tachypnea with inadequate tidal volumes, which in turn leads to alveolar hypoventilation.

In the uncomplicated Pickwickian syndrome, there is no evidence of increased resistance to air flow. There is generally a decreased ventilatory response to CO_2 inhalation. This finding is consistent with a decrease in respiratory center sensitivity and tends to accentuate alveolar hypoventilation.

Intrapulmonary gas mixing may be entirely normal. Occasionally there is maldistribution of inspired air, presumably caused by the exaggeration of hypoventilation which occurs in the less distensible perihilar areas, producing ventilation-perfusion abnormalities and accentuating arterial oxygen unsaturation.

In occasional patients, the Pickwickian syndrome is associated with diffuse obstructive disease or myxedema. Pulmonary vascular occlusion, resulting from either embolism or thrombosis, is common. Its pathogenesis is undoubtedly related to the relative immobility of these patients, the high viscosity of their blood, and the presence of congestive failure.

Several clinical features of this syndrome require additional emphasis. Alveolar hypoventilation is relatively uncommon in even massively obese patients. Normal pulmonary function has been found in patients whose weight exceeded 400 lb. The exact factors which determine the development of pulmonary failure in some obese patients are not entirely understood. Among the factors favoring the development of alveolar hypoventilation are the pattern of distribution of the fat and its rate of accumulation. Pulmonary-cardiac failure occurs most commonly when the excess fat is packed tightly under the diaphragm, restricting its range of motion. Not infrequently there is a history of rapid weight gain in the immediate period preceding the development of frank pulmonary insufficiency. In some patients the rapid accumulation of intraabdominal fluid, rather than fat, may precipitate the full-blown syndrome.

The degree of somnolence is usually more severe in this syndrome than in other diseases associated with alveolar hypoventilation. At times the somnolence is truly extraordinary and the patient may find it impossible to distinguish between the waking and sleeping state. Somnolence occasionally antedates the appearance of respiratory insufficiency and may be present with only minor elevations of arterial CO_2 tension, suggesting the importance of independent central nervous system disease in the pathogenesis of the syndrome. Normal sleep is known to be associated with a rise in CO_2 tension and a decrease in respiratory center sensitivity. For this reason somnolence per se may increase the blood gas abnormalities.

The most remarkable aspect of both the clinical and physiologic abnormalities is that they may be completely reversed by simple loss of weight. With weight reduction, somnolence and the ventilatory abnormalities may disappear, blood gases may become normal, and pulmonary hypertension and cor pulmonale may disappear. Because of such dramatic changes, the Pickwickian syndrome represents an important example of curable lung and heart disease. However, in some patients, complicating obstructive pulmonary disease, independent heart disease, or pulmonary vascular occlusion limits reversibility.

The most important aspect of therapy is weight reduction. It is generally not necessary for the patient to lose weight to the predicted or "ideal" level. Often the loss of only 25 or 30 lb is sufficient to restore normal pulmonary function. However, excessive appetite is frequently a fundamental part of the illness (or of the patient's personality) and recurrent gain of weight is not uncommon.

Restrictive Diseases Rarely Associated with Alveolar Hypoventilation. A number of primary restrictive diseases are rarely or never associated with alveolar hypoventilation. Pulmonary collapse (atelectasis) and pleural fibrosis are discussed in Chap. 264. *Pectus excavatum* (funnel chest) is a congenital malformation consisting of a depression of the lower portion of the sternum and the adjacent costal cartilages. The depressed sternum may compress and restrict the lower portions of the lung or may produce restriction by distortion of the diaphragm. Restriction due to pleural fibrosis is limited to the areas of lung involved in fibrosis. Bilateral constrictive calcific fibrosis may result in virtually complete loss of thoracic motion and even limitation of diaphragmatic motion. Rheumatoid spondylitis has been shown to result in loss of chest expansion because of immobility of the costovertebral and costosternal joints. Reduction of vital capacity and total lung capacity with a normal residual volume result from this immobility. An interesting aspect of the impaired thoracic mobility is that painful or difficult sneezing is a common complaint. However, there is a striking absence of pulmonary signs and of pulmonary infections.

DISORDERS OF PULMONARY DIFFUSION

Diffusion is the statistical movement of molecules from a region of relatively high concentration to a region of low concentration. As already described (p. 110), it is believed to be the sole process responsible for the movement of oxygen from the alveolar air across the alveolar–pulmonary capillary membrane to pulmonary capillary blood and for the movement of CO_2 in the reverse direction.

The movement of oxygen takes place across the alveolar–pulmonary capillary membrane, and the volume of oxygen which diffuses across this membrane per unit time depends on the difference in partial pressure of oxygen between alveolar air and pulmonary capillary blood, its solubility in the pulmonary membrane, the molecular weight of the gas, the time available for diffusion, the area of contact between gas and blood, the thickness and physicochemical properties of the membrane, the pulmo-

Table 261-1. ETIOLOGIC AND PATHOLOGIC CLASSIFICATION OF DISORDERS OF PULMONARY DIFFUSION

I. Diseases associated with anatomic alterations of the diffusing membranes (alveolar-capillary block)
   A. Sarcoidosis (p. 1246)
   B. Miliary granulomatoses of infectious origin
      1. Tuberculosis (p. 999)
      2. Histoplasmosis (p. 1059)
   C. Berylliosis (p. 1547)
   D. Asbestosis (p. 1547)
   E. Silicosis (p. 1544)
   F. Lymphangitic carcinomatosis (p. 1562)
   G. Bronchiolar carcinoma (p. 1561)
   H. Pulmonary scleroderma
   I. Pulmonary involvement in "collagen" diseases (p. 1893)
   J. Reticuloendotheliosis of lung
   K. Diffuse interstitial fibroses and granulomatoses of lung of unknown etiology (including Hamman-Rich syndrome)
   L. Eosinophilic pneumonia (p. 1556)
   M. Leukemic infiltration of lung
   N. Postradiation fibrosis
II. Disorders of impaired diffusion associated with intraalveolar fluid accumulation and relatively normal diffusing membranes (alveolar block)
   A. Pulmonary edema
   B. Pulmonary alveolar proteinosis
   C. Influenzal pneumonia (p. 1125)
   D. Pneumocystis carinii plasma cell pneumonia
   E. Phosgene poisoning
III. Disorders associated with a decrease in total pulmonary-capillary bed
   A. Pulmonary resection
   B. Chronic obstructive emphysema
   C. Pulmonary embolism (p. 1535)
IV. Disorders associated with decreased red cell mass
   A. Anemia

nary capillary blood volume, and the reaction rate between oxygen and hemoglobin. The diffusing capacity of the lung may be quantitatively defined as the volume of gas in milliliters which crosses the membrane per minute for 1 mm Hg partial pressure difference between mean alveolar and mean pulmonary capillary blood oxygen tensions.

Pulmonary diseases characterized by diffuse pulmonary infiltration with adequate alveolar ventilation and associated with abnormalities of the diffusion capacity of the lung have been given the generic name of "alveolar-capillary block syndrome."

In many situations, increased membrane thickness cannot be implicated in the pathogenesis of impaired diffusion. Loss of total surface area available for diffusion is thought to represent one of the mechanisms for the decrease in diffusing capacity observed in patients after pneumonectomy and in patients with obstructive emphysema. Diffusion defects may occur in the presence of relatively normal alveolar-capillary membranes when there is an intraalveolar accumulation of protein-rich fluid which offers an additional resistance to the diffusion of oxygen. This situation, for example, appears to apply to patients with pulmonary alveolar proteinosis. Finally, diffusion may be impaired by a reduction of the amount of hemoglobin available in the pulmonary capillaries, as in anemia.

Table 261-1 summarizes the etiologic background of the various disorders which are associated with abnormalities of pulmonary diffusion. The individual etiologies will be discussed at greater length, either below or elsewhere (see accompanying page references).

Diffusion Defects Associated with Anatomic Alteration of the Diffusing Membrane

The radiologic, clinical, and physiologic features of primary diffusion defect include the following: (1) diffuse, finely dispersed pulmonary lesions shown on x-ray, (2) reduction of arterial oxygen tension and saturation either at rest or during exercise, (3) reduced lung volumes, (4) maintenance of a relatively normal maximal breathing capacity, (5) hyperventilation at rest and during exercise, (6) normal or supranormal alveolar oxygen tension, (7) reduced diffusing capacity of the lung, (8) variable degrees of polycythemia, (9) dyspnea, (10) cyanosis, (11) pulmonary hypertension, and (12) cor pulmonale.

The physiologic basis of these features has been discussed (p. 110). Several points are worthy of note: (1) radiographic examination is an important diagnostic aid in this group of diseases—x-ray abnormalities are often the first indication that a diffusion defect is present; (2) with severe degrees of lung involvement, abnormal ventilation-perfusion relations become increasingly important; (3) for reasons not entirely known, the degree of polycythemia observed is often small in comparison with the degree of hypoxic stimulus; (4) the type of hyperventilation observed characteristically consists of tachypnea rather than hyperpnea—perhaps because of the increased elastic work of breathing necessitated by the stiffened lung.

The findings on physical examination of the lung in this group of diseases are rather nonspecific and relatively unimportant. Extensive disease may be present without frank abnormality. Indeed, an important clue to the possible presence of a diffusion defect may be the presence of severe pulmonary insufficiency in the absence of gross abnormalities of pulmonary function as judged by physical examination.

Therapy. Specific aspects of therapy will be discussed under the various etiologic entities. However, there are several nonspecific aspects of therapy. The inhalation of air containing high concentrations of oxygen is frequently useful in patients with impaired diffusion. Such therapy markedly increases alveolar oxygen tension, thereby increasing the gradient which is available for driving oxygen across the diffusing membranes.

Adrenal steroids may be useful in many of these diseases. Although the mechanism of action is poorly understood, they occasionally produce subjective and objective improvement of pulmonary function. It is generally believed that these drugs should be administered before advanced pulmonary fibrosis has occurred.

Cor pulmonale frequently occurs during the end stage of these disorders; suitable therapy for this manifestation is useful (see p. 1539).

Pulmonary Sarcoidosis. The etiologic background and general features of sarcoidosis are discussed elsewhere (p. 1246). This section will deal specifically with the pulmonary forms of the disease.

The lung is the organ most often involved in sarcoidosis. The pattern of pulmonary involvement varies. Granulomatous and/or fibrotic infiltration may be found involving hilar and mediastinal lymph nodes, peribronchial parenchyma, interstitial parenchyma, the pleura (very rarely), and pulmonary vasculature. Each of these areas may be involved alone or in combination.

Because of this diversity of anatomic involvement, the physiologic and clinical pictures tend to be rather diverse. Although a subdivision into distinct groups is somewhat arbitrary, patients with pulmonary sarcoidosis generally fall into three groups: (1) those without physiologic abnormalities; (2) those with increased airflow resistance; and (3) those with restrictive disease with or without diffusion impairment.

Patients with sarcoidosis may show *no* abnormalities of pulmonary function on careful testing. This may occur, not only with isolated hilar or mediastinal lymphadenopathy, but also with fairly extensive intraalveolar infiltration, replacing both alveoli and pulmonary blood vessels with sparing of the airways and interstitial areas of the lung. Aside from abnormality of the chest x-ray, such patients commonly show no clinical evidence of lung disease. Indeed the finding of marked pulmonary infiltration in the absence of clinical symptoms should raise the possibility of sarcoid. Isolated adenopathy is the most favorable form of this disease from the prognostic standpoint. A large percentage of such patients will show no progression of lesions and may have complete resolution of x-ray densities.

Involvement of the tracheobronchial tree produces an increase in airflow resistance leading to obstructive disease and ultimately obstructive emphysema. The major physiologic abnormalities of obstructive disease have already been discussed (p. 1520). In general, the most favorable response to steroid therapy in pulmonary sarcoidosis is seen in this group of patients.

Diffuse interstitial involvement by granulomatous or fibrotic tissue leads to restrictive disease with or without abnormalities of pulmonary diffusion. This form of pulmonary sarcoid produces the physiologic and clinical abnormalities which have already been described.

There may be poor correlation between physiologic abnormalities, as demonstrated by functional measurements, and the clinical status of the patient. In general, physiologic abnormalities tend to antedate frank clinical symptoms. Scalene lymph node or lung biopsy may be required for diagnosis.

The natural life history of pulmonary sarcoidosis is characterized by variability. Remissions and exacerbations, as judged by radiologic appearance, signs, and symptoms and physiologic measurements, are not uncommon. Steroid therapy is frequently effective in inducing a clinical and physiologic remission.

Miliary Granulomatoses of Infectious Origin. The development of abnormalities of pulmonary diffusion has been documented in patients with diffuse miliary tuberculosis and presumably can occur in other diffuse infectious miliary granulomatoses— e.g., histoplasmosis. Such patients show dyspnea, tachypnea, and cyanosis during the acute phase of their illness. Function measurements are consistent with the thesis that the major physiologic abnormality is difficulty with the transfer of oxygen across the alveolar–pulmonary capillary membrane. Once an etiologic diagnosis is established, prompt specific chemotherapy, when available, together with adrenal steroid therapy, is appropriate.

Chronic pulmonary fibrosis and insufficiency may develop in the late stages of these disorders.

Chronic Beryllium Disease of the Lung. The inhalation of certain salts of beryllium by human beings (p. 1547) leads to the development of pulmonary lesions. In the acute form of the disease there is the development of a chemical pneumonia, characterized by cough, with occasional blood-streaking of the sputum, substernal burning pain, dyspnea, cyanosis, anorexia with weight loss, progressive fatigue, and diffuse radiologic densities. In patients who recover, the lung fields generally clear after several months.

Beryllium exposure is also capable of producing a chronic form of lung disease. This disorder develops insidiously months to years after the initial exposure. The clinical picture is that associated with diffusion defects. Pathologically the pulmonary lesions are indistinguishable from those seen in sarcoidosis, and indeed beryllium, like sarcoidosis, may be associated with granulomatous and fibrotic lesions involving lymph nodes, liver, spleen, and heart. Definitive diagnosis is generally based on a history of exposure to beryllium, together with suitable histologic changes on lung biopsy. The chemical demonstration of beryllium in lung or urine may help to reinforce the diagnosis. Therapy includes the use of adrenal steroids, oxygen, and measures designed to relieve cor pulmonale.

Asbestosis. The inhalation of asbestos dust (hydrated calcium-magnesium silicate) may lead to the development of a diffuse interstitial pulmonary fibrosis known as *asbestosis* (p. 1547). A striking feature of the reaction to asbestos is the development of marked pleural fibrosis. Significant physiologic derangements indicating abnormalities of diffusion have been noted even in the absence of x-ray changes.

Silicosis. Silicosis, the disease resulting from the inhalation of silicon dioxide dust, is described elsewhere (p. 1544). Usually this disease gives rise to an obstructive ventilatory defect whose end stage is chronic obstructive emphysema. Occasionally, patients with silicosis present with physiologic abnormalities consistent with impaired diffusion and without significant obstruction.

Lymphangitic Carcinomatosis. Lymphangitic carcinomatosis (see also p. 1562) may be defined as a process in which there are widespread neoplastic metastases throughout the lymphatics of both lungs. It differs from the more common varieties of pulmonary metastases in that it causes severer symptoms and is the direct cause of death in most patients.

The primary tumor may arise from any site, but bronchogenic carcinoma and carcinoma of the stomach are the most common primary tumors. The primary tumor may be small and clinically inapparent during life. The outstanding symptom is severe and rapidly progressive dyspnea. The characteristic radiologic appearance is that of fine stringlike shadows distinct from vascular markings, stretching from the hila to the periphery of all lung zones. Rarely the chest x-ray may be normal despite severe dyspnea. The possibility of lymphangitic carcinomatosis should be considered in older patients with marked dyspnea for which no other cause can be determined.

Postradiation Fibrosis of the Lung. Pulmonary fibrosis resulting from x-ray radiation of the lung is a somewhat uncommon but definite clinical entity. It occurs as a complication of radiation therapy directed against neoplasms of thoracic structures such as carcinoma of the breast, lung, or esophagus or pulmonary lymphoma. Ordinarily, pulmonary fibrosis following therapeutic radiation is insignificant. Occasionally, marked fibrosis and severe pulmonary insufficiency may result.

The reaction to x-ray occurs in two stages. The initial stage is the development of acute radiation pneumonitis. There is damage to alveolar cells and capillary endothelium, with resultant swelling and necrosis of the capillary endothelium. Fibroblastic proliferation occurs relatively early and is especially severe in alveolar walls. The late reaction is characterized by a vascular hyaline fibrosis with thickening of alveolar walls and septums. Peribronchial and perivascular fibrosis are also present.

The clinical picture is so variable that a typical syndrome cannot be defined. Most patients with localized fibrosis are entirely asymptomatic. In others, mild dyspnea and cough may be present for limited periods. In a small number of patients with extensive bilateral involvement, there may be high fever, severe dyspnea, hyperventilation, cyanosis, and progressive pulmonary insufficiency. Pulmonary function studies in these patients suggest that the major defect present is impaired membrane diffusion.

It has been claimed that adrenal steroids may cause marked symptomatic improvements in patients with severe forms of the disease and may be useful prophylactically.

Pulmonary Reticuloendothelioses (Eosinophilic Granuloma, Hand-Schüller-Christian Disease, Letterer-Siwe Disease). Pulmonary involvement in these diseases produces a diffuse fibrosis associated with formation of multiple small cysts (honeycomb lungs). The clinical course varies. The occurrence of spontaneous pneumothorax is frequent. Diabetes insipidus or bone lesions are commonly associated findings. In severe forms, impaired diffusion is a major physiologic abnormality. Diagnosis in general depends on the presence of other stigmata of the disease as well as pulmonary involvement. Radiation and/or steroid therapy has been advocated.

Pulmonary Scleroderma. Its general manifestations are described elsewhere (p. 1896). Pulmonary involvement in scleroderma is common. The manifestations vary depending on the site and extent of the disease. With extensive involvement of the skin of the thorax, there may be an inability to expand the chest adequately, leading to restrictive disease. Diffuse peribronchial fibrosis may lead to an obstructive pulmonary defect and to marked distortions of pulmonary parenchyma with the development of honeycombing of the lung. Pleural fibrosis may produce pulmonary restriction. Diffuse interstitial fibrosis may produce abnormalities of diffusion leading to the clinical and physiologic abnormalities of impaired diffusion which have already been described. With esophageal involvement, there may be "spillover" of esophageal contents, leading to recurrent bronchopneumonia. There may be direct involvement of the pulmonary vasculature by fibrosis, leading ultimately to the development of cor pulmonale. It has also been suggested that the proclivity of systemic vessels to show abnormal vasospasm may be shared by pulmonary vessels, thereby producing pulmonary hypertension and eventually cor pulmonale. Rarely, pulmonary manifestations may antedate the appearance of skin or esophageal lesions (scleroderma *sine* scleroderma). Under this circumstance, diagnosis is difficult since the histologic appearance of the pulmonary lesions is not specific. The coexistence of scleroderma and bronchiolar (alveolar cell) carcinoma occurs with sufficient frequency to suggest more than a coincidental relationship between the two diseases.

Diffuse Interstitial Fibroses and Granulomatoses of Unknown Etiology (Including Hamman-Rich Syndrome). Granulomatous and/or fibrotic involvement of pulmonary interstitium occurs in a number of disease states the etiologic nature of which is not well established. Obscure pulmonary infections, viral pneumonias, pulmonary venous occlusion and hypertension, and allergic reactions may all be associated with interstitial infiltration. Such infiltration may be localized or diffuse and may regress quickly or may persist indefinitely. When such infiltrates are extensive and persist for relatively long periods, the familiar clinical manifestations of diffusion abnormalities may appear. Despite exhaustive diagnostic studies, frequently no etiologic basis is found and only a descriptive pathologic diagnosis is possible. Of this indefinite group of entities, the best characterized is the Hamman-Rich syndrome. In 1935 and again in 1944, Hamman and Rich reported four patients with an unusual form of pneumonia characterized by progressive interstitial fibrosis of both lungs. The disease was accompanied by progressive hypoxia and the ultimate development of right ventricular failure. The disease in

each patient ended fatally within a year of onset. Since this original description a relatively large number of patients have been described who more or less fit into this diagnostic category.

The histologic abnormality consists of a bilateral, diffuse interstitial infiltrate resulting from the successive deposition of abnormal inflammatory cells, fibroblasts, hyaline, and collagen, in alveolar septums. Clinical features include dyspnea, cough, and cyanosis, terminating in many patients with intractable pulmonary insufficiency and cor pulmonale. Physiologically, there is evidence not only of abnormal diffusion but of abnormal ventilation-perfusion relations as well.

The etiology of this disorder is unknown and indeed it seems likely that a number of different processes may have as their end result the development of Hamman-Rich changes. Etiologic theories include viral infection with an unknown agent, infection caused by the pleuropneumonia group, the failure of resolution of acute interstitial pneumonia, a hypersensitivity reaction, and a form of collagen disease. Germane to the last two possibilities is that hypergammaglobulinemia, splenomegaly, and eosinophilia have been reported in some patients with Hamman-Rich syndrome.

The radiographic signs vary, and severe physiologic involvement has been reported in patients with only moderate x-ray abnormalities. The chest films in some patients resemble those found in congestive heart failure with marked cardiomegaly, and lung lesions resembling pulmonary edema; or the chest x-ray may resemble those found in diffuse bronchopneumonia; or the films may reveal diffuse interstitial fibrosis. Adrenal steroids apparently have induced remissions in some patients. Such remissions tend to be rather limited in time. Hormone withdrawal may produce a severe and unrelenting relapse.

Disorders of Impaired Diffusion Associated with Intraalveolar Fluid Accumulation and Relatively Normal Diffusing Membranes (Alveolar Block)

Pulmonary Edema. The general subject of pulmonary edema is discussed elsewhere (p. 1382). A priori, it might be expected that edema of interstitial tissue and edema fluid inside alveoli would tend to act as a diffusion barrier. Indeed, a decrease in diffusing capacity has been reported in some patients with pulmonary edema. However, a decrease in diffusing capacity is not found in all patients with pulmonary edema, nor does the decrease correlate well with the extent of pulmonary edema.

The major gas exchange abnormality in pulmonary edema appears to be based on rather complete exclusion of air from bubble-filled alveoli (ventilation-perfusion imbalance). In addition the stiff lungs of acute pulmonary edema lead to abnormal ventilatory mechanics. The difference between the physiologic abnormalities seen in simple pulmonary edema and in alveolar proteinosis suggests that not only the location and extent of fluid but also the nature of the fluid is important in determining the type of physiologic defect.

Pulmonary Alveolar Proteinosis. The name *pulmonary alveolar proteinosis* has been applied to a syndrome of unknown etiology with a fairly specific histologic pattern. The typical lesion consists of the deposition of eosinophilic proteinaceous material within the alveoli without serious alteration of the lung tissue structure. There is usually proliferation of the alveolar septal cells. The disease had not been recognized before 1953, and the total number of reported cases is less than 50. The chief clinical symptom is that of progressive dyspnea associated with the signs and sequelae of hypoxia, including cyanosis, clubbing, and polycythemia. Few or no abnormal physical signs are found on physical examination of the chest. Laboratory findings aside from those related to the pulmonary abnormality are not remarkable. X-ray examination usually reveals a diffuse, hazy, ground-glass appearance of the lung. In several asymptomatic patients, the disease was discovered on routine chest film. Physiologically, these patients show the classical hallmarks of impaired diffusion, although ventilation-perfusion abnormalities are also present. Histologically the alveolar walls are relatively normal, and the diffusion block is presumably related to the presence of fluid of high protein content within the alveoli. Death usually occurs as a result of pulmonary insufficiency, but there have been instances of spontaneous and complete recovery. The etiologic basis of this disorder is unknown. In some patients coexistent cryptococcal infection of the lung has been reported. The relationship between the two diseases is not clear. Specific diagnosis requires lung biopsy.

Phosgene Poisoning. Phosgene gas is carbonyl chloride ($COCl_2$). It may be considered as a prototype of gases whose inhalation leads to intense respiratory tract irritation. Following exposure there is an intense outpouring of protein-rich fluid, which ultimately fills the alveoli. The source of this fluid is not clear. It may originate from bronchiolar glands as a result of chemical bronchiolitis, or from pulmonary capillaries as a result of increased capillary permeability produced by the toxic effect of the agent, or from both sites. In any case, the basic abnormality is related to the large quantity of intraalveolar fluid, and post-mortem examination reveals diffuse pulmonary edema. Following exposure, patients develop dyspnea, chest pain, tachypnea, and cyanosis. It seems likely, therefore,

that the intraalveolar fluid may serve as a diffusion barrier.

Disorders Associated with a Decrease in Total Pulmonary-Capillary Bed

Pulmonary Resection. Patients undergoing pulmonary resection may show significant decreases in the diffusion capacity of the lung. Even with complete removal of a single lung, the decrease in diffusing capacity is moderate; indeed, the *resting* diffusing capacity may be normal and only the maximal diffusing capacity (diffusing capacity during severe exercise) may be reduced. This observation emphasizes the large functional reserve available for the diffusion function in the normal lung. It suggests that involvement of more than 50 per cent of the total anatomic area available for diffusion is present in disorders associated with impaired diffusion at rest. In simple, uncomplicated pulmonary resection, limitation of diffusion is not clinically significant.

Chronic Obstructive Emphysema. Significant decreases in diffusing capacity are invariably seen in patients with advanced obstructive emphysema. It is believed that this decrease is related to the loss of pulmonary vascular bed. For example, it has been suggested that the differential diagnosis between bronchial asthma (a disease in which there is presumably no loss of vascular bed) and obstructive emphysema can be established by the presence of a normal diffusing capacity in asthma as compared with a low diffusing capacity in emphysema. It has also been suggested that measurements of diffusing capacity have prognostic implications for the patient with emphysema. Unfortunately, maldistribution of air and ventilation-perfusion imbalance almost certainly affect clinical measurements of diffusing capacity, and a given reduction in diffusing capacity cannot be equated with a given loss of pulmonary vascular bed. There is little doubt that the decrease in diffusing capacity in this disorder in some measure reflects the loss of normally ventilated and perfused alveolar-pulmonary capillary units.

Diffusion Disorders Associated with Decreased Red Cell Mass

Cyanosis is unusual in the anemic patient because with a decrease in total hemoglobin concentration, there is a decrease in the amount of reduced hemoglobin. However, recent studies have suggested that in the severely anemic patient, there may be an impairment of oxygen diffusion. This impairment is located not in the pulmonary "membrane" itself but in the red blood cell. An ingenious technique has been devised by which the total resistance to diffusion of gas can be quantitatively subdivided into the resistance offered by the membranes and that offered by the red cell. With a decrease in red cell mass, the latter resistance may be substantially increased and, hence, the total diffusing capacity of lung (which measures both membrane and red cell resistance) may be decreased. This impairment of diffusion has no known clinical significance but illustrates the complexity of the processes involved in pulmonary diffusion and their aberrations in disease.

THE DIFFUSE PULMONARY INFILTRATE

The preceding section has dealt with a group of diseases in which the functional abnormalities are more or less specifically defined. Not infrequently, the physician is faced with the problem of the patient whose chest x-ray shows the presence of diffuse pulmonary infiltrations of varying sizes, shapes, and degrees of opacity. Such patients represent a heterogeneous group clinically, physiologically, and etiologically. The patient may be entirely asymptomatic and have as his only abnormality the presence of abnormal x-ray densities. Or the patient may have high-grade pulmonary insufficiency.

The differential diagnosis involved in this group of diseases is vast. Frequently, a diagnosis can be made only by means of lung biopsy, and occasionally even lung biopsy does not permit accurate diagnosis. Table 261-2 is a partial list of the entities which may produce diffuse pulmonary infiltrations. This list comprises 111 different diseases. Some of these have been discussed in the previous section. The remainder of this section will be devoted to a description of a few of the more important entities that have not been previously discussed.

Table 261-2. THE ETIOLOGIC BASIS OF DIFFUSE
PULMONARY INFILTRATION

I. Infections
   A. Bacterial
      1. Miliary tuberculosis
      2. Staphylococcal
      3. Streptococcal
      4. Salmonellosis
      5. Shigellosis
      6. Infectious bronchiolitides
      7. Brucellosis
      8. Tularemia
      9. Glanders
      10. Plague
   B. Mycotic
      1. Histoplasmosis
      2. Blastomycosis
      3. Coccidioidomycosis
      4. Cryptococcosis
      5. Aspergillosis

Table 261-2. THE ETIOLOGIC BASIS OF DIFFUSE
PULMONARY INFILTRATION (*Continued*)

      6. Moniliasis
      7. Sporotrichosis
      8. Actinomycosis
      9. Streptotrichosis
      10. Nummulariasis
   C. Viral and rickettsial
      1. Chickenpox
      2. Measles
      3. Psittacosis (ornithosis)
      4. Influenza
      5. Lymphopathia venereum
      6. Rocky Mountain spotted fever
      7. Q fever
   D. Parasitic
      1. Schistosomiasis
      2. Toxoplasmosis
      3. Pneumocystis carinii
      4. Trichinosis
   E. Possibly infectious but etiology unknown
      1. Primary atypical pneumonia
      2. Acute miliary pneumonia
      3. Diffuse miliary granulomatous pneumonia
      4. Acute diffuse interstitial fibrosis (Hamman-Rich)
      5. Infectious mononucleosis
      6. Inclusion body pneumonia
      7. Erythema nodosum
      8. Pulmonary-alveolar proteinosis
II. Pneumoconiosis
   A. Berylliosis
   B. Asbestosis
   C. Silicosis
   D. Shaver's disease
   E. Bagassosis
   F. Byssinosis
   G. Tin
   H. Siderosis
   I. Barium
   J. Welder's lung
   K. Baratosis
   L. Talc
   M. Vanadium
   N. Silver
   O. Aluminum
III. Systemic of unknown etiology
   A. "Collagen" diseases
      1. Scleroderma
      2. Lupus erythematosus
      3. Polyarteritis
      4. Wegner's granulomatosis
      5. Rheumatoid arthritis
      6. Rheumatic fever pneumonia
      7. Weber-Christian disease
   B. Sarcoidosis
   C. Amyloidosis
   D. Reticuloendotheliosis
      1. Eosinophilic granuloma
      2. Hand-Schüller-Christian disease
      3. Letterer-Siwe disease

Table 261-2. THE ETIOLOGIC BASIS OF DIFFUSE
PULMONARY INFILTRATION (*Continued*)

  E. Hexamethonium fibrosis
  F. Idiopathic pulmonary hemosiderosis
 IV. Allergic
  A. Eosinophilic pneumonia
   1. Loeffler's syndrome
   2. Tropical eosinophilia
 V. Congenital or familial (possibly hereditary)
  A. Congenital cystic disease of the lung
  B. Pneumatocele
  C. Tuberous sclerosis
  D. Mucoviscidosis (cystic fibrosis of the pancreas)
  E. Pulmonary alveolar microlithiasis
 VI. Inhalational
  A. Farmer's lung
  B. Silo-filler's lung
  C. Sulfur dioxide
  D. Phosgene
  E. Lipiodol pneumonia
  F. Lipid pneumonia
  G. Acetylene
  H. Carbon tetrachloride
  I. Nitric acid
  J. Vomitus
 VII. Metabolic
  A. Uremic pneumonia
  B. Hyperparathyroidism
 VIII. Neoplastic
  A. Bronchiolar carcinoma
  B. Hematogenous metastatic malignancy
  C. Lymphangitic carcinomatosis
  D. Leukemia
  E. Lymphoma
  F. Polycythemia vera
  G. Sarcomatosis
  H. Multiple myeloma
 IX. Physical agents
  A. Postradiation fibrosis
  B. Uranium exposure
  C. Thermal
 X. Circulatory
  A. Pulmonary edema
  B. Multiple pulmonary emboli
  C. Chronic congestive failure with secondary hemosiderosis
   1. Mitral stenosis
   2. Left ventricular failure
  D. Bronchial artery occlusion
  E. Fat embolism
  F. Sickle-cell anemia with multiple pulmonary infarcts

Idiopathic Pulmonary Hemosiderosis. Idiopathic pulmonary hemosiderosis is a relatively uncommon pulmonary disease that results from recurrent hemorrhages into the lung. Most of the reported cases have been in children, but it is also found in the adult.

The clinical picture is relatively characteristic.

These patients have recurrent febrile episodes of cough, dyspnea, severe hemoptysis, hypochromic anemia, and diffuse pulmonary mottling. The chest x-ray usually shows diffuse shadows which suggest edema or hemorrhage. These shadows may clear or change rapidly, leaving multiple nodular areas behind. Following repeated episodes, there may be progressive increase in nodularity. The disease may also be associated with the development of diffuse myocardial fibrosis without iron deposition. Heart failure from this cause is one of the mechanisms of death.

The anemia found in these patients is related to the pulmonary hemorrhages. Although a shortened life span of red cells in these patients has been reported, it has been established that this finding is caused by loss of red cells inside the pulmonary parenchyma.

The mechanism of the pulmonary hemorrhages is not known. Various suggestions have been advanced, including the possibility that the disorder represents an immunoallergic disease. This hypothesis suggests that an unknown sensitizing agent produces autoantibody formation and that the hemorrhages result from an immunoallergic reaction with the lung as the shock organ. In line with this possibility are the reports of rather remarkable improvements produced by adrenal steroid therapy. Unless the disease is ameliorated by steroids, its outcome is frequently fatal.

Farmer's Lung. Farmer's lung is a disease of unknown etiology whose pathogenesis is related in some fashion to the inhalation of spoiled ("moldy") hay. Clinically, the disease is characterized by the sudden onset of dyspnea within hours of exposure to moldy hay or other vegetable matter, including silage. In addition to dyspnea, there may be fever, chills, and cyanosis. The disease usually lasts from several days to several weeks and is followed, as a rule, by complete recovery. However, subacute and chronic forms of the disease have been described.

The histologic picture of this disease consists of numerous granulomas involving the pulmonary interstitium, containing histiocytes, foreign-body-type giant cells, and occasional fibrotic strands. Many of these are located within alveolar walls. There may also be an obliterative bronchiolitis and pleuritis as well. The histologic picture is similar to that of sarcoidosis. It has been suggested that hypersensitivity to moldy hay dust may be an important element in the pathogenesis of the disease. The disease differs histologically and clinically from silo-filler's disease (see below). Most patients show spontaneous improvement.

Silo-filler's Disease. Silo-filler's disease results from the inhalation of the oxides of nitrogen (primarily nitrogen dioxide). Evolution of the various oxides of nitrogen dioxide starts within a few hours after silo filling, reaches a maximum between 1 and 2 days later, and continues at a decreasing rate for a week or longer. The disease is limited to individuals who enter silos within a day or two after filling. The clinical picture is as follows: (1) cough and dyspnea immediately after exposure; (2) relative remission of symptoms during the next 2 to 3 weeks but with some dyspnea, cough, malaise, and weakness; (3) onset of a second phase of the illness with fever, chills, progressively severe dyspnea, and cyanosis. During this phase of the illness numerous bubbling rales are heard over the entire extent of the lungs, and there is wheezing during expiration consistent with respiratory tract obstruction. X-ray examination during this phase reveals generalized infiltration of the lung with innumerable discrete nodular densities. Blood gas studies show arterial oxygen unsaturation and respiratory acidosis. If the patient survives this phase, he may go on to develop diffuse obstructive emphysema.

Histologic examination during the acute phase reveals diffuse pulmonary edema. As the disease progresses, pathologic examination shows the lung to be filled with innumerable grossly visible, uniformly distributed lesions. Each nodule consists of a small bronchus or bronchiole filled with fibrotic exudate. This exudate becomes organized, obliterating the bronchiolar lumen. The pathologic picture is typical for what has been called bronchiolitis obliterans fibrosa. This entity is composed of a group of diseases whose end stage is the fibrotic obliteration of significant portions of the bronchiolar tree resulting from inhalation of toxic gases, from infection of the bronchial tree, and in some patients from unknown causes.

The basic physiologic defect in fibrosing bronchiolitis is that many areas of the lung have a marked reduction in ventilation although perfusion is *relatively* well maintained. Under these circumstances total effective ventilation is inadequate and hypoxia and hypercapnia result. The marked decrease in airway diameter produces greatly augmented air flow resistance during both inspiration and expiration, resulting in severe respiratory tract obstruction. Silo-filler's disease appears to be a classical example of this disorder.

An important aspect of the therapy of this disease is its prevention. Freshly filled silos should not be entered during the first 7 to 10 days after filling. Special precautions such as fences should be established to prevent children from straying into silos. Adequate ventilation should be maintained inside the silo.

The use of adrenal steroids has proved extremely valuable in the acute phase of the disease. Other measures already outlined in the general section for treating respiratory tract obstruction and blood gas abnormalities are applicable.

Pulmonary Alveolar Microlithiasis. Pulmonary alveolar microlithiasis is a disease of unknown etiology characterized by familial occurrence and the deposition of laminated calcium stones within alveoli.

The intraalveolar concretions are similar in appearance to the corpora amylacea found in the prostate. The alveoli containing concretions are themselves normal although there may be some small degree of interstitial cellular infiltration or fibrosis. The number of alveoli containing stones may vary from 25 to 80 per cent of the total number. It seems probable that both the number of calculi and the amount of interstitial reaction increase with the age of the patient or the known duration of the disease. At post-mortem examination, there may be startling increases of lung weight (to over 4,000 Gm) because of the accumulated mass of small stones.

The most specific diagnostic technique available is radiologic examination of the chest by means of overpenetrated (Bucky) films. On such films the x-ray appearance is pathognomonic, since it shows the fine sandlike particles spread uniformly through both lungs. There is little variation in particle size, and the calcific nature of the particles is unmistakable. The total density of the millions of stones may be sufficient to obscure cardiac and diaphragmatic outlines. Chemical analysis of the alveolar microliths reveals that they consist of calcium and phosphorus, with smaller amounts of magnesium and aluminum and traces of silicon and iron. The nature of the process leading to the precipitation of calcium inside apparently normal alveoli is unknown.

Although the etiologic basis of the disease is unknown, approximately 50 per cent of cases have been associated with familial incidence, suggesting a hereditary basis.

The disease is usually asymptomatic for years and most commonly discovered on routine chest film. With progressive alveolar involvement, there is the ultimate development of pulmonary insufficiency, characterized by dyspnea, cyanosis, cor pulmonale, and a fatal outcome. There is no known specific therapy for the disorder.

REFERENCES

Alexander, J. K., J. R. West, J. A. Wood, and D. W. Richards: Analysis of the Respiratory Response to Carbon Dioxide Inhalation in Varying Clinical States of Hypercapnia, Anoxia and Acid-Base Derangements, J. Clin. Invest., 34:511, 1955.

Banyai, A. L.: Collapse of the Lung, in "Clinical Cardio-pulmonary Physiology," B. L. Gordon (Ed.), 2d ed., p. 681, New York, Grune & Stratton, Inc., 1960.

Benaim, S., and C. Worster-Drought: Dystrophica Myotonica with Myotonia of the Diaphragm Causing Pulmonary Hypoventilation with Anoxemia and Secondary Polycythemia, Med. Illus., 8:221, 1954.

Bergofsky, E. H., M. Turino, and A. P. Fishman: Cardiorespiratory Failure in Kyphoscoliosis, Medicine, 38:263, 1959.

Brown, A., and O. Cook: Cardio-respiratory Studies in Pre- and Postoperative Funnel Chest (Pectus Excavatum), Diseases of Chest, 20:378, 1958.

Burwell, C. S., E. D. Robin, R. D. Whaley, and A. G. Bickelmann: Extreme Obesity Associated with Alveolar Hypoventilation: A Pickwickian Syndrome, Am. J. Med., 21:811, 1956.

Feltman, J., W. Newman, A. Schwartz, D. Stone, and F. Lovelock: Cardiac Failure Secondary to Ineffective Bellows Action of the Chest Cage, J. Clin. Invest., 31:762, 1952.

Fishman, A. P., G. M. Turino, and E. H. Bergofsky: The Syndrome of Alveolar Hypoventilation, Am. J. Med., 23:333, 1957.

Forster, R. E.: Exchange of Gases between Alveolar and Pulmonary-Capillary Blood: Pulmonary Diffusing Capacity, Physiol. Revs., 37:391, 1957.

Ratto, O., W. A. Briscoe, J. W. Morton, and J. H. Comroe, Jr.: Anoxemia Secondary to Polycythemia and Polycythemia Secondary to Anoxemia, Am. J. Med., 19:958, 1955.

Robin, E. D., C. H. Crump, and R. J. Wagman: Low Sedimentation Rate, Hypofibrinogenemia and Restrictive Pseudo-obstructive Pulmonary Disease Associated with Trichinosis, New Engl. J. Med., 262:758, 1960.

Sarnoff, S. J., J. L. Whittenberger, and J. E. Affeldt: Hypoventilation Syndrome in Bulbar Poliomyelitis, J.A.M.A., 147:30, 1951.

Travis, D. M., C. D. Cook, D. M. Julian, C. H. Crump, P. Helliesen, E. D. Robin, T. B. Bayles, and C. S. Burwell: The Lungs in Rheumatoid Spondylitis, Am. J. Med., 29:623, 1960.

Turner, W. A., and McD. Critchley: Respiratory Disorders in Epidemic Encephalitis, Brain, 48:72, 1925.

Wilson, W. R., and G. N. Bedell: The Pulmonary Abnormalities in Myxedema, J. Clin. Invest., 39:42, 1960.

262 CIRCULATORY DISORDERS OF THE LUNG (Including Cor Pulmonale)

T. R. Harrison,
William H. Resnik, and
Ben V. Branscomb

The most frequent disturbances of the pulmonary vascular bed are congestion and edema, which have been discussed in Chap. 249.

Anatomic and Physiologic Considerations. The vascular bed of the lungs is very large and, compared to the systemic circuit, is an area of low pressure and low resistance. As long as it is free of disease, even large increments in blood flow, such as accompany vigorous exercise, cause relatively little rise in pressure. Resection of an entire lung, with reduction of the circulatory channels by approximately one-half, likewise causes no elevation of pressure if the blood vessels of the remaining lung are normal. The several factors that may produce increased pulmonary resistance will be considered later.

Although there are some normal collateral pathways between the bronchial and the pulmonary arterioles, these are very small and carry no significant amount of blood in healthy persons. When, because of certain congenital lesions, the normal pulmonary circulation is seriously restricted, the bronchial flow may be markedly increased and may become the chief perfusion system of the lungs. In certain acquired pulmonary diseases, especially bronchiectasis and emphysema, pulmonary-capillary blood passing through poorly ventilated areas or even bypassing the alveoli entirely through shunts between arteries and veins is inadequately oxygenated, thus leading to cyanosis and/or clubbing of the fingers.

Conditions, such as mitral stenosis, which produce long-standing and pronounced elevation of pressure in the pulmonary veins may cause large varicose communications with the bronchial veins, and these may be the source of massive hemoptysis. When portal venous pressure is markedly elevated, anastomotic communications with the pulmonary veins may develop, and here again, either cyanosis or slight clubbing of the fingers may occur.

The congenital anomalies of the pulmonary circulation are closely allied with congenital heart disease, and the more important ones are considered in Chap. 252. One should remember that anomalous pulmonary venous drainage into the right atrium may closely simulate interatrial septal defect both clinically and in the catheterization findings, while congenital fistulas between the pulmonary arteries and veins mimic the cyanotic types of congenital heart disease. The latter condition should be suspected when a young individual with cyanosis, polycythemia, and clubbing of the fingers has negative cardiac findings, and especially if there are one or more discrete shadows in the x-ray, or a faint continuous murmur in the area of the shadow (p. 1462), or cutaneous angiomas.

Pulmonary Sequestration. Occasionally, portions of the embryonic lung obtain their principal arterial supply not from the pulmonary artery, which is derived from the ventral aorta, but from anomalous branches of the dorsal aorta. These usually arise from the upper abdominal or lower thoracic portions, or from branches of the celiac axis, and enter the lung through the pulmonary ligament. The involved region is commonly near the cardiophrenic angle, and the bronchi to it usually are tortuous, cystic, and irregular, though they may be entirely normal or completely absent. The area may remain within the rest of the lung (intrapulmonary sequestration) or may be enclosed in its own pleural sac (extrapulmonary sequestration).

If the bronchi in the area are normal, the only danger may be unexpected arterial bleeding during pulmonary resection for some unrelated process. More often, the bronchi are grossly irregular but communicate with the trachea, and then the area becomes a site of chronic infection. The occurrence of bright-red hemoptysis and the bronchographic demonstration of an extreme degree of distortion in a well-localized area that contrasts with entirely normal bronchi in immediately adjacent segments may suggest that the problem is not simply that of bronchiectasis. If the bronchi contain little air or if the sequestration is complete and the area gasfree, the resulting mass is usually confused with neoplasm or abscess.

Angiographic demonstration of the abnormal vascular pattern is the definitive diagnostic method. The condition ordinarily calls for resection of the involved areas.

Acquired disorders of the lung, such as primary or metastatic carcinoma, bronchiectasis, or lung abscess, may also lead to arteriovenous communications. If the shunts are sufficiently large, arterial anoxia may occur.

EMBOLISM AND INFARCTION

Under exceptional circumstances, these disorders may be due to air, fat, or amniotic fluid. Blood clots are usually responsible. These commonly arise from the deep veins of the legs or pelvis, and occasionally from the right atrial appendage. Much less frequently, thrombosis of veins of the arms is responsible, and this usually follows intravenous therapy with irritating solutions.

Although embolism and infarction are closely associated phenomena, either may occur without the other. Following massive embolism, the survival time may be too short for necrosis to develop, or effective collateral flow may prevent infarction. Very rarely the latter disorder may occur because of thrombosis *in situ* rather than embolism. In the absence of congestive failure and preexisting pulmonary congestion, very small emboli are not usually followed by infarction, which is especially apt to occur when medium-sized arteries (lobar or lobular) are occluded.

In a physiologic sense, infarction, which causes decline in both perfusion and ventilation of the involved area, is analogous to resection of a portion

of the lung. However, embolism without infarction impairs circulation only. The resulting ventilation of nonperfused lung increases the physiologic dead space. This leads to excessive ventilation in relation to oxygen absorption and to a discrepancy between the carbon dioxide concentration of terminal expired air and of arterial blood. Thus an excess arterial CO_2 tension of 5 mm Hg or more as compared to end tidal air constitutes strong evidence for a large or medium-sized embolus, provided the patient does not have emphysema or some other disorder affecting the ventilation-perfusion relationship. A smaller difference indicates that embolism is either absent or, if present, has occluded a relatively small fraction of the pulmonary arterial system. The larger the area of ventilated but unprefused lung, the greater will be the lowering of the end tidal as compared to the arterial carbon dioxide tension.

Arterial hypoxia may develop following embolism. This is not completely alleviated by breathing oxygen and hence appears to depend, in part, on pulmonary arteriovenous shunts through small, normally functionless, channels which bypass the capillaries.

Clinical Picture. A *single massive embolus* induces a state which mimics closely that of myocardial infarction. The pain is likely to have the same substernal location and tight quality. It is probably the result of hypoxia of the right ventricle because both the increased systolic pressure in this chamber and the decline in systemic arterial pressure decrease the coronary flow to the right ventricle. Other clinical features which are similar to those occurring in myocardial infarction are dyspnea, venous distention, and sudden death. Both conditions are commonly followed by a transient elevation of the leukocyte count, temperature, and sedimentation rate. The electrocardiographic alterations ("right ventricular strain pattern"), consisting of depression of the S-T segments in leads II, III, AVF, and V_2 and V_3, may be similar in the two conditions. Finally, although pulmonary infarction per se does not cause much elevation of the serum transaminase, the associated injury to skeletal muscle from the coexisting (and often silent) thrombophlebitis may cause marked elevation. When evidence of a local thrombotic process in the veins is absent, and when the comparison of carbon dioxide tensions in the arterial blood and terminal expired air (see above) yields no decisive information, the distinction between pulmonary embolism and myocardial infarction may be well-nigh impossible. However, the combination of elevated lactic dehydrogenase, normal level of transaminase, and elevated serum bilirubin is strongly suggestive of pulmonary infarction.

More commonly, the embolus is not sufficiently

large to cause marked elevation of pulmonary pressure, and both clinical and radiologic manifestations may be absent. When symptoms do occur, they are the result of the associated infarct. Here, the pain has the typical pleuritic character and its sudden onset, with local alteration in breath sounds, and rales, and the associated hemoptysis, cough, and fever produce a picture which closely resembles that of lobar pneumonia (p. 889). In both disorders the acceleration of breathing is disproportionately great in relation to the degree of tachycardia and fever. The pleural fluid which often develops is frequently bloody and may be confused with effusions due to tuberculosis or neoplasm.

When recurrent small emboli lead to multiple small infarctions, the condition mimics that of bronchopneumonia, or pulmonary carcinomatosis or other rapidly progressive parenchymal disorders. Such patients may exhibit increasing dyspnea with cough and irregular fever, and both the pleural pain and the hemoptysis may be absent. However, the diagnosis is facilitated when typical pleuritic pain is present and associated with a friction rub and local tenderness. In any patient with evidence of recent pulmonary hypertension, a negative chest x-ray does not preclude multiple pulmonary emboli as the cause. The distinction between multiple pulmonary emboli and the syndrome of alveolocapillary block is considered in Chap. 261.

Diagnosis. The recognition of pulmonary infarction depends, in the main, on the combination of a high index of suspicion, with repeated careful examination of the legs for evidence of venous thrombolic disease (p. 1375). The disorder usually occurs in patients with disorders which predispose to phlebothrombosis. Thus it is common in persons with congestive failure or polycythemia, or during the postoperative or post-partum state, or in elderly persons who are bedridden for any reason. It is not rare in healthy individuals following long automobile trips or airplane rides associated with immobility and dependency of the legs. In any such person, the occurrence of pleural pain, sudden dyspnea, hemoptysis, syncope, or of a bloody pleural effusion should arouse the suspicion of pulmonary infarction.

Congestive heart failure is the most common of the several predisposing conditions. In the absence of anticoagulant therapy, about 60 per cent of the patients with mitral stenosis and 40 per cent of individuals dying of congestive heart failure due to other causes can be demonstrated at autopsy to have had one or more pulmonary infarctions. The sole clinical clues in such patients may be a sudden worsening of the clinical state, with increase in dyspnea and refractoriness to therapy, accompanied by transient elevations of leukocyte count,

temperature, and sedimentation rate. Slight jaundice occasionally occurs and is due not to increased destruction of erythrocytes but to sudden impairment of liver function because of increasing congestion brought on by the rise in pulmonary pressure. Although daily examination of the calves will often display some of the signs of venous thrombosis, these phenomena may be completely absent, despite the most careful search.

Usually, the radiologic findings are entirely normal or nonspecific, or delayed for several days. The finding of transient enlargement of some of the vascular shadows may be helpful. Physical signs may also be completely absent, or may be indistinguishable from those due to pneumonia or to the commonly preceding pulmonary congestion and edema. Under these circumstances it is usually wise to treat the patient for phlebothrombosis and pulmonary infarction, even though one cannot always establish the diagnosis beyond question.

Prevention. Conditions which predispose to venous stagnation should be combated. Predisposed patients should wear elastic stockings and, in the absence of compelling contraindications, should walk for a few minutes several times each day. When this is undesirable, massage of the calves with passive or active motions of the legs should be instituted every few hours. It is highly probable that these measures reduce the frequency of phlebothrombosis (p. 1375).

Treatment. The treatment of anoxia, of any complicating pulmonary infection, or of heart failure is essentially the same as under other circumstances. The specific measures aimed toward the thromboembolic disease per se are concerned not with the treatment of the infarction which has already occurred, but toward prevention of recurrences. Here, the first consideration is vigorous anticoagulation therapy (p. 1455). Hemoptysis, unless massive, does not constitute a contraindication for such therapy. In most instances, anticoagulation will prevent recurrences. When the latter do develop despite adequate anticoagulation, venous ligation becomes imperative. It may be necessary to tie both femoral veins, or even the inferior vena cava, because the demonstration in one calf of evidence of thrombophlebitis does not necessarily mean that the emboli are arising from that side. They frequently come from the other silent opposite extremity.

There is some evidence that the increase in pulmonary vascular resistance following embolism is due, in part, to release of serotonin from the blood clot and that heparin tends to neutralize this effect. Therefore, heparin is preferable to other anticoagulants during the initial phase of treatment.

The value of the new fibrinolytic drugs has not yet been clearly defined.

Rarer Causes of Embolism. *Air* may enter the vascular system as a consequence of thoracentesis or of open-heart operations. Under such circumstances the emboli involve the systemic rather than the pulmonary vessels, and the chief manifestations are likely to be those of cerebral or coronary arterial occlusion. Pulmonary embolism may occur as the result of technical errors during intravenous therapy, or because of the rupture of a cervical vein at operation. *Amniotic fluid* with its contained debris may cause emboli during delivery.

Fat embolism is usually the sequence of fracture of the femur or of other large bones. However, it may occur following injury to small bones or even to soft adipose tissue. When it results from sternotomy in patients having cardiac surgery and cardiopulmonary bypass, the temporary absence of the filtering function of the lungs increases the likelihood of cerebral fat embolism. The manifestations may be mainly pulmonary or systemic as the result of passage of the fat masses through the capillaries of the lungs, with embolization in various organs. The presence of the fat globules in the retinal arteries, in the sputum, and especially in the urine may offer a clue to the diagnosis. This is frequently difficult because the clinical picture may be bizarre and resemble that of a collagen or other multiple organ system disorder. In some instances, the chief manifestations are those of an acute multifocal disease of the central nervous system. The diagnosis of fat embolism is usually not difficult *if one thinks of it* as a possibility in a patient presenting evidence of bizarre pulmonary and/or systemic disease following trauma.

Embolism of the lungs, as well as of other organs, may also occur during the acute crises of sickle-cell disease.

Infection may be superimposed on pulmonary infarction and may lead to lung abscess. The therapeutic implications are obvious.

Hemosiderosis of the Lungs. This is usually a complication of mitral stenosis and is due to the long-standing pulmonary congestion. The chief features are diffuse nodular changes in the x-ray, associated with the presence in the sputum of phagocytes containing hemosiderin crystals (*Herzfehlenzellen*). However, these cells may be encountered in the sputum of any patient with long-standing congestive heart failure. Primary or idiopathic hemosiderosis of the lungs is discussed elsewhere (p. 1532).

PULMONARY HEART DISEASE
(Cor Pulmonale)

Read

Definition. As here employed, this term designates those clinical conditions characterized by hypertrophy and/or failure of the right ventricle due to disorders of the lungs, of the pulmonary vessels, or of the chest wall. Hence the group includes right ventricular disorders due to primary pulmonary hypertension as well as those secondary to pulmonary embolism or thrombosis. However, the most common causes are extensive emphysema or infiltration of the pulmonary parenchyma. Excluded from this group are disorders involving pulmonary hypertension and right ventricular hypertrophy due to left ventricular failure, mitral stenosis, or left-to-right shunts.

Pulmonary hypertension due to disease of the lungs is one of the commonest causes of congestive heart failure in the United States, and it is even more common in Britain. As persons live longer and the incidence of long-standing severe bronchitis associated with emphysema rises, it is probable that the frequency of cor pulmonale will also increase.

Mechanisms of Elevation of the Pulmonary Arterial Pressure. Of the two factors—blood flow and the size of the vascular bed in the lungs—that influence the pulmonary arterial pressure, the second is the more important. Increase in cardiac output may cause a slight rise in the mean pressure in the pulmonary arteries. However, unless there is also an elevated resistance, the increment in pressure is small because of the compensatory effect of vascular dilatation. When the resistance is high and fixed, the absolute level of the pulmonary pressure will tend to vary directly with the cardiac output. Therefore, any condition such as anoxia, exercise, emotional stress, or fever, which increases the latter function, becomes especially important in a person with narrowed pulmonary arteries (see p. 93 for discussion of relationship between pressure, flow, and resistance).

Increased pulmonary resistance may be due to several factors. Of especial importance are those which are *reversible*. These include capillary narrowing when the alveoli are distended because of *bronchial obstruction*, arteriolar constriction due to *anoxia* or *hypercapnia*, and increased viscosity resulting from *polycythemia*. The partially or completely *irreversible* causes of increased resistance include obliteration of the vascular bed due to parenchymal destruction, distortion of the smaller vessels with turbulent rather than laminar flow, abnormal anastomoses between the bronchial and pulmonary arterial channels, and various structural intraluminal changes. Among these are thromboses *in situ*, embolism, arteritis, necrotizing arteriolitis, and intimal hyperplasia. The two latter lesions, themselves probably secondary to elevated flow or pressure, cause increased resistance with further rise in pulmonary pressure and thus tend to perpetuate a vicious cycle. The elevation of resistance caused by embolism may be partially due to release of serotonin, and heparin is believed to be an antidote for this effect.

In certain tropical regions schistosomiasis with obstructive inflammation of the pulmonary vessels is a common cause of cor pulmonale. This disorder is occasionally seen in the United States in immigrants from Puerto Rico or other tropical regions.

Chest deformities may produce heart failure without significant parenchymal disease of the lungs. When there is extreme obesity, hypoventilation is the major factor (p. 1524). Kyphoscoliosis causes interference with gas exchange plus turbulent flow through distorted vessels.

There is a serious disorder known as "primary pulmonary hypertension" which is associated with increased resistance of unknown cause. Most of the patients are young women who have recently passed through pregnancy. Multiple embolism of the small pulmonary branches, possibly due to amniotic fluid, has been considered by some observers to be the responsible factor.

Passive congestion of the lungs also tends to elevate resistance. Aside from the mechanical increase of pulmonary capillary pressure due to left ventricular failure or to mitral stenosis, there is some evidence that congestion of one portion of the lung leads to reflex vasoconstriction in other areas. However, the quantitative significance of such a reflex effect is not established.

Increased pulmonary blood flow may result from anoxia, which thus has a doubly harmful effect because it also produces constriction of the arterioles. Acute respiratory infections not only may aggravate anoxia but also tend to increase cardiac output because of fever, tachycardia, emotional stress, and the elevation of metabolism incident to labored breathing.

Those congenital anomalies associated with large left-to-right shunts (p. 1423) may produce striking increase in blood flow through the lungs, and this in turn tends to lead to slowly progressive and eventually irreversible thickening of the smaller branches of the pulmonary arteries.

The precise quantitative significance of these several factors which increase pulmonary arterial pressure varies according to the type and severity of the underlying disease process.

Clinical Manifestations. The *signs of the primary underlying disorder* will naturally vary according to whether emphysema, infiltration of the lung, chest deformity, or extreme obesity (the Pickwickian syndrome) is responsible. In the absence of manifestations of some such underlying disorder, a patient presenting evidence of cor pulmonale should be subjected to the most careful search for some possible area of clinically silent venous thrombosis from which emboli might have arisen.

The second group of phenomena, which are characteristic of pulmonary heart disease, are the *signs of right ventricular hypertrophy* (p. 1406). This is commonly overlooked in the x-ray but will usually be made apparent by an exaggerated systolic lift of the precordium or of the epigastric area. Most of the patients exhibit a narrow spiked P wave in leads II and AVF (P pulmonale), and many of them display electrocardiographic signs of right ventricular hypertrophy.

The *signs of anoxia* are often pronounced. Thus cyanosis is more striking than in other patients with right ventricular failure, while clubbing of the fingers is relatively common, as contrasted to its rarity in patients with other types of acquired heart disease. Marked fatigability is usually present, and drowsiness is pronounced in the advanced stages.

A few of the patients exhibit the *clinical phenomena of elevated cardiac output,* with a wide pulse pressure, loud heart sounds, and exaggerated peripheral pulsations. These signs are most likely to be seen in the presence of anoxia or of fever and in patients with minimal or no signs of congestive failure.

The *manifestations of right ventricular failure* due to any one of this group of disorders are essentially the same as those due to other causes (p. 1381).

Natural History and Prognosis. The outlook depends on the cause and on the physiologic disturbances. When a reversible condition, such as prolonged severe asthma, is at fault, complete recovery may occur. *Acute cor pulmonale* due to a single massive embolus may likewise be followed by complete recovery if the patient survives the initial insult.

Regardless of the underlying cause, bronchial obstruction, infection, anoxia, and the increased blood viscosity due to polycythemia are partially reversible in most instances.

The subacute type of the disorder is most likely to occur when there is some rapidly progressive disease such as miliary carcinosis or tuberculosis, a spreading fungous infection, or progressive interstitial fibrosis. Unless the underlying cause is subject to therapeutic control, such patients usually expire within a few weeks.

Once right-sided failure has appeared as the result of primary pulmonary hypertension, the outlook is also grave. Such individuals rarely live for more than a year or two.

The most common clinical picture is that of chronic cor pulmonale due to bronchitis and emphysema. In these individuals heart failure occurs at first only when there is a complicating respiratory infection and improves as this is controlled. After some years of such an intermittent course, the patient may expire either of pulmonary or of cardiac failure. However, even with advanced emphysema, complicated by failure of the right side of the heart, vigorous treatment will often result in remarkable improvement in a patient who at first appeared to be hopelessly ill (p. 1573).

Diagnosis. The chief problem is the separation from right ventricular hypertrophy or failure, due to pulmonary hypertension caused by mitral stenosis or by failure of the left ventricle. When congenital disorders can be excluded, the presence of the typical manifestations of anoxia, i.e., excessive fatigue, cyanosis, polycythemia, and clubbing of the fingers, constitutes strong evidence in favor of cor pulmonale as compared to other types of acquired heart disease. Other valuable guides are the history of long-standing cough, clinical or x-ray phenomena pointing toward emphysema, extensive infiltrative or fibrotic disease of the lungs, the relatively small heart, and the absence of clinical, electrocardiographic, and radiologic evidence of left ventricular hypertrophy. Carbon dioxide retention is the rule in patients with cor pulmonale due to emphysema or chest deformities but is usually absent when other conditions are responsible.

The arm-to-tongue circulation time is likely to be prolonged in both conditions, but the abnormality affects particularly the arm-to-lung time in the patient with cor pulmonale, who may have a normal lung-to-tongue time because the pulmonary vascular bed is not widened.

When pulmonary heart disease is caused by an infiltrative or fibrotic disorder, total vital capacity is likely to be more reduced for a given degree of dyspnea than in the case of an individual with pulmonary congestion due to left ventricular failure or to mitral stenosis. On the other hand, when emphysema or some other basically obstructive disorder is mainly responsible for cor pulmonale, the total vital capacity may be relatively high, even though the timed vital capacity and similar measurements are reduced as compared to comparably severe cardiac dyspnea secondary to pulmonary congestion.

The considerations which are important in the differentiation of cor pulmonale from those exceptional instances of mitral stenosis, in which a clear diastolic rumble is lacking, have been considered in some detail on p. 1438.

Pain resembling that of angina pectoris in its relation to exertion is not uncommon in patients with cor pulmonale. The duration may be much longer, and episodes lasting for several hours may occur and be confused with myocardial infarction. Although this type of pain responds poorly to nitroglycerin, it is probably related to ischemia of the right ventricle, induced by diminished systolic perfusion as the result of the abnormal elevation

of the intramural pressure in this chamber (p. 33).

Attacks of syncope are not unusual in patients with cor pulmonale and with the exception of heart block and aortic stenosis are more frequent than with other types of acquired cardiac disease.

In summary, it may be said that the diagnosis of cor pulmonale will usually depend on the demonstration of clear evidence of diffuse pulmonary disease in association with the signs of anoxia, of right ventricular hypertrophy, and of systemic congestion.

Treatment. The principles involved are (1) prevention and vigorous management of chronic and recurrent acute respiratory infections (p. 1576); (2) use of bronchodilator drugs, expectorants, steam inhalations (p. 1574), enzymes to thin sputum, and, under appropriate circumstances, of steroids; (3) management of anoxia and of hypercapnia, with due consideration of the dangers of aggravation of these disturbances by morphine and other respiratory depressants (p. 1575); (4) reduction of blood viscosity by venesection when the hematocrit is greater than 50 to 55 per cent; (5) management of congestive heart failure with digitalis and diuretics (p. 1386); and (6) utilization of mechanical aids to breathing when such adjuvants are needed (p. 1576). Each of these therapeutic problems is discussed in detail in other chapters, and especially in those concerned with pneumonia, respiratory failure, and congestive heart failure. There is some evidence that Isuprel, Priscoline, and rauwolfia derivatives may lower pulmonary vascular resistance.

REFERENCES

Cobb, B., and E. M. Nanson: Further Studies with Serotonin and Experimental Pulmonary Embolism, Ann. Surg., 151:501, 1960.

Comroe, J. H., Jr., et al.: "The Lung," Chicago, The Year Book Publishers, Inc., 1955.

Cournand, Andre: Some Aspects of the Pulmonary Circulation in Normal Man and in Chronic Cardiopulmonary Diseases, Circulation, 2:641, 1950.

Fleischner, F. G.: Pulmonary Embolism, Can. Med. Assoc., 78:653, 1958.

Harvey, R. M., D. W. Richards, Jr., and A. Cournand: The Influence of Chronic Pulmonary Disease on the Heart and Circulation, Am. J. Med., 10:719, 1951.

Knowles, John H.: "Respiratory Physiology and Its Clinical Application," Cambridge, Mass., Harvard University Press, 1959.

Robin, Eugene D.: Some Aspects of the Physiologic Disturbances Associated with Pulmonary Embolism, Med. Clin. N. Am., Semptember, 1960.

Stuart-Harris, C. H., and T. Hanby: "Chronic Bronchitis, Emphysema and Cor Pulmonale," Bristol, John Wright & Sons, Ltd., 1957.

Wacker, W. E. C., M. Rosenthal, P. J. Snodgrass, and E. Amador: A Triad in the Diagnosis of Pulmonary Embolism and Infarction, J.A.M.A., 178:9, 1961.

Wood, Paul: Pulmonary Hypertension, Modern Concepts Cardiovascular Disease, 28:513, 1959.

263 PULMONARY DISORDERS DUE TO INHALATION OF NOXIOUS AGENTS

George W. Wright

AIR POLLUTION AND LUNG CLEANSING

That the air environment of specific work places may constitute a potential health hazard has long been recognized. The health hazard posed by urban air pollution and airborne infection has become a matter of increasing concern because of changing industrial practice, augmented use of petroleum products, and an increasing population density. Chronic bronchitis in England has been shown to be more common in urban than rural populations and far more common over all than in countries where home heating and industry cast fewer solids into the air. Cancer of the lung is statistically linked with population density and "air pollution." An augmented population density brings with it an increased discharge of incompletely burned automobile as well as home heating fuels and an increase in the number of persons exposed. The fumes of burning cigarette tobacco, an intense form of local air pollution, is linked statistically as a cause with both lung cancer and chronic bronchitis. The incidence and spread of airborne infection have been shown to be related to population density. Information regarding these extremely complex problems is meager and daily leads to conflicts of interest based on misinformation by both the laity and physicians. In spite of our comparative ignorance concerning important details of these problems, some valid information does exist which is of practical use to the physician in evaluating these health hazards.

Three facts explain why we survive so well under circumstances which, on superficial examination, one would think should cause grave consequences. The first of these is that, because of certain physical characteristics of airborne particulates, many never have an opportunity to enter the respiratory orifices or penetrate into the deeper parts of the lung. Secondly, the body possesses a remarkable ability to rid itself rapidly of particles deposited within the respiratory system. Third,

many things that are inhaled are biologically inert.

Particles discharged into still air will settle out with a speed dependent upon diameter, shape, and density. For example, quartz particles 200, 50, and 10 μ in diameter have a terminal settling velocity of 100, 20, and 0.5 cm per sec, respectively. It is apparent, therefore, that only particles of a size smaller than 10 μ stay suspended long enough to move very far from their points of origin. The bulk of heavy, visible industrial dusts are larger than 20 μ in diameter and settle out rapidly. Of great importance is the fact that particles smaller than 0.3 μ in diameter tend to remain permanently airborne. Smokes are generally in this latter class. Particles larger than 0.3 μ in diameter move only by virtue of motion of the air in which they are suspended, whereas those smaller than this tend to diffuse like gases. Because air is virtually never "still," there is constant mixing with progressive dilutions of contaminated by uncontaminated air. It is obvious that polluted air is being constantly changed in its character so that the farther one is from the source of contamination, the smaller and the fewer the particles in the air will be.

Of the particles present in the air entering the nose, those larger than 10 μ are almost completely removed along with 10 to 20 per cent of the smaller particles (down to a fraction of a micron) during transit from the nasal orifice to the larynx. The deposition within the nasopharynx occurs by reason of the effects of gravity, direct impingement, and to some degree, electrostatic precipitation. Particles smaller than 10 μ penetrate the larynx, but of these the larger ones are deposited on the surface of the bronchial system, with the net effect that 80 per cent or more of all particles larger than 3 μ are deposited in the upper respiratory tract. The smaller the size of the particle, the farther it tends to penetrate the air passages. Those larger than 5 μ penetrate deeply only in small numbers, while those smaller than 1 μ make up the majority of those penetrating farthest and in largest numbers.

Mass movement of air probably does not extend to the alveoli, and perhaps not even to the respiratory bronchioles. This means that practically all the deposited particulates larger than 0.3 μ fall on the mucociliary apparatus of the nose, pharynx, and tracheobronchial system. This remarkable apparatus comprises the surface of the area from the respiratory bronchioles up to and from the nasal orifice down to the oral pharynx. There is a constant movement of the mucous escalator toward the oral pharynx at a speed such that particles deposited anyplace on that surface reach the oral pharynx in less than 30 min. The material brought to the oral pharynx is either swallowed or expectorated.

Some particles of all sizes do reach the alveoli and nonciliated air tubes, though the majority are less than 3 μ in diameter. The effects of gravity on larger particles and diffusion of submicroscopic particles account for this deposit. What is their fate? Most, and perhaps all, are ultimately phagocytized by macrophages. Recent studies indicate that the majority are soon engulfed, and the loaded macrophages then move out onto the mucociliary escalator where they are subsequently disposed of. This process takes days rather than minutes. Some of the loaded macrophages apparently move into the interstitial tissues of the lung and thence via the lymphatics to the regional and more distal nodes of the lymphoid tissue or even into the blood stream. This process takes months. Naked particles can be seen upon the alveolar surface and in the interstitial tissue, a fact that has led some to believe that these particles move through the alveolar membrane by purely mechanical forces. It has been shown that particles taken up by macrophages may be discharged from or left behind by death of the macrophage only to be taken up again. This seems a more reasonable explanation of the naked particles seen within the interstitial tissues.

The clearance of particulates from the lungs has been extensively studied by using radioactive materials. The time course of removal of inhaled particles indicated above has been confirmed. As would be expected, on the basis of the preceding discussion, particles larger than 1 μ are almost completely removed in hours, smaller particles in days, and there is a small residuum that remains permanently.

Thus far, the fate of inanimate particulates has been discussed. What about living particulates? Evidence in this regard is meager. Fungi, bacteria, and viruses can become directly airborne by sneezing, coughing, and other subtle ways of creating aerosols. The individual droplets making up liquid aerosols are rapidly dehydrated, leaving behind droplet nuclei composed of the organisms and proteinaceous material. The size of these airborne droplet nuclei varies between 0.1 and 3.0 μ. These could be expected readily to penetrate into the sublaryngeal parts of the respiratory tract. Considering the number of persons who sneeze and cough and contaminate the atmosphere with respirable sized particles, why are the deeper parts of our lung sterile and why is transmission of infection relatively infrequent except under certain circumstances? Infection depends upon the number of *viable* organisms inhaled, the duration of residence within the body thus permitting time for propagation, and the favorableness of the environment where the organisms are deposited. These are complex factors, especially the third one. Organisms suspended in the relatively unfavorable environ-

ment of ambient air show great variation of viability; spores live a long time, but some bacteria survive less than a minute. The number of *living* organisms in the inhaled air will, therefore, be highly dependent on the proximity of the inhaler to the dispenser. Hence, crowding of populations is a prime factor in airborne spread of disease. Since many droplet nuclei are larger than 1 μ, the majority will fall on the mucociliary escalator and be removed too quickly to permit colonization. Because of macrophage activity, plus mechanisms of immunity and perhaps direct antibacterial substances such as lysozyme, the human respiratory tract presents an adverse environment for propagation of living particulates.

The ability of the lung to cleanse itself is maintained at a high level of efficiency in normal persons. Precise quantitative data relating total deposition to permanent retention are not available. Analysis of the lungs of hard rock miners after more than 30 years of work usually reveals no more than 5 Gm of silicon dioxide as having been retained in the total lung tissue. On the basis of reasonable calculations, it can be assumed that such workers may have inhaled 500 Gm or more of silicon dioxide during this entire period. An upper limit of permanent retention of approximately 1 per cent seems reasonable but may be in considerable error. In any event, it gives a rough estimate of the effectiveness of the cleansing mechanism under circumstances of rather high loading.

If the cleansing capacity of the lung is so great, one can properly ask why it is that disease ever develops. That the inhalation of biologically inert materials fails to cause disease is easy to understand in the light of the fact that the material is inert and so little is retained over many years of exposure. It seems reasonable to assume, however, that whenever biologically active particulates of either inanimate or animate materials can accumulate in sufficient quantities in the lung, disease will ensue. Two factors are thus important. The first is that the materials must be biologically active, and second, a sufficient quantity must either be retained in the lung or be permitted to grow in the lung. The following factors are known to favor accumulation of particulates in the lung. Overloading doubtless plays a major role. A strong relationship between intensity and duration of exposure and subsequent disease has been repeatedly shown in numerous different circumstances. The corollary of this is that a load considered tolerable for a normal may be intolerable for a subnormal cleansing mechanism. Anything known to interfere with the effectiveness of the mucociliary apparatus or of the macrophage system or of immune reactions could hence be expected to favor the development of disease. Cigarette smoke, sulfur dioxide, nitrogen dioxide, drying, and numerous other agents are known to impair mucociliary action. When these factors coexist in the inspired air with known injurious particulates such as silicon dioxide or carcinogenic hydrocarbons, the intensity-duration relationship must be augmented. Other factors undoubtedly play a role. For example, the virus of influenza is known directly to injure and destroy the cells of the tracheal mucosa, leaving such tissue vulnerable to infestation and infection by bacteria. Infection, either bacterial or viral, established in the supralaryngeal regions leads to copious production of secretions of a mucous and serous nature. These secretions are apt to be loaded with viable organisms. Normally, swallowing or expectoration disposes of these secretions. When, however, the pharynx is painful and swallowing is impaired or when drugs or sleep reduce the swallowing reflex, these bacteria-laden materials may often be, and often are, aspirated into the trachea and bronchi. The consequent introduction of viable organisms in a liquid medium may rapidly overload and impair the sublaryngeal mucociliary escalator and promote the development of pneumonia or acute bronchitis.

The degree to which permanent impairment of lung cleansing might follow acute inflammatory disease of the tracheobronchial system is not clearly known. Acute pneumonias caused by the pneumococcus do not appear to be followed by such impairment. The same can be said to be generally true for chemical pneumonias. The ability of the respiratory apparatus to regenerate normal functioning tissues after repeated acute injury is probably great.

TYPES OF RESPONSE

For centuries it has been recognized that certain particulate substances cause no untoward effects even when inhaled for many years, whereas others may rapidly or gradually cause pulmonary changes that vary considerably in degree of severity and seriousness. The number of known pathogenic substances continues to increase with the recognition of previously obscured relationships and with the development of new substances or new situations to which men may be exposed.

The body response to these noxious agents is of two broad categories, acute pneumonitis and chronic granuloma with fibrosis. The acute response may be immediate or delayed hours or even days after the contact; in the chronic form there is, with one exception, a history of prolonged exposure and a delay in development of the body reaction. Because of the trend toward a delayed reaction, the inciting cause may be difficult to discover except by the most painstaking anamnesis. In no other category of disease is the past history more important and at the same time apt to be so poorly explored. Most physicians have little contact with and knowledge of specific working conditions in industry and, hence, they are likely to be ill prepared to take an occupational history. No occupational history is adequate until the activities and surroundings of the patient during every year of his life are accounted for and the potential for hazard of each specific occupation is known.

Acute Reactions. The acute pulmonary injuries usually arise from the inhalation of irritant, vesicatory, or necrotizing gases or fumes. Certain gases have an immediate powerful irritating action which is characterized by lachrymation, burning and pain of the nose, pharynx, and trachea, and by severe cough. Strong concentrations may cause such severe irritation as to bring about prompt cessation of respiration, allegedly by laryngeal spasm. If the subject survives the immediate effects of the gas, pulmonary edema may ensue with subsequent recovery, or death may occur in spite of all efforts to provide relief. Other gases, for example, the nitrous fumes of detonated blasting powder or burning celluloid, may not cause such severe immediate reactions as to be unduly alarming, but after a delay of several hours, the patient may rather rapidly develop severe respiratory distress, cyanosis, and shock, with all the signs of pulmonary edema and exudate. Because serious delayed reaction is possible, it is wise to keep all persons who have been exposed to unusual concentrations of the irritating gases under close scrutiny for at least 24 hr. Some degree of inflammation and necrosis of tissue always occurs following severe pulmonary reactions, and during this period, the lungs are unusually susceptible to bacterial infection. Recovery may occur by resolution of the edema and inflammatory products or by fibrous replacement. Commonly there are no recognizable residua or sequelae.

That certain gases act primarily on the upper respiratory tract, whereas others affect chiefly the deeper structures of the lung, is partly attributable to their varying solubility in water. Ammonia, formaldehyde, hydrofluoric and hydrochloric acid are so soluble as to attack the first moist surface with which contact is made. The concentration of these chemicals in the air going to the deep parts of the lung is thus reduced to some extent on the way through the upper passages, and pulmonary injury is lessened. In contrast, nitrogen dioxide (nitrous fume), phosgene, and cadmium oxide fumes are relatively less soluble and hence less irritating to the upper respiratory tract. They can be respired without great discomfort and reach the deeper parts of the lung in atmospheric concentration that may be exceedingly injurious. The reaction to these chemicals is delayed but often far more serious than that to those causing more immediate discomfort. In fact, the lack of distress immediately upon inhalation makes these gases especially dangerous. Midway between these two groups in solubility and action are sulfur dioxide, the halogens, and hydrogen sulfide.

Treatment of the acute reaction depends little or not at all upon the recognition of the specific noxious agent responsible for the event. Therapy is directed first at overcoming the alterations of physiology. Shock must often be combated. Oxygen in concentrations of 50 per cent or more is imperative. There is little scientific support for the use of positive pressure by mask although a priori reasoning has prompted its use. Practical experience has shown that physical struggle and unrest may cause sudden death. If positive pressure during inspiration makes breathing less of an effort and is tolerated without restlessness, it is not contraindicated except in shock. In the hypotensive state due to poor venous return, positive pressure breathing is contraindicated. The use of agents which lower the surface tension of serum might be useful when administered via the airway as recommended in pulmonary edema of circulatory origin, but the author has no information on this point. Sedation is very important. Bromides appear to be preferable to barbiturates. Morphine is contraindicated. The prophylactic use of antibacterials is recommended throughout the period of pulmonary inflammation.

Other relatively acute reactions of the lung to inhaled material are noteworthy because of the long delay between initial contact and the reaction. Although exposure to high concentrations of a fume thought to be anhydrous beryllium sulfate may cause a violent chemical pneumonitis in a few to 72 hr, a much more insidious chemical pneumonia (not to be confused with the chronic granuloma discussed later) is also known to occur in the beryllium extraction industry and in other exposures where beryllium fluoride and beryllium oxide are inhaled. In this reaction, which develops weeks or even months after exposure begins, the symptoms of dyspnea on exertion, paroxysmal cough, substernal pain, weakness, and weight loss may precede the development of any abnormal shadows seen in the roentgenogram of the chest by 1 to 3 weeks. When abnormal shadows develop, they are characterized by a granular haziness of a diffuse patchy distribution which, in some instances, may be fluffy in appearance. The pathologic change is that of a true chemical pneumonia. Treatment is the same as for the acute reactions described before. This disease is apt to persist for several weeks, and treatment must be continued throughout. The use of ACTH or cortisone has not received adequate trial but should be explored. Recovery is the rule, but fatalities do occur.

A rather rare disease brought about by the inhalation of bagasse dust has been described in workers preparing bagasse from sugar cane or using it in manufacture. The true etiologic factor is unknown, but its association with bagasse seems established, and for the present, the disease might be properly included under the heading of this chapter. Weeks to months after the beginning of exposure to bagasse dust, the disease makes its presence known by severe paroxysmal cough and dyspnea. Fever may persist for weeks or months. The lung shows evidence of resistance to expansion. Cyanosis may be present. The white blood count is elevated, the polymorphonuclear cells forming 70 to 90 per cent of the total. The clinical picture is that of a diffuse pneumonia which persists for weeks. The scant tissue available for study shows an interstitial fibroelastic reaction. The pulmonary roentgenogram shows an abnormal diffuse pattern of fine stippling. Recovery is slow but usually occurs, and few if any sequelae remain. Treatment is symptomatic. The use of ACTH or cortisone has not been reported.

Chronic Reactions. As mentioned earlier, the majority of the various kinds of material inhaled and deposited in the lung cause no tissue reaction. Particles larger than 10 μ in size are not found in the deeper parts of the lung, but those of smaller size do reach the alveoli where they are engulfed by phagocytes. Soluble particles such as marble or gypsum disappear entirely, while those less soluble or insoluble particles are carried by the phagocytes to the lymphoid collection of the lung and mediastinum and there deposited. Many of the insoluble varieties of dust are inert so far as tissue reaction is concerned and do not cause significant fibrosis. The particles of such substances as iron, soot, etc., simply remain in the lymphoid tissue along the course of the lymphatic and blood vessels that accompany the bronchial tree. If present in large enough quantities, these inert substances may stimulate sufficient proliferation of fibrous tissue along the lymphatic channels to cause the shadows cast by normal pulmonary vascular markings to be exaggerated as to size, density, and projection toward the periphery. Indeed if the inert material is dense enough—as is iron, for example—the concentrated metallic deposits may themselves cause a shadow easily seen in the roentgenogram. Although these inert substances do cause a slight proliferation of fibrous tissue in their immediate vicinity, the reaction is mild, and there do not appear to be any recognizable evidences of interference with either the physiologic or immunologic functions of the respiratory apparatus from their retention. In contrast to these so-called "inert" particulate substances, there are others which when inhaled cause definite tissue reaction.

PNEUMOCONIOSIS

Pneumoconiosis is a generic term embracing all chronic changes in the lung induced by the prolonged inhalation of dust of a nonliving character, with no implication as to the type or severity of the change. This definition is so broad that the term no longer connotes disease. The necessity for some such term is obvious when one realizes that only a few of the inhalable substances truly cause a pulmonary change that results in sufficient dysfunction to warrant the appellation of disease. The pneumoconioses of importance to health are silicosis, asbestosis, coal worker's pneumoconiosis (South Wales), pulmonary granulomatosis of beryllium workers, Shaver's disease, and diatomaceous earth pneumoconiosis. Of these, silicosis, asbestosis, and coal worker's pneumoconiosis (South Wales) have broad socioeconomic implications in addition.

Siderosis. Siderosis, one of the pneumoconioses generally termed benign because it has no demonstrable significance as regards health, nevertheless has definite economic implications because its pulmonary radiographic appearance mimics simple silicosis. Since it may occur in conjunction with industries which also are known to produce silicosis, the differential diagnosis is of considerable importance. A detailed history indicating heavy exposure to inhalation of iron oxide rather than free crystalline silica will usually establish the diagnosis. When pulmonary nodulation develops in a person who has done welding, oxyacetylene cutting of iron, or mining of hematite in atmospheres heavily contaminated with crystalline silica particles, the differential diagnosis may require lung biopsy.

Silicosis. Silicosis is a disease of the lungs caused by the prolonged inhalation of fine particles (less than 5 μ) of free crystalline silica (SiO_2) in quantities sufficient to produce the characteristic fibrosis. It is manifested clinically by the development of discrete nodules confined to the lung and lymph nodes of the mediastinum, by an increased susceptibility to tuberculosis, and by a paucity of symptoms and signs during the discrete nodular phase of the disease. Severe evidences of respiratory embarrassment are likely to develop when conglomerate masses and secondary emphysema develop in the lungs.

With the exception of asbestos, the various silicates and amorphous silicas produce little or no reaction in the lungs. Silicosis, therefore, is associated only with those pursuits which expose one to the inhalation of naturally occurring or artificially produced forms of free crystalline silica. The common form of free silica is quartz, which is abundantly distributed in the earth's surface. Mining, tunneling, rock-cutting, sandblasting, abrasive manufacture and use, ceramic manufacture, foundry work, and glass manufacture are among those industries associated in certain jobs with the production or handling of finely divided free crystalline silica. Not all jobs or locations in these industries expose the worker to hazardous quantities of silica. For example, coremakers in most foundries have little exposure to silica, whereas the sand reconditioner or shake-out operator may have considerable. If, however, the coremaker works in a common room he may be exposed to an adjacent silica hazard. One can readily understand that an occupational history disclosing only that the occupation was miner or foundryman is entirely inadequate. Intimate knowledge of the job, working place, duration of various jobs, and even the actual place in which the work is done is an absolute necessity. Anything less provides inadequate data on which to evaluate the exposure of a given individual.

The silica particles that enter the alveoli and respiratory bronchioles are 10 μ or under. Most visible dusts are made up of particles larger than this. It has also been shown that silica particles between 5 and 10 μ act only as a foreign body and that the active or fibrogenic component of hazardous silica dust is 1 to 5 μ. Many extremely "dusty" atmospheres as tested visually are really quite harmless so far as the lung is concerned. The reverse may be equally true, some very harmful exposures being where there is little visible dust. The occupational history must therefore elicit information about particle size as well as about the chemical nature of the dust.

It has been amply demonstrated that the total number of particles of hazardous size inhaled is an important consideration in determining the severity of pulmonary injury. Contrary to popular belief, the black native labor of the South African gold fields has a relatively low incidence of silicosis. This is thought to be attributable to the fact that the individual usually works only 9 to 18 months underground. The whites working in the same areas have a much higher incidence because they are employed on a long-term basis.

It is obvious from these considerations that the size and concentrations of hazardous particles and the duration of exposure are important determinants of whether or not silicosis will develop in a given individual. There is also a factor of individual variation that is related to the effectiveness of the individual's "air filter" and lung-cleansing mechanism. There is acceptable experimental and clinical evidence to show that, when the reticuloendothelial system of the lung is saturated with inert foreign material, less than the usual amounts of silica will produce silicosis. This has an obvious practical implication.

Experience has shown that dusts containing fewer than 5 million particles of free silica 10 μ or less in size per cubic foot will rarely cause silicosis in the normal working span of a man. Concentrations above 100 million are considered very unsafe for more than a few months of exposure. Under most working conditions of the past, it took 10 to 20 years of exposure to produce recognizable silicosis. Exceptional circumstances have been reported where unusual exposures of 2 or 3 years' duration produced the disease. Men exposed approximately a year to high concentrations of virtually pure silica develop a nonnodular change having more the appearance of a chemical pneumonia.

In most occupations, the inhaled dusts are a mixture of silica and other substances. There is no doubt that these accompanying dusts, as for example gypsum or iron, are capable of modifying the activity of the silica in such a way as to diminish and delay its fibrogenic action. In the experimental animal, finely divided aluminum hydrate and "metallic" aluminum have both been shown capable of so modifying the action of silica as to prevent the development of significant fibrosis.

After the silica particles reach the alveoli, they are picked up by phagocytes. These migratory cells carry their engulfed particles to regional lymphoid clusters and to the large nodes of the hilum and mediastinum. The actual process whereby the silica particles stimulate cell proliferation and fibrosis is unknown but appears to be a physicochemical process associated with surface phenomena. In the areas where the particles accumulate, fibroblastic proliferation and hyaline formation produce nodules of a characteristic whorled appearance. At first these silicotic nodules are found only in the larger lymph nodes; but as lymph drainage becomes progressively more impaired, the particles accumulate in the peripheral lymph channels along the course of the blood vessels, especially those of the pulmonary artery. The tissue reaction in these areas gives the vessels a beaded appearance which can be recognized in a pulmonary roentgenogram but not differentiated from the beading caused by dusts which are entirely free of silica. As more and more silica is accumulated in the periphery of the lung, the tissue reaction increases to form nodules which alone or by merging with other nodules achieve a size and density sufficient to cast a shadow on the roentgenogram. Reconstruction of the nodules in man has demonstrated that they usually form around, compress, and finally close off a blood vessel of the pulmonary artery tree. Around each nodule there is a zone of dilated air spaces described as focal emphysema. At this stage the nodules are discrete and comprise a relatively small amount of the total lung tissue. The lung between the nodules has a normal appearance. This stage of silicosis has been categorized as simple discrete nodular silicosis. Some subdivide this group on the basis of the size of the nodules seen in the roentgenogram.

In many individuals, the reaction does not progress beyond the discrete nodular stage. In others, large irregular masses of very dense fibrous tissue with irregular radiating strands develop. As a rule this occurs in the upper parts of both lungs. In advanced stages the entire upper part of both lungs may be a dense shrunken mass of fibrous tissue firmly adherent to the chest wall, with the lower parts of the lung the site of severe diffuse emphysema. In some instances, it appears that these masses form by a shrinking together of the lung and conglomeration of the nodules. In others, there is little shrinkage but rather an extraordinary proliferation of fibrous tissue. When massive or conglomerate shadows appear in the roentgenogram, the disease is categorized as complicated or *conglomerate silicosis*. Rarely the conglomerate form appears with little or no discoverable accompanying discrete nodulation.

Histologic study reveals that, in 60 to 70 per cent of those persons exhibiting the conglomerate form of silicosis, evidences of tuberculosis can be found associated with the pulmonary masses. In the remainder, nontuberculous infection may have played a role in causing the intense proliferation of fibrous tissue. It seems logical to believe that previous nontuberculous infection may so damage the self-cleansing mechanism of the lung that unusual amounts of silica are likely to be retained at the site of previous infections and thus cause unusual fibrotic response in these areas.

The diagnosis of silicosis requires that one see nodulation characteristically distributed throughout the lungs in the roentgenogram, that other causes of the nodular pattern be ruled out, and that a history of exposure to the inhalation of free crystalline silica of particle size and amount capable of causing the nodular fibrosis be obtained. These requirements may seem unduly strict in view of the fact that a histologic stage of the disease must precede the clinical manifestations. The tendency to make a diagnosis of silicosis solely on the basis of a history of exposure to silica is certainly not realistic, because in actual practice the majority of persons so exposed never develop clinically significant evidences of the disease. To make the diagnosis on the basis of a positive occupational history and the presence or development of exaggerated bronchovascular shadows will lead to frequent false diagnoses. Many persons who have inhaled non-silica dust and some with no history of any dust exposure at all will be found to have markedly exaggerated bronchovascular markings. To require nodulation demonstrable by roentgenogram in order to establish a diagnosis is justifiable both from a medicolegal point of view and from that of the person's health since no clinical significance is attached to the prenodular stage of silicosis.

In the simple discrete nodular stage of silicosis there are few related symptoms. Numerous investigators studying silicotic persons from several industries have found only slight evidences of impaired cardiorespiratory function. Many silicotics show entirely normal measurements during this stage. In others there is a moderate reduction of maximal breathing capacity and an absolute increase of residual air. These findings are evidence of slight diffuse obstructive emphysema. When conglomerate masses develop, these evidences of emphysema are likely to become more severe and may lead to complete respiratory crippling. In the simple discrete nodular stage there is no impairment of gas diffusion between the atmosphere and pulmonary blood. In the conglomerate stage, poor mixing and distribution associated with emphysema lead to a lowered alveolar pO_2, and some degree of arterial hypoxia may develop during exercise. The physiologic abnormalities of conglomerate silicosis are caused primarily by the diffuse obstructive emphysema which accompanies this stage of silicosis. The complaint of exertional dyspnea is due almost entirely to a reduction in the ability to pump air into and out of the lungs. At this stage the clinical symptoms in addition to dyspnea on exertion are cough, expectoration, chest pain, and weakness. Cor pulmonale is a late complication and is the cause of death in many instances.

Discrete nodular silicosis appears to be progressive for a year or two after the individual is removed from exposure but then stabilizes, and life expectancy appears normal. The conglomerate form progresses slowly even after removal from exposure, and life expectancy is diminished.

Tuberculosis is the most feared complication of silicosis. Some individuals having simple discrete nodular silicosis may develop active tuberculosis, the characteristic infiltrates or cavities going through the conventional pattern that eventuates in subsequent spontaneous healing. This combination is best referred to as silicosis *with* tuberculosis and is reported to respond favorably to antibacterial therapy for tuberculosis. More often than not, however, active tuberculosis is prone to pursue one of three courses in the person with silicosis. In the unusual circumstance of a primary or hematogenous infection occurring in lungs already the site of silicosis, one finds that the peripheral zone of the silicotic nodule is a preferred site for the development of the tuberculous lesion. Previously sharp borders of the shadow of the nodule in a roentgenogram become blurred, and the nodule enlarges. The tuberculous process proceeds with enhanced speed and practically always ends fatally. Reactivation of a preexisting tuberculous focus or the occurrence of exogenous reinfection may lead to rapidly developing cavitation. The disease may then become widely disseminated and will run a rampant and fatal course. In these two types of reaction, the tuberculosis is the most prominent feature. Spontaneous recovery is so unusual and the clinical course so adverse that this modification of tuberculosis warrants the designation of silicotuberculosis.

A third combination occurs when silicosis and tuberculosis exist together in such a way as to produce massive fibrosis. The presence of conglomerate shadows in the silicotic person is assumed on statistical grounds to indicate complicating tuberculosis, although tuberculosis can be proved in only about 70 per cent of the cases. The silicosis and tuberculosis both are modified to the extent that they produce massive fibrotic conglomerates in which silicotic nodules and the granuloma of tuberculosis can be recognized histologically. Clinically the tuberculosis is modified by becoming very indolent and losing all or most of its invasive and disseminating character. This combination is termed tuberculosilicosis and can exist for many years with few if any symptoms other than cough and dyspnea on exertion.

Anthracosilicosis is a variant caused by the inhalation of a mixture of coal dust and free crystalline silica. In essence its course is very similar to conventional silicosis. It appears that emphysema may develop earlier and be more of a complication in the simple discrete nodular phase in anthracosilicosis.

The type of pathologic process which characterizes silicosis affords little hope of any form of effective treatment for the patient having well-established disease. Prevention by adequate control of all dust hazards is the answer to the problem. Aluminum powder has definite prophylactic action in animals, and presumably would also be effective in human beings unavoidably exposed to silica. No critical data on this point are available. Aluminum by inhalation has been recommended and tried as an agent to relieve the symptoms of silicosis. Critical data fail to support its effectiveness except as a form of psychotherapy. When active tuberculosis is a complication, antimicrobial therapy may be effective in the discrete nodular stage but has little if any influence on the massive conglomerate stage. Experience suggests that in the simple discrete nodular stage continued employment is well tolerated. It has been argued that in the conglomerate stage physical work is deleterious. No critical evidence bears on this important point. The silicotic man should of course be protected from any additional silica hazard in the environment.

Coal Worker's Pneumoconiosis. Exposure to the inhalation of coal dust without substantial quantities of silica appears to be rare, at least in the United States. Because of this and the fact that pure coal dust or carbon inhalation by animals produced no reaction similar to silicosis, it has been accepted that the nodulation and conglomerate masses seen in coal miners is in reality a modified form of silicosis. Recently the Pneumoconiosis Research Unit of Cardiff, South Wales, has reported studies strongly suggesting that in the miners of that area pulmonary injury occurs from the inhalation of coal per se rather than from the inhalation of silica. Histologic studies show that the earliest change is the deposition of pigment in a stellate-shaped discrete macule about which is a zone of emphysema. There is a delicate network of reticular fibers in these pigmented areas, but characteristically there is no hyaline deposition or extensive fibrosis such as typifies the silicotic nodule. These macules with their zone of focal emphysema are numerous and scattered throughout both lungs. This stage of the disease is categorized as simple pneumoconiosis of coal workers and is recognized in the roentgenogram by tiny nodulations which may coalesce into larger nodules or mottlings. The disease remains at this stage if no further exposure occurs and is characterized by a lack of symptoms. Physiologic studies show little or no abnormality of function in spite of the focal emphysema. When, as happens occasionally, a person with evidence of severe emphysema is seen at this stage, a nonindustrial or spontaneous origin of the emphysema must be strongly considered.

In certain cases of simple pneumoconiosis, irregular, large localized masses appear and progress in size. This stage is termed *progressive massive fibrosis* or *complicated pneumoconiosis* of coal workers. This stage is thought to be caused by coexistent infection, and tuberculosis is implicated in a high proportion of the cases. As the massive fibrosis develops, severe obstructive emphysema usually but not always becomes apparent.

It is of interest that this entity so closely parallels conventional silicosis, differing chiefly in that the focal emphysema is said to be more severe and the degree of fibrosis much less severe in the simple uncomplicated stage of coal worker's pneumoconiosis than is true of silicosis. Also, a high incidence of active tuberculosis and its rapid progression have not been reported in coal worker's pneumoconiosis. Typical changes have been reported in coal trimmers where silica exposure is considered nonexistent, hence the conclusion that they are the result solely of coal dust. There is a divergence of incidence in different geographic locations of South Wales, and the incidence for South Wales is much higher than in other coal fields of Great Britain.

There are no critical studies to demonstrate whether or not this entity exists in other coal mining areas. Similar cases, both radiographically and histologically, are alleged to have been demonstrated in the United States. Many questions remain to be studied before the proper meaning of this interesting study from South Wales can be assessed in terms of the coal workers of other areas.

Asbestosis. The prolonged inhalation of sufficient quantities of asbestos fiber produces a diffuse fibrosis of the lung which may be extremely severe. The disease offers a contrast to silicosis in many features. Long fibers (20 to 50 μ) rather than short fibers evoke the tissue response; the irritant is mechanical rather than chemical; the lymphatic system is involved only slightly and late, the early lesion being a peribronchial fibrosis; the fibrosis is diffuse rather than nodular in character; severe pleural changes are common; interference with the passage of oxygen from the alveolus to the blood because of thickened alveolar walls is the characteristic physiologic alteration; diffuse obstructive emphysema is not manifested clinically or physiologically; clinical symptoms and physiologic abnormalities may precede unequivocal roentgenographic evidences of asbestosis; there is no alteration of susceptibility to tuberculosis. The diseases are similar in that the quantity of proper-sized particulates inhaled is the chief determinant of the development of diseases. Under usual working conditions, years of exposure are required to produce the disease. Severe disability (entirely different in fundamental character from that of silicosis) is likely to be present only in advanced cases; cor pulmonale, though a common cause of death in both, is more frequent in asbestosis. There is no effective form of treatment for the disease per se.

Pulmonary Granulomatosis of Beryllium Workers. An unusual chronic granuloma of the lung has been described in persons working where they may be exposed to the inhalation of beryllium and its compounds. Although an association with industries using beryllium compounds has been proved, the etiologic factors have not been determined. The disease is characterized in the severe form by extreme exertional dyspnea, paroxysmal cough, marked loss of weight, and cyanosis; the roentgenogram shows a diffuse ground-glass appearance of the lungs plus enlargement of the hilar lymph nodes. Interference with diffusion of oxygen across the alveolar membrane is the underlying physiologic defect and cor pulmonale the usual cause of death. Minute exposures to the chemical and a delay of months to years between exposure and onset of the disease make this a most bizarre entity. The disease has more than just industrial implications, since bona fide cases have developed following the inhalation of exceedingly minute quantities of beryllium under nonindustrial circumstances. The number of cases is increasing. Differential diagnosis from other nodular granulomas is at times most difficult. No authentic spontaneous complete recovery has been reported. The mortality rate is high, but many persons remain in an arrested state of the disease for years. ACTH and cortisone have produced dramatic but not permanent remissions.

Byssinosis. This is a remarkable disorder of cotton mill workers exposed to high concentrations of cotton dust. It is characterized by chest tightness, wheezing, dyspnea, and cough. The symptoms recur each Monday (in those workers who have a Sunday holiday), are less intense on Tuesday, and then gradually disappear during the remainder of the week only to recur the next Monday. The cause of this peculiar and specific fluctuation is unknown.

After one or more decades, the symptoms may become persistent but still with exacerbation each Monday. Respiratory failure and/or cor pulmonale may ultimately occur.

During its early years, the disease is cured by cessation of exposure to cotton dust. However, this measure may be ineffective if instituted after irreversible pulmonary or cardiac changes have occurred.

Byssinosis is common in British workers and is occasionally seen in the United States.

REFERENCES

Baetjer, A. M.: Chronic Exposures to Air Pollutants and Acute Infectious Respiratory Diseases, A.M.A. Arch. Indust. Hyg. and Occupational Med., 2:400, 1950.

Cotter, L. H., and B. H. Cotter: Cadmium Poisoning, A.M.A. Arch. Indust. Hyg. and Occupational Med., 3:495, 1951.

Denardi, J. M., H. S. van Ordstrand, and C. H. Curtis: Berylliosis: Summary and Survey of All Clinical Types in Ten-year Period, Cleveland Clinic Quart., 19:171, 1952.

Furness, G., and H. B. Maitland: Studies on Cotton Dust in Relation to Byssinosis; Bacteria and Fungi in Cotton Dust, Brit. J. Indust. Med., 9:138, 1952.

Gardner, L. U.: The Pathology and Roentgenographic Manifestations of Pneumoconiosis, J.A.M.A., 114:535, 1940.

Gilson, J. C., and P. Hugh-Jones: "Lung Function in Coalworker's Pneumoconiosis," Medical Research Council, Special Report, ser. 290, London, Her Majesty's Stationery Office, 1955.

Gregoire, F., and G. W. Wright: "The Pathologic Physiology of Asbestosis in Humans," Seventh Saranac Symposium, Saranac Lake, N.Y., Saranac Laboratory, 1952.

Henderson, Y., and H. W. Haggard: "Noxious Gases," New York, Reinhold Publishing Corporation, 1943.

Kerr, Louis E.: Coal Workers' Pneumoconiosis, Ind. Med. and Surg., 25:355, 1956.

Motley, H. L., L. P. Land, and B. Gordon: Pulmonary Emphysema and Ventilation Measurements in 100 Anthracite Coal Miners with Respiratory Complaints, Am. Rev. Tuberc., 59:270, 1949.

Patty, F. A.: "Industrial Hygiene and Toxicology," vol. I, New York, Interscience Publishers, Inc., 1948. (Vols. II and III, in preparation.)

Perry, K. M. A.: Diseases of the Lung Resulting from Occupational Dusts Other than Silica, Thorax, 2:91, 1947.

Rossier, P. H., H. Bucher, and K. Wiesinger: Die Lungenfunktion in Ruhe bei der Silikose, Vierteljahrsschr. naturforsch. Ges. Zürich, 92 (Supp. 3–4):83, 1947.

Sanders, O. A.: Benign Pneumoconiosis Due to Metal Fumes and Dust, Am. J. Roentgenol. Radium Therapy, 58:277, 1947.

Sayers, R. R.: "Anthracosilicosis," U.S. Public Health Bull. 41, Washington, 1943.

Shaver, C. G.: Further Observations of Lung Changes Associated with the Manufacture of Alumina Abrasives, Radiology, 50:760, 1948.

Smart, R. H., and W. M. Anderson: Pneumoconiosis Due to Diatomaceous Earth, Ind. Med. and Surg., 21:509, 1952.

Sterner, J. H., and M. Eisenbud: Epidemiology of Beryllium Intoxication, Arch. Indust. Hyg. and Occupational Med., 4:123, 1951.

Stoll, R., R. Bass, and A. Angrist: Asbestosis Associated with Bronchogenic Carcinoma, A.M.A. Arch. Internal Med., 88:831, 1951.

Symposia on Chronic Beryllium Poisoning, A.M.A. Arch. Indust. Hyg. and Occupational Med., 3:543, 1951.

Vorwald, A. J., T. Durkan, and P. C. Pratt: Experimental Studies of Asbestos, A.M.A. Arch. Indust. Hyg. and Occupational Med., 3:1, 1951.

Wegelius, C.: Changes in the Lungs in 126 Cases of Asbestosis Observed in Finland, Acta Radiol., 28:139, 1947.

Wright, G. W.: Chronic Pulmonary Granulomatosis of Beryllium Workers, Trans. Am. Clin. Climat. Assoc., 61:166, 1949.

—— and G. Filley: Pulmonary Fibrosis and Respiratory Function, Am. J. Med., 10:642, 1951.

264 BRONCHIECTASIS, LUNG ABSCESS, AND MISCELLANEOUS DISORDERS

John H. Knowles

BRONCHIECTASIS

The term bronchiectasis refers to a state of dilatation of the bronchial tree. The disease was first described by Laennec in 1819. Extensive clinical study and description were made possible with the introduction of bronchography in 1922 by Sicard and Forestier. The incidence, prognosis, and severity of the disease have been radically altered with the advent of chemotherapy.

Bronchiectasis is a disease of *patchy* distribution in the lung. The affected segmental or subsegmental bronchus may undergo a tubular (cylindrical) or saccular dilatation. *Generalized* tubular dilatation of smaller (more peripheral) bronchi may be seen in chronic bronchitis and obstructive emphysema, but this is not of the same significance as the *localized*, more striking dilatation of larger (more proximal) bronchi seen in bronchiectasis. The differentiation of bronchitis and bronchiectasis is discussed below and on p. 1510.

Pathogenesis. Prolonged bronchial obstruction and infection must be present to cause irreversible dilatation of the bronchial tubes. If uncontrolled, the infection extends into the bronchial wall, with disruption of smooth muscle and elastic tissue, and invades the adjacent peribronchial tissue. Ciliated columnar epithelium is replaced by nonciliated cuboidal epithelium, and in some instances the entire bronchial wall may be replaced by fibrous tissue, with resultant formation of saccules. With damage or loss of ciliated epithelium and loss of bronchial tone and peristaltic action there is further stasis of infected secretions. Traction by peribronchial and parenchymal scars distorts the diseased bronchus. In the region of third order bronchi, large (up to 1 mm in size) anastomotic communications between bronchial artery and pulmonary artery may be seen.

The posterior basal segments of the lower lobes are the most commonly involved. More than half of patients with left lower lobe disease also have involvement of the lingular segment of the left upper lobe. Upper lobe bronchiectasis is usually seen in the posterior or apical segment and is likely to be secondary to (old) tuberculous endobronchitis or to healed lung abscess.

Etiology. Prior to the introduction of antibiotics and extensive immunization programs, the commonest precursors of bronchiectasis were pertussis, measles, and influenza, and more than 50 per cent of patients dated the onset of their symptoms from the first decade. By giving rise to peripheral bronchial obstruction and stasis, these infections set the stage for superimposition of suppurative infection and bronchiectasis. At present *bronchopneumonia* is the most likely precursor of bronchiectasis. When drainage is hindered by inspissation of secretions or treatment is inadequate, there is delay in resolution and bronchial infection persists. Similarly, aspiration of a foreign body, particularly in children, and bronchogenic carcinoma and bronchial

adenoma by partially obstructing the bronchial lumen lead to chronic infection and the development of bronchiectasis distally.

Kartagener's syndrome consists of a triad of dextrocardia, sinusitis, and bronchiectasis. The incidence of bronchiectasis in patients with congenital dextrocardia is 15 to 20 per cent. The disease may never supervene in subjects with dextrocardia or it may develop late in life, depending probably on the element of infection. The reasons for the association are obscure.

Cystic fibrosis of the pancreas is a congenital disease characterized by exocrine pancreatic insufficiency and chronic obstructive pulmonary disease. Ninety per cent of deaths in cystic fibrosis are directly attributable to the pulmonary complication of obstructive emphysema, atelectasis, and bronchiectasis. Thick, tenacious secretions obstruct the bronchial lumen, resulting in atelectasis distally. If infection is superimposed (commonly with the staphylococcus or *Pseudomonas aeruginosa*), the ground is set for the development of bronchiectasis.

Bronchiectasis is a frequent complication of congenital *agammaglobulinemia* and results presumably from recurrent pulmonary infection. Only rare instances of bronchiectasis have been reported in adults in association with acquired agammaglobulinemia.

The right middle lobe bronchus is particularly vulnerable to compression by lymph nodes situated at its origin from the right bronchus. With enlargement of the peribronchial lymph nodes because of tuberculosis or nonspecific infection the right middle lobe bronchus is compressed and stasis and infection occur distally. This has been called the *middle lobe syndrome*.

Primary tuberculosis can lead to bronchiectasis via enlarged, obstructing lymph nodes at the root of a lobar bronchus. Secondary or reinfection tuberculosis may lead to a state of bronchiectasis by (1) distortion of subsegmental bronchi adjacent to a healing cavitary or granulomatous lesion, or (2) destruction secondary to endobronchial tuberculosis.

Bronchiectasis, usually of the tubular type, may occasionally be seen in long-standing cases of bronchial asthma, chronic bronchitis, and obstructive emphysema. Presumably this has resulted from bronchial obstruction and infection due to viscid secretions and is patchy in distribution. Generalized dilatation of smaller bronchi may be seen in chronic bronchitis and emphysema (see below).

Bronchiectatic changes can frequently be demonstrated in the area of a healed lung abscess. Reepithelization of lung abscess cavities and extension of suppurative disease to surrounding segmental bronchi result in their permanent dilatation.

Anomalous pulmonary arteries arising from the

aorta may be associated with sequestration of a lobe and resulting bronchiectasis commonly in the region of the posterior segment of the left lower lobe and close to the diaphragm.

Because of the frequent association of sinusitis with bronchiectasis, an etiologic role was assigned with the notion that chronic aspiration of infected sinus contents led to bronchiectasis. Similar reasoning has been applied to poor oral hygiene because of the rarity of healthy teeth and gingiva in patients with bronchiectasis. Perhaps this mechanism applies in a few individuals, but the association of upper and lower respiratory tract disease has not offered a convincing clue to the etiology of disease in either area.

Clinical Manifestations. *Symptoms of bronchiectasis depend on superimposed infection and not the bronchial dilatation per se.* Thus bronchiectasis may be continuously or intermittently symptomatic. Some individuals known to have bronchial dilatation in a lower lobe for many years have symptoms only after an upper respiratory tract infection. Upper lobe lesions may remain permanently asymptomatic because stasis and infection of secretions do not occur.

The *cardinal manifestations* are *cough, mucopurulent sputum, hemoptysis,* and *recurrent pneumonitis.* The cough is particularly severe and productive when the subject lies down, thereby emptying the contents of the dependent lower lobes into the larger bronchi. The morning production of sputum is large, and the patient may have syncopal episodes (cough syncope) or vomit (emetic cough) as he struggles to rid his bronchi of the overnight accumulation.

The sputum is mucopurulent and varies from 1 to 8 oz a day. It initially settles into three and finally into two layers as the frothy top layer subsides. The final two layers consist of an upper watery saline component and a lower heavier part consisting mainly of pus cells, and includes various organisms, Dietrich's plugs, and elastic tissue. The sputum (and breath) is occasionally foul smelling but usually has a sickish sweet odor and a pea-soup appearance.

Hemoptysis varies from blood-streaking of the sputum to massive and rarely exsanguinating amounts. In the former instance the blood has arisen from granulation tissue in the chronically infected bronchial wall and in the latter instance from erosion of a bronchial artery or a bronchial-pulmonary arteriolar anastomosis. Commonly in upper lobe bronchiectasis and occasionally with lower lobe disease, the initial symptom may be that of hemoptysis, so-called "dry bronchiectasis." Here cough and sputum production have been minimal (or minimized by the patient) and a subclinical, smoldering infection in a bronchiectatic segment has finally eroded a vessel. Hemoptysis is said to be more common with saccular than tubular disease.

Recurrent pneumonitis commonly punctuates the course of bronchiectasis. A high index of suspicion should be aroused when recurrent pneumonia involves the same lobe repeatedly. In this case the reservoir of infection is the underlying infected bronchiectasis, and extension from here into the surrounding parenchyma has developed. Occasionally intrapulmonary aspiration of infected secretions from a diseased area into a healthy lobe has occurred.

More than 60 per cent of patients will have associated symptoms of sinusitis with postnasal drip and sinus headaches.

Dyspnea may be a prominent complaint in some patients, particularly older adults with extensive bilateral disease or an additional element of diffuse chronic bronchitis and obstructive emphysema.

On physical examination, the patient appears chronically ill. His wet cough frequently interrupts the examination. Sinus tenderness may be elicited. Clubbing of the fingers and toes is observed in 50 per cent of the patients. The chest may have the emphysematous configuration if accompanying diffuse chronic bronchitis is present. The most important finding is the auscultation of persistent, wet, coarse inspiratory rales at either or both posterior lung bases, more frequently the left, and over the right middle lobe or lingular segment of the left upper lobe. The breath sounds may be coarse and bronchial. The findings of diffuse chronic bronchitis may also exist (see Chap. 260). Examination of the heart may rarely reveal the findings of pulmonary hypertension. One should also be alert to the possibility of dextrocardia. There may be *no* abnormal physical findings in the chest in some patients.

Laboratory Findings. There is mild normocytic normochromic anemia if infection has been prolonged and severe. Leukocytosis may be seen if acute bacterial infection with pneumonitis is superimposed on the chronic infection. Urinalysis may reveal persistent albuminuria if the rare complication of secondary amyloidosis has occurred. The characteristics of the sputum have been alluded to above. Only occasionally do cultures reveal a predominant pathogen, particularly during an acute pneumonitis. Study of plasma protein electrophoretic pattern and of sweat electrolyte excretion may be useful in excluding agammaglobulinemia and cystic fibrosis, respectively (pp. 752 and 1666).

Pulmonary function is not measurably altered until the disease involves more than three segments or is bilateral. Decrease in vital capacity correlates with the extent of the disease. Some patients will show the pattern of obstructive emphysema, and their dyspnea correlates well with the reduction in ventilatory reserve. Abnormalities of distribution as regards venous admixture effect (resulting in arterial oxygen unsaturation) may be minimized by the effect of the bronchial artery–pulmonary artery precapillary anastomoses in shunting returning venous blood away from diseased, poorly ventilated areas to normally ventilated areas where gas exchange is normally maintained. Pulmonary hypertension and cor pulmonale result when extensive bilateral disease destroys excessive parenchymal vascular bed.

Although the conventional x-ray of the chest may be normal in some cases, it is usually abnormal. Linear shadows extending from the hilum into the periphery of the lung field probably represent peribronchial thickening. Triangular shadows of lobar collapse may be seen at either lung base, particularly in children. So-called ring shadows— air-filled areas with thin or thick walls—may represent bronchiectatic sacs or local overdistention emphysema adjacent to atelectatic areas. With lobar collapse and in the rare instance of massive whole lung involvement, mediastinal contents will be shifted toward the diseased area and the homolateral hemidiaphragm will be elevated.

Bronchoscopy is ordinarily done prior to bronchography. It is an important diagnostic adjunct and helps in localization of the disease. It is also used to rule out bronchostenosis by external compression or by intrinsic tumor, foreign body, or endobronchial tuberculosis.

Bronchography is necessary to define the extent of the disease. The bronchial tree is outlined by the use of an aqueous iodine preparation called Dionosil. This is completely absorbed in several days in contrast to older oily preparations (Lipiodol) which might remain at the lung bases permanently. The bronchogram generally reveals a tubular or saccular dilatation of several or more of the proximal (second or third order) bronchi in the lung. The affected lobe is atelectatic, and the dilated bronchi are squeezed together.

A problem frequently arises in the differential diagnosis of bronchiectasis and chronic bronchitis, both of which may have the same symptoms and very similar bronchographic patterns and frequently coexist. Clinically sinus disease, copious amounts of sputum, hemoptysis, clubbing, wet rales which persist in a localized area of the lung over long periods of time, all seen in a youth or young adult patient, are highly suggestive of bronchiectasis. The middle-aged or elderly man with the chronic, poorly productive "cigarette" cough, signs of hyperinflated chest with quiet breath sounds, and *generalized* squeaks but no local wet bubbling rales more likely has chronic bronchitis and emphysema. There are several important radiographic points which may help in diagnosis: in bronchitis the volume of the lung (or lobe) is increased, whereas in bronchiectasis it is decreased even though there may be emphysematous changes peripherally. In bronchitis the bronchi fill out more peripherally, whereas in bronchiectasis only the larger and more proximal bronchi fill. Bronchial diverticula, representing filling of the dilated ducts of mucous glands, are diffuse and sparse in chronic bronchitis. In bronchiectasis they are numerous and localized to the bronchus of the involved lobe. If both situations exist, then both diseases may be present.

The *diagnosis* of bronchiectasis should be suspected in any patient complaining of chronic and usually productive cough or hemoptysis or recurrent episodes of pneumonia. The suspicion is strengthened if clubbing is found along with persistent, wet inspiratory rales at the lung bases posteriorly or over the lingular segment or right middle lobe. If radiographic abnormalities are also seen on the plain film, the diagnosis is almost certain. It is strengthened by the bronchoscopic findings and confirmed by bronchography.

The *course* of the disease is extremely variable. Known bronchial dilatation may exist without symptoms for years only to become suddenly and persistently symptomatic. As a general rule, saccular bronchiectasis is a more serious disease than the tubular form, and bilateral involvement carries a worse prognosis than unilateral disease. It is of utmost importance to note that bronchiectasis is an acquired disease that is not, except in rare instances, progressive. It does not commonly spread and is ordinarily maximal when first seen. The typical patient *prior to the antibiotic era* was between fifteen and thirty years of age. His symptoms extended over 10 to 20 years, and their onset was usually dated from an episode of pneumonia or pertussis during the first decade of life. He was incapacitated by his foul sputum, general debility, and malnutrition. The individual whose illness began before ten years of age rarely lived beyond the age of forty, and the mortality of hospital cases followed for any length of time was 30 to 50 per cent. The usual causes of death were pneumonia, overwhelming sepsis, brain abscess, hemorrhage, and cor pulmonale. In addition to the complications, an occasional instance of secondary amyloidosis was recorded. More recent studies have shown that those complications now are exceedingly rare and that the prognosis has improved considerably, partly because of antibiotics and partly because more recent studies have considered ambulatory groups of clinic patients. Bilateral disease, persistent large amounts of fetid sputum, frequent bouts of fever, and clubbing of the fingers are poor prognostic signs. The presence of chronic bronchitis and obstructive emphysema also worsens the prognosis. The mortality is now approximately 10 per cent over a 10-year period. The cause of death may be pulmonary insufficiency and cor pulmonale, but intercurrent and unrelated disease are also frequent causes. Surviving subjects rarely show progression of disease and fairly frequently show improvement.

Treatment. The treatment of bronchiectasis combines the judicious use of antibiotics, postural drainage (see Chap. 268, Therapy), and in certain patients resection of diseased areas. Antibiotic therapy is guided during periods of acute infection by the results of sputum (or blood) cultures. In patients who suffer repeated episodes of acute infection, small doses of antibiotics can be given prophylactically during the winter months. Periodic culture of the sputum should be obtained during such therapy to detect the emergence of other, sometimes resistant, organisms.

Because the disease is usually not a progressive or spreading process, every patient at least initially deserves a course of conservative medical therapy under close observation before a decision for or against surgery is made. The most dramatic surgical cures are effected by the excision of localized, unilateral disease which has remained symptomatic despite medical therapy. Massive and recurrent hemoptysis may also necessitate surgical removal. The poorest results are obtained with the excision of local disease in the face of bilateral, extensive disease and coexistent diffuse chronic bronchitis or bronchial asthma. Bronchitis or bronchial asthma is not cured by excision of bronchiectatic segments. Surgical therapy in general is not indicated where there is too little or too much disease. A period of conservative medical therapy is nearly always indicated, perhaps even for as long as a year, not only to judge its success or failure, but to avoid the mistake of resecting reversible or pseudobronchiectasis, recalling that the bronchial tree following the expansion of a collapsed lobe or the resolution of atypical pneumonia may take months and even a year to revert to normal with disappearance of bronchial dilatation.

BRONCHIAL OBSTRUCTION AND PULMONARY ATELECTASIS

Atelectasis refers to a state of incomplete expansion of the lung, due to failure to expand at birth (atelectasis of the newborn) or to collapse of pulmonary alveoli. This results from external compression (pleural effusion or pneumothorax) or bronchial obstruction. Collapse from external compression is ordinarily readily reversible with removal of fluid, air, or fibrous tissue (decortication) from the intrapleural space provided the underlying lung is normal. Atelectasis distal to bronchial obstruction is important for several reasons: (1) its discovery aids considerably in diagnosis as, for example, the lobar atelectasis seen in infancy associated with cystic fibrosis of the pancreas, and in childhood associated with compression of lobar bronchi by caseous nodes, or in adult life associated with bronchogenic carcinoma; (2) it is one of the prevalent causes of postoperative morbidity, and (3) it predisposes to lung abscess and bronchiectasis.

Bronchial obstruction with atelectasis may be caused by endobronchial disease such as tumor, stenosing inflammatory disease such as tuberculosis, foreign body, broncholiths, or inspissated mucous plugs; or it may be caused by extrabronchial compression by enlarged lymph nodes (middle-lobe syndrome), neoplasm, or aneurysm. Inspissation of mucus to form an obstructing plug is particularly common in patients with bronchial asthma, cystic fibrosis of the pancreas, or chronic bronchitis, in conditions associated with decreased movement of the chest wall, e.g., poliomyelitis, and in the early postoperative period.

Aspiration of foreign body, gastric contents, or of infected material from the upper respiratory tract occurs commonly and may result in pneumonia or abscess formation (see pp. 1554 and 1556) because of bronchial obstruction with distal infection. The defenses against aspiration of cough, laryngeal closure, and ciliary motion are impaired by sleep, alcohol, anesthesia, immersion and exposure, epilepsy, or coma from any cause. Aging per se results in a lessening of the airway's protective reflexes. Blood, mucus, dental deposits, or food may be aspirated, and the infected plug occludes the segmental bronchus. The right lung is more commonly involved because the right main bronchus is the straightest route for aspiration. The parts of the lung affected most often are the posterior segments of the upper lobes and superior segments of the lower lobes as these are the most dependent areas when in the supine or lateral decubitus positions, respectively. Foreign body, lung abscess, and aspiration pneumonia are discussed further below.

Obstruction of a main stem bronchus which develops gradually may give rise to mild, vague discomfort in the chest and little or no dyspnea. Acute obstruction of the same bronchus in the postoperative period (acute massive collapse of the lung) may be accompanied by anxiety, agitation, dyspnea, tachypnea, fever, and tachycardia.

Postoperative atelectasis occurs in about 5 per cent of patients, most commonly following upper abdominal procedures. It is more likely to be found in men, in smokers, in chronic bronchitics, in the aged, obese, and debilitated, and in patients incapable of early ambulation. Minimal degrees of atelectasis are heralded by mild fever (temperatures to 101°F), tachycardia, and tachypnea within 48 hr after operation. Vague chest discomfort and mild respiratory distress and a cough, first nonproductive but later yielding tenacious mucus or mucopurulent sputum, are usual. If the collapse increases, expansion of the chest may be diminished on the affected side, and hyporesonance, inspiratory rales, and depressed breath sounds may be heard. The chest x-ray reveals linear shadows, usually in the lower lung fields, segmental or lobar atelectasis, or merely increased density of pulmonary parenchyma. If lobar or whole lung collapse has occurred acutely, it is heralded by severe agitation and anxiety, dyspnea and tachypnea. Hypoxia leads to cyanosis and acute systemic hypertension, and there may be substernal oppression if the mediastinum shifts toward the affected side. The percussion note may not be dull if the lung has not had time to lose enough air, but the hemithorax moves poorly and the trachea and heart are shifted *toward* the collapsed side. The x-ray shows the mediastinal shift, narrowing of the intercostal spaces, a high diaphragm, and a dense lobe or lung on the affected side. If the inspissated secretions are not removed, pneumonia may develop.

Treatment of atelectasis depends on the cause of the obstruction, and for this reason diagnostic bronchoscopy is always indicated in obscure cases. This procedure is also therapeutic in instances where removal of a foreign body or inspissated secretions is feasible. Therapeutic bronchoscopy may be necessary in postoperative cases if suctioning, percussion therapy, and coughing do not relieve the situation. The best treatment is preventive, however, and careful pre- and postoperative care will be amply rewarded.

FOREIGN BODIES IN THE AIR PASSAGES

The importance of aspiration of a foreign body in the genesis of pulmonary disease is frequently overlooked. The physician fails to elicit the history, the patient may have forgotten the event because of a symptomless interval following aspiration, and the various clinical syndromes produced are more readily explained by invoking the commoner disease processes which are mimicked, such as asthma, lung abscess, or bronchiectasis.

In order of frequency, the foreign bodies found are nuts, hardware, pins and needles, dental material, safety pins, and bone. A variety of predisposing factors are known, such as weakening of the defenses against aspiration, bad personal hygiene (loose teeth), or hasty eating. Inhalation of vegetable material such as a peanut causes a severe local and systemic reaction because its shape allows complete occlusion of a bronchus and it also incites

a chemical bronchitis. Irregular metallic objects usually produce only incomplete blockage.

A foreign body may shift its location in the lung or be passed to the opposite lung. Those which lodge in the trachea give rise to a palpable thud, an audible slap, and loud wheeze when expiration or cough forces the object against the inferior surface of the vocal cords. Death from asphyxia may occur. When a bronchus is occluded so that there is a "check-valve" effect with expiratory trapping of air, there will be distal emphysema, but complete obstruction leads to atelectasis and, finally, to drowned lung.

The initial episode may be violently symptomatic with severe cough, wheezing, dyspnea, and cyanosis. Bronchoscopy is an immediate necessity and is successful in removing the foreign body in most cases. If the level of obstruction is in a lobar or segmental bronchus, the initial fit of coughing may be followed by a symptomless interval of days or weeks after which chronic suppurative disease (lung abscess, bronchiectasis) develops. The patient may finally show the clinical picture of "asthma" and localized hyperinflation of the lung, lung abscess, or bronchiectasis. Bronchoscopy may not reveal the foreign body as overgrowth of granulation tissue may have obscured it. X-ray may show the radiopaque object which may also be confused with calcified hilar lymph nodes. Even though symptoms have been present for several years, removal of the foreign body can lead to complete restoration of apparently damaged lung. Therefore after removal, observation under medical therapy is advisable before deciding about the need for lobectomy.

BRONCHOLITHIASIS

Broncholithiasis refers to calcified concretions occurring in the tracheobronchial tree. They may arise in three ways: (1) by calcification of tracheobronchial cartilage and subsequent sequestration, (2) by secondary calcification of an exogenous foreign body, or (3) most commonly by migration and erosion of calcified material from hilar and paratracheal nodes into the tracheobronchial tree. The calcified node is the "tombstone" of the original disease, usually tuberculosis or histoplasmosis.

The condition occurs in both sexes equally and is most common between the ages of forty and sixty years. Cough and hemoptysis are the commonest manifestations and are due to bronchial ulceration or to intrabronchial location of the stone, with resultant obstruction and bronchiectasis. Recurrent chills and fever and purulent sputum may be noted, and 50 per cent of patients give a history of coughing up one or more stones. Some complain of wheezing or "asthma" which is due to partial bronchial obstruction by the concretion. The right bronchial tree is involved twice as often as the left. Rarely, active tuberculosis is found distal to such an obstruction, and careful examination for tubercle bacilli is essential.

The x-ray reveals calcification of hilar or paratracheal nodes, atelectasis or pneumonitis with dense calcification at the apex of the affected lobe, or bronchiectasis on plain film or bronchography. Tomography may be necessary to delineate the relationship of calcification and bronchus.

The broncholith can be removed occasionally through the bronchoscope, but thoracotomy and broncholithotomy are usually necessary. Lobectomy is reserved for those patients who have persistent or recurrent symptoms or localized bronchiectasis.

LUNG ABSCESS

Etiology and Pathogenesis. The commonest etiologic factor in the development of primary lung abscess is aspiration of infected material from the upper respiratory tract, such as dental deposits (see above under Bronchial Obstruction). The virulence of the organisms and their ability to cause necrosis of tissue, the development of vascular occlusion due to septic endarteritis, and the pressure of increasing exudation combine to cause liquefaction of tissue within a few days. If the bronchus is eroded, partial drainage will lead to the formation of an air-fluid level. New abscesses or suppurative pneumonia can occur by direct extension or aspiration of pus into another segment. If healing is delayed, the cavity is lined by a downgrowth of cuboidal or squamous epithelium from connecting bronchi. Formerly, the differentiation of putrid (anaerobic) and nonputrid (aerobic) abscesses was stressed, but this is no longer regarded as important in therapy.

The following conditions predispose to abscess formation in the lung and should be considered in any patient with localized pulmonary suppuration:

Bronchial Obstruction. Most lung abscesses are initiated by bronchial occlusion, either by virtue of aspiration of infected material from the upper airway or the occurrence of an obstructing lesion, such as a tumor or postinflammatory bronchostenosis. Foreign body and bronchostenosis are relatively unusual. *Bronchogenic carcinoma* may be even commoner than aspiration as a condition leading to lung abscess in men beyond the age of forty-five. The abscess may be produced either by obstruction of the bronchus with distal stasis and infection of secretions or, more commonly, by necrosis and excavation within the tumor mass. Radiologically, the wall of the cavity is thick and irregular, the most important clue to the correct diagnosis.

Bacterial Pneumonia. Pneumonias due to the Friedländer bacillus, *actinomyces bovis,* pneumococcus type III, *Staphylococcus aureus,* and *Streptococcus hemolyticus* are occasionally complicated by true abscess formation because of the ability of these organisms to cause necrosis.

Vascular Embolism. Pulmonary infarction is a rare cause of abscess formation; less than 5 per cent of bland pulmonary infarcts are secondarily infected. Vascular embolization of infected material from osteomyelitis, suppurative pelvic disease (postabortal), or phlebitis (for example, in a drug addict) can result in multiple small pulmonary abscesses.

Other Causes. Trauma to the chest may result in abscess formation by penetration of the chest wall by an infected foreign body, by infection superimposed on a traumatic pulmonary hematoma—a very rare event—or because of retained secretions due to reduced cough following rib fracture.

Stasis of secretions or aspiration of infected secretions into a congenital or acquired cyst may result in localized suppuration and accumulation of pus. The finding of a very thin wall with minimal surrounding inflammation may be a radiologic clue.

Amebic or pyogenic abscesses in the liver or beneath the right diaphragm may extend into the right lower lobe of the lung and result in abscess formation.

Clinical Description. The patient may present himself to the physician with acute or chronic symptoms. Following the initiating event, such as tooth extraction or an alcoholic debauch, there is a several day period of fever and malaise (representing segmental atelectasis and pneumonitis) followed by chest pain, usually pleuritic (extension of suppurative pneumonitis to pleural surface), and a dry cough. Anywhere from 4 to 10 days after the onset, the cough and fever become more severe (gangrene of lung). Scanty amounts of purulent blood-streaked sputum (erosion of bronchus) precede acute rupture of the abscess into the bronchial tree. When this occurs, the sputum becomes copious, and up to a liter of purulent and sometimes bloody sputum may be produced for the next several days. As free drainage continues, illness begins to abate, although the temperature may not become normal for several more days. When severe respiratory distress and prostration occur suddenly after the onset of pleural pain, rupture of the abscess into the pleural space with the formation of a pyopneumothorax has probably occurred. In acute lung abscess, if drainage of the area and antibiotic treatment are adequate, the patient will be free of cough and sputum production and constitutional debility after 10 days to 3 weeks of treatment, although complete clearing by x-ray and closure of the cavity may take anywhere from 10 days to 4 months. If drainage is inadequate, the organism is resistant, or treatment is delayed, a necrotic slough forms in the cavity. Chronic cough and purulent sputum persist with intermittent fever and cachexia.

In the acute disease physical examination reveals a febrile, anxious patient with rapid pulse and respiratory rate. The oral hygiene is usually bad, and the gag reflex may be absent or diminished. Dullness and bronchial breath sounds and rarely a pleural friction rub may be heard over the diseased segment. Exquisite tenderness to palpation of the chest wall over the diseased area may be elicited because of pleural involvement. After bronchial communication has been established, amphoric breath sounds may be heard. Clubbing of fingers and toes is present within weeks of the onset in 10 to 20 per cent of cases and regresses with resolution of the disease. Rarely painful hypertrophic osteoarthropathy may occur, although this usually signifies underlying bronchogenic carcinoma.

Laboratory findings show a polymorphonuclear leukocytosis in the acute phase. With chronic lung abscess a normocytic normochromic anemia may develop.

The sputum is purulent and frequently bloody. Elastic fibers are present, indicating tissue destruction. Culture is essential and may reveal a single organism or varying combinations of beta- and alpha-hemolytic streptococci, staphylococci, occasionally pneumococci, *Hemophilus influenzae,* and *Escherichia coli.* Sensitivity to antibiotics must be determined. Anaerobic cultures will reveal the anaerobic streptococcus, fusiform bacilli, and spirochetal organisms. Sputum should also be examined for tubercle bacilli and malignant cells. Blood cultures obtained during the acute disease may yield the predominant pathogen.

Early in the disease the x-ray reveals segmental or lobar consolidation which assumes a spherical shape as the area distends with pus. Localization in the posterior segment of the right upper lobe or superior segment of the lower lobes should suggest the possibility of lung abscess. With rupture into the bronchial tree, an air fluid level appears. The wall of the abscess cavity should be inspected carefully. If very thin, with minimal surrounding pneumonitis, the process may represent infection of a preexisting congenital cyst or bulla. If irregular and thick, cavity formation in a bronchogenic carcinoma may be at fault. Abscess due to Friedländer's bacilli may be multiloculated with many fluid levels, and staphylococcic abscess is frequently multiple, small, and thin-walled in a peripheral, subpleural location.

Bronchoscopic examination is necessary, particularly in the patient past forty or in any patient with atypical features or delayed resolution, to rule out neoplasm as the underlying cause. In the child, foreign body must be considered.

Complications of lung abscess are very rare at present, with the exception of pyopneumothorax, and include exsanguinating hemorrhage, metastatic brain abscess, and secondary amyloidosis.

Differential diagnosis of the primary lung abscess includes tuberculosis, empyema with bronchopleural fistula, infected lung cyst, and peripheral carcinoma. Abscess formation must not be confused with the rarefied areas seen in a pneumonic consolidation undergoing normal resolution. Also transient ball-valve occlusion of the bronchus in an area of pneumonia may lead to acute tension cysts distinguished from lung abscess by their rapid onset and disappearance.

Treatment. The principles of treatment of lung abscess are similar to those involved in any suppuration—the establishment of adequate drainage and the eradication of infection (see also Chronic Empyema). Antibiotics and postural drainage are the mainstays of treatment. The longer the duration of symptoms prior to therapy, the less likely is medical cure, although every case deserves a trial of medical therapy initially. Treatment is begun with 2 million units of penicillin daily. The urgency of the situation and the results of culture dictate the need for an additional antibiotic to cover gram-negative organisms (see Chap. 268). Postural drainage is instituted, and its practice guided by the segmental localization of the abscess. A record of sputum volume is kept to follow the course of healing. Bronchoscopy may rarely be of therapeutic benefit. Tracheostomy and suctioning of secretions may be necessary in the weak or paralyzed patient. Clinical improvement occurs within days, and radiologic clearing usually becomes complete within 3 to 6 weeks. Segmental resection and lobectomy are reserved for those individuals who remain symptomatic and without continuous radiologic clearing during 3 to 6 weeks of continuous medical therapy.

MISCELLANEOUS TYPES OF PNEUMONIA

Aspiration Pneumonia

Aspiration pneumonia usually refers to the acute parenchymal inflammation associated with aspiration of infected material from the upper respiratory passages and to the condition associated with aspiration of water, food, or vomit. The same etiologic and pathogenic considerations described for lung abscess apply here, and indeed aspiration pneumonia will result in an abscess if necrosis is extensive. Aspiration of food and drink is particularly common in debilitated, elderly individuals. Patients with obstructing esophageal disease often develop chronic, bilateral lower lobe pneumonitis because of repeated aspiration.

Aspiration of gastric contents may occur in infancy and old age, in alcoholics and epileptics, and in subjects with head injuries, after the administration of drugs such as morphine, and during anesthesia. Maternal death during or following delivery may be due to aspiration of gastric contents. Rapid onset of acute toxemia occurs with high fever, tachycardia, cyanosis, tachypnea, and extreme dyspnea. Rhonchi and bubbling rales may be heard over the lower lobes. The x-ray shows bilateral lower lobe infiltrates with indistinct borders. There is necrotizing bronchopneumonia with hemorrhage, edema, and often multiple abscess. Treatment consists of immediate suctioning of the tracheobronchial tree and bronchoscopy as soon as possible. Penicillin and streptomycin should be given. Corticosteroids have been advocated to quell the chemical inflammation, although their effectiveness is not established.

Lipid Pneumonia

Lipid pneumonia is due to the repeated aspiration of animal oil (halibut and cod liver oil, milk, and egg yolk), vegetable oil (castor, olive, and wheat germ oil), or mineral oil. In the adult subject, the condition is almost invariably due to the chronic administration of mineral oil as a laxative or to drugs administered in an oily vehicle, such as nose drops. The condition is seen most frequently in elderly, bedridden, and chronically ill individuals, in short, those apt to have difficulty swallowing and to suffer from constipation necessitating the use of laxatives. Mineral oil apparently incites no cough reflex and moves unimpeded into the tracheobronchial tree. As it is chemically inert, it acts as a foreign body and incites a chronic inflammatory and granulomatous reaction. The disease is usually seen as a bilateral, lower lobe process but may rarely be confined to one lobe and simulate neoplasm (paraffinoma).

Clinically, nonspecific symptoms of mild cough and signs of scattered rales at the lung bases may be elicited. Most frequently the condition is asymptomatic and is discovered unexpectedly on routine x-ray examination.

The x-ray reveals increased lung markings, most notable at the lung bases early in the disease and scattered nodular and irregular infiltrates which become confluent in more advanced cases. Sometimes a local circumscribed density simulates bronchogenic carcinoma. The right lower lobe is the most frequent site of such a paraffinoma; hilar lymph nodes are not enlarged.

Examination of fresh sputum reveals characteristic macrophages filled with vacuoles which stain positively for fat with Sudan III or IV. Their appearance may be intermittent, however, and several sputum examinations should be done.

The vital capacity is reduced in cases with extensive involvement, indicating a restrictive ventilatory defect due to replacement of air spaces with fat-laden inflammatory tissue.

The only treatment is cessation of the use of oil. When the disease is localized, pulmonary neoplasm must be excluded and exploratory thoracotomy may be necessary; when the disease is diffuse, tuberculosis and the diseases associated with interstitial fibrosis should be ruled out. One should not confuse cholesterol (or lipid) pneumonitis of endogenous origin (see p. 1528) with lipid pneumonia of exogenous origin.

Loeffler's Pneumonia and Pulmonary Eosinophilia

In 1932, Loeffler described a syndrome of transient pulmonary infiltration associated with peripheral blood eosinophilia and minimal or no symptoms. Mild cough, lassitude, and low-grade fever were associated with migrating, fleeting nodular pulmonary densities and mild leukocytosis with eosinophiles to 20 per cent of the total differential count. The disease was benign and self-limited, rarely lasted more than 3 weeks, and left no residual lesion. Although Loeffler initially thought this might be a manifestation of tuberculosis, subsequent studies by himself and others revealed infestation by ascaris in some patients.

Since that time the association of pulmonary infiltration and peripheral eosinophilia has been described in a wide variety of conditions, and the term PIE syndrome (pulmonary infiltration with eosinophilia) has been used. Thus collagen disease, such as polyarteritis nodosa, malignant neoplastic disease, bronchial asthma, tropical eosinophilia, the Hamman-Rich syndrome, sarcoidosis, allergic reactions to drugs such as penicillin, the sulfonamides, PAS, organic arsenicals, barbiturates, and thiouracil, certain infectious diseases such as tuberculosis, coccidiodomyocosis, brucellosis, or exposure to the privet plant, mite infection, and parasitic infestation have all been described as causes. The following parasites have been associated with the syndrome: *Ascaris lumbricoides*, *Necator americanus*, *Trichinella spiralis*, *Fasciola hepatica*, *Strongyloides stercoralis*, and *Ancylostoma brasiliense*. In the case of some of these parasites, such as ascaris, larval migration through the lung doubtless gives rise to the syndrome and explains its transient, benign, and self-limited course.

The diagnosis of Loeffler's syndrome should be limited to cases conforming to his original description. In cases associated with persistence of symptoms and recurrence of x-ray abnormalities with marked systemic reaction, a hypersensitivity angiitis such as polyarteritis nodosa must be considered.

Tropical eosinophilia should be considered under similar circumstances, particularly in India and Ceylon or in natives from these countries. The condition consists of cough, paroxysmal dyspnea with bronchospastic, asthmatic attacks, splenomegaly in 50 per cent of cases, a positive Wassermann or Kahn reaction (which reverts after specific therapy), a high titer of cold agglutinins, and an x-ray showing bilateral mottled shadows. The sputum may contain many eosinophils. The white blood cell count ranges from 12,000 to 80,000, with 20 to 80 per cent eosinophils. A curious subacute degenerative syndrome affecting the cerebellum has been associated with the condition, being especially well documented in the French medical literature. Over 35 per cent of the cases respond to arsenical therapy, and this has been considered a diagnostic feature. It differs from Loeffler's syndrome in the presence of marked systemic reaction, persistence and chronicity of symptoms and x-ray findings, the striking response to arsenical therapy, and the occurrence of relapse in occasional cases.

Present theories of the causation of Loeffler's syndrome favor a local hypersensitivity state in the lung. Bronchial asthma, hypersensitivity angiitis, or polyarteritis nodosa may represent other more dire manifestations of similar immunologic processes.

CYSTIC DISEASE OF THE LUNG

Cysts of the lung may be either congenital or acquired, solitary or multiple. The congenital origin of cystic disease has been presumed because of its occurrence in infancy and childhood and its association with congenital heart disease, polycystic disease of the liver or kidneys, dextrocardia, and aberrant pulmonary vessels (pulmonary sequestration). Congenital cysts are of bronchial origin. Presumably, maldevelopment and failure of maturation of the terminal bronchial passages result in blind rests lined with bronchial epithelium, which usually communicate with the bronchial tree.

Acquired cysts develop from the rupture and coalescence of alveoli and are thus "alveolar in origin." When the air collection lies between visceral pleura and lung substance it is termed a *bleb*. They occur commonly at the apices and ordinarily have little functional significance. The term *bulla* refers to an air space more than 1 cm in diameter, situated in the substance of the lung, and frequently seen in association with obstructive pulmonary emphysema. Acquired cysts may be seen as a sequel to lung abscess (due to epithelialization of the cavity), pneumonia, tuberculosis,

fungous disease such as coccidiodomycosis, or echinococcus disease.

Air cysts are ordinarily asymptomatic. The patient may suffer one or more of the complications which are (1) infection, (2) hemorrhage, (3) rupture of blebs or subpleural cysts with pneumothorax formation or rupture of bullae with interstitial and mediastinal emphysema, and (4) respiratory insufficiency. Repeated infection is what usually necessitates surgical removal of the diseased area. Communication with the bronchial tree determines the clinical behavior and functional deficit. The cyst may be air filled and remain stable in size over long periods if it communicates freely. If the opening is small and is intermittently occluded, the cyst may enlarge progressively as air trapping occurs on expiration and may intermittently become infected and fluid filled. In infancy large unilateral cysts called pneumatoceles may develop rapidly in association with pneumonia and occupy the entire hemithorax. In adults, a progressively enlarging bullous lesion may replace an entire lung and is referred to as the "vanishing lung syndrome." Multiple cysts are usually bilateral and may simulate bronchiectasis in their clinical course.

The development of respiratory insufficiency depends on the communication of the cyst, its size and the degree of parenchymal replacement or compression, and the presence of obstructive emphysema. If the cyst is large and communicates freely with the bronchial tree, the effect is an increase in dead space ventilation, as the wall of the cyst is poorly vascular and gas exchange does not occur. If the cyst communicates poorly or intermittently with the respiratory tree, air trapping and, as the cyst grows larger, compression of the surrounding parenchyma occur. Obstruction to air flow and reduction in lung volume may be seen, and dyspnea is thus due to both obstructive and restrictive ventilatory defects. Arterial oxygen unsaturation occurs if ventilation to surrounding parenchyma is reduced more than perfusion, leading to a venous admixture effect.

The presence of associated obstructive emphysema must be detected prior to surgical removal of pulmonary cysts. Fluoroscopic demonstration of contralateral air trapping and restriction of diaphragmatic motion, great reduction in maximal breathing capacity, and large increase in residual lung volume may be helpful differential points. The finding of respiratory acidosis with an elevated CO_2 tension in the arterial blood nearly always indicates the presence of underlying, severe obstructive emphysema and virtually precludes surgical therapy. This is not true of oxyhemoglobin unsaturation as an isolated abnormality of the blood gases, as this may be relieved by surgical excision of a large cyst.

Physical examination may be unremarkable. Tracheal deviation may be seen with large unilateral, poorly communicating cysts as well as mediastinal shifting toward the lesion on inspiration and away on expiration. Rales may be heard if there is infection or bronchiectasis adjacent to the cyst. Large unilateral air cysts simulate pneumothorax with hyperresonance, decreased or absent breath sounds, and tracheal deviation.

Radiologically the cysts are usually thin-walled and multiple but may be solitary and easily confused with lung abscess, bronchiectasis, chronic nonspecific pneumonitis, staphylococcic pneumonia, and tuberculosis. Pneumothorax and encapsulated empyema with bronchopleural fistula must also be differentiated. Generally the same principles of medical treatment apply here as in lung abscess (see p. 1555).

CHRONIC EMPYEMA

Chronic empyema is a persistent collection of pus or fibropurulent material in the pleural space. In over 75 per cent of cases, the cause is inadequate treatment of acute empyema. Underlying lung disease such as bronchiectasis, lung abscess, tuberculosis, mycotic infection such as actinomycosis, and bronchogenic carcinoma may be the initiating process which has rendered the condition chronic and difficult to treat. Other causes for chronicity include the formation of a bronchopleural fistula leading to repeated infection of the area. Occasionally a foreign body is present in the empyema cavity, such as a rubber drain or a sponge left behind from previous drainage.

The pathologic change is essentially one of intense fibrous thickening of visceral and parietal pleura due to chronic fibrin deposition and organization. The cavity may be multiloculated because of formation of fibrous septums. If the underlying lung is diseased, as in tuberculosis or bronchiectasis, fusion of the visceral pleura with parenchyma may be such that separation is impossible.

The history may extend anywhere from 6 weeks to 20 years or more. It is of utmost importance to obtain details of the diagnosis and treatment of the acute illness, usually pneumonia. A history of tuberculosis, previous thoracic surgery, bronchiectasis, or in the case of older subjects, one suggestive of bronchogenic carcinoma may provide the etiologic clue and thus direct management. The symptoms of chronic empyema may be surprisingly few as in tuberculosis where the pleural infection may remain latent for years. A poorly productive cough with recurrent febrile episodes, chronic fatigue and malnutrition, intermittent drainage of pus from the scarred site of previous drainage, and moderate dyspnea may occur. Intermittent expectoration of purulent sputum may indicate the presence of bronchopleural fistula.

The physical signs depend on the duration of the process. The scar of a previous drainage site may contain a small cutaneous fistula and intermittently discharge pus and air. The hemithorax is contracted and poorly expansile. Its muscles are wasted. Scoliosis may be present, with the convexity toward the normal hemithorax. The percussion note is dull and the breath sounds are decreased or bronchial if underlying lung is sufficiently compressed. Amphoric breath sounds and air bubbling through fluid may be heard in the presence of a bronchopleural fistula. Clubbing may occur. Secondary amyloidosis and cerebral abscess are unusual complications. Penetration of the chronic infection through the intercostal soft tissue with spontaneous drainage through the skin of the chest wall may occur rarely (empyema necessitatis), but particularly with mycotic infection.

The normochromic, normocytic anemia of chronic infection may be seen along with the hypoproteinemia of malnutrition. Persistent albuminuria may be found if secondary amyloidosis has involved the kidneys.

Roentgenograms of the chest reveal an asymmetrically small hemithorax with crowded ribs which may appear to overlap ("tiling"). An area of rib resection and bizarre, irregular periosteal proliferation may be seen in previously treated cases. The area of empyema may be represented by radiopacity of the entire hemithorax, or there may only be a basilar density obscuring the hemidiaphragm with a rim of thickened pleura extending to the apex of the lung. An air-fluid level may be seen if a bronchopleural fistula is present. A grid film may reveal the condition of the underlying lung as well as demonstrating the thickness of the pleural walls of the empyema cavity. Calcification of the pleura may be seen in cases due to tuberculosis or infected hemothorax.

The thickened pleura encases and compresses the lung, preventing its expansion and contraction. The vital capacity is reduced in proportion to the severity of the restrictive ventilatory defect and accurately mirrors its extent. Dyspnea of more than a mild degree is unusual when the contralateral lung is normal. When extensive underlying pulmonary disease is present (e.g., tuberculosis, bronchiectasis), the entire lung may be nearly functionless and represents a "physiologic autopneumonectomy." The extent of the underlying lung disease and the duration of the empyema determine the degree of functional improvement following therapy (e.g., pleural decortication). The disease may have been present for years, and still reexpansion and excellent return of function may occur following surgery.

The management of chronic empyema depends on the etiology and the presence or absence of underlying pulmonary disease. Thoracentesis with withdrawal of fluid for examination and culture (routine as well as for tubercle bacilli and fungi) is necessary. The fluid is purulent or fibropurulent and has a high specific gravity (>1.028) and protein content (>4.5 Gm per 100 ml). Varying numbers of polymorphonuclear leukocytes and lymphocytes may be present along with much amorphous debris. Lymphocytic effusions with absence or paucity of mesothelial cells should arouse suspicion of tuberculosis. A pleural biopsy should be done at the time of thoracentesis with the Vim-Silverman needle. If this is unrevealing (as regards fungous disease or tuberculosis), a generous biopsy should be obtained at the time of surgical therapy. The extent of the empyema sac should be determined by introducing air or radiopaque material after diagnostic thoracentesis. If there is any suggestion of underlying lung disease, bronchoscopy and bronchography should be considered, as the results will have a direct bearing on therapy and prognosis. Culture of secretions obtained at bronchoscopy should be done both routinely and for tubercle bacilli. Tuberculin and fungus skin testing as well as gastric aspiration for culture of the tubercle bacillus should be done where indicated.

The principles of successful treatment are eradication of infection and obliteration of the empyema space, with freeing of the underlying lung. Thoracotomy with local rib resection and drainage of the empyema sac under cover of appropriate antibiotic therapy is usually the first step. Excision of the empyema sac and pleural decortication may be necessary ultimately. Drainage and local thoracoplasty are occasionally employed to obliterate the cavity. In some cases with extensive parenchymal disease, pneumonectomy is performed.

It is important to distinguish the postpneumonic empyema, now sterile and resolving slowly in a clinically well individual, from the chronically infected collection adversely affecting the patient. Very frequently persistence with conservative therapy will result in complete resolution in the former, while it may do great harm in the latter situation.

REFERENCES

BRONCHIAL OBSTRUCTION
AND PULMONARY ATELECTASIS

Churchill, E. D.: The Architectural Basis of Pulmonary Ventilation, Ann. Surg., 137:1, 1953.

Dripps, R. D., and M. V. Deming: Postoperative Atelectasis and Pneumonia, Ann. Surg., 124:94, 1946.

Knowles, J. H.: Pulmonary Function Tests and Thoracic Surgery, pp. 228–243, in "Surgery: A Concise Guide to Clinical Practice," G. L. Nardi and G. D.

Zuidema (Eds.), Boston, Little, Brown & Company, 1961.

Spain, D. M.: Acute Nonaeration of Lung: Edema Versus Atelectasis, Diseases Chest, 25:550, 1954.

BRONCHIECTASIS

Mallory, T. B.: The Pathogenesis of Bronchiectasis, New Engl. J. Med., 237:795, 1947.

Perry, K. M. A., and D. S. King: Bronchiectasis: Study of Prognosis Based on a Follow-up of 400 Patients, Am. Rev. Tuberc., 41:531, 1940.

Wynn-Williams, N.: Bronchiectasis: A Study Centered on Bedford and Its Environs, Brit. Med. J., 1:1194, 1953.

——: Observations on the Treatment of Bronchiectasis and Its Relation to Prognosis, Tubercle, 38:133, 1957.

BRONCHOLITHIASIS

Moersch, H. J., and H. W. Schmidt: Broncholithiasis, Ann. Otol., Rhinol. & Laryngol., 68:548, 1959.

CHRONIC EMPYEMA

Lindskog, G. E., and A. A. Liebow: Chronic Empyema, p. 62, in "Thoracic Surgery and Related Pathology," New York, Appleton-Century-Crofts, Inc., 1953.

Sellors, T. H., and G. Cruickshank: Chronic Empyema, Brit. J. Surg., 38:411, 1951.

CYSTIC DISEASE OF THE LUNG

Baldwin, E. deF., K. A. Harden, D. C. Greene, A. Cournand, and D. W. Richards, Jr.: Pulmonary Insufficiency IV. A Study of 16 Cases of Large Pulmonary Air Cysts or Bullae, Medicine, 29:169, 1950.

Sellors, T. H.: Congenital Cystic Disease of the Lung, Tubercle, 20:49, 114, 1938.

Siebens, A. A., A. R. Grant, D. C. Kent, R. Klopstock, and J. J. Cincotti: Pulmonary Cystic Disease: Physiologic Studies and Results of Resection, J. Thoracic Surg., 33:185, 1957.

FOREIGN BODIES IN THE AIR PASSAGES

Jackson, C., and C. L. Jackson: "Bronchoesophagology," Sec. III, pp. 13, 106, Foreign Bodies in the Air and Food Passages, Philadelphia, W. B. Saunders Company, 1950.

Linton, J. S. A.: Long-standing Intrabronchial Foreign Bodies, Thorax, 12:164, 1957.

LUNG ABSCESS

Amberson, J. B.: A Clinical Consideration of Abscesses and Cavities of the Lung, Bull. Johns Hopkins Hosp., 94:227, 1954.

Brock, R. C.: "Lung Abscess," Oxford, Blackwell Scientific Publications, 1952.

MISCELLANEOUS TYPES OF PNEUMONIA

Berg, J. R., and T. H. Burford: Pulmonary Paraffinoma (Lipoid Pneumonia), A Critical Study, J. Thoracic Surg., 20:418, 1950.

Gardner, A. M. N.: Aspiration of Food and Vomit, Quart. J. Med. (n.s.), 27:227, 1958.

Loeffler, W.: Die fluchtigen lungen Infiltrate mit Eosinophile, Schweiz. med. Wochschr., 66:1069, 1936.

Reader, W. H., and B. E. Goodrich: Pulmonary Infiltration with Eosinophilia (PIE Syndrome), Ann. Internal Med., 36:1217, 1952.

Viswanathan, R.: Pulmonary Eosinophilosis, Quart. J. Med., (n.s.), 17:257, 1949.

Volk, B. W., L. Nathanon, S. Sosner, W. B. Slade, and M. Jacobi: Incidence of Lipoid Pneumonia in a Survey of 389 Chronically Ill Patients, Am. J. Med., 10:316, 1951.

265 NEOPLASMS OF THE LUNG

Champ Lyons

CARCINOMA OF THE BRONCHUS

The great majority of the neoplasms of the lung arise within the wall or epithelial lining of the bronchus, either centrally or peripherally. About half of all bronchogenic carcinomas are squamous cell types. About one-third are highly anaplastic and are designated as undifferentiated carcinoma. These two types occur predominantly in males. There is considerable sentiment to indict the smoking of cigarettes in the genesis of lung cancer, but there are still two sides to the question. More clearly carcinogenic are the industrial exposures in the mining of radioactive ores, the refining of nickel, the manufacture of chromates and coal gas, and the processing of arsenic and asbestos. The siliceous dusts, as encountered in mining, do not seem to increase the vulnerability of the lung to cancer.

About one-fifth of bronchogenic cancers are adenocarcinoma. These occur with almost equal frequency in females, and it has been suggested that they arise from embryonic bronchial buds. They are usually highly malignant.

Early lymphatic and vascular invasion are so constantly a feature of bronchogenic carcinoma that initial symptoms in many cases are attributable to metastases. These involve the mediastinal and supraclavicular lymph nodes, brain, bone, adrenal cortex, liver, and subcutaneous tissues. Tumors arising in the apex of the lung may invade directly the brachial plexus and subclavian vessels producing neuritic pain, Horner's syndrome, and vasomotor crises in the hand and arm, the *Pancoast syndrome*

of superior sulcus tumor. Secondary involvement of the superior mediastinum may compress the superior vena cava, with resulting edema and venous suffusion of the face, neck, and arms, the *superior vena caval syndrome.* Less frequently, direct invasion of the esophagus behind the heart may be responsible for obscure dysphagia.

Another pattern of symptoms is to be attributed to the encroachment of the tumor upon the lumen of the bronchus or bronchiole. With partial occlusion of the lumen there is persistent cough, asthmatic breathing, and x-ray evidence of localized emphysema. As the obstruction becomes complete, there is atelectasis, recurrent pneumonitis, distal bronchiectasis, and occasionally, lung abscess. Hemoptysis is fairly common in both the early and the late stages.

Extrapulmonary manifestations unrelated to metastatic spread may dominate the initial symptomatology. Clubbing of the fingers, with or without painfully swollen joints (pulmonary osteoarthropathy), is the most frequent peripheral sign of bronchogenic carcinoma. Migratory phlebitis and peripheral neuropathy are similarly associated as are, less commonly, hypercalcemia and Cushing's syndrome.

Apart from the demonstration of localized emphysema and segmental atelectasis, the most suggestive x-ray finding is that of a hilar density extending peripherally (see Fig. 265-1). Bronchoscopy permits visualization and biopsy of the primary tumor in 40 to 60 per cent of the cases. Cytologic study of the sputum, in expert hands, may permit diagnosis in 85 per cent, and is especially useful for peripheral tumors. Early recourse to exploratory thoracotomy with biopsy of the primary tumor or regional nodes is the procedure of choice in any controversial diagnosis. Contrast bronchography is rarely indicated.

The treatment of choice for bronchogenic carcinoma is radical pneumonectomy. It is of great clinical concern that about one-half of the symptomatic patients, presenting at an average lapse of 5 months from onset, are rejected for operation on the basis of local extension or distant metastases. About one-third of the symptomatic cases prove to be resectable, and the 5-year survival rate is about 6 per cent. In older patients with reduced respiratory reserve, less radical resections, such as lobectomy or partial pneumonectomy with plastic reconstruction of the bronchus, have proved practical without apparent reduction in the salvage rate. X-ray treatment and nitrogen mustard therapy occasionally retard the rate of growth and spread.

Identification of the presence of a tumor *before the onset of symptoms* remains the chief hope for greater salvage. Mass radiography for tuberculosis has provided numerous instances of the silent and "solitary nodule." Many of these have proved to be totally resectable cancers. The problem of early recognition of cancer of the lung is now so pressing that all males over forty should have x-ray examination of the chest at intervals of 6 months. It is to be expected that refinement of cytologic techniques may contribute to early diagnosis.

Carcinoma of the bronchus should also be suspected whenever any individual in the susceptible age group shows delayed resolution of any intrapulmonary inflammation. The unresolved pneumonia or a lung abscess or pneumonia recurrent in the same lobe in males over forty should invite immediate study for tumor.

The Problem of the Solitary Pulmonary Nodule. Occasionally, a roentgenogram of the chest may reveal a nodule, less than 6 cm in diameter, which is fairly sharply delineated from adjacent pulmonary tissue. Such lesions have been designated *solitary pulmonary nodules,* in preference to the term *coin lesions.* About one-third of these are peripheral bronchogenic carcinomas, demonstrable as such only after excision. (Simple lobectomy can be expected to result in a cure in 75 per cent of these patients.) In the absence of other diagnostic aids, thoracotomy is indicated by the x-ray findings in most cases. Ten per cent of such lesions are metastatic neoplasms, and about half are granulomas, with histoplasma, tuberculosis, and coccidioidomycosis responsible in that order. Hamartomas, lipid granulomas, lipid granulomas from oily nose drops, and pulmonary sequestrations also produce this picture. A nonoperative program of continued observation may be elected when a review of earlier films demonstrates no change over a period of 5 years, but it should be realized that such nodules have been followed for 8 years, only to declare themselves as cancers. Considerable interest in radiologically demonstrable calcium deposits has demonstrated that "flecks" of calcium may occur in bronchogenic cancers. A central core or concentric lamellations of calcium are indicative of granuloma. (See also Table p. 1509, Some of the Causes of Puzzling Radiologic Pulmonary Shadows.)

BRONCHIOLAR CARCINOMA

This disease has been known as *pulmonary adenomatosis,* but the ultimately fatal outcome and the increasing recognition of regional and distant metastases render suspect the identity of completely benign pulmonary adenomatosis. It is not certain whether the tumor cells are derived from the basal cells of the terminal bronchioles or from the lining membrane of the alveoli. Usage dictates preference for *alveolar cell carcinoma,* or *bronchiolar carcinoma.* There occurs in sheep a contagious

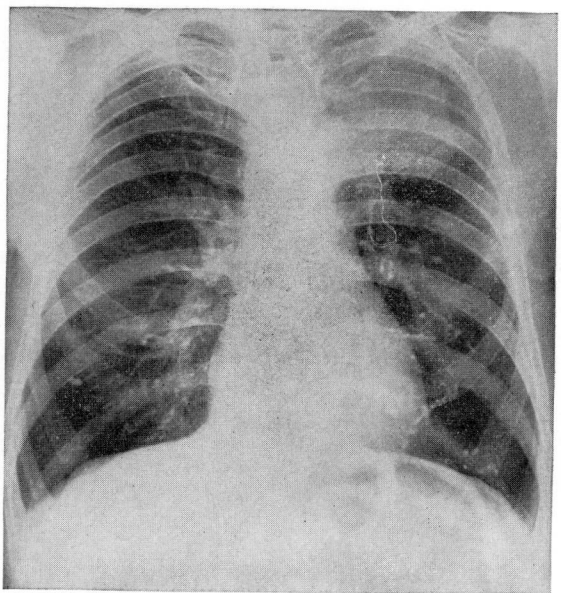

FIG. 265-1. Carcinoma of the bronchus.

disease, of presumptive viral etiology, known as *jaagziekte* in South Africa, and as *Montana chronic progressive pneumonia* in the United States. This disease is not transmissible to man, but is characterized by hyperplasia of cuboidal epithelial cells within the alveoli in striking similarity to the neoplastic disease of man.

The tumor appears to arise from multicentric foci, and ultimately involves both lungs. Both sexes are susceptible, and the usual age of onset is in the fourth and fifth decades. Symptoms begin insidiously, often following an acute respiratory infection. Cytologic examination of the sputum, even in early cases, frequently reveals tumor cells. Dyspnea, because of faulty gas exchange, is out of proportion to x-ray findings. Cough productive of the typically viscid pinkish sputum is a manifestation of the tumor. Terminally, there is frank hemoptysis with clubbing, intense cyanosis, recurrent pneumonitis, and evidence of metastasis. Nodular and confluent patterns of the disease are recognized.

The treatment of choice is surgical excision of the initially involved lobe or lobes, when practical. There is some hope of palliation by x-ray therapy, but nitrogen mustard appears useless.

ADENOMA OF THE BRONCHUS

The bronchial adenoma is a locally invasive and occasionally metastasizing tumor derived from the mucous glands of the bronchus and requiring separate classification from the more rapidly growing bronchogenic carcinomas. It constitutes about 3 per cent of all lung tumors and differs from

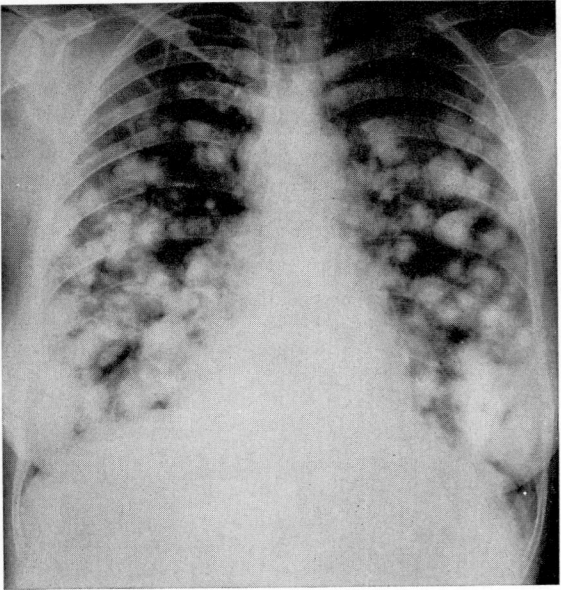

FIG. 265-2. Hematogenous metastasis from sarcoma of the ileum marked by intense dyspnea and cyanosis. (*Courtesy, Dr. C. L. Martin.*)

bronchogenic carcinoma in that it is usually apparent before the fifth decade, lacks sexual predilection, and develops metastases persisting for long periods without apparent change.

Histologically the adenomas show a peculiar epithelial proliferation and an equally peculiar stroma. Inclusions of bone are thought to represent metaplasia from chronic infection. The mixed tumor (cylindroma) type (10 per cent) is somewhat more invasive than the carcinoid adenoma (90 per cent). There is still controversy about these tumors as regards etiology, the occurrence of mixed types, the absence of argentaffin granules in the types designated as carcinoid, and their relationship to other polypoid tumors of the bronchial wall.

The adenoma syndrome is the clinical consequence of the slow growth of a vascular tumor producing major bronchial occlusion in a young person, i.e., hemoptysis, asthmatic wheezes, obstructive emphysema, recurrent pneumonitis, and the complications therefrom: bleeding, atelectasis, bronchiectasis, pleuritis, lung abscess, and empyema. The lower lobes are more often affected, and there is a slightly greater incidence on the right side. Contrast radiography (bronchography or tomography) often demonstrates the tumor, but routine x-rays are noncontributory in about one-fifth of the cases. About 90 per cent of the tumors may be recognized bronchoscopically by their polypoid appearance, mobility, vascularity, and absence of ulcerations. The vascularity dictates caution in the indicated biopsy. The lack of ulceration explains

the absence of tumor cells in sputum and bronchial washings.

Older methods of piecemeal excision by repeated bronchoscopic nibblings have largely been replaced by direct surgical removal of the primary tumor, the involved hilar lymph nodes, and the secondarily diseased lung. Exceptions to pneumonectomy consist of lobectomy for the more peripheral tumor without involvement of hilar nodes, and bronchotomy for the small tumor with a tiny stalk. Long term survival is the rule, especially for the carcinoid adenomas. Mediastinal recurrence and hepatic metastases are an especial hazard of the mixed tumor adenomas (cylindromas). There is some evidence to suggest that true bronchogenic carcinoma may occasionally develop within an adenoma.

METASTATIC TUMORS OF THE LUNG

Metastasis to the lung results from infarction with tumor emboli carried by the peripheral veins. The x-ray appearance is frequently characteristic and may appear as a solitary "cannonball" nodule, multiple nodules (see Fig. 265-2), or miliary dissemination known as *lymphangitic carcinomatosis* (see Fig. 265-3). It is hazardous to make an x-ray diagnosis of lymphangitic carcinomatosis of the lung in the absence of clinical evidence of alveolar capillary block, namely, severe dyspnea and obvious cyanosis. Sarcomas, hypernephromas, melanomas,

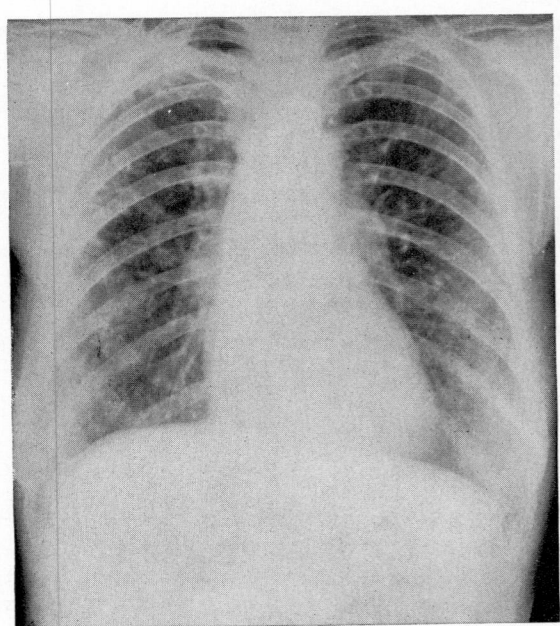

FIG. 265-3. So-called "lymphangitic carcinomatosis," metastatic from a carcinoma of the cervix. (*Courtesy, Dr. C. L. Martin.*)

and tumors of the testicle, breast, thyroid, and pancreas seem to find the lung an especially favorable site for the growth of metastases.

Dyspnea and pleuritic pain are the cardinal symptoms of lung metastases. Erosion into the bronchial tree may be associated with cough, hemoptysis, and occasionally, with tumor cells in the sputum. Treatment is largely palliative, with opiates and repeated thoracenteses to relieve the pain and dyspnea. Irradiation may prove helpful for sensitive tumors, but more reliance is placed upon hormonal or isotope approaches for specific tumors.

In the course of exploratory thoracotomy for asymptomatic solitary nodules, it occasionally happens that a metastasis from a previously unidentified primary tumor is found. The ground rules for deliberate surgical excision of solitary lung metastases include prior control of the primary focus, lapse of a reasonable length of time between initial treatment and appearance of the lung metastasis, and absence of other areas of tumor recurrence.

PRIMARY TUMORS OF THE PLEURA

Localized pleural tumors are usually proved to be mesenchymonas of subpleural mesodermal elements or granulomatous inclusion cysts complicating interlobular inflammation. Primary pleural neoplasms are restricted to the mesothelioma. This may occur as a localized tumor, frequently arising from the visceral pleura or embedded in the lung and distinctively associated with clubbing and arthralgia which disappear after removal of the tumor. The diffuse mesotheliomas require difficult differentiation from metastatic anaplastic carcinoma with pleural effusion and are characterized by a comparably intractable course. Treatment is limited to repeated thoracenteses, radiation therapy, and instillation of radioactive gold as palliative procedures.

REFERENCES

Benoit, H. W., Jr., and L. V. Ackerman: Solitary Pleural Mesotheliomas, J. Thoracic Surg., 25:346, 1953.

Churchill, E. D.: Primary Carcinoma of the Lung, J.A.M.A., 137:455, 1948.

Davis, E. W., J. W. Peabody, Jr., and S. Katz: The Solitary Pulmonary Nodule—A Ten-year Study Based on 215 Cases, J. Thoracic Surg., 32:728, 1956.

Habein, H. C., Jr., O. T. Clagett, and J. R. McDonald: Pulmonary Resection for Metastatic Tumors, A.M.A. Arch. Surg., 78:716, 1959.

Knowles, J. H., and L. H. Smith, Jr.: Medical Progress: Extrapulmonary Manifestations of Bronchogenic Carcinoma, New Engl. J. Med., 262:505, 1960.

Lawrence, G. H., J. H. Walker, and L. Pinkers: Extended Resection of Bronchogenic Carcinoma, New Engl. J. Med., 263:615, 1960.

Soutter, L., R. C. Sniffen, and L. L. Robbins: Clinical Survey of Adenomas of Trachea and Bronchus in General Hospital, J. Thoracic Surg., 28:412, 1954.

Storey, C. F., K. P. Knudtson, and B. J. Lawrence: Bronchiolar (Alveolar Cell) Carcinoma of Lung, J. Thoracic Surg., 26:331, 1953.

Editorial: Cancer of the Lung in Industry. Brit. Med. J., Sept. 24, 1955, p. 780.

266 DISEASES OF THE PLEURA, MEDIASTINUM, AND DIAPHRAGM

Ben V. Branscomb and T. R. Harrison

THE PLEURA

Hydrothorax

The typical physical signs of the accumulation of noninflammatory fluid in the pleural cavity include prominence of the interspaces on the affected side, which displays a dull to flat percussion note with diminution of breath sounds and of spoken and whispered voice. The heart and trachea tend to be displaced toward the normal side of the chest, and the circumference of the involved side may be demonstrably greater by measurement. Certain aspects of this disorder have been considered in the chapter dealing with congestive heart failure, which is much the commonest cause. Less frequently, hydrothorax may occur in persons with hypoproteinemia due to nephrosis or cirrhosis, or it may be caused by neoplastic or traumatic disorders involving the thoracic duct. In the latter instance the fluid is chylous, with a milky appearance due to the presence of fat droplets. The mechanism of the accumulations of pleural fluid associated with benign tumors of the ovary (Meig's syndrome) remains to be clarified.

An unusual variety of hydrothorax is that due to an interlobar effusion. The resulting rounded mass is likely to be confused with a neoplastic shadow but tends to disappear as cardiac failure improves (phantom tumor). The distinction of the noninflammatory hydrothorax from effusions due to pleuritis is discussed below. The treatment is that of the underlying cause of the condition plus the withdrawal of fluid by puncture when this is needed for the relief of dyspnea (p. 1564).

Pleuritis

The widespread radiation of pain arising from pleural irritation has been previously considered

(p. 15). The cardinal feature of the pain is its sharp stabbing quality, with aggravation by deep inspiration and, particularly, by the more sudden respiratory acts such as coughing and sneezing.

Inflammation of the pleura is commonly due to infections, the most frequent being tuberculous, the bacterial pneumonias, and the various viral diseases which affect the respiratory tract. Much less frequently pleuritis is the result of the spread from below of a subdiaphragmatic or hepatic abscess. Ischemic pleuritis consequent to pulmonary infarction is perhaps the second commonest cause. However, pleural involvement due to collagen disease, especially by rheumatic fever or disseminated lupus, or to neoplasm is not unusual. Trauma is an occasional cause.

Fibrinous Pleurisy. Acute fibrinous or dry pleurisy occurs in most persons at some time in their lives and is rarely serious. The clinical manifestations are those of the associated causative disease, which is usually a respiratory infection, pleural pain, and the characteristic friction rub, which is absent in many instances. This pleural friction sound must be distinguished from respiratory wheezes.

Fibrinous pleurisy must be distinguished from pain arising in the structures of the chest wall and, particularly, from fractured rib. The latter condition may also produce pain on breathing but is especially apt to be accompanied by discomfort on specific motions of the body, such as turning or twisting, and may be associated with exquisite tenderness over a sharply localized area.

The treatment of dry pleurisy is largely that of the causative disorder. If pain persists despite voluntary restriction of respiratory excursion, mechanical measures which limit chest motion may be used. These include lying on the affected side, the use of chest binders to limit intercostal and promote diaphragmatic excursion, and strapping of the affected area with adhesive plaster. If a productive cough is present, binders should not be used. Here, application of heat, spraying the chest with ethyl chloride, or occasionally intercostal nerve block will be helpful.

Pleuritis with Effusion (Serofibrinous Pleurisy). In general, the seriousness of pleural effusion depends on that of the underlying cause. However, the effusion itself may produce dyspnea due either to the marked encroachment on lung volume or to the shallow breathing made necessary by the pain. Pronounced pleural reaction, such as sometimes occurs with effusions, may cause permanent impairment of pulmonary function with constrictive pleuritis, which increases the work of breathing and interferes with filling of the lung in the same way that constrictive pericarditis hampers filling of the heart.

Three diagnostic problems are involved in patients with pleural effusion. The first is the recognition of the presence of the fluid in the chest. This depends on the radiologic and physical findings which have been mentioned in relation to hydrothorax. The second problem is the distinction of inflammatory from noninflammatory effusions. This depends in large measure on the associated findings such as pleural pain and friction, which are absent in patients with simple hydrothorax. The character of the pleural fluid (see below) is also of great importance in this distinction.

The third diagnostic problem is that of the detection of the underlying cause, once an effusion has been recognized to be of the inflammatory type. Here, the total clinical picture will often be decisive, as when rheumatic fever or typical lupus erythematosus is the cause. Similarly, there will be no doubt when the patient presents the classic evidences of lobar pneumonia or those of phlebothrombosis plus pulmonary infarction. However, in many instances the cause of the effusion will not be immediately apparent, and the diagnosis will depend in large measure on careful examination of the fluid itself.

When pleural fluid is removed, a portion should be drawn into a vessel containing an anticoagulant. Otherwise, clotting may prevent its careful study, which is often essential for diagnosis. The examination should include gross inspection, measurement of specific gravity, cell content, and the utilization of appropriate staining and culture methods for tubercle bacilli, fungi, aerobic and anaerobic bacteria. The content of protein should be measured, and cytologic examination for malignant cells should be made. If the fluid is withdrawn and discarded, it may subsequently be difficult to obtain a sufficient quantity for study and the opportunity for diagnosis will have been lost.

Gross inspection may reveal the obviously purulent fluid of empyema (p. 889) or the milky appearance of chylothorax—usually the result of traumatic or neoplastic damage to the thoracic duct. Blood is usually present in fluid due to carcinoma or infarction but may also be seen in the effusions of tuberculosis, congestive failure, and other diseases.

The specific gravity is helpful in separating the transudates from the exudates. About three-fourths of the patients with congestive failure have fluids with specific gravity of less than 1.016, and a similar percentage of patients with tumor or tuberculosis have values greater than 1.016. The separation of the transudates from the exudates is somewhat more precise when a protein concentration of 3 Gm per 100 ml of fluid is used as the dividing value.

The organisms can be recovered by smear or

culture in about two-thirds of the tuberculous fluids. The leukocyte and differential counts are of little value in establishing the etiology of nonpurulent effusion.

Needle biopsy is simple and often provides early histologic diagnosis. However, it must be carried out when sufficient effusion of air is present to separate the pleural surfaces. For this reason, the procedure should be considered early—prior to aspiration of all the fluid. In the hands of a pathologist skilled in the distinction between malignant and inflammatory endothelial cells, a correct cytologic diagnosis of neoplastic disease may be made in more than half the patients with malignant effusions. This finding seems to be independent of the presence of blood.

Tumors of the pleura cause massive and often rapidly recurring effusion. The x-ray frequently shows masses or sheets of tissue implanted on the pleura, especially if the fluid is removed and air injected into the space. The most common neoplasms are carcinoma of the lung and breast, lymphomas, and less often, primary pleural mesothelioma. Benign pleural fibroma is a rare but curable cause of effusion.

In a considerable proportion of patients with pleural effusion, doubt as to the cause will remain even after the most thorough consideration of the total clinical picture and the most meticulous examination of the fluid. The tendency to designate such patients as having "idiopathic pleural effusions" should be condemned. It has been properly said that the term idiopathic applied to such a patient is idiotic from the standpoint of the physician and pathetic from that of the patient. Such confusion of a name with an explanation may lead to a false sense of security and a failure to pursue the careful future following which is necessary in all patients with effusions of undiagnosed cause. It is likely but as yet unproved that viral infections are responsible in many instances, and in these, no further complications are to be expected. However, pleural effusion may be the earliest and the sole manifestation of tuberculosis, and many such patients will subsequently develop lesions in the lungs or elsewhere. Therefore, repeated subsequent careful examinations are essential. One or more attacks of pleuritis with effusion may be the sole manifestation of pulmonary infarction.

The first principle in the management of the patient with pleuritis and effusion is the treatment of the underlying causative disorder. The second is the appropriate utilization of thoracentesis. This procedure is indicated for diagnosis in almost all instances, and is frequently needed for the relief of dyspnea. Thoracentesis is likewise indicated to promote reexpansion of the lung and prevent its future mechanical deformity when spontaneous resolution of the fluid fails to occur within a few weeks. The purulent fluids constitute special problems, and these have been considered in a previous chapter (p. 893).

Chronic Adhesive Pleuritis. All degrees of this disorder exist. A few small adhesions between the parietal and visceral layers is a routine autopsy finding and ordinarily carries no clinical significance. Such adhesions are not detectable by physical examination and may or may not be seen in the x-ray as "tenting" of the diaphragm or thin shadows at the apex or in the interlobar fissures. These minor lesions are presumably the result of the minor episodes of dry pleuritis, which most persons have in association with one or more respiratory infections at some time during their lives.

Widespread and marked pleural thickening sufficient to interfere with pulmonary function is usually the end result of empyema or of tuberculous effusions. The physical signs resemble those of effusion in the presence of dullness and diminished breath sounds. However, the affected side of the chest is smaller than the normal opposite side, and the mediastinum is shifted toward rather than away from the disease process. In the earlier stages there may be a combination of extensive pleural thickening in some areas, with localized accumulations of fluid in others, and during this phase the mediastinum may be shifted in either direction, depending on which process predominates.

The distinction of pleural thickening from pulmonary atelectasis may be difficult or impossible by physical examination but will usually be resolved by the x-ray.

Advanced pleural thickening with or without calcification compromises the excursion of the affected lung and also interferes with bronchial drainage, thus promoting stasis and infection and favoring progressive pulmonary damage and further pleural injury. When the disorder is advanced, medical management is ineffective and decortication of the lung by an extensive surgical procedure, with resection of the diseased pleura, may be indicated. However, it is much better to prevent this disorder by the early recognition and proper management of empyema and of tuberculous effusions (pp. 893 and 1014).

Pneumothorax

Spontaneous Pneumothorax. This is a frightening emergency which often affects apparently healthy young men. There may be a history of some unusual exertion, but the rupture of the lung, ordinarily assumed to occur in a small subpleural bleb, usually does not accompany the exercise. Older patients with pulmonary emphysema are also prone to develop pneumothorax. In these individuals the lack of retractive force of the lung may result in a collapse of only a limited extent. However, the gravity of pneumothorax in such patients is enhanced by the underlying limitation of pulmonary reserve and also by the avascular character of the pulmonary surface, with consequent slow healing of the leak. Spontaneous pneumothorax is occasionally seen in sarcoidosis, silicosis, and in miscellaneous fibrotic or infectious disorders of the lung; when rupture occurs through an infected area as in patients with tuberculosis, carcinoma, or lung abscess, *pyopneumothorax* or an infected *hemopneumothorax* usually ensues. Here the management must include that of the underlying pulmonary disease, and of the resulting empyema, as well as maneuvers designed first to prevent pleural scarring and later to restore ventilatory function. Persistent *bronchopleural fistula* is a common and distressing problem in such patients.

Tension pneumothorax consists of the progressive increment of positive pressure in the pleural space by a ball-valve action of the air leak. Deep, gasping inspirations, which are common in the anxious and dyspneic victim of a spontaneous pneumothorax, serve to aspirate large volumes of air into the pleural cavity. During expiration the leak becomes obstructed. Cyanosis is often intense, and failure to decompress the pleural space within a few minutes may result in death.

The diagnosis of spontaneous pneumothorax is suggested by sudden severe dyspnea with unilateral chest pain, usually pleuritic in character, plus tachycardia and shock in some patients. Physical findings may include cyanosis and displacement of the trachea and mediastinum as well as the classic signs of air in the pleural cavity. A small pneumothorax may be overlooked in the x-ray and may produce only minimal signs. Thus the physician must be skilled in physical diagnosis. Recognition of pneumothorax is especially treacherous in the presence of emphysema, which itself may cause wide flat interspaces, increased resonance, distant bronchial breathing, or absent breath sounds.

X-ray demonstration of pneumothorax is best obtained during full expiration which sharpens the contrast between the lung and the pleural air.

Spontaneous pneumothorax is often a recurrent disorder. Adhesions acquired as a result of spontaneous pneumothorax may prevent total collapse of the lung at the time of a subsequent episode. However, although dyspnea may thereby be lessened, these adhesions may increase the pain. In order to prevent recurrent pneumothorax, several operations have been devised, all of which depend on the production of pleural symphysis. Most satisfactory is probably the decortication of the pleura combined with resection of blebs. Opinion is divided concerning the number of pneumothoraxes which should be permitted before these operations are attempted.

The management of a spontaneous pneumothorax with only slight retraction of the lung from the chest wall and minimal symptoms should consist in observation alone. When the findings are more compelling, a needle should be inserted immediately into the pleural space. If the pressure is positive throughout most of the respiratory cycle, which may be detected by observing the plunger to be blown back in the syringe, the latter should be removed until atmospheric pressure is attained. A thoracic pump or, if this is not available, an underwater trap is then attached.

Once the tension pneumothorax is controlled, the decision must be made whether tubes are to be inserted into the chest for further decompression or whether simple aspiration will suffice. Tubes attached to a pump should always be employed when there is a tension pneumothorax, when there is respiratory insufficiency, when there is fluid and therefore the likelihood of infection, and when there is a history of pneumothorax on the opposite side. Otherwise, a needle should be inserted and air aspirated until a mean negative pressure of 3 or 4 cm of water is attained. If, after a few moments of waiting, the pressure has crept back to an atmospheric level, the leak is still open and a tube should be inserted. If the pressure remains negative, the needle may be removed. From 12 to 24 hr later a needle is again inserted and the pressure again measured. If the lung has not leaked, the pressure will now be more negative than previously and as much air as possible should be removed. The remaining air is allowed to absorb. If, on the other hand, the pressure indicates continued leakage into the pleural space, one should not delay longer the insertion of a tube.

Hemothorax. Hemothorax or blood in the pleural space may accompany pneumothorax, as discussed above, may be associated with a broken rib, or may occur as a result of a neoplasm. Diagnosis may be aided by cytologic examination and by x-ray after removal of the blood, perhaps with instillation of air to demonstrate the pleural surfaces. If blood is allowed to remain, the likelihood of empyema and also of fibrothorax is increased. Ventilatory function is often preserved after traumatic hemothorax by early thoracotomy for decortication of the restricting layer of organizing thrombus.

DISORDERS OF THE MEDIASTINUM

Tumors and aneurysms within the mediastinum are discussed on pp. 1365 and 1568, respectively. All the disorders of the pleura may at times involve the mediastinal surfaces, and a collection of pleural fluid lodged between the lung and the mediastinum may resemble a mediastinal mass.

Displacement. When a major bronchus on one side is completely obstructed, the mediastinum will move to the opposite side during expiration, remain there until inspiration, and then return. In partial bronchial obstruction the structures shift similarly during expiration but then begin to drift back toward the midline prior to inspiration. During inspiration the mediastinum is then pulled toward the obstructed side, but if the breath is then held at full inspiration, it drifts back to the center.

Other common causes of mediastinal displacement include (1) various types of chest deformity, (2) hydrothorax and pneumothorax, which push the mediastinum away from the lesion, and (3) atelectasis and pleural adhesions which pull the mediastinum toward the diseased side. Scars in the apex of the lung, such as in old fibrotic tuberculosis, may lead to sharp angulation of the trachea, with obstructive dyspnea.

Herniation. The parietal pleurae of the two lungs are in apposition in the anterior superior mediastinum and also in the posterior inferior (retrocardiac) area. At these sites the lung of a patient with bullous emphysema may herniate from one side far into the contralateral hemithorax.

Acute Mediastinitis. This may be associated with deep pharyngeal, thyroid, or cervical infection, with pyogenic pneumonia, and with many viral and rickettsial diseases. Retroxiphoidal pain, aggravated by breathing, by extension of the head, and by yawning, is a common manifestation. The problems are analogous to acute pleuritis except that residuals of infection may obstruct the venous return, may damage the phrenic or recurrent laryngeal nerve, and may involve the pericardium.

Rupture of the esophagus which produces acute mediastinal necrosis and constitutes a grave emergency is discussed on p. 1589.

Spontaneous Mediastinal Emphysema. This condition may occur following rupture of a pulmonary alveolus, with dissection of air along the vessels and extension to the mediastinum. The tight retrosternal pain accompanied by venous distention and cyanosis may lead to an erroneous diagnosis of myocardial infarction. However, the pain is more likely to be sharply aggravated by breathing, a systolic popping, clicking, or crunching sound (Hamman's sign) is often heard, cervical subcutaneous emphysema may be present, and the x-ray may demonstrate air in the mediastinum.

Other causes of mediastinal emphysema include tension pneumothorax, thoracentesis, tracheotomy, thoracotomy, and pneumoperitoneum. The outlook is usually good, but rarely convulsions or even death from air embolism may occur. The likelihood of subcutaneous and mediastinal emphysema with pneumothorax or following thoracotomy is greatly lessened by the use of the Emerson high flow, low pressure thoracic pump, emptying the pleural space through adequately large tubes.

DISORDERS OF THE DIAPHRAGM

Displacement. Because of the liver, the right hemidiaphragm is normally about 4 cm higher than the left. Upward displacement of a localized area may be caused by a subdiaphragmatic mass such as an abscess or by an adhesion within the thorax. Less commonly, it is the result of a congenital weakness of a small area of diaphragm. Upward displacement of both sides is common in disorders associated with high intraabdominal pressure, such as pregnancy, extreme obesity, or ascites. When the total lung capacity is reduced as with diffuse pulmonary fibrosis, the diaphragm may be pulled upward to its normal expiratory position. Conversely, the loss of pulmonary retractive force associated with emphysema causes an abnormally low position, and the liver may be palpable even though it is not enlarged.

Unilateral downward displacement results from pleural effusion. Occasionally, pleural fluid may collect entirely between the diaphragm and the inferior aspect of the lung, rather than in the lateral and posterior aspects of the pleural cavity, thus causing both physical examination and the x-ray to give the erroneous impression of a high position.

The diaphragm normally moves 4 to 10 cm with deep breathing. Scarring following empyema, hemothorax, or long-standing effusion not only limits excursion but may produce a fixed high position, simulating paralysis. Injury to the phrenic nerve results in variable degrees of elevation and reduced motion. The high completely paralyzed diaphragm moves paradoxically upward during quick inspiration. Partial injury to the phrenic nerve—which may be important in the evaluation of a mediastinal mass—sometimes can be detected only by fluoroscopic demonstration of a lag in the descent of the diaphragm during inspiration or a failure to move either way. The usual cause of phrenic paresis or paralysis is invasion by tumor; less frequent causes are mediastinitis or extensive scarring of the adjacent pleura. Therapeutic phrenic crush is now rarely done, but trauma to the nerve may occur with thoracic or cervical injury.

Singultus, or Hiccup. This is a quick involuntary contraction of the diaphragm with a closed glottis and may be of central origin, as in persons with encephalitis or brain-stem injury. More commonly, it appears to be initiated by reflexes arising from neighboring organs. Thus it may be present in patients with myocardial infarction, pneumonia, gastric distention, pancreatitis, or peritonitis. Prolonged singultus is exhausting and interferes with nutrition as well as with respiration. When gastric suction, antiemetic drugs, carbon dioxide breathing or rebreathing in a paper bag fail, the phrenic nerve may be anesthetized. The nerve also can be rendered refractory by rapid stimulation over its source in the neck, using an electrophrenic respirator.

Diaphragmatic Flutter. Diaphragmatic flutter is a rapid regular or irregular contraction of the diaphragm, continual or in paroxysms. It may be painful. The cause is usually obscure but in some instances appears to be hysterical. Often only a small portion of the diaphragm is involved, and if this area is on the left, the repetitive audible sound of the contraction may lead to an erroneous impression of cardiac arrhythmia.

Herniation. Herniation of the abdominal viscera through the diaphragm may occur in several locations, including the anterior substernal space (foramen of Morgagni), the pleuroperitoneal hiatus, and through defects in the posterior portion of the diaphragm near the esophagus. By far the most frequent site is through the esophageal hiatus itself (p. 1584). Fluoroscopic examination of the barium-filled stomach with the patient in the head-down position is the best means of demonstrating a diaphragmatic hernia. When a portion of the fundus of the stomach lies above the diaphragm, one must ascertain whether in addition an abnormally short esophagus is also present because of the more difficult surgical correction of this condition.

Eventration. Eventration of the diaphragm consists of an extreme upward displacement of a congenitally thin, often membranous, hemidiaphragm and must be distinguished from a large hernia or total absence of the hemidiaphragm since the surgical management is quite different. These disorders may cause digestive symptoms, dyspnea and cough, recurrent pulmonary infections, or may be asymptomatic. They may be suspected only when abdominal sounds are heard in the thorax of the recumbent patient, thus representing an exception to the rule that the sitting or standing position is best for physical examination. The diaphragm in eventration can often be seen, even though it is thin on the radiograph, but for a positive diagnosis one may have to instill a few hundred milliliters of air into the abdominal cavity and then determine by x-ray whether the air collects under the diaphragm or at the apex of the lung.

REFERENCES

Cardon, L.: Significance of Small Pleural Effusions in Cardiopulmonary Disease, and Some Other Observations on Pleural Fluid in General, Ann. Internal Med., 53:765, 1960.

Gaensler, E. A.: Parietal Pleurectomy for Recurrent Spontaneous Pneumothorax, Surg. Gynecol. Obstet., 102:293, 1956.

Harrington, S. W.: Various Types of Diaphragmatic Herniae Treated Surgically: Report of 430 Cases, Surg. Gynecol. Obstet., 86:735, 1948.

Kjaergaard, H.: Spontaneous Pneumothorax in the Apparently Healthy, Acta Med. Scand., Suppl. 43, p. 1, 1932.

Leuallen, E. C., and D. T. Carr: Pleural Effusion; Statistical Study of 436 Patients, New Engl. J. Med., 252:79, 1955.

267 TUMORS OF THE MEDIASTINUM

Gustaf E. Lindskog

Mediastinal tumefactions may be classified according to their pathogenesis as follows: true neoplasms (e.g., thymoma), congenital malformations (e.g., bronchogenic cysts), infections (e.g., tuberculomas), and degenerative lesions (e.g., arteriosclerotic aneurysms). True neoplasms may be primary or secondary and benign or malignant.

Within the narrow confines of the mediastinum even the most benign and slowly growing tumor can on occasion produce irreparable damage to the host by mechanical encroachment, compression, and obstruction of vascular channels, the esophagus, and the tracheobronchial tree. Infection may develop in cystic lesions from blood-borne sources or by direct extension after erosion into the bronchi or into the esophagus. A comprehension of mediastinal anatomy is therefore essential to the study of mediastinal tumors; furthermore, any attempt to define the pathologic nature of these lesions before surgical excision must lean heavily on their location in the mediastinal compartments, since the different varieties of tumor have definite sites of predilection (Fig. 267-1).

Anatomy of the Mediastinum. The mediastinum, as the name implies, is a space lying between the right and left pleurae in or near the median sagittal plane of the thorax. More for clinical purposes than for anatomic reasons, the mediastinum has been divided into four compartments: superior, anterior, middle, and posterior.

The *superior* mediastinum is bounded in front by the manubrium and behind by the upper four thoracic vertebras. Inferiorly, it is demarcated by an imaginary line extending from the manubriogladiolar juncture to the fourth vertebral body. This space contains the aortic arch and its major branches (innominate, left subclavian, and left common carotid origins), the innominate veins, and the upper half of the superior vena cava, the trachea, esophagus, thoracic duct, thymus gland, some lymph nodes, and the vagus, phrenic, left recurrent, and cardiac sympathetic nerves.

To be found in the superior compartment are bronchogenic cysts, tuberculomas, thyroid and parathyroid adenomas, teratomas, and metastatic tumors.

The *anterior* mediastinum is demarcated in front by the sternum, posteriorly by the pericardium, and below by the diaphragm. It is a very meager space and contains normally only some areolar tissue, lymphatics, lymph nodes, and branches of the internal mammary arteries.

In this space may be located teratomas, thymomas, lymphangiomas, and any of those listed for the superior mediastinal space.

The *middle* mediastinum comprises the heart and its pericardial covering, the ascending aorta, the lower portion of the superior vena cava and its junction with the azygos vein, the bifurcation of the trachea, the proximal pulmonary arteries and veins, the phrenic nerves, and some lymph nodes.

In this compartment may be found bronchogenic cysts and pericardial cysts or diverticula.

The *posterior* mediastinum is bounded in front by the heart, in back by the lower eight thoracic vertebras and the shelving posterior portion of the diaphragm. It contains the thoracic descending aorta, the azygos and hemiazygos veins, the esophagus, the thoracic duct, the vagus and splanchnic nerves, and some lymph glands.

In the posterior mediastinal compartment are typically found neurogenic tumors and also certain bronchogenic, esophageal, and gastroenteric cysts.

Symptomatology. A majority of benign mediastinal tumors are asymptomatic and are discovered in the course of routine roentgenograms or those done for other purposes. With very few exceptions, symptoms are not specific and are caused by complications which include pressure necrosis, secondary infection, hemorrhage, and rupture of cystic lesions into a neighboring viscus. Thus fever, cough, dyspnea, wheezing, chest pain, and hemoptysis may occur in any combination and sequence. Dysphagia is not a very common symptom.

Malignant tumors which invade extensively in the mediastinum tend to produce the so-called *syndrome of the superior vena cava.* This is manifested by edema of the neck, face, and conjunctiva, together with distention and increased pressure in the veins of the neck, chest, and upper extremities. Epistaxis may occur, and also hoarseness from laryngeal edema or paralysis of the recurrent nerve. The patient may have severe headache, fainting spells, and vertigo. This syndrome sometimes occurs with very large benign tumors, such as thyroid

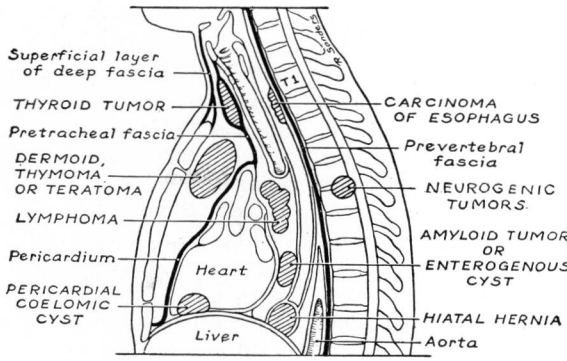

FIG. 267-1. A simplified lateral projection of the chest showing sites of predilection of various mediastinal tumefactions. (*Courtesy, Dr. John Chapman.*)

adenoma, located in the superior aperture of the thorax.

One pathognomonic symptom of a particular mediastinal tumor is *trichoptysis* or the spitting up of hair, usually accompanied by sebaceous material. This occurs in the case of dermoid cysts, but only when fistulization into the tracheobronchial tree has taken place.

Differential Diagnosis. Certain lesions originating in structures outside the mediastinum proper can intrude themselves secondarily and give rise to confusion in diagnosis. Such include (1) substernal goiter, (2) diaphragmatic hernias, (3) tumors arising in the thoracic skeleton, and (4) thoracic meningocele. In addition, aneurysms of the heart, aorta, and great vessels and pericardial effusion may simulate tumor.

Substernal goiter usually arises as a nodular downward extension from a lower thyroid pole. There may be a palpable mass in the neck; the trachea tends to be compressed and deviated away from the side of the lesion. Radiographic continuity of the mediastinal mass with a cervical thyroid shadow is commonly seen under fluoroscopy, most substernal goiters move freely and downward during deglutition, just as the normal thyroid gland does. Radioactive iodine tracer techniques may be useful in doubtful cases.

The *diaphragmatic hernias* most likely to be confused with mediastinal tumor are those located in the parasternal foramen of Morgagni. These may be essentially solid lesions consisting of herniated omental fat. In the lateral radiographic projection, they are based strictly in the anterior cardiophrenic angle. The air pattern of the transverse colon may be abnormally elevated; this can be further demonstrated by barium enema. Esophageal hiatal hernias also may present a homogeneous tumefaction in the lower middle mediastinum when the content of the hernial sac is principally omentum. A barium swallow is therefore an important procedure with supradiaphragmatic lesions.

Chondroma, chondrosarcoma, and *Ewing's sarcoma* arising in rib or vertebra may grow internally and expansively in certain cases. Careful roentgenologic study of the involved bone should lead to the detection of some changes, but these may be quite inconspicuous. Pain is likely to be severe with malignant bone tumors and can simulate that caused by neurogenic tumors when it is segmental in type.

Thoracic meningocele is a very rare lesion seen chiefly in middle-aged women and associated with von Recklinghausen's disease (*café-au-lait* spots and multiple neurofibromatosis). Radiographic examination of the spine shows enlargement of several intervertebral foramina.

Aneurysms of the aorta and its major branches are of great concern in the differential diagnosis of mediastinal tumors. They are discussed in Chap. 247.

Large *pericardial effusions, pericardial cysts,* and *idiopathic cardiac hypertrophy* may be confused radiologically and clinically with mediastinal neoplasms. Chronic lymphadenopathy related, for example, to tuberculosis or fungous infection may produce mediastinal tumefactions readily confused with tumors. In the condition known as giant lymph node hyperplasia, discrete masses of thickly encapsulated lymphoid tissue may occur in the upper and anterior mediastinum and persist in the absence of any recognized infectious or malignant process. Some cases are associated with accumulation of plasmocytes and reticular cells.

In the lower posterior mediastinum, extramedullary hematopoiesis may result in a lobulated tumefaction large enough to be recognized radiographically.

Diagnostic Methods. Physical examination should include a careful study for enlarged peripheral lymph nodes, especially in the supraclavicular and axillary groups, and for splenomegaly and hepatomegaly in connection with the malignant lymphomas. Recurrent nerve paralysis should be ruled out by indirect laryngoscopy. *Horner's syndrome* is usually a stigma of malignant infiltration of the upper dorsal sympathetic chain, but may occur as a pressure effect from discrete and benign tumors. This syndrome is characterized by narrowing of the palpebral fissure, recession of the eyeball, a contracted pupil, and absence of sweating on the ipsilateral side of the face.

Bronchoscopy is rarely of definitive value in the diagnosis of primary mediastinal tumors but may be required to rule out lesions such as bronchogenic carcinoma. Bronchography employing iodized oil is neither helpful nor necessary unless obstructive complications in the lung require evaluation.

Sometimes the latter are at least as demanding of therapy as the causative tumor.

A complete radiologic study includes fluoroscopy, lateral and oblique roentgenograms, as well as the standard PA projection. A barium study of the esophagus should be carried out in every case of aneurysm and in the case of all tumors of the middle and posterior compartments. Laminagrams may be very helpful. The radiologist tries to determine, among other things, the presence or absence of encapsulation, the existence of calcifications, air and fluid levels, intrinsic or extrinsic pulsations, and the movement of the lesion during respiration and deglutition. Of greatest importance is the position of the lesion in the mediastinal compartments; characteristic locations are described under Anatomy.

Surgical excision of a cervical, axillary, or other enlarged lymph nodes may be of great diagnostic value particularly when such diseases as Hodgkin's, tuberculosis, and Boeck's sarcoid enter the differential diagnostic picture.

Even when lymph node enlargement is not detectable, it is sometimes possible to establish a tissue diagnosis after *en bloc* resection of the small lymph nodes in the fatty tissue overlying the scalenus anticus muscle near its insertion.

The commoner types of mediastinal tumors will be discussed briefly in terms of their special characteristics.

Teratoid Tumors. Benign teratoid tumors are commonly called dermoids. They are usually large when first recognized, ordinarily in the third and fourth decades. More often unilocular than multilocular, they contain sebaceous material and hair. Dental structures and bone are sometimes present and cause characteristic radiographic densities. The more complex teratomas are fleshy and contain tissue recognizable as nervous system, intestinal tract, pancreas, kidney or testis, and the like. The capsules may be ill-defined and infiltrated by carcinomatous or sarcomatous cells. A predominantly unilateral development may lead to confusion with such tumors as seminoma and chorionepithelioma. The complex teratomas have a very high incidence of malignant change with local invasion and metastases.

Bronchogenic, Esophageal, and Gastroenteric Cysts. These are developmental anomalies of the primitive foregut and bronchial buds. Commonly unilocular, they are chiefly located in relation to the trachea, upper bronchi, and esophagus; rarely they are found in the periphery of the lung or upon the diaphragm. Communication with the air passages may preexist or develop later because of pressure. The result is *pyocyst,* and this may be associated radiographically with an air-fluid level simulating pulmonary abscess.

The majority of these cysts have a respiratory type of epithelial lining with ciliated columnar cells and pseudostratified basilar nuclei; smooth muscle, cartilage, and mucous glands may be present. Squamous and gastrointestinal types of lining cells are occasionally encountered, principally in the cysts located about the distal esophagus. The gastrointestinal types are prone to give rise to serious symptoms in the first year of life, the others in adult life.

Neurogenic Tumors. Neurogenic tumors are the most frequently encountered of primary mediastinal neoplasms. Several pathologic types are recognized: (1) neurilemmomas, derived from the sheath cells of Schwann; (2) neurofibroma, a more complex but usually benign lesion showing, in addition to Schwann cells, neuraxones and proliferated connective tissue; (3) ganglioneuroma, with ganglion cells in variable stages of maturity interspersed in a stroma of neurofibromatous type; (4) sympathicoblastoma, derived from primitive cells which are small, round, densely nucleated, and with a tendency to pseudorosette patterns; (5) paraganglioma, including the rare hypersecreting variant, pheochromocytoma.

About 95 per cent of posterior mediastinal tumors are neurogenic in derivation, but neurilemmoma and neurofibroma may occur in a more lateral or peripheral situation in relation to the intercostal nerves. An expansile growth located in an intervertebral foramen may enlarge the latter as demonstrated in roentgenograms; by intrusion into the epidural space it can produce symptoms of spinal cord compression, the so-called "dumbbell" tumor. Other histologic types of tumor, such as benign lipoma, may produce these same effects.

Ganglioneuromas exist principally in relation to the sympathetic chain and can produce the typical Horner's syndrome and sweating changes of the ipsilateral upper extremity. Neurofibroma may be a local manifestation of von Recklinghausen's disease.

Tumors of the Thymus. Tumors arising in the thymus gland are frequently difficult to identify and classify. The two main cell types, thymocyte (lymphocyte?) and reticulum (epithelial?) may be present in varying proportions. Thymomas tend to be heavily encapsulated and lobulated, fleshy or solid. Microcyst formation is common, but gross cystic changes can occur. Microscopically perithelial arrangement of tumor cells around vascular, lymphatic, or tissue spaces is rather characteristic. Hassal's corpuscles are found in only about 25 per cent.

Malignant change in a thymic tumor is signaled by capsular infiltration and invasion of contiguous structures, such as pericardium, trachea, large vessels, and pleura. Remote metastases are uncommon even in fatal cases.

Thymic tumors are found in 15 to 20 per cent of myasthenia gravis cases, and a significant number of patients with thymic tumors on careful analysis are noted to have myasthenic symptoms. Thymectomy and excision of thymic tumors have an unpredictable effect upon the course of myasthenia gravis, ranging from cure to no effect.

Thymomas are known to occur in not infrequent association with aregenerative anemias, but the surgical ablation of the tumor, again, does not necessarily cure the hematologic disorder.

Other Generally Benign Tumors of the Mediastinum. Lipomas and fibromas are relatively rare. They occur anywhere in the mediastinum and furnish the largest specimens; some as heavy as 17 lb have been reported. Pressure symptoms are disproportionately mild.

Lymphangiomas are typically cystic and located in the anterior mediastinum and cardiophrenic angle. They are multilocular and demonstrate elastic tissue and smooth muscle in association with the mesothelium-lined channels. Cervical and mediastinal locations may be combined in the same case. Spontaneous chylothorax has been reported, and secondary infection, but ordinarily these are asymptomatic tumors.

Parathyroid adenomas usually occur in the expected distribution of the normal parathyroid glands. In perhaps 20 per cent of cases they are located ectopically in the mediastinum. Such adenomas are ordinarily quite small and are not often visualized by radiographic methods. An outline of the esophagus with barium may be helpful. The surgical treatment of hyperparathyroidism requires a complete search of the cervical area before the mediastinum is explored, ideally in a single operation.

Pericardial (Pericardiodiaphragmatic) Cysts and Diverticula. Aberrations in the development of the pericardial sac may lead to the formation of pericardial diverticula or cysts. These are unilocular, thin-walled sacs containing clear colorless fluid. A simple endothelium lines the thin connective tissue wall. Diverticula are rarer than cysts; they communicate by a narrow ostium with the main pericardial sac, whereas the cysts are separate and may even be at some distance from the pericardium. They produce no symptoms as a rule and are removed only for diagnostic purposes.

Primary Malignant Tumors. The lymphoblastic series of tumors (lymphoma, Hodgkin's disease, and lymphosarcoma) constitute about 70 per cent of this category. Various types of connective tissue malignancies also occur, such as fibrosarcoma. Epithelial neoplasms independent of any demonstrable extramediastinal focus (such as the peripheral lung) are least common. Some of these rarities may arise from the thymus, from pharyngeal pouch remnants, or from degenerating teratoid lesions.

Hodgkin's disease (see Chap. 243) may begin in the mediastinal nodes and remain apparently localized there. More commonly, there is relatively early involvement of the cervical, axillary, or other peripheral lymph nodes; this enlargement may constitute the first clinical evidence of the disease. Splenomegaly occurs in about 70 per cent of Hodgkin's cases at some time in the course. There may be itching of the skin. Systemic manifestations such as periodic fever, malaise, anorexia, and weight loss are more common with Hodgkin's disease than with lymphosarcoma and reticulum cell sarcoma. The latter is sometimes confined to the region of the thymus when first recognized, only to spread later and produce the clinical picture of superior vena caval obstruction. Pleural effusion may develop.

Secondary Malignant Tumors. The commonest tumor of the mediastinum is undoubtedly metastatic carcinoma. The site of origin may be an intrathoracic organ such as esophagus, trachea, or bronchi. Mammary cancer is a frequent invader, however, and remote neoplasms such as renal and ovarian carcinoma may metastasize to lymph nodes and subsequently extend more diffusely in the mediastinal tissues.

Extension to mediastinal lymph nodes is an important limiting factor in the surgical treatment of mammary carcinoma. Its frequency has led to the recommendation that preliminary biopsy of the internal mammary chain of nodes be performed in cases where the primary breast lesion is situated in the medial quadrants, and when the axillary lymph nodes are palpably involved.

Isolated lymph node metastases in the mediastinum may be quite asymptomatic. As enlargement and infiltration occur, manifestations of pressure and pain may develop, and the syndrome of superior vena caval obstruction (p. 1560) is not infrequently observed.

Treatment of Mediastinal Tumors. Benign mediastinal neoplasms cannot be differentiated accurately by clinical and radiographic methods from localized malignant forms. Therefore, the indicated therapy is surgical exploration and excision, unless there exists some compelling reason to the contrary, such as extreme old age, or coexisting disease which itself has a lethal prognosis.

The most useful exploratory incision is a long posterolateral one with rib resection, since technical problems may be considerable. Certain anterior tumors can be reached by medium sternotomy or parasternal chondrectomy. Ideally the tumor should be totally extirpated in a single stage.

Certain large and infected cystic tumors in poor-risk patients may be marsupialized for drainage and resected at a later date.

The mortality rate for excision of benign and localized malignant mediastinal tumors is less than 5 per cent and in some reported series approaches zero.

Invasive malignant neoplasms can only be biopsied or partially resected. An attempt should be made to recognize these unfavorable cases by careful physical examination and to obtain tissue for microscopic study by simple techniques such as needle biopsy and the like. When these fail, a mediastinotomy may be required. It is important not to treat a suspected lymphoma or other mediastinal neoplasm by radiation until a tissue diagnosis is established. There are many pitfalls in so-called diagnostic radiotherapy.

Hodgkin's disease confined to a local area should be treated with heavy doses of radiation, and in a rare case this may be combined with surgical excision. Widely disseminated tumors must be palliated with smaller doses of roentgen rays and such chemotherapeutic agents as the nitrogen mustards.

REFERENCES

Blades, B.: Mediastinal Tumors: Report of Cases Treated at Army Thoracic Surgical Centers in the United States, Ann. Surg., 123:749, 1946.

Clagett, O. T., and L. M. Eaton: Surgical Treatment of Myasthenia Gravis, J. Thoracic Surg., 16:62, 1947.

Clarkson, B., and D. J. Prockop: Aregenerative Anemia Associated with Benign Thymoma, New Engl. J. Med., 259:253, 1958.

Hartfall, S. J., and M. J. Stewart: Massive Paravertebral Heteropia of Bone Marrow in a Case of Acholuric Jaundice, J. Pathol. Bacteriol., 37:455, 1933.

Kent, E. M., B. Blades, A. B. Valle, and E. A. Graham: Intrathoracic Neurogenic Tumors, J. Thoracic Surg., 13:116, 1944.

Lindskog, G. E., and A. A. Liebow: "Thoracic Surgery and Related Pathology," chap. 29, New York, Appleton-Century-Crofts, Inc., 1953.

Morrison, I. M.: Tumors and Cysts of the Mediastinum, Thorax, 13:294, 1958.

Ringertz, N., and S. O. Lidholm: Mediastinal Tumors and Cysts, J. Thoracic Surg., 31:458, 1956.

Rives, J. D.: Mediastinal Aberrant Goitre, Ann. Surg., 126:797, 1947.

Schechter, M. M.: The Superior Vena Cava Syndrome, Am. J. Med. Sci., 227:46, 1954.

268 THERAPY OF RESPIRATORY INSUFFICIENCY

Eugene Robin and
John H. Knowles

The numerous physiologic defects present in chronic pulmonary disease have already been discussed (pp. 104 to 124). Regardless of etiology, these defects are found to a greater or lesser degree in most forms of chronic pulmonary disease. Effective therapy must obviously be based on an understanding of the physiologic aberration present and should be guided by the fact that the defects due to infection, excessive secretions, bronchospasm, and alteration of the blood gases are potentially reversible. The physiologic abnormalities and their therapy are considered below. Generally the discussion applies to chronic bronchitis and obstructive emphysema, the commonest forms of chronic pulmonary disease.

AIRWAY OBSTRUCTION

Airway obstruction in chronic pulmonary disease results from the presence of thick, viscid respiratory tract secretions; from bronchial edema, from bronchospasm, from bronchial or peribronchial fibrosis; and from parenchymal destruction with the development of bronchiolar check valves.

Secretions. The patient with chronic pulmonary disease commonly suffers from hypersecretion of mucus in the tracheobronchial tree, which leads to chronic cough, dyspnea by virtue of airway obstruction, and recurrent infection. He may be unable to dispose of such secretions because of ineffective mechanics of coughing and inadequate ciliary activity. The first principle of treatment is the avoidance of irritants, the chief offender being tobacco smoke. Complete cessation of smoking should be advised. Careful inquiry into the presence of noxious environmental gases and dusts, both at work and in the vicinity of the patient's home, must be undertaken. A change of job or home might be indicated. Similarly, a change of climate, from one with wide swings of temperature and humidity to one which is warm and dry the year around, may be beneficial if the patient can undertake the financial and emotional burden of moving. A trial period in the chosen area should precede the patient's final decision.

Periodic increase in cough and in the volume of secretions is commonly due to superimposed bacterial infection, particularly during the winter months (see also below). Both cough and sputum production may be markedly diminished by full courses of the appropriate antibiotic dictated by the result of sputum culture.

During periods of acute infection, secretions may become particularly thick, tenacious, and viscid (in addition to their volume increase) and therefore difficult to remove. The sputum of the ambulatory patient without obvious infection may have similar characteristics, although in lesser degree. Measures to liquefy the sputum should be employed in either instance. The inhalation of warm, moist air (steam) is probably the single most effective measure in decreasing sputum viscosity. Other measures include close attention to the general hydration of the patient; the use of iodides orally or parenterally; the use of detergents by inhalation ("Alevaire," which consists of glycerin, sodium bicarbonate, and Triton A-20) to lower sputum viscosity; and the attempted enzymatic digestion of sputum by the inhalation of aerosolized enzymes such as trypsin (Tryptar) or pancreatic dornase. Iodides are the most effective measure and are usually given as saturated solution of potassium iodide, 10 drops by mouth, three or four times a day. Definite evidence is lacking that the use of detergents and enzymes aids measurably in the removal of secretions except for the resultant local hydration per se. In addition, the enzymes may give rise to considerable local irritation of the pharynx. In a small number of patients with chronic pulmonary disease, the volume of secretions is so excessive that drugs, such as terpin hydrate or guaiacol, that diminish the amount of sputum may be usefully employed.

Special measures designed to assist in removing secretions may be necessary. In the patient who is not acutely ill, a consistent program of postural drainage may be helpful, particularly if the volume of secretions is continuously large. The patient should be carefully instructed in the proper technique of performing postural drainage. During its performance the patient should assume the head-down position, the prone position, right and left lateral decubitus, and the sitting position, so that all lobes are drained. Coughing in explosive style during drainage should be avoided, to prevent further lung damage. During acute respiratory infections, postural drainage may not suffice; mechanical removal of secretions is then necessary. This may take the form of tracheal suction by means of a soft catheter passed through the naso- or oropharynx. If this is not successful in the emergency situation, therapeutic bronchoscopy may be required. Finally, if none of the above measures is effective, or if they are of only transient benefit in the severely ill patient, a tracheostomy may be necessary for the purpose of frequent and efficient suctioning of secretions. Tracheostomy also decreases the respiratory dead space, thereby facilitating improvement in the level of alveolar ventilation. Exact indications for tracheostomy are difficult to outline. Certainly, inability to control secretions by more conservative methods is one indication. Continued deterioration despite intensive therapy is another indication. Such deterioration may be defined by either clinical criteria or by a rising arterial CO_2 tension. The patient with severe pulmonary insufficiency, who is about to undergo thoracic surgery, may be considered as a candidate for prophylactic tracheostomy. In general, if any doubt exists as to the necessity for this procedure, it should be resolved by having the procedure performed. Preferably then, if indicated, the tracheostomy should be instituted early rather than late, should be done in a slow, unhurried manner, and should be performed in the operating room rather than at the bedside.

After the tracheostomy, a number of precautions are necessary to prevent complications. To avoid infection, tracheal suction should be performed with sterile precautions and disposable catheters. To prevent trauma to the tracheal mucosa, the catheter should be moistened before use. A T-tube arrangement should be placed in the suction line so that negative pressure is applied only when the catheter has been positioned inside the lumen of the trachea. The catheter should not be vigorously thrust up and down within the tracheal lumen. The patient's head should be turned to the right and left during suction, so that the left and right main-stem bronchi can be reached. If available, a curved catheter for entering the left main-stem bronchus is desirable. To prevent hypoxia, hypercapnea, and fatigue, suctioning periods should be limited to 15 to 30 sec at a time. The use of very high expiratory flow rates to dislodge retained secretions (exsufflation with negative pressure) has been of value in some patients with postoperative atelectasis, but only rarely in those with chronic pulmonary disease.

Decreased Cross-sectional Area of the Bronchial Tree. The degree of reversible luminal narrowing of the bronchial tree due to bronchospasm and bronchial edema varies widely from patient to patient. It is not sufficiently appreciated that many patients with chronic obstructive ventilatory disease have a component of bronchospasm as a factor in their airflow obstruction. This may be impossible to detect clinically. For this reason, the routine use of bronchodilators is useful in the therapy of chronic pulmonary disease. Their use need not be entirely empiric. The 1-sec timed vital capacity or maximal midexpiratory flow rate should be determined before and after the inhalation of aerosolized bronchodilator and any increase noted.

The drugs may be administered orally (ephedrine, 15 to 25 mg three or four times a day, usu-

ally combined with 15 mg phenobarbital), rectally (0.5 Gm aminophylline suppository at bedtime), by aerosol inhalation [1:200 isoproterenol hydrochloride (Isuprel) or 2.25 per cent racemic epinephrine hydrochloride (Vaponephrin)], or parenterally (intravenous aminophylline). (Parenteral epinephrine is not ordinarily used in the older patient with chronic lung disease as it is in bronchial asthma.) The aim of therapy is to relieve bronchospasm for as much of each 24 hr as possible. For this reason, bronchodilators should be administered on a consistent schedule, and around the clock, if possible; the dosage should be increased during periods of increased bronchospasm.

Corticosteroids may be useful in the control of bronchospasm and bronchial edema in some patients. In the life-threatening situation, they may be used empirically if the condition does not respond to the usual measures outlined above and a reversible bronchospastic element is suspected. Similarly, in the occasional patient with chronic pulmonary disease whose clinical state suggests the possibility of bronchial asthma or at least a large reversible obstructive element which is not improved by the usual therapy, a diagnostic and therapeutic trial with corticosteroids may be indicated. Careful evaluation by serial test (e.g., timed vital capacity) is necessary to determine the ultimate need for such therapy. The hazards of peptic ulceration and reactivation of pulmonary tuberculosis must be recognized in such patients.

Since it has been demonstrated that cigarette smoke and other respiratory tract irritants produce an increase of resistance to airflow, cigarette smoking should be interdicted and the patient removed from exposure to irritant fumes to whatever degree possible.

More difficult to treat than the functional decreases in bronchial cross-sectional area are those based on anatomic damage to the bronchial tree or its loss. One major factor in this form of respiratory tract obstruction is that the application of high positive pressure across the thorax tends to collapse bronchioles and, hence, increases the degree of obstruction. Breathing exercises teach the patient to prolong expiration using lower intrapleural pressures. Pursed-lip breathing—pursing the lips and making an "F" sound on expiration—is taught. Expiration is made an active, prolonged effort; active use of abdominal muscles is stressed. The pressure gradient across the thoracic cage is lessened, and the amount of air trapping and of airway resistance due to early closure of bronchioles is decreased. The inhalation of gas mixtures that are less dense than air (80 per cent helium 20 per cent oxygen) may decrease the resistance to turbulent flow, although resistance to laminar flow may be increased because the mixture is more viscid than air.

HYPOXIA

Hypoxia in patients with chronic pulmonary disease may result from generalized alveolar hypoventilation, from regional hypoventilation, or from a decrease in the diffusing capacity of the lung. Aside from measures designed to produce an overall increase in total ventilation and to improve regional hypoventilation by decreasing airflow resistance, the most effective measure in therapy of hypoxia is the inhalation of oxygen-enriched mixtures. The inhalation of high concentrations of oxygen will produce an increase in the alveolar tension of oxygen in all ventilated alveoli (i.e., those that are not totally occluded). The increase in alveolar oxygen tension will be reflected in an increase of oxygen tension in the pulmonary-capillary blood supplying these alveoli and will ultimately be reflected in an increased tissue oxygen supply (provided cardiac output remains constant). Oxygen administration also permits an adequate supply of oxygen at a minimal work cost of breathing to the patient. This factor tends to decrease the over-all oxygen consumption of the patient and may partially explain the decrease in dyspnea that occurs during oxygen inhalation. Oxygen-enriched mixtures may be supplied by nasal catheter, oxygen tent, face mask, or by means of an intermittent positive-pressure apparatus. The exact technique of administration will depend on individual circumstances. The oxygen stream must be kept moist to prevent drying of the respiratory mucosa and secretions. This may be accomplished by bubbling the oxygen through properly warmed water.

In some patients with extremely severe pulmonary disease with acute or chronic hypercapnia and hypoxemia, there may be a loss of the normal respiratory center responsiveness to CO_2-pH stimulation, presumably because of narcotic levels of CO_2 tension in the blood. In such patients the ventilatory drive appears to depend chiefly on impulses arising from the chemoreceptors of the aortic and carotid bodies, which respond chiefly to hypoxemia. Removal of the hypoxemic drive by means of oxygen inhalation may result in increasingly severe hypoventilation with a precipitous rise in arterial blood CO_2 tension and drop in pH. Drowsiness and disorientation occur, and in severe cases convulsions, coma, and even apnea ensue. In such patients, oxygen administration must be carefully controlled. However, it should be emphasized that the relief of profound hypoxia is essential in the treatment of such patients. The problem, therefore, is not whether they should be treated with oxygen but how to treat them with oxygen and maintain ventilation while doing so. The dilemma may be resolved in one of several ways. It may be possible to wean the patient back to the continuous use of oxygen by giving it intermittently at first, or in concentrations less than 100 per cent (e.g., a 40 per cent oxygen mixture; or reduction in the flow rate of 100 per cent oxygen given by nasal catheter). If these measures are unsuccessful, mechanical ventilators are necessary in patients developing life-threatening hypoventilation during oxygen administration.

RESPIRATORY ACIDOSIS

The basic mechanism producing respiratory acidosis is always inadequate alveolar ventilation. Such inadequacy may result from an over-all decrease in ventilation or from severe regional hypoventilation of sufficient magnitude so that CO_2 being produced metabolically cannot be disposed of in adequate amounts. Carbon dioxide retention may be treated by two general techniques: (1) reduction of the amount of CO_2 being produced metabolically, and (2) increased CO_2 excretion by the lungs.

The following techniques are available for reducing CO_2 production:

1. Reduction in the work cost of breathing. In normal subjects the work cost of breathing amounts to less than 2 per cent of total metabolism. In patients with chronic pulmonary disease, this value may increase to as much as 40 per cent. Indeed, it has been suggested that the CO_2 cost of breathing may be so high in some patients with chronic pulmonary disease that further increase in ventilation actually causes a rise and not a fall in CO_2 tension. The measures which have been outlined above result in more efficient ventilation and, hence, in a decreased work cost of breathing.

2. Reduction in physical activity. Obviously a reduction in over-all activity will result in a decrease of metabolism. Such reduction in activity during periods of acute illness is usually provided by hospitalization. In nonacute periods, the avoidance of severe overexertion and periodic rest intervals may help to accomplish the same purpose.

3. Reduction of total metabolism by means of induced hypothyroidism. Radioactive iodine administration has been employed in an effort to induce some degree of hypothyroidism in patients with chronic pulmonary disease and in this manner to limit their metabolic requirements. This approach is as yet experimental and has not enjoyed widespread use. The unpleasant symptoms and appearance of hypothyroidism may be intolerable to the patient and his family.

The following techniques are available for increasing CO_2 output by the lung:

1. Improving the ventilatory status of the lungs by removal of secretions, treatment of infection,

and the liberal use of bronchodilators, as outlined above.

2. Attempted stimulation of the respiratory center by drugs in order to induce hyperventilation. Such drugs as Coramine, progesterone, and Vandid are capable of increasing alveolar ventilation. In general, these drugs have limited usefulness because regardless of central drive, the degree of hyperventilation is limited by the underlying abnormalities of the peripheral ventilatory mechanism, i.e., the disease of the lungs and thoracic cage. The same is true of the use of salicylates and acetazolamide (Diamox).

In this regard it is useful to point out that one of the most important aids in restoring respiratory center sensitivity is to improve the blood gas composition by elevating ventilation. Either increasing oxygenation or reducing CO_2 retention (or both) of the arterial blood may result in resumption of rhythmic and efficient respiratory movement in the patient nearly apneic with uncoordinated respiratory muscle activity. It is *mandatory* to withhold any drugs, such as morphine, Demerol, and the barbiturates, that are capable of accentuating respiratory center depression.

3. In the acutely ill patient, assisted ventilation by means of one or another type of mechanical ventilator offers the best method of increasing alveolar ventilation and decreasing CO_2 tension, thus increasing the excretion of CO_2. A number of different respirators are available. The one most commonly used at present employs intermittent positive pressure (IPPB). With this apparatus the lungs are periodically inflated by means of positive pressure and expiration takes place passively. Such apparatus also provides facilities for the humidification of inspired air and for the administration of bronchodilators in the form of aerosol deep into the tracheobronchial tree. This type of apparatus is generally designed so that it may be activated by the patient's own respiratory efforts or may function automatically in the patient whose spontaneous respiratory drive is not sufficient to maintain ventilation.

There is no general agreement on the value of IPPB as a *routine* measure in the day-to-day treatment of patients with chronic obstructive disease. Some workers believe that such therapy has great value in increasing alveolar ventilation, and others feel that it may represent a potentially useful technique for administering bronchodilator aerosols.

COR PULMONALE

The treatment of this complication is considered in some detail on p. 1539. The problem is basically that of the vigorous management of both congestive heart failure (Chap. 249) and of pulmonary failure, as discussed above.

INFECTION

Because of the difficulties of proper drainage of secretions, the problem of recurrent infection in patients with chronic pulmonary disease is serious. Either frankly pathogenic organisms or bacteria of relatively low virulence, such as *Hemophilus influenzae*, may be responsible. Severe pulmonary infection may occur in this group of patients without the usual systemic indications such as fever or leukocytosis. For this reason early and vigorous chemotherapy is important. Such chemotherapy should be guided by careful bacteriologic examination. Less well established is the use of prophylactic chemotherapy during infection-free periods. This problem is currently under study. It should also be reiterated that postural drainage, bronchodilators, and steam inhalation are important adjuvants to the therapy of recurrent pulmonary infection.

SURGICAL THERAPY

The operative treatment of chronic pulmonary disease involves the excision of blebs and bullae which have compressed normal lung. Resection of such lesions allows adjacent normal lungs to reexpand and, depending on the size and location, will allow greater excursion of the diaphragm and relieve distortion of the mediastinal contents. The poorest results are achieved when a severe degree of underlying obstructive emphysema exists which has accounted for the dyspnea and disability experienced by the patient. Indications and contraindications for the removal of cysts have been discussed on p. 1557.

Direct approach to the problem of obstructive pulmonary emphysema per se has centered on surgery of the autonomic nervous system and on efforts to increase the blood supply of the lung. Dorsal sympathectomy, vagal denervation, dissection of perivascular and peribronchial tissues, and parietal pleurectomy with talc poudrage have all been tried, alone or in combination. The evidence is slim that any of these maneuvers gives lasting benefit to subjects with chronic pulmonary disease, and the hazards involved do not usually justify the attempts.

The use of pneumoperitoneum and of abdominal binders, in the hope of increasing the excursion of the diaphragm by upward displacement, has largely been abandoned.

THE ACUTE RESPIRATORY EMERGENCY

A number of different diseases may produce such interference with the process of ventilation that the patient's life is threatened by the resultant hypoventilation or apnea. Under these circumstances, artificial maintenance of ventilation is mandatory. The initial step is to ensure a patent airway. The patient's neck should be hyperextended and, if available, either an oropharyngeal airway or, preferably, a cuffed endotracheal tube inserted. While equipment is mobilized, adequate ventilation may be maintained by means of mouth-to-mouth breathing. As soon as possible, suction should be performed to clear respiratory secretions. Artificial ventilation over a prolonged period can be successfully carried out by a number of techniques. One commonly employed method uses an intermittent positive-pressure apparatus (IPPB). This apparatus is powered by compressed air or oxygen. The lungs are inflated by positive pressure and deflate passively. Preferably, the instrument should have an automatic cycling device so that if the patient's respiratory efforts are too feeble to trigger the mechanism, ventilation will continue. Also desirable in such instruments are independent controls for the regulation of air flow and pressure, so that these parameters may be tailored to the patient's requirements. All such apparatus provides means of humidifying the inspired gas before it reaches the patient. Another commonly used variety of respirator is the piston type (Moersch), in which fixed volumes of moistened and heated air or oxygen are driven into the lung by means of a piston powered by a motor.

Ventilation may also be accomplished by means of a tank (Drinker) respirator. The patient's body (except for head and neck) is enclosed in a chamber, in which subatmospheric and supraatmospheric pressures are generated to produce volume flow of air into and out of the patient's respiratory tract.

As indicated above, when cough or swallowing is impaired, tracheostomy should be performed for the control of secretions.

Meticulous attention to hydration, electrolytes, care of bowel and bladder, infections, and orthopedic and psychologic problems is required. The patient's survival frequently depends on the degree of excellence of the nursing care provided.

REFERENCES

Comroe, J. H., Jr., and R. D. Dripps: "The Physiological Basis for Oxygen Therapy," (American Lecture Series, 42) Springfield, Ill., Charles C Thomas, Publisher, 1950.

Mushin, W. W., L. Rendell-Baker, and P. W. Thompson: "Automatic Ventilation of the Lungs," Springfield, Ill., Charles C Thomas, Publisher, 1959.

Pridie, R. B., N. Dotte, D. G. Massey, G. W. Poole, J. Schneeweiss, and P. Stradling: A Trial of Continuous Winter Chemotherapy in Chronic Bronchitis, Lancet, 2:723, 1960.

Sieker, H. O., and J. B. Hickam: Carbon Dioxide Intoxication: The Clinical Syndrome, Its Etiology and Management with Particular Reference to the Use of Mechanical Respirators, Medicine, 35:389, 1956.

Snider, G. L., H. K. Barnett, D. B. Radner, and M. M. Mosko: The Evaluation of Bronchodilator Drugs in the Treatment of Asthma, J. Lab. Clin. Med., 46: 348, 1955.

Thacker, E. W.: "Postural Drainage and Respiratory Control," 2d ed., London, Lloyd-Luke, Publisher, 1959.

Section 5: The Alimentary Tract

269 GENERAL CONSIDERATIONS

Franz J. Ingelfinger

The evaluation of gastrointestinal complaints is becoming harder and knottier as the diagnostic techniques available become more numerous and intricate. This paradox, in view of the contributions made to the diagnosis of gastrointestinal disorders by roentgen rays, biochemistry, and endoscopy, may be challenged as hyperbole, but it sets in focus a disturbing question: To what extent is diagnosis today a human or mechanical function? The problem is particularly acute for the physician trying to diagnose an abdominal disorder. Aware of human error, and his confidence circumscribed because he must decide on the condition of viscera that he often can neither see nor feel, the physician turns for help to the laboratory or the machine, to which he imputes an unwarranted objectivity and accuracy. The more elaborate and complex the technical method, moreover, the more the ordinary physician is unaware of its limitations, and the more he stands in awe of the results it bears. Thus any student or physician preparing himself to handle gastrointestinal problems (or any medical problem for that matter) must decide whether it is better to run or to be run by a technology that is superb but strange to him. Put in another way, he must decide between a purposefully eclectic and routinely comprehensive approach.

The comprehensive routine is the method of the survey: it rigorously pursues an unvarying check list of questions, orders a complete "battery" of laboratory tests and extensive radiologic studies, viz., pyelography, cholecystography, upper gastrointestinal series, and barium enema. The routinely comprehensive approach thus provides automatic safeguards; it protects against ignorance, negligence, and forgetfulness. It also detects the unexpected: the colonic polyp, for example, in the patient whose symptoms of heartburn direct attention to the esophagus and stomach. It even permits the physician—if he orders blood calcium determinations (at $5 a test) routinely—to exhibit a somewhat spurious serendipity in finding the rare patient with hyperparathyroidism among the many patients with digestive complaints.

An elevated serum calcium level, however, does not necessarily signify hyperparathyroidism; it may be the result of vitamin D intoxication, of excessive milk-alkali therapy, or perhaps merely of laboratory error. The trouble with the routine mill is that its products—whether hypercalcemia, an x-ray report of diaphragmatic hernia, or the patient's insistence that certain foods give her indigestion—tumble forth in haphazard and unrelated fashion. So unrelated, indeed, are the results that it makes little difference if x-rays or history are obtained first, and adherents of the comprehensive survey might indeed perform more efficiently by reversing the usual sequence. Eventually, of course, all the findings have to be assembled into a meaningful whole, but it takes time to put together a jigsaw puzzle, and completion of the picture is easily prevented by a big piece which does not fit but which seems important because it originated in the laboratory or in the x-ray dark room.

The eclectic method uses the chief complaint to orient the line of study and then purposefully proceeds to elicit points of information specifically designed to support or to weaken the various diagnoses possible. This means that the chief complaint immediately should suggest a list of differential diagnoses. Historical data, physical findings, x-rays, and laboratory examination are thereupon sought and analyzed to create a framework that has meaning at all stages of its development. As points of information become available, they are evaluated for significance on the basis of their interrelationship: do they make sense within the diagnostic framework being erected? Or perhaps they are sufficiently cogent to undermine its foundations and thus to necessitate a new start. In the end, the structure created should form a compact and reasonable whole with as few extra pieces lying around as possible.

The gastrointestinal complaints of many a patient are in great part determined by the kind of individual he is. Ulcerative colitis flourishes in individuals of certain emotional make-up and family background, psychologic stress intensifies the symptoms of sprue, and the anxious cancerophobe fearfully mulls over the meaning of her aerophagic belching. A knowledge of the patient's character is therefore highly desirable, and it is obtainable only by conversation. Thus, a careful and purposefull exploration of the chief complaint, performed with a full realization of the close interrelationship of psyche and gut, almost automatically provides the physician with the character insight he needs to handle his patient not only sympathetically but also effectively.

THE INTERPRETATION OF SYMPTOMS

Pain of all varieties, ranging from vague discomfort to excruciating colic, is the most common of digestive tract symptoms. To distinguish such pain from painful conditions of other organs, its location and quality serve some purpose; but the prime consideration in deciding whether or not abdominal, thoracic, or back pain is of alimentary tract origin is its relation, or lack of relation, to some gastrointestinal function. Thus the man with colonic pain may experience relief after passing gas or stool, or he may feel worse, or a desire to defecate may accompany his distress. If a patient has esophageal pain, its incidence and intensity are usually related to swallowing. In other instances, the relationship is less obvious and depends upon interpretive use of medical knowledge, as, for example, in the case of the patient with duodenal ulcer who has pain at times when his gastric pH may be assumed to be at its lowest.

Correlation between a pain and a gastrointestinal function must of necessity be chronologic and hence susceptible to the fallacies of *post hoc–propter hoc* reasoning. A meticulous inquiry as to the frequency, specificity, and chronology of the relationship serves, however, to reduce the likelihood of error. When the patient says, as he so often does, that "the pain comes on after meals," find out exactly *when* (while eating dessert, immediately after finishing, within 15 min, or later, while at work or watching television); find out after *what* meals and *how often* after given meals. Such questioning, the heart of the eclectic method, serves not only to determine the degree and nature of the relationship between eating and pain, but also helps to distinguish the organic from the functional complaint. The man with cancer of the esophagus or duodenal ulcer has relatively little difficulty in describing the chronologic relationships of his complaints, but the person with functional complaints[1] cannot be pinned down. A relationship between meals, particularly between certain kinds of foods and symptoms, may be vigorously claimed by the patient with functional disorders, but lawyer-like cross examination reveals a witness who cannot describe consistent or specific relationships.

Caution is of course also necessary. Some digestive tract pain, as from pancreatic cancer, for example, may appear totally unrelated to any alimentary tract activity. Conversely, copious eructations after meals may mark the pure neurotic or the man with serious coronary insufficiency. Renal colic may wear the costume of paralytic ileus, and endocrine disorders may present as abdominal pain with deranged bowel habits. Such pitfalls and exceptions notwithstanding, the rule stands: gastrointestinal pain usually has something to do with gastrointestinal function.

Nausea and vomiting are such frequent manifestations of all kinds of diseases—or of injudicious therapy—that their relatively limited significance as symptoms of digestive tract disease deserves emphasis. If some cases of gastric retention are excluded, painless nausea and vomiting (the "painless" is crucial) do not indicate major disease of the alimentary tube, gallbladder, or pancreas. Much more likely to be responsible are functional disorders, central nervous system disease, cardiovascular-renal disease, endocrine abnormalities, or drugs. Painless nausea and vomiting, of course, are frequent symptoms of hepatic disorders.

INTERPRETATION OF REPORTS FROM THE LABORATORY, THE RADIOLOGIST, AND THE ENDOSCOPIST

Whether the average physician attempting the diagnosis of a gastrointestinal complaint uses the eclectic or routine approach, he depends for help on the specialized skill of others and must accept, perforce, the results of a serum transaminase determination, a gastroscopy, or a barium enema at their face value. The problem presented by the x-ray examination of the gastrointestinal tract is particularly troublesome. With the knowledge, skill, and technical facilities now in his hands, the expert radiologist can detect a host of variations from normal, and as is his duty, he reports them. If the physician

---

[1] "Organic" and "functional" are frequently used words, but with nuances and implications that vary from user to user. To the author, an organic disease is one with recognizable structural changes. A functional disorder is literally a disorder of function, a change in "how an organ works." According to this view, functional is a descriptive term, not etiologic. Thus a functional disorder, e.g., simple constipation, may or may not be psychogenic in etiology.

receiving these reports makes diagnoses by using the comprehensive survey method, if his x-ray requests are not dictated by a specific diagnostic question, he is apt to be overwhelmed. After all, here is a report in black and white of something clearly pictured in white and black. His unorganized clinical investigation offers little resistance, and the x-ray report becomes the final diagnosis by subtle metamorphosis. Thus the patient's real trouble may be relegated or even obliterated by the x-ray findings. A combination of x-ray findings may, indeed, be confused with clinical syndromes, and the patient in whom the astute radiologist finds a coexistence of gallstones, diaphragmatic hernia, and diverticulosis may be portentously diagnosed as suffering from Saint's triad, a "syndrome" which from the clinical viewpoint is unadulterated nonsense. (If among women aged fifty or more, gallstones occur in 20 per cent, diaphragmatic hernia in another 20 per cent, and diverticulosis in 50 per cent, a combination of these conditions will unavoidably exist in two out of every 100 such women examined.)

The physician with the eclectic approach is better prepared. Having a diagnostic pattern in mind, he tests the fit of laboratory, x-ray, endoscopic, cytologic, and biopsy findings. If the fit is bad but the finding weighty, he does not insist on his clinical judgment; he is well aware, for example, that a vague and nonspecific clinical picture in no way contravenes an x-ray diagnosis of gastric cancer. On the other hand, he also knows that x-rays are not infallible, and if a patient has typical ulcer symptoms or a classic history of biliary colic, the physician does not permit his clinical case to collapse merely because of a negative x-ray report. Nor is he necessarily content with the diagnosis of diaphragmatic hernia in a patient who has a radiologically demonstrated hernia and unimpressive electrocardiographic findings, but who gives a history of squeezing substernal distress coming on with exercise and promptly relieved by rest or nitroglycerin.

Exceptions and atypy confuse the path, but to reach correct gastroenterologic diagnosis most consistently, it pays to insist (1) that gastrointestinal symptoms and gastrointestinal function evidence some interrelationship, (2) that the clinical picture and the results of technical diagnostic procedures jibe, and (3) that all information, whatever its source and nature, create a reasonable whole.

EVALUATION OF TREATMENT

Some years ago, an English physician named Gill treated 20 patients with gastric ulcer by giving them a daily injection of 1 ml of sterile water. As judged by gastroscopic criteria, the ulcers healed in 4 to 8 weeks, the time usually required under conventional therapy. In a study organized on statistical principles, Doll, Jones, and Pygott observed the rate of gastric ulcer healing in three groups: nonsmokers, smokers who continued to smoke, and smokers who stopped smoking. Decrease of ulcer size by two-thirds or more was attained within 28 days in 75 per cent of the smokers who stopped smoking, as opposed to 58 per cent of those who did not stop; but the proportion of nonsmokers showing comparable ulcer healing was also 58 per cent, i.e., no better than the results obtained in the unregenerate. Such observations highlight the problem of rational treatment of gastrointestinal disorders. Except in cases where surgical intervention is either mandatory or highly effective (e.g., appendicitis, cholelithiasis with biliary colic, intestinal obstruction, ulcerative colitis refractory to medical treatment), the specific effects of therapeutic procedures, whether medical, dietary, or surgical, are assessed with great difficulty.

Enthusiasm, of course, may run high, and the medical literature is swollen by reports vigorously advocating this or that treatment. The fact remains, however, that if surgical procedures and specific infections and infestations are excluded, no gastrointestinal condition exists that is susceptible to dependably curative medical management. To be sure, symptomatic or partial improvement is possible. Elimination of gluten arrests the steatorrhea in many cases of idiopathic sprue; stretching the gastroesophageal junction decreases the dysphagia of the patient with cardiospasm; intensive neutralization of gastric juice heals the peptic ulcer; and adrenocortical therapy may induce remission in ulcerative colitis; but these methods provide alleviation, not cure of the condition. In the case of more vaguely defined entities, gastritis and irritable colon, for example, the efficacy of any therapeutic endeavor is even more difficult to evaluate.

These points are not meant to inculcate a pessimistic attitude toward gastrointestinal therapy. They do mean, however, that the student or the practitioner of gastroenterology must maintain an objective attitude concerning the regimen he advocates. If he insists on rigid dietary injunctions, he should have some rationale beyond reliance upon routine practice. When antacids are prescribed, he should have some reason for prescribing an elaborate (and expensive) concoction of aluminum hydroxide, magnesium salt, sedative, and a so-called antispasmodic, as opposed to giving much cheaper and often equally effective calcium salts and tincture of belladonna. In deciding on an anticholinergic agent, he should be aware of exactly what such agents may do to gastrointestinal motility and

secretion and that these agents are not necessarily beneficial under all conditions. A potent anticholinergic, for example, may reduce the volume of gastric secretion, but this possibly beneficial effect may be offset by the increased gastric retention that also results from vagal inhibition. Furthermore, the claims that synthetic anticholinergic agents are so selective that only the gastrointestinal tract is affected must be judged in the light of evidence suggesting that individuals vary tremendously in terms of dose response and that, as of the moment, specific gastrointestinal effects without side effects are more of a hoped-for ideal than an accomplished fact.

The patient with gastrointestinal complaints obviously requires therapy, but in view of the uncertain state of many of the measures employed, a number of generalizations are offered to guide treatment along an honest path.

1. To the extent that treatment is nonspecific, the art of medicine becomes important. Thus the care, sympathy, and enthusiasm with which treatment is administered clearly influence the results.

2. Traditional treatment is tested by experience and hence safe in the eyes of the public and the medical profession. By and large, it is also safe for the patient, but not always so, as, for example, the not-so-old practice of forcing large amounts of protein on the semistuporous patient with advanced liver disease. Thus the alert physician, aware of the deficiencies of traditonal gastrointestinal treatment, may use its principles as a therapeutic base line but is constantly looking for and receptive to new approaches.

3. Before a new regimen or approach is used, it deserves analysis. A new medicine should obviously not be employed merely because it is new ("the latest development") and insistently distributed by its maker. If a new method is recommended in the medical literature, the basis for such recommendation is examined with profit. Is it rational in terms of what is known concerning gastrointestinal physiology, pharmacology, and pathology? Has the investigation of the new treatment's efficacy been distinguished by adequate control studies with proper checks on the subjective influences of the investigator? Is there real evidence that the new method or agent is better than existing methods?

The generalizations made concerning treatment are of course not peculiar in their application to gastroenterology. On the other hand, the fact that treatment of gastroenterologic conditions is so limited to a symptomatic plane makes such treatment highly susceptible, on one hand to hasty innovations and ill-considered enthusiasms, and on the other to stubborn adherence to practice sanctified by no more than tradition. The best thing a physician can do to avoid these extremes is to ask himself, as he instructs the patient, "Why am I doing this?"

REFERENCES

Doll, R., F. Avery Jones, and F. Pygott: Effect of Smoking on Production and Maintenance of Gastric and Duodenal Ulcers, Lancet, 1:657, 1958.

Gill, A. M.: Pain and the Healing of Peptic Ulcers, Lancet, 1:291, 1947.

270 DISEASES OF THE MOUTH
E. Cheraskin

Significant diagnostic information can be obtained from simple inspection of the oral cavity. This is possible because the mouth is a very sensitive barometer of systemic balance.

Oral symptoms and signs fall into two groups. Some of these findings are highly characteristic, though generally not pathognomonic, of a specific disease state or a family of disorders. Others reflect, through nonspecific clues, simply the presence of chronic disease.

SPECIFIC ORAL FINDINGS OF SYSTEMIC DISEASE

The oral symptoms and signs of about 50 systemic disorders are characteristic enough to warrant special mention. These conditions include the active participation of biologic agents, chemical intoxication, hormonal imbalance, nutritional deficiency, developmental factors, and the lack of adaptation to stress.

In the main, the oral clues may be divided into the following categories: (1) pigmentation, (2) ulceration, (3) salivary changes, (4) dental pathosis, and (5) miscellaneous findings.

Pigmentation. Congenital lues is characterized by red or copper-colored necrotic crusts on the lips which, with healing, leave linear scars radially arranged and perpendicular to the mucocutaneous junction (rhagades). Thrush is noted by a soft, painless, pearly-white elevated patch. Some of the common viral diseases are associated with oral signs. Koplik's spots are blue-white specks surrounded by a red border on the buccal mucosa just opposite the maxillary first molars. These lesions appear about 24 to 48 hr prior to the onset of the rash of measles. Occasionally, one may observe early in mumps, inflammation of the buccal mucosa surrounding the opening of Stensen's duct. Characteristic yellow to gray palatal papules, 2 to 20 in number, which form vesicles and quickly rupture

may be observed in herpangina. Gingival and palatine petechiae have been described in infectious mononucleosis. Argyria is associated with generalized mucosal darkening and possibly a violet line at the free marginal gingiva. Bismuthism, mercurialism, thallotoxicosis, and plumbism all show a pigmented line in the free gingival margin. With cadmium intoxication there is a yellow to gold ring about the cervixes of the teeth. The most suggestive oral finding of Addison's disease is generalized mucosal melanin pigmentation. The tongue in many of the vitamin B–deficiency states may become red or magenta. One of the highly characteristic findings in pernicious anemia is the red inflamed dorsum of the tongue. In the Peutz-Jeghers syndrome, there are often melanin macules upon the lips, buccal mucosa, tongue, and hard palate. Wickham's striae (thin white strands of lacelike arrangement on the buccal mucosa) are considered typical of lichen planus. Finally, primary or secondary polycythemia may be recognized by the generalized deepening of the color (blue-red) of the entire oral mucosa.

Ulceration. The two most common extragenital sites for the luetic chancre are the lips and tongue. Secondary syphilis is recognized by oral mucous patches. A cardinal sign of agranulocytosis is pleomorphic dirty-gray or black ulcers which are not surrounded by the erythematous margin that is generally observed bordering most oral ulcers. Riboflavin, nicotinic acid, and pyridoxine deficiency can contribute to the development of angular cheilosis.

Salivary Changes. Sialorrhea (an increase in saliva) is commonly associated with arsenism, bismuthism, mercurialism, thallotoxicosis, plumbism, and cadmium intoxication. An increase in salivary flow has also been described with cretinism and vitamin B–deficiency states. On the other hand, asialorrhea is encountered with hyperthyroidism, diabetes mellitus, Sjögren's disease, and hereditary ectodermal dysplasia.

Dental Pathoses. In about one-third of the cases of congenital syphilis, Hutchinsonian incisors and mulberry molars are present. Slight to moderate enamel chalkiness which becomes exogenously pigmented is fairly common with chronic fluorosis. When hyperactivity of the anterior lobe of the hypophysis commences early in life, the end result (gigantism) may include generalized macrodontia. On the other hand, the oral picture of the acromegalic patient shows macroglossia, prognathism, and malocclusion. Hypophyseal dwarfism demonstrates delayed exfoliation of the primary teeth, retarded eruption of the permanent dentition, possibly microdontia, and commonly malocclusion. In the cretin, there is macroglossia, retarded eruption of the permanent teeth, and delayed exfoliation of the primary dentition as well as malocclusion. Loosening of the teeth and disappearance of the lamina dura, as observed in the roentgenogram, are sometimes seen with hyperparathyroidism. In the case of hypoparathyroidism, there is enamel hypoplasia and possibly delayed eruption; the lamina dura, however, remains intact. With vitamin A deficiency there is sometimes enamel hypoplasia. One very glaring clue of Cooley's anemia is malocclusion of the medial open-bite type, where the teeth posteriorly are in contact but are not in occlusion anteriorly. This is due to maxillary overdevelopment. Osteogenesis imperfecta is notable for the opalescent color of the teeth. In addition, the crowns are disproportionately larger than the roots and the pulps are completely obliterated at an early age. Cleidocranial dysostosis may be recognized by a reduced number of teeth, lack of dental eruption, and the presence of a host of unerupted malformed teeth. Finally, a reduction in the number of teeth is a cardinal sign of hereditary ectodermal dysplasia. The developing teeth of the child with erythroblastosis fetalis may show a yellow to green endogenous pigment. Juvenile rheumatoid arthritis frequently includes destruction of the growth centers in the mandibular condyles. Hence, the end result is underdevelopment of the mandible, leading to severe malocclusion. Serial roentgenographic study of the jaws of the sclerodermic patient will disclose periodic thickening and thinning of the periodontal membranes. A fairly constant observation in mongolian idiocy is malformation or absence of the maxillary lateral incisor.

Miscellaneous Findings. In scarlet fever the fungiform papillae become enlarged (raspberry tongue). Sometimes there follows desquamation of the papillary tips (strawberry tongue). The most common oral stigma of tertiary syphilis is palatal perforation secondary to gumma formation. Fungi may invade the mouth. Actinomycosis is often recognizable by a yellow, purulent, granular drainage. Diphenylhydantoin (Dilantin) frequently results in the development of a painless, mulberry-shaped gingival hyperplasia. Fine tongue tremor is included in the classical description of hyperthyroidism. Hyperkeratosis is now regarded as sometimes indicative of a vitamin A deficiency. Thickening of the tongue and reduced lingual activity are observed frequently in patients with scleroderma.

NONSPECIFIC ORAL FINDINGS

More common, if not as dramatic, are the nonspecific oral symptoms and signs. These do not provide the examiner with immediate clues to a specific systemic problem. However, they do supply evidence of chronic debilitation.

Oral Symptoms. A number of symptoms are peculiar to the oral cavity by virtue of its special structural design. Included in this group are gingival tenderness, xerostomia (dry mouth), and stomatopyrosis (burning mouth). The presence of this triad usually signifies a metabolic disturbance. For example, these three oral symptoms occur earlier and with greater regularity than polyphagia, polydipsia, and polyuria in the patient with diabetes mellitus. As a matter of fact, as evidence of their relationship to metabolic imbalance, these three oral symptoms may signify hypo- as well as hyperglycemia, and both hypo- and hyperproteinemia.

Oral Signs. Significant, though nonspecific, information can be derived from the presence of gingival bleeding and clinically demonstrable tooth mobility. Gingival bleeding occurs in approximately two-thirds of the population. Though it is usually attributed to faulty toothbrushing, there is the strong possibility that it may be a measure of increased vascular fragility and permeability.

Under physiologic conditions, the teeth are not clinically mobile. Clinical tooth mobility is a sensitive measure of metabolism. For example, it appears in the presence of carbohydrate, protein, and vitamin imbalance. Thus, clinical tooth mobility may be the first expression of diabetes mellitus, scurvy, protein deficiency, and the vitamin B–complex syndrome.

Oral Roentgenographic Findings. In the physiologic state, the alveolar bone should extend almost up to the cervixes of the teeth. Alveolar bone loss occurs with defective osteoid matrix formation (osteogenesis imperfecta, protein and ascorbic acid deficiency, alarm syndrome), reduced matrix mineralization (rickets and osteomalacia), and increased bone resorption (hyperparathyroidism).

REFERENCES

Burket, L. W.: "Oral Medicine," 3d ed., Philadelphia, J. B. Lippincott Company, 1957.
Cheraskin, E., and L. L. Langley: "Dynamics of Oral Diagnosis," Chicago, Year Book Publishers, Inc., 1956.

271 DISEASES OF THE ESOPHAGUS

Franz J. Ingelfinger

Although the anatomy of the swallowing tube is still controversial, the structural definitions indicated in Fig. 271-1 are used in this discussion. The esophagus proper, with principally propulsive functions, is regarded as lying between two sphincteric segments at its upper and lower ends. The upper segment comprises the cricopharyngeus muscle and the highest circular muscles of the esophagus. The lower sphincteric mechanism is believed to lie in the upper part of the vestibule. It normally remains closed except during swallowing and regurgitation, and acts, in conjunction with the diaphragm and a possible flap-valve mechanism provided by the angle of His, to prevent gastroesophageal reflux. Compression of the intraabdominal portion of the vestibule by intraperitoneal pressure may provide another barrier against reflux.

Symptomatology. *Dysphagia.* Although esophageal disease accounts for no more than one-tenth of all gastrointestinal complaints, it is characterized by one of the most specific symptoms in medicine: the sensation of food sticking on its way from the mouth to the stomach. This dysphagia of esophageal origin can usually be distinguished from oropharyngeal dysphagia, which is characterized by inability to move a bolus out of the mouth, by nasal regurgitation, or by tracheal aspiration. Esophageal dysphagia, since it occurs only with swallowing, also differs from the persistent sensation of globus hystericus. Esophageal dysphagia may be painless, more often it is distressing, and sometimes it causes pain of alarming proportions. Whatever its concomitants, the complaint of food sticking somewhere behind the sternum signifies that some process—whether functional spasm or organic stricture—is occluding the esophageal lumen.

The level of the sticking sensation, corresponding to the most frequent site of esophageal disease, is usually under the lower end of the sternum. In other instances dysphagia is localized higher in the chest or at the base of the neck, either because the responsible lesion is situated higher or because sensations from the distal esophagus are referred to the sternal notch by approximately one-fourth of adult patients.

Dysphagia occasionally begins abruptly and reaches maximum intensity at the onset, but more commonly it appears gradually in intermittent attacks precipitated by the ingestion of certain foods. Beef and fresh bread are notorious offenders, probably because these elastic solids are wedged by peristalsis into the esophageal area narrowed by disease. If this happens, the patient may be able to force the offending morsel past the obstructing point by rapidly gulping water or may be able to regurgitate it by forceful retching. With progressive disease, however, the swallowing of liquid as well as solid becomes difficult. Liquids of low viscosity, as a matter of fact, are regurgitated too readily, and the peristaltic action of the esophagus is used to best advantage when the patient takes food of pultaceous consistency.

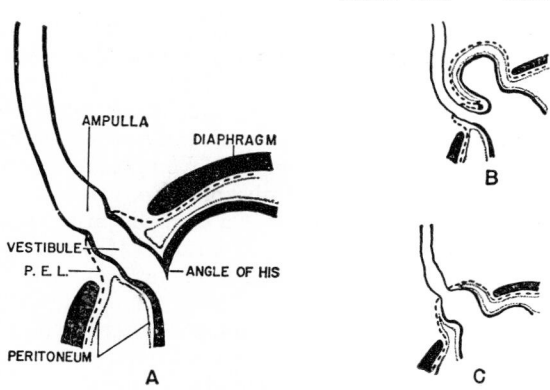

Fig. 271-1. Diagrammatic representation of the structure and relations of the lower esophagus. *A.* Normal esophagus. *B.* Parahiatal hernia. *C.* Sliding hernia. In this type of hernia the distinction between the vestibule and the herniated cardia is lost, and the angle of His has become obtuse. P.E.L. = phrenoesophageal ligament. The location of the gastroesophageal junction is a matter of opinion. It may be defined as located at the level where the tube of the esophagus widens into the sac of the stomach, but sometimes the transition from one shape to the other is gradual rather than abrupt. Alternatively, the junction is placed at the serrated line where squamous esophageal and glandular gastric mucosas meet, but this epithelial boundary may be located somewhat above the level of the angle of His and thus does not necessarily coincide with a division of stomach and esophagus based on gross shape and muscular function.

Pain. Pain, a common symptom of esophageal disease, may be persistent and unrelated to swallowing or intermittent and intimately associated with dysphagia; often it is precipitated by the ingestion of acid, spicy, carbonated, very cold, or very hot substances. The mechanisms underlying esophageal pain are two: (1) ulceration or inflammation of the mucosa, and (2) increased intramural tension produced by violent peristalsis or stationary muscular spasm. Esophageal pain is usually felt anteriorly under the sternum at a level corresponding to the position of the lesion, but it may also be referred to the upper back, the neck, the jaws, and into both arms, particularly their inner aspects. Anatomically and functionally, therefore, the transmission and reference of pain from the esophagus and from the heart may be the same.

Heartburn. Heartburn, pyrosis, and water brash mean different things to different people, and it is important to determine what heartburn signifies to the patient with this complaint. Here the term heartburn is used to denote an intermittent symptom complex which begins with a burning, tight sensation under the sternum, and then travels upwards, wavelike, to reach its scalding, acid maximum in the neck or throat. Salivation is often part of the picture. The cause of heartburn may be muscular spasm, reflux of gastric contents, or both, but its exact pathogenesis is still uncertain.

Belching. Many a belch is forceful regurgitation of air that has been sucked or swallowed into the esophageal lumen. Although belching, therefore, is frequently an esophageal phenomenon, it is, except in diaphragmatic hernia, not a common manifestation of esophageal disease. More often it is a functional disorder or is indicative of gastric, cardiac, or biliary tract disease.

Regurgitation. Regurgitation, as opposed to vomiting, means the effortless appearance of esophageal or gastric contents in the mouth. A functional disorder of gastroesophageal motility, a retrograde flow of material forced by normal esophageal peristalsis against a stenotic area, or as in the case of the dilated esophagus of cardiospasm, a gravitational effect may be responsible for regurgitation.

CANCER

Symptoms. The importance of dysphagia as a symptom and the urgent necessity of determining its cause are no better exemplified than by the patient with esophageal cancer. Difficulty in swallowing is often the patient's first, and at times his only, complaint as the growth encroaches upon the lumen. Although intermittent initially, the dysphagia is inexorably progressive over the course of months. In fungating tumors, the commonest gross variety of esophageal cancer, pain under the sternum, in the back, or in the neck, is usual and sometimes precedes dysphagia. In some cases an early symptom not to be ignored is substernal burning on swallowing hot liquids. Slow oozing of blood is a frequent complication, and brisk bleeding a rare one. In about 25 per cent of cases, however, particularly with infiltrative or polypoid cancers, symptoms other than dysphagia appear only terminally. When esophageal stenosis is severe, regurgitation of esophageal contents, sometimes blood-flecked, is common.

Approximately 20 per cent of esophageal cancers are in the upper third, 30 per cent in the middle, and 50 per cent in the lower third of the organ. The lesions in the upper two-thirds are derived from squamous esophageal mucosa. In the distal esophagus over half the cases prove to be adenocarcinomas, indicating that many cancers in this area are gastric in origin. A gastric origin is, as a matter of fact, often evident on operation in cases which radiologically appear to be purely esophageal.

Course. Physical examination is usually negative and even those patients with advanced disease may present no more than the signs of malnutrition. Although metastases to lymph nodes occur in three-fourths of the cases, only 5 per cent have palpable nodes in the supraclavicular or other accessible areas. Since the liver and lung are each involved eventually in 20 to 25 per cent of the cases, hepatomegaly or pulmonary lesions may be evident. Other organs subject to metastatic foci are bone, kidneys, and adrenal glands. Sometimes direct invasion of adjoining structures leads to dramatic complications: (1) mediastinitis with subcutaneous emphysema in the neck, (2) tracheo- or bronchoesophageal fistula, with an apoplectic cough induced by swallowing liquids, or (3) aortic perforation with precipitous exsanguination.

Diagnosis. Esophageal cancer occurs in the usual cancer age groups, and males preponderate 4:1. It is about one-tenth as common as cancer of the stomach in either sex. X-ray often reveals the irregular and sometimes surprisingly long luminal defect caused by esophageal cancer, but supplemental diagnostic information must usually be sought by esophagoscopy with biopsy. The initial examination with either procedure is not, however, invariably adequate in differentiating cancer from inflammatory stricture. In these cases, cytologic examination of material obtained by esophageal lavage is indicated. This procedure yields 75 per cent positive results in patients with esophageal cancer.

Treatment. Lesions that appear to be resectable are usually treated surgically. Calculated on the basis of all esophageal cancer patients who enter a hospital, the 5-year cure rate is still a disappointing 0 to 7 per cent. In some hands, however, 5-year cure rates in patients who at operation have no gross evidence of extension are over 30 per cent for cancers in the lower third of the esophagus. Successful resection of higher cancers is more difficult. In patients with inoperable tumors of the fungating variety, palliation of dysphagia may be achieved to a remarkable degree by deep radiotherapy delivered by high voltage x-ray apparatus and Co^{60} bombs.

DIAPHRAGMATIC HERNIA

A common abnormality affecting the esophagus but, strictly speaking, of gastric origin is herniation of the stomach through the esophageal hiatus of the diaphragm. Two types of hernia are described. In one, the paraesophageal or parahiatal type, the gastric cardia rolls through the muscular aperture beside a gastroesophageal junction that is still normally situated with respect to the level of the diaphragmatic hiatus (Fig. 271-1*B*). In the other, the sliding, axial, concentric, or short esophagus type, both the stomach and the gastroesophageal junction slip up into the chest, thereby placing the gastroesophageal junction above the diaphragmatic hiatus (Fig. 271-1*C*). This position of the junction makes the esophagus appear shortened, and actual shortening may be caused by chronic esophageal inflammation. A congenitally short esophagus, however, is rare. Many hernias are mixed in that they present features of both types.

The incidence of diaphragmatic hernia is debated, since its radiologic differentiation from a prominent vestibule is a matter of individual interpretation. In elderly persons, the incidence of sliding hernia exceeds 50 per cent, men appearing to be somewhat more susceptible; paraesophageal hernia, predominantly a disorder of women, is only one-tenth as common. Both types of hernia are more prevalent in stocky and obese individuals.

Symptoms. Both parahiatal and sliding hernias may give rise to symptoms when the herniated pouch is irritated or injured by the mechanical disadvantages of its position or when it is sufficiently large to affect adjoining viscera. These complications characteristically affect the paraesophageal variety of hernia. The most common complaint is high epigastric or low midthoracic pressure or a pain which may radiate along the left costal margin, to the top of the left shoulder or down the arms. Belching is copious and hiccoughing occasional. By and large, the symptoms are moderately distressing, but a rare case may suffer acute prostration should strangulation of the herniated stomach take place. If the mucosa of the hernia becomes eroded, acute or chronic blood loss is possible, but the importance of diaphragmatic hernia as a source of gastrointestinal blood loss is usually exaggerated. Large hernias rarely cause intermittent acute dysphagia by angulating, twisting, or compressing the esophagus, or they may sufficiently displace the lungs or heart to cause cardiorespiratory symptoms. Whatever the clinical manifestations of diaphragmatic hernia, they are characteristically precipitated by eating and aggravated by lying down, both of which actions tend to force more of the stomach into the thoracic cavity.

The principal complication affecting sliding diaphragmatic hernias is peptic esophagitis. This is discussed below.

Diagnosis. Diagnosis is made by radiologic means. Once a diaphragmatic hernia is radiologically identified, however, its relation to the patient's symptoms poses a nice problem. On one hand, the symptoms of diaphragmatic hernia are so diverse that they may resemble the symptoms of coronary insufficiency, biliary colic, pancreatitis, gastric or duodenal ulcers, esophageal diseases, or functional digestive disorders. On the other hand, diaphragmatic hernias are diagnosed so frequently by the radiologist that many hernias must be considered as incidental findings unrelated to the patient's complaints. As a rule upper abdominal or lower thoracic symptoms should not be ascribed to a radiologically demonstrated diaphragmatic hernia unless (1) other possible causes are excluded with reasonable certainty and (2) some evidence exists that the symptoms are intensified when the patient eats or lies down. A particularly difficult problem in differential diagnosis is substernal distress in the elderly patient with both electrocardiographic abnormalities and diaphragmatic hernia. Although coronary pain is usually related to exercise and that of hernia precipitated by lying down, these associations are not constant, and both conditions may be aggravated by a full meal. When the evidence is conflicting, the wiser course is to assume that coronary disease is the principal offender.

Treatment. Most patients can become fairly comfortable but not entirely symptom-free by eating small meals of low fat content (fat retards gastric evacuation), by avoiding food entirely for 3 hr before going to bed, and by sleeping with the upper half of the body elevated. Additional symptomatic relief may be afforded by sedatives and antispasmodics. Weight loss is imperative for the obese. With respect to surgery, sliding hernias with esophagitis present a special problem, which is discussed later. Operative repair of paraesophageal hernias is indicated if they have been identified as causing intermittent esophageal obstruction, respiratory disease, perforation, strangulation, repeated or chronic bleeding, or severe distress not affected by intensive use of medical measures. If surgery is risky because of age or other illness, symptoms can be partially controlled by crushing the left phrenic nerve to paralyze the left diaphragm.

ACUTE ESOPHAGITIS

Acute esophagitis in a mild form, with substernal pain aggravated by swallowing, may complicate upper respiratory infections. More violent forms with variable necrosis may occur in moribund states, in diseases of the central nervous system, after extensive burns or trauma, after operations, especially if vomiting is pronounced or gastric intubation prolonged, and with specific infections such as scarlet fever, diphtheria, typhoid, and viral diseases with herpetic oral lesions that extend into the esophagus. Monilial esophagitis may appear in those weakened by chronic disease, especially if antibiotics or adrenocortical therapy has been used. In many of these conditions, debility, ischemia, the trauma of vomiting, or exposure of the esophageal mucosa to acid gastric contents must be important pathogenic factors.

The ingestion of alkaline corrosive agents produces a classic variety of acute esophagitis which, if not immediately fatal, may terminate in extensive esophageal stenosis. Immediate treatment depends on giving parenteral analgesics as needed for pain and antibiotics (e.g., aqueous penicillin, 600,000 units, and streptomycin, 250 mg, intramuscularly, four times daily for an adult) for fear of an impending mediastinitis. Oral intake is avoided for 3 to 7 days. After approximately one week, if no extraesophageal infection is apparent, adrenocortical therapy in full doses is recommended to contain the tissue reaction believed responsible for the ensuing stricture. The use of intubation is controversial; if undertaken, it should be performed by expert and cautious hands; the corroded esophagus is easily lacerated.

CHRONIC PEPTIC ESOPHAGITIS

Chronic esophagitis is an inflammatory reaction of the esophageal wall with erosions or frank ulceration of the mucosa and narrowing of the lumen by muscular spasm and fibrotic stricture. Although the etiology of some cases is obscure, the great majority are the result of excessive reflux of acid gastric juice. Peptic esophagitis and the acid-peptic factor appear to be causally related since the disorder occurs predominantly in those with high gastric acidity, is more common in males, and is associated in over one-third of the cases with former or concurrent duodenal ulcer. The abnormality that permits the excessive reflux is usually a sliding diaphragmatic hernia, which obtunds the flap valve created by the angle of His and eliminates both the intraabdominal segment of the vestibule and whatever contribution the diaphragmatic hiatus makes toward maintaining the competence of the normal gastroesophageal barrier (Fig. 271-1C). Occasionally a chronic esophagitis makes its sudden and discouraging appearance in an elderly patient following a severe vomiting episode or after intubation has been used as a postoperative measure or to treat gastrointestinal distention. In these cases, debility and local trauma presumably enhance esophageal susceptibility to refluxed gastric material.

Symptoms. The patient may or may not have had a past history of duodenal ulcer, but almost invariably he has been a long sufferer from heartburn. At first this symptom troubles the patient only after overeating, soon after retiring to bed, or when bending over. Intermittently and progressively, however, the heartburn worsens, cold and hot foods and slightly acid foods are increasingly painful to swallow, and eventually dysphagia appears. With advancing disease, malnutrition is inevitable and slow blood loss occasional.

Diagnosis. Diagnosis is made principally by x-ray, which in cases with stricture shows a gradual and funnel-shaped narrowing of the distal esophagus. The esophagus appears shortened and terminates in a tentlike supradiaphragmatic projection of the stomach characteristic of a sliding hernia. Early cases, with minimal x-ray findings, may be recognized by the fiery, oozing, and mucus-flecked appearance of the distal esophagus seen through the esophagoscope. Patients with esophagitis are also apt to experience typical pain within 30 min when 0.1 N hydrochloric acid is dripped into the esophagus at a rate of 100 drops per minute (Bernstein acid test). The normal esophagus is said not to be sensitive to this procedure, but care must be taken to differentiate esophageal pain from any gastric pain that might be elicited by the acid drip. In the differential diagnosis, cancer, cardiospasm, diffuse spasm, and scleroderma must be considered. In the attempt to exclude cancer, examination of cells obtained by biopsy, esophageal washings, or both is essential.

Treatment. Medical management aims to protect the esophagus, reduce gastric acidity, and prevent gastric reflux. To protect the esophagus, the patient takes 1 tbs of a liquid, viscous antacid preparation, such as an aluminum hydroxide gel, at hourly intervals between meals while he is awake. The medication is taken "straight" and not followed by other material. To enhance its viscosity and emollient properties, the antacid gel may be mixed with 1 tsp of a vegetable oil. If pain is marked, additional symptomatic relief is achieved by giving an aluminum hydroxide gel containing a surface-active anesthetic such as oxethazine. Anticholinergics are as a rule not indicated, since any advantage they might gain by reducing gastric secretion is offset by their disadvantageous action of increasing gastric retention as well. A bedtime anticholinergic is, however, reasonable for those who suffer nocturnal heartburn. A moderately bland diet is desirable, but more important is the avoidance of large meals at all times, and of any food or drink after the evening meal. In stocky or obese patients, weight loss is beneficial since abdominal fat may increase the degree of gastric herniation and reflux. Finally, 6- to 8-in. blocks are placed under the head of the bed to lessen nocturnal gastroesophageal regurgitation.

Medical management of peptic esophagitis may relieve esophageal pain and the dysphagia produced by edema and spasm, but it is ineffective when dysphagia is caused by fibrous stricture. This must be treated by cautious dilatation. If dysphagia persists or recurs in spite of medical measures and dilatation, surgical intervention is indicated. In an early case, repair of the sliding hernia may be sufficient, but in most instances some type of operation designed to reduce gastric acidity (subtotal gastrectomy, vagotomy *with* a drainage procedure) is carried out at the same time. Such surgical effort is unfortunately not much more than 75 per cent successful. Resection of the involved area, as may be necessitated by uncontrollable stenosis, is also not too rewarding; since all barriers to gastric reflux are removed, recurrence of esophagitis proximal to the gastroesophageal anastomosis is likely. Progress is being made in overcoming this difficulty by replacing the resected gastroesophageal section with a segment of small or large bowel.

PEPTIC ULCER

A solitary peptic ulcer is occasionally found in the distal esophagus. This lesion differs from peptic esophagitis in that the ulcer is more sharply localized, penetrates more deeply, and is more apt to perforate or to cause massive bleeding. On the other hand the ulcer is more susceptible to standard medical antacid management (Chap. 272), produces less extensive stricture on healing, and causes less chronic dysphagia than peptic esophagitis. The solitary peptic ulcer in the distal esophagus thus resembles a benign gastric ulcer in many respects. Indeed many ulcers at the lower end of the gullet actually involve either a herniated portion of stomach or a section of the esophagus—perhaps the vestibule—that is lined with gastric mucosa.

CARDIOSPASM (Achalasia)

The term *cardiospasm* does not describe the nature of the disorder accurately but is well established by custom. Actually cardiospasm is a motor disorder involving the entire distal two-thirds of the esophagus. In the esophagus above the vestibule, the normal propulsive pattern of peristalsis is replaced by nonprogressive and uncoordinated contractions. For this reason the name *aperistalsis* is used in Brazil. The massive esophageal dilatation seen in some cases has, in turn, given rise to the name *megaesophagus*. Finally, the term *achalasia* (literally, "not relaxation") is popular because the lower esophageal sphincter, i.e., the vestibular area, does not relax normally in response to swallowing and thus creates an obstructing segment at the distal end of the esophagus.

The motor disorders of cardiospasm appear to reflect an impaired cholinergic innervation of the esophagus. Histologically the cells of the myenteric plexus, i.e., the parasympathetic ganglions, are damaged or absent. Pharmacologic studies have shown that administration of a cholinergic agent produces a tetanic, specific, and often violent contraction of the affected esophagus. This response, when interpreted in the light of Cannon's finding that denervated structures respond maximally to neurohumoral stimulation, provides additional evidence that the cholinergic innervation of the esoph-

agus is deficient in cardiospasm. The ultimate etiology, however, is unknown. In Brazil, the remarkable prevalence of cardiospasm in areas where Chagas disease is endemic has fostered the strong conviction that the intrinsic esophageal denervation is a late result of esophageal infestation by the responsible agent, *Trypanosoma cruzi*.

Symptoms. Cardiospasm affects all ages of both sexes. Its course is usually chronic, with dysphagia gradually worsening over months to years. In some patients, the process is painless; in others spasms of substernal pain may follow eating. Occasionally the initial episode of dysphagia appears with dramatic suddenness, either after bolting food or after an emotional upset. In either case, however, the condition has probably been present in latent form before the acute episode. As the disease progresses, extreme and tortuous dilatation of the esophagus may develop. When the patient lies down, the copious amount of food residue, saliva, and other secretions contained in the spacious esophageal sac runs freely back into the pharynx and mouth. If the regurgitated material is aspirated, chronic infection of the lung bases is a potential complication. Stagnation of food also leads to a chronic inflammatory reaction of the esophageal mucosa and submucosa. Obviously, weight loss is common.

Diagnosis. Diagnosis is usually made without difficulty on the basis of the history and the characteristic radiologic findings of abnormal esophageal motor function with a smooth, beaklike narrowing of the distal esophageal segment. In some cases, cancer originating in the gastric cardia, but infiltrating the esophagus, may present a somewhat similar x-ray appearance, and a variety of motor disorders of the lower esophagus has been confused with cardiospasm. These problems in differential diagnosis should be less frequent if it is remembered that the radiologic abnormalities of cardiospasm consist of deranged peristalsis as well as narrowing in the area of the vestibule.

Treatment. Medical treatment, symptomatic at best, consists of the use of sedatives and bland, semisolid foods warmed to body temperature. Smooth-muscle relaxants such as nitrites are often used to open the vestibule, but the effect is too transient to permit the patient to enjoy a meal. Anticholinergics may lessen oral and esophageal secretions and may inhibit painful spasms; in view of the basic neurologic defect, however, they potentiate rather than alleviate the dysphagia. The best available therapy is forceful dilatation of the narrowed vestibule, with the specific purpose of tearing some of the muscle fibers in this area. Passing graduated mercury-tipped bougies does not accomplish this and therefore relieves dysphagia only briefly. It is necessary to use bags that can be inflated under pressure or a mechanical

(Starck) dilator. In experienced hands, these instruments, when positioned under fluoroscopic control, rarely cause complete esophageal rupture, and dysphagia is relieved successfully for years, or even permanently, in over 75 per cent of cases. Forceful dilatation does not restore normal esophageal motility, but it impairs the contractile power of the vestibule and thus permits the esophagus to empty under the influence of hydrostatic and transmitted oropharyngeal pressures. Improved esophageal emptying, in turn, prevents further esophagitis and distention of the lumen.

When the esophagus is extremely dilated and sufficiently tortuous to warrant the adjective *sigmoid*, mechanical dilatation of the narrowed area is often not feasible. Surgery is then necessary. Unfortunately any procedure that creates a new opening between the dilated esophagus and the stomach permits, when the patient lies down, reflux of gastric contents into an already damaged esophagus which cannot muster the peristaltic force necessary to return the gastric contents where they belong. The consequence is severe esophagitis, often more distressing than the cause of the operation and a major source of blood loss. If technically feasible, the surgical procedure favored at present is the Heller myotomy, which is based on the same principle as forceful dilatation: the contractile power of the vestibule is destroyed by placing a longitudinal cut through the muscle, but not the mucosa, of the narrowed segment. Myotomy is, however, not invariably successful in alleviating dysphagia or preventing reflux esophagitis. In advanced cases, with unsuccessful previous operative procedures, jejunal interposition may have to be used to replace the hopelessly malfunctioning gastroesophageal segment.

DIVERTICULA

Diverticula are found in the esophagus in about 5 per cent of older patients who are given a swallow of barium. Most of these pouches occur in the mid- and distal esophagus, but they are usually small (1 to 4 cm in diameter) and do not cause symptoms. Extremely rarely an esophageal diverticulum is subject to ulceration or becomes large enough to cause dysphagia. A diverticulum of great clinical importance, however, is Zenker's diverticulum, a pouch which actually arises in the posterior aspect of the hypopharynx but which extends downward between the spine and the esophagus. Patients with this condition—elderly men for the most part—suffer dysphagia because swallowed material tends to fill the diverticular sac, which then compresses the esophagus. Regurgitation of food fouled by stagnation and nocturnal fits of coughing may complicate the picture. Diagnosis can usually be made by x-ray provided the pharynx is adequately studied as the patient swallows barium. Surgical treatment is necessary to relieve the symptoms of a Zenker's diverticulum but may be complicated by mediastinal infection, disorders of pharyngeal function during swallowing, or recurrence of the diverticulum.

OTHER ESOPHAGEAL DISORDERS

Disorders of Motor Function. In elderly persons normal peristalsis in the lower esophagus above the vestibule may be replaced by so-called "curling," a type of motility which on radiologic study imparts a peculiar beaded appearance to the contracting organ. The condition is usually asymptomatic but may be confused radiologically with esophageal varices. Occasionally the abnormality is sufficiently severe to cause dysphagia and pain on swallowing. The disorder is then known as diffuse spasm of the esophagus or corkscrew esophagus, because the contracting esophagus appears by x-ray to have assumed a bizarre corkscrew pattern. As treatment is relatively unsatisfactory, patients with this disorder may have to subsist on liquid and semisolid food. A longitudinal myotomy of the entire distal esophagus has recently been introduced as a sometimes successful surgical treatment.

The lower esophageal ring is a thin, symmetrical, annular narrowing located 1 to 4 cm above the diaphragmatic hiatus. The ring is caused by a diaphragm-like structure containing strands of connective and muscular tissue. It is covered in some cases by esophageal mucosa on its upper aspect and gastric mucosa on its under aspect. In other cases, the covering epithelium is entirely esophageal. Its etiology is unknown, but the ring is found with increasing frequency in the older age groups and often appears associated with a small sliding hernia. Some 10 to 20 per cent of adults have asymptomatic rings, but if the residual lumen is less than 12 mm in diameter, the ring may cause a highly characteristic syndrome consisting of intermittent attacks of dysphagia, recurring over years, unassociated with any other esophageal abnormality, and precipitated only when the patient swallows meat or other elastic chunks without proper chewing. Treatment usually consists of avoiding such haste. Dilatation is inconstantly successful. In a few, unusually severe cases, surgery with direct cutting or fracture of the responsible diaphragm is indicated as an effective procedure.

In infants with chalasia, the normal tonic contraction of the lower sphincter between swallows is absent and free regurgitation from the stomach occurs. The condition also affects an occasional adult.

About 20 per cent of patients with scleroderma

suffer esophageal involvement with moderate dilatation of the lumen, absent motor function, and variable dysphagia. In doubtful cases the esophageal changes may be the means of diagnosing scleroderma. An almost invariable late complication is a distal esophagitis producing ulceration, stricture, or both just above the gastroesophageal junction.

Perforation and Rupture. Perforation of the esophagus may complicate esophagitis, peptic ulcer, or neoplasm. Rupture may be induced by external trauma or, more commonly, during instrumentation of the esophagus. Sometimes it develops spontaneously in a previously healthy organ. The consequences are a syndrome comprising (1) severe pain, usually substernal, but occasionally epigastric or precordial, and intensified by swallowing; (2) free air in the mediastinum, producing a mediastinal crunch and subcutaneous emphysema palpable within 1 to 12 hr above the collarbones; (3) digestion of mediastinal pleura by pressure and gastric juice with resultant hydro- or hemopneumothorax and respiratory embarrassment; (4) shock; and (5) secondary infection.

Spontaneous rupture is a specific entity that develops suddenly during vomiting or coughing, or occasionally merely after injudicious gluttony. The tear, 1 to 8 cm in length, almost invariably is in the posterolateral portion of the esophagus immediately proximal to the diaphragmatic hiatus. The diagnosis is to be suspected in elderly men (80 per cent of cases) who are suddenly seized by the typical syndrome while vomiting or coughing; it is established by x-ray (air in mediastinum or neck, demonstration of laceration by having the patient swallow radiopaque material, pleuropulmonary abnormalities), thoracentesis revealing gastric contents, and exclusion of myocardial infarction, pancreatitis, and ruptured abdominal viscus. Air under the diaphragm is never found in spontaneous esophageal rupture.

Perforation of the esophagus is highly lethal if not treated vigorously. In early cases, constant esophageal suction and parenteral administration of penicillin (600,000 units) and streptomycin (250 mg) intramuscularly every 6 hr is immediately urgent. If sepsis or signs of increasing mediastinal reaction are not thereby controlled, surgical drainage and repair of the laceration are indicated.

A disorder closely allied to spontaneous esophageal rupture is vertical laceration of the gastroesophageal junction producing, since local vessels are involved, severe and usually exsanguinating hemorrhage. This so-called Mallory-Weiss syndrome usually develops when prolonged vomiting follows an alcoholic bout.

Foreign Bodies. Foreign bodies may cause dysphagia, pain, or perforation of the esophagus. Rigid bodies usually are arrested above the aortic arch, and elastic material in the distal esophagus. Not infrequently a structural abnormality or disease of the esophagus is responsible for stopping the foreign body.

Varices. Esophageal varices are discussed in Chap. 19, p. 156, and Chap. 280, p. 1686. They do not cause dysphagia or other esophageal symptoms. Radiologically, however, their appearance may be confused with that of cancer or esophagitis.

Plummer-Vinson Syndrome. This syndrome, also known as sideropenic dysphagia, is a cause of dysphagia in women with hypochromic anemia. Often a crescentic web indents the anterior aspect of the cricopharyngeal area; in other cases mucosal atrophy and inflammation appear prominent at the same site. A good diet and iron are usually therapeutic, but sometimes supplemental instrumental dilatation is required. The lesion is regarded as predisposing to pharyngeal carcinoma.

Benign intramural tumors of the esophagus, such as cyst (usually of respiratory tract origin), leiomyoma, fibroma, and neurofibroma, may cause intermittent dysphagia and sharply defined radiologic defects with smooth margins. Some benign tumors, especially adenomas, may produce intraluminal polyps.

The esophagus may be affected by leukoplakia, acanthosis nigricans, sarcoma, Hodgkin's disease, and leukemia.

Extrinsic Disease. Diseases of the aorta, heart, respiratory tract, or mediastinal lymph nodes often displace the esophagus and may appear to narrow the lumen, at least in one diameter. Aneurysms of the aortic arch may compress the esophageal lumen against the spine; otherwise, however, dysphagia is rarely produced by extrinsic esophageal masses. Invasion of the esophagus by bronchogenic carcinoma is possible.

For further discussion of problems considered in this chapter, the reader is referred to Chap. 5, Pain in the Chest, and Chap. 16, Indigestion, Dysphagia, Nausea, and Vomiting.

REFERENCES

Allison, P. R.: Reflux Esophagitis, Sliding Hiatal Hernia, and the Anatomy of Repair, Surg., Gynecol. Obstet., 92:419, 1951.

Code, C. F., B. Creamer, J. F. Schlegel, A. M. Olsen, J. E. Donoghue, and H. A. Andersen: "An Atlas of Esophageal Motility in Health and Disease," Springfield, Ill., Charles C Thomas, Publisher, 1958.

Derbes, V. J., and R. E. Mitchell, Jr.: Rupture of the Esophagus, Surgery, 39:688, 865, 1956.

Evans, J. A.: Sliding Hiatus Hernia, Am. J. Roentgenol., 68:754, 1952.

Ingelfinger, F. J.: Esophageal Motility, Physiol. Rev., 38:533, 1958.

——: The Physiologic Background of Heartburn, Esophagitis and Cardiospasm, A.M.A. Arch. Internal Med., 105:770, 1960.

MacMahon, H. E., R. Schatzki, and J. E. Gary: Pathology of a Lower Esophageal Ring: Report of a Case with Autopsy Observed for 9 Years, New Engl. J. Med., 259:1, 1958.

Palmer, E. D.: "The Esophagus and Its Diseases," New York, Paul B. Hoeber, Inc., Medical Department of Harper & Brothers, 1952.

Terracol, J., and R. H. Sweet: "Diseases of the Esophagus," Philadelphia, W. B. Saunders Company, 1958.

Wolf, B. S.: Roentgen Features of the Normal and Herniated Esophagogastric Region: Problems in Terminology, Am. J. Digest. Diseases, 5:751, 1960.

272 DUODENAL ULCER
Marvin H. Sleisenger

INTRODUCTION TO THE STUDY OF GASTRODUODENAL DISEASE

Serious disease and disorder of the stomach and duodenum, particularly inflammation, ulceration, and malignancy, are extremely common. Although in most instances these processes are not directly related, they give rise to a number of overlapping symptoms and demonstrate characteristic alterations in gastric secretory capacity. Knowledge of pain patterns, of the motor and secretory behavior of the stomach, of the response of the stomach to stress, and of the influences of the neuroendocrine system and of heredity is essential for the proper clinical study of these ailments. Such information provides not only a basis for rational diagnosis and therapy, but a framework on which to build a better understanding of pathogenesis of these diseases, particularly *peptic ulcer* and *gastric cancer*.

Pain. Pain originating in the stomach or duodenum, respectively, is referred to the midepigastrium or subxyphoid. Pain of the second and third portions of the duodenum is low epigastric. Some overlapping, of course, may be encountered. *Timing* of pain is also important. Distress which is felt while the stomach is empty (except on arising) usually reflects stimuli generated by acid peptic activity; that which appears while eating or immediately thereafter indicates a local disturbance, perhaps inflammation and/or abnormal motor activity, and is often relieved by emesis.

Secretory and Motor Activity. The principal gastric secretions are *hydrochloric acid, pepsin, intrinsic factor,* and a variety of mucoproteins and mucopolysaccharides. Clinically, measurement of acid is the most informative and important test. Normally, gastric juice is highly acid, with a pH 1.0 to 1.5; the secretion of the resting stomach averages about 17 mEq of acid in about 500 ml of fluid over 12 hr. The various influences upon acid production—the vagi, eating, stress, neuroendocrine stimuli, etc.—are complex and interrelated (Fig. 272-1); an understanding of their effects is important for intelligent study and management of patients with ulcer disease.

Of all the stimuli of gastric secretion which are sketched in Fig. 272-1, the best established and most important are the *vagus nerves,* the *antral mechanism,* and *histamine.* The production of acid during interdigestive periods, i.e., overnight, in response to sight, smell, or memory of food, and following insulin hypoglycemia, results from vagal activity. Outpouring of acid during meals is due to the release of *gastrin* by the *antrum* when food comes in contact with it. Fall in pH below about 1.5 in the antrum leads, in some unknown manner, to a diminution of acid secretion by the fundus. Other factors which depress acid output include contact of the upper duodenum with acid (? mediated by secretin) and the effect of intense fear.

Histamine is the most powerful stimulant of the parietal cell; however, complete understanding of its endogenous activity is lacking. The integrity of the vagi or of the antral mechanism, respectively, is tested when gastric acid is measured in the basal state or after feeding a "test meal" such as gruel or alcohol. Responsiveness of the parietal cell, however, is best tested by histamine injection. The other stimuli shown in Fig. 272-1 will be discussed in later sections of this chapter. Regardless of the relative importance of the roles of these stimuli, measurement of acid secretion is vital to correct clinical diagnosis of the important gastroduodenal diseases.

Methods and Significance of Acid Measurement. Aspiration of gastric juice by nasogastric tube after an overnight fast is the standard method of obtaining samples for determination of acidity. The appearance of a red color upon addition of Töpfer's reagent indicates the presence of free acid. If no free acid is present, 0.3 to 0.5 mg histamine base is injected subcutaneously and three 15-min collections are obtained. Again, if no free acid is present in any sample and it is imperative to know whether absolute (true) achlorhydria exists, maximal histamine stimulation should be given. A suitable antihistamine preparation—20 mg chlorpheniramine maleate—is given subcutaneously to minimize side effects, and about 20 min later 0.04 mg histamine per kilogram is also injected subcutaneously. Juice is collected during the 15- to 45-min period after injection of the stimulant and is tested for free acid.

Despite the availability of antihistaminic agents, maximal stimulation should not be given patients with severe allergy, or with pulmonary disease, asthma, hypertension, or significant cardiovascular disease.

Failure to secrete acid after maximal stimulation indicates *absolute (true) achlorhydria;* whereas absence of acid or a lower than normal amount either basally and/or after routine histamine stimulation (0.3 to 0.5 mg) signifies only a *relative hypochlorhydria.* Although values tend to be high for duodenal ulcer, they overlap the normal considerably. Secretion in gastric ulcer has been variously reported as normal or, on the average, slightly below normal. Acid secretion in carcinoma is, on the average, below normal in both the basal and post-stimulation states (Chap. 273). *Absolute achlorhydria,* never encountered in benign peptic ulcer, is common in gastric cancer.

Acid may also be measured, both basally and after stimulation, by means of a "tubeless" method. This procedure consists of administration, following stimulation by caffeine, of resins that exchange a cation, quininium, or azure A for hydrogen. The cation or dye is absorbed and excreted in the urine, where its concentration reflects semiquantitatively the amount of gastric acid which has been exchanged. With the azure A method, 0.6 mg of dye in the urine, determined colorimetrically, signifies the presence of free acid. In a small percentage of instances, when gastric secretion is temporarily diminished, false negatives may be found. If doubt exists, the intubation method should be employed. The cation exchange method is suitable for individuals in whom intubation is unfeasible and for screening large populations for relative hypochlorhydria. A positive test excludes complete (true) achlorhydria. The "tubeless" method, of course, should not be employed in patients with pyloric or esophageal obstruction, malabsorption, severe liver or kidney disease and in those who are vomiting. As with intubation, a negative result is unreliable in patients with gastroenterostomy or pyloroplasty.

The finding of relative hypochlorhydria is of some importance only in ruling out a diagnosis of duodenal ulcer in a patient with suggestive symptoms. Absolute (true) achlorhydria, on the other hand, is an essential point in the diagnosis of pernicious anemia; it also dictates the decision to operate upon patients with gastric ulcer and early or suspicious gastric carcinoma.

Measurement of gastric pepsin is much more difficult and at present has no practical advantage in clinical medicine. In some institutions, urinary pepsin—uropepsin—is measured when pernicious anemia or carcinoma is suspected, but is significant only when absent in more than one specimen. Further, correlation of urinary level with either gastric

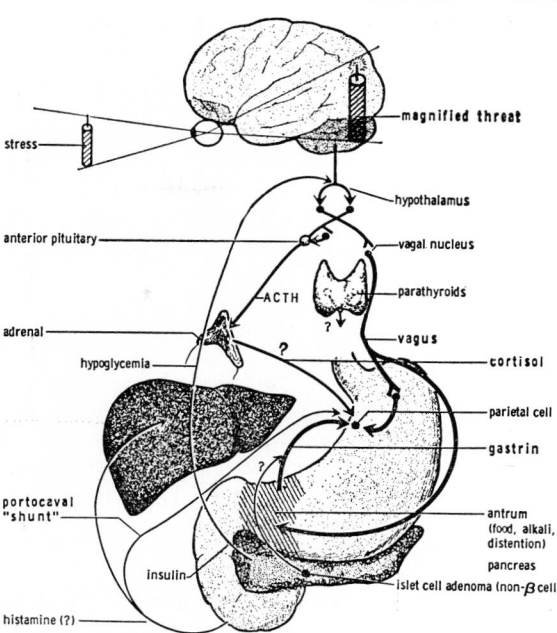

FIG. 272-1. Known and possible stimuli of gastric acid secretion. (*Based upon an idea of Dr. T. P. Almy.*)

acidity or even gastric pepsin secretion is not good, and collection and measurement of 24-hr urine specimens is more troublesome than gastric analysis for acid. Like uropepsin, blood pepsin is usually elevated in duodenal ulcer; it may be high, low, or normal in gastric ulcer; and usually is low in gastric cancer and very low to absent in pernicious anemia. However, as with measurement of gastric acidity, overlap among the categories is so great that a single determination is of limited value. Although study of the mucoproteins of gastric juice has increased greatly, analysis of these constituents has not reached the stage of clinical applicability.

Other Tools of Investigation. ROENTGENOGRAPHIC. In the vast majority of instances, the diagnosis of gastroduodenal disease is confirmed by roentgenographic examination with the barium meal. This must be carried out in all instances of upper abdominal distress, particularly in patients of middle age, those with digestive symptoms lasting longer than a week or two, and those who have bled, grossly or occultly.

DETERMINATION OF BLOOD LOSS. Routinely, determination of hematocrit and test for blood in the stool should be carried out in all patients. Anemia or other evidence of blood loss must be explained, and roentgenographic examination is required.

EXFOLIATIVE CYTOLOGY. The study of exfoliated gastric mucosal cells, obtained in a variety of ways and prepared and stained by the technique of Papanicolaou, has become increasingly accurate in the diagnosis of gastric cancer. This approach has special applicability in the study of those gastric diseases—polyps and atrophy—which are precursors of cancer.

Endoscopy. Gastroscopy is helpful in establishing the diagnosis of diffuse gastritis, carcinoma, lymphoma, and a variety of benign tumors. It may also aid in the differential diagnosis of benign and malignant ulcer and of upper gastrointestinal bleeding of unknown cause, as well as in evaluation of questionable roentgenographic findings.

Limitations of the procedure are: (1) technical inadequacies resulting from "blind areas" which include a small strip of the posterior wall in contact with the instrument, a small portion of the lower pole of the stomach, the lesser curvature of the antrum, and part of the cardia immediately adjacent to the esophagus; and (2) difficulties in interpretation except by operators who have had vast experience.

Gastric biopsy obtained with an appropriate gastroscopic attachment or by a flexible suction tube inserted into the stomach has contributed further to the differential diagnosis of stomach disease. Biopsy is of value, however, in diagnosis of suspected tumor only if histologic proof is obtained. Biopsy is also extremely helpful in diagnosis of diffuse disease, particularly gastritis and, occasionally, lymphoma.

Response to Stress. The clinician quickly learns that emotional reactions have their effects on the upper gastrointestinal tract. The observations of Wolf and Wolff have led to a better understanding of the effect of stress upon gastric function. Hypersecretion, mucosal hyperemia, and heightened motor activity accompany rage and hostility. In contrast, fear and dejection are associated with hyposecretion and hypomotility. While we cannot conclude that peptic ulcer represents a direct response to emotion, we must recognize emotional influences in its pathogenesis. Stress is also important in the appearance of symptoms which result from delayed gastric emptying and hyposecretion.

Hereditary Influences. Evidence is gradually accumulating of a familial influence in such diseases as duodenal ulcer and gastric carcinoma. Their relationship to "precursor" states such as hypersecretion of gastric acid and pepsin in the former and mucosal atrophy and hyposecretion in the latter is now recognized. The clinician must realize the need for constant surveillance of both the patient with pernicious anemia who may develop a gastric cancer and the young man with a strong family history of duodenal ulcer disease who has recurrent epigastric pain and hypersecretion.

Associated Neuroendocrine Disturbances. Knowledge constantly grows of the number of influences upon gastric secretion and function. In addition

to the role of the vagus and the antrum, the endocrine glands, particularly the adrenals and the parathyroids, and the pancreas appear to affect secretory activity. While the relationship of the central nervous system to the action of these organs is not clear, it is possible that impulses from the hypothalamus via the pituitary may be important. In any event, the clinician who deals with ulcer disease must think about calcium metabolism and be well versed in steroid excretion and pancreatic function (Fig. 272-1).

DUODENAL ULCER

Definition. Duodenal ulcer, the commonest form of peptic ulceration, is an acute and chronic recurrent disorder affecting all ages of the population, but predominantly men from the third to fifth decades. The ulcer is usually circumscribed and located in the first portion of the duodenum and extends to the level of the muscularis. The crater generally has rather sharp edges. About 50 per cent of duodenal ulcers are less than 1 cm in size, the remainder being larger; only about 10 per cent, however, are greater than 3 cm in diameter. Microscopically, the lesion is characterized by coagulation necrosis at the base with infiltration and accumulation of acute and chronic inflammatory cells. Often the ulcer is covered with a thin layer of serofibrinous exudate.

Incidence. The distribution in the population is not exactly known. Estimates of the incidence of the disease, based on necropsy studies, run from 7 to 10 per cent; the ratio of men to women is about 3.4:1. The incidence of this disease varies according to race, and for the sexes within the races; the total incidence of ulcer for Negro men is lower than for whites—again, Chinese have 10 times as many ulcers as Javanese, as noted in a survey from Java.

The only conclusion that can be drawn from a study of geographic and occupational factors in the twentieth century is that the incidence varies from place to place and from time to time in the same place. Over all, the disease does not predominate in any single occupational group—professional, skilled, semiskilled, heavy laboring, or agricultural.

Etiology and Pathophysiology

The cause of duodenal ulcer is unknown. However, much information has been accumulated about gastric secretion in this disease. Whatever the ultimate cause, abnormal elaboration of acid must play a part. Figure 272-1 is a diagram of the various stimuli, established and implicated, which increase acid production. A review of these influences is helpful for a better understanding of this disease.

Secretory Pattern. The outstanding feature of the secretory pattern of the stomach of patients with duodenal ulcer is the basal hypersecretion of acid and pepsin. In addition, all the common stimuli—vagal, food (particularly alcohol, coffee, and beef broth), stress, insulin, and histamine—elicit a greater than normal acid secretion. However, despite the significantly increased mean rate of secretion in patients with duodenal ulcer, in only a minority does the response to the standard secretory tests exceed the upper normal limit. Hence, measurement of secretory rates has only a limited value for identification of duodenal ulcer.

The reason for the increased rate of acid secretion in duodenal ulcer is not altogether clear. Perhaps the most important factor is heightened vagal activity which may explain the high rate of acid secretion during the cephalic and interdigestive phases and its marked reduction after vagotomy. Others consider the dominant cause to be the increased parietal cell mass, since the maximum acid output of the stomach may be quantitatively related to the total number of parietal cells. Whether the number of parietal cells increases before or after ulceration has occurred is not definitely known.

Despite the experimental production of peptic ulcer in animals by continuous stimulation of acid secretion, the hypersecretion of the stomach per se in duodenal ulcer may not be the cause of the disease. The persistence of elevated secretion of pepsin and acid after the healing of a duodenal ulcer is evidence that the abnormal secretion is not solely responsible for the disease. Proper understanding of the secretory pattern of these patients is, nevertheless, necessary for intelligent treatment, since the cornerstone of therapy rests upon continuous suppression of acid-peptic activity.

Heredity. A hereditary predisposition seems apparent from the family histories of these patients. Pertinent, perhaps, is the association between the incidence of blood group O and duodenal ulcer. Further, there is a significant coincidence of blood group O and of nonsecretion of ABH substances in duodenal ulcer patients. Since the ability to secrete these substances into the gastrointestinal tract is inherited independently of the ABO groups, the effects of nonsecretion and of the occurrence of blood group O are not only coincidental but also additive. That this association of various genetic factors is causal in duodenal ulceration remains, however, to be proved.

Effect of Stress. Although much has been written of the personality of the patient with duodenal ulcer, no completely acceptable prototype has emerged. We are prone to characterize him as an individual who is hard-driving, conscientious, ambitious, and, in general, successful. Plainly, this is at once exaggeration and oversimplification. While many duodenal ulcer patients fit this description, it is equally true that a large number are rather shy, soft-spoken, unaggressive, and even withdrawn.

From the time of Beaumont's classical study on the gastric secretion of Alexis St. Martin, increasing attention has been paid to the role of emotional stress in gastric secretion and, in turn, in the genesis of duodenal ulcer. One cannot doubt, on the one hand, an association between anger and hostility and increased acid secretion and, on the other, a frequent temporal relationship between emotional turmoil and the onset of reactivation of duodenal ulcer. Indeed, in this area rather elaborate, but conflicting, theories have been proposed which attempt to relate definite personality patterns and/or environmental influences to the genesis of this disease. These remain, for the most part, unsubstantiated.

Studies in monkeys and man both indicate that behavioral reaction patterns are quite important. However, it is impossible to achieve an acceptable definition of stress which may be universally applicable, and this failure renders difficult the assessment of this factor in an individual case. While stress may lead to hypersecretion of acid, it is important to remember that these patients are capable of hyperresponding in this way to many stimuli of acid secretion.

Neuroendocrine Influences. Some investigators believe that stress affects gastric secretion partly via the anterior hypothalamic and vagal pathway and partly through the posterior hypothalamus–anterior pituitary–adrenal axis. Insulin hypoglycemia can increase secretion of acid in man, as in the monkey, presumably via these pathways. Further, the peaks of secretion which are noted at 1 hr and 3 to 4 hr after insulin are thought ultimately to be due to the action of the vagus and the adrenal glands, respectively. With the available information, however, it is impossible to draw an analogy between effects of hypoglycemia and the stress of daily living.

Adrenal. The virtual absence of duodenal ulcer disease in patients with untreated adrenal insufficiency and the appearance of such ulceration in a number of individuals receiving adrenal corticosteroid therapy has focused a great deal of attention on the possible role of adrenal cortical secretions in the genesis of duodenal ulcer disease. Although patients with adrenal insufficiency secrete less than normal amounts of acid and pepsin, in individuals who develop peptic ulcer while receiving either ACTH or adrenal corticosteroids, acid and pepsin secretion is increased inconsistently. Indeed, in many of these instances there is hyposecretion or even achlorhydria. Studies of urinary 17-OH-corticoids during periods of activity and quiescence in patients with duodenal ulcer indicate no variation in the normal function of the adrenal cortex. Indeed, several studies demonstrate that ulcers in rats may be induced by techniques involving stress only in the absence of normal adrenal function.

Parathyroid Glands. Recent studies have demonstrated that incidence of duodenal ulcer is slightly increased in patients with hyperparathyroidism although gastric secretion is normal. Subcutaneous injection of parathyroid hormone—1,000 units—increases volume and pepsin secretion, but not acid; indeed, animal experiments indicate that long-term administration of this hormone depresses secretion, possibly by the inhibiting action of hypercalcemia on the vagus. The mechanism of peptic ulcer formation in hyperparathyroidism, therefore, is unknown.

Hypoparathyroidism is associated with depressed gastric secretion, which, however, is corrected when the serum calcium returns to normal, either by the administration of calcium or parathormone. Thus, the parathyroids seem to influence gastric secretion solely through their effect on serum calcium, since a certain level of serum calcium seems necessary for normal gastric secretion.

Pancreatic Adenomas and Multiple Endocrine Adenomas. The reports of unusually severe recurrent peptic ulceration in the duodenum or jejunum associated with noninsulin secreting islet cell adenomas of the pancreas have aroused a great deal of interest. In addition to the fulminating ulcer diathesis, these individuals secrete excessive quantities of gastric juice, 12-hr collections ranging from 2,000 to 14,000 ml, with a total acid output as great as 10 mEq per hr, about four times the normal mean rate. Ulcerations recur, despite high subtotal gastrectomy and removal of the pancreatic tumor, because this neoplasm often either is malignant with functioning metastases or is scattered diffusely through the pancreas. In almost all instances, total gastrectomy must be carried out in order to prevent recurrent ulceration. Some evidence exists that a gastrinlike substance, produced by the adenoma, is responsible for the gastric hypersecretion which accompanies the severe recurrent ulcerations. Some of these patients may also have diarrhea, steatorrhea, and hypopotassemia.

In approximately one-fifth of these individuals, multiple endocrine adenomas are present involving parathyroid, adrenal, pituitary, and thyroid glands. Since the nonpancreatic adenomas are functioning in only 20 per cent of instances, it is unlikely that the ulcerative process is related in some way to multiple endocrine dysfunction. It is quite difficult to ascribe either the hypersecretory state of the stomach or the severe peptic ulcerations *directly* to the pancreatic adenomas for two reasons: (1)

significant reduction in gastric secretion following removal of a tumor *alone* has not yet been shown; (2) some patients with duodenal ulcer secrete as much gastric juice and acid as those with ulcer and adenomas.

Relationship of Disorders of Other Tissues to Peptic Ulcer. *Liver.* The incidence of peptic ulcer is increased in cirrhosis of the liver for reasons which are not clear. Recent observations in patients after portocaval anastomosis for portal hypertension indicate a hepatic role both in control of gastric secretion and in the appearance of peptic ulcer since there is an increase after operation not only in gastric acid output but also in the incidence of peptic ulcer. The increased frequency of ulcer may be related to the former phenomenon, but the reason for the increased acid production is not evident. Perhaps it is due to absorbed histamine which is not detoxified by the liver because of the shunt.

Malignant Carcinoid. Reports indicate that duodenal ulcer is frequently noted in patients with metastatic malignant carcinoid tumor. Increased acid secretion has not been found and, indeed, 5-hydroxytryptamine (Serotonin) which is produced in tremendous amounts by the tumor has been shown to inhibit acid secretion.

Although the incidence of duodenal ulcer is alleged to be increased in *pulmonary emphysema* and *polycythemia vera,* acceptable supporting evidence is lacking.

Clinical Picture

Classical Picture. The symptoms of duodenal ulcer are fairly characteristic and easily recognized. Among them, *pain* predominates; it is usually well localized to an area a few centimeters in diameter, high in the epigastrium or subxyphoid, but sometimes in the midepigastrium or to the right of the midline in this area. The pain is steady, deep, and nonfluctuating and is described as gnawing, but it may be dull, aching, or burning. An outstanding feature of the distress is its *rhythmicity,* since it appears about 1 to 3 hr after meals, when the stomach is empty; it also often awakens the patient from sleep about midnight to 2:00 A.M. However, the pain rarely is noted on arising in the morning. This distress is almost always alleviated by eating. Milk is particularly effective. Nausea and vomiting are uncommon in uncomplicated duodenal ulcer. These symptoms may predominate, however, when ulcer cicatrix has narrowed the pyloroduodenal segment. Occasionally, the pain may radiate into the midback or, indeed, be felt only in this area or in the right flank, indicating possible penetration of a duodenal ulcer (see pp. 18 and 1605).

Occurrence of ulceration varies according to season in certain parts of the world, being greater in the spring and autumn in the temperate zones.

This *periodicity* has been attributed to seasonal changes in atmospheric pressure, dietary habits, incidence of respiratory infection, and stressful situations; however, substantiation is lacking.

The basis for the pain of duodenal ulcer has not been clearly defined. Some observers feel that it is due to the action of acid upon exposed nerve fibers at the edge or base of the ulcer, the pain threshold of which has been lowered by the inflammatory reaction to the erosion. Cited in support of this is the relief from pain which follows ingestion of substances that neutralize acid. Others believe that increased muscular activity initiates pain, stressing the effectiveness of administration of substances (anticholinergics) which greatly reduce smooth muscle spasm. Possibly both mechanisms are interrelated; that is, hydrochloric acid on an inflamed surface leads to direct stimulation of nerve fibers as well as heightened intragastric pressure.

Ulcer of the Pyloric Canal and Postbulbar Ulcer. Variants of the usual clinical picture may be due to location of the ulcer in the *pyloric canal* or *postbulbar segment* (Fig. 272-2). Although patients with the lesion in the pyloric canal often have the same complaints as those with duodenal ulcer, the history may be atypical in 20 to 50 per cent of these individuals. Prominent complaints, not usually encountered with uncomplicated duodenal ulcer, include nausea, vomiting, and other symptoms related to gastric retention. Delay in gastric emptying stems from the spasm and edema of the pyloric canal in which the crater is situated. Because of these symptoms, the patient's appetite may decline and he may lose a considerable amount of weight. In the patient with *postbulbar ulcer*, pain may be felt lower in the epigastrium, be more severe and less responsive to food, milk, and alkali than in a typical duodenal ulcer. Also, ulcer in this location bleeds more readily. Jaundice due to obstruction of the ampulla by edema and spasm is a rare complication.

Duodenal Ulcer of Childhood. The clinical picture of duodenal ulcer in children differs greatly from its counterpart in the adult. In the former group, the location and character of the pain may not be so precise, the child often complaining of diffuse, poorly localized upper abdominal distress, without the rhythmicity of the adult form and often made *worse* rather than better by eating. Thus, attention may be drawn initially by the child's refusal to eat for fear of discomfort. Bleeding commonly is the presenting complaint. A significant difference between the juvenile and adult forms of the disease is the greater resistance of the child's symptoms to classical therapy, which may be partially due to the difficulty in instituting a dietary regimen; nevertheless, every effort should be made

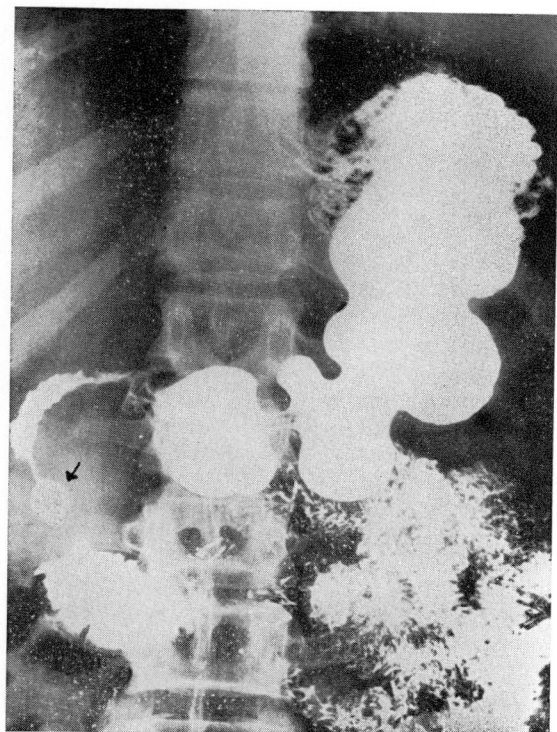

Fig. 272-2. Postbulbar peptic ulcer in second part of duodenum.

to maintain young patients on a medical regimen (see below). The indications for surgical intervention in this age group are the same as for adults, and, on the whole, results of subtotal gastric resection are good. However, the hazard of resection is somewhat greater in juveniles, since impaired nutrition, which occasionally follows such procedures, may have a very serious effect upon growth and development.

Diagnosis

Physical examination in uncomplicated duodenal ulcer is quite unrevealing, with occasional patients exhibiting variable tenderness in a localized area in the epigastrium. Diagnosis may often be made from the history of the patient; however, confirmation must rest upon radiographic demonstration of the disease. This examination is carried out in most instances using a barium sulfate–water mixture after an overnight fast. The key to the diagnosis is the proper use of compression spot films of the duodenal bulb; one cannot accept inability to demonstrate a filled duodenal bulb with a normal contour or rapid emptying of the bulb as evidence for duodenal ulceration. Conversely, a filled bulb cannot be considered normal unless it has no crater on compression (Fig. 272-3). Even in patients with long-standing disease, a crater may

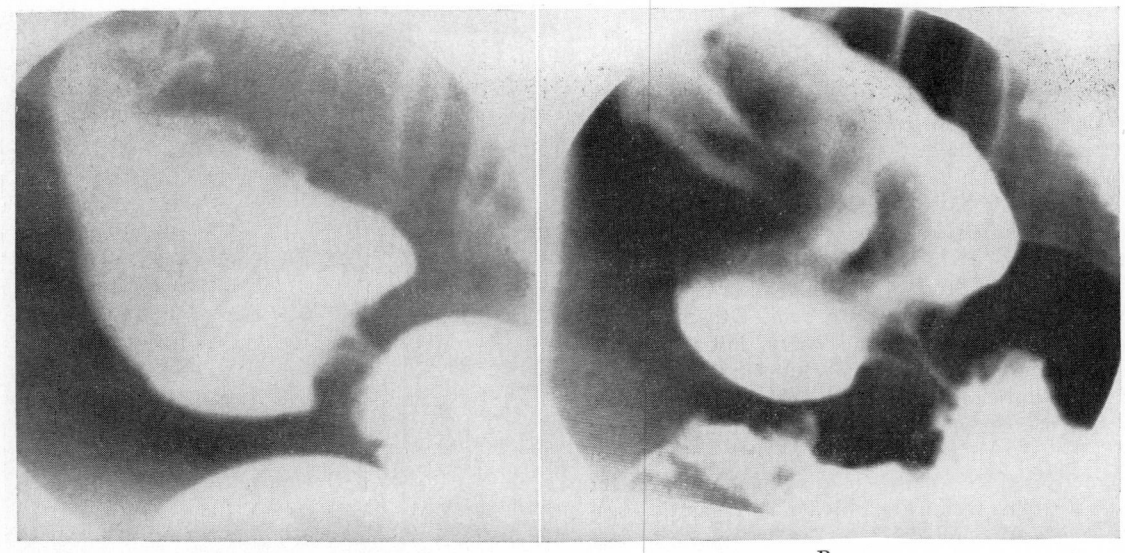

A   B

FIG. 272-3. The importance of compression over the duodenal bulb in demonstration of an ulcer crater. A. Routine film; B, "spot" film with compression.

be demonstrated despite the distortion of the bulb by scars of previous ulcerations (clover-leaf deformity) (Fig. 272-4). Occasionally, however, the distortion of the bulb obscures the crater; in such instances the history of symptoms of an active ulcer may be considered diagnostic. Another radiologic feature of duodenal ulcer may be an abnormal amount of fluid (gastric juice) in the stomach at the outset of the examination, attributable either to hypersecretion or to partial obstruction, provided the patient has fasted overnight.

Occasionally, the measurement of gastric acid in a single random fasting specimen, or in a 1- to 4-hr or overnight collection, may be helpful in supporting a diagnosis of duodenal ulcer in doubtful cases. The average volume and amount of acid secreted by normal individuals is roughly 500 ml and 15 mEq, respectively, over a 12-hr period. In the patients with duodenal ulcer, the average value for acid secretion is about twice normal. Only about 50 per cent of duodenal ulcer patients, however, secrete more acid than the upper limit of normal.

Response to therapy (see below) may also help substantially in the diagnosis of duodenal ulcer. Any individual who gives a history compatible with this disorder and who is relieved of the symptoms in a period of a day or two after institution of therapy for peptic ulcer should be suspected of having this disease. In addition, in some instances of duodenal ulcer disease with gastric retention, intubation of the stomach, with a Levine or Rehfus tube each night or several times daily, with emptying of the gastric contents, may provide dramatic relief from symptoms. At the same time, this provides valuable information about the secretory state as well as the degree of gastric obstruction.

Differential Diagnosis

The differential diagnosis of duodenal ulcer may be difficult. A great many common disorders are characterized by pain in the epigastrium which may be compatible with, albeit not characteristic of, duodenal ulcer. However, it must be emphasized that, with rare exceptions, the distress of such disorders is *not* relieved by the ingestion of food, milk, or alkali, nor are these disorders apt to become symptomatic when the stomach is empty. The commonest conditions which may be confused with duodenal ulcer disease are referred to as "functional dyspepsia," or "nervous stomach," and chronic gastritis. In these disorders, the patient complains of burning epigastric distress, often of a dull, "heavy" quality which is almost always noted immediately after meals. The symptoms which often make the physician think of duodenal ulcer disease are: heartburn, "sourness," belching, and "gas." While occasionally patients with duodenal ulcer disease complain of heartburn (particularly those who also have an associated reflux of acid gastric juice into the lower esophagus due to hiatus hernia or incompetency of the gastroesophageal sphincter), the other symptoms are relatively rare in duodenal ulcer. These patients are apt to indicate the site of reference with the entire palm of the hand, moving it back and forth and up and down over the entire epigastric area in contrast to the rather circumscribed area delineated in duodenal ulcer. Moreover, this distress is most often brought on by eating. Often the patients with these disorders will indicate that they feel best "on an empty stomach." The association of stress with the onset or reappearance of symptoms in functional dyspepsia and gastritis is often as striking as in duodenal disease. Most of these patients also note improvement coinciding with relief of tension.

The history of a patient with a *benign gastric ulcer* may be identical with that of one with duodenal ulcer. Frequently, however, patients with gastric ulcer are apt to have distress following meals and may not have as dramatic relief with food (see Chap. 273, Benign Gastric Ulcer). Upper gastrointestinal x-ray examination is, of course, necessary for differential diagnosis.

The distress of *gallbladder colic* differs from that of duodenal ulcer. The former is usually steady and is localized in the midepigastrium or in the right upper quadrant; at times it radiates to the tip of the right scapula; it comes on *after* ingestion of food, particularly a heavy meal, is accompanied by nausea and vomiting, and lasts for hours. Occasionally, the patient has chills or fever and may note dark urine, pruritus, or jaundice if the common duct is obstructed. Such an individual has no desire to eat and almost certainly will obtain no relief from so doing. The pain of *acute cholecystitis* or *common duct obstruction* may be similar to that of posterior penetration of a duodenal ulcer, particularly when the latter involves the pancreas. The pain will be intense, located in the deep epigastrium, often with radiation into the back.

Acute Pancreatitis. When duodenal ulcer is advanced sufficiently to penetrate into the pancreas, the clinical pictures may be identical. Usually the symptomatology of the two disorders differs. Pain of pancreatitis typically is deeper, more constant, and lasts for many hours to days, often with radiation into the back. Some degree of relief is obtained by bending forward or by compression on the abdomen and not by the ingestion of food. Perhaps most important, the onset of pancreatitis is rather dramatic and is often associated with the ingestion of excessive amounts of alcohol and/or food (see below).

Treatment

Peptic ulceration occurs via the action of an acid-peptic juice on susceptible mucosa. Because the factors determining mucosal susceptibility are still poorly understood, treatment is chiefly directed toward reduction of the volume, acidity, and pepsin content of gastric juice. Therapy is further complicated by the fact that in duodenal ulcer the stomach tends to empty more rapidly than normally, thus shortening the effect of the neutralizing

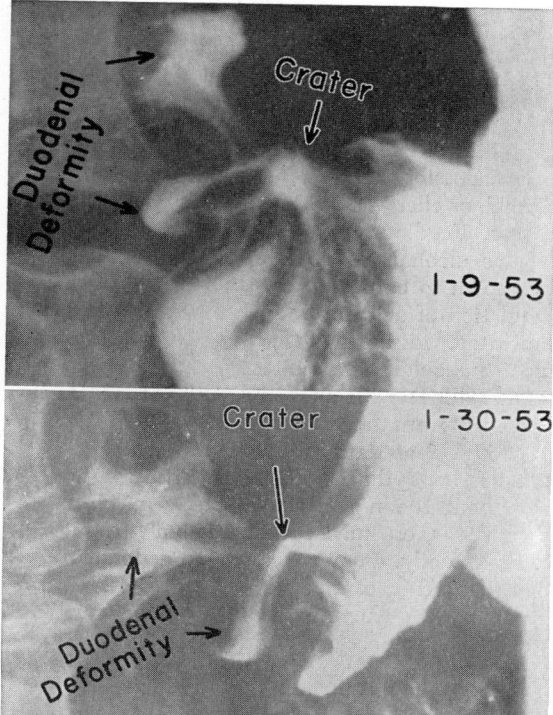

FIG. 272-4. Large duodenal ulcer crater in a 52-year-old woman, demonstrating radiating folds, duodenal deformity, and pseudodiverticulum formation. The crater healed in approximately 3 weeks.

power of ingested food and milk. The therapeutic armamentarium includes diet, a number of antacids, and anticholinergic, tranquilizing, and sedative drugs. To use these to the best effect, singly or in combinations, it is necessary to know in what manner and to what degree a particular agent modifies the composition of gastric juice, as well as the cost in side effects, money, and inconvenience to the patient.

While effective acid neutralization which diminishes peptic activity is possible, there is little at hand to increase the resistance of the tissues to ulceration. It is known, however, that healing is more likely to occur at a satisfactory rate if defects in protein intake are corrected and if certain drugs such as adrenal corticosteroids, salicylates, etc., are forbidden. Physical and mental rest are also important adjuncts to therapy.

Diet. The diet features soft, well-cooked, nonfibrous, nonfried foods with liberal amounts of dairy products. The rationale for such a regimen rests upon its increased neutralizing power and the empirical observation that the patient's symptoms respond more quickly than when normal fare is offered. However, the beneficial effect of food may be due more to frequency than to content of feedings. Although coarse vegetables, condiments, fried food, and pork products do not stimulate gastric secretion excessively, nevertheless, a great many patients with ulcer will complain of distress after eating these foods as well as after hot or cold liquids. Possibly this effect is related to mechanical, thermal, or chemical irritation of the gastroduodenal mucosa. Feedings should be *frequent*. Substances such as alcohol, coffee, and beef extracts, which are known to cause not only irritation but marked stimulation of acid production, must be completely eliminated. Because of its effect upon secretion, smoking should be prohibited.

The patient with an active ulcer should be fed frequently from the very onset of treatment. During the initial few days, diet should include hourly milk feedings during the day and every 2 hr throughout the night, as well as semisolids such as puddings, creamed soups, soft-boiled eggs, etc., six times daily. In most cases, broiled and boiled meat, cooked or canned vegetables, and fruit juice may be added. The milk feeding between meals and at bedtime may be given with cheese and crackers. When the patient has been asymptomatic for a few days or so, he may omit hourly milk feedings, but should be maintained on three regular meals and three small, between-meal feedings of milk with crackers or small sandwiches. If weight gain is a problem, or if the patient is obese, or if some predisposition to or evidence of coronary artery disease is recognized, skimmed milk may be used and the amount of starch in the diet reduced.

After there is radiologic evidence of healing, usually in several months or less, the diet may be liberalized to include raw fruit and vegetables, coffee with milk once a day, fried foods, and even small amounts of alcohol before dinner. The diet should be outlined carefully since cooperation is more likely when patients understand the principles of therapy.

Antacids. Antacids reduce peptic digestion of gastric and intestinal mucosa by elevating the pH of the gastric juice. For this purpose, pH levels above 3.5 are desirable, since pepsin shows a maximal activity at pH 1 to 2. To accomplish this aim requires frequent and adequate antacid dosage over periods of weeks or months. The sporadic use of antacids cannot maintain any significant pH elevation and is, therefore, of little therapeutic value.

Calcium carbonate is probably the most effective antacid, and it has no significant effect on acid-base balance. Laxatives may be required to counteract the constipation often associated with its use. With an hourly dose of 2 to 4 Gm, it should be possible to maintain a pH in the vicinity of 4.0, well within desired therapeutic limits. *Aluminum*

hydroxide also tends to cause constipation and has no beneficial effects not exhibited by the use of calcium carbonate. Of occasional clinical importance is the diminished absorption of the tetracycline drugs which are bound by the aluminum ion. It is possible to achieve a pH above 2 to 3 only with a 30 ml per hr dose, alternating on the half hour with 120 ml milk. This program is usually adequate for ulcer healing, even though it does not effect an optimal neutralization of free hydrochloric acid.

Sodium bicarbonate is both rapidly acting and highly effective as an antacid. It has, however, serious limitations because of its ability to produce a marked systemic alkalosis. The alkalosis may be clinically significant and produce a variety of signs and symptoms including anorexia, nausea, vomiting, headache, muscle aches, and tetany. By decreasing the solubility of calcium phosphate, it may lead to the formation of renal calculi and thus seriously affect renal function. The consequence of ingestion of large amounts of both milk and alkali may be a marked rise in blood calcium, and the hypercalcemia may lead to nephrocalcinosis and impairment of renal function. This "milk-alkali" syndrome (p. 607) may be treated effectively by discontinuance of the milk and absorbable alkali. Because of its systemic action and the availability of other agents, sodium bicarbonate has little place in the treatment of peptic ulcer.

Antisecretory Compounds. These parasympathetic blocking agents decrease gastric and intestinal motility and the volume, pepsin content, and acidity of the gastric juice. Their effectiveness is frequently limited by the associated side effects: blurring of vision, dry mouth, tachycardia, and in the presence of prostatic hypertrophy, urinary obstruction. In susceptible patients, an attack of acute glaucoma may be precipitated.

It is difficult to obtain clinical evidence sufficient to justify the selection of one anticholinergic drug, natural or synthetic, over another. As a general rule, it may be said of all anticholinergic drugs that the dosage that produces a satisfactory depression in acid secretion also causes one or more of the side effects mentioned above.

Although anticholinergics in effective dosage at bedtime suppress the basal (nocturnal) acid secretion, these drugs do not significantly affect acid secretion in response to feeding or hypoglycemia. During the day, therefore, when given before meals, anticholinergics in themselves are of little use in raising the pH to therapeutic levels. They may, however, delay gastric emptying and prolong the action of simultaneously administered antacids and, therefore, are recommended. The decrease in gastrointestinal motility and spasm may be a factor in relieving the pain of peptic ulceration, although the mechanisms remain unclear. The exact role of anticholinergic drugs in the therapy of peptic ulcer is still uncertain; comparable results have been obtained in controlled series with placebos. To date there is no evidence that their long-term administration alters recurrence rate, incidence of complications, or the eventual need for surgery.

The action of *sedatives, tranquilizers,* and *antihistamines* upon gastric secretion is also important. Often the agitated and hyperirritable peptic ulcer patient will benefit from mild sedation in clinically applicable dosage. However, there are no adequately controlled studies which show that tranquilizing drugs promote more rapid healing or prevent complications or recurrences. *Reserpine* in usual oral dosage (approximately 1 mg per day) has no significant effect on the volume and acidity of gastric juice. With 2.0 to 3.0 mg orally, or 1 to 2.5 mg intramuscularly, however, marked increase in both of these parameters may result. Other tranquilizers such as the *phenothiazines* have not been shown to have any effect on gastric secretion other than some diminution in total volume.

Antihistamines have been disappointing, and most studies have shown no significant effect on gastric secretion in man.

Attention to Psychologic Factors. Despite lack of precise psychiatric information about the personality structure and reaction patterns of the patient with duodenal ulcer, the physician must pay attention to these factors. Unquestionably, onset and exacerbation of this disease can often be temporally related to emotional upheavals. While in most instances the physician cannot hope to alter the life situation of his patient appreciably, he can, by close inquiry and attention, seek personality and environment factors which may contribute to anxiety and hostility. Often he is able to give the patient some insight into the nature of his disturbance and, at all times, to afford him sympathy and understanding. Knowledge of the important factors of personality and environment will enable the physician to guide his medical therapy more intelligently with particular reference to prophylaxis, i.e., to institute a more stringent regimen at times when the patient will be under greater emotional strain. Caution must be observed in handling emotional problems, particularly in such matters as encouraging the patient to make dramatic changes in his home or occupational life and in probing deeply into the personal problems which are uncovered. If the need for psychiatric help is apparent, or if the patient expresses a desire for such therapy, appropriate arrangements should then be made.

Use of X-ray Therapy. X-ray therapy of the stomach has been successfully employed in the treatment of duodenal ulcer when response to medical therapy has been poor. This form of treatment is especially applicable to individuals for whom immediate surgical intervention is not mandatory or to those who are deemed fair to poor risks for surgical intervention. The goal of radiation therapy is temporary destruction of the parietal cells, thus rendering the patient anacidic for periods ranging up to a year. Usually 2,000 to 2,400 roentgen units, total depth dose through anterior and posterior ports, is administered over a course of 15 treatments. It has been found that the ulcers will heal in almost all patients in whom x-ray treatment reduces acid secretion by 50 per cent. Among those whose acid secretion returns in less than a year, the recurrence rate is nevertheless reduced to one-sixth of that in the preradiation period. Hemorrhage and perforation are also reduced by 75 and 50 per cent, respectively. However, secretory levels usually return to normal after a year, and this makes it questionable whether the long-term beneficial results which have been reported are due to x-ray treatment or to close medical supervision.

COMPLICATIONS OF DUODENAL ULCER

The complications of peptic ulcer disease are four in number and broadly constitute the basis for surgical management of this disease. They are: intractability, bleeding, obstruction, and perforation or penetration.

Intractability

The most frequent complication of this disease is intractability. It is characterized by lengthy and frequently recurring periods of moderate to severe activity which render the patient either partially or completely incapacitated. One must be sure of two points before operation is recommended: (1) that the patient indeed *has* an active ulcer, since some ulcer patients may continuously complain of symptoms, obtain little or no relief from medical therapy, and yet will not have an ulcer crater demonstrable on x-ray examination. In this circumstance the physician must exercise the greatest amount of caution in recommending surgical intervention, since this group of patients contributes the greatest number of individuals with complaints following gastrectomy. (2) One must be sure that the patient has had a fair trial of good medical care, preferably in the hospital, directed by an interested, informed physician. In the initial phase of treatment of an active ulcer, feedings of milk and antacid should be alternated half hourly during the day, and milk (4 to 6 oz) is given every 2 hr at night. In addition to this "around the clock" program, the patient is sedated with phenobarbital and given an antisecretory compound as already outlined. If the patient does not respond to this program in 5 to 7 days, surgery should be carried out.

Bleeding and Massive Hemorrhage

From 15 to 20 per cent of ulcer patients have bleeding as an initial symptom of their disease, and of these, a significant percentage will have this complication as the only evidence of activity throughout the course of their disease. It is most often manifested by the passage of black or tarry stools and on occasion, if the bleeding is very severe, by dark red blood per rectum. Less frequently, the patient will have hematemesis, but this is more characteristic of bleeding from the stomach or esophagus.

Since duodenal ulcer is responsible for at least 60 per cent of upper gastrointestinal bleeding, extra consideration will be given to the problem of massive upper gastrointestinal bleeding. Factors contributing to massive hemorrhage include alcoholism, undue physical or emotional stress, hypertension and arteriosclerosis, excessive salicylate ingestion, infection, fatigue, dietary indiscretion, and prolonged use of the adrenal corticosteroids or phenylbutazone (see below).

In cases of fatal hemorrhage, a branch of the pancreaticoduodenal, gastroduodenal, or gastric coronary artery has usually been involved, in which instance the vessel is often markedly arteriosclerotic and rigid.

Clinical Picture. The signs and symptoms depend upon the degree of blood loss, the rate of bleeding, and the suddenness of onset. Hematemesis is commonly observed in bleeding from gastric ulcer, esophageal varices, and duodenal ulcer, although bleeding from the latter is much more likely to appear as melena (see Chap. 18).

Symptoms following massive bleeding usually include faintness, weakness, dizziness, headache, perspiration, thirst, syncope, pallor, and shock (see p. 100, Chap. 13). A persistently low blood pressure and a weak, rapid pulse signify a dangerous degree of hemorrhage.

On physical examination, signs should be sought which would indicate less common causes of bleeding. These include telengiectasia of lips, tongue, and buccal mucosa (Weber-Rendu-Osler disease); pigmented spots of the same structures associated with polyposis of the gastrointestinal tract (Puetz-Jeghers syndrome); petechiae, purpura and/or splenomegaly without liver disease, findings which suggest a bleeding diathesis and a blood dyscrasia. Liver disease and possibly esophageal varices are indicated by hepatomegaly, splenomegaly, jaundice, and spider angiomas.

The initial *hematocrit* value may be normal or elevated in spite of considerable blood loss, since plasma and red blood cells are lost simultaneously. The magnitude of the hemorrhage may not become evident for at least 12 hr, depending upon the state of hydration and the rapidity with which the total blood volume is restored by hemodilution (see Chap. 18).

Diagnosis. When the diagnosis is uncertain or the source of bleeding has not been established, several procedures should be employed. Among these, gastric intubation, the fluorescein string test, flexible esophagoscopy, and early upper gastrointestinal series have been useful. Initially, a small-bore soft polyethylene nasogastric tube should be introduced into the stomach. If no blood or guaiac positive material can be aspirated, *bleeding has either ceased or originates distal to the pylorus.* In this instance, a string, to the end of which is attached a mercury bag containing a radiopaque monofilament and with similar markers spaced transversely at 1-in. intervals, may be passed through the mouth into the upper small bowel. A flat film of the abdomen is then obtained to identify the position of the string with reference to the esophagogastric junction, body of the stomach, duodenum, etc. Then 20 ml of sodium fluorescite is injected intravenously, and 4 min later the string is withdrawn and examined under ultraviolet light. The site of active bleeding will fluoresce, and its measured distance from the mercury bag will allow identification of the site on the flat film. Should bleeding have ceased, a site may be discovered by the presence of blood or guaiac positive material on a localized segment of the string. Esophageal varices are not a contraindication to either intubation or passage of the string (Fig. 272-5).

Following the "string test" an upper gastrointestinal series should be obtained, provided that the patient is not in shock or bleeding massively. Information obtained beforehand from both intubation and the string test may be of great value to the radiologist. If blood is aspirated from the stomach, indicated diagnostic maneuvers are flexible esophagoscopy and gastroscopy, before barium studies. The former may verify the presence of bleeding varices and may be carried out by a skilled operator before other procedures in cases strongly suspected of having portal hypertension. Before insertion of the instrument, the stomach should be lavaged with cold saline in order to clear the field and perhaps reduce the bleeding. Gastroscopy is most useful when the diagnosis of bleeding from erosions of acute gastritis or from gastric ulcer is suspected. If endoscopy fails to reveal the source of bleeding, and, if the patient's condition is stable, upper gastrointestinal series should be done.

Of major importance is the differential diagnosis of *bleeding esophageal varices.* In the majority of instances the physician will be able quickly to

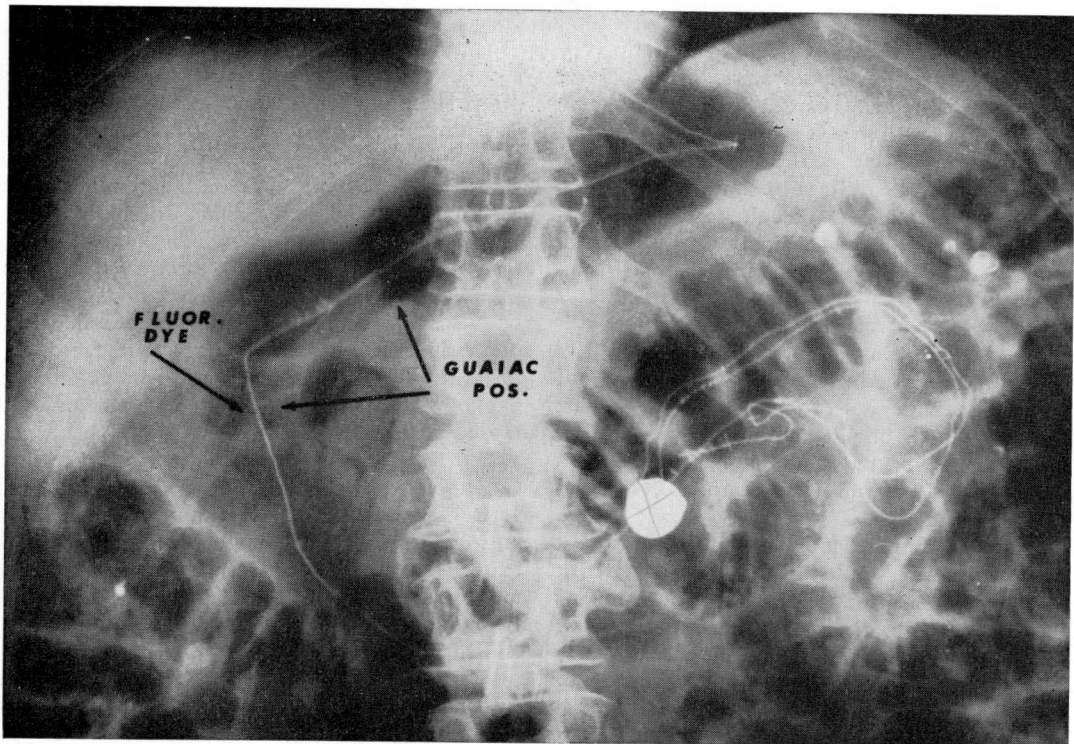

FIG. 272-5. A 77-year-old white man with gastrointestinal hemorrhage. Upper gastrointestinal series failed to reveal an ulcer crater. Fluorescein string test localized bleeding site to the first part of the duodenum. At operation a deep perforating ulcer in the first part of the duodenum was found. (*Courtesy, Dr. Fred Pittman.*)

ascertain that the patient has liver disease (history of poor nutrition and alcoholism, or of postnecrotic cirrhosis with enlarged or shrunken liver, spider angiomas, jaundice, etc.) and portal hypertension (splenomegaly, abdominal venous pattern). Bleeding may, nevertheless, still be due to ulcer or erosion which occurs in 10 to 15 per cent of cirrhotics. Accordingly, balloon tamponade is best employed when bleeding from varices is established by flexible esophagoscopy. In many instances, however, the patient's condition or unavailability of a skilled operator does not favor use of the procedure. A trial of compression is indicated if the diagnosis of varices had been previously established in an individual who is vomiting blood or if bleeding is massive in a patient with evidence of cirrhosis. When it is employed, the stomach should be aspirated continuously. If blood is returned after several hours of tamponade, bleeding may be presumed to arise from a cause other than esophageal varices, and the apparatus is removed. The measurement of elevated portal pressure by percutaneous splenic puncture supports the decision to undertake a trial of tamponade if esophagoscopy has not been done or is inconclusive (Chap. 18). This procedure should be undertaken only by a

person thoroughly familiar with the technique. Under these circumstances, measurement of the splenic pulp pressure and injection of radiopaque dyes to obtain splenoportograms may provide information that is decisive in the differentiation of bleeding from peptic ulcer or esophageal varices.

Principles of Management of Massive Hemorrhage from Duodenal Ulcer. Treatment of massive bleeding from peptic ulcer includes blood replacement, treatment of shock, acid neutralization, maintenance of nutrition, and reduction of the motor and secretory activity of the stomach. The keystone of therapy, however, is close surveillance of the patient. Since the pulse rate and blood pressure reflect the rate and severity of the bleeding, they should be determined at 30- to 60-min intervals until bleeding has ceased. To ensure a route for possible transfusion of blood, a No. 18 needle should be inserted immediately into a suitable vein and an infusion of glucose and water begun. If the patient is in shock, the foot of the bed should be elevated. Blood transfusions are given until the pulse rate stabilizes at 100 or less, or the blood pressure at 90 to 100 mm Hg, or the hematocrit is maintained at approximately 35 per cent. If there is extreme restlessness or pain, meperidine,

75 to 100 mg may be given. Ordinarily, parenteral sodium phenobarbital, 32.0 to 96.0 mg given every 4 to 6 hr as needed, is sufficient to allay anxiety. Urinary output should be carefully observed, since oliguria or anuria may result from prolonged hypotension. Continuous lavage of the stomach with cold saline solution may help to slow the bleeding.

Since it is technically difficult to perform repeated blood volume determinations during the course of therapy, the total volume of transfusion has to be estimated. Assessment of the blood loss is difficult in view of variability in rate of hemodilution. In general, the patient whose pulse is 100 or over, or whose blood pressure is 100 or less, and who has other evidences of shock has lost at least 1,500 ml of blood; one who has vomited a large amount of coffee-ground material has sustained a loss of at least 1,000 ml (see Chap. 13, Circulatory Failure).

In any event, if pulse and blood pressure do not return toward normal and stabilize, or if hematocrit determinations performed at 4- to 6-hr intervals show no rise or the rise is not maintained after transfusion, it may be concluded that bleeding continues. If this situation obtains after 24 hr of replacement therapy, or if the bleeding has proceeded so briskly within this period of time that 5 units or more of blood (2,500 ml) is required, surgical intervention should be carried out forthwith.

This approach has reduced the mortality from bleeding, particularly in the group of patients over age fifty. The need for rapid blood replacement in the older age group is more urgent since ischemia of the heart, brain, or kidneys may result in fatal myocardial infarction, cerebral vascular accident, or renal failure. Special care must be taken with patients who have heart disease. Packed red cells may be given slowly to such individuals, if shock is not present. When whole blood must be administered, the rate must be adjusted constantly. In this regard, frequent checks of venous pressure should be made via a manometer attached to the transfusion system by a three-way stopcock.

When vital signs have stabilized, whole milk in amounts varying from 90 to 120 cc is administered hourly from 7 A.M. to 10 P.M. and 120 cc at 2-hr intervals throughout the night. An initial period of continuous gastric aspiration may be necessary for 24 to 48 hr, if the patient is persistently nauseated and vomiting, during which parenteral fluids are given. Small feedings of warm skimmed milk are then offered, and these are gradually increased as tolerated.

The hourly regimen is maintained for approximately 24 to 48 hr after active bleeding has ceased. Then the usual routine ulcer management is instituted, consisting of six feedings of a diet from which fried food, spices, coffee, fresh fruits and vegetables are omitted. Antacids are continued hourly between feedings. At this time, antisecretory drugs such as the quaternary amines (methanthaline, propanthaline, etc.) or atropine may be given to reduce gastric H+, particularly nocturnally. Thus, 15 to 30 mg propanthaline may be given before meals and at bedtime. In this regard, use of these drugs is unwise while the patient is actively bleeding, since dosages required to suppress secretion would affect pulse rate, possibly interfere with bladder function, and promote ileus. Since neutralization of acid by frequent feedings appears to be adequate, added benefit from anticholinergic drugs at this stage does not justify their attendant risks.

Sedation is a most important part of therapy. Often the patient is anxious, worried, and restless. It is essential that these symptoms be alleviated and that he be maintained in a calm to drowsy state. The effect of anxiety upon gastric secretion and emptying can be detrimental. Phenobarbital by mouth, 32.0 to 96.0 mg, every 4 to 6 hr will suffice in most instances.

A word of caution about the use of morphine is in order. While it may be of great benefit in allaying anxiety, its use generally in therapy of gastrointestinal tract bleeding is to be condemned, since the drug may seriously depress respiration and blood pressure. Further, it is spasmogenic for smooth muscle of the gut and often causes nausea and vomiting. Barbiturates in adequate doses will effect satisfactory sedation without these undesirable reactions.

Emergency Surgery. Every effort is made to terminate the bleeding by conservative means, yet avoid delay of emergency surgery in those who will not respond to medical management. While the mortality rate with conservative treatment (2 to 5 per cent) is lower than that for surgery performed during active bleeding (8 to 15 per cent), the latter figures, however, are derived from a group of severe bleeders for whom medical therapy had already been ineffectual. Further, the mortality for those individuals over age fifty who continue to bleed after 24 hr of medical therapy exceeds 15 per cent.

The ulcer should be removed surgically, if possible. If this is not feasible, the ulcer bed can be transfixed with sutures or the branches of the gastroduodenal artery leading to the ulcer ligated. Subtotal gastric resection is then performed.

Elective Surgery. Elective surgery is recommended when the patient has suffered one severe or two mild hemorrhages while on satisfactory medical management and is strongly indicated when such an individual fails to follow a medical ulcer regimen. The procedures of choice are then a standard 75 per cent subtotal gastric resection, hemigastrectomy (50 per cent) with vagotomy, or gastroenterostomy with vagotomy.

Obstruction

Spasm, edema, or cicatrix of a peptic ulcer of the antrum, pylorus, or duodenum may obstruct the stomach. Often a combination of these factors is responsible.

The symptoms of gastric obstruction include progressive fullness after meals, voluntary restriction of food, nausea, and eventually, vomiting of partly undigested food. At first vomiting occurs sporadically, perhaps once in 24 to 36 hr and, characteristically, after the evening meal. As the degree of obstruction increases, vomiting becomes more frequent, despite considerable dilation of the stomach. Distress is almost always relieved by emesis. Occasionally, the patient has typical ulcer pain which is not relieved effectively by food. It must be remembered, however, that prolonged and severe vomiting may occur without organic obstruction.

Diagnosis. The diagnosis is best established by gastric aspiration and roentgenologic examination. Initial aspiration will reveal the degree of obstruction. Not uncommonly, 4 to 5 liters of undigested food may be obtained; however, the volume of aspirate may be small despite complete obstruction if the patient has been constantly vomiting. To ascertain the degree of obstruction in such a situation, the patient should be put on milk feedings, 90 cc every hour from 8 A.M. to 6 P.M., and aspirations may be carried out at 8 A.M. and at 10 P.M. Normally, 100 cc or less of gastric juice is present. If the amount exceeds this, then the difference represents the degree of obstruction. Quantities over 500 cc usually signify cicatricial obstruction. If the nightly retention of gastric juice gradually falls to normal after 3 to 4 days of medical management, spasm or edema is likely. In the presence of cicatricial stenosis, high levels of gastric retention persist. An exception to this formulation is the patient with cicatricial narrowing whose obstruction subsides under therapy. Failure of motility of the antrum, the so-called "antral pump," in the face of organic obstruction is believed to be the cause.

Delay in gastric emptying may be demonstrated on physical examination by a succession splash or by large gastric peristaltic waves moving from the left rib margin toward the right midabdomen. Physical evidences of dehydration include poor skin turgor, dry mucous membranes, and sunken eyes.

The roentgenologic examination gives the most accurate evidence of obstruction and should be made soon after initial decompression of the stomach. The site, nature, and extent of the obstructive lesion may be determined and the degree of retention and stenosis evaluated. Cicatricial stenosis (lumen 3 mm or less) of the duodenal bulb or pyloric canal can be seen on spot films of these segments and is frequently, but not always, accompanied by dilation of the stomach and hyperperistalsis. Other evidences of marked obstruction, in all probability cicatricial, include oliguria with urine of high specific gravity, dehydration, high hematocrit, and a metabolic alkalosis, occasionally aggravated by ingestion of alkali.

Treatment. Patients with prolonged vomiting and dehydration must be given 3 liters or more of normal saline with added potassium, 40 mEq per liter, intravenously, in the first 24 hr, in addition to a volume equal to total gastric aspirate and urinary output. If renal function is normal, alkalosis will thus be readily corrected.

In those patients in whom the pyloroduodenal channel is patent on x-ray, and in whom the stomach is only slightly or moderately dilated, hourly feedings of 120 cc milk may be started, 6 A.M. to 6 P.M. The stomach is then aspirated at 10 P.M., the degree of obstruction ascertained as outlined and, if mild, this program may be continued. Obstruction which is due to edema and/or spasm, associated with pyloric canal or prepyloric ulcer, will subside in 4 to 5 days; however, normal emptying may also be restored in a patient with cicatricial narrowing which will be noted on subsequent gastrointestinal series. If retention of over 150 cc is found after 5 to 7 days, surgery is indicated.

When the obstruction is marked on admission, decompression by continuous gastric aspiration up to 72 hr is advisable. Thereafter, the tube may be clamped, and milk may be either fed or instilled through the tube at the rate of 100 cc hourly for 7-hr periods. Following an additional ½ hr during which the tube is clamped, suction is reinstituted for ½ hr. If the residual for each 7-hr period progressively decreases over 72 hr to 100 cc or less, then the obstruction may be presumed to have been due principally to spasm or edema. If, however, 150 cc or more is aspirated on each occasion, cicatricial stenosis is very likely the cause, and operation is indicated. In this instance, continuous aspiration is reinstituted for 48 hr and definitive surgery carried out.

Each day the volume of the aspirate is replaced by intravenous administration of 5 per cent glucose and 0.9 per cent saline with 20 mEq K+ per liter to which soluble vitamin B complex is added. In addition, 500 ml of 5 per cent glucose and water per 24 hr are given for insensible loss. *Anticholinergic drugs must not be administered, since they delay gastric emptying.* Adequate sedation must be ensured, as already outlined. Urinary output and blood urea nitrogen must be carefully checked, particularly in those patients with renal disease. Since obstructing ulcers also tend to bleed, stools and hematocrit must be carefully evaluated during treatment.

Subtotal gastric resection is the procedure of choice for cicatricial obstruction, but it should not be performed until the stomach has been adequately decompressed and any acid-base derangement corrected. In some instances a posterior gastroenterostomy is preferable, particularly in elderly patients who are not good surgical risks. This procedure should, if possible, be combined with vagotomy.

Perforation and Penetration

Perforation is the most dramatic complication of duodenal ulcer. It is most frequent in men under the age of forty-five and is rare in women. Typically, the anterior wall is the site of rupture. Although in most instances there is an antecedent history of duodenal ulcer, acute perforation occasionally is the initial manifestation of this disease.

Since rupture of the anterior wall of the duodenum is attended by free release of intestinal contents into the peritoneal cavity, the patient complains of sudden, excruciating epigastric pain, rapidly becomes weak to faint, perspires freely, is nauseated, and often vomits. Because of irritation of the diaphragmatic pleura, pain aggravated by inspiration may be felt over the area of the trapezius ridge.

Physical examination will reveal a pale or gray individual, exhibiting marked diaphoresis, a pronounced preference for remaining still in order to minimize peritoneal irritation, and a normal or elevated pulse rate. The blood pressure is usually normal or only slightly reduced. Examination of the abdomen reveals marked rigidity, particularly in the upper quadrants, and palpation or movement causes the patient to complain of increased pain. If gastric contents have drained into the lower abdomen, there will be tenderness and some guarding in the right lower quadrant or in the flank.

Several hours later the patient may regain normal color, cease to perspire, and be more comfortable, although tenderness and spasm in the upper abdomen persist. This change in the picture signifies only that homeostatic mechanisms have compensated for the initial reaction to stress and in no way signifies that the patient is recovering. The peritoneal irritation will doubtless progress to frank peritonitis attended by fever, tachycardia, and progressive abdominal distention.

Diagnosis is usually made by the characteristic history, together with the findings of a rigid or boardlike abdomen with loss of normal liver dullness to percussion. A flat film of the abdomen taken in a sitting position or lateral decubitus will show free air beneath the diaphragm or lateral abdominal wall, respectively (Fig. 272-6).

Anterior perforation of a duodenal ulcer must be distinguished from several common intraabdominal inflammatory states, particularly acute pancreatitis, acute appendicitis, acute cholecystitis or cholangitis associated with choledocholithiasis, acute intestinal obstruction, mesenteric arterial occlusion, myocardial infarction, ruptured ectopic pregnancy, dissecting aneurysm of the aorta, and inflammatory diseases of the diaphragmatic pleura and lungs.

Of these diagnoses, the one which most simulates perforation is acute pancreatitis. The principal points of differential diagnosis are: pancreatitis typically has a rather gradual onset, the pain often is felt predominantly in the back, is diminished by abdominal compression or bending forward, and lasts for many hours to a day or so. In severe hemorrhagic pancreatitis, however, the onset may be as dramatic and the collapse as complete as in perforation. Indeed, shock is much more likely to occur in the former condition. Abdominal examination reveals tenderness usually over the upper abdomen with some muscle resistance, but nothing approximating boardlike rigidity. Again, there is no obliteration of liver dullness, and an upright film of the abdomen shows no free air. In acute pancreatitis the serum amylase will show elevation, usually over 350 units and, if the patient is seen within a few hours of the onset of the attack, often in the range of 600 to 700 units. While a rise in amylase may attend anterior perforation, due to the escape of pancreatic juice into the peritoneal cavity, it frequently is no higher than 200 to 300 units. Also, a significant rise in serum lipase and some elevation of serum bilirubin and alkaline phosphatase often attend acute pancreatitis.

With *acute appendicitis,* onset of symptoms is insidious, with localization of pain in the right lower quadrant after a period of hours. On examination there is both direct and rebound tenderness in the right lower quadrant as well as rectal tenderness on the right.

In *biliary colic* the pain almost invariably is steady, but rarely may wax and wane, and the episode is more frequently associated with nausea and vomiting. Chills, fever, and jaundice are common. If, however, the acutely inflamed gallbladder perforates, upper abdominal rigidity may be found associated with other evidences of peritoneal irritation which may later become generalized. However, in this instance, a history of acute cholecystitis in the very recent past can be obtained.

The other conditions mentioned in the differential diagnosis are usually clearly distinguished from acute anterior perforation of a duodenal ulcer by differences in characteristics of pain, location of tenderness or rigidity, and in the case of myocardial infarction, by the abnormalities of the electrocardiogram. With diaphragmatic irritation due to basal pneumonia, the upper abdomen is not usually tender despite rigidity. Of course, confusion will not exist if the patient also has significant cough, sputum, and fever.

Relation of Penetration and Perforation to Intractability. In many instances of "intractability" the basis for the persistence of severe pain which does not respond to usual medical measures is posterior penetration of the ulcer into a neighboring viscus, commonly the pancreas. Often the process culminates in a small perforation which is quickly walled off so that recovery ensues without surgical intervention. When there is penetration into the pancreas, considerable back pain and associated evidences of acute pancreatitis are present.

Continued ulcer distress with localization of pain in the epigastrium and right upper quadrant associated with tenderness may be indicative of a small lateral duodenal perforation which has sealed. In such instances, tenderness, perhaps even with rebound, can be elicited because of the leakage of a small amount of fluid. Usually free air within the peritoneal cavity cannot be demonstrated, and abscess is a rare complication. Once the diagnosis of localized perforation is reasonably suspected, surgical intervention should be undertaken, although in many instances it need not be immediate.

Treatment. If the diagnosis of perforation is established within the first 24 to 36 hr after onset, immediate surgical intervention is indicated. Preoperatively, constant gastric suction, adequate replacement of fluids and electrolytes, broad-spectrum antibiotic therapy (penicillin, 1.2×10^6 units, and streptomycin, 1.0 Gm, daily in divided doses) all should be instituted. In perforations of 36 hr or more duration, conservative therapy may be undertaken. This regimen includes continuous gastric suction, vigorous treatment with broad-spectrum antibiotics, adequate fluid replacement, and administration of blood and albumin as needed.

THE SURGICAL APPROACH TO DUODENAL ULCER

For many years the surgical techniques for the treatment of duodenal ulcer have been constantly revised, based on continuing additions to knowledge of the various roles which parietal cell mass, the vagus, and the antrum play in gastric hypersecretion. It is now generally accepted that no procedure is satisfactory unless it significantly reduces the secretion of hydrochloric acid and pepsin

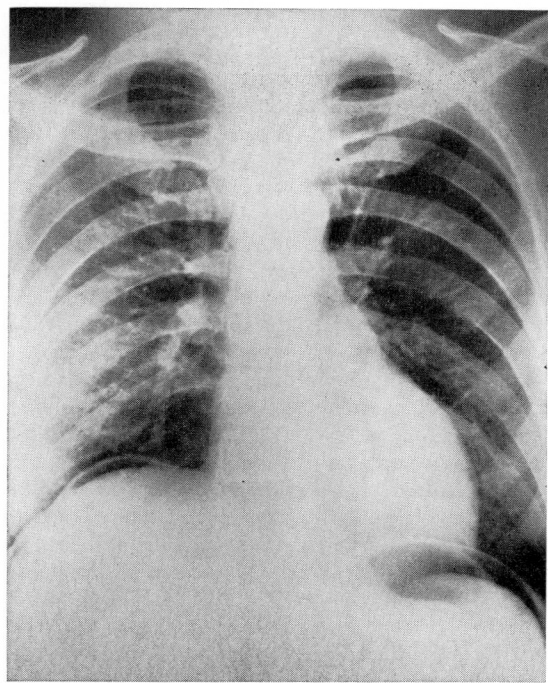

FIG. 272-6. Upright (sitting) abdominal film of a patient with an anterior perforation of a duodenal ulcer, demonstrating air beneath the diaphragm.

by the stomach. This may be accomplished in a number of different ways. All the procedures to be discussed were developed after the earliest operations of simple gastroenterostomy or "antral exclusion."

Gastroenterostomy and antral exclusion were designed to permit the patient to retain most or all of the stomach; however, the rate of recurrent jejunal peptic ulceration has been prohibitively high (about 35 to 50 per cent) following these procedures. As a result, more radical resections have been done. With bolder resection have come several important inverse relationships. As the amount removed approaches 75 per cent of the organ, the incidence of recurrent ulcer drops; however, as size of the remnant diminishes, the incidence of digestive and nutritional disturbances increases. Reaction to the latter sequence has led many surgeons either to resect less stomach and perform simultaneous vagotomy or to preserve the duodenum, i.e., to do gastroduodenostomy (Billroth I) rather than gastrojejunostomy (Billroth II).

Although a great experience with all varieties of surgical correction has been accumulated, it must be emphasized that the ideal procedure has not yet been developed.

Subtotal Gastric Resection. In this now classic operation for duodenal ulcer, two-thirds to three-quarters of the distal stomach is removed along with the ulcer in most instances. A loop of jejunum is anastomosed to the resected end of the stomach according to the methods and modifications of Polya or Hofmeister. When performed in this fashion, the incidence of recurrent jejunal ulcer is low, of the order of 3 to 5 per cent at most. Nevertheless, this operation leaves about 15 to 20 per cent of individuals with significant weight loss resulting from serious disorders of digestion, which include anorexia, postprandial fullness, nausea and vomiting, postprandial "dumping" symptoms, and diarrhea.

The "Dumping Syndrome." This syndrome may be described as follows: toward the end of the meal or within a few minutes of its completion, the patient complains of some warmth, a feeling of weakness, often with lightheadedness and palpitations, begins to perspire, feels faint, is apprehensive, and frequently has to lie down. This sequence is most likely to appear after ingestion of carbohydrates which are rapidly hydrolyzed. This disorder is probably related to shift of intravascular fluid into the jejunum in order to dilute hyperosomotic contents; often as much as 20 per cent of plasma volume is thus displaced within a short period of time. The rapid pulse and lightheadedness or syncope are due to hypovolemia; the apprehension,

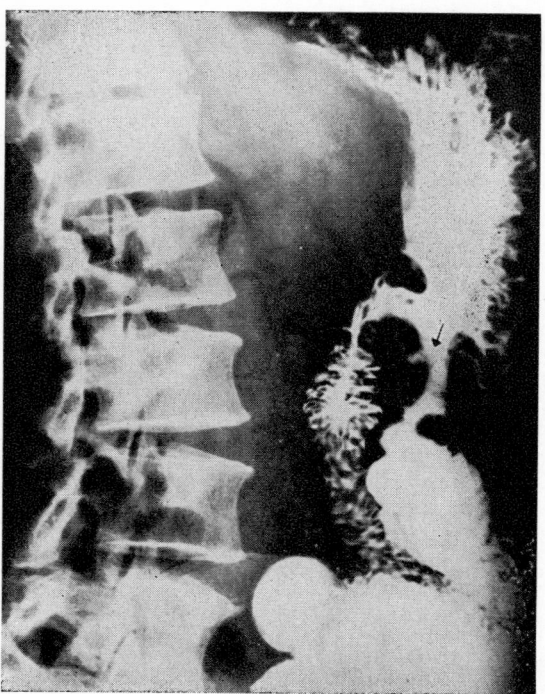

FIG. 272-7. Recurrent peptic ulcer (marginal ulcer) of jejunum in a patient after subtotal gastrectomy and gastrojejunostomy (Billroth II).

pallor, and sweating, to sympathetic response. However, a relationship between diminished plasma volume and the symptoms has not been consistently demonstrated. Perhaps the symptoms in some instances are due to autonomic overreaction, based as much upon psychologic factors as upon response to rapid jejunal filling. The management of this distressing condition consists of frequent small feedings which are low in carbohydrate.

The basis for impaired absorption and diarrhea following subtotal gastrectomy has not been established. Factors to be considered include inadequate mixing of food with the digestive ferments from the liver and pancreas due both to bypass of the duodenum and to rapid dispersion over most of the small bowel. In these instances there is significant steatorrhea, with 10 to 20 per cent and occasionally as much as 40 per cent of ingested fat appearing in the stool. Up to 30 per cent of the preoperative body weight may be lost after gastrectomy. Indeed, after high subtotal gastrectomy, a definite malabsorption syndrome may be seen, including symptoms and signs of deficiency of fat-soluble vitamins (paresthesias and tetany due to hypocalcemia; bleeding due to hypoprothrombinemia), vitamin B complex, iron and vitamin B_{12}, etc. (see Chap. 62). Perhaps as a consequence of their poor nutritional status, these individuals have an increased incidence of tuberculosis. Recent evidence indicates that bacterial contamination of the afferent loop is another cause for steatorrhea and malabsorption following Billroth II procedures. Correction may follow a course of broad-spectrum antibiotic therapy such as tetracycline. (Neomycin should not be used, since its administration may be associated with steatorrhea.) Of interest, biopsy specimens of the upper jejunum in patients with steatorrhea following gastrectomy and with gastrojejunostomies reveal atrophic changes of columnar epithelium resembling nontropical sprue. (For discussion of therapy of postgastrectomy problems, see Chap. 274.)

In order to preserve enough stomach to lessen the occurrence of these distressing complications, hemigastrectomy with gastroduodenostomy (Billroth I) is now being performed. Several reports indicate that digestive disturbances are fewer and nutrition is better after this procedure, attributable to better reservoir function and mixing of food with duodenal juices. However, the rate of recurrence of ulcer seems to be higher than after standard high subtotal resection and gastrojejunostomy.

A number of investigators feel that maximum protection against both recurrent ulceration and digestive problems can be assured if the distal half of the stomach including the antrum and pylorus is resected and a vagotomy performed. As indicated, there is some evidence that nutrition is better after low than after high subtotal gastrectomy. The incidence of diarrhea and dumping syndrome may be less, particularly if gastroduodenostomy is done. Theoretically, then, when the antrum is resected and the vagi are cut, the operation should be satisfactory. However, if vagotomy is complete, there is no evidence that antrectomy will add protection against recurrent jejunal ulceration. If vagotomy is incomplete, one is left with a simple resection of the antrum, an operation known to be inadequate. The rationale of this operation will be established only when it has been shown that the good results reported are not the result of the vagotomy.

Vagotomy alone is unsatisfactory, since it is attended by gastric stasis which stimulates the gastric antrum with release of gastrin, leading to further hypersecretion and reulceration. Therefore, when it is done, a procedure to ensure adequate drainage must accompany it. If the low recurrence rate of ulcer after hemigastrectomy and vagotomy is due principally to the latter, then vagotomy with pyloroplasty or gastroenterostomy will be preferable to vagotomy with resection, since the former combination will ensure retention of a greater amount of reservoir function of the stomach.

Recurrent (Marginal) Ulceration. Following simple gastroenterostomy, and much less commonly after high subtotal gastrectomy or partial gastrectomy with vagotomy, a marginal ulcer may appear on the efferent side of the anastomosis at any time (even up to 30 years), but most often occurs within a year of the procedure (Fig. 272-7). The pain is much like that of duodenal ulcer except that it is located more to the left of the midline in the midepigastrium rather than being high midline or subxyphoid. While it is relieved by eating and by drinking milk or alkali, the response to such measures is less satisfactory than with duodenal ulcer and, in general, the healing of such craters is more difficult.

The diagnosis is often suggested by the history, but frequently there is no pain, and bleeding is the only manifestation. Often these bleeding episodes can be severe, and in many instances the crater will not be demonstrable by x-ray. Whether the marginal ulcer presents with pain or bleeding, intensive management is required. If satisfactory evidence of healing is not obtained, further surgery must be undertaken. If the patient has had only a simple gastroenterostomy, then subtotal gastrectomy with vagotomy is recommended; if the patient has had a subtotal gastrectomy, then vagotomy should be done; if, rarely, the patient has had subtotal gastrectomy and vagotomy, a high subtotal gastrectomy should be performed. In all instances of recurrent ulceration, search for tumor of the pancreas must be made.

REFERENCES

Allen, J. G.: "The Physiology and Treatment of Peptic Ulcer," Chicago, University of Chicago Press, 1959.

Card, W. I., and I. N. Marks: The Relationship between the Acid Output of the Stomach Following "Maximal" Histamine Stimulation and the Parietal Cell Mass, Clin. Sci., 19:147, 1960.

Kay, A. W.: Effect of Large Doses of Histamine on Gastric Secretion of HCl: An Augmented Histamine Test, Brit. Med. J., 2:77, 1953.

Kirsner, J. B., and W. L. Palmer (Eds.): Symposium on Peptic Ulcer, Am. J. Med., 29:723, 1960.

Sleisenger, M. H., C. M. Lewis, M. Lipkin, and C. Wierum: Uropepsin and 17-Hydroxycorticoid Excretion in Normal Subjects and Patients with Peptic Ulcer during Both States of Activity and Quiescence, Am. J. Med., 25:395, 1958.

Weiner, H., M. Thaler, M. F. Reiser, and I. A. Mirsky: Etiology of Duodenal Ulcer: I. Relation of Specific Psychological Characteristics to Rate of Gastric Secretion (Serum Pepsinogen), Psychosomat. Med., 19:1, 1957.

Wolf, S., and H. Wolff: "Human Gastric Function," New York, Oxford University Press, 1943.

273 BENIGN GASTRIC ULCER
Marvin H. Sleisenger

Pathology and Clinical Picture. Benign peptic ulceration of the stomach, like duodenal ulcer, is a chronic, recurrent disease in which there is a localized erosion of the mucosa, extending into the submucosa and averaging 10 to 20 mm in diameter; occasionally, it may be as great as 50 mm (Fig. 273-1). The ulcer usually is single, but occasionally dual or multiple. In most instances the edges of the ulcer crater are sharply defined, with a surrounding area of inflammatory edema, hyperemia, and infiltration. The base of the ulcer is generally covered with a small amount of fibrinous or fibropurulent exudate which overlies zones of necrosis, granulation, and fibrosis, depending upon the degree of healing which has occurred. In the more chronic penetrating variety, the muscle coats may be interrupted and interspersed with fibrosis; in these instances, blood vessels may become thrombosed or eroded.

The *clinical picture* is variable. Epigastric pain is the prominent presenting symptom. As in duodenal ulcer, it is gnawing or aching, varies from mild discomfort to severe distress, appears one to several hours after meals, lasts 30 min or more with prompt relief upon ingestion of food or alkali. Distress at night seems to be rare. Frequently,

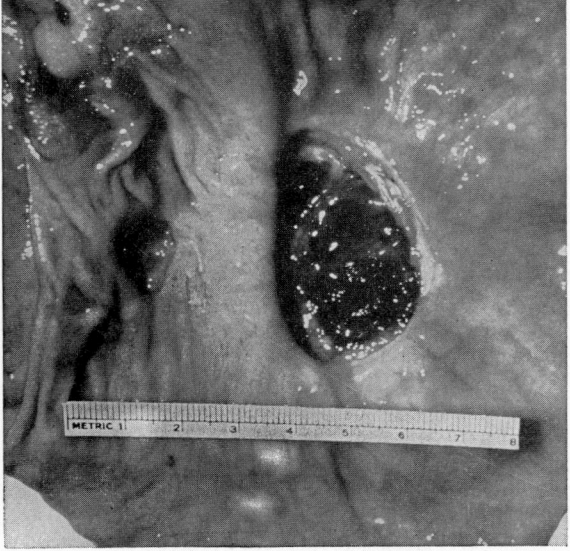

FIG. 273-1. Large chronic gastric ulcer 4.1 × 2.5 cm in diameter and 8 mm in depth on the posterior wall of the stomach, lower third, producing a massive fatal hemorrhage. A second smaller ulcer is seen on the left.

however, the story is different. The discomfort may be burning or cramplike, may not be relieved by food or alkali, and in fact may be aggravated by eating. Also, the area of the distress is apt to be more diffuse than for duodenal ulcer, covering the major part of the epigastric area and often extending over the left lower anterior rib cage. Periodicity of gastric ulcer activity is not nearly so striking as that of duodenal ulcer, in which recurrences are most common in the spring and autumn.

As with duodenal ulcer, radiation of the pain to the back is not uncommon and suggests penetration of the lesion beyond the serosa into adjacent organs, particularly the pancreas.

The exact clinical incidence of gastric ulcer is unknown, but it is thought to be about one-tenth as common as duodenal ulcer. Accurate determination is difficult, since small and/or rapidly healing ulcerations are extremely difficult to demonstrate. As with duodenal ulcer, this disorder occurs more commonly in men than in women, the ratio in most large series varying from 2:1 to 4:1.

The majority of gastric ulcers occur at two sites: the prepyloric area and along the lesser curvature. About 90 per cent of lesser curvature ulcers are located in mucosa containing pyloric glands, suggesting that the latter is less resistant than mucosa with acid and pepsin secreting cells. Less common sites include the posterior wall of the body of the stomach, along the greater curvature, and the area of the cardia and cardioesophageal junc-

tion. A gastric ulcer may occasionally appear in association with either an active or a healed duodenal ulcer.

Etiology and Pathogenesis. In benign gastric ulcer, unlike duodenal ulcer, gastric secretion rarely is above normal. Aside from the digestive action of acid peptic juice upon the mucosa and its underlying layers, little is known of the etiology and pathogenesis of gastric ulceration. Nevertheless, certain facts are available which suggest that this disease is different from duodenal ulcer. The incidence appears to be higher in patients with chronic pulmonary disease and rheumatoid arthritis and in those treated with certain drugs, particularly adrenal steroids (see below). Since the secretion of acid is often normal or, as found in other studies, slightly depressed, ulceration may be due to some defect either in the protective mucus of gastric juice or in tissue resistance, or both. Since a normal regenerative capacity is important for adequate resistance, it is possible that impaired protein metabolism may play a role in the genesis of gastric ulcer. The importance of mucosal regeneration in relation to mucosal integrity is suggested by the frequency of atrophic changes adjacent to the ulcer area of the stomach, perhaps resulting from an antecedent gastritis.

The increased incidence of gastric ulcers in patients with gastric retention due to pyloric obstruction or following vagotomy alone or combined with high lying gastroenterostomy has stimulated interest in the role of the antrum in the genesis of gastric ulcer. Evidence obtained from experiments with dogs indicates that antral stimulation by contact with food or by distention results in hypersecretion of acid mediated by gastrin (Chap. 272). In addition, reflux of alkaline fluid into the antrum after gastroenterostomy abolishes the normal antral inhibition of gastrin release, thereby promoting acid secretion. A clinical observation which supports the importance of the antrum is the healing of proximal gastric ulcers after simple antrectomy. Although psychologic factors may play a significant role in the genesis of gastric ulcer, helpful studies of the personality patterns of patients with gastric ulcer or of the role of emotional trauma are not available.

Acute Gastric Ulcer. Gastric ulceration may develop acutely. A major difference between the acute ulcer and the more common variety is the lack of fibrosis and of endarteritic vascular thrombosis in the former which renders these craters more liable to perforation and bleeding. Indeed, one of these complications may be the presenting symptom in many instances. Acute gastric ulcer is likely to occur in the situations discussed below.

Drug-induced Gastric Ulcer. A large number of drugs, particularly the *adrenal steroids,* may induce

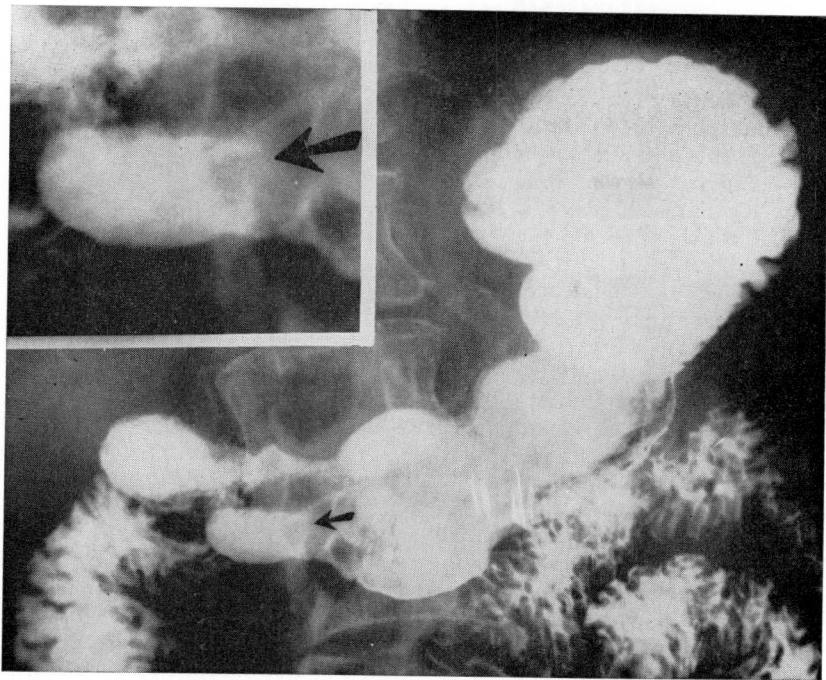

FIG. 273-2. Large gastric ulcer of the antrum in a 56-year-old woman with rheumatoid arthritis treated with adrenal corticosteroids for 6 years. This is a common location and appearance for "steroid ulcers." (*From W. H. Kammerer, R. H. Freiberger, and A. Rivelis: Arthritis and Rheumatism, 1:122, 1958. Reprinted with permission of the author and publisher.*)

gastric ulceration (Fig. 273-2). The incidence of peptic ulcer in patients receiving adrenal steroids varies from 7 to 32 per cent, depending upon the length of administration, the dosage employed, and the nature of the underlying disease being treated with the steroids. The highest incidence is recorded when patients receiving steroids are subjected to routine roentgenographic examination, thus revealing asymptomatic ulcers. Steroid ulcer seems to occur more frequently in patients with rheumatoid arthritis, lupus erythematosis, and certain skin diseases, and less frequently in those with ulcerative colitis and malignant diseases. Whether duodenal or gastric in location, these ulcers may be asymptomatic, may often bleed severely, and occasionally perforate without prior symptoms. Although they are not generally associated with elevated secretion of acid and pepsin, nevertheless, they frequently heal on a regimen of a high protein diet and frequent feedings, with antacids and antisecretory drugs (see below).

The appearance of benign gastric ulcer of the stomach, frequently severe enough to bleed or perforate, may be associated with the administration of certain other therapeutic agents. Drugs which block adrenergic activity, such as *tolazoline hydrochloride* (Priscoline), *hydralazine* (Apreso-

line), and *hexamethonium*, are thought to induce ulceration by augmenting gastric acid secretion via a relatively greater vagal influence. Two other agents, *phenylbutazone* (Butazolidine) and *reserpine*, stimulate acid production, the former by direct action on the parietal cells, and the latter by central suppression of sympathetic stimuli. In this regard, the usual therapeutic dose of reserpine, 1.0 mg daily, does not increase acid secretion, but 2.0 mg or more may elevate both the volume of secretion and the total acid. To some extent these drugs probably act by local irritation. It is likely that *cincophen* and *salicylates* also cause acute inflammation and erosion by their irritative action, although salicylates may also increase secretion. The ulcerogenic effect of *caffeine* probably arises as a result of increased acid secretion and local mucosal irritation. It is also possible that the ulcerogenic potential of some or all of these agents results partly from an adverse effect upon the blood flow to the mucosa.

The role of *salicylate* ingestion in upper gastrointestinal bleeding has received considerable attention of late. Data which suggest that salicylates cause upper gastrointestinal bleeding, particularly in patients with preexisting peptic ulcer disease, are sufficiently impressive to restrict the use of these agents, as much as possible, in such individuals and in those without known ulcer disease who have bled following their use. The quantity of salicylate required to induce bleeding in susceptible individuals varies, but may be as little as 0.6 Gm three to four times daily for several days. Chronic occult bleeding has also been observed. The "buffering" of aspirin with alkali does not prevent this type of bleeding. Perhaps administration of salicylates in either dispersed or enteric-coated forms may reduce the incidence of this effect; however, evidence at present is inconclusive on this point.

Ulcer Associated with Stress. Peptic ulceration may occur during acutely or chronically stressful situations. In many instances these ulcers are associated with cerebral vascular lesions, particularly subarachnoid and intracerebral hemorrhage and thrombosis. Documentation of stress ulcers may be difficult; indeed, suspicion of their presence may be aroused only by a severe or exsanguinating hemorrhage. Such ulcerations are also associated with burns, multiple injuries, fulminating sepsis, snake bite, exposure, and many other stressful situations.

Diagnosis of Gastric Ulcer. Although variable, the history in gastric ulcer may be highly suggestive; the physical examination, except possibly for some tenderness in the epigastrium, is usually unrevealing. Generally, also, there is no anemia and the stools are often negative for occult blood. The diagnosis of gastric ulcer can be established with certainty only by radiologic examination, gastroscopy, or surgical exploration.

Radiographically, the benign gastric ulcer of the stomach appears as a discrete punched-out crater which, if located on the curvature, extends beyond its margin. Characteristically, radiating mucosal folds extend to the crater. Benign gastric ulcers are smooth or only slightly irregular; a rim or "halo" of radiolucency, due to inflammatory edema of the margins of the crater, separates the crater from the remainder of the barium-filled stomach (Fig. 273-3).

Differentiation of Benign and Malignant Gastric Ulcer. The clinical history does not usually distinguish the benign from malignant ulcer. It is generally thought that carcinoma of the stomach is rare in the third and fourth decades; however, enough exceptions have been encountered to make the age factor unreliable in differential diagnosis. A long history of recurrent symptoms is more characteristic of benign gastric ulcer, but certainly this disease process may be acute in onset and brief in course. Loss of appetite and significant loss of weight are more characteristic of malignancy, but these symptoms are not specific for it. The pain may be identical in both conditions if peptic ulcer-

ation occurs within the malignancy. In this situation, *relief with milk or alkali may not distinguish between the two conditions.* Frequently, pain in malignant gastric ulcer is due to neoplastic involvement of dorsal root nerve fibers; in this instance food and antacids are, of course, ineffective in relieving it. Anemia or occult blood in the stool suggests a malignant process.

The vast majority of gastric ulcers are benign. In order to differentiate the ulcer from ulcerated malignancy, five diagnostic criteria should be routinely employed. These are: determination of capacity for acid secretion, careful study of the upper gastrointestinal x-ray, cytologic study of exfoliated cells, gastroscopy and biopsy, and response to therapy as measured roentgenographically.

The *x-ray appearance* of the lesion is one of the most important aids in differentiating benign from malignant gastric ulcer. Presence or absence of a tumor mass at the margins of the ulcer crater or evidence that the ulcer is in the midst of a tumor is crucial in this matter. Some of the features of benign gastric ulcer which have already been alluded to, such as presence of radiating folds and extension beyond the contour of the curvature, may be present in a malignant ulcer. Conversely, the large translucent shadow between the barium-filled crater and the stomach, reflecting edema of benign gastric ulcer, may be confused with a corresponding one in carcinoma. This latter crescentic shadow between the gastric wall and lumen is due to tumor infiltration about an ulcer which does not project beyond the contour of the curvature (Carmen's meniscus sign) (Fig. 273-4). Although it has long been alleged that ulcers of the greater curvature and the prepyloric area are more likely to be malignant, careful analysis of such craters in these areas does not support the contention. Therefore, diagnosis must not be made on the basis of location.

While both conditions may be associated with a relative hypochlorhydria, the likelihood of malignancy is increased if the patient has complete (true) achlorhydria, for such a secretory response is very rare in benign gastric ulcer. Indeed, this finding necessitates surgical exploration. The converse, i.e., that the capacity to secrete free acid indicates a benign process, does not hold and, per se, should never be a criterion for excluding malignancy.

Several additional aids in laboratory diagnosis are very helpful. One of these has been the study of exfoliated cells from the gastric mucosa, prepared according to the method of Papanicolaou. Techniques for obtaining such cells include lavage with saline or chymotrypsin or mucosal abrasion with a brush or balloon covered by a net. Accuracy of cytologic diagnosis of carcinoma varies from 60 to

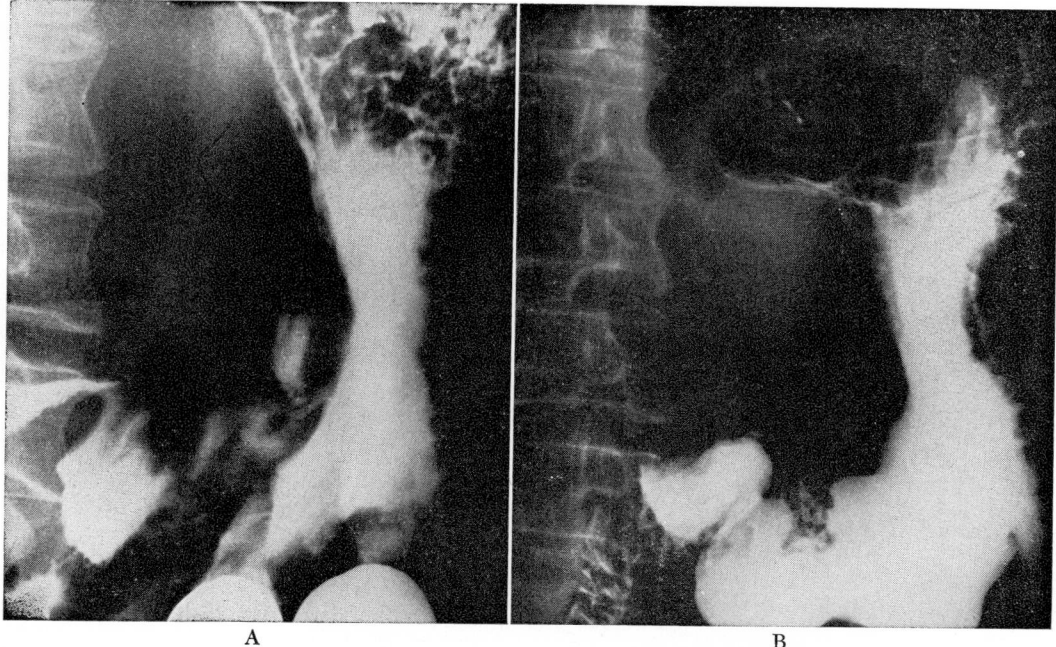

Fig. 273-3. A. Large benign gastric ulcer on the lesser curvature of the stomach of a 42-year-old woman. Note the projection of the crater beyond the contour of the curvature and the prominent area of radiolucency which separates the crater from the stomach lumen. (Compare with Fig. 273-4.) B. After 3 weeks of therapy the ulcer has healed.

80 per cent. When combined with radiology, the percentage of positive diagnosis of carcinoma approaches 90 per cent (Table 273-1). If the results of either of these procedures indicate malignancy, operation should be performed without delay.

Gastroscopy with or without *biopsy* may contribute to correct diagnosis. Gastroscopic differentiation of the lesion alone is not completely reliable. Differentiation of benign from malignant gastric ulcer must not rest on gastroscopic features alone, since often even at operation the surgeon is unable to tell whether or not the lesion is malignant. Also, "blind areas" in the cardia and antrum escape the view of the endoscopist. Biopsy is decisive only when positive.

Finally, the *behavior of the lesion during intensive medical therapy,* perferably in the hospital, is a most important criterion in the differential diagnosis. While it is alleged that malignant gastric ulcer may heal completely during a trial of medical therapy, such an event is rare. The incidence of complete healing of malignant ulcer is probably no greater than 1 per cent. Most benign ulcers either heal completely or nearly completely in a period of 4 to 6 weeks. Failure to respond in this manner must be considered presumptive evidence of malignancy (Fig. 273-5). Nonetheless, one must remember that ulcers in older individuals, as well as in individuals with moderate to severe nutri-

Table 273-1. COMPARISON OF CYTOLOGY AND X-RAY IN DIAGNOSIS OF GASTRIC CANCER AND ULCER

114 CASES OF CARCINOMA

X-ray	Cytology		
	I–II (benign)	III (suspicious)	IV–V (malignant)
Normal 4 (3.4%)	0	0	4
Benign 12 (10.5%)	4	3	5
Equivocal 20 (17.6%)	3	3	14
Positive 78 (68.5%)	11	14	53

By combining all positive reports (not including equivocal or class III), correct diagnosis made in 88.7 per cent.

421 CASES WITHOUT CARCINOMA

Procedure	Correct report (%)
X-ray	368 (88)
Cytology	398 (94.5)

SOURCE: From Seybolt, J., and G. Papanicolaou: The Value of Cytology in Diagnosis of Gastric Cancer, Gastroenterol., 33:369, 1957. By permission of the authors and publisher.

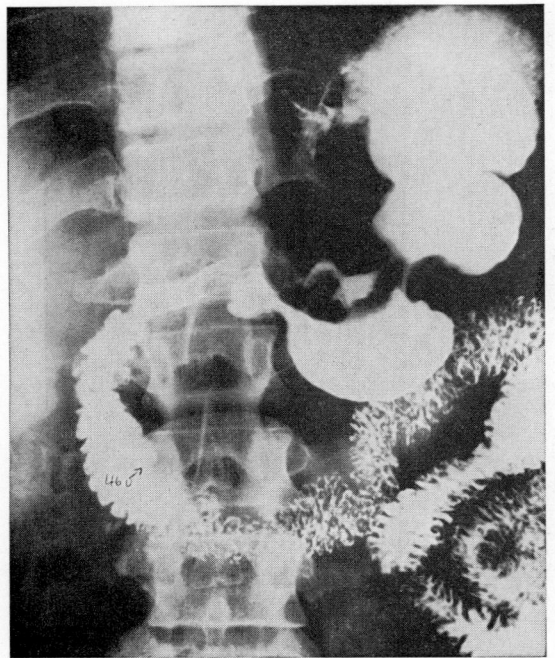

FIG. 273-4. An ulcerated carcinoma in a 46-year-old man, demonstrating both crescentic crater within the contour of the lesser curvature and the area of radiolucency between the gastric wall and lumen. (Carmen's sign.) (Compare with Fig. 273-3.)

tional problems, may heal more slowly. Conversely, it is astonishing how rapidly large ulcers may disappear (Fig. 273-3).

If one uses all these criteria, including the trial of therapy, the incidence of erroneous diagnosis in malignant gastric ulcer will be less than 5 per cent and, in institutions where great experience has accumulated, will probably be about 2 or 3 per cent. This is a wholly acceptable approach, since the delay of 3 to 4 weeks in operating has not been satisfactorily demonstrated to affect the prognosis of malignant ulcer. Indeed, several studies of patients with gastric ulcer have shown that operative mortality in benign ulcers, suspected preoperatively of being malignant, was higher than that from cancer which had been misdiagnosed as benign ulceration.

The surgical approach to uncomplicated, nonrecurrent gastric ulcer should not be based upon the possibility of malignancy in the face of criteria which indicate that the process is benign; rather, it should be based primarily upon either unequivocal or strongly suggestive evidence of cancer derived from careful studies and observation. Conservative medical treatment demands that the patient be kept under close surveillance and that decision regarding surgery be made promptly after the trial period. However, since the prognosis for small gastric carcinoma which has ulcerated is vastly better than that for gastric cancer in general (5-year cure rates of 25 per cent versus 5 to 10 per cent), the physician should decide in favor of surgical intervention in unresolved or doubtful cases. The rare occurrence of marginal ulceration after subtotal gastrectomy for gastric ulcer as well as the lower incidence of dumping syndrome and other nutritional problems further support this attitude.

The possible relationship between benign gastric ulcer and the subsequent development of stomach cancer is pertinent to this discussion. In five reported studies, 0.4 to 3.0 per cent of patients with benign gastric ulcer developed carcinoma of the stomach within 10 years. The average was 1.5 per cent. These figures per se do not warrant gastrectomy for benign ulcer as a cancer prophylaxis. In many instances the carcinoma is located at a site different from the antecedent ulcer, which had long since completely healed, making it difficult to accept a cause-effect relationship.

Treatment. The management of the patient with benign peptic ulcer of the stomach follows the same general principles outlined for duodenal ulcer. The major difference is that, if possible, the patient should be hospitalized during the period of treatment to afford maximum opportunity for the ulcer to heal. Obviously, this is of great importance, since the extent of healing will determine whether operation will be performed. Removal of the patient from his environment will provide mental as well as physical rest and will promote the strong doctor-patient relationship so important to good management.

Naturally, all drugs which might contribute to the ulcerative process such as adrenal steroids, salicylates, Butazolidine, etc., should be discontinued as rapidly as possible. Occasionally, however, adrenal steroid therapy will have to be maintained or reduced very slowly. The ulcers will often heal even with continued steroid administration.

Although secretion of acid and pepsin may be subnormal in the patient with benign gastric ulcer, healing is slow when nutrition is poor and nitrogen balance is negative, as is commonly the case in chronic pulmonary or rheumatic diseases, or with adrenal steroid therapy. Accordingly, *diet* should consist of frequent feedings of foods with high protein content as well as substantial buffering power. At onset of therapy, 4 to 6 oz milk is given hourly. After a few days, three regular meals and a bedtime feeding may be added. Several times daily milk feedings may be supplemented with protein hydrolysates. (For further details of diet, see Chap. 272.)

Antacid and antisecretory drugs are also benefi-

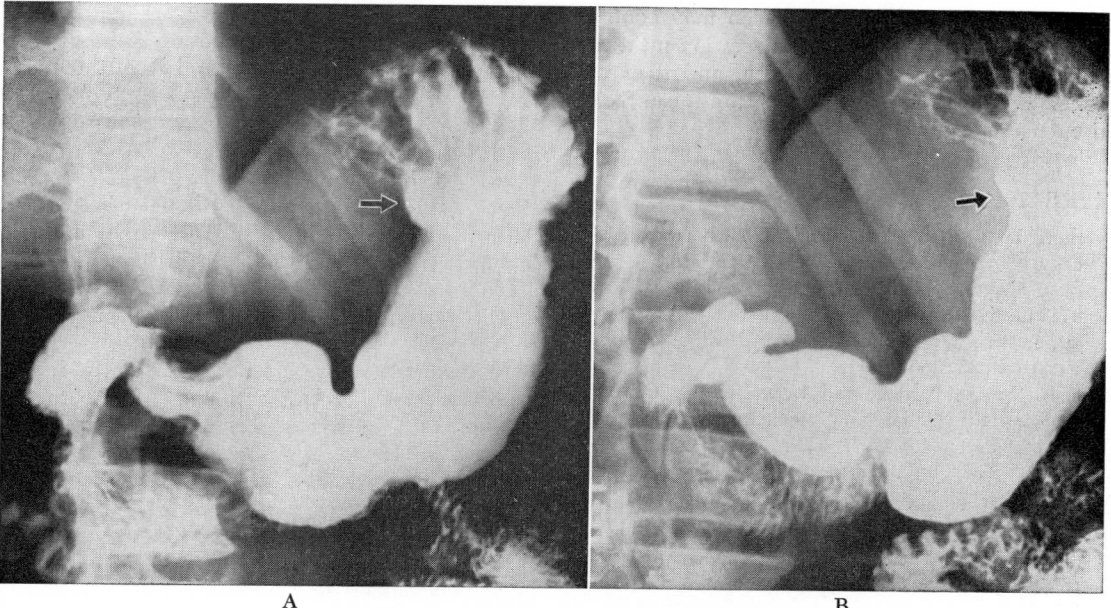

Fig. 273-5. Large lesser curvature ulcer in a 42-year-old man which appeared benign (*A*) but which showed incomplete healing in 5 weeks (*B*). At operation an ulcerated carcinoma with metastases was found.

cial. Since relief from anxiety is essential to optimum healing, sedatives should be given in the same manner as for duodenal ulcer. (For details of use of all these drugs as well as tranquilizers, antacids, and antisecretory compounds, refer to Chap. 272.)

Indications for Surgery. The most compelling indication for surgery in gastric ulcer is the suspicion of malignancy which arises from the demonstration of either histamine fast achlorhydria, exfoliated malignant cells, evidence of tumor by x-ray, or failure of the ulcer to heal in a 4- to 6-week period of optimum therapy (Fig. 273-5). Other common indications for surgical intervention include recurrence, bleeding, and perforation. Special mention must be made of these conditions.

Bleeding gastric ulcer carries a graver risk than its duodenal counterpart. Indeed, the single greatest cause of mortality from upper gastrointestinal bleeding, aside from esophageal varices, is gastric ulcer. This is particularly true in the age group over fifty, especially in the presence of hypertension or other cardiovascular disease. Should bleeding persist despite transfusion and supportive measures, early operation is advisable (see the section on upper gastrointestinal bleeding in Chap. 272, Duodenal Ulcer).

Recurrence of benign gastric ulcer has been estimated to be as high as 25 to 55 per cent. Since the disease is disabling and increasingly hazardous as the patient grows older, surgical intervention is recommended for recurrence.

Free perforation of a benign gastric ulcer is unusual, but *penetration* into the pancreas is not. The signs and symptoms of these complications are similar to those which are outlined in the chapter on duodenal ulcer. Surgery is also indicated in these instances.

Indications for X-ray Therapy. When strong contraindications to surgery exist in elderly and/or chronically ill individuals with gastric ulcer, radiation of the stomach, which diminishes gastric secretion by its effect upon secretory cells and also induces a vascular fibrosis, may be employed. Recurrence rate, though reduced, is still high (40 per cent). (For details of treatment and its effect upon secretion, see Chap. 272.)

Long-term Management. In the long-term medical management of the patient with a healed benign gastric ulcer, the following program is usually employed. The patient should be seen routinely at regular 3- to 4-month intervals. An upper gastrointestinal tract series should be done routinely once each year and at any other time that symptoms reappear, to determine whether or not recurrence has taken place. While the patient need not be on a "strict" dietary regimen, he should *avoid* black coffee, alcohol, fried and spicy foods and should be encouraged to continue to eat between meals, usually a milk feeding with crackers and cheese. At appropriate times of stress, the physician should employ sedatives and tranquilizers and antisecretory (anticholinergic) drugs, as already outlined in Chap. 272. Certain drugs (adrenal steroids, salicylates, phenylbutazone, etc.) which may contribute to the recurrence of gastric ulceration must not be utilized without clear indication, and their use necessitates concomitant administration of antacids and antisecretory drugs.

REFERENCES

Dworken, H. J., H. P. Roth, and H. Duber: The Efficacy of Medical Criteria in Differentiating Benign from Malignant Gastric Ulcers, Ann. Internal Med., 47:711, 1957.

Kirsner, J. B.: Drug-induced Peptic Ulcer, Ann. Internal Med., 47:666, 1957.

Levin, E., W. L. Palmer, and J. B. Kirsner: Observations on the Diagnosis, Treatment and Course of Gastric Ulcer, J.A.M.A., 156:1383, 1954.

Seybolt, J., and G. Papanicolaou: The Value of Cytology in Diagnosis of Gastric Cancer, Gastroenterol., 33:369, 1957.

Wolf, S., and H. Wolff: "Human Gastric Function," London, Oxford University Press, 1943.

274 GASTRIC CARCINOMA AND OTHER DISEASES OF THE STOMACH

Marvin H. Sleisenger

GASTRIC CARCINOMA

Incidence. The over-all incidence of gastric carcinoma is not accurately known, but the disease seems to be decreasing in recent years. It occurs in all races of man, although there is some difference in racial predisposition. For example, it is at least twice as common in Japanese as in Caucasians. In Java, gastric cancer accounted for only 1 per cent of all malignancies seen among the Javanese, whereas it accounted for 19 per cent among the Chinese. The disease is several times more common in men than women in the United States, where it is responsible for approximately 10 per cent of all deaths from cancer. It occurs rarely in the first and second decades, sporadically in the third and fourth decades, and the incidence increases sharply in the fifth and sixth decades.

Predisposing Factors. *Antecedent alteration* of the gastric mucosa, probably genetically determined, plays an important role in the genesis of carcinoma of the stomach. Several studies have indicated a familial incidence two to four times greater than that in a normal population controlled for sex, age, race, etc. That specific genetic factors may have a role is suggested by an apparently increased incidence of gastric cancer in persons with blood group A. This association has been noted in Great Britain, Denmark, Switzerland, and the United States; yet, no such difference between the incidence in blood groups O and A in this disease has been discovered in Glasgow, Sydney, and Vienna. The importance of blood group substances in the genesis of gastric carcinoma is unknown. Persons of blood group O usually secrete one substance (H), whereas persons of groups A, B, and AB usually secrete their specific group substance in addition. These substances, which are mucopolysaccharides, are important constituents of the mucus of the stomach and, in some way, may protect the mucosa.

In regard to antecedent changes of the mucosa, reports during the last 10 years indicate that the incidence of gastric carcinoma in patients with *pernicious anemia* ranges from 7 to 12 per cent. It is to be expected that, with the increased survival of these patients as a result of better and more widespread medical care, and the availability of specific replacement therapy (vitamin B_{12}), the incidence of gastric carcinoma will increase. Indeed, it is in this group of patients that the greatest effort must be made to discover an early polypoid or infiltrative lesion. Such prophylaxis may be accomplished by routine cytologic and roentgenologic examinations, in rotation, at 6-month intervals. The hazard of leukemia or serious suppression of the bone marrow from yearly radiologic examinations is not known. At present, such a program appears to be worth the risk in this group of individuals, particularly those over age fifty. Patients with *gastric atrophy* and relative or complete (true) hypochlorhydria, but without pernicious anemia, also have a higher incidence of gastric carcinoma. In the combined group (gastric atrophy and pernicious anemia), gastric cancer is at least five times more frequent than in normal subjects.

Gastric polyps, unassociated with pernicious anemia, may also undergo malignant degeneration. Such carcinomatous changes have often been observed in individual polyps; the frequency of such malignant change lies between 7 to 22 per cent. Whether single or multiple, associated with pernicious anemia or not, excision must, therefore, be advised, unless there is a specific contraindication (see Fig. 274-4). The low or absent acid secretion in patients with carcinoma probably precedes the appearance of the malignancy in most instances and is not due to an inhibitory effect of the malignancy upon distant parietal cell activity.

Some investigators believe that *chronic gastritis* causes the gastric atrophy which is a precursor of gastric cancer. While it is known that superficial inflammation of the mucosa, if severe and/or prolonged, may lead to atrophy and hypo- or anacidity, the incidence of this sequence of events is not known. Again, debate continues concerning the possibility of malignant degeneration of a benign gastric ulcer. This hypothesis is supported entirely by studies of pathologic specimens of malignant ulcerations. Based upon such observation, the contention is not acceptable, since a lesion combining features of a benign gastric ulcer with carcinomatous change in a surgical specimen could result from acid-peptic erosion of devitalized malignant tissue and adjacent uninvolved tissue. Evidence for malignant change in long-standing gastric ulcers is almost impossible to obtain at present.

Clinical Picture. The clinical picture of carcinoma of the stomach is highly variable. Unfortunately, the patient often will suffer no indisposition whatever for many weeks or months. When symptomatic, the patient usually complains of upper abdominal distress which ranges from rather typical peptic ulcer symptoms (uncommon) to a feeling of epigastric heaviness or discomfort following meals. The former symptoms are usually associated with an ulcerated lesion and the latter with encroachment upon the lumen by the tumor. Frequently, the distress radiates to the back or beneath the left lower rib cage and is accompanied by an early sense of fullness during meals. With advanced disease, the patient progressively loses appetite and weight, and may show evidences of anemia.

Symptoms may vary considerably in duration, but the average is several months. A feature which distinguishes gastric cancer from benign peptic ulcer is that often the distress or discomfort is precipitated, not relieved, by ingestion of food. Nausea and vomiting, which also may be prominent symptoms, are generally associated with those lesions which are situated more distally and, therefore, tend to obstruct early. In a small percentage of patients, presenting symptoms of hematemesis or melena may result from invasion of a major blood vessel.

Physical examination may be negative or reveal pallor, a mass in the upper abdomen, or evidence of metastasis either to the liver or to a supraclavicular lymph node (Virchow's node). Rarely, metastatic lesions to the lower abdominal organs such as the ovaries (Krukenberg tumor) or rectum (Blumer's shelf) or to the peritoneum (ascites) may be found.

Roentgenologic examination is a most important method for diagnosing gastric carcinoma. In the barium-filled stomach, one may recognize several kinds of gross tumors. These include: the polypoid growth which protrudes into the lumen; the annular and locally infiltrative type of cancer which occurs most commonly in the distal portion of the stomach and which obstructs early (Fig. 274-1); the diffuse infiltrating type, often associated with rigidity and constriction (linitis plastica or "leather bottle") (Fig. 274-2), which is sometimes ulcer-

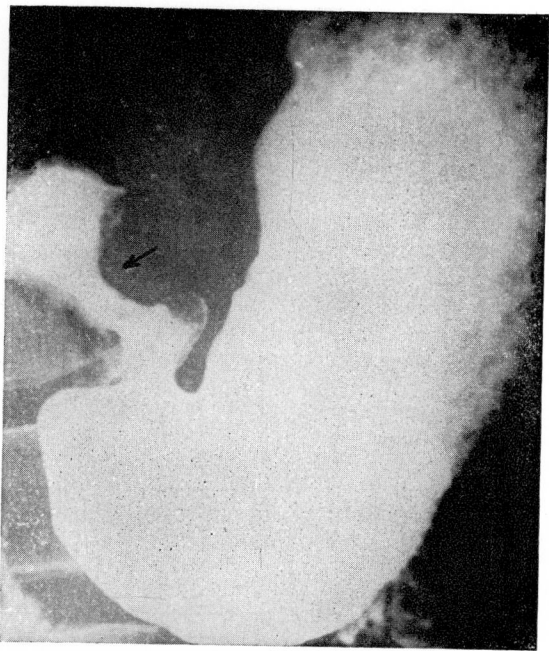

Fig. 274-1. Annular adenocarcinoma of the stomach involving the antrum, producing a narrowed lumen in a 60-year-old man with a 10-year history of pernicious anemia.

ated superficially; and finally, the tumor mass which is irregular and which may be deeply ulcerated (Fig. 274-3). In addition, a small group of patients presents no clear evidence of infiltration or of tumor of the stomach, but only an ulcerated area (Fig. 273-5). It is in such instances that the differentiation between a benign and malignant process must be made according to the criteria already outlined in Chap. 273.

Laboratory examination usually reveals a mild to moderate anemia of the iron deficient type, and frequently stools will be found to contain occult blood. Attention has been drawn to low levels of serum albumin which may be found in these patients, an abnormality due to exudation of plasma into the gastric lumen. Gastric analysis will reveal achlorhydria after maximal histamine stimulation in about half the cases and submaximal responses to this agent in about 30 per cent. Thus, a minority (20 per cent) of patients with carcinoma of the stomach will have a normal basal secretion of acid and normal response to histamine stimulation. Therefore, the presence of gastric acid does not eliminate the possibility of malignancy. On the other hand, the absence of free acid and, more particularly, failure to secrete after maximal histamine stimulation, should lead the physician to this diagnosis in any patients whose history, physical examination, or x-ray examination arouses the suspicion.

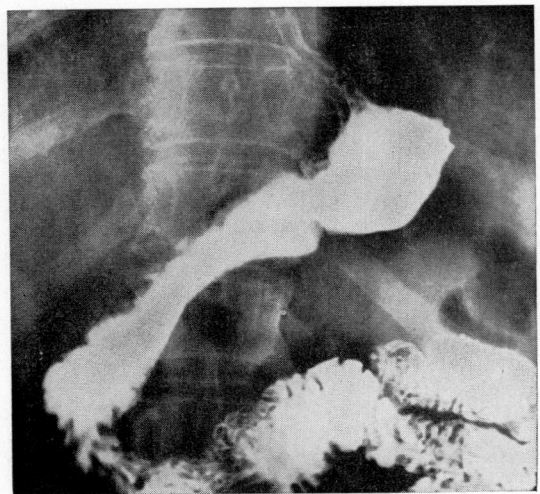

FIG. 274-2. Diffusely infiltrative carcinoma of the stomach ("linitis plastica").

With good reason *cytologic examination* of gastric washings has become increasingly widespread. As already pointed out, this method alone is 60 to 80 per cent accurate in the diagnosis of stomach cancer, and when combined with x-ray, the figure rises to about 90 per cent (Table 273-1). Further, such study may occasionally be useful in detecting malignant transformation of the stomach mucosa in patients with diseases which are known precursors of cancer such as pernicious anemia or in patients with polyps who are reluctant to undergo surgery (Fig. 274-4).

Occasionally, gastroscopy alone may reveal the tumor, since in some instances it will be obscured in the roentgenogram. Its reliability, however, in the differentiation of benign and malignant ulcer is limited.

Screening for Asymptomatic Gastric Carcinoma. In several studies thousands of asymptomatic individuals have undergone an upper gastrointestinal x-ray examination either by standard or photofluorometric techniques in an effort to detect stomach cancer. The incidence of previously undetected neoplasm was shown to vary from 0.08 to 0.3 per cent. An x-ray study of over 3,000 adult patients who could reasonably be suspected of harboring a stomach cancer revealed lesions in only 15. Thus, the yield for a selected group is also extremely low. Nevertheless, of 13 patients operated upon, 12 had resectable lesions and 6 of these had no spread, a considerably higher proportion than is usual.

On the other hand, annual routine gastrointestinal x-rays of patients with no free acid in the basal state or subnormal response to histamine injection will show carcinoma in about 1 per cent and polyps in about 3 per cent. This incidence of "unsus-

pected" cancer is five times that in a normal population. When compared with gastric cancer in general, tumors discovered in this way are only half as likely to have local spread. Annual "screening" of these patients alternately by cytologic and radiologic methods is to be recommended. Gastroscopy has been advised by some as an additional procedure for following such patients.

Surgical Management. The 5-year cure rate following surgical treatment of gastric carcinoma has risen slowly in recent years; in the large metropolitan institutions, it is of the order of 5 to 10 per cent, and in some large private clinics has been reported to be as high as 14 per cent. It must be stated, however, that the latter statistics have been influenced by varying degrees of selectivity. Higher cure rates have been reported for the small ulcerated carcinoma in a stomach able to secrete free acid and for antral carcinomas in individuals in whom the radiologic diagnosis was doubtful. Mortality rates for "curative" procedures have steadily dropped and at present are in the range of 5 to 10 per cent.

A number of important factors affect the cure rate in gastric carcinoma. These include: duration of symptoms, location and extent of the tumor, its morphologic characteristics, general condition of the patient, and presence or absence of lymph node metastases at the time of operation. As stated, lesions which are small, have some ulceration, and are associated with capacity to secrete acid and

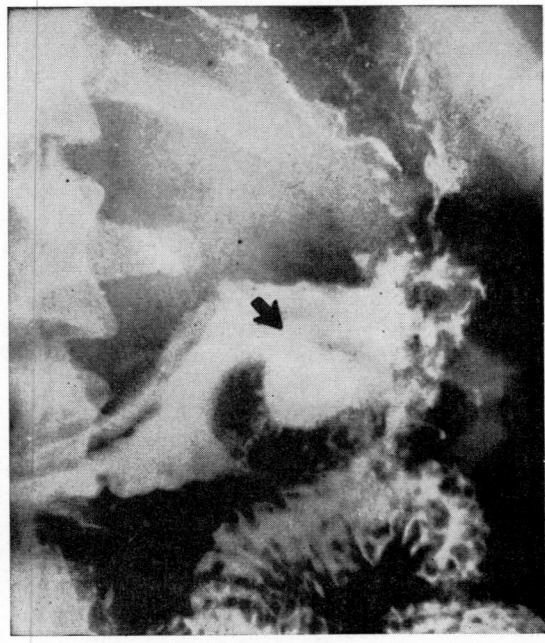

FIG. 274-3. Large carcinoma of the stomach with ulceration.

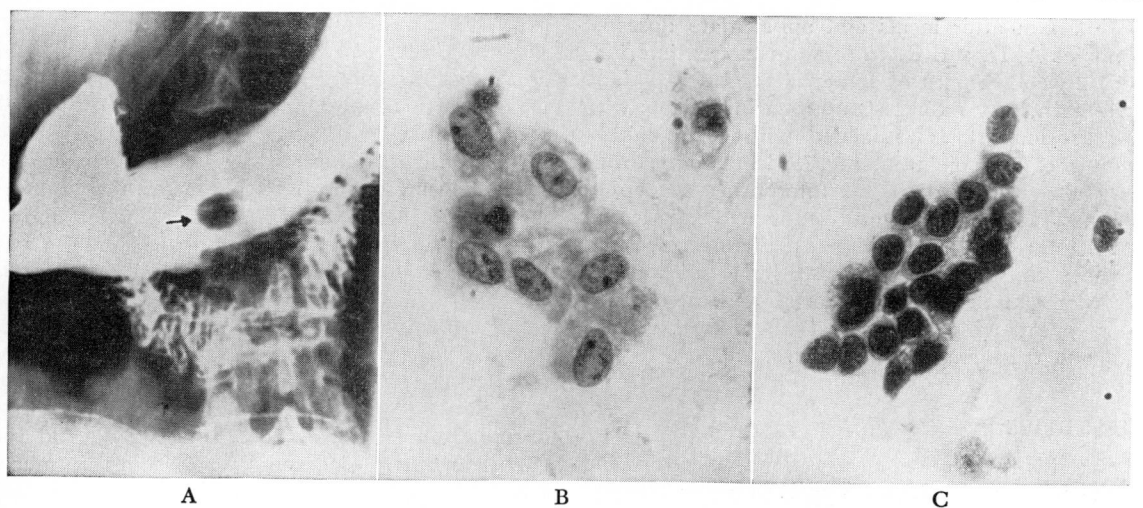

A   B   C

Fig. 274-4. *A.* Gastric polyp discovered in 1955 at yearly x-ray examination in 69-year-old patient with pernicious anemia for 19 years. Patient refused operation. *B.* Benign ("bland") cells obtained from chymotrypsin lavage, February, 1956. *C.* Malignant cells obtained in September, 1956. Threefold increase in size of polyp. Surgical removal of carcinoma resulted in apparent cure (4½ years).

those which occur more distally in the stomach are more amenable to surgical cure. Surgical curability does not necessarily depend upon the duration of preceding symptoms; indeed, some workers feel that those inherent biologic characteristics of the tumor such as slowness of growth, lack of invasiveness, etc., predetermine prognosis. In many instances those cancers which have produced symptoms for the longest periods of time are the least aggressive. The most important factor in prognosis is the presence or absence of lymph node metastases. When no metastases are found, subtotal resection results in a 5-year survival rate ranging between 40 and 50 per cent.

Percentages of 5-year survivors based on gross appearance are about as follows: superficial spreading, 54 per cent; fungating, 36 per cent; penetrating, 12 per cent; and linitis plastica, 0 per cent.

Effect of Gastrectomy. Following partial and particularly total resection of the stomach, the patient frequently fails to gain weight and develops diarrhea, anorexia, weakness, and symptoms of anemia, avitaminosis, and malnutrition. The diarrhea and steatorrhea reflect malabsorption, which is responsible for a great deal of the patient's malnutrition (p. 141).

Absorption and utilization of vitamins are also impaired following gastrectomy, particularly total gastrectomy. This is, of course, true of vitamin B_{12}, the absorption of which requires combination with intrinsic factor produced by the stomach. Total gastrectomy in the absence of parenteral B_{12} therapy must inevitably result in pernicious anemia. The delayed appearance of this type of ane-

mia after total gastrectomy is related to the variable hepatic stores of the vitamin present in a particular individual. Such stores may be sufficient to assure adequate red cell maturation in the marrow for periods up to 5 years. Evidences of other B complex deficiency may appear and are almost invariably encountered in individuals who have markedly reduced their caloric intake and/or have diarrhea or rapidly advancing malignancy. Nutritional inadequacy is also partially the result of loss of appetite or fear of symptoms following meals. These symptoms constitute the "dumping syndrome," which has been discussed in Chap. 272.

Other problems arise postoperatively, particularly in the patient with total gastrectomy or high subtotal resection. Regurgitant esophagitis results from removal of the esophagogastric sphincter, which permits regurgitation of alkaline jejunal fluids. Another troublesome symptom may be postprandial (2 to 4 hr) hypoglycemia, which is due to excessive insulin secretion stimulated by an abnormally rapid rise in blood sugar after meals.

Management of Patients with Partial or Total Gastrectomy. The management of the patient who has had a partial or total gastrectomy of the stomach should, therefore, include frequent small feedings high in fat and protein, since carbohydrate is the principal offending food in the dumping syndrome. Administration of iron orally is indicated for hypochromic anemia. If total resection has been done, vitamin B_{12} must be given parenterally—100 μg monthly—to prevent macrocytic anemia. Steatorrhea may often be partially corrected by the oral administration of concentrated pancreatic extract

3 to 7 Gm after meals and appropriate doses of vitamins A, D, and K. In some instances, intermittent 2-week courses of tetracycline, 1.0 Gm daily by mouth, may reduce steatorrhea in patients with afferent loop stasis associated with gastrojejunostomy or esophagojejunostomy. Anticholinergic drugs may also reduce diarrhea. Interposing a loop of jejunum between the esophagus and duodenum after total gastrectomy creates a "reservoir" and reduces the incidence of disturbing postprandial symptoms, nutritional problems, and regurgitant esophagitis, which are noted after the standard Roux-en-Y esophagojejunostomy.

GASTRITIS

Gastritis is an inflammation of the mucosa of the stomach with or without hypertrophy or atrophy and may be associated with distressing symptoms of indigestion. Clinically, it may be conveniently divided into the acute and chronic forms.

Acute Gastritis. Although the epithelium of the gastric mucosa is capable of rapid regeneration, noxious stimuli may cause diffuse hyperemia, edema, exudation, and if sufficiently severe, erosion and bleeding. Rarely, the erosive process may penetrate the muscularis mucosa to become an ulcer. Although regeneration takes place, some glandular elements may disappear and the submucosa may become scarred. Contributory factors include malnutrition, infection (virus, staphylococcus, salmonella), ethyl alcohol, many drugs (aspirin, Butazolidin, etc.), and a wide variety of chemicals (caustic soda, phenol, acids, etc.).

Symptoms. Anorexia, nausea, diffuse epigastric discomfort ("heaviness" and "burning") are the cardinal symptoms; occasionally, vomiting and profuse bleeding complicate the picture. In the event of bleeding, the clinical picture depends largely upon the amount and rapidity of blood loss and may vary, therefore, from slight pallor to marked diaphoresis and shock. (In this regard, diffuse acute gastritis per se is not so common a cause of bleeding as acute erosion or ulcer without diffuse inflammation.) If vomiting is severe, sufficiently prolonged, or untreated, the patient may rapidly become weak and dehydrated, and he may suffer shock. The abdomen is usually flat, but in those who are very ill, it may be distended.

Diagnosis may be confirmed only by gastroscopy. The mucosa usually heals completely in 3 to 4 days; however, repeated episodes may lead to permanent damage.

Treatment. Management of gastritis depends upon the cause. Withdrawal of the offending agent is necessary. If the patient is seen early, the stomach should be lavaged with saline. Fluids, electrolytes (Na+, K+ particularly), and blood are given as indicated. Staphyloccocal food poisoning and salmonellosis may be treated with broad-spectrum antibiotics in severe cases; however, supportive measures are usually sufficient.

Chronic Gastritis. In chronic gastritis, the recurrence of inflammation is often superficial and affects the surface of the mucosa without causing atrophy of the glands. The mucosa is of normal depth, and although the inflammatory changes may be slight, moderate, or severe, the lesion is capable of complete resolution. However, irreversible changes may occur which progress to atrophic gastritis. Atrophic gastritis is characterized by a more diffuse inflammation of the mucosa combined with varying degrees of atrophy of mucosal elements. Complete resolution is not likely, and the condition frequently progresses to complete mucosal atrophy. It must be emphasized, however, that the degree and extent of inflammation and atrophy often overlap.

The typical clinical picture of chronic gastritis is that of a middle-aged patient with a history of indigestion extending over several years. Symptoms are usually intermittent and consist of distress in the epigastrium occurring almost always immediately after meals, particularly if the patient has partaken of a great deal of fried or spicy food, often with alcoholic beverages, or if he has overeaten. Nausea and vomiting may be a feature.

Bleeding occasionally occurs in chronic gastritis, but is rarely of sufficient magnitude to warrant emergency surgical intervention. It seems to be associated in most instances with "spree" drinking of alcohol.

Physical examination of these patients is unrevealing. A small number may have diffuse epigastric tenderness. Rarely, there will be some evidences of anemia or of vitamin deficiency.

Laboratory investigation of these complaints reveals varying secretory patterns which depend mainly upon the degree of atrophy of the gastric mucosa and its parietal cells. About 25 per cent of patients with superficial gastritis will have a normal response to histamine, whereas an equal number will show hyposecretion, and about 45 per cent will not respond at all. As atrophy progresses, the incidence of histamine fast achlorhydria arises steeply, with only about 5 per cent of these individuals capable of secreting any acid after such maximum stimulation. Radiologically, no abnormalities may be detected and gastric emptying is normal.

Relationship to Peptic Ulcer and Carcinoma. Studies on the relationship between chronic gastritis and peptic ulcer indicate that this entity is more closely related to gastric than duodenal ulcer. Gastritis initially may be patchy and limited, and the involved area may be digested by acid-peptic juice. The zone which ulcerates and its surrounding mucosa are incapable of normal secretion, which perhaps explains the reduced acidity in a large number of patients with benign gastric ulcer. Several studies of gastric mucosa in duodenal ulcer revealed that gastritis is associated in only a minority of instances.

The role of chronic gastritis is also pertinent in the genesis of carcinoma of the stomach. An old theory holds that gastric carcinoma has its origins superimposed upon inflammatory changes, since pathologists have reported that carcinoma is frequently associated with such changes. Yet, limited studies of patients with chronic gastritis have revealed no definite relationship to gastric carcinoma, and none of the patients in several series has developed the latter disease. However, it is noteworthy that as chronic gastritis progresses the same secretory pattern characteristic of gastric carcinoma, that is, hyposecretion or achlorhydria, develops.

The anemia of chronic gastritis is usually of the iron-deficiency type, and several factors probably contribute to this; anorexia leads to a diminished food intake, which is often low in iron and protein; in a minority of instances, iron absorption may be impaired; the anemia may result from repeated small hemorrhages. In some instances atrophy may be complete, resulting in failure of absorption of vitamin B_{12} and in pernicious anemia.

Treatment. The treatment for chronic gastritis consists of encouragement of a satisfactory caloric intake and of a relaxed atmosphere at mealtime, abstinence from foods which are prone to cause difficulty, such as fried food and alcohol, and the administration of nonabsorbable antacids, which are somehow effective in the face of hypochlorhydria or even achlorhydria. Little basis exists for the belief that dilute hydrochloric acid with meals is beneficial. If the blood smear, red blood cell indices, and if necessary, serum iron and iron binding capacity reveal an iron-deficiency anemia, ferrous salts should be given by mouth. Often, however, response is poor despite apparently normal absorption and the absence of occult blood loss. If complete gastric atrophy and achlorhydria are present, the anemia may be megaloblastic, in which instance parenteral vitamin B_{12} should be administered. One of the most important aspects of therapy is to reassure the patient and to explain the nature of the symptoms and their relationship both to inflammation of the mucosa of the stomach and to stressful situations. It should be emphasized that there is no known relationship to future development of cancer. Often such reassurance brings dramatic relief.

Diffuse Giant Hypertrophic Gastritis. Another variety of "gastritis" may be associated with the same symptoms found in chronic superficial or atrophic gastritis. This entity is called "diffuse giant hypertrophic gastritis" and was first described by Menetrier in 1888. It is a rare disease of the stomach characterized by the presence of very prominent folds with profuse epithelial proliferation and some inflammatory reaction. The lesion may diffusely involve the whole gastric mucosa, or it may be localized in distribution, particularly in the antrum. The folds may be swollen and tortuous so as to appear polypoid and may be as great as 3.5 cm in diameter. The mucosa is soft and pliable, but may become relatively fixed if inflammation is great. Histologically, changes consist of hyperplasia of the surface epithelium and infiltration of the interstitium by inflammatory cells.

This disease or condition appears principally in men from the fourth to the sixth decade who complain of the same postprandial epigastric pain and distress as do most patients with chronic gastritis. In addition, they may also note vomiting, weight loss, and bleeding.

The disease may be strongly suspected from the radiologic appearance of the stomach, which is characterized by very large, tortuous, often polypoid, folds in one or more areas of the stomach (Fig. 274-5). Since carcinoma, granulomas, and lymphosarcoma may be indistinguishable on roentgenogram, further studies are strongly indicated.

Gastric analysis reveals a normal or nearly nor-

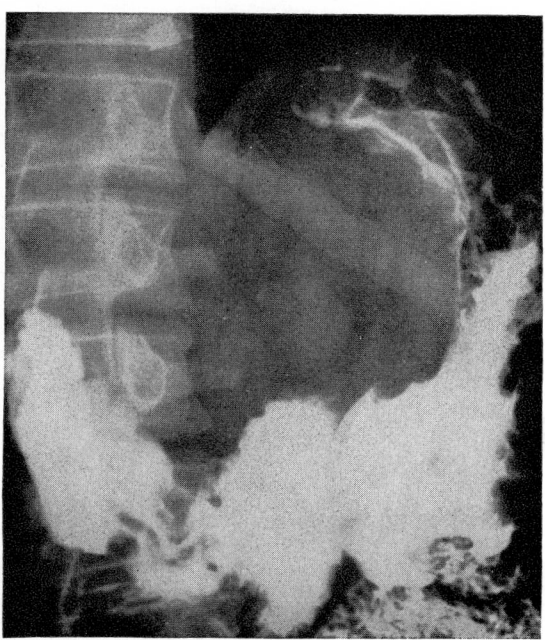

Fig. 274-5. Giant rugal hypertrophy presenting the appearance of a neoplasm in a 47-year-old man with melena. Microscopic examination revealed a thickened mucosa with elongated, cystically dilated gastric glands. There was no evidence of malignancy.

mal response to histamine. The diagnosis may be confirmed by biopsy, either by suction tube or in conjunction with gastroscopy. As in carcinoma of the stomach, these patients may have significant hypoalbuminemia due to exudation of serum albumin from the hypertrophic rugae into the lumen of the stomach. In many instances, differential diagnosis cannot be made without laparotomy.

FUNCTIONAL DYSPEPSIA

While it is true that a high percentage of patients with symptoms of indigestion demonstrate gross and microscopic evidences of chronic, superficial, or atrophic gastritis, many individuals with these complaints have no alteration of the mucosa at all; conversely, many individuals with no complaints are found to have changes of acute or chronic inflammation.

Repeated studies have shown that emotion has a powerful effect upon the motor activity of the stomach, which raises the question of the relationship of emotional factors to the symptoms of patients with chronic gastritis. Reaction to life stress may satisfactorily explain the symptoms in many patients who are able to relate them to periods of emotional strain. Perhaps the fullness or heaviness is due to failure of normal gastric emptying. Scant data are available on this point; however, from Wolf and Wolff's studies on the fistula subject, Tom, we have learned that during periods of fear, dejection, or sadness gastric activity was diminished (see Chap. 272). Such decrease in gastric motor function also is an accompaniment of nausea, which, with increased pressure in the duodenum, has been provoked by the technique of "stressful interview." Although no evidence exists that prolonged tension induces changes of superficial gastritis, intense resentment and anger may be associated with marked hyperemia and friability.

Functional dyspepsia is usually chronic; the majority of these patients will be plagued by their symptoms indefinitely, but will respond at times to strong reassurance, judicious sedation, and empiric alteration of diet.

OTHER MALIGNANT TUMORS OF THE STOMACH

Sarcoma. These malignancies comprise about 3 per cent of all stomach tumors; the *lymphoma* group (lymphosarcoma, reticulum-cell sarcoma, Hodgkin's disease, and "lymphoblastoma") is about three to four times as common as the rest. The mean age of onset is about 10 years younger than for carcinoma, but the symptoms are quite similar —pain, anorexia, weight loss, and anemia due to blood loss. Physical examination may reveal a mass; a differential point is the splenomegaly which is present in some, but not in the majority, of instances of primary gastric lymphoma. Massive bleeding complicates the course more commonly than it does in carcinoma. Achlorhydria is found in 60 to 70 per cent.

The lymphomas tend to be locally invasive, and blood-borne metastases are less likely than for the other sarcomas.

Differential diagnosis of lymphoma may occasionally be aided by the occurrence of other systemic symptoms and signs of the process, particularly fever and lymphadenopathy.

X-ray appearance of sarcoma is easily confused with that of carcinoma, since infiltration, ulceration, distortion, etc., are commonly found in this condition; however, these lesions, particularly lymphosarcoma, may appear in a minority of instances—about 20 per cent—only as enlarged folds, without a discrete mass (Fig. 274-6). Occasionally, a submucosal tumor mass may indicate presence of a malignancy of smooth muscle origin. Diagnosis of lymphosarcoma may be made occasionally either by gastroscopic or suction biopsy; however, resection of the tumor is, of course, the principal method of diagnosis.

Surgical excision, followed by irradiation, is the treatment of choice. Such combined therapy results in 5-year cures in excess of 25 per cent. It is well to remember that not all lymphomas are equally radiosensitive; for example, reticulum-cell sarcoma is more resistant than the small-cell variety.

Leiomyosarcoma, fibrosarcoma, neurogenic sarcoma, neurofibrosarcoma, and *myxosarcoma* comprise a group of rare malignant tumors of the stomach. Leiomyosarcoma is the most common and constitutes 1 per cent of all malignancies of the stomach. The others are all very rare tumors.

These lesions most often involve the greater or lesser curvature and are usually well circumscribed and pedunculated. Radiologically, they may appear as circumscribed globular filling defects or submucosal tumors with ulceration of the overlying mucosa.

Melena or hematemesis is the most common presenting complaint. Anorexia, indigestion, weight loss, and obstruction may be present, but much less often than in carcinoma or lymphoma. A mass is frequently palpable.

Leiomyosarcoma does not appear to arise from a preexisting benign leiomyoma. Clinically and grossly it is difficult to distinguish between leiomyoma and leiomyosarcoma. Histologic study is necessary.

These tumors metastasize locally and less frequently than carcinoma. The treatment of these sarcomas is radical surgical removal. A great majority of cases undergoing exploratory laparotomy are found to be operable, and the 5-year survival rate after surgery is between 45 and 55 per cent. Ten-year survivals are not at all uncommon.

BENIGN TUMORS OF THE STOMACH

The incidence of benign tumors of the stomach in an adult population is estimated at about 0.4 per cent. These neoplasms may be divided according to origin into epithelial (60 per cent), mesenchymal (32 per cent), and ectodermal (8 per cent).

Epithelial. These tumors are polypoid adenomas, most of which are asymptomatic. The majority are located in the antrum and frequently are multiple. Over 75 per cent of cases have associated achlorhydria (following test meal or histamine). Clinical importance centers upon potentiality for malignant degeneration, particularly when associated with pernicious anemia (Fig. 274-4), which is present in about 10 per cent of the entire group. The exact incidence of malignant transformation is not precisely known; however, evidence indicates it to vary from 7 to 22 per cent. In those patients with symptoms, pain and bleeding are most prominent. Preoperatively, diagnosis may be made only by

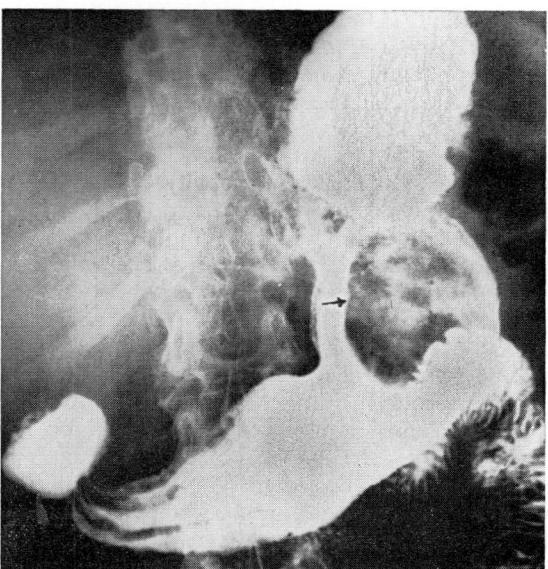

Fig. 274-7. Large leiomyoma of the stomach.

x-ray or gastroscopy. Local resection of the lesion is the treatment of choice. If large, multiple, or malignant, partial or total resection becomes necessary.

Mesenchymal. These include *leiomyoma, fibroma,* and *lipoma.* Leiomyoma is the commonest of this group, comprising 25 per cent of all benign tumors. It may be situated in any area, is always submucosal, frequently ulcerates, and may bleed massively. Occasionally, the patient will complain of pain in the epigastrium. Diagnosis is established by x-ray; however, small tumors may easily be overlooked. Indeed, tiny mesenchymal tumors are found commonly at autopsy. The typical appearance of such a neoplasm is illustrated in Fig. 274-7. A small percentage seem to undergo malignant change, but proof on this point is lacking. Treatment is surgical removal, necessitating local or partial gastric resection in all instances.

Fibroma is a rare benign gastric tumor constituting about 5 per cent of the group, and in the vast majority of cases is asymptomatic and, therefore, is an incidental finding at laparotomy or autopsy. *Lipoma* is an extremely rare and usually asymptomatic tumor.

Ectodermal. *Neurofibroma* is the principal ectodermal tumor. Pain and/or bleeding are often noted. Diagnosis is frequently made only by surgical exploration.

MISCELLANEOUS DISEASES OF THE STOMACH

Prolapse of the Gastric Mucosa. Prolapse of the gastric mucosa is a herniation of a portion of gastric

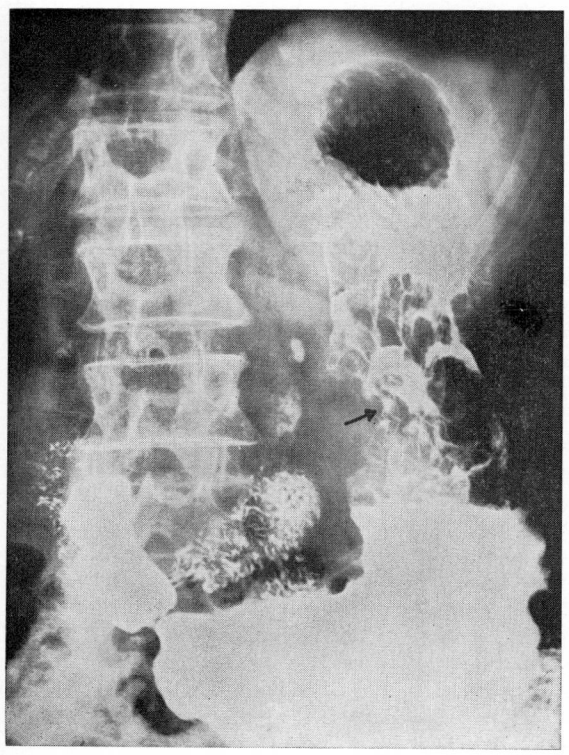

Fig. 274-6. Lymphosarcoma of the stomach. Note infiltration, enlargement of folds of this tumor.

mucosa through the pylorus, resulting in a characteristic roentgen appearance. It may occur at any age, but is usually seen in the fifth decade, and is seen in 2 to 14 per cent of patients subjected to examination. The cause is unknown but is thought to be due to hyperperistalsis associated with local inflammation and excessive mobility of the mucosa upon the muscularis.

This condition usually is asymptomatic and is discovered as an incidental finding. The symptoms attributed to this condition—epigastric distress, nausea, vomiting, weakness, weight loss, and occasionally bleeding—are nonspecific and are probably caused by an accompanying gastritis, peptic ulcer, or spasm.

The diagnosis of prolapse is suggested by the roentgen demonstration of (1) an "umbrella" or "mushroomlike" filling defect in the base of the duodenal bulb and (2) rugae extending through the pylorus into the duodenal cap. If symptoms are present, a bland diet with antispasmodics may be prescribed, but frequently is ineffective. Results of surgery are not clear. Subtotal gastric resection is occasionally necessary if bleeding is severe.

Foreign Bodies in the Stomach. A wide variety of foreign bodies may be found in the stomach. Small objects such as coins and marbles accidentally swallowed by children rarely cause symptoms and eventually pass through the gastrointestinal tract. Sharp-pointed objects (pins, needles) may penetrate the wall of the stomach or intestine, producing peritonitis or an abscess. Large foreign bodies (spoons, knives, forks) found in the stomachs of the insane usually produce no symptoms, although ulceration, perforation, or obstruction may occur.

Bezoars are conglomerations of swallowed foreign material consisting of hair (trichobezoar), hair and vegetable fiber (trichophytobezoar), or vegetable fiber alone (phytobezoar). The prolonged use of calcium or magnesium powders may give rise to concretions in the stomach (gastroliths). Bezoars may attain a large size, producing symptoms simulating gastritis, peptic ulcer, cancer, or pyloric obstruction. They may occasionally simulate malignancy during roentgen examination. Significantly, these masses are found almost exclusively in severely disturbed or psychotic individuals.

Treatment is indicated only when definite symptoms are present or when the foreign body presents a mechanical hazard. Laparotomy with surgical removal may then be necessary.

Syphilis of the Stomach. Although extremely rare, this disease must be considered in any individual with active or latent lues who has epigastric pain, vomiting, weight loss, or bleeding. X-ray of the stomach may reveal one of several abnormalities: (1) filling defect or localized infiltration without a mass, (2) "hourglass" stomach, and (3) diffuse involvement of the wall. Differentiation, therefore, from carcinoma of the stomach is almost impossible, and surgical exploration is recommended. Response to antiluetic therapy is dramatic, but the x-ray appearance may change only very slowly.

Tuberculosis of the Stomach. Tuberculosis infection of the stomach is rare and is almost always associated with disease in other organs, particularly the lungs. The lesion may be infiltrative, granulomatous, or ulcerative. Symptoms are the same as those noted in carcinoma, benign ulcer, syphilis, etc. Diagnosis can be made only by examination of tissue obtained at laparotomy. Antituberculosis therapy (isonicotinic acid hydrochloride and streptomycin) is usually effective in those rare instances in which the diseased portion is not resected.

Mycotic Infections of the Stomach. Mycotic infections of the stomach include actinomycosis, moniliasis (*Candida albicans*), aspergillosis, and many others. These infections frequently produce superficial or deep ulcerations of the stomach, which may be single or multiple, although they rarely penetrate or perforate. The symptoms simulate those of gastritis, ulcer, or malignant disease of the stomach. Examination of the vomitus or the gastric contents may reveal the fungus. Treatment is that for fungus infections in general.

Acute Dilatation of the Stomach. Acute dilatation of the stomach is characterized by a rapid accumulation of large quantities (2,000 to 4,000 ml) of gastric and intestinal juices with marked gaseous distention of the stomach.

Etiology. The cause of the disorder is unknown. It usually occurs as a sequela of abdominal or pelvic operations, or it may follow abdominal trauma, severe injury, parturition, or overeating. At times it is associated with severe diabetic acidosis. It may complicate an acute infectious disease or be associated with uremia or marked electrolyte disturbances, particularly potassium deficiency. Since gastric intubation, particularly after abdominal surgery, has become widely used, acute dilatation is rarely encountered after laparotomy.

Acute dilatation of the stomach has been attributed to the reflex inhibition of the gastric motor mechanism through efferent impulses reaching the stomach by way of the vagi and splanchnics. The primary defect appears to be a loss of gastric tone followed by the swallowing of air and the accumulation of gastric and duodenal secretions which cannot be reabsorbed.

The onset is often insidious. During the first 24 to 48 hr there is marked apathy and listlessness or epigastric fullness and constipation, rarely with severe pain. The epigastrium progressively increases in size, but regurgitation and vomiting **may not** appear until tremendous distention has developed. Although vomiting may be copious, the stomach cannot empty completely. Visible gastric peristalsis is absent because of gastric atony; a succussion splash may be elicited. Dehydration ensues, associated with hypochloremic alkalosis, tetany, and uremia as a result of electrolyte imbalance. Profound prostration, collapse, shock, delirium, coma, and death follow.

The flat film of the abdomen reveals a markedly dilated stomach filled with air and fluid. Treatment consists of continuous gastric suction for one day or more, administration of parenteral fluids, and correction of serum electrolytes, particularly potassium deficiency, as discussed in the section on pyloric obstruction. The patient usually recovers if treatment is instituted promptly.

CONGENITAL ANOMALIES OF THE STOMACH

Congenital Hypertrophic Pyloric Stenosis of Infancy and Adulthood. This disease is characterized by (1) hypertrophy of the pyloric muscle, particularly the circular muscle layer; and (2) spasm resulting in narrowing of the pyloric channel. There is no histologic evidence of inflammation. Boys are affected four times as commonly as girls. Rarely, incomplete congenital stenosis may become asymptomatic in adults.

Symptoms. Regurgitation and periodic vomiting herald the onset, usually from 2 to 3 weeks to 2 to 4 months after birth. The vomiting is often projectile, without retching, and is followed by rapid weight loss, constipation, and dehydration. In the adult form, intermittent but progressive vomiting, which may appear at any age, dominates the clinical picture.

Diagnosis. Physical examination reveals visible hyperperistalsis, dehydration, and malnutrition. In infants, a mass the size of an olive may be felt at the right rectus border beneath the costal margin. In doubtful cases, that is, when a tumor is not palpable, x-ray examination should be done, using water-soluble radiopaque substances such as Myokon, which, unlike barium, will not plug the pylorus or cause serious pulmonary damage if aspirated. This usually demonstrates some enlargement of the stomach with delayed gastric emptying and an elongated, narrowed, pyloric segment. Diagnosis is made in adults by roentgenographic examination, which reveals the same changes of the pyloric canal as noted in infants. Figure 274-8 is the roentgenogram of a middle-aged woman with recurrent vomiting of many years' duration, which had never previously been investigated. Pyloroplasty resulted in complete relief.

Treatment. A trial of medical management with

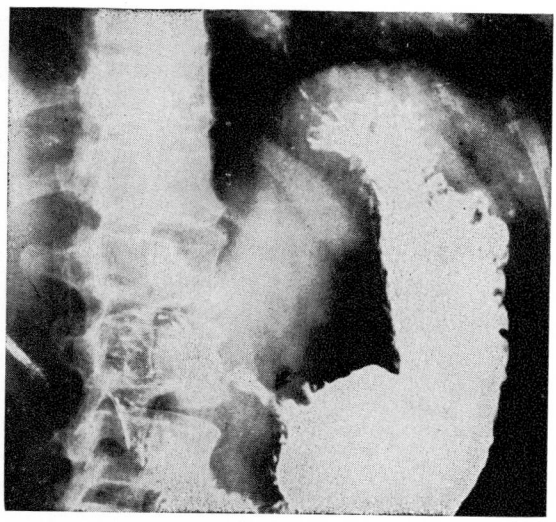

FIG. 274-8. Congenital hypertrophic stenosis in a 53-year-old woman with recurrent vomiting.

frequent small feedings, antispasmodics, and correction of electrolyte and fluid imbalance may be instituted when the history is not clear and if a mass is not palpable. Once the diagnosis is made, however, the Ramstedt operation, which consists of a longitudinal incision through the pyloric muscle to the mucosa, and which is uniformly successful, should be performed. The same approach is recommended when the diagnosis of pyloric stenosis is made in an adult.

Diverticula of the Stomach. A gastric diverticulum is an outpouching or protrusion of the stomach wall, forming a permanent sac. True diverticula contain all the muscular coats within the wall of the pouch and are usually congenital. False diverticula are acquired, and they lack the muscular coats.

Incidence. Both congenital and acquired gastric diverticula are most often seen in middle-aged women. The posterior wall of the cardia near the lesser curvature is the most common site for the congenital type. Acquired gastric traction diverticula are found most often near the pylorus and are caused by inflammatory or malignant involvement of adjacent organs. The former variety is almost always asymptomatic. Surgery may be required for the condition which underlies the acquired type.

REFERENCES

Amberg, J. R., E. N. Gipson, A. R. Margulis, and L. G. Rigler: Yield of Gastric Carcinoma from Radiologic Screening, Gastroenterol., 36:796, 1959.

Eklöf, O., E. Eriksson, and O. Sahlin: Benign Epithelial Tumors of the Stomach and Duodenum—Diagnosis and Treatment, Acta Chir. Scand., Suppl. 255, 1960.

Flood, C. A.: Carcinoma of the Stomach, Ann. Internal Med., 48:919, 1958.

Hitchcock, C. R., W. A. Sullivan, and O. H. Wangensteen: Value of Achlorhydria as a Screening Test for Gastric Cancer: 10 Year Report, Gastroenterol., 29:621, 1955.

Kaplan, H. S., and L. G. Rigler: Pernicious Anemia and Carcinoma of Stomach—Autopsy Studies Concerning Their Interrelationship, Am. J. Med. Sci., 209:339, 1945.

Wood, I. J., and L. I. Taft: "Diffuse Lesions of the Stomach," Baltimore, The Williams & Wilkins Company, 1958.

275 DISEASES OF THE DUODENUM AND SMALL INTESTINE

Albert I. Mendeloff

DIVERTICULOSIS

It is usually impossible on clinical grounds to decide whether diverticula of the intestinal tract are congenital or acquired. The rarer congenital diverticula contain the entire thickness of the intestinal wall, whereas acquired diverticula consist of mucosa and serosa alone. Probably the defect in the muscular wall through which the mucosa herniates is always potentially present, usually at the points where the nutrient arteries perforate the serosal and muscular layers. As with other forms of herniations, these potential tunnels are widened as life proceeds, so that all forms of diverticulosis are more common among persons in the later decades of life. Some individuals display great numbers of diverticula of the gastrointestinal tract, from esophagus to anus, but more often diverticula of the stomach and small intestine are solitary; they are more common in the duodenum (possibly 5 per cent of all persons having barium studies of this area), next most frequent in the jejunum, and rare in the ileum, except for Meckel's diverticulum. Colonic diverticula are more common than small intestinal diverticula, and are always multiple.

Diverticula of the Duodenum. These are most commonly found on the medial surface of the second portion of the duodenum, in close proximity to the entrance of the pancreatic and common ducts. They are usually wide-necked, about 1 cm in diameter, and appear to fill with and expel intestinal contents with ease. Occasionally on intubation studies of the second duodenum one aspirates undigested food particles, which must of necessity represent gastric chyme trapped in these diverticula and protected from digestive action.

The location of duodenal diverticula constitutes the main reason for suspecting their pathogenicity. Although statistically few patients harboring these common outpouchings suffer any misfortune from their presence, there are documented cases in which obstruction to the neck of the diverticulum has led to acute diverticulitis, hemorrhage, and necrosis of the wall; pressure exerted by obstructed diverticula on pancreatic ducts has definitely resulted in acute pancreatitis, pressure on the common duct in obstructive jaundice. When diverticula occur along the third portion of the duodenum they have occasionally been the site of acute inflammation and free perforation, with consequent peritonitis.

Diverticula of the Jejunum. Although less common, these seem to be more subject to the development of acute inflammation and necrosis of the wall, with severe upper abdominal pain and occasionally massive intestinal hemorrhage ensuing. The acute process may go on to suppurate; a definite mass and localized peritonitis are the accompanying physical findings. Another way in which multiple diverticula of the jejunum may result in disease is the effective replacement of normal absorbing jejunal surface by multiple bacteria-filled sacs, resulting in a characteristic malabsorption syndrome due to loss of surface and competitive loss of nutrients to the saprophytic bacteria in the diverticula (Fig. 275-1) (see Chap. 62).

Meckel's Diverticulum. Resulting from persistence of the omphalomesenteric duct, this diverticulum is reasonably common, occurring in about 3 per cent of all laparotomized children in whom a definite search is made and in about 2 per cent of autopsied adults. Even though only a small percentage of these diverticula cause trouble, the possibility must be thought of in every case of gastrointestinal hemorrhage and obstruction. The diverticula are usually found on the antimesenteric border within the last 90 cm of the ileum, and most frequently within 50 cm of the ileocecal valve. They may be wide-mouthed or narrow, short or long, sometimes a nubbin hard to find on the smooth surface of the ileum, occasionally a long 10- to 20-cm funnel attached like a stout pipe to the umbilicus. Diverticula lying within the mesentery are rare and do not arise from the omphalomesenteric duct. The diverticulum may be lined with normal ileal mucosa, or it may contain varying amounts of ectopic gastric, pancreatic, duodenal, or colonic epithelium. Symptoms are more common in males by at least 3:1. Coincident malformations are infrequently met. There is no hereditary pattern. In children and adolescents, bleeding from this epithelium is the striking clinical feature, with or without the presence of a palpable mass. The source of bleeding is almost invariably an ulceration, and this is generally of peptic origin. The gastric mucosa in the Meckel's diverticulum has been shown to secrete acid peptic juice, which acts on bordering ileal epithelium to produce the ulcer. Pathologically the ulcer is always near the junction of gastric and ileal mucosa, on the ileal side; it thus resembles the usual anastomotic ulcer occurring after gastrojejunostomy. In the young adult the clinical picture begins to change, inflammatory processes becoming more prominent, and varying degrees of intestinal obstruction, either of the ileum proximal to the diverticulum or of neighboring loops of bowel trapped behind the inflammatory mass, constitute the most serious presenting symptoms. Free perforation of Meckel's diverticulum is relatively uncommon, but sealed-off localized perforations are very common once the initial inflammatory process has distorted the bowel enough to set up the pathologic requisites for cyclical bouts of inflammation. A number of these patients have repeated bouts of low-grade abdominal cramps referred to the infraumbilical area, usually aggravated by eating. The diagnosis is rarely made by x-ray studies of the small or large intestine, but these are necessary in order to eliminate other possible lesions. The treatment is entirely surgical.

DUODENITIS

When a patient presents the symptoms and signs of peptic ulcer (Chap. 272) but the radiologic examination of the duodenum demonstrates no localized ulceration or deformity, but rather coarsely irregular mucosal folds from the duodenal bulb well down into the junction of the second and third portions of the duodenum, with irritability of the area, that patient is said to be suffering from peptic duodenitis. The incidence of this disease is not known, since radiologists vary in their willingness to apply the label to persons displaying minimal abnormalities of this type, but it is probably a common disorder, closely related in every way to the classical disorder—duodenal ulcer—of which it is the frequent precursor. Often the irritability and edema of the area prevent visualization by x-ray of a small ulcer crater, which may be the source of a severe hemorrhage, and thus the duodenitis is said to be the source of the hemorrhage. In terms of the host factors and the environmental stresses now well-identified as important in the genesis of peptic ulcer of the duodenum, these patients are in no way different from those suffering from the latter disease and respond in characteristically favorable ways to the medical regimen employed in treating the patient with duodenal ulcer.

Occasionally one notes on radiologic examination a cobble-stoned appearance of the duodenal bulb caused by hypertrophy of Brunner's glands,

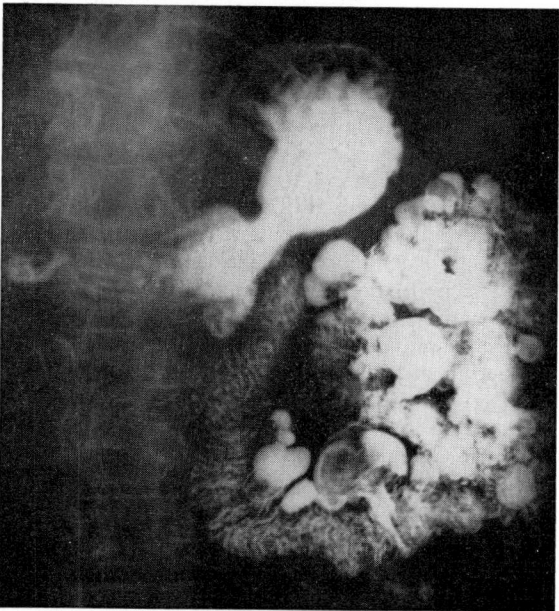

FIG. 275-1. Multiple diverticula of jejunum in 55-year-old man with macrocytic anemia.

deep structures secreting an alkaline mucoid material of unknown function. Most authorities regard this hypertrophy as of no clinical significance, but occasionally it is associated with the symptoms of duodenitis.

MOTOR DISTURBANCES

Obstructive Syndromes. The natural tendency of smooth muscle when operating against a pressure gradient is to stretch and contract forcibly. This increased distention is pain-producing (see Chap. 6, Acute Abdominal Pain). Thus all syndromes in which normal small bowel is trying to force luminal contents past nonrelaxing segments of more distal bowel, whether occasioned by a tumor, a stricture, an occluding gallstone, or a constricting band, are primarily characterized by painful cramps at the onset, progressing to loss of pain sensation as the bowel loses its viability. Associated with the progress of events are many others which may assume prominent roles in coloring the symptoms evoked. Intermittent jejunal or ileal obstruction, with poor maintenance of oil-water interfaces, will lead to malabsorption (see Chaps. 62 and 276).

Motor abnormalities of the duodenum associated with many psychic disturbances (e.g., anorexia nervosa) or with generalized disorders such as lupus erythematosus may result in severe bouts of nausea and vomiting. The radiologist may get the impression of an organic obstruction of the third portion of the duodenum at the point at which the superior mesenteric vessels cross anterior to the gut. Such impressions have given rise to many diagnoses of "mesenteric root compression syndrome" which fail to be borne out on surgical exploration to remove the source of the obstruction. It is important to understand that an atonic or sluggish duodenum proximal to this "compressed" area will of itself produce the apparent obstructive picture, just as gastric atony may make a normal pyloric area appear to be "obstructing." Only if the peristaltic activity of the first and second portions of the duodenum is normal or hyperactive can one suspect an organic obstruction of the third portion of the duodenum. If this is identified, exploration is indicated and a bypassing operation justified.

Stasis. Complete stasis of the duodenum occurs rarely, usually in association with mesenteric vascular catastrophes. On x-ray examination, dilatation of the duodenum with a peculiar churning of the barium meal is characteristically noted in the patient with anorexia nervosa and, occasionally, in those suffering from severe ulcerative colitis. Elsewhere in the small intestine, stasis is the result of loss of vascular integrity, an exhaustion following mechanical or paralytic ileus (Chap. 276).

Spasm. Spasm of the duodenum occurs in peptic disorders, acute pancreatitis, or in various conditions associated with severe nausea. Experimental nausea, as, for example, that produced by vestibular stimulation, gives characteristically a tetanic spasm of the duodenum.

Pain. Migratory or steady pain around the umbilicus may result from *insufficiency of the mesenteric vessels,* usually as a result of degenerative aortic disease encroaching on the lumina of the vessels.

REGIONAL ENTERITIS

The most disabling and discouraging affliction of the small intestine known to the internist is regional enteritis, an unpredictable granulomatous response of the submucosa to an unknown agent or agents, in which damage is done by encroachment upon the lumen, scarring of the muscle, ulceration of the mucosa, and necrotic breakdown with fistula formation between loops of bowel, bowel and skin, and bowel and perirectal spaces. Any, all, or none of these sequelae may follow the initial bout of the disease, and single attacks are well documented. Much more common, however, is recurrence and slow spread of the lesion to involve contiguous areas of the intestine, including occasionally the duodenum. Involvement of the antrum of the stomach by a similar process has been described.

Since the original description by Crohn, Ginz-burg, and Oppenheimer in 1932, in which this disorder was localized to the terminal ileum, a number of different clinical syndromes have been distinguished from the classical forms, but our knowledge is far from satisfactory as to causes, course, and proper management.

Epidemiology. The disorder is world-wide in distribution, and occurs among all races. In the United States its exact incidence is unknown, but it appears to be about one-fifth as common as chronic ulcerative colitis. It has been reported as having its onset in every decade of life, but it is characteristically a disorder of young adults, the peak incidence being between the ages of fifteen and thirty-five. Both sexes are affected with equal frequency; Negroes are less commonly affected than whites.

The affected subjects are more often of Jewish origin than one would expect by chance; in some series Jews appear to be about three times as commonly involved as their distribution in the population at large would suggest. The patients show urban backgrounds more commonly than rural, reach higher levels of schooling than usual and slightly higher economic status than ordinarily encountered. Despite some evidence to the contrary, severely disturbed personalities are not routinely met with in these patients, particularly early in the course of the disease or antedating the onset of the disease. Many such patients show remarkable fortitude in meeting the innumerable difficulties wrought by progressive destruction of the intestine; a number have distinguished themselves in the arts, sciences, professions, and business despite prolonged and progressive disease.

Familial occurrence of the disease has been recognized from the onset. In various series the percentage of cases occurring in siblings ranges from 2 to 10; father-daughter, mother-son, and father-son patterns are recorded in all large series of cases. The onset of disease in the child does not exhibit anticipation, and other associated stigmas are so rare as to make it unlikely that genetic factors are of more than predisposing importance.

Etiology and Pathogenesis. No specific cause of this disease has been identified. Investigations have been carried out on the possible etiologic relationship of bacterial and viral organisms identified more frequently in the gastrointestinal tract of these patients than in normal subjects, but all such studies have been fruitless. Certain disorders of the mesenteric arteries seen in the aging population have occasionally given rise to a submucosal inflammatory and cicatricial reaction producing a picture similar to that of regional enteritis, but in the majority of cases of regional enteritis no such arterial lesions can be found. The enlarged and succulent lymph nodes of the mesentery seem to result from the submucosal inflammation rather

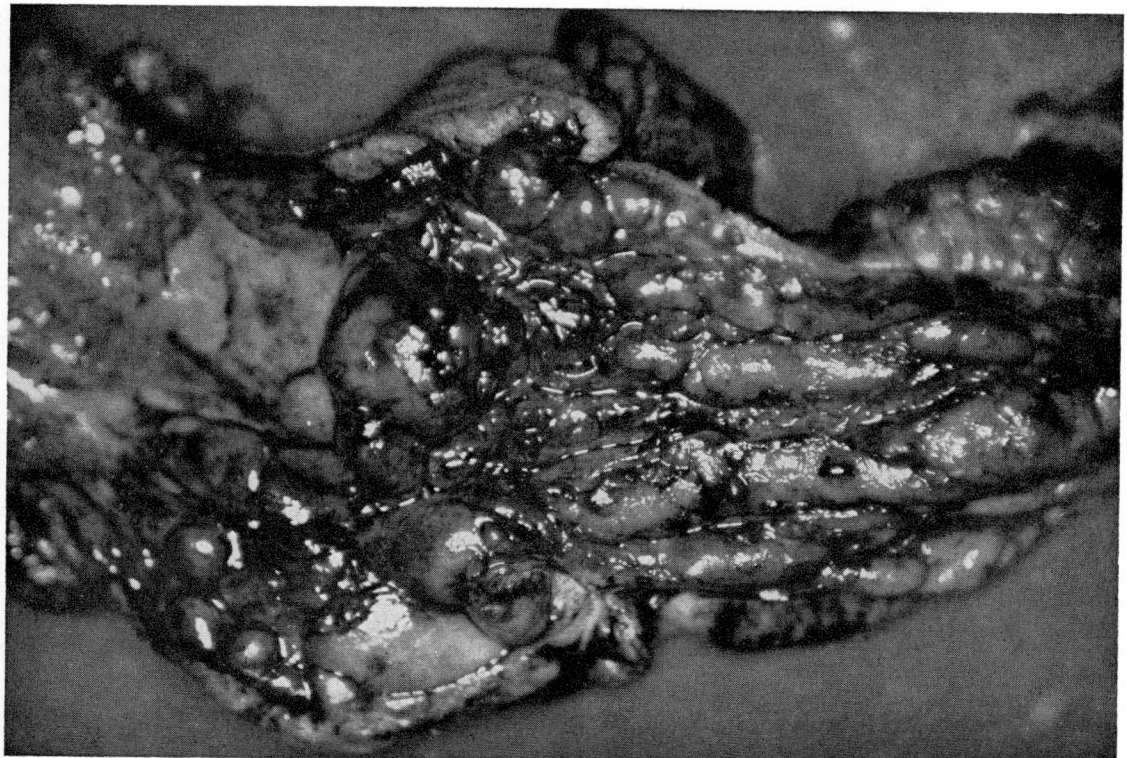

FIG. 275-2. Regional enteritis: resected specimen of ileocecal area demonstrating the hypertrophy of ileal submucosa (*right*), with nodular encroachment on the lumen and minute areas of mucosal hemorrhage.

than to be its cause; remarkable alterations in the autonomic ganglia of the bowel wall, frequently seen in excised specimens, are rarely present early in the course of the disease. Histochemical studies are remarkably normal, particularly with respect to the columnar epithelium of the bowel luminal surface. Granulomatous tubercles are characteristically encountered in the submucosa, in the peritoneal reactions of serosa, and in fistulous tracts; these show giant cells in the center, but no caseation and no evidences of fungi or inclusion bodies.

The earliest lesions, as seen in the terminal ileum, are rarely minute, and more usually involve appreciable (6 to 20 cm) lengths of gut in a swollen beefy glistening mass, occasionally rather purplish, but more often intensely red. The serosa is often injected and the mesenteric fat edematous. Large lymph nodes in the mesentery nearby are commonly noted. The luminal surface of the bowel is thrown up into injected folds stretched over the heaped-up submucosal hypertrophy (Fig. 275-2). Ulceration of this mucosa, although common, is usually superficial in the early stages of the disease, when microscopically the nonulcerated areas of mucosa appear healthy.

There is usually a definite demarcation between the diseased and healthy bowel; the appendix may be involved by a similar process or may merely show lymphoid hyperplasia and venous congestion as a result of the adjacent inflammatory reaction. The initial process may disappear rather quickly, may remain indolent only to flare up months or years later, or may slowly progress to involve ileal segments more cephalad. "Skips" are well-documented, in which an initial ileal lesion subsides, and a midjejunal lesion of similar character develops later, the intervening area remaining uninvolved. Adjacent or contiguous small or large intestine may be involved, if not invaded, by this inflammatory process; cicatrization, local perforations, abscesses, and fistulas commonly characterize the development of such a process. The fistulas may go from intestine to colon, from intestine to skin, or from one loop of intestine to another. Loops low in the pelvis or involving sigmoid colon often produce perirectal or ischiorectal abscesses, perirectal nodular masses seen on proctoscopy, or proctitis. A number of changes—endothelial cell proliferation in lymphatics, giant cell aggregations in the edematous submucosa, ischemic contraction of smaller arterioles, and increased numbers of ganglion cells and neurofibrillar accumulations—occur characteristically in surgical and autopsy material and in such profusion as to render the pathologic diagnosis of the disease easy to make. How-ever, the primacy of any one of these changes, or even the proper sequence of lesions, is not clear.

The endothelial reaction in lymphatics and the presence of granulomas as the principal tissue reaction have suggested to many that the disease must be a reaction to some irritant absorbed in the lymphatics; the absence of foreign bodies in the giant cells would lead one not to suspect particulate foreign matter as the offending agent; attempts have been made to produce the disease experimentally by abnormal fatty substances, but so far these studies have been fruitless. There is little evidence that the succulent lymph nodes seen in the mesentery of cases of early acute ileitis are more than a phase of acute secondary lymphadenitis, rather than a reflection of an etiologic primary lymphangitis. Sarcoidosis, tuberculosis, and reaction to abdominal trauma seem unrelated to the characteristic forms of this disease, even though some of the granulomas may be indistinguishable from the characteristic lesions of these processes.

Symptoms. These depend on the location of the inflammatory lesion, its extent, its acuteness, the amount of obstruction it produces, the peritoneal reaction, if any, and its relationship to contiguous structures. A certain number of such patients may present only with the systemic features of a febrile illness without localizing symptoms or signs. Even in these cases, a careful history will often document abdominal discomfort, loose stools, rectal urgency, and mild anorexia made worse by the feeling that abdominal discomfort increases after eating.

Acute ileitis presents as the sudden development of right lower quadrant pain and tenderness, with fever, localized guarding, and some disturbance of bowel motility—either diarrhea or constipation. It thus presents the clinical picture of appendicitis, and the differential diagnosis can be made only at laparotomy, when the characteristic beefy red terminal ileum, boggy mesenteric fat, and succulent lymph nodes of the mesentery tell the surgeon that appendicitis alone could not produce the picture. The appendix also may be involved in the primary lesion, or may be obstructed secondarily by the acute submucosal edema of the adjacent ileitis.

In one large series, diarrhea, colicky pain, and weight loss were encountered as presenting symptoms in over two-thirds of 600 patients. Fever occurred in one-third, and a history of bright red rectal bleeding or melena in less than one-sixth. Symptoms related to rectal and anal complications predominated in about 10 per cent.

Approximately half the patients have initial involvement of the terminal ileum, another 15 per cent have both ileum and cecum affected at the onset, and less than 4 per cent present initial symptoms due exclusively to jejunal or duodenal involvement. Various other combinations of jejunal, ileal, and colonic lesions may be seen at the time the patient first consults the physician.

Variants of this picture include (1) a full-blown *malabsorption syndrome* (Chap. 62) with any one or many malnutritive derangements capturing the spotlight, (2) *acute perforation and generalized peritonitis* (less than 1 per cent), or (3) *massive melena*, seen in less than 2 per cent of cases. The advanced case, with cutaneous fistulas, easily appreciable masses throughout the abdomen, increased pigmentation, and severe proctitis, presents little difficulty in diagnosis. Amyloidosis due to regional enteritis is becoming a more frequent complication and may be responsible for the patient's death in renal failure.

As experience with the disease as a whole has expanded, a certain number of patients have been encountered who present a diffuse involvement of jejunum and ileum when first seen. These patients have been described by Crohn as having a subtype of regional enteritis in which the lesions are more superficial but much more extensive, less prone to suppurative complications and fistula formations, but likely to lead to malabsorptive symptoms, fever, splenomegaly, and clubbing of the fingers, the reasons for which are not understood.

On physical examination these patients with enteritis characteristically display various evidences of undernutrition and malnutrition if the symptoms are of long standing. Clubbing of the fingers is frequent in this group. Special attention to the abdominal examination is necessary, since a definite mass or doughy aggregations of bowel loops can be felt in one-third of the patients. Fistulous tracts between the involved bowel and the abdominal skin are classical complications of the disease and are easily appreciated. More readily overlooked are the perirectal and ischiorectal fistulas found in nearly 10 per cent of chronic cases; rectal digital examination will disclose an anorectal stricture in half of these cases and in 3 to 4 per cent of those without fistulas. Proctoscopic examination is abnormal in 10 to 15 per cent; the abnormalities may include nodular submucosal masses, acute proctitis, ulceration, or stricture in the rectosigmoid junction. Rectovaginal fistulas are noted in a small percentage of cases.

Diagnosis. Regional enteritis should be suspected on clinical grounds in most instances when a patient presents with a history of intermittent chronic diarrhea, fever, weight loss, crampy pain or distention, and on physical examination shows perianal suppuration, anal strictures, and abdominal masses. It should be part of the differential diagnosis of all types of malabsorption (Chap. 62), fever of unexplained origin, intermittent small bowel obstruction, and secondary amyloidosis.

Laboratory features of regional enteritis parallel the severity of the (1) inflammatory reaction: leukocytosis, elevated sedimentation rate; (2) blood loss by ulceration: iron deficiency anemia; (3) undernutrition and malabsorption: hypoalbuminemia, hypocalcemia, hypokalemia, elevated serum alkaline phosphatase, hypoprothrombinemia, and macrocytic anemia; (4) possibly more specific changes related to disturbed protein metabolism: elevated seromucoids in the serum and hypergammaglobulinemia. None of these laboratory tests is diagnostic.

The most helpful adjunct to the clinician suspicious of regional enteritis is the radiologist, who generally establishes the diagnosis short of histologic confirmation. Marshak and Wolf have tried to separate the nonstenotic phase of regional enteritis from the stenotic phase on radiologic grounds, despite the fact that occasionally both phases may be encountered in the same patient. In the nonstenotic phase the principal changes are loss of detail in the mucosa, stiffening of the submucosa to form a tubular pattern on the radiograph, and separation of the tubular loops by inflammation in the mesentery. The stenotic phase is characterized by narrowing of the lumen, with dilatation of normal bowel proximally. In the dilated area poor oil-water interfaces and retained mucus secretions produce abnormal puddling of the barium. Fistulous tracts are often seen, particularly in the ileocecal area, and are practically diagnostic, the only other disease likely to produce a similar picture being actinomycosis. When the duodenum or upper jejunum is involved by regional enteritis, the stenotic phase predominates from the onset, whereas ileal involvement characteristically is nonstenotic and ulcerative early in its course (Fig. 275-3). The unoperated case usually demonstrates little radiologic change after the first studies are completed, except for fistula formation.

Definitive diagnosis on histologic grounds is established under the microscope, although most surgeons can make an accurate diagnosis by inspection at the operating table of the beefy reddish-to-bluish serosa, edematous mesentery, and large lymph nodes. Differential diagnosis in the operating room includes tuberculosis, various lymphomas, sarcoidosis, and fungous diseases. Biopsies of the bowel and lymph nodes provide adequate bases for histologic diagnosis.

Course and Prognosis. Acute regional ileitis apparently is self-limited in about a third of the cases; the other two-thirds go on to develop chronic enteritis, and it is possible that 10 to 15 per cent of all cases of regional enteritis are outgrowths of an original acute ileitis.

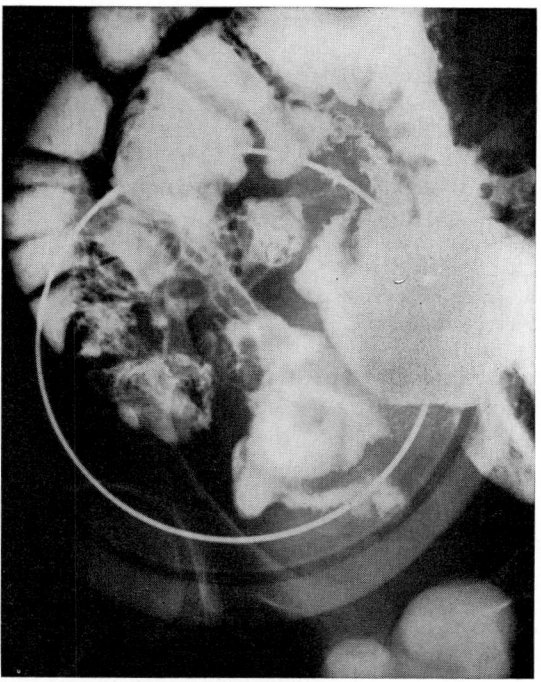

FIG. 275-3. Regional enteritis: several involved loops of ileum communicate via multiple fistulous tracts. Small bowel proximal to involved areas is dilated (*upper*).

Accurate prognostication in this disease is at present impossible, largely because there exists no large body of cases treated entirely supportively in the atmosphere of a sanatorium. Almost every large series of cases consists of a heterogeneous population of enteritis of different longevity, severity, and past nutritional and pharmaceutical experience, 90 per cent of whom require surgery for some complication of the original disease. Our prognostications, then, must be made on the basis of surgically treated patients subjected to a wide variety of therapeutic procedures at widely varying periods of disease, with interim periods of varying supportive therapy. The extent of the intestinal lesions in an unoperated case tends to remain that present when the patient was first seen, except for the development of fistulas. If operation is carried out to remove the entire diseased bowel, as was the custom soon after the disease was first identified, approximately half the cases have a recurrence of the disease within a few years of the operation. Whether this is due to failure at operation to recognize "skip" areas of enteritis proximal to the resected area, or whether new foci of enteritis develop in hitherto normal bowel is not clear. In any case, the physician should expect a patient with regional enteritis to have exacerbations and remissions over a period of many years; these exacerbations usually involve the same areas of bowel established as diseased in the first attack, but ulceration, fistulas, and stenosis may supervene at any time. Extension of these suppurative and necrotic lesions to neighboring loops of small bowel, colon, bladder, and perirectal tissues may be constantly suspected and looked for by the physician.

Involvement of the colon by a granulomatous inflammatory process is reported by some workers in half their cases of enteritis, but most investigators believe that a true granulomatous colitis is seen in only a small percentage of enteritis cases. Minimal involvement of the colon by fistulas and masses does not produce granulomatous reactions in the colon, but occasionally true ulcerative colitis is seen in the colon when indubitable regional enteritis is present in the small intestine.

Involvement of more distant organs and organ systems unrelated to the intestine has been reported with increasing frequency as these patients have been studied more closely over a long time span. Liver abnormalities and nodular pancreatitis have been reported, but their relation to the primary disease is dubious in view of the transfusions, injections, and drugs these patients receive and of the many nutritional deficiencies they incur. More significant is the incidence of arthritic symptoms which also are noted in a proportion of cases of ulcerative colitis. The arthritis involves larger joints and is often of the spondylitis type; under any circumstances it is not accompanied by the laboratory data suggestive of rheumatoid disease.

Treatment. In a chronic disease of unknown cause and unpredictable course, medical management of the most comprehensive type is mandatory. Regardless of the validity of the theory that psychiatric disorder underlies or determines the onset and progression of this disease, it is clear that careful attention to personality factors must proceed *pari passu* with meticulous attempts to meet the nutritional requirements of these patients. These must be combined to assure physical and mental rest as part of the program for combating the discouraging periods during which all efforts of physician and patient seem unable to slow the progress of the process. Psychiatric assistance will be needed in evaluating a number of these cases and should form the principal management in a small percentage. Supportive care consists first of all in explaining to the patient the problem which faces him, the relatively limited areas in which pharmacologic and surgical maneuvers can aid him, and yet at the same time repeatedly pointing out that adequate hyperalimentation, rest, and the more specific measures can enable him to "ride out" the disease; it is generally true that the activity of the disease does slow down after a number of years, at which time the patient will have residua demonstrable on x-ray and physical examination, but will be able to lead a reasonably normal life. For women it should be made clear that pregnancy is not something to avoid; many women with severe ileitis but with a genuine wish to have children have produced normal offspring without undue hazard to themselves. Even menstrual function seems preserved better in the women with ileitis than in those with ulcerative colitis.

Specific Measures. Chemotherapeutic and antibiotic drugs are of assistance in managing the purulent complications of enteritis but have little or no effect on the primary disease process. Nonabsorbable sulfonamides have been the most beneficial of these agents.

Hormonal treatment with ACTH and with various adrenal steroids has been largely unavailing. Although many of the secondary manifestations of the disease, in particular arthritis, erythema nodosum, iritis, have cleared up quickly after the institution of such therapy, the primary intestinal lesion remains unaffected. Their use may be highly efficacious in managing the rare toxic episodes characterized by high fever, severe anorexia, and depression, but constant caution must be exercised that perforations and peritonitis are not masked by this therapy.

Radiation therapy was originally proposed to control the inflammation and suppuration in patients whose disease was too generalized or whose condition too poor to tolerate resective surgery. In some cases dramatic improvement has been reported following general abdominal irradiation, and it is possibly a measure which has not been used sufficiently often as a therapeutic adjunct. No series have yet been reported which include a large number of early cases of the disease treated in this way.

Surgical therapy, originally used solely for the complications of a then little-understood process, has gone through a number of stages only to return full circle to its original status. In the 15 years, 1932 to 1947, surgery was thought to effect a cure of the disease; radical resection of the involved ileocecal area in the original group of patients with disease localized there was advocated as curative. As the years went by, however, not only did a high percentage of these patients return with a recurrent disease, but more diffuse lesions were encountered than at the first operation, making eradication surgically impossible. A more conservative surgical approach was then devised, essentially consisting of enterocolostomy without resection. Although the operative mortality and immediate postoperative morbidity from this procedure has been satisfactorily low, it is difficult to state that the recurrence rate among these patients is much lower (about 33 per cent) than among those treated with radical excision (about 40 per cent). Whether these recurrences result from spread outward of foci of disease not seen at the time of operation or from some ill-understood activation of the disease process by newly contiguous bowel is not clear. Unfortunately, once a recurrence has occurred following surgery, every subsequent surgical maneuver tends to result in recurrence.

Since surgery is not curative, it has now returned to its original place in the therapy of enteritis, as a means of eliminating complications of the disease which are producing serious symptoms on their own. Among these are intermittent intestinal obstruction, blind loops leading to macrocytic anemia, ulcerating lesions in fixed stenotic bowel, and fistulas between the bowel and adjacent hollow viscera.

The sequelae of resections of the small intestine have been of considerable interest in throwing light on the mechanisms of nutrient absorption. The physician taking care of a patient with unoperated enteritis must have a good understanding of the nutritional derangements produced by the disease; when that patient has lost, in addition, a sizable segment of his small intestine by resection, the physician must be very much more alert in detecting and correcting the multitude of nutritional defects which inevitably result (see Chap. 62).

UNUSUAL DISORDERS OF THE SMALL INTESTINE

Pneumatosis Cystoides Intestinalis

This is a rare disease involving small or large intestine, predominantly the former, in a process characterized by numerous nitrogen-filled cysts under the serosa. These cysts are lined by endothelium and vary in size from 1 to 3 cm. It is generally assumed that the gas has arrived subserosally from the retroperitoneal space; presumably intestinal gas has penetrated lymphatics from the luminal surface, passed retroperitoneally, then dissected along the mesentery until it again reaches the subserosa. Obstructive lesions of the bowel are common precursors of the condition—pyloric stenosis, tumors, regional enteritis, have been specifically described.

Symptoms are primarily abdominal pain, bloody diarrhea, or the sudden onset of pneumoperitoneum from rupture of a cyst. Diagnosis is usually made radiologically, the cysts deforming the bowel lumen in a characteristic way.

Treatment is that of the underlying disease, which is generally surgical.

Whipple's Disease

In 1907, G. H. Whipple described a new disease entity marked clinically by progressive wasting, diarrhea, arthritis, and skin pigmentation. At autopsy the patient displayed a diffusely edematous small and large intestine supported by a mesentery full of enlarged lymph nodes. The microscopic and chemical analyses of the tissues disclosed a great increase in fat content, but Whipple noted especially the presence of large macrophages throughout the lamina propria of the gut and in the lymph nodes; these macrophages were filled with a foamy material which did not stain with lipophilic dyes; he also noted small sickle-form particles in the macrophages which took a silver stain. He called the disease "intestinal lipodystrophy."

Since 1907 the disease has been reported in increasing numbers. The clinical course is quite variable, the multiplicity of organs and tissues involved suggesting that this is indeed a generalized disturbance. The material in the macrophages is a mucoprotein; such cells have been identified in all portions of the intestinal tract, in peripheral lymph nodes, liver, pancreatic acini, spleen, bone marrow, myocardium, lungs and pleura, adrenal glands, and the hypothalamus.

The reported cases have occurred almost entirely in men; there may be a familial predisposition. The disturbed mucoproteins noted in the histochemical preparations may also be found in the serum. The disease should be thought of in any adult patient presenting with diarrhea, malabsorption syndrome, pigmentation, or polyarthritis. Diagnosis is made by biopsy of small intestine, colon, or peripheral nodes, or at laparotomy. There is no therapy of proved efficacy, although steroids and tetracycline compounds have been of temporary benefit. Spontaneous remissions have been described, but generally the disease is progressive and leads to the death of the patient.

TUMORS OF THE SMALL INTESTINE

Generally, this is an infrequently occurring group of lesions, but because of the variety of symptoms they produce, they may be very difficult to diagnose. It is perhaps best to describe them according to their pathology, since any or all of them may produce identical symptoms.

Benign Tumors

Leiomyomas of clinical significance are rare in the small intestine, but they may produce intussusception with obstruction, ulceration and hemorrhage, with fatal outcome, or varying degrees of intestinal obstruction alone. The mucosa becomes stretched tightly over these solid tumors and frequently ulcerates to produce gastrointestinal hemorrhage of mild to fatal severity. Malignant change may occur at any time.

Hemangiomas of the small intestine, although rare, are very difficult to identify by clinical methods or radiologic examination. When they bleed suddenly into the bowel wall they often collapse, so that they do not present to radiologic study any space-occupying defect in the barium-filled bowel. They may be multiple. The occurrence of these various syndromes as hereditary disorders is well documented, and a hint as to the existence of an intestinal hemangioma may well be gleaned from identification of hemangiomas of the skin or mucous membrane (see Chap. 238).

Lipomas are more common than leiomyomas or hemangiomas in the small intestine and, like them, may be involved in developmental anomalies of supporting tissues in the bowel and elsewhere. Although a number of these could be considered to be hamartomas, they do exhibit the neoplastic ability to grow and expand. Characteristically, they are found in middle adult life, although they may have been growing slowly for many years before making clinical mischief. Sex incidence is probably equal. It is probable that they arise from adipose tissue anywhere in the body. Since the mesentery of the small intestine contains a large amount of such tissue, a variety of lipomas involving the wall of the bowel to produce obstruction have been documented.

Polypoid tumors of the small intestine usually turn out to be hamartomas. These have been thoroughly studied as part of the Peutz-Jeghers syndrome (see Chap. 98). Such tumors are rarely malignant, but may cause intussusception and hemorrhage.

Malignant Tumors

Malignant tumors of the small intestine are not common in the United States, accounting for less than 1 per cent of all digestive tract cancers. In Africa, on the other hand, primary tumors of the small intestine have been described among some races as more common than carcinoma of the stomach.

Adenocarcinoma of the duodenum is more frequent as an independent lesion than is carcinoma of the jejunum or ileum. However, in recent years diffuse carcinomas of the small bowel have been described in patients with long-standing regional enteritis. The most frequently involved area of duodenum is the second, near the papilla of Vater. The tumor usually causes ulceration with hemorrhage or high obstruction and may be easily confused radiologically with chronic peptic ulcer in the same area. Carcinoma of the jejunoileum may present as diffuse foci of intestinal obstruction due to early metastases to the peritoneum, as ascites, or as a malabsorption syndrome.

Argentaffine tumors are found in 0.5 per cent of all surgically removed appendixes, as a yellowish indurated area. They are the commonest epithelial tumors of the small intestine, and may appear anywhere from the duodenum to the colon. They arise from argentaffin cells in the crypts of Lieberkühn, and grow as clumps or strands of small closely packed polyhedral cells. The degree to which these tumors are regarded as malignant varies among pathologists, but there is increasing recognition of their invasive tendencies. They are often multiple, but when solitary some 60 per cent arise in the ileum, enlarging to form plaques projecting into the muscularis and serosa. Adenofibrosis of the surrounding tissues accompanies this spread so that ulceration from the luminal spread and compromise of the lumen by pressure of the inflammatory reaction may produce the symptoms. They are tumors of middle age, more common in men. Remote spread is infrequent and late. For some reason, lesions of the duodenum tend less to invade surrounding tissues. When metastases invade the liver, a characteristic syndrome results (see Chap. 90).

Lymphosarcoma, which may develop in any region where lymphoid tissue is present, is an important invader of the small intestine. Reticulum cell sarcoma usually develops in retroperitoneal lymph nodes, secondarily involving the bowel; localized lymphosarcoma usually involves the ileum as a solid bulky tumor which may cause ileal obstruction. It may remain stationary for a long time and can produce an x-ray picture simulating that of localized ileitis. When it spreads, it does so slowly, to regional lymph nodes. Hodgkin's granuloma and sarcoma may invade any organ in the body, but they rarely cause localized lesions in the small intestine. Enlarged retroperitoneal nodes may distort the x-ray picture of the upper small intestine, but localized infiltrations are uncommon.

Both *liposarcoma* and *leiomyosarcomas* are infrequently encountered in the small intestine. The symptoms may be the same as those of the benign tumors or of any malignant lesion.

Diagnosis. Tumors of the small intestine should be thought of in the differential diagnosis of obstructive syndromes of any type, of gastrointestinal bleeding, and of malabsorptive states. They are less likely to cause fever than is regional enteritis or tuberculosis, but in all other respects benign inflammatory disease, benign tumors, and malignant tumors of this organ can produce identical clinical syndromes. The reason for this is not hard to find, since most symptoms are due to: (1) ulceration of mucosa with bleeding; (2) obstruction of the lumen behind which mucosal bowel wall contracts forcibly, giving rise to crampy pain; (3) necrosis and inflammation of the wall, giving rise to persistent pain and tender masses; (4) interference with intraluminal, mucosal, and lymphatic aspects of digestion and absorption of nutrients, producing abnormal stools, weight loss, anorexia, vomiting, and occasionally intestinal obstruction.

Radiologic techniques designed to differentiate localized from generalized lesions, pressure of enlarged nodes or inflammatory abscesses on the intestines, "deficiency patterns" and flocculation of barium in the bowel lumen, distortion of outlines of the bowel by stiffened mesentery—all these may be of the greatest diagnostic assistance, or may indicate only in a general way the nature of the underlying disease.

Localization of a specific bleeding point may be carried out by use of the long intestinal tube, through which luminal contents are aspirated and tested for blood, or by the use of a string test; in the latter maneuver, injection of fluorescein intravenously during active bleeding will stain the string at the site of bleeding; fluorescence of the stained area is proof positive of locus of bleeding.

Careful microscopic and chemical testing of the stools may confirm the presence or absence of an inflammatory exudate, cancer cells, and malabsorbed or maldigested foodstuffs, as well as blood, abnormal concretions, or parasites.

If a diagnosis of tumor is made presumptively or if symptoms persist and no diagnosis can be arrived at, laparotomy is indicated. Therapy for most of the tumors described is entirely surgical. In the case of lymphoma and lymphosarcomas, local removal and general radiation or chemotherapy are employed.

REFERENCES

Chanoine, F.: Contribution à l'étude des tumeurs malignes primitives du jéjuno-ileon, Acta Gastroenterol. Belge., 18:163, 1955.

Corhn, B. B., and H. Yarnis: "Regional Ileitis," 2d ed., New York, Grune & Stratton, Inc., 1958.

Soderlund, S.: Meckel's Diverticulum, Acta Chir. Scand., Suppl. 248, 1959.

Van Patter, W. N., J. A. Bargen, M. B. Dockerton, D. V. M. Feldman, C. W. Mayo, and J. M. Waugh: Regional Enteritis, Gastroenterol., 26:347, 1954.

Whipple, G. H.: Bull. Johns Hopkins Hosp., 18:382, 1907.

276 ACUTE INTESTINAL OBSTRUCTION

Albert I. Mendeloff and Arnold M. Seligman

Definition. Acute intestinal obstruction may be defined as a failure of progression of intestinal con-

tents, whether due to mechanical causes or to inadequacy of intestinal muscular activity.

Etiology. The most useful classification is based on the immediate need for surgical or medical therapy. The *mechanical type* of intestinal obstruction usually requires surgical intervention for its correction. This type is due either to intraluminal obstruction by foreign bodies, gallstones, meconium, bezoars, enteroliths, and worms; or to mural obstruction due to encroachment by compression of the intestinal wall, such as in adhesions, stenosis, hernia, volvulus, intussusception, tumors, and atresia. *Nonmechanical obstruction* is referred to as *ileus.* Ileus is either adynamic (paralytic) or dynamic (spastic).

Adynamic ileus occurs (1) reflexly after certain surgical manipulations, diagnostic studies such as retrograde pyelography, or trauma; (2) secondary to peritoneal insult by chemical agents (hydrochloric acid or blood), pancreatic enzymes or bacterial agents; (3) as the result of metabolic changes, secondary to generalized dislocation of electrolyte equilibrium, especially abnormally low serum potassium levels, interference with the enzymes and coenzymes involved in acetylocholine synthesis (pantothenic acid), or due to drug effects (especially ganglionic blocking agents); (4) following mechanical *hypoactivity* in which the musculature of the intestinal wall loses its functional integrity on the basis of localized hypoxia secondary to compromised blood supply. This can happen suddenly as a result of arterial spasm secondary to venous or arterial thrombosis or embolism of intestinal vasculature, or more slowly when obstructing factors progress to a degree that embarrasses the arterial or venous blood flow through localized portions of the bowel.

Spastic ileus is an uncommon form of mechanical *hyperactivity* of the normal bowel behind a spastic segment or segments of the gut. It is seen in toxic conditions such as uremia, heavy metal poisoning, porphyria, infections, and extensive ulcerations.

Untreated ileus with progressive distention enhances mechanical obstruction as well as circulatory embarrassment in the wall of the involved lumen. In this way partial mechanical occlusion may progress to complete obstruction and eventually strangulation.

Symptoms. Acute mechanical intestinal obstruction is characterized by colicky pain, nausea, vomiting, distention, and constipation or obstipation. Obstruction high in the intestinal tract produces earlier and more severe vomiting, whereas obstruction low in the intestinal tract produces earlier obstipation, more distention, and later vomiting. When obstruction is accompanied by strangulation, the pain is more severe and constant, and the patient soon develops evidence of sepsis. Diagnosis of the strangulation is relatively easy when a large segment of bowel is involved, but the diagnosis of devitalized bowel, although equally important, is difficult when only a few centimeters of bowel are involved. When the obstruction is primarily due to adynamic ileus, pain is absent, obstipation is present, and discomfort results when distention is severe enough to cause a tight abdomen, at which time tachypnea, tachycardia, and oliguria are the result of pooling of fluids in the intestinal lumen.

Pain in acute mechanical obstruction of the small bowel is referred to the midabdomen and occurs in severe paroxysms that reach a crescendo and cease abruptly. In acute mechanical obstruction of the large bowel, colicky pain is less severe and is referred to the lower abdomen. When the ileocecal valve is competent, distention is confined to the colon and vomiting occurs late if at all. As distention progresses, the intensity of the pain decreases and the paroxysms become less frequent. When strangulation supervenes, the discomfort becomes constant and pain becomes more localized to the quadrant of the abdomen in which the strangulated loop of bowel resides.

Vomiting occurs earlier and is more severe, the higher the obstruction in the intestinal tract. High obstructions result in earlier dehydration and alkalosis due to loss of hydrochloric acid, whereas lower obstructions result in slower dehydration, loss of alkaline fluid, and produce acidosis. Vomitus at first contains bile and mucus, but later becomes brown and fecal in odor because of putrefaction of protein in the small bowel. When the ileocecal valve is competent, little or no vomiting occurs in colonic obstruction.

Obstipation results in all cases of complete obstruction after the intestinal tract distal to the obstruction is emptied. In high obstruction, the lower bowel may function quite well for a time, e.g., expelling an enema readily, whereas in low intestinal obstruction and colonic obstruction obstipation occurs early. Blood in the scanty stool suggests strangulation in low lesions. Diarrhea is not encountered, except in those rare situations where mechanical obstruction is precipitated by gastroenteritis in already mechanically embarrassed loops of intestine. When the onset of constipation is gradual but steadily increasing in severity, chronic intestinal obstruction due to encroachment on the lumen of bowel by the growth of neoplasm should be suspected. The progression of symptoms may be marked by bouts of obstipation, distention, and cramps, only to be relieved by purgation with the passage of a fecal impaction. Eventually these measures fail to give relief and complete obstruction supervenes, with the added hazard of perforation into the peritoneal cavity of bowel proximal to the obstruction.

Physical Findings. The physical findings vary from very little at the onset, to severe dehydration and alkalosis or acidosis from continued vomiting, to localized or generalized distention with abdominal tenderness after several hours of obstruction. Severe sepsis and shock revealed by pallor, sweating, cold and clammy extremities, rapid pulse, hypotension, and stupor supervene when strangulation and perforation occur. Disorientation may be one of the earliest evidences of peritonitis, especially in older persons, occurring before shock becomes manifest. Clinical evidences of shock indicate extensive fluid and blood loss into bowel lumen, bowel wall, and peritoneal cavity as well as loss of fluid by vomiting. Shock is seen early when the intestine is infarcted, whether due to vascular occlusion or strangulation of bowel wall. Involuntary spasm of the abdominal muscles is noted only when strangulation with local peritonitis occurs and is not a prominent feature of acute obstruction. During paroxysmal painful contractions of small intestine, proximal to the point of obstruction, there is noted voluntary rigidity of the abdominal wall, but this subsides when the contraction subsides. These paroxysms of bowel contraction are accompanied by auscultatory sounds that are exaggerated, gurgle more than normal due to the abnormal amounts of fluid in the bowel, and become more high pitched as gaseous distention increases. Sometimes one can locate the noisy proximal bowel in one quadrant of the abdomen by auscultation with a stethoscope. The sounds become more tinkling in character as the ileus progresses, and the abdomen is silent when ileus becomes adynamic, such as occurs when peritonitis is superimposed or when large segments of bowel are infarcted.

Distention in high obstruction may be limited to the upper abdomen and in low colonic obstruction may outline the colon. Most of the gas in the distention that accompanies acute intestinal obstruction is from swallowed air. In those who tend to swallow air readily and unconsciously, gaseous distention may develop very rapidly indeed and to a degree not only to aggravate mechanical obstruction but to endanger life by respiratory embarrassment, cardiac arrhythmias, and the precipitation of vascular insufficiency of the gut with perforation. When perforation results, it usually occurs on the antimesenteric surface.

Detection of a large heart with irregular rhythm, or the definitive finding of mitral stenosis, may suggest that an embolus to the superior mesenteric artery has occurred. Embolism to that artery is also rendered possible by a history of recent myocardial infarction, subacute bacterial endocarditis, or other embolic phenomena. In an older patient, palpation of an abdominal aortic aneurysm, evidence of defective arterial circulation to the legs, or history of diffuse abdominal pain exacerbated by eating all suggest diffuse aortic arteriosclerosis with encroachment on the lumina of vessels supplying the intestine. Rarely, periarteritis nodosa will cause thrombosis of the superior mesenteric artery or one of its branches. When portal hypertension is present, thrombosis of the portal venous bed may occur, with resultant mesenteric venous thrombosis. Polycythemia vera, postsplenectomy states, and disorders of the coagulating mechanism such as thrombotic thrombocytopenic purpura are rare but documented causes of venous mesenteric thrombosis.

Reontgenographic Findings. An x-ray is a very valuable adjunct to the physical examination in demonstrating whether gas is present in loops of small bowel with or without fluid levels, whether gas is in the upper or entire small bowel, or in single loops of intestine, or primarily in the colon. A clue to the point of obstruction may be obtained often by a flat film together with a film of the patient sitting up or lying on his side. Classical radiologic evidence of obstruction of the small intestine is seen in Fig. 276-1, the stepladder distribution of distended small bowel loops being readily identified. Distention of the large bowel is usually recognized on the flat films from the distribution of the air-filled colon, the haustral markings extending not entirely down the lumen. Volvulus of the sigmoid colon presents a very characteristic radiologic picture, and various forms of internal or sliding hernias give characteristic radiologic patterns. The diagnosis may be much more difficult when low-grade or early obstruction is present or when large fecal masses obscure the picture. In acute obstructions it is not wise to give barium by mouth, although in chronic situations contrast media can sometimes be injected through a tube in the intestinal tract to visualize the point of obstruction. If evidence points to colonic obstruction, a carefully administered barium enema will often demonstrate the point of obstruction and reveal its cause.

Laboratory Findings. Laboratory findings are usually related to the amount of necrosis, the presence of peritonitis, and other chronic diseases which may underly the catastrophe. Leukocytosis is usually of moderate degree, the hematocrit may be high, and electrolytes are disturbed to various degrees. Lactic dehydrogenase levels in the serum are often very high in intestinal infarction. The stool may be grossly bloody if a large area of small bowel has been infarcted.

Treatment. Therapy consists in (1) correcting fluid and electrolyte imbalance, (2) alleviating vomiting and distention by intubation and decompression, (3) control of peritonitis if present and blood transfusion for shock if present, and (4)

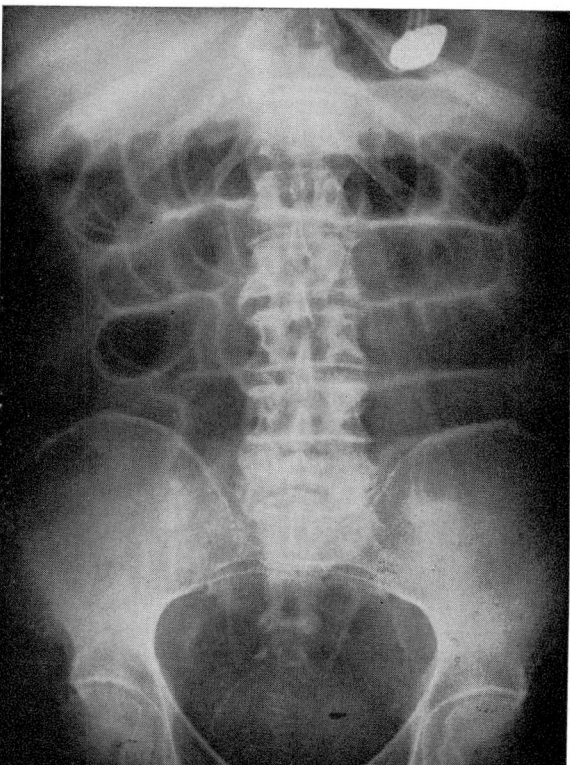

Fig. 276-1. Paralytic ileus due to thrombosis of superior mesenteric artery.

removal of the obstruction and restoration of bowel continuity and function.

Since the efflux of fluid into the dilated gut and peritoneal cavity results in dehydration and often hemoconcentration, and since chloride is lost in high obstructions, and both sodium chloride and potassium chloride in lower obstructions, the administration of saline and potassium chloride is indicated. Extra water should also be given in the form of 5 per cent glucose. Because these patients have not taken anything by mouth and will continue not to do so for several days, caloric requirements (2,000 per day) must be met by continuous infusion of glucose and parenteral vitamin preparations should be given. Adequate hydration can be gauged by measuring urinary excretion, which should be kept near a liter per day. The hematocrit is also useful in determining the results of combating hemoconcentration. Determination of sodium, chloride, potassium, and bicarbonate ionic levels in the serum twice a day in very sick patients serves as a useful guide to electrolyte therapy and control of acidosis or alkalosis. No attempt to maintain nitrogen equilibrium other than by blood and plasma infusion is indicated in short periods of disability.

Decompression is best achieved by intubation with one of the long, weighted intestinal tubes attached to gentle continuous suction. Single lumen tubes drain more effectively than double lumen tubes. This method of decompression, supplemented with pantothenic acid parenterally, is useful in adynamic ileus. However, there is great danger in relying solely on this means of relieving mechanical obstruction whenever there is any question of strangulation of bowel or when large bowel obstruction occurs in the presence of a competent ileocecal valve. Early operative intervention is required in all such cases.

In the majority of cases, surgical intervention is necessary to remove the obstructing agent and restore normal bowel continuity and function. In some cases due to adhesions and hernia, relief by decompression suffices, and in some cases of intussusception or volvulus, a barium enema under fluoroscopy restores normal continuity. Many cases of adynamic ileus are cured by tube decompression alone. However, if the patient does not improve rapidly on such conservative measures, operation within 24 hr is indicated to establish an accurate evaluation of the cause of obstruction and to effect a cure. When *severe* distention is not relieved *promptly* by intubation, surgical intervention is required for immediate decompression by means of enterostomy or colostomy. However, treatment of shock and dehydration should be instituted before surgery is undertaken in order to lessen the operative risk.

Prognosis. The prognosis is always guarded, depending upon the level of obstruction, being poorer in high obstruction than in low intestinal obstruction, and upon the viability of the bowel wall, the length of time the bowel has been obstructed and strangulated, and the amount of bowel involved in the strangulation. Patients with complicating peritonitis from perforation have a poor prognosis, and this is especially true in very young infants or in elderly patients with complicating cardiovascular or renal disease.

REFERENCES

DeMuth, W. E., W. T. Fitts, Jr., and L. T. Patterson: Mesenteric Vascular Occlusion, Surg., Gynecol. Obstet., 108:209, 1959.

Elman, R., B. A. Shatz, R. E. Keating, and T. E. Weichselbaum: Intracellular and Extracellular Potassium Deficits in Surgical Patients, Ann. Surg., 136:111, 1952.

Wangensteen, O. H. (Ed.): "Intestinal Obstructions," 3d ed., Springfield, Ill., Charles C Thomas, 1955.

277 ACUTE APPENDICITIS

Albert I. Mendeloff and Arnold M. Seligman

Inflammation of the vermiform appendix constitutes one of the commonest and most important acute disease processes. Although descriptions of isolated cases of the disease had been written in the seventeenth and eighteenth centuries, and appendiceal abscesses had been described at autopsy, it was Reginald Fitz in 1886 who first collected a series of cases in which clinicopathologic correlations were established.

Epidemiology. The disease occurs in all age groups, but appears to be productive of higher mortality rates in the group aged five to fourteen and after age fifty-five. It is estimated that in 1946, in England and Wales, one case occurred every year for every 700 of the population. The incidence of the disease is somewhat higher in males, and the death rates for the period prior to 1946 were 40 per cent higher in males. A consistent feature of the disease has been its greater incidence and mortality in the upper socioeconomic stratum and its tendency to decline in frequency during periods of food shortages. In Western Europe and in the United States, the death rates for the disease have shown a steady decline, ranging from 8.1 per 100,000 population in 1941 to 1.3 per 100,000 in 1956. There is also definite evidence that the incidence of the disease has recently decreased; despite great increases in the number of admissions of surgical patients to American hospitals since the Second World War, the absolute number of acutely inflamed appendixes removed has steadily declined by 30 to 60 per cent, and approximately at the same rates in urban and rural institutions. It is difficult to explain this decrease by single causation. Possible factors are the greater use of effective antibiotics and chemotherapeutic agents to treat upper respiratory infections, some of which undoubtedly have been associated with appendicitis, and a lessened infestation with helminths. Changes in diet have also occurred, changes which many feel have increased the incidence of degenerative disease, but may have sharply reduced the incidence and the mortality from appendicitis. Surgeons are also probably more careful about removing nearly normal appendixes now than heretofore. None of these explanations is adequate to clarify in its totality what appears to be a progressive and definite decrease in the incidence of one of our most important acute inflammatory diseases.

Pathogenesis. Appendicitis is an inflammation of the vermiform appendix involving all layers of the organ, beginning either as a focal ulceration or as a diffuse phlegmon. Evidence of a focal point of obstruction due to fecalith or stricture is sometimes found. The appendiceal artery is an end artery, and its tributaries are susceptible to occlusion from the increased pressure within the lumen of the obstructed appendix or direct pressure of a fecalith. Infections lead to vascular thrombosis, local necrosis, and infarction resulting in perforation. Streptococcal involvement, which rises in frequency when acute respiratory infections are prevalent, adds to the necrotic process and to the virulence of the disease. The process either subsides early or progresses to gangrene or perforation with abscess or peritonitis. Chronic inflammation occurs only with the granulomatous infections such as tuberculosis, amebas, or actinomycosis. Recurring appendicitis due to spontaneous subsidence of acute attacks should not be considered chronic appendicitis. Recognition of the disease as an entity was first made by Fitz, and treatment by appendectomy was introduced thereafter by Morton, Ochsner, Murphy, McBurney, and Deaver. Since then to the present time, acute appendicitis is the most common major surgical disease.

Clinical Picture. The history of onset should be carefully obtained, for the history may be the *only* clue to a correct diagnosis of retrocecal appendicitis, when abdominal signs are absent. The first symptom in an otherwise well individual is acute periumbilical or epigastric pain. In young children the abdominal pain cannot be localized and is usually generalized. Pain varies from mild or vague to quite severe and is followed by anorexia, nausea, or vomiting. The sequence of these symptoms is very important. When the illness is initiated by nausea and vomiting, which is then followed by abdominal pain, one should suspect an infection capable of producing extensive toxic absorption such as noted in cases of gastroenteritis, tonsillitis, scarlet fever, and pneumonia, rather than the early stage of appendiceal inflammation. Pain is the first symptom of appendicitis and is due to distention of the appendiceal serosa by edema. Stretching of the serosa stimulates sympathetic nerve endings in the wall of the appendix, producing pain first and, because of continued stimuli, anorexia, nausea, and vomiting afterward. For this reason it is important to determine whether abdominal pain preceded the nausea and vomiting. The only other mechanism for producing pain is by the acute contractions of the appendiceal musculature which occurs in appendiceal colic, when the lumen is obstructed by stricture, fecalith, worms, or foreign bodies. Since the sensory innervation of the appendix corresponds to the tenth spinal segment, the pain is referred to the periumbilical region like sensory impulses originating anywhere in the entire small bowel.

At the time of the initial symptoms, inflammation is confined to the appendix. Fever and abdominal signs are not prominent at the onset. High fever, like vomiting, as an initial symptom is suggestive of some other diagnosis. Within a few hours, when the inflammatory process has begun to involve peritoneal surfaces of neighboring loops of bowel, omentum, and the anterior parietal peritoneum, pain shifts to the right lower quadrant of the abdomen and tenderness, spasm, and rebound tenderness become increasingly prominent. In a sixth of the patients, diarrhea may appear owing to irritation of bowel, but constipation is more common. Contralateral rebound tenderness, like pain in the right lower quadrant on sneezing, is a particularly reliable sign of peritoneal inflammation. Although direct pressure of the examining hand produces pain, it may do so in the distended gut of gastroenteritis as well. However, release of tension by the examining hand, as in demonstrating rebound tenderness, can produce pain only when peritoneal surfaces are inflamed. Sudden cessation of abdominal pain some hours after onset signifies perforation of a distended appendix, infarction of the appendix, or the accumulation of enough peritoneal fluid to lubricate the moving inflamed surfaces.

In the absence of anterior abdominal signs and a history of onset consistent with appendicitis, one must suspect that the appendix is in the retrocecal position. Evidence for inflammation in this area may be obtained by stretching the iliopsoas muscle either by passive hyperextension of the legs on the torso or by actively flexing the iliopsoas by straight leg raising. When the appendix lies over the brim of the pelvis, evidence of inflammation is more striking on rectal examination than on abdominal examination. After 24 hr, progressive appendicitis results in localized peritonitis and abscess formation, when the signs remain confined to the right lower quadrant with the appearance of a tender mass. Diffuse peritonitis develops as a result of perforation before adequate adhesions by omentum and neighboring loops of bowel have been able to form. This is more common in children than in adults. Tenderness and spasm are generalized, ileus becomes evident, and the patient develops progressively severe toxicity, with high fever, severe leukocytosis, vomiting, dehydration, rapid pulse, and shock. When a history of illness for 2 to 3 days is obtained, one should expect to find evidence of appendiceal abscess with mass or more generalized peritonitis with ileus, rather than signs of appendicitis alone.

Atypical clinical pictures of appendicitis are distressingly common and difficult to identify. If one remembers that appendicitis is the most common acute intraabdominal focal inflammation, the onset of unexplained weakness, anorexia, and tachycardia in the elderly may lead the physician to suspect the appendix; similarly, in patients obtunded by cerebral disease, or whose pain pathways are disturbed by neurologic degeneration, or whose appreciation of pain is blunted by sedatives or ganglionic blocking agents, the objective signs of early peritonitis may be the only clue that an acute appendicitis has occurred. Retrocecal appendicitis can easily be confused with disease of the right kidney or ureter or with colonic disease, as noted above.

Differential Diagnosis. *Gastroenteritis* may produce vomiting, abdominal pain, and fever that are difficult to distinguish from those of acute appendicitis. However, vomiting is often the first and predominating symptom in the former and is later followed by diarrhea. Sometimes diarrhea ushers in the illness. Although tenderness is sometimes present, especially after considerable retching has occurred, spasm and rebound tenderness are absent. Systemic muscle aching and prostration are common, and bowel sounds are loud and "whooshing." The illness may occur in epidemics or affect several members of a family, making diagnosis somewhat easier.

Referred pain from diaphragmatic irritation in *pneumonia* may simulate appendicitis, especially in children. This is especially the case when the signs of appendicitis are found to be higher in the abdomen than usual and are attributed to malrotation of the colon. However, fever and vomiting are more prominent at the onset of abdominal symptoms and respiration is more rapid in pneumonia. Abdominal spasm and rebound tenderness should be absent in pneumonia, unless pneumococcal peritonitis has occurred.

Abdominal pain from mesenteric *lymphadenitis* is very difficult to distinguish from acute appendicitis and is frequently a cause of illness in children. Less spasm and rebound tenderness, lower leukocytosis, and more gradual onset of symptoms help distinguish it from appendicitis.

Since free blood in the peritoneal cavity produces the symptoms and signs of peritoneal irritation, a *ruptured graafian follicle* or a *ruptured tubal pregnancy* will simulate the acute abdomen of appendicitis. The signs are less localized, however. Other acute processes accompanied by a mass are *torsion of an ovarian cyst* and *acute salpingitis*. These conditions are usually readily distinguished on vaginal examination by noting tenderness mainly on movement of the cervix. The local signs are usually more pronounced than the general illness of the patient would warrant.

Other acute processes such as *acute cholecystitis*, *diverticulitis* of the *colon*, and *perforation* of *carcinoma* of the *colon* are often difficult to distinguish, especially in older patients. The history is the most helpful means of making a correct diagnosis. Urologic conditions such as *stone* and *pyelonephritis*

of the right kidney may give symptoms referred to the right lower quadrant. The urine is usually abnormal, and pain begins in the costovertebral angle and radiates to the groin or pubic area. However, a retrocecal appendicitis may also cause the appearance of blood cells in the urine.

In all these conditions, with the exception of pneumonia, it is usually safer to operate in the suspected case of acute appendicitis than to wait until the signs and symptoms of peritonitis make diagnosis relatively easy. The more patients who are operated upon after peritonitis has occurred, the higher the mortality will be.

Treatment. If appendicitis is considered a possible diagnosis, cathartics are absolutely contraindicated.

Once the diagnosis of acute appendicitis is made, the patient is prepared for surgery by initiating parenteral administration of fluid and electrolytes, and surgical removal of the appendix is performed as soon as possible, at any hour of the day or night. Uncomplicated appendicitis results in prompt recovery; with early ambulation, the patient may be able to eat within 2 days and be discharged within a few days thereafter. The complications of appendicitis such as local abscess, peritonitis with ileus, and intestinal obstruction require surgical intervention such as drainage or lysis of adhesions, prolonged hospitalization, energetic treatment with gastrointestinal intubation, antibiotics, and careful control of fluid, glucose, and electrolyte balance by parenteral means.

REFERENCES

Bowers, W. F.: Appendicitis, with Especial Reference to Its Pathogenesis, Bacteriology, and Healing, Arch. Surg., 39:362, 1939.

Castleton, K. B., C. D. Puestow, and D. Sauer: Is Appendicitis Decreasing in Frequency? A.M.A. Arch. Surg., 78:794, 1959.

Fitz, Reginald: Perforating Inflammation of the Vermiform Appendix, Am. J. Med. Sci., 92:321, 1886.

Moloney, G. E., W. T. Russell, and D. C. Wilson: Appendicitis—A Report on Its Social Pathology and Recent Surgical Experience, Brit. J. Surg., 38:52, 1950.

278 DISEASES OF THE COLON AND RECTUM
Albert I. Mendeloff

Symptoms of Colonic and Rectal Disease. Man can exist without a colon or rectum, although with some difficulty. This basic fact has allowed important observations to be made regarding the functions carried on by the large bowel and the adjustments which result when it is no longer present. The increasing freedom with which resections of the organ, bypassing operations, and colostomies have been carried out has led to significant advances in our understanding of normal activities of the colon, although our comprehension of many of its diseased states is still rudimentary.

Pain Reference. Anatomists, experimentally minded surgeons, and gastroenterologists have established that pain of colonic origin, unlike small intestinal pain, is lateralized by the brain to the right or left sides of the abdomen. Pain fibers from the cecum and ascending colon accompany sympathetic fibers to the lower ganglions of the celiac plexus; fibers from the transverse colon, sigmoid, and rectum accompany fibers passing into the inferior mesenteric ganglions. Interconnections of these fibers with somatic nerves permit a considerable amount of localization of pain by the brain, roughly corresponding to the festoon distribution of the colon in the peritoneal cavity. Pain from the rectum is projected low on to the sacral nerve distribution; the lower it arises, the more accurate is the localization. Anal pain has the exquisite tactile discriminative accuracy expected of skin near a mucocutaneous junction.

Pain stimuli from the noninflamed large bowel, as from other areas of the normal intestinal tract, consist almost exclusively of distention of the bowel musculature. In the uninflamed gut most forms of trauma result in no appreciable pain, stretching of the muscularis layer of the bowel wall being alone adequate to excite this sensation. When the wall is stiffened by an inflammatory response, however, the threshold for pain stimuli is lowered, and many previously subliminal impulses are perceived as pain. In the presence of peritoneal inflammation, pain previously lateralized on the abdominal wall in a general way becomes much more sharply localized and may be accompanied by spasm of the abdominal muscles and rebound tenderness to pressure.

Thus it is evident that pain from the uninflamed colon really results from distention of normal bowel proximal to an unrelaxing segment. If the unrelaxing segment is inflamed or infiltrated, pain arises from this area as well as from the contraction of the normal bowel proximal to it; if the inflammation or infiltration penetrates through the serosa of the gut to involve the parietal peritoneum, the more localized and sharper pain of spastic striated muscle and overlying skin becomes prominent.

Motor Disorders. The colon is a rather sluggish organ, contracting desultorily at rates not exceeding 1 per minute, compared to regular contraction frequencies in the small intestine ranging from 10 to 12 per minute in the duodenum to 3 to 4 per minute in the ileum. The transition between the innervation of the ascending colon and that of the transverse colon occurs just distal to the hepatic flexure, where radiologists often note irregular propulsion of barium (Cannon's point). The colon husbands its motor activity for the processing of ileal contents, waiting until a certain volume has accumulated in the cecum. Gas delivered into the cecum from the small intestine, which is intolerant of air and passes it rapidly downward, diffuses into the colon and distributes itself along the length of that organ. A liter of gas ordinarily is found in the large intestine, obeying the law of gravity, rising to the most superior portion of the colon— the flexures—when the subject is erect, the transverse colon when he is supine, the rectum when he is in the knee-chest position. Since most colonic motility is uncoordinated segmental churning of the fecal contents for the purpose of their partial desiccation, symptomatic disturbances of motor activity tend to be related rather to the infrequent mass propulsive waves which deliver the fecal bolus to an adjacent and more distal colonic region. The same types of disturbance which cause motor difficulties in the small intestine are also seen in the colon—intraluminal obstruction, destruction or paralysis of muscle, compromise of vascular integrity, pressure from neighboring masses, or infectious processes. The colon differs from the small intestine, however, in its more successful accommodation to these processes, distending to much greater degrees without serious symptoms than the small bowel can accomplish. In particular, obstructive lesions of the left colon characteristically produce gradual enlargement of the right colon of astonishing magnitude, occasionally to the point of cecal perforation.

Defecation Patterns. These have been described in Chap. 17. It is still not common knowledge among physicians how varied are the defecatory habits of their fellow citizens, how fanciful their interpretation of deviations from those habits. It is well to ask the patient to describe in some detail what he regards as his normal defecatory pattern, with particular attention to time of day or night, relation to meals, sensation during actual expulsion of stool, and aftersensations. Cardinal symptoms of serious disease are the inability to exert adequate expulsive pressure, a sense of incomplete evacuation, an intolerable urgency, and the presence of blood or of mucopus in the stools.

Bleeding. Bleeding from the colon may be occult, massive, or of any grade between. Most often it is occult, an important early sign of malignancy, often of the right colon. Melena and tarry stools rarely result from colonic bleeding. Bright red blood, either by itself or coating the stools, may originate from any portion of the lower ileum as well as from the colon. Bleeding results from localized lesions such as polyps, Meckel's diverticulum, hemangiomas, other tumors, from generalized blood dyscrasias, from uremic states, from inflammatory lesions—ulcerative colitis, regional enteritis, bacillary dysentery, diverticulitis—from diverticulosis on occasion, or from vascular anomalies such as hereditary telangiectasia. Hemorrhoids are so common that their presence can never allow the physician to abandon the search for other bleeding lesions.

Diagnostic Procedures. *Examination of the Abdomen.* Careful examination will often disclose masses or palpable colonic contents strongly suggesting more distal narrowing. Colonic outlines distended by gas have similar significance in leading one to the diagnosis of a more distal obstructing lesion. Spasm and guarding in the left lower quadrant are characteristic of an acute diverticulitis; a distended loop of sigmoid percussed in the midline at the level of the umbilicus may represent a sigmoid volvulus. Generalized hypogastric tenderness is associated with acute inflammations of the colon, the dysenteries and ulcerative colitis, both of which may also be accompanied by abdominal distention out of proportion to the habitus of the patient.

Digital Examination. This is a cheap and highly efficient procedure provided that the finger's education is maintained by steady use. Proper routinization of this examination should permit recognition of perianal, sphincteric, and ampullary lesions, gross deformities of prostate and cervix, and perception of even small neoplastic masses in the rectum. Two-thirds of all rectal carcinomas lie within reach of the inquiring index finger; when one considers that these cancers not only account for 12 per cent of all gastrointestinal cancers, but have a favorable prognosis if removed early, the importance of digital rectal examination is easily appreciated. Examination of the material coating the gloved finger on its withdrawal from the rectum is often of diagnostic importance, and all physicians should form the habit of routine testing of the finger specimen for occult blood.

Proctosigmoidoscopy. The proctosigmoidoscope is an inexpensive instrument of extraordinary importance in the detection of colonic disease. Contrary to the general impression, it is not difficult to master, and it can be introduced into the rectum as the examining finger is removed without discomfort to the patient. As experience accrues in its use, this examination becomes a very informative one. The physician should learn to evaluate friability of the mucosa, one of the earliest signs of proctitis and colitis, abnormal vascular patterns, edema, ulcerations, and polyps. Ninety per cent of tumors

of the rectum and rectosigmoid can be directly visualized with this instrument; 70 per cent of all tumors of the large intestine lie within the terminal 25 cm of the colon which it can bring into view. This area is particularly difficult to visualize radiographically, so that the proctosigmoidoscope is the most important diagnostic instrument in this region. In addition, radiography in the pelvis carries a radiation hazard to the gonads which can frequently be minimized or avoided by making the diagnosis endoscopically.

In addition to the visual inspection of the area, bacteriologic, parasitologic, and cytologic studies can be made on washings obtained through the instrument, and biopsy of a suspicious lesion is easy to perform. Routine proctosigmoidoscopy of all patients past the age of forty produces a substantial yield of "precancerous" lesions, since most such surveys have identified adenomatous polyps in 5 to 8 per cent of these individuals.

Stool Examination. Stools constitute important objective evidence of disease processes; some of the difficulties in obtaining them and describing them are discussed in Chap. 17. One must distinguish blood streaking on otherwise normal stools from dark stools containing blood, tarry stools from the gray-black formed stools passed by patients ingesting iron, and most importantly, the inflammatory mucopurulent exudate passed by patients with inflammatory rectal and sigmoid disease from true diarrheal stools. Microscopic examination of the freshly passed stool or rectal swab is useful not only for parasitologic study but for demonstration of the characteristic exudate of ulcerative colitis and bacillary dysentery and the presence of malignant cells (Papanicolaou technique). Tests for occult blood employ gum guaiac, benzidine base or benzidine dihydrochloride, or orthotolidine. Of these, the modified Gregersen test using benzidine dihydrochloride, barium peroxide, and 50 per cent acetic acid is the most satisfactory screening test, being roughly five times as sensitive as the guaiac test, and yet not producing a significant number of false positive reactions.

To summarize, the digital examination should be a routine feature of the general physical examination of all adults. Finger specimens obtained during the examination should be inspected and tested for blood. Whenever abdominal complaints, stool abnormalities, unexplained weight loss, changes in defecation patterns, or a strong family history of colonic disease are features of the history, proctosigmoidoscopy should be carried out. Any patient with anorectal disease should have routine proctosigmoidoscopy prior to surgery for the same.

When these procedures have been carried out, it is usually necessary to visualize the colon proximal to the rectosigmoid by radiologic techniques.

The routine barium enema is a very accurate diagnostic tool for the identification of structural abnormalities of the colon; for detection of mucosal abnormalities such as small polyps or early ulcerative colitis, it is often necessary to follow it with an air contrast enema. The combined use of the digital examination, proctosigmoidoscope, and radiologic investigation of the colon will identify 95 per cent of inflammatory, neoplastic, congenital, and vascular diseases of this organ. Negative results of these procedures constitutes strong evidence that disorders of a functional type are producing symptoms. Routine employment of these measures in the periodic health examination of all persons over forty years of age will disclose frequent evidence of serious disease in an early and treatable stage.

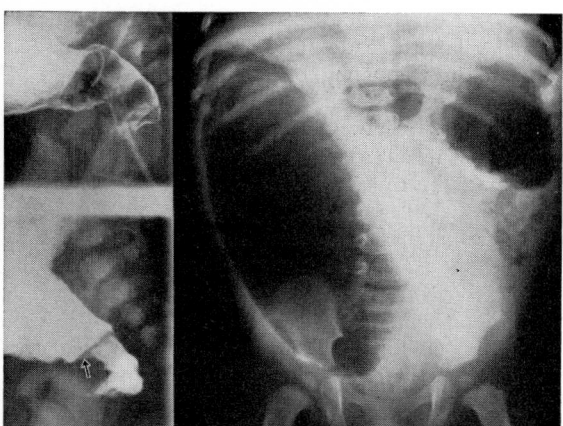

Fig. 278-1. Aganglionic megacolon: the contracted rectal segment is seen on the left, the dilated colon on the right.

DEVELOPMENTAL DISORDERS

Malrotations of the colon produce no disease states, but the abnormal location of the organ and its attachments (e.g., appendix) produces serious confusion in the pain reference pattern when any of the usual colonic diseases are present. Barium enema studies are usually necessary to identify the abnormally placed organ and make possible a more rational interpretation of the symptoms and physical findings.

Megacolon

Aganglionic megacolon, or Hirschsprung's disease, is a congenital disorder manifesting symptoms in early infancy, occurring more often in boys, often in familial clusters. There is abdominal distention occasionally reaching massive proportions; the sigmoid colon is the earliest segment to be distended, and visible peristalsis is common. The stools consist of characteristically very small pellets or ribbons of pasty consistency. On rectal examination the ampulla is empty of feces, and the anal sphincter feels normal. X-ray examination, when properly carried out, shows a narrowed lumen in the rectosigmoid area, with a distended sigmoid colon above the constricted area. Swenson and others have now established that the narrowed area results from a lack of functioning ganglion cells in Auerbach's plexus; this area is thus unable to relax in advance of the normal peristaltic activity of the colon proximal to it (Fig. 278-1).

The condition may also be acquired; in Brazil a large number of acquired megacolon cases have been reported in the aged; pathologic specimens show all degrees of degeneration of the ganglion cells of Auerbach's plexus, and in some cases a relationship to infection with *Trypanosoma cruzi* (Chagas disease) has been demonstrated. In a small number of patients generalized aganglionosis of the esophagus, ureters, and colon has been described, and thiamine deficiency has been incriminated as the etiologic agent.

Treatment of this condition is largely surgical, although a number of borderline cases may be carried along on measures designed to empty the colon. Definitive diagnosis is made by a rectal biopsy deep enough to include the muscularis layer of the rectum; failure to find adequate numbers of ganglion cells indicates that the most effective treatment is resection of the aganglionic segment and a "pull-through" anastomosis to the intact anal sphincter.

Chronic idiopathic megacolon has its onset later in childhood, usually at the time toilet training begins, is characterized more by constipation than distention, and the rectal ampulla is invariably found distended with feces. X-ray examination shows the entire colon to be distended from the anal sphincter cephalad; no narrowed segment is seen, and rectal biopsy discloses the normal complement of ganglion cells in Auerbach's plexus. The treatment is based on education in normal bowel habits, but a long course of enemas may have to be carried out concomitantly. It should be pointed out that water intoxication may occur in small children whose enormously dilated colons are vigorously irrigated with tap water; saline enemas are probably safe.

Diverticulosis

Saccular outpouchings of the colon are more common than those of the small intestine, occurring probably in 10 per cent of all persons over fifty years of age. The outpouchings are nearly always made up of mucosa and serosa following the course of a nutrient artery perforating the muscularis layer of the organ. There is a definite increase in the frequency of the findings as one follows patients into the later decades of life; indeed, there is an increase in frequency of diverticula in the same individual as he ages. It is probable that straining at stool has some role in increasing the rate at which diverticula develop, since the potential tunnel along the nutrient arteries is present in everyone. Diverticula are most frequently found in the sigmoid colon, least commonly in the ascending colon.

These diverticula are occasionally associated with diverticula elsewhere in the stomach or small intestine (see Chap. 275); in themselves they can hardly be called pathologic, but the peculiarities of their structure and location provide the basis for two serious complications.

1. Acute inflammation of the diverticular sac, known as diverticulitis (see below).

2. Hemorrhage into the colon. This may occur in the absence of an acute diverticulitis, although the association is much more common. The anatomic basis for the bleeding in uninflamed diverticulosis consists of the glomuslike capillary and arteriolar vascular network left unprotected in the lumen of the colon when the diverticular sac pushes out along the nutrient artery of the mucosa and serosa. In older patients these vessels, presumably damaged by contact with hard fecal aggregates, may be ruptured and bleed furiously. Such catastrophes, seen with increasing frequency as the population ages, often require emergency surgery for their amelioration.

Polyposis

Single polyps are identified in some 5 to 8 per cent of the adult population subjected to sigmoidoscopy as a routine screening procedure. They occur more often in men than in women (2:1) and increase in frequency with increasing age. In children polyps are frequently large, vascular, on long pedicles, and may produce intussusception or massive hemorrhage. In adults the polyps are more frequently sessile, arise from the glandular epithelium of the crypts, and bleed less frequently. Less often, polyps arising from the surface epithelium may form villous masses which secrete watery discharges rich in potassium. Such villous adenomas, although infrequent, can lead to watery diarrhea of remarkable magnitude, but the primary danger they pose is their high capacity for malignant transformation. (Probably 75 per cent of these polypoid tumors will become cancers if not totally removed; fulguration is usually followed by prompt recurrence.)

Adenomatous polyps, whether sessile or pedunculated, have a distribution in the colon which most pathologists, but not all, consider to parallel the distribution of rectal and colonic cancer. Colonic specimens resected for cancer frequently show adenomatous polyps in close proximity to the malignant tissue; polyps removed from noncancerous patients have been observed to show all grades of differentiation known to occur in the progression from benignancy to frank malignancy (Fig. 278-2).

Clinically, polyps are usually silent. When they do give rise to symptoms, these are either intermittent episodes of bleeding, manifest or occult, or of intermittent obstruction. The latter occurs when a large sessile polypoid mass weakens the wall to which it is attached or a pedunculated polyp flips caudad, causing the wall from which it arises to buckle. In either case a partial intussusception may result, with the production of crampy pain, occasionally an abdominal mass, and often a bloody exudate.

Treatment of polyps in adults is influenced by the fear of their malignant transformation. The diagnostic sigmoidoscopy which identifies adenomatous polyps will often permit the fulguration or excision of small lesions. Larger lesions, *all* villous adenomas, or lesions above the reach of the sigmoidoscope will require laparotomy and resection of the involved bowel. Inspection by sigmoidoscopy at the operating table of the area above and below

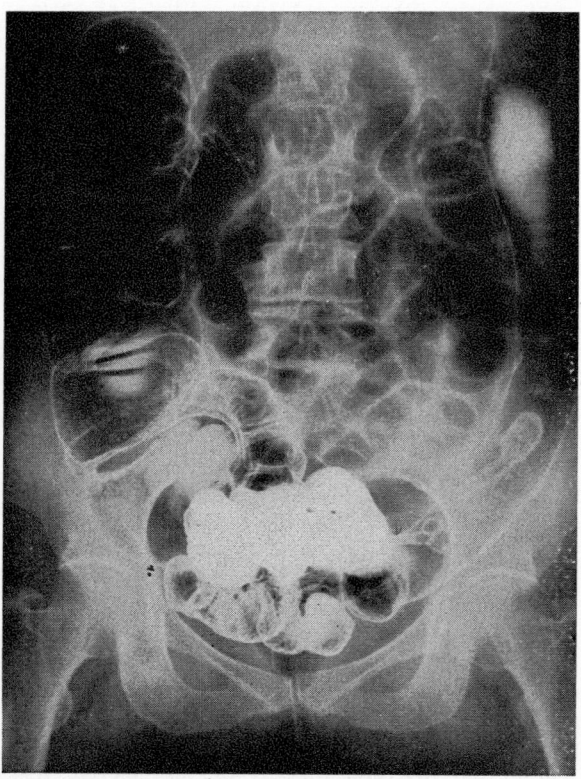

FIG. 278-2. Two adenomatous polyps in the sigmoid.

the resected bowel will often reveal hitherto unrecognized lesions, although it should be said that often small polyps readily demonstrated by barium enema prove hard to find in the operating room.

Sufficient information is now at hand to disclose the remarkably high incidence of recurrence of adenomatous polyps after fulguration and excision. Approximately 40 to 50 per cent of patients who have had polyps removed from the colon and rectum will develop new polyps in the decade following the polypectomies. Although most of the new polyps will be of the same type as the original polyps, about 15 to 20 per cent of the new polyps will be malignant when the original polyps were benign.

Multiple congenital polyposis of the colon, inherited as a simple dominant gene and thus characterizing many members of the families affected, is a disorder in which many adenomatous polyps are found from ileocecal valve to anus (Fig. 278-3). These usually give rise to some symptoms, usually diarrhea or bleeding, but once such a disorder has been identified in a patient, it is imperative that the entire family be examined sigmoidoscopically and radiologically to detect the characteristic polyps. The probability of malignancy supervening in these polypoid colons is so high that present reasoning requires each sufferer from this disorder to have a total colectomy; since sigmoidoscopic follow-up can be effectively and easily carried out, some surgeons elect to perform ileoproctostomy, leaving the rectum intact.

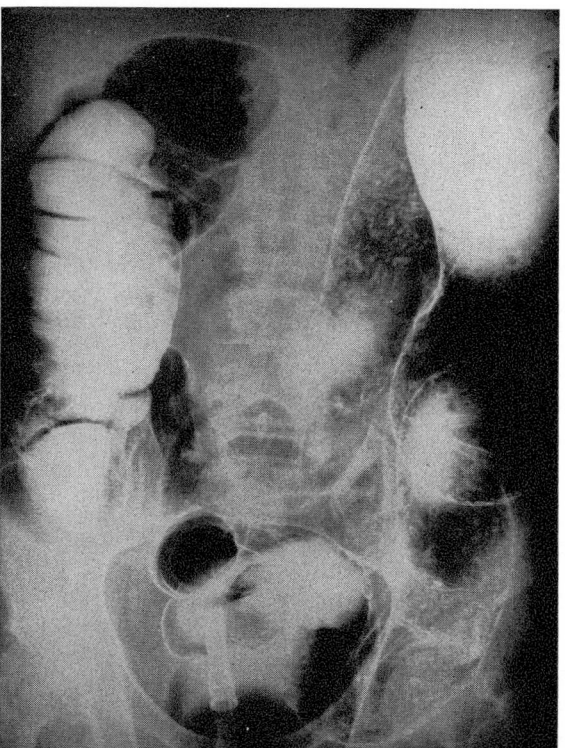

FIG. 278-3. Multiple congenital polyposis of the entire colon.

FUNCTIONAL DISTURBANCES

Irritable Colon Syndrome

This name is applied to a triad of symptoms—abdominal distress following the colonic distribution of pain, variations in defecatory habits from constipation to diarrhea, and the passage of stools which are of small caliber at the time abdominal distress is at its worst. The stools may be hard and pellet-like, or soft and pasty, but they are characteristically of smaller size than when the patient is not complaining of distress. The physiologic basis for most of these symptoms has been dealt with in Chap. 17. Over the years many different terms have been applied to this syndrome: some, such as "unstable colon" or "colonic neurosis," stress the anxiety which characterizes those patients; others, like "spastic colitis," lay emphasis on the pain and distress experienced by these patients; still others, such as "mucous colitis," describe the increased mucus content of the stools and the pain which is usually relieved by defecation. In its milder forms the syndrome is extremely common, being more frequently seen in women

aged fifteen to forty-five, but commonly observed in both sexes under conditions of emotional tension. Constipation, with pain in the left lower quadrant relieved by defecation, is the commonest symptom when the disorder is mild. Extremely severe pain, diarrheal stools accompanied by much mucus, and various degrees of generalized disability are much less common and carry a rather serious prognosis, patients with such complaints being severely psychoneurotic. Vasomotor instability and disabling headaches are frequently noted to occur in many patients even when the colonic symptoms are minimal. Aerophagia is a frequent accompaniment of the attacks, the swallowed air producing further difficulties when irregularly handled by the "irritable" colon. Bloating, borborygmi, explosive flatulence, and low backache are often described during the days or weeks when the symptoms are at their worst.

On *physical examination* these patients are anxious, often sweaty, but otherwise normal. During intense pain the abdomen may be distended, but no visible peristalsis is noted, the abdominal musculature is relaxed, and in the left lower quadrant a tender sigmoid full of feces may be palpated. Characteristically, the rectal ampulla is empty of feces. Proctoscopic examination usually is entirely normal or may show prominent vascular patterns in an otherwise unremarkable mucosa. Large amounts of clear mucus are frequently encountered during the examination, and there is often difficulty in negotiating the rectosigmoid curve at 13 to 15 cm from the anus because of violent spasm of the rectosigmoid.

The *diagnosis* of the irritable colon syndrome is suggested by the length of the history without obvious signs of physical deterioration, the intermittent character of the disability, and the relationship of distress to periods of environmental or emotional stress. Nevertheless, each patient presenting such symptoms deserves not only a careful history but also a complete physical examination including proctosigmoidoscopy, stool examinations for blood parasites and pathogenic bacteria; a barium enema is also indicated. The radiographic study serves to rule out other lesions, since there are no findings diagnostic for this syndrome, although spasticity of the sigmoid, accentuated haustrations, and tubular descending colon may be observed if the patient is having symptoms at the time of the examination.

The *differential diagnosis* includes all disorders of the colon, female genital tract diseases, regional enteritis, malignancies of stomach or pancreas, and those common disorders which are often associated with the irritable colon—gastric and duodenal ulcer and cholelithiasis.

Treatment of the irritable colon syndrome is that of any chronic anxiety neurosis with more specific symptomatic medication. The relationship between patient and physician can be established on the firm grounds of reassurance that the syndrome does not lead to the development either of ulcerative colitis or colonic malignancy, although it should be stated that it confers no protection against these eventualities. From this point the patient should receive a sympathetic ear from the physician as he talks over the circumstances surrounding the onset of his symptoms and those characterizing his present difficulties. Attempts should be made to discover in what way situational and emotional stresses differ when symptoms are present and when they are absent. The emphasis is placed on the patient and his relationship to others in his environment rather than on the symptoms and long discussions of what is "normal" bowel physiology. Repeated x-ray examinations are avoided in so far as possible, but general physical examinations, hemograms, and stool examinations are carried out at regular intervals.

During the acute attacks it is generally best to limit the diet to frequent bland feedings, with emphasis upon relatively even temperatures of liquids. Many patients find sweet whole milk troublesome at these times; skimmed milk, buttermilk, and cheeses are better tolerated. The cabbage and turnip families should be avoided, as well as coffee, alcoholic drinks, and tobacco. Bulk laxatives employing *Plantago ovata* powders are often remarkably helpful. Other laxatives and cathartics are best interdicted. Fecal impaction is a very infrequent complication of this syndrome unless the patient has taken to his bed unexpectedly for some disorder which prevents his customary posture at stool.

Medications of proved value include antispasmodics of the anticholinergic type; it is unlikely that any of those available are as effective in controlling colonic motility as they are in decreasing the tone of the stomach and small intestine, and it is necessary to push the dosage to the point of dry mouth or blurring of visual accommodation. Sedation with phenobarbital is probably as satisfactory as with various tranquilizing drugs, doses of 15 to 30 mg three to four times a day being adequate. For the temporary control of severe diarrhea, the combination of an anticholinergic drug with deodorized tincture of opium (8 to 10 drops in water four or five times a day) is very satisfactory.

Constipation and Urgency of Rectal Origin

In Chap. 17 the mechanism of defecation is discussed. Disorders involving the sensory or motor components of this mechanism may arise from destruction of the nerves subserving these functions, from invasion or inflammation of the rectosigmoid itself, or from central nervous system dysfunctions based on conditioning abnormalities or structural disorganization. If the afferent stimulus from the rectal wall cannot reach the brain, or if, upon reaching it, no efferent action occurs, defecation is not initiated. If defecation is initiated, but muscular power is lessened or lost, the act is not carried to completion. If all anatomic pathways are intact, but habitual neglect of the afferent impulses is established, defecation is not initiated. The result of all these disorders, regardless of etiology, is failure of the rectum to empty its contents. Accordingly, physical examination of such patients reveals the rectal ampulla to be full of stool, often to the astonishment of the patient.

Aside from degenerative disease of the central nervous system, severe psychoses, the use of ganglionic blocking drugs, and morphine addiction, the commonest cause of this type of rectal or "simple" constipation is voluntary suppression of the defecation reflex. Such inhibitory activity is essential in the daily routines of civilized society; disordered bowel habits are therefore very common in civilized life. Toilet training in infancy leads to a powerful development of these inhibitory actions; repeated experiences in suppressing defecation because of social impropriety, unaccustomed surroundings, uncomfortable commodes, or intercurrent factors lead to a habit pattern in which suppression of defecation becomes simpler than its achievement. When constant distention of the rectum with feces becomes habitual, anorectal disorders, in particular hemorrhoidal itching and bleeding and anal fissures, make defecation painful, thus reinforcing the inhibitory impulses. The next step for the patient is the use of laxatives, which soon becomes as much a constant feature of the regimen as is the voluntary suppression of defecation.

Treatment. The principal bulwark of therapy for rectal constipation is education. The chain of events leading up to the ineffective rectum is evaluated by careful physical examination of the status of the abdominal musculature, neurologic defects, drug effects, postural abnormalities, and accompanying local lesions of the anus and rectum. Such lesions as can be treated are taken care of, but the therapy may take a long time, and usually must be carried out concomitantly with efforts to modify anal sphincteric spasm when it is present. Attention to regular habits of diet and time of defecation is most important; although defecation for most persons is best accomplished following meals, particularly breakfast, in these patients it is more important to select for evacuation whatever time is as free as possible from the pressure of daily events. Habit patterns of many years' standing may have to be altered, one may need to force the patient to get up earlier in the morning, to take some form of physical exercise—for older patients walking briskly outdoors is often helpful—to abandon the usual laxatives and cathartics, to pay more attention to defecatory urges (without becoming excessively bowel-conscious), and to space out the workday in such a way as to honor these urges when they arise.

The elderly patient may be feebly motivated to make such sweeping changes; under such circumstances one must proceed cautiously, making sure impactions are broken up by the physician's finger, that oil retention enemas at night are utilized, that sigmoidoscopy above the impaction reveals no tumor or diverticulitic encroachment on the lumen. The use of hydrophilic colloid laxatives or enemas of tap water may be required for the remainder of the patient's life, if motivation for more drastic alteration of living, eating, and defecatory habits cannot be stimulated, or if poor muscle tone, difficulties in ambulation and in achieving a comfortable posture at stool, or cerebral arteriosclerosis are major factors.

As described in Chap. 17, the presence of unaccustomed fecal masses in the rectosigmoid may produce rectal urgency in the patient who has always had normal defecatory responses to such masses. Sudden onset of rectal urgency in a previously healthy person demands immediate investigation. Usually it is seen in young adults required by emergency surgical indications to lie very still in bed (classically, in ophthalmologic, orthopedic, or neurosurgical disorders); intolerable urgency accompanied by the passage of watery exudate of small quantity suggests that an impaction has occurred. Severe urgency accompanied by the frequent passage of an exudate rich in blood, pus, or mucus usually signifies the presence of an acute proctitis (see below).

INFLAMMATORY DISORDERS

Acute Diverticulitis

Acute diverticulitis is an acute inflammation of colonic diverticula, the origin of which has been described above. (Inflammation of a Meckel's diverticulum has been discussed in Chap. 275.) The causes of the acute inflammation of single or multiple diverticula usually are mechanical, related to the plugging of the neck of the outpouching by undigested food residues. Under such conditions the blood supply to the thin wall of the diverticular sac, made up of mucosa and serosa only, is easily compromised, and colonic bacteria can invade these tissues and produce a purulent reaction. Mild attacks of this type are probably quite frequent in the elderly population; dislodgment of the obstructing plug by the increased pressure in the sac is followed by evacuation of its contents into the bowel lumen, thus resolving the process uneventfully. When this does not occur, however, the purulent sac enlarges and causes an inflammatory reaction in neighboring structures, including the colonic wall. As this latter becomes edematous, other diverticular necks are blocked, and a number of adjacent diverticula become the site of abscess formation. If no other egress is afforded, and the process enlarges, the sacs may rupture into other hollow viscera to which the inflammatory reaction has attached them; fistula formation follows, most frequently into the bladder in men, into the bladder and pelvic organs in women. Not only is diverticulitis of the colon more common in men, but it is at least three times as often encountered in the descending colon as in the right colon. This is probably explainable because of the higher intraluminal pressures developed in the sigmoid and rectosigmoid, the less fluid character of the fecal contents in this area, and the anatomic fixation of the organ at the apex of an intraperitoneal pressure cone during defecation.

The *clinical features* of acute diverticulitis are lower abdominal pain, made worse by defecation, and the signs of peritoneal irritation—muscle spasm, guarding, fever, and leukocytosis. The disease has long been called "left-sided appendicitis," with good reason; diverticulitis of the transverse colon or ascending colon, although less common, presents similar findings; such a process in the cecal area may be impossible to distinguish from true appendicitis. The attendant spasm of the colonic wall in patients with diverticulitis usually produces constipation; the stools may be fluid or pasty. Rectal bleeding occurs in one-fourth the cases of sigmoid diverticulitis, and is usually gross. Occasionally it is massive and life-threatening. As the process develops, the inflammatory reaction produces a tender mass appreciated on abdominal examination; behind the obstructing mass partial large bowel obstruction may develop, and in low-grade or recurrent diverticulitis the entire picture cannot be distinguished from that due to a rectosigmoid carcinoma.

The *differential diagnosis* is principally that of neoplasm in the area of known or detected diverticulosis. Proctoscopy may show an acutely inflamed mucosa pushed into the lumen by an extrinsic mass; it is usually impossible to force the instrument through the spastically contracted lumen. Cytologic studies of rectal exudate may show carcinoma cells. Radiologic findings on barium enema may be diagnostic (see Fig. 278-4), but often the distortion of the area by the inflammation prevents a clear distinction between cancer and diverticulitis. The same difficulty confronts the surgeon at operation; he sometimes cannot make this distinction even when looking directly at the specimen. Occasionally a patient presents with generalized peritonitis, acute paralytic ileus, and shock. Differential diagnosis here is that of any ruptured viscus, or of any intraabdominal catastrophe producing such manifestations—acute pancreatitis, mesenteric infarction, mechanical forms of intestinal obstruction, or acute pyelophlebitis.

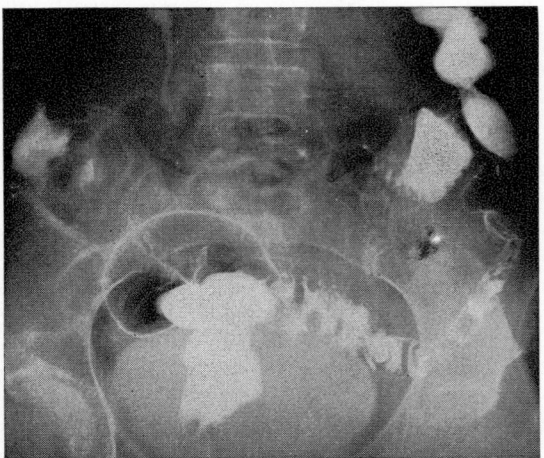

FIG. 278-4. Diverticulitis of the sigmoid colon.

Treatment in the usual case comprises bed rest, heat to the tender abdominal area, and the administration of antibiotics, usually penicillin plus tetracycline or chloramphenicol. Warm cottonseed oil enemas and a very soft diet complete the management of the mild acute attack. Once the attack is over the patient is cautioned to avoid eating nuts, seeds, and fibrous foods, and any constipation is treated as described previously.

The principal danger of such repeated attacks is the development of fistulous tracts between the diverticula and neighboring structures, in particular the bladder and vagina. These are extremely difficult to manage surgically. A preliminary colostomy has to be created before any attack on the primary disease can be undertaken; the ensuing postoperative period may be prolonged, numerous surgical attempts may have to be made, and the general health of the patient may deteriorate, thus preventing adequate healing.

Because of the dangers of such complications, as well as the possibility of peritonitis and acute perforation, current opinion is in favor of primary resection of the diverticulitic segment of colon if it is subject to recurrence of the disease despite adequate medical management.

Chronic Nonspecific Ulcerative Colitis

This disorder or group of disorders is characterized pathologically by an inflammatory reaction involving the mucosa and submucosa of the colon and/or rectum, not ascribable to invasion of these tissues by specific bacteria, parasites, or viruses. The clinical expression of the inflammatory response is the passage of an inflammatory exudate—blood, pus, fibrin, and mixtures thereof—into the lumen, where it may coat an otherwise normal stool, be admixed with unformed stools, or be excreted as a pure exudate. The absence of parasites (*Endomoeba histolytica* in particular), bacteria (of the genus *Shigella* or *Salmonella* in particular), mycobacteria (*Mycobacterium tuberculosis* in particular), and the virus of lymphogranuloma venereum in stools, exudates, or biopsies of the colonic mucosa suggests the diagnosis, although certain characteristic findings allow the experienced physician to classify the disorder in the idiopathic group *despite* the presence of these organisms.

The disease is world-wide in distribution, although there are marked differences in the reported frequency from country to country. The reported mortality from the disease is remarkably similar in the United States, Canada, and Denmark, about 0.5 per 100,000 population. It is much higher in England and Wales, and distinctly lower in Norway. All ages are affected, from infancy to the ninth decade, and both sexes are affected approximately equally; the greatest number of cases is recognized between the ages of fifteen and forty. In the United States the disease is more common in the city than in the country, in the north than in the south, in the wards of private voluntary hospitals than in those of city and county hospitals, among those of better-than-average incomes and educational backgrounds. As with regional enteritis, the frequency with which the disease is seen in the United States in those of Jewish faith is three times the expected incidence; the disease is about one-third as frequent among Negroes as among whites. A family history of ulcerative colitis can be elicited in 5 to 10 per cent of all cases. The number of reported cases is highest where the reported frequency of shigellosis and salmonellosis is least. There is little doubt that it is becoming increasingly frequent, so that it now constitutes one of the most commonest forms of severe chronic diarrhea encountered in American medical practice.

Etiology and Pathogenesis. There is no known single cause of ulcerative proctitis or colitis. Not only are no specific viruses or bacteria associated with its onset, but no other disorders—irritable colon syndrome, long-standing constipation, attacks of gastroenteritis—seem to predispose the patient to the later development of ulcerative colitis. The amount of mucosal destruction noted in the disease has led to emphasis on the proteolytic quality of the fecal contents or the secretions of the bowel; over the years such a proteolytic enzyme as lysozyme has been shown to increase in concentration in colonic inflammatory exudates paralleling the degree of inflammation, but not at the time of onset of the disease, prior to the occurrence of the secondary infection so commonly noted in all progressive cases. A filtrable proteolytic factor from the stools of patients with ulcerative colitis which is capable of producing acantholysis in formalin-fixed human skin was studied by Stoughton; more recent evidence discloses that the same factor is found in diseases other than ulcerative colitis. Exogenous food allergy is not generally regarded as of etiologic significance, nor do various nutritional deficiencies play a causative role.

The primary pathologic lesion in this disease is not understood. Far-advanced lesions removed by colonic resection or at autopsy show varying degrees of abscesses in the crypts of Lieberkühn and some degree of vascular injury, expressed as thrombosis, hyaline change, or perivascular inflammation. Some pathologists believe there is evidence of defective epithelial regeneration. Specimens removed from less ill patients by rectal or colonic biopsy show principally an intense inflammatory reaction, acute, chronic, or mixed; in early acute cases the lamina propria is often full of eosinophils, the basement membrane of the glandular epithelium is disrupted, and the goblet cells appear abnormal. In recurrent cases of longer duration, such biopsies often reveal plasma cell infiltration, small granulomas, dilatation of lymphatics, and vascular thrombosis.

In *all* stages of the disease, however, small abscesses just beneath the mucosa are seen breaking through the epithelium, leaving an ulceration. The nature of the exudate seen in the colonic lumen reflects accurately the primacy of this ulcerative process, which spews forth blood, pus, fibrin, and mucus. As the disease waxes, wanes, and becomes chronic granulomatous responses, plasma cell invasion, histiocytes, and crypt abscesses are seen. The mucosa and submucosa take on the general characteristics of granulation tissue—telangiectasis, fibrosis, conversion of columnar to cuboidal epithelium, and disappearance of the crypts. As this process becomes generalized, the total colonic bulk shrinks, is replaced by fibrous tissue, and the mucosa exhibits the characteristic pseudopolypoid appearance of normal or abnormal mucosa projecting from the diseased bowel.

Attempts to produce experimental ulcerative colitis have employed chronic overstimulation of the parasympathetic nervous system, postganglionic splanchnicectomy, inoculations with many different bacteria, and a variety of hyperimmunizing systems. All these have been followed irregularly by a hemorrhagic colitis which resembles to some degree the human lesion.

The systemic effects of the disease in patients carefully followed for a number of years, plus the tissue eosinophilia and granulomas, have led many investigators to postulate an autoimmune origin for the disease, but at this writing no such hypothesis has been proved. Nevertheless, circulating antibodies to colonic antigen have been demonstrated in an appreciable percentage of patients with chronic ulcerative colitis, and it is possible that this concept may prove to be the most fruitful lead yet uncovered to our understanding of the pathogenesis of the process.

Hay fever, asthma, and drug sensitivity seem to be more common among these patients than among controls.

Classification. *Clinical classifications* of ulcerative colitis have been based on the presenting features —these depend on the area of the colon or rectum involved—and the acuteness of the inflammatory process. Thus a sudden *acute ulcerative proctitis* involving the lower rectum might be manifest solely by a bloody exudate on otherwise normal stools, unaccompanied by fever, anorexia, or any signs of systemic toxicity. Proctoscopy reveals an intensely red and edematous mucous membrane, the normal vascular pattern completely disappearing from view until the proctoscope reaches 10 to 12 cm from the anal margin, at which point all inflammatory changes subside. The intense friability of the involved mucosa, bleeding at the slightest touch of a cotton swab, cannot be identified above this point; biopsies from the involved and uninvolved areas are strikingly different. If the proctitis is most active in the upper rectum, intolerable rectal urgency may be the presenting sign. Under such circumstances the rectal mucosa may not appear so abnormal near the anus, but reaches its most friable and edematous appearance at 5 cm or so from the skin, abruptly receding at 15 cm, so that the visible rectosigmoid appears normal.

Patients with this type of ulcerative proctitis have been considered to differ from those patients whose colons are the site of disease, although the appearance of the lesions in the rectum via proctoscopy and on microscopic inspection via biopsy cannot be distinguished. It is generally agreed that the course of the disease is definitely milder, systemic symptoms being absent, and response to local therapeutic measures more gratifying, but recent follow-up studies suggest that these patients have the same familial aggregates of colitis, similar age and sex distribution, and similar types and degrees of personality maladjustments. It is the feeling of most authorities in the field that at least 10 per cent of these patients will develop the complete clinical picture of ulcerative colitis.

Acute ulcerative colitis is the term given to an acutely developing pancolitis, characterized by toxicity, fever, abdominal pain, distention, and tenesmus. The sigmoidoscopic picture shows uniform involvement for the length of the instrument (25 cm); the mucosa bleeds easily and is covered by a purulent exudate full of neutrophils and eosinophils. When the rectum and rectosigmoid are both involved maximally, as is most frequently the case, diarrhea and tenesmus are usually present, and the sigmoidoscopic appearance is similar throughout. The muscular contractions of the sigmoid make sigmoidoscopy above 13 cm difficult to perform; ulcerations are usually quite evident under the exudate one swabs away, and friability is extreme.

As a general rule, the larger the area of involvement, the greater the systemic toxicity, the more diffuse the cramps, and the more abnormal the stools. Exceptions are not rare, however; *an ulcerative pancolitis* from the ileocecal valve to the anus, demonstrable by barium enema in terms of innumerable ulcerations, spasm, and contraction, may rarely be accompanied by little clinical evidence of active inflammation; conversely, some patients are prostrated despite the involvement of only a few inches of colon in a segmental or regional colitic process.

The clinical course is sometimes used as the basis for classification of this disease, but this is, naturally, not known when the patient is first seen. The only rationale for this is to characterize those few unfortunate patients who suffer from *fulminant ulcerative colitis;* in these the disease is maximal at its onset, and literally overwhelms the patient with the dissolution of his colon, massive colonic hemorrhage, or generalized sepsis. Such patients, accounting for perhaps 1 per cent of all cases of the disease, either die within 1 to 8 weeks of the onset or survive emergency colectomy and ileostomy.

Chronic Intermittent Colitis. The course of the disease is unpredictable, but the majority of patients have a chronic intermittent colitis once the initial episode has been weathered. As described above, of this group the majority presents with disease localized in the descending colon and rectum; no evidences of toxicity may ever be noted, and blood on the stool, rectal urgency, and the characteristic proctoscopic findings may constitute all the evidence of disease. For *most* patients the initial bout is accompanied by fever, malaise, anorexia, and weight loss; the stools contain blood before they become unformed. Cramping abdominal pain aggravated by eating, severe urgency, and tenesmus are more prominent than nausea and vomiting. If properly managed medically, such patients undergo a slow subsidence of symptoms over a period of weeks or months; usually a definite remission of months or years ensues before another exacerbation comes on to plague them. The recurrences may be as severe or more severe than the original bout and may follow an upper respiratory infection or an emotional upset. The succession of remissions and exacerbations over the years often results in a prematurely aged appearance of the patient, in the production of damage to other organ systems, in conditioned malnutrition, and in severe depression. Specific complications are considered below.

About 10 per cent of all severe cases have a *segmental* or *regional colitis* in which the disease is confined to an area above the rectosigmoid, the sigmoidoscopy being normal or minimally abnormal.

Ileocolitis. Ulcerative colitis may predominantly involve the ascending colon, as a form of "regional colitis"; occasionally it will also invade the terminal ileum to produce an ileocolitis in which the primary pathologic lesion is that of ulcerative colitis, i.e., thinning of the submucosa, ulceration of the mucosa, and dilatation of the lumen. On the other hand, as noted in Chap. 275, regional enteritis may involve the ascending colon, the pathologic lesion being identical in both organs, i.e., hypertrophy of the submucosa, minimal ulceration, narrowing of the lumen, and enlarged mesenteric nodes. An acute form of ulcerative colitis involving ileum and ascending colon has been described.

If the ileum and ascending colon are ulcerated and thinned, there may be abnormal motor and absorptive function of the ileum, with production of steatorrhea. A few of these cases have severe systemic complications and are more prone to hepatic abnormalities. Pseudopolyposis is less frequent than in other forms of ulcerative colitis.

Psychologic Features. The psychologic features of patients with ulcerative colitis, although largely ignored in the medical literature prior to 1932, have enlisted intense interest in recent years. It is probably correct to say that a larger proportion of patients with ulcerative colitis resemble each other psychologically, and even physically, than is the case with many other chronic disorders. The patients who fall into this category are juvenile in appearance, hostile and depressed, guarded in their relationships with physicians, and very easily wounded by verbal and attitudinal disparagement. They seem to maintain their interpersonal contacts only by devious and tenuous means, erecting a system of interdependent relationships which seem preposterous to the physician and disheartening to the psychiatrist. On the other hand, nearly half the patients with this disorder cannot be distinguished from the general population; these subjects have a resilient personal and work history, often have been successful at school, trade, or profession, have maintained strong interpersonal attractions and defenses, and to the careful historian present many facets of character which provide clear guides to proper supportive psychotherapy. The disease itself, however, with its chronicity, relapses, and remissions and cost in time and money, usually, is associated in all patients with some degree of depression and anxiety, and these reactions influence both the course of the disease and its therapy.

Laboratory Studies. These comprise radiologic, chemical, and bacteriologic techniques. Sigmoidoscopy usually makes the diagnosis, but the barium enema is employed to determine the extent of the lesions above the reach of that instrument, to identify regional or segmental disease when the sigmoidoscopy is negative, and to follow the course of the disease and detect the presence of complications. No formal preparations are needed before sigmoidoscoping a patient with ulcerative colitis; for the barium enema any preparation more violent than a low-pressure warm saline enema is best avoided. It is important to obtain good delineation of mucosal relief by the barium enema; air-contrast studies are helpful if the patient is not too spastic

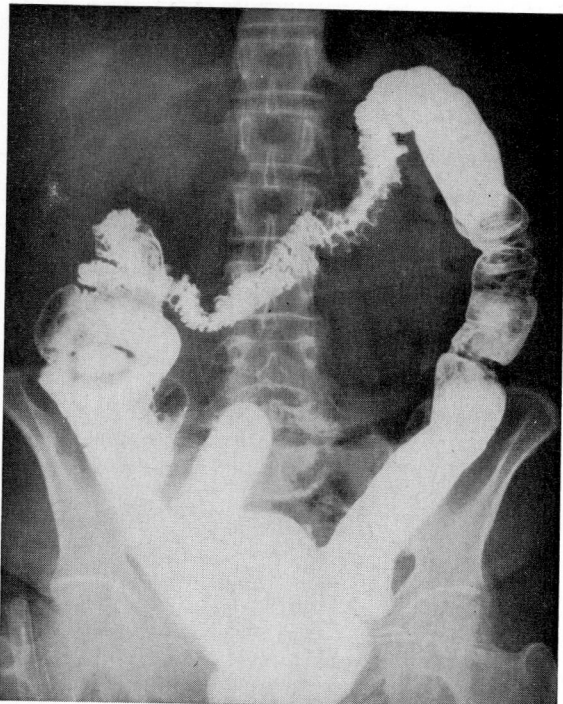

FIG. 278-5. Regional colitis (early) of the transverse colon.

to prevent a successful visualization of pseudopolyps and other abnormalities often overlooked in the routine examination.

The radiologic findings in the disease may bear little relationship to the clinical severity or course of the patient (Fig. 278-5). Characteristically, in early ulcerative colitis irritability of the rectosigmoid is combined with demonstrations of hairline projections of barium from the wall of this spastic area; more irregular serrations and even flask-shaped ulcerations may be seen as the disease progresses. The entire colon is abnormal on barium examination in a large number of patients, even though their symptoms may be minimal or confined to the rectosigmoid. In patients with fulminant colitis, or in aged persons who display rather marked lack of resistance to the process, the entire colon may be dilated—so-called "toxic megacolon." In long-standing disease the entire organ may appear contracted, irregular, with a totally disorganized mucosal pattern. Pseudopolyps, which may occasionally be visualized sigmoidoscopically, more often are in the descending and transverse colon and seen only in the barium enema (Fig. 278-6). The terminal ileum may be involved in an ulcerative process which renders it dilated and patulous in contrast to the constricted lumen noted in regional enteritis. Localized masses may be fecaliths,

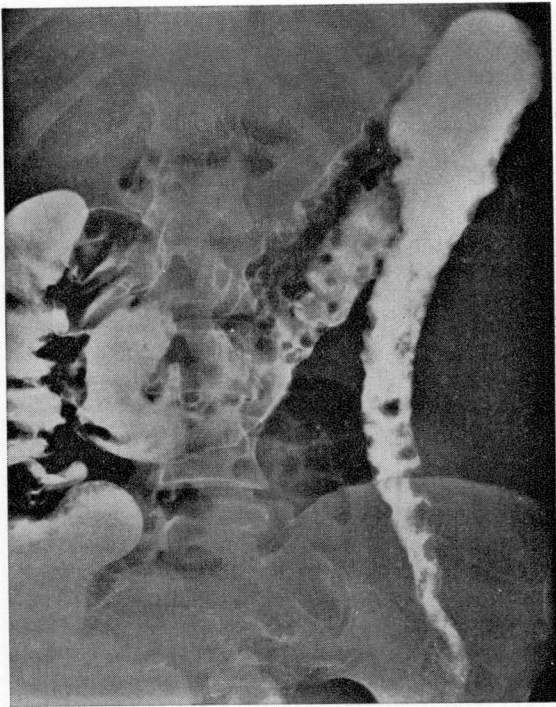

FIG. 278-6. Pseudopolyposis of the entire colon secondary to chronic ulcerative colitis of 12 years' duration.

localized constrictions, or carcinoma of the colon, a recognized complication of this disorder. When the right side of the colon and the terminal ileum bear the brunt of the disease process, a small intestinal barium series is mandatory to investigate the jejunoileal area.

Chronic intermittent forms of colitis are identified primarily by history and radiologic abnormalities, as above described. On sigmoidoscopy these patients usually show at all times the scars of their disease, presenting an abnormal mucous membrane which bleeds very easily, has lost its normal vascular patterns, and may vary in consistency from an edematous beefy involvement of superficial submucosa and mucosa to a leathery violaceous colonic wall, studded with scar tissue and pseudopolyps. Characteristically there is a fibrinopurulent exudate present, and broad flat ulcerations may be seen. Biopsies in this stage usually reveal areas of granulation tissue, containing very few crypts; the lamina propria is thickened and infiltrated with plasma cells and lymphocytes. Small blood vessels are prominent.

Strictures of the rectum are frequent in the long-standing case, being encountered just inside the anus or about midrectum. Perianal suppurative processes are common; both perirectal abscesses and fistula in ano derive from the prolonged suppurative involvement of the rectosigmoid.

Differential Diagnosis. This includes the following entities: Specific colonic infections are identified by culture and examination of the stools or rectal exudate and by sigmoidoscopic appearance. *Amebic disease* characteristically presents as deep ulcerations in an otherwise nearly normal mucosa, which is not friable or granular. Swabs or biopsies from the edges of these ulcers give a good yield of the trophozoites of *Endamoeba histolytica;* the exudate contains few neutrophils but much frank blood. *Bacillary dysentery* can present as an acute ulcerative colitis; the exudate is very rich in neutrophils, but friability is not striking in the rectum. Cultural identification of the organisms makes the diagnosis. *Tuberculosis* involves the cecum and ileum; if ulcerative it is usually associated with active pulmonary tuberculosis; if hyperplastic it produces obstructive symptoms rather than bloody diarrhea, and the sigmoidoscopy is negative. *Lymphogranuloma venereum* can rarely produce a mild acute colitis, but under such circumstances the venereal characteristics of the disease are prominent. The proctitis associated with the long-standing case is secondary to chronic lymphadenitis; it is thus more common in women and associated with rectal stricture, usually just inside the anus; the blood shows hyperglobulinemia, and the skin gives a positive reaction to the Frei antigen.

Nonspecific involvement of the colon may be produced by *regional enteritis*, in which case the colon is infiltrated by a hyperplastic submucosal granulomatous process, friability of mucous membrane is absent, and small intestinal disease is identified by radiologic examination. The *uremic patient* may have a bloody rectal or colonic discharge, because of the vascular fragility produced by that condition; there is little difficulty in identifying the accompanying stigmas of uremia. *Diverticulitis* of the sigmoid may cause spasm, fever, and rectal bleeding, but the sigmoidoscopic appearance is entirely unlike that of ulcerative colitis, and the exudate usually is much less purulent. A segmental colitis localized to the rectosigmoid may, however, be impossible to differentiate from this disorder. Cancer of the colon may give many of the symptoms of colitis, but usually is easy to distinguish from it. However, cancer of the colon supervening on a chronic colitis may be impossible to identify short of surgical biopsy, and rarely a mild ulcerative colitis seems to occur proximal and secondary to a slowly obstructing carcinoma of the left colon.

Complications, Sequelae, and Associated Disorders. These may be *local:* perianal abscesses, fistulas in ano, strictures, sealed-off perforations, pseudopolyposis, localized peritonitis, and carcinomatous changes; if one excludes those patients presenting ulcerative proctitis alone, the incidence of carcinoma of the colon in patients with chronic ulcerative colitis is 3 to 5 per cent, or an incidence 40 to 50 times that of the general population. Or they may be *systemic*: patients with colitis may have all their disease confined to the colon or may exhibit a wide range of symptoms and signs, suggesting that many distant organ systems reflect to some degree the underlying inflammation. Such occurrences are considered evidence of an underlying systemic hyperimmune response of patients with this disorder. The most important of these is arthritis, particularly of the large joints in both sexes, and the spine in men. The symptoms primarily are those of periarthritis; rheumatoid factor is absent from the serum, and the severity of the process usually parallels that of the colitis. The skin shows a number of abnormalities, usually forms of erythema nodosum, erythema multiforme, and rarely, the very dangerous pyoderma gangrenosum. The eyes may be the seat of chorioretinitis or iridocyclitis; thrombophlebitis may be present in a migratory form, and endocrine abnormalities, particularly amenorrhea, are common. It is thought by some that cirrhosis of the liver is more common in this group of patients than one would expect, and varying degrees of pancreatic fibrosis have also been described. Most of the patients with these complications have had a severe illness, characterized by long periods of malnutrition, have received multiple transfusions and intensive chemotherapeutic regimens, and have suffered severe electrolyte disturbances. Amyloid disease may also complicate the course of patients with long-standing and severe colitis.

Treatment. The treatment of patients with this disease comprises both medical and surgical management. Since there is no truly specific form of therapy, medical regimens of treatment aim to correct nutritional and electrolyte loss, control diarrhea, discourage bacterial invasion, and minister to the psychologic needs of the patient. When fever, anorexia, severe diarrhea, and increasing blood loss are present, hospitalization is necessary, and a very careful watch over daily changes in status must be maintained. The disease is very treacherous in that perforations and massive hemorrhage may occur without warning.

Most ill patients are best treated by parenteral alimentation on admission to a hospital. Complete parenteral supplementation can be achieved for 3 or 4 days, at which time a low residue but highly nutritious regimen is instituted.

Oftentimes it is wise to allow the patient to eat foods he particularly craves. There is no evidence that any articles of food influence the disease, but it is felt that some foods increase diarrhea and abdominal gaseousness. Small frequent feedings are usually better tolerated than larger meals, but this is not always the case. It is best not to give very cold liquids, which stimulate small bowel propulsive activity. Vitamin preparations should be added to both the parenteral and oral intakes; preparations containing fat-soluble vitamins dispersed in watery vehicles are preferred to capsules or tablets. Blood transfusions should be given for anemia and hypoproteinemia. Anabolic steroid preparations are often useful (testosterone propionate in men, 25 mg two to three times weekly; norethandrolone, 30 mg daily).

The diarrhea is most effectively controlled by opiates; laudanum is the most convenient preparation, 8 to 10 drops four or five times daily usually sufficing to make the patient comfortable during the phase of intense discomfort. Antispasmodics have the disadvantage of producing upper intestinal hypomotility without greatly affecting the colon and are therefore not very useful in acutely ill patients. As toxicity abates, the opiates are reduced in dosage and sedatives plus antispasmodics are more vigorously employed.

Chemotherapeutic and antibiotic drugs are very useful in managing certain stages and complications of ulcerative colitis. In milder forms of colitis, wherein high fever and toxicity are not prominent, salicylazosulfapyridine (Azulfidine) (1.0 Gm six times a day) has been proved able to control friability and bleeding and to lessen markedly the rectosigmoid irritability responsible for urgency and tenesmus. It can be given in courses lasting 3 to 6 weeks, followed by intervals of several months, then reinstituted as a prophylactic; many patients do very well on such a regimen, taking the drug for one month out of every four for many years. In the acutely ill patient in the hospital, penicillin and chloramphenicol are usually administered concomitantly in an attempt to halt or prevent acute peritonitis. Other sulfonamide drugs and broad-spectrum antibiotics, although not without usefulness, have been less specific than those described.

Adrenal steroid hormones and ACTH have become very important in the medical management of ulcerative colitis. For acute proctitis and proctosigmoiditis, where urgency is very severe despite the absence of generalized illness, rectal instillations of soluble corticosteroids have been remarkably effective. They are usually given as retention enemas of small volume (100 ml of an aqueous solution containing 20 mg prednisolone) morning and at night until symptoms have been brought under control; then only the nightly instillation is continued, the frequency of administration gradually diminishing. In the acutely ill patient with life-threatening colitis, parenteral administration of ACTH (40 to 80 mg daily) for a 10-day period usually effects an improvement in appetite, a decrease in toxicity, and a gradual improvement in sigmoidoscopic appearance of the involved bowel. Cortisone, hydrocortisone, or prednisolone in adequate doses may produce similar effects in the acutely ill patient, but seem rather less reliable than ACTH. On the other hand, in the less severely toxic patient, or in the toxic patient as he recovers, oral steroids are easy to administer and are quite effective. Many patients have now been maintained for years on oral doses of these hormones, either alone or combined with Azulfidine, with a low incidence of complications of therapy. The hormones are also useful in preparing patients for colectomy.

Psychiatric approaches to the patient with ulcerative colitis are not generally agreed upon. It is the opinion of most psychiatrists that the acutely ill patient is approachable only by the most superficial forms of supportive psychotherapy. In the more usual types of the disease the physician managing the case can supply the needed support by searching the patient's history and behavior for indications of inner resources and motivations which can be converted to therapeutic use. Attempts to manipulate the immediate home and work environment of the patient are necessary, but may require professional assistance beyond the scope of the physician's training and resources. Pregnancy frequently mobilizes severe stress and can aggravate or ameliorate the disease. When ulcerative colitis begins during pregnancy it is usually very severe.

Professional psychiatric assistance should not be neglected when indicated. An attitude of optimism, warm concern, and patience, tempered with frequent medical examinations of the patient, his rectum, and his stools seems the best armamentarium of the physician caring for patients suffering from this disorder.

Surgical measures are absolutely indicated for several local complications and for certain catastrophic events which may complicate the course of the disease. In the presence of a diseased colon it is almost impossible to heal perianal and perirectal abscesses, fistulas, and rectal strictures. Furthermore, it is not possible to make use of a rectum deformed by these processes after localized lesions of the colon have been resected, so that ileostomy and total colectomy are the treatment of choice. Similarly, massive hemorrhage from the diseased bowel and acute toxic dilatation of the colon are best handled as emergencies by ileostomy and colectomy. Segmental colitis can be successfully treated by resection of the diseased portion and primary anastomosis.

The principal areas of disagreement as to the proper time for or advisability of surgical therapy concern patients with chronic recurrent disease of more than 2 years' duration and those who are dis-

abled by chronic anemia, arthritis, or pseudopolyposis. Increasingly, and in particular as surgical techniques for ileostomy and colectomy have improved, more of these patients are being subjected to this treatment earlier in the course of their disease. Attempts to preserve the rectal area by ileorectal anastomosis and the French techniques for electrocoagulative prefrontal lobotomy are new but as yet unproved methods to modify the surgical approach. Any patient with ulcerative colitis of 10 years' activity must be considered to have a 3 to 5 per cent risk of malignancy of the colon; the presence of pseudopolyposis or the slightly less common adenomatous polyposis complicating the disease is probably an indication for colectomy. The ileostomized patient has now a much better outlook for a normal life than ever before; the formation of ileostomist clubs has stimulated interest in the intelligent design and management of ileostomy appliances; reanastomosis of the ileum to partially resected colons has proved so often disastrous that it is better to offer the patient no unrealizable picture of the ileostomy as a temporary measure, but rather to concentrate his attention on the fuller life he will be able to lead with his diseased bowel totally removed.

Summary. Ulcerative colitis is, then, a progressive inflammatory disease of the colon, encountered in all age groups, affecting any portion or all of the large bowel. About 75 to 80 per cent of all patients with the disease will be able to cope medically with its ravages, despite the remissions and exacerbations which characterize its course. There is some evidence that the disease is more severe when its onset is in young children or in those over sixty. The case fatality rate is hard to determine, since so many patients with ulcerative proctitis alone never come into hospitals, but for those ill enough to warrant hospitalization, approximately 10 per cent now die of the disease or its complications, including carcinoma of the colon. Surgery at present is necessary for approximately 20 per cent of patients with the disease involving more than the rectum. Unless some newer medical or psychiatric therapy is devised, it is probable that this figure will increase.

TUMORS OF THE COLON AND RECTUM

In 1958, neoplasms of the large intestine and rectum accounted for 38,000 deaths in the United States, or 15 per cent of all deaths due to malignant disease. These lesions represented 42 per cent of all deaths due to neoplasms of the digestive tract, being nearly twice as frequent as the number of deaths due to cancer of the stomach. They occur equally among males and females, and in all age groups, but of course are most frequently encountered in persons forty-five to seventy-five years of age.

Etiology. Although the true causes of colonic malignancy are not established, there appears to be an intimate relation between the adenomatous polyp and the development of carcinoma. All stages of carcinomatous change have been recognized in polyps, and there appears to be a definite risk of malignant polypoid growth and of malignancy in the colons of patients who have polyps, whether or not the tumor originates in or near the polyps. Congenital multiple polyposis of the colon has an astonishingly high malignant potential; chronic inflammatory disease of the colon, as seen in ulcerative colitis, also seems to potentiate or stimulate the development of carcinoma in the diseased bowel. Other lesions of the large intestine seem to bear no relationship to cancer, although in no case is it possible to demonstrate that they offer protection against its development. As with malignant disease generally, familial aggregates of the disease are well documented, and multiple malignancies have been shown to occur in certain members of such families.

Pathology. The vast majority of tumors originating in the colon and rectum are of epithelial origin. Those which are not are usually benign; they include lipomas, endometriosis, benign lymphomas, leiomyomas, enterocytomas, and hemangiomas. Nonepithelial malignant lesions are infrequent, but should be mentioned because of the necessity for recognizing them in a treatable stage of their development. *Carcinoids* of the rectosigmoid and rectum ordinarily form yellowish elevations between the muscularis mucosae and mucosa; they are usually discovered by chance sigmoidoscopy, although a few have been indicted as causing bleeding. If the muscularis is invaded, the tumor is malignant and will require wide excision. It is estimated that 10 per cent of rectal carcinoids will metastasize. Those beginning in the ileocecal valve or in the cecum, although not ulcerating deeply, metastasize early to regional nodes and the liver; radiologically they may present as a rounded filling defect. *Leiomyosarcomas* are almost never found elsewhere in the colon than in the sigmoid or rectum, where they may grow to large size and produce mucosal ulceration with bleeding. *Lymphosarcomas* of the colon and rectum may present exactly as do carcinomas, but there is less fixation of the wall as the tumor grows, so that intussusception is occasionally the presenting syndrome.

Carcinoma of the colon and rectum together account for 15 per cent of all carcinomas, and for approximately 50 per cent of all digestive tract cancers. Colon carcinomas affect women more often than men, whereas rectal carcinomas are seen more commonly in men. They have been re-corded at all ages, but with their peak incidence in the fifth, sixth, and seventh decades. The cecum and ascending colon are involved in 15 per cent of all carcinomas of the large bowel and rectum, the transverse colon in 10 per cent, and the sigmoid colon, rectosigmoid, and rectum in 75 per cent. Thus, nearly two-thirds of all cancers of the large intestine are within reach of the sigmoidoscope. In most series of cases, multiple primary colonic cancers are found in about 3 per cent of operated or autopsied patients. Lesions of the colon which seem statistically to favor the development of carcinoma are multiple polyposis, adenomatous polyposis, and chronic ulcerative colitis of over 10 years' duration. In addition to the statistical "precancerousness" of these lesions, indubitable malignant transformation of villous adenomas, single adenomatous polyps, multiple adenomatous polyps, and multicentric foci in ulcerative colitis have been observed.

In the colon above the rectum, adenocarcinoma is the common cell type. Classifications of the tumors according to their microscopic appearance —papillary, medullary, scirrhous, or colloid—is not of great assistance to the physician. Obviously, scirrhous carcinomas tend to constrict the lumen of the bowel, thereby producing obstructive syndromes, especially in the sigmoid area. Colloid tumors, most common in the right colon, can grow to enormous bulky mucinous masses, often forming mucous fistulas to the overlying skin. The common medullary tumor grows as a solid mass, the bulk of which may produce intermittent obstructive symptoms. Papillary tumors of the distal colon usually bleed early. All these tumors invade the regional lymph nodes and spread through the lymphatics and portal veins to the liver; direct spread into the paravertebral venous plexus is occasionally seen.

Symptoms of colonic carcinoma are usually vague and nonspecific at the outset. Rarely an acute perforation with peritonitis or a massive hemorrhage will call attention to the disease while it is still in an early stage, but much more often many months elapse before the symptoms finally bring the patient to the physician.

1. Changes in bowel habits are most frequent when carcinoma affects the left colon; these changes are often minimal but progressive alterations in frequency or in time of evacuation, in the size of the stool, and most significantly, in a sensation that evacuation has been incomplete.

2. Bleeding is complained of by the patient with a left-sided lesion in about 70 per cent of cases; when the lesion is in the ascending colon or cecum, less than 25 per cent of patients notice any blood in or with the stools, owing no doubt to the fact that the blood is thoroughly admixed with the fecal

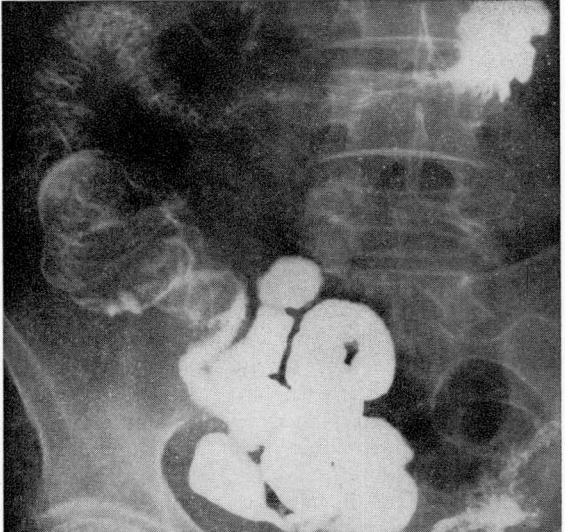

FIG. 278-7. Filling defect in the cecum produced by a carcinoma.

slurry in the right colon. It is urgently important that the physician *not* attribute to hemorrhoids or anal fissures bleeding that is dark, associated with clots, well-mixed with mucus, or adherent to the stool.

3. Pain in the lower abdomen is common in lesions of the cecum or ascending colon; the pain is characteristically severe on climbing stairs or on bending forward; pain in left colonic lesions is often felt in the right side as a vague distention, or as a dragging sensation low in the pelvis toward the left inguinal ligament. Low-back pain is frequently present later in the course of the disease.

4. Pallor and anemia are classical presenting syndromes of right-sided colonic cancer; cardiac insufficiency and angina may be striking manifestations of the anemia, which reaches a remarkably severe degree in the absence of symptoms calling attention to the diseased bowel.

5. Anorexia, weight loss, and malaise may occur at any time or be absent.

Physical Examination. As with most malignancies, early signs are not found. Aside from the characteristic pallor of anemia and the wasting suggestive of chronic disease, the signs are principally those due to masses, partial obstruction of the bowel, fistulas, and invasion of abdominal wall, bladder, uterus, and liver. Fecal masses are often felt behind partially obstructing neoplasms or inflammatory aggregates which have surrounded a perforation due to tumor. Rectal examination with the patient in the lithotomy or right decubitus position will often detect an intussuscepting lesion of the rectosigmoid. Marked distention in the right

lower quadrant may represent an accommodation of bowel contents to incomplete obstruction by carcinoma of the left colon; caution should be exercised in palpating the cecal area under such circumstances, as perforation, always imminent, may be precipitated by digital manipulation either from the abdominal or intrarectal areas.

Laboratory Findings. There are no diagnostic laboratory procedures. Detection of occult blood or gross blood in the stools is the most important laboratory technique for early identification of the possibility that malignancy of the colon exists. Other findings occur as the tumor spreads locally to provoke an inflammatory response (increased sedimentation rate, leukocytosis), invasion of the liver (increased serum alkaline phosphatase, Bromsulphalein retention), hemolytic anemia, or direct bone marrow invasion. The anemia is usually hypochromic and is present in over half the patients with right-sided lesions, even when occasional stool specimens do not contain occult blood. Patients with left-sided lesions may also be anemic, but to a much less severe degree, and not so frequently, since their blood loss is more easily appreciated in the appearance of the stools, and they see physicians earlier.

Diagnosis. Carcinoma of the colon is one of the commonest malignancies and therefore must be thought of whenever a patient complains of changes in bowel habits, regardless of the kind of change. The finding of gross or occult blood in the stools, or of a mass or distended colon on routine physical examination, or of definite abnormalities on rectal examination, or of evidences of weight loss and chronic illness should make one consider the diagnosis very seriously. Vague dyspeptic symptoms, especially when hypochromic anemia is present, also should lead the physician to investigate the right colon in particular.

The combination of digital and proctosigmoidoscopic examination should bring two-thirds of all cancers of the colon and rectum into direct view. The lesion may present itself directly as a polypoid or solid mass, frequently ulcerated, or as a large ulcer with a rolled margin, or as a deformity of the colonic wall producing obstruction to the passage of the instrument. Instillation of Ringer's solution through the sigmoidoscope and centrifugation of the returning fluid will yield exfoliative cytologic smears of diagnostic value in many cases. Biopsy of suspicious lesions should be carried out whenever possible.

Radiologic diagnosis of lesions above the peritoneal reflection is highly accurate, but not infallible. In the presence of rectal bleeding it is important to follow a barium enema which has been reported as normal with an air-contrast study; such air-contrast enemas may reveal small lesions (greater than 5 mm in diameter) as well as non-distensible portions of the bowel wall. A cecal area which does not respond satisfactorily to preparative enemas and laxatives and shows poor radiologic detail should be particularly suspected of harboring a tumor.

The radiologist looks for structural and physiologic abnormalities reflecting the various ways these tumors may present, as described above under Pathology. (1) Tumors may project into the bowel, giving rise to a filling defect in the barium column (Fig. 278-7). (2) They may partially or completely encircle the bowel, producing a narrowing of the barium column proximal to which the bowel is often dilated (Fig. 278-8). (3) They may, by contiguous infiltration, distort the position of the colon, so that it is not free to follow gravity during the radiologist's maneuvering of the patient. (4) After the patient has expelled the barium, films of the mucosal relief may show defects due to tumor which has not penetrated the muscular coat. (5) Some tumors give rise to no defects as such, but interfere with neuromuscular integration, so that irritability, fluid retention, and spasticity may be noted.

Differential diagnosis of carcinoma of the ascending colon includes: (1) benign lesions: gastric and duodenal ulcer, cholecystitis and cholelithiasis, liver disease; (2) inflammatory processes: appendiceal abscess, amebiasis, regional enteritis, segmental colitis, tuberculosis; (3) other tumors, such as carcinoids, lymphomas, lipomas, gastric cancer, renal cancer; (4) blood dyscrasias and uremia. In the descending colon carcinomas must be distinguished from diverticulitis, endometriosis, ulcerative colitis, lymphogranuloma venereum, and benign tumors.

Carcinoma of the rectum and anus presents more specific early symptomatology than is the case with the lesions discussed above. Bleeding, intolerable rectal urgency, pain, and soiling are the most frequent symptoms. The principal difficulty occurs when preexisting abnormalities have been present for so long a time that the patient and his physician do not detect subtle changes in them. Most frequently such problems arise when the patient has had an irritable colon syndrome, ulcerative colitis, simple constipation, or a variety of anorectal disorders, often complicated by surgery.

These carcinomas are more frequent in men than in women (5:4) and comprise both adenocarcinoma in the rectum and squamous carcinoma in the anal skin, as well as mixed tumors in the anal canal. Malignant melanoma and basal-cell carcinoma may arise in the anal skin, and lymphoma, carcinoids, tumors arising from neighboring structures—prostate, cervix, ovary—as well as the seeding of upper abdominal carcinoma into the pelvic peritoneum

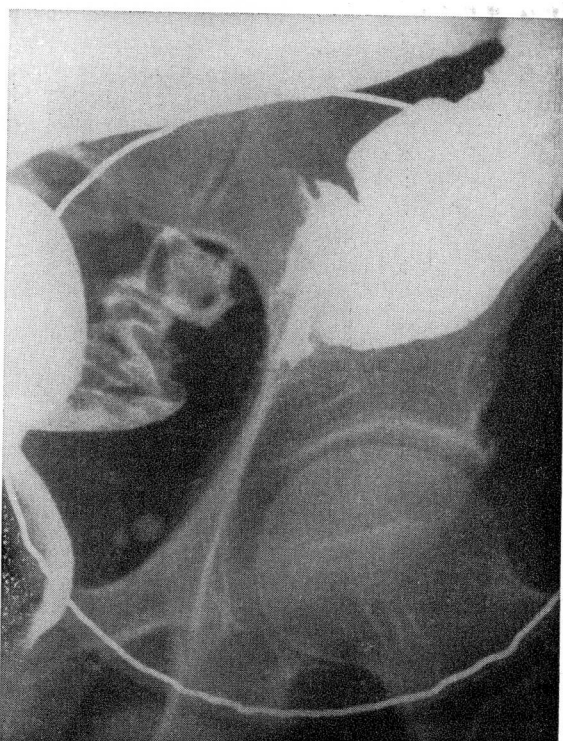

FIG. 278-8. Obstructing carcinoma of the sigmoid.

may present as though they were primary lesions of the rectum.

Diagnosis is made by inspection, digital examination, anoscopy, proctoscopy, biopsy, and exfoliative cytology. Radiologic accuracy in the rectum is only fair and should not be necessary for identification of these low lesions.

Complications. Since it is the character of tumors to invade, many tumors of the colon, like tumors elsewhere, may first be diagnosed because of a complication of the original lesion; that is, the tumor may perforate the bowel wall giving rise to acute peritonitis, may perforate slowly and wall itself off, giving rise to local inflammatory mass and localized peritonitis, or may invade blood vessels to produce a brisk episode of rectal bleeding. More often, the tumor partially obstructs the bowel lumen for a long period of time, during which the colon proximal to the tumor dilates slowly without dramatic change in symptoms until a fecal impaction occurs, converting the proximal bowel into a large distended sac which may very well produce symptoms in the right lower quadrant, as noted previously. This occurs most often when the tumor is in the sigmoid, where the stool is driest. Tumors also weaken the colonic wall in such a way that an intussusception may occur, the tumor leading the intussusceptum. Similarly, fixation of the bowel wall by a tumor may produce a volvulus, which is most frequently seen in the sigmoid colon. Very large and slowly growing tumors may produce symptoms by pressure on neighboring organs; in particular, the uterus and the ureters may be involved, and conversely, tumors of the uterus may compress the colon. Inguinal hernias may become apparent as the first sign of such increased pressure. Fistulas between the colon and pelvic organs suggest a thorough search for an underlying neoplastic infiltration. Abscesses inside the peritoneal cavity and cellulitis of the abdominal wall secondary to tumor infiltration are not infrequent.

Treatment. Although the only readily available therapeutic techniques are surgical, there are indications that radiotherapy combined with surgery and some new chemotherapeutic means may significantly improve the outlook for patients with colonic and rectal cancer. Surgeons generally prefer abdominoperitoneal resection and colostomy for tumors located below the peritoneal reflections; above this area there is considerably more freedom of choice, depending primarily on the size and extent of the lesions. It is important to realize that good preoperative management and skillful work at the table will ensure that 70 to 80 per cent of all cases can receive either extirpative or palliative surgery with an operative mortality under 10 per cent; the operative mortality is somewhat higher for lesions in the left colon. On the other hand, the survival rate for tumors of the left colon which can be resected is slightly higher than that for right colon cancers. There has been an impressive improvement in the 5-year survivals since 1930; in 1960 approximately half of all patients who can be resected are expected to survive this length of time. Of the 20 to 30 per cent who are first seen with extensive lymphatic or perineural spread, a few will survive 5 years without surgery. When patients without any evidence of lymphatic or distant spread of cancer are subjected to radical operations, the 5-year survival in some series has been as high as 80 per cent. It is important that palliative surgical attempts not be discouraged, as the symptomatic relief they bring may allow the patient to live in comfort the shortened terminal months of his life.

The complications of surgery and the management of colostomies can best be found discussed in surgical texts.

OBSTRUCTION OF THE COLON AND RECTUM

Chronic colonic obstruction has been dealt with above in the sections dealing with its principal causes—tumors, diverticulitis, and megacolon. Additional disorders which may present as chronic large bowel obstruction are strictures resulting from inflammatory processes (ulcerative colitis, lymphogranuloma venereum, perirectal abscesses), from pelvic disease (endometriosis, tumors), from traumatic scarring either postoperative or crushing, or from radiation necrosis, secondary to treatment of pelvic cancer.

The presenting symptoms in all cases are similar, the diagnosis is made clinically and radiologically, and the treatment is surgical.

Acute colonic obstruction has been discussed briefly in Chap. 276. Whereas acute small bowel obstruction is more often due to mechanical and vascular causes, colonic obstruction occurring suddenly is statistically most often a result of neoplastic disease; other major causes of this process in adults are volvulus, diverticulitis, and intussusception.

Volvulus is a twisting of a portion of the colon on its mesentery, with trapping of air in the affected segment and progressive circulatory embarrassment as a result of the compression of the vascular pedicle to the segment. The two areas of colon most subject to this complication are the cecum and the sigmoid. *Cecal volvulus* is due to abnormal fixation of the cecum, associated with malrotation of the right colon. Severe volvulus of the cecum is uncommon except in Sweden; in the United States it accounts for less than 0.2 per cent of all adult intestinal obstruction. Minor degrees of volvulus leading to recurrent right lower quadrant pain may be more common since it is thought that 10 to 15 per cent of the population have right colons sufficiently mobile to permit at least some degree of volvulus. The *symptoms* of acute cecal volvulus are severe, continuous right lower quadrant abdominal pain, followed by vomiting, constipation, and rapid intestinal distention. Treatment is surgical.

Sigmoid volvulus is more common than cecal volvulus and is especially common among persons of eastern European ancestry. It is predominantly a disease of elderly persons with chronic constipation who eat food containing much roughage. The symptoms are usually those of increasing constipation for a few days preceding the first attack of hypogastric pain; this pain is usually colicky and discontinuous for a few hours, but then becomes more severe and unremitting, as vascular supply to the twisted loop is throttled. The twisted loop enlarges enormously, rising up in the midline of the lower abdomen to produce the characteristic radiologic picture (Fig. 278-9). In contrast to acute small bowel obstruction, vomiting is rarely encountered; shock is generally absent unless gangrene and perforation of the loop have supervened.

Treatment is decompression. Although occasionally this can be done by a tube inserted via the sigmoidoscope, most of these patients require laparotomy, with decompression under direct vision, and whatever other extirpative surgical means are deemed necessary. Since sigmoid volvulus is known to recur in the same patient, it is probably wisest to resect the entire twisted loop at the time of operation.

Intussusception is the term applied to the invagination of one segment of intestine into another. *Primary intussusception,* which occurs without antecedent cause, is rarely seen after the third year of life; in infants it is a common cause of rectal bleeding. *Secondary intussusception* is seen at all ages and anywhere in the gut, from esophagogastric junction to rectum. It usually occurs when an intraluminal neoplasm, benign or malignant, bulges out into the lumen, often buckling the wall from which it arises, and is propelled caudad by peristaltic activity. The tumor acts as the leading portion of the full thickness of the intestinal wall, producing a partial or complete obstruction to the propulsion of intestinal contents. The doubling over of the entire thickness of the gut wall leads to impairment of blood supply and eventual gangrene.

Symptoms are those of sudden abdominal pain and distention, with passage of blood-tinged rectal discharge. Low-lying intussusceptions may be felt on rectal examination, but usually a careful barium enema reveals the site and the characteristic "coiled-spring" appearance produced when the barium outlines the space between the intussuscepted bowel and the outer intussuscipiens.

Treatment is surgical removal of the underlying abnormality.

Subacute and Chronic Colonic Obstruction

Much more difficult to identify are the insidious forms of subacute obstruction of the large bowel, which usually present as (1) intermittent lower abdominal pain of the colicky type, (2) gradually progressive constipation, (3) distention, or (4) a combination of these. The failure of the patient to complain actively or to appear very ill makes it easy for the physician to overlook the possible cecal twist or the obstructing tumor in the left colon. Very often it is the additional impetus provided by a fecal impaction which converts the vague symptoms into those of a definite closed-loop obstruction, with marked distention of the cecal area; in the elderly patient the distended bowel may rupture and produce an acute peritonitis, treatment of which uncovers the underlying tumor, diverticulitis, or volvulus.

Diagnostic aids consist of abdominal palpation and auscultation, which may identify markedly different patterns during the several days of such an episode, and digital examination, which may disclose an impaction, or an intussuscepting tumor, or blood on the stool. Roentgen examination is important in demonstrating on the open film unusual gas collections which define an obstruction and on

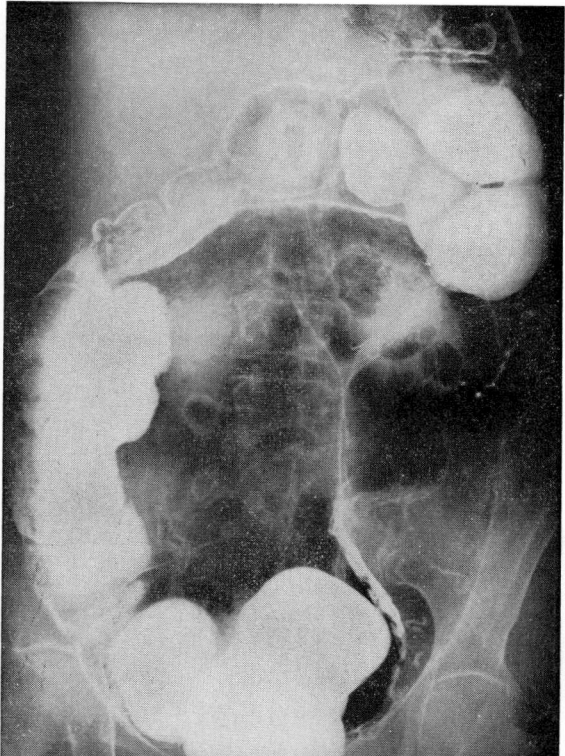

FIG. 278-9. Volvulus of the sigmoid.

the barium enema a definite obstacle to the passage of barium (Fig. 278-10). *Treatment* is that of the underlying lesion and is therefore usually surgical.

ACUTE NECROTIZING (MEMBRANOUS) ENTEROCOLITIS

This severe necrotizing lesion of large and small intestine has been known under a variety of names. It almost always occurs in association with a massive insult to the circulation (myocardial infarction with shock) in the otherwise well patient, in debilitated elderly patients who suffer mechanical trauma or undergo surgery, and more recently in severely ill patients receiving antibiotic therapy.

The pathologic features are those of a coagulative necrosis of the mucosa of the small and large intestine; thrombosed capillaries and venules underlie the necrosis; a pseudomembrane may be present in patchy distribution. Staphylococci may be found in large quantities but are not necessary for the diagnosis.

Symptoms are those of severe shock, accompanied by variable degrees of abdominal distention, high fever, and diarrhea. If the condition follows an operation, it usually occurs between the third and fifth postoperative day. The stools often con-

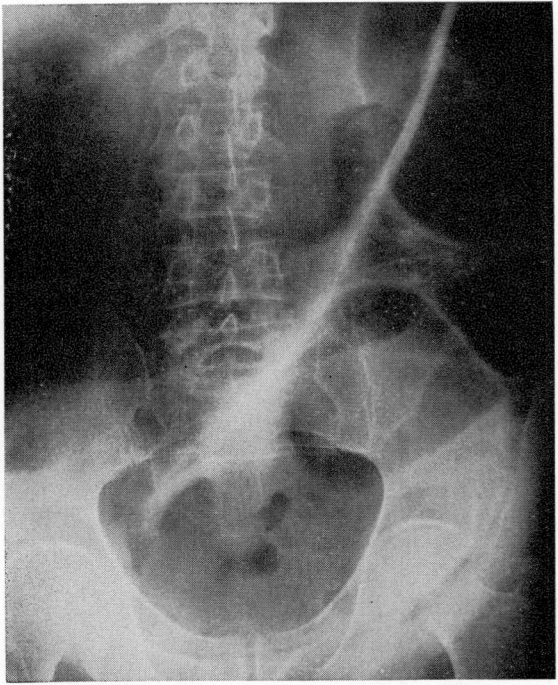

FIG. 278-10. Enormous dilatation of the cecum secondary to sigmoid cancer.

tain whitish collections of exudate and staphylocci; the latter may be cultured by rectal swab if no stool is passed.

Treatment is that of shock, with special emphasis on blood, plasma, and adrenal steroids. If staphylococci are isolated from the stools, erythromycin or vancomycin are given in large doses. If no staphylococci are cultured, most authorities advise the use of polyvalent serum against clostridia. The case fatality rate is extremely high despite these measures, and intensive medical and nursing care is critical.

ANORECTAL PROBLEMS

Complaints centered in this area are among the commonest and most troublesome encountered by the physician. Because of failure to understand the anatomy and function of perianal skin, anal sphincters, lower rectal mucosa, and levator muscles many misdiagnoses are made and therapy based on these misconceptions prolongs or even aggravates the difficulties. There is no way in which the physician can move with assurance in evaluating these complaints unless he learns the anatomy and constantly performs careful and thorough physical examinations directed to an appreciation of the disturbed physiology.

Pruritus Ani

Itching of the perianal skin is a very frequent and usually mild complaint, but it can be so severe and persistent as to deprive the patient of sleep and lead him to thoughts of suicide. The first step in diagnosis is to examine the skin for evidence of a dermatosis, to culture the area, and if necessary to biopsy it. Anoscopic and proctoscopic examinations follow. The most important preventive measure is careful cleansing of fecal residues from the skin. In elderly persons, obese persons, and those with joint difficulties, efficient wiping after defecation is difficult to achieve. Simple cleansing techniques using cotton balls rather than toilet tissue often remove or greatly ameliorate the symptoms. Specific dermatoses, parasitic infestations, folliculitis, and fungous infections may cause the symptom. Drugs taken orally or parenterally rarely produce pruritus ani, but antibiotics may do so, and any ointments or medications applied to the perineal area may give rise to it. Diabetes mellitus, although often responsible for pruritus vulvae, is a rare cause of pruritus ani. Psychogenic pruritus ani is difficult to define, since secondary dermatitis and excoriations often can be greatly improved by conservative palliative methods and better postdefecation hygiene; bland or hydrocortisone ointments are also utilized in the psychotherapy of reported cases.

Fistulas and Abscesses

These septic disorders may be the first signs of primary colitis, enteritis, or diverticulitis, as previously discussed, or may be complications of surgical procedures employed for these or other conditions. *Fistula in ano,* a tract leading from the rectal lumen to the perianal skin, usually results from local anal crypt abscesses; less than 5 per cent of such lesions found in medical practice in the United States are due to tuberculosis or cancer. The fistula is a chronically inflamed tube made up of fibrous tissue surrounding granulation tissue, the lumen of which may be difficult to demonstrate. *Perirectal abscesses* often represent the tracking down into the anal area of purulent material escaping from the rectosigmoid; diverticulitis, enteritis, or colitis may be the source. Previous anal or rectal surgery may be causal. *Fistulas* between the rectum and vagina and between the rectum and bladder represent serious complications of granulomatous, septic, or malignant disorders and require that the patient be hospitalized for definitive diagnostic and therapeutic procedures.

Anal Lesions

These lesions comprise a wide variety of distressing inflammatory, traumatic, and neoplastic disorders. *Anal fissures* represent superficial erosions of the anal canal epithelium which can heal rapidly on conservative therapy. *Anal ulcers* are more chronic and deep and give symptoms largely as the result of painful spasm of the external anal sphincter during and after defecation. Bleeding may occur with either fissure or ulcer; healing of the ulcer often is associated with a hypertrophied anal papilla and some degrees of anal contracture. Crypt abscesses may produce pain early and should be treated promptly.

Hemorrhoids

The internal hemorrhoidal plexus of veins is located in the submucosal space above the valves of Morgagni; the anal canal separates it from the external hemorrhoidal venous plexus, but the two spaces communicate under the anal canal, the submucosa of which is attached to underlying tissue to form the interhemorrhoidal depression. Whenever the internal hemorrhoidal plexus is enlarged, there is associated increase in supporting tissue mass, and the resultant venous swelling is called an internal hemorrhoid. When veins in the external hemorrhoidal plexus become enlarged or thrombosed, the resultant bluish mass is called an external hemorrhoid.

Both types of hemorrhoids are very common and are associated with increased hydrostatic pressure in the portal venous system, characteristically noted during pregnancy, straining at stool, chronic liver disease, and sudden increases of intraabdominal pressure, or with local factors associated with diarrhea, tumors, or incomplete evacuation of feces. When internal hemorrhoids enlarge, pain is not a usual feature until complicated by thrombosis, infection, or erosion of the overlying mucosal surface. Most persons complain of bright red blood on the toilet tissue or coating the stool, with a feeling of vague disquiet about the state of their anus. The discomfort is increased when the hemorrhoidal enlargement becomes great or prolapses through the anus; prolapse is often accompanied by edema and sphincteric spasm. Prolapse if not treated usually becomes chronic as the muscularis stays stretched, and the patient complains of constant soiling of underclothing with very little pain. Prolapsed hemorrhoids may become infected or thrombosed; the overlying mucous membrane may bleed profusely as the result of the trauma of defecation.

External hemorrhoids, lying as they do under the skin, are quite often painful, particularly if there is a sudden increase in their mass. These episodes result in a tender blue swelling at the anal verge due to thrombosis of a vein in the external plexus, and need not be associated with enlargement of the internal veins. Since the thrombus usually lies at the level of the sphincteric muscles, anal spasm often occurs.

The diagnosis of internal and external hemorrhoids is made by inspection, digital examination, and direct vision through the anoscope and proctoscope. Since such lesions are very common, they must not be regarded as the cause of rectal bleeding or chronic hypochromic anemia until a thorough investigation has been made of the more proximal gastrointestinal tract. Acute blood loss to shock levels can more certainly be attributed to internal hemorrhoids seen to be bleeding actively than can lesser degrees of chronic anemia in the presence of large but not definitely bleeding hemorrhoids.

Most hemorrhoids respond to conservative therapy, employing sitz baths or other forms of moist heat, compresses, suppositories, medications to soften the stool, and bed rest. Internal hemorrhoids which remain permanently prolapsed are best treated by surgery; milder degrees of prolapse or enlargement with pruritus ani or intermittent bleeding can be successfully handled by the injection of sclerosing solutions. External hemorrhoids which become acutely thrombosed are treated by incision, extraction of the clot, and compressing the incised area following clot removal. No surgery should be carried out in the presence of acute inflammation of the anus, ulcerative proctitis, or ulcerative colitis, and both proctoscopy and barium enema should always be performed before a patient is subjected to hemorrhoidectomy.

REFERENCES

Brown, D. B., and W. F. Toomey: Diverticular Disease of the Colon, Brit. J. Surg., 47:485, 1960.

Helwig, E. B.: Adenomas and Pathogenesis of Cancer of Colon and Rectum, Diseases Colon and Rectum, 2:5, 1959.

Jackman, R. J.: Lesions of the Lower Bowel, Springfield, Ill., Charles C Thomas, Publisher, 1958.

Jones, F. Avery (Ed.): "Modern Trends in Gastroenterology," 2d series, Chap. 19, Ulcerative Colitis, New York, Paul B. Hoeber, Inc., Medical Department of Harper & Brothers, 1958.

Kay, A. W., R. I. Richards, and A. J. Watson: Acute Necrotizing (Pseudomembranous) Enterocolitis, Brit. J. Surg., 46:45, 1958.

Kirsner, J. B., J. A. Rider, H. C. Moeller, W. L. Palmer, and S. S. Gold: Polyps of the Colon and Rectum, Gastroenterol., 39:178, 1960.

Lockhart-Mummery, H. E., C. E. Dukes, and H. S. R. Bussey: Multiple Congenital Polyposis, Brit. J. Surg., 43:476, 1956.

Swenson, O.: Hirschsprung's Disease (Aganglionic Megacolon), New Engl. J. Med., 260:272, 1959.

The Colon: Its Normal and Abnormal Physiology and Therapeutics, Ann. N.Y. Acad. Sci., July 15, 1954.

Wangensteen, O. (Ed.): "Intestinal Obstructions," 3d ed., Springfield, Ill., Charles C Thomas, Publisher, 1955.

279 DISEASES OF THE PANCREAS

Franz J. Ingelfinger

Symptomatology. The outstanding symptom of pancreatic disease is pain. In addition, pancreatic disorders may produce symptoms by altering the structure and function of any of the following systems: (1) the pancreatic acini and ducts, (2) the islands of Langerhans, (3) the biliary passages, (4) the gastrointestinal tract, (5) the portal circulation, and (6) the lung and pleural cavity on the left.

Pain. The pain of pancreatic disease roughly corresponds in location to the position of the lesion, but its character is capricious and its borders are indeterminate. Presumably made up of both true visceral and referred somatic components, pancreatic pain is felt between the xiphoid and umbilicus in front, and between the tenth thoracic and second lumbar vertebras in back. Frequently it bores through the body from front to back, or vice versa, but superficial radiation along the costal margin is unusual. Because of the central position of the pancreas and its bilateral sensory innervation, pain from a lesion confined to the head or tail tends to be felt centrally, but with increased emphasis to right or left, depending on the position of the lesion.

Abnormalities of External Secretion. The pancreatic juice, amounting approximately to 1,500 ml per day, contains water, bicarbonate (60 to 120 mEq per liter), sodium (140 mEq per liter), potassium (4 mEq per liter), smaller quantities of other ions, and numerous digestive ferments classified under the broad headings of trypsin, amylase (diastase is used as an equivalent term), and lipase. Loss of this entire secretion through an external pancreatic fistula leads to dehydration and electrolyte depletion. In addition, deviation of the pancreatic enzymes from the gut causes a fecal loss of about half the fat and 30 per cent of the protein ingested. Carbohydrate is also digested poorly, but hydrolysis by intestinal bacteria prevents its loss in the feces. Similar absorptive defects follow total pancreatectomy, complete obstruction of the ducts, or extensive destruction of the gland by disease. On the other hand, subtotal resection of the pancreas or incomplete involvement by disease usually does not bring about obvious steatorrhea (fecal fat loss) or creatorrhea (fecal protein loss), since the reserve capacity of the surviving

pancreatic acini is tremendous. In dogs, digestion may be unimpaired after resection of four-fifths of the pancreas.

Abnormalities of Internal Secretion. The islands of Langerhans often remain relatively unaffected by inflammatory or neoplastic lesions of acinar tissue. Consequently, diabetes may be mild or even absent in the face of extensive pancreatic disease. Total pancreatectomy in man is compatible with life, provided that insulin requirements (about 50 units per day) are met and digestion is aided by oral administration of pancreatic material. The suggestion that the islet cells elaborate a lipotropic hormone (lipocaic) has not been accepted; inadequate digestion and absorption of nitrogenous substances probably account for the fatty liver that attends total pancreatectomy in dogs.

Disorders of the Biliary Passages. Lesions in the head of the pancreas may obstruct the common bile duct, producing jaundice. Without a complicating infection, such purely mechanical obstruction of 3 weeks' duration or less rarely affects the liver seriously, especially if a normal gallbladder is present (see p. 1713). It is possible, but not established, that reflux of normal or infected pancreatic juice into the biliary system may initiate disease in this organ.

Gastrointestinal Disorders. Nausea, vomiting, belching, bloating, distention, or diarrhea are caused partly by direct irritation or reflex stimulation of gastrointestinal motor function and partly by fermentation of undigested food residues. Digestive disorders also arise if the alimentary organs are displaced or compressed by pancreatic tumor; and direct invasion of the stomach, duodenum, or transverse colon by cancer of the pancreas may lead to mechanical obstruction or bleeding.

Disorders of the Portal Venous System. Because of the intimate anatomic relationship of the splenic and portal veins and the pancreas, hematogenous metastases to the liver are an early possibility in pancreatic cancer; and neoplastic obstruction of the portal venous system may produce portal hypertension, gastric varices, and congestive splenomegaly. Thrombosis or erosion of the splenic vein is an occasional complication of pancreatitis.

Pancreatic Function Tests. These depend on analyzing the blood, the intestinal contents, or both for pancreatic secretory products. Pancreatic abnormality is in general indicated by excessive amounts of such products in the blood and insufficient amounts in the digestive tract. In the serum, normal amylase concentration is less than 150 Somogyi units per 100 ml, and lipase is less than 1.5 Cherry-Crandall units per 1.0 ml. Inhibitor substances interfere with the satisfactory measurement of pancreatic proteases in the blood. When the outflow of pancreatic secretion is blocked, amylase and lipase tend to regurgitate into the blood, in part via lymphatic routes, and serum levels of these enzymes rise. Necrosis with disruption of cellular membranes may presumably enhance this trend and also permits pancreatic deoxyribonuclease to escape and accumulate in the serum.

Latent pancreatic disease causing partial secretory block may sometimes be brought to light by evocative tests. If the normal pancreas is stimulated by intravenous secretin (increases pancreatic output of water and bicarbonate), by intravenous pancreozymin or intramuscular cholinergic drugs (increase pancreatic output of enzymes), or by a combination of such agents, serum levels of amylase and lipase change but little. In some cases of pancreatic cancer or chronic inflammation, however, pancreatic stimulation produces serum enzyme concentrations exceeding control values by 100 per cent. If the gland is extensively destroyed, stimulation of pancreatic secretion is patently incapable of causing increased serum enzyme levels. In this case, evocative tests yield falsely normal results in that serum enzyme concentrations remain at basal levels, but it is said that patients with such extensive pancreatic destruction also have some diabetic tendency and hence can be recognized by glucose tolerance tests.

Urinary concentrations of diastase reflect serum amylase changes. The most informative test of urinary amylase is measurement of its 24-hr output; values above 6,000 Somogyi units per 24 hr are considered abnormal, and above 15,000 as indicative of pancreatitis. An increased output of urinary amylase may persist longer than increased serum amylase levels following an attack of pancreatitis.

Direct measurement of pancreatic secretion is accomplished by quantitative collection of duodenal contents after stimulation with secretin, pancreozymin, or cholinergic drugs. Following secretin stimulation, the normal pancreas puts out a minimum of 2 ml per kg juice per 80 min, and a concentration of 90 mEq $NaHCO_3$ per liter. Accurate results are not obtained unless contamination of duodenal by gastric contents is prevented by simultaneous and independent gastric suction. Rough tests for the presence of pancreatic ferments in the feces (i.e., gelatin film test) are not useful in adult patients.

Indirect evidence of pancreatic exocrine function is obtained by various tests of absorption. When pancreatic disease is advanced, microscopic examination of the stools shows abundant fat droplets and meat fibers with sharp edges; and the administration of test substances that require digestion prior to their absorption is followed by a subnormal appearance of their products in the blood. Such fecal examinations and "tolerance" tests are not adequate, however, to detect borderline pancreatic

insufficiency. For this purpose, it is necessary to use balance studies, comparing the oral intake and fecal elimination of substances which are measured chemically or, more simply, by isotopic techniques. Unfortunately early or limited pancreatic disease may fail to alter absorption as measured by even the most meticulous methods. To differentiate malabsorption of pancreatogenous and of other origin, the absorption of a whole food and of its digestion product may be compared. Thus I^{131}-labeled triglyceride may be poorly absorbed in various malabsorption states, but absorption of I^{131}-labeled oleic acid is much more normal when the pancreas rather than the intestine is at fault.

Although abnormal glucose metabolism is a frequent manifestation of pancreatic disease, evidence of such an abnormality is obviously not specific for infections or tumors of the pancreas. Xylose absorption is relatively unaffected by pancreatic insufficiency.

ACUTE PANCREATITIS

Acute pancreatitis is divided into the edematous, hemorrhagic, and necrotic varieties according to the pathologic change that predominates. Although the clinical and pathologic features of the three types vary, their pathogenesis is presumably the same, and such differences as exist are attributable to the degree of pancreatic damage.

Etiology. Acute pancreatitis tends to occur in patients with alcoholism, gallstones, and peptic ulcer; occasionally it appears as a complication of pregnancy, essential hyperlipemia, and diffuse vascular disease such as periarteritis nodosa. Metabolic and possibly genetic disorders that at times appear associated with pancreatitis are essential hyperlipemia, aminoaciduria, especially an increased urinary output of lysine, and hyperparathyroidism. A not-infrequent cause is trauma, either indirect, as from a heavy abdominal blow, or direct, as from surgery in the upper abdomen. Pancreatitis also appears in normal persons following a heavy meal and sometimes has no recognizable antecedent.

The pathogenesis of pancreatitis presumably depends on intrapancreatic activation of proteolytic enzymes with consequent digestion of pancreatic tissue and blood vessels. Such pancreatic autodigestion apparently may develop under two general conditions: (1) when pancreatic secretion is obstructed, either by a solitary lesion of a major duct or by diffuse blockage of many tiny ductules; or (2) when acinar tissue is exposed to direct injury by toxins, ischemia, inflammation, or trauma. Experimentally, for example, pancreatitis can be initiated by the combined procedure of obstructing the pancreatic ducts and injecting agents such as bile or bacteria to activate proteolysis. This fact lends credence to the hypothesis that pancreatitis may develop if a stone in the ampulla of Vater or a spasm of the sphincter of Oddi impedes pancreatic secretion, with reflux of bile into the pancreatic ducts. Arguments against this theory are as follows: reflux of bile into the pancreatic ducts may occur without untoward effects; the secretory pressure of the pancreas equals or exceeds that of the biliary system; and a common channel of pancreatic and common ducts long enough to permit reflux probably exists in less than 50 per cent of all persons.

Direct injury to acinar tissue would appear to be responsible for the pancreatitis that follows pancreatic trauma or a penetrating peptic ulcer. In animals, the tissue damage and ischemia produced by a local Shwartzman reaction or by injection of staphylococcal toxin into the pancreatic ducts induces a fulminating pancreatitis. The nature of alcoholic pancreatitis is obscure; alcohol does not appear to have a direct effect on pancreatic function. It has, however, been suggested that chronic pancreatitis in alcoholics may be a deficiency disease because chronic pancreatic changes characterize the deficiency disease kwashiorkor, and because degenerative lesions can be induced in the pancreas of rats exposed to the methionine antagonist ethionine.

Incidence. Except for the occasional case exposed to abdominal trauma, or with an ascaris in the duct of Wirsung, pancreatitis is rare in children; but it affects adults of any age. As might be anticipated from the incidence of the antecedent disorders, pancreatitis associated with alcoholism, duodenal ulcer, or trauma is vastly more common in men than in women; but even pancreatitis associated with gallstones is as common in men as in women in spite of women's greater tendency to form gallstones.

Symptoms. Severe upper abdominal pain, usually beginning with catastrophic suddenness, is the outstanding symptom. Its degree varies with the violence of the pancreatic insult, but it is rarely less than agonizing. In mild (edematous) pancreatitis, the patient may content himself with demanding analgesic medication; in the hemorrhagic form, he is anxious and restless even though motion may aggravate his suffering; whereas the pain of necrotic pancreatitis is so severe as to produce shock. Though centered initially in the upper midabdomen, the violent pain of acute pancreatitis usually diffuses to the back, chest, and the lower abdomen.

Nausea and vomiting, abdominal bloating, and constipation are frequent complaints. Mild jaundice may be detected clinically or biochemically within 1 to 3 days of the onset in 25 per cent of cases. In those with alcoholism, psychotic episodes may complicate the picture.

Physical Examination. The patient is obviously distressed and anxious. In some patients, beads of sweat emphasize an underlying pallor; in others, subject to severe shock, the face is livid and the extremities are clammy. Fever is usually not present initially, and the pulse, subject to a variety of defense mechanisms, may be slow or fast, strong or imperceptible. The blood pressure reflects the degree of shock. Tenderness, voluntary resistance, and spasm in the upper abdomen are present to a variable degree, but these signs, in striking contrast to the intense pain, may be remarkably unimpressive. Moderate abdominal distention and suppression of peristaltic sounds are frequent findings.

Laboratory Data. Urinary output is depressed in shock. One out of four cases has glucosuria, and the incidence of choluria is the same. The white count ranges from 8,000 to 20,000, with increased polymorphonuclear cells. A striking finding in severe cases is hemoconcentration, with hematocrit values at times exceeding 60 per cent. Mild hyperglycemia is common, not only because of islet cell damage but also because of the patient's reaction to violent stress.

The concentration of pancreatic enzymes in the blood provides the most specific laboratory information. Within 8 hr of the onset of acute pancreatitis, serum amylase values rise in 80 per cent of the cases to values exceeding 250 Somogyi units. After 48 hr, even in the face of clinical evidence of continuing pancreatitis, amylase values tend to return to normal. As amylase decreases, blood lipase values rise in about half the patients to exceed 2.0 Cherry-Crandall units and then subside slowly over a period of days to weeks. In severe cases, blood calcium levels fall 3 to 10 days after the onset, presumably because calcium soaps form with the fatty acids liberated by lipolytic destruction of abdominal and retroperitoneal fat.

X-ray. Abdominal films may reveal moderately distended gas-filled loops of intestine; the paralytic ileus particularly affects the jejunal coils near the pancreas ("sentinel loops").

Course. Hemorrhagic or necrotic pancreatitis is fatal in over 50 per cent of the cases. Almost all cases with edematous pancreatitis recover. In the most severe cases, death occurs within hours. The mildest forms, on the contrary, subside completely with equal rapidity. Most clinically recognized attacks run a course between these extremes. Abdominal pain and distention persist or may reappear in bouts of renewed intensity, expressing not only further pancreatic injury but also chemical peritonitis which develops as peripancreatic, mesenteric, and omental tissues are digested. Concurrent with fat necrosis, a dark, bloody, and cloudy peritoneal exudate accumulates in amounts ranging from 500 to 2,000 ml. The patient at this point is no longer in shock but appears toxic and febrile. Hypocalcemic tetany occurs in some cases.

Hemorrhagic phenomena manifest at the onset of pancreatitis and reflecting proteolytic injury to clotting mechanisms are seen but rarely. From 3 to 6 days later, however, edema and the typical blue-green-brown discoloration of a hematoma may appear on the abdominal wall, either about the umbilicus or in the flanks (Grey-Turner sign). The source of the blood is the hemorrhagic pancreas, whence blood seeps by retroperitoneal routes to reach the abdominal wall.

Late complications of pancreatitis are the formation of abscesses or pseudocysts (see Pseudocysts), an increased susceptibility to further attacks of pancreatitis, and chronic pancreatitis. The abscesses, usually sterile, are essentially collections of pancreatic secretions, necrotic debris, inflammatory cells, and tissue fluids. Pain, fever, chills, and left-sided pleural effusions are often evident. The process may subside spontaneously or may drain by rupturing into the alimentary tract, but surgical drainage is usually required. Serious and life-threatening complications are secondary bacterial infections, at times by gas-forming anaerobes, perforation with retroperitoneal sepsis, rupture into a major blood vessel with internal hemorrhage, and persistent external pancreatic fistula following drainage procedures. The disease may run a slow downhill course characterized by malnutrition, ileus, and diarrhea.

Differential Diagnosis. Any severe pain in the middle of the body should suggest pancreatitis. A history of previous attacks of pain is common but also characterizes important differential diagnoses. Once pancreatitis is suspected, its diagnosis can usually be established by measurement of pancreatic enzymes in the blood, by exclusion of the conditions most likely to simulate pancreatitis, and by the course of the disease. In considering the differential diagnoses (Table 279-1), it is well to remember that coronary occlusion and biliary colic are approximately twenty times as common as acute pancreatitis, that perforated ulcer is three times as common, that mesenteric vascular occlusion is, except in postoperative cases, somewhat less common, and that a dissecting aneurysm is rarely seen.

Elevation of serum amylase levels, as occurs in pancreatitis, sometimes is seen in mumps, in patients given morphine (presumed reason: contraction of sphincter of Oddi with temporary "backing up" of pancreatic juice), in perforated ulcer (presumed reason: leakage of pancreatic enzymes from duodenal lumen into peritoneal cavity and thence absorption into blood), in some cases of acute cholecystitis unaccompanied by pancreatic reaction, and in isolated instances of various other conditions, particularly mesenteric vascular occlusion.

Treatment. Direct surgical attack with incision and drainage of the inflamed pancreas has been generally abandoned as ineffective and as incurring the risk of external pancreatic fistula. Surgeons who believe that pancreatitis is caused by biliary reflux favor drainage of the common bile duct or the gallbladder in the hope of achieving "decompression," but the preponderant tendency at present is to treat pancreatitis conservatively.

The rationale of therapy is (1) to keep pancreatic secretory activity at a minimum, (2) to avoid any increase in ductal obstruction, and (3) to prevent potential and treat actual complications. Shock and hemoconcentration are treated with parenteral water, electrolytes, and human albumin. Since opiates increase the resistance of the sphincter of Oddi, meperidine is recommended on theoretical grounds for relief of pain but proves inadequate in many severe cases. In such cases, morphine or its derivatives may have to be used. Nothing is given by mouth, and constant gastric suction is used for several days to reduce intestinal distention and secretin production by the duodenum. Fluid, salt, and small quantities of glucose are given intravenously with temporary disregard of caloric requirements. Because secondary infection of necrotic tissue, of partially obstructed biliary passages, or of atelectatic lung is a dangerous possibility, prophylactic daily doses of parenteral penicillin (1,000,000 units or more) and streptomycin (1 Gm) are advisable.

Other, less routine measures may be used. Anticholinergics, in full parenteral doses (e.g., 30 mg of propantheline bromide, 0.5 to 1.0 mg of methscopolamine bromide) are given every 6 hr to inhibit the vagal phase of pancreatic secretion, but the rationale of such therapy in massive necrosis of the pancreas is questionable. Although experimental evidence suggests that inhibition of carbonic anhydrase with acetazoleamide (Diamox) decreases secretin-stimulated pancreatic secretion, the efficacy of Diamox in the management of pancreatitis is not striking. Numerous case reports assert that ACTH or parenterally administered adrenal glucocorticoids are lifesaving when given to the desperate case of acute pancreatitis, but such apparent salutory effects are difficult to evaluate, and it is quite clear that acute pancreatitis may suddenly strike a patient receiving adrenocortical therapy for other reasons. Paravertebral, splanchnic, or epidural procaine block sometimes relieves pain dramatically, and some investigators believe that these procedures not only are symptomatic but also actually help the injured pancreas by augmenting its blood supply. Hyperglycemia may require control with insulin. Hypocalcemia is treated by injections of calcium gluconate, 10 ml of a 10 per cent solution (90 mg Ca) being given slowly by vein. The total amount

Table 279-1. DIFFERENTIAL DIAGNOSIS OF ACUTE PANCREATITIS*

Disease	History	Physical examination	Laboratory findings
Acute pancreatitis......	Sudden onset, often with immediate maximal development of pain Past or recent history of gallstones, alcoholism, peptic ulcer, dietary debauch, trauma, or upper abdominal surgery	Abdominal findings moderate as compared to violence of pain Tenderness extends to left of epigastrium Abdominal distention moderate or absent Peristaltic noises diminished or absent Shock and cyanosis may be striking Patient may be restless	Elevation of amylase in serum and urine Hypocalcemia in severe cases Paracentesis: evidence of fat necrosis, sometimes sanguineous fluid, high amylase levels X-ray may show fluid at base of left pleural cavity
Perforated viscus, especially peptic ulcer	History of ulcer	Boardlike spasm and tenderness in epigastrium Patient fears movement and jarring Shock rare	X-ray shows free intraperitoneal air
Mesenteric vascular occlusion	Elderly patient with cardiovascular disease or recent operation Development of pain may be gradual	. . . .	WBC over 20,000 Paracentesis: sanguineous fluid Stool may contain blood
Acute intestinal obstruction	Intermittent colics with relative comfort between pains Past history of abdominal operation or of inguinal or femoral hernia	Abdominal distention with loud peristalsis Shock rare Patient moves around with colic	X-ray of abdomen shows characteristics of mechanical obstruction
Biliary colic............	Pain more right-sided, more gradual in onset, and less prostrating than that of pancreatitis	Tenderness maximal on right side of abdomen	
Coronary occlusion.....	Pain usually maximal in chest, neck, or arms	Relatively few abdominal findings Shock and restlessness often present	Electrocardiographic abnormalities
Dissecting aneurysm of aorta	. . . .	Impaired femoral pulsations Shock and restlessness often present	Hematuria

* The points listed are, if present, important guides toward the correct diagnosis, but they are not invariable features of the diseases under which they are grouped.

needed is determined by the patient's clinical response and his serum calcium level.

As the patient improves, foods may be given slowly, beginning with a low fat, low caloric intake which is increased according to individual tolerance. Residual intraperitoneal collections may have to be drained eventually.

PSEUDOCYSTS

Sometimes the collections of fluid and cellular debris that may follow pancreatitis produce only moderate inflammatory reaction but persist in chronic form for weeks to months. Usually situated in the middle or left upper abdomen, these pseudo-

cysts may fluctuate in size or may form tremendous masses which create symptoms by pushing the duodenum to the right, the stomach forward (Fig. 279-1), the left diaphragm and lung upward, and the transverse colon downward. Aching distress rather than acute pain is the usual presenting complaint.

Pancreatic pseudocysts are tender and usually are readily palpable. Their cystic nature, however, is difficult to ascertain, for the mass, as palpated through muscles tensed by considerable guarding, may give the impression of hardness. Signs of fluid or atelactasis at the left lung base are common. X-rays establish the location of the tumor and exclude lesions of the gastrointestinal tract and kidneys. Jaundice occurs in about 10 per cent of the cases.

The principal differential diagnosis is upper abdominal neoplasm, particularly of the pancreas. If an attack consistent with pancreatitis has occurred within months, the history is helpful, but in approximately one out of three pseudocysts, the initiating pancreatitis is mild, atypical, and unrecognized. In these instances, the existence of conditions predisposing to pancreatitis, such as gallstones, alcoholism, duodenal ulcer, or trauma, provides a basis for suspecting a pseudocyst. On the whole, the patient with pseudocyst, though perhaps febrile and distressed, is not so debilitated as one would expect were his huge abdominal mass composed of neoplastic cells.

In case of doubt, exploratory surgery is always warranted. Surgical treatment of a pancreatic pseudocyst consists of external or internal drainage or of removal with or without simultaneous resection of pancreatic tissue.

CHRONIC RELAPSING AND CALCAREOUS PANCREATITIS

Chronic relapsing pancreatitis sometimes is initiated by a clear-cut attack of acute pancreatitis; at other times it begins insidiously with atypical and relatively mild pains. Whatever the onset, the pancreas undergoes chronic changes consisting of acinar destruction, inflammatory reaction, interstitial fibrosis, and variable damage to the islet cells. In about half the cases, calcific deposits form in the tubules, the pancreatic substance, or both (Fig. 279-2). The name *calcareous* or *calcific* pancreatitis is often applied when the pancreas is irregularly calcified, but the clinical characteristics are similar to those of chronic relapsing pancreatitis without calcific deposits. The formation of pseudocysts is a common complication.

As is true of acute pancreatitis, the chronic varieties tend to appear in alcoholic patients, those with gallstones or peptic ulcer, and in those who have had upper abdominal trauma. In the past, gallstones have been considered as the principal antecedent, but at present, particularly in males with calcareous pancreatitis, chronic alcoholism is the commonest background condition.

Although chronic pancreatitis occasionally runs a painless course, the outstanding symptoms are recurrent bouts of pain, interspersed by periods either asymptomatic or characterized by persistent distress. The episodic pains, probably caused by limited but acute pancreatic inflammation, resemble the pains of acute edematous pancreatitis in their character, location, and radiation. The nature of the chronic distress is unpredictable, partly because the patient with relapsing pancreatitis, sometimes

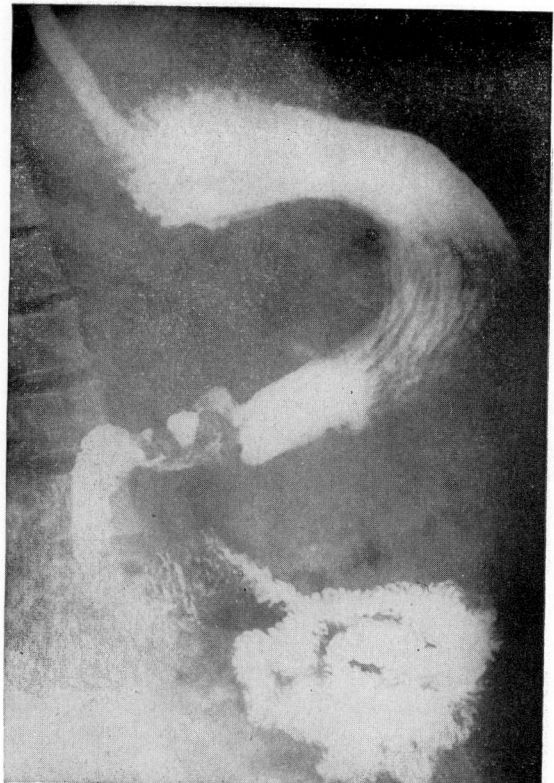

FIG. 279-1. Pancreatic pseudocyst. In this lateral view the body of the stomach appears to be pushed forward by a large mass between it and the spine. The cause of the pseudocyst is well shown: a large penetrating duodenal ulcer.

an alcoholic and sometimes addicted to narcotics after months of agonizing pain, is a poor describer of his pains.

The changes of chronic pancreatitis are so diffuse that some degree of pancreatic insufficiency is often manifest. Because of impaired lipolytic and proteolytic activity, digestion is impaired, weight loss is striking, and fatty and nitrogenous foods are lost in the stools. The patient may consider his bowel movements normal, but direct questioning reveals that they are bulky, light and greasy in appearance, and tend to float, all indications of steatorrhea. Although the absorption of vitamins D and K is impaired, tetany and purpura, such as occur in sprue, are extremely unusual. Frank diabetes occurs in only 10 to 15 per cent of the cases, but impaired glucose tolerance is found in 75 per cent. A few patients, for unknown reasons, manifest hyperlipemia, either persistently or only during the acute attacks.

Diagnosis. Chronic relapsing pancreatitis is a good diagnostic possibility in all patients suffering from recurrent upper abdominal pain, especially if (1) pain and tenderness extend to the left of the

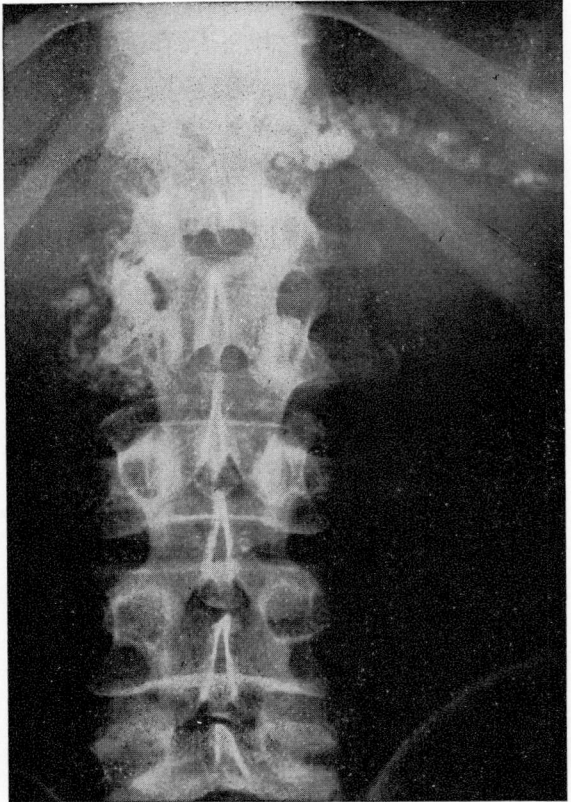

FIG. 279-2. Chronic relapsing pancreatitis. In this film of the upper abdomen the entire pancreas is shown outlined by extensive calcific deposits.

midline, (2) alcoholism is present, or gallstones, and (3) more common abdominal disorders have been excluded. The disease also may explain mild or recurrent jaundice, diabetes, or vague symptoms of indigestion, particularly if these phenomena are accompanied by low-grade fever or a persistently elevated sedimentation rate, otherwise unexplained. If pancreatic calcification is present, its radiologic demonstration permits ready diagnosis, but specially positioned oblique views in a patient who has not been given barium in the immediate past may be necessary to demonstrate small calcareous deposits. In patients without such calcification, diagnosis is best achieved by serum amylase determinations taken within 8 hr of a major attack. Repeated attempts may be necessary, however, for the levels of amylase do not rise with each episode. The bicarbonate concentration of secretin-stimulated pancreatic juice is said to be reduced in 95 per cent of cases of chronic pancreatitis. Absorption tests may reveal impairment of this function, but it is not certain that they reveal early or mild disease of the pancreas.

Treatment. The consequences of pancreatic insufficiency can be controlled with moderate success by dietary restriction of fats and calories and by oral administration of 10 to 20 Gm pancreatin daily. Medical control of pain, on the other hand, is desultory. Manipulation of diet, anticholinergics, and ulcer-type regimens, given in the hope of controlling gastric acidity and thereby lessening the stimulus for secretin production, are all more or less ineffective. ACTH, cortisone, and similar agents are of doubtful benefit and may cause harm because of their effect on gastric secretion. Surgery must therefore be tried when pain is disabling, but its results, too, are far from satisfactory. Surgery is most successful if a responsible biliary tract abnormality, such as stone, can be corrected; or if obstruction of a major pancreatic duct exists and can be eliminated by cutting a stenotic sphincter of Oddi, removing an obstructing lesion near the sphincter, or establishing reverse drainage by resecting the pancreatic tail with anastomosis of the severed duct to the jejunum. Vagotomy, subtotal gastrectomy to reduce gastric secretion, and cutting a normal or "spastic" sphincter of Oddi to prevent biliary reflux in the pancreatic ducts have produced erratically successful results. Bilateral sympathectomy and splanchnicectomy may be used as symptomatic procedures to relieve pain, but the relief is only temporary in most of the cases. If the process is localized, partial pancreatectomy may prove successful; total pancreatectomy relieves pain but results in other disabilities.

FIBROCYSTIC DISEASE

In this perhaps genetically transmitted disorder of infancy and childhood, several organ systems are affected. (1) The pancreatic acini are replaced by fibrotic tissue, multiple cysts, and inspissated mucus. The clinical manifestations of the consequent pancreatic insufficiency are malnutrition and bulky and greasy stools. (2) Somewhat similar pathologic changes affect the lungs so that the patient suffers from obstructive emphysema and is susceptible to chronic bronchopneumonia. (3) The sweat and the saliva contain high concentrations of chloride and sodium; in hot weather this abnormality may cause acute salt depletion and at times death. (4) In a few cases, the smaller hepatic biliary channels are plugged, with the consequent development of cirrhosis and portal hypertension. (5) In the newborn infant a thick meconium, presumably viscous because pancreatic juice is absent, may cause meconium ileus. (6) Retinal changes have been described.

The etiology is obscure. One hypothesis holds that abnormally viscid mucus blocks small tubular structures in the various organs involved. This concept of "mucoviscidosis," however, does not explain the abnormalities of sweat, since sweat glands secrete no mucus. Diagnosis is made on the basis of the clinical picture, deficiency of pancreatic ferments, and high sweat electrolytes. A simplified method to detect abnormal electrolyte concentrations in sweat is provided by an agar plate containing silver nitrate and potassium chromate or by modifications of this technic. If the palm is placed on the plate, a white imprint of the hand develops, the degree of whiteness corresponding to the amount of silver chloride formed, which in turn depends on the amount of chloride in the sweat. Treatment consists of pancreatic substitution therapy and, for the pulmonary complications, potassium iodide to loosen bronchial secretions, postural drainage, and a combination of penicillin and streptomycin.

Because of longer survival of moderate cases, and because mild cases may pass through childhood unrecognized, adult cases of cystic fibrosis may be more prevalent than heretofore appreciated. Thus some adults regarded as having "idiopathic" pancreatitis, bronchitis, cor pulmonale, or hepatic cirrhosis may in fact be the victims of cystic fibrosis. Some reports also suggest that borderline cases of adult cystic fibrosis, recognized on the basis of family history and sweat electrolyte tests, are prone to peptic ulceration.

CANCER

Incidence. Cancer of the pancreas predominantly affects patients over forty-five, attacks men twice as frequently as women, and accounts for about one out of every two to three hundred deaths. It is seen about one-tenth as often as gastric cancer in men and one-fortieth as often as mammary cancer in women. Diabetic patients are believed to have an increased susceptibility to the disease.

Symptoms. Weight loss, pain, and jaundice are the outstanding symptoms. Digestive disorders, including anorexia, nausea, loose stools, or, more commonly, constipation, are prevalent. The site of the lesion, however, to a great extent influences the character of the symptoms, their time of onset, and their correct interpretation.

Considering the total course of all types of pancreatic cancer, jaundice occurs less frequently than weight loss or pain, but diagnostically it is the most important symptom. It points specifically to the biliary passages, and in lesions near the ampulla of Vater gives early warning before extensive growth or metastasis has taken place. The course and intensity of the jaundice depend on the degree of biliary obstruction (Table 279-2). In advanced cases of cancer of the head of the pancreas, it

assumes a deep, greenish-brown hue. Itching is an associated symptom in three-fourths of the cases.

Literally painless jaundice characterizes cancer in the head of the pancreas in only a few cases. More frequently, the patient suffers from vague abdominal distress and fullness, sometimes worse, sometimes better after eating. The severe pain of cancer in the body or tail may, however, be diagnostic: it bores through to the midback when the patient lies supine, and he obtains relief only by standing or by sitting hunched up with arms clasped about the knees.

Physical Examination. Physical examination may reveal nothing except jaundice and the excoriations produced by scratching. In spite of biliary obstruction, hepatic enlargement is not striking unless the liver is involved by metastases or cholangitis, or the gallbladder is not functioning. In protecting the liver from back pressure, however, the gallbladder is itself enlarged in nearly all malignant obstructions of the common duct, but it can be palpated in only half the cases. A definite finding of an enlarged, nontender gallbladder in a jaundiced patient may therefore be taken as a reliable sign of malignant choledochal obstruction (Courvoisier's law). No diagnostic inference is warranted if the gallbladder is not palpable.

In advanced cases, abdominal masses, enlarged supraclavicular nodes, a liver hardened and enlarged by metastases, or evidences of ascites may be found. Splenomegaly does not occur except in the rare case of occlusion of the splenic vein by cancer arising in the pancreatic body or tail. In 20 per cent of the cancers at this site, spontaneous venous thromboses of the extremities, particularly the legs, take place.

Laboratory Data. The urine, blood, and feces of nonicteric patients are often normal. Those with icterus manifest persistent and progressive bilirubinemia and choluria. The stools may be greasy, "abundant, of a pultaceous consistence, very deficient in bile, and most dreadfully foetid" (Richard Bright, 1883). In at least half the cases, however, the clay-colored stools are not grossly fatty and are more like putty than butter. Since bile salts are necessary for the absorption of vitamin K, hypoprothrombinemia develops with prolonged biliary obstruction.

Since neoplastic cells are in general nonfunctioning, and since the functional capacity of surviving acinar cells is tremendous, serum enzyme values are normal in three-fourths of the cases. Except in case of very small and nonobstructing lesions, the volume of pancreatic juice in response to secretin stimulation is usually reduced. Glucose tolerance tests are abnormal in 40 per cent of the cases, but the patient's age or an antecedent diabetes may account for this finding. Many patients with pancreatic cancers have increased serum values of leucine amino peptidase, but such increases are principally the nonspecific result of hepatic metastasis or of biliary tract obstruction.

Because ampullary cancers tend to ulcerate and form fistulas between the biliary and alimentary tracts, the results of laboratory tests may differ from those usually obtaining in jaundiced patients with cancer in the head of the pancreas (Table 279-2).

Course. Pancreatic cancer leads to death by inanition, biliary obstruction, local extension, or distant metastases. By direct extension, the cancer may invade the liver, spleen, stomach, duodenum, colon, portal venous system, or peritoneum. Invasion of the gut or development of varices following malignant occlusion of the portal or splenic vein can cause moderate to severe gastrointestinal blood loss. Peritoneal seeding or, very rarely, portal obstruction is responsible for ascites. Metastatic lesions develop in the regional lymph nodes, liver, lungs, mediastinal and cervical lymph nodes, and bones.

Diagnosis. In jaundiced patients, differential diagnosis from liver disease or gallstones depends on the clinical picture and on laboratory tests showing, in pancreatic cancer, regurgitation jaundice (Chap. 19) and normal hepatic metabolic function (Chap. 19). Favoring pancreatic cancer is a gradual onset of symptoms in elderly patients without antecedent acute malaise, intermittent colics, or chills and fever. If itching is noticed before jaundice, mechanical obstruction of the biliary passages is likely. In early cases, before diagnosis is made obvious by massive or metastatic growth, cancer is indicated by finding an enlarged gallbladder and a nontender liver not more than moderately enlarged, and by not finding such stigmas of liver disease as spider angiomas, dilated abdominal veins, and splenomegaly.

Radiologic procedures may show the effect of the pancreatic lesion on other organs. Changes in the mucosa or configuration of the duodenal loop or stomach may sometimes appear as early phenomena, but secondary gastrointestinal abnormalities are usually signs of advanced disease. Applica-

Table 279-2. CLINICAL FEATURES AND LABORATORY FINDINGS IN CANCER OF THE BILE DUCTS AND PANCREAS*

	Cancer of ampulla of Vater	Cancer of bile ducts	Cancer of head of pancreas	Cancer of body and tail of pancreas
Pain.................	Absent—60% Moderate—40%	Absent—40% Moderate to severe—60%	Absent to mild—15% Moderate to severe—85%	Almost invariably present Agonizing and boring Often worse in back and accentuated when patient is supine
Jaundice:				
Onset..............	Early	Early	Variable	Late to terminal
Character..........	Progressive and marked—80% Fluctuating—20%	Progressive and marked—90% Fluctuating—10%	Progressive and marked	Mild to moderate
Weight loss before onset of jaundice†	None to mild	None to moderate	Occasionally none, but often 10 to 20 lb	Marked, 10 to 60 lb
Fever and chills........	20%	10%	None	May have low-grade fever No chills
Hepatomegaly.........	None to slight	Slight in some cases, but may be extreme	Moderate Marked only if metastases present	None to marked Size depends on degree of metastatic involvement
Enlarged gallbladder palpable or visible....	50%	20%	50%	0
Splenomegaly.........	None	None	None	Occasional
Bile in stools and urobilinogen in urine	Absent—80% Fluctuating—20%	Absent—90% Fluctuating—10%	Absent	Present
Occult blood in stools...	50%	15%	Rare	Rare

* Because of their anatomic proximity, advanced cancers of the ampulla of Vater, the bile ducts, and the pancreatic head at times cannot be distinguished clinically.

† All these cancers cause impressive weight loss sooner or later.

tion of newer x-ray techniques, such as aortograms and splenoportograms, rarely proves fruitful; percutaneous cholangiography via the gallbladder or the liver may be diagnostic but is risky (see Chap. 281).

When the patient is not jaundiced, early diagnosis is difficult, particularly since the patient may exhibit psychoneurotic tendencies. Persistent pain and progressive weight loss with negative radiologic studies of the alimentary, renal, and biliary passages should raise the suspicion of pancreatic cancer. In patients with ascites, the character of the fluid and its cellular content often permit the diagnosis of cancer, but differential diagnosis from ovarian, gastric, or primary hepatic cancer is not easy. Duodenal drainage may reveal neoplastic cells in the cellular sediment.

Treatment. Resection of lesions confined to the ampullary area is successful in terms of 5-year cures in 15 per cent of the cases. In cancers located elsewhere in the pancreas, extensive pancreatic-duodenal resection, including total pancreatectomy, is feasible in many instances, but the patient almost invariably succumbs to local or distant recurrence. In jaundiced patients, however, palliative anastomosis of the gallbladder to the intestinal tract affords relief from the intolerable itching. Before operation is undertaken, any existing deficiencies of water, electrolytes, red cells, and vitamin K should be corrected.

OTHER CONDITIONS

The pancreas is often involved by mumps, but only rarely is pancreatitis the sole manifestation of the disease. Like other viscera, the pancreas may be affected by periarteritis nodosa.

Ectopically placed pancreatic tissue may be found in the gastrointestinal tract, Meckel's diverticulum, and various other areas. Nearly all pancreatic rests radiologically discovered in adults, however, occur in the distal stomach and duodenum. Rarely the rest creates an annular constriction of the duodenum.

Unusual pancreatic neoplasms are cystadenomas, cystadenocarcinomas, and hemangiomas. Benign and malignant growths of the islet cells are discussed in Chap. 71.

The reader is referred to Chap. 6, Acute Abdominal Pain; Chap. 17, Constipation and Diarrhea; Chap. 19, Jaundice and Other Manifestations of Liver Disease; Chap. 70, Diabetes Mellitus; and Chap. 94, Disorders of Carbohydrate Metabolism, for further consideration of problems discussed in this chapter.

REFERENCES

Bachrach, W. H., and M. I. Grossman: The Medical Management of Acute and Chronic Pancreatitis, M. Clin. N. Am., 43:1101, 1959.

Bockus, H. L., M. H. Kalser, J. L. A. Roth, A. L. Bogoch, and G. Stein: Clinical Features of Acute Inflammation of the Pancreas, A.M.A. Arch. Internal Med., 96:308, 1955.

Burton, P., E. M. Hammond, A. A. Harper, H. T. Howat, J. E. Scott, and H. Varley: Serum Amylase and Serum Lipase Levels in Man after Administration of Secretin and Pancreozymin, Gut, 1:125, 1960.

Comfort, M. W., E. E. Gambill, and A. H. Baggenstoss: Chronic Relapsing Pancreatitis: A Study of Twenty-nine Cases without Associated Disease of the Biliary or Gastro-intestinal Tract, Gastroenterol., 6:239, 376, 1946.

di Sant'Agnese, P. A.: Fibrocystic Disease of the Pancreas, a Generalized Disease of Exocrine Glands, J.A.M.A., 160:846, 1956.

Dreiling, D. A., and H. D. Janowitz: "The Pathophysiology of the Pancreas," p. 65, vol. VII, in "Advances in Internal Medicine," Chicago, Year Book Publishers, Inc., 1955.

Elliott, D. W., R. D. Williams, and R. M. Zollinger: Alterations in the Pancreatic Resistance to Bile in the Pathogenesis of Acute Pancreatitis, Ann. Surg., 146:669, 1957.

Grossman, M. I., et al.: Symposium: Exocrine Pancreatic Function, Gastroenterol., 36:362, 1959.

Ingelfinger, F. J.: The Diagnosis of Cancer of the Pancreas, New Engl. J. Med., 235:653, 1946.

Shwachman, H., and N. Gahm: Studies in Cystic Fibrosis of the Pancreas: A Simple Test for the Detection of Excessive Chloride on the Skin, New Engl. J. Med., 255:999, 1956.

Thomas, J. E.: "The External Secretion of the Pancreas," Springfield, Ill., Charles C Thomas, Publisher, 1950.

Section 6: The Liver, Gallbladder, and Bile Ducts

280 DISEASES OF THE LIVER
Gerald Klatskin

In trying to establish the nature of any hepatic disorder it is helpful to begin with a consideration of the probable anatomic localization and morphologic character of the underlying lesion before proceeding to the identification of its etiology. Despite the intimate interrelationships between the major functional components of the liver and the tendency for lesions in one to affect the others secondarily, it is possible usually to distinguish among diseases that arise in the hepatic parenchyma, biliary tree, and vasculature. In many instances the etiology is unknown, while in others the etiology must be inferred from the character of the lesions. For that reason a morphologic classification of liver disease (Table 280-1) is more practical than one based on etiologic factors.

Table 280-1. CLASSIFICATION OF LIVER DISEASE

I. Parenchymal
    A. Hepatitis: viral, "lupoid" toxic and drug-induced, associated with systemic infections, granulomatous
    B. Cirrhosis: Laennec's, postnecrotic, biliary, cardiac, hemochromatosis, Wilson's disease, rare types
    C. Infiltrations: fat, iron, glycogen, amyloid, lymphoma, Gaucher's disease, Niemann-Pick disease
    D. Space-occupying lesions: tumors, amebic abscess, pyogenic abscess, gummas, echinococcus cyst
    E. Functional disorders accompanied by jaundice: Gilbert's syndrome, Dubin-Johnson syndrome, Rotor syndrome, Crigler-Najjar syndrome
II. Hepatobiliary
    A. Extrahepatic biliary obstruction: stone, stricture, malignancy
    B. Cholangitis
III. Vascular
    A. Chronic passive congestion
    B. Cardiac cirrhosis
    C. Budd-Chiari syndrome
    D. Portal vein thrombosis
    E. Pylephlebitis
    F. Cruveilhier-Baumgarten syndrome

To avoid unnecessary duplication, the clinical manifestations and functional abnormalities shared by many diseases of the liver are considered together in Chap. 19. The latter is intended to serve as an introduction and should be read in conjunction with the discussion of the individual diseases in the section to follow.

HEPATITIS

Viral Hepatitis

Viral hepatitis is an acute systemic infection that affects the liver predominantly, giving rise to highly characteristic hepatic lesions. The disease occurs in two forms due to closely related but distinct etiologic agents known as *virus IH* and *SH*, or *A* and *B*, respectively. The two infections are indistinguishable on the basis of their clinical and morphologic manifestations, but they exhibit differences in their epidemiologic and immunologic behavior. The IH type is known as *infectious* or *epidemic hepatitis*, the SH type as *homologous serum, post-transfusion, inoculation,* or *syringe-transmitted hepatitis*. Since both viruses may be transmitted by the parenteral route, the terms indicated may be confusing. There is a growing tendency, therefore, to supplant them with the terms IH and SH or A and B viral hepatitis. Before the pathogenesis of viral hepatitis was understood, the IH type was called *catarrhal jaundice* in the mistaken belief that the symptoms were due to an inflammatory obstruction of the common duct. There is no justification for the continued use of this obsolete term.

Etiology. The agents responsible for this form of hepatitis have not been identified microscopically or serologically and have not been propagated in tissue culture, embryonated eggs, or experimental animals. However, they have been shown to be filtrable through a Seitz EK filter and are readily transmitted to susceptible human volunteers, suggesting very strongly that they are viral in nature. What little is known about the properties and behavior of these viruses has been derived from transmission experiments in man. Since of necessity these experiments have been limited in number, there are still a great many gaps in our knowledge of the viruses. The absence of a susceptible animal host or a suitable serologic technique for identifying these agents has been a stumbling block in the study of viral hepatitis, not only for the virologist, but also for the clinician, pathologist, and epidemiologist. From a diagnostic point of view the clinician is obliged to depend on clinical and laboratory features, which, while highly characteristic, are never pathognomonic. Even the histologic changes in the liver, which are more specific, cannot be considered unequivocal evidence of infection, particularly in the more unusual and late forms of the disease, in which the morphologic features are less distinctive.

Both the IH and SH viruses are peculiarly resistant to heat (56°C for 30 min and 60 min, respectively), prolonged storage in the cold (−10 to −20°C for 1½ and 4½ years, respectively), and the action of chemical agents (chlorine 1:1,000,-000 for the IH virus; and merthiolate 1:2,000, tricresol 2:1,000, and equal parts of phenol and ether 5:1,000 for the SH virus).

The principal differences between the two viruses may be summarized as follows: (1) the IH virus has been recovered from both blood and feces, the SH virus from the blood only; (2) the IH virus may be transmitted to man by either the oral or the parenteral route, the SH virus by the parenteral route only; (3) the incubation period is 2 to 6 weeks for the IH virus, irrespective of the route of administration, and 6 weeks to 6 months for the SH virus; (4) the IH virus has been found in the blood from 3 days before to 8 days after the onset of jaundice, while the SH virus has been recovered at intervals throughout the long incubation period and during the acute phase of the disease; with the rare exceptions to be mentioned, in neither case has the agent been demonstrated during convalescence; (5) the asymptomatic carrier state appears to be more common and prolonged in the SH type, virus having been demonstrated in the blood for periods up to 5 years in individuals with no history of hepatitis; the IH type has been recovered from the feces during convalescence in only two instances, 4 and 15 months following infection, but never from blood or feces in individuals with no history of hepatitis; (6) both viruses confer homologous but not heterologous immunity; (7) γ-globulin isolated from large pools of plasma collected from randomly selected donors protects against IH but not against SH infection; (8) IH infections occur at an earlier age, tend to be less severe, and are more likely to be accompanied by preicteric constitutional symptoms. It is still not clear whether these two types of virus represent distinct species or merely strain variants of the same species. Moreover, it is not known whether all the strains belonging to each type are antigenically identical. Clinical and epidemiologic studies and transmission experiments have failed to demonstrate any significant differences between the behavior of the strains of each type isolated in various areas of the world. However, more precise information will have to await the development of better methods of isolating and identifying these agents.

Epidemiology. *IH viral hepatitis* occurs both sporadically and in epidemic form. The latter is seen particularly under conditions of crowding and poor sanitation. Infection is usually acquired through the oral route by close personal contact with individuals passing virus in their feces. It is presumed that the occurrence of many unapparent infections in the population accounts for the infrequency with which definite exposure to the disease can be established. Young children, and especially infants, appear to be an important reservoir for this type of infection. Explosive epidemics may follow exposure to feces-contaminated water or food supplies, and occasionally infections are acquired by the parenteral route following the transfusion of blood or the use of blood-contaminated instruments. In many areas infections are more prevalent in the autumn and early winter months, but in others there appears to be no seasonal fluctuation.

The disease may occur at any age but is most common in children and young adults. After the age of thirty the incidence is relatively low, apparently because of immunity acquired in early life. No doubt this accounts also for the effectiveness of pooled γ-globulin in preventing infection following exposure. The immunity that follows infection is usually lifelong in duration but may be less sustained in some individuals, so that reinfection is possible.

In *SH virus infections* the virus gains entry to the body by the parenteral route as a result of transfusions or injections of infected blood, plasma, or serum, or the use of improperly sterilized blood-contaminated needles, syringes, or other surgical equipment. Occasionally handlers of blood and blood products become infected, presumably through nicks in the skin. The disease may occur also following the use of topical thrombin. However, other blood products prepared by the ethanol fractionation method, such as γ-globulin, serum albumin, and antihemophiliac globulin, appear to be noninfectious. Recent evidence suggests that the transplacental transmission of virus to the fetus in pregnant asymptomatic carriers may be responsible for neonatal hepatitis and that this may be an important mode of propagating the virus from one generation to the next.

Asymptomatic carriers play a key role in the spread of this disease. Estimates of their prevalence are not available, but on the basis of the number of infections that follow a single blood transfusion they would appear to comprise approximately 1 per cent of the population. Very few of these individuals have had a clinically recognizable infection, but some exhibit minor alterations in liver function, and a few have significant hepatic lesions, suggesting that some carriers, at least, have active but subclinical disease.

Since a large number of bloods is used to make up a single pool of plasma, the recipient of a plasma infusion is exposed to numerous potentially infected donors. As a result the risk is very much greater than that following a single blood transfusion. The virus may be present in high concentration. In some instances as little as 0.00005 ml is infectious, which explains why needles, syringes, and other instruments inconspicuously contaminated with blood may serve as vehicles for infection.

Pathology. The lesions of viral hepatitis, which are uniformly distributed throughout the liver, are characterized by degeneration and necrosis of parenchymal cells, proliferation and swelling of the reticuloendothelium, and cellular infiltration of the sinusoids and portal triads. Scattered groups of hepatic cells undergo rapid lysis, especially in the pericentral areas of the lobules, while many of the remaining cells show degenerative changes characterized by ballooning, or hyalinization to form densely stained acidophilic bodies. Almost from the beginning there are signs of active regeneration, including mitotic figures, hyperchromatism, and numerous binucleate cells. As a result of these changes, the liver cords are disrupted and distorted, leading to disorganization of the normal lobular pattern. The intervening sinusoids contain clumps of swollen Kupffer cells and numerous lymphocytes, plasma cells, wandering macrophages, and occasional eosinophils and polymorphonuclear cells. A similar exudate is seen in the portal triads. Many of the macrophages adjacent to necrotic areas contain lipofuscin, a yellow, acid-fast pigment presumably derived from broken-down hepatic cells. Occasionally some of the canaliculi are filled with inspissated bile.

The reticulum fibers are spared and serve an important function in providing a framework for the orderly reorganization of the lobules. As long as the areas of necrosis, whatever their size, are limited to the confines of the individual lobules, local regeneration and restitution of the normal architecture are assured. In contrast, when the necrotic zones encompass whole lobules this is not possible, since regeneration must proceed from distant unaffected lobules. This leads to the formation of large regenerating nodules, which compress the intervening reticulum of the completely destroyed lobules into bands containing the remaining blood

vessels, regenerating ducts, and exudate. This variant of the disease is known as *subacute necrosis of the liver*. Ultimately, if the patient survives, the collapsed reticulum undergoes collagenization, giving rise to *postnecrotic cirrhosis*. However, even in the healed state, signs of varying degrees of active parenchymal inflammation and necrosis may be evident for long periods of time. When the areas of necrosis are extensive, the liver tends to be small and coarsely nodular, with broad intervening bands of collapse and fibrosis, the usual picture in this type of cirrhosis. However, if the necrosis involves limited numbers of adjacent lobules, a finely nodular cirrhosis may ensue. Fine nodulation may occur also as a result of progressive degeneration and collapse of large nodules, because of either continued inflammatory activity or the tendency of the nodules to outgrow their circulatory supply. At this stage it may be difficult to distinguish the lesion from that of Laennec's cirrhosis.

Occasionally the hepatitis virus produces *massive necrosis of the liver*. In this condition there are large areas of necrosis and collapse, as in subacute necrosis, but death ensues before signs of regeneration appear. Since the liver tends to shrink in size and is often bile stained, at least early in the disease, the lesion was once termed *acute yellow atrophy*.

It should be noted that, while the hepatitis virus is the most common cause of subacute and massive necrosis, certain drugs and poisons are capable of producing a very similar lesion.

Although restoration of the normal architecture and resolution of the inflammatory reaction are the rule following recovery from *uncomplicated* viral hepatitis, mild degrees of periportal fibrosis and round-cell infiltration are common residuals. They bear no relationship to the minor symptoms and alteration in function that may be present at this time and are *not* to be interpreted as evidence of chronic hepatitis.

Clinical Manifestations. Usually the clinical manifestations follow a highly characteristic pattern and subside without residuals within a period of 4 months. For purposes of identification and further discussion this form of the disease will be designated as *typical acute viral hepatitis*. In approximately 15 per cent of patients the clinical course is atypical, in that it terminates fatally, is greatly prolonged, or is characterized by unusual manifestations. These features are sometimes considered complications of the disease, but it should be emphasized that the basic lesion is the same in all instances.

The mortality rate, based usually on the number of fatalities from subacute and massive necrosis that occur within the first few months of the disease, is said to lie between 0.2 and 0.4 per cent.

This does not take into account the late deaths that follow residual postnecrotic cirrhosis. However, since the number of unrecognized mild and non-icteric infections is probably large, the over-all mortality rate may be considerably lower than that indicated.

Little is known about the factors responsible for the variations in the severity and clinical course of viral hepatitis. Complicating malnutrition, alcoholism, intercurrent infection, physical exhaustion, and inadequate therapy are thought to be important, but the evidence implicating these factors is inconclusive. The severity of the disease and its mortality rate appear to be greater in older persons and in those infected with the SH virus, possibly because of the higher incidence of complicating disease in such individuals. An autoimmune mechanism has been invoked to explain the chronicity of the disease in some patients, but this remains to be established.

Typical Acute Viral Hepatitis. *Symptoms and Signs.* In approximately 80 per cent of IH but in only 20 per cent of SH viral infections, the onset of jaundice is preceded by a period of nonspecific constitutional and gastrointestinal symptoms that may last from a few days up to 2 weeks. Often these symptoms are mistaken for signs of a respiratory infection or acute gastroenteritis.

Usually the onset of the *preicteric phase* is abrupt. *Fever,* marked *anorexia,* and *weakness* are the outstanding symptoms, and often a sudden distaste for cigarettes is a striking feature. These symptoms may be accompanied by nausea and vomiting, indigestion, abdominal pain, headache, pain on moving the eyes, arthralgia, and myalgia. Occasionally there is an erythematous or urticarial rash. As a rule, the fever is remittent and only moderate in degree, but in severe infections it may be high and associated with marked prostration. Chilly sensations are relatively common in such cases, but *frank shaking chills are rare.* When abdominal pain is present, it is usually dull and aching in character and located in the epigastric area or right upper quadrant. Rarely, it is severe and may be accompanied by marked abdominal tenderness and spasm, suggesting an acute surgical emergency. In some individuals upper respiratory symptoms are a prominent feature.

Often at this stage the liver is slightly enlarged and tender, but even if it is not, percussion over the hepatic region may provoke pain. In about 20 per cent of patients a mild degree of splenomegaly can be demonstrated, and in a somewhat smaller number the posterior cervical lymph nodes are enlarged.

Within a few days to a week of the onset, and sometimes even before the appearance of jaundice, the urine darkens, owing to the presence of bilirubin. This may be the first clue to the true nature of an otherwise obscure febrile illness. Usually icterus of the skin and scleras becomes evident within a day or two.

Early in the *icteric phase* the jaundice deepens, hepatic enlargement and tenderness become more evident, and the patient's general condition worsens. However, within a few days the fever and preicteric symptoms usually abate, even though the icterus is still increasing. Occasionally the fall in temperature and clinical improvement coincide with the appearance of clinical jaundice, but in severely ill patients prostration, anorexia, nausea, and vomiting may persist, or even increase, after subsidence of the fever. Unless measures are taken to maintain food intake, marked weight loss may ensue.

Characteristically the jaundice increases rapidly, reaching a maximum in 3 to 14 days, and then recedes at a somewhat slower rate, clearing up completely in 1 to 6 weeks. If the serum bilirubin level is followed closely, it can be shown that in typical cases there is no plateau at the peak, although one may occur during convalescence as the serum bilirubin approaches the normal concentration. The intensity of the jaundice at its maximum tends to mirror the extent of the hepatic damage, so that usually it provides some indication of the expected severity and duration of the disease. However, there are many exceptions; minimal jaundice, therefore, does not exclude the possibility of severe hepatic injury, nor does deep jaundice necessarily imply a protracted or severe illness.

Immediately following the subsidence of jaundice the patient usually feels well, but recovery is seldom complete at this stage. The liver may be enlarged and tender, abnormalities of hepatic function are often evident, and histologic studies usually show incomplete resolution of the lesion. Of even greater importance, resumption of full activity at this time may precipitate a relapse, with a recrudescence of any or all of the previous symptoms. The duration of this *posticteric phase* varies from 2 to 6 weeks but may be longer in some instances. However, full clinical and biochemical recovery is to be expected within 4 months.

Laboratory Features. The *leukocyte count* is normal but may be low during the preicteric phase. Occasionally, atypical lymphocytes, indistinguishable from those of infectious mononucleosis, are present in small numbers. The *sedimentation rate* is high in the preicteric stage, falls to normal during the icteric stage, and rises again during convalescence.

The *urine* may contain traces of bilirubin even before jaundice appears. As jaundice deepens, the amount of bilirubin increases, but during convalescence bilirubin excretion often ceases before the serum bilirubin has returned to normal. During the preicteric phase urine urobilinogen may be increased, but as jaundice and light-colored feces appear the amount of urobilinogen falls to the normal level. Often a secondary increase in urine urobilinogen occurs when the jaundice begins to fade and the stools return to their normal color. Finally, the level falls to normal when recovery has occurred.

Early in the course of the jaundice the stools may be light or clay-colored for a few days to a week. Later their appearance is normal. In many cases there is no change in color despite the presence of overt jaundice.

The *direct and total serum bilirubin* levels rise and fall together and reflect the depth of jaundice. The direct fraction usually constitutes 50 to 75 per cent of the total early in the course of the disease, but may be relatively lower later. An increase in the direct fraction without a concomitant rise in the total bilirubin may be seen both in the preicteric phase and late in convalescence. In a few individuals the indirect fraction remains slightly elevated for long periods following apparent recovery (see Gilbert's syndrome, p. 1699).

Bromsulphalein retention is increased during the preicteric phase and remains so for some time after the subsidence of jaundice. It returns to normal when healing is complete, but occasionally mild retention persists despite apparent full recovery.

The *cephalin-cholesterol flocculation* and *thymol turbidity* tests usually become positive toward the end of the preicteric phase or shortly thereafter. They tend to revert to normal late in convalescence but often persist for long periods following apparent recovery. Occasionally one or both tests remain normal throughout the course of the disease.

The *serum alkaline phosphatase* level tends to rise slightly, but occasionally it reaches the concentration seen in extrahepatic obstructive jaundice.

The *serum protein* pattern is normal early in the disease but may show a fall in albumin and a rise in globulin if the disease is prolonged or severe.

Usually the *serum cholesterol* concentration is normal, but during the icteric phase the percentage of esters tends to fall. In a few individuals a high total cholesterol is seen transiently during the phase of increasing jaundice.

Characteristically, the serum transaminase levels (GOT and GPT) rise sharply. Values in excess of 500 units are common but may be lower in some cases. Frequently, the serum GOT is high before jaundice is evident clinically.

Diagnosis. During the preicteric phase, viral hepatitis may be difficult to differentiate from a number of other infections, but marked anorexia out of proportion to the degree of fever, subcostal tenderness, and the occurrence of dark urine should alert the clinician to the possibility of viral hepatitis and call for investigation of the liver by appropriate tests.

Once jaundice has appeared it becomes necessary to exclude other forms of hepatitis, an exacerbation of a chronic hepatic disorder, and extrahepatic biliary obstruction. A careful history will usually suffice to rule out toxic and drug hepatitis, but the appearance of renal failure or signs of a hypersensitivity reaction should call for further inquiry. Marked myalgia, nuchal rigidity, conjunctival injection, and leukocytosis should suggest the possibility of leptospirosis. A severe sore throat and marked cervical adenopathy may be indicative of infectious mononucleosis with jaundice. The presence of spider nevi, ascites, or edema early in the disease usually denotes an underlying cirrhosis, but later it may be indicative of subacute necrosis of the liver. Shaking chills, colicky pain, significant leukocytosis, and a past history of dyspepsia usually point to a common duct stone.

Even in the most typical case of viral hepatitis, the clinical course should be scrutinized with care, since any deviation from the usual pattern may indicate an error in diagnosis or the occurrence of a complication. The particular points to note are the duration of the preicteric phase, the time it takes for jaundice to reach its maximum, the presence or absence of a pleateau at the peak of the serum bilirubin curve, and the occurrence of ascites, edema, or spider nevi.

Variants of Acute Viral Hepatitis. *Acute Anicteric Hepatitis.* A number of individuals infected with the hepatitis virus fail to develop jaundice. In some patients the clinical features are otherwise identical with those of the icteric form of the disease, although they tend to be somewhat milder. However, there is reason to believe, on the basis of transmission experiments, that the disease may present as a nonspecific illness without localizing signs. In infants and young children a mild gastroenteritis or diarrhea may be the only manifestation. Liver function tests may show the same pattern seen in icteric hepatitis, but often the changes are less striking. Occasionally the direct and total serum bilirubin levels are slightly elevated, and traces of bile can be demonstrated in the urine.

Diagnosis is difficult in this group unless an epidemic is in progress, or the clinical and laboratory features closely resemble those of the icteric form of the disease. Under other conditions the diagnosis can seldom be made with confidence, since the symptoms and changes in liver function are nonspecific.

The high incidence of immunity to IH virus infections in adults with no history of hepatitis suggests that anicteric infections are common. However, relatively few are recognized clinically.

Fulminant Hepatitis (Massive Necrosis of the Liver). This form of the disease is usually fatal within 10 days, some deaths occurring as early as the second day. In the preicteric and early icteric phases, the clinical and laboratory features may be identical with those in the more benign type. However, nausea, vomiting, and abdominal pain tend to be more severe, and jaundice is likely to appear earlier and to deepen more rapidly. Usually the first clue of an impending fatal outcome is the appearance of cerebral manifestations indicating the onset of hepatic coma. Occasionally the disease is ushered in with neurologic manifestations and progresses rapidly to deep coma and death. Other features seen in many, but not all, cases include a sharp terminal rise in temperature, significant leukocytosis, a rapid decrease in the size of the liver, coffee grounds vomitus or gross hemorrhage into the gastrointestinal tract, purpura, and ascites. Terminally the patient lapses into deep coma and may exhibit muscular twitchings, convulsions, shock, oliguria, and azotemia. Occasionally the course of the disease is so rapid that death occurs before jaundice develops. It may be difficult to establish the diagnosis in such cases, unless the possibility of viral hepatitis is considered and appropriate laboratory studies are carried out.

Subacute Hepatitis (Subacute Necrosis of the Liver). The clinical course in subacute necrosis of the liver varies, depending on the extent of the necrosis, the degree of healing, and the amount of regeneration. As in the fulminant form of the disease, the illness often begins as an uncomplicated viral hepatitis, only to go on to progressive hepatic failure and death. Many patients die within 2 to 12 weeks, but some survive for a period of a year or more, and a few go on to apparent clinical recovery. In the latter group postnecrotic scarring and cirrhosis are inevitable, but the outcome depends on the activity of the associated parenchymal inflammatory process and the degree of portal hypertension that develops. Relapses with jaundice and other signs of hepatic failure are common in those with active inflammatory lesions, and may terminate fatally after one or more such episodes. Not infrequently the first recognizable signs of subacute necrosis of the liver make their appearance during a relapse following what was believed to be an uncomplicated attack of acute viral hepatitis. There is reason to believe that the apparent progression in such cases merely represents the recrudescence of a lesion incurred during the initial infection. Occasionally the same picture is seen following an attack of anicteric hepatitis. In cases with postnecrotic scarring, there may be a long asymptomatic interval between the initial infection and the accidental discovery of cirrhosis or the occurrence of bleeding from esophageal varices. Biopsy studies of the liver indicate that mild forms of subacute necrosis and postnecrotic fibrosis occur more frequently than is evident clinically. It is possible, therefore, that viral hepatitis may be responsible for many instances of cirrhosis discovered years after the initial infection.

The clinical features that should suggest the possibility of subacute hepatic necrosis in patients with acute viral hepatitis include (1) jaundice that increases progressively for more than 2 weeks, remains stationary at a high level, or shows recurrent remissions and relapses, (2) fever and leukocytosis that appear after jaundice has developed, (3) ascites, edema, and numerous large spider nevi, (4) the appearance of splenomegaly late in the course of the disease, (5) severe and persistent vomiting, particularly if accompanied by coffee grounds vomitus, (6) severe abdominal pain, (7) a hemorrhagic tendency as evidenced by epistaxis, hematemesis, melena, hematuria, or purpura, and (8) fetor hepaticus and other signs of impending coma. Not infrequently the serum albumin falls and the globulin increases. When the clinical course is prolonged, hyperglobulinemia may be extreme. As hepatocellular function fails, the serum cholesterol may fall to abnormally low levels.

Terminally the patient lapses into hepatic coma and dies of advanced hepatocellular failure. However, in patients with a prolonged course, death may be due to intercurrent infection or massive bleeding from esophageal varices.

Cholestatic ("Cholangiolitic") Hepatitis. Occasionally patients with a typical onset of acute viral hepatitis develop clinical and laboratory features suggestive of biliary obstruction. It has been postulated that the inflammatory reaction in such cases involves the terminal perilobular cholangioles, permitting the regurgitation of bile as a result of compression by exudate or abnormal permeability. For that reason the syndrome has been called *cholangiolitic* hepatitis. However, there is no histologic evidence that the cholangiolar involvement is any more severe or qualitatively different from that in the usual form of hepatitis, so that the theory of increased cholangiolar permeability or obstruction rests solely on circumstantial clinical evidence. Most pathologists do not consider "cholangiolitic" hepatitis a distinct pathologic entity, but the unusual clinical manifestations of the syndrome warrant its classification as an atypical variant of acute viral hepatitis.

The distinctive features of the disease are prolonged jaundice, often accompanied by pruritus, significant hepatomegaly, a sustained and marked increase in the percentage of direct-reacting serum bilirubin, high levels of serum alkaline phosphatase and cholesterol, and a negative or only weakly positive cephalin-cholesterol flocculation reaction. Despite the obstructive-like chemical pattern, the *serum transaminase* levels tend to be high, as in other forms of acute hepatocellular disease. Usually the serum albumin concentration is normal or only slightly depressed, but the globulin fraction is almost always increased. Early in the disease the histologic features are indistinguishable from those of typical acute viral hepatitis, but later they may be difficult to differentiate from those of an extra-hepatic biliary obstruction, the principal findings being bile staining of the parenchyma, intracanalicular bile thrombi, and a mononuclear periportal exudate without hepatocellular changes.

Except for unusual fatigability and pruritus, the patient often feels remarkably well and goes on to an uneventful recovery after a period of sustained or fluctuating jaundice lasting from a few months to a year. In some instances, however, the disease appears to be progressive, giving rise to "cholangiolitic" cirrhosis, an entity thought to be closely related to primary biliary cirrhosis (p. 1691).

The differentiation between cholangiolitic hepatitis and extrahepatic biliary obstruction may be exceedingly difficult, even after the most exhaustive investigation including liver biopsy, so that exploratory laparotomy may be necessary. However, a careful history will often reveal the typical symptoms of viral hepatitis at the onset, and the results of liver function tests carried out early in the course of the disease are likely to be more typical of hepatocellular disease. Certain drugs, and particularly chlorpromazine (Thorazine) and methyltestosterone, are capable of producing an identical picture. It is essential, therefore, that the possibility of a drug reaction be excluded with certainty in all instances of suspected "cholangiolitic" hepatitis.

Sequelae. Occasionally signs or symptoms of liver disease persist or recur beyond the 4-month period during which recovery is to be expected. This may be because of slow resolution and healing, progressive inflammation and destruction of the parenchyma, postnecrotic scarring, functional disorders of the parenchyma, or even complicating psychogenic disturbances. It is misleading, therefore, to classify all forms of delayed recovery as "chronic viral hepatitis." Moreover, the term has the additional disadvantage that it is sometimes used in a more specific sense to indicate posthepatitic cirrhosis or chronic parenchymal destruction leading to cirrhosis. Wherever possible an attempt should be made to determine the anatomic and physiologic basis for the persistence of abnormal findings. Unfortunately this is not always feasible without re-

sort to liver biopsy, but prolonged observation and serial laboratory studies often suffice to distinguish between the several types of prolonged or recurrent hepatitis to be discussed.

Minor Residuals without Clinical Significance. A significant number of patients with acute viral hepatitis exhibit minor abnormalities of hepatic function or slight nontender hepatomegaly for periods of several months to a year following apparent clinical recovery. Slight increases in thymol turbidity and cephalin-cholesterol flocculation are the most common findings, but serum bilirubin levels of 1.2 to 2 mg per 100 ml and Bromsulphalein retention of 6 to 10 per cent are not rare. Liver biopsy in this group invariably reveals complete healing. It should be noted, however, that both in this group and in patients without residuals the portal triads may show a mild degree of fibrosis and mononuclear cellular infiltration. In the absence of parenchymal changes, there is no evidence that either the histologic or functional residuals described are forerunners of progressive disease or relapse.

Prolonged Convalescence. In this group any or all of the clinical or laboratory features of the acute disease may persist for long periods, but usually full recovery ensues within a year. On histologic examination the liver shows incomplete healing of the parenchymal lesions, as in the convalescent stage of the uncomplicated form of the disease. In the author's experience this lesion shows no tendency to progress to subacute necrosis of the liver or to posthepatitic cirrhosis. However, it is in this group that recrudescences may occur, either spontaneously or following premature return to full activity.

Subacute Hepatic Necrosis and Posthepatitic Cirrhosis. Before signs of overt hepatic failure or portal hypertension appear, it may be impossible to distinguish between the clinical and laboratory manifestations of persistent liver disease due to subacute hepatic necrosis and posthepatitic cirrhosis and those due to prolonged convalescence from the uncomplicated form of viral hepatitis. However, the two can be differentiated readily on the basis of their histologic features.

Relapses and Recurrence. Not infrequently there is a transient recurrence of symptoms or an increase in functional abnormalities during convalescence. Usually this is the result of premature ambulation and resumption of full activity, but it may occur also without provocation. The manifestations may be identical with those of the initial attack, or even more severe, but usually they are milder and of shorter duration. When the interval between the two attacks is less than 6 months the recurrence almost invariably represents a recrudescence of an unrecognized, incompletely healed lesion of either the prolonged convalescent or subacute necrotic type. The possibility of reinfection with the heterologous strain of the hepatitis virus or of an error in diagnosis must be considered when the interval is longer. However, the relapses in posthepatitic cirrhosis, which may resemble those of acute hepatitis, often occur at long intervals.

"Posthepatitis" Syndrome. Occasionally patients complain of unusual fatigability, vague discomfort in the right upper quadrant, anorexia, and indigestion for long periods following complete subsidence of all clinical, laboratory, and histologic evidence of active liver disease. Psychogenic factors are thought to be responsible for this syndrome. However, in the author's experience, the syndrome is rare in individuals who have had adequate bed rest during convalescence, which suggests that it may represent a type of postinfectional asthenia.

The Carrier State. The importance of carriers in the spread of viral hepatitis has been touched on under Epidemiology. Only rarely does the carrier state follow a clinically recognizable attack of acute viral hepatitis, which suggests that it is usually the result of an asymptomatic infection. However, in a few instances, virus has been recovered from the feces of infants convalescing from a prolonged but mild illness. Since parenteral injections can hardly account for the unusually large number of SH virus carriers in the population, serious consideration must be given to the suggestion that the virus may be acquired transplacentally before birth. The question of whether the carrier harbors the virus in a diseased liver or merely permits its propagation without incurring any hepatic injury is still under study. A significant number of carriers show minor abnormalities of hepatic function, and in a few, significant histologic changes have been demonstrated in the liver. However, many carriers show no clinical, chemical, or histologic evidence of liver disease.

"Lupoid" Hepatitis and Cirrhosis of Possible Viral Etiology. See pp. 1675 and 1679.

Treatment. Rest. It is the opinion of many that strict bed rest is indicated until the signs of active hepatic disease have subsided. However, on the basis of an experimental study carried out under carefully controlled conditions in military personnel, it has been recommended that patients be allowed up as soon as the acute symptoms abate, and that further physical activity be limited to the confines of a hospital ward until full recovery ensues. It is difficult to reconcile the results of this investigation with the experience of most clinicians indicating that the incidence of recrudescences, prolonged convalescence, and postinfectional asthenia is significantly reduced by enforced bed rest. Until this difference of opinion is resolved, the clinician would be well advised to err on the

side of conservatism, particularly since complete bed rest does not entail any greater loss of time from work than limiting activity to the confines of the patient's home or hospital ward. Moreover, the increase in the length of time required for recuperation following a regime of strict bed rest reported in military personnel has not been observed in civilian patients.

The patient may be allowed out of bed when (1) all symptoms have subsided, (2) the liver is no longer significantly enlarged or tender, and (3) the levels of total serum bilirubin, serum GOT, and Bromsulphalein retention have fallen below 2 mg per 100 ml, 40 units, and 10 per cent, respectively. Residual abnormalities in cephalin-cholesterol flocculation and thymol turbidity may be disregarded. Activity should be increased slowly and a close watch kept for signs of clinical or laboratory relapse. If these signs appear, bed rest should be reinstituted. Resumption of full activity is permitted when the patient's strength has returned to normal. In those with residual hepatomegaly or minor alterations in liver function, further follow-up studies at monthly intervals are advisable. The physician should exercise great care in reassuring the patient that such studies are a precautionary measure and that most minor residuals have no clinical significance. For that reason it is unwise, and usually unnecessary, to limit the patient's activity or diet during this period.

Obviously there are limits to the benefits to be derived from bed rest in the more prolonged forms of viral hepatitis. An attempt should be made, therefore, to determine when maximum benefit has been achieved. This can be accomplished by delaying ambulation until the levels of serum bilirubin and Bromsulphalein retention have been stable for at least a week. The patient is then allowed increasing activity under supervision. If there is any tendency for the clinical signs or laboratory abnormalities to worsen, bed rest should be resumed.

Diet. Patients with viral hepatitis may lose considerable weight. If this is prevented by feeding sufficient calories, convalescence may be shortened. *An intake of 2500 to 3000 Cal* is usually adequate, but this may be difficult to achieve for short periods during the acute phase of the disease, particularly if parenteral feeding becomes necessary.

The *optimal protein requirement* is still a matter of debate. Many, including the author, believe that positive nitrogen balance can be achieved with an intake of 70 to 100 Gm, and that the regenerative rate of the liver cannot be accelerated by providing an excess. However, in the military study previously mentioned, an intake of 150 to 200 Gm appeared to shorten the period of convalescence significantly, but these results are difficult to reconcile with those previously reported by others. Except in patients with subacute or massive hepatic necrosis and impending coma, in whom the protein intake must be sharply curtailed, there is no harm in forcing protein to this extreme, but it is difficult to do so, and the physician need not be concerned if he fails.

The *fat content* of the diet need not be limited. There is no evidence that fats are harmful, and, indeed, they are useful in enriching the caloric value and palatability of the diet. However, while milk, butter, and eggs are usually well tolerated, fried and cooked fats often produce gastrointestinal distress and, therefore, should be restricted.

Once the protein requirement has been satisfied, and fat has been added as tolerated, the remaining caloric needs are made up with *carbohydrate*. A high carbohydrate intake has no special virtue, and the outmoded practice of forcing sweets throughout the day is to be condemned, since it often spoils the patient's appetite for other foods and may provoke fatty infiltration of the liver if the patient's protein intake is not increased proportionately.

There is no convincing evidence to show that vitamin supplements are of value in the treatment of viral hepatitis, although they may be indicated if there was antecedent malnutrition, or if prolonged parenteral feeding becomes necessary. Similarly, there is no logical reason for adding lipotropic substances, like choline and methionine, to a balanced diet, particularly since fatty infiltration is not a feature of viral hepatitis.

Severe anorexia, nausea, and vomiting may necessitate resort to parenteral feeding. A slow drip of 15 per cent glucose, providing 300 to 400 Gm per day, will usually suffice to maintain the patient in a reasonable state of nutrition and hydration over the brief period usually required before oral feedings can be resumed. The amount of sodium, potassium, and chloride to be added to the solution will depend on the losses in the urine, feces, vomitus, and sweat and may be estimated from the state of hydration and the serum electrolyte pattern. Parenteral amino acid supplements have been advocated, but there is no evidence that they are of special benefit. Moreover, they frequently cause reactions and are contraindicated in patients with impending coma.

Antibiotics. The antibiotics do not appear to be of any value in the treatment of acute viral hepatitis. However, broad-spectrum antibiotics, and especially neomycin, may be useful in the management of coma complicating massive and subacute hepatic necrosis.

ACTH and Prednisone. These agents are capable of inducing a prompt clinical remission in acute viral hepatitis. However, the length of the convalescent period is not shortened in the uncompli-

cated form of the disease, and relapses are common unless treatment is prolonged. It is deemed inadvisable, therefore, to subject patients to the possible hazards of ACTH and prednisone therapy unless there are clear-cut indications for it. Certainly this form of treatment is warranted when the symptoms are severe and do not respond to conservative measures, and when there are signs of subacute hepatic necrosis. There is a clinical impression that the duration of the disease is shortened and that residual lesions are minimized under these conditions, but the evidence for this is still inconclusive. Not infrequently a course of steroid therapy is effective in terminating prolonged convalescence, particularly in patients with chronic "cholangiolitic" hepatitis, and occasionally large doses appear to be lifesaving in comatose patients with massive hepatic necrosis. Although it is worth trying these agents in the treatment of postnecrotic cirrhosis with evidence of active inflammatory disease, the results are usually disappointing and complications are frequent.

In using ACTH and prednisone, treatment should be continued until the serum bilirubin drops to a normal level or reaches a stable plateau, but in either event for a period of not less than 3 weeks. In *acutely ill* patients an infusion of 25 to 50 units of ACTH daily administered over an 8- to 10-hr period appears to yield the most satisfactory results, although orally administered prednisone in doses of 60 to 100 mg per day may be equally effective in some instances. If the expected response is not obtained, the dose of ACTH may be increased to 100 units. As soon as the patient shows marked improvement, usually in 2 or 3 days, the dose of ACTH is reduced to 10 units and ultimately to 5 units. To avoid the inconvenience of repeated infusions, oral prednisone may be substituted for ACTH at any time during convalescence. Similarly, in less acutely ill patients, prednisone may be used from the beginning, starting with large doses and reducing them as rapidly as the clinical condition permits. As indicated elsewhere, sodium and potassium intake must be regulated, and a watch must be kept for signs of toxicity.

In the *fulminant* form of the disease with coma, doses of ACTH and hydrocortisone up to 1,000 mg daily have been recommended. However, too few cases of this type have been treated in this manner to know whether massive therapy has any advantage over the usual dose levels employed.

Treatment of Postnecrotic Cirrhosis and Its Complications. The problems of therapy in this condition are very similar to those in Laennec's cirrhosis (p. 1688).

Prevention. Since the patient with an IH viral infection passes the virus in his stools, the usual sanitary measures employed in other enteric diseases must be initiated to prevent spread of the infection to others. Unfortunately, the duration of fecal infectivity is not known, so that precise recommendations cannot be made regarding the length of the period during which precautionary measures must be followed. However, it is customary to carry them out until clinical recovery has been achieved.

The blood is a source of infection in both types of viral hepatitis, so that special care must be taken to avoid the transfer of virus to other patients through the agency of improperly sterilized, blood-contaminated instruments. Preliminary washing followed by boiling for 10 min or, preferably, autoclaving for 15 min will ensure destruction of the virus. The practice of using a single syringe with a change of needles for multiple injections in groups of patients is dangerous and is to be condemned.

The selection of donors in blood banks is a difficult problem. It is customary to eliminate individuals who have had viral hepatitis within a year. However, such persons appear to be a less dangerous source of infection than asymptomatic carriers with no history of previous disease. Unfortunately, there is no assured method of detecting such individuals. Various methods of chemical treatment have been recommended to sterilize blood, but none has proved satisfactory. Since the possibility of infection cannot be eliminated with certainty, the clinician would be well advised to limit the use of transfusions to conditions in which they are unequivocally indicated.

Commercially available plasma is even more dangerous than blood, since large numbers of donors are used in making up a single pool. If plasma must be used it should be obtained from as small a pool of donors as possible. There is suggestive evidence that storage of plasma in the liquid state at room temperature for periods of 6 months or longer greatly reduces the risk of infection, but other methods of sterilization that have been recommended are of little value.

Individuals exposed to the IH type of viral hepatitis may be immunized passively by administering normal human γ-globulin at any time up to within 6 days of the expected onset of the disease. The usual dose is 10 ml. However, recent evidence suggests that with very much smaller doses, 0.01 ml per lb body weight, it may be possible to achieve a more prolonged type of active-passive immunity. It is believed that under these conditions the γ-globulin suppresses the symptoms but does not prevent infection, so that a natural acquired immunity develops. It is doubtful that γ-globulin is of prophylactic value in SH viral infections, although it has been reported that two injections of 10 ml each given at monthly intervals may be partially protective.

Although γ-globulin is of particular value in the control of institutional and family epidemics, there is no reason why it should not be used in any individual who has been exposed. However, the disease is so mild in healthy young children that it may be better to allow them to become infected and acquire a natural immunity.

"Lupoid Hepatitis"

Occasionally the LE cell test is positive in liver disease. This occurs most frequently in subacute hepatic necrosis and its sequela postnecrotic cirrhosis and, rarely, in Laennec's cirrhosis. In many cases the disease starts acutely with a typical attack of viral hepatitis, but in others the onset is insidious and the etiology is uncertain. Anicteric infections with the hepatitis virus may be responsible for some of the latter, but this has not been established. Because the LE phenomenon in such cases may be accompanied by clinical features suggestive of disseminated lupus erythematosus (DLE), and is considered by some as evidence of an underlying autoimmune mechanism responsible for the progressive nature of the hepatic disease, such cases have been grouped in the special category of "lupoid hepatitis."

Although this syndrome may occur in either sex and at any age, it is seen most frequently in young women. Characteristically the disease runs a chronic or intermittently active progressive course, ultimately terminating in hepatic failure or massive hemorrhage from esophageal varices. Cortisone and its derivatives in large doses often induce a remission, but relapses are common. Although it is possible to maintain some patients in a good state of health for long periods of time with prolonged steroid therapy, many either fail to respond or become refractory and ultimately succumb.

Apart from the clinical manifestations of chronic or intermittently active progressive liver disease, which are not distinctive, most patients show a greatly increased serum concentration of γ-globulin, and some exhibit facial rash, arthralgia, signs of renal disease, pleural effusion, hemolytic anemia or thrombocytopenia. Although these features are suggestive of disseminated lupus erythematosus, the characteristic lesions of that disease are rarely, if ever, demonstrable at autopsy. Another point of difference is that in lupoid hepatitis in contrast to disseminated lupus erythematosus, the LE cell phenomenon usually is only weakly and intermittently positive. In addition, it should be noted that the features generally considered distinctive of lupoid hepatitis are commonly seen in subacute hepatic necrosis and posthepatitic cirrhosis in the absence of the LE cell phenomenon. These apparent contradictions suggest that there may be no connection between lupoid hepatitis and disseminated lupus erythematosus and that the LE phenomenon in the former may represent a false positive test related to the production of some unusual serum protein. However, there are two observations that are difficult to account for on this basis. (1) Postnecrotic cirrhosis of the type that occurs in lupoid hepatitis is seen occasionally in patients with classical disseminated lupus erythematosus. In such cases the sequence in which the two diseases appeared can seldom be determined. (2) Attacks of what appear to be typical acute viral hepatitis occasionally occur as a late complication of disseminated lupus erythematosus, and when they do they almost invariably follow the chronic or intermittently progressive course seen in lupoid hepatitis. The hypothesis that disseminated lupus erythematosus and lupoid hepatitis are both manifestations of an autoimmune reaction triggered usually by different types of injury, but occasionally by the same type, is an attractive one and would account for the apparent interrelationships between the two diseases and their tendency to run a chronic progressive course. However, the evidence on which it is based is far from conclusive. A possibility that merits consideration, but which is equally speculative, is that the development of disseminated lupus erythematosus and lupoid hepatitis is dependent upon some constitutional (? hereditary) determinant of tissue reactivity.

Toxic and Drug-induced Hepatitis

The type of liver injury known as toxic hepatitis occurs following exposure to certain poisons and drugs or during the course of some systemic infections and metabolic disturbances. True hepatotoxins, such as carbon tetrachloride and phosphorus, are tissue poisons that damage the liver by inactivating essential protoplasmic enzyme systems. In contrast, most drugs that produce hepatic injury, such as cinchophen and the sulfonamides, exert their effects by inducing a hypersensitivity reaction. However, a few, like chloroform, are truly hepatotoxic, while others, such as the arsenicals, may behave both as hepatotoxins and sensitizing agents. A number of parenterally administered drugs, once considered hepatotoxic because of their apparent tendency to produce jaundice, are now known to serve as innocuous vehicles in the transmission of the hepatitis virus by means of inadequately sterilized blood-contaminated syringes. The type of hepatitis that accompanies certain systemic infections and metabolic disturbances is thought to be the consequence of an endogenous intoxication. However, little is known about the nature of the presumed toxins involved or the manner in which they exert their deleterious effects, so that this form of hepatitis will be considered separately.

The clinical and pathologic features of the hepatitis produced by hepatotoxins and sensitizing drugs are sufficiently different to warrant their consideration as separate entities. Since space does not permit a detailed discussion of the individual agents in each group, Table 280-2 is appended at the end of this chapter to indicate their probable mode of action.

Toxic Hepatitis. Characteristically the liver lesions produced by true hepatotoxins make their appearance within a day or two of exposure, are readily reproducible in most, if not all, species, and exhibit morphologic features distinctive for each of the agents. In many instances there are accompanying toxic lesions in other organs, especially in the kidney.

The *histologic changes* in the liver vary not only with the agent involved but also with the dose and route of administration. In general, however, the acute lesions tend to be distributed uniformly throughout the lobules in either a central or a periportal zonal pattern, and show all stages of parenchymal degeneration from simple swelling to acute necrosis with little or no inflammatory reaction. Often fatty infiltration is a prominent feature. Usually the lesion is reversible, but death may occur before healing takes place. Some poisons, such as the *Amanita phalloides* toxin and the chlorinated naphthalenes, produce subacute and massive hepatic necrosis, which, if not fatal, leads to the development of postnecrotic cirrhosis. Even the agents that produce reversible lesions, such as carbon tetrachloride, may give rise to cirrhosis if the exposures are repeated at close enough intervals to prevent normal healing.

Usually the *clinical picture* resembles that of acute viral hepatitis, except for the absence of preicteric fever and constitutional symptoms. Anorexia, nausea, and vomiting are the principal symptoms, while jaundice and hepatomegaly are the major physical findings. It should be noted, however, that significant liver damage may occur without producing jaundice. The *laboratory features* also are similar to those in viral hepatitis, although the changes in cephalin-cholesterol flocculation and thymol turbidity tend to be less striking.

In addition to the symptoms of liver injury, there may be others referable to the extrahepatic pharmacologic and toxic effects of the offending agent. Often it is difficult to distinguish between these two groups, but renal failure and severe gastrointestinal irritation usually are due to extrahepatic lesions.

As a rule, recovery occurs more rapidly and residuals are less common than in acute viral hepatitis. However, subacute or massive hepatic necrosis may be fatal or may give rise to postnecrotic cirrhosis. Occasionally death occurs as a result of an accompanying renal lesion despite satisfactory healing of the liver.

The *diagnosis* is seldom difficult. However, errors are inevitable unless a specific inquiry about possible exposure to hepatotoxins is made in every case of hepatitis. The sudden occurrence of oliguria and azotemia during an attack of acute hepatitis should always arouse suspicion of an intoxication, even if there is no history of exposure, since poisoning may occur without the patient's knowledge.

Treatment is very much like that described for acute viral hepatitis. However, greater consideration must be given to the status of the kidneys, since hepatotoxins not infrequently produce acute renal tubular necrosis. In such cases measures designed to reduce nitrogen retention and to attain a normal internal environment take precedence over the less urgent needs of the liver. This usually entails marked restriction or actual omission of protein, provision of sufficient carbohydrate and fat calories to minimize protein catabolism, and careful regulation of fluid and electrolyte balance.

Hepatitis Due to Drug Hypersensitivity. The features that characterize this type of hepatic damage and serve to distinguish it from that produced by true hepatotoxins include the following: (1) the hepatitis occurs in only a small proportion of individuals exposed, (2) neither the incidence nor the severity of the injury can be correlated with the amount of drug consumed, (3) the lesion is not reproducible in animals, (4) the onset of hepatitis bears no constant temporal relationship to the institution of drug therapy, occurring with dramatic suddenness after the first dose in some individuals, and only after prolonged administration, or even following its withdrawal, in others, (5) the lesions are more variable than in toxic hepatitis, and (6) signs of liver disease often are accompanied by other manifestations of hypersensitivity.

Two generalizations are worth bearing in mind in interpreting the role of drugs in the pathogenesis of hepatitis: (1) if a drug produces liver injury in man but fails to do so in other species, it almost certainly is a sensitizing agent; (2) if a drug gives rise to any other manifestations of hypersensitivity, it can be predicted that sooner or later it will produce hepatitis in some individuals.

Experimentally it has been shown that simple chemical compounds by combining with proteins may serve as antigens and induce hypersensitivity. Also the striking clinical similarities between drug reactions and serum sickness suggest that the former are allergic in nature. However, drug reactions differ from the classical types of anaphylactic and tuberculin hypersensitivity in that (1) circulating antibodies and skin sensitivity can rarely be demonstrated, (2) the interval between the first exposure to a drug and the appearance of a reaction is inconstant, and (3) the manifestations of the reaction are unpredictable, varying not only in different individuals but also with the particular drug involved. It is especially difficult to explain why a single drug may produce fever and rash in one individual, hepatitis in another, or a depression of myelopoiesis in a third, and why different drugs vary with respect to the frequency with which they induce one or another manifestation of hypersensitivity.

The *morphologic changes* in the liver vary from case to case but, in general, fall into one of two patterns. In the first, *the hepatocellular type*, there are irregularly distributed focal areas of parenchymal degeneration and necrosis, and an intense portal inflammatory reaction with little or no fatty infiltration. Occasionally the lesions are difficult to distinguish from those of acute viral hepatitis, and rarely they are sufficiently extensive to produce the picture of subacute hepatic necrosis. As a rule, the lesions regress when the offending agent is withdrawn, but occasionally the hypersensitivity reaction appears to trigger a progressive inflammatory process which may result in cirrhosis.

The second or *cholestatic type*, seen following reactions to drugs such as chlorpromazine, is characterized by marked intralobular bile stasis and significant, predominantly mononuclear and eosinophilic inflammatory reaction in the portal triads. In contrast, the parenchymal cells show little or no change. These features bear a striking resemblance to those of "cholangiolitic" hepatitis and extrahepatic biliary obstruction. Occasionally the disease runs a long course despite the cessation of drug administration, and rarely a type of biliary cirrhosis develops.

The *clinical and laboratory features* of the *hepatocellular type* of drug hepatitis resemble those of acute viral hepatitis. However, the signs of liver disease are often preceded or accompanied by other manifestations of hypersensitivity, such as fever, rash, arthralgia, lymphadenopathy, and signs of renal or hematopoietic injury. Also there is a tendency for the serum alkaline phosphatase to be higher and the cephalin-cholesterol and thymol turbidity reactions to be weaker than in viral hepatitis.

In the *cholestatic type* of hepatitis produced by drugs such as chlorpromazine, symptoms suggesting an extrahepatic biliary obstruction appear following a brief episode of fever and other constitutional symptoms. The latter may or may not be associated with more distinctive signs of hypersensitivity. Often the icterus is accompanied by dark urine and clay-colored stools, and pruritus may be a prominent feature. The serum bilirubin and alkaline phosphatase levels tend to be as high as in obstructive jaundice, while the cephalin-cholesterol floc-culation and thymol turbidity reactions are normal.

It should be noted that in some drug reactions, features of hepatocellular and cholestatic hepatitis coexist.

Usually the hepatitis subsides within a few weeks following withdrawal of the offending drug. How-ever, it may run a more chronic course, occasionally terminating in a form of biliary cirrhosis (p. 1691).

The *diagnosis* may be exceedingly difficult if there are no other manifestations of hypersensitiv-ity. A history of drug ingestion is helpful, but obvi-ously it does not exclude the possibility of an un-related viral hepatitis or biliary obstruction. Eosino-philia is an inconstant finding but when present favors a drug reaction. Unfortunately, even a liver biopsy may be inconclusive, so that exploratory laparotomy may be indicated in cases with pro-longed cholestatic jaundice of doubtful etiology.

In patients receiving a number of drugs it may be difficult to determine which is responsible for the reaction. Even a clinical trial following recov-ery may be misleading, since multiple sensitivities may develop as a result of a reaction to a single drug. Moreover, it is unwise to carry out such tests, since severe and even fatal reactions may ensue.

The principles of *treatment* are the same as for toxic hepatitis. In addition, ACTH and prednisone may be useful adjuvants in severe illnesses. Ob-viously, at the first sign of a reaction the offend-ing drug should be withdrawn. However, this may fail to abort the reaction. Occasionally, spontaneous or induced desensitization permits resumption of drug therapy following recovery. However, unless the drug is urgently needed it is unwise to use it again.

Hepatitis Associated with Systemic Infections

Bacterial Infections. Many systemic infections are accompanied by minor functional and struc-tural changes in the liver that have little clinical significance. Occasionally, however, severe bacterial infections give rise to sufficiently extensive hepatic lesions to produce jaundice and, in rare instances, may be responsible for progressive hepatocellular failure.

Although the liver plays an important role in removing bacteria that gain access to the blood, the parenchyma seldom becomes infected in the process. More often the signs of hepatic damage which accompany systemic infections are due to circulating toxins or to the effects of such nonspe-cific factors as fever, anemia, hypoxia, and malnu-trition. Some of the infectious agents involved are known to have in vitro hemolytic properties. How-ever, except in the case of *Clostridium welchii* (*C. perfringens*) sepsis, it is doubtful that hemolysis

plays a significant role in the production of jaun-dice.

Almost any severe bacterial infection may give rise to toxic hepatitis, but the organisms implicated most frequently include pneumococci, streptococci, gonococci, *Escherichia coli,* and the salmonella group. While bacteremia is often present in such infections, it does not appear to be essential for the development of toxic hepatitis, as for example in pneumococcal pneumonia, scarlet fever, typhoid fever, and food poisoning with *Salmonella typhi-murium* and *Salmonella enteritidis.*

The *pathologic changes* in the liver are nonspe-cific. They may include focal areas of hepatocellu-lar degeneration and necrosis, signs of regeneration, and an inflammatory reaction in the portal triads.

The *clinical and laboratory features* resemble those in toxic hepatitis. As a rule, the signs of hepatic damage subside promptly as the underly-ing infection is brought under control. In most cases the hepatitis does not appear to add materially to the severity of the illness. However, in rare in-stances severe hepatocellular failure may be con-tributory to a fatal outcome.

Not all forms of jaundice accompanying severe infections can be attributed to toxic hepatitis. In *E. coli* bacteremia and in typhoid and paratyphoid fever it may be due to a complicating acute chol-angitis, while in *C. welchii* sepsis it is usually the result of acute intravascular hemolysis and the destructive action of the invading organisms on the hepatic parenchyma. Occasionally the jaundice that occurs in salmonella and shigella infections is due to a coincidental acute viral hepatitis. Double in-fections of this type are not rare during concurrent epidemics of the two diseases. Finally, the possi-bility of a drug-induced hepatitis must not be for-gotten in evaluating the pathogenesis of any hepa-titis that occurs during an infection.

Infectious Mononucleosis. On the basis of histo-logic studies and tests of hepatic function, it would appear that the liver almost always participates in the generalized inflammatory reaction of the reticu-loendothelial system that characterizes infectious mononucleosis. However, overt clinical manifesta-tions of hepatic involvement are relatively uncom-mon, jaundice occurring in 5 to 10 per cent of cases, and hepatomegaly only slightly more fre-quently.

The outstanding finding in the liver is an intense inflammatory reaction involving the sinusoids and portal triads. The exudate is largely mononuclear, consisting of atypical lymphocytes, monocytes, plasma cells, and swollen proliferating Kupffer cells. Occasionally the latter are arrayed in rosettes, forming small granulomatous nodules in the sinus-oids. A few scattered parenchymal cells may exhibit early degenerative changes, but hepatocellular necrosis is unusual, despite the fact that the parenchymal cells often show evidence of active regeneration. In jaundiced cases the canaliculi not infrequently contain bile thrombi. Except for swelling and cellular infiltration, the portal triads are not altered.

Abnormalities of "liver function" are demonstrable in most cases, those depending on alterations in the serum protein pattern, such as the cephalin-cholesterol flocculation and thymol turbidity reactions, predominating. Since the latter can seldom be correlated with evidence of hepatocellular injury histologically, and since they often persist long after clinical recovery, it is highly probable that they are, in part at least, due to nonspecific changes in serum protein related to the underlying infection. Characteristically the serum albumin level falls, while the γ-globulin concentration rises. Occasionally there is a less pronounced increase in α_1- and β-globulin. Strongly positive cephalin-cholesterol flocculation reactions and increased levels of thymol turbidity are seen in at least 80 per cent of cases. Bromsulphalein retention, high levels of serum alkaline phosphatase, increased serum transaminase activity, increased urine urobilinogen, and decreases in prothrombin and serum cholesterol esters are less common findings. Hyperbilirubinemia and bilirubinuria occur in 10 to 30 per cent of cases.

In general, the histologic changes and alterations in hepatic function parallel the severity of the underlying infection. What role the former play in producing clinical manifestations is difficult to assess. However, it is doubtful that the minor changes in the liver that occur in most anicteric cases contribute significantly to the symptomatology or clinical course of the disease. When the hepatic lesions are more extensive, and particularly when jaundice occurs, the symptoms may resemble those of acute viral hepatitis, suggesting that they are of hepatic origin.

The jaundice that occurs in infectious mononucleosis tends to be mild and usually clears up within a few weeks. Its appearance may precede or coincide with the onset of lymphadenopathy. Occasionally the lymph nodes fail to enlarge, in which case the etiology of the fever and jaundice may be more difficult to identify. Often the jaundice is accompanied by slight tenderness and enlargement of the liver and by splenomegaly. The other clinical manifestations of infectious mononucleosis are described elsewhere (p. 1249).

The biochemical changes suggesting hepatic involvement usually return to normal by the end of the second month, but in occasional instances they persist for many months. However, there is no convincing evidence that infectious mononucleosis gives rise to cirrhosis or to any other form of chronic hepatic disease.

In the presence of jaundice it may be difficult to differentiate infectious mononucleosis from acute viral hepatitis. The occurrence of sore throat, significant lymphadenopathy, or chills favors the former. Atypical lymphocytes may appear in the blood in both diseases but seldom exceed 10 per cent of the total leukocyte count in acute viral hepatitis. In the last analysis the diagnosis must be established serologically (p. 1250).

The hepatic lesions of infectious mononucleosis require no special treatment. There is no convincing evidence to indicate that dietary measures shorten the course of the disease or have any effect on the symptoms.

Leptospirosis. See p. 1084.

Granulomatous Hepatitis

The liver often participates in generalized granulomatous reactions of such varied etiology as sarcoidosis, tuberculosis, brucellosis, certain mycoses, and berylliosis. The lesions, which consist of discrete collections of epithelioid and giant cells apparently derived from the reticuloendothelium, tend to displace adjacent hepatic cells as they expand. However, they usually remain quite small, so that the loss of parenchyma is minimal even when the lesions are numerous. Rarely, they coalesce to form large lesions, in which case they may produce signs and symptoms of liver disease.

As a rule, it is difficult to distinguish between the hepatic granulomas of different diseases on a morphologic basis alone. Central necrosis is more common in tuberculosis, brucellosis, and mycotic infection than in sarcoidosis and berylliosis, but it is an inconstant finding, and caseation, which is such a common feature in tuberculous lesions elsewhere in the body, is rare in the liver. Occasionally, by means of special stains or cultural methods, it is possible to demonstrate the underlying etiologic agent.

Sarcoidosis. In approximately 70 per cent of patients with sarcoidosis it is possible to demonstrate the presence of hepatic granulomas by means of needle biopsy. Since this approaches the incidence found at autopsy it may be inferred that usually the lesions are numerous and uniformly distributed. Nevertheless, they seldom give rise to symptoms, although mild degrees of hepatomegaly and minor alterations of function are common. The high serum alkaline phosphatase level seen in this disease appears to be more closely related to the presence of hepatic granulomas than to the occurrence of lesions in bone. Rarely, the granulomatous reaction and the fibrosis that follows are so extensive that overt signs of liver disease appear. These signs may include marked hepatomegaly, jaundice, ascites, splenomegaly, and bleeding esophageal varices, and they may be mistaken for evidence of other types of cirrhosis, especially if there are no extrahepatic manifestations of sarcoidosis. As a rule, the diagnosis depends on liver biopsy, although it may be suspected when there are other signs of the disease.

Tuberculosis. Needle biopsy studies indicate that hepatic granulomas can be demonstrated in most patients with acute miliary tuberculosis and in approximately half of those with other forms of the disease. Presumably the lesions are indicative of a hematogenous spread of the infection, but, since acid-fast organisms can seldom be demonstrated, the question arises whether the granulomas may not represent a nonspecific response to the infection. In addition to the granulomas, fatty infiltration, portal fibrosis, and, less commonly, Laennec's cirrhosis may be found. These appear to be related to the malnutrition which may accompany this disease.

Occasionally the number of hepatic granulomas in acute miliary tuberculosis is so great that significant hepatomegaly and jaundice develop. In most other forms of tuberculosis, however, signs of liver disease are unusual, except for slight hepatomegaly and nonspecific minor alterations in function, which may be unrelated to the presence of hepatic granulomas.

Three rare forms of hepatic tuberculosis are characterized by marked enlargement and tenderness of the liver, chills and fever, jaundice, and a rapid downhill course. They are (1) pylephlebogenous tuberculosis, in which there is massive dissemination of tubercle bacilli to the liver by way of the portal vein from an intraabdominal focus; (2) hepatic tuberculomas, which are large caseating masses or abscesses of tuberculous origin; and (3) tuberculous cholangitis, or tubular tuberculosis of the liver, a condition which arises as a result of rupture of a caseating tuberculoma or abscess into the biliary tract, and subsequent spread of the infection along its course.

Brucellosis. Granulomas can be demonstrated in the liver in a high proportion of patients with active *Brucella abortus* infections; they are relatively uncommon in *Brucella suis* and *Brucella melitensis* infections.

The lesions seldom give rise to clinical manifestations, although hepatomegaly is common. Several instances of jaundice have been reported, but they are rare. Hepatic function is little impaired and may be normal even in the presence of granulomas.

Occasionally cirrhosis is a late complication of brucellosis.

CIRRHOSIS

Any diffuse fibrosis that destroys the normal lobular architecture of the liver may be properly classified as a form of cirrhosis. Characteristically the parenchymal cells lying between the connective tissue septums are arranged in islands that differ from normal lobules not only in size and shape but also in their lack of normally oriented central veins and portal triads. They may represent segments of lobules isolated by encircling fibrous bands, or nodules of regenerating parenchyma, and may vary in size from less than a millimeter to several centimeters in diameter. Other features seen in many but not all cases of cirrhosis include degeneration, atrophy and necrosis of parenchymal cells, an inflammatory reaction, usually most marked in the periportal areas, proliferation of the small perilobular bile ducts, and alterations in the intrahepatic vasculature characterized by compression, distortion, and reduction in the size of either the portal or hepatic venous bed, and the occurrence of abnormal shunts between the major vascular components of the lobules. In addition, there may be a number of changes related to the specific effects of certain etiologic factors. The deposition of iron-containing pigment in hemochromatosis may be cited as an example.

Although there are well-defined differences in the pathogenesis of the several known types of cirrhosis, the basic fibrotic process in all appears to be the consequence of hepatocellular necrosis or atrophy resulting in collapse and condensation of the normal supporting reticulum, followed by deposition of collagen. It is doubtful that the apparent proliferation of connective tissue from periportal and pericentral foci is the primary cause of parenchymal replacement, although it may contribute to the process by compressing adjacent hepatic cells or by reducing their blood supply.

As the cirrhotic process advances, signs of hepatocellular failure and portal hypertension appear, owing to progressive degeneration and obliteration of the parenchyma and to obstruction to the outflow of portal blood. However, cirrhosis is not always progressive. Indeed, the disease may remain asymptomatic, or may regress once overt manifestations have appeared. Although experimental evidence suggests that even fibrosis may diminish under certain conditions, the improvement that occurs in man appears to be due to the recovery of injured liver cells, the replacement of lost cells by active regeneration, and the resolution of inflammatory exudates.

Occasionally the etiology of the cirrhotic process may be inferred from the morphologic changes in the liver, but more often the differentiation among the several known types of cirrhosis depends, in part at least, on collateral historical and clinical evidence. This is not surprising, considering the limited number of ways in which the liver can react to diverse types of injury.

The forms of cirrhosis that are recognized clinically include the following: (1) Laennec's, (2) postnecrotic, (3) biliary, (4) cardiac, (5) hemochromatosis, (6) hepatolenticular degeneration (Wilson's disease), (7) cirrhosis due to schistosomiasis, and (8) rarer types.

Laennec's Cirrhosis

Definition. Laennec's cirrhosis, by far the most common type encountered, is characterized by a fine diffuse fibrosis of the liver, often accompanied by fatty infiltration and degeneration of the parenchyma. Malnutrition and chronic alcoholism are the major factors involved in its pathogenesis, but in some instances the etiology is obscure. Occasionally the hepatitis virus and certain poisons give rise to lesions which in their late stages closely resemble those of Laennec's cirrhosis. However, because of the manner in which they develop, such lesions are usually classified as forms of postnecrotic cirrhosis.

Laennec's cirrhosis is known also as *alcoholic, fatty, portal,* or *atrophic* cirrhosis. These terms would appear to be inappropriate, since (1) alcohol is not always an etiologic factor, (2) fatty infiltration is not demonstrable in all cases, (3) the fibrous septums radiate not only from the portal triads but also from the central veins, and (4) the liver may be either large or small, depending on the relative degrees of fatty infiltration, fibrosis, and hepatocellular necrosis and regeneration.

Etiology. Laennec's cirrhosis is thought to be the consequence of a specific type of malnutrition usually related to chronic alcoholism and/or faulty dietary habits. In this country and in many parts of Europe, chronic alcoholism is a major etiologic factor in approximately 75 per cent of cases, but in England and in other parts of the world it plays a relatively unimportant role. A faulty diet probably accounts for the prevalence of the disease among nonalcoholics in certain tropical and subtropical areas but does not appear to be a significant factor in the pathogenesis of cirrhosis among nonalcoholics in the Temperate Zone. On the basis of indirect evidence, it has been suggested that viral hepatitis may be of etiologic importance in such cases. To be sure, the hepatitis virus is capable of producing a finely nodular cirrhosis, but the resulting lesion differs from that in the usual form of Laennec's cirrhosis not only in its mode of development but also in many of its histologic features and, hence, should be classified as postnecrotic, along with other forms of posthepatitic cirrhosis.

Occasionally Laennec's cirrhosis is a complication of other diseases. In a few instances the lesion appears to be the consequence of malnutrition, due either to an absorptive defect, as in pancreatic insufficiency, or to a poor dietary intake, as in ulcerative colitis, chronic malaria, and chronic dysentery, but in other conditions, such as diabetes mellitus, galactosemia, and thyrotoxicosis, the pathogenesis of the cirrhosis is obscure.

It is generally believed that alcohol is not a hepatotoxin and that its effects on the liver are secondary to an associated nutritional disturbance. However, the nature of the deficiency and the precise mechanism responsible for the development of cirrhosis are still uncertain. According to one widely held theory, excessive drinking merely reduces food intake and, thus, leads to a deficiency of lipotropic substances, including choline, its precursor methionine, vitamin B_{12}, folic acid, and possibly some of the other amino acids, like threonine, lysine, and tryptophan, that affect the lipid content of the liver. As a result, the liver becomes fatty and ultimately undergoes fibrosis. It is believed that the accumulation of fat under these conditions may be due to a reduced rate of fatty acid oxidation in the liver, but it is not known whether the fibrosis is the direct consequence of fatty infiltration or is an independent sequela of the lipotropic deficiency. In support of the lipotrope theory, it has been shown that (1) diets rich in protein, and, hence, high in lipotropic activity, are effective in the treatment of Laennec's cirrhosis, (2) it is possible to produce a similar lesion in animals by reducing the intake of protein and other lipotropic substances, and (3) the diet in tropical and subtropical areas, where Laennec's cirrhosis is common, is low in protein content. However, it has been found that in animals on low protein diets, and in children with kwashiorkor, a form of malignant malnutrition seen in the tropics, supplements of protein are far more effective in reversing the associated hepatic lesions than equivalent amounts of choline or methionine, suggesting that the injurious effects of low protein diets on the liver are due to more than a simple deficiency in lipotropic activity. Moreover, since the hepatic lesions of uncomplicated protein deficiency show few of the characteristic degenerative and inflammatory changes seen in Laennec's cirrhosis, the question arises whether nondietary factors may not be involved in their pathogenesis.

A number of clinical observations cast doubt on the concept that the effects of chronic alcoholism on the liver are due solely to a reduction in food consumption. In particular it should be noted that alcoholics occasionally develop Laennec's cirrhosis despite an apparently adequate dietary intake, and that simple undernutrition, such as occurs in many chronic illnesses, seldom gives rise to cirrhosis. In animal experiments it has been shown that while the ingestion of alcohol leads to a decrease in food consumption, apparently in response to the homeostatic mechanism controlling the caloric intake, it also raises the requirement for lipotropic substances, first, by increasing the total caloric intake and, second, by some other as yet unidentified mechanism not dependent on the calorigenic activity of alcohol. This may explain why apparently adequate diets occasionally fail to protect against the development of cirrhosis in individuals who consume a large number of alcohol calories, and why the natives of tropical and subtropical areas, whose diets are low in protein but high in carbohydrate calories, are more likely to develop cirrhosis than undernourished invalids whose diets are likely to be deficient in both protein and calories.

It should be noted that, while chronic alcoholism may be an important factor in the pathogenesis of cirrhosis, only a small proportion of chronic users of alcohol actually develop cirrhosis. No doubt differences in dietary habits play a role, but marked differences in individual susceptibility appear to be an equally important factor. This has been confirmed in animal experiments.

Pathology. In the incipient stage of the disease, the liver is enlarged and pale, owing to the presence of large fat globules in the parenchymal cells. As these become more numerous, stellate-shaped areas of fibrosis appear in the portal areas and, to a lesser extent, around the central veins. Later, thin connective tissue septums join the portal triads and traverse the lobules, breaking them up into islands of cells, which tend to proliferate, forming small nodules or pseudolobules. As the disease progresses, the fibrous bands become thicker and more numerous, are infiltrated by mononuclear cells, and incorporate an increasing number of blood vessels and regenerating perilobular bile ducts. At the same time foci of degeneration and necrosis infiltrated with mononuclear and polymorphonuclear cells appear in the parenchyma, while the amount of fatty infiltration tends to decline. Often the cytoplasm of the hepatic cells contains highly characteristic eosinophilic droplets and club-shaped masses of hyalinelike material known as *Mallory bodies*. These are especially common when chronic alcoholism is an etiologic factor and may be very numerous when the disease is severe. In jaundiced patients the canaliculi may contain plugs of inspissated bile, and occasionally there is bile staining of the parenchymal and Kupffer cells.

Late in the disease the liver is firm and finely nodular or granular, but occasionally it is coarsely nodular with broad intervening connective tissue septums, very much as in postnecrotic cirrhosis. Whether this represents a morphologic variant of Laennec's cirrhosis dependent on a more acute patchy type of necrosis with more active regeneration than in the usual case, or whether it is the sequela of an unrecognized intercurrent infection with the hepatitis virus is still uncertain. The size of the liver is variable, being small in some cases and large in others.

As previously indicated, the fibrosis in Laennec's cirrhosis appears to be the consequence of hepatocellular necrosis and collapse of normal supporting reticulum. Whether fatty infiltration plays an important role in this process is still uncertain, particularly since fatty livers do not necessarily become fibrotic. In animal experiments it has been shown that large fat globules in adjacent cells tend to coalesce, forming large cysts, and that, as the fat is reabsorbed, the reticulum fibers derived from the original cells collapse to form a network of fine septums which ultimately undergo collagenization. It is doubtful that this is the only way in which fibrosis can develop.

In the florid form of Laennec's cirrhosis, which occurs exclusively in alcohol addicts, the predominant findings are extensive hepatocellular degeneration and necrosis with numerous Mallory bodies and infiltrating polymorphonuclear cells. Fatty infiltration and fibrosis vary in extent and may be negligible.

Clinical Features. Usually the onset is insidious with nonspecific complaints, including anorexia, weakness, and unusual fatigability, that relate both to early hepatic dysfunction and to the accompanying underlying malnutrition and chronic alcoholism. Although weight loss is common late in the disease, it may be absent in its early phases. This relates to the fact that while the alcoholic is malnourished, in the sense that the quality of his diet is poor, he frequently obtains a sufficient number of calories in the form of alcohol to maintain or even gain weight. Similarly, the natives of tropical areas who develop nutritional cirrhosis often show no evidence of wasting, since their caloric intake in the form of carbohydrate tends to be high despite a deficiency of protein.

As the disease advances, signs of frank hepatocellular failure and portal hypertension appear. The former include jaundice, ascites, edema, pleural effusion, alterations in serum electrolytes, spider nevi, palmar erythema, gynecomastia, testicular atrophy, impotence, loss of axillary and pubic hair, and a bleeding tendency; the latter splenomegaly, esophageal varices with or without massive bleeding, and a visible venous collateral circulation over the abdomen (p. 156). Usually the above symptoms of hepatocellular failure dominate the clinical picture, but not infrequently the signs of portal hypertension can be demonstrated even before symptoms appear, and occasionally massive bleeding from esophageal varices is the initial manifestation.

Low-grade fever, nausea, vomiting, diarrhea, and abdominal pain are common complaints in the stage of advanced hepatic failure. As indicated previously, the pathogenesis of these symptoms is uncertain. Usually the pain is mild and aching in character, but occasionally, and especially in the florid form of the disease, it may be severe and may be mistaken for biliary colic or a sign of ruptured peptic ulcer. Hepatomegaly is an inconstant but fairly frequent finding. When palpable, the liver usually is firm; occasionally it is slightly tender. The nodules on its surface can rarely be felt.

Impending and overt hepatic coma usually are signs of terminal hepatocellular failure. However, they may be indicative of portacaval shunting of nitrogenous substances from the intestine as a consequence of massive hemorrhage or the ingestion of excessive amounts of protein (p. 157), and they may be reversible.

In the florid form of the disease, the onset tends to be more acute and the progression of symptoms more rapid and less responsive to treatment. Often nausea, vomiting, abdominal pain, high fever, and marked leukocytosis are prominent features.

Usually hepatic decompensation is the consequence of progressive hepatocellular failure resulting from prolonged malnutrition and overindulgence in alcohol. However, it may be precipitated acutely by massive gastrointestinal bleeding, intercurrent infection, surgical trauma, or the development of a complicating hepatoma.

The principal complications of Laennec's cirrhosis include bleeding from esophageal varices, hepatoma, portal vein thrombosis, and intercurrent infection. Bacteremia, apparently arising in the tributaries of the portal vein, is an occasional terminal event. Peptic ulcer and acute pancreatitis are common complications but appear to be more closely related to the accompanying chronic alcoholism than to the cirrhosis.

Laboratory Features. The results of *liver function tests* point to hepatocellular damage. Bromsulphalein retention is an almost invariable finding, even when other tests are negative. The serum albumin level falls progressively as the disease advances, while the serum globulin, and especially the gamma fraction, tends to rise. The direct and total serum bilirubin concentrations may be normal but often are increased to a variable degree. The cephalin-cholesterol flocculation test usually is positive, but thymol turbidity often remains normal. The serum alkaline phosphatase concentration tends to increase slightly but occasionally it rises to the levels seen in obstructive jaundice. In most cases there is no change in the total serum cholesterol, but often the unesterified fraction is increased, especially when jaundice is present. A subnormal cho-

lesterol concentration usually signifies advanced hepatocellular failure and is a bad prognostic sign. The *serum transaminase* levels tend to rise when the disease is active. Usually they remain below 500 units, but in the florid type higher levels may be seen. All these changes tend to revert toward normal under treatment, although Bromsulphalein retention usually persists.

Moderate *anemia* is a common finding. Usually it is normocytic or slightly macrocytic in character, and often it is accompanied by a hyperactive normoblastic bone marrow, mild reticulocytosis, and a decrease in the red cell survival time, features suggesting a hemolytic basis possibly related to overactivity of the spleen, although other factors cannot be excluded. A few instances of frank hemolytic anemia with a positive Coombs test have been reported. These have been attributed to "hypersplenism." Occasionally the anemia is microcytic and hypochromic, as a result of chronic blood loss from esophageal varices or hemorrhoids. Rarely the anemia is megaloblastic and responds to vitamin B_{12} or folic acid, suggesting a nutritional basis.

Slight *leukopenia* and *thrombocytopenia* are common and probably represent manifestations of "hypersplenism." As previously mentioned, *leukocytosis* is the rule in florid cirrhosis, the count often ranging between 20,000 and 50,000 per cu mm. In other cases lesser degrees of leukocytosis may occur when there is active hepatocellular necrosis and degeneration.

Diagnosis. With a history of chronic alcoholism and/or malnutrition, a firm liver and signs of hepatocellular failure and portal hypertension, the diagnosis of Laennec's cirrhosis presents no problem. However, in the absence of any one or several of these features, the differentiation from other diseases may be difficult. The particular disorders to be considered in any given case will depend on the presenting manifestations; they include such diverse conditions as other forms of cirrhosis, hepatitis, intrahepatic malignancy, portal and hepatic vein obstruction, congestive heart failure, constrictive pericarditis, various infiltrative and granulomatous diseases that involve the liver and spleen, and bleeding peptic ulcer. Usually a thorough clinical investigation, including tests of liver function, will serve to distinguish among these disorders, but in doubtful cases a biopsy of the liver may be required.

Prognosis. There is no doubt that the modern therapeutic attack on Laennec's cirrhosis is effective in restoring many patients to good health, provided vigorous treatment is begun at an early stage of the disease. This is reflected in the increased life expectancy reported by several investigators. However, the mortality rate is still distressingly high in patients with advanced hepatocellular failure or bleeding esophageal varices. Thus, of patients with ascites, approximately 35 per cent are dead in 1 year, 50 per cent in 2 years, and 70 per cent in 5 years. Even more alarming statistics may be cited for the group with massive bleeding, but there is some hope that recently developed surgical techniques for controlling portal hypertension may reduce these figures.

The improvement in the outlook for the cirrhotic patient usually is credited to the introduction of modern dietary therapy. However, while this represents an important advance, there is little doubt that more effective methods of combating infection and controlling hemorrhage and more stringent control over the patient's drinking habits and physical activity have contributed to the results. It should be noted in this connection that intercurrent infection and hemorrhage still account for almost half the deaths that occur, which emphasizes the need for meticulous care and close supervision of the cirrhotic patient.

Treatment. A nutritious diet, strict prohibition of alcohol, judicious regulation of salt and water balance, prompt control of hemorrhage and replacement of lost blood, a prompt and vigorous attack on all intercurrent infections, and provision for adequate rest are the mainstays of treatment in Laennec's cirrhosis.

A palatable *diet* containing 80 to 120 Gm protein and 2500 to 3000 Cal, depending on the patient's size and degree of malnutrition, appears to be adequate for the needs of the liver and the replenishment of depleted tissue stores. There is no convincing evidence that a larger intake of protein is more effective as far as the recovery of the liver is concerned, but it may restore the wasted tissues more rapidly. However, it usually is difficult to get sick patients to consume such large amounts of food, and there is the potential hazard of precipitating hepatic coma in those with extensive portacaval shunting. There is no need to restrict fat, so that the patient's personal preferences and tolerance may be used as a guide in adjusting the ratio of fat to carbohydrate calories.

Vitamin supplements are indicated in patients with overt signs of deficiency and in those who will not or cannot eat, but they are an unnecessary expense to patients who are consuming a well-balanced diet. Similarly, *choline* and *methionine* supplements may be helpful in individuals with fatty livers who are poor eaters, but they are of no value if the protein intake is adequate. Moreover, methionine may be toxic in some individuals (p. 158).

Prednisone in small doses (15 to 20 mg per day) may be useful in the management of Laennec's cirrhosis since it often stimulates the appetite, induces a sense of well-being, and potentiates the action of diuretics. According to some authorities it also facilitates healing of the hepatic lesions, but this has not been established. Prednisone must be used with caution since it occasionally accentuates salt and water retention, may lead to potassium depletion, and predisposes to bleeding from esophageal varices and peptic ulcer.

Salt restriction is the simplest and one of the most effective means of managing fluid retention and should be the first employed when ascites, edema, and hydrothorax appear (p. 154). Often limitation of the sodium intake to 500 mg (22 mEq) a day will suffice, but it may be necessary to reduce the intake to 200 mg (10 mEq) to promote a diuresis. Unfortunately, restricting salt makes it difficult to prepare diets that are palatable and rich in protein. The use of salt substitutes, salt-poor derivatives of milk protein, such as Lanolac, and salt-free bread is helpful in this connection.

If salt restriction is ineffective in relieving ascites and edema, *diuretics*, such as the mercurials, chlorothiazide, and the aldosterone antagonist, Aldactone, may be used either singly or in combination, due care being taken to avoid sodium and potassium depletion. Potassium supplements are almost always required with prolonged diuretic therapy. These not only prevent hypopotassemia but also potentiate diuresis and prevent the development of diuretic-induced impending hepatic coma.

Intravenous infusions of *concentrated salt-poor human albumin* may be helpful in producing a diuresis when other measures have failed, and occasionally, for reasons that are not clear, they appear to improve the general clinical status of severely ill patients. Unfortunately, they may produce bleeding from esophageal varices or may precipitate pulmonary edema if given too rapidly, so that they must be used with caution and only when other therapeutic measures have been ineffective.

Paracentesis and *thoracentesis* are indicated whenever the amount of fluid accumulated is sufficiently great to produce symptoms. Their number should be kept to a minimum, since they waste protein and subject the patient to the hazards of the salt depletion syndrome. Application of a tight abdominal binder and restriction of water for a period of 24 hr following paracentesis will do much to prevent the latter. If this fails, a slow infusion of albumin to maintain the blood volume may be more effective. Obviously sodium administration is indicated once the salt depletion syndrome has appeared.

The occurrence of massive bleeding from esophageal varices calls for prompt action including: (1) intravenous replacement of losses in blood, water, and electrolytes, (2) balloon tamponade of the esophagus and cardia with a Sengstaken-Blakemore tube, (3) lowering of portal venous pressure by the use of diuretics and intravenous surgical Pituitrin (20 units in 100 ml of 5 per cent glucose every 4 hr), (4) suppression and neutralization of gastric acid secretion with Banthine and antacids to prevent further erosion of the esophageal mucosa and digestion of newly formed clots, (5) correction, if possible, of any defect in the clotting mechanism, and (6) removal of blood from the intestinal tract to prevent coma by means of gastric aspiration, catharsis, and enemas. Although balloon tamponade is an effective method for controlling active bleeding from esophageal varices, it may give rise to such complications as ulceration and rupture of the esophagus, aspiration of esophageal or gastric contents with resultant pneumonia, and asphyxia as a consequence of aspiration of gastric contents or accidental dislodgment of the balloon into the pharynx. Accordingly it is advisable to try diuretics and intravenous Pituitrin before resorting to tamponade. These agents are known to lower portal venous pressure, and not infrequently they stop esophageal bleeding in this way. Should they prove ineffective and it becomes necessary to use tamponade, the balloon should be deflated at the end of 48 hr and removed 24 hr later unless bleeding recurs in the interim, necessitating further tamponade. In using the Sengstaken-Blakemore tube, (1) check the pressures in both balloons at frequent intervals to ensure that they are intact and in proper position, (2) have a nurse well trained in the management of esophageal tamponade in constant attendance if the patient is unconscious or disoriented, (3) fix the tube at the external nares with adhesive tape, do not use a suspended weight for traction, (4) use hand restraints if the patient is uncooperative or disoriented, and (5) be on the alert for possible dislodgment of the balloon into the pharynx; transect the tube with scissors and immediately withdraw the balloons at the first sign of inspiratory distress; under these conditions do not attempt to deflate the balloons in the usual way since their removal may be delayed and result in a fatality.

If hemorrhage from esophageal varices cannot be controlled by conservative measures, emergency surgical intervention may become necessary. The procedures used include resection of the cardia and lower esophagus, transthoracic-transesophageal suture of the varices, and portacaval shunt. Of these the last two appear to be the most effective and least hazardous. However, the mortality following any of these procedures is high, so that none should be undertaken unless it is certain that tamponade and transfusion are ineffective and that the degree of hemorrhage is a threat to life.

Once a patient has had a massive hemorrhage from esophageal varices, the risk of recurrence is great, even after ligation of the vessels and strict adherence to a good medical regime, and with each subsequent hemorrhage the chances of survival diminish. For this reason there is a growing tendency to advise a surgical attack on either the underlying portal hypertension or the site of varix formation as soon after the first hemorrhage as the patient's condition permits. The most impressive results have been obtained with *portacaval shunts.* Recurrences of massive hemorrhage have been infrequent, and there is suggestive evidence that longevity has been increased. However, while it has been shown that 70 per cent of the patients operated upon are alive after 2 years, as against only 20 per cent for randomly collected untreated cases, little attention has been paid to the fact that the patients selected for surgery have, in general, been the ones in the best condition and, hence, the ones most likely to survive multiple hemorrhages if left untreated. Nevertheless, it cannot be denied that if hemorrhage is prevented the chances of survival for the cirrhotic patient must be improved. Unfortunately, the postoperative mortality rate following portacaval shunt is still 10 to 20 per cent, so that the decision whether to operate and when requires fine judgment.

Ligation of the hepatic and splenic arteries with splenectomy, in the hope of reducing portal pressure, is less effective than portacaval shunt and carries an even higher mortality rate. *Resection of the cardia and lower esophagus,* in an attempt to remove the site of varix formation, is used but cannot be recommended, since recurrences of varices and hemorrhage are common. Recently there has been a renewal of interest in the *injection of esophageal varices* with sclerosing solutions. While this is not the treatment of choice, since varices are likely to recur, it may be useful in patients whose physical condition contraindicates a surgical procedure, or in individuals in whom thrombosis of the portal and splenic veins makes portacaval shunt impossible.

A period of *bed rest* is strongly recommended for the sick cirrhotic patient. Not infrequently it is followed by striking improvement in individuals who have done poorly on an otherwise exemplary regime. Similarly, in ambulatory patients physical activity should be regulated in an attempt to avoid undue fatigue and exhaustion. The basis for the efficacy of rest is not known; it may be related to the increase in hepatic blood flow and decrease in over-all metabolic activity that accompany inactivity and recumbency.

The principles of treatment in hepatic coma are based on current concepts of its pathogenesis (p. 157). They include (1) restriction or omission of protein and provision for maintenance of caloric needs in the form of carbohydrate and fat; in the comatose patients 2 to 2.5 liters of intravenously administered 15 per cent glucose will suffice; (2) correction of any deficits in water, blood, or electrolytes; (3) intravenous administration of L-arginine monohydrochloride, 25 Gm in 500 ml distilled water, repeated once or twice daily depending upon the response of the blood ammonia level; (4) neomycin, by mouth or tube, 8 to 12 Gm daily; and (5) clearing the intestinal tract of blood, if present, by means of gastric aspiration, catharsis, and enemas. Neomycin may cause diarrhea and occasionally leads to the development of staphylococcal enteritis, so that it should be used with caution and for only limited periods of time.

Postnecrotic Cirrhosis

Definition. In contrast to Laennec's cirrhosis, which is characterized by the gradual disintegration of cells in small symmetrical foci giving rise to a fine diffuse fibrosis with small nodules, postnecrotic cirrhosis is the result of a more acute type of necrosis involving larger areas of parenchyma in a more irregular pattern, which produces a characteristic picture of large nodules separated by broad bands of stromal collapse and fibrosis. The size of the nodules and the breath of the connective tissue septums vary, depending on the distribution and extent of the original necrosis. In typical cases, broad zones of necrosis traverse the parenchyma, subdividing it into large lobular aggregates which tend to proliferate, thereby increasing the size and distorting the architecture of their constituent lobules. Occasionally the necrosis is so extensive that an entire lobe, usually the left, is destroyed, leaving nothing but stroma. A finely nodular or granular cirrhosis may be produced if the zones of necrosis and collapse are diffusely distributed in a fine pattern. This type may be difficult to distinguish from Laennec's cirrhosis, unless the process is active and some of the characteristic histologic features of the underlying acute disease are still evident. Although there is reason to believe that postnecrotic cirrhosis represents the healed stage of acute hepatic necrosis, the initial inflammation and necrosis may persist so that not infrequently the disease runs a chronic or intermittently active progressive course.

Postnecrotic cirrhosis is known by a variety of other names, including *postnecrotic scarring, toxic cirrhosis, posthepatitic cirrhosis, coarsely nodular cirrhosis, healed yellow atrophy,* and *Marchand's multiple nodular hyperplasia.*

Etiology. Many instances of postnecrotic cirrhosis represent the sequelae of subacute hepatic necrosis due to the hepatitis virus (p. 1675). In some the manifestations of cirrhosis follow so closely on the heels of a typical attack of acute viral hepatitis that there can be little doubt about the etiology, but in others the onset is insidious, so that the viral origin of the lesion must be inferred from either the character of the histologic changes in the liver or a history suggestive of infection in the past. Less commonly, postnecrotic cirrhosis is the consequence of subacute hepatic necrosis due to poisoning with carbon tetrachloride, chloroform, the chlorinated naphthalenes and diphenyls, tetrachlorethane, TNT, or mushrooms (*Amanita phalloides*), or to the administration of drugs like cinchophen.

Late in the disease there may be none of the earmarks of the acute necrosis responsible for the fibrosis, so that the etiology of the lesion may be difficult to establish, especially if the nodules are of the small variety. Many instances of cirrhosis seen among nonalcoholics fall into this group.

Although diets deficient in selenium and tocopherol lead to subacute hepatic necrosis and postnecrotic cirrhosis in rats, there is no convincing evidence that nutritional factors are involved in the pathogenesis of postnecrotic cirrhosis in man.

Pathology. The evolution of the lesion in the viral type of postnecrotic cirrhosis has been described elsewhere (p. 1686). Except for the occurrence of fatty infiltration early in the course of the disease, the zonal distribution of the necrosis, and the character of the inflammatory reaction, which tends to be less extensive but more polymorphonuclear in type, the toxic form of postnecrotic cirrhosis develops in the same manner.

The features that distinguish the posthepatitic type from Laennec's cirrhosis include the following: (1) the nodules usually are larger, vary more in size and shape, and often contain several intact, but abnormally oriented central veins and portal triads; (2) the septums tend to be broader, show a more intensive mononuclear inflammatory reaction, and contain many more blood vessels, regenerating bile ducts, and collapsed and thickened reticulum fibers but fewer collagen fibers; (3) the parenchyma shows a more active type of regeneration, with the appearance of bizarrely shaped, multinucleated cells, and often exhibits eosinophilic Councilman-like hyaline bodies (p. 1672), scattered foci of necrosis and degeneration, and a mononuclear exudate; (4) often the veins show an inflammatory reaction in their walls; and (5) fatty infiltration and Mallory bodies (p. 1501) are rare.

Clinical Features. Often the overt manifestations of cirrhosis appear insidiously (1) during convalescence from an otherwise uncomplicated, and sometimes very mild, attack of acute viral or toxic hepatitis, (2) after one or more relapses following an attack of acute hepatitis, (3) following a vague anicteric illness, presumably due to the hepatitis virus, or (4) in an individual in apparent good health who may or may not give a history of previous hepatitis. Occasionally the onset is acute and severe with signs of subacute hepatic necrosis (p. 1675), following which, progression to the stage of fibrosis may be remarkably rapid.

The clinical features are very much like those of Laennec's cirrhosis (p. 1686), except that (1) jaundice appears at an earlier phase and is more likely to be persistent or to recur at intervals, (2) abdominal pain and gastrointestinal symptoms are more frequent and tend to be more severe, (3) purpura, epistaxis, and other hemorrhagic phenomena are more common, (4) the liver tends to be smaller and is more often nodular on palpation, (5) once ascites appears the life expectancy is very much shorter, and (6) therapy is far less effective.

Laboratory Features. The results of liver function tests are like those in Laennec's cirrhosis, except that (1) the serum globulin level tends to be higher, occasionally reaching concentrations of 8 or 9 Gm per 100 ml, while the serum albumin level tends to be lower, (2) hypocholesteremia is more common, and (3) thymol turbidity is increased with greater regularity, and higher values are more frequent.

Treatment. The principles of treatment outlined for Laennec's cirrhosis (p. 1688) are equally applicable in this disease. Although dietary therapy is less effective as far as recovery of the liver is concerned, it is, nevertheless, important in maintaining the patient's nutritional status during his prolonged illness and in controlling water and salt retention. Bed rest is particularly important during the early phase of the disease and during periods of acute progression. ACTH and prednisone may be helpful, and should be tried in all cases with evidence of active hepatocellular necrosis and inflammation. Usually prolonged therapy is indicated, so that the dose must be reduced to low maintenance levels as soon as maximum benefit has been achieved in order to minimize undesirable side effects.

Biliary Cirrhosis

Definition. While it may be difficult to differentiate between biliary and other forms of cirrhosis on morphologic grounds alone, especially late in the disease, the clinical manifestations and laboratory features of biliary cirrhosis are highly characteristic. They include (1) the early appearance and persistence of an obstructive-like jaundice, with pruritus, dark urine, and high levels of serum alkaline phosphatase, cholesterol, and phospholipid; (2) marked hepatomegaly; (3) a tendency to develop xanthomas of the skin as the serum lipids increase progressively; and (4) a relatively benign course for a number of years, during which there are few if any clinical or laboratory signs of hepatocellular failure, followed ultimately by terminal hepatic decompensation or massive bleeding from esophageal varices.

Etiology and Classification. There are two major types of biliary cirrhosis: one develops following prolonged obstruction of the extrahepatic bile ducts; the other is the consequence of a chronic intrahepatic inflammatory reaction due to a variety of factors, some of which are still unknown. These two types may be conveniently classified as follows:

CLASSIFICATION OF BILIARY CIRRHOSIS

I. Extrahepatic—due to partial or complete occlusion of the major bile ducts
II. Intrahepatic
    A. Primary—etiology unknown
    B. Secondary—due to:
        1. Viral hepatitis
        2. Drug sensitization reactions

The *extrahepatic* type is seen most frequently following prolonged partial occlusion of the common bile duct by postoperative stricture or stone. However, it may be the result of congenital atresia, carcinoma, or benign cysts anywhere along the course of the biliary tract from the ampulla of Vater to the bifurcation of the hepatic duct in the porta hepatis, provided the patient survives sufficiently long and the obstruction is not relieved. There appear to be marked differences in individual susceptibility, biliary cirrhosis occurring within a few months of obstruction in some instances, and not for several years, or not at all, in others. The question of whether biliary tract infection is a contributory factor is still unsettled.

The *primary type of intrahepatic biliary cirrhosis* occurs almost exclusively in women. Neither the etiology nor the reason for the unusual sex distribution is known. However, it is noteworthy that many of the patients have an allergic background, and that the number of cases reported has increased since the introduction of the sulfonamides and other sensitizing drugs. Since some of the latter have been implicated in the pathogenesis of the secondary type of intrahepatic biliary cirrhosis, it is conceivable that unrecognized drug reactions are a more important etiologic factor in the primary type than is generally recognized. Similarly, unrecognized infections with the hepatitis virus may be a factor in some cases, since it is known that they are capable of producing biliary cirrhosis.

The *secondary type of intrahepatic biliary cirrhosis* appears to be the end stage of a progressive "cholangiolitic" hepatitis, due either to the hepatitis virus (p. 1675) or to drug hypersensitivity (p. 1681). Thus, typical cases have been reported following acute viral hepatitis and reactions to neoarsphenamine, neocinchophen and chlorpromazine.

At one time the primary intrahepatic type of

biliary cirrhosis was called *xanthomatous biliary cirrhosis* in the belief that the xanthomatosis was a manifestation of a primary disturbance in lipid metabolism, and that the hepatic lesion was secondary to xanthomatous obstruction of the biliary tract. However, it is now known that the hypercholesteremia and xanthomatosis in both extra- and intrahepatic biliary cirrhosis are manifestations of the underlying liver disease and bear no relationship to familial hypercholesteremia and xanthomatosis, and that xanthomatous deposits in the biliary tract play no role in the pathogenesis of cirrhosis. It should be emphasized that not all cases of biliary cirrhosis develop xanthomatosis, the occurrence of such lesions depending on the magnitude and duration of the serum lipid elevation. In general, xanthomas occur more frequently in the primary intrahepatic type than in any of the other forms of biliary cirrhosis. The longer duration of the disease in the former and the greater delay in the appearance of hepatocellular failure, which tends to lower the serum lipids, probably account for this difference.

Other synonyms sometimes applied to the primary type of intrahepatic biliary cirrhosis include *Hanot's hypertrophic, pericholangiolitic, cholangiolitic,* and *nonobstructive cholangitic biliary cirrhosis.*

Pathology. Following occlusion of the extrahepatic bile ducts the liver shows a number of characteristic changes, which include (1) signs of bile stasis, as evidenced by the presence of bile thrombi in the central canaliculi, and bile staining of scattered parenchymal and Kupffer cells, (2) foci of parenchymal necrosis in the periportal and midzonal areas, presumably due to the effects of escaped bile, (3) elongation, dilatation, and proliferation of the interlobular and perilobular bile ducts, (4) exudation of polymorphonuclear, eosinophilic, and mononuclear cells in the portal triads, and (5) thickening of the portal triads due to edema, exudate, duct proliferation, and fibrosis. If the obstruction is not relieved, the portal triads continue to thicken and extend farther and farther into the parenchyma, ultimately bridging adjacent portal triads and giving rise to a perilobular fibrosis. At this stage the lobular pattern is still evident, but extension of the fibrotic and inflammatory process to the parenchyma ultimately destroys the normal lobular pattern, producing the full-blown picture of biliary cirrhosis. The liver is enlarged, finely granular, firm, and bile stained. Large nodules are unusual, since the regenerative response of the parenchyma is limited in the face of bile stasis. It should be noted that the transition from simple bile stasis to outspoken cirrhosis is a very gradual one and seldom can be recognized clinically, except late in the disease.

Early in *primary intrahepatic biliary cirrhosis* there is a low-grade chronic inflammatory reaction centered about the small perilobular cholangioles. This is accompanied by perilobular bile stasis and degenerative changes in the adjacent parenchymal cells. As the disease advances, fibrosis and inflammation extend into the parenchyma, bridging adjacent portal triads and producing the type of perilobular fibrosis seen in early obstructive biliary cirrhosis. However, the reduplication of the terminal cholangioles is less striking, the large interlobular ducts tend to diminish in number, and evidence of bile stasis is less prominent. Later, as the fibrotic process progresses, the lobular pattern is obliterated and the picture of cirrhosis emerges. At this stage the liver is enlarged, bile stained, and finely granular.

The evolution of the lesion in *posthepatitic biliary cirrhosis* has been described elsewhere (p. 1675).

In *drug-induced* biliary cirrhosis the pathogenesis of the lesions closely resembles that of the primary intrahepatic type.

It should be emphasized that, while it may be possible to distinguish between the lesions in the various forms of biliary cirrhosis early in the course of the disease, it is rarely possible to do so by the time the full-blown picture of cirrhosis has developed.

The pathogenesis of the jaundice in the intrahepatic type of biliary cirrhosis is uncertain. Obstruction of the cholangioles by inflammatory exudate and fibrosis, and increased cholangiolar permeability with regurgitation of bile are thought to be the principal factors involved, but the evidence for this is indirect and inconclusive.

Clinical Features. In the *primary intrahepatic type* of biliary cirrhosis the onset is insidious, with pruritus or, less commonly, with jaundice. As the disease advances, pruritus becomes more troublesome, jaundice deepens slowly, bile appears in the urine, and the stools tend to lighten in color. Often these signs of biliary "obstruction" fluctuate in intensity. Progressive enlargement and induration of the liver occurs and usually is accompanied by significant splenomegaly. Many patients develop a striking melanotic pigmentation of the skin, and occasionally this is associated with vitiligo. Generalized lymphadenopathy is common, and occasionally clubbing of the fingers is seen.

Some months to years after onset a certain number of patients develop xanthomatosis. Usually this can be correlated with a sustained elevation of the serum lipids. It has been found that if the total lipids exceed 1,800 mg, or if the total cholesterol exceeds 500 mg per 100 ml for a period in excess of 3 months, xanthomas may be expected to appear. This occurs first as typical xanthelasma of the eyelids, and then as flat planus lesions in the palmar creases and over the skin of the neck, chest, and back. Later, more nodular tuberous lesions appear over the extensor surfaces of the knuckles, elbows, knees, and ankles, and over the buttocks.

Another striking feature of this disease is steatorrhea, due apparently to malabsorption of fat related to a decrease in bile salt excretion. The stools tend to increase in frequency and occasionally are bulky, foul, and loose. A more important complication is decalcification of bone, which often is accompanied by compression of the vertebral bodies and back pain. This appears to be the consequence of excessive fecal losses of vitamin D and calcium in relation to the steatorrhea, but a postmenopausal defect in bone matrix formation may be involved in some cases. It has been suggested that losses of other fat-soluble vitamins, and especially vitamin A, may play a role in the pigmentation and thickening of the skin that occurs in this disease.

In contrast to other forms of cirrhosis, the patient feels remarkably well and loses little or no weight over a period of years, despite the fact that the disease is progressive. Also, there is a striking absence of anorexia, indigestion, abdominal pain and tenderness, chills, and fever. Ultimately, however, signs of hepatic failure (p. 1686) or massive bleeding from esophageal varices appear. Death may occur within 2 years, but many patients live as long as 10 years. Of interest is the fact that, as hepatocellular failure develops, there is a fall in the serum lipids and a disappearance or decrease in the size of the xanthomatous lesions.

The clinical course in the other forms of biliary cirrhosis is very similar, except that attacks of abdominal pain, chills and fever, and a history of antecedent gallbladder disease or biliary tract surgery are common in the extrahepatic type, while an onset with typical acute viral hepatitis or a drug sensitization reaction is characteristic of the secondary intrahepatic type.

Laboratory Features. Early in the disease the principal findings are those of obstructive jaundice, viz., an elevated direct and total serum bilirubin, a high serum alkaline phosphatase level, slightly raised levels of serum transaminase, increased serum cholesterol and phospholipid, and a decrease in fecal urobilinogen. Characteristically the serum is clear despite its high lipid content, apparently because the concentration of neutral fat is not increased. The serum albumin level is normal or only slightly decreased but falls when hepatocellular failure occurs. However, the serum globulins, and especially the β- and γ-fractions, are increased from the beginning. The cephalin-cholesterol flocculation reaction may be positive or negative, but thymol turbidity is increased with regularity, high values being especially common in patients with marked hypercholesteremia. Despite steatorrhea and jaundice, the prothrombin level is normal, or if depressed, is readily corrected by the parenteral administration of vitamin K.

Diagnosis. The possibility of biliary cirrhosis must be considered in any case of prolonged "obstructive" jaundice accompanied by significant hepatomegaly. Once signs of portal hypertension or xanthomatosis appear the diagnosis can be made clinically with reasonable assurance, but earlier in the disease biopsy of the liver may be necessary. Usually the most difficult problem is the distinction between the extra- and intrahepatic types. Since this can seldom be made with certainty on clinical or even histologic grounds, every patient with biliary cirrhosis deserves a thorough surgical exploration with cholangiography to exclude the presence of a remediable obstruction in the extrahepatic biliary tree.

Treatment. Surgical relief of biliary obstruction is essential in those with extrahepatic biliary cirrhosis. If this can be accomplished, remarkable improvement may be expected, even when the disease is advanced.

The objectives of treatment in the intrahepatic type of cirrhosis are the maintenance of nutrition, the control and prevention of complications, and the relief of pruritus.

While a high protein, high caloric diet is of value in maintaining weight and strength, it appears to have little effect on the underlying hepatic lesion. Fats need not be restricted unless steatorrhea becomes troublesome. There is no evidence that limitation of dietary fat alters the course of the disease or the accompanying hypercholesteremia and xanthomatosis. Daily supplements of vitamins A and D and a high calcium intake are indicated to compensate for fecal losses. Vitamin K is administered if the prothrombin level is low. It may be necessary to administer the fat-soluble vitamins by the parenteral route if steatorrhea is severe.

The management of ascites and bleeding esophageal varices is the same as in Laennec's cirrhosis (p. 1688).

Pruritus is a difficult therapeutic problem. Occasionally soothing lotions and baths and the antihistamine drugs are helpful, but when itching is severe only methyltestosterone in daily doses of 25 to 50 mg sublingually appears to be effective. Although it usually produces an increase in jaundice, it has no long-term ill effects. Moreover, it tends to lower the serum cholesterol and phospholipid levels and may thus prevent further xanthoma formation.

A course of prednisone is worth trying, particularly in patients whose biliary cirrhosis is thought to be posthepatitic, since it occasionally suppresses the activity of the disease and induces a partial remission.

Cardiac Cirrhosis

Pathology. Characteristically the liver enlarges in congestive heart failure. Microscopically there is engorgement of the pericentral sinusoids with atrophy, degeneration, and necrosis of the intervening parenchymal cells, and little or no inflammatory reaction. The central veins are dilated and thickened, and occasionally there is hemorrhage into the pericentral zone of degenerating liver cells. Usually these changes are the consequence of the increase in hepatic venous pressure, the stasis of blood, and the hypoxia that follow congestive heart failure. However, very similar changes may be produced by occlusion of the hepatic veins (Chiari's syndrome), constriction of the pericardium, and vascular shock.

If congestion is prolonged and severe, the pericentral zones of parenchymal atrophy and necrosis extend until adjacent central veins are bridged. Since hepatocellular regeneration is relatively ineffective under these conditions, the stroma tends to collapse, forming bands of condensed and thickened reticulum fibers, which ultimately undergo collagenization. This gives rise to a reversal of the normal lobular pattern, with centrally placed portal triads and perilobular rings of fibrous tissue joining adjacent central veins. Later, the zones of congestion, atrophy, and reticular collapse extend to the portal triads, so that ultimately the lobular architecture is destroyed, resulting in the development of cirrhosis. As a rule, there is little active regeneration, so that the liver is finely granular and tends to diminish in size. Occasionally, however, particularly when bouts of severe congestion alternate with periods of compensation, regenerative nodules of varying size may be formed.

Clinical Features. In uncomplicated *chronic passive congestion,* the liver is enlarged and tender, and in long-standing cases it may be firm, even in the absence of fibrosis. Pulsation of the liver is characteristic of tricuspid valvular disease. Pressure over the liver often produces a significant increase in the distention of the jugular veins (hepatojugular reflux). Occasionally the spleen is enlarged, but other signs of portal hypertension are rare, although small asymptomatic esophageal varices may be observed at autopsy. Many patients with congestive failure exhibit mild hyperbilirubinemia, but frank jaundice and bilirubinuria are unusual, except in patients with severe tricuspid valvular disease or in those with complicating pulmonary infarction. The jaundice is primarily of hepatocellular origin, but increased hemolysis may be a factor in cases with pulmonary infarction. Ascites is a common finding in advanced congestive failure. No doubt the increase in hepatic venous pressure plays a role in its pathogenesis, as it does in other conditions (p. 154), but how much the accompanying hepatocellular injury contributes to the general phenomenon of salt and water retention in cardiac failure is still a matter of conjecture.

The transition from chronic passive congestion of the liver to *cardiac cirrhosis* is a very gradual one and difficult to recognize clinically, since the signs and symptoms in the two conditions are very much the same. However, intractable ascites, a firm, nontender liver, absence of a demonstrable hepatojugular reflux, and progressive splenomegaly are features that should suggest the diagnosis. In contrast to other forms of cirrhosis, deep jaundice, spider nevi, bleeding from esophageal varices, and hepatic coma are unusual.

While cardiac cirrhosis may occur in any type of heart disease, it is seen most frequently in rheumatic heart disease, severe cor pulmonale, and constrictive pericarditis.

Laboratory Features. The most frequent functional abnormalities associated with congestion of the liver include Bromsulphalein retention, a slight rise in the serum bilirubin level, an increase in urine urobilinogen, and a fall in the serum albumin. These parallel the severity of the hepatocellular changes. However, there is some evidence to indicate that Bromsulphalein retention may, in part at least, be a function of reduced hepatic blood flow. In patients with overt jaundice the urine may contain bile. Occasionally there is an increase in serum globulin, cephalin-cholesterol flocculation, and thymol turbidity.

The changes in cardiac cirrhosis are very similar, but the serum albumin concentration tends to fall to a lower level.

Diagnosis. The recognition of congestive hepatomegaly and cardiac cirrhosis is seldom difficult. However, they may be mistaken for other forms of cirrhosis when the signs of heart disease are masked, as in constrictive pericarditis.

Hemochromatosis

See p. 785.

Hepatolenticular Degeneration (Wilson's Disease)

See p. 768.

Cirrhosis Due to Schistosomiasis

Infestations with *Schistosoma mansoni* or *Schistosoma japonicum* may give rise to an unusual type of cirrhosis. Although the disease is not indigenous to this country, it is very common among Puerto Rican immigrants, and is seen occasionally in veterans of the Second World War who served in the Pacific area.

Pathology. Some of the schistosome ova deposited in the distal tributaries of the portal vein are swept back into the liver, where they produce a granulomatous reaction in the portal triads, the periportal parenchyma, and the intrahepatic portal radicles themselves. As the lesions age and become fibrotic, the encapsulated ova degenerate. Occasionally the process is confined to the larger intrahepatic periportal areas, giving rise to so-called "white, pipestem fibrosis," which mimics cirrhosis clinically but differs from it in that the remaining parenchyma is intact. However, patients with hepatic schistosomiasis may develop a fine nodular cirrhosis of the Laennec's type. In some, this appears to be the consequence of a widespread granulomatous reaction to ova, but in others the etiology is uncertain and may be related to accompanying malnutrition.

Clinical Features. The principal findings in hepatic schistosomiasis are progressive enlargement of the liver and signs of portal hypertension. Bleeding from esophageal varices is a frequent complication, while signs of hepatocellular failure are relatively uncommon, except in patients with malnutrition, in whom the disease behaves more like Laennec's cirrhosis.

Some patients have frank signs of intestinal schistosomiasis, but many of the Puerto Ricans seen in this country, who present with hepatomegaly or esophageal bleeding, have no other clinical manifestations of the disease. Often rectal biopsy is positive for ova, but if not the diagnosis can usually be established by means of needle biopsy of the liver.

For a more complete discussion of schistosomiasis see p. 1225.

Rare Forms of Cirrhosis

Granulomatous Cirrhosis. Occasionally, granulomatous diseases are accompanied by cirrhosis. In the case of sarcoidosis (p. 1683) and brucellosis (p. 1684) it is reasonably certain that the cirrhosis follows healing of extensive granulomatous lesions, but in tuberculosis (p. 1684) it is doubtful that the cirrhosis is of granulomatous origin.

Cirrhosis Associated with Metabolic Disorders. A significant number of patients with *diabetes mellitus* have fatty livers, and a few develop a lesion resembling Laennec's cirrhosis. Many authorities attribute the fatty infiltration to obesity, starvation, or poor regulation of the diabetes and regard the association of diabetes and cirrhosis as fortuitous. However, this opinion is not shared by all investigators, so that the pathogenesis of cirrhosis in diabetes is still an unsettled problem.

Rarely, *hyperthyroidism* is accompanied by cirrhosis. It is generally believed that the cirrhosis is the consequence of congestive heart failure, but it

has been suggested that in some instances it may be the result of a specific circulatory disturbance, an induced nutritional deficiency, or a relative hypoxia related to the hyperthyroid state.

Not infrequently infants with *galactosemia*, a congenital disease in which galactose cannot be metabolized, develop an hepatic lesion resembling Laennec's cirrhosis. This has been attributed to the toxic action of galactose or to a nutritional deficiency related to the inability to utilize the galactose in milk. However, neither of these theories has been established.

Rarely *von Gierke's disease* (p. 772) is associated with cirrhosis.

Occasionally the *de Toni-Fanconi syndrome* is accompanied by a coarsely nodular cirrhosis. The pathogenesis of the hepatic lesion is unknown. A nutritional deficiency related to the loss of amino acids has been postulated, but the evidence for this is not convincing.

Erythroblastosis Fetalis. Often the liver is severely injured in erythroblastosis, and rarely cirrhosis is a sequela. On the basis of indirect evidence it has been suggested that other forms of infantile or juvenile cirrhosis may be the consequence of other unrecognized maternal blood incompatibilities.

INFILTRATIONS OF THE LIVER

Fatty Liver

Usually fatty infiltration of the liver is due to a deficiency of lipotropic substances secondary to faulty dietary habits, chronic alcoholism, absorptive defects, or the malnutrition of certain chronic wasting diseases. However, it is seen also in metabolic disorders such as diabetes mellitus and galactosemia, in obesity, and as a transient phenomenon in poisoning with agents like carbon tetrachloride and phosphorus. The pathogenesis in the latter group is uncertain. Except in the case of obesity, long-continued fatty infiltration appears to predispose to the development of cirrhosis.

Often the fatty liver is enlarged to palpation, and not infrequently there is mild Bromsulphalein retention. Other signs of hepatocellular failure and portal hypertension do not occur unless there is accompanying hepatic necrosis or fibrosis.

Hemosiderosis

Usually abnormal deposits of hemosiderin in the liver are a sign of increased total body stores of iron. This may be the result of an excessive uptake of iron from the gastrointestinal tract due to (1) a congenital absorptive defect, as in hemochromatosis, (2) the stimulus of chronic anemia with failure to utilize the absorbed iron, as in certain hemolytic states, (3) an excessive intake of iron, (4) the use of low protein, low phosphate diets that enhance iron absorption, or (5) the transfusion of large amounts of blood.

Uncomplicated hemosiderosis of the liver produces no symptoms. The question of whether the fibrosis seen in advanced cases is the result of hepatocellular degeneration related to excessive storage of iron is still unsettled.

The reader is referred to the chapter on hemochromatosis (p. 785) for a more complete discussion of this subject.

Glycogen Storage (von Gierke's) Disease

See p. 772.

Amyloidosis

The liver is involved in a high proportion of patients with secondary amyloidosis, and somewhat less frequently in those with primary amyloidosis and the type associated with multiple myeloma. Amyloid is deposited between the sinusoids and the parenchymal cells, slowly obliterating the former and causing atrophy of the latter. In addition, the walls of the blood vessels may be infiltrated, especially in the primary type.

The liver is enlarged, smooth, and firm. Jaundice, spider nevi, and ascites are rare, except in advanced cases. Portal hypertension is not a feature, but the spleen may be enlarged as a result of amyloid deposition. The remaining clinical signs and symptoms relate to involvement of other tissues and are described elsewhere (p. 783).

Despite extensive infiltration of the liver, hepatocellular function tends to be little deranged, except for slight Bromsulphalein retention. Hypoalbuminemia and hypercholesteremia, common in advanced cases, appear to be more closely related to the accompanying nephrotic syndrome. Hyperglobulinemia is an inconstant finding, and usually the cephalin-cholesterol and thymol turbidity reactions are normal. Occasionally high levels of serum alkaline phosphatase are seen.

Lymphomatous and Other
Reticuloendothelial Infiltrations

Not infrequently the liver participates in the abnormal generalized reticuloendothelial reactions that characterize leukemia, Hodgkin's disease, and lymphosarcoma. Whether the hepatic lesions represent infiltrations from without or a local reticuloendothelial reaction to the underlying stimulus is not clear. Hepatomegaly is the principal finding, apart from the other manifestations of the underlying disease, and, except for jaundice, rarely is accompanied by other signs or symptoms of hepatocellular failure. While jaundice may occur in any

of these conditions, it is most common in Hodgkin's disease, where it usually is due to a combination of biliary obstruction and parenchymal destruction. Occasionally a hemolytic process is involved.

In *extramedullary hematopoiesis* the liver may be enlarged owing to infiltration of the sinusoids and portal triads with megakaryocytes and immature erythrocytes and leukocytes. Marked splenomegaly is an invariable accompaniment. The disease represents a reversion to a fetal type of hematopoietic activity in response to aplasia or replacement of the normal bone marrow. The hepatic lesions seldom give rise to any symptoms, the principal manifestations being related to the underlying bone marrow disease.

Gaucher's disease and *Niemann-Pick disease* are hereditary disorders characterized by a generalized proliferation of abnormal reticuloendothelial cells containing lipid, a cerebroside (kerasin) in the former, and a phospholipid (sphingomyelin) in the latter. In both diseases the liver and spleen are infiltrated with these cells, resulting in hepatomegaly and splenomegaly. The hepatic lesions give rise to no symptoms, the clinical manifestations being due to involvement of other tissues (p. 780).

SPACE-OCCUPYING LESIONS

Primary Carcinoma of the Liver

Carcinomas that arise in the liver may be derived from either the parenchymal cells or the intrahepatic bile duct epithelium, and are known respectively as *hepatomas* and *cholangiomas*. The former are twice as common as the latter. Occasionally tumors show features of both types.

Males are affected more frequently than females, and the onset is more common after the age of fifty, although the disease may occur in children and young adults. The incidence is particularly high in areas where nutritional and parasitic disease of the liver is endemic. Thus, in this country primary hepatic carcinomas comprise only 2.5 per cent of all malignancies, while in South Africa, China, and Malaya the incidence among natives ranges from 30 to 50 per cent.

Cirrhosis appears to be an important predisposing factor and is found in approximately 75 per cent of patients with hepatoma and 50 per cent of those with cholangioma. While the incidence of primary hepatic carcinoma is only 0.3 per cent in routine autopsies, it varies between 2 and 8 per cent in the cirrhotic group, being highest in the postnecrotic and hemochromatotic types.

Often the clinical picture is that of the underlying cirrhosis, so that the presence of a complicating hepatoma may be overlooked. In patients known to have cirrhosis, the possibility of this complication should be considered when (1) jaundice, ascites, or bleeding from esophageal varices occurs without provocation, (2) abdominal pain is a prominent feature, (3) the liver is unusually large and tender, has large palpable nodules on its surface, is enlarged asymmetrically, or has an overlying friction rub or vascular bruit, (4) there is rapid weight loss out of keeping with the dietary intake, (5) high fever and leukocytosis are present, (6) the serum alkaline phosphatase level is unusually high, or (7) the ascitic fluid is bloody. It must be emphasized that these features are not seen in all cases, and, indeed, some are relatively uncommon. Jaundice occurs in only half the patients and may be due to obstruction of bile ducts or to extensive destruction of the parenchyma. Ascites and esophageal bleeding are frequent but inconstant features. While they may be related to the accompanying cirrhosis, the tendency of the tumor to invade the hepatic and portal veins appears to be an important factor in many cases. High fever, marked leukocytosis, friction rubs, and bruits are unusual but are important clues when present. A high alkaline phosphatase level is not a constant finding but is highly suggestive of intrahepatic malignancy, particularly in the absence of jaundice. Bloody ascitic fluid is seen occasionally in uncomplicated Laennec's cirrhosis but is more common in the presence of malignancy.

In the absence of overt signs of cirrhosis, the diagnosis may be very difficult, since cachexia, abdominal pain, jaundice, ascites, and hepatomegaly are features common to other forms of intraabdominal malignancy with metastases to the liver and peritoneum. There is a clinical impression that hepatomas rarely metastasize. However, this is not borne out by autopsy studies, which indicate that metastases occur in approximately 65 per cent of cases, the sites of predilection being the periportal and peripancreatic lymph nodes, the lungs and pleura, the peritoneum, the bones, the brain, and the adrenal glands. Occasionally symptoms referable to bony metastases are the first to appear.

Needle biopsy of the liver is an important diagnostic aid and is positive in a high proportion of cases. X-ray studies are useful in excluding primary carcinomas in other sites and, occasionally, are helpful in establishing the presence of an intrahepatic mass by demonstrating a localized elevation of the right leaf of the diaphragm.

The outlook is virtually hopeless, most patients dying within a few months to a year. Successful excision of carcinoma localized to a single lobe has been reported, but this is a rarity, since the tumor has usually spread by way of the intrahepatic vessels to involve the entire liver by the time the disease is recognized clinically.

Other Primary Tumors of the Liver

Hemangiomas are common in the liver. Usually they are small and asymptomatic, but occasionally they are large or very numerous, producing hepatic enlargement or localized swelling of the liver. Females are affected more frequently than males, and left lobe involvement is more common than right. When the tumor is large it may produce pain or may give rise to a fatal hemorrhage into the peritoneal cavity, either spontaneously or following trauma. Occasionally, obstructive jaundice is a complication, and, rarely, congestive heart failure is the result of extensive arteriovenous shunting of blood through the tumor. An hepatic bruit is audible in some cases, and not infrequently calcification is demonstrable radiographically. Successful surgical removal of localized hemangiomas is possible and is generally recommended to prevent massive hemorrhage and to relieve pressure symptoms.

Malignant *hemangioendotheliomas* and other forms of *sarcoma* are very rare.

Metastatic Neoplasms of the Liver

These occur at least twenty times as frequently as primary carcinoma of the liver and are found in approximately one-third of all malignancies.

The liver appears to provide a peculiarly favorable environment for the growth of tumor cells, and by virtue of its double circulation is in a strategic position to trap metastasizing cells gaining access to either the portal venous or hepatic arterial blood stream. In addition, retrograde invasion of its lymphatics from adjacent organs is possible. As might be expected, tumors arising in the distribution of the portal vein, such as gastrointestinal and pancreatic carcinoma, metastasize to the liver more commonly than to the lung. However, it is surprising to find that the same is true of tumors arising in the breast, uterus, ovary, and kidneys, whose venous drainage reaches the lungs first. Only in the case of thyroid and prostatic carcinoma is pulmonary involvement more common. Whether tumor cells pass through the lung and reach the liver by way of the arterial circulation or extend to contiguous tissues drained by the portal vein is uncertain. In the case of the breast, it is believed that metastasis occurs by way of lymphatics.

Metastases are usually multiple and, once implanted, tend to grow rapidly, invading blood vessels and lymphatics and extending to other parts of the liver. Not infrequently the growth of tumor tissue in the liver is far more conspicuous than at the primary site, and, indeed, the clinical manifestations may be predominantly hepatic at a time when the primary lesion is not detectable. This is particularly true of carcinomas arising in the pancreas, gallbladder, kidney, and lung, and of mela-nosarcomas.

The clinical features vary, depending on the extent and location of the lesion. At one extreme, there may be no signs or symptoms suggestive of metastasis, while at the other, invasion may be so extensive that signs of hepatocellular failure and portal obstruction are produced.

Sooner or later, weight loss, anorexia, abdominal pain, and hepatomegaly develop. Usually the liver is very hard, because of the fibrotic reaction frequently associated with malignant infiltration, and often nodules are palpable. Although the liver is not palpable in all instances, it tends to enlarge progressively as the disease advances, and occasionally it grows to tremendous size. Rarely, an overlying friction rub may be audible. Jaundice is an inconstant and late finding and may be due to obstruction of major bile ducts, either within the liver or at the porta hepatis, or, less commonly, to hepatocellular failure. Usually ascites follows spread of the tumor to the peritoneum, but it may be the result of invasion of the hepatic or portal vein, severe hypoalbuminemia, or hepatic decompensation. Splenomegaly occurs in 10 to 15 per cent of cases. It is said to be especially common in pancreatic carcinoma because of splenic vein obstruction, but in the author's experience splenomegaly has not been limited to this particular type of tumor and usually has been due to massive invasion of the liver producing portal hypertension. Esophageal varices and massive upper gastrointestinal bleeding may be complications in such cases.

Hepatocellular function may be completely normal, even in the face of extensive metastasis. However, Bromsulphalein retention and a significant elevation of serum alkaline phosphatase are common findings. Usually cephalin-cholesterol flocculation and thymol turbidity are normal, except very late in the disease. Often the serum albumin level is lowered, but this may be the consequence of malnutrition. The high alkaline phosphatase level is of particular diagnostic significance in the absence of jaundice and signs of bone involvement; it should suggest the possibility of hepatic malignancy or some other type of infiltration.

Short of surgical exploration, needle biopsy of the liver is by far the most useful and accurate diagnostic aid in this disease. Approximately 80 per cent of hepatic metastases can be demonstrated by this technique, not infrequently in the absence of any overt signs of the disease. Considering the focal character of the gross lesions seen at the autopsy and their scattered distribution, this incidence appears incredible. However, the infiltration usually is much more diffuse than is evident on macroscopic examination, because of the tendency of the tumor to spread along vascular channels.

Amebic Abscess

See p. 1197.

Pyogenic Abscess

The incidence of pyogenic abscess, which has always been lower than that of the amebic variety, has declined appreciably since the introduction of antibiotic therapy in the management of infections that predispose to abscess formation.

Almost always, pyogenic abscess of the liver is the result of parenchymal invasion by organisms stemming from an adjacent or distant septic focus. However, the source of infection may be difficult to detect, and rarely the infection is primary in the liver as a result of a penetrating or crushing wound. Organisms may gain access to the liver via the portal vein, hepatic artery, or lymphatics, or by direct extension from the biliary tract or other contiguous structures.

Any suppurative focus in the drainage area of the portal vein may give rise to an hepatic abscess. At one time acute appendicitis was the most frequent offender, but it has been superseded by biliary tract infection, probably because the latter is less amenable to chemotherapy. Usually there is an initial local thrombophlebitis, from which organisms are fed into the liver, either by embolization or by direct extension of the phlebitic process to the portal vein and its intrahepatic radicles (pylephlebitis).

Direct extension of infection to the hepatic parenchyma occurs most commonly in suppurative cholangitis associated with biliary obstruction, but it may also follow rupture of the gallbladder, perforation of a peptic ulcer, pancreatic abscess, or other conditions leading to subhepatic or subphrenic suppuration. No doubt spread of infection by way of the lymphatics or portal radicles is an additional factor in many such cases.

Rarely, pyogenic infections are the result of bacterial embolization by way of the hepatic artery in hematogenous infections associated with osteomyelitis, bacterial endocarditis, or pulmonary disease.

The lesions may be single or multiple, the latter occurring more frequently when the infection has spread by way of the biliary tract or the vessels. Occasionally small abscesses coalesce to form a large solitary lesion. The right lobe is involved more often than the left.

Most pyogenic abscesses of the liver are due to infection with *Escherichia coli*, streptococci, staphylococci, or Friedländer's bacilli, but occasionally *Clostridium welchii* (*C. perfringens*), *Pseudomonas aeruginosa*, salmonellas, gonococci, *Bacteroides fundiliformis*, and other agents are implicated.

The principal symptoms are those of sepsis, namely, recurrent chills and fever, sweats, prostration, anorexia, nausea, vomiting, and weight loss.

In addition, there are signs pointing to involvement of the liver, including abdominal pain, distention, and hepatic enlargement and tenderness. Usually the pain is aching in character and localized over the hepatic area or epigastrium, and not infrequently it radiates to the right shoulder and is aggravated by respiration. Percussion and compression of the liver are painful. Occasionally a large abscess may be palpable as a localized mass beneath the costal margin, or may cause fullness and tenderness of the intercostal spaces. When the abscess is located high in the right lobe, secondary involvement of the diaphragm and pleura may ensue, giving rise to cough, splinting of the chest, pleural effusion, and signs of atelectasis. On x-ray examination the diaphragm is elevated and fixed, the cardiophrenic angle is blunted, and occasionally a local bulge can be made out. If a gas-producing organism is present, it may be possible to demonstrate fluid levels within the abscess. Jaundice is not a prominent feature, except in multiple abscess associated with suppurative cholangitis or pylephlebitis. Usually its presence denotes a grave prognosis.

In addition to the signs of hepatic abscess, there may be others related to (1) the underlying source of infection, such as acute appendicitis, (2) concomitant metastatic suppurative foci in the lungs, spleen, kidney, or brain, or (3) any of the complications of hepatic abscess, including peritonitis, subphrenic abscess, empyema, lung abscess, and bronchohepatic fistula.

Usually the patient is acutely ill, but solitary abscesses may encapsulate and run a more indolent course, characterized by low-grade fever, sweats, wasting, and abdominal pain.

Marked leukocytosis and an increase in the percentage of polymorphonuclear cells are the outstanding laboratory features. Liver function test results may be normal, but in patients with jaundice the concentrations of serum bilirubin and alkaline phosphatase are increased. With prolonged infection the serum albumin level falls and the globulin rises.

Most pyogenic abscesses of the liver can be prevented by prompt use of antibiotics and appropriate surgical measures in the treatment of intraabdominal infections. Once the abscess has developed, surgical drainage and intensive antibiotic therapy are indicated. Unfortunately, drainage is seldom successful when multiple abscesses are present. However, in those abscesses associated with suppurative cholangitis, drainage of the extrahepatic bile ducts may be effective.

Gumma

Gummas, the necrotic masses of conglomerate granulomas seen in late syphilis, are rare at present.

In the liver they give rise to deep scars as they heal and, if multiple, may produce the type of deformity known as *hepar lobatum*. Solitary lesions seldom produce symptoms. However, hepar lobatum, while not a form of cirrhosis since the lobular pattern of the remaining parenchyma is normal, occasionally produces signs of portal hypertension, ascites, and jaundice. Pain and low-grade fever are prominent in some cases. Usually the liver is palpable and coarsely nodular. Predominant involvement of the left lobe is said to be characteristic, but this is denied by many authorities. Liver function is little deranged, except terminally.

Echinococcus Cyst

See p. 1234.

Polycystic Disease

As a result of a congenital developmental defect, isolated segments of the intrahepatic bile ducts may undergo cystic change within the trabeculae of the liver. The cysts vary in size and number and, if numerous, may cause great enlargement and honeycombing of the liver. In approximately half the cases there are associated polycystic lesions in other organs, including the kidney, spleen, pancreas, and lungs.

As a rule, hepatic cysts give rise to no symptoms. Occasionally, however, the liver enlarges during middle age and, by exerting pressure on adjacent structures, produces pain and gastrointestinal symptoms. Rarely, portal hypertension is a complication.

FUNCTIONAL DISORDERS ACCOMPANIED BY JAUNDICE

Gilbert's Syndrome (Constitutional Hyperbilirubinemia, Congenital Hyperbilirubinemia, Familial Nonhemolytic Jaundice, Chronic Intermittent Juvenile Jaundice)

This is a disorder of varied etiology characterized by a mild fluctuating hyperbilirubinemia of the indirect-reacting type in the absence of *overt* hemolytic or hepatic disease. In most cases the disturbance in pigment metabolism is attributable to impairment of the uptake and/or transport of bilirubin by the hepatic cells. Usually the etiology is unknown, but in some instances the defect appears to be the sequela of an antecedent attack of viral hepatitis or is due to underlying chronic biliary disease. Less commonly the hyperbilirubinemia is related to (1) a hereditary deficiency of glucuronyl transferase activity in the liver, (2) a well-compensated hemolytic process with increased bilirubin production, or (3) nonhemolytic overproduction of bilirubin from sources other than circulating hemoglobin, as in the familial disorder described by

Israels and his associates, and in some forms of posthepatitic hyperbilirubinemia. To distinguish between the various forms of Gilbert's syndrome requires an exhaustive investigation, including measurement of the red cell survival time, reticulocyte count, fecal urobilinogen excretion, and the capacity of the liver to conjugate test compounds with glucuronide; examination of the bone marrow; liver biopsy; and tests of liver function.

In the *idiopathic* type, jaundice usually is first noted in adolescence or early adult life, although it may appear at any age. Thereafter it runs an intermittent course, often tending to regress with advancing age. Characteristically the jaundice is mild; the serum bilirubin level rarely exceeding 5 mg per 100 ml. In some individuals, the exacerbations are accompanied by lassitude and vague digestive complaints. However, not infrequently the jaundice is asymptomatic, and is discovered quite by accident during an unrelated illness or in the course of a routine physical examination. Occasionally exacerbations can be related to overindulgence in alcohol, intercurrent infection, or excessive physical exertion. The liver and spleen are not enlarged, and on biopsy the liver usually shows no abnormalities. Except for impaired bilirubin tolerance, tests of hepatic function yield normal results. The capacity to conjugate N-acetyl-*p*-aminophenol, menthol, and other compounds with glucuronide is normal. Fecal urobilinogen excretion, the reticulocyte count, and the life span of the red cell are normal.

The clinical and laboratory features in cases with impaired uptake and/or transport of bilirubin following viral hepatitis are similar to those described. Occasionally, however, there is splenomegaly, and the liver may show residuals of the antecedent infection on histologic examination.

The *hereditary type* associated with a deficiency of hepatic glucuronyl transferase activity probably represents a nonlethal variant of the Crigler-Najjar syndrome without kernicterus (see p. 152). Its distinguishing features include (1) a family history of jaundice, (2) onset in infancy, (3) levels of serum bilirubin that often exceed 5 mg per 100 ml, and (4) impairment of the capacity to conjugate compounds that are excreted as glucuronides.

In cases with chronic hyperbilirubinemia associated with a *compensated hemolytic process,* the erythrocyte and reticulocyte counts may be normal, but the red cell survival time is reduced, fecal urobilinogen excretion is increased, and often the bone marrow shows erythroid hyperplasia. As a rule the degree of hemolysis is insufficient to account for the hyperbilirubinemia, so that it must be assumed that such patients also have a defect in bilirubin uptake and/or transport or are producing an excess of bilirubin from sources other than circulating hemoglobin. In some cases the spleen is slightly enlarged.

The distinguishing features of *nonhemolytic overproduction hyperbilirubinemia* are (1) increased fecal urobilinogen, (2) a normal red cell life span, and (3) a normal reticulocyte count. In the familial type described by Israels and his associates the bone marrow shows erythroid hyperplasia. Splenomegaly and minor histologic changes in the liver are common in cases of nonhemolytic overproduction hyperbilirubinemia attributable to antecedent viral hepatitis.

Dubin-Johnson Syndrome (Chronic Idiopathic Jaundice with Pigmentation of the Liver)

As in Gilbert's syndrome, this disease affects young individuals and is characterized by a chronic intermittent jaundice. However, in contrast, the increase in serum bilirubin is of the direct-reacting type, there are other associated abnormalities of hepatic function, and histologically the liver shows a curious type of pigmentation which is pathognomonic.

Usually the onset is insidious, but in approximately a third of the cases it is acute and simulates an attack of acute viral hepatitis. The chief complaints are jaundice, right upper quadrant pain, anorexia, nausea, vomiting, weakness, and fatigability. The liver may be enlarged and tender and, when inspected during surgical exploration, appears dark brown or green-black in color. On histologic examination, a highly characteristic, coarsely brown pigment is found in the centrolobular parenchymal cells. The nature of this pigment is not known, but it does not appear to be bilirubin, hemosiderin, ceroid, or any of the known lipochromes. In many respects its staining properties resemble those of the fine granular pigment found in many normal livers, but in very much smaller amounts. Usually the liver shows no other abnormalities, although the portal triads may contain a small number of mononuclear cells.

The principal laboratory findings are a slight to moderate increase in serum bilirubin and a mild degree of Bromsulphalein retention. Approximately half the bilirubin reacts directly and is made up of a mixture of pigments I and II. The capacity of the liver to conjugate bilirubin and other aglycones with glucuronide is unimpaired, but its capacity to clear the serum of injected bilirubin is reduced. Often at the height of the jaundice the urine contains bile and an increased amount of urobilinogen. Occasionally, cephalin-cholesterol flocculation and thymol turbidity are abnormal, but usually the levels of serum protein, cholesterol, and alkaline phosphatase remain within normal limits. On cholecystography the gallbladder usually fails to fill with dye.

In the cases reported thus far, there has been no evidence of progressive hepatic damage, although the disease has shown no tendency to abate over a period of years.

The jaundice appears to be due to a defect in the transport mechanism of the hepatic cells, resulting in impaired excretion not only of bilirubin, but also of Bromsulphalein, cholecystogram dye, and possibly the pigment that accumulates in the parenchymal cells.

Although the disorder is familial in some instances, sporadic cases are more common. The suggestion that the disease is hereditary in nature has not been established. The possibility that it may be acquired, in some instances at least, following an attack of acute viral hepatitis has not been excluded.

It is difficult, if not impossible, to differentiate this condition from the various forms of chronic hepatitis and low-grade extrahepatic biliary obstruction on clinical grounds alone, so that liver biopsy is essential for diagnosis.

Rotor and Related Syndromes

The Rotor syndrome is a rare familial form of chronic jaundice accompanied by increased levels of conjugated bilirubin in the serum in which neither biliary nor hepatocellular lesions can be demonstrated. It closely resembles the Dubin-Johnson syndrome, except for the absence of pigment in the parenchymal cells, and shows the same defects in pigment metabolism. Whether or not the disorder is hereditary is not known. Of interest is the fact that in two reported families with the Dubin-Johnson syndrome some affected members exhibited no abnormal pigment in their livers. This suggests the possibility that the Rotor syndrome may be a variant of the Dubin-Johnson syndrome.

Similar nonfamilial cases of unknown etiology have been reported.

Crigler-Najjar Syndrome (Familial Nonhemolytic Jaundice in the Newborn)

See p. 152.

HEPATOBILIARY DISEASE

Extrahepatic Biliary Obstruction

Any obstruction to the outflow of bile from the ampulla of Vater to the bifurcation of the common hepatic duct in the hilum of the liver will result in jaundice. Since the excretory capacity of the liver for bilirubin greatly exceeds the normal demands made upon it, uncomplicated occlusion of the right or left hepatic duct alone does not produce jaundice. The pathogenesis of the jaundice and the nature of the associated hepatic lesions have been described elsewhere (p. 149).

The most frequent causes of obstruction include stone, stricture, congenital atresia, carcinoma of the bile duct, and carcinoma of the head of the pancreas. Extrinsic pressure by malignant, cystic, or inflammatory masses, enlarged hepatic hilar lymph nodes, or inflammatory reactions in the pancreas may constrict the duct, but this occurs less frequently than is generally believed. Even in the case of carcinoma of the head of the pancreas, invasion of the duct wall appears to be a more important factor than extrinsic pressure. Choledochal cyst and invasion of the biliary tree by *Ascaris lumbricoides* are rare causes of obstructive jaundice.

The obstruction is rarely complete, except in the case of congenital atresia and malignancy, and even in the latter it may be incomplete for some time and may fluctuate in degree, as a result of inflammatory swelling and necrosis of the tumor.

Usually the *onset* of obstructive jaundice is gradual, but it may be sudden when the common duct is occluded by stone or when a partial obstruction is complicated by an acute cholangitis. Nevertheless, the jaundice rarely deepens with the rapidity seen in acute viral hepatitis, since the interruption of bile flow is seldom so sudden or complete. The depth of jaundice ultimately attained depends on the degree and duration of the obstruction and, to some extent, on the presence or absence of complicating cholangitis and hepatocellular injury. The most intense forms of jaundice are seen in malignant obstruction and not infrequently are associated with a greenish tint to the skin and sclerae due to the presence of biliverdin. The course of the jaundice is variable, depending on the nature of the obstruction. However, it seldom follows the regular pattern seen in acute viral hepatitis (p. 1673).

Pruritus is a common feature but is not pathognomonic of obstructive jaundice, occurring as a transient phenomenon in viral hepatitis and as a more persistent symptom in primary hepatic biliary cirrhosis. Usually the *urine darkens*, because of the presence of bilirubin, and if the obstruction is reasonably complete the *stools* become *clay-colored*.

If the obstruction is sustained, the *liver enlarges*, and may be *tender*. Often in carcinomatous obstruction of the common duct the *gallbladder* is *distended* and *palpable*. This is unusual when stone or stricture is present, since the gallbladder is apt to be contracted as a result of chronic inflammation and scarring (Courvoisier's law). Occasionally the gallbladder is palpable because it contains numerous large stones, is distended by an impacted stone in the cystic duct (hydrops), or is the site of carcinomatous infiltration. Splenomegaly is unusual, except when the obstruction is due to carcinoma of the pancreas or is associated with extensive intrahepatic metastases.

Fever, particularly if accompanied by recurrent *chills,* usually indicates the presence of a complicating ascending cholangitis. However, it may be related to an underlying malignancy.

Pain is an inconstant feature in obstructive jaundice and may be due to the presence of stone, acute cholangitis, carcinoma, or other complicating disease. The occurrence of typical biliary colic almost always points to a common duct stone. However, not infrequently stones produce obstruction without inducing pain. In acute cholangitis, which may accompany either a common duct stone or a stricture, the pain tends to be more constant and is located either in the epigastrium or over the liver itself. As a rule, the onset of carcinomatous obstructive jaundice is painless, but frequently as the disease progresses and the underlying tumor invades adjacent structures, pain is produced.

Other clinical and diagnostic features related to the specific diseases that give rise to obstructive jaundice are described in the chapter that follows.

The principal *laboratory features* include hyperbilirubinemia with a high proportion of the direct-reacting fraction, bilirubinuria, and significant elevation of the serum alkaline phosphatase and cholesterol levels, Usually the transaminase level rises, but seldom exceeds 200 to 300 units. Fecal urobilinogen is decreased, and if the obstruction is complete, as in carcinoma, the daily excretion is less than 5 mg. Usually urine urobilinogen is decreased or absent, but if cholangitis is present, it may be increased, owing to the production and reabsorption of urobilinogen in the biliary tract. Cephalin-cholesterol flocculation and thymol turbidity are normal early in uncomplicated biliary obstruction, but often they are abnormal, and may be accompanied by hypoalbuminemia and hyperglobulinemia, when acute cholangitis is present or when the obstruction is prolonged. These changes relate both to infection and to hepatocellular injury. The prothrombin concentration tends to fall; it will usually rise following the parenteral administration of vitamin K.

Acute cholangitis, biliary cirrhosis, and hepatic abscess are the chief complications of biliary obstruction.

Once the diagnosis of extrahepatic biliary obstruction is firmly established, the *treatment* of choice is surgical relief of the obstruction and antibiotic therapy for any accompanying inflammatory process. A brief period of watchful waiting is warranted in the case of common duct stone, since the latter may pass spontaneously, and in the case of certain inflammatory obstructive lesions, such as pancreatitis, which may subside spontaneously or following appropriate chemotherapy. Conservative

therapy is indicated also in patients with common duct stricture who have been subjected to repeated plastic procedures and who are not likely to benefit from further attempts at repair. Not infrequently the obstructive symptoms in such cases are due to a superimposed cholangitis which may respond to antibiotics.

Cholangitis

Acute cholangitis of bacterial origin is almost always a complication of (1) bile stasis due to extrahepatic biliary obstruction by stone, stricture, or carcinoma, (2) spread of infection from adjacent structures, such as the gallbladder and pancreas, (3) enteric infections such as typhoid and paratyphoid fever, or (4) parasitic invasion of the bile ducts with *Ascaris lumbricoides,* liver flukes (*Clonorchis sinensis* and *Fasciola hepatica*), or *Giardia lamblia.* Common duct stone is by far the most frequent cause of acute cholangitis, while enteric infections and parasitic infestations are of little etiologic importance in this part of the world. The relationship between cholangitis and pancreatitis is a curious one, since each may be a complication of the other. As a result, it may be difficult in any given case to determine which is the primary disorder.

Escherichia coli and enterococci are the organisms most frequently recovered from infected bile ducts, but a wide variety of other bacteria are capable of inducing acute cholangitis. Most infections appear to be of the ascending type, organisms gaining entrance to the common duct in the duodenum. However, hematogenous infections are known to occur and are of special importance in bacteremic diseases like typhoid and paratyphoid fever.

It is doubtful that acute cholangitis occurs as a primary disease of the bile ducts. In the curious syndrome known as *cholangitis lenta,* it is alleged that the protracted *Streptococcus viridans* bacteremia, which characterizes the disease, is the result of a primary infection of a previously normal biliary tract. However, in most cases that have been investigated thoroughly, an underlying biliary stone or tumor has been found.

Often extrahepatic biliary obstruction is accompanied by an inflammatory reaction within the walls of the ducts and their supporting stroma in the liver, even when there is no accompanying infection (p. 1701). Similar, but less acute reactions, are seen in chronic cholecystitis and a wide variety of nonbacterial hepatocellular diseases. Often these are classified on an anatomic basis as forms of cholangitis. However, the term, as used clinically, implies a bacterial infection of the bile ducts, often accompanied by a purulent exudate.

Chills, fever, and jaundice are the outstanding *clinical features* in acute cholangitis. Jaundice is not a constant finding, although an increase in serum bilirubin can almost always be demonstrated. When present it may be due to (1) an underlying calculous or malignant biliary obstruction, (2) increase of a previously asymptomatic partial occlusion by inflammatory edema, or (3) hepatocellular injury as a result of the infection spreading to the parenchyma. Often the liver enlarges and is painful, but biliary colic is unusual, except in those with an underlying common duct stone. Anorexia, nausea, and vomiting are frequent complaints.

If the cholangitis is secondary to an unrelieved partial biliary obstruction, and especially a common duct stone, chills and fever may recur at intervals of a few days to a few months, a syndrome known as Charcot's intermittent biliary fever.

Bacteremia, liver abscess, and pylephlebitis are the major complications. Rarely chronic infection leads to contracture and occlusion of the extrahepatic bile ducts.

Laboratory studies usually reveal marked leukocytosis, hyperbilirubinemia, bilirubinuria, and a high serum alkaline phosphatase level. Often the latter is present even in the absence of jaundice, and this may be of considerable diagnostic value. Not infrequently there is a modest increase in serum transaminase, as in extrahepatic biliary obstruction.

Treatment depends on the underlying etiology but in general consists of surgical relief of biliary obstruction and the administration of antibiotics.

VASCULAR DISEASE OF THE LIVER

Chronic Passive Congestion

See p. 1694.

Occlusion of the Hepatic Veins (Budd-Chiari Syndrome)

The hepatic veins may be occluded by thrombus or tumor arising either locally or by extension from the inferior vena cava. Rarely a congenital or acquired stricture is responsible.

Hepatic vein thrombosis may be the result of (1) hepatic cirrhosis, suppuration, or malignancy, (2) congenital stricture, (3) polycythemia, (4) crushing injury to the abdomen, (5) local or generalized phlebitis, (6) poisoning with senecio, a weed found in South Africa, or (7) thrombosis of the inferior vena cava secondary to intraabdominal suppuration, malignancy, or trauma. Occlusion of the hepatic veins by tumor usually follows carcinomatous invasion of the vessels, either directly from the liver, or indirectly by way of the inferior vena cava from the kidney.

The changes produced in the liver are those of severe congestion or cardiac cirrhosis (p. 1694), depending on the duration of the disease.

The *clinical course* is variable, depending on the extent of the occlusion, the rapidity with which it develops, and the nature of the underlying etiology. Occasionally the onset is abrupt, with abdominal pain, vomiting, progressive enlargement and tenderness of the liver, and rapid accumulation of ascites. Jaundice is an inconstant finding and when present is mild. Patients with an acute and complete occlusion may go on to shock and die within a few days. Others may survive for months or even years. In the more chronic form of the disease, ascites, hepatomegaly, and signs of portal hypertension predominate. Ultimately the patient dies of hepatocellular failure, mesenteric thrombosis, hemorrhage from esophageal varices, or as a result of the underlying disease responsible for the thrombosis. Signs of inferior vena caval obstruction may antedate or accompany those pointing to occlusion of the hepatic veins.

Occasionally hepatic vein thrombosis is discovered as an incidental finding at autopsy in individuals who allegedly have had no symptoms. Presumably incomplete occlusion, recanalization of the thrombus, and the development of a collateral circulation account for the absence of symptoms in such cases.

The *laboratory findings* are very much like those in chronic passive congestion and cardiac cirrhosis.

Occlusion of the Portal Vein

Most occlusions of the portal vein are the result of thrombosis, but a few are of congenital origin, due either to anomalous development of the vein or to neonatal extension of the obliterative fibrotic process in the ductus venosus and umbilical vein to the portal vein. Occasionally, the portal vein is replaced by a mass of thin-walled vessels, a condition known as *cavernomatous transformation*. When it occurs in young individuals it usually is regarded as a congenital anomaly resulting from failure of the portal vein to canalize normally. However, since recanalization of an obstructed portal vein and the development of centripetal collateral vessels produces a similar picture, cavernomatous transformation of the portal vein may represent an acquired anomaly even in children.

Usually *acute thrombosis* is a complication of suppurative pylephlebitis or of surgical manipulation of the portal vein during splenectomy or portacaval anastomosis. Less commonly, it occurs during the course of a prolonged febrile illness such as typhoid fever, or following abdominal trauma. *Chronic thrombosis*, which is more common, is seen in approximately 10 per cent of cirrhotic patients and may be a complication of polycythemia vera

Table 280-2. CHEMICAL AGENTS AND DRUGS KNOWN TO PRODUCE HEPATITIS IN MAN

Agent	Toxic	Drug hypersensitivity	
		Hepatocellular	Cholestatic
Industrial and plant poisons:			
Carbon tetrachloride....................	+		
Chlorinated naphthalenes and diphenyls...............	+		
Dimethylnitrosamine....................	+		
Mushroom poisoning (*Amanita phalloides*).............	+		
Phosphorus............................	+		
Senecio (ragwort poison)................	+		
Tetrachlorethane......................	+		
Trinitrotoluene......................	+		
Anesthetic agents:			
Chloroform..........................	+		
Divinyl ether........................	P		
Ether (diethylether)..................	±		
Tribromethanol......................	P		
Antiarthritic agents:			
Cinchophen and related derivatives....................	......	+	
Desacetylmethylcolchicine (Colcemide).................	......	......	+
Gold compounds........................	......	......	+
Phenylbutazone (Butazolidin)...............	......	+	
Probenecid (Benemid).....................	......	+	
Antibiotics:			
Chloramphenicol (Chloromycetin)....................	......	+ (?)	
Chlortetracycline (Aureomycin).....................	......	+ (?)	
Novobiocin............................	+ (?)		
Oxytetracycline (Terramycin)...............	+ (?)		
Penicillin..........................	......	+	
Streptomycin.........................	......	+ (?)	
Anticonvulsants and sedatives:			
Sodium diphenylhydantoinate (Dilantin)...............	......	+	
Phenobarbital........................	......	+	
Phenylacetylurea (Phenurone).................	......	+	
Trimethadione (Tridione)................	......	+	
Chemotherapeutic agents used in infection:			
Antimony compounds (pentavalent).................	P		
Arsenicals (inorganic)....................	+		
Arsenicals (organic)....................	+	+	+
Quinacrine (Atabrine)................	......	+	
Isoniazid (isonicotinic acid hydrazide).............	......	+	
Para-aminosalicylic acid..................	......	+	
Pyrazinamide (Aldinamide)...............	......	+	
Stilbamidine and related stilbenes.................	......	+	
Sulfonamides..........................	+	+	
Chemotherapeutic agents used in malignant disease:			
Aminopteroylglutamate sodium (Aminopterin).........	+ (?)		
Chlorambucil (Leukeran)....................	......	+	
6-Mercaptopurine.....................	+	+ (?)	+ (?)
Nitrogen mustard.....................	P		
Urethane............................	+		
Hormonal and metabolic agents:			
Carbutamide (BZ-55)...................	......	......	+
Chlorpropamide (Diabenese)................	......	......	+
Dinitrophenol........................	±	......	+
Metahexamide (Euglycin)................	......	+	

Table 280-2. CHEMICAL AGENTS AND DRUGS KNOWN TO PRODUCE HEPATITIS IN MAN (continued)

Agent	Type of injury		
	Toxic	Drug hypersensitivity	
		Hepatocellular	Cholestatic
Methimazole (Tapazole)................................	......	......	+
Methyl testosterone..................................	......	......	+ (?)
Nicotinic acid.....................................	......	......	+
Norethandrolone (Nilevar)............................	......	......	+ (?)
Tranquilizers and psychic energizers:			
Chlorpromazine (Thorazine)...........................	......	......	+
Iproniazid (Marsilid)................................	......	+	
Mepazine (Pacatal).................................	......	......	+
β-Phenylisopropylhydrazine (Catron)...................	......	+	
Promazine (Sparine)................................	......	+ (?)	+ (?)
Miscellaneous:			
Apiol...	+ (?)		
Chlorthiazide (Diuril)...............................	......	......	+ (?)
Phenindione (Hedulin)...............................	......	+	+
Tannic acid.......................................	+		

+, frank hepatitis; ±, minor hepatic injury; P, potential hazard, produces injury in animals, but not as yet reported in man; ?, hepatitis reported, but etiology and pathogenesis uncertain.

or of carcinomatous invasion of the vein from any of the structures that it drains.

The principal *clinical manifestations* relate to the development of portal hypertension and congestion. In addition there may be signs pointing to the underlying disease responsible for the thrombosis. The liver is not affected by the thrombosis per se but may be involved as a result of other concomitant factors.

In acute thrombosis the early signs include abdominal pain, ileus, vomiting, and diarrhea. Later, there may be ascites and splenomegaly, and if the thrombosis spreads to the tributaries of the portal vein, gastrointestinal infarction may ensue, resulting in hematemesis, melena, and peritonitis.

The signs of chronic thrombosis are those of portal hypertension, which have been discussed elsewhere (p. 155). Often the occurrence of thrombosis is overlooked, particularly in patients with an underlying cirrhosis. The possibility of this complication should be considered whenever sudden ascites or hematemesis occurs in a previously well-compensated case of cirrhosis.

Acute Pylephlebitis. Acute bacterial infections of the portal vein are always secondary to suppurative foci in tissues drained by its tributaries, or to suppuration in contiguous structures. As previously noted (p. 1698), acute appendicitis and biliary tract infections are the most common causes.

The portal vein and its intrahepatic radicles show an acute inflammatory reaction and not infrequently contain pus or thrombi. Hepatic abscess, peritonitis, and septicemia are common complications.

The *clinical features* resemble those of pyogenic hepatic abscess and include chills, fever, nausea and vomiting, abdominal pain, and enlargement and tenderness of the liver. Jaundice is an inconstant finding and, if present, is usually mild. Signs of hepatic abscess or acute portal vein thrombosis may complicate the picture.

Recovery may follow antibiotic therapy and surgical drainage of septic foci, but the mortality rate is still high in the suppurative type of pylephlebitis. Portal thrombosis and hypertension may be important sequelae.

Curveilhier-Baumgarten Syndrome

The outstanding feature in this condition is a periumbilical or epigastric venous bruit, often accompanied by a thrill, and usually associated with dilatation of the abdominal veins, especially around the umbilicus, where they form a rosette of vessels known as a *caput medusae*.

Originally it was believed that the syndrome was always due to a congenital anomaly characterized by patency of the umbilical vein, hypoplasia of the portal vein, and secondary atrophy of the liver. However, it is now known that the dilated vessels and bruit usually are due to a greatly increased venous collateral circulation reaching the abdominal wall by way of the falciform ligament as a result of an acquired portal hypertension. Both the umbilical and paraumbilical veins may participate in this process. The syndrome occurs most frequently in cirrhosis but may be seen in any other form of portal hypertension.

To distinguish between the congenital type due to failure of the umbilical vein to close, and the acquired type related to portal hypertension, it is customary to designate the former as Cruveilhier-Baumgarten *disease* and the latter as the Cruveilhier-Baumgarten *syndrome*. However, some authorities believe that the condition is always the result of portal hypertension and that patency of the umbilical vein in the congenital type is the result rather than the cause of the associated hypoplasia of the portal vein.

REFERENCES

GENERAL

Schiff, L.: "Diseases of the Liver," Philadelphia, J. B. Lippincott Company, 1956.

Sherlock, S.: "Diseases of the Liver and Biliary System," Springfield, Ill., Charles C Thomas, Publisher, 1955.

CIRRHOSIS

Ahrens, E. H., Jr., M. A. Payne, H. G. Kunkel, W. J. Eisenmenger, and S. H. Blondheim: Primary Biliary Cirrhosis, Medicine, 29:299, 1950.

Baggenstoss, A. H., and M. H. Stauffer: Posthepatitic and Alcoholic Cirrhosis: Clinicopathologic Study of 43 Cases of Each, Gastroenterol., 22:157, 1952.

Finch, S. C., and C. A. Finch: Idiopathic Hemochromatosis, and Iron Storage Disease, Medicine, 34:381, 1955.

Klatskin, G.: Subacute Hepatic Necrosis and Postnecrotic Cirrhosis Due to Anicteric Infections with the Hepatitis Virus, Am. J. Med., 25:333, 1958.

——: Effect of Alcohol on the Liver, J.A.M.A., 170:1671, 1959.

FUNCTIONAL DISORDERS
OF PIGMENT METABOLISM

Billing, B. H., and G. H. Lathe: Bilirubin Metabolism in Jaundice, Am. J. Med., 24:111, 1958.

Crigler, J. F., Jr., and V. A. Najjar: Congenital Familial Nonhemolytic Jaundice with Kernicterus, Pediatrics, 10:169, 1952.

Dubin, I. N., and F. B. Johnson: Chronic Idiopathic Jaundice with Unidentified Pigment in the Liver Cells: A New Clinico-pathological Entity with a Report of Twelve Cases, Medicine, 33:155, 1954.

Foulk, W. T., H. R. Butt, C. A. Owen, Jr., F. F. Whitcomb, Jr., and H. L. Mason: Constitutional Hepatic Dysfunction (Gilbert's Disease): Its Natural History and Related Syndromes, Medicine, 38:25, 1959.

Israels, L. G., H. J. Suderman, and S. E. Ritzmann:

Hyperbilirubinemia Due to an Alternate Path of Bilirubin Production, Am. J. Med., 27:693, 1959.

Schiff, L., B. H. Billing, and Y. Oikawa: Familial Nonhemolytic Jaundice with Conjugated Bilirubin in the Serum, New Engl. J. Med., 260:1315, 1959.

HEPATITIS

Havens, W. P., Jr.: Infectious Hepatitis, Medicine, 27:279, 1948.

Klatskin, G.: Toxic Hepatitis, and Hepatitis Associated with Systemic Infections, in "Diseases of the Liver," Schiff, L. (Ed.), Philadelphia, J. B. Lippincott Company, 1956.

Kunkel, H. G., and D. H. Labby: Chronic Liver Disease Following Infectious Hepatitis: II. Cirrhosis of the Liver, Ann. Internal Med., 32:433, 1950.

——, ——, and C. Hoagland: Chronic Liver Disease Following Infectious Hepatitis: I. Abnormal Convalescence from Initial Attack, Ann. Internal Med., 27:202, 1947.

Lucké, B.: Pathology of Fatal Epidemic Hepatitis, Am. J. Pathol., 20:471, 1944.

—— and T. B. Mallory: Fulminant Form of Epidemic Hepatitis, Am. J. Pathol., 22:867, 1946.

Watson, C. J., and F. W. Hoffbauer: The Problem of Prolonged Hepatitis with Particular Reference to the Cholangiolitic Type and to the Development of Cholangiolitic Cirrhosis of the Liver, Ann. Internal Med., 25:195, 1946.

SPACE-OCCUPYING LESIONS

Hoyne, R. M., and J. W. Kernohan: Primary Carcinoma of the Liver: A Study of 31 Cases, Arch. Internal Med., 79:532, 1947.

Ochsner, A., M. E. DeBakey, and S. Murray: Pyogenic Abscess of the Liver: An Analysis of Forty-seven Cases with Review of the Literature, Am. J. Surg., 40:292, 1938.

VASCULAR DISORDERS

Armstrong, E. L., W. L. Adams, Jr., L. J. Tragerman, and E. W. Townsend: The Cruveilhier-Baumgarten Syndrome: Review of the Literature and Report of Two Additional Cases, Ann. Internal Med., 16:113, 1942.

Hunt, A. H., and B. R. Whittard: Thrombosis of the Portal Vein in Cirrhosis Hepatitis, Brit. Med. J., 2:4, 1954.

Kelsey, M. P., and M. W. Comfort: Occlusion of the Hepatic Veins: A Review of 20 Cases, Arch. Internal Med., 75:175, 1945.

281 DISEASES OF THE GALLBLADDER AND BILE DUCTS
Franz J. Ingelfinger

Symptomatology. The outstanding symptoms of disorders affecting the extrahepatic biliary system are pain and jaundice. Very common but less specific symptoms are fever, chills, and a variety of digestive disturbances.

Pain. As is true of digestive viscera in general, the major cause of pain in the biliary tract is an abrupt increase in intramural tension. Thus any process which suddenly tenses the wall of the gallbladder or bile ducts—whether spasm or obstruction by stone—may precipitate biliary tract pain, usually known as *biliary colic.* To the patient biliary colic is severe and disabling, a grinding pain that builds up rapidly, persists maximally for 10 to 40 min, tapers off gradually over hours, and then terminates in a residual soreness lasting a day or more. Although produced by smooth muscle and given the name *colic,* biliary colic is a relatively steady pain without the extreme fluctuations characteristic of colic arising in the intestine. Biliary colic originating in the hepatic or common duct is located high in the midepigastrium initially but spreads, as the attack develops, to the right and straight through the body to an area bounded by the vertebral column and the inferior angle of the right scapula. If the gallbladder or cystic duct is the source of trouble, colic is felt predominantly in the right epigastrium and tends to radiate along the costal margin to the right scapula. Variants, however, do occur, and in one out of ten cases, pain extends principally to the left upper or right lower abdominal quadrant. Biliary colic is not intensified by moving about—in fact, the patient is often restless—but lifting the right arm or taking a deep breath may hurt, presumably because of reflex spasm of upper abdominal and lower intercostal muscles.

Gradual stenosis of the biliary passages, as opposed to sudden obstruction, is relatively painless. Under such conditions an increase in intramural tension apparently is prevented by progressive atony of the biliary tract and diminished hepatic secretion.

Biliary tract pain can also be caused by inflammation. Slower in onset and duller in character, this pain is also more persistent than biliary colic. Because the inflammatory process usually irritates nearby parietal peritoneum, pain of this type often becomes quite sharply localized in the right hypochondrium, but patients with a markedly distended gallbladder or inflammatory mass projecting down to the level of the umbilicus place the maximum distress correspondingly lower.

Jaundice. Obstruction of the hepatic or common bile ducts leads to jaundice with regurgitation of conjugated bilirubin and bile salts into the blood. The rate at which jaundice appears and its degree depend upon the nature of the obstruction and the function of the gallbladder. In gradual obstruction of the common duct, as by neoplasm for example,

biliary congestion is initially cushioned by the storing and concentrating functions of the gallbladder, which becomes greatly enlarged and filled with a thick and viscid concentrate of bile. Jaundice usually does not become noticeable until considerable dilatation of both the extra- and intrahepatic biliary tract has taken place. In spite of the dilated bile channels within the liver, however, marked hepatic enlargement rarely occurs on the basis of bile stasis alone, at first because of the safety valve function of the gallbladder, and later because hepatic secretion is increasingly inhibited in the face of progressive biliary stasis. With prolonged biliary obstruction, indeed, resorption of pigment from the stagnant bile takes place and may leave a clear and mucoid residue in the common duct.

The situation is vastly different when the gallbladder is nonfunctioning or absent. Under these conditions, an acute obstruction of the common duct, as by stone, can produce slight icterus and choluria within hours, and prolonged obstruction may lead to considerable enlargement of the liver, particularly if biliary stasis is complicated by chronic infection. Enlargement of the gallbladder is, on the contrary, unlikely since the nonfunctioning gallbladder usually has lost its elasticity and cannot take up bile.

Complete occlusion of the cystic duct has little effect on a gallbladder permanently scarred by fibrosis, but if the viscus is elastic, it enlarges progressively to form a huge cystlike mass: hydrops of the gallbladder. The contents of a hydropic gallbladder gradually become colorless, and occasionally calcium salts precipitate to form a turbid fluid known as *milk of calcium bile.*

Fever and Chills. These symptoms result from a combination of two factors: biliary stasis and some mechanism permitting infection of the biliary passages. Either condition alone is not enough. For example, patients with free regurgitation of chyme into the biliary radicles of the liver because of surgical anastomosis of hepatic duct to duodenum do not have fever or chills if the stoma is widely patent. Biliary stasis without infection, as is characteristic of cancer in the head of the pancreas, is likewise insufficient to cause fever and chills. When biliary stasis occurs as a complication of gallstones, however, or when ulcerating cancers in the area of the ampulla of Vater allow bacteria to enter the common duct, cholangitis develops, and the patient is shaken by intermittent agues (Charcot's intermittent hepatic fever). The chills probably represent bouts of transient bacteremia.

Disorders of the Gastrointestinal Tract. Common manifestations of biliary tract disease include nausea, vomiting, belching, epigastric bloating, flatulence, and constipation. With severe biliary pain or inflammation, intestinal distention and obstipation may be sufficiently marked to mimic obstruction of the gut. Diarrhea is rare but may occur if an inflammatory cholecystic mass irritates the contiguous colon.

If an obstruction of the biliary channels prevents bile from entering the intestine, the digestion and absorption of fats is impaired, and 10 to 40 per cent of the fat intake may be lost in the feces. Fat-soluble vitamins are similarly lost, but the adult patient with biliary obstruction tolerates the loss of vitamins A, D, and E without serious consequences. Decreased absorption of vitamin K, however, may rapidly induce hypoprothrombinemia.

Impaired function of the gallbladder, unlike obstruction of the common duct, does not affect intestinal digestion or absorption, and symptoms such as belching, bloating, and regurgitation are caused, not by indigestion, but by reflex disorders of gastrointestinal motility. Thus the epigastric "lump" which distresses some patients after a fatty meal is not fat intolerance in the sense of impaired digestion of fat; it is fat intolerance characterized by abnormal gastroduodenal motor mechanisms. Since there are many extrabiliary causes for deranged gastroduodenal motility, the symptoms of "indigestion" are not specific for gallbladder disease. A patient with postcibal epigastric distress may have gallbladder disease or, more likely, a functional disorder unrelated to the biliary tract.

Bleeding. The question is often asked whether or not gallstones and their complications can cause bleeding into the gastrointestinal tract. A few case reports exist of biliary tract bleeding caused by stones eroding into the hepatic artery or a minor vessel, but as a general rule gallstones, if not complicated by hypoprothrombinemia, do not cause clinically significant blood loss.

Biliary Tract Radiology

Radiopaque gallstones may be observed by plain films of the right upper abdomen. To opacify various portions of the biliary system, iodinated organic compounds excreted by the liver are used. In routine cholecystography the compound is given by mouth. Some 12 hr later, the gallbladder contains sufficient dye to render it radiopaque, provided that (1) gastrointestinal motility and absorption are normal, (2) hepatic function is normal, (3) the biliary channels are free of obstruction, and (4) the gallbladder takes up, concentrates, and stores bile. A gallbladder well filled with radiopaque dye indicates a normal viscus. If radiolucent stones are present, they are silhouetted against the contrast medium, but small stones may at times be obscured by the very density of the dye. This error may be avoided to a great extent by taking pictures with the patient standing, or by taking successive pictures after evacuation of the gallbladder has been

stimulated by a fatty meal (Fig. 281-1). As better preparations of cholecystokinin become available, this humoral agent is also being used to promote emptying of the gallbladder.

Failure to visualize the gallbladder suggests an abnormal viscus provided the first three of the four conditions listed above are fulfilled. At times, even a normal gallbladder may fail to take up, concentrate, or store the dye. This, however, happens only sporadically; if the gallbladder fails to fill in each of two attempts at cholecystography, the likelihood of gallstones is 90 per cent. Poor concentration of the dye, or increased or decreased rate of gallbladder evacuation in response to a fatty meal has little diagnostic significance. Because of the enterohepatic circulation, indeed, a gallbladder may contain dye for many days following cholecystography.

The dyes used for oral cholecystography are not sufficiently radiopaque to outline the biliary passages before concentration by the gallbladder. The development of compounds which contain over 60 per cent by weight of iodine and which are excreted by the liver (and in part by the kidney) within 5 to 50 min of their intravenous injection has permitted moderately satisfactory visualization of the larger biliary channels independent of gallbladder function. Intravenous cholangiography is thus used to study patients whose gallbladders have been removed or are nonfunctioning because of disease. A radiolucent stone in the common duct may at times be outlined by this procedure; more often the partial obstruction produced by various choledochal lesions causes widening of the common duct (usual diameter less than 10 mm; diameter over 15 mm definitely abnormal, but magnification by x-ray technique must be taken into account) and imparts a blunted, dilated, and tortuous appearance to the intrahepatic radicles. Like oral cholecystography, intravenous cholangiography is unsuccessful in the face of hepatic disease or advanced biliary obstruction. Failure to produce visualization with either procedure therefore has no diagnostic significance in a patient with an increased serum level of conjugated bilirubin. On the other hand, visualization of either the gallbladder or the bile ducts is at times possible in patients with bilirubinemia up to 5 mg per 100 ml, especially if jaundice is subsiding.

Direct cholangiography consists of injecting an iodinated water- or oil-soluble medium into the common duct, either at the time of surgery or subsequently while a T tube is maintained in the common duct. In intact patients, radiopaque substances may be injected into the biliary passages, especially the gallbladder, by means of a needle percutaneously inserted and guided, once in the abdomen, under peritoneoscopic control. A more hazardous procedure is puncture of the liver with

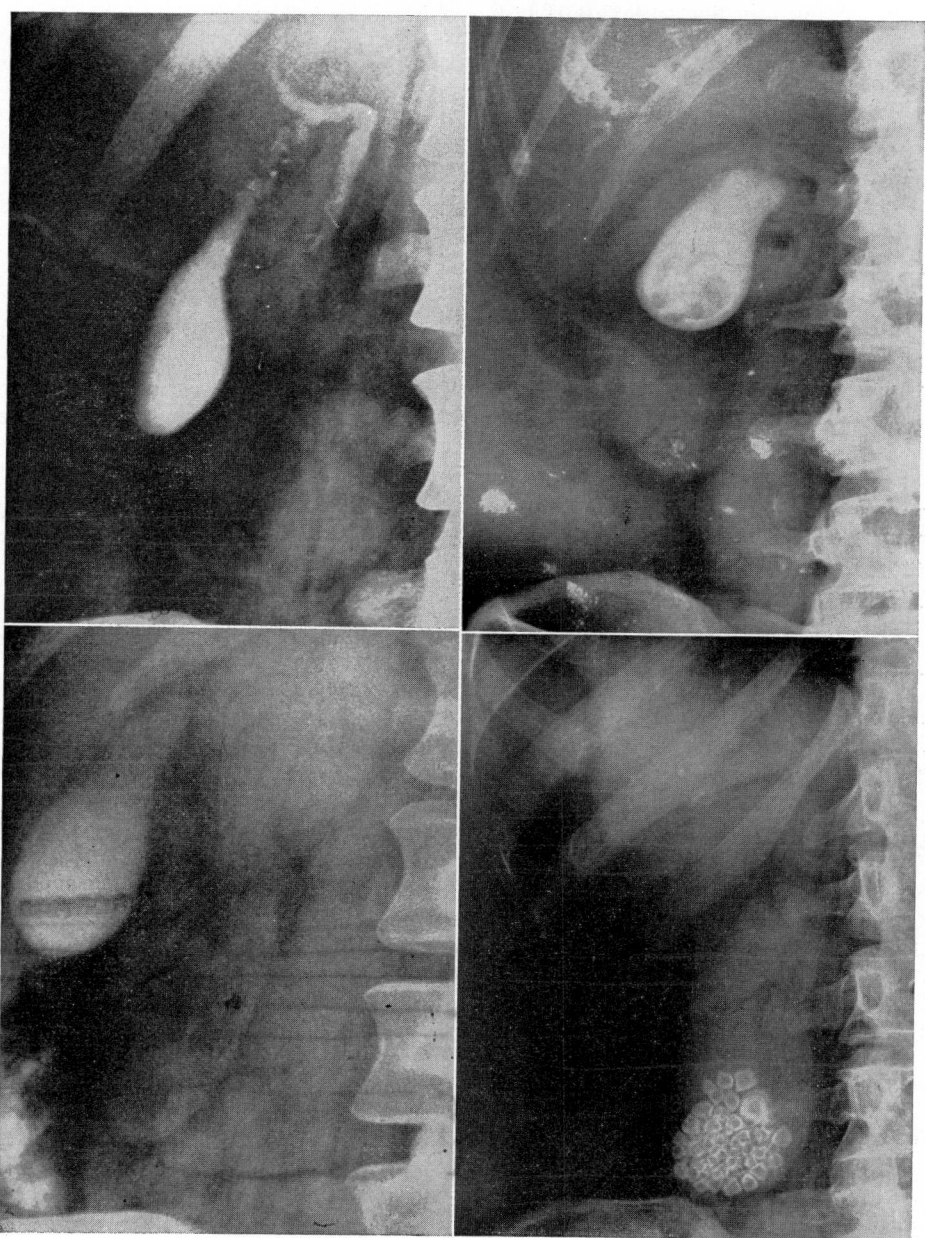

FIG. 281-1. Results of cholecystography. (*Upper left*) Normal gallbladder. The concentrated radiopaque dye outlines the gallbladder and cystic, hepatic, and common ducts. The dye appears in the ducts because this picture was taken after gallbladder evacuation had been stimulated by a fatty meal. (*Upper right*) Cholelithiasis. Nonopaque stones of varying sizes are shown as negative shadows within a gallbladder outlined by concentrated dye. (*Lower left*) Cholelithiasis. Numerous small stones are grouped in a layer near the bottom of the gallbladder. This picture was taken with the patient standing. Small stones such as these are dispersed when the patient is in a horizontal position and may be difficult to see. (*Lower right*) Cholelithiasis. Multiple radiopaque stones in a gallbladder with impaired concentrating ability.

a percutaneously inserted needle that is advanced until bile is aspirated; at this point, the radiopaque dye is injected. These last two techniques obviously entail risks and are indicated only in jaundiced patients presenting difficult problems in differential diagnosis and not considered candidates for exploratory laparotomy.

Biliary Tract Manometry

In many European and Latin American countries, biliary tract dynamics are studied at laparotomy by measuring basal intraluminal pressure, the resistance to perfused fluid, and the response to drugs such as morphine and nitrites. The purpose is to detect abnormal motor function of the gallbladder and bile ducts or increased or decreased resistance of the sphincter of Oddi. Such tests have found little favor elsewhere, partly because biliary pressure readings taken during laparotomy are probably not representative of pressures existing under usual conditions, and partly because surgical attacks (e.g., section of autonomic nerves, sphincterotomy) undertaken to correct real or fancied abnormalities do not appear to yield substantial benefit.

GALLSTONES

At the age of thirty a few women and a rare man have gallstones; by the time they die, 25 per cent of women and 10 per cent of men are so afflicted. Why or how these stones form is still unknown. Cholesterol and pigments in the bile are normally kept in solution by the action of bile salts, phospholipids, and perhaps lipoprotein aggregates. When this physicochemical equilibrium is disrupted by changes in hepatic bile, by deranged function of the gallbladder mucosa, or by infection of the bile itself, cholesterol, bile pigment, and sometimes calcium may precipitate. Thus, as in the case of pigment (bilirubin) stones found in patients with chronic hemolytic anemia, the high concentration of bilirubin in the bile is said to cause precipitation of pigment. Similarly, a postulated but unproved abnormality in the biliary excretion of lipids may explain why cholesterol stones are alleged to be more common in multiparous women, in diabetic patients, and in the obese.

A patient may have one gallstone, or she may have over 200. Multiple stones are usually small and faceted; sometimes they occur in groups of several sizes as if produced in successive crops. Larger stones, commonly one to three in number, tend to be round or elliptical. Pure pigment or pure cholesterol stones are rare; usually both substances make up a gallstone, and approximately 50 per cent of stones contain sufficient calcium to make them radiopaque.

Symptoms and Signs. Half of all persons with gallstones have no biliary symptoms. The other half suffer distress ranging from mild postprandial belching and bloating to full-blown attacks of biliary colic. The episodes of colic occur intermittently, each attack presumably representing the reaction of the biliary tract as a stone passes through the common duct or is wedged into the entrance of the cystic duct. As might be expected, therefore, stimulation of the gallbladder by a fatty meal may precipitate biliary colic, but many an attack seizes the patient in the middle of the night without any obvious dietary reason. At the height of the colic, nausea, vomiting, and difficulty in taking a deep breath are frequent but not invariable complaints. Tenderness and spasm in the right upper abdomen are present when pain is maximal but thereafter recede rapidly. Residual sensitivity to fist percussion over the ribs may, however, persist for several days. Transient bilirubinuria and mild bilirubinemia probably follow biliary colic caused by stone in about one-third the cases, but the icterus is usually imperceptible and the darkening of the urine unnoticed by the patient. Between attacks the patient may feel in the best of health.

Diagnosis. Characteristic biliary colic, typical in location and radiation, is usually recognized without difficulty. Though intense, it is less disabling and prostrating than the pains of intestinal perforation, mesenteric occlusion, severe myocardial infarction, or hemorrhagic pancreatitis. Less severe forms of myocardial infarction or pancreatitis may, however, cause pain not easily distinguished from biliary colic. As a rule biliary colic is briefer than the pain of pleurisy but lasts much longer than each fluctuating wave of intestinal colic. Both biliary colic and peptic ulcer pain may occur during the night, but biliary colic tends to strike in irregular and isolated attacks, whereas the pain of severe peptic ulcer returns regularly night after night.

X-ray examination (see above) is the most fruitful method of establishing the diagnosis of gallstones. Duodenal drainage serves as a supplemental procedure when cholecystograms are inconclusive, as in jaundiced cases with nonfilling of the gallbladder; or when radiologic and clinical indications are contradictory, as in the case of patients who have typical biliary colic but apparently normal x-ray findings. The identification of cholesterol crystals in bile obtained by duodenal drainage is strong but not unequivocal evidence for cholelithiasis. Granules of calcium bilirubinate in duodenal aspirate indicate gallstones with an accuracy of about 50 per cent in patients who are not icteric; in jaundiced patients, these granules have little significance as they may precipitate as a result of prolonged hepatogenous jaundice.

Course and Indications for Surgical Treatment. The possible complications of gallstones are many: acute and chronic cholecystitis, choledocholithiasis, cholangitis, hepatic abscesses, biliary cirrhosis, fistulas from the biliary tract to adjoining viscera, and gallstone ileus. In addition, gallstones appear to predispose the gallbladder to cancer. Although the likelihood of these complications is greatest in those who develop gallstones at an early age, have many small stones, or suffer repeatedly from biliary colic, any gallstone, including so-called silent stones (i.e., asymptomatic stones discovered accidentally by x-ray or at operation), must be regarded as a potential source of trouble.

Patients with gallstones and one or more attacks of biliary colic should be treated by cholecystectomy; there is no medical means of cure, and the probability of further colics and worse complications is great. Patients with stones who suffer merely from "indigestion" also deserve to have the gallbladder removed, but the complaints may not be alleviated completely because their relation to the gallstones may be merely coincidental. Finally, a middle-aged woman with a "silent" stone faces the following choice:

1. Do nothing. In this case, the chances are approximately even that she will develop symptoms warranting cholecystectomy later. Furthermore, because she faces the risks of serious complications, surgical fatality, and cancer of the gallbladder, the chances are about six out of a hundred that the "silent" gallstone eventually will cause her death.

2. Immediate elective cholecystectomy. The mortality risk varies widely, but it probably averages about 1 per cent throughout the country. In addition there is a 0.5 per cent risk of a surgical accident leading to stricture of the common duct, a crippling and potentially fatal complication.

Most surgeons, pointing to the 4:1 ratio of mortality risks between these alternatives, recommend immediate cholecystectomy. These statistics, however, give only a two-dimensional picture. The 1.5 per cent risk is immediate and threatens a woman just beyond middle age. The 6 per cent risk is usually incurred when the patient is sixty-five to seventy-five years old, an age when her life expectancy is threatened by many disorders. In other words, in terms of patient *years*, nothing is gained by elective cholecystectomy, and it appears reasonable to follow the patient with "silent" stone and to recommend surgery if and when the first biliary colic takes place.

ACUTE CHOLECYSTITIS

Acute inflammation of the gallbladder is associated with gallstones nine times out of ten. The part played by biliary calculi in precipitating acute cholecystitis is not clear, but in some cases sudden occlusion of the cystic duct by a gallstone produces biliary stasis and thus promotes an eruptive growth of the few bacteria that indolently inhabit many calculous gallbladders. In nearly half the cases, however, bile removed from an acutely inflamed gallbladder contains neither bacteria nor pus: the evidence for a primary bacterial infection is not good. To explain these cases, it has been suggested that a stone in the cystic duct causes enough spasm and edema to compromise the nearby cystic artery, with resultant ischemic damage to the gallbladder wall. Acute cholecystitis has also been attributed to chemical irritants in the bile and, in the case of noncalculous varieties, to bacterial infection reaching the gallbladder by vascular or lymphatic routes.

Symptoms. Upper abdominal pain and fever are the outstanding symptoms. The pain either may begin gradually or may explode with biliary colic; thereafter it settles as a chronic but severe distress in the right upper abdomen. Ten per cent of cases, however, usually comprising those of advanced age, suffer relatively little pain. Nearly all patients have fever, not necessarily striking, but often spiking to 101°F at least once in 24 hr. Chills may precede the febrile peaks. Nausea and vomiting are common, but clinically perceptible jaundice appears in no more than 25 per cent of patients. If icterus is severe, an associated choledocholithiasis may be responsible; milder and more transient bouts of jaundice can probably be ascribed to spasm, edema, or inflammation of the ducts draining the liver.

Signs. In addition to fever, local signs ranging from slight muscular guarding and sensivity on fist percussion to acute tenderness and boardlike spasm are found almost invariably in the right upper abdomen. A tender, vague mass comprising the swollen gallbladder and adherent omentum is palpable in roughly half the cases.

Laboratory and X-ray. A quite consistent finding is polymorphonuclear leukocytosis ranging between 10,000 and 20,000. The results of other blood and urine tests are not remarkable except for the evidences of regurgitation jaundice in the icteric cases. Bromsuphalein retention and increased serum alkaline phosphatase may be noted even in the absence of bilirubinemia, and the gallbladder usually fails to opacify if cholecystography is attempted.

Diagnosis. The differential diagnosis includes coronary, pleural, and pulmonary diseases, right-sided heart failure, perforated peptic ulcer, pancreatitis, mesenteric occlusion, appendicitis, acute salpingitis, pyelitis, intestinal obstruction, and in jaundiced cases, liver disease, hemolytic crises, and malignancy affecting the extrahepatic biliary system. Pancreatitis presents a special problem not only because many clinical and laboratory findings are common to both conditions, but also because pancreatitis may ensue as a complication of gallbladder infection. Otherwise the typical case of acute cholecystitis is readily differentiated from the conditions listed, particularly if clinical judgment can be supported by x-rays, electrocardiograms, and appropriate examinations of blood and urine. The atypical, relatively painless case, however, may go undiagnosed. To avoid this error, any elderly patient with unexplained fever and leukocytosis should be suspected of biliary tract disease, and extra care is warranted in examining the right upper abdomen for slight guarding, minimal tenderness, or a vague mass. Sometimes a difficult diagnostic problem is presented by acute colonic obstruction which may closely simulate acute cholecystitis, particularly if the responsible lesion is an ulcerated cancer near the hepatic flexure. Although many cases of cholecystitis are nonicteric, early and repeated examinations of blood and urine for even fleeting signs of jaundice are invaluable in the correct interpretation of acute abdominal disorders. During the acute episode, intravenous cholangiography may be used to advantage. If the common duct is opacified, indicating adequate hepatobiliary excretion of the dye, and the gallbladder does not fill, cholecystitis is a good possibility. Conversely, filling of the gallbladder under such conditions tends to rule out disease of this viscus. If neither duct nor gallbladder are shown to contain dye, no diagnostic inferences are possible.

Course. Many attacks of acute cholecystitis subside within 1 to 4 days, but in some 40 per cent of cases the process either does not abate or is progressive. It is then that the danger of empyema, gangrene, or perforation of the gallbladder becomes acute. Other threatening complications are cholangitis, liver abscesses, pancreatitis, and pylephlebitis. An occasional sequel of acute cholecystitis is erosion of the damaged gallbladder wall by a gallstone, which thereafter may continue to lie outside the gallbladder but in 90 per cent of these cases escapes into the gastrointestinal tract by means of a fistula between the gallbladder and duodenum.

CHRONIC CHOLECYSTITIS

Two types of chronic cholecystitis must be distinguished: that which is clinically a bona fide entity and that which is not. The bona fide variety presents the symptoms of acute cholecystitis in dilute and chronic form. These include upper abdominal distress ranging from epigastric pressure to biliary colic, indolent bouts of fever, intermittent mild jaundice, and various digestive complaints. The right hypochondrium is often tender and almost invariably sensitive to fist percussion. Cholecystography reveals nonfilling of the gallbladder. In the

vast majority of cases with these clinical and radiologic findings, the pathologist finds a thick-walled, contracted gallbladder containing stones. Rarely, however, no stones are found. Under such circumstances, the origin of the chronic inflammatory process is obscure. Some cases may be the residuals of an acute hematogenous cholecystitis; in other instances, it is probable that stones were present initially but were then passed via the bile ducts or fistulous communications into the intestinal tract. Bona fide chronic cholecystitis with the clinical and radiologic criteria here defined warrants cholecystectomy.

The bogus variety of chronic cholecystitis is a straw man conveniently erected to explain functional digestive complaints and waiting to be felled by useless operation. The patient usually has a large variety of digestive and systemic complaints, but belching, bloating, and epigastric pressure after meals are predominant. Fat intolerance, in the sense that these symptoms are aggravated by a fatty meal, is typical. Tenderness may be elicited in many spots, but objective abnormalities on physical examination are nil. On cholecystography the gallbladder is outlined and shows no stones, but the concentration of the dye or its evacuation in response to a fatty meal may not satisfy the radiologist.

Patients with this clinical picture have been and are labeled as having chronic cholecystitis on the grounds that improper cholecystic function literally causes indigestion with deficient exposure of chyme to bile, that variations in the concentration and evacuation of cholecystographic dyes provide a satisfactory index of gallbladder morphology and function, and that chronic inflammatory and degenerative changes in the gallbladder wall furnish substantial evidence that the viscus causes clinical symptoms. Actually patients with alleged chronic cholecystitis have no demonstrable digestive or absorptive defect, the concentration and evacuation of gallbladder dyes are variable phenomena, and in very few fields is correlation between structural change and clinical symptomatology so poor as in disorders of the gallbladder. Many an oldster has pathologic evidence of advanced cholecystitis but never a biliary symptom, and conversely, the gallbladder affected by acute cholecystitis may reveal few of the pathologic changes usually expected of inflammatory disease. The "strawberry gallbladder" with its prominent mucosal and submucosal deposits of cholesterol is another entity which is striking pathologically but of nebulous significance clinically.

Perhaps the best evidence that this variety of noncalculous chronic cholecystitis is not a real clinical entity is found in its treatment. Those who treat the condition medically advise antispasmodics, antacids, laxatives, rest, and sedatives for the insomnia of which a majority of these patients complain, measures that are usually marshaled to treat functional disorders of the alimentary tract. Those who go further and remove an allegedly poorly functioning but stoneless gallbladder account for many of the failures of cholecystectomy. Since the gallbladder is not the cause of the symptoms, the patient can hardly be expected to benefit from its removal.

CHOLEDOCHOLITHIASIS

Gallstones are found in the common duct in one out of every seven patients operated on for biliary tract symptoms. Most of these stones originate in the gallbladder and become arrested as they pass from gallbladder to duodenum, but under some conditions biliary "mud" (precipitated bile pigment) and even larger concretions form in the hepatic and common ducts. It is therefore possible that stones found in the common duct of a patient who previously had a cholecystectomy were deposited *de novo*, but it is more likely that the stones were already in the biliary channels at the time of surgery but escaped detection.

Symptoms and Signs. Gallstones in the common duct cause biliary colic, jaundice, fever and chills, but the pattern of these symptoms is variable. A stone rapidly passed from gallbladder to duodenum may prostrate the patient with colic, but the attack is brief, afebrile, and jaundice if present at all is light and evanescent. Two out of every five patients with common duct stones removed at surgery have had no evidence of jaundice. If stones pass more slowly or become lodged in the common duct, biliary colic may be accompanied by chills and fever and is usually followed by a definite wave of jaundice with dark urine and light stools. Nausea and vomiting are more prominent than with colic originating in the gallbladder. Within 24 to 48 hr many attacks subside, and the patient, in spite of the continued presence of stones in the duct, is quite well until movement of the stones, spasm, or inflammatory edema precipitates the next bout. Though choledocholithiasis may thus be silent between attacks, both extra- and intrahepatic biliary passages are exposed to progressive dilatation and to smoldering infection by such organisms as *Escherichia coli, Aerobacter aerogenes,* and *Streptococcus fecalis.*

Some attacks of colic are followed by persistent jaundice, which may be constant or may fluctuate as the stones in the common duct shift position or as the inflammatory reaction waxes and wanes. During this period deep discomfort in the right hypochondrium gradually replaces the initial colicky pains, presumably because choledochal motility be-comes fatigued in the face of continuing obstruction and inflammation. In some patients with chronic distention and infection of the choledochal wall, pain is never prominent, and about 5 per cent of patients chronically jaundiced because of choledocholithiasis have painless jaundice. Fever and chills indicate that an ascending cholangitis is flourishing in the obstructed biliary passages and give warning that multiple hepatic abscesses or pylephlebitis may ensue if biliary stasis is unrelieved. Other symptoms are anorexia, meteorism, constipation, and pruritus.

On physical examination, tenderness and some muscular guarding are usually found in the right hypochondrium. In chronically jaundiced cases, the liver is enlarged 1 to 4 cm below the costal margin because of biliary stasis, ascending cholangitis, or both. The skin is often excoriated and may show the purpuric manifestation of hypoprothrombinemia.

Diagnosis. When the whole clinical triad of biliary colic, jaundice, and spiking fever characterizes choledocholithiasis, differential diagnosis from the other major causes of persistent jaundice, i.e., liver disease and neoplastic biliary obstruction, is not difficult. By contrast, jaundiced patients with little pain or fever present knotty diagnostic problems. In these, a past history of coliclike pain or a shaking chill points to choledocholithiasis. Itching and failure to palpate the gallbladder should also characterize the jaundice of choledocholithiasis but often are relatively unreliable guides. Splenomegaly argues against calculous biliary obstruction, as does a history of colicless jaundice appearing after exposure to chlorpromazine or other drugs producing intrahepatic but cholestatic jaundice. Intravenous cholangiography (see Biliary Tract Radiology, above) in patients who are minimally or not icteric helps to establish or exclude the diagnosis of common duct stones when biliary colic occurs after cholecystectomy. Other findings that suggest choledocholithiasis are leukocytosis, bilirubinemia, bilirubinuria, or increased amylase values in blood or urine samples taken within 3 to 12 hr of an attack of colic. The diagnosis of choledocholithiasis is also supported by the discovery of abnormal biliary sediment on duodenal drainage and, in jaundiced patients, by a pattern of liver function and bile pigment tests indicative of a fluctuating regurgitation jaundice. In the face of persistent cholangitis, however, flocculation tests may yield increasingly positive values.

GALLSTONE ILEUS

Fistulous tracts formed by gallstones eroding through a chronically diseased gallbladder or common duct may enter any adjoining viscus, but by far the most common route leads into the duodenum. Large stones, "hen's egg" size, are most apt to be responsible, and, strangely enough, stones like this may erode into the gut without producing acute symptoms. Hours to days later, however, an escaped gallstone, sometimes enlarged by layers of inspissated intestinal material, may suddenly cause gallstone ileus; i.e., it may acutely obstruct the distal ileum or, very rarely, the sigmoid. Gallstone ileus accounts for only 1 to 2 per cent of all small-bowel obstructions but should be suspected whenever an elderly woman who has had biliary symptoms for years suddenly experiences ileal obstruction. The suspicion is changed to certainty if x-rays show gas shadows outlining the biliary passages, clear evidence of an abnormal communication between the biliary and enteric tracts.

STRICTURE

One of the most distressing disorders of the biliary tract is chronic stricture of the hepatic or common duct. Perhaps one-tenth of such strictures are spontaneous, in the sense that they appear mysteriously or are the direct results of choledocholithiasis. In most cases, however, accidental injury of the common duct during gallbladder surgery is the cause. Sometimes the surgeon recognizes that he has cut the duct and attempts repair; more often, he is unaware of the accident until the patient becomes jaundiced or develops an external biliary fistula some days after operation. The exact incidence of such common duct injuries is unknown; in experienced hands it is very rare, but throughout the United States accidental injury of the common duct probably occurs in one out of every 200 cholecystectomies.

Stricture, whether spontaneous or surgically induced, causes partial biliary obstruction usually complicated by chronic infection. The biliary tree behind the stricture becomes progressively dilated, its branches tortuous and damaged by varying degrees of cholangitis. With virulent infection multiple hepatic abscesses may develop, but the more common end result is biliary cirrhosis. Clinically the patient exhibits a course slowly carrying him downhill over months to years. Much of the time he suffers only from mild jaundice, itching, lassitude, and digestive disorders, but at irregular intervals he is suddenly seized by rigors and headache followed by sharp increases in jaundice. These bouts probably are caused by transient exacerbations of the chronic cholangitis, with bacteremia and increased biliary obstruction produced by the inflammatory reaction in the common duct.

The only effective therapy is surgical correction of the partial obstruction, sometimes with the creation of new biliary-intestinal anastomoses. This is surgery that requires a master, but if repair is successful in the sense that bile flow is unimpeded, not only is the patient symptomatically relieved, but even advanced grades of biliary cirrhosis recede miraculously.

TREATMENT OF GALLSTONES AND THEIR COMPLICATIONS

The only definitive treatment of a gallstone is its surgical removal. Medical measures, however, are necessary to relieve pain, to tide the patient over attacks, and to prepare him for surgery. For the relief of pain, often the patient's first need, meperidine (Demerol) is usually recommended, on the premise that this narcotic analgesic, unlike morphine, does not cause spasm of the sphincter of Oddi. Unfortunately this agent may not provide the necessary relief, in which case an opiate may become mandatory. The dramatic benefit which patients with biliary tract pain often obtain from morphine or one of its derivatives suggests that the harm done by morphine-induced spasm of the sphincter of Oddi is of greater theoretical than real importance.

During acute attacks of painful or inflammatory nature, nothing is given by mouth and meteorism is forestalled by constant gastric suction. Fluids, glucose, and electrolytes are provided parenterally. In patients with fever (i.e., those with acute cholecystitis, choledocholithiasis with cholangitis, stricture) antibiotics are indicated. Although it is true that antibiotics will not appear in static bile dammed up behind an obstruction, their dissemination by the blood tends to prevent the spread of infection and decreases the dangers of bacteremia. Broad-spectrum antibiotics are often used, but the combination of parenteral penicillin (1 to 2 million units per day) and streptomycin (1.0 to 2.0 Gm per day) appears preferable from the viewpoint of wide effectiveness and low toxicity. Of crucial importance is the parenteral administration of vitamin K preparations to any patient who is jaundiced or has had jaundice recently, for the prothrombin resources of such patients may be unexpectedly low.

When biliary obstruction is prolonged, as in the case of certain strictures or neoplasms of the common duct, the patient is given a low fat diet, water-soluble or water-miscible preparations of vitamins K, A, D, and E by mouth, and sulfonamides or antibiotics as needed for the control of cholangitis. One of the most distressing symptoms is apt to be itching, which is only partially controlled by local applications. Calcium gluconate injections may afford relief, but their effect is only temporary. Methyltestosterone, 25 mg daily, has been used to control the itching of regurgitation jaundice. Bile salts have been made unnecessary by the availability of fat-soluble vitamins in water-miscible form; in fact, since bile salts may increase pruritus, their use is inadvisable.

Dietotherapy. From many points of view, a diet low in fats (40 to 75 Gm per day) appears suitable for all types of biliary tract disorders. For those with gallbladder stones, one object of therapy is not to provoke movement of the stones into a position where they might produce symptoms. Since the ingestion of fats is a stimulus for gallbladder motility, the dietary restriction of fats appears rational, even though many colics and other complications of cholelithiasis have no clear-cut relation to the size and composition of antecedent meals. For those who suffer from belching, epigastric pressure, and bloating, a diet relatively low in fats is also recommended, partly on empirical grounds, and partly because fats are particularly instrumental in affecting the gastroduodenal motor mechanisms that are responsible for many of the symptoms of "indigestion."

As far as the surgical treatment of biliary tract disorders is concerned, the following principles pertain to most cases:

1. If gallstones are to be removed, the gallbladder is if possible removed as well. Sometimes the condition of the patient or a technical difficulty precludes cholecystectomy, and the surgeon must content himself with cholecystostomy to drain the gallbladder of stones, fluid, or pus. The disadvantage of this procedure is that the gallbladder remains behind to serve as a further seat of inflammation and stone formation. On the other hand, removal of the gallbladder incurs no disability. Except for an irregularly occurring and mild dilatation of the common duct, the structure of the biliary channels remains unaltered, and the digestion and absorption of fats are not impaired. Cholecystectomy, as far as the patient is concerned, need not interfere with normal living and a normal diet.

2. Every effort is made to free the common duct of calculi or crystals that might serve as a nucleus for further stones. For this reason the common duct is explored not only in patients who have had obvious symptoms of choledocholithiasis, but also in those who have a good probability of choledocholithiasis as indicated by a past history of jaundice, the presence of many small stones in the gallbladder, or the operative finding of choledochal dilatation. The careful search for common duct stones often entails the meticulous probing and flushing of the duct. After the common duct has been inspected and cleared of stones, it is the usual practice to drain the duct by means of a T tube for several weeks. During and after operation, direct cholangiography is used to advantage to ensure that no stones remain.

3. The acutely inflamed gallbladder is ideally removed at a time when technical difficulties are minimal but before perforation or gangrene develop. Nearly all surgeons agree that these ideals are fulfilled if cholecystectomy is performed immediately in patients seen within 48 hr of the onset of symptoms, but the management of patients seen later in the course of their disease is subject to sharp controversy. Some operate as soon as the patient can be prepared for surgery. Others prefer to wait 1 to 3 weeks until inflammatory reaction and tissue friability subside. Surgeons in this group intervene only if increasing fever, pain, leukocytosis, and general evidences of toxicity suggest impending necrosis or perforation of the gallbladder.

4. In jaundiced patients with choledocholithiasis, a waiting period is usually indicated before surgery is undertaken. This gives the obstruction an opportunity to subside spontaneously, or, if jaundice persists, time is available for carrying out the repeated tests often necessary to establish the correct diagnosis.

BILIARY DYSKINESIA

Disorders of gastrointestinal motor function are generally accepted as adequate causes of abdominal pain. The underlying mechanisms, although not well understood, are believed to consist of muscular spasms and lack of coordination between motor functions that normally are smoothly integrated. Even more obscure are the nonorganic disorders that affect the extrahepatic biliary tract, but it is reasonable that pain may arise here, as in the gut, on the basis of spasm and incoordination.

The dynamics of the biliary tract are normally regulated by a coordinated inverse relationship between hepatic secretion, cholecystic evacuation, and choledochal tone on one hand, and sphincteric mechanisms on the other. This relationship, however, may be replaced under the influence of certain pharmacologic, neurogenic, or locally irritative stimuli by uncoordinated activity, usually referred to as *biliary dyskinesia.* The gallbladder, for example, may ineffectually attempt evacuation against a cystic duct tightly closed by spasm. Alternatively a contracted sphincter of Oddi and duodenal musculature may oppose forces actively promoting bile flow. In either case intraluminal pressure between the opposing forces is increased, the wall of a hollow viscus is tensed, and pain ensues.

The archtype of biliary dyskinesia is provided by the spasmogenic effect of morphine on the duodenum and sphincter of Oddi. To some extent this effect of opiates takes place in everyone, but in hypersensitive patients, opiates induce intense nausea, vomiting, and a violent contraction of the duodenum and sphincter of Oddi with biliary colic. A similar though less well-documented dyskinetic mechanism may account for the biliary type of pain that sometimes occurs during migrainous attacks, for neurogenic nausea is usually accompanied by considerable duodenal spasm. Finally it may be postulated that biliary dyskinesia is caused by cholinergic or adrenergic imbalance, by reflexes from other organs, and by a locally irritative focus, such as a cystic duct remnant following cholecystectomy or the scar of a spontaneous or operative injury.

Symptoms and Signs. Clinically, the pain, tenderness, nausea, and vomiting of biliary dyskinesia closely mimic organic disease of the gallbladder and bile ducts, but jaundice, fever, chills, and leukocytosis do not occur, and tests that reflect hepatic, biliary, and pancreatic secretory function (see below, Postcholecystectomy Syndrome) reveal no abnormalities. X-rays of the biliary system show no structural abnormalities, but disorders of function, such as failure of cholecystic evacuation after a fatty meal, may occasionally be seen. Those who practice biliary tract manometry insist that this technique provides the only method for diagnosing dyskinetic syndromes accurately; and if such manometry were only safely feasible under basal, nonoperative conditions, the soundness of this view could hardly be contradicted.

Typically, biliary dyskinesia appears as part of a more general syndrome in which various autonomic phenomena may be prominent. The patient, a woman nine times out of ten, usually has had a stoneless gallbladder removed. Headache, giddiness, scotomas, nausea, or some other aura may *precede* the biliary colic (in organic biliary tract disease, pain is usually the first symptom), sweating and pallor may accompany it, and loose bowel movements may follow. A careful history may reveal that the attack has been precipitated by the ingestion of a minute quantity of opiate, as may be found in many analgesics or cough medicines. If this clinical picture is accompanied by completely negative laboratory and radiologic studies, particularly a normal intravenous cholangiogram, the diagnosis of biliary dyskinesia can be made with some assurance. If the biliary symptoms occur by themselves, unaccompanied by signs of a diffuse reaction of the autonomic nervous system, diagnosis is more difficult. In patients who still have the gallbladder in place, a cholecystogram during an attack may show good filling of the viscus, but its evacuation cannot be induced for the duration of the painful episode.

Treatment. The treatment of biliary dyskinesis is medical. In essence, it consists of (1) reassurance, (2) avoidance of opiates in all forms, (3) elimination of fats and alcohol from the diet, and (4) a combination (admittedly "shot gun" in character) of sedatives and antispasmodics to be taken at the very first sign of the attack; e.g., salicylates, anti-

cholinergics, and barbiturates or phenothiazine derivatives are given in combination and maximal oral doses in an effort to abort the attack and put the patient to sleep. Rectal suppositories containing sedatives or tranquilizers are useful if vomiting contraindicates oral medication. Once the attack is well on its way, a sedative or meperidine has to be given subcutaneously.

POSTCHOLECYSTECTOMY SYNDROME

The term *postcholecystectomy syndrome* is often used in referring to real or alleged biliary symptoms which persist after cholecystectomy but which cannot be explained on the basis of residual or new biliary calculi. It thus serves as a scrap-basket term which comprises a number of conditions:

1. Organic abnormalities of the bile ducts such as stricture, fibrosis of the sphincter of Oddi, cystic duct stump, and tumors of nerve tissue. A cystic stump remaining after cholecystectomy has become a more important entity since the advent of intravenous cholangiography. Such stumps may enlarge and may serve as a site for new gallstone formation. Some surgeons hold cystic stumps responsible for symptoms whether or not additional disorders are present, but this view appears untenable because uncomplicated cystic duct stumps are seen as often in normal postcholecystectomy patients as in those complaining of symptoms.

2. Chronic relapsing pancreatitis.

3. Biliary dyskinesia. The operative record in most of these cases shows that no stones were found at cholecystectomy, and it may be assumed that biliary dyskinesia accounts for both pre- and postoperative symptoms. In a few cases, however, biliary dyskinesia appears to affect patients who underwent cholecystectomy because of the sound indication of cholelithiasis.

4. Functional gastrointestinal disorders. In this, the largest group of postcholecystectomy syndromes, symptoms persist after operation for the obvious reason that removal of a noncalculous gallbladder, falsely incriminated under the diagnosis of chronic cholecystitis, cannot be expected to alter upper abdominal distress produced by an irritable colon or some other disorder of gastrointestinal function.

When the postcholecystectomy syndrome is caused by organic disease of the bile ducts, sphincter of Oddi, or pancreas, surgical exploration is usually indicated. If biliary dyskinesia or functional gastrointestinal disorders are responsible, surgical intervention is to be deplored. Fever, chills, jaundice, and a history of gallstones having been found at the time of cholecystectomy favor an organic disorder. If a stoneless gallbladder was removed, and the patient has headache, sweating, giddiness, and diarrhea with the attack, a functional disorder should be strongly suspected. In any case, however, intravenous cholangiography is indicated; and within 24 hr of an attack some or all of the following measurements should be performed: leukocyte count, bile pigment in urine, serum bilirubin, serum amylase and lipase, serum alkaline phosphatase, Bromsulphalein excretion, and 24-hr output of urine diastase. If these tests are performed repeatedly on blood and urine samples obtained immediately after attacks, some abnormal results will usually be observed if the underlying cause is an organic change susceptible to surgical correction. If the patient has biliary dyskinesia or an extrabiliary functional disorder, consistently normal results will be obtained.

CANCER OF THE GALLBLADDER

As far as the general population goes, cancer of the gallbladder is a rare and unimportant disease. For those who develop gallstones before the seventh decade, however, the picture is different, for unless cholecystectomy is performed, 3 per cent of this group will succumb to this cancer.

The early symptoms of cholecystic cancer usually go unrecognized and are attributed to a benign biliary disorder, particularly since two-thirds of the patients with this cancer give a history of biliary symptoms extending over years. In any elderly patient with clinical or radiologic evidence of gallstones, however, the diagnosis may be suspected if pain becomes boring and persistent rather than acute and episodic, and if weight loss occurs because of anorexia rather than because of voluntary restriction of food intake. Moderate to severe jaundice, usually stable or progressive, is seen on admission in half the cases. Because of associated infection of the biliary tract, or because of tissue destruction within or by the tumor, fever is common and chills not rare. In 50 to 75 per cent of the cases, a hard and tender mass is palpable in the right upper quadrant, but this may be confused with inflammatory tumor of the gallbladder, with biliary cirrhosis, and with metastatic nodules in the liver.

Cancer of the gallbladder usually spreads by direct invasion of the liver and the vital structures of the hepatic porta. Its successful surgical extirpation, consequently, is well-nigh impossible, and 5-year cures are reportable rarities.

CANCER OF THE BILE DUCTS

Adenocarcinoma may grow in any portion of the bile ducts: occasionally in the right or left hepatic duct, sometimes in the common duct close to the ampulla of Vater, but most frequently near the junction of the hepatic and cystic ducts. It is not a common cancer. In men, who appear to be more frequently affected than women, it occurs about one-fifth as often as pancreatic cancer. The clinical manifestations are similar to those of cancer in the head of the pancreas but may be modified by superimposed infection or by elimination of cholecystic function. Thus cancers situated at or above the junction of the cystic and hepatic ducts produce hepatomegaly rather than enlargement of the gallbladder (Table 279-2). Although resection of early cancer in the distal common duct is possible, the prognosis is usually hopeless, as the growth spreads and secondary infection as well as persistent biliary obstruction impair hepatic function. Examination of the duodenal contents for exfoliated neoplastic cells should make possible earlier diagnosis of some of these growths.

UNUSUAL CONDITIONS

Congenital abnormalities of the gallbladder include complete absence of the viscus, anomalous structure such as double gallbladder, and unusual position within the liver or the anterior abdominal wall. The bile ducts are also subject to numerous congenital defects, among which atresia and cystic dilatation are the most prominent.

Cholecystitis due to *Salmonella* is rare in areas where salmonella infections are controlled, but formerly typhoidal infection of the gallbladder was responsible for many typhoid carriers. Very infrequent causes of biliary tract infection are tuberculosis, syphilis, actinomycosis, and septic emboli. The characteristic lesions of periarteritis nodosa are sometimes exceptionally prominent in the walls of the gallbladder.

The biliary tract may be infested by *ascarids, liver flukes,* and *echinococcus cysts.* These parasites may cause biliary obstruction with cholangitis and jaundice. A parasite found in the United States in about 0.5 per cent of patients examined by duodenal drainage is *Giardia lamblia,* but the pathogenicity of this organism is variable.

With improved cholecystography, *small polypoid masses* are discovered not infrequently in the gallbladder, but their clinical significance is controversial. Many of these polyps are merely mucosal prominences containing localized cholesterol deposits; much more rarely true adenomatous growths occur. In either case, the lesion cannot be held responsible for symptoms. That the adenomatous polyps progress to cancer is a vehement but unproved assertion used by those who insist on cholecystectomy whenever a polyp is discovered radiologically in the gallbladder.

Traumatic rupture of the gallbladder with bile

peritonitis occasionally is a serious complication of abdominal injuries.

REFERENCES

Arminski, T. C.: Primary Carcinoma of the Gallbladder, Cancer, 2:379, 1949.

Comfort, M. W., H. K. Gray, and J. M. Wilson: The Silent Gallstone: A Ten to Twenty Year Follow-up Study of 112 Cases, Ann. Surg., 128:931, 1948.

Neibling, H. A., M. B. Dockerty, and J. M. Waugh: Carcinoma of the Extrahepatic Bile Ducts, Surg., Gynecol. Obstet., 89:429, 1949.

Newman, H. F., and J. D. Northup: Hydrodynamics of the Human Common Duct, Surg., Gynecol. Obstet., 105:355, 1957.

Robertson, H. E.: The Preponderance of Gallstones in Women, Surg., Gynecol. Obstet. (Internat. Abstr. Surg.), 80:1, 1945.

Walters, W., and A. M. Snell: "Diseases of the Gallbladder and Bile Ducts," Philadelphia, W. B. Saunders Company, 1940.

Zollinger, R. M.: Significance of Pain and Vomiting in Cholelithiasis, J.A.M.A., 105:1647, 1935.

Zollinger, R. M., E. T. Boles, and G. B. Crawford: The Diagnosis and Management of Biliary-tract Disease, New Engl. J. Med., 252:203, 1955.

Section 7: The Nervous System

282 APPROACH TO THE PATIENT WHO HAS A NEUROLOGIC PROBLEM

Raymond D. Adams

Neurology is often regarded as one of the most difficult and exacting specialties of medicine. The student coming to the neurology clinic for the first time tends to be easily discouraged by what he sees. Already he is somewhat intimidated by the complexity of the nervous system through his brief contact with neuroanatomy, neurophysiology, and neuropathology, and often has a defeatist attitude. The ritual he then witnesses, of putting the patient through a series of maneuvers designed to evoke certain mysterious signs named after famous neurologists or called by unpronounceable terms, does not reassure him. In fact it often appears to conceal the very intellectual processes by which neurologic diagnosis is attained. Moreover, the student has no aptitude for the many special tests which are used, such as the lumbar puncture and cerebrospinal fluid examination and the electroencephalographic, pneumoencephalographic, and arteriographic examinations, and he does not know how to interpret the results of such tests when they are given him. Neurologic textbooks only confirm his fears as he reads the details of the countless rare diseases of the nervous system.

THE CLINICAL METHOD

The author believes that many of the students' difficulties with neurology may be overcome by proper instruction in the basic principles of clinical medicine. First and foremost he must know and acquire facility in the use of the *clinical method*. Without a clear comprehension of this method he is virtually as helpless with a new problem as would be the botanist or chemist who attempted to do research without having learned the essentials of the scientific method.

The importance of the clinical method stands out more clearly in the study of neurologic diseases than in certain other fields of medicine, but the following remarks nevertheless have universal application. The solution of any clinical problem is reached by a series of inferences and deductions, each an attempt to explain an item in the history of an illness or a physical finding. Diagnosis is the mental act of selecting the one explanation most compatible with all the facts of clinical observation. Probably no two minds function exactly alike in this process, and indeed one physician may not reason the same way on two different clinical problems. Yet an analysis of the clinical method used will show that it generally consists of an orderly series of steps, as follows:

1. The essential clinical data are secured by history and physical examination.

2. Those clinical data which are considered relevant to the current problem are interpreted and translated in terms of anatomy and physiology. Certain complexes of symptoms and signs are recognized as having a meaningful relationship. This may be called *syndrome diagnosis*.

3. From these data the physician is able to determine the anatomic localization that best explains these findings. This may be called the *anatomic diagnosis*.

4. The course of the illness, the associated medi-

cal findings, and the accessory laboratory data are then ascertained.

5. And finally the *etiologic diagnosis* is educed from these data and from the location of the disease process.

The elicitation of accurate and reliable data concerning the disordered functioning of the nervous system is the first step in diagnosis. If these data are incorrect, the diagnosis will surely be erroneous. The taking of the history and the performance of the physical examination, then, are the primary and fundamental methods in diagnosis. Where there is disagreement as to diagnosis it will often be discovered that the source of the difficulty is an uncertainty as to the significant items in the history or physical examination. Repeated examination may be necessary in order to establish them beyond doubt. This is why it is said that the second examination is the most helpful diagnostic method in a difficult case.

Different disease processes may cause identical symptoms, which is understandable from the fact that several diseases may involve the same parts of the nervous system. For example, a spastic paraplegia may result from spinal cord tumor, syphilitic meningomyelitis, or multiple sclerosis. Conversely, one disease may cause several different symptoms. Despite the almost infinite number of possible combinations of symptoms and signs, a few occur with greater frequency than others in a given disease, and indeed some do not occur at all; and these can be recognized as the characteristic symptom complexes or syndromes. The experienced clinical worker acquires the habit of attempting to categorize every clinical case by placing it under one or another syndrome. In doing so he more or less determines the anatomic basis of the illness in question and at the same time narrows the range of possible etiologic factors.

The final diagnosis must state the locality of the disease as well as its nature and, to be complete, should express the degree of functional impairment as well. Anatomic diagnosis has precedence over etiologic diagnosis. To seek the cause of a disease without first ascertaining the part or parts of the nervous system which are affected would be analogous in internal medicine to an attempt at etiologic diagnosis without knowledge of whether the disease involved the lungs, stomach, or kidneys.

The study of neurology should always proceed from the general to the specific. The student must learn the identity and differential diagnosis of the common syndromes before the details of individual diseases. It should be kept clearly in mind, however, that syndromes are not diseases but rather abstractions set up by clinical workers in order to facilitate the diagnosis of disease. The inherent danger in the method is that it may inculcate a rigidity of thinking and keep one from conceiving of diseases in new relationships.

TAKING THE HISTORY

Skill in taking a clear, meaningful history of an illness is the mark of an able clinician. In fact, this faculty more than any other distinguishes the competent from the incompetent clinical worker. The following three points about history taking in neurology deserve comment.

1. Special care must be exercised to avoid suggesting to the patient the symptoms that one seeks. The clinical interview is a bipersonal engagement, and the conduct of the examiner has a great influence on the patient. Psychiatrists have talked and written about this so much that the repetition may seem tedious, but it is evident that many of the conflicting histories presented on ward rounds can be traced to leading questions that have suggested to the patient the symptoms that the examiner expects to find or to an unconscious distortion of the patient's story. Errors and inconsistencies in recording the history are as often the fault of the physician as of the patient. Here the practice of making bedside notes is particularly to be recommended. Considerable experience may be necessary to keep a suggestible and highly circumstantial patient on the subject of his illness, and of course discreet questions are always necessary to draw out certain important points.

2. The mode of onset and the course of the illness are of paramount importance. Often the nature of the disease process can be decided by these facts alone. One must know how each symptom began and progressed from the onset of the illness to the present. If the patient cannot supply this information, it may be necessary to judge the course of the symptoms by what he was able to do at different times, i.e., how far he could walk, whether he could carry on his work, etc., or by changes in the clinical findings between successive examinations. Following a case and allowing time for a disease to evolve, a method relied upon by all astute physicians, takes advantage of the latter procedure.

3. Since neurologic diseases often derange the patient's mind, it is necessary in every case to decide by assessment of the mental status and the circumstances under which symptoms occurred whether or not he is competent to give the story of his own illness. If not, the history must be obtained from an outside source such as a relative, friend, or employer. The nature of certain illnesses, such as a convulsion, obviously precludes the patient's knowledge of all the details of that part of his illness. In general, students and some physicians, as well, tend to be careless in the estimation of the mental capacities of their patients. An attempt is

sometimes made to take a history from a patient who is feebleminded or so confused that he has no idea why he is in a doctor's office or a hospital, or from one who could not possibly have been aware of the details of the illness.

THE NEUROLOGIC EXAMINATION

The neurologic examination begins always with the history. The manner in which the patient tells the story of his illness may betray lack of coherence or confusion in thinking, defection of memory, faultiness of judgment, or difficulty in comprehending or in expressing ideas. This is an essential part of the examination of every medical case and provides information as to the adequacy of cerebral function. Usually this type of information can be obtained without embarrassment to the patient. The physician should maintain the same objective attitude toward the verbal responses of his patient and the thoughts expressed as he does in auscultation of the chest. A common error is to pass over inconsistencies in history and inaccuracies about dates and symptoms as being unimportant, only to discover later that these are the major symptoms of the illness.

The remainder of the neurologic examination should be performed as part of the general physical examination and not as a special procedure, to be done later if indicated. It should always be carried out in an orderly, systematic manner, proceeding from the examination of the cranial nerves, to the upper extremities, trunk, and lower extremities, in order to avoid omissions. The cranial nerves can be tested along with the examination of the eyes, ears, nose, and throat. The arms should be examined after the cervical structures and before the heart and lungs, and the legs before the pelvic and rectal examination. Gait and station should be observed at some time during the procedure, usually before or after the rest of the examination.

The thoroughness of the examination of the nervous system must of necessity depend on the type of clinical problem presented by the patient. To spend a half-hour testing motor and sensory function in a patient seeking treatment for a sprained ankle is pointless and uneconomical. Furthermore, the procedure must be varied according to the condition of the patient. If he is comatose, obviously many tests cannot be done; infants and small children and psychotic patients must be examined in special ways. The following comments about the examination procedure apply to these particular clinical circumstances.

The Average Medical or Surgical Patient without Neurologic Symptoms. Brevity is desirable in the neurologic examination, but any test that is undertaken should be done well and recorded accurately on the patient's chart. In the examination of the cranial nerves, the pupil size, reaction to light, ocular movements, visual acuity and auditory acuity (by question), movements of face, jaw, palate, and tongue should be scrutinized. Observing the bare, outstretched arms for atrophy, weakness, tremor, or abnormal movements, inquiring about strength and subjective sensory disturbances, and tapping the supinator, biceps, and triceps tendons to evoke reflexes are usually sufficient for the upper extremities. The abdominal reflexes should be tested when the abdomen is examined. Inspection of the legs as the feet, toes, and knees are actively flexed and extended, elicitation of the knee and ankle jerks, and stroking the lateral border of the foot for the plantar reflexes complete the essential part of the neurologic examination. The only sensory tests that should be attempted are vibration and position in the fingers, ankles, and feet. Coordination may be tested by watching the patient place his finger on the tip of his nose and run the heel up and down the front of his leg. This entire procedure does not add more than 3 or 4 min to the physical examination. The routine performance of these few simple tests may offer clues as to the presence of diseases of which the patient is not aware. For example, by finding Argyll Robertson pupils, absent tendon reflexes, and diminished vibratory and position sense in the legs the surgeon is alerted to the possibility of the gastric crises of tabes when there are no other symptoms of neurosyphilis.

An accurate record of the results of these tests should be kept. Even if the tests are negative and do not aid in understanding the present illness, a neurologic disease developing later may be more accurately dated.

Patients Who Present Symptoms of a Disease of the Nervous System. Several monographs have been written on the neurologic examination of such patients. For a full account of the methods the reader is referred to Denny-Brown, Monrad-Krohn, Wartenberg and DeJong, each of whom approaches the subject from a special point of view. A large number of tests have been devised, and it is not proposed to review them. Many are of doubtful value and should not be taught to students of neurology. Merely to perform all these tests on any one patient would require several hours, and probably the examiner would in many instances be none the wiser. The danger in all clinical tests is that the student and physician may regard them as the inscrutable symbols of disease rather than manifestations of disordered functioning of the nervous system. In general the tests which provide the most useful information are few in number and relatively simple. The student should be taught to do these few tests well and to understand their meaning. The entire examination procedure should never require more than 15 or 20 min, because if it does, the patience of both examiner and patient are likely to be exhausted and the results then become inaccurate.

Testing of Cerebral Function. Cerebral function is tested in detail only if there is reason to suspect some defect from the patient's behavior during the general examination. Questions should then be directed toward determining orientation in time and place and insight into the current medical problem. Attention, speed of response, ability to give relevant answers to simple questions, and in general the capacity for sustained mental effort, all lend themselves to straightforward observation. Useful bedside tests of attention, memory, and clarity of thought are the repetition of a series of digits in forward or reverse order, serial subtraction of 7s from 100, the recall of the names of three objects after an interval of 3 min, and the solution of simple problems and riddles. Day-to-day recollection of the medical procedures and incidents in the hospital is an excellent test of memory. Other tests can be devised for the same purpose. Often the examiner can obtain a better idea of the clearness of the patient's sensorium and the soundness of his intellect by giving him a few tests and noting the manner in which he deals with them than by relying on a crude score of a formal intelligence or achievement test (see Chap. 37).

If there is any suggestion of aphasia, a record of the patient's spontaneous speech should be made. In addition, accuracy in the naming of objects, in the execution of spoken commands, and the ability to read and write should also be noted (see Chap. 40).

Testing the Cranial Nerves. The function of the cranial nerves must be investigated more fully than in the previous examination procedure. Tests of smell are carried out only if one suspects a lesion in the anterior fossa, and then it usually suffices to determine whether odors are perceived in each nostril. In every case of brain disease the visual fields should be outlined by a perimeter and scotomas sought on the Bjerrum screen. The careful use of a small white test object in a confrontation test of the visual fields is a useful method and should suffice in cases of spinal cord and peripheral nerve disease. It may at times, however, reveal or localize a scotoma more accurately than the use of the Bjerrum screen.

Sensation over the face should be tested with a pin and wisp of cotton, and the corneal reflexes should be tried. Facial movements should be observed as the patient speaks and smiles, for a slight weakness may be more evident then than during voluntary movement. Audiograms and special tests of auditory recruitment and labyrinthine tests are needed if there is suspicion of disease of the eighth nerve. The vocal cords should be inspected in cases of medullary disease, especially when there is hoarseness. Corneal and pharyngeal reflexes are usually of value only if there is a difference on the two sides; bilateral absence of gag and corneal reflexes is seldom significant. Inspection of the protruded tongue is helpful; atrophy, fibrillation, weakness, and instability of posture may be seen. Deviation of the protruded tongue to one or the other side as a solitary finding may usually be disregarded. Articulation and the pronunciation of words should be noted. The jaw jerk and buccal and sucking reflexes should be elicited particularly if there is suspicion of dysphagia or dysarthria (see Chap. 40).

Tests of Motor Function. In the assessment of motor function the student must remind himself that observations of the speed and strength of movements of muscle bulk and of tone and coordination are usually more informative than the tendon reflexes. It is essential to have the limbs fully exposed and to watch the patient maintain the arms in the outstretched position; to perform simple tasks, such as touching first the examiner's finger and his own nose; to make rapid alternating movements that necessitate sudden acceleration and deceleration and changes in direction; and to do simple tasks such as buttoning clothes, opening a safety pin, or handling common tools. Estimates of the strength of leg muscles with the patient in bed are often unreliable; there may seem to be no weakness even though the patient cannot step up on a chair or arise from a squatting position. Running the heel down the front of the other shin, and alternately touching the examiner's finger with the toe, then the opposite knee with the heel is the only test of coordination that can be carried out in bed. The maintenance of both arms or both legs against gravity is a useful test; the weak one, tiring first, soon begins to sag. Also abnormalities of movement and posture and tremors may appear (see Chap. 27).

Tests of Reflex Function. A large variety of tests of reflex function have been devised. There are 20 or 30 special tests that can be performed on the foot alone. Most of them can be ignored for all practical purposes; it is recommended that only the response to stroking the outer part of the sole or lateral surface of the foot be used. If the plantar reflex is extensor, the others are superfluous; if it is equivocal or flexor in type, the other tests cannot be taken as substitutes. When in doubt as to the nature of the response, an involuntary flexion of the leg at the hip, knee, and ankle after a series of pinpricks is a valuable confirmation of an extensor plantar reflex. The Hoffmann reflex in the hand, better called the finger jerk, is merely a tendon reflex and is not equivalent to the Babinski sign. The biceps, triceps, and supinator or radial-periosteal reflexes, the knee and ankle reflexes, and the cutaneous abdominal and plantar reflexes permit an adequate sampling of reflex activity of the spinal cord.

Testing of Sensory Function. The testing of sensory function is undoubtedly the most difficult part of the neurologic examination. If the findings are to be reliable, it should be reserved for the end of the examination procedure and not prolonged for more than a few minutes. Usually an explanation of the purpose of the test should be given; yet too much discussion of it with a meticulous, introspective patient may encourage the reporting of useless minor variations of stimulus intensity. It is well to ask whether or not stimuli on opposite sides of the body feel the same, not if they feel different. If the patient is highly suggestible, in which case sensory tests are unreliable, differences that demand further investigation will not then be reported.

The skin surface of the body is large, and it is not necessary to examine all areas. A quick survey of the face, neck, arms, trunk, and legs with a pin takes only a few seconds. One is of course usually seeking differences between the two sides of the body, a level below which sensation is lost, or a zone of relative or absolute anesthesia. Regions of sensory deficit can then be tested more carefully and mapped out. Hyperesthetic zones are usually not of much help in diagnosis and more often than not are the result of faulty technique; nevertheless they may call attention in some patients to areas of peripheral sensory disturbance. Variations in the sensory findings from one examination to another reflect differences in technique of examination as well as inconsistency in the responses of the patient.

Light touch, pain, temperature, vibratory, and position sense should be examined systematically in every neurologic case. Stereognosis, tactile localization, two-point discrimination, and the recognition of numbers written on the skin afford the means of evaluating cutaneous perception. If the patient is an unreliable witness, only a few tests such as position and vibratory sense in the fingers and toes, pinprick in hands, trunk, and feet, and stereognostic sense in hands are worthwhile (see Chap. 28).

Testing Gait and Stance. No examination is complete without seeing the patient on his feet and walking. An ataxia of gait may be the only neurologic abnormality, as in certain cases of cerebellar tumor. And, the stance, posture, and lack of certain highly automatic adaptive movements may be the most definite finding in an early case of paralysis agitans.

The Comatose Patient. Although subject to obvious limitations, examination of the stuporous or comatose patient may yield considerable information concerning the function of the nervous system. The special techniques involved have been presented in Chap. 34, Coma and Related Disturbances of Consciousness.

The demonstration of signs of focal brain disease or of meningeal irritation is of aid in the differential diagnosis of the diseases which cause coma and are the basis of the three syndromes outlined in Chap. 34.

The Psychiatric Patient. One is compelled in the examination of psychiatric cases to rely less on the cooperation of the patient and to be unusually critical of his statements and opinions. The depressed patient for example may declare that his limbs are weak or useless when actually there is little or no diminution in muscular power, or the psychopathic patient may feign paralysis. The opposite is sometimes true—that the most psychotic patient may make accurate observations of his own symptoms, only to have them ignored because the attending physician has been in the habit of disregarding his complaints.

If the patient will speak and cooperate to the slightest degree, much may be learned as to the functional integrity of different parts of the nervous system. Aphasia can, in nearly every instance, be diagnosed by the manner in which the patient uses words in phrases and sentences, or responds to spoken or written commands. Often it is possible to determine whether there are hallucinations, defective memory, or other symptoms of recognizable brain disease merely by watching and listening to the patient. The visual fields can often be tested with fair accuracy by observing the patient's response to a moving stimulus or threat in all four quadrants of the fields. The tests of cranial nerve, motor, and reflex function in the legs, already outlined for the examination of the stuporous and comatose patient, can be carried out even better if minimal cooperation is obtained from the patient. It must be remembered, however, that the neurologic examination is never complete unless the patient will speak and carry out the usual tests. On numerous occasions mute patients, judged to be schizophrenic, have had some widespread cerebral disease such as hypoxic or hypoglycemic encephalopathy, a brain tumor, a vascular lesion, or extensive demyelinative lesions.

Infants and Small Children. At an early age, before a child has learned to speak or carry out spoken commands, neurologic disease manifests itself almost exclusively as a disturbance of sensorimotor reactions. Many parts of the neurologic examination which are of value in testing nervous function in adults are of little use in infants. For example, the tendon and plantar reflexes are seldom of much help. The examination of the optic fundi rarely is of value except in amaurotic familial idiocy, toxoplasmosis, or tuberous sclerosis. Sensory tests, except response to painful stimulation, are not worthwhile. More can be learned by merely sitting at the bedside for a few minutes and observing the activity of the patient than by attempting special tests. Within a few minutes the average infant who is awake will move every muscle in the body. Rigidity or spasticity of the limbs or paralysis of a muscle or group of muscles is easily discovered by merely observing these motor performances and by manipulating the limbs.

The neurologic examination of the infant and small child should always begin with careful inspection of the head and palpation of the anterior fontanel. Peculiarities in the shape and size of the skull are often found with brain disease. The head is unnaturally small in many cases of amentia with gross brain lesions, and unilaterally small with hemiatrophy of the brain. Premature closure of sutures, which accounts for odd shapes of the skull, is frequently associated with brain disease and developmental retardation. And, of course, enlargement of the head may occur with hydrocephalus, chronic subdural hematoma, and rarely macrocephaly. Retarded children who remain in one position because of a postural abnormality due to nervous disease may show flattening of the skull on one side. A bony defect, a tuft of hair or a peculiarity in the skin over neck and spine permit diagnosis of a cranium bifidum or spina bifida (see Chap. 283).

The condition of the infant during the examination of sensorimotor functions must be taken into account for behavior is variable according to whether he is asleep, drowsy, wakeful, hungry, contented, premature, frail, sick, or injured. Most of the examination procedure should be conducted with the infant lying supine, but later some of the same tests are performed in the prone, sitting, suspended prone or supine, or vertical positions. The degree of motor activity is observed and recorded, and also the predominant postures and reactions to direct and indirect passive movement of the limbs (resistance to passive movement and tone). The ciliary reflex (homolateral or bilateral blink to stroking the eyelashes), the blinking reflex and pupillary reflexes to a light, the nasopalpebral and McCarthy reflexes (homolateral or bilateral blinking to tapping eyebrow or root of nose, respectively), the auriculocephalic reaction (rotation of head to the opposite side when touching the ear), the cardinal points sign (lip and tongue movements and head rotation toward a stimulus which touches successively the two angles of mouth and center of upper and lower lips), doll's eyes phenomenon on rotating or tilting the

head, tonic grasp reaction and tonic reactions of plantar flexors and Moro reflex (extension and abduction of arms and extension of fingers and wrists followed by flexion when the supine infant is lifted by arms and then released) should be elicited. Evaluation of righting, standing, and walking reactions and tendon and plantar reflexes (triceps and ankle reflexes often absent) complete the examination.

Visual activity assumes particular importance after the first 2 or 3 weeks of life. Conjugate movements of the eyes in fixating and following a visual stimulus develop early. The coordination of hand and eye and alertness to a moving stimulus introduced in various parts of the visual field are normally acquired in the first 1 to 3 months. Retardation in these activities suggests a specific visual defect or a general disturbance in nervous development. Attentiveness and response to sounds also constitute a good test of sensorimotor organization and of adaptive behavior.

The organization of motor activity in head control, in grasping and reaching for objects, in sitting, crawling, standing, walking, and vocalizing are reliable indices of the functional activity of the nervous system. Social behavior may later be used in the same way as a sign of nervous organization. These motor skills and items of adaptive and social behavior develop in an orderly sequence; a timetable has been established by Gesell and other workers. The developmental quotient, a figure arrived at by comparing chronologic age with developmental age, expresses the degree to which motor development is retarded. Unless conditioned by psychologic factors, a significant degree of retardation of development signifies a disease of the brain which may prove, as time passes, to be regressive, stationary, or progressive. The subsequent course of the illness should distinguish these three classes of disease. A progressive brain disease not only interferes with the normal processes of maturation but may cause an actual regression in behavior.

Neurologic diseases in infancy may be extensive without causing obvious focal neurologic signs, and it must be assumed that the functions of a large part of the cerebrum and basal ganglions are inactive during the early months of life. Cerebellar ataxia and motor and sensory paralysis from cerebral lesions may not be recognizable at this time. In fact, seizures, general motor inactivity, lack of startle reaction, opisthotonos and abnormal postures, poor regulation of breathing, and inability to suckle are the only dependable neurologic signs during the first days and weeks of life.

The author has found the methods of examination outlined by Gesell and Amatruda and by André Thomas and his associates to be of far greater value in infants than those customarily employed by neurologists. However, the limitations of a clinical method that depends largely on assessment of the strictly motor aspects of behavior are obvious. Experience in pediatric neurology dictates caution in prognosticating the potential mental capacities of an infant until there is a sufficient degree of maturation to permit the testing of the more specific sensorial and intellectual faculties of the mind.

IMPORTANCE OF A WORKING KNOWLEDGE OF NEUROANATOMY AND NEUROPHYSIOLOGY

Once the technique of obtaining reliable clinical data is mastered, the student may find himself handicapped in the interpretation of the findings by a lack of facility in neuroanatomy and neurophysiology. These are highly complex subjects, and to acquire a practical working knowledge of them is time consuming. Fortunately these subjects are taught well in most schools, and those principles which are immediately applicable to the clinical neurologic problem are to be found in most textbooks.

DIFFERENTIAL DIAGNOSIS

The differential diagnosis of the cause of a clinical syndrome requires knowledge of an entirely different order. One must be conversant with the clinical details and the course and natural history of the more common disease entities. Many of these facts are simple and well known and can be found in any standard textbook on neurology. For instance, the distinguishing characteristic of vascular disease of the brain is its sudden onset and, if death does not occur, the improvement in the patient's neurologic status. Similarly, insidious onset and slow progression often punctuated by convulsions are typical of brain tumor.

The findings in the general medical examination are of importance; the fallacy of studying nervous symptoms and disregarding the general medical findings must be obvious. To illustrate: low-grade fever, anemia, heart murmur, and splenomegaly indicate that in a case of unexplained apoplexy subacute bacterial endocarditis with embolic occlusion of a brain artery is the most likely cause. Pleocytosis in the cerebrospinal fluid with elevated protein, abnormal gold sol, and a positive Wassermann test reaction establish a syphilitic etiology in a case with symptoms of apoplexy, a progressive dementia, or blindness.

The anatomic diagnosis may suggest the etiology of a disease. Thus when a unilateral Horner's syndrome, cerebellar ataxia, paralysis of a vocal cord, and analgesia of the face are combined with loss of pain and temperature sensation in the opposite arm, trunk, and leg, an occlusion of the posterior inferior cerebellar artery is suggested, because all the involved structures lie within the territory of this artery. In a sense the anatomic diagnosis determines and limits the possible disease entities. If the signs point to disease of the peripheral nerves, it is not necessary to consider the causes of disease of the spinal cord. Some signs themselves are almost specific, e.g., Argyll Robertson pupils for neurosyphilis or oculogyric crises for postencephalitic parkinsonism.

If one adheres faithfully to the method of making these clinical observations, and to the interpretations and methods of reasoning, neurologic diagnosis becomes relatively simple. In nearly every case it will be possible to reach an anatomic diagnosis. The etiology of the disease may prove more elusive. Even the most experienced neurologist is unable to ascertain the cause of many neurologic syndromes.

THE PURPOSE OF THE CLINICAL METHOD OF NEUROLOGY

Finally, a word about the main purposes of the clinical method of neurology. Actually, diagnosis accomplishes two purposes. First it enables the physician to decide on the proper method of treating the ailing patient; and second, it serves as an essential method in the scientific study of disease by permitting the identification and segregation of clinical phenomena. The medical profession is primarily concerned with the prevention and cure of illness, and all our knowledge is applied to this well-defined end. The practical physician applies himself to the diagnosis of diseases for which he has an effective treatment. Each of the treatable causes of a given syndrome must be carefully considered and excluded by clinical and laboratory methods. In the study of a case of disease of the spinal cord one must take special care to diagnose a tumor, subacute combined degeneration, spinal syphilis, or epidural abscess, for these are the treatable spinal cord diseases. Failure to recognize amyotrophic lateral sclerosis is a less serious error as far as the patient is concerned. The failure to diagnose one case of chronic subdural hematoma is more serious than the incorrect diagnosis of several cases of brain tumor.

One cannot agree with those who hold that neurologic diagnosis is merely an intellectual pastime. It is true that means are available for treating only a few of the many diseases known to affect the nervous system. But there is no doubt that the first step in the scientific study of a disease process is the identification of it in the living patient. Until this is achieved it is impossible to apply adequately the "master method of controlled experiment." The clinical method of neurology thus serves both the physician in the practical diagnosis and treatment of a patient and the clinical scientist who seeks the ultimate cause of the disease.

REFERENCES

DeJong, Russell, N.: "Neurologic Examination: Including the Fundamentals of Neuroanatomy and Neurophysiology," New York, Paul B. Hoeber, Inc., Medical Department of Harper & Brothers, 1950.

Denny-Brown, D.: "Handbook of Neurology and Case Recording," Cambridge, Mass., Harvard University Press, 1942.

Gesell, A., and C. S. Amatruda: "Developmental Diagnosis," New York, Paul B. Hoeber, Inc., Medical Department of Harper & Brothers, 1941.

Monrad-Krohn, G. H.: "The Clinical Examination of the Nervous System," New York, Paul B. Hoeber, Inc., Medical Department of Harper & Brothers, 1947.

Thomas, André, Yves Chesin, and Saint-Anne Dargassies: "The Neurological Examination of the Infant," National Spastics Society, London, 1960.

283 DEVELOPMENTAL ABNORMALITIES OF THE NERVOUS SYSTEM

Philip R. Dodge and Raymond D. Adams

The human nervous system is subject to a variety of developmental abnormalities which may be traced to genetic faults or to diseases acquired in utero, at birth, or during the early years of life. Some of these conditions are manifest at birth; others may be recognized only in late infancy and early childhood, after some degree of maturation is attained. Together these diseases comprise a large segment of pediatric neurology, and to discuss them fully it would be necessary to touch upon the entire field of nervous disease in infancy and childhood. However, in a textbook of medicine, limitations of space prevent the full presentation of pediatric disease, and for this reason only those conditions which are likely to come to the attention of the internist and general physician are considered.

MAJOR PROBLEMS OF PEDIATRIC NEUROLOGY

The diseases included in this chapter differ from most of those acquired in late childhood, adoles-

cence, and adult life in that they are likely to cause (1) deformity of the skull, spine, and limbs, (2) delayed or abnormal motor and speech development, (3) or mental retardation. The corollary of this axiom is that when any one of these abnormalities is observed in the adult there is a strong probability of a disease of the nervous system that had its onset before birth or during infancy or early childhood. Understanding fully the significance of these three types of abnormality will enable the student or physician to deal effectively with the majority of patients who suffer from developmental abnormalities. For this reason this chapter is devoted to an exposition of these topics. In addition, certain seizure problems peculiar to the pediatric age group deserve special consideration here.

Malformations of the Cranium, Spine, and Limbs

A congenital abnormality may be defined as a structural defect in some tissue or organ of the body, which is present at birth. It may be "gross or microscopic, on the surface of the body or within it, familial or sporadic, hereditary or nonhereditary, single or multiple" (Warkany).

Estimates as to the incidence of congenital abnormalities of the nervous system vary substantially, depending upon the definition adopted by the reporter and the time in life when the survey was made. Malpas found a congenital malformation of the nervous system in approximately 1 per cent of 13,000 births, and McIntosh and his associates give a figure of 1.3 per cent of total births, 7.2 per cent of stillbirths, 6.1 per cent of infants dying in the first days of life, and 1.1 per cent of live births. Malformations of the central nervous system are of importance in stillbirth and infantile mortality. They cause 76 per cent of all fetal deaths prior to birth and 39 per cent of deaths in the first year of life according to Record and McKeown. As was pointed out by Murphy, the nervous system is involved in 60 per cent of all patients with a congenital malformation.

General understanding of these malformations has been advanced by experimental teratology, a branch of biology that seeks the causes of abnormalities of structural development. In the progeny of animals possessing certain abnormal genes, developmental abnormalities can be predicted in ratios that agree with established genetic laws. Equally predictable results have been obtained by subjecting the embryo or fetus, under controlled conditions, to certain environmental stresses. X-ray, hypoxia, deficient diet, viral infections, and toxic substances have been shown to induce a variety of defects in the central nervous system, depending on the stage of embryogenesis at which the noxious agent is applied to the pregnant animal. These genetically and environmentally determined malformations serve as experimental models which can be investigated to great advantage.

In human beings both genetic and environmental factors have been established in the production of congenital defects. Neurofibromatosis (von Recklinghausen), craniofacial dysostosis (Crouzon), optic atrophy (Leber), and craniostenosis with syndactylism (Apert) have a dominant pattern of inheritance, whereas the lipid storage diseases (Tay-Sachs) and gargoylism (Hurler), phenylketonuria, hepatolenticular degeneration (Wilson), Hallevorden-Spatz disease, and galactosemia are examples of disease inherited according to a recessive pattern. Specific enzymes are found to be lacking in some of these diseases and are suspected of being absent in others. Examples of malformations due to the action of a noxious agent during human development are less numerous. Exposure to roentgen radiation during the first trimester of pregnancy is said to produce microcephaly and mental defect. Maternal infection with German measles (rubella) during the first trimester of pregnancy may result in mental defect, deafness, cataracts, and heart disease in the newborn. Toxoplasmosis, cytomegalic inclusion disease, and syphilis may damage the fetal nervous system in the latter half of the period of intrauterine life. Isoimmunization by Rh and ABO blood factors may affect the nervous system during the first days of postnatal life, leaving in its wake a permanent mental defect, choreoathetosis, and deafness.

Abnormalities of the Head

Alterations in the size and shape of the head, when observed in the adult, can usually be traced to infancy. At least three separate factors are operative: (1) the growth thrust of the developing brain and the intracranial pressure, (2) the time at which the suture lines close, (3) the existence of external pressures against the skull. In addition a depressed fracture, cephalohematoma, craniocele, or tumor may cause a localized cephalic deformity.

It is the constant outward pressure of the developing brain which under normal circumstances causes the head to enlarge rapidly in the first months and years of life. Any disease which destroys a substantial portion of the cerebral hemispheres in infancy will usually result in microcephaly. Excessive intracranial pressure, as from hydrocephalus or chronic subdural hematomas, will enlarge the head to an abnormal degree. Focal lesions, e.g., destruction of one hemisphere, result in smallness of the skull on that side, just as a unilateral subdural hematoma enlarges it. Regarding premature closure of the sutures (synostosis), it should be noted that this may occur without abnormality of the brain. If all sutures close, cranial expansion is prevented; or if some sutures close

and others remain open, enlargement will occur only at the latter sites, and the skull then becomes deformed. A flattening of one side of the head (plagiocephaly) often is found in defective or sick infants who lie in one position for prolonged periods of time. The weight of the head against the bed prevents part of the skull from expanding but the cranial capacity is usually undiminished, for there is a bulge in another direction; for example, flattening in one occipital region is usually associated with frontal prominence on the same side. This deformity will persist, if the abnormal positioning continues beyond the period of maximal brain growth. Congenital depressions have been observed to result from the prolonged pressure of a fetal hand or foot against the cranial bones in utero.

Macrocephaly (Enlargement of the Head). A general enlargement of the head must be distinguished from a misshapen head, one that is enlarged in one direction only. Three different conditions must be considered in the differential diagnosis—infantile hydrocephalus, infantile chronic subdural hematoma, and macroencephaly.

Hydrocephalus. This most frequent cause of enlargement of the head is the only condition in which there is enormous enlargement. The majority of severely hydrocephalic infants die within a few months or years and are not seen by internists, but a few linger on. Sometimes the hydrocephalus becomes arrested and there is a long-term survival. Hydrocephalus was discussed in Chap. 32.

Hydrocephalus due to congenital causes may appear years after birth. If the sutures have already closed (after the twelfth year), the head cannot enlarge and the hydrocephalus is poorly tolerated. Increased intracranial pressure with papilledema, vomiting, and mental dullness are the usual signs.

The usual causes of hydrocephalus are:

1. *Arnold-Chiari malformation with spina bifida and meningomyelocele.*

2. *Atresia or stenosis of the aqueduct of Sylvius* with obstructive hydrocephalus and a small, normal-appearing posterior fossa. This may be an inherited abnormality, an accompaniment of an Arnold-Chiari malformation or of neurofibromatosis, or the result of a chronic meningoependymal inflammation.

3. *Atresia of the foramens of Luschka and Magendie (Dandy-Walker syndrome)* with obstructive hydrocephalus and enlargement of the posterior fossa. Here the basal foramens fail to form or are sealed off, and the cerebrospinal fluid cannot enter the subarachnoid space.

4. *Chronic meningitis* with communicating or obstructive hydrocephalus. This is due to obliteration of the subarachnoid space over the brain stem and/or obstruction of the foramens of Luschka and Magendie. The meningitis may be due to syphilis,

toxoplasmosis, a chronic pyogenic or other infection.

5. *A tumor* of the fourth ventricle (medulloblastoma, ependymoma, or teratoma), of the third ventricle (craniopharyngioma), or of the pineal body (teratoma) may cause obstructive hydrocephalus (see Chap. 286).

6. Other conditions such as hypertrophy of the choroid plexuses and achondroplastic dwarfism with hydrocephalus are occasionally observed; and finally there is always a large number of patients with hydrocephalus, particularly of the communicating type, in which a cause can never be established.

Subdural Hematoma and Effusion in Infancy. This is a not infrequent cause of a symmetric enlargement of the skull. It may occur in several circumstances: (1) trauma to the head at birth or later, (2) with bleeding diseases or in poorly nourished, sickly infants, some of whom are said to have had scurvy, (3) in association with pyogenic meningitis, and (4) secondary to encephaloclastic disease processes with brain atrophy or rarely the result of rapid shrinkage due to hypertonicity. In acute subdural hematoma the symptoms are the same as those described in Chap. 285 on head injury. In the chronic subdural hematoma of infancy the initial symptoms are usually irritability, vomiting, and seizures. Later the cranium enlarges, symmetrically as a rule, even though the subdural hematoma is unilateral. X-rays of the skull even years later will reveal that a characteristic enlargement of the middle cranial fossa has occurred, followed later, after resorption or removal of the clot, by thickening of the skull and enlargement of the frontal and ethmoidal sinuses (Davidoff and Dyke).

Macroencephaly. This is a rare cause of enlargement of the head. The brain is malformed and greatly increased in size; specimens weighing over 2,500 Gm have been recorded. Mental retardation, feebleness of movement, and enlargement of the head with small ventricles are the criteria for clinical diagnosis. Macroencephaly is characteristically found in chronic Tay-Sachs disease, gargoylism, spongy degeneration of the brain (Canavan), some cases of achondroplastic dwarfism, and the leukodystrophy associated with hyalin bodies.

The *diagnosis* of hydrocephalus is usually established by injecting air directly into the dilated ventricles. In the infant this is usually done by inserting a needle through the lateral border of the anterior fontanel. The subdural space can also be entered during this maneuver, and the aspiration of it will rule out chronic subdural hematoma. If the cortical mantle is thin or the subarachnoid space dilated, cerebrospinal fluid may be obtained and mistaken for subdural fluid. The latter is usually xanthochromic, with a total protein content of 300 to 2,000 mg per 100 ml. In the older child or adult, pneumoencephalography, burr holes, and inspection of the dura must be used. Macroencephaly is distinguished by the small lateral and third ventricles. The entrance into the ventricles of air that has been introduced into the lumbar subarachnoid space, or the passage of a dye such a phenolsulfonphthalein, injected into the lateral ventricles, to the lumbar subarachnoid space, is of help in determining whether or not the hydrocephalus is due to an obstruction in the ventricular system (*obstructive* hydrocephalus) or is *nonobstructive* (also called *communicating* hydrocephalus). The latter is usually due to obliteration of subarachnoid space over the medulla, pons, and midbrain by a fibrosing meningitis. Thrombosis of the superior sagittal sinus may cause headache and elevated intracranial pressure but does not expand the ventricles.

The *treatment* of these conditions is relatively unsatisfactory. If the hydrocephalus has stabilized, i.e., the head is no longer enlarging, no treatment should be undertaken. If the head is large and the patient is mentally enfeebled or has other serious malformations, surgical therapy is ill-advised. If the hydrocephalus is definitely progressive but the patient's neurologic status is good, operative treatment is indicated. The introduction of ventriculoatriostomy in which the cerebrospinal fluid is shunted from the occipital horn of the lateral ventricle of the brain to the right atrium of heart by a tube with one-way valves is applicable to the treatment of all types of hydrocephalus and has largely replaced other forms of surgical treatment. In certain instances of obstructive hydrocephalus, the Torkildsen procedure (short-circuiting the fluid through a tube from the occipital horn of the lateral ventricle to the cisterna magna) may be used. The treatment of chronic subdural effusion is repeated percutaneous aspiration by needle; and in some cases removal of the membranes enclosing the subdural hematoma must be carried out at a later stage. Nothing can be done about macroencephaly.

Deformity of the Skull. The usual cause of a severely misshapen head in the adolescent or adult is cranial dysostosis. The cause of this premature fusion, or synostosis, of one or several cranial sutures is unknown, but the most plausible explanation is that the mesenchymal tissues which form the cranial bones are defective, the premature ossification being secondary. The occasional association of cranial synostosis with syndactylism (Apert's syndrome) has been cited in support of this hypothesis. The developmental defect and synostosis are believed to date from intrauterine life. Closure of the sagittal suture results in an elongated, dolichocephalic head to which the term *scaphocephaly* is applied. When the coronal suture fuses prematurely, the growth is restricted in the anteroposterior diameter, and only lateral and, to a lesser extent, vertical enlargement may occur. This condition is called *brachycephaly* (wide skull) or *acrobrachycephaly*. Synostosis of all sutures leaves the cranium small but usually with the greatest growth in the vertical direction, the so-called *oxycephaly* or *turrencephaly*. *Plagiocephaly* refers to an asymmetric deformity of the skull which may be due to synostosis of a single coronal suture or to the application of some external force. *Crouzon's craniofacial dysostosis scaphocephaly* is associated with a "beak nose." This condition is inherited as a mendelian dominant. In *Apert's syndrome* webbed or "mitten" fingers and toes are combined with acrobrachycephaly. *Hypertelorism,* as described by Greig in 1924, is a rare deformity characterized by wide separation of the eyes and a flat, retracted bridge of the nose. Mental retardation frequently accompanies the deformity. The primary abnormality has usually been ascribed to an abnormally large lesser wing of the sphenoid bone. In several instances a dominant mode of inheritance has been found.

The most serious complication of synostosis of sutures is a gradual increase in intracranial pressure which occurs during the most active growth period of the brain. This tends to be less marked in patients with scaphocephaly than in those with acrobrachycephaly. In these patients the orbits are shallow and the eyes bulge. Headache, divergent strabismus, papilledema, optic atrophy and later blindness, nystagmus, mental retardation, and behavioral abnormalities are the most striking clinical manifestations. Usually the patients require medical attention within the first 2 or 3 years of life, though it may be needed later. In roentgenograms of the skull one observes the primary suture involvement, prominence of convolutional markings, and a depression and smallness of the sella turcica.

In the absence of increased intracranial pressure, the diagnosis of premature closure of the sutures should always raise the suspicion of defective growth of the brain (see below, Microcephaly).

The treatment of primary craniosynostosis is surgical, and if it is to be effective in preventing permanent injury to the brain, it should probably be carried out early in life, particularly if one has any intention of lessening the skull deformity. The operative procedure is one of making artificial suture lines by removing pieces of bone and inserting a plastic material in their place to prevent regrowth. Occasionally this results in a striking improvement in mental function and behavior, even in an older child in whom the diagnosis had not been made early in life. In other cases progression of the illness is halted. Failure to improve even when surgery has been performed early suggests that the brain defect is independent of the cranial abnormality.

Microcephaly. This term is used to designate any condition in which there is an abnormally small head. An occipitofrontal circumference of less than 19 in. beyond the age of ten years is given as the dividing line between normal and abnormal. Microcephaly is accompanied by a reduction in the mass of the brain, and two types of pathologic change have been reported. There is one form in which the growth disturbance appears to be the sole factor; the brain, except for its smallness, has a normal appearance. This is called *microcephaly vera.* The other is a focal arrest of growth due either to embryonal failure in development of a part of the cerebral hemisphere (*schizencephaly*) or to an acquired disease which has resulted in destruction of one, or both, of the cerebral hemispheres (*encephaloclastic microcephaly*).

Microcephaly vera may occur in several members of one generation of a family and can often be linked to a recessive gene. The head tends to be extraordinarily small, usually measuring 15 in. or less in circumference. It is usually of symmetric shape and owing to the lack of frontal prominence resembles the skull of a monkey. The ears are large and often malformed. The neurologic picture varies. All patients show simple mental retardation of moderate or severe degree. Seizures and quadriparesis have been described in some patients but in the authors' experience are much less frequent than in the other forms of microcephaly. Those cases with focal arrest of growth or destruction of cerebral tissue, *schizencephaly,* and *encephaloclastic microcephaly* exhibit a wide variety of clinical findings. The mental state in the most severe cases is usually that of an idiot, and all cerebral functions fail to develop. In fact the cerebral hemispheres may be represented only by membranes filled with clear or yellowish fluid, *hydranencephaly.* In others, in which the cerebral defect is restricted to one cerebral hemisphere or part of a hemisphere, there may be hemiplegia with a small arm and leg, gross hemianesthesia, homonymous hemianopia, and seizures with lesser degrees of mental backwardness. The skull on the side of the damaged hemisphere is smaller, and in roentgenograms the frontoparietal bones are thick, the middle fossa is shallow, and the paranasal sinuses are enlarged.

Abnormalities of the Spine of Neurologic Significance

There is a remarkable variety of neurologic syndromes which include an abnormality of the vertebral column. Some of these, like hemivertebra, platybasia, fusion of the atlas and occiput or of vertebras (Klippel-Feil syndrome), or congenital dislocation of the atlas, are the consequence of a malformation of the spine itself, and the enclosed spinal cord may or may not be involved. Others, such as spina bifida occulta, spinal meningocele or myelomeningocele, or dysraphism, involve the whole neural tube, including spinal cord, investing meninges, vertebral bodies, and even the overlying skin and subcutaneous tissues.

In many of these patients the neurologic defect which appears in infancy does not shorten life; in others it may be recognized only during adult life.

Primary Malformations of Vertebras. These are most frequent in the cervico-occipital region.

The Klippel-Feil Deformity. This abnormality consists of maldevelopment and fusion of two or more cervical vertebras, resulting in a short neck of limited mobility. The hairline is low, often at the level of the first thoracic vertebra. There may or may not be associated neurologic symptoms or signs. The importance of the spinal deformity lies in its frequent association with other abnormalities, especially platybasia and syringomyelia.

Platybasia (Basilar Impression). In this maldevelopment of the base of the skull there is invagination of the occiput and upper cervical spine into the posterior fossa. Often the foramen magnum itself is imperfectly developed or the atlas and occiput are fused. The exact teratogenesis of this anomaly is uncertain. It may in some instances be asymptomatic, but frequently there is "crowding," distortion, or compression of the spinal cord, medulla, and cranial and spinal nerves. The resulting clinical picture is variable. Symptoms may be present from early life or may begin in late childhood, adolescence, or even adult years. Early symptoms, in patients old enough to give a history, consist of "dizzy" or "weak" spells, occipital neuralgia, transient paresthesias in the occipital region, neck, or arm, double vision, facial paresthesias and deafness, cerebellar ataxia, and spastic weakness of the legs. The symptoms may at first be intermittent and at any time in the course of the illness may be aggravated by straining, moving the head, or placing the head and neck in certain positions. Inspection alone provides a clue to diagnosis. The whole configuration of the head and neck is unnatural. The neck is short; the ears and hairline are low; neck movements are obviously restricted; and the normal cervical lordosis is lost or greatly exaggerated, sometimes to the extent that the occiput lies almost on the upper dorsal spine and shoulders.

Platybasia and these related anomalies of the spine should be suspected in all cases presenting progressive cerebellar, brain stem, and cervical cord syndromes. Many of these patients have been diagnosed as having multiple sclerosis. The clinical suspicion of platybasia can be confirmed by a true lateral roentgenogram of the skull. In such a projection the extension of a line drawn from the hard palate and posterior border of the foramen magnum (Chamberlain's line) and another through the spine and body of the first cervical vertebra (Bull's line), instead of being more or less parallel as they normally are, intersect when extended. This has proved to be the most useful measurement. Chamberlain's basal angle, obtained by drawing lines along the hard palate and clivus, is greater than 135° in platybasia. Also, when visible, the odontoid process may project above Chamberlain's line. In Towne's view of the skull, a malformation or coarctation of the foramen magnum is occasionally found. An acquired form of platybasia occurs with rickets and Paget's disease. It is usually asymptomatic.

The Arnold-Chiari Malformation. This condition, in which medulla and inferior-posterior portions of the cerebellar hemispheres project caudally through the foramen magnum, often to the level of the second cervical vertebra, has already been mentioned as a cause of hydrocephalus. When present it is nearly always associated with a spinal meningocele or myelomeningocele, and often there are deformities of the cervical spine and cervico-occipital junction. The symptoms of hydrocephalus dominate the clinical picture in infants, but in milder cases, there may develop during adolescence or adult years any one of the several syndromes already described under platybasia. When platybasia and the Arnold-Chiari malformation coexist, it is generally impossible to decide which of the two is responsible for the clinical findings.

The cause of the Arnold-Chiari malformation itself has been the subject of speculation. It has been suggested that the hydrocephalus is primary and that the displacement of the medulla and cerebellum through the foramen magnum is secondary to pressure from above. The close relationship to spinal myelomeningocele casts doubt on this explanation. The more generally accepted hypothesis is that the associated myelomeningocele causes downward traction on structures in the posterior fossa because of fixation of the cord to the vertebral column prior to the period when the growth of the vertebral column outstrips that of the spinal cord. The cerebrospinal fluid then flows from the fourth ventricle into the cervical canal, cannot reenter the cranial cavity, and therefore is not reabsorbed. Also the aqueduct of Sylvius is elongated and sometimes critically narrowed (traction stenosis), which may itself account for the hydrocephalus. This is not the mechanism in all cases, however, for examples of the Arnold-Chiari malformation have been observed without evidence of myelomeningocele or hydrocephalus. Dysraphism of the spinal cord, which resembles syringomyelia, may accompany both platybasia and Arnold-Chiari malformation and manifests itself by segmental weakness, atrophy, areflexia, and sensory loss in the arms and hands. Syringomyelia may also occur.

Methods of treatment of platybasia and the Arnold-Chiari malformation have not been entirely satisfactory. If clinical progression is slight or uncertain, it is probably advisable to do nothing. If progression is certain and disability is increasing, upper cervical laminectomy and enlargement of the foramen magnum are indicated. Sometimes these procedures halt the course of the illness or result in improvement. The surgical procedure must be done cautiously, however, for extensive manipulation of these structures may aggravate the symptoms or even cause death.

Malformations Associated with a Defect in Closure of the Neural Arch. There are many deformities along the posterior surface of the body that are accompanied by an abnormality in the formation of the posterior aspect of the neural arch and closure of the primitive neural tube. The entire neural canal, including the cranium, may fail to close (*craniorhachischisis totalis*), or there may be only a minute defect in one or more of the vertebral arches, demonstrable by roentgenograms (*spina bifida occulta*). The latter is said to occur in one-quarter of the population. It has been estimated that in approximately one of every 900 births there is a serious closure defect in the spine, or more rarely in the cranium.

The neural tube is closed and has been separated completely from the anlage of the skeleton by approximately the third week of intrauterine life; and by three months the neural arches are completely fused along their dorsal aspect. The defects under discussion must, then, have originated during the early weeks of embryonic life, in all probability by the middle of the first month. The skeletal malformations may arise at any time prior to the end of the third month. The not infrequent occurrence of some of these defects in several siblings suggests a genetic origin with a recessive mode of inheritance.

Defects of this type may be found at any point along the neuraxis. They are most frequent in the lumbosacral and cranial regions, less frequent in the cervical region, and rare in the thoracic region. The character of the abnormality varies. There may be an outpouching of neural elements (nerve root and cord) through a defect in mesenchymal tissue and skin (*myelomeningocele*); less often, actually in less than one-fifth of all cases, only a thin-walled cyst composed of meninges and containing no neural tissue can be found. The cranial defect similarly may consist of an encephalocele with evagination of cerebral tissue and meninges through a midline defect in the membranous bones of the skull. These are most often occipital in location, though a few may be frontal, presenting either anteriorly or inferiorly into the nasal cavity. Probably the most astonishing cranial defect of all, and one nearly as frequent as the myelomeningocele, is *anencephaly.* In this condition there is a gross defect or absence of the membranous bones of the skull; the cerebral hemispheres and corpus striatum are also absent, and the remainder of the brain is grossly malformed. Patients with severe defects of this type usually do not survive.

MENINGOCELE AND MYELOMENINGOCELE. Meningocele may exist alone and unaccompanied by any symptoms or signs. Myelomeningocele, in contrast, is associated with some dysfunction of those nervous structures that lie within the wall of the sac. The signs may be minimal, limited to sensorimotor dysfunction of a few segments, or pronounced, with total paraplegia and incontinence of urine and feces. Severe paralysis and wasting of muscles in the legs may result in contractures and various skeletal deformities such as *clubfoot* or *arthrogryposis multiplex congenita* (see Malformations of the Extremities, further on in this chapter). Such cases show a susceptibility to decubitus ulcers, and not infrequently there is infection of the sac and neighboring tissues. When the defect involves only the meninges or a few roots, the neurologic defect may not be apparent at birth. After a year or two attention is directed toward this possibility by the discovery of contracture, feebleness of movement, smallness of muscles of the legs, or by some urologic disorder.

The decision to operate upon these infants with total paralysis of the legs and of the rectal and bladder sphincters may be questioned. One must be alert to the development of hydrocephalus, either before or after operation on the spinal lesion. This almost always means an associated Arnold-Chiari malformation, as already stated. Some of these cases can be helped by craniocervical decompression.

SINUS TRACTS AND CONGENITAL CYSTS. These are often indicated by a small dimple in the skin or by a tuft of hairs along the posterior surface of the body in the midline. These signs occur most often in the lumbosacral and occipital regions and are thought to represent failure of closure of the anterior or posterior neuropores. (The pilonidal sinus, in the opinion of the authors, should not be included in this group.) Small *sinus tracts* may exist at these points and are of clinical importance because they frequently connect with the central nervous system or its coverings and are not uncommonly associated with dermoid cysts at the central end of the tract. These cysts most often occur in the cerebellum or in the lumbosacral regions, and the sinus tracts which connect them to the skin provide free access for bacteria and are often a source of abscess and recurrent meningitis. Evidence of such tracts should be sought in every instance of meningitis in children and adolescents, especially when infection has recurred.

There are in addition other *congenital cysts* and *tumors* which may produce progressive symptoms and signs by compressing the spinal cord or by implicating nerve roots.

DIASTEMATOMYELIA. This is another unusual abnormality of the spinal cord. Here a bony spicule or ridge protrudes into the spinal canal from the body of one of the thoracic or upper lumbar vertebras. If the bony abnormality is in the thoracic region, there will be duplication of, or splitting of, the spinal cord (diplomyelia). As the vertebral column grows, traction is exerted on the less rapidly growing cord. The stretched spinal cord is injured ("traction myelopathy"), with classical manifestations of urinary and fecal incontinence and sensorimotor dysfunction in the legs. A patch of hair and some degree of spina bifida is reported to overlie the lesion in more than half the cases. The diagnosis can be made by roentgenograms and myelogram and the bony spicule removed by surgery.

These spinal abnormalities are of particular interest to internists when they begin to produce symptoms for the first time in an adolescent or adult. Several clinical syndromes have been delineated: (1) Progressive spastic weakness of the legs during late childhood or adolescence in a patient known to have had a meningocele or myelomeningocele. Presumably the spinal cord, which is securely attached to the lumbar vertebras, is stretched during the period of rapid lengthening of the vertebral column. (2) An acute cauda equina syndrome following some unusual activity or incident, e.g., rowing or a fall in a sitting position, in patients who have had an asymptomatic or symptomatic spina bifida or meningocele. The implicated sensory and motor roots are believed to be injured by sudden or repeated stretching. Weakness of bladder control, impotence (in the male), numbness of feet and legs, or foot drop comprise the clinical syndrome. (3) Syringomyelia. (4) Progressive cauda equina syndrome due to a lipoma or dermoid in the lumbosacral region.

SYRINGOMYELIA. This term refers to a cavity (Greek *syrinx* meaning pipe or tube). The cavity occupies the central parts of the spinal cord in the cervical region but may extend upward into the medulla oblongata (syringobulbia) or downward into thoracic or even lumbar segments. In approximately 15 per cent of cases studied post mortem an intramedullary tumor (hemangioblastoma or glioma) has been found in or near some part of the syrinx. The syrinx is independent of the central canal and replaces the gray matter of the posterior or anterior horns of the spinal cord and also interrupts the crossing pain and temperature fibers in the anterior commissure in several successive cord segments. The cavity is lined with astrocytic glia and thick-walled blood vessels. It may enlarge the spinal cord and even widen the interpedicular spaces, but the cerebrospinal fluid in the cavity always has a relatively low protein. The cause is unknown. Familial incidence is rare. A blastomatous formation akin to tuberous sclerosis or central von Recklinghausen's disease but with tendency for the abnormal tissue to cavitate is the most plausible explanation.

The clinical triad upon which the diagnosis is based consists of (1) segmental sensory loss or dissociation (loss of pain and temperature and preservation of touch) over neck, shoulders, and arms, (2) amyotrophy, and (3) thoracic scoliosis. Symptoms usually begin in late childhood, adolescence, or adult life and progress irregularly, often being arrested for long periods of time. The segmental sensory loss or dissociation and amyotrophy are caused by cavitation of the gray matter of the posterior columns or ventral commissure, respectively. Analgesia and thermanesthesia account for severe painless ulcers, injuries, and burns so often sustained by patients with syringomyelia; Charcot joints, also common in this disease, result from painless injury of the joint tissue. Areflexia without atrophy may be due to involvement of the afferent limb of the reflex arc; destruction of anterior horn cells is probably the more frequent cause, particularly if accompanied by muscle atrophy. A useful clinical rule is that a neurologic disease which leaves all deep tendon reflexes in the arms intact is probably not syringomyelia. A Horner's syndrome on the affected side may result from involvement of cells of the intermedial lateral cell column of the eighth cervical to first thoracic segments of the spinal cord. Pyramidal tract signs in the legs tend to appear late in the course of the disease and are attributable to extension of the syrinx into the lateral columns of the cord, the decussation of corticospinal tracts at the first cervical segment, or compression of these tracts by a distended syrinx. If the cavity enlarges the spinal cord, a spinal subarachnoid block may result, and prolonged pressure may cause widening of the spinal canal and erosion of pedicles. The kyphoscoliosis, which may antedate other evidence of disease by several years, is thought to result from weakness due to asymmetrical involvement of anterior horns in the thoracic region.

A syrinx in the brain stem (syringobulbia) usually extends into the lateral tegmentum of the medulla, being so placed as to result in nystagmus and sensory impairment over one or both sides of the face. Unilateral palatal and vocal cord paralysis as well as weakness and atrophy of one side of the tongue are other clinical signs which call attention to lesions at this level of the neuraxis.

The association of cavitation of the spinal cord with myelomeningocele (so-called myelodysplasia), Arnold-Chiari malformation, platybasia, and other congenital defects about the cervicocranial junction has been commented on in previous sections.

The treatment of syringomyelia is unsatisfactory. The fact that the disease process may remain stationary for some months or years before progressing makes evaluation of any mode of therapy difficult. Decompression of a distended syrinx may alleviate temporarily those symptoms and signs resulting from local compression of ascending and descending spinal tracts, but relief is seldom lasting. The results of x-ray treatment, based on the belief that symptoms result from a gliomatous malformation of the cord which subsequently cavitates, have been difficult to evaluate. It is worth a trial.

Malformations of the Extremities

A variety of primary skeletal defects, such as absence of or increase in number of digits or extremities, fusion or webbing of digits (syndactylism), deformity of digits or limbs or abnormalities of size have neurologic import, for they tend to be associated with malformations of the central nervous system. For example, *syndactylism* is frequently combined with oxycephaly (*Apert's syndrome*). In *mongolism* the fifth digit is usually short and curved, the hands are broad and simian-like, and there is usually only a single transverse crease in the palm. In arachnodactyly the digits are long and tapering, a condition frequently linked to disease of the aorta and congenital heart disease and to dislocation of the lens (cf. Marfan's syndrome, Chap. 292).

Shortening of all the extremities with normal growth of the trunk is characteristic of achondroplasia. In Morquio's syndrome both the trunk and the limbs are short and deformed. Thus dwarfism may be importantly linked in this condition with a neurologic abnormality, just as it is in cretinism, mongolism, and gargoylism. The sufferers from these several neurologic diseases in which growth is stunted may be referred to collectively as "amented midgets"; and since many of them reach adult years, they must be treated by general practitioners, internists, and surgeons for other diseases which develop during this age period.

In some cases the deformity of the extremities is the direct consequence of a congenital neuromuscular defect. In fact this happens so often that whenever deformities of the limbs are known to have begun early in life one should at once evaluate the status of the nervous system. In most cases of *clubfoot* (talipes equinovarus), no abnormality of the nervous system can be ascertained. In a few,

however, the deformity results from paralysis of the anterior tibial and peroneal muscles due to a primary defect in the anterior horn cells of the lumbo-acral segments of the spinal cord. The contracture of calf muscles is secondary. Widespread weakness and contractures of many limb muscles may cause extensive deformities (*arthrogryposis multiplex* or *amyoplasia congenita*). This syndrome may also be the result of any one of several other primary neural or muscular diseases such as congenital absence of muscles, muscular dystrophy, and rarely from infantile motor neurone disease (*Werdnig-Hoffmann infantile muscular atrophy*). Reconstructive surgery and the techniques of physical medicine may permit a certain measure of rehabilitation in those cases with nonprogressive diseases. However, severe mental defect, which is frequent in these conditions, tends to discourage elaborate programs of therapy.

Birthmarks and Associated Neurologic Conditions

A number of neurologic abnormalities are combined with congenital defects of skin or retina, explained usually by their common ectodermal origin. The terms *congenital ectodermal dysplasias, congenital neurocutaneous syndromes,* or *phacomatoses* (*phakos,* birthmark) are used frequently to designate this general class of disorders. The major syndromes include *neurofibromatosis, tuberous sclerosis, encephalotrigeminal syndrome,* and rarely the *cerebelloretinal hemangioblastomatosis.* Another variant of the latter is the *myelocutaneous syndrome,* in which a vascular malformation of spinal cord and meninges is associated with a vascular nevus within the area of skin innervated by the involved spinal segments. Recently it has been suggested that *ataxia telangiectasia* be included with this group of conditions.

Neurofibromatosis (von Recklinghausen's Disease). This is an inherited disease (mendelian dominant) in which spots of increased skin pigmentation are combined with multiple neurofibromas. The pigmented spots are irregular in shape with relatively even borders, vary in size from a few millimeters to several centimeters, and are of brownish-coffee color (*café-au-lait*). They are most prominent over the trunk and especially about the pelvis. Similar lesions occur in individuals without neurofibromatosis but in such instances are generally smaller than 2 cm in diameter and fewer than five in number. The tumors arise from the neurilemmal sheath (Schwann cells) and fibroblasts of the peripheral nerve. They are usually multiple and vary in size from minute lesions to large tumors several centimeters in diameter. The majority are smoothly rounded or lobulated, soft or firm, and can sometimes be seen or felt along the course of a peripheral nerve. Often they sink into the subcutaneous fat on gentle pressure. Like the pigmented lesions, the tumors are more frequent over the trunk than on the extremities. The pigmented areas of skin may be visible in infancy, though usually they become increasingly apparent with age; the tumors of nerve sheaths are often not demonstrable early in life. Most of the tumors in neurofibromatosis are asymptomatic; but occasionally, if they attain a large size or occupy an unusual position, they may produce symptoms by pressing upon contiguous structures. Tumors of the spinal nerves may compress the spinal cord and at the same time extend through the intervertebral foramens to form a large mass in the posterior mediastinum (dumbbell tumors). Acoustic neurinomas, usually bilateral in patients with neurofibromatosis, may produce deafness and symptoms and signs of a cerebellopontine angle tumor. Other histopathologic types of tumor (meningioma, glioma) are encountered more frequently in neurofibromatosis than in the general population. Most of these tumors are rare in infancy and childhood, though pontine glioma and glioma of the optic nerve are exceptions to this clinical rule. The latter condition should always be considered in the differential diagnosis of unilateral (rarely bilateral) blindness, proptosis, and extraocular muscle paralysis in childhood, especially if there are signs of von Recklinghausen's disease. Enlargement of the optic foramens, demonstrable by roentgenogram, is a valuable aid in diagnosis. Pulsating exophthalmos may result from congenital absence of part of the sphenoid bone. Pheochromocytoma is an infrequent accompaniment of the disease. In about 5 to 10 per cent of cases of neurofibromatosis one of the tumors will become sarcomatous.

Fibrous dysplasia, congenital vertebral anomalies, local gigantism of an extremity, subperiosteal bone cysts, and pseudoarthrosis of the tibia may be associated with neurofibromatosis. Any of these can lead to scoliosis, a common skeletal deformity in children with this disease, so that neurofibromatosis must be added to the list of neurogenic kyphoscolioses (the others are syringomyelia, Friedreich's ataxia, and poliomyelitis). Stenosis of the aqueduct with obstructive hydrocephalus is at times observed in neurofibromatosis. Also, mental retardation is rather common in families with von Recklinghausen's disease, though its pathogenesis is not at all understood. Spina bifida, hypospadias, glaucoma, and elephantiasis are occasionally seen.

There is no treatment for the disease other than excision of symptomatic tumors.

Tuberous Sclerosis (Bourneville's Disease). This curious disease, of dominant inheritance, is manifested by the clinical triad of convulsive seizures, progressive mental deficiency, and adenoma sebaceum. The latter are fine, wartlike lesions predominantly in a butterfly distribution over the cheeks and forehead. The individual adenomas vary in size from 0.1 to 1.0 cm and are elevated and pinkish or pinkish yellow in color. In addition, the skin over the lower back may be thick, rough, and of yellowish color (sharkskin patch, shagreen). The mental deficiency may be relatively stationary or progressive. The seizures are usually generalized but may be focal. Retinal tumors, optic atrophy, cataracts and hyperonchomas, syndactylism, spina bifida, and other visible malformations may be conjoined.

The lesions of the skin are pathologically fibromas and not true adenomas. Some are rather vascular and suggest telangiectasia. The brain lesions consist of areas of malformed cortex with extensive astrogliosis and a curious mixture of glioblasts and monster nerve cells. Calcification may or may not be present. Masses of subependymal glial tissue account for nodules which project into and form the "candle gutterings" on the walls of the ventricles that are often seen in pneumograms. In Bourneville's original case, death was due to rhabdomyoma of the heart. This lesion has been combined in some cases with vascular malformations of kidney, liver, adrenal glands, and pancreas.

The diagnosis is aided by roentgenograms of the skull. Calcified nodules occur particularly in the temporal lobe. The center of the nodule tends to be more densely radiopaque than the periphery. The electroencephalogram is usually abnormal but without specific pattern. The cerebrospinal fluid may be normal; rarely the total protein is elevated.

The only treatment is symptomatic. The prognosis for life beyond the third decade is poor. Death may be due to seizures, associated tumors (glioma), or intercurrent diseases.

Cerebelloretinal Hemangioblastomatosis (Lindau's and von Hippel's Disease). This condition is discussed here though the skin is seldom involved. As the name implies, the syndrome consists of a vascular malformation of retina and cerebellum. The retinal lesion usually has the characteristics of a malformation, whereas the cerebellar lesion consists of a slowly growing cystic tumor. The clinical symptoms and signs consist of progressive cerebellar ataxia, headache, and papilledema. Polycythemia of undetermined etiology has been observed in many cases and has in a few instances disappeared after excision of the tumor. Rarely do these tumors appear before adolescence. Some cases are familial.

This condition is often associated with malformation of other organs, especially with visceral tumors. Angiomas of the liver, cysts of the pancreas and kidneys, and tumors of the epididymis and kidney, which have been the cause of death in some cases, are the major parts of the syndrome. Pheochromocytomas have been described in this and in other of the phakomatoses. Syringomyelia has been observed in a few cases, and if a careful search is made, a hemangioblastoma can often be found in relation to the syrinx at some level.

The cerebellar hemangioblastoma demands surgical treatment, and if the nodule of tumor is found in the wall of the cyst and is excised, the results can be excellent.

Encephalotrigeminal Syndrome (Sturge-Weber-Dimitri Disease). This curious disease consists of capillary or cavernous hemangiomas within the cutaneous distribution of the trigeminal nerve and of a predominantly venous hemangioma of the leptomeninges. If the skin lesion is within the area of supply of the ophthalmic division of the trigeminal nerve, the occipital lobes are more commonly involved, whereas a facial nevus is more often associated with involvement of the parietal and frontal lobes. The intracranial or cutaneous lesion may occur separately.

Pathologically, in addition to the large number of abnormal blood vessels in the meninges, the cortex is destroyed, and in some cases a band of calcium develops within the lesion. This band, following the convolutional pattern as it does, is responsible for the characteristic roentgenographic picture.

The first neurologic symptom is usually a focal seizure on the side opposite the skin lesion. Transient postictal (Todd's) paralysis or permanent paralysis may follow the seizure. Sensorimotor paralysis or permanent visual field defect, the most frequent findings, may be either of insidious onset with slow progression or apoplectic. Hemorrhage into the meninges has been reported, but this must be a rare event. Possibly occlusion of cortical vessels will, in certain instances, be responsible for neurologic deficits. Blindness in the eye on the side of the nevus is frequent and is nearly always due to glaucoma. Most patients with this malformation survive for many years, often with residual mental and other neurologic defects.

The lesions are usually too extensive to be treated surgically, though hemispherectomy has been advised by some surgeons. Anticonvulsant medication is indicated, but the seizures may be difficult to control.

Ataxia Telangiectasia. Only recognized as a disease entity recently, this condition has attracted considerable interest. It is characterized neurologically by a progressive cerebellar ataxia, apraxia of ocular movement, and choreoathetosis beginning during the early years of life. Telangiectasias of bulbar conjunctivas and skin, especially about the ears, neck, and in flexor creases at the elbows and knees, appear somewhat later. Recurring pulmonary and sinus infections have been prominent in many cases. The cause of this disease is unknown, but more than one child in a family may be affected. The associated pathologic changes must still be clarified; Courville has described an extensive loss of Purkinje cells of the cerebellum in one case.

Abnormalities of Motor Function (Cerebral Palsy)

In this category of neurologic defect a major disturbance of motor function, usually nonprogressive, has been present since infancy or childhood. The popular term for these conditions is *cerebral palsy*. The name is not altogether appropriate, nor is such a crude classification of nervous disorders particularly useful from the viewpoint of the physician, because it results in a collocation of diseases of widely differing etiologic and anatomic types. The hereditary and acquired, the intrauterine, natal, and postnatal diseases lose their identity. Nevertheless, the term has been adopted as a slogan for fundraising societies and for a major rehabilitation movement throughout the United States, and it will not soon disappear from medical terminology.

Clinical Approach to Motor Disturbances Which Have Developed in Infancy or Childhood

Motor abnormalities which have their onset early in life are so numerous and diverse that it is necessary to acquire some knowledge of the motor system in order to interpret them. Also, a classification is useful in guiding one's thinking. It is helpful

Table 283-1. CLASSIFICATION OF DEVELOPMENTAL MOTOR ABNORMALITIES

I. Spastic or rigid paralyses
  A. Cerebral spastic diplegia and paraplegia
  B. Infantile hemiplegia
  C. Double hemiplegia
  D. Quadriplegic states
II. Extrapyramidal syndromes
  A. Choreoathetosis and dystonia
  B. Cerebellar ataxia
III. Flaccid paralyses
  A. Generalized
    1. Cerebral type—cerebral atonic diplegia (of Foerster)
    2. Spinal type
      a. Infantile muscular atrophy of Werdnig-Hoffmann
      b. Traumatic necrosis of spinal cord
    3. Other types
      a. Infantile muscular dystrophy
      b. Lipoid and glycogen storage diseases
      c. Infantile polymyositis
      d. The "slack child" and amyotonia congenita of Oppenheim
  B. Localized (nerve)
    1. Brachial plexus palsies of Erb and Klumpke
    2. Facial palsy
    3. Other peripheral nerve palsies

to attempt to categorize a given case according to the extent and nature of the abnormality.

These motor abnormalities of infancy and childhood are relatively frequent, and many of the affected children reach adult years.

Special Types

Infantile Spastic and Rigid Paralyses. The pattern of paralysis or rigidity is important, for it provides information as to the etiology and possible pathogenetic mechanism.

Cerebral Spastic Diplegia (Little's Disease). In 1862 Little called attention to the concurrence of "Abnormal Parturition, Difficult Labours, Premature Birth, and Asphyxia Neonatorum" and of a spastic weakness that affected legs more than arms. He emphasized the prenatal or natal origin, the diplegic (legs > arms) distribution of the paralysis, and the nonprogressive course. Little was of the opinion that asphyxia caused the cerebral damage, but the present view is that it represents a syndrome of multiple etiology and of diverse pathology.

S. A. K. Wilson distinguishes three types, the paraplegic, diplegic, and the generalized and pseudobulbar. These differ from one another only in respect to the severity of affection of the arms and bulbar musculature. Pure paraplegias and pure pseudobulbar cases are relatively rare. Usually all four extremities are involved, the legs much more than the arms. As a rule the abnormality is recognized at birth or soon thereafter by some abnormality of breathing, sucking and swallowing, color of mucous membranes, or responsiveness. These latter signs may indicate either a congenital defect of the nervous system or birth injury. The stiff, awkward movements of the legs, maintained in an extended, adducted posture, attract attention at this time or in the ensuing weeks. Seizures occur in some cases, and it is not uncommon to observe a delay in all the normal developmental sequences, especially those which depend on the motor system. Once walking is attempted the characteristic stance and gait become manifest. The legs are advanced stiffly in short steps, each describing part of the arc of a circle; adduction is often so strong as to lead to actual crossing (scissors gait) with lower legs slightly splayed out and the feet flexed and turned in, the heels no longer touching the ground. The legs tend to be thin, but the muscles are not markedly atrophic, as in infantile muscular atrophy and dystrophy. Passive manipulation of the limbs reveals marked spasticity in the extensors and adductors and also slight contracture of calf muscles. The hands and arms may be little if at all affected, but in many cases there is awkwardness and stiffness of the fingers and in a few, pronounced weakness and spasticity. Speech may be well articulated or noticeably slurred, and often the face is set in a spastic smile. The deep tendon reflexes are exaggerated, those in the legs more than in the arms, and the plantar reflexes are extensor. Usually there is no disturbance of sphincteric function, though delay in acquiring voluntary function is usual. Athetotic postures and movements of the face, tongue, and hands are present in some cases and may actually conceal the pyramidal weakness. Ataxic and hypotonic forms also exist. The mentality ranges from normal to idiocy.

Surprisingly little information has been obtained concerning the cause, mechanism, and morbid anatomy of this syndrome. The claim that birth injury is responsible has been challenged, and the existence of an antenatal lesion can no longer be doubted. The association of cerebral spastic diplegia with abnormality of the placenta and prematurity is striking and suggests a possible causative relationship. A familial variety of spastic diplegia is now well documented, but such a genetic determination applies to only a minority of cases, and the progressive nature of the illness readily distinguishes this disease from the conditions under discussion (see p. 1870). The brain has appeared grossly normal in some instances, and the only microscopic abnormality has been an absence of Betz cells and a poorly myelinated corticospinal tract. It is as though the corticospinal system had failed to develop. In others a diffuse loss of nerve cells and gliosis of cerebral cortex (mantle sclerosis) has been found. Shrunken, atrophic convolutions with or without cavitation of white matter (ulegyria), a restricted form of which may involve only a few convolutions, has probably been the most frequent pathologic finding. The pathologic findings give little information as to the original process except that it must have occurred after cerebral development was nearly complete.

Infantile Hemiplegia. In this not uncommon condition of infancy and childhood, a functional difference between the two sides may be noticed at birth or during the first 6 to 12 months of life. Acquired forms following an infection or thrombosis of cerebral arteries or veins usually develop later. The parents may be the first to notice that movements of prehension and exploration are carried out with only one arm. The affection of the leg is usually recognized later, i.e., during the first attempts to walk.

The cardinal feature of a cerebral hemiplegia, and this also applies to diplegia, is that it is partial; the limbs will always move under certain circumstances. The most satisfactory tests are the facility with which the two arms engage in manipulative, prehensile, and exploratory movements. The latter may be examined in the first weeks of life by placing the infant on his feet and making him step forward by advancing and tipping the trunk from side to side. Hand preference during the first 1 to 2 years of life should always raise a suspicion of a motor defect on the opposite side.

If the brain lesion responsible for the hemiplegia is of recent onset (at birth or shortly before) and the cerebral lesion extensive, one may observe sluggishness of all motor responses, poor sucking reflexes, difficulty in breathing, and irregular pulse. The tendon reflexes tend to be more active on the affected side and the plantar reflexes more definitely extensor in type than on the normal side. There may be a homonymous visual field defect, as shown by a neglect of dangling objects on one side, or a unilateral somatic sensory loss, indicated by a lesser response to tickle, a vibrating tuning fork, and painful stimuli. The muscular tone is usually normal.

An assessment of the neurologic status at the end of the first and second years reveals more clearly the extent of the motor defect. The hand and fingers are clumsy and slow. Often the fingers are hyperextensible, and in one-third of cases they exhibit athetotic movements and postures, in which the wrist is strongly flexed, metacarpal-phalangeal joints are extended, and phalangeal joints are variably flexed or extended in various sequences. The adult hemiplegic attitude, i.e., the arm adducted at the shoulder, flexed, and internally rotated at the elbow, pronated and flexed at wrist and fingers with the thumb adducted and covered by the fingers, and the leg adducted and internally rotated at the hip with the foot inverted and plantar flexed, is evident at this time. Contractures may be found in the hip flexors, hamstrings, and plantar flexors of the foot. Sitting, standing, and walking are delayed but not so frequently as in cases of cerebral diplegia. Improvement may be noticed as the child grows and matures, especially if there has been a severe sensory defect. Impaired sensation appears to retard motor development early in life but later is compensated for, even though such patients retain their sensory defects. At a more advanced age when sensory testing can be done, specific difficulties of proprioception, two-point localization, recognition of form by feeling an object, and failure to appreciate a stimulus on the involved side when one is simultaneously applied to the other side can be demonstrated in about a fourth of these cases. Smallness or hypoplasia of the hemiplegic extremities (hemiatrophy) is another common finding especially during adolescent and adult years. The use of a limb appears to be a necessary stimulus to its growth. Hemiatrophy in the adult always means that the neurologic deficit began before growth had proceeded very far, usually in childhood or before.

Mental defect may be associated with infantile hemiplegia but is much more common with cerebral diplegia and with bilateral hemiplegia. Convulsions occur in 35 to 50 per cent of children with congenital hemiplegia. They may commence at any time of life but more often in infancy or early childhood, if the disease was congenital. If the hemiplegia was acquired during infancy, seizures often accompany the onset. They may be generalized but are frequently unilateral and limited to the hemiplegic side. Often, after a series of seizures the affected side will be weak for several hours or longer (Todd's paralysis).

Double Hemiplegia. This term is applied to bilateral weakness of face, arms, and legs. The arms are severely affected, in contrast to their minimal affection in cerebral diplegia. Difficulty with breathing, sucking, and swallowing is usually noted in the neonatal period, if the illness began at or before birth. Weakness and spasticity are apparent at an early age. Opisthotonos with flexed arms and extended legs is the usual attitude and is exaggerated during periods of crying. The cry itself tends to be high-pitched and shrill. Mental development is almost invariably retarded, and such children usually never learn to sit, walk, or develop any effective use of the limbs. The bulbar musculature is also affected. Choreoathetosis, blindness, and seizures occur in many of the patients. The head tends to be small in children with double hemiplegia, reflecting the small size of the brain. In other respects bilateral hemiplegia does not differ from unilateral hemiplegia.

Quadriplegic States. Differing from bilateral hemiplegias in that the bulbar musculature is not involved, this condition is relatively rare but may result from a bilateral cerebral lesion. However, a spastic quadriplegia should always alert one to the possibility of a high cervical cord lesion. Although this may occasionally result from cysts, tumors, and other malformations, it is usually produced in the infant by a fracture-dislocation of the cervical spine, incurred during a difficult breech delivery. Crothers and Putnam state that an audible snap may be heard at the time of fracture. If the condition goes unrecognized, recurrent contusion of the spinal cord may result from handling the infant, there being excessive mobility of the vertebral column. If the upper cervical cord is severely damaged, respirations may be difficult and signs of lower brain stem dysfunction may also appear. Traction and stabilization of the cervical spine by orthopedic measures may prevent further damage and some improvement may occur, but complete recovery is unusual with this condition.

Similarly in *paraplegia* with weakness or paralysis limited to the legs, the lesion may be cerebral or spinal. Sphincter disturbances and a definite loss of somatic sensation below a certain level on the trunk should always favor a spinal localization. Congenital cysts, tumors, and diastematomyelia are more frequently found in cases of paraplegia than of quadriplegia.

The *etiology, pathogenesis,* and *morbid anatomy* of infantile cerebral hemiplegia, bilateral hemiplegia, and quadriplegia are not well understood. Birth injury has been invoked as a leading cause, and there is no doubt that prolonged labor, delay in breathing, bulging fontanel, bloody cerebrospinal fluid, periods of apnea and cyanosis occur with greater frequency in a series of hemiplegic infants than in any other group of infants. Also birth injury is more frequent in hemiplegic than in diplegic cases. The mechanism of the injury is not known. In the majority of patients the birth trauma is not due simply to the direct application of force to the cerebral hemispheres. Hypoxia due to cardiac arrest or interference with fetal circulation at the time when the brain was compressed may be responsible for the lesions. The hemisphere opposite the hemiplegia may be small, a veritable miniature of normal; the cortex is thin, depleted of nerve cells, and gliotic, and the thalamus and corticospinal tract are reduced in size. In others, a circumscribed encephalomalacia with shrinkage of convolutions, gliosis, or cavitation of white matter and basal ganglions have been found. Central *lobar sclerosis* with destruction of the white matter and sparing of the cortex or multiple cavities in the white matter have been observed in a few cases. It must be assumed that many of these abnormalities have been acquired during intrauterine life or at birth, but their cause and pathogenesis are unknown. They appear to represent forms of *porencephaly* or *pseudoporencephaly.* Some may be due to narrowing or occlusion of the carotid artery (sometimes demonstrated in an arteriogram) or Sylvian vein. Congenital neurosyphilis and toxoplasmosis have been established in others. Prematurity may be a contributing factor, and in some a history of vaginal bleeding during pregnancy has been recorded. Developmental abnormalities of the brain have been discovered in a few cases.

Congenital Extrapyramidal Syndromes in Infancy and Childhood. The spastic and rigid cerebral diplegias discussed above shade almost imperceptibly into the extrapyramidal syndromes. Many such cases can be found in every cerebral palsy clinic, and they appear from time to time in adult medical clinics. Pyramidal tract signs may be completely absent, and the inexperienced student, familiar only with the pure cerebral spastic diplegia syndrome, is always puzzled as to their classification. Some extrapyramidal cases of this type undoubtedly are attributable to the same pathologic processes as cerebral spastic diplegia and attest to the diverse clinical manifestations of these states; others represent separate diseases such as erythroblastosis fetalis with kernicterus. In the interest of being able to state accurately the probable pathologic basis and future course of these illnesses, it is desirable to separate the extrapyramidal syndromes due to prenatal and natal diseases, which usually become manifest during the first year of life, from the acquired postnatal syndromes such as familial athetosis, dystonia musculorum deformans, and cerebellar ataxia. The latter will be discussed in Chap. 290, Degenerative Diseases of the Nervous System.

Congenital Choreoathetosis (Double Athetosis). Probably the most frequent representative of this group, this condition is like the spastic states in that it may not be recognized at birth but only after several months have elapsed. The nature of chorea and athetosis has been discussed in Chap. 27, Disturbances of the Motor System. All combinations of chorea, athetosis, hemiballismus, and even dystonia may be found in a single case, or one or another type of movement disorder may predominate. However, in all instances there is a defect in voluntary movement.

Choreoathetosis in infants and children varies in severity. In some the disorder is so mild that the abnormal movements are misinterpreted as restlessness or the "fidgets"; in others every voluntary act is rendered ineffective by these involuntary movements, leaving the patient nearly helpless. The tongue may extrude itself from the mouth with constant drooling, and the face is contorted in a never-ending series of grimaces. Speech is slurred, inarticulate, and punctuated by grunts and hideous throat sounds. The hands and arms are engaged in a constant play of writhing, twisting movements, and all attempts to use the limbs result in a slow, spreading spasm of the entire limb or all the musculature (intention spasm). Bizarre postures may be assumed. The arms may be carried in a flexed or extended position in front of or behind the body, and the legs may be extended. The feet may be deformed; walking on the heels or side of the foot is more common than the "toe walking" of the cerebral diplegic. Movements may also be ataxic, and tremors are not uncommon. A retardation of motor development is the rule in these cases. Upright posture and walking may, in fact, never be acquired or may be delayed until the age of three to five years in severe cases, but thereafter more or less effective locomotion is possible. Tonic neck reflexes or fragments thereof are commonly noted. The tendon reflexes are not consistently abnormal; plantar reflexes are characteristically flexor, though they may be difficult to interpret because of the continuous play of flexion and extension of the toes. The various sensory pathways usually function normally.

It is because of the motor and speech impairment that patients are many times erroneously classified as mentally defective. No doubt in some patients this evaluation is correct, but others retain adequate intellectual function and can be educated. With growth and development new postures and new motor capacities are acquired. The less severely affected patients can make successful occupational adjustments. However, the severely handicapped patients, even with the help of rehabilitation clinics and corrective orthopedic operations, rarely achieve a degree of motor control that will permit them to lead an independent existence. One sees these unfortunate individuals in public places bobbing and weaving as they walk along.

The most frequently observed pathologic change in the brain has been a curious whitish marblelike appearance of the putamen, thalamus, and cerebral cortex. These whitish strands represent foci of nerve cell destruction and gliosis with a peculiar condensation or formation of myelinated fibers (hypermyelination). Oscar and Cecile Vogt, who first described this condition, called it *état marbré* or *status marmoratus*. They attributed it to neonatal asphyxia, but the hypoxic factor is far from established.

The *neurologic sequelae* of *kernicterus* are of importance here and are encountered not infrequently in adults. It is true that the majority of infants who suffer this disease die within the first week or two of life, and those who survive are mentally retarded, deaf, and totally unable to sit, stand, or walk, so that the tendency is always to put them in homes for the feebleminded. It is only the exceptional patient, obviously less damaged, who is mentally normal or at most only slightly backward. These are the ones who exhibit a variety of motor disorders as they grow older, the most frequent being mild ataxia or choreoathetosis, which involves the face and arms. A few have also shown rigid limbs and a picture not too different from that of cerebral spastic diplegia with involuntary movements. Kernicterus should always be suspected if an extrapyramidal syndrome is accompanied by bilateral deafness and ocular palsies. The neuropathology in these milder surviving cases consists of nerve cell loss and gliosis in the subthalamic nucleus of Luys, the globus pallidus, thalamus, Ammon's horn, and oculomotor and cochlear nuclei. No one explanation of the neurologic lesion has been accepted. Elsewhere we have postulated severe liver damage and hyperbilirubinemia as a cause of the brain disease, but this hypothesis is unproved. Others attribute the brain damage to hypoxia.

Congenital Ataxia. The combination of cerebral diplegia with cerebellar ataxia has already been mentioned. These are cases in whom difficulty in standing and walking cannot be attributed to spas-

ticity or paralysis. Incoordination similar to that seen in cerebellar disease and hypotonia are the principal findings. The motor defect may be so great that the child is never able to sit or stand; the muscles are of normal size, and voluntary movements, though weak, are possible in all the limbs. In less severe cases sitting, standing, and walking are merely delayed, and, with advancing years, cerebellar ataxia and tremor become manifest. Relative improvement may occur as the child grows older. The tendon reflexes are present, and the plantar reflexes are either flexor or extensor. Many of these patients suffer a degree of amentia and retardation of speech development that results in their placement in homes for the feebleminded. In relatively few of the recorded cases have the pathologic changes of this condition been studied. Aplasia or hypoplasia of the cerebellum has been reported only a few times. Radiation of the abdomen of a parturient woman during the first trimester of pregnancy is said to have resulted in cerebellar hypoplasia in a few cases. A cerebral and cerebellar lesion may coexist, which is the reason for their classification as cerebrocerebellar diplegias.

Aside from the congenital ataxias, some of which are cerebellar, others probably of cerebral type, there are other forms of ataxia which have an acute onset and which persist during adolescence and adult life. Batten has written informatively on this subject, calling those forms the acute cerebellar ataxias of childhood. Some are sequelae of an infection (a postinfectious encephalitis especially postvaricella), and a few may be due to virus infections which affect the cerebellum more than other parts of the nervous system. Hyperthermia, with temperatures over 106°F, may result in extensive destruction of Purkinje cells and ataxia. Cerebellar tumors and demyelinative and lipid storage diseases also occur at this age and may at times give rise to cerebellar ataxia. Labyrinthine injury resulting from streptomycin therapy and polyneuritis or mumps are the common causes of noncerebellar ataxia, which must be differentiated from the above condition.

The hereditary ataxias are likely to begin at a later age and are progressive. They are discussed in Chap. 290.

In all these congenital diseases of the brain, once the symptoms and signs are well established, there is no progression of the illness. In fact, with further maturation and training there may be improvement. The clinical course thus distinguishes this whole group of diseases from those of delayed onset and progressive course (see Schilder's disease, lipid storage diseases, congenital neurosyphilis, and toxoplasmosis which are described in Chaps. 290 and 163).

The Flaccid Paralyses of Infancy and Childhood. The cerebral form, first described by Foerster and called *cerebral atonic diplegia*, has already been mentioned in connection with congenital cerebellar ataxia. It can usually be distinguished from spinal and peripheral nerve paralysis by the retention of postural reflexes (flexion of the legs at the knee and hip when the patient is lifted by placing the hands in the axillas), the preservation of tendon reflexes, and the failure of mental development.

The syndrome of *infantile muscular atrophy* (Werdnig-Hoffmann disease) is the leading example of the category of infantile spinal muscular atrophies. These little patients are usually brought to the clinic by their parents because of a difficulty with feeding and a delay of motor development. About half of them are said to have been normal at birth and during the first weeks of life. Others have been slack, feeble infants from the day they were born and even before, since some mothers recall a weakness also of fetal movement. Slowness in feeding, frequent choking, constant drooling, recurrent respiratory infections due to weak respiratory movements, and aspiration of milk are troublesome in early life. As a rule the patient prefers a supine posture; his motor deficit is manifested by an inability to maintain the head in stable balance and also by the absence of the usual twisting, squirming movements of the trunk. The arms tend to be kept at the sides and flexed at the elbows, bringing the hands over the chest. The legs are characteristically abducted and flexed at the hips and knees so that the soles of the feet oppose one another ("frog posture"). When the infant is pulled to a sitting position, the head lolls and all but the most feeble support reactions in the legs are absent. Despite this profound weakness, all muscle groups are capable of feeble movement until late in the course of the illness. The tendon reflexes are invariably absent in those cases in which the disease begins before birth or during the early months of life. Tendon reflexes may rarely be preserved if the disease has an onset at a later age. A remarkable action tremor of the arms may then be observed. Atrophy of muscle is obscured by subcutaneous fat tissues ("puppy fat"), and fascicular twitches, though detectable in an electromyogram, are invisible to the naked eye except in the tongue. In contrast to their feeble movements these patients usually are attractive, with bright, sparkling eyes and lively countenance, which attest to normal brain development. All sensory functions are likewise retained. The illness progresses slowly over a period of months or a few years, and few of these patients survive until puberty. Several members of a sibship may suffer the same illness, but never the antecedents, the pattern of inheritance usually being autosomal recessive. In biopsy ma-

terial or at autopsy the muscles are thin and the majority of their fibers are atrophic, preserving their fetal dimensions as though improperly innervated or denervated. The anterior horn cells in the spinal cord and brain stem have disappeared or are in process of degenerating and are replaced by fibrous astrocytes. There is no known treatment for the disease.

A few patients suspected of having infantile muscular atrophy prove with the passage of time to be merely rather inactive, "slack" children, and their motor development later proceeds at the usual rate. A few may remain rather weak with thin musculature. Such cases fall into the vague category of *amyotonia congenita* described by Oppenheim, Brandt, and others, or into the group called *benign congenital hypotonia* (Walton) or *benign congenital myopathy* (Turner). Probably several types of myopathy are being included in this category. Muscle biopsy usually reveals no definite abnormality, and the electromyogram is often normal. Polymyositis and acute idiopathic polyneuritis may rarely manifest themselves as a syndrome of amyotonia congenita.

Infantile muscular dystrophy and lipoid and glycogen storage diseases may also produce a clinical picture of progressive atrophy and enfeeblement of muscles. The diagnosis of *glycogen storage disease* (von Gierke's disease) should be entertained when the syndrome of infantile muscular atrophy is associated with clinical enlargement of heart, liver, or spleen. The motor disturbance in this condition may be related in some way to the abnormal deposits of glycogen found in skeletal muscle, though it is more likely due to the degeneration of the anterior horn cells of the spinal cord, which are distended with glycogen and other substances. Lipoid storage disease of *Tay-Sachs* and the variants which occur later in life may also cause thinness of limb musculature, feebleness of movement, and diminution or loss of tendon reflexes. Regression of mental development, blindness, macular degeneration, which are almost always present to some degree, should leave little doubt as to the nature of the illness. Also muscular dystrophy, either familial or nonfamilial, may begin during fetal life or during infancy and childhood. There is obvious palsy of the limbs, with proximal and trunk muscles more involved than distal ones. Contractures are frequent, with a leg or arm held in a curious abducted or extended posture. This state of contracture of the limbs in infants is called *arthrogryposis*, already referred to above. It may be caused by either a primary muscular disease or a defect of the central nervous system.

Brachial plexus palsies, well-known complications of dystocia, usually result from forcible extraction of the fetus by downward traction on the shoulder in a breech presentation, or from traction and tipping of the head in a shoulder presentation. The upper brachial plexus and roots of the fifth cervical or the lower plexus and roots of the seventh and eighth cervical and first thoracic nerves suffer the brunt of the injury. Sometimes the entire plexus is involved. The upper plexus injuries (*Erb's plexus syndrome*) are estimated to be twenty times more frequent than lower (*Klumpke plexus syndrome*), according to Ford, who has examined more than 200 cases of this type. There should be no difficulty in distinguishing these plexus injuries from the preceding motor disorders. The paralysis is restricted and complete. The condition is nearly always unilateral, though a few cases with bilateral involvement have been reported. The infant with Erb's palsy lies in a characteristic position: the affected arm is adducted and internally rotated at the shoulder and extended at the elbow. The deltoid, spinati, biceps, brachioradialis, and upper pectoral muscles are paralyzed. The diaphragm on the side of the palsy, instead of descending with each inspiration, moves paradoxically, and the efficiency of pulmonary ventilation may be greatly reduced. During spontaneous movements and in the Moro reflex the affected limb is motionless. The grasp reflex is preserved in upper plexus injuries. The biceps and supinator reflexes are absent, and the triceps is present, but one cannot count on these reflexes for they may normally be difficult to elicit. In the Klumpke plexus injury the muscles of the hand and forearm are paralyzed, whereas the function of the shoulder abductor and external rotators and elbow flexors is preserved. The limb reposes in a flexed position across the trunk, and the grasp reflex is absent. There is often an associated Horner's syndrome. The remainder of the musculature is active. The pathologic change associated with these plexus injuries has not been carefully studied. From the few reports it appears that the traumatic lesion involves motor roots at their junction with the brachial plexus. In some cases the roots are torn from the spinal cord, and the latter may be damaged. The treatment of Erb's palsy is immobilization of the affected arm in an abducted and flexed position. Prognosis is good in the majority of cases, but in severe injuries paralysis may be permanent, in which instance the hand or arm fails to develop.

Facial paralysis, due to injury of the facial nerve immediately distal to its exit from the stylomastoid foramen by the application of forceps, is another common peripheral nerve affection in the newborn. The failure of one eye to close and the difficulty in suckling make this condition easy to recognize. It must be distinguished from congenital facial paralysis or facial diplegia with or without weakness of the abducens muscles (*Moebius' syndrome*), in which the facial nerve cells fail to develop. In most cases of facial paralysis function is recovered after a few weeks; in some the paralysis is permanent and may account for an asymmetry observed in later life.

The Retarded Child (*Feeblemindedness*)

Mental retardation has been commented upon in the discussion of many of the craniospinal malformations and in the several varieties of cerebral palsy. However, it may also occur as the only neurologic abnormality and must therefore be discussed separately.

To the pediatrician the clinical problem of mental retardation is one of the most difficult and to the parents it is one of the most dreadful of all conditions. The intelligent father and mother are alert to every sign of possible brain injury, and often they become alarmed about trivial deviations from their standard of normal development. Slowness in sitting, standing, walking, delay in speech, any difficulty in acquiring toilet training may be seized upon as an indication of feeblemindedness. The internist and general physician are apt to see only the milder noninstitutionalized patients who reach adolescence and adult years and then develop other diseases.

The primary responsibility of the physician in cases of this type is to determine whether there is unmistakable evidence of maldevelopment or disease of the brain. The uncertainty in evaluating cerebral function during early infancy has already been discussed. From experience one learns that successive examinations, over a period of months or years, may be required in order to evaluate the infant's or child's capacity for mental development. Above all, the physician should not permit himself to be forced into a hasty or premature judgment. Deafness, blindness, congenital speech defects (word deafness and word blindness), and motor defects must be searched for with particular care, for they may account for an apparent delay in mental development by interfering with the learning processes. Emotional privation and neglect may also lead to some degree of backwardness. However, mental retardation of significant degree cannot be explained in this way.

The student confronted with a backward infant is likely to be rather bewildered by the vast array of developmental abnormalities and diseases which may affect the brain at an early age and prevent normal mental development. It becomes necessary to acquire a way of thinking about these problems. The authors' bedside approach has been to attempt to categorize each case according to the scheme presented in Table 283-2. This can be done by obtaining the necessary clinical data—a careful history, in order to determine whether or not the condition is progressive, and a physical examination in which one searches for evidences of cranial, skeletal, ectodermal, cardiac, and other developmental abnormalities. Once a patient is categorized, it is less difficult to decide which of several diseases is present.

Table 283-2. CLINICAL CLASSIFICATION OF THE VARIETIES OF NONPROGRESSIVE MENTAL RETARDATION

I. Mental defect with associated developmental abnormalities in nonnervous structures
   A. Those affecting cranioskeletal structures

1. Microcephaly	8. Cretinism
2. Macroencephaly	9. Cleidocranial
3. Hydrocephalus	dysostosis
4. Craniostenosis	10. Achondroplasia
5. Morquio's disease	11. Gonadal dysgenesis
6. Gargoylism	(Bonnevie-Ullrich-
7. Mongolian idiocy	Turner syndrome)

   B. Those affecting nonskeletal structures
      1. Phacomatoses (tuberous sclerosis, von Recklinghausen's disease, Sturge-Weber syndrome, etc.)
      2. Ectodermal dysplasia
      3. Congenital heart disease
      4. Deafness and congenital heart disease following maternal rubella
II. Mental defect without developmental anomalies in nonnervous structures, but with focal cerebral and other neurologic abnormalities[1]
   A. Cerebral spastic diplegia with or without involuntary movements (rarely associated ichtyosis)
   B. Cerebral hemiplegia, unilateral or bilateral
   C. Congenital choreoathetosis or ataxis
      1. Kernicterus
      2. Status marmoratus (hypoxia?)
   D. Congenital atonic diplegia
   E. Rarely with other inherited neuromuscular abnormalities (muscular dystrophy, Friedreich's ataxia, etc.)
III. Mental defect without signs of other developmental abnormality or neurologic disorder
   A. Simple mental retardation
   B. Kernicterus
   C. Hypoxia
   D. Heller's disease, variably progressive, may affect nonnervous structures
   E. Mental defect associated with inborn errors of metabolism (e.g., galactosemia, phenylketonuria, hypothyroidism, maple syrup urine disease, etc.)
   F. Congenital infections (e.g., cytomegalic inclusion disease, syphilis, toxoplasmosis, etc.)

[1] A number of progressive neurologic diseases—chronic subdural hematoma, lipidoses, and cerebral scleroses—may be confused with these static defects.

Clinical Characteristics. As an aid to the general physician who must undertake the diagnosis and management of backward children, the following comments may be of some value. Mental retardation manifests itself in the spheres of motor, language, social, and intellectual development. The severely retarded child at idiot level with an intelligence quotient (IQ) of less than 20 and unable to look after himself often does not sit up, walk, or stand, and if any of these motor activities is acquired, it appears late and is imperfectly performed. Language is not mastered, or at most only a few words are understood and uttered. Physical growth is usually retarded; nutrition may be poor, and susceptibility to respiratory infections is common. Sphincteric control is never accomplished. Most of these severe aments never learn to dress, bathe, or feed themselves or to use implements and common tools. Physical deformities are common in this group, and they always suggest that the brain disease began in the antenatal period, because of either a genetic disorder or a disease which occurred during the first 12 weeks of pregnancy. Affections of the nervous system which have their onset later in life are usually not attended by bodily disfigurement.

If the mental defect is less pronounced, with the IQ 20 to 50 (i.e., imbecile), or 50 to 70 (i.e., moron), and if specific motor defects do not coexist, then sitting, walking, and speech are acquired but only after a delay, in many cases. The existence of a cerebral defect may be noted for the first time when the child fails to speak normally during the second and third years of life and seems not to be able to learn the usual household tasks as well as other children. However, delay in language development must not by itself be taken as a mark of mental retardation, for many bright children who are obviously intelligent and who show remarkable talent in communicating by gesture are slow in talking. Toilet training also may be difficult to accomplish in the retarded child, but again it may be delayed in an otherwise normal child because of incorrect parental attitudes and emotional problems. The appearance of these retarded children is revealing, for many have a dull, apathetic appearance and their motor activity may be either reduced or excessive. Some are very docile and affectionate; others display a curious inquisitiveness, irritability, and destructiveness. The most extreme degree of this overactivity is seen in the patient with "organic driveness," a term introduced by Eugene Kahn to designate the incessantly moving, incorrigible child who strikes at or bites every person or object which thwarts him in any way and who demolishes every object which he can reach. Some of these children seem strangely impervious to injury, and neither reward nor punishment influences them. This organic driveness is perhaps more commonly observed in acquired postnatal encephalitis than with congenital diseases.

Rhythmic rocking, rolling, head banging, and bouncing movements are common in retarded children and may be performed hour after hour, often to the accompaniment of bleating sounds, squeals, and other ejaculations. Here the abnormality is not the appearance of rhythmic movements of the body, which are observed at one period in the development of many normal children, but their persistence. Music may encourage rhythmic movement and gives pleasure to many retarded children.

The least severely retarded child (IQ 50 to 70) grows and develops in many ways not different from normal, and he can be taught useful occupational skills. A few can work under careful supervision.

Special Varieties of Mental Retardation. Several of the special types of mental retardation are being discussed in this and other chapters (see lipidoses and cerebral sclerosis, in Chap. 290). In the following pages are presented only those with special features.

Mongolism. This is a unique condition, and although accounting for only about 1 per cent of all mental defectives, it is the reason for one-third to one-half the admissions to state schools. Mental retardation which varies from mild to severe, a curious facial configuration with an Oriental cast to the eyes, and a dwarfed physical stature constitute a clinical triad. Many of the stigmas of mongolism can be recognized in the neonatal period. The head tends to be small and oval, with the forehead sloping. The ears are set low on the scalp and are oval with small lobules. The eyes slant slightly upward and outward owing to the presence of an epicanthal fold, which covers the medial angle of the palpebral fissure. The bridge of the nose is generally absent or poorly developed, and the crest of the nose small. The mouth tends to hang open, and the tongue is usually enlarged, heavily fissured, and protruding. Gray-white specks of depigmentation are seen in the iris (Brushfield's spots). The little fingers are often short and curved, owing to a hypoplastic middle phalanx. The hands are broad and simianlike, with a single transverse palmar crease. Lenticular opacities and congenital heart lesions are found in some cases. At birth the mongoloid child is of average size, but at later periods of life he is characteristically small. Benda estimates that the average adult person with mongolism, of whom there are many, never exceeds the stature of a ten-year-old boy. The resemblance to the Oriental is at most superficial; in fact the differences are so striking that it is quite easy to recognize the condition in those of Oriental heritage.

The cause of mongolism is not known. It has been suggested that the defects arise as a result of some metabolic abnormality which occurs late in the second or early third month of pregnancy. Older mothers are more apt to have mongoloid babies than are young mothers. The mean age of the mother at the time of birth of the mongoloid child is thirty-seven. It is thought by some workers that a genetic factor is responsible, but familial incidence is rare. Aside from a rather rounded brain, which conforms to the shape of the skull, a subnormal weight, and a relatively simple convolutional pattern, with particular smallness of the superior temporal convolutions, no abnormalities can be seen in the brain of the mongolian idiot. Of great interest has been the demonstration of abnormal chromosomal patterns in these children (Lejeune). Trisomy of chromosome pair 21 has been found repeatedly by many workers; the rare concurrence of mongolism with Klinefelter's syndrome is explained by this and an additional X chromosome. Translocations of chromosomal parts has been reported in a few mongols of younger mothers.

Cretinism. This is due to congenital deficiency of thyroid secretion and is distinguished from myxedema, a form of hypothyroidism acquired later in life (see Chap. 66).

Gargoylism (Hunter-Hurler Disease). This condition is discussed in Chap. 290. Mental development may be normal or retarded to a variable degree and hydrocephalus may occur. Postmortem examination has shown the nerve cells to be swollen with inclusion material, which chemical analysis shows to be a ganglioside like that found in the nerve cells of Tay-Sachs, infantile Gaucher's, and Niemann-Pick diseases. There are also fat-laden macrophages in the perivascular spaces, and in the meninges both macrophages and an increase in fibrous tissue. Glycogen and a peculiar lipoprotein material are also found in liver cells and the Kupffer cells and macrophages in a fashion reminiscent of von Gierke's disease.

Osteochondrodystrophy (Morquio's Disease). Sometimes confused with gargoylism, this is a nonprogressive osseous disorder with a cranial appearance similar to that of gargoylism. Some patients have a normal mind, others have a stationary mental defect, but in the latter none of the typical brain lesions of gargoylism have been found and the nature of the anatomic defect remains unknown. No visceral lesions have been observed. The primary defect is believed to be one of the chondroblasts.

Phenylketonuria (Phenylpyruvic Oligophrenia). This condition is discussed in Chap. 98.

Galactosemia. Another congenital metabolic disease, galactosemia is thought to be transmitted by a single, autosomal recessive gene. It is characterized clinically by mental defect, cataract, nausea, vomiting, hepatomegaly, jaundice, and the excretion of large quantities of galactose in the urine. The biochemical defect is discussed in Chap. 94.

Anhidrotic Ectodermal Dysplasia. This is a congenital disorder in which there are anhidrosis, defects in salivation, lacrimation, sparse hair, and faulty dentition. Heat intolerance with paroxysmal fever, unrelated to infection, may occur. Several of the reported cases have been feebleminded. A sex-linked inheritance pattern has been reported. The neuropathologic basis for this disease is unknown. There is no treatment.

Heller's Disease (Dementia Infantilis). This condition is of uncertain status. Neurologists and some psychiatrists look upon it as a cerebral disease of undetermined cause. Other psychiatrists believe it to be a form of precocious schizophrenia. As a rule the onset is in about the third or fourth year of life. At this age, usually without previous illness, a change in character is noted. Irritability, negativism, disobedience, and outbursts of unprovoked temper become manifest. Restlessness and destructiveness are other prominent symptoms. Toys with which the child had played normally are now senselessly destroyed. Within a few months there is complete loss of speech, and also failure in the understanding of words. Grimacing and ticlike movements appear, but motor and sensory functions are preserved. Continence of sphincters is lost. The mental regression continues to a stage of idiocy, but all through the illness the patient continues to give an impression of greater intelligence than do most feebleminded individuals. Many patients of this type reach adult life but remain in institutions. The pathology of the disease is unknown. A few of the reports state the brain to be abnormal and suggest that there may be degeneration of ganglion cells like that of Tay-Sachs disease, but the illustrations are unconvincing. There is no treatment. The relationship of this disease to cases of so-called "childhood schizophrenia" and infantile autism is not always clear. It is said that the patient with childhood schizophrenia, although withdrawn and mute, maintains an inquisitive interest in his surroundings and is clever in handling tools and in manipulating objects. A clinical distinction between these entities has not proved possible in the authors' experience.

Simple Mental Retardation. Although presented last, this category includes the great bulk of children with mental defect of indeterminate etiology who exhibit neither craniovertebral or neurologic abnormality. The degree of mental impairment tends to be mild (moron, feebleminded, educable) or moderate (imbecile, trainable). Penrose found that this group of aments comprised 24 per cent of 1,280 institutionalized children, and of course those who are in institutions represent only the more severely damaged individuals in our society. The physical appearance of these children is usually not strikingly abnormal; yet many of the aforementioned characteristics of the mentally retarded child are to be observed. Seizures occur in a significant number, being several times more frequent than in a normal population. Within the limits of their intelligence, the success of these children in learning to look after themselves is often determined by the effectiveness of their teachers and the suitability of the environment in which they are placed. The brighter ones can profit to some extent from formal education. Those less well endowed may be trained to care for their personal wants and needs and may profit from a limited amount of manual training. Special schools and classes are of great help.

Society, in the final analysis, determines the eventual disposition of these unfortunates. Many of them, being not unattractive and giving less trouble than many other defective children, may adjust to foster families and live in a community. They need protection, for they are easily led astray and may commit infractions of the law, usually of a minor sort. Sexual offenses are common in the girls. Institutionalization is required when family and society cannot or do not wish to look after them. Reproductivity is frequently impaired in those with severe mental defect but may be distressingly undisturbed in many of the less defective individuals.

The problem of eugenics assumes great importance. This type of mental defect is often seen in families where one or both parents are dull or retarded. The term *familial* may be applied to this group. However, the majority of cases are sporadic. Probably there are multiple etiologic factors which may lead to simple mental retardation. The pathologic change is variable, ranging from "no demonstrable lesion" to several different gross and microscopic abnormalities.

Management of the Retarded Child and His Parents. It is an unpleasant task to inform parents that their child is abnormal in any respect, and many, if not most, parents find it difficult to accept a mental defect without much self-recrimination and feelings of guilt. To give an honest statement of the degree of the child's retardation and, based on the nature of the problem, some professional estimate of the likelihood of future growth and development, once one is sure of the status and potentialities of the child, require tact and sympathetic understanding. The family must eventually be told to what extent the child is likely to be trainable or educable. Obviously this can often be no more than an educated guess, and if there is still reasonable doubt about the future, this fact should be so stated. In general it should be possible to give at least a rough approximation of the child's capabilities and likely attainments. Frequently the parents themselves are well aware of the child's limitations, and then a useful technique is to ask the parents to estimate the nature of the problem. The physician is in this way informed of the degree of their insight and their general attitudes. He may then agree with them or may amplify and clarify any misconceptions.

The parents will want to know the probable cause of the defect and the likelihood of subsequent children being affected. In most instances the answer to the second question will depend on the etiology. If the abnormality is determined by known genetic factors, as in congenital microcephaly, phenylpyruvic oligophrenia, or tuberous sclerosis, there is of course a strong likelihood of other children being abnormal. If on the other hand the abnormality is due to specific environmental influences peculiar to the pregnancy, as in the case of maternal rubella or excessive radiation to the pelvis, the prospects of having other normal children are good. Unfortunately in the great majority of cases the etiology will not be certain, and advice must be tendered cautiously. It is quite clear from the studies of Penrose, Halperin, and others that the chance of parents of normal intelligence with one defective child having other subnormal children is greater than that of the general population. If one or both parents is of less than normal intelligence, or if there is consanguinity in the parents, then the risk is considerably greater. A recessive trait in a first child, which is inherited in only one of four children and cannot be passed on in overt form to succeeding generations, need not discourage a family from "taking a chance" on having other normal children.

Special Paroxysmal Disorders of Nervous Function in Infancy and Childhood

The convulsive disorders have been discussed in Chap. 36, Recurrent Convulsions, and all that was said there applies to infants and children as well as adults. There are, however, many special problems raised by the child who is having spells or seizures, and these must be known and properly interpreted by the physician, who upon seeing the patient at a more advanced age obtains the history of these spells.

The incidence of convulsions is known to be high in infancy and early childhood, and seizures at that age may have an altogether different significance than in the adult. All the seizure patterns that may be witnessed in the adult may also occur in infancy and childhood—i.e., focal motor and Jacksonian as well as petit mal and psychomotor seizures—but certain ones appear at this age which are not often observed in the adult. These are the petit mal and its variants and massive myoclonus. Then, too,

there are other types of spells, unique to infancy and childhood, which must be distinguished from convulsions, i.e., breath-holding spells and the congestive attacks that accompany congenital heart disease.

Seizures have different meanings at different periods of infancy and childhood. A series of seizures that occurred during the neonatal period must always be regarded as an omen of cerebral damage. It may have been due to subdural and subarachnoid hemorrhage, in which unresponsiveness, pallor, periods of apnea, bulging fontanel, and grossly bloody cerebrospinal fluid clarify the diagnostic problem. It may reflect a congenital brain disease, sometimes of such major proportions as to have prevented further development, or it may have been so slight as not to disturb the normal maturation processes. Actually very little is known of the import of seizures at this period with reference to prognosis for mental development. Infantile tetany during the first 2 to 3 weeks of life may have been the cause of seizures as well as of a remarkable stiffness of limbs and carpal spasms. (The Chvostek sign is misleading at this age, being present in many normal babies.) Only the blood calcium and phosphorus levels and the response to intravenous calcium would have confirmed the diagnosis. A single outburst of seizures in a previously healthy infant may have been merely an expression of the low convulsive threshold of the infantile nervous system, as in febrile convulsions, or may signify a mortal process such as acute toxic encephalopathy, thrombosis of the superior sagittal sinus or cerebral veins, meningitis, hypoglycemia, brain hemorrhage from an angioma, or massive arterial infarction. Idiopathic epilepsy also begins during infancy and childhood and may interfere relatively little with normal development. Brain tumors are an infrequent cause of seizures during infancy and childhood.

Febrile Fits

Certain infants and children are disposed to convulsions with fever. Lennox estimates that approximately 2 per cent of all children have one or more convulsions with fever at one time or another during infancy or childhood. In some 20 per cent of these cases it can be decided in retrospect that fever has served merely to precipitate a seizure in an individual who has suffered a cerebral disease or who has idiopathic epilepsy. Such individuals will continue to have seizures, unassociated with fever. In the other 80 per cent of cases, seizures occur only during febrile episodes and never recur beyond early childhood. The reason for this low seizure threshold in the infantile brain is unknown, but a family history of similar febrile fits in other members of the family can be obtained in about 50 per cent of cases.

From the history it can usually be learned that febrile convulsions have occurred between the ages of one and three years; only a few cases are seen earlier or later—up until the age of seven or eight years. Any febrile illness may have been provocative, but usually a rapid ascent of temperature to 103°F or higher was responsible. The seizures themselves are generalized and of short duration and may have occurred singly or in a cluster of two or three. The postictal coma is of short duration. No record of focal or lateralizing neurologic signs can be obtained. The cerebrospinal fluid is clear and acellular and the total protein normal. The electroencephalogram is diffusely abnormal, with theta and delta waves predominating in all leads immediately after the seizure, with rapid return to normal at the termination of the illness. After the illness there should be no residual signs of brain disease.

It must be remembered that there are certain sources of error in the diagnosis of febrile convulsions. The fever may have been caused by convulsions, as so often happens in idiopathic epilepsy, especially with status epilepticus. Some primary inflammatory disease of the brain or meninges may have been responsible for both fever and convulsions. Meningitis, for example, may have begun in this way but would probably have ended fatally if not diagnosed and treated.

Massive Myoclonus

This syndrome, known also by the names *infantile muscular spasm, Blitzkrampf, myoclonic seizure,* "Salaam fit," "flexor spasm," and "jackknife seizure," has been recognized recently and should be known to general physicians and internists for they may see the patient long after the seizures have stopped. In essence it is a sudden synchronous contraction of many muscle groups. Contraction of flexor muscles usually predominates, and there is a sudden flexion of trunk, neck, and extremities, often accompanied by a cry or occasionally by a laugh. In some patients there is a combination of flexor and extensor movements, and least often the contraction of extensor muscles predominates, with a straightening of the body and a fall backward. The spasm itself is usually momentary but often recurs one or several times, with each spasm separated from the next by an interval of a few seconds. There may be only a few spasms in a cluster or upward of a hundred or more in a series. They are especially frequent as the patient is falling off to sleep or upon awakening. The patient may fall, if he is standing at the time of the spasm. Sensory precipitation by handling, feeding, noise, and fever have been noted.

Massive myoclonic spasms usually begin during the first few months of life and tend to disappear or to be replaced by other seizure patterns between the second and third years of age. The pathophysiology is not well understood, and the neuropathology of the condition has not been studied systematically.

However, massive myoclonus has been observed in a number of clinical states including mongolism, congenital malformation, and disorders of amino acid metabolism such as phenylketonuria and maple syrup urine disease. The frequent association of mental retardation (over half the cases) and the consistent diffusely abnormal electroencephalogram with bursts of high-voltage slow waves, referred to as *hypsarrhythmia* by Gibbs, suggest a diffuse neuronal pathology. It is of interest that the seizures may become less frequent as the dementia progresses.

In early life parents may mistake the flexor spasm for colic. This is especially true when feeding is a precipitating stimulus. Colic, however, is never associated with even a transient loss of consciousness. Associated seizure phenomena, such as rolling up of the eyes and pupillary dilatation, may be helpful points. In the young infant this condition may also be confused with the Moro reflex, but such an error is avoided if one gives attention to the precipitating sensory stimulus, which is different in the two conditions, and to the movements, which usually occur in series. Nevertheless, the similarity of the movement pattern suggests that massive myoclonus and the Moro response probably both utilize the same physiologic mechanisms.

The treatment of the seizures is difficult. Some respond dramatically to the first drug tried but soon become resistant to it. Several authors have reported recently that treatment with adrenocorticotropic hormone is beneficial, especially if it is begun in the first 2 to 3 weeks of the illness.

"Breath-holding Spells"

This is a special type of attack peculiar to young children. Anger or a mild injury is the precipitating factor. The patient begins to cry or scream. After a few moments he suddenly stops breathing and remains apneic for many seconds to as long as a minute. During this period there is a color change from an initial redness to cyanosis, presumably as the result of hypoxia. If this persists for a short period, the patient suddenly becomes limp and is unresponsive for some seconds. Convulsive twitching may occur, but rarely is there a sustained convulsion. The whole attack is over in one to a few minutes. The child may then be drowsy and sleep for a short while thereafter or may be at once as alert as before. Such attacks usually begin late in the first year of life and rarely after the third year. They are outgrown, so to speak. The mechanism is unclear; in breath holding the infant may perform the Valsalva maneuver and then faint, as in tussive syncope. The treatment consists of reassurance and a careful explanation of the spells to the family. It should be pointed out that in certain instances a child may seem to "use" the attacks to obtain what he wishes and that by ignoring them they may be eliminated or reduced in number.

Apnea may be observed as a fragment of a generalized seizure and must be differentiated from breath holding. The sequence of events is so characteristic in breath holding that the diagnosis is usually not difficult.

Congestive Attacks with Congenital Cardiac and Pulmonary Disease

This condition has been described only recently and is of importance in the histories of cases of congenital heart disease. Cyanotic infants and children with gravely limited cardiopulmonary function may, upon some unusual exertion or excitement or while crying, momentarily lose consciousness and twitch a few times. Presumably the spell depends on hypoxia or inadequacy of cerebral blood flow. It must be distinguished from seizures which occur with a higher than normal frequency in patients with congenital heart disease.

Hypoglycemia

As stated in Chap. 34, Coma and Related Disturbances of Consciousness, hypoglycemia may cause seizures and unresponsiveness, but as a rule the seizure does not interrupt a normal state of consciousness. An unexpected convulsion is almost never due to hypoglycemia alone. When this state is encountered in infants, it is sometimes traceable to a hepatic form of glycogen storage disease in which there is an inherited defect of an enzyme system necessary in the synthesis or breakdown of glycogen. These children tend to be obese. Hepatomegaly and splenomegaly are important clinical features. The failure of epinephrine to produce a significant rise in the blood sugar levels is diagnostic of glycogen storage disease. Treatment consists of a regular diet supplemented by carbohydrate about 45 min after each meal to offset the fall in blood sugar.

Older children are prone to attacks of idiopathic hypoglycemia. They tend to be thin rather than obese, and the attacks occur on a background of relatively poor intake of food or actual fasting for 12 to 36 hr. Occasionally the child has engaged in unusually strenuous and prolonged exercise prior to an attack. The mechanism is not clearly understood, but depletion of glycogen stores and lack of available sugar due to fasting have been suggested. The symptomatology is fairly characteristic. The child is noted to be apathetic or mentally dull and pale. Vomiting occurs early, and there may be a complaint of hunger despite the vomiting. If no food is ingested, stupor, coma, or convulsions may develop. The seizures tend to consist of irregular, poorly synchronized twitchings that may shift from side to side. They may continue for long periods. A well-circumscribed, isolated convulsion, however, is uncommon.

Hypoglycemia as a result of hypopituitarism, Addison's disease, and renal glucosuria, as in the de Toni-Fanconi syndrome, is occasionally seen in children. Pancreatic adenomas are rare in this age group.

CONCLUSION

A knowledge of these special neurologic problems of infancy and childhood is of value to the student, as well as to the general physician or internist; it enables him to understand the nature of such illnesses when they are encountered in adults and permits better evaluation of their role in any new illness. Also, the habit of making observations on the level of native intellectual endowment is of importance. The histories given by patients with neurologic problems must always be carefully checked against an outside source; in planning for therapy one must always enlist the aid of the responsible member of the family or, if the patient is institutionalized, of the nurse or attendant. Finally, problems in eugenics are likely to arise, and the physician is often asked to advise the family or health agencies in the community on such matters. Accurate diagnosis and a carefully established genealogy usually permit a separation of a genetic from an acquired disease and are of some value in predicting the occurrence of such diseases in the progeny of the afflicted individual.

REFERENCE

Ford, F. R.: "Diseases of the Nervous System in Infancy, Childhood and Adolescence," 4th ed., Springfield, Ill., Charles C Thomas, Publisher, 1959.

284 CEREBROVASCULAR DISEASE AND THE STROKE SYNDROME

C. Miller Fisher, Praful M. Dalal, and Raymond D. Adams

Vascular diseases of the nervous system rank first among all the diseases of the nervous system. The recognition of this fact and of the need of careful investigation of the causes and mechanisms of these diseases has aroused increasing interest in this subject in the past 10 years, and for the first time the common "stroke case" is being made the object of systematic study. Furthermore, it is evident to all who work in this field of medicine that the cerebrovascular diseases provide one of the best approaches to the study of neurology. No other group of diseases creates with such precision a localized brain lesion of comprehensible type or permits a nervous disorder to unfold with such clarity. In the past the neurologist, in attempting to learn the secrets of the function of the human brain, has depended heavily on the focal ischemic lesion, and there is no reason to doubt that cerebrovascular disease will continue to offer instructive examples of disorders of nervous function, the assiduous study of which will be well repaid.

Every neurologic disease may be said to involve the vasculature of the nervous system in one way or another, and it is necessary at the very outset to delineate the boundaries of the subject. The term *cerebrovascular disease* is intended here to denote any disease in which a derangement of the circulation to any part of the brain is the primary disorder. The responsible pathologic process may be an abnormality of the vessel wall, an occlusion by thrombus or embolus, rupture of a vessel, a failure of cerebral blood flow due to a fall in blood pressure, a change in the caliber of the lumen, altered permeability of the vascular wall, or increased viscosity of the blood. The pathologic process affecting the vessel can be described not only in terms of thrombosis, embolism, rupture of a vessel, etc., but also according to the more basic aspects of the vascular disorder, e.g., atherosclerosis, hypertensive arteriolosclerosis, arteritis, trauma, aneurysm, developmental malformation, etc. Furthermore, in studying cerebrovascular diseases one must consider not only the vascular lesion but also the resultant changes in brain tissue. The pathologic changes in the brain are limited to two types, ischemia with or without infarction and hemorrhage. This is the sum total, and aside from these the vascular lesion is silent, the only exceptions being the local pressure effects of an aneurysm, vascular headache (migraine, hypertension, arteritis), and occasionally increased intracranial pressure as in hypertensive encephalopathy and venous thrombosis.

Brain tissue is dependent for its existence on the moment-to-moment supply of oxygenated blood. In Stokes-Adams attacks unconsciousness occurs within 10 sec of cardiac arrest. In animal experiments stoppage of blood flow for longer than 3 min produces irreversible damage. When brain tissue is deprived of blood and oxygen, it undergoes ischemic necrosis (infarction) and is destroyed. Obstruction of the nutrient artery by thrombus or embolus is the usual cause, but failure of the systemic circulation and hypotension, if severe and prolonged enough, can also produce infarction. Cerebral infarcts vary greatly in the amount of congestion and hemorrhage found within the softened tissue. Some infarcts are strikingly pallid (*pale infarction*), others show mild congestion (dilatation of vessels and some extravasation of red blood cells), and still others show an extensive scattering of petechial hemorrhages throughout the damaged gray matter (*red infarction*). Thrombotic infarcts are usually pale, while embolic infarcts are sometimes pale, sometimes red; i.e., red infarction is usually a sign of embolism. The reason for the different coloration of softenings is not known, although one hypothesis attributes it to the fragmentation and migration of embolic material from its original site of arrest, the movement distally allowing blood to enter the part of the infarct lying more proximally.

A *hemorrhage* consists of an extravasation of blood into the parenchyma or the subarachnoid space or both. The blood is slowly resorbed over a period of weeks and months. Damage to the brain results from the pressure of the mass of blood on the surrounding tissue combined with physical disruption of the region directly involved.

In classifying cerebrovascular diseases it is most practical from a clinical viewpoint to preserve the three classical divisions, thrombosis, embolism, and hemorrhage, listing the causes of each in the corresponding section. This method has some disadvantages in not providing a precise niche for disorders such as reversible ischemia, hypertensive encephalopathy, venous thrombosis, etc. These latter will be discussed separately.

THE STROKE SYNDROME

The clinical picture resulting from vascular disease is in most instances so distinctive that the diagnosis is more readily made than any other in the realm of neurology. The cardinal feature is the *stroke,* a term which connotes the sudden and dramatic development of a focal neurologic deficit. In the severest form of a stroke, the patient falls hemiplegic and even unconscious—an event so striking as to deserve its own separate designation, viz., apoplexy, stroke, shock, or cerebrovascular accident. In its mildest form, it may consist of only a trivial neurologic disorder insufficient to disturb the customary activities of the patient or to demand medical attention.

Undoubtedly, the most characteristic feature is the sequence of events which may be called the *temporal profile* of the stroke. It is the suddenness with which the neurologic deficit develops that especially stamps the disorder as vascular. The speed of evolution, though variable, depending on the cause, is comparatively rapid, and the deficit appears in a matter of seconds, minutes, hours, or at most a few days. When a thrombotic stroke develops over a period of several days, it usually progresses in a stepwise fashion, i.e., in a series of sudden changes, rather than smoothly. A slow, gradual downhill course over a period of several days to a few weeks or more indicates that the process is probably not vascular in nature. Later in the course of the illness, if the attack is not fatal, some stabilization occurs followed by some degree of recovery. Not infrequently an extensive deficit reverses itself dramatically within a few hours or a day. More often, however, the improvement is gradual, taking place over weeks and months.

It must not be supposed that every neurologic abnormality in patients with cerebrovascular disease can be related by the patient or his family to a stroke. Often the exact date of onset of a given symptom cannot be remembered. One has the impression that some of the vascular incidents, especially in the hypertensive patient, are so mild that they do not attract notice until their cumulative effects become manifest as a neurologic deficit of indeterminate date. Furthermore, patients with lesions in the right (nondominant) parietal region often have anosognosia and cannot be depended upon to give any of the important details of their illness. In dominant hemispheral lesions, aphasia hampers history-taking.

The neurologic deficit in a stroke depends, of course, on the location of the infarct or hemorrhage in the brain and the size of the lesion. Hemiplegia is the classical sign of vascular disease and occurs chiefly with massive lesions of either cerebral hemisphere, but it also occurs with lesions of the brain stem. In the most serious cases of hemorrhage, the patient literally falls in his tracks, paralyzed on one side, and soon passes into deep coma and dies within a few hours. In other cases, more commonly in infarction, the patient, although hemiplegic, remains alert, and from the beginning it is obvious that he will survive his illness whether or not neurologic recovery occurs. A stroke, however, may give rise to many manifestations other than a hemiplegia, e.g., numbness, sensory deficit, dysphasia, blindness, diplopia, dizziness, dysarthria, etc. In the following paragraphs these manifestations will be emphasized equally with hemiplegia.

To summarize briefly, it might be said that the stroke syndrome is the common denominator of all cerebrovascular disease and is recognized chiefly by its temporal profile and characteristic focal neurologic deficit.

In practice, however, the diagnosis of cerebrovascular disease is established by the entire constellation of clinical features. Often the patient is elderly and arterial hypertension is present. There may be evidence of vascular disease at other sites, e.g., heart, lower limbs, and aorta; or the patient may have diabetes mellitus and thereby be predisposed to atherosclerosis. A source of emboli may be present (atrial fibrillation, myocardial infarction, subacute bacterial endocarditis, etc.). Many strokes are preceded by transient warning episodes of weakness, numbness, dizziness, etc., and these attacks, if they are nonconvulsive in nature, should always suggest thrombotic cerebrovascular disease. The neurologic signs may occur in certain combinations having a neurovascular relationship; i.e., they may depend on structures which lie within a given vascular territory, as in the lateral medullary syndrome, and thus suggest occlusive vascular disease. And last but not least, the presence of blood in the cerebrospinal fluid signifies that the process is vascular, and diagnostic deductions can proceed from that vantage point.

CEREBRAL THROMBOSIS

Table 284-1. CAUSES OF CEREBRAL THROMBOSIS

I. Atherosclerosis
II. Ruptured saccular aneurysm
III. Cerebral thrombophlebitis: secondary to infection of ear, paranasal sinus, face, etc.; with meningitis and subdural empyema; debilitating states, post partum, postoperative, cardiac failure, hematologic disease (polycythemia, sickle-cell disease), and of undetermined cause
IV. Arteritis
  A. Meningovascular syphilis, arteritis secondary to pyogenic and tuberculous meningitis, rare types [typhus, schistosomiasis mansoni, malaria (?), trichinosis (?), mucormycosis, etc.]
  B. *Connective tissue diseases:* polyarteritis (necrotizing, granulomatous, allergic, Wegner's), temporal arteritis, Takayasu's disease, granulomatous arteritis of aorta, lupus erythematosus
V. Hematologic disorders: polycythemia, sickle-cell disease, thrombotic thrombopenia, etc.
VI. Trauma to carotid
VII. Dissecting aortic aneurysm
VIII. Systemic hypotension: "simple faint," acute blood loss, myocardial infarction, Stokes-Adams syndrome, traumatic and surgical shock, sensitive carotid sinus, severe postural hypotension
IX. Complications of arteriography
X. Migrainous aura with persistent deficit
XI. With tentorial, foramen magnum, and subfalcial herniation
XII. Hypoxia

XIII. Miscellaneous rare types: radioactive or x-ray radiation, lateral pressure of intracerebral hematoma, unexplained middle cerebral infarction in closed head injury, pressure of unruptured saccular aneurysm, mural thrombus in fusiform aneurysm, local dissection of carotid or middle cerebral artery

XIV. Undetermined cause

Of these many causes, thrombosis with atherosclerosis accounts for the overwhelming majority of cases seen clinically. Several others (hypotension, cerebral herniation, with ruptured aneurysm) are conveniently included here although they are really examples of infarction without actual thrombosis.

Thrombosis with Atherosclerosis

Atherosclerosis in the arteries of the brain is similar to that elsewhere in the body. The atheromatous plaques tend to form at branchings and curves. The severity of the process runs parallel to but is somewhat less severe than that of other arteries—aorta, lower limbs, and heart. Thrombosis is most likely to occur where the plaque narrows the lumen to the greatest degree. The commonest sites of thrombosis are the internal carotid artery at the carotid sinus in the neck, at the main bifurcation of the middle cerebral artery, in the vertebral and basilar arteries in the region of their junction, in the posterior cerebral artery as it winds round the cerebral peduncle, and in the anterior cerebral artery as it cuves upward over the corpus callosum. Occlusion of the common carotid, innominate, or subclavian arteries in the upper thorax occasionally is responsible for cerebral ischemia, and the vertebral arteries may be narrowed at their origins from the subclavian. Hypertension aggravates the atherosclerotic process and leads to deposition of atheromatous material in smaller vessels (1 mm and less), and thrombosis will then occur in the penetrating branches of the middle, posterior cerebral, and basilar arteries, producing small infarcts, called *lacunes,* in the deeper parts of the basal ganglions and brain stem. In hypertension the cerebellar and ophthalmic arteries also are liable to involvement. It is extremely rare for the cerebral arteries to be significantly affected beyond their first major branching; i.e., thrombotic occlusion over the convexities seldom occurs. The details of the process by which thrombosis becomes superimposed on atherosclerosis are poorly understood.

The effect of atherosclerotic thrombosis on the brain is not easy to predict accurately, and this is also true of embolic occlusion. If the obstruction lies proximal to the circle of Willis, collateral flow via the circle may be and often is adequate to prevent infarction. If the occlusion is distal to the circle of Willis, i.e., in the stem of one of the cerebral or cerebellar arteries, a series of subarachnoid interarterial anastomoses which join many of the branches of the major cerebral arteries end-to-end may carry sufficient blood into the compromised territory to prevent or lessen the ischemic damage (Fig. 284-4). There is a capillary anastomotic system between adjacent brain arteries, and although it appears always to be the source of some collateral supply it is probably inconsequential. The collateral flow is occasionally so great that a major arterial trunk can be entirely occluded without visible damage to the parenchyma. In other cases, occlusion may lead to softening throughout a vast area which extends to the outermost boundaries of the territory nourished by the affected vessel. In between these two extremes there are countless variations in the size, shape, and completeness of an infarct, depending on factors such as the availability of collateral flow, the speed of occlusion (time for compensation), and the level of the systemic blood pressure. For convenience, these factors (the most important of which is the anastomotic circulation) may be called the *ischemia-modifying factors.* These factors and possibly others such as hypoxia and altered physical state of the blood may also at times operate adversely to produce ischemia in the territory of partially occluded vessels.

The actual condition of the arterial lumen during the period when the stroke is evolving varies from case to case, and as yet the spectrum of pathologic changes is not fully known. Judging from arteriographic and surgical findings in the carotid and vertebral arteries in the neck, it is likely that when prodromal transient ischemic attacks are occurring, atherosclerosis and superimposed thrombus only incompletely occlude the affected artery; blood flow for reasons not yet understood is intermittent in the territory distal to the stenosis. Or the main vessel is totally occluded while the compensating collateral channel is stenotic. By the time the neurologic deficit persists and is advancing, the superimposed thrombus will in the majority of cases have progressed to block completely the main vessel of supply. When the stroke has become fully established, complete occlusion is the rule. It is common to find more than one vessel affected by stenosis or occlusion, and then it is especially difficult to decipher the interplay of hemodynamic factors leading to symptoms, transitory or persistent. It must be pointed out, too, that it is by no means uncommon for stenosis or occlusion of the carotid and vertebral arteries to be "silent."

Clinical Picture. In general, the evolution of the total clinical picture in cerebral thrombosis is much more variable than in embolism and hemorrhage. In approximately 80 per cent of cases, the main part of the stroke (paralysis or other deficit) is preceded by minor signs or by one or more transient, warning ischemic attacks, which in a sense herald the oncoming vascular catastrophe. *A history of such prodromal episodes is of paramount importance in establishing the diagnosis of cerebral thrombosis.* Such episodes are extremely uncommon preceding intracerebral hemorrhage and embolism. Transient warning attacks in carotid–middle cerebral disease consist of hemiplegia, hemiparesis, blindness in one eye, aphasia, confusion, etc., and in the vertebral-basilar system of unilateral numbness, dizziness, diplopia, impaired vision in one or both visual fields, dark vision, dysarthria, headache, head pain, deafness, etc. The attacks last from a few seconds to an hour or so, and the final stroke may be preceded by hundreds of attacks or by only a single one. The stroke may come within a day of the first one or may be delayed for weeks or even months, and sometimes the attacks die away without leading to a stroke. When these minor ischemic attacks are not part of the picture, one must depend on other factors in identifying the cerebrovascular process as one of cerebral thrombosis.

The main part of the thrombotic stroke, whether or not it is preceded by warning attacks, develops in one of several ways. There may be but a single attack, the whole illness developing in a few hours. The patient may awaken in the morning with a full-blown paralysis (or other deficit) or have it come on shortly after arising, perhaps while eating breakfast. Another pattern is for the stroke, once it commences, to have a stuttering intermittent progression in the next several hours or days. Or a partial stroke may develop, and after the patient has improved for several hours a full paralysis may develop. Again, after one or more fleeting episodes, there may be a longer-lasting attack, succeeded in a day or two by the occurrence of a complete and permanent paralysis. The affection may involve several parts of the body simultaneously or, as not infrequently happens, one part, such as a limb or one side of the face, is first paralyzed and the other parts become involved serially in steplike fashion until the stroke is fully developed. This may take several days or weeks, during which time there may be superimposed *transient* episodes of improvement or worsening. All these various modes of development bespeak cerebral thrombosis, and the whole process may be referred to as *thrombosis in evolution.* It might be commented that in the transitory attacks and the abrupt episodes of progression we are really witnessing the temporal profile of the stroke syndrome in miniature. The principle of intermittency seems to characterize the thrombotic process from the beginning to the end. In thrombotic strokes either the onset or progression of the stroke is particularly common during sleep or shortly after arising (60 per cent of cases). Occasionally a thrombotic stroke comes on in what appears to be a slow, gradual fashion, but in most of these cases careful inquiry will reveal an uneven or saltatory progression, and actually there are only a few patients in whom it can be said that the evolution of the thrombotic stroke was truly gradual over a period of several days. Table 284-2 shows the way in which the clinical picture developed in 125 cases of cerebral thrombosis diagnosed clinically, for the most part.

Headache although absent in the majority of cases is not uncommon in cerebral thrombosis, generally being on one side in the front part of the head in occlusion of the carotid system and at the back of the head or in the forehead in basilar disease. The headache is usually not so violent as in cases of intracranial hemorrhage. Its cause is unknown. Presumably it is related in some way to the disease process within the vessel, since it may antedate the other symptoms of the stroke. Stiffness of the neck rarely occurs with cerebral infarction.

The patient, although usually elderly, is not invariably so, and persons in the fourth decade or even younger may be stricken. Hypertension, an important aggravating factor in atherosclerosis, is more often present than not. Diabetes is not uncommon. Often there is evidence of vascular disease elsewhere, e.g., angina pectoris, electrocardiographic abnormality, myocardial infarction, absence of one or several peripheral pulses in the lower limbs, or intermittent claudication. The retinal arteries may show uniform or focal narrowing, increase and irregularity of the light reflex, or displacement of the veins, but these alterations cannot be correlated with cerebral atherosclerosis, and thus fundoscopic examination is at present of little or no help in assessing the state of the intracranial arteries.

The *specific neurologic abnormality* depends, of course, on the location and size of the infarct, or the focus of ischemia. The territory of any vessel may be affected, large or small, deep or superficial. The carotid and basilar systems are approximately equally affected. In involvement of the carotid system, *unilateral* signs predominate: hemiplegia, hemihypesthesia, hemianopia, aphasia, and agnosia. In the basilar system, hemiplegia may also be found, but more commonly involvement here results in the occurrence of *bilateral* signs, motor and/or sensory, in combination with a disturbance of cranial nerves, cerebellum, or other structures localized in or related to the brain stem. In order that carotid occlusion cause bilateral signs, the vessels to both hemispheres would have to be affected at the same time (bilateral carotid occlusion), and this is uncommon. Therefore, in identifying vascular syndromes it is important to determine if the signs and symptoms indicate unilateral or bilateral lesions.

In order to understand the particular groupings of neurologic symptoms and signs, the student must be familiar with certain points of neurovascular anatomy which will now be presented. The clinical syndrome associated with occlusion of each of the cerebral and cerebellar arteries will then become clear. It has already been pointed out that, because of differences in collateral blood flow, speed of occlusion, etc., the effect of occlusion at any one site is highly variable, and therefore partial syndromes and notable variations are extremely common; indeed, they are in the majority. The following descriptions apply particularly to infarction and ischemia due to thrombosis or embolism. While hemorrhage in the same sites may give rise to many of the same effects, the total clinical picture is apt to differ, because in its deep extension the hemorrhage may involve the territory of more than one vessel. Also it displaces tissues and causes an increase in intracranial pressure.

Vascular Ischemic Syndromes. *Middle Cerebral Artery.* The middle cerebral artery through its cortical branches supplies the lateral surface of the hemisphere except for the frontal pole, a strip along the superomedial border irrigated by the anterior cerebral, and the lowermost temporal convolution, which is in the territory of the posterior cerebral artery.

Table 284-2. DEVELOPMENT OF THE CLINICAL PICTURE
IN 125 CASES OF CEREBRAL THROMBOSIS

Clinical development	No. of cases	Per- centage
Transient ischemic attacks progress- ing to a persistent neurologic defi- cit, major or minor................	53	42
Stepwise development of a stroke, with or without transient ischemic attacks.......................	23	18
Stroke developing as a single event	21	17
Abrupt (hours), with or without fluctuations.................	*14*	
Slow, gradual (a few days), with or without minor fluctuations...	*7*	
Transient ischemic attacks only.....	17	14
Development of a limited stroke fol- lowed by transient ischemic at- tacks........................	11	9

Its area includes the cortex and white matter of the lateral and inferior aspects of the frontal lobe,

the motor cortex (areas 4 and 6, the centers for contraversive eye movements, and in the dominant hemisphere, the motor speech area of Broca), the cortex and white matter of the lateral parietal lobe (sensory cortex, angular and supramarginal convolutions), the lateral and superior parts of the temporal lobe, and the insula. The penetrating branches of the middle cerebral artery supply the putamen, outer globus pallidus, the posterior limb of the internal capsule above the plane of the upper border of the globus pallidus, the adjacent part of the corona radiata, the body of the caudate nucleus, and the superior portion of the head of the caudate nucleus (Fig. 284-1).

The middle cerebral territory is the region most frequently affected in embolic and thrombotic cerebrovascular disease. The artery may be occluded in its stem,[1] blocking the mouths of the penetrating vessels as well as the flow to the superficial (cortical) vessels, or its major branches can be involved individually. Foix and Levy recognized eight territorial syndromes: (1) total middle cerebral infarction (deep and superficial), (2) major deep middle cerebral infarction, (3) partial deep middle cerebral infarction, (4) major superficial middle cerebral infarction, (5) major posterior middle cerebral infarction, (6) partial posterior middle cerebral infarction, (7) partial anterior middle cerebral infarction, (8) multiple infarction, unilateral and bilateral. This list has little practical use but emphasizes the numerous possibilities.

The classical picture of total superficial and deep middle cerebral infarction is a contralateral hemiplegia, hemianesthesia, and homonymous hemianopia (Fig. 284-2). If the dominant hemisphere is involved, global or total sensorimotor aphasia also is present. If the nondominant hemisphere is affected, speech is spared but apractognosia of the minor hemisphere is added to the clinical syndrome (see below).

In the middle cerebral territory the motor and sensory cortical zones are spread out over a large area, and hence an infarct of restricted size can produce paralysis of the face alone or of only one limb or even part of a limb. This restricted deficit is referred to as a *monoplegia* or *monoparesis* (facial, brachial, crural).

An infarct which lies posteriorly in the superficial

[1] The term *stem* refers to the section of artery lying between the origin of the middle cerebral and the first major branching. The stem of the anterior cerebral artery lies between its origin and the junction with the anterior communicating artery. The stem of the posterior cerebral stretches from its origin to the posterior communicating artery. The stem of the internal carotid artery extends from the region of the clinoid process to the bifurcation into the middle and anterior cerebral arteries.

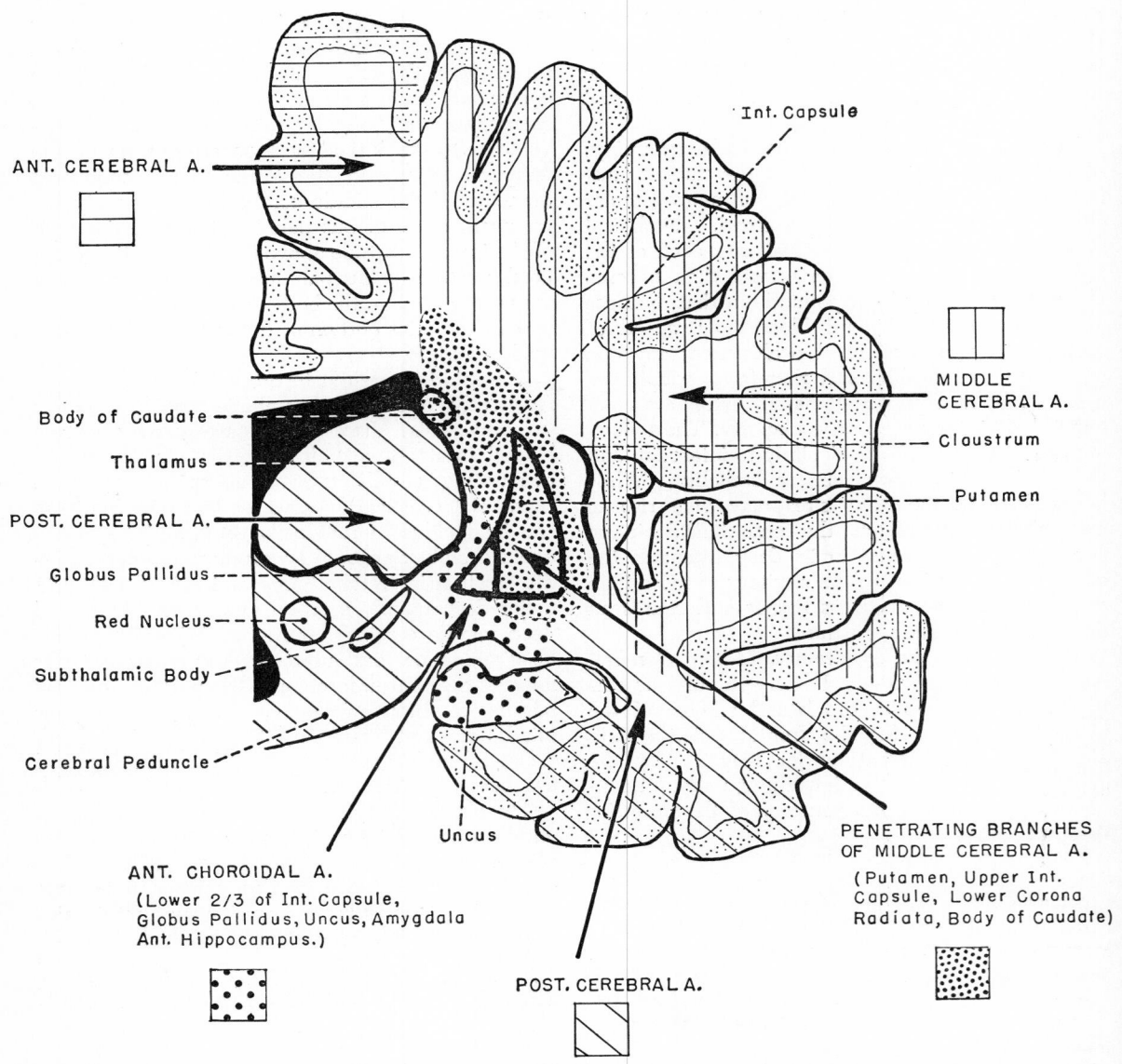

FIG. 284-1. Diagram of a cross section of cerebral hemisphere to show the deep and superficial territories of the major cerebral vessels.

middle cerebral territory of the dominant hemisphere may cause hemianopia, sensory aphasia [auditory verbal agnosia, jargon speech, anomia, agraphia, alexia (visual verbal agnosia)], acalculia (inability to calculate), finger agnosia (inability to recognize fingers and parts of the body), and right-left disorientation (inability to tell right from left). The last four of these symptoms comprise the well-known *Gerstmann's syndrome* (see Chap. 37). Ideational apraxia is another common finding. This is an inability to carry out a purposeful act, presumably because of the faulty function of that part of the brain which conceives and initiates a desired performance, with the result that the motor apparatus is not guided through the proper series of movements. In partial lesions these symptoms may occur singly or in various combinations. When the nondominant hemisphere is involved posteriorly, apractognosia of the minor hemisphere (a combination of apraxias and agnosias) may dominate the picture or be the only finding. This includes anosognosia (unawareness of the illness or disability), left asomatognosia (unawareness of the left side), constructional apraxia (inability to construct a simple object from its parts), dressing apraxia (inability to dress), etc.

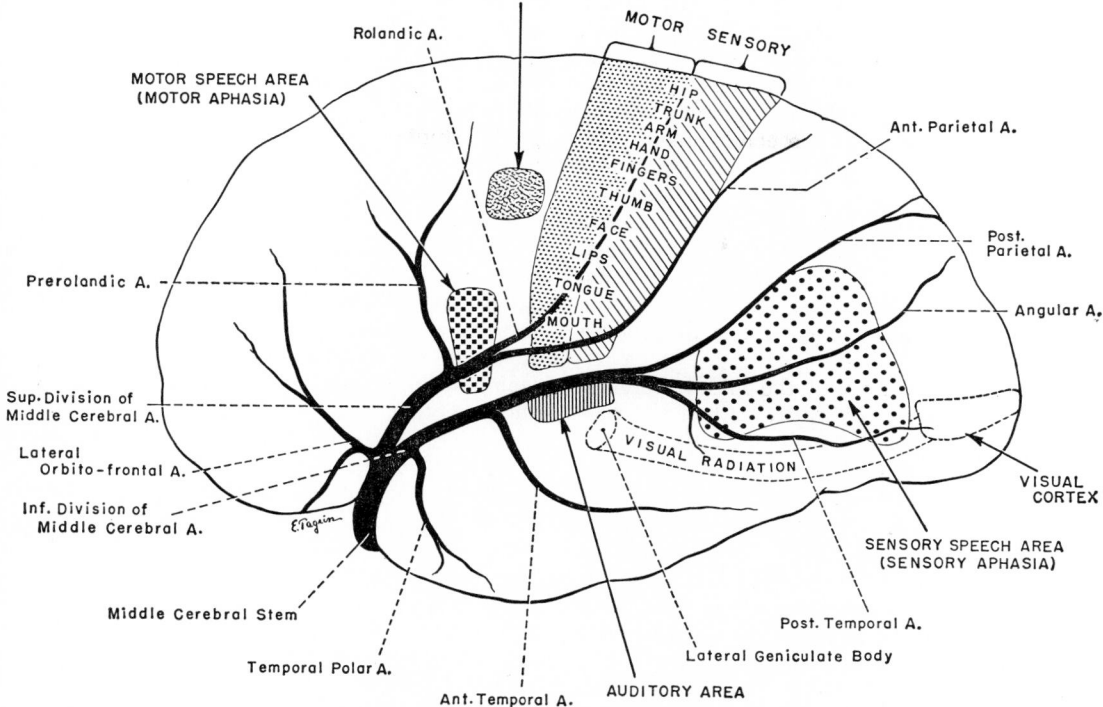

AREA FOR CONTRAVERSION
OF EYES AND HEAD

Rolandic A.

MOTOR SPEECH AREA
(MOTOR APHASIA)

MOTOR SENSORY

HIP
TRUNK
ARM
HAND
FINGERS
THUMB
FACE
LIPS
TONGUE
MOUTH

Ant. Parietal A.

Post. Parietal A.

Angular A.

Prerolandic A.

Sup. Division of
Middle Cerebral A.

Lateral
Orbito-frontal A.

Inf. Division of
Middle Cerebral A.

VISUAL RADIATION

VISUAL
CORTEX

SENSORY SPEECH AREA
(SENSORY APHASIA)

Middle Cerebral Stem

Temporal Polar A.

Ant. Temporal A. AUDITORY AREA

Post. Temporal A.

Lateral Geniculate Body

FIG. 284-2. Diagram of the lateral aspect of the cerebral hemisphere showing the branches and distribution of the middle cerebral artery and the principal regions of cerebral localization. Below is a list of the clinical manifestations produced by infarction in the territory of the middle cerebral artery and the corresponding regions of cerebral damage. In each case the signs and symptoms are separated from the anatomic area by a colon (:).

Paralysis of the contralateral face, arm, and leg: Somatic motor area for face and arm and the fibers descending from the leg area to enter the corona radiata.

Sensory impairment over the contralateral face, arm, and leg (pinprick, cotton touch, vibration, position, two-point discrimination, stereognosis, tactile localization, barognosis, cutaneographia): Somatic sensory system corresponding to motor involvement described above.

Motor aphasia (speech apraxia): Motor speech area of the dominant hemisphere.

Sensory aphasia (word deafness, anomia, jargon speech, sensory agraphia, amusia, acalculia, alexia, finger agnosia, right-left confusion [the last four comprise the Gerstmann syndrome]): Sensory speech area and parieto-occipital cortex of the dominant hemisphere.

Ideational apraxia: Sensory speech area (parietal portion).

Apractognosia of the minor hemisphere (amorphosynthesis), anosognosia, hemiasomatognosia, unilateral neglect, agnosia for the left half of external space, dressing "apraxia," constructional "apraxia," distortion of visual coordinates, inaccurate localization in the half field, impaired ability to judge distance, upside down reading, visual illusions (e.g., it may appear that another person walks through a table): Nondominant supersensory zone (area corresponding to speech area in dominant hemisphere). Loss of topographic memory is usually due to a dominant lesion, occasionally to a nondominant one.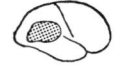

Homonymous hemianopia (often homonymous inferior quadrantanopia): Optic radiation deep to second temporal convolution.

Paralysis of conjugate gaze to the opposite side: Frontal contraversive field or fibers projecting therefrom.

Repellent kinetic apraxia (Denny-Brown) of individual limb or of gait: Parietal lobe lesion.

Miscellaneous: Frontal ataxia due to lesion of frontopontine tract, loss or impairment of optokinetic nystagmus due to lesion of supramarginal or angular gyrus; disturbance of caloric nystagmus due to posterior temporal lobe lesion; limb-kinetic apraxia (?) related to premotor cortical damage; asymbolia for pain due to lesion of dominant parietal lobe; intellectual deterioration, mirror movement, Cheyne-Stokes respiration, contralateral hyperhidrosis, occasionally mydriasis: the localization of the responsible lesions for the last five is not known. Acute lesions of the nondominant hemisphere may cause severe amnesia and confabulation mimicking Korsakoff's syndrome.

Capsular hemiplegia: This results usually from a softening of the upper portion of the posterior limb of the internal capsule and the adjacent corona radiata. Motor paralysis is the chief sign, and dysphasia, homonymous hemianopia, and significant sensory loss seldom occur in the syndrome.

If the infarct lies centrally in the motor-sensory strip, hemiplegia with sensory change will be the chief finding; and if situated farther anteriorly, paralysis often of the monoplegic form with little or no sensory deficit will predominate. On the dominant side, motor aphasia and agraphia will be present (see Chap. 40). On the nondominant side, motor impersistence (inability to maintain eyes closed or tongue out or to fix gaze, etc.) may be noted. Deviation of the eyes and head to the side of the lesion (i.e., paralysis of conjugate lateral gaze to the opposite side) is extremely common with acute lesions of the anterior part of the middle cerebral territory or the motor tracts descending therefrom.

When the deep territory of the middle cerebral artery is involved, i.e., the upper part of the posterior limb of the internal capsule, the adjacent part of the corona radiata, the putamen, and the outer part of globus pallidus, a total hemiplegia usually results, face, arm, and leg being affected together rather than in monoplegic form. This is because the motor fibers lie closely packed in the capsule and destruction is less likely to single out the fibers to only one limb than it is in the cortex, where the motor area extends over a wide territory. The aphasic disorder, if any, which results from these deep lesions has not been sufficiently studied. Sensory loss is minimal or absent.

Damage to the basal ganglions (putamen, caudate) produces no specific clinical effects which have so far been recognized. A hemianopia does not occur as a rule in lesions in the territory of the penetrating arteries, since the optic radiation lies at a more inferior level.

Hypertension combined with atherosclerosis results in thrombotic occlusion of individual penetrating branches running to the internal capsule and putamen, and the resultant small infarctions, 2 to 8 mm in extent, are called *lacunes*. When they involve the internal capsule, a hemiplegia results, recovery from which is often nearly complete. Multiple *lacunes* involving the corticospinal and corticobulbar motor tracts cause the clinical picture of "pseudobulbar palsy" (more appropriately called *bipyramidal palsy*), featuring bilateral upper motor neurone signs, i.e., spasticity, increased tendon reflexes, Babinski sign, dysarthria, and dysphagia. Spasms of excessive crying or laughing, marche à petit pas, and mental impairment are also part of the picture. *Lacunes* are sometimes said to be the basis of so-called "arteriosclerotic parkinsonism," but proof that such an entity exists is wanting.

Anterior Cerebral Artery. The anterior cerebral artery, through its cortical branches, supplies the anterior four-fifths of the medial surface of the cerebral hemisphere, the medial part of the orbital surface of the frontal lobe, the frontal pole, a strip of the lateral surface along the superomedial border, and the anterior seven-eighths of the corpus callosum. The deep branches, which arise near the circle of Willis, run chiefly to the anterior limb of the internal capsule and inferior part of the head of the caudate nucleus (see Fig. 284-3).

Well-studied cases of infarction of the territory of the anterior cerebral artery are not common, and the syndrome of this artery has not been clearly determined as yet. Again the clinical picture will depend on the size and location of the infarct, which in turn depend on the site of the occlusion, the pattern of the circle of Willis, and the other ischemia-modifying factors. Occlusion of the stem of the anterior cerebral artery proximal to the anterior communicating artery is usually well tolerated, since collateral flow will come from its mate of the opposite side. The maximal disturbance occurs when both anterior cerebral arteries happen to arise from one anterior cerebral stem, occlusion of which then results in a devastating infarction of the anterior cerebral territory of both hemispheres. This may include bilateral pyamidal signs with paraplegia and profound mental symptoms. The typical syndrome resulting from occlusion of one anterior cerebral artery distal to the circle of Willis includes paralysis and a cortical sensory deficit of the opposite lower limb (paracentral sensorimotor area) and possibly involvement of the opposite arm (fibers descending from the arm area through the central white matter to the internal capsule), mental changes such as forgetfulness, akinetic mutism (lack of impulse and animation), motor apraxia (a localized inability to use a limb or a part to carry out a simple coordinated act) of the nondominant upper extremity, grasping and sucking reflexes, a special type of resistance to passive movement of the limbs (counterholding or *gegenhalten*), and incontinence of bowel and bladder. The degree of impairment of sensory and motor function is variable. Occlusion of individual branches of the anterior cerebral artery causes only a part of the total syndrome. Hemianopia does not occur in anterior cerebral lesions, nor has an aphasic difficulty been reported, except in rare instances where a softening in the central white matter supplied by the penetrating or deep branches has been held responsible for a partial motor-speech deficit. Occasionally the speechlessness of marked abulia may mimic aphasia.

Anterior Choroidal Artery. A few incomplete clinicopathologic studies have been the basis of present knowledge of the syndrome of the anterior choroidal artery. It is said to consist of contralateral hemiplegia, hemianesthesia (hypesthesia), and homonymous hemianopia, all due to involvement of the posterior limb of the internal capsule and the white matter posterolateral to it, through which

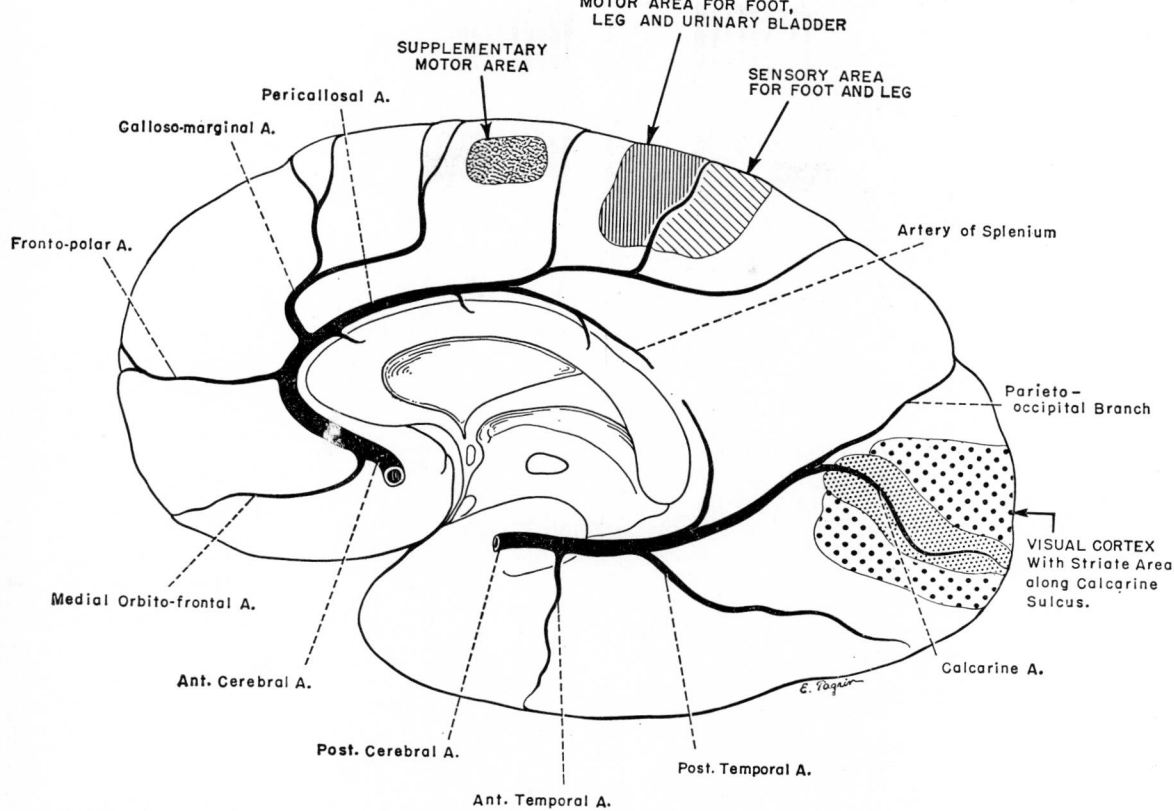

MOTOR AREA FOR FOOT, LEG AND URINARY BLADDER

SUPPLEMENTARY MOTOR AREA

Pericallosal A.

Calloso-marginal A.

SENSORY AREA FOR FOOT AND LEG

Fronto-polar A.

Artery of Splenium

Parieto-occipital Branch

VISUAL CORTEX With Striate Area along Calcarine Sulcus.

Medial Orbito-frontal A.

Calcarine A.

Ant. Cerebral A.

Post. Cerebral A.

Post. Temporal A.

Ant. Temporal A.

FIG. 284-3. Diagram of the medial aspect of the cerebral hemisphere to show the branches and distribution of the anterior cerebral artery and the principal regions of cerebral localization. Below is a list of the clinical manifestations produced by infarction in the territory of the anterior cerebral artery and the corresponding regions of cerebral damage. In each case signs and symptoms are separated from the anatomic area by a colon (:).

Paralysis of opposite foot and leg: Motor leg area.

A lesser degree of paresis of opposite arm: Involvement of arm area of cortex or fibers descending to corona radiata therefrom.

Cortical sensory loss over toes, foot and leg: Sensory area for foot and leg.

Urinary incontinence: Sensorimotor area in paracentral lobule.

Magnetic apraxia of limb (Denny-Brown) or of gait (gait apraxia): Lesion of the cortex of the frontal lobe or of the anterior limb of internal capsule.

Grasp reflex, sucking reflex, Gegenhalten (paratonic rigidity), "frontal tremor": Medial surface of the posterior frontal lobe (?) supplementary motor area.

Loss of memory, mental impairment: Localization not known.

Akinetic mutism: Bilateral frontal-cingulate lesions (?). (Note that aphasia and hemianopia do not occur.)

Miscellaneous: Frontal ataxia (the occurrence of such a disorder mimicking cerebellar ataxia is disputed) has not been reported with vascular lesions; cerebral paraplegia may be due to bilateral anterior cerebral artery occlusion; the present nosologic position of limb-kinetic apraxia in frontal lobe (corpus callosum) lesions is uncertain.

the first part of the geniculocalcarine fibers pass. In the reported cases, however, the clinical syndrome usually fell far short of what was expected on anatomic grounds. Furthermore, the practice of surgically occluding the anterior choroidal artery in the treatment of parkinsonism has shown that hemiplegia, hemianesthesia, and hemianopia rarely occur; in the pathologically studied surgical cases, the lesions have been most capricious, and, indeed, in some no lesion at all has been found. Because of the present uncertainty surrounding the syndrome, it will not be further discussed here except to say that at autopsy on very rare occasions one finds a major infarct in the posterior limb of the internal capsule in the anterior choroidal territory. In one of our cases the only vessel occluded was the cervical portion of the internal carotid artery.

Internal Carotid Artery. The clinical picture of occlusion of the internal carotid artery is very variable. Not infrequently occlusion is completely asymptomatic, while in other cases it produces a devastating massive infarction which leads to death in a few days. Between these two extremes lies every shade of variation. As a rule, the infarct involves some part of the middle cerebral territory, but when the anterior communicating artery is very small, the ipsilateral anterior cerebral territory may be affected, too, in which case the anterior part of the hemisphere (the frontal lobe) bears the brunt of the insult, while the region posterior to the rolandic fissure tends to be spared. When both anterior cerebral arteries arise from a common stem on one side, infarction may involve the anterior cerebral territory bilaterally. Likewise, the posterior cerebral artery may be supplied from the internal carotid rather than from the basilar artery, in which case its territory, too, may be softened, and thus the entire hemisphere and even part of the other may be involved. Not infrequently the territory of the anterior choroidal artery is also infarcted. When one carotid has been asymptomatically occluded at a previous time, occlusion of the other can result in bilateral hemispheric infarction.

In symptomatic occlusion of the internal carotid artery, the picture usually resembles that of middle cerebral occlusion with a contralateral hemiplegia and hemihypesthesia and aphasia when the dominant hemisphere is involved. The relative sparing of the posterior part of the hemisphere is reflected in a low incidence of homonymous hemianopia. When the anterior cerebral territory is also involved, the clinical picture will include some or all of the features already mentioned under anterior cerebral territory. Patients with infarction in the combined territories of the middle and anterior cerebral arteries are much less responsive than those with lesions in only one territory, and often they are in a state of light coma. No special signs attributable to anterior choroidal involvement have so far been identified.

In addition to supplying the brain, the internal carotid artery supplies the optic nerve and retina via the ophthalmic artery (Fig. 284-4). Transient monocular blindness occurs intermittently as a warning symptom prior to the onset of the stroke in almost 50 per cent of cases of symptomatic carotid occlusion. However the picture of central retinal artery occlusion rarely develops at the time of the stroke.

Whereas most cerebral vessels are inaccessible within the skull and topical diagnosis is made only by inference, in carotid occlusion more direct diagnostic tests are available. Pulsation may be lacking in the internal or common carotid arteries in the neck, in the external carotid branch in front of the ear, or in the internal carotid artery when palpated in the pharynx. Also, pressure in the central retinal artery is often reduced on the side of the carotid occlusion, and a pressure difference in the two eyes on careful ophthalmodynamometry will point strongly to carotid occlusion. Another test consists of compressing the patent opposite carotid artery in the neck, precipitating unconsciousness, seizures, or an electroencephalographic change, but such a maneuver cannot be recommended for routine use. An additional sign of carotid occlusion is the presence on the *opposite* side of an intracranial murmur, heard best by placing the bell of the stethoscope over the eyeball. The murmur is presumably due to enhanced blood flow through the remaining patent vessel. Headache associated with cerebral thrombosis or embolism in the carotid artery is situated just above the eyebrow, while in the middle cerebral artery, it is usually more lateral, at the temple. Severe stenosis within the carotid sinus due to an atherosclerotic plaque—with or without superimposed thrombus—may give rise to a local bruit which can be an important finding in assessing the carotid circulation. Occasionally the murmur results from stenosis at the mouth of the external carotid artery and can then be misleading. Stenosis of the carotid sinus with an accompanying murmur may be present bilaterally or may occur lower in the neck along the common carotid arteries, the subclavians, or the innominate. Propagation distally of an aortic valvular murmur must be distinguished from carotid bruits.

The common carotid arteries may be occluded at their origin, as in "pulseless disease" or the *aortic arch syndrome.* The neurologic symptoms and signs of carotid occlusion, just discussed, may or may not be present, depending on the adequacy of the circle of Willis and of the vertebral-basilar system. The following manifestations, for the most part nonneurologic, have been reported in the aortic arch syndrome: absence of pulsation in carotid and radial arteries, faintness on arising from the horizontal position, recurrent loss of consciousness, headache, neck pain, paresthesias of various parts of the body, transient blindness (unilateral or bilateral), dimness of vision with exercise, premature cataracts, retinal atrophy and pigmentation, atrophy of the iris, leukomas, peripapillary arteriovenous anastomoses, optic atrophy, claudication of the jaw muscles, perforation of the nasal septum, saddle nose deformity, trophic ulceration of the face, facial atrophy (unilateral or bilateral), indolent infections of the face, abnormal facial pigmentation, and loss of hair. This condition was originally described in Japan, particularly in young women who were found to be suffering from a granulomatous arteritis involving all three major trunks arising from the aortic arch (Takayasu's disease, see Chap. 247). An incomplete aortic arch syndrome consisting of various combinations of carotid, subclavian, and innominate occlusion or stenosis is not uncommon. The majority of the authors' cases of pulseless disease, both the partial and the complete syndrome, have been due to severe atherosclerosis.

Vertebral-Basilar-Posterior Cerebral System. *Posterior Cerebral Artery.* The terminal or cortical branches of this vessel supply the undersurface of the temporal and occipital lobes, as well as the entire medial surface of the occipital lobe including the visual area (areas 17, 18, and 19). From

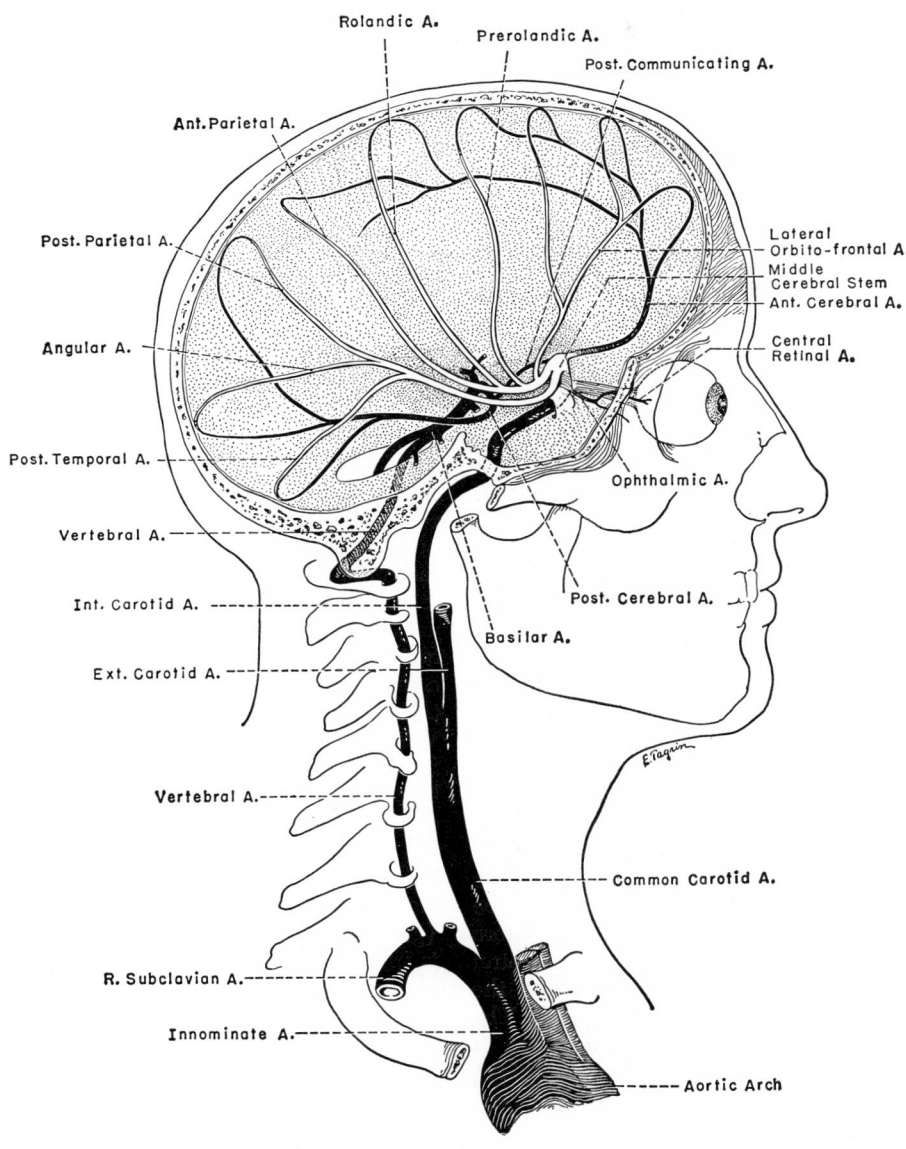

Fig. 284-4. Drawing to illustrate the arrangement of the major arteries carrying blood from the heart to the brain (only the right side is shown). The posterior communicating artery connects the internal carotid and the posterior cerebral arteries, forming an important anastomosis between the carotid and basilar systems. Further distally, the subarachnoid interarterial anastomoses which link the middle cerebral with the anterior and posterior cerebral arteries are shown. The ophthalmic and central retinal arteries have been included to remind the student that observations and measurements of the retinal circulation provide information concerning the carotid circulation.

the more proximal part of the artery between its origin at the bifurcation of the basilar artery and the cortical distribution many important branches arise.

The interpeduncular branches arising near its origin penetrate the brain stem to supply the red nucleus, subthalamic nucleus of Luys, substantia nigra, the most medial part of the cerebral peduncle, the oculomotor nucleus, the reticular substance of the midbrain, the decussation of the superior cerebellar peduncles, rubrothalamic tract, medial longitudinal fasciculus, and the medial lemniscus. The thalamoperforating branches also arise here and pass to the inferior mesial and anterior parts of the thalamus. Branches arising serially along the parent vessel as it encircles the midbrain supply the cerebral peduncle, lateral part of the medial lemniscus, corpora quadrigemina, pineal gland, lateral geniculate bodies, choroid plexus, and hippocampus. The thalamogeniculate branches supply the pulvinar and the lateral nuclei of the thalamus (Fig. 284-5).

Again the clinical picture resulting from occlusion will depend on the site of the obstruction, the site and size of the infarct, and the ischemia-modifying factors. Occlusion proximal to the posterior communicating artery may be tolerated if collateral flow via that vessel is adequate; however, the penetrating branches arising from the stem of the posterior cerebral artery may be occluded at their mouths. Even distal to the posterior communicating artery, occlusion may cause no damage if collateral flow via the subarachnoid interarterial anastomoses is sufficient.

Classically, occlusion of the cortical or superficial branches of the posterior cerebral artery gives rise to a contralateral homonymous hemianopia because of involvement of the primary visual area in the calcarine region. Partial visual field defects are common, and posterior cerebral lesions are likely to cause a superior homonymous quadrantanopia, whereas middle cerebral lesions (involving the superior portion of the optic radiation) tend to be associated with an inferior quadrantanopia. More often the defect is hemianopic. Only the central part of the visual field may be affected, with the production of a hemianopic central scotoma. The patient's awareness of the visual disturbance is variable. He may be totally unaware of the defect, which is discovered for the first time by the examiner, or he may have vaguely appreciated that something was wrong with one eye. In the acute stage of large temporo-occipital lesions, the opposite extreme may be encountered, the patient reporting that he is able to see only one-half of objects or words, or that he is totally blind when he obviously is not. Scintillating phenomena, i.e., flashes of light, crude white or colored figures appearing in the

affected part of the visual field, are not uncommon. When the lesion lies in the dominant hemisphere, a dysphasic disturbance, not yet clearly delineated, may result. The most prominent feature is alexia, the patient reading very laboriously and having great difficulty in perceiving letters and numbers although in some cases comprehending what he reads, when given sufficient time. The reading material may be held at an angle, and in rare instances the patient may read better when the lines are placed vertically. Copying print and script is impaired. The capacity for revisualization of spatial relationships (the ability to imagine the topography of home or town) may be impaired. There may be color blindness, total or in the half-field, as well as visual-object agnosia (inability to recognize objects), and simultanagnosia (inability to synthesize the elements of a scene into a whole). Involvement of the minor hemisphere brings prosopagnosia (difficulty in recognizing faces) often in association with topographic disorientation, simultagnosia, and achromatopsia. Temporary disorientation and memory loss attributable to damage to the hippocampal and lingual gyri may occur with lesions on either side but are more prominent with involvement of the dominant hemisphere.

Bilateral lesions of the occipital lobes, if extensive, cause total blindness of the cortical type, because of a bilateral homonymous hemianopia. The pupillary reflexes are retained, and funduscopically the optic nerves are normal, unlike blindness from retinal and optic nerve or tract disease. Often the patient is unaware of the blindness and may in fact deny it when questioned specifically. More commonly the bilateral lesions are incomplete, and the patient is left with a sector of visual field intact. When the remnant is very restricted, vision may fluctuate greatly from minute to minute, suggesting hysteria. In small calcarine lesions there may be loss of central vision only (bilateral homonymous central scotomas); on the other hand, in larger calcarine lesions, only central vision may be spared and vision is likened to looking through a narrow pipe (gun-barrel vision). With bilateral lesions, there is usually a loss of memory, the severity of which varies from case to case. There may or may not be the various cortical disturbances described under unilateral lesions.

When occlusion of the posterior cerebral artery occurs more proximally (one might speak of anterior syndromes), the clinical picture will comprise signs of damage to thalamus, cerebral peduncle, midbrain, and hypothalamus, and possibly in addition, the manifestations just described (hemianopia, etc.), depending on the collateral inflow of blood. Best known is the *thalamic syndrome* of Déjerine and Roussy, which results from infarction of the region of the sensory nucleus in the posterolateral

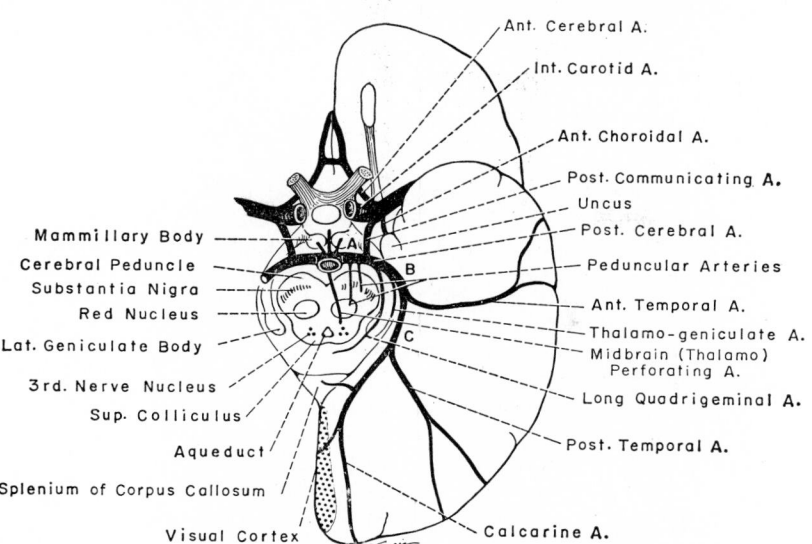

Labels on diagram (top to bottom, right side):
Ant. Cerebral A.
Int. Carotid A.
Ant. Choroidal A.
Post. Communicating A.
Uncus
Post. Cerebral A.
Peduncular Arteries
Ant. Temporal A.
Thalamo-geniculate A.
Midbrain (Thalamo) Perforating A.
Long Quadrigeminal A.
Post. Temporal A.
Calcarine A.

Labels on diagram (left side):
Mammillary Body
Cerebral Peduncle
Substantia Nigra
Red Nucleus
Lat. Geniculate Body
3rd. Nerve Nucleus
Sup. Colliculus
Aqueduct
Splenium of Corpus Callosum
Visual Cortex

Fig. 284-5. Diagram of the inferior aspect of the brain to show the branches and distribution of the posterior cerebral artery and the principal anatomic structures. Below is a list of the clinical manifestations produced by infarction in the territory of the posterior cerebral artery and the corresponding regions of damage. In each case the signs and symptoms are separated from the anatomic area by a colon (:).

Peripheral territory

Homonymous hemianopia (often upper quadrantic): Calcarine cortex or optic radiation nearby. Hemiachromatopsia may be present. Macular or central vision tends to be preserved because occipital polar striate cortex is spared.

Bilateral homonymous hemianopia, cortical blindness, unawareness or denial of blindness; apraxia of ocular movements, failure to see to-and-fro movements, inability to perceive objects not centrally located, inability to count or enumerate objects, tendency to run into things which the patient sees and tries to avoid: Bilateral calcarine cortex (possibly the parietal lobe is involved also).

Dyslexia, visual object agnosia, associated tactile agnosia, achromatopsia, topographic disorientation, simultanagnosia, perseveration: Calcarine and pericalcarine cortex of dominant hemisphere. Prosopagnosia usually occurs with nondominant lesion.

Unformed visual hallucinations, peduncular hallucinosis, metamorphopsia, teleopsia, illusory visual spread, irreminiscence, paliopsia, distortion of outlines: Calcarine cortex.

Memory defect: Hippocampal lesion bilaterally or the dominant side only; or involvement of hippocampal system at another level (mammillary bodies, psalterium, etc.).

Central territory

Thalamic syndrome—sensory loss (all modalities), spontaneous pain and dysesthesias, sensory or pseudoathetosis, intention tremor, spasms of hand, mild hemiparesis: Posteroventral nucleus of thalamus in territory of thalamogeniculate artery. Involvement of the adjacent subthalamic body or its afferent tracts results in hemiballismus and choreoathetosis.

Thalamoperforate syndrome—(a) *superior,* crossed cerebellar ataxia; (b) *inferior,* crossed cerebellar ataxia with ipsilateral third nerve palsy (Claude's syndrome): Dentatorubrothalamic tract and issuing third nerve.

Weber's syndrome—third nerve palsy and contralateral hemiplegia: Third nerve and cerebral peduncle.

Contralateral hemiplegia: Cerebral peduncle.

Paralysis or paresis of vertical eye movement, skew deviation, sluggish pupillary responses to light, slight miosis and a trace of ptosis (retraction nystagmus and "tucking" of the eyelids may be associated): Supranuclear fibers to third nerve, interstitial nucleus of Cajal, nucleus of Darkschewitsch, and posterior commissure.

Contralateral rhythmic ataxic action tremor; rhythmic postural or "holding" tremor (rubral tremor): Dentatothalamic tract (?) after decussation. The site of the lesion is actually unknown.

Coma: Damage to upper brain stem (midbrain, thalamus).

Decerebrate attacks: Damage to upper brain stem (especially motor tracts).

Resting tremor or tremor not easily abolished by relaxation has been omitted because of the uncertainty of its occurrence in the posterior cerebral artery syndrome.

Peduncular hallucinosis may occur in thalamic-subthalamic *ischemic* lesions, but the exact location of the lesion is unknown.

part of the thalamus (supplied by the thalamogeniculate vessel). The lesion may be so small as to be overlooked on pathologic examination. The central feature is a sensory loss on the opposite side of the body, usually affecting deep and superficial sensation (pain, temperature, touch, proprioception); or rarely, it may be of the dissociated type, either pain and temperature or vibratory and position sense being affected while the other sensory modalities are relatively spared. It may take a monoplegic pattern. Sometimes there is an associated intractable agonizing pain in the affected parts of the body (thalamic pain), occurring spontaneously and augmented by all types of stimulation of the affected parts. Hyperpathia and taste disorders are common. Often spontaneous pain is entirely missing. In the motor sphere there may be a mild evanescent hemiparesis, and in some patients the affected limbs show hemiballismus, choreoathetosis, incoordination, intention tremor, asynergy, cramplike spasms, and a postural abnormality of the hand (cf. Chap. 28). The mind is usually strikingly spared.

Occlusion of the stem of the posterior cerebral artery may lead to a hemiplegia owing to infarction of the cerebral peduncle, but this is rather rare. Occlusion of the thalamoperforate branches which originate from the most medial part of the posterior cerebral stem gives rise to several different syndromes, depending on the branches involved: (1) a superior syndrome in which the upper part of the red nucleus or rubrothalamic tract is involved, producing on the opposite side of the body a gross ataxia (see Chap. 30); (2) an inferior syndrome (Claude's syndrome), in which a third nerve palsy and contralateral cerebellar signs are combined; (3) Weber's syndrome, i.e., a third nerve palsy combined with a contralateral hemiplegia (see Chap. 31); (4) *hemiballismus,* which probably arises also from an occlusion of the branch of the posterior cerebral artery running to the subthalamic nucleus of Luys; (5) Parinaud's syndrome, paralysis of conjugate vertical gaze and at times of lateral gaze, which results from damage to the region of the posterior commissure; (6) peduncular hallucinosis (visual hallucinations of brightly colored scenes and objects) has been observed in occlusion of the posterior cerebral artery, but the site of the lesion has not been determined. More often an intracerebral hemorrhage is responsible. All these abnormalities are relatively uncommon in cerebrovascular disease. Finally, (7) extensive infarction of the upper midbrain results in deep coma and "decerebrate rigidity" (reflex extensor posture).

Vertebral Artery. The vertebral arteries are the chief arteries of the medulla, and each supplies the lower three-fourths of the pyramid, the medial lemniscus, all or nearly all of the retro-olivary region (the lateral medullary region), the restiform body, and the posteroinferior part of the cerebellar hemisphere (see Fig. 284-6). The relative size of the vertebral arteries varies a good deal, and in approximately 10 per cent of cases, one vessel is so small that the other can be considered the only artery of supply to the brain stem. In this case, depending on collateral inflow from the carotid system via the circle of Willis, occlusion would be equivalent to occlusion of the total vertebral-basilar system, including the posterior cerebral arteries. The posterior inferior cerebellar artery is usually a branch of the vertebral artery, but not infrequently it has a common origin with the anterior inferior cerebellar artery from the basilar artery. It is necessary to keep these anatomic variations in mind when visualizing the effects of vertebral artery occlusion.

The results of vertebral occlusion are quite variable. When there are two good-sized vertebral arteries, occlusion on one side occurs not infrequently without any recognizable symptoms and signs or pathologic changes. If the occlusion of the vertebral artery is so situated as to block the mouth of one or more arteries supplying the lateral medulla, the lateral medullary syndrome may be precipitated, and this is probably the commonest picture in vertebral occlusion (see below). When the branch to the anterior spinal artery is blocked, collateral influx from the spinal artery branch of the opposite side is usually sufficient to prevent infarction. If the branch to the pyramid is occluded, that part of the corticospinal tract may be infarcted unless collateral flow is adequate. Of course, any of these branches may become occluded in its course after leaving the vertebral artery and produce similar effects. Rarely, occlusion of the vertebral artery or one of its medial branches produces an infarct which involves the medullary pyramid, the medial lemniscus, and the emergent hypoglossal fibers [contralateral paralysis of arm and leg (face spared), contralateral loss of touch and vibration sense, and ipsilateral paralysis and atrophy of the tongue]. This is the medial medullary syndrome (see Fig. 284-6D). Finally, vertebral occlusion can lead to symptoms by blocking the posterior inferior cerebellar artery.

The posterior inferior cerebellar artery supplies the inferior portion of the lateral medullary region, the restiform body, and the inferior surface of the cerebellar hemisphere. It may be occluded at its mouth, i.e., by thrombosis of the vertebral artery —or anywhere along its course. Some patients tolerate obstruction of the vessel with little or no ill effect; in others an extensive infarct results in the cerebellum and/or the posterolateral medulla. It should be pointed out that the various cerebellar arteries are connected to their neighbors by sub-

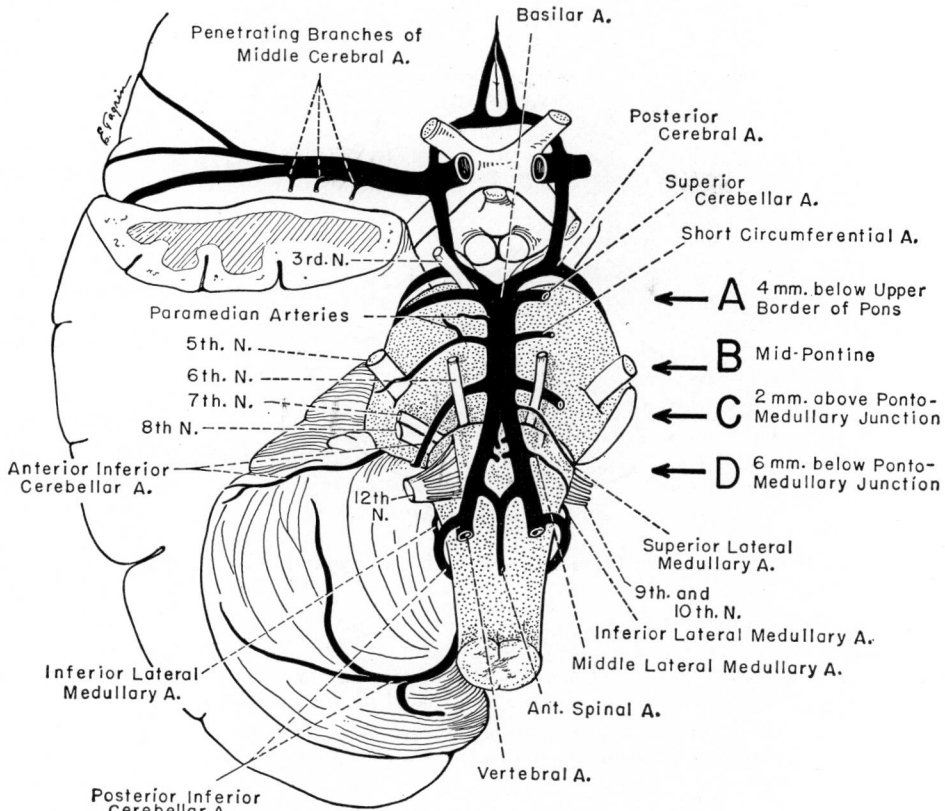

Fig. 284-6. Diagram of the brain stem showing the principal vessels of the vertebral-basilar system. The letters and arrows on the right indicate the levels of the four cross sections A, B, C and D which follow. Although typical vascular syndromes of the pons and medulla have been designated by sharply outlined shaded areas, the student must appreciate that since satisfactory clinicopathologic studies are far from numerous, the diagrams are not necessarily accurate nor do they always represent established fact. The great frequency with which infarcts fail to produce a well-recognized syndrome and the special tendency for syndromes to merge with one another must be emphasized.

arachnoid interarterial anastomoses, in the same way as the main arteries of the cerebrum, and the potential for collateral flow to a compromised territory is excellent.

The clinical picture resulting from occlusion of the posterior inferior cerebellar artery is highly variable. Often no serious damage results. At other times, there may be dizziness, homolateral cerebellar ataxia, nystagmus, and loss of equilibrium (due to involvement of the inferior surface of the cerebellum and its connections with the brain stem. Or, the *lateral medullary syndrome* may be evoked through blockage of flow along the inferior artery of the lateral medulla. While occlusion of the posterior inferior cerebellar artery is usually stated to be the cause of the lateral medullary syndrome, this appears to be true in only a minority of patients; more careful studies have shown that in 8 out of 10 cases the vertebral artery is occluded, and in the other 2 cases either the posterior in-

ferior cerebellar artery is occluded or no arterial occlusion is found.

The *lateral medullary syndrome* is produced by infarction of a small wedge of lateral medulla lying posterior to the inferior olivary nucleus (see Fig. 284-6D). The classical syndrome consists of pain and numbness of the ipsilateral face (descending tract and nucleus of the trigeminal nerve), dizziness, nausea, vomiting, nystagmus (vestibular nucleus or fibers), dysarthria, dysphagia, ipsilateral palatal weakness, hoarseness, ipsilateral paralysis of vocal cord, weakness of the sternocleidomastoid muscle (nucleus ambiguus or issuing fibers), homolateral cerebellar ataxia of arm and leg, disequilibrium with falling to the side of the lesion (inferior cerebellar peduncle, olivocerebellar fibers, or cerebellum), dissociated sensory deficit consisting of loss of pain and temperature sensation on the opposite side of the body below the neck—sometimes the face is included (spinothalamic tract), ipsilateral

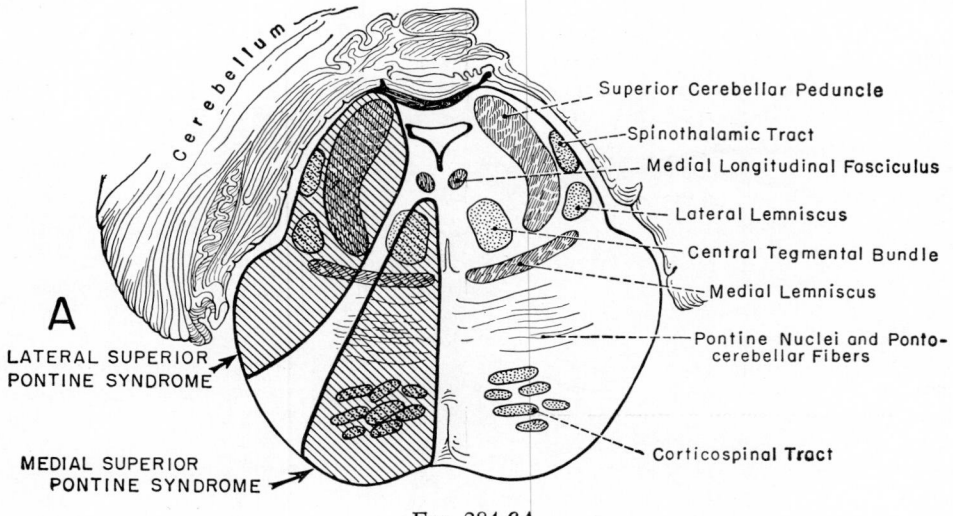

FIG. 284-6A.

1. MEDIAL SUPERIOR PONTINE SYNDROME (paramedian branches of upper basilar artery)

Signs and symptoms	Structures involved
On side of lesion	
Cerebellar ataxia (probably)	Superior and/or middle cerebellar peduncle
Internuclear ophthalmoplegia	Medial longitudinal fasciculus
Myoclonic syndrome, palate, pharynx, vocal cords, respiratory apparatus, face, oculomotor apparatus, etc.	Localization uncertain—central tegmental bundle (?), dentate projection (?), inferior olivary nucleus (?)
On side opposite lesion	
Paralysis of face, arm, and leg	Corticobulbar and corticospinal tract
Rarely touch, vibration, and position are affected	Medial lemniscus

2. LATERAL SUPERIOR PONTINE SYNDROME (syndrome of superior cerebellar artery)

On side of lesion	
Ataxia of limbs and gait, falling to side of lesion	Middle and superior cerebellar peduncles, superior surface of cerebellum, dentate nucleus
Dizziness, nausea, vomiting,	Vestibular nucleus ⎤
Horizontal and vertical nystagmus	Vestibular nucleus ⎥ Territory of descending branch to
Paresis of conjugate gaze (ipsilateral)	Uncertain ⎬ middle cerebellar peduncle from
Loss of optokinetic nystagmus	Uncertain ⎥ superior cerebellar artery
Skew deviation	Uncertain ⎦
Miosis, ptosis, decreased sweating over face (Horner's syndrome)	Descending sympathetic fibers
Static tremor reported in one case	Dentate nucleus (?), superior cerebellar peduncle (?)
On side opposite lesion	
Impaired pain and thermal sense on face, limbs, and trunk	Spinothalamic tract
Impaired touch, vibration, and position sense, more in leg than arm. (There is therefore a tendency to syringomyelic dissociation in upper extremity and face)	Medial lemniscus (lateral portion)

Horner's syndrome (descending sympathetic tract), and hiccups. Added to the basic picture, there may be ipsilateral loss of taste (tractus solitarius), diplopia, skew deviation, internuclear ophthalmoplegia (the medial longitudinal fasciculus-vestibular connections or perhaps the sixth nerve), contralateral corticospinal signs (pyramid), ipsilateral Babinski sign, loss of the knee jerks, ipsilateral peripheral facial palsy, paresthesias of the ipsilateral side, carotid sinus sensitivity, incontinence, hippus, and trophic ulceration. Some of these additional signs may indicate extension of the lesion to a slightly higher level. This syndrome, one of the most striking in neurology, is almost always due to infarction. It should be emphasized that very frequently the syndrome is present only in part.

Basilar Artery. The basilar artery supplies not only the pons and upper part of the cerebellum but also in most cases both posterior cerebral territories. Occlusion may occur in the trunk of the basilar artery or in any one of its branches.

The branches of the basilar artery may be conveniently grouped as follows: (1) paramedian, seven to ten in number, supplying a wedge of pons on either side of the midline; (2) the short circumferential branches, five to seven in number, supplying the lateral two-thirds of the pons and the middle and superior cerebellar peduncles; and (3) the long circumferential, two in number on each side running laterally across the pons to reach the cerebellar hemispheres (the superior cerebellar artery and the anterior inferior cerebellar artery).

Occlusion of the basilar artery evokes a vast array of clinical manifestations reflecting involvement of a large number of structures [corticospinal and corticobulbar tracts, cerebellum, middle and superior cerebellar peduncles, medial and lateral lemnisci, spinothalamic tracts, medial longitudinal fasciculi, pontine nuclei, vestibular and cochlear nuclei, descending hypothalamospinal sympathetic fibers, the upper medulla and the third, fourth, fifth, sixth, seventh, and eighth cranial nerves (including the nuclei, the segment within the brain stem, and the peripheral nerve itself); see Fig. 284-6].

The picture of basilar occlusion due to thrombosis may arise in several ways: (1) occlusion in the basilar artery itself usually in the lower portion near its origin, at the site of an atherosclerotic plaque; (2) both vertebral arteries may become occluded, closure of the second amounting to basilar obstruction; (3) occlusion of a single vertebral, when there is only one of good size, is equivalent to basilar occlusion. It must be em-

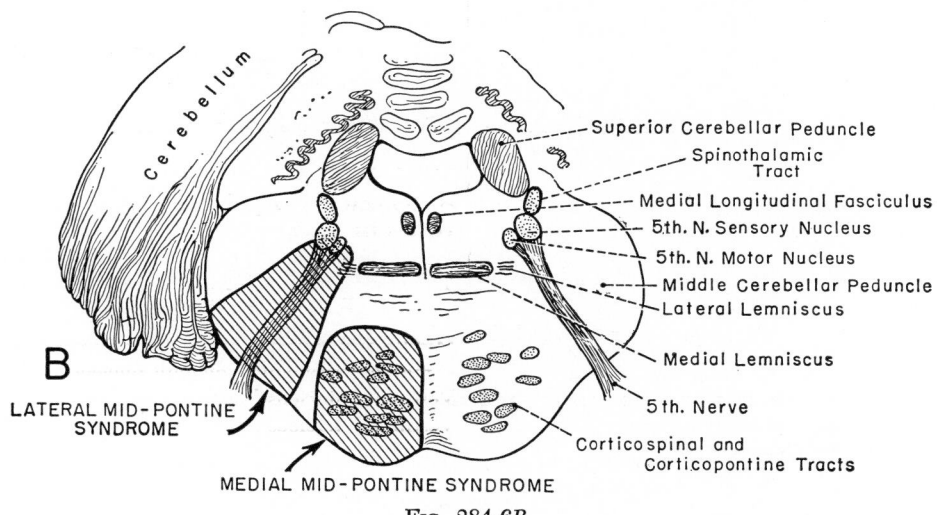

FIG. 284-6*B*.

1. MEDIAL MIDPONTINE SYNDROME (paramedian branch of midbasilar artery)

Signs and symptoms	*Structures involved*
On side of lesion	
Ataxia of limbs and gait (more prominent in bilateral involvement)	Middle cerebellar peduncle
On side opposite lesion	
Paralysis of face, arm, and leg	Corticobulbar and corticospinal tract
Variable and transient impaired touch and proprioception (this has not been clearly established)	Medial lemniscus

2. LATERAL MIDPONTINE SYNDROME (short circumferential artery)

On side of lesion	
Ataxia of limbs	Middle cerebellar peduncle
Paralysis of muscles of mastication	Motor fibers or nucleus of fifth nerve
Impaired sensation over side of face	Sensory fibers or nucleus of fifth nerve

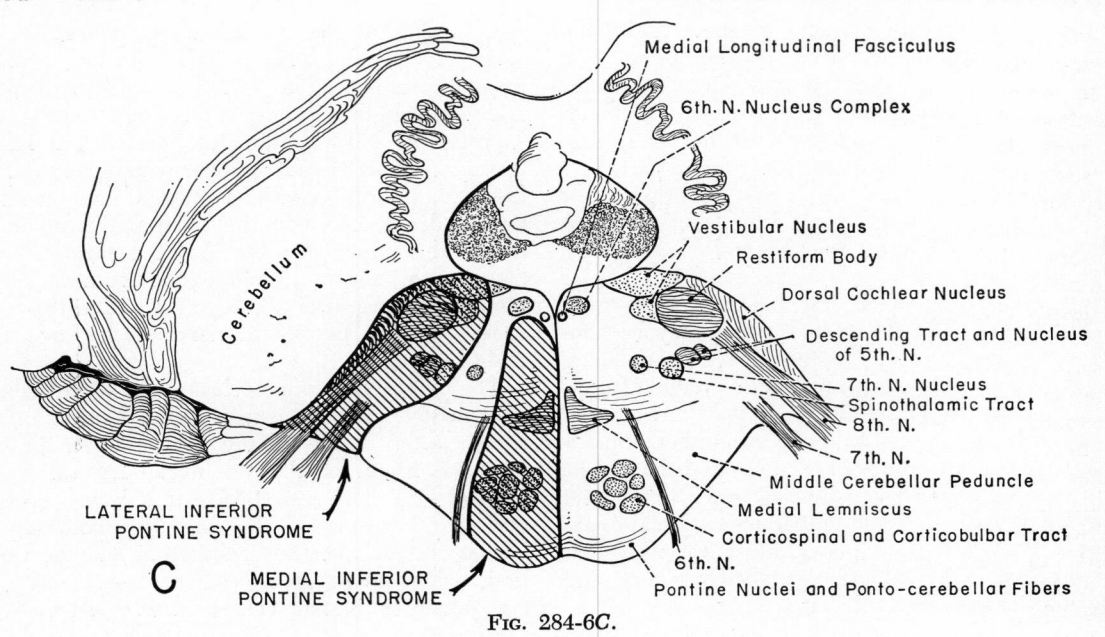

Medial Longitudinal Fasciculus

6th. N. Nucleus Complex

Vestibular Nucleus

Restiform Body

Dorsal Cochlear Nucleus

Descending Tract and Nucleus of 5th. N.

7th. N. Nucleus
Spinothalamic Tract
8th. N.

7th. N.

Middle Cerebellar Peduncle

Medial Lemniscus

Corticospinal and Corticobulbar Tract

6th. N.

Pontine Nuclei and Ponto-cerebellar Fibers

Cerebellum

LATERAL INFERIOR
PONTINE SYNDROME

C

MEDIAL INFERIOR
PONTINE SYNDROME

FIG. 284-6C.

1. MEDIAL INFERIOR PONTINE SYNDROME (occlusion of paramedian branch of basilar artery)

Signs and symptoms	Structures involved
On side of lesion	
Paralysis of conjugate gaze to side of lesion (preservation of convergence)	"Center" for conjugate lateral gaze
Nystagmus	Vestibular nucleus
Ataxia of limbs and gait	Middle cerebellar peduncle (?)
Diplopia on lateral gaze	Abducens nerve
On side opposite lesion	
Paralysis of face, arm, and leg	Corticobulbar and corticospinal tract in lower pons
Impaired tactile and proprioceptive sense over half of the body	Medial lemniscus

2. LATERAL INFERIOR PONTINE SYNDROME (occlusion of anterior inferior cerebellar artery)

On side of lesion	
Horizontal and vertical nystagmus, vertigo, nausea, vomiting	Vestibular nerve or nucleus
Facial paralysis	Seventh nerve
Paralysis of conjugate gaze to side of lesion	"Center" for conjugate lateral gaze
Deafness, tinnitus	Auditory nerve or cochlear nucleus
Crossed diplopia	Uncertain
Ataxia	Middle cerebellar peduncle and cerebellar hemisphere
Impaired sensation over face (uncommon)	Descending tract and nucleus fifth nerve
On side opposite lesion	
Impaired pain and thermal sense over half the body (may include face)	Spinothalamic tract

3. TOTAL UNILATERAL INFERIOR PONTINE SYNDROME (occlusion of anterior inferior cerebellar artery). Combination of lateral and medial syndromes.

phasized that thrombosis may involve only a branch rather than the trunk of the basilar artery, and this is probably the commonest cause of basilar symptomatology. When the obstruction is embolic, the embolus usually lodges at the upper bifurcation of the basilar or in one or other posterior cerebral artery, since if it is small enough to pass through the vertebral artery, it should easily traverse the length of the basilar artery, which is usually of greater diameter than either vertebral artery.

In the complete basilar syndrome, there will be paralysis of all four extremities (often one side is more affected than the other) and the bulbar musculature, dysarthria, dysphagia, diplopia, sensory loss for pain, temperature, touch, and vibration (motor paralysis usually predominates over sensory deficit), and perhaps impaired vision. At the most advanced stage of the illness, the patient is deeply comatose, both voluntary and reflex eye movements are absent, the pupils usually but not always are fixed to light and may be dilated, respirations are irregular, the systemic blood pressure fluctuates, and accesses of extensor rigidity may occur spontaneously or be evoked by pinch or other stimuli. Occasionally, with low pontine lesions, the patient, although totally paralyzed and subject to violent extensor spasms, may be relatively alert but physically powerless to evince signs of it, except by signaling with upward eye movements (see Chap. 34).

In the presence of the full syndrome, it is usually not difficult to make the correct diagnosis. The aim should be, however, to recognize basilar insufficiency long before the stage of total deficit has been reached. The early manifestations occur in many combinations, and it would be difficult to list all the possibilities. Most commonly the following will be encountered: weakness or paralysis of one or both sides of the body, occasionally a monoplegia only; numbness and a corresponding sensory loss involving one or both sides of the face, or both hands, or both legs; or numbness of one side can be combined with paralysis of the other; dysarthria, speechlessness, stuttering, and dysphagia; dizziness of a vestibular type, either in spontaneous attacks or upon change of posture, often associated with nausea and vomiting; diplopia, due to a disturbance of the third or sixth nerves, or resulting from faulty conjugate lateral gaze or internuclear ophthalmoplegia (see Chap. 31); paralysis of conjugate lateral gaze to the side of the *lesion* (this is the reverse of a hemispheric lesion, in which the patient is unable to turn his eyes toward the side of the *paralysis*); paralysis of vertical gaze upward and downward due to a subthalamic lesion; forced deviation of the eyes; loss of ability to accommodate for near and far vision; cerebellar ataxia involving the limbs of one or both sides, or affecting chiefly walking and standing; infranuclear palsy of the seventh nerve (facial paralysis) or the motor part of the fifth nerve (weakness of masseter muscle and deviation of the jaw to the side of the lesion); impaired vision, blurred vision, dark vision, or scintillating scotomas; loss of hearing, either unilateral or bilateral, and rarely tinnitus; headache, head pain, or peculiar head sensations (like a cord being drawn tightly around the head); confusion and impaired memory; drowsiness (the patient may, however, be lucid). Other phenomena include rhythmic bulbar myoclonus, bilateral internuclear ophthalmoplegia, hemiballismus, choreoathetosis, Cheyne-Stokes respiration, facial fasciculations or twitchings, simple auditory hallucinations, and distortions of taste.

In regard to occlusion of individual basilar branches, the main signs of occlusion of the *superior cerebellar artery* are severe ipsilateral cerebellar ataxia (middle and/or superior cerebellar peduncles), nausea and vomiting, slurred speech, and loss of pain and temperature over the extremities, body, and face of the opposite side (spinothalamic tract). Partial deafness, a static tremor of the ipsilateral upper extremity, Horner's syndrome, and bulbar myoclonus have also been reported. In occlusion of the *anterior inferior cerebellar artery* the extent of the infarct is extremely variable. The size of this artery and the territory it supplies vary inversely with that of the posterior inferior cerebellar artery. The principal findings are ipsilateral cerebellar ataxia (middle cerebellar peduncle), Horner's syndrome, ipsilateral deafness, whirling dizziness, facial palsy, and sensory loss over the face. Nausea, vomiting, tinnitus, and nystagmus may be associated. Pain and temperature sensation may be lost on the opposite side of the body. If the occlusion is close to the origin of the artery, the corticospinal fibers may also be involved, producing a hemiplegia. Occlusion of the *artery to the retro-olivary space* will produce the lateral medullary syndrome. Occlusion of a *paramedian branch* will result in infarction of the corticospinal fibers, the adjacent pontine nuclei, and the pontocerebellar fibers on one side of the pons. If the infarct extends deeply to reach the tegmentum as it occasionally does, paralysis of conjugate lateral gaze and a sensory deficit will result. Occlusion of smaller branches in patients with hypertension and atherosclerosis results in small infarcts (lacunes) which may be responsible for or contribute to the syndrome of pseudobulbar palsy.

One of the hallmarks of a brain stem lesion is the occurrence of *bilateral* motor and/or sensory signs; within the brain stem, tracts descending to and ascending from each side of the body either cross each other or run in close proximity, in contrast to the cerebral hemispheres where the motor and sensory tracts subserving the two sides of the body are distantly separated. While it is correct to emphasize that bilaterality of a lesion strongly suggests brain stem involvement, it must be pointed out with equal force that unilaterality of a lesion by no means precludes a brain stem site. On the contrary, in many instances of infarction within the basilar territory the lesion is strictly

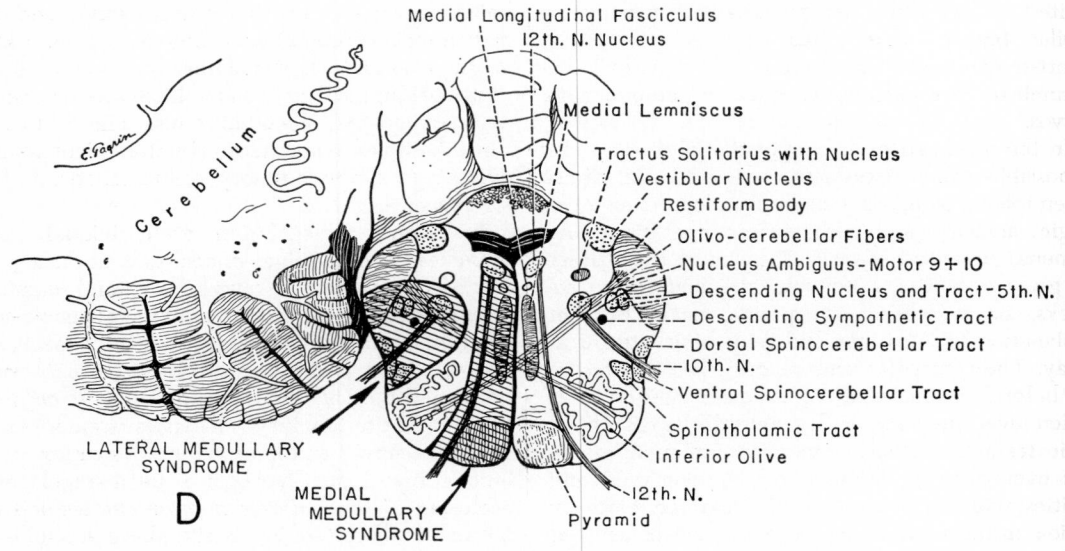

FIG. 284-6D.

1. MEDIAL MEDULLARY SYNDROME (occlusion of vertebral artery or of branch of vertebral or lower basilar artery)

Signs and symptoms	Structures involved
On side of lesion	
Paralysis with atrophy of half the tongue	Issuing twelfth nerve
On side opposite lesion	
Paralysis of arm and leg sparing face	Pyramidal tract
Impaired tactile and proprioceptive sense over half the body	Medial lemniscus

2. LATERAL MEDULLARY SYNDROME (occlusion of any of five vessels may be responsible—vertebral, posterior inferior cerebellar, or superior, middle, or inferior lateral medullary arteries)

On side of lesion	
Pain, numbness, impaired sensation over half the face	Descending tract and nucleus fifth nerve
Ataxia of limbs, falling to side of lesion	Uncertain restiform body, cerebellar hemisphere, olivocerebellar fibers, spinocerebellar tract (?)
Vertigo, nausea, vomiting	Vestibular nucleus
Nystagmus	Vestibular nucleus
Miosis, ptosis, decreased sweating (Horner's syndrome)	Descending sympathetic tract
Dysphagia, hoarseness, paralysis of palate, paralysis of vocal cord, diminished gag reflex	Issuing fibers ninth and tenth nerves
Loss of taste	Nucleus and tractus solitarius
Numbness of arm, trunk, or leg	Cuneate and gracile nuclei
Hiccups	Uncertain
On side opposite lesion	
Impaired pain and thermal sense over half the body, sometimes face	Spinothalamic tract

3. TOTAL UNILATERAL MEDULLARY SYNDROME (occlusion of vertebral artery). Combination of medial and lateral medullary syndromes.

4. LATERAL PONTOMEDULLARY SYNDROME (occlusion of anterior inferior cerebellar artery or superior lateral medullary artery). Combination of lateral medullary and lateral inferior pontine syndromes.

limited to one side, bespeaking occlusion of a basilar branch rather than of the main trunk. Another cardinal brain stem sign is nuclear or infranuclear involvement of one or more cranial nerves.

In the diagnosis of disease of the brain stem it is impossible from motor signs alone to distinguish a hemiplegia of pontine origin from one of cerebral origin, and we are dependent on coexisting phenomena. As with cerebral lesions, a flaccid paralysis gives way to spasticity in the following days, weeks, or months; and there is no satisfactory explanation for the variability in this period of delay. The pattern of sensory disturbance may also be helpful in localization. A dissociated sensory deficit over the face or one-half the body usually indicates a lesion within the brain stem; a sensory loss over one side of the body involving all modalities with no suggestion of dissociation in any region indicates a lesion at the thalamic level or higher. When position sense, two-point discrimination, and tactile localization are affected relatively more than pain, temperature, and tactile sense, a cortical lesion is suggested; the reverse suggests a brain stem location of the lesion. When both motor and sensory manifestations are bilateral, it is almost unequivocal evidence that the lesion lies infratentorially. When hemiplegia or hemiparesis and sensory loss are coextensive, the lesion lies supratentorially. Additional manifestations which point unequivocally to a brain stem site are whirling dizziness, diplopia, cerebellar ataxia, Horner's syndrome, and deafness. The several brain stem syndromes illustrate the important point that the cerebellar system, spinothalamic tract, trigeminal nucleus, and sympathetic fibers can be involved at different levels, and neighborhood phenomena are necessary in order to identify the exact level.

A myriad of eponymic brain stem syndromes, e.g., Weber, Claude, Benedict, Foville, Raymond-Cestan, Millard-Gubler, etc., already mentioned in pp. 295 to 297, have been described in relation to brain stem lesions. In their classical descriptions most of them relate to cases of tumor and other nonvascular diseases, and only occasionally is one of these syndromes encountered in association with vascular disease. The diagnosis of vascular disorders in this region of the brain is not greatly facilitated by these syndromes, and it is preferable to memorize the neuroanatomy of the brain stem.

The great desirability of being able to categorize brain stem vascular cases with accuracy hardly need be mentioned. Nonetheless, an analysis of the authors' experience with a large number of these cases shows that too often it has been impossible either to designate the vessel involved or to fit the clinical picture to an eponym. A survey of the literature indicates that complete neuropathologic studies in this territory are so few that reliable rules for the exact identification of the vessel or vessels involved are not available except for a few of the major syndromes. It seemed more practical, therefore, to classify the cases according to the topography of the lesions within the brain stem, and the classification shown in Fig. 284-6 was drawn up. There are some 12 syndromes in all, the principal eight being medial and lateral lesions at four different levels of the brain stem, upper pons, midpons, lower pons, and midmedulla. Three are combinations of two or more of the eight syndromes just mentioned, while the final syndrome represents a full brain stem infarction. This list of syndromes has been useful to the authors in cataloguing day-to-day clinical cases, but there are patients who do not fit the classification.

Further Remarks Concerning Symptomatology. In addition to the neurologic manifestations which can be assigned to one or another region of the brain, many phenomena whose origin is still obscure are encountered in stroke cases of all types. The following remarks relate chiefly to infarction, but for the most part they apply also to hemorrhage. Cheyne-Stokes respiration or a variant thereof is an extremely common finding, especially with supratentorial lesions, unilateral or bilateral. Incontinence of bladder and/or bowel is a regular

---

5. BASILAR ARTERY SYNDROME (the syndrome of the lone vertebral artery is equivalent). A combination of the various brain stem syndromes plus those arising in the posterior cerebral artery distribution. The clinical picture comprises bilateral long-tract signs (sensory and motor) with cerebellar and peripheral cranial nerve abnormalities.

Signs and symptoms	*Structures involved*
Paralysis or weakness of all extremities, plus all bulbar musculature	Corticobulbar and corticospinal tracts bilaterally
Diplopia, paralysis of conjugate lateral and/or vertical gaze, internuclear ophthalmoplegia, horizontal and/or vertical nystagmus	Ocular motor nerves, apparatus for conjugate gaze, medial longitudinal fasciculus, vestibular apparatus
Blindness, impaired vision, various visual field defects	Visual cortex
Bilateral cerebellar ataxia	Cerebellar peduncles and the cerebellar hemispheres
Coma	Tegmentum of midbrain, thalami
Sensation may be strikingly intact in the presence of almost total paralysis. Sensory loss may be syringomyelic or the reverse or involve all modalities	Medial lemniscus, spinothalamic tracts or thalamic nuclei

accompaniment of strokes of moderate to severe degree. Vomiting once or twice at the onset of a stroke is frequent. Sucking and grasping reflexes are extremely common on the side opposite the hemiplegia, i.e., the supposedly unaffected side, the grasp reflex showing itself in several ways, e.g., the patient's tendency to palpate the folds of the bedclothes or rubber tubing. The temperature and the pulse, although often not altered to any extent in cerebral thrombosis, may in basilar artery occlusion undergo a terminal rise, the temperature reaching 104 to 106°F. The blood pressure fluctuates but seldom falls to low levels.

It is difficult to make broadly applicable statements about mental change, stupor, and coma in cerebral thrombosis, for they are in large part related to both the site of the lesion and its size; massive lesions in addition may induce pressure secondarily on diencephalic, midbrain, and pontine structures. Drowsiness, apathy, impairment of memory, and mild degrees of confusion are extremely common in brain infarction due to cerebral thrombosis, especially when the lesion is situated supratentorially. However, a patient with a complete hemiplegia, right or left, due to a hemispheral lesion may remain relatively alert and may be found propped up in bed reading, or pretending to read, the morning newspaper. With small lesions of the motor system there may be no discernible intellectual change whatsoever. Spasmodic crying or laughing is frequently seen in unilateral lesions and is not always to be taken as a sign of bipyramidal palsy. When both the middle and anterior cerebral territories on one side are involved, responsiveness is conspicuously reduced, although the patient is generally awake or can be aroused. Extensive bilateral lesions of the cerebral hemispheres precipitate deep coma. In bilateral lesions of the *basis pontis,* almost total paralysis of the entire body musculature may be combined with a surprising degree of awareness; but if the tegmentum of the upper brain stem is softened, deep coma results.

When a massive hemispheral infarct has occurred, there is always the possibility that severe cerebral swelling will follow in the next few days. When this happens, tentorial, subfalcial, or cerebellar herniation may occur, and if the midbrain is seriously compressed, deep coma, dilated fixed pupils, respiratory embarrassment, and rising temperature presage a hopeless outcome. In milder cases the patient passes through an extremely drowsy period, and transient papilledema, raised spinal fluid pressure, and a marked shift of the pineal gland or the anterior cerebral artery in the arteriogram may be encountered. *Decerebrate posture* (reflex extensor rigidity) usually reflects irreversible damage to the midbrain or pons, either by softening or as the result of Duret hemorrhages

secondary to tentorial herniation and midbrain compression. *Unilateral decerebrate posture* is seen not infrequently and does not carry with it the poor prognosis of the bilateral variety.

Laboratory Findings. Renal function is not altered in cerebral infarction, and any urinary abnormalities are to be attributed to concomitant renal disease. A significant leukocytosis does not occur. The cerebrospinal fluid pressure is normal in patients with cerebral thrombosis, unless the infarct is large and associated with severe swelling of the damaged tissue. Cerebral thrombosis never causes blood in the spinal fluid, which is "crystal clear" unless the infarct is especially congested, when a very faint xanthochromia (1 to 2 on a scale of 10) may occur. A slight increase in the leukocytes of the spinal fluid (3 to 8 polymorphonuclears) is common in the first few days of the illness. Rarely, and for unexplained reasons, a brisk, transient pleocytosis (400 to 2,000 polymorphonuclears per cu mm) occurs on about the third day. A persistent increase in the white blood cells of the cerebrospinal fluid suggests the presence of chronic meningitis (syphilis, tuberculosis, torula), granulomatous arteritis, septic embolism, cerebral thrombophlebitis, or a nonvascular process. The total protein may be normal, but frequently it is raised to 50 to 80 mg per 100 ml. Rarely is it over 100, in which case some other diagnosis should be seriously considered. A Wassermann or some other specific test for syphilis is still routinely made in many clinics but can be dispensed with unless the rest of the clinical and laboratory picture points toward neurosyphilis. A positive test in a bloody fluid is not valid, since syphilitic reagin may have been carried into the fluid by the contaminating blood. Skull x-rays are not remarkable, and the pineal gland will not be shifted unless severe cerebral swelling has occurred, in which case the patient will usually be stuporous or comatose. The use of ophthalmodynomometry in the diagnosis of carotid obstruction has already been referred to.

The electroencephalogram is still of limited value in indicating infarction or distinguishing it from hemorrhage and from nonvascular conditions. Generally speaking, in cerebral infarction the electrical activity is found to be of a slightly slower frequency and lower voltage than normal. High-voltage slow waves (3 to 5 per second) are evidence in favor of hemorrhage or tumor. In brain stem and capsular infarction the tracing is usually within normal limits. In distinguishing a vascular lesion from brain tumor, serial electroencephalograms may be useful in that in the former the tracing tends to improve, in the latter to worsen. The detection of latent cerebral ischemia, using the electroencephalogram in conjunction with tilting the body or compressing one carotid artery, has not attained wide popularity. The pneumoencephalo-gram may be normal or show local swelling in the acute stages of arterial occlusion, but in the healed stages local ventricular dilatation may occur at the site of tissue loss due to infarction. This procedure is not recommended as a diagnostic laboratory test in patients with occlusive cerebrovascular disease, because of the danger of precipitating progression of the neurologic syndrome, due to the hypotensive state which so often attends the introduction of air. Carotid arteriography, a procedure widely used in many clinics to visualize the site of the vascular occlusion, will demonstrate the blocked artery if it is in the carotid or in the proximal parts of the middle cerebral or anterior cerebral stems. To detect occlusion of the proximal parts of the common carotid or vertebral arteries or of the innominate and subclavian trunks, injection via the subclavian route or into the arch of the aorta itself is necessary. Arteriography is not without risk, and in patients with vessels narrowed by atherosclerosis the infarction may be extended. It is not to be recommended as a routine measure in cerebral thrombosis but should be used only if the diagnosis of vascular disease is uncertain, if vascular surgery is contemplated, or as part of a scientific investigation of cerebrovascular disease. Radioactive concentration studies (arsenic scan) used for the detection of tumor, abscess, etc., often show a mildly positive picture over infarcts. Scintillation counting over the two sides of the skull after the intravenous injection of radioactive material may provide a comparative index of circulation in the two carotid systems.

Course and Prognosis. In the introduction it was pointed out that in the characteristic temporal profile of a vascular lesion improvement is the rule if the patient survives. When the patient is seen early in the course of his illness, it is extremely difficult to generalize about the *immediate prognosis*. This raises a crucial question in cerebral thrombosis: Where does the patient stand in his stroke process when first examined? Is worsening to be anticipated or not? No rules have yet been laid down which allow one to predict the course. A mild paralysis today may become a disastrous hemiplegia tomorrow, or the patient's condition may only worsen temporarily for a day or two. In basilar artery occlusion, dizziness and dysphagia may progress in a few days to total paralysis and deep coma. The course of the deficit is so often progressive that a pessimistic attitude on the part of the physician is justified in what appears to be a mild case.

Progression of the stroke is probably due to increasing stenosis of the involved artery by mural thrombus and to extension of the thrombus along the artery to block side branches or hinder anasto-

motic flow. In the basilar artery, thrombus may gradually build up along its entire length. In the carotid system, thrombus at times propagates distally from the site of origin in the neck, to the intracranial supraclinoid portion, and possibly into the anterior cerebral artery, preventing collateral flow from the opposite side. In middle cerebral occlusion, retrograde thrombosis may occur back to the mouth of the anterior cerebral, perhaps secondarily infarcting the territory of that vessel. Some of the ischemia-modifying factors already referred to probably also play a part in the progression.

Several circumstances influence the *immediate prognosis* in cerebral thrombosis. In the case of large infarcts, swelling of the infarcted tissue occurs, tentorial herniation follows, and the patient dies in 2 to 4 days. On the other hand, milder degrees of swelling and increased intracranial pressure, though causing an apparent progression for 2 to 3 days, may not prove fatal. In extensive basilar infarction associated with deep coma, the patient seldom lives for more than a few days. If coma or stupor is present in a case from the beginning, survival may be largely determined by the success in keeping the airways clear and maintaining fluid and electrolyte balance (see Chap. 34). Respiratory and urinary infections are a constant danger, and once they begin there is usually a rapid decline in the patient's condition with rise in temperature.

As for the *eventual or long-term prognosis* of the neurologic deficit, there are too many possibilities to recount them in detail. In the case of small infarcts, recovery may start within hours or a day or two, and restoration may be complete. In severe cases there may be no significant recovery whatsoever, and after months of assiduous efforts at rehabilitation, the patient may remain bereft of speech, with the upper extremity still totally useless and the lower extremity serving only as an uncertain prop in attempting to walk. Between these two extremes there is every shade of recovery. It is safe to say that the longer the delay before movement begins, the poorer the prognosis becomes. If recovery is not started in 1 or 2 weeks, the outlook is gloomy both for motor activity and speech, and in general it may be said that whatever motor paralysis remains after 5 to 6 months will probably be permanent. Aphasia, dysarthria, and cerebellar ataxia may improve for a year or longer, and sensory improvement has been detected for up to 2 years. A hemianopia which has not cleared in a few weeks will often remain permanently, although reading, color discrimination, and object recognition may continue to improve. Lateral medullary infarction might be regarded as an exception to the above rule, for difficulty in swallowing may be protracted (4 to 7 weeks), and yet relatively normal function may be restored finally.

The question of recovery after cerebral lesions raises the broad problem of the functional substitution of one part of the brain for another. At present it is the consensus of opinion that one region does not take over the function of another unless those parts normally worked in close cooperation. For example, musculature which is subserved by both hemispheres, e.g., the face, eyes, throat, etc., may resume functionally normal activity after an extensive hemispheral lesion. It has not been proved that recovery from expressive or receptive aphasia is due to the assumption of speech function by the intact nondominant cerebral hemisphere; some part of the damaged speech areas will usually have escaped destruction.

Characteristically, the paralyzed muscles are flaccid in the first days or weeks following a stroke, but gradually spasticity develops and the tendon reflexes become brisker. The arm tends to assume a flexed adducted posture, whereas the leg is usually extended and adducted. Function is rarely if ever restored after the slow evolution of spasticity. Conversely, the early development of spasticity in the hand, or the appearance of a grasp reflex, and other postural reactions may presage a favorable outcome. Bowel and bladder control usually returns as mental clarity is regained, and sphincteric disorders persist only in patients with the most severe hemiplegia or bilateral motor deficit. Not uncommonly the hemiplegic limbs are at first tender and ache on manipulation, interfering with the physical therapy program. Nevertheless, physiotherapy should be initiated early in order to prevent contracture of muscles at shoulder, elbow, wrist, knuckles, knee, and ankle, a frequent complication and often the source of pain and added disability, particularly in relation to the shoulder. An annoying, unsteady, "dizzy" feeling in the head often persists after damage to the vestibular system in brain stem infarcts.

Recurrent cerebral (epileptic) seizures are a complication in some 20 per cent of cases of infarction in which the cerebral cortex has been involved. They are infrequent during the evolution of a thrombotic stroke and usually appear within a few weeks or months. The occurrence of a seizure followed by postictal (Todd's) paralysis must not be construed as extension of an infarct.

Many patients complain of fatigability and are depressed. The explanation of these symptoms is uncertain; psychologic factors may be important. Only a few patients become serious *behavior problems* or psychotic after a stroke, but paranoid trends, ill temper, stubbornness, and peevishness are common.

Finally, in regard to prognosis, it must be mentioned that having had one thrombotic stroke, the patient is in danger in the ensuing months and years of suffering delayed progression of his deficit or having a stroke at another site. The latter is especially true in hypertension.

Treatment of Cerebral Thrombosis. The treatment of cerebrovascular disease and strokes may be divided into four parts: (1) general medical management in the acute phase, (2) measures to restore the circulation and arrest the pathologic process, (3) physical therapy and rehabilitation, (4) preventive measures against strokes and vascular disease.

General Medical Management in the Acute Phase. In essence, this is the care of the comatose or helpless patient (see Chap. 34). Maintenance of the airway is of great importance. The only real danger is pooling of secretions in the pharynx, and to avoid this the patient must be nursed on his side or in the semiprone position. *Pharyngeal suction* is often necessary; the larynx or trachea is touched by the tip of the suction tube to stimulate coughing. Respiratory exchange may be insufficient if the jaw is tightly clenched and one nostril is blocked by a nasal feeding tube. A mouth airway, as employed in administering anesthesia, can be used if the patient is sufficiently stuporous to tolerate it. A *tracheostomy* will have to be performed if suction via the pharynx is ineffectual and coughing is in abeyance. Oxygen therapy, preferably by nasal tube, is advisable if aeration of the lungs is compromised in any way. *Prevention of pulmonary complications* is best achieved by turning the patient every hour, by strict avoidance of oral feeding if the slightest dysphagia exists, and by the use of prophylactic penicillin therapy. Constant urinary bladder drainage, with daily irrigation, regular changing of catheters, and urinary antibacterial agents (1.0 Gm Gantrisin per day), is necessary if coma is protracted. Intravenous fluids for the first 2 to 3 days followed by transnasal stomach tube feedings are the best means of providing adequate fluid intake and nourishment. Other measures include elastic stockings on the legs and treatment of cardiac failure.

Measures to Restore the Circulation and Arrest the Pathologic Process. Once a thrombotic stroke has developed fully, no therapy so far devised is of any value in restoring the cerebral tissue or its function. *Therapy to be effective must be preventive.* The diagnosis of thrombosis must be made at the earliest possible stage and the full catastrophe circumvented by every means. It will be appreciated, therefore, that all the measures used in combating a stroke in so far as they are designed to alleviate, check, or prevent the cerebral ischemic process are really preventive in nature. They will be instituted at various stages of the process— when only transient ischemic attacks are occurring or at any point in the progression of a thrombosis-in-evolution or when almost the full neurologic deficit has appeared. Even when persistent signs and symptoms have appeared it is conceivable that some of the tissues affected, particularly at the edges of the infarct or islands within, have not been irreversibly damaged and will survive if blood flow can be increased.

The following therapeutic methods are being tried at present or have been tried in the recent past:

MEDICAL MEASURES TO IMPROVE THE BLOOD SUPPLY TO THE BRAIN. Clinical observation indicates that strokes and ischemic attacks in many cases develop when the patient gets up from his bed, particularly in the morning or postoperatively. On the assumption that decrease in the cerebral circulation resulting from the upright position can aggravate cerebral ischemia, it is recommended that patients with a stroke as the result of ischemic infarction should remain horizontal in bed for 7 to 10 days initially and that, when ambulation starts, special attention should be given to preservation of the systemic circulation (avoid standing quietly for prolonged periods, sit with the feet up, etc.). Elevating the foot of the bed 14 in. or more in the acute stage appears to be beneficial. In stroke cases it is of great importance that the systemic blood pressure be maintained (correction of blood loss, use of Levophed in myocardial infarction with vascular collapse, avoidance of autonomic blocking agents, etc.). Injections of epinephrine have been recommended as a means of raising the systemic blood pressure above the usual levels. Although this enhances cerebral blood flow and might be beneficial, a systematic trial in thrombotic cases has not been undertaken. Anemia must be corrected. Polycythemia may slow the circulation locally and must be treated.

ANTICOAGULATION. According to present reports anticoagulant therapy prevents transient ischemic attacks and postpones the arrival of an impending stroke whether the carotid or vertebral system is involved. Anticoagulants also halt the advance of a progressive thrombotic stroke but not in all cases. In assessing anticoagulant therapy one faces the crucial question of where in the course of the stroke the patient stands when he is first examined. Will his course be benign or disastrous? There are no reliable rules for prediction at the present time. Anticoagulants are not of value in the fully developed stroke. Whether when given for a prolonged period of time they prevent the recurrence of a thrombotic stroke is still under study, but the incidence of severe hemorrhagic complications appears to limit their value in these cases.

When *anticoagulant therapy* is instituted in stroke cases, Dicumarol or a drug of similar action is usually used. If an anticoagulant effect appears to be urgently required, heparin is administered, concomitantly, intravenously in doses of 50 to 75 mg every 3 to 5 hr until the Dicumarol becomes effective. Dicumarol alone is sufficient in patients with transient ischemic attacks, repeated thrombotic strokes, or cerebral embolism (see p. 1779). Heparin is used in addition when in thrombotic cases worsening in the clinical picture is occurring from hour to hour or day to day.

The use of anticoagulant drugs makes an accurate clinical diagnosis imperative. Intracranial hemorrhage must be ruled out, by relying primarily on examination of the cerebrospinal fluid; it is to be remembered, however, that a clear fluid does not necessarily exclude hemorrhage (see p. 1782). A control prothrombin concentration and coagulation time are desirable before therapy is started, but if this is not feasible, the initial doses of anticoagulant drugs can usually be given safely if there is no evidence of active bleeding anywhere in the body. The question of whether or not severe hypertension is a contraindication to anticoagulant therapy has not been accurately answered. There is no reliable evidence that complications are more frequent in the presence of hypertension if the prothrombin activity is maintained at 15 per cent or higher, and therefore the authors have not withheld anticoagulant therapy in these patients; however, when the diastolic blood pressure is in the range of 130 mm Hg or more an attempt is made at the same time to lower the pressure gradually with hypotensive agents, exercising great care not to prejudice further the circulation in the region of the infarct by too great a reduction in the systemic pressure. It is preferable to avoid reduction of the blood pressure in the 2-week period immediately following a thrombotic stroke.

Anticoagulant therapy is relatively safe provided the prothrombin concentration is determined regularly (once a day, for the first 10 days, thence thrice a week, and finally every week or 10 days) at a laboratory using reliable methods. Therapy can be prolonged for months and years, and only occasionally is it necessary to interrupt treatment because of unexplained disturbances of coagulation. Dicumarol overdosage will cause hemorrhage from the kidney, nose, bowel, skin, or into muscle, as well as subdurally and into brain. Although most of these accidents are not serious, vitamin K_1 should be administered immediately.

SURGERY. In recent years surgical management of the arterial obstruction in the neck and thorax has been used with increasing frequency employing thrombendarterectomy or bypass grafts. The region of the carotid sinus is most frequently amenable to such therapy, but operation must be carried out at the stage of carotid stenosis rather than total occlusion; otherwise secondary clot will have formed in the distal reaches of the artery from whence removal is impossible. Other sites suitable for surgical management include the origin of the vertebral arteries from the subclavians, and the common carotid, innominate, and subclavian trunks. Before operation the existence of the lesion and its extent must be determined by arteriography. Surgery is undertaken at the stage of transient ischemic attacks or early in the course of thrombosis-in-evolution. When total infarction has occurred, surgery will be ineffective even though patency of the vessel is restored. The early reports of surgical results are extremely promising —ischemic attacks are abolished, incipient strokes are halted, and the occurrence of another stroke is averted—but surgery is not without risk, and its place in the treatment of cerebrovascular diseases has not been fully determined. To be sure, in only a small minority of the total number of thrombotic strokes are the lesions situated extracranially and hence suitable for surgery.

CEREBRAL VASODILATORS. Despite experimental evidence that these agents increase the cerebral blood flow, as measured by the nitrous oxide method, they have not proved beneficial in careful studies in human stroke cases at the stage of transient ischemic attacks, thrombosis-in-evolution, or in the established stroke. This is true of nicotinic acid, Priscoline, alcohol, papaverine, and inhalation of 5 per cent carbon dioxide. A few clinical trials have indicated that histamine, aminophylline, and intraarterial papaverine have some merit. In opposition to the use of these methods is the suggestion that vasodilators are harmful rather than beneficial, since by lowering the systemic blood pressure the intracranial anastomotic flow may be reduced.

CERVICAL SYMPATHETIC BLOCK. This procedure fell into discard after careful clinical studies failed to confirm initial reports of beneficial effects. Its use was based on the suggestion that widespread vasoconstriction is precipitated by a vascular occlusion.

THROMBOLYTIC AGENTS. Presently, the efficacy of various preparations of fibrinolysin and profibrinolysin activator is being tested in cases of transient ischemia, thrombosis-in-evolution, and the established stroke.

Physical Therapy and Rehabilitation. Beginning within a few days, the joints of the paralyzed limbs should be passively carried through a full range of movement fifty times a day. Contracture (shortening of muscle) must be avoided, especially at the shoulder, elbow, and ankle. Pain, soreness, and aching in the paralyzed limbs may temporarily interfere with exercises. The patient can be placed in a chair after 2 weeks or so, depending on the severity of his illness. Nearly all hemiplegics can learn to walk again to some extent, usually within a 3- to 6-month period, and this should be a primary aim in rehabilitation. A short or long leg brace is often required. Speech therapy is of questionable value but should be tried. At least it is of value psychologically. Physical therapy seems not to benefit patients with cerebellar ataxia. As the hemiplegic patient improves and if mentality is preserved, instruction in the activities of daily living, using various special devices, can assist him in becoming at least partially independent in the home.

General Preventive Measures against Strokes and Vascular Disease. AVOIDING SITUATIONS IN WHICH STROKES ARE LIKELY TO OCCUR. (1) Particular care should be taken to maintain the systemic blood pressure, oxygenation, and intracranial blood flow during surgical procedures, especially in elderly patients; (2) hypotensive agents, whether given therapeutically or for diagnostic procedures, should be administered with great care; (3) in the elderly patient in whom deep sleep might help to precipitate cerebral ischemia, oversedation should be avoided; (4) systemic hypotension, severe anemia, and polycythemia should be treated promptly.

FACTORS WHICH DETERMINE ULTIMATE OUTCOME. The ultimate solution of the problem of cerebrovascular disease lies in more fundamental fields. Atherosclerosis and hypertension must be prevented or alleviated (see Chap. 246 for prophylaxis of atherosclerosis, and Chap. 245 for the treatment of hypertension). Another factor possibly of great importance in contributing to vascular disease is the smoking of cigarettes; the authors advise all patients with cerebral atherothrombotic disease to stop smoking. Hypercoagulability of the blood has been suggested as the explanation for the fact that some atherosclerotic patients are more disposed to thrombotic episodes than others. Correction of such an abnormality would be highly advantageous, but at present there is no reliable method of detecting intravascular hypercoagulability if such a disorder exists.

RECURRENT FOCAL CEREBRAL ISCHEMIA

It has already been pointed out that, when transient ischemic attacks precede a stroke, they stamp the process as thrombotic. Furthermore, neuropathologic studies indicate that these attacks are linked almost exclusively to atherosclerotic thrombosis. They belong therefore under the heading of cerebral thrombosis, but here they are discussed separately because of their importance clinically and therapeutically. Recurrent ischemic cerebral attacks consist of repeated transient episodes of focal cerebral disturbance, e.g., weakness, numbness, dizziness, etc., and are most commonly encountered in the days or weeks preceding the onset of a thrombotic stroke, occurring as a sort of a warning that disaster threatens. In recent years increasing attention has been directed to these attacks, with the purpose of averting the threatening stroke by administering anticoagulant drugs or performing surgical endarterectomy at the stage of prodromal symptoms. There would seem to be little doubt that they are due to transient focal ischemia, and they might be referred to as temporary strokes which fortunately reverse themselves. Corresponding to the higher incidence of atherosclerosis in hypertension and in the male population, about two-thirds of all patients with transient ischemic attacks are men and/or hypertensive.

Clinical Picture. Transient ischemic attacks can occur by themselves, or they may precede, accompany, or follow the development of a stroke. So far, it has not been possible to distinguish the early cases destined to do well from those in which a full-blown stroke will develop. Thrombosis of virtually any cerebral or cerebellar artery, deep or superficial, can be associated with transient ischemic attacks, e.g., common carotid, internal carotid, middle cerebral, anterior cerebral, ophthalmic, vertebral, basilar, posterior cerebral, the cerebellar arteries, and the penetrating branches to the deep structures of the basal ganglions and brain stem. If the posterior cerebral arteries are included in the vertebral-basilar system, ischemic episodes are slightly more common in that system than in the carotid.

The neurologic features of the transient episode indicate the territory or artery involved and are fragments borrowed from the stroke which often is approaching. In the carotid system the episodes commonly take the form of unilateral weakness or numbness of the side of the body opposite the lesion. The entire side may be involved, or the parts in various combinations: face and lips, or lips and fingers, fingers alone, hand and foot, etc. Other manifestations include aphasia, difficulty in calculation and other temporal-parietal-occipital disturbances (when the dominant hemisphere is involved), confusion, veering to one side, transient monocular blindness or blurring of vision, headache, and occasionally jerking or twitching mimicking a focal epileptic seizure. Lack of pulsation in the internal carotid artery in the neck or pharynx, reduced pressure in the appropriate central retinal artery, and a carotid bruit in the neck indicate carotid disease.

The clinical picture in the vertebral-basilar system is exceedingly diverse, since so much motor and sensory traffic is sustained by the blood carried in these vessels. Occurring in the most varied combinations, the following manifestations may be recognized (the more common ones are italicized):

weakness of part or all of one side of the body, or both sides; *numbness* of part or all of one side, or both sides, or crossed numbness (one side of face and opposite limbs); *dizziness, diplopia* (vertical or horizontal); dark vision, *blurred vision;* tunnel vision; partial or complete blindness; scintillating scotomas; pupillary change; ptosis; paralysis of gaze; *dysarthria; speechlessness; dysphagia; staggering gait;* veering to one side; and *headache.* Less common symptoms include noise or pounding in the ear or in the head, head or face pain, peculiar head sensations, vomiting, hiccups, memory lapse, confused behavior, drowsiness, unconsciousness (rare), impaired hearing, deafness, a feeling of movement of a part, hemiballismus, peduncular hallucinosis, forced deviation of the eyes, sweating, and facial redness.

It is not always easy to identify the territory affected. However, the occurrence of receptive or sensory aphasia always points to the carotid system, as does monocular blindness with or without contralateral weakness or numbness. The hallmarks of vertebral-basilar involvement are (1) bilateral weakness and/or numbness, i.e., a disturbance of the long motor or sensory tracts bilaterally, (2) involvement of the infranuclear portion of one or more cranial nerves, (3) disturbance of cerebellum and tegmental structures, subserving equilibrium, ocular mechanisms, posture, and autonomic functions. Perioral numbness is not an infrequent complaint, and the patient may not be certain whether it is equally bilateral, bilateral with unilateral preponderance, or mostly unilateral with spread slightly to the other side of the midline. Whirling dizziness and diplopia are of particular importance in indicating a brain stem localization, and they are rarely if ever associated with occlusion of the carotid system. The most frequent complaints in our material were dizziness, numbness, diplopia, dysarthria, staggering, hemiparesis, quadriparesis, dim vision, headache, pain in the head, and scintillating scotomas in approximately that order. Unilateral weakness and unilateral numbness as isolated phenomena are difficult to localize, since they can occur in both carotid and basilar occlusion.

The following manifestations are either very rare or occur not at all in ischemic attacks: unconsciousness, frank convulsive movements, fecal or urinary incontinence, tongue-biting, and the manifestations of temporal lobe seizures.

Transient ischemic attacks last a few seconds up to several hours, the most common duration being a few seconds up to 5 to 10 min. It is uncommon for recurrent discrete attacks to last more than 30 min. There may be only a few attacks or several hundred. Between attacks, the neurologic examination may disclose no abnormalities. A stroke may ensue after the second episode or may be postponed until hundreds of attacks have occurred over a period of weeks or months. Not infrequently the attacks gradually cease and no important paralysis occurs, a fact which makes any form of therapy difficult to evaluate. The attacks may all take approximately the same pattern or they may vary considerably in detail, although maintaining the same basic pattern. For example, weakness or numbness may involve fingers and face in some episodes and fingers only in others; or dizziness alone may occur in some attacks, while in others diplopia is added to the picture. In basilar artery disease each side of the body may be affected alternately. All the involved parts may be affected simultaneously, or a definite march or spread from one region to another can occur in a period of 10 to 60 sec, or even a few minutes; e.g., numbness may spread from the hand to the face, or the reverse. The individual attack may cease abruptly or fade gradually.

Mechanism. The onset of attacks in some patients is clearly related to standing up after lying or sitting. In general, attacks are likely to occur when the patient is up and around rather than lying down, but in many cases the episodes bear no relation to position or activity. They have been encountered in relation to exercise, exertion, emotional outbursts of anger or joy, and during bouts of coughing. Transient symptoms present on awakening from sleep usually indicate that a stroke is in the offing.

Ophthalmoscopic observations of the retinal vessels made during episodes of transient monocular blindness show either arrest of the blood flow in the retinal arteries and breaking up of the venous column to form the well-known "boxcar" pattern or white material temporarily blocking the retinal arteries. This indicates that in ischemic attacks a temporary complete or relatively complete cessation of blood flow occurs locally, possibly with associated microembolism.

The pathogenesis of transient ischemic attacks is still not clear. In the past they have been attributed to cerebral vasospasm or to transient episodes of systemic arterial hypotension with resulting compromise of the intracranial circulation. Neither of these factors has been established. Although dropping the blood pressure to 90 or even 80 mm Hg by tilting the patient upright on a tilt table may cause electroencephalographic changes, it has not in the authors' experience reproduced the attacks. Vasodilator drugs have been without effect. There is good evidence that the attacks are abolished by anticoagulant drugs, but the mechanism of this is not known. Whatever their exact cause, they are closely related to vascular stenosis due to atherosclerosis and thrombosis. A proper recognition of the transient ischemic episode is of importance, since the use of anticoagulant drugs may prove of value in warding off an oncoming stroke.

The differential diagnosis of recurrent cerebral ischemic attacks raises special problems. The following conditions must be differentiated: cerebral seizures (epileptic seizures), Ménière's syndrome, paralytic migraine, Stokes-Adams attacks, hypersensitive carotid sinus reflex, transient global amnesia, insulin reactions, complaints associated with anxiety and depression, akinetic falling spells of the aged, and recurrent cerebral embolism.

Frank motor *convulsions* rarely if ever occur in ischemic attacks. The patient may report a feeling of movement, distortion, drawing, jumping, or jerking, but an isolated frank focal seizure has not been encountered. On the other hand, a cerebral seizure rarely if ever displays as its only manifestation a temporary paralysis of a limb or of one side of the body. Unconsciousness is rare in ischemic attacks, and its occurrence even in only a few attacks indicates another diagnosis (seizure, Stokes-Adams attacks, etc.). Incontinence of bowel and bladder, tongue biting, cyanosis, and residual sleepiness or muscle soreness are indicative of a seizure rather than an ischemic episode. In the sensory sphere, the distinction between ischemic episodes and seizures is less clear, for numbness or scintillating visual phenomena are seen in both conditions, and therefore in making a differentiation one must rely on the presence of associated phenomena (dizziness, diplopia, etc.). When numbness appears simultaneously in face, hand, and leg, i.e., when there is no "march," ischemia rather than a seizure is probably responsible. When a sensory march occurs, it will not serve to distinguish the two, for while it is more characteristic of a seizure, it may also occur in ischemic episodes, being then very slow.

The type of dizziness associated with brain stem ischemia has no characteristics which allow it to be distinguished from that seen in *Ménière's syndrome* or labyrinthitis. Therefore, in making a diagnosis one depends on the presence of associated symptoms and signs. It is a simple matter to decide that the dizziness is of central origin when there are other evidences of brain stem involvement, by history or on neurologic examination: diplopia, numbness, weakness, dysphagia, dysarthria, cerebellar ataxia, vertical nystagmus, persistent horizontal nystagmus, etc. On the other hand, the isolated presence of the triad—recurrent dizziness, tinnitus, and chronic deafness (i.e., signs of both auditory and vestibular involvement)—is almost certain evidence of Ménière's syndrome. However, in the early stages the pictures at times resemble each other closely, and only an especially thorough search will reveal signs indicating that the disorder is due to ischemia of the brain stem. Tinnitus of a constant hissing or ringing type is a rare complaint in brain stem vascular disease. When dizziness is the sole symptom in an elderly person, it is often impossible to make an accurate diagnosis, and only after observing the patient for a period of time will the nature of the underlying disease be disclosed. Finally, it must be remembered that since both basilar artery disease and Ménière's syndrome are common conditions the two may coexist.

The visual, sensory, and motor phenomena which precede the headache in some cases of *migraine* bear a close resemblance to ischemic manifestations, but since migraine originates in early life, only occasionally does its differentiation from ischemic attacks pose a problem. When vascular disease has its onset during the period of life when migraine is prevalent, the two may be confused until the history is carefully taken. Occasionally a migrainous paralytic aura returns after a headache-free interval of 10 to 20 years. It has already been pointed out that headache, at times of great intensity, frequently accompanies cerebral thrombosis; therefore in the elderly person the occurrence for the first time of periodic headache associated with scintillations or numbness should always suggest atherothrombosis rather than migraine. *Stokes-Adams attacks* and *hypersensitivity* of the *carotid sinus reflex* cause "collapsing spells" with unconsciousness, confusion, and jerking, but almost never do they produce focal neurologic manifestations such as numbness, weakness, diplopia, etc. Difficulty in differentiation of these conditions will arise only when the clinical details of the episode are not available, and usually a careful minute-by-minute description of the attack will enable the correct diagnosis to be reached. Only in an occasional case of basilar artery insufficiency will an ischemic episode result in unconsciousness, usually accompanied by other symptoms such as weakness, numbness, blindness, or dysarthria. In *akinetic falling spells of the aged,* a rather vague entity, the patient falls unconscious without convulsive movements, color change, or alteration in pulse, blood pressure, or respiration. Within a few seconds or a minute or two consciousness is restored.

Occasionally ischemic attacks may be confused with tussive syncope, multiple sclerosis, ulnar neuropathy, carpal tunnel syndrome, overhydration (hyponatremia), cataplexy with narcolepsy, brachial discomfort with hiatus hernia, cervical disk disease, severe postural hypotension, unusual symptomatology in angina pectoris, hemangioma of brain stem (especially in pregnancy), recurrent pulmonary embolism, etc.

Cerebral embolism is frequently suggested as an explanation for recurrent cerebrovascular episodes. However, this seems unlikely if all the attacks are of approximately identical pattern, for successive emboli coming from a distance could not be expected to enter the same arterial branch. Moreover, the involved cerebral tissue would be at least partially damaged, leaving some residual signs. When only a single transient episode has occurred, the factor of recurrence does not assist in the diagnosis, and cerebral embolism must then be strongly considered. Single transitory episodes and multiple episodes of different pattern must be clearly distinguished from recurrent attacks of the same pattern.

Treatment. The therapy of transient ischemic attacks has already been discussed under cerebral thrombosis (p. 1771), where it was pointed out that anticoagulants or surgical endarterectomy usually stop the attacks and prevent indefinitely the onset of a threatening stroke. In many patients the attacks cease spontaneously and therapy can be withheld if the episodes are few and spaced at long intervals. However, anticoagulants are indicated if the attacks are becoming more frequent, more severe, or of longer duration, or if each attack no longer clears away completely and a persistent neurologic deficit is accumulating.

Other measures that have been recommended include administration of phenobarbital, papaverine, or nicotinic acid, inhalation of 5 per cent carbon dioxide, breathing into a paper bag, and stellate block or cervical sympathectomy, but none of these has proved effective under careful clinical testing. On several occasions the authors have been impressed with the salutary effect of having the patient stop smoking cigarettes. For the more general therapeutic measures applicable in these cases, see pp. 1771 and 1772.

OTHER CAUSES OF CEREBRAL THROMBOSIS (Infarction)

It will be seen from the list at the beginning of this chapter that there are few causes of cerebral thrombosis other than atherosclerosis. There are fewer still that are important in the stroke picture. In some of those included the mechanism is ischemia without actual thrombosis. *Venous thrombosis* is a rather uncommon condition and rarely mimics a cerebrovascular stroke. Arising in relation to extracranial and intracranial sepsis, surgical operations, parturition, and chronic wasting illnesses particularly in children, it can cause a relatively mild neurologic illness with raised intracranial pressure, headache, visual obscurations, and focal seizures, or on the other hand, it can lead to extensive cerebral infarction and hemorrhage, with grave neurologic manifestations.

Systemic hypotension usually results in unconsciousness (syncope) without focal motor and sensory signs, but in the presence of vascular narrowing from any cause, weakness or numbness may be precipitated, and if the state of vascular collapse persists for a sufficient length of time, local infarction will occur distal to the point of stenosis. It has already been mentioned that transient ischemic attacks and persistent strokes often develop under circumstances which suggest that a fall of the systemic blood pressure was the precipitating factor. Hypotension occurs in "simple faint," acute blood loss, myocardial infarction, Stokes-Adams syndrome, traumatic and surgical shock, cardiac arrest or anesthetic accident during surgery, hypersensitivity of the carotid sinus reflex, and in the several types of postural hypotension [idiopathic, post-sympathectomy, tabetic, diabetic, with autonomic blocking agents, with reserpine (Serpasil), and on getting up and around after surgical operations].

Arteriography occasionally results in cerebral infarction. In some cases this is because of cerebral thrombosis, but the pathogenesis of other cases requires further study. Arteritis is no longer a common cause of cerebral thrombosis, at least in North America, owing to the present satisfactory treatment of syphilis. This is to be contrasted with the period up to 10 years ago when meningovascular syphilis had to be seriously considered in every stroke case; "hemiplegia in the young" especially was strongly indicative of syphilis. Necrotizing or granulomatous arteritis, whether limited to the cerebral vessels or occurring as part of a polyarteritis, has usually produced a slowly progressive neurologic deficit and has only rarely mimicked a stroke. Idiopathic giant-cell arteritis involving the large arteries arising from the aortic arch is a rare cause of unilateral or bilateral carotid occlusion but must be kept in mind. It appears to be much more common in young women in Japan, the aforementioned Takayasu's syndrome or "pulseless disease." Cranial arteritis or temporal arteritis is almost always limited to the extracranial arteries except for the small vessels supplying the optic and oculomotor nerves. Unfortunately, in over 50 per cent of cases permanent blindness or a severe impairment of vision results. When the process has involved the internal or common carotid arteries, it has usually not caused a stroke (see p. 1899, Chap. 300).

Polycythemia, sickle-cell disease, and thrombotic thrombopenia are stated to be causes of cerebral thrombosis, but further study of the matter is required. A dissecting aortic aneurysm may involve the large vessels arising from the arch and result in carotid occlusion and hemiplegia, a concomitant fall in systemic blood pressure probably contributing to the picture. Carotid occlusion may be the result of direct trauma to the neck, or it may be precipitated by a "closed head injury," sometimes of a seemingly trivial nature. Hypoxia usually produces a diffuse destruction of neurones rather than frank infarction, but bilateral softening of the globus pallidus is a classical feature. Tentorial and subfalcial herniation and sometimes a cerebellar pressure cone can cause infarction by compression of the posterior cerebral, anterior cerebral, and inferior cerebellar arteries, respectively. Under the rare types of infarction, it should be mentioned that carotid occlusion has been described following tonsillectomy, in association with cavernous sinus thrombophlebitis, and the trigeminal ganglionitis of herpes zoster. Also, a previously transient and harmless migrainous aura is occasionally transformed into a persistent deficit, presumably because of infarction as the result of excessive ischemia. This complication most frequently takes the form of a homonymous hemianopia. Finally, a category for cerebral infarction of undetermined cause is included, for it must be admitted that in some cases even at neuropathologic examination it is impossible to determine the exact cause of an infarct.

Omitted here is Binswanger's chronic progressive subcortical encephalitis, a rare disease of cerebral white matter tentatively attributed by Binswanger to atherosclerosis. The status of the disease is uncertain at present, and further investigation of the problem is warranted before the disease can be accepted as a separate entity.

CEREBRAL EMBOLISM

In most cases of cerebral embolism, the embolic material consists of a fragment which has broken away from a thrombus within the heart. Embolism due to fat, tumor cells, or air is a rare occurrence and seldom enters into the differential diagnosis of strokes. The embolus usually becomes arrested at a bifurcation or other site of narrowing of the lumen. Ischemic infarction usually follows and is pale, red, or mixed, red infarction as pointed out earlier nearly always indicating embolism. Any region of the brain may be affected, but the territory of the middle cerebral artery is most frequently involved. The two hemispheres are approximately equally affected. Large embolic masses will block larger vessels (sometimes the carotids in the neck), while tiny fragments may reach vessels as small as 0.2 mm, in which case the resultant infarct might be so small as almost to escape detection at autopsy. The exact behavior of embolic material is not fully understood. Often, it remains arrested and plugs the lumen solidly, but in many cases it breaks up into fragments which enter smaller vessels or even disappear completely, so that careful pathologic examination fails to reveal their final location. The anatomic diagnosis must then be made by inference, e.g., the absence of a vascular occlusion at the proper site to explain the infarct, the absence of atherosclerosis or other cause for thrombosis in

Table 284-3. CAUSES OF CEREBRAL EMBOLISM

I. Cardiac origin
  A. Atrial fibrillation and other arrhythmias (with rheumatic, atherosclerotic, hypertensive, or congenital heart disease)
  B. Myocardial infarction with mural thrombus
  C. Acute and subacute bacterial endocarditis
  D. Heart disease without arrhythmia or mural thrombus (mitral stenosis, etc.)
  E. Complications of cardiac surgery
  F. Nonbacterial thrombotic (marantic) endocardial vegetations
  G. Paradoxical embolism with congenital heart disease
  H. Trichinosis
II. Noncardiac origin
  A. Atherosclerosis of aorta and carotid arteries (mural thrombus, atheromatous material)
  B. From sites of cerebral artery thrombosis (basilar, vertebral, middle cerebral)
  C. Thrombus in pulmonary veins
  D. Fat
  E. Tumor
  F. Air
  G. Complications of neck and thoracic surgery
III. Undetermined origin

the cerebral vessel, a ready source of embolus, infarcts in other organs such as kidney and spleen, the occurrence of hemorrhagic infarction, and last, but not least, the clinical history.

Because of the rapidity with which occlusion develops in embolism, there is not much time for collateral influx to become established. Thus sparing of territory distal to the site of occlusion is not so common as in thrombosis. However, all the ischemia-modifying factors mentioned under thrombosis are still operative and will influence the size, shape, and severity of the infarct.

Brain embolism is essentially a manifestation of heart disease. Many kinds of heart disease can be associated with embolism. The commonest direct cause is *chronic atrial fibrillation* due to atherosclerotic or rheumatic heart disease, the source of the embolus being mural thrombus deposited within the atrial appendage. Atrial fibrillation due to other types of heart disease can, of course, also lead to embolism, e.g., hypertensive, congenital, thyrotoxic, syphilitic, etc. Embolism probably occurs also during paroxysmal atrial fibrillation or flutter, but there is need for further exact documentation of such cases. Mural thrombus deposited on the damaged endocardium overlying a myocardial infarct is the second most frequent source of cerebral emboli. Emboli can also arise from atrial thrombus associated with severe mitral stenosis without atrial fibrillation. Cardiac surgery, especially valvoplasty, may disseminate fragments of

thrombus or particles of a calcified valve leaflet. Subendocardial fibroelastosis, idiopathic myocardial hypertrophy, and cardiac tumors are rare causes of embolism.

The vegetations of acute and subacute bacterial endocarditis, being infected, give rise to septic embolism, which results in several different pathologic pictures in the brain. In some cases the infarcts (they are usually multiple) do not differ from those due to bland emboli; in others, tiny septic infarcts develop or, as in acute bacterial endocarditis, there may be miliary abscesses into which a small amount of hemorrhage may occur (focal embolic encephalitis) and even meningitis. Mycotic aneurysm, now seen infrequently, is another complication of septic embolism and may be a source of intracerebral or subarachnoid hemorrhage.

Marantic or nonbacterial endocarditis occasionally causes cerebral embolism and can produce a most baffling clinical picture, especially when associated, as it often is, with carcinomatosis. The diagnosis can only be suspected in life. Paradoxic embolism can occur when an abnormal communication exists between the right and left sides of the heart, or when both ventricles communicate with the aorta. Thus embolic material arising in the veins of the lower extremity or, indeed, anywhere in the systemic venous tree can bypass the pulmonary circulation and reach the cerebral vessels.

The following sources of embolic material are less frequent or more difficult to prove: (1) Mural thrombus, deposited upon ulcerated atheroma in the arch of the aorta or in the carotid arteries, may break loose and find its way into brain arteries. Massage of the carotid sinus, a favorite site for atherosclerosis, may dislodge mural thrombus, with the production of a hemiplegia. This is one of the reasons why carotid massage should always be carried out gently. (2) Atheromatous material may be washed out of a large plaque in the aorta or carotid arteries and carried distally into the branches of the cerebral tree. (3) The pulmonary veins are a source of cerebral emboli, as indicated by the occurrence of cerebral abscesses in association with pulmonary suppurative processes and by the high incidence of carcinoma of the brain secondary to pulmonary deposits. (4) Surgery of the neck and thorax can be complicated by cerebral embolism. A rare type is that which follows thyroidectomy, in which thrombosis in the stump of the superior thyroid artery extends proximally until a section of it, protruding into the lumen of the carotid, is carried away into the cerebral arteries.

Cerebral embolism must always have occurred when secondary tumor is deposited in the brain, and cerebral embolism must regularly accompany septicemia. However, it is rare for a mass of tumor cells or bacteria to be large enough to occlude a cerebral artery and produce the picture of a stroke. Nevertheless tumor embolism has been reported secondary to cardiac myomyxomas and occasionally with other tumors. It must be distinguished from the marantic endocarditis and embolism which occasionally complicate carcinomatosis. Embolism in the course of septicemia usually means that a vegetative endocarditis is present with thrombus formation. Cerebral fat embolism is usually related to trauma. As a rule the emboli are minute and widely dispersed, giving rise to multiple petechial hemorrhages in white matter; accordingly the clinical picture is usually not focal, as in a stroke. Cerebral air embolism is a rare complication of criminal abortion or of cervical and thoracic operations and was formerly encountered as a complication of pneumothorax therapy.

Not infrequently at autopsy the diagnosis of cerebral embolism is made with full justification without finding a source. The same is true of embolism elsewhere in the body. Possibly the routine search for a thrombotic nidus is not sufficiently thorough, and small thrombi in the atrial appendage, the pulmonary veins, or the endocardium between the papillary muscles of the heart may be overlooked. Nevertheless, in some cases studied most carefully, no source of embolic material has been discovered.

Clinical Picture. Of all strokes, those due to cerebral embolism develop most rapidly. "Like a bolt from the blue," the full-blown picture evolves within several seconds or a minute, exemplifying most strikingly the temporal profile of a stroke. The neurologic deficit comes in a single sudden attack, scarcely ever in stuttering fashion. As a rule, there are no warning episodes whatsoever. These statements are possibly too stringent, for in occasional cases the picture may take several hours to develop or a transient episode may precede the final arrival of the stroke. However, any emphasis on these few exceptions is entirely misleading. The embolus strikes at any time of the day or night. When the stroke develops during sleep, its exact mode of development will not be known.

The neurologic picture will depend on the artery involved and where the obstruction lies. The syndromes related to each cerebrovascular territory are the same as those outlined under thrombosis (see p. 1751). A large embolus may plug the internal carotid artery or the stem of the middle cerebral artery, producing a severe hemiplegia. Or the embolus may be smaller and pass into one of the branches of the middle cerebral artery, producing a strikingly focal disorder: motor aphasia, a monoplegia (or part thereof), a receptive type of aphasia with little or no motor paralysis, or a sensorimotor paralysis with little or no involvement of the supersensory zone. It is important to realize

that an embolus in its passage along an artery may produce a severe neurologic deficit which is only temporary and which clears up almost as quickly as it came, as the embolus finally passes into a small branch supplying a relatively silent part of the hemisphere. In other words, embolism is one of the causes of a single evanescent stroke and a not uncommon one. Also it can give rise to multiple transient attacks of differing pattern. It has already been pointed out that recurrent transient ischemic attacks of the same pattern are not likely to be embolic, since successive emboli would hardly lodge at identical sites. Embolic material entering the vertebral-basilar system occasionally lodges in the vertebral artery just below its union with the basilar, but more often it traverses the vertebral and also the basilar which is larger and is not held up until it reaches the upper bifurcation. If arrested here, it abruptly produces deep coma and total paralysis. More often the embolus enters one or other posterior cerebral artery, or both, and by infarcting the visual cortex, causes a unilateral or bilateral homonymous hemianopia. Embolic infarction of the undersurface of the cerebellum is extremely common, whereas embolic material rarely enters the penetrating branches of the pons.

The general neurologic disturbance associated with embolic strokes is not significantly different from that seen in thrombotic cases, and the reader is referred to the description of the changes in consciousness, respiration, etc., on p. 1768. Again the patient may have a most devastating hemiplegia and yet be quite alert. Headache is not uncommon.

Although the abruptness with which the stroke develops and the lack of prodromal symptoms point strongly to embolism, it is the total clinical picture upon which the diagnosis is based. If hemorrhage is ruled out, there remains only thrombosis to be excluded. The presence of atrial fibrillation, a history of myocardial infarction (recent or in the preceding months), or the occurrence of embolism to other regions of the body all support the diagnosis of embolism. Embolism merits the most careful consideration in young persons in whom atherosclerosis is rather unlikely. Not infrequently the first sign of myocardial infarction is the occurrence of embolism; therefore, it is advisable that *an electrocardiogram be made in all cerebrovascular strokes of uncertain origin.*

Acute and subacute bacterial endocarditis do not usually present as a stroke due to infarction, although this happens occasionally. The cardiac signs of endocarditis, anemia, splenomegaly, and often a pleocytosis in the cerebrospinal fluid should point to the correct diagnosis.

The diagnosis of the other causes of cerebral embolism—cardiac surgery, neck surgery, pulmonary vein thrombosis, marantic endocarditis, paradoxic embolism, tumor, fat, and air—need not be enlarged upon here.

Laboratory Findings. The description under thrombosis (p. 1768) applies for the most part to embolism except in so far as hemorrhagic infarction and septic embolism (focal embolic encephalitis) are concerned. Cerebral embolism in some 30 per cent of cases produces a hemorrhagic infarct, which in most instances does *not* cause the cerebrospinal fluid to be bloody. However, in some excessively hemorrhagic infarcts, the fluid may be grossly bloody and contain as high as 10,000 or more red cells per cu mm. In the milder cases of hemorrhagic infarction, a slight xanthochromia (grade 1 to 3 on the scale of 1 to 10) may appear after a few days. The possibility that an embolic infarct is unusually bloody underlines the danger of administering anticoagulants routinely in cases of cerebral embolism without a careful examination of the cerebrospinal fluid. Also, it is the single exception to the rule that blood in the spinal fluid is unequivocal evidence that the stroke is due primarily to a hemorrhage.

In septic embolism resulting from subacute bacterial endocarditis the white blood cells in the cerebrospinal fluid are increased, usually numbering up to 200 per cu mm and occasionally reaching several hundred; the proportion of lymphocytes and polymorphonuclears varies with the acuteness of the septic process. There may also be several hundred or more red blood cells, and a faint xanthochromia is often present. However, a pleocytosis is not invariably seen in this condition. The protein values are elevated, and the sugar content is within normal limits. No bacteria are seen or obtained by culture. In acute bacterial endocarditis there may be either the cerebrospinal fluid formula of subacute endocarditis or a frank purulent meningitis.

Course and Prognosis. The remarks made concerning the *immediate prognosis* in cerebral thrombosis apply as well here. Life is threatened in patients who have massive cerebral swelling, inadequate airway, and respiratory or urinary infection. As a rule, all but the most aggravated cases survive the initial insult. Massive brain stem infarction as a result of basilar embolism is almost always fatal. The *eventual prognosis* as to survival is determined by the occurrence of further emboli and the gravity of the underlying illness—cardiac failure, rheumatic heart disease, myocardial infarction, bacterial endocarditis, malignant growth, etc. The threat of an early recurrence of embolism is very real, and it is not uncommon to have the second embolus strike within a few days or weeks of the first. The urgency of anticoagulant therapy is thereby emphasized. The *eventual prognosis* regarding the neurologic deficit is not different from that given for cerebral thrombosis (p. 1769). The

fact that an embolic episode may last only minutes or hours before clearing up should be stressed, especially in estimating the effect of any therapeutic measure.

Treatment. The first three phases of therapy—(1) general medical management in the acute phase, (2) measures directed to restoring the circulation, and (3) rehabilitation—are much the same as described under cerebral thrombosis (see p. 1770). Attempted embolectomy at the bifurcation of the common carotid artery has usually failed but should be considered. If pulsation in the temporal artery in front of the ear is present, it means the embolus is not at that bifurcation but has passed up into the internal carotid system and embolectomy will probably be unsuccessful. Rarely embolectomy of the middle cerebral artery has been attempted. Recently, fibrinolysin therapy has been tried but with conflicting results. In the field of prophylaxis there is strong evidence that the use of long-term anticoagulant therapy is effective in the prevention of embolism in cases of atrial fibrillation and myocardial infarction. After cerebral embolism has occurred, the question arises as to the necessity of delaying anticoagulant therapy for several days to avoid precipitating bleeding into a hemorrhagic infarct. It is the authors' practice always to perform a lumbar puncture first in order to rule out gross hemorrhage from the infarct. If the cerebrospinal fluid is clear, the authors proceed with anticoagulant therapy, since there is the constant danger of another embolus breaking away from the heart. We have not encountered a case in which the use of anticoagulant drugs has seemed to increase the degree of hemorrhage within a hemorrhagic infarct, and indications are that such therapy is relatively safe. Rare exceptions to this statement may be expected. The use of anticoagulant therapy in cases of acute myocardial infarction, including those judged to be in the "good risk" category, is advisable. In cerebral embolism associated with subacute bacterial endocarditis, anticoagulant therapy is usually held to be contraindicated because of the danger of intracranial bleeding, but this viewpoint is not well founded. Nevertheless caution is advisable in this matter, and it is preferable to rely on a rapid sterilization of the blood stream.

Valvoplasty and amputation of the atrial appendage have substantially reduced the incidence of embolism in rheumatic heart disease. The need for special care in preventing emboli from entering the carotid arteries during the performance of cardiac valvoplasty is appreciated by all thoracic surgeons.

INTRACRANIAL HEMORRHAGE

Although more than a dozen causes of intracranial hemorrhage have been listed, the first two, hypertensive intracerebral hemorrhage and ruptured saccular aneurysm, are much more important than the others and account for most of the hemorrhages which give rise to the clinical picture of a stroke. Duret hemorrhages, hypertensive encephalopathy, and idiopathic brain purpura will not simulate a stroke and are included only for the sake of completeness.

Hypertensive Intracerebral Hemorrhage

Hypertensive intracerebral hemorrhage is the ordinary, well-recognized brain hemorrhage. Although sometimes the levels of blood pressure are only in the range of 160 to 170/90, in most cases they are much higher. Hypertensive hemorrhage occurs within brain tissue, and rupture of the arteries lying in the subarachnoid space is practically unknown, apart from aneurysm. It is a mistake to think of hypertensive hemorrhage as arising from the large arteries at the base of the brain. The extravasation which results from rupture of an artery forms a roughly circular or oval mass, which grows in volume as the bleeding continues. Adjacent brain tissue is displaced and compressed. If the hemorrhage is large, midline structures are displaced to the opposite side and vital centers are compromised, leading to coma and death. Rupture or seepage into the ventricular system usually occurs, and the spinal fluid becomes bloody in more than 90 per cent of cases. A hemorrhage of this type almost never ruptures directly into the subarachnoid space through the cerebral cortex, and the blood reaches the subarachnoid spinal fluid via the ventricular system. When the hemorrhage is small and placed at a distance from the ventricles, the cerebrospinal fluid may remain clear even on repeated examinations.

Extravasated blood undergoes a series of changes beginning with phagocytosis at the outer rim producing a brown-orange zone of hemosiderin-filled macrophages. The mass gradually decreases in size, and after a period of some 2 to 6 months only an orange-stained cleft is left at the site of the hemorrhage.

Hemorrhages might be classified as massive, small, slit, and petechial. "Massive" refers to huge hemorrhages several centimeters in diameter; "small" to those 1 to 2 cm in diameter; "slit" applies to a special type of hypertensive hemorrhage which lies subcortically at the junction of white and gray matter and which in the healing stage becomes narrowed to an orange slit.

In order of frequency, the commonest sites for hypertensive hemorrhage are (1) the putamen and adjacent internal capsule (50 per cent of cases), (2) thalamus, (3) cerebellar hemisphere, (4) pons, and (5) various parts of the central white matter (frontal lobe, corona radiata, etc., probably exten-

Table 284-4. CAUSES OF INTRACRANIAL HEMORRHAGE
(Including Intracerebral, Subarachnoid, Ventricular, and Rarely Subdural)

1. Hypertensive intracerebral hemorrhage
2. Ruptured saccular aneurysm
3. Ruptured angioma
4. Trauma including posttraumatic delayed apoplexy
5. Hemorrhagic disorders: leukemia, aplastic anemia, thrombopenic purpura, liver disease, complication of anticoagulant therapy, hyperfibrinolysis, hypofibrinogenemia, hemophilia, Christmas disease
6. Undetermined cause (normal blood pressure and no angioma)
7. Hemorrhage into primary and secondary brain tumors
8. Septic embolism, mycotic aneurysm
9. With hemorrhagic infarction, arterial or venous
10. Hypertensive encephalopathy
11. Idiopathic brain purpura
12. Secondary brain-stem hemorrhage
13. With inflammatory disease of the arteries and veins
14. Miscellaneous rare types: after vasopressor drugs, upon exertion, during arteriography, during painful urologic examination, as a late complication of early-life carotid occlusion, complication of carotid-cavernous arteriovenous fistula, with anoxemia, migraine, teratomatous malformations. (Acute inclusion body encephalitis produces xanthochromia and up to 2,000 red blood cells or more in the cerebrospinal fluid; acute necrotizing hemorrhagic encephalopathy may be associated with up to 100 red blood cells in the cerebrospinal fluid; tularemia and snake venom poisoning may cause bloody cerebrospinal fluid.)

sions from the putamen). The vessel involved is usually a penetrating artery. The nature of the vascular lesion which leads to arterial rupture is not known, and, indeed, the site of the rupture has not often been identified. Atherosclerosis is held by many to be a factor, but there is no proof for this view, and hemorrhages are encountered in the absence of grossly visible atherosclerosis. Small aneurysmal dilatations were reported by Charcot and Bouchard to be the basis for the rupture. They may be responsible for hemorrhage in some instances, but their occurrence only in arterioles and frequently in the cerebral cortex makes it unlikely that they explain the majority of massive cerebral hemorrhages. Hyalinosis and necrotizing change in the small arteries due to hypertension have also been described as the precursor of hemorrhage. Another hypothesis attributes the hemorrhage to a confluence of myriads of smaller diapedetic hemorrhages rather than a single extravasation, but this is entirely without grounds and represents a confusion of hemorrhagic infarction and massive hemorrhage.

Clinical Picture. The clinical picture conforms accurately to the temporal profile of a cerebrovascular stroke, viz., it has an abrupt onset and rather rapid evolution. The stroke usually evolves gradually and steadily over an appreciable length of time, taking minutes, hours, or occasionally days (average of 1 to 6 hr) to reach its peak, depending on the speed of bleeding. Usually there are no recognizable warning or prodromal symptoms, the patient being stricken "out of the blue." Often the patient has been astonishingly well and headache, dizziness, and epistaxis have not occurred with any consistency as prodromal symptoms. There is no sex or age predilection except that the younger are usually spared. In the great majority of cases, the hemorrhage comes on while the patient is up and active, and onset during sleep is a great rarity. Hypertension is by definition always present, and the elevation is maintained early in the course of the stroke or may even rise higher, so that the existence of hypertension will be easily established when the patient is first examined. Hypertension is usually of the "essential" type, but other causes must always be considered—renal disease, toxemia of pregnancy, pheochromocytoma, ACTH overdosage, injection of excessive amounts of epinephrine, and rarely, violent exertion or an intense emotional experience. Cardiomegaly is usually present.

There is usually only one episode of hemorrhage, and recurrence of bleeding from the same site, as occurs in cases of saccular aneurysm, is not encountered. Once bleeding has become arrested, rebleeding in the near future, that is, after the first few days, is not to be anticipated. Once blood is spilled into the tissues, it is removed only slowly, over a period of weeks and months, during which time symptoms and signs persist. Hence neurologic deficit is never transitory in intracerebral hemorrhage, as it so often is in thrombosis and embolism and, for the same reason, rapid fluctuations in the neurologic deficit from one examination to another are not to be expected.

The neurologic signs and symptoms vary with the site and size of the extravasation. The commonest picture is that associated with a *putaminal hemorrhage* in which the adjacent internal capsule is implicated. The patient complains of something going awry within the head. In a few minutes the face sags on one side, speech becomes slurred or aphasic, the arm and leg gradually weaken, and the eyes tend to deviate away from the side of the paretic limbs. A carefully taken history often reveals that these events occurred gradually over a period of 5 to 30 min. This type of evolution is virtually diagnostic of intracerebral bleeding. Gradually the paralysis worsens, the affected limbs become flaccid, pinprick is not appreciated, a Babinski sign appears, speaking becomes impossible, and confusion gives way to stupor. In the worst cases,

signs of upper brain stem compression appear—coma, Babinski sign bilaterally, deep, irregular or intermittent respiration and dilated fixed pupils.

Thalamic hemorrhage of moderate size also produces a hemiplegia or hemiparesis via pressure on the adjacent internal capsule. The sensory deficit equals or outstrips the motor weakness. Dysphasia may be present with lesions of the dominant side and apractognosia on the nondominant. A homonymous field defect if present usually clears in a few days. Thalamic hemorrhage by virtue of its extension medially and into subthalamus causes a series of ocular disturbances, including paralysis of vertical gaze, forced deviation of the eyes downward, inequality of pupils, with absence of light reaction, skew deviation with the eye opposite the hemorrhage being displaced downward and medially, ipsilateral ptosis and miosis, absence of convergence, an assortment of lateral gaze abnormalities (paresis or pseudoparesis of the sixth nerve), retraction nystagmus, and tucking of the eyelids. Another unusual sign is so-called peduncular hallucinosis. Neck retraction may be prominent. Hemorrhage into the nondominant thalamus is liable to produce mutism.

Cerebellar hemorrhage usually develops over a period of several hours and loss of consciousness at the onset is almost unknown. Repeated vomiting is a hallmark of cerebellar hemorrhage alone with occipital headache, vertigo, and inability to walk or stand. In the acute illness there may be little or no evidence of cerebellar disease and only a minority of cases show nystagmus or cerebellar ataxia of the limbs, although these signs must always be sought for. Contralateral hemiplegia and facial weakness do not occur. Ocular signs are prominent including small pupils which continue to react until very late in the illness, slight inequality of the pupils, paralysis of conjugate lateral gaze to the side of the lesion, forced deviation of the eyes, palsy or pseudopalsy of the sixth nerve, "ocular bobbing," blepharospasm, involuntary closure of one eye, skew deviation, and maintenance of vertical eye movements. Occasionally at the onset there is a quadriplegia with preservation of consciousness or a spastic paraparesis. Plantar reflexes are flexor early, extensor late. Dysarthria and dysphagia may be prominent. As the hours pass the patient becomes stuporous, then comatose as a result of brain stem compression.

In *pontine hemorrhage,* consciousness is lost rather promptly, and death usually occurs within a few hours. There are rare exceptions, however, where consciousness is retained, and the clinical manifestations indicate a lesion in the tegmentum of the pons, e.g., disturbances of lateral ocular movements, crossed sensory or motor disturbances, small pupils, cranial nerve palsies, and bilateral signs of pyramidal tract disease. Lateral eye movements, evoked by head turning or irrigation of the ears with ice water, are impaired. The cerebrospinal fluid will be sanguineous.

At each of these sites the hemorrhage is usually massive, and the patient survives only a few hours or a few days, succumbing as a result of secondary brain stem insult. Rarely does a patient survive once deep stupor supervenes, although in some cases the patient may linger in an unresponsive state for a week or two. However, in some 30 per cent of cases, the hemorrhage is less extensive and survival is possible, hemorrhage into the thalamus especially tending to be somewhat smaller than putaminal or cerebellar hemorrhage.

A *severe headache* is considered to be a constant accompaniment of intracerebral hemorrhage, and while it is prominent in many cases and a helpful diagnostic point, in almost 50 per cent of our cases headache has been absent or insignificant. *Nuchal rigidity* is frequently found, but again it is so often absent that failure to find it must by no means detract from the diagnosis. If the neck becomes stiff it will become supple again as coma deepens. *Vomiting* occurs once or twice at the onset of intracerebral hemorrhage, and repeated *vomiting* should always suggest a cerebellar location. *Coma* is said to be a sign of cerebral hemorrhage, and generally speaking it is more frequent in hemorrhage than in infarction, but of equal importance is the fact that the patient often is far from comatose and may even be alert and responding accurately. This is true with grossly bloody spinal fluid, and thus the adage that hemorrhage into the ventricular system always precipitates coma is quite incorrect. Only if bleeding into the ventricles is massive will coma result. *Cerebral seizures*, usually focal, occur in some 10 per cent of cases of supratentorial hemorrhage in the first few days, especially as the result of a "slit" hemorrhage. The fundi often show hypertensive changes in the arteries, and occasionally fresh preretinal hemorrhages occur, although the latter are much more common in ruptured aneurysm or angioma. Grade 4 hypertension (malignant) with papilledema need by no means be present for cerebral hemorrhage to occur.

Many of the less precisely localized neurologic manifestations described under cerebral thrombosis are also encountered in intracerebral hemorrhage, including coma, stupor, drowsiness, confusion, delirium, Cheyne-Stokes respiration, grasping and sucking reflexes, incontinence of bowel and bladder, and unilateral and bilateral extensor rigidity.

Although the proper interpretation of this array of clinical data allows the correct diagnosis to be established in most cases, the examination of the cerebrospinal fluid for blood is the single most important step in the detection of intracranial bleeding.

Laboratory Findings. Any urinary abnormalities will for the most part reflect coexisting renal disease, although transient glucosuria has been reported to result specifically from intracranial hemorrhage. The white blood cell count often rises to 15,000 to 20,000, a higher figure than in thrombosis. The sedimentation rate is elevated. In cases of massive hemorrhage, the cerebrospinal fluid is often under increased pressure but in almost half of our cases readings under 200 mm were obtained. The fluid is usually grossly bloody, although not so bloody as in ruptured saccular aneurysm (the count ranging from a few thousand cells up to one million). In smaller hemorrhages into central structures the cerebrospinal fluid contains a lesser amount of blood, and in occasional cases of intracerebral hemorrhage, particularly in those of the "slit" type, between cortex and white matter, it remains free of blood and clear of xanthochromia despite repeated taps. In these latter cases, slight xanthochromia may appear after a few days to a week. At times the spinal fluid may appear clear grossly but contain some 200 to 400 red cells, and it is then difficult to decide if this represents intracranial bleeding or a traumatic tap. These details are mentioned because they are of great importance in the essential task of making an accurate diagnosis of the type of stroke prior to the use of therapeutic measures such as anticoagulant drugs, surgical exploration, hypothermia, etc. *A traumatic bloody spinal tap* greatly complicates the diagnostic problem. In a bloody tap the pressure tends to be low, the fluid that first flows from the needle is more bloody than that which comes later (third tube less bloody than the first), the fluid often clots in the test tube, and xanthochromia is either absent or at most present only in proportion to the amount of serum bilirubin admixed with the fluid. Bloody fluid due to cerebral hemorrhage is often under increased pressure, there is an even admixture of blood in all samples, the cerebrospinal fluid will not clot, and if more than 8 to 12 hr has elapsed since the hemorrhage, a definite xanthochromia will be present in the supernatant fluid after centrifugation, which should always be carried out if there is any question of the reliability of the tap. However, the presence of xanthochromia after centrifugation may be due to the bilirubin contained in the blood spilled by a traumatic tap and therefore is not an infallible index of subarachnoid or brain hemorrhage. The white blood cells of the cerebrospinal fluid are accounted for by the amount of hemorrhage, and their ratio to red cells is usually the same as in the circulating blood. After hemolysis of red blood cells, the white cell count in the cerebrospinal fluid may be disproportionately increased. Sometimes after a questionably traumatic tap it is worth while to perform another puncture immediately at a higher level.

Lumbar puncture is not completely innocuous, since temporal lobe or cerebellar herniation may be aggravated in cases of massive supratentorial hemorrhage or softening and in cerebellar hemorrhage. Despite this danger, the procedure is necessary if specific therapeutic measures are contemplated or if any doubt exists as to the diagnosis of cerebrovascular disease. X-ray of the skull early in the stroke may show a shift of the calcified pineal gland to the side of the cranium opposite the lesion, a change not seen in infarction. The electroencephalogram does not show a typical or diagnostic pattern, but high-voltage, slow waves are the commonest finding with hemorrhage into the cerebral hemisphere. X-ray of the chest will often show cardiomegaly, and after coma has persisted for a time, there may be pulmonary congestion and edema.

Course and Prognosis. The immediate prognosis is grave, some 70 to 75 per cent of cases dying in 1 to 30 days. Either the hemorrhage ruptures under pressure into the ventricular system, or temporal lobe herniation and midbrain compression occur. Sometimes the hemorrhage appears to seep gradually into vital centers. Gastric erosion and gastrointestinal hemorrhage of neurogenic origin may occur at any time within the first week or two. When the hemorrhage is smaller, survival is possible, and the restitution of motor function, speech, etc., can be excellent, since, in contrast to infarction, the hemorrhage has to some extent pushed brain tissue aside instead of destroying it. Function may be slow to return, because extravasated blood is slow to be resorbed or removed from the tissues. Since rebleeding from the same site is unlikely, the patient may live for many years. In some instances of medium-sized cerebral and cerebellar hemorrhages the patient survives and his condition gradually stabilizes, but definite papilledema appears after several days of increased intracranial pressure (socalled pseudotumorous hemorrhage). Healed scars impinging on the cortex are liable to be epileptogenic.

Treatment. *The general medical management of the comatose, apoplectic patient is the same as that outlined under thrombosis.* Measures to stem the hemorrhage and restore the integrity of damaged tissue have been relatively ineffective up to the present. *Surgical removal of the clot* in the acute stage, either by aspiration or evacuation, has seldom proved successful except in patients with a hemorrhage lying near the surface and who are not comatose. Recently the prospect that acute cere-

bellar hemorrhage may be amenable to surgical therapy is being explored. In the smaller hemorrhages that reach a subacute stage, papilledema may appear, and this in many instances has dictated surgical evacuation of the hemorrhage when the patient's condition stabilized. Under these circumstances the operative procedure has often been successful, but the prognosis in hemorrhage into the cerebral hemisphere is probably little altered by surgery although the outlook for cerebellar cases seems to have improved. Attempts to halt the hemorrhage by lowering the systemic blood pressure through the use of autonomic blocking agents have not been effective, and in many instances the inadvertent occurrence of disastrously low levels of blood pressure has complicated the illness. Artificial hypothermia has been used sporadically, but there are insufficient data to permit appraisal of this procedure. Intermittent compression of the ipsilateral carotid in the neck may be beneficial in acute putaminal cases.

The *only preventive measure* is lowering the blood pressure in cases of essential hypertension by every possible means. If ACTH or one of the adrenal steroids is being given, toxicity must be watched for. When hypotension threatens during surgical procedures, injections of excessive amounts of epinephrine or ephedrine must be avoided. Toxemia of pregnancy must be detected early.

Ruptured Saccular Aneurysm

This is the fourth most frequent of the cerebrovascular disorders after thrombosis with atherosclerosis, embolism, and hypertensive intracerebral hemorrhage. Saccular aneurysms take the form of small, thin-walled blisters protruding from the arteries of the circle of Willis or the major branches arising therefrom. These saccules or "berries," as they have been called, are located for the most part at bifurcations and branchings and are presumed to be the result of developmental defects in the media and elastica. A small number of aneurysms have been attributed to incomplete involution of embryonic vessels. Owing to the local weakness, the intima bulges outward, covered by adventitia; the sac gradually enlarges, until finally dissolution of the wall and rupture occur. Saccular aneurysms vary in size from tiny nubbins 2 mm in diameter up to spherical masses 2 or 3 cm in diameter, averaging 8 to 10 mm. Aneurysms vary greatly in form, some being round and connected to the parent artery by a narrower stalk, others are broad-based without a stalk, and still others are narrow cylinders. The site of rupture is always the dome of the aneurysm, which may present one or more secondary sacculations. In routine autopsies the incidence of ruptured aneurysms is 1.8 per cent, of unruptured aneurysms, 2.0 per cent.

Saccular aneurysms are rare in childhood, even at routine postmortem examination, and increase in frequency to reach their highest plateau of incidence in the age period of thirty-five to sixty-five years. Therefore, they are not congenitally formed anomalies but develop over the years on the basis of a developmental arterial defect. There is an increased incidence of congenital polycystic disease of the kidney and of coarctation of the aorta in association with saccular aneurysm. Hypertension is more frequently present than in the average population, but aneurysms occur in persons with perfectly normal blood pressure. Atherosclerosis, although present in the walls of about 50 per cent of aneurysms, probably plays no part in their formation or enlargement.

From 85 to 90 per cent of saccular aneurysms lie on the anterior part of the circle of Willis. The four commonest sites are (1) in relation to the anterior communicating artery, (2) at the origin of the posterior communicating artery from the stem of the internal carotid, (3) at the first major bifurcation of the middle cerebral artery, and (4) at the bifurcation of the internal carotid into middle and anterior cerebral arteries (see Fig. 284-7). Other sites include the internal carotid in the cavernous sinus, at the origin of the ophthalmic artery, at the junction of the posterior communicating artery with the posterior cerebral, at the bifurcation of the basilar artery, and at the origins of the three cerebellar arteries. In 8 per cent of cases there is more than one aneurysm, and they may be situated unilaterally or bilaterally.

Several types of aneurysm other than saccular occur, e.g., mycotic, fusiform, diffuse, and globular. The last three are named for their predominant morphologic aspects and consist of enlargement or dilatation of the entire circumference of the involved vessels, usually the internal carotid, vertebral, or basilar arteries. Frequently showing atherosclerotic deposition in their walls, they are often referred to as arteriosclerotic, but most likely they are at least partly developmental in nature. They press on neighboring structures or become occluded by thrombosis and rupture only infrequently, usually after lumbar puncture.

Clinical Picture. Prior to rupture, saccular aneurysms are usually asymptomatic and rarely cause even headache. Occasionally, large aneurysms immediately distal to the cavernous sinus may compress the optic nerves or chiasm, third nerve, hypothalamus, or pituitary gland. In the posterior fossa, one or more of the cranial nerves may be compressed adjacent to the brain stem.

When rupture occurs, blood under high pressure is discharged into the subarachnoid space (the circle of Willis lies in the subarachnoid space), and the resulting clinical events fall into one of three

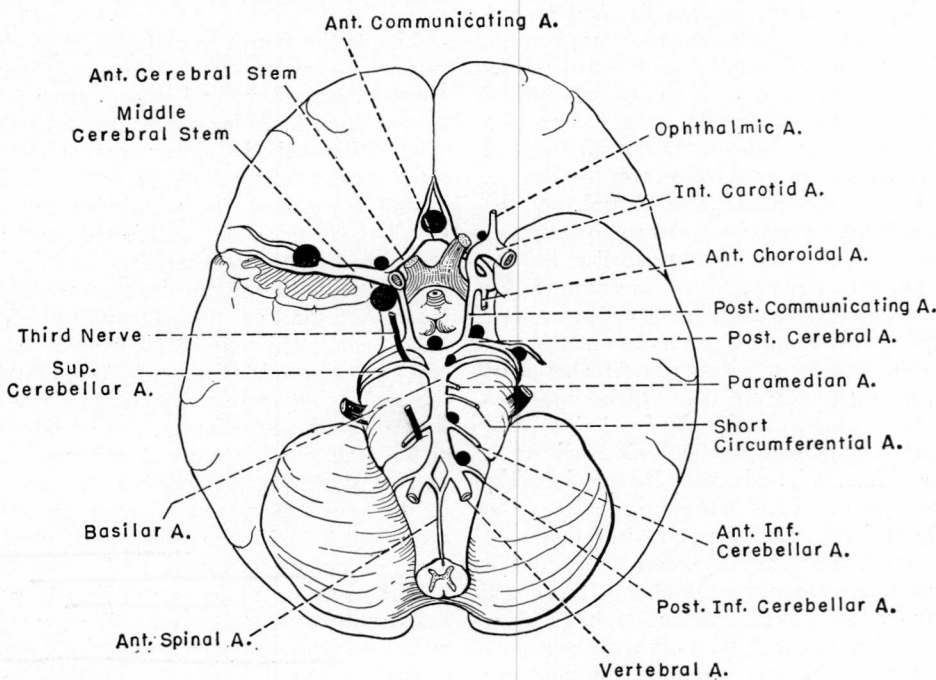

Fig. 284-7. Diagram of the circle of Willis to show the principal sites of saccular aneurysm. Approximately 90 per cent of aneurysms are on the anterior half of the circle.

patterns: (1) the patient may be stricken with an excruciating generalized headache and fall unconscious almost immediately; (2) headache may develop as in (1), but the patient remains relatively lucid; (3) consciousness may be lost quickly without any preceding complaint. Convulsive seizures occur at the onset of hemorrhage in about 10 per cent of patients. If the hemorrhage is massive, a fatal issue may ensue in a matter of minutes, hours, or a day or two, deep coma persisting in association with irregular respiration, attacks of extensor rigidity, and finally respiratory arrest and circulatory collapse. In these rapidly fatal cases, the blood has usually dissected intracerebrally and entered the ventricular system. Death occasionally occurs within 5 to 10 min, and ruptured aneurysm must be considered in the differential diagnosis of sudden death.

In mild cases, consciousness, if lost, may be regained within a few minutes, but a residuum of confusion and amnesia persists for a day or two thereafter, accompanied by an excruciating headache and stiff neck. It is not uncommon for drowsiness and confusion to last 7 to 10 days or longer. If the hemorrhage is confined to the subarachnoid space, there are few or no lateralizing neurologic signs.

In most patients there are no warning symptoms whatsoever; in some, however, minor leakage from the aneurysm sometimes precedes devastating rupture by a few days or weeks, headache being the chief sign of such an event. Aneurysmal rupture usually occurs while the patient is active rather than during sleep, and sexual intercourse or other exertion precipitates the ictus in many instances.

Gross lateralizing signs in the form of hemiplegia, hemiparesis, or aphasia are absent in the majority of cases, but can occur and are usually due to the presence of an intracerebral clot. In this case the aneurysm will have ruptured partly into the subarachnoid space and partly into brain tissue (subarachnoid-cerebral hemorrhage) even reaching the ventricular system (subarachnoid cerebroventricular hemorrhage), rendering the patient stuporous or comatose. The initial neurologic deficit may clear in a matter of days, indicating that hemorrhage into tissues was not responsible for the focal signs. The pathogenesis of the manifestations in such cases is not fully understood, and vasospasm produced by the presence of subarachnoid blood has, without good evidence, been invoked as the cause. Areas of ischemic necrosis of tissue in the territory of the vessel bearing the aneurysm, usually without thrombosis of the vessel, may be found postmortem. Transient deficits which are still more evanescent are by no means uncommon, and motor paralysis or aphasia, for example, may be present for only a few minutes or so after the onset of bleeding, con-

stituting reliable telltales of ruptured aneurysm. The deficits may be due to a transitory fall in pressure in the circulation distal to the aneurysmal perforation.

Although in most patients the neurologic manifestations do not point to the exact site of the aneurysm, in many instances there are clues to the localization. For example: (1) third nerve palsy (ptosis, diplopia, mydriasis, and oculomotor paralysis) usually indicates an aneurysm at the junction of the posterior communicating artery and the internal carotid stem. The third nerve passes immediately lateral to this point. (2) Transient paresis of one or both of the lower limbs at the onset of the hemorrhage is suggestive of an anterior communicating aneurysm which has interfered with the circulation in the anterior cerebral arteries, causing ischemia of the motor areas for the lower extremities. (3) Hemiparesis or aphasia often points to an aneurysm at the bifurcation of the middle cerebral artery which has critically reduced the circulation in the middle cerebral system. (4) Unilateral blindness or amblyopia indicates an aneurysm which lies anteromedially in the circle of Willis (at the origin of the ophthalmic artery, at the bifurcation of the internal carotid artery, or in the anterior communicating region). (5) A curious state of retained consciousness with akinetic mutism, abulia, or adynamia favors an aneurysm of the anterior communicating artery which has caused ischemia of or hemorrhage into one or both of the frontal lobes, hypothalamus, or corpus callosum. (6) The side on which the aneurysm lies may be indicated by a unilateral preponderance of headache or preretinal hemorrhages, by the occurrence of monocular pain, or by the lateralization of an intracranial sound heard at the time of rupture of the aneurysm. Sixth nerve palsy, unilateral or bilateral, results from the presence of subarachnoid blood and raised intracranial pressure and is seldom of localizing value. Other neurologic signs which have relatively little localizing value include sucking and grasping reflexes, choreoathetosis, and extensor rigidity.

In summary, the clinical sequence of sudden violent headache, collapse, brief unconsciousness and confusion, combined with an absence of prodromal symptoms and a paucity of lateralizing signs is diagnostic of a ruptured saccular aneurysm (or angioma).

Other clinical data may be of assistance in reaching a correct diagnosis. Nuchal rigidity is usually present. Examination of the fundi not infrequently reveals smooth-surfaced, sharply outlined collections of blood which cover the retinal vessels—the so-called "preretinal" or "subhyaloid" hemorrhages. These are usually a sign of ruptured aneurysm or angioma but can occur with hypertensive hemorrhage and in cranial trauma. Bilateral Babinski signs are found in the early days following rupture, especially if there is impairment of consciousness. The patient may appear to be normally alert; yet impairment of memory and confabulation may be present on more careful testing. A fever with the temperature rising to 102°F is common in the first week. A faint intracranial bruit, the mechanism of which is not clear, may rarely be heard in ruptured aneurysm but is much more common in angioma. The escaping blood occasionally enters the subdural space and produces a subdural hematoma, evacuation of which may be lifesaving. Aneurysmal rupture may complicate pregnancy, but pregnancy is not associated with an increased incidence of aneurysmal rupture. The association of polycystic kidneys or coarctation of the aorta has been mentioned. Spontaneous intracranial bleeding with normal blood pressure should always suggest ruptured aneurysm, ruptured angioma, or hemorrhage into a cerebral tumor.

Laboratory Findings. Any urinary abnormality is usually due to concomitant renal disease. Rarely diabetes insipidus occurs. A leukocytosis of 15,000 to 18,000 is common. The cerebrospinal fluid is usually extremely bloody, with red cell counts reaching to 1 million per cu mm or higher. When the hemorrhage is very slight there may be only a few thousand cells. It is unlikely that an aneurysm can rupture entirely into brain tissue without some leakage of blood into the subarachnoid fluid, and therefore the diagnosis of ruptured saccular aneurysm must never be made unless blood is present in the spinal fluid. Only expanding saccular aneurysms which either compress the optic nerves and chiasm or cranial nerves or lie within the cavernous sinus produce symptoms without hemorrhage. Usually deep xanthochromia is found after centrifugation. The cerebrospinal fluid is under greatly increased pressure, as high as 1,000 mm (see p. 1782 regarding traumatic tap). The white blood cells in the spinal fluid are usually present in the same proportion to red blood cells as in the circulating blood, but within 48 hr a brisk leukocytosis appears, reaching 2,000 to 3,000 cells per cu mm in some patients.

X-rays of the skull are usually negative, though in a few patients one or both of the anterior clinoid processes has been eroded by the pressure of an adjacent aneurysm, or calcification has occurred in the region of a previous hemorrhage. A calcified pineal gland may be displaced by an intracerebral or subdural clot.

Acute subarachnoid hemorrhage may be associated with electrocardiographic abnormalities suggestive of myocardial ischemia. The electroencephalogram is of little help in localizing the lesion unless a gross neurologic deficit is present, in which case the lateralization is probably already evident clinically. The abnormality usually consists of slow waves.

Carotid and vertebral angiography, using Diodrast or Hypaque, will demonstrate the aneurysm in some 70 per cent of patients in which aneurysm appears to be the correct diagnosis on clinical grounds, i.e., in cases of so-called "spontaneous subarachnoid hemorrhage."

Course and Prognosis. The outstanding characteristic of this condition is the tendency for the hemorrhage to recur. This threat colors all prognostications, and unfortunately there appears to be no way of determining reliably which cases will rebleed.

Patients with the typical clinical picture of spontaneous subarachnoid hemorrhage but in whom the angiogram shows no aneurysm or angioma have a better prognosis than those in whom the lesion is demonstrated. The cause of the intermittency of bleeding is not understood.

McKissock et al. found that the patient's state of consciousness at the time of arteriography was the best single criterion of prognosis. Using their data as representative of any large medical center, it can be shown that of every 100 patients coming to arteriography, 17 will be stuporous or comatose, and 83 will appear to be recovering from the ictus. At the end of the next 6 months, of the first 17, 7 will have died from the original hemorrhage and 7 more will have had a fatal recurrence, making a total of 14 deaths and 3 survivors. Of the other 83, one will have died of the original hemorrhage, 52 will have had a recurrence of whom 33 will have died, making a total of 34 deaths and 49 survivors. Thus, of the total of 100, at the end of 6 months, 8 will have died of the original hemorrhage, 59 more will have had a recurrence with 40 deaths, making a total of 48 deaths and 52 survivors. The gravity of the illness is immediately apparent. In regard to the recurrence of bleeding, of every 50 patients seen on the first day of the illness, 5 will rebleed in the first week (all fatal), 8 in the second week (5 fatal), 6 in the third and fourth weeks (4 fatal), and 2 in the next 4 weeks (2 fatal), making a total of 21 recurrences in 8 weeks (16 fatal). Rerupture did not occur in the first 2 days; thereafter it occurred at a steady rate for the next 19 days and tapered off abruptly.

Of the survivors in the first group, all but one returned to work, and in the second group, 36 went back to full work, 12 were partly disabled, and 4 were totally disabled. The disability was due to paralysis, mental deterioration, or epilepsy.

Treatment. General medical management in the acute stage is similar to that described under cerebral thrombosis (p. 1770). Any specific medical measures are based on the assumption that decreasing the arterial blood pressure is the most reasonable way of arresting the hemorrhage and preventing recurrence. Absolute bed rest for 4 to 8 weeks is prescribed, with the head of the bed raised some 15 to 20°. Straining during bowel movement is forbidden, and laxatives or gentle enemas are administered. Coughing and all forms of exertion are carefully avoided. The patient is fed. The duration of the period of bed rest is empirical and not founded on any reliable clinical observations or the formation of scar tissue around aneurysms. Sedatives (barbiturates) and analgesics (opiates, acetylsalicylic acid) are important in aiding relaxation. The use of hypotensive agents has been widely suggested, but no proof of their efficacy has been presented. In the presence of severe hypertension, hexamethonium, orally or by injection, may be cautiously used to lower the blood pressure to 160/100, great care being exercised not to precipitate excessive hypotension and cerebral infarction. Hexamethonium and chlorpromazine are usually not very effective in lowering the blood pressure of normotensives confined to bed. Chlorpromazine intramuscularly is used to control nausea and vomiting. Dilantin or phenobarbital is prescribed routinely to prevent cerebral seizures.

The place of repeated drainage of the cerebrospinal fluid by lumbar puncture is still uncertain, although several workers have concluded that it does not affect the outcome of the illness. At present, one lumbar puncture is usually carried out for diagnostic purposes, and thereafter it is performed only for the relief of intractable headache, to detect recurrence of bleeding, or to measure the intracranial pressure prior to surgery.

In maintaining fluid balance, intravenous fluids should be used sparingly and in the proper electrolyte combination (a mixture of equal parts of 5 per cent glucose in water and normal saline solution or balanced electrolytes) in order to minimize the danger of aggravating brain swelling. Any abnormality of concentration of electrolytes in the blood must be corrected. Diabetes insipidus is treated with Pitressin. Disorders of blood coagulation should be amended. Vitamins C and K have been recommended, but there is no evidence that they are beneficial. The use of body hypothermia for 2 to 5 days in the stage of acute hemorrhage has been used but remains to be scientifically evaluated. Intravenous hypertonic urea may be effective in temporarily reducing the intracranial pressure.

After resting in bed for 6 weeks, the patient is gradually allowed to resume activity and may return to work in 4 months. It seems logical to advise that heavy labor not be resumed.

Surgical Therapy. Apart from occasionally evacuating an associated intracerebral clot, surgical treatment is for the most part directed to the prevention of recurrence of the hemorrhage. The procedures are either *extracranial* (ligation of the common carotid in the neck) or *intracranial* (resection of the aneurysm, ligation of the neck of the aneurysm, wrapping or tamponade of the aneurysmal sac by muscle, fascia, plastic coating or arterial graft, trapping the aneurysm, ligation of the main vessel proximal to the aneurysm). Occasionally extracranial and intracranial procedures are combined. Because of the high operative mortality if surgery is undertaken early, operation has usually been delayed until the patient's condition has stabilized following the first hemorrhage. During the waiting period, however, the patient is liable to suffer a further hemorrhage, and in an effort to intervene before this happens neurosurgeons are now attempting to operate much earlier than formerly, sometimes using hypothermia and hypotension during surgery. Before treatment is undertaken, the site, size, and form of the aneurysm must be determined by at least bilateral carotid angiography. At the same time the pattern of the anterior half of the circle of Willis is noted, as it may influence the choice of operative procedure. That surgery is useful in some cases seems incontrovertible, and at present the indications, time, and operative methods are being gradually deduced. After aneurysmal rupture a chronic obstructive or communicating hydrocephalus may develop causing persistent headache and stupor which are relieved by ventricular drainage.

OTHER CAUSES OF INTRACRANIAL HEMORRHAGE

Angioma. An angioma or hemangioma consists of a tangle of abnormal vessels forming an abnormal communication between the arterial and venous systems, really an arteriovenous fistula. It is a developmental abnormality and not a neoplasm, but the constituent vessels enlarge with growth and the passage of time. Angiomas vary in size from a small blemish a few millimeters in diameter lying in the cortex to a huge mass of tortuous channels comprising an arteriovenous shunt of sufficient magnitude to raise the cardiac output. Hypertrophic dilated arterial "feeders" approach the main lesion, disappear below the cortex, and break up into a network of thin-walled blood vessels which connect directly with draining veins. The latter often form huge, dilated, pulsating channels, carrying away arterial blood. The blood vessels forming the tangle interposed between arteries and veins are usually abnormally thin and do not have the normal structure of arteries or veins. Angiomas occur in all parts of the brain, brain stem, and spinal cord, but the larger ones are more frequently found in the middle and anterior cerebral territories, commonly forming a wedge-shaped lesion extending from the cortex to the ventricular lining.

Angiomas predominate in males over females about 2:1. Although the lesion is present from birth, the onset of complaints is most common between the ages of ten and thirty, but occasionally it is delayed as late as the fifties. The chief clinical features are epileptic seizures and cerebral or cerebral-subarachnoid hemorrhage occurring in a child or young adult. In 50 per cent the first manifestation is a seizure, in 20 per cent an intracerebral hemorrhage with hemiplegia, and in 20 per cent a typical subarachnoid hemorrhage. The seizure pattern depends on the site of the lesion; when focal motor in type the seizure may be followed by a temporary postictal paralysis. When hemorrhage occurs, blood may enter the subarachnoid space almost exclusively, producing a picture identical with that of ruptured saccular aneurysm, or since the angioma lies within the cerebral tissue, the bleeding is liable to be partly intracerebral, causing hemiparesis, hemiplegia, or death. Before rupture, chronic nondescript headache is a frequent complaint. Occasionally typical migraine is associated, but whether it is the result of the angioma or a coincidence is not known. Huge angiomas may produce a slowly progressive neurologic deficit due to depletion of blood from adjacent brain tissue. Proptosis has been encountered. When the vein of Galen is involved, hydrocephalus may result. Not infrequently one or both carotid arteries pulsate unusually forcefully in the neck. A systolic bruit heard over the carotid in the neck, the mastoid process, or the eyeballs in young adults is almost pathognomonic of angioma. The patient should be exercised in order to bring out a bruit if none is present at rest. A bruit may be heard over a spinal angioma of large size. The blood pressure may be raised or normal, and it is axiomatic that the occurrence of intracranial bleeding with normal blood pressure should lead to the suspicion of an angioma, ruptured saccular aneurysm, or hemorrhage into a tumor. The eye grounds may reveal a retinal vascular abnormality. Preretinal hemorrhages may be found after hemorrhage has occurred. X-ray of the skull occasionally shows crescentic linear calcification in the vicinity of larger angiomas. Pneumoencephalography may show the picture of an expanding lesion combined with cerebral atrophy, a combination typical of angioma. Arteriography is necessary to establish the diagnosis with certainty and will demonstrate angiomas larger than 1.5 cm in diameter. Small angiomas may be obscured by the resulting hemorrhage, and even at autopsy a careful microscopic search may be necessary to find them.

Most angiomas bleed sooner or later. The first hemorrhage may be fatal, but in more than 90 per cent of cases bleeding stops, and the patient survives. Recurrence of hemorrhage with a fatal outcome is a constant danger. In recent years it has been the practice of neurosurgeons to perform a block dissection of angiomas of suitable size and location.

Trauma. Although intracranial bleeding due to head trauma does not rightfully fall within the scope of the stroke problem, it must be mentioned here because of the great frequency with which it enters into the differential diagnosis, especially in cases in which the history is inadequate or the patient falls and injures himself at the onset of the stroke. *Acute extradural* and *acute subdural hemorrhage* must always be considered in the patient who under unknown circumstances has rather abruptly developed a neurologic deficit such as hemiparesis or confusion, whether the spinal fluid is bloody or not. In *chronic subdural hemorrhage,* which can occur without known trauma, the indefinite picture of drowsiness, confusion, and mild hemiparesis may be erroneously attributed to a stroke, especially in elderly persons. These three conditions must be constantly kept in mind, since failure to make the correct diagnosis deprives the patient of lifesaving surgical intervention. There should be no hesitation in carrying out arteriography or placing diagnostic burr holes in all patients in whom subdural hemorrhage cannot be excluded on clinical grounds. *Cerebral contusion and laceration* may be a cause of subarachnoid hemorrhage, and if the patient has fallen and struck his head at the time of the onset of the stroke, it may be difficult or impossible to decide if the red blood cells in the cerebrospinal fluid are due to a cerebrovascular stroke or to cerebral contusion. Trauma may also cause *acute* or *delayed intracerebral hemorrhage, acute intracerebellar hemorrhage, acute infratentorial subdural hemorrhage, acute brain swelling,* and on rare occasions, extensive *focal infarction* of undetermined pathogenesis.

Several *hemorrhagic hematologic disorders* are not infrequently complicated by hemorrhage into the brain. The most frequent of these are leukemia, aplastic anemia, and thrombopenic purpura. As a rule this complication signals a fatal issue. Any part of the brain may be involved, and not infrequently the lesions are multiple. Usually there is already evidence of abnormal bleeding elsewhere (skin, mucous membranes, kidney) by the time cerebral hemorrhage occurs. Intracranial bleeding is a complication of anticoagulant therapy.

Hemorrhages of undetermined origin are of importance since both clinically and pathologically hemorrhages are found in which the blood pressure is normal and neither an aneurysm nor angioma can be demonstrated. In some postmortem cases a careful microscopic search discloses a small angioma in the cerebral tissue at one side of the hemorrhage, and on this basis it is suspected that in other cases, too, an overlooked angioma may have been the cause of the extravasation of blood. Primary intraventricular hemorrhage, a rare event, is at times due to angioma or neoplasm of the choroid plexus, which may not have been seen by the prosector.

Hemorrhage into primary and secondary brain tumors is not rare, and when it is the first manifestation of the neoplasm, the correct diagnosis may be extremely obscure. Chorionephithelioma, melanotic carcinoma, renal cell carcinoma, bronchogenic carcinoma, pituitary adenoma, glioblastoma multiforme, and medulloblastoma may present in this way. Careful inquiry will usually disclose the fact that signs of a neurologic disorder compatible with intracranial tumor growth have preceded the onset of hemorrhage. Examination clinically and by x-ray may reveal evidence of intracranial tumor or of secondary tumor deposits in other organs. A chest film will frequently show metastatic or primary neoplasm and should be performed in all cases of obscure intracerebral hemorrhage.

Septic embolism may lead to massive fatal intracranial bleeding via a *mycotic aneurysm*. Any part of the circulatory tree may be involved, but usually the aneurysm lies at a branching or forking of a small vessel (about 0.5 mm in diameter) within the subarachnoid space.

On infrequent occasions bleeding within an area of *hemorrhagic infarction* as a result of cerebral embolism or venous thrombosis reaches major proportions, forming an intracerebral hematoma, and the cerebrospinal fluid becomes bloody.

Hypertensive encephalopathy may in its most advanced stage result in intracerebral hemorrhages, which can vary in size from petechial to massive.

Idiopathic brain purpura, or hemorrhagic encephalitis, consists of multiple petechial hemorrhages scattered throughout the white matter of the brain. The picture is that of a diffuse cerebral disease. There is never blood in the spinal fluid, and the condition should never be confused with a typical stroke.

Brain stem hemorrhages secondary to temporal lobe herniation are extremely common but never present as a cerebrovascular stroke.

Inflammatory disease of arteries and veins, especially polyarteritis nodosa and lupus erythematosus, occasionally cause hemorrhage into the nervous system. In polyarteritis rupture of a vessel may occur on the basis of a concomitant hypertension or local vascular disease. In lupus erythematosus —if it can be included in the arteritides—hemorrhage is attributable to hypertension, agamma-globulinemia, or disease of the vascular wall of undetermined nature. Bleeding nearly always occurs into the parenchyma rather than the subarachnoid space.

The rarer types of hemorrhage listed in the classification are largely self-explanatory.

HYPERTENSIVE ENCEPHALOPATHY

This term refers to an acute syndrome in which severe hypertension is associated with headache, nausea, vomiting, convulsions, confusion, stupor, and coma. Focal or lateralizing neurologic signs, either transitory or lasting, are rare and always suggest some other form of vascular disease (hemorrhage, embolism, atherosclerotic thrombosis). By the time the neurologic manifestations appear, the hypertension has usually reached the malignant stage, with retinal hemorrhages, exudates, papilledema (*hypertensive retinopathy* grade IV), and evidence of renal and cardiac disease. In many but not all of the cases, the cerebrospinal fluid pressure and the protein values are both elevated, the latter sometimes over 100 mg per 100 ml. The hypertension may be essential or due to chronic renal disease, acute glomerulonephritis, acute toxemia of pregnancy, pheochromocytoma, Cushing's syndrome, or ACTH toxicity. Lowering of the blood pressure with hypotensive drugs may reverse the picture in a day or two. If the hypertension cannot be controlled, the outcome is fatal. Neuropathologic examination may reveal a rather normal-looking brain, but usually cerebral swelling and/or hemorrhages of various sizes will be found from massive to petechial. Microscopically there are clusters of glial cells, necrosis of arterioles, and minute cerebral infarcts.

The term *hypertensive encephalopathy* should be reserved for the above syndrome and not used to refer to chronic recurrent headaches, dizziness, epileptic seizures, recurrent transient ischemic attacks, or small strokes which often occur in association with high blood pressure. For further discussion, see p. 1774.

INFLAMMATORY DISEASES OF BRAIN ARTERIES

Inflammatory diseases of the vessels of the brain have been mentioned on several occasions in the preceding paragraphs, and here they are reviewed and discussed briefly.

Meningovascular syphilis, formerly one of the most frequent causes of occlusive vascular disease in patients of all ages, has become a rarity since the introduction of penicillin therapy. Neurosyphilis is basically a chronic treponemal cerebrospinal meningitis and, as in all forms of chronic meningitis, the subarachnoid vessels become involved in the inflammatory process. This is the reason for calling syphilitic vascular disease of the brain *meningo-vascular*. If the arteritis is active and symptoms of vascular occlusion are of recent origin, there are almost invariably signs of meningitis, as evidenced by an increase in the cerebrospinal fluid protein and cells; and its syphilitic nature is revealed by the positive Wassermann reaction. Syphilis must still be considered as a diagnostic possibility in all patients who suffer a brain infarct, particularly at an early age. In the experience of the authors, however, the usual error is to assume that a stroke is syphilitic when in fact some other arterial disease is the cause. If the cerebrospinal fluid is normal or "inactive," meaning that the cell and protein values are normal, a stroke will nearly always prove to be nonsyphilitic even when the blood Wassermann reaction is positive. Formerly syphilis was errone-ously assumed to be the cause of cerebral aneurysms or rupture of vessels with intracerebral or meningeal hemorrhage, but now this formulation is rarely entertained.

Tuberculous meningitis, fungous meningitis, and the subacute forms of bacterial meningitis (in-fluenzal bacillus, staphylococcus, pneumococcus) may also be accompanied by vascular disorders of the occlusive type, in either the cerebral arteries or veins. Occasionally in tuberculous meningitis a stroke may be the first clinical sign of meningitis; more often it develops after the meningeal symp-toms are well established. The diagnosis of these meningeal diseases is relatively simple, for the cerebrospinal fluid contains the essential clues. A treatment which suppresses the meningitis also controls the arteritis. *Septic embolism* may be a source of arteritis and sometimes of mycotic aneu-rysm formation. The latter may rupture and cause either cerebral or subarachnoid hemorrhage, but more often the clinical manifestations are those of arterial occlusion.

Typhus, schistosomiasis mansoni, mucormycosis, malaria, and *trichinosis* are rare types of infective inflammatory diseases of the arteries and, unlike the above, are not secondary to meningeal inflam-mation. The cerebrospinal fluid may be normal or abnormal. In typhus and other rickettsial diseases, capillary and arteriolar changes and perivascular inflammatory cells are found in the brain, and presumably they underlie the convulsions, acute psychoses, and coma which reflect the central nervous system involvement. The internal carotid artery may be occluded in diabetic patients during orbital and cavernous sinus infections with mu-cormycosis. In trichinosis the sudden onset of con-vulsions, aphasia, hemiplegia, and coma may either accompany or, as happens more often, follow the systemic and muscular symptoms. The cause of the

cerebral symptoms has not been established. Para-sites have been found in the brain; in one case known to the authors the cerebral lesions were pro-duced by bland emboli arising in the heart and related to a severe myocarditis. Malaria of the malignant or falciparum variety is frequently at-tended by a clinical state known as "cerebral malaria," in which convulsions and coma and some-times focal symptoms appear to be due to blockage of capillaries and precapillaries by masses of para-sitized red blood corpuscles.

The *arteritides of obscure origin* include poly-arteritis nodosa, disseminated lupus erythematosus, granulomatous arteritis, giant-cell arteritis, temporal (cranial) arteritis, and rheumatic arteritis.

Polyarteritis nodosa frequently involves the small blood vessels in the peripheral nerves, giving rise to a clinical picture of a multiple asymmetric sen-sorimotor *polyneuropathy*, and cerebral vessels usu-ally escape. If hypertension becomes severe, as it often does, brain hemorrhage or hypertensive en-cephalopathy may occur. More recently a granu-lomatous form of polyarteritis nodosa has been delineated in which the neurologic syndrome has been more "encephalitic" than "vascular," with headache, ataxia, confusion, convulsions, hemi-paresis, etc. In these latter cases a moderate in-crease in white blood cells and total protein of the cerebrospinal fluid provides further evidence that the illness is not an ordinary type of vascular disease.

In *systemic lupus erythematosus* delirium, con-fusional states, convulsions, hemiplegia and aphasia, and brain stem or cerebellar syndromes may be traced to small infarcts or hemorrhages of obscure pathogenesis. If renal hypertension develops, intra-cerebral hemorrhage and hypertensive encephalop-athy may terminate the illness.

Temporal arteritis (cranial arteritis) is an un-common affliction of elderly persons in which the external carotid system, particularly the temporal branches, is the seat of a subacute granulomatous inflammation with an exudate of lymphocytes, monocytes, neutrophilic leukocytes, and giant cells. Usually the most severely affected parts of the artery become thrombosed. This aspect of the disease is distressingly painful. The inflammatory nature of the illness is indicated by the occurrence of fever, slight leukocytosis, increased sedimentation rate, and anemia. Occlusion of branches of the ophthalmic artery results in blindness in one or both eyes in over 50 per cent of patients, and occasionally an ophthalmoplegia due to involvement of ocular nerves occurs. An arteritis of the aorta and its major branches, including carotid, subclavian, coro-nary, and femoral arteries, is found at postmortem examination. Strokes occur occasionally, probably due to occlusion of the extracranial arteries for significant inflammatory involvement of intracranial arteries has rarely been demonstrated. The diagnosis depends on the finding of a tender thrombosed or thickened cranial artery and the demonstration of the lesion in a biopsy. Meticorten and ACTH bring striking subjective relief, but whether or not they prevent blindness has not been clearly determined. See p. 1899 for further discussion.

There is another type of *giant-cell arteritis* which occurs in younger people, and although the pathologic process is somewhat similar to that of temporal arteritis, the biology of the illness is entirely different. All branches of the aorta, including the common carotid arteries, may become occluded. This disease, commonly referred to as "pulseless disease," was described long ago in Japan (Takayasu) and in Norway (Harbitz). The vascular pathology is not well defined, but chronic inflammation with destruction of all coats of the vessel, infiltrates of lymphocytes, plasma cells, and mononuclear leukocytes, the presence of giant cells, and thrombosis comprise the lesion. The cause of the disease is unknown. Extracranial thromboendarterectomy may be helpful in treatment. See Chap. 284 and p. 1771.

Rheumatic arteritis is still a highly debatable subject. Pathologic studies have not provided convincing evidence of a primary arteritis. In many of the reported cases, infarction, which has been the usual parenchymal brain lesion, was due to embolism from a rheumatic endocarditis. However, the close relationship of lupus erythematosus, in which there is an arterial lesion, and rheumatic fever offers a plausible basis for a primary involvement of cerebral vessels.

Thromboangiitis obliterans of cerebral vessels (Winiwarter-Buerger disease) has not been included in the foregoing list. Despite the large amount of literature on the subject, the pathology is so dubious that it does not merit further exposition. All the patients that the authors have studied proved to have had either atherosclerosis of the carotid or cerebral arteries with "statis thrombosis" of more distant cerebral branches. Buerger's disease of the legs has an equally uncertain status.

THE DIAGNOSIS OF CEREBROVASCULAR DISEASE

There are two separate aspects of the problem of differential diagnosis: (1) vascular disease must be distinguished from other neurologic illnesses, and (2) the different kinds of vascular diseases must be separated from one another. In the following pages many of the important points discussed in the body of the chapter will be recapitulated.

Differentiation of Vascular Disease from Other Neurologic Illnesses. It has already been stated that the diagnosis of a vascular lesion rests solely on recognition of the stroke syndrome, and that without evidence of this the diagnosis must always be in doubt. Three useful criteria in the identification of the stroke have already been emphasized: (1) the temporal profile of the clinical syndrome, (2) evidence of focal brain disease, and (3) the clinical setting. The temporal profile can usually be defined by means of a clear history of premonitory phenomena, the mode of the onset, and the evolution of the neurologic disturbance taken in relationship to the medical status at the time of examination. If these data are lacking, the course may still be determined by extending the period of observation for a few more days or weeks, thus resorting to the clinical rule that the physician's best diagnostic tool is the second and third examination. An inadequate history is probably the most frequent cause of diagnostic errors.

As stated above, the neurologic deficit in a cerebrovascular stroke develops relatively suddenly, and later in the illness, if death does not occur, stabilization and some degree of recovery take place. There are few neurologic illnesses whose temporal profile mimics that of the cerebrovascular disorders. Tumor, infection, inflammation, degeneration, and nutritional disorders are not likely to manifest themselves precipitously. In trauma, of course, a sudden insult occurs, but usually injury is readily recognizable as the cause. In multiple sclerosis and other demyelinative diseases, abrupt episodes of exacerbation occur, but for the most part they occur in a different age group and clinical setting.

Many thrombotic strokes are preceded by transient ischemic episodes which, if they are nonconvulsive in nature, are almost diagnostic of vascular disease. Their differentiation from cerebral seizures, attacks of Ménière's syndrome, and paralytic migraine was discussed in the description of intermittent cerebral ischemia. A stroke developing over a period of several days rather than evolving smoothly usually progresses in a stepwise fashion, increments of additional deficit being added serially from time to time. A slow gradual downhill course over a period of 2 weeks or more indicates that the lesion is probably not vascular, but rather a tumor, abscess, granuloma, or subdural hematoma.

In regard to the focal neurologic deficit, many nonvascular neurologic diseases (tumor, abscess, etc.) produce manifestations which are not strikingly different from those resulting from vascular disease, and the diagnosis usually cannot rest solely on this aspect of the clinical picture. Nonetheless, certain combinations of neurologic signs which conform to the neurovascular pattern, e.g., the lateral medullary syndrome, are seen almost exclusively in occlusive vascular disease.

The presence of *blood in the cerebrospinal fluid* always points to a cerebrovascular lesion, provided that trauma and a "bloody tap" can be excluded. *Headache* is common in cerebrovascular disease, not only in hemorrhage but also in thrombosis and embolism. *Cerebral seizures* are almost never the premonitory, first, or only manifestation of a stroke but can occur in the first few hours after infarction or intracranial bleeding. *Brief unconsciousness* (5 to 10 min) is rare in stroke cases, being seen only in ruptured aneurysm and basilar artery insufficiency. The presence of certain neurologic disturbances which are scarcely ever attributable to cerebrovascular disorder, e.g., diabetes insipidus, bitemporal hemianopia, classical parkinsonism, generalized myoclonus, and isolated cranial nerve palsies, may be of help in ruling out vascular disease.

Finally, the diagnosis of cerebrovascular disease should always be made on positive data, and diagnosis by exclusion is to be deprecated.

A few conditions are so often confused with the cerebrovascular diseases that they merit further consideration. When a history of trauma is absent, the headache, drowsiness, and mild hemiparesis accompanying a *subdural hematoma* may all too easily be ascribed to a "slight stroke," and the patient may fail to receive immediate surgical therapy. In classic subdural hematoma the symptoms and signs will usually develop gradually over a period of days or weeks. The degree of obtundation and confusion will often be disproportionately great in comparison with the focal neurologic deficit, which tends to be indefinite and variable. In addition to arteriography, pneumoencephalography, or operation, a subdural hematoma may be indicated by finding a fracture line or a displacement of the pineal gland in the x-ray of the skull. The cerebrospinal fluid may be blood-tinged or xanthochromic when the type of stroke under suspicion would not be expected to show this. The electroencephalogram occasionally is strikingly silent over a subdural hematoma, and this may be of help. If the patient has fallen and injured his head at the onset of the stroke, it may be impossible to rule out a complicating subdural hematoma on clinical grounds alone.

The reverse diagnostic error of mistaking a stroke for a subdural hematoma is also often made. Here it is helpful to remember that patients with subdural hematoma rarely exhibit a complete hemiplegia, monoplegia, hemianesthesia, homonymous hemianopia, or well-developed aphasia. If these focal signs are present and particularly if they developed suddenly, subdural hematoma is not likely to be the explanation.

A *brain tumor,* especially a rapidly growing glioblastoma multiforme which may produce a severe hemiplegia within a week or two, can be mistaken for a stroke. Secondary carcinoma also may quickly lead to a marked neurologic deficit. However, in both conditions, a detailed history will show that the course was gradual; and if the symptoms progressed in saltatory fashion, seizures will usually have occurred. A chest film will be of great help in detecting a primary or secondary source of cancer in the lung. An increased blood sedimentation rate may suggest that a concealed systemic disease process is at work. Rarely, a *brain abscess* occurs without an evident antecedent focus of infection and may escape consideration in the differential diagnosis, especially if the patient is elderly.

Senile dementia, with a progressive loss of memory and enfeeblement of the intellect, is often ascribed on insufficient grounds to multiple small strokes, possibly in silent areas of the brain. If vascular lesions are responsible, evidence of a stroke will be disclosed by the history (sudden onset, episodic development) and by examination (a focal neurologic deficit—motor or sensory aphasia, visual field defect, etc.). The commonest cause of mental deterioration in the elderly patient is Alzheimer's disease or related degenerative processes, and in the absence of focal neurologic signs, it is unwarranted to attribute this syndrome to cerebral vascular disease—in particular, small strokes in silent areas. Cerebral arteriosclerosis is another term used too loosely as an explanation for such mental changes, the inference being that multiple areas of focal ischemia irreparably damage the nervous system, producing loss of memory but no other focal neurologic signs. If cerebral arteriosclerosis (atherosclerosis) is actually responsible, there should be evidence of it in the brain (strokes), heart (myocardial infarction, angina pectoris), or legs (intermittent claudication, loss of pulses).

Chronic cerebral seizures occur as the result of the stroke (*poststroke seizures*) in some 20 per cent of cases. When the seizures are infrequent or not properly observed, or when they leave behind a temporary increase in the neurologic deficit (Todd's paralysis), the diagnosis of another stroke may be made in error.

Fear, anxiety, and depression in patients who have had one small stroke may lead to additional symptoms, such as alterations in the paresthesias, headache, or disequilibrium, which suggest to the patient and his physician that further vascular lesions have occurred or threaten.

Miscellaneous conditions which occasionally lead to the suspicion of a stroke are Bell's palsy, Stokes-Adams attacks, diabetic ophthalmoplegia, acute ulnar, radial, or peroneal palsy, embolism to a limb, and temporal arteritis associated with blindness.

Strokes may be wrongly diagnosed as other neurologic illnesses. This happens under a variety of circumstances, but often it is due to an inadequate history and incomplete knowledge of the evolution of the illness. Unfortunately some of the patients who are subjected to pneumoencephalography for the diagnosis of these other conditions develop widespread brain infarction during the fall in blood pressure accompanying the procedure. In the lateral medullary syndrome, *dysphagia* may be the outstanding feature, and if the syndrome is not kept in mind, a fruitless surgical investigation may be undertaken looking for an esophageal neoplasm. *Headache* at times occurs as the prodrome of an oncoming thrombotic stroke, and unless this is appreciated a diagnosis of migraine may be made. In the elderly patient, *vertiginous attacks* due to vascular disease of the brain stem may be diagnosed as labyrinthine disease or Ménière's syndrome (see Chap. 31). Dizzy spells or brief lapses or intermittent loss of equilibrium due to cerebrovascular disease may be ascribed to Stokes-Adams syncope or paroxysmal tachycardia. A detailed account of the attack will usually serve to avert this error. A strikingly focal monoplegia of cerebral origin causing only weakness of the fingers or foot drop is not infrequently misdiagnosed as a peripheral lesion.

The differentiation of vascular disease from other neurologic illnesses in the presence of coma offers special problems. If the patient is comatose when first seen and an adequate history is not available, cerebrovascular lesions will have to be differentiated from all the other causes of coma described on p. 317. In most cases some history will be at hand to assist in the series of diagnostic deductions described below. The cerebrovascular causes of coma are as follows: hypertensive intracerebral hemorrhage, ruptured saccular or mycotic aneurysm, ruptured angioma, basilar artery embolism or thrombosis, acute hypertensive encephalopathy with brain edema, extensive infarction involving most of one cerebral hemisphere due to occlusion of a major arterial trunk, bilateral occlusion of the internal carotid arteries, bilateral cerebral embolism, multiple septic emboli, and widespread cerebral ischemia due to systemic hypotension (shock due to gastrointestinal bleeding, myocardial infarction, ruptured aneurysm, Stokes-Adams attacks, syncope). Nearly all these forms of cerebrovascular coma are accompanied by either changes in the cerebrospinal fluid or focal or lateralizing neurologic signs, which aid in separating them from toxic and metabolic abnormalities (see Chap. 289).

Differentiation of Thrombosis, Embolism, Hypertensive Hemorrhage, and Ruptured Saccular Aneurysm. Although it is difficult to lay down simple, hard and fast rules, usually it is possible to distinguish the four conditions at the bedside.

The most important criteria of *atherosclerotic thrombosis* are (1) a history of prodromal transient ischemic attacks; (2) an intermittent or stepwise evolution of the neurologic deficit, with recovery or improvement between worsenings, rather than a steady progression; (3) relative preservation of consciousness unless the upper part of the basilar territory is infarcted; (4) clear cerebrospinal fluid (except in meningovascular syphilis, intracranial arteritis, and occasionally an idiopathic pleocytosis with bland infarction); (5) the occurrence of rapid improvement at times; (6) onset during sleep or shortly after arising or during a period of hypotension; (7) certain constellations of symptoms and signs, e.g., the lateral medullary syndrome; (8) evidence of atherosclerosis elsewhere, especially in the coronary and peripheral vessels and the aorta; (9) the advancing age of the patient and the presence of disorders usually associated with atherosclerosis (hypertension, diabetes mellitus, and xanthomatosis); (10) headache of moderate severity (either as prodromal warning or accompanying the stroke); (11) carotid bruit in the neck, indicating carotid stenosis; (12) contralateral cranial bruit may indicate carotid occlusion of thrombotic type; (13) occlusion of the internal carotid artery in the neck (atherothrombotic or posttraumatic) as determined by palpation, auscultation, and ophthalmodynamometry.

Cerebral embolism is characterized by (1) sudden development of the clinical picture within a period of a few seconds or minutes; (2) the absence of prodromal transient ischemic attacks (rarely, one or two transitory episodes occur in the hours before the stroke especially if the embolus lodges in the carotid artery); (3) a source of embolus, usually in the heart, i.e., atrial fibrillation or other arrhythmia, myocardial infarction, subacute bacterial endocarditis, mitral stenosis, valvulotomy, marantic endocarditis associated with carcinoma; (4) evidence of recent embolism in other organs, i.e., spleen, kidney, extremities, gastrointestinal tract, or lungs; (5) evidence of recent involvement of several regions of the brain in different cerebrovascular territories; (6) clear cerebrospinal fluid except in those cases in which extensive bleeding occurs into an area of hemorrhagic infarction (most often in hemorrhagic infarction the cerebrospinal fluid is clear or at most faintly xanthochromic); (7) rapid improvement (many embolic strokes produce persistent deficits, but it is not uncommon for an extensive focal deficit to reverse itself in minutes or hours); (8) relative preservation of consciousness in the presence of extensive neurologic deficit, unless the upper part of the basilar territory is involved or massive brain swelling has occurred with temporal lobe tentorial herniation; (9) occurrence at an age when atherosclerosis is usually not a factor and in the absence of hypertension, arteritis, or infection; (10) localized headache of moderate severity, not infrequently accompanies cerebral embolism.

Other causes of cerebral infarction: The *diagnosis of arteritis* as a cause of infarction is justifiable only in the following circumstances: (1) evidence of an arteritis elsewhere, (2) in young individuals who manifest neither hypertension nor signs of cardiovascular disease, (3) in individuals with a meningeal infection which could affect the meningeal vessels (syphilis, tuberculosis). *Venous thrombosis with infarction* should be especially considered when focal neurologic signs develop after an operation or in the period following parturition, in the course of meningeal infection, ear or sinus suppuration, diseases which result in cachexia, and in congenital heart disease, polycythemia, or sickle-cell disease.

In *hypertensive cerebral hemorrhage* the diagnosis rests on (1) presence of hypertension; (2) grossly bloody spinal fluid under elevated pressure due to rupture of the hemorrhage into the ventricles (this is not invariable, for rarely the hemorrhage does not extend to the ventricular system and thus does not reach the cerebrospinal fluid); accurate diagnosis is difficult in these patients; (3) history of the gradual development of a deficit over a period of 10 min up to several hours (sometimes the onset appears to have been abrupt); (4) absence of prodromal phenomena; (5) deepening stupor or coma (generally speaking a patient with an extensive paralysis will be stuporous, and a hemiplegic stroke which leaves the patient alert and the mind relatively clear proves in nearly all instances to be due to an infarct); (6) onset during waking hours rather than in sleep; (7) severe headache is often but not invariably present; (8) nuchal rigidity; (9) preretinal hemorrhages; (10) a lateral displacement of the pineal gland (evidence of a hemorrhage rather than of an infarct, provided that massive brain swelling can be excluded). Absence of rapid fluctuation in the clinical course and persistence of the neurologic deficit in an evanescent stroke are never due to a hemorrhage, since extravasated blood is removed very slowly from the brain tissues.

The chief clinical features of *ruptured saccular aneurysm* are (1) sudden onset of severe headache; (2) brief or prolonged loss of consciousness at onset (in the most severe cases coma persists and the patient dies within a few hours); (3) grossly bloody spinal fluid under increased pressure (rupture of a saccular aneurysm without subarachnoid hemorrhage rarely if ever occurs, except in the case of aneurysms within the cavernous sinus; grossly bloody cerebrospinal fluid in the presence

of a third nerve palsy indicates a ruptured aneurysm at the origin of the posterior communicating artery from the internal carotid artery); (4) a relative absence of focal neurologic signs; (5) preretinal (subhyaloid) hemorrhages (these suggest ruptured aneurysm or angioma, although they can occur in massive intracerebral hemorrhage) and after trauma; (6) stiff neck on forward bending, Kernig and Brudzinski signs; (7) transient weakness, numbness, or aphasia at onset; (8) palsy of third nerve; (9) convulsion at onset; (10) usually an absence of prodromal warnings, although there may be a history of one or more premonitory "leaks" associated with transient headache; (11) onset during exertion, sexual intercourse, etc.; (12) absence of hypertension in many cases. Saccular aneurysm is likely to produce a diffuse subarachnoid hemorrhage without causing significant damage to the cerebral hemispheres. If the cerebrospinal fluid is bloody and the patient retains mental clarity or is only mildly confused, aneurysm or cerebellar hemorrhage is the diagnosis of choice. If the aneurysm bleeds into the brain tissue (subarachnoid-cerebral hemorrhage) or into the ventricular system also (subarachnoid-cerebroventricular hemorrhage), focal neurologic signs and coma ensue, as in intracerebral hemorrhage. Cerebral infarction associated with ruptured aneurysm, not an uncommon event, is another cause for a focal neurologic deficit. In the latter circumstance often the patient will remain alert.

Coarctation of the aorta and polycystic disease of the kidneys may be present.

Intracranial hemorrhage from an angioma is a tenable diagnosis under the following circumstances: (1) stroke in a young patient with bloody cerebrospinal fluid in the absence of hypertension; (2) antecedent epilepsy, often with transient postictal paralysis; (3) presence of a cranial or cervical bruit sometimes heard by the patient as well; (4) repeated subarachnoid hemorrhages (sometimes more than five); (5) calcification in the region of the lesion in x-ray of the skull; (6) lateralizing neurologic signs are more frequent than with aneurysm.

LABORATORY METHODS OF DIAGNOSIS

A number of special laboratory tests are of value in the diagnosis of cerebrovascular disease, but none of them can approach in general usefulness a careful history and physical examination. The importance of lumbar puncture has already been mentioned. If a fine needle is used, No. 20, and the jugular veins are not compressed, there is probably little danger in doing a "spinal tap" in most cases. Nevertheless, the procedure should not be routine; in every case a decision should be reached at the time of the first examination as to the necessity of the procedure and as to the most appropriate time. If cerebellar or temporal lobe herniation is threatening, the lumbar puncture may contribute to a fatal issue and should be deferred unless absolutely necessary. This is especially so in cerebral hemorrhage, cerebellar hemorrhage, massive cerebral infarction, cerebellar infarction, and hypertensive encephalopathy. In primary subarachnoid hemorrhage, the lumbar puncture, although necessary for diagnosis, should not be repeated except to investigate the possibility of further hemorrhage or in order to alleviate severe headache.

Many cases of apoplexy should have x-rays of the skull en route to a hospital bed, especially if there is any suspicion of trauma. The finding of unexpected fractures, a displaced pineal gland, or calcification in an aneurysm or vascular malformation will be helpful in diagnosis. X-ray of the chest is useful as part of the cardiac examination and sometimes will disclose a pulmonary neoplasm or a dissecting aortic aneurysm.

Blood cell counts also provide useful information. A high hematocrit suggests that polycythemia is a factor; a severe anemia and greatly increased sedimentation rate might provide a clue to the existence of subacute bacterial endocarditis and should lead to a blood culture. Leukemia and thrombopenia, of course, must be diagnosed from the blood examination. Serologic tests for syphilis should be done on the blood and spinal fluid. In aneurysmal rupture there may be a transient albuminuria and hyperglycemia with glucosuria. Hypertensive hemorrhage, too, can cause hyperglycemia.

An electrocardiogram should be obtained in all cases of cerebral infarction. Occasionally it will establish the presence of a recent, silent myocardial infarct or provide correlative evidence of hypertension. An electroencephalogram will be abnormal in most major strokes and is a useful means of following the course of the illness. However, its value in the diagnosis of cerebrovascular diseases has yet to be determined.

Carotid arteriography is indispensable in the diagnosis of aneurysms and vascular malformations. Some 75 to 80 per cent of such lesions within the territory of the carotid arteries are revealed by this method. With recent interest in vascular surgery of the carotid and vertebral systems, *arteriography* will have to be used with increasing frequency but by no means should it be routine. Retinal arterial pressure measurements have been of great help in detecting occlusion of the internal carotid artery.

CONCLUSION

Of all the forms of neurologic disease, those described in this chapter are of the greatest impor-

tance to the practicing physician. The assiduous application of clinical method and laboratory test will permit diagnosis of the type of cerebrovascular disease with approximately 75 per cent accuracy, enabling the physician to use a sensible therapeutic measure in many of the cases. Future developments, it is hoped, will improve both the accuracy of diagnosis and the effectiveness of therapy.

REFERENCES

Field, W. S.: "Pathogenesis and Treatment of Cerebrovascular Disease," Springfield, Ill., Charles C Thomas, Publisher, 1961.

Foix, C., and M. Levy: Les ramollissements sylviens: Syndromes des lesions en foyer du territoire de l'artère sylviennes et ses branches, Rev. neurol., 2:1, 1927.

Kubik, C. S., and R. D. Adams: Occlusion of Basilar Artery—Clinical and Pathologic Study, Brain, 69: 73, 1946.

McKissock, W., L. Walsh, and J. C. Richardson: Paper read at Massachusetts General Hospital, March, 1959.

Walton, J.: "Subarachnoid Hemorrhage," Edinburgh, E. and S. Livingstone, Ltd., 1956.

285 TRAUMATIC DISEASES OF THE BRAIN AND SPINAL CORD

Karl-Erik Åström,
Henri vander Eecken, and
Raymond D. Adams

TRAUMATIC DISEASES OF THE BRAIN

Head injury, which is the basis of some of the most frequent and serious neurologic disorders in these times of high-velocity transport and mechanization in industry, poses many problems to the practicing physician. To deal with them effectively demands a knowledge of the clinical manifestations as well as a sound grasp of fundamental physiologic mechanisms. The physician must stand prepared at all times, for he may at any moment be summoned to render aid or to assess the clinical status of a person who has suffered an injury of the head or spine. The present chapter undertakes to review the salient facts concerning these injuries of the nervous system and to outline an approach to these problems that has been useful to the authors.

Physiologic and Pathologic Considerations

The very language with which certain types of head injury are discussed divulges a number of misconceptions that have been inherited from previous generations of physicians. Words have crept into medical vocabulary and have often been retained long after the ideas for which they stood have been refuted—clear evidence of the disadvantage of prematurely adopting explanatory rather than descriptive terms. The word *concussion,* for example, implies the violent shaking and agitation of an organ or the functional impairment which results therefrom. Yet despite numerous experiments intended to demonstrate these physical changes within nerve cells (vibration effects, formation of intracellular vacuoles, etc.), no confirmation of their existence has been possible. Similarly the word *contusion,* meaning a bruising or crushing without interruption of physical continuity, is applied rather indiscriminately to a variety of clinical states, some of which could not depend on a pathologic change of this type, e.g., "minor contusion state or syndrome"—an expression introduced by Wilfred Trotter, who was himself most critical of words that "embalm a fallacious theory."

In all attempts to analyze the mechanism of brain damage in head injury one fact stands preeminent—that there must be the sudden application of a physical force of considerable magnitude to the head. Unless the head is struck, the brain suffers no injury—except in the rare and somewhat controversial cases of crush injury to the chest or explosive injury with raised intrapulmonary pressure, in which petechial hemorrhages are said to have been found in the brain. A second fact, also susceptible of easy verification, is that the size of the area on the skull over which the force is exerted is of importance. High-velocity missiles destroy a small part of the skull and penetrate the cranial cavity without significant displacement of the head or brain; and heavy, crushing injuries which result from the skull being compressed between two converging objects may crush the brain. In these two circumstances it is interesting to note that the patient may suffer severe and often fatal injury without immediate loss of consciousness. Hemorrhage, destruction of brain tissue, and if the patient survives for a time, meningitis or abscess, are the principal pathologic changes created by injuries of this type. They offer little difficulty to understanding.

The common civilian injury is one in which a rapidly moving blunt object strikes the head or the head is flung against a hard surface. Injuries of this type, often termed *blunt head injuries,* are remarkable in two respects: (1) they almost always induce at least a temporary loss of consciousness; (2) even though the skull is not penetrated and fragments of bone are not driven into its cavity, the brain may suffer gross damage, i.e., contusion, laceration, hemorrhage, swelling, herniation, etc.

Clinicians as well as experimental physiologists have sought a theory which would bring into plausible form all gross neuropathologic changes, the skull fracture and the transient paralysis of nervous function (concussion) or prolonged coma, so often observed in fatal cases. It may be said that a comprehensive theory, acceptable to all workers in this field, has not been developed as yet.

The relation of skull fracture to injury of the cerebral tissues has been viewed in changing perspective through the entire history of this subject. In earliest times fractures dominated the thinking of the medical profession, and cerebral lesions were regarded as secondary. Some of the best articles on the location of fractures and their relationship to anatomic peculiarities of the cranial bones were written in the eighteenth and nineteenth centuries. Later it became known that the skull, although rigid, is still flexible enough to yield to a severe blow without fracture. Therefore, the presence of a fracture, although a rough measure of the violence to which the brain has been exposed, is not an infallible index; and even in fatal head injury, autopsy may reveal an intact skull in 20 to 30 per cent of cases. Also many patients suffer skull fracture without serious disorder of cerebral function.

The modern trend is to be interested more in the presence or absence of brain injury than in the fracture of the skull itself. Nevertheless fractures cannot be dismissed without a few comments, for they assume importance in indicating the site and possible severity of brain damage, in providing an explanation for cranial nerve palsies, and in affording potential pathways for the ingress of bacteria and air or the egress of cerebrospinal fluid.

The existence of a basal skull fracture may be indicated by signs of cranial nerve damage. Cranial nerves which are particularly liable to injury are the olfactory, optic, oculomotor, first and second branches of the trigeminal, the facial, and the auditory. Anosmia and an apparent loss of taste (actually a loss of aromatic flavors, elementary tastes—salt, sweet, bitter, sour—being retained) are frequent sequelae of head injury, especially of falls on the back of the head. In the majority of cases the anosmia is permanent or the patient may have some perversion of smell (parosmia). The anosmia may be unilateral and not noticed by the patient. The mechanism of these disturbances is believed to be displacement of the brain and tearing of the olfactory nerve filaments. A fracture in or near the sella may tear the stalk of the pituitary gland, with resulting diabetes insipidus. A fracture of sphenoid bone may lacerate the optic nerve, with complete blindness from the beginning. The pupil is dilated and unreactive to a direct light stimulus but still takes part in the consensual reflex.

The optic disk becomes pale, i.e., atrophic, after an interval of several weeks. Partial injuries may result in a troublesome blurring of vision. Injury to the eighth cranial nerve with petrosal fractures causes loss of hearing and/or dizziness, immediately after injury. The deafness due to nerve injury must be distinguished from that caused by rupture of the eardrum or the presence of blood in the middle ear, and the vertigo, from posttraumatic giddiness. In oculomotor nerve injury there is a divergent squint, with loss of internal and vertical movement of the eye and a fixed, dilated pupil. Diplopia only on looking down suggests trochlear nerve affection. Direct injury of the facial nerve by a basal fracture may be present immediately after the injury or may be delayed, coming on after several days. This delayed form is usually transitory, and its mechanism is not known. It may be misinterpreted as an important progression of the traumatic intracranial lesion. Injury to the ophthalmic or maxillary divisions of the trigeminal nerve may be the result either of a basal fracture across the middle cranial fossa or of a direct extracranial injury to the branches of these nerves. Numbness and paresthesias over the area of skin supplied by the nerve or a troublesome neuralgia are the sequelae of these injuries.

If the skin is lacerated over the skull fracture and the underlying meninges are torn, or if the fracture passes through the posterior wall of a nasal sinus, bacteria or air may enter the cranial cavity with resulting meningitis, abscess, and aerocele. Cerebrospinal fluid may also leak into the sinus and present as a watery discharge from the nose (cerebrospinal fluid rhinorrhea). Persistence of the rhinorrhea or the occurrence of episodes of recurrent meningitis (headache, convulsions, fever, and stiff neck with pleocytosis and sometimes bacteria) are often indications for a repair of the torn dura mater over the fissure. Depressed fractures are of significance only if the underlying dura is lacerated by spicules of bone or the brain is compressed.

Much has been written about the mechanism of coma in closed or blunt head injury. Two facts concerning this condition stand out clearly: (1) it bears no relationship to skull fracture; (2) the optimal conditions for its production are those in which there is some change in the momentum of the head; i.e., movement is suddenly imparted to it by a blow, or its movement is suddenly arrested. Striking the stationary head of an experimental animal will cause a loss of brain stem reflexes only if the head was free to move; not if it is clamped in one position (Denny-Brown and Russell). This finding alone would stand in refutation of such theories of concussion as a wave of high intracranial pressure due to the indentation of the skull or a subsequent wave of negative pressure (Kahn,

Ward, and Clark), cerebral anemia (Trotter), or a general vibration or agitation transmitted via the skull. The speed of acceleration or deceleration of the head necessary for this concussive effect must exceed 28 ft per sec. The initial action of the blunt injury of this type is to excite the nervous system (the "stars" that one sees with a minor injury, the gasp of the animal); and this is followed by transient paralysis of cerebral function, i.e., abolition of consciousness, suppression of reflexes, arrest of respiration, etc. The means whereby the latter effects are produced is not known. The old studies of Fischer and Alquie show that in most head injuries there is displacement of the brain within the skull. The brain, being suspended in a water jacket of cerebrospinal fluid, tends not to follow movements of the cranium but to lag, because of its own inertia. The superior parts of the cerebral hemispheres are free to move more than the lower parts, which are attached to the relatively fixed brain stem. There is the possibility, then, of stretch or torsion on midbrain and subthalamic structures, and indeed temporary paralysis of the reticular activating mechanism, which is located in these parts of the brain, has recently been demonstrated. This could account for both the unconsciousness and suppression of reflexes and also the electroencephalographic changes (relative electrical silence followed by slow waves). It would appear, however, that the cerebrum itself does not escape damage, for Meyer and Denny-Brown have found evidence of an electrical "injury potential" and reduction in oxygen uptake in the cerebral cortex. The changes, whatever and wherever they may be, are for the most part transitory and would be expected to have no visible structural basis. Pathologic changes, such as have been described in several published accounts of experimental concussion, are difficult to evaluate. The report of diffuse degeneration of the cerebral white matter in rabbits and monkeys which were repeatedly struck on the head (Jakob), the observation of petechial hemorrhages in the cervical cord and medulla in the cat, dog, and monkey (Denny-Brown and Russell), and the demonstration of chromatolysis of large nerve cells in the brain stem of concussed animals (Windle et al.) have not been verified. It is unlikely that any of them could be the pathologic basis of the concussive state.

In fatal cases of severe head injury, where this concussive injury must also have existed, the brain is almost invariably bruised or lacerated, and often there is hemorrhage, either meningeal or intracerebral. The observation of these gross pathologic findings had led to the widely prevalent view that head injuries are largely matters of bruises and hemorrhages and of urgent operations. That this can hardly be the case is suggested by the fact that some patients survive head injuries almost as severe as the fatal ones and yet make an excellent recovery. At autopsy years later old contusions (*plaques jaunes*) and hemorrhages of approximately the same distribution and extent as those observed in some of the immediately fatal cases are found. One can only conclude, therefore, that most of the immediate symptomatology of severe head injury, both general and localized, depends on invisible and highly reversible change in the brain, probably of the same nature as that which underlies concussion. Nevertheless these bruises, lacerations, hemorrhages, and localized swellings of tissues cannot be disregarded, because they are probably responsible for many of the fatalities that occur 12 to 72 hr or more after the injury. Of these lesions the most important is the surface bruising of the brain beneath the point of impact (*coup* injury) and the more extensive lacerations and contusions on the opposite side of the brain (*contrecoup* injuries). The inertia of the brain, which causes it to be flung against the side of the skull that was struck and to be pulled away from the contralateral side, has been invoked to explain these coup-contrecoup contusions. This theory has been further elaborated by Holburn, who points out that the brain is roughly spherical and that all movements of the head describe an arc with its axis at the point of attachment of skull to spine. Sudden changes in the momentum of the head, therefore, induce a swirling motion to the brain, which may then suffer injury against all rough, bony prominences (wings of sphenoid bones, petrous parts of temporal bones, rough surfaces of orbital and frontal bones). The lacerations and hemorrhages are based on a similar mechanism, the latter being due merely to the tearing of larger vessels. Also extensive infarction of the brain may occur when cerebral arteries are compressed between a herniating mass of brain and the dura, e.g., the posterior cerebral artery in temporal lobe herniations. An important fact from the standpoint of the clinician is that these contusions, hemorrhages, and extensive necrotic lesions, whatever their mechanism may be, may occur without a penetrating head injury; and under these circumstances they and their clinical effects are engrafted upon the traumatic paralysis of cerebral function which is called *concussion*. They are in a sense epiphenomena which nonetheless may unfavorably tip the balance of life and death. The most compelling evidence of the correctness of this view is that head injury may end fatally without any visible structural change in the nervous system. However, in most fatal cases a significant degree of bruising, edema, hemorrhage, and herniation is also present.

Clinical Manifestations of Head Injury

The physician upon being called to see a patient who has had a head injury will generally find him in one of three clinical conditions; each, as Trotter, Symonds, and Rowbotham have pointed out, must be dealt with differently. It is usually possible to place the patient in one of the following three categories by assessing the mental and general neurologic status when the patient is first seen and at intervals of time after the accident.

Patients Who Are Conscious or Are Rapidly Regaining Mental Clarity When First Seen (Minor Head Injury). The typical example is a patient who was rendered unconscious by a knock on the head and then regained his senses within seconds, minutes, or hours. Roughly two degrees of disturbance of consciousness may have occurred. First, there is the patient who was never unconscious at all. He was observed to have struck his head and was stunned or "saw stars." By all criteria his head injury was insignificant when judged in terms of life and death and severe brain damage, though in exceptional cases there is always the possibility of skull fracture or epidural or subdural hematoma. Nevertheless, a troublesome group of symptoms may have developed at once or within a few days. The patient may begin to complain of headache, dizziness, loss of confidence in himself, inability to concentrate, nervousness, poor sleep, fatigue, and depression. The headache is of a pressing, aching type and is characteristically worsened by any physical and mental effort, stooping, and excitement. No clue is provided as to the mechanism of these symptoms. The possibility that they represent a traumatic or compensation neurosis is suggested because of the purely subjective nature of the symptoms and lack of abnormal neurologic signs and the absence of change in cerebrospinal fluid or alteration of the EEG. In recent years a better appreciation of the constancy of this clinical syndrome has favored the view first put forward by Wilfred Trotter that they are the direct physical effects of injury, incorrectly designated by him *minor cerebral contusion* state. The severity of these symptoms is not clearly related to the severity of the head injury. Their persistence constitutes a most vexatious therapeutic problem.

If consciousness was temporarily abolished, the patient is said to have suffered a *concussion*, defined by Trotter as "an essentially transient state due to head injury which is instantaneous in onset, manifests widespread symptoms of a purely paralytic kind, does not as such comprise any evidence of structural cerebral injury and is always followed by amnesia for the actual moment of the impact." The patient, if observed immediately after the injury, shows a complete paralysis of nervous function. In a few instances death has occurred at this time, from respiratory arrest or cardiac arrhythmia, and no lesion was found at postmortem examination. However, the usual sequela is for the pulse and respiration (if they were depressed or arrested) to return at once and for muscle tone, reflexes, voluntary movement, and mental clarity to be regained within a few minutes. Only an amnesia for the accident and the events that immediately preceded (retrograde amnesia) and followed it (anterograde amnesia) will remain. Thereafter the patient may suffer the same headaches, giddiness, and nervousness described above.

These relatively trivial head injuries may rarely be followed by a number of other puzzling features all of which indicate the occurrence of some process in addition to concussion: (1) *Delayed traumatic collapse:* following an accident a few patients, after walking about and seeming to be mentally normal, will turn pale and fall unconscious for a few minutes. This is a vasomotor syncopal attack and is probably related to injury, pain, and emotional upset. Rarely does the patient exhibit any focal or lateralizing neurologic signs. The suggestion that this represents medullary edema is hardly tenable. (2) *Immediate traumatic paraplegia:* with falls on top of the head, which may injure the motor areas for the lower extremities, both legs may become temporarily weak and numb, sometimes with bilateral Babinski signs and sphincteric incontinence. Concussion of the cervical segments of the spinal cord is another possible mechanism of this paraplegia. (3) *Immediate hemiplegia* or *monoplegia:* these conditions may develop immediately after a minor injury, with or without blood in the cerebrospinal fluid, and are commonly attributed to a relatively circumscript injury with minimal concussion and a direct contusion or laceration of the underlying brain (cerebrospinal fluid is sanguineous). (4) *Immediate traumatic epilepsy:* a series of focal seizures may occur with a minor bruise of the cortex and may be followed by a postepileptic paralysis of short duration. (5) *Delayed hemiplegia* or *monoplegia:* an "interval" paralysis in cases of minor or major injury usually signifies an epidural hemorrhage, a subdural hemorrhage or hygroma, arterial thrombosis, spreading venous thrombosis, or intracerebral hemorrhage. (6) *Acute drowsiness, confusion,* and *headache* or *coma,* due presumably to localized and generalized traumatic brain edema: children who have had concussion are especially liable to headache, drowsiness, and vomiting which may have its onset some hours after the injury. In these children infusions and clyses of water and 5 per cent glucose are particularly dangerous; such treatment may prove fatal, owing to a water intoxication and severe brain swelling. Apparently an excessive output of antidiuretic hormone and water retention occur under these circumstances.

Patients Who Are and Have Been Unconscious Since the Time of the Accident (Major Head Injury). *The Clinical State.* In this group, which includes the patients with the more severe head injuries, the outlook is obviously less favorable and one is concerned at first for their life. However, within this group there is still a wide variation in the severity of the traumatic brain disease. A certain number of patients die at once or within a few minutes, and it may be assumed that the direct injury to the brain or some other organ was incompatible with life. Other patients in this group recover consciousness rapidly after several hours, but a few remain deeply comatose for days or even weeks. The mortality rate in those who reach a hospital in coma is approximately 20 per cent, and most of them die within the first 12 to 24 hr. Of those alive after 24 hr, the mortality is 7 to 8 per cent, and after 48 hr the figure falls to 1 per cent.

In the patient whose prognosis is favorable, the coma is less deep; i.e., they are confused, stuporous, or semicomatose (see Chap. 34). For a time he may be restless and difficult to control. The reflexes are normal, as are pulse, blood pressure, and respiration. He is able to swallow and may or may not speak. There are no obvious neurologic signs. In contrast, those patients whose illness will end fatally may be moribund from the beginning. Their coma is profound. The limbs may be flaccid and without reflexes. The corneal and pharyngeal (gag) reflexes are absent. The pupils are small and unreactive to light, or dilated and fixed, or unequal. The ocular axes are divergent or askew. The jaw sags, the tongue falls back in the throat, saliva drools from the mouth, and swallowing is obviously lost. There may be surgical shock at first for a brief period, with the usual findings of pale and moist skin, weak and rapid pulse, subnormal temperature, and a blood pressure that is difficult to obtain. Within a few hours, however, the temperature usually rises, and this may continue until death. The breathing may be stertorous and later feeble and irregular. The state of consciousness and the temperature chart provide information of great value in appraising the status of the patient. An ascending pulse rate, possibly interspersed by short periods in which there is a bounding, slow pulse, and rising temperature or a combination of fast pulse and subnormal temperature, is a sign of a grave prognosis.

In the group of patients whose outlook is less bleak, deep coma soon gives way to semicoma. The blood pressure stabilizes, and the temperature and pulse, having risen to 101 to 102°F and 100 to 110 per min, respectively, remain at these levels. Muscular tone is regained in the limbs, and the tendon reflexes are present. This is a critical period, for a sudden rise in temperature, cyanosis, and increasing respiratory difficulty may result in a fatal issue. Once the patient regains full consciousness sufficiently to respond to a spoken command, the physician no longer needs to be concerned about survival and may begin to think about the possibility of focal brain damage and prospects for recovery. There is still a substantial risk in the first 2 or 3 weeks, however, from pneumonia, meningitis, or epidural and subdural hemorrhage, which may intervene and impair the chances of survival. It is often said that death during the first 12 hr is the result of the direct injury of the brain; that which occurs later is usually the result of some complication of cranial trauma (intracerebral or subarachnoid hemorrhage, herniation of the temporal lobe, localized or generalized edema, epidural or subdural hemorrhage, meningitis, pneumonia).

There is another group of patients to which some reference must be made for they represent difficult problems in diagnosis and therapy. Here a known or evident head injury is not followed by deep and lasting coma, but instead the patient is awake and able to respond moderately well upon arrival at the hospital. Yet as the hours pass it is apparent that his condition is deteriorating, and within a day or two he lapses into coma. A sanguineous cerebrospinal fluid under slightly elevated pressure attests to the existence of contusion. The progressive nature of the illness suggests intracerebral, epidural, or subdural hemorrhage; yet at postmortem examination only contusion, localized edema (sometimes generalized), and temporal lobe pressure cone are found to be the basis of the clinical syndrome. The point to remember is that consciousness may return early, i.e., within minutes or hours, after a head injury severe enough seriously to contuse the brain, and yet may lead to death, after some few days.

The course of clinical events in those who survive the first 24 to 48 hr is much like that in patients with type I injury, except that it is likely to be more prolonged so that one may witness all the varying stages of recovery. As coma lessens, the patient opens his eyes; he may pause in his restless activity and seem to listen to what is said. He reacts briskly to painful stimuli applied to the face, passive manipulations of the head, and pinching the inner surface of the arms or legs. Moaning and groaning are the first vocal activities to return; their absence in patients who are beginning to respond always suggests aphasia. Restlessness, irritability, and hyperactivity may assume such proportions that the patient must be restrained. For example, he may resist all attempts to help him, struggle against restraints, yell, talk incessantly and

without sense, strike at everyone near the bed, etc. This state, sometimes called *traumatic delirium,* may last hours or days but eventually is replaced by a more quiet confusional state. Then the patient speaks, unless lacking in impulse to act (abulia) or capacity for speech (aphasia), and is variably able to engage in conversation. His thinking processes are slow and inefficient, and his thoughts are likely to be incoherent. Often he cannot understand the purposes of his splints, bandages, catheters, etc., and will remove them even when asked repeatedly not to do so. Movements and reactions to stimuli are more or less automatic, and if conversation is possible it is repetitious and often incoherent. Also, memory is obviously faulty. As confusion lessens, there may be a brief period when mental function is nearly normal; yet later there will be little or no memory for what transpired. From a close study of this clinical sequence it is obvious that the capacity to form, retain, and reproduce new experiences is one of the best tests of the mental status. Not until the patient reaches the stage of continuous anterograde memory will he regard himself as fully normal. In looking back upon this period the patient can recall only a few events and has the impression that he was unconscious all this time. Retrograde amnesia for the accident and for the events which preceded it, which often extends over a period of minutes, hours, or even days, is another invariable accompaniment of severe head injury. This period of retrograde memory defect shortens as convalescence proceeds.

Focal and lateralizing neurologic symptoms and signs, as would be anticipated, will be observed with notable frequency in this group of patients. These abnormalities are presumably related to hemorrhage and contusion; and in as much as they are usually engrafted on a severe concussive injury, they become manifest as consciousness is regained. Local injury to the brain without a disturbance of consciousness occurs exceptionally, and then more often with the penetration of the skull by missiles or a direct or glancing blow by a relatively small object (golf ball, stone), sometimes with depression fractures. Of the focal symptoms, hemiparesis is probably the most frequent. The weakness of arm and leg may be evident even during coma by the hypotonia, the less frequent movement of the limbs, inequality of tendon reflexes, and a more persistent Babinski sign on one side. Complete hemiplegia is rarely observed. Hemihypesthesia, although occasionally found, is less common, possibly because sensory tests are difficult to interpret until mental clarity is regained. Homonymous hemianopia is not at all infrequent and may present early as an inattentiveness to visual stimuli on one side. Aphasia, usually of mixed type, may be noted in a number of the cases. A series of focal seizures may occur within a few days of the time of injury and, as said before, are probably due to cortical contusion. They usually cease after a few days and do not necessarily signify that epilepsy is to be a sequel to the trauma. Diabetes insipidus, disturbances of sleep (reversal of rhythm, somnolence, later narcolepsy), diplopia, heteronymous visual field defects, gastrointestinal hemorrhage, amenorrhea, and impotence in the male indicate damage to the hypothalamus and walls of the third ventricle. Midbrain or diffuse cerebral lesions are evidenced by ocular palsies, protracted coma (weeks, months, or years), decerebrate rigidity, crossed ocular-limb paralyses, bilateral Babinski signs, and later dysarthria, ataxia of limbs on one side, and sensory disturbances.

Laboratory Findings. In this group of patients with severe head injury there is a high incidence of skull fracture. The cerebrospinal fluid is usually sanguineous (red blood cells usually 100,000 per cu mm or less) and under elevated pressure (between 200 and 300 mm) in the majority of patients. The prognosis is distinctly less good in those with more than 100,000 red cells per cu mm and pressures in excess of 300 mm. Nevertheless death may occur in patients who have no skull fracture, a subnormal intracranial pressure, and relatively clear cerebrospinal fluid. The electroencephalogram regularly shows focal and diffuse abnormalities.

Neuropathologic Findings. In patients who die during the first few hours or days after a severe head injury, hemorrhage and necrosis of tissue will frequently be observed. In 50 consecutive autopsies summarized in Rowbotham's excellent monograph, only two showed no macroscopic change. Lacerations of cerebral cortex (28 per cent), surface contusions (48 per cent), subarachnoid hemorrhage (72 per cent), acute subdural hemorrhage (16 per cent), extradural hemorrhage (20 per cent) were the usual findings. As a rule, several of these pathologic changes were found in the same case. Skull fractures were discovered in 72 per cent. With such striking gross lesions there is a great temptation to assume that they account for the deep coma and the other general neurologic findings, though, as already pointed out, this assumption may be erroneous. The basis of at least part of the general symptoms (coma, stupor, delirium, confusion) is usually the initial concussion itself, which is nearly always of greater magnitude than that seen in cases of the first group. Recovery from hemiplegia, aphasia, etc., must indicate some reversible process near the contusions and hemorrhages (localized cerebral edema?). This use of the term *concussion* to refer to a prolonged instead of transient (usually defined as less than 5 min) traumatically induced loss of consciousness has been criticized by many physicians. Nevertheless, there is no reason to be-

lieve that the same forces which cause a brief cerebral disorder could not, when acting more forcibly, cause a more protracted one. This is not to deny, of course, that expanding clots, cerebral herniations, midbrain hemorrhages, and high intracranial pressure, so frequent in this group, are responsible for the most prolonged states of coma.

Patients Who Are Unconscious When First Seen but Who Are Said to Have Been Conscious after the Accident (Presence of Lucid Interval). This group of patients is smaller than the other two but is of great importance because it includes many who are in urgent need of surgical treatment. The initial coma may have been brief or there may have been none at all, in which instance one may conclude that there was neither concussion nor contusion. The following conditions must be considered in every case of this type.

Acute Epidural Hemorrhage. This condition is due as a rule to a temporal or parietal fracture with laceration of the middle meningeal artery and vein. Less often there is a tear in a dural venous sinus. The injury, even when it fractures the skull, may not have produced coma. A typical example is a child who has fallen from a bicycle or a swing or has suffered a hard blow to the head in a fight and was only momentarily unconscious. A few hours or a day or two later (the interval may be as long as several days or a week, especially with venous bleeding), he develops headache of increasing severity, vomiting, drowsiness, confusion, seizures (which may be one-sided), hemiparesis, with slightly increased tendon reflexes and Babinski sign. As coma develops, the hemiparesis with Babinski sign may give way to flaccid or spastic limbs and Babinski signs bilaterally. There may be aphasia. Respirations become deeper and stertorous, then shallow and irregular, and finally stop. The pulse is often slow (below 60) and bounding, with a concomitant rise in systolic blood pressure. The pupil may dilate on the side of the hematoma. The cerebrospinal fluid is usually under increased pressure, though normal and subnormal pressures do not exclude the possibility of an epidural hematoma. The fluid may be clear or sanguineous, depending on whether or not there is an associated contusion, laceration, or subarachnoid hemorrhage. Death, which is almost invariable if the clot is not removed surgically, comes at the end of a comatose period, rarely if ever in a conscious patient, and is due to respiratory arrest. The visualization of a fracture line across the groove of the middle meningeal artery and a knowledge of the side of the head struck (the clot is usually on that side) are of aid in diagnosis and of lateralization of the lesion. The surgical procedure is placement of several burr holes (a single one may miss the clot), drainage, identification of the bleeding vessel, and ligation. The operative results are excellent, except in the cases with extensive fractures and laceration of the dural venous sinuses, in which instance the epidural hematoma may be bilateral rather than unilateral, as it ordinarily is. If coma, bilateral Babinski signs, spasticity, or decerebrate rigidity supervene before operation, the prognosis for life becomes poor. This usually means that a temporal lobe herniation and crushing of the midbrain have already occurred.

Acute and Chronic Subdural Hematoma. The problems created by the acute and the chronic subdural hematoma are so different that they must be discussed separately. In *acute subdural hematomas,* which may be unilateral or bilateral, the latent interval is usually longer than in epidural hemorrhage—many days or 1 to 2 weeks. Headaches, drowsiness, sometimes agitation, slowness in thinking, and confusion, all of which progressively worsen, are the most frequent symptoms. Focal or lateralizing signs (hemiplegia) are late and tend to be less prominent than the disturbance of consciousness. Frequently the acute subdural hematoma is combined with cerebral contusion and laceration, so that the clinical effects of these several lesions are difficult to distinguish; and there are some patients in whom it is impossible before operation to state whether the surface clot is epidural or subdural in location. The treatment is bilateral temporal burr holes, and this is also one of the most certain diagnostic procedures. If the clot that is found is too small to explain the symptoms, the surgeon usually proceeds to do a right subtemporal decompression.

In chronic subdural hematoma, mentioned in the differential diagnoses in Chaps. 34, 37, and 38, the traumatic etiology is less clear. The head injury, especially in the elderly person, may be trivial (striking the head against a branch of a tree, or on the mantel of a fireplace during a faint, etc.), and it may have been forgotten completely. A period of weeks then follows when headaches (not invariable), giddiness, slowness in thinking, confusion, exaggeration of certain personality traits, and rarely a seizure or two are the main symptoms. The initial impression may be that the patient has a brain tumor, a drug intoxication, or a depressive, senile, or other psychosis. As with acute subdural hematoma, the disturbance of consciousness (drowsiness, inattentiveness, incoherence of thought, stupor, or coma) is more prominent than focal or lateralizing signs. The latter usually consist of hemiparesis and rarely of an aphasic disturbance. Hemianesthesia and homonymous hemianopia are seldom observed, probably because the anatomic structures subserving these functions are deep and not easily compressed (in the case of the geniculocalcarine pathway) and sensory changes are likely to be overlooked in a stuporous, confused patient. Hemiplegia, i.e., complete paralysis of one arm and leg, is usually indicative of an intracerebral lesion rather than of a compressive surface lesion. Another important feature of the hemiparesis is that it may be contralateral or ipsilateral, depending on whether or not herniation of the temporal lobe through the notch of the tentorium into the posterior fossa and compression of the contralateral cerebral peduncle are present; if they are present, pyramidal signs are then ipsilateral to the clot or bilateral. As the condition progresses, the patient becomes comatose but often with striking fluctuations of awareness. The ipsilateral pupil dilates (Hutchinson's pupillary sign), owing, it is believed, to direct pressure of the herniating temporal lobe upon the oculomotor nerve. The dilated pupil and aptotic eyelid are more reliable indicators of the side of the hematoma than the hemiparesis, though they too can be misleading in certain cases. Convulsions are usually seen only in alcoholics or cases with a contusion and cannot be regarded as a cardinal sign of subdural hematoma, even though they are not infrequent. Roentgenograms of the skull are usually negative except for a shift of a calcified pineal to one side or an occasional unexpected fracture line. The electroencephalogram is usually bilaterally abnormal, sometimes with reduced voltage or electrical silence over the subdural hematoma or high-voltage slow waves over the same and opposite sides because of the damping effects of the clot and displacement of the brain. The anterior and middle cerebral arteries are seen to be displaced in an arteriogram. The cerebrospinal fluid may be clear, bloody, or xanthochromic, depending on the presence or absence of recent or old contusion and subarachnoid hemorrhage, and the pressure may be elevated, normal, or subnormal. Of all these diagnostic procedures, direct burr hole exploration is the most reliable.

The acute, rapidly evolving subdural hematomas are due to tearing of bridging veins and direct compression of the brain by an expanding clot of fresh blood. Unlike the epidural arterial hemorrhage, which is progressive, the bleeding is usually arrested by the rising intracranial pressure. The chronic subdural hematoma is believed to cause symptoms by becoming encysted by fibrous membranes (pseudomembranes) which grow from the dura. In its encysted state, as red corpuscles hemolyze and blood proteins disintegrate, the osmotic pressure rises and fluid enters the hematoma, with the result that the hematoma enlarges and the compressive effects increase. Severe cerebral compression and displacement with temporal lobe–tentorial herniation are the usual causes of death. Treatment consists of placing burr holes and evacuating the clot before deep coma has developed.

Subdural hygromas (collections of blood and cerebrospinal fluid in the subdural space) may also form after an injury, as well as after meningitis (in an infant) and pneumoencephalography. It is said that a tear of the arachnoid permits the accumulation of cerebrospinal fluid into the subdural space, where it becomes trapped. The patient may complain of severe headache, drowsiness, and confusion, which are relieved when the subdural fluid is drained.

Cerebral Hemorrhage (Immediate and Delayed). Acute, massive brain hemorrhages are more frequent in elderly than in young patients and are usually fatal within a few hours. The clinical picture is similar to that of hypertensive brain hemorrhage (deepening coma with hemiplegia, a dilating pupil, bilateral Babinski signs, stertorous and irregular respirations). Indeed the problem that often cannot be solved even at postmortem examination is whether the patient had a hemorrhagic type of stroke and then fell, or a fall that caused the hemorrhage. If the bleeding is slow, there may be an interval of 2 to 3 days between injury and the symptoms of the oncoming hemorrhage. Coma or confusion, if present from the time of the injury, may obscure the signs of the intracerebral hemorrhage. Craniotomy with evacuation of the clot has given a successful result in a few cases.

Repeated Concussion (Punch Drunk). The cumulative effects of repeated injuries, observed almost exclusively in professional boxers, constitute a type of head injury difficult to classify for it has never been well studied pathologically. It is a common observation that, after a number of years in the ring, pugilists often become forgetful, slow in thinking, and slightly dysarthric. Their movements are stiff and uncertain, especially those involving the legs, there is unsteadiness of gait, and occasionally there may be involuntary movements. The plantar reflexes may be extensor on one or both sides. The electroencephalogram shows slow waves of theta and sometimes of delta type. The anatomic basis of this disease is unknown. The postulation of showers of petechial hemorrhages from repeated blows on the jaws should not be given credence until demonstrated pathologically. The findings of diffuse degeneration of the cerebral white matter in rabbits and monkeys which have been subjected to repeated concussions (Jakob) offer a more acceptable possibility.

Sequelae of Severe Head Injury

The signs of focal brain disease, whether due to open and penetrating or closed head injuries, tend always to ameliorate as the months pass. A hemiplegia is often reduced to a minimal hemiparesis or ineptitude of voluntary motor function with exaggerated reflexes and an equivocal Babinski sign on that side, and aphasia improves to become a stuttering or hesitant paraphasia which is not disabling except in a professional worker or writer. Many of the signs of brain stem disease improve, often to an astonishing degree.

Protracted Traumatic Coma and Pseudocoma. Of particular interest is the outcome of those few patients who remain comatose for weeks or months or even years. The authors have examined the brains of nearly a dozen cases of this type, and nearly all have shown numerous foci of hemorrhage and ischemic necrosis in the midbrain and subthalamus, especially in the tegmentum and tectum. These were probably due in most instances to temporal lobe herniation and midbrain compression, for one could see where one side of the base and tegmentum had been indented by the free edge of the tentorium. In others there may have been direct injury to the midbrain and pons, with numerous small hemorrhages. Presumably these pathologic changes are not constant, for scattered lesions in the cerebral cortex (contusions of the summits of convolutions, ischemia with necrosis in the depths of sulci) and a remarkable diffuse degeneration of cerebral white matter have also been observed in cases of this type (Strich). These patients, while comatose (i.e., unreceptive to stimuli and unresponsive) or while in a state of pseudocoma (receptive and capable of signaling by blinking their eyes but otherwise unresponsive), usually exhibit a variety of neurologic abnormalities: unequal pupils; dilated, fixed pupil and oculomotor palsy on one side and hemiplegia on the other; disturbances of gaze; bilateral pyramidal paralysis with Babinski signs; extensor postures of arm and leg on one side and flexed arm and extended leg on the other; brain stem attacks (extension of limbs, increased respiration, blood pressure, and sweating on stimulation of any kind); and involuntary movements (tremor, chorea, athetosis). Some remain in this reduced mental state until death (nearly 10 years in one of the authors' cases, but usually a few months or a year or two). The majority, however, may regain enough function to leave the hospital; a few, surprising as it may seem, are restored to full alertness and adequate mental function. Residual weakness of limbs, slurred speech, ocular palsies, ataxia of an arm or leg, or involuntary movements are frequent. During convalescence, language mechanisms may be disturbed in various ways. There may be mutism, akinesia or adynamia (lack of volition or impulse to speak or move), dysarthria, and, if there are contusions of the cortex of the dominant hemisphere, an aphasia as well. Any one or a combination of these abnormalities may be present.

Epilepsy. Posttraumatic epilepsy, which occurs in 20 to 40 per cent of patients, is one of the most dreaded complications of head injury. Its basis is nearly always a contusion or laceration of the cortex. The likelihood of epilepsy is said to be greater in parietal and posterior frontal lesions, but it may arise from lesions in any area of the cerebral cortex. The incidence of epilepsy is much greater in "open" than in "closed" head injuries. Indeed, in cases of pure concussion without contusion or laceration, seizures are not much more frequent than in the general population. The interval between the head injury and the first seizure averages about 9 months, but it may be much longer, i.e., many years, particularly in children. The longer the interval, the less certain one is of its relationship to the traumatic incident. There is a slightly greater tendency for those patients who had seizures at the time of head injury to become subject to recurrent seizures later. The seizures are always of focal character, or grand mal; petit mal is rarely if ever due to trauma. The significance of the different patterns of focal seizures, which varies according to the location of the lesion, has been worked out in detail by Penfield and his associates (see Chap. 36) and by Russell et al. The frequency of seizures in any given patient varies widely; some patients have only a few, others many, with episodes of status epilepticus. The electroencephalogram is of value in diagnosis; a focus of spike or sharp waves is the characteristic finding. Usually the seizures can be controlled by anticonvulsant medications, and only the recalcitrant cases are likely to require excision of the epileptic focus. The surgical results vary according to the methods of selection and technique of operation. Seizures are abolished in approximately 50 per cent by excision of the focus.

Impairment of Mental Function. Fortunately this is a rare sequela to head trauma. Although mental function may be disturbed by focal lesions which produce dysphasia, agnosia, apraxia, etc., intellectual functions and memory are usually preserved. This is true of even the most severe head injuries and is understandable when one considers the relatively small amount of brain tissue destroyed by the traumatic process. The only exceptions to this statement are the few patients who survive a severe compression of the midbrain by a herniating temporal lobe and those with extensive degeneration of the cerebral white matter. Children previously of low-average or borderline intelligence and the aged who, unnoticed, had developed senile mental changes constitute other exceptions. The aging person may have worked and functioned reasonably well until the time of the injury and afterward is found to have a grave impairment of memory, thinking, and emotional control that permanently disables him. That this is not simply a traumatic effect is indicated by the fact that the severity of the mental defect does not seem to parallel the severity of the head injury, and, as the months and years pass, the mental disorder may progress (the natural course of brain trauma is one of sudden onset with maximal functional disturbance within minutes or hours, and then improvement). This is one of the reasons why the prognosis in elderly adults is less good than for younger individuals.

Posttraumatic Nervous Instability. Undoubtedly the most troublesome sequela of head injury is that alluded to in the discussion of group 1 cases—*headache, giddiness,* and *nervous instability.* This has been called the *postconcussional syndrome* or the *minor contusion syndrome* (Trotter), or *posttraumatic vasomotor neurosis* (Friedmann). All these terms are objectionable on the grounds that they suggest an explanatory hypothesis, as yet unproved. Headache is the central symptom, usually, at times localized to the part struck. It is variously described as an aching, throbbing, pounding, stabbing, pressing pain and is remarkable for its variability. The intensification of symptoms by mental and physical effort, straining, stooping, and emotional excitement has already been mentioned. Rest and quiet may relieve it. Thus it becomes a major obstacle to convalescence, which demands always a resumption of normal activities. The dizziness is usually not a true vertigo but a giddiness. The patient feels suddenly unsteady, dazed, weak, or faint. However, a certain number of patients report symptoms which suggest a labyrinthine disorder. For example, objects in the environment are said to move momentarily, and looking upward or to the side may cause a sense of unbalance. Labyrinthine tests may show either hypo- or hyperreactivity, or the results may prove to be normal. The data are usually so indefinite that it is impossible to state whether or not the labyrinth and vestibular mechanisms have been injured. Exceptionally, vertigo is accompanied by diminished excitability of both the labyrinth and the cochlea, and one may assume the existence of direct injury to the nerve or end organ. The giddy patient usually is intolerant of noise, emotional excitement, and crowds. Tenseness, restlessness, inability to concentrate, a feeling of nervousness, fatigue, worry, apprehension, and an inability to tolerate the usual amount of alcohol complete the clinical picture. In contrast to the multiple subjective symptoms, detailed tests of intellectual functions and memory show little or no impairment. This syndrome, once established, may persist for months or even years, but usually the symptoms lessen as time passes. It occurs in both sexes, all races, and at all ages, excepting childhood. There has been much controversy over its cause, and to the present time its anatomic and physiologic basis has not been settled. The constancy of the symptoms, their appearance in individuals who have had no trace of neurosis prior to the accident, and their relationship to physical and mental activity have led most neurologists to view this syndrome as a manifestation of a specific morbid process in cranial structures. Nevertheless, the striking reduction in disability when the physician gives firm reassurance and encourages early rehabilitation leaves little doubt as to the existence of important psychologic mechanisms, at least for the maintenance of the symptoms. And if compensation is involved, the motivation to return to previous activities is still further impaired.

Extrapyramidal and Cerebellar Disorders. The question of *posttraumatic Parkinson's syndrome* has been discussed many times, usually with the general conclusion that a true traumatic parkinsonism does not exist. Most patients have merely had paralysis agitans or postencephalitic Parkinson's disease brought to light by head injury. The head injury may have been severe or trivial, and the course of the illness is usually progressive, just as it is in the nontraumatic cases. Patients who survive a severe midbrain syndrome manifested in the beginning by protracted coma, may have a clinical picture which bears some similarity to Parkinson's syndrome, but the presence of ocular palsies, nystagmus, and unilateral or bilateral pyramidal signs should permit easy distinction. One should be equally skeptical regarding the existence of a posttraumatic cerebellar ataxia.

Posttraumatic Hydrocephalus. Rare examples of posttraumatic hydrocephalus with intermittent headaches, vomiting, confusion, and drowsiness have been reported, and autopsy has demonstrated an adhesive basilar meningitis, attributed to subarachnoid or ventricular hemorrhage. Since a symptomatology like this has been observed occasionally after the rupture of a saccular aneurysm with massive subarachnoid hemorrhage, due presumably to blocking of the aqueduct and fourth ventricle by blood clot, this mechanism has also been suggested as a possible explanation of traumatic hydrocephalus in patients with cerebral contusion. However, there are other patients with enlarged ventricles who probably at no time had a significant degree of subarachnoid and ventricular hemorrhage. The mechanism of the hydrocephalus in these cases is not known.

Posttraumatic Psychiatric Disorders. In contrast to nervousness and nervous instability, which are common sequelae of injuries of all types, posttraumatic psychoses are relatively infrequent. Adolph Meyer, whose study of traumatic insanity is still a standard reference, encountered this type of illness in approximately 1 per cent of admissions to a state hospital. Statistics from military files and civilian hospitals show that about 1 of

every 100 patients with a head injury exhibits a behavioral change which requires commitment to a mental hospital (the figure is lower for military head injuries: 1 in every 1,000 cases). These terms, traumatic psychosis and insanity, have been used in various ways, which makes any summary of data and opinion difficult. From the psychiatric standpoint, many of the posttraumatic states already described (traumatic stupor, delirium, confusion, or dementia) would be classified as "defect psychoses." Other physicians use this term, as it is used here, to designate aberrations of behavior which prevent the patient from resuming his place in society. The most distressing psychiatric syndromes have been suspiciousness and paranoid delusions, unaccountable outbursts of violent temper, sometimes with homicidal or suicidal tendencies, progressive hyperactivity, delirium, and mania, and episodes of bizarre behavior with subsequent amnesia, reminiscent of temporal lobe seizures. Alcoholism may provoke some of these behavioral abnormalities. Some of these illnesses are undoubtedly due to residual brain damage in individuals of peculiar personality make-up. However, attempts to account for psychoses of this type by reference to constitutional peculiarities and predisposition, laid bare, so to speak, by head injury, have not been convincing. They may be said to represent first attempts to find working hypotheses. Some patients afflicted with these psychoses remain helplessly disabled. In others the outcome has been surprisingly good, and the patient, after some months in a psychiatric hospital, has been able to return to his home and his former job.

Clinical Approach to the Patient Who Has Suffered Head Injury; Suggested Plan for Management

The physician who undertakes to treat the "head injury case" must at all times bear in mind that assiduous attention to detail may prove to be lifesaving, and that accurate documentation of all diagnostic findings and therapy is desirable if the medical data are later to be used in the arbitration of insurance claims, worker's unemployment compensation, etc. The suggestions which follow can do no more than serve as guides, for every patient presents a combination of problems that the physician has not encountered before and may not observe again in identical form.

Exact data concerning the patient's medical status before the accident (previous illnesses, work and social record, emotional stability), the nature and precise circumstances of the accident, the duration of retrograde and anterograde amnesia, and all that transpired afterward should be obtained and recorded. Verbatim statements should be written down whenever possible.

The treatment problems presented by each of the three groups of clinical cases discussed above are as follows.

Minor Head Injury. In this group are included patients who (1) were never unconscious at any time, (2) were briefly unconscious but are mentally clear at the time of the first examination, (3) are rapidly regaining consciousness.

Circumstances dictate how each case is managed. If the injury was trivial and the scalp was not lacerated, and if the patient is entirely clear mentally, little or nothing need be done. When the patient is unable to give an accurate account of what has happened and appears still to be somewhat confused or incoherent, he should be compelled to lie down or at least remain in one place. It often happens that the confusion is not detected and the patient is permitted to resume activity while still acting in an irrational manner. He may get into his car and attempt to drive, only to have another accident; or if an athlete he may continue to play a game and make a series of errors.

When a conscious or nearly conscious patient is admitted to a general hospital, it is tempting to let him go his way. Experience teaches caution, however. A complete examination, with the patient fully undressed, should be carried out. It is well, if there is any likelihood of litigation, to obtain x-rays of the skull and an electroencephalogram. The question of lumbar puncture will usually depend on how serious the injury was, on the prominence of posttraumatic headache, etc. The patient should probably be detained for a few hours or overnight in order to make sure that he is not merely in a lucid interval. The first few hours or days may be spent in the hospital. If this cannot be arranged and he is sent home, a member of the family should be charged with the responsibility of reporting any important change, such as increasing headache, vomiting, drowsiness, confusion, or seizure. Its occurrence would dictate hospital entry for further examination, an x-ray of the skull, and possibly a lumbar puncture. A posttraumatic headache and drowsiness may be the first signs of an oncoming epidural or subdural hematoma. On the other hand, they may reflect only what is presumed to be a localized edema. Further observation will usually distinguish between these conditions. Observation may be safely continued as long as the patient remains conscious. Here one may proceed on the rule that the life of the patient with a head injury is never in jeopardy as long as he is mentally clear and responsive. The only exceptions to this statement are rare instances of severe cerebral contusion with minimal concussion (cf. pp. 1799 and 1800) or fracture through the foramen magnum with contusion of the inferior surface of the cerebellum and with swelling of

tissue and herniation through the foramen magnum. Two of the authors' patients with this condition died unexpectedly after a period of intense occipital headache, at a time when they were quite alert. The management of posttraumatic headache, dizziness, and nervous instability, which often follow relatively minor injuries to the head, will be discussed below. A simple fracture without involvement of paranasal sinuses requires no special treatment but is believed to contraindicate vigorous athletic activities for several months or a year.

Patients Who Are Unconscious When First Seen. If the physician arrives on the scene of the accident, a hurried examination should be made before the patient is moved in order to determine whether there is dangerous hemorrhage from a laceration of the scalp or other parts of the body and whether there is likelihood of a fracture-dislocation of the cervical spine, which is occasionally associated with head injury. If the patient is in shock, with cold clammy skin and feeble pulse, he should be covered with warm blankets. In moving an individual with a potential cervical spine injury, the spine should be kept straight at all times and flexion of the neck should be avoided. This can best be done by placing sand bags or firm pillows on either side of the head and warning everyone against neck flexion. An even safer method is to place the patient on a stretcher face down and arrange pillows to assure a clear airway. Bleeding from the scalp can usually be controlled with a firm pad unless an artery is divided, and then a suture becomes necessary.

In the hospital, where all such patients should be taken, the first steps should be to control shock. This can usually be done by the application of warmth, keeping the head low and leaving the patient alone for a few minutes. The shock will usually come under control in a few minutes with or without vasopressor drugs or transfusions. Persistent shock is rare in head injury and always raises the suspicion of a ruptured viscera with internal bleeding, extensive fractures, or traumatism of the cervical spinal cord. A quick survey will enable one to estimate the depth of coma, size of pupils, and presence of obvious fractures; and if shock is not present, or after the blood pressure has stabilized, a more detailed examination can be performed. The skull should be carefully inspected and palpated. The hair should be cut off around the scalp wound. A bogginess of the temporal or postauricular region (Battle's sign), bleeding from the nose or ear, extensive conjunctival edema and hemorrhage are useful signs of underlying skull fracture. However, it should be remembered that rupture of the eardrum or a blow on the nose may also cause bleeding from the ear and nose, respectively. Fractures of the orbital bones may cause displacement of the eye, with resulting diplopia, and fracture of the jaws, disalignment of the teeth, and great discomfort on attempting to open the mouth. Careful notes should be made regarding temperature, pulse, blood pressure, state of consciousness, pupil size, ocular movements, corneal reflexes, facial movements during grimace, swallowing, tone of limb muscles, movements of limbs, predominant postures, and reflexes. Vital signs and consciousness should be checked and recorded by the nurse or physician every 2 hr. A proper airway must be maintained. The best position for the patient is semisupine, with the head on a pillow and turned to one side. If urine is retained and the bladder distended, a catheter should be inserted and kept there. If coma persists for more than 12 to 24 hr, a nasal tube should be passed and fluids and nourishment given by that route. Intravenous fluids should be administered slowly and not in excessive amounts; even hypertonic glucose may increase oncoming pulmonary and cerebral edema, the danger of the latter being especially great in children. Lumbar puncture should be done as soon as practicable for diagnostic purposes (immediately if bacterial meningitis is suspected), and if the pressure is elevated it should be lowered to 100 to 150 mm. The practice of daily lumbar punctures has its advocates and its opponents. The authors have tended to use them only if the pressure is elevated and the patient's condition is not improving. Hypertonic solutions ($MgSO_4$, 90 Gm, and water, 180 ml) may be given per rectum, after a cleansing enema, and held for 30 min; or if the patient can swallow, 60 ml of this solution may be given by mouth every hour until a loose bowel movement is obtained. Hypertonic solutions intravenously are of less certain therapeutic value. One hundred millimeters of hypertonic urea, or if not available, 50 to 100 ml of 50 per cent glucose, or hypertonic sucrose, may be injected intravenously if operation is to follow within a few hours, but otherwise should probably not be given, for there may be an even higher cerebrospinal fluid pressure after its hypertonic effect wears off. X-rays of skull and other parts should be taken after the first day or two, unless there is a suspicion of an epidural hemorrhage, in which case they should be made at once, to visualize a crack across the course of the middle meningeal artery. Restlessness is controlled by sodium phenobarbital or paraldehyde, but only if careful nursing does not quiet the patient and permit him to sleep for a few hours at a time.

Once the patient has regained consciousness, the danger of suffocation, aspiration pneumonia, bronchopneumonia, thrombophlebitis, and pulmonary embolism has usually passed, and therapy can proceed along the lines indicated for the first group.

It is often stated that death from head injury during the first 12 to 24 hr is the direct effect of primary brain injury and cannot be prevented. The advisability of any surgical procedure during this period is much debated. If the patient survives for one, two, or more days and remains in coma, the control of brain swelling and hemorrhage by surgical means must be considered. Should the condition of the patient then begin to deteriorate (pulse rising, temperature subnormal or rising, state of consciousness worsening, hemiplegia more obvious, plantar reflexes more clearly extensor), a decision must be made concerning an epidural or subdural hemorrhage and of increasing brain edema with temporal lobe herniation. Rowbotham, who has had a large experience with cases of this type, recommends a right-sided temporal decompression and two inspection burr holes in the left, one at the Sylvian point and one at the parietal eminence, for some of these patients. In his opinion the indications for surgery are (1) retrogression following a period of improvement, which cannot be controlled by lumbar puncture and oral and rectal hypertonic solutions or intravenous dehydration measures; (2) decerebrate rigidity which has its onset after an interval of 24 hr (early decerebrate rigidity implies primary brain stem injury) if meningitis is ruled out; (3) a dilated fixed pupil on one side, with no improvement after 12 hr; (4) prolonged unconsciousness associated with a persistently high cerebrospinal fluid pressure. Not all neurologists and neurosurgeons are agreed on the value of surgical decompression, but certainly the removal of a large epidural or subdural hemorrhage, which cannot be diagnosed easily in the comatose patient, may be a lifesaving procedure.

The treatment of the patient with protracted coma is too complex to be outlined in detail here. The reader should refer to p. 318. Every patient presents special problems which must be dealt with individually.

Patients Who Temporarily Recovered Consciousness (Lucid Interval) and Then Became Stuporous or Comatose. The treatment is that of epidural, subdural, and delayed cerebral hemorrhage. This has already been discussed.

General Convalescence

A head injury carries dire import to most lay individuals, who often fear for their mind and are concerned about their capacity to resume their place in society. In former times, therapeutic measures often involved long discussions of the seriousness of the injury, protracted bed rest, and inactivity, all of which served only to engender greater anxiety. Even worse, these measures were not of proved value. It is now widely acknowledged that the patient does better if his physician tends to minimize the seriousness of his head injury and to reassure him that he will recover. Early rehabilitation should be encouraged. It may safely begin as soon as the cerebrospinal fluid becomes clear, usually within a few days or 1 to 2 weeks at the most, except of course in the rare cases of protracted coma.

Posttraumatic headache, dizziness, and nervousness are the most difficult symptoms to manage during this period. Careful explanation of the symptoms, an optimistic prognosis, and the institution of a program of graded mental and physical activities to the point of tolerance stand the best chance of restoring the patient to a useful life. The patient should be told that he must expect a certain amount of headache and should carry on in spite of it. Meprobamate, 200 mg t.i.d., is useful for anxiety, and a non-habit-forming analgesic medication should be given for the more severe headaches (Empirin or aspirin). Insomnia may require a barbiturate medication or chloral hydrate at first, but they should be discontinued as soon as possible. Any litigation that may be involved should be settled within 6 to 9 months. To delay settlement usually works against the best interests of the patient. The severity of his injury can be ascertained within this period of time, and a longer period of observation only enhances his worries and fears and reduces his motivation to return to work.

The prognosis of head injury, in good hands, is influenced by several variables. Elderly patients often remain disabled, especially when compensation is involved. Young and middle-aged adults do better if they are not entitled to compensation (Russell's figures: 70 per cent of compensation cases back at work in 18 months; 83 per cent of noncompensation cases working at the end of this period). Russell also pointed out that the severity of the injury as measured by the duration of traumatic amnesia was a factor. If the period of amnesia was less than 1 hr, 95 per cent of cases were back at work within 2 months; if longer than 24 hr, only 80 per cent had returned to work in 6 months. About 60 per cent, however, still had symptoms at the end of 2 months, and 40 per cent at the end of 18 months.

INJURIES OF THE SPINE AND SPINAL CORD

Injury to the spinal cord is not infrequent in both civilian and military life. It may be the sole complication of an injury, or, as indicated above, it may be combined with head injury. Although the primary consideration is whether the spinal cord or spinal roots have been damaged, some reference to the nature of vertebral injury is necessary for an understanding of this type of traumatic disease.

Varieties of Spinal Injury

A useful classification of spinal injuries is one which divides them into fracture-dislocations, pure fractures, and pure dislocations. The relative frequency of these types is about 3:1:1. Direct violence to the spine is an uncommon cause of vertebral disruption; except for stab and bullet wounds, most spine injuries are the result of force "applied at a distance." All three types of injury are produced by a similar mechanism, usually a vertical compression of the spinal column to which flexion is almost immediately added. The two important variables in the mechanics of vertebral injury are the nature of the bones and the strength, direction, and point of impact of the force.

The Nature of the Vertebral Body and Other Spinal Structures. It was pointed out in Chap. 7 that the vertebral column consists of two parallel, fused cylinders of different structure and serving different purposes, the anterior column comprised of the vertebral bodies and intervertebral cartilages whose general purpose is weight bearing, the posterior cylinder an articulated column of neural arches giving protection to the spinal cord. Of these two columns or cylinders, the anterior is more compressible, being constituted of very little compact and much cancellous bone. Thus a compressive force usually causes wedging of a vertebral body, and is followed by flexion. Wedging or collapse of vertebral bodies is most to be expected where they are high and spongy and separated by thick intervertebral disks, i.e., in the lower thoracic and lumbar spine. Wedging is seldom complete in the cervical region because violence to the neck in a vertical direction is not applicable without movement of the spine, part of the force of the blow being converted into a movement of flexion.

Strength, Direction, and Point of Impact of the Force. If the injuring body striking the cranium is hard and the velocity is high, a skull fracture occurs, the elastic quality of the skull absorbing the force of the injury. If the injuring body is soft yet heavy, the spine and particularly its cervical portion will be the part injured. If the neck happens to be rigid and straight and the force is quickly applied to the head, the atlas and the odontoid process of the axis may break. If the force is not so quickly applied and removed, an element of flexion occurs. Flexion movement plus a vertical force constitute the essential factors in fracture-dislocation or pure dislocation. These types of injury are most frequent in the cervical region.

Another mechanism of spinal injury, occurring most often in military life, is that in which missiles of high velocity pass through the vertebral canal and destroy the spinal cord. In some cases they may strike the vertebral column without entering the spinal canal and agitate it so violently that the cord suffers injury. The term given the temporary spinal paralysis which results is *spinal concussion.* This condition may also be produced by violent falls flat on the back.

A study of 2,006 cases collected from the literature by Jefferson shows that most vertebral injuries occur at the first to second cervical, fourth to sixth cervical, and eleventh thoracic to second lumbar vertebras. Industrial accidents most often involve the dorsolumbar vertebras, and those caused by falling, either in a sitting position or with head down as in diving accidents, affect the cervical region. In the authors' neuropathologic material, which contains 26 cases, the usual circumstances of spinal injury were a state of alcoholic intoxication and a fall down a flight of stairs, automobile accidents, crushing industrial accidents, gunshot or stab wounds, and birth injury in that order of frequency. The majority of these fatal cases were fracture-dislocations or· dislocations of the cervical spine.

Mechanism of Spinal Cord Injury

The spinal cord may escape injury even though there is vertebral dislocation, especially in regions where the spinal canal is large, i.e., in the cervical and lumbar regions. Or the spinal cord may be damaged without radiologic evidence of fracture or dislocation. One cannot easily determine the full extent of spinal injury, however, even at autopsy, because of difficulty in examining the vertebras. By far the most satisfactory technique for demonstrating the degree of spine injury and the presence of a tearing of ligaments with dislocation is the x-ray, taken laterally with the neck flexed and extended. The most frequently established mechanism is a vertebral dislocation with or without fracture. The upper vertebras are displaced anteriorly, and there is a break in posterior longitudinal ligament and intervertebral disk. The spinal cord is most often subjected to a shearing force between the pedicles of the vertebra above and the body and laminas of the vertebra below the dislocation, or is sharply angulated in violent extension of the neck. Agitation of the spine, as when it is struck in some part by a bullet, has been postulated as a means of spinal concussion. This has led to much confusion, because the term is not employed here in the usual sense of a transient interruption of neural function by trauma without perceptible structural change.

Pathology of Spinal Cord Injury

As a result of squeezing or shearing of the cord, there are necrosis of fiber tracts and gray matter and a variable amount of hemorrhage, chiefly in the more vascular gray matter. These changes are maximum at the point of injury and one or two segments above and below it. Rarely is the cord cut in two, and seldom is the pia-arachnoid lacerated. This condition is best designated as *traumatic necrosis of the spinal cord.* Separation of such pathologic entities as hematomyelia, concussion, contusion, and hematorrhachis is rarely of value, either clinically or pathologically. As with most lesions, the total disease picture is compounded of an irreversible structural lesion and a disorder of function, each of which may vary in degree. The extent and permanence of the clinical manifestations are determined by the relative amounts of these two. An exception to this statement might be made for gunshot wounds of vertebras. Here the explosive force of the missile may shatter myelinated fibers without dislocation of vertebras. A blow from behind may cause sudden extension of the neck (so-called "whiplash" injury). As a rule this does not injure the spinal cord, but it does damage the cervical ligaments and muscles. Theoretically it may affect the vertebral arteries, but this is unproved. (See Chap. 7 for discussion of lumbar injury.)

Clinical Effects of Spinal Cord Damage

The description of traumatic paraplegia by Riddock cannot be excelled. He divides the clinical picture into two stages, as follows:

Muscular Flaccidity or "Spinal Shock." The loss of function which is inflicted at the time of injury, i.e., fourth to fifth cervical quadriplegia; thoracic paraplegia; paralysis of bladder and bowel sphincters (and loss of sensibility below the level corresponding to the spinal lesion), is accompanied by a complete or almost complete suppression of reflex activity of all spinal segments below the lesion. This condition is the so-called "spinal shock." The plantar reflexes are at first variable and may be flexor or extensor. The lower extremities lose heat if left uncovered, and swell if dependent. Sweating is abolished. Cutaneous ulcerations may develop over bony prominences. Urine and feces are retained to the point where involuntary overflow or leakage results. Occasionally there is priapism because of venous congestion. A paralytic ileus may occur.

Reflex Activity. If the lumbosacral segments are undamaged, spinal shock wears off in 2 to 3 weeks. The first sign of this is contraction of the hamstrings, with flexion or extension of the toes on plantar stimulation. Then gentle and later strong involuntary flexor spasms make their appearance. Ankle jerks and then knee jerks return. Retention of urine and feces becomes less complete, and at irregular intervals urine is expelled by active contraction of the detrusor muscle. Reflex defecation and sweating also return. At times flexor spasms and later extensor spasms, with sweating and micturition, all occur after stimulation of the skin, viz., the *mass reflex*. This stage of reflex activity may last for years unless sepsis intervenes, in which case the state of spinal shock may return.

Less complete lesions of the spinal cord may result in little or no spinal shock or extensor spasm; incomplete voluntary motor paralysis, a flaccid atrophic paralysis, variable sensory impairment in the arms, and a spastic weakness of the legs, and a partial or complete Brown-Séquard syndrome are some of the resulting clinical pictures.

The final result may be permanent and complete disability, rarely consistent with survival for more than a short time (days to weeks); or a gradual improvement and complete or almost complete recovery may occur. Any residual symptoms after 6 months are likely to be more or less permanent.

The level of the cord lesion can be determined by the clinical picture. A complete paralysis of arms and legs usually indicates a dislocation at the fourth to fifth cervical. If legs are paralyzed and arms can be abducted and flexed, the dislocation is likely to be at the fifth to sixth cervical. Paralysis only of hands and of legs indicates the level of vertebral disorder to be the sixth to seventh cervical. When the motor paralysis involves muscles above the knees and sensory loss includes the twelfth thoracic dermatome, the site is the eleventh to twelfth thoracic. If the paralysis is below the knees and the first lumbar escapes, the lesion is at the twelfth thoracic, first lumbar vertebras. Prognosis for the latter, preponderately a cauda equina lesion, is better than for the former.

Treatment

In general, the treatment of spinal cord injuries is conservative and symptomatic. When there is x-ray evidence of bony displacement or of bone fragments pressing on the cord, or when spinal subarachnoid block is present, the cord should be decompressed by laminectomy. This should not be undertaken, however, until the patient has recovered from shock. If the spinal cord injury is associated with dislocation of the vertebras, traction on the neck is necessary to secure proper realignment. This is accomplished by a head halter attached through the head of the bed over a pulley to a weight of 10 to 15 lb. There are other more complicated techniques, such as tongs which fasten onto the skull (Crutchfield). In thoracic crush injuries, hyperextension can be maintained by placing a narrow pillow under the affected area. Traction should be continued for 4 to 6 weeks, and then a brace may be substituted. The aftercare of patients with paraplegia and disturbance of vesical or rectal function is similar to that of patients with like symptoms from other causes (see Chap. 29). Tidal drainage is a valuable adjunct in preventing infection, stone formation, and contracture and in securing return of function. Daily enemas are usually the most effective means of controlling fecal incontinence. Physiotherapy, muscle reeducation, and the application of proper braces are all important in the rehabilitation of the patient.

INJURIES TO SPINAL ROOTS, PLEXUSES, AND PERIPHERAL NERVES

Discussions of these subjects will be found in Chaps. 26 and 291. Ruptured intervertebral disk is presented in Chap. 7.

CONCLUSION

Head and spine injuries should invite the attention of general physicians, internists, and neurologists. There are many important lessons to be learned about the function of the human nervous system from following these cases. Their treatment, except in a minority of cases, where there is laceration of scalp, depressed fracture, epidural and subdural hemorrhage, or compression of the spinal cord, must be conducted largely along medical lines.

REFERENCES

Brock, S. (Ed.): "Injuries of the Brain and Spinal Cord and Their Coverings," 3d ed., p. 71, Baltimore, The Williams & Wilkins Company, 1949.

Denny-Brown, D. E., and W. R. Russell: Experimental Concussion, Proc. Roy. Soc. Med., 34:691, 1941.

Kuhn, W. G., Jr.: Care and Rehabilitation of Patients with Injuries to the Spinal Cord and Cauda Equina: Preliminary Report on 113 Cases, J. Neurosurg., 4:40, 1947.

Merritt, H. H.: Diagnostic Considerations in Patients with Head Injury, Research Publs., Assoc. Research Nervous Mental Disease, 24:379, 1943.

Meyer, A.: The Anatomical Facts and Clinical Varieties of Traumatic Insanity: Am. J. Psychiat., 60:373, 1903–1904.

Munro, D.: "The Treatment of Injuries to the Nervous System," Philadelphia, W. B. Saunders Company, 1952.

Prather, G. C., and F. H. Mayfield: "Injuries of the Spinal Cord," Springfield, Ill., Charles C Thomas, Publisher, 1953.

Rowbotham, G. F.: "Acute Injuries of the Head," Baltimore, The Williams & Wilkins Company, 1945.

Russell, W. R.: Cerebral Involvement of Head Injury, Brain, 55:549, 1932.

———: The After-effects of Head Injury, Trans. Med. Chir. Soc., Edinburgh, 113:129, 1933–1934.

Strich, S.: Diffuse Degeneration of the Cerebral White Matter in Severe Dementia Following Head Injury, J. Neurol. Neurosurg. Psychiat., 19:163, 1956.

Symonds, C. P.: The Effects of Injury on the Brain, Lancet, I:820, 1932.

286 TUMORS OF THE BRAIN AND SPINAL CORD

Henry deF. Webster and Raymond D. Adams

Tumors of the central nervous system play a very important part in neurologic medicine and occupy a distinct field by themselves. It may be said of them generally that they occur in great variety; are dangerous (malignant) because of size, location, and invasive qualities; usually destroy the tissues in which they are situated and displace those around them; are a frequent cause of increased intracranial pressure; and are often lethal.

During the first half of the twentieth century a great deal was learned about the gross and microscopic features of these tumors. Also a number of classifications were introduced, the most notable being those of Bailey and Cushing, Hortega, and Kernohan. However, little has been found out about their fundamental nature. The experimental work done in animals in which tumors have been induced by chemical substances and the bacteriologic, biochemical, histologic, and tissue culture studies of tumor tissue obtained from human beings during operation or postmortem have, unfortunately, shed little light on the fundamental problems of etiology and pathogenesis. Trauma, viruses, chemical irritation, and heredity have been suggested as causative agents, but no convincing evidence on these points has been accumulated.

Probably the most singular advances in this field during the present century concern diagnosis and treatment. The standard textbooks of neurology written before 1900 by Osler, Strümpell, Oppenheim, Gowers and the monographs containing the brilliant lectures on nervous disease by Hammond, Charcot, Romberg, Duchenne, and Gowers reveal that tumor of the brain and spinal cord rarely figured in the thinking of these great clinicians. Moreover it was not until 1879 that Macewen diagnosed and operated on the first intracranial tumor and shortly thereafter that Sir Victor Horsley explored the possibilities of intracranial surgery. By the turn of the last century barely 50 cases had been operated upon successfully. The great developments achieved within the modern era of medicine must be credited largely to Harvey Cushing and his students, who showed the feasibility of removing intracranial growths and who worked out the necessary technical details of diagnosis and operative surgery. Their work was aided immeasurably by the use of air to visualize the ventricular system and subarachnoid spaces [the pneumoencephalogram (PEG) and ventriculogram of Dandy], the development of arteriography (Moniz), and the invention of electrocoagulation, the "sucker," and the Gigli saw. More recently radioactive isotopes have been exploited by a number of American investigators (Moore, Sweet, and others) for the purpose of localizing tumor growths.

CLASSIFICATION

The classification of the tumors of the nervous system, like that of tumors of other viscera, is primarily regional and histogenetic. Subdivisions are based on the cells of origin. The embryologic studies of His, Cajal, Hortega, and their students established the existence of 14 important cell types within the cranial cavity: the astrocyte, oligodendrocyte, microgliacyte, ependymal cell, choroidal epithelial cell, nerve cell, fibroblast, specialized arachnoidal fibroblast, Schwann cell, histiocyte, vascular endothelial cell, pituitary epithelial cell, pineal epithelial cell, and meningeal melanophore cell. Each of these basic "type cells" is capable of giving origin to a series of tumors which grow at various rates of speed, and all gradations can usually be found between the slowest and fastest growing. The tumor cells tend to differentiate, as do the cells from which they arise. If the growth rate is slow, differentiation may be perfect, just as it is in normal tissues, and there is no difficulty in determining the type. If the growth rate is rapid, the differentiation is less complete or entirely lacking and recognition of the "type cell" in microscopic sections may be nearly impossible.

In the first part of the classification given below the tumors are arranged in order of frequency and their terms are formed by affixing "oma" to the name of the cell of origin, viz., astrocytoma, oligodendrocytoma, microglioblastoma, neurocytoma, fibroblastoma, histiocytic sarcoma, etc. However, if the tumor cell is poorly differentiated, it has become the accepted practice to denominate the tumor by the name of the embryologic precursor of that cell. A poorly differentiated astrocytoma thus is called a glioblastoma; an oligodendrocytoma becomes an oligodendroblastoma; a neurocytoma is referred to as a neuroblastoma. Special terms have had to be introduced to denote tumors whose cell of origin is uncertain but has resemblance to some particular embryologic element; e.g., the medulloblastoma is used to designate the small-cell tumor of the cerebellum in children, believed to be derived from the "indifferent" cells of Schaper. In general, as with all tumors, the less the degree of differentiation, the greater the malignancy.

In addition to the tumors derived from these 14 "type cells," others originate from cells ordinarily not part of the nervous system. They may arise from "cell rests" that are left in the meninges or substance of the brain owing to some fault in embryologic development, e.g., ectodermal cells from skin or mucous membranes which give rise to Rathke pouch cysts, craniopharyngiomas, and cholesteatomas, or lipocytes from which the rare lipomas arise.

Finally there is a group of tumors which affect the brain secondarily, that is, they arise in some other tissue and extend to the brain and, rarely, the spinal cord. Of these there are two groups—those which reach the nervous tissues via the blood stream, i.e., metastasize, such as the carcinoma and the sarcoma; and those which have their source in the epidural and osseous tissues that envelop the brain and which invade the meninges and cerebral tissues by direct extension, e.g., chordoma, osteoblastic sarcoma, lymphocytoma, lymphoblastoma, plasmocytoma, Hodgkin's granuloma and sarcoma, etc.

For the student of medicine the most important facts to know are (1) that many types of tumor occur in the cranial cavity and spinal canal and that certain ones are much more frequent than others (pp. 1813 and 1814); (2) that some of these tumors, such as the craniopharyngioma, meningioma, and schwannoma, have a disposition to grow in certain parts of the cranial cavity; (3) that their growth rates vary, some like the glioblastoma being highly malignant, others like the meningioma being benign; and (4) that there are differences in the growth behavior of these several tumors, some being invasive, others compressive. These pathologic peculiarities are important for they have valuable clinical correlations, providing the explanation of slowly or rapidly progressive clinical states, excellent or poor prognosis after surgical excision, etc. It is for these reasons that the clinician is encouraged to learn a histologic classification and to think always in terms of particular types of intracranial and intraspinal tumors.

The one place where these pathologic-clinical correlations tend to fail is in the glioma group of tumors, i.e., astrocytoma—glioblastoma series; and this is regrettable because tumors of this type are so common. Often these gliomas are of mixed cell type. For example, one part of the tumor may be a typical astrocytoma and another an oligodendrocytoma. Also the degree of differentiation or its opposite, the degree of anaplasia, varies from one part of the tumor to another. As would be expected with such heterogeneous growths, a biopsy sample

Table 286-1. CLASSIFICATION OF INTRACRANIAL AND INTRASPINAL TUMORS

I. Primary tumors of
  A. Nervous parenchyma
    1. Blastomas of glial origin
      a. Glioblastomas (isomorphic, heteromorphic)
      b. Astroblastomas
      c. Astrocytomas
      d. Ependymoma (glioepitheliomas)
      e. Oligodendrocytomas
    2. Blastomas of neuronal origin
      a. Neuroblastomas (some medulloblastomas)
      b. Neurocytomas
  B. Meninges
    1. Meningioma or arachnoidal fibroblastoma (meningoexothelioma)
    2. Fibroblastomas
    3. Reticulum cell sarcomas
    4. Hemangioblastomas (including Lindau's cyst)
    5. Other, e.g., melanocarcinomas
  C. Hypophysis and Rathke's pouch
    1. Chromophobe, chromophil adenomas of pituitary gland
    2. Craniopharyngiomas, etc.
  D. Developmental origin ("rest cell" tumors)
    1. Teratomas
    2. Epidermoids (cholesteatomas) and dermoids
    3. Lipomas
    4. Angiomas (vascular malformations)
  E. Adnexal organs in the brain
    1. Choroidal tumors (papillomas, epitheliomas, adenocarcinomas)
    2. Pineal tumors or pinealomas (pineocytomas, pineoblastomas)
  F. Nerves
    1. Neurinomas
    2. Neurofibromas
    3. Plexiform neuromas
II. Secondary tumors (cranial, spinal, extracranial, extraspinal)
  A. Those arising outside the central nervous system and metastasizing via the blood stream
    1. Carcinoma (most frequent: lung, breast, kidney, colon; infrequent: stomach, bile ducts, liver, thyroid, testicle, ovary, uterus; hardly ever metastasizing to the brain: prostate, esophagus, pancreas, skin, mucous membranes)
    2. Sarcoma (rhabdomyosarcoma, osteogenic sarcoma, leiomyosarcoma, fibrosarcoma)
  B. Those arising in cranial bones and enclosed paranasal sinuses, vertebral bodies, and epidural tissues
    1. Carcinoma of paranasal sinuses
    2. Transitional cell epitheliomas from tissue of pharynx
    3. Metastatic carcinomas which metastasize to bone (prostate, breast, thyroid, etc.)
    4. Multiple myeloma and plasmacytoma, and other lymphomas including Hodgkin's disease
    5. Chloroma
    6. Chordoma
    7. Osteogenic and fibrosarcoma of bone

is often quite misleading with reference to the expected clinical behavior of the tumor. For example, the clinician may be led to believe that a tumor which in a biopsy is composed of astrocytes is benign, whereas actually the main mass of it still in the brain is a glioblastoma; or a small nodule of glioblastoma in an excised specimen may suggest a hopeless prognosis when actually the remainder of the tumor in the brain is a well-differentiated astrocytoma.

The classification on p. 1812 is modified from that of the Spanish histologist Rio del Hortega. It represents his last great contribution to medical science and is based on a meticulous study by silver impregnation methods of the cell types of nearly a hundred brain tumors.

Implicit in the histogenetic theory is the notion first advanced by Cohnheim—that the type cell from which the tumor originates is a primitive undifferentiated element that has resided within the nervous system since the earliest embryonal period. This is a likely explanation of certain teratomas, dermoids, hamartomas, and other tumors apparently derived from "cell rests," but there is no evidence that this hypothesis is applicable to the gliomas and meningiomas. Indeed the careful studies of experimental tumors suggest that under certain conditions normal-appearing, well-differentiated glial cells may be induced to undergo neoplastic metamorphosis. And the more malignant forms of tumor appear to be due to anaplasia and not to failure of differentiation. These facts can also be established when a succession of biopsies of any one tumor is arranged in a series according to cell type (cf. Kernohan) and in the study of the histopathology of tumors by whole-brain sections which show the relation of the differentiated to the nondifferentiated parts (Scherer).

INCIDENCE

Most of the available statistics on tumors of the central nervous system have been collected in special neurosurgical clinics and are somewhat misleading, for they fail to reveal their natural incidence in an unselected population. The figures in Table 286-2, compiled by Peer, are thus rather exceptional, for they avoid this error of selection and represent the natural incidence of these tumors in postmortem material during the period 1900–1930, at a time when very little neurosurgery was being performed in the hospital from which they were taken (Boston City Hospital).

These data reveal that the central nervous system and its enveloping tissues are fruitful soil for tumor growth and, further, that the bulk of these tumors are gliomas, metastatic tumors, and meningiomas. The increasing rarity of gummas and tuberculomas, noted in all pathologic material from

Table 286-2. INCIDENCE OF INTRACRANIAL AND INTRASPINAL TUMORS AT BOSTON CITY HOSPITAL, 1900–1930

Total autopsies	10,592
Total number of tumors	1,458
Tumors of other organs	1,270
Intracranial and intraspinal tumors	188 (12.7%)
Gliomas	81 (43.1%)
Pituitary adenomas	6 (3.2%)
Sheath tumors	22 (11.7%)
Meningioma	18
Acoustic neuroma	4
Metastatic tumors	29 (15.4%)
Blood vessel tumors	6 (3.0%)
Congenital tumors	8 (4.3%)
Granulomas	19 (10.1%)
Spinal cord tumors	4 (2.1%)
Unclassified	13 (7.1%)

the United States during the past two decades, leads to the belief that far less than 10 per cent of intracranial growths are of granulomatous nature; and the rising age of the population and the increasing frequency of all types of tumors would probably raise the figures for secondary tumors. Of the gliomas, approximately half are glioblastoma multiforme, and the remainder are divided between astrocytoma, oligodendroglioma, ependymoma, medulloblastoma, and undiagnosed gliomas. All statistics show the peak age incidence to be the fifth decade of life, with a fairly symmetric curve which reflects the lessening incidence at the extremes of age—infancy and the senescent period. In children, tumors of the posterior fossa (medulloblastomas, ependymomas, and gliomas) predominate; in adults, supratentorial tumors (glioblastomas, meningiomas, and metastatic carcinomas) are more frequent. Males appear to be more susceptible to intrinsic tumors of the brain (gliomas) than females, the ratio being 2:1. In contrast the meningioma occurs more frequently in elderly women.

INTRACRANIAL TUMORS

Pathophysiology

The cranium, according to the Monro-Kellie law, contains three elements—nervous tissue, blood, and cerebrospinal fluid—the total bulk of which must always be constant. Any increase in the volume of the brain, for example, can take place only at the expense of one of the other elements, and a diminished volume of brain is compensated by an increase in the amount of cerebrospinal fluid. The cerebrospinal fluid pressure, while reflecting the volume of the intracranial mass, is largely maintained by the pressure under which the blood is delivered to the skull. In profound shock the cerebrospinal fluid pressure falls, and at death it is zero.

When a tumor or other space-occupying mass forms in the cranial cavity, the volume of cerebrospinal fluid within the subarachnoid and ventricular spaces is reduced and the cerebrospinal fluid is displaced into the spinal and perioptic subarachnoid spaces. Soon, however, the limits of these adjustments are surpassed, and the pressure throughout the ventricles and in all parts of the subarachnoid space rises. Presumably the veins in the cerebral tissues adjacent to the tumor are compressed, with resulting increase in capillary pressure locally—the conditions necessary for *regional swelling,* or *edema.* Inasmuch as any general increase in venous pressure results in retarded absorption of cerebrospinal fluid and an increase in its volume, the pressure in the subarachnoid space and veins is nearly the same at all times. If the rise in cerebrospinal fluid pressure is slow, the stasis of blood resulting from this elevated venous pressure can be compensated for by vasodilatation of arteries and arterioles, and cerebral circulation is unimpaired. If the rise is rapid and to high levels approaching diastolic blood pressure, the blood pressure must rise, usually the systolic more than the diastolic, in order to maintain cerebral blood flow. As a rule this is accompanied by a slow, bounding pulse. Under these conditions, the velocity of cerebral blood flow again approaches normal. Presumably these circulatory reflexes, which result in the rise of blood pressure and bradycardia, are initiated by venous stasis and accumulation of carbon dioxide in the vasomotor center in the medulla oblongata. The respiratory centers also become affected, for increases in intracranial pressure usually cause an irregularity and finally a cessation of respiration.

These changes in blood pressure, pulse, and respiration, which were studied by Kocher and by Cushing in 1901, are of the greatest importance in the clinic, for they may afford valuable clues as to the existence of increased intracranial pressure. Not less valuable is the papilledema, or "choked disk," that can be seen with an ophthalmoscope in the optic fundi of most patients who have elevated intracranial pressure of more than a few days' standing. The papilledema is best accounted for by the high pressure in the subarachnoid space surrounding the optic nerves. The veins that drain the retina, as they course back along the optic nerves en route to the cavernous sinuses, are blocked, creating a lymphedema of the nerve head.

Raised intracranial pressure due to a mass or enlargement of the ventricles (blockage of cerebrospinal fluid circulation), when severe, causes obtundation of cerebral function. This is manifested clinically by a number of characteristic symptoms (see p. 303) and electroencephalographically by diffuse slowing of the electrical activity of the cortex.

Another extremely important anatomic fact is that the closed cranial "box" is subdivided into fairly rigid compartments by two infoldings of dura mater, one the falx, which lies between the two cerebral hemispheres, and the other the tentorium, which separates the cerebellum from the occipital lobes. These anatomic arrangements and the opening at the base of the skull through which the spinal cord and medulla are joined leave three important apertures, the foramen magnum, the tentorial opening or "notch," and the subfalcial or supracallosal space. A tumor growth in one compartment, say the right middle cranial fossa, raises the pressure in that compartment more than in the others, and either brain or tumor tissue tends to be displaced along lines of least resistance, i.e., through the subfalcial space to the left half of the cranial cavity and through the tentorial opening into the posterior fossa on the right side. These brain displacements are exceedingly dangerous and contribute, as a rule, to the death of the patient in most cases of intracranial tumor, abscess, trauma, and subdural and epidural hemorrhage. The temporal lobe–tentorial hernia is said to stretch the ipsilateral oculomotor nerve (Hutchinson's pupil—a dilated pupil on the side of a lesion, and also a drooping eyelid); to displace and compress the midbrain with resulting stupor or coma, bilateral pyramidal signs (often greater on the side of the hernia), decerebrate postures of extension of all four extremities, and perhaps irregularity and final arrest of respiration; and to distort and partially block the aqueduct of Sylvius and to narrow the perimesencephalic subarachnoid space with hydrocephalus and rising intracranial pressure. Also, the posterior cerebral arteries may be occluded on one side or both sides, with infarction of the occipital lobes. The cerebellar–foramen magnum pressure cone (herniation of cerebellar tonsils), in which the cerebellar tissue or tumor mass is displaced into the cervical spinal canal with compression of the medulla oblongata, results in tilting or altered posture of the head, dilated pupils, impairment of consciousness, and death due to respiratory arrest. The physiologic and clinical effects of subfalcial herniation are not known.

Herniation of the floor of the third ventricle and adjacent parts of the brain into the sella turcica may, if acute, be accompanied by marked reduction in vision and, if chronic, cause enlargement of the sella and atrophy of the pituitary gland.

A knowledge of these effects of elevated intracranial pressure and of the herniations and displacements of tissue is necessary if one is to understand the clinical behavior of intracranial growths. Symptoms and signs of brain tumor depend not on the invasion and destruction of important nervous structures alone but also on the pressure phenomena.

Clinical and Pathologic Characteristics

As was pointed out by Bailey, the intracranial tumors are far too heterogeneous to be treated as a whole. The origin, structure, symptoms, and treatment of each pathologic entity must be considered separately. This can be done in either of two ways—by taking up seriatim each of the special types of tumor, i.e., following a scheme based on pathology with the clinical manifestations of each tumor type being added; or by making a purely clinical approach, presenting the common syndromes created by intracranial tumors and then offering only a few relevant points with respect to pathology. The latter scheme is followed here.

It may be said at the very outset that tumors of the brain may exist with hardly any symptoms. Often only a slight deficiency in mental power, a slowness in comprehension, or a loss of capacity in sustaining continuous mental activity suggests any deviation from normal health. Specific signs that would lead to a suspicion of any real cerebral disease may be wholly wanting. In some patients, on the other hand, there is evidence of cerebral disease in the form of a seizure or some other symptom, but the evidence is not clear enough to warrant the diagnosis of a cerebral tumor. In a third group, the existence of a new growth in the brain may be determined with much probability by the presence of signs of elevated intracranial pressure, but there are no symptoms which warrant localization of the growth. Lastly, the symptoms may be so clear and definite as to make it probable not only that there is a new growth within the cranium but that it is located in one particular region. In fact these localized growths may create unique tumor syndromes, unlike those of any other disease.

These are the plain facts of clinical observation; in the further exposition of this subject, therefore, all intracranial tumors are considered in relation to the common clinical circumstances in which they are likely to be encountered, as follows:

1. The patient whose presenting symptom is either a decline in general mental ability or a seizure.

2. The patient with unmistakable evidence of raised intracranial pressure.

3. Specific intracranial tumor syndromes.

The Patient with General Symptoms of Cerebral Disease or a Seizure as the Main Complaint. In general practice or on the wards of the hospital, these are the patients who give the most trouble in diagnosis and about whom decisions are often made with a great degree of uncertainty. Their symptoms are general, as a rule, and not until some time has elapsed will signs of focal brain disease be added; and when they do, they are not always of accurate localizing value. Altered psychic function, headache, giddiness, and seizures comprise the usual symptomatology in this group of patients.

As pointed out by Knapp, some *change in mental function* may be found in nearly every patient of this type, but it may be necessary to obtain observations of a person who knows the patient intimately to learn of it. A lack of power of persistent application to the tasks of the day, an undue irritability, emotional lability, a "peculiar inertia," faulty insight, forgetfulness, inability to retain impressions, indifference to social practices, lack of initiative and spontaneity, all of which may be attributable to worry, anxiety, or depression, are the usual symptoms. Much of this behavior is accepted by the patient with forbearance, and if he has any complaint it is of being weak, tired, dizzy (nonrotational), or "queer in the head." Inordinate drowsiness, a remarkable equanimity, and stoicism may be prominent findings. These symptoms become more persistent and obtrusive with the passage of time. Usually within a few weeks or months the drowsiness and mental dullness increase. This curious inertia and lack of spontaneity then become even more conspicuous and are evident during the interview. The patient seems strangely indifferent to the questions of the examiner. A long pause precedes each reply, and at times he may not bother to respond at all. Or at the very moment when the examiner has decided that the patient has not heard the question and prepares to repeat it, an appropriate, sensible answer is given, usually in relatively few words. The responses are usually much more intelligent than would be expected from the torpid mental state. There are, in addition, patients who are confused or demented (see Chap. 37). The dullness and somnolence may gradually increase and finally, as increased intracranial pressure supervenes, end in coma.

Mental symptoms of this type cannot be ascribed to disease in any particular part of the brain. S. A. K. Wilson has expressed the opinion that tumors are most likely to be accompanied by intellectual disturbance when they interfere with large association fiber systems such as the corpus callosum, inferior and superior longitudinal fasciculi, etc.; growths limited to the cortex and subcortical white matter are less likely to affect the mind. The drowsiness, torpor, inertia, lack of spontaneity, and general restriction of mental horizon are usually related to increased intracranial pressure and are unrelated to the site and nature of the lesion.

The *headaches* in the "tumor patient" may vary exceedingly. In some the pain is slight, temporary, and dull in character; in others it may be severe and unendurable, being either dull or sharp, but as a rule transitory or intermittent. If there are any characteristics of the headache, they are its nocturnal occurrence, its presence on first awakening, and its deep nonpulsatile quality. However, these are not specific attributes, since migraine, hypertensive vascular headaches, etc., may also begin early in the morning on first awakening. The patient does not always complain of the pain even when it is present, and often he betrays its existence by placing his hand on his forehead and looking distressed.

The mechanism of the headache is not known. In the majority of instances, the intracranial pressure is normal during the first weeks when the headache is present, and one can attribute it only to distortion or alteration of blood vessels in or around the tumor. Later the headache appears to be related to rises in intracranial pressure. The location of the headache bears some relation to the situation of the growth. Tumors above the tentorium cause headache on the side of and in the vicinity of the tumor, usually in the orbital, frontal, temporal, or parietal regions. Tumors in the posterior fossa usually cause ipsilateral retroauricular or occipital headache. With elevated intracranial pressure, bifrontal and biooccipital headache is the rule, regardless of the location of the tumor.

Vomiting appears in about one-third of the patients with tumor syndromes of this type and usually accompanies the headache. It is more frequent with tumors of the posterior fossa. Some patients may vomit unexpectedly and forcibly, without preceding nausea (projectile vomiting), but others suffer both nausea and great pain. Usually the vomiting is not related to the ingestion of food, often occurring before breakfast.

No less frequent is the complaint of *giddiness* or *dizziness*. As a rule it is not described with accuracy and consists of a more or less confused sensation in the head, coupled with feelings of strangeness and insecurity when its position is altered. As such it can be assigned little or no localizing value. Its alleged relationship to labyrinthine stasis, or "choked ear," is difficult to verify. The labyrinthine function in such cases is usually normal. True rotational vertigo may also occur and usually signifies disease of the eighth nerve, medulla, or cerebellum.

One or more generalized *convulsions* is the other major symptom which calls attention to the existence of cerebral tumor. Their frequency in various statistical analyses is 20 to 50 per cent of all patients with cerebral tumors. The onset of a seizure during adult years and the existence of a localizing aura are always suggestive of tumor. The localizing significance of seizure patterns has already been discussed (see Chap. 36). The seizures may occur once or many times and may precede other symptoms for as long as 10 years or more in cases of astrocytoma or meningioma. The manner in which

a cerebral tumor can cause a seizure is not known. The majority of the tumors involve the cerebral cortex, though a few cerebellar tumors will be accompanied in the late stages by a generalized seizure for a reason that usually cannot be determined.

The management of patients who present any one of the afore-mentioned symptoms requires brief discussion. The physician is well advised, whenever he encounters any clinical problem of this type, to consider the possibility of a cerebral tumor in its early stages. A careful inquiry should then be made concerning the rest of the symptoms of this complex. In other words, if either a recurrent headache, of a type which the patient recognizes as different from his customary headaches, or a seizure, appearing for the first time, has occurred, there is indication for a careful review of the patient's general behavior. In obtaining further data, one must rely heavily on the observations of other members of the family. A thorough neurologic examination with careful inspection of optic fundi, a test of visual fields, motor, reflex, and sensory functions in the limbs, alertness, memory, facility in language (speaking, reading, writing, and understanding the spoken word), calculation, tests of visuospatial orientation must follow. Sooner or later other regional or localizing symptoms and signs will be discovered, and it is only by repeated examinations that one will note the earliest stages of a hemiparesis, aphasia, visual field defect, hemianesthesia, etc. (For the interpretation of these localizing symptoms and signs the reader is referred to Chaps. 37, 38, and 40.) Unmistakable signs of increased intracranial pressure may become manifest and establish the diagnosis of tumor with reasonable certainty (see Astrocytoma, below).

The necessity of performing confirmatory diagnostic tests will be realized sooner or later, and the decision as to the appropriate time for doing them requires balanced clinical judgment. Since many of the symptoms described above are in no way specific, one should rely on repeated and thorough examinations and should not proceed too quickly to expensive and difficult diagnostic tests. Watchful waiting without unduly alarming the patient is the best plan for a certain period. As more of the clinical picture unfolds, however, there comes a time when x-rays of the skull and chest (always done to help rule out metastatic carcinoma), lumbar puncture (for pressure, cells, protein, and Wassermann), and localizing electroencephalogram should be made, preferably by admitting the patient to a hospital. Perimetry, audiograms, vestibular tests, and psychometric tests are also helpful in the study of many of these patients. Pneumoencephalography and carotid arteriography are reserved in most medical neurologic clinics for those in whom the total clinical syndrome is already strongly suggestive of tumor. These procedures are too costly and hazardous to be used routinely in every "tumor suspect." One proceeds on the basic assumptions that tumor symptoms and signs are progressive and that the treatment of tumors of the brain may proceed satisfactorily from the point at which diagnosis becomes fairly obvious from the clinical facts alone. Experience teaches that little gain comes from attempting early diagnosis and early operation before signs are well established. This point will be further discussed under Treatment.

Tumors Which Tend to Produce General Cerebral Symptoms or Seizures. The following tumors are most likely to produce initial convulsions or a vague syndrome of headache, giddiness, vomiting, dull or stuporous state, and psychic changes: glioblastoma multiforme, astrocytoma, oligodendroglioma, metastatic carcinoma, meningioma, and primary reticulum cell sarcoma of the cerebrum.

GLIOBLASTOMA MULTIFORME. In all statistic analyses of surgical and postmortem material, glioblastoma multiforme is responsible for more than 25 per cent of intracranial gliomas and for more than 90 per cent of gliomas of the cerebral hemispheres in adults. Approximately 20 to 30 per cent of the cerebral tumors are bilateral, occupy more than one lobe of a hemisphere, or show multicentric foci of growth. Although predominantly cerebral in location, similar tumors may be observed in the brain stem, cerebellum, or spinal cord. The peak incidence is in middle adult life, but no age group is spared.

The glioblastoma is a highly malignant tumor which infiltrates the brain extensively and may attain enormous size. It may extend to the meningeal surface or the ventricular wall, which probably accounts for the elevation of protein (often over 100 mg per 100 ml) in many cases and sometimes a pleocytosis of 10 to 100 cells or more, mostly lymphocytes. The tumor has a variegated appearance, being a mottled gray, red, orange, or brown, depending on the degree of necrosis and whether hemorrhage is recent or old. It is highly vascular, and in an arteriogram one can often see a network of abnormal vessels, mistaken at times for a hemiangioma, and the displacement of normal vessels which may result from any "mass lesion." Some part of one lateral ventricle is often distorted, and both lateral and third ventricles are displaced contralaterally, which may be demonstrated by pneumoencephalography or ventriculography. The vessels in the tumor are excessively permeable to fluorescein, P^{32}, radioactive arsenic, etc., which is the basis for radioactive scanning techniques. Calcification and cavity formation are not prominent. The characteristic microscopic pathologic findings are great cellularity with pleomorphism of cells and hyperchromatism of nuclei; identifiable astrocytes with fibrils in combination with astroblasts, tumor giant cells, and cells in mitosis; a curious neoplastic proliferation of the cells of small vessels (adventitial and endothelial); necrosis, pseudopalisading of viable cells, hemorrhage, and thrombosis of vessels. Temporal lobe–tentorial herniation, midbrain compression, midbrain and pontine hemorrhages, and increased intracranial pressure are usually the immediate causes of death. At autopsy the tumor is often seen spreading along cerebrospinal fluid pathways (seedings around spinal cord and cauda equina), but metastasis outside the craniovertebral cavity is almost unheard of except postoperatively when dura, scalp, and draining cervical nodes are invaded.

Clinically the diffuse cerebral symptoms and seizures (present in 30 to 40 per cent of cases) usually give way to a more definite frontal, temporal, parietooccipital, or callosal syndrome in a few weeks or months. Seldom, however, do the symptoms and signs point to one lobe, and often one is satisfied to be able to specify the region of the hemisphere which is involved. When the corpus callosum is invaded, as it so often is, the so-called "callosal syndrome" (apathy, drowsiness, forgetfulness, apractic and agnostic disturbance) may precede or follow other lateralizing signs. Increased intracranial pressure usually follows the other neurologic signs. There are no other important clinical abnormalities. The sedimentation rate, white cell count, and hemoglobin remain normal. Survival for more than a few months or a year after operation is exceptional and should lead one to question the accuracy of histologic diagnosis.

ASTROCYTOMA. The astrocytoma may occur anywhere in the brain or spinal cord. Favored sites are cerebrum, cerebellum, thalamus, optic chiasm, and pons. It is a slowly growing tumor of infiltrative character with a marked tendency to undergo some type of degeneration, with the formation of large cavities or pseudocysts. In some instances much of the tumor may be composed of a pseudocyst surrounded by a thin border of astrocytic tissue, and the only sizable mass of tumor tissue may be a mural nodule. Others of these tumors are noncavitating, grayish-white, firm, and relatively avascular, almost indistinguishable from normal white matter, with which they may merge imperceptibly. Calcium deposits may occur in parts of the tumor and may be seen in a plain x-ray of the skull. The cerebrospinal fluid is acellular, the only abnormality being the increased pressure and elevated protein in some cases. The tumor by its mass may distort the lateral and third ventricles (seen in pneumoencephalogram or ventriculogram) and may be seen to displace the anterior and middle cerebral arteries in a carotid arteriogram. Microscopically the tumor tissue is composed of well-differentiated astrocytes of fibrillary, protoplasmic, or transitional type.

The majority of cerebral astrocytomas undergo malignant degeneration and present as mixed astrocytomas and glioblastomas. In 94 gliomas studied post mortem by Scherer, of which 18 were astrocytomas, all but 5 showed areas of glioblastoma multiforme. This fact, as well as the frequent finding of fiber-forming astrocytes throughout the tumor (obviously tumor cells and not reacting astrocytes), has led Kernohan and his associates to conclude that the glioblastoma, astroblastoma, and astrocytoma are all derived from mature astrocytes which have undergone various degrees of anaplasia. Thus the glioblastoma is an astrocytoma of grade 4 malignancy, and the astroblastoma is of grade 2 or grade 3 malignancy. The authors' observations are, for the most part, in agreement with this opinion, though one must admit the possibility that glial tumors of other cell types upon becoming anaplastic might occasionally give rise to a glioblastoma. The astroblastomas fall between the astrocytoma and glioblastoma in both clinical and pathologic characteristics.

The astrocytoma may cause trivial symptoms for a long period of time. Seizures, headaches, and bizarre mental symptoms may be present for several years, in a few instances more than 10, before the diagnosis is made. The average survival period after the first symptom is 67 months in cerebral growths and 89 months in cerebellar ones. The cystic astrocytoma of the cerebellum is particularly benign, and some patients are alive and well as long as 20 years after part of the cyst was excised. Here of course accuracy of the original diagnosis of neoplasm is always open to question. The astrocytoma of the pons, optic nerves, and chiasm will be discussed in more detail later on in this chapter.

OLIGODENDROCYTOMA. The oligodendrocytoma is a relatively rare cerebral tumor (5 to 10 per cent of gliomas) and is usually slow in its rate of growth (average span of evolution is 66 months). It is generally a soft solid tumor, rarely cystic or hemorrhagic, and through its tendency to calcify (spherules and particles of calcium in microscopic sections) often casts a shadow in the roentgenogram of the skull. Microscopically it is composed of small round cells with spherical nuclei and cytoplasm that stains poorly, forming a halo around the nucleus. Seizures are uncommon, and generalized or focal cerebral symptoms may be present for a long time before the mass of the tumor declares its presence by increased intracranial pressure.

EPENDYMOMA AND EPENDYMOBLASTOMA. Although occasionally this tumor presents as a solitary mass in a cerebral hemisphere in adults, presumably arising from the ependymal wall of the lateral ventricle, its most distinctive form is a papillary growth filling the fourth ventricle of children. It will be discussed further on p. 1821.

MENINGIOMA (ARACHNOIDAL FIBROBLASTOMA AND ENDOTHELIOMA). This is a benign tumor composed of specialized arachnoidal lining cells, arising usually in places where there are arachnoidal villi. Since these clusters of arachnoidal cells penetrate the dura in the vicinity of the venous sinuses, they often appear to originate from the dura itself, hence the old term "dural endothelioma." Grossly the tumors are firm, gray-white lobulated, bulbous, or plaquelike masses which indent or compress but do not invade brain tissue. Many of them are highly vascular. In size they are variable; some are only a centimeter or two in size and are turned up as incidental findings at autopsy. Others, usually those which have produced symptoms, have attained a size of 3 to 4 cm or more. The cellular composition permits easy identification. The cells are of uniform type and have the peculiar disposition to encircle one another and to form characteristic whorls and psammoma bodies. The common sites of these tumors are the olfactory groove, tuberculum sellae, parasagittal region, Sylvian fissure, cerebellopontine angle, and spinal canal. Inasmuch as they lie on the surface of the brain or in next to the dura, changes in the skull are frequent. The skull may be eroded over the tumor and the diploic vessels, which provide part of the blood supply of the tumor, dilate, and are unusually prominent in an x-ray. Or the tumor cells may invade the bone and stimulate osteoblastic activity, as a consequence of which a bony bulge may be seen and felt, or an endostosis is visualized on the inner table of the skull in an x-ray. The meningioma must be listed with metastatic carcinoma and the true cholesteatoma as the three tumors most likely to cause a visible cranial boss in relation to cerebral symptoms (benign exostoses are neurologically asymptomatic). Offering a broad vascular meningeal surface as they do, these tumors often elevate the protein of the cerebrospinal fluid. Their striking vascularity accounts for a characteristic "blush" seen in arteriograms; and the excessive permeability of the vessels, as well as the superficial location of the tumors, make them ideal subjects for localization with radioactive isotopes. The displacement without invasion of cerebral tissue probably explains the interruption locally of normal alpha frequencies in the electroencephalogram with sharp waves or theta waves, in contrast to the delta waves so often found in infiltrative gliomas. Multiple meningiomas may be found, particularly in cases of neurofibromatosis.

These tumors may be found at any age but are more frequent in advanced years, especially in women. Their slow growth is reflected in the long duration of symptoms in many cases, and their indentation of cerebral cortex explains the high incidence of focal convulsions. Aside from the general cerebral disorder and seizures, those tumors which occupy special locations create unique syndromes. Some of these will be discussed later, starting on p. 1823.

METASTATIC CARCINOMA. Of the secondary tumors of the brain only metastatic carcinoma will be discussed here because the other tumors that metastasize to the brain are decidedly rare. Carcinomas reach the brain by hematogenous spread. Probably 35 to 40 per cent come from the lung, and approximately 15 per cent each from the breast, gastrointestinal tract (usually colon or rectum), and kidney. Melanotic carcinoma of the skin, carcinoma of the stomach, gallbladder, liver, thyroid, testicle, uterus, ovary, etc., account for the remainder, no one of them usually being responsible for more than 3 or 4 per cent of secondary tumors of the brain. Carcinoma of the prostate, esophagus, oropharynx, or skin (except for melanocarcinoma) rarely if ever is disseminated in the brain. In more than 75 per cent of cases the metastases are multiple and are scattered through both the cerebrum and cerebellum, often near the surface and involving white matter, cortex, and meninges. The hypernephroma and thyroid carcinoma have a greater tendency to form solitary metastases than other tumors, and as with the chorioepithelioma and some lung tumors, the metastases are likely to be hemorrhagic. The tumor tissue generally has all the gross and microscopic features of any carcinomatous implant and excites rather little glial reaction but much edema.

The usual clinical picture in metastatic carcinoma of the brain has already been described under Glioblastoma Multiforme. However, a number of other rather striking clinical neurologic syndromes also occur. One that is particulary difficult to diagnose is a widespread *carcinomatous meningoencephalopathy* with headache, nervousness, depressed mood, trembling, mental confusion, and forgetfulness, the whole picture looking very much like that of general paresis. Carcinomatosis of the cerebellum with headache, dizziness, and ataxia, the ataxia being brought out only by having the patient walk, is another difficult condition to diagnose during life. Such patients may be regarded as hysterical until sudden death due to a cerebellar pressure cone terminates the illness. Here the metastases may be more or less limited to the midline structures of the cerebellum. Symptoms and signs referable to one or several cranial and spinal nerve roots may be combined with headache and confusion in widespread *carcinomatosis of the craniospinal meninges* (carcinomatous meningitis). Usually the cerebrospinal fluid contains a few white blood cells (lymphocytes) and an elevated protein. Tumor cells can often be identified in Papanicolaou stains of cerebrospinal fluid sediment, and if many are present in the meninges, the sugar values may be subnormal, even as low as 0.

When the syndromes due to these several varieties of metastatic tumor are fully developed, diagnosis is relatively easy. If only headache and vomiting are present, a common error is to explain these symptoms on a psychologic basis. One should make a psychiatric diagnosis only if the patient has the standard symptoms of the mental illnesses (see p. 369). A lumbar puncture, with a chest x-ray (positive in 75 per cent of cases of metastatic tumor of brain), and other x-rays (gastrointestinal series, barium enema, and pyelograms if symptoms point to these organs) are advisable. The metabolic neurologic syndromes which accompany carcinoma but which are not due to tumor invasion of the central nervous system (multiple neuropathy, especially with carcinoma of the lung), polymyositis, and spinocerebellar degeneration (ovarian and other carcinomas) should also be kept in mind.

TUMORS OF INFECTIVE ORIGIN (GRANULOMAS AND PARASITIC CYSTS). Tuberculoma is much less frequent in the United States than it was 20 years ago, and gumma has become almost nonexistent. In fact a patient with serologic syphilis and a positive Wassermann reaction of the cerebrospinal fluid has a greater chance of having two diseases, a cerebral tumor and asymptomatic neurosyphilis, than a gumma. The tuberculoma may occur in any part of the brain, but in children it is more likely to develop in the posterior fossa, i.e., in the cerebellum or brain stem, than in the cerebrum. Often there are a small number of cells and an increased protein content in the cerebrospinal fluid because the lesion frequently lies contiguous to the meninges; and it may at any time give rise to a tuberculous meningitis with typical cerebrospinal fluid formula (50 to 300 cells, increased protein, decreased sugar content and decreased chloride content).

In South America tuberculoma and gumma are much more frequent, and one can usually depend on evidence of disease in other parts of the body, especially the lungs, and characteristic changes in the cerebrospinal fluid (see Chap. 32) to indicate the nature of the lesion. In addition, cysticercus cellulosae and hydatid cysts are common lesions and should always be suspected when seizures, increased intracranial pressure, or diffuse cerebral symptoms develop in the adult. X-rays of the skull and skeletal muscles (e.g., thigh) may reveal characteristic calcific deposits in cysticercosis. Torula and other fungous granulomas and *Schistosoma japonicum* infection may also present as space-occupying cerebral lesions.

Patients with Unmistakable Signs of Increased Intracranial Pressure When First Seen. A certain number of patients show all the characteristic symptoms and signs of increased intracranial pressure [periodic bifrontal and bioccipital headaches which awaken him during the night or are present upon awakening, vomiting that may or may not be expected and projectile, mental torpor, and papilledema (see Chap. 32)] when first seen. The physician confronted with this clinical problem is forced to take immediate action, for the condition is potentially dangerous. A critical rise in intracranial hypertension may occur at any time and result in coma, respiratory arrest, and death. Admission to a hospital with a neurosurgical service is therefore usually urgent. Nevertheless all the medical aspects of the patient's problem should first be worked out.

Three questions demand immediate answers: (1) Does the patient have a space-occupying intracranial lesion? (2) Where in the cranial cavity is it situated? (3) What is its nature? With respect to the first question it is well to keep in mind that a number of medical conditions may simulate an intracranial growth that causes only the general symptoms of increased intracranial pressure. These are (1) "pseudotumor cerebri," (2) hypertensive encephalopathy, (3) chronic pulmonary disease with hypercapnia and hypoxia, (4) chronic adhesive arachnoiditis and/or aqueductal stenosis, (5) thrombosis of cerebral veins and dural sinuses, (6) Addison's disease with encephalopathy or hypoparathyroidism with papilledema. Several of these conditions have been discussed elsewhere in this book, and it is sufficient to mention them briefly; others have not been considered before and will be discussed in detail.

Pseudotumor Syndromes. In the condition of *pseudotumor cerebri* (meningeal hydrops) the patient, more often than not a young woman, complains of headaches of some weeks' standing and when first examined is found to have papilledema, or choked disk, with slightly constricted visual fields and enlarged blind spots. Other neurologic signs, with the occasional exception of a vague dizziness, diplopia due to a slight abducens weakness, or paresthesias of some part of the body, are conspicuously absent, and the patient appears remarkably "bright" and well. The cerebrospinal fluid is acellular with normal protein content, and a ventriculogram reveals small or normal-sized ventricles. With daily, then biweekly, then weekly lumbar punctures to lower the cerebrospinal fluid pressure, most of the patients gradually recover over a period of weeks to months. Extremely high cerebrospinal fluid pressure with episodes of cloudy vision (obscurations) may herald the onset of blindness and require a right subtemporal decompression as an emergency measure. The cause of the condition is unknown. Extreme hypertension (diastolic pressures of 120 mm or over), retinal arteriolar changes with hemorrhages and exudates in the periphery of the optic fundi, signs of renal disease, and headache, convulsions, confusion, stupor, or coma are the basis of the diagnosis of *hypertensive encephalopathy* (see p. 1789). *Chronic emphysema or other lung disease*, with cyanosis, dyspnea, cough, signs of cor pulmonale with right-sided congestive heart failure and secondary polycythemia, may be attended by bilateral papilledema, elevated cerebrospinal fluid pressure, high venous pressure, severe headache, drowsiness, stupor, or coma and a peculiar lapse in the posture of the outstretched limbs and other contracted skeletal muscles (flapping movements or asterixis similar to the flap in impending liver coma). The finding of an elevated carbon dioxide–combining power and diminished arterial oxygen concentration substantiate the diagnosis. *Chronic adhesive arachnoiditis* due to chronic fibrosing meningeal diseases such as syphilis, postspinal anesthesia arachnoiditis, and cryptogenic meningeal diseases may be attended by headache, papilledema, seizures, blindness, paraplegia, or quadriplegia. The cerebrospinal fluid protein may be normal or elevated, with or without a "dynamic block"; and the lateral and third ventricles are enlarged in the ventriculogram. Syphilis and the other chronic meningitides may also cause *aqueductal stenosis* owing to a proliferative gliotic ependymitis, with enlargement of the lateral and third ventricles (see Chap. 32). *Thrombosis of the jugular veins and of the lateral and posterior parts of the superior sagittal sinus* may result in increased intracranial pressure, with otherwise normal cerebrospinal fluid and small ventricles (see Chap. 284). Several cases of unexplained papilledema with headache, drowsiness, and confusion and elevated cerebrospinal fluid pressure have been observed in conjunction with *Addison's disease* (Jefferson) and also in rare cases of hypoparathyroidism. The mechanism is not known. *Retrobulbar neuritis of demyelinative type*, if it extends to the optic nerve head, may cause a papillitis with elevation and edema of the optic disk and even hemorrhages around the disk. There is invariably an early development of a marked impairment of vision and large central scotomas. The prominent visual change and the absence of clinical and laboratory evidence of increased intracranial pressure distinguish this condition from true papilledema, and also from pseudopapilledema (spurious papilledema) and tortuosity of retinal veins—a normal ophthalmoscopic picture in some patients, especially those with marked hyperopia. Severe anemia may also cause hemorrhages, exudates, and a suspicion of papilledema, which may at times be confused with the retinal picture of neoplasm.

"False Localizing Signs." If the clinical findings permit the exclusion of the afore-mentioned conditions, there is reasonable certainty that the patient has an intracranial growth. The problem then is to search for signs that will localize the lesion. In doing this, several pitfalls must be avoided. One common source of error is to place undue reliance on a sign which proves to have no localizing value whatsoever. With experience in this field one comes to distrust any symptom or sign which develops late, after headache and increased intracranial pressure have been established, for it often turns out to be a "false localizing sign." Under these circumstances drowsiness, slowness in response, inattentiveness, and emotional blunting can be found as often with cerebellar as with cerebral growths. Unilateral or bilateral abducens palsy is another common false localizing sign (Collier), and reference has already been made to the drooping eyelid, dilated pupil, ipsilateral hemiparesis and bilateral Babinski signs, and coma in temporal lobe herniation. Jacksonian and generalized seizures and ipsilateral or bilateral pyramidal signs may be observed in the advanced stages of a cerebellar tumor. On the other hand, relatively slight focal signs that may be easily overlooked are sometimes the only clues as to the localization of the tumor. Examples are ataxia of gait (but not of limbs) and head tilt in cerebellar tumors, paralysis of upward gaze with the Argyll Robertson pupillary phenomenon in pinealomas, pale optic disks and chiasmal field defects in craniopharyngiomas, homonymous visual inattentiveness and sensory extinction (see pp. 1823 and 1824) in posterior cerebral tumors, and a facial asymmetry in emotional expression in frontal tumors.

Tumors Which Tend to Produce Elevated Intracranial Pressure without Conspicuous Localizing Signs. The tumors most likely to cause increased intracranial pressure with few or no focal or lateralizing signs are medulloblastoma, ependymoma of the fourth ventricle, hemangioblastoma, pinealoma, colloid cysts of the third ventricle, gliomas of tegmentum of the midbrain blocking the aqueduct, and craniopharyngioma. In addition, in many of the cerebral gliomas discussed above, particularly those of the corpus callosum and frontal lobes, increased intracranial pressure may precede focal cerebral signs.

MEDULLOBLASTOMA. This is a rapidly growing tumor which arises in the posterior part of the vermis of children. The midline part of the cerebellum may be invaded and completely destroyed. The tumor also fills the fourth ventricle and com-

presses the medulla. The tonsils of the cerebellum are forced down into the cervical spinal canal (cerebellar pressure cone) in fatal cases. Seedings of the tumor may be seen on the walls of the third and lateral ventricles, on the meningeal surfaces of the brain, and around the spinal cord. The tumor is solid, reddish gray in color, and poorly demarcated from the adjacent brain tissue. It is very cellular, and the cells are small, closely packed with little cytoplasm, many mitoses, scant stroma, and a tendency to form clusters or pseudorosettes. As already stated, these cells resemble the "indifferent cells" which may be observed in the embryonic or fetal brain and are thought to be capable of differentiation into either glial cells or neuroblasts. Bailey and Cushing introduced the name *medulloblastoma* in 1925. Although medulloblasts as such have not been described in the fetal or adult human brain and the cell type is not known for certain, the term is retained if for no other reason than its familiarity. In adults a somewhat similar neuroblastoma of less malignant character may arise in the cerebral hemisphere.

The clinical picture is distinctive. Typically, the patient, a child of five to ten years, becomes listless, vomits repeatedly, and has a morning headache. The first diagnosis which suggests itself may be gastrointestinal disease or abdominal migraine. Soon, however, a stumbling gait, frequent falls, and a squint lead to a neurologic examination and the discovery of papilledema. Ataxia of the limbs may be absent at all times (see Chap. 27 on the syndrome of flocculonodular lobe). Decerebrate attacks (tonic cerebellar fits) may occur in the late stages of the disease. The tumor is highly radiosensitive, and surgery with x-ray treatment may prolong life for several years.

EPENDYMOMA AND PAPILLOMA OF THE FOURTH VENTRICLE. This tumor also arises from the walls of the fourth ventricle in children. It is a firm, whitish lobulated growth composed of small cells arranged in the form of small rosettes around vessels or central clear areas and containing blepharoplasts in their cytoplasm. Mitoses are absent; if present, they mark the tumor as an ependymoblastoma. The clinical syndrome is much like that of the medulloblastoma except for the absence of ataxia of gait. The tumor is not very sensitive to x-ray, and surgical removal offers the only hope of survival. The papilloma or papillary adenocarcinoma of the choroid plexus of the fourth ventricle gives rise to a similar syndrome but tends to occur later in life.

HEMANGIOBLASTOMA OF THE CEREBELLUM. The disease of Lindau was described in Chap. 283. Dizziness, ataxia of gait or of the limbs on one side, symptoms and signs of increased intracranial pressure, and in some instances a retinal angioma (von

Hippel's disease) and polycythemia constitute the neurologic syndrome. Familial incidence is well known. Craniotomy with opening of the cerebellar cyst and excision of the mural hemangioblastomatous nodule may be curative.

PINEALOMA. This may be either a teratoma or a glioma of the pineal gland. The teratoma is a firm, discrete noninvasive mass which usually reaches 3 to 4 cm in greatest diameter. It compresses the superior colliculi and sometimes the superior surface of the cerebellum, with narrowing of the aqueduct of Sylvius. Often it extends anteriorly into the third ventricle and may then compress the hypothalamus. Microscopically it is composed of large, spherical epithelial cells (much like those of a seminoma), separated by a network of reticular connective tissue which contains many lymphocytes. The gliomas have the usual morphology of an astrocytoma of varying degrees of malignancy. Children, adolescents, and young adults, either male or female, may be affected. In some cases the clinical syndrome consists solely of symptoms and signs of increased intracranial pressure, and the diagnosis can be made only by a ventriculogram which reveals the tumor. The most characteristic symptom, however, is an inability to look upward (Parinaud's syndrome), with slightly dilated pupils which react on accommodation but not to light. Sometimes ataxia of the limbs, choreatic movements, or spastic weakness appears in the later stages of the illness. A Torkildsen ventriculo-cisterna magna shunt of cerebrospinal fluid and x-ray therapy have been remarkably successful in controlling the symptoms. Attempts at surgical removal of the tumor have usually proved fatal.

COLLOID (PARAPHYSEAL) CYST OF THE THIRD VENTRICLE. This is a papillomatous structure always situated in the anterior extremity of the third ventricle between the interventricular foramens and attached to the roof of the ventricle. Usually it is about a centimeter in diameter, is oval or round with a smooth external surface, and is filled with a glairy colloid material. The wall is composed of a layer of epithelial cells surrounded by a capsule of fibrous connective tissue. These benign cysts may exist for long periods of time; they produce neurologic symptoms by blocking the third ventricle and causing an obstructive hydrocephalus. This tumor should be suspected when the following clinical syndromes are found: dementia with or without headache, intermittent severe bifrontal-biooccipital headaches, sometimes modified by posture (ballvalve obstruction of the third ventricle), crises of headache with obtundation, bilateral paresthesias, dim vision, and weakness of legs with sudden falls.

CRANIOPHARYNGIOMA (SUPRASELLAR OR RATHKE'S POUCH CYST, HYPOPHYSEAL DUCT TUMORS, ADAMANTINOMAS, AMELOBLASTOMAS). This is a benign congenital or "rest cell" tumor. By the time it has grown to a diameter of 3 to 4 cm it is almost always cystic. Usually it lies above the sella turcica, depressing the optic chiasm and extending up into the third ventricle. Less often it is subdiaphragmatic, i.e., within the sella, where it compresses the pituitary body, erodes one part of the wall of the sella or a clinoid process but seldom balloons the sella like a pituitary adenoma. The tumor is oval, round, or lobulated and has a smooth surface. The wall of the cyst and the solid parts of the tumor consist of cords and whorls of epithelial cells, often with intercellular bridges and keratohyalin, separated by a loose network of stellate cells. The cyst contains dark albuminous fluid and cholesterol crystals. Calcium deposits are found in nearly all of them and can be seen in plain x-rays of the suprasellar region in about 40 per cent of cases. The sella beneath the tumor tends to be flattened and enlarged. This is more often a tumor of children than of adults, but patients of all ages may be seen with it. In children, adiposity, delayed or infantile physical and sexual development (Froehlich's syndrome or Lorain syndrome—see Chap. 283), headaches, vomiting, dim vision with chiasmal field defects (see p. 274), optic atrophy or papilledema comprise the clinical picture. In adults, waning libido, amenorrhea, slight spastic weakness of the legs, headache without papilledema, and mental dullness and confusion are often found. Later drowsiness, diabetes insipidus, and disturbances of temperature regulation may occur, indicating hypothalamic involvement (see p. 274).

In the differential diagnosis of these several tumor syndromes a careful clinical analysis is often more important than laboratory procedures. Arteriography and electroencephalography are not so helpful as in cerebral tumors. The tests which, though somewhat hazardous, are likely to give the most useful information are the air ventriculogram or a combined ventriculogram-pneumoencephalogram and the Pantopaque ventriculogram (injection of radiopaque fluid).

Tumors of the Posterior Fossa and Third Ventricle in Infancy and Early Childhood. Any discussion of tumors of the brain would be incomplete if some reference were not made to intracranial tumors of infancy and childhood, for they often create clinical problems of a special type. Fully two-thirds of tumors before the age of puberty are medulloblastomas, ependymomas, cerebellar astrocytomas, and pontine gliomas, are situated in the posterior fossa, and produce increased intracranial pressure. Hence this brief digression is appropriate at this point in the general exposition.

As stated in Chap. 283 in the section on congenital hydrocephalus, the cranial sutures do not close until about the time of puberty, and an elevation of intracranial pressure, especially if it occurs in the first months and years of life, results in separation of sutures and enlargement of the head. This is evident by inspection, by head measurement, and in x-rays, and it is also demonstrated by finger percussion of the parietal eminence of the skull, which produces a peculiar sound as though a cracked cup or bowl were being tapped (Macewen's sign). The separation of sutures by enlarging the intracranial cavity permits temporary restitution of intracranial pressure and amelioration of symptoms. Papilledema does not develop if the head enlarges.

The cardinal symptoms of a posterior fossa tumor in an infant or small child are different from those of the adult. They consist of weakness, vomiting, and unsteadiness of gait. These symptoms may fluctuate in severity, tending to subside temporarily with further separation of sutures. The vomiting may be prominent and occur at any time of day. Often is it not preceded by nausea. An erroneous diagnosis of "cyclic vomiting" or vomiting due to an emotional disturbance may be made. Unlike vomiting due to intraabdominal disease, this vomiting is not accompanied by abdominal pain. Weakness and listlessness are also present but are more difficult to interpret. Headache is seldom a complaint, and seizures are rare.

In tumors of the vermis of the cerebellum (medulloblastoma), the ataxia of gait and disinclination to walk (see Chap. 27 on the vermis syndrome), without evident incoordination of the movements of arms or legs, can usually be demonstrated by careful observation. In astrocytoma or hemangioblastoma of one cerebellar hemisphere, the ipsilateral arm and leg are ataxic (see Chap. 27 on the syndrome of neocerebellum), and a nystagmus which is much coarser on looking to the side of the lesion than to the opposite side is present. Also, the head is often tilted with tumor of the cerebellar hemisphere, the ear on the side of the tumor being brought toward the shoulder. The ipsilateral arm is hypotonic and swings less than the contralateral one in walking. General hypotonia and bilateral extensor plantar reflexes are late signs and are of less value in localization.

These cerebellar signs, when added to the general picture described above, regardless of whether or not papilledema is present, point to the posterior fossa as the site of a tumor. More difficult to diagnose are the patients with only signs of hydrocephalus. This condition may come about with a medulloblastoma arising in the upper vermis and filling the fourth ventricle or with an ependymoma arising from either the roof or the floor of the fourth ventricle. Occasionally a craniopharyngioma may cause only hydrocephalus, but then a peculiar docility, an appearance of maturity due to greater inter-

est in mental than physical activities, and a retardation of growth may be helpful signs in identifying a lesion within the walls of the third ventricle.

In later childhood, separation of sutures and head enlargement are slight, and headache and papilledema are the common signs of increased intracranial pressure, just as in the adult.

Patients with Symptoms and Signs of a Slowly Progressive Lesion in a Particular Region of the Cranial Cavity. In this condition general cerebral symptoms and the signs of increased intracranial pressure occur late or not at all. The physician arrives at the correct diagnosis by being able to make an anatomic or regional diagnosis from a set of neurologic findings and by reasoning that the etiology must be neoplastic because of the slowly progressive nature of the illness. Special x-rays of the skull, cerebrospinal fluid examination, and depending on the location of the disease, either pneumoencephalography or arteriography will usually confirm the clinical impression.

The following tumors produce unique syndromes usually diagnostic of a special type of tumor.

ACOUSTIC NEUROFIBROMA OR NEURINOMA. This slowly growing benign tumor may occur as a solitary lesion or as a part of the syndrome of neurofibromatosis. By the time of operation the tumor has usually attained a size of 4 to 6 cm in diameter. It arises from the extramedullary part of the eighth cranial nerve, usually within the internal auditory meatus, where the intracranial part of the nerve first acquires the histologic character of a peripheral nerve, i.e., has Schwann cells and fibroblasts. The space in which it lies is the cerebellopontine angle, i.e., between the cerebellum, pons, and medulla posteriorly, the petrous pyramid anteriorly, and the tentorium above. The internal auditory meatus is usually enlarged (visible in x-rays), the middle cerebellar peduncle and the anterolateral part of the cerebellum are depressed, and the trigeminal, facial, glossopharyngeal, and vagus nerves are displaced and stretched over the surface of the growth. The fourth ventricle is deformed, displaced, and narrowed (visible in a pneumoencephalogram), and there is hydrocephalic enlargement of the aqueduct and of the third and lateral ventricles in the late stages. The tumor is vascular, and the surrounding cerebrospinal fluid has a high protein content (cerebrospinal fluid protein of 300 mg per 100 ml or over is not infrequent). The microscopic picture is that of a typical neurofibroma (axis cylinders mixed with masses of fibrous connective tissue in interlacing strands, palisaded nuclei, and mononuclear giant cells without mitoses). The typical clinical syndrome, which usually occurs in adult men or women, is tinnitus, deafness, and rotational vertigo [seldom in discrete attacks as in Ménière's syndrome (see p. 293)] of several years' standing, followed by stiff neck and postauricular or suboccipital pain, spasms and twitching or slight weakness of the face, paresthesias or pain in the face, dysphonia and dysphagia, and homolateral cerebellar ataxia of the arm and leg. Headache, vomiting, and choked disk are late findings. Variations of this syndrome are numerous. Early in its development only progressive deafness, tinnitus, and vague vertigo may be present, and the abnormal audiogram, impaired vestibular function, elevated cerebrospinal fluid protein, widened internal auditory meatus, and obliteration of the lateral recess of the fourth ventricle in a pneumoencephalogram must be depended upon for diagnosis. Dementia may later be the presenting syndrome, and the deaf ear may be overlooked. Unilateral cerebellar ataxia and dizziness may predominate, and definite signs of involvement of the fifth, seventh, and eighth cranial nerves may not be found. The treatment is surgical excision.

The *trigeminal* or *gasserian ganglion neurinoma* and *meningioma* of the *cerebellopontine angle* may be indistinguishable from an acoustic neurinoma. They should always be considered if early tinnitus and deafness and an unresponsive labyrinth ("dead labyrinth") are not the initial symptoms of the cerebellopontine angle syndrome. A true *cholesteatoma of the temporal bone* may simulate this clinical picture, but usually the facial weakness is early and severe, the ear is deaf, and labyrinthine function is absent, whereas the other cranial nerve signs, cerebellar ataxia, and increased intracranial pressure are absent. The *tumor of the glomus jugulare* (a flat ovoid body, found in the adventitia of the jugular bulb, immediately below the floor of the middle ear and near the ramus tympanicus of the ninth cranial nerve) may, like the acoustic neurofibroma, basal meningioma, metastatic cancer, syphilitic meningitis, neurofibroma of other cranial nerves, and vascular malformation, cause unilateral lower cranial nerve palsies (see p. 295). It is a purplish-red, highly vascular tumor composed of large epithelioid cells in an alveolar pattern and an abundant capillary network. Partial deafness, facial palsy, dysphagia, and unilateral atrophy of the tongue, combined with a vascular polyp in the auditory meatus and a palpable mass below and anterior to the mastoid eminence, often with a bruit, comprise the syndrome. The jugular foramen is eroded (visible by x-ray), and the cerebrospinal fluid protein may be elevated. Women are affected more than men, and the peak incidence is during middle adult life. The tumor grows slowly over a period of many years, sometimes 10 or more. The treatment is x-ray radiation.

THE PITUITARY ADENOMAS. These tumors, which are so common, particularly in late adult life, often are discovered when a patient begins to complain of a visual disturbance. A unilateral or bilateral temporal hemianopia progressing to blindness, with optic atrophy, is the usual finding and, with x-ray evidence of an expanded sella turcica, leads to a diagnosis of pituitary adenoma. As the growth enlarges and extends laterally, an oculomotor palsy is occasionally seen, and large suprasellar extensions may involve the hypothalamus or temporal lobe. If there are signs of acromegaly, one may assume that an eosinophilic adenoma is present; if not, and signs of pituitary insufficiency are present (amenorrhea without "hot flashes," sexual impotence, etc.—see Chap. 69), there is usually a chromophobe adenoma. Basophilic adenomas, one of the causes of Cushing's syndrome, rarely if ever produce enlargement of the sella or visual symptoms. The diagnosis is made from the endocrine picture (see Chap. 69). The cerebrospinal fluid is usually under normal pressure, and protein is elevated only in exceptional cases. Other tumors may rarely expand the sella (craniopharyngioma), and there are also rather wide normal variations in its size. Hence the diagnosis of pituitary adenoma should not be made because of minor enlargements in the absence of neighborhood neurologic signs. In doubtful cases a pneumoencephalogram permits visualization of the suprasellar extension of the tumor. Treatment is x-ray radiation and, if vision is threatened despite x-ray therapy, either transnasal or transfrontal surgical excision.

MENINGIOMA OF THE SELLAR TUBERCLE. This tumor arises from the region of tuberculum sellae, and as it grows it lifts the optic chiasm upward and backward. The optic nerves become stretched and separated. With further increases in size, it may expand anteriorly, compressing the olfactory bulbs, or posteriorly, compressing the hypothalamus. When the tumor is small, the only symptom is bitemporal hemianopia; later, blindness with optic atrophy, anosmia, mental deterioration, hemiparesis, uncinate seizures, oculomotor palsy, and amenorrhea are added. The diagnosis is made when a middle-aged person is found to have a bitemporal hemianopia, normal-sized sella, and no signs of hypothalamic or pituitary involvement. Saccular aneurysm of the carotid artery and rarely craniopharyngioma, extrasellar pituitary adenoma, and Boeck's sarcoid may be confused with it. The treatment is surgical excision.

MENINGIOMA OF THE SPHENOID RIDGE. This tumor arises from arachnoid cap cells over the lesser wing of the sphenoidal bone. As it increases in size, it may expand medially to encroach on structures in the wall of the cavernous sinus, anteriorly to invade the orbit, or laterally to erode or invade the temporal bone. Most prominent among the symptoms are a slowly developing unilateral exophthalmos, slight bulging of the bone in the temporal region, and roentgenologic evidence of thickening or erosion of the lesser wing of the sphenoid bone. Variants of the clinical syndrome include oculomotor palsy or syndrome of Foix (p. 297), blindness in one eye with optic atrophy, anosmia (and sometimes the Kennedy syndrome—see below), mental changes, uncinate fits, and increased intracranial pressure. Sarcomas arising from the skull bones, metastatic carcinoma, orbitoethmoidal osteoma, tumors of the optic nerve, and angiomas of the orbit must be considered in the differential diagnosis. Auscultation of the skull, x-ray of the skull, and carotid arteriography are helpful in differentiating these lesions.

MENINGIOMA OF THE OLFACTORY GROOVE. This tumor is a growth derived from arachnoidal cap cells along the cribriform plate. The diagnosis depends on the finding of ipsilateral or bilateral anosmia, ipsilateral or bilateral blindness, often with optic atrophy on one side and papilledema without atrophy on the other (Kennedy syndrome), and mental changes. The tumors may reach enormous size before coming to the attention of the physician. The anosmia, if unilateral, is rarely if ever reported by the patient. The unilateral visual disturbance may consist of a slowly developing unilateral central scotoma. Confusion, forgetfulness, inappropriate jocularity (*Witzelsucht*) are the usual psychic disturbances. The patient is indifferent to or jokes about blindness. Usually there are x-ray changes along the cribriform plate and an extremely high cerebrospinal fluid protein (200 to 400 mg).

GLIOMA OF THE BRAIN STEM. Astrocytomas of the brain stem (formerly called "bipolar spongioblastomas") are slow-growing, firm, white infiltrating growths which insinuate themselves between tracts and nuclei. They produce a variable clinical picture, depending on their exact location in the medulla, pons, and midbrain (see Chaps. 31 and 26 for syndromes). The characteristic features, in the early stages, are signs of crossed motor or sensory disturbances, which always indicate brain stem disease, and, as the lesion advances, an orderly succession of new signs due to involvement of neighboring structures, and finally signs of bilateral disease in the brain stem. Headache, vomiting, and papilledema occur late. The course is slowly progressive over years unless some part of the tumor becomes more malignant (glioblastoma multiforme), in which instance the illness may terminate fatally within months. The main clinical problem is to differentiate between this disease, multiple sclerosis, and vascular malformations of the pons. These so-called "intramedullary" or intrinsic brain stem lesions may usually be distinguished from extramedullary compressive ones by (1) predominance of both tract and nuclear involvement in the former and of cranial nerve involvement in the latter; (2) signs of involvement of special intramedullary structures, e.g., internuclear ophthalmoplegia due to affection of medial longitudinal fasciculi, or vertical nystagmus, which are rarely observed in compressive lesions of the brain stem. Pneumoencephalography to visualize the fourth ventricle and aqueduct and occasionally vertebral arteriography are helpful in diagnosis. The treatment is x-ray radiation and if intracranial pressure is increased, a Torkildsen ventriculo-cisterna magna shunt.

GLIOMA OF THE OPTIC NERVES AND CHIASM. This tumor is often found in patients with von Recklinghausen's disease and, like the glioma of the brain stem, arises most frequently during the period of childhood and adolescence. The initial symptoms are dimness of vision with constricted fields, bizarre bilateral field defects of homonymous, heteronymous, sometimes bitemporal type, blindness, and optic atrophy with or without papilledema. Hypothalamic signs (infantilism, adiposity, polyuria, somnolence, and genital atrophy) are common. X-rays reveal an enlargement of the optic foramen. With this finding and the lack of ballooning of the sella or suprasellar calcification, pituitary adenoma, Hand-Schüller-Christian disease, and craniopharyngioma can be excluded. The treatment is surgical excision or x-ray, depending on the exact location.

CHORDOMA. This is a soft, jellylike gray-pink growth composed of cords or masses of large cells with granules of glycogen in their cytoplasm and often multiple nuclei and intercellular mucoid material. They are locally invasive but do not metastasize. They may arise from any part of the base of the cranium or vertebral column, but the commonest sites are the base of the skull (from physaliphora ecchondrosis) or lumbosacral region (giving rise to a cauda equina syndrome). Those in the base of the skull create a remarkable clinical picture in which all or any combination of cranial nerve palsies from the second to twelfth on one or both sides are combined with a retropharyngeal mass and erosion of the clivus of sphenoid bone and the occiput. It is one of the five tumors that may present both as an intracranial and as an extracranial mass. (The other four are the meningioma, neurofibroma, glomus jugulare tumor, and carcinoma of sinuses or pharynx.) The treatment is x-ray therapy.

NASOPHARYNGEAL GROWTHS WHICH ERODE THE BASE OF THE SKULL. These are rather common in a general hospital and arise from the mucous membrane of the paranasal sinuses or the nasopharynx near the eustachian tube, i.e., the fossa of Rosenmueller (*transitional cell carcinoma, Schmincke tumor*). In addition to symptoms of nasopharyngeal or sinus disease, which may not be prominent, facial pain and numbness (trigeminal), abducens palsy (sixth cranial nerve), and other cranial nerve palsies may occur. Diagnosis depends on inspection and biopsy of a nasopharyngeal mass, biopsy of an involved cervical gland, and x-ray evidence of erosion of the base of the skull. The treatment is x-ray therapy.

Prognosis

The prognosis of intracranial tumor is influenced by the nature of the growth, its location, and other factors. As a general rule unless an operation is performed almost all intracranial tumors end fatally. Death in most instances is preceded by a critical rise in intracranial pressure and tentorial or foramen magnum herniation. The more malignant tumors, such as the glioblastoma multiforme, medulloblastoma, and metastatic carcinoma, end fatally within a year, as a rule, whereas the slowly growing meningiomas and astrocytomas often permit survival for many years.

The prospects for recovery after surgery depend largely upon the type of tumor. With meningiomas and acoustic neurofibromas, if completely excised, there may be a complete cure. In gliomas the outlook is more bleak. Cure is rare, for seldom can complete excision be accomplished. Nevertheless with the slow-growing gliomas, partial excision, the marsupialization of a cyst, the relief of increased intracranial pressure may lead to improvement and resumption of a useful life for many years. With metastatic growths the outlook is dismal, though if there are no metastases in other organs and the cerebral deposit appears to be solitary, operation has occasionally resulted in temporary recovery for a few months or a year or two.

Treatment

The treatment of primary intracranial tumors is surgical removal. Unless the patient is old or suffers some other disease which threatens to take his life within a few months, the brain tumor should be exposed by craniotomy and biopsied. This craniotomy, which usually carries a mortality rate of 2 to 5 per cent, should be undertaken only when the diagnosis of an intracranial space-occupying lesion is clearly established by clinical symptoms and signs and confirmed by one or more special diagnostic procedures. The latter should be kept at a minimum; arteriography and ventriculography are in themselves hazardous, particularly if done when intracranial pressure is high; and they add to the mortality from craniotomy.

The premium on early diagnosis is not so great as in tumors elsewhere in the body. In the vast majority of patients there is little prospect that an early diagnosis and operation will improve the surgical result or effect a cure. The benign surface tumors grow so slowly that one can usually temporize for weeks or months, if diagnosis is uncer-

tain, without significantly worsening the surgical outcome, provided of course that the operation is not delayed until high intracranial pressure has developed. If the tumor is a glioma, the prospect of complete eradication, even with early operation, is almost nil; hence little is lost by waiting a few weeks or months, provided the patient is not permitted to become comatose before being transferred to the neurosurgeon, in which instance the chances of surviving the operative procedure are poor. By waiting for the clinical syndrome to evolve one avoids diagnostic errors (confusion of tumors with other diseases).

The physician's responsibilities in this field of intracranial tumors are (1) diagnosis—he must separate the tumor cases from all the others which pass through his hands; (2) exclusion of the possibility that the intracranial mass is part of a general disease which would contraindicate surgery, i.e., metastatic carcinoma, syphilis, tuberculosis, parasitic infections, etc.; (3) exclusion of the several pseudotumor syndromes; (4) maintenance of the patient in the best possible condition, until surgery can be undertaken (fluids, electrolytes, etc.); (5) assisting the surgeon in the postoperative medical management. Dehydration, i.e., use of hypertonic solutions [$MgSO_4$ by mouth or rectally or 33 per cent urea or 50 per cent sucrose by vein (see p. 1807)], may be of help as a palliative measure in tiding the patient over a bout of intracranial hypertension. In inoperable cases the objectives are to maintain the morale of the family and patient as long as possible and to provide intelligent supportive therapy.

In general, although the results of therapy are frequently disappointing, there are always the few dramatic successes that serve as a perpetual stimulus to the physician, and so it is always with the next patient that he hopes to achieve a cure.

SPINAL CORD TUMORS

Growths and other space-occupying lesions within the spinal canal can be conveniently divided into two groups, those which arise within the substance of the spinal cord and invade and destroy tracts and central gray structures (intramedullary) and those which arise outside the spinal cord (extramedullary) from the vertebral bodies and epidural tissues (extradural), the meninges or roots (intradural). The relative frequency of spinal tumors in these different locations in a general hospital is about 5 per cent intramedullary, 40 per cent intradural-extramedullary, and 55 per cent extradural. The percentage of extradural lesions in a general hospital population is usually higher than in most neurosurgical series (e.g., Elsberg's figures of 10, 67, and 15 per cent respectively), which often do not include many of the lymphomas, metastatic carcinomas, etc., most of which are extradural.

The cellular origin of the intramedullary gliomas has been mentioned in the section on intracerebral tumors. The proportions of the different cell types differ, however. Kernohan, who has had one of the largest series of pathologic cases, found all the gliomas represented in the spinal cord, but ependymoma was noted to make up 40 per cent, and the remainder were more or less evenly distributed amongst astrocytomas, glioblastomas, oligodendrogliomas, ganglioneuromas, medulloblastomas, hemangiomas, and hemangioblastomas. The hemangioma is the common source of spontaneous hematomyelia, and the hemangioblastoma may give rise to a syringomyelia.

Pathologic Anatomy and Physiology

Peculiarities of anatomic structure are decisive factors in determining the symptomatology of tumor growths. The structure of the spine was described in Chap. 7, Pain in the Back, and Chap. 285, Traumatic Diseases of the Brain and Spinal Cord. The spinal cord hangs as a cylinder within it, being moored by the denticulate ligaments and spinal roots. There is a small space between the dura and vertebral column which contains fat and a venous plexus and is in communication with extradural tissues through the intervertebral foramens. Epidural growth—whether arising as direct extensions from the vertebral bodies, by hematogenous dissemination in epidural fat, or extension through intervertebral foramens from an extraspinal tumor—may displace and finally compress the spinal cord. Masses within the spinal canal may also interfere with its circulation, either by blocking the collateral vessels which enter through the intervertebral foramen along the roots or by direct compression of the veins which course longitudinally on the surface of the spinal cord.

Intramedullary growths both invade as well as compress and distort fasciculi in the adjacent white matter. As the cord enlarges from the tumor growing within it or is compressed from a tumor growing without, the free space around the cord is consumed, and the cerebrospinal fluid below the lesion becomes isolated or loculated from the rest of the so-called "circulating cerebrospinal fluid" above. This can be demonstrated by a positive Queckenstedt test (Chap. 32), Froin's syndrome, and interruption of the flow of Pantopaque in the subarachnoid space (myelogram).

Symptomatology

Patients with spinal cord tumor are likely to manifest one of two clinical pictures, one a radicular-spinal syndrome, nearly always painful, the other

a purely sensorimotor spinal tract or rarely a syringomyelic syndrome.

Spinal Cord Compression. The predominant clinical syndrome relates to spinal cord compression. With intraspinal tumors the onset of the compressive symptoms is usually gradual, over a period of weeks or months, and the course is progressive. The initial disturbance is likely to be motor, and often the distribution is asymmetric. With cervical lesions the order of motor impairment is first the arm, then the leg on the same side, next the opposite leg, and finally the opposite arm. With thoracic lesions one leg usually becomes weak and stiff before the other one. Subjective sensory symptoms (tingling paresthesias) of spinal tract type take the same pattern. Pain and temperature are more likely to be affected than touch, vibration, and position senses and are contralateral to the maximum motor weakness (Brown-Séquard syndrome). Nevertheless the posterior columns are also frequently involved. The bladder and bowel usually become paralyzed coincident with motor paralysis of the legs. If the compression is relieved, there is recovery of these members of the body in the reverse order of their affection, the first part affected being the last to recover and sensory symptoms disappearing before motor.

Compressive-irritative Radicular Syndrome. This syndrome of spinal cord compression is often combined with radicular pain, i.e., pain in the distribution of a spinal root. It is described as knifelike or as merely a dull ache with superimposed sharp pains which are intensified by cough, sneeze, or strain and radiation in a distal direction, i.e., away from the spine. Segmental sensory changes (paresthesias, hyperalgesia, impairment of pain and touch) or motor disturbances (spasm, cramp, twitching, atrophy, fascicular twitching, and loss of tendon reflex) and an ache in the spine are the usual manifestations of a compressive-irritative lesion of roots. Tenderness of spinous processes over the growth is found in half the patients. These segmental changes, particularly the sensory ones, often precede the signs of spinal cord compression by months or years, if the lesion is benign. Sphincter disturbances usually appear late.

The clinical findings upon examination are spastic weakness of the legs, in one leg more than in the other, with thoracolumbar lesions, and of the arms and legs with cervical lesions; a sensory level for pain on the trunk, below which pain sense is reduced or lost; posterior column signs; and a spastic bladder under weak voluntary control.

The diagnosis is established by x-rays of the spine (erosion of vertebras, widened spinal canal), lumbar puncture, and electromyography to demonstrate the fasciculations resulting from involvement of motor roots. But the most important diagnostic test of all is Pantopaque myelography for the direct visualization of the compressive lesion. Although necessary procedures, lumbar puncture and myelography may occasionally exacerbate the symptoms and signs.

Special Spinal Syndromes. Unusual clinical syndromes may be found in patients with tumors near the foramen magnum. They may produce a quadriparesis with pains in the back of the head and stiff neck, a weakness and atrophy of the hands and dorsal neck muscles, and either bizarre sensory changes or no sensory loss whatsoever. Lesions of the tenth, eleventh, and twelfth thoracic and the first lumbar vertebras may result in a curious syndrome of mixed cauda equina and spinal cord symptoms. Lesions of the cauda equina alone, always difficult to separate from diseases of the plexus and multiple nerves, are usually attended in the early stages by pain which is variously combined with an asymmetric, atrophic, areflexic paralysis, radicular sensory loss, and later sphincteric disorder. This must be distinguished from tumors of the conus medullaris (lower sacral segments of spinal cord), in which there are early disturbances of sphincters of the bladder and bowel, back pain, hypesthesia and anesthesia over the sacral dermatomes, a lax anal sphincter with loss of anal and bulbocavernosus reflexes, and sometimes weakness of lower leg muscles. A Babinski sign means that the spinal cord is involved above the fifth lumbar segment.

Diagnosis

Several problems may arise in the diagnosis of patients with spinal cord tumors. First, in the early stages spinal tumor must be distinguished from other diseases which cause pain over certain segments of the body, i.e., those affecting the gallbladder, kidney, stomach and intestinal tract, pleura, etc. Here the localization of the pain to a dermatome, its intensification by effort, segmental sensory changes, and minor alterations of motor, reflex, or sensory function in the legs will usually provide the clues to the compressive-irritative radicular lesion. Examination of the cerebrospinal fluid, x-ray of the spine, and myelography will settle the diagnosis in most instances.

If symptoms and signs of disorder of sensory and motor tracts of the spinal cord are present, there is still the problem of determining the segmental level of the lesion. At first the sensory and motor deficiencies may be most pronounced in those parts of the body farthest removed from the lesion, i.e., in feet or lumbosacral segments. Later these sensory and motor levels may rise, but at any time they may continue to be far below the lesion. Of greatest help here are the locality of the root pains and atrophic paralysis and lastly the upper level of hypalgesia. Again, myelography is necessary to determine the exact level of the cord compression. If localization of the cord lesion in terms of spinal segments has been established, there is still the problem of ascertaining the vertebral localization, for the two do not correspond (see Chap. 26 for a statement of the relationship of spinal segment to vertebras).

Once vertebral and segmental levels are settled, there is still the necessity of determining whether the lesion is neoplastic and is extradural, intradural-extramedullary, or intramedullary. This is important from the standpoint of etiologic diagnosis. If there is a visible or palpable spinal deformity or x-ray evidence of vertebral destruction, one may confidently assume an extradural localization. Without x-ray changes one still suspects extradural lesion if root pain developed early and is bilateral, spine ache is prominent, and percussion tenderness is marked. Motor symptoms below the lesions precede sensory changes, and sphincter disturbances are late. The distinction between intradural-extramedullary and intramedullary lesions is almost impossible. Radicular pain, asymmetry of signs of motor and sensory tract involvement, and early cerebrospinal fluid blockage (positive Queckenstedt test and high protein) favor the extramedullary localization. With extradural lesions one must differentiate between ruptured disk, spondylosis (hypertrophic spurring and osteophyte formation in cervical spinal canal), tuberculous caries, other pyogenic, fungous, or syphilitic granulomatous lesions, secondary carcinoma or lymphoma. With intradural-extramedullary lesions, meningioma, neurofibroma, meningeal carcinomatosis, cholesteatoma, teratomatous cyst, or meningomyelitic process is most likely. Intramedullary lesions are usually gliomas or vascular malformations. A negative Queckenstedt test, normal or relatively low protein in cerebrospinal fluid, and a negative myelogram will serve to rule out intraspinal tumors or granulomatous lesions, in most instances.

In conclusion, it is well always to remind oneself that of the more than 30 diseases of the spinal cord there are available effective means of treating only a few—extramedullary spinal cord tumors, syphilis (meningomyelitis and tabes), epidural granulomas (pyogenic, tuberculous, fungous), subacute combined degeneration and nutritional myelopathy. The physician's major responsibility is to determine whether or not his patient has one of the treatable diseases.

Treatment

This varies with the nature of the lesion and the clinical condition of the patient. Intradural-extramedullary tumor should be removed. Laminectomy, decompression, marsupialization of cysts, and x-ray therapy is the treatment of intramedullary gliomas. Extradural malignant growths are best managed by the use of opiates for pain, x-ray therapy, endocrine therapy (for carcinoma of breast and prostate), nitrogen mustard (for certain lymphomas). Sometimes laminectomy and decompression are necessary for diagnosis and prevention of irreversible compressive effects and infarction of the spinal cord. With tuberculous caries, immobilization of the spine in hyperextension and streptomycin therapy are indicated, and laminectomy should be reserved for exceptional cases with complete and irreversible spinal block. Immobilization of the neck and later a collar (Thomas or other) is the treatment of choice in spondylosis. Only in a rapidly advancing compressive spinal cord syndrome in a relatively young person should there be a laminectomy and cutting of the denticulate ligaments.

TUMORS OF THE PERIPHERAL NERVES

These tumors are discussed in Chap. 291.

REFERENCES

Bailey, P.: "Intracranial Tumors," 2d ed., Springfield, Ill., Charles C Thomas, Publisher, 1948.
——, D. N. Buchanan, and P. C. Bucy: "Intracranial Tumors in Infancy and Childhood," Chicago, University of Chicago Press, 1939.
—— and H. Cushing: "A Classification of Tumors of The Glioma Group," London, 1926.
Brain, W. R., D. W. C. Northfield, and M. Wilkinson: The Neurological Manifestations of Cervical Spondylosis, Brain, 75:187, 1952.
Elsberg, C. A.: "Tumors of the Spinal Cord," London, Paul B. Hoeber, 1925.
Kernohan, J. W., H. W. Wolkman, and A. W. Adson: Intramedullary Tumors of the Spinal Cord, Arch. Neurol. Psychiat., 25:679, 1931.
Knapp, P. C.: "Intracranial Growths," Boston, 1891.
Peers, J. H.: Occurrence of Tumors of Central Nervous System in Routine Autopsies, Am. J. Pathol., 12:911, 1936.
Seddon, H. J.: Pott's Paraplegia: Prognosis and Treatment, Brit. J. Surg., 22:769, 1934–1935.
Wyburn-Mason, R.: "Vascular Abnormalities and Tumours of the Spinal Cord," London, Kimpton, 1943.

287 DEMYELINATING DISEASES

John N. Walton

It is well recognized that there exists a large and important group of diseases of the nervous system all of which are characterized pathologically by a destructive process involving the myelin sheaths of nerve fibers. Despite this single common feature, there are numerous variations in the clinical manifestations and in the severity and distribution of the pathologic changes which serve, in typical cases, to distinguish the several disease entities within the group. Nevertheless, it may at times be impossible to classify an individual case with certainty, so ill-defined are the clinical and pathologic margins which separate the constituent disorders.

CLASSIFICATION

Any classification of diseases in medicine must depend upon a combination of evidence from three sources—etiologic, clinical, and pathologic. The lack of clear definition in any one of these three fields has led to the difficulties now experienced when attempting to classify the demyelinating diseases. Although a familial incidence has been observed occasionally, there is no clear evidence to suggest that genetic factors play a fundamental part in their causation. It is also true that while many theories of etiology—infective, metabolic, allergic, and vascular—have been invoked, none conforms entirely to the observed facts. An allergic process seems very probable in acute disseminated encephalomyelitis and may well be the basis of the disease state in other conditions within the group, but knowledge is still incomplete so that in most instances the etiology remains obscure. Clinically there is no doubt that the natural history of the illness in a chronic relapsing case of multiple sclerosis is entirely different from that observed in, say, acute disseminated encephalomyelitis following measles. On the other hand, a distinction on purely clinical grounds between acute multiple sclerosis and subacute encephalomyelitis may be impossible; the existence of such transitional and borderline cases precludes a classification based entirely upon clinical criteria.

Similar difficulties arise in considering pathologic data. In general, the basic process is one of destruction of myelin sheaths with relative sparing of nerve cells, axis cylinders, and supporting structures; however, the distribution and severity of the lesions vary greatly. In one disease the foci may be multiple, small, and widely disseminated, in another they are large and spreading outward from one or a few centers; sometimes they are all perivenous, but in other cases this is only partially true. Whereas in one instance the axis cylinders are virtually intact despite severe myelin destruction, in another they may suffer to an almost equal extent. From the pathologic as well as the clinical standpoint, intermediate or transitional changes may be seen bridging the gap between disease entities which have been customarily though artificially defined. The source of these difficulties springs from the probability that myelin destruction is not the primary process but merely a response of the nervous system to a variety of noxae. Definition of such etiologic factors, if achieved, must surely lead to a clearer understanding of the clinical and pathologic changes observed and in turn to a firm classification. In the meantime, correlation of the available information from all sources would support the following classification as the most practical:

1. Acute disseminated encephalomyelitis
2. Acute necrotizing hemorrhagic encephalomyelopathy (acute hemorrhagic leukoencephalitis)
3. Multiple sclerosis
4. The neuromyelitis optica syndrome
5. Diffuse cerebral sclerosis

Future investigation may reveal that necrotizing encephalomyelopathy is merely a severe form of disseminated encephalomyelitis and that the neuromyelitis optica syndrome is a variant of the latter disease or of multiple sclerosis. It is also possible that in due course certain cases now regarded as acute multiple sclerosis may come to be recognized as constituting another form of disseminated encephalomyelitis. However, the above disorders are here considered individually, although it is recognized that at least some of them may be artificially defined.

ACUTE DISSEMINATED ENCEPHALOMYELITIS

This term includes cases of postexanthematous, postvaccinal, and postinfective encephalomyelitis; the condition may also be referred to as acute perivascular myelinoclasis. In its most typical form it follows vaccination against smallpox and inoculation against rabies. In such cases the clinical manifestations follow a relatively stereotyped pattern; this is much less true of the encephalomyelitic complications of the exanthems of childhood, in which, in addition, the time relationship to the onset of the exanthem is not so clearly defined. Within recent years this group has been broadened to include cases showing encephalitic and/or myelitic manifestations after nonspecific infective illnesses; in such cases the pathologic changes are essentially the same as those in the more clearly defined syndromes referred to above.

Definition. Acute disseminated encephalomyelitis may therefore be defined as an acute encephalitic and/or myelitic disorder of variable course and severity, which is characterized clinically by symptoms indicating damage chiefly to the white matter of the brain and/or spinal cord and pathologically by perivascular cellular infiltration and perivenous demyelination. The syndrome may follow smallpox

vaccination, antirabic inoculation, or a nonspecific infective illness (sometimes vaguely referred to as "influenzal"), or may develop during the course of an exanthem; occasionally it may occur with no clear history of preceding or concurrent infection.

Pathology. Naked-eye examination of the brain and spinal cord reveals no distinctive changes. Microscopically the white matter shows innumerable small zones of demyelination, from 0.1 to 1.0 mm in diameter, which invariably surround small or medium-sized veins. Conspicuous subpial demyelination is a prominent feature and is probably related to the profusion of small veins in these situations; a similar relationship can also be adduced to explain the areas of subependymal demyelination that are frequently seen around the third and lateral ventricles. Silver stains generally demonstrate the integrity of the axis cylinders within the lesions, though they may be damaged, as shown by their tortuosity and thickening. Reacting microglial cells are seen in the demyelinated areas, and there is also perivascular infiltration with lymphocytes, histiocytes, and plasma cells, sometimes slight and sometimes massive. Meningeal infiltration, although invariable, is rarely marked. Detailed observation reveals that nearly all the lesions are of the same age, and that they are usually scattered throughout the length and breadth of the nervous system, indicating simultaneous involvement of the entire neuraxis. In other instances, however, they may be more severe in one part of the nervous system than in another, thus determining the primarily encephalitic or myelitic nature of the illness. In patients who recover the pathologic changes are probably less widespread and severe; and it seems that they may be almost, if not entirely, reversible.

Etiology. In this form of demyelinating disease above all, there is much evidence to suggest that one is dealing with an allergic response of the nervous system to an unidentified antigenic agent. The main support for this hypothesis lies in the close resemblance of the pathologic findings in such cases to those observed in experimental allergic encephalomyelitis.

Clinical Manifestations. In view of the pleomorphism of the clinical picture of disseminated encephalomyelitis, depending as it does upon the nature of the primary disease which it complicates, it will be convenient to subdivide this section with reference to identity of the preceding or concurrent infection.

Postvaccinal Encephalomyelitis. Encephalomyelitis following antismallpox vaccination is by far the commonest disorder of this type, though an identical syndrome may follow inoculation against rabies, and a similar illness may rarely occur after smallpox itself. A number of epidemics of the postvaccinal type occurred in Holland and England in the

1920s, when it became evident that the disorder affected both sexes equally, was commonest in children of school age, and was much more frequent after primary vaccination than after revaccination. In Holland it affected roughly one person in every 2,300 primary vaccinations and one in every 50,000 revaccinations.

In most instances the disease develops between the seventh and twelfth days after vaccination, though the period may be shorter after revaccination. The onset is generally abrupt, with headache, drowsiness, fever, and vomiting. There may be neck stiffness and other signs of meningeal irritation at this stage, while convulsions are occasionally seen. Soon afterwards signs of spinal cord involvement usually appear with flaccid paralysis of the limbs, which may be hemiplegic in distribution but more commonly involves all four limbs. Tendon reflexes disappear and the plantar responses become extensor. Sphincter control is generally lost, and sensory loss, though variable, may be extensive and severe. Nystagmus, ocular palsies, pupillary changes, and sometimes trismus may give evidence of brain stem involvement, while extension of the cerebral affection may lead to stupor and deepening coma. Despite these general features of the typical case, numerous variations occur less commonly, so that one patient may suffer a predominantly encephalitic illness with little evidence of cord damage, another may have a hemiplegia, while sometimes a purely myelitic syndrome may occur with no headache, neck stiffness, or clouding of consciousness. Less frequently still a syndrome suggesting involvement of nerve roots or even peripheral nerves may develop. Usually the site of vaccination is not remarkable, although a few patients show a generalized erythematous rash and others generalized vaccinia. The cerebrospinal fluid almost invariably shows an increase in protein and lymphocytes, but in rare cases it is normal.

DIAGNOSIS. The association with vaccination or inoculation will usually leave the diagnosis in little doubt, and the characteristic combination of encephalitic and myelitic features will readily distinguish the condition from meningitis, virus encephalitis, tetanus, and poliomyelitis. Rarely an atypical case may mimic any one of these disorders. In the radicular form there may be difficulty in differentiating the condition from idiopathic polyneuritis (the Guillain-Barré syndrome).

PROGNOSIS. Between 30 and 50 per cent of patients reported have died within 4 to 5 days of the ictus, usually in deep coma with terminal evidence of medullary paralysis. Improvement, with recovery of consciousness and regression of neurologic signs, takes place in the remaining cases and may be surprisingly complete. Miller has shown, however, that a significant proportion of patients show residual neurologic signs, intellectual impairment, and/or psychoneurotic sequelae many years after the illness.

Postexanthematous Encephalomyelitis. More cases of encephalomyelitis have been described after measles than after any other exanthem, but occasionally rubella and chickenpox have been complicated in this way. The exact status of the neurologic complications of scarlatina, whooping cough, and mumps has yet to be defined. Miller, Stanton, and Gibbons have shown that lymphocytic meningitis is the principal complication of scarlatina and mumps, and in the latter condition it is probably due to invasion of the nervous system by the virus. However, in a proportion of cases of mumps and very rarely in scarlatina a true demyelinating encephalomyelitis may occur. The encephalopathy of pertussis, which is fatal in over a third of cases and may leave disabling sequelae in many others, is entirely different pathologically and may be hypoxic in origin.

Encephalomyelitis complicating *measles* generally begins 2 to 4 days after the appearance of the rash but may antedate it and may even occur in patients with a history of contact who do not develop a rash. The clinical picture is variable but like that of postvaccinal encephalomyelitis, it indicates the presence of widespread lesions throughout the white matter of the neuraxis. The most common clinical syndrome is one dominated by convulsions and deepening coma; most fatal cases fall into this group. Less commonly the patient may suddenly develop a hemiplegia as if from a cerebral vascular accident, or show evidence of severe cerebellar disease, while occasionally there develops the clinical picture of transverse myelitis or that of polyradiculitis. Athetoid movements resulting from involvement of the basal ganglia are also seen infrequently. In many cases, however, the disease is much less severe, and the patient suffers a transient encephalitic illness with headache, confusion, and signs of meningeal irritation. About a tenth of the patients succumb to the disease or to intercurrent infection; however, less than half the remainder recover completely and the others remain more or less severely disabled with hemiplegia, paraplegia, cerebellar ataxia, fits, or mental impairment. It is not entirely certain that all the neurologic complications described are truly encephalomyelitic; in some cases cerebral vascular disease, particularly thrombophlebitis, may be responsible.

In *rubella* a diffuse and fatal encephalomyelitic illness may rarely occur, and in other uncommon cases a syndrome suggestive of polyradiculitis has been described, but more often a mild and transient encephalitic illness develops. The neurologic complications of *chickenpox* are similarly benign and usually occur in the second week after the rash has appeared, though they can arise at the onset of the illness. It is possible that in some cases the varicella virus, which is closely related to that of herpes zoster, is directly responsible for the patient's symptoms. There is no doubt that in others characteristic perivenous lesions, unlike those of virus infection, have been observed. In most cases a transient illness occurs with headache, drowsiness, and neck stiffness; in others there may be a severe ataxia and occasionally athetotic movements, while in yet others the typical picture of transverse myelitis develops. Whatever the clinical manifestations, the prognosis is good; death is uncommon and over 90 per cent of patients make a complete recovery.

In postexanthematous cases, as in the postvaccinal, the cerebrospinal fluid may rarely be normal but usually contains an excess of lymphocytes and protein. Diagnosis is comparatively easy in the presence of the exanthem.

Postinfective Encephalomyelitis. This group includes a heterogeneous collection of cases in which an encephalomyelitic illness succeeds a respiratory tract infection or an influenza-like illness; it probably embraces cases of similar clinical course, showing identical pathologic features, in which there is no history of a preceding illness.

The clinical manifestations in cases in this group may vary from the typical picture of severe disseminated encephalomyelitis, with deepening coma and flaccid paraplegia on the one hand, to a mild illness with headache, drowsiness, fever, and perhaps transient limb or bulbar pareses on the other. Myelitic syndromes may occur, though in a considerable proportion of these cases the disease process also affects the brain stem, giving nystagmus, impairment of ocular movement, dysphagia, facial weakness, and variable long tract signs. Evidence of nerve root involvement is common in cases where the disorder is primarily spinal, and the condition may then resemble the closely related idiopathic polyneuritis (Guillain-Barré syndrome). In many other cases there will be a striking resemblance to the accepted clinical manifestations of acute multiple sclerosis. However, a follow-up study carried out by Miller and Evans on cases of this type has shown that they do not develop further neurologic episodes during the succeeding years.

Cerebrospinal fluid changes, as in the other forms of acute encephalomyelitis, are not diagnostic, and in these cases, particularly those with no history of preceding infection, diagnosis may be very difficult. The development of coma and flaccid quadriplegia following an influenza-like illness is distinctive, but on other occasions virus encephalitis, multiple sclerosis, and bulbospinal poliomyelitis may be mimicked. Indeed, accurate diagnosis may depend in the last resort upon pathologic evidence,

and even this may fail to distinguish the condition from multiple sclerosis. It is difficult to glean accurate information about prognosis. A considerable proportion of comatose and quadriplegic patients die; those in whom the neurologic signs are relatively mild usually recover, but in the intermediate group it is impossible to predict with certainty which patients will be left with residual evidence of neurologic deficit.

Treatment. In an attempt to prevent the occurrence of postvaccinal encephalomyelitis some authorities consider it unwise to carry out primary vaccination in a young adult unless he has been in contact with a case of smallpox, or during an epidemic. This view is not generally accepted. Other prophylactic measures are probably of little avail.

Benefit has been claimed for the administration of immune human serum, 10 ml intravenously, both in cases appearing after vaccination and in those following or complicating the exanthems; if this administration is impossible, an intramuscular injection of immune citrated whole blood may be given. Recent work, however, indicates that administration of steroid drugs or ACTH is the treatment of choice, though controlled trials of treatment in this condition are difficult.

ACUTE NECROTIZING HEMORRHAGIC ENCEPHALOMYELITIS

In a small number of patients dying from a fulminating encephalopathic illness, certain distinctive pathologic features may be found. On section of the brain, the white matter of one or both hemispheres is seen to be destroyed almost to the point of liquefaction. The involved tissue is pink or yellowish gray and flecked with multiple small hemorrhages. Sometimes similar changes are localized to the brain stem. On histologic examination one finds widespread necrosis of small blood vessels, necrosis of brain tissue around the vessels with intense cellular infiltration, multiple small hemorrhages, and a violent inflammatory reaction in the meninges. The pathologic picture resembles disseminated encephalomyelitis in its perivascular distribution and diffuse sclerosis in its tendency to congregate into large foci in the cerebral hemispheres.

The clinical course of the illness resembles that of acute disseminated encephalomyelitis save for its apoplectiform onset and rapidity of progress, leading often to death within 48 hr; it is also true that neurologic signs are frequently unilateral or purely bulbar in type, reflecting the localized nature of the pathologic process. It is probable that certain patients showing an explosive myelitic illness are suffering from a necrotizing myelitis of similar type, but pathologic evidence in support of this view has been difficult to obtain. The cerebrospinal fluid reveals a more intense reaction than in other demyelinating diseases, showing a polymorphonuclear pleocytosis and a considerable increase in protein.

The etiology of this condition remains obscure, but the resemblance to the other demyelinating diseases should be noted, a resemblance which is strengthened by the fact that certain patients showing the typically fulminating clinical picture have recovered, some completely, others with neurologic sequelae of variable severity. The points of similarity are sufficient to suggest that steroid drugs should be tried in such cases.

MULTIPLE SCLEROSIS

Multiple sclerosis, commonly termed *disseminated* or *insular sclerosis* or *sclérose en plaque*, is one of the commonest chronic neurologic diseases. While pleomorphic in its clinical presentation, numerous symptom complexes have come to be recognized as characteristic of the disease so that usually diagnosis is a matter of little difficulty. On the other hand many acute cases show notable clinical and pathologic affinities with disseminated encephalomyelitis and with the syndrome of neuromyelitis optica. Despite this lack of definition of the borderline case, much less is known concerning the etiology of multiple sclerosis than of the acute demyelinating disorders previously described.

Definition. Multiple sclerosis is a disease of obscure etiology, characterized clinically by symptoms indicating the presence of multiple lesions in the white matter of the brain and spinal cord. In most cases there are relapses interspersed with long periods of remission, but in others it presents as an intermittently progressive disease with paraplegia and added cerebellar and brain stem signs; the latter state is also the eventual outcome of the relapsing cases. Pathologically there are multiple plaques of demyelination and gliosis, of varying age, throughout the central nervous system.

Pathology. Since the original description of the pathologic changes in this disease by Cruveilhier in 1835 and Carswell in 1838 there have been numerous valuable presentations, notably those of Dawson, Hassin, Zimmermann and Netzky, and Adams and Kubik. Macroscopically the brain before sectioning generally shows no evidence of disease, but the surface of the spinal cord may feel uneven. On section, numerous scattered lesions are seen which are slightly depressed and which, by virtue of their pinkish-gray appearance (due to loss of myelin), stand out in contrast with the surrounding white matter. The lesions may vary in diameter from 1 mm to several centimeters; they affect principally the white matter and the roots of cranial nerves but also encroach frequently on cerebral gray matter; much less often spinal roots and spinal gray matter are involved. The lesions appear to have a predilection for the optic nerves and chiasm and the paraventricular areas of the brain; in the spinal cord the subpial region is often predominantly affected.

The histologic appearances depend upon the age of the lesion. Relatively recent lesions show a predominantly perivenous distribution of the demyelination, with sparing of axis cylinders, degeneration of oligodendroglia, neuroglial reaction, and perivascular infiltration with mononuclear cells. Later large numbers of microglial phagocytes infiltrate the lesion and astrocytes in and around it increase in number and size. A long-standing lesion, on the other hand, will show thickly matted, relatively acellular fibroglial tissue, with only occasional perivascular macrophages; in such a lesion intact axis cylinders may still be discovered but many are destroyed, and this in turn leads to descending and ascending degeneration of long-fiber tracts. All gradations of pathologic change between these two extremes may be found in lesions of variegated size and shape. Except in the most acute cases the distribution is not so strikingly perivenous as in disseminated encephalomyelitis.

Etiology. Little concrete information is available concerning the etiology of this disease except for its occasional familial incidence. Pratt, Compston, and McAlpine have shown conclusively that it occurs in more than one member of a family more often than could be accounted for by chance. This should not be taken to indicate that the disease is transmitted as a genetic trait; rather it suggests that an inherited predisposition may make an individual more susceptible to the unknown agent or agents responsible for the demyelinating process.

None of the numerous theories advanced to explain this disease has been validated. Infection by a spirochete or filtrable virus has been adduced, only to be refuted by later work; thrombosis of venules, copper deficiency (suggested by analogy with sway-back disease of sheep), and abnormal enzymes or poisoning with lead have all been considered. The very multiplicity of theories pays tribute to the lack of concrete evidence, and recent experimental work has added little that is conclusive. Lumsden believes that degeneration of the oligodendrocytes may be the primary factor in producing demyelination, but this too is open to confirmation. There is far less evidence to support the role of allergy as a causative agent in multiple sclerosis than in disseminated encephalomyelitis.

Precipitating Factors. It has been suggested frequently that various infective and traumatic agencies have provoked the initial symptoms of multiple sclerosis or that in other cases they have been responsible for producing a relapse. Nonspecific and specific febrile illnesses, pregnancy, surgical operations, trauma, lumbar puncture, and many other factors have been invoked from time to time. An increasing volume of statistical evidence suggests that pregnancy and lumbar puncture have no influence upon the course of the disease, but Mc-Alpine and Compston believe that there is sometimes a significant relationship between infective illness or local trauma on the one hand and onset or relapse on the other. The onset of the disease, or a relapse, may occasionally seem to be precipitated by emotional stress.

Incidence. Multiple sclerosis is common in Europe, being particularly prevalent in Switzerland and Scandinavia. It occurs less frequently on the American continent and is rare in Africa and Asia. Recent epidemiologic work indicates clearly that it occurs predominantly in areas of temperate climate. It is commonest in the white races, but does occur in the Negro.

It affects the two sexes approximately equally and usually begins between the ages of twenty and forty; some cases develop in the second decade, and an increasing number are being reported with onset in the forties and fifties.

Clinical Manifestations. *Chronic Relapsing Type.* Given a clear understanding of the pathologic changes outlined, it will be evident that the clinical features of the disease may vary greatly, depending upon the situation and intensity of the lesions. If it begins with a single discrete lesion, there may be a great variety of presenting symptoms, depending upon its site; on the other hand if multiple lesions occur simultaneously in eloquent areas of the nervous system, a much more specific clinical picture will result. This variation in spatial distribution of the areas of demyelination is responsible for the remarkable clinical pleomorphism of the disease. Symptoms attributable to a single lesion almost invariably remit, to be followed by other manifestations at a later date; the same is largely true of other cases in which there is clinical evidence of multiple lesions initially but in which the onset is acute. In these two types numerous relapses may occur, each followed by a remission, but each leaving in its wake further evidence of permanent neurologic deficit upon which every succeeding acute manifestation is superimposed. As a rule such a patient eventually reveals a clinical state indistinguishable from that observed in another type of case which from the start can be recognized as harboring multiple disseminated lesions, all progressing inexorably at much the same rate. The relapsing type with multiple acute and subacute episodes is of course commoner in younger patients, while the slowly progressive form is most frequent in patients whose disease begins in middle age; in these latter individuals the major burden of the disease process generally falls upon the spinal cord.

Numerous characteristic symptom complexes may be recognized as occurring within the structure of the disease process and are best classified according to the mode of onset. Despite the variability of initial expression of the disease, most cases after a greater or lesser period of time follow a final common path of increasing spasticity, immobility, respiratory or urinary infection, and death. McAlpine believes that in a small proportion of cases the disease may be arrested spontaneously.

The more common symptom complexes observed in this disease are outlined below.

1. **TRANSIENT WEAKNESS OR LOSS OF CONTROL OF THE LIMBS.** This symptom may involve one limb (monoparesis) or both limbs on the same side (hemiparesis), but more often both lower limbs are involved (paraparesis). The patient has difficulty in walking or in using the affected limbs, and physical examination during the episode reveals evidence of corticospinal tract and/or cerebellar disease. These early manifestations frequently resolve completely only to be succeeded by others after months or years.

2. **VISUAL SYMPTOMS.** Sudden loss of vision in one eye (because of retrobulbar neuritis) or diplopia are common initial symptoms of this disease and invariably remit; sometimes as long as 20 years may elapse before other features develop.

3. **SENSORY SYMPTOMS.** The disease may begin with numbness and paresthesias in a limb or limbs, and these symptoms, being transient, may well be overlooked. The so-called "useless hand" syndrome, in which the patient complains of clumsiness or uselessness of the hand lasting for some days or weeks, must be included in this group, being generally due to impairment of position sense from a lesion in the posterior column of the cord. Less frequently, there may be symptoms to suggest loss of temperature sensation in one lower limb and the patient is found to have a partial Brown-Séquard syndrome due to a plaque in one lateral column. These manifestations, too, almost invariably remit.

4. **SLOWLY PROGRESSIVE CLUMSINESS AND WEAKNESS OF LIMBS.** In certain young patients the disease may be slowly progressive without clinical remission, and in such individuals there is usually evidence of widespread lesions; most often they show temporal pallor of the optic disks, nystagmus, cerebellar ataxia, and weakness and spasticity of the limbs. In the commoner intermittently progressive type which begins in middle life the corticospinal tracts are predominantly affected, though there is usually some loss of position and vibration sense in the lower limbs, indicating posterior column in addition to lateral column disease.

5. **SYMPTOMS OF PRIMARY BRAIN STEM INVOLVEMENT.** Some patients may present evidence of predominantly cerebellar disease, and it is often these

individuals who show Charcot's triad of nystagmus, "scanning" or "syllabic" speech, and intention tremor; this form is somewhat uncommon. Other patients may suffer a transient episode of severe vertigo and vomiting, because of a lesion affecting the vestibular connections, and may then go for years before other symptoms develop. The same is generally true of patients showing evidence of a pontine lesion, some of whom may have transient facial anesthesia followed months later by tic douloureux and later still by evidence of spinal cord disease; on other occasions tic douloureux may develop in a patient showing overt manifestations of the disease.

Acute Multiple Sclerosis. Occasionally multiple sclerosis runs an acute or subacute course leading to death in weeks or months, or else a series of symptoms may develop rapidly and then remit partially or completely to be followed by characteristic relapses. In some of these cases the onset is marked by headache, vomiting, and delirium and by a succession of symptoms indicating severe involvement of the brain stem as described above, or of the brain, optic nerves, or spinal cord. In the so-called "cerebral" cases there may be mental changes, convulsions, aphasia, hemianopia, and variable long-tract signs; the spinal type may show the picture of a transverse myelitis. These forms of the disease are uncommon and may be very difficult to distinguish from disseminated encephalomyelitis and neuromyelitis optica.

Motor symptoms are generally due to corticospinal tract or cerebellar involvement or to a combination of the two. Corticospinal tract disease gives a spastic gait and muscular weakness of upper motor neurone type, with exaggeration of tendon reflexes in the affected limbs and extensor plantar responses. Cerebellar disease results in intention tremor and clumsiness in the performance of fine coordinated movements, and the gait is often characteristically broad-based and ataxic. Involvement of central cerebellar connections gives nystagmus on lateral gaze, with the quick phase in a lateral direction.

Sensory symptoms, such as paresthesias and uselessness of the limbs, are due to posterior column involvement; in such cases loss of position sense, of two-point and tactile discrimination, and of vibration sense will be observed, and if the changes are extensive Romberg's sign will be positive.

Visual loss is due to retrobulbar neuritis, which may produce pain in the eye and sometimes disk swelling; vision gradually returns after weeks or months and central scotomas may persist, while the temporal half of the optic disk becomes pale. Such pallor is frequently seen in the absence of any history to suggest an acute neuritic episode. Diplopia is occasionally due to selective involvement of one of the oculomotor nerves but more often is of central origin, occurring without objective ocular palsy. Paralysis of conjugate ocular deviation, particularly internuclear ophthalmoplegia, is frequent. Horner's syndrome occurs rarely, but the pupils are usually unaffected.

Hysterical features are not uncommon in patients with multiple sclerosis and may make diagnosis difficult; some individuals eventually show evidence of dementia. Although euphoria, or pathologic cheerfulness, is generally regarded as characteristic, many patients are depressed.

The sphincters are often involved; precipitancy of micturition is characteristic in the early stages, but later there may be both fecal and urinary retention. Rarely fecal incontinence occurs alone.

CEREBROSPINAL FLUID. A small proportion of cases, particularly the more acute ones, show a slight mononuclear pleocytosis. The protein content may be normal, but there often is slight excess of globulin. The latter is most characteristic, occurring in perhaps 50 per cent of cases, and is indicated by an abnormal colloidal gold curve, usually paretic, generally first-zone, but occasionally mid-zone, in type, in the presence of a negative Wassermann reaction. When γ-globulin forms 20 per cent or more of the total protein, multiple sclerosis is the probable diagnosis.

DIAGNOSIS. In a characteristic case the evidence of wide dissemination of lesions throughout the neuraxis leaves the diagnosis in little doubt. Indeed it is an axiom that the disease should not be diagnosed when all the patient's symptoms and signs can be explained by a single lesion. Occasionally this rule must be ignored in the presence of one of the characteristic symptom complexes already described, but it is a valuable guide. For reasons already given, distinction from disseminated encephalomyelitis and neuromyelitis optica is particularly difficult in the acute case, but bilateral visual loss as well as stupor and coma are rare in multiple sclerosis, while disseminated encephalomyelitis is a self-limiting monophasic disease. Other acute manifestations may mimic labyrinthitis, meningovascular syphilis, and encephalitis; the first may be recognized only by the course of the disease and then not with certainty, but cerebrospinal fluid examination will generally identify the other conditions.

Confusion may occasionally arise with the familial ataxias, which are generally distinguished by their familial incidence, the occurrence of skeletal abnormalities and other associated genetic traits, and by their stereotyped clinical pattern. Amyotrophic lateral sclerosis and subacute combined degeneration may be closely mimicked, but muscle wasting and fasciculations will identify the former and the latter can be confirmed by the absence of acid from the gastric juice, by the anemia in most cases, by the presence of megaloblasts in the bone marrow, and by a low level of vitamin B_{12} in the serum.

Patients with a progressive spastic paraplegia may have an intrathecal neoplasm or cervical spondylosis. Pain and extensive sensory loss are common in the former and rare in multiple sclerosis, in which muscle wasting due to anterior horn or spinal root involvement (as sometimes seen in spondylosis) is almost unknown. Basilar impression of the skull, or platybasia, must also be considered, but in such patients there is characteristic shortening of the neck and radiographs of the base of the skull are diagnostic. Careful clinical appraisal will usually lead to accurate diagnosis, but occasionally the problem can be resolved only by recourse to cerebrospinal fluid examination, radiography of the spinal canal, and myelography.

PROGNOSIS. The duration of the disease is variable. Some patients die within a few months, others live 30 years or longer. In general, patients whose disease runs a relapsing course live longer, but accurate prediction of the progress in an individual case is difficult. The average total duration from the time of the first symptom is 15 to 20 years. The final state of the bedridden, incontinent patient, racked by painful flexor spasms of the lower limbs and shaken by febrile episodes of intercurrent infection, is one of the most distressing in medicine; it is fortunate that many individuals retain their euphoria to the end.

TREATMENT. Despite the large number of remedies which have been tried, no drug therapy appears to have any influence on the course of the disease. Claims for the efficacy of arsenicals, vasodilators, and a low fat diet have not been substantiated. Recent work suggests that treatment with steroid drugs may be useful in acute episodes and that long-term treatment may reduce the frequency of relapses. Intrathecal tuberculin has recently been tried, but is not of proven value. Claims made by Shubladze for the efficiency of a vaccine recently developed in Russia are also unsupported by scientific evidence.

The most that can be done is to encourage and reassure the patient through moderate exercise and supportive measures and to keep him mobile and actively employed for as long as possible. During an acute episode of the type which invariably remits it is surely preferable to assure the patient that he will recover and to preserve silence on the subject of relapse, in view of the long periods of remission which may occur. No patient with this disease should be told its nature until the fact becomes self-evident, and even when all hope of remission seems past the patient should be advised that improvement is still possible.

In the late bedridden stage little can be done beyond meticulous care of the skin, bladder, and bowels, but vigorous administration of analgesics or sometimes even rhizotomy or cordotomy may be required to ease the pain of flexor spasms in the legs. Sometimes these may be abolished by means of intrathecal injections of 5 per cent phenol in glycerin around the second and third lumbar roots.

THE NEUROMYELITIS OPTICA SYNDROME

This disorder, also referred to as *diffuse* or *disseminated myelitis with optic neuritis, ophthalmoneuromyelitis,* and *Devic's disease,* is probably not a distinct nosologic entity, as it resembles on the one hand multiple sclerosis and on the other disseminated encephalomyelitis and necrotizing encephalomyelopathy. Clinical surveys of patients presenting with this syndrome tend to favor its identification as a form of multiple sclerosis, but pathologic studies of fatal cases, particularly those in which cavitation of white matter is found, have often revealed a more acute and uniformly severe destructive process than is usually seen in the latter disease. In the absence of any authoritative evidence to indicate in which group the condition rightly belongs, it will be considered as a clinical syndrome with full recognition of the fact that its exact nature is not yet established.

Definition. Neuromyelitis optica is a syndrome produced by a subacute demyelinating process involving the optic nerves and spinal cord; this process may be self-limiting and reversible or may be progressive.

Pathology. To the naked eye the optic nerves and spinal cord are often soft, swollen, and congested. Microscopy reveals extensive demyelination in the optic nerves and chiasm, and a similar process is seen in the spinal cord, sometimes localized to a few cervical segments and sometimes more extensive. Axis cylinders are relatively intact, though swollen and irregular; there is microglial reaction in and around the demyelinated areas, and perivascular infiltration with mononuclear cells is seen.

Clinical Manifestations. The syndrome affects the sexes equally and can probably occur at any age, even during the first decade of life. In the so-called typical case there is often pain in the eyes, followed by impairment of vision first in one eye but affecting the other within a few hours or days. Visual loss is variable in extent; characteristically there are bilateral central scotomas, but total blindness may occur, or one eye may be more severely affected. Papilledema is sometimes seen, but the optic disks often look normal. Soon afterwards the characteristic picture of a transverse myelitis appears, with flaccid paralysis, loss of sphincter control, absence of tendon reflexes and extensor plantar responses, and variable sensory loss in the extremities, depending on the level of the lesion. The sensorium is not affected. Occasionally the spinal cord syndrome precedes the visual disturbance. It is possible that certain cases of bilateral optic neuritis without signs of cord damage may be abortive examples of this syndrome, and the same may well be true of a proportion of cases of transverse myelitis.

Cerebrospinal fluid changes are not distinctive; the fluid may occasionally be normal but more often shows a moderate increase in protein and mononuclear cells.

Diagnosis. The relationship of this syndrome to disseminated encephalomyelitis and multiple sclerosis has already been mentioned; the main reasons for considering it separately are that visual loss is rare in the former and not often bilateral in the latter. In cases with optic disk swelling, intracranial tumor may be considered in differential diagnosis, but this problem will rarely present serious difficulty; similarly, distinction from optic neuritis of diverse etiology will usually be straightforward, since in the latter condition usually only one eye is affected. In cases without spinal cord involvement, temporal arteritis may come to mind as a possible cause of visual loss, but it affects a different age group and the appearance of the temporal arteries is characteristic. In other cases the distinction from syphilitic meningomyelitis or cord tumor will generally be made with ease by spinal fluid examination.

Prognosis. About half the patients die, usually from intercurrent infection, but the others may recover to a remarkable extent, some apparently completely. A significant number are left with permanent severe visual loss and paraplegia.

Treatment. There is no specific therapy for this condition; treatment must be directed to palliation of pain and other symptoms, and as in any case of paraplegia, meticulous nursing care is required.

DIFFUSE CEREBRAL SCLEROSIS

In 1912 Schilder first called attention to a disease in which progressive massive demyelination of the white matter of the cerebral hemispheres occurred, and the condition was later referred to as *Schilder's disease* or *encephalitis periaxialis diffusa.* Since that time many other cases have been described, some resembling Schilder's original description, others differing in certain specific details. An attempt has been made by Krabbe, Pelizaeus, Merzbacher, and others to define certain clinical subgroups on the basis of variations in age of onset, familial incidence, and clinical course. Three broad pathologic types have been distinguished, one corresponding to Schilder's original description and another showing changes that cannot be distinguished from those of cerebral multiple sclerosis.

The third type, which has been reviewed in detail by Brain and Greenfield, under the name *late infantile metachromatic leukoencephalopathy,* is probably a separate disease entity related to lipidosis, and it may be that the cases of Krabbe and those of Pelizaeus and Merzbacher were examples of this or a fourth condition (see Chap. 290, Leukodystrophy).

Definition. The diffuse cerebral scleroses are a group of conditions of unknown etiology, some occurring sporadically, others running in families, which are characterized clinically by progressive visual failure, mental deterioration, and spastic paralysis, and pathologically by massive demyelination of the white matter of the cerebral hemispheres.

Pathology. On inspection the brain often appears somewhat shrunken and feels firmer than usual. On section the white matter is seen to be largely replaced by a brownish-gray, rubbery, translucent material which may occasionally show small cavities. Usually the process spares the subcortical arcuate fibers. The changes are generally most advanced in the occipital lobes and involve the parietal and frontal areas to a variable extent, but occasionally they may begin frontally; the two hemispheres are often not affected symmetrically. Baló has described certain cases in which demyelination occurs in concentric rings surrounding normal areas of white matter; Adams and Kubik believe this appearance to be an occasional feature of multiple sclerosis but not of diffuse sclerosis.

Histologic examination usually reveals that all myelin has disappeared from the affected areas and that axis cylinders have been involved to an almost equal extent. In the older parts of the lesion there is proliferation of fibrous astrocytes, but in the more recent areas swollen astrocytes are seen and around the margins of the lesion macrophages are plentiful. The oligodendrocytes are almost completely destroyed. Perivascular infiltration is minimal, but in the vicinity of the more recent lesions the perivascular spaces may contain numerous fat-filled macrophages.

In the metachromatic form of diffuse sclerosis (Brain and Greenfield), the macroscopic appearances are similar though more symmetric, but there is severe degeneration of the interfascicular oligodendroglia, and large granular bodies, staining metachromatically with thionine, are frequent.

Clinical Manifestations. In about half the cases the condition begins in the first decade; Schilder's original description was of a disease occurring in early childhood, but it is now recognized that this pathologic process may occur at any age. More males than females suffer in childhood, but in later years the sexes are equally affected.

The disorder often begins with slowly progressive visual failure, usually affecting both eyes simultaneously but occasionally beginning unilaterally. These features are succeeded by focal or general fits, dysphasia, mental deterioration, and variable weakness of the limbs, leading eventually to total blindness, dementia, and spastic quadriplegia. On occasion the onset may be sudden, with headache, stupor, and convulsions, in which case visual failure develops later. Nystagmus is common but other ocular signs are rare; if the pathologic change spreads to the temporal lobe, deafness may result.

The cerebrospinal fluid is generally normal but may show a slight increase in protein and mononuclear cells.

Diagnosis. In a child presenting with visual loss, fits, progressive dementia, and spasticity the diagnosis is often self-evident, but even in such cases there may be difficulty in differentiation from cerebral lipidosis or subacute inclusion encephalitis. In lipidosis, e.g., Tay-Sachs disease, there will generally be a history of affection of other members of the family, but diagnosis from subacute encephalitis may be impossible clinically; differentiation is only of academic interest since all these disorders are progressive and ultimately fatal. The electroencephalogram, which shows paroxysmal and bilaterally synchronous slow-wave complexes in subacute encephalitis and almost continuous irregular spike-and-wave activity in lipidosis, may be of great value in making the distinction, since cases of Schilder's disease show only diffuse slow rhythms. Cases arising in later life may be confused with intracranial tumor, necrotizing hemorrhagic encephalopathy, and presenile or atherosclerotic dementia; few cases in this age group, save those showing the classical clinical picture, are diagnosed during life.

Prognosis. The disease is steadily progressive, usually leading to death within 3 years; but uncommonly patients may survive, though progressively disabled, for longer periods.

Treatment. No treatment is known to influence the course of the disease, though vigorous anticonvulsant therapy may be required for the control of seizures.

REFERENCES

Adams, R. D., J. Cammermeyer, and D. Denny-Brown: Acute Necrotizing Hemorrhagic Encephalopathy, J. Neuropathol. Exptl. Neurol., 8:1, 1949.

—— and C. S. Kubik: The Morbid Anatomy of the Demyelinative Diseases, Am. J. Med., 12:510, 1952.

Bastiaanse, F. S., and B. Bastiaanse: Encéphalite consécutive à la vaccination antivariolique, Bull. acad. méd. (Paris), 94:815, 1925.

Brain, W. R., and J. G. Greenfield: Late Infantile Metachromatic Leucoencephalopathy with Primary Degeneration of the Interfascicular Oligodendroglia, Brain, 73:291, 1950.

Dawson, J. W.: The Histology of Multiple Sclerosis, Edinburgh Med. J., 17:229, 311, 377, 1916.

Ferraro, A.: Primary Demyelinating Processes of the Central Nervous System, Arch. Neurol. Psychiat., 37:1100, 1937.

Ford, F. R.: The Nervous Complications of Measles with a Summary of the Literature and Publication of 12 Additional Case Reports, Bull. Johns Hopkins Hosp., 43:140, 1928.

Hassin, G. B.: Pathological Studies on the Pathogenesis of Multiple Sclerosis, Research Publs. Assoc. Research Nervous Mental Disease, 2:144, 1921.

——: Neuroptic Myelitis versus Multiple Sclerosis, Arch. Neurol. Psychiat., 37:1083, 1937.

Krabbe, K.: A New Familial Form of Diffuse Brain Sclerosis, Brain, 39:74, 1916.

McAlpine, D., N. D. Compston, and C. E. Lumsden: "Multiple Sclerosis," Edinburgh and London, E. & S. Livingstone, 1955.

Merritt, H. H., and Y. D. Koskoff: Encephalomyelitis Following German Measles, Am. J. Med. Sci., 191:690, 1936.

Miller, H. G.: Prognosis of Neurologic Illness Following Vaccination against Smallpox, A.M.A. Arch. Neurol. Psychiat., 69:695, 1953.

—— and M. J. Evans: Prognosis in Acute Disseminated Encephalomyelitis, with a Note on Neuromyelitis Optica, Quart. J. Med., 22:347, 1953.

——, J. B. Stanton, and J. L. Gibbons: Para-infectious Encephalomyelitis and Related Syndromes, Quart. J. Med., 25:427, 1956.

Pratt, R. T. C., N. D. Compston, and D. McAlpine: The Familial Incidence of Disseminated Sclerosis and Its Significance, Brain, 74:191, 1951.

Wolf, A., E. A. Kabat, and A. E. Bezer: The Pathology of Acute Disseminated Encephalomyelitis Produced Experimentally in the Rhesus Monkey and Its Resemblance to Human Demyelinative Disease, J. Neuropathol. Exptl. Neurol., 6:333, 1947.

Zimmermann, H. M., and M. G. Netzky: The Pathology of Multiple Sclerosis, Research Publs. Assoc. Research Nervous Mental Disease, 28:271, 1950.

—— and H. Yannet: Nonsuppurative Encephalomyelitis Accompanying Chickenpox, Arch. Neurol. Psychiat., 26:322, 1931.

288 NUTRITIONAL DISORDERS OF THE NERVOUS SYSTEM

Maurice Victor and Raymond D. Adams

The general principles of deficiency disease have been presented in Chap. 57, and the reader should review them as an introduction to this discussion of deficiency diseases of the nervous system. It is noteworthy that many of these principles were derived from the study of disordered nervous function consequent upon dietary inadequacy.

Of the known vitamin deficiencies only those of the B group are of importance in neurology. A lack of the other known vitamins does not appear to have any effect on the brain, spinal cord, peripheral nerves, or muscles of man. Thiamine chloride, nicotinic acid, pyridoxine, pantothenic acid, and riboflavin all play a role in carbohydrate metabolism upon which the central nervous system depends for its principal source of energy. These vitamins are essentially coenzymes mainly in the Krebs citric acid cycle. Vitamin B_{12} is also of importance, but little is known of its mode of action.

The history of our knowledge of the human B vitamin deficiencies in man is an interesting one, and the discovery of the effects of a deficiency of these vitamins represents one of the most brilliant achievements in neurologic medicine in the twentieth century. The action of single vitamins in neuronal metabolism has been investigated in experimental animals, but our knowledge of these processes is still incomplete. Limitations of space do not permit a detailed review of these experiments nor of the experimentally induced deficiency states in man.

Except for subacute combined degeneration of the spinal cord (vitamin B_{12} deficiency) and certain instances of Wernicke's disease (vitamin B_1 deficiency), it is not possible to relate the clinical vitamin deficiency syndromes in man to a lack of single vitamins. For example, polyneuropathy may result from one of several vitamin deficiencies [thiamine chloride, pyridoxine (vitamin B_6), and pantothenic acid]. Moreover such conditions as pellagra and beriberi consist of syndromes which are often the result of a simultaneous deficiency of multiple vitamins.

VITAMIN DEFICIENCIES OF THE HUMAN NERVOUS SYSTEM

Wernicke's disease and Korsakoff's psychosis
Nutritional polyneuropathy (neuritic beriberi)
Nutritional amblyopia (retrobulbar neuropathy)
Pellagra
Strachan's syndrome
Subacute combined degeneration of the cord

With the exception of subacute combined degeneration of the cord, these syndromes are rarely seen in pure form. In patients with nutritional disease, it is usual for both the central and peripheral nervous systems to be involved, a clinical situation found in few other circumstances. Also, the examination of these patients frequently discloses nonneurologic signs of malnutrition such as general wasting, mucocutaneous lesions, circulatory abnormalities, and skin lesions.

In this country the nutritional disorders of the nervous system are most often observed in the alcoholic population of the large urban centers. Alcohol plays a major role mainly by displacing food in the diet. It is also possible that excessive ingestion of alcohol impairs the absorption of nutrients and increases the need for thiamine by adding nonvitamin calories to the diet.

WERNICKE'S DISEASE

In 1881 Carl Wernicke described an illness of sudden onset, characterized by mental disturbance, paralysis of eye movements, and ataxic gait. Swelling of the optic disks with retinal hemorrhages was also said to be present, and in all three of his patients there was a progressive depression of the state of consciousness, and death. A fatal outcome was at one time regarded as a universal feature of this disease. Wernicke described focal vascular lesions, primarily affecting the gray matter around the third and fourth ventricles and aqueduct of Sylvius. He regarded the disease as inflammatory in nature, and suggested the name *acute superior hemorrhagic polioencephalitis.*

Since Wernicke's time, views regarding this disease have undergone considerable modification, clinically, pathologically, and etiologically.

Symptoms and Signs. The crux of the clinical picture is the ocular disturbance; and the clinical diagnosis of Wernicke's disease can hardly be made without it. The usual ocular motor signs consist of (1) nystagmus, both horizontal and vertical, (2) paralysis of the external recti, and (3) paralysis of conjugate gaze. These signs show a considerable diversity. The paralysis of conjugate movement varies from merely a nystagmus on extreme gaze in one direction to a complete loss of ocular movement in that direction. Also, vertical movements may be affected, though abnormalities of the horizontal movement are commoner. Paralysis of downward gaze is an unusual manifestation of Wernicke's or, in fact, of any neuroophthalmic disease. Next to nystagmus, one most frequently encounters a lateral rectus muscle weakness or paralysis. The sixth nerve palsy is always bilateral, though not always symmetric, and is accompanied by diplopia and internal strabismus. With complete paralysis nystagmus is absent, but it becomes evident as the weakness improves. In advanced stages of the disease there may be a complete loss of ocular movement, and the pupils, which ordinarily are spared, may become miotic and nonreacting. Other ocular disturbances, such as ptosis, retrobulbar neuropathy, retinal hemorrhages, involvement of the near-far focusing mechanism, and internuclear ophthalmoplegia are decidedly rare, although they do occur on occasion. The authors have never observed papilledema in this disease.

The ataxia affects stance and gait predominantly. In its severest form the patient is unable to stand or walk without support. The mildest degree of ataxia may be brought out only by special tests, such as heel-to-toe walking. In contrast to the gross disorder of locomotion is the relative infrequency of a clear-cut intention tremor. When present, it affects the legs more than the arms. Scanning speech is present only in isolated instances. The ataxia of gait is cerebellar in origin, but it is often mistakenly attributed to a polyneuropathy.

Affection of the peripheral nerves is common in Wernicke's disease, occurring in over half the patients; in the majority of these patients, however, the signs of neuropathy are slight and could not account for the disordered gait. Nevertheless, in a small proportion the neuropathy is so severe that stance and gait cannot be tested.

The third consistent clinical feature of Wernicke's disease is the mental disturbance. Several distinct groups of symptoms can be recognized.

1. A small proportion of patients show the symptoms of delirium tremens or its variants, i.e., hallucinations and other disorders of sense perception, confusion, agitation, and autonomic overactivity. The symptoms are evanescent in nature and may clear without any treatment.

2. The majority of patients are apathetic, listless, and severely confused. Unconsciousness as part of the initial episode is distinctly rare, but mild drowsiness is common. The patient's mental state is best described as one of disinterest or indifference. His spontaneous speech is minimal, and he is inattentive and cannot concentrate on the simplest task. Many questions directed to him go unanswered, or he may suspend conversation in the middle of a sentence, to turn over and sleep. He is readily roused from this state, however. Whatever questions the patient answers betray disorientation in time and place, misidentification of those around him, and an inability to grasp the meaning of his illness or immediate situation. Many of his remarks are irrational and show no consistency from one moment to another. Under these circumstances a proper evaluation of the mental status is seldom possible. When the patient's interest and attention can be maintained for a long enough period to ensure adequate testing, one usually finds an impairment of retentive memory and of other cognitive functions. If these patients are given thiamine or simply an adequate diet, they lose most of these symptoms in a matter of days. They become more alert, attentive, and responsive, and in general more able to take part in mental testing. At this time it becomes evident that the most prominent abnormality is one of retentive memory, or what is ordinarily regarded as Korsakoff's psychosis.

3. Some patients, from the time they are first seen show a disorder of retentive memory and other cognitive functions characteristic of Korsakoff's psychosis.

The symptoms of Wernicke's disease all appear at the same time and rather abruptly, but more frequently the ophthalmoplegia and ataxia precede the mental signs by a few days or a week or two. The patient may also show other stigmas of malnutrition, the most frequent of which is polyneuropathy. Occasionally, amblyopia or spinal spastic ataxia may be added to the clinical picture. Although neuropathy is common in Wernicke's disease, the advanced stages of beriberi heart disease are rarely observed. There are, however, indications of disordered cardiovascular function in these patients, such as tachycardia, exertional dyspnea, postural hypotension, and minor electrocardiographic abnormalities. Occasionally the patient may die suddenly, the mode of death suggesting "cardiovascular collapse." It has been shown that Wernicke's disease is characterized by a state of high cardiac output, out of proportion to the oxygen consumption. This is probably due to an abnormal state of vasodilatation, which in turn may be related specifically to thiamine deficiency. Death occurs in about 15 per cent of hospitalized patients and is usually due to some serious complication, such as cirrhosis of the liver or tuberculosis.

Pathologic Changes. Postmortem examination reveals symmetrically located lesions in the paraventricular regions of the thalamus and hypothalamus, the mammillary bodies, the periaqueductal region of the midbrain, the floor of the fourth ventricle, and the anterior lobe of the cerebellum, particularly the vermis. The lesions are invariably found in the mammillary bodies and less consistently in the other areas. Microscopically the principal change consists of varying degrees of necrosis of parenchymal structures. Many nerve cells and fibers are destroyed; others remain intact and are seen against a background of reactive glial elements, both astrocytes and microgliacytes. The blood vessels are prominent, owing to adventitial and endothelial proliferation. Hemorrhagic lesions, as the original name suggests, are not present in all instances, and when they are give the appearance of being of recent origin. The oculomotor nuclei and the medial longitudinal fasciculi are involved only to a mild degree, which is consistent with the rapid clinical improvement in oculomotor function.

Etiology. Wernicke's disease is no longer regarded as inflammatory in nature or as the result of the neurotoxic effects of alcohol. Nutritional deficiency is now established as the causal factor. Outbreaks have been encountered in prisoner-of-war camps, and occasional cases have been reported in wasting diseases of varied origin, where alcohol played no part. The specific nutritional factor in most, if not all, of the symptomatology of Wernicke's disease is thiamine. The experimental evidence for this statement, both in animals and in man, is quite certain. This idea has received confirmation through numerous clinical observations. The marked sensitivity of the ophthalmoplegia to the administration of thiamine accounts for the rapid disappearance of this sign following the ingestion of one or two meals. The quality of prompt reversibility suggests that these symptoms are due to a biochemical abnormality and not to structural change. On the other hand, the memory loss responds slowly or not at all, suggesting that this symptom is the result of structural changes, presumably in the mammillary bodies and adjacent areas in the walls of the third ventricle.

KORSAKOFF'S PSYCHOSIS

Korsakoff's psychosis is generally defined as a state of "memory defect with confabulation." These features alone, however, fail to characterize this disease adequately. It is apparent from Korsakoff's writings that his patients displayed a much wider range of symptoms, including those of delirium and what he termed "irritable weakness" (anxiety, fear, and depression). Furthermore, if one subjects these patients to formal psychologic testing, they are found defective in concentration, verbal and visual abstraction, visual-motor coordination, and learning ability, i.e., in cognitive functions which depend little or not at all on memory functions. Nevertheless, as has been repeatedly stressed, memory is disproportionately disturbed. Thus a patient may be capable of performing adequately the problems posed by a standard intelligence test and yet, within a few minutes of completing the test, be unable to recall either the examiner or having taken the test. Although it is recent memory that suffers most, the memory of events preceding the illness is always defective, and even remote memory is defective in all but the mildest cases.

Hand in hand with the disorder of memory function is a persistent inability to learn newly presented material, i.e., to make "new memories." Since the adaptation to every new situation requires the forming of new memories or at least combining new and old ones, it is the defect in this function which renders the patient helpless in society and capable of performing only the most routine tasks. Moreover, when the patient attempts to reconstruct the recent past, there are large gaps in the recounted material. Only isolated facts are retained, and these are not combined in proper chronology, so that the whole is distorted. Or new material may be introduced, drawn from the patient's own experience and having some logical relation to the story. This defect becomes obvious after the acute stage

of the illness has passed and some improvement in function has occurred, and it remains the dominant disturbance in all but the few patients who make a complete recovery.

Confabulation is widely regarded as a specific symptom of Korsakoff's psychosis, but it is found in many other confusional states as well. Although this symptom is frequently present in the early stages of the disease, it is not discerned in all the patients and is characteristically absent in the chronic stages of the disease.

The outcome of Korsakoff's psychosis varies. In a small proportion of patients complete recovery occurs. More commonly there is slow and incomplete recovery over a year or longer. Depending on the severity of the residual symptoms, the patient may or may not be able to lead an independent existence out of a hospital. The residual mental state is usually one in which the patient shows large gaps in memory and the inability to sort out events in their proper temporal sequence. If the patient is seen for the first time during this stage, the diagnosis of "alcoholic deteriorated state" or "organic brain syndrome due to alcohol" is commonly made.

The Unity of Wernicke's Encephalopathy and Korsakoff's Psychosis. Several allusions have already been made to the relation between these two syndromes. Clinically, the majority of patients with Wernicke's disease show signs of Korsakoff's psychosis, either from the time they are first seen or following a period of apathy and drowsiness. Conversely, the vast majority of patients with an amnestic-confabulatory psychosis show the stigmas of Wernicke's disease (slight nystagmus and ataxia) even years after the onset of the illness. The pathologic changes in the brain are very much the same whether the patient dies in the acute stages of Wernicke's disease or in the chronic phase of the illness, when the ocular palsies have cleared and the amnestic symptoms predominate. It would appear that in the nutritionally deficient alcoholic patient, Wernicke's disease and Korsakoff's psychosis represent but different facets of the same disease process.

NUTRITIONAL POLYNEUROPATHY
(Neuritic Beriberi)

For many years it was believed that dry or neuritic beriberi was exclusively a disease of the Orient. Now it is established that no essential difference exists, clinically or pathologically, between the neuropathy of beriberi and that which occurs among alcoholics in the Western Hemisphere. Even the cardiovascular manifestations of beriberi have their counterpart in the alcoholic populations. The following description, therefore, applies both to alcoholic neuropathy and dry (neuritic) beriberi.

Symptoms and Signs. The symptomatology of nutritional polyneuropathy is remarkably diverse. In fact, many patients are asymptomatic. Only on examination will thinness of the leg muscles and loss or depression of the knee and ankle jerks or of the ankle jerks alone be detected. Less frequently, calf tenderness, somewhat diminished muscle power in the feet and legs, or a patchy blunting of pain and touch sensation over the feet and shins are also found.

Patients with the manifest form of polyneuropathy report a variety of symptoms consisting of weakness, paresthesias, and sometimes pain. The symptoms are usually insidious and slowly progressive over a period of a few weeks, although at times there may be a rapid progression of the weakness. In a small group the transition from an asymptomatic state to one of virtual paralysis occurs in a matter of several days. The symptoms are at first referred to the distal portions of the limbs and progress proximally if the illness remains untreated. The legs are affected earlier than the arms and practically always more severely. Motor and sensory symptoms tend to occur concomitantly, although the patient may complain much more of one than the other. Usually weakness constitutes the source of disability. Sensory symptoms may, however, be troublesome; they consist mainly of numbness, prickly feelings, coldness, deadness, tenderness of the calf and plantar musculature, or unusual sensitivity to contact. In a minority of patients, pain and paresthesias constitute the chief complaints. The pain may take the form of a dull constant ache in the feet, sometimes of the entire leg; often the pains are sharp and lancinating, momentary in duration, like the lightning pains of tabes dorsalis. Complaints of coldness are common, but they are purely subjective, the feet feeling warm to touch. Much more distressing and incapacitating are the "burning" feelings and sensations of heat; usually these affect the soles, and less frequently the dorsal aspects of the feet as well. They fluctuate in intensity or may be clearly intermittent in nature. Characteristically, a patient afflicted with pains and paresthesias suffers not one but all of the symptoms enumerated. Although the painful symptoms may arise spontaneously, they are made much worse by contact. The amount of pressure required to produce discomfort varies; in severe cases the patient cannot bear to have the bedclothes touch his feet or to touch an eating utensil. Because of these dysesthesias he may be unable or unwilling to walk, despite the preservation of motor power.

The examination reveals varying degrees of motor, reflex, and sensory loss. As the symptoms would suggest, the signs are symmetric, usually more prominent in the distal portions of the limbs, and often confined to the legs. The weakness varies greatly in degree. It may be evident only with muscular exertion, or it may take the form of a foot and wrist drop or even of a complete paralysis of the limb. The deep reflexes in the legs are almost universally lost, even with the mildest degrees of weakness. In the arms the tendon reflexes may occasionally be retained despite serious loss of power in the hands. In a small number of patients, particularly those with pain and paresthesias, the reflexes may be brisk. The sensory loss usually involves all the modalities. Although one cannot adequately equate touch, pain, and temperature, and vibratory and position sense, some patients seemingly show an impairment or loss of one modality out of proportion to the others. There is no sharp border between normal and impaired sensation; the sensory loss, which is most profound distally, shades off gradually, the transition to normal sensation occurring over a long vertical extent of the limb.

As a rule, only the limbs are affected, and the abdominal, thoracic, and bulbar musculature are intact. In some instances of Oriental beriberi, sensory loss has reportedly involved the face and abdomen as well. Tinnitus, vertigo, nerve deafness, aphonia due to vocal cord paralysis (particularly in infants), and retrobulbar neuropathy may also complicate beriberi in rare instances. The relation of these disturbances to beriberi has been a point of contention that cannot be settled with finality, since the specific cause of neither is known. Far more frequently, they are engrafted on the syndrome of ataxia and burning, tender feet and are therefore appropriately considered as a part of Strachan's syndrome.

The *spinal fluid* in these nutritional neuropathies and in Wernicke-Korsakoff disease is usually normal, although some cases show a modest elevation of the protein content. Normal spinal fluid findings may be helpful in distinguishing the rapidly evolving form of nutritional neuropathy from infectious polyneuritis.

Recovery is invariably a slow process. In the mildest cases there may be considerable restoration of motor power in a few weeks; in the severest forms several weeks may pass before the first signs of recovery become manifest, and up to a year before the patient is able to walk unaided. Recovery in severely affected patients is often incomplete, and they may be left with some weakness of the feet and an absence of the knee and ankle jerks. Contractures may develop because of inadequate physiotherapy, which greatly prolongs convalescence.

Pathologic Changes. Pathologically, there is a degeneration of the peripheral nerves, and in advanced cases, of the anterior and posterior nerve roots. The degenerative process is more intense in the distal portions of the nerves than in the proximal ones. Both the myelin and the axis cylinders are destroyed, the former probably earlier and to a greater extent than the latter. The degeneration is Wallerian in type in some places, whereas in others there may be short segments of nerve in which the myelin is lost and the bare axis cylinders remain (the segmental demyelination of Gombault). Dorsal root ganglion cells may be lost to a variable extent, and the anterior horn cells of the spinal cord show an axonal reaction. The latter change is probably secondary to the axis cylinder damage in the anterior roots and peripheral nerves.

The "Burning Feet" Syndrome. The term *burning feet* is frequently applied to a state in which pain in the extremities is the outstanding symptom and in which the advanced signs of neuropathy may be absent. It was the subject of many reports from the prisoner-of-war and internment camps of the Far East. The pain was variously described as tingling, burning, aching, shooting, cramplike, or resembling the lightning pains of tabes. The pain was often very severe; it was greatest at night and interfered with sleep. Some patients found relief from the application of cold; others only in movement. The presence of associated neuritic signs was a variable matter. In some patients, wasting, dropped foot, reflex loss, and sensory changes were completely wanting; in a significant proportion the tendon reflexes were exaggerated, but without clonus or extensor plantar responses. However, in other patients, the painful feet were but one stage in the evolution of a peripheral neuropathy characterized by tenderness of the calves, reflex and sensory loss, and ataxia, and complicated in many cases by retrobulbar neuropathy.

In alcoholic polyneuropathy, pain is the outstanding symptom in a relatively small number of patients; however, these do not constitute a distinct group in terms of their neurologic signs. In some cases the pain and dysesthesia may be associated with a severe degree of motor, reflex, and sensory loss. In others the weakness may be slight or absent, and in rare instances reflexes may be retained. However, in all cases there is some degree of sensory loss, even where the slightest stimulus appears intolerable. The term *hyperesthetic* is not well chosen to describe such cases; since it implies a heightened receptiveness of the nervous system or an increased response of the receptors to tactile and painful stimuli. Actually, there is an underlying sensory deficit or an elevated threshold to various stimuli; once the stimulus is perceived, however, it may have a severely painful or unpleasant quality (hyperpathia). The term *burning* is also not particularly applicable, considering the wide variety of symptoms apart from thermal dysesthesias. Because of this, as well as the fact that the hands may be involved, the term *acrodysesthesias*, or *painful extremities*, seems preferable.

The specific deficiency responsible for the dysesthesias has not been clearly established. The pathophysiology is likewise unknown. Spillane suggests that this affection represents an early stage of the nutritional disturbance in the nerves to the lower limbs. He draws an analogy to the burning pains produced by the interruption of conduction in large nerve fibers by rendering a limb ischemic. The authors have been impressed by the similarity of the pain to causalgia and in several patients have succeeded in abolishing the pain for several hours to days by paravertebral sympathetic block. These observations require confirmation.

NUTRITIONAL AMBLYOPIA

This term refers to the visual failure which occurs in nutritional disease and which is not due to a lesion of the cornea or other parts of the eye concerned with refraction. Since the primary lesion is probably in the retina, the term *retrobulbar neuropathy* is not a suitable synonym. The optic nerve lesion consists of a degeneration of myelinated fibers of the zone and the papillomacular bundle.

Clinically the characteristic symptom is a blurring of vision for near and distant objects, usually developing gradually over a period of several weeks. Examination discloses a reduction in visual acuity, the presence of central and centrocecal scotomas, larger for red than for white test objects. A mild pallor of the temporal portion of the optic disk is a common finding. Retinal hemorrhages may be seen occasionally. These changes are always bilateral, and more or less symmetrical. Untreated, the disease may progress to irreversible optic atrophy. With nutritious diet and vitamin supplements, improvement occurs in all instances, though to a variable extent.

Deficiency amblyopia was particularly prevalent during the last war in the prisoner-of-war and civilian internment camps of the Far East. Although it had previously been described in association with beriberi and pellagra, the peak incidence did not coincide with that of either of these syndromes but with the mucocutaneous lesions in orogenital regions and "burning feet" syndromes. In this country many, if not all, of the cases of retrobulbar neuropathy attributed to the toxic effects of alcohol or tobacco are probably of nutritional origin. Retrobulbar neuropathy may occur as the only manifestation of deficiency, but far more frequently it is combined with other nutritional syndromes, such as peripheral neuropathy, the Wernicke-Korsakoff syndrome, or rarely by a spinal spastic and ataxic syndrome (Strachan's disease).

Treatment

In all the acute neurologic disturbances outlined in the preceding pages it is essential to administer an adequate supply of B vitamins at the earliest possible moment. A delay of a few hours may be crucial in determining whether the patient with Wernicke-Korsakoff disease may be restored to a state of mental competency. Fifty milligrams of thiamine chloride may be given intramuscularly and repeated each day until the patient resumes a normal diet. The other B vitamins (nicotinic acid, pantothenic acid, and B_6) may be given by mouth in dosages outlined in Chaps. 59 and 60. A particular danger attends the administration of intravenous glucose solution to a severely depleted patient, for this may exhaust his last reserve of B vitamins and result in circulatory collapse and death. In this weakened state bed rest is advisable, and if signs of cardiac weakness are betrayed by pulmonary edema, feeble heart sounds, tachycardia, and low blood pressure, rapid digitalization should be undertaken. Since these patients are confused and forgetful, their medical care must be supervised continuously by nurse and attendant, preferably on a medical ward.

If the patient is in good physical condition when first seen, it will prove sufficient merely to insist that he eat a balanced diet supplemented by B vitamins, though the latter are probably not necessary. If alcoholic the patient must be made to abstain completely from all alcoholic beverages. Should the intake have been high until the day of hospital entry, it is best gradually to reduce the daily quota over a period of a week in order to avoid convulsions or delirium tremens. If hepatosis or cirrhosis exists, it requires a program of treatment outlined in Chap. 280. For deficiency polyneuropathy, pain and sensitivity of the feet require a foot cradle and cock-up splints, and codeine and acetylsalicylic acid may be given in the first week or two. If the patient's legs are too weak to support him and he is bedfast, one can expect upright stance and locomotion to be regained in 3 to 6 months. Burning pain if persistent and severe may be relieved by sympathetic lumbar blocks and possibly by sympatholytic agents. Physiotherapy in the form of gentle massage, stretching of muscles, and graded resistance exercises is useful during this period. As health improves the physician should remain alert to the appearance of depressive symptoms and anxiety, which may retard the rehabilitation program.

Nutritional amblyopia will respond to normal diet and vitamin B supplements.

Prognosis

The outcome of these illnesses is always uncertain. Usually there is almost complete symptomatic recovery from a nutritional polyneuropathy, the patient being in the end left only with diminished or absent ankle and knee reflexes and slight blunting of sensation over feet and shins. As the nutritional amblyopia improves, central scotomas and diminished visual acuity may persist and the temporal sectors of optic disks become pale. The memory and learning defects of Korsakoff's psychosis usually improves to some degree but if severe at first a permanent disability requiring institutionalization is not infrequent. Nystagmus may also persist, but usually the disorder of gait subsides as do the ocular palsies.

Although the nutritional origin of this type of amblyopia seems established, the specific nutrient responsible is uncertain. Isolated reports have implicated riboflavin, thiamine, and vitamin B_{12}, but the evidence provided is inconclusive.

PELLAGRA

This discussion is concerned only with the neurologic manifestations, which in themselves are extremely diverse. Pellagra is essentially an encephalopathy, although involvement of other parts of the nervous system may occur. The mental symptoms may be mistaken for those of a psychoneurosis. Insomnia, fatigue, nervousness, irritability, or feelings of depression are common complaints. Examination may reveal retardation of mental processes and impairment of memory. Sometimes an acute confusional psychosis combined with changing rigidity of the limbs, grasping and sucking reflexes, and Babinski signs, dominates the clinical picture. Pellagra not only may produce insanity but occasionally may result from it because of the anorexia and refusal of food that accompany certain mental illnesses. The manifestations of spinal cord involvement have not been clearly delineated, perhaps because the mental state of the patients has precluded accurate testing. In general, they are referable to both the posterior columns and the lateral column, predominantly the former. Neuritic signs are common and are often difficult to distinguish from affection of the posterior columns. Signs such as tremors, extrapyramidal rigidity, sucking and grasping reflexes, and coma have often been included in the pellagrous syndrome, as have various disorders of the special senses.

The distinctive *pathologic changes* in pellagra are most readily discerned in the large cells of the motor cortex, the cells of Betz, which appear swollen and rounded, with eccentric nuclei and loss of the Nissl particles. This change was first described by Adolf Meyer as *central neuritis* and is frequently referred to as *axonal reaction* because of the similarity to the nerve cell change which occurs in the anterior horn cells when their axons are severed. The central neuritis of pellagra is probably not dependent on injury to the axones of the Betz cells, but appears to represent a primary affection of the whole motor cell. The spinal cord lesions take the form of a symmetric degeneration of the dorsal columns, especially of Goll, and to a lesser extent of the pyramidal tracts. The posterior column degeneration affects a specific system of fibers and is secondary to the degeneration of the posterior roots. The nature of the pyramidal tract lesion in pellagra is not known; one can only speculate that this change is secondary to the pyramidal cell degeneration.

A *spinal spastic syndrome*, apart from the other symptoms and signs of pellagra, may be a rare manifestation of deficiency disease. The chief clinical signs are spastic weakness of the legs with absent abdominal and increased tendon reflexes, clonus, and extensor plantar responses. These signs are usually accompanied by other signs of nutritional deficiency, such as Wernicke's disease and retrobulbar and peripheral neuropathy.

Treatment. If there is an acute nicotinic acid encephalopathy, prompt administration of nicotinic acid or nicotinamide in a dose of 50 to 100 mg intravenously, in 1,000 to 1,500 ml of normal saline, is indicated. Otherwise the oral administration of either of these drugs in a dose of 50 to 100 mg per day and a balanced ration of green vegetables, lean meat, and fruit will be adequate.

Prognosis. Improvement may be dramatic and recovery complete if the neurologic symptoms were not too severe or long-standing before treatment was started. Many patients appear to be left with a curious psychic weakness in which irritability, mild suspiciousness, moodiness, lack of power of concentration, and indisposition to work are the main symptoms. The signs of pyramidal tract disease nearly always disappear.

STRACHAN'S SYNDROME

Beginning with the report of Strachan in 1888 and culminating with the recent observations among prisoners of war and civilian internees, there has appeared a large number of reports concerning a nutritional disorder of the nervous system which cannot be forced into the boundaries of the classical syndromes described above. Strachan was the first to describe this syndrome, although he did not recognize its nutritional etiology.

Strachan's syndrome is essentially a disorder of the peripheral and optic nerves. Clinically, sensory symptoms and signs dominate the picture; in this respect the syndrome differs from beriberi. Paresthesias of the extremities, face, and trunk, painful "hyperesthesia" of the feet, loss of superficial and deep sensation, and ataxia are the common manifestations. On the other hand, foot drop and muscle

weakness occur very rarely. A frequent associated disorder is failing vision, which may go on to complete blindness and pallor of the optic disks. In general, deafness and vertigo are rare complications, but in some outbreaks these symptoms were so common as to earn the epithet "camp dizziness." In some patients, as in the group described by Cruikshank, spasticity, increased tendon reflexes, and Babinski signs are prominent, indicating involvement of the pyramidal tracts. Along with the neurologic signs there may be varying degrees of stomatoglossitis, corneal degeneration, and genital dermatitis; these mucocutaneous lesions are often spoken of together as the *orogenital syndrome* and are quite distinct from those of pellagra.

There have been only a few pathologic studies of this syndrome. Aside from the damage to the papillomacular bundle in the optic nerve, the most consistent abnormality has been a loss of medullated fibers in each column of Goll adjacent to the midline. This indicates a systematized degeneration of the central process of the bipolar sensory neurone of the lumbosacral spinal ganglions. The fact that the primary sensory neurone is the chief site of disease is consistent with the predominant sensory symptomatology. Cases with pyramidal tract signs have not been examined pathologically.

SUBACUTE COMBINED DEGENERATION OF THE SPINAL CORD AND BRAIN

Subacute combined degeneration of the spinal cord, the neurologic component of pernicious anemia, is due to vitamin B_{12} deficiency but is clearly different from the other nutritional diseases. The disease results not from the lack of vitamin B_{12} in the food but from the inability to transfer minute amounts of this nutrient across the intestinal mucosa. Such "starvation in the midst of plenty" has been called *conditioned deficiency disease*, since it depends on the lack of an intrinsic factor in the gastric secretion. The general features of pernicious anemia are fully discussed in Chap. 235; here only the neurologic manifestations will be considered.

Clinical Manifestations. Symptoms of nervous system disease are present in the large majority of patients with pernicious anemia. The patient first notices general weakness and paresthesias consisting of tingling, "pins and needles" feelings, or other vaguely described sensations. The paresthesias tend to be constant, to progress steadily, and to be the source of much distress. They are localized to the distal parts of all four limbs in a symmetric distribution, the lower extremities usually being involved before the upper ones. As the illness progresses, stiffness and weakness of the limbs develop, especially of the legs, which combined with a defect in postural sensation produce a weak, unsteady gait and awkwardness of the limbs. If the disease remains untreated, an ataxic paraplegia with variable degrees of spasticity and contracture may develop.

Early in the course of the illness, when only paresthesias are present, there may be no objective signs. Later, the neurologic examination discloses a disorder of the posterior and lateral columns of the spinal cord, predominantly of the former. Loss of vibration sense is by far the most consistent sign; it is more pronounced in the legs than in the arms, and frequently it extends over the trunk. Position sense is involved somewhat less frequently. The motor signs include loss of power, spasticity, changes in the tendon reflexes, clonus, and extensor plantar responses. These signs are practically limited to the legs. At first the patellar and Achilles reflexes are found to be diminished in activity as frequently as they are increased, and may even be absent. With treatment the reflexes may return to normal or even become hyperactive. The gait at first is predominantly ataxic, later ataxic and spastic.

Isolated instances of loss of superficial sensation below a segmental level on the trunk do occur, implicating the spinothalamic tracts, but such a finding should always suggest the possibility of some other disease of the spinal cord. The defect of cutaneous sensation takes the form of a mild blunting of touch, pain, and temperature sensation over the limbs in a distal distribution, but such a finding is also uncommon.

The nervous system involvement in subacute combined degeneration is characteristically, although not always, symmetric. A definite asymmetry of motor or sensory findings maintained over a period of weeks or months should always cast doubt on the diagnosis of subacute combined degeneration of the spinal cord.

Mental signs are frequent, ranging from irritability, apathy, somnolence, suspiciousness, and emotional instability to a marked confusional or depressive psychosis, or intellectual deterioration. Signs of visual impairment are distinctly rare; when present, they take the form of centrocecal scotomas. If involvement of the optic nerve is severe, optic atrophy may occur.

Neuropathologic Changes. The pathologic process takes the form of diffuse, although uneven, degeneration of the white matter. There are multiple foci of spongy degeneration, often in relation to small blood vessels. The myelin sheaths and the axis cylinders are both affected, the former perhaps earlier and to a greater extent than the latter. There is relatively little fibrous gliosis in the early lesions, but in the older treated cases, gliosis is pronounced. The changes begin in the posterior columns of the thoracic cord and spread from this region up and down the cord, as well as forward into the lateral columns. The lesions are not limited to specific systems of fibers within the posterior and lateral funiculi but are scattered irregularly through the latter.

The paresthesias, impairment of vibratory and position sense, ataxia, and the Romberg sign are due to affection of the posterior columns, and lesions here may also account for loss of tendon reflexes. Weakness, spasticity, increased tendon reflexes, and Babinski signs depend on involvement of the pyramidal tracts in the lateral columns. The spinothalamic tract may be involved in the pathologic process, which explains the occasional clinical finding of loss of pain and temperature sensation at a segmental level on the trunk. In advanced forms of the disease, pathologic changes similar to those in the spinal cord may be found in the white matter of the brain and the optic nerves.

There is no unanimity of opinion regarding the occurrence of lesions in the peripheral nerves in pernicious anemia. The evidence is largely inferential. The distal and symmetric blunting to pain, touch, and temperature that occurs in many cases is certainly a point in favor of peripheral nerve disease. It has been shown that there is a loss of myelin in peripheral nerves, but there is no convincing evidence that axis cylinders are affected.

The *spinal fluid* is usually normal, although occasionally there may be a slight elevation of the protein content. See Chap. 235 for other laboratory findings in pernicious anemia.

Efficacy of Liver and Vitamin B$_{12}$. At first it was believed that the spinal cord and blood changes were due to separate deficiencies, and for this reason treatment with liver extract was supplemented with crude liver. However, it is now known that the response to vitamin B$_{12}$ alone is in all ways comparable to that from refined liver extract or crude liver. One microgram of parenterally administered vitamin B$_{12}$ daily is theoretically an adequate dosage in the treatment of subacute combined degeneration of the cord, but in practice much larger amounts should be used.

The most important factor influencing the response to treatment is the duration of the disease, which for practical purposes may be measured by the duration of difficulty in walking. The greatest improvement occurs in those whose difficulty in walking is of less than 3 months' duration; in fact, it may be complete if therapy is instituted soon after the onset of symptoms. For this reason, the diagnosis of subacute combined degeneration is a matter of great urgency. Conversely, the least improvement occurs in those with difficulty in walking of longer than 2 years' duration. In practically all instances at least partial improvement is effected, although in long-standing cases often the best that can be be accomplished is arrest of progression. Other factors such as age, sex, severity, arteriosclerosis, hypertension, and the degree of anemia are relatively unimportant. Neurologic relapses during therapy are usually associated with infections and can be corrected by increasing the dose of vitamin B_{12}. All neurologic symptoms and signs may be improved; extensor plantar responses are as responsive to treatment as paresthesias and loss of vibratory sense. The return of absent deep reflexes is commonly observed, although at times it may take longer than a year. Improvement occurs mostly during the first 3 to 6 months of therapy and then continues at a slower tempo for a year and frequently longer.

Diagnosis. The chief obstacle in the early diagnosis of subacute combined degeneration of the cord is the lack of parallelism between the hematologic remission for an indefinite period, while the neurologic signs worsen, often to an irreversible stage. Other problems concern the difficulty of distinguishing between intrinsic spinal cord disease of nonpernicious anemia type from posterior and lateral column disease due to pernicious anemia, and of distinguishing pernicious anemia and subacute combined degeneration from other macrocytic anemias and their associated neurologic disturbances.

In most instances the diagnosis can be made by utilizing the standard methods for the diagnosis of pernicious anemia (see Chap. 235), the examination of the blood, gastric acidity, and the bone marrow. These methods are of limited value when the anemia is mild or absent or when the anemia has been corrected by folic acid. A therapeutic trial of vitamin B_{12} may be employed, but recourse to such a procedure means that therapy must be continued indefinitely, and the diagnosis may remain in doubt. Under these circumstances a number of refined diagnostic aids may be employed, such as the Schilling test or the microbiologic assay of B_{12} utilizing the organism *Euglena gracilis*.

REFERENCES

Adams, R. D., and C. S. Kubik: Subacute Degeneration of the Brain in Pernicious Anemia, New Engl. J. Med., 231:2, 1944.

Victor, M., and R. D. Adams: The Effect of Alcohol on the Nervous System, Research Publs. Assoc. Research Nervous Mental Disease, vol. 32 (Metabolic and Toxic Diseases of the Nervous System), 1953.

—— and A. A. Lear: Subacute Combined Degeneration of the Spinal Cord, Am. J. Med., 20:6, 896, 1956.

Spillane, J. D.: "Nutritional Disorders of the Nervous System," Baltimore, The Williams & Wilkins Company, 1947.

289 METABOLIC DISEASES OF THE BRAIN
Raymond D. Adams

Some of the most exciting developments in the whole history of neurologic medicine loom in fair prospect before us because of recent advances in our knowledge of metabolism. Already it has become apparent that many diseases of the nervous system, formerly classed as degenerative, are more properly to be comprehended in terms of subtle derangements of the liver and endocrine glands, which in turn have acted on the nervous system through the blood. As would be expected some of these disorders of metabolism are of rather general nature and exert their effects on many organs, including the nervous system. It has been expedient to group them together in a category of general metabolic disease, as was done in Part Four, Section 5. In others the brain is so clearly the target organ and the principal manifestations are so uniquely neurologic that it has been more appropriate to consider them with the other diseases of the nervous system. To place them here also serves other purposes—to underscore once again the inseparability of neurology and internal medicine and the probability that the cause of most diseases of the nervous system lies outside it and to dispel the belief that present concepts of "degenerative" or abiotrophic possess any essential validity as explanations of disease.

SPECIAL METABOLIC REQUIREMENTS OF THE BRAIN

Much that has been presented in Chaps. 51 to 54 is relevant to the understanding of the structure and function of the neurones of the central nervous system, just as it is to the cells of other organs and tissues. But as neurochemistry has progressed in recent years, several special ways in which the chemistry of the brain and probably the spinal cord differ from other viscera have been discovered. Some of these are pertinent to neuropathology.

One of the first and most essential facts about the chemistry of the nervous system is its continuously high metabolic rate, during both waking and sleeping hours; this is expressed in terms of oxygen consumption per minute, the requirement of the brain being approximately 50 cc per min in the adult and 65 cc in a six-year-old child (the equivalent of 20 per cent of the total oxygen consumption of the body in the adult and 50 per cent in the child). To supply this amount of oxygen the cerebral blood flow, which is determined at any one moment by the effective arterial pressure, blood volume, peripheral vasomotor tone, and the cerebral vascular resistance, must be maintained at approximately 750 cc per min in the adult (20 per cent of total cardiac output) and 1,250 cc in the child (40 per cent of total cardiac output). Since the brain can store no oxygen and the net yield of energy in its absence is relatively small, this organ more than any other is absolutely dependent upon a steady supply of oxygen to maintain cellular metabolism. A critical fall in the oxygenation of arterial blood, or in the blood levels of hemoglobin, or in the red blood cells, or in the effective arterial blood pressure may impair the function and even destroy parts of the brain.

A second special feature of brain metabolism is the importance of glucose as its principal nutrient. Of the many available raw materials such as carbohydrate, lipid, and proteins only glucose crosses the blood-brain barrier in sufficient quantity to maintain cerebral oxidative metabolism. The adult brain needs approximately 75 mg of glucose per minute, about 65 per cent of all that is available to the body; and since there is no significant store of glucose in the form of glycogen, it is dependent upon that which is delivered from minute to minute. In keeping with its exclusive use of glucose as a nutrient, the respiratory quotient (RQ) of the brain is 0.99. Insulin, strangely enough, plays no part in cerebral oxidative metabolism. Complete oxidation of glucose to CO_2 and H_2O occurs in three interrelated stages: (1) glycolysis, (2) Krebs citric acid cycle, and (3) the cytochrome or electron transport system. These have been described in Chap. 52. The glycolytic process is anaerobic but yields only a small amount of energy in the form of ATP. The tricarboxylic cycle is aerobic, but again the energy yield is too small for cerebral demands. The great source of energy comes from the electron transport system, three energy-rich phosphate bonds being formed for each hydrogen pair. Cellular metabolism has adapted itself to the utilization of such phosphate-stored energy. If the cytochrome transport system, an aerobic process, should fail for lack of oxygen the Krebs citric acid cycle is stalled. In vivo experiments have recently revealed a surprising finding—that of all the glucose used only about 35 per cent is directly oxidized. An almost equal amount is converted into amino acids and the remainder into lipids and proteins. This means that these latter constituents of the brain are constantly being metabolized and renewed, in contrast to certain of the complex lipids and proteolipids of myelin which remain relatively stable for years. It explains the fact that under conditions of hypoglycemia within a period of 60 to 90 min cerebral metabolism (O_2 utilization) not only is reduced but brain structure is destroyed as essential substances such as lipids and proteins are called upon to sustain metabolism.

The third and last peculiarity of cerebral metabolism which will be mentioned is the important role played by glutamic acid, glutamine, γ-aminobutyric acid (GABA), and aspartic acid. Glutamic acid or its amide, glutamine, is present in higher concentration in the brain than in any other organ, and it has been shown that it is the only amino acid capable of sustaining oxidative metabolism in tissue slices. The majority of free amino acids in the brain are derived from the same group. Pyridoxal phosphate (vitamin B_6) or pyridoxine is the coenzyme which catalyzes these amino acid reactions. A closely related substance γ-aminobutyric acid is entirely unique to the mammalian nervous system. These four amino acids are localized principally in the gray matter in varying amounts. In vivo experiments have shown that relatively little glutamic acid, aspartic acid, and γ-aminobutyric acid can penetrate the blood-brain barrier, but glutamine may do so freely as does also the amide of aspartic acid, asparagine. However, glucose is probably the main source of cerebral glutamate, being provided as a by-product of the Krebs tricarboxylic cycle via a-ketoglutarate. This latter reaction is of major importance in ammonia and amino acid metabolism; it utilizes two enzymes, glutamic dehydrogenase and glutamic transaminase, and pyridoxine is the coenzyme. Essentially glutamic acid synthesis involves the addition of another amine or NH_3 group to glutamic acid. Hence it is one of the principal means of removing or detoxifying excess ammonia. γ-Aminobutyric acid is formed from glutamic acid, a reaction which has not been demonstrated in any other organ. Both glutamic acid and γ-aminobutyric acid could serve as substrates for oxidative metabolism, but their importance cannot be stated as this time.

CLASSIFICATION OF METABOLIC DISEASES OF THE NERVOUS SYSTEM

One large category of these metabolic diseases of the nervous system are those in which the cerebral disorder is related to a demonstrated fault in general metabolism, the latter traceable to a disease of the heart and circulation, lungs, liver, kidneys, and endocrine glands. In this group may be included acute hypoxia, hypercapnia, acute hepatic stupor or coma, uremia, hypoglycemia, acidosis (diabetic, uremic, and other), Addison's disease, Cushing's syndrome, hyper- and hypothyroidism, and hypoparathyroidism. A second category comprises disorders of the nervous system and also other organs, in which a metabolic abnormality of obscure nature may explain both the lesions in the brain and other organs. Here reference is made to such conditions as hepatolenticular degeneration, porphyria, galactosemia, glycogen storage diseases, phenylpyruvic oligophrenia and several of the syndromes of aminoaciduria with mental defect, and most recently the Kornzweig-Bassen syndrome. Some of these are familial as are many of those of the third category which encompasses cerebral disorders of assumed metabolic origin in which no evidence of disease in other viscera or in blood can presently be evoked. Representatives of this third class of disease are: the leukodystrophies, lipid storage diseases, Friedreich's ataxia, dystonia musculorum deformans, Jakob-Creutzfeldt-Heidenhain's disease, and many others discussed in the chapter on degenerative diseases.

A classification of this type provides a conceptual locus for all the known varieties of nervous disease and ultimately will bring them into orderly relationship to the chemistry of the nervous system. However, it leaves the clinician without a practical approach to the subject, until he has been able to reach a diagnosis. Only then is it possible to turn to the relevant published literature for detailed information concerning his patient. More helpful, it would seem, would be clinical classification in which diseases with similar clinical manifestations are grouped together. Final diagnosis depends then on the differentiation by clinical and laboratory methods of the several diseases subsumed in a single syndrome. Such is the scheme which follows.

Table 289-1. CLASSIFICATION OF METABOLIC DISEASES OF THE BRAIN

I. Metabolic diseases presenting as a syndrome of acute impairment of consciousness (confusion, stupor, and coma, with or without seizures)
   A. Hypoxia
   B. Hypercapnia
   C. Hypoglycemia
   D. Acidosis
   E. Uremia
   F. Hepatic failure
   G. Addison's disease
II. Metabolic diseases presenting as chronic dementia (mental retardation in childhood) or extrapyramidal or cerebellar motor disorder or other neurologic abnormality
   A. Liver disease or Eck fistula and hepatolenticular degeneration of Wilson
   B. Porphyria
   C. Cushing's disease
   D. Hypothyroidism
   E. Hypoparathyroidism and Fahr's syndrome
   F. Aminoacidurias
   G. Lipid storage diseases
   H. Leukodystrophies
   I. Kornzweig-Bassen syndrome

Here only a few of these many diseases will be considered in detail, and the reader is referred to other sections of the book for the definitive discussion of the metabolic aberration and its main clinical expression, if generalized.

Syndrome of Impaired Consciousness

The character of these types of derangement have been described in detail in Chap. 34, and it was therein stated that a metabolic disorder of the brain should be considered when there was an acute disturbance of consciousness without localizing or lateralizing signs and without change in the cerebrospinal fluid. An intoxication with alcohol or other drug enters prominently in the differential diagnosis, as does also a nutritional disorder due to lack of B vitamins.

Acute Hypoxic Encephalopathy. The hypoxic states have already been described in Chap. 14. But it is important for the clinician to realize that a hypoxic accident so often encountered in the emergency room or on the wards of a general hospital is one of the more frequent causes of death or even worse, the cause of the tragedy of permanent coma or mental enfeeblement. The medical situations which most often have led to this have been strangulation (blood, surgical pack or sponge, foreign body), respiratory-cardiac arrest during inhalation, spinal or intravenous anesthesia, cardiac disease with arrest, disease which causes paralysis of respiratory muscles such as poliomyelitis or acute idiopathic polyneuritis, central nervous system disease [cerebrovascular lesions, acute toxic encephalopathy (in children), epilepsy, head injury, etc., with respiratory arrest]. Carbon monoxide intoxication has similar effects. Mild hypoxia induces only inattentiveness, poor judgment, and motor incoordination and has no lasting effects if corrected. Severe hypoxia causes coma within less than a minute, but again recovery will be complete if breathing, oxygenation of blood, or cardiac action is restored within 3 to 5 min. Periods of hypoxia with coma that exceed 7 to 8 min usually result in serious and permanent injury to the brain, particularly in those parts most susceptible to injury because of the marginal efficiency of their circulation (globus pallidus, cerebral cortex, especially that of the hippocampus and parietal-occipital regions, and cerebellar cortex). However, it is difficult to judge the degree of hypoxia accurately since slight heart action or an imperceptible blood pressure may serve to maintain some degree of circulation. Hence some individuals have made an excellent recovery after alleged cerebral hypoxia of 8 to 10 min or longer. Degrees of hypoxia which do not at any time abolish consciousness rarely if ever cause permanent damage to the nervous system.

The patient who has suffered a serious hypoxic episode is often breathing normally and has good color and normal heart action when first seen. The hypoxic crisis has already terminated. Yet he may be profoundly comatose with dilated, fixed pupils, eyes slightly divergent and motionless or roving from side to side, and limbs and tendon reflexes diminished or absent. Within a few minutes after cardiac action and breathing have been restored, generalized convulsions and also isolated or grouped twitches of muscles (myoclonus) supervene. If the damage is severe coma persists and decerebrate postures may be present or occur upon pinching the limbs, and bilateral Babinski signs can be evoked. In the first 24 to 48 hr death may terminate this state, in a setting of rising temperature, deepening coma, and circulatory collapse. If the patient survives this period he usually begins to respond in varying degrees. A period of restlessness and chaotic movement, sometimes clearly revealing ataxia, and myoclonic jerks or choreoathetosis appear. Again improvement may be arrested at this point; some patients remain unresponsive with bizarre postures until their death several weeks, months, or years later. No electrical activity is seen in their electroencephalogram, and at autopsy nearly all cerebral and cerebellar cortex is found to have been destroyed. If further improvement takes place, as it usually does in the less damaged patients, consciousness may be regained and then confusion, visual agnosia, or any one of several types of abnormal movement becomes manifest. Some of these patients quickly pass through this phase and proceed to make a full recovery; others are left with some disabling syndrome. Seizures may or may not continue to be a problem. One unexplained phenomenon is an initial improvement for 1 to 2 days followed by a relapse, a further progression of the neurological syndrome, and death after 1 to 2 weeks.

The permanent neurologic sequelae, which may be classed as the posthypoxic syndromes are: dementia with or without extrapyramidal signs, visual agnosia with variable rigidity of limbs and slowness of movement, Parkinsonian syndrome, choreoathetosis, cerebellar ataxia, and myoclonic epilepsy. In the latter conditions the mental capacities may be intact.

The essential mechanism in hypoxic encephalopathy is a lack of oxygen and an arrest of all aerobic metabolic processes necessary for the Krebs tricarboxylic cycle and the hydrogen transport system. Neurones are injured to such a degree they cannot survive. The phenomenon of delayed progression is not understood but may be due to the blockage or exhaustion of some enzymatic process during the period when brain metabolism is restored or even increased (as in hyperthermia).

Diagnosis depends on (1) the history of the hypoxic event and evidence of reduced oxygenation of arterial blood or CO (the latter is indicated by its cherry red color or spectroscopic band only for a few minutes to hours after the spisode), blood pressures below 70 systolic, or cardiac arrest; (2) the typical sequence of events outlined above after the episode has terminated. Renal damage (anuria) and injury to the myocardium may also have occurred and provide corroborative evidence.

Treatment is mainly the prevention of a critical degree of hypoxic injury. Quickly securing a clear airway, artificial respiration, external thoracic cardiac massage and open-chest surgery, the use of a cardiac defibrillator or pacemaker all have their place and every second counts in their prompt utilization. Once cardiac and pulmonary function are restored there is some evidence from the work of Blalock and his associates that reducing cerebral metabolic requirements by continuous hypothermia for 48 to 72 hr may prevent the progressive changes referred to above. Oxygen may be of value during the first hours and days but probably is of little use after the blood becomes well oxygenated. Seizures should be controlled by intramuscular Dilantin sodium 100 mg every 6 hr, and sodium phenobarbital 120 mg every 4 hr by mouth or stomach tube or parenterally four times a day. Mebaral 500 mg per day or phenobarbital 300 mg per day in several divided doses controls the myoclonic seizures better than other anticonvulsants.

Hypercapnia (and Hypoxia) in Pulmonary Disease. Chronic emphysema, chronic fibrosing lung disease, and in some instances a seeming inadequacy disorder of the respiratory center (Chap. 14) lead to respiratory acidosis, with an elevation of P_{CO_2} and a reduction in arterial oxygen tension. Secondary polycythemia, cor pulmonale, and heart failure often accompany these diseases of the lungs, and pulmonary infection may be superimposed. Brief reference to the clinical syndrome was made in Chap. 34, but it is sufficiently complex to merit elaboration. It is comprised of an action tremor and a coarse twitching of all muscles sustained in a state of contraction (termed *asterixis*), headache and papilledema and mental dullness, drowsiness, confusion, and coma. The cerebrospinal fluid is under increased pressure. P_{CO_2} may exceed 75 mm of Hg, and the oxygen concentration of arterial blood ranges from 85 per cent to as low as 40 per cent. The danger of administering morphine which depresses the respiratory center or the inhalation of oxygen which removes the sole stimulus to the respiratory center is now widely recognized, for many patients so treated have lapsed into coma (CO_2 narcosis) and have died.

Forced ventilation with a Benedict positive-pressure respirator, with inhalation of room air or oxygen if hypoxia is severe, the treatment of heart failure with digitalis and diuretic measures, vene-section to reduce the viscosity of the blood, and antibiotics to combat pulmonary infection has been the most effective program of therapy and has often resulted in a surprising degree of improvement that may be maintained for months or years.

Unlike pure hypoxic encephalopathy, in hyper-capnia prolonged coma is exceptional and the pa-pilledema and the jerky, intermittent postures or asterixis, the latter characteristic only of liver fail-ure and hypercapnia and rare instances of meta-bolic acidosis, are features of diagnostic import. The syndrome is apt to be mistaken for brain tumor or a confusional psychosis of nondescript type or a disease causing chorea or myoclonus. In the latter instance it must be distinguished from a chronic extrapyramidal syndrome, as outlined be-low.

Hypoglycemic Encephalopathy. This condition has been discussed in Chaps. 70 and 71. None-theless it is a rather frequent cause of profound coma, episodic confusion, and convulsions and merits separate consideration as a metabolic dis-order of brain function. The essential biochemical datum is a blood sugar level of less than 25 to 30 mg per 100 ml, lasting 1 to 2 hr and leading to ex-haustion of the store of cerebral glucose and glyco-gen. Within this brief span of time, as cerebral oxidation proceeds without exogenous glucose, the structural components of neurones in the form of lipids and proteins are metabolized and irreversi-ble damage occurs.

Clinically the most common situations in which severe hypoglycemia develops are: (1) accidental or deliberate overdose of insulin or one of the oral antidiabetic agents in the diabetic patient, (2) insulin therapy in schizophrenia, (3) an islet cell insulin-secreting tumor of the pancreas, (4) glyco-gen storage disease in infancy, and (5) rarely some form of liver disease. In functional hyperinsulinism the hypoglycemia is rarely of sufficient severity or duration to damage the central nervous system.

The clinical picture has already been sketched. The initial symptoms, as the level of blood glucose descends, are nervousness, hunger, and cold and these gradually give way to confusion, drowsiness, and occasionally excitement or overactivity. In the next stage forced sucking, grasping, motor restless-ness, muscular spasms, and finally decerebrate ri-gidity occur in that sequence. Myoclonic twitching and convulsions may develop in some patients but are by no means the rule. Deepening coma is at-tended by dilatation of pupils, pale skin, shallow respiration, slow heart, and hypotonicity of limb musculature—the so-called medullary phase of hy-poglycemia. Should glucose be administered before this medullary phase appears, the patient is re-stored to normalcy, retracing the afore-mentioned steps in reverse order. However, once this medul-lary phase is reached, and particularly if it persists for a time before the hypoglycemia is corrected therapeutically by intravenous glucose or spontane-ously by the so-called gluconeogenic activities of the adrenal glands and liver, recovery may be de-layed over a period of days or weeks and may be incomplete. A huge dose of insulin with intense hypoglycemia, even of relatively brief duration (30 to 60 min), is more dangerous than smaller ones, even though the lowering of blood sugar is equally severe in both, because it impairs or ex-hausts essential enzymes; and this cannot be over-come by large quantities of glucose intravenously. The cerebral cortex suffers major damage; cortical nerve cells degenerate and are replaced by micro-gliacytes and astrocytes. The distribution of lesions is not quite the same as in hypoxic encephalopathy.

The major difference, clinically, between hypo-glycemia and hypoxia lies in the clinical setting of the illness and the mode of evolution of the neuro-logic disorder. Hypoglycemia usually unfolds slowly over a period of 30 to 60 min, instead of suddenly within seconds or a few minutes. The recovery phase and sequelae of the two conditions bear close resemblance and may not be possible of dif-ferentiation. Recurrent hypoglycemia, as with an islet cell tumor, may masquerade for some time as a recurrent confusional psychosis or convulsive ill-ness, and diagnosis awaits the demonstration of low blood sugar or hyperinsulinism.

The correction of the hypoglycemia at the ear-liest moment is the obvious therapy. It is not known whether or not hypothermia or other measures will increase the tolerance or safety period in hypo-glycemia or alter the outcome.

Hepatic Stupor and Coma. Chronic hepatic in-sufficiency with portocaval shunting of blood is often punctuated by episodes of mental dullness, drowsiness, confusion, stupor or coma, flapping of outstretched limbs, or intermittency of sustained postures (asterixis). This condition has been de-scribed fully in Chap. 19. Less widely known is the fact that a pure Eck fistula may be attended by a similar clinical picture.

In many patients the syndrome does not advance beyond the stage of flapping and confusion with mild electroencephalographic changes. In this mild form it must be distinguished from the chronic extrapyramidal syndromes.

Reducing the protein intake, ridding the intesti-nal tract of blood, suppressing the bacterial action in protein in the intestinal tract with neomycin or kanamycin, and the administration of sodium glu-tamate intravenously which tends to lower the NH_3 levels of the blood have been found in recent years to restore many of these patients to a relatively normal state. Although the biochemical mechanism is not fully understood, the most plausible hypothesis is that the levels of blood NH_3 are elevated because the diseased or by-passed liver fails to convert it into urea; glucose metabolism of the brain at the Krebs cycle stage is disturbed by withdrawing alpha-ketoglutaric acid from the metabolic pool as the cerebral tissues attempt to remove the NH_3 formed in situ. Should these measures not control NH_3 production, death is inevitable.

In acute hepatitis delirious and confusional reactions of slightly different type may develop, and their mechanism is still obscure. NH_3 may be elevated but not often to a degree that would be expected to affect central nervous system function.

Other Metabolic Encephalopathies. Limitations of space permit only brief reference to other important metabolic disturbances of the brain. Metabolic *acidosis*, such as that due to diabetes mellitus or renal failure, produces the typical drowsiness, stupor, and coma with dry skin and Kussmaul breathing as described in Chap. 70. There is no recognizable neuropathologic change, high-voltage, fast electrical activity predominates in the electroencephalogram, and correction of the acidosis restores nervous function to a normal level, provided coma has not persisted for too long a time, in which instance death supervenes. *Uremic encephalopathy* remains confused because of the existence of two neurologic syndromes, one of hypertensive encephalopathy, the other a somnolent-twitching-convulsive syndrome (uremic twitching) which is highly characteristic of renal failure but still of obscure cause (see Chap. 20). Its recent ascription to magnesium depletion is interesting but has not been substantiated. Encephalopathy due to *Addison's adrenal insufficiency* may be attended by episodic confusion, stupor, or coma, usually of nondescript type without special identifying features. Its basis remains unclear. Hypotension and diminished cerebral circulation and hypoglycemia are the principal hypotheses presently being entertained, and measures which correct these conditions appear to have been beneficial in some instances. In *Cushing's disease* an obscure encephalopathy manifested by a complex psychosis may arise (see Chap. 68). Brain atrophy, demonstrated during life by enlarged ventricles in a pneumoencephalogram, has been demonstrated in some patients, but its cause, mechanism, and pathology have not been subjected to systematic study. A sudden lowering of serum calcium after operation for a parathyroid adenoma may be attended by drowsiness and confusion with electroencephalographic changes; and the administration of calcium salts has seemed to correct the neurologic syndrome. *Hypercalcemia* of extreme degrees is also associated with confusion.

Syndrome of Dementia with Extrapyramidal Motor Disorder or Other Neurologic Signs

Chronic Hepatic Failure. Two chronic, progressive hepatic-cerebral syndromes have now been delineated, (1) *Wilson's familial progressive hepatolenticular degeneration* (see Chap. 93) and (2) *a chronic progressive, nonfamilial encephalopathy.* The latter resembles Wilson's disease but shows no disturbance of copper metabolism or marked aminoaciduria. In chronic progressive, nonfamilial encephalopathy, which is more frequent than Wilson's disease, the patient usually has had episodes of coma, though a few patients have never been comatose at any time. In either case they undergo a slow, intermittently progressive dementia with the added features of slurred speech, tremor of limbs (both simple and intention type), cerebellar ataxia, and choreoathetosis. This picture is almost identical with that of Wilson's disease save for the absence of Kayser-Fleischer corneal rings. As with hepatic coma there may be any type of chronic liver disease (postnecrotic or alcoholic cirrhosis, biliary cirrhosis, or hemachromatosis, or any one of these with hepatoma), or an Eck fistula may produce the same syndrome, the liver being altogether normal in the latter instance. Although not fully understood, chronic NH_3 intoxication seems to be the most likely explanation and should be corrected by measures described in Chap. 280.

Chronic hypercapnia may cause protracted confusion and action tremor with flapping movements of outstretched limbs.

In *hypoparathyroidism*, tetany, convulsions, cerebral calcification (lenticular and dentatic nuclei and cerebellar cortex) may occur, and with the passage of time a mild choreoathetosis on one or both sides of the body or cerebellar ataxia may develop insidiously. This condition may respond to the administration of vitamin D (see Chap. 67). A similar cerebral calcification and neurologic syndrome (except for tetany) but without evidence of disturbed calcium metabolism occurs in Fahr's syndrome (see Chap. 290) and is not at all understood. There is no treatment.

Hallervorden-Spatz Disease. This is a curious siderosis of the basal ganglions attended by progressive rigidity of the legs and later arms, athetosis, and respiratory and other spasms. It begins in late childhood and progresses slowly. A hereditary disposition is established. No disturbance in serum iron or iron metabolism in other organs has been established. (See Chap. 290.)

Leukodystrophies and the lipid storage diseases are representative of two important categories of metabolic diseases of the brain. They are discussed in Chap. 290, pending further clarification.

Aminoacidurias of several types are just now

emerging as a new class of biochemical abnormalities with prominent neurologic aspects, particularly in infants and children (see Chap. 283). *Hartnup's disease,* consisting of hereditary pellagra-like skin rash, a temporary cerebellar ataxia, and aminoaciduria, is a prominent member of this group.

Kornzweig-Bassen Syndrome. This is a familial disease, recently come into prominence by virtue of being the first of the chronic hereditary ataxias to have a possible biochemical basis. The syndrome consists of abnormal erythrocytes of thorny appearance (acanthrocytes), an ataxia which resembles that of Friedreich, and retinitis pigmentosa. In three closely studied patients (only seven have been reported) there was a marked deficiency of serum beta-lipoprotein and serum cholesterol, an abnormal pattern of erythrocyte phospholipids, and marked impairment of gastrointestinal absorption of fat. The neurologic disorder is typified by proprioceptive deficit in the limbs (with sensory ataxia) and loss of tendon reflexes. Weakness with myopathic features is also suspected, and an ophthalmoplegia is found in some patients.

Acquired porphyria which declares itself usually by a neurologic syndrome—thoracic or abdominal pain, acute psychosis, and polyneuropathy—has no established biochemical basis, at least as far as the lesions in the brain, autonomic and peripheral nervous system are concerned (see Chap. 91).

In the diagnosis of this second category of metabolic diseases of the brain, their clinical attributes alone are of importance, but they are readily confused with some of the chronic forms of encephalitis, chronic drug intoxications and withdrawal therefrom, and several varieties of degenerative diseases. But more important, if the clinical manifestations are accurately interpreted and the patient in question recognized as having a metabolic disorder, appropriate biochemical tests of blood and urine may now provide reliable confirmation of diagnosis.

These latter examples of dementia, extrapyramidal motor disorder, and other neurologic abnormality are but a few examples of a widening circle of metabolic diseases of the nervous system. They are not clearly separated at the moment from the larger group of nutritional and degenerative diseases described in Chaps. 288 and 290. It is hoped that by the time of the next edition this section may be expanded to include many more diseases and that a more selective and useful syndromic approach can replace the crude one offered above.

REFERENCES

Courville, C. B.: "Contributions to the Study of Cerebral Anoxia," Los Angeles, Calif., San Lukas Press.

Merritt, H. H., and C. C. Hare: Metabolic and Toxic Diseases of the Nervous System, Research Publications of the Association for Research in Nervous and Mental Disease, vol. 32, Baltimore, The Williams & Wilkins Company, 1953.

Himwich, H. E.: "Brain Metabolism and Cerebral Disorders," Baltimore, The Williams & Wilkins Company, 1951.

290 DEGENERATIVE DISEASES OF THE NERVOUS SYSTEM

Edward P. Richardson, Jr., and Ansgar Torvik

The term degenerative as applied to diseases of the nervous system is used to designate a group of disorders in which there is gradual, generally symmetric, relentlessly progressive wasting away of structural elements of the nervous system, for reasons still unknown. Many of the conditions so designated depend upon abnormal genetic factors and thus appear in more than one member of the same family; this general group of diseases is therefore frequently referred to as heredodegenerative. A number of other conditions not apparently differing in any fundamental way from the hereditary disorders occur only sporadically, i.e., as isolated instances in a given family. Sir William Gowers in 1902 suggested the now familiar term *abiotrophy,* by which he meant that diseases of this class were the result of "defective vital endurance" of the structures affected, leading to their premature death. This term of course tells nothing of the true nature of the defects. It is to be assumed that the basis for these diseases must be found in some disorder of the metabolism of the parts involved.

Within relatively recent times there has been some elucidation of the nature of a number of nervous disorders which, in their symmetric distribution and gradually progressive course, resemble the class of diseases under discussion. Examples of these are the deficiency diseases, such as subacute combined degeneration of the spinal cord with pernicious anemia, deficiency neuropathy, pellagra, and the Wernicke-Korsakoff syndrome, in which disease or death of neural structures results from impaired function of enzyme systems required in the metabolism of the cells concerned. In hepatolenticular degeneration (Wilson's disease), long classed with the heredodegenerative disorders, significant defects in copper and protein metabolism have been discovered, which may well be of fundamental importance in its pathogenesis (see Chap. 93). Furthermore, chronic exposure to a number of toxic substances may produce effects on the nervous system closely resembling those encountered in the spontaneously occurring degenerative diseases. This is seen, for instance, in the chronic peripheral neuropathy of arsenic intoxication, the neuropathy and myelopathy from poisoning with triorthocresyl phosphate (Jamaica ginger paralysis), or the tremor and rigidity that have been seen with chronic manganese intoxication. It seems reasonable to expect that further advances in knowledge of the metabolism of the nervous system will do much to disclose the underlying abnormalities in the disease states at present under consideration.

The large group of the degenerative diseases of the nervous system can be divided into a number of syndromes by means of various distinguishing clinical and pathologic features. Nevertheless, there are certain aspects common to all, the recognition of which can assist the clinician in arriving at the diagnosis of a disorder of this class. Some of these are summarized in the following paragraphs.

General Considerations. It is a characteristic of the degenerative diseases that they begin insidiously and run a gradually progressive course which may extend over many years. The earliest changes may be so slight that it is frequently impossible to assign any precise time of onset. As with other gradually developing conditions, the patient or his family may give a history implying an abrupt appearance of disability. This is particularly likely to occur if there has been an injury, or if some other dramatic event has taken place in the patient's life to which illness might conceivably be related. In such a case, skillful taking of the history may bring out that the patient or family has suddenly become aware of a condition which had, in fact, already been present for some time but had passed unnoticed. Whether or not trauma or other stress may bring on or aggravate one of the degenerative diseases is still a question that cannot be answered with certainty. It would seem highly improbable from all that is known. In any event, it must be kept in mind that the disease processes under discussion by their very nature develop spontaneously without relationship to external factors.

The family history is of great importance, but one cannot always be immediately satisfied with that obtained on first contact with the patient. One reason for this is that patients or their relatives may be ashamed to disclose that a neurologic disease occurs in the family. Another is that it may not be realized that an illness is hereditary when other members of the family have a much less severe form of the disorder than the patient and have themselves been unaware of the abnormality—as not infrequently occurs in the hereditary ataxias and related conditions. However, in modern western families the small sibships may prevent even well-established hereditary diseases from expressing themselves. It must, of course, be remembered that familial occurrence of a disease does not always mean that it is hereditary; it may indicate instead that more than one member of a family has been exposed to the same infectious or toxic agent.

Another significant feature of the degenerative nervous diseases is that in general their ceaselessly progressive course is uninfluenced by all medical or surgical measures. Dealing with a case of this kind is often, therefore, an anguishing experience for all concerned. Yet symptoms can often be alleviated by wise and skillful management, and the physician's kindly interest may be of great help to a patient even when curative measures cannot be offered.

The bilaterally symmetric distribution of the changes brought about by these diseases has already been mentioned. This feature alone may serve to distinguish conditions in this group from many other diseases of the nervous system. At the same time, it should be pointed out that, in the earliest stages, greater involvement on one side or in one limb is not uncommon. Sooner or later, however, despite the asymmetric beginning, the inherently symmetric nature of the process asserts itself.

A striking feature of a number of disorders of this class is the almost selective involvement of anatomically or physiologically related systems of neurones. This is clearly exemplified in amyotrophic lateral sclerosis, in which the process is almost entirely limited to cortical and spinal motor neurones, and in the cases of progressive ataxia, in which the Purkinje cells of the cerebellum are alone affected. Many other examples could be cited (e.g., Friedreich's ataxia) in which certain neuronal systems disintegrate, leaving others perfectly intact. An important group of the degenerative diseases has therefore been called "system diseases" ("progressive cerebrospinal system atrophies"—Spatz), and many of these are strongly hereditary. It must be realized, however, that selective involvement of neuronal systems is not exclusively a property of the degenerative group, since several disease processes of known cause have similarly circumscribed effects on the nervous system. Diphtheria toxin, for instance, selectively attacks the myelin of the peripheral nerves, and triorthocresyl phosphate affects particularly the corticospinal tracts in the spinal cord as well as the peripheral nerves. Another example is the special vulnerability of the Purkinje cells of the cerebellum to hyperthermia. On the other hand, several of the conditions included among the degenerative diseases are characterized by pathologic changes that are diffuse and unselective. These exceptions nevertheless do not detract from the importance of affection of particular neuronal systems as a distinguishing feature of many of the diseases under discussion.

Typically, the pathologic process in the nervous system is one of slow involution of nerve cell bodies or their prolongations as nerve fibers, unaccompanied by any intense tissue reaction or cellular response. The cerebrospinal fluid, therefore, shows little if any change—at most a slight elevation of protein, without abnormalities in pressure, cell count, or in other constituents. Moreover, since these diseases invariably result in tissue loss, rather than in new tissue formation (as with neoplasms or inflammation), x-ray visualization of the ventricular system or subarachnoid space shows either no change or an enlargement of these compartments. These negative laboratory findings thus help to distinguish the degenerative disorders from the other large classes or progressive disease of the nervous system—tumor and infections.

Classification. Since etiologic classification is impossible, subdivision of the degenerative diseases into individual syndromes rests on descriptive criteria, based largely upon pathologic anatomy, but to some extent on clinical aspects as well. In the terms used to designate many of these syndromes, the names of a number of distinguished neurologists and neuropathologists are commemorated. A useful way of keeping in mind the various disease states is to group them according to the outstanding clinical features that may be found in an actual case. The following classification, intended to be of practical help to the physician, is based on such a plan.

Table 290-1. CLASSIFICATION OF THE DEGENERATIVE
DISEASES OF THE NERVOUS SYSTEM

I. Syndrome in which progressive dementia is an outstanding feature, in the absence of other prominent neurologic signs
  A. Diffuse cerebral atrophy
    1. Senile dementia
    2. Alzheimer's disease
  B. Pick's disease (circumscribed cerebral atrophy)
II. Syndrome in which progressive dementia is combined with other neurologic signs
  A. Principally in adults
    1. Huntington's chorea
    2. Cerebrocerebellar degeneration
    3. Jakob-Creutzfeldt disease
  B. In children and adults
    1. Amaurotic family idiocy (neuronal lipidoses)
    2. Leukodystrophy
    3. Familial myoclonus epilepsy
    4. Hallervorden-Spatz disease
    5. Wilson's disease (hepatolenticular degeneration; Westphal-Strümpell pseudosclerosis)
III. Syndrome chiefly manifested by gradual development of abnormalities of posture or involuntary movements
  A. Paralysis agitans (Parkinson's disease)

Table 290-1. CLASSIFICATION OF THE DEGENERATIVE
DISEASES OF THE NERVOUS SYSTEM (*Continued*)

  B. Dystonia musculorum deformans (torsion dystonia)
  C. Spasmodic torticollis
IV. Syndrome chiefly manifested by slowly developing ataxia
  A. Cerebellar degenerations
  B. Spinocerebellar degenerations (Friedreich's ataxia; Marie's hereditary ataxia)
V. Syndrome with slowly developing muscular weakness and wasting
  A. Without sensory changes: motor system disease
    1. In adults
      a. Amyotrophic lateral sclerosis
      b. Progressive muscular atrophy
      c. Progressive bulbar palsy
      d. Primary lateral sclerosis
    2. In children or young adults
      a. Infantile muscular atrophy (Werdnig-Hoffmann disease; amyotonia congenita)
      b. Hereditary spastic paraplegia
  B. With sensory changes
    1. Progressive neural muscular atrophy
      a. Peroneal muscular atrophy (Charcot-Marie-Tooth)
      b. Hypertrophic interstitial neuropathy (Déjerine-Sottas)
    2. Miscellaneous forms of chronic progressive neuropathy
VI. Syndrome chiefly manifested by progressive visual loss
  A. Hereditary optic atrophy (Leber)
  B. Pigmentary degeneration of the retina (retinitis pigmentosa)

SYNDROME IN WHICH PROGRESSIVE DEMENTIA ALONE PREDOMINATES

In the disease entities about to be discussed, the clinical picture is dominated by gradual loss of intellectual capacities, i.e., by dementia. Other neurologic abnormalities, except in the terminal stages, are absent or relatively insignificant. (For further discussion of dementia, including its clinical evaluation, Chap. 37 should be consulted.)

Diffuse Cerebral Atrophy: Senile Dementia; Alzheimer's Disease

Some degree of shrinkage in size and weight of the brain, i.e., "atrophy," has been shown to be the inevitable accompaniment of advancing age. In many instances, this is of no clinical significance, and there are many very old people who remain alert and perceptive, with keen intellect, to the end. Nevertheless, severe degrees of diffuse cerebral atrophy are as a general rule associated with some evidence of dementia. When these changes occur in old age (and the definition of when old age begins is largely a subjective one), it is usual to speak of *senile dementia*. That this is a fairly frequent condition is common experience. Much more infrequent is a pathologically identical progressive dementia with diffuse brain atrophy coming on well before the senile period—a presenile dementia. This condition, classically described in 1906 by Alois Alzheimer, has since become generally known as *Alzheimer's disease*. The distinction between the two conditions is purely a clinical one; pathologically, they differ only in that the characteristic abnormalities tend to be more severe and widespread in cases beginning at an earlier age than at the senile period. It is to be presumed that the basic underlying derangement is the same but that its effects differ somewhat, depending on the age of the patient.

Pathology. The brain presents a generally shrunken appearance, with atrophy of the convolutions and symmetric enlargement of the lateral and third ventricles. Frequently, these changes are especially pronounced in the frontal and temporal lobes. Microscopically, there is widespread loss of nerve cells, most apparent in the cerebral cortex, but often present likewise in the basal ganglia, with secondary glial proliferation. In addition, two types of lesions give this disease process its distinctive character. First, scattered throughout the cerebral cortex are microscopic deposits of amorphous material, most easily seen with silver staining methods. These are the so-called "senile plaques," which have been known for almost 70 years. They are generally considered to be an abnormal deposition or precipitation of material in the brain tissue, rather than the remains of diseased nerve cells. Despite numerous investigations and an extensive literature devoted to them, their origin and nature still remain uncertain. The other characteristic histopathologic feature is the Alzheimer fibrillary change in nerve cells. This striking abnormality, first clearly described by Alzheimer in his publication on presenile dementia, consists of the presence, within the cytoplasm, of thick fiberlike strands of silver staining material, often in the form of loops, coils, or tangled masses. This is a cytologic derangement which apparently ends in death of the cell, for clumps of these fibrils can often be seen even after the cell bodies within which they arose have disappeared. Despite ingenious attempts to explain them (cf. von Braunmühl, 1957), the true nature and meaning of these remarkable appearances have yet to be learned. Senile plaques and fibrillary changes occur most abundantly in the cortex and are widely distributed, although they are most frequent in the frontal lobes and hippocampal gyri. They have been encountered in all regions of the brain, but almost never occur in the spinal cord. In rare instances of otherwise typical diffuse cerebral atrophy, these characteristic tissue changes may be absent. Abundant pathologic evidence clearly establishes that the neuropathologic alterations just described are not related to vascular disease or to any known systemic disorder.

Clinical Aspects. Although Alzheimer's disease has been described as occurring during every age period, it is most frequently a disease of the later decades of life. A number of well-documented familial cases have been recorded, but there is not sufficient evidence to indicate that this is truly a hereditary disorder. Most of the cases actually seen in practice are sporadic. The onset is insidious and subtle, with changes first most noticeable in memory for recent happenings and in over-all judgment of situations. Emotional disturbances such as depression or anxiety states, or odd, unpredictable quirks of behavior, may be salient features in the early stages. Progression is very slow and gradual, and unless the condition is earlier brought to a close by the effects of advanced age, it may linger on for some 10 to 15 years.

In the milder cases, including those of the senile period, the noteworthy features are those of simple dementia, as described in Chap. 37. More unusual disorders of thought and intellect, including aphasia, apraxialike disturbances, and abnormalities of space perception, may be seen in the more severe forms, such as occur in the presenile group. Not infrequently, the patient walks in a shuffling manner with short steps, and there is a generalized stiffness of the musculature with slowness and awkwardness of all movements; these abnormalities have been attributed to involvement of the basal ganglia. Neurologic examination characteristically discloses no other significant findings. Additional investigative procedures, including the usual blood and cerebrospinal fluid determinations and electroencephalography, do not yield any conclusive or pertinent data. The enlargement of the ventricular system and subarachnoid space resulting from the diffuse brain atrophy can be demonstrated by pneumoencephalography; otherwise, no characteristic roentgenographic findings are seen. During the course of the illness, occasional convulsive seizures may occur, but they do not always accompany the disorder. Terminally, a state of total helplessness is reached, and the patient dies from intercurrent disease. Usually, long before the end, institutional care is necessary.

Differential Diagnosis. Several disease states for which effective treatment is available may give rise to progressive intellectual deterioration closely resembling what may be seen with the diffuse cerebral atrophy above described. It is imperative that these be looked for. Specific examples include chronic subdural hematoma, frontal meningioma, bromide intoxication, myxedema, pernicious anemia (vitamin B_{12} deficiency), and neurosyphilis. Various other forms of intoxication, infection, metabolic disorder, or neoplasm may have to be considered. Thus, in addition to careful clinical assessment, and whatever laboratory investigations may be indicated to exclude the various possibilities listed above, special procedures such as pneumoencephalography or carotid angiography may be necessary. Vascular disease of the brain is often included in the differential diagnosis, but dementia on the basis of cerebrovascular disorders characteristically progresses in a halting or stepwise fashion, whereas progression in senile dementia or Alzheimer's disease is gradual and steady.

No specific therapy is known. The management should be along the lines of that described in Chaps. 37 and 38 for the delirious and demented patient.

Pick's Disease (*Circumscribed Cerebral Atrophy*)

This remarkable form of cerebral disease characterized by the circumscription of the atrophy, a lobar sclerous, was first described in a series of publications by Arnold Pick in Prague, around the turn of the past century. In the differential diagnosis of dementia in the presenile period, it is often mentioned in the same breath with Alzheimer's disease. It is, however, an extremely rare condition as compared with diffuse cerebral atrophy of the Alzheimer type.

Pathology. So striking are the gross pathologic changes in the brain that in typical cases the diagnosis can be made at a glance. One sees severe atrophy of the anterior portions of the frontal and temporal lobes, and there is a curiously sharp line of demarcation between the atrophied portions and the remainder of the brain, which appears normal or nearly so. In some cases, the frontal atrophy is more prominent; in others, the temporal lobes are more severely involved; in general, both regions are affected. Not infrequently the process extends to the Rolandic and parietal regions, but the occipital lobes are spared. In many of the reported cases, the changes have been considerably more pronounced on one side of the brain than the other, an exception to the general rule of symmetry in degenerative nervous disease, but bilaterality is the rule. Characteristically, there likewise are atrophic changes in a number of subcortical structures: caudate nucleus, putamen, thalamus, and substantia nigra, and in the descending frontopontine fiber system. In the diseased regions, there is local destruction of central and convolutional white matter out of proportion to the degree of loss of nerve cell bodies in corresponding areas of the cortex; this finding has suggested that the peripheral axonal processes of the nerve cells, together with their myelin sheaths, may atrophy first, consequently that there may be a gradual "dying back" of the neurone from the periphery to the center. A noteworthy histologic feature of this condition is the occurrence of numerous swollen "ballooned-out" nerve cells in the atrophic regions, a finding which has been interpreted as an axonal reaction or retrograde cell change secondary to the degenerative process in the periphery. Another frequent cell nerve change is the presence of spherical intracytoplasmic inclusions that stain deeply with silver impregnation methods; the significance of these is unknown. The peculiarly selective nature of the degenerative process in Pick's disease has led some to classify it with the system diseases, although not all observers adhere to this view. Since the distribution of the brain atrophy is not related in any way to territories of vascular supply, it is to be presumed that this condition is not in any way the result of a disorder of cerebral circulation.

Clinical Aspects. There is no satisfactory way of differentiating between Alzheimer's and Pick's disease during life, nor is this of any practical importance. Early dilapidation of personality with relative preservation of such intellectual faculties as memory and gross reasoning ability are considered to be particularly characteristic of Pick's disease. Involvement of areas related to language function in the posterior frontal and anterior temporal regions of the dominant cerebral hemisphere may lead to pronounced aphasia. The disease is one of adult years, especially of the presenile period (with onset at age fifty to sixty). A considerable number of cases with earlier onset have been reported (the youngest at twenty-two); in these, the condition tends to be somewhat more severe than in older individuals, as in Alzheimer's disease. Familial occurrence is on record in a number of instances. Progression is slow and relentless, with an average duration of about 7 years.

Differential Diagnosis. The considerations noted above with respect to Alzheimer's disease apply to Pick's disease as well. The circumscribed frontotemporal atrophy can at times be demonstrated by pneumoencephalography. As with Alzheimer's disease there is no known treatment, but the principles of management are the same as those outlined above.

SYNDROME COMBINING DEMENTIA WITH OTHER NEUROLOGIC SIGNS

Huntington's Chorea (*Chronic Progressive Hereditary Chorea*)

This condition, which genetically follows the pattern of a mendelian dominant, was classically described in 1872 by George Huntington, who, with his father and grandfather, both physicians, observed cases in members of a family living near their home on Long Island. Unmistakable in its typical form, the affliction combines progressive dementia with bizarre involuntary movements and odd postures. Atypical cases have also been recognized (see below), but in general the disorder runs true to form.

Pathology. The brain has a generally atrophic appearance, especially noticeable in the frontal lobes. Particularly characteristic is severe bilateral atrophy of the caudate nucleus, which becomes flattened and concave instead of projecting as a convex rounded eminence into the anterior horn of the lateral ventricle. The putamen likewise is shrunken, although not to the same extent as the caudate nucleus. The globus pallidus is generally involved to some degree, but less severely than the caudate nucleus and putamen. Microscopically, the affected regions show severe nerve cell loss with reactive glial changes. The small nerve cells of the caudate nucleus and putamen appear to be more affected than the large ones. The disease process may likewise involve the thalamus, subthalamic nucleus (corpus Luysii), and dentate nucleus of the cerebellum. The cerebral cortex regularly shows loss of nerve cells, but other portions of the nervous system are usually spared, and there are no characteristic visceral lesions.

Clinical Aspects. This distressing condition generally makes its appearance in early to middle adult years, in what ordinarily would be the most effective and productive period of a person's existence. Its typical hereditary nature has been emphasized, but it is not at all rare for sporadic cases to occur. The involuntary movements (bizarre grimacing, respiratory irregularity, faulty articulation of speech, and irregular, arrhythmic, unpatterned movements of the limbs imparting to the gait a peculiar dancing quality) tend to be less quick and more athetoid than in Sydenham's chorea (see Chap. 26). A few reported cases which on genealogic and pathologic grounds must be classified with Huntington's chorea have shown progressive rigidity, rather than choreiform movements. As a general rule, dementia runs parallel with the motor disorder. Occasionally it may appear before or after chorea; very rarely it may be lacking altogether. The advance of the disease is slow. There is increasing disability both from involuntary movements and mental changes, terminated after many years by death from intercurrent infection or, not rarely, by suicide.

Differential Diagnosis. There is no difficulty in the recognition of typical cases. The relatively late onset, the slowly progressive course, the prominent dementia, and lack of association with rheumatic fever, help to exclude Sydenham's chorea. Hepatolenticular degeneration (Wilson's disease) may display clinical abnormalities resembling those of Huntington's chorea, but the specific changes characteristic of that disorder, including liver disease, corneal Kayser-Fleischer rings, and typical biochemical abnormalities (increased copper excretion, aminoaciduria), are absent in Huntington's chorea. Sporadic cases of choreiform movements beginning in middle or late life may present a difficult problem in exact diagnosis. The occasional cases of violent choreiform movements produced by vascular lesions, classically in the subthalamic region, are characterized by sudden onset, unilateral distribution (hemiballismus), and a tendency to improve after a period of initial severity. Virus encephalitis may occasionally be associated with choreiform movements; acute development, fever, and pleocytosis in the cerebrospinal fluid help in recognizing such cases, which can further be identified by appropriate virologic studies. Although it occurs rarely, self-limited chorea may appear in older persons without identifiable cause.

Treatment. It is impossible to halt the progress of this disease by any of the suggested forms of treatment. Chlorpromazine has been proposed as a means of controlling the chorea but has not been successful in the authors' hands.

Cerebrocerebellar Degeneration

The progressive cerebellar degenerations of late life, and some cases of spinocerebellar degeneration, may be accompanied by significant dementia, the pathologic basis for which is not always easily demonstrated. These disorders are dealt with more fully below in the section devoted to conditions manifested by ataxia.

Jakob-Creutzfeldt Disease

This name serves to identify a group of cases characterized by relatively rapid progression and widespread neuronal degeneration occurring in adult life. The original descriptions were by H. G. Creutzfeldt (1920) and A. M. Jakob (1921 and later). Since then additional studies of similar cases by a number of authors have led to the emergence of a more or less well-defined syndrome, within which there is, however, considerable variability both clinically and pathologically. Although most cases occur sporadically, the disease appears to be hereditary in one family on record.

Pathology. This condition is distinguished by widespread neuronal destruction and extensive astroglial proliferation chiefly involving the cerebral and cerebellar cortex. Subcortical nuclei are variably affected; the spinal cord, in the authors' experience, is spared. Although typically the pathologic changes affect all parts of the cerebral cortex, the characteristic changes may be virtually restricted to the occipitoparietal regions, as in the cases described by Heidenhain (1929) and Meyer, Leigh, and Bagg (1954). The lesions do not in any way suggest an inflammatory process. There are no significant vascular changes and no relevant abnormalities in other organs.

Clinical Aspects. Most of the cases described have begun between the ages of fifty and sixty, but the disorder may occur in young adults. In the early stages, a great variety of clinical manifestations may be seen, but those most frequently observed are changes in behavior, emotional responses, memory, and reasoning, together with abnormalities of vision such as peculiar distortions of the appearance of objects or actual impairment of visual acuity. The disease characteristically progresses with great rapidity, so that obvious deterioration may be seen from day to day. Sooner or later, in all cases, sudden myoclonic contractions of various muscle groups appear, perhaps unilaterally at first, but later becoming generalized. These generally are brought on by sudden sensory stimuli of all sorts, but they occur spontaneously as well, particularly in the late stages. Sudden jerks of individual fingers are typical. Ataxia and dysarthria are likewise prominent. Hallucinations, confusion, delusional ideas, and other evidences of delirium are frequently seen as the disease progresses. These changes gradually give way to stupor and coma, but the myoclonic contractions may continue to the end. Although abnormalities in the tendon and plantar reflexes may occur, they are not constant. In all cases, however, the electroencephalogram shows distinctive abnormalities, especially when the disease is fully developed. The total course of the illness is generally less than a year from onset; it may be confined to a few weeks or months. The outcome is invariably fatal, with death from intercurrent infection. Investigations of blood and cerebrospinal fluid consistently show no significant findings. A few cases have been extensively studied in an attempt to discover a toxic substance, infectious agent, or identifiable metabolic abnormality that might account for the pathologic changes, but without success.

Differential Diagnosis. In the earliest stages, the mental changes resulting from this disease may be misinterpreted as an atypical or unusually intense emotional reaction to environmental factors or as one of the major psychoses. Intoxication, as with bromides or other central nervous system depressants, or infection, such as neurosyphilis, may have to be considered, but none of these is likely to produce so dramatic a clinical picture. In its fully developed form, the only other disease process in adults that resembles it is a rare form of encephalitis thought (but not yet proved) to be due to viral infection ("subacute sclerosing encephalitis," see Chap. 287). The cerebrospinal fluid examination may help in differentiating these conditions, in that it is invariably normal in Jakob-Creutzfeldt disease, whereas the fluid may contain cells, or at least an abnormal colloidal gold reaction, in subacute encephalitis. In children or young adults, cerebral lipidosis (see below) may result in a similar combination of myoclonus and dementia, but there are typical retinal changes that do not occur in Jakob-Creutzfeldt disease. The other forms of presenile dementia do not display such a bewildering array of neurologic signs, and in them the course is much slower.

No treatment is known.

Amaurotic Family Idiocy and Other Lipidoses

The conditions to be considered here differ from other degenerative disorders in that the underlying biochemical abnormality is better defined. They are characterized by a more or less widespread derangement of lipid metabolism, which results in abnormal accumulations of lipids in the cytoplasm of cells of the nervous system and often of other organs as well. (For information relating to the problem of the lipidoses in general, Chaps. 95 and 283 should be consulted.) This process leads to abnormal function and, eventually, to death of the affected nerve cells. There is ample evidence for hereditary transmission of these disorders, the basis for which is presumed to be a genetically determined abnormality of enzymes concerned with intracellular lipid metabolism. What specific enzymes are abnormal and how disease results from their biochemical derangement have yet to be discovered, although considerable progress has been made in identifying the lipids involved. As far as is known, these substances are not foreign to the body or even to the cells in which they accumulate, but instead are normally present there although in much smaller quantities.

Special Clinical Types. The forms of lipidosis which affect the nervous system exclusively are generally classified together as "amaurotic family idiocy." This term emphasizes the important hereditary aspect, but it is not entirely satisfactory, since it can be correctly applied only to cases occurring in infancy. In the cases occurring in older children and adults, blindness (amaurosis) may never develop, and "idiocy," strictly speaking, implies defective intelligence existing from earliest infancy. Another name frequently given to this group of lipidoses is "cerebromacular degeneration," but it is accurate only for infantile cases and for patients with the combination of cerebral lesions and degeneration of the macular part of the retina.

Within the group designated as amaurotic family idiocy, the following varieties are generally distinguished:

Tay-Sachs Disease. This is the classic form of

amaurotic family idiocy occurring in infants, almost exclusively in Jewish families. It is characterized by extremely widespread neuronal involvement. In the retina, the lipid accumulation is especially pronounced in the nerve cells of the region surrounding the macula, so that this region appears pale on ophthalmoscopy. The normal red color of the macula thus stands out, giving the characteristic "cherry red spot." Typically, the affected children are normal at birth and for a few months thereafter. Then, generally between the third and tenth month of life, the infant becomes sluggish and apathetic. This is followed by obvious psychomotor regression. Simultaneously, there is progressive impairment of vision, leading finally to complete blindness. As the disease advances, convulsive seizures occur frequently, and the infant shows an abnormally active startle response to sounds. Eventually, there is a stage of complete dementia and paralysis (with hypotonia), and death, from intercurrent infection, usually occurs before the third year of age. Aronson (1959) has pointed out that if the child survives longer, as may result from skillful nursing care and vigorous treatment of infections, progressive enlargement of the head, simulating hydrocephalus, is to be expected.

Late Infantile Form (Bielschowsky). This variety, which is rare, begins at a somewhat later age than Tay-Sachs disease (age three to four) and has a more chronic course. Optic atrophy, rather than the macular red spot, is typical, and unsteadiness of gait with tremulous ataxia on attempted movements of the limbs (cerebellar ataxia) are prominent. In other respects, the clinical manifestations resemble those seen in Tay-Sachs disease. Death occurs after a total course of about 4 to 5 years.

Juvenile Form (Spielmeyer-Vogt). This form of lipidosis is not confined to patients of Jewish parentage. Clinically, the onset is between the ages of five to ten, and the course is relatively prolonged, with death at the time of adolescence or early adulthood. The disorder may begin with progressive visual impairment, or with personality changes and intellectual deterioration, and progresses gradually to blindness and dementia. On ophthalmoscopy, the retina shows the lesions of pigmentary degeneration (a form of retinitis pigmentosa). Additional clinical abnormalities which are useful in diagnosis are convulsions, myoclonic jerks, tremors at rest and on movement, rigidity, and dysarthria. Eventually a state of total helplessness is reached, and death soon follows.

Adult Form (Kufs). This is an extremely rare disorder with a very prolonged course. In all essential respects, it is identical to the juvenile form, except that retinal lesions may be completely absent. Progressive dementia combined with convulsive seizures and tremors or other involuntary movements is characteristic of this group. Late in the course, generalized rigidity may supervene. A duration of up to 20 years has been described.

Generalized Lipidoses with CNS Involvement. In addition to the group of lipidoses exclusively affecting the nervous system, there are a number of more generalized disorders of lipid metabolism in which the nervous system participates.

Niemann-Pick Disease. This disease has already been discussed in Chap. 95. The typical accumulation of large amounts of lipid in macrophages (reticuloendothelial cells) in many organs, including particularly the liver and spleen, is accompanied in almost all cases by lipidosis of the nervous system, similar to that occurring in the various forms of amaurotic family idiocy. The clinical abnormalities referable to the nervous system involvement consist chiefly of mental retardation and visual impairment. Convulsive seizures do not occur regularly, and the patients do not show the exaggerated startle response to sounds that is characteristic of Tay-Sachs disease. Other neurologic changes occur late. The disorder is considered to be a recessive hereditary trait. In most cases it becomes clinically apparent within the first year of life. The duration is variable; survival into adult years has been reported, but is extremely rare.

Gargoylism. This likewise is a metabolic abnormality affecting many organs. Affection of the nervous system is manifested clinically by mental retardation and pathologically by neuronal lipidosis.

For further information, Chap. 296 should be consulted.

Gaucher's Disease. This generalized metabolic disorder of childhood, already described in Chap. 95, resembles Niemann-Pick disease in many respects, inasmuch as it likewise is characterized by extensive lipid accumulations in various organs, especially the spleen, liver, and bone marrow. The nervous system, however, is much less regularly affected; it may be entirely normal in cases occurring in late childhood or adult life, although it usually is involved in infants. In infantile cases with involvement of the nervous system, the earliest stages are characterized by abnormalities referable to impaired function of cranial nerves, such as strabismus, dysphagia, weakness of the face and jaws, and extension of neck (opisthotonic postures). These changes are followed later by mental retardation, spasticity, and convulsions. Retinal lesions are not a constant feature, but have been described. Elevation of serum acid phosphatase, for unexplained reasons, is frequently found in Gaucher's disease but not in the other lipidoses.

Pathology. The characteristic neuropathologic change in all types of nervous system lipidosis is engorgement and distention of nerve cell bodies with the lipids concerned, resulting finally in death and disappearance of the diseased cells. Abundant chemical evidence indicates that in Tay-Sachs disease the abnormal lipid accumulation consists chiefly of gangliosides (Klenk). In the various other forms of amaurotic family idiocy, the histochemical findings (Diezel, 1960) suggest that gangliosides predominate in the diseased nerve cells, but quantitative chemical proof is lacking. Although in any one variety of neuronal lipidosis a particular form of lipid may be the one chiefly present, available evidence suggests that the abnormal accumulations are composed of a mixture of lipids in differing proportions, depending upon the particular type of disorder. Some of these differences are pointed out below.

In Tay-Sachs disease, the changes are of extreme degree and involve nerve cells at all levels, central and peripheral, including those in the walls of the viscera. In addition, the white matter, particularly in cases with prolonged survival, shows widespread devastation of myelinated fibers, more extensive than can be accounted for by loss of nerve cell bodies and the attendant degeneration of their axons. These white matter changes suggest that this variety of lipidosis may include a primary disorder of myelin and axons of the sort that characterizes the leukodystrophies to be discussed below.

In the forms of nervous system lipidosis occurring at later ages, the neuronal abnormalities are less severe and widespread than in infants. It can be stated as a general rule that the older the patient and the more chronic the course, the less pronounced are the neuronal changes. It is typical in the late infantile and juvenile forms for the cerebellum to be severely affected. In some adult cases the principal location of the pathologic alterations has been in the basal ganglions.

In gargoylism, the changes in the nerve cells are morphologically and histochemically identical with those found in the juvenile (Spielmeyer-Vogt) form of amaurotic family idiocy and are of similar distribution. The identity of the substances in the nerve cells has not been established chemically.

The lipid found to be in excessive amounts in the brain in Niemann-Pick disease is chiefly sphingomyelin rather than gangliosides, although these also may be increased. The histologic appearance of the nerve cells is indistinguishable from that in the other forms of neuronal lipidosis, although a difference can be shown histochemically.

Infantile Gaucher's disease is characterized by a considerable degree of nerve cell destruction in the cerebral cortex and brain stem and relatively slight amounts of intraneural lipid accumulation. Glycolipid-laden macrophages, resembling those seen in other organs, may be found in the brain. Cerebro-sides constitute the largest proportion of the abnormally accumulating lipids in this disease.

Differential Diagnosis. Typical instances of neuronal lipidosis in infancy or childhood are so distinctive as to be readily recognizable. The diagnosis of the Tay-Sachs form of the disease may be established by a biopsy of the rectal mucosa which demonstrates the typical nerve cell changes in the Meissner plexus. Diagnostic difficulties may arise, however, in atypical cases, or in those occurring during late childhood or adult life. Under such circumstances, other forms of progressive neurologic disease, such as neoplasms, chronic infective meningoencephalitis, or encephalopathy due to nutritional deficiency or heavy metal poisoning may have to be considered. In children, it may be difficult to distinguish during life between neuronal lipidosis and one of the progressive diseases of white matter (leukodystrophies) to be discussed below. In the latter group, however, convulsive seizures are met with less frequently and myoclonic jerks do not usually occur; furthermore, there are no visible retinal lesions. Subacute sclerosing encephalitis (of van Bogaert) may closely resemble juvenile amaurotic family idiocy, but is characteristically associated with a first zone elevation of the colloidal gold curve in the cerebrospinal fluid, whereas the cerebrospinal fluid is normal in the neuronal lipidoses. Jakob-Creutzfeldt disease must be mentioned because of some clinical similarities, but it affects a much older age group.

There is no known treatment. Families with one child must be warned of the strong likelihood of having other similar children since a recessive inheritance from both parents is the rule.

Leukodystrophy (Degenerative Diffuse Cerebral Sclerosis)

This rare group of conditions, in which familial incidence has frequently been observed, is characterized by a widespread disintegration of white matter in association with a remarkable sparing of the nerve cell bodies in the gray matter. There is thus a superficial resemblance to Schilder's disease ("encephalitis periaxialis diffusa"), which is best considered as an unusual variant of multiple sclerosis; in fact, the leukodystrophies have frequently been grouped together as "familial Schilder's disease." The best evidence at present indicates, however, that the leukodystrophies represent disorders of the metabolism of the myelin sheath lipids, and thus are probably most closely related to the neuronal lipidoses previously discussed. The leukodystrophies can be further classified on the basis of histopathologic and histochemical differences into a number of subtypes, which are considered below.

Pathology. The distinguishing feature is diffuse, symmetric breakdown of the white matter of the cerebral hemispheres, in which, as a rule, axones suffer damage to approximately the same degree as the myelin sheaths. Also characteristic is the presence, within the devastated regions, of lipid breakdown products of myelin which show distinct histochemical differences from the familiar lipid products met with in all the other disease processes destroying myelin, such as infarction, traumatic necrosis, secondary fiber tract degeneration, demyelinative lesions in multiple sclerosis or Schilder's disease, and so on. The relative intactness of the nerve cell bodies forms a striking contrast to the extensive white matter lesions.

Metachromatic Leukoencephalopathy. In an important group of cases, the lipid breakdown products display the staining reaction called metachromasia to a degree and intensity encountered in no other nervous system disease. Myelin at every level in the central and peripheral nervous system is involved in this variety of leukodystrophy, and engorgement of nerve cell bodies with similar metachromatic lipid has regularly been found in anterior horn cells of the spinal cord, dentate nuclei of the cerebellum, and in some of the nuclei of the brain stem and basal ganglions, but not in the cerebral cortex. The appearance of such cells is reminiscent of that in conditions such as amaurotic family idiocy (see above), but the location and histochemical behavior of the involved cells are different. Recent investigations (e.g., Austin, 1960) indicate that the metachromatic lipid is chiefly composed of cerebroside–sulfuric acid esters (sulfatides), which are a normal component of myelin. Possibly this material accumulates in abnormal amounts because of a failure of its utilization during the processes of myelin metabolism, an abnormality which in turn could well lead to breakdown of the myelin. It is noteworthy that similar metachromatic material is regularly found in kidney tubule cells and in Kupffer cells of the liver, unaccompanied by any functional disorder or tissue destruction in these organs. It seems most likely that the changes in these organs are a secondary phenomenon, resulting from the excretion of substances originating in the nervous system, rather than that the liver and kidneys are primarily involved in the metabolic disorder.

This form of leukodystrophy with metachromatic breakdown products has been encountered in infants, children, and young adults, occurring in a familial or sporadic pattern. It has not so far been found in old age. The familial diffuse cerebral sclerosis of Scholz has clearly been shown to belong to the group, and the similar familial cases of Bielschowsky and Henneberg almost surely do.

Krabbe Form of Leukodystrophy. In this variety, first described by Knud Krabbe in 1916 as a familial

disorder of infants, the lipid breakdown products also are atypical as compared with those occurring in most pathologic processes which destroy myelin. They differ histochemically from the metachromatic material just described in several ways, including absence of metachromasia. Typical of this disorder is the presence of unusual multinucleated phagocytic cells resembling foreign body giant cells, within which the lipid breakdown products are contained. Recent studies suggest that cerebrosides may predominate in the phagocytosed lipid (Cumings, 1960).

Late Life Leukodystrophy. In recent years, a few cases have been described of a very chronic form of white matter degeneration occurring in the presenile period, in which the atypical lipid products most closely resemble the lipofuscins, the "wear-and-tear" lipid pigment of advancing age. This is an extremely rare condition, about which very little so far is known.

Pelizaeus-Merzbacher Disease. In this condition, which is characterized clinically by a pronounced familial tendency and a very chronic course, the white matter lesions are patchy and irregular, rather than evenly distributed as in the other forms of leukodystrophy. Furthermore, there is relative sparing of axones. Another distinguishing feature of this disorder is that the breakdown products of the myelin, although very sparse (as would be expected from the prolonged course), are of the usual sort regularly seen with myelin destruction, rather than being atypical as in the conditions described above.

Clinical Aspects. The symptoms and signs in all the forms of leukodystrophy are mainly those of a progressive dementia, often associated in the early stages with weakness and unsteadiness of gait. Likewise prominent are spasticity and exaggeration of tendon reflexes, referable to the destructive lesions in the corticospinal motor system. Generalized convulsive seizures may occur but are not invariable. No clinical phenomena clearly serve to differentiate leukodystrophy from other diffuse progressive cerebral diseases. In the form with metachromatic breakdown products of myelin, it is possible to demonstrate metachromatic lipids in the urine which do not occur normally or in other diseases (Austin, 1957, cf. 1960). In this way, the diagnosis can be made during life.

Differential Diagnosis. Familial occurrence, signs referable to a disorder of long projection and associative fiber systems, and relative lack of convulsive manifestations may suggest the diagnosis during life. Otherwise, the identification of these conditions requires pathologic examination, except in so far as it may be possible to identify the metachromatic variety by appropriate examination of urinary sediment.

Progressive Familial Myoclonic Epilepsy

This rare disorder forms a distinct clinicopathologic syndrome characterized by recessive heredity. Typically, it appears in childhood or early adult life, beginning with generalized convulsive seizures, which are followed after an interval of years by myoclonic jerks of increasing frequency and severity and progressive dementia, with death before middle age. The pathologic features suggest a disorder of nerve cell metabolism, the nature of which remains unidentified.

Pathology. In many of the cases on record, there are distinctive intracytoplasmic inclusion bodies within nerve cells which may be found at all levels in the central nervous system, although they are most frequent in the dentate nucleus of the cerebellum, substantia nigra, and thalamus. These bodies, which have the histochemical properties of acid mucopolysaccharides, were initially described by Gonzalo Lafora (1911) and are generally known as Lafora bodies. In addition to these inclusions, there is always some degree of nerve cell loss in gray matter structures, together with some reactive gliosis. In a recently described case with typical clinical findings and numerous Lafora bodies in the brain and spinal cord, material histochemically similar to the Lafora bodies was found in heart muscle fibers and liver cells (Harriman and Millar, 1956). Some otherwise typical cases have been described in which Lafora bodies were absent. A few cases are on record in which the disorder was associated with the pathologic findings of amaurotic family idiocy.

Clinical Aspects. The onset in most cases is at about the time of puberty. The convulsive seizures, with which the disorder usually begins, are in no way distinctive. The myoclonic jerks are sudden, asymmetric or symmetric brief contractions of muscle groups of the limbs, face, and trunk, occurring arrhythmically and unpredictably, usually with sufficient force to displace the parts affected. They characteristically are provoked by all sorts of stimuli, but occur spontaneously as well. The sudden contractions may interfere seriously with willed movements, or may cause the patient to fall abruptly. The disorder progresses gradually, running a course over several years, with terminal stages characterized by profound dementia and total helplessness. Treatment with anticonvulsant medication may relieve the generalized convulsive seizures and reduce the frequency of the myoclonic jerks, but has no effect on the dementia.

Differential Diagnosis. Other forms of progressive dementia with myoclonus may have to be considered. These are discussed above under Jakob-Creutzfeldt disease and the lipidoses. In familial myoclonic epilepsy, convulsive seizures are more prominent than in the other disorders mentioned. The diagnosis may be suspected during life but can be confirmed only by autopsy.

There is no treatment.

Hallervorden-Spatz Disease

This unusual disorder, often familial, is associated with a rather variable clinical picture in which abnormalities of posture and muscle tone, involuntary movements, and progressive dementia predominate. Pathologically, there are characteristic abnormalities in the basal ganglions, suggesting a localized disorder of metabolism. The features of the condition were classically described in an affected family by Hallervorden and Spatz (1922).

Pathology. Distinctive of this condition is the accumulation of large amounts of pigmented material in the globus pallidus and zona reticulata of the substantia nigra, resulting in grossly visible brownish discoloration of these regions. Microscopically, there are irregular pigmented concretions and granules of varying brownish or greenish hues, depending upon the stains used. A considerable number of these show the presence of iron, and the local tissue iron is increased in amount. It is generally believed that these deposits of material consist of substances normally present in the regions affected, but greatly increased in quantity. There is no systemic disorder of iron metabolism. Nerve cell loss occurs in these regions and likewise to some extent in the cerebral cortex, although it generally is not so severe as in other forms of degenerative brain disease and is overshadowed by the pigmentary disorder in the basal ganglions.

Clinical Aspects. The disorder typically makes its appearance in childhood or adolescence, with abnormalities in muscle tone and movements such as rigidity and choreoathetosis. Abnormal postures of the trunk characteristic of torsion spasm (dystonia) may be seen. Cerebellar ataxia is also present in some cases. The tongue may protrude involuntarily from the mouth. Speech becomes indistinct, and there is progressive intellectual impairment. Eventually, the involuntary movements give way to increasing generalized rigidity, and death comes as a rule about 10 years after onset.

Differential Diagnosis. No feature of the clinical picture serves to distinguish this particular disorder from other conditions showing dementia with extrapyramidal motor abnormalities. Hepatolenticular degeneration must be excluded by appropriate laboratory tests. The clearly progressive course sets this condition apart from clinically similar abnormalities resulting from accidents or illnesses at birth or in the neonatal period. The disease is probably linked to the Kufs' type of lipidosis, at least in some patients.

There is no treatment.

Wilson's Disease (Hepatolenticular Degeneration)

This condition is discussed in Chap. 93.

SYNDROME CHIEFLY MANIFESTED BY SLOW DEVELOPMENT OF ABNORMAL POSTURES OR INVOLUNTARY MOVEMENTS

Paralysis Agitans (Parkinson's Disease)

This by no means rare conditions was named and classically described by James Parkinson in 1817. His remarkably complete account gives this definition: "Involuntary tremulous motion, with lessened muscular power, in parts not in action and even when supported; with a propensity to bend the trunk forward, and to pass from a walking to a running pace, the senses and intellects being uninjured."

Typically, paralysis agitans is a disorder of middle or late life, with very gradual progression and a prolonged course. Although it has been seen to occur in families (the estimated familial incidence is 6 per cent), it usually is sporadic. It bears no consistent relationship to any known disease process such as arteriosclerosis, trauma, or intoxication, although such conditions have often been invoked as etiologically significant and may at times produce somewhat similar clinical manifestations. It is well recognized, however, that the epidemic encephalitis of von Economo, which occurred in a world-wide distribution in the years following the First World War, was followed in a considerable number of cases by a syndrome clinically indistinguishable from paralysis agitans. It is usual in such instances to speak of postencephalitic parkinsonism, whereas the term Parkinson's disease should be reserved for true paralysis agitans of unknown cause.

Pathology. Despite the general familiarity with the condition and an extensive literature on the subject, it cannot be said that the pathologic changes of paralysis agitans are yet fully understood. The only regularly observed changes have been in the aggregates of melanin-containing nerve cells in the brain stem (substantia nigra, locus caeruleus, dorsal motor nucleus of the vagus), where varying degrees of nerve cell loss with reactive gliosis, most pronounced in the substantia nigra, along with distinctive eosinophilic intracytoplasmic inclusions (Lewy bodies, after their description by F. H. Lewy in 1913) are a consistent finding. Changes have also been described in other structures of the basal ganglions, but they are not clearly different in nature or degree from what may be encountered in other patients of similar age without extrapyramidal motor disorders. It is tempting, therefore, to consider paralysis agitans as belonging with the system diseases, the affected "system" being that of the pigmented nuclei of the brain stem. It is noteworthy that similar changes in the same groups of melanin-containing cells are likewise found in postencephalitic parkinsonism, which pathologically, as well as clinically, may be extremely difficult to distinguish from paralysis agitans.

Clinical Aspects. In its fully developed form, this disorder cannot be mistaken for any other. The stooped posture, the stiffness and slowness of movement, the rigidity of facial expression, and the rhythmic tremor of the limbs which subsides on active willed movement or complete relaxation are familiar to every clinician. Although symmetric in the later stages, the disorder typically begins asymmetrically, e.g., as a slight tremor of the fingers of one hand or in one leg. Also typical is more or less general stiffness of the musculature so that even where tremor is inapparent, the disease may betray itself by a somewhat staring and immobile facial expression, a monotonous voice, a general slowness of all motor activity, and a curious lack of the little spontaneous movements of postural change that are so characteristic of the normal individual. When tremor is minimal, patients often are able to alleviate it by resting their hands on a table or the arms of a chair or by keeping them in their pockets. The tremor, although fluctuating from moment to moment in amplitude and distribution, is perfectly regular, at a rate of about 4 to 6 per second. A fine, more rapid (action) tremor may be seen in the early stages of the disease, whereas a more violent trembling of greater amplitude characterizes the later course. The tremor is generally most pronounced in the hands but may involve also the legs (and thus secondarily the trunk), lips, tongue, and neck muscles, and is easily seen in the eyelids when they are lightly closed. There is no total paralysis, although general enfeeblement of voluntary movement is characteristic of the fully developed disorder. Together with the stooped attitude, there is the typical "festinating" gait, whereby the patient, prevented by the abnormaliy of postural tone from making the appropriate reflex adjustments required for effective walking, progresses with quick shuffling steps at an accelerating pace as if to catch up with his center of gravity. Clinical examination of the tendon and plantar reflexes discloses no abnormalities. There are no sensory changes, although deep aching in joints and muscles is common. Eventually, the patient may become so incapacitated by rigidity and tremor as to be helpless in caring for himself.

It has often been observed, however, that even severely disabled patients may under great emotional stress perform complex motor acts quickly and efficiently in a manner that ordinarily would be impossible for them. Thus, a patient may be able to jump up and run out of a burning building on hearing the call of "Fire"—only to be helpless as before once the crisis is past. Although the temporary alleviation under extreme provocation can never be long maintained, it is nevertheless true that the severity of the symptoms is considerably influenced by emotional factors, being aggravated by anxiety, tension, and unhappiness, and minimal when the patient is in a contented frame of mind. Despite the inherently progressive nature of the condition, much can be achieved with good medical management, and patients may continue for years to live effective, happy lives in spite of this affliction. Intellectual deterioration is not a consistent feature of paralysis agitans, but it must be conceded that in very advanced stages of the condition in some cases, dementia may be encountered.

Differential Diagnosis. In typical cases, this is not difficult. The extrapyramidal syndromes associated with most diseases of known cause or established nature such as cerebral vascular disease, cerebral hypoxia (including carbon monoxide asphyxia), or metallic poisoning differ from paralysis agitans in a number of respects, such as atypical behavior of tremor, presence of signs of pyramidal tract deficit, or early onset of dementia. The differentiation from postencephalitic parkinsonism may be impossible; a clear history of an attack of epidemic encephalitis (prolonged somnolence, disturbance of consciousness, diplopia) and relatively early age of onset of the disorder and the presence of tics, localized spasms, and oculogyric crises may be the only clues to this diagnosis. In recent years, a neurologic disorder strikingly similar to Parkinson's disease has been seen following the prolonged administration of large amounts of reserpine and similar drugs, which subsides on withdrawal of the offending drug—a matter of considerable theoretic and practical importance. Parkinsonism is rarely if ever produced by cerebral neoplasms.

Treatment. Although no known treatment influences the underlying disease process, patients with paralysis agitans can often be greatly helped by well-managed symptomatic therapy. An important part of any such program is to help the patient by means of sympathetic understanding to comprehend the nature of his illness and to carry on courageously in spite of it. The constant tremor and rigidity result in physical fatigue; thus patients generally require more rest than previously. Physical measures, such as massage, active exercises, and passive manipulations may promote greater muscular relaxation, alleviate the muscle and joint aching which

may be prominent and early symptoms of the disease, and help to prevent contractures.

Along with these general supportive measures, optimum treatment in most cases requires the wise use of antispasmodic drugs, singly or in combination. The program of medication in each case must be on an individual basis, with choice of drugs and adjustment of dosages under close medical supervision until a maximum of therapeutic benefit with a minimum of toxic side effects is achieved. At best, only a partial relief of symptoms can be expected, with rigidity in general responding better than tremor, although even the latter may be considerably allayed in some cases; but even partial relief may make the difference between effective living and incapacity.

The drug treatment of paralysis agitans (and postencephalitic parkinsonism) is on a purely empirical basis. It has long been known that some relief can be obtained with drugs of the belladonna group (atropine, scopolamine, stramonium), and these substances are still extensively used. A number of synthetic antispasmodics have become available and appear to be more effective in many instances than the older forms of medication. Preparations of this kind are trihexyphenidyl (Artane), ethopropazine hydrochloride (Parsidol, Lysivane), procyclidine hydrochloride (Kemadrin), cycrimine hydrochloride (Pagitane), benzatropine methanesulfonate (Cogentin), and caramiphen hydrochloride (Panparnit). Some of the antihistamines, such as phenindamine (Thephorin) and diphenhydramine (Benadryl), have likewise been shown to be helpful. A combination of drugs is often better than one alone. A recommended program is to begin with Parsidol, 10 to 20 mg, three to four times daily, and to increase this gradually at 3-day intervals to a maximum of one 100-mg tablet four times daily. If the patient already is taking one form of medication for this condition and it is desired to substitute another form, the older medication must be discontinued gradually by small decrements, rather than abruptly, while the newer one is being increased to full dosage; otherwise a severe increase of rigidity or tremor may occur. Toxic effects include nausea, lightheadedness, drowsiness, and particularly in older patients, mental confusion, often at night. These effects subside rapidly when smaller dosage is resumed. Once the optimum dosage with this preparation is reached, further therapeutic benefit may be achieved by adding other drugs, such as Artane (2- or 5-mg tablets, three to four times daily) or Thephorin (25 to 50 mg, three to four times daily), or both. It is to be emphasized that any of these drugs should be given to the threshold of toxicity before being discontinued as ineffective and that dryness of the mouth is an unavoidable side effect. Occasional patients, with drowsiness or sluggishness, are helped by the additional use of analeptics (dextroamphetamine, 5 mg, two to three times daily) but not late in the day so that sleep is not disturbed. Patients who are tense and restless may require judicious use of sedatives.

In recent years, surgical measures have been developed for the relief of parkinsonism and have been attended by very gratifying results in well-selected cases. The procedure consists of producing carefully localized focal destructive lesions in or near the globus pallidus or in the ventrolateral nucleus of the thalamus on the side opposite the tremor and rigidity. The anatomic and physiologic reasons for the effectiveness of these surgical lesions are still very poorly known. The best results are obtained in relatively young patients with normal intellectual faculties in whom the disease is chiefly unilateral; under such circumstances, dramatic benefit may be obtained by a correctly placed contralateral lesion. Bilateral operations are carried out, sometimes with excellent results, but the risks of mental and physical crippling are greater. Advanced stages of the disease and dementia are absolute contraindications for surgical treatment. Any surgery for this disease must, of course, be carried out by a neurosurgeon who is particularly trained in and competent in these special techniques.

Dystonia Musculorum Deformans (Torsion Spasm)

This is a clinical term, denoting a state characterized by slow, nonrhythmic involuntary movements which produce abnormal, at times bizarre, postures of the trunk and limbs. With passage of time, these postures tend to become more or less fixed. Underlying the clinical disorder may be any of several pathologic conditions, such as the residual lesions of epidemic encephalitis, the pigmented deposits of Hallervorden-Spatz disease (described above), hepatolenticular degeneration (Wilson's disease), or the scars of cerebral birth injury in the broad sense, or kernicterus. In addition, there are a few rare cases with relatively early onset and progressive course and, in some instances, familial occurrence.

Pathology. Very few cases have been studied pathologically. In some, the caudate nucleus and putamen were the chief sites of disease; in others, the globus pallidus was affected without significant alteration of other parts of the corpus striatum. In addition, lesions have been found in the thalamus and subthalamic nucleus in a few instances. The abnormalities have consisted of simple cell loss with reactive gliosis, without specific features. Because of the variability in the location of lesions, it has not been possible to relate the motor abnormalities to disease in any specific anatomic structures.

Clinical Aspects. The motor abnormalities are described in Chap. 26. In the early stages, the involuntary muscular contractions are intermittent and variable in location and severity, but typically interfere with motor performance by superimposing an unwanted posture upon parts in use. Progression may be relatively rapid in cases with onset during early childhood, but is slow in those beginning in late childhood or adult life. The end-result is extreme disability, with grossly distorted postures of the trunk and contractures of the limbs. Affection of face and tongue muscles results in faulty articulation of speech, which eventually becomes incomprehensible. The tendon and plantar reflexes, which can be assessed only during moments of relaxation of the affected parts, are characteristically normal.

Dementia is not a necessary accompaniment of the condition, except perhaps in the terminal stages; but with severe derangement of all available methods of communication, an adequate evaluation of mental capacity may be impossible.

Spasmodic torticollis (see Chap. 26) may well be a form of dystonia, but it typically does not progress to involve the musculature generally. However, torticollis may be an early symptom in cases later showing the typical generalized motor abnormalities.

Differential Diagnosis. Hepatolenticular degeneration should be seriously considered in any case presenting these motor symptoms, and appropriate measures should be undertaken for its investigation (see Chap. 93). The progressive course, and possibly the family history, differentiate the degenerative group from the "symptomatic" dystonias resulting from infections or metabolic disorders occurring at birth or later.

Treatment. This is most unsatisfactory. Dystonia is notoriously unresponsive to drug therapy, although antispasmodic drugs such as those used for parkinsonism should be tried. Surgical relief has been attempted in a few cases, with some promising early results in approximately 80 per cent and a 5.6 per cent mortality. This is the only treatment of any real value. Pending decision to operate it is worthwhile to try the drugs used in the treatment of Parkinson's disease.

SYNDROME CHIEFLY MANIFESTED BY SLOWLY DEVELOPING ATAXIA

The conditions about to be considered are distinguished clinically by progressive unsteadiness in standing and walking, along with more or less impairment of the coordination of other motor acts. Pathologically, they are characterized by degeneration of the cerebellum and/or its related fiber systems, and thus constitute classic examples of the system diseases. Although sporadic instances occur, hereditary transmission is an outstanding feature in many cases; thus, this group of disorders is often referred to as the hereditary ataxias. Their subdivision into more or less separate entities is largely arbitrary, with pathologic changes of varying distribution underlying clinically indistinguishable symptom complexes. Furthermore, there is considerable overlapping with other forms of hereditary nervous disease, so that in a given case a remarkable combination of defects may be encountered. These facts have led to the idea that in the ataxias there is a group of closely related genetically determined abnormalities that may occur together in an almost infinite series of combinations, so that it is not possible to separate out well-defined disease pictures. Nevertheless, certain constellations of symptoms and pathologic findings occur with sufficient regularity to warrant their separation for purposes of discussion. The classification about to be given is not entirely satisfactory but is designed to be of practical help to the physician confronted with a case.

Cerebellar Degenerations

To be discussed are the forms of progressive ataxia which are associated with pathologic changes predominantly in the cerebellum. These include both hereditary and sporadic cases and comprise, in addition, the rather rare subacute spinocerebellar degeneration associated with the presence of carcinoma of various types elsewhere in the body. The hereditary and sporadic forms of cerebellar degeneration resemble one another so closely that, for the purposes of the present discussion, they will all be referred to as "hereditary cerebellar degeneration." Most cases are seen in adults, with the onset occurring in middle life.

Pathology. In hereditary cerebellar degeneration the cerebellum is obviously atrophied. In one group of cases, these changes are chiefly localized to the superior vermis and adjacent parts of the cerebellar cortex, whereas in an even larger group, the entire cerebellar cortex is affected. Microscopically there is loss of nerve cells principally affecting the Purkinje cells, although the granule cells are often involved as well. In most cases, there is an associated atrophy of nerve cells in the inferior olivary nuclei in a distribution dependent upon the location and extent of the changes in the cerebellar cortex. It no longer seems justifiable to separate the cases with associated olivary degeneration from the rest and to designate them as "cerebello-olivary degeneration," as has been done in the past. In *olivopontocerebellar degeneration,* there are extensive degenerative changes in the pontine nuclei, middle cerebellar peduncles, and olivary nuclei. In addi-

tion changes in the cerebellar cortex such as have been noted above may or may not be present. In all varieties of cerebellar degeneration, affection of other neuronal systems—as, for instance, the cerebral cortex and basal ganglions—may be encountered. In some cases, there are changes in the dentate and roof nuclei of the cerebellum and their projections in the superior cerebellar peduncles (*dentatorubral atrophy*), but these are always found in association with more diffuse cerebellar or spinocerebellar degeneration. *Carcinomatous cerebellar (spinocerebellar) degeneration* is characterized by extensive cell loss in all parts of the cerebellar cortex, often associated with inflammatory (lymphocytic) infiltrations in the perivascular and subarachnoid spaces. In addition there are degenerative changes in the long fiber tracts of the spinal cord. These lesions do not depend upon the presence of tumor implants anywhere in the nervous system or its coverings, but rather are thought to be due to a metabolic abnormality somehow resulting from the presence of carcinoma.

Clinical Aspects. In the hereditary form of cerebellar degeneration the abnormality appears first in the legs, resulting in unsteadiness of stance and gait of the peculiar wavering, lurching character so typical of cerebellar ataxia (see Chap. 26). This has been correlated with the localization of changes in the superior vermis of the cerebellum and adjacent parts of the cerebellar cortex. With more extensive cerebellar involvement, a disturbance in articulation and rhythm of speech occurs that may progress to total incomprehensibility, and the arms likewise become ataxic. There may be nystagmus, but it is often absent. Where there is affection of other neuronal systems, additional neurologic abnormalities, such as exaggerated tendon reflexes, extensor plantar responses, rigidity, tremor, and dementia, may be encountered (*cerebrocerebellar degeneration*). Progression is gradual and slow, being measured in decades, and may not necessarily shorten life. There is no specific treatment available for any of the progressive ataxias, although encouragement and gait training may enable a patient to overcome his disability to some extent.

In the cases associated with carcinoma, the tempo of evolution of the process is relatively rapid, with severe disability coming on within a period of months. Vertigo, diplopia, and nausea may be prominent. In an occasional case, the neurologic symptoms have appeared before there was any obvious evidence of carcinoma. In contrast to the consistently normal cerebrospinal fluid findings in the forms of cerebellar degeneration noted above, the cerebrospinal fluid may show increased lymphocytes and protein in carcinomatous spinocerebellar degeneration.

Differential Diagnosis. The slow but relentless

progression in the absence of abnormalities in the cerebrospinal fluid distinguishes the hereditary group from other forms of cerebellar ataxia such as may occur with neoplastic, infectious, or demyelinative disease, with drug intoxications (e.g., barbiturates), or with hyperpyrexia. The degenerative disorders under discussion tend to occur in a setting of otherwise good general health; this, together with other clinical differences, distinguishes them from the ataxia of deficiency disease, as in the Wernicke-Korsakoff syndrome (see Chap. 288). The form of spinocerebellar degeneration associated with carcinoma may be distinguished from direct carcinomatous involvement of the nervous system by the symmetry of the findings and the absence of increased intracranial pressure. Alcoholic cerebellar degeneration usually develops rapidly, and then may remain more or less stationary for the remainder of the patient's life (Chap. 288).

Hereditary Ataxia of Pierre Marie

This designation has been applied to cases of hereditary progressive ataxia with onset in early adulthood. Considerable doubt has been raised as to the validity of retaining the concept of Marie's hereditary ataxia, because pathologically this is by no means a uniform group. When Pierre Marie wrote about the subject in 1893, Friedreich's ataxia (to be described below) had relatively recently become recognized as a distinct entity. Marie pointed out, on the basis of case reports in the literature, that there were other cases of hereditary ataxia, of later onset, which could not be fitted into Friedreich's description. He offered the suggestion that the cerebellum itself was the major site of disease in these cases. Subsequent pathologic examination of the cases he reviewed have shown that he was partly in error in this supposition; nevertheless, following his report, the concept of Marie's ataxia has appeared repeatedly in the writings on hereditary ataxia. Cases that might be classified with this group either are indistinguishable from those discussed above under the cerebellar degenerations or are variants of Friedreich's ataxia.

Friedreich's Ataxia

This classic form of hereditary ataxia, first clearly depicted by Nikolaus Friedreich of Heidelberg in 1863, forms a relatively distinct symptom complex which generally runs true to form, although it overlaps other heredodegenerative syndromes, particularly the chronic peripheral neuropathies and progressive optic atrophy, conditions to be discussed subsequently. Friedreich's ataxia is typically a disease of childhood or adolescence, although onset at a somewhat later age has occasionally been seen. In some families, the disorder occurs with dominant inheritance; it is a recessive trait in others.

Pathology. The principal changes are in the spinal cord and peripheral nerves; they are typical of a chronic degenerative process. In the cord the disease affects chiefly the sensory fibers of the posterior columns, the spinocerebellar tracts, and the corticospinal (pyramidal) tracts. Additional lesions of varying extent may be found in the brain stem and in the cerebellum itself, although the latter structure occasionally is intact. Involvement of other parts of the central nervous system at higher levels occasionally occurs. In the peripheral nerves the lesions vary likewise in severity and extent. They resemble those encountered in the chronic peripheral neuropathies to be described below. In addition to the neuropathologic changes, there is in some cases a peculiar form of myocardial degeneration resulting in thickening and fibrosis of the myocardium. There are no other associated visceral lesions.

Clinical Aspects. As with other progressive ataxias, the disorder first appears in the legs. Thus, the child patient, previously healthy, begins to stagger and lurch in walking and is unsteady, often in a tremulous fashion, on standing. Clumsiness and intention tremor of the hands and arms appear later, along with faulty articulation and abnormal rhythm (scanning) of speech. These symptoms usually result from changes in the cerebellum. The limbs, in addition to being ataxic, generally show considerable weakness. Examination usually discloses nystagmus and skeletal deformities: kyphoscoliosis, the basis for which is not certain, and a peculiar foreshortening and high arching of the feet (pes cavus) with cocking up of the toes (sometimes called the "Friedreich foot"), best ascribed to atrophy and contractures of the musculature of the feet. Typically, there is the unusual combination of total absence of tendon reflexes with extensor plantar reflexes (Babinski sign). This results from the presence of pyramidal tract degeneration together with peripheral neuropathy. The presence of a peripheral neuropathy is further indicated by impairment of position and vibration sense in the extremities and, in some patients, by impairment of the sensations of pain, temperature, and light touch in a roughly glove-and-stocking distribution. The optic disks may be pale, indicating optic atrophy, although actual blindness is relatively rare. Some patients are of low intelligence or may become demented in the course of the disease. Survival beyond early adult life is rare, with death frequently the result of associated myocardial disease.

Occasionally very mild or fragmentary forms of the disorder (such as pes cavus and absent or hyperactive tendon reflexes) may be encountered, with little if any disability or progression. Such abnormalities are most likely to be seen in other members of the family of a patient afflicted with the fully developed form of the disease.

Differential Diagnosis. The classic form of Friedreich's ataxia is readily recognizable and cannot easily be confused with other conditions. It is to be expected, however, that variations in the clinical manifestations may occur because of the variable pathologic changes. One particularly well-known variant was described in 1926 by Levy and Roussy, in which the muscle wasting of the legs is severe and is combined with areflexia and a sensory ataxia. There have been reports of Friedreich's ataxia in some members of a family and of the Levy-Roussy syndrome in others. In the absence of a family history, and with atypical clinical findings, further diagnostic studies to exclude tumor, chronic basal meningitis, intoxication, or congenital malformation will be necessary.

No treatment is known. Physical medicine and rehabilitation measures are of little value in cerebellar ataxia.

SYNDROME WITH SLOW DEVELOPMENT OF MUSCULAR WEAKNESS AND WASTING, WITHOUT SENSORY CHANGES

Motor System Disease

This general term is used to designate a progressive disorder of motor neurones in the cerebral cortex, brain stem, and spinal cord, manifested clinically by muscular weakness, with muscle atrophy and spasticity with exaggeration of tendon reflexes in varying combinations. It is a disease of middle life, generally appearing in the fifth or sixth decades. Customarily a subdivision is made on the basis of the particular grouping of symptoms and signs observed. Thus, the most frequent form, in which muscular atrophy and hyperreflexia are combined, is called *amyotrophic lateral sclerosis.* Rather more rare are the cases in which weakness and atrophy alone exist without clinical evidence of corticospinal tract dysfunction; for these, the term *progressive muscular atrophy* is used. Where the disorder affects predominantly the musculature innervated by the cranial nerves, it is usual to speak of *progressive bulbar palsy.* Very rarely, the clinical state is dominated by spasticity and hyperreflexia without obvious muscular wasting; such cases are classed as *primary lateral sclerosis.* There is no reason to believe that these subgroupings are anything other than clinical variants of the same disease process, which is another classic example of a system disease. Most cases are sporadic, but occasionally this disorder occurs in families in a manner suggesting genetic transmission.

Pathology. There is widespread selective atrophy and loss of motor nerve cells at all levels of the central nervous system, including the Betz cells in the motor areas of the cerebral cortex. Some evidence of disease in the corticospinal motor system is usually found pathologically, even when physical signs referable to such changes were not observed during life. The atrophy of fibers in skeletal muscles is typically that due to loss of motor innervation.

Clinical Aspects. The disease begins insidiously and may be well advanced before the patient is aware of it. Although often asymmetric initially, the weakness and muscular wasting gradually become symmetric and widespread. Classically, the disorder becomes first evident in the small muscles of the hands, but it may begin in one or both legs, or in muscles supplied by cranial nerves. Vague feelings of discomfort in the muscles, tightness, numbness (without objective sensory changes), and recurrent cramps may be early symptoms. The progressive atrophy of the musculature is accompanied by widespread visible fascicular twitchings of groups of muscle fibers, a classic feature that can be related to degeneration of the motor nerve cells supplying the involved muscles. Despite extensive involvement of skeletal muscles generally, sphincter control remains intact. Sooner or later the disease affects muscles supplied by the brain stem, resulting in weakness, atrophy, and fasciculations in the tongue and facial musculature associated with dysarthria and impairment of chewing or swallowing. The functions of the ocular muscles, oddly enough, are invariably spared. In most cases, the weakness and muscular wasting are accompanied by exaggeration of tendon reflexes, extensor plantar reflexes and spasticity, to a degree dependent upon the severity of degeneration in the corticospinal (pyramidal) motor system. Affection of corticobulbar fibers results in manifestations of pseudobulbar palsy such as involuntary weeping or laughter, exaggerated reflex movements of the facial muscles of expression, and sucking reflexes. Progression is unhalting and relatively rapid, leading to extensive paralysis, with death from respiratory weakness or aspiration pneumonia, generally within about 2 to 5 years or more from onset. Intelligence and awareness are typically preserved to the end.

Differential Diagnosis. Spinal cord compression from tumors in the cervical region or from cervical spondylosis with osteophytes projecting into the vertebral canal can at times give rise to weakness, wasting, and fasciculations in the upper limbs and spasticity in the legs, thus closely resembling amyotrophic lateral sclerosis. The absence of cranial nerve involvement may be helpful in differentiation, although some compressive lesions at the foramen magnum may implicate the twelfth cranial (hypoglossal) nerve, with resulting affection of the tongue. Absence of pain or of sensory changes, normal function of bowels and bladder, normal roentgenographic studies of the spine, and absence of changes in the composition or dynamics of the cerebrospinal fluid are all points in favor of motor system disease and against spinal cord compression. Where doubt exists, contrast myelography should be performed and the cervical region should be visualized.

Chronic inflammatory disorders of the meninges and spinal cord, exemplified by syphilitic meningomyelitis or some cases of adhesive arachnoiditis, may have to be considered. These conditions can readily be recognized by cerebrospinal fluid changes and, if necessary, by abnormal myelographic findings. Nutritional myelopathy can be excluded by history and on other clinical grounds.

Although fasciculations are a prominent feature of motor system disease, they are not, in the absence of weakness, muscle atrophy, or loss of tendon reflexes, valid signs of it, for they may occur in a variety of metabolic or toxic disorders (e.g., thyrotoxicosis, salt depletion) as well as in otherwise healthy individuals. Careful clinical evaluation suffices in such instances to exclude serious neurologic disease.

Progressive weakness from intrinsic disease of muscle (myopathy, polymyositis) may occasionally be difficult to distinguish from progressive muscular atrophy of the type under discussion; yet the differentiation is important from the standpoint of prognosis or treatment. Under such circumstances, the diagnosis can be made by muscle biopsy and electromyography.

There is no known treatment for any form of motor system disease.

Infantile Muscular Atrophy (Werdnig and Hoffmann), Amyotonia Congenita (Oppenheim)

The form of progressive muscular atrophy described by Werdnig and Hoffmann is a disease of infants and young children, typically afflicting several members of a family. Pathologically, it closely resembles the adult disease described above. Amyotonia congenita is a purely clinical term, used to designate abnormal laxness of somatic musculature observed at birth or in early infancy; it may occur in a number of different pathologic processes, including Werdnig-Hoffmann disease. For further details of these conditions, Chap. 283 should be consulted.

Hereditary Spastic Paraplegia

This very rare disorder is characterized by weakness and spasticity of the legs, with early onset (childhood or adolescence) and slow progression. Later the arms may be affected, but usually to a lesser degree. The pathologic changes closely resemble those of Friedreich's ataxia, and there is reason now to believe that this condition is in fact an incomplete form of Friedreich's disease in which spastic weakness overshadows minimal or absent ataxia and sensory changes. The diagnosis is made by the family history and by excluding other possible causes of bilateral spastic weakness of the limbs. The relationship to Friedreich's ataxia is further confirmed by the occurrence of pes cavus and optic atrophy in some cases. One group of patients also has progressive dementia.

SYNDROME COMBINING WEAKNESS AND WASTING WITH SENSORY CHANGES

Progressive Neural Muscular Atrophy

The degenerative disorders characterized by progressive weakness and wasting of skeletal muscles combined with sensory changes are chronic diseases of peripheral nerves, often occurring as hereditary conditions. Although clinical and pathologic subvarieties exist, there is no sharp dividing line between them and they are best considered together under the designation given above, in which the term "neural" emphasizes the peripheral nerve affection. As already pointed out above, chronic peripheral neuropathy is an associated disorder in some of the hereditary ataxias and is regularly encountered in the classic form of Friedreich's ataxia. An additional connecting link with other genetically determined nervous diseases is the occurrence of progressive optic atrophy or pigmentary degeneration of the retina in some cases. Common to all is for the peripheral neuropathy to begin distally and to progress in a centripetal fashion and for the feet and legs to become first affected, with involvement of the hands and more proximal parts only after a considerable interval.

The variety most usually seen is that generally called *peroneal muscular atrophy* (*Charcot-Marie-Tooth disease*), a name which draws attention to the changes in the lower legs, although the disorder affects far more than the peroneal muscle groups or nerves. This condition was first clearly differentiated from other forms of muscular atrophy by Charcot and Marie in France, and independently by H. H. Tooth in England, in 1886. In rare cases which are otherwise similar, there is a remarkable palpable thickening of peripheral nerve trunks. Such cases are generally designated as *hypertrophic interstitial neuropathy* (of *Déjerine and Sottas*, the French neurologists who, in 1893, first described the condition clinically and pathologically). In a few cases, there are pronounced trophic and vasomotor abnormalities of the affected parts, chiefly the feet, which may lead to chronic poorly healing perforating ulcers on the ball of the foot among other abnormalities (*familial neuro-vascular dystrophy,* Wadulla, 1949, Krücke, 1955; *hereditary sensory neuropathy,* Denny-Brown, 1951). Probably related is the unusual condition described by Refsum (1946) and called by him *heredopathia atactica polyneuritiformis,* in which peripheral neuropathy and ataxia are associated with progressive nerve deafness, retinitis pigmentosa, and a high cerebrospinal fluid protein, and possibly familial amyloid polyneuropathy.

Pathology. The lesions are typical of a chronic multiple peripheral neuropathy with secondary atrophic changes in muscles. The degenerative process in the nerve fibers is associated with abortive regenerative phenomena and with proliferation of connective tissue and Schwann cells which, in the hypertrophic variety, may reach extreme degrees. In the central nervous system, there are varying degrees of overlap with the lesions found in the various forms of hereditary ataxia already discussed.

Clinical Aspects. The disorder usually begins in childhood and progresses very slowly. In the classic cases of peroneal muscular atrophy, the combination of pes cavus with extreme atrophy of the anterior tibial and calf muscles ("stork legs") and wasting of the lower thigh musculature (giving an appearance like an "inverted champagne bottle") presents a striking picture. There is total absence of deep reflexes, and sensation is altered as described above under Friedreich's ataxia. The possibility of combinations with other hereditary neurologic syndromes has already been pointed out. Although death in a state of extreme debility in early adult life is common, progression in some cases may be extremely slow and may lead to very little disability.

Differential Diagnosis. It may be necessary to consider various other forms of chronic polyneuropathy (toxic, metabolic, nutritional), described in Chap. 29. However, the familial incidence, early onset, very slow progression, and absence (usually) of significant cerebrospinal fluid changes, except for increased protein in some patients, are generally sufficient for the accurate recognition of the hereditary neuropathies under discussion. In occasional sporadic or atypical cases, biopsy of muscle and of a small cutaneous nerve twig (most conveniently the sural cutaneous nerve) will be necessary.

Treatment. Although no specific treatment is available, patients whose disease is of slow progression and in whom conditions are otherwise favorable may be greatly helped by measures to ensure a stable walking surface, such as corrective shoes, braces to prevent foot drop, and even orthopedic procedures to stabilize the joints.

SYNDROME CHIEFLY MANIFESTED BY PROGRESSIVE VISUAL LOSS

As already stated in previous sections, progressive impairment or loss of vision, due to degenerative changes in the visual system (retinas and optic nerves), may be an accompaniment of morbid processes affecting the nervous system diffusely— in particular, the nervous system lipidoses and the hereditary ataxias. Occasionally, however, the peripheral visual system is the major, or only, site of disease. In such cases, the disorders are strongly hereditary. For detailed discussion of these conditions, standard reference works on ophthalmology should be consulted. Nevertheless, two entities, because of their close relationship with other degenerative diseases of the nervous system, warrant some discussion here.

Hereditary Optic Atrophy (Leber)

This rare condition is characterized by the relatively rapid development of bilateral blindness with optic atrophy, coming on in early adult life. It was first thoroughly described by Leber in 1871. Typically, it occurs as a sex-linked recessive trait, chiefly affecting men; but it likewise may be seen in women.

Pathology. In the only recorded case with autopsy, the changes occurred primarily in the ganglion cells of the retina, with secondary degeneration in optic nerve fibers. Because of the limited examination in this case, it is not known whether there were lesions in other parts of the nervous system.

Clinical Aspects. The condition often begins asymmetrically, with blurring of vision in one eye followed in days or weeks by similar affection of the other eye. Vision then deteriorates rapidly over ensuing weeks or months, generally with eventual total blindness as a result, although arrest before this stage has been seen, or even a little improvement after initial steady progression. In the early stages, examination of the visual fields shows large central scotomas. The optic disks may be normal at first, or may be swollen (optic neuritis); later, the appearance is typically that of optic atrophy, with pale, clearly outlined disks.

Differential Diagnosis. Multiple sclerosis may at times act in a manner identical to that just described, but without a definite hereditary background and with a much better outlook for improvement of vision. Toxic or nutritional amblyopia can generally be excluded by history and associated clinical findings. In some cases it may be necessary to eliminate the possibility of a tumor compressing the chiasmal region and optic nerves, although some evidence of bitemporal defects would be then expected, rather than bilateral central scotomas alone. In addition to careful roentgenograms of the skull and cerebrospinal fluid examination, pneumoencephalographic visualization of the chiasmal region may be indicated in cases of serious doubt.

Pigmentary Degeneration of the Retina (Retinitis Pigmentosa)

This may at times occur as a relatively independent disorder, although it is often associated with other abnormalities, of which cataracts, deafness, and mental deficiency are outstanding. It is strongly hereditary, chiefly as a recessive trait, although dominant inheritance has been seen. Pigmentary degeneration of the retina is one of the features of the Laurence-Moon-Biedl syndrome (Chap. 29). Special varieties of the condition also accompany some cases of neuronal lipidosis or hereditary ataxia, as already noted.

Pathology. The principal lesion is a degeneration of the rods and cones, associated with displacement of melanin-containing cells from the pigment epithelium into more superficial parts of the retina. Other retinal structures are relatively intact.

Clinical Aspects. The disorder typically begins in childhood, first as night blindness. The visual fields become concentrically narrowed from the periphery to the center, until eventually (by adolescence, or perhaps not until middle age) very little useful vision remains. Ophthalmoscopic examination may be normal at first, but generally discloses irregular patches of dark pigment in the periphery of the retina. When cataracts are likewise present, as sometimes is the case, visual acuity may be significantly improved by their removal. The frequent association of the retinal lesions with other abnormalities has been mentioned in previous paragraphs.

Differential Diagnosis. Chorioretinitis from other causes (e.g., syphilis) may present a similar ophthalmoscopic appearance and should be excluded. The hereditary background and the progressive course, with night blindness and peripheral constriction of the visual fields, may lead to the diagnosis even in the rare cases where pigmentary deposits in the retina are absent. In most instances, the opinion of a qualified ophthalmologist must be obtained.

REFERENCES

Aronson, S. M., A. Lewitan, A. M. Rabiner, N. Epstein, and B. W. Volk: The Megalencephalic Phase of Infantile Amaurotic Familial Idiocy, A.M.A. Arch. Neurol. Psychiat., 79:151, 1958.

Austin, J. H.: Observations on the Syndrome of Hypertrophic Neuritis (the Hypertrophic Interstitial Radiculo-neuropathies), Medicine, 35:187, 1956.

——: Metachromatic Form of Diffuse Cerebral Sclerosis: I. Diagnosis during Life by Urine Sediment Examination, Neurology, 7:415, 1957; II. Diagnosis during Life by Isolation of Metachromatic Lipids from Urine, Neurology, 7:716, 1957; III. Significance of Sulfatide and Other Lipid Abnormalities in White Matter and Kidney, Neurology, 10:470, 1960.

Critchley, M. (Ed.): "James Parkinson 1755–1824," New York, The Macmillan Company, 1955.

Crocker, A. C., and S. Farber: Niemann-Pick Disease: A Review of Eighteen Patients, Medicine, 37:1, 1958.

Diezel, P. B.: Lipidoses of the Central Nervous System, chap. 3 in "Modern Scientific Aspects of Neurology," J. N. Cumings (Ed.), London, Edward Arnold Ltd., 1960.

Doshay, L. J.: Treatment of Parkinson's Disease: I. Medicinal Therapy, New Engl. J. Med., 264:988, 1097, 1961.

Gowers, W. R.: A Lecture on Abiotrophy: Diseases from Defect of Life, Lancet, I:1003, 1902.

Greenfield, J. G.: "The Spino-Cerebellar Degenerations," Springfield, Ill., Charles C Thomas, Publisher, 1954.

—— et al.: "Neuropathology," London, Edward Arnold Ltd., 1958.

Harriman, D. G. F., and J. H. D. Millar: Progressive Familial Myoclonic Epilepsy in Three Families: Its Clinical Features and Pathological Basis, Brain, 78:325, 1955.

Lubarsch, Henke, and Rössle (Eds.): "Handbuch der speziellen pathologischen Anatomie und Histologie," vol. 13, "Nervensystem," Berlin, Springer-Verlag OHG, 1956–1957. (Cf. review articles by von Braunmühl; Eicke; Friedreich; Hallervorden; Krücke; Lüers and Spatz; Noetzel; Ule.)

Meyer, A., D. Leigh, and C. E. Bagg: A Rare Presenile Dementia Associated with Cortical Blindness (Heidenhain's Syndrome), J. Neurol., Neurosurg. Psychiat., 17:129, 1954.

Reese, H., and J. Bareta: Heredopathia Atactica Polyneuritiformis, J. Neuropathol. Exptl. Neurol., 9:385, 1950.

Schwab, R. S., and A. C. England, Jr.: Newer Preparations in the Treatment of Parkinsonism, Med. Clin. N. Am., 1957:369.

Walsh, F. B.: "Clinical Neuro-ophthalmology," 2d ed., Baltimore, The Williams & Wilkins Company, 1957.

Wilson, S. A. K. (A. N. Bruce, Ed.): "Neurology," Baltimore, The Williams & Wilkins Company, 1957.

291 DISEASES OF THE PERIPHERAL NERVES

Vincent Perlo and
Raymond D. Adams

Diseases of the peripheral nervous system constitute a unique field of neurology. Except for vitamin deficiency states, diffuse vascular diseases, and cerebrospinal meningeal diseases there is usually no overlap between pathologic states which involve the peripheral nerves and spinal cord or brain. In other words the causes and pathogenetic mechanisms of peripheral nerve diseases, which are not at all infrequent, are different from those which involve the brain and spinal cord, and their clinical manifestations are also different.

Definition. According to common clinical usage, multiple symmetric involvement of peripheral nerves resulting in varying degrees of muscular weakness and sensory impairment is termed *polyneuritis. Mononeuritis* indicates involvement of single nerves. *Neuritis* implies inflammatory disease of nerves, but inflammatory reactions in the neuritides are uncommon compared with the incidence of toxic, metabolic, or ischemic processes. The terms *neuropathy, polyneuropathy,* and *mononeuropathy* are considered preferable in describing noninflammatory conditions.

General Considerations. The peripheral nervous system includes 12 pairs of cranial nerves originating from the brain and 31 pairs of segmentally arranged spinal nerves arising from the spinal cord. The parts of the spinal nerves within the spinal canal and attached to the ventral and dorsal surfaces of the cord are called *roots.* The dorsal roots contain afferent fibers, of which the cells of origin are in the dorsal root ganglions, while ventral root fibers arise from anterior horn cells in the gray matter of the cord. The dorsal and ventral roots join to form the spinal nerves just outside the intervertebral foramens. Each spinal nerve receives fibers from the sympathetic trunk of its own side.

The peripheral nerves are composed of myelinated and unmyelinated nerve fibers bound together by endoneural connective tissue. Each fiber bundle is surrounded by a connective tissue sheath, or perineurium, and groups of bundles are enveloped by epineurium, forming nerve trunks. The nerve fibers, or axones, vary in size and in the number of myelinated fibers. The myelinated fibers are surrounded by a sheath of myelin, and this in turn is invested by a thin, membranous neurilemma sheath. The myelin sheaths are interrupted by nodes of Ranvier, and each segment of myelin contains a single Schwann cell. Motor fibers are generally large and myelinated, while sensory branches are composed mainly of smaller myelinated and unmyelinated fibers. Each nerve has its own vascular, lymphatic, and nerve supply. Affection of single or multiple nerves or roots results in varying degrees of sensory loss, motor weakness, and autonomic disturbance, depending on the severity of the lesion and the type of fibers involved.

Pathologically the different diseases of the peripheral nerves have certain points in common. Degeneration of medullated nerve fibers is found in all, though it varies in degree and site of the primary damage. The myelin sheaths are most susceptible. The sheath disintegrates and forms ovoid masses or balls and often fine droplets. These excite a reaction in the histiocytes, which are converted into fatty macrophages as they phagocytize particles of myelin. This myelin change may be limited to a few segments of the myelinated fiber, a condition sometimes referred to as the *periaxial degeneration of Gombault;* or the entire nerve distal to the point of damage may be affected (so-called *Wallerian degeneration*). The axis cylinders swell and undergo fragmentation in the latter instance. But as a rule, axis cylinder damage is less pronounced than that of the myelin sheath.

The location of the primary damage varies. In acute idiopathic and diphtheritic polyneuritis, the dorsal and ventral roots, spinal ganglions, and spinal nerves bear the brunt of the damage; and the more peripheral parts of the nerve are affected only very slightly, if at all. In diabetic polyneuropathy, ganglions, root, and proximal nerves are involved; and this may extend secondarily to the spinal cord. In alcoholic and arsenical polyneuropathy and many cases of porphyria, the changes are mostly in the peripheral segments of the nerves. Very commonly the axis cylinders are affected relatively little in comparison with the myelin sheaths. The degeneration of dorsal root ganglion cells occurs in only a few types of polyneuritis, such as diabetic, idiopathic, and diphtheritic polyneuritis. When the ganglion cell is destroyed, there is invariably a degeneration of the axis cylinder and myelin sheath in the peripheral nerve, dorsal root, and posterior column of the spinal cord. Whenever the motor nerve fibers degenerate, the anterior horn cells within the spinal cord swell and undergo chromatolysis (axonal reaction).

The various types of polyneuritis are distinguished, then, by the character and extent of the nerve fiber changes. However, certain other pathologic changes also serve to differentiate them. In idiopathic polyneuritis there is an infiltration of inflammatory cells, i.e., lymphocytes, plasma cells, and mononuclears in the roots, spinal ganglions, and nerves. In polyarteritis nodosa not only is the nerve degeneration distributed in foci according to the location of vascular occlusion, but there is a unique necrotizing panarteritis. Amyloid neuritis is identified by the deposits of material staining like amyloid in the intraneural blood vessels and connective tissue.

The pathogenesis of diseases of the peripheral nervous system is largely unexplored. In some diseases the primary disorder appears to be a direct affection of Schwann cells and the myelin sheath segments which they control (diphtheria toxin). In others the sensory and motor nerve cells are involved, and changes in the myelin sheath may be secondary (beriberi?). Inflammatory or other alterations in the connective tissues of the nerves may be the mechanism of another type of peripheral neuropathy (lupus erythematosus?). Ischemia resulting from occlusion of the nutrient arteries, e.g., polyarteritis nodosa, is still another mode of nerve fiber damage. Stretch, laceration, compression, and other mechanical factors are operative in injuries of peripheral nerves.

There is often a remarkable discrepancy between the degree of functional impairment before death and the degree of nerve fiber degeneration at autopsy, particularly in the acute cases. With complete paralysis there may be degeneration of only a few fibers, or nearly every one may be involved. This fact undoubtedly explains differences in the recovery rate from acute polyneuropathy.

CLASSIFICATION

Table 291-1. PRINCIPAL CAUSES OF
PERIPHERAL NEUROPATHY

I. Polyneuropathy (generalized neuropathy)
  A. Poisons
    1. Metals: arsenic, lead, mercury, antimony, bismuth, copper, phosphorus, thallium
    2. Organic substances: carbon monoxide, carbon disulfide, trichloroethylene, methyl alcohol, triorthocresylphosphate, immune serums, benzene and derivatives
  B. Deficiency states and metabolic disorders: chronic alcoholism, beriberi, pellagra, combined system disease, pregnancy, chronic gastrointestinal disease, carcinoma of lung, diabetes mellitus, porphyria, amyloid disease
  C. Nonspecific inflammatory states and infections
    1. Acute idiopathic polyneuritis (acute febrile polyneuritis of Osler, Landry-Guillain-Barre syndrome)
    2. Polyneuropathy complicating acute or chronic infection: diphtheria, Boeck's sarcoid, infectious mononucleosis
    3. Local infection of nerves: leprosy
  D. Vascular disease: polyarteritis nodosa, arteriosclerosis
  E. Familial polyneuropathy: progressive hypertrophic polyneuropathy, peroneal muscular atrophy
  F. Polyneuropathy of obscure origin: chronic progressive or recurrent polyneuropathy

Table 291-1. PRINCIPAL CAUSES OF
PERIPHERAL NEUROPATHY (*Continued*)

II. Mononeuropathy (localized neuropathy)
  A. Infections: diphtheria, leprosy, herpes zoster, sarcoid, local sepsis, Bornholm disease (epidemic pleurodynia and coxackie virus infection)
  B. Trauma: including stretching, laceration, and contusion, external pressure, compression by tumor, herniated disk, or cervical rib, injection of medication into nerve
  C. Tumors: neurofibroma, neurofibrosarcoma, von Recklinghausen's neurofibromatosis
  D. Idiopathic: Bell's palsy, brachial and sciatic neuritis
  E. Serum neuritis
  F. Vascular disease: polyarteritis nodosa, diabetes mellitus

GENERAL SYMPTOMS AND SIGNS OF POLYNEUROPATHY

Multiple peripheral nerve involvement is characterized by varying degrees of symmetric or asymmetric sensory impairment and motor weakness, as a rule most pronounced over the distal portions of the extremities.

Numbness and tingling of the hands and feet are frequent subjective symptoms. They are variously described as prickling, formication, and "sleepy feeling"; in medical terminology they are called *paresthesias*. They nearly always indicate involvement of fibers which convey the senses of touch, vibration, and position; and impairment of these sensory modalities is usually found. The skin may be exquisitely tender to touch, pressure, and pricking or pinching, which produce a disagreeable sensation (dysesthesia) that may last for some time after the removal of the stimulus. Marked tenderness to palpation over nerve trunks or muscles is common. There may be hyperpathia, or excessive reaction with raised threshold to painful stimulation and persistence of severe discomfort after removal of the stimulus. Some degree of objective sensory impairment in the extremities is usually present. Perception of light touch and pain is characteristically impaired in a distal distribution, sometimes referred to as glove-and-stocking, but is unlike hysterical sensory loss in that there is a gradual change to normal sensation proximally. Position and vibratory sensation are diminished in the toes and fingers to varying degrees, and these changes underlie the sensory ataxia and stereoanesthesia commonly observed with involvement of these modalities. Impairment of temperature sensation frequently occurs, and heat or cold may produce altered, disagreeable sensations, i.e., burning, painful coldness (thermal dysesthesias) (see Chap. 28, Disorders of Sensation).

Muscular weakness varies from slight involvement of distal muscle groups to complete, symmetric paralysis of all muscles in the extremities and face. In milder forms of weakness, foot and wrist drop are common. Muscle groups involved become flabby and undergo atrophy fairly rapidly. Of the muscles innervated by cranial nerves, bilateral facial involvement is most frequent, followed by paralysis of bulbar muscles, i.e., tongue, pharynx, larynx. Paralysis of the external ocular muscles may occur in exceptional cases.

The tendon reflexes are occasionally retained in the early stages of polyneuropathy; but by the time sensory and motor paralysis has developed, they are nearly always lost. Reflex loss may be restricted to the legs—absent knee and ankle jerks —or there may be generalized areflexia. Cutaneous reflexes, i.e., abdominal and plantar, are not affected.

In certain cases vasomotor changes in the skin occur. These include excessive sweating, mottling, cyanosis, and edema. Vasomotor paralysis resulting in hot, dry skin is less frequently observed. In chronic forms of polyneuropathy postural syncope may occur as a consequence of this vasomotor paralysis.

CLINICAL VARIETIES OF POLYNEUROPATHY

Acute Polyneuritis

Acute Idiopathic Polyneuritis. Acute idiopathic polyneuritis (infectious polyneuritis, Landry's paralysis, Guillain-Barré syndrome, acute polyneuritis with facial diplegia, polyradiculoneuritis) is confined to the peripheral nervous system and is usually characterized by symmetric, ascending motor weakness, areflexia, distal sensory impairment, and albuminocytologic dissociation of the spinal fluid. The various designations given above are felt to be different names for the same condition, first described by Landry in 1859. Although the clinical picture may vary considerably, the pathologic changes are relatively constant. When death occurs, a week or more following the onset of symptoms, there is marked degeneration of spinal nerves, roots, and ganglions, with infiltration of inflammatory cells. There is usually no evidence that the process extends to the central nervous system. In view of the acute nature of the disease and the inflammatory character of the lesions, an infectious etiology has been assumed, but no evidence of virus or other infectious agent has been demonstrated.

The condition often begins within a week or two following an acute febrile illness, most commonly an upper respiratory infection. In some cases, however, there is no history of prior illness.

Initial symptoms usually develop rapidly; symmetric weakness of the lower extremities is accompanied by paresthesias in the fingers and toes. Over a period of several days to a week, weakness may progress to involve the trunk, upper extremities, face, and bulbar muscles. In the extremities both the distal and the proximal muscle groups are involved. However, the degree of weakness is variable, at times reaching almost total voluntary paralysis. Although the lower extremities tend to be involved first, followed by upward spread of paralysis, occasionally the arms or the muscles supplied by cranial nerves may be affected initially. There is usually some impairment of position and vibratory sensation in the toes and fingers, with relative sparing of other sensory modalities. Pain is usually not a prominent symptom; but in some cases it may be conspicuous, and there may be tenderness of muscles and nerve trunks. The muscles become flaccid, and the tendon reflexes disappear as weakness increases. Sphincter impairment is uncommon, but transitory urinary retention may occur. The motor weakness reaches a peak and remains unchanged for days or weeks. If the patient survives the initial acute phase, the prognosis for recovery is good; and improvement, once started, usually progresses rapidly, although occasionally convalescence may be prolonged. During the acute phase, mortality due to respiratory and vasomotor paralysis is as high as 30 per cent. A characteristic finding in the spinal fluid is an elevated protein with a normal cell count (albuminocytologic dissociation). This spinal fluid formula appears in most cases, but occasionally the protein is not elevated, and rarely there is a significant number of lymphocytes in the spinal fluid. A moderate polymorphonuclear leukocytosis may be found in the peripheral blood.

Variants of this syndrome, separable by their descending march or slower course or asymmetry, are also known and usually have a good prognosis with complete recovery after 6 to 12 months. Other special types are those associated with infections mononucleosis (often with cerebrospinal fluid pleocytosis) and infectious hepatitis.

The treatment is symptomatic, with the use of the respirator in the acute phase, if respiratory paralysis occurs. Adrenal steroids have been used in a few cases with encouraging results but have had no effect in others. A trial of these hormones is indicated in critically ill patients in a dosage of 300 mg per day for 2 days and 150 mg daily thereafter for at least 2 to 3 weeks (Meticorten, 25 to 40 mg per day).

Diphtheritic Polyneuritis. In the course of diphtheria various localized neuritic manifestations occur early in the disease and may be followed by the later development of generalized polyneuritis with degenerative changes in the spinal ganglions, roots, and peripheral nerves. These complications occur more frequently in children than in adults. Palatal paralysis occurs during the second or third week and occasionally earlier. It is characterized by nasal speech and regurgitation of fluids through the nose. Paralysis of accommodation with inability to focus on near objects may occur at the same time. During the fifth to seventh weeks of the illness, generalized sensorimotor polyneuritis develops, but it may be delayed up to 2 or 3 months from the onset of diphtheria. It may occur without evidence of a preceding pharyngitis or localized neuritis. The progression and course of diphtheritic polyneuritis are similar in many respects to those of idiopathic polyneuritis, and clinically it may be difficult to distinguish between the two conditions. The generalized symptoms and signs progress for a week or two, then become stationary, and gradually subside. The lower limbs tend to be more involved than the upper, and distal muscle weakness is more pronounced than proximal. Paresthesias in the fingers and toes are prominent, and sensory impairment conforms to a distal distribution. Position sense is often greatly impaired. The tendon reflexes disappear. The spinal fluid protein is usually elevated and always without increase in cells. Improvement usually begins within a few weeks but may be delayed for months. Prognosis for complete recovery is usually good. Fatalities have usually been due to myocarditis or respiratory paralysis. Treatment is symptomatic. Administration of antitoxin is of no value once paralysis has developed. Antitoxin given within several days of the onset of diphtheria usually prevents the development of polyneuritis.

Pink Disease (Erythredema Polyneuropathy). This syndrome of obscure etiology occurs in young children and is characterized by chronic polyneuropathy with generalized weakness, muscular hypotonia, areflexia, and distal sensory impairment. Typical associated findings are swelling and erythema of the face, hands, trunk, and feet, irritability, insomnia, anorexia, alopecia, and trophic changes of the skin. Fever is usually absent. The peripheral nerves show degenerative changes. Improvement occurs slowly over a period of months. Treatment is symptomatic, with vitamin supplements on the assumption that the condition may represent a deficiency disease. A similar clinical picture has been produced by mercury intoxication in children. In some of these cases, rapid improvement resulted following administration of BAL.

Leprous Polyneuritis. In leprosy there is marked, irregular thickening of peripheral nerves owing to formation of leprous nodules, i.e., aggregations of inflammatory cells and Hansen bacilli surrounded by a connective tissue capsule. Secondary degeneration of myelin and axones occurs. Multiple peripheral nerves are involved, producing symmetric distal weakness and sensory impairment. Leprous nodules in the skin of the face are common, and in many cases there is facial anesthesia. Trophic changes with necrosis of phalanges are observed in some patients. The greatly thickened, nodular nerves are frequently palpable. The diagnosis can be proved by demonstrating bacilli in nasal scrapings or by biopsy of a leprous nodule.

Deficiency and Metabolic Disorders

Alcoholic Polyneuropathy. This is described in Chap. 288, Nutritional Disorders of the Nervous System. Other conditions caused by thiamine deficiency are beriberi, polyneuropathy of pregnancy, and chronic deficiency syndromes due to gastrointestinal disease. The symptoms of polyneuropathy in these conditions are similar to those encountered in the alcoholic variety.

Polyneuropathy due to degeneration of peripheral nerves occurs also in pellagra and is said to occur in combined system disease. The latter responds to administration of liver extract or vitamin B_{12}.

Recently cases of sensory and sensorimotor polyneuropathy have been discovered in association with bronchogenic carcinoma and multiple myeloma. The mechanism of the neuropathy in these conditions is obscure.

Diabetic Polyneuropathy. About 50 per cent of older diabetic patients have a mild and relatively asymptomatic neuropathy with absent ankle jerks and impaired vibratory sensation in the toes as the only signs. Symptomatic neuropathy, on the other hand, occurs in about 4 per cent of diabetic patients and is more frequent among patients with poorly controlled diabetes, i.e., prolonged hyperglycemia and weight loss. There are burning, tearing, or lancinating pains in the calves and paresthesias in the feet. The pains occur frequently during the night. Motor weakness is not prominent in some cases but dominates the clinical picture in others (diabetic amyotrophy). Sensory impairment involves mainly pain with only slight loss of touch and pressure sensation. Occasionally, vibratory and position senses alone may be impaired (diabetic tabes). The arms are infrequently involved. The reflexes in the legs are sluggish or absent. The spinal fluid protein is frequently elevated, without increase in the cell count. There is, rarely, a generalized polyneuropathy involving all extremities and producing symmetric atrophy, weakness, and sensory impairment. A mononeuropathic form of diabetic neuropathy may occur, in which single nerve trunks are involved, e.g., sciatic or femoral, with symptoms referable to the distribution of the involved nerve. Involvement of autonomic nerves occurs occasionally, resulting in the loss of sweating, impaired vasomotor control, dependent edema, gastrointestinal disturbance, and sphincter impairment. Cranial nerve lesions may occur, unilateral third or sixth nerve palsy being most frequent; but this is nearly always an isolated phenomenon unrelated to peripheral neuropathy. The pathogenesis is unknown. Vitamin deficiency or the vascular changes of Kimmelstiel-Wilson disease have been suggested as the basis of the pathologic changes but are unproved. The prognosis for improvement of diabetic neuropathy is usually good. Treatment consists in rigid control of the diabetes with maintenance of relatively normal levels of blood sugar. Vitamin supplements of the B group are usually added. Pregnant mammalian liver extract has been ineffective in the experience of the authors.

Porphyric Polyneuropathy. This subject has been presented in Chap. 91 on porphyria. It is a more or less symmetrical sensorimotor neuropathy which may begin in the legs and ascend or in the arms and trunk and descend. The peripheral nerve disorder may or may not be preceded by abdominal or thoracic pain, convulsions and a confusional or schizophrenic-like psychosis. The polyneuropathy may be severe and rapidly fatal or may lead to a prolonged atrophic paralysis from which there is slow recovery over 1 to 2 years. The cerebrospinal fluid is usually normal. Porphyria excretion does not coincide in all patients with the clinical course. Recently promising results have been claimed for BAL, used as in Wilson's disease (Chap. 93).

Amyloid Polyneuropathy. Primary amyloidosis is a rare condition in which amyloid is deposited in blood vessels, connective tissue, and (rarely) in nerves. A clinical picture of slowly progressive sensorimotor polyneuropathy is produced which may resemble beriberi or hypertrophic polyneuropathy. Electrocardiographic changes and anemia are found in some patients. The diagnosis is established by finding amyloid in a biopsy of skin and muscle. Many of these cases have a plasmocytoma or multiple myeloma. The clinical picture must be distinguished from that of a toxic polyneuropathy due to stilbamidine treatment or a compression myelopathy (myelomatous paraplegia).

Vascular Disease

Polyneuropathy Associated with Periarteritis Nodosa. Multiple ischemic involvement of peripheral nerves secondary to damage to nutrient arteries occurs frequently in periarteritis nodosa. Occasionally only single nerves may be involved, resulting in mononeuropathy with sensory and motor symptoms restricted to the distribution of the damaged nerve. Usually the nerves are involved diffusely and produce a clinical picture of subacute polyneuropathy with pain, muscular wasting, areflexia, and peripheral sensory impairment. Although at times

symmetric in distribution, its most distinctive features are its asymmetry and its intermittently progressive course. The neurologic manifestations occur in association with the usual syndrome of fever, cachexia, hypertension, abdominal pain, focal visceral symptoms, and eosinophilia. See Chap. 297 for treatment.

Poisons

Arsenical Polyneuropathy. Polyneuropathy resulting from chronic arsenical poisoning is relatively infrequent. The involved nerves show nonspecific degenerative changes. The symptoms develop rather slowly and are of both sensory and motor type, like those of alcoholic polyneuropathy. Pain and paresthesias in the legs and feet are prominent. Weakness in the lower extremities is more pronounced than in the upper ones. Disturbance of the mental functions, convulsions, and coma due to arsenical encephalopathy may occur. The subacute course of the illness, in conjunction with certain other findings, is of importance in diagnosis. These other findings include gastrointestinal irritation, brownish cutaneous pigmentation most marked about normally pigmented areas, hyperkeratosis of the palms and soles and white transverse bands in the nails (Mees lines), anemia, and signs of liver disease. The diagnosis is confirmed by demonstration of arsenic in the hair, nails, urine, or feces. Treatment consists of withdrawal from exposure and administration of BAL in doses of 3 mg per kg body weight every 4 to 6 hr for 3 days and then twice daily for 10 days. The prognosis is usually good but depends on the duration of symptoms prior to treatment. Recovery of motor power may require months or a year or more.

Poisoning due to mercury, thallium, and antimony may also cause a polyneuropathy which may respond to the administration of BAL.

Lead Neuropathy. Lead neuropathy occurs following chronic exposure to lead, and its most characteristic feature is the predominantly motor affection involving mainly the upper extremities. The radial nerves are most frequently involved, producing wrist and finger drop with little or no sensory manifestations. Less commonly, weakness of proximal shoulder-girdle muscle occurs, and in the lower extremities foot drop may appear. Clinically the paralyzed muscles are those which are most used. Important associated findings are anemia, basophilic stippling of red blood cells, lead line along the gingival margins, colicky abdominal pain, and constipation. Neuropathy occurs usually in adults and is infrequent in children. In contrast, lead encephalopathy, manifested by increased intracranial pressure, convulsions, blindness, and coma, occurs more frequently in children. The diagnosis of lead neuropathy is established by the history of lead intoxication, the characteristic motor involvement, associated findings, and increased urinary excretion of lead. Treatment consists of withdrawal from exposure to lead and measures to eliminate lead from the blood stream (see Chap. 102). The prognosis for recovery of motor power is good, although in chronic cases recovery may be slow.

Triorthocresylphosphate Polyneuropathy (Jamaica Ginger Paralysis). Periodic outbreaks of polyneuropathy have occurred because of ingestion of triorthocresylphosphate. The largest number of cases occurred in 1930, following consumption of adulterated extract of ginger. Recent cases have occurred because of the contamination of cooking oil. Pathologically, there are degeneration of peripheral nerves and also destruction of white matter and anterior horn cells in the spinal cord. The initial symptomatology is that of gastrointestinal irritation, followed in about 10 days by the development of a severe motor neuropathy involving distal muscles. Wrist and foot drop occur. Pain is common, but there is usually no sensory impairment. Later, extensor plantar reflexes appear. In many cases the paralysis fails to improve. The treatment is symptomatic.

Familial Polyneuropathy

Peroneal Muscular Atrophy (Charcot-Marie-Tooth Disease). This is a hereditary disease with onset during adolescence or adult years. There is chronic degeneration of peripheral nerves and roots, resulting in distal muscle atrophy, beginning in the feet and legs and later in the hands. Early symptoms are muscular wasting and weakness affecting the extensor and abductor muscles of the feet and producing an equinovarus deformity. Later, all muscles below the middle third of the thigh may be affected, resulting in a "stork leg" appearance of the legs. After a period of years, atrophy of hand and forearm muscles develops. The wasting never extends above the elbows or above the middle third of the thighs. Perforating ulcers may occur in the feet. Pain, paresthesias, and cramps are common. The sensory disorder is usually rather slight. Often there is some impairment of position and vibratory sensation in the feet, and touch and pain sensation are lost in the feet in some cases. Reflexes are lost in the involved limbs. The progression of the illness is very slow and may be arrested at any stage. (See Chap. 290 for more complete description.)

Progressive Hypertrophic Polyneuropathy (Déjerine-Sottas Disease). This type of neuropathy is uncommon and is frequently familial. It begins usually in childhood and is slowly progressive. Pain and paresthesias in the feet are early symptoms, followed by development of symmetric weakness and wasting of the distal portion of the limbs. Sensation is impaired in a distal distribution, and the tendon reflexes are absent. Miotic pupils, nystagmus, and kyphoscoliosis have been observed in some cases. A characteristic finding is the enlargement of the peripheral nerves because of hypertrophy and proliferation of the cells of the sheath of Schwann and fibroblasts. Palpable thickening of the ulnar and peroneal nerves may be conspicuous. In the absence of palpable enlargement of nerves, the diagnosis can be established by biopsy of a cutaneous nerve. The treatment is symptomatic.

Polyneuropathy of Obscure Origin

Chronic Progressive Polyneuropathy. Not infrequently one encounters patients with a slowly progressive polyneuropathy in whom no etiologic factor can be found. There are weakness and wasting of the limbs, areflexia, and peripheral sensory impairment. Pain is less prominent than in the acute forms of neuropathy and is often absent altogether. Progression occurs over a period of months, occasionally with fatal termination, but may be followed by recovery or arrest of the condition. The peripheral nerves show evidence of widespread degeneration. Without knowledge of etiology and lacking a specific therapy, one can only resort to the usual symptomatic treatment of polyneuropathy. A course of BAL may be tried on empirical grounds.

Acute idiopathic polyneuritis must be distinguished from other acute affections of peripheral nerves and roots, poliomyelitis, and acute ascending myelitis. Postdiphtheritic polyneuritis produces a somewhat similar picture and may be identified by the recent history of diphtheria and transitory paralysis of palate or accommodation. A positive Schick test is evidence against a preceding diphtheritic infection. Acute porphyric polyneuropathy is distinguished by a recent history of abdominal symptoms, normal spinal fluid protein, and presence of porphyrins in the urine. In acute idiopathic polyneuritis, the features of acute onset following a febrile episode, the rapid development of symptoms, and the more prominent involvement of motor nerve fibers can help distinguish it from deficiency and toxic forms of polyneuropathy. Meningeal carcinomatosis with multiple involvement of nerve roots is characterized by less acute onset, steady progression of symptoms, and frequently, by inflammatory and neoplastic cells in the spinal fluid. Poliomyelitis is distinguished by the asymmetric paralysis, absence of sensory impairment, and the pleocytosis of the cerebrospinal fluid. Acute ascending myelitis may cause widespread flaccid paralysis, but in this condition sphincter disturbance is usually severe, sensory loss is more extensive, involving the whole body below the level of the cord lesion, and plantar responses are later extensor. See Chap. 287 for further discussion.

Once the neuropathic nature of the disease is established, then the specific type of the neuropathy must be ascertained.

Chronic polyneuropathy (usually separable from distal myopathy and spinal muscular atrophy) leads to consideration of the four familial peripheral nerve diseases—Charcot-Marie-Tooth, Déjerine-Sottas, familial amyloidosis (Portuguese polyneuropathy), and Refsum's syndrome of polyneuropathy, deafness, and retinitis pigmentosa—and also several acquired types such as chronic beriberi, diabetic polyneuropathy, polyneuropathy with carcinoma or multiple myeloma, and idiopathic polyneuropathy. These are distinguished on the grounds of familial history as well as the details of the clinical picture and biochemical findings. The cause and mechanism of as many as 50 per cent of all cases of chronic polyneuropathy cannot be determined at this time.

LOCALIZED NEUROPATHY

The Common Brachial and Crural Mononeuropathies

Brachial Palsies. The fifth to eighth cervical and first thoracic spinal nerves innervate the muscles of the shoulder girdles and upper extremities. The brachial plexus is formed by components of these nerves, and lesions of the nerves or their branches result in characteristic palsies. The following are the brachial palsies most likely to be observed on the medical wards of a hospital.

Long Thoracic Nerve. This nerve is derived from the fifth, sixth, and seventh cervical nerves and supplies the serratus magnus muscle. Paralysis of the serratus magnus muscle results in inability to raise the arm over the head from a forward position, and there is winging of the inner border of the scapula on pushing forward against resistance. It is injured most commonly by pressure on the shoulder, from either a sudden blow or prolonged pressure from carrying heavy weights. It is also involved at times in diabetic patients and as a manifestation of brachial and serum neuritides and in other idiopathic forms of neuritis (pleurodynia, Coxsackie).

Suprascapular Nerve. This nerve is derived from the fifth and sixth cervical nerves and supplies the supra- and infraspinatus muscles. Lesions may be diagnosed from the presence of weakness of abduction and external rotation of the arm and atrophy of the supra- and infraspinatus muscles. The nerve may be injured by blows on top of the shoulder and fracture-dislocations of the shoulder joint.

Upper Brachial Plexus Paralysis. This is due to injury to the fifth cervical nerve, caused most commonly by forceful separation of the head and shoulder during difficult delivery or by pressure in the supraclavicular region during anesthesia. The muscles affected are the biceps, deltoid, brachialis anticus, supinator longus, supra- and infraspinatus, and rhomboids. The arm hangs at the side, internally rotated, with the elbow extended. The forearm is pronated. Hand motion is unaffected. The prognosis for spontaneous recovery is generally good, especially in cases of birth injury. This condition as a result of birth injury (Erb-Duchenne brachial plexus palsy) is discussed in Chaps. 26 and 283.

Lower Brachial Plexus Paralysis. This is due to injury to the eighth cervical and first thoracic roots as a result of traction on the abducted arm in falls, during operation, and with tumors of the apex of the lung (superior sulcus or Pancoast syndrome). Injury may occur during birth (Déjerine-Klumpke brachial plexus injury). There are paralysis and wasting of the small muscles of the hand and a characteristic claw-hand deformity. Sensory loss is limited to the ulnar border of the hand, and there may be an associated paralysis of the cervical sympathetic nerve with a Horner's syndrome.

Lesions of the Cords of the Brachial Plexus. The outer and inner cords are most commonly affected. Dislocation of the head of the humerus, pressure of the cervical rib, and stab wounds are the most frequent causes. Injury to the outer cord results in paralysis of the biceps and coracobrachialis muscles and all muscles supplied by the median nerve except the intrinsic hand muscles. There is some loss of sensation over the radial aspects of the forearm. Involvement of the inner cord, as may occur in compression by cervical rib, results in paralysis of the muscles supplied by the ulnar nerve together with the median-innervated intrinsic muscles of the hand and sensory loss over the ulnar aspect of the hand and forearm.

Axillary Nerve. This nerve arises from the posterior cord of the brachial plexus and supplies the teres minor and deltoid muscles. It may be involved in injuries resulting from fractures of the neck of the humerus, serum neuritis, brachial neuritis, or as part of a disease of unknown etiology. The anatomic localization depends on the recognition of a paralysis of abduction of the arm, wasting of the deltoid muscle, and slight impairment of sensation over the outer aspect of the shoulder.

Musculocutaneous Nerve. This nerve is derived from the fifth and sixth cervical nerves and is a branch of the outer cord of the brachial plexus. It innervates the biceps and brachialis anticus muscles. Lesions of the nerve result in weakness of elbow flexion. This nerve is rarely injured alone.

Radial Nerve. This nerve is derived from the fifth to eighth cervical nerves and is the termination of the posterior cord of the brachial plexus. It innervates the triceps muscle and the supinator and extensor muscles of the forearm and hand. Complete radial paralysis results in inability to extend the elbow, paralysis of supination of the forearm, and complete wrist and finger drop. Sensation is impaired over the posterior aspect of the forearm and a small area over the radial aspect of the dorsum of the hand. The nerve may be injured in the axilla, for example, in "crutch" palsy, but most commonly traumatism occurs in the lower arm where the nerve winds around the humerus. Common types of injury at this site are fractures and pressure palsies during sleep.

Median Nerve. This nerve is derived from the sixth cervical to the first thoracic root and is formed by the union of two heads from the inner and outer cords of the brachial plexus. It innervates the pronators of the forearm, long finger flexors, and abductor and opponens muscles of the thumb and is a sensory nerve to the palmar aspect of the hand. Complete median nerve paralysis results in wasting of the affected muscles and inability to pronate the forearm or deviate the hand in an ulnar direction, paralysis of flexion of the index finger and terminal phalanx of the thumb, weakness of flexion of the remaining fingers, weakness of abduction and opposition of the thumb, and sensory impairment over the radial two-thirds of the palmar aspect of the hand and over the distal phalanges of the dorsum of the index and third fingers. The nerve may be injured in the axilla by shoulder dislocation and in any part of its course by laceration, stab, or gunshot wounds. The wrist is the most common site of external injury. Compression of the nerve at the wrist (carpal-tunnel syndrome) may occur secondary to prolonged occupational pressure or local infiltration, for example, by a thickening of connective tissue and deposit of amyloid with multiple myeloma. Incomplete lesions of the median nerve between the axilla and wrist may result in *causalgia*.

Ulnar Nerve. This nerve is derived from the eighth cervical and first thoracic roots. It innervates the ulnar flexor of the wrist, the inner half of the deep finger flexors, the adductors and abductors of the fingers, adductor of the thumb, the two medial lumbricales, and muscles of the hypothenar eminence. It is the sensory nerve to the fifth and ulnar half of the fourth fingers and ulnar border of the hand. Complete ulnar paralysis results in a characteristic claw-hand deformity owing to wasting of the small hand muscles and hyperextension of the fingers at the metacarpophalangeal joints and flexion at the interphalangeal joints. The flexion deformity is most pronounced in the fourth and fifth fingers. Sensory loss occurs over the fifth finger, the ulnar aspect of the fourth finger, and the ulnar border of the palm. The ulnar nerve is most commonly injured at the elbow because of fracture or dislocation involving the joint. *Delayed ulnar palsy* may occur many years after an injury to the elbow joint which has resulted in a cubitus valgus deformity of the joint. Because of the deformity, the nerve is stretched in its course over the ulnar condyle. The superficial location of the nerve at the elbow makes it a common site of pressure palsy. Prolonged pressure on the outer part of the palm may result in damage to the deep palmar branch of the ulnar nerve, causing weakness of small hand muscles but on sensory loss.

Crural Palsies. The twelfth thoracic, first to fifth lumbar, and first, second, and third sacral spinal nerve roots compose the lumbosacral plexuses and innervate the muscles of the lower extremities and "saddle" region. The following are the common crural palsies.

Lateral Femoral Cutaneous Nerve. This nerve is derived from the second and third lumbar roots. It is a sensory nerve supplying the lateral aspect of the thigh. The nerve enters the thigh beneath the lateral end of the inguinal ligament and then enters the fascia lata, where it may become constricted. Compression of the nerve results in uncomfortable paresthesias along its cutaneous distribution and in sensory impairment. The condition is called *meralgia paresthetica* (mentioned below).

Obturator Nerve. This nerve is derived from the second, third, and fourth lumbar roots. It supplies the adductor muscles of the thigh, and injury to the nerve results in almost complete paralysis of adduction of the thigh. The nerve is most frequently injured during the course of a difficult labor and also as a result of dislocation of the hip or an obturator hernia. It may be affected in diabetes, polyarteritis nodosa, retroperitoneal cervical carcinoma and other tumors, etc.

Femoral Nerve. This nerve is derived from the second, third, and fourth lumbar roots. It supplies the iliacus, pectineus, sartorius, and quadriceps muscles and carries sensory impulses from the anteromedial aspect of the thigh and medial side of the lower leg. Following injury to the nerve, there is paralysis of extension of the knee, with wasting of the quadriceps muscle and also some weakness of hip flexion. The knee jerk is abolished. The nerve may be involved in fractures and dislocation of the hip and in fractured pelvis. It may be affected in diabetes, polyarteritis nodosa, and in retroperitoneal pelvic or abdominal lesions such as psoas abscess or tumor. Because of the proximity of the femoral artery to the nerve in the femoral triangle, wounds in this region may be fatal.

Sciatic Nerve. This nerve is derived from the fourth and fifth lumbar and first, second, and third sacral roots. It provides the motor innervation of the hamstring muscles and all those below the knee; and it carries sensory impulses from the posterior aspect of the thigh and posterior and lateral aspects of the leg and entire sole. In complete sciatic paralysis, the knee cannot be flexed and all muscles below the knee are paralyzed. The sciatic nerve is commonly injured in fractures of the pelvis or femur and in gunshot wounds of the buttock and thigh. It may also be involved by pelvic tumors and in both diabetes mellitus and polyarteritis nodosa. Cryptogenic forms also occur and are actually more frequent than the identifiable types of disease. A ruptured lumbar disk often simulates sciatic neuropathy. Incomplete lesions of the sciatic nerve occasionally result in causalgia.

Common Peroneal Nerve. This nerve is one of the terminal divisions of the sciatic nerve in the popliteal fossa. It supplies the dorsiflexors of the foot and toes and everters of the foot, and sensation to the dorsum of the foot and lateral aspect of the lower half of the leg. These functions are lost with lesions which completely interrupt the nerves. Pressure or sleep palsy is one of the most frequent types of injury, the compression being of that part of the nerve which passes over the head of the fibula. It is also commonly involved by fractures involving the upper end of the fibula and in diabetic polyarteritis.

Tibial Nerve. This nerve is the other of the two terminal divisions of the sciatic nerve in the popliteal fossa. It supplies all the calf muscles and the flexors of the foot. Complete paralysis of the nerve results in a calcaneovalgus deformity of the foot, which no longer can be plantar flexed. There is loss of sensation over the plantar aspect of the foot.

The Diseases Which Involve Single Nerves or Plexuses

Infections. In faucial diphtheria, selective involvement of the vagi and nerves to the ciliary muscles of the eye results in palatal paralysis and paralysis of accommodation. The palatal palsy occurs in the first 2 weeks of infection and the loss of accommodation about a week later. Both tend to improve rapidly. In cutaneous diphtheria, involvement of nerves locally results in paralysis of the muscles supplied by the spinal segment from which the infected region is innervated. In leprosy, granulomatous infection of multiple peripheral nerves usually takes place simultaneously, producing symptoms of polyneuritis rather than localized asymmetric neuritis, but the latter may be found in the early stages of leprous neuritis. Herpes zoster is a sensory neuritis of virus etiology, characterized by acute inflammation of one or more posterior root ganglions, spinal nerves, and roots and gray matter of the spinal cord. Lancinating pain and hyper-

algesia over the skin surface supplied by affected roots occur for 3 or 4 days, followed by the appearance of a segmental herpetic eruption. If the inflammatory process spreads to involve adjacent motor roots of anterior horns of the cord, segmental motor weakness and wasting appear. Paralysis of the oculomotor nerves may occur in conjunction with involvement of the gasserian ganglion (ophthalmoplegic zoster). Facial paralysis may occur with involvement of the geniculate ganglion (Ramsay Hunt syndrome) but has accompanied zoster of other ganglions as well. Sarcoidosis can involve single or multiple peripheral nerves, producing asymmetric mononeuritis or polyneuritis. Unilateral or bilateral facial paralysis is common in association with parotitis and uveitis in sarcoidosis.

Trauma. External trauma may result in complete transection of a peripheral nerve or may impair conduction without interrupting the anatomic continuity of the involved nerve. Complete division of a mixed peripheral nerve results in paralysis and sensory loss corresponding to the region supplied by the damaged nerve. Recovery of function after complete division can take place only when the divided ends lie in apposition or have been sutured. Growth of nerve fibers from the central end proceeds at a rate of 1 to 2 mm a day, and the recovery time can be estimated by the distance between the site of injury and destination of the nerve. An early indication of regeneration is the presence of tingling sensation on tapping the nerve below the lesion (Tinel's sign). Sensory recovery precedes the return of motor power. All forms of cutaneous sensation begin to return together. Appreciation of pain and temperature improves, but the stimuli are poorly localized for some time. Eventually there is recovery of the discriminative aspects of sensation, including localization of sensory stimuli, postural sense, recognition of slight differences in temperature, and appreciation of very light touch.

Pressure Palsy. This results in temporary paralysis owing to local compression. Mild degrees of compression are followed by fairly rapid recovery. Severe compression, such as may occur during a bout of alcoholic intoxication, deep sleep, or anesthesia, may result in focal disintegration of myelin, damage to axis cylinders, and Wallerian degeneration of distal segments. Recovery is slow and must await regeneration. Common varieties of pressure palsy are radial nerve paralysis with wrist drop due to prolonged pressure against the back of the arm (Saturday-night palsy), ulnar palsy due to repeated trauma to the nerve at the elbow, especially after an old fracture that changes the relation of the nerve to the bicipital groove, and peroneal nerve palsy with foot drop caused by compressing the nerve against the fibula, as in sitting with legs crossed or during obstetric procedures with legs in stirrups.

Meralgia paresthetica is a sensory neuropathy characterized by pain and paresthesia over the lateral aspect of the thigh because of compression of the lateral femoral cutaneous nerve in the fascia lata. Pressure on nerve roots in the cervical and lumbar regions by *herniated intervertebral disks* results in pain, sensory impairment, and variable motor weakness corresponding to the area supplied by the involved root (see Chap. 7). Compression of the inner cord of the brachial plexus by a *cervical rib or by some other malformation of the thoracic outlet* (thoracic outlet syndrome) results in atrophy of small hand muscles and sensory impairment over the ulnar and sometimes median nerve distribution (see Chap. 7). The median nerve may be compressed at the wrist beneath the transverse carpal ligament (carpal-tunnel syndrome). There are pain and paresthesias in the palmar surface of the hand and first three fingers, thenar atrophy, weakness in flexor of thumb and opponens muscle, and sensory impairment over the median nerve distribution.

Tumor. Peripheral nerves may be compressed or invaded by primary or metastatic tumors arising in other tissues. Solitary tumors of nerve sheaths, or neuromas, commonly occur along the roots of spinal nerves, chiefly in the thoracic and lumbar regions. Compression of the nerve root and adjacent spinal cord may occur. Root compression causes pain referred to the distribution of the involved nerve, and there may be associated sensory impairment and motor weakness. Lymphomatosis and carcinomatosis of the cranial and spinal meninges may implicate single or multiple cranial and spinal nerve roots and give rise to confusing clinical syndromes. Tumor cells may be found in the cerebrospinal fluid. Solitary neuromas may involve any of the peripheral nerves, producing local pain and tenderness to palpation. Multiple neuromas occur in von Recklinghausen's disease and are associated in this condition with multiple congenital anomalies, as well as kyphoscoliosis, cutaneous pigmentation, and cutaneous fibromas. The treatment of solitary expanding nerve tumors of the limbs is wide excision with nerve graft or suture, if that is possible.

Idiopathic Neuropathy. *Bell's palsy* is due to compression of the facial nerve in the fallopian canal as a result of an acute inflammatory process involving the nerve. Edema leads to compression of nerve fibers, with resulting unilateral paralysis of facial muscles (see Chap. 31).

Brachial neuritis is an acute affection of the brachial plexus, characterized by the acute or subacute onset of severe pain in the neck, arm, and hand, followed by moderate muscle weakness, slight impairment of sensation in the fingers and hand,

numbness or hyperesthesia, and depressed reflexes in the involved arm. The pain is usually severe and constant and is aggravated by moving the arm or stretching the brachial plexus. Muscle wasting is rarely severe, but some cases of brachial neuritis, especially those described by the term *neuralgic amyotrophy,* may be followed by localized paralysis and atrophy of the shoulder-girdle and arm muscles. Recovery slowly occurs over a period of several weeks to months. Symptomatic treatment, including complete rest of the involved arm and analgesics in the acute phase, followed by mild massage and exercise, usually suffices.

Sciatic neuritis causes pain in the lumbar region and behind the leg from buttock to ankle. The pain is aching or burning in quality and is aggravated by movement or straining. The sciatic nerve is tender to palpation or stretching. There may be slight weakness of the hamstrings and muscles below the knee. The ankle jerk is absent. Sensory impairment is usually slight. It is necessary to distinguish the symptoms of sciatic neuritis from those of sciatic compression. In compression (e.g., by tumor) the onset is more gradual, symptoms are progressive, muscle wasting is more conspicuous, the nerve is less tender to palpation, and sensory loss is greater. The course of sciatic neuritis is stationary at first, followed by slow improvement. Treatment is symptomatic.

Serum neuritis develops several days after the onset of serum sickness. The fifth cervical nerve is most commonly involved, with pain, paralysis, and atrophy corresponding to the distribution of the nerve. Occasionally the entire brachial plexus may be involved, and there is sometimes, but rarely, a generalized polyneuritis. The etiology is not known but is attributed to perineural edema comparable to the urticaria of serum sickness, with compression of affected roots or nerves. Recovery is usually complete but occurs slowly.

TREATMENT

In addition to measures already mentioned, general principles in the treatment of polyneuropathy include removal of any known toxic factor, correction of nutritional deficiency, rest of affected nerves and muscles, maintenance of muscle tone by heat, massage, and electrical stimulation, and the prevention of joint fixation and contractures. Bed rest is indicated for generalized weakness, to relax involved muscles, and to avoid cardiac strain. Pain in the acute stage is relieved by analgesics and the use of moist, hot packs, if tolerated. Pressure of bedclothes is avoided by cradle support, and foot drop is prevented by sand bags beneath the soles. Passive movement and gentle massage are started as soon as tolerated in order to maintain tone and prevent contracture. After the acute, painful stage, appropriate splints can be worn and more intensive physiotherapy carried out. Adequate nutrition must be maintained, with vitamin supplements of the B group added. In the nutritional polyneuropathies, a high calorie, high vitamin diet with 50 mg thiamine daily and 15 Gm of brewer's yeast, t.i.d., are prescribed. On the basis of blood pyruvate levels following glucose administration, it is said that three main groups of peripheral neuropathy can be distinguished. One group shows no impairment of pyruvate metabolism and is not affected by thiamine treatment. In the second group, there is a block in pyruvate oxidation that responds to thiamine, and in the third group, a block in pyruvate oxidation that is not changed by thiamine. The latter group includes cases of arsenic intoxication which respond to treatment with BAL. In cases of polyneuropathy of obscure origin in which pyruvate metabolism is impaired, if there is no response to thiamine, a short trial of BAL is indicated. The authors have been unable to verify this subdivision of cases of polyneuropathy, and the efficacy of the therapeutic methods which follow from it has not been substantiated.

Treatment in localized neuropathy is directed toward maintaining tone and preventing stretching of paralyzed muscles, preventing contractures, and keeping joints mobile while nerve regeneration is taking place. Heat, massage, passive movement, and electrical stimulation are employed. Operative repair is necessary in cases of complete nerve transection, and surgical treatment is required in some but by no means all cases of chronic compression by tumor, cervical rib, or herniated intervertebral disk.

REFERENCES

Brain, W. R.: "Diseases of the Nervous System," New York, Oxford University Press, 1951.

Cobb, S., and H. C. Coggeshall: Neuritis, J.A.M.A., 103:1608, 1934.

Denny-Brown, D., and D. Sciarra: Changes in the Nervous System in Acute Porphyria, Brain, 68:1, 1945.

Haymaker, W., and J. Kernohan: The Landry-Guillain-Barré Syndrome, Medicine, 28:59, 1949.

Jonier, C. L., B. McArdle, and R. H. S. Thompson: Blood Pyruvate Estimation in the Diagnosis and Treatment of Polyneuritis, Brain, 73:431, 1950.

Merritt, H. H.: Corticotropin and Cortisone in Diseases of the Nervous System, Yale J. Biol. and Med., 24:466, 1952.

Rundles, R. W.: Diabetic Neuropathy, Medicine, 24: 111, 1945.

Watson, C., and S. Schwartz: A Simple Test for Urinary Porphobilinogen, Proc. Soc. Exptl. Biol. Med., 47:393, 1951.

Section 8: Diseases of Supporting Tissues Other than Bone

INTRODUCTION

Ivan L. Bennett, Jr.

This section contains descriptions of diseases which damage the body's "soft skeleton," the skin and connective tissue. Although this categorization is arbitrary, it possesses advantages. Generally, common or related etiology is the basis for classification, and, ideally, similarity in manifestations is the most useful clinical criterion for grouping diseases. Here, we are dealing for the most part with diseases of obscure etiology; many of the disorders are actually known to occur in association with a variety of infections and hypersensitivity states. Furthermore, because injury to connective tissue can produce structural or functional abnormalities in almost any organ system or anatomic site, it is difficult to select a few predominant symptoms and signs from the diversity of manifestations that can accompany such diseases and to rely on them as a logical starting point in grouping. If they are considered by the clinician as generalized disorders of connective tissues, however, they are less perplexing. For example, several genetically determined diseases, once looked upon as rare and esoteric "syndromes" composed of a peculiar hodgepodge of unrelated abnormalities, are discussed in the next five chapters. They are now known to be relatively common. When viewed as disorders of connective tissue, such associations as ectopia lentis, inguinal hernia, and aortic dissection in the Marfan syndrome or angioid streaks and melena in pseudoxanthoma elasticum are logical and expected.

In addition to the major "collagen vascular diseases," a few relatively unusual diseases of uncertain etiology but closely related histologic manifestations are included: relapsing panniculitis and scleredema. Because rheumatic fever and acute hemorrhagic glomerulonephritis are known to be related etiologically to group A streptococcal infection, they are discussed in another part of the book as complications of streptococcal disease. Dermatomyositis has been included elsewhere along with other diseases of muscle. All these disorders might well have been included in this section.

The two most important afflictions of the joints, rheumatoid arthritis and degenerative joint disease, are included in this section along with a detailed discussion of the problem of rheumatism and arthritis. Finally, some of the more important problems of dermatology are presented from the point of view of the patient with skin disease or with systemic disease manifested by cutaneous lesions.

292 THE MARFAN SYNDROME
Victor A. McKusick

Definition. The Marfan syndrome [synonyms: arachnodactyly, dolichostenomelia (long thin

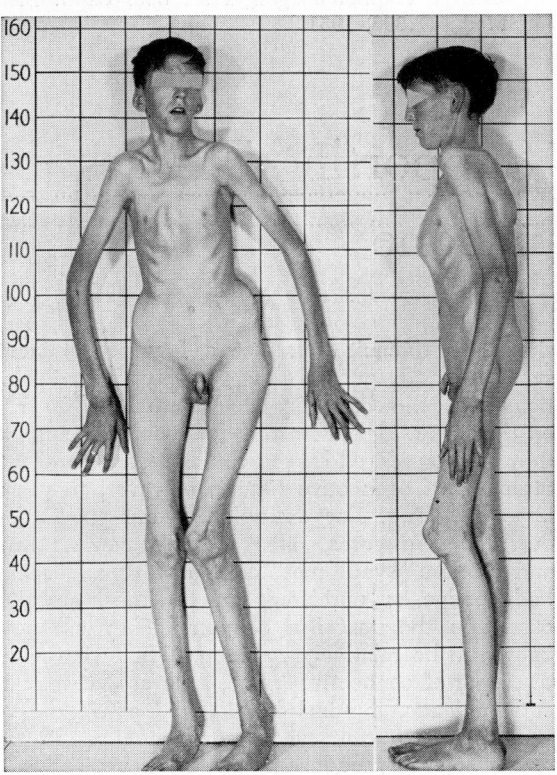

FIG. 292-1. Typical features of the Marfan syndrome in an 11-year-old boy.

limbs), dystrophia mesodermalis congenita, typus Marfanis] is a heritable, generalized disorder of one element of connective tissue, clinically manifested by abnormalities of the eye (especially ectopia lentis), of the skeletal system (especially excessive length of the long bones), and of the cardiovascular system (especially diffuse and/or dissecting aneurysm of the ascending aorta).

Clinical Manifestations. *Skeleton.* Characteristically, the tubular bones are excessively long, resulting in arachnodactyly and in anomalous proportions. Normally after puberty the ratio of upper segment (pubic symphysis to crown) to the lower segment (pubic symphysis to sole) is about 0.92 (SD = 0.04) in whites and 0.85 (SD = 0.03) in Negroes. Because of the excessively long lower segment the ratio is usually lower in patients with the Marfan syndrome. The arm span exceeds the height. The patient with the Marfan syndrome is taller than the average for his age and family; however, the deviation from the normal skeletal proportion is of more specific diagnostic significance. Excessive longitudinal growth of ribs may result in outward displacement of the sternum (pigeon breast, pectus carinatum) or inward displacement (pectus excavatum, *Trichterbrust*). Redundant ligaments, tendons, and joint capsules result in loose-jointedness, hyperextensibility of joints, genu recurvatum (backward curvature of the legs at the knees), flat feet, kyphoscoliosis, and habitual dislocation of the hips, patella, clavicles, mandible, and other joints. Hernia occurs with increased frequency. In general, patients with the Marfan syndrome display a sparsity of subcutaneous fat (see Fig. 292-1).

Eye. Ectopia lentis (subluxation of the lens, dislocated lens) is the ocular hallmark of the Marfan syndrome. Iridodonesis, tremor of the iris, is occasionally a clue to the presence of dislocated lenses. Occasionally the margin of a dislocated lens is visible through the undilated pupil, and occasionally there may be a total dislocation of the lens into the anterior chamber. To exclude minor subluxation, it is necessary to dilate the pupil maximally and perform a careful slit-lamp examination. Under these circumstances one sees in the severely affected person that the suspensory ligaments are redundant, attenuated, and fragmented.

Myopia, often of high grade, is usually present; a long orbit usually occurs as an integral part of the syndrome. Spontaneous detachment of the retina is frequent.

Cardiovascular System. The principal cardiovascular manifestation of the Marfan syndrome is a weakness of the aortic media such that the portion subject to greatest hemodynamic stress of certain types—the ascending aorta—tends to undergo progressive dilation or acute dissection. The dilation,

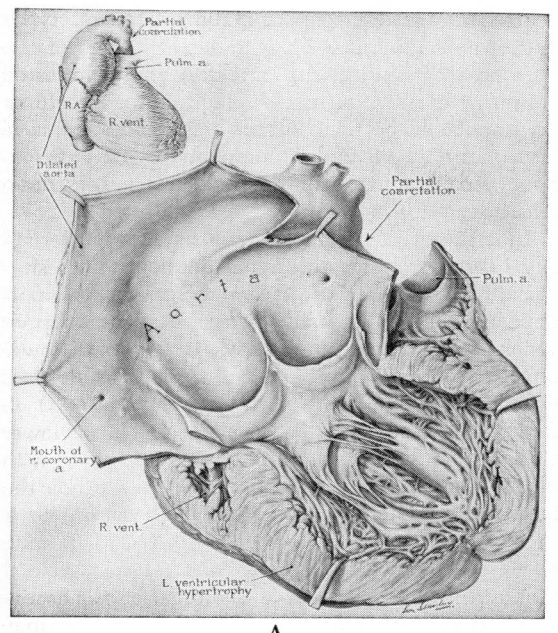

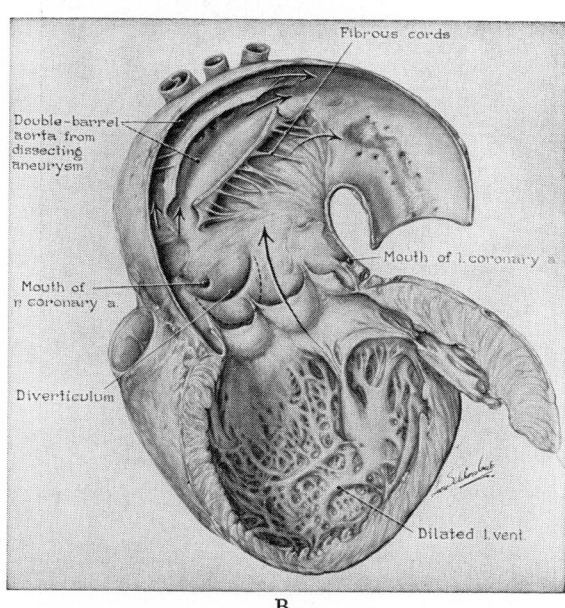

A   B

Fig. 292-2. The aorta in two instances of the Marfan syndrome. A. Diffuse aneurysm of the ascending aorta. B. Dissecting aneurysm.

beginning as early as the first or as late as the fifth decade, occurs first in the coronary sinuses. Profound aortic regurgitation may precede evidence of dilation of the aorta on ordinary radiographic study. The clinical features of acute dissection are discussed on p. 1365 (see Fig. 292-2).

Less common cardiovascular complications are bacterial endocarditis superimposed on minor changes of the heart valves, interatrial septal defect, and incomplete coarctation.

Other internal ramifications include cystic disease of the lung and recurrent spontaneous pneumothorax.

Differential Diagnosis. Given cardiovascular and skeletal manifestations consistent with the Marfan syndrome, one cannot be certain of the diagnosis unless ectopia lentis, the most specific of the components of the syndrome, can be demonstrated, or unless close relatives display unmistakable evidence of the disease. Confusion results from the fact that there is wide variability in the clinical severity of this syndrome, and its individual components display some independence in their severity ("expressivity") or even in whether they are present at all ("penetrate"). When the mutant gene for this syndrome occurs in pyknic stock, the affected person is likely to display less impressive skeletal abnormalities. The patient must be judged against the background of his family.

Intrauterine insults to the embryo, such as maternal rubella, can produce changes in the eye, heart, and skeleton (including arachnodactyly) which superficially suggest the Marfan syndrome.

Inheritance. The Marfan syndrome is usually inherited as an autosomal dominant.

Pathology and Basic Defect. The main histologic abnormality is that of the aortic media. Probably in most cases normal at birth by the usual pathologic techniques, it undergoes changes which in the mildest form are identical with Erdheim's cystic medial necrosis seen in other settings (p. 1365). In its advanced form, there are loss of elastic fibers, scarring, hyperplasia of smooth muscle in large whorls, and dilation of the vasa vasorum. What element of connective tissue is fundamentally defective is unknown. The elastic fiber is under suspicion.

REFERENCE

McKusick, V. A.: "Heritable Disorders of Connective Tissue," 2d ed., St. Louis, The C. V. Mosby Company, 1960.

293 THE EHLERS-DANLOS SYNDROME

Victor A. McKusick

Definition. The Ehlers-Danlos syndrome (synonyms: cutis hyperelastica, "India rubber men,"

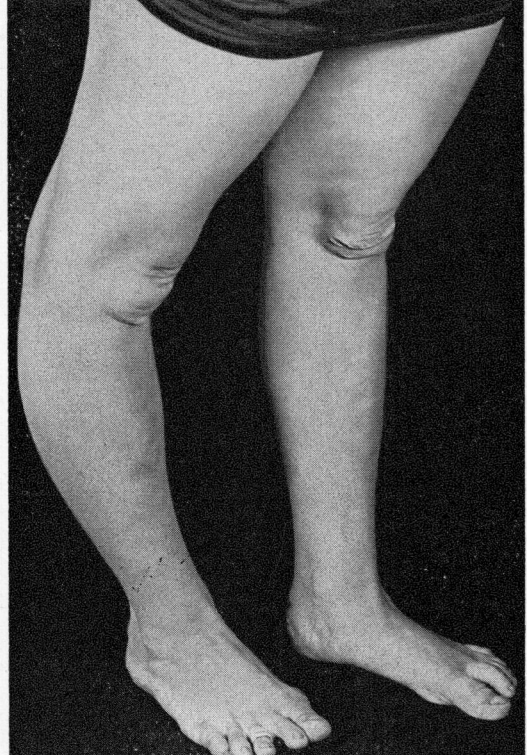

FIG. 293-1. Both the loose-jointedness and the "cigarette-paper" scarring of the Ehlers-Danlos syndrome are demonstrated.

dermatorrhexis with dermatochalasis and arthrochalasis) is a heritable and generalized disorder of one element of connective tissue, clinically manifested by fragility and hyperelasticity of the skin and loose-jointedness.

Clinical Manifestations. Characteristically, the skin can be stretched through an unusually great range, but returns promptly to its normal position on release. Later on, the skin may lose its elasticity, become truly cutis laxa, and hang in flabby folds or wrinkles. The skin is fragile, so that minor trauma is likely to produce gaping, "fish-mouth" wounds which bleed little and hold sutures poorly. There is easy bruisability. Firm spherules up to about 1 cm in diameter develop subcutaneously, can be moved about through a considerable range, and can be demonstrated radiographically because of calcification. "Cigarette paper" scars develop over the knees, shins, etc. So-called "molluscoid pseudotumors" develop on the knees, ankles, and elbows as soft, poorly outlined swellings that can be several centimeters in diameter.

The loose-jointedness results in genu recurvatum, habitual dislocation of various joints, flat feet, etc. Recurrent hydrarthrosis may result from the re-

peated trauma due to poor stabilization, especially in the knees (Fig. 293-1).

Internal ramifications include diaphragmatic hernia or eventration of the diaphragm, ectasia or diverticula of portions of the gastrointestinal and respiratory tracts, and spontaneous pneumothorax. Spontaneous rupture of the bowel is a rare complication.

Inheritance. The Ehlers-Danlos syndrome is usually inherited as an autosomal dominant.

Pathology and Basic Defect. The basic defect appears to be abnormality in the way the collagen "wickerwork" is arranged such that excessive extensibility of collagenous structures is possible (see Fig. 293-2). The normal elastic tissues appear to function in restoring structures to their normal position; the elastic fibers may, in fact, be hyperplastic, possibly in response to the repeated stimulus of extra stretching.

REFERENCE

McKusick, V. A.: "Heritable Disorders of Connective Tissue," 2d ed., St. Louis, The C. V. Mosby Company, 1960.

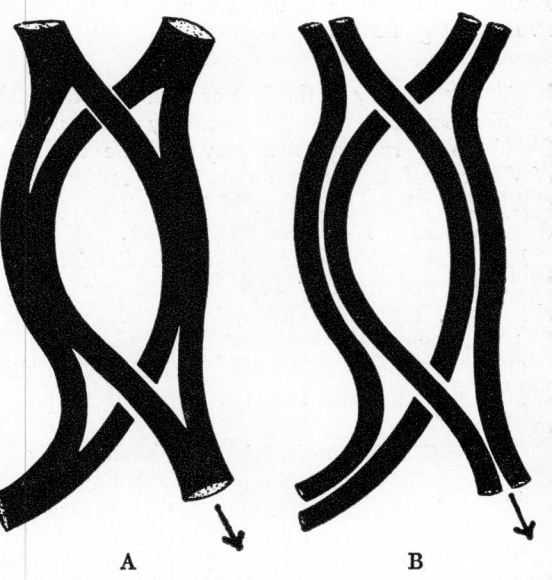

FIG. 293-2. Schematic representation of the postulated nature of the defect in the collagen basketry in the Ehlers-Danlos syndrome. *A.* Normal. *B.* Ehlers-Danlos syndrome. (*After Jansen.*)

294 OSTEOGENESIS IMPERFECTA

Victor A. McKusick

Definition. Osteogenesis imperfecta (synonyms: fragilitas ossium, osteopsathyrosis idiopathica, disease of Eddowes, Lobstein, van der Hoeve, Vrolik) is a heritable, generalized disorder of one element of connective tissue with clinical manifestations in the eye (blue scleras), the ear (progressive deafness), the skeleton (especially multiple fractures; see p. 705), the joints (loose-jointedness), and the skin. The nosography of this syndrome has been much confused because of this wide variability in its clinical expression. Osteogenesis imperfecta congenita and tarda have been separated. A further separation of the tarda type into levis and gravis forms has been suggested. A hereditary disease characterized by fragility of bones, without blue scleras, has been claimed as a separate entity and called specifically osteopsathyrosis idiopathica. Until there is convincing evidence to the contrary, however, the information available leads the author to maintain that all the several clinical pictures which have been described, and which go by separate names in many instances, are one and the same disease which has wide systemic ramifications and an exceedingly great range of clinical severity.

Clinical Manifestations. Skeleton. Multiple fractures with trivial trauma are a main feature. Intrauterine fractures may permit antenatal diagnosis. Usually after puberty, the victim of this disease becomes less subject to fractures; susceptibility may return in later life, especially after the menopause in the female. Bowing of bones, porotic appearance by x-ray, without fracture, "codfish" or "hourglass" vertebras, platybasia (basilar impression of the skull, p. 1729), are all features. Dwarfism with short legs and relatively large head may be confused with achondroplasia. The French artist Toulouse-Lautrec is thought to have had osteogenesis imperfecta. The calvarium tends to bulge laterally, and the head and face have a triangular configuration which often permits diagnosis from photographs alone.

Eye. The change in the sclera, which may be various shades of blue, is the only important ocular feature.

Ear. The deafness has the clinical features of conventional otosclerosis: variable age of onset, steady progression, and likelihood to begin during pregnancy. The tympanic membrane may be blue like the sclera.

Joints. Loose-jointedness is one of the four cardinal features of the disease. It is responsible, at least in part, for the flat feet, kyphoscoliosis, and habitual dislocation of joints. Weakness of ligaments and tendons responsible for the loose-jointedness sometimes results in rupture of tendons from relatively minor stress.

Others. Hernia is frequent. The teeth are characteristically small, misshapen, and bluish-yellow. Kyphoscoliosis can lead in later life to cardiorespiratory complications.

Inheritance. Usually, osteogenesis imperfecta is clearly inherited as an autosomal dominant. Some aspects of its genetics are still confused. Certain features, especially those concerning sporadic cases and the so-called congenital form, suggest a recessive mode of inheritance in a portion of cases.

Pathology and Basic Defect. In the bones, peculiar basophilic-staining material is found in place of osteoid. In other tissues, there is a sparsity of collagen fibers and replacement by fibers with tinctorial and other characteristics of reticulin. There appears to be a generalized defect in maturation of collagen.

REFERENCE

McKusick, V. A.: "Heritable Disorders of Connective Tissue," 2d ed., St. Louis, The C. V. Mosby Company, 1960.

295 PSEUDOXANTHOMA ELASTICUM

Victor A. McKusick

Definition. Pseudoxanthoma elasticum (synonyms: PXE, Groenblad-Strandberg syndrome) is a hereditary, generalized disorder of one element of connective tissue, resulting in premature breakdown of the skin in exposed areas, angioid streaks in the fundus oculi, and hemorrhage from arterial degeneration.

Clinical Manifestations. Skin. In the second, third, or fourth decade of life, patients affected by PXE are likely to develop changes in the skin of the neck, axillas, inguinal areas, and periumbilical zone, consisting of thickening, grooving, and formation of yellowish, diamond-shaped, rectangular, and polygonal nodules (Fig. 295-1). The skin in involved areas becomes inelastic, lax, and redundant. In women, the changes in the neck may be cosmetically disturbing.

Eye. Angioid streaks develop at a variable time, often as early as the second decade. They are brownish or gray and four or five times wider than the veins but resemble vessels in the manner in which they course over the fundus. Proliferative changes occur in the retina, with angioid streaks as points of origin. Hemorrhage contributes further to the ocular damage which may progress to near blindness (see Fig. 295-2).

Arterial Tree. Weak or absent pulses may be found in the extremities. Calcification of arteries is often demonstrable by radiography early in life. Intermittent claudication and easy fatigability of the arms and legs occur. Many of the affected

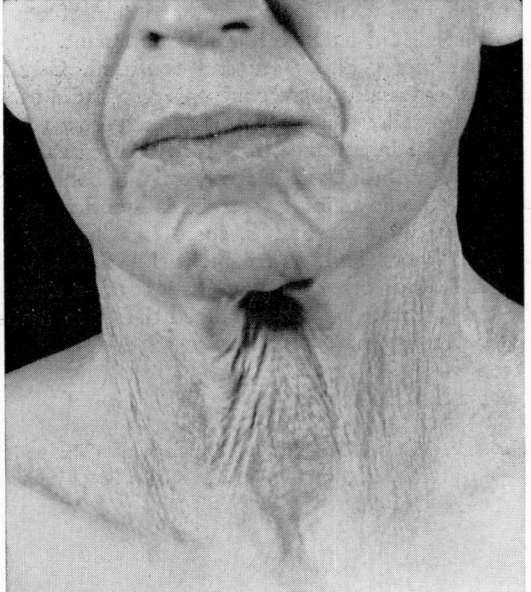

FIG. 295-1. The skin in pseudoxanthoma elasticum.

persons suffer from angina pectoris and hypertension. Recurrent gastrointestinal hemorrhage is the problem which most often brings the patient to the attention of the internist. Occasionally, some lesion such as peptic ulcer or hiatus hernia is discovered and the vascular disease of PXE is considered only an aggravating factor. More often, no such lesion is found. Hemorrhage from other sites—uterine, urinary, nasal, or subarachnoid—may occur.

Inheritance. Pseudoxanthoma elasticum behaves genetically like an autosomal recessive.

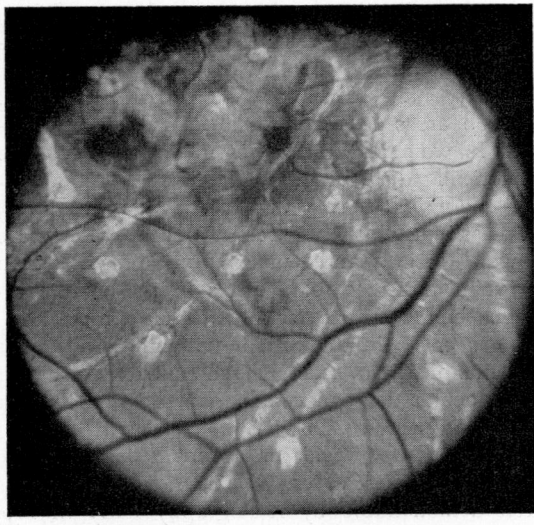

FIG. 295-2. The fundus oculi in pseudoxanthoma elasticum.

Pathology and Basic Defect. The skin and media of arteries of intermediate and smaller size (and occasionally the endocardium and pericardium) become the site of markedly altered connective tissue fibers which are basophilic, have an affinity for calcium, and display the tinctorial characteristics of elastic fibers. In some areas, material of this description is reduced to amorphous or granular accumulations. The basis for angioid streaks appears to be basophilic change and subsequent crazing (cracking) of Bruck's membrane behind the retina. A growing body of evidence suggests that, fundamentally, PXE is a hereditary weakness of collagen fibers which renders them prone to undergo what some call "elastotic degeneration" under stress. Others ascribe the fundamental defect to the elastic fiber.

REFERENCE

McKusick, V. A.: "Heritable Disorders of Connective Tissue," 2d ed., St. Louis, The C. V. Mosby Company, 1960.

296 THE HURLER SYNDROME
Victor A. McKusick

Definition. The Hurler syndrome (synonyms: gargoylism, Hunter-Hurler-Pfaundler syndrome, lipochondrodystrophy, dysostosis multiplex) is thought to be a generalized, heritable disorder of one element of connective tissue, manifested by a characteristic malformation of the skeleton, stiff joints, deafness, lesions of the arterial retina and heart valves, hepatosplenomegaly, corneal clouding, and impairment of intellect.

Clinical Manifestations. Although previously considered the exclusive property of the pediatrician, this syndrome is coming more to the attention of the internist. Milder forms of the disease are consistent with survival to adulthood (Fig. 296-1), and improved supportive measures permit longer survival of more severely affected cases. The child is often considered normal at birth; with time, the abnormality in pattern of growth of the skeleton becomes evident, and slowing of intellectual development, deafness, enlargement of the liver and spleen, and clouding of the cornea set in. The deformity of the facial bones results in stertorous respiration, frequent upper respiratory infection, and mouth breathing which creates an appearance superficially suggesting cretinism. Virtually all joints of the body display reduced mobility. Dyspnea, precordial pain, and congestive heart failure develop. Murmurs referable to any of the four valves of the heart can develop. The mitral and

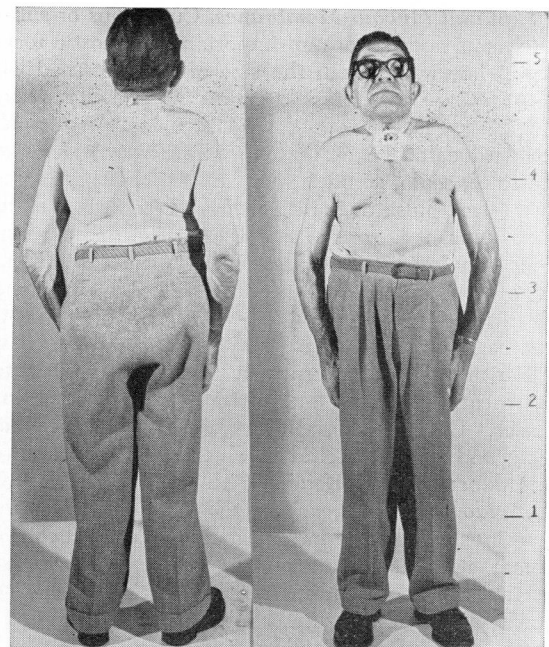

FIG. 296-1. The Hurler syndrome in a 46-year-old man. (*Courtesy, Dr. John F. Murray and New England Journal of Medicine.*)

aortic valves are most often affected. Sudden death, seemingly cardiac in origin, is frequent. Intercurrent respiratory infection is also a common cause of death.

Inheritance. There are at least two genetic variants of this disease—one inherited as an autosomal recessive and one as a sex-linked inheritance—the cornea is less likely to be affected, intellect is less severely impaired, gibbus (or lumbar kyphosis) is less frequent, and survival to a later age, even the forties, is possible. Otherwise, the clinical features of the two varieties are identical.

Pathology and Basic Defect. Cartilage, fascia, tendons, periosteum, blood vessels, heart valves, meninges, and cornea show characteristic cells which are thought to arise from fibroblasts; these are distended by a substance with properties of a mucopolysaccharide and have been designated as "gargoyle cells." Material presumably identical with that in the fibroblasts "balloons" the nerve cells of the central nervous system, peripheral ganglions, and retina, the Kupffer and parenchymal cells of the liver, the reticulum cells of spleen and lymph nodes, and the epithelial cells of endocrine glands. Extensive deposits may be found in the intima of coronary arteries, aorta, and pulmonary artery. The heart valves become scarred and deformed.

Two mucopolysaccharides are excreted in the urine in appreciable amounts and are identified in various organs: chondroitin sulfate B and sulfate. There is no qualitative difference in the mucopolysaccharides excreted in the two genetic forms of the disease.

The basic defect is thought to concern mucopolysaccharide metabolism. To account for the excess of two mucopolysaccharides on the basis of a single gene defect, one is forced to conclude that some step common to the metabolism of the two is defective. The biochemical basis of the progressive mental defect is not clear. Hydrocephalus resulting from meningeal deposits undoubtedly contributes to the mental defect.

REFERENCE

McKusick, V. A.: "Heritable Disorders of Connective Tissue," 2d ed., St. Louis, The C. V. Mosby Company, 1960.

297 POLYARTERITIS NODOSA
Philip A. Tumulty

Definition. Polyarteritis nodosa is characterized by focal and diffuse inflammatory damage to blood vessels, especially small and medium arteries, with resulting altered function of the organs involved. The disease runs a subacute or chronic course, and its clinical manifestations are often confusingly diverse.

Incidence and Etiology. Polyarteritis is relatively uncommon. It is most often seen in the fourth decade, although it has occurred in infants and the aged. The disease is two to three times as frequent in males as in females. There is no known racial or familial predisposition.

In the past, many possible etiologies have been considered, including specific infectious agents, "toxins" of several types, and neurogenic disturbance. Necrotizing arteritis morphologically similar to that of polyarteritis in man has been produced in rabbits by sensitization to proteins and in rats by several procedures that induce hypertension.

In many cases of polyarteritis nodosa, the onset of symptoms has followed closely on serum sickness or sensitivity reaction to sulfonamides, iodides, penicillin, thiouracil, or other drugs. Furthermore, there is a close association between chronic bronchial asthma and polyarteritis. While the possibility of diverse etiologies cannot be excluded, it seems certain that hypersensitivity is one cause of the disease in man.

Pathology. The principal lesion is an inflammation of small and medium arteries, including the vasa vasorum. Veins and capillaries are sometimes involved also. The entire thickness of the vessel wall is inflamed with necrosis and destruction of all coats. Involvement is usually segmental, and only a portion of the circumference of the artery may be attacked. Eosinophils are usually prominent in the acute lesions. The consequences of the injury vary; there may be rupture, healing with fibrosis, or thrombosis and recanalization, or an aneurysm can develop. It is common to find lesions in all stages of inflammation and repair in biopsy or autopsy specimens; this is in keeping with the subacute or chronic intermittent clinical course. Granulomatous nodules that seem unrelated to vessels may occur in various organs or on serosal surfaces, and focal or diffuse glomerulonephritis is a frequent feature of the disease.

It is important to realize that arteritis is a feature of many diseases, including lupus erythematosus, rheumatoid arthritis, serum sickness, and rheumatic fever. Furthermore, arterial changes morphologically indistinguishable from those of polyarteritis can be found in the intestinal submucosa of some patients with uremia or at the periphery of necrotizing or suppurative bacterial lesions. Therefore, the presence of arteritis, especially in the absence of a prominent eosinophilic component in the inflammation, is not diagnostic of polyarteritis nodosa, and biopsy findings must be interpreted in light of the entire clinical picture.

Manifestations. The initial manifestations are so variable that it is impossible to describe a "typical" mode of onset. Symptoms sometimes appear abruptly in an individual who has previously been entirely well; more often, the process seems to begin as the second chapter of a recent illness. The primary incident may be some banal disorder (pulmonary infection, cholecystitis) with apparent recovery or a period of vague indisposition and the subsequent development of new manifestations and overt disability, hard to interpret in terms of what has previously transpired.

Disease of an organ system such as nephritis or neuritis is not at all infrequent in polyarteritis, but, initially, the patient more often gives the impression that he is suffering from some subacute febrile disease, perhaps infectious in origin, without localizing signs. Frequent early complaints are weakness, myalgia, fatigability, anorexia, weight loss (sometimes striking), headache, chilliness or chills, and fever. There may be afebrile intervals, but patients usually continue to feel ill; a few patients never have fever. Drenching sweats are common, and disproportionate tachycardia is frequent.

Past emphasis on the "triad" of fever, abdominal pain, and hypertension in a young man as typical of polyarteritis was probably unjustified. Certainly, the vast majority of cases fail to show this picture in any clear-cut fashion.

Skin and Mucous Membranes. Cutaneous or subcutaneous nodules are an important diagnostic feature. They range from the size of a millet seed to that of a pea, occur singly or in crops, regress very quickly (repeated examination is mandatory), and can be located on any part of the body, including the soles, scalp, scrotum, and tongue. Occasionally, they are pulsatile and clearly represent small aneurysms; it is rare to find these. The nodular lesions may be distributed linearly along vessels, and the overlying skin can be normal, reddened, or even ulcerated. Unfortunately, only a minority of patients will be found to have these striking lesions.

Far more frequent are such nonspecific eruptions as urticaria, purpura, and a variety of erythematous rashes. Occasionally, Raynaud's phenomenon is seen, and rarely, arterial involvement will simulate thromboangiitis obliterans with acrogangrene.

Livido racemosa, arborescent red or purplish markings which fade into normal skin without sharp demarcation, is an unusual but diagnostically important cutaneous finding in polyarteritis. Mucosal lesions are unusual in this disease.

Musculoskeletal. Tenderness and aching in muscles and arthralgia are often prominent early features. Occasionally, trichinosis or primary myositis are suggested by the severity of pain. Later, weakness and atrophy can be so profound that a primary disorder of muscle seems likely. Frank arthritis is relatively unusual, although deformities indistinguishable from rheumatoid disease have been noted.

Eyes. Ocular manifestations are common, arising in four ways: (1) direct involvement of retinal vessels with exudation, hemorrhage, "cytoid" bodies, retinal detachment, arterial occlusion, papilledema, and optic atrophy; (2) exudative lesions of mesenchymal elements leading to episcleritis, iridocyclitis, or tenonitis; (3) cerebral arterial disease with extraocular palsy or pupillomotor disturbances and visual field defects; (4) hypertensive retinopathy associated with renal impairment.

Lungs and Pleura. Pulmonary alterations occur in about 25 per cent of patients with polyarteritis. Because histologic changes may be present without symptoms and because the roentgenographic findings and clinical manifestations are rarely diagnostic, it suffices to realize that the lungs may be involved in this disease. The observed changes range from nodular opacities resembling miliary tuberculosis or carcinomatosis to confluent pneumonic consolidation, usually basilar or extending fanlike from the hilum. There may be cavitation if larger vessels are involved, and pulmonary infarcts or rupture of vessels can lead to hemoptysis. Lesions in the submucosal vessels can result in tracheobronchial ulceration, with cough and bloody sputum.

Secondary bacterial infection may lead to pneumonitis, lung abscess, or emphysema.

The relationship of polyarteritis to *bronchial asthma* has long been stressed. A history of typical asthmatic attacks may precede the onset of systemic arteritis by many years. Whether the asthma indicates the early onset of pulmonary arteritis or is of the ordinary type is not known.

An attempt has been made to characterize a group of patients with polyarteritis nodosa whose illness is primarily pulmonary. The individuals all have chronic pulmonary alterations of long standing, develop what appears to be a respiratory infection, and then are found to have high blood eosinophilia, numerous eosinophils in acute arteritic lesions, and many focal necrotic or granulomatous lesions unrelated to blood vessels in the liver, spleen, kidneys, lymph nodes, and heart.

Pleurisy occurs with or without effusion, occasionally bloody and, at times, secondarily infected.

Serial x-rays of the lungs may help somewhat in establishing a diagnosis of polyarteritis if they show regression of earlier lesions, appearance of new infiltrates and, in general, a continuous flux. The instability of the findings contrasts with those in lupus erythematosus which are likely to remain stable for many months.

Cardiovascular. Episodes of pericarditis with or without small effusions are frequent; a massive bloody effusion may result from a ruptured vessel. The myocardium is affected by coronary arteritis and, rarely, the clinical picture may be dominated by coronary insufficiency and terminate with massive infarction. Focal granulomatous myocarditis is sometimes severe enough to produce congestive failure or conduction defects. With the onset of renal insufficiency and hypertension, cardiac enlargement and failure are even more likely. Warty, abacterial vegetations sometimes appear on the endocardium. They may be a locus of bacterial endocarditis.

The concurrent existence of rheumatic heart disease and polyarteritis has been recognized for many years and, of course, is one of the arguments for hypersensitivity as a common factor in the etiology of these two diseases.

Gastrointestinal. Abdominal pain, nausea, vomiting, diarrhea, and intestinal bleeding are often early and outstanding manifestations. Features of "multisystem" disease are sometimes preceded by an episode of clinically uncomplicated appendicitis, cholecystitis, or pancreatitis. Later, confusing indications of systemic disease appear or abdominal pain continues. Recognition that it is associated with disease in other organs may lead to the correct diagnosis.

Depending upon the extent and localization of vascular disease, many intraabdominal disturbances occur: focal pain; acute diffuse pain without findings at laparotomy; focal or diffuse bleeding, sometimes massive; intraabdominal hematomas mistaken for tumor, cyst, or aneurysm; perforation of a viscus (especially the gallbladder); mucosal ulcerations; infarction of the gut.

A moderate degree of hepatomegaly is usual. Because the hepatic arterial and venous radicles can be involved in the disease, there may ensue enough vascular insufficiency to produce true infarction of the liver parenchyma. Indeed, polyarteritis is the most frequent cause of large hepatic infarcts. Pain, friction rubs, and jaundice signal massive infarction. Smaller foci of destruction heal with scarring that, in a single biopsy specimen, resembles a cirrhosis.

Spleen and Lymph Nodes. Lymphadenopathy is not characteristic of polyarteritis. Mild splenic enlargement is present in about one-third of the cases. Rarely, splenic infarction or hemorrhage around the spleen has been observed, the latter simulating a large tumor.

Genitourinary. Some type of renal involvement occurs in at least 80 per cent of patients. Often this becomes clinically evident only late in the disease.

Rupture of a renal artery can produce a large *perirenal hematoma*, and on many occasions, this has been mistaken for a tumor or cyst. Renal *infarcts* are not infrequent. However, focal or diffuse glomerulonephritis is by far the most important renal lesion in polyarteritis. It can be severe and progressive, is often accompanied by hypertension, and leads to death in uremia or congestive heart failure.

Hypertension sometimes fluctuates so strikingly that pheochromocytoma is suspected.

The vessels of the bladder may be affected, producing changes resembling "hemorrhagic cystitis." The testes and epididymis are frequently involved; testicular infarction with severe pain and subsequent atrophy is more frequent in polyarteritis nodosa than in any other single condition.

Nervous System. *Peripheral neuritis,* a result of inflammation of nutrient vessels, is the most commonly encountered abnormality of nervous function. It is often one of the first and most marked disabilities. Indeed, in any obscure illness, the appearance of neuritis should immediately call to mind the possibility of polyarteritis. In about half the affected cases, involvement is mononeural; in the others a symmetrical polyneuritis, more severe in the lower extremities, is seen. Severe pain is common, and the sensory deficit frequently exceeds the motor. Regression of the neuritis is characteristic.

Involvement of carotid, vertebral, meningeal, or deep cerebral vessels can lead to hemiplegia, transverse myelitis, convulsions, cerebellar dysfunction, extrapyramidal disorders, optic atrophy, or subarachnoid hemorrhage.

Cranial palsies are not common; the facial nerve is most frequently involved. Implication of the meninges may result in changes in the spinal fluid suggesting aseptic or lymphocytic meningitis.

Laboratory Findings. Polymorphonuclear leukocytosis is the rule, total counts of 40,000 or more being seen. Mild eosinophilia occurs in 20 to 30 per cent, and striking eosinophil counts are occasionally found. The sedimentation rate is elevated; mild anemia, even in the absence of uremia, is frequent. It may be hemolytic and associated with a positive Coombs test.

The urine may show protein, erythrocytes, leukocytes, and a variety of cellular and noncellular casts, so-called "telescoping" of the sediment.

False positive serologic tests for syphilis are found in a small number of cases, and many serum protein changes including hyperglobulinemia, cryoglobulinemia, macroglobulinemia, as well as circulating anticoagulants have been reported.

Diagnosis. Abdominal pain, muscular aches, peripheral neuritis, evidence of renal disease, or hypertension in a setting of weight loss, fever, and leukocytosis are the predominant clinical features, but variation is endless. The process may run an acute, subacute, or chronic course over a period of months or years. Spontaneous recovery can occur. Periods of remission of varying length may punctuate the indolent evolution of a bewildering array of seemingly unrelated disorders. Careful search for cutaneous nodules and repeated attempts to confirm the diagnosis by biopsy examination are essential. Skin or muscle is probably the best tissue for examination. Lymph nodes will rarely give the diagnosis. Renal biopsy often shows glomerular disease, but the specific diagnosis of polyarteritis is difficult to establish on this basis. Liver biopsy is very unlikely to show the vascular lesion, although, on rare occasions, the diagnosis has come from examination of this tissue alone. It is important to take skin and muscle from an area of tenderness, where possible. Because the demonstration of arteritis is the only method for establishing the presence of polyarteritis, repeated biopsy examinations are in order.

Treatment. The long-term use of corticosteroids as outlined in the section on systemic lupus erythematosus (p. 1896) is the only presently available therapy of any value. Although use of these agents may result in further injury to tissues by virtue of occlusion of vessels secondary to the healing process, this also happens spontaneously, and there is no choice. While on corticosteroids, the patient's adherence to a modified ulcer program is essential. One must be constantly on the lookout for secondary bacterial and other infections which not infrequently complicate the disease and which may easily be overlooked as a part of the primary disease process.

REFERENCES

Nuzum, J. W., Jr., and J. W. Nuzum: Polyarteritis Nodosa: A Statistical Review of 175 Cases from Literature and Report of "Typical" Case, A.M.A. Arch. Internal Med., 94:942, 1954.

Rose, G. A.: The Natural History of Polyarteritis, Brit. Med. J., 5054:1148, 1957.

——, and H. Spencer: Polyarteritis Nodosa, Quart. J. Med., Oxford, 26:43, 1957.

Zeek, P. M.: Medical Progress: Periarteritis Nodosa and Other Forms of Necrotizing Angiitis, New Engl. J. Med., 248:764, 1953.

298 SYSTEMIC LUPUS ERYTHEMATOSUS

Philip A. Tumulty

Definition. Systemic lupus erythematosus (SLE) is manifested by characteristic inflammation of the skin, mucosal surfaces, serous membranes, and singly or in combination, other organs including the kidney, heart, lung, and brain. The disorder tends to evolve episodically over a span of years, although it may run an acute, fulminating course.

Incidence and Etiology. Systemic lupus erythematosus is three to four times more frequent in women especially during the third and fourth decades. It appears at any age, in Negroes and whites and, while familial occurrence of the full-blown disease is rare, there is some evidence implicating a congenital susceptibility to the disease. Systemic lupus erythematosus is not uncommon; indeed, its incidence seems to be increasing at a rate that cannot be explained solely by better diagnosis. Exposure to sunlight; various stresses, such as surgery, trauma, and pregnancy; and taking of drugs have often seemed to precipitate an exacerbation of the disease. A lupuslike illness may follow the chronic administration of hydralazine. Upper respiratory infections sometimes precede the initial appearance of symptoms. An allergic mechanism has been suggested, and the frequency with which patients with SLE develop hypersensitivity to drugs and other substances is impressive. There is abundant evidence for a peculiar alteration in immune mechanisms as a major feature of the disease, and it is possible that so-called autoimmunity may prove to be important etiologically. In almost all patients with lupus, the serum eventually shows abnormal γ-globulins which behave as antibodies. Serum factors that interact with erythrocytes, white cells, platelets, kidney, heart, liver, and thyroglobulin have been demonstrated. The Wassermann reaction is frequently positive, and the rheumatoid factor (see p. 1911) is found in approximately 20 per cent of lupus serums.

The LE factor which promotes phagocytosis of nucleoprotein is the basis for the convenient diagnostic test. However, many patients also possess serum antibodies to whole nuclei and nucleoprotein, to DNA, to histone, and to a water-soluble extract of cells (perhaps RNA). Anticytoplasmic factors may be present, as well. Whether these abnormal substances have a direct causal relationship to lupus or are merely manifestations of some more fundamental disorder is still obscure. There is no consistent correlation between their presence and the manifestations or activity of the disease.

Pathology. The typical histologic alteration is swelling of the collagen, "fibrinoid" changes in the ground substance, and infiltration of polymorphonuclear leukocytes, plasma cells, and lymphocytes. Such connective tissue lesions have been observed in almost all structures of the body, the more striking examples being found in the walls of small arteries and arterioles, the skin, spleen, glomeruli, endocardium, and serous membranes. Hematoxylin bodies, remnants of injured nuclei closely resembling the inclusions in LE cells, may occur in association with these lesions and are pathognomonic.

Manifestations. Fever, malaise, weakness, anorexia, weight loss, and other evidences of debility without apparent localization of the disease are very common.

Skin and Mucous Membranes. Cutaneous lesions occur in 85 per cent of patients, usually early in the course but sometimes late. They may appear alone, or with disorders of other organ systems. The lesions have been confused with lichen planus, seborrhea, sarcoidosis, psoriasis, scleroderma, erythema multiforme, dermatomyositis, eczema, rosacea, and drug reactions. Pleomorphic erythematous maculopapular eruptions, often symmetrical, appear most commonly on the face, neck, and extremities. The "typical" malar butterfly appears less often. Quite characteristic of lupus are vascularized lesions round the nail beds and the tips of the digits, with eventual thinning and atrophy of the skin in these locations. Patchy edema, blebs and bullae, or small areas of ulceration may appear. In chronic lesions the skin becomes thickened, scaly, and atrophic. Urticaria, altered pigmentation, and alopecia are common. Erythema nodosum and purpura are frequent, and the patient may be thought to have idiopathic thrombocytopenic purpura.

The mucous membranes are usually involved only during severe exacerbations of the disease, showing ulceration or hemorrhagic foci.

Raynaud's phenomenon sometimes precedes other evidences of SLE by several years, although this is noted more frequently in scleroderma.

Approximately 1 per cent of patients who are believed to have "discoid lupus" of the skin eventually develop manifestations of SLE.

Lymphatics and Spleen. Lymphadenopathy, especially cervical and axillary, is sometimes so prominent that the diagnosis of lymphoma or tuberculous adenitis (which sometimes complicates SLE) is suggested. Mild splenomegaly is frequent, but very large spleens are rare.

Musculoskeletal. It is unusual for SLE to run its course without involvement of the joints, which is often the earliest and only abnormality, sometimes for a prolonged period. Acute migratory polyarthritis closely simulating rheumatic fever even in its dramatic response to salicylates, arthralgias without objective changes, and deforming arthropathy indistinguishable from rheumatoid arthritis are all seen. The concomitant occurrence of SLE and rheumatoid disease cannot be excluded in many patients, but it can be stated that deformities once considered to be characteristic of rheumatoid arthritis are frequent in patients with unequivocal SLE.

Muscle atrophy and weakness can be so pronounced that patients may be suspected of having dermatomyositis or dystrophy. It may be difficult or impossible to distinguish lupus from dermatomyositis on either clinical or histologic grounds.

Aseptic necrosis of bone, particularly of the femoral head, has been noted in SLE, although the role of long-term adrenal steroid treatment in its genesis remains to be worked out.

Eyes. Nonspecific retinal hemorrhages and exudates are not rare, and conjunctivitis is common. More helpful diagnostically is the finding in 10 to 20 per cent of patients of small, round or oval, white opacities adjacent to vessels in the central fundus. These "cytoid bodies" are believed to represent foci of retinal neural degeneration secondary to occlusion of small vessels.

Lungs and Pleura. Recurrent episodes of pleurisy are very common. Effusions are usually small; massive hydrothorax should suggest a complicating infection such as tuberculosis.

Pulmonary infiltrates, especially in the basilar segments, can be a direct result of SLE, as can more extensive involvement which may mimic miliary tuberculosis or lymphangitic carcinomatosis, and lead to respiratory insufficiency or cor pulmonale. However, no pulmonary lesion in a patient with SLE should be accepted as primary until complicating infection has been excluded. Lupus infiltrates may persist without changes for many months. The finding by x-ray of the combination of multiple platelike areas of atelectasis at the bases, elevation of the diaphragm, and pleuritis is probably the one that is most suggestive of SLE. Abnormal physical signs are not prominent. Arteritis of pulmonary vessels may result in hemoptysis, cavity formation, or lung abscess, if secondary infection occurs.

Cardiovascular. Pericarditis is very frequent, but significant effusions are unusual although tamponade has been observed. A complicating bacterial pericarditis requires exclusion.

Typical flat vegetations occur on the heart valves, especially the mitral. Unlike the lesions of rheumatic fever which follow the line of closure, lupus vegetations are found under the valve leaflets, in the commissure. These so-called Libman-Sacks vegetations do not usually interfere with valve function, but rare instances of mitral stenosis or insufficiency attributable to SLE are known. They may form a nidus for bacterial endocarditis.

Myocarditis is not evident clinically in most patients but may result in congestive failure and various conduction abnormalities.

Lesions of the arteries indistinguishable histologically from those of polyarteritis nodosa save for a paucity of eosinophils are frequent in SLE. This type of vascular change can lead to disordered function of any organ system sometime during the course of the disease and is responsible for many puzzling clinical manifestations.

Gastrointestinal. Any portion of the esophagus, stomach, or intestine may be involved by infarcts or ulcerations, the majority of which are initiated by arterial changes. The result may be dysphagia and changes simulating scleroderma, or massive hemorrhage, diarrhea, or focal abdominal pain. A malabsorption syndrome may be consequent to diffuse intestinal changes.

Mild hepatomegaly is frequent, but jaundice or overt evidence of disordered liver function is rare. So-called lupoid hepatitis is discussed on p. 1679.

Kidneys. Focal or diffuse glomerulonephritis with or without classic "wire loop" changes is present in the kidneys of a majority of patients who die with SLE. The basic renal alteration is a glomerulitis.

Episodes of acute nephritis, a typical nephrotic syndrome, and varying degrees of chronic renal impairment are very common. Microscopic hematuria, red blood cell casts, and proteinuria are the usual urinary findings, but occasional patients may show heavy pyuria without hematuria. It is not unusual for patients with relatively normal urine and renal function as measured by the usual tests to show extensive histologic alterations in renal biopsy specimens. This clinical-pathological paradox in which abnormal urinary findings appear late in the course of the renal lesion probably explains the apparent abruptness of renal failure in some individuals with SLE.

Recovery from episodes of acute nephritis is common, but the appearance of renal impairment of significant degree is an ominous sign. In the absence of renal failure, sustained hypertension is unusual in uncomplicated SLE.

It is appropriate to mention the relative frequency of complicating pyelonephritis in SLE and the consequent necessity of differentiating bacterial infection from the primary disease.

Central Nervous System. Many abnormalities can occur; because these are produced by vascular lesions of varying extent and location, no typical pattern results. Psychotic episodes, convulsions, hemipareses, and transient cranial palsies are relatively common. Peripheral neuritis and spinal cord lesions are extremely rare. Epileptiform seizures in patients with SLE have often been mistaken initially for the idiopathic variety, and similarly, SLE may be recognized only after a patient has been treated for several episodes of psychotic behavior of unknown etiology.

Sterile meningitis with fever, headache, and polymorphonuclear pleocytosis can occur in SLE, sometimes in the absence of other distinctive signs of this disease. Cryptococcosis and tuberculosis may complicate the course of SLE and require exclusion.

Generally, significant disorders of the nervous system signify a severe exacerbation of the disease and demand immediate therapy.

Other Organs. Systemic lupus erythematosus is associated with the Sjögren syndrome (p. 1917) and Hashimoto's disease of the thyroid (p. 598) with considerable frequency. It is not surprising that this has led to much discussion of autoimmune mechanisms in the etiology of all three diseases.

Laboratory Findings. The *peripheral leukocyte count* is usually normal or depressed, although complicating bacterial infection may induce a brisk leukocytosis. Even with marked leukopenia, the differential count remains normal; appreciable neutropenia is not characteristic of SLE.

Moderate anemia is common, but severe anemia is not. *Hemolytic anemia* can occur and may dominate the clinical course; the Coombs test is sometimes positive, and a primary hematologic disorder is often suspected initially in such cases.

Thrombocytopenia with purpura is a rather frequent presenting manifestation. Splenectomy has led to amelioration of the platelet deficiency in these patients. In one well-studied group of patients with "idiopathic" thrombocytopenic purpura, splenectomy was effective but, in subsequent years, other stigmas of SLE made their appearance. A review of the histologic sections of the spleens showed the typical "onion-peel" lesion of small arteries in every case. Underlying SLE should be suspected in any patient with thrombocytopenia and, of course, if splenectomy is done, a careful search for these diagnostic lesions is in order.

In a few instances circulating anticoagulants have been demonstrated.

About 15 per cent of patients with SLE show chronic *biologic false positive tests for syphilis*. It is now well recognized that this finding may precede the onset of overt symptoms by many years. The etiologic significance of false positive serologic tests and of the even more frequent elevation in serum globulin, usually the gamma portion, in terms of a basic abnormality of immune mechanisms is strongly suspected but not yet completely established.

Approximately 80 per cent of patients with SLE will eventually be found to have positive LE cell tests. The cells are often present intermittently during the course of the disease, or more properly, the plasma LE factor responsible for the formation of the cells is present intermittently, and repeated tests are indicated in any case of suspected SLE. There are scattered reports of the occurrence of LE cells in other disorders (hepatitis, cirrhosis, drug reactions, rheumatoid arthritis). However, the relatively rare exceptions in no way detract from the great diagnostic significance of the test for SLE. The presence or number of LE cells in the blood at any given time is not correlated with activity of the disease and is not an index of therapeutic effect.

Finally, it is not surprising that such tests as those of cephalin flocculation and thymol turbidity are frequently positive in patients with SLE; this is nearly always a result of abnormalities in serum proteins which are unrelated to any disease or dysfunction of the liver.

Diagnosis. The course of SLE may be short and fulminant. More often, it is prolonged for several or many years. The characteristic feature of its natural course is episodicity, periods of activity of the process of varying length and severity being followed by periods of remission for months or years. During episodes of activity one or more of the organ systems may be involved, either singly or in a wide variety of confusing combinations. This can make diagnosis exceedingly difficult. Not only is the physician who is confronted by an isolated exacerbation of pleurisy or febrile lymphadenopathy likely to conclude that he is dealing with a disorder that affects those tissues only, but the significance of past bouts of seemingly unrelated illness is difficult to appreciate. The common clinical manifestations of SLE are fever, malaise, anorexia, etc., which, of course, are completely nonspecific. Therefore, in few other circumstances is it more important to interpret a patient's complaints in terms of his past history. Previous episodes of pneumonia, pleurisy, purpura, or dermatitis (especially following exposure to sunlight) would certainly give new meaning to a current attack of arthritis. When confronted by an illness with a confusing array of

disorders, one must realize that this is typical of SLE. Among the diseases that have been confused with SLE are:

Rheumatic fever	Nephrosis
Rheumatoid arthritis	Ulcerative colitis
Felty's syndrome	Meningitis
Various skin disorders	Cerebrovascular accident
Dermatitis medicamentosa	Epilepsy
Syphilis	Psychosis
Idiopathic thrombopenic purpura	Drug reaction
	Septicemia
Hemolytic or other obscure anemias	Dermatomyositis
	Scleroderma
Leukopenia due to other causes	Tuberculosis
	Trichinosis
Virus pneumonia	Brucellosis
Chronic basilar infection	Bacterial endocarditis
Raynaud's syndrome	Lymphoma
Fever of undetermined origin	Sjögren's syndrome
	Periarteritis
Acute or chronic nephritis	Hepatitis

In addition to the LE test, biopsy examination of skin lesions or a lymph node may establish the diagnosis. Muscle or renal biopsy is less likely to be diagnostic, although valuable additional evidence in support of SLE is often found.

Treatment. No curative therapy is known. However, with judicious management, the disease can often be controlled well enough for patients to lead active lives with a minimum of disability or discomfort.

General. Direct exposure to sunlight should be shunned. Also to be avoided in so far as possible are elective surgery, trauma, emotional stress, nonessential drugs, and serum products, including transfusions, all of which appear to be capable of "triggering" an exacerbation of SLE. The role of *pregnancy* is not clear cut; in some patients it appears to activate the disease, in others not. One can advise a patient only by balancing the severity and extent of illness against her desire for a family.

For many patients, the unqualified term "lupus" has come to have as bad a connotation as "cancer" or "leukemia," and thoughtless use of it should be avoided. The physician must use all his ingenuity in maintaining the patient's morale during the course of SLE, which can encompass many years.

For reasons not yet clear (perhaps related to dysproteinemia or to adrenal steroid therapy) patients with SLE seem prone to *bacterial infections,* which they resist poorly. The therapeutic implications of realizing that all manifestations of illness in these patients are not necessarily directly attributable to SLE are obvious.

Specific. Antimalarial drugs sometimes help to control discoid skin lesions, but their relative ineffectiveness and untoward side effects limit their usefulness in systemic lupus. Hydroxychloroquine (Plaquenil) may be given in a dosage of 200 mg three or four times daily; the dose of chloroquine (Aralen) is 250 mg twice daily; and that of amodiaquin (Camoquin) 200 mg twice daily. These agents have largely replaced atabrine (100 mg twice daily). Anorexia, nausea, and diarrhea are not rare with these drugs, and dermatitis has been reported in 10 to 15 per cent of patients who take them over prolonged periods.

Nitrogen mustards have been advocated for the nephrotic syndrome of SLE, but results are unimpressive and they should be tried only under the rarest of circumstances.

Salicylates are very helpful in controlling musculoskeletal pain; they may obviate the need for steroids or enable the use of smaller maintenance doses of these hormones.

Both *ACTH* and the *corticosteroids* are highly effective in controlling the inflammatory manifestations of SLE. There is no clear-cut evidence that any one of the many steroid compounds now available is superior for SLE. Prednisone is preferred by many because of wide experience with it. A program employing moderate dosage is usually effective, and it is rarely necessary to make patients "Cushingoid." An exception is the rare "lupus crisis" in which an overwhelming exacerbation of the disease has been controlled by massive administration of steroids within hours or days. From 40 to 60 mg prednisone in divided doses four times daily almost invariably brings about prompt subsidence of symptoms in SLE. As soon as fever, pain, etc., are controlled, the dosage should be reduced slowly over a period of a few weeks until a maintenance level (usually 10 to 20 mg daily) is found. If the disease flares up, the dosage is increased again. The maintenance may have to be continued for months or years, but in all patients, the amount of steroid taken should be reduced cautiously at regular intervals to see if a lower dose will maintain the remission.

Renal insufficiency is no longer regarded as a contraindication to steroids, which should be continued along with other appropriate measures (see p. 1496). The confusion between effects of SLE and of steroids upon the central nervous system can be troublesome, but the nervous system alterations caused by SLE are usually found only when other organ systems are actively involved and will often be benefited by increased dosage of steroid.

A modified regimen for peptic ulcer is extremely important in patients given steroids for SLE and should be maintained strictly.

Prognosis. Because of previous failure to recognize the episodic recurrences of illness in SLE, accurate information about the natural history of the disease is scanty. Similarly, definite evidence that steroids alter the duration of life in any significant fashion is lacking. It appears that the duration of illness in SLE is a function of the wide spectrum of the disease's severity, ranging from death in a few weeks with fulminant lupus to reasonable good health for 15 or even 20 years despite occasional episodes of active disease.

A deciding factor in prognosis, of course, is the amount of irreversible damage to essential organs. It is probably that the control of inflammation by adrenal steroids can minimize this damage and prolong life. Of importance in considering this matter also are the antibiotics, which now prevent many deaths from complicating infection.

REFERENCES

Deicher, H. R., H. R. Holman, and H. G. Kunkel: The Precipitin Reaction between DNA and a Serum Factor in SLE, J. Exptl. Med., 109:97, 1959.

Friedman, E. A., W. A. Bardawil, J. P. Merrill, and E. Hanan: "Delayed" Cutaneous Hypersensitivity to Leukocytes in SLE, New Engl. J. Med., 262:486, 1960.

Harvey, A. M., L. E. Shulman, P. A. Tumulty, and C. L. Conley: Systemic Lupus Erythematosus: Review of the Literature and Clinical Analysis of 138 Cases, Medicine, 33:291, 1954.

Miescher, P.: The Immunopathology of Lupus Erythematosus, Brit. J. Dermatol., 72:221, 1960.

Moore, J. E., and W. B. Lutz: The Natural History of Systemic Lupus Erythematosus: Approach to Its Study through Chronic Biologic False Positive Reactors, J. Chron. Diseases, 1:297, 1955.

Muehrcke, R. C., R. M. Kark, C. L. Pirani, and V. E. Pollak: Lupus Nephritis: A Clinical and Pathologic Study Based on Renal Biopsies, Medicine, 36:1, 1957.

Systemic Lupus Erythematosus: Combined Staff Clinic, Am. J. Med., 28:416, 1960.

299 SCLERODERMA (Progressive Systemic Sclerosis)

Philip A. Tumulty

Definition. Scleroderma is a chronic disease of unknown etiology characterized by diffuse sclerosis of the connective tissue of the integument and many other organs. While it occurs at almost any age, the majority of patients are between thirty and fifty years of age, and women are affected twice as frequently as men.

Pathology. The etiology is unknown; suggestions have included neurotropic disturbance, "endocrine imbalance," toxins, and altered immune response.

The principal change is swelling, hypertrophy, and condensation of collagen with the formation of dense, compact connective tissue. Early, there is variable inflammation, but this rarely persists. In the skin, there is atrophy of the epidermis and appendages, increase or decrease in pigment, and often, calcinosis. The increased connective tissue leads to atrophy of skeletal, smooth, and even cardiac muscle. The walls of small arteries and arterioles undergo "fibrinoid" changes leading to occlusion and secondary ischemic alterations.

Manifestations. Depending upon the site of predominant involvement, patients with scleroderma may present in many guises: (1) local or diffuse thickening of the skin, with pigmentary changes or telangiectasis, (2) Raynaud's syndrome with sclerodactylia, (3) diffuse calcinosis, (4) dysphagia, dyspepsia, abnormal intestinal motility, or the malabsorption syndrome, (5) pulmonary cysts, fibrosis, bronchiectasis, or cor pulmonale, (6) hypertension and uremia, (7) myocardial failure or pericardial disease, (8) arthritis, muscle weakness and atrophy, (9) subarachnoid hemorrhage, focal cerebral disease, (10) neurasthenia.

The skin and subcutaneous tissues may be involved in a diffuse or focal manner. The focal form may occur as patches, often about the neck (morphea), as linear streaks sometimes following the course of nerves or blood vessels, or as sclerodactylia. The process may start as the focal type, later becoming diffuse. Either may become associated with visceral involvement, which likewise may be focal or diffuse. Sometimes the visceral component is clinically hidden and is brought to light only by special studies, or is revealed at postmortem examination. Generally, the integumentary changes precede the visceral, sometimes by many years, but occasionally the reverse happens. Constitutional symptoms such as fever are not prominent. Progressive weakness, weight loss, and musculoskeletal aching are early accompaniments, and Raynaud's phenomena may precede other manifestations by many years.

Integument. The evolution of the changes in skin and subcutaneous tissue is usually edema and induration progressing to atrophy, but in the individual patient, these are seen singly or in combination. Alterations in pigment and a variety of vascular lesions such as telangiectasis and currant-like dilatations of vessels in the skin or mucous membranes are common. The upper extremities, trunk, head, and lower extremities tend to be involved in sequence. The skin develops a waxy hardness and luster. The face becomes expressionless, and the nose, ears, and lips appear smaller, thinner, and sharper. If the process extends to the buccal mucosa, talking and swallowing may be difficult. The finger tips thicken and shorten, the overlying skin atrophies, and often, numerous tiny, painful, pitted ulcers appear. These may heal with scarring but can become chronic, with deposition of calcium and extrusion of chalky material. Calcium may be laid down elsewhere in the skin and subcutaneous tissues. Axillary and pubic hair are usually lost, but except for atrophy, the nails are usually spared.

Gastrointestinal Tract. The replacement of smooth muscle by overgrowth of dense fibrous tissue which can occur segmentally or diffusely eventually leads to motor disturbances, loss of propulsive power, and dilatation. Changes in submucosal blood vessels may cause ulcerative lesions. The frequency of involvement is in the following order: esophagus, duodenum, jejunum, and colon. The severity of these visceral changes is unrelated to the degree of dermal involvement; esophageal or intestinal symptoms may precede or follow the external alterations. They are often asymptomatic and unnoted unless disclosed by x-rays or other special studies.

The *esophagus* becomes stiffened, wide, and patulous with diminished or absent peristalsis. Reflux of gastric contents can lead to esophagitis and distal narrowing. While patients may complain of dysphagia, heartburn, etc., striking functional derangement is often disclosed by appropriate x-ray studies in an individual who has had no symptoms, and when scleroderma is suspected, the esophagus should be investigated. The typical functional changes are best demonstrated by intubation with balloons.

The *small intestine* is more often affected than has heretofore been recognized. X-ray findings are marked dilatation of affected segments with adynamic function. Intestinal loops may be dilated from the normal of 2 to 3 cm to more than 5 cm. Clinically, there may be diarrhea, constipation, bloating, episodes simulating obstruction, or frank malabsorption with all the usual nutritional complications (see p. 554).

The *colon* may be affected by similar organic and functional changes, resulting in a large sacculated organ with decreased motility.

Lungs. Diffuse fibrosis with obliteration of alveoli and distortion of the air passages and, occasionally, the development of multiple small cysts is directly attributable to the basic disease process. Additionally, limitation of movements of the chest wall and weakness of the diaphragm can aggravate the alveolocapillary block by superimposing hypoventilation. A third source of pulmonary disease is aspiration of ingested food as esophageal dysfunction progresses. Widespread histologic changes may be present in the lungs even though x-rays of the chest show surprisingly little, or the patient may have few symptoms and a normal physical examination despite widespread fibroses shown by x-ray. The x-ray appearance of the lung is nonspecific, but because extensive pulmonary lesions may antedate the skin changes, scleroderma should be considered in any case of unexplained fibrosis of the lung, especially with cystic changes. Cor pulmonale is a common late sequel to the lung disease. Acute or chronic secondary bacterial infections may be very important.

Heart. Fibrinous pericarditis and hydropericardium are rare, but both have been observed with enough frequency to make it clear that they are a part of the disease. In some instances, the myocardium becomes infiltrated by large bands of vascular connective tissue, independent of any alteration in coronary arterial flow. Cardiomegaly, conduction defects, arrhythmias, and frank congestive heart failure can result. Fibrotic nodules, sometimes calcified, are found along the line of closure of the valves in occasional cases. Clinically, these may produce murmurs that mimic mitral stenosis, and rarely, bacterial endocarditis has arisen at these sites.

Kidney. The course of scleroderma may be dominated by manifestations of hypertensive cardiovascular renal disease. Characteristic histologic lesions in the kidney consist of intimal proliferation and fibrinoid necrosis of interlobular arteries with afferent arteriolonecrosis and focal, necrotizing glomerulitis. Sizable cortical infarcts may occur. It is probable that these lesions can exist focally for a long time without appreciable clinical evidence of renal abnormality. Some patients slowly develop uremia and finally die after many months. In others, however, evidence of renal disease appears abruptly, hypertension and uremia are acute, and the patient dies within a short period. There is nothing characteristic about renal function tests or the urinary sediment. Renal biopsy is helpful in diagnosis. The onset of renal disease is a grave prognostic sign.

While it has been suggested that the administration of adrenal steroids may increase the likelihood of abrupt renal failure, it is clear that sudden hypertension and uremia have occurred terminally in many individuals with scleroderma who were not receiving hormonal treatment.

Musculoskeletal. Muscle weakness and atrophy may be widespread. Myositis that is clinically and histologically similar to dermatomyositis may occur. Arthralgia or arthritis may be prominent.

Central Nervous System. Focal vascular lesions of the brain, cord, and peripheral nerves result in mental aberrations, convulsions, hemorrhage (sometimes subarachnoid), pareses, neuritis, and other nonspecific neurologic complaints.

Endocrine Glands. The adrenal, thyroid, and parathyroid glands are rarely affected, although formerly dysfunction of these glands was considered to have an etiologic role.

Laboratory Findings. None is diagnostic of or specific for scleroderma. The hemogram is usually normal but for an elevated sedimentation rate. The serum γ-globulins may be increased.

Biopsy may be helpful in establishing the diagnosis, although at times the changes are disappointingly nonspecific, particularly early in the disease.

Course. The disease may progress relentlessly, reach a plateau, or partially regress over a period of months and years. The visceral lesions seem less likely to remit than do those in the skin. Death is usually attributable to aspiration pneumonia, pulmonary failure, heart failure, uremia, or general inanition secondary to gastrointestinal malfunction or inability to ingest.

Treatment. Of the many agents that have been tried, only adrenal steroids appear to have any value. Eradication of established sclerotic and atrophic changes is not to be expected, but steroids may halt and reverse the edematous inflammatory phase. From 40 to 60 mg daily of prednisone should be given initially in divided dosage. Depending upon clinical response, this may be gradually reduced to a maintenance level of 15 to 20 mg daily which should be continued until maximum regression of the process has been achieved. Many months and even years of continuous treatment may be required. These patients *must* be placed on a six feeding modified ulcer diet with antacids after meals and at bedtime to avoid peptic ulceration.

Esophagitis may be ameliorated by elevating the head of the bed on 6-in. blocks, and atropine derivatives should be tried although sometimes they increase bloating by further depressing motility. Physiotherapy in the form of heat and massage may be comforting and also prevent fixation of the affected parts. As in systemic lupus (p. 1895) one must be constantly on the lookout for complicating bacterial infections which may be mistaken for manifestations of the primary process.

The treatment of Raynaud's syndrome is described on p. 1374. Long-term anticoagulant therapy might be tried for the vascular components of the disease.

REFERENCES

Abrahms, H. L., W. H. Carnes, and J. Eaton: Alimentary Tract in Disseminated Scleroderma with Emphasis on Small Bowel, A.M.A. Arch. Internal Med., 94:61, 1954.

Leinwand, I., A. W. Duryee, and M. N. Richter: Scleroderma (Based on Study of Over 150 Cases), Ann. Internal Med., 41:1003, 1954.

Rodnan, G. P., G. E. Schreiner, and R. L. Black:

Renal Involvement in Progressive Systemic Sclerosis (Generalized Scleroderma), Am. J. Med., 23: 445, 1957.

Spain, D. M., and A. G. Thomas: Pulmonary Manifestations of Scleroderma: Anatomic-Physiological Correlation, Ann. Internal Med., 32:152, 1950.

Symposium on Manifestations of Scleroderma: Proc. Staff Meet., Mayo Clinic, 34:53, 1957.

300 MISCELLANEOUS AND RARER DISEASES OF CONNECTIVE TISSUE

Philip A. Tumulty

TEMPORAL ARTERITIS

Definition. Temporal arteritis is a disease of unknown etiology characterized by granulomatous inflammation of the temporal arteries, headache, blindness or lesser visual disturbances, and associated systemic reactions such as fever, malaise, and weight loss. Other cranial and systemic arteries may be involved.

Individuals in the age group fifty to eighty are principally affected, women preponderantly. No familial or other predisposing factors are recognized, although occasionally the disease has seemed to follow respiratory infections.

Pathology. The histologic alterations involve the entire arterial wall, particularly the media. Areas of necrosis are accompanied by diffuse infiltration of cells, predominantly mononuclear. Giant cells are conspicuous. The vessel may become thrombosed, but aneurysms are rare. Veins are occasionally affected. These changes are often segmental, an important consideration in obtaining adequate material for biopsy examination.

Manifestations. The disease may run its course in a few months or may last for 3 years or more. The mortality is estimated at 10 or 15 per cent. The principal *systemic manifestations* are fever, malaise, weakness, anorexia, weight loss, and musculoskeletal aching, the latter sometimes accompanied by muscular atrophy or peripheral neuropathy. Some patients are confused or disoriented.

A mild leukocytosis with shift to the left, increased sedimentation rate, and moderate anemia are common. There may be striking rouleaux formation of the red blood cells. Eosinophilia is not prominent. An abnormal serum electrophoretic pattern with hypergammaglobulinemia may be present.

Severe throbbing *headache* associated with a red, swollen, tender, nodular, and thrombosed temporal artery or arteries is one of the chief local manifestations. The vessel may remain normally pulsatile although involved histologically. There may also be pain in the scalp, the face, the eyes, or the temperomandibular joints. The last may cause difficulty with eating and speech.

Of great importance are the *visual complications* which occur in about one-half the patients. While these changes are usually closely associated in time with the local manifestations of temporal arteritis, they occasionally precede it, or follow after a period of prolonged remission and appear to be primary. One or both eyes may be affected. There is no clear-cut relationship between the degree of involvement of the temporal or other arteries and the eyes. Ophthalmoplegias and transient diplopia may occur. Impairment of vision may be partial or complete, transient, or permanent, and usually occurs in the first 10 months of the disease. The onset may be sudden or gradual, and although there is usually some residual defect, surprising recovery of vision may take place, even after as long as 5 days of total blindness. The loss of vision is often strikingly out of proportion to changes visible ophthalmoscopically. An ischemic optic neuritis and closure of the central retinal artery or its branches are the changes most often seen, but the retina may be normal in appearance. The repeated episodes of transient loss of vision in older individuals may be confused with atherosclerotic blockage of the internal carotid arteries. The correct diagnosis may be made difficult in the absence of local indications of a temporal arteritis.

There may be other localized manifestations, depending upon the arterial segments involved. There are reports of similar granulomatous changes occurring in various branches of the cranial, coronary, renal, mesenteric, and other vessels.

Treatment. Adrenal corticosteroids have been effective in suppressing (though not eradicating) the inflammatory process, relieving local and systemic symptoms, usually within a few days. Treatment may be required for many months, depending upon the degree of continued activity of the process, and a program similar to that outlined for systemic lupus should be followed (p. 1896). The use of adrenal steroids has been so effective in preventing blindness or other permanent visual disability in temporal arteritis that treatment should be begun whenever there is reasonable evidence for the diagnosis. Procaine block or surgical resection of the affected segment of the temporal artery may be of benefit in relieving the local pain due to this process.

RELAPSING FEBRILE NODULAR NONSUPPURATIVE PANNICULITIS (Weber-Christian Disease)

Definition. Relapsing febrile nodular nonsuppurative panniculitis (Weber-Christian disease) is characterized by recurrent tender or painless inflammatory and necrotic nodules in the panniculus adiposus, fever, malaise, and other systemic manifestations.

Pathology. The nodules consist of necrotic fatty tissue infiltrated with lymphocytes, plasma cells, and macrophages. Foreign body giant cells are often present, and a few vessels may show a perivasculitis. Healing occurs with scarring and atrophy, resulting in characteristic areas of depression in the skin. Similar alterations have also been noted in the epicardial, peripancreatic, periadrenal, perirenal, and mesenteric fat. A fatty liver has been observed in a few patients and fat emboli in the lungs of at least one. The spleen is sometimes enlarged. The cause of these changes is unknown. Possibilities include a response to some primary disturbance of fat metabolism and injury produced by an infection, toxic states, drug reactions, or trauma.

Manifestations. This disease usually occurs between the ages of twenty and forty. Formerly regarded as primarily a disease of women (often obese), it is now known to affect men with considerable frequency.

The illness commonly begins insidiously, with the appearance of subcutaneous nodules. These may occur on any part of the body, but are usually confined to the thighs, buttocks, legs, abdomen, breasts, and arms. The lesions vary from 0.5 to more than 10 cm in diameter and are usually very tender but, in rare cases, are painless. They are freely movable, and the overlying skin is usually red or violaceous.

With the appearance of the nodules, the patient generally develops chills, fever, malaise, nausea, and musculoskeletal aching. Splenomegaly and regional adenopathy are not rare. The nodules do not suppurate, but in some instances an oily liquid is extruded from them.

The process subsides spontaneously after days or weeks, only to recur in weeks, months, or years. The only residua are concave or dimpled areas in the skin. These atrophic depressions are characteristic and form an important diagnostic feature. Death due to the uncomplicated disease is unusual. The white blood cell count may be moderately elevated, or there may be a leukopenia. Sometimes there is a mild anemia.

This condition must be distinguished from lipomatosis, adiposis dolorosa (Dercum's disease), erythema nodosum, erythema induratum (p. 1924), sarcoid (p. 1246), and insulin atrophy. A biopsy may be helpful, but biopsy wounds are said to heal slowly.

Treatment. Present methods are unsatisfactory. Sulfonamides and antibiotics are of no benefit. In some cases, adrenal corticosteroids have produced transient symptomatic relief with disappearance of fever and nodules, and this therapy should be tried.

WEGENER'S GRANULOMATOSIS

Definition. Wegener's granulomatosis is a syndrome of unknown etiology characterized by necrotizing granulomatous lesions, generalized arteritis, and glomerulonephritis. Klinger reported the first case in 1931, and Wegener described the features which distinguish this syndrome from other forms of angiitis.

Individuals of any age may be affected, most commonly those in the fourth and fifth decades. Their past health has generally been good, with no unusual allergic background. The outcome of the disease has been fatal in most recognized cases, generally after 6 to 8 months, although occasionally the course is intermittent or subacute for 2 years or more.

Pathology. There are three features of the histologic alterations: (1) necrotizing granulomas in the upper and/or lower respiratory tract, (2) focal inflammatory lesions of arteries and veins, usually widely disseminated, (3) focal glomerulitis. Because similar changes occur in hypersensitivity states and also in those produced experimentally, this process has been regarded as a manifestation of abnormal immune mechanisms.

Manifestations. The characteristic clinical triad consists of intractable rhinitis and sinusitis, nodular pulmonary lesions, and terminal uremia. The first symptoms are usually respiratory, the patient complaining of persistent rhinitis or sinusitis, chronic cough, hemoptysis, pleuritis, or pneumonia. Sometimes, however, the initial features are fever, weakness, malaise, and weight loss, the respiratory disorder becoming prominent somewhat later. The course is usually relentlessly progressive. Ulceration and erosion of cartilage and bone may occur in the nasal passages and sinuses, resulting in saddle nose deformity. There may be orbital extension with papillitis, chemosis, and exophthalmos. Any portion of the lungs may become implicated by nodular densities, irregular infiltrates, or cavitation, and secondary bacterial infection may complicate these changes.

Other organs which may be affected include the heart, brain, meninges, peripheral nerves, joints, muscles, skin, liver, pancreas, intestine, adrenals, prostate, and testes.

In time, renal involvement becomes evident, with the appearance of protein, red cells, and red cell casts in the urine. Renal failure is often rapid, the patient dying in uremia in a matter of weeks. The terminal phase may be dominated by uremia or by the effect of the generalized arteritis upon a variety of organ systems. High fever, arthritis, and hemorrhagic lesions of the skin and mucous membranes may be prominent.

Anemia, leukocytosis, occasionally with a mild eosinophilia, are common accompaniments. Hyperglobulinemia is frequent.

This syndrome is to be distinguished from other conditions in which vasculitis and granuloma formation may occur in varying combinations. Included among these are tuberculosis, sarcoidosis, lethal midline granuloma (p. 1253), polyarteritis nodosa, allergic angiitis, and macroglobulinemia of Waldenstrom (p. 1344).

Treatment. There is no effective management. Adrenal steroid therapy has at times appeared to repress the advancement of the process. Antibiotics are useful in combating bacterial complications. X-ray therapy for the lesions in the nose or lung has been tried occasionally, but evidence for any benefit is doubtful.

SCLEREDEMA

Definition. Scleredema is a disease of unknown etiology characterized by benign, spreading swelling and induration of the skin and subcutaneous tissues. It occurs at any age, most commonly in childhood and young adulthood. It may be seen in the neonatal period. Females are twice as often affected as males.

Pathology. The chief histologic alteration is pronounced swelling of the collagen of the skin and subcutaneous tissues with deposition between the bundles and about the vessels of a peculiar mucinous material. There is moderate infiltration by lymphocytes and plasma cells, but no intense inflammation. The process subsides without residuum.

Scleredema often follows bacterial or viral infections, particularly of the respiratory tract. The nature of this relationship remains obscure.

Manifestations. The disease begins with swelling and induration of the skin and subcutaneous tissues. The swelling does not pit, and the skin feels as though it had been infiltrated with wax. These changes may be preceded by a blotchy erythematous or livid rash and, at times, by a short period of malaise, low fever, and musculoskeletal aching. The swelling usually starts in the neck, spreading in turn to the face, scalp, shoulders, trunk, and abdomen. The hands and feet are spared entirely or, at most, show only slight swelling. The face becomes mask like and the patient appears "hidebound." Involvement of the eyelids can lead to pronounced chemosis, and the tongue and pharynx may be affected so extensively that dysarthria and dysphagia result. Additional features include sterile effusions in the pleura, pericardium, abdomen or joints, and muscle weakness. Histologic alterations

in the viscera comparable to the changes in the skin have been described in one patient.

The swelling may spread rapidly and reach its maximum in a matter of days or a few weeks. This is followed by very slow regression, many months or even years being required for complete healing. The areas of initial involvement, the face and the neck, often are the last to clear. Residual patches may persist for many years. Relapses are not common, but recurrence after a prolonged free period has been observed.

The white blood cell count is usually normal as is the sedimentation rate. Elevated serum γ-globulin has been recorded in a few instances.

Differential Diagnosis. It is most important to distinguish this relatively benign disease from scleroderma (p. 1896). Sometimes it is quite impossible to separate the two diseases on clinical grounds or even by biopsy examination, the distinction becoming clear only from patient's clinical course. The following points are often helpful in differentiation: In scleredema the hands and feet are relatively unaffected and, while there may be mild thickening of the skin of the extremities, there is no atrophy or Raynaud's phenomenon, commonly noted in scleroderma. Furthermore, in scleredema there is no pigmentation or calcinosis of the skin, the process involutes completely without residuum, and abnormalities in the esophagus, lungs, kidneys, or other viscera are not encountered.

Treatment. There is no satisfactory method of treatment, and supportive measures only are indicated. Adrenal steroids have been used in a few instances, with equivocal results.

REFERENCES

SCLEREDEMA

Leinwand, I.: Generalized Scleredema: Report with Autopsy Findings, Ann. Internal Med., 34:226, 1951.

O'Leary, P. A., M. Waisman, and M. W. Harrison: Scleredema Adultorum, Am. J. Med. Sci., 199: 458, 1940.

Vallee, B. L.: Scleredema: A Systemic Disease, New Engl. J. Med., 235:207, 1946.

TEMPORAL ARTERITIS

Birkhead, N. C., H. P. Wagener, and R. M. Shick: Treatment of Temporal Arteritis with Adrenal Corticosteroids: Results in Fifty-five Cases in Which Lesion Was Proved at Biopsy, J.A.M.A., 163:821, 1957.

Crosby, R. C., and R. C. Wadsworth: Temporal Arteritis: Review of Literature and Report of Five Additional Cases, Arch. Internal Med., 81:431, 1948.

Harrison, C. V.: Giant-cell or Temporal Arteritis: Review, J. Clin. Pathol., 1:197, 1948.

Hollenhorst, R. W., J. R. Brown, H. P. Wagener, and R. M. Shick: Neurologic Aspects of Temporal Arteritis, Neurology, 10:490, 1960.

Russell, R. W.: Giant-cell Arteritis: A Review of 35 Cases, Quart. J. Med., 28:471, 1959.

WEBER-CHRISTIAN DISEASE

Beerman, H.: Weber-Christian Syndrome, Am. J. Med. Sci., 225:446, 1953.

Hallahan, J. D., and T. Klein: Relapsing Febrile Nodular Non-suppurative Panniculitis (Weber-Christian Disease): Review of Literature and Report of Case, Ann. Internal Med., 34:1179, 1951.

Shuman, C. R.: Relapsing Panniculitis (Weber-Christian Disease): Review of Literature and Report of Case Including Treatment with Cortisone, A.M.A. Arch. Internal Med., 87:669, 1951.

WEGENER'S GRANULOMATOSIS

Fahey, J. L., E. Leonard, J. Chrug, and G. C. Godman: Wegener's Granulomatosis, Am. J. Med., 17:168, 1954.

Godman, G. C., and J. Chrug: Wegener's Granulomatosis: Pathology and Review of Literature, A.M.A. Arch. Pathol., 58:533, 1954.

Walton, E. W.: Giant-cell Granuloma of the Respiratory Tract (Wegener's Granulomatosis), Brit. Med. J., 5091:265, 1958.

301 DISORDERS OF THE JOINTS

Lawrence E. Shulman and Joseph J. Bunim

Terms used to designate abnormal conditions of the joints are numerous and frequently ambiguous. *Rheumatism* is used mostly as a generic term to indicate pain, stiffness, or deformity of joints, muscles, and related structures. The *rheumatic diseases* embrace a large group of diseases of the musculoskeletal system in which alterations take place in the articular structures (synovial tissue, joint capsule, cartilage, and bone) and/or in the connective tissue surrounding the joints, as in tendons. Because of the prominent involvement of this tissue in these disorders it is becoming more fashionable to designate them *diseases of connective tissue*. The term *arthritis* is usually used to denote any disorder of joints, although properly it should be restricted to those disorders of joints which are inflamed. A joint disorder, unaccompanied by grossly evident inflammation, is frequently called an *arthropathy*. If pain, tenderness, or stiffness originates from a nonarticular structure, such as muscle, tendon, ligament, or bursa, the condition is often labeled "*fibro-*

sitis." Wherever possible, more specific terminology, such as *tendinitis* or *bursitis*, should be used.

Prevalence. Surveys conducted by the Public Health Service show that over 10 million persons suffer from some form of rheumatism, indicating that it is one of the most common causes of chronic illness in the United States, ranking second to nervous and mental diseases as a cause of disability. Of the 10 million people with rheumatic complaints, 4.5 million have arthritis; over 10 per cent, or 1,143,000, are partially disabled; and almost 2 per cent, 190,000, are completely disabled. More than half the disabled are under forty-five years of age. In other countries, the toll from rheumatism is even greater. In Great Britain, for example, half the population suffers from nondisabling rheumatism; 7 per cent are incapacitated by it for at least 1 day each year, and one-sixth of the total industrial disability is ascribed to rheumatism. In Switzerland, arthritis is responsible for 16 per cent of all sickness reports to insurance companies and the same proportion of total absence from work. Among the major categories of chronic disease, rheumatism cripples most and kills least. Much of the crippling occurs in young people during their productive years.

Classification. A workable and logical classification of joint diseases cannot be constructed satisfactorily on etiologic grounds when the cause of so many forms of joint disease is unknown. Separation on the basis of pathologic change is often helpful, yet it may actually restrict knowledge, since the connective tissues are capable of reacting to injurious stimuli in only a limited number of ways. Differentiation on clinical grounds alone may be similarly unsatisfactory because widely divergent pathologic forces may give rise to an identical clinical picture. Division into acute and chronic categories is also hazardous because acute arthritides may become chronic, and chronic arthritides may begin acutely or have acute exacerbations.

Thus, it is clear that the state of our knowledge, or lack of it, permits no complete or satisfactory classification. Most attempts at clarifying joint diseases include etiologic, pathologic, and clinical factors. The American Rheumatism Association has approved a classification which conforms to the phraseology of "The Standard Nomenclature of Disease," thus providing uniformity. Wherever possible, its use is recommended. The accompanying outline (Table 301-1), however, is offered as a more useful guide to differential diagnosis because it is based largely on pathogenetic features.

Approach to the Patient with Joint Disease. *History.* The *age* of the patient is not so important in diagnosis as was formerly thought. In the elderly, arthritis was assumed to be degenerative joint disease; in the young or middle-aged, rheumatoid

Table 301-1. CLASSIFICATION OF DISORDERS OF JOINTS

I. Arthritis caused by specific infection
    A. Pyogenic arthritis
        1. Staphylococcus
        2. Streptococcus
        3. Pneumococcus
        4. Gonococcus
        5. Meningococcus
    B. Brucellosis (arthritis rare; arthralgia common)
    C. Tuberculosis
        1. Arthritis
        2. Spondylitis (Pott's disease)
    D. Syphilis
        1. Congenital
            a. Symmetric synovitis (Clutton's joints)
            b. Osteochondritis (Parrot's pseudoparalysis)
        2. Acquired (tertiary)
            a. Synovitis
            b. Gummatous
    E. Less common infectious arthritides
        1. Bacteria
        2. Fungi
        3. Viruses
II. Arthritis possibly caused by specific infection
    A. Reiter's syndrome
III. Arthritis as a sequel to specific infection
    A. Rheumatic fever
IV. Arthritis caused by hypersensitivity to foreign agent
    A. Drug reactions
    B. Serum sickness
    C. Anaphylactoid purpura
V. Arthritis in widespread inflammatory connective tissue disease, cause unknown
    A. Rheumatoid arthritis and variants
        1. Adult peripheral type
        2. Juvenile rheumatoid arthritis (Still's disease)
        3. Ankylosing spondylitis (Marie-Strümpell disease)
        4. Psoriatic arthritis
        5. Felty's syndrome
        6. Arthritis with ulcerative colitis and other gastrointestinal diseases
        7. Sjögren's syndrome
    B. Collagen vascular disorders
        1. Systemic (disseminated) lupus erythematosus
        2. Polyarteritis (periarteritis nodosa)
        3. Progressive systemic sclerosis (scleroderma)
        4. Dermatomyositis
    C. Granulomatous reactions
        1. Sarcoidosis
        2. Erythema nodosum
VI. Arthritis caused by metabolic or endocrine disorders
    A. Gout
    B. Ochronosis
    C. Acromegaly
VII. Degenerative joint disease (osteoarthritis)
    A. Generalized
    B. Localized
        1. Hereditary (such as Heberden's nodes)
        2. Secondary to previous trauma or infection
        3. Secondary to faulty body mechanics
        4. Unknown cause
VIII. Arthritis caused by trauma to joints
    A. Direct trauma
    B. Internal mechanical derangement of joint
IX. Neurogenic arthropathy (Charcot joint)
    A. Tabes dorsalis
    B. Syringomyelia
    C. Neuropathy of diabetes mellitus
    D. Peripheral nerve injuries
    E. Leprosy
X. Arthritis caused by bleeding into joints
    A. Direct trauma
    B. Disorders of blood coagulation
        1. Hemophilia and variants
XI. Neoplasms of joints
    A. Cyst
    B. Lipoma
    C. Hemangioma
    D. Synovioma
    E. Giant-cell tumor
XII. Arthritis secondary to lesions of bone
    A. Aseptic necrosis of bone
        1. Primary, of unknown cause
        2. Secondary to
            a. Trauma
            b. Vascular occlusion
    B. Neoplasms of bone
        1. Primary
        2. Metastatic to bone
    C. Osteochondromatosis
    D. Osteochondritis dissecans
    E. Endocrine diseases of bone
XIII. Hypertrophic osteoarthropathy
XIV. Miscellaneous arthritis
    A. Shoulder-hand syndrome
    B. Palindromic rheumatism
    C. Intermittent hydrarthrosis
    D. Psychogenic rheumatism (hysterical "arthritis")
XV. Paraarticular conditions ("nonarticular rheumatism")
    A. "Fibrositis"
    B. Tendinitis
    C. Bursitis
    D. Tendon sheath cyst (ganglion)
    E. Myositis
    F. Neuritis
    G. Panniculitis

arthritis. Actually, the chance of a person's having rheumatoid arthritis increases up to the age of fifty-five years, after which it remains stationary; conversely, degenerative joint disease can begin as early as the second decade.

Females are more likely to have Heberden's nodes (10:1), systemic lupus erythematosus (8:1), or peripheral rheumatoid arthritis (2:1), whereas rheumatoid spondylitis is decidedly more common in men (9:1).

It is important to know the *occupation* and *avocations* of the arthritic patient. Injury at work or at play gives rise to such conditions as "housemaid's knee," "nurse's feet," "boxer's bursitis," "student's elbow," "baseball fingers," and "weaver's bottom." Trauma can also play an important role in the selection of the sites affected in degenerative joint disease.

Careful attention must also be paid to the *family history*. The family incidence of gout varies from 10 to 18 per cent.

"Growing pains" in childhood may direct one's attention to rheumatic fever or juvenile rheumatoid arthritis. Repeated throat infections, especially if known to be caused by the beta-hemolytic streptococcus, also point to rheumatic fever. A history of unexplained fever, skin disorders, serositis, and hematologic abnormalities may suggest that the arthritis is merely one manifestation of a collagen vascular disorder. Urethritis may precede arthritis and conjunctivitis in Reiter's syndrome or gonorrhea. At times, renal calculi may appear before gouty arthritis. Nephritis may antedate arthralgia in systemic lupus erythematosus. Clearly, a history of trauma to a joint or arthritis in the remote past must be sought, because such an event may be related to the present rheumatic illness.

Meticulous inquiry into *events immediately preceding the onset* of the arthritis yields important clues to diagnosis. An antecedent infection of one or more organs, especially if accompanied by bacteremia, indicates that the arthritis may be infectious. Streptococcal tonsillitis or pharyngitis preceding the arthritis by 1 to 4 weeks strongly suggests rheumatic fever. Prior injections of penicillin or foreign protein, especially if accompanied by fever or urticaria, bring to mind the arthritis of serum sickness. Frequently, rheumatoid arthritis is preceded by overwork, emotional stress, or exposure to a cold, damp environment and is ushered in by constitutional symptoms—feverishness, malaise, fatigability, anorexia, paresthesias, and weight loss. Such constitutional symptoms do not antedate the onset of degenerative joint disease.

The *mode of onset* of the arthritis should be ascertained. A joint disorder may appear explosively (as in rheumatic fever), subacutely (as in rheumatoid arthritis), or insidiously (as in degenerative joint disease). There are many exceptions, however, and the interpretation by patients of the acuteness of an illness varies greatly.

It is also important to obtain a full characterization of the patient's joint *pain*. The pain of acute gouty arthritis, for example, is constant, severe, boring, and not influenced by position or time of day. In contrast, the discomfort in degenerative joint disease is usually transient, mild, and superficial; it emerges with attempted movement after a period of rest in one position and disappears readily after brief exercise. In a different manner, the patient with rheumatoid arthritis complains of morning stiffness which disappears gradually only after activity for several hours, whereas the pains in the affected joints may become more severe as the day progresses.

The patient should also be asked about the occurrence of other signs which reflect articular inflammation, viz., excessive *heat, discoloration of the skin, tenderness,* or *swelling* of the involved joint.

Valuable diagnostic information may come from ascertaining which joint was first involved, i.e., the proximal interphalangeal joint in rheumatoid arthritis, the sacroiliac in ankylosing spondylitis, the distal interphalangeal in degenerative joint disease, the great toe in gout, or the shoulder in bursitis. One should find out whether the arthritis is *migratory* and, if it is, the *nature of its spread*. In degenerative joint disease, for example, the sites of arthritic symptoms do not tend to change; whereas migration of the arthritis is characteristic of rheumatic fever, where it is rapid and transient, and of rheumatoid arthritis, where it tends to be slower and additive. Rheumatoid arthritis is noted for the *symmetry* of involvement of joints.

The *course* of the disease may provide additional diagnostic clues. Acute exacerbations with complete remissions are characteristic of intermittent hydrarthrosis, where the flare-ups occur regularly, and of the early stage of gout, where they occur irregularly. Over-all progression with partial remissions is the most common course in rheumatoid arthritis; whereas in degenerative joint disease, the illness is usually static or slowly progressive.

The presence and extent of *deformities* and the *functional capacity* of the patient may also aid in diagnosis. Some disorders, such as rheumatoid arthritis, are notoriously deforming and crippling; others, such as rheumatic fever, produce no residual articular disability.

The details of *previous management and its effect* should be carefully recorded. The daily dosage and duration of administration of a given agent are important, for the program may not have been sufficient to constitute a valid therapeutic trial. An illustration of the potential usefulness of knowing the previous response to therapy is in so-called "psychogenic rheumatism," where the diagnosis is said to be confirmed by a reportedly complete lack of response to salicylates or physical therapy.

Physical Examination. All accessible joints should be systematically and meticulously examined for heat or discoloration of the overlying skin, swelling, tenderness, limitation of motion, deformity, and crepitation. The *temperature* and *color* of the skin proximal and distal to the joint should be compared with those over the joint. *Swelling* of the joint may result from one or more of the following pathologic conditions: (1) the accumulation within the joint space of fluid, demonstrable by fluctuation, as in the "patellar click"; (2) thickening of the soft tissue (synovia, capsule, ligament, or adipose tissue), in which case there is no fluctuation; (3) localized periarticular effusion in a tendon sheath or a bursa; (4) diffuse periarticular subcutaneous edema; or (5) bony enlargement, as in acromegaly, tumors of bone, or the osteophytes of degenerative joint disease. One must be sure that the joint is really enlarged, since atrophic muscles may falsely give the impression of joint swelling. The degree of *tenderness* should be recorded and subsequently interpreted with the help of the sensory examination and an evaluation of the emotional state of the patient.

Limitation of motion of a joint may result from (1) sufficiently painful inflammation to cause muscular spasm or guarding, (2) effusions large enough to distend the capsule tightly, (3) fibrosis of the capsule, (4) fibrosis across the joint space from one synovial surface to another (fibrous ankylosis), (5) bony bridging across the space (bony ankylosis), or (6) various disorders of tendon, muscle, or nerve. One should try to determine whether the *deformity* results from effusion or pain, and thus is possibly reversible, or from irreversible destruction of joint structures.

Crepitation, a grating feeling or noise, results from the rubbing together of opposing joint surfaces on motion of the joint. The character of the crepitation varies with the joint disorder: fine, or "rubbing," in rheumatoid arthritis, where the abrasive surface is villous granulation tissue; coarse, or "crunching," from the osteophytes and disorganized cartilage in degenerative joint disease. These forms of crepitation should be distinguished from "cracking" or "snapping," which is caused by tendons slipping over bony prominences.

A few instruments are available for quantitating the degree of disability of joints and related structures. Simplest, and perhaps most important, is a tape measure with which the circumference of large joints and certain muscle groups is recorded. It should also be used to measure the chest expansion in patients with rheumatoid spondylitis. With a jeweler's ring sizer one can determine the size of the smaller joints of the fingers and toes. A dynamometer is used to record grip strength; the range of motion of a joint can be ascertained with a goniometer. These instruments are useful in following the course of the patient's illness and particularly in studies designed to test the efficacy of a therapeutic agent.

The *functional capacity* of the patient, with special reference to tasks performed by the extremities, should also be carefully recorded. Can the patient get out of bed, walk, or climb stairs? Can he comb his hair, tie his shoelaces, unscrew a bottle cap, or sweep the floor?

Organs, other than the joints, which deserve special attention in the physical examination of the arthritis patient include the skin, subcutaneous tissue, eyes, pharynx, lymph nodes, lungs, heart, liver, spleen, muscles, and nerves.

Valuable clues to the diagnosis of the joint disorder come from abnormalities of the *skin.* Associated urticarial wheals point to serum sickness. Petechiae and ecchymoses suggest meningococcemia or a defect of blood coagulation; a "butterfly rash," systemic lupus erythematosus; and erythema marginatum, rheumatic fever.

The patient complaining of arthritis of the hands may exhibit no evidence of arthritis but rather diffuse swelling of the subcutaneous tissue as seen in the early stages of scleroderma. *Subcutaneous nodules* are frequently encountered in patients with various forms of arthritis. Those occurring on the extensor surfaces of the forearms just distal to the elbows are thought to be the hallmark of rheumatoid arthritis, although sarcoid or lupus nodules or gouty tophi may occasionally occur in the same location. A striking feature of the nodules of rheumatoid arthritis is their symmetry. The nodules in rheumatic fever are more transitory, less symmetric, softer, and not so frequently near joints; the distribution of those of polyarteritis nodosa and amyloidosis tends to be linear, along the course of affected arteries. The external ears should be carefully searched for gouty tophi. Tophi or nodules near joints are usually fixed to the periosteum or the joint capsule. Synovial cysts, *ganglions,* should not be mistaken for nodules or tophi.

The *ocular* examination may yield useful information in differential diagnosis. Conjunctivitis may suggest Reiter's syndrome; keratitis, gonococcal arthritis or Clutton's joints; uveitis, rheumatoid arthritis or sarcoid; "cytoid bodies," systemic lupus erythematosus; and retinal arterial thromboses, polyarteritis nodosa.

Similar differential diagnostic analyses may be constructed for the other extraarticular organs previously listed.

Laboratory Tests. After a careful history has been recorded and a thorough physical examination performed, the aid of certain appropriate laboratory studies should be obtained. The *hematologic examination* should be performed in all arthritic patients. In rheumatoid arthritis, rheumatic fever, or sarcoid, anemia may be mild or moderate; in some patients with collagen vascular disease, it may be more severe. In rheumatoid arthritis, the anemia is typically hypochromic and normocytic, whereas in systemic lupus erythematosus, it is usually normochromic and normocytic but may be hemolytic. The white blood cell count is usually slightly elevated in serum sickness, rheumatic fever, many cases of active rheumatoid arthritis, and some infectious arthritides; it may be greatly elevated in other infections, polyarteritis nodosa, and leukemia. Conversely, leukopenia frequently accompanies tuberculous arthritis, Felty's syndrome, systemic lupus erythematosus, and sarcoid. In purpuric states, the platelets should be counted and, when indicated, further special studies on blood coagulation performed.

The erythrocyte *sedimentation rate* is one of the more important laboratory determinations in rheumatology. It is particularly useful in (1) the differential diagnosis of the mild early case; (2) estimating the severity of the inflammation in those conditions, such as rheumatic fever or rheumatoid arthritis, where the rate is known to be elevated; and (3) determining by serial tests the course of the arthritis and the effect of therapy. Among the disorders of joints the rate is usually high in infectious arthritis, serum sickness, acute phases of rheumatic fever, rheumatoid arthritis and variants, and collagen vascular disorders, acute gouty arthritis, and neoplasms in or near joints. Normal values are recorded in degenerative joint disease, traumatic arthritis, neurogenic arthropathy, "fibrositis," psychogenic rheumatism, and between acute attacks of inflammatory or gouty arthritis. The test is nonspecific. A normal rate cannot be relied upon to rule out such diseases as rheumatic fever or rheumatoid arthritis because the disease may be only minimally active or there may have been technical difficulties. In such cases, the determination should be repeated. Various nonspecific "acute phase reactions," such as that to *C-reactive protein,* may also help to estimate the activity of the arthritis.

Other *serologic* tests may also aid in diagnosis. One or more of the serologic tests for syphilis (STS) may not only indicate that the patient has one of the several rheumatic sequelae of this infection, but also augment the physician's alertness to the possibility of gonococcal arthritis. If the STS is positive, a *Treponema pallidum* immobilization test (TPI) should also be performed, since it has been shown that many patients with a false positive STS have some form of connective tissue disease. The antistreptolysin O titers of serum help greatly to confirm the diagnosis of rheumatic fever, being elevated in more than 85 per cent of patients with active polyarthritis caused by this disease.

The sheep cell agglutination test is positive in approximately 75 per cent of patients with active peripheral rheumatoid arthritis unaccompanied by psoriasis or spondylitis and in over 90 per cent of patients with subcutaneous nodules. It is not entirely specific for rheumatoid arthritis, however, and positive tests may be found in patients with systemic lupus erythematosus or progressive systemic sclerosis (scleroderma). Other serologic agglutination tests for brucellosis or tularemia are occasionally useful.

If possible, *LE cell* preparations should also be made in arthritic patients, especially those in whom the diagnosis is in doubt. The importance of this test is readily grasped when one realizes that arthralgia or arthritis is the presenting manifestation in one-third of patients with systemic lupus erythematosus.

Since the rheumatic manifestations of gout are so pleomorphic, all patients with joint complaints should have a blood *uric acid* determination.

Urinalysis and tests of renal function may help in difficult diagnostic situations by focusing one's attention on the possibilities of Reiter's syndrome, gout, one of the collagen vascular disorders, or amyloidosis secondary to rheumatoid arthritis.

X-ray findings also aid materially when interpreted in the light of clinical and other laboratory information. They should not be considered the final arbiter, however, since different types of arthritis may produce identical roentgenographic changes. Furthermore, even in obviously inflamed joints, the x-ray findings may be totally negative in the early stages of illness.

Bacteriologic, cytologic, and chemical examination of *synovial fluid* may provide further information of diagnostic and prognostic importance. The splendid monograph by Ropes and Bauer has done much to increase our knowledge of the characteristics of joint fluid, both in normal persons and in those with various pathologic states.

Normal synovial fluid is small in volume, clear, pale yellow, sticky, and relatively acellular. It is essentially a dialysate of blood plasma, the albumin passing through readily but the globulin passing through with difficulty. The fluid, which helps to lubricate the articulating surfaces, contains mucin, a protein-polysaccharide complex similar to that found in the ground substance of connective tissue.

A proper examination of joint fluid should include all those features recorded in the analysis of fluid from other body cavities, i.e., volume, appearance, specific gravity, reaction, cell counts including a differential, and concentrations of protein and sugar (with comparative blood levels). Anaerobic as well as aerobic cultures should be planted immediately. A Gram stain of the centrifuged sediment should also be carried out. If tuberculosis is suspected, an aliquot of the fluid should be inoculated into a guinea pig. The turbidity should be estimated and the fluid observed for clot formation. The diluting medium for white cell counts should be physiologic saline solution, not acetic acid, because the addition of acetic acid to normal joint fluid so precipitates, or denatures, the mucin that a ropy clot is formed. An icteric index of the joint fluid may be helpful when traumatic arthritis is suspected.

Fluids obtained from patients with joint disorders fall into two antagonistic groups, and there is a third group with intermediate findings. Diseases included within the first group are degenerative joint disease, traumatic arthritis, neurogenic arthropathy, osteochondromatosis, and osteochondritis dissecans. In these disorders the amount of fluid is usually increased, but the changes from normal are small: slightly more polymorphonuclear leukocytes, slightly less mucin, and therefore, slightly reduced viscosity.

The second group comprises all the specific infectious arthritides, Reiter's syndrome, rheumatoid arthritis, and intermittent hydrarthrosis. The aspirated fluids in this group appear turbid, clot readily, and have a low viscosity. Although there is considerable variation, the white cell count is elevated, largely as a result of a polymorphonuclear response. Sugar concentration is usually reduced, and the protein concentration is elevated, with a considerable contribution from the globulin fraction.

Among the disorders which fall in the intermediate group, the findings in systemic lupus erythematosus, hemophilia, and hypertrophic osteoarthropathy more closely resemble those in the first group; those of the second are more frequently seen in the synovial fluids of rheumatic fever, gout, and synovial tumors.

It is thus clear that in many situations where diagnosis is difficult, such as between rheumatoid and gonococcal arthritis, the solution may not be found by cytologic or chemical analysis of the synovial fluid. On the other hand, in many other situations, as in the patient who has either a Charcot joint or gonococcal arthritis, or others in whom the choice lies between traumatic or rheumatoid arthritis, the diagnostic dilemma may be resolved by such an analysis. Moreover, uric acid crystals may be seen in synovial fluid examined under a polarizing microscope.

When all the above methods have failed to clarify the diagnostic problem, a *biopsy* specimen of an affected joint may be obtained. The value of the histologic method in the diagnosis of rheumatic disease, however, is somewhat limited by the paucity of accumulated experience, not only in diseased joints, but in normal ones as well. This deficiency exists largely because in this country dissection of joint structures at post-mortem examination is illegal, unless special permission is obtained, and joint biopsies have been performed infrequently. In doing the latter procedure, strict aseptic precautions should be observed. A method of securing a punch biopsy of the synovial membrane of the knee has been introduced, but its usefulness is limited, as in punch biopsy of the liver, by the small amount of tissue for examination. This deficiency is significant in light of studies describing, in several rheumatic disorders, great variability in pathologic change from place to place in the same specimen. Nevertheless, synovial biopsy can answer various diagnostic problems by differentiating gout from rheumatoid arthritis (by revealing urate crystals) or rheumatoid from tuberculous arthritis (by demonstrating acid-fast bacilli). Moreover, biopsy findings have added to our knowledge of the rheumatic diseases by showing, for example, that sarcoid or progressive systemic sclerosis (scleroderma) may involve the synovium as well as other, more usual, sites.

REITER'S SYNDROME

Definition. Reiter's syndrome (Reiter's disease, venereal arthritis, infectious uroarthritis, idiopathic blenorrheal arthritis, arthritis urethritica) is recognized strictly by the triad of arthritis, nongonococcal urethritis, and conjunctivitis. Most patients, however, also exhibit one or more characteristic mucocutaneous manifestations. Although the complete triad (or tetrad) is relatively uncommon, the combination of arthritis and urethritis (and/or prostatitis) is especially frequent in young men. Although there is a strong clinical impression that Reiter's syndrome is infectious, attempts to isolate a specific microorganism have been unsuccessful and the etiology remains obscure.

Epidemiology and Pathogenesis. Reiter's syndrome is largely a disorder of young adult males, although it has been reported in children, in older persons, and in females. The incidence is especially high in military populations.

In Britain and the United States the disease is considered by many investigators to be of venereal origin. In Scandinavia and France, the syndrome is considered a complication of bacillary dysentery. Support of this thesis was obtained from a report from Finland in 1948 of 334 cases of Reiter's syndrome, occurring for the most part during an epidemic of dysentery from Flexner bacillus. However, only 0.2 per cent of those with dysentery were estimated to have developed Reiter's syndrome.

Extensive microbiologic investigations have failed to uncover a specific pathogen. The organisms of greatest pathogenetic interest have been the pleuropneumonia-like organisms (PPLO), variant forms of common bacteria, on the basis of (1) their identification from the genital secretions of 115 males, 27 of whom also had arthritis, and (2) their presence in the joints of certain animals with spontaneous polyarthritis. However, PPLO organisms have also been isolated from the majority of patients with gonococcal or nongonococcal urethritis unassociated with arthritis or conjunctivitis.

Clinical Features. The triad of Reiter's syndrome usually evolves over a 3- to 4-week period, although this varies from days to months. The symptoms of urethritis usually appear first, followed by conjunctivitis and arthritis, in that order. Although all three manifestations vary in severity and duration from one patient to another, in most cases the arthritis is the most severe and prolonged of the three. At onset there may be fever (to 103°F), malaise, anorexia, or weight loss.

The initial attack is typically self-limited. The urethritis and conjunctivitis usually disappear after days or a few weeks, but the arthritis may last for several months, even 1 to 4 years. Recurrences are very common, as many as eight episodes having been recorded in a single individual.

The first attack of *arthritis* is likely to be explosive. Typically, it is a migratory polyarthritis, usually symmetric. The most commonly affected joints are the knees, ankles, metatarsophalangeal joints, and wrists, in order of decreasing frequency. However, any peripheral joint may be involved, or the disease may affect only one joint, such as a knee or ankle. Pain, often severe, in one or both heels is a common complaint which is helpful in diagnosis. The affected joints are usually hot, tender, and swollen, often with demonstrable fluid; these inflammatory signs subside slowly over months. Lateral compression or pressure over the plantar surfaces of the heels often elicits pain. Evidence of spondylitis, such as low-back pain and stiffness or tenderness over spinous processes, usually appears late, if at all. Subsequent attacks of arthritis often develop more slowly than the initial attack. The feet and the spine are the most common sites of permanent joint deformity.

Although the *genitourinary* involvement is usually obvious, with dysuria and urethral discharge, it may be necessary to "milk" the urethra or massage the prostate to establish the diagnosis. The urethral meatus is frequently red and edematous. At the same time there may be (1) nonbacterial cystitis manifested by frequency of urination, suprapubic pain, and terminal hematuria, (2) prostatitis, or (3) seminal vesiculitis. Urethral stricture is an uncommon late complication.

The most common *ocular* manifestation is conjunctivitis, which usually starts in one eye, then spreads to the other. Photophobia, burning pain, and hyperemia may be intense; they subside in 1 to 2 weeks. Other ocular lesions include superficial keratitis, corneal ulcers, episcleritis, and iritis.

Mucocutaneous lesions are an important feature of the syndrome, facilitating diagnosis. Usually they appear early in the disease; they may even precede other manifestations. The most common locations are the glans penis (80 per cent), mouth (50 per cent), and the soles and palms (30 per cent). The lesions on the *glans penis* begin as small blebs, which later coalesce into large patches with sharply defined borders ("balanitis circinata"); in the circumcised individual, they may be hyperkeratotic.

The *oral* lesions, found on the palate, buccal mucosa, tongue, and pharynx, consist of small papules or vesicles which coalesce to form irregular gray patches demarcated by a serpiginous red border.

The lesions on the *soles and palms* consist of keratoderma blennorrhagica, beginning as red-purple papules, often in clusters, which may later coalesce. No specific microorganism has been recovered from these lesions, and there is no evidence that they are the result of gonorrheal infection, as considered previously. Hyperkeratoses may cover the entire soles. Accumulations of keratotic material beneath the fingernails and toenails are characteristic.

An unusual feature is *pericarditis,* diagnosed on an electrocardiographic basis alone, although transient pericardial friction rubs have been detected in a few patients.

Laboratory Findings. None is diagnostic. There may be a moderate normochromic anemia and a neutrophilic leukocytosis of 10,000 to 20,000 per cu mm. The erythrocyte sedimentation rate parallels the clinical course.

The radiologic signs, which may be helpful, consist of juxtaarticular periosteal proliferation and, less frequently, erosions at joint margins. Irregular periosteal thickening over calcaneal spurs is a common finding.

Diagnosis. It is important to distinguish Reiter's syndrome from gonococcal arthritis, which, strictly, should be diagnosed only by identifying gonococci from the synovial fluid or membrane. Many cases formerly considered gonorrheal arthritis were, in all likelihood, Reiter's syndrome, especially in males. The distinction is important in prognosis; untreated gonococcal arthritis is often rapidly destructive, and Reiter's syndrome is unresponsive to antibiotics. Separation from rheumatoid arthritis or spondylitis is usually not difficult. The mucocutaneous lesions may resemble erythema multiforme exudativum (Stevens-Johnson syndrome) or Behcet's syndrome, but arthritis in these conditions is unusual. Reiter's syndrome may be differentiated from psoriasis by the absence of mucosal lesions in the latter and the self-limited course of the former.

Treatment. Treatment is palliative since there is no specific therapy. Corticoids may be necessary to suppress symptoms in the acute fulminant phase.

RHEUMATOID ARTHRITIS

Definition. Rheumatoid arthritis (atrophic arthritis, chronic proliferative arthritis, chronic infectious arthritis) is a systemic disease of unknown etiology in which symptoms and inflammatory change predominate in articular and related structures. The course is variable but tends to be chronic and to result in characteristic deformities.

Epidemiology. Rheumatoid arthritis is a common disorder. Its prevalence, estimated by population surveys, in Pittsburgh, Pennsylvania, and Lancashire, England, among those fifteen years of age or older is 2.7 and 3.5 per cent, respectively. A large proportion of patients become incapacitated; in one study, 58 per cent were unable to carry out their ordinary occupations or duties.

The disease may begin in infancy or in the ninth decade. In the United States the *onset* of the disease is most frequent in the fourth decade.

Most studies indicate that the disease occurs three times more commonly in women than in men, but this does not apply at all ages; in older patients, if more definite criteria such as x-ray changes are used, neither sex predominates. There is no racial predisposition.

There seems to be a familial tendency in rheumatoid arthritis. One study concludes that this is the result not of common environmental factors, but rather of a genetically determined susceptibility. Two independent studies concur that the rheumatoid factor is four times more prevalent in blood relatives of seropositive rheumatoid arthritic patients than in controls; other studies have failed to confirm this.

Rheumatoid arthritis is most prevalent in the Temperate Zones, especially in cold, damp climates.

Pathology. There is virtually no specificity to the histologic changes in the joints, and it is only by the fairly characteristic distribution of the lesions that the disease is discernible. The lesions include the usual changes of chronic inflammation: edema, proliferation of capillaries and fibroblasts, and infiltration, at first with round cells and a few polymorphonuclears, and later with plasma cells. This progresses to the formation of granulation tissue

containing islands of fibrinoid change and necrosis.

The consequences are thickening of the synovial membrane, destruction of cartilage and bone, and ankylosis. The layer of granulation tissue, called *pannus,* begins to invade and destroy cartilage, presumably by interfering with its proper nutrition. The villi of the pannus may interdigitate with corresponding villi on the opposing pannus, forming the nidus for fibrous ankylosis. When ossification takes place in the adhesions, bony ankylosis ensues. Subchondral granulation may be so extensive that bony trabeculae may be resorbed. Changes similar to those in the synovial membrane described above take place in the joint capsule, tendon sheaths, and bursae.

Rheumatoid nodules consist of clusters of granulation tissue in which foci of fibrinoid material and necrosis are surrounded by "palisading" mononuclear cells. Whereas an old subcutaneous nodule is an avascular structure with central necrosis, the young nodule consists of vascular granulation tissue, the small arteries often undergoing active inflammatory change (arteritis).

Cardiac lesions occur in different forms. Healed pericarditis, usually focal, is seen in as many as 40 per cent of cases at necropsy. Granulomatous lesions, morphologically similar to those of the subcutaneous nodule, are found infrequently in the myocardium and the aortic and mitral valves. Lesions indistinguishable from those of rheumatic heart disease are reported to occur in 12 to 66 per cent of autopsied cases of rheumatoid arthritis. Although these figures are probably excessive, the relationship between these two diseases seems to involve more than coincidence.

The arteritis that is sometimes found in synovium, nodule, muscle, heart, and other organs constitutes a common link with the lesions of rheumatic fever and the collagen disorders (systemic lupus erythematosus, progressive systemic sclerosis, and polyarteritis nodosa).

Secondary amyloidosis is found in as many as 26 per cent of severely disabled individuals at postmortem examination.

Etiology. Both cause and pathogenesis of rheumatoid arthritis remain unknown. Many hypotheses have been put forth, only to be discarded because of lack of convincing evidence.

A few adherents of the "focus of infection" school persist in having their patients free of teeth, tonsils, and paranasal sinus mucosa. Neither removal of the offending focus nor chemotherapy has altered the course of the disease, and most patients do not appear to harbor such foci.

A currently popular concept of the pathogenesis of rheumatoid arthritis maintains that the lesions result from some derangement of the immunologic mechanism of the host. Evidence that the rheumatoid factor originates in the cytoplasm of plasma cells in the lymph nodes and synovia supports an immunologic significance. When rheumatoid factor was passively transferred by repeated plasma transfusions to normal volunteers, no lesions developed. Patients with agammaglobulinemia who are unable to produce either rheumatoid factor or plasma cells develop rheumatoid arthritis with unusual frequency. Moreover the rheumatoid factor does not meet all the criteria of classical antibodies. The common occurrence of granulomatous lesions (subcutaneous nodules), vasculitis, and dense infiltration of lymphocytes and plasma cells is consistent with a hypersensitivity tissue reaction, but the antigen that evokes this reaction has not been identified. In summary, the provocative concept that the pathogenesis of rheumatoid arthritis may result from an abnormal immunologic response requires proof.

After Hench revealed the beneficial effects of ACTH and cortisone, the inference was drawn by many investigators that patients with rheumatoid arthritis were adrenocortically deficient. However, production, metabolism, and excretion of endogenous corticosteroids in patients with rheumatoid arthritis are normal.

Clinical Features. In some patients, the illness may be acute and fulminating, with high fever, intense joint inflammation, and the rapid evolution of severe deformities; in others, mild deformities develop insidiously and with little discomfort.

The earliest symptoms are frequently fatigability, anorexia, and weight loss; later, patients notice evanescent aches and pains in muscles and joints.

The great majority of patients seek the help of the physician only after the joint pain, swelling, redness, heat, or deformity has appeared. Although virtually any joint in the body may be involved first, the knees, hands, and feet are the most common sites of initial attack. Rheumatoid arthritis is characteristically migratory. Once affected, a joint tends to remain inflamed for weeks, months, or years. Symmetry of joint involvement is characteristic. Joint deformities are caused by intrinsic articular disease, shortening of tendons, and the muscle imbalance which results from involuntary splinting or from a true myositis. Deformities usually consist of flexion contractures. Favorite sites for flexion deformities include the metacorpophalangeals, wrists, elbows, and knees. Ulnar deviation is very common and is one of the hallmarks of rheumatoid arthritis.

The *skin,* especially over the extremities and more so distally, is cool, pale, and clammy. Excessive sweating of the palms and soles is characteristic. Over the fingers, the skin appears taut and shiny, and erythema of the hypothenar eminences, identical with "liver palms," is a common finding.

Fleeting erythematous blotches may be present on other areas.

Subcutaneous nodules are found in 10 to 20 per cent of patients with rheumatoid arthritis. They are firm, nontender, round or ovoid masses varying from 2 mm to 2 cm in diameter. The overlying skin slides over them easily, and they may or may not be attached to underlying structures. They are located usually over pressure points and near bones and joints. The most common site is the extensor surface of the forearm just below the elbow. In the bedridden patient, they may appear over the scapulae or the buttocks. In general, patients with nodules have active and severe disease. Nodules are rare in juvenile rheumatoid arthritis, ankylosing spondylitis, and psoriatic arthropathy. Characteristically, the nodules persist for months or years. The nodules of many other diseases (gout, sarcoid, xanthomatosis, syphilis, etc.) may resemble those of rheumatoid arthritis clinically.

Muscle aching, tenderness, and stiffness occur early in rheumatoid arthritis and are prominent throughout the course of the disease. Morning stiffness and stiffness after inactivity are common complaints. Muscular atrophy and weakness may be striking. To what extent these changes in muscle are due to direct inflammatory disease or disuse is not known. Increased urinary creatine excretion has been recorded in some bedridden patients with severe muscle wasting.

Among the various *ocular lesions* in rheumatoid arthritis, the most common are kerotoconjunctivitis sicca (see Sjögren's Syndrome) in 15 per cent of patients, and an anterior, nongranulomatous, usually bilateral uveitis in approximately 5 per cent. Episcleritis and scleritis may·also appear, sometimes as nodules which are histologically similar to the subcutaneous nodule. Rarely, these perforate the sclera and cause extrusion of the uveal tract, a condition called *scleromalacia perforans.*

During active phases of the disease, the lymph nodes may be so prominently enlarged that the patient is thought to have a lymphoma.

Clinical manifestations of heart disease probably do not occur more frequently in patients with rheumatoid arthritis than in the general population. Such a view contrasts sharply with the high incidence of cardiac lesions—granulomatous and fibrotic—reported in postmortem examinations of patients who have had rheumatoid arthritis.

Clinical features which are encountered not infrequently in the course of rheumatoid arthritis (but which are not specific for this disease) include pleuritis (with or without effusion), splenomegaly, peripheral neuropathy, chronic leg ulcers, and Baker's cysts.

Laboratory Findings. A moderate normocytic, hypochromic anemia may be found in active rheumatoid arthritis. It does not usually respond to iron therapy, and folic acid or vitamin B_{12} never affects it. Transfusions are rarely indicated. Splenectomy is ineffective.

The white cell count is within normal limits in 80 per cent of cases. A mild leukocytosis is common in early active disease.

The erythrocyte sedimentation rate is almost always elevated during active disease and is valuable as a rough index of activity. Other nonspecific host responses which may be used to estimate disease activity include C-reactive protein and hyperglobulinemia, with elevations predominantly in the alpha-2 and gamma fractions.

Serologic tests for rheumatoid factor are positive in 75 per cent of adult patients with "classical" or "definite" rheumatoid arthritis, as defined by the criteria of the American Rheumatism Association. Since these tests are negative in almost all cases of rheumatic fever, gout, osteoarthritis, ankylosing spondylitis, or suppurative arthritis, they are useful in differential diagnosis and are of special value in clinical investigations, where comparability of groups of cases is required. The rheumatoid factor tests also have prognostic significance: patients with consistently positive tests generally follow a progressively unfavorable course as compared with those whose tests are repeatedly negative.

The rheumatoid factor is a γ-globulin with a molecular weight of about 1,000,000. It circulates in the plasma as a soluble complex, combined with smaller γ-globulins of 160,000 molecular weight.

Several serologic tests for rheumatoid factor are in common use, but the basic principle of all is the same: the test serum is added in serial dilutions to a suspension of particles which have been coated with a "sensitizing" substance. The particles may be sheep or human red blood cells, latex (a synthetic polystyrene), or bentonite (a natural clay). In the sheep cell agglutination test the red cells are coated with a subagglutinating dose of rabbit antiserum against sheep erythrocytes; in the latex or bentonite tests the inert particles are coated with aggregated human γ-globulin. The test is considered positive when a serum agglutinates sensitized sheep cells or bentonite particles at a dilution of 1:32 or higher, or latex particles at 1:160 or higher.

In the first few months of rheumatoid arthritis these tests are likely to be negative; most cases become positive after 6 months. The tests are positive in 95 per cent of rheumatoid patients who have subcutaneous nodules. Especially high titers are found in those with splenomegaly, vasculitis, or neuropathy. Contrariwise, only 10 to 20 per cent of those with juvenile rheumatoid arthritis have positive tests. In two allied diseases—systemic lupus erythematosus and progressive systemic sclerosis—

the test is commonly positive. In random samples of the population the frequency of positive tests ranges from 1 to 5 per cent.

Synovial fluid findings, discussed previously, are usually not specific.

Radiologic examination of the affected joints is helpful in diagnosis and in charting the course of rheumatoid arthritis. The earliest changes, which are subtle and should be sought meticulously, consist of soft-tissue swelling, osteoporosis, periosteal elevation, erosions and narrowing of joint space. Osteoporosis is due to disuse and is at first juxtaarticular (paraepiphyseal). Later it becomes diffuse and characterized by narrowing of shaft cortices and coarsened trabeculations. Erosions are the most characteristic radiologic feature of chronic rheumatoid arthritis. *Surface erosions* are recognized early by the loss of the delicate white line of the articular cortex and are especially well visualized in the hands and feet. Enclosed erosions may attain sizes of several centimeters and must be distinguished from pseudocysts and the "punched-out" areas of gout. Narrowed joint space results from destruction of articular cartilage, and is therefore nonspecific.

Diagnosis. In the patient who gives a history of prodromal symptoms, paresthesias, weight loss, repeated episodes of acute migratory polyarthritis, and who exhibits on examination symmetric deforming arthritis with flexion contractures, ulnar deviation, and subcutaneous nodules, a diagnosis of rheumatoid arthritis may be readily made. However, the help of a physician is usually sought at an earlier stage of the disease when the clinical picture may be that of an acute febrile polyarthritis or merely monarticular disease.

Many syndromes may mimic rheumatoid arthritis in its early phases. One of these is *rheumatic fever* (p. 914); another is *systemic lupus erythematosus* (p. 1892). An acute attack of *gout* may closely resemble early rheumatoid arthritis but may be ruled out by a normal blood uric acid concentration and by a failure to respond promptly to colchicine. *Reiter's syndrome* may be differentiated from rheumatoid arthritis by (1) its prevalence in young men; (2) history of recent urethritis; (3) predominance of arthritis in the lower extremities; and (4) its mucocutaneous manifestations.

Degenerative joint disease is distinguished from rheumatoid arthritis by the presence of Heberden's nodes, involvement of the distal rather than the proximal interphalangeal joints, infrequent involvement of the wrist and metacarpophalangeal joints, and the lack of muscular wasting.

In the last analysis, the most helpful diagnostic aids are certain physical signs (sustained symmetric inflammatory polyarthritis, ulnar deviation, and subcutaneous nodules), positive tests for rheumatoid factor, and characteristic roentgenographic abnormalities.

Management. Efforts are directed toward (1) assuring proper amounts of rest and exercise, (2) the relief of pain, (3) combating the rheumatoid process, (4) preventing deformities, (5) correcting deformities which have developed, (6) controlling complications, (7) maintaining nutrition, and (8) rehabilitating the patient.

It is generally agreed that the earlier the therapeutic efforts, the more salutary the outcome. The patient should be helped to develop a degree of optimism and confidence but should under no circumstances be led to expect a rapid cure. He should be told that much can be done to relieve pain and prevent crippling but that the course of his disease cannot be predicted with precision and that medical care may be required for months or years.

Rest and Exercise. Most investigators agree that in certain stages of rheumatoid arthritis, rest is beneficial. In general, patients with acute polyarthritis and fever should be at complete bed rest. In milder cases, 8 to 10 hr of sleep at night and brief rest periods during the day should be advised. Excessive fatigue should be avoided. In order to maintain the patient's morale, he should be encouraged to continue work as long as it is not tiring or traumatizing to joints. In mild and moderate cases, special exercises should be prescribed along with rest to obtain the fullest possible range of joint motion, but these should not be so severe that joint pains persist for more than 1 hr thereafter. During the periods of severe disease, and especially in the early case, hospitalization is highly desirable to establish the optical medical regimen, to institute physiotherapy, and to instruct the patient so that he can continue physiotherapy at home.

Relief of Pain. Pain relief is important in itself and must be achieved before active physical therapy can be undertaken. Many of the physical measures to be described, such as the application of heat, may help to alleviate pain. Drugs such as morphine and Demerol should be strictly avoided because of the danger of addiction. Codeine may be used in unusual circumstances for brief periods. Since pain is largely the result of inflammation, the drug of choice should be anti-inflammatory rather than strictly analgesic. Three widely used groups of agents help to combat inflammation; salicylates, phenylbutazone (Butazolidin) or its analogues, and adrenocortical steroids.

Salicylates should be tried first; they frequently achieve the desired result and are least toxic and least costly. Acetylsalicylic acid (aspirin) and sodium salicylate seem to be equally effective, but care should be taken not to give sodium salicylate to patients with cardiac or renal disease, in whom

sodium restriction is desired. Aspirin should not be given only "as needed for pain" but regularly and frequently "around the clock" in doses to maximal benefit or to tolerance. Administration with meals and at bedtime often suffices. Gastric disturbances may be overcome by using buffered aspirin or an enteric-coated preparation. The coated tablets sometimes traverse the gastrointestinal tract unaltered.

The initial dose of aspirin in ambulatory patients is usually 2.4 Gm daily, but if the response is unsatisfactory, the dose should be increased until the desired response is achieved or side reactions supervene.

Salicylate therapy should be given the fullest possible trial before turning to other agents. In those cases not alleviated by salicylates there is considerable disagreement as to whether one should next try antimalarials, gold therapy, adrenocortical steroid therapy, or phenylbutazone.

Phenylbutazone (Butazolidin) has had widespread clinical trial in various rheumatic states. Curiously, its effectiveness in rheumatoid spondylitis and acute gouty arthritis seems more striking and more predictable than in peripheral rheumatoid arthritis, where major clinical improvement has been reported in approximately 25 to 40 per cent of cases. The erythrocyte sedimentation rate does not decrease consistently with its administration, and it is potentially dangerous. The incidence of side reactions varies considerably. In one large series of 800 cases, side reactions appeared in 40 per cent of patients, and in 15 per cent the drug had to be discontinued. Toxic effects include agranulocytosis, hypoplastic or hemolytic anemia, thrombocytopenia, peptic ulceration, and retention of sodium and water. Because of side reactions doses of no more than 300 to 400 mg daily are now recommended, but hematopoietic disorders may occur even at this level. In view of the toxicity of phenylbutazone, it should not be given until after other less hazardous measures have failed; it is contraindicated in patients with a history of allergy, peptic ulcer, or cardiovascular renal disease. If after 7 to 10 days of administration the patient does not improve, the drug should be discontinued.

Antimalarials. Both chloroquine phosphate and hydroxychloroquine sulfate have been shown recently by "double-blind" therapeutic trials in rheumatoid arthritis to have a significant antirheumatic effect. Improvement is slower and less dramatic than with corticoid therapy; benefit begins in 2 to 10 weeks. It is administered orally, 250 to 500 mg chloroquine or 200 to 400 mg hydroxychloroquine daily. Side reactions occur in up to 50 per cent of patients but are usually not serious, consisting of lichenoid and other types of dermatitis, anorexia, nausea, vomiting, loss or blanching of hair, corneal infiltration, mental disturbances, and anemia or leukopenia.

Adrenocortical Hormones. A full and detailed discussion of adrenocortical steroid therapy in clinical medicine, including the various types of steroid hormones, dosage, route of administration, contra-indications, complications, and precautions, appears elsewhere (p. 625). In 1949 when Hench and his associates first demonstrated the prompt and striking subjective improvement in patients with active rheumatoid arthritis given cortisone or corticotropin, hopes for its use were high. It was not long, however, before the limitations and dangers of these agents began to be recognized. Considerable disagreement prevails upon such issues as whether or not they should be used at all in rheumatoid arthritis, when to administer them, which of the many steroids to select, in what doses, for how long, and in conjunction with what other therapeutic measures.

After several years of experience with these agents, certain general conclusions may be drawn. (1) Prednisone, singled out for this discussion, is a potent, nonspecific, anti-inflammatory agent. It does not act in rheumatoid arthritis as replacement therapy in a deficiency state, as insulin does in diabetes mellitus. (2) In the vast majority of patients with active rheumatoid disease, prednisone in adequate dosage can induce rapid suppression of the symptoms and signs, as shown by regression of fever, joint manifestations, size of enlarged lymph nodes, scleral nodules, and other signs of ocular inflammation and pericarditis. Synovial fluid findings may revert to or toward normal. (3) On the other hand, in spite of clinical improvement, anemia may not be completely corrected, the erythrocyte sedimentation rate may not be reduced to normal levels, the serum protein abnormalities may persist, and the sheep cell agglutinating titer may remain unaltered. None of these tests should in itself serve as a guide to therapy. (4) The results of prednisone treatment are better in patients with severe inflammation. Other variables important in the outcome are dose and duration of administration, other concomitant therapeutic efforts, and psychologic factors. (5) Some patients fail to improve. In many instances, this may be attributed to irreversible changes, severe contractures, or ankylosis which had taken place prior to therapy, or to insufficient dosage. (6) Subjective and functional improvement usually exceed objective improvement. Joint destruction, as shown by serial roentgenographic studies, usually progresses. (7) Prednisone therapy by itself is insufficient and should be combined with the usual conservative program—rest, physical therapy, and salicylates. Actually, steroids have proved exceedingly helpful adjuncts to both physical therapy and orthopedic surgical correction.

It should be strongly emphasized that the corticosteroids are hazardous and should be withheld until the fullest possible trial with rest, physical therapy, and salicylates regularly given has failed to modify the course of the disease. Nevertheless, the concept that corticoid therapy should be a measure of last resort can be carried too far. Time is important in rheumatoid arthritis: the patient should not be allowed to become irreversibly incapacitated by his disease before prednisone is tried. Rapidly progressing articular or systemic disease, intractable pain requiring narcotics for control, and the patient's economic and social situation should also play a role in deciding when to institute steroid therapy.

In such a chronic disease long-term therapy will probably be required. Therefore, large initial doses are no longer given; one starts with a lower, safer dose—10 to 15 mg or less prednisone daily. After manipulation, a "maintenance" dosage is determined, but every effort should be made to keep this at a minimum, and one may have to compromise one's therapeutic efforts, if the dosage required to suppress symptoms is high and, therefore, hazardous. Under any circumstances, gradual dose reduction should be carried out periodically, at least every 6 months, in the hope that the patient may be entering a remission spontaneously.

The complications of corticosteroid administration and the contraindications to such therapy are discussed on p. 625. Those complications to which patients with rheumatoid arthritis are specially subject include (1) gastric and duodenal ulcers (more common in persons with untreated rheumatoid arthritis than in the general population); (2) osteoporosis and fractures, commonly of the vertebral bodies of the thoracic and lumbar spine, especially in postmenopausal women; and (3) necrotizing arteritis (also a feature of the untreated disease and resulting at times in neuropathy or ulcers of the extremities).

Intraarticular injections of suspensions of corticosteroid esters are useful when only a few easily accessible joints are involved. The amount injected varies from 10 to 50 mg, depending on size of joints. In most cases substantial relief of pain and stiffness lasts for 1 to 2 weeks. The procedure is then repeated as indicated.

Chrysotherapy. Until the advent of adrenocortical steroid therapy, gold compounds were perhaps the most popular of the specific agents in the treatment of rheumatoid arthritis. The mechanism of their action has not been elucidated. They are not effective in any other rheumatic disease. Significant improvement has taken place in 40 to 60 per cent of patients among the reported series. It appears from a few well-controlled clinical trials that gold is beneficial, although its advantage over more routine measures is moderate. It is given over several months, and the reported improvement characteristically occurs gradually. The remissions seen after a single course (total dosage of 1 Gm) are usually temporary. The value of maintenance therapy has not yet been fully determined but thus far seems impressive.

Several gold compounds are available; most of them contain approximately 50 per cent of metallic gold, are water-soluble, and are given intramuscularly. The usual regimen consists of an initial test dose of 10 mg, a second injection of 25 mg 1 week later, and 50 mg weekly thereafter until a total dose of 1.0 Gm has been given. Maintenance therapy is usually 50 mg every second or third week.

Toxic reactions occur frequently (in up to 50 per cent of patients), vary in severity, and are rarely fatal (in less than 1 per cent of patients). They include skin disorders, varying from pruritus to severe exfoliative dermatitis, stomatitis, hematopoietic disturbances—hypoplastic anemia, agranulocytosis, or thrombocytopenia—and nephritis. With the exception of the hematopoietic damage, which may not respond to any form of therapy, these toxic reactions usually disappear after gold is discontinued or, if severe, during treatment with BAL (British anti-lewisite) or adrenocortical steroids. Prior to each injection, the patient should be carefully interviewed and examined for symptoms and signs suggesting gold toxicity. There is neither synergism nor antagonism between gold and adrenocortical steroids.

Physical Therapy. A primary objective is *prevention of loss of normal joint motion* which ultimately leads to crippling. Therapeutic exercises, essentially nontiring movement to carry the joints through their normal range of motion daily, are prescribed. Active exercise is preferable; assistance may be given when needed.

Prevention of deformity requires attention to positioning in bed and to posture in general. Use of a board beneath the mattress prevents sagging. The patient should be encouraged to lie flat on his back when resting or sleeping, to use as small a pillow as possible under the head and neck, to avoid altogether the use of pillows under the knees, and to sit in a chair with a firm seat and straight back.

Graded exercises are given to *increase or maintain muscle power.* For patients confined to bed and unable to perform strengthening exercises, "muscle setting" (isometric contraction) is prescribed for the quadriceps and gluteals, which tend to weaken rapidly on bed rest.

Heat is generally used preceding exercise to diminish pain and muscle spasm and permit increased range of motion. The hot tub bath is indicated when involvement is extensive. For one or two joints, hot compresses or a heat bulb may be used. The par-

affin bath, which can be set up at home, is particularly effective for hands and wrists.

Canes and crutches are prescribed as assistive devices when it is necessary to reduce stress on hips, knees, and feet.

Ambulation is frequently aided by properly designed and well-fitted shoes. A straight last is generally recommended in contrast to a style which crowds the toes and ultimately causes deformity. A long counter and Thomas heel will provide helpful additional support to the patient whose foot tends to pronate, or roll inwards. The metatarsal bar is a simple and effective device for relieving painful pressure in the area of the metatarsal heads.

Splints and casts, properly applied, immobilize an inflamed and painful joint more completely than it can be immobilized by general limitation of the patient's activity. Particularly useful are "gutter splints" and long leg cylinder casts. Worn at night, they can prevent threatened flexion contracture of the knee. To correct a flexion contracture, a series of cylinder casts may be needed, each gaining a few degrees of extension. Functional wrist splints, which immobilize and protect the painful or deformed wrist while permitting active use of fingers and hands, have also proved to be effective. All splints and casts are made removable to enable the joint to be put through its range of motion daily.

The physical therapy program usually will have to be continued over a long period of time, making it important to prescribe measures which are readily carried out in the home.

Therapists also give specific training to increase the patient's capacity to perform activities of daily living such as bathing, dressing, and eating, and in the case of the housewife, to improve function in kitchen and household routines. In addition, appropriate simple and inexpensive devices, such as a long-handled shoe horn, a bathtub seat, and a built-up knife and fork, are recommended to enable the patient to become self-sufficient despite weakness and fixed joint deformities.

VARIANTS OF RHEUMATOID ARTHRITIS

Juvenile Rheumatoid Arthritis

Commonly called "Still's disease," this disorder begins in children before puberty and comprises 4 per cent of all cases of rheumatoid arthritis.

Systemic symptoms and signs are more severe in the juvenile than in the adult form. Fever often spikes daily to 105°F and may continue for months. Lymphadenopathy occurs in 60 per cent of cases and splenomegaly in 30 per cent. A transient and recurrent rash, consisting usually of small, erythematous, macular or maculopapular lesions, is seen in one-fourth of cases. Pericarditis, pleuritis, and pneumonitis are common features. Subcutaneous nodules are relatively rare. The juvenile form tends to affect the larger joints, especially in the earlier stages, and spondylitis is common. Growth and development may be impaired. Leukocyte count is often as high as 50,000 per cu mm. Rheumatoid serologic tests are positive in only 10 to 20 per cent of patients; a special inhibition technique increases this in about 80 per cent of cases.

Early in the disease, differentiation from acute rheumatic fever or systemic lupus erythematosus may be difficult. When juvenile rheumatoid arthritis presents monarticularly, as in the hip or the knee, tuberculous arthritis must be carefully ruled out.

The natural history of juvenile rheumatoid arthritis has not been fully charted. Contrary to earlier beliefs, the disease may be mild and result in little deformity. Satisfactory functional recovery occurs in three-fourths of the patients. Also contrary to earlier tenets, the disease process does not terminate with puberty. In cases with prolonged and severe involvement, secondary amyloidosis may appear. Management is generally similar to that for adult rheumatoid arthritis.

Ankylosing Spondylitis

This disorder (also called *Marie-Strümpell arthritis* or *rheumatoid spondylitis*) is a chronic arthritis involving the spine, sacroiliac joints, and in a minority of cases, peripheral joints as well. Some investigators believe it to be a variant of rheumatoid arthritis; others think it is a separate and distinct, but homogeneous, disease; still others look on it as a heterogeneous group of diseases with a common symptomatology. Those who propose that it is merely a variant point to the pathologic similarities in the two diseases and the fact that involvement of the peripheral joints in spondylitis is clinically indistinguishable from classical rheumatoid arthritis. The separatists can marshal several supporting arguments. Eighty to 90 per cent of spondylitics are men, whereas 60 to 70 per cent of rheumatoids are women. Spondylitis usually begins at a younger age. Subcutaneous nodules are almost never found in spondylitis. When the peripheral joints are involved in spondylitis, the common sites are the shoulders, hips, and knees; in rheumatoid arthritis, fingers, wrists, toes, and ankles predominate. Serologic reactions, such as sheep cell agglutination, are usually negative in spondylitis. Other points include the tendency for spondylitis to produce calcification of ligaments (absent in rheumatoid arthritis), to respond to x-ray therapy, and to fail to respond to gold. Lastly, the role of inheritance has been more firmly established in spondylitis. It has occurred in identical twins and is apparently inherited through an autosomal dominant gene with a penetrance of 70 per cent for the male and 10 per cent for the female.

The basic pathologic lesion is a synovitis similar to that of peripheral rheumatoid arthritis. The disease usually begins in the sacroiliac joints. Initially, these exhibit condensation of bone; later, they show erosions, articular narrowing, and in most instances, obliteration of the joint space with bony ankylosis. The next event is involvement of the spine where synovitis is confined to the posterior intervertebral joints, the only true diarthrodeses of the vertebral column. Later the spinal ligaments become calcified. Demineralization of the vertebral bodies may appear during any phase of the disease.

Spondylitis usually begins insidiously, with stiffness of the back after inactivity, lumbar pain with root radiation, often sciatic, and limitation of forward bending. The lumbar spine gradually loses its normal lordosis. With progressive involvement of the costovertebral joints, chest expansion diminishes and pain may be elicited by deep inspiration, coughing, or sneezing. As the spine fuses it may be held erect, the so-called "poker spine," but more frequently, the pull of the spinal muscles results in dorsal kyphosis and scoliosis. Frequently the head becomes fixed in forward displacement. Peripheral joint involvement may either precede or follow spinal disease. In many instances it is brief and intermittent, but in one-fourth of the patients it persists, characteristically in the "root joints" (shoulders and hips). About 3 per cent of patients develop aortitis and aortic insufficiency.

Although the course of the disease may vary a great deal, the usual pattern is persistent activity for 2 or 3 years, with pain, low-grade fever, weight loss, anemia, and a high sedimentation rate. As the spine fuses, pain disappears, on the average 10 years after onset. In contrast to patients with rheumatoid arthritis, the majority (roughly three-fourths) of those with spondylitis continue to lead relatively normal lives; less than 10 per cent become totally incapacitated. The average duration of life after clinically detectable aortic insufficiency develops is 10 years.

The general principles of management are similar to those employed in rheumatoid arthritis—the relief of pain and the preservation of the best possible skeletal function. For analgesia, salicylates in the fullest tolerable doses should be tried first. X-ray therapy affords pain relief to many patients. Since the incidence of leukemia after radiotherapy is at least twenty times that in the general population or in those with spondylitis without radiotherapy, this form of treatment may be unjustifiable. Phenylbutazone (Butazolidin) appears to be more effective in spondylitis than in peripheral rheumatoid arthritis. It is particularly helpful in minimizing periodic painful attacks in ambulatory patients. The contraindications, complications, and appropriate prophylactic measures are described in the section on peripheral rheumatoid arthritis. The indications for adrenocortical steroid therapy are fewer than in rheumatoid arthritis, being largely confined to patients with severe, sustained disease in whom the peripheral joints are also seriously affected.

Special attention should be paid to keeping deformities to a minimum by seeing that fusion takes place in the optimal position. The bed should be kept flat, by placing a board underneath a firm mattress, and the head pillow small to prevent kyphosis and neck flexion. A small pillow under the lumbar spine may preserve the normal lordotic curvature. Exercises of the paravertebral, abdominal, and respiratory muscles are designed to maintain a straight back and neck and to retain ventilatory sufficiency. Muscle relaxants may be useful in the early phases of the disease. Back braces may help to combat thoracic kyphosis. Rarely, in the extremely deformed patient, lumbar osteotomy may be indicated.

Psoriatic Arthritis (or Arthropathy)

The incidence of arthritis is greater in patients with psoriasis than in the general population. In a minority of those with psoriasis and arthritis, there is striking involvement of the distal interphalangeal joints, often with marked destruction and psoriatic changes in the adjacent nails. Some investigators consider this true "psoriatic arthropathy." The majority of cases resemble clinically rheumatoid arthritis. However, several features distinguish both forms from rheumatoid arthritis: the conspicuous absence of subcutaneous nodules, high incidence of sacroiliac involvement, and a low incidence of positive rheumatoid factor tests (perhaps no greater than in the population at large). The psoriasis usually antedates the arthritis by months or years, although they may appear simultaneously or the arthritis may come first. The principles and details of management are similar to those of rheumatoid arthritis, although *chloroquine* should be avoided for it may precipitate a severe attack of psoriasis. Contrary to earlier reports, triamcinolone has no advantage over other corticosteroids.

Felty's Syndrome

In 1924, Felty reported a series of five patients with febrile migratory polyarthritis, splenomegaly, and leukopenia. Subsequently, many other such cases have been described and the disease presenting with this triad has since borne his name. Three of his five patients also exhibited brown hyperpigmentation over the exposed surfaces. This syndrome is usually encountered in far-advanced rheumatoid disease; its separation as a syndrome is perhaps unwarranted. The serum may contain unusually large amounts of rheumatoid factor. Lupus erythematosus (LE) cells and antinuclear antibodies are more frequent than in rheumatoid arthritis in general. There may be anemia and thrombocytopenia, in addition to the neutropenia. The hematologic abnormalities respond to splenectomy, but the arthritis is unaffected.

ARTHRITIS AND GASTROINTESTINAL DISEASE

Ulcerative Colitis

Rheumatic complaints are common in ulcerative colitis, occurring in as many as half the cases. After excluding degenerative joint disease, traumatic arthritis, rheumatic fever, and gout, three groups remain: (1) "colitic arthritis," 10 to 20 per cent of cases; (2) ankylosing spondylitis, 5 to 10 per cent; and (3) definite rheumatoid arthritis, 2 to 3 per cent (an incidence perhaps no greater than in the general population).

Colitic arthritis is an acute synovitis which is mostly monarticular; if polyarticular, it is usually asymmetric. The joints involved are knee, ankle, elbow, and proximal interphalangeal joint, in order of decreasing frequency. Attacks last only a few weeks; the recurrence rate is high. Histologically, the synovitis resembles that of rheumatoid arthritis. The arthritis usually develops during exacerbations of colitis and late in the disease; it is more common in those with perianal suppuration, pseudopolyposis, and/or erythema nodosum. Features which help to distinguish colitic arthritis from rheumatoid arthritis are (1) younger age at onset, (2) absence of residual deformity, (3) absence of subcutaneous nodules or tendon sheath lesions, (4) paucity of radiologic changes, (5) negative tests for rheumatoid factor, and (6) an apparent cure after colectomy. Moreover, patients with rheumatoid arthritis develop ulcerative colitis only rarely.

The majority with spondylitis and colitis are men. Symptoms of spondylitis may antedate (by several years), coincide with, or follow the onset of colitis; they may persist after colectomy. In most patients the x-ray changes are confined to the sacroiliac joints, but other portions of the spine may be involved. Certain patients complain of low-back pain during attacks of colitis, but have no radiologic evidence of spondylitis.

Regional Enteritis

As with the other systemic "complications" of regional enteritis, both peripheral arthritis and spondylitis are less frequent than in ulcerative colitis, the incidences being estimated at 2 to 6 per cent and 1 to 2 per cent, respectively. Most patients have ileocolitis, the distribution of the acute or sub-acute arthritis resembles that in ulcerative colitis, and the severity of the arthritis parallels the activity of the enteritis.

Whipple's Disease

This disorder, first described by Whipple in 1907, and also known as intestinal lipodystrophy or lipogranulomatosis, is a systemic disorder of middle-aged men, manifested by intermittent arthritis, weight loss, cutaneous hyperpigmentation, lymphadenopathy, abdominal pain, diarrhea, and intestinal malabsorption. Diagnosis may be made by finding periodic acid–Schiff (PAS)–positive material in lymph node or jejunal biopsy.

The joint involvement, which usually antedates other manifestations by months or years, consists of a migratory polyarthralgia or polyarthritis affecting any joint. Articular recurrences accompany exacerbations of abdominal symptoms, but joint deformities do not develop.

SJÖGREN'S SYNDROME

In 1933, Sjögren, a Swedish ophthalmologist, reported among patients with keratoconjunctivitis sicca the additional findings of xerostomia, enlargement of the lacrimal and salivary glands, and rheumatoid arthritis. Since then, he and others have extended these observations and emphasized the systemic nature of the disorder. The syndrome is defined variously by the presence of two or more of these manifestations. Recent clinical, histologic, and laboratory investigations have provided information possibly of considerable pathogenetic significance for this and related disorders. The majority of patients are women with a mean age of 50 years.

Clinical Features. In the fully developed case, the disorder involves virtually all the exocrine glands of the body. Keratoconjunctivitis sicca is recognized by (1) stinging and grittiness of the eyes, (2) reduced lacrimal secretion as measured by the Schirmer test (p. 418), (3) desquamation of corneal or conjunctival epithelium as demonstrated by rose bengal staining, and (4) filamentary keratitis (slit lamp examination). With xerostomia, there are dry mouth, decreased salivary flow, and abnormal sialogram. The lacrimal and/or parotid glands are enlarged in one-half the cases. The mucosa of nose, pharynx, and larynx may be dry and atrophic. There may be a dry cough, with tracheobronchitis, pneumonitis, and/or pleuritis. Involvement of the alimentary tract results in dysphagia, achlorhydria, or constipation. Many patients have atrophic vaginitis.

Half the patients have definite rheumatoid ar-thritis; a few, transitory polyarthritis. Felty's syndrome is occasionally encountered. Conversely, 13 per cent of patients with rheumatoid arthritis have keratoconjunctivitis sicca. Less frequently seen in Sjögren's syndrome are purpura (usually nonthrombocytopenic), Raynaud's phenomenon, thyroid enlargement, lymphadenopathy, splenomegaly, hepatomegaly, focal myositis, arteritis, and peripheral neuropathy. Sjögren's syndrome has been associated with each of the collagen disorders (systemic lupus erythematosus, progressive systemic sclerosis, polyarteritis, and polymyositis) and with purpura hyperglobulinemia (of Waldenström) (p. 1344).

Laboratory Findings. One-third of patients with Sjögren's syndrome have anemia, which is usually mild. A leukopenia, with fewer than 4,000 leukocytes per cu mm, is also found in one-third of patients; rarely is it severe. One-fourth have eosinophilia. The erythrocyte sedimentation rate is usually raised.

Most patients have hyperglobulinemia, mainly from an increase in γ-globulin of the 7S type. Tests for rheumatoid factor by several different methods (sheep cell agglutination, bentonite flocculation, latex fixation) are positive in the vast majority of cases, even in those having no joint symptoms. Similarly, most patients, with or without arthritis, have antinuclear factor (p. 1893), although LE cells are found in only a few, with severe rheumatoid arthritis. There is an appreciable incidence of complement-fixing antibodies to suspensions of homogenates from various tissues; these antigens are neither organ- nor species-specific.

Abnormalities on urinalysis are unusual but several patients have shown an unexplained inability to concentrate urine. Chest x-rays may reveal pleural thickening or atelectasis.

Pathology. Characteristically, the salivary and lacrimal glands reveal massive dense infiltration with lymphocytes and plasma cells (as in the thyroid of Hashimoto's disease), atrophy of acini, proliferation of the duct-lining cells, and myoepithelial islands. This is the histologic picture of Mikulicz's disease, and on the basis of this and other evidence Morgan and Castleman in 1953 concluded that Sjögren's syndrome and primary Mikulicz's disease were the same. Muscle biopsy may reveal a widespread acute myositis or a mild chronic focal myositis.

Etiology. The etiology of Sjögren's syndrome, as defined here, is unknown. Because of the striking similarity of the histopathologic changes in the salivary and lacrimal glands to those in the thyroid gland in Hashimoto's disease, and moreover, in view of the abundance of abnormal serum factors (rheumatoid and antinuclear factors) and circulating antibodies to tissue components, the possibility has been entertained that Sjögren's syndrome may be the result of autoimmunity. This, however, remains to be substantiated.

Diagnosis. Clearly, Sjögren's syndrome is more common than has been generally realized. The generous use of such techniques as the Schirmer test, rose bengal staining, slit lamp examination, sialography, serologic testing, and biopsies facilitates diagnosis. Every effort should be made to rule out other causes of Mikulicz's syndrome (salivary gland enlargement), such as lymphoma, leukemia, tuberculosis, sarcoid, hepatic cirrhosis, and malnutrition.

Treatment. Many patients need no systemic therapy. Local measures, such as methylcellulose (artificial tears) for keratoconjunctivitis sicca are often very beneficial; methylcellulose swab or spray is effective in xerostomia. There should be frequent search for complicating infection, especially in the salivary glands and lower respiratory tract. Antimalarials, such as chloroquine, are at times helpful for arthritis but have little or no effect on the glandular abnormalities. In view of the usually benign course, corticosteroids are rarely indicated, except in the patient with concomitant systemic or articular disease. In cases of severe enlargement of the parotids, the response to radiotherapy is often striking. Surgical excision should be discouraged because of recurrences and the risk of injury to the facial nerve.

DEGENERATIVE JOINT DISEASE

Definition. Degenerative joint disease (DJD), otherwise known as *osteoarthritis, hypertrophic arthritis,* or *senescent arthritis,* is a chronic disorder characterized pathologically by degeneration of articular cartilage and hypertrophy of bone, clinically by pain which appears with use and subsides with rest, and by typical roentgenographic findings. It occurs more commonly in older people, usually affecting weight-bearing joints and the distal interphalangeal joints of the fingers. It may develop spontaneously with advancing age (primary osteoarthritis) or at an earlier age as a sequel to articular injury of various kinds (secondary osteoarthritis). The pathologic changes begin early in life and increase in frequency with each successive decade. Pathologic joint changes may not give rise to articular symptoms. There are no systemic manifestations as in rheumatoid arthritis.

Epidemiology. Degenerative joint disease is world-wide although it is best known in temperate climates, reflecting perhaps the longer life span of the populations in these areas. It is an ancient disease. In human beings it dates back to Neanderthal man (40,000 B.C.).

Roentgenographic abnormalities usually do not appear until the third or fourth decade, but after the age of fifty, virtually everyone has some charac-

teristic x-ray changes. Nevertheless, only a minority experience symptoms. Although this disorder is not so disabling as rheumatoid arthritis, it has economic importance, as revealed by the results of an industrial survey which showed that 14 per cent of all patients exhibiting objective evidence of musculoskeletal disease had DJD. It is largely a disorder of middle and late life, often appearing in women at the time of the menopause. Most studies reveal that DJD is divided equally between the sexes, although for a variety of reasons (occupational, genetic, etc.) the distribution of joint involvement does differ between them.

Etiology. It is generally held that DJD is related to the physiologic process of aging. Many anatomic studies, including the excellent one of Bennett, Waine, and Bauer in which knee joints from persons one month to ninety years of age were examined, reveal that alterations in the articular cartilage characteristic of DJD begin to appear as early as the second decade of life and increase in frequency and severity with advancing age. The most commonly held view is that these changes result from ordinary "wear and tear," i.e., from cumulative trauma.

Although there is little doubt that repeated injury of one form or another frequently plays a role in this disorder, this concept does not explain the disease completely. A striking exception to this hypothesis is the common involvement of the distal interphalangeal joints (Heberden's nodes). These joints are not subject to any more frequent or severe mechanical injury than others, such as the metacarpophalangeals, which are rarely involved in DJD. Necropsy studies have failed to uncover any difference in the incidence of this disorder between laborers and sedentary workers.

Heredity clearly plays a role in the pathogenesis of Heberden's nodes. They are ten times more common in women than in men. Stecher showed that they are inherited as a sex-influenced characteristic, dominant in the female and recessive in the male. However, the importance of heredity or constitution in the pathogenesis of DJD at other sites has not been demonstrated.

Pathology. The initial step in the chain of pathologic events in DJD is degeneration of articular hyaline cartilage. Grossly, the cartilage becomes less elastic, yellow, and more opaque. Under the microscope, the surface is made uneven by the appearance of shallow linear furrows which later deepen into clefts, or fissures, running perpendicular to the surface of the cartilage. At this stage, the articular surface appears much like velvet on gross examination. The cartilage cells form clusters. Later, there is fraying and then ulceration. In this manner, the hyaline cartilage is gradually destroyed.

In response to this primary injury, certain secondary productive or hypertrophic changes ensue. In areas where the articular cartilage becomes thin, the underlying calcified cartilage becomes thick and dense. In the neighboring subchondral bone there is proliferation of fibroblasts, endosteal cells, and blood vessels. This subchondral granulation tissue then breaks through the calcified cartilage to reach the surface of the joint space. This surfacing of new bone, which later thickens and becomes highly polished, is called *eburnation*. As a result, perhaps, of the response to injured cartilage and blood vessel proliferation, bony excrescences, or osteophytes, begin to form at the joint margin. These consist of cancellous bone, the marrow spaces of which are continuous with those of epiphyseal marrow.

Synovial changes occur late and consist of a tissue response to the deposition of debris such as fragments of degenerating cartilage or bone. The synovial membrane may appear slightly hypertrophic, mostly from fibrosis, and with little cellular reaction. In advanced cases, fibrous thickening and contraction of the joint capsule may be intense. Although the mechanism of pain production in this disease is not well understood, it is possible that this shrinkage of the joint capsule, supplied as it is with somatic and autonomic fibers, may be responsible.

Clinical Features. Only a small proportion of patients with DJD have symptoms from the disease. Symptoms develop insidiously and consist chiefly of joint pain and stiffness. The pain is characteristically aching and mild; it appears with exercise of the part and abates with rest. The stiffness, or articular "jelling," develops after prolonged rest in a fixed position and disappears a few minutes after resuming activity, in contrast to that of rheumatoid arthritis which may last for hours. Although the disorder is frequently progressive, it rarely causes the degree of discomfort and invalidism encountered in rheumatoid arthritis.

Objectively the joints may appear entirely normal, even in the patient with symptoms. Joint enlargement, when present, is the result of secondary hypertrophy of bone. The enlarged joints feel hard and knobby, unlike the soft, fluctuant swelling in rheumatoid disease. There may be tenderness but rarely excessive warmth or erythema. In the later stages a grating sensation, or crepitus, may be felt on moving the affected joint. There are no diagnostic laboratory abnormalities or changes in the synovial fluid.

In the symptomatic patient, the roentgenographic appearance may be normal or there may be one or more abnormalities. These include (roughly in order of advancing disease) unevenness and narrowing of the joint space, secondary to destruction of cartilage; sharpening of the articular margins; irregularity and widening of the articulating surfaces; bony sclerosis, or eburnation, as shown by heightened radiopacity at the ends of bone; osteophytes, or marginal lipping; and bone cysts. Osteoporosis does not result from DJD; when it is present, other causes should be sought.

The most commonly involved joints are those that bear weight (knees, hips, and lumbar spine) and also the cervical spine, shoulders, and distal interphalangeal joints of the fingers.

Diagnosis. Since DJD and rheumatoid arthritis, the two most common forms of chronic joint disease in the middle-aged and the elderly, differ so widely in both prognosis and management it is important to distinguish one disorder from the other. In virtually every instance, this is readily accomplished. Differentiation should never be made on the basis of age alone. In contrast to rheumatoid arthritis, DJD is confined to the joint structures and is not a widely disseminated systemic disease. There are no constitutional symptoms and signs such as fever, weakness, fatigability, anorexia, weight loss, or muscular wasting; nor are there laboratory abnormalities such as anemia, leukocytosis, elevated sedimentation rate, or hyperglobulinemia. The joints are not hot or red and there are no subcutaneous nodules. The sheep cell agglutination test is negative.

Even though x-ray changes of an affected joint may be those of DJD, the articular symptoms and signs may be caused by a coexistent joint disorder such as rheumatoid arthritis or gout. In such cases, objective evidence of inflammation may have great diagnostic significance. Errors of overdiagnosis are commonly made in cases demonstrating osteophytosis of the spine; this rarely gives rise to symptoms. In patients with back symptoms, some other process, such as a herniated nucleus pulposus, and not the DJD, may be responsible. At any rate, if pain believed to be attributable to DJD is severe and fails to respond to the usual measures, one must rule out other diseases such as metastasis of a malignancy to bone, multiple myeloma, or osteomyelitis.

Management. The most important feature in the care of the patient with DJD is to advise him that although his disease is annoying and at times uncomfortable it is not serious and not the kind (like rheumatoid arthritis) that causes severe pain, disability, and crippling. By such reassurance, the patient is spared the anguish of the pronouncement that he has "arthritis" and "nothing can be done." Conservative measures—adequate rest of the involved joints, physical therapy including corrective exercises, and safe analgesics such as salicylates—usually suffice. Attention should be directed toward eliminating or minimizing secondary traumatic influences. Obese patients should lose weight. Certain occupational adjustments may be made. Abdominal supports for lumbar spine disease aggravated by a sagging abdomen, and a Thomas collar or head traction for cervical spine involvement are other examples of ways to eliminate precipitating influences. Repeated intraarticular injections of hydrocortisone are beneficial only in those patients with a superimposed, nonspecific inflammatory response to fragmented cartilage or bone. The systemic use of such potentially hazardous agents as adrenocortical steroids or phenylbutazone should be discouraged. Corrective orthopedic surgical methods are useful for severely disabled and painful hips and knees unresponsive to conservative management.

HYPERTROPHIC OSTEOARTHROPATHY

Definition. This disorder, also known as *hypertrophic pulmonary osteoarthropathy, osteoarthropathie hypertrophiante pneumique, secondary hypertrophic osteoarthropathy*, and *Marie-Bamberger syndrome,* is characterized by (1) clubbing of the fingers and toes, (2) chronic periostitis with new bone formation at the distal ends of the long bones, and (3) arthritis. In the vast majority of cases, this syndrome is secondary to one of several diverse, serious chronic illnesses in other parts of the body; in the remainder, it is hereditary or idiopathic. Because of its frequent association with diseases of the lung, the disorder is often called "hypertrophic pulmonary osteoarthropathy," but this is a restrictive designation in that the primary disease may reside elsewhere, as in the heart, liver, or gastrointestinal tract.

Formerly, chronic suppurative conditions, such as bronchiectasis, were the most common underlying diseases, but now pulmonary neoplasms head the list. Osteoarthropathy may appear several months before the first symptom or sign of bronchogenic carcinoma.

Classification. Hypertrophic osteoarthropathy occurs either *symmetrically,* all four extremities usually being involved, or *unilaterally,* affecting only one extremity, more commonly an upper. Symmetric disease is subdivided into *acquired, hereditary,* and *idiopathic* forms. The acquired form is further categorized according to the location of the underlying condition:

1. *Pulmonary.* Various pulmonary, pleural, and mediastinal disorders lead to this syndrome. It occurs in 5 to 10 per cent of cases of bronchogenic carcinoma; it has a high incidence in pleural tumors but is rare in tumors which have metastasized to lung. Chronic infections include bronchiectasis, lung abscess, and empyema. It is rare in tuberculosis. Arthropathy has occurred with Hodgkin's disease,

aortic aneurysm, and other disorders of the mediastinum.

2. *Cardiac.* Hypertrophic osteoarthropathy occurs in cyanotic forms of congenital heart disease but is not seen in noncyanotic forms. It is sometimes present in subacute bacterial endocarditis.

3. *Hepatic.* The incidence of this syndrome is high in cholangiolitic biliary cirrhosis, but much lower in obstructive biliary, portal, and postnecrotic cirrhosis.

4. *Gastrointestinal.* Most of the intraabdominal conditions leading to osteoarthropathy are characterized by chronic diarrhea. They include ulcerative colitis and regional enteritis, amebic and bacillary dysentery, intestinal tuberculosis, polyposis of the colon, neoplasms, and idiopathic steatorrhea.

5. *Miscellaneous.* Although it is very rare in spontaneous myxedema (and cretinism), several cases of osteoarthropathy have developed following thyroidectomy for Graves' disease. Isolated cases have been described in chronic urinary tract infections, syringomyelia, and various other disorders.

The *hereditary* form of osteoarthropathy is rare and is distinguished from the acquired form by remarkable thickening of the skin over the face and limbs and by little bone or joint pain. It is inherited as a mendelian dominant trait, appears shortly after puberty, progresses for about 10 years, and remains stationary thereafter.

Many cases designated as *idiopathic* are examples of the hereditary form or acquired disease in which the primary condition is unrecognized. A few cases of typical osteoarthropathy are, however, unexplainable.

Unilateral clubbing and osteoarthropathy are most commonly caused by aneurysm of the aorta, innominate, or subclavian. Other causes are apical lung cancer, axillary tumors, subluxation of the shoulder, and brachial arteriovenous anastomoses.

Pathology. The basic lesion is chronic inflammation of periosteum, synovial membrane, joint capsule, and adjacent subcutaneous tissue. The periosteum early in the disease exhibits edema and round-cell infiltration and, at its inner margin, osteoid matrix. Initially, only scattered foci of new bone appear; later, the distal segments may become completely encased by new bone.

The synovial membrane, articular capsule, and the subcutaneous tissue about the affected bones and joints become thickened and chronically inflamed. There may be an intermittent hydrarthrosis. Rarely, the synovitis goes on to pannus formation, ankylosis, and degeneration of cartilage.

Pathogenesis. Theories advanced for the mechanism of osteoarthropathy include (1) chronic infection, (2) action of toxins absorbed from the primary focus, (3) capillary stasis caused by elevated venous pressure, (4) arterial hypoxemia, (5) local hypoxia, (6) action of local toxins formed as a result of circulatory disturbances, (7) anterior pituitary overactivity, (8) thyroid underactivity, and (9) the elaboration by pleural mesothelial cells of an osteoblast-stimulating substance. None of these hypotheses accounts for more than a small proportion of cases.

The first and only experimental reproduction of this condition was achieved by Mendlowitz and Leslie in the dog by anastomosing the left pulmonary artery to the left auricle, thus creating a situation similar to cyanotic congenital heart disease. As the osteoarthropathy developed, the systemic cardiac output increased (the pulmonary blood flow remaining normal).

After resection of a lung abscess or tumor, symptoms and signs of osteoarthropathy frequently subside within a few days. The speed of this improvement suggests that the alterations in the peripheral circulation are corrected rapidly, perhaps by interrupting an abnormal pulmonary-vascular reflex. This hypothesis is supported by a recent report of prompt improvement in hypertrophic osteoarthropathy after dividing the vagus in five patients with inoperable lung cancer. Thoracotomy alone is ineffective.

Manifestations. In clubbing, the fingertips feel warm and slightly burning but pain is unusual. The first change is thickening about the nail bed, which can be detected by a reduction in the angle made by the nail and the dorsal plane of the distal phalanx, normally about 15°. Profuse sweating of the hands and feet is common.

Rheumatic complaints vary greatly in severity. There may be deep-seated burning pain and exquisite tenderness over the distal ends of the bones in acute and advanced cases. About the affected bones and joints, the skin may be dusky red, warm, and tender, and the subcutaneous tissue thickened. The joints may be swollen and their mobility restricted. Most commonly involved are the knees, ankles, wrists, elbows, and metacarpophalangeal joints. There may be slight fever.

In the early stages of clubbing, the terminal phalanges appear normal on x-ray, but with advancing disease they reveal flaring of the ungual process and osteoporosis. The x-ray evidence of osteoarthropathy consists of periosteal thickening along the shafts of the long bones, appearing first and being thickest in the region of the distal epiphyses, especially at the points of musculotendinous insertion. The periosteal elevation spreads proximally as the disease progresses. Later, the cancellous portion of the involved bone becomes osteoporotic and the cortex becomes thin.

The course of hypertrophic osteoarthropathy reflects the activity of the underlying disease. In cases where it waxes and wanes with exacerbations and remissions of the primary condition, the roentgenograms show a tree trunk-like layering of thin sheets of newly formed bone. In cases secondary to chronic suppuration, the osteoarthropathy emerges insidiously and is usually mild. In cases secondary to lung tumors, the clubbing and arthropathy may appear very suddenly. Articular symptoms and signs sometimes antedate clubbing of the fingers, but this is unusual.

Diagnosis. When clubbing, arthritic symptoms, and periosteal proliferation by x-ray are all present, this syndrome is easily recognized. The patient in whom arthritic symptoms predominate is often thought to have rheumatoid or some other form of polyarthritis. In patients with erythema and superficial tenderness, especially about the ankles, thrombophlebitis is a frequent diagnosis. Differentiation from acromegaly is usually not difficult. The diagnosis cannot rest on evidence of periosteal proliferation alone because scurvy, syphilis, trauma, lymphangitis, varicose veins, and other conditions give rise to periosteal disorders.

Treatment. Therapeutic efforts in hypertrophic osteoarthropathy should be directed toward the elimination of the underlying condition or its amelioration. In cases where the osteoarthropathy is severe and a satisfactory attack on the primary disorder is not possible, relief of disabling symptoms has been obtained by intrathoracic vagotomy or adrenocortical steroid therapy.

MISCELLANEOUS ARTHRITIDES

Palindromic Rheumatism

This controversial syndrome of unknown cause consists of recurring afebrile attacks of acute arthritis with pain, swelling, erythema, heat, and tenderness. The arthritis appears suddenly, usually involves a single joint, and lasts a few hours or days. Attacks are numerous and irregularly spaced; during the intervals between them, the joints appear normal and function properly. Essential to the diagnosis is the absence of residual arthritis, even after hundreds of attacks, and normal values for the hematocrit and blood uric acid concentration. The sedimentation rate may be elevated. Some patients demonstrate paraarticular involvement but without constitutional symptoms or signs. Many patients diagnosed as having palindromic rheumatism eventually develop typical rheumatoid arthritis or gout.

Intermittent Hydrarthrosis

This uncommon idiopathic condition consists of joint effusions recurring regularly every 7 to 11 days over several years. It is seen mostly in adolescents and young adults. Typically, it affects the knee (ankle or hip less commonly) and is unilateral. The joints, in addition to being swollen, are often painful and restricted in mobility but not hot or red. It is not a systemic disease; there is no fever, weight loss, or muscular wasting; there is no anemia and the sedimentation rate is normal. Strictly defined, it is not a simple hydrarthrosis because biopsy usually reveals a villous synovitis indistinguishable from that of rheumatoid arthritis. There is a leukocytosis in the synovial fluid, polymorphonuclears predominating. Most patients with this diagnosis subsequently prove to have rheumatoid arthritis. However, 150 cases have been reported with these characteristic periodic effusions over periods as long as 22 years with no residual deformity. The disease is refractory to salicylates and physical therapy. Some workers believe this condition to be an unusual form of allergy because, in a few patients, elimination of a food item has coincided with cessation of attacks. Antihistaminics are ineffective. The response to the intraarticular injection of hydrocortisone is usually favorable. Careful exclusion of other rheumatic disorders is essential.

Psychogenic Rheumatism

This term refers to the rheumatic manifestations of psychoneurosis, in which patients undergoing psychic trauma complain of stiffness, pains in joints, tendons, or muscles, and limitation of joint motion. In the United States Armed Forces during the Second World War, psychogenic rheumatism was thought to be the most common rheumatic disease; in the British forces such cases were labeled "fibrositis." Essential for this diagnosis are good general health, emotional instability, absence of objective joint changes clinically and radiologically, normal laboratory findings, vacillating complaints, and failure to respond to analgesics and physical therapy. Some investigators feel that a category of psychogenic rheumatism is unjustified and that there is probably some organic basis for the symptoms.

NONARTICULAR RHEUMATISM

The patient complaining of "rheumatism" often is referring to symptoms resulting not from joint disease per se but from dysfunction of other tissues near joints. These include tendons, bursae, bones, muscles, nerves, and adipose tissue. This heterogeneous group of extraarticular disorders is probably responsible for more rheumatic complaints than any one of the various intrinsic joint disorders. Approximately 30 per cent of patients who attend arthritis clinics in the United States have nonarticular rheumatism.

Fibrositis

This is a controversial, unfortunate term which Gowers introduced in 1904 to describe the chronic inflammation of fibrous tissue which he believed to be responsible for "lumbago." This concept was avidly adopted to explain the various aches and stiffness appearing in various sites of the body, and "fibrositis" has become a wastebasket term to cover many forms of nonarticular rheumatism. In addition to stiffness and soreness, there are often tenderness and limitation of motion of the affected part. The presence of nodules has been overemphasized; in many instances, these are really fat hernias. The frequent sites of pain are the lower back, gluteal region, neck, shoulder, and chest. Fatigability is the only constitutional manifestation. Precipitating factors include infections such as malaria, influenza, or pleurodynia; trauma; overexposure to cold, dampness, or drafts; and more specific connective tissue disorders, such as bursitis or tenosynovitis.

Tendinitis and Tenosynovitis

Inflammation of tendons and tendon sheaths may be associated with various types of arthritis or may occur independently. It is more frequent in gonococcal arthritis (present in 48 per cent of cases in one series) than in any other form of arthritis. Occasionally, one finds gonococcal tenosynovitis without arthritis. Tuberculous tenosynovitis is chronic and destructive. The most common site is the wrist. Tenosynovitis also occurs in rheumatoid arthritis, gout, and palindromic rheumatism.

Nonspecific tenosynovitis is thought to be a consequence of single or repeated injuries incurred during movements demanding strength and speed. The wrist and ankle tendons and sheaths are most commonly involved. If conservative therapy (immobilization, heat, and analgesics) fails, local injection of hydrocortisone or surgical excision of the sheath may be helpful.

Bursitis

This term is used loosely by patients to signify pain in one shoulder or both. To the physician, it denotes pain in the region of one of the 140 or more bursae in the body. The most commonly affected deep bursae (those situated between bony prominences and muscle or tendon) include the subacromial, subgluteal, supratrochanteric, and Achilles bursae. The most frequently involved superficial bursae (those situated between bony prominences and skin) are the olecranon and prepatellar. Subacromial bursitis is estimated to be the cause of shoulder pain in 80 per cent of patients who do not have evidence of rheumatic disease elsewhere. Its numerous synonyms include subdeltoid bursitis, calcific bursitis, calcific tendinitis, periarthritis of the shoulder, and *Duplay's disease.*

The pathogenesis of subacromial bursitis is obscure. The generally held concept is that acute or chronic trauma leads to rupture of a calcium "abscess" which has formed in the tendon of one of the short rotator shoulder muscles (supraspinatus, infraspinatus, teres minor, or subscapularis). Inflammation within and about the bursa is thought to be secondary to the tendinous necrosis and calcification.

In acute subacromial bursitis, agonizing pain appears suddenly in the region of the shoulder joint and is aggravated by motion, especially by abduction of the arm. The pain often radiates into the neck or down the lateral aspect of the arm, even to the fingertips. There is exquisite tenderness over the greater tuberosity of the humerus. In approximately half the cases, roentgenograms of the shoulder reveal a calcific deposit, or more than one, over the greater tuberosity and localized atrophy of adjacent bone. The acute attack subsides completely or passes into a chronic phase, which is usually mild.

Adhesive capsulitis (also called *adhesive tendinitis, chronic adhesive bursitis,* or "frozen shoulder") is distinguished from subacromial bursitis by a more insidious onset, less pain, and more stiffness. Dense adhesions form between the opposing surfaces of the subacromial bursa. Some investigators believe that the initial change is degeneration of the biceps tendon. It is thought to result from prolonged immobilization, senescent change, or trauma. In advanced cases, the arm becomes locked at the side and the shoulder muscles become atrophic.

Therapeutically the acute attack of bursitis may require no more than rest, immobilization with slings or splints, physical therapy, and analgesic drugs. The local injection of procaine and/or hydrocortisone sometimes affords prompt relief. Aspiration or surgical removal of the calcific deposit is recommended for persistent disabling disease. In adhesive capsulitis, manipulation of the shoulder under anesthesia may become necessary.

REFERENCES

GENERAL

Copeman, W. S. C. (Ed.): "Textbook of Rheumatic Diseases," 2d ed., Baltimore, The Williams & Wilkins Company, 1955.
Hollander, J. L. (Ed.): "Comroe's Arthritis and Allied Conditions," 6th ed., Philadelphia, Lea & Febiger, 1960.

Rheumatism Reviews, First through Thirteenth: Ann. Internal Med., 8–15, 28, 39, 45: 1935–1960. (Excellent and comprehensive periodic review of the American and British literature in rheumatic disease; prepared by the Editorial Committee of the American Rheumatism Association.)
Ropes, M. W., and W. Bauer: "Synovial Changes in Joint Disease," Cambridge, Harvard University Press, 1953.

DEGENERATIVE JOINT DISEASE

Bennett, G. A., H. Waine, and W. Bauer: "Changes in the Knee Joint at Various Ages with Particular Reference to the Nature and Development of Degenerative Joint Disease," New York, The Commonwealth Fund, 1942.
Bunim, J. J.: Arthritis in the Elderly Patient (Osteoarthritis), Bull. N.Y. Acad. Med., 32:102, 1956.
Kellgren, J. H., and R. Moore: Generalized Osteoarthritis and Heberden's Nodes, Brit. Med. J., 1952, I: 181.
Stecher, R. M.: Heberden's Nodes: A Clinical Description of Osteoarthritis of the Finger Joints, Ann. Rheumatic Diseases, 14:1, 1955.

HYPERTROPHIC OSTEOARTHROPATHY

Mendlowitz, M.: Clubbing and Hypertrophic Osteoarthropathy, Medicine, 21:269, 1942.

RHEUMATOID ARTHRITIS

Bunim, J. J. (Ed.): Symposium, Rheumatoid Arthritis, J. Chron. Dis., 5:609, 1957.
Kellgren, J. H., and J. S. Lawrence: Rheumatoid Arthritis in a Population Sample, Ann. Rheumatic Diseases, 15:1, 1956.
Ragan, C., and A. I. Synder: "Rheumatoid Arthritis," Disease-a-Month Series, Chicago, Year Book Publishers, Inc., November, 1955.
Short, C. L., W. Bauer, and W. E. Reynolds: "Rheumatoid Arthritis," Cambridge, Harvard University Press, 1957.
Ward, L. E., H. F. Polley, C. H. Slocumb, and P. S. Hench: Cortisone in Treatment of Rheumatoid Arthritis, J.A.M.A., 152:119, 1953.

VARIANTS OF RHEUMATOID ARTHRITIS

Blumberg, B., and C. Ragan: The Natural History of Rheumatoid Spondylitis, Medicine, 35:1, 1956.
Bunim, J. J.: Heberden Oration: A Broader Spectrum of Sjögren's Syndrome and Its Pathogenetic Implications, Ann. Rheumatic Diseases, 20:1, 1961.
Farnan, P.: Whipple's Disease: The Clinical Aspects, Quart. J. Med. (New Series), 28:163, 1959.
Felty, A. R.: Chronic Arthritis in the Adult, Associated with Splenomegaly and Leucopenia, Bull. Johns Hopkins Hosp., 35:16, 1924.
Wright, V., and G. Watkinson: The Arthritis of Ulcerative Colitis, Medicine, 38:243, 1959.

302 THE ERYTHEMAS
*Donald M. Pillsbury and
Walter B. Shelley*

ERYTHEMA MULTIFORME

Erythema multiforme is a symptom complex characterized by vivid, erythematous, urticarial, bullous, and at times purpuric lesions. Distinctive in its symmetrical acral distribution, it appears suddenly, is self-limited, but often recurrent. Commonly regarded as a bullous disease, it may still appear without this change. Mucous membrane involvement is a significant accompaniment of the syndrome. The oral membranes and the lips usually show erosions, but the penis or vagina may also show inflammatory areas. On the skin, the initial change is an erythematous plaque with sharp margination. In the center of this papules or vesicles may arise, with later clearing. Subsequent changes often lead to a diagnostic multiringed "target" lesion. This may have dramatic coloring due to the varied states of dilatation, stasis, exudation, and purpura. Coalescence of lesions may lead to bizarre, gyrate, serpiginous arrangements. The associated skin and constitutional symptoms are often minor, except for the discomfort of the mucosal erosions. Usually appearing in the spring or the fall, an attack lasts for several weeks.

Erythema multiforme is actually a reaction pattern so that there is no single cause. It may result from or be associated with any one of the following:

1. Systemic infection: pneumonia, meningitis, measles, dental sepsis
2. Viral infection of the skin: herpes simplex
3. Drug intolerance: antipyrine, arsenic, belladonna, Butazolidin, mercury, phenobarbital, quinine, sulfonamides
4. Pregnancy
5. Foods: allergic reaction
6. Deep x-ray therapy
7. Malignancy

Treatment of erythema multiforme is less than satisfactory. Corticosteroids offer the greatest promise, but often the eruption proceeds at its own pace to a spontaneous involution.

Erythema multiforme exudativum is simply an extremely serious variant of erythema multiforme. As described by pediatricians (Stevens-Johnson syndrome), it ordinarily affects the younger age group and is ushered in by high fever, headache, and a fulminant stomatitis. Ulcers may develop in all the mucous membranes so that the patient presents conjunctivitis, rhinitis, stomatitis, urethritis, and balanitis. Shortly thereafter the vesiculobullous reaction arises on the skin. The patients are obviously in a toxic state with prostration, arthralgia, and myalgia. Crops of lesions continue to assail the patient, and the eye itself may be involved with keratitis iritis, uveitis, and even panophthalmitis occurring. The prognosis for life as well as vision is a guarded one. Treatment with intensive systemic steroid therapy is always indicated, and ophthalmologic consultation should be obtained.

ERYTHEMA NODOSUM

Erythema nodosum is another reaction pattern of the skin. It is characterized by bright red tender and painful nodules, usually of the anterior surface of both lower legs. These lesions never suppurate or ulcerate, normally undergoing slow resolution over a period of several weeks. Often in crops they may be associated with mild constitutional malaise, joint pain, and fever.

Usually these changes are the cutaneous manifestations of infection or a drug intolerance. Thus it is seen in association with

Ascariasis	Pharyngitis
Cat-scratch fever	Rheumatic fever
Chancroid	Sarcoidosis
Coccidioidomycosis	Scarlet fever
Diphtheria	Streptococcal infections
Leprosy	Syphilis
Lymphogranuloma venereum	Tonsillitis
	Trichophyton infection
Meningococcemia	Tuberculosis

In addition, many drugs may trigger this reaction, e.g., sulfonamides, iodides, or bromides. Thus careful medical studies are indicated in any patient with erythema nodosum.

Erythema nodosum, of and by itself, requires little specific treatment. It is self-limited, but bed rest may be indicated in severe cases. Local heat and salicylates may also be considered.

ERYTHEMA INDURATUM

Erythema induratum is another nodular eruption of the legs, but one which can be clinically distinguished from erythema nodosum. Thus, although occurring in young adult women, it appears on the calves and may lead to ulceration. The lesions, notoriously chronic and recurrent, begin as deep subcutaneous nodules or infiltrations, later showing necrotic change, and finally end in scarring. Cold weather often acts as a precipitating factor.

Erythema induratum is defined as a form of tuberculosis of the skin and hence is rather rare. The tuberculin test should be positive, and evidence of tuberculosis elsewhere must be sought. Appropriate treatment includes antitubercular measures.

Actually most of the cases which match the clinical and histologic criteria for erythema induratum are not seen in tuberculous individuals and do not represent a tuberculoid granuloma. Rather, they are of unknown origin. Some have called this non-tuberculous erythema induratum or nodular vasculitis. It would seem appropriate to consider erythema induratum as a reaction pattern in which tuberculosis is just one cause. Just as erythema nodosum may be due to tuberculosis, as well as numerous other conditions, so may erythema induratum. The authors prefer not to use additional terms for the description of subcutaneous lesions which are, by virtue of their very location, obscure and not susceptible to fine clinical distinctions as are their counterparts in the surface epithelium.

REFERENCES

Scott, T. F. M.: Hypersensitivity Syndromes, Erythema Multiforme, Erythema Nodosum, Urticaria, Pediat. Clinics N. Am. 3:771, 1956.

Vesey, C. M. R., and D. S. Wilkinson: Erythema Nodosum; A Study of Seventy Cases, Brit. J. Dermatol., 71:139, 1959.

303 DISEASES AFFECTING THE SKIN

Donald M. Pillsbury and
Walter B. Shelley

The physician possessed of reasonable familiarity with the principles of applied anatomy, physiology, and chemistry of the skin and with the dozen or so chief patterns of disease which it presents, will be able to classify over 90 per cent of all dermatologic syndromes with reasonable accuracy and to treat most of them effectively. If, in the course of the initial examination, the skin lesions of a patient can be classified as representative of a common or uncommon disease, as banal or serious, as a local disturbance, or a manifestation of systemic disease, much has been accomplished. Many diseases of the skin can be diagnosed with accuracy on inspection, provided the examination is adequate and complete, as surely as the pathologist recognizes a characteristic cytologic picture. Others require further study utilizing all the resources of general medicine and of special laboratory procedures.

Dermatologic diseases are encountered rather frequently by the general physician and by all medical specialists. On the basis of the enormous United States Armed Forces' experience during the Second World War, it is clear that any general physician who is practicing in a Temperate Zone will find that some 7 to 15 per cent of his patients present themselves with a chief complaint of a disease affecting the skin. In warm, humid, tropical climates this incidence rises to 25 per cent or more. Under con-

ditions of disaster and war the skins of the affected population offer a particularly fertile field for micro-organisms and parasites. In industry various dermatoses comprise by far the largest group of occupational medical diseases. The scope of internal medicine and its subspecialties is so broad and complex as to make it impossible for any physician to be familiar with all of them in any detail. In dermatology, as in other medical specialties, however, the most rewarding initial approach is through an understanding of the general principles of anatomy, physiology, and pathology which have useful clinical application to both diagnosis and treatment.

It is essential for the internist to gain an understanding of the characteristics of the principal syndromes which affect the skin. In a number of these, experience has shown that involvement is almost entirely mucocutaneous, and there is no need for extensive procedures of examination other than an adequate general physical evaluation and a few key laboratory studies, as in pityriasis rosea, certain types of dermatitis, acne, dermatotropic viral infections (warts, molluscum contagiosum), vitiligo, most diseases of the hair and nails, moderate genetic changes such as mild ichthyosis, and benign tumors which may be recognized on clinical examination. In most patients these diseases are not particularly disabling, and the eventual outcome is ordinarily good. Disability and subsequent systemic disease most commonly *result from mistreatment,* e.g., the application of known sensitizing topical agents such as sulfonamides, certain antibiotics and antihistaminics, the excessive use of ionizing radiation therapy, and more and more prominently, from the prolonged administration of corticosteroids in doses which are almost certain to produce undesirable physiologic effects.

In a second group of diseases affecting only the skin during the initial phase, lack of recognition of the nature of the process may be followed by the progression of systemic disease. Examples of this group of dermatoses include mild drug reactions, the initial manifestations of atopy, mild contact dermatitis with continued exposure to the offending allergen, bacterial infections which are initially superficial (impetigo and acute folliculitis) but which may produce irreversible systemic infection if not promptly dealt with, parasitic infestations such as scabies and pediculosis, certain tumors such as active junction type nevi or basal cell and prickle cell epitheliomas, in which cure is almost always possible by early treatment, and a wide variety of industrial dermatoses, hyperpigmentary disorders, and photosensitivity reactions.

A third group of diseases affecting the skin with which some familiarity is essential includes many conditions which are relatively uncommon but in which an early diagnosis may sometimes lead to complete cure or at least a slower progression of the disease. In this group may be included pemphigus, syphilis, discoid lupus and system lupus erythematosus, scleroderma, miliaria (in which extension of the poral closure may lead to marked disturbances in heat regulation), tuberculosis, deep fungous infections, sarcoid, various purpuras, some xanthomas, diphtheria cutis, many parasitic infestations, cutaneous manifestations of lymphomas, angiomas, acanthosis nigricans, psychocutaneous syndromes (especially factitial dermatitis), and chronic effects of physical agents, particularly sunlight and cold.

In a fourth large group of diseases in which the skin is affected, the mucocutaneous manifestations are variable and often incidental, though frequently they represent the chief sign through which the nature of the disease may be suspected. Examples include the viral exanthems, rickettsioses, sarcoidosis, erythema nodosum, leprosy, dermatomyositis, peripheral vascular diseases, erythema multiforme, several metabolic diseases, neurocutaneous syndromes (adenoma sebaceum), spider angiomas in hepatic disease, pruritus, as the initial sign of lymphomas or hepatic disease, etc.

In addition to these there are a considerable number of localized banal conditions in which patients have a consuming interest, though they are of no general medical importance. A reasonable interpretation of these may often be given, not necessarily in terms of any specific syndrome, on the basis of the etiologic and physiologic forces involved, e.g., in disturbances of growth or pigmentation of hair and nails. Of all the sources of interest and concern of patients about their skin that of possible cancer is paramount, and this is constantly increasing as cancer education campaigns and publicity increase. An assessment of dermal neoplasms, examples of which will be found in every patient examined, is a requisite of every general medical evaluation. Fortunately, the vast majority of tumors and excrescences of the skin are benign and can be recognized as such on close inspection. Others must be suspected of being malignant or are patently so. In the latter circumstance, the sooner the tumor is classified accurately, the better.

In a short chapter of this type it is not feasible to include detailed descriptions of the wide variety of changes to which the skin is subject. This discussion will, therefore, be confined to a brief summary of the means by which a diagnosis may be established.

DERMATITIS AND ECZEMA

Various types of acute and chronic dermatitis constitute over 50 per cent of all clinical dermatology. While the changes in the skin follow a basic pattern which is reasonably constant, the factors which may initiate or prolong a dermatitis are numerous.

The morphologic changes of acute and chronic dermatitis are clear cut and not easy to confuse with other patterns of skin reactions. The signs of dermatitis, in the order of their evolution, are as follows: (1) erythema and swelling, (2) oozing and/or vesiculation, (3) crusting and scaling, (4) thickening and evidence of repeated excoriation, (5) hyperpigmentation, scratch papule formation, and lichenification. The first three changes are those of an acute dermatitis; the latter two are seen only if the process persists for several weeks or longer. While there is no entirely satisfactory classification which will include all variants of a dermatitis-eczema group of diseases, some categorization is helpful. Separate classification of a particular group is justified and helpful if one or more of the following criteria are satisfied: (1) it is a type in which a definite cause can be determined, (2) it occurs in a fairly regular pattern which (3) is helpful in determining the prognosis in the individual patient, gives clear indication for certain types of treatments, or indicates the need for further allergic and other medical studies. The following main groups exist:

Acute Contact Dermatitis. In this type of dermatitis the change may be due either to primary irritation from toxic substances or to true allergic sensitization (see p. 1266). Contact dermatitis is the prototype of all dermatitic reactions in the skin and by far the most satisfactory to manage therapeutically. In a very high proportion of patients the responsible substance may be determined accurately and the cause removed. It is essential that this be done as quickly as possible because persistence of the reaction will lead to "trailing" complications which may be self-perpetuating.

Atopic Dermatitis. This exceedingly chronic dermatitis possesses distinctive features in respect to localization of lesions, personal and familial evidence of allergy, and a characteristic though often erratic course. It produces more chronic disability than any other disease in which the chief manifestations are in the skin. This, plus the fact that the affected patient frequently has other evidences of atopy, makes the disease of considerable medical importance. In addition, because corticosteroid therapy is often rapidly effective in relieving the inflammatory changes, the problem of untoward physiologic effects arising from prolonged therapy of this type given for atopic dermatitis is assuming increasing importance. Atopic dermatitis of and by itself is not a fatal disease, but the suddenly developing complication of secondary infection by the virus either of herpes simplex or of vaccinia may sometimes lead to death.

Seborrheic Dermatitis. This form of dermatitis is also quite clear cut in respect to localization of lesions, frequent association with evidence of sebaceous dysfunction, increased vulnerability to secondary bacterial infection, and a course which is often chronic. In widespread forms it may be very disabling.

Nummular Dermatitis. This type of dermatitis has a distinctive morphologic pattern (nummular, coinlike). The lesions are frankly dermatitic, round, and usually vary in size from 2 to 4 cm in diameter. Low-grade secondary infection is common. The distribution is chiefly to the extensor surfaces of the extremities and the posterior shoulders and back, though any site may be affected. The dermatitis is most common in patients above middle age, and may follow an acute contact dermatitis, or occur as an "id" complication of chronic stasis dermatitis. It is possibly seen more frequently in individuals with atopic backgrounds. The causative factors are poorly understood, but a psychosomatic component is often prominent. The lesions commonly recur at the same site, and the outlook for immediate cure of the disease is poor, though permanent remission may ordinarily be anticipated eventually.

Lichen Simplex Chronicus (Circumscribed Neurodermatitis). This is a clear-cut and very common condition in which the changes are due almost entirely to scratching and rubbing. The lesions are usually sharply circumscribed. Any site may be affected, but common ones are in the occipital region in women, on the neck, and on the lower legs. Many cases of vulvar and anal pruritus fall into the group of circumscribed neurodermatitis. The area involved becomes itchy either as a result of some preceding irritation or often without any previous lesion. The scratch-itch-scratch cycle becomes firmly established. Psychosomatic factors are often prominent, and many patients frequently admit to indulging in scratching as a means of relieving nervous tension. In such persons, if the patch is not too troublesome, such a lesion is probably to be preferred to some psychosomatic manifestation affecting another organ system.

Stasis Dermatitis. This is another clear-cut type of dermatitis in which the basic etiologic factors are peripheral venous disease and tissue edema (see p. 1374). It is important that prompt measures to control the dermatitis be undertaken before it has become severe and chronic. Stasis dermatitis is characterized by greatly increased vulnerability to primary irritant or sensitization reactions to topical medication.

These are the reasonably clear-cut syndromes in the dermatitis-eczema group. There are three other well-defined large groups, as follows:

Chronic Eczematous Dermatitis. This is a group in which, often, the original cause and initial pattern of the disease have long been lost sight of, and in which various secondary factors are playing a predominant role. It is frequently the end point of a contact dermatitis in which the causative factor was not recognized promptly. The extent and distribution of the dermatitis may vary greatly. There are no constant associated systemic factors, though sensitivity to particular foods or drugs must always be kept in mind. In such patients there is temptation to use a wide variety of topical measures or to resort to systemic corticosteroid therapy without careful study of the patient as a whole and painstaking analysis of the various etiologic factors which might be playing a role, including vasomotor disturbances, sweating dysfunction, low-grade bacterial infection, and psychosomatic factors.

Infantile Eczema. This is a classification based entirely on the age and the peculiarities of dermatitic reactions of the infantile skin. These differ considerably from those of the adult.

Chronic Dermatitis of Hands and/or Feet. This is a classification based entirely upon the region involved, but it is justified because it is such a common problem. The etiologic factors are often complex. Contact, atopic, and nummular dermatitis not infrequently are localized to the hands and feet. Certain forms of psoriasis and of "id" reactions may appear in this fashion. For all practical purposes, superficial acute fungous infections may be included in this group. This condition may be exceedingly chronic and at times highly disabling.

Generalized Exfoliative Dermatitis

A chronic dermatosis which affects all or nearly all the skin surface is a general medical problem of considerable importance and much difficulty. Though examples of such conditions are seen in all age groups, the incidence is highest in persons above middle age. In some instances the early origins of the exfoliative dermatitis, in terms of the type or etiology of the inflammatory changes, are fairly clear. Not infrequently, however, the generalized dermatitis arises for no apparent cause. The changes may prove to be completely intractable, especially in older patients.

In the chronic phase of a generalized exfoliative process, the skin is red, thickened, and scaling. There may be oozing, but vesicles are rarely seen. A variety of disease conditions may give rise to this process. It is fortunately very rare after acute contact dermatitis, localized neurodermatitis, nummular dermatitis, and eruptions of the hands and feet. Seborrheic dermatitis and atopic dermatitis may sometimes eventuate in a chronic exfoliative process. Drugs may produce a chronic generalized reaction; this was seen frequently when trivalent arsenical compounds were used in the treatment of syphilis. Prolonged extensive contact with a sensitizing agent, particularly an airborne one, may occasionally induce an irreversible generalized dermatitis.

Certain nevoid changes may produce chronic redness and exfoliation. The most common of these are severe ichthyosis or congenital ichthyosiform erythroderma. Psoriasis may, at any age, but most frequently in adults, become completely generalized. In this phase, it is frequently accompanied by rheumatoid arthritic changes.

In any patient with a generalized exfoliative process, but particularly those above middle age, the possibility of a lymphoma must receive serious consideration. Mycosis fungoides is frequently preceded, prior to the development of frank skin tumors, by a dry, patchy dermatitis which, with each recurrence, becomes more severe and extensive. Such lesions may recur for as long as a decade. Repeated biopsies over a period of years may be required before the characteristic cellular infiltrate of mycosis fungoides is demonstrable.

Senile involution of the skin may produce a severe and extensive erythroderma. Such changes have been designated by a variety of terms based on morphologic variations, but these are of little value to the general clinician. The syndrome may be designated as *exfoliative erythroderma,* and the patient then studied further for any dermatologic or general medical criteria which will provide a more useful and precise classification.

Management. Patients with generalized inflammatory exfoliative dermatoses deserve the most searching study. They are often relatively or completely disabled, and their appearance may bring about social ostracism.

Biopsy of the skin, often with repetition at intervals of weeks or months, is an essential feature of the study of such patients. The most careful hematologic studies are indicated. In such patients, varying degrees of generalized lymphadenopathy are almost always present, either in response to the chronic inflammatory changes of the skin or as part of an underlying lymphoma. Lymph node biopsy obviously will be required at times but should not be undertaken without due consideration because the healing after deep surgical biopsy is often very protracted, especially in the inguinal or axillary regions. Chemical studies of the blood, with particular reference to serum protein levels and electrolytes, may at times be revealing. It is particularly important to keep in mind that the protein losses from exfoliation may be significant.

The heat regulatory mechanisms of such patients are greatly disturbed. A moderately cool environment may often induce a chill because of increased radiation from the vascular bed. Because of the marked decrease in sweating which may be present, sometimes amounting to complete anhidrosis,

increase in the environmental temperature is poorly tolerated and may induce febrile episodes.

Skilled nursing care is of the utmost importance in such patients but may be a disagreeable and taxing task. Topical therapy, other than with very bland and inexpensive agents, is not feasible. As a rule, petroleum or equal parts of water and Aquaphor or ordinary hydrogenated vegetable oils are best tolerated. Care should be employed in the widespread use of compounds which may be toxic on absorption, e.g., salicylic acid, mercury, phenol, and strong concentrations of tar and resorcin.

Systemic corticosteroid therapy is almost always indicated in patients with severe intractable exfoliative dermatitis, but such therapy must sometimes be very prolonged. In exfoliative psoriasis the author has found the steroid triamcinolone of considerable value in comparison with the steroids previously available. Occasional transfusions of whole blood may be indicated. Fever therapy by foreign protein injections is sometimes worthwhile. The condition sometimes justifies a trial of x-ray therapy, preferably to a restricted portion of the skin initially. This must be given with the greatest care and expertness, however, if extensive areas are to be exposed to ionizing radiation.

Patients with generalized exfoliative dermatitis may be highly susceptible to infection of localized superficial type, to cellulitis, to deep cutaneous abscesses, and to thrombophlebitis. Intermittent or prolonged administration of appropriate antibiotics may be necessary.

PEMPHIGUS

Pemphigus is an uncommon relapsing disease which affects the mucocutaneous surface initially. There are no signs of systemic diseases at the onset, but these soon develop secondarily. Pemphigus is invariably fatal within a few months or years if adequate treatment is not instituted. The disease is ordinarily controllable with corticoid therapy.

The most common type of pemphigus (pemphigus vulgaris) is characterized by tense or flaccid bullae of varying size. They appear without symptoms, as a rule, on skin or mucous membranes which had seemed entirely normal. Occasional slight itching or burning may be noted. The bullae rupture quite readily, especially in the mouth, pharynx, and vagina, leaving denuded areas. These erosions or superficial ulcers are very slow to heal and often enlarge gradually. When healing occurs, no scarring results if there has not been secondary infection. In some patients, particularly those with brunet skins, there may be marked residual hyperpigmentation.

The distribution of lesions in pemphigus is variable, though areas which are subject to rubbing, pressure, or stretching are more prone to develop lesions. In pemphigus, the epidermis readily detaches upon lateral tension, and this phenomenon (Nikolsky's sign) may be demonstrated by drawing the finger over the surface of the skin with firm pressure. The epidermis slides off much like a piece of wet tissue paper. Though this sign is almost always present in pemphigus, it may be seen in other bullous diseases as well, e.g., epidermolysis bullosa and widespread bullous drug eruptions.

The lesions of pemphigus usually involve the mucous membranes as well as the skin. In many patients the initial lesions are entirely oral and/or vaginal. The disease attacks adults of any age. It is not seen in children and is rare during adolescence. Members of the Jewish race are most commonly afflicted. There is no sex predisposition.

Secondary bacterial infection of the bullae or of denuded skin occurs commonly, producing the rather characteristic "mousy" odor of the disease, and frequently gives rise to septicemia which is a characteristic complication.

Certain variations from the most common morphologic type of pemphigus occur.

Pemphigus Foliaceus. This is a rare member of the pemphigus group in which the lesions are predominantly those of exfoliative dermatitis. Because of the very extensive cutaneous involvement, signs of systemic disease may develop rapidly. The disease begins with the appearance of small vesicles in which scaling and crusting develop, producing a flaky surface similar to that seen in exfoliative dermatitis. This is in contrast to the characteristic raw denuded areas seen in pemphigus vulgaris. Slow symmetric spread of the lesions occurs, and within a period of months the entire body may be covered with exfoliative lesions. The hair and nails commonly are lost. The histologic picture is characteristic. The odor in exfoliative pemphigus is offensive. The response of this form of pemphigus to corticosteroid therapy is less favorable than in common pemphigus.

In *pemphigus vegetans,* many of the bullous lesions are succeeded by hypertrophic vegetative masses in intertriginous areas such as the axillas, groin, and inframammary region. These may later become dry and verrucose. The vegetative lesions do not occur on the mucous membranes with the exception of the vermilion border of the lip and sometimes on the vulvar labia. The lesions are malodorous, and evidence of secondary bacterial infection is always present. The process may suggest a fungating iododerma or bromoderma grossly or may even mimic the condylomas of secondary syphilis or the lesions of granuloma inguinale. In this type, as in exfoliative pemphigus, the response to corticosteroid therapy may be poor and massive doses are often required.

In another type of pemphigus, not uncommon, the distribution and morphology of the lesions are suggestive of a mixture of pemphigus, seborrheic dermatitis, and lupus erythematosus (Senear-Usher syndrome). Erythematous, scaling, and crusted lesions develop on the nose and malar areas in a butterfly distribution, and similar lesions, with or without bullae, may also appear on the anterior chest, interscapular area, and the scalp. The mucous membranes show involvement only occasionally. The general health of the patient is ordinarily good for some time after the onset of the disease. The course of the eruption is insidious and slow, but frank fatal pemphigus usually develops.

Brazilian Pemphigus (Fogo Selvagem). This disease, which is endemic in Brazil, is clinically and histologically identical with pemphigus foliaceus. The endemic nature of the disease makes it impossible to state with certainty that it is similar to pemphigus foliaceus, since the latter has never been seen in endemic form in the United States or in Europe. The best opinion would indicate that fogo selvagem is an infectious contagious disease. About 3,000 cases are on record in Brazil, and convincing evidence of transmission from person to person is available. The disease almost always begins before the age of thirty, is frequently associated with endocrine disturbances, and does not involve the mucous membranes.

Histologic Diagnosis. The histologic features of common pemphigus are highly characteristic, and the changes seen in smears or biopsies of early lesions are diagnostic. There is a disturbance of the epidermal cells in which the fundamental change is a disruption of the intercellular connections of the epidermis (acantholysis) seen in either biopsies or material taken by a special scraping (see p. 79).

The course of pemphigus is variable. The untreated patient may show occasional remissions, but recurrences invariably develop, each a little more severe than the previous one. Death may occur 2 to 3 months following the initial lesion, or the disease may continue for years. If corticosteroid therapy is not administered, death within 2 years may be anticipated. This occurs as a result of shock, toxemia, a cachectic state, or some secondary complication, such as septicemia or bronchopneumonia. It is important to keep in mind that the skin and mucous membranes are the primary tissues involved, and if these lesions can be controlled, signs of systemic disease will remain absent or very moderate. In uncontrolled pemphigus, marked secondary anemia may develop. Hypoalbuminemia may also be present because of the negative nitrogen balance resulting from loss of protein to denuded areas of skin and from the inability of some patients to ingest solid foods. In widespread severe pemphigus the patients are extremely ill. There may be a marked leukocytosis, at times eosinophilia, and the general picture is one of serious toxicity. The temperature is ordinarily not markedly elevated unless extensive secondary bacterial infection has occurred. Routine laboratory studies do not yield characteristic or constant findings. However, in advanced cases, the sedimentation rate is increased, anemia is constant, the total serum proteins are almost invariably lowered, and marked disturbance of serum electrolytes may be seen.

Treatment. Corticosteroid therapy is the only means by which true pemphigus may be controlled; it is one of the few diseases in which such therapy is justified as soon as the diagnosis is established even though the presenting signs and symptoms are mild. Conditions which might ordinarily be regarded as contraindications to corticosteroid therapy must often be waived if the diagnosis of pemphigus is established. It is too early to suggest that actual cures of pemphigus have been achieved, but considerable numbers of patients have been maintained in a state of remission for the several years since corticosteroid therapy became available. As a rule such therapy must be continued indefinitely; very few patients have found it possible to remain in remission in the absence of continued treatment.

It is advisable to start treatment with rather large doses of corticosteroids; the authors prefer ACTH, ordinarily in the gel form. If the patient is critically ill, ACTH in a dose of 25 to 40 units should be given daily by 8-hr intravenous drip. In many patients subsidence of the eruption will be noted in a few days, and reduction of the dose of corticotropin may then be possible, ordinarily by lowering the daily dose to 15 to 20 units and then giving such a dose less frequently. No set rules for this can be put down. In some patients the dose may be reduced to a surprisingly low level, as little as 10 or 15 units of ACTH every 2 weeks. If cortisone or its analogues are used, the initial dose required may sometimes be so high as to be unfeasible economically. However, later in the course of treatment, trial of such therapy may ordinarily be undertaken safely.

The corollary medical and nursing care of extensive pemphigus is a formidable problem in some patients. The supervision required is not dissimilar to that of an extensive burn, and close check for evidence of local or systemic infection, of protein and electrolyte balance, and of the nutritional and hematologic status must be kept. Blood transfusions are sometimes of critical value. If there is evidence of bacterial infection of the skin, even in the absence of a systemic response, it is rarely possible to control it by topical therapy. It is of the greatest importance to conserve the accessible veins as much as possible because they may be few in number if the cutaneous lesions are extensive.

ACNE

This is the classic stigma of adolescence, almost a normal physiologic reaction in the skin. The various clinical manifestations of acne have been designated by a variety of terms. Most of these have little meaning or usefulness to nonspecialists, but it is convenient to grade the severity of acne from I to IV as a guide in selecting the types of therapy which are most likely to be helpful. Hereditary determinants condition the follicular orifice "target organ" response, yet fundamentally the excitant is hormonal. At least 75 per cent of both sexes show some evidence of acne at the age of puberty. There is no significant sex difference in incidence or severity.

In some patients comedones may begin to develop at the age of nine or ten, and if these patients are from a family stock in which acne has appeared frequently, the outlook is disquieting. The evidence of acne may persist for a variable period of time, probably never less than a year, but sometimes spanning the entire teens, with extension well into the twenties. The precise hormonal excitation of acne is not understood in complete detail. ACTH injections in *susceptible individuals* of any age may produce acne. Eunuchs do not develop the disease.

The treatment of acne is not always satisfactory. Although the hormonal stimulus is basic to the development of the disease, there are no regularly effective means of combating it from this etiologic standpoint. The routine administration of estrogenic hormones is illogical, though there are selected cases in which a striking menstrual periodicity of the eruption seems to make such treatment advisable. The therapeutic attack on acne must be on the fringes: (1) local therapy which may help in relieving the plugging and rupture of the follicular orifice, (2) control of contributing factors such as food or drugs, (3) judicious drainage of purulent lesions by means which are least likely to produce scarring, (4) combating infection with appropriate antibacterial measures, and (5) taking advantage of natural aids, such as sunlight, as fully as possible. None of these measures is curative in the strict sense; all are palliative and serve only to keep the acne in check and to prevent undue scarring until the hormonal and, sometimes, emotional storm of adolescence has subsided.

The treatments used for acne are extraordinarily numerous. In assessing the value of some of them, no particular attention seems to be paid to the associated factor of the passage of time in judging the true curative influence of a particular method. There are some methods, moreover, such as stringent restrictions of diet, the prolonged administration of antibacterial preparations, and the use of x-ray therapy which may have bad effects if employed overzealously and without good medical judgment.

Preparations containing sulfur and resorcin are undoubtedly useful in mild acne, particularly if the lesions are superficial. They should be used to the point of producing a mild chapping effect. Regular removal of comedones is helpful in some patients and with proper instruction may be done safely at home. Drainage of frankly pustular lesions requires judgment. It should not be done too early in the course of the lesion but may promote more rapid healing if performed when the nodule is fully fluctuant and the infection near the surface.

The restriction of foods and drugs is important in many patients with acne but should not be done on any routine basis. It can be shown, without question, that iodides, bromides, and Tridione make acne worse. Foods such as chocolate, nuts, and coffee so frequently cause exacerbations as to make routine elimination justifiable. From this point on, it is advisable to individualize dietary elimination. It should be kept in mind that in most patients with acne juvenile growth is rapid and energy output high so that dietary restrictions should be advised with care and good reason.

Trauma to the skin may induce and perpetuate inflammatory acne lesions. Constant pinching, rubbing, and picking of the face may become a subconscious habit and lead to much scarring because the acne lesions are not given a chance to heal spontaneously. Violent traumatic exercise, such as wrestling or football, sometimes produces inflammatory acne lesions, as does the rubbing of sweaters, dirty sweat shirts, or bacteria-laden shoulder pads and other gear.

In chronic severe acne in which there is unmistakable evidence of bacterial infection, antibacterial therapy is often effective and justified. As is the case with many chronic bacterial infections of the skin, particularly if there is a tendency to formation of minute to larger abscesses within the skin, such therapy must often be continued for long periods of time and should be initiated and supervised with good medical judgment. Though penicillin is useful at times, the incidence of acquired or potential allergic sensitivity to it is high. Sulfonamide therapy is sometimes adequate, but it may be necessary to employ broad-spectrum antibiotics. In general, the drug should be given in full dosage initially to determine whether or not it will be effective, following which the dose may be reduced to the lowest level which appears to keep the infection under control.

Hormonal therapy of many types has been used in acne usually with indifferent results. The routine administration of thyroid extract has long been a favorite treatment, but the authors are not convinced of its effectiveness. Mention has been made of the occasional use of estrogenic hormones both topically and systemically. Though such therapy may sometimes appear to be helpful, it should be used on the basis of adequate endocrinologic study and supervision. More recently, the administration of corticosteroids systemically has enjoyed a considerable vogue. In the authors' experience there can be no question whatever that the anti-inflammatory effect of such treatment on acne lesions may be marked, sometimes with very small doses, but the inherent physiologic risks of such therapy must be very carefully weighed against the fact that acne is a purely local disease with no systemic manifestations.

Sunlight and vacation have a good effect in acne and may provide a striking demonstration of the inadequacies of previous treatment. In so-called "tropical acne," a very widespread and severe pustular eruption may develop on the face and entire trunk, usually in persons who have had some evidence of acne previously, but not infrequently in those in whom there has been no previous sign of the disease. Treatment is futile until the patient can be placed in a cool, dry environment.

X-ray Therapy. The opinion expressed here on x-ray therapy for acne is at variance with almost every textbook of dermatology or radiotherapy with which the authors are familiar. It is the authors' belief that the value of such treatment has been greatly overrated, but this is a controversial matter. The authors do not administer x-ray therapy for acne.

Acne was one of the first diseases of the skin for which x-ray therapy was used. Its popularity was based upon a supposed specific selective effect on the sebaceous glands. The rather limited and surprisingly few controlled studies which have been done on the therapeutic effects of x-ray therapy in acne have failed to demonstrate any immediate good effects with doses which may be regarded as comparatively safe in so far as late effects on the skin are concerned. In these studies varying amounts of ionizing irradiation in divided doses have been administered to one side of the face while the other side was left untreated. No difference in the progress of the acne of the two sides has been demonstrated.

Acne Scarring. The treatment of acne scars has long been considered unsatisfactory, but the technique known as skin planing, or surgical planing or dermabrasion, is useful. The most popular method involves freezing the skin with an ethyl chloride or Freon refrigerant spray followed by mechanical removal of the epidermis and upper dermis by means of a high-speed rotary steel brush. The epidermis then regenerates rapidly from the numerous pilosebaceous and sweat gland units which remain. The rotating wire brush has almost completely replaced the sandpapering method formerly in vogue, both because the technique is simpler and because of the occasional development of small foreign-body granulomas from embedded silicate granules after sandpapering.

SKIN GROWTHS

Hemangiomas

One of the most common skin tumors is the hemangioma. Over one-third of all newborn infants present this problem for evaluation. These lesions are best grouped into three classes for prognosis and therapy. The first is the *port-wine stain* (nevus flammeus). This lesion appears as a perfectly flat blue-red patch of variable size. It represents a diffuse telangiectasis of mature vessels in the dermis. No form of treatment is satisfactory. These lesions are of cosmetic significance only, so that potentially harmful or scarring modalities should not be employed. The parents should be acquainted with the fact that the lesion will neither extend nor fade. All efforts must be directed toward methods of obscuring lesion if it is in a distressing location. Several commercially available cosmetic products are suitable for this.

The second major type of hemangioma is the *immature angioma* (strawberry mark). This lesion is usually seen at birth, may show dramatic enlargement, and then undergoes spontaneous involution in a matter of months or years. The lesions are red to blue and consist of compressible vascular tumors. Over one-half are on the face. During the period of enlargement the temptation to treat vigorously is strong, but this should be resisted in view of the excellent cosmetic appearance associated with spontaneous resolution. Rare exceptions are made in the case of a bleeding angioma, an extending ulcer, or interference with the function of an eye or body orifice, e.g., the urethra and anus. In such instances, one has a choice of treatments: low-dosage radiotherapy, local freezing, surgical excision, injection of sclerosing solution, electrocoagulation, or compression. The immature angioma is made up of immature vessels which may show sclerosing changes at any time. In two-thirds of the cases this occurs before the age of one year, but in some the involution is not complete until the child is seven years old. The signs of disappearance are subtle at first, but later one sees white or gray islands appearing in the crimson lesion.

Mature angioma, the rarest form, shows no tendency to involution, nor is it radiosensitive. The lesion is made up of adult type venous channels. Much of the tumor is in the subcutaneous tissue, but parts may be raised in nodules or plaques. These lesions are distinguished from the immature type by the fact that they show no relative increase in size with age. The only definitive treatment is excision and grafting. Often such radical treatment is inadvisable and the lesion is left alone.

The Evaluation of Pigmented Nevi

It may be stated at the outset that it is impossible to examine any single pigmented nevus and state positively that it will *never* undergo a malignant change. On the other hand, it is neither feasible not justifiable to undertake wholesale excision of pigmented moles; some degree of clinical judgment must be exercised.

Pigmented nevi are often not manifest at birth but characteristically develop during infancy and childhood, and a few do not appear until adulthood. Nevi first appear as macules. These lesions are ordinarily of two histologic types: (1) those in which the skin appears normal histologically except for increased deposition of melanin and a greater number of melanocytes at the *epidermal-dermal junction* and (2) lesions which show clumps or aggregations of nevus cells apparently "dropping off" or being extruded from the epidermal-dermal junction into the underlying corium. The first type is known as an *inactive junction nevus;* the second may be active or inactive. As the child becomes older, these macules may become thickened and slightly elevated, and the histologic picture changes, with cords or bands of nevus cells becoming aggregated in the corium. This lesion is called a compound nevus, *part epidermal and part dermal.* With the further passage of time, more elevation of the lesion occurs and the nevus cells aggregate *entirely within the corium.* This is the intradermal nevus, a mature lesion which is almost always benign.

In children a pigmented nevus can evolve rapidly with cellular features of hyperplasia and anaplasia resembling a malignant melanoma of the adult. To this lesion the term *juvenile melanoma* has been applied. However, true malignant melanomas are so rare in childhood that it is often justifiable to delay decision about removal of a suspicious nevus until puberty.

The presence of pigment alone does not indicate that a papule or tumor of the skin is a melanocytic nevus. Certain entirely unrelated tumors, many of them benign, may show marked hyperpigmentation. The seborrheic keratosis or wart, a very common lesion, is the best example of this. Histiocytoma, a common fibromatous lesion arising from the corium (seen on the lower legs of women) may also be pigmented. Senile or actinic keratoses are sometimes dark, and pigmentation is frequent in basal cell epitheliomas (see Fig. 303-1).

Flat Lesions. These are simply macular, pigmented spots. On histologic examination they show junctional activity in over two-thirds of instances. In such lesions *even pigmentation* and *sharp definition* of the border are reassuring. In adults a very high proportion of such lesions will prove to be lentigines and of little significance in regard to potential malignancy. However, *if the pigmentation becomes speckled and the border more hazy and irregular,* the odds are in favor of junctional activity, and the lesion must be regarded with suspicion.

Slightly Elevated Lesions. Such moles are intermediate between flat pigmented and those which are raised above the surface of surrounding skin. The lesion is clearly palpable. Most will prove to be compound nevi and will give some evidence of junctional activity. Many of them, particularly in younger patients, will evolve in time into "pure" intradermal nevi. They need not be excised routinely.

Nevi with Pigmented Halo. These are ordinarily slightly elevated lesions the base of which is surrounded by a flat pigmented ring with a border that is sometimes irregular. These lesions are very likely to show junctional activity and should be adequately excised.

Verrucoid Lesions. Pigmented nevi with a markedly verrucose surface are raised and often very dark. Some three-fourths of such lesions show histologic evidence of junctional activity while the rest are intradermal.

Raised nevi take other forms; these include lesions with a polyploid or raspberry-like surface, a dome-shaped flat lesion, a lesion attached to the skin by a thick pedicle, and lesions definitely papillomatous, sometimes attached only by a thin stalk. These four types of lesions tend to be of the intradermal type and need not be excised unless definite changes are noted in them.

Certain general considerations in the assessment of nevi apply to all morphologic types. A *sudden change in the pigmentation,* either to more marked pigmentation, to splotchy irregular character, or to fuzziness at the border of the lesion must be regarded with suspicion, particularly in flat lesions. However, it must be kept in mind that melanocytic nevi show variations in pigment at puberty and during pregnancy and, to some degree, after exposure to sunlight.

The presence of fully developed, stiff hairs in the nevus is a reassuring sign. While it is not an absolute dictum that hairy moles do not precede melanocarcinoma, it can be said that they rarely do. Such lesions are often frequently traumatized by repeated pulling of the hair or during shaving. We have never observed an instance of melanoma arising from such a lesion, though there are isolated reports of this.

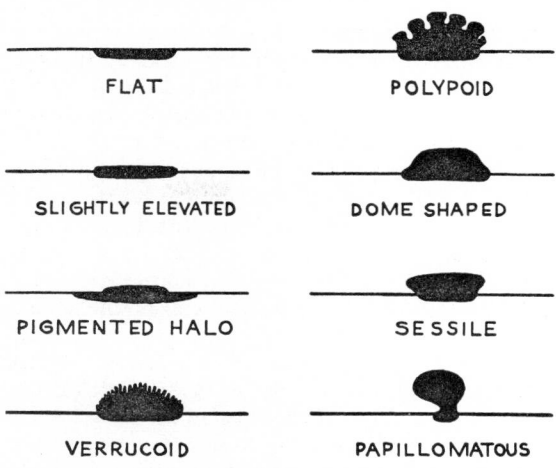

FIG. 303-1. Various morphologic patterns in pigmented nevi. The lesions in the left column are, in general, more likely to be junction nevi. (*After B. Shaffer, A.M.A. Arch. Dermatol.,* 72:120, 1955.)

Changes in Size. *A significant change in size* of a pigmented nevus in adults must almost always be regarded as a basis for excision. The one exception to this is the common occurrence of acute or chronic follicular infection in hairy nevi with the development of tenderness and swelling. Such inflammatory changes are no cause for alarm, but if the mole becomes repeatedly infected, excision is advisable.

Ulceration and/or bleeding of previously quiescent moles are two signs of melanocarcinoma which are most commonly mentioned in cancer propaganda. However, these are late changes, and it is essential to recognize the more subtle prodromal changes in moles if melanocarcinoma is to be controlled.

Pigmented Lesions of the Mucous Membranes. Melanocytic nevi may involve the stratified epithelium of the mouth and mucocutaneous junction of the anus. Such lesions are usually flat and may be exceedingly difficult to interpret clinically. The decision is often crucial because melanocarcinoma arising in the mucous membranes is rarely cured. Pigmentation of the mouth in Negroes is common and is ordinarily blotchy and fairly diffuse. Hyperpigmentation from chronic irritation, e.g., along the bite margin, is also common and need not be a cause for worry. In the Peutz-Jeghers syndrome, pigmented macules of the mouth, lips, and/or digits may be associated with intestinal polyposis. The most difficult lesions to interpret are freckles on the lips or dilated superficial blood vessels, usually veins, which are commonly blue-black and may become sclerosed. While these latter lesions are usually recognizable, punch biopsy may occasionally be indicated.

Cancer of the Skin

The majority of skin cancers arise in the epidermis and are known as *basal cell epitheliomas*. Long known for their chronic tendency to enlarge and ulcerate, they are responsible for the public injunction, "See your doctor about any sore which doesn't heal." It is a destructive tumor which presents no immediate or direct threat to life, but which if not removed completely will progress relentlessly, possibly killing by invasion into underlying structures. The typical basal cell epithelioma is recognizable as a discrete pale waxy nodule. However, the range of appearances is so great that histologic study is regularly demanded of any suspicious growth or ulcer. Crusted bleeding lesions, pearly borders, and telangiectasia, all suggest an epithelioma. The lesions may be of any size and may be multiple, but over 90 per cent are on the exposed areas, viz., head and neck. Treatment may be surgical excision, curettage, electrocoagulation (these two only for small early lesions), or x-ray therapy. In every instance, however, tissue must be presented for histologic study.

Squamous cell carcinoma is the active, invasive, metastasizing form of cancer of the epidermis. It commonly arises on the face and neck, one-third being found on the lower lip. All these areas are overexposed to the elements or are sites of chronic irritation. Often the precancerous change of *leukoplakia* is the warning signal. Treatment again is complete eradication of all tumor cells. Surgery and/or roentgen therapy should be employed. Where there is reason to suspect regional lymph node metastasis or subcutaneous extension, radical dissection may be necessary.

Lymphomas

Cutaneous lesions accompanying lymphomatous disease are either specific or nonspecific. In the specific lesions, e.g., papules, the lymphoma cells are found in the skin on biopsy. In the nonspecific lesions or leukemids, toxic or allergic factors are responsible. Of particular note are certain cutaneous reactions incited by lymphomas:

Generalized pruritus	Purpura
Edematous plaques	Herpes zoster
Erythema multiforme	Acquired ichthyosis
Exfoliative dermatitis	

Any of these demand a careful medical examination.

Mycosis fungoides stands apart, although it is a member of the lymphoma group. It has a distinctive cutaneous evolution and can often be recognized clinically before histologic proof is forthcoming. The course is ultimately fatal, although usually slow and protracted. It evolves in three distinctive phases:

1. Premycotic (erythematous) stage characterized by scattering pruritic patches on the body may be present for a score of years. The skin changes resemble psoriasis or neurodermatitis and are well demarcated. Itching is the predominant sign. Histologic study is not diagnostic.

2. The plaque or infiltrative stage is associated with lymphadenopathy and infiltrative lesions. In this stage there may be associated skin changes such as erythema multiforme. The biopsy gives a distinctive diagnostic patterning of mycosis fungoides.

3. The tumor stage presents numerous tumors (1 to 15 cm), reddish-brown, and at times ulcerative. Again the histologic picture is clearly diagnostic. The end is near at this stage. Treatment is usually by roentgen rays or radiomimetic drugs.

PHOTOSENSITIVE STATES

Discoid Lupus Erythematosus. From a practical clinical standpoint discoid lupus erythematosus is to be sharply differentiated from systemic lupus erythematosus (p. 1892). Although transitions in these diseases may occur, they are unusual and should not influence the general nosologic distinctions. Discoid lupus presents a pathognomonic clinical, as well as histologic, pattern. Occurring more often in women between the ages of twenty and forty, the disease begins as erythematous scaling lesions, commonly of the cheeks and the bridge of the nose. The scalp, mucous membranes, and V of the chest, are often involved as well. As the lesions extend, they show evidence of depigmentation, alopecia, and true atrophy. Telangiectasia is an especially prominent finding. In nearly all cases, sensitivity to sunlight is a primary finding. Exposure to ultraviolet light therapy may set off an explosive flare. Treatment centers on the antimalarial compounds. In most instances avoidance of sunlight, coupled with chloroquine (250 to 500 mg a day), affords the patient protection from extension, and reduces the acute inflammatory element, but does not erase the atrophy or depigmentation.

Other Photosensitive Syndromes

Although marked sunburn, freckles, aging, keratoses, herpes simplex, and epitheliomas follow excessive sun exposure in sensitive individuals, there are two major classes of cutaneous reaction to sunlight.

Photosensitization Reaction. This is receiving considerable attention now because some of the newer drugs induce this sensitivity to sunlight. These include demethyl-chlortetracycline, the psoralens, sulfonamides (including the antidiuretic derivatives, Chlorothiazide), and phenothiazines. These compounds, acting as photodynamic agents, make the patient more sensitive to ultraviolet radiation. The photodynamic action is a primary physicochemical phenomenon wherein radiant energy is captured in the skin and produces toxic effects. Clinically, one sees a brisk and prolonged accentuation of the sunburn reaction.

Polymorphic Light Eruption. In certain individuals, exposure to sunlight may induce a wide range of eczematous or papular and inflammatory changes. Unlike the photosensitizer reaction, the cause here is entirely unknown. Clinically, suspicion is aroused by the history of sun intolerance and appearance of the eruption in the exposed areas. Chloroquin therapy is remarkably specific and effective. Indeed, a therapeutic trial may be used as a diagnostic test at times.

SUPERFICIAL FUNGOUS INFECTIONS (Ringworm)

The resident cutaneous flora is predominantly bacterial, but a single fungous genus, *Pityrosporum,* with two species, is also represented. *Pityrosporum ovale,* a yeastlike budding organism, occurs in abundance in the scalp and in areas of high sebaceous gland activity, but its etiologic relationship to dandruff or seborrheic dermatitis has never been proved. *Pityrosporum orbiculare,* while normally a skin resident, may play a part in the development of the common banal disease tinea versicolor. Saprophytic mold fungi are numerous in the atmosphere, and spores contaminate the cutaneous surface more or less continuously. For the most part they remain dormant on the skin but are problems in mycologic diagnostic work because of their tendency to overgrow culture plates. Common weed fungi, such as species of *Penicillium* and *Aspergillus,* proliferate on diseased skin and have often been wrongly incriminated as the primary cause of cutaneous disease. Weed fungi are particularly prone to colonize necrotic ulcers, the inflamed ear canal, and disease of the subungual skin, but recovery of these fungi from such areas should not be interpreted as signifying pathogenicity.

The importance of the superficial fungi as a cause of many cutaneous diseases has been considerably exaggerated and has led to many unnecessary reactions from treatment by irritating so-called "fungicidal compounds." It is worthy of emphasis that inflammatory reactions on the feet are by no means always due to fungi, and even if the pathogenic fungus is recovered, this may be only a minor contributor to the inflammatory changes which may be present.

The superficial ringworm infections may be divided into two main groups: (1) the keratinolytic and (2) the nonkeratinolytic, a miscellaneous group. The distinctive property of the ringworm fungi is the possession of an enzyme which enables them to digest keratin. With this biochemical equipment, the nails can be disintegrated, hair dissolved, and the scaffolding of the stratum corneum, the keratinized cells, demolished. The matrix of the hair and nails is not attacked nor the epidermis itself. Except in unusual instances, there is no tendency whatever for these fungi to invade living tissue, nor has any toxin been isolated. However, sensitization to ringworm fungi may be induced. This is seen most strikingly in inflammatory reactions occurring during the course of ringworm of the scalp or in some instances of acute inflammatory eruptions of the feet.

The ringworm fungi, or dermatophytes, are divided among three genera, *Trichophyton, Microsporum,* and *Epidermophyton.* At least one pathogenic ringworm organism (*M. gypseum*) has been repeatedly isolated from the soil, which it presumably inhabits as a saprophyte. By and large, however, human infections are contracted either from infected animals or from other human beings. Certain species, the so-called *anthropophilic organisms,* show a distinct preference for human beings, occurring rarely or not at all in animals. The best example of this is the organism which commonly causes ringworm of the scalp, especially in urban areas, *M. audouini.* The *zoophilic ringworm* fungi, on the other hand, are frequent pathogens of domestic animals from which they may be transmitted to human beings. The anthropophilic species have the clinical peculiarity of causing relatively noninflammatory and often very persistent types of ringworm while the zoophilic organisms tend to incite short-lived inflammatory diseases in man.

The transmissibility of ringworm infections has been greatly overrated. It can be demonstrated regularly only in certain types of ringworm infections of the scalp occurring almost entirely in children. In adults, the transmission of the common types of ringworm infections of the feet, groin, and nails remains to a great extent a mystery. It is difficult to produce an infection with superficial ringworm fungi experimentally in man regardless of the conditions of exposure. It is a curious fact that ordinary ringworm infections of the feet, though common in young men, are relatively uncommon to rare in children, in women, and in the aged. Familial infections with superficial ringworm fungi, with the exception of tinea capitis, are very uncommon. This is in contrast to some other infections such as the virus of warts in which infection of all members of the family living together is sometimes observed.

An important principle that provides much insight into certain peculiarities of the host-parasite relationship in ringworm infections is that if superficial ringworm infections become markedly inflammatory, there is a tendency toward spontaneous cure. Marked inflammation is incompatible with the continued proliferation of the fungus because it is either desquamated along with other products in the wake of the inflammatory reaction or finds itself in an inhospitable environment owing to interference with normal keratin synthesis. The success of the ringworm parasite in entrenching itself on the surface is dependent on its *not* provoking much reaction in the host. This is particularly well seen in one of the most chronic of all common ringworm infections of adults, that due to *Trichophyton rubrum,* in which the inflammatory changes may be minimal, but in which the infection, once established, may persist for many years. On the other hand, when the parasite injures the host to the point of provoking a significant tissue reaction, it seals its own doom, and the infection is almost always short-lived. This type of spontaneous cure is the basis for a clinical rule that such lesions should be treated conservatively. Antifungous agents become superfluous and unnecessary; the treatment is essentially that which might be applied to an acute or chronic dermatitic process of any type.

In an inflammatory change affecting the skin in which a diagnosis of superficial ringworm is suspected, there are three essential considerations:

1. *Is a fungus present?* This may be determined easily by obtaining an adequate scraping from an active portion of the lesion and examination of the scales in a potassium hydroxide preparation. Precise cultural identification of the fungus present is by no means always necessary to intelligent treatment, though it is of value if the facilities for this are readily available.

2. *Is the process acute, subacute, or chronic?* In the presence of an acute reaction, the inflammatory changes will ordinarily subside spontaneously provided chemical or physical trauma to the affected skin is avoided. In subacute or chronic ringworm infections nothing can be accomplished in terms of a compound which is specifically fungicidal in vivo; there are no such compounds available. The therapeutic attack must be by way of making conditions less favorable for the proliferation of the fungi, by combating inflammation, by assisting the exfoliation of infected skin, and by preventing secondary bacterial invasion.

3. *Are factors other than fungi contributing to the inflammatory changes seen?* Examples include excessive sweating and maceration, primary irritations or sensitizations from applied medication, and physical trauma from shoes or clothing.

Specific Treatment

The clinical use of the antifungous antibiotic, griseofulvin, dates from 1958. The experimental and

clinical studies with the compound have now been sufficient to permit certain conclusions as to its efficacy in various types of superficial fungous infections. Though griseofulvin has, to date, proved to be a very safe drug, its final capacity for adverse reactions must await further widespread clinical use under varying conditions. Also, though acquired resistance of fungi to the antibiotic does not yet seem to be a significant clinical problem, further experience may require some revision of this view.

Griseofulvin is water insoluble and thermostable and is obtained as an antibiotic by fermentation of several species of penicillia. It is chemically unrelated to any other antibiotic now in use, and no cross-sensitization reactions with other medicaments have been observed. Following oral administration, the peak concentration occurs in the blood in 4 hr, but traces persist for 72 to 96 hr. Active material is apparently concentrated in the stratum corneum, the hair, and the nails, as these structures are formed, and is transferred to the periphery at the same rate as the normal growth of the keratinous structure. It is clinically important to recognize that the antibiotic does not penetrate to infected dead keratinous structures, particularly nails and hairs, but is deposited only as new keratin is formed.

Griseofulvin is highly active against all known species of *Trichophyton, Microsporum,* and *Epidermophyton.* It is *not effective* against *Candida albicans,* the organisms causing tinea versicolor or erythrasma, and the deep fungi pathogens. The antibiotic is fungistatic and not fungicidal. Some antibiotic resistance has been induced in vitro, but this is of a low order, and has not proved to have clinical significance as yet.

Toxic reactions resulting from therapeutic doses of griseofulvin in man are uncommon, and to date none of them has proved life-threatening. They include: (1) gastrointestinal distress or loose stools, (2) headaches, (3) urticaria, (4) an erythematous morbilliform eruption. All these reactions disappear promptly on cessation of the drug, or even while it is being continued.

Possibly the most significant, though very rare, reaction to griseofulvin is an ill-defined slowing of reaction time and interference with coordinated movements, particularly if the dose of the drug is raised to 2.0 Gm per day. This may be of importance in the driving of automobiles, the flying of aircraft, and other activities requiring well-coordinated reactions. In the few patients who have experienced this reaction, lowering of the dose to 1.0 Gm per day has resulted in its disappearance. The mechanism is unknown.

Hematologic studies, and determinations of liver and kidney function, in patients receiving prolonged griseofulvin therapy, have not yielded any convincing evidence of toxicity on these organs. Neverthe-

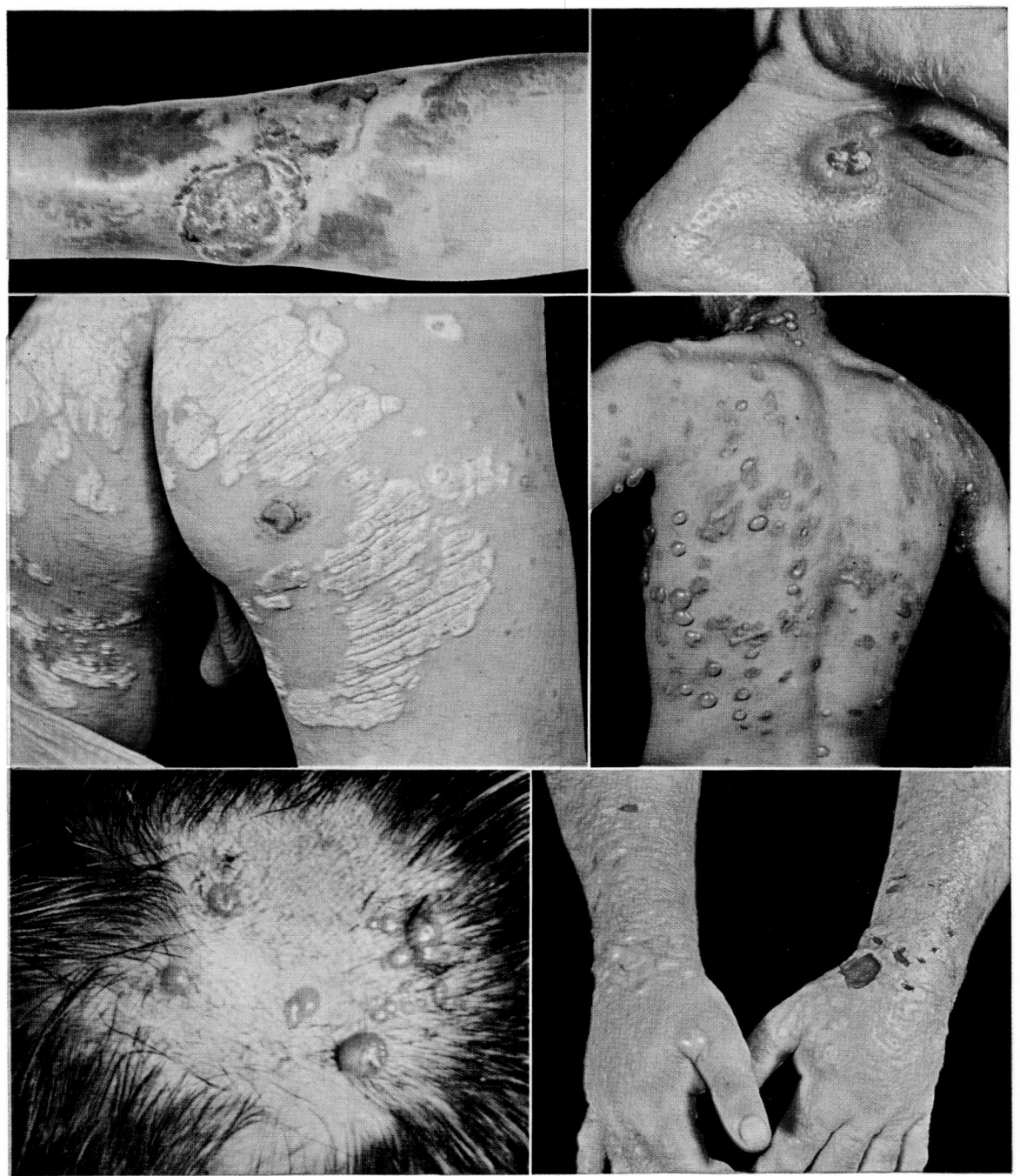

PLATE III

(*Upper left*) Epidermoid carcinoma developing in scar of burn on lower leg. Any persistent ulcerative or proliferative process in a scar should be subjected to biopsy. (*Upper right*) Basal cell epithelioma. This is a relatively neglected lesion. Surgical excision was curative. (*Center left*) Chronic psoriasis and amelanotic melanoma. In extensive chronic dermatoses the development of other significant unrelated skin lesions, particularly tumors, may easily go unnoted. (*Center right*) Severe bullous reaction to sulfathiazole. The lesions are very similar to those seen in pemphigus. This patient had been sensitized by previous prolonged topical sulfonamide therapy. (*Lower left*) Nodules of melanocarcinoma of scalp occurring around scar of previously excised nevus. Wide excision was not curative. (*Lower right*) Severe industrial contact dermatitis.

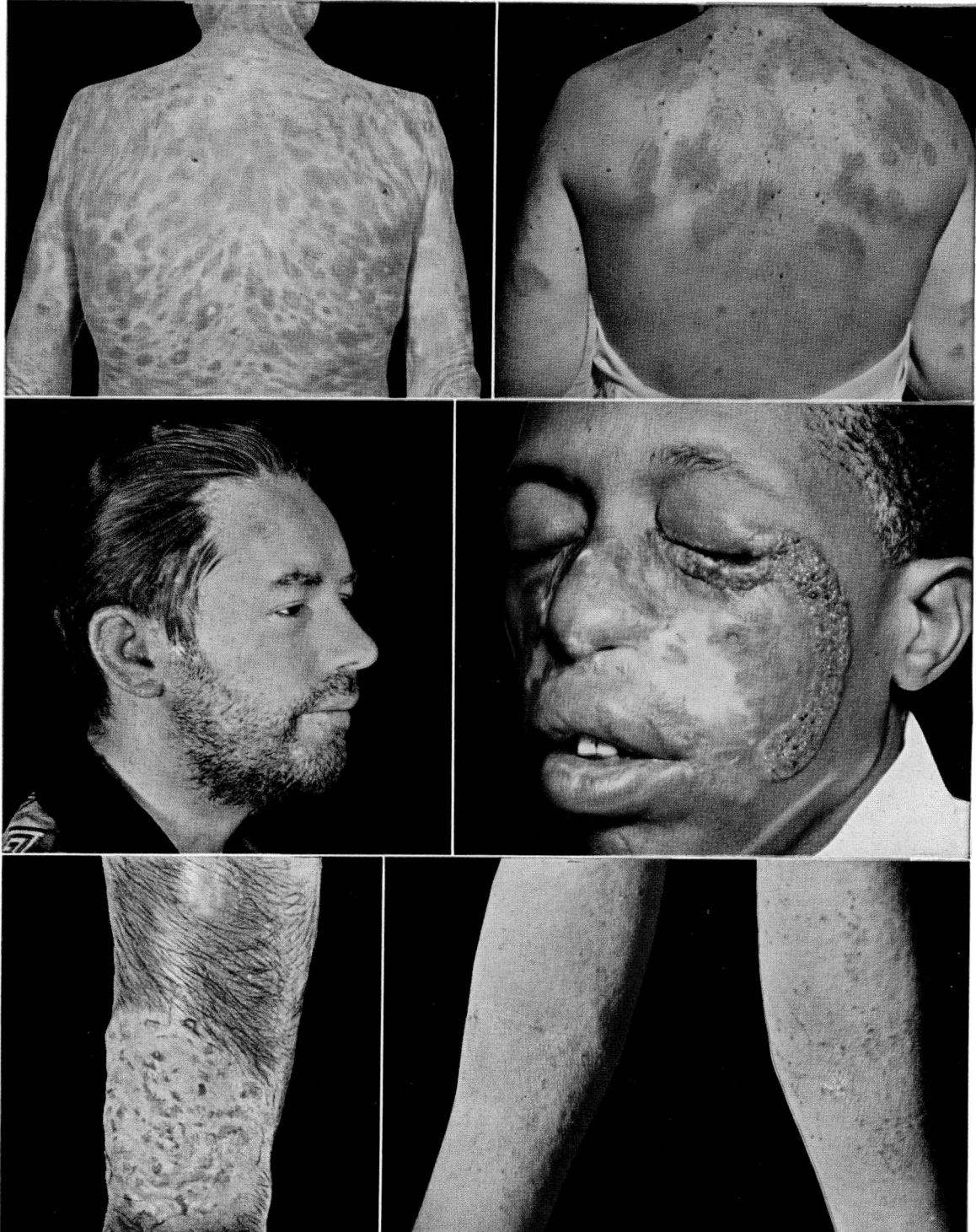

PLATE IV

(*Upper left*) Widespread mycosis fungoides. This is the only lymphoma which produces characteristic skin lesions. (*Upper right*) Leukemid eruption in a patient with rapidly fatal acute myelogenous leukemia. This was the initial sign of illness. The skin lesions showed no leukemic infiltrate. (*Center left*) Severe seborrheic dermatitis with otitis externa and secondary streptococcal infection. (*Center right*) Longstanding blastomycosis. The patient's general health was excellent. (*Lower left*) Inflammatory tinea profunda (*Trichophyton mentagrophytes*) infection acquired from a cow. No systemic reaction. This lesion involuted spontaneously. (*Lower right*) Atopic dermatitis. Involvement of the antecubital fossa and surrounding skin is characteristic. The changes seen are almost entirely due to scratching and rubbing.

less, as has been the case with many drugs in the past, isolated serious reactions involving these organ systems may not be seen until hundreds of thousands of patients have been treated. The extensive initial experience has, however, been extremely encouraging.

Griseofulvin when taken by mouth is effective against skin, nail, and hair infection produced by the dermatophytic fungi. It has shown no effectiveness whatever against other diseases which clinically resemble such infections, and the diagnosis should be firmly established before the drug is given. Because, in the majority of cases, prolonged therapy is necessary for cure, the advisability of avoiding futile administration for nondermatophytic diseases of the skin becomes particularly important.

The average dose advised for griseofulvin for adult patients is 1.0 Gm daily. There seems little to be gained by dividing this into four equal doses of 250 mg each, and it may be fully effective if the daily dose is taken all at once. In occasional patients, a lack of clinical response may dictate an increase in the dose to 2.0 Gm daily. With doses of less than 1.0 Gm daily, relapse of the infection or partial failure of treatment is common.

Ringworm of the Feet. This is the most common type of ringworm infection and is largely a penalty for wearing shoes. The majority of young American adult males acquire fungous infections of the feet, the incidence being between 40 and 80 per cent. The rate is highest in semitropical to tropical climates. Fungous infections of the feet are extremely rare in children and are not common in women.

The favorite sites of involvement in ringworm of the feet are the interdigital spaces, especially the third and fourth, the inner side of the arch, and the toenails. Scaling is a constant feature of subacute or chronic fungous infections of the feet. Inflammation in interdigital spaces may be variously caused by fungi, by *Monilia,* by simple maceration, or may be due to psoriasis or some other disease of the skin. If inflamed fissures are present, secondary bacterial infection may be suspected. The fungus most commonly cultured is *Trichophyton mentagrophytes.* The intertriginous involvement may remain chronic and localized or may sometimes show acute exacerbations, with the formation of vesicles and bullae extensively over the feet and with vesicular lesions elsewhere on the body, particularly the hands ("id" reaction).

Ringworm infections of the feet may persist as occasional patches of vesicles which tend to localize on the instep portion of the sole and on the heel and ball of the foot. In severe cases the entire sole may be involved. The process does not commonly extend over the dorsum of the foot. If the dorsal surface of the toes is involved, a contact dermatitis from applied medication or from footgear should be suspected.

During exacerbations of the vesicular type of ringworm infection, the lesions frequently fuse and contain a yellowish, gelatinous fluid. Fungi are often not demonstrable at this phase because they are being cast off so rapidly. Vesicles on the sole may be so deep as to appear papular and may not rupture spontaneously.

The most chronic type of ringworm infection of the feet is caused by *T. rubrum.* This is frequently unilateral. It is characterized by diffuse scaling, often of a fine, branny character, by relative lack of inflammation, and by extreme chronicity. The process may become diffuse over the entire plantar surface and extend over the sides of the foot in a "moccasin" distribution. The condition is sometimes difficult to differentiate from ichthyosis, from a congenital keratosis, or from psoriasis.

Involvement of the toenails is almost inevitable in any long-standing fungous infection of the feet. This may be difficult to differentiate from the traumatic distortion which occurs inevitably in the toenails of older persons, particularly men. Fungi are hard to isolate in scrapings taken from the nails because they are overshadowed by keratinous debris, bacteria, and molds. It is probable that fungi in and under the nails are the chief source of what appear to be reinfections of other parts of the foot.

Griseofulvin is of considerable value in the treatment of the dry scaling fungous infections of the feet, but it is of lesser help in approaching the problem of vesicular fungous infections of the feet.

1. *Dryness* is the most important single factor, especially in intertriginous involvement. A patient with subacute or chronic ringworm should be most meticulous and careful about drying the toes after bathing. It is helpful to do this with a dry, crash washcloth, with friction sufficient to remove scales and mascerated skin. The wearing of tight occlusive footgear should be avoided whenever possible, and during warm weather the wearing of sandal-type or aerated shoes is worthwhile. If there is excessive perspiration, the use of a nonabrasive foot powder is helpful; it may be found advisable to change the socks once or twice daily. Socks of an absorbent variety are best, though they should not be too heavy during warm weather. An elaborate ritual of boiling socks has no demonstrable value; the sources of reinfection are numerous enough on the foot itself.

2. *Rest* is helpful in the treatment of inflammation of the feet due to fungi. In severe exacerbations bed rest may be essential. In less severe forms the patient should restrict walking and athletic activity.

The actual treatment of the infection is dependent upon the degree of inflammation. In acute bullous exacerbations, foot soaks of any bland solution, either hot or cold, are helpful. Vesicles and bullae should be opened; this may be done safely by the patient himself, with a needle or with curved manicure scissors. Tops of bullae should not be cut away completely because this exposes the underlying epidermis. A shake lotion may be used sparingly to advantage, and in this phase hydrocortisone in a lotion is often helpful. Ointments should be used only after the process becomes less acute and should be applied at night rather than in the morning. It is of particular importance that evidence of secondary bacterial infection be watched for. For very severe acute attacks a short course of systemic corticosteroid therapy may be justified.

In subacute or chronic types of fungous infection, whether intertriginous, vesicular, or dry scaling type, several preparations are useful. The fatty acids are helpful and rarely cause irritation. Castellani's paint is especially good for intertriginous areas and for patches of vesicles. If there is thickened skin on the soles or macerated debris between the toes, a preparation which will increase exfoliation should be prescribed. Care must be taken, however, that it is not applied in a concentration which will produce damage. Between the toes, a preparation containing 3 per cent salicylic acid and 6 per cent benzoic acid in 70 per cent propyl alcohol is useful. The same chemicals may be incorporated in an ointment-type base yielding a half-strength Whitfield ointment. Some patients may find fatty acid ointments more helpful. An alternate type of preparation is one containing salicylic acid and sulfur, usually in a concentration of 2 or 3 per cent each. *Treatment should be directed toward making the conditions for the growth of the fungi less optimal, toward allowing the skin to recover as rapidly as possible during acute exacerbations, and toward assisting the skin to cast off the fungi which are present entirely in the stratum corneum or in the nails.*

It has been suggested, though on debatable evidence, that the presence of a ringworm infection of the feet, particularly that caused by *T. rubrum*, may induce peripheral vascular disease in the feet and lower legs. The authors are not convinced that this is true, but, in any event, a ringworm infection of the feet becomes of increased importance in patients with peripheral vascular disease or with diabetes. The scrupulousness of foot hygiene must be redoubled, and particular care should be taken not to use chemicals with possible cauterant effects on the skin because a very slowly healing ulcer may result. The services of a competent chiropodist are helpful to such patients, not only from the standpoint of maintaining good foot hygiene, but in an effort to remove irritation from toenails, calluses, and footgear.

Majocchi's granuloma is a distinctive manifestation of ringworm infection in the form of a granulomatous folliculitis and perifolliculitis. It occurs most frequently in women who shave their legs and who have a diffuse *T. rubrum* infection of the feet. Indefinite and rather indistinct scaling patches develop on the lower half of the lower leg, and inflammatory nodules develop at the borders of these patches. The nodules rarely exceed a centimeter in diameter and are flat or only slightly elevated. If the lesion is observed early, it may be seen to be centered by a hair. The nodules are not pruritic and usually only slightly tender. They do not progress to suppuration and persist as long as 3 or 4 months. They may then become slowly absorbed or undergo necrosis and heal with a depressed scar. Histopathologic examination reveals a characteristic foreign-body granuloma; degenerating fungous elements may be demonstrated by the Hotchkiss-McManus method.

Certain other puzzling conditions of the lower extremities are seen in association with fungous infections of the feet, though the precise relation is difficult to establish. One is an erysipelas-like process of the lower extremities occurring in the form of a recurrent superficial cellulitis of brief duration and apparently representing an "id" reaction. On the legs and elsewhere, the following reaction patterns may be in some cases representative of an allergic sensitivity to ringworm: (1) erythema nodosum, (2) erythema multiforme (rare), and (3) indefinite macular rashes.

Ringworm of the Nails. When a superficial ringworm infection involves the toenails and/or fingernails, topical therapy becomes quite useless. Cure may sometimes be effected by removal of the nail plate, and careful scraping away of all debris in the lateral gutters and in the nail base. However, this procedure is rarely successful in the toenails and is not advised. Reinfection is usually prompt. In fingernails, successful cure of the ringworm infection by surgical avulsion is more frequent, though probably less than 50 per cent. It is more likely to be helpful if only one or two fingernails are involved and if there is not an extensive focus of ringworm infection on the skin of the hand. Care must be taken not to confuse other nail dystrophies with a ringworm infection. The most common of these are psoriasis, chronic dermatitis of the distal phalanges, chronic paronychial infection, and arthritis involving the distal joint.

Griseofulvin has revolutionized the treatment of fungous infections of the fingernails. Cure can be obtained by the administration of griseofulvin over long periods. Because of the slow growth rate, it is necessary to administer the drug daily for periods of as long as 5 or 6 months in the treatment of fingernail infections. The toenail grows even more slowly.

Clinical cure of toenail infections may require a period of treatment of 18 months. Hence griseofulvin is rarely recommended for treatment of ringworm of the toenails.

Ringworm of the Groin. This is a common affliction, especially in males during the summer months. The characteristic lesions are seen in the crural folds and the upper inner thigh, usually with an annular, scaling ring in the latter area. Several other conditions may be confused, particularly psoriasis and seborrheic dermatitis. Anal and vulvar pruritus are not, per se, commonly due to fungi, though *Candida* may sometimes play a role. In tinea cruris it is particularly important not to use compounds which will produce any reaction because the male genitalia are very susceptible to irritation, and a chronic dermatitis which is protracted by scratching may result.

Ringworm of the Body. Extensive ringworm infections of the trunk or extremities are uncommon in temperate climates, though they are seen with some frequency in the tropics. In the presence of a ring-shaped, moderately inflamed lesion, the odds are generally in favor of some condition other than a fungous infection, e.g., pityriasis rosea, seborrheic dermatitis, or psoriasis. In those instances in which a proved extensive fungous infection of the skin of the trunk and extremities is observed in patients in temperate climates, patients should be subjected to careful study for hematologic disease or diabetes.

Ringworm of the Hands. Though fungous infections of the hands are by no means rare, this diagnosis is made with too great frequency. The infection in this area has so much in common with infections of the feet that it need not be considered in any great detail. There are two main types: (1) the inflammatory vesicular and (2) the noninflammatory squamous. The former is uncommon in temperate climates, though dermatophytids associated with infections of the feet are common. *Trichophyton mentagrophytes* is the organism usually recoverable from the acute vesicular type. The course is one of spontaneous healing provided the hands are not subjected to constant chemical or traumatic irritation.

Ringworm of the Scalp. Tinea capitis is predominantly a disease of children and will not be considered in detail herein. It is caused by a variety of fungi. In cases which are transmitted from man to man, and in which the most common causative organism is *Microsporum audouini,* the course is one of great chronicity; healing does not occur unless increased resistance of the host becomes evident in the form of inflammatory changes. Such a local response may become quite severe and produce the lesion called a kerion. This has the appearance of a bacterial infection and in time involutes spontaneously with cure of the ringworm

infection, usually without permanent alopecia. In ringworm of the scalp acquired by children from animals, in which *M. canis* is the most common causative organism, the process is ordinarily inflammatory from the onset and is self-limited.

Ringworm of the scalp in children is a considerable public health problem, and the incidence of the infection rises and falls in urban centers for reasons which are not readily apparent. Treatment with griseofulvin has been remarkably effective. Some clinicians favor a *single* curative dose of 3 Gm.

Various fungi are capable of producing chronic infection of the scalp in adults. Favus, caused by *T. schoenleini,* is relatively common in eastern Europe, but is rare in the United States. Another type of adult ringworm of the scalp, that due to *T. tonsurans,* has long been seen with considerable frequency in Mexico and is being encountered increasingly in the southwestern United States and California. The condition resembles seborrheic dermatitis or psoriasis, and there is usually moderate to marked loss of hair. It cannot be detected easily because there is no fluorescence on Wood's light examination as is the case with almost all ringworm infections in childhood. The proper diagnosis is made, in most cases, only if the clinical acuity of the examiner is high and if adequate mycologic studies are done.

REFERENCES

ACNE

Baer, R. L., and V. H. Witten: Acne Vulgaris, in "Year Book of Dermatology," Chicago, Year Book Publishers, Inc., 1959–1960.

Strauss, J. S., and A. M. Kligman: The Pathologic Dynamics of Acne Vulgaris, Arch. Dermatol., 88: 779, 1960.

CANCER

Belisario, J. C.: "Cancer of the Skin," London, Butterworth & Co. (Publishers) Ltd., 1959.

DERMATITIS AND ECZEMA

Kligman, A. M.: Poison Ivy (Rhus) Dermatitis, Arch. Dermatol., 77:149, 1958.

Loewenthal, L. J. A.: "The Eczemas," London, E. & S. Livingstone, Ltd., 1954.

Wilson, H. T. H.: Exfoliative Dermatitis: Its Etiology and Prognosis, Arch. Dermatol., 69:577, 1954.

FUNGOUS INFECTIONS

Blank, H., and F. J. Roth: The Treatment of Dermatomycoses with Orally Administered Griseofulvin, Arch. Dermatol., 79:259, 1959.

Moss, E. S., and A. L. McQuown: "Atlas of Medical Mycology," 2d ed., Baltimore, The Williams & Wilkins Company, 1960.

HEMANGIOMAS

Bean, W. B.: "Vascular Spiders and Related Lesions of the Skin," Springfield, Ill., Charles C Thomas, Publisher, 1958.

Bowers, R. E., E. A. Graham, and K. M. Tomlinson: The Natural History of the Strawberry Nevus, Arch. Dermatol., 82:667, 1960.

LYMPHOMAS

Bluefarb, S. M.: "Cutaneous Manifestations of the Malignant Lymphomas," Springfield, Ill., Charles C Thomas, Publisher, 1959.

———: "Leukemia Cutis," Springfield, Ill., Charles C Thomas, Publisher, 1960.

PEMPHIGUS

Lever, W. F.: Pemphigus, Medicine, 32:1, 1953.

PHOTOSENSITIVE STATES

Kesten, B. M.: Photosensitivity in Various Dermatoses, Lupus Erythematosus, Urticaria Due to Light and Polymorphic Light Eruptions, Arch. Dermatol., 74:40, 1956.

PIGMENTED NEVI

Baer, R. L., and V. H. Witten: Selected Benign Pigmented Cutaneous Lesions, in "Year Book of Dermatology," Chicago, Year Book Publishers, Inc., 1958–1959.

TREATMENT

Lerner, M. R., and A. B. Lerner: "Dermatologic Medications," Chicago, Year Book Publishers, Inc., 1960.

Sternberg, T. H., and V. D. Newcomer: "Modern Dermatologic Therapy," New York, McGraw-Hill Book Company, Inc., 1959.

APPENDIX
Laboratory Values of Clinical Importance

Laboratory Values of Clinical Importance

BODY FLUIDS AND OTHER MASS DATA

Body fluid, total volume: 56% (in obese) to 70% (lean)
of body weight
  Intracellular: Approximately 67% of total
  Extracellular: 16–20% of body weight

Blood:
  Total volume: Male: 75 ml/kg body weight
    Female: 67 ml/kg body weight
  Plasma volume: Male: 44 ml/kg body weight
    Female: 43 ml/kg body weight
  Red cell volume: Male: 30 ml/kg body weight (1.15–
    1.21 L per sq m surface area)
    Female: 24 ml/kg body weight

$$mEq \text{ (milliequivalent)} = \frac{mg/100 \text{ ml} \times 10 \times valence}{atomic\ weight}$$

$$mg/100 \text{ ml} = \frac{mEq \times atomic\ weight}{10 \times valence}$$

Atomic Weights of Elements Commonly Encountered in Clinical Medicine

Calcium	40.08	Magnesium	24.32
Carbon	12.01	Nitrogen	14.008
Chlorine	35.46	Oxygen	16.00
Copper	63.54	Phosphorus	30.98
Hydrogen	1.008	Potassium	39.100
Iodine	126.91	Sodium	22.997
Iron	55.85	Sulfur	32.07

CEREBROSPINAL FLUID

Cells: <5 per cu mm, all lymphocytes
Pressure, initial (horizontal position): 70–200 mm water
Calcium*: 1.13–1.30 mEq/L
Chloride,* as Cl⁻: 118–127 mEq/L
Cholesterol: 0.06–0.22 mg/100 ml
Colloidal gold test: Not more than two in any tube
Creatinine: 0.4–1.5 mg/100 ml
Glucose*: 44–100 mg/100 ml
pH*: 7.35–7.70
Magnesium (average)*: 0.82–1.08 mEq/L
Nonprotein nitrogen*: 12–30 mg/100 ml
Phosphorus (inorganic)*: 1.2–2.1 mg/100 ml
Potassium*: 2.18–3.38 mEq/L
Protein:
  (Total): 14–45 mg/100 ml
  Lumbar: 14–45 mg/100 ml
  Cisternal: 15 mg/100 ml
  Ventricular: 10 mg/100 ml
Sodium*: 217–237 mEq/L
Urea nitrogen*: 6–28 mg/100 ml

* Since the cerebrospinal fluid concentrations are equilibrium values, measurement of blood plasma obtained at the same time is recommended.

CHEMICAL CONSTITUENTS OF BLOOD

Albumin, serum: 4.0–5.2 Gm/100 ml
Ammonia, whole blood, venous: 30–70 μg/100 ml
Amylase, whole blood (Somogyi): 60–180 units/100 ml
Ascorbic acid, whole blood: 0.4–1.0 mg/100 ml
  Leukocytes: 25–40 mg/100 ml
Base, total, serum: 145–155 mEq/L
Bilirubin, total, serum (Malloy-Evelyn):
  0.1–0.8 mg/100 ml
  Direct, serum: 0.1–0.2 mg/100 ml
  Indirect, serum: 0.1–0.6 mg/100 ml
Calcium, serum: 4.5–6.0 mEq/L; 9–11 mg/100 ml
Carbon dioxide–combining power, serum (sea level):
  21–28 mEq/L; 50–65 vol %
Carbon dioxide content, blood (sea level):
  21–30 mEq/L; 50–70 vol %
Carbon dioxide tension, arterial blood (sea level):
  42 ± 4 mm Hg
Carotenoids, serum: 100–200 μg/100 ml
Chlorides, serum (as Cl): 98–106 mEq/L;
  355–376 mg/100 ml
Cholesterol: Total, serum (Man-Peters method)
  (mean ± 1 SD): 194 ± 36 mg/100 ml
  Esters, serum: 100–180 mg/100 ml
Cholesterol ester fraction of total cholesterol, serum:
  68–72%
Copper, serum (mean ± 1 SD): 114 ± 14 μg/100 ml
Corticoids, plasma (Porter-Silber) (mean ± 1 SD):
  13 ± 6 μg/100 ml
Creatinine, serum (Peters): 1–1.5 mg/100 ml
Fat, neutral, serum: 150–250 mg/100 ml
Fatty acids, serum: 380–465 mg/100 ml
Fibrinogen, plasma: 0.2–0.4 Gm/100 ml
Globulins, serum: 1.3–2.7 Gm/100 ml
Glucose (fasting), blood (Nelson-Somogyi):
  60–90 mg/100 ml
Hemoglobin, blood (sea level):
  Males: 14–18 Gm/100 ml
  Females: 12–16 Gm/100 ml
Icterus index, serum: 4–6 units
Iodine, protein-bound, serum: 4–8 μg/100 ml
Iron, serum, males and females (mean ± 1 SD):
  105 ± 32.8 μg/100 ml
Iron-binding capacity, serum (mean ± 1 SD):
  359 ± 30.8 μg/100 ml
Ketones, total: 0.5–1.5 mg/100 ml
Lipase, serum (Cherry-Crandall): 1.5 ml N/20 NaOH
  (upper limit of normal). (However, values above 1.0
  should be regarded with suspicion.)
Lipid phosphorus (Man-Peters) (mean ± 1 SD):
  9.2 ± 1.4 mg/100 ml
Lipids, total, serum: 500–600 mg/100 ml
Magnesium, serum: 1.5–3.0 mEq/L; 2–3 mg/100 ml
Methemoglobin: <1.8 %
Nitrogen, nonprotein, serum: 15–35 mg/100 ml

Oxygen capacity, blood: 18–22 vol %
Oxygen content: Arterial blood (sea level): 17–21 vol %
Venous blood, arm (sea level): 10–16 vol %
Oxygen per cent saturation (sea level):
Arterial blood: 97 vol %
Venous blood, arm: 60–85 vol %
Oxygen tension, blood: 95–100 mm Hg
pH blood: 7.38–7.44
Phosphatase, acid, total serum: Bodansky method:
0.2–0.8 unit/100 ml
Gutman or King-Armstrong method:
1–4 units/100 ml
Phosphatase, acid, tartrate sensitive (Fishman-Lerner):
<0.6 unit/100 ml
Phosphatase, alkaline, serum: Bodansky method:
1–4 units/100 ml
King-Armstrong method: 8–13 units/100 ml
Phospholipids, serum: 150–250 mg/100 ml
Phosphorus, inorganic, serum: 1–1.5 mEq/L;
3–4.5 mg/100 ml
Potassium, serum: 3.5–5.0 mEq/L; 13.7–20.0 mg/100 ml
Proteins, total, serum: 6.5–8.0 Gm/100 ml
Proteins, electrophoretic fractions:

	Plasma, %	Serum, %	Serum, % (paper)
	(Tiselius)	(Tiselius)	
Albumin	55.2	58 ± 3	45–55
Globulins: α_1	5.3	5 ± 2	5–8
α_2	8.7	12 ± 3	8–13
β	13.4	11 ± 4	11–17
Fibrinogen:	6.5		
Globulins: γ_1	11.0	2 ± 2	15–25
γ_2		12 ± 3	

Prothrombin, plasma (Quick method):
11–12 sec (cf. control)
Sodium, serum: 132–142 mEq/L;
303–327 mg/100 ml (as sodium)
771–832 mg/100 ml (as sodium chloride)
Sulfates, inorganic, serum: 0.5–1.5 mg/100 ml
Urea nitrogen, whole blood: 10–20 mg/100 ml
Uric acid, serum, enzymatic method (Praetorius)
(mean ± 1 SD):
Males: 5.0 ± 1.2 mg/100 ml
Females: 3.8 ± 0.9 mg/100 ml
Uric acid, serum (Talbot): 2.5–5.0 mg/100 ml
Vitamin A, serum: 50–100 μg/100 ml

FUNCTION TESTS

Liver

Bromsulphalein (5 mg/kg body weight, IV):
5% or less retention at end of 45 min
Cephalin-cholesterol flocculation: 0 or + at 48 hr
Galactose tolerance, after ingestion of 40 Gm:
Excretion of not more than 3 Gm in urine in 5 hr

Hippuric acid: After ingestion of 6 Gm sodium benzoate:
Excretion of 3–3.5 Gm hippuric acid in urine in
4 hr
After injection of 1.77 Gm sodium benzoate, IV:
Excretion of 0.70 Gm hippuric acid in urine in
1 hr
Prothrombin test: Increase of 15% or more in prothrom-
bin concentration in blood in 24 hr after injection
of synthetic vitamin K
Serum glutamic oxalacetic transaminase (SGOT)
(mean ± 1 SD): 22 ± 7 units/ml/min
Serum glutamic pyruvic transaminase (mean ± 1 SD):
16 ± 9 units/ml/min
Thymol turbidity: 0–4 units
Urobilinogen:
Urine: Semiquantitative (2 hr): 0.5–1.5 units
Quantitative: 1–3.5 mg/24 hr
Stool: Semiquantitative (per 100 Gm): <350 units
Quantitative: 40–280 mg/24 hr
Zinc sulfate turbidity: <4 units

Circulation

Cardiac output (Fick): 2.2–4.0 L/sq m/min
Circulation time: Arm to lung, ether: 4–8 sec
Arm to tongue, calcium gluconate: 12–18 sec
Decholin: 10–16 sec
Saccharin: 9–16 sec
Pressures, intracardiac and intraarterial:
Aorta: Systole: 120 mm Hg
Diastole: 80 mm Hg
Atrium: Left (mean): 5 mm Hg
Right (mean): 2 mm Hg
Pulmonary artery: Systole: 25 mm Hg
Diastole: 10 mm Hg
Wedge (mean): 9 mm Hg
Ventricle, left: Systole: 120 mm Hg
Diastole: 5 mm Hg
Ventricle, right: Systole: 25 mm Hg
Diastole: 0 mm Hg
Venous (antecubital): 70–140 mm H_2O

Gastrointestinal

Gastric juice:

	Fasting	Basal	Maximum response in 10 min following administration of		
			Alcohol or broth	Hista-mine	Insulin
Volume, ml	10–25	0–10	10–25	15–30	10–30
Free acid, units	0–30	10–30	30–60	70–110	50–100
Total acid, units	5–40	15–35	40–80	80–120	60–110

Chlorides (as Cl) (mean and range): 104 (24–127)
mEq/L

Reaction, as pH: 1.6–1.8
Volume, 24 hr: 2–3 L
Nocturnal secretion, 600–700 ml
Jejunal secretion, fasting: Chloride: 80–140 mEq/L
HCO$_3$: 2–32 mEq/L
Total base: 110–160 mEq/L
Tubeless gastric analysis with azure A dye: HCl acid present if more than 0.6 mg dye is excreted in urine over a 2-hr period. (CAUTION: A negative test is meaningless and requires performance of the ordinary test with a gastric tube.)

Pulmonary

Maximum Breathing Capacity (MBC) (*the higher values are for taller individuals*)

Males, age 20..................... 180–200 L/min
Males, age 60..................... 125–150 L/min
Females, age 20.................. 100–125 L/min
Females, age 60.................. 65–85 L/min

Formula: *MBC*, L/min = 3.39 *H* (height in in.) − 1.26 *A* (age, yr) − 21.4 ± 29 (males)

Vital Capacity (VC) (*the higher values are for taller subjects*)

Males, age 20....................... 4.5–5.5 L
Males, age 60....................... 3.8–4.6 L
Females, age 20..................... 3.0–3.5 L
Females, age 60..................... 2.5–3.0 L

Formula: *VC*, L = 0.133 *H* − 0.22 *A* − 3.60 ± 0.6 (males)

Timed Vital Capacity

1 sec: 72 ± 5% of total vital capacity
3 sec: 95 ± 5% of total vital capacity

Total Capacity (TC) (*supine*), *in ml*

$\dfrac{VC}{80} \times 100$ at 16–34 yr; $\dfrac{VC}{76.6} \times 100$ at 35–49 yr

$\dfrac{VC}{69.2} \times 100$ at 50–59 yr; $\dfrac{VC}{60} \times 100$ at 60 yr and older

Residual Volume (RV), *in ml*

$\dfrac{RV}{TC} \times 100 = 20 \pm 4\%$ at 16–34 yr
$25 \pm 4\%$ at 35–40 yr
$39 \pm 5\%$ over 60 yr

Dead Space

150–200 cc during tidal breathing (roughly equal to the body weight in pounds)

Kidney

Clearances (corrected to 1.73 sq m body surface area):
Measures of glomerular filtration rate:
Inulin clearance (C_I): Males: 124 ± 25.8 ml/min
Females: 119 ± 12.8 ml/min
Endogenous creatinine: 91–130 ml/min
Urea: 60–100 ml/min

Measures of effective renal plasma flow and tubular function:
Para-aminohippuric acid (C_{PAH}):
Males: 654 ± 163 ml/min
Females: 594 ± 102 ml/min
Tubular maximum for *PAH*, males and females: 77.2 mg/min
Diodrast: 600–800 ml/min;
20–30% excretion in 15 min
Concentration and dilution test:
Specific gravity of urine: After 12 hr fluid restriction: 1.025 or more
After 12 hr water intake: 1.003 or less
Phenolsulfonphthalein: After intramuscular injection:
Excretion in urine in 15 min: 25% or more
Excretion in urine in 2 hr: 55–75%
After intravenous injection:
Excretion in urine in 2 hr: 55–75%
Specific gravity, maximal: 1.022–1.028
Tubular reabsorption, phosphorus:
79–94% of filtered load

Metabolic

Basal metabolic rate: −10% to +10% of mean standard
Creatine tolerance: 70% ingested creatine retained in adults
Glucose tolerance, 100 Gm glucose or 1.75 Gm glucose/kg body weight, p.o.: Blood sugar not more than 180 mg/100 ml after ½ hr; return to normal in 2 hr; sugar not present in any urine specimen
Radioactive iodine (I[131]): Uptake: 20–50% of administered dose
Excretion: 30–70% of administered dose in 24 hr following tracer dose, provided renal function is normal
Protein-bound, serum or plasma: <0.3% of administered dose per liter of plasma at 72 hr following tracer dose
Conversion ratio: <35% at 24 hr
Water test (Soffer): 80% excretion of a 1,500 ml water load in 4 hr

HEMATOLOGIC EXAMINATIONS

(See also Chemical Constituents of Blood)

Bone Marrow (see Table 23-3, p. 213)

Erythrocytes (see table below)

Fragility, osmotic: Slight hemolysis: 0.45–0.39%
Complete hemolysis: 0.33–0.30%
Hemochromogens in plasma: 3–5 mg/100 ml
"Life span": Normal survival: 120 days
Chromium, half-life (T ½): 28 days
Plasma iron turnover rate: 38 mg/24 hr (0.47 mg/kg)
Protoporphyrin, free erythrocyte (E.P.):
20–38 μg/100 ml RBCs
Reticulocytes: 0.5–2.0% of red cells
Sedimentation rate: Westergren: <15 mm/1 hr
Wintrobe: Male: 0–9 mm/1 hr
Female: 0–20 mm/1 hr

NORMAL VALUES AT VARIOUS AGES

Age	Red cell count, millions/cu mm	Hemoglobin, Gm/100 ml	Vol. packed RBC, ml/100 ml	Corpuscular values			
				MCV, cuμ	MCH, γγ	MCHC, %	MCD, μ
First day........	5.1 ± 1.0*	19.5 ± 5.0*	54.0 ± 10.0*	106	38	36	8.6
2–3 days........	5.1	19.0	53.5	105	37	35	
4–8 days........	5.1	18.3 ± 4.0	52.5	103	36	35	
9–13 days.......	5.0	16.5	49.0	98	33	34	
14–60 days......	4.7 ± 0.9	14.0 ± 3.3	42.0 ± 7.0	90	30	33	8.1
3–5 mo..........	4.5 ± 0.7	12.2 ± 2.3	36.0	80	27	34	7.7
6–11 mo........	4.6	11.8	35.5 ± 5.0	77	26	33	7.4
1 yr............	4.5	11.2	35.0	78	25	32	7.3
2 yr............	4.6	11.5	35.5	77	25	32	
3 yr............	4.5	12.5	36.0	80	27	35	7.4
4 yr............	4.6 ± 0.6	12.6	37.0	80	27	34	
5 yr............	4.6	12.6	37.0	80	27	34	
6–10 yr........	4.7	12.9	37.5	80	27	34	7.4
11–15 yr........	4.8	13.4	39.0	82	28	34	
Adults:							
Females.......	4.8 ± 0.6	14.0 ± 2.0	42.0 ± 5.0	87 ± 5	29 ± 2	34 ± 2	7.5 ± 0.3
Males........	5.4 ± 0.8	16.0 ± 2.0	47.0 ± 7.0	87 ± 5	29 ± 2	34 ± 2	7.5 ± 0.3

MCV = mean corpuscular volume. MCH = mean corpuscular hemoglobin. MCHC = mean corpuscular hemoglobin concentration. MCD = mean corpuscular diameter. (*Wintrobe: "Clinical Hematology,"* 5th ed., *Philadelphia, Lea & Febiger,* 1961.)

* The range of values represents almost the extremes of observed variations (93 per cent or more) at sea level. The blood values of healthy persons should fall well within these figures.

Leukocytes

NORMAL VALUES

	Per cent	Average	Minimum	Maximum
Total number, per cu mm........	...	7,000	5,000	10,000
Neutrophils:				
Juvenile........	3–5	300	150	400
Segmented......	54–62	4,000	3,000	5,800
Eosinophils........	1–3	200	50	250
Basophils.........	0–0.75	25	15	50
Lymphocytes......	25–33	2,100	1,500	3,000
Monocytes........	3–7	375	285	500

Platelets and Coagulation

Platelets, per cu mm, direct counting method: 200,000–300,000

Bleeding time (Ivy method), majority and range: 1–5 mm, 0–12 min

Clot retraction time: Begins in 30 min, complete in less than 24 hr, usually <6 hr

Coagulation time (Lee-White method), majority and range: 5–15 min, 2–19 min

Schilling Test

Excretion in urine of orally administered, radioactive vitamin B_{12} following "flushing" parenteral injection of B_{12}: 7–22%

SEROUS FLUIDS (pleural, pericardial, peritoneal)

pH: 6.80–7.60
Specific gravity: 1.010–1.026
Protein:
  Total: 0.30–4.10 Gm/100 ml
  Albumin: 50.5–69.8%
  Globulin: 29.5–45.8%
  Fibrinogen: 0.3–4.5%

STOOL

Bulk: Wet weight: <197.5 Gm/day (mean 115 ± 41)
  Dry weight: <66.4 Gm/day (mean 34 ± 16)
Fat, on diet containing at least 50 Gm fat: <7.2 Gm/day when measured on a 3-day (or longer) collection (mean 4.0 ± 1.6)
  As percentage of dry weight:
    <30.4 (mean 13.3 ± 8.07)
  Coefficient of fat absorption: >93%
Fatty acid: Free: 1–10% of dry matter
  Combined as soap: 0.5–12% of dry matter

Nitrogen: <2.2 Gm/day (mean 1.8 ± 0.2)
Protein content: Minimal
Water: Approximately 65%
Urobilinogen: 40–280 mg/24 hr
Coproporphyrin: 400–1,000 µg/24 hr

URINE

Acidity, titratable: 125–150 mEq/24 hr
α-Amino nitrogen: 0.4–1.0 Gm/24 hr
Ammonia: 30–50 mEq/24 hr
Amylase (Somogyi): 260–950 mg glucose/24 hr
Calcium, 10 mEq or 200 mg calcium diet:
     <7.5 mEq/24 hr or <0.15 Gm/24 hr
Copper: 0–25 µg/24 hr
Coproporphyrins (types I and III): 100–300 µg/24 hr

Creatine, as creatinine: Adult males: <50 mg/24 hr
     Adult females: <100 mg/24 hr
Creatinine: 1.0–1.6 Gm/24 hr
D-Xylose excretion: 5–8 Gm/5 hr after oral dose of 25 Gm
Estrogens (Jailer method): Male: 5–20 µg/24 hr
     Female (nonpregnant):
          15–100 µg/24 hr depending on time of menstrual cycle
Glucose, true (oxidase method): 50–300 mg/24 hr
Ketones, total (mean ± 1 SD): 50.5 ± 30.7 mg/24 hr
17-Ketosteroids (Holtorf-Koch method):
     Male: 8–20 mg/24 hr
     Female: 6–15 mg/24 hr
11-Oxysteroids or corticoids (Porter-Silber method):
     2.2–8.0 mg/24 hr
Protein: <50 mg/24 hr
Urobilinogen: 1–3.5 mg/24 hr

Index